Goodman & Gilman's

The
Pharmacological
Basis of
THERAPEUTICS

eleventh edition

EDITOR

Laurence L. Brunton, PhD

Professor of Pharmacology and Medicine
University of California San Diego School of Medicine
La Jolla, California

ASSOCIATE EDITORS

John S. Lazo, PhD

Allegheny Foundation Professor of Pharmacology
University of Pittsburgh School of Medicine
Pittsburgh, Pennsylvania

Keith L. Parker, MD, PhD

Professor of Internal Medicine and Pharmacology
Wilson Distinguished Professor of Biomedical Research
Chief, Division of Endocrinology and Metabolism
University of Texas Southwestern Medical Center
Dallas, Texas

Goodman & Gilman's

The
Pharmacological
Basis of
THERAPEUTICS

eleventh edition

McGRAW-HILL
MEDICAL PUBLISHING DIVISION

New York Chicago San Francisco Lisbon London Madrid Mexico City Milan New Delhi
San Juan Seoul Singapore Sydney Toronto

HEAL ADDL
0 14772152

GOODMAN AND GILMAN'S
THE PHARMACOLOGICAL BASIS OF THERAPEUTICS, 11/E

1234567890 DOW/DOW 098765

ISBN 0-07-142280-3

Digital Edition Set ISBN: 0-07-146804-8
Digital Edition Jacket ISBN: 0-07-146891-9
Digital Edition Subscription Access Card ISBN: 0-07-146892-7

This book was set in Times Roman and Formata by Silverchair Science + Communications, Inc.
The editors were James F. Shanahan, Janet Foltin, Karen Edmonson, and Regina Y. Brown.
The production manager was Philip Galea.
The illustration manager was Charissa Baker.
The cover designer was Libby Pisacreta.
The indexer was Coughlin Indexing Services.
RR Donnelley was printer and binder.

This book is printed on acid-free paper.

Library of Congress Cataloging-in-Publication Data

Goodman & Gilman's the pharmacological basis of therapeutics.-- 11th ed. / editor,
    Laurence L. Brunton ; associate editors, John S. Lazo, Keith L. Parker.
        p. cm.
    Includes index.
    ISBN 0-07-142280-3
    1. Pharmacology. 2. Therapeutics. I. Title: Pharmacological basis of therapeutics. II. Title: Goodman and Gilman's the pharmacological basis of therapeutics. III. Goodman, Louis Sanford, 1906- IV. Gilman, Alfred, 1908- V. Brunton, Laurence L. VI. Lazo, John S. VII. Parker, Keith L.

RM300.G644 2005
615'.7--dc22
                                                                    2004063122

Cover illustration: Imposed on the cover is a schematic rendering of the alpha subunit of the heterotrimeric G protein G_s as determined by x-ray crystallography (Sunahara, R.K., Tesmer, J.J.G., Gilman, A.G., and Sprang, S.R., Science vol 278, p 1943–1947, [1997]). Figure credit to Mark Wall, PhD.

CONTENTS

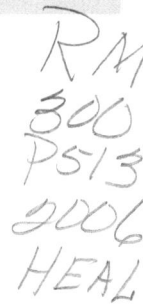

SECTION I

GENERAL PRINCIPLES   1

SECTION II

DRUGS ACTING AT SYNAPTIC AND NEUROEFFECTOR JUNCTIONAL SITES   137

SECTION III

DRUGS ACTING ON THE CENTRAL NERVOUS SYSTEM

317

SECTION IV

AUTACOIDS: DRUG THERAPY OF INFLAMMATION

629

SECTION XIII
DERMATOLOGY

SECTION XIV
OPHTHALMOLOGY

SECTION XV
TOXICOLOGY

APPENDICES

CONTRIBUTORS

Huda Akil, MD

Co-Director, Mental Health Research Institute;
University of Michigan
Ann Arbor, Michigan

Philip C. Amrein, MD

Assistant Professor of Medicine, Harvard Medical School;
Physician, Massachusetts General Hospital
Boston, Massachusetts

Ross J. Baldessarini, MD

Professor of Psychiatry (Neuroscience)
Harvard Medical School
Boston, Massachusetts;
Director, Neuropharmacology Laboratory & Psychopharmacology
    Program
McLean Division of Massachusetts General Hospital
Belmont, Massachusetts

Jeffrey R. Balser, MD, PhD

Associate Vice Chancellor for Research
The James Tayloe Gwathmey Professor of Anesthesiology and
    Pharmacology
Vanderbilt University Medical Center
Nashville, Tennessee

William M. Bennett, MD

Medical Director, Transplant Services
Legacy Transplant Services
Portland, Oregon

John E. Bennett, MD

Head, Clinical Mycology Section
Laboratory of Clinical Infectious Diseases, NIAID
National Institutes of Health
Bethesda, Maryland

Thomas P. Bersot, MD, PhD

Professor of Medicine
University of California, San Francisco;
Associate Investigator
Gladstone Institute of Cardiovascular Disease
San Francisco, California

David R. Bickers, MD

Carl Truman Nelson Professor/Chair
Department of Dermatology
Columbia University Medical Center
New York, New York

Floyd E. Bloom, MD

Professor Emeritus
Department of Neuropharmacology
The Scripps Research Institute
La Jolla, California

Lewis E. Braverman, MD

Chief, Section of Endocrinology, Diabetes,
    and Nutrition
Boston Medical Center
Professor of Medicine
Boston University School of Medicine
Boston Massachusetts

Joan Heller Brown, PhD

Chair and Professor of Pharmacology
Department of Pharmacology
University of California, San Diego
La Jolla, California

Anne Burke, MB, BCh, BAO

Assistant Professor of Medicine
Hospital of the University of Pennsylvania
Philadelphia, Pennsylvania

Iain L. O. Buxton, DPh

Professor of Pharmacology
University of Nevada School of Medicine
Reno, Nevada

William A. Catterall, PhD

Professor and Chair
Department of Pharmacology
University of Washington
Seattle, Washington

Bruce A. Chabner, MD

Professor of Medicine, Harvard Medical School
Clinical Director, Massachusetts General Hospital Cancer Center
Boston, Massachusetts

Henry F. Chambers, MD

Professor of Medicine, University of California, San Francisco
Chief, Division of Infectious Diseases
San Francisco General Hospital
San Francisco, California

Dennis S. Charney, MD

Dean of Research
Anne and Joel Ehrenkranz Professor
Departments of Psychiatry, Neuroscience, and Pharmacology &
    Biological Chemistry
Mount Sinai School of Medicine
New York, New York

C. Michael Crowder, MD, PhD

Associate Professor of Anesthesiology and Molecular Biology/
    Pharmacology
Washington University School of Medicine
St. Louis, Missouri

Stephen N. Davis, MD

Chief, Division of Diabetes, Endocrinology & Metabolism;
Rudolph Kampmeier Professor of Medicine,
Professor of Molecular Physiology & Biophysics
Vanderbilt University Medical Center
Nashville, Tennessee

Brian Druker, MD

Investigator, Howard Hughes Medical Institute
JELD-WEN Chair of Leukemia Research
Oregon Health & Science University Cancer Institute
Portland, Oregon

Ervin G. Erdös, MD

Professor of Pharmacology and Anesthesiology
University of Illinois at Chicago College of Medicine
Chicago, Illinois

Alex S. Evers, MD

Henry E. Mallinckrodt Professor and Head of Anesthesiology
Professor of Internal Medicine and Molecular Biology and
    Pharmacology
Washington University School of Medicine
Anesthesiologist-in-Chief
Barnes-Jewish Hospital
St. Louis, Missouri

James C. Fang, MD

Medical Director of Heart Transplantation and Circulatory
    Assistance
Brigham and Women's Hospital
Associate Professor of Medicine
Harvard Medical School
Boston, Massachusetts

Alan P. Farwell, MD

Associate Professor of Medicine
Division of Endocrinology
University of Massachusetts Medical School
Worcester, Massachusetts

Garret A. FitzGerald, MD

Chair, Department of Pharmacology
Director, Institute for Translational Medicine and Therapeutics
University of Pennsylvania
Philadelphia, Pennsylvania

Michael F. Fleming, MD, MPH

Professor of Family Medicine
University of Wisconsin
Madison, Wisconsin

Charles Flexner, MD

Associate Professor of Medicine, Pharmacology and Molecular
    Sciences, and International Health
Johns Hopkins University
Baltimore, Maryland

Lindy P. Fox, MD

Instructor in Dermatology
Department of Dermatology
Yale University School of Medicine
New Haven, Connecticut

Peter A. Friedman, PhD

Professor of Pharmacology
University of Pittsburgh School of Medicine
Pittsburgh, Pennsylvania

Kathleen M. Giacomini, PhD

Professor and Chair, Department of Biopharmaceutical
    Sciences
School of Pharmacy
University of California, San Francisco
San Francisco, California

Daniel E. Goldberg, MD, PhD

Professor of Medicine and Molecular Microbiology
Washington University School of Medicine
Investigator, Howard Hughes Medical Institute
St. Louis, Missouri

Frank J. Gonzalez, PhD

Chief, Laboratory of Metabolism
Center for Cancer Research
National Cancer Institute
Bethesda, Maryland

Paul E. Goss, MD, PhD, FRCPC, FRCP (UK)

Professor of Medicine, Harvard Medical School;
Director of Breast Cancer Research, MGH Cancer Center;
Co-Director of the Breast Cancer Disease Program, DF/HCC;
Avon Foundation Senior Scholar
Boston, Massachusetts

Howard B. Gutstein, MD

Associate Professor of Anesthesiology and Molecular Genetics
MD Anderson Cancer Center
Houston, Texas

R. Adron Harris, PhD

Director, Waggoner Center for Alcohol and Addiction
    Research
University of Texas, Austin
Austin, Texas

Frederick G. Hayden, MD

Richardson Professor of Clinical Virology
Professor of Internal Medicine and Pathology
University of Virginia School of Medicine
Charlottesville, Virginia

Jeffrey D. Henderer, MD

Assistant Professor of Ophthalmology
Thomas Jefferson University School of Medicine and
Assistant Surgeon
Wills Eye Hospital
Philadelphia, Pennsylvania

Brian B. Hoffman, MD

Professor of Medicine
Harvard Medical School;
Chief of Medicine
VA Boston Health Care System
Boston, Massachusetts

Willemijntje A. Hoogerwerf, MD

Assistant Professor of Medicine
University of Texas Medical Branch
Galveston, Texas

Peter J. Hotez, MD, PhD

Professor and Chair, Department of Microbiology, Immunology
    and Tropical Medicine
The George Washington University
Washington, DC

Nina Isoherranen, PhD

Acting Assistant Professor
Department of Pharmaceutics
University of Washington
Seattle, Washington

Edwin K. Jackson, PhD

Professor of Pharmacology
Associate Director, Center for Clinical Pharmacology
University of Pittsburgh School of Medicine
Pittsburgh, Pennsylvania

Roger A. Johns, MD, MHS

Professor of Anesthesiology & Critical Care Medicine
Johns Hopkins University School of Medicine
Baltimore, Maryland

Kenneth Kaushansky, MD

Helen M. Ranney Professor and Chair
Department of Medicine
University of California, San Diego
San Diego, California

Thomas J. Kipps, MD, PhD

Professor of Medicine
Deputy Director of Research, Moores Cancer Center
University of California, San Diego
La Jolla, California

Curtis D. Klaassen, PhD

University Distinguished Professor and Chair
Department of Pharmacology, Toxicology & Therapeutics
University of Kansas Medical Center
Kansas City, Kansas

Alan M. Krensky, MD

Shelagh Galligan Professor of Pediatrics
Chief, Division of Immunology and Transplantation
    Biology
Associate Dean for Children's Health
Stanford University School of Medicine
Stanford, California

David S. Loose, PhD

Associate Professor & Director
Department of Integrative Biology and Pharmacology
University of Texas - Houston Medical School
Houston, Texas

Alex Loukas, PhD

Senior Research Fellow
Queensland Institute of Medical Research
Australia

Ken Mackie, MD

Professor of Anesthesiology
Adjunct Professor of Physiology & Biophysics
University of Washington
Seattle, Washington

Robert W. Mahley, MD, PhD

President, The J. David Gladstone Institutes
Director, Gladstone Institute of Cardiovascular Disease
Senior Investigator, Gladstone Institute of Neurological Disease
San Francisco, California

Philip W. Majerus, MD

Professor of Medicine;
Co-Chairman, Division of Hematology
Washington University School of Medicine
St. Louis, Missouri

Steven E. Mayer, MD

Emeritus Professor of Pharmacology
University of California, San Diego
La Jolla, California

James O. McNamara, MD

Carl R. Deane Professor and Chair
Department of Neurobiology
Professor of Medicine (Neurology)
Director, Center for Translational Neuroscience
Duke University Medical Center
Durham, North Carolina

Hans F. Merk, MD

Professor of Dermatology & Allergology
University Hospital - RWTH Aachen
Aachen, Germany

M. Dror Michaelson, MD

Instructor in Medicine
Harvard Medical School;
Physician, Massachusetts General Hospital
Boston, Massachusetts

Thomas Michel, MD, PhD

Professor of Medicine, Harvard Medical School
Chief of Cardiology, VA Boston Healthcare System
Senior Physician, Brigham & Women's Hospital
Boston, Massachusetts

S. John Mihic, PhD

Associate Professor
Section of Neurobiology and Waggoner Center for Alcohol &
    Addiction Research
University of Texas at Austin
Austin, Texas

Constantine S. Mitsiades, MD, PhD

Instructor in Medicine
Department of Medical Oncology
Dana Farber Cancer Institute
Department of Medicine
Harvard Medical School
Boston, Massachusetts

Eric J. Moody, MD

Associate Professor
Department of Anesthesiology and Critical Care Medicine
Johns Hopkins University
Baltimore, Maryland

John A. Oates, MD

Professor of Medicine and Pharmacology
Vanderbilt University School of Medicine
Nashville, Tennessee

Charles P. O'Brien, MD, PhD

Professor of Psychiatry
University of Pennsylvania
Philadelphia, Pennsylvania

Keith L. Parker, MD, PhD

Professor of Internal Medicine & Pharmacology
Wilson Distinguished Professor of Biomedical Research
Chief, Division of Endocrinology & Metabolism
University of Texas Southwestern Medical Center
Dallas, Texas

Pankaj Jay Pasricha, MD

Chief, Division of Gastroenterology and Hepatology
Bassel and Frances Blanton Distinguished Professor of Internal
    Medicine
Professor of Neuroscience & Cell Biology and Biomedical
    Engineering
University of Texas Medical Branch
Galveston, Texas

William A. Petri, Jr., MD, PhD

Wade Hampton Frost Professor of Epidemiology
Professor of Medicine, Microbiology, and Pathology
Chief, Division of Infectious Diseases and International Health
University of Virginia Health System
Charlottesville, Virginia

Margaret A. Phillips, PhD

Professor of Pharmacology
University of Texas Southwestern Medical Center
Dallas, Texas

Sumant Ramachandra, MD, PhD

Vice President, Global Development-Oncology
Schering-Plough
Kenilworth, New Jersey

Christopher J. Rapuano, MD

Co-Director and Attending Surgeon, Cornea Service
Co-Director, Refractive Surgery Department
Wills Eye Hospital
Professor, Jefferson Medical College of Thomas Jefferson
    University
Philadelphia, Pennsylvania

Mary V. Relling, PharmD

Chair, Pharmaceutical Sciences
St. Jude Children's Research Hospital
Professor, University of Tennessee Colleges of Pharmacy and
    Medicine
Memphis, Tennessee

Paul G. Richardson, MD

Clinical Director, Jerome Lipper Multiple Myeloma Center;
Assistant Professor in Medicine, Harvard Medical School
Boston, Massachusetts

Thomas P. Rocco, MD

Director, Clinical Cardiology
VA Boston Health Care System
West Roxbury, Massachusetts
Assistant Professor of Medicine
Harvard Medical School
Boston, Massachusetts

Dan M. Roden, MD, CM

Director, Oates Institute for Experimental Therapeutics
William Stokes Professor of Experimental Therapeutics
Vanderbilt University Medical Center
Nashville, Tennessee

David P. Ryan, MD

Clinical Director, Tucker Gosnell Center for Gastrointestinal
    Cancers
Massachusetts General Hospital
Assistant Professor of Medicine, Harvard Medical School
Boston, Massachusetts

Elaine Sanders-Bush, PhD

Professor of Pharmacology and Psychiatry
Vanderbilt University School of Medicine
Nashville, Tennessee

Bernard P. Schimmer, PhD

Professor of Medical Research and Pharmacology
Banting & Best Department of Medical Research
University of Toronto
Toronto, Ontario, Canada

Joseph H. Sellin, MD

Professor of Medicine
Director, C²CREATE
Inflammatory Bowel Disease Center
Division of Gastroenterology
University of Texas Medical Branch
Galveston, Texas

Theresa A. Shapiro, MD, PhD

Wellcome Professor and Director
Division of Clinical Pharmacology
Departments of Medicine and Pharmacology and Molecular
    Sciences
Johns Hopkins University School of Medicine
Baltimore, Maryland

Danny D. Shen, PhD

Professor & Chair, Department of Pharmacy
University of Washington
Seattle, Washington

Brett A. Simon, MD, PhD

Associate Professor of Anesthesiology/Critical Care Medicine and
    Medicine
Vice Chair for Faculty Development
Chief, Division of Adult Anesthesia
Department of Anesthesiology and Critical Care Medicine
Johns Hopkins University
Baltimore, Maryland

Randal A. Skidgel, PhD

Professor of Pharmacology
University of Illinois at Chicago College of Medicine
Chicago, Illinois

Helen E. Smith, RPh, PhD

Clinical Pharmacist/Research Associate
University of Washington
Seattle, Washington

Emer M. Smyth, PhD

Research Assistant Professor of Pharmacology
University of Pennsylvania
Philadelphia, Pennsylvania

Peter J. Snyder, MD

Professor of Medicine
University of Pennsylvania
Philadelphia, Pennsylvania

George M. Stancel, PhD

Dean, Graduate School of Biomedical Sciences
University of Texas Health Science Center at Houston and
M.D. Anderson Cancer Center
Houston, Texas

David G. Standaert, MD, PhD

Associate Professor of Neurology
Massachusetts General Hospital
Harvard Medical School
Boston, Massachusetts

Samuel L. Stanley, Jr., MD

Professor of Medicine and Molecular Microbiology
Director, Midwest Regional Center of Excellence for
    Biodefense and Emerging Infectious Diseases Research
Washington University School of Medicine
St. Louis, Missouri

Yuichi Sugiyama, PhD

Professor and Chair
Department of Molecular Pharmacokinetics
Graduate School of Pharmaceutical Sciences
University of Tokyo
Tokyo, Japan

Jeffrey G. Supko, PhD

Director, Clinical Pharmacology Laboratory
Massachusetts General Hospital Cancer Center
Associate Professor of Medicine
Harvard Medical School
Boston, Massachusetts

Frank I. Tarazi, PhD, MSc

Associate Professor of Psychiatry and Neuroscience
Harvard Medical School;
Director, Psychiatric Neuroscience Laboratory
Mailman Research Center
McLean Division of Massachusetts General Hospital
Belmont, Massachusetts

Palmer Taylor, PhD

Sandra and Monroe Trout Professor of Pharmacology
Dean, Skaggs School of Pharmacy and Pharmaceutical Sciences
Associate Vice Chancellor, Health Sciences
University of California, San Diego
La Jolla, California

Kenneth E. Thummel, MD

Professor of Pharmaceutics
Associate Dean for Research and New Initiatives
University of Washington, School of Pharmacy
Seattle, Washington

Douglas M. Tollefsen, MD, PhD

Professor of Medicine
Washington University Medical School
St. Louis, Missouri

Robert H. Tukey, PhD

Professor of Chemistry & Biochemistry and Pharmacology
University of California, San Diego
La Jolla, California

Bradley J. Undem, PhD

Professor of Medicine
Johns Hopkins Asthma and Allergy Center
Baltimore, Maryland

Flavio Vincenti, MD

Professor of Clinical Medicine
University of California, San Francisco
San Francisco, California

Thomas C. Westfall, PhD

William Beaumont Professor and Chairman
Department of Pharmacological and Physiological Science
Saint Louis University School of Medicine
St. Louis, Missouri

David P. Westfall, PhD

Dean, College of Science
University of Nevada, Reno;
Foundation Professor of Pharmacology
University of Nevada School of Medicine
Reno, Nevada

Wyndham H. Wilson, MD, PhD

Senior Investigator and Chief, Lymphoma Section
Experimental Transplantation and Immunology Branch
National Cancer Institute
Bethesda, Maryland

Anne B. Young, MD, PhD

Julieanne Dorn Professor of Neurology
Harvard Medical School
Cambridge, Massachusetts

CONSULTANTS TO THE EDITORS

Jeffrey R. Balser, MD, PhD
Vanderbilt University

Donald K. Blumenthal, PhD
University of Utah

Douglas Brown, MD
Vanderbilt University

John M. Carethers, MD
University of California, San Diego

William R. Crowley, PhD
University of Utah

Wolfgang Dillmann, MD
University of California, San Diego

Merrill J. Egorin, MD
University of Pittsburgh

Joshua Fierer, MD
University of California, San Diego

Michael B. Gorin, MD, PhD
University of Pittsburgh

Glen R. Hanson, PhD, DDS
University of Utah

Raymond Harris, MD
Vanderbilt University

J. Harold Helderman, MD
Vanderbilt University

Charles L. James, PharmD
University of California, San Diego

Matthew A. Movsesian, MD
University of Utah

Nelda Murri, PharmD, MBA
University of Washington

Paul Ragan, MD
Vanderbilt University

Sharon L. Reed, MD
University of California, San Diego

George M. Rodgers, MD, PhD
University of Utah

Douglas E. Rollins, MD, PhD
University of Utah

David M. Roth, PhD, MD
University of California, San Diego

Richard Shelton, MD
Vanderbilt University

Lawrence Steinman, MD
Stanford University

Stephen I. Wasserman, MD
University of California, San Diego

H. Steve White, PhD
University of Utah

Joseph L. Witztum, MD
University of California, San Diego

John J. Zone, MD
University of Utah

PREFACE

Upon learning that I was assuming the editorship of this book, a senior colleague warned, "Be careful. Don't tamper lightly with the bible." This reputation of "G & G" as the "bible of pharmacology" is a tribute to the ideals and writing of the original authors, Alfred Gilman and Louis Goodman. In 1941, they set forth the principles that have guided this book through ten prior editions and that the associate editors and I have continued to use: to correlate pharmacology with related medical sciences, to reinterpret the actions and uses of drugs in light of advances in medicine and the basic biomedical sciences, to emphasize the applications of pharmacodynamics to therapeutics, and to create a book that will be useful to students of pharmacology and physicians alike.

As with all editions since the second, expert scholars have written the individual chapters, a number of which are new to this edition. We have emphasized basic principles, adding chapters on drug transporters and drug metabolism; the material covered in these chapters explains many prominent drug-drug interactions and adverse drug responses. We have also added a chapter on the emerging field of pharmacogenetics, looking toward the individualization of therapy and an understanding of how our genetic make-up influences our responses to drugs. A chapter entitled "The Science of Drug Therapy" describes how basic principles of pharmacology apply to the care of the individual patient. Most other chapters have been extensively revised; a few have been condensed or eliminated.

Assembling a multi-author pharmacology book challenges contributors and editors in different ways. Among the apparently irresistible and understandable temptations in writing a chapter are the desire to cover everything, the urge to explain G-protein coupled signaling, and the inclination to describe in detail the history of the field in which one is an expert, citing all relevant papers from Claude Bernard to the present. These hazards, plus the continuing advance of knowledge, produce considerable pressure to increase the length of the book. As an anti-dote, the associate editors and I have worked to eliminate repetition and extraneous text. We have pressed contributors hard, using the communicative rapidity and ease of e-mail to interact with them, to clarify and condense, and to re-write while adhering to the principles of the original authors and retaining the completeness for which the book is known. We have tried to standardize the organization of chapters; thus, students should easily find the physiology and basic pharmacology set forth in regular type in each chapter, and the clinician and expert will find details in extract type under identifiable headings. We have also tried to improve the clarity of tables and figures to provide summaries of concepts and large amounts of information. Although this 11th edition is slightly shorter than its predecessor, we believe that it is every bit as thorough.

Many deserve thanks for their contributions to the preparation of this edition. Professors Keith Parker (UT Southwestern) and John Lazo (U. Pittsburgh) have lent their considerable energy and expertise as associate editors. Professor Nelda Murri (U. Washington) has read each chapter with her keen pharmacist's eye. Two Nashville novelists played essential roles: Lynne Hutchison again served ably as managing editor, coordinating the activities of contributors, editors, and word processors; and, for the second time, Chris Bell checked references and assembled the master copy. Each chapter has been read by an expert in addition to the editors, and the editors thank those readers. We also express our appreciation to former contributors, who will, no doubt, recognize some of their best words from previous editions. We are grateful to our editors at McGraw-Hill, Janet Foltin and James Shanahan, who have shepherded the edited text into print, and to our wives, whose support and forbearance are gifts beyond reckoning.

Lastly, I would like to pay tribute to my friend, Alfred G. Gilman. As a teacher, mentor, researcher, editor of several editions of this book, Nobel laureate, chair of a distinguished pharmacology department, and now dean of a medical school, he has enriched every aspect of our field.

Laurence Brunton

SAN DIEGO, CALIFORNIA
JULY 1, 2005

PREFACE TO THE FIRST EDITION

Three objectives have guided the writing of this book—the correlation of pharmacology with related medical sciences, the reinterpretation of the actions and uses of drugs from the viewpoint of important advances in medicine, and the placing of emphasis on the applications of pharmacodynamics to therapeutics.

Although pharmacology is a basic medical science in its own right, it borrows freely from and contributes generously to the subject matter and technics of many medical disciplines, clinical as well as preclinical. Therefore, the correlation of strictly pharmacological information with medicine as a whole is essential for a proper presentation of pharmacology to students and physicians. Furthermore, the reinterpretation of the actions and uses of well-established therapeutic agents in the light of recent advances in the medical sciences is as important a function of a modern textbook of pharmacology as is the description of new drugs. In many instances these new interpretations necessitate radical departures from accepted but outworn concepts of the actions of drugs. Lastly, the emphasis throughout the book, as indicated in its title, has been clinical. This is mandatory because medical students must be taught pharmacology from the standpoint of the actions and uses of drugs in the prevention and treatment of disease. To the student, pharmacological data per se are valueless unless he/she is able to apply this information in the practice of medicine. This book has also been written for the practicing physician, to whom it offers an opportunity to keep abreast of recent advances in therapeutics and to acquire the basic principles necessary for the rational use of drugs in his/her daily practice.

The criteria for the selection of bibliographic references require comment. It is obviously unwise, if not impossible, to document every fact included in the text. Preference has therefore been given to articles of a review nature, to the literature on new drugs, and to original contributions in controversial fields. In most instances, only the more recent investigations have been cited. In order to encourage free use of the bibliography, references are chiefly to the available literature in the English language.

The authors are greatly indebted to their many colleagues at the Yale University School of Medicine for their generous help and criticism. In particular they are deeply grateful to Professor Henry Gray Barbour, whose constant encouragement and advice have been invaluable.

Louis S. Goodman
Alfred Gilman

NEW HAVEN, CONNECTICUT
NOVEMBER 20, 1940

CHAPTER

1

PHARMACOKINETICS AND PHARMACODYNAMICS
The Dynamics of Drug Absorption, Distribution, Action, and Elimination

Iain L. O. Buxton

Numerous factors in addition to a known pharmacological action in a specific tissue at a particular receptor contribute to successful drug therapy. When a drug enters the body, the body begins immediately to work on the drug: absorption, distribution, metabolism (biotransformation), and elimination. These are the processes of *pharmacokinetics*. The drug also acts on the body, an interaction to which the concept of a drug receptor is key, since the receptor is responsible for the selectivity of drug action and for the quantitative relationship between drug and effect. The mechanisms of drug action are the processes of *pharmacodynamics*. The time course of therapeutic drug action in the body can be understood in terms of pharmacokinetics and pharmacodynamics (Figure 1–1).

I. PHARMACOKINETICS: THE DYNAMICS OF DRUG ABSORPTION, DISTRIBUTION, METABOLISM, AND ELIMINATION

PHYSICOCHEMICAL FACTORS IN TRANSFER OF DRUGS ACROSS MEMBRANES

The absorption, distribution, metabolism, and excretion of a drug all involve its passage across cell membranes. Mechanisms by which drugs cross membranes and the

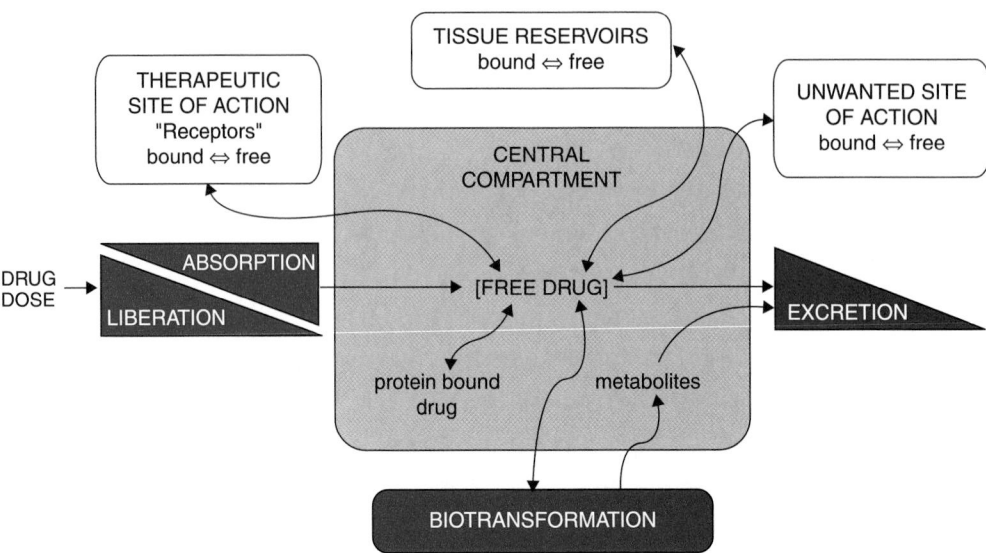

Figure 1–1. *The interrelationship of the absorption, distribution, binding, metabolism, and excretion of a drug and its concentration at its sites of action.* Possible distribution and binding of metabolites in relation to their potential actions at receptors are not depicted.

physicochemical properties of molecules and membranes that influence this transfer are critical to understanding the disposition of drugs in the human body. The characteristics of a drug that predict its movement and availability at sites of action are its molecular size and shape, degree of ionization, relative lipid solubility of its ionized and nonionized forms, and its binding to serum and tissue proteins.

In most cases, a drug must traverse the plasma membranes of many cells to reach its site of action. Although barriers to drug movement may be a single layer of cells (intestinal epithelium) or several layers of cells and associated extracellular protein (skin), the plasma membrane represents the common barrier to drug distribution.

Cell Membranes. The plasma membrane consists of a bilayer of amphipathic lipids with their hydrocarbon chains oriented inward to the center of the bilayer to form a continuous hydrophobic phase and their hydrophilic heads oriented outward. Individual lipid molecules in the bilayer vary according to the particular membrane and can move laterally and organize themselves with cholesterol (*e.g.,* sphingolipids), endowing the membrane with fluidity, flexibility, organization, high electrical resistance, and relative impermeability to highly polar molecules. Membrane proteins embedded in the bilayer serve as receptors, ion channels, or transporters to transduce electrical or chemical signaling pathways and provide selective targets for drug actions. These proteins may be associated with caveolin and sequestered within caveolae, they may be excluded from caveolae, or they may be organized in signaling domains rich in cholesterol and sphingolipid not containing caveolin.

Cell membranes are relatively permeable to water either by diffusion or by flow resulting from hydrostatic or osmotic differences across the membrane, and bulk flow of water can carry with it drug molecules. However, proteins with drug molecules bound to them are too large and polar for this type of transport to occur; thus, transmembrane movement generally is limited to unbound drug. Paracellular transport through intercellular gaps is sufficiently large that passage across most capillaries is limited by blood flow and not by other factors (*see* below). As described later, this type of transport is an important factor in filtration across glomerular membranes in the kidney. Important exceptions exist in such capillary diffusion, however, because "tight" intercellular junctions are present in specific tissues, and paracellular transport in them is limited. Capillaries of the central nervous system (CNS) and a variety of epithelial tissues have tight junctions (*see* below). Bulk flow of water can carry with it small water-soluble substances, but bulk-flow transport is limited when the molecular mass of the solute exceeds 100 to 200 daltons. Accordingly, most large lipophilic drugs must pass through the cell membrane itself.

Passive Membrane Transport. Drugs cross membranes either by passive processes or by mechanisms involving the active participation of components of the membrane. In passive transport, the drug molecule usually penetrates by diffusion along a concentration gradient by virtue of its solubility in the lipid bilayer. Such transfer is directly proportional to the magnitude of the concentration gradient across the membrane, to the lipid–water partition coefficient of the drug, and to the membrane surface area exposed to the drug. The greater the partition coefficient, the higher is the concentration of drug in the membrane, and the faster is its diffusion. After a steady state is attained, the concentration of the unbound drug is the same on both sides of the membrane if the drug is a nonelectrolyte. For ionic compounds, the steady-state concentrations depend on the electrochemical gradient for the ion and on differences in pH across the membrane, which may influence the state of ionization of the molecule disparately on either side of the membrane.

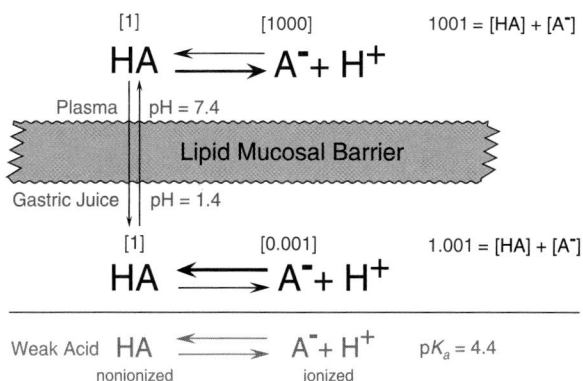

Figure 1–2. *Influence of pH on the distribution of a weak acid between plasma and gastric juice separated by a lipid barrier.*

Weak Electrolytes and Influence of pH. Most drugs are weak acids or bases that are present in solution as both the nonionized and ionized species. The nonionized molecules usually are more lipid-soluble and can diffuse readily across the cell membrane. In contrast, the ionized molecules usually are unable to penetrate the lipid membrane because of their low lipid solubility.

Therefore, the transmembrane distribution of a weak electrolyte is determined by its pK_a and the pH gradient across the membrane. The pK_a is the pH at which half the drug (weak electrolyte) is in its ionized form. To illustrate the effect of pH on distribution of drugs, the partitioning of a weak acid (pK_a = 4.4) between plasma (pH = 7.4) and gastric juice (pH = 1.4) is depicted in Figure 1–2. It is assumed that the gastric mucosal membrane behaves as a simple lipid barrier that is permeable only to the lipid-soluble, nonionized form of the acid. The ratio of nonionized to ionized drug at each pH is readily calculated from the Henderson–Hasselbalch equation:

$$\log \frac{[\text{protonated form}]}{[\text{unprotonated form}]} = pK_a - pH \qquad (1-1)$$

This equation relates the pH of the medium around the drug and the drug's acid dissociation constant (pK_a) to the ratio of the protonated (HA or BH^+) and unprotonated (A^- or B) forms, where $HA \leftrightarrow A^- + H^+$ ($K_a = [A^-][H^+]/[HA]$) describes the dissociation of an acid, and $BH^+ \leftrightarrow B + H^+$ ($K_a = [B][H^+]/[BH^+]$) describes the dissociation of the pronated form of a base.

Thus, in plasma, the ratio of nonionized to ionized drug is 1:1000; in gastric juice, the ratio is 1:0.001. These values are given in brackets in Figure 1–2. The total concentration ratio between the plasma and the gastric juice therefore would be 1000:1 if such a system came to a steady state. For a weak base with a pK_a of 4.4, the ratio would be reversed, as would the thick horizontal arrows in Figure 1–2, which indicate the predominant species at each pH. Accordingly,

at steady state, an acidic drug will accumulate on the more basic side of the membrane and a basic drug on the more acidic side—a phenomenon termed *ion trapping*. These considerations have obvious implications for the absorption and excretion of drugs, as discussed more specifically below. The establishment of concentration gradients of weak electrolytes across membranes with a pH gradient is a physical process and does not require an active electrolyte transport system. All that is necessary is a membrane preferentially permeable to one form of the weak electrolyte and a pH gradient across the membrane. The establishment of the pH gradient, however, is an active process.

Carrier-Mediated Membrane Transport. While passive diffusion through the bilayer is dominant in the disposition of most drugs, carrier-mediated mechanisms also play an important role. *Active transport* is characterized by a direct requirement for energy, movement against an electrochemical gradient, saturability, selectivity, and competitive inhibition by cotransported compounds. Na^+,K^+-ATPase is an active transport mechanism. Secondary active transport uses the electrochemical energy stored in a gradient to move another molecule against a concentration gradient; *e.g.,* the Na^+–Ca^{2+} exchange protein uses the energy stored in the Na^+ gradient established by the Na^+,K^+-ATPase to export cytosolic Ca^{2+} and maintain it at a low basal level, approximately 100 nM in most cells (*see* Chapter 33); similarly, the Na^+-dependent glucose transporters SGLT1 and SGLT2 move glucose across membranes of gastrointestinal (GI) epithelium and renal tubules by coupling glucose transport to downhill Na^+ flux. *Facilitated diffusion* describes a carrier-mediated transport process in which there is no input of energy, and therefore, enhanced movement of the involved substance is down an electrochemical gradient as in the permeation of glucose across a muscle cell membrane mediated by the insulin-sensitive glucose transporter protein GLUT4. Such mechanisms, which may be highly selective for a specific conformational structure of a drug, are involved in the transport of endogenous compounds whose rate of transport by passive diffusion otherwise would be too slow. In other cases, they function as a barrier system to protect cells from potentially toxic substances. Pharmacologically important transporters may mediate either drug uptake or efflux and often facilitate vectorial transport across polarized cells. An important efflux transporter present at many sites is the P-glycoprotein encoded by the multidrug resistance-1 (*MDR1*) gene. P-glycoprotein localized in the enterocyte limits the oral absorption of transported drugs because it exports compounds back into the GI tract subsequent to their absorption by passive diffusion. The P-glycoprotein also can confer resistance to some cancer chemotherapeutic agents (*see* Chapter 51). The importance of P-glycoprotein in the elimination of drugs is underscored by the presence of genetic polymorphisms in *MDR1* (*see* Chapters 2 and 4 and Marzolini *et al.*, 2004) that can affect therapeutic drug levels. Transporters and their roles in drug action are presented in detail in Chapter 2.

DRUG ABSORPTION, BIOAVAILABILITY, AND ROUTES OF ADMINISTRATION

Absorption is the movement of a drug from its site of administration into the central compartment (Figure 1–1)

Table 1–1
Some Characteristics of Common Routes of Drug Administration*

ROUTE	ABSORPTION PATTERN	SPECIAL UTILITY	LIMITATIONS AND PRECAUTIONS
Intravenous	Absorption circumvented Potentially immediate effects Suitable for large volumes and for irritating substances, or complex mixtures, when diluted	Valuable for emergency use Permits titration of dosage Usually required for high-molecular-weight protein and peptide drugs	Increased risk of adverse effects Must inject solutions *slowly* as a rule Not suitable for oily solutions or poorly soluble substances
Subcutaneous	Prompt, from aqueous solution Slow and sustained, from repository preparations	Suitable for some poorly soluble suspensions and for instillation of slow-release implants	Not suitable for large volumes Possible pain or necrosis from irritating substances
Intramuscular	Prompt, from aqueous solution Slow and sustained, from repository preparations	Suitable for moderate volumes, oily vehicles, and some irritating substances Appropriate for self-administration (*e.g.*, insulin)	Precluded during anticoagulant therapy May interfere with interpretation of certain diagnostic tests (*e.g.*, creatine kinase)
Oral ingestion	Variable, depends on many factors (*see* text)	Most convenient and economical; usually more safe	Requires patient compliance Bioavailability potentially erratic and incomplete

*See text for more complete discussion and for other routes.

and the extent to which this occurs. For solid dosage forms, absorption first requires dissolution of the tablet or capsule, thus liberating the drug. The clinician is concerned primarily with bioavailability rather than absorption. *Bioavailability* is a term used to indicate the fractional extent to which a dose of drug reaches its site of action or a biological fluid from which the drug has access to its site of action. For example, a drug given orally must be absorbed first from the stomach and intestine, but this may be limited by the characteristics of the dosage form and the drug's physicochemical properties. In addition, drug then passes through the liver, where metabolism and biliary excretion may occur before the drug enters the systemic circulation. Accordingly, a fraction of the administered and absorbed dose of drug will be inactivated or diverted before it can reach the general circulation and be distributed to its sites of action. If the metabolic or excretory capacity of the liver for the drug is large, bioavailability will be reduced substantially (the *first-pass effect*). This decrease in availability is a function of the anatomical site from which absorption takes place; other anatomical, physio-

logical, and pathological factors can influence bioavailability (*see* below), and the choice of the route of drug administration must be based on an understanding of these conditions.

Oral (Enteral) *versus* Parenteral Administration. Often there is a choice of the route by which a therapeutic agent may be given, and knowledge of the advantages and disadvantages of the different routes of administration is then of primary importance. Some characteristics of the major routes employed for systemic drug effect are compared in Table 1–1.

Oral ingestion is the most common method of drug administration. It also is the safest, most convenient, and most economical. Disadvantages to the oral route include limited absorption of some drugs because of their physical characteristics (*e.g.*, water solubility), emesis as a result of irritation to the GI mucosa, destruction of some drugs by digestive enzymes or low gastric pH, irregularities in absorption or propulsion in the presence of food or other drugs, and the need for cooperation on the part of the patient. In addition, drugs in the GI tract may be metabolized by the enzymes of the intestinal flora, mucosa, or liver before they gain access to the general circulation.

The parenteral injection of drugs has certain distinct advantages over oral administration. In some instances, parenteral administration is essential for the drug to be delivered in its active form, as in the case of monoclonal antibodies such as *infliximab,* an antibody against tumor necrosis factor α (TNF-α) used in the treatment of rheumatoid arthritis. Availability usually is more rapid, extensive, and predictable when a drug is given by injection. The effective dose therefore can be delivered more accurately. In emergency therapy and when a patient is unconscious, uncooperative, or unable to retain anything given by mouth, parenteral therapy may be a necessity. The injection of drugs, however, has its disadvantages: Asepsis must be maintained, and this is of particular concern when drugs are given over time, such as in intravenous or intrathecal administration; pain may accompany the injection; and it is sometimes difficult for patients to perform the injections themselves if self-medication is necessary.

Oral Ingestion. Absorption from the GI tract is governed by factors such as surface area for absorption, blood flow to the site of absorption, the physical state of the drug (solution, suspension, or solid dosage form), its water solubility, and the drug's concentration at the site of absorption. For drugs given in solid form, the rate of dissolution may be the limiting factor in their absorption, especially if they have low water solubility. Since most drug absorption from the GI tract occurs by passive diffusion, absorption is favored when the drug is in the nonionized and more lipophilic form. Based on the pH–partition concept (Figure 1–2), one would predict that drugs that are weak acids would be better absorbed from the stomach (pH 1 to 2) than from the upper intestine (pH 3 to 6), and *vice versa* for weak bases. However, the epithelium of the stomach is lined with a thick mucous layer, and its surface area is small; by contrast, the villi of the upper intestine provide an extremely large surface area (approximately 200 m²). Accordingly, the rate of absorption of a drug from the intestine will be greater than that from the stomach even if the drug is predominantly ionized in the intestine and largely nonionized in the stomach. Thus, any factor that accelerates gastric emptying will be likely to increase the rate of drug absorption, whereas any factor that delays gastric emptying is expected to have the opposite effect, regardless of the characteristics of the drug. Gastric emptying is influenced in women by the effects of estrogen (*i.e.,* slower than in men for premenopausal women and those taking estrogen in replacement therapy).

Drugs that are destroyed by gastric secretions or that cause gastric irritation sometimes are administered in dosage forms with an enteric coating that prevents dissolution in the acidic gastric contents. However, some enteric-coated preparations of a drug also may resist dissolution in the intestine, reducing drug absorption. The use of enteric coatings is nonetheless helpful for drugs such as *aspirin* that can cause significant gastric irritation in many patients.

Controlled-Release Preparations. The rate of absorption of a drug administered as a tablet or other solid oral dosage form is partly dependent on its rate of dissolution in GI fluids. This is the basis for *controlled-release, extended-release, sustained-release,* and *prolonged-action* pharmaceutical preparations that are designed to produce slow, uniform absorption of the drug for 8 hours or longer. Such preparations are offered for medications in all major drug categories. Potential advantages of such preparations are reduction in the frequency of administration of the drug as compared with conventional dosage forms (possibly with improved compliance by the patient), maintenance of a therapeutic effect overnight, and decreased incidence and/or intensity of both undesired effects (by elimination of the peaks in drug concentration) and nontherapeutic blood levels of the drug (by elimination of troughs in concentration) that often occur after administration of immediate-release dosage forms.

Many controlled-release preparations fulfill these expectations and may be preferred in some therapeutic situations such as antidepressant therapy (Nemeroff, 2003) or treatment with dihydropyridine Ca^{2+} entry blockers (*see* Chapter 32). However, such products have some drawbacks. Generally, interpatient variability in terms of the systemic concentration of the drug that is achieved is greater for controlled-release than for immediate-release dosage forms. During repeated drug administration, trough drug concentrations resulting from controlled-release dosage forms may not be different from those observed with immediate-release preparations, although the time interval between trough concentrations is greater for a well-designed controlled-release product. It is possible that the dosage form may fail, and "dose dumping" with resulting toxicity can occur because the total dose of drug ingested at one time may be several times the amount contained in the conventional preparation. Factors that may contribute to dose dumping for certain controlled-release preparations include stomach acidity and administration along with a high-fat meal. Controlled-release dosage forms are most appropriate for drugs with short half-lives (<4 hours). So-called controlled-release dosage forms are sometimes developed for drugs with long half-lives (>12 hours). These usually more expensive products should not be prescribed unless specific advantages have been demonstrated.

Sublingual Administration. Absorption from the oral mucosa has special significance for certain drugs despite the fact that the surface area available is small. Venous drainage from the mouth is to the superior vena cava, which protects the drug from rapid hepatic first-pass metabolism. For example, *nitroglycerin* is effective when retained sublingually because it is nonionic and has very high lipid solubility. Thus, the drug is absorbed very rapidly. Nitroglycerin also is very potent; relatively few molecules need to be absorbed to produce the therapeutic effect. If a tablet of nitroglycerin were swallowed, the accompanying hepatic metabolism would be sufficient to prevent the appearance of any active nitroglycerin in the systemic circulation.

Transdermal Absorption. Not all drugs readily penetrate the intact skin. Absorption of those that do is dependent on the surface area over which they are applied and their lipid solubility because the epidermis behaves as a lipid barrier (*see* Chapter 63). The dermis, however, is freely permeable to many solutes; consequently, systemic absorption of drugs occurs much more readily through abraded, burned, or denuded skin. Inflammation and other conditions that increase cutaneous blood flow also enhance absorption. Toxic effects sometimes are produced by absorption through the skin of highly lipid-soluble substances (*e.g.,* a lipid-soluble insecticide in an organic solvent). Absorption through the skin can be enhanced by suspending the drug in an oily vehicle and rubbing the resulting preparation into the skin. Because hydrated skin is more permeable than dry skin, the dosage form may be modified or an occlusive dressing may be used to facilitate absorption. Controlled-release topical patches have become increasingly available, including *nicotine* for tobacco-smoking withdrawal, *scopolamine* for motion sickness, nitroglycerin for angina pectoris, *testosterone* and *estrogen* for replacement therapy, and various estrogens and progestins for birth control.

Rectal Administration. The rectal route often is useful when oral ingestion is precluded because the patient is unconscious or when vomiting is present—a situation particularly relevant to young children. Approximately 50% of the drug that is absorbed from the rectum will bypass the liver; the potential for hepatic first-pass metabolism thus is less than that for an oral dose. However, rectal absorption often is irregular and incomplete, and many drugs can cause irritation of the rectal mucosa.

Parenteral Injection. The major routes of parenteral administration are intravenous, subcutaneous, and intramuscular. Absorption from subcutaneous and intramuscular sites occurs by simple diffusion along the gradient from drug depot to plasma. The rate is limited by the area of the absorbing capillary membranes and by the solubility of the substance in the interstitial fluid. Relatively large aqueous channels in the endothelial membrane account for the indiscriminate diffusion of molecules regardless of their lipid solubility. Larger molecules, such as proteins, slowly gain access to the circulation by way of lymphatic channels.

Drugs administered into the systemic circulation by any route, excluding the intraarterial route, are subject to possible first-pass elimination in the lung prior to distribution to the rest of the body. The lungs serve as a temporary storage site for a number of agents, especially drugs that are weak bases and are predominantly nonionized at the blood pH, apparently by their partition into lipid. The lungs also serve as a filter for particulate matter that may be given intravenously, and they provide a route of elimination for volatile substances.

Intravenous. Factors relevant to absorption are circumvented by intravenous injection of drugs in aqueous solution because bioavailability is complete and rapid. Also, drug delivery is controlled and achieved with an accuracy and immediacy not possible by any other procedure. In some instances, as in the induction of surgical anesthesia, the dose of a drug is not predetermined but is adjusted to the response of the patient. Also, certain irritating solutions can be given only in this manner because the drug, if injected slowly, is greatly diluted by the blood.

There are both advantages and disadvantages to the use of this route of administration. Unfavorable reactions can occur because high concentrations of drug may be attained rapidly in both plasma and tissues. There are therapeutic circumstances where it is advisable to administer a drug by bolus injection (small volume given rapidly, *e.g., tissue plasminogen activator* immediately following an acute myocardial infarction) and other circumstances where slower administration of drug is advisable, such as the delivery of drugs by intravenous "piggy-back" (*e.g.,* antibiotics). Intravenous administration of drugs warrants close monitoring of the patient's response. Furthermore, once the drug is injected, there is often no retreat. Repeated intravenous injections depend on the ability to maintain a patent vein. Drugs in an oily vehicle, those that precipitate blood constituents or hemolyze erythrocytes, and drug combinations that cause precipitates to form must not be given by this route.

Subcutaneous. Injection of a drug into a subcutaneous site can be used only for drugs that are not irritating to tissue; otherwise, severe pain, necrosis, and tissue sloughing may occur. The rate of absorption following subcutaneous injection of a drug often is sufficiently constant and slow to provide a sustained effect. Moreover, altering the period over which a drug is absorbed may be varied intentionally, as is accomplished with *insulin* for injection using particle size, protein complexation, and pH to provide short- (3 to 6 hours), intermediate- (10 to 18 hours), and long-acting (18 to 24 hours) preparations. The incorporation of a vasoconstrictor agent in a solution of a drug to be injected subcutaneously also retards absorption. Thus, the injectable local anesthetic *lidocaine* incorporates *epinephrine* into the dosage form. Absorption of drugs

implanted under the skin in a solid pellet form occurs slowly over a period of weeks or months; some hormones (*e.g.,* contraceptives) are administered effectively in this manner.

Intramuscular. Drugs in aqueous solution are absorbed quite rapidly after intramuscular injection depending on the rate of blood flow to the injection site. This may be modulated to some extent by local heating, massage, or exercise. For example, while absorption of insulin generally is more rapid from injection in the arm and abdominal wall than the thigh, jogging may cause a precipitous drop in blood sugar when insulin is injected into the thigh rather than into the arm or abdominal wall because running markedly increases blood flow to the leg. A hot bath accelerates absorption from all these sites owing to vasodilation. Generally, the rate of absorption following injection of an aqueous preparation into the deltoid or vastus lateralis is faster than when the injection is made into the gluteus maximus. The rate is particularly slower for females after injection into the gluteus maximus. This has been attributed to the different distribution of subcutaneous fat in males and females and because fat is relatively poorly perfused. Very obese or emaciated patients may exhibit unusual patterns of absorption following intramuscular or subcutaneous injection. Slow, constant absorption from the intramuscular site results if the drug is injected in solution in oil or suspended in various other repository (*depot*) vehicles. Antibiotics often are administered in this manner. Substances too irritating to be injected subcutaneously sometimes may be given intramuscularly.

Intraarterial. Occasionally, a drug is injected directly into an artery to localize its effect in a particular tissue or organ, such as in the treatment of liver tumors and head/neck cancers. Diagnostic agents sometimes are administered by this route (*e.g., technetium-labeled human serum albumin*). Intraarterial injection requires great care and should be reserved for experts. The first-pass and cleansing effects of the lung are not available when drugs are given by this route.

Intrathecal. The blood–brain barrier and the blood–cerebrospinal fluid (CSF) barrier often preclude or slow the entrance of drugs into the CNS. Therefore, when local and rapid effects of drugs on the meninges or cerebrospinal axis are desired, as in spinal anesthesia or treatment of acute CNS infections, drugs sometimes are injected directly into the spinal subarachnoid space. Brain tumors also may be treated by direct intraventricular drug administration.

Pulmonary Absorption. Provided that they do not cause irritation, gaseous and volatile drugs may be inhaled and absorbed through the pulmonary epithelium and mucous membranes of the respiratory tract. Access to the circulation is rapid by this route because the lung's surface area is large. The principles governing absorption and excretion of anesthetic and other therapeutic gases are discussed in Chapters 13 and 15.

In addition, solutions of drugs can be atomized and the fine droplets in air (aerosol) inhaled. Advantages are the almost instantaneous absorption of a drug into the blood, avoidance of hepatic first-pass loss, and in the case of pulmonary disease, local application of the drug at the desired site of action. For example, owing to the ability to meter doses and create fine aerosols, drugs can be given in this manner for the treatment of allergic rhinitis or bronchial asthma (*see* Chapter 27). Pulmonary absorption is an important route of entry of certain drugs of abuse and of toxic environmental substances of varied composition and physical states. Both local and systemic reactions to allergens may occur subsequent to inhalation.

Topical Application. *Mucous Membranes.* Drugs are applied to the mucous membranes of the conjunctiva, nasopharynx, oropharynx, vagina, colon, urethra, and urinary bladder primarily for their local effects. Occasionally, as in the application of synthetic *antidiuretic hormone* to the nasal mucosa, systemic absorption is the goal. Absorption through mucous membranes occurs readily. In fact, local anesthetics applied for local effect sometimes may be absorbed so rapidly that they produce systemic toxicity.

Eye. Topically applied ophthalmic drugs are used primarily for their local effects (*see* Chapter 63). Systemic absorption that results from drainage through the nasolacrimal canal is usually undesirable. Because drug that is absorbed *via* drainage is not subject to first-pass hepatic metabolism, unwanted systemic pharmacological effects may occur when β adrenergic receptor antagonists or corticosteroids are administered as ophthalmic drops. Local effects usually require absorption of the drug through the cornea; corneal infection or trauma thus may result in more rapid absorption. Ophthalmic delivery systems that provide prolonged duration of action (*e.g.,* suspensions and ointments) are useful additions to ophthalmic therapy. Ocular inserts, such as the use of *pilocarpine*-containing inserts for the treatment of glaucoma, provide continuous delivery of small amounts of drug. Very little is lost through drainage; hence systemic side effects are minimized.

Novel Methods of Drug Delivery. Drug-eluting stents and other devices are being used to target drugs locally and minimize systemic exposure. The toxicity of potentially important compounds can be decreased significantly by combination with a variety of drug carrier vehicles that modify distribution. For example, the cytotoxic agent *calicheamicin,* when linked to an antibody directed to an antigen found on the surface of certain leukemic cells, can target drug to its intended site of action, improving the therapeutic index of calicheamicin.

Recent advances in drug delivery include the use of biocompatible polymers with functional monomers attached in such a way as to permit linkage of drug molecules to the polymer.

A drug–polymer conjugate can be designed to be a stable, long-circulating prodrug by varying the molecular weight of the polymer and the cleavable linkage between the drug and the polymer. The linkage is designed to keep the drug inactive until it released from the backbone polymer by a disease-specific trigger, typically enzyme activity in the targeted tissue that delivers the active drug at or near the site of pathology.

Bioequivalence. Drug products are considered to be pharmaceutical equivalents if they contain the same active ingredients and are identical in strength or concentration, dosage form, and route of administration. Two pharmaceutically equivalent drug products are considered to be *bioequivalent* when the rates and extents of bioavailability of the active ingredient in the two products are not significantly different under suitable test conditions. In the past, dosage forms of a drug from different manufacturers and even different lots of preparations from a single manufacturer sometimes differed in their bioavailability. Such differences were seen primarily among oral dosage forms of poorly soluble, slowly absorbed drugs such as the urinary antiinfective *metronidazole* (FLAGYL). When first introduced, the generic form was not bioequivalent because the generic manufacturer was not able to mimic the proprietary process used to microsize the drug for absorption initially. Differences in crystal form, particle size, or other physical characteristics of the drug that are not rigidly controlled in formulation and manufacture affect disintegration of the dosage form and dissolution of the drug and hence the rate and extent of drug absorption.

The potential nonequivalence of different drug preparations has been a matter of concern. Strengthened regulatory requirements have resulted in few, if any, documented cases of nonequivalence between approved drug products in recent years. The significance of possible nonequivalence of drug preparations is further discussed in connection with drug nomenclature and the choice of drug name in writing prescription orders (*see* Appendix I).

DISTRIBUTION OF DRUGS

Following absorption or systemic administration into the bloodstream, a drug distributes into interstitial and intracellular fluids. This process reflects a number of physiological factors and the particular physicochemical properties of the individual drug. Cardiac output, regional blood flow, capillary permeability, and tissue volume determine the rate of delivery and potential amount of drug distributed into tissues. Initially, liver, kidney, brain, and other well-perfused organs receive most of the drug, whereas delivery to muscle, most viscera, skin, and fat is slower. This second distribution phase may require minutes to several hours before the concentration of drug in tissue is in equilibrium with that in blood. The second phase also involves a far larger fraction of body mass than does the initial phase and generally accounts for most of the extravascularly distributed drug. With exceptions such as the brain, diffusion of drug into the interstitial fluid occurs rapidly because of the highly permeable nature of the capillary endothelial membrane. Thus, tissue distribution is determined by the partitioning of drug between blood and the particular tissue. Lipid solubility and transmembrane pH gradients are important determinants of such uptake for drugs that are either weak acids or bases. However, in general, ion trapping associated with transmembrane pH gradients is not large because the pH difference between tissue and blood (approximately 7.0 *versus* 7.4) is small. The more important determinant of blood–tissue partitioning is the relative binding of drug to plasma proteins and tissue macromolecules.

Plasma Proteins. Many drugs circulate in the bloodstream bound to plasma proteins. Albumin is a major carrier for acidic drugs; α_1-acid glycoprotein binds basic drugs. Nonspecific binding to other plasma proteins generally occurs to a much smaller extent. The binding is usually reversible; covalent binding of reactive drugs such as alkylating agents occurs occasionally. In addition to the binding of drugs to carrier proteins such as albumin, certain drugs may bind to proteins that function as specific hormone carrier proteins, such as the binding of estrogen or testosterone to sex hormone–binding globulin or the binding of *thyroid hormone* to thyroxin-binding globulin.

The fraction of total drug in plasma that is bound is determined by the drug concentration, the affinity of binding sites for the drug, and the number of binding sites. Mass-action relationships determine the unbound and bound concentrations (*see* below). At low concentrations of drug (less than the plasma protein binding dissociation constant), the fraction bound is a function of the concentration of binding sites and the dissociation constant. At high drug concentrations (greater than the dissociation constant), the fraction bound is a function of the number of binding sites and the drug concentration. Therefore, plasma binding is a nonlinear, saturable process. For most drugs, the therapeutic range of plasma concentrations is limited; thus the extent of binding and the unbound fraction are relatively constant. The percentage values listed for protein binding in Appendix II refer to binding in the therapeutic range unless otherwise indicated. The extent of plasma protein binding also may be affected by disease-related factors. For example, hypoalbuminemia secondary to severe liver disease or the nephrotic syndrome results in reduced binding and an increase in the unbound fraction. Also, conditions resulting in the acute-phase reaction response (*e.g.,* cancer, arthritis, myocardial infarction, and Crohn's disease) lead to elevated levels of α_1-acid glycoprotein and enhanced binding of basic drugs.

Because binding of drugs to plasma proteins such as albumin is nonselective, and because the number of binding sites is relatively large (high capacity), many drugs with similar physicochemical characteristics can compete with each other and with endogenous substances for these binding sites, resulting in noticeable displacement of one drug by another. For example, displacement of unconjugated bilirubin from binding to albumin by the sulfonamides and other organic anions is known to increase the risk of bilirubin encephalopathy in the newborn. Drug toxicities based on competition between drugs for binding sites is not of clinical concern for most therapeutic agents. Since drug responses, both efficacious and toxic, are a function of the concentrations of unbound drug, steady-state unbound concentrations will change significantly only when either drug input (dosing rate) or clearance of unbound drug is changed [*see* Equation (1–2) and discussion below]. Thus, steady-state unbound concentrations are independent of the extent of protein binding. However, for narrow-therapeutic-index drugs, a transient change in unbound concentrations occurring immediately following the dose of a competing drug could be of concern, such as with the anticoagulant *warfarin.* A more common problem resulting from competition of drugs for plasma protein binding sites is misinterpretation of measured concentrations of drugs in plasma because most assays do not distinguish free drug from bound drug.

Importantly, binding of a drug to plasma proteins limits its concentration in tissues and at its site of action because only unbound drug is in equilibrium across membranes. Accordingly, after distri-

bution equilibrium is achieved, the concentration of active, unbound drug in intracellular water is the same as that in plasma except when carrier-mediated transport is involved. Binding of a drug to plasma protein also limits the drug's glomerular filtration because this process does not immediately change the concentration of free drug in the plasma (water is also filtered). However, plasma protein binding generally does not limit renal tubular secretion or biotransformation because these processes lower the free drug concentration, and this is followed rapidly by dissociation of drug from the drug–protein complex, thereby reestablishing equilibrium between bound and free drug. Drug transport and metabolism also are limited by binding to plasma proteins, except when these are especially efficient, and drug clearance, calculated on the basis of unbound drug, exceeds organ plasma flow.

Tissue Binding. Many drugs accumulate in tissues at higher concentrations than those in the extracellular fluids and blood. For example, during long-term administration of the antimalarial agent *quinacrine,* the concentration of drug in the liver may be several thousandfold higher than that in the blood. Such accumulation may be a result of active transport or, more commonly, binding. Tissue binding of drugs usually occurs with cellular constituents such as proteins, phospholipids, or nuclear proteins and generally is reversible. A large fraction of drug in the body may be bound in this fashion and serve as a reservoir that prolongs drug action in that same tissue or at a distant site reached through the circulation. Such tissue binding and accumulation also can produce local toxicity, as in the case of the accumulation of the aminoglycoside antibiotic *gentamicin* in the kidney and vestibular system.

Fat as a Reservoir. Many lipid-soluble drugs are stored by physical solution in the neutral fat. In obese persons, the fat content of the body may be as high as 50%, and even in lean individuals it constitutes 10% of body weight; hence fat may serve as a reservoir for lipid-soluble drugs. For example, as much as 70% of the highly lipid-soluble barbiturate *thiopental* may be present in body fat 3 hours after administration. Fat is a rather stable reservoir because it has a relatively low blood flow. However, among highly lipophilic drugs (*e.g.,* remifentanil and some β blockers), the degree of lipophilicity does not predict their distribution in obese individuals.

Bone. The *tetracycline* antibiotics (and other divalent metal-ion chelating agents) and heavy metals may accumulate in bone by adsorption onto the bone crystal surface and eventual incorporation into the crystal lattice. Bone can become a reservoir for the slow release of toxic agents such as lead or radium into the blood; their effects thus can persist long after exposure has ceased. Local destruction of the bone medulla also may lead to reduced blood flow and prolongation of the reservoir effect because the toxic agent becomes sealed off from the circulation; this may further enhance the direct local damage to the bone. A vicious cycle results, whereby the greater the exposure to the toxic agent, the slower is its rate of elimination. The adsorption of drug onto the bone crystal surface and incorporation into the crystal lattice have therapeutic advantages for the treatment of osteoporosis. Phosphonates such as *sodium etidronate* bind tightly to hydroxyapatite crystals in mineralized bone matrix. However, unlike naturally occurring pyrophosphates, etidronate is resistant to degradation by pyrophosphatases and thus stabilizes the bone matrix.

Redistribution. Termination of drug effect after withdrawal of a drug usually is by metabolism and excretion but also may result from redistribution of the drug from its site of action into other tissues or sites. Redistribution is a factor in terminating drug effect primarily when a highly lipid-soluble drug that acts on the brain or cardiovascular system is administered rapidly by intravenous injection or by inhalation. A good example of this is the use of the intravenous anesthetic thiopental, a highly lipid-soluble drug. Because blood flow to the brain is so high, the drug reaches its maximal concentration in brain within a minute of its intravenous injection. After injection is concluded, the plasma concentration falls as thiopental diffuses into other tissues, such as muscle. The concentration of the drug in brain follows that of the plasma because there is little binding of the drug to brain constituents. Thus, in this example, the onset of anesthesia is rapid, but so is its termination. Both are related directly to the concentration of drug in the brain.

Central Nervous System and Cerebrospinal Fluid. The distribution of drugs into the CNS from the blood is unique. One reason for this is that the brain capillary endothelial cells have continuous tight junctions; therefore, drug penetration into the brain depends on transcellular rather than paracellular transport. The unique characteristics of brain capillary endothelial cells and pericapillary glial cells constitute the blood–brain barrier. At the choroid plexus, a similar blood–CSF barrier is present except that it is epithelial cells that are joined by tight junctions rather than endothelial cells. The lipid solubility of the nonionized and unbound species of a drug is therefore an important determinant of its uptake by the brain; the more lipophilic a drug is, the more likely it is to cross the blood–brain barrier. This situation often is used in drug design to alter drug distribution to the brain; *e.g.,* the so-called second-generation antihistamines, such as *loratidine,* achieve far lower brain concentrations than do agents such as *diphenhydramine* and thus are nonsedating. Drugs may penetrate into the CNS by specific uptake transporters normally involved in the transport of nutrients and endogenous compounds from blood into the brain and CSF.

Another important factor in the functional blood–brain barrier involves membrane transporters that are efflux carriers present in the brain capillary endothelial cell and capable of removing a large number of chemically diverse drugs from the cell. P-glycoprotein (P-gp, encoded by the *MDR1* gene) and the organic anion–transporting polypeptide (OATP) are two of the more notable of these. The effects of these exporters are to dramatically limit access of the drug to the tissue expressing the efflux transporter. Together, P-gp and the OATP family export a large array of structurally diverse drugs (Kim, 2003) (*see* Chapter 2). Expression of OATP isoforms in the GI tract, liver, and kidney, as well as the blood–brain barrier, has important implications for drug absorption and elimination, as well as tissue penetration. Expression of these efflux transporters accounts for the relatively restricted pharmacological access to the brain and other tissues such as the testes, where drug concentrations may be below those necessary to achieve a desired effect despite adequate blood flow. This situation occurs with HIV protease inhibitors and with *loperamide,* a potent, systemically active opioid that lacks any central effects characteristic of other opioids (*see* Chapter 21). Efflux transporters that actively secrete drug from the CSF into the blood also are present in the choroid plexus (*see* Chapters 2 and 3 for details of the contribution of drug transporters to barrier function). Drugs also may exit the CNS along with the bulk flow of CSF through the arachnoid villi. In general, the blood–brain barrier's function is well maintained; however, meningeal and encephalic inflammation increase local permeability. Recently, blood–brain barrier disruption has emerged as a treatment for certain brain tumors such as primary CNS lymphomas (Tyson *et al.*, 2003). The goal of this treatment is to enhance delivery of chemotherapy to the brain tumor while maintaining cognitive function that is often damaged by conventional radiotherapy (Dahlborg *et al.*, 1998).

Placental Transfer of Drugs. The transfer of drugs across the placenta is of critical importance because drugs may cause anomalies in the developing fetus. Administered immediately before delivery, as is often the case with the use of tocolytics in the treatment of preterm labor, they also may have adverse effects on the neonate. Lipid solubility, extent of plasma binding, and degree of ionization of weak acids and bases are important general determinants in drug transfer across the placenta. The fetal plasma is slightly more acidic than that of the mother (pH 7.0 to 7.2 *versus* 7.4), so that ion trapping of basic drugs occurs. As in the brain, P-gp and other export transporters are present in the placenta and function to limit fetal exposure to potentially toxic agents. The view that the placenta is an absolute barrier to drugs is, however, completely inaccurate (Holcberg *et al.*, 2003), in part because a number of influx transporters are also present (Unadkat *et al.*, 2004). The fetus is to some extent exposed to all drugs taken by the mother.

EXCRETION OF DRUGS

Drugs are eliminated from the body either unchanged by the process of excretion or converted to metabolites. Excretory organs, the lung excluded, eliminate polar compounds more efficiently than substances with high lipid solubility. Lipid-soluble drugs thus are not readily eliminated until they are metabolized to more polar compounds.

The kidney is the most important organ for excreting drugs and their metabolites. Substances excreted in the feces are principally unabsorbed orally ingested drugs or drug metabolites excreted either in the bile or secreted directly into the intestinal tract and not reabsorbed. Excretion of drugs in breast milk is important not because of the amounts eliminated, but because the excreted drugs are potential sources of unwanted pharmacological effects in the nursing infant. Excretion from the lung is important mainly for the elimination of anesthetic gases (*see* Chapter 13).

Renal Excretion. Excretion of drugs and metabolites in the urine involves three distinct processes: glomerular filtration, active tubular secretion, and passive tubular reabsorption. Changes in overall renal function generally affect all three processes to a similar extent. Even in healthy persons, renal function is not constant. In neonates, renal function is low compared with body mass but matures rapidly within the first few months after birth. During adulthood, there is a slow decline in renal function, about 1% per year, so that in elderly patients a substantial degree of functional impairment may be present.

The amount of drug entering the tubular lumen by filtration depends on the glomerular filtration rate and the extent of plasma binding of the drug; only unbound drug is filtered. In the proximal renal tubule, active, carrier-mediated tubular secretion also may add drug to the tubular fluid. Transporters such as P-gp and the multidrug-resistance–associated protein type 2 (MRP2), localized in the apical brush-border membrane, are responsible for the secretion of amphipathic anions and conjugated metabolites (such as glucuronides, sulfates,

and glutathione adducts), respectively (*see* Chapters 2 and 3). ATP-binding cassette (ABC) transporters that are more selective for organic cationic drugs are involved in the secretion of organic bases. Membrane transporters, mainly located in the distal renal tubule, also are responsible for any active reabsorption of drug from the tubular lumen back into the systemic circulation. However, most of such reabsorption occurs by nonionic diffusion.

In the proximal and distal tubules, the nonionized forms of weak acids and bases undergo net passive reabsorption. The concentration gradient for back-diffusion is created by the reabsorption of water with Na^+ and other inorganic ions. Since the tubular cells are less permeable to the ionized forms of weak electrolytes, passive reabsorption of these substances depends on the pH. When the tubular urine is made more alkaline, weak acids are largely ionized and thus are excreted more rapidly and to a greater extent. When the tubular urine is made more acidic, the fraction of drug ionized is reduced, and excretion is likewise reduced. Alkalinization and acidification of the urine have the opposite effects on the excretion of weak bases. In the treatment of drug poisoning, the excretion of some drugs can be hastened by appropriate alkalinization or acidification of the urine. Whether or not alteration of urine pH results in a significant change in drug elimination depends on the extent and persistence of the pH change and the contribution of pH-dependent passive reabsorption to total drug elimination. The effect is greatest for weak acids and bases with pK_a values in the range of urinary pH (5 to 8). However, alkalinization of urine can produce a four- to sixfold increase in excretion of a relatively strong acid such as salicylate when urinary pH is changed from 6.4 to 8.0 and the fraction of nonionized drug is reduced from 1% to 0.04%.

Biliary and Fecal Excretion. Transporters analogous to those in the kidney also are present in the canalicular membrane of the hepatocyte, and these actively secrete drugs and metabolites into bile. P-gp transports a plethora of amphipathic lipid-soluble drugs, whereas MRP2 is mainly involved in the secretion of conjugated metabolites of drugs (*e.g.*, glutathione conjugates, glucuronides, and some sulfates). Ultimately, drugs and metabolites present in bile are released into the GI tract during the digestive process. Because secretory transporters also are expressed on the apical membrane of enterocytes, direct secretion of drugs and metabolites may occur from the systemic circulation into the intestinal lumen. Subsequently, drugs and metabolites can be reabsorbed back into the body from the intestine, which, in the case of conjugated metabolites such as glucuronides, may require their enzymatic hydrolysis by the intestinal microflora. Such enterohepatic recycling, if extensive, may prolong significantly the presence of a drug (or toxin) and its effects within the body prior to elimination by other pathways. For this reason, drugs may be given orally to bind substances excreted in the bile. For example, in the case of mercury poisoning, a resin can be administered orally that binds with dimethylmercury excreted in the bile, thus preventing reabsorption and further toxicity. Enterohepatic recycling also can be an advantage in the design of drugs. *Ezetimibe* is the first of a new class of drugs that specifically reduces the intestinal absorption of cholesterol (Lipka, 2003). The drug is absorbed into the intestinal epithelial cell, where it is believed to interfere with the sterol transporter system. This prevents both free cholesterol and plant sterols (phytosterols) from being transported into the cell from the intestinal lumen. The drug is absorbed rapidly and glucuronidated in the intestinal cell before secretion into the blood. Ezetimibe is avidly taken up by the liver from the portal blood and excreted into the bile, resulting in low peripheral blood concentrations. The glucuronide conjugate is hydrolyzed and absorbed and is equally effective in inhibiting sterol absorption. This enterohepatic recycling is responsible for a half-life in the body of more than 20 hours. The principal benefit is a reduction in low-density lipoprotein cholesterol (*see* Chapter 35).

Excretion by Other Routes. Excretion of drugs into sweat, saliva, and tears is quantitatively unimportant. Elimination by these routes depends mainly on diffusion of the nonionized lipid-soluble form of drugs through the epithelial cells of the glands and depends on the pH. Drugs excreted in the saliva enter the mouth, where they are usually swallowed. The concentration of some drugs in saliva parallels that in plasma. Saliva therefore may be a useful biological fluid in which to determine drug concentrations when it is difficult or inconvenient to obtain blood. The same principles apply to excretion of drugs in breast milk. Since milk is more acidic than plasma, basic compounds may be slightly concentrated in this fluid; conversely, the concentration of acidic compounds in the milk is lower than in plasma. Nonelectrolytes, such as *ethanol* and urea, readily enter breast milk and reach the same concentration as in plasma, independent of the pH of the milk. Thus, the administration of drugs to breast-feeding women carries the general caution that the suckling infant will be exposed to some extent to the medication and/or its metabolites. In certain cases, such as treatment with the β blocker *atenolol*, the infant may be exposed to significant amounts of drug (Ito and Lee, 2003). Although excretion into hair and skin is quantitatively unimportant, sensitive methods of detection of drugs in these tissues have forensic significance.

METABOLISM OF DRUGS

The lipophilic characteristics of drugs that promote their passage through biological membranes and subsequent access to their site of action also serve to hinder their excretion from the body. Renal excretion of unchanged drug plays only a modest role in the overall elimination of most therapeutic agents because lipophilic compounds filtered through the glomerulus are largely reabsorbed into the systemic circulation during passage through the renal tubules. The metabolism of drugs and other xenobiotics into more hydrophilic metabolites is essential for their elimination from the body, as well as for termination of their biological and pharmacological activity. In general, biotransformation reactions generate more polar, inactive metabolites that are readily excreted from the body. However, in some cases, metabolites with potent biological activity or toxic properties are generated. Many of the enzyme systems that transform drugs to inactive metabolites also generate biologically active metabolites of endogenous compounds, as in steroid biosynthesis.

Drug metabolism or biotransformation reactions are classified as either phase I functionalization reactions or phase II biosynthetic (conjugation) reactions. Phase I reactions introduce or expose a functional group on the parent compound such as occurs in hydrolysis reactions. Phase I reactions generally result in the loss of pharmacological activity, although there are examples of retention or enhancement of activity. In rare instances, metabolism is associated with an altered pharmacological activity. *Prodrugs* are pharmacologically inactive compounds designed to maximize the amount of the active species that reaches its site of action. Inactive prodrugs are converted rapidly to biologically active metabolites often by the hydrolysis of an ester or amide linkage. Such is the case with a number of angiotensin-converting enzyme (ACE) inhibitors employed in the management of high blood pressure. *Enalapril,* for instance, is relatively inactive until converted by esterase activity to the diacid enalaprilat. If not excreted rapidly into the urine, the products of phase I biotransformation reactions then can react with endogenous compounds to form a highly water-soluble conjugate.

Phase II conjugation reactions lead to the formation of a covalent linkage between a functional group on the parent compound or phase I metabolite and endogenously derived glucuronic acid, sulfate, glutathione, amino acids, or acetate. These highly polar conjugates generally are inactive and are excreted rapidly in the urine and feces. An example of an active conjugate is the 6-glucuronide metabolite of *morphine,* which is a more potent analgesic than its parent.

The enzyme systems involved in the biotransformation of drugs are localized primarily in the liver, although every tissue examined has some metabolic activity. Other organs with significant metabolic capacity include the GI tract, kidneys, and lungs. Following oral administration of a drug, a significant portion of the dose may be metabolically inactivated in either the intestinal epithelium or the liver before the drug reaches the systemic circulation. This so-called first-pass metabolism significantly limits the oral availability of highly metabolized drugs. Within a given cell, most drug-metabolizing activity is found in the smooth endoplasmic reticulum and the cytosol, although drug biotransformations also can occur in the mitochondria, nuclear envelope, and plasma membrane. The enzyme systems involved in phase I reactions are located primarily in the endoplasmic reticulum, whereas the phase II conjugation enzyme systems are mainly cytosolic. Often, drugs biotransformed through a phase I reaction in the endoplasmic reticulum are conjugated at this same site or in the cytosolic fraction of the same cell in a sequential fashion. These biotransforming reactions are carried out by cytochrome P450 isoforms (CYPs) and by a variety of transferases. These enzyme families, the major reactions they catalyze, and their role in drug metabolism and adverse drug responses are presented in detail in Chapter 3.

CLINICAL PHARMACOKINETICS

The fundamental tenet of clinical pharmacokinetics is that a relationship exists between the pharmacological effects of a drug and an accessible concentration of the drug (*e.g.*, in blood or plasma). This relationship has been documented for many drugs and is of benefit in the therapeutic management of patients. For some drugs, no clear or simple relationship has been found between pharmacological effect and concentration in plasma, whereas for other drugs, routine measurement of drug concentration is impractical as part of therapeutic monitoring. In most cases, as depicted in Figure 1–1, the concentration of drug at its sites of action will be related to the concentration of drug in the systemic circulation. The pharmacological effect that results may be the clinical effect desired, a toxic effect, or in some cases an effect unrelated to the known therapeutic efficacy or toxicity. Clinical pharmacokinetics attempts to provide both a quantitative relationship between dose and effect and a framework within which to interpret measurements of concentrations of drugs in biological fluids for the benefit of the patient. The importance of pharmacokinetics in patient care is based on the improvement in therapeutic efficacy and the avoidance of unwanted effects that can be attained by application of its principles when dosage regimens are chosen and modified.

The physiological and pathophysiological variables that dictate adjustment of dosage in individual patients often do so as a result of modification of pharmacokinetic parameters. The four most important parameters governing drug disposition are *clearance,* a measure of the body's efficiency in eliminating drug; *volume of distribution,* a measure of the apparent space in the body available to contain the drug; *elimination half-life,* a measure of the rate of removal of drug from the body; and *bioavailability*, the fraction of drug absorbed as such into the systemic circulation.

Clearance

Clearance is the most important concept to consider when designing a rational regimen for long-term drug administration. The clinician usually wants to maintain steady-state concentrations of a drug within a *therapeutic window* associated with therapeutic efficacy and a minimum of toxicity for a given agent. Assuming complete bioavailability, the steady-state concentration of drug in the body will be achieved when the rate of drug elimination equals the rate of drug administration. Thus:

$$\text{Dosing rate} = CL \cdot C_{ss} \qquad (1\text{–}2)$$

where *CL* is clearance of drug from the systemic circulation and C_{ss} is the steady-state concentration of drug. If the desired steady-state concentration of drug in plasma or blood is known, the rate of clearance of drug by the patient will dictate the rate at which the drug should be administered.

The concept of clearance is extremely useful in clinical pharmacokinetics because its value for a particular drug usually is constant over the range of concentrations encountered clinically. This is true because systems for elimination of drugs such as metabolizing enzymes and transporters (*see* Chapters 2 and 3) usually are not saturated, and thus the *absolute* rate of elimination of the drug is essentially a linear function of its concentration in plasma. That is, the elimination of most drugs follows first-order kinetics, where a constant *fraction* of drug in the body is eliminated per unit of time. If mechanisms for elimination of a given drug become saturated, the kinetics approach zero order, in which a constant *amount* of drug is eliminated per unit of time. Under such a circumstance, clearance (*CL*) will vary with the concentration of drug, often according to the equation

$$CL = v_m / (K_m + C) \qquad (1\text{–}3)$$

where K_m represents the concentration at which half the maximal rate of elimination is reached (in units of mass/volume) and v_m is equal to the maximal rate of elimination (in units of mass/time). Thus, clearance is derived in units of volume/time. This equation is analogous to the Michaelis–Menten equation for enzyme kinetics. Design of dosage regimens for drugs with zero-order elimination kinetics is more complex than when elimination is first-order and clearance is independent of the drug's concentration (*see* below).

Principles of drug clearance are similar to those of renal physiology, where, for example, creatinine clearance is defined as the rate of elimination of creatinine in the urine relative to its concentration in plasma. At the simplest level, clearance of a drug is its rate of elimination by all routes normalized to the concentration of drug *C* in some biological fluid where measurement can be made:

$$CL = \text{rate of elimination} / C \qquad (1\text{–}4)$$

Thus, when clearance is constant, the rate of drug elimination is directly proportional to drug concentration. It is important to recognize that clearance does not indicate how much drug is being removed but rather the volume of biological fluid such as blood or plasma from which drug would have to be completely removed to account for the clearance (*e.g.,* milliliters per minute per kilogram). Clearance can be defined further as blood clearance (CL_b), plasma clearance (CL_p), or clearance based on the concentration of unbound drug (CL_u), depending on the measurement made (C_b, C_p, or C_u).

Clearance of drug by several organs is additive. Elimination of drug may occur as a result of processes that occur in the GI tract, kidney, liver, and other organs. Division of the rate of elimination by each organ by a concentration of drug (*e.g.,* plasma concentration) will yield the respective clearance by that organ. Added together, these separate clearances will equal systemic clearance:

$$CL_{renal} + CL_{hepatic} + CL_{other} = CL \qquad (1-5)$$

Other routes of elimination could include loss of drug in saliva or sweat, secretion into the GI tract, volatile elimination from the lung, and metabolism at other sites such as skin.

Systemic clearance may be determined at steady state by using Equation (1–2). For a single dose of a drug with complete bioavailability and first-order kinetics of elimination, systemic clearance may be determined from mass balance and the integration of Equation (1–4) over time:

$$CL = \text{Dose} / AUC \qquad (1-6)$$

where *AUC* is the total area under the curve that describes the measured concentration of drug in the systemic circulation as a function of time (from zero to infinity) as in Figure 1–5.

Examples. In Appendix II, the plasma clearance for the antibiotic *cephalexin* is reported as 4.3 ml/min per kilogram, with 90% of the drug excreted unchanged in the urine. For a 70-kg man, the clearance from plasma would be 301 ml/min, with renal clearance accounting for 90% of this elimination. In other words, the kidney is able to excrete cephalexin at a rate such that the drug is completely removed (cleared) from approximately 270 ml of plasma per minute (renal clearance = 90% of total clearance). Because clearance usually is assumed to remain constant in a medically stable patient, the rate of elimination of cephalexin will depend on the concentration of drug in the plasma (Equation 1–4).

The β adrenergic receptor antagonist *propranolol* is cleared from the blood at a rate of 16 ml/min per kilogram (or 1120 ml/min in a 70-kg man), almost exclusively by the liver. Thus the liver is able to remove the amount of propranolol contained in 1120 ml of blood in 1 minute. Even though the liver is the dominant organ for elimination, the plasma clearance of some drugs exceeds the rate of blood flow to this organ. Often this is so because the drug partitions readily into red blood cells (RBCs), and the rate of drug delivered to the eliminating organ is considerably higher than suspected from measurement of its concentration in plasma. The relationship between plasma (p) and blood (b) clearance at steady state is given by

$$\frac{CL_p}{CL_b} = \frac{C_b}{C_p} = 1 + H\left[\frac{C_{rbc}}{C_p} - 1\right] \qquad (1-7)$$

Clearance from the blood therefore may be estimated by dividing the plasma clearance by the drug's blood-to-plasma concentra-

tion ratio, obtained from knowledge of the hematocrit ($H = 0.45$) and the red cell–to–plasma concentration ratio. In most instances, the blood clearance will be less than liver blood flow (1.5 L/min) or, if renal excretion also is involved, the sum of the blood flows to each eliminating organ. For example, the plasma clearance of the immunomodulator *tacrolimus,* about 2 L/min, is more than twice the hepatic plasma flow rate and even exceeds the organ's blood flow despite the fact that the liver is the predominant site of this drug's extensive metabolism. However, after taking into account the extensive distribution of tacrolimus into red cells, its clearance from the blood is only about 63 ml/min, and it is actually a low- rather than high-clearance drug, as might be interpreted from the plasma clearance value alone. Sometimes, however, clearance from the blood by metabolism exceeds liver blood flow, and this indicates extrahepatic metabolism. In the case of the β_1 receptor antagonist *esmolol,* the blood clearance value (11.9 L/min) is greater than cardiac output (approximately 5.3 L/min) because the drug is metabolized efficiently by esterases present in red blood cells.

A further definition of clearance is useful for understanding the effects of pathological and physiological variables on drug elimination, particularly with respect to an individual organ. The rate of presentation of drug to the organ is the product of blood flow (Q) and the arterial drug concentration (C_A), and the rate of exit of drug from the organ is the product of blood flow and the venous drug concentration (C_V). The difference between these rates at steady state is the rate of drug elimination by that organ:

$$\text{Rate of elimination} = Q \cdot C_A - Q \cdot C_V \qquad (1-8)$$
$$= Q(C_A - C_V)$$

Division of Equation (1–8) by the concentration of drug entering the organ of elimination C_A yields an expression for clearance of the drug by the organ in question:

$$CL_{organ} = Q\left[\frac{C_A - C_V}{C_A}\right] = Q \cdot E \qquad (1-9)$$

The expression $(C_A - C_V)/C_A$ in Equation (1–9) can be referred to as the *extraction ratio (E)* of the drug. While not employed in general medical practice, calculations of a drug's extraction ratio are useful for modeling the effects of disease of a given metabolizing organ on clearance and in the design of ideal therapeutic properties of drugs in development.

Hepatic Clearance. The concepts developed in Equation (1–9) have important implications for drugs that are eliminated by the liver. Consider a drug that is removed efficiently from the blood by hepatic processes—metabolism and/or excretion of drug into the bile. In this instance, the concentration of drug in the blood leaving the liver will be low, the extraction ratio will approach unity, and the clearance of the drug from blood will become limited by hepatic blood flow. Drugs that are cleared efficiently by the liver (*e.g.,* drugs in Appendix II with systemic clearances greater than 6 ml/min per kilogram, such as *diltiazem, imipramine,* lidocaine, morphine, and propranolol) are restricted in their rate of elimination not by intrahepatic processes, but by the rate at which they can be transported in the blood to the liver.

Additional complexities also may be considered. For example, the equations presented earlier do not account for drug binding to components of blood and tissues, nor do they permit an estimation of the intrinsic capacity of the liver to eliminate a drug in the absence of limitations imposed by blood flow, termed *intrinsic clearance*. In biochemical terms and under first-order conditions, intrinsic clearance is a measure of the ratio of the Michaelis–Menten kinetic parameters for the eliminating process (*i.e.*, v_m/K_m) and thus reflects the maximum metabolic or transport capability of the clearing organ. Extensions of the relationships of Equation (1–9) to include expressions for protein binding and intrinsic clearance have been proposed for a number of models of hepatic elimination (Kwon and Morris, 1997). All these models indicate that when the capacity of the eliminating organ to metabolize the drug is large in comparison with the rate of presentation of drug to the organ, clearance will approximate the organ's blood flow. In contrast, when the drug-metabolizing capacity is small in comparison with the rate of drug presentation, clearance will be proportional to the unbound fraction of drug in blood and the drug's intrinsic clearance. Appreciation of these concepts allows understanding of a number of possibly puzzling experimental results. For example, enzyme induction or hepatic disease may change the rate of drug metabolism in an isolated hepatic microsomal enzyme system but not change clearance in the whole animal. For a drug with a high extraction ratio, clearance is limited by blood flow, and changes in intrinsic clearance owing to enzyme induction or hepatic disease should have little effect. Similarly, for drugs with high extraction ratios, changes in protein binding owing to disease or competitive binding interactions by other drugs should have little effect on clearance. By contrast, changes in intrinsic clearance and protein binding will affect the clearance of drugs with low intrinsic clearances such as warfarin, and thus extraction ratios, but changes in blood flow will have little effect.

Renal Clearance. Renal clearance of a drug results in its appearance in the urine. In considering the impact of renal disease on the clearance of a drug, complications that relate to filtration, active secretion by the kidney tubule, and reabsorption from it must be considered along with blood flow. The rate of filtration of a drug depends on the volume of fluid that is filtered in the glomerulus and the unbound concentration of drug in plasma because drug bound to protein is not filtered. The rate of secretion of drug by the kidney will depend on the drug's intrinsic clearance by the transporters involved in active secretion as affected by the drug's binding to plasma proteins, the degree of saturation of these transporters, and the rate of delivery of the drug to the secretory site. In addition, processes involved in drug reabsorption from the tubular fluid must be considered. The influences of changes in protein binding and blood flow and in the number of functional nephrons are analogous to the examples given earlier for hepatic elimination.

DISTRIBUTION

Volume of Distribution. Volume is a second fundamental parameter that is useful in considering processes of drug disposition. The volume of distribution (*V*) relates the amount of drug in the body to the concentration of drug (*C*) in the blood or plasma depending on the fluid measured. This volume does not necessarily refer to an identifiable physiological volume but rather to the fluid volume that would be required to contain all the drug in the body at the same concentration measured in the blood or plasma:

$$\text{Amount of drug in body}/V = C \quad \text{or}$$
$$V = \text{amount of drug in body}/C \quad (1\text{–}10)$$

A drug's volume of distribution therefore reflects the extent to which it is present in extravascular tissues and not in the plasma. The plasma volume of a typical 70-kg man is 3 L, blood volume is about 5.5 L, extracellular fluid volume outside the plasma is 12 L, and the volume of total-body water is approximately 42 L.

Many drugs exhibit volumes of distribution far in excess of these values. For example, if 500 μg of the cardiac glycoside *digoxin* were in the body of a 70-kg subject, a plasma concentration of approximately 0.75 ng/ml would be observed. Dividing the amount of drug in the body by the plasma concentration yields a volume of distribution for digoxin of about 667 L, or a value approximately 10 times greater than the total-body volume of a 70-kg man. In fact, digoxin distributes preferentially to muscle and adipose tissue and to its specific receptors (Na^+,K^+-ATPase), leaving a very small amount of drug in the plasma to be measured. For drugs that are bound extensively to plasma proteins but that are not bound to tissue components, the volume of distribution will approach that of the plasma volume because drug bound to plasma protein is measurable in the assay of most drugs. In contrast, certain drugs have high volumes of distribution even though most of the drug in the circulation is bound to albumin because these drugs are also sequestered elsewhere.

The volume of distribution may vary widely depending on the relative degrees of binding to high-affinity receptor sites, plasma and tissue proteins, the partition coefficient of the drug in fat, and accumulation in poorly perfused tissues. As might be expected, the volume of distribution for a given drug can differ according to patient's age, gender, body composition, and presence of disease. Total-body water of infants younger than 1 year of age, for example, is 75% to 80% of body weight, whereas that of adult males is 60% and that of females is 55%.

Several volume terms are used commonly to describe drug distribution, and they have been derived in a number of ways. The volume of distribution defined in Equation (1–10) considers the body as a single homogeneous compartment. In this *one-compartment model*, all drug administration occurs directly into the central compartment, and distribution of drug is instantaneous throughout the volume (*V*). Clearance of drug from this compartment occurs in a first-order fashion, as defined in Equation (1–4); *i.e.,* the amount of drug eliminated per unit of time depends on the amount (concentration) of drug in the body compartment. Figure 1–3A and Equation (1–11) describe the decline of plasma concentration with time for a drug introduced into this central compartment:

$$C = (\text{dose}/V) \cdot \exp(-kt) \quad (1\text{–}11)$$

where *k* is the rate constant for elimination that reflects the fraction of drug removed from the compartment per unit of time. This

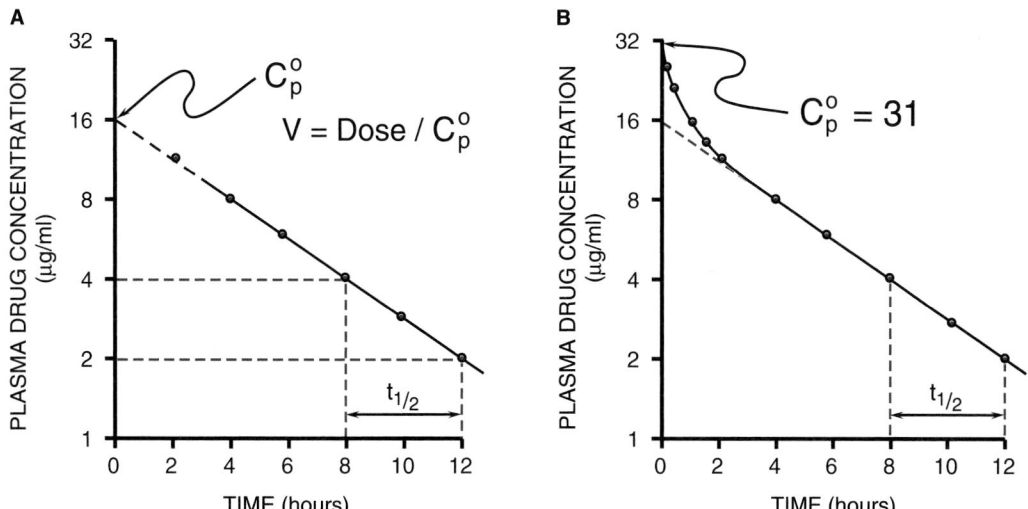

Figure 1–3. *Plasma concentration–time curves following intravenous administration of a drug (500 mg) to a 70-kg patient.* **A.** Drug concentrations are measured in plasma at 2-hour intervals following drug administration. The semilogarithmic plot of plasma concentration (C_p) *versus* time appears to indicate that the drug is eliminated from a single compartment by a first-order process (Equation 1–11) with a half-life of 4 hours ($k = 0.693/t_{\frac{1}{2}} = 0.173$ h^{-1}). The volume of distribution (*V*) may be determined from the value of C_p obtained by extrapolation to $t = 0$ ($C_p^o = 16$ μg/ml). Volume of distribution (Equation 1–10) for the one-compartment model is 31.3 L, or 0.45 L/kg ($V = \text{dose}/C_p^o$). The clearance for this drug is 90 ml/min; for a one-compartment model, $CL = kV$. **B.** Sampling before 2 hours indicates that, in fact, the drug follows multiexponential kinetics. The terminal disposition half-life is 4 hours, clearance is 84 ml/min (Equation 1–6), V_{area} is 29 L (Equation 1–11), and V_{ss} is 26.8 L. The initial or "central" distribution volume for the drug ($V_1 = \text{dose}/C_p^o$) is 16.1 L. The example chosen indicates that multicompartment kinetics may be overlooked when sampling at early times is neglected. In this particular case, there is only a 10% error in the estimate of clearance when the multicompartment characteristics are ignored. For many drugs, multicompartment kinetics may be observed for significant periods of time, and failure to consider the distribution phase can lead to significant errors in estimates of clearance and in predictions of the appropriate dosage. Also, the difference between the "central" distribution volume and other terms reflecting wider distribution is important in deciding a loading dose strategy.

rate constant is inversely related to the half-life of the drug ($k = 0.693/t_{\frac{1}{2}}$).

The idealized one-compartment model discussed earlier does not describe the entire time course of the plasma concentration. That is, certain tissue reservoirs can be distinguished from the central compartment, and the drug concentration appears to decay in a manner that can be described by multiple exponential terms (Figure 1–3B). Nevertheless, the one-compartment model is sufficient to apply to most clinical situations for most drugs. Indeed, appreciation of the drug half-life in the central compartment has a direct and significant impact on the appropriate dosing interval for the drug.

Rate of Drug Distribution. The multiple exponential decay observed for a drug that is eliminated from the body with first-order kinetics results from differences in the rates at which the drug equilibrates to and within tissues. The rate of equilibration will depend on the ratio of the perfusion of the tissue to the partition of drug into the tissue. In many cases, groups of tissues with similar perfusion–partition ratios all equilibrate at essentially the same rate such that only one apparent phase of distribution is seen (rapid initial fall of concentration of intravenously injected drug, as in Figure 1–3B). It is as though the drug starts in a "central" volume (Figure 1–1), which consists of plasma and tissue reservoirs that are in rapid equilibrium with it, and distributes to a "final" volume, at which point

concentrations in plasma decrease in a log-linear fashion with a rate constant of k (Figure 1–3B). The multicompartment model of drug disposition can be viewed as though the blood and highly perfused lean organs such as heart, brain, liver, lung, and kidneys cluster as a single central compartment, whereas more slowly perfused tissues such as muscle, skin, fat, and bone behave as the final compartment (*i.e.,* the tissue compartment).

If the pattern or ratio of blood flow to various tissues changes within an individual or differs among individuals, rates of drug distribution to tissues also will change. However, changes in blood flow also may cause some tissues that were originally in the "central" volume to equilibrate sufficiently more slowly so as to appear only in the "final" volume. This means that central volumes will appear to vary with disease states that cause altered regional blood flow (such as would be seen in cirrhosis of the liver). After an intravenous bolus dose, drug concentrations in plasma may be higher in individuals with poor perfusion (*e.g.,* shock) than they would be if perfusion were better. These higher systemic concentrations, in turn, may cause higher concentrations (and greater effects) in tissues such as brain and heart, whose usually high perfusion has not been reduced by the altered hemodynamic state. Thus, the effect of a drug at various sites of action can vary depending on perfusion of these sites.

Multicompartment Volume Terms. Two different terms have been used to describe the volume of distribution for drugs that follow multiple exponential decay. The first, designated V_{area}, is calculated as the ratio of clearance to the rate of decline in concentration during the elimination (final) phase of the logarithmic concentration *versus* time curve:

$$V_{area} = \frac{CL}{k} = \frac{\text{dose}}{k \cdot AUC} \tag{1-12}$$

The estimation of this parameter is straightforward, and the volume term may be determined after administration of a single dose of drug by intravenous or oral route (where the value for the dose must be corrected for bioavailability). However, another multicompartment volume of distribution term may be more useful, especially when the effect of disease states on pharmacokinetics is to be determined. The volume of distribution at steady state (V_{ss}) represents the volume in which a drug would appear to be distributed during steady state if the drug existed throughout that volume at the same concentration as that in the measured fluid (plasma or blood). V_{ss} also may be appreciated as shown in Equation (1–13), where V_C is the volume of distribution of drug in the central compartment and V_T is the volume term for drug in the tissue compartment:

$$V_{ss} = V_C + V_T \tag{1-13}$$

Although V_{area} is a convenient and easily calculated parameter, it varies when the rate constant for drug elimination changes, even when there has been no change in the distribution space. This is so because the terminal rate of decline of the concentration of drug in blood or plasma depends not only on clearance but also on the rates of distribution of drug between the "central" and "final" volumes. V_{ss} does not suffer from this disadvantage. When using pharmacokinetics to make drug dosing decisions, the differences between V_{area} and V_{ss} usually are not clinically significant. Nonetheless, both are quoted in the table of pharmacokinetic data in Appendix II, depending on the availability of data in the published literature.

Half-Life

The half-life ($t_{\frac{1}{2}}$) is the time it takes for the plasma concentration or the amount of drug in the body to be reduced by 50%. For the simplest case, the one-compartment model (Figure 1–3A), half-life may be determined readily by inspection and used to make decisions about drug dosage. However, as indicated in Figure 1–3B, drug concentrations in plasma often follow a multiexponential pattern of decline; two or more half-life terms thus may be calculated.

In the past, the half-life that was usually reported corresponded to the terminal log-linear phase of elimination. However, as greater analytical sensitivity has been achieved, the lower concentrations measured appeared to yield longer and longer terminal half-lives. For example, a terminal half-life of 53 hours is observed for gentamicin (*versus* the more clinically relevant 2- to 3-hour value in Appendix II), and biliary cycling probably is responsible for the 120-hour terminal value for *indomethacin* (as compared with the 2.4-hour half-life listed in Appendix II). The appreciation of longer terminal half-lives for some medications may relate to their accumulation in tissues during chronic dosing or shorter periods of high-dose treatment. Such is the case for gentamicin, where the terminal half-life is associated with renal and ototoxicities. The relevance of a particular half-life may be defined in terms of the fraction of the clearance and volume of distribution that is related to each half-life and whether plasma concentrations or amounts of drug in the body are best related to measures of response. The single half-life values given for each drug in Appendix II are chosen to represent the most clinically relevant half-life.

In studies of pharmacokinetic properties of drugs in disease, the half-life is a derived parameter that changes as a function of both clearance and volume of distribution. A useful approximate relationship between the clinically relevant half-life, clearance, and volume of distribution at steady state is given by

$$t_{1/2} \cong 0.693 \cdot V_{ss}/CL \tag{1-14}$$

Clearance is the measure of the body's ability to eliminate a drug; thus, as clearance decreases, owing to a disease process, for example, half-life would be expected to increase. However, this reciprocal relationship is valid only when the disease does not change the volume of distribution. For example, the half-life of *diazepam* increases with increasing age; however, it is not clearance that changes as a function of age but rather the volume of distribution. Similarly, changes in protein binding of a drug may affect its clearance as well as its volume of distribution, leading to unpredictable changes in half-life as a function of disease. The half-life of *tolbutamide,* for example, decreases in patients with acute viral hepatitis in a fashion opposite from what one might expect. The disease alters the drug's protein binding in both plasma and tissues, causing no change in volume of distribution but an increase in clearance because higher concentrations of unbound drug are present in the bloodstream.

Although it can be a poor index of drug elimination from the body *per se* (disappearance of drug may be the result of formation of undetected metabolites that have therapeutic or unwanted effects), half-life does provide a good indication of the time required to reach steady state after a dosage regimen is initiated or changed (*i.e.,* four half-lives to reach approximately 94% of a new steady state), the time for a drug to be removed from the body, and a means to estimate the appropriate dosing interval (*see* below).

Steady State. Equation (1–2) (dosing rate = $CL \cdot C_{ss}$) indicates that a steady-state concentration eventually will be achieved when a drug is administered at a constant rate. At this point, drug elimination [the product of clearance and concentration; Equation (1–4)] will equal the

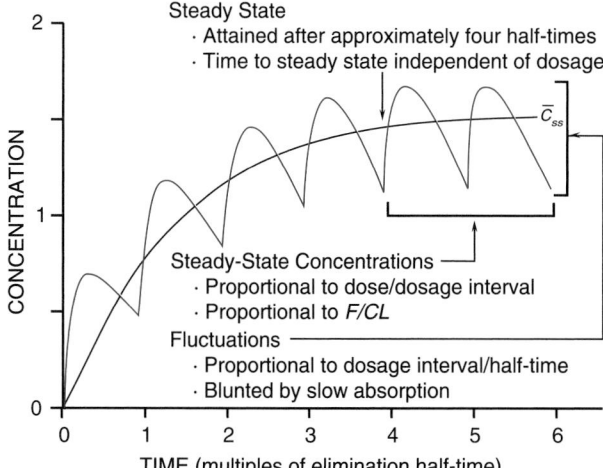

Figure 1–4. Fundamental pharmacokinetic relationships for repeated administration of drugs. The blue line is the pattern of drug accumulation during repeated administration of a drug at intervals equal to its elimination half-time when drug absorption is 10 times as rapid as elimination. As the rate of absorption increases, the concentration maxima approach 2 and the minima approach 1 during the steady state. The black line depicts the pattern during administration of equivalent dosage by continuous intravenous infusion. Curves are based on the one-compartment model. Average concentration ($\bar{C}_{ss}$) when the steady state is attained during intermittent drug administration is

$$\bar{C}_{ss} = \frac{F \cdot \text{dose}}{CL \cdot T}$$

where F is fractional bioavailability of the dose and T is dosage interval (time). By substitution of infusion rate for $F \cdot \text{dose}/T$, the formula is equivalent to Equation (1–2) and provides the concentration maintained at steady state during continuous intravenous infusion.

rate of drug availability. This concept also extends to regular intermittent dosage (*e.g.,* 250 mg of drug every 8 hours). During each interdose interval, the concentration of drug rises with absorption and falls by elimination. At steady state, the entire cycle is repeated identically in each interval (*see* Figure 1–4). Equation (1–2) still applies for intermittent dosing, but it now describes the average steady-state drug concentration (C_{ss}) during an interdose interval.

Extent and Rate of Bioavailability

Bioavailability. It is important to distinguish between the rate and extent of drug absorption and the amount of drug that ultimately reaches the systemic circulation. The amount of the drug that reaches the systemic circulation depends not only on the administered dose but also on the

fraction of the dose (F) that is absorbed and escapes any first-pass elimination. This fraction is the drug's *bioavailability*. Reasons for incomplete absorption were discussed earlier. Also, as noted previously, if the drug is metabolized in the intestinal epithelium or the liver or excreted in bile, some of the active drug absorbed from the GI tract will be eliminated before it can reach the general circulation and be distributed to its sites of action.

Knowing the extraction ratio (E_H) for a drug across the liver (*see* Equation 1–9), it is possible to predict the maximum oral availability (F_{max}), assuming that hepatic elimination follows first-order processes:

$$F_{max} = 1 - E_H = 1 - (CL_{hepatic}/Q_{hepatic}) \qquad (1\text{–}15)$$

Thus, if the hepatic blood clearance for the drug is large relative to hepatic blood flow, the extent of availability will be low when the drug is given orally (*e.g.,* lidocaine or propranolol). This reduction in availability is a function of the physiological site from which absorption takes place, and no modification of dosage form will improve the availability under conditions of linear kinetics. Incomplete absorption and/or intestinal metabolism following oral dosing will, in practice, reduce this predicted maximal value of F.

When drugs are administered by a route that is subject to first-pass loss, the equations presented previously that contain the terms *dose* or *dosing rate* (Equations 1–2, 1–6, 1–11, and 1–12) also must include the bioavailability term F such that the available dose or dosing rate is used. For example, Equation (1–2) is modified to

$$F \cdot \text{dosing rate} = CL \cdot C_{ss} \qquad (1\text{–}16)$$

where the value of F is between 0 and 1. The value of F varies widely for drugs administered by mouth. Etidronate, a bisphosphonate used to stabilize bone matrix in the treatment of Paget's disease and osteoporosis, has an F of 0.03, meaning that only 3% of the drug appears in the bloodstream following oral dosing. In the case of etidronate, therapy using oral administration is still useful, and the dose of the drug administered per kilogram is larger than would be given by injection.

Rate of Absorption. Although the rate of drug absorption does not, in general, influence the average steady-state concentration of the drug in plasma, it may still influence drug therapy. If a drug is absorbed rapidly (*e.g.,* a dose given as an intravenous bolus) and has a small "central" volume, the concentration of drug initially will be high. It will then fall as the drug is distributed to its "final" (larger) volume (Figure 1–3B). If the same drug is absorbed more slowly (*e.g.,* by slow infusion), it will be distributed while it is being administered, and peak concentrations will be lower and will occur later. Controlled-release preparations are designed to provide a slow and sustained rate of absorption in order to produce smaller fluctuations in the plasma concentration–time profile during the dosage interval compared with more immediate-release formulations. A given drug may act to produce both desirable and undesirable effects at several sites in the body, and the rates of distribution of drug to these sites may not be the same. The relative intensities of these different effects of a drug thus may vary transiently when its rate of administration is changed. Since the beneficial, nontoxic effects of drugs are based on knowledge of an ideal or desired plasma concentration range, maintaining that range while avoiding large swings between peak and trough concentrations can improve therapeutic outcome.

Nonlinear Pharmacokinetics

Nonlinearity in pharmacokinetics (*i.e.,* changes in such parameters as clearance, volume of distribution, and half-life as a function of dose or concentration of drug) usually is due to saturation of either protein binding, hepatic metabolism, or active renal transport of the drug.

Saturable Protein Binding. As the molar concentration of drug increases, the unbound fraction eventually also must increase (as all binding sites become saturated). This usually occurs only when drug concentrations in plasma are in the range of tens to hundreds of micrograms per milliliter. For a drug that is metabolized by the liver with a low intrinsic clearance–extraction ratio, saturation of plasma-protein binding will cause both V and CL to increase as drug concentrations increase; half-life thus may remain constant (Equation 1–14). For such a drug, C_{ss} will not increase linearly as the rate of drug administration is increased. For drugs that are cleared with high intrinsic clearance–extraction ratios, C_{ss} can remain linearly proportional to the rate of drug administration. In this case, hepatic clearance will not change, and the increase in V will increase the half-time of disappearance by reducing the fraction of the total drug in the body that is delivered to the liver per unit of time. Most drugs fall between these two extremes, and the effects of nonlinear protein binding may be difficult to predict.

Saturable Elimination. In this situation, the Michaelis–Menten equation (Equation 1–3) usually describes the nonlinearity. All active processes are undoubtedly saturable, but they will appear to be linear if values of drug concentrations encountered in practice are much less than K_m. When drug concentrations exceed K_m, nonlinear kinetics are observed. The major consequences of saturation of metabolism or transport are the opposite of those for saturation of protein binding. Saturation of protein binding will lead to increased CL because CL increases as drug concentration increases, whereas saturation of metabolism or transport may decrease CL. When both conditions are present simultaneously, they may virtually cancel each others' effects, and surprisingly linear kinetics may result; this occurs over a certain range of concentrations for *salicylic acid,* for example.

Saturable metabolism causes oral first-pass metabolism to be less than expected (higher F), and there is a greater fractional increase in C_{ss} than the corresponding fractional increase in the rate of drug administration. The latter can be seen most easily by substituting Equation (1–3) into Equation (1–2) and solving for the steady-state concentration:

$$C_{ss} = \frac{\text{dosing rate} \cdot K_m}{v_m - \text{dosing rate}} \qquad (1\text{--}17)$$

As the dosing rate approaches the maximal elimination rate (v_m), the denominator of Equation (1–17) approaches zero, and C_{ss} increases disproportionately. Because saturation of metabolism should have no effect on the volume of distribution, clearance and the relative rate of drug elimination decrease as the concentration increases; therefore, the log C_p time curve is concave-decreasing until metabolism becomes sufficiently desaturated and first-order elimination is present. Thus, the concept of a constant half-life is not applicable to nonlinear metabolism occurring in the usual range of clinical concentrations. Consequently, changing the dosing rate for a drug with nonlinear metabolism is difficult and unpredictable because the resulting steady state is reached more slowly, and importantly, the effect is disproportionate to the alteration in the dosing rate.

The antiseizure medication *phenytoin* provides an example of a drug for which metabolism becomes saturated in the therapeutic range of concentrations (*see* Appendix II), and half-life can vary between 7 and 42 hours. K_m (5 to 10 mg/L) is typically near the lower end of the therapeutic range (10 to 20 mg/L). For some individuals, especially young children and newborns being treated for emergent seizures, K_m may be as low as 1 mg/L. If, for an adult, the target concentration is 15 mg/L and this is attained at a dosing rate of 300 mg/day, then from Equation (1–17), v_m equals 320 mg/day. For such a patient, a dose that is 10% less than optimal (*i.e.,* 270 mg/day) will produce a C_{ss} of 5 mg/L, well below the desired value. In contrast, a dose that is 10% greater than optimal (330 mg/day) will exceed metabolic capacity (by 10 mg/day) and cause a long and slow but unending climb in concentration during which toxicity will occur. Dosage cannot be controlled so precisely (<10% error). Therefore, for patients in whom the target concentration for phenytoin is more than tenfold greater than the K_m, alternating between inefficacious therapy and toxicity is almost unavoidable. For a drug such as phenytoin that has a narrow therapeutic index and exhibits nonlinear metabolism, therapeutic drug monitoring (*see* below) is most important. When the patient is a neonate, appreciation of this concept is of particular concern because signs and symptoms of toxicity are particularly difficult to monitor. In such cases, a pharmacokinetic consult may be appropriate.

Design and Optimization of Dosage Regimens

Following administration of a dose of drug, its effects usually show a characteristic temporal pattern (Figure 1–5). Onset of the effect is preceded by a lag period, after which the magnitude of the effect increases to a maximum and then declines; if a further dose is not administered, the effect eventually disappears as the drug is eliminated. This time course reflects changes in the drug's concentration as determined by the pharmacokinetics of its absorption, distribution, and elimination. Accordingly, the intensity of a drug's effect is related to its concentration above a minimum effective concentration, whereas the duration of this effect reflects the length of time the drug level is above this value. These considerations, in general, apply to both desired and undesired (adverse) drug effects, and as a result, a *therapeutic window* exists reflecting a concentration range that provides efficacy without unacceptable toxicity. Similar considerations apply after multiple dosing associated with long-term therapy, and they determine the amount and frequency of drug administration to achieve an optimal therapeutic effect. In general, the lower limit of the therapeutic range appears to be approximately equal to the drug concentration that produces about half the greatest possible therapeutic effect, and the upper limit of the therapeutic range is such that no

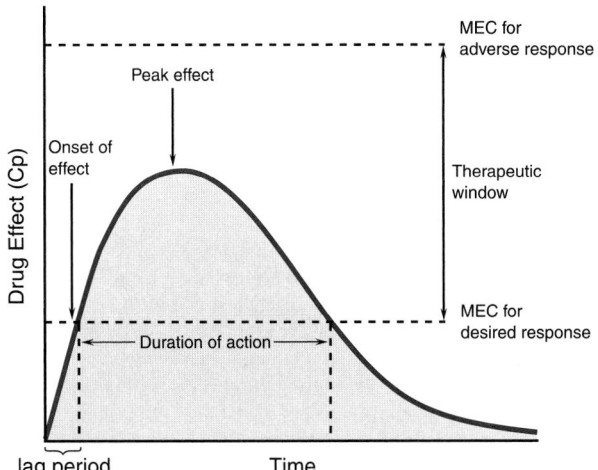

Figure 1–5. *Temporal characteristics of drug effect and relationship to the therapeutic window (e.g., single dose, oral administration).* A lag period is present before the plasma drug concentration (Cp) exceeds the minimum effective concentration (MEC) for the desired effect. Following onset of the response, the intensity of the effect increases as the drug continues to be absorbed and distributed. This reaches a peak, after which drug elimination results in a decline in Cp and in the effect's intensity. Effect disappears when the drug concentration falls below the MEC. Accordingly, the duration of a drug's action is determined by the time period over which concentrations exceed the MEC. An MEC exists for each adverse response, and if drug concentration exceeds this, toxicity will result. The therapeutic goal is to obtain and maintain concentrations within the therapeutic window for the desired response with a minimum of toxicity. Drug response below the MEC for the desired effect will be subtherapeutic; above the MEC for an adverse effect, the probability of toxicity will increase. Increasing or decreasing drug dosage shifts the response curve up or down the intensity scale and is used to modulate the drug's effect. Increasing the dose also prolongs a drug's duration of action but at the risk of increasing the likelihood of adverse effects. Unless the drug is nontoxic (*e.g.,* penicillins), increasing the dose is not a useful strategy for extending the duration of action. Instead, another dose of drug should be given, timed to maintain concentrations within the therapeutic window. The area under the blood concentration–time curve (*area under the curve,* or AUC, shaded in gray) can be used to calculate the clearance (*see* Equation 1–6) for first-order elimination. The AUC is also used as a measure of bioavailability (defined as 100% for an intravenously administered drug). Bioavailability will be <100% for orally administered drugs, due mainly to incomplete absorption and first-pass metabolism and elimination.

more than 5% to 10% of patients will experience a toxic effect. For some drugs, this may mean that the upper limit of the range is no more than twice the lower limit. Of course, these figures can be highly variable, and some patients may benefit greatly from drug concen-

trations that exceed the therapeutic range, whereas others may suffer significant toxicity at much lower values (*e.g.,* digoxin).

For a limited number of drugs, some effect of the drug is easily measured (*e.g.,* blood pressure, blood glucose), and this can be used to optimize dosage using a trial-and-error approach. Even in an ideal case, certain quantitative issues arise, such as how often to change dosage and by how much. These usually can be settled with simple rules of thumb based on the principles discussed (*e.g.,* change dosage by no more than 50% and no more often than every three to four half-lives). Alternatively, some drugs have very little dose-related toxicity, and maximum efficacy usually is desired. For these drugs, doses well in excess of the average required will both ensure efficacy (if this is possible) and prolong drug action. Such a "maximal dose" strategy typically is used for *penicillins.*

For many drugs, however, the effects are difficult to measure (or the drug is given for prophylaxis), toxicity and lack of efficacy are both potential dangers, or the therapeutic index is narrow. In these circumstances, doses must be titrated carefully, and drug dosage is limited by toxicity rather than efficacy. Thus, the therapeutic goal is to maintain steady-state drug levels within the therapeutic window. For most drugs, the actual concentrations associated with this desired range are not and need not be known. It is sufficient to understand that efficacy and toxicity generally depend on concentration and how drug dosage and frequency of administration affect the drug level. However, for a small number of drugs for which there is a small (two- to threefold) difference between concentrations resulting in efficacy and toxicity (*e.g.,* digoxin, *theophylline,* lidocaine, aminoglycosides, *cyclosporine,* warfarin, and anticonvulsants), a plasma concentration range associated with effective therapy has been defined. In these cases, a target-level strategy is reasonable, wherein a desired (target) steady-state concentration of the drug (usually in plasma) associated with efficacy and minimal toxicity is chosen, and a dosage is computed that is expected to achieve this value. Drug concentrations are subsequently measured, and dosage is adjusted if necessary to approximate the target more closely (*see* below).

Maintenance Dose. In most clinical situations, drugs are administered in a series of repetitive doses or as a continuous infusion to maintain a steady-state concentration of drug associated with the therapeutic window. Calculation of the appropriate maintenance dosage is a primary goal. To maintain the chosen steady-state or target concentration, the rate of drug administration is adjusted such that the rate of input equals the rate of loss. This relationship was defined previously in Equations (1–2) and (1–16) and is expressed here in terms of the desired target concentration:

$$\text{Dosing rate} = \text{target } C_p \cdot CL/F \qquad (1\text{–}18)$$

If the clinician chooses the desired concentration of drug in plasma and knows the clearance and bioavailability for that drug in a particular patient, the appropriate dose and dosing interval can be calculated.

Example. Oral digoxin is to be used as a maintenance dose to gradually "digitalize" a 69-kg patient with congestive heart failure. A steady-state plasma concentration of 1.5 ng/ml is selected as an appropriate target based on prior knowledge of the action of the drug in patients with heart failure. Based on the fact that the patient's creatinine clearance (CL_{Cr}) is 100 ml/min, digoxin's clearance may be estimated from data in Appendix II.

$$CL = 0.88\, CL_{CR} + 0.33\ \text{ml} \cdot \text{min}^{-1} \cdot \text{kg}^{-1}$$
$$= 0.88 \times 100/69 + 0.33\ \text{ml} \cdot \text{min}^{-1} \cdot \text{kg}^{-1}$$
$$= 1.6\ \text{ml} \cdot \text{min}^{-1} \cdot \text{kg}^{-1}$$
$$= 110\ \text{ml} \cdot \text{min}^{-1} = 6.6\ \text{liters} \cdot \text{hr}^{-1}$$

Equation (1–18) then is used to calculate an appropriate dosing rate knowing that the oral bioavailability of digoxin is 70% ($F = 0.7$).

$$\text{Dosing rate} = \text{Target } C_p \cdot CL/F$$
$$= 1.5\ \text{ng} \cdot \text{ml}^{-1} \times 1.6/0.7\ \text{ml} \cdot \text{min}^{-1} \cdot \text{kg}^{-1}$$
$$= 3.43\ \text{ng} \cdot \text{ml}^{-1} \cdot \text{min}^{-1} \cdot \text{kg}^{-1}$$
$$\text{or } 236\ \text{ng} \cdot \text{ml}^{-1} \cdot \text{min}^{-1} \text{ for a 69-kg patient}$$
$$= 236\ \text{ng} \cdot \text{ml}^{-1} \times 60\ \text{min} \times 24\ \text{hr}$$
$$= 340\ \mu g = 0.34\ \text{mg}/24\ \text{hr}$$

In practice, the dosing rate would be rounded to the closest dosage size, either 0.375 mg/24 h, which would result in a steady-state plasma concentration of 1.65 ng/ml ($1.5 \times 375/340$), or 0.25 mg/24 h, which would provide a value of 1.10 ng/ml ($1.5 \times 250/340$).

Dosing Interval for Intermittent Dosage. In general, marked fluctuations in drug concentrations between doses are not desirable. If absorption and distribution were instantaneous, fluctuations in drug concentrations between doses would be governed entirely by the drug's elimination half-life. If the dosing interval T were chosen to be equal to the half-life, then the total fluctuation would be twofold; this is often a tolerable variation.

Pharmacodynamic considerations modify this. If a drug is relatively nontoxic such that a concentration many times that necessary for therapy can be tolerated easily, the maximal-dose strategy can be used, and the dosing interval can be much longer than the elimination half-life (for convenience). The half-life of *amoxicillin* is about 2 hours, but dosing every 2 hours would be impractical. Instead, amoxicillin often is given in large doses every 8 or 12 hours. For some drugs with a narrow therapeutic range, it may be important to estimate the maximal and minimal concentrations that will occur for a particular dosing interval. The minimal steady-state concentration $C_{ss,min}$ may be reasonably determined by the use of Equation (1–19):

$$C_{ss,\,min} = \frac{F \cdot \text{dose}/V_{ss}}{1 - \exp(-kT)} \cdot \exp(-kT) \tag{1–19}$$

where k equals 0.693 divided by the clinically relevant plasma half-life and T is the dosing interval. The term $\exp(-kT)$ is, in fact, the fraction of the last dose (corrected for bioavailability) that remains in the body at the end of a dosing interval.

For drugs that follow multiexponential kinetics and are administered orally, estimation of the maximal steady-state concentration $C_{ss,max}$ involves a complicated set of exponential constants for distribution and absorption. If these terms are ignored for multiple oral dosing, one easily may predict a maximal steady-state concentration by omitting the $\exp(-kT)$ term in the numerator of Equation (1–19) [*see* Equation (1–20) below]. Because of the approximation, the predicted maximal concentration from Equation (1–20) will be greater than that actually observed.

Example. In the patient with congestive heart failure discussed earlier, an oral maintenance dose of 0.375 mg digoxin per 24 hours

was calculated to achieve an average plasma concentration of 1.65 ng/ml during the dosage interval. Digoxin has a narrow therapeutic index, and plasma levels between 0.8 and 2.0 ng/ml usually are associated with efficacy and minimal toxicity. What are the maximum and minimum plasma concentrations associated with the preceding regimen? This first requires estimation of digoxin's volume of distribution based on available pharmacokinetic data (Appendix II).

$$V_{ss} = 3.12\, CL_{CR} + 3.84\ \text{liters} \cdot \text{kg}^{-1}$$
$$= 3.12 \times (100/69) + 3.84\ \text{liters} \cdot \text{kg}^{-1}$$
$$= 8.4\ \text{liters} \cdot \text{kg}^{-1}, \text{ or } 580\ \text{liters for a 69-kg patient}$$

Combining this value with that of digoxin's clearance provides an estimate of digoxin's elimination half-life in the patient (Equations 1–2 through 1–14).

$$t_{1/2} = 0.693\, V_{ss}/CL$$
$$= \frac{0.693 \times 580\ \text{liters}}{6.6\ \text{liters} \cdot \text{hr}^{-1}} = 61\ \text{hr}$$

Accordingly, the fractional rate constant of elimination is equal to $0.01136\ \text{h}^{-1}$ (0.693/61 h). Maximum and minimum digoxin plasma concentrations then may be predicted depending on the dosage interval. With T = 48 hours (i.e., 2×0.375 mg given every other day):

$$C_{ss,\,max} = \frac{F \cdot \text{dose}/V_{ss}}{1 - \exp(-kT)} \tag{1–20}$$
$$= \frac{0.7 \times 0.375 \times 2\ \text{mg}/580\ \text{liters}}{0.42}$$
$$= 2.15\ \text{ng/ml}$$

$$C_{ss,\,min} = C_{ss,\,max} \cdot \exp(-kT) \tag{1–21}$$
$$= (2.15\ \text{ng/ml})(0.58) = 1.25\ \text{ng/ml}$$

Thus, the plasma concentrations would fluctuate about twofold, consistent with the similarity of the dosage interval to digoxin's half-life. Also, the peak concentration would be above the upper value of the therapeutic range, exposing the patient to possible adverse effects, and at the end of the dosing interval, the concentration would be above but close to the lower limit. By using the same dosing rate but decreasing the dosing interval, a much smoother plasma concentration *versus* time profile would be obtained while still maintaining an average steady-state value of 1.65 ng/ml. For example, with T = 24 hours, the predicted maximum and minimum plasma concentrations would be 1.90 and 1.44 ng/ml, respectively, which are in the upper portion of the therapeutic window. By contrast, administering a more conservative dosing rate of 0.25 ng every 24 hours would produce peak and trough values of 1.26 and 0.96 ng/ml, respectively, which would be associated with a steady-state value of 1.10 ng/ml. Of course, the clinician must balance the problem of compliance with regimens that involve frequent dosage against the problem of periods when the patient may be subjected to concentrations of the drug that could be too high or too low.

Loading Dose. The *loading dose* is one or a series of doses that may be given at the onset of therapy with the aim of achieving the target concentration rapidly. The appropriate magnitude for the loading dose is

$$\text{Loading dose} = \text{target } C_p \cdot V_{ss}/F \qquad (1\text{--}22)$$

A loading dose may be desirable if the time required to attain steady state by the administration of drug at a constant rate (four elimination half-lives) is long relative to the temporal demands of the condition being treated. For example, the half-life of lidocaine is usually 1 to 2 hours. Arrhythmias encountered after myocardial infarction obviously may be life-threatening, and one cannot wait 4 to 8 hours to achieve a therapeutic concentration of lidocaine by infusion of the drug at the rate required to attain this concentration. Hence, use of a loading dose of lidocaine in the coronary care unit is standard.

The use of a loading dose also has significant disadvantages. First, the particularly sensitive individual may be exposed abruptly to a toxic concentration of a drug. Moreover, if the drug involved has a long half-life, it will take a long time for the concentration to fall if the level achieved is excessive. Loading doses tend to be large, and they are often given parenterally and rapidly; this can be particularly dangerous if toxic effects occur as a result of actions of the drug at sites that are in rapid equilibrium with plasma. This occurs because the loading dose calculated on the basis of V_{ss} subsequent to drug distribution is at first constrained within the initial and smaller "central" volume of distribution. It is therefore usually advisable to divide the loading dose into a number of smaller fractional doses that are administered over a period of time. Alternatively, the loading dose should be administered as a continuous intravenous infusion over a period of time. Ideally, this should be given in an exponentially decreasing fashion to mirror the concomitant accumulation of the maintenance dose of the drug, and this is accomplished using computerized infusion pumps.

Example. Administration of digitalis ("digitalization") in the patient described earlier is gradual if only a maintenance dose is administered (for at least 10 days based on a half-life of 61 hours). A more rapid response could be obtained (if deemed necessary by the physician; *see* Chapter 33) by using a loading-dose strategy and Equation (1–22):

$$\begin{aligned}\text{Loading dose} &= 1.5 \text{ ng} \cdot \text{ml}^{-1} \times 580 \text{ liters}/0.7 \\ &= 1243 \text{ } \mu g \sim 1 \text{ mg}\end{aligned}$$

To avoid toxicity, this oral loading dose, which also could be administered intravenously, would be given as an initial 0.5-mg dose followed by a 0.25-mg dose 6 to 8 hours later, with careful monitoring of the patient. It also would be prudent to give the final 0.25-mg fractional dose, if necessary, in two 0.125-mg divided doses separated by 6 to 8 hours to avoid overdigitalization, particularly if there were a plan to initiate an oral maintenance dose within 24 hours of beginning digoxin therapy.

Individualizing Dosage. A rational dosage regimen is based on knowledge of F, CL, V_{ss}, and $t_{\frac{1}{2}}$ and some information about rates of absorption and distribution of the drug together with potential effects of the disease on these parameters. Recommended dosage regimens generally are designed for an "average" patient; usual values for the important determining parameters and appropriate adjustments that may be necessitated by disease or other factors are presented in Appendix II. This "one size fits all" approach, however, overlooks the considerable and unpredictable interpatient variability that usually is present in these pharmacokinetic parameters. For many drugs, one standard deviation in the values observed for F, CL, and V_{ss} is about 20%, 50%, and 30%, respectively. This means that 95% of the time the C_{ss} that is achieved will be between 35% and 270% of the target; this is an unacceptably wide range for a drug with a low therapeutic index. Individualization of the dosage regimen to a particular patient therefore is critical for optimal therapy. The pharmacokinetic principles described earlier provide a basis for modifying the dosage regimen to obtain a desired degree of efficacy with a minimum of unacceptable adverse effects. In situations where the drug's plasma concentration can be measured and related to the therapeutic window, additional guidance for dosage modification is obtained from blood levels taken during therapy and evaluated in a pharmacokinetic consult available in many institutional settings. Such measurement and adjustment are appropriate for many drugs with low therapeutic indices (*e.g.,* cardiac glycosides, antiarrhythmic agents, anticonvulsants, theophylline, and warfarin).

Therapeutic Drug Monitoring

The major use of measured concentrations of drugs (at steady state) is to refine the estimate of CL/F for the patient being treated [using Equation (1–16) as rearranged below:

$$CL/F(\text{patient}) = \text{dosing rate}/C_{ss}(\text{measured}) \qquad (1\text{--}23)$$

The new estimate of CL/F can be used in Equation (1–18) to adjust the maintenance dose to achieve the desired target concentration.

Certain practical details and pitfalls associated with therapeutic drug monitoring should be kept in mind. The first of these relates to the time of sampling for measurement of the drug concentration. If intermittent dosing is used, when during a dosing interval should samples be taken? It is necessary to distinguish between two possible uses of measured drug concentrations to understand the possible answers. A concentration of drug measured in a sample taken at virtually any time during the dosing interval will provide information that may aid in the assessment of drug toxicity. This is one type of therapeutic drug monitoring. It should be stressed, however, that such use of a measured concentration of drug is fraught with difficulties because of interindividual variability in sensitivity to the drug. When there is a question of toxicity, the drug concentration is just one of many items used to interpret the clinical situation.

Changes in the effects of drugs may be delayed relative to changes in plasma concentration because of a slow rate of distribution or pharmacodynamic factors. Concentrations of digoxin, for example, regularly exceed 2 ng/ml (a potentially toxic value) shortly after an oral dose, yet these peak concentrations do not cause toxicity; indeed, they occur well before peak effects. Thus, concentrations of drugs in samples obtained shortly after administration can be uninformative or even misleading.

When concentrations of drugs are used for purposes of adjusting dosage regimens, samples obtained shortly after administration of a dose almost invariably are misleading. The purpose of sampling during supposed steady state is to modify the estimate of *CL/F* and thus the choice of dosage. Early postabsorptive concentrations do not reflect clearance; they are determined primarily by the rate of absorption, the "central" (rather than the steady-state) volume of distribution, and the rate of distribution, all of which are pharmacokinetic features of virtually no relevance in choosing the long-term maintenance dosage. When the goal of measurement is adjustment of dosage, the sample should be taken well after the previous dose, as a rule of thumb, just before the next planned dose, when the concentration is at its minimum. The exceptions to this approach are drugs that are eliminated nearly completely between doses and act only during the initial portion of each dosing interval. If it is questionable whether efficacious concentrations of such drugs are being achieved, a sample taken shortly after a dose may be helpful. On the other hand, if a concern is whether low clearance (as in renal failure) may cause accumulation of drug, concentrations measured just before the next dose will reveal such accumulation and are considerably more useful for this purpose than is knowledge of the maximal concentration. For such drugs, determination of both maximal and minimal concentrations is recommended. These two values can offer a more complete picture of the behavior of the drug in a specific patient (particularly if obtained over more that one dosing period) can better support pharmacokinetic modeling.

A second important aspect of the timing of sampling is its relationship to the beginning of the maintenance-dosage regimen. When constant dosage is given, steady state is reached only after four half-lives have passed. If a sample is obtained too soon after dosage is begun, it will not reflect this state and the drug's clearance accurately. Yet, for toxic drugs, if sampling is delayed until steady state is ensured, the damage may have been done. Some simple guidelines can be offered. When it is important to maintain careful control of concentrations, the first sample should be taken after two half-lives (as calculated and expected for the patient), assuming that no loading dose has been given. If the concentration already exceeds 90% of the eventual expected mean steady-state concentration, the dosage rate should be halved, another sample obtained in another two (supposed) half-lives, and the dosage halved again if this sample exceeds the target. If the first concentration is not too high, the initial rate of dosage is continued; even if the concentration is lower than expected, it is usually reasonable to await the attainment of steady state in another two estimated half-lives and then to proceed to adjust dosage as described earlier.

If dosage is intermittent, there is a third concern with the time at which samples are obtained for determination of drug concentrations. If the sample has been obtained just prior to the next dose, as recommended, concentration will be a minimal value, not the mean. However, as discussed earlier, the estimated mean concentration may be calculated by using Equation (1–16).

If a drug follows first-order kinetics, the average, minimum, and maximum concentrations at steady state are linearly related to dose and dosing rate [*see* Equations (1–16), (1–19), and (1–20)]. Therefore, the ratio between the measured and desired concentrations can be used to adjust the dose, consistent with available dosage sizes:

$$\frac{C_{ss}(\text{measured})}{C_{ss}(\text{desired})} = \frac{\text{dose (previous)}}{\text{dose (new)}} \qquad (1\text{–}24)$$

In the previously described patient given 0.375 mg digoxin every 24 hours, for example, if the measured steady-state concentration were found to be 1.65 ng/ml rather than a desired level of 1.3 ng/ml, an appropriate, practical change in the dosage regimen would be to reduce the daily dose to 0.25 mg digoxin.

$$\text{Dose (new)} = \frac{C_{ss}(\text{measured})}{C_{ss}(\text{desired})} \times \text{dose (previous)}$$

$$= \frac{1.3}{1.65} \times 0.375 = 0.295 \sim 0.25 \text{ mg}/24 \text{ hr}$$

Compliance

Ultimately, therapeutic success depends on the patient actually taking the drug according to the prescribed dosage regimen—"Drugs don't work if you don't take them." Noncompliance with the prescribed dosing schedule is a major reason for therapeutic failure, especially in the long-term treatment of disease using antihypertensive, antiretroviral, and anticonvulsant agents. When no special efforts are made to address this issue, only about 50% of patients follow the prescribed dosage regimen in a reasonably satisfactory fashion, approximately one-third comply only partly, and about 1 in 6 patients is essentially noncompliant. Missed doses are more common than too many doses. The number of drugs does not appear to be as important as the number of times a day doses must be remembered (Farmer, 1999). Reducing the number of required dosing occasions can improve adherence to a prescribed dosage regimen. Equally important is the need to involve patients in the responsibility for their own health using a variety of strategies based on improved communication regarding the nature of the disease and the overall therapeutic plan (*see* Appendix I).

II. PHARMACODYNAMICS

MECHANISMS OF DRUG ACTION AND THE RELATIONSHIP BETWEEN DRUG CONCENTRATION AND EFFECT

Pharmacodynamics deals with the study of the biochemical and physiological effects of drugs and their mechanisms of action. A thorough analysis of drug action can provide the basis for both the rational therapeutic use of a drug and the design of new and superior therapeutic agents. Basic research in pharmacodynamics also provides fundamental insights into biochemical and physiological regulation.

Mechanisms of Drug Action

The effects of most drugs result from their interaction with macromolecular components of the organism.

These interactions alter the function of the pertinent component and thereby initiate the biochemical and physiological changes that are characteristic of the response to the drug. The term *receptor* denotes the component of the organism with which the chemical agent is presumed to interact.

The concept of drugs acting on receptors generally is credited to John Langley (1878). While studying the antagonistic effects of *atropine* against *pilocarpine*-induced salivation, Langley observed, "There is some substance or substances in the nerve ending or gland cell with which both atropine and pilocarpine are capable of forming compounds." He later referred to this factor as a "receptive substance." The word *receptor* was introduced in 1909 by Paul Ehrlich. Ehrlich postulated that a drug could have a therapeutic effect only if it has the "right sort of affinity." Ehrlich defined a receptor in functional terms: ". . . that combining group of the protoplasmic molecule to which the introduced group is anchored will hereafter be termed *receptor*."

The notion that the receptor for a drug can be any functional macromolecular component of the organism has several fundamental corollaries. One is that a drug potentially is capable of altering both the extent and rate at which any bodily function proceeds. Another is that drugs do not create effects but instead modulate intrinsic physiological functions.

Drug Receptors

From a numerical standpoint, proteins form the most important class of drug receptors. Examples include the receptors for hormones, growth factors, transcription factors, and neurotransmitters; the enzymes of crucial metabolic or regulatory pathways (*e.g.*, dihydrofolate reductase, acetylcholinesterase, and cyclic nucleotide phosphodiesterases); proteins involved in transport processes (*e.g.*, Na^+,K^+-ATPase); secreted glycoproteins (*e.g.*, Wnts); and structural proteins (*e.g.*, tubulin). Specific binding properties of other cellular constituents also can be exploited for therapeutic purpose. Thus nucleic acids are important drug receptors, particularly for cancer chemotherapeutic agents.

A particularly important group of drug receptors consists of proteins that normally serve as receptors for endogenous regulatory ligands (*e.g.*, hormones and neurotransmitters). Many drugs act on such physiological receptors and often are particularly selective because physiological receptors are specialized to recognize and respond to individual signaling molecules with great selectivity. Drugs that bind to physiological receptors and mimic the regulatory effects of the endogenous signaling compounds are termed *agonists*. Other drugs bind to receptors without regulatory effect, but their binding blocks the binding of the endogenous agonist. Such compounds with no stimulatory action of their own that still may produce useful

effects by inhibiting the action of an agonist (*e.g.*, by competition for agonist-binding sites) are termed *antagonists*. Agents that are only partly as effective as agonists no matter the amount employed are termed *partial agonists,* and those which stabilize the receptor in its inactive conformation are termed *inverse agonists* (*see* "Quantitation of Drug–Receptor Interactions and Elicited Effect," below).

The binding of drugs to receptors can involve all known types of interactions—ionic, hydrogen bonding, hydrophobic, van der Waals, and covalent. Most interactions between drugs and their receptors involve bonds of multiple types. If binding is covalent, the duration of drug action is frequently, but not necessarily, prolonged. Noncovalent interactions of high affinity also may be essentially irreversible.

Structure–Activity Relationship and Drug Design. The strength of the reversible interaction between a drug and its receptor, as measured by their dissociation constant, is defined as the *affinity* of one for the other. Both the affinity of a drug for its receptor and its intrinsic activity are determined by its chemical structure. This relationship frequently is quite stringent. Relatively minor modifications in the drug molecule may result in major changes in its pharmacological properties based on altered affinity for one or more receptors.

The stringent nature of chemical structure to specificity of binding of a drug to its receptor is illustrated by the capacity of receptors to interact selectively with optical isomers, as described for the antimuscarinic actions of L-hyoscyamine *versus* DL-hyoscyamine (atropine) by the classic studies of Arthur Cushney.

Exploitation of structure–activity relationships on many occasions has led to the synthesis of valuable therapeutic agents. Because changes in molecular configuration need not alter all actions and effects of a drug equally, it is sometimes possible to develop a congener with a more favorable ratio of therapeutic to adverse effects, enhanced selectivity among different cells or tissues, or more acceptable secondary characteristics than those of the parent drug. Therapeutically useful antagonists of hormones or neurotransmitters have been developed by chemical modification of the structure of the physiological agonist. Minor modifications of structure also can have profound effects on the pharmacokinetic properties of drugs. Addition of a phosphate ester, for example, at the N3 position in the antiseizure drug phenytoin (5,5-diphenyl-2,4-imidazolidinedione) produces a prodrug (*fosphenytoin*) that is more soluble in intravenous solutions than its parent. The modification results in far more reliable distribution in the body and a drug that must be cleaved by esterase to become active.

Given adequate information about both the molecular structures and the pharmacological activities of a relatively large group of congeners, it is possible to identify the chemical properties (*i.e.*, the pharmacophore) required for optimal action at the receptor: size, shape, position and orientation of charged groups or hydrogen bond donors, and so on. Advances in molecular modeling of organic compounds and the methods for drug target (receptor) discovery and biochemical measurement of the primary actions of drugs at their receptors have enriched the quantitation of structure–activity relationships and its use in drug design (Carlson and McCammon, 2000). The importance of specific drug–receptor interactions can be evaluated further by analyzing the responsiveness of receptors that have been selectively mutated at individual amino acid residues. Such information increasingly is allowing the optimization or design of chemicals that can bind to a receptor with improved affinity, selectivity, or regulatory effect. Similar structure-based approaches also are used to improve pharmacokinetic properties of drugs, particularly with respect to knowledge of their metabolism. Knowledge of the structures of receptors and of drug–receptor complexes, determined at atomic resolution by x-ray crystallography, is even more helpful in the design of ligands and in understanding the molecular basis of drug resistance and circumventing it (*i.e., imatinib*). Emerging technology in the fields of *pharmacogenetics* and *pharmacoproteomics* (Chapter 4) is improving our understanding of the nature of and variation in receptors and is positioned to permit molecular diagnostics in individual patients to predict those who will benefit from a particular drug (Jain, 2004).

Advances in combinatorial chemistry contribute to structure-motivated drug design through powerful, if random, generation of new drugs. In this approach, huge libraries of randomly synthesized chemicals are generated either by combining chemical groups in every possible combination by various chemical methodologies or by genetically engineered microbes. A library that can include proteins and even oligonucleotides then is screened for pharmacologically active agents using mammalian cells or microorganisms that have been engineered to express the receptor of therapeutic interest and the associated biochemical machinery necessary for detection of the response to receptor activation. Although libraries can contain on the order of a million compounds, automated high-throughput screening methods permit rapid assessment of putative new drugs. Active compounds initially discovered by such random screens then can be modified and improved using knowledge of their target receptor and essential principles of structure–function relationships.

Cellular Sites of Drug Action. Because drugs act by altering the activities of their receptors, the sites at which a drug acts and the extent of its action are determined by the location and functional capacity of its receptors. Selective localization of drug action within an organism therefore does not necessarily depend on selective distribution of the drug. If a drug acts on a receptor that serves functions common to most cells, its effects will be widespread. If the function is a vital one, the drug may be particularly difficult or dangerous to use. Nevertheless, such a drug may be important clinically. Digitalis glycosides, classically employed in the treatment of heart failure, are potent inhibitors of an ion transport process that is vital to most cells, Na^+,K^+-ATPase. As such, cardiac glycosides can cause widespread toxicity, and their margin of safety is dangerously low. Indeed, some drugs are intentional poisons, such as the antifolate cancer drug *methotrexate*, which, when used in high dose for the treatment of osteo-

sarcoma, requires rescue with *leucovorin* (5-formyl tetrahydrofolic acid). If a drug interacts with receptors that are unique to only a few types of differentiated cells, its effects are more specific. Hypothetically, the ideal drug would cause its therapeutic effect by such a discrete action. Side effects would be minimized, but toxicity might not be. If the differentiated function were a vital one, this type of drug also could be very dangerous. Some of the most lethal agents known (*e.g., botulinum toxin*) show such specificity. Even if the primary action of a drug is localized, the consequent physiological effects of the drug may be widespread.

Receptors for Physiological Regulatory Molecules

The term *receptor* has been used operationally to denote any cellular macromolecule to which a drug binds to initiate its effects. Among the most important drug receptors are cellular proteins, whose normal function is to act as receptors for endogenous regulatory ligands—particularly hormones, growth factors, and neurotransmitters. The function of such physiological receptors consists of binding the appropriate endogenous ligand and, in response, propagating its regulatory signal in the target cell.

Identification of the two functions of a receptor, ligand binding and message propagation (*i.e.,* signaling), correctly suggests the existence of functional domains within the receptor: a *ligand-binding domain* and an *effector domain*. The structure and function of these domains often can be deduced from high-resolution structures of receptor proteins and by analysis of the behavior of intentionally mutated receptors. Increasingly, the mechanism of intramolecular coupling of ligand binding with functional activation also can be learned. A case in point is knowledge of the crystal structure of the receptor/visual pigment *rhodopsin* that reveals details of the structure of the protein not expected from chemical modeling (Patel *et al.,* 2004). The biological importance of these functional domains is further indicated by the evolution both of different receptors for diverse ligands that act by similar biochemical mechanisms and of multiple receptors for a single ligand that act by unrelated mechanisms.

The regulatory actions of a receptor may be exerted directly on its cellular target(s), *effector protein(s),* or may be conveyed by intermediary cellular signaling molecules called *transducers*. The receptor, its cellular target, and any intermediary molecules are referred to as a *receptor–effector system* or *signal-transduction pathway*. Frequently, the proximal cellular effector protein is not the ultimate physiological target but rather is an enzyme or transport protein that creates, moves, or degrades a small metabolite (*e.g.*, a cyclic nucleotide or inositol-trisphosphate) or ion (*e.g.*, Ca^{2+}) known as a *second messenger*. Second messengers can diffuse in the proximity of their binding sites and convey information to a variety of targets, which can respond simultaneously to the output of a single receptor binding a single agonist molecule. Even though these second messengers originally were thought of as freely diffusible molecules within the cell, their diffusion and their intracellular actions are constrained by compartmentation—selective localization of receptor–transducer–effector–signal termination complexes—established *via* protein–lipid and protein–protein interactions (Buxton and Brunton, 1983; Wong and Scott, 2004; Baillie and Houslay, 2005).

Receptors and their associated effector and transducer proteins also act as integrators of information as they coordinate signals from multiple ligands with each other and with the metabolic activities of the cell (*see* below). This integrative function is particularly evident when one considers that the different receptors for scores of chemically unrelated ligands use relatively few biochemical mechanisms to exert their regulatory functions and that even these few pathways may share common signaling molecules.

An important property of physiological receptors that also makes them excellent targets for drugs is that they act catalytically and hence are biochemical signal amplifiers. The catalytic nature of receptors is obvious when the receptor itself is an enzyme, but all known physiological receptors are formally catalysts. For example, when a single agonist molecule binds to a receptor that is an ion channel, hundreds of thousands to millions of ions flow through the channel every second. The number of ions moving through the channel depends on the characteristic conductance of the channel, a property analogous to amplifier gain. Physiological receptor channels display conductance in the range of tens to hundreds of picosiemens. Similarly, a single steroid hormone molecule binds to its receptor and initiates the transcription of many copies of specific mRNAs, which, in turn, can give rise to multiple copies of a single protein.

Drug–Receptor Binding and Agonism. A receptor can exist in at least two conformational states, active (R_a), and inactive (R_i). If these states are in equilibrium and the inactive state predominates in the absence of drug, then the basal signal output will be low. The *extent* to which the equilibrium is shifted toward the active state is determined by the *relative* affinity of the drug for the two conformations (Figure 1–6). A drug that has a higher affinity for the active conformation than for the inactive conformation will drive the equilibrium to the active state and thereby activate the receptor. Such a drug will be an agonist. A full agonist is sufficiently selective for the active conformation that at a saturating concentration it will drive the receptor essentially completely to the active state (Figure 1–6). If a different but perhaps structurally similar compound binds

to the same site on R but with only moderately greater affinity for R_a than for R_i, its effect will be less, even at saturating concentrations. A drug that displays such intermediate effectiveness is referred to as a *partial agonist* because it cannot promote a full biological response at any concentration. In an absolute sense, all agonists are partial; selectivity for R_a over R_i cannot be total. A drug that binds with equal affinity to either conformation will not alter the activation equilibrium and will act as a competitive antagonist of any compound, agonist or antagonist, that does. A drug with preferential affinity for R_i actually will produce an effect opposite to that of an agonist; examples of such *inverse agonists* at G protein–coupled receptors (GPCRs) do exist (*e.g.*, *famotidine, losartan, metoprolol*, and *risperidone*) (Milligan, 2003).

Inverse agonism may be measurable only in systems in which an equilibrium between R_i and R_a exists in the absence of drug such that a decrease in physiological or biochemical response can be measured in the presence of drug with a higher affinity for R_i than R_a. If the *preexisting* or basal equilibrium for unliganded receptors lies far in the direction of R_i, negative antagonism may be difficult to observe and to distinguish from simple competitive antagonism.

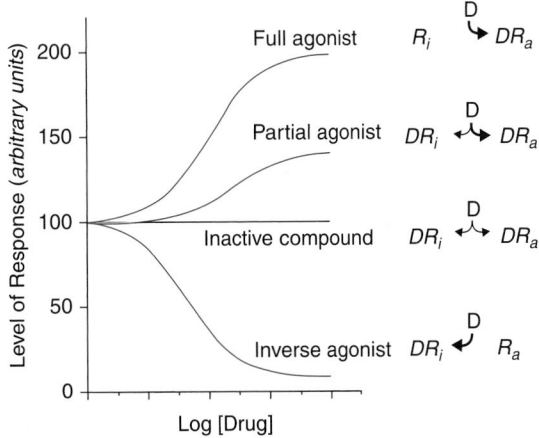

Figure 1–6. Regulation of the activity of a receptor with conformation-selective drugs. The ordinate is some activity of the receptor produced by R_a, the active receptor conformation (*e.g.*, stimulation of adenylyl cyclase). If a drug D selectively binds to R_a, it will produce a maximal response. If D has equal affinity for R_i and R_a, it will not perturb the equilibrium between them and will have no effect on net activity; D would appear as an inactive compound. If the drug selectively binds to R_i, then the net amount of R_a will be diminished. If there is sufficient R_a to produce an elevated basal response in the absence of ligand (agonist-independent constitutive activity), then activity will be observably inhibited; D will be an inverse agonist. If D can bind to receptor in an active conformation R_a but also bind to inactive receptor R_i with lower affinity, the drug will produce a partial response; D will be a partial agonist.

Careful biochemical studies of receptor–drug interactions, coupled with the analysis of receptors in which the intrinsic R_a/R_i equilibrium has been shifted by mutation, have supported this general model of drug action. The model is readily applicable to experimental data through the use of appropriate computer-assisted analysis of the laws of mass action and is used frequently as a guide to understanding drug action. This approach has been particularly useful in understanding the interaction of agonists and antagonists with GPCRs and ion channels. Indeed, electrophysiological measurements, particularly those of single-channel behavior, create a moment-to-moment analysis of receptor function that permits detailed modeling of intermediate states of receptor conformation that have led to the design of more selective drugs (*e.g.,* antiarrhythmics).

Current models for GPCR activation assume that receptors are in equilibrium between inactive (R_i) and active (R_a) conformations (Milligan, 2003). R_a is promoted by agonists but also may occur in their absence, leading to constitutive activity. In order to explain the behavior of recombinant receptors in model systems however, it is necessary to consider additional receptor conformations. The term *protean agonist* has been used to explain reversal from agonism to inverse agonism when an agonist produces an active conformation of lower efficacy than the constitutively active conformation of the receptor (Kenakin, 1995). Apparent protean agonism has been observed recently for native receptors under physiological conditions (Gbahou *et al.*, 2003).

Physiological Receptors: Structural and Functional Families. We have witnessed both an explosion in our appreciation of the number of physiological receptors and, in parallel, the development of our understanding of the fundamental structural motifs and biochemical mechanisms that characterize them. Molecular cloning has identified both completely novel receptors (and their regulatory ligands) and numerous isoforms, or subtypes, of previously known receptors. There now exist data banks devoted exclusively to structures of single classes of receptors. Members of various classes of receptors, transducers, and effector proteins have been purified, and their mechanisms of action are understood in considerable biochemical detail. Receptors, transducers, and effectors can be expressed or, conversely, repressed *via* molecular genetic strategies and the consequence of their alteration studied in cultured mammalian cells or systems of convenience such as yeast or *Candida elegans*. Furthermore, it is now possible to produce transgenic knockout animals (notably mice) that lack a particular receptor. Providing that the deletion is not lethal and that the resulting offspring can breed, much can be learned about the role of the missing receptor.

Receptors for physiological regulatory molecules can be assigned to a relatively few functional families whose members share both common mechanisms of action and similar molecular structures (Figure 1–7). For each receptor superfamily, there is now a context for understanding

the structures of ligand-binding domains and effector domains and how agonist binding influences the regulatory activity of the receptor. The relatively small number of biochemical mechanisms and structural formats used for cellular signaling is fundamental to the ways in which target cells integrate signals from multiple receptors to produce additive, sequential, synergistic, or mutually inhibitory responses.

Receptors as Enzymes: Receptor Protein Kinases and Guanylyl Cyclases. The largest group of receptors with intrinsic enzymatic activity consists of cell surface protein kinases, which exert their regulatory effects by phosphorylating diverse effector proteins at the inner face of the plasma membrane. Protein phosphorylation can alter the biochemical activities of an effector or its interactions with other proteins. Indeed, of all the possible reversible covalent modifications of proteins that regulate their function, phosphorylation is the most common. Most receptors that are protein kinases phosphorylate tyrosine residues in their substrates; these include receptors for insulin and diverse polypeptides that direct growth or differentiation, such as epidermal growth factor and nerve growth factor. A few receptor protein kinases phosphorylate serine or threonine residues. The most structurally simple receptor protein kinases are composed of an agonist-binding domain on the extracellular surface of the plasma membrane, a single membrane-spanning element, and a protein kinase domain on the inner membrane face. Many variations on this basic architecture exist, including assembly of multiple subunits in the mature receptor, obligate oligomerization of the liganded receptor, and the addition of multiple regulatory or protein-binding domains to the intracellular protein kinase domain that permit association of the liganded receptor with additional effector molecules (frequently *via* interaction of phosphotyrosine residues and SH$_2$ domains) and with substrates. Drugs designed to act at receptors in this diverse family include *insulin* for the treatment of diabetes mellitus and imatinib, designed to inhibit both receptor and nonreceptor tyrosine kinases and approved for the treatment of chronic myelogenous leukemia.

Another family of receptors that are functionally linked to protein kinases contains a modification of the structure just described. Protein kinase–associated receptors lack the intracellular enzymatic domains but, in response to agonists, bind or activate distinct protein kinases on the cytoplasmic face of the plasma membrane. Receptors of this group include the cytokine receptors, several receptors for neurotrophic peptides, the growth hormone receptor, the multisubunit antigen receptors on T- and B-lymphocytes, and the interferon-γ receptor.

The domain structure described for cell surface protein kinases is varied in other receptors to use other signaling outputs. A family of protein tyrosine phosphatases has extracellular domains with a sequence reminiscent of cellular adhesion molecules. Although the extracellular ligands for many of these phosphatases are not known, the importance of their enzymatic activity has been demonstrated through genetic and biochemical experiments. Indeed, these receptor protein tyrosine phosphatases (RPTPs) appear to be activated by each other and by extracellular matrix proteins expressed by particular cell types, consistent with their role in regulating cell–cell interactions and tissue organization. For the receptors that bind atrial natriuretic peptides and the peptides guanylin and uroguanylin, the intracellular domain is not a protein kinase but rather a guanylyl

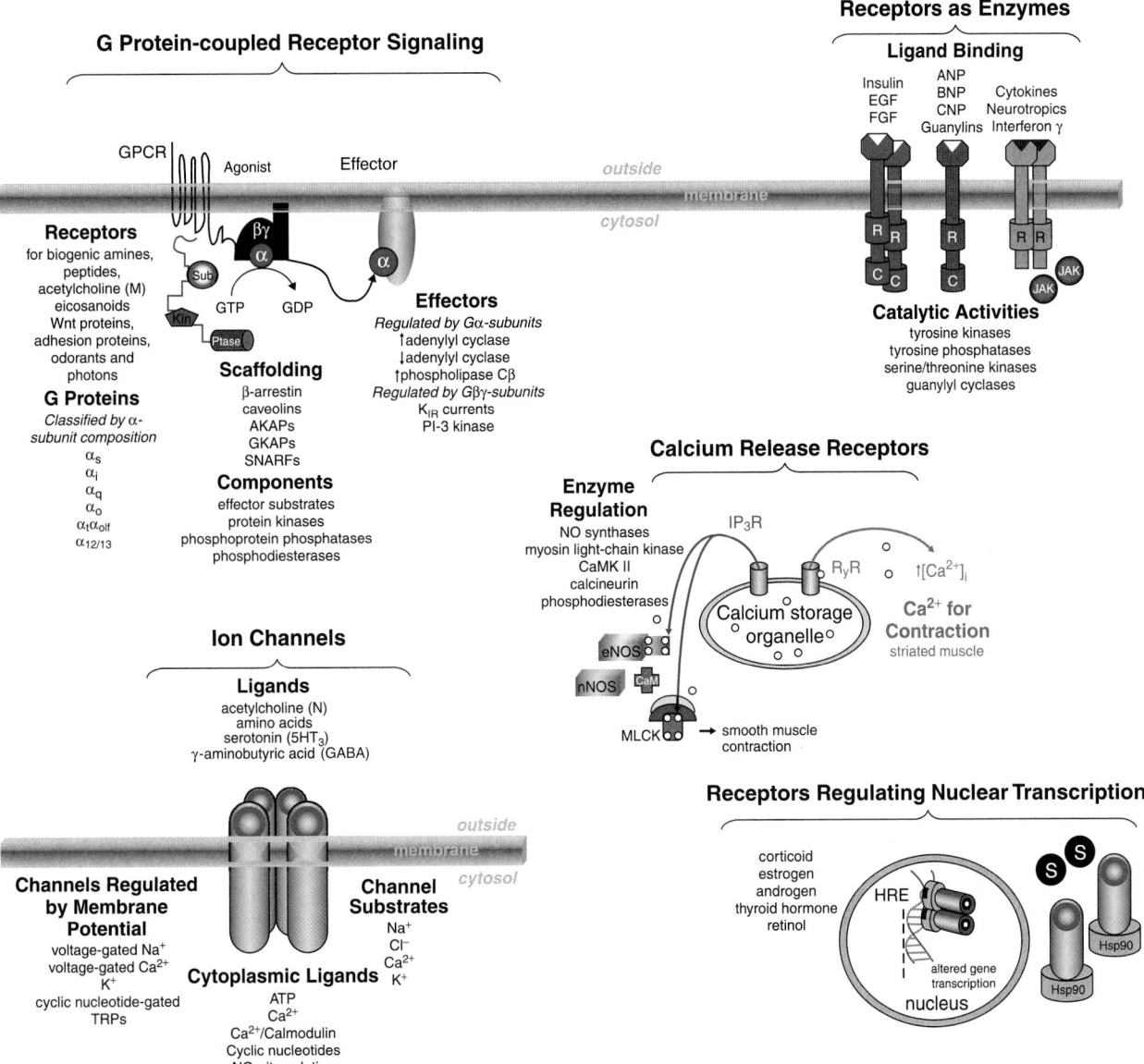

Figure 1–7. ***Structural motifs of physiological receptors and their relationships to signaling pathways.*** Schematic diagram of the diversity of mechanisms for control of cell function by receptors for endogenous agents acting *via* the cell surface or at calcium storage sites or in the nucleus. Detailed descriptions of these signaling pathway are given throughout the text in relation to the therapeutic actions of drugs affecting these pathways.

cyclase that synthesizes the second messenger cyclic guanosine monophosphate (GMP), which activates a cyclic GMP–dependent protein kinase (PKG) and modulates the activities of several nucleotide phosphodiesterases.

Protease-Activated Receptor Signaling. Some receptors are not presented by the cell in a form readily accessible to agonist. Proteases that are anchored to the plasma membrane or that are soluble in the extracellular fluid (*e.g.,* thrombin) can cleave ligands or receptors at the surfaces of cells to either initiate or terminate signal transduction. Peptide agonists often are processed by proteolysis to become active at their receptors. Tumor necrosis factor α (TNF-α)–

converting enzyme (TACE) cleaves the precursor of TNF-α at the plasma membrane, releasing a soluble form of this pro-inflammatory cytokine. Similarly, angiotensin-converting enzyme (ACE), which is also an integral membrane protein preferentially expressed by endothelial cells in the blood vessels of the lung, converts angiotensin I to angiotensin II (Ang II), thereby generating the active hormone near receptors for Ang II on vascular smooth muscle. In contrast, neutral endopeptidase degrades and inactivates the neuropeptide substance P (SP) in the vicinity of its receptors and thus terminates the biological effects of SP. Some GPCRs (*see below*) also can be activated or inactivated by proteases at the cell surface. For example, the coagulation factor thrombin cleaves protease-activated platelet receptor 1 (PAR1), activating it to induce platelet aggregation. On the other hand, neutrophil-derived cathepsin G cleaves PAR1 at a site distinct from that of thrombin, generating a thrombin-insensitive receptor. Targeting the proteolytic regulation of receptor mechanisms has produced successful therapeutic strategies, such as the use of ACE inhibitors in the treatment of hypertension (*see* Chapters 30 and 32) and the generation of new anticoagulants targeting the action of thrombin (*see* Chapter 54).

Ion Channels. Receptors for several neurotransmitters form agonist-regulated ion-selective channels in the plasma membrane, termed *ligand-gated ion channels* or *receptor operated channels*, that convey their signals by altering the cell's membrane potential or ionic composition. This group includes the nicotinic cholinergic receptor, the γ-aminobutyric acid A (GABA$_A$) receptor, and receptors for glutamate, aspartate, and glycine (*see* Chapters 9, 12, and 16). They are all multisubunit proteins, with each subunit predicted to span the plasma membrane several times. Symmetrical association of the subunits allows each to form a segment of the channel wall, or pore, and to cooperatively control channel opening and closing. Agonist binding may occur on a particular subunit that may be represented more than once in the assembled multimer (*e.g.*, the nicotinic acetylcholine receptor) or may be conferred by a separate single subunit of the assembled channel, as is the case with the so-called sulfonylurea receptor (SUR) that associates with a K$^+$ channel (Kir$_{6.2}$) to regulate the ATP-dependent K$^+$ channel (K$_{ATP}$). The K$_{ATP}$ channel is a receptor for compounds such as *glibenclamide* (a channel antagonist) in the treatment of diabetes type 2 (*see* Chapter 60). Openers of the same channel (*minoxidil*) are used as vascular smooth muscle relaxants. Receptor-operated channels also are regulated by other receptor-mediated events, such as protein kinase activation following activation of GPCRs (*see* below). Phosphorylation of the channel protein on one or more of its subunits can confer both activation and inactivation depending on the channel and the nature of the phosphorylation.

G Protein–Coupled Receptors. A large superfamily of receptors that accounts for many known drug targets interacts with distinct heterotrimeric GTP-binding regulatory proteins known as *G proteins*. G proteins are signal transducers that convey information (*i.e.*, agonist binding) from the receptor to one or more effector proteins. GPCRs include those for a number of biogenic amines, eicosanoids and other lipid-signaling molecules, peptide hormones, opioids, amino acids such as GABA, and many other peptide and protein ligands. G protein–regulated effectors include enzymes such as adenylyl cyclase, phospholipase C, phosphodiesterases, and plasma membrane ion channels selective for Ca^{2+} and K$^+$ (Figure 1–7). Because of their number and physiological importance, GPCRs are widely used targets for drugs; perhaps half of all nonantibiotic prescription drugs are directed toward these receptors that make up the third largest family of genes in humans.

GPCRs span the plasma membrane as a bundle of seven α-helices. Agonists bind to a cleft within the extracellular face of the bundle or to a globular ligand-binding domain sometimes found at the amino terminus. G proteins bind to the cytoplasmic face of the receptors. Receptors in this family respond to agonists by promoting the binding of GTP to the G protein α subunit. GTP activates the G protein and allows it, in turn, to activate the effector protein. The G protein remains active until it hydrolyzes the bound GTP to GDP and returns to its ground (inactive) state. G proteins are composed of a GTP-binding α subunit, which confers specific recognition by receptor and effector, and an associated dimer of β and γ subunits

that can confer both membrane localization of the G protein (*e.g.*, *via* myristoylation) and direct signaling such as activation of inward rectifier K$^+$ (GIRK) channels and binding sites for G protein receptor kinases (GRKs). Activation of the G$_\alpha$ subunit by GTP allows it to both regulate an effector protein and drive the release of G$_{\beta\gamma}$ subunits, which can, in addition to regulating their own group of effectors, reassociate with GDP-liganded G$_\alpha$, returning the system to the basal state.

A cell may express as many as twenty different GPCRs, each with distinctive specificity for one or several of half a dozen G proteins. Each subunit of the G protein complex is encoded by a member of one of three corresponding gene families. Currently, 16 different members of the α-subunit family, 5 different members of the β-subunit family, and 11 different members of the γ-subunit family have been described in mammals. A G protein can regulate one or more effectors, and multiple GPCRs can activate the same G protein. A receptor also may generate multiple signals by activating more than one G protein species. GPCRs can activate several signal-transduction systems as a consequence of G protein activation. From the classical view of G protein activation of adenylyl cyclase, accumulation of cyclic adenosine monophosphate (cAMP), and activation of cAMP-dependent protein kinase (PKA), we now know that the consequences of G protein activation have both direct and indirect effects on multiple pathways.

Central to the effect of many GPCRs is release of calcium (Ca^{2+}) from intracellular stores. For example, α receptors for norepinephrine activate G$_q$ specific for the activation of phospholipase C$_\beta$. Phospholipase C$_\beta$ (PLC$_\beta$) is a membrane-bound enzyme that hydrolyzes a membrane phospholipid, phosphatidylinositol-4,5-bisphosphate, to generate inositol-1,4,5-trisphosphate (IP$_3$) and the lipid, diacylglycerol. IP$_3$ binds to receptors on Ca^{2+} release channels in the IP$_3$-sensitive Ca^{2+} stores of the endoplasmic reticulum, triggering the release of Ca^{2+} and rapidly raising [Ca^{2+}]$_i$ from approximately 100 nM into the micromolar range. When Ca^{2+} levels rise following release from intracellular stores, the elevation of Ca^{2+} is transient owing to avid reuptake of Ca^{2+} into stores. Ca^{2+} can bind to and directly regulate ion channels (*e.g.*, large conductance Ca^{2+}-activated K$^+$ channels), or Ca^{2+} can bind to calmodulin, and the resulting Ca^{2+}–calmodulin complex then can bind ion channels (*e.g.*, small conductance Ca^{2+}-activated K$^+$ channels) or to intracellular enzymes such as Ca^{2+}–calmodulin–dependent protein kinases (*e.g.*, CaMKII, MLCK, and phosphorylase kinase).

Diacylglycerol (DAG), formed by the action of PLC$_\beta$, also participates in the response to G protein activation by binding to protein kinase C (PKC), thereby promoting its association with the cell membrane and lowering its requirement for activation by Ca^{2+}. DAG binds to other proteins with cysteine-rich (C-1) domains that participate in non-kinase-mediated regulation of processes such as neurotransmitter release. PKC can regulate numerous cellular events by activating members of the mitogen-activated kinase (MAPK) family, which, depending on the cell type, includes extracellular signal-regulated kinases (ERKs), c-Jun N-terminal kinases (JNKs), and p38 MAPKs. The initial increase in intracellular diacylglycerol can be sustained by its activation of phospholipase D, which hydrolyzes membrane phosphatidylcholine to generate phosphatidic acid and choline. Phosphatidic acid, in turn, can be converted enzymatically to diacylglycerol or serve as a substrate for phospholipase A$_2$ (PLA$_2$), which generates lysophosphatidic acid (LPA) and frees 20-carbon fatty acids (*e.g.*, C20:4, 5,8,11,14-eicosatetraenoic acid) for eicosanoid synthesis. Eicosanoids act as autocrine and paracrine agents frequently *via* specific GPCRs (*see* Chapters 26 and 35).

LPA can bind to specific GPCRs of the endothelial differentiating gene family (Edg receptors) that signal cell growth and differentiation and can regulate transcription factors such as the peroxisome proliferator–activated receptors (PPARs) that modulate nuclear transcription and are the receptors (PPARγ) for the glitazones, newer oral hypoglycemic agents (*see* Chapter 60).

While the complexity of receptor signaling through G proteins is clear from the abundance of GPCRs present on a single cell, receptor–ligand interactions alone do not regulate all GPCR signaling. It is now clear that GPCRs undergo both homo- and heterodimerization and possibly oligomerization (Kroeger *et al.*, 2003; Milligan, 2004). Evidence of therapeutic importance for dimerization is suggested by many recent studies; heterodimerization can result in receptor units with altered pharmacology compared with either individual receptor. For example, heterodimerization between the γ-aminobutyric acid receptor subunit protein $GABA_{B1}$ and $GABA_{B2}$ is required for receptor binding of agonist ($GABA_{B1}$) and trafficking ($GABA_{B2}$) to the cell surface and receptor function (these receptors mediate the metabotropic actions of the inhibitory neurotransmitter GABA). Dimerization also appears to be important in the actions of dopamine receptors (D_2 homodimers), where ligand preference appears to be conferred by dimerization, a finding that could have therapeutic implications. Evidence also is emerging that dimerization of receptors may regulate the affinity and specificity of the complex for G protein and regulate the sensitivity of the receptor to phosphorylation by receptor kinases and the binding of arrestin, events important in termination of the action of agonists and removal of receptors from the cell surface. Dimerization also may permit binding of receptors to other regulatory proteins such as transcription factors. Thus, the receptor–G protein effector systems are complex networks of convergent and divergent interactions involving both receptor–receptor and receptor–G protein coupling that permits extraordinarily versatile regulation of cell function.

Transcription Factors. Receptors for steroid hormones, thyroid hormone, vitamin D, and the retinoids are soluble DNA-binding proteins that regulate the transcription of specific genes (Wei, 2003). They are part of a larger family of transcription factors whose members may be regulated by phosphorylation, association with other cellular proteins, or binding to metabolites or cellular regulatory ligands (*e.g.,* heat shock proteins). These receptors act as dimers—some as homodimers and some as heterodimers—with homologous cellular proteins, but they may be regulated by higher-order oligomerization with other modulator molecules. Often bound to proteins in the cytoplasm that retain them in an inactive state, they provide examples of conservation of structure and mechanism in part because they are assembled as three largely independent domains. The region nearest the carboxyl terminus binds hormone and is called the *ligand-binding domain* (LBD) that confers a negative regulatory role; hormone binding relieves this inhibitory constraint. The central region of the receptor is the *DNA binding domain* (DBD) that mediates binding to specific sites on the genome to activate or inhibit transcription of the nearby gene. These regulatory sites in DNA are likewise receptor-specific: the sequence of a "glucocorticoid-response element," with only slight variation, is associated with each glucocorticoid-response gene, whereas a "thyroid-response element" confers specificity of the actions of the thyroid hormone nuclear receptor. The amino-terminal region of the receptor provides the activation function (AF) domain essential for transcriptional regulation.

Steroid hormone receptors undergo a complex interaction with themselves and coregulators. There are at least three subfamilies of proteins that form the steroid receptor coactivator (SRC) family. The specific set of proteins that assemble with a particular steroid hormone–liganded receptor in the regulation of transcription varies with the receptor in question (*see* Chapters 57 through 59). In general, the members of this family serve functions essential for DNA binding such as acetylation of histone proteins [*e.g.,* histone acetyl transferase activity (HAT)] that permit interaction of the receptor with the hormone response element to initiate transcription. Steroid hormone receptor regulation of transcription does not always result in transcriptional activation; in some cases, as in glucocorticoid action, the effect of the hormone is to decrease the production of steroid-responsive protein transcription.

Cytoplasmic Second Messengers. Binding of an agonist to a receptor provides the first message in receptor signal transduction to effector pathways and an eventual physiological outcome. The first messenger promotes the cellular production or mobilization of a second messenger, which initiates cellular signaling through a specific biochemical pathway. Physiological signals are integrated within the cell as a result of interactions between and among second-messenger pathways. Compared with the number of receptors and cytosolic signaling proteins, there are relatively few recognized cytoplasmic second messengers. However, their synthesis or release and degradation or excretion reflects the activities of many pathways. Well-studied second messengers include cyclic AMP, cyclic GMP, cyclic ADP–ribose, Ca^{2+}, inositol phosphates, diacylglycerol, and nitric oxide. Second messengers influence each other both directly, by altering the other's metabolism, and indirectly, by sharing intracellular targets. This pattern of regulatory pathways allows the cell to respond to agonists, singly or in combination, with an integrated array of cytoplasmic second messengers and responses.

Cyclic AMP. Cyclic AMP, the prototypical second messenger, remains a good example for understanding the regulation and function of most second messengers (for an overview of cyclic nucleotide action, *see* Beavo and Brunton, 2002). Cyclic AMP is synthesized by adenylyl cyclase under the control of many GPCRs; stimulation is mediated by G_s; inhibition, by G_i.

There are nine membrane-bound isoforms of adenylyl cyclase (AC) and one soluble isoform found in mammals (Hanoune and Defer, 2001). The membrane-bound ACs are glycoproteins of approximately 120 kDa with considerable sequence homology: a small cytoplasmic domain; two hydrophobic transmembrane domains, each with six membrane-spanning helices; and two large cytoplasmic domains. Membrane-bound ACs exhibit basal enzymatic activity that is modulated by binding of GTP-liganded α subunits of the stimulatory and inhibitory G proteins (G_s and G_i). Numerous other regulatory interactions are possible, and these enzymes are catalogued based on their structural homology and their distinct regulation by G protein α and βγ subunits, Ca^{2+}, protein kinases, and the actions of the diterpene forskolin. Because each AC isoform has its own tissue distribution and regulatory properties, different cell types respond differently to similar stimuli.

The role of agonists interacting at GPCRs is to accelerate the exchange of GDP for GTP on the α subunits of these G proteins, thereby promoting the dissociation of the heterotrimeric G proteins into α-GTP and βγ subunits and resulting in modulation of adenylyl cyclase activity. Once activated by $α_s$-GTP, AC remains activated until $α_s$ hydrolyses the bound GTP to GDP, which returns the system to its ground state (*see* Ross and Wilkie, 2000). As a consequence, there is amplification at this step, a single activation producing numerous molecules of cyclic AMP, which, in turn, can activate PKA. Cyclic AMP is eliminated by a combination of hydrolysis, catalyzed by cyclic nucleotide phosphodiesterases, and extrusion by several plasma membrane transport proteins.

Phosphodiesterases (PDEs) form yet another family of important signaling proteins whose activities are regulated by controlled transcription as well as by second messengers (cyclic nucleotides and Ca^{2+}) and interactions with other signaling proteins such as β-arrestin and protein kinases (Brunton, 2003; Maurice *et al.*, 2003). PDEs are enzymes responsible for the hydrolysis of the cyclic $3',5'$-phosphodiester bond found in cyclic AMP and cyclic GMP. PDEs comprise a superfamily with 11 subfamilies, having been characterized on the basis of amino acid sequence, substrate specificity, pharmacological properties, and allosteric regulation. The PDE superfamily encompasses 25 genes that are thought to give rise to more than 50 different PDE proteins. PDEs share a conserved catalytic domain at the carboxyl terminus, regulatory domains located most often at the amino terminus, and targeting domains that are the subject of active investigation. The substrate specificities of the PDEs include enzymes that are specific for cyclic AMP hydrolysis, cyclic GMP hydrolysis, and those that hydrolyze both. PDEs play a highly regulated role that is important in controlling the intracellular levels of cyclic AMP and cyclic GMP. The importance of the PDEs as regulators of signaling is evident from their development as drug targets in diseases such as asthma and chronic obstructive pulmonary disease, cardiovascular diseases such as heart failure and atherosclerotic peripheral arterial disease, neurological disorders, and erectile dysfunction (Mehats *et al.*, 2002).

Cyclic GMP. Cyclic GMP is generated by two distinct forms of guanylyl cyclase (GC). Nitric oxide (NO) stimulates soluble guanylyl cyclase (sGC), and the natriuretic peptides, guanylins, and heat-stable *Escherichia coli* enterotoxin stimulate members of the membrane-spanning GCs (*e.g.*, particulate GC).

Actions of Cyclic Nucleotides. In most cases, cyclic AMP functions by activating the isoforms of cyclic AMP–dependent protein kinase (PKA), and cyclic GMP activates a cGMP-dependent protein kinase (PKG). Recently, a number of additional actions of cyclic nucleotides have been described, all with pharmacological relevance.

Cyclic Nucleotide–Dependent Protein Kinases. PKA holoenzyme consists of two catalytic (C) subunits reversibly bound to a regulatory (R) subunit dimer. The holoenzyme is inactive. Binding of four cyclic AMP molecules, two to each R subunit, dissociates the holoenzyme, liberating two catalytically active C subunits that phosphorylate serine and threonine residues on specific substrate proteins.

PKA diversity lies in both its R and C subunits. Molecular cloning has revealed α and β isoforms of both the classically described PKA regulatory subunits (RI and RII), as well as three C subunit isoforms Cα, Cβ, and Cγ. The R subunits exhibit different binding affinities for cyclic AMP, giving rise to PKA holoenzymes with different thresholds for activation. In addition to differential expression of R and C isoforms in various cells and tissues, PKA function is modulated by subcellular localization mediated by A-kinase-anchoring proteins (AKAPs) (*see* Wong and Scott, 2004).

PKA can phosphorylate both final physiological targets (metabolic enzymes or transport proteins) and numerous protein kinases and other regulatory proteins in multiple signaling pathways. This latter group includes transcription factors that allow cyclic AMP to regulate gene expression in addition to more acute cellular events. For instance, phosphorylation by PKA of serine 133 of CREB (the cyclic AMP response element–binding protein) recruits CREB-binding protein (CBP), a histone acetyltransferase that interacts with

PNA polymerase II (POLII0) and leads to enhanced transcription of approximately 105 genes containing a cyclic AMP response element motif (CRE) in the promoter region (*e.g.*, tyrosine hydroxylase, iNOS, AhR, angiotensinogen, insulin, the glucocorticoid receptor, BCl2, and CFTR) (*see* Mayr and Montminy, 2001).

Cyclic GMP activates a protein kinase, PKG, that phosphorylates some of the same substrates as PKA and some that are PKG-specific. Unlike PKA, PKG does not disassociate on binding cyclic GMP. PKG is known to exist in two homologous forms. PKGI, with an acetylated N terminus, is associated with the cytoplasm and known to exist in two isoforms (Iα and Iβ) that arise from alternate splicing. PKGII, with a myristylated N terminus, is membrane-associated and may be compartmented by PKG-anchoring proteins (Vo *et al.*, 1998) in a manner similar to that known for PKA. Pharmacologically important effects of elevated cyclic GMP include modulation of platelet activation and regulation of smooth muscle contraction (Rybalkin *et al.*, 2003; Buxton, 2004).

Cyclic Nucleotide–Gated Channels. In addition to activating a protein kinase, cyclic AMP also directly regulates the activity of plasma membrane cation channels referred to as *cyclic nucleotide–gated* (CNG) *channels*. CNG ion channels have been found in kidney, testis, heart, and the CNS (for a review, *see* Beavo and Brunton, 2002). These channels open in response to direct binding of intracellular cyclic nucleotides and contribute to cellular control of the membrane potential and intracellular Ca^{2+} levels. The CNG ion channels are multisubunit pore-forming channels that share structural similarity with the voltage-gated K^+ channels. Modulation of channel activity is the result of binding of as many as four molecules of cyclic nucleotide to the channel.

Cyclic AMP–Regulated GTPase Exchange Factors (GEFs). The small GTP-binding proteins are monomeric GTPases and key regulators of cell function. They integrate extracellular signals from membrane receptors with cytoskeletal changes and activation of diverse signaling pathways, regulating such processes as phagocytosis, progression through the cell cycle, cell adhesion, gene expression, and apoptosis (Etienne-Manneville and Hall, 2002). The small GTPases operate as binary switches that exist in GTP- or GDP-liganded conformations. The switch is activated when an upstream signal activates a GTPase exchange factor (GEF) that, on binding to the GDP-liganded GTPase, promotes the exchange of GDP for GTP. A number of extracellular stimuli signal to the small GTPases through second messengers such as cyclic AMP, Ca^{2+}, and DAG that regulate GEFs. Two of these proteins involved in the regulation of the Ras protein, termed *exchange proteins activated by cyclic AMP* (EPAC-1 and -2), are cyclic AMP GEFs. The EPAC pathway provides an additional effector system for cyclic AMP signaling and drug action. When GTP binds to the small GTP-binding protein, it induces a conformational change that promotes binding and modification of the activities of effector proteins. The switch is terminated by hydrolysis of GTP by the GTPase activity of the small GTP-binding protein. The rate of GTP hydrolysis is accelerated by interaction with GTPase-activating proteins (GAPs).

GAF Domains. GAF domains are a phylogenetically broad family of proteins that bind cyclic GMP and other ligands. In mammalian cells, GAF domains confer on a protein sensitivity to cyclic GMP. For instance, cyclic GMP binding to GAF domains activates PDE2, renders PDE5 phosphorylatable (and activatable) by PKG, and regulates the affinity of PDE6 for its autoinhibitory domain. Given the myriad important roles of PDE activities in physiology, GAF domains may be therapeutically useful drug targets (Martinez *et al.*, 2002).

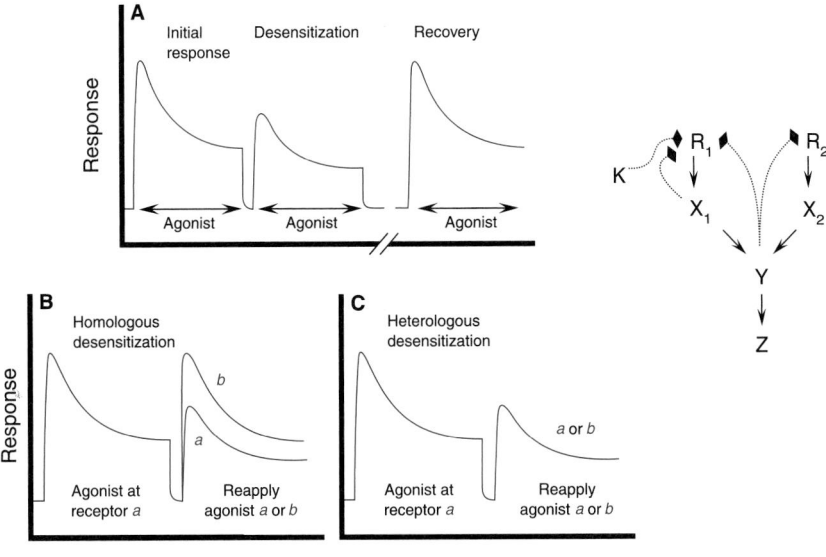

Figure 1–8. *Desensitization in response to an agonist.* **A.** After exposure to an agonist, the *initial response* usually peaks and then decreases to approach some tonic level elevated but below the maximum. If the drug is removed for a brief period, the state of *desensitization* is maintained such that a second addition of agonist also provokes a diminished response. Removal of the drug for a more extended period allows the cell to recover its capacity to respond. **B, C.** Desensitization may be *homologous* (**B**), affecting responses elicited only by the stimulated receptor, or *heterologous* (**C**), acting on several receptors or on a pathway that is common to many receptors. Agonist *a* acts at receptor *a* and agonist *b* at receptor *b*. Homologous desensitization can reflect feedback from a transducer (or effector) unique to the pathway of the receptor (X_1) or from an off-pathway component (K) that is sensitive to the activation state of the receptor. Heterologous desensitization is initiated by transducers or effectors common to multiple receptor signaling pathways (Y or Z).

Calcium. The entry of Ca^{2+} into the cytoplasm is mediated by diverse channels: Plasma membrane channels regulated by G proteins, membrane potential, K^+ or Ca^{2+} itself, and channels in specialized regions of endoplasmic reticulum that respond to IP_3 or, in excitable cells, to membrane depolarization and the state of the Ca^{2+} release channel and its Ca^{2+} stores in the sarcoplasmic reticulum. Ca^{2+} is removed both by extrusion (Na^+–Ca^{2+} exchanger and Ca^{2+} ATPase) and by reuptake into the endoplasmic reticulum (SERCA pumps). Ca^{2+} propagates its signals through a much wider range of proteins than does cyclic AMP, including metabolic enzymes, protein kinases, and Ca^{2+}-binding regulatory proteins (*e.g.*, calmodulin) that regulate still other ultimate and intermediary effectors that regulate cellular processes as diverse as exocytosis of neurotransmitters and muscle contraction. Drugs such as *chlorpromazine* (an antipsychotic agent) are calmodulin inhibitors.

Regulation of Receptors

Receptors not only initiate regulation of biochemical events and physiological function but also are themselves subject to many regulatory and homeostatic controls. These controls include regulation of the synthesis and degradation of the receptor by multiple mechanisms, covalent modification, association with other regulatory proteins, and/or relocalization within the cell. Transducer and effector proteins are regulated similarly. Modulating

inputs may come from other receptors, directly or indirectly, and receptors are almost always subject to feedback regulation by their own signaling outputs.

Continued stimulation of cells with agonists generally results in a state of *desensitization* (also referred to as *adaptation, refractoriness,* or *down-regulation*) such that the effect that follows continued or subsequent exposure to the same concentration of drug is diminished (Figure 1–8). This phenomenon known as *tachyphylaxis* occurs rapidly and is very important in therapeutic situations; an example is attenuated response to the repeated use of β receptor agonists as bronchodilators for the treatment of asthma (*see* Chapters 10 and 27).

Desensitization can be the result of temporary inaccessibility of the receptor to agonist or the result of fewer receptors synthesized and available at the cell surface. Down-regulation of receptor number best describes this latter accommodation of the cell to the chronic presence of excess agonist. Agonist stimulation of GPCRs initiates regulatory processes that are often rapid, leading to desensitization to subsequent stimulation by agonist without immediately changing the total number of receptors. Phosphorylation of the receptor by specific GPCR kinases (GRKs) plays a key role in triggering rapid desensitization. Phosphorylation of agonist-occupied GPCRs by GRKs facilitates the binding of cytosolic proteins termed *arrestins* to the receptor, resulting in the uncoupling of G protein from the receptor. The β-arrestins recruit proteins such as PDE4 (which limits cyclic AMP signaling), and others such as clathrin and β_2-adaptin, promoting sequestration of receptor from the membrane (internalization) and providing a scaffold that permits additional signaling steps such as activation of the ERK/MAPK cascade associated with activation of some GPCRs (Baillie and Houslay, 2005; Tan *et al.*, 2004).

Feedback inhibition of signaling may be limited to output only from the stimulated receptor, a situation known as *homologous desensitization*. Attenuation extending to the action of all receptors that share a common signaling pathway is called *heterologous desensitization* (Figure 1–8). Homologous desensitization indicates feedback directed to the receptor molecule itself (*e.g.,* phosphorylation, internalization and proteolysis, decreased synthesis, etc.), whereas heterologous desensitization may involve inhibition or loss of one or more downstream proteins that participate in signaling from other receptors as well. Mechanisms involved in homologous and heterologous desensitization of specific receptors and signaling pathways are discussed in greater detail in later chapters related to individual receptor families.

Predictably, supersensitivity to agonists also frequently follows chronic reduction of receptor stimulation. Such situations can result, for example, following withdrawal from prolonged receptor blockade (*e.g.,* the long-term administration of β receptor antagonists such as propranolol (*see* Chapter 10) or in the case where chronic denervation of a preganglionic fiber induces an increase in neurotransmitter release per pulse, indicating postganglionic neuronal supersensitivity. Supersensitivity can be the result of tissue response to pathological conditions such as happens in cardiac ischemia and is due to synthesis and recruitment of new receptors to the surface of the myocyte.

Diseases Resulting from Receptor Malfunction. Considering the roles of receptors in mediating the actions of regulatory ligands acting on cells, it is not surprising that alteration in receptors and their immediate signaling effectors can be the cause of disease. The loss of a receptor in a highly specialized signaling system may cause a relatively limited, if dramatic, phenotypic disorder such as the genetic deficiency of the androgen receptor in the testicular feminization syndrome (*see* Chapter 58). Deficiencies in more widely used signaling systems have a broader spectrum of effects, as are seen in myasthenia gravis and some forms of insulin-resistant diabetes mellitus, which result from autoimmune depletion of nicotinic cholinergic receptors (*see* Chapter 9) or insulin receptors (*see* Chapter 60), respectively. A lesion in a component of a signaling pathway that is used by many receptors can cause a generalized endocrinopathy, as is seen in pseudohypoparathyroidism-1a owing to mutations in maternally inherited $G_s\alpha$. Heterozygous deficiency of $G_s\alpha$, the G protein that activates adenylyl cyclase, causes multiple endocrine disorders (Spiegel and Weinstein, 2004). Homozygous deficiency in G_s presumably would be lethal.

The expression of aberrant or ectopic receptors, effectors, or coupling proteins potentially can lead to supersensitivity, subsensitivity,

or other untoward responses. Among the most significant events is the appearance of aberrant receptors as products of *oncogenes* that transform otherwise normal cells into malignant cells. Virtually any type of signaling system may have oncogenic potential. The *erb*A oncogene product is an altered form of a receptor for thyroid hormone, constitutively active because of the loss of its ligand-binding domain. The *ros* and *erb*B oncogene products are activated, uncontrolled forms of the receptors for insulin and epidermal growth factor, respectively, both known to enhance cellular proliferation. The *Mas* oncogene product is a GPCR that may regulate responses to angiotensins. Constitutive activation of GPCRs owing to subtle mutations in receptor structure has been shown to give rise to retinitis pigmentosa, precocious puberty, and malignant hyperthyroidism. G proteins themselves can be oncogenic when either overexpressed or constitutively activated by mutation (Spiegel and Weinstein, 2004).

Mutation of receptors can alter either acute responsiveness to drug therapy or its continuing efficacy. For example, a mutation of β_2 receptors, which mediate airway smooth muscle relaxation and bronchial airflow, accelerates desensitization to β_2 receptor agonists used to treat asthma (*see* Chapter 27). The cloning of mutant genes that mediate pathophysiological conditions should speed the development of suitable drugs to target them specifically. Ultimately, designing therapeutic agents that can be useful at mutant receptors will require the crystal structure of these altered proteins as well as their normal counterparts. To date, the only liganded GPCR to be crystallized is rhodopsin (Palczewski *et al.*, 2000).

Classification of Receptors and Drug Effects

In the years between editions of this book, pharmaceutical firms have invested heavily in high-throughput screening systems that rely on ligand binding rather than function to discover potential medicines. This investment has not paid off as handsomely as predicted, and the industry is now placing increased value on functional pharmacological assays that have been the cornerstone of pharmacology since its inception.

Traditionally, drug receptors have been identified and classified primarily on the basis of the effect and relative potency of selective agonists and antagonists. For example, the effects of acetylcholine that are mimicked by the alkaloid muscarine and that are selectively antagonized by atropine are termed *muscarinic effects*. Other effects of acetylcholine that are mimicked by nicotine are described as *nicotinic effects*. By extension, these two types of cholinergic effects are said to be mediated by muscarinic or nicotinic receptors. Although it frequently contributes little to delineation of the mechanism of drug action, such categorization provides a convenient basis for summarizing drug effects. A statement that a drug activates a specified type of receptor is a succinct summary of its spectrum of effects and of the agents that will regulate it. However, the accuracy of this statement may be altered when new receptors or receptor subtypes are identified or additional drug mechanisms or side effects are revealed.

Significance of Receptor Subtypes. As the diversity and selectivity of drugs increase, it is evident that multiple subtypes of receptors exist within many previously defined classes. Molecular cloning has further accelerated discovery of novel receptor subtypes, and their expression as recombinant proteins has facilitated discovery of subtype-selective drugs. Distinct but related receptors may, but may not, display distinctive patterns of selectivity among agonist or antagonist ligands. When selective ligands are not known, the receptors are more commonly referred to as *isoforms* rather than as *subtypes*. Receptor subtypes may display different mechanisms of signal output. For example, M_1 and M_3 muscarinic receptors activate the G_q–PLC–IP_3–Ca^{2+} pathway, and M_2 and M_4 muscarinic receptors activate G_i to reduce the activity of adenylyl cyclase. The distinction between classes and subtypes of receptors, however, often is arbitrary or historical. The α_1, α_2, and β receptors differ from each other both in ligand selectivity among drugs and in coupling to G proteins (G_q, G_i, and G_s, respectively), yet α and β are considered receptor classes and α_1 and α_2 are considered subtypes. The α_{1A}, α_{1B}, and α_{1C} receptor isoforms differ little in their biochemical properties, although their tissue distributions are distinct. The β_1, β_2, and β_3 adrenergic receptor subtypes exhibit both differences in tissue distribution; *e.g.*, β_3 receptors are localized to adipose tissue and are not phosphorylated by either GRKs or PKA, both known to phosphorylate β_1 and β_2 receptor subtypes (Hall, 2004).

Pharmacological differences among receptor subtypes are exploited therapeutically through the development and use of receptor-selective drugs. Such drugs may be used to elicit different responses from a single tissue when receptor subtypes initiate different intracellular signals, or they may serve to differentially modulate different cells or tissues that express one or another receptor subtype. Increasing the selectivity of a drug among tissues or among responses elicited from a single tissue may determine whether the drug's therapeutic benefits outweigh its unwanted effects.

The molecular biological search for novel receptors has moved well beyond the search for isoforms of known receptors toward the discovery of hundreds of genes for completely novel human receptors. Many of these receptors can be assigned to known families based on sequence, and their functions can be confirmed with appropriate ligands. However, many are "orphans," the designation given to receptors whose ligands are unknown. Discovery of the endogenous ligands and physiological functions of orphan receptors may lead to new drugs that can modulate currently intractable disease states.

The discovery of numerous receptor isoforms raises the question of their importance to the organism, particularly when their signaling mechanisms and specificity for endogenous ligands are indistinguishable. Perhaps this multiplicity of genes facilitates the independent, cell-specific, and temporally controlled expression of receptors according to the developmental needs of the organism. Regardless of their mechanistic implications (or lack thereof), discovery of isoform-selective ligands may improve our targeting of therapeutic drugs substantially.

Actions of Drugs Not Mediated by Receptors

If one restricts the definition of receptors to macromolecules, then several drugs may be said not to act on receptors as such. Some drugs specifically bind small molecules or ions that are found normally or abnormally in the body. One example is the therapeutic neutralization of gastric acid by a base (antacid). Another example is the use of *2-mercaptoethane sulphonate (mesna)*, a free-radical scavenger eliminated rapidly by the kidneys, to bind to reactive metabolites associated with some cancer chemotherapeutic agents and thus to minimize their untoward effects on the urinary tract. Other agents act according to nonpharmacological colligative properties without a requirement for highly specific chemical structure. For example, certain relatively benign compounds, such as *mannitol,* can be administered in quantities sufficient to increase the osmolarity of various body fluids and thereby cause appropriate changes in the distribution of water (*see* Chapter 28). Depending on the agent and route of administration, this effect can be exploited to promote diuresis, catharsis, expansion of circulating volume in the vascular compartment, or reduction of cerebral edema. In a similar fashion, the introduction of cholesterol-binding agents orally (*e.g., cholestyramine resin*) can be used in the management of hypercholesterolemia to decrease the amount of cholesterol absorbed from the diet.

Certain drugs that are structural analogs of normal biological chemicals may be incorporated into cellular components and thereby alter their function. This property has been termed a *counterfeit incorporation mechanism* and has been particularly useful with analogs of pyrimidines and purines that can be incorporated into nucleic acids; such drugs have clinical utility in antiviral and cancer chemotherapy (*see* Chapters 49 and 51).

QUANTITATION OF DRUG–RECEPTOR INTERACTIONS AND EFFECTS

Receptor Pharmacology

Receptor occupancy theory, in which it is assumed that response emanates from a receptor occupied by a drug, has its basis in the law of mass action, with modifying constants added to accommodate experimental findings. Receptor theory was originated by A.J. Clark, who was the first to apply mathematical rigor to the notions of drug action. Ariëns (1954) modified this model to describe the range of drug effect between full agonist and antagonist as a proportionality factor called *intrinsic activity.* Stephenson (1956) added the notion of stimulus–response to understanding drug efficacy, and Furchgott (1966) contributed a method of measuring the affinity of an agonist by comparing its concentration–response curve before and

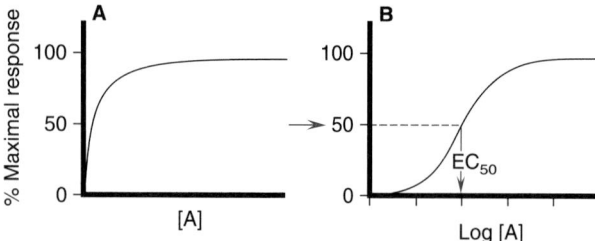

Figure 1–9. *Graded responses (y axis as a percent of maximal response) expressed as a function of the concentration of drug A present at the receptor.* The hyperbolic shape of the curve in panel *A* becomes sigmoid when plotted semi-logarithmically, as in panel *B*. The concentration of drug that produces 50% of the maximal response quantifies drug activity and is referred to as the EC_{50} (effective concentration for 50% response).

after inactivating a proportion of the receptors with an irreversible antagonist. Antagonism was modeled by Gaddum (1937, 1957) and Schild (1957) to determine the affinity of antagonists. The history and principles of receptor pharmacology have been well reviewed by Limbird (2005).

The basic currency of receptor pharmacology is the dose–response curve, a depiction of the observed effect of a drug as a function of its concentration in the receptor compartment. Figure 1–9A shows a typical dose–response curve; it reaches a maximal asymptote value when the drug occupies all the receptor sites. The range of concentrations needed to fully depict the dose–response relationship (approximately $3\log_{10}[D]$) usually is too wide to be useful in the linear format shown in Figure 1–9A; thus most dose–response curves are constructed with the logarithm of the concentration plotted on the *x* axis (Figure 1–9B). Dose–response curves presented in this way are sigmoidal in shape and have three basic properties: threshold, slope, and maximal asymptote. These parameters characterize and quantitate the activity of the drug. As noted below, this sigmoidal curve also depicts the law of mass action in its simplest form.

The response to drugs in biological systems does not always follow the classic concentration–response curve shown in Figure 1–9. On occasion, some drugs cause low-dose stimulation and high-dose inhibition of response. These U-shaped relationships for some receptor systems are said to display *hormesis*. Several drug–receptor systems can display this property (*e.g.,* prostaglandins, endothelin, and purinergic and serotonergic agonists, among others). While no one mechanism can be used to explain this phenomenon or a particular patient type be described to judge the clinical relevance of the effect, hormesis is likely to be at the root of the toxicity of drugs in patients (Calabrese and Baldwin, 2003).

Potency and Relative Efficacy

In general, the drug–receptor interaction is characterized first by binding of drug to receptor and second by generation of a response in a biological system. The first function is governed by the chemical property of *affinity,* ruled by the chemical forces that cause the drug to associate reversibly with the receptor.

$$D + R \underset{k_2}{\overset{k_1}{\rightleftarrows}} DR \rightarrow Response \qquad (1\text{–}25)$$

This simple relationship, derived for drug–receptor interactions from the Langmuir absorption isotherm, permits an appreciation of the reliance of the interaction of drug (D) with receptor (R) on both the forward or association rate constant (k_1) and the reverse or dissociation rate constant (k_2). At any given time, the concentration of agonist–receptor complex [DR] is equal to the product of $k_1[D][R]$ minus the product $k_2[DR]$. At equilibrium (*i.e.* when $\delta[DR]/\delta\tau = 0$), $k_1[D][R] = k_2[DR]$. The equilibrium dissociation constant (K_D) is then described by ratio of the off-rate and the on-rate (k_2/k_1).

$$At\ equilibrium,\qquad K_D = \frac{[D][R]}{[DR]} = \frac{k_2}{k_1} \qquad (1\text{–}26)$$

The affinity constant is the reciprocal of the equilibrium dissociation constant (affinity constant = $K_D = 1/K_A$). A high affinity means a small K_D. As a practical matter, the affinity of a drug is influenced most often by changes in its off-rate (k_2) rather than its on-rate (k_1). Although a number of assumptions are made in this analysis, it is generally useful for considering the interactions of drugs with their receptors. Using this simple model of Equation (1–26) permits us to write and expression of the fractional occupancy (f) of receptors by agonist:

$$f = \frac{[\text{drug-receptor complexes}]}{[\text{total receptors}]} = \frac{[DR]}{[R] + [DR]} \qquad (1\text{–}27)$$

This can be expressed in terms of K_A (or K_D) and [D]:

$$f = \frac{K_A[D]}{1 + K_A[D]} = \frac{[D]}{[D] + K_D} \qquad (1\text{–}28)$$

Thus, when [D] = K_D, a drug will occupy 50% of the receptors present. From this analysis, it is possible to relate a drug's potency in a particular receptor system to its K_D. Potent drugs are those which elicit a response by binding to a critical number of a particular receptor type at low concentrations (high affinity) compared with other drugs acting on the same system and having lower affinity and thus requiring more drug to bind to the same number of receptors.

The generation of a response from the drug–receptor complex is governed by a property described as *efficacy*. Where *agonism* is the information encoded in a drug's chemical structure that causes the receptor to change conformation to produce a physiological or biochemical response when the drug is bound, *efficacy* is that property *intrinsic* to a particular drug that determines how "good" an agonist the drug is. Historically, efficacy has been treated as a proportionality constant that quantifies the extent of functional change imparted to a receptor-mediated response system on binding a drug. Thus, a drug with high efficacy may be a full agonist eliciting, at some concentration, a full response, whereas a drug with a lower efficacy at the same receptor may not elicit a full response at any dose. When it is possible to describe the relative efficacy of drugs at a particular receptor, a drug with a low intrinsic efficacy will be a partial agonist.

Since the effects of drugs in the human body often are compared as the physiological outcome of treatment (*e.g.,* diuresis) rather than comparisons of drugs at the same receptor, the term *relative efficacy* can be used to characterize one drug *versus* another. Thus, the relative efficacy of loop diuretics in the treatment of heart failure is high, making them therapeutically useful; the relative efficacy of thiazide diuretics (their capacity to produce significant diuresis) in this setting is low, and they are of no therapeutic value.

Quantifying Agonism. Drugs have two observable properties in biological systems: potency and magnitude of effect (when a biological response is produced). Potency is controlled by four factors: Two relate to the biological system containing the receptors (receptor density and efficiency of the stimulus–response mechanisms of the tissue), and two relate to the interaction of drug with its receptor (affinity and efficacy). When the relative potency of two agonists of equal efficacy is measured in the same biological system, downstream signaling events are the same for both drugs, and the comparison yields a relative measure of the affinity and efficacy of the two agonists (Figure 1–10A). It is convenient to describe agonist response by determining the half-maximally effective concentration (EC_{50}) for producing a given effect. Thus, measuring agonist potency by comparison of EC_{50} values is one method of measuring the capability of different agonists to induce a response in a test system and for predicting comparable activity in another. Another method of estimating agonist activity is to compare maximal asymptotes in systems where the agonists do not produce maximal response (Figure 1–10B). The advantage of using maxima is that this property depends solely on efficacy, whereas potency is a mixed function of both affinity and efficacy.

Quantifying Antagonism. Characteristic patterns of antagonism are associated with certain mechanisms of blockade of receptors. One is simple *competitive antagonism*, whereby a drug that lacks intrinsic efficacy but retains affinity competes with the agonist for the binding site on

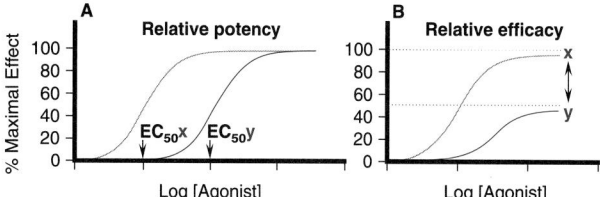

Figure 1–10. *Two ways of quantifying agonism.* ***A.*** The relative potency of two agonists (drug **x**, *gray line;* drug **y**, *blue line*) obtained in the same tissue is a function of their relative affinities and intrinsic efficacies. The half-maximal effect of drug **x** occurs at a concentration that is one-tenth the half-maximally effective concentration of drug **y**. Thus, drug **x** is more potent than drug **y**. ***B.*** In systems where the two drugs do not both produce the maximal response characteristic of the tissue, the observed maximal response is a nonlinear function of their relative intrinsic efficacies. Drug **x** is more efficacious than drug y; their asymptotic fractional responses are 100% (drug **x**) and 50% (drug **y**).

the receptor. The characteristic pattern of such antagonism is the concentration-dependent production of a parallel shift to the right of the agonist dose–response curve with no change in the maximal asymptotic response. Competitive antagonism is surmountable by a sufficiently high concentration of agonist (Figure 1–11A). The magnitude of the rightward shift of the curve depends on the concentration of the antagonist and its affinity for the receptor. The affinity of a competitive antagonist for its receptor therefore can be determined according to its concentration-dependent capacity to shift the concentration–response curve for an agonist rightward, as analyzed by Schild (1957).

Note that a partial agonist similarly can compete with a "full" agonist for binding to the receptor. However, increasing concentrations of a partial agonist will inhibit response to a finite level characteristic of the drug's intrinsic efficacy; a competitive antagonist will reduce the response to zero. Partial agonists thus can be used therapeutically to buffer a response by inhibiting untoward stimulation without totally abolishing the stimulus from the receptor. The β receptor agent *pindolol* is an example; it is a very weak partial agonist, a β-antagonist with "intrinsic sympathomimetic activity" (*see* Chapters 10 and 31 through 33).

An antagonist may dissociate so slowly from the receptor as to be essentially irreversible in its action. Under these circumstances, the maximal response to the agonist will be depressed at some antagonist concentrations (Figure 1–11B). Operationally, this is referred to as *noncompetitive antagonism,* although the molecular mechanism of action really cannot be inferred unequivo-

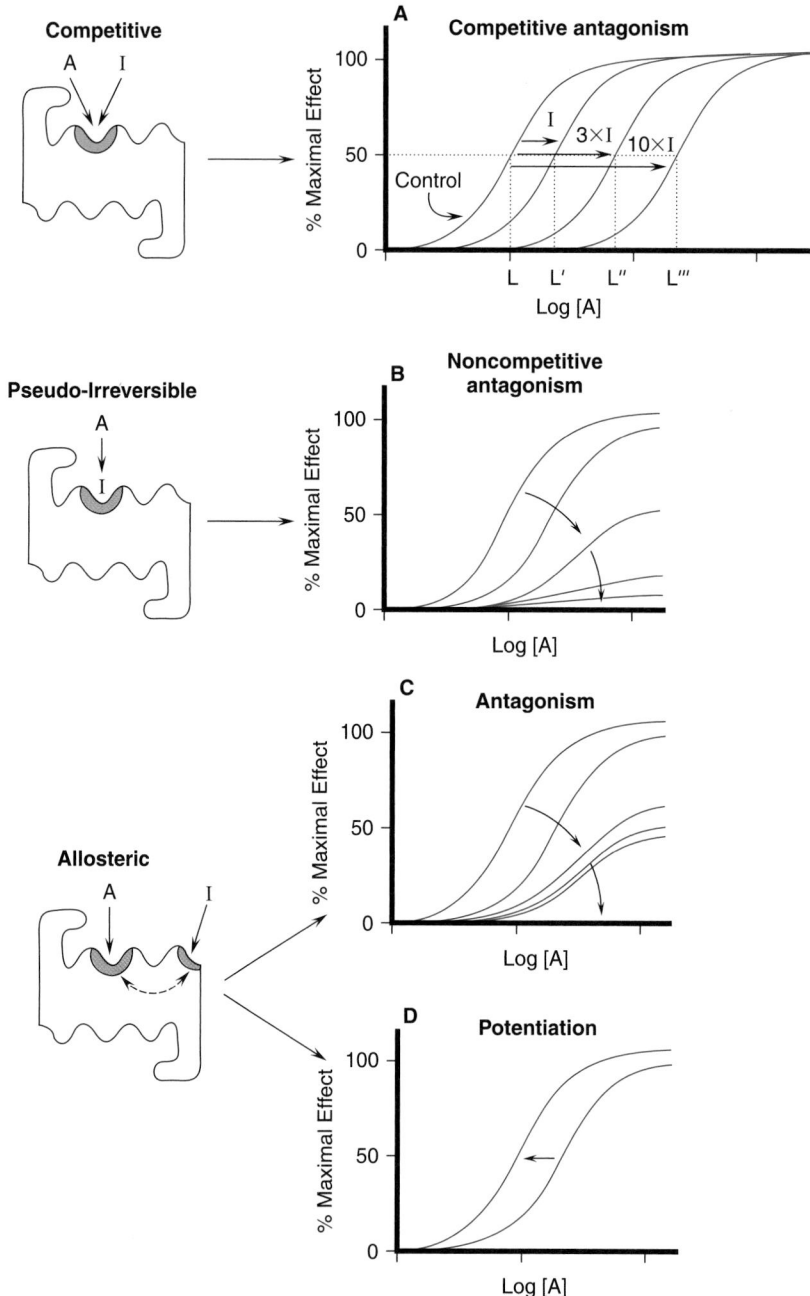

Figure 1–11. *Mechanisms of receptor antagonism.* **A.** Competitive antagonism occurs when the agonist A and antagonist I compete for the same binding site on the receptor. Response curves for the agonist are shifted to the right in a concentration-related manner by the antagonist such that the EC_{50} for the agonist increases (*e.g.,* L *versus* L', L", and L'") with the concentration of the antagonist. **B.** If the antagonist binds to the same site as the agonist but does so irreversibly or pseudo-irreversibly (slow dissociation but no covalent bond), it causes a shift of the dose–response curve to the right, with further depression of the maximal response. Allosteric effects occur when the ligand I binds to a different site on the receptor to either inhibit response (*see* panel ***C***) or potentiate response (*see* panel ***D***). This effect is saturable; inhibition reaches a limiting value when the allosteric site is fully occupied.

cally from the effect. An irreversible antagonist competing for the same binding site as the agonist also can produce the pattern of antagonism shown in Figure 1–11B.

Noncompetitive antagonism can be produced by another type of drug, referred to as an *allosteric antagonist*. This type of drug produces its effect by binding a site on the receptor distinct from that of the primary agonist and thereby changing the affinity of the receptor for the agonist. In the case of an allosteric antagonist, the affinity of the receptor for the agonist is decreased by the antagonist (Figure 1–11C). In contrast, some allosteric effects could potentiate the effects of agonists (Figure 1–11D). The interaction of benzodiazepines (anxiolytics) with the $GABA_A$ receptor to increase the receptor's affinity for GABA is an example of allosteric potentiation.

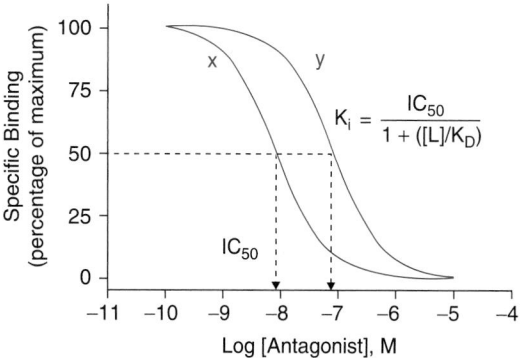

Figure 1–12. *Radioligand binding method for determining antagonist affinity.* Binding of a radioligand (L) to receptors in the presence of increasing concentrations of a nonradioactive competitive antagonist results in a competition curve, in this case, a curve consistent with binding to a single population of identical receptors. Determining the concentration of antagonist competing for 50% of the receptors present (IC_{50}) and knowing the concentration of radioligand [L] and its affinity (K_D) for the receptor permits calculation of the antagonist affinity (K_i) for more (x) and less (y) potent antagonists. A constant amount of radioligand and equal portions of cellular material (receptor source) were placed in each reaction. Data are amount of radioligand bound, expressed as a percentage of maximal binding (*i.e.*, in the absence of any competing ligand).

The quantification of drug–receptor interactions in a binding assay can be used to estimate the affinity of agonist (K_D) and antagonist drugs (K_i) for receptors. In this approach, receptors are partially purified from a given cell or tissue (*e.g.*, as membrane preparations) and studied directly *in vitro* using a radioactive form of a drug with known specificity for the receptor. In the most straightforward use of the method for the quantification of antagonist affinity (K_i), a series of competition studies is performed at equilibrium in the presence of a single K_D concentration of radioligand (*e.g.*, that occupying 50% of the receptors present). Addition of the nonradioactive drug to be studied at increasing concentrations and then separating bound and free drug at equilibrium permit direct measurement of the amount of radioligand bound in the presence of increasing concentrations of the antagonist. When the interaction is a bimolecular competition between the radioligand and antagonist for binding to the same site on the receptor, a sigmoid competition curve is obtained (Figure 1–12). The antagonist concentration competing for 50% of the binding of the radioligand (IC_{50}) can be determined from inspection or mathematically from curve fitting, whereas the K_i for an antagonist can be determined knowing the concentration of the radioligand ([L]) employed and its K_D for the receptor.

$$K_i = \frac{IC_{50}}{1 + \dfrac{[L]}{K_D}} \tag{1–29}$$

This relationship, known as the *Cheng–Prusoff equation* (Cheng and Prusoff, 1973), can be employed for determining the potency of antagonists at a given receptor and, when performed using subtype-selective antagonists and nonselective radioligands, can quantify the presence of receptor subtypes and the relative affinity of various antagonists for them. Although the Cheng–Prusoff analysis assumes a bimolecular reaction obeying the laws of mass action, mathematical approaches are also available for cases where cooperativity rather than the presence of multiple receptor subtypes causes the Hill coefficient to differ from unity (Cheng, 2004).

A similar analysis can be performed in experiments measuring a functional response of a system to a drug and a competitive antagonist or inhibitor. Concentration curves are run with the agonist alone and with the agonist plus an effective concentration of the antagonist (Figure 1–11A). As noted in the figure, as more antagonist (I) is added, a higher concentration of the agonist (A) is needed to pro-

duce an equivalent response (the half-maximal, or 50%, response is a convenient and accurately determined level of response). The extent of the rightward shift of the concentration-dependence curve is a measure of the effect of the inhibitor, and a more potent inhibitor will cause a greater rightward shift than a less potent inhibitor at the same concentration. One may write expressions of fractional occupancy (f) of the receptor by agonist for the control curve and each of the other curves.

For an agonist drug (D) alone,

$$f_{control} = \frac{[D]}{[D] + K_D} \tag{1–30}$$

For the case of agonist plus antagonist (I),

$$f_{+I} = \frac{[D]}{[D] + K_D\left(1 + \dfrac{[I]}{K_i}\right)} \tag{1–31}$$

Assuming that equal responses result from equal fractional receptor occupancies in both the absence and presence of antagonist, one can set the fractional occupancies equal at agonist concentrations (L and L′) that generate equivalent responses in Figure 1–11A. Thus,

$$\frac{L}{L + K_D} = \frac{L'}{L' + K_D\left(1 + \dfrac{[I]}{K_i}\right)} \tag{1–32}$$

Simplifying, we get:

$$\frac{L'}{L} - 1 = \frac{[I]}{K_i} \tag{1–33}$$

where all values are known except K_i. Thus, one can determine the K_i for a reversible, competitive antagonist without knowing the K_D for the agonist and without needing to define the precise relationship between receptor and response.

Inverse Agonists. The overexpression of wild-type receptors and the creation of constitutively active mutant receptors have facilitated the study of a novel class of functional antagonists, the inverse agonists. As discussed earlier, receptors can adopt active conformations that produce a cellular response spontaneously. The fraction of unoccupied receptors in the active conformation usually is too low to allow observation of their agonist-independent activity, but this activity sometimes can be observed, especially when the receptor is expressed heterologously at high levels or when mutation shifts the conformational equilibrium toward the active form. In these situations, the tissue behaves as if there were an agonist present, and a conventional competitive antagonist has no effect. However, certain agents are capable of inhibiting agonist-independent or constitutive signaling. These agents are termed *inverse agonists*. Inverse agonists selectively bind to the inactive form of the receptor and shift the conformational equilibrium toward the inactive state. In systems that are not constitutively active, inverse agonists will behave like competitive antagonists, which in part explains why the properties of inverse agonists and the number of such agents previously described as competitive antagonists were not appreciated until recently. Milligan (2003) and Kenakin (2004) recently have reviewed inverse agonism.

It is not known to what extent constitutive receptor activity is a physiologically or pathologically important phenomenon, and it is therefore unclear to what extent inverse agonism is a therapeutically relevant property. In some cases, however, the preferability of an inverse agonist over a competitive antagonist is obvious. For example, the human herpesvirus KSHV encodes a constitutively active chemokine receptor that generates a second messenger that drives cell growth and viral replication (Verzijl *et al.*, 2004). In such a case, a conventional antagonist would not be useful because no chemokine agonist is involved; however, an inverse agonist could be an effective intervention. In most cases, the role of inverse agonists is less clear but may be of therapeutic benefit as we discover the importance of the various conformations in which receptors can exist. In this regard, there are two important examples to consider. First is the discovery that GPCRs exist in multiple states, as revealed by inverse agonists such as propranolol. In cells overexpressing the human β_2 adrenergic receptor (Azzi *et al.*, 2003), it is possible to measure both the antagonism of receptor activation of adenylyl cyclase produced by propranolol and the activation of extracellular signal-regulated kinase (ERK1/2). These data reveal that the inverse agonistic activity of propranolol puts the receptor in a conformation that is unable to interact with G_s protein but is capable of interacting with proteins such as β-arrestin to cause ERK activation. Similar conclusions are drawn by studies with histamine H_3 receptors and *proxyfan* (Gbahou *et al.*, 2003). It is conceivable that the discovery of drugs that select a particular conformation of a receptor (*e.g.*, a ligand-directed conformation) can be used to select the profile of effect desired in a patient to improve therapy.

BIBLIOGRAPHY

Ariëns, E.J. Affinity and intrinsic activity in the theory of competitive inhibition: I. Problems and theory. *Arch. Intern. Pharmacodyn. Ther.,* **1954**, *99*:32–49.

Azzi, M., Charest, P.G., Angers, S., *et al.* Beta-arrestin-mediated activation of MAPK by inverse agonists reveals distinct active conformations for G protein–coupled receptors. *Proc. Natl. Acad. Sci. U.S.A.,* **2003**, *100*:11406–11411.

Baillie, G.S., and Houslay, M.D., Arrestin times for compartmentalised cAMP signalling and phosphodiesterase-4 enzymes. *Curr. Opin. Cell Biol.,* **2005**, *17*:1–6

Beavo, J.A., and Brunton, L.L. Cyclic nucleotide research: Still expanding after half a century. *Nature Rev. Mol. Cell. Biol.,* **2002**, *3*:710–718.

Brunton, L.L. PDE4: arrested at the border. *Sci. STKE.,* **2003**, 2003:PE44.

Buxton, I.L. Regulation of uterine function: A biochemical conundrum in the regulation of smooth muscle relaxation. *Mol. Pharmacol.,* **2004**, *65*:1051–1059.

Buxton, I.L., and Brunton, L.L. Compartments of cyclic AMP and protein kinase in mammalian cardiomyocytes. *J. Biol. Chem.,* **1983**, *258*:10233–10239.

Calabrese, E.J., and Baldwin, L.A. Hormesis: The dose–response revolution. *Annu. Rev. Pharmacol. Toxicol.,* **2003**, 43:175–197.

Carlson, H.A., and McCammon, J.A. Accommodating protein flexibility in computational drug design. *Mol. Pharmacol.,* **2000**, *57*:213–218.

Cheng, H.C. The influence of cooperativity on the determination of dissociation constants: examination of the Cheng–Prusoff equation, the Scatchard analysis, the Schild analysis and related power equations. *Pharmacol. Res.,* **2004**, *50*:21–40.

Cheng, Y.-C., and Prusoff, W.H. Relationship between the inhibition constant (K_i) and the concentration of inhibitor which causes 50 percent inhibition (IC$_{50}$) of an enzymatic reaction. *Biochem. Pharmacol.,* **1973**, *1973*:3099–3108.

Dahlborg, S.A., Petrillo, A., Crossen, J.R., *et al.* The potential for complete and durable response in nonglial primary brain tumors in children and young adults with enhanced chemotherapy delivery. *Cancer J. Sci. Am.,* **1998**, *4*:110–124.

Etienne-Manneville, S., and Hall, A. Rho GTPases in cell biology. *Nature,* **2002**, *420*:629–635.

Farmer, K.C. Methods for measuring and monitoring medication regimen adherence in clinical trials and clinical practice. *Clin. Ther.,* **1999**, *21*:1074–1090.

Furchgott, R.F. The use of β-haloalkylamines in the differentiation of receptors and in the determination of dissociation constants of receptor–agonist complexes. In, *Advances in Drug Research,* Vol. 3. (Harper, N.J., and Simmonds, A.B., eds.) Academic Press, London, **1966**, pp. 21–55.

Gaddum, J.H. The quantitative effects of antagonistic drugs. *J. Physiol.,* **1937**, *89*:7P–9P.

Gaddum, J.H. Theories of drug antagonism. *Pharmacol. Rev.,* **1957**, *9*:211–218.

Gbahou, F., Rouleau, A., Morisset, S. *et al.* Protean agonism at histamine H_3 receptors *in vitro* and *in vivo*. *Proc. Natl. Acad. Sci. U.S.A.,* **2003**, *100*:11086–11091.

Hall, R.A. Beta-adrenergic receptors and their interacting proteins. *Sem. in. Cell Dev. Biol.,* **2004**, *15*:281–288.

Holcberg, G., Tsadkin-Tamir, M., Sapir, O., *et al.* New aspects in placental drug transfer. *Isr. Med. Assoc. J.,* **2003**, *5*:873–876.

Hanoune, J., and Defer, N. Regulation and role of adenylyl cyclase isoforms. *Ann. Rev. Pharmacol. Toxicol.,* **2001**, *41*:145–174.

Ito, S., and Lee, A. Drug excretion into breast milk: Overview. *Adv. Drug Deliv. Rev.,* **2003**, *55*:617–627.

Jain, K.K. Role of pharmacoproteomics in the development of personalized medicine. *Pharmacogenomics,* **2004**, *5*:331–336.

Kenakin, T. Pharmacological proteus? *Trends Pharmacol. Sci.,* **1995,** *16*:256–258.

Kenakin, T. Efficacy as a vector: The relative prevalence and paucity of inverse agonism. *Mol. Pharmacol.,* **2004,** *65*:2–11

Kim, R.B. Organic anion-transporting polypeptide (OATP) transporter family and drug disposition. *Eur. J. Clin. Invest.,* **2003,** *33*(suppl 2):1–5.

Kroeger, K.M., Pfleger, K.D., and Eidne, K.A. G protein–coupled receptor oligomerization in neuroendocrine pathways. *Front. Neuroendocrinol.,* **2003,** *24*:254–278.

Kwon, Y., and Morris, M.E. Membrane transport in hepatic clearance of drugs: I. Extended hepatic clearance models incorporating concentration-dependent transport and elimination processes. *Pharm. Res.,* **1997,** *14*:774–779.

Limbird, L.E. *Cell Surface Receptors: A Short Course on Theory and Methods,* 3d ed. Springer-Verlag , New York, **2005.**

Lipka, L.J. Ezetimibe: A first-in-class, novel cholesterol absorption inhibitor. *Cardiovasc. Drug Rev.,* **2003,** *21*:293–312.

Martinez, S.E., Wu, A.Y., Glavas, N.A., *et al.* The two GAF domains in phosphodiesterase 2A have distinct roles in dimerization and in cGMP binding. *Proc. Natl. Acad. Sci. U.S.A.,* **2002,** *99*:13260–13265.

Marzolini, C., Paus, E., Buclin, T., and Kim, R.B. Polymorphisms in human MDR1 (P-glycoprotein): Recent advances and clinical relevance. *Clin. Pharmacol. Ther.,* **2004,** *75*:13–33.

Maurice, D.H., Palmer, D., Tilley, D.G., *et al.* Cyclic nucleotide phosphodiesterase activity, expression and targeting in cells of the cardiovascular system. *Mol. Pharmacol.,* **2003,** *64*:533–546.

Mayr, B., and Montiminy, M. Transcriptional regulation by the phosphorylation-dependent factor CREB. *Nature Rev. Mol. Cell Biol.,* **2001,** *2*:599–609.

Mehats, C., Andersen, C.B., Filopanti, M., *et al.* Cyclic nucleotide phosphodiesterases and their role in endocrine cell signaling. *Trends Endocrinol. Metab.,* **2002,** *13*:29–35.

Milligan, G. Constitutive activity and inverse agonists of G protein–coupled receptors: A current perspective. *Mol. Pharmacol.,* **2003,** *64*:1271–1276.

Nemeroff, C.B. Improving antidepressant adherence. *J. Clin. Psychiatry,* **2003,** *64*(suppl 18):25–30.

Palczewski, K., Kumasaka, T., Hori, T., *et al.* Crystal structure of rhodopsin: A G protein–coupled receptor. *Science,* **2000,** *289*:739–745.

Patel, A.B., Crocker, E., Eilers, M., *et al.* Coupling of retinal isomerization to the activation of rhodopsin. *Proc. Natl. Acad. Sci. U.S.A.,* **2004,** *101*:10048–10053.

Ross, E.M., and Wilkie, T.M. GTPase-activating proteins for heterotrimeric G proteins: Regulators of G protein signaling (RGS) and RGS-like proteins. *Annu. Rev. Biochem.,* **2000,** *69*:795–827.

Rybalkin, S.D., Yan, C., Bornfeldt, K.E., and Beavo, J.A. Cyclic GMP phosphodiesterases and regulation of smooth muscle function. *Circ. Res.,* **2003,** *93*:280–291.

Schild, H.O. Drug antagonism and pA2. *Pharmacol. Rev.,* **1957,** *9*:242–246.

Spiegel, A.M., and Weinstein, L.S. Inherited diseases involving G proteins and G protein–coupled receptors. *Annu. Rev. Med.,* **2004,** *55*:27–39.

Stephenson, R.P. A modification of receptor theory. *Br. J. Pharmacol.,* **1956,** *11*:379–393.

Tan, C.M., Brady, A.E., Nickols, H.H., *et al.* Membrane trafficking of G protein–coupled receptors. *Annu. Rev. Pharmacol. Toxicol.,* **2004,** *44*:559–609.

Tyson, R.M., Siegal, T., Doolittle, N.D., *et al.* Current status and future of relapsed primary central nervous system lymphoma (PCNSL). *Leuk. Lymphoma,* **2003,** *44*:627–633.

Unadkat, J.D., Dahlin, A., and Vijay, S. Placental drug transporters. *Curr. Drug Metab.,* **2004,** *5*:125–131.

Vo, N.K., Gettemy, J.M., and Coghlan, V.M. Identification of cGMP-dependent protein kinase anchoring proteins (GKAPs). *Biochem. Biophys. Res. Commun.,* **1998,** *246*:831–835.

Verzijl, D., Fitzsimons, C.P., Van, D.M., *et al.* Differential activation of murine herpesvirus 68– and Kaposi's sarcoma–associated herpesvirus-encoded ORF74 G protein–coupled receptors by human and murine chemokines. *J. Virol.,* **2004,** *78*:3343–3351.

Wei, L.N. Retinoid receptors and their coregulators. *Annu. Rev. Pharmacol. Toxicol.,* **2003,** *43*:47–72.

Wong, W., and Scott, J.D. AKAP signaling complexes: Focal points in space and time. *Nature Rev. Mol. Cell Biol.,* **2004,** *5*:959–970.

MEMBRANE TRANSPORTERS AND DRUG RESPONSE

Kathleen M. Giacomini and Yuichi Sugiyama

Transporters are membrane proteins that are present in all organisms. These proteins control the influx of essential nutrients and ions and the efflux of cellular waste, environmental toxins, and other xenobiotics. Consistent with their critical roles in cellular homeostasis, approximately 2000 genes in the human genome ~7 of the total number of genes code for transporters or transporter-related proteins. The functions of membrane transporters may be facilitated (equilibrative, not requiring energy) or active (requiring energy).

In considering the transport of drugs, pharmacologists generally focus on transporters from two major superfamilies, ABC (*ATP binding cassette*) and SLC (*solute carrier*) transporters. Most ABC proteins are primary active transporters, which rely on ATP hydrolysis to actively pump their substrates across membranes. There are 49 known genes for ABC proteins that can be grouped into seven subclasses or families (ABCA to ABCG) (Borst and Elferink, 2002). Among the best recognized transporters in the ABC superfamily are P-glycoprotein (P-gp, encoded by *ABCB1*, also termed *MDR1*) and the cystic fibrosis transmembrane regulator (CFTR, encoded by *ABCC7*). The SLC superfamily includes genes that encode facilitated transporters and ion-coupled secondary active transporters that reside in various cell membranes. Forty-three SLC families with approximately 300 transporters have been identified in the human genome (Hediger, 2004). Many serve as drug targets or in drug absorption and disposition. Widely recognized SLC transporters include the serotonin and dopamine transporters (SERT, encoded by *SLC6A4*; DAT, encoded by *SLC6A3*).

Drug-transporting proteins operate in pharmacokinetic and pharmacodynamic pathways, including pathways involved in both therapeutic and adverse effects (Figure 2–1).

MEMBRANE TRANSPORTERS IN THERAPEUTIC DRUG RESPONSES

Pharmacokinetics. Transporters that are important in pharmacokinetics generally are located in intestinal, renal, and hepatic epithelia. They function in the selective absorption and elimination of endogenous substances and xenobiotics, including drugs (Dresser *et al.*, 2001; Kim, 2002). Transporters work in concert with drug-metabolizing enzymes to eliminate drugs and their metabolites (Figure 2–2). In addition, transporters in various cell types mediate tissue-specific drug distribution (drug targeting); conversely, transporters also may serve as protective barriers to particular organs and cell types. For example, P-glycoprotein in the blood–brain barrier protects the central nervous system (CNS) from a variety of structurally diverse compounds through its efflux mechanisms. Many of the transporters that are relevant to drug response control the tissue distribution as well as the absorption and elimination of drugs.

Pharmacodynamics: Transporters as Drug Targets. Membrane transporters are the targets of many clinically used drugs. For example, neurotransmitter transporters are the targets for drugs used in the treatment of neuropsychiatric disorders (Amara and Sonders, 1998; Inoue *et al.*, 2002). SERT (*SLC6A4*) is a target for a major class of antidepressant drugs, the serotonin selective reuptake inhibitors (SSRIs). Other neurotransmitter reuptake transporters serve

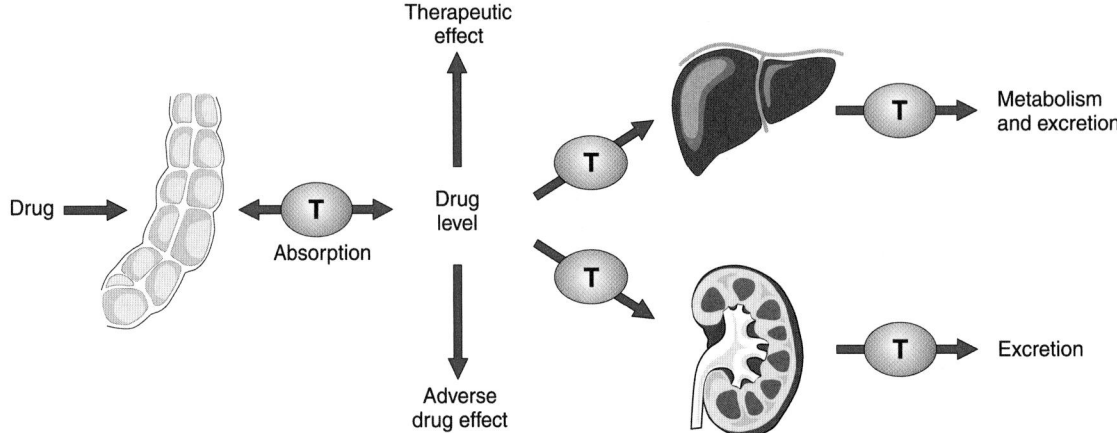

Figure 2–1. *Roles of membrane transporters in pharmacokinetic pathways.* Membrane transporters (T) play roles in pharmacokinetic pathways (drug absorption, distribution, metabolism, and excretion), thereby setting systemic drug levels. Drug levels often drive therapeutic and adverse drug effects.

as drug targets for the tricyclic antidepressants, various amphetamines (including amphetaminelike drugs used in the treatment of attention deficit disorder in children), and anticonvulsants (Amara and Sonders, 1998; Jones *et al.*, 1998; Elliott and Beveridge, 2005). These transporters also may be involved in the pathogenesis of neuropsychiatric disorders, including Alzheimer's and Parkinson's diseases (Shigeri *et al.*, 2004). Transporters that are nonneuronal also may be potential drug targets, *e.g.,* cholesterol transporters in cardiovascular disease, nucleoside transporters in

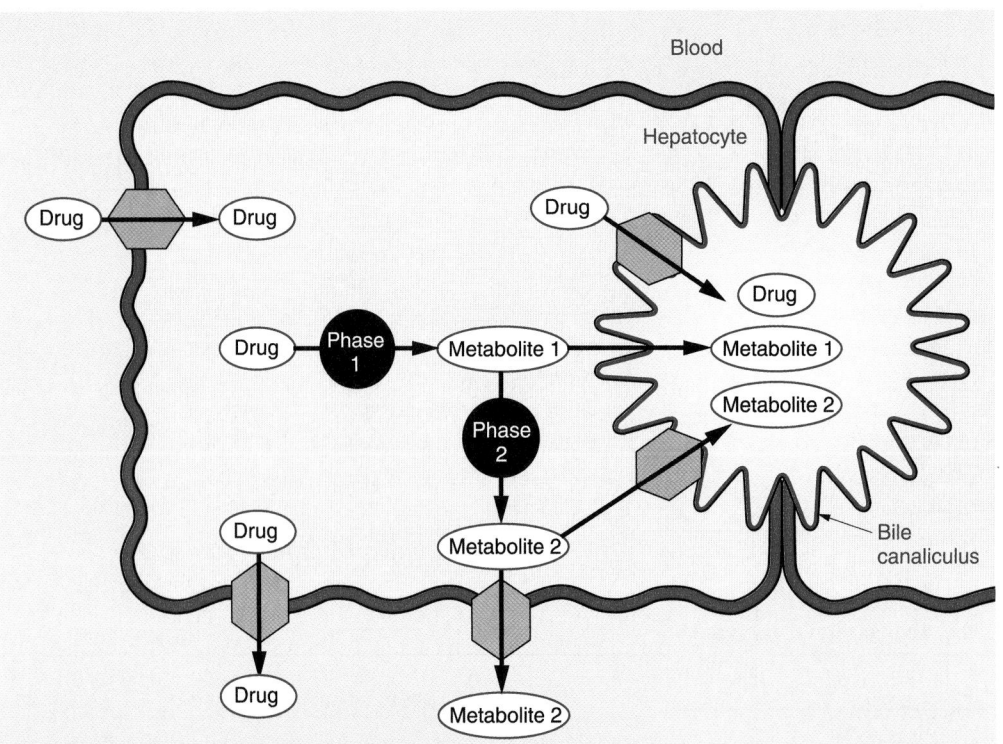

Figure 2–2. *Hepatic drug transporters.* Membrane transporters, shown as hexagons with arrows, work in concert with phase 1 and phase 2 drug-metabolizing enzymes in the hepatocyte to mediate the uptake and efflux of drugs and their metabolites.

cancers, glucose transporters in metabolic syndromes, and Na$^+$-H$^+$ antiporters in hypertension (Damaraju *et al.*, 2003; Pascual *et al.*, 2004; Rader, 2003; Rosskopf *et al.*, 1993).

Drug Resistance. Membrane transporters play a critical role in the development of resistance to anticancer drugs, antiviral agents, and anticonvulsants. For example, P-glycoprotein is overexpressed in tumor cells after exposure to cytotoxic anticancer agents (Gottesman *et al.*, 1996; Lin and Yamazaki, 2003; Leslie *et al.*, 2005). P-glycoprotein pumps out the anticancer drugs, rendering cells resistant to their cytotoxic effects. Other transporters, including breast cancer resistance protein (BCRP), the organic anion transporters, and several nucleoside transporters, also have been implicated in resistance to anticancer drugs (Clarke *et al.*, 2002; Suzuki *et al.*, 2001). The overexpression of multidrug-resistance protein 4 (MRP4) is associated with resistance to antiviral nucleoside analogs (Schuetz *et al.*, 1999).

MEMBRANE TRANSPORTERS AND ADVERSE DRUG RESPONSES

Through import and export mechanisms, transporters ultimately control the exposure of cells to chemical carcinogens, environmental toxins, and drugs. Thus, transporters play critical roles in the cellular toxicities of these agents. Transporter-mediated adverse drug responses generally can be classified into three categories, as shown in Figure 2–3.

Transporters in the liver and kidney affect the exposure of drugs in the toxicological target organs. Transporters expressed in the liver and kidney, as well as metabolic enzymes, are key determinants of drug exposure in the circulating blood (Mizuno *et al.*, 2003) (Figure 2–3, *top panel*). For example, after oral administration of an HMG-CoA reductase inhibitor (*e.g.*, pravastatin), the efficient first-pass hepatic uptake of the drug by the organic anion–transporting polypeptide OATP1B1 maximizes the effects of such drugs on hepatic HMG-CoA reductase. Uptake by OATP1B1 also minimizes the escape of these drugs into the systemic circulation, where they can cause adverse responses such as skeletal muscle myopathy. Transporters in the liver and kidney, which control the total clearance of drugs, thus have an influence on the plasma concentration profiles and subsequent exposure to the toxicological target.

Transporters in toxicological target organs or at barriers to such organs affect drug exposure by the target organs. Transporters expressed in tissues that may be targets for drug toxicity (*e.g.*, brain) or in barriers to such tissues

[*e.g.*, the blood–brain barrier (BBB)] can tightly control local drug concentrations and thus control the exposure of these tissues to the drug (Figure 2–3, *middle panel*). For example, to restrict the penetration of compounds into the brain, endothelial cells in the BBB are closely linked by tight junctions, and some efflux transporters are expressed on the blood-facing (luminal) side. The importance of the ABC transporter multidrug-resistance protein (*ABCB1*, MDR1; P-glycoprotein, P-gp) in the BBB has been demonstrated in *mdr1a* knockout mice (Schinkel *et al.*, 1994). The brain concentrations of many P-glycoprotein substrates, such as *digoxin,* used in the treatment of heart failure (*see* Chapters 33 and 34), and *cyclosporin A* (*see* Chapter 52), an immunosuppressant, are increased dramatically in *mdr1a*(–/–) mice, whereas their plasma concentrations are not changed significantly.

Another example of transporter control of drug exposure can be seen in the interactions of *loperamide* and *quinidine.* Loperamide is a peripheral opioid used in the treatment of diarrhea and is a substrate of P-glycoprotein. Coadministration of loperamide and the potent P-glycoprotein inhibitor quinidine results in significant respiratory depression, an adverse response to the loperamide (Sadeque *et al.*, 2000). Because plasma concentrations of loperamide are not changed in the presence of quinidine, it has been suggested that quinidine inhibits P-glycoprotein in the BBB, resulting in an increased exposure of the CNS to loperamide and bringing about the respiratory depression. Inhibition of P-glycoprotein-mediated efflux in the BBB thus would cause an increase in the concentration of substrates in the CNS and potentiate adverse effects.

Drug-induced toxicity sometimes is caused by the concentrative tissue distribution mediated by influx transporters. For example, biguanides (*e.g.*, metformin and phenformin), widely used as oral hypoglycemic agents for the treatment of type II diabetes mellitus, can produce lactic acidosis, a lethal side effect. Phenformin was withdrawn from the market for this reason. Biguanides are substrates of the organic cation transporter OCT1, which is highly expressed in the liver. After oral administration of metformin, the distribution of the drug to the liver in *oct1*(–/–) mice is markedly reduced compared with the distribution in wild-type mice. Moreover, plasma lactic acid concentrations induced by metformin are reduced in *oct1*(–/–) mice compared with wild-type mice, although the plasma concentrations of metformin are similar in the wild-type and knockout mice. These results indicate that the OCT1-mediated hepatic uptake of biguanides plays an important role in lactic acidosis (Wang *et al.*, 2003).

The organic anion transporter 1 (OAT1) provides another example of transporter-related toxicity. OAT1 is expressed

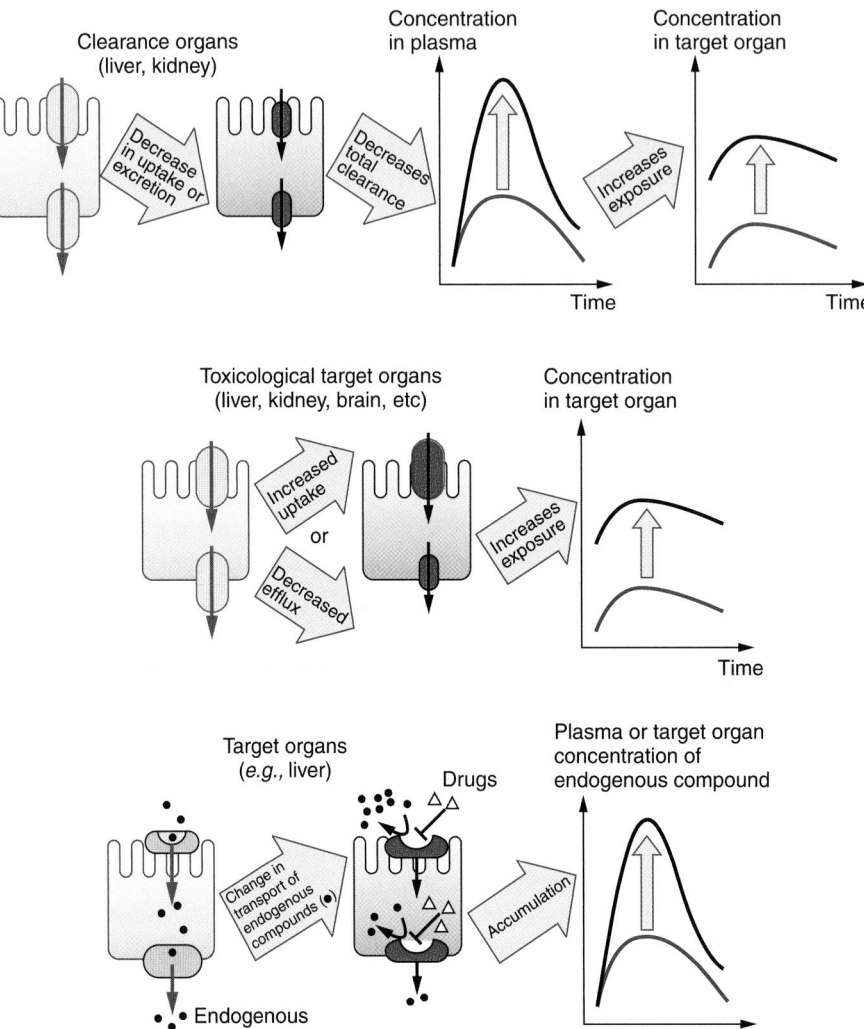

Figure 2–3. ***Major mechanisms by which transporters mediate adverse drug responses.*** Three cases are given. The *left panel* of each case provides a cartoon representation of the mechanism; the *right panel* shows the resulting effect on drug levels. (*Top panel*) Increase in the plasma concentrations of drug due to a decrease in the uptake and/or secretion in clearance organs such as the liver and kidney. (*Middle panel*) Increase in the concentration of drug in toxicological target organs due either to the enhanced uptake or to reduced efflux of the drug. (*Bottom panel*) Increase in the plasma concentration of an endogenous compound (*e.g.*, a bile acid) due to a drug's inhibiting the influx of the endogenous compound in its eliminating or target organ. The diagram also may represent an increase in the concentration of the endogenous compound in the target organ owing to drug-inhibited efflux of the endogenous compound.

mainly in the kidney and is responsible for the renal tubular secretion of anionic compounds. Some reports have indicated that substrates of OAT1, such as *cephaloridine,* a β-lactam antibiotic, sometimes cause nephrotoxicity. *In vitro* experiments suggest that cephaloridine is a substrate of OAT1 and that OAT1-expressing cells are more susceptible to cephaloridine toxicity than control cells.

Transporters for endogenous ligands may be modulated by drugs and thereby exert adverse effects (Figure 2–3, *bottom panel*). For example, bile acids are taken up

mainly by *N*a+-*t*aurocholate *c*otransporting *p*olypeptide (NTCP) (Hagenbuch *et al.*, 1991) and excreted into the bile by the *b*ile *s*alt *e*xport *p*ump (BSEP, *ABCB11*) (Gerloff *et al.*, 1998). Bilirubin is taken up by OATP1B1 and conjugated with glucuronic acid, and bilirubin glucuronide is excreted by the *m*ultidrug-*r*esistance-*a*ssociated *p*rotein (MRP2, *ABCC2*). Inhibition of these transporters by drugs may cause cholestasis or hyperbilirubinemia. *Troglitazone,* a thiazolidinedione insulin-sensitizing drug used for the treatment of type II diabetes mellitus, was withdrawn from the market because it caused hepatotoxicity. The mechanism for this troglitazone-induced hepatotoxicity remains unclear. One hypothesis is that troglitazone and its sulfate conjugate induced cholestasis. Troglitazone sulfate potently inhibits the efflux of taurocholate (K_i = 0.2 μM) mediated by the ABC transporter BSEP. These findings suggest that troglitazone sulfate induces cholestasis by inhibition of BSEP function. BSEP-mediated transport is also inhibited by other drugs, including cyclosporin A and the antibiotics *rifamycin* and *rifampicin* (Stieger *et al.*, 2000).

Thus, uptake and efflux transporters determine the plasma and tissue concentrations of endogenous compounds and xenobiotics and thereby can influence the systemic or site-specific toxicity of drugs.

BASIC MECHANISMS OF MEMBRANE TRANSPORT

Transporters *versus* Channels. Both channels and transporters facilitate the membrane permeation of inorganic ions and organic compounds (Reuss, 2000). In general, channels have two primary states, *open* and *closed,* that are totally stochastic phenomena. Only in the open state do channels appear to act as pores for the selected ions, allowing their permeation across the plasma membrane. After opening, channels return to the closed state as a function of time. In contrast, a transporter forms an intermediate complex with the substrate (solute), and subsequently a conformational change in the transporter induces translocation of the substrates to the other side of the membrane. Therefore, there is a marked difference in turnover rates between channels and transporters. The turnover rate constants of typical channels are 10^6 to 10^8 s^{-1}, whereas those of transporters are, at most, 10^1 to 10^3 s^{-1}. Because a particular transporter forms intermediate complexes with specific compounds (referred to as *substrates*), transporter-mediated membrane transport is characterized by saturability and inhibition by substrate analogs, as described below.

The basic mechanisms involved in solute transport across biological membranes include passive diffusion, facilitated diffusion, and active transport. Active transport can be further subdivided into primary and secondary active transport. These mechanisms are depicted in Figure 2–4 and described below.

Passive Diffusion. Simple diffusion of a solute across the plasma membrane consists of three processes: partition from the aqueous to the lipid phase, diffusion across the lipid bilayer, and repartition into the aqueous phase on the opposite side. Diffusion of any solute (including drugs) occurs down an electrochemical potential gradient $\Delta\mu$ of the solute, given by the equation:

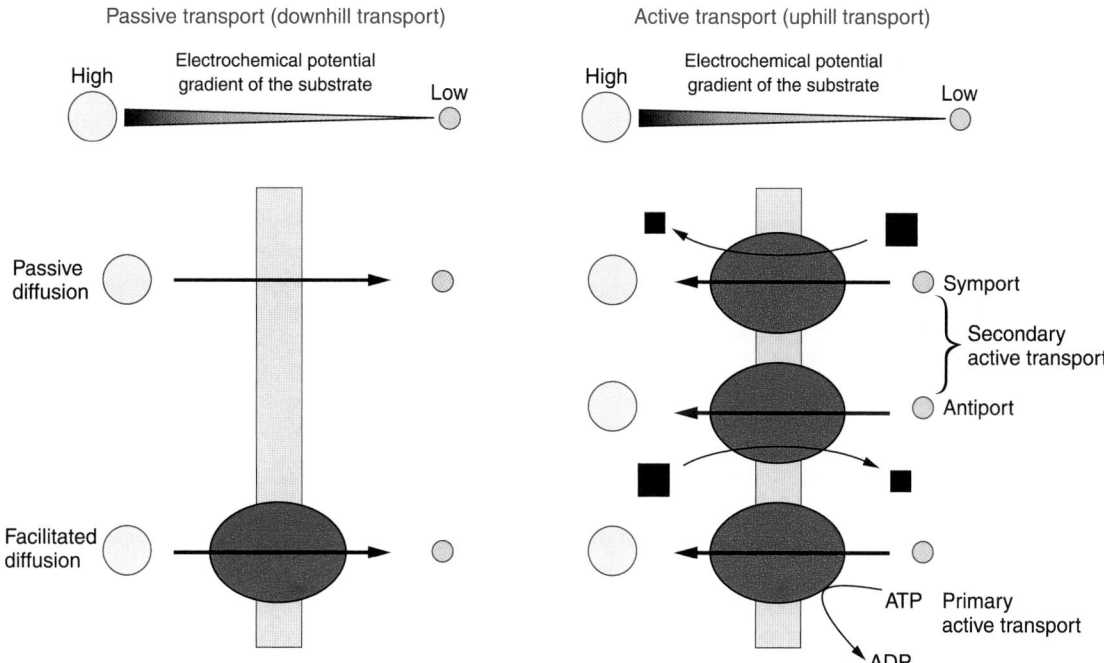

Figure 2–4. *Classification of membrane transport mechanisms.* *Light blue circles* depict the substrate. Size of the circles is proportional to the concentration of the substrate. *Arrows* show the direction of flux. *Black squares* represent the ion that supplies the driving force for transport (size is proportional to the concentration of the ion). *Dark blue ovals* depict transport proteins.

$$\Delta\mu = zE_mF + RT\ln\left(\frac{C_i}{C_o}\right) \qquad (2\text{--}1)$$

where z is the charge valence of the solute, E_m is the membrane voltage, F is the Faraday constant, R is the gas constant, T is the absolute temperature, C is the concentration of the solute inside (i) and outside (o) of the plasma membrane. The first term on the right side in Eq. (2–1) represents the electrical potential, and the second represents the chemical potential.

For nonionized compounds, the flux J owing to simple diffusion is given by Fick's first law (permeability multiplied by the concentration difference). For ionized compounds, the difference in electrical potential across the plasma membrane needs to be taken into consideration. Assuming that the electrical field is constant, the flux is given by the Goldman–Hodgkin–Katz equation:

$$J = -P\frac{zE_mF}{RT}\left[\frac{C_i - C_o\exp(E_mF/RT)}{1 - \exp(E_mF/RT)}\right] \qquad (2\text{--}2)$$

where P represents the permeability. The lipid and water solubility and the molecular weight and shape of the solute are determinants of the flux in passive diffusion; they are incorporated in the permeability constant P. The permeability constant positively correlates with the lipophilicity, determined by the partition between water and organic solvents, such as octanol, and is also related to the inverse of the square root of the molecular weight of the solute. At steady state, the electrochemical potentials of all compounds become equal across the plasma membrane. In the case of nonionized compounds, the steady-state concentrations are equal across the plasma membrane. For ionized compounds, however, the steady-state concentration ratio across the plasma membrane is affected by the membrane voltage and given by the Nernst equation (Eq. 2–3).

$$\frac{C_i}{C_o} = \exp\left(\frac{-zE_mF}{RT}\right) \qquad (2\text{--}3)$$

The membrane voltage is maintained by the ion gradients across the membrane.

Facilitated Diffusion.

Diffusion of ions and organic compounds across the plasma membrane may be facilitated by a membrane transporter. Facilitated diffusion is a form of transporter-mediated membrane transport that does not require energy input. Just as in passive diffusion, the transport of ionized and un-ionized compounds across the plasma membrane occurs down their electrochemical potential gradient. Therefore, steady state will be achieved when the electrochemical potentials of the compound on both sides of the membrane become equal.

Active Transport.

Active transport is the form of membrane transport that requires the input of energy. It is the transport of solutes against their electrochemical gradients, leading to the concentration of solutes on one side of the plasma membrane and the creation of potential energy in the electrochemical gradient formed. Active transport plays an important role in the uptake and efflux of drugs and other solutes. Depending on the driving force, active transport can be subdivided into primary and secondary active transport (Figure 2–4).

Primary Active Transport. Membrane transport that directly couples with ATP hydrolysis is called *primary active transport*. ABC transporters are examples of primary active transporters. They contain one or two ATP binding cassettes and a highly conserved domain in the intracellular loop region that exhibits ATPase activity. In mammalian cells, primary active transporters mediate the unidirectional efflux of solutes across biological membranes. The molecular mechanism by which ATP hydrolysis is coupled to the active transport of substrates by ABC transporters is a subject of current investigation.

Secondary Active Transport. In secondary active transport, the transport across a biological membrane of one solute S_1 against its concentration gradient is energetically driven by the transport of another solute S_2 in accordance with its concentration gradient. The driving force for this type of transport therefore is stored in the electrochemical potential created by the concentration difference of S_2 across the plasma membrane. For example, an inwardly directed Na^+ concentration gradient across the plasma membrane is created by Na^+,K^+-ATPase. Under these conditions, inward movement of Na^+ produces the energy to drive the movement of a substrate S_1 against its concentration gradient by a secondary active transporter as in Na^+/Ca^{2+} exchange.

Depending on the transport direction of the solute, secondary active transporters are classified as either symporters or antiporters. *Symporters,* also termed *cotransporters,* transport S_2 and S_1 in the same direction, whereas *antiporters,* also termed *exchangers,* move their substrates in opposite directions (Figure 2–4). The free energy produced by one extracellular sodium ion (Na^+) is given by the difference in the electrochemical potential across the plasma membrane:

$$\Delta\mu_{Na} = E_mF + RT\ln\left(\frac{C_{Na,i}}{C_{Na,o}}\right) \qquad (2\text{--}4)$$

The electrochemical potential of a nonionized compound $\Delta\mu_s$ acquired from one extracellular Na^+ is less than this value:

$$\Delta \mu_S + \Delta \mu_{Na} \leq 0 \qquad (2-5)$$

Therefore, the concentration ratio of the compound is given by the following equation:

$$\frac{S_i}{S_o} \leq \left(\frac{C_{Na,o}}{C_{Na,i}} \right) \exp \left(\frac{-E_m F}{RT} \right) \qquad (2-6)$$

Assuming that the concentration ratio of Na^+ is 10 and that E_m is –60 mV, ideally, symport of one nonionized organic compound with one Na^+ ion can achieve a one hundredfold difference in the intracellular substrate concentration compared with the extracellular concentration. When more than one Na^+ ion is coupled to the movement of the solute, a synergistic driving force results. For the case in which two Na^+ ions are involved,

$$\frac{S_i}{S_o} \leq \left(\frac{C_{Na,o}}{C_{Na,i}} \right)^2 \exp \left(\frac{-2E_m F}{RT} \right) \qquad (2-7)$$

In this case, the substrate ideally is concentrated intracellularly one thousandfold relative to the extracellular space under the same conditions. The Na^+/Ca^{2+} antiporter shows the effect of this dependence in the square of the concentration ratio of Na^+; Ca^{2+} is transported from the cytosol (0.1 μM < $[Ca^{2+}]$ < 1 μM) to the plasma $[Ca^{2+}]_{free}$ ~ 1.25 mM.

KINETICS OF TRANSPORT

The flux of a substrate (rate of transport) across a biological membrane *via* transporter-mediated processes is characterized by saturability. The relationship between the flux v and substrate concentration C in a transporter-mediated process is given by the Michaelis–Menten equation:

$$v = \frac{V_{max} C}{K_m + C} \qquad (2-8)$$

where V_{max} is the maximum transport rate and is proportional to the density of transporters on the plasma membrane, and K_m is the Michaelis constant, which represents the substrate concentration at which the flux is half the V_{max} value. K_m is an approximation of the dissociation constant of the substrate from the intermediate complex. When C is small compared with the K_m value, the flux is increased in proportion to the substrate concentration (roughly linear with substrate concentration). However, if C is large compared with the K_m value, the flux approaches a constant value (V_{max}). The K_m and V_{max} values can be determined by examining the flux at different substrate concentrations. The Eadie–Hofstee plot often is used for graphical interpretation of satura-

tion kinetics. Plotting clearance v/C on the y axis and flux v on the x axis gives a straight line. The y intercept represents the ratio V_{max}/K_m, and the slope of the line is the inverse of the K_m value:

$$\frac{v}{C} = \frac{V_{max}}{K_m} - \frac{C}{K_m} \qquad (2-9)$$

Involvement of multiple transporters with different K_m values gives an Eadie–Hofstee plot that is curved. In algebraic terms, the Eadie–Hofstee plot of kinetic data is equivalent to the Scatchard plot of equilibrium binding data.

Transporter-mediated membrane transport of a substrate is also characterized by inhibition by other compounds. The manner of inhibition can be categorized as one of three types: competitive, noncompetitive, and uncompetitive.

Competitive inhibition occurs when substrates and inhibitors share a common binding site on the transporter, resulting in an increase in the apparent K_m value in the presence of inhibitor. The flux of a substrate in the presence of a competitive inhibitor is

$$v = \frac{V_{max} C}{K_m (1 + I/K_i) + C} \qquad (2-10)$$

where I is the concentration of inhibitor, and K_i is the inhibition constant.

Noncompetitive inhibition assumes that the inhibitor has an allosteric effect on the transporter, does not inhibit the formation of an intermediate complex of substrate and transporter, but does inhibit the subsequent translocation process.

$$v = \frac{V_{max}/(1 + I/K_i) \cdot C}{K_m + C} \qquad (2-11)$$

Uncompetitive inhibition assumes that inhibitors can form a complex only with an intermediate complex of the substrate and transporter and inhibit subsequent translocation.

$$v = \frac{V_{max}/(1 + I/K_i) \cdot C}{K_m/(1 + I/K_i) + C} \qquad (2-12)$$

VECTORIAL TRANSPORT

The SLC type of transporter mediates either drug uptake or efflux, whereas ABC transporters mediate only unidirectional efflux. Asymmetrical transport across a monolayer of polarized cells, such as the epithelial and endothelial cells of brain capillaries, is called *vectorial transport* (Figure 2–5). Vectorial transport is important in

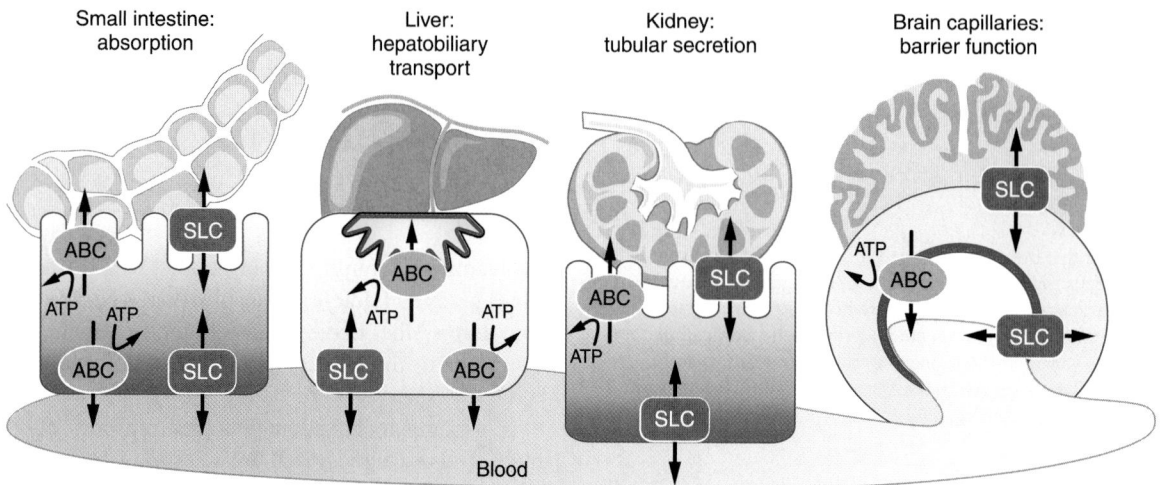

Figure 2–5. *Transepithelial or transendothelial flux.* Transepithelial or transendothelial flux of drugs requires distinct transporters at the two surfaces of the epithelial or endothelial barriers. These are depicted diagrammatically for transport across the small intestine (absorption), the kidney and liver (elimination), and the brain capillaries that comprise the blood–brain barrier.

the efficient transfer of solutes across epithelial or endothelial barriers. For example, vectorial transport is important for the absorption of nutrients and bile acids in the intestine. From the viewpoint of drug absorption and disposition, vectorial transport plays a major role in hepatobiliary and urinary excretion of drugs from the blood to the lumen and in the intestinal absorption of drugs. In addition, efflux of drugs from the brain *via* brain endothelial cells and brain choroid plexus epithelial cells involves vectorial transport.

For lipophilic compounds that have sufficient membrane permeability, ABC transporters alone are able to achieve vectorial transport by extruding their substrates to the outside of cells without the help of influx transporters (Horio *et al.*, 1990). For relatively hydrophilic organic anions and cations, coordinated uptake and efflux transporters in the polarized plasma membranes are necessary to achieve the vectorial movement of solutes across an epithelium. Common substrates of coordinated transporters are transferred efficiently across the epithelial barrier (Sasaki *et al.*, 2002). In the liver, a number of transporters with different substrate specificities are localized on the sinusoidal membrane (facing blood). These transporters are involved in the uptake of bile acids, amphipathic organic anions, and hydrophilic organic cations into the hepatocytes. Similarly, ABC transporters on the canalicular membrane (facing bile) export such compounds into the bile. Overlapping substrate specificities between the uptake transporters (OATP family) and efflux transporters (MRP family) make the vectorial transport of organic

anions highly efficient. Similar transport systems also are present in the intestine, renal tubules, and endothelial cells of the brain capillaries (Figure 2–5).

Regulation of Transporter Expression. Transporter expression can be regulated transcriptionally in response to drug treatment and pathophysiological conditions, resulting in induction or downregulation of transporter mRNAs. Recent studies have described important roles of type II nuclear receptors, which form heterodimers with the 9-cis-retinoic acid receptor (RXR), in regulating drug-metabolizing enzymes and transporters (Kullak-Ublick *et al.*, 2004; Wang and LeCluyse, 2003). Such receptors include pregnane X receptor (PXR/NR1I2), constitutive androstane receptor (CAR/NR1I3), farnesoid X receptor (FXR/NR1H4), PPARα (peroxisome proliferator-activated receptor α), and retinoic acid receptor (RAR). Except for CAR, these are ligand-activated nuclear receptors that, as heterodimers with RXR, bind specific elements in the enhancer regions of target genes. CAR has constitutive transcriptional activity that is antagonized by inverse agonists such as *androstenol* and *androstanol* and induced by barbiturates. PXR, also referred to as *steroid X receptor* (SXR) in humans, is activated by synthetic and endogenous steroids, bile acids, and drugs such as *clotrimazole, phenobarbital, rifampicin, sulfinpyrazone, ritonavir, carbamazepine, phenytoin, sulfadimidine, taxol,* and *hyperforin* (a constituent of St. John's wort). Table 2–1 summarizes the effects of drug activation of type II nuclear receptors on expression of transporters. The potency of activators of PXR varies among species such that rodents are not necessarily a model for effects in humans. There is an overlap of substrates between CYP3A4 and P-glycoprotein, and PXR mediates coinduction of CYP3A4 and P-glycoprotein, supporting their synergetic cooperation in efficient detoxification. *See* Table 3–4 and Figure 3–13 for information on the role of type II nuclear receptors in induction of drug-metabolizing enzymes.

Table 2–1
Regulation of Transporter Expression by Nuclear Receptors

TRANSPORTER	SPECIES	TRANSCRIPTION FACTOR	LIGAND (DOSE)	EFFECT OF LIGAND
MDR1 (P-gp)	Human	PXR		↑ Transcription activity (promoter assay)
			Rifampicin (600 mg/day, 10 days)	↑ Expression in duodenum in healthy subjects
			Rifampicin (600 mg/day, 10 days	↓ Oral bioavailability of digoxin in healthy subjects
			Rifampicin (600 mg/day, 9 days)	↓ AUC of talinolol after IV and oral administration in healthy subjects
MRP2	Human	PXR	Rifampicin (600 mg/day, 9 days)	↑ Expression in duodenum in healthy subjects
			Rifampicin/hyperforin	↑ Expression in human hepatocytes
		FXR	GW4064/chenodeoxy-cholate	↑ Expression in HepG2 cells
	Mouse	PXR	PCN/dexamethasone	↑ Expression in mouse hepatocyte
		CAR	Phenobarbital	↑ Expression in hepatocyte of PXR KO mice (promoter assay)
	Rat	PXR/FXR/CAR	PCN/GW4064/phenobar-bital	↑ Expression in rat hepatocytes
		PXR/FXR/CAR		↑ Transcription activity (promoter assay)
BSEP	Human	FXR	Chenodeoxycholate, GW4064	↑ Transcription activity (promoter assay)
Ntcp	Rat	SHP1		↓ RAR mediated transcription
OATP1B1	Human	SHP1		Indirect effect on HNF1a expression
OATP1B3	Human	FXR	Chenodeoxycholate	↑ Expression in hepatoma cells
MDR2	Mouse	PPARa	Ciprofibrate (0.05% w/w in diet)	↑ Expression in the liver

See Geick *et al.*, 2001; Greiner *et al.*, 1999; Kok *et al.*, 2003.

MOLECULAR STRUCTURES OF TRANSPORTERS

Predictions of secondary structure of membrane transport proteins based on hydropathy analysis indicate that membrane transporters in the SLC and ABC superfamilies are multi-membrane-spanning proteins. A typical predicted secondary structure of the ABC transporter MRP2 (*ABCC2*) is shown in Figure 2–6. However, understanding the secondary structure of a membrane transporter provides little information on how the transporter functions to translocate its substrates. For this, information on the tertiary structure of the transporter is

needed, along with complementary molecular information about the residues in the transporter that are involved in the recognition, association, and dissociation of its substrates.

To obtain high-resolution structures of membrane proteins, the proteins first must be crystallized, and then the crystal structure must be deduced from analysis of x-ray diffraction patterns. Crystal structures generally are difficult to obtain for membrane proteins primarily because of their amphipathic needs for stabilization. Further, membrane proteins generally are in low abundance, so obtaining sufficient quantities for structural determination is difficult. The few membrane transporters that have been crystallized are bacterial proteins that can be expressed in high abundance. Information on two representative membrane transporters that have been crystallized and analyzed at relatively high resolu-

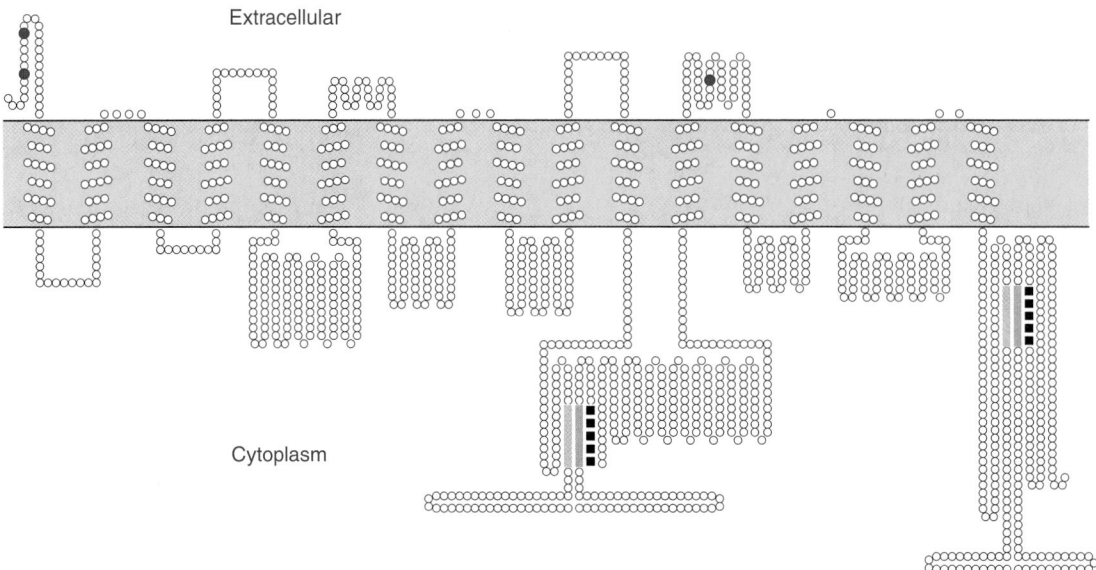

Extracellular

Cytoplasm

Figure 2–6. *Predicted secondary structure of MRP2 based on hydropathy analysis.* The *dark blue circles* depict glycosylation sites; Walker A motif is colored *light blue; black* boxes represent the Walker B motif. *Light gray* is the middle region between the two motifs. The Walker A motifs interact with α and β phosphates of di- and tri-nucleotides; the Walker B motifs help to coordinate Mg^{2+}.

tion (<4 Å) serves to illustrate some basic structural properties of membrane transporters. One of the transporters, MsbA, is an ABC transporter from *E. coli* with homology to multidrug-resistance efflux pumps in mammals. The second transporter, LacY, is a proton symporter, also from *E. coli*, that translocates lactose and other oligosaccharides. Each of these transporters is illustrative of a different transport mechanism.

Lipid Flippase (MsbA). MsbA is an ABC transporter in *E. coli* that, like other ABC transporters, hydrolyzes ATP to export its substrate. Based on an x-ray crystal structure, MsbA forms a homodimer consisting of two six-transmembrane units, each with a nucleotide-binding domain on the cytoplasmic surface (Chang and Roth, 2001) (Figure 2–7). The hexaspanning unit consists of six α-helices. There is a central chamber with an asymmetrical distribution of charged residues. A transport mechanism that is consistent with this asymmetrical distribution of charges is a "flippase" mechanism. That is, substrates in the inner leaflet of the bilayer are recognized by MsbA and then flipped to the outer leaflet of the bilayer. This hypothetical mechanism, although intriguing, leaves many questions unanswered. For example, how is the energy of ATP hydrolysis coupled to the flipping process? Once in the outer leaflet, how are substrates translocated to the extracellular space? Nevertheless, from this structure and other structures, we now know that transmembrane domains form α-helices, that six-unit dimers are central to the transport mechanism, and that there is an asymmetrical distribution of charged residues in a central chamber.

Lactose Permease Symporter (LacY). Lactose permease is a bacterial transporter that belongs to the *m*ajor *f*acilitator *s*uperfamily (MFS). This transporter is a proton-coupled symporter. A high-resolution X-ray crystal structure has been obtained for the proto-

nated form of a mutant of LacY (C154G) at a 3.5-Å α-resolution (Abramson *et al.*, 2003) (Figure 2–8). In brief, LacY is comprised of two units of six membrane-spanning α-helices. The crystal structure showed substrate located at the interface of the

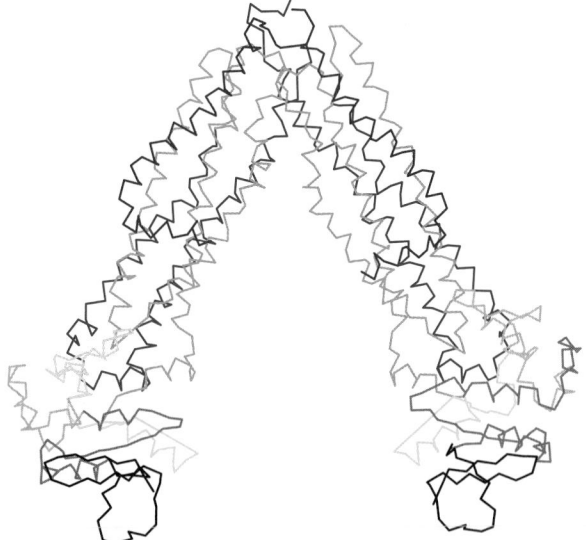

Figure 2–7. *Structure showing the backbone of MsbA from E. coli.* The structure shows a central chamber and a homodimer formed by units of six-transmembrane α-helices. Structure was reconstructed by Libusha Kelly using the coordinates deposited in the Protein Data Bank (PDB; *http://www.rcsb.org/pdb/*).

two units and in the middle of the membrane. This location is consistent with an alternating-access transport mechanism in which the substrate recognition site is accessible to the cytosolic and then the extracellular surface but not to both simultaneously. Eight helices form the surface of the hydrophilic cavity, and each contains proline and glycine residues that result in kinks in the cavity. From LacY, we now know that as in the case of MsbA, six membrane-spanning α-helices are critical structural units for transport by LacY.

TRANSPORTER SUPERFAMILIES IN THE HUMAN GENOME

Two major gene superfamilies play critical roles in the transport of drugs across plasma and other biological membranes: the SLC and ABC superfamilies. Web sites that have information on these families include *http://nutrigene.4t.com/humanabc.htm* (ABC superfamily), *http://www.biopara-digms.org/slc/intro.asp* (SLC superfamily), *http://www.pharmaconference.org/slctable.asp* (SLC superfamily), and *http://www.TP_Search.jp/* (drug transporters). Information on pharmacogenetics of these transporters can be found in Chapter 4 and at *http://www.pharmgkb.org* and *http://www.pharmacogenetics.ucsf.edu.*

SLC Transporters. The solute carrier (SLC) superfamily includes 43 families and represents approximately 300 genes in the human genome. The nomenclature of the transporters within each family is listed under the Human Genome Organization (HUGO) Nomenclature Committee database at *http://www.gene.ucl.ac.uk/nomenclature/.* Table 2–2 lists the families in the human SLC superfamily and some of the genetic diseases that are associated with members of selected families. The family name provides a description of the function(s) of each family. However, some caution should be exercised in interpretation of family names because individual family members may have vastly different specificities or functional roles. All the SLC families with members in the human genome were reviewed recently (Hediger, 2004). In brief, transporters in the SLC superfamily transport diverse ionic and nonionic endogenous compounds and xenobiotics. SLC superfamily transporters may be facilitated transporters or secondary active symporters or antiporters. The first SLC family transporter was cloned in 1987 by expression cloning in *Xenopus laevis* oocytes (Hediger *et al.*, 1987). Since then, many transporters in the SLC superfamily have been cloned and characterized functionally. Predictive models defining important characteristics of substrate binding and knockout mouse models defining the *in vivo* role of specific transporters

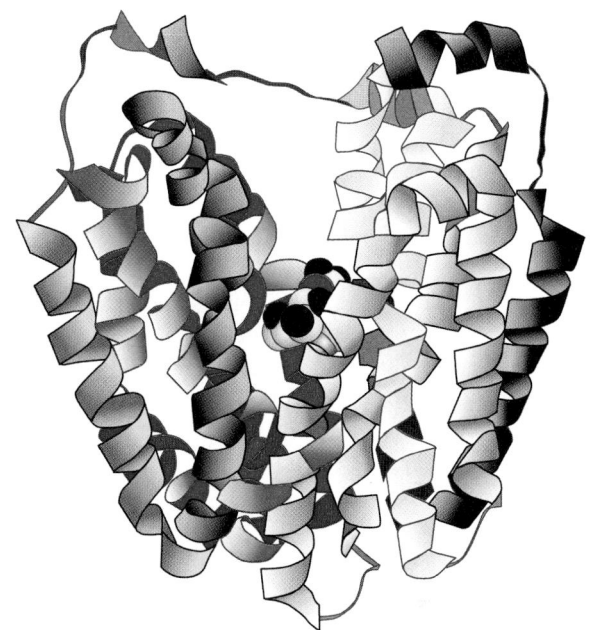

Figure 2–8. *Structure of the protonated form of a mutant of LacY.* Two units of six-membrane-spanning α-helices (shown as *colored ribbons*) are present. Substrate (depicted as *gray and black balls*) is bound to the interface of the two units and in the middle of the membrane. Structure has been redrawn from coordinates in Protein Data Bank (*http://www.rcsb.org/pdb/*).

have been constructed for many SLC transporters (Chang *et al.*, 2004; Ocheltree *et al.*, 2004). In general, in this chapter we focus on SLC transporters in the human genome, which are designated by capital letters (SLC transporters in rodent genomes are designated by lowercase letters).

ABC Superfamily. In 1976, Juliano and Ling reported that overexpression of a membrane protein in *colchicine*-resistant Chinese hamster ovary cells also resulted in acquired resistance to many structurally unrelated drugs (*i.e.*, multidrug resistance) (Juliano and Ling, 1976). Since the cDNA cloning of this first mammalian ABC protein (P-glycoprotein/MDR1/ABCB1), the ABC superfamily has continued to grow; it now consists of 49 genes, each containing one or two conserved ABC regions (Borst and Elferink, 2002). The ABC region is a core catalytic domain of ATP hydrolysis and contains Walker A and B sequences and an ABC transporter-specific signature C sequence (Figure 2–6). The ABC regions of these proteins bind and hydrolyze ATP, and the proteins use the energy for uphill transport of their substrates across the membrane. Although

Table 2–2
Families in the Human Solute Carrier Superfamily

GENE NAME	FAMILY NAME	NUMBER OF FAMILY MEMBERS	SELECTED DRUG SUBSTRATES	EXAMPLES OF LINKED HUMAN DISEASES
SLC1	High-affinity glutamate and neutral amino acid transporter	7		Amyotrophic lateral sclerosis
SLC2	Facilitative GLUT transporter	14		
SLC3	Heavy subunits of the heteromeric amino acid transporters	2	Melphalin	Classic cystinuria type I
SLC4	Bicarbonate transporter	10		Hemolytic anemia, blindness–auditory impairment
SLC5	Na$^+$ glucose cotransporter	8	Glucosfamide	Glucose–galactose malabsorption syndrome
SLC6	Na$^+$- and Cl$^-$-dependent neurotransmitter transporter	16	Paraoxetine, fluoxetine	X-linked creatine deficiency syndrome
SLC7	Cationic amino acid transporter	14	Melphalin	Lysinuric protein intolerance
SLC8	Na$^+$/Ca^{2+} exchanger	3	Asymmetrical dimethylarginine	
SLC9	Na$^+$/H$^+$ exchanger	8	Thiazide diuretics	Congenital secretory diarrhea
SLC10	Na$^+$ bile salt cotransporter	6	Benzothiazepine	Primary bile salt malabsorption
SLC11	H$^+$ coupled metal ion transporter	2		Hereditary hemochromatosis
SLC12	Electroneutral cation–Cl$^-$ cotransporter family	9		Gitelman's syndrome
SLC13	Na$^+$–sulfate/carboxylate cotransporter	5	Sulfate, cysteine conjugates	
SLC14	Urea transporter	2		Kidd antigen blood group
SLC15	H$^+$–oligopeptide cotransporter	4	Valacyclovir	
SLC16	Monocarboxylate transporter	14	Salicylate, atorvastatin	Muscle weakness
SLC17	Vesicular glutamate transporter	8		Sialic acid storage disease
SLC18	Vesicular amine transporter	3	Reserpine	Myasthenic syndromes
SLC19	Folate/thiamine transporter	3	Methotrexate	Thiamine-responsive megaloblastic anemia
SLC20	Type III Na$^+$–phosphate cotransporter	2		
SLC21/ SLC0	Organic anion transporter	11	Pravastatin	
SLC22	Organic cation/anion/zwitterion transporter	18	Pravastatin, metformin	Systemic carnitine deficiency syndrome
SLC23	Na$^+$-dependent ascorbate transporter	4	Vitamin C	
SLC24	Na$^+$/(Ca^{2+}-K$^+$) exchanger	5		
SLC25	Mitochondrial carrier	27		Senger's syndrome
SLC26	Multifunctional anion exchanger	10	Salicylate, ciprofloxacin	Congenital Cl$^-$-losing diarrhea
SLC27	Fatty acid transporter protein	6		

(Continued)

Table 2–2
Families in the Human Solute Carrier Superfamily (Continued)

GENE NAME	FAMILY NAME	NUMBER OF FAMILY MEMBERS	SELECTED DRUG SUBSTRATES	EXAMPLES OF LINKED HUMAN DISEASES
SLC28	Na$^+$-coupled nucleoside transport	3	Gemcitabine, cladribine	
SLC29	Facilitative nucleoside transporter	4	Dipyridamole, gemcitabine	
SLC30	Zinc efflux	9		
SLC31	Copper transporter	2	Cisplatin	
SLC32	Vesicular inhibitory amino acid transporter	1	Vigabatrin	
SLC33	Acetyl-CoA transporter	1		
SLC34	Type II Na$^+$–phosphate cotransporter	3		Autosomal-dominant hypo-phosphatemic rickets
SLC35	Nucleoside-sugar transporter	17		Leukocyte adhesion deficiency type II
SLC36	H$^+$-coupled amino acid transporter	4	D-Serine, D-cycloserine	
SLC37	Sugar-phosphate/phosphate exchanger	4		Glycogen storage disease non-1a
SLC38	System A and N, Na$^+$-coupled neutral amino acid transporter	6		
SLC39	Metal ion transporter	14		Acrodermatitis enteropathica
SLC40	Basolateral iron transporter	1		Type IV hemochromatosis
SLC41	MgtE-like magnesium transporter	3		
SLC42	Rh ammonium transporter (pending)	3		Rh-null regulator
SLC43	Na$^+$-independent system-L-like amino acid transporter	2		

some ABC superfamily transporters contain only a single ABC motif, they form homodimers (BCRP/ABCG2) or heterodimers (ABCG5 and ABCG8) that exhibit a transport function. ABC transporters (*e.g.,* MsbA) (Figure 2–7) also are found in prokaryotes, where they are involved predominantly in the import of essential compounds that cannot be obtained by passive diffusion (sugars, vitamins, metals, etc.). By contrast, most ABC genes in eukaryotes transport compounds from the cytoplasm to the outside or into an intracellular compartment (endoplasmic reticulum, mitochondria, peroxisomes).

ABC transporters can be divided into seven groups based on their sequence homology: ABCA (12 members), ABCB (11 members), ABCC (13 members), ABCD (4 members), ABCE (1 member), ABCF (3 members), and ABCG (5 members). ABC genes are essential for many cellular processes, and mutations in at least 13 of these genes cause or contribute to human genetic disorders (Table 2–3).

In addition to conferring multidrug resistance (Sadee *et al.,* 1995), an important pharmacological aspect of these transporters is xenobiotic export from healthy tissues. In particular, MDR1/ABCB1, MRP2/ABCC2, and BCRP/ABCG2 have been shown to be involved in overall drug disposition (Leslie *et al.,* 2005).

Properties of ABC Transporters Related to Drug Action

The tissue distribution of drug-related ABC transporters in the body is summarized in Table 2–4 together with information about typical substrates.

Tissue Distribution of Drug-Related ABC Transporters. MDR1 (*ABCB1*), MRP2 (*ABCC2*), and BCRP (*ABCG2*) are all expressed in the apical side of the intestinal epithelia, where they serve to

Table 2–3

The ATP Binding Cassette (ABC) Superfamily in the Human Genome and Linked Genetic Diseases

GENE NAME	FAMILY NAME	NUMBER OF FAMILY MEMBERS	EXAMPLES OF LINKED HUMAN DISEASES
ABCA	ABC A	12	Tangier disease (defect in cholesterol transport; ABCA1), Stargardt syndrome (defect in retinal metabolism; ABCA4)
ABCB	ABC B	11	Bare lymphocyte syndrome type I (defect in antigen-presenting; ABCB3 and ABCB4), progressive familial intrahepatic cholestasis type 3 (defect in biliary lipid secretion; MDR3/ABCB4), X-linked sideroblastic anemia with ataxia (a possible defect in iron homeostasis in mitochondria; ABCB7), progressive familial intrahepatic cholestasis type 2 (defect in biliary bile acid excretion; BSEP/ABCB11)
ABCC	ABC C	13	Dubin–Johnson syndrome (defect in biliary bilirubin glururonide excretion; MRP2/ABCC2), pseudoxanthoma (unknown mechanism; ABCC6), cystic fibrosis (defect in chloride channel regulation; ABCC7), persistent hyperinsulinemic hypoglycemia of infancy (defect in inwardly rectifying potassium conductance regulation in pancreatic B cells; SUR1)
ABCD	ABC D	4	Adrenoleukodystrophy (a possible defect in peroxisomal transport or catabolism of very long-chain fatty acids; ABCD1)
ABCE	ABC E	1	
ABCF	ABC F	3	
ABCG	ABC G	5	Sitosterolemia (defect in biliary and intestinal excretion of plant sterols; ABCG5 and ABCG8)

pump out xenobiotics, including many clinically relevant drugs. The kidney and liver are major organs for overall systemic drug elimination from the body. The liver also plays a role in presystemic drug elimination. Key to the vectorial excretion of drugs into urine or bile, ABC transporters are expressed in the polarized tissues of kidney and liver: MDR1, MRP2, and MRP4 (*ABCC4*) on the brush-border membrane of renal epithelia, and MDR1, MRP2, and BCRP on the bile canalicular membrane of hepatocytes. Some ABC transporters are expressed specifically on the blood side of the endothelial or epithelial cells that form barriers to the free entrance of toxic compounds into naive tissues: the BBB (MDR1 and MRP4 on the luminal side of brain capillary endothelial cells), the blood–cerebrospinal fluid (CSF) barrier (MRP1 and MRP4 on the basolateral blood side of choroid plexus epithelia), the blood–testis barrier (MRP1 on the basolateral membrane of mouse Sertoli cells and MDR1 in several types of human testicular cells), and the blood–placenta barrier (MDR1, MRP2, and BCRP on the luminal maternal side and MRP1 on the antiluminal fetal side of placental trophoblasts).

Substrate Specificity of ABC Transporters. MDR1/ABCB1 substrates tend to share a hydrophobic planar structure with positively charged or neutral moieties as described in Table 2–4 (*see also* Ambudkar *et al.*, 1999). These include structurally and pharmacologically unrelated compounds, many of which are also substrates of CYP3A4, a major drug-metabolizing enzyme in the human liver and GI tract. Such overlapping substrate specificity implies a synergistic role for MDR1 and CYP3A4 in protecting the body by reducing the intestinal absorption of xenobiotics (Zhang and Benet, 2001). After being taken up by enterocytes, some drug molecules are metabolized by CYP3A4. Drug molecules that escape metabolic conversion are eliminated from the cells *via* MDR1 and then reenter the enterocytes. The intestinal residence time of the drug is prolonged with the aid of MDR1, thereby increasing the chance of local metabolic conversion by the CYP3A4 (*see* Chapter 3).

MRP/ABCC Family. The substrates of transporters in the MRP/ABCC family are mostly organic anions. The substrate specificities of MRP1 and MRP2 are similar: Both accept glutathione and glucuronide conjugates, sulfated conjugates of bile salts, and nonconjugated organic anions of an amphipathic nature (at least one negative charge and some degree of hydrophobicity). They also transport neutral or cationic anticancer drugs, such as *vinca alkaloids* and *anthracyclines*, possibly *via* a cotransport or symport mechanism with reduced glutathione (GSH).

MRP3 also has a substrate specificity that is similar to that of MRP2 but with a lower transport affinity for glutathione conjugates compared with MRP1 and MRP2. Most characteristic MRP3 substrates are monovalent bile salts, which are never transported by MRP1 and MRP2. Because MRP3 is expressed on the

Table 2–4
ABC Transporters Involved in Drug Absorption, Distribution, and Excretion

TRANSPORTER NAME	TISSUE DISTRIBUTION	PHYSIOLOGICAL FUNCTION	SUBSTRATES
MDR1 (ABCB1)	Liver Kidney Intestine BBB BTB BPB	Detoxification of xenobiotics?	**Characteristics:** Neutral or cationic compounds with bulky structure **Anticancer drugs:** etoposide, doxorubicin, vincristine **Ca^{2+} channel blockers:** diltiazem, verapamil **HIV protease inhibitors:** indinavir, ritonavir **Antibiotics/antifungals:** erythromycin, ketoconazole **Hormones:** testosterone, progesterone **Immunosuppressants:** cyclosporine, FK506 (tacrolimus) **Others:** digoxin, quinidine
MRP1 (ABCC1)	Ubiquitous (kidney, BCSFB, BTB)	Leukotriene (LTC$_4$) secretion from leukocyte	**Characteristics:** Amphiphilic with at least one negative net charge **Anticancer drugs:** vincristine (with GSH), methotrexate **Glutathione conjugates:** LTC$_4$, glutathione conjugate of ethacrynic acid **Glucuronide conjugates:** estradiol-17-D-glucuronide, bilirubin mono(or bis)glucuronide **Sulfated conjugates:** estrone-3-sulfate (with GSH) **HIV protease inhibitors:** saquinavir **Antifungals:** grepafloxacin **Others:** folate, GSH, oxidized glutathione
MRP2 (ABCC2)	Liver Kidney Intestine BPB	Excretion of bilirubin glucuronide and GSH into bile	**Characteristics:** Amphiphilic with at least one negative net charge (similar to MRP1) **Anticancer drugs:** methotrexate, vincristine **Glutathione conjugates:** LTC$_4$, GSH conjugate of ethacrynic acid **Glucuronide conjugates:** estradiol-17-D-glucuronide, bilirubin mono(or bis)glucuronide **Sulfate conjugate of bile salts:** taurolithocholate sulfate **HIV protease inhibitors:** indinavir, ritonavir **Others:** pravastatin, GSH, oxidized glutathione
MRP3 (ABCC3)	Liver Kidney Intestine	?	**Characteristics:** Amphiphilic with at least one negative net charge (Glucuronide conjugates are better substrates than glutathione conjugates.) **Anticancer drugs:** etoposide, methotrexate **Glutathione conjugates:** LTC$_4$, glutathione conjugate of 15-deoxy-delta prostaglandin J2 **Glucuronide conjugates:** estradiol-17-D-glucuronide, etoposide glucuronide **Sulfate conjugates of bile salts:** taurolithocholate sulfate **Bile salts:** glycocholate, taurocholate **Others:** folate, leucovorin

(Continued)

Table 2–4
ABC Transporters Involved in Drug Absorption, Distribution, and Excretion (Continued)

TRANSPORTER NAME	TISSUE DISTRIBUTION	PHYSIOLOGICAL FUNCTION	SUBSTRATES
MRP4 (ABCC4)	Ubiquitous (kidney, prostate, lung, muscle, pancreas, testis, ovary, bladder, gallbladder, BBB, BCSFB)	?	**Characteristics:** Nucleotide analogues **Anticancer drugs:** 6-mercaptopurine, methotrexate **Glucuronide conjugates:** estradiol-17-D-glucuronide **Cyclic nucleotides:** cyclic AMP, cyclic GMP **HIV protease inhibitors:** adefovir **Others:** folate, leucovorin, taurocholate (with GSH)
MRP5 (ABCC5)	Ubiquitous	?	**Characteristics:** Nucleotide analogues **Anticancer drugs:** 6-mercaptopurine **Cyclic nucleotides:** cyclic AMP, cyclic GMP **HIV protease inhibitors:** adefovir
MRP6 (ABCC6)	Liver Kidney	?	**Anticancer drugs:** doxorubicin*, etoposide* **Glutathione conjugate of:** LTC_4 **Other:** BQ-123 (cyclic peptide ET-1 antagonist)
BCRP (MXR) (ABCG2)	Liver Intestine BBB	Normal heme transport during maturation of erythrocytes	**Anticancer drugs:** methotrexate, mitoxantrone, camptothecin analogs (SN-38, etc.), topotecan **Glucuronide conjugates:** 4-methylumbelliferone glucuronide, estradiol-17-D-glucuronide **Sulfate conjugates:** dehydroepiandrosterone sulfate, estrone-3-sulfate **Others:** cholesterol, estradiol
MDR3 (ABCB4)	Liver	Excretion of phospholipids into bile	**Characteristics:** Phospholipids
BSEP (ABCB11)	Liver	Excretion of bile salts into bile	**Characteristics:** Bile salts
ABCG5 and ABCG8	Liver Intestine	Excretion of plant sterols into bile and intestinal lumen	**Characteristics:** Plant sterols

NOTE: Representative substrates and cytotoxic drugs with increased resistance (*) are included in this table (cytotoxicity with increased resistance is usually caused by the decreased accumulation of the drugs). Although MDR3 (ABCB4), BSEP (ABCB11), ABCG5, and ABCG8 are not directly involved in drug disposition, inhibition of these physiologically important ABC transporters will lead to unfavorable side effects.

sinusoidal side of hepatocytes and is induced under cholestatic conditions, backflux of toxic bile salts and bilirubin glucuronides into the blood circulation is considered to be its physiological function.

MRP4 and MRP5 have narrower substrate specificities. They accept nucleotide analogues and clinically important anti–human immunodeficiency virus (HIV) drugs. Although some transport substrates have been identified for MRP6, no physiologically important endogenous substrates have been identified that explain the mechanism of the MRP6-associated disease pseudoxanthoma.

BCRP/ABCG2. BCRP accepts both neutral and negatively charged molecules, including cytotoxic compounds (*e.g., mitoxantrone, topotecan, flavopiridol,* and *methotrexate*), sulfated conjugates of therapeutic drugs and hormones (*e.g., estrogen sulfate*), and toxic compounds found in normal food [2-amino-1-methyl-6-phenylimidazo[4,5-*b*]pyridine (PhIP) and pheophorbide A, a chlorophyll catabolite].

Physiological Roles of ABC Transporters. The physiological significance of the ABC transporters is illustrated by studies involving knockout animals or patients with genetic defects in these transporters. Mice deficient in MDR1 function are viable and fertile and do not display obvious phenotypic abnormalities other than hypersensitivity to toxic drugs, including the neurotoxic pesticide ivermectin (one hundredfold) and the carcinostatic drug *vinblastine* (threefold) (Schinkel *et al.*, 1994). *mrp1* (–/–) mice are also viable and fertile without any obvious difference in litter size. However, these mice are hypersensitive to the anticancer drug *etoposide*. Damage is especially severe in the testis, kidney, and oropharyngeal mucosa, where MRP1 is expressed on the basolateral membrane. Moreover, these mice have an impaired response to an arachidonic acid–induced inflammatory stimulus, which is likely due to a reduced secretion of leukotriene C4 from mast cells, macrophages, and granulocytes. MRP2-deficient rats (TR– and EHBR) and Dubin–Johnson syndrome patients are normal in appearance except for mild jaundice owing to impaired biliary excretion of bilirubin glucuronide (Ito *et al.*, 1997; Paulusma *et al.*, 1996).

BCRP knockout mice are viable but highly sensitive to the dietary chlorophyll catabolite phenophorbide, which induces phototoxicity. These mice also exhibit protoporphyria, with a tenfold increase in protoporphyrin IX accumulation in erythrocytes, resulting in photosensitivity. This protoporphyria is caused by the impaired function of BCRP in bone marrow: Knockout mice transplanted with bone marrow from wild-type mice become normal with respect to protoporphyrin IX level in the erythrocytes and photosensitivity.

As described earlier, complete absence of these drug-related ABC transporters is not lethal and even can remain unrecognized without exogenous perturbation owing to food, drugs, or toxins. Inhibition of physiologically important ABC transporters (especially those related directly to the genetic diseases described in Table 2–3) by drugs should be avoided to reduce the incidence of drug-induced side effects.

ABC Transporters in Drug Absorption and Elimination. With respect to clinical medicine, MDR1 is the most important ABC transporter yet identified, and digoxin is one of the most widely studied of its substrates. The systemic exposure to orally administered digoxin (as assessed by the area under the plasma digoxin concentration–time curve) is increased by coadministration of *rifampin* (an MDR1 inducer) and is negatively correlated with the MDR1 protein expression in the human intestine. MDR1 is also expressed on the brush-border membrane of renal epithelia, and its function can be monitored using digoxin as a probe drug. Digoxin undergoes very little degradation in the liver, and renal excretion is the major elimination pathway (>70%) in humans. Several studies in healthy subjects have been performed with MDR1 inhibitors (*e.g.*, quinidine, *verapamil, vaspodar, spironolactone, clarithromycin,* and *ritonavir*) with digoxin as a probe drug, and all resulted in a marked reduction in the renal excretion of digoxin. Similarly, the intestinal absorption of *cyclosporine* is also related mainly to the MDR1 level rather than to the CYP3A4 level, although cyclosporine is a substrate of both CYP3A4 and MDR1.

Alteration of MDR1 activity by inhibitors (drug–drug interactions) affects oral absorption and renal clearance. Drugs with narrow therapeutic windows (such as the cardiac glycoside digoxin and the immunosuppressants cyclosporine and *tacrolimus*) should be used with great care if MDR1-based drug–drug interactions are likely.

Despite the broad substrate specificity and distinct localization of MRP2 and BCRP in drug-handling tissues (both expressed on the canalicular membrane of hepatocytes and the brush-border membrane of enterocytes), there has been very little integration of clinically relevant information. Part of the problem lies in distinguishing the biliary transport activities of MRP2 and BCRP from the contribution of the hepatic uptake transporters of the OATP family. Most MRP2 or BCRP substrates also can be transported by the OATP family transporters on the sinusoidal membrane. The rate-limiting process for systemic elimination is uptake in most cases. Under such conditions, the effect of drug–drug interactions (or genetic variants) in these biliary transporters may be difficult to identify. Despite such practical difficulties, there is a steady increase in the information about genetic variants and their effects on transporter expression and activity *in vitro*. Variants of BCRP with high allele frequencies (0.184 for V12M and 0.239 for Q141K) have been found to alter the substrate specificity in cellular assays. The clinical impact of these variants and drug–drug interactions needs to be studied in more detail in humans and under *in vivo* conditions using appropriate probe drugs.

GENETIC VARIATION IN MEMBRANE TRANSPORTERS: IMPLICATIONS FOR CLINICAL DRUG RESPONSE

Inherited defects in membrane transport have been known for many years, and the genes associated with several inherited disorders of membrane transport have been identified [Table 2–2 (SLC) and Table 2–3 (ABC)]. Reports of polymorphisms in membrane transporters that play a role in drug response have appeared only recently, but the field is growing rapidly. Cellular studies have focused on genetic variation in only a few drug transporters, but progress has been made in characterizing the functional impact of variants in these transporters. Further, large-scale studies in the area of single-nucleotide polymorphisms (SNPs) in membrane transporters and cellular characterization of transporter variants have been performed (Burman *et al.*, 2004; Gray *et al.*, 2004; Leabman *et al.*, 2003; Osato *et al.*, 2003; Shu *et al.*, 2003) (*see* Chapter 4). The clinical impact of membrane transporter variants on drug response has been studied only recently. Like the cellular studies, the clinical studies have focused on a limited number of transporters.

The most widely studied drug transporter is P-glycoprotein (MDR1, *ABCB1*), and results from clinical studies have been controversial. Associations of the *ABCB1* genotype with responses to anticancer drugs, antiviral agents, immunosuppressants, antihistamines, cardiac glycosides, and anticonvulsants have been described (Anglicheau *et al.*, 2003; Drescher *et al.*, 2002; Fellay *et al.*, 2002; Hoffmeyer *et al.*, 2000; Illmer *et al.*, 2002; Johne *et al.*, 2002; Macphee *et al.*, 2002; Pauli-Magnus *et al.*, 2003; Sai *et al.*, 2003; Sakaeda *et al.*, 2003; Siddiqui *et al.*,

2003; Verstuyft *et al.*, 2003). *ABCB1* SNPs also have been associated with tacrolimus and *nortriptyline* neurotoxicity (Roberts *et al.*, 2002; Yamauchi *et al.*, 2002) and susceptibility for developing ulcerative colitis, renal cell carcinoma, and Parkinson's disease (Drozdzik *et al.*, 2003; Schwab *et al.*, 2003; Siegsmund *et al.*, 2002).

Recently, two common SNPs in *SLCO1B1* (OATP1B1) have been associated with elevated plasma levels of pravastatin, a widely used drug for the treatment of hypercholesterolemia (Mwinyi *et al.*, 2004; Niemi *et al.*, 2004) (*see* Chapter 35).

TRANSPORTERS INVOLVED IN PHARMACOKINETICS

Hepatic Transporters

Drug transporters play an important role in pharmacokinetics (Koepsell, 1998; Zamek-Gliszczynski and Brouwer, 2004) (Figure 2–1). Hepatic uptake of organic anions (*e.g.*, drugs, leukotrienes, and bilirubin), cations, and bile salts is mediated by SLC-type transporters in the basolateral (sinusoidal) membrane of hepatocytes: OATPs (SLCO) (Abe *et al.*, 1999; Konig *et al.*, 2000) and OATs (SLC22) (Sekine *et al.*, 1998), OCTs (SLC22) (Koepsell, 1998) and NTCP (SLC10A1) (Hagenbuch *et al.*, 1991), respectively. These transporters mediate uptake by either facilitated or secondary active mechanisms.

ABC transporters such as MRP2, MDR1, BCRP, BSEP, and MDR2 in the bile canalicular membrane of hepatocytes mediate the efflux (excretion) of drugs and their metabolites, bile salts, and phospholipids against a steep concentration gradient from liver to bile. This primary active transport is driven by ATP hydrolysis. Some ABC transporters are also present in the basolateral membrane of hepatocytes and may play a role in the efflux of drugs back into the blood, although their physiological role remains to be elucidated. Drug uptake followed by metabolism and excretion in the liver is a major determinant of the systemic clearance of many drugs. Since clearance ultimately determines systemic blood levels, transporters in the liver play key roles in setting drug levels.

Vectorial transport of drugs from the circulating blood to the bile using an uptake transporter (OATP family) and an efflux transporter (MRP2) is important for determining drug exposure in the circulating blood and liver. Moreover, there are many other uptake and efflux transporters in the liver (Figure 2–9). Two examples illustrate the

importance of vectorial transport in determining drug exposure in the circulating blood and liver: HMG-CoA reductase inhibitors and angiotensin-converting enzyme (ACE) inhibitors.

HMG-CoA Reductase Inhibitors. Statins are cholesterol-lowering agents that reversibly inhibit HMG-CoA reductase, which catalyzes a rate-limiting step in cholesterol biosynthesis (*see* Chapter 35). Statins affect serum cholesterol by inhibiting cholesterol biosynthesis in the liver, and this organ is their main target. On the other hand, exposure of extrahepatic cells in smooth muscle to these drugs may cause adverse effects. Among the statins, pravastatin, *fluvastatin, cerivastatin, atorvastatin, rosuvastatin,* and *pitavastatin* are given in a biologically active open-acid form, whereas *simvastatin* and *lovastatin* are administered as inactive prodrugs with lactone rings. The open-acid statins are relatively hydrophilic and have low membrane permeabilities. However, most of the statins in the acid form are substrates of uptake transporters, so they are taken up efficiently by the liver and undergo enterohepatic circulation (Figures 2–5 and 2–9). In this process, hepatic uptake transporters such as OATP1B1 and efflux transporters such as MRP2 act cooperatively to produce vectorial transcellular transport of bisubstrates in the liver. The efficient first-pass hepatic uptake of these statins by OATP1B1 after their oral administration helps to exert the pharmacological effect and also minimizes the escape of drug molecules into the circulating blood, thereby minimizing the exposure in a target of adverse response, smooth muscle. Recent studies indicate that the genetic polymorphism of OATP1B1 also affects the function of this transporter (Tirona *et al.*, 2001).

Temocapril. *Temocapril* is an ACE inhibitor (*see* Chapter 30). Its active metabolite, temocaprilat, is excreted both in the bile and in the urine *via* the liver and kidney, respectively, whereas other ACE inhibitors are excreted mainly *via* the kidney. The special feature of temocapril among ACE inhibitors is that the plasma concentration of temocaprilat remains relatively unchanged even in patients with renal failure. However, the plasma area under the curve *AUC* of *enalaprilat* and other ACE inhibitors is markedly increased in patients with renal disorders. Temocaprilat is a bisubstrate of the OATP family and MRP2, whereas other ACE inhibitors are not good substrates of MRP2 (although they are taken up into the liver by the OATP family). Taking these findings into consideration, the affinity for MRP2 may dominate in determining the biliary excretion of any series of ACE inhibitors. Drugs that are excreted into both the bile and urine to the same degree thus are expected to exhibit minimum interindividual differences in their pharmacokinetics.

Irinotecan (CPT-11). *Irinotecan hydrochloride* (CPT-11) is a potent anticancer drug, but late-onset gastrointestinal toxic effects, such as severe diarrhea, make it difficult to use CPT-11 safely. After intravenous administration, CPT-11 is converted to SN-38, an active metabolite, by carboxy esterase. SN-38 is subsequently conjugated with glucuronic acid in the liver. SN-38 and SN-38 glucuronide are then excreted into the bile by MRP2. Some studies have shown that the inhibition of MRP2-mediated biliary excretion of SN-38 and its glucuronide by coadministration of *probenecid* reduces the drug-induced diarrhea, at least in rats. For additional details, *see* Figures 3–5 and 3–7.

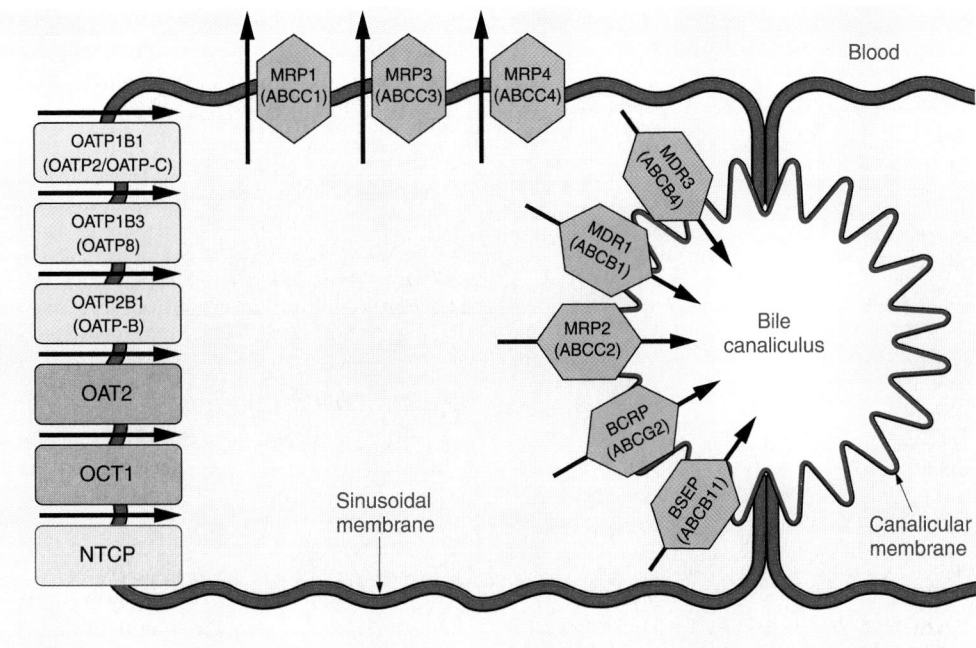

Figure 2–9. *Transporters in the hepatocyte that function in the uptake and efflux of drugs across the sinusoidal membrane and efflux of drugs into the bile across the canalicular membrane.* *See* text for details of the transporters pictured.

Drug–Drug Interactions Involving Transporter-Mediated Hepatic Uptake. Since drug transporters are determinants of the elimination rate of drugs from the body, transporter-mediated hepatic uptake can be the cause of drug–drug interactions involving drugs that are actively taken up into the liver and metabolized and/or excreted in the bile.

Cerivastatin (currently withdrawn), an HMG-CoA reductase inhibitor, is taken up into the liver via transporters (especially OATP1B1) and subsequently metabolized by CYP2C8 and CYP3A4. Its plasma concentration is increased four- to fivefold when coadministered with cyclosporin A. Transport studies using cryopreserved human hepatocytes and OATP1B1-expressing cells suggest that this clinically relevant drug–drug interaction is caused by inhibition of OATP1B1-mediated hepatic uptake (Shitara *et al.*, 2003). However, cyclosporin A inhibits the metabolism of cerivastatin only to a limited extent, suggesting a low possibility of serious drug–drug interactions involving the inhibition of metabolism. Cyclosporin A also increases the plasma concentrations of other HMG-CoA reductase inhibitors. It markedly increases the plasma *AUC* of pravastatin, pitavastatin, and rosuvastatin, which are minimally metabolized and eliminated from the body by transporter-mediated mechanisms. Therefore, these pharmacokinetic interactions also may be due to transporter-mediated hepatic uptake. However, the interactions of cyclosporin A with prodrug-like statins (lactone form) such as simvastatin and lovastatin are mediated by CYP3A4.

Gemfibrozil is another cholesterol-lowering agent that acts by a different mechanism and also causes a severe pharmacokinetic interaction with cerivastatin. *Gemfibrozil glucuronide* inhibits the CYP2C8-mediated metabolism and OATP1B1-mediated uptake of cerivastatin more potently than does gemfibrozil. Laboratory data show that the glucuronide is highly concentrated in the liver *versus* plasma probably owing to transporter-mediated active uptake and intracellular formation of the conjugate. Therefore, it may be that gemfibrozil glucuronide, concentrated in the hepatocytes, inhibits the CYP2C8-mediated metabolism of cerivastatin. Gemfibrozil markedly (four- to fivefold) increases the plasma concentration of cerivastatin but does not greatly increase (1.3 to 2 times) that of unmetabolized statins pravastatin, pitavastatin, and rosuvastatin, a result that also suggests that this interaction is caused by inhibition of metabolism. Thus, when an inhibitor of drug-metabolizing enzymes is highly concentrated in hepatocytes by active transport, extensive inhibition of the drug-metabolizing enzymes may be observed because of the high concentration of the inhibitor in the vicinity of the drug-metabolizing enzymes.

The Contribution of Specific Transporters to the Hepatic Uptake of Drugs. Estimating the contribution of transporters to the total hepatic uptake is necessary for understanding their importance in drug disposition. This estimate can help to predict the extent to which a drug–drug interaction or a genetic polymorphism of a transporter may affect drug concentrations in plasma and liver. The contribution to hepatic uptake has been estimated successfully for CYP-mediated metabolism by using neutralizing antibody and specific chemical inhibitors. Unfortunately, specific inhibitors or antibodies for important transporters have not been identified yet, although some *relatively specific* inhibitors have been discovered.

The contribution of transporters to hepatic uptake can be estimated from *in vitro* studies. Injection of cRNA results in transporter expression on the plasma membrane of *Xenopus laevis* oocytes (Hagenbuch *et al.*, 1996). Subsequent hybridization of the cRNA with its antisense oligonucleotide specifically reduces its expression. Comparison of the drug uptake into cRNA-injected oocytes in the presence and absence of antisense oligonucleotides clarifies the contribution of a specific transporter. Second, a method using reference compounds for specific transporters has been proposed. The reference compounds should be specific substrates for a particular transporter. The contribution of a specific transporter can be calculated from the uptake of test compounds and reference compounds into hepatocytes and transporter-expressing systems (Hirano *et al.*, 2004):

$$\text{Contribution} = \frac{CL_{\text{hep,ref}}/CL_{\text{exp,ref}}}{CL_{\text{hep,test}}/CL_{\text{exp,test}}} \qquad (2\text{–}13)$$

where $CL_{\text{hep,ref}}$ and $CL_{\text{exp,ref}}$ represent the uptake of reference compounds into hepatocytes and transporter-expressing cells, respectively, and $CL_{\text{hep,test}}$ and $CL_{\text{exp,test}}$ represent the uptake of test compounds into the corresponding systems. For example, the contributions of OATP1B1 and OATP1B3 to the hepatic uptake of pitavastatin have been estimated using estrone 3-sulfate and cholecystokinine octapeptide (CCK8) as reference compounds for OATP1B1 and OATP1B3, respectively. However, for many transporters, reference compounds specific to the transporter are not available.

Renal Transporters

Secretion in the kidney of structurally diverse molecules including many drugs, environmental toxins and carcinogens is critical in the body's defense against foreign substances. The specificity of secretory pathways in the nephron for two distinct classes of substrates, organic anions and cations, was first described decades ago, and these pathways were well characterized using a variety of physiological techniques including isolated perfused nephrons and kidneys, micropuncture techniques, cell culture methods, and isolated renal plasma membrane vesicles. However, not until the mid-1990s were the molecular identities of the organic anion and cation transporters revealed. During the past decade, molecular studies have identified and characterized the renal transporters that play a role in drug elimination, toxicity, and response. Thus, we now can describe the overall secretory pathways for organic cations and their molecular and functional characteristics. Although the pharmacological focus is often on the kidney, there is useful information on the tissue distribution of these transporters. Molecular studies using site-directed mutagenesis have identified substrate-recognition and other functional domains of the transporters, and genetic studies of knockout mouse models have been used to characterize the physiological roles of individual transporters. Recently, studies have identified and functionally analyzed genetic polymorphisms and haplotypes of the relevant transporters in humans. Our understanding of organic anion transport has progressed in a similar fashion. In some cases, transporters that are considered organic anion or organic cation transporters have dual specificity for anions and cations. The following section summarizes recent work on human transporters and includes some information on transporters in other mammals. An excellent review of renal organic anion and cation transport has been published recently (Wright and Dantzler, 2004).

Organic Cation Transport. Structurally diverse organic cations are secreted in the proximal tubule (Dresser *et al.*, 2001; Koepsell and Endou, 2004; Wright and Dantzler, 2004). Many secreted organic cations are endogenous compounds (*e.g.*, choline, *N*-methylnicotinamide, and dopamine), and renal secretion appears to be important in eliminating excess concentrations of these substances. However, a primary function of organic cation secretion is ridding the body of xenobiotics, including many positively charged drugs and their metabolites (*e.g.*, *cimetidine, ranitidine,* metformin, *procainamide,* and *N-acetylprocainamide*), and toxins from the environment (*e.g., nicotine*). Organic cations that are secreted by the kidney may be either hydrophobic or hydrophilic. Hydrophilic organic drug cations generally have molecular weights of less than 400 daltons; a current model for their secretion in the proximal tubule of the nephron is shown in Figure 2–10.

For the transepithelial flux of a compound (*e.g.*, secretion), it is essential for the compound to traverse two membranes sequentially, the basolateral membrane facing the blood side and the apical membrane facing the tubular lumen. Distinct transporters on each membrane mediate each step of transport. Organic cations appear to cross the basolateral membrane by three distinct transporters in the SLC family 22 (SCL22): OCT1 (*SLC22A1*), OCT2 (*SLC22A2*), and OCT3 (*SLC22A3*). Organic cations are transported across this membrane down their electrochemical gradient (–70 mV). Previous studies in isolated basolateral membrane vesicles demonstrate the presence of a potential-sensitive mechanism for organic cations. The cloned transporters OCT1, OCT2, and OCT3 are all potential sensitive and mechanistically coincide with previous studies of isolated basolateral membrane vesicles.

Transport of organic cations from cell to tubular lumen across the apical membrane occurs *via* an electroneutral proton–organic cation exchange mechanism in a variety of species, including human, dog, rabbit, and cat. Transporters assigned to the apical membrane are in the SLC22 family and termed *novel organic cation transporters* (OCTNs). In humans, these include OCNT1 (*SLC22A4*) and OCTN2 (*SLC22A5*). These bifunctional transporters are involved not only in organic cation secretion but also in carnitine reabsorption. In the reuptake mode, the transporters function as Na^+ cotransporters, relying on the inwardly driven Na^+ gradient

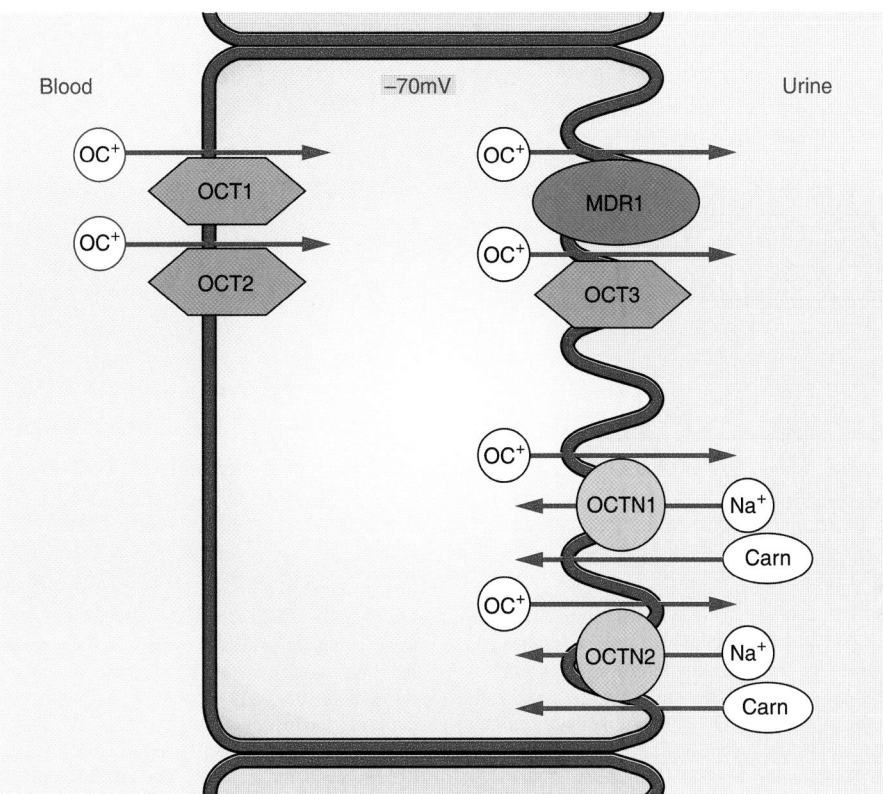

Figure 2–10. *Model of organic cation secretory transporters in the proximal tubule.* *Hexagons* depict transporters in the SLC22 family, *SLC22A1* (OCT1), *SLC22A2* (OCT2), and *SLC22A3* (OCT3). *Circles* show transporters in the same family, *SLC22A4* (OCTN1) and *SLC22A5* (OCTN2). MDR1 (*ABCB1*) is depicted as a *dark blue oval.* Carn, carnitine; OC⁺, organic cation.

created by Na⁺,K⁺-ATPase to move carnitine from tubular lumen to cell. In the secretory mode, the transporters appear to function as proton–organic cation exchangers. That is, protons move from tubular lumen to cell interior in exchange for organic cations, which move from cytosol to tubular lumen. The inwardly directed proton gradient (from tubular lumen to cytosol) is maintained by transporters in the SLC9 family (NHEs), which are Na⁺/H⁺ exchangers (antiporters). The bifunctional mechanism of OCTN1 and OCTN2 may not totally explain the organic cation–proton exchange mechanism that has been described in many studies in isolated plasma membrane vesicles. Of the two steps involved in secretory transport, transport across the luminal membrane appears to be rate-limiting.

OCT1 (SLC22A1). OCT1 (*SLC22A1*) was first cloned from a rat cDNA library (Koepsell and Endou, 2004). Subsequently, orthologs were cloned from mouse, rabbit, and humans. Mammalian isoforms of OCT1, which vary in length from 554 to 556 amino acids, have 12 putative transmembrane domains (Figure 2–11) and include several *N*-linked glycosylation sites. A long extracellular loop between transmembrane domains 1 and 2 is characteristic of the OCTs. The gene for the human OCT1 is mapped to chromosome 6 (6q26). There are four splice variants in human tissues, one of which is functionally active, OCT1G/L554 (Hayer *et al.*, 1999). In humans, OCT1 is expressed primarily in the liver, with some expression in heart, intestine, and skeletal muscle. In mouse

and rat, OCT1 is also abundant in the kidney, whereas in humans, very modest levels of OCT1 mRNA transcripts are detected in kidney. The transport mechanism of OCT1 is electrogenic and saturable for transport of model small-molecular-weight organic cations including tetraethylammonium (TEA) and dopamine. Interestingly, OCT1 also can operate as an exchanger, mediating organic cation–organic cation exchange. That is, loading cells with organic cations such as unlabeled TEA can trans-stimulate the inward flux of organic cations such as MPP⁺. It also should be noted that organic cations can transinhibit OCT1. In particular, the hydrophobic organic cations quinine and quinidine, which are poor substrates of OCT1, when present on the cytosolic side of a membrane, can inhibit (*trans*inhibit) influx of organic cations *via* OCT1.

The human OCT1 generally accepts a wide array of monovalent organic cations with molecular weights of less than 400 daltons, including many drugs (*e.g.,* procainamide, metformin, and *pindolol*) (Dresser *et al.,* 2001). Species differences in the substrate specificity of OCT1 mammalian orthologs have been described. Inhibitors of OCT1 are generally more hydrophobic. Detailed structure–activity relationships have established that the pharmacophore of OCT1 consists of three hydrophobic arms and a single cationic recognition site. The kinetics of uptake and inhibition of model compounds with human OCT1 differ among studies and may be related to experi-

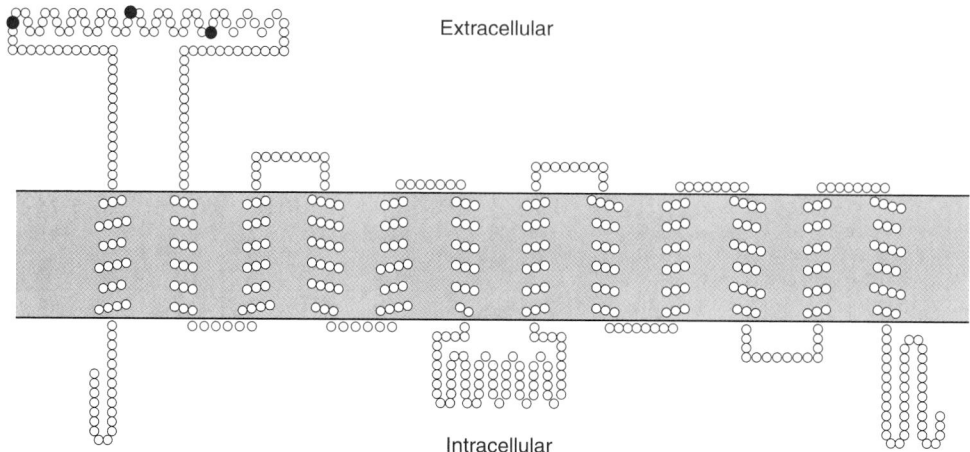

Figure 2–11. *Secondary structure of OCT1* (**SLC22A1**) *constructed from hydropathy analysis.* The transmembrane topology diagram was rendered using transmembrane protein display software available at the UCSF Sequence Analysis Consulting Group Web site, *http://www.sacs.ucsf.edu/TOPO/topo.html.* The *blue circles* show putative *N*-glycosylation sites.

mental techniques, including a range of heterologous expression systems. Key residues that contribute to the charge specificity of OCT1 have been identified by site-directed mutagenesis studies and include a highly conserved aspartate residue (corresponding to position 475 in the rat ortholog of OCT1) that appears to be part of the monoamine recognition site. Since OCT1 mammalian orthologs have greater than 80% amino acid identity, evolutionarily nonconserved residues among mammalian species clearly are involved in specificity differences (Wright and Dantzler, 2004).

OCT2 (SLC22A2). OCT2 (*SLC22A2*) was first cloned from a rat kidney cDNA library in 1996 (Okuda *et al.*, 1996). Human, rabbit, mouse, and pig orthologs all have been cloned. Mammalian orthologs range in length from 553 through 555 amino acids. Similar to OCT, OCT2 is predicted to have 12 transmembrane domains, including one *N*-linked glycosylation site. OCT2 is located adjacent to OCT1 on chromosome 6 (6q26). A single splice variant of human OCT2, termed *OCT2-A,* has been identified in human kidney. OCT2-A, which is a truncated form of OCT2, appears to have a lower K_m (or greater affinity) for substrates than OCT2, although a lower affinity has been observed for some inhibitors (Urakami *et al.*, 2002). Human, mouse, and rat orthologs of OCT2 are expressed in abundance in human kidney and to some extent in neuronal tissue such as choroid plexus. In the kidney, OCT2 is localized to the proximal tubule and to distal tubules and collecting ducts. In the proximal tubule, OCT2 is restricted to the basolateral membrane. OCT2 mammalian species orthologs are greater than 80% identical, whereas OCT1 and OCT2 paralogs are approximately 70% identical. The transport mechanism of OCT2 is similar to that of OCT1. In particular, OCT2-mediated transport of model organic cations MPP+ and TEA is electrogenic, but like OCT1, OCT2 can support organic cation–organic cation exchange (Koepsell *et al.*, 2003). Some studies show modest proton–organic cation exchange. More hydrophobic organic cations may inhibit OCT2 but may not be translocated by it.

Like OCT1, OCT2 generally accepts a wide array of monovalent organic cations with molecular weights of less than 400 daltons. The apparent affinities of the human OCT1 and OCT2 paralogs for some organic cation substrates and inhibitors have been shown to be different in side-by-side comparison studies. Isoform-specific inhibi-

tors of the OCTs are needed to determine the relative importance of OCT1 and OCT2 in the renal clearance of compounds in rodents, in which both isoforms are present in kidney. OCT2 is also present in neuronal tissues. However, studies with monoamine neurotransmitters demonstrate that dopamine, serotonin, histamine, and norepinephrine have low affinities for OCT2. These studies suggest that OCT2 may play a housekeeping role in neurons, taking up only excess concentrations of neurotransmitters. OCT2 also may be involved in recycling of neurotransmitters by taking up breakdown products, which in turn enter monoamine synthetic pathways.

OCT3 (SLC22A3). OCT3 (*SLC22A3*) was cloned initially from rat placenta (Kekuda *et al.*, 1998). Human and mouse orthologs have also been cloned. OCT3 consists of 551 amino acids and is predicted to have 12 transmembrane domains, including three *N*-linked glycosylation sites. hOCT3 is located in tandem with OCT1 and OCT2 on chromosome 6. Tissue distribution studies suggest that human OCT3 is expressed in liver, kidney, intestine, and placenta, although it appears to be expressed in considerably less abundance than OCT2 in the kidney. Like OCT1 and OCT2, OCT3 appears to support electrogenic potential-sensitive organic cation transport. Although the specificity of OCT3 is similar to that of OCT1 and OCT2, it appears to have quantitative differences in its affinities for many organic cations. Some studies have suggested that OCT3 is the extraneuronal monoamine transporter based on its substrate specificity and potency of interaction with monoamine neurotransmitters. Because of its relatively low abundance in the kidney, OCT3 may play only a limited role in renal drug elimination.

OCTN1 (SLC22A4). OCTN1, cloned originally from human fetal liver, is expressed in the adult kidney, trachea, and bone marrow (Tamai *et al.*, 1997). The functional characteristics of OCTN1 suggest that it operates as an organic cation–proton exchanger. OCTN1-mediated influx of model organic cations is enhanced at alkaline pH, whereas efflux is increased by an inwardly directed proton gradient. OCTN1 contains a nucleotide-binding sequence motif, and transport of its substrates appears to be stimulated by cellular ATP content. OCTN1 also can function as an organic cation–organic cation exchanger. Although the subcellular localization of OCTN1 has not been demonstrated clearly, available data collectively suggest that OCTN1 functions as a bidirectional pH- and

ATP-dependent transporter at the apical membrane in renal tubular epithelial cells. Its physiological role is not yet known because studies in *octn1* knockout mice are not available.

OCTN2 (SLC22A5). OCTN2 was first cloned from human kidney and determined to be the transporter responsible for systemic carnitine deficiency (Tamai *et al.*, 1998). Rat OCTN2 mRNA is expressed predominantly in the cortex, with very little expression in the medulla, and is localized to the apical membrane of the proximal tubule.

OCTN2 is a bifunctional transporter. That is, it transports L-carnitine with high affinity in an Na$^+$-dependent manner, whereas, Na$^+$ does not influence OCTN2-mediated transport of organic cations such as TEA. Thus, OCTN2 is thought to function as both an Na$^+$-dependent carnitine transporter and an Na$^+$-independent organic cation transporter. Similar to OCTN1, OCTN2 transport of organic cations is sensitive to pH, suggesting that it may function as an organic cation exchanger. Studies in mice containing a missense mutation in Slc22a5 suggest that organic cations are transported in a secretory direction by OCTN2, whereas carnitine is transported in a reabsorptive direction (Ohashi *et al.*, 2001). Therefore, transport of L-carnitine by OCTN2 is an Na$^+$-dependent electrogenic process. Mutations in OCTN2 have been found to be the cause of primary systemic carnitine deficiency (OMIM 212140) (Nezu *et al.*, 1999).

Polymorphisms of OCTs. Polymorphisms of OCTs have been identified in large post–human genome SNP discovery projects (Kerb *et al.*, 2002; Leabman *et al.*, 2003; Shu *et al.*, 2003). OCT1 exhibits the greatest number of amino acid polymorphisms, followed by OCT2 and then OCT3. Furthermore, allele frequencies of OCT1 amino acid variants in human populations generally are greater than those of OCT2 and OCT3 amino acid variants. Functional studies of OCT1 and OCT2 polymorphisms have been performed. OCT1 exhibits five variants with reduced function. These variants may have important implications clinically in terms of hepatic drug disposition and targeting of OCT1 substrates. In particular, individuals with OCT1 variants may have reduced liver uptake of OCT1 substrates and therefore reduced metabolism. Clinical studies need to be performed to ascertain the implications of OCT1 variants to drug disposition and response. For OCT2, several polymorphisms exhibited altered kinetic properties when expressed in *Xenopus laevis* oocytes. These variants may lead to alterations in renal secretion of OCT2 substrates.

Organic Anion Transport. A wide variety of structurally diverse organic anions are secreted in the proximal tubule (Burckhardt and Burckhardt, 2003; Dresser *et al.*, 2001; Wright and Dantzler, 2004). As with organic cation transport, the primary function of organic anion secretion appears to be the removal from the body of xenobiotics, including many weakly acidic drugs [*e.g., pravastatin, captopril, p-aminohippurate* (PAH), and penicillins] and toxins (*e.g.,* ochratoxin). Organic anion transporters move both hydrophobic and hydrophilic anions but also may interact with cations and neutral compounds.

A current model for the transepithelial flux of organic anions in the proximal tubule is shown in Figure 2–12. Two primary transporters on the basolateral membrane mediate the flux of organic anions from interstitial fluid to tubule cell: OAT1 (*SLC22A6*) and OAT3 (*SLC22A8*). Energetically, hydrophilic organic anions are transported across the basolateral membrane against an electrochemical gradient in exchange with intracellular α-ketoglutarate, which moves down its concentration gradient from cytosol to blood. The outwardly directed gradient of α-ketoglutarate is maintained at least in part by a basolateral Na$^+$-dicarboxylate transporter (NaDC3). The Na$^+$ gradient that drives NaDC3 is maintained by Na$^+$,K$^+$-ATPase. Transport of small-molecular-weight organic anions by the cloned transporters OAT1 and OAT3 can be driven by α-ketoglutarate. Coupled transport of α-ketoglutarate and small-molecular-weight organic anions (*e.g., p-aminohippurate*) has been demonstrated in many studies in isolated basolateral membrane vesicles. The molecular pharmacology and molecular biology of OATs have recently been reviewed (Eraly *et al.*, 2004).

The mechanism responsible for the apical membrane transport of organic anions from tubule cell cytosol to tubular lumen remains controversial. Some studies suggest that OAT4 may serve as the luminal membrane transporter for organic anions. However, recent studies show that the movement of substrates *via* this transporter can be driven by exchange with α-ketoglutarate, suggesting that OAT4 may function in the reabsorptive, rather than secretory, flux of organic anions. Other studies have suggested that in the pig kidney, OATV1 serves as an electrogenic facilitated transporter on the apical membrane (Jutabha *et al.*, 2003). The human ortholog of OATV1 is NPT1, or NaPi-1, originally cloned as a phosphate transporter. NPT1 can support the low-affinity transport of hydrophilic organic anions such as PAH. Other transporters that may play a role in transport across the apical membrane include MRP2 and MRP4, multidrug-resistance transporters in the ATP binding cassette family C (ABCC). Both transporters interact with some organic anions and may actively pump their substrates from tubule cell cytosol to tubular lumen.

OAT1 (SLC22A6). OAT1 was cloned from rat kidney (Sekine *et al.*, 1997; Sweet *et al.*, 1997). This transporter is greater than 30% identical to OCTs in the SLC22 family. Mouse, human, pig, and rabbit orthologs have been cloned and are approximately 80% identical to human OAT1. Mammalian isoforms of OAT1 vary in length from 545 to 551 amino acids, with features similar to those shown in Figure 2–11. The gene for the human OAT1 is mapped to chromosome 11 and is found in an SLC22 cluster that includes OAT3 and OAT4. There are four splice variants in human tissues, termed *OAT1-1, OAT1-2, OAT1-3,* and *OAT1-4.* OAT1-2, which includes a 13-amino-acid deletion, transports PAH at a rate comparable with OAT1-1. These two splice variants use the alternative 5′-splice sites in exon 9. OAT1-3 and OAT1-4, which result from a 132-bp (44-amino-acid) deletion near the carboxyl terminus of OAT1, do not transport PAH. In humans, rat, and mouse, OAT1 is expressed primarily in the kidney, with some expression in brain and skeletal muscle.

Immunohistochemical studies suggest that OAT1 is expressed on the basolateral membrane of the proximal tubule in human and rat, with highest expression in the middle segment, S2. Based on a quantitative polymerase chain reaction (PCR), OAT1 is expressed at a third of the level of OAT3, the other major basolateral membrane organic anion transporter. OAT1 exhibits saturable transport of organic anions such as PAH. This transport is trans-stimulated by

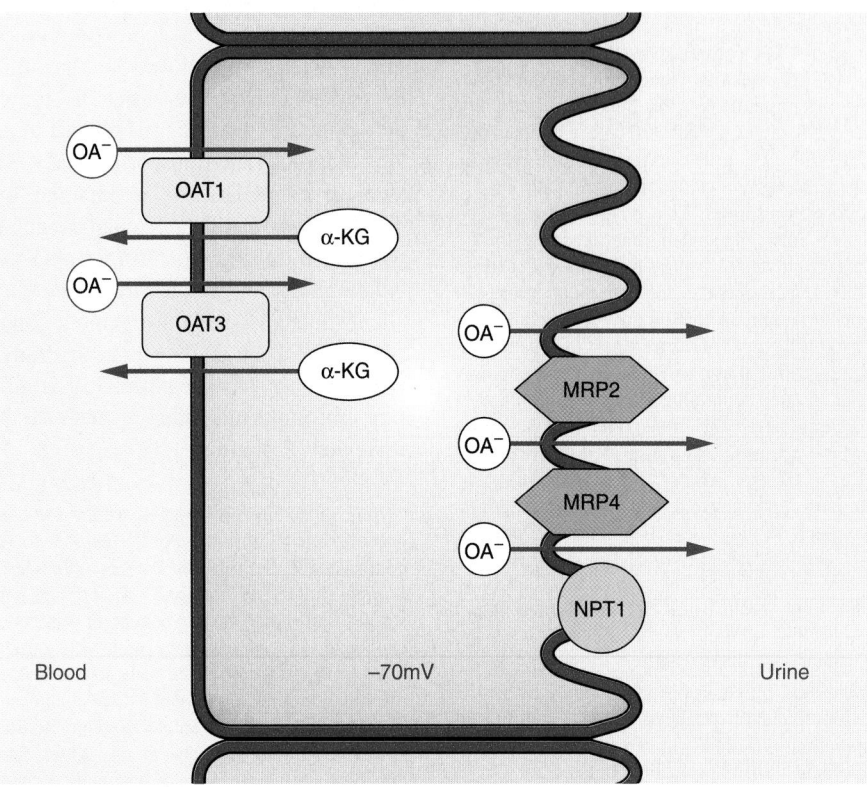

Figure 2–12. *Model of organic anion secretory transporters in the proximal tubule.* *Rectangles* depict transporters in the SLC22 family, OAT1 (*SLC22A6*) and OAT3 (*SLC22A8*), and *hexagons* depict transporters in the ABC superfamily, MRP2 (*ABCC2*) and MRP4 (*ABCC4*). NPT1 (*SLC17A1*) is depicted as a *circle*. OA⁻, organic anion; α-KG, α-ketoglutarate.

other organic anions, including α-ketoglutarate. Thus, the inside negative-potential difference drives the efflux of the dicarboxylate α-ketoglutarate, which, in turn, supports the influx of monocarboxylates such as PAH. Regulation of expression levels of OAT1 in the kidney appears to be controlled by sex steroids.

OAT1 generally transports small-molecular-weight organic anions that may be endogenous (*e.g.,* PGE_2 and urate) or ingested drugs and toxins. Some neutral compounds are also transported by OAT1 at a lower affinity (*e.g.,* cimetidine). Key residues that contribute to transport by OAT1 include the conserved K394 and R478, which are involved in the PAH–*glutarate* exchange mechanism.

OAT2 (SLC22A7). OAT2 was cloned first from rat liver (and named *NLT* at the time) (Sekine *et al.,* 1998; Simonson *et al.,* 1994). This transporter has a gender-based tissue distribution between the liver and the kidney in rodents but not in humans, OAT2 is present in both kidney and liver. In the kidney, the transporter is localized to the basolateral membrane of the proximal tubule. Efforts to stimulate organic anion–organic anion exchange *via* OAT2 have not been successful, leading to the speculation that OAT2 is a basolateral membrane transporter that serves in the reabsorptive flux of organic anions from tubule cell cytosol to interstitial fluids. OAT2 transports many organic anions, including PAH, methotrexate, *ochratoxin A,* and glutarate. Human, mouse, and rat orthologs of OAT2 have high affinities for the endogenous prostaglandin, PGE_2.

OAT3 (SLC22A8). OAT3 (*SLC22A8*) was cloned originally from rat kidney (Kusuhara *et al.,* 1999). Human OAT3 consists of two variants, one of which transports a wide variety of organic anions, including PAH and *estrone sulfate.* The longer OAT3 in humans, a 568-amino-acid protein, does not support transport. It is likely that the two OAT3 variants are splice variants. Northern blotting suggests that the human ortholog of OAT3 is primarily in the kidney. Mouse and rat orthologs show some expression in the brain and liver. OAT3 mRNA levels are higher than those of OAT1, which in turn are higher than those of OAT2 or OAT4. Human OAT3 is confined to the basolateral membrane of the proximal tubule.

OAT3 clearly has overlapping specificities with OAT1, although kinetic parameters differ. For example, estrone sulfate is transported by both OAT1 and OAT3, but OAT3 has a much higher affinity in comparison with OAT1. The weak base cimetidine (an H_2-receptor antagonist) is transported with high affinity by OAT1, whereas the cation TEA is not transported. Domains and residues involved in the charge specificity of OAT3 have been identified in several studies. Interestingly, changing two basic amino acid residues in OAT3 (R454D and K370A) shifts the charge specificity of OAT3 from anionic to cationic. Like OAT1, OAT3 appears to be an exchanger that couples the outward flux of α-ketoglutarate to the inward flux of organic anions: The inside negative-potential difference repels α-ketoglutarate from the cells *via* OAT3, which in turn transports its substrates against a concentration gradient into the tubule cell cytosol.

OAT4 (SLC22A9). OAT4 (*SLC22A9*) was cloned from a human kidney cDNA library (Cha *et al.*, 2000). Quantitative PCR indicates that the expression level of OAT4 in human kidneys is approximately 5% to 10% of the level of OAT1 and OAT3 and is comparable with OAT2. OAT4 is expressed in human kidney and placenta; in human kidney, OAT4 is present on the luminal membrane of the proximal tubule. At first, OAT4 was thought to be involved in the second step of secretion of organic anions, *i.e.,* transport across the apical membrane from cell to tubular lumen. However, recent studies demonstrate that organic anion transport by OAT4 can be stimulated by transgradients of α-ketoglutarate (Ekaratanawong *et al.*, 2004), suggesting that OAT4 may be involved in the reabsorption of organic anions from tubular lumen into cell. The specificity of OAT4 is narrow but includes estrone sulfate and PAH. Interestingly, the affinity for PAH is low (>1 mM). Collectively, emerging studies suggest that OAT4 may be involved not in secretory flux of organic anions but in reabsorption instead.

Other Anion Transporters. URAT1 (*SLC22A12*), first cloned from human kidney, is a kidney-specific transporter confined to the apical membrane of the proximal tubule (Enomoto *et al.*, 2002). Data suggest that URAT1 is primarily responsible for urate reabsorption, mediating electroneutral urate transport that can be trans-stimulated by Cl⁻ gradients. The mouse ortholog of URAT1 is involved in the renal secretory flux of organic anions including *benzylpenicillin* and urate.

NPT1 (*SLC17A1*), cloned originally as a phosphate transporter in humans, is expressed in abundance on the luminal membrane of the proximal tubule as well as in the brain (Werner *et al.*, 1991). NPT1 transports PAH, probenecid, and *penicillin G*. It appears to be part of the system involved in organic anion efflux from tubule cell to lumen.

MRP2 (*ABCC2*), an ABC transporter, initially called the *GS-X pump* (Ishikawa *et al.*, 1990), has been considered to be the primary transporter involved in efflux of many drug conjugates such as glutathione conjugates across the canalicular membrane of the hepatocyte. However, MRP2 is also found on the apical membrane of the proximal tubule, where it is thought to play a role in the efflux of organic anions into the tubular lumen. Its role in the kidney may be to secrete glutathione conjugates of drugs, but it also may support the translocation (with glutathione) of various nonconjugated substrates. In general, MRP2 transports larger, bulkier compounds than do most of the organic anion transporters in the SLC22 family.

MRP4 (*ABCC4*) is found on the apical membrane of the proximal tubule and transports a wide array of conjugated anions, including glucuronide and glutathione conjugates. However, unlike MRP2, MRP4 appears to interact with various drugs, including methotrexate, cyclic nucleotide analogs, and antiviral nucleoside analogs. It is possible that MRP4 is involved in the apical flux of many drugs from cell to tubule lumen. Other MRP efflux transporters also have been identified in human kidney, including MRP3 and MRP6, both on the basolateral membrane. Their roles in the kidney are not yet known.

Polymorphisms of OATs. Polymorphisms in OAT1 and OAT3 have been identified in ethnically diverse human populations. Two amino acid polymorphisms (allele frequencies greater than 1%) in OAT1 have been identified in African-American populations (OAT1-R50H). Three amino acid polymorphisms and seven rare amino acid variants in OAT3 have been identified in ethnically diverse U.S. populations (*see www.pharmgkb.org*).

TRANSPORTERS INVOLVED IN PHARMACODYNAMICS: DRUG ACTION IN THE BRAIN

Neurotransmitters are packaged in vesicles in presynpatic neurons, released in the synapse by fusion of the vesicles with the plasma membrane, and, excepting acetylcholine, are then taken back into the presynaptic neurons or postsynaptic cells (*see* Chapter 6). Transporters involved in the neuronal reuptake of the neurotransmitters and the regulation of their levels in the synaptic cleft belong to two major superfamilies, SLC1 and SLC6. Transporters in both families play roles in reuptake of γ-aminobutyric acid (GABA), glutamate, and the monoamine neurotransmitters norepinephrine, serotonin, and dopamine. These transporters may serve as pharmacologic targets for neuropsychiatric drugs.

SLC6 family members localized in the brain and involved in the reuptake of neurotransmitters into presynaptic neurons include the norepinephrine transporters (NET, *SLC6A2*), the dopamine transporter (DAT, *SLC6A3*), the serotonin transporter (SERT, *SLC6A4*), and several GABA reuptake transporters (GAT1, GAT2, and GAT3) (Chen *et al.*, 2004; Hediger, 2004; Elliott and Beveridge, 2005). Each of these transporters appears to have 12 transmembrane secondary structures and a large extracellular loop with glycosylation sites between transmembrane domains 3 and 4. These proteins are typically approximately 600 amino acids in length. SLC6 family members depend on the Na⁺ gradient to actively transport their substrates into cells. Cl⁻ is also required, although to a variable extent depending on the family member. Residues and domains that form the substrate recognition and permeation pathways are currently being identified.

Through reuptake mechanisms, the neurotransmitter transporters in the SLC6A family regulate the concentrations and dwell times of neurotransmitters in the synaptic cleft; the extent of transmitter uptake also influences subsequent vesicular storage of transmitters. It is important to note that many of these transporters are present in other tissues (*e.g.,* kidney and platelets) and may serve other roles. Further, the transporters can function in the reverse direction. That is, the transporters can export neurotransmitters in an Na⁺-independent fashion. The characteristics of each member of the SLC6A family of transporters that play a role in reuptake of monoamine neurotransmitters and GABA merit a brief description.

SLC6A1 (GAT1), SLC6A11 (GAT3), and SLC6A13 (GAT2). GAT1 (599 amino acids) is the most important GABA transporter in the brain, expressed in GABAergic neurons and found largely on presynaptic neurons (Chen *et al.*, 2004). GAT1 is found in abundance in the neocortex, cerebellum, basal ganglia, brainstem, spinal cord, retina, and olfactory bulb. GAT3 is found only in the brain, largely in glial cells. GAT2 is found in peripheral tissues, including the kidney and liver, and within the CNS in the choroid plexus and meninges.

GAT1, GAT2, and GAT3 are approximately 50% identical in amino acid sequence. Functional analysis indicates that GAT1 transports GABA with a 2:1 Na^+:$GABA^-$ stoichiometry. Cl^- is required. Residues and domains responsible for the recognition of GABA and subsequent translocation have been identified: Tyr140 appears to be crucial for binding GABA. Physiologically, GAT1 appears to be responsible for regulating the interaction of GABA at receptors. The presence of GAT2 in the choroid plexus and its absence in presynaptic neurons suggest that this transporter may play a primary role in maintaining the homeostasis of GABA in the CSF. GAT1 and GAT3 are drug targets. GAT1 is the target of the antiepileptic drug *tiagabine,* which presumably acts to increase GABA levels in the synaptic cleft of GABAergic neurons by inhibiting the reuptake of GABA. GAT3 is the target for the nipecotic acid derivatives that are anticonvulsants.

SLC6A2 (NET). NET (617 amino acids) is found in central and peripheral nervous tissues as well as in adrenal chromaffin tissue (Chen *et al.*, 2004). In the brain, NET colocalizes with neuronal markers, consistent with a role in reuptake of monoamine neurotransmitters. The transporter functions in the Na^+-dependent reuptake of norepinephrine and dopamine and as a higher-capacity norepinephrine channel. A major role of NET is to limit the synaptic dwell time of norepinephrine and to terminate its actions, salvaging norepinephrine for subsequent repackaging. NET knockout mice exhibit a prolonged synaptic half-life of norepinephrine (Xu *et al.*, 2000). Ultimately, through its reuptake function, NET participates in the regulation of many neurological functions, including memory and mood. NET serves as a drug target; the antidepressant *desipramine* is considered a selective inhibitor of NET. Other drugs that interact with NET include other tricyclic antidepressants and *cocaine.* Orthostatic intolerance, a rare familial disorder characterized by an abnormal blood pressure and heart rate response to changes in posture, has been associated with a mutation in NET.

SLC6A3 (DAT). DAT is located primarily in the brain in dopaminergic neurons. Although present on presynaptic neurons at the neurosynapatic junction, DAT is also present in abundance along the neurons, away from the synaptic cleft. This distribution suggests that DAT may play a role in clearance of excess dopamine in the vicinity of neurons. The primary function of DAT is the reuptake dopamine, terminating its actions, although DAT also weakly interacts with norepinephrine. Physiologically, DAT is involved in the various functions that are attributed to the dopaminergic system, including mood, behavior, reward, and cognition. The half-life of dopamine in the extracellular spaces of the brain is prolonged considerably in DAT knockout mice (Uhl, 2003), which are hyperactive and have sleep disorders. Drugs that interact with DAT include cocaine and its analogs, *amphetamines,* and the neurotoxin *MPTP.*

SLC6A4 (SERT). SERT is located in peripheral tissues and in the brain along extrasynaptic axonal membranes (Chen *et al.*, 2004; Olivier *et al.*, 2000). SERT clearly plays a role in the reuptake and clearance of serotonin in the brain. Like the other SLC6A family members, SERT transports its substrates in an Na^+-dependent fashion and is dependent on Cl^- and possibly on the countertransport of K^+. Substrates of SERT include serotonin (5-HT), various tryptamine derivatives, and neurotoxins such as *3,4-methylene-dioxymethamphetamine* (MDMA; ecstasy) and *fenfluramine.* The serotonin transporter has been one of the most widely studied proteins in the human genome. First, it is the specific target of the antidepressants in the selective serotonin reuptake inhibitor class (*e.g., fluoxetine* and *paroxetine*) and one of several targets of tricyclic antidepressants (*e.g., amitriptyline*). Further, because of the important role of serotonin in neurological function and behavior, genetic variants of SERT have been associated with an array of behavioral and neurological disorders. In particular, a common promoter region variant that alters the length of the upstream region of *SLC6A4* has been the subject of many studies. The short form of the variant results in a reduced rate of transcription of SERT in comparison with the long form. These differences in the rates of transcription alter the quantity of mRNA and, ultimately, the expression and activity of SERT. The short form has been associated with a variety of neuropsychiatric disorders (Lesch *et al.*, 1996). The precise mechanism by which a reduced activity of SERT, caused by either a genetic variant or an antidepressant, ultimately affects behavior, including depression, is not known.

BLOOD–BRAIN BARRIER AND BLOOD–CSF BARRIER

Drugs acting in the CNS have to cross the BBB or blood–CSF barrier. These two barriers are formed by brain capillary endothelial cells and epithelial cells of the choroid plexus, respectively. Recent studies have shown that this is not only a static anatomical barrier but also a dynamic one in which efflux transporters play a role (Begley and Brightman, 2003; Sun *et al.*, 2003). P-glycoprotein was identified initially as an efflux transporter, and it extrudes its substrate drugs on the luminal membrane of the brain capillary endothelial cells into the blood. Thus, recognition by P-glycoprotein as a substrate is a major disadvantage for drugs used to treat CNS diseases. In addition to P-glycoprotein, there is accumulating evidence for the presence of efflux transport systems for anionic drugs. The transporters involved in the efflux transport of organic anions from the CNS are being identified in the BBB and the blood–CSF barrier and include the members of organic anion transporting polypeptide (OATP1A4 and OATP1A5) and organic anion transporter (OAT3) families (Kikuchi *et al.*, 2004; Mori *et al.*, 2003). They facilitate the uptake process of organic compounds such as β-lactam antibiotics, statins, *p*-aminohippurate, H_2 antagonists, and bile acids on the plasma membrane facing the brain–CSF. The transporters involved in the efflux on the membranes that face the blood still remain to be identified, although several candidate primary active transporters, such as MRP and BCRP, already have been proposed. Members of the organic anion transporting polypeptide family also mediate uptake from the blood on the plasma membrane facing blood. Further clarification of influx and efflux transporters in the barriers will enable delivery of CNS drugs efficiently into the brain while avoiding undesirable CNS side effects and help to define the mechanisms of drug–drug interactions and interindividual differences in the therapeutic CNS effects.

BIBLIOGRAPHY

Abe, T., Kakyo, M., Tokui, T., *et al.* Identification of a novel gene family encoding human liver-specific organic anion transporter LST-1. *J. Biol. Chem.,* **1999,** *274*:17159–17163.

Abramson, J., Smirnova, I., Kasho, V., *et al.* Structure and mechanism of the lactose permease of *Escherichia coli. Science,* **2003,** *301*:610–615.

Amara, S.G., and Sonders, M.S. Neurotransmitter transporters as molecular targets for addictive drugs. *Drug Alcohol Depend.,* **1998,** *51*:87–96.

Ambudkar, S.V., Dey, S., Hrycyna, C.A., *et al.* Biochemical, cellular, and pharmacological aspects of the multidrug transporter. *Annu. Rev. Pharmacol. Toxicol.,* **1998,** *39*:361–398.

Anglicheau, D., Verstuyft, C., Laurent-Puig, P., *et al.* Association of the multidrug resistance-1 gene single-nucleotide polymorphisms with the tacrolimus dose requirements in renal transplant recipients. *J. Am. Soc. Nephrol.,* **2003,** *14*:1889–1896.

Begley, D.J., and Brightman, M.W. Structural and functional aspects of the blood–brain barrier. *Prog. Drug Res.,* **2003,** *61*:39–78.

Borst, P., and Elferink, R.O. Mammalian ABC transporters in health and disease. *Annu. Rev. Biochem.,* **2002,** *71*:537–592.

Burckhardt, B.C., and Burckhardt, G. Transport of organic anions across the basolateral membrane of proximal tubule cells. *Rev. Physiol. Biochem. Pharmacol.,* **2003,** *146*:95–158.

Burman, J., Tran, C.H., Glatt, C., Freimer, N.B. and Edwards, R.H. The effect of rare human sequence variants on the function of vesicular monoamine transporter 2. *Pharmacogenetics,* **2004,** *14*:587-594.

Cha, S.H., Sekine, T., Kusuhara, H., *et al.* Molecular cloning and characterization of multispecific organic anion transporter 4 expressed in the placenta. *J. Biol. Chem.,* **2000,** *275*:4507–4512.

Chang, C., Swaan, P.W., Ngo, L.Y., *et al.* Molecular requirements of the human nucleoside transporters hCNT1, hCNT2, and hENT1. *Mol. Pharmacol.,* **2004,** *65*:558–570.

Chang, G., and Roth, C.B. Structure of MsbA from *E. coli:* A homolog of the multidrug resistance ATP binding cassette (ABC) transporters. *Science,* **2001,** *293*:1793–1800.

Chen, N.H., Reith, M.E., and Quick, M.W. Synaptic uptake and beyond: the sodium- and chloride-dependent neurotransmitter transporter family SLC6. *Pflugers Arch.,* **2004,** *447*:519–531.

Clarke, M.L., Mackey, J.R., Baldwin, S.A., Young, J.D. and Cass, C.E. The role of membrane transporters in cellular resistance to anticancer nucleoside drugs. *Cancer Treat. Res.,* **2002,** *112*:27–47.

Damaraju, V.L., Damaraju, S., Young, J.D., *et al.* Nucleoside anticancer drugs: The role of nucleoside transporters in resistance to cancer chemotherapy. *Oncogene,* **2003,** *22*:7524–7536.

Drescher, S., Schaeffeler, E., Hitzl, M., *et al.* MDR1 gene polymorphisms and disposition of the P-glycoprotein substrate fexofenadine. *Br. J. Clin. Pharmacol.,* **2002,** *53*:526–534.

Dresser, M.J., Leabman, M.K., and Giacomini, K.M. Transporters involved in the elimination of drugs in the kidney: organic anion transporters and organic cation transporters. *J. Pharm. Sci.,* **2001,** *90*:397–421.

Drozdzik, M., Bialecka M, Mysliwiec K, *et al.* Polymorphism in the P-glycoprotein drug transporter MDR1 gene: A possible link between environmental and genetic factors in Parkinson's disease. *Pharmacogenetics,* **2003,** *13*:259–263.

Ekaratanawong, S., Anzai, N., Jutabha, P., *et al.* Human organic anion transporter 4 is a renal apical organic anion/dicarboxylate exchanger in the proximal tubules. *J. Pharmacol. Sci.,* **2004,** *94*:297–304.

Elliott, J., and Beveridge, T. Psychostimulants and monoamine transporters: Upsetting the balance. *Curr. Opin. Pharmacol.,* **2005,** *5*:94–100.

Enomoto, A., Kimura, H., Chairoungdua, A., *et al.* Molecular identification of a renal urate anion exchanger that regulates blood urate levels. *Nature,* **2002,** *417*:447–452.

Eraly, S., Bush, K., Sampogna, R., Bhatnagar, V., and Nigam, S. The molecular pharmacology of organic ion transporters: From DNA to FDA? *Mol. Pharmacol.,* **2004,** *65*:479–487.

Fellay, J., Marzolini, C., Meaden, E.R., *et al.* Response to antiretroviral treatment in HIV-1-infected individuals with allelic variants of the multidrug resistance transporter 1: A pharmacogenetics study. *Lancet,* **2002,** *359*:30–36.

Gerloff, T., Stieger, B., Hagenbuch, B., *et al.* The sister of P-glycoprotein represents the canalicular bile salt export pump of mammalian liver. *J. Biol. Chem.,* **1998,** *273*:10046–10050.

Gottesman, M.M., Pastan, I., and Ambudkar, S.V. P-glycoprotein and multidrug resistance. *Curr. Opin. Genet. Dev.,* **1996,** *6*:610–617.

Gray, J.H., Mangravite, L.M., and Owen, R.P. Functional and genetic diversity in the concentrative nucleoside transporter, CNT1, in human populations. *Mol. Pharmacol.,* 2004, *65*:512–519.

Greiner, B., Eichelbaum, M., Fritz, P., *et al.* The role of intestinal P-glycoprotein in the interaction of digoxin and rifampin. *J. Clin. Invest.,* 1999, *104*:147–153.

Hagenbuch, B., Scharschmidt, B.F., and Meier, P.J. Effect of antisense oligonucleotides on the expression of hepatocellular bile acid and organic anion uptake systems in *Xenopus laevis* oocytes. *Biochem. J.,* 1996, *316*:901–904.

Hagenbuch, B., Stieger, B., Foguet, M., Lubbert, H., and Meier, P.J. Functional expression cloning and characterization of the hepatocyte Na⁺/bile acid cotransport system. *Proc. Natl. Acad. Sci. U.S.A.,* 1991, *88*:10629–10633.

Hayer, M., Bonisch, H., and Bruss, M. Molecular cloning, functional characterization and genomic organization of four alternatively spliced isoforms of the human organic cation transporter 1 (hOCT1/SLC22A1). *Ann. Hum. Gene.,* 1999, *63*:473–482.

Hediger, M.A. (ed.). In, *Special Issue: The ABCs of Solute Carriers: Physiological, Pathological and Therapeutic Implications of Human Membrane Transport Proteins.* Springer-Verlag, Berlin, 2004.

Hediger, M.A., Coady, M.J., Ikeda, T.S., and Wright, E.M. Expression cloning and cDNA sequencing of the Na⁺/glucose co-transporter. *Nature,* 1987, *330*:379–381.

Hirano, M., Maeda, K., Shitara, Y., and Sugiyama, Y. Contribution of OATP2 (OATP1B1) and OATP8 (OATP1B3) to the hepatic uptake of pitavastatin in humans. *J. Pharmacol. Exp. Ther.,* 2004, *311*:139–146.

Hoffmeyer, S., Burk, O., von Richter, O., *et al.* Functional polymorphisms of the human multidrug-resistance gene: Multiple sequence variations and correlation of one allele with P-glycoprotein expression and activity in vivo. *Proc. Natl. Acad. Sci. U.S.A.,* 2000, *97*:3473–3478.

Horio, M., Pastan, I., Gottesman, M.M., and Handler, J.S. Transepithelial transport of vinblastine by kidney-derived cell lines: Application of a new kinetic model to estimate in situ K_m of the pump. *Biochem. Biophys. Acta,* 1990, *1027*:116–122.

Illmer, T., Schuler, U.S., Thiede, C., *et al.* MDR1 gene polymorphisms affect therapy outcome in acute myeloid leukemia patients. *Cancer Res.,* 2002, *62*:4955–4962.

Inoue, T., Kusumi, I., and Yoshioka, M. Serotonin transporters. *Curr. Drug Targets CNS Neurol. Disord.,* 2002, *1*:519–529.

Ishikawa, T., Muller, M., Klunemann, C., *et al.* ATP-dependent primary active transport of cysteinyl leukotrienes across liver canalicular membrane: Role of the ATP-dependent transport system for glutathione *S*-conjugates. *J. Biol. Chem.,* 1990, *265*:19279–19286.

Ito, K., Suzuki, H., Hirohashi, T., *et al.* Molecular cloning of canalicular multispecific organic anion transporter defective in EHBR. *Am. J. Physiol.,* 1997, *272*:G16–22.

Johne, A., Kopke, K., Gerloff, T., *et al.* Modulation of steady-state kinetics of digoxin by haplotypes of the P-glycoprotein MDR1 gene. *Clin. Pharmaco.l Ther.,* 2002, *72*:584–594.

Jones, S.R., Gainetdinov, R.R., Wightma, R.M., *et al.* Mechanisms of amphetamine action revealed in mice lacking the dopamine transporter. *J. Neurosci.,* 1998, *18*:1979–1986.

Juliano, R.L., and Ling, V. A surface glycoprotein modulating drug permeability in Chinese hamster ovary cell mutants. *Biochem. Biophys. Acta,* 1976, *455*:152–162.

Jutabha, P., Kanai, Y., Hosoyamada, M., *et al.* Identification of a novel voltage-driven organic anion transporter present at apical membrane of renal proximal tubule. *J. Biol. Chem.,* 2003, *278*:27930–27938.

Kekuda, R., Prasad, P.D., Wu, X., *et al.* Cloning and functional characterization of a potential-sensitive polyspecific organic cation transporter (OCT3) most abundantly expressed in placenta. *J. Biol. Chem.,* 1998, *273*:15971–15979.

Kerb, R., Brinkmann, U., Chatskaia, N., *et al.* Identification of genetic variations of the human organic cation transporter hOCT1 and their functional consequences. *Pharmacogenetics,* 2002, *12*:591–595.

Kikuchi, R., Kusuhara, H., Abe, T., *et al.* Involvement of multiple transporters in the efflux of 3-hydroxy-3-methylglutaryl-CoA reductase inhibitors across the blood–brain barrier. *J. Pharmacol. Exp. Ther.,* 2004, *311*:1147–1153.

Kim, R.B. Transporters and xenobiotic disposition. *Toxicology,* 2002, *181–182*:291–297.

Koepsell, H. Organic cation transporters in intestine, kidney, liver, and brain. *Annu. Rev. Physiol.,* 1998, *60*:243–266.

Koepsell, H., and Endou, H. The SLC22 drug transporter family. *Pflugers Arch.,* 2004, *447*:666–676.

Koepsell, H., Schmitt, B.M., and Gorboulev, V. Organic cation transporters. *Rev. Physiol. Biochem. Pharmacol.,* 2003, *150*:36–90.

Kok, T., Wolters, H., Bloks, V.W., *et al.* Induction of hepatic ABC transporter expression is part of the PPARα-mediated fasting response in the mouse. *Gastroenterology,* 2003, *124*:160–171.

Konig, J., Cui, Y., Nies, A.T., and Keppler, D. Localization and genomic organization of a new hepatocellular organic anion transporting polypeptide. *J. Biol. Chem.,* 2000, *275*:23161–23168.

Kullak-Ublick, G,A., Stieger, B., and Meier, P.J. Enterohepatic bile salt transporters in normal physiology and liver disease. *Gastroenterology,* 2004, *126*:322–342.

Kusuhara, H., Sekine, T., Utsunomiya-Tate, N., *et al.* Molecular cloning and characterization of a new multispecific organic anion transporter from rat brain. *J. Biol. Chem.,* 1999, *274*:13675–13680.

Leabman, M.K., Huang, C.C., DeYoung, J., *et al.* Natural variation in human membrane transporter genes reveals evolutionary and functional constraints. *Proc. Natl. Acad. Sci. U.S.A.,* 2003, *100*:5896–5901.

Lesch, K.P, Bengel, D., Heils, A., *et al.* Association of anxiety-related traits with a polymorphism in the serotonin transporter gene regulatory region. *Science,* 1996, *274*:1527–1531.

Leslie, E., Deeley, R., and Cole, S. Multidrug resistance proteins: role of P-glycoprotein, MRP1, MRP2 and BCRP (ABCG2) in tissue defense. *Toxicol. Appl. Pharmacol.,* 2005, *204*:216–237.

Lin, J.H., and Yamazaki, M. Clinical relevance of P-glycoprotein in drug therapy. *Drug Metab. Rev.,* 2003, *35*:417–454.

Macphee, I.A,, Fredericks, S., Tai, T., *et al.* Tacrolimus pharmacogenetics: Polymorphisms associated with expression of cytochrome P4503A5 and P-glycoprotein correlate with dose requirement. *Transplantation,* 2002, *74*:1486–1489.

Mizuno, N., Niwa, T., Yotsumoto, Y., and Sugiyama, Y. Impact of drug transporter studies on drug discovery and development. *Pharmacol. Rev.,* 2003, *55*:425–461.

Mori, S., Takanaga, H., Ohtsuki, S., *et al.* Rat organic anion transporter 3 (rOAT3) is responsible for brain-to-blood efflux of homovanillic acid at the abluminal membrane of brain capillary endothelial cells. *J. Cereb. Blood Flow Metab.,* 2003, *23*:432–440.

Mwinyi, J., Johne, A., Bauer, S., *et al.* Evidence for inverse effects of OATP-C (SLC21A6) 5 and 1b haplotypes on pravastatin kinetics. *Clin. Pharmacol. Ther.,* 2004, *75*:415–421.

Nezu, J., Tamai, I., Oku, A., *et al.* Primary systemic carnitine deficiency is caused by mutations in a gene encoding sodium ion–dependent carnitine transporter. *Nature Genet.,* 1999, *21*:91–94.

Niemi, M., Schaeffeler, E., Lang. T., *et al*. High plasma pravastatin concentrations are associated with single nucleotide polymorphisms and haplotypes of organic anion transporting polypeptide-C (OATP-C, SLCO1B1). *Pharmacogenetics*, **2004**, *14*:429–440.

Ocheltree, S.M., Shen, H., Hu, Y., *et al*. Mechanisms of cefadroxil uptake in the choroid plexus: Studies in wild-type and PEPT2 knockout mice. *J. Pharmacol. Exp. Ther.*, **2004**, *308*:462–467.

Ohashi, R., Tamai, I., Nezu Ji, J., *et al*. Molecular and physiological evidence for multifunctionality of carnitine/organic cation transporter OCTN2. *Mol. Pharmacol.*, **2001**, *59*:358–366.

Okuda, M., Saito, H., Urakami, Y., *et al*. cDNA cloning and functional expression of a novel rat kidney organic cation transporter, OCT2. *Biochem. Biophys. Res. Commun.*, **1996**, *224*:500–507.

Olivier, B., Soudijn, W., and van Wijngaarden, I. Serotonin, dopamine and norepinephrine transporters in the central nervous system and their inhibitors. *Prog. Drug Res.*, **2000**, *54*:59–119.

Osato, D.H., Huang, C.C., Kawamoto, M., *et al*. Functional characterization in yeast of genetic variants in the human equilibrative nucleoside transporter, ENT1. *Pharmacogenetics*, **2003**, *13*:297–301.

Pascual, J.M., Wang, D., Lecumberri, B., *et al*. GLUT1 deficiency and other glucose transporter diseases. *Eur. J. Endocrinol.*, **2004**, *150*:627–633.

Pauli-Magnus, C., Feiner, J., Brett C, *et al*. No effect of MDR1 C3435T variant on loperamide disposition and central nervous system effects. *Clin. Pharmacol. Ther.*, **2004**, *74*:487–498.

Paulusma, C.C., Bosma, P.J., Zaman, G.J., *et al*. Congenital jaundice in rats with a mutation in a multidrug resistance-associated protein gene. *Science*, **1996**, *271*:1126–1128.

Rader, D.J. Regulation of reverse cholesterol transport and clinical implications. *Am. J. Cardiol.*, **2003**, *92*:42J–49J.

Reuss, L. Basic mechanisms of ion transport. In, *The Kidney Physiology and Pathophysiology*. (Seldin, D., and Giebisch, G., eds.), Lippincott Williams & Wilkins, Baltimore, **2000**, pp. 85–106.

Roberts, R.L., Joyce, P.R., Mulder, R.T., *et al*. A common P-glycoprotein polymorphism is associated with nortriptyline-induced postural hypotension in patients treated for major depression. *Pharmacogenomics J.*, **2002**, *2*:191–196.

Rosskopf, D., Dusing, R., and Siffert, W. Membrane sodium–proton exchange and primary hypertension. *Hypertension*, **1993**, *21*:607–617.

Sadee, W., Drubbisch, V., and Amidon, G.L. Biology of membrane transport proteins. *Pharm. Res.*, **1995**, *12*:1823–1837.

Sadeque, A.J., Wandel, C., and He, H., Increased drug delivery to the brain by P-glycoprotein inhibition. *Clin. Pharmacol. Ther.*, **2000**, *68*:231–237.

Sai, K., Kaniwa, N., and Itoda, M., Haplotype analysis of ABCB1/MDR1 blocks in a Japanese population reveals genotype-dependent renal clearance of irinotecan. *Pharmacogenetics*, **2003**, *13*:741–757.

Sakaeda, T., Nakamura, T., Horinouchi, M., *et al*. MDR1 genotype-related pharmacokinetics of digoxin after single oral administration in healthy Japanese subjects. *Pharm. Res.*, **2003**, *18*:1400–1404.

Sasaki, M., Suzuki, H., and Ito, K. Transcellular transport of organic anions across a double-transfected Madin-Darby canine kidney II cell monolayer expressing both human organic anion-transporting polypeptide (OATP2/SLC21A6) and multidrug resistance-associated protein 2 (MRP2/ABCC2). *J. Biol. Chem.*, **2002**, *277*:6497–6503.

Schinkel, A.H., Smit, J.J., and van Tellingen, O. Disruption of the mouse mdr1a P-glycoprotein gene leads to a deficiency in the blood–brain barrier and to increased sensitivity to drugs. *Cell*, **1994**, *77*:491–502.

Schuetz, J.D., Connelly, M.C., and Sun, D. MRP4: A previously unidentified factor in resistance to nucleoside-based antiviral drugs. *Nature Med.*, **1999**, *5*:1048–1051.

Schwab, M., Schaeffeler, E., Marx, C., *et al*. Association between the C3435T MDR1 gene polymorphism and susceptibility for ulcerative colitis. *Gastroenterology*, **2003**, *124*:26–33.

Sekine, T., Cha, S.H., Tsuda, M., *et al*. Identification of multispecific organic anion transporter 2 expressed predominantly in the liver. *FEBS Lett.*, **1998**, *429*:179–82.

Sekine, T., Watanabe, N., Hosoyamada, M., *et al*. Expression cloning and characterization of a novel multispecific organic anion transporter. *J. Biol. Chem.*, **1997**, *272*:18526–18529.

Shigeri, Y., Seal, R.P., and Shimamoto, K. Molecular pharmacology of glutamate transporters, EAATs and VGLUTs. *Brain Res. Rev.*, **2004**, *45*:250–265.

Shitara, Y., Itoh, T., Sato, H., *et al*. Inhibition of transporter-mediated hepatic uptake as a mechanism for drug–drug interaction between cerivastatin and cyclosporin A. *J. Pharmacol. Exp. Ther.*, **2003**, *304*:610–616.

Shu, Y., Leabman, M.K., Feng, B., *et al*. Evolutionary conservation predicts function of variants of the human organic cation transporter, OCT1. *Proc. Natl. Acad. Sci. U.S.A.*, **2003**, *100*:5902–5907.

Siddiqui, A., Kerb, R., Weale, M.E., *et al*. Association of multidrug resistance in epilepsy with a polymorphism in the drug-transporter gene ABCB1. *New Engl. J. Med.*, **2003**, *348*:1442–1448.

Siegsmund, M., Brinkmann, U., Schaffeler, E., *et al*. Association of the P-glycoprotein transporter MDR1(C3435T) polymorphism with the susceptibility to renal epithelial tumors. *J. Am. Soc. Nephrol.*, **2002**, *13*:1847–1854.

Simonson, G.D., Vincent, A.C., Roberg, K.J., *et al*. Molecular cloning and characterization of a novel liver-specific transport protein. *J Cell Sci.*, **1994**, *107*:1065–1072.

Stieger, B., Fattinger, K., Madon, J., *et al*. Drug- and estrogen-induced cholestasis through inhibition of the hepatocellular bile salt export pump (BSEP) of rat liver. *Gastroenterology*, **2000**, *118*:422–430.

Sun, H., Dai, H., Shaik, N., and Elmquist, W.F. Drug efflux transporters in the CNS. *Adv. Drug Deliv. Rev.*, **2003**, *55*:83–105.

Suzuki, T., Nishio, K., and Tanabe, S. The MRP family and anticancer drug metabolism. *Curr. Drug Metab.*, **2001**, *2*:367–377.

Sweet, D.H., Wolff, N.A., and Pritchard, J.B. Expression cloning and characterization of ROAT1: The basolateral organic anion transporter in rat kidney. *J. Biol. Chem.*, **1997**, *272*:30088–30095.

Tamai, I., Ohashi, R., Nezu, J., *et al*. Molecular and functional identification of sodium ion–dependent, high affinity human carnitine transporter OCTN2. *J. Biol. Chem.*, **1998**, *273*:20378–20382.

Tamai, I., Yabuuchi, H., Nezu, J., *et al*. Cloning and characterization of a novel human pH-dependent organic cation transporter, OCTN1. *FEBS Lett.*, **1997**, *419*:107–111.

Tirona, R.G., Leake, B.F., Merino, G., and Kim, R.B. Polymorphisms in OATP-C: Identification of multiple allelic variants associated with altered transport activity among European- and African-Americans. *J. Biol. Chem.*, **2001**, *276*:35669–35675.

Uhl, G.R. Dopamine transporter: basic science and human variation of a key molecule for dopaminergic function, locomotion, and parkinsonism. *Mov. Disord.*, **2003**, *18*:S71–80.

Urakami, Y., Akazawa, M., Saito, H., *et al*. cDNA cloning, functional characterization, and tissue distribution of an alternatively spliced variant of organic cation transporter hOCT2 predominantly expressed in the human kidney. *J. Am. Soc. Nephrol.*, **2002**, *13*:1703–1710.

Verstuyft, C., Schwab, M., Schaeffeler, E., *et al.* Digoxin pharmacokinetics and MDR1 genetic polymorphisms. *Eur. J. Clin. Pharmacol.,* **2003,** *58*:809–812.

Wang, D.S., Kusuhara, H., Kato, Y., *et al.* Involvement of organic cation transporter 1 in the lactic acidosis caused by metformin. *Mol. Pharmacol.,* **2003,** *63*:844–848.

Wang, H., and LeCluyse, E.L. Role of orphan nuclear receptors in the regulation of drug-metabolising enzymes. *Clin. Pharmacokinet.,* **2003,** *42*:1331–1357.

Werner, A., Moore, M.L, Mantei, N., *et al.* Cloning and expression of cDNA for a Na/P$_i$ cotransport system of kidney cortex. *Proc. Natl. Acad. Sci. U.S.A.,* **1991,** *88*:9608–9612.

Wright, S.H., and Dantzler, W.H. Molecular and cellular physiology of renal organic cation and anion transport. *Physiol. Rev.,* **2004,** *84*:987–1049.

Xu, F., Gainetdinov, R.R., Wetsel, W.C., *et al.* Mice lacking the norepinephrine transporter are supersensitive to psychostimulants. *Nature Neurosci.,* **2000,** *3*:465–471.

Yamauchi, A., Ieiri, I., Kataoka, Y., *et al.* Neurotoxicity induced by tacrolimus after liver transplantation: Relation to genetic polymorphisms of the ABCB1 (MDR1) gene. *Transplantation,* **2002,** *74*:571–572.

Zamek-Gliszczynski, M., and Brouwer, K. In vitro models for estimating hepatobiliary clearance. In, *Biotechnology: Pharmaceutical Aspects,* Vol. 1: *Pharmaceutical Profiling in Drug Discovery for Lead Selection.* (Borchardt, R., Kerns, E., Lipinski, C., *et al.,* eds.) AAPS Press, Arlington, VA **2004,** pp. 259–292.

Zhang, Y. and Benet, L.Z. The gut as a barrier to drug absorption: Combined role of cytochrome P450 3A and P-glycoprotein. *Clin. Pharmacokinet.,* **2001,** *40*:159–168.

DRUG METABOLISM

Frank J. Gonzalez and Robert H. Tukey

How Humans Cope with Exposure to Xenobiotics. The ability of humans to metabolize and clear drugs is a natural process that involves the same enzymatic pathways and transport systems that are utilized for normal metabolism of dietary constituents. Humans come into contact with scores of foreign chemicals or xenobiotics (substances foreign to the body) through exposure to environmental contaminants as well as in our diets. Fortunately, humans have developed a means to rapidly eliminate xenobiotics so they do not cause harm. In fact, one of the most common sources of xenobiotics in the diet is from plants that have many structurally diverse chemicals, some of which are associated with pigment production and others that are actually toxins (called phytoallexins) that protect plants against predators. A common example is poisonous mushrooms that have many toxins that are lethal to mammals, including amanitin, gyromitrin, orellanine, muscarine, ibotenic acid, muscimol, psilocybin, and coprine. Animals must be able to metabolize and eliminate such chemicals in order to consume vegetation. While humans can now choose their dietary source, a typical animal does not have this luxury and as a result is subject to its environment and the vegetation that exists in that environment. Thus, the ability to metabolize unusual chemicals in plants and other food sources is critical for survival.

Drugs are considered xenobiotics and most are extensively metabolized in humans. It is worth noting that many drugs are derived from chemicals found in plants, some of which had been used in Chinese herbal medicines for thousands of years. Of the prescription drugs in use today for cancer treatment, many derive from plant species (*see* Chapter 51); investigating folklore claims led to the discovery of most of these drugs. It is therefore not surprising that animals utilize a means for disposing of human-made drugs that mimics the disposition of chemicals found in the diet. This capacity to metabolize xenobiotics, while mostly beneficial, has made development of drugs very time consuming and costly due in large part to (1) interindividual variations in the capacity of humans to metabolize drugs, (2) drug-drug interactions, and (3) species differences in expression of enzymes that metabolize drugs. The latter limits the use of animal models in drug development.

A large number of diverse enzymes have evolved in animals that apparently only function to metabolize foreign chemicals. As will be discussed below, there are such large differences among species in the ability to metabolize xenobiotics that animal models cannot be relied upon to predict how humans will metabolize a drug. Enzymes that metabolize xenobiotics have historically been called drug-metabolizing enzymes, although they are involved in the metabolism of many foreign chemicals to which humans are exposed. Dietary differences among species during the course of evolution could account for the marked species variation in the complexity of the drug-metabolizing enzymes.

Today, most xenobiotics to which humans are exposed come from sources that include environmental pollution, food additives, cosmetic products, agrochemicals, processed foods, and drugs. In general, these are lipophilic chemicals, that in the absence of metabolism would not be efficiently eliminated, and thus would accumulate in the body, resulting in toxicity. With very few exceptions, all xenobiotics are subjected to one or multiple pathways that constitute the phase 1 and phase 2 enzymatic systems. As a general paradigm, metabolism serves to convert these hydrophobic chemicals into derivatives that can easily be eliminated through the urine or the bile.

In order to be accessible to cells and reach their sites of action, drugs generally must possess physical properties that allow them to move down a concentration gradient into the cell. Thus, most drugs are hydrophobic, a property that allows entry through the lipid bilayers into cells where drugs interact with their target receptors or proteins. Entry into cells is facilitated by a large number of transporters on the plasma membrane (*see* Chapter 2). This property of hydrophobicity would render drugs difficult to eliminate, since in the absence of metabolism, they would accumulate in fat and cellular phospholipid bilayers in cells. The xenobiotic-metabolizing enzymes convert drugs and xenobiotics into compounds that are hydrophilic derivatives that are more easily eliminated through excretion into the aqueous compartments of the tissues. Thus, the process of drug metabolism that leads to elimination plays a major role in diminishing the biological activity of a drug. For example, *(S)-phenytoin*, an anticonvulsant used in the treatment of epilepsy, is virtually insoluble in water. Metabolism by the phase 1 cytochrome P450 isoenzymes (CYPs) followed by phase 2 uridine diphosphate-glucuronosyltransferase (UGT) enzymes produces a metabolite that is highly water soluble and readily eliminated from the body (Figure 3–1). Metabolism also terminates the biological activity of the drug. In the case of phenytoin, metabolism also increases the molecular weight of the compound, which allows it to be eliminated more efficiently in the bile.

While xenobiotic-metabolizing enzymes are responsible for facilitating the elimination of chemicals from the body, paradoxically these same enzymes can also convert certain chemicals to highly reactive toxic and carcinogenic metabolites. This occurs when an unstable intermediate is formed that has reactivity toward other compounds found in the cell. Chemicals that can be converted by xenobiotic metabolism to cancer-causing derivatives are called carcinogens. Depending on the structure of the chemical substrate, xenobiotic-metabolizing enzymes produce electrophilic metabolites that can react with nucleophilic cellular macromolecules such as DNA, RNA, and protein. This can cause cell death and organ toxicity. Reaction of these electrophiles with DNA can sometimes result in cancer through the mutation of genes such as oncogenes or tumor suppressor genes. It is generally believed that most human cancers are due to exposure to chemical carcinogens. This potential for carcinogenic activity makes testing the safety of drug candidates of vital importance. Testing for potential cancer-causing activity is particularly critical for drugs that will be used for the treatment of chronic diseases. Since each species has evolved a unique combination of xenobiotic-metabolizing enzymes, nonprimate rodent models cannot be solely used during drug development for testing the safety of new drug candi-

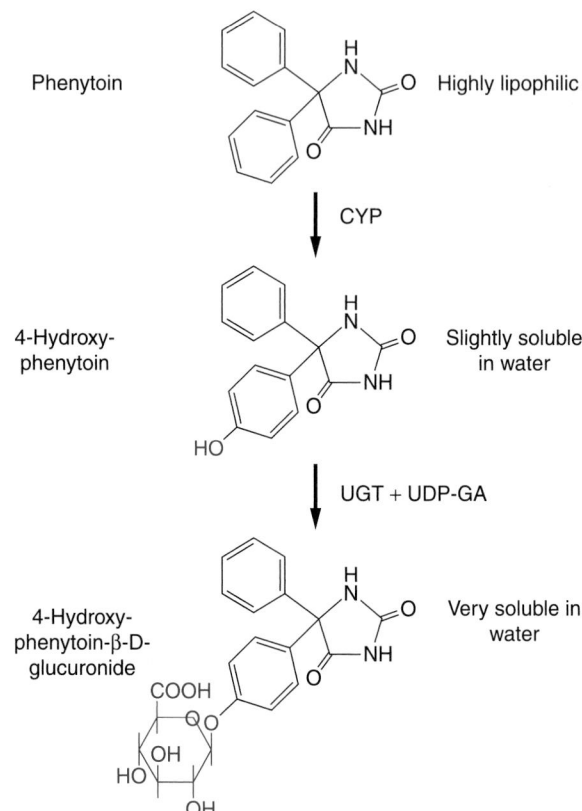

Figure 3–1. *Metabolism of phenytoin by phase 1 cytochrome P450 (CYP) and phase 2 uridine diphosphate-glucuronosyltransferase (UGT).* CYP facilitates 4-hydroxylation of phenytoin to yield 5-(-4-hydroxyphenyl)-5-phenylhydantoin (HPPH). The hydroxy group serves as a substrate for UGT that conjugates a molecule of glucuronic acid using UDP-glucuronic acid (UDP-GA) as a cofactor. This converts a very hydrophobic molecule to a larger hydrophilic derivative that is eliminated *via* the bile.

dates targeted for human diseases. Nevertheless, testing in rodent models such as mice and rats can usually identify potential carcinogens.

The Phases of Drug Metabolism. Xenobiotic metabolizing enzymes have historically been grouped into the phase 1 reactions, in which enzymes carry out oxidation, reduction, or hydrolytic reactions, and the phase 2 reactions, in which enzymes form a conjugate of the substrate (the phase 1 product) (Table 3–1). The phase 1 enzymes lead to the introduction of what are called functional groups, resulting in a modification of the drug, such that it now carries an –OH, -COOH, -SH, -O- or NH$_2$ group. The addition of functional groups does little to increase the water solubility of the drug, but can dra-

Table 3–1
Xenobiotic Metabolizing Enzymes

ENZYMES	REACTIONS
Phase 1 "oxygenases"	
Cytochrome P450s (P450 or CYP)	C and O oxidation, dealkylation, others
Flavin-containing monooxygenases (FMO)	N, S, and P oxidation
Epoxide hydrolases (mEH, sEH)	Hydrolysis of epoxides
Phase 2 "transferases"	
Sulfotransferases (SULT)	Addition of sulfate
UDP-glucuronosyltransferases (UGT)	Addition of glucuronic acid
Glutathione-S-transferases (GST)	Addition of glutathione
N-acetyltransferases (NAT)	Addition of acetyl group
Methyltransferases (MT)	Addition of methyl group
Other enzymes	
Alcohol dehydrogenases	Reduction of alcohols
Aldehyde dehydrogenases	Reduction of aldehydes
NADPH-quinone oxidoreductase (NQO)	Reduction of quinones

mEH and sEH are microsomal and soluble epoxide hydrolase. UDP, uridine diphosphate; NADPH, reduced nicotinamide adenine dinucleotide phosphate.

matically alter the biological properties of the drug. Phase 1 metabolism is classified as the functionalization phase of drug metabolism; reactions carried out by phase 1 enzymes usually lead to the inactivation of an active drug. In certain instances, metabolism, usually the hydrolysis of an ester or amide linkage, results in bioactivation of a drug. Inactive drugs that undergo metabolism to an active drug are called prodrugs. An example is the antitumor drug *cyclophosphamide*, which is bioactivated to a cell-killing electrophilic derivative (*see* Chapter 51). Phase 2 enzymes facilitate the elimination of drugs and the inactivation of electrophilic and potentially toxic metabolites produced by oxidation. While many phase 1 reactions result in the biological inactivation of the drug, phase 2 reactions produce a metabolite with improved water solubility and increased molecular weight, which serves to facilitate the elimination of the drug from the tissue.

Superfamilies of evolutionarily related enzymes and receptors are common in the mammalian genome; the enzyme systems responsible for drug metabolism are good examples. The phase 1 oxidation reactions are carried out by CYPs, flavin-containing monooxygenases (FMO), and epoxide hydrolases (EH). The CYPs and FMOs are composed of superfamilies of enzymes. Each superfamily contains multiple genes. The phase 2 enzymes include several superfamilies of conjugating enzymes. Among the more important are the glutathione-S-transferases (GST), UDP-glucuronosyltransferases (UGT), sulfotransferases (SULT), *N*-acetyltransferases (NAT), and methyltransferases (MT). These conjugation reactions usually require the substrate to have oxygen (hydroxyl or epoxide groups), nitrogen, and sulfur atoms that serve as acceptor sites for a hydrophilic moiety, such as glutathione, glucuronic acid, sulfate, or an acetyl group, that is covalently conjugated to an acceptor site on the molecule. The example of phase 1 and phase 2 metabolism of phenytoin is shown in Figure 3–1. The oxidation by phase 1 enzymes either adds or exposes a functional group, permitting the products of phase 1 metabolism to serve as substrates for the phase 2 conjugating or synthetic enzymes. In the case of the UGTs, glucuronic acid is delivered to the functional group, forming a glucuronide metabolite that is now more water soluble with a higher molecular weight that is targeted for excretion either in the urine or bile. When the substrate is a drug, these reactions usually convert the original drug to a form that is not able to bind to its target receptor, thus attenuating the biological response to the drug.

Sites of Drug Metabolism. Xenobiotic metabolizing enzymes are found in most tissues in the body with the highest levels located in the tissues of the gastrointestinal tract (liver, small and large intestines). Drugs that are orally administered, absorbed by the gut, and taken to the liver, can be extensively metabolized. The liver is considered the major "metabolic clearing house" for both endogenous chemicals (*e.g.,* cholesterol, steroid hormones, fatty acids, and proteins), and xenobiotics. The small intestine plays a crucial role in drug metabolism since most drugs that are orally administered are absorbed by the gut and taken to the liver through the portal vein. The high concentration of xenobiotic-metabolizing enzymes located in the epithelial cells of the GI tract is responsible for the initial metabolic processing of most oral medications. This should be considered the initial site for first-pass metabolism of drugs. The absorbed drug then enters the portal circulation for its first pass through the liver, where metabolism may be prominent, as it is for β adrenergic receptor antagonists, for example. While a portion of active drug escapes this first-pass metabolism in the GI tract and liver, subsequent passes through the liver result in more metabolism of the parent drug until the agent is eliminated. Thus, drugs that are poorly metabolized remain in the body for longer periods of time and their pharmacokinetic profiles show much longer elimination

half-lives than drugs that are rapidly metabolized. Other organs that contain significant xenobiotic-metabolizing enzymes include the tissues of the nasal mucosa and lung, which play important roles in the first-pass metabolism of drugs that are administered through aerosol sprays. These tissues are also the first line of contact with hazardous chemicals that are airborne.

Within the cell, xenobiotic-metabolizing enzymes are found in the intracellular membranes and in the cytosol. The phase 1 CYPs, FMOs, and EHs, and some phase 2 conjugating enzymes, notably the UGTs, are all located in the endoplasmic reticulum of the cell (Figure 3–2). The endoplasmic reticulum consists of phospholipid bilayers organized as tubes and sheets throughout the cytoplasm of the cell. This network has an inner lumen that is physically distinct from the rest of the cytosolic components of the cell and has connections to the plasma membrane and nuclear envelope. This membrane localization is ideally suited for the metabolic function of these enzymes: hydrophobic molecules enter the cell and become embedded in the lipid bilayer where they come into direct contact with

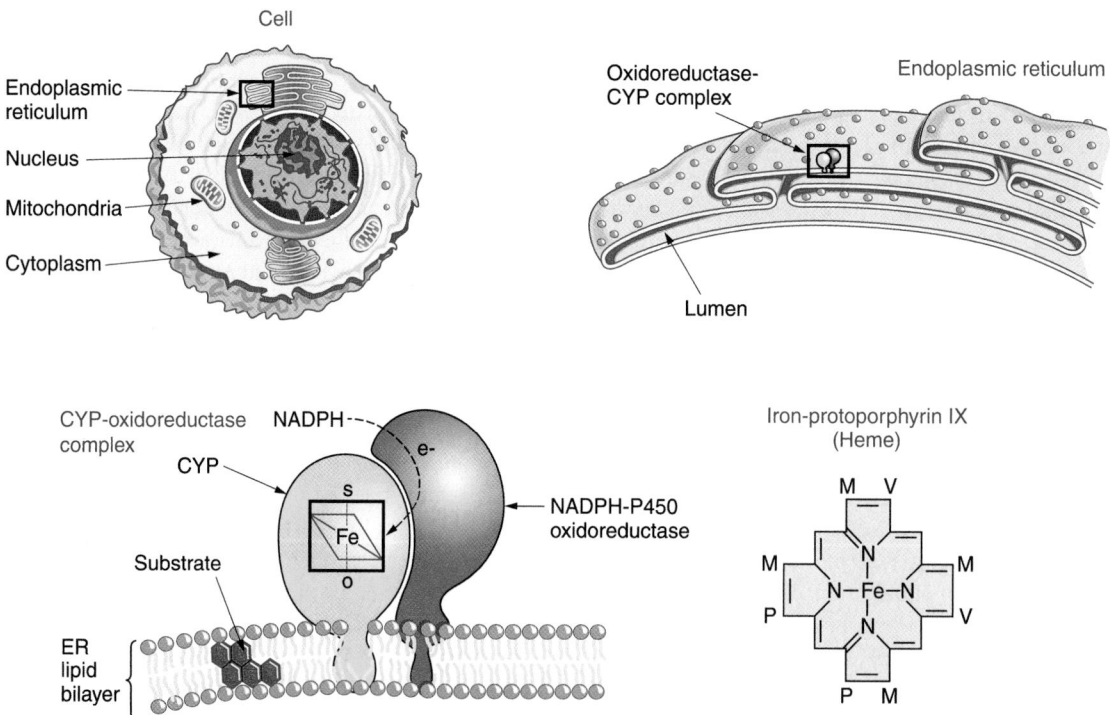

Figure 3–2. *Location of CYPs in the cell.* The figure shows increasingly microscopic levels of detail, sequentially expanding the areas within the black boxes. CYPs are embedded in the phospholipid bilayer of the endoplasmic reticulum (ER). Most of the enzyme is located on the cytosolic surface of the ER. A second enzyme, NADPH-cytochrome P450 oxidoreductase, transfers electrons to the CYP where it can, in the presence of O_2, oxidize xenobiotic substrates, many of which are hydrophobic and dissolved in the ER. A single NADPH-CYP oxidoreductase species transfers electrons to all CYP isoforms in the ER. Each CYP contains a molecule of iron-protoporphyrin IX that functions to bind and activate O_2. Substituents on the porphyrin ring are methyl (M), propionyl (P), and vinyl (V) groups.

the phase 1 enzymes. Once subjected to oxidation, drugs can be conjugated in the membrane by the UGTs or by the cytosolic transferases such as GST and SULT. The metabolites can then be transported out of the cell through the plasma membrane where they are deposited into the bloodstream. Hepatocytes, which constitute more than 90% of the cells in the liver, carry out most drug metabolism and can produce conjugated substrates that can also be transported though the bile canalicular membrane into the bile from which they are eliminated into the gut (*see* Chapter 2).

The CYPs. The CYPs are a superfamily of enzymes, all of which contain a molecule of heme that is noncovalently bound to the polypeptide chain (Figure 3–2). Many other enzymes that use O_2 as a substrate for their reactions contain heme. Heme is the oxygen-binding moiety, also found in hemoglobin, where it functions in the binding and transport of molecular oxygen from the lung to other tissues. Heme contains one atom of iron in a hydrocarbon cage that functions to bind oxygen in the CYP active site as part of the catalytic cycle of these enzymes. CYPs use O_2, plus H^+ derived from the cofactor-reduced nicotinamide adenine dinucleotide phosphate (NADPH), to carry out the oxidation of substrates. The H^+ is supplied through the enzyme NADPH-cytochrome P450 oxidoreductase. Metabolism of a substrate by a CYP consumes one molecule of molecular oxygen and produces an oxidized substrate and a molecule of water as a by-product. However, for most CYPs, depending on the nature of the substrate, the reaction is "uncoupled," consuming more O_2 than substrate metabolized and producing what is called activated oxygen or O_2^-. The O_2^- is usually converted to water by the enzyme superoxide dismutase.

Among the diverse reactions carried out by mammalian CYPs are *N*-dealkylation, *O*-dealkylation, aromatic hydroxylation, *N*-oxidation, *S*-oxidation, deamination, and dehalogenation (Table 3–2). More than 50 individual CYPs have been identified in humans. As a family of enzymes, CYPs are involved in the metabolism of dietary and xenobiotic agents, as well as the synthesis of endogenous compounds such as steroids and the metabolism of bile acids, which are degradation by-products of cholesterol. In contrast to the drug-metabolizing CYPs, the CYPs that catalyze steroid and bile acid synthesis have very specific substrate preferences. For example, the CYP that produces estrogen from testosterone, CYP19 or aromatase, can metabolize only testosterone and does not metabolize xenobiotics. Specific inhibitors for aromatase, such as *anastrozole*, have been developed for use in the

treatment of estrogen-dependent tumors (*see* Chapter 51). The synthesis of bile acids from cholesterol occurs in the liver, where, subsequent to CYP-catalyzed oxidation, the bile acids are conjugated and transported through the bile duct and gallbladder into the small intestine. CYPs involved in bile acid production have strict substrate requirements and do not participate in xenobiotic or drug metabolism.

The CYPs that carry out xenobiotic metabolism have a tremendous capacity to metabolize a large number of structurally diverse chemicals. This is due both to multiple forms of CYPs and to the capacity of a single CYP to metabolize many structurally distinct chemicals. A single compound can also be metabolized, albeit at different rates, by different CYPs. In addition, CYPs can metabolize a single compound at different positions on the molecule. In contrast to enzymes in the body that carry out highly specific reactions involved in the biosynthesis and degradation of important cellular constituents in which there is a single substrate and one or more products, or two simultaneous substrates, the CYPs are considered promiscuous in their capacity to bind and metabolize multiple substrates (Table 3–2). This property, which is due to large and fluid substrate binding sites in the CYP, sacrifices metabolic turnover rates; CYPs metabolize substrates at a fraction of the rate of more typical enzymes involved in intermediary metabolism and mitochondrial electron transfer. As a result, drugs have, in general, half-lives of the order of 3 to 30 hours, while endogenous compounds have half-lives of the order of seconds or minutes (*e.g.,* dopamine and insulin). Even though CYPs have slow catalytic rates, their activities are sufficient to metabolize drugs that are administered at high concentrations in the body. This unusual feature of extensive overlapping substrate specificities by the CYPs is one of the underlying reasons for the predominance of drug-drug interactions. When two coadministered drugs are both metabolized by a single CYP, they compete for binding to the enzyme's active site. This can result in the inhibition of metabolism of one or both of the drugs, leading to elevated plasma levels. If there is a narrow therapeutic index for the drugs, the elevated serum levels may elicit unwanted toxicities. Drug-drug interactions are among the leading causes of adverse drug reactions.

The CYPs are the most actively studied of the xenobiotic metabolizing enzymes since they are responsible for metabolizing the vast majority of therapeutic drugs. CYPs are complex and diverse in their regulation and catalytic activities. Cloning and sequencing of CYP complementary DNAs, and more recently total genome sequencing, have revealed the existence of 102 putatively functional genes and 88 pseudogenes in the mouse, and 57 putatively functional

Table 3–2
Major Reactions Involved in Drug Metabolism

REACTION		EXAMPLES
I. *Oxidative reactions*		
N-Dealkylation	$RNHCH_3 \rightarrow RNH_2 + CH_2O$	Imipramine, diazepam, codeine, erythromycin, morphine, tamoxifen, theophylline, caffeine
O-Dealkylation	$ROCH_3 \rightarrow ROH + CH_2O$	Codeine, indomethacin, dextromethorphan
Aliphatic hydroxylation	$RCH_2CH_3 \rightarrow RCHOHCH_3$	Tolbutamide, ibuprofen, phenobarbital, meprobamate, cyclosporine, midazolam
Aromatic hydroxylation		Phenytoin, phenobarbital, propanolol, ethinyl estradiol, amphetamine, warfarin
N-Oxidation		Chlorpheniramine, dapsone, meperidine
S-Oxidation		Cimetidine, chlorpromazine, thioridazine, omeprazole
Deamination		Diazepam, amphetamine
II. *Hydrolysis reactions*		
		Carbamazepine
		Procaine, aspirin, clofibrate, meperidine, enalapril, cocaine
		Lidocaine, procainamide, indomethacin
III. *Conjugation reactions*		
Glucuronidation	UDP-glucuronic acid	Acetaminophen, morphine, oxazepam, lorazepam

(Continued)

Table 3–2
Major Reactions Involved in Drug Metabolism (Continued)

	REACTION		EXAMPLES
Sulfation	PAPS + ROH $\rightarrow$ R—O—SO$_2$—OH + PAP		Acetaminophen, steroids, methyldopa
	3'-phosphoadenosine-5' phosphosulfate	3'-phosphoadenosine-5'- phosphate	
Acetylation	CoAS—CO—CH$_3$ + RNH$_2$ $\rightarrow$ RNH—CO—CH$_3$ + CoA-SH		Sulfonamides, isoniazid, dapsone, clonazepam (*see* Table 3–3)
Methylation	RO-, RS-, RN- + AdoMet $\rightarrow$ RO-CH$_3$ + AdoHomCys		L-Dopa, methyldopa, mercaptopurine, captopril
Glutathione conjugation	GSH + R $\rightarrow$ R-GSH		Adriamycin, fosfomycin, busulfan

genes and 58 pseudogenes in humans. These genes are grouped, based on amino acid sequence similarity, into a large number of families and subfamilies. CYPs are named with the root CYP followed by a number designating the family, a letter denoting the subfamily, and another number designating the CYP form. Thus, CYP3A4 is family 3, subfamily A, and gene number 4. While several CYP families are involved in the synthesis of steroid hormones and bile acids, and the metabolism of retinoic acid and fatty acids, including prostaglandins and eicosanoids, a limited number of CYPs (15 in humans) that fall into families 1 to 3 are primarily involved in xenobiotic metabolism (Table 3–1). Since a single CYP can metabolize a large number of structurally diverse compounds, these enzymes can collectively metabolize scores of chemicals found in the diet, environment, and administered as drugs. In humans, 12 CYPs (CYP1A1, 1A2, 1B1, 2A6, 2B6, 2C8, 2C9, 2C19, 2D6, 2E1, 3A4, and 3A5) are known to be important for metabolism of xenobiotics. The liver contains the greatest abundance of xenobiotic-metabolizing CYPs, thus ensuring efficient first-pass metabolism of drugs. CYPs are also expressed throughout the GI tract, and in lower amounts in lung, kidney, and even in the CNS. The expression of the different CYPs can differ markedly as a result of dietary and environmental exposure to inducers, or through interindividual changes resulting from heritable polymorphic differences in gene structure, and tissue-specific expression patterns can impact on overall drug metabolism and clearance. The most active CYPs for drug metabolism are those in the CYP2C, CYP2D, and CYP3A subfamilies. CYP3A4 is the most abundantly expressed and involved in the metabolism of about 50% of clinically used drugs (Figure 3–3A). The CYP1A, CYP1B, CYP2A, CYP2B, and CYP2E subfamilies are not significantly involved in the metabolism of therapeutic drugs, but they do catalyze the metabolic activation of many protoxins and procarcinogens to their ultimate reactive metabolites.

There are large differences in levels of expression of each CYP between individuals as assessed both by clinical pharmacologic studies and by analysis of expression in human liver samples. This large interindividual variability in CYP expression is due to the presence of genetic polymorphisms and differences in gene regulation (*see* below). Several human CYP genes exhibit polymorphisms, including *CYP2A6, CYP2C9, CYP2C19,* and *CYP2D6.* Allelic variants have been found in the *CYP1B1* and *CYP3A4* genes, but they are present at low frequencies in humans and appear not to have a major role in interindividual levels of expression of these enzymes. However, homozygous mutations in the *CYP1B1* gene are associated with primary congenital glaucoma.

Drug-Drug Interactions. Differences in the rate of metabolism of a drug can be due to drug interactions. Most commonly, this occurs when two drugs (*e.g.,* a statin and a macrolide antibiotic or antifungal) are coadministered and are metabolized by the same enzyme. Since most of these drug-drug interactions are due to CYPs, it becomes important to determine the identity of the CYP that metabolizes a particular drug and to avoid coadministering drugs that are metabolized by the same enzyme. Some drugs can also inhibit CYPs independently of being substrates for a CYP. For example, the common antifungal agent, *ketoconazole* (NIZORAL), is a potent inhibitor of CYP3A4 and other CYPs, and coadministration of ketoconazole with the anti-HIV viral protease inhibitors reduces the clearance of the protease inhibitor and increases its plasma concentration and the risk of toxicity. For most drugs, descriptive information found on the package insert lists the CYP that carries out its metabolism and the potential for drug interactions. Some drugs are CYP inducers that can induce not only their own metabolism, but also induce metabolism of other coadministered drugs (*see* below and Figure 3–13). Steroid hormones and herbal products such as St. John's wort can increase hepatic levels of CYP3A4, thereby increasing the metabolism of

A

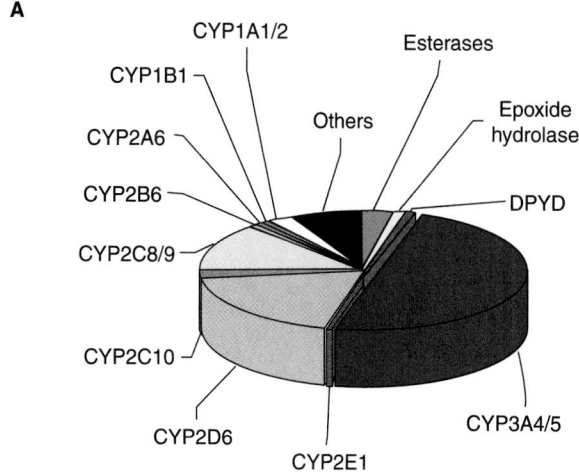

B

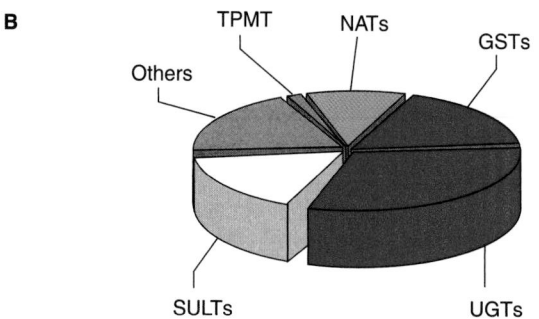

Figure 3–3. ***The fraction of clinically used drugs metabolized by the major phase 1 and phase 2 enzymes.*** The relative size of each pie section represents the estimated percentage of drugs metabolized by the major phase 1 (panel ***A***) and phase 2 (panel ***B***) enzymes, based on studies in the literature. In some cases, more than a single enzyme is responsible for metabolism of a single drug. CYP, cytochrome P450; DPYD, dihydropyrimidine dehydrogenase; GST, glutathione-S-transferase; NAT, N-acetyltransferase; SULT, sulfotransferase, TPMT, thiopurine methyltransferase; UGT, UDP-glucuronosyltransferase.

many orally administered drugs. Drug metabolism can also be influenced by diet. CYP inhibitors and inducers are commonly found in foods and in some cases these can influence the toxicity and efficacy of a drug. Components found in grapefruit juice (*e.g.,* naringin, furanocoumarins) are potent inhibitors of CYP3A4, and thus some drug inserts recommend not taking medication with grapefruit juice because it could increase the bioavailability of a drug.

Terfenadine, a once popular antihistamine, was removed from the market because its metabolism was blocked by CYP3A4 sub-

strates such as *erythromycin* and grapefruit juice. Terfenadine is actually a prodrug that requires oxidation by CYP3A4 to its active metabolite, and at high doses the parent compound caused arrhythmias. Thus, elevated levels of parent drug in the plasma as a result of CYP3A4 inhibition caused ventricular tachycardia in some individuals, which ultimately led to its withdrawal from the market. In addition, interindividual differences in drug metabolism are significantly influenced by polymorphisms in CYPs. The CYP2D6 polymorphism has led to the withdrawal of several clinically used drugs (*e.g., debrisoquine* and *perhexiline*) and the cautious use of others that are known CYP2D6 substrates (*e.g., encainide* and *flecainide* [antiarrhythmics], *desipramine* and *nortriptyline* [antidepressants], and *codeine*).

Flavin-Containing Monooxygenases (FMOs). The FMOs are another superfamily of phase 1 enzymes involved in drug metabolism. Similar to CYPs, the FMOs are expressed at high levels in the liver and are bound to the endoplasmic reticulum, a site that favors interaction with and metabolism of hydrophobic drug substrates. There are six families of FMOs, with FMO3 being the most abundant in liver. FMO3 is able to metabolize nicotine as well as H_2-receptor antagonists (*cimetidine* and *ranitidine*), antipsychotics (*clozapine*), and antiemetics (*itopride*). A genetic deficiency in this enzyme causes the fish-odor syndrome due to a lack of metabolism of trimethylamine *N*-oxide (TMAO) to trimethylamine (TMA); in the absence of this enzyme, TMAO accumulates in the body and causes a socially offensive fish odor. TMAO is found at high concentrations, up to 15% by weight, in marine animals where it acts as an osmotic regulator. FMOs are considered minor contributors to drug metabolism and they almost always produce benign metabolites. In addition, FMOs are not induced by any of the xenobiotic receptors (*see* below) or easily inhibited; thus, in distinction to CYPs, FMOs would not be expected to be involved in drug-drug interactions. In fact, this has been demonstrated by comparing the pathways of metabolism of two drugs used in the control of gastric motility, itopride and *cisapride*. Itopride is metabolized by FMO3 while cisapride is metabolized by CYP3A4; thus, itopride is less likely to be involved in drug-drug interactions than is cisapride. CYP3A4 participates in drug-drug interactions through induction and inhibition of metabolism, whereas FMO3 is not induced or inhibited by any clinically used drugs. It remains a possibility that FMOs may be of importance in the development of new drugs. A candidate drug could be designed by introducing a site for FMO oxidation with the knowledge that selected metabolism and pharmacokinetic properties could be accurately calculated for efficient drug-based biological efficacy.

Hydrolytic Enzymes. Two forms of *epoxide hydrolase* carry out hydrolysis of epoxides produced by CYPs. The soluble epoxide hydrolase (sEH) is expressed in the cytosol while the microsomal epoxide hydrolase (mEH) is localized to the membrane of the endoplasmic reticulum. Epoxides are highly reactive electrophiles that can bind to cellular nucleophiles found in protein, RNA, and DNA, resulting in cell toxicity and transformation. Thus, epoxide hydrolases participate in the deactivation of potentially toxic derivatives generated by CYPs. There are a few examples of the influence of mEH on drug metabolism. The antiepileptic drug *carbamazepine* is a prodrug that is converted to its pharmacologically active derivative, carbamazepine-10,11-epoxide by CYP. This metabolite is efficiently hydrolyzed to a dihydrodiol by mEH, resulting in inactivation of the drug (Figure 3–4). Inhibition of mEH can cause an elevation in plasma concentrations of the active metabolite, causing side effects. The tranquilizer *valnoctamide* and anticonvulsant *valproic acid* inhibit mEH, resulting in clinically significant drug interactions with carbamazepine. This has led to efforts to develop new antiepileptic drugs such as *gabapentin* and *levetiracetam* that are metabolized by CYPs and not by EHs.

The *carboxylesterases* comprise a superfamily of enzymes that catalyze the hydrolysis of ester- and amide-

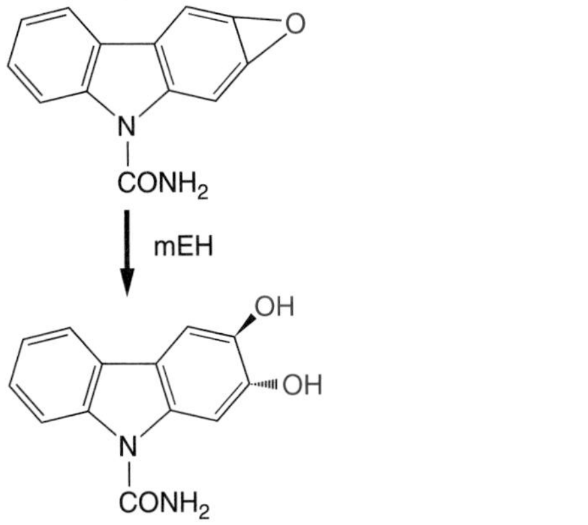

Figure 3–4. *Metabolism of carbamazepine by CYP and microsomal epoxide hydrolase (mEH).* Carbamazepine is oxidized to the pharmacologically-active metabolite carbamazepine-10,11-epoxide by CYP. The epoxide is converted to a trans-dihydrodiol by mEH. This metabolite is biologically inactive and can be conjugated by phase 2 enzymes.

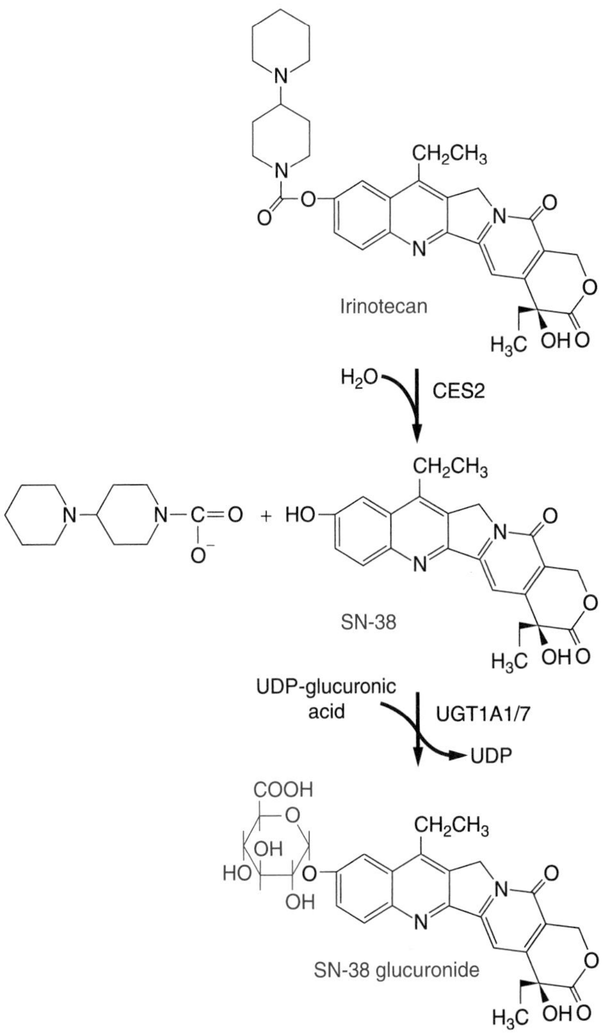

Figure 3–5. *Metabolism of irinotecan (CPT-11).* The prodrug CPT-11 is initially metabolized by a serum esterase (CES2) to the topoisomerase inhibitor SN-38, which is the active camptothecin analog that slows tumor growth. SN-38 is then subject to glucuronidation, which results in loss of biological activity and facilitates elimination of the SN-38 in the bile.

containing chemicals. These enzymes are found in both the endoplasmic reticulum and the cytosol of many cell types and are involved in detoxification or metabolic activation of various drugs, environmental toxicants, and carcinogens. Carboxylesterases also catalyze the activation of prodrugs to their respective free acids. For example, the prodrug and cancer chemotherapeutic agent *irinotecan* is a *camptothecin* analog that is bioactivated by plasma and intracellular carboxylesterases to the potent topoisomerase inhibitor SN-38 (Figure 3–5).

Conjugating Enzymes. There are a large number of phase 2 conjugating enzymes, all of which are considered to be synthetic in nature since they result in the formation of a metabolite with an increased molecular mass. Phase 2 reactions also terminate the biological activity of the drug. The contributions of different phase 2 reactions to drug metabolism are shown in Figure 3–3B. Two of the phase 2 reactions, glucuronidation and sulfation, result in the formation of metabolites with a significantly increased water-to-lipid partition coefficient, resulting in hydrophilicity and facilitating their transport into the aqueous compartments of the cell and the body. Glucuronidation also markedly increases the molecular weight of the compound, a modification that favors biliary excretion. While sulfation and acetylation terminate the biological activity of drugs, the solubility properties of these metabolites are altered through minor changes in the overall charge of the molecule. Characteristic of the phase 2 reactions is the dependency on the catalytic reactions for cofactors such as UDP-glucuronic acid (UDP-GA) and 3'-phosphoadenosine-5'-phosphosulfate (PAPS), for UDP-glucuronosyltransferases (UGT) and sulfotransferases (SULT), respectively, which react with available functional groups on the substrates. The reactive functional groups are often generated by the phase 1 CYPs. All of the phase 2 reactions are carried out in the cytosol of the cell, with the exception of glucuronidation, which is localized to the luminal side of the endoplasmic reticulum. The catalytic rates of phase 2 reactions are significantly faster than the rates of the CYPs. Thus, if a drug is targeted for phase 1 oxidation through the CYPs, followed by a phase 2 conjugation reaction, usually the rate of elimination will depend upon the initial (phase 1) oxidation reaction. Since the rate of conjugation is faster and the process leads to an increase in hydrophilicity of the drug, phase 2 reactions are generally considered to assure the efficient elimination and detoxification of most drugs.

Glucuronidation. Among the more important of the phase 2 reactions in the metabolism of drugs is that catalyzed by UDP-glucuronosyltransferases (UGTs) (Figure 3–3B). These enzymes catalyze the transfer of glucuronic acid from the cofactor UDP-glucuronic acid to a substrate to form β-D-glucopyranosiduronic acids (glucuronides), metabolites that are sensitive to cleavage by β-glucuronidase. The generation of glucuronides can be formed through alcoholic and phenolic hydroxyl groups, carboxyl, sulfuryl, and carbonyl moieties, as well as through primary, secondary, and tertiary amine linkages. Examples of glucuronidation reactions are shown in Table 3–2 and Figure 3–5. The structural diversity in the many different types of drugs and xenobiotics that are processed through

glucuronidation assures that most clinically efficacious therapeutic agents will be excreted as glucuronides.

There are 19 human genes that encode the UGT proteins. Nine are encoded by the *UGT1* locus and 10 are encoded by the *UGT2* family of genes. Both families of proteins are involved in the metabolism of drugs and xenobiotics, while the UGT2 family of proteins appears to have greater specificity for the glucuronidation of endogenous substances such as steroids. The UGT2 proteins are encoded by unique genes on chromosome 4 and the structure of each gene includes six exons. The clustering of the UGT2 genes on the same chromosome with a comparable organization of the regions encoding the open reading frames is evidence that gene duplication has occurred, a process of natural selection that has resulted in the multiplication and eventual diversification of the potential to detoxify the plethora of compounds that are targeted for glucuronidation.

The nine functional UGT1 proteins are all encoded by the *UGT1* locus (Figure 3–6), which is located on chromosome 2. The *UGT1* locus spans nearly 200 kb, with over 150 kb encoding a tandem array of cassette exonic regions that encode approximately 280 amino acids of the amino terminal portion of the UGT1A proteins. Four exons are located at the 3' end of the locus that encode the carboxyl 245 amino acids that combine with one of the consecutively numbered array of first exons to form the individual *UGT1* gene products. Since exons 2 to 5 encode the same sequence for each UGT1A protein, the variability in substrate specificity for each of the UGT1A proteins results from the significant divergence in sequence encoded by the exon 1 regions. The 5' flanking region of each first-exon cassette contains a fully functional promoter capable of initiating transcription in an inducible and tissue-specific manner.

From a clinical perspective, the expression of UGT1A1 assumes an important role in drug metabolism since the glucuronidation of bilirubin by UGT1A1 is the rate-limiting step in assuring efficient bilirubin clearance, and this rate can be affected by both genetic variation and competing substrates (drugs). Bilirubin is the breakdown product of heme, 80% of which originates from circulating hemoglobin and 20% from other heme-containing proteins such as the CYPs. Bilirubin is

UGT1 Locus

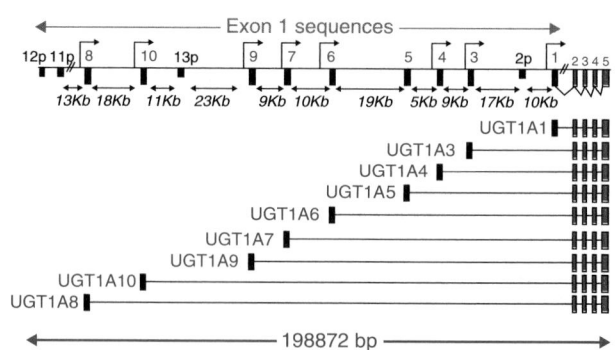

Figure 3–6. Organization of the UGT1A Locus. Transcription of the *UGT1A* genes commences with the activation of PolII, which is controlled through tissue-specific events. Conserved exons 2 to 5 are spliced to each respective exon 1 sequence resulting in the production of unique *UGT1A* sequences. The *UGT1A* locus encodes nine functional proteins.

hydrophobic, associates with serum albumin, and must be metabolized further by glucuronidation to assure its elimination. The failure to efficiently metabolize bilirubin by glucuronidation leads to elevated serum levels and a clinical symptom called hyperbilirubinemia or jaundice. There are more than 50 genetic lesions in the *UGT1A1* gene that can lead to inheritable unconjugated hyperbilirubinemia. Crigler-Najjar syndrome type I is diagnosed as a complete lack of bilirubin glucuronidation, while Crigler-Najjar syndrome type II is differentiated by the detection of low amounts of bilirubin glucuronides in duodenal secretions. Types I and II Crigler-Najjar syndrome are rare, and result from genetic polymorphisms in the open reading frames of the *UGT1A1* gene, resulting in abolished or highly diminished levels of functional protein.

Gilbert's syndrome is a generally benign condition that is present in up to 10% of the population; it is diagnosed clinically because circulating bilirubin levels are 60% to 70% higher than those seen in normal subjects. The most common genetic polymorphism associated with Gilbert's syndrome is a mutation in the *UGT1A1* gene promoter, which leads to reduced expression levels of UGT1A1. Subjects diagnosed with Gilbert's syndrome may be predisposed to adverse drug reactions resulting from a reduced capacity to metabolize drugs by UGT1A1. If a drug undergoes selective metabolism by UGT1A1, competition for drug metabolism with bilirubin glucuronidation will exist, resulting in pronounced hyperbilirubinemia as well as reduced clearance of metabolized drug. *Tranilast* [N-(3′4′-demethoxycinnamoyl)-anthranilic acid] is an investigational drug used for the prevention of restenosis in patients that have undergone transluminal coronary revascularization (intracoronary stents). Tranilast therapy in patients with Gilbert's syndrome has been shown to lead to hyperbilirubinemia as well as potential hepatic complications resulting from elevated levels of tranilast.

Gilbert's syndrome also alters patient responses to irinotecan. Irinotecan, a prodrug used in chemotherapy of solid tumors (*see* Chapter 51), is metabolized to its active form, SN-38, by serum carboxylesterases (Figure 3–5). SN-38, a potent topoisomerase inhibitor, is inactivated by UGT1A1 and excreted in the bile (Figures 3–7 and 3–8). Once in the lumen of the intestine, the SN-38 glucuronide undergoes cleavage by bacterial β-glucuronidase and re-enters the circulation through intestinal absorption. Elevated levels of SN-38 in the blood lead to hematological toxicities characterized by leukopenia and neutropenia, as well as damage to the intestinal epithelial cells (Figure 3–8), resulting in acute and life-threatening diarrhea. Patients with Gilbert's syndrome who are receiving irinotecan therapy are predisposed to the hematological and gastrointestinal toxicities resulting from elevated serum levels of SN-38, the net result of insufficient UGT1A activity and the consequent accumulation of a toxic drug in the GI epithelium.

The UGTs are expressed in a tissue-specific and often inducible fashion in most human tissues, with the highest concentration of enzymes found in the GI tract and liver. Based upon their physicochemical properties, glucuronides are excreted by the kidneys into the urine or through active transport processes through the apical surface of the liver hepatocytes into the bile ducts where they are transported to the duodenum for excretion with components of the bile. Most of the bile acids that are glucuronidated are reabsorbed back to the liver for reutilization by "enterohepatic

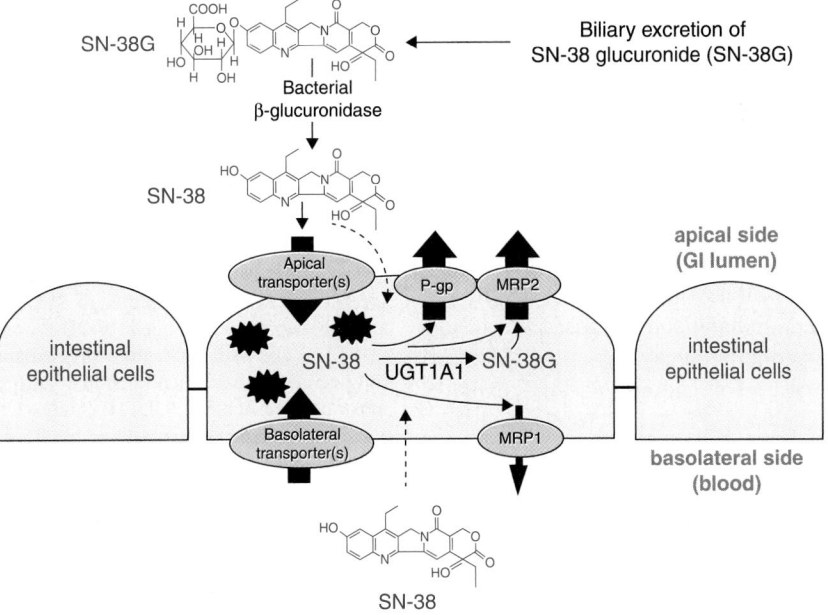

Figure 3–7. Routes of SN-38 transport and exposure to intestinal epithelial cells. SN-38 is transported into the bile following glucuronidation by liver UGT1A1 and extrahepatic UGT1A7. Following cleavage of luminal SN-38 glucuronide (SN-38G) by bacterial β-glucuronidase, reabsorption into epithelial cells can occur by passive diffusion (indicated by the dashed arrows entering the cell) as well as by apical transporters. Movement into epithelial cells may also occur from the blood by basolateral transporters. Intestinal SN-38 can efflux into the lumen through P-glycoprotein (P-gp) and multidrug resistance protein 2 (MRP2) and into the blood *via* MRP1. Excessive accumulation of the SN-38 in intestinal epithelial cells, resulting from reduced glucuronidation, can lead to cellular damage and toxicity (Tukey *et al.*, 2002).

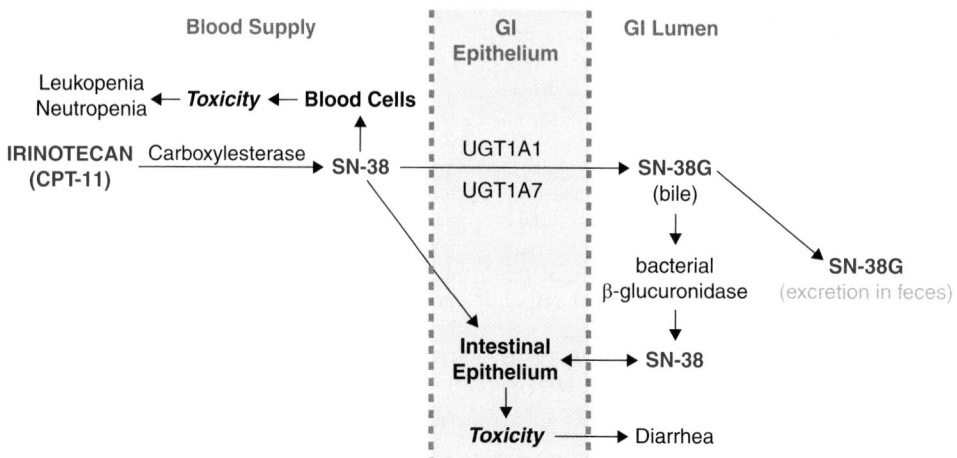

Figure 3–8. *Cellular targets of SN-38 in the blood and intestinal tissues.* Excessive accumulation of SN-38 can lead to blood toxicities such as leukopenia and neutropenia, as well as damage to the intestinal epithelium. These toxicities are pronounced in individuals that have reduced capacity to form the SN-38 glucuronide, such as patients with Gilbert's syndrome. Note the different body compartments and cell types involved (Tukey *et al.*, 2002).

recirculation"; many drugs that are glucuronidated and excreted in the bile can re-enter the circulation by this same process. The β-D-glucopyranosiduronic acids are targets for β-glucuronidase activity found in resident strains of bacteria that are common in the lower GI tract, liberating the free drug into the intestinal lumen. As water is reabsorbed into the large intestine, free drug can then be transported by passive diffusion or through apical transporters back into the intestinal epithelial cells, from which the drug can then re-enter the circulation. Through portal venous return from the large intestine to the liver, the reabsorption process allows for the re-entry of drug into the systemic circulation (Figures 3–7 and 3–8).

Sulfation. The sulfotransferases (SULTs) are located in the cytosol and conjugate sulfate derived from 3'-phosphoadenosine-5'-phosphosulfate (PAPS) to the hydroxyl groups of aromatic and aliphatic compounds. Like all of the xenobiotic metabolizing enzymes, the SULTs metabolize a wide variety of endogenous and exogenous substrates. In humans, 11 SULT isoforms have been identified, and, based on evolutionary projections, have been classified into the SULT1 (SULT1A1, SULT1A2, SULT1A3, SULT1B1, SULT1C2, SYLT1C4, SULT1E1), SULT2 (SULT2A1, SULT2B1-v1, SULT2B1-v2), and SULT4 (SULT4A1) families. SULTs play an important role in normal human homeostasis. For example, SULT1B1 is the predominant form expressed in skin and brain, carrying out the catalysis of cholesterol and thyroid hormones. Cholesterol sulfate is an essential metabolite in regulating keratinocyte differentiation and skin development. SULT1A3 is highly selective for catecholamines, while estrogens are sulfated by SULT1E1 and dehydroepi-

androsterone (DHEA) is selectively sulfated by SULT2A1. In humans, significant fractions of circulating catecholamines, estrogens, iodothyronines, and DHEA exist in the sulfated form.

The different human SULTs display a variety of unique substrate specificities. The SULT1 family isoforms are considered to be the major forms involved in drug metabolism, with SULT1A1 being the most important and displaying extensive diversity in its capacity to catalyze the sulfation of a wide variety of structurally heterogeneous xenobiotics. The isoforms in the SULT1 family have been recognized as phenol SULTs, since they have been characterized to catalyze the sulfation of phenolic molecules such as *acetaminophen, minoxidil,* and *17α-ethinyl estradiol.* While two SULT1C isoforms exist, little is known about their substrate specificity toward drugs, although SULT1C4 is capable of sulfating the hepatic carcinogen N-OH-2-acetylaminofluorene. Both SULT1C2 and SULT1C4 are expressed abundantly in fetal tissues and decline in abundance in adults, yet little is known about their substrate specificities. SULT1E catalyzes the sulfation of endogenous and exogenous steroids, and has been found localized in liver as well as in hormone-responsive tissues such as the testis, breast, adrenal gland, and placenta.

The conjugation of drugs and xenobiotics is considered primarily a detoxification step, assuring that these agents are compartmented into the water compartments of the body for targeted elimination. However, drug metabolism through sulfation often leads to the generation of chemically reactive metabolites, where the sulfate is electron withdrawing and may be heterolytically cleaved, leading to the formation of an electrophilic cation. Most examples of the generation by sulfation of a carcinogenic or toxic response in animal or test mutagenicity assays have been documented with chemicals derived from the environment or from food mutagens generated from well-cooked meat. Thus, it is important to understand whether genetic linkages can be made by associating known human SULT polymorphisms to cancer episodes that are felt to originate from environmental sources. Since SULT1A1 is the most abundant in human tissues and displays broad substrate specificity, the polymorphic profiles associated with this gene and the onset of various human cancers is of considerable interest. An appreciation of the structure of the proteins of the SULT family will aid in drug design and advance an understanding of the linkages relating sulfation to cancer susceptibility, reproduction, and development. The SULTs from the SULT1 and SULT2 families were among the first xenobiotic-metabolizing enzymes to be crystallized and the data indicate a highly conserved catalytic core (Figure 3–9A). The structures reveal the role of the co-substrate PAPS in catalysis, identifying the conserved amino acids that facilitate the $3'$ phosphate's role in sulfuryl transfer to the protein and in turn to the substrate (Figure 3–9B). Crystal structures of the different SULTs indicate that while conservation in the PAPS binding region is maintained, the organization of the substrate binding region differs, helping to explain the observed differences in catalytic potential displayed with the different SULTs.

Glutathione Conjugation. The glutathione-S-transferases (GSTs) catalyze the transfer of glutathione to reactive electrophiles, a function that serves to protect cellular macromolecules from interacting with electrophiles that contain electrophilic heteroatoms (-O, -N, and -S) and in turn protects the cellular environment from damage. The co-substrate in the reaction is the tripeptide glutathione, which is synthesized from γ-glutamic acid, cysteine, and glycine (Figure 3–10). Glutathione exists in the cell as oxidized (GSSG) or reduced (GSH), and the ratio of GSH:GSSG is critical in maintaining a cellular environment in the reduced state. In addition to affecting xenobiotic conjugation with GSH, a severe reduction in GSH content can predispose cells to oxidative damage, a state that has been linked to a number of human health issues.

In the formation of glutathione conjugates, the reaction generates a thioether linkage with drug or xenobiotic to the cysteine moiety of the tripeptide. Characteristically, all GST substrates contain an electrophilic atom and are hydrophobic, and by nature will associate with cellular proteins. Since the concentration of glutathione in cells is usually very high, typically ~7 μmol/g of liver, or in the 10 mM range, many drugs and xenobiotics can react nonenzymatically with glutathione. However, the GSTs have been found to occupy up to 10% of the total cellular protein concentration, a property that assures efficient conjugation of glutathione to reactive electrophiles. The high concentration of GSTs also provides the cells with a sink of cytosolic protein, a property that facilitates noncovalent and sometimes covalent interactions with compounds that are not substrates for glutathione conjugation. The cytosolic pool of GSTs, once identified as *ligandin*, has been

shown to bind steroids, bile acids, bilirubin, cellular hormones, and environmental toxicants, in addition to complexing with other cellular proteins.

Over 20 human GSTs have been identified and divided into two subfamilies: the cytosolic and the microsomal forms. The major differences in function between the microsomal and cytosolic GSTs reside in the selection of substrates for conjugation; the cytosolic forms have more importance in the metabolism of drugs and xenobiotics, whereas the microsomal GSTs are important in the endogenous metabolism of leukotrienes and prostaglandins. The cytosolic GSTs are divided into seven classes termed alpha (GSTA1 and 2), mu (GSTM1 through 5), omega (GSTO1), pi (GSTP1), sigma (GSTS1), theta (GSTT1 and 2), and zeta (GSTZ1). Those in the alpha and mu classes can form heterodimers, allowing for a large number of active transferases to form. The cytosolic forms of GST catalyze conjugation, reduction, and isomerization reactions.

The high concentrations of GSH in the cell, as well as the overabundance of GSTs, means that few reactive molecules escape detoxification. However, while there appears to be an overcapacity of enzyme and reducing equivalents, there is always concern that some reactive intermediates will escape detoxification, and by nature of their electrophilicity, will bind to cellular components and cause toxicity. The potential for such an occurrence is heightened if GSH is depleted or if a specific form of GST is polymorphic. While it is difficult to deplete cellular GSH levels, therapeutic agents that require large doses to be clinically efficacious have the greatest potential to lower cellular GSH levels. Acetaminophen, which is normally metabolized by glucuronidation and sulfation, is also a substrate for oxidative metabolism by CYP2E1, which generates the toxic metabolite *N*-acetyl-*p*-benzoquinone imine (NAPQI). An overdose of acetaminophen can lead to depletion of cellular GSH levels, thereby increasing the potential for NAPQI to interact with other cellular components. Acetaminophen toxicity is associated with increased levels of NAPQI and tissue necrosis.

Like many of the enzymes involved in drug and xenobiotic metabolism, all of the GSTs have been shown to be polymorphic. The mu (GSTM1*0) and theta (GSTT1*0) genotypes express a null phenotype; thus, individuals that are polymorphic at these loci are predisposed to toxicities by agents that are selective substrates for these GSTs. For example, the GSTM1*0 allele is observed in 50% of the Caucasian population and has been linked genetically to human malignancies of the lung, colon, and bladder. Null activity in the GSTT1 gene has been associated with adverse side effects and toxicity in cancer chemotherapy with cytostatic drugs; the toxicities result from insufficient clearance of the drugs *via* GSH conjugation. Expression of the null genotype can be as high as 60% in Chinese and Korean populations. Therapies may alter efficacies, with an increase in severity of adverse side effects.

While the GSTs play an important role in cellular detoxification, their activities in cancerous tissues have been linked to the development of drug resistance toward chemotherapeutic agents that are both substrates and nonsubstrates for the GSTs. Many anticancer drugs are effective because they initiate cell death or apoptosis, which is linked to the activation of mitogen-activated protein (MAP) kinases such as JNK and p38. Investigational studies have demonstrated that overexpression of GSTs is associated with resistance to apoptosis and the inhibition of MAP kinase activity. In a variety of tumors, the levels of GSTs are overexpressed, which

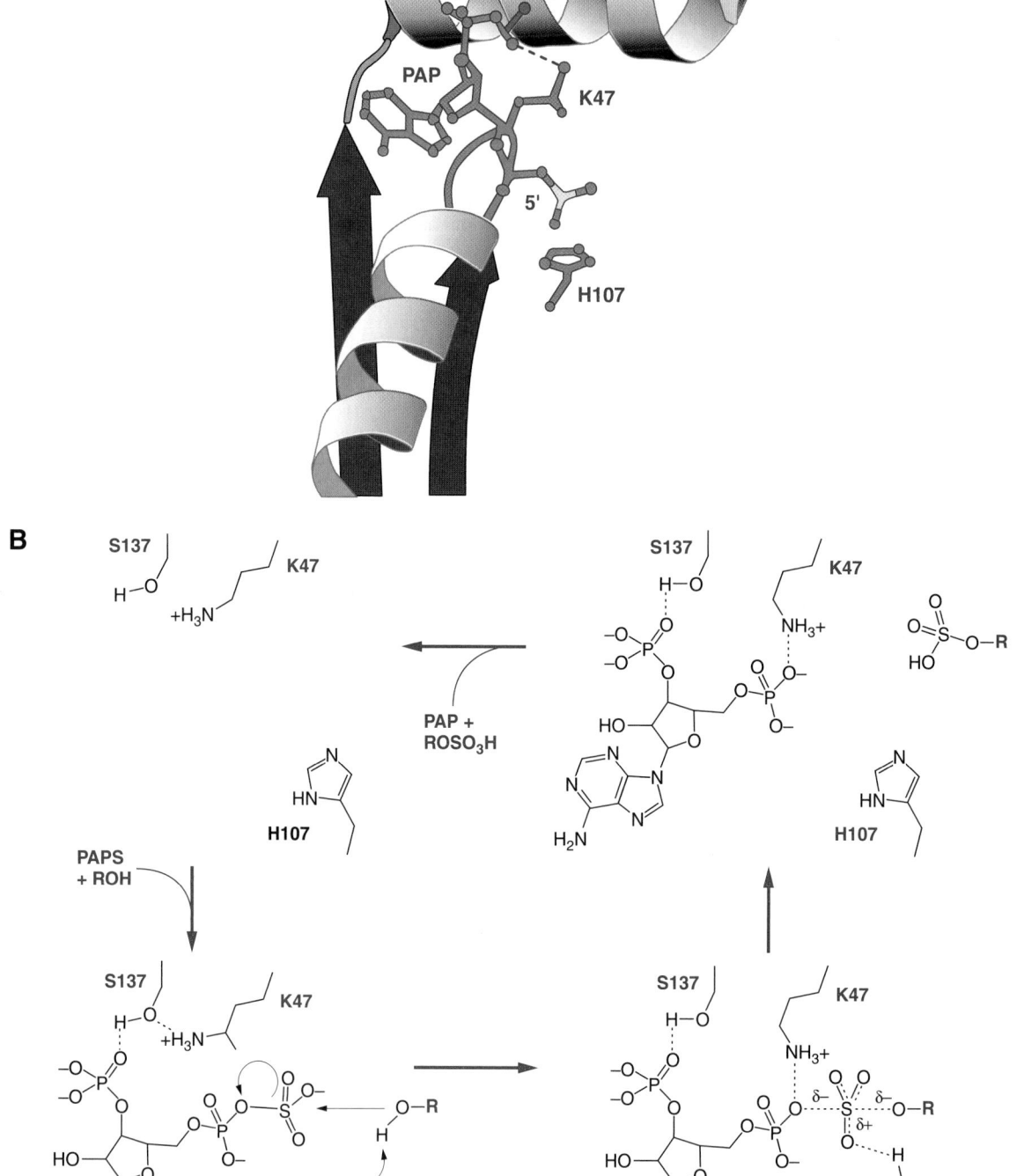

Figure 3–9. *The proposed reaction mechanism of sulfuryl transfer catalyzed by the sulfotransferases (SULTs).* **A.** Shown in this figure are the conserved strand-loop-helix and strand-turn-helix structure of the catalytic core of all SULTs where PAPS and xenobiotics bind. Shown is the hydrogen bonding interaction of PAPS with Lys[47] and Ser[137] with His[107] which complexes with substrate (xenobiotic). **B.** The proposed reaction mechanism shows the transfer of the sulfuryl group from PAPS to the OH-group on the substrate and the interactions of the conserved SULT residues in this reaction. (For additional information *see* Negishi *et al.*, 2001.)

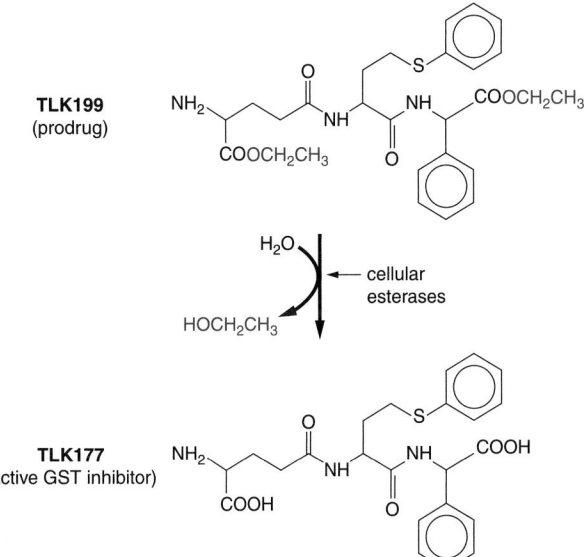

Figure 3–10. *Glutathione as a co-substrate in the conjugation of a drug or xenobiotic (X) by glutathione-S-transferase (GST).*

leads to a reduction in MAP kinase activity and reduced efficacy of chemotherapy. Taking advantage of the relatively high levels of GST in tumor cells, inhibition of GST activity has been exploited as a therapeutic strategy to modulate drug resistance by sensitizing tumors to anticancer drugs. TLK199, a glutathione analog, serves as a prodrug that undergoes activation by plasma esterases to a GST inhibitor, TLK117, which potentiates the toxicity of different anticancer agents (Figure 3–11). Alternatively, the elevated level of GST activity in cancerous cells has been utilized to develop prodrugs that can be activated by the GSTs to form electrophilic intermediates. TLK286 is a substrate for GST that undergoes a β-elimination reaction, forming a glutathione conjugate and a nitrogen mustard (Figure 3–12) that is capable of alkylating cellular nucleophiles, resulting in antitumor activity.

N-Acetylation. The cytosolic N-acetyltransferases (NATs) are responsible for the metabolism of drugs and environmental agents that contain an aromatic amine or hydrazine group. The addition of the acetyl group from the cofactor acetyl-coenzyme A often leads to a metabolite that is less water soluble because the potential ionizable amine is neutralized by the covalent addition of the acetyl group. NATs are among the most polymorphic of all the human xenobiotic drug-metabolizing enzymes.

The characterization of an acetylator phenotype in humans was one of the first hereditary traits identified, and was responsible for the development of the field of pharmacogenetics (*see* Chapter 4). Following the discovery that isonicotinic acid hydrazide (*isoniazid*) could be used in the cure of tuberculosis, a significant proportion of the patients (5% to 15%) experienced toxicities that ranged from numbness and tingling in their fingers to CNS damage. After finding that isoniazid was metabolized by acetylation and excreted in the urine, researchers noted that individuals suffering from the toxic effects of the drug excreted the largest amount of unchanged drug and the least amount of acetylated isoniazid. Pharmacoge-

netic studies led to the classification of "rapid" and "slow" acetylators, with the "slow" phenotype being predisposed to toxicity. Purification and characterization of N-acetyltransferase and the eventual cloning of its RNA provided sequence characterization of the gene for slow and fast acetylators, revealing polymorphisms that correspond to the "slow" acetylator phenotype. There are two functional NAT genes in humans, *NAT1* and *NAT2*. Over 25 allelic variants of *NAT1* and *NAT2* have been characterized, and in individuals in whom acetylation of drugs is compromised, homozygous genotypes for at least two variant alleles are required to predispose a patient to lowered drug metabolism. Polymorphism in the *NAT2* gene and its association with the slow acetylation of isoniazid was one of the first completely characterized genotypes shown to impact drug metabolism, thereby linking pharmacogenetic phenotype to a genetic polymorphism. Although nearly as many mutations have been identified in the *NAT1* gene as the *NAT2* gene, the frequency of the *slow* acetylation patterns are attributed mostly to polymorphism in the *NAT2* gene.

A list of drugs that are subject to acetylation and their known toxicities are listed in Table 3–3. The therapeutic relevance of NAT polymorphisms is in avoiding drug-induced toxicities. The adverse drug response in a slow acetylator resembles a drug overdose; thus, reducing the dose or increasing the dosing interval is recommended. Drugs containing an aromatic amine or a hydrazine group

Figure 3–11. *Activation of TLK199 by cellular esterases to the glutathione-S-transferase (GST) inhibitor TLK117.* (For additional information, *see* Townsend and Tew, 2003.)

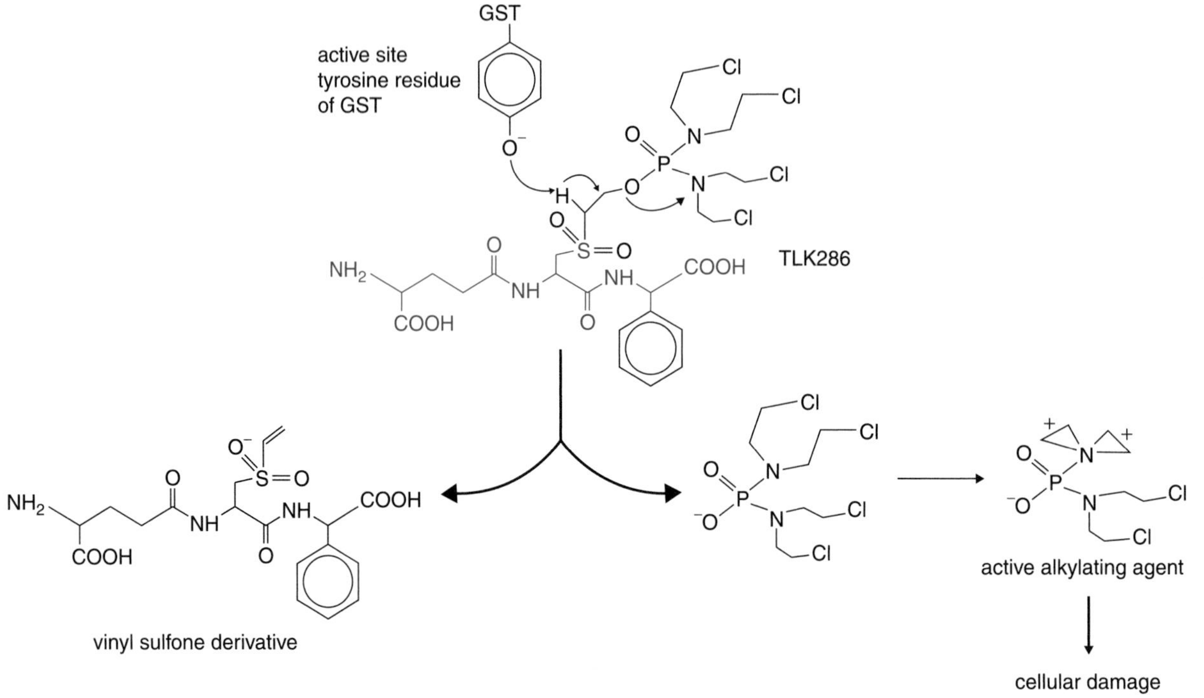

Figure 3–12. *Generation of the reactive alkylating agent following the conjugation of glutathione to TLK286.* GST interacts with the prodrug and GSH analog, TLK286, *via* a tyrosine in the active site of GST. GSH portion is shown in blue. The interaction promotes β-elimination and cleavage of the prodrug to a vinyl sulfone and an active alkylating fragment. (*See* Townsend and Tew, 2003.)

exist in many classes of clinically used drugs, and if a drug is known to be subject to drug metabolism through acetylation, confirming an individual's phenotype can be important. For example, *hydralazine*, a once popular orally active antihypertensive (vasodilator) drug, is metabolized by NAT2. The administration of therapeutic doses of hydralazine to a slow acetylator can result in extreme hypotension and tachycardia. Several drugs, such as the sulfonamides, that are known targets for acetylation have been implicated in idiosyncratic hypersensitivity reactions; in such instances, an appreciation of a patient's acetylating phenotype is particularly important. Sulfonamides are transformed into hydroxylamines that interact with cellular proteins, generating haptens that can elicit autoimmune responses. Individuals who are slow acetylators are predisposed to drug-induced autoimmune disorders.

Tissue-specific expression patterns of NAT1 and NAT2 have a significant impact on the fate of drug metabolism and the potential for eliciting a toxic episode. NAT1 seems to be ubiquitously expressed among most human tissues, whereas NAT2 is found in liver and the GI tract. Characteristic of both NAT1 and NAT2 is the ability to form N-hydroxy–acetylated metabolites from bicyclic aromatic hydrocarbons, a reaction that leads to the nonenzymatic release of the acetyl group and the generation of highly reactive nitrenium ions. Thus, N-hydroxy acetylation is thought to activate certain environmental toxicants. In contrast, direct N-acetylation of the environmentally generated bicyclic aromatic amines is stable and leads to detoxification. Individuals who are NAT2 fast acetylators are able to efficiently metabolize and detoxify bicyclic aromatic amine through liver-dependent acetylation. Slow acetylators (NAT2 deficient), however, accumulate bicyclic aromatic amines, which then become substrates for CYP-dependent N-oxidation. These N-OH metabolites are eliminated in the urine. In tissues such as bladder epithelium, NAT1 is highly expressed and can efficiently catalyze the N-hydroxy acetylation of bicyclic aromatic amines, a process that leads to de-acetylation and the formation of the mutagenic nitrenium ion, especially in NAT2-deficient subjects. Epidemiological studies have shown that slow acetylators are predisposed to bladder cancer if exposed environmentally to bicyclic aromatic amines.

Methylation. In humans, drugs and xenobiotics can undergo O-, N-, and S-methylation. The identification of the individual methyltransferase (MT) is based on the substrate and methyl conjugate. Humans express three N-methyltransferases, one catechol-O-methyltransferase (COMT) a phenol-O-methyltransferase (POMT), a thiopurine S-methyltransferase (TPMT), and a thiol methyl-

Table 3–3
Indications and Unwanted Side Effects of Drugs Metabolized by N-Acetyltransferases

DRUG	INDICATION	MAJOR SIDE EFFECTS
Acebutolol	Arrhythmias, hypertension	Drowsiness, weakness, insomnia
Amantadine	Influenza A, parkinsonism	Appetite loss, dizziness, headache, nightmares
Aminobenzoic acid	Skin disorders, sunscreens	Stomach upset, contact sensitization
Aminoglutethimide	Adrenal cortex carcinoma, breast cancer	Clumsiness, nausea, dizziness, agranulocytosis
Aminosalicylic acid	Ulcerative colitis	Allergic fever, itching, leukopenia
Amonafide	Prostate cancer	Myelosuppression
Amrinone	Advanced heart failure	Thrombocytopenia, arrhythmias
Benzocaine	Local anesthesia	Dermatitis, itching, rash, methemoglobinemia
Caffeine	Neonatal respiratory distress syndrome	Dizziness, insomnia, tachycardia
Clonazepam	Epilepsy	Ataxia, dizziness, slurred speech
Dapsone	Dermatitis, leprosy, AIDS-related complex	Nausea, vomiting, hyperexcitability, methemoglobinemia, dermatitis
Dipyrone, metamizole	Analgesic	Agranulocytosis
Hydralazine	Hypertension	Hypotension, tachycardia, flush, headache
Isoniazid	Tuberculosis	Peripheral neuritis, hepatotoxicity
Nitrazepam	Insomnia	Dizziness, somnolence
Phenelzine	Depression	CNS excitation, insomnia, orthostatic hypotension, hepatotoxicity
Procainamide	Ventricular tachyarrhythmia	Hypotension, systemic lupus erythematosus
Sulfonamides	Antibacterial agents	Hypersensitivity, hemolytic anemia, fever, lupuslike syndromes

For details, *see* Meisel, 2002.

transferase (TMT). All of the MTs exist as monomers and use S-adenosyl-methionine (SAM; AdoMet) as the methyl donor. With the exception of a signature sequence that is conserved among the MTs, there is limited conservation in sequence, indicating that each MT has evolved to display a unique catalytic function. Although the common theme among the MTs is the generation of a methylated product, substrate specificity is high and distinguishes the individual enzymes.

Nicotinamide N-methyltransferase (NNMT) methylates serotonin and tryptophan, and pyridine-containing compounds such as nicotinamide and nicotine. Phenylethanolamine N-methyltransferase (PNMT) is responsible for the methylation of the neurotransmitter norepinephrine, forming epinephrine; the histamine N-methyltransferase (HNMT) metabolizes drugs containing an imidazole ring such as that found in histamine. COMT methylates neurotransmitters containing a catechol moiety such as dopamine and norepinephrine, drugs such as *methyldopa*, and drugs of abuse such as *ecstasy* (MDMA; 3,4-methylenedioxymethamphetamine).

From a clinical perspective, the most important MT may be TPMT, which catalyzes the S-methylation of aromatic and hetero-

cyclic sulfhydryl compounds, including the thiopurine drugs *azathioprine* (AZA), *6-mercaptopurine* (6-MP), and *thioguanine*. AZA and 6-MP are used for the management of inflammatory bowel disease (*see* Chapter 38) as well as autoimmune disorders such as systemic lupus erythematosus and rheumatoid arthritis. Thioguanine is used in acute myeloid leukemia, and 6-MP is used worldwide for the treatment of childhood acute lymphoblastic leukemia (*see* Chapter 51). Because TPMT is responsible for the detoxification of 6-MP, a genetic deficiency in TPMT can result in severe toxicities in patients taking these drugs. When given orally at clinically established doses, 6-MP serves as a prodrug that is metabolized by hypoxanthine guanine phosphoribosyl transferase (HGPRT) to 6-thioguanine nucleotides (6-TGNs), which become incorporated into DNA and RNA, resulting in arrest of DNA replication and cytotoxicity. The toxic side effects arise when a lack of 6-MP methylation by TPMT causes a buildup of 6-MP, resulting in the generation of toxic levels of 6-TGNs. The identification of the inactive TPMT alleles and the development of a genotyping test to identify homozygous carriers of the defective allele have now made it possible to identify individuals who may be predisposed to the toxic side effects of 6-MP therapy. Simple adjustments in the patient's dosage regiment have been shown to be a life-saving intervention for those with TPMT deficiencies.

The Role of Xenobiotic Metabolism in the Safe and Effective Use of Drugs. Any compound entering the body must be eliminated through metabolism and excretion *via* the urine or bile/feces. This mechanism keeps foreign compounds from accumulating in the body and possibly causing toxicity. In the case of drugs, metabolism results in the inactivation of their therapeutic effectiveness and facilitates their elimination. The extent of metabolism can determine the efficacy and toxicity of a drug by controlling its biological half-life. Among the most serious considerations in the clinical use of drugs are adverse drug reactions. If a drug is metabolized too quickly, it rapidly loses its therapeutic efficacy. This can occur if specific enzymes involved in metabolism are overly active or are induced by dietary or environmental factors. If a drug is metabolized too slowly, the drug can accumulate in the bloodstream; as a consequence, the pharmacokinetic parameter AUC (area under the plasma concentration–time curve) is elevated and the plasma clearance of the drug is decreased. This increase in AUC can lead to overstimulation of some target receptors or undesired binding to other receptors or cellular macromolecules. An increase in AUC often results when specific xenobiotic-metabolizing enzymes are inhibited, which can occur when an individual is taking a combination of different therapeutic agents and one of those drugs targets the enzyme involved in drug metabolism. For example, the consumption of grapefruit juice with drugs taken orally can inhibit intestinal CYP3A4, blocking the metabolism of many of these drugs. The inhibition of specific CYPs in the gut by dietary consumption of grapefruit juice alters the oral bioavailability of many classes of drugs, such as certain antihypertensives, immunosuppressants, antidepressants, antihistamines, and the statins, to name a few. Among the components of grapefruit juice that inhibit CYP3A4 are naringin and furanocoumarins.

While environmental factors can alter the steady-state levels of specific enzymes or inhibit their catalytic potential, these phenotypic changes in drug metabolism are also observed clinically in groups of individuals that are genetically predisposed to adverse drug reactions because of pharmacogenetic differences in the expression of xenobiotic-metabolizing enzymes (*see* Chapter 4). Most of the xenobiotic-metabolizing enzymes display polymorphic differences in their expression, resulting from heritable changes in the structure of the genes. For example, as discussed above, a significant population was found to be hyperbilirubinemic, resulting from a reduction in the ability to glucuronidate circulating bilirubin due to a lowered

expression of the *UGT1A1* gene (Gilbert's syndrome). Drugs that are subject to glucuronidation by UGT1A1, such as the topoisomerase inhibitor SN-38 (Figures 3–5, 3–7, and 3–8), will display an increased AUC because individuals with Gilbert's syndrome are unable to detoxify these drugs. Since most cancer chemotherapeutic agents have a very narrow therapeutic index, increases in the circulating levels of the active form can result in significant toxicities. There are a number of genetic differences in CYPs that can have a major impact on drug therapy.

Nearly every class of therapeutic agent has been reported to initiate an adverse drug response (ADR). In the United States, the cost of such response has been estimated at $100 billion and to be the cause of over 100,000 deaths annually. It has been estimated that 56% of drugs that are associated with adverse responses are subjected to metabolism by the xenobiotic-metabolizing enzymes, notably the CYPs, which metabolize 86% of these compounds. Since many of the CYPs are subject to induction as well as inhibition by drugs, dietary factors, and other environmental agents, these enzymes play an important role in most ADRs. Thus, it has become mandatory that before a new drug application (NDA) is filed with the Food and Drug Administration, the route of metabolism and the enzymes involved in the metabolism must be known. As a result, it has become routine practice in the pharmaceutical industry to establish which enzymes are involved in metabolism of a drug candidate and to identify the metabolites and determine their potential toxicity.

Induction of Drug Metabolism. Xenobiotics can influence the extent of drug metabolism by activating transcription and inducing the expression of genes encoding drug-metabolizing enzymes. Thus, a foreign compound may induce its own metabolism, as may certain drugs. One potential consequence of this is a decrease in plasma drug concentration over the course of treatment, resulting in loss of efficacy, as the auto-induced metabolism of the drug exceeds the rate at which new drug enters the body. A list of ligands and the receptors through which they induce drug metabolism is shown in Table 3–4. A particular receptor, when activated by a ligand, can induce the transcription of a battery of target genes. Among these target genes are certain CYPs and drug transporters. Thus, any drug that is a ligand for a receptor that induces CYPs and transporters could lead to drug interactions. Figure 3–13 shows the scheme by which a drug may interact with nuclear receptors to induce its own metabolism.

The aryl hydrocarbon receptor (AHR) is a member of a superfamily of transcription factors with diverse roles in mammals, such as a regulatory role in the development of the mammalian CNS and modulating the response to chemical and oxidative stress. This

Table 3–4
Nuclear Receptors That Induce Drug Metabolism

RECEPTOR	LIGANDS
Aryl hydrocarbon receptor (AHR)	Omeprazole
Constitutive androstane receptor (CAR)	Phenobarbital
Pregnane X receptor (PXR)	Rifampin
Farnesoid X receptor (FXR)	Bile acids
Vitamin D receptor	Vitamin D
Peroxisome proliferator activated receptor (PPAR)	Fibrates
Retinoic acid receptor (RAR)	*all-trans*-Retinoic acid
Retinoid X receptor (RXR)	9-*cis*-Retinoic acid

superfamily of transcription factors includes Per and Sim, two transcription factors involved in development of the CNS, and the hypoxia-inducible factor 1α (HIF1α) that activates genes in response to low cellular O_2 levels. The AHR induces expression of genes encoding CYP1A1 and CYP1A2, two CYPs that are able to metabolically activate chemical carcinogens, including environmental contaminants and carcinogens derived from food. Many of these substances are inert unless metabolized by CYPs. Thus, induction of these CYPs by a drug could potentially result in an increase in the toxicity and carcinogenicity of procarcinogens. For example, *omeprazole*, a proton pump inhibitor used to treat gastric and duodenal ulcers (*see* Chapter 36), is a ligand for the AHR and can induce CYP1A1 and CYP1A2, with the possible consequences of toxin/carcinogen activation as well as drug-drug interactions in patients receiving agents that are substrates for either of these CYPs.

Another important induction mechanism is due to type 2 nuclear receptors that are in the same superfamily as the steroid hormone receptors. Many of these receptors, identified on the basis of their structural similarity to steroid hormone receptors, were originally termed "orphan receptors," because no endogenous ligands were known to interact with them. Subsequent studies revealed that some of these receptors are activated by xenobiotics, including drugs. The type 2 nuclear receptors of most importance to

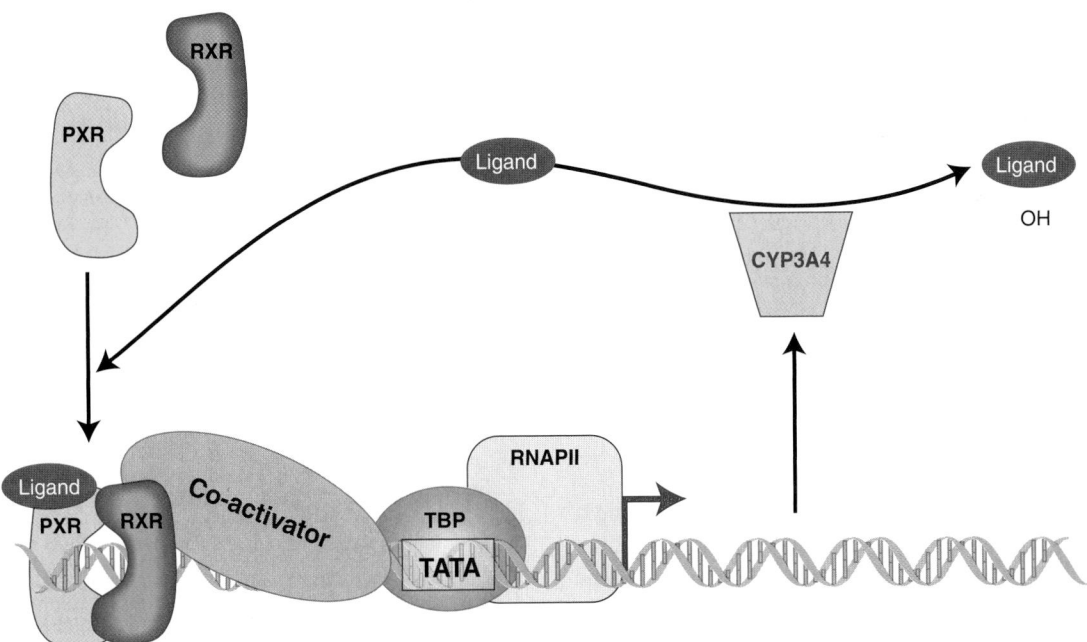

Figure 3–13. *Induction of drug metabolism by nuclear receptor–mediated signal transduction.* When a drug such as atorvastatin (Ligand) enters the cell, it can bind to a nuclear receptor such as the pregnane X receptor (PXR). PXR then forms a complex with the retinoid X receptor (RXR), binds to DNA upstream of target genes, recruits coactivator (which binds to the TATA box binding protein, TBP), and activates transcription. Among PXR target genes are CYP3A4, which can metabolize the atorvastatin and decrease its cellular concentration. Thus, atorvastatin induces its own metabolism. Atorvastatin undergoes both ortho and para hydroxylation. (*See* Handschin and Meyer, 2003.)

drug metabolism and drug therapy include the pregnane X receptor (PXR), constitutive androstane receptor (CAR), and the peroxisome proliferator activated receptor (PPAR). PXR, discovered based on its ability to be activated by the synthetic steroid pregnane 16α-carbonitrile, is activated by a number of drugs including, antibiotics (*rifampicin* and *troleandomycin*), Ca^{2+} channel blockers (*nifedipine*), statins (*mevastatin*), antidiabetic drugs (*troglitazone*), HIV protease inhibitors (*ritonavir*), and anticancer drugs (*paclitaxel*). Hyperforin, a component of St. John's wort, an over-the-counter herbal remedy used for depression, also activates PXR. This activation is thought to be the basis for the increase in failure of oral contraceptives in individuals taking St. John's wort: activated PXR is an inducer of CYP3A4, which can metabolize steroids found in oral contraceptives. PXR also induces the expression of genes encoding certain drug transporters and phase 2 enzymes including SULTs and UGTs. Thus, PXR facilitates the metabolism and elimination of xenobiotics, including drugs, with notable consequences (Figure 3–13).

The nuclear receptor CAR was discovered based on its ability to activate genes in the absence of ligand. Steroids such as *androstanol*, the antifungal agent *clotrimazole*, and the antiemetic *meclizine* are inverse agonists that inhibit gene activation by CAR, while the pesticide 1,4-bis[2-(3,5-dichloropyridyloxy)]benzene, the steroid 5β-pregnane-3,20-dione, and probably other endogenous compounds, are agonists that activate gene expression when bound to CAR. Genes induced by CAR include those encoding several CYPs (CYP2B6, CYP2C9, and CYP3A4), various phase 2 enzymes (including GSTs, UGTs, and SULTs), and drug and endobiotic transporters. CYP3A4 is induced by both PXR and CAR and thus its level is highly influenced by a number of drugs and other xenobiotics. In addition to a potential role in inducing the degradation of drugs including the over-the-counter analgesic acetaminophen, this receptor may function in the control of bilirubin degradation, the process by which the liver decomposes heme.

Clearly, PXR and CAR have a capacity for binding a great variety of ligands. As with the xenobiotic-metabolizing enzymes, species differences also exist in the ligand specificities of these receptors. For example, rifampicin activates human PXR but not mouse or rat PXR. Meclizine preferentially activates mouse CAR but inhibits gene induction by human CAR. These findings further establish that rodent model systems do not reflect the response of humans to drugs.

The peroxisome proliferator activated receptor (PPAR) family is composed of three members, α, β, and γ.

PPARα is the target for the fibrate class of hyperlipidemic drugs, including the widely prescribed *gemfibrozil* and *fenofibrate*. While activation of PPARα results in induction of target genes encoding fatty acid metabolizing enzymes that result in lowering of serum triglycerides, it also induces CYP4 enzymes that carry out the oxidation of fatty acids and drugs with fatty acid–containing side chains, such as *leukotriene* and *arachidonic acid* analogs.

Role of Drug Metabolism in the Drug Development Process. There are two key elements associated with successful drug development: efficacy and safety. Both depend on drug metabolism. It is necessary to determine how and by which enzymes a potential new drug is metabolized. This knowledge allows prediction of whether the compound may cause drug-drug interactions or be susceptible to marked interindividual variation in metabolism due to genetic polymorphisms.

Historically, drug candidates have been administered to rodents at doses well above the human target dose in order to predict acute toxicity. For drug candidates to be used chronically in humans, such as for lowering serum triglycerides and cholesterol or for treatment of type 2 diabetes, long-term carcinogenicity studies are carried out in rodent models. For determination of metabolism, the compound is subjected to analysis by human liver cells or extracts from these cells that contain the drug-metabolizing enzymes. Such studies determine how humans will metabolize a particular drug, and to a limited extent, predict the rate of metabolism. If a CYP is involved, a panel of recombinant CYPs can be used to determine which CYP predominates in the metabolism of the drug. If a single CYP, such as CYP3A4, is found to be the sole CYP that metabolizes a drug candidate, then a decision can be made about the likelihood of drug interactions. Interactions become a problem when multiple drugs are simultaneously administered, for example in elderly patients, who on a daily basis may take prescribed antiinflammatory drugs, cholesterol-lowering drugs, blood pressure medications, a gastric acid suppressant, an anticoagulant, and a number of over-the-counter medications. Ideally, the best drug candidate would be metabolized by several CYPs so that variability in expression levels of one CYP or drug-drug interactions would not significantly impact its metabolism and pharmacokinetics.

Similar studies can be carried out with phase 2 enzymes and drug transporters in order to predict the metabolic fate of a drug. In addition to the use of recombinant human xenobiotic-metabolizing enzymes in predicting drug metabolism, human receptor–based (PXR and CAR) systems should also be used to determine whether a particular drug candidate could be a ligand for PXR, CAR, or PPARα.

Computer-based computational (*in silico*) prediction of drug metabolism may also be a prospect for the future, since the structures of several CYPs have been determined, including those of CYPs 2A6, 2C9, and 3A4. These structures may be used to predict metabolism of a drug candidate by fitting the compound to the enzyme's active site and determining oxidation potentials of sites on the molecule. However, the structures, determined by x-ray analysis of crystals of enzyme-substrate complexes, are static, whereas enzymes are flexible, and this vital distinction may be limiting. The large size of the CYP active sites, which permits them to metabolize many different compounds, also renders them difficult to model. The potential for modeling ligand or activator for the nuclear receptors also exists with limitations similar to those discussed for the CYPs. With refinement of structures and more powerful modeling software, *in silico* drug metabolism may be a reality in the future.

BIBLIOGRAPHY

Blanchard, R.L., Freimuth, R. R., Buck, J., *et al.* A proposed nomenclature system for the cytosolic sulfotransferase (SULT) superfamily. *Pharmacogenetics,* **2004,** *14*:199–211.

Cashman, J.R. The implications of polymorphisms in mammalian flavin-containing monooxygenases in drug discovery and development. *Drug Discov. Today,* **2004,** *9*:574–581.

Coughtrie, M.W. Sulfation through the looking glass—recent advances in sulfotransferase research for the curious. *Pharmacogenomics J.,* **2002,** 2:297–308.

Dutton, G.J. Glucuronidation of drugs and other compounds. *CRC Press, Inc.,* Boca Raton, **1980.**

Evans, W.E., and Relling, M.V. Pharmacogenomics: translating functional genomics into rational therapeutics. *Science,* **1999,** *286*:487–491.

Glatt, H. Sulfotransferases in the bioactivation of xenobiotics. *Chem. Biol. Interact.,* **2000,** *129*:141–170.

Golka, K., Prior, V., Blaszkewicz, M. and Bolt, H.M. The enhanced bladder cancer susceptibility of NAT2 slow acetylators towards aromatic amines: a review considering ethnic differences. *Toxicol. Lett.,* **2002,** *128*:229–241.

Gong Q.H., Cho J.W., Huang T., *et al.* Thirteen UDP glucuronosyltransferase genes are encoded at the human UGT1 gene complex locus. *Pharmacogenetics,* **2001,** *11*:357–368.

Hayes, J.D., Flanagan, J.U., and Jowsey, I.R. Glutathione transferases. *Annu. Rev. Pharmacol. Toxicol.,* **2004.**

Handschin, C., and Meyer, U.A. Induction of drug metabolism: the role of nuclear receptors. *Pharmacol. Rev.,* **2003,** *55*:649–673.

Kadakol, A., Ghosh, S.S., Sappal, B.S., *et al.* Genetic lesions of bilirubin uridine-diphosphoglucuronate glucuronosyltransferase (UGT1A1) causing Crigler-Najjar and Gilbert syndromes: correlation of genotype to phenotype. *Hum. Mutat.,* **2000,** *16*:297–306.

Kobayashi, K., Bouscarel, B., Matsuzaki, Y., *et al.* PH-dependent uptake of irinotecan and its active metabolite, SN-38, by intestinal cells. *Int. J. Cancer,* **1999,** *83*:491–496.

Krynetski, E.Y., and Evans, W.E. Pharmacogenetics of cancer therapy: getting personal. *Am. J. Hum. Genet.,* **1998,** *63*:11–16.

Landi, S. Mammalian class theta GST and differential susceptibility to carcinogens: a review. *Mut. Res.,* **2000,** *463*:247–283.

Lee, K.A., Fuda, H., Lee, Y.C., *et al.* Crystal structure of human cholesterol sulfotransferase (SULT2B1b) in the presence of pregnenolone and 3'- phosphoadenosine 5'-phosphate. Rationale for specificity differences between prototypical SULT2A1 and the SULT2BG1 isoforms. *J. Biol. Chem.,* **2003,** *278*:44593–44599.

Meisel, P. Arylamine N-acetyltransferases and drug response. *Pharmacogenomics,* **2002,** *3*:349–366.

Negishi, M., Pederson L. G., Petrotchenko, E., *et al.* Structure and function of sulfotransferases. *Arch. Biochem. Biophys.,* **2001,** *390*:149–157.

Nelson, D.R., Zeldin, D.C., Hoffman, S.M., *et al.* Comparison of cytochrome P450 (CYP) genes from the mouse and human genomes, including nomenclature recommendations for genes, pseudogenes and alternative-splice variants. *Pharmacogenetics,* **2004,** *14*:1–18.

Pedersen, L.C., Petrotchenko, E., Shevtsov, S., and Negishi, M. Crystal structure of the human estrogen sulfotransferase-PAPS complex: evidence for catalytic role of Ser137 in the sulfuryl transfer reaction. *J. Biol. Chem.,* **2002,** *277*:17928–17932.

Townsend, D.M., and Tew, K.D. The role of glutathione-S-transferase in anti-cancer drug resistance. *Oncogene,* **2003,** *22*:7369–7375.

Tukey, R.H., and Strassburg, C.P. Human UDP-glucuronosyltransferases: metabolism, expression, and disease. *Annu. Rev. Pharmacol. Toxicol.,* **2000,** 40:581–616.

Tukey, R.H., Strassburg, C.P., and Mackenzie, P.I. Pharmacogenomics of human UDP-glucuronosyltransferases and irinotecan toxicity. *Mol. Pharmacol.,* **2002,** *62*:446–450.

Vatsis, K.P., Weber, W.W., Bell, D.A., *et al.* Nomenclature for N-acetyltransferases. *Pharmacogenetics,* **1995,** *5*:1–17.

Weinshilboum, R.M., Otterness, D.M., and Szumlanski, C.L. Methylation pharmacogenetics: catechol O-methyltransferase, thiopurine methyltransferase, and histamine N-methyltransferase. *Annu. Rev. Pharmacol. Toxicol.,* **1999,** *39*:19–52.

Yamamoto, W., Verweij, J., de Bruijn, P., *et al.* Active transepithelial transport of irinotecan (CPT-11) and its metabolites by human intestinal Caco-2 cells. *Anticancer Drugs,* **2001,** *12*:419–432.

Williams, P.A., Cosme, J., Vinkovic, D.M., *et al.* Crystal structures of human cytochrome P450 3A4 bound to metyrapone and progesterone. *Science,* **2004,** *305*:683–686.

PHARMACOGENETICS

Mary V. Relling and Kathleen M. Giacomini

Pharmacogenetics is the study of the genetic basis for variation in drug response. In this broadest sense, pharmacogenetics encompasses pharmacogenomics, which employs tools for surveying the entire genome to assess multigenic determinants of drug response. Until the technical advances in genomics of the last few years, pharmacogenetics proceeded using a forward genetic, phenotype-to-genotype approach. Drug response outliers were compared to individuals with "normal" drug response to identify the pharmacologic basis of altered response. An inherited component to response was demonstrated using family studies or imputed through intra- *vs.* intersubject reproducibility studies. With the explosion of technology in genomics, a reverse genetic, genotype-to-phenotype approach is feasible whereby genomic polymorphisms can serve as the starting point to assess whether genomic variability translates into phenotypic variability.

Historical Context. In the pre-genomics era, the frequency of genetic variation was hypothesized to be relatively uncommon, and the demonstration of inherited drug-response traits applied to a relatively small number of drugs and pathways (Eichelbaum and Gross, 1990; Evans and Relling, 2004; Johnson and Lima, 2003). Historically, uncommon severe drug-induced phenotypes served as the triggers to investigate and document pharmacogenetic phenotypes. Prolonged neuromuscular blockade following normal doses of *succinylcholine*, neurotoxicity following *isoniazid* therapy (Hughes *et al.*, 1954), and methemoglobinemia in glucose-6-phosphate dehydrogenase (G6PD) deficiency (Alving *et al.*, 1956) (*see* Chapter 39) were discovered to have a genetic basis in the first half of the 20th century. In the 1970s and 1980s, *debrisoquine* hydroxylation and exaggerated hypotensive effects from that drug were related to an autosomal recessive inherited deficiency in the cytochrome P450 isoenzyme 2D6 (CYP2D6) (Evans and Relling, 2004). Since the elucidation of the molecular basis of the phenotypic polymorphism in CYP2D6 (Gonzalez *et al.*, 1988), the molecular bases of many other monogenic pharmacogenetic traits have been identified (Meyer and Zanger, 1997).

Individuals differ from each other approximately every 300 to 1000 nucleotides, with an estimated total of 3.2 million single nucleotide polymorphisms (SNPs; single base pair substitutions found at frequencies ≥1% in a population) in the genome (Sachidanandam *et al.*, 2001; The International SNP Map Working Group, 2001). Identifying which of these variants or combinations of variants have functional consequence for drug effects is the task of modern pharmacogenetics.

Importance of Pharmacogenetics to Variability in Drug Response

Drug response is considered to be a gene-by-environment phenotype. That is, an individual's response to a drug depends on the complex interplay between environmental factors and genetic factors (Figure 4–1). Variation in drug response therefore may be explained by variation in environmental and genetic factors, alone or in combination. What proportion of drug-response variability is likely to be genetically determined? Classical family studies provide some information (Weinshilboum and Wang, 2004). Because estimating the fraction of phenotypic variability that is attributable to genetic factors in pharmacogenetics usually requires administration of a drug to twins or trios of family members, data are somewhat limited. Twin studies have shown that drug metabolism is highly heritable, with genetic factors accounting for most of the variation in metabolic rates for many drugs (Vesell, 2000). Results from a twin study in which the half-life of *antipyrine* was measured are typical (Figure 4–2). Antipyrine, a pyrazolone analgesic, is eliminated exclusively by metabolism and is a substrate for multiple CYPs. There is considerably greater concordance in the half-life of antipyrine between the monozygotic (identical) twin pairs in comparison to the dizygotic (fraternal) twin pairs. Comparison of intra-twin *vs.* inter-pair variability suggests that approximately 75% to 85% of the variability in pharmacokinetic half-lives for drugs that are eliminated by metabolism is heritable (Penno *et al.*, 1981). It has also

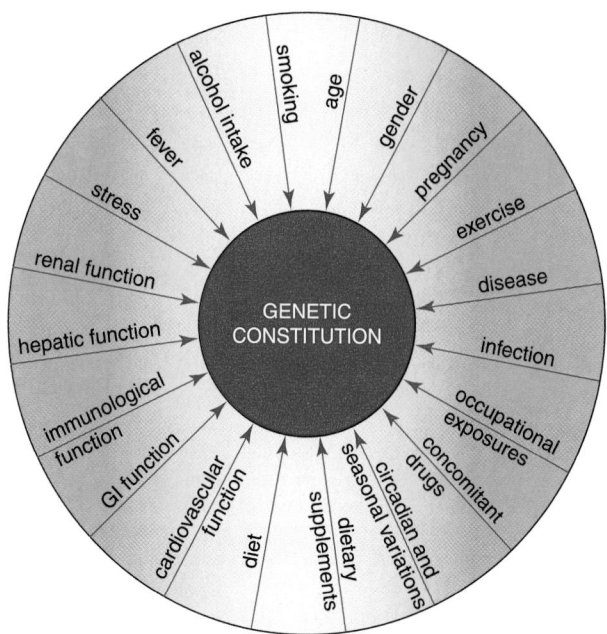

Figure 4–1. Exogenous and endogenous factors contribute to variation in drug response. (Reproduced with permission from Vesell, 1991.)

tance to the phenotype; because multiple gene products contribute to antipyrine disposition, most of which have unelucidated mechanisms of genetic variability, the predictability of antipyrine disposition based on known genetic variability is poor.

Another approach to estimating the degree of heritability of a pharmacogenetic phenotype uses *ex vivo* experiments with cell lines derived from related individuals. Inter- *vs.* intrafamily variability and relationships among members of a kindred are used to estimate heritability. Using this approach with lymphoblastoid cells, cytotoxicity from chemotherapeutic agents was shown to be heritable, with about 20% to 70% of the variability in sensitivity to *5-fluorouracil* and *docetaxel* estimated as inherited, depending upon dose (Watters *et al.*, 2004).

For the "monogenic" phenotypic traits of G6PD deficiency, CYP2D6 or thiopurine methyltransferase (TPMT) metabolism, it is possible to predict phenotype based on genotype. Several genetic polymorphisms of drug metabolizing enzymes result in monogenic traits. Based on a retrospective study, 49% of adverse drug reactions were associated with drugs that are substrates for polymorphic drug metabolizing enzymes, a proportion larger than estimated for all drugs (22%) or for top-selling drugs (7%) (Phillips *et al.*, 2001). Prospective genotype determinations may result in the ability to prevent adverse drug reactions (Meyer, 2000).

Defining multigenic contributors to drug response will be much more challenging. For some multigenic phenotypes, such as response to antihypertensives, the large numbers of candidate genes will necessitate a large patient sample size to produce the statistical power required to solve the "multigene" problem.

been proposed that heritability can be estimated by comparing intra-subject *vs.* inter-subject variability in drug response or disposition in unrelated individuals (Kalow *et al.*, 1998), with the assumption that high intra-subject reproducibility translates into high heritability; the validity of this method across pharmacologic phenotypes remains to be established. In any case, such studies provide only an estimate of the overall contribution of inheri-

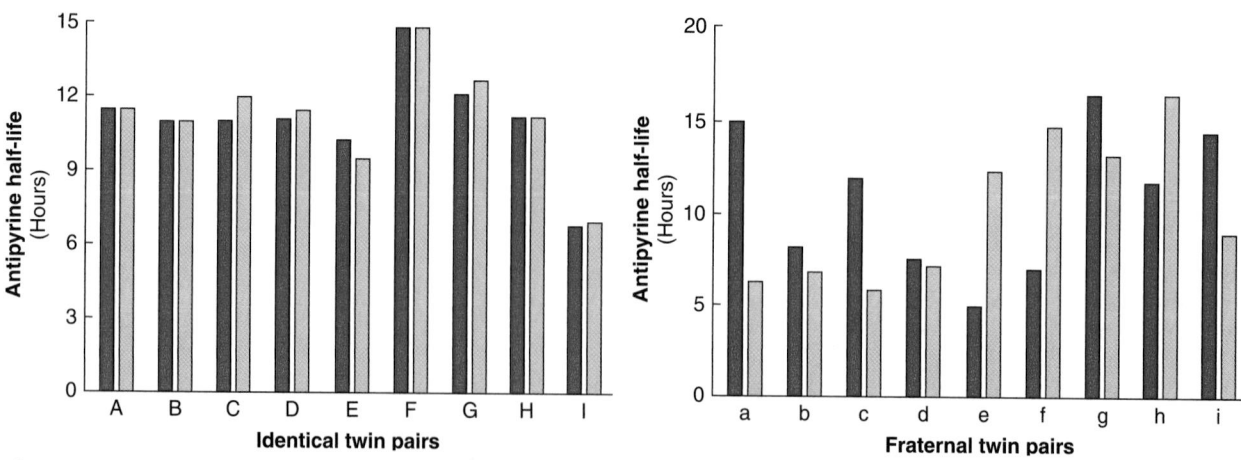

Figure 4–2. Pharmacogenetic contribution to pharmacokinetic parameters. Half-life of antipyrine is more concordant in identical in comparison to fraternal twin pairs. Bars show the half-life of antipyrine in identical (monozygotic) and fraternal (dizygotic) twin pairs. (Redrawn from data in Vesell and Page, 1968.)

GENOMIC BASIS OF PHARMACOGENETICS

Phenotype-Driven Terminology

Because initial discoveries in pharmacogenetics were driven by variable phenotypes and defined by family and twin studies, the classic genetic terms for monogenic traits apply to some pharmacogenetic polymorphisms. A trait (*e.g.*, CYP2D6 "poor metabolism") is deemed autosomal recessive if the responsible gene is located on an autosome (*i.e.*, it is not sex-linked) and a distinct phenotype is evident only with nonfunctional alleles on both the maternal and paternal chromosomes. For many of the earliest identified pharmacogenetic polymorphisms, phenotype did not differ enough between heterozygotes and homozygous "wild-type" individuals to distinguish that heterozygotes exhibited an intermediate (or codominant) phenotype (*e.g.,* for CYP2D6-mediated debrisoquine metabolism). Other traits, such as TPMT, exhibit three relatively distinct phenotypes, and thus were deemed codominant even in the premolecular era. With the advances in molecular characterization of polymorphisms and a genotype-to-phenotype approach, additional polymorphic traits (*e.g.,* CYP2C19 metabolism of drugs such as *mephenytoin* and *omeprazole*) are now recognized to exhibit some degree of codominance. Some pharmacogenetic traits, such as the long QT syndrome, segregate as dominant traits; the long QT syndrome is associated with heterozygous loss-of-function mutations of ion channels. A prolonged QT interval is seen on the electrocardiogram, either basally or in the presence of certain drugs, and the individual is predisposed to cardiac arrhythmias (*see* Chapter 34).

In an era of detailed molecular characterization, two major factors complicate the historical designation of recessive, codominant, and dominant traits. First, even within a single gene, a vast array of polymorphisms (promoter, coding, noncoding, completely inactivating, or modestly modifying) are possible, making the assignment of "variant" *vs.* "wild-type" to an allele a designation that depends upon a complete survey of the gene's polymorphisms and is not necessarily easily assigned. Secondly, most traits (pharmacogenetic and otherwise) are multigenic, not monogenic. Thus, even if the designations of recessive, codominant, and dominant are informative for a given gene, their utility in describing the genetic variability that underlies variability in drug response phenotype is diminished, because most phenotypic variability is likely to be multigenic.

Types of Genetic Variants

A *polymorphism* is a variation in the DNA sequence that is present at an allele frequency of 1% or greater in a population. Two major types of sequence variation have been associated with variation in human phenotype: *single nucleotide polymorphisms* (SNPs) and *insertions/deletions* (indels) (Figure 4–3). In comparison to base pair substitutions, indels are much less frequent in the genome and are of particularly low frequency in coding regions of genes (Cargill *et al.*, 1999; Stephens *et al.*, 2001). Single base pair substitutions that are present at frequencies of 1% or greater in a population are termed single nucleotide polymorphisms (SNPs) and are present in the human genome at approximately 1 SNP every few hundred to a thousand base pairs, depending on the gene region (Stephens *et al.*, 2001).

SNPs in the coding region are termed *cSNPs*. cSNPs are further classified as nonsynonymous (or *missense*) if the base pair change results in an amino acid substitution, or synonymous (or *sense*) if the base pair substitution within a codon does not alter the encoded amino acid. Typically, substitutions of the third base pair, termed the *wobble position*, in a three base pair codon, such as the G to A substitution in proline shown in Figure 4–3, do not alter the encoded amino acid. Base pair substitutions that lead to a stop codon are termed *nonsense* mutations. In addition, about 10% of SNPs can have more than two possible alleles (*e.g.,* a C can be replaced by either an A or G), so that the same polymorphic site can be associated with amino acid substitutions in some alleles but not others.

Polymorphisms in noncoding regions of genes may occur in the 3' and 5' untranslated regions, in promoter or enhancer regions, in intronic regions, or in large regions between genes, intergenic regions (Figure 4–4). Polymorphisms in introns found near exon-intron boundaries are often treated as a separate category from other intronic polymorphisms since these may affect splicing, and thereby affect function. Noncoding SNPs in promoters or enhancers may alter *cis*- or *trans*-acting elements that regulate gene transcription or transcript stability. Noncoding SNPs in introns or exons may create alternative exon splicing sites, and the altered transcript may have fewer or more exons, or shorter or larger exons, than the wild-type transcript. Introduction or deletion of exonic sequence can cause a frame shift in the translated protein and thereby change protein structure or function, or result in an early stop codon, which makes an unstable or nonfunctional protein. Because 95% of the genome is intergenic, most polymorphisms are unlikely to directly affect the encoded transcript or protein. However, intergenic polymorphisms

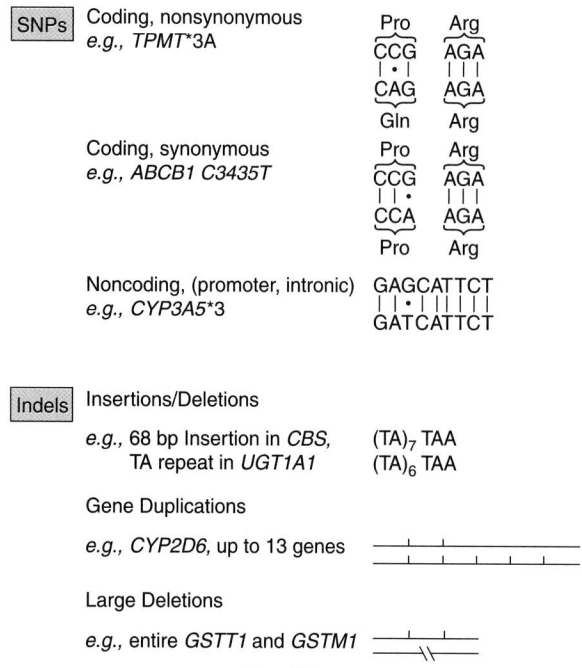

Figure 4–3. **Molecular mechanisms of genetic polymorphisms.** The most common genetic variants are single nucleotide polymorphism substitutions (SNPs). *Coding nonsynonymous* SNPs result in a nucleotide substitution that changes the amino acid codon (here proline to glutamine), which could change protein structure, stability, substrate affinities, or introduce a stop codon. *Coding synonymous* SNPs do not change the amino acid codon, but may have functional consequences (transcript stability, splicing). Noncoding SNPs may be in promoters, introns, or other regulatory regions that may affect transcription factor binding, enhancers, transcript stability, or splicing. The second major type of polymorphism is *indels (insertion/deletions).* SNP indels can have any of the same effects as SNP substitutions: short repeats in the promoter (which can affect transcript amount), or larger insertions/deletions that add or subtract amino acids. Indels can also involve gene duplications, stably transmitted inherited germline gene replication that causes increased protein expression and activity, or gene deletions that result in the complete lack of protein production. All of these mechanisms have been implicated in common germline pharmacogenetic polymorphisms. TPMT, thiopurine methyltransferase; ABCB1, the multidrug resistance transporter (P-glycoprotein); CYP, cytochrome P450; CBS, cystathionine β-synthase; UGT, UDP-glucuronyl transferase; GST, glutathione-S-transferase.

may have biological consequences by affecting DNA tertiary structure, interaction with chromatin and topoisomerases, or DNA replication. Thus, intergenic polymorphisms cannot be assumed to be without pharmacogenetic importance.

A remarkable degree of diversity in the types of insertions/deletions that are tolerated as germline polymorphisms is evident. A common glutathione-S-transferase M1 (*GSTM1*) polymorphism is caused by a 50-kilobase (kb) germline deletion, and the null allele has a population frequency of 0.3 to 0.5, depending on race/ethnicity. Biochemical studies indicate that livers from homozygous null individuals have only ~50% of the glutathione conjugating capacity of those with at least one copy of the *GSTM1* gene (Townsend and Tew, 2003a). The number of TA repeats in the *UGT1A1* promoter affects the quantitative expression of this crucial glucuronosyl transferase in liver; although 4 to 9 TA repeats exist in germline-inherited alleles, 6 or 7 repeats constitute the most common alleles (Monaghan *et al.*, 1996). Cystathionine β-synthase has a common 68 base pair insertion/deletion polymorphism that has been linked to folate levels (Kraus *et al.*, 1998). Although in many of these cases the local sequence context of these insertions/deletions strongly suggests mechanisms underlying the genomic alterations (*e.g.*, homologous recombination sites bracket the *GSTM1* deletion), high allele frequencies are maintained due to Mendelian inheritance.

A *haplotype*, which is defined as a series of alleles found at a linked locus on a chromosome, specifies the DNA sequence variation in a gene or a gene region on one chromosome. For example, consider two SNPs in *ABCB1*, which encodes for the multidrug resistance protein, P-glycoprotein. One SNP is a T to A base pair substitution at position 3421 and the other is a C to T change at position 3435. Possible haplotypes would be $T_{3421}C_{3435}$, $T_{3421}T_{3435}$, $A_{3421}C_{3435}$, and $A_{3421}T_{3435}$. For any gene, individuals will have two haplotypes, one maternal and one paternal in origin, which may or may not be identical. Haplotypes are important because they are the functional unit of the gene. That is, a haplotype represents the constellation of variants that occur together for the gene on

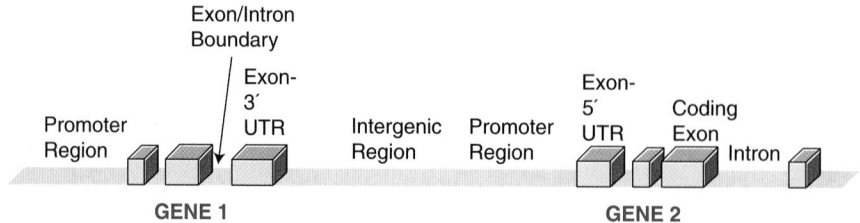

Figure 4–4. *Nomenclature of genomic regions.*

each chromosome. In some cases, this constellation of variants, rather than the individual variant or allele, may be functionally important. In others, however, a single mutation may be functionally important regardless of other linked variants within the haplotype(s).

Ethnic Diversity

Polymorphisms differ in their frequencies within human populations (Burchard *et al.*, 2003; Rosenberg *et al.*, 2002; Rosenberg *et al.*, 2003). Among coding region SNPs, synonymous SNPs are present, on average, at higher frequencies than nonsynonymous SNPs. Thus, for most genes, the nucleotide diversity, which reflects the number of SNPs and the frequency of the SNPs, is greater for synonymous than for nonsynonymous SNPs. This fact reflects selective pressures (termed *negative* or *purifying selection*), which act to preserve the functional activity of proteins, and therefore the amino acid sequence. Frequencies of polymorphisms in ethnically or racially diverse human populations have been examined in whole genome scanning studies (Cargill *et al.*, 1999; Stephens *et al.*, 2001). In these studies, polymorphisms have been classified as either cosmopolitan or population (or race and ethnic) specific. Cosmopolitan polymorphisms are those polymorphisms present in all ethnic groups, although frequencies may differ among ethnic groups. Cosmopolitan polymorphisms are usually found at higher allele frequencies in comparison to population-specific polymorphisms. Likely to have arisen before migrations of humans from Africa, cosmopolitan polymorphisms are generally older than population-specific polymorphisms.

The presence of ethnic and race-specific polymorphisms is consistent with geographical isolation of human populations (Xie *et al.*, 2001). These polymorphisms probably arose in isolated populations and then reached a certain frequency because they are advantageous (positive selection) or more likely, neutral, conferring no advantage or disadvantage to a population. Large-scale sequence studies in ethnically diverse populations in the United States demonstrate that African Americans have the highest number of population-specific polymorphisms in comparison to European Americans, Mexican Americans, and Asian Americans (Leabman *et al.*, 2003; Stephens *et al.*, 2001). Africans are believed to be the oldest population and therefore have both recently derived, population-specific polymorphisms, and older polymorphisms that occurred before migrations out of Africa.

Consider the coding region variants of two membrane transporters identified in 247 ethnically diverse DNA samples (Figure 4–5). Shown are nonsynonymous

and synonymous SNPs; population-specific nonsynonymous cSNPs are indicated in the figure. The multidrug resistance associated protein, MRP2, has a large number of nonsynonymous cSNPs. There are fewer synonymous variants than nonsynonymous variants, but the allele frequencies of the synonymous variants are greater than those of the nonsynonymous variants (Leabman *et al.*, 2003). By comparison, DAT, the dopamine transporter, has a number of synonymous variants but no nonsynonymous variants, suggesting that selective pressures have acted against substitutions that led to changes in amino acids.

In a survey of coding region haplotypes in 313 different genes in 80 ethnically diverse DNA samples, most genes were found to have between 2 and 53 haplotypes, with the average number of haplotypes in a gene being 14 (Stephens *et al.*, 2001). Like SNPs, haplotypes may be cosmopolitan or population specific and about 20% of the over 4000 identified haplotypes were cosmopolitan (Stephens *et al.*, 2001). Considering the frequencies of the haplotypes, cosmopolitan haplotypes actually accounted for over 80% of all haplotypes, whereas population-specific haplotypes accounted for only 8%.

Polymorphism Selection

Genetic variation that results in penetrant and constitutively evident biological variation sometimes causes a "disease" phenotype. Cystic fibrosis, sickle-cell anemia, and Crigler-Najjar syndrome are examples of inherited diseases caused by single gene defects (Pani *et al.*, 2000). In the case of Crigler-Najjar syndrome, the same gene (*UGT1A1*) that is targeted by rare inactivating mutations (and associated with a serious disease) is also targeted by modest polymorphisms (and associated with modest hyperbilirubinemia and altered drug clearance) (Monaghan *et al.*, 1996). Due to the disease, some evolutionary selection against these single-gene polymorphisms is present. Polymorphisms in other genes have highly penetrant effects in the drug-challenged but not in the constitutive state, which are the causes of monogenic pharmacogenetic traits. There is unlikely to be any selective pressure for or against these polymorphisms (Evans and Relling, 2004; Meyer, 2000; Weinshilboum, 2003). The vast majority of genetic polymorphisms have a modest impact on the affected genes, are part of a large array of multigenic factors that impact on drug effect, or affect genes whose products play a minor role in drug action relative to a large nongenetic effect. For example, phenobarbital induction of metabolism may be such an overwhelming "environmental" effect that polymorphisms in the

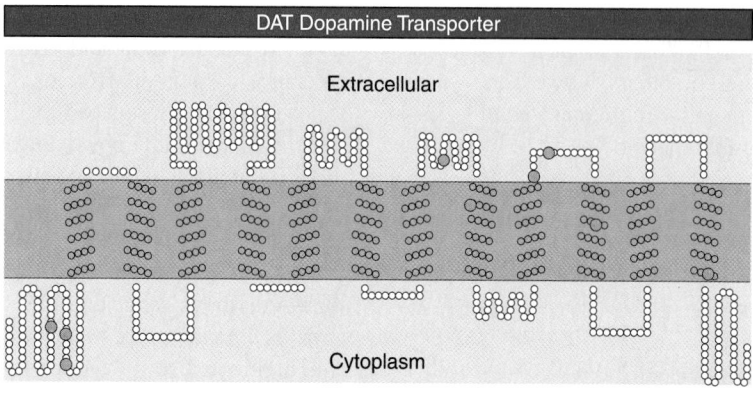

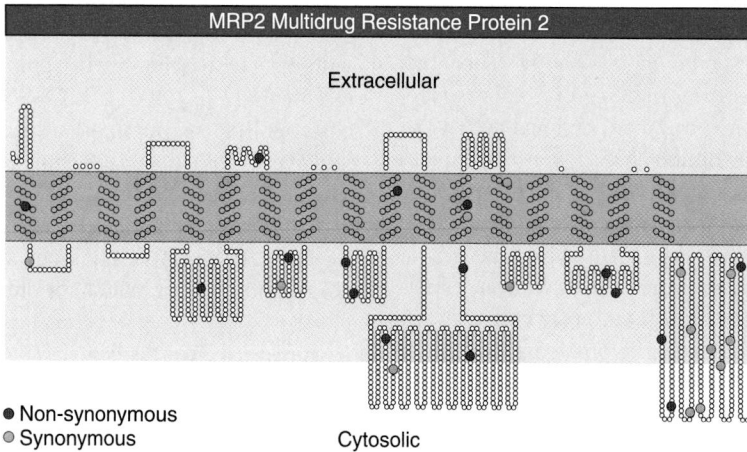

● Non-synonymous
● Synonymous

Figure 4–5. Coding region polymorphisms in two membrane transporters. Shown are the dopamine transporter, DAT (encoded by *SLCGA3*) and multidrug resistance associated protein, MRP2 (encoded by *ABCC2*). Coding region variants were identified in 247 ethnically diverse DNA samples (100 African Americans, 100 European Americans, 30 Asians, 10 Mexicans, and 7 Pacific Islanders). Shown in light gray are synonymous variants, and in black, nonsynonymous variants. (Reproduced with permission from Shu *et al.,* 2003.)

affected transcription factors and drug-metabolizing genes have modest effects in comparison.

PHARMACOGENETIC STUDY DESIGN CONSIDERATIONS

Pharmacogenetic Measures

What are pharmacogenetic traits and how are they measured? A *pharmacogenetic trait* is any measurable or discernible trait associated with a drug. Thus, enzyme activity, drug or metabolite levels in plasma or urine, blood pressure or lipid lowering produced by a drug, and drug-induced gene expression patterns are examples of pharmacogenetic traits. Directly measuring a trait (*e.g.,* enzyme activity) has

the advantage that the net effect of the contributions of all genes that influence the trait is reflected in the phenotypic measure. However, it has the disadvantage that it is also reflective of nongenetic influences (*e.g.,* diet, drug interactions, diurnal or hormonal fluctuation) and thus, may be "unstable." For CYP2D6, if a patient is given an oral dose of *dextromethorphan*, and the urinary ratio of parent drug to metabolite is assessed, the phenotype is reflective of the genotype for CYP2D6 (Meyer and Zanger, 1997). However, if dextromethorphan is given with *quinidine,* a potent inhibitor of CYP2D6, the phenotype may be consistent with a poor metabolizer genotype, even though the subject carries wild-type CYP2D6 alleles. In this case, quinidine administration results in a drug-induced haplo-insufficiency, and the assignment of a CYP2D6 poor metabolizer phenotype would not be accurate for that subject in the absence of quinidine. If a phenotypic measure, such as the erythromycin

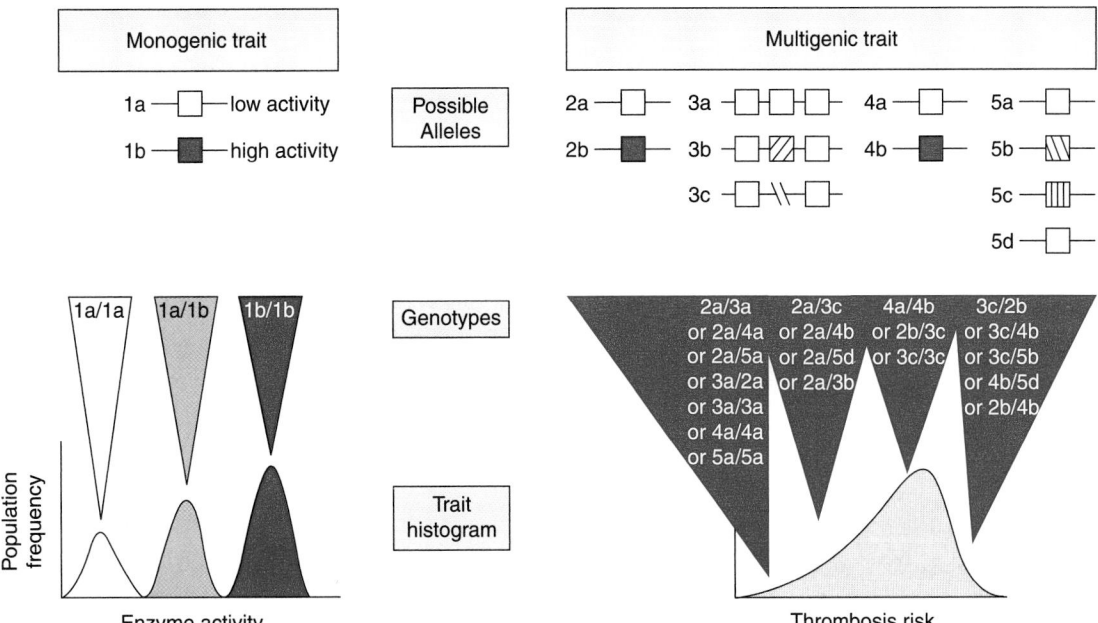

Figure 4–6. *Monogenic* **versus** *multigenic pharmacogenetic traits.* Possible alleles for a monogenic trait (*upper left*), in which a single gene has a low-activity (1a) and a high-activity (1b) allele. The population frequency distribution of a monogenic trait (*bottom left*), here depicted as enzyme activity, may exhibit a trimodal frequency distribution with relatively distinct separation among low activity (homozygosity for 1a), intermediate activity (heterozygote for 1a and 1b), and high activity (homozygosity for 1b). This is contrasted with multigenic traits (*e.g.*, an activity influenced by up to four different genes, genes 2 through 5), each of which has 2, 3, or 4 alleles (a through d). The population histogram for activity is unimodal-skewed, with no distinct differences among the genotypic groups. Multiple combinations of alleles coding for low activity and high activity at several of the genes can translate into low-, medium-, and high-activity phenotypes.

breath test (for CYP3A), is not stable within a subject, this is an indication that the phenotype is highly influenced by nongenetic factors, and may indicate a multigenic or weakly penetrant effect of a monogenic trait. Because most pharmacogenetic traits are multigenic rather than monogenic (Figure 4–6), considerable effort is being made to identify the important genes and their polymorphisms that influence variability in drug response.

Most genotyping methods use germline DNA, that is, DNA extracted from any somatic, diploid cells, usually white blood cells or buccal cells (due to their ready accessibility). DNA is extremely stable if appropriately extracted and stored, and unlike many laboratory tests, genotyping need be performed only once, because DNA sequence is generally invariant throughout an individual's lifetime. Although tremendous progress has been made in molecular biological techniques to determine genotypes, relatively few are used routinely in patient care. Genotyping tests are directed at each specific known polymorphic site using a variety of strategies that generally depend at some level on the specific and avid annealing of at least one oligonucleotide to a region of DNA flanking or overlapping

the polymorphic site (Koch, 2004). Because genomic variability is so common (with polymorphic sites every few hundred nucleotides), "cryptic" or unrecognized polymorphisms may interfere with oligonucleotide annealing, thereby resulting in false positive or false negative genotype assignments. Full integration of genotyping into therapeutics will require high standards for genotyping technology, perhaps with more than one method required for each polymorphic site.

One method to assess the reliability of genotype determinations in a group of individuals is to assess whether the relative number of homozygotes to heterozygotes is consistent with the overall allele frequency at each polymorphic site. *Hardy-Weinberg equilibrium* is maintained when mating within a population is random and there is no natural selection effect on the variant. Such assumptions are described mathematically when the proportions of the population that are observed to be homozygous for the variant genotype (q^2), homozygous for the wild-type genotype (p^2), and heterozygous ($2*p*q$) are not significantly different from that predicted from the overall allele frequencies (p = fre-

Table 4–1
Databases Containing Information on Human Genetic Variation

DATABASE NAME	URL (*Agency*)	DESCRIPTION OF CONTENTS
Pharmacogenetics and Pharmacogenomics Knowledge Base (PharmGKB)	www.pharmgkb.org (NIH Sponsored Research Network and Knowledge Database)	Genotype and phenotype data related to drug response
Single Nucleotide Polymorphism Database (dbSNP)	www.ncbi.nlm.nih.gov/entrez/query.fcgi?db=snp (National Center for Biotechnology Information, NCBI)	SNP
Human Genome Variation Database (HGVbase)	hgvbase.cgb.ki.se/	Genotype/phenotype associations
Human Gene Mutation Database (HGMD)	www.hgmd.org/	Mutations/SNPs in human genes
Online Mendelian Inheritance in Man	www.ncbi.nlm.nih.gov/entrez/query.fcgi?db=OMIM (NCBI)	Human genes and genetic disorders

quency of wild-type allele; q = frequency of variant allele) in the population. If proportions of the observed three genotypes, which must add up to one, differ significantly from those predicted, it may indicate that a genotyping error may be present.

Because polymorphisms are so common, haplotype (the allelic structure that indicates whether polymorphisms within a gene are on the same or different alleles) may also be important. Thus far, experimental methods to unambiguously confirm whether polymorphisms are allelic has proven to be feasible but technically challenging (McDonald *et al.*, 2002). Most investigators use statistical probability to assign putative or inferred haplotypes; *e.g.,* because the two most common SNPs in *TPMT* (at 460 and 719) often are allelic, a genotyping result showing heterozygosity at both SNPs will have a >95% chance of reflecting one allele wild-type and one allele variant at both SNP positions (resulting in a "heterozygote" genotype for *TPMT*). However, the remote prospect that each of the two alleles carries a single SNP variant, thereby conferring a homozygous variant/deficient phenotype, is a theoretical possibility.

Candidate Gene *versus* Genome-Wide Approaches

Because pathways involved in drug response are often known or at least partially known, pharmacogenetic studies are highly amenable to candidate gene association studies. After genes in drug response pathways are identified, the next step in the design of a candidate gene association pharmacogenetic study is to identify the genetic polymorphisms that are likely to contribute to the therapeutic and/or adverse responses to the drug. There are several databases that contain information on polymorphisms and mutations in human genes (Table 4–1), which allow the investigator to search by gene for polymorphisms that have been reported. Some of the databases, such as the Pharmacogenetics and Pharmacogenomics Knowledge Base (PharmGKB), include phenotypic as well as genotypic data.

Because it is currently not practical to analyze all polymorphisms in a candidate gene association study, it is important to select polymorphisms that are likely to be associated with the drug-response phenotype. For this purpose, there are two categories of polymorphisms. The first are polymorphisms that do not, in and of themselves, cause altered function of the expressed protein (*e.g.,* an enzyme that metabolizes the drug or the drug receptor). Rather, these polymorphisms are linked to the variant allele that produces the altered function. These polymorphisms serve as biomarkers for drug-response phenotype. However, their major shortcoming is that unless they are in 100% linkage with the causative polymorphism, they are not the best markers for the drug-response phenotype.

The second type of polymorphism is the *causative polymorphism,* which directly precipitates the phenotype. For example, a causative SNP may change an amino acid residue at a site that is highly conserved throughout evolution. This substitution may result in a protein that is nonfunctional or has reduced function. Whenever possible, it is desirable to select polymorphisms for pharmacogenetic studies that are likely to be causative (Tabor *et al.*, 2002). If biological information indicates that a particular polymorphism alters function, for example, in cellular assays of nonsynonymous variants, this polymorphism is an excellent candidate to use in an association study.

A potential drawback of the candidate gene approach is that the wrong genes may be studied. Genome-wide approaches, using gene expression arrays, genome-wide scans, or proteomics, can complement the candidate gene approach by providing a relatively unbiased survey of the genome to identify previously unrecognized candidate genes. For example, RNA, DNA, or protein from patients who have unacceptable toxicity from a drug can be compared with identical material from identically treated patients who did not have such toxicity. Patterns of gene expression, clusters of polymorphisms or heterozygosity, or relative amounts of proteins can be ascertained using computational tools, to identify genes, genomic regions, or proteins that can be further assessed for germline polymorphisms differentiating the phenotype. Gene expression and proteomic approaches have the advantage that the abundance of signal may itself directly reflect some of the relevant genetic variation; however, both types of expression are highly influenced by choice of tissue type, which may not be available from the relevant tissue; for example, it may not be feasible to obtain biopsies of brain tissue for studies on CNS toxicity. DNA has the advantage that it is readily available and independent of tissue type, but the vast majority of genomic variation is not in genes, and the large number of SNPs raises the danger of type I error (finding differences that are false-positives). Nonetheless, technology is rapidly evolving for genome-wide surveys of RNA, DNA, and protein, and such approaches hold promise for future pharmacogenomic discoveries.

Functional Studies of Polymorphisms

For most polymorphisms, functional information is not available. Therefore, to select polymorphisms that are likely to be causative, it is important to predict whether a polymorphism may result in a change in protein function, stability, or subcellular localization. One way that we can gain an understanding of the functional effects of various types of genomic variations is to survey the

mutations that have been associated with human Mendelian disease. The greatest number of DNA variations associated with diseases or traits are missense and nonsense mutations, followed by deletions (Figure 4–7). Further studies have suggested that of amino acid replacements associated with human disease, there is a high representation at residues that are most evolutionarily conserved (Miller and Kumar, 2001; Ng and Henikoff, 2003). These data have been supplemented by a large survey of genetic variation in membrane transporters important in drug response (Leabman *et al.*, 2003). That survey shows that nonsynonymous SNPs that alter evolutionarily conserved amino acids are present at lower allele frequencies on average than those that alter residues that are not conserved across species. This suggests that SNPs that alter evolutionarily conserved residues are most deleterious. The nature of chemical change of an amino acid substitution determines the functional effect of an amino acid variant. More radical changes in amino acids are more likely to be associated with disease than more conservative changes. For example, substitution of a charged amino acid (Arg) for a nonpolar, uncharged amino acid (Cys) is more likely to affect function than substitution of residues that are more chemically similar (*e.g.,* Arg to Lys).

Among the first pharmacogenetic examples to be discovered was glucose-6-phosphate dehydrogenase (G6PD) deficiency, an X-linked monogenic trait that results in severe hemolytic anemia in individuals after ingestion of fava beans or various drugs, including many antimalarial agents (Alving *et al.*, 1956). G6PD is normally present in red blood cells and helps to regulate levels of glutathione (GSH), an antioxidant. Antimalarials such as *primaquine*

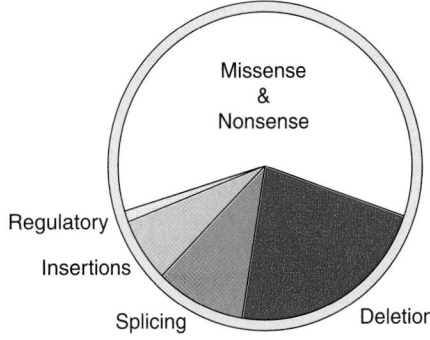

Figure 4–7. *DNA mutations associated with human diseases.* Among the 27,027 DNA variations studied, 1,222 were associated with diseases. These 1,222 are sorted into functional groups in the proportions indicated by the pie chart. Missense and nonsense mutations account for the greatest fraction of DNA variations associated with Mendelian disease (Botstein and Risch, 2003).

Table 4–2
The Predicted Functional Effect and Relative Risk That a Variant Will Alter Function of SNP Types in the Human Genome

TYPE OF VARIANT	LOCATION	FREQUENCY IN GENOME	PREDICTED RELATIVE RISK OF PHENOTYPE	FUNCTIONAL EFFECT
Nonsense	Coding region	Very low	Very high	Stop codon
Nonsynonymous Evolutionarily conserved	Coding region	Low	High	Amino acid substitution of a residue conserved across evolution
Nonsynonymous Evolutionarily unconserved	Coding region	Low	Low to moderate	Amino acid substitution of a residue not conserved across evolution
Nonsynonymous Radical chemical change	Coding region	Low	Moderate to high	Amino acid substitution of a residue that is chemically dissimilar to the original residue
Nonsynonymous Low to moderate chemical change	Coding region	Low	Low to high	Amino acid substitution of a residue that is chemically similar to the original residue
Insertion/deletion	Coding/noncoding region	Low	Low to high	Coding region: can cause frameshift
Synonymous	Coding region	Medium	Low	Can change mRNA stability or affect splicing
Regulatory region	Promoter, 5'UTR, 3'UTR	Medium	Low	Can affect the level of mRNA transcript by changing rate of transcription or stability of transcript
Intron/exon boundary	Within 8 bp of intron	Low	High	May affect splicing
Intronic	Deep within intron	Medium	Very low	No known function; may affect mRNA transcript levels through enhancer mechanism
Intergenic	Noncoding region between genes	High	Very low	No known function

Data adapted from Tabor *et al.*, 2002.

increase red blood cell fragility in individuals with G6PD deficiency, leading to profound hemolytic anemia. Interestingly, the severity of the deficiency syndrome varies among individuals and is related to the amino acid variant in G6PD. The severe form of G6PD deficiency is associated with changes at residues that are highly conserved across evolutionary history. Chemical change is also more radical on average in mutations associated with severe G6PD deficiency in comparison to mutations associated with milder forms of the syndrome. Collectively, studies of Mendelian traits and polymorphisms suggest that nonsynonymous SNPs that alter residues that are highly conserved among species and those that result in more radical changes in the nature of the amino acid are likely to be the best candidates for causing functional changes. The infor-

mation in Table 4–2 (categories of polymorphisms and the likelihood of each polymorphism to alter function) can be used as a guide for prioritizing polymorphisms in candidate gene association studies.

With the increasing number of SNPs that have been identified in large-scale SNP discovery projects, it is clear that computational methods are needed to predict the functional consequences of SNPs. To this end, predictive algorithms have been developed to identify potentially deleterious amino acid substitutions. These methods can be classified into two groups. The first group relies on sequence comparisons alone to identify and score substitutions according to their degree of conservation across multiple species; different scoring matrices have been used (*e.g.*, BLOSUM62 and SIFT)

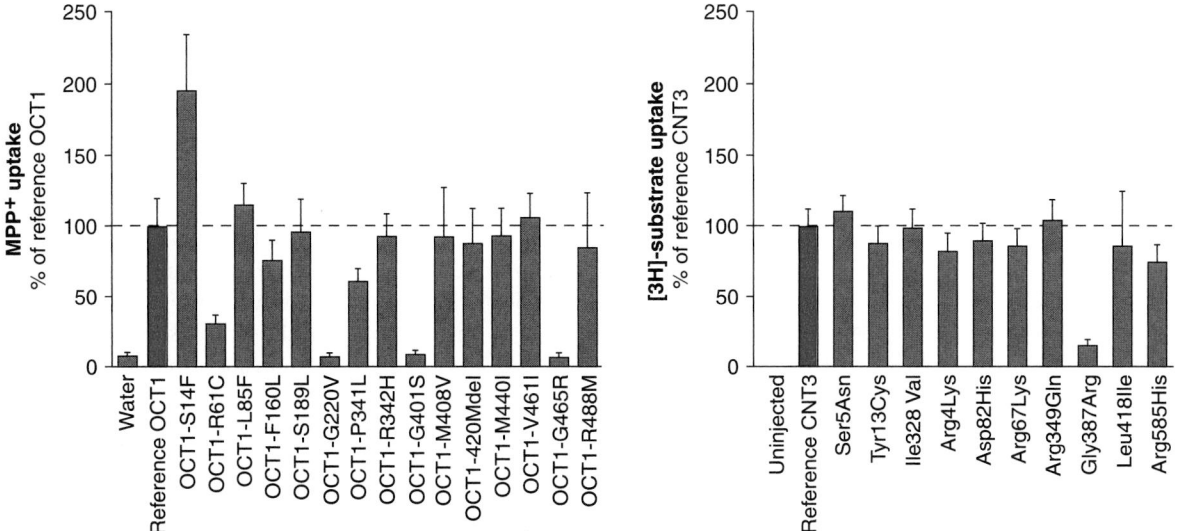

Figure 4–8. *Functional activity of natural variants of two membrane transporters.* Data for the organic cation transporter (OCT1, *left panel*) and the nucleoside transporter (CNT3, *right panel*). Variants, identified in ethnically diverse populations, were constructed by site-directed mutagenesis and expressed in *Xenopus laevis* oocytes. Dark shaded bars represent uptake of the model compounds by variant transporters. Blue bars represent uptake of the model compounds by reference transporters (Shu *et al.*, 2003).

(Henikoff and Henikoff, 1992; Ng and Henikoff, 2003). The second group of methods relies on mapping of SNPs onto protein structures, in addition to sequence comparisons (Mirkovic *et al.*, 2004). For example, rules have been developed that classify SNPs in terms of their impact on folding and stability of the native protein structure as well as shapes of its binding sites. Such rules depend on the structural context in which SNPs occur (*e.g.,* buried in the core of the fold or exposed to the solvent, in the binding site or not), and are inferred by machine learning methods from many functionally annotated SNPs in test proteins.

Functional activity of amino acid variants for many proteins can be studied in cellular assays. An initial step in characterizing the function of a nonsynonymous variant would be to isolate the variant gene or construct the variant by site-directed mutagenesis, express it in cells, and compare its functional activity to that of the reference or most common form of the protein. In the past few years, large-scale functional analyses have been performed on genetic variants in membrane transporters and phase II enzymes. Figure 4–8 shows the function of all nonsynonymous variants and coding region insertions and deletions of two membrane transporters, the organic cation transporter, OCT1 (encoded by *SLC22A1*) and the nucleoside transporter, CNT3 (encoded by *SLC28A3*). As shown, most of the naturally occurring variants have similar functional activity as that of

the reference transporters. However, several variants exhibit reduced function; in the case of OCT1, a gain-of-function variant is also present. Results such as these indicate heterogeneity exists in the functionality of natural amino acid variants in normal healthy human populations.

For many proteins, including enzymes, transporters, and receptors, the mechanisms by which amino acid substitutions alter function have been characterized in kinetic studies. Figure 4–9 shows simulated curves depicting the rate of metabolism of a substrate by two amino acid variants of an enzyme and the most common genetic form of the enzyme. The kinetics of metabolism of substrate by one variant enzyme, Variant A, is characterized by an increased K_m. Such an effect can occur if the amino acid substitution alters the binding site of the enzyme leading to a decrease in its affinity for the substrate. An amino acid variant may also alter the maximum rate of metabolism (V_{max}) of substrate by the enzyme, as exemplified by Variant B. The mechanisms for a reduced V_{max} are generally related to a reduced expression level of the enzyme, which may occur because of decreased stability of the protein or changes in protein trafficking or recycling (Shu *et al.*, 2003; Tirona *et al.*, 2001; Xu *et al.*, 2002).

In contrast to the studies with SNPs in coding regions, predicting the function of SNPs in noncoding regions of genes represents a major new challenge in

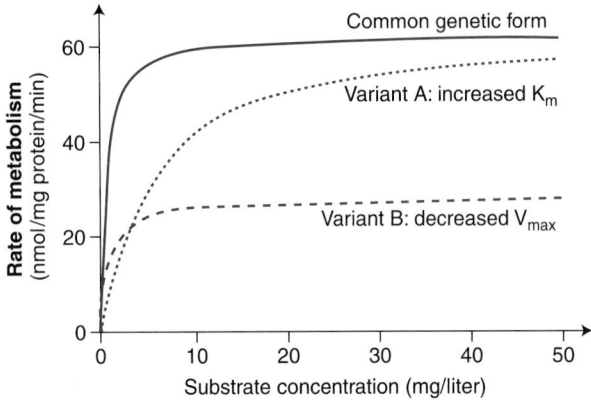

Figure 4–9. *Simulated concentration–dependence curves showing the rate of metabolism of a hypothetical substrate by the common genetic form of an enzyme and two nonsynonymous variants.* Variant A exhibits an increased K_m and likely reflects a change in the substrate binding site of the protein by the substituted amino acid. Variant B exhibits a change in the maximum rate of metabolism (V_{max}) of the substrate. This may be due to reduced expression level of the enzyme.

human genetics and pharmacogenetics. The principles of evolutionary conservation that have been shown to be important in predicting the function of nonsynonymous variants in the coding region need to be refined and tested as predictors of function of SNPs in noncoding regions. New methods in comparative genomics are being refined to identify conserved elements in noncoding regions of genes that may be functionally important (Bejerano *et al.*, 2004; Boffelli *et al.*, 2004; Brudno *et al.*, 2003).

Pharmacogenetic Phenotypes

Candidate genes for therapeutic and adverse response can be divided into three categories: pharmacokinetic, receptor/target, and disease-modifying.

Pharmacokinetics. Germline variability in genes that encode determinants of the pharmacokinetics of a drug, in particular enzymes and transporters, affect drug concentrations, and are therefore major determinants of therapeutic and adverse drug response (Table 4–3; Nebert *et al.*, 1996). Multiple enzymes and transporters may be involved in the pharmacokinetics of a single drug. Several polymorphisms in drug metabolizing enzymes were discovered as monogenic phenotypic trait variations, and thus may be referenced using their phenotypic designations (*e.g.*, slow *vs.* fast acetylation, extensive *vs.* poor metabolizers of debrisoquine or *sparteine*) rather

than their genotypic designations that reference the gene that is the target of polymorphisms in each case (NAT2 and CYP2D6 polymorphisms, respectively) (Grant *et al.*, 1990). CYP2D6 is now known to catabolize the two initial probe drugs (sparteine and debrisoquine), each of which was associated with exaggerated responses in 5% to 10% of treated individuals. The exaggerated responses are an inherited trait (Eichelbaum *et al.*, 1975; Mahgoub *et al.*, 1977). At present, a very large number of medications (estimated at 15% to 25% of all medicines in use) have been shown to be substrates for CYP2D6 (Table 4–3). The molecular and phenotypic characterization of multiple racial and ethnic groups has shown that seven variant alleles account for well over 90% of the "poor metabolizer" low-activity alleles for this gene in most racial groups; that the frequency of variant alleles varies with geographic origin; and that a small percentage of individuals carry stable duplications of CYP2D6, with "ultra-rapid" metabolizers having up to 13 copies of the active gene (Ingelman-Sundberg and Evans, 2001). Phenotypic consequences of the deficient CYP2D6 phenotype include increased risk of toxicity of antidepressants or antipsychotics (catabolized by the enzyme), and lack of analgesic effects of codeine (anabolized by the enzyme); conversely, the ultra-rapid phenotype is associated with extremely rapid clearance and thus inefficacy of antidepressants (Kirchheiner *et al.*, 2001).

A promoter region variant in the enzyme UGT1A1, UGT1A1*28, which has an additional TA in comparison to the more common form of the gene, has been associated with a reduced transcription rate of *UGT1A1* and lower glucuronidation activity of the enzyme. This reduced activity has been associated with higher levels of the active metabolite of the cancer chemotherapeutic agent *irinotecan* (*see* Chapters 3 and 51). The metabolite, SN38, which is eliminated by glucuronidation, is associated with the risk of toxicity (Iyer *et al.*, 2002), which will be more severe in individuals with genetically lower UGT1A1 activity.

CYP2C19 codes for a cytochrome P450, historically termed mephenytoin hydroxylase, that displays penetrant pharmacogenetic variability, with just a few SNPs accounting for the majority of the deficient, poor metabolizer phenotype (Mallal *et al.*, 2002). The deficient phenotype is much more common in Chinese and Japanese populations. Several proton pump inhibitors, including omeprazole and *lansoprazole,* are inactivated by CYP2C19. Thus, the deficient patients have higher exposure to active parent drug, a greater pharmacodynamic effect (higher gastric pH), and a higher probability of ulcer cure than

Table 4–3

Examples of Genetic Polymorphisms Influencing Drug Response

GENE PRODUCT (GENE)	DRUGS	RESPONSES AFFECTED
Drug metabolizers		
CYP2C9	Tolbutamide, warfarin, phenytoin, nonsteroidal antiinflammatories	Anticoagulant effect of warfarin (Aithal *et al.*, 1999; Roden, 2003; Weinshilboum, 2003)
CYP2C19	Mephenytoin, omeprazole, hexobarbital, mephobarbital, propranolol, proguanil, phenytoin	Peptic ulcer response to omeprazole (Kirchheiner *et al.*, 2001)
CYP2D6	β blockers, antidepressants, antipsychotics, codeine, debrisoquine, dextromethorphan, encainide, flecainide, fluoxetine, guanoxan, N-propylajmaline, perhexiline, phenacetin, phenformin, propafenone, sparteine	Tardive dyskinesia from antipsychotics, narcotic side effects, codeine efficacy, imipramine dose requirement, β blocker effect (Kirchheiner *et al.*, 2001; Weinshilboum, 2003)
CYP3A4/3A5/3A7	Macrolides, cyclosporine, tacrolimus, Ca^{2+} channel blockers, midazolam, terfenadine, lidocaine, dapsone, quinidine, triazolam, etoposide, teniposide, lovastatin, alfentanil, tamoxifen, steroids	Efficacy of immunosuppressive effects of tacrolimus (Evans and Relling, 2004)
Dihydropyrimidine dehydrogenase	Fluorouracil	5-Fluorouracil neurotoxicity (Chibana *et al.*, 2002)
N-acetyltransferase (*NAT2*)	Isoniazid, hydralazine, sulfonamides, amonafide, procainamide, dapsone, caffeine	Hypersensitivity to sulfonamides, amonafide toxicity, hydralazine-induced lupus, isoniazid neurotoxicity (Roden, 2003; Grant *et al.*, 1990)
Glutathione transferases (*GSTM1, GSTT1, GSTP1*)	Several anticancer agents	Decreased response in breast cancer, more toxicity and worse response in acute myelogenous leukemia (Townsend and Tew, 2003b)
Thiopurine methyltransferase (*TPMT*)	Mercaptopurine, thioguanine, azathioprine	Thiopurine toxicity and efficacy, risk of second cancers (Relling and Dervieux, 2001; Weinshilboum, 2003)
UDP-glucuronosyl-transferase (*UGT1A1*)	Irinotecan, bilirubin	Irinotecan toxicity (Iyer *et al.*, 1998; Relling and Dervieux, 2001)
P-glycoprotein (*ABCB1*)	Natural product anticancer drugs, HIV protease inhibitors, digoxin	Decreased CD4 response in HIV-infected patients, decreased digoxin AUC, drug resistance in epilepsy (Fellay *et al.*, 2002; Quirk *et al.*, 2004; Roden, 2003; Siddiqui *et al.*, 2003)
UGT2B7	Morphine	Morphine plasma levels (Sawyer *et al.*, 2003)
COMT	Levodopa	Enhanced drug effect (Weinshilboum, 2003)
CYP2B6	Cyclophosphamide	Ovarian failure (Takada *et al.*, 2004)
Targets and receptors		
Angiotensin-converting enzyme (ACE)	ACE inhibitors (*e.g.*, enalapril)	Renoprotective effects, hypotension, left ventricular mass reduction, cough (van Essen *et al.*, 1996; Roden, 2003)

(Continued)

Table 4–3
Examples of Genetic Polymorphisms Influencing Drug Response (Continued)

GENE PRODUCT (GENE)	DRUGS	RESPONSES AFFECTED
Thymidylate synthase	Methotrexate	Leukemia response, colorectal cancer response (Krajinovic *et al.*, 2002; Relling and Dervieux, 2001)
β_2 Adrenergic receptor (*ADBR2*)	β_2 Antagonists (*e.g.*, albuterol, terbutaline)	Bronchodilation, susceptibility to agonist-induced desensitization, cardiovascular effects (*e.g.*, increased heart rate, cardiac index, peripheral vasodilation) (Roden, 2003; Tan *et al.*, 1997)
β_1 Adrenergic receptor (*ADBR1*)	β_1 Antagonists	Response to β_1 antagonists (Johnson and Lima, 2003)
5-Lipoxygenase (ALOX5)	Leukotriene receptor antagonists	Asthma response (Drazen *et al.*, 1999)
Dopamine receptors (D_2, D_3, D_4)	Antipsychotics (*e.g.*, haloperidol, clozapine, thioridazine, nemonapride)	Antipsychotic response (D_2, D_3, D_4), antipsychotic-induced tardive dyskinesia (D_3) and acute akathisia (D_3), hyperprolactinemia in females (D_2) (Arranz *et al.*, 2000; Evans and McLeod, 2003)
Estrogen receptor α	Estrogen hormone replacement therapy	High-density lipoprotein cholesterol (Herrington *et al.*, 2002)
Serotonin transporter (5-HTT)	Antidepressants (*e.g.*, clomipramine, fluoxetine, paroxetine, fluvoxamine)	Clozapine effects, 5-HT neurotransmission, antidepressant response (Arranz *et al.*, 2000)
Serotonin receptor (5-HT$_{2A}$)	Antipsychotics	Clozapine antipsychotic response, tardive dyskinesia, paroxetine antidepression response, drug discrimination (Arranz *et al.*, 2000) (Murphy *et al.*, 2003)
HMG-CoA reductase	Pravastatin	Reduction in serum cholesterol
Modifiers		
Adducin	Diuretics	Myocardial infarction or strokes (Roden, 2003)
Apolipoprotein E	Statins (*e.g.*, simvastatin), tacrine	Lipid-lowering; clinical improvement in Alzheimer's (Evans and McLeod, 2003)
Human leukocyte antigen	Abacavir	Hypersensitivity reactions (Mallal *et al.*, 2002)
Cholesteryl ester transfer protein	Statins (*e.g.*, pravastatin)	Slowing atherosclerosis progression (Evans and McLeod, 2003)
Ion channels (*HERG*, *KvLQT1*, *Mink*, *MiRP1*)	Erythromycin, cisapride, clarithromycin, quinidine	Increased risk of drug-induced *torsades de pointes*, increased QT interval (Roden, 2003; Roden, 2004)
Methylguanine-deoxy-ribonucleic acid methyltransferase	Carmustine	Response of glioma to carmustine (Evans and McLeod, 2003)
Parkin	Levodopa	Parkinson's disease response (Evans and McLeod, 2003)
MTHFR	Methotrexate	Gastrointestinal toxicity (Ulrich *et al.*, 2001)
Prothrombin, factor V	Oral contraceptives	Venous thrombosis risk (Evans and McLeod, 2003)
Stromelysin-1	Statins (*e.g.*, pravastatin)	Reduction in cardiovascular events and in repeat angioplasty (Evans *et al.*, 2003)
Vitamin D receptor	Estrogen	Bone mineral density (Hustmyer *et al.*, 1994)

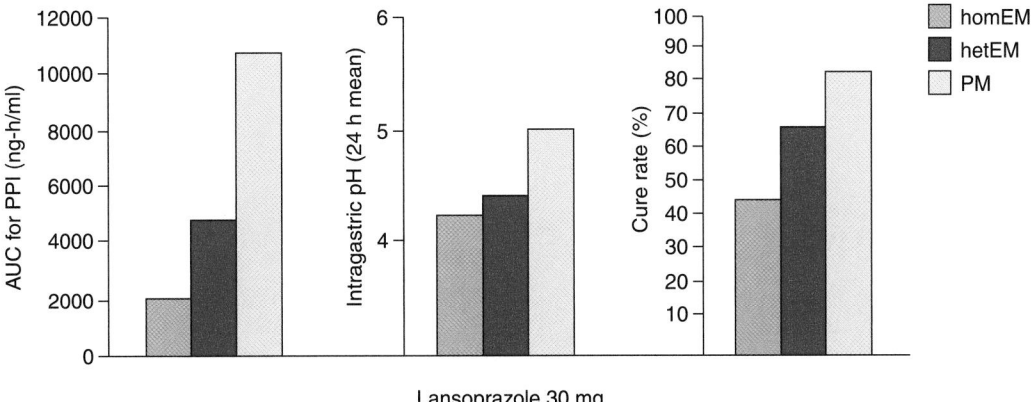

Figure 4–10. *Effect of CYP2C19 genotype on proton pump inhibitor (PPI) pharmacokinetics (AUC), gastric pH, and ulcer cure rates.* Depicted are the average variables for *CYP2C19* homozygous extensive metabolizers (homEM), heterozygotes (hetEM), and poor metabolizers (PM). (Reproduced with permission from Furuta *et al.*, 2004.)

heterozygotes or homozygous wild-type individuals (Figure 4–10).

The anticoagulant *warfarin* is catabolized by CYP2C9. Inactivating polymorphisms in *CYP2C9* are common (Goldstein, 2001), with 2% to 10% of most populations being homozygous for low-activity variants, and are associated with lower warfarin clearance, a higher risk of bleeding complications, and lower dose requirements (Aithal *et al.*, 1999).

Thiopurine methyltransferase (TPMT) methylates thiopurines such as *mercaptopurine* (an antileukemic drug that is also the product of *azathioprine* metabolism). One in 300 individuals is homozygous deficient, 10% are heterozygotes, and about 90% are homozygous for the wild-type alleles for *TPMT* (Weinshilboum and Sladek, 1980). Three SNPs account for over 90% of the inactivating alleles (Yates *et al.*, 1997). Because methylation of mercaptopurine competes with activation of the drug to thioguanine nucleotides, the concentration of the active (but also toxic) thioguanine metabolites is inversely related to TPMT activity and directly related to the probability of pharmacologic effects. Dose reductions (from the "average" population dose) may be required to avoid myelosuppression in 100% of homozygous deficient patients, 35% of heterozygotes, and only 7% to 8% of those with homozygous wild-type activity (Relling *et al.*, 1999). The rare homozygous deficient patients can tolerate 10% or less of the mercaptopurine doses tolerated by the homozygous wild-type patients, with heterozygotes often requiring an intermediate dose. Mercaptopurine has a narrow therapeutic range, and dosing by trial and error can place patients at higher risk of

toxicity; thus, prospective adjustment of *thiopurine* doses based on *TPMT* genotype has been suggested (Lesko and Woodcock, 2004). Life-threatening toxicity has also been reported when azathioprine has been given to patients with nonmalignant conditions (such as Crohn's disease, arthritis, or for prevention of solid organ transplant rejection) (Evans and Johnson, 2001; Evans and Relling, 2004; Weinshilboum, 2003).

Pharmacogenetics and Drug Targets. Gene products that are direct targets for drugs have an important role in pharmacogenetics (Johnson and Lima, 2003). Whereas highly penetrant variants with profound functional consequences in some genes may cause disease phenotypes that confer negative selective pressure, more subtle variations in the same genes can be maintained in the population without causing disease, but nonetheless causing variation in drug response. For example, complete inactivation *via* rare point mutations in methylenetetrahydrofolate reductase (MTHFR) causes severe mental retardation, cardiovascular disease, and a shortened lifespan (Goyette *et al.*, 1994). MTHFR reduces 5,10-CH$_2$- to 5-CH$_3$-tetrahydrofolate, and thereby interacts with folate-dependent one-carbon synthesis reactions, including homocysteine/methionine metabolism and pyrimidine/purine synthesis (*see* Chapter 51). This pathway is the target of several antifolate drugs (Figure 4–11). Whereas rare variants in *MTHFR* may result in early death, the 677C→T SNP causes an amino acid substitution that is maintained in the population at a high frequency (variant allele, q, frequency in most white populations = 0.4). This variant is associated with modestly lower MTHFR

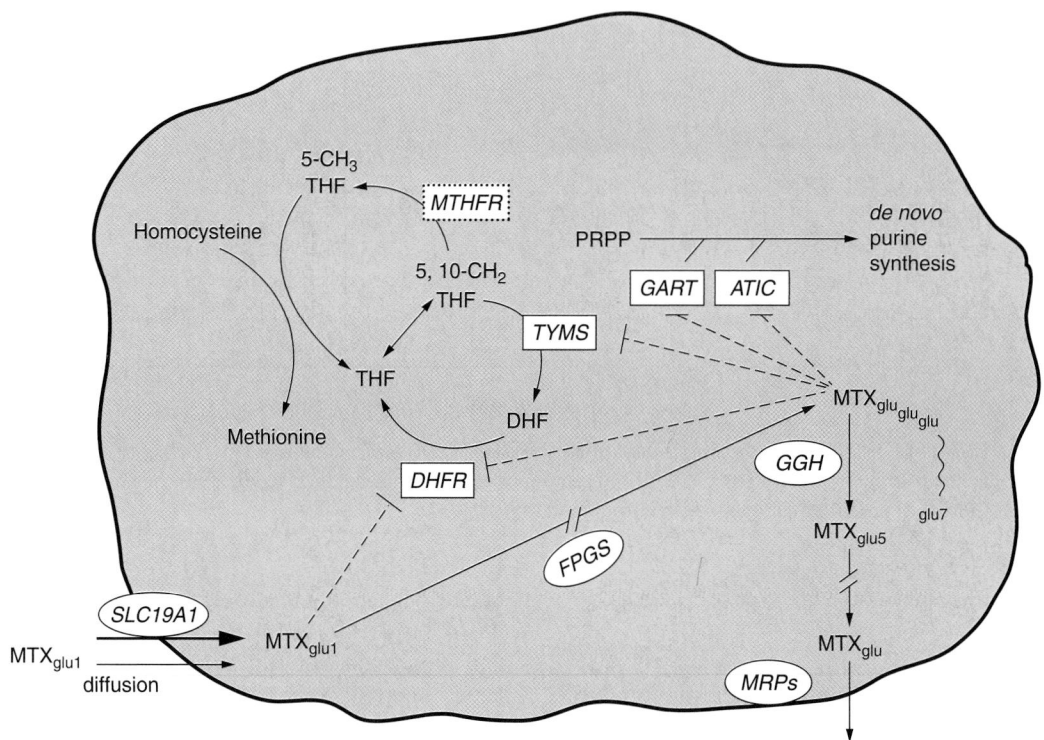

Figure 4–11. *Gene products involved in the pharmacogenetics of a single drug, methotrexate.* Those involved directly in pharmacokinetics (transport and metabolism) of methotrexate are circled (*e.g., SLC19A1, FPGS, MRPs, GGH*); direct targets of the drug are outlined in solid rectangles (*e.g., DHFR, TYMS, GART, ATIC*); and a gene product that may indirectly modulate the effect of methotrexate (*e.g.,* MTHFR) is outlined with a dotted line. DHFR, dihydrofolate reductase; TYMS, thymidylate synthetase; GART, glycinamide ribonucleotide transformylase; ATIC, aminoimidazole carboxamide transformylase; MTHFR, methylenetetrahydrofolate reductase.

activity (about 30% less than the 677C allele) and modest but significantly elevated plasma homocysteine concentrations (about 25% higher) (Klerk *et al.*, 2002). This polymorphism does not alter drug pharmacokinetics, but does appear to modulate pharmacodynamics by predisposing to gastrointestinal toxicity to the antifolate drug *methotrexate* in stem cell transplant recipients. Following prophylactic treatment with methotrexate for graft-*versus*-host disease, mucositis was three times more common among patients homozygous for the 677T allele than those homozygous for the 677C allele (Ulrich *et al.*, 2001).

Methotrexate is a substrate for transporters and anabolizing enzymes that affect its intracellular pharmacokinetics and that are subject to common polymorphisms (Figure 4–11). Several of the direct targets (dihydrofolate reductase, purine transformylases, and thymidylate synthase [*TYMS*]) are also subject to common polymorphisms. A polymorphic indel in *TYMS* (two *vs.* three repeats of a 28–base pair repeat in the enhancer) affects the amount of enzyme expression in both normal and

tumor cells. The polymorphism is quite common, with alleles equally split between the lower-expression two-repeat and the higher-expression three-repeat alleles. The *TYMS* polymorphism can affect both toxicity and efficacy of anticancer agents (*e.g.,* fluorouracil and methotrexate) that target *TYMS* (Krajinovic *et al.*, 2002). Thus, the genetic contribution to variability in the pharmacokinetics and pharmacodynamics of methotrexate cannot be understood without assessing genotypes at a number of different loci.

Many drug target polymorphisms have been shown to predict responsiveness to drugs (Table 4–3). Serotonin receptor polymorphisms predict not only the responsiveness to antidepressants (Figure 4–12), but also the overall risk of depression (Murphy *et al.*, 2003). β adrenergic receptor polymorphisms have been linked to asthma responsiveness (degree of change in one-second forced expiratory volume after use of a β agonist) (Tan *et al.*, 1997), renal function following angiotensin-converting enzyme (ACE) inhibitors (van Essen *et al.*, 1996), and heart rate following β-blockers (Tay-

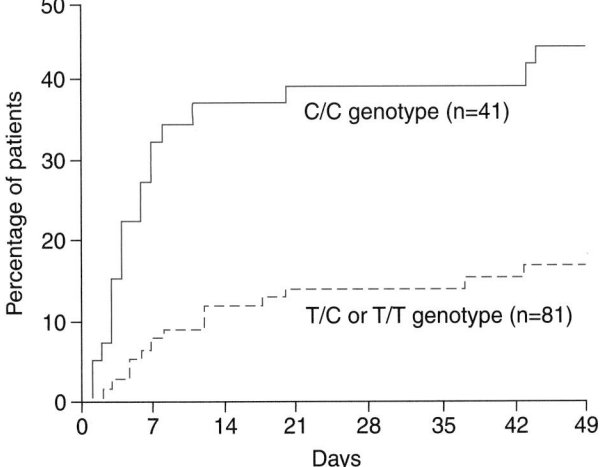

Figure 4–12. *Pharmacodynamics and pharmacogenetics.* The proportion of patients requiring a dosage decrease for the antidepressant drug paroxetine was greater ($p = 0.001$) in the approximately one-third of patients who have the C/C genotype for the serotonin 2A receptor ($5HT_{2A}$) compared to the two-thirds of patients who have either the T/C or T/T genotype at position 102 (Murphy *et al.*, 2003). The major reason for dosage decreases in paroxetine was the occurrence of adverse drug effects. (Reproduced with permission from Greer *et al.*, 2003.)

lor and Kennedy, 2001). Polymorphisms in 3-hydroxy-3-methylglutaryl coenzyme A (HMG-CoA) reductase have been linked to the degree of lipid lowering following statins, which are HMG-CoA reductase inhibitors (*see* Chapter 35), and to the degree of positive effects on high-density lipoproteins among women on estrogen replacement therapy (Herrington *et al.*, 2002; Figure 4–13). Ion channel polymorphisms have been linked to a risk of cardiac arrhythmias in the presence and absence of drug triggers (Roden, 2004).

Polymorphism-Modifying Diseases and Drug Responses. Some genes may be involved in an underlying disease being treated, but do not directly interact with the drug. Modifier polymorphisms are important for the *de novo* risk of some events and for the risk of drug-induced events. The *MTHFR* polymorphism, for example, is linked to homocysteinemia, which in turn affects thrombosis risk (den Heijer, 2003). The risk of a drug-induced thrombosis is dependent not only on the use of prothrombotic drugs, but on environmental and genetic predisposition to thrombosis, which may be affected by germline polymorphisms in *MTHFR*, factor V, and prothrombin (Chanock, 2003). These polymorphisms do not directly act on the pharmacokinetics or pharmacodynamics of prothrombotic drugs, such as glucocorticoids, estrogens, and asparaginase, but may modify the risk of the phenotypic event (thrombosis) in the presence of the drug.

Likewise, polymorphisms in ion channels (*e.g., HERG*, KvLQT1, Mink, and *MiRP1*) may affect the overall risk of cardiac dysrhythmias, which may be accentuated in the presence of a drug that can prolong the QT interval in some circumstances (*e.g.,* macrolide antibiotics, antihistamines) (Roden, 2003). These modifier polymorphisms may impact on the risk of "disease" phenotypes even in the absence of drug challenges; in the presence of drug, the "disease" phenotype may be elicited.

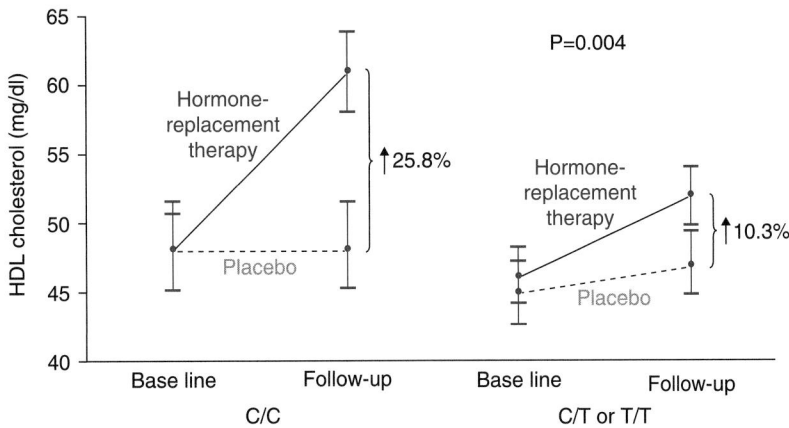

Figure 4–13. *Effect of genotype on response to estrogen hormone replacement therapy.* Depicted are pretreatment (base line) and posttreatment (follow-up) high-density lipoprotein (HDL) cholesterol levels in women of the C/C *vs.* C/T or T/T HMG-CoA reductase genotype. (Reproduced with permission from Herrington *et al.*, 2002.)

Cancer pharmacogenetics have an unusual aspect in that tumors exhibit somatically-acquired mutations in addition to the underlying germline variation of the host. Thus, the efficacy of some anticancer drugs depends on the genetics of both the host and the tumor. For example, non-small-cell lung cancer is treated with an inhibitor of epidermal growth factor receptor (EGFR), *gefitinib* (*see* Chapter 51). Patients whose tumors have activating mutations in the tyrosine kinase domain of *EGFR* appear to respond better to gefitinib than those without the mutations (Lynch *et al.*, 2004). Thus, the receptor is altered, and at the same time, individuals with the activating mutations may be considered to have a distinct category of non-small-cell lung cancer. As another example, the *TYMS* enhancer repeat polymorphism affects not only host toxicity, but also tumor susceptibility to thymidylate synthase inhibitors (Evans and McLeod, 2003; Villafranca *et al.*, 2001; Relling and Dervieux, 2001).

Pharmacogenetics and Drug Development

Pharmacogenetics will likely impact drug regulatory considerations in several ways (Evans and Relling, 2004; Lesko and Woodcock, 2004; Weinshilboum and Wang, 2004). Genome-wide approaches hold promise for identification of new drug targets and therefore new drugs. In addition, accounting for genetic/genomic interindividual variability may lead to genotype-specific development of new drugs, and to genotype-specific dosing regimens.

Pharmacogenomics can identify new targets. For example, genome-wide assessments using microarray technology could identify genes whose expression differentiates inflammatory processes; a compound could be identified that changes expression of that gene; and then that compound could serve as a starting point for anti-inflammatory drug development. Proof of principle has been demonstrated for identification of antileukemic agents (Stegmaier *et al.*, 2004) and antifungal drugs (Parsons *et al.*, 2004), among others.

Pharmacogenetics may identify subsets of patients who will have a very high or a very low likelihood of responding to an agent. This will permit testing of the drug in a selected population that is more likely to respond, minimizing the possibility of adverse events in patients who derive no benefit, and more tightly defining the parameters of response in the subset more likely to benefit. Somatic mutations in the *EGFR* gene strongly identify patients with lung cancer who are likely to respond to the tyrosine kinase inhibitor gefitinib (Lynch *et al.*, 2004); germline variations in 5-lipoxygenase (*ALOX5*) determine

which asthma patients are likely to respond to ALOX inhibitors (Drazen *et al.*, 1999); and vasodilation in response to β_2 agonists has been linked to β_2 adrenergic receptor polymorphisms (Johnson and Lima, 2003).

A related role for pharmacogenomics in drug development is to identify which genetic subset of patients is at highest risk for a serious adverse drug effect, and to avoid testing the drug in that subset of patients (Lesko and Woodcock, 2004). For example, the identification of HLA subtypes associated with hypersensitivity to the HIV-1 reverse transcriptase inhibitor *abacavir* (Mallal *et al.*, 2002) could theoretically identify a subset of patients who should receive alternative therapy, and thereby minimize or even abrogate hypersensitivity as an adverse effect of this agent. Children with acute myeloid leukemia who are homozygous for germline deletions in GSH transferase (*GSTT1*) are almost three times as likely to die of toxicity as those patients who have at least one wild-type copy of *GSTT1* following intensively timed antileukemic therapy but not after "usual" doses of antileukemic therapy (Davies *et al.*, 2001). These latter results suggest an important principle: pharmacogenetic testing may help to identify patients who require altered dosages of medications, but will not necessarily preclude the use of the agents completely.

Pharmacogenetics in Clinical Practice

Despite considerable research activity, pharmacogenetics is rarely utilized in clinical practice (Evans and Johnson, 2001; Weinshilboum and Wang, 2004). There are three major types of evidence that should accumulate in order to implicate a polymorphism in clinical care (Figure 4–14): screens of tissues from multiple humans linking the polymorphism to a trait; complementary preclinical functional studies indicating that the polymorphism is plausibly linked with the phenotype; and multiple supportive clinical phenotype/genotype studies. Because of the high probability of type I error in genotype/phenotype association studies, replication of clinical findings will generally be necessary. Although the impact of the polymorphism in TPMT on mercaptopurine dosing in childhood leukemia is a good example of a polymorphism for which all three types of evidence are available, proactive individualized dosing of thiopurines based on genotype has not been widely incorporated into clinical practice (Lesko *et al.*, 2004).

Most drug dosing takes place using a population "average" dose of drug. Adjusting dosages for variables such as renal or liver dysfunction is often accepted in drug dosing, even in cases in which the clinical outcome

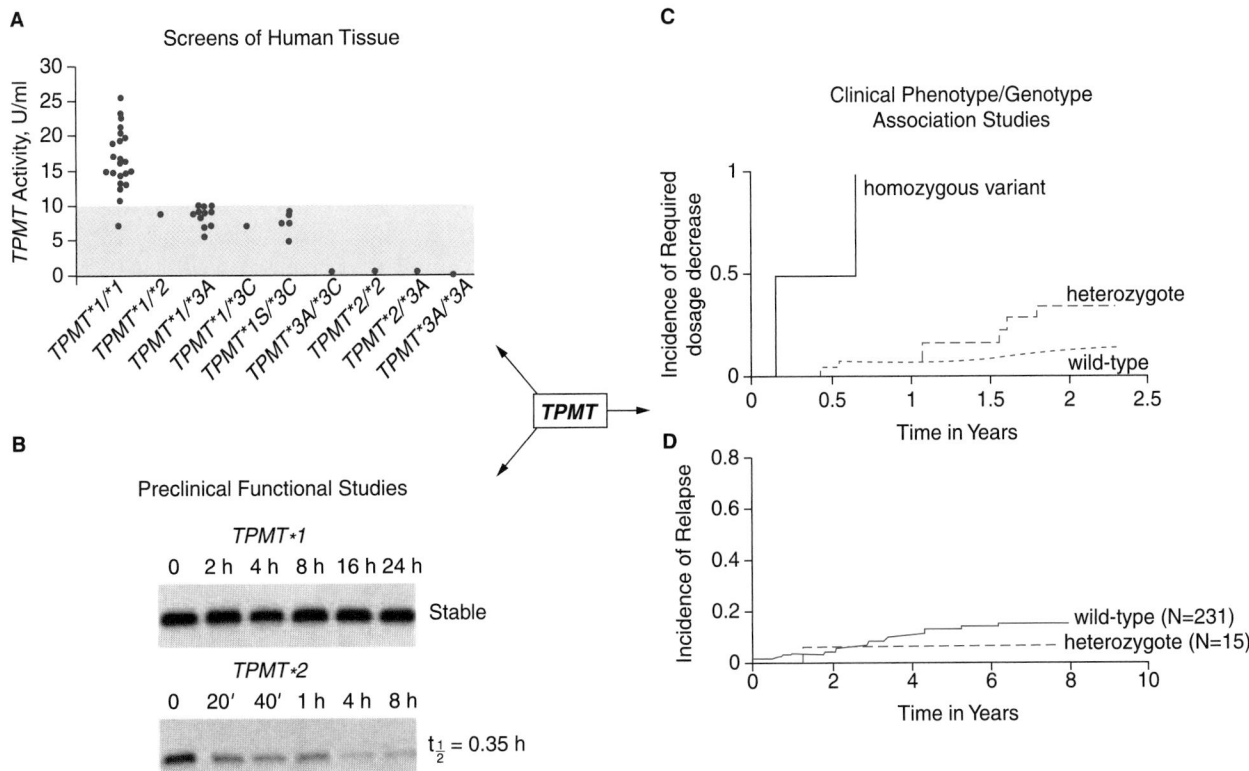

Figure 4–14. *Three primary types of evidence in pharmacogenetics.* Screens of human tissue (***A***) link phenotype (thiopurine methyltransferase activity in erythrocytes) with genotype (germline *TPMT* genotype). The two alleles are separated by a slash (/); the *1 and *1S alleles are wild-type, and the *2, *3A, and *3C are nonfunctional alleles. Shaded areas indicate low and intermediate levels of enzyme activity: those with the homozygous wild-type genotype have the highest activity, those heterozygous for at least one *1 allele have intermediate activity, and those homozygous for two inactive alleles have low or undetectable TPMT activity (Yates *et al.*, 1997). Directed preclinical functional studies (***B***) can provide biochemical data consistent with the *in vitro* screens of human tissue, and may offer further confirmatory evidence. Here, the heterologous expression of the *TPMT*1* wild-type and the *TPMT*2* variant alleles indicate that the former produces a more stable protein, as assessed by Western blot (Tai *et al.*, 1997). The third type of evidence comes from clinical phenotype/genotype association studies (***C*** and ***D***). The incidence of required dosage decrease for thiopurine in children with leukemia (***C***) differs by *TPMT* genotype: 100%, 35%, and 7% of patients with homozygous variant, heterozygous, or homozygous wild-type, respectively, require a dosage decrease (Relling *et al.*, 1999). When dosages of thiopurine are adjusted based on *TPMT* genotype in the successor study (***D***), leukemic relapse is not compromised, as indicated by comparable relapse rates in children who were wild-type *vs.* heterozygous for *TPMT*. Taken together, these three data sets indicate that the polymorphism should be accounted for in dosing of thiopurines. (Reproduced with permission from Relling *et al.*, 1999.)

of such adjustments has not been studied. Even though there are many examples of significant effects of polymorphisms on drug disposition (*e.g.*, Table 4–3), there is much more hesitation from clinicians to adjust doses based on genetic testing than on indirect clinical measures of renal and liver function. Whether this hesitation reflects resistance to abandon the "trial-and-error" approach that has defined most drug dosing, distrust of the genetic tests (which are constantly being refined), or unfamiliarity with the principles of genetics is not clear. Nonetheless, broad public initiatives, such as the NIH-funded Pharmacogenetics and Pharmacogenomics

Knowledge Base (www.pharmGKB.org), provide useful resources to permit clinicians to access information on pharmacogenetics (*see* Table 4–1).

The fact that functionally important polymorphisms are so common means that complexity of dosing will be likely to increase substantially in the postgenomic era. Even if every drug has only one important polymorphism to consider when dosing, the scale of complexity could be large. Many individuals take multiple drugs simultaneously for different diseases, and many therapeutic regimens for a single disease consist of multiple agents. This situation translates into a large number of possible drug-dose combina-

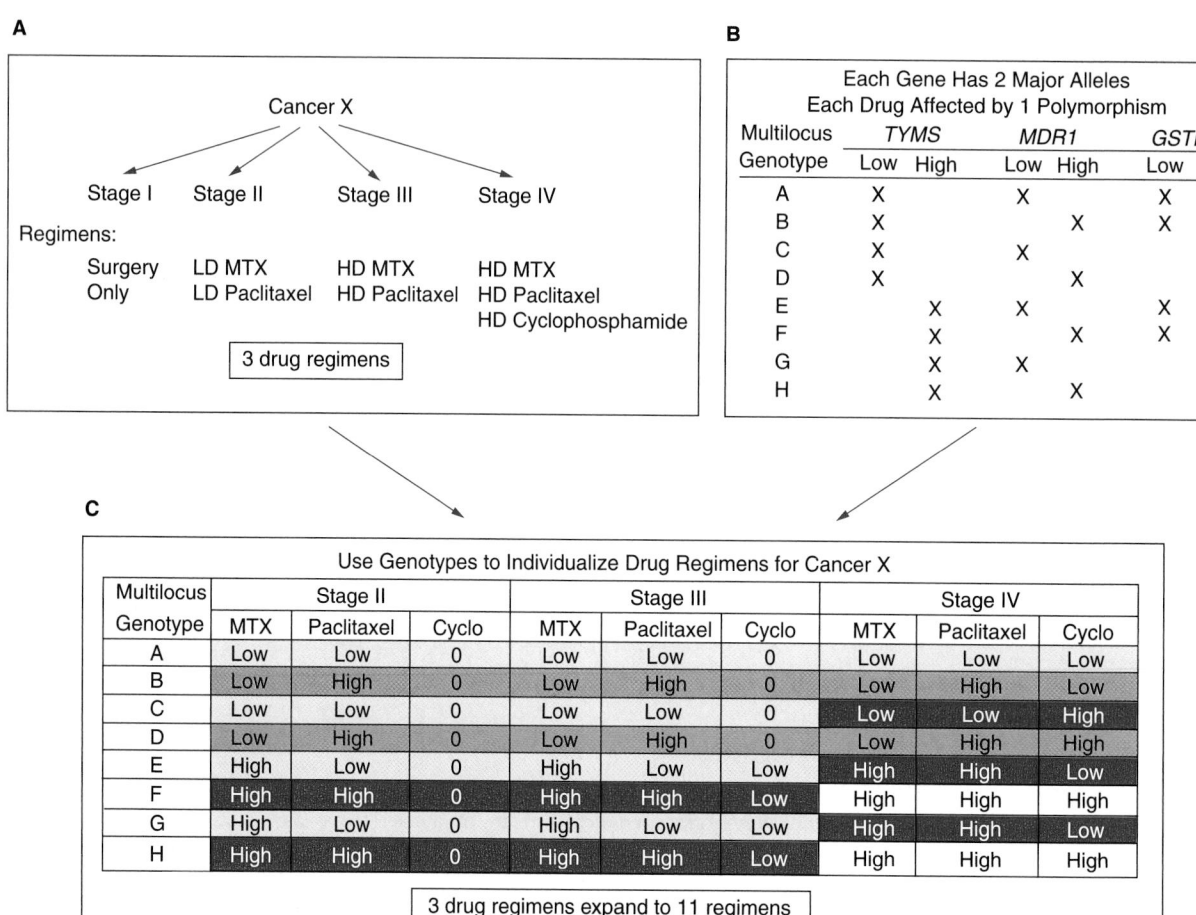

A

Cancer X

Stage I   Stage II   Stage III   Stage IV

Regimens:

Surgery   LD MTX   HD MTX   HD MTX
Only   LD Paclitaxel   HD Paclitaxel   HD Paclitaxel
                                           HD Cyclophosphamide

3 drug regimens

B

Each Gene Has 2 Major Alleles
Each Drug Affected by 1 Polymorphism

Multilocus Genotype	TYMS		MDR1		GSTM1	
	Low	High	Low	High	Low	High
A	X		X		X	
B	X			X	X	
C	X		X			X
D	X			X		X
E		X	X		X	
F		X		X	X	
G		X	X			X
H		X		X		X

C

Use Genotypes to Individualize Drug Regimens for Cancer X

Multilocus Genotype	Stage II			Stage III			Stage IV		
	MTX	Paclitaxel	Cyclo	MTX	Paclitaxel	Cyclo	MTX	Paclitaxel	Cyclo
A	Low	Low	0	Low	Low	0	Low	Low	Low
B	Low	High	0	Low	High	0	Low	High	Low
C	Low	Low	0	Low	Low	0	Low	Low	High
D	Low	High	0	Low	High	0	Low	High	High
E	High	Low	0	High	Low	Low	High	High	Low
F	High	High	0	High	High	Low	High	High	High
G	High	Low	0	High	Low	Low	High	High	Low
H	High	High	0	High	High	Low	High	High	High

3 drug regimens expand to 11 regimens

Figure 4–15. Potential impact of incorporation of pharmacogenetics into dosing of drugs for a relatively simple therapeutic regimen. The traditional approach to treatment for a disease (*A*), in this case a cancer, is based purely on stage of the cancer. Up to three different drugs are used in combination, with intensity of dosing dependent on the stage of the cancer. With this strategy, some with stage II disease are not receiving as much drug as they could tolerate; some patients with stage III or IV disease are undertreated and some are overtreated. *B* illustrates a hypothetical patient population with eight different multilocus genotypes. It is assumed that each of the three drugs is affected by just one genetic polymorphism (*TYMS* for methotrexate [MTX], *MDR1* for paclitaxel, and *GSTM1* for cyclophosphamide), and each polymorphism has just two important genotypes (one coding for low and one for high activity). The possible multilocus genotypes are designated by the letters A to H, and the combinations of *TYMS*, *MDR1* and *GSTM1* genotypes giving rise to those multilocus genotypes are indicated in the table. If these three genotypes, along with stage of cancer, are used to individualize dosages (*C*), so that those with low activity receive lower doses (LD) and those with higher activity receive higher doses (HD) of the relevant drug, what began as a total of three drug regimens in the absence of pharmacogenetics becomes 11 regimens by using pharmacogenetics for dosage individualization.

tions. Much of the excitement regarding the promise of human genomics has emphasized the hope of discovering individualized "magic bullets," and ignored the reality of the added complexity of additional testing and need for interpretation of results to capitalize on individualized dosing. This is illustrated in a potential pharmacogenetic example in Figure 4–15. In this case, a traditional anticancer treatment approach is replaced with one that incorpo-

rates pharmacogenetic information with the stage of the cancer determined by a variety of standardized pathological criteria. Assuming just one important genetic polymorphism for each of the three different anticancer drugs, 11 individual drug regimens can easily be generated.

Nonetheless, the potential utility of pharmacogenetics to optimize drug therapy is great. Once adequate genotype/phenotype studies have been conducted, molecular diagnostic tests will be developed that detect >95% of the important genetic variants for the majority of polymorphisms, and genetic tests have the advantage that they need only be conducted once during an individual's lifetime. With continued incorporation of pharmacogenetics into clinical trials, the important genes and polymorphisms will be identified, and data will demonstrate whether dosage individualization can improve outcomes and decrease short- and long-term adverse effects. Significant covariates will be identified to allow refinement of dosing in the context of drug interactions and disease influences. Although the challenges are substantial, accounting for the genetic basis of variability in response to medications is likely to become a fundamental component of diagnosing any illness and guiding the choice and dosage of medications.

BIBLIOGRAPHY

Aithal, G.P., Day, C.P., Kesteven, P.J., and Daly, A.K. Association of polymorphisms in the cytochrome P450 CYP2C9 with warfarin dose requirement and risk of bleeding complications. *Lancet,* **1999,** *353:*717–719.

Alving, A.S., Carson, P.E., Flanagan, C.L., and Ickes, C.E. Enzymatic deficiency in primaquine-sensitive erythrocytes. *Science,* **1956,** *124:*484–485.

Arranz, M.J., Munro, J., Birkett, J., *et al.* Pharmacogenetic prediction of clozapine response [letter]. *Lancet,* **2000,** *355:*1615–1616.

Bejerano, G., Pheasant, M., Makunin, I., *et al.* Ultraconserved elements in the human genome. *Science,* **2004,** *304:*1321–1325.

Boffelli, D., Nobrega, M.A., and Rubin, E.M. Comparative genomics at the vertebrate extremes. *Nat. Rev. Genet.,* **2004,** *5:*456–465.

Botstein, D., and Risch, N. Discovering genotypes underlying human phenotypes: past successes for mendelian disease, future approaches for complex disease. *Nat. Genet.,* **2003,** *33*(suppl):228–237.

Brudno, M., Do, C.B., Cooper, G.M., *et al.* LAGAN and Multi-LAGAN: efficient tools for large-scale multiple alignment of genomic DNA. *Genome Res.,* **2003,** *13:*721–731.

Burchard, E.G., Ziv, E., Coyle, N., *et al.* The importance of race and ethnic background in biomedical research and clinical practice. *N. Engl. J. Med.,* **2003,** *348:*1170–1175.

Cargill, M., Altshuler, D., Ireland, J., *et al.* Characterization of single-nucleotide polymorphisms in coding regions of human genes. *Nat. Genet.,* **1999,** *22:*231–238.

Chanock, S. Genetic variation and hematology: single-nucleotide polymorphisms, haplotypes, and complex disease. *Semin. Hematol.,* **2003,** *40:*321–328.

Chibana, K., Ishii, Y., and Fukuda, T. Tailor-made medicine for bronchial asthma. *Nippon Rinsho,* **2002,** *60:*189–196.

Davies, S.M., Robison, L.L., Buckley, J.D., *et al.* Glutathione S-transferase polymorphisms and outcome of chemotherapy in childhood acute myeloid leukemia. *J. Clin. Oncol.,* **2001,** *19:*1279–1287.

Drazen, J.M., Yandava, C.N., Dube, L., *et al.* Pharmacogenetic association between ALOX5 promoter genotype and the response to anti-asthma treatment. *Nat. Genet.,* **1999,** *22:*168–170.

Eichelbaum, M., and Gross, A.S. The genetic polymorphism of debrisoquine/sparteine metabolism—clinical aspects. *Pharmacol. Ther.,* **1990,** *46:*377–394.

Eichelbaum, M., Spannbrucker, N., and Dengler, H.J. Proceedings: N-oxidation of sparteine in man and its interindividual differences. *Naunyn Schmiedebergs Arch. Pharmacol.,* **1975,** *287*(suppl):R94.

van Essen, G.G., Rensma, P.L., de Zeeuw, D., *et al.* Association between angiotensin-converting-enzyme gene polymorphism and failure of renoprotective therapy. *Lancet,* **1996,** *347:*94–95.

Evans, W.E., and Johnson, J.A. Pharmacogenomics: the inherited basis for interindividual differences in drug response. *Annu. Rev. Genomics Hum. Genet.,* **2001,** *2:*9–39.

Evans, W.E., and McLeod, H.L. Pharmacogenomics—drug disposition, drug targets, and side effects. *N. Engl. J. Med.,* **2003,** *348:*538–549.

Evans, W.E., and Relling, M.V. Moving towards individualized medicine with pharmacogenomics. *Nature,* **2004,** *429:*464–468.

Fellay, J., Marzolini, C., Meaden, E.R., *et al.* Response to antiretroviral treatment in HIV-1-infected individuals with allelic variants of the multidrug resistance transporter 1: a pharmacogenetics study. *Lancet,* **2002,** *359:*30–36.

Furuta, T., Shirai, N., Sugimoto, M., *et al.* Pharmacogenomics of proton pump inhibitors. *Pharmacogenomics,* **2004,** *5:*181–202.

Goldstein, J.A. Clinical relevance of genetic polymorphisms in the human CYP2C subfamily. *Br. J. Clin. Pharmacol.,* **2001,** *52:*349–355.

Gonzalez, F.J., Skoda, R.C., Kimura, S., *et al.* Characterization of the common genetic defect in humans deficient in debrisoquine metabolism. *Nature,* **1988,** *331:*442–446.

Goyette, P., Sumner, J.S., Milos, R., *et al.* Human methylenetetrahydrofolate reductase: isolation of cDNA, mapping and mutation identification. *Nat. Genet.,* **1994,** *7:*195–200.

Grant, D.M., Morike, K., Eichelbaum, M., and Meyer, U.A. Acetylation pharmacogenetics. The slow acetylator phenotype is caused by decreased or absent arylamine N-acetyltransferase in human liver. *J. Clin. Invest.,* **1990,** *85:*968–972.

Greer, M., Murphy, J., *et al.* Pharmacogenomics of antidepressant medication intolerance. *Am. J. Psychiatry,* **2003,** *160:*1830–1835.

den Heijer, M. Hyperhomocysteinaemia as a risk factor for venous thrombosis: an update of the current evidence. *Clin. Chem. Lab. Med.,* **2003,** *41:*1404–1407.

Henikoff, S., and Henikoff, J.G. Amino acid substitution matrices from protein blocks. *Proc. Natl. Acad. Sci. U.S.A.,* **1992,** *89:*10915–10919.

Herrington, D.M., Howard, T.D., Hawkins, G.A., *et al.* Estrogen-receptor polymorphisms and effects of estrogen replacement on high-density lipoprotein cholesterol in women with coronary disease. *N. Engl. J. Med.,* **2002,** *346:*967–974.

Hughes, H.B., Biehl, J.P., Jones, A.P., and Schmidt, L.H. Metabolism of isoniazid in man as related to occurrence of peripheral neuritis. *Am. Rev. Tuberc.,* **1954,** *70:*266–273.

Hustmyer, F.G., Peacock, M., Hui, S., *et al.* Bone mineral density in relation to polymorphism at the vitamin D receptor gene locus. *J. Clin. Invest.,* **1994,** *94:*2130–2134.

Ingelman-Sundberg, M., and Evans, W.E. Unravelling the functional genomics of the human CYP2D6 gene locus. *Pharmacogenetics,* **2001,** *7:*553–554.

Iyer, L., Das, S., Janisch, L., *et al.* UGT1A1*28 polymorphism as a determinant of irinotecan disposition and toxicity. *Pharmacogenomics J.,* **2002,** *2:*43–47.

Iyer, L., King, C.D., Whitington, P.F., *et al.* Genetic predisposition to the metabolism of irinotecan (CPT-11). Role of uridine diphosphate glucuronosyltransferase isoform 1A1 in the glucuronidation of its active metabolite (SN-38) in human liver microsomes. *J. Clin. Invest.*, **1998,** *101:*847–854.

Johnson, J.A., and Lima, J.J. Drug receptor/effector polymorphisms and pharmacogenetics: current status and challenges. *Pharmacogenetics,* **2003,** *13:*525–534.

Kalow, W., Tang, B.K., and Endrenyi, L. Hypothesis: comparisons of inter- and intra-individual variations can substitute for twin studies in drug research. *Pharmacogenetics,* **1998,** *8:*283–289.

Kirchheiner, J., Brosen, K., Dahl, M.L., *et al.* CYP2D6 and CYP2C19 genotype-based dose recommendations for antidepressants: a first step towards subpopulation-specific dosages. *Acta. Psychiatr. Scand.,* **2001,** *104:*173–192.

Klerk, M., Verhoef, P., Clarke, R., *et al.* MTHFR 677C→T polymorphism and risk of coronary heart disease: a meta-analysis. *JAMA,* **2002,** *288:*2023–2031.

Koch, W.H. Technology platforms for pharmacogenomic diagnostic assays. *Nat. Rev. Drug Discov.,* **2004,** *3:*749–761.

Krajinovic, M., Costea, I., and Chiasson, S. Polymorphism of the thymidylate synthase gene and outcome of acute lymphoblastic leukaemia. *Lancet,* **2002,** *359:*1033–1034.

Kraus, J.P., Oliveriusova, J., Sokolova, J., *et al.* The human cystathionine beta-synthase (CBS) gene: complete sequence, alternative splicing, and polymorphisms. *Genomics,* **1998,** *52:*312–324.

Leabman, M.K., Huang, C.C., DeYoung, J., *et al.* Natural variation in human membrane transporter genes reveals evolutionary and functional constraints. *Proc. Natl. Acad. Sci. U.S.A.,* **2003,** *100:*5896–5901.

Lesko, L.J., and Woodcock, J. Opinion: Translation of pharmacogenomics and pharmacogenetics: a regulatory perspective. *Nat. Rev. Drug Discov.,* **2004,** *3:*763–769.

Lynch, T.J., Bell, D.W., Sordella, R., *et al.* Activating mutations in the epidermal growth factor receptor underlying responsiveness of non-small-cell lung cancer to gefitinib. *N. Engl. J. Med.,* **2004,** *350:*2129–2139.

McDonald, O.G., Krynetski, E.Y., and Evans, W.E. Molecular haplotyping of genomic DNA for multiple single-nucleotide polymorphisms located kilobases apart using long-range polymerase chain reaction and intramolecular ligation. *Pharmacogenetics,* **2002,** *12:*93–99.

Mahgoub, A., Idle, J.R., Dring, L.G., *et al.* Polymorphic hydroxylation of debrisoquine in man. *Lancet,* **1977,** *2:*584–586.

Mallal, S., Nolan, D., Witt, C., *et al.* Association between presence of HLA-B*5701, HLA-DR7, and HLA-DQ3 and hypersensitivity to HIV-1 reverse-transcriptase inhibitor abacavir. *Lancet,* **2002,** *359:*727–732.

Meyer, U.A. Pharmacogenetics and adverse drug reactions. *Lancet,* **2000,** *356:*1667–1671.

Meyer, U.A., and Zanger, U.M. Molecular mechanisms of genetic polymorphisms of drug metabolism. *Annu. Rev. Pharmacol. Toxicol.,* **1997,** *37:*269–296.

Miller, M.P., and Kumar, S. Understanding human disease mutations through the use of interspecific genetic variation. *Hum. Mol. Genet.,* **2001,** *10:*2319–2328.

Mirkovic, N., Marti-Renom, M.A., Weber, B.L., *et al.* Structure-based assessment of missense mutations in human BRCA1: implications for breast and ovarian cancer predisposition. *Cancer Res.,* **2004,** *64:*3790–3797.

Monaghan, G., Ryan, M., Seddon, R., *et al.* Genetic variation in bilirubin UPD-glucuronosyltransferase gene promoter and Gilbert's syndrome. *Lancet,* **1996,** *347:*578–581.

Murphy, G.M. Jr., Kremer, C., Rodrigues, H.E., and Schatzberg, A.F. Pharmacogenetics of antidepressant medication intolerance. *Am. J. Psychiatry,* **2003,** *160:*1830–1835.

Nebert, D.W., McKinnon, R.A., and Puga, A. Human drug-metabolizing enzyme polymorphisms: effects on risk of toxicity and cancer. *DNA Cell Biol.,* **1996,** *15:*273–280.

Ng, P.C., and Henikoff, S. SIFT: Predicting amino acid changes that affect protein function. *Nucleic Acids Res.,* **2003,** *31:*3812–3814.

Pani, M.A., Knapp, M., Donner, H., *et al.* Vitamin D receptor allele combinations influence genetic susceptibility to type 1 diabetes in Germans. *Diabetes,* **2000,** *49:*504–507.

Parsons, A.B., Brost, R.L., Ding, H., *et al.* Integration of chemical-genetic and genetic interaction data links bioactive compounds to cellular target pathways. *Nat. Biotechnol.,* **2004,** *22:*62–69.

Penno, M.B., Dvorchik, B.H., and Vesell, E.S. Genetic variation in rates of antipyrine metabolite formation: a study in uninduced twins. *Proc. Natl. Acad. Sci. U.S.A.,* **1981,** *78:*5193–5196.

Phillips, K.A., Veenstra, D.L., Oren, E., *et al.* Potential role of pharmacogenomics in reducing adverse drug reactions: a systematic review. *JAMA,* **2001,** *286:*2270–2279.

Quirk, E., McLeod, H., and Powderly, W. The pharmacogenetics of anti-retroviral therapy: a review of studies to date. *Clin. Infect. Dis.,* **2004,** *39:*98–106.

Relling, M.V., and Dervieux, T. Pharmacogenetics and cancer therapy. *Nat. Rev. Cancer,* **2001,** *1:*99–108.

Relling, M.V., Hancock, M.L., Rivera, G.K., *et al.* Mercaptopurine therapy intolerance and heterozygosity at the thiopurine S-methyltransferase gene locus. *J. Natl. Cancer Inst.,* **1999,** *91:*2001–2008.

Roden, D.M. Cardiovascular pharmacogenomics. *Circulation,* **2003,** *108:*3071–3074.

Roden, D.M. Drug-induced prolongation of the QT interval. *N. Engl. J. Med.,* **2004,** *350:*1013–1022.

Rosenberg, N.A., Li, L.M., Ward, R., and Pritchard, J.K. Informativeness of genetic markers for inference of ancestry. *Am. J. Hum. Genet.,* **2003,** *73:*1402–1422.

Rosenberg, N.A., Pritchard, J.K., Weber, J.L., *et al.* Genetic structure of human populations. *Science,* **2002,** *298:*2381–2385.

Sachidanandam, R., Weissman, D., Schmidt, S.C., *et al.* A map of human genome sequence variation containing 1.42 million single nucleotide polymorphisms. *Nature,* **2001,** *409:*928–933.

Sawyer, M.B., Innocenti, F., Das, S., *et al.* A pharmacogenetic study of uridine diphosphate-glucuronosyltransferase 2B7 in patients receiving morphine. *Clin. Pharmacol. Ther.,* **2003,** *73:*566–574.

Shu, Y., Leabman, M.K., Feng, B., *et al.* Evolutionary conservation predicts function of variants of the human organic cation transporter, OCT 1. *Proc. Natl. Acad. Sci. U.S.A.,* **2003,** *100:*5902–5907.

Siddiqui, A., Kerb, R., Weale, M.E., *et al.* Association of multidrug resistance in epilepsy with a polymorphism in the drug-transporter gene ABCB1. *N. Engl. J. Med.,* **2003,** *348:*1442–1448.

Stegmaier, K., Ross, K.N., Colavito, S.A., *et al.* Gene expression-based high-throughput screening (GE-HTS) and application to leukemia differentiation. *Nat. Genet.,* **2004,** *36:*257–263.

Stephens, J.C., Schneider, J.A., Tanguay, D.A., *et al.* Haplotype variation and linkage disequilibrium in 313 human genes. *Science,* **2001,** *293:*489–493.

Tabor, H.K., Risch, N.J., and Myers, R.M. Opinion: Candidate-gene approaches for studying complex genetic traits: practical considerations. *Nat. Rev. Genet.,* **2002,** *3:*391–397.

Tai, H.L., Krynetski, E.Y., Schuetz, E.G., *et al.* Enhanced proteolysis of thiopurine S-methyltransferase (TPMT) encoded by mutant alleles in humans (TPMT*3A, TPMT*2): mechanisms for the genetic polymorphism of TPMT activity. *Proc. Natl. Acad. Sci. U.S.A.,* **1997,** *94:*6444–6449.

Takada, K., Arefayene, M., Desta, Z., *et al*. Cytochrome P450 pharmacogenetics as a predictor of toxicity and clinical response to pulse cyclophosphamide in lupus nephritis. *Arthritis Rheum.,* **2004,** *50:*2202–2210.

Tan, S., Hall, I.P., Dewar, J., *et al*. Association between β_2-adrenoceptor polymorphism and susceptibility to bronchodilator desensitisation in moderately severe stable asthmatics. *Lancet,* **1997,** *350:*995–999.

Taylor, D.R., and Kennedy, M.A. Genetic variation of the β_2-adrenoceptor: its functional and clinical importance in bronchial asthma. *Am. J. Pharmacogenomics.,* **2001,** *1:*165–174.

The International SNP Map Working Group. A map of human genome sequence variation containing 1.4 million single nucleotide polymorphisms. *Nature,* **2001.**

Tirona, R.G., Leake, B.F., Merino, G., and Kim, R.B. Polymorphisms in OATP-C: identification of multiple allelic variants associated with altered transport activity among European- and African-Americans. *J. Biol. Chem.,* **2001,** *276:*35669–35675.

Townsend, D., and Tew, K. Cancer drugs, genetic variation and the glutathione-S-transferase gene family. *Am. J. Pharmacogenomics,* **2003a,** *3:*157–172.

Townsend, D.M., and Tew, K.D. The role of glutathione-S-transferase in anti-cancer drug resistance. *Oncogene,* **2003b,** *22:*7369–7375.

Ulrich, C.M., Yasui, Y., Storb, R., *et al*. Pharmacogenetics of methotrexate: toxicity among marrow transplantation patients varies with the methylenetetrahydrofolate reductase C677T polymorphism. *Blood,* **2001,** *98:*231–234.

Vesell, E.S. Advances in pharmacogenetics and pharmacogenomics. *J. Clin. Pharmacol.,* **2000,** *40:*930–938.

Vesell, E.S. Genetic and environmental factors causing variation in drug response. *Mutat. Res.,* **1991,** *247:*241–257.

Vesell, E.S., and Page, J.G. Genetic control of drug levels in man: antipyrine. *Science,* **1968,** *161:*72–73.

Villafranca, E., Okruzhnov, Y., Dominguez, M.A., *et al*. Polymorphisms of the repeated sequences in the enhancer region of the thymidylate synthase gene promoter may predict downstaging after preoperative chemoradiation in rectal cancer. *J. Clin. Oncol.,* **2001,** *19:*1779–1786.

Watters, J.W., Kraja, A., Meucci, M.A., *et al*. Genome-wide discovery of loci influencing chemotherapy cytotoxicity. *Proc. Natl. Acad. Sci. U.S.A.,* **2004,** *101:*11809–11814.

Weinshilboum, R. Inheritance and drug response. *N. Engl. J. Med.,* **2003,** *348:*529–537.

Weinshilboum, R.M., and Sladek, S.L. Mercaptopurine pharmacogenetics: monogenic inheritance of erythrocyte thiopurine methyltransferase activity. *Am. J. Hum. Genet.,* **1980,** *32:*651–662.

Weinshilboum, R., and Wang, L. Pharmacogenomics: bench to bedside. *Nat. Rev. Drug Discov.,* **2004,** *3:*739–748.

Xie, H.G., Kim, R.B., Wood, A.J., and Stein, C.M. Molecular basis of ethnic differences in drug disposition and response. *Annu. Rev. Pharmacol. Toxicol.,* **2001,** *41:*815–850.

Xu, Z.H., Freimuth, R.R., Eckloff, B., *et al*. Human 3'-phosphoadenosine 5'-phosphosulfate synthetase 2 (PAPSS2) pharmacogenetics: gene resequencing, genetic polymorphisms and functional characterization of variant allozymes. *Pharmacogenetics,* **2002,** *12:*11–21.

Yates, C.R., Krynetski, E.Y., Loennechen, T., *et al*. Molecular diagnosis of thiopurine S-methyltransferase deficiency: genetic basis for azathioprine and mercaptopurine intolerance. *Ann. Intern. Med.,* **1997,** *126:*608–614.

THE SCIENCE OF DRUG THERAPY

John A. Oates

Drug therapy affords an expanding opportunity for preventing and treating disease and for alleviating symptoms. Pharmacologic agents also expose patients to risk. Basic principles of drug therapy provide a conceptual framework for deploying drugs with maximal efficacy while minimizing the risk of adverse effects.

Optimal therapeutic decisions are based on an evaluation of the individual patient in concert with assessment of the evidence for efficacy and safety of the treatment under consideration. An understanding of the pharmacokinetics and pharmacodynamics of the drug should be integrated with this patient-focused information to guide implementation of therapy.

EVALUATION OF THE EVIDENCE

Initial determination of the effectiveness and safety of drugs is based predominantly on evaluation of experimental interventions in *clinical trials*. Well-designed and effectively executed clinical trials provide the scientific evidence that informs most therapeutic decisions. Evidence from clinical trials may be supplemented by *observational studies*, particularly in assessing adverse effects that elude detection in clinical trials designed to determine efficacy and that do not occur frequently or rapidly enough.

Clinical Trials

Similarity of the control group with the group receiving the intervention is key to obtaining valid information in all experimental science. In clinical trials, this similarity is best achieved by random assignment of patients or volunteers to the control group or the group receiving the experimental therapy. Such randomization is the optimal method for distributing between the treatment and control groups the known and unknown variables that could affect outcome. Recognizing that a randomized clinical trial is the "gold standard" of clinical trials, it nonetheless may be impossible to use this design to study all disorders; for patients who cannot—by regulation, ethics, or both—be studied with this design (*e.g.*, children, fetuses, or some patients with psychiatric disease) or for disorders with a typically fatal outcome (*e.g.*, rabies), it may be necessary to resort to historical controls.

A second important element of study design is *concealment* of the outcome of randomization from the study participants and investigators. Concealing whether participants are assigned to the control or the treatment group is referred to as *blinding* or *masking* the study. In therapeutic investigations, participants in the control group will receive an inactive replica of the drug, *e.g.*, a tablet or capsule containing inert ingredients that is identical in appearance to the active agent. This inert replica of the drug is designated as a *placebo*. When only the study participants are blinded to treatment assignment but investigators know whether the active agent is being given, this is designated as a *single-blind study*. In a *double-blind study*, neither the study participants nor the investigators knows whether the active agent is being given. Blinding the investigators not only removes bias in interpreting the outcomes and in decisions regarding management of the patient but also eliminates selectivity in the enthusiasm for therapy typically conveyed by clinicians. By eliminating participant and observer bias, the randomized, double-blind, placebo-controlled trial provides the highest likelihood of revealing the truth about the effects of a drug (Temple, 1997). The double-blind, placebo-controlled design permits evaluation of subjective end points, such as pain, that are powerfully influenced by the administration of placebo. Striking instances in which placebo effects are observed include pain in labor, where a placebo produces approximately 40% of the relief provided by the opioid analgesic *meperidine* with a remarkably similar time course, and angina pectoris, where as much as a 60% improvement in symptoms is achieved with placebo. The response to placebo in patients with depression is often 60% to 70% as great as that of an active antidepressant drug; as described below, this complicates clinical trials of efficacy.

Benjamin Franklin pioneered the blinded study design. The king of France appointed him to a commission to evaluate the claims of the flamboyant healer Friedrich Anton Mesmer, who employed magnetized iron rods to heal illnesses. Franklin and the commission conducted an experiment in which patients were blindfolded to conceal whether or not they received Mesmer's treatment and found that the healing effects were independent of exposure to the magnetized rods.

The existence of a therapy already known to improve disease outcome may provide an ethical basis for comparing a new drug with the established treatment rather than placebo (Passamani, 1991). If the aim is to show that the new drug is as effective as the comparator, then the size of the trial must be sufficiently large to have the statistical power to demonstrate a meaningful difference between the two groups if such a difference were to exist. Trials conducted against comparators as controls can be misleading if they claim equal effectiveness based on the lack of a statistical difference between the drugs in a trial that was too small to demonstrate such a difference. When trials against comparator drugs examine the relative incidence of side effects, it also is important that the doses of the drugs are equally effective.

A clear hypothesis for the trial should guide the selection of a *primary end point*, which should be specified before the trial is initiated. Ideally, this primary end point should measure a clinical outcome, either a disease-related outcome, such as improvement of survival or reduction of myocardial infarction, or a symptomatic outcome, such as pain relief or quality of life. Examination of a single, prospectively selected end point is most likely to yield a valid result from the study. A few additional (secondary) end points also may be designated in advance; the greater the number of end points that are examined, the greater is the likelihood that apparently significant changes in one of them will occur by chance. The least rigorous examination of trial results comes from retrospective selection of end points after viewing the data. Because this introduces a selection bias and increases the probability of a chance result, retrospective selection should be used only as the basis to generate hypotheses that then can be tested prospectively.

In some instances, therapeutic decisions must be based on trials evaluating surrogate end points—measures such as clinical signs or laboratory findings that are correlated with but do not directly measure clinical outcome. Such surrogate end points include measurements of blood pressure (for antihypertensive drugs), plasma glucose (for diabetic drugs), and levels of viral RNA in plasma (for antiretroviral drugs). The extent to which surrogate end points predict clinical outcomes varies, and two drugs with the same effect on a surrogate end point may have different effects on clinical outcome. Of greater concern, the effect of a drug on a surrogate end point may lead to erroneous conclusions about the clinical consequences of drug administration. One compelling example of the danger of reliance on surrogate end points emerged from the Cardiac Arrhythmia Suppression Trial (CAST). Based on their ability to suppress the surrogate markers of ventricular premature contractions and nonsustained ventricular tachycardia, antiarrhythmic drugs such as *encainide*, *flecanide*, and *moricizine* frequently were used in patients with ventricular ectopy after myocardial infarction (*see* Chapter 33). The CAST study showed that despite their ability to suppress ventricular ectopy, the drugs actually increased the frequency of sudden cardiac death (Echt *et al.*, 1991). Thus, the ultimate test of a drug's efficacy must arise from actual clinical outcomes rather than surrogate markers (Bucher *et al.*, 1999).

The *sample* of patients selected for a clinical trial may not be representative of the entire *population* of patients with that disease who may receive the drug. The patients entered into a trial usually are selected according to the severity of their disease and other characteristics (*inclusion criteria*) or are excluded because of coexisting disease, concurrent therapy, or specific features of the disease itself (*exclusion criteria*). It always is important to ascertain that the clinical characteristics of an individual patient correspond with those of patients in the trial (Feinstein, 1994). For example, the Randomized Aldactone Evaluation Study (RALES) showed that treatment with the mineralocorticoid-receptor antagonist *spironolactone* was associated with a 30% reduction in death in patients with severe congestive heart failure (Pitt *et al.*, 1999). The potential adverse effect of hyperkalemia was seen only rarely in this study, which excluded patients with serum creatinine levels of greater than 2.5 mg/dl. With the expanded use of spironolactone after the RALES results were published, numerous patients, many of whom did not meet the criteria for inclusion that minimized the risk in the RALES trial, have developed severe hyperkalemia on spironolactone (Jurlink *et al.*, 2004). Knowledge of the criteria for selecting the patients in a trial must inform the application of study results to an individual patient.

Determination of efficacy and safety is an ongoing process that usually is based on the results of more than one randomized, double-blind, controlled trial. Because the trials may not all provide the same results, and some may show an apparent effect that does not achieve statistical significance, it may be useful to aggregate the results of several similarly designed drug trials that examined the same clinical end point into an overview termed a *meta-analysis*. The larger numbers of patients and controls in such a meta-analysis can yield narrower confidence limits and strengthen the likelihood that an apparent effect is (or is not) due to the drug rather than chance. In one example, a meta-analysis of 65 randomized trials involving nearly 60,000 patients strongly supported the current use of low-dose aspirin to prevent death, myocardial infarction, and stroke in high-risk patients (Antiplatelet Trialists' Collaboration, 2002).

Observational Studies

Important but infrequent adverse drug effects may escape detection in the randomized, controlled trials that demonstrate efficacy. In controlled trials that form the basis for approval of drugs for marketing, the number of patient-years of exposure to a drug is small relative to exposure after it is marketed. Also, some adverse effects may have a long latency or may affect patients excluded from the controlled trials. Therefore, nonexperimental or observational studies are used to examine those adverse effects that only become apparent with widespread, prolonged use of the drug in the practice of medicine. For example, such observational studies identified peptic ulcers and gastritis as serious adverse effects of nonsteroidal anti-inflammatory drugs and aspirin.

The quality of information derived from observational studies varies with the design and depends highly on the selection of controls and the accuracy of the information on medication use (Ray, 2004; Sackett, 1991). Automated prescription databases provide a relatively reliable measure of drug exposure for such studies. *Cohort studies* compare the occurrence of events in users and nonusers of a drug; this is the more powerful of the observational study designs. *Case-control studies* compare drug exposure among patients with an adverse outcome with that in control patients. Because the control and treatment groups in an observational study are not selected randomly, there may be unknown differences between the groups that determine outcome independent of drug use. Because of the limitations of observational studies, their validity cannot be equated with that of randomized, controlled trials (Table 5–1). Rather, the role of observational studies is to raise questions and pose hypotheses about adverse reactions. However, if it is not feasible to test these hypotheses in controlled clinical trials, then replicated findings from observational studies may form the basis for clinical decisions.

Table 5–1
A Ranking of the Quality of Comparative Studies

Randomized, controlled trials
Double blinded
Single blinded
Unblinded
Observational studies
Prospective cohort study
Prospective case-control study
Retrospective cohort study
Retrospective case control study

PATIENT-CENTERED THERAPEUTICS

Optimal treatment decisions are based on an understanding of the characteristics of the individual patient that will determine the response to the drug. Interindividual differences in drug delivery to its site(s) of action can profoundly influence therapeutic effectiveness and adverse effects. Pharmacodynamic differences in the response to a drug may result from alterations in the effect on the target organ or from differences in the body's adaptation to the target-organ response owing to disease or other drugs. Moreover, precision in diagnosis and prognosis governs the type of therapy and the therapeutic regimen, as well as the urgency and intensity of treatment. Some of the determinants of interindividual variation are indicated in Figure 5–1. Thus, therapeutic success and safety are determined by integration of evidence of efficacy and safety with knowledge of the individual factors that determine response in a particular patient.

Drug History

A thorough drug history is a key element in individualizing therapy, and information on concurrent therapy must be accessible at each encounter to guide safe and effective treatment. Documentation of current prescription drug use is a starting point in the drug history. Despite increasing use of computerized drug lists, it often is very helpful for patients to bring all current medications with them to the clinical encounter. Specific prompting is required to elicit the use of over-the-counter drugs and herbal medications, both of

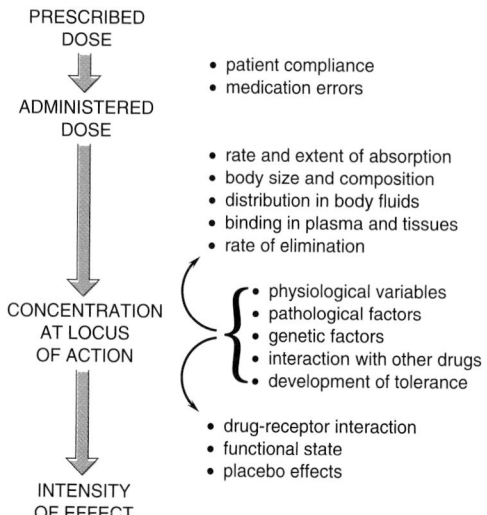

Figure 5–1. *Factors that determine the relationship between prescribed drug dosage and drug effect.* (Modified from Koch-Weser, 1972.)

which may affect therapeutic decisions. Information about medications that are used only sporadically (*e.g., sildenafil* for erectile dysfunction) may not be volunteered without a specific query. With cognitively impaired patients, it may be necessary to go beyond the interview to include caregivers and pharmacy records; as noted earlier, requests to examine the actual medications also can be invaluable.

Adverse reactions to drugs, allergic or otherwise, should be documented with specifics regarding severity. Full elucidation of adverse effects is aided by asking whether patients or their physicians have discontinued any medications in the past.

An accessible current drug profile and list of adverse effects are required for each patient encounter. Review of the medication list on hospital rounds and during outpatient visits is essential to maximize effectiveness and safety of treatment. With electronic medical records, the medication list can be printed for the patient to optimize communication about therapy and adherence to the regimen.

DETERMINANTS OF INTERINDIVIDUAL VARIATION IN RESPONSE TO DRUGS

Disease-Induced Alterations in Pharmacokinetics

Knowledge of the pathway of a drug's disposition is key to predicting how a disease process will alter delivery of the drug to its site of action.

Impaired Renal Clearance of Drugs. If a drug is cleared primarily by the kidney, and if adverse effects result from elevated levels of the drug, then dose modification should be considered in patients with renal dysfunction. There are many such drugs, including *vancomycin, aminoglycoside antibiotics,* and *digoxin.* When renal clearance of a drug is diminished, the desired pharmacological effect can be maintained either by decreasing the dose or lengthening the interval between doses. Estimation of the glomerular filtration rate (GFR) provides an approximation of the extent to which renal drug clearance is impaired; this index of renal function is applicable to assessing decreases in elimination of drugs cleared by either glomerular filtration or tubular secretion. GFR can be measured by the iothalamate clearance method. Alternatively, creatinine clearance can be used, as estimated from serum creatinine by the formula of Cockcroft and Gault:

$$\frac{\text{creatinine}}{\text{clearance}} = \frac{(140 - \text{age}) \times \binom{\text{ideal body}}{\text{weight in kg}}}{72 \times \text{serum creatinine (mg/dl)}} \times 0.85 \text{ for women}$$

Ideal body weight for men = 50 kg + 2.3 kg/in over 5 ft in height. Ideal body weight for women = 45.5 kg + 2.3 kg/in over 5 feet in height. The 0.85 multiplier for women accounts for their reduced muscle mass. The serum creatinine concentration may be a misleading indicator of renal impairment because it does not reflect GFR in states where the GFR is changing or in elderly or emaciated patients whose decreased muscle mass is associated with decreased creatinine formation.

With knowledge of the GFR, initial dosing reductions can be estimated from tables provided in the package insert or from other published tables (*e.g.,* Aronoff, 1999). The accuracy of the estimated initial dosing regimen should be monitored by clinical assessment and by analysis of plasma drug concentration where feasible.

Drug metabolites that may accumulate with impaired renal function may be pharmacologically active or toxic. Although *meperidine* is metabolized extensively and is not dependent on renal function for elimination, its metabolite, *normeperidine,* is cleared by the kidney and accumulates when renal function is impaired. Because normeperidine has greater convulsant activity than meperidine, its high levels in renal failure probably account for the central nervous system (CNS) excitation with irritability, twitching, and seizures that can occur when multiple doses of meperidine are given to patients with impaired renal function (*see* Chapter 21).

Impaired Hepatic Clearance of Drugs. The effect of liver disease on the hepatic biotransformation of drugs cannot be predicted from any measure of hepatic function.

Thus, even though the metabolism of some drugs is decreased with impaired hepatic function, there is no quantitative basis for dose adjustment other than assessment of the clinical response and plasma concentration. The oral bioavailability of drugs may be increased in liver disease, and a marked increase may occur with drugs that normally have high first-pass hepatic clearance. In patients with cirrhosis, the oral availability of drugs that have high first-pass clearance (*e.g.*, morphine, meperidine, *midazolam,* and *nifedipine*) is almost doubled. Portosystemic shunting will further reduce first-pass clearance and lead to high plasma drug levels with the potential for adverse effects.

Circulatory Insufficiency Owing to Cardiac Failure or Shock. In circulatory failure, neuroendocrine compensation can reduce renal and hepatic blood flow substantially. Accordingly, elimination of many drugs is reduced. Particularly affected are drugs with high hepatic extraction ratios, such as *lidocaine,* whose clearance is a function of hepatic blood flow; in this setting, only half the usual infusion rate of lidocaine is required to achieve therapeutic plasma levels.

Altered Drug Binding to Plasma Proteins. When a drug is highly bound to plasma proteins, its egress from the vascular compartment is limited largely to the unbound (free) drug. Thus, the therapeutic response should be related to the level of unbound drug in plasma rather than to the total drug concentration. Hypoalbuminemia owing to renal insufficiency, hepatic disease, or other causes can reduce the extent of binding of acidic and neutral drugs; in these conditions, measurement of free drug provides a more accurate guide to therapy than does analysis of total drug. Because a small change in the extent of binding produces a large change in the level of free drug, drugs for which changes in protein binding are particularly important are those that are more than 90% bound to plasma protein. *Phenytoin* is one such drug, and measurement of unbound phenytoin is used to guide dosing in patients with renal failure or other conditions that reduce protein binding (*see* Chapter 19).

Metabolic clearance of such highly bound drugs also is a function of the unbound fraction of drug. Thus, clearance is increased in those conditions that reduce protein binding; shorter dosing intervals therefore must be employed to maintain therapeutic plasma levels.

INTERACTIONS BETWEEN DRUGS

Marked alterations in the effects of some drugs can result from coadministration with another agent. Such interactions can increase the drug effect to the level of toxicity, or they can inhibit the drug effect and deprive the patient of therapeutic benefit. Drug interactions always should be considered when unexpected responses to drugs occur. Whereas the sheer number of drug interactions defies memorization, understanding their mechanisms provides a conceptual framework for preventing them.

Drug interactions may be *pharmacokinetic* (*i.e.*, the delivery of a drug to its site of action is altered by a second drug) or *pharmacodynamic* (*i.e.*, the response of the drug target is modified by a second drug).

Pharmacokinetic Interactions Caused by Diminished Drug Delivery to the Site of Action

A number of mechanisms may affect drug delivery to the site of action. Impaired gastrointestinal absorption is an important consideration for drugs administered orally. For example, aluminum ions in certain antacids or ferrous ions in oral iron supplements form insoluble chelates of the *tetracycline antibiotics,* thereby preventing their absorption. The antifungal *ketoconazole* is a weak base that is only soluble at acid pH. Drugs that raise gastric pH, such as the protein pump inhibitors and histamine H_2-receptor antagonists, impair the dissolution and absorption of ketoconazole.

An especially prominent form of drug interaction involves the cytochrome P450 enzymes (CYPs). As described in detail in Chapter 3, the hepatic CYPs play a key role in the metabolism of a large number of drugs, and their expression can be induced or their activity inhibited by a diverse array of drugs. Examples of drugs that induce these enzymes include antibiotics (*e.g.*, rifampin), anticonvulsants (*e.g.*, *phenobarbital,* phenytoin, and *carbamazepine*), nonnucleoside reverse transcriptase inhibitors (*e.g.*, efavirenz and *nevirapine*), and herbal drugs (*e.g.*, *St. John's wort*). Although these drugs most potently induce CYP3A4, the expression of CYPs in the 1A, 2B, and 2C families also can be increased. Induction of these enzymes accelerates the metabolism of drugs that are their substrates and notably decreases oral bioavailability by increasing first-pass metabolism in the liver. The inducing drugs lower the plasma levels of drugs that are metabolized predominantly by these enzymes, including *cyclosporine, tacrolimus, warfarin, verapamil, methadone, dexamethasone, methylprednisolone, low-dose oral contraceptives,* and the *HIV protease inhibitors.* Loss of efficacy is the unfortunate but predictable consequence of these interactions.

Pharmacokinetic Interactions That Increase Drug Delivery to the Site of Action

Inhibition of Drug-Metabolizing Enzymes. For drugs whose clearance depends primarily on biotransformation, inhibition of a metabolizing enzyme leads to reduced clearance, prolonged half-life, and drug accumulation during maintenance therapy, sometimes with severe adverse effects. The prominent role of CYPs in drug metabolism makes them key effectors of such interactions, and knowledge of the CYP isoforms that catalyze the principal pathways of drug metabolism provides a basis for understanding and even predicting drug interactions (*see* Chapter 3).

Hepatic CYP3A isozymes catalyze the metabolism of many drugs that are subject to significant drug interactions owing to inhibition of metabolism. Drugs metabolized predominantly by CYP3A isozymes include immunosuppressants (*e.g.,* cyclosporine and tacrolimus), HMG-CoA reductase inhibitors (*e.g., lovastatin, simvastatin,* and *atorvastatin*), HIV protease inhibitors (*e.g., indinavir, nelfinavir, saquinavir, amprinavir,* and *ritonavir*), Ca^{2+} channel antagonists (*e.g., felodipine, nifedipine, nisoldipine,* and *diltiazem*), glucocorticoids (*e.g.,* dexamethasone and *methylprednisolone*), benzodiazepines (*e.g., alprazolam,* midazolam, and *triazolam*), and lidocaine.

The inhibition of CYP3A isoforms may vary even among structurally related members of a given drug class. For example, the antifungal azoles ketoconazole and *itraconazole* potently inhibit CYP3A enzymes, whereas the related *fluconazole* inhibits minimally except at high doses or in the setting of renal insufficiency. Similarly, certain macrolide antibiotics (*e.g., erythromycin* and *clarithromycin*) potently inhibit CYP3A isoforms, but *azithromycin* does not. In one instance, the inhibition of CYP3A4 activity is turned to therapeutic advantage. The HIV protease inhibitor ritonavir inhibits CYP3A4 activity; when administered in combination with other protease inhibitors metabolized by this pathway, it increases their half-lives and permits less frequent dosing.

Drug interactions mediated by inhibition of CYP3A can be severe. Examples include nephrotoxicity induced by cyclosporine and tacrolimus and severe myopathy and rhabdomyolysis resulting from increased levels of HMG-CoA reductase inhibitors. Whenever an inhibitor of the CYP3A isoforms is administered, the clinician must be cognizant of the potential for serious interactions with drugs metabolized by CYP3A.

Drug interactions also can result from inhibition of other CYPs. *Amiodarone* and its active metabolite *desethylamiodarone* promiscuously inhibit several CYPs, including CYP2C9, the principal enzyme that eliminates the active *S*-enantiomer of warfarin. Because many patients treated with amiodarone are also receiving warfarin (*e.g.,* subjects with atrial fibrillation), the potential exists for major bleeding complications.

Knowledge of the specific pathways of metabolism of a drug and the molecular mechanisms of enzyme induction can help to identify potential interactions; thus the pathways of drug metabolism often are determined during preclinical drug development (Yuan *et al.,* 1999; Peck, 1993). If *in vitro* studies indicate that a compound is metabolized by CYP3A4, for example, studies can focus on commonly used drugs that either inhibit (*e.g.,* ketoconazole) or induce (*e.g.,* rifampin) this enzyme. Other probes for the evaluation of potential drug interactions targeted at CYPs in human beings include midazolam or erythromycin for CYP3A4 and *dextromethorphan* for CYP2D6.

Inhibition of Drug Transport. Drug transporters are key determinants of the availability of certain drugs to their site(s) of action, and clinically significant drug interactions can result from inhibition of drug transporters (*see* Chapter 2). The best-studied drug transporter is the P-glycoprotein, which initially was defined as a factor that actively transported multiple chemotherapeutic drugs out of cancer cells, thereby rendering them resistant to drug action. P-glycoprotein is expressed on the luminal aspect of intestinal epithelial cells (where it functions to inhibit xenobiotic absorption), on the luminal surface of renal tubular cells, and on the canalicular aspect of hepatocytes; inhibition of P-glycoprotein-mediated transport at these sites results in increased plasma levels of drug at steady state. Digoxin is largely dependent on transport by P-glycoprotein for elimination, and drugs that inhibit the transporter can elevate plasma digoxin levels to the toxic range. Inhibitors of P-glycoprotein include verapamil, diltiazem, amiodarone, *quinidine,* ketoconazole, itraconazole, and erythromycin; as discussed earlier, many of these drugs also inhibit CYP3A4 (Kim *et al.,* 1999). P-glycoprotein on the capillary endothelium that forms the blood–brain barrier exports drugs from the brain, and inhibition of P-glycoprotein enhances CNS distribution of some of these drugs (*e.g.,* some HIV protease inhibitors).

Pharmacodynamic Interactions

Combinations of drugs often are employed to therapeutic advantage either because their beneficial effects are additive or synergistic or because therapeutic effects can be achieved with fewer drug-specific adverse effects by using submaximal doses of drugs in concert. As discussed in more detail in specific chapters, combination therapy constitutes optimal treatment for many conditions, including heart failure (*see* Chapter 33), severe hypertension (*see* Chapter 32), and cancer (*see* Chapter 51). This section addresses pharmacodynamic interactions that produce adverse effects.

Nitroglycerin, related *nitrates,* and *nitroprusside* produce vasodilation by nitric oxide–dependent elevation of cyclic GMP in vascular smooth muscle. The pharmacologic effects of sildenafil, *tadalafil,* and *vardenafil* result from inhibition of the type 5 isoform of phosphodiesterase that inactivates cyclic GMP in the vasculature. Thus, coadministration of a nitric oxide donor such as nitroglycerin with a phosphodiesterase 5 inhibitor can cause profound and potentially catastrophic hypotension.

The oral anticoagulant warfarin has a narrow margin between therapeutic inhibition of clot formation and bleeding complications and is subject to several important drug interactions (*see* Chapter 54). Nonsteroidal antiinflammatory drugs cause gastric and duodenal ulcers (*see* Chapter 36), and their concurrent administration with warfarin increases the risk of gastrointestinal bleeding almost fourfold compared with warfarin alone. By inhibiting platelet aggregation, *aspirin* increases the incidence of bleeding in warfarin-treated patients. Finally, antibiotics that alter the intestinal flora reduce the bacterial synthesis of vitamin K, thereby enhancing the effect of warfarin.

A subset of nonsteroidal antiinflammatory drugs, including *indomethacin, ibuprofen, piroxicam,* and the *cyclooxygenase-2 inhibitors,* can antagonize antihypertensive therapy, especially with regimens employing angiotensin-converting enzyme inhibitors, angiotensin-receptor antagonists, and β adrenergic receptor antagonists. The effect on arterial pressure ranges from trivial to severe. Interestingly, these cyclooxygenase inhibitors do not reverse the hypotensive effect of Ca^{2+} channel blockers. Aspirin and *sulindac,* in contrast, produce little, if any, elevation of blood pressure when used concurrently with these antihypertensive drugs.

Antiarrhythmic drugs that block potassium channels, such as *sotalol* and quinidine, can cause the polymorphic ventricular tachycardia known as *torsades de pointes* (*see* Chapter 34). The abnormal repolarization that leads to polymorphic ventricular tachycardia is potentiated by hypokalemia, and diuretics that produce potassium loss increase the risk of this drug-induced arrhythmia.

Age as a Determinant of Response to Drugs. Most drugs initially are evaluated in young and middle-aged adults, and data on their use in children and the elderly frequently are sparse and become available only belatedly.

At the extremes of age, individuals differ in the way that they handle drugs (pharmacokinetics) and in their response to drugs (pharmacodynamics). These differences may require substantial alteration in the dose or dosing regimen to produce the desired clinical effect in children (Kearns *et al.,* 2003) or in the very old.

Children. Drug disposition in childhood does not vary linearly with either body weight or body surface area, and there are no reliable, broadly applicable principles or formulas for converting doses of drugs used in adults to doses that are safe and effective in children. An important generality is that variability in pharmacokinetics is likely to be greatest at times of physiological change (*e.g.,* the newborn or premature baby or at puberty) such that dosing adjustment, often aided by therapeutic drug monitoring for drugs with narrow therapeutic indices, becomes critical for safe, effective therapeutics.

Most drug-metabolizing enzymes are expressed at low levels at birth, followed by an isozyme-specific postnatal induction of CYP expression. CYP2E1 and CYP2D6 appear in the first day, followed within 1 week by CYP3A4 and the CYP2C subfamily. CYP2A1 is not expressed until 1 to 3 months after birth. Some glucuronidation pathways are decreased in the newborn, and an inability of newborns to glucuronidate *chloramphenicol* was responsible for the "gray baby syndrome" characterized by vomiting, neonatal hypothermia, flaccidity, cyanosis, and cardiovascular collapse (*see* Chapter 46). When adjusted for body weight or surface area, hepatic drug metabolism in children after the neonatal period often exceeds that of adults. Studies using *caffeine* as a model substrate illustrate the developmental changes in CYP1A2 that occur during childhood (Figure 5–2). The mechanisms regulating such developmental changes are uncertain, and other pathways of drug metabolism probably mature with different patterns (deWildt *et al.,* 1999).

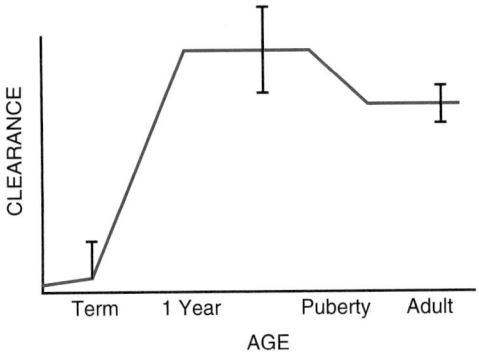

Figure 5–2. *Developmental changes in CYP1A2 activity, assessed as caffeine clearance.* (*See* Lambert *et al.,* 1986.)

Renal elimination of drugs also is reduced in the neonatal period. Neonates at term have markedly reduced GFRs (2 to 4 ml/min/1.73 m²), and prematurity reduces renal function even further. As a result, neonatal dosing regimens for a number of drugs (*e.g.*, aminoglycosides) must be reduced to avoid toxic drug accumulation. GFR (corrected for body surface area) increases progressively to adult levels by 8 to 12 months of age.

Based on these nonlinear changes in drug disposition that differ depending on the mode of elimination, dosing guidelines for children—where they exist—are drug- and age-specific, as detailed in drug labeling and in handbooks (Taketomo *et al.*, 2000). The need for attention to dosing guidelines is not eliminated by topical drug administration; severe hypoadrenal crisis in children has resulted from the use of adult doses of inhaled glucocorticoids.

Drug pharmacodynamics in children also may differ from those in adults. *Antihistamines* and *barbiturates* that generally sedate adults may cause children to become "hyperactive." The enhanced sensitivity to the sedating effects of *propofol* in children has led to the administration of excessive doses that produced a syndrome of myocardial failure, metabolic acidosis, and multiorgan failure. Unique features of childhood development also may provide special vulnerabilities to drug toxicity; for example, tetracyclines can permanently stain developing teeth, and glucocorticoids can attenuate linear growth of bones.

The Elderly. As adults age, gradual changes in pharmacokinetics and pharmacodynamics increase the interindividual variability of doses required for a given effect. Pharmacokinetic changes result from changes in body composition and the function of drug-eliminating organs. The reduction in lean body mass, serum albumin, and total-body water, coupled with the increase in percentage of body fat, alters distribution of drugs in a manner dependent on their lipid solubility and protein binding. The clearance of many drugs is reduced in the elderly. Renal function declines at a variable rate to about 50% of that in young adults. Hepatic blood flow and drug metabolism also are reduced in the elderly, but the variability of these changes is great. In general, the activities of hepatic CYPs are reduced, but conjugation mechanisms are relatively preserved. Frequently, the elimination half-lives of drugs are increased as a consequence of larger apparent volumes of distribution of lipid-soluble drugs and/or reductions in the renal or metabolic clearance.

Changes in pharmacodynamics also are important factors in treating the elderly. Drugs that depress the CNS produce increased effects at any given plasma concentration. Even if the dosage is decreased appropriately to account for age-related pharmacokinetic changes, physiological changes and loss of homeostatic resilience can result in increased sensitivity to unwanted effects of drugs (*e.g.*, hypotension from psychotropic medications and hemorrhage from anticoagulants).

The proportion of the elderly and very old in the population of developed nations is increasing rapidly. These individuals have more illnesses than younger people and consume a disproportionate share of prescription and over-the-counter drugs. These factors, combined with age-related changes in pharmacokinetics and pharmacodynamics, make the elderly a population in whom drug use is especially likely to be marred by serious adverse effects and drug interactions. They therefore should receive drugs only when absolutely necessary for well-defined indications and at the lowest effective doses. Prospectively defined end points, appropriate monitoring of drug levels, and frequent reviews of the patient's drug history, with discontinuation of those drugs that did not achieve the desired end point or are no longer required, would greatly improve the health of the elderly population. On the other hand, *appropriate* therapy should not be withheld because of these concerns; outcomes data with several drug interventions for chronic conditions (*e.g.*, hypertension and dyslipidemia) have proven that the elderly benefit at least as much as, and often more than, the young (LaRosa *et al.*, 1999). Furthermore, several chronic diseases that predominantly affect the elderly, such as osteoporosis and prostatic hypertrophy, can be halted or reduced by appropriate drug therapy.

GENETIC DETERMINANTS OF THE RESPONSE TO DRUGS

Allelic variations in the genes encoding drug-metabolizing enzymes, drug transporters, and receptors can be responsible for striking differences in pharmacological activity. A variation in DNA sequence that occurs with a frequency of more than 1% is termed a *polymorphism*. Polymorphisms in the enzymes responsible for drug disposition can produce major alterations in the delivery of a drug or its active metabolite to the pharmacologic target.

Mercaptopurine, an antileukemia drug, also is the active metabolite of the immunosuppressant *azathioprine.* Mercaptopurine is inactivated by thiopurine *S*-methyltransferase (TPMT). Genetic polymorphisms in this enzyme lead to differences in inactivation of mercaptopurine and to vast interindividual differences in toxic and therapeutic responses. Homozygotes for alleles encoding inactive

TPMT (0.3% to 1% of patients) experience severe pancytopenia on the "usual" dose of mercaptopurine or azathiopurine, and even heterozygotes experience more bone marrow suppression. Importantly, the occurrence of bone marrow toxicity in heterozygotes has resulted in the selection of a standard dose of the drugs that probably undertreats patients homozygous for TPMT alleles with full catalytic activity. The genotype for TPMT polymorphisms is highly concordant with phenotype, providing a basis for genotyping patients to direct safer and more effective therapy with these drugs (*see* Chapter 4).

The proton pump inhibitor *omeprazole* is metabolized almost entirely by CYP2C19, and polymorphisms of this isoform determine the rate of omeprazole elimination. After the recommended drug doses, patients homozygous for the polymorphism that confers the highest rate of elimination (*extensive metabolizers*) have drug levels that are too low to inhibit gastric acid secretion, whereas those homozygous for the poor metabolizer polymorphism respond with suppression of acid secretion. Predictably, the efficacy of omeprazole in eradication of *Helicobacter pylori* infection is markedly reduced in the extensive metabolizer phenotype.

Activity of the CYP2D6 isoform is polymorphically distributed in the population, and 8% to 10% of Caucasians are deficient in the enzyme (*poor metabolizers*). CYP2D6 is the principal pathway for the metabolism of many drugs, including selective serotonin-reuptake inhibitors (*e.g., fluoxetine* and *paroxetine*), tricyclic antidepressants (*e.g., nortriptyline, desipramine, imipramine,* and *clomipramine*), and certain opiates (*e.g., codeine* and dextromethorphan). Because the analgesic effect of codeine depends on its metabolism to morphine by CYP2D6, patients who are poor metabolizers respond poorly to the analgesic effect of codeine. At the other extreme, patients who have a gene duplication of CYP2D6 exhibit an exaggerated response to codeine. Poor metabolizers and extensive metabolizers differ substantially in their therapeutic and adverse responses to many of the CYP2D6 substrates; as a consequence, there is an active attempt in drug development programs to avoid candidate drug molecules that depend on CYP2D6 for metabolism.

CYP2C9 catalyzes the major pathway of metabolism of warfarin and phenytoin. Certain allelic variants of CYP2C9 are devoid of catalytic function, and the required doses of warfarin and phenytoin are much reduced in these patients. Initiation of therapy with the usual dose of warfarin in such CYP2C9-deficient patients puts them at risk of bleeding complications.

Genetic polymorphisms also influence the response of the target organs to drugs. The antiarrhythmic drugs that act by prolonging repolarization (*e.g.,* quinidine and sotalol) can prolong repolarization markedly in some patients and induce polymorphic ventricular tachycardia. Allelic variants of genes encoding ion channels also are associated with prolonged repolarization, and patients with these polymorphism are highly susceptible to arrhythmias when treated with these drugs (*see* Chapter 34).

Altered drug response has been associated with allelic variants of genes encoding the molecular targets of drugs or of key proteins in the pathophysiologic system affected by the drug. For example, the effect of β-adrenergic receptor antagonists on blood pressure has been shown to be associated with β_1-receptor polymorphisms, and the action of β adrenergic receptor agonists in asthma has been related to variants in the β_2 adrenergic receptor gene. With the availability of the human genomic database and the identification of multiple single-nucleotide polymorphisms, associations between drug effect and genetic polymorphisms will be reported increasingly. The initial reports undoubtedly will yield a number of false-positive associations and will require confirmation in prospective studies. Even if an association between a polymorphism and drug response is confirmed, it may reflect a haplotype effect or linkage of the polymorphism with another genetic determinant.

Some general principles of pharmacogenetics and additional examples are presented in Chapter 4.

THE PHARMACODYNAMIC CHARACTERISTICS OF A DRUG THAT DETERMINE ITS USE IN THERAPY

When drugs are administered to patients, there is no single characteristic relationship between the drug concentration in plasma and the measured effect; the concentration–effect curve may be concave upward, concave downward, linear, sigmoid, or an inverted-U shape. Moreover, the concentration–effect relationship may be distorted if the response being measured is a composite of several effects, such as the change in blood pressure produced by a combination of cardiac, vascular, and reflex effects. However, such a composite concentration–effect curve often can be resolved into simpler curves for each of its components. These simplified concentration–effect relationships, regardless of their exact shape, can be viewed as having four characteristic variables: *potency, maximal efficacy, slope,* and *individual variation*. These are illustrated in Figure 5–3 for the common sigmoidal log dose–effect curve.

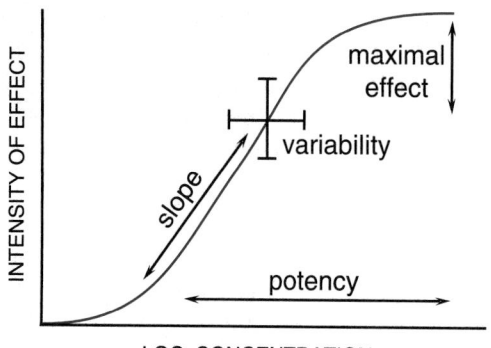

Figure 5–3. *The log concentration–effect relationship.* Representative log concentration–effect curve illustrating its four characterizing variables. Here, the effect is measured as a function of increasing drug concentration in the plasma. Similar relationships also can be plotted as a function of the dose of drug administered. These plots are referred to as dose–effect curves. (*See* text for further discussion.)

Potency. The location of the concentration–effect curve along the *concentration axis* is an expression of the potency of a drug. Although often related to the dose of a drug required to produce an effect, potency is more properly related to the concentration of the drug in plasma to approximate more closely the situation in isolated systems *in vitro* and to avoid the complicating factors of pharmacokinetic variables. Although potency obviously affects drug dosage, potency *per se* is relatively unimportant in the clinical use of drugs, provided that the required dose can be given conveniently and that there is no toxicity related to the chemical structure of the drug rather than to its mechanism. There is no justification for the view that more potent drugs are superior therapeutic agents. However, if the drug is to be administered by transdermal absorption, a highly potent drug is required because the capacity of the skin to absorb drugs is limited (*see* Chapter 62).

Maximal Efficacy. The maximal effect that can be produced by a drug is its *maximal,* or *clinical, efficacy* (which is related to, but not precisely the same as, the term *efficacy* as discussed in Chapter 1). Maximal efficacy is determined principally by the properties of the drug and its receptor–effector system and is reflected in the plateau of the concentration–effect curve. In clinical use, however, undesired effects may limit a drug's dosage such that its true maximal efficacy may not be achievable. The maximal efficacy of a drug is clearly a major characteristic—of much greater clinical importance than its potency. Furthermore, the two properties are not related and should not be confused. For instance, although some thiazide diuretics have similar or

greater potency than the loop diuretic *furosemide,* the maximal efficacy of furosemide is considerably greater.

Slope. The *slope* of the concentration–effect curve reflects the mechanism of action of a drug, including the shape of the curve that describes drug binding to its receptor (*see* Chapter 1). The steepness of the curve dictates the range of doses that are useful for achieving a clinical effect. Aside from this fact, the slope of the concentration–effect curve has more theoretical than practical usefulness.

Pharmacodynamic Variability

Individuals vary in the magnitude of their response to the same concentration of a single drug or to similar drugs when the appropriate correction has been made for differences in potency, maximal efficacy, and slope. In fact, a single individual may not always respond in the same way to the same concentration of drug. A concentration–effect curve applies only to a single individual at one time or to an average individual. The intersecting brackets in Figure 5–3 indicate that an effect of varying intensity will occur in different individuals at a specified concentration of a drug or that a range of concentrations is required to produce an effect of specified intensity in all of the patients.

Attempts have been made to define and measure individual "sensitivity" to drugs in the clinical setting, and progress has been made in understanding some of the determinants of sensitivity to drugs that act at specific receptors. For example, responsiveness to β adrenergic receptor agonists may change because of disease (*e.g.,* thyrotoxicosis or heart failure) or because of previous administration of either β adrenergic receptor agonists or antagonists that can cause changes in the concentration of the β adrenergic receptor and/or coupling of the receptor to its effector systems (Iaccarino *et al.*, 1999) (*see* Chapter 10). Receptors are not static components of the cell; rather, they are in a dynamic state, and their concentration and function may be up-regulated and down-regulated by endogenous and exogenous factors.

Data on the association of drug levels with efficacy and toxicity must be interpreted in the context of the pharmacodynamic variability in the population. The plasma concentration of phenobarbital required to control seizures, for example, is higher in children than in adults. Variability in pharmacodynamic response can result from any of the factors responsible for altering drug effect that include genetics, age, disease, and other drugs. The variability in pharmacodynamic response in the population may be analyzed by constructing a quantal concentration–effect curve (Figure 5–4A). The concentration of a drug that produces a specified effect in a single patient is called

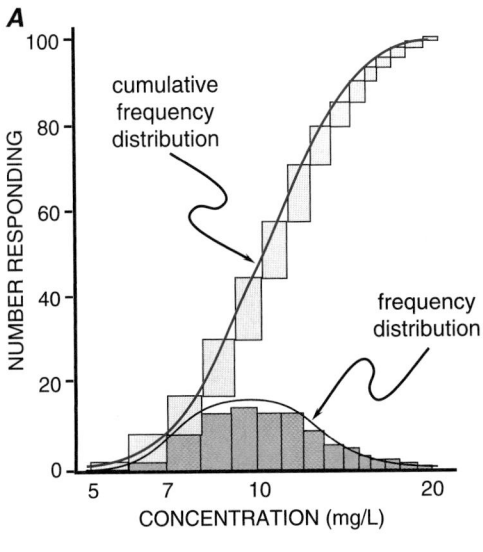

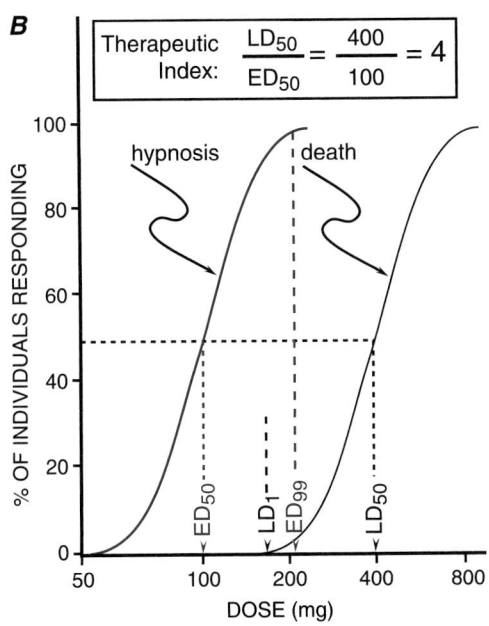

*Figure 5–4. Frequency distribution curves and quantal concentration–effect and dose–effect curves. **A.** Frequency distribution curves. An experiment was performed on 100 subjects, and the effective plasma concentration that produced a quantal response was determined for each individual. The number of subjects who required each dose is plotted, giving a log-normal frequency distribution (colored bars). The gray bars demonstrate that the normal frequency distribution, when summated, yields the cumulative frequency distribution—a sigmoidal curve that is a quantal concentration–effect curve. **B.** Quantal dose–effect curves. Animals were injected with varying doses of sedative-hypnotic, and the responses were determined and plotted. The calculation of the therapeutic index, the ratio of the LD_{50} to the ED_{50}, is an indication of how selective a drug is in producing its desired effects relative to its toxicity. (See text for additional explanation.)*

the *individual effective concentration.* This is a quantal response because the defined effect is either present or absent. Individual effective concentrations usually are log normally distributed, which means that a normal variation curve is the result of plotting the logarithms of the concentration against the frequency of patients achieving the defined effect. A cumulative frequency distribution of individuals achieving the defined effect as a function of drug concentration is the concentration–percent curve or the quantal concentration–effect curve. The slope of the concentration–percent curve is an expression of the pharmacodynamic variability in the population.

The Therapeutic Index

The dose of a drug required to produce a specified effect in 50% of the population is the *median effective dose,* abbreviated as the ED_{50} (Figure 5–4B). In preclinical studies of drugs, the *median lethal dose,* as determined in experimental animals, is abbreviated as LD_{50}. The ratio of the LD_{50} to the ED_{50} is an indication of the *therapeutic index,* which is a statement of how selective the drug is in producing its desired *versus* its adverse effects. In clinical studies, the dose, or preferably the concentration, of a drug required to produce toxic effects can be compared with the concentration required for the therapeutic effects in the population to evaluate the *clinical therapeutic index.* However, since pharmacodynamic variation in the population may be marked, the concentration or dose of drug required to produce a therapeutic effect in most of the population usually will overlap the concentration required to produce toxicity in some of the population, even though the drug's therapeutic index in an individual patient may be large. Also, the concentration–percent curves for efficacy and toxicity need not be parallel, adding yet another complexity to determination of the therapeutic index in patients. Finally, no drug produces a single effect, and depending on the effect being measured, the therapeutic index for a drug will vary. For example, much less codeine is required for cough suppression than for control of pain in 50% of the population, and thus the margin of safety, selectivity, or therapeutic index of codeine are much greater as an antitussive than as an analgesic.

ADVERSE DRUG REACTIONS AND DRUG TOXICITY

Any drug, no matter how trivial its therapeutic actions, has the potential to do harm. Adverse reactions are a cost of modern medical therapy. Although the mandate of the Food and Drug Administration (FDA) is to ensure that drugs are safe and effective, these terms are relative. The anticipated benefit from any therapeutic decision must be balanced by the potential risks.

The magnitude of the problem of adverse reactions to marketed drugs is difficult to quantify. It has been estimated that 3% to 5% of all hospitalizations can be attributed to adverse drug reactions, resulting in 300,000 hospitalizations annually in the United States. Once hospitalized, patients have about a 30% chance of an untoward event related to drug therapy, and the risk attributable to each course of drug therapy is about 5%. The chance of a life-threatening drug reaction is about 3% per patient in the hospital and about 0.4% per each course of therapy (Jick, 1984). *Adverse reactions to drugs are the most common cause of iatrogenic disease* (Leape *et al.*, 1991).

Mechanism-based adverse drug reactions are extensions of the principal pharmacological action of the drug. These would be expected to occur with all members of a class of drugs having the same mechanism of action. Hyperkalemia, for example, is a mechanism-based adverse effect of all mineralocorticoid-receptor antagonists. Adverse effects that are not a consequence of the drug's primary mechanism of action are considered to be *off-target reactions* and are a consequence of the particular drug molecule. The hepatotoxicity of *acetaminophen* is an off-target toxicity.

When an adverse effect is encountered infrequently, it may be referred to as *idiosyncratic,* meaning that it results from an interaction of the drug with unique host factors and does not occur in the population at large. Idiosyncratic adverse effects may be mechanism-based (*e.g.,* angioedema on angiotensin-converting enzyme inhibitors) or off-target reactions (*e.g.,* anaphylaxis to *penicillin*). Investigations of idiosyncratic reactions often have identified a genetic or environmental basis for the unique host factors leading to the unusual effects.

THERAPEUTIC DRUG MONITORING

Given the multiple factors that alter drug disposition, measurement of the concentration in body fluids can assist in individualizing therapy with selected drugs. Determination of the concentration of a drug in blood, serum, or plasma is particularly useful when well-defined criteria are fulfilled:

1. A demonstrated relationship exists between the concentration of drug in plasma and the desired therapeutic effect or the toxic effect to be avoided. The range of plasma levels between that required for efficacy and that at which toxicity occurs for a given individual is designated the *therapeutic window* (Figure 5–5).
2. There is sufficient variability in plasma level that the level cannot be predicted from the dose alone.
3. The drug produces effects, intended or unwanted, that are difficult to monitor.
4. The concentration required to produce the therapeutic effect is close to the level that causes toxicity (*i.e.,* there is a low therapeutic index).

A clear demonstration of the relation of drug concentration to efficacy or toxicity is not achievable for many drugs; even when such a relationship can be determined, it usually predicts a probability of efficacy or toxicity. In trials of antidepressant drugs, for example, such a high proportion of patients respond to placebo that it is difficult to determine the plasma level associated with efficacy. The end points defining drug effect may not prove to be relevant. A digoxin level of 2 ng/ml initially was selected as the threshold of toxicity based on the surrogate marker of electrocardiographic evidence of ventricular arrhythmias at higher concentrations. A subsequent retrospective examination of the data from a clinical trial of the effect of digoxin *versus* placebo on clinical outcome in patients with heart failure revealed that patients with digoxin levels exceeding 1.1 ng/ml had a higher risk of cardiac mortality. Like most data that link plasma levels with effect, this was not a randomized, controlled evaluation of the consequences of drug level but rather a retrospective examination of trial data, and an alternative explanation is that impaired clearance of digoxin *via* P-glycoprotein is an indicator of a poor prognosis in cardiac failure. Nonetheless, these data provide evidence based on clinical outcome that will guide the adjustment of digoxin dosing until controlled data become available.

There is a quantal concentration–response curve for efficacy and adverse effects (Figure 5–5), and for many drugs, the concentration that achieves efficacy in all the population may produce adverse effects in some individuals. Thus, a *population therapeutic window* expresses a range of concentrations in which the likelihood of efficacy is high and the probability of adverse effects is low. It is not a guarantee of either efficacy or safety. *Therefore, use of the population therapeutic window to adjust dosage of a drug should be complemented by monitoring appropriate clinical and surrogate markers for drug effect.*

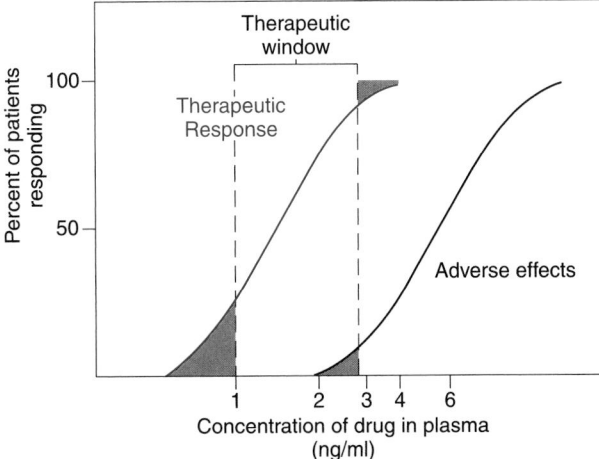

Figure 5–5. *The relation of the therapeutic window of drug concentrations to the therapeutic and adverse effects in the population.* Ordinate is linear; abcissa is logarithmic.

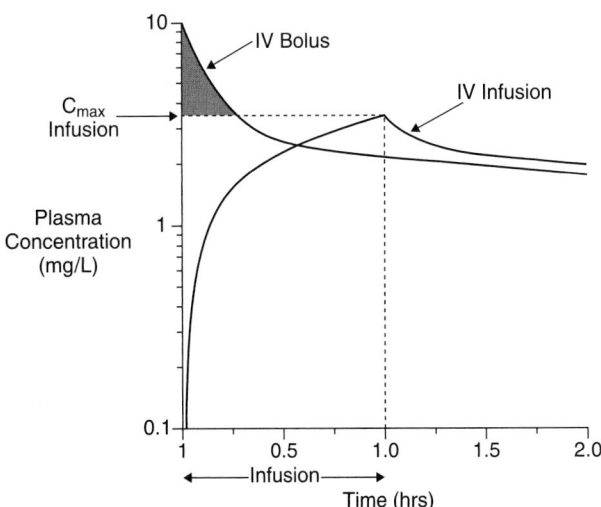

Figure 5–6. *High concentrations of drug in the plasma after rapid (bolus) intravenous administration.* The plasma levels achieved after intravenous administration of procainamide (500 mg) as a rapid bolus compared with an infusion over 1 hour. The shaded area depicts the excess exposure to the drug in the plasma compartment when a rapid bolus instead of an infusion is administered. Scale on ordinate is logarithmic.

Intravenous Administration of Drugs

Rapid intravenous administration produces an abrupt rise in the concentration of drug in the plasma compartment (Figure 5–6). The concentration then falls rapidly as the drug distributes to the extravascular compartments, after which the plasma and extravascular compartments are in equilibrium during the phase of drug elimination. By contrast, when the same dose is infused more slowly (*e.g.*, over 1 hour), as illustrated in Figure 5–6, distribution takes place concurrently with delivery of drug into the plasma compartment, and concentrations of drug in plasma do not rise much above the level achieved at equilibrium. Thus the slower intravenous administration never produces the high plasma concentration that follows the intravenous bolus. The shaded area in Figure 5–6 indicates the excess exposure to drug in the plasma compartment during the distribution phase after intravenous bolus compared with the peak level after the slower infusion. The excessive levels after intravenous bolus could yield either therapeutic advantage or a catastrophic outcome depending on the drug and the target organs that are immediately affected by the concentration of drug in plasma.

If the drug in the plasma compartment is immediately available to an organ to which the higher levels are toxic, then an adverse outcome rapidly ensues. Thus bolus or even very rapid intravenous administration of drugs such as *procainamide, phenytoin,* or *potassium* can produce cardiovascular collapse. However, if the same intravenous doses were given slowly, the continuous distribution of the infused drug would prevent the excessively high plasma levels and would be safe. Thus, the rate of intravenous administration is of crucial importance for drugs that could produce toxicity from high plasma levels.

By contrast, some sedative drugs are distributed rapidly from plasma to the brain, and relatively rapid intravenous administration will produce prompt sedation as the brain extracts the drug from plasma. In this case, the high concentration of drug in plasma during the distribution phase after rapid intravenous administration is therapeutically advantageous for use in anesthesiology.

When considering administration of a drug by intravenous bolus, a full understanding of the safety of this mode of administration is required.

THE DYNAMIC INFORMATION BASE

With the development of new drugs, the accrual of new information on marketed agents, the findings emerging from clinical trials, ongoing regulatory decisions, and the updated guidelines for disease management, the information base available to guide drug therapy is in a state of constant and brisk evolution. Among the available sources are textbooks of pharmacology and therapeutics, medical journals, published guidelines for treatment of specific diseases, analytical evaluations of drugs, drug compendia, professional seminars and meetings, and advertising. Developing a strategy to extract objective and unbiased data is required for the practice of rational therapeutics. As is the case with all continuing medical education, patient-centered acquisition of the relevant information is a centerpiece of such a strategy. This requires access to the information in the practice setting and increasingly is facilitated by electronic availability of information resources. Facile online access to the primary medical literature that forms the basis for therapeutic decisions is available *via* PubMed, a search and retrieval system of the National Center for Biotechnology Information (*www.ncbi.nlm.nih.gov/entrez/query.fcgi*).

Depending on their aim and scope, textbooks of pharmacology may provide, in varying proportions, basic pharmacological principles, critical appraisal of useful categories of therapeutic agents, and detailed descriptions of individual drugs or prototypes that serve as standards of reference for assessing new drugs. In addition, pharmacodynamics and pathophysiology are correlated. Therapeutics is considered in virtually all textbooks of medicine, but often superficially.

A source of information often used by physicians is the *Physicians' Desk Reference* (PDR), available in printed form and online (*www.pdr.net*). The brand-name manufacturers whose products appear support this book. No comparative data on efficacy, safety, or cost are included. The information is identical to that contained in drug package inserts, which are largely based on the results of phase 3 testing; its value includes designation of the FDA-approved indications for use of a drug and summaries of pharmacokinetics, contraindications, adverse reactions, and recommended doses; some of this information is not available in the scientific literature. Many commonly used drugs that are no longer patent-protected are not covered by the PDR.

Several unbiased sources of information on the clinical uses of drugs provide balanced and comparative data. All recognize that the clinician's legitimate use of a drug in a particular patient is not limited by FDA-approved labeling in the package insert. The *Medical Letter* (*www.medletter.com*) provides objective summaries in a biweekly newsletter of scientific reports and consultants' evaluations of the safety, efficacy, and rationale for use of drugs. The "Drug Therapy" section of the *New England Journal of Medicine* provides timely evaluations of specific drugs and areas of therapeutics. The *United States Pharmacopeia Dispensing Information* (USPDI) comes in two volumes. One, *Drug Information for the Health Care Professional,* consists of drug monographs that contain clinically

significant information aimed at minimizing the risks and enhancing the benefits of drugs. Monographs are developed by USP staff and are reviewed by advisory panels and other reviewers. The *Advice for the Patient* volume is intended to reinforce, in lay language, the oral consultation with the physician and may be provided to the patient in written form. *Drug Facts and Comparisons* also is organized by pharmacological classes and is updated monthly (online at *www.factsandcomparisons.com*). Information in monographs is presented in a standard format and incorporates FDA-approved information, which is supplemented with current data obtained from the biomedical literature. A useful feature is the comprehensive list of preparations with a "Cost Index," an index of the average wholesale price for equivalent quantities of similar or identical drugs. Other online resources that can bring data to the practice setting include *Epocrates* (*www2.epocrates.com*) and *UpToDate* (*www.uptodateonline.com*).

Particularly helpful in obtaining a comprehensive overview of therapy for specific diseases are the guidelines published by a number of professional organizations. These can be accessed by judicious use of a search engine; for example, a search for *heart failure guidelines* on Google will yield the Web address for the American College of Cardiology/American Heart Association Guidelines for the Evaluation and Management of Chronic Heart Failure in the Adult.

Industry promotion—in the form of direct-mail brochures, journal advertising, displays, professional courtesies, or the detail person or pharmaceutical representative—is intended to be persuasive rather than educational. The pharmaceutical industry cannot, should not, and indeed does not purport to be responsible for the education of physicians in the use of drugs.

More than 1500 medical journals are published regularly in the United States. However, of the two to three dozen medical publications with circulations in excess of 70,000 copies, the great majority are sent to physicians free of charge and paid for by the industry. In addition, special supplements of some peer-reviewed journals are entirely supported by a single drug manufacturer whose product is featured prominently and described favorably. Objective journals that are not supported by drug manufacturers include *Clinical Pharmacology and Therapeutics,* which is devoted to original articles that evaluate the actions and effects of drugs in human beings, and *Drugs,* which publishes timely reviews of individual drugs and drug classes. The *New England Journal of Medicine, Annals of Internal Medicine, Journal of the American Medical Association, Archives of Internal Medicine, British Medical Journal,*

Lancet, and *Postgraduate Medicine* offer timely therapeutic reports and reviews.

DRUG NOMENCLATURE

The existence of many names for each drug, even when the names are reduced to a minimum, has led to a lamentable and confusing situation in drug nomenclature. In addition to its formal *chemical* name, a new drug is usually assigned a *code* name by the pharmaceutical manufacturer. If the drug appears promising and the manufacturer wishes to place it on the market, a *U.S. adopted name* (USAN) is selected by the USAN Council, which is jointly sponsored by the American Medical Association, the American Pharmaceutical Association, and the United States Pharmacopeial Convention, Inc. This *nonproprietary* name often is referred to as the *generic name.* If the drug is eventually admitted to the *United States Pharmacopeia* (*see* below), the USAN becomes the *official name.* However, the nonproprietary and official names of an older drug may differ. Subsequently, the drug also will be assigned a *proprietary name,* or *trademark,* by the manufacturer. If more than one company markets the drug, then it may have several proprietary names. If mixtures of the drug with other agents are marketed, each such mixture also may have a separate proprietary name.

There is increasing worldwide adoption of the same *nonproprietary name* for each therapeutic substance. For newer drugs, the USAN is usually adopted for the nonproprietary name in other countries, but this is not true for older drugs. International agreement on drug names is mediated through the World Health Organization and the pertinent health agencies of the cooperating countries.

One area of continued confusion and ambiguity is the designation of the stereochemical composition in the name of a drug. The nonproprietary names usually give no indication of the drug's stereochemistry except for a few drugs such as *levodopa* and *dextroamphetamine.* Even the chemical names cited by the USAN Council often are ambiguous. Physicians and other medical scientists frequently are ignorant about drug stereoisomerism and are likely to remain so until the system of nonproprietary nomenclature incorporates stereoisomeric information (Gal, 1988). This issue becomes especially important when a drug's different diastereomers produce different pharmacologic effects, as is the case with *labetalol,* for instance (*see* Chapters 10 and 32).

The nonproprietary or official name of a drug should be used whenever possible, and such a practice has been adopted in this textbook. The use of the nonproprietary name is clearly less confusing when the drug is available under multiple proprietary names and when the nonproprietary name more readily identifies the drug with its pharmacological class. The facile argument for the proprietary name is that it is frequently more easily pronounced and remembered as a result of advertising. *For purposes of identification, representative proprietary names, designated by* SMALLCAP TYPE, *appear throughout the text and in the index.* Not all proprietary names for drugs are included because the number of proprietary names for a single drug may be large and because proprietary names differ from country to country.

The Drug Price Competition and Patent Term Restoration Act of 1984 allows more generic versions of brand-name drugs to be approved for marketing. When the physician prescribes drugs, the question arises as to whether the nonproprietary name or a proprietary name should be employed. A pharmacist may substitute a preparation that is equivalent unless the physician indicates "no substitution" or specifies the manufacturer on the prescription. In view of the preceding discussion on the individualization of drug therapy, it is understandable why a physician who has carefully adjusted the dose of a drug to a patient's individual requirements for chronic therapy may be reluctant to surrender control over the source of the drug that the patient receives (Burns, 1999). In the past, there was concern that prescribing by nonproprietary name could result in the patient's receiving a preparation of inferior quality or uncertain bioavailability; indeed, such therapeutic failures owing to decreased bioavailability have been reported (Hendeles *et al.,* 1993). To address this issue, the FDA has established standards for bioavailability and compiled information about the interchangeability of drug products, which are published annually (*Approved Drug Products with Therapeutic Equivalence Evaluations*). Because of potential cost savings to the individual patient and simplification of communication about drugs, nonproprietary names should be used when prescribing except for drugs with a low therapeutic index and known differences in bioavailability among marketed products (Hendeles *et al.,* 1993).

DRUG DEVELOPMENT AND ITS REGULATION

Drug Regulation

The history of drug regulation in the United States reflects the growing involvement of governments in most countries to ensure some degree of efficacy and safety in marketed medicinal agents. The first legislation, the Federal Food and Drug Act of 1906, was concerned with the interstate transport of adulterated or misbranded foods and drugs. There were no obligations to establish drug efficacy and safety. This act was amended in 1938, after the deaths of 105 children that resulted from the marketing of a solution of *sulfanilamide* in diethylene glycol, an excellent but highly toxic solvent. The amended act, the enforcement of which was entrusted to the FDA, was concerned primarily with the truthful labeling and safety of drugs. Toxicity studies, as well as approval of a new drug application (NDA), were required before a drug could be promoted and distributed. However, no proof of efficacy was required, and extravagant claims for therapeutic indications were made commonly (Wax, 1995).

In this relatively relaxed atmosphere, research in basic and clinical pharmacology burgeoned in industrial and academic laboratories. The result was a flow of new drugs, called "wonder drugs" by the lay press. Because efficacy was not rigorously defined, a number of therapeutic claims could not be supported by data. The risk-to-benefit ratio was seldom mentioned, but it emerged in dramatic fashion early in the 1960s. At that time, *thalidomide,* a hypnotic with no obvious advantage over other drugs in its class, was introduced in Europe. After a short period, it became apparent that the incidence of a relatively rare birth defect, phocomelia, was increasing. It soon reached epidemic proportions, and retrospective epidemiological research firmly established the causative agent to be thalidomide taken early in the course of pregnancy. The reaction to the dramatic demonstration of the teratogenicity of a needless drug was worldwide. In the United States, it resulted in the Harris-Kefauver Amendments to the Food, Drug, and Cosmetic Act in 1962.

The Harris-Kefauver Amendments require sufficient pharmacological and toxicological research in animals before a drug can be tested in human beings. The data from such studies must be submitted to the FDA in the form of an application for an investigational new drug (IND) before clinical studies can begin. Three phases of clinical testing (*see* below) have evolved to provide the data that are used to support an NDA. Proof of efficacy is required, as is documentation of relative safety in terms of the risk-to-benefit ratio for the disease entity to be treated.

To demonstrate efficacy, "adequate and well-controlled investigations" must be performed. This generally has been interpreted to mean two replicate clinical trials that are usually, but not always, randomized, double-blind, and placebo-controlled. Safety is demonstrated by having a sufficiently large database of patients/subjects who have received the drug at the time of filing an NDA with the FDA for approval. As a result of these requirements, the number of patients on the drug, the number of studies, the development cost, and the time required for the clinical studies to complete the NDA increased. The regulatory review time also increased as a result of the mass and complexity of the data so that by 1990 the average review time was approaching 3 years. This increased the inherent tension that exists between the FDA, which is motivated to protect the public health, and the drug developers, who are motivated to market effective and profitable drugs. Competing pressures also exist in the community, where medical practitioners and patient activist groups have criticized the FDA for delaying approval, whereas some "watchdog" groups criticize the FDA for allowing drugs on the market that occasionally cause unexpected problems after they are marketed. The FDA has the difficult task of balancing the requirement that drugs be safe and effective and yet allowing useful medications to be made available in a timely manner.

Beginning in the late 1980s with pressure from AIDS activists, the FDA undertook a number of initiatives that have had profound effects in streamlining the process of regulatory approval. These initiatives have all but eliminated the concern about the "drug lag," where drugs were available in other countries significantly sooner than in the United States (Kessler *et al.*, 1996). First, the FDA initiated new "treatment" IND regulations that allow patients with life-threatening diseases for which there is no satisfactory alternative treatment to receive drugs for therapy prior to general marketing if there is limited evidence of drug efficacy without unreasonable toxicity (Figure 5–5). Second, the agency has established expedited reviews for drugs used to treat life-threatening diseases. Congress has enacted the Prescription Drug User Fee Act, whereby the FDA collects a fee from drug manufacturers that is to be used to help fund the personnel required to speed the review process (Shulman and Kaitin, 1996). Finally, the FDA is becoming involved more actively in the drug development process in order to facilitate the approval of drugs. A priority review system has been established for drugs in new therapeutic classes and drugs for the treatment of life-threatening or debilitating diseases. By working with the pharmaceutical industry throughout the period of clinical drug development, the FDA attempts to reduce the time from submission of an IND application to approval of an NDA. This streamlining process is accomplished by the interactive design of well-planned, focused clinical studies using validated surrogate markers or clinical end points other than survival or irreversible morbidity. Sufficient data then will be available earlier in the development process to allow a risk-benefit analysis and a possible decision for approval. In some cases, this system may reduce or obviate the need for phase 3 testing prior to approval. Coupled with this expedited development process is the requirement, when appropriate, for restricted distribution to certain specialists or facilities and for postmarketing studies to answer remaining issues of risks, benefits, and optimal uses of the drug. If postmarketing studies are inadequate or demonstrate lack of safety or clinical benefit, approval for the new drug may be withdrawn. In 1997, these changes were codified in the FDA Modernization Act (Suydam and Elder, 1999). As a result of these initiatives, the review time at the FDA has been reduced dramatically to a period of less than 1 year, with an ultimate goal of 10 months. Details of this act, which includes a variety of other initiatives, such as those discussed earlier for pediatric drug development, are available on the Internet at *www.fda.gov/opacom/7modact.html*. These new initiatives by the FDA are based on the assumption that society is willing to accept unknown risks from drugs used to treat life-threatening or debilitating diseases. Some worry that such shortcuts in the drug approval process will result in the release of drugs without sufficient information to determine their utility and proper use. A seemingly contradictory directive to the FDA also is contained in the Food, Drug, and Cosmetic Act: The FDA cannot interfere with the practice of medicine. Thus, once the efficacy of a new agent has been proven in the context of acceptable toxicity, the drug can be marketed. The physician then is allowed to determine its most appropriate use. Physicians must realize that new drugs are inherently more risky because of the relatively small amount of data about their effects, yet there is no practical way to increase knowledge about a drug before it is marketed. Thus, a systematic method for postmarketing surveillance is an indispensable requirement for early optimization of drug use.

Before a drug can be marketed, a package insert for use by physicians must be prepared. This is a cooperative effort between the FDA and the pharmaceutical company. The insert usually contains basic pharmacological information, as well as essential clinical information in regard to approved indications, contraindications, precautions, warnings, adverse reactions, usual dosage, and available preparations. Promotional materials cannot deviate from information contained in the insert.

One area in which the FDA does not have clear authority is in the regulation of "dietary supplements," including vitamins, minerals, proteins, and herbal preparations. Until 1994, the FDA regulated such supplements as either food additives or drugs depending on the substance and the indications that were claimed. However, in 1994, Congress passed the Dietary Supplement Health and Education Act (DSHEA), which weakened the authority of the FDA. The act defined *dietary supplement* as a product intended to supplement the diet that contains "*(a) a vitamin; (b) a mineral; (c) an herb or other botanical; (d) an amino acid; (e) a dietary substance for use by humans to supplement the diet by increasing the total daily intake; or (f) a concentrate, metabolite, constituent, extract or combination of an ingredient described in clause (a), (b), (c), (d), or (e).*" Such products must be labeled as *dietary supplement.* The FDA does not have the authority to require approval prior to marketing of such supplements unless the supplements make specific claims relating to the diagnosis, treatment, prevention, or cure of a disease. However, the common conditions associated with natural states, such as pregnancy, menopause, aging, and adolescence, will not be treated as diseases by the FDA. Treatment of hot flashes, symptoms of the menstrual cycle, morning sickness associated with pregnancy, mild memory problems associated with aging, hair loss, and noncystic acne are examples of claims that can be made without prior FDA approval. Also, health maintenance and other "nondisease" claims such as "helps you relax" or "maintains a healthy circulation" are allowed without approval. Many supplements with such claims are labeled as follows: "*This statement has not been evaluated by the FDA. This product is not intended to diagnose, treat, cure, or prevent any disease.*" The FDA cannot remove such products from the market unless it can prove that there is a "significant or unreasonable risk of illness or injury" when the product is used as directed or under normal conditions of use. It is the manufacturer's responsibility to ensure that its products are safe.

As a result of the DSHEA legislation, a large number of unregulated products that have not been demonstrated to be safe or effective are widely available. There have been several occasions where such products have been associated with serious adverse effects or have been shown to interact with prescription drugs (*see* Fugh-Berman, 2000). Under these circumstances, the FDA can act, but the burden is on the FDA to prove that the supplements are not safe.

The presence of *ephedrine* in weight-loss supplements is a recent case in point (*see* Chapter 10). In many ways, this situation is analogous to the lack of regulation of drugs that existed before the 1938 disaster involving elixir of sulfanilamide (described earlier). Physicians and patients alike should be aware of the lack of regulation of dietary supplements. Adverse reactions or suspected interactions with such substances should be reported to the FDA using the same mechanisms as for adverse drug reactions (*see* below).

Drug Development

Understanding the process of drug development and realizing the type and limitations of the data that support the efficacy and safety of a marketed product are necessary in estimating the risk-to-benefit ratio of a new drug.

By the time an investigational new drug (IND) application has been initiated and a drug reaches the stage of testing in humans, its pharmacokinetic, pharmacodynamic, and toxic properties have been evaluated *in vivo* in several species of animals in accordance with regulations and guidelines published by the FDA. Although the value of many requirements for preclinical testing is self-evident, such as those that screen for direct toxicity to organs and characterize dose-related effects, the value of others is controversial, particularly because of the well-known interspecies variation in the effects of drugs.

Trials of drugs in human beings in the United States generally are conducted in three phases, which must be completed before an NDA can be submitted to the FDA for review; these are outlined in Figure 5–7. Although assessment of risk is a major objective of such testing, this is far more difficult than is the determination of whether a drug is efficacious for a selected clinical condition. Usually about 2000 to 3000 carefully selected patients receive a new drug during phase 3 clinical trials. At most, only a few hundred are treated for more than 3 to 6 months regardless of the likely duration of therapy that will be required in practice. Thus, the most profound and overt risks that occur almost immediately after the drug is given can be detected in a phase 3 study if they occur more often than once per 100 administrations. Risks that are medically important but delayed or less frequent than 1 in 1000 administrations may not be revealed prior to marketing. Consequently, a number of unanticipated adverse and beneficial effects of drugs are detectable only after the drug is used broadly. The same can be more convincingly stated about most of the effects of drugs on children or the fetus, where premarketing experimental studies are restricted. For these reasons, many countries, including the United States, have established systematic methods for the surveillance of the effects of drugs after they have been approved for distribution (Brewer and Colditz, 1999; *see* below).

Postmarketing Surveillance for Adverse Reactions

Because of the limitations in the capacity of the premarketing phase of drug development to define uncommon but significant risks of new drugs, postmarketing surveillance of drug usage is imperative to detect such adverse effects.

Mechanism-based adverse drug reactions are relatively easily predicted by preclinical and clinical pharmacology studies. For idiosyncratic adverse reactions, current approaches to "safety assessment," preclinically and in clinical trials, are problematic.

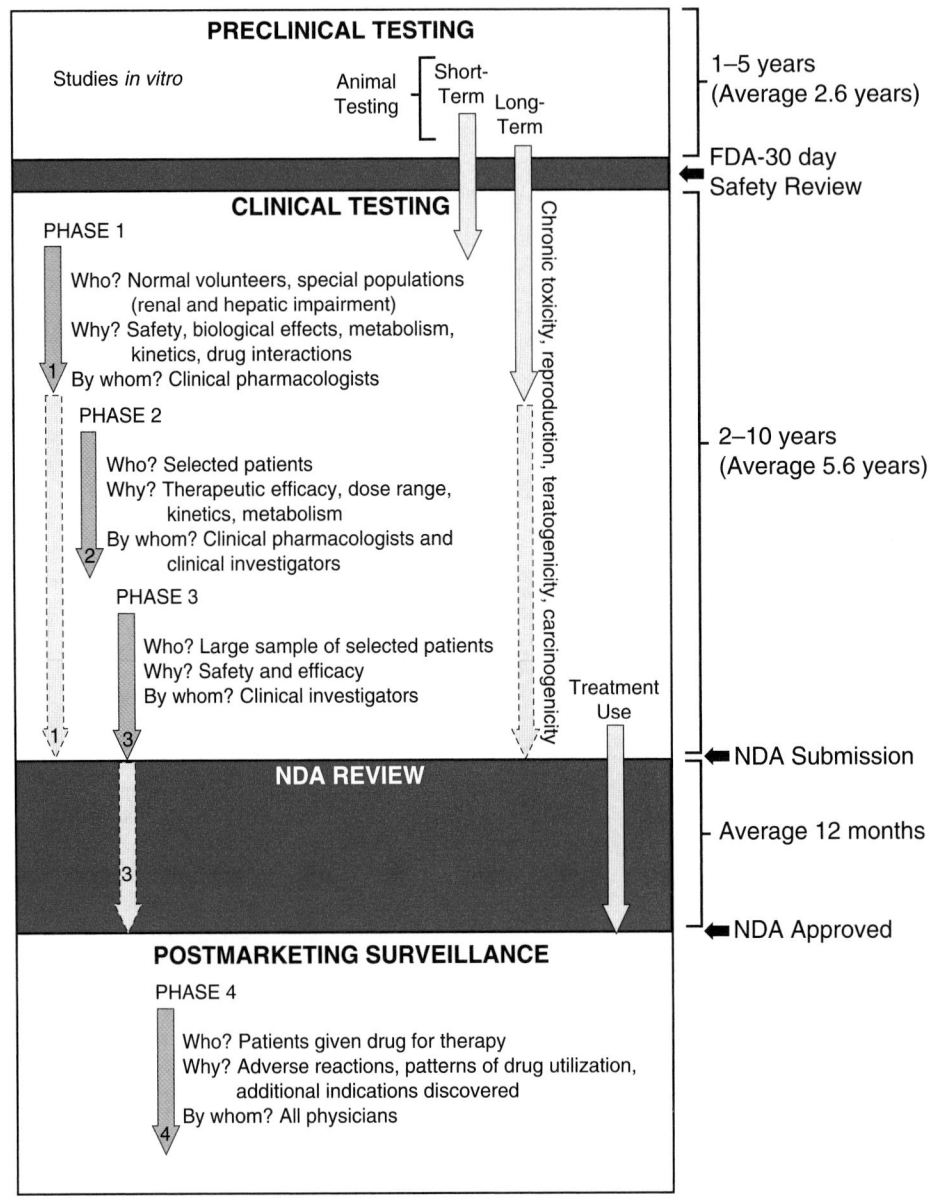

Figure 5–7. *The phases of drug development in the United States.*

The relative rarity of severe idiosyncratic reactions (*e.g.,* severe dermatological, hematological, or hepatological toxicities) presents epidemiological ascertainment issues. In addition, it is clear that a risk of 1 in 1000 is not distributed evenly across the population; some patients, because of unique genetic or environmental factors, are at an extremely high risk, whereas the remainder of the population may be at low or no risk. In contrast to the human heterogeneity underlying idiosyncratic risk, the standard process of drug development, particularly the preclinical safety assessment using inbred healthy animals maintained in a defined environment on a defined diet and manifesting predictable habits, limits the identification of risk for idiosyncratic adverse drug reactions in the human population. Understanding the genetic and environmental bases of idiosyncratic adverse events holds the promise of assessing individual rather than population risk, thereby improving the overall safety of pharmacotherapy.

Several strategies exist to detect adverse reactions after marketing of a drug, but debate continues about the most efficient and effective method. Formal approaches for estimation of the magnitude of an adverse drug effect are the *follow-up* or *cohort* study of patients who are receiving a particular drug, the *case-control study,* where the frequency of drug use in cases of adverse reactions is compared with controls, and *meta-analyses* of pre- and postmarketing studies. Cohort studies can estimate the incidence of an adverse reaction but cannot, for practical reasons, discover rare events. To have any significant advantage over the premarketing studies, a cohort study must follow at least 10,000 patients who are receiving the drug to detect with 95% confidence one event that occurs at a rate of 1 in 3300, and the event can be attributed to the drug only if it does not occur spontaneously in the control population. If the adverse event occurs spontaneously in the control population, substantially more patients and controls must be followed to establish the drug as the cause of the event (Strom and Tugwell, 1990). Meta-analyses combine the data from several studies in an attempt to discern benefits or risks that are sufficiently uncommon that an individual study lacks the power to discover them (Temple, 1999). Case-control studies also can discover rare drug-induced events. However, it may be difficult to establish the appropriate control group (Feinstein and Horwitz, 1988), and a case-control study cannot establish the incidence of an adverse drug effect. Furthermore, the suspicion of a drug as a causative factor in a disease must be the impetus for the initiation of such case-control studies.

The Key Role of the Clinician in Surveillance for Adverse Reactions

Because of the shortcomings of cohort and case-control studies and meta-analyses, additional approaches must be used. Spontaneous reporting of adverse reactions has proven to be an effective way to generate an early signal that a drug may be causing an adverse event. It is the only practical way to detect rare events, events that occur after prolonged use of drug, adverse effects that are delayed in appearance, and many drug–drug interactions. In the past few years, considerable effort has gone into improving the reporting system in the United States, which is now called MEDWATCH (Brewer and Colditz, 1999). Still, the voluntary reporting system in the United States is deficient compared with the legally mandated systems of the United Kingdom, Canada, New Zealand, Denmark, and Sweden. Most physicians feel that detecting adverse reactions is a professional obligation, but relatively few actually report such reactions. Many physicians are not aware that the FDA has a reporting system for adverse drug reactions, even though the system has been repeatedly publicized in major medical journals.

The most important spontaneous reports are those that describe serious reactions, whether they have been described previously or not. Reports on newly marketed drugs (within the past 5 years) are the most significant, even though the physician may not be able to attribute a causal role to a particular drug. The major use of this system is to provide early warning signals of unexpected adverse effects that can then be investigated by more formal techniques. However, the system also serves to monitor changes in the nature or frequency of adverse drug reactions owing to aging of the population, changes in the disease itself, or the introduction of new, concurrent therapies. *The primary sources for the reports are responsible, alert physicians; other potentially useful sources are nurses, pharmacists, and students in these disciplines.* In addition, hospital-based pharmacy and therapeutics committees and quality assurance committees frequently are charged with monitoring adverse drug reactions in hospitalized patients, and reports from these committees should be forwarded to the FDA. *The simple forms for reporting may be obtained 24 hours a day 7 days a week by calling (800)-FDA-1088; alternatively, adverse reactions can be reported directly on the Internet (www.fda.gov/medwatch).* Additionally, health professionals may contact the pharmaceutical manufacturer, who is legally obligated to file reports with the FDA. With this facile reporting system, the clinician can serve as a vital sentinel in the detection of unexpected adverse reactions to drugs.

BIBLIOGRAPHY

Antiplatelet Trialists' Collaboration. Collaborative meta-analysis of randomized trials of antiplatelet therapy for prevention of death, myocardial infarction and stroke in high risk patients. *Br. Med. J,* **2002,** *324*:71–86.

deWildt, S.N., Kearns, G.L., Leeder, J.S., and van den Anker, J.N. Cytochrome P450 3A: Ontogeny and drug disposition. *Clin. Pharmacokinet.,* **1999,** *37*:485–505.

Echt, D.S., Liebson, P.R., Mitchell, L.B., *et al.* Mortality and morbidity in patients receiving encainide, flecainide, or placebo. The Cardiac Arrhythmia Suppression Trial. *New Engl. J. Med.,* **1991,** *324*:781–788.

Jurlink, D.N., Mamdani, M., Lee, D.S., *et al.* Rates of hyperkalemia after publication of the randomized aldactone evaluation Study. *New Eng. J. Med.,* **2004,** *351*:543–531.

Kim, R.B., Wandel, C., Leake, B., *et al.* Interrelationship between substrates and inhibitors of human CYP3A and P-glycoprotein. *Pharm. Res.,* **1999,** *16*:408–414.

Lambert, G.H., Schoeller, D.A., Kotake, A.N., Flores, C., and Hay, D. The effect of age, gender, and sexual maturation on the caffeine breath test. *Dev. Pharmacol. Ther.,* **1986,** *9*:375–388.

LaRosa, J.C., He, J., and Vupputuri, S. Effect of statins on risk of coronary disease: A meta-analysis of randomized controlled trials. *JAMA,* **1999,** *282*:2340–2346.

Leape, L.L., Brennan, T.A., Laird, N., *et al.* The nature of adverse events in hospitalized patients: Results of the Harvard Medical Practice Study II. *New Engl. J. Med.,* **1991,** *324*:377–384.

Taketomo, C.K., Hodding, J.H., and Kraus, D.M. *Pediatric Dosage Handbook,* 6th ed. Lexi-Comp, Hudson, Ohio, **2000.**

Yuan, R., Parmelee, T., Balian, J.D., *et al.* In vitro metabolic interaction studies: Experience of the Food and Drug Administration. *Clin. Pharmacol. Ther.,* **1999,** *66*:9–15.

MONOGRAPHS AND REVIEWS

Aronoff, G.R. *Drug Prescribing in Renal Failure,* 4th ed. American College of Physicians, Philadelphia, **1999.**

Brewer, T., and Colditz, G.A. Postmarketing surveillance and adverse drug reactions: Current perspectives and future needs. *JAMA,* **1999,** *281*:824–829.

Bucher, H.C., Guyatt, G.H., Cook, D.J., Holbrook, A., and McAlister, F.A. Users' guides to the medical literature: XIX. Applying clinical trial results A. How to use an article measuring the effect of an intervention on surrogate endpoints. Evidence-Based Medicine Working Group. *JAMA,* **1999,** *282*:771–778.

Burns, M. Management of narrow therapeutic index drugs. *J. Thromb. Thrombolysis,* **1999,** *7*:137–143.

Feinstein, A.R. "Clinical judgment" revisited: The distraction of quantitative models. *Ann. Intern. Med.,* **1994,** *120*:799–805.

Feinstein, A.R., and Horwitz, R.I. Choosing cases and controls: The clinical epidemiology of "clinical investigation." *J. Clin. Invest.,* **1988,** *81*:1–5.

Fugh-Berman, A. Herb–drug interactions. *Lancet,* **2000,** *355*:134–138.

Gal, J. Stereoisomerism and drug nomenclature. *Clin. Pharmacol. Ther.,* **1988,** *44*:251–253.

Hendeles, L., Hochhaus, G., and Kazerounian, S. Generic and alternative brand-name pharmaceutical equivalents: Select with caution. *Am. J. Hosp. Pharm.,* **1993,** *50*:323–329.

Iaccarino, G., Lefkowitz, R.J., and Koch, W.J. Myocardial G protein–coupled receptor kinases: Implications for heart failure therapy. *Proc. Assoc. Am. Phys.,* **1999,** *111*:399–405.

Jick, H. Adverse drug reactions: The magnitude of the problem. *J. Allergy Clin. Immunol.,* **1984,** *74*:555–557.

Kearns, G.L., Abdel-Rahman, S.M., Alander, S.W. Developmental pharmacology—drug disposition, action, and therapy in infants and children. *New Engl. J. Med.,* **2003,** *349*:1157–1167.

Kessler, D.A., Hass, A.E., Feiden, K.L., Lumpkin, M., and Temple, R. Approval of new drugs in the United States: Comparison with the United Kingdom, Germany, and Japan. *JAMA,* **1996,** *276*:1826–1831.

Koch-Weser, J. Serum drug concentrations as therapeutic guides. *New Engl. J. Med.,* **1972,** *287*:227–231.

Passamani, E. Clinical trials—are they ethical? *New Engl. J. Med.,* **1991,** *324*:1589–1592.

Peck, C.C. Understanding consequences of concurrent therapies. *JAMA,* **1993,** *269*:1550–1552.

Pitt, B., Zannad, Z., Remme, W.J., *et al.* The effect of spironolactone on morbidity and mortality in patients with severe heart failure. *New Eng. J. Med.,* **1999,** *341*:709–717.

Ray, W.A. Population-based studies of adverse effects. *New Eng J. Med.,* **2004,** *349*:1592–1594.

Sackett, D.L. *Clinical Epidemiology: A Basic Science for Clinical Medicine.* Little, Brown, Boston, **1991.**

Shulman, S.R., and Kaitin, K.I. The Prescription Drug User Fee Act of 1992: A 5-year experiment for industry and the FDA. *Pharmacoeconomics,* **1996,** *9*:121–133.

Smith, W.M. Drug choice in disease states. In, *Clinical Pharmacology: Basic Principles in Therapeutics,* 2d ed. (Melmon, K.L., and Morelli, H.F., eds.) Macmillan, New York, **1978,** pp. 3–24.

Strom, B.L., and Tugwell, P. Pharmacoepidemiology: Current status, prospects, and problems. *Ann. Intern. Med.,* **1990,** *113*:179–181.

Suydam, L.A., and Kubic, M.J. FDA's implementation of FDAMA: an interim balance sheet. *Food Drug Law J.,* **2001,** *56*:131–135.

Temple, R. Meta-analysis and epidemiologic studies in drug development and postmarketing surveillance. *JAMA,* **1999,** *281*:841–844.

Temple, R.J. When are clinical trials of a given agent vs. placebo no longer appropriate or feasible? *Control. Clin. Trials,* **1997,** *18*:613–620.

Wax, P.M. Elixirs, diluents, and the passage of the 1938 Federal Food, Drug, and Cosmetic Act. *Ann. Intern. Med.,* **1995,** *122*:456–461.

SECTION II

Drugs Acting at Synaptic and Neuroeffector Junctional Sites

CHAPTER

6

NEUROTRANSMISSION

The Autonomic and Somatic Motor Nervous Systems

Thomas C. Westfall and David P. Westfall

ANATOMY AND GENERAL FUNCTIONS OF THE AUTONOMIC AND SOMATIC MOTOR NERVOUS SYSTEMS

The autonomic nervous system, also called the *visceral, vegetative,* or *involuntary nervous system,* is distributed widely throughout the body and regulates autonomic functions that occur without conscious control. In the periphery, it consists of nerves, ganglia, and plexuses that innervate the heart, blood vessels, glands, other visceral organs, and smooth muscle in various tissues.

Differences between Autonomic and Somatic Nerves. The efferent nerves of the involuntary system supply all innervated structures of the body except skeletal muscle, which is served by somatic nerves. The most distal synaptic junctions in the autonomic reflex arc occur in ganglia that are entirely outside the cerebrospinal axis. These ganglia are small but complex structures that contain axodendritic synapses between preganglionic and postganglionic neurons. Somatic nerves contain no peripheral ganglia, and the synapses are located entirely within the cerebrospinal axis. Many autonomic nerves form extensive peripheral plexuses, but such networks are absent from the somatic system. Whereas motor nerves to skeletal muscles are myelinated, postganglionic autonomic nerves generally are nonmyelinated. When the spinal efferent nerves are interrupted, the denervated skeletal muscles lack myogenic tone, are paralyzed, and atrophy, whereas smooth muscles and glands generally retain some level of spontaneous activity independent of intact innervation.

Visceral Afferent Fibers. The afferent fibers from visceral structures are the first link in the reflex arcs of the autonomic system. With certain exceptions, such as local axon reflexes, most visceral reflexes are mediated through the central nervous system (CNS).

Information on the status of the visceral organs is transmitted to the CNS through two main sensory systems: the cranial nerve (parasympathetic) visceral sensory system and the spinal (sympathetic) visceral afferent system (Saper, 2002). The cranial visceral sensory system carries mainly mechanoreceptor and chemosensory information, whereas the afferents of the spinal visceral system principally convey sensations related to temperature and tissue injury of mechanical, chemical, or thermal origin. Cranial visceral sensory information enters the CNS *via* four cranial nerves: the trigeminal (V), facial (VII), glossopharyngeal (IX), and vagus (X). These four cranial nerves transmit visceral sensory information from the internal face and head (V), tongue (taste, VII), hard palate and upper part of the oropharynx (IX), and carotid body, lower part of the oropharynx, larynx, trachea, esophagus, and thoracic and abdominal organs, with the exception of the pelvic viscera

(X). The pelvic viscera are innervated by nerves from the second through fourth sacral spinal segments.

The visceral afferents from these four cranial nerves terminate topographically in the solitary tract nucleus (STN) (Altschuler *et al.*, 1989). The most massive site for termination of the fibers from the STN is the parabrachial nucleus, which is thus the major relay station. The parabrachial nucleus consists of at least 13 separate subnuclei, which in turn project extensively to a wide range of sites in the brainstem, hypothalamus, basal forebrain, thalamus, and cerebral cortex. Other direct projections from the STN also innervate these brain structures.

Sensory afferents from visceral organs also enter the CNS *via* the spinal nerves. Those concerned with muscle chemosensation may arise at all spinal levels, whereas sympathetic visceral sensory afferents generally arise at the thoracic levels where sympathetic preganglionic neurons are found. Pelvic sensory afferents from spinal segments S2–S4 enter at that level and are important for the regulation of sacral parasympathetic outflow. In general, visceral afferents that enter the spinal nerves convey information concerned with temperature as well as nociceptive visceral inputs related to mechanical, chemical, and thermal stimulation. The primary pathways taken by ascending spinal visceral afferents are complex and controversial (Saper, 2002). Most probably converge with musculoskeletal and cutaneous afferents and ascend *via* the spinothalamic and spinoreticular tracts. Others ascend *via* the dorsal column. An important feature of the ascending pathways is that they provide collaterals that converge with the cranial visceral sensory pathway at virtually every level (Saper, 2000). At the brainstem level, collaterals from the spinal system converge with the cranial nerve sensory system in the STN, the ventrolateral medulla, and the parabrachial nucleus. At the level of the forebrain, the spinal system appears to form a posterolateral continuation of the cranial nerve visceral sensory thalamus and cortex (Saper, 2000).

The neurotransmitters that mediate transmission from sensory fibers have not been characterized unequivocally. Substance P and calcitonin gene–related peptide, which are present in afferent sensory fibers, in the dorsal root ganglia, and in the dorsal horn of the spinal cord, are leading candidates for neurotransmitters that communicate nociceptive stimuli from the periphery to the spinal cord and higher structures. Other neuroactive peptides, including somatostatin, vasoactive intestinal polypeptide (VIP), and cholecystokinin, also have been found in sensory neurons (Lundburg, 1996; Hökfelt *et al.*, 2000), and one or more such peptides may play a role in the transmission of afferent impulses from autonomic structures. Adenosine triphosphate (ATP) appears to be a neurotransmitter in certain sensory neurons, including those that innervate the urinary bladder. Enkephalins, present in interneurons in the dorsal spinal cord (within an area termed the *substantia gelatinosa*), have antinociceptive effects that appear to arise from presynaptic and postsynaptic actions to inhibit the release of substance P and diminish the activity of cells that project from the spinal cord to higher centers in the CNS. The excitatory amino acids glutamate and aspartate also play major roles in transmission of sensory responses to the spinal cord.

Central Autonomic Connections. There probably are no purely autonomic or somatic centers of integration, and extensive overlap occurs. Somatic responses always are accompanied by visceral responses, and *vice versa*. Autonomic reflexes can be elicited at the level of the spinal cord. They clearly are demonstrable in experimental animals or humans with spinal cord transection and are manifested by sweating, blood pressure alterations, vasomotor responses

to temperature changes, and reflex emptying of the urinary bladder, rectum, and seminal vesicles. Extensive central ramifications of the autonomic nervous system exist above the level of the spinal cord. For example, integration of the control of respiration in the medulla oblongata is well known. The hypothalamus and the STN generally are regarded as principal loci of integration of autonomic nervous system functions, which include regulation of body temperature, water balance, carbohydrate and fat metabolism, blood pressure, emotions, sleep, respiration, and reproduction. Signals are received through ascending spinobulbar pathways, the limbic system, neostriatum, cortex, and to a lesser extent other higher brain centers. Stimulation of the STN and the hypothalamus activates bulbospinal pathways and hormonal output to mediate autonomic and motor responses (Andresen and Kunze, 1994) (*see* Chapter 12). The hypothalamic nuclei that lie posteriorly and laterally are sympathetic in their main connections, whereas parasympathetic functions evidently are integrated by the midline nuclei in the region of the tuber cinereum and by nuclei lying anteriorly.

The CNS can produce a wide range of patterned autonomic and somatic responses from discrete activation of sympathetic or parasympathetic neurons to more generalized activation of these nerves with highly integrated patterns of response. There are highly differentiated patterns of activity during a wide range of physiological conditions consistent with the need for modulation of different organ functions. There is evidence for organotropical organization of neuronal pools at multiple levels of the CNS that generate these various patterns of sympathetic and parasympathetic responses. The pattern generators at these different levels of the neuroaxis are often organized in a hierarchical manner that allows individual response or larger responses made up of multiple individual units.

As mentioned earlier, highly integrated patterns of response generally are organized at a hypothalamic level. These integrated patterns of response involve autonomic, endocrine, and behavioral components. On the other hand, more limited patterned responses are organized at other levels of basal forebrain, brainstem, and spinal cord.

Divisions of the Peripheral Autonomic System. On the efferent side, the autonomic nervous system consists of two large divisions: (1) the sympathetic or thoracolumbar outflow and (2) the parasympathetic or craniosacral outflow. A brief outline of those anatomical features is necessary for an understanding of the actions of autonomic drugs.

The arrangement of the principal parts of the peripheral autonomic nervous system is presented schematically in Figure 6–1. The neurotransmitter of all preganglionic autonomic fibers, all postganglionic parasympathetic fibers, and a few postganglionic sympathetic fibers is *acetylcholine* (ACh). The adrenergic fibers comprise the majority of the postganglionic sympathetic fibers; here the transmitter is *norepinephrine (noradrenaline, levarterenol)*. The terms *cholinergic* and *adrenergic* were proposed originally by Dale to describe neurons that liberate ACh or norepinephrine, respectively. As noted earlier, not all the transmitter(s) of the primary afferent fibers, such as those from the mechano- and chemo-receptors of the carotid body and aortic arch, have been identified conclusively. Substance P and glutamate are thought to mediate many afferent impulses; both are present in high concentrations in the dorsal spinal cord.

Sympathetic Nervous System. The cells that give rise to the preganglionic fibers of this division lie mainly in the intermediolateral columns of the spinal cord and extend from the first thoracic to the second or third lumbar segment. The axons from these cells are carried in the anterior (ventral) nerve roots and synapse, with neurons lying in sympathetic ganglia outside the cerebrospinal axis. Sympathetic ganglia are found in three locations: paravertebral, prevertebral, and terminal.

The 22 pairs of paravertebral sympathetic ganglia form the lateral chains on either side of the vertebral column. The ganglia are connected to each other by nerve trunks and to the spinal nerves by *rami communicantes*. The white rami are restricted to the segments of the thoracolumbar outflow; they carry the preganglionic myelinated fibers that exit the spinal cord *via* the anterior spinal roots. The gray rami arise from the ganglia and carry postganglionic fibers back to the spinal nerves for distribution to sweat glands and pilomotor muscles and to blood vessels of skeletal muscle and skin. The prevertebral ganglia lie in the abdomen and the pelvis near the ventral surface of the bony vertebral column and consist mainly of the celiac (solar), superior mesenteric, aorticorenal, and inferior mesenteric ganglia. The terminal ganglia are few in number, lie near the organs they innervate, and include ganglia connected with the urinary bladder and rectum and the cervical ganglia in the region of the neck. In addition, small intermediate ganglia lie outside the conventional vertebral chain, especially in the thoracolumbar region. They are variable in number and location but usually are in close proximity to the communicating rami and the anterior spinal nerve roots.

Preganglionic fibers issuing from the spinal cord may synapse with the neurons of more than one sympathetic ganglion. Their principal ganglia of termination need not correspond to the original level from which the preganglionic fiber exits the spinal cord. Many of the preganglionic fibers from the fifth to the last thoracic segment pass through the paravertebral ganglia to form the splanchnic nerves. Most of the splanchnic nerve fibers do not synapse until they reach the celiac ganglion; others directly innervate the adrenal medulla (*see* below).

Postganglionic fibers arising from sympathetic ganglia innervate visceral structures of the thorax, abdomen, head, and neck. The trunk and the limbs are supplied by the sympathetic fibers in spinal nerves, as described earlier. The prevertebral ganglia contain cell bodies whose axons innervate the glands and smooth muscles of the abdominal and the pelvic viscera. Many of the upper thoracic sympathetic fibers from the vertebral ganglia form terminal plexuses, such as the cardiac, esophageal, and pulmonary plexuses. The sympathetic distribution to the head and the neck (vasomotor, pupillodilator, secretory, and pilomotor) is *via* the cervical sympathetic chain and its three ganglia. All postganglionic fibers in this chain arise from cell bodies located in these three ganglia; all preganglionic fibers arise from the upper thoracic segments of the spinal cord, there being no sympathetic fibers that leave the CNS above the first thoracic level.

The adrenal medulla and other chromaffin tissue are embryologically and anatomically similar to sympathetic ganglia; all are derived from the neural crest. The adrenal medulla in humans and many other species differs from sympathetic ganglia in that its principal catecholamine is *epinephrine (adrenaline)*, whereas norepinephrine is released from postganglionic sympathetic fibers. The chromaffin cells in the adrenal medulla are innervated by typical preganglionic fibers that release ACh.

Parasympathetic Nervous System. The parasympathetic nervous system consists of preganglionic fibers that originate in the CNS and their postganglionic connections. The regions of central origin are the midbrain, the medulla oblongata, and the sacral part of the spinal cord. The midbrain, or tectal, outflow consists of fibers arising from the Edinger–Westphal nucleus of the third cranial nerve and going to the ciliary ganglion in the orbit. The medullary outflow consists of the parasympathetic components of the seventh, ninth, and tenth cranial nerves. The fibers in the seventh (facial) cranial nerve form the chorda tympani, which innervates the ganglia lying on the submaxillary and sublingual glands. They also form the greater superficial petrosal nerve, which innervates the sphenopalatine ganglion. The autonomic components of the ninth (glossopharyngeal) cranial nerve innervate the otic ganglia. Postganglionic parasympathetic fibers from these ganglia supply the sphincter of the iris (pupillary constrictor muscle), the ciliary muscle, the salivary and lacrimal glands, and the mucous glands of the nose, mouth, and pharynx. These fibers also include vasodilator nerves to these same organs. The tenth (vagus) cranial nerve arises in the medulla and contains preganglionic fibers, most of which do not synapse until they reach the many small ganglia lying directly on or in the viscera of the thorax and abdomen. In the intestinal wall, the vagal fibers terminate around ganglion cells in the myenteric and submucosal plexuses. Thus, preganglionic fibers are very long, whereas postganglionic fibers are very short. The vagus nerve also carries a far greater number of afferent fibers (but apparently no pain fibers) from the viscera into the medulla; the cell bodies of these fibers lie mainly in the nodose ganglion.

The parasympathetic sacral outflow consists of axons that arise from cells in the second, third, and fourth segments of the sacral cord and proceed as preganglionic fibers to form the pelvic nerves (*nervi erigentes*). They synapse in terminal ganglia lying near or within the bladder, rectum, and sexual organs. The vagal and sacral outflows provide motor and secretory fibers to thoracic, abdominal, and pelvic organs, as indicated in Figure 6–1.

Enteric Nervous System. The processes of mixing, propulsion, and absorption of nutrients in the GI tract are controlled locally through a restricted part of the peripheral nervous system called the *enteric nervous system* (ENS). The ENS is involved in sensorimotor control and thus consists of both afferent sensory neurons and a number of motor nerves and interneurons that are organized principally into two nerve plexuses: the myenteric (Auerbach's) plexus and the submucosal (Meissner's) plexus. The myenteric plexus, located between the longitudinal and circular muscle layers, plays an important role in the contraction and relaxation of gastrointestinal smooth muscle (Kunze and Furness, 1999). The submucosal plexus is involved with secretory and absorptive functions of the gastrointestinal epithelium, local blood flow, and neuroimmune activities (Cooke, 1998). Although originally classified by Langley in the 1920s as a third division of the autonomic nervous system, the ENS is actually comprised of components of the sympathetic and parasympathetic nervous systems and has sensory nerve connections through the spinal and nodose ganglia (*see* Chapter 37).

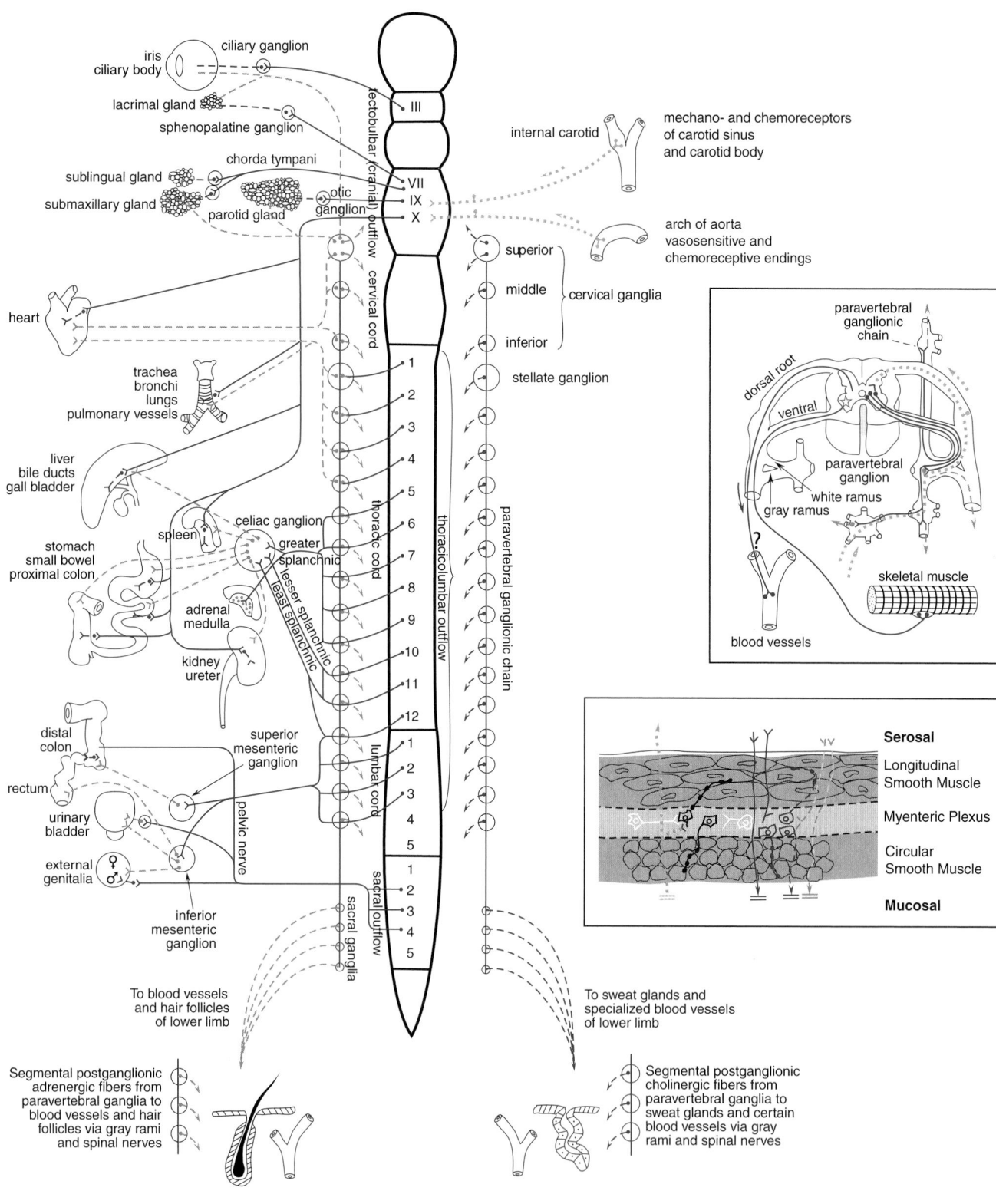

Parasympathetic input to the GI tract is excitatory; preganglionic neurons in the vagus innervate the parasympathetic ganglia of the enteric plexuses. Postganglionic sympathetic nerves also synapse with the intramural enteric parasympathetic ganglia. Sympathetic nerve activity induces relaxation primarily by inhibiting the release of ACh from the preganglionic ganglia (Broadley, 1996).

The intrinsic primary afferent neurons are present in both the myenteric and submucosal plexuses. They respond to luminal chemical stimuli, to mechanical deformation of the mucosa, and to stretch (Costa *et al.*, 2000). The nerve endings of the primary afferent neurons can be activated by a number of endogenous substances (*e.g.*, serotonin) arising from enterochromaffin cells in the wall of the gut or possibly from serotonergic nerves.

The muscle layers of the GI tract are dually innervated by excitatory and inhibitory motor neurons whose cell bodies are in the gut wall (Kunze and Furness, 1999). ACh, in addition to being the transmitter of parasympathetic nerves to the ENS, is the primary excitatory transmitter acting on nicotinic acetylcholine receptors (nAChRs) in ascending intramural pathways. Pharmacological blockade of cholinergic neurotransmission, however, does not completely abolish this excitatory transmission because tachykinin cotransmitters, such as substance P and neurokinin A, are coreleased with ACh and contribute to the excitatory response (Costa *et al.*, 1996). Although ACh also may play a role in descending motor pathways, another important excitatory neurotransmitter in such pathways is ATP acting through P2X receptors (Galligan, 2002).

◀────────────────────────────

Figure 6–1. The autonomic nervous system. Schematic representation of the autonomic nerves and effector organs based on chemical mediation of nerve impulses. Blue, cholinergic; gray, adrenergic; dotted blue, visceral afferent; solid lines, preganglionic; broken lines, postganglionic. In the upper rectangle at the right are shown the finer details of the ramifications of adrenergic fibers at any one segment of the spinal cord, the path of the visceral afferent nerves, the cholinergic nature of somatic motor nerves to skeletal muscle, and the presumed cholinergic nature of the vasodilator fibers in the dorsal roots of the spinal nerves. The asterisk (*) indicates that it is not known whether these vasodilator fibers are motor or sensory or where their cell bodies are situated. In the lower rectangle on the right, vagal preganglionic (*solid blue*) nerves from the brainstem synapse on both excitatory and inhibitory neurons found in the myenteric plexus. A synapse with a postganglionic cholinergic neuron (*blue with varicosities*) gives rise to excitation, whereas synapses with purinergic, peptide (VIP), or an NO-generating neuron (*black with varicosities*) lead to relaxation. Sensory nerves (*dotted blue lines*) originating primarily in the mucosal layer send afferent signals to the CNS but often branch and synapse with ganglia in the plexus. Their transmitter is substance P or other tachykinins. Other interneurons (*white*) contain serotonin and will modulate intrinsic activity through synapses with other neurons eliciting excitation or relaxation (*black*). Cholinergic, adrenergic, and some peptidergic neurons pass through the circular smooth muscle to synapse in the submucosal plexus or terminate in the mucosal layer, where their transmitter may stimulate or inhibit gastrointestinal secretion.

Similar to excitatory intramural neurons, inhibitory neurons of the ENS exhibit a variety of transmitters and cotransmitters, including nitric oxide (NO), ATP acting on P2Y receptors, VIP, and pituitary adenylyl cyclase–activating peptide (PACAP) (Kunze and Furness, 1999). NO seems to be the primary inhibitory transmitter (Stark and Szurszewski, 1992).

The interstitial cells of Cajal (ICC) are one component of the excitatory and inhibitory pathways in the GI tract. These cells appear to relay signals from the nerves to the smooth muscle cells to which they are electrically coupled. The ICC have receptors for both the inhibitory transmitter NO and the excitatory tachykinins. Disruption of the ICC impairs excitatory and inhibitory neurotransmission (Horowitz *et al.*, 1999).

Differences among Sympathetic, Parasympathetic, and Motor Nerves. The sympathetic system is distributed to effectors throughout the body, whereas parasympathetic distribution is much more limited. Furthermore, the sympathetic fibers ramify to a much greater extent. A preganglionic sympathetic fiber may traverse a considerable distance of the sympathetic chain and pass through several ganglia before it finally synapses with a postganglionic neuron; also, its terminals make contact with a large number of postganglionic neurons. In some ganglia, the ratio of preganglionic axons to ganglion cells may be 1:20 or more. This organization permits a diffuse discharge of the sympathetic system. In addition, synaptic innervation overlaps, so one ganglion cell may be supplied by several preganglionic fibers.

The parasympathetic system, in contrast, has terminal ganglia very near or within the organs innervated and thus is more circumscribed in its influences. In some organs, a 1:1 relationship between the number of preganglionic and postganglionic fibers has been suggested, but the ratio of preganglionic vagal fibers to ganglion cells in the myenteric plexus has been estimated as 1:8000. Hence this distinction between the two systems does not apply to all sites.

The cell bodies of somatic motor neurons reside in the ventral horn of the spinal cord; the axon divides into many branches, each of which innervates a single muscle fiber, so more than 100 muscle fibers may be supplied by one motor neuron to form a motor unit. At each neuromuscular junction, the axonal terminal loses its myelin sheath and forms a terminal arborization that lies in apposition to a specialized surface of the muscle membrane, termed the *motor end plate.* Mitochondria and a collection of synaptic vesicles are concentrated at the nerve terminal. Through trophic influences of the nerve, those cell nuclei in the multinucleated skeletal muscle cell lying in close apposition to the synapse acquire the capacity to activate specific genes that express synapse-localized proteins (Hall and Sanes, 1993; Sanes and Lichtman, 1999).

Details of Innervation. The terminations of the postganglionic autonomic fibers in smooth muscle and glands form a rich plexus, or terminal reticulum. The terminal reticulum (sometimes called the *autonomic ground plexus*) consists of the final ramifications of the postganglionic sympathetic, parasympathetic, and visceral afferent fibers, all of which are enclosed within a frequently interrupted sheath of satellite or Schwann cells. At these interruptions, varicosities packed with vesicles are seen in the efferent fibers. Such varicosities occur repeatedly but at variable distances along the course of the ramifications of the axon.

"Protoplasmic bridges" occur between the smooth muscle fibers themselves at points of contact between their plasma membranes. They are believed to permit the direct conduction of impulses from cell to cell without the need for chemical transmission. These structures have been termed *nexuses,* or *tight junctions,* and they enable the smooth muscle fibers to function as a syncytial unit.

Sympathetic ganglia are extremely complex anatomically and pharmacologically (*see* Chapter 9). The preganglionic fibers lose their myelin sheaths and divide repeatedly into a vast number of end fibers with diameters ranging from 0.1 to 0.3 μm; except at points of synaptic contact, they retain their satellite cell sheaths. The vast majority of synapses are axodendritic. Apparently, a given axonal terminal may synapse with one or more dendritic processes.

Responses of Effector Organs to Autonomic Nerve Impulses.
From the responses of the various effector organs to autonomic nerve impulses and the knowledge of the intrinsic autonomic tone, one can predict the actions of drugs that mimic or inhibit the actions of these nerves. In most instances, the sympathetic and parasympathetic neurotransmitters can be viewed as physiological or functional antagonists. If one neurotransmitter inhibits a certain function, the other usually augments that function. Most viscera are innervated by both divisions of the autonomic nervous system, and the level of activity at any moment represents the integration of influences of the two components. Despite the conventional concept of antagonism between the two portions of the autonomic nervous system, their activities on specific structures may be either discrete and independent or integrated and interdependent. For example, the effects of sympathetic and parasympathetic stimulation of the heart and the iris show a pattern of functional antagonism in controlling heart rate and pupillary aperture, respectively, whereas their actions on male sexual organs are complementary and are integrated to promote sexual function. The control of peripheral vascular resistance is primarily, but not exclusively, due to sympathetic control of arteriolar resistance. The effects of stimulating the sympathetic and parasympathetic nerves to various organs, visceral structures, and effector cells are summarized in Table 6–1.

General Functions of the Autonomic Nervous System.
The integrating action of the autonomic nervous system is of vital importance for the well-being of the organism. In general, the autonomic nervous system regulates the activities of structures that are not under voluntary control and that function below the level of consciousness. Thus, respiration, circulation, digestion, body temperature, metabolism, sweating, and the secretions of certain endocrine glands are regulated, in part or entirely, by the autonomic nervous system. Thus, the autonomic nervous system in the primary regulator of the constancy of the internal environment of the organism.

The sympathetic system and its associated adrenal medulla are not essential to life in a controlled environment, but the lack of sympatho-adrenal functions becomes evident under circumstances of stress. Body temperature cannot be regulated when environmental temperature varies; the concentration of glucose in blood does not rise in response to urgent need; compensatory vascular responses to hemorrhage, oxygen deprivation, excitement, and exercise are lacking; resistance to fatigue is lessened; sympathetic components of instinctive reactions to the external environment are lost; and other serious deficiencies in the protective forces of the body are discernible.

The sympathetic system normally is continuously active; the degree of activity varies from moment to moment and from organ to organ. In this manner, adjustments to a constantly changing environment are accomplished. The sympathoadrenal system also can discharge as a unit. This occurs particularly during rage and fright, when sympathetically innervated structures over the entire body are affected simultaneously. Heart rate is accelerated; blood pressure rises; red blood cells are poured into the circulation from the spleen (in certain species); blood flow is shifted from the skin and splanchnic region to the skeletal muscles; blood glucose rises; the bronchioles and pupils dilate; and the organism is better prepared for "fight or flight." Many of these effects result primarily from or are reinforced by the actions of epinephrine secreted by the adrenal medulla (*see* below). In addition, signals are received in higher brain centers to facilitate purposeful responses or to imprint the event in memory.

The parasympathetic system is organized mainly for discrete and localized discharge. Although it is concerned primarily with conservation of energy and maintenance of organ function during periods of minimal activity, its elimination is not compatible with life. Sectioning the vagus, for example, soon gives rise to pulmonary infection because of the inability of cilia to remove irritant substances from the respiratory tract. The parasympathetic system slows the heart rate, lowers the blood pressure, stimulates gastrointestinal movements

Table 6–1
Responses of Effector Organs to Autonomic Nerve Impulses

ORGAN SYSTEM	SYMPATHETIC EFFECT[a]	ADRENERGIC RECEPTOR TYPE[b]	PARASYMPATHETIC EFFECT[a]	CHOLINERGIC RECEPTOR TYPE[b]
Eye				
Radial muscle, iris	Contraction (mydriasis)++	α_1		
Sphincter muscle, iris			Contraction (miosis)+++	M_3, M_2
Ciliary muscle	Relaxation for far vision[+]	β_2	Contraction for near vision+++	M_3, M_2
Lacrimal glands	Secretion+	α	Secretion+++	M_3, M_2
Heart[c]				
Sinoatrial node	Increase in heart rate++	$\beta_1 > \beta_2$	Decrease in heart rate+++	$M_2 \gg M_3$
Atria	Increase in contractility and conduction velocity++	$\beta_1 > \beta_2$	Decrease in contractility++ and shortened AP duration	$M_2 \gg M_3$
Atrioventricular node	Increase in automaticity and conduction velocity++	$\beta_1 > \beta_2$	Decrease in conduction velocity; AV block+++	$M_2 \gg M_3$
His–Purkinje system	Increase in automaticity and conduction velocity	$\beta_1 > \beta_2$	Little effect	$M_2 \gg M_3$
Ventricle	Increase in contractility, conduction velocity, automaticity and rate of idioventricular pacemakers+++	$\beta_1 > \beta_2$	Slight decrease in contractility	$M_2 \gg M_3$
Blood vessels				
(Arteries and arterioles)[d]				
Coronary	Constriction+; dilation[e]++	$\alpha_1, \alpha_2; \beta_2$	No innervation[h]	—
Skin and mucosa	Constriction+++	α_1, α_2	No innervation[h]	—
Skeletal muscle	Constriction; dilation[e,f]++	$\alpha_1; \beta_2$	Dilation[h] (?)	—
Cerebral	Constriction (slight)	α_1	No innervation[h]	—
Pulmonary	Constriction+; dilation	$\alpha_1; \beta_2$	No innervation[h]	—
Abdominal viscera	Constriction +++; dilation +	$\alpha_1; \beta_2$	No innervation[h]	—
Salivary glands	Constriction+++	α_1, α_2	Dilation[h]++	M_3
Renal	Constriction++; dilation++	$\alpha_1 \alpha_2; \beta_1, \beta_2$	No innervation[h]	
(Veins)[d]	Constriction; dilation	$\alpha_1, \alpha_2; \beta_2$		
Endothelium			Activation of NO synthase[h]	M_3
Lung				
Tracheal and bronchial smooth muscle	Relaxation	β_2	Contraction	$M_2 = M_3$
Bronchial glands	Decreased secretion, increased secretion	α_1 β_2	Stimulation	M_3, M_2
Stomach				
Motility and tone	Decrease (usually)[i]+	$\alpha_1, \alpha_2, \beta_1, \beta_2$	Increase[i]+++	$M_2 = M_3$
Sphincters	Contraction (usually)+	α_1	Relaxation (usually)+	M_3, M_2
Secretion	Inhibition	α_2	Stimulation++	M_3, M_2

(Continued)

Table 6–1
Responses of Effector Organs to Autonomic Nerve Impulses (Continued)

ORGAN SYSTEM	SYMPATHETIC EFFECT[a]	ADRENERGIC RECEPTOR TYPE[b]	PARASYMPATHETIC EFFECT[a]	CHOLINERGIC RECEPTOR TYPE[b]
Intestine				
Motility and tone	Decrease[h]+	$\alpha_1, \alpha_2, \beta_1, \beta_2$	Increase[i]+++	M_3, M_2
Sphincters	Contraction+	α_1	Relaxation (usually)+	M_3, M_2
Secretion	Inhibition	α_2	Stimulation++	M_3, M_2
Gallbladder and ducts	Relaxation+	β_2	Contraction+	M
Kidney				
Renin secretion	Decrease+; increase++	$\alpha_1; \beta_1$	No innervation	—
Urinary bladder				
Detrusor	Relaxation+	β_2	Contraction+++	$M_3 > M_2$
Trigone and sphincter	Contraction++	α_1	Relaxation++	$M_3 > M_2$
Ureter				
Motility and tone	Increase	α_1	Increase (?)	M
Uterus	Pregnant contraction;	α_1		
	Relaxation	β_2	Variable[j]	M
	Nonpregnant relaxation	β_2		
Sex organs, male	Ejaculation+++	α_1	Erection+++	M_3
Skin				
Pilomotor muscles	Contraction++	α_1		
Sweat glands	Localized secretion[k]++	α_1		
	Generalized secretion+++			M_3, M_2
Spleen capsule	Contraction+++	α_1	—	—
	Relaxation+	β_2	—	—
Adrenal medulla	—			$N (\alpha_3)_2(\beta_4)_3; M$
	Secretion of epinephrine and norepinephrine			(secondarily)
Skeletal muscle	Increased contractility; glycogenolysis; K^+ uptake	β_2	—	—
Liver	Glycogenolysis and gluconeogenesis+++	$\alpha_1,$ β_2	—	—
Pancreas		α		
Acini	Decreased secretion[+]	α	Secretion[++]	M_3, M_2
Islets (β cells)	Decreased secretion[+++]	α_2	—	
	Increased secretion[+]	β_2		
Fat cells[l]	Lipolysis+++; (thermogenesis)	$\alpha_1, \beta_1, \beta_2, \beta_3$	—	—
	Inhibition of lipolysis	α_2		
Salivary glands	K^+ and water secretion+	α_1	K^+ and water secretion+++	M_3, M_2
Nasopharyngeal glands	—		Secretion++	M_3, M_2
Pineal glands	Melanton synthesis	β	—	
Posterior pituitary	Antidiuretic secretion	β_1	—	

(Continued)

Table 6–1
Responses of Effector Organs to Autonomic Nerve Impulses (Continued)

ORGAN SYSTEM	SYMPATHETIC EFFECT[a]	ADRENERGIC RECEPTOR TYPE[b]	PARASYMPATHETIC EFFECT[a]	CHOLINERGIC RECEPTOR TYPE[b]
Autonomic nerve endings				
Sympathetic terminals				
Autoreceptor	Inhibition of NE release	$\alpha_{2A} > \alpha_{2C}\ (\alpha_{2B})$		
Heteroreceptor	—		Inhibition of NE release	M_2, M_4
Parasympathetic terminal	—			
Autoreceptor			Inhibition of ACh release	M_2, M_4
Heteroreceptor	Inhibition ACh release	$\alpha_{2A} > \alpha_{2C}$		

[a]Responses are designated + to +++ to provide an approximate indication of the importance of sympathetic and parasympathetic nerve activity in the control of the various organs and functions listed. [b]Adrenergic receptors: α_1, α_2 and subtypes thereof; β_1, β_2, β_3. Cholinergic receptors: nicotinic (N); muscarinic (M), with subtypes 1–4. The receptor subtypes are described more fully in Chapters 7 and 10 and in Tables 6–2, 6–3 and 6–8. When a designation of subtype is not provided, the nature of the subtype has not been determined, unequivocally. Only the principal receptor subtypes are shown. Transmitters other than acetylcholine and norepinephrine contribute to many of the responses. [c]In the human heart, the ration of β_1 to β_2 is about 3:2 in atria and 4:1 in ventricles. While M_2 receptors predominate, M_3 receptors are also present (Wang *et al.*, 2004). [d]The predominant α_1 receptor subtype in most blood vessels (both arteries and veins) is α_{1A} (see Table 6–8), although other α_1 subtypes are present in specific blood vessels. The α_{1D} is the predominant subtype in the aorta (Michelotti *et al.*, 2000). [e]Dilation predominates *in situ* owing to metabolic autoregulatory mechanisms. [f]Over the usual concentration range of physiologically released circulating epinephrine, the β-receptor response (vasodilation) predominates in blood vessels of skeletal muscle and liver; α-receptor response (vasoconstriction) in blood vessels of other abdominal viscera. The renal and mesenteric vessels also contain specific dopaminergic receptors whose activation causes dilation (see review by Goldberg *et al.*, 1978). [g]Sympathetic cholinergic neurons cause vasodilation in skeletal muscle beds, but this is not involved in most physiological responses. [h]The endothelium of most blood vessels releases NO, which causes vasodilation in response to muscarinic stimuli. However, unlike the receptors innervated by sympathetic cholinergic fibers in skeletal muscle blood vessels, these muscarinic receptors are not innervated and respond only to exogenously added muscarinic agonists in the circulation. [i]While adrenergic fibers terminate at inhibitory β-receptors on smooth muscle fibers and at inhibitory α-receptors on parasympathetic (cholinergic) excitatory ganglion cells of the myenteric plexus, the primary inhibitory response is mediated *via* enteric neurons through NO, P2Y receptors, and peptide receptors. [j]Uterine responses depend on stages of menstrual cycle, amount of circulating estrogen and progesterone, and other factors. [k]Palms of hands and some other sites ("adrenergic sweating"). [l]There is significant variation among species in the receptor types that mediate certain metabolic responses. All three β adrenergic receptors have been found in human fat cells. Activation of β_3 adrenergic receptors produces a vigorous thermogenic response as well as lipolysis. The significance is unclear. Activation of β adrenergic receptors also inhibits leptin release from adipose tissue.

and secretions, aids absorption of nutrients, protects the retina from excessive light, and empties the urinary bladder and rectum. Many parasympathetic responses are rapid and reflexive in nature.

NEUROTRANSMISSION

Nerve impulses elicit responses in smooth, cardiac, and skeletal muscles, exocrine glands, and postsynaptic neurons by liberating specific chemical neurotransmitters. The processes are presented in some detail because an understanding of the chemical mediation of nerve impuls-

es provides the framework for our knowledge of the mechanism of action of drugs at these sites.

Historical Aspects

The earliest concrete proposal of a neurohumoral mechanism was made shortly after the turn of the twentieth century. Lewandowsky and Langley independently noted the similarity between the effects of injection of extracts of the adrenal gland and stimulation of sympathetic nerves. A few years later, in 1905, T. R. Elliott, while a student with Langley at Cambridge, England, postulated that sympathetic nerve impulses release minute amounts of an epinephrine-like substance in immediate contact with effector cells. He considered this substance to be the chemical step in the process of transmission. He also noted that long after sympathetic nerves had degenerated, the effector organs still responded characteristically to the hormone of the adrenal medulla. In 1905, Langley suggested that effector cells have excitatory and inhibitory "receptive substances" and that the response to epinephrine depended on which type of substance was present. In 1907, Dixon, impressed by the correspondence between the effects of the alkaloid *muscarine* and the responses to vagal stimulation, advanced the concept that the vagus nerve liberated a muscarine-like substance that acted as a chemical transmitter of its impulses. In the same year, Reid Hunt described the actions of ACh and other choline esters. In 1914, Dale investigated the pharmacological properties of ACh and other choline esters and distinguished its nicotine-like and muscarine-like actions. Intrigued with the remarkable fidelity with which this drug reproduced the responses to stimulation of parasympathetic nerves, he introduced the term *parasympathomimetic* to characterize its effects. Dale also noted the brief duration of action of this chemical and proposed that an esterase in the tissues rapidly splits ACh to acetic acid and choline, thereby terminating its action.

The studies of Loewi, begun in 1921, provided the first direct evidence for the chemical mediation of nerve impulses by the release of specific chemical agents. Loewi stimulated the vagus nerve of a perfused (donor) frog heart and allowed the perfusion fluid to come in contact with a second (recipient) frog heart used as a test object. The recipient frog heart was found to respond, after a short lag, in the same way as the donor heart. It thus was evident that a substance was liberated from the first organ that slowed the rate of the second. Loewi referred to this chemical substance as *Vagusstoff* ("vagus substance," "parasympathin"); subsequently, Loewi and Navratil presented evidence to identify it as ACh. Loewi also discovered that an accelerator substance similar to epinephrine and called *Acceleranstoff* was liberated into the perfusion fluid in summer, when the action of the sympathetic fibers in the frog's vagus, a mixed nerve, predominated over that of the inhibitory fibers. Feldberg and Krayer demonstrated in 1933 that the cardiac "vagus substance" also is ACh in mammals.

In addition to its role as the transmitter of all postganglionic parasympathetic fibers and of a few postganglionic sympathetic fibers, ACh has been shown to function as a neurotransmitter in three additional classes of nerves: preganglionic fibers of both the sympathetic and the parasympathetic systems, motor nerves to skeletal muscle, and certain neurons within the CNS.

In the same year as Loewi's discovery, Cannon and Uridil reported that stimulation of the sympathetic hepatic nerves resulted in the release of an epinephrine-like substance that increased blood pressure and heart rate. Subsequent experiments firmly established that this substance is the chemical mediator liberated by sympathetic nerve impulses at neuroeffector junctions. Cannon called this substance "sympathin." In many of its pharmacological and chemical properties, "sympathin" closely resembled epinephrine but also differed in certain important respects. As early as 1910, Barger and Dale noted that the effects of sympathetic nerve stimulation were reproduced more closely by the injection of sympathomimetic primary amines than by that of epinephrine or other secondary amines. The possibility that demethylated epinephrine (norepinephrine) might be "sympathin" had been advanced repeatedly, but definitive evidence for its being the sympathetic nerve mediator was not obtained until specific assays were developed for the determination of sympathomimetic amines in extracts of tissues and body fluids. In 1946, von Euler found that the sympathomimetic substance in highly purified extracts of bovine splenic nerve resembled norepinephrine by all criteria used. Norepinephrine is the predominant sympathomimetic substance in the postganglionic sympathetic

nerves of mammals and is the adrenergic mediator liberated by their stimulation. Norepinephrine, its immediate precursor *dopamine,* and epinephrine also are neurotransmitters in the CNS (*see* Chapter 12).

Evidence for Neurohumoral Transmission

The concept of neurohumoral transmission or chemical neurotransmission was developed primarily to explain observations relating to the transmission of impulses from postganglionic autonomic fibers to effector cells. Evidence supporting this concept includes (1) demonstration of the presence of a physiologically active compound and its biosynthetic enzymes at appropriate sites; (2) recovery of the compound from the perfusate of an innervated structure during periods of nerve stimulation but not (or in greatly reduced amounts) in the absence of stimulation; (3) demonstration that the compound is capable of producing responses identical to responses to nerve stimulation; and (4) demonstration that the responses to nerve stimulation and to the administered compound are modified in the same manner by various drugs, usually competitive antagonists.

While these criteria are applicable for most neurotransmitters, including norepinephrine and ACh, there now are exceptions to these general rules. For instance, NO has been found to be a neurotransmitter in nonadrenergic, noncholinergic neurons in the periphery, in the ENS, and in the CNS. However, NO is not stored in neurons and released by exocytosis. Rather, it is synthesized when needed and readily diffuses across membranes.

Chemical rather than electrogenic transmission at autonomic ganglia and the neuromuscular junction of skeletal muscle was not generally accepted for a considerable period because techniques were limited in time and chemical resolution. Techniques of intracellular recording and microiontophoretic application of drugs, as well as sensitive analytical assays, have overcome these limitations.

Neurotransmission in the peripheral and central nervous systems once was believed to conform to the hypothesis that each neuron contains only one transmitter substance. However, peptides such as enkephalin, substance P, neuropeptide Y, VIP, and somatostatin; purines such as ATP and adenosine; and small molecules such as NO have been found in nerve endings. These substances can depolarize or hyperpolarize nerve terminals or postsynaptic cells. Furthermore, results of histochemical, immunocytochemical, and autoradiographic studies have demonstrated that one or more of these substances is present in the same neurons that contain one of the classical biogenic amine neurotransmitters (Bartfai *et al.,* 1988; Lundberg *et al.,* 1996). For example, enkephalins are found in postganglionic sympathetic neurons and adrenal medullary chromaffin cells. VIP is localized selectively in peripheral cholinergic neurons that innervate exocrine glands, and neuropeptide Y is found in sympathetic nerve endings. These observations suggest that synaptic transmission in many instances may be mediated by the release of more than one neurotransmitter (*see* below).

Steps Involved in Neurotransmission

The sequence of events involved in neurotransmission is of particular importance because pharmacologically active agents modulate the individual steps.

The term *conduction* is reserved for the passage of an impulse along an axon or muscle fiber; *transmission* refers to the passage of an impulse across a synaptic or neuroeffector junction. With the exception of the local anesthetics, very few drugs modify axonal conduction in the doses employed therapeutically. Hence this process is described only briefly.

Axonal Conduction. Current knowledge of axonal conduction stems largely from the work of Hodgkin and Huxley.

At rest, the interior of the typical mammalian axon is approximately 70 mV negative to the exterior. The resting potential is essentially a diffusion potential based chiefly on the 40 times higher concentration of K^+ in the axoplasm as compared with the extracellular fluid and the relatively high permeability of the resting axonal membrane to K^+. Na^+ and Cl^- are present in higher concentrations in the extracellular fluid than in the axoplasm, but the axonal membrane at rest is considerably less permeable to these ions; hence their contribution to the resting potential is small. These ionic gradients are maintained by an energy-dependent active transport mechanism, the Na^+K^+-ATPase (*see* Hille, 1992; Hille *et al.*, 1999).

In response to depolarization to a threshold level, an action potential or nerve impulse is initiated at a local region of the membrane. The action potential consists of two phases. Following a small gating current resulting from depolarization inducing an open conformation of the channel, the initial phase is caused by a rapid increase in the permeability of Na^+ through voltage-sensitive Na^+ channels. The result is inward movement of Na^+ and a rapid depolarization from the resting potential, which continues to a positive overshoot. The second phase results from the rapid inactivation of the Na^+ channel and the delayed opening of a K^+ channel, which permits outward movement of K^+ to terminate the depolarization. Inactivation appears to involve a voltage-sensitive conformational change in which a hydrophobic peptide loop physically occludes the open channel at the cytoplasmic side. Although not important in axonal conduction, Ca^{2+} channels in other tissues (*e.g.*, L-type Ca^{2+} channels in heart) contribute to the action potential by prolonging depolarization by an inward movement of Ca^{2+}. This influx of Ca^{2+} also serves as a stimulus to initiate intracellular events (Hille, 1992; Catterall, 2000).

The transmembrane ionic currents produce local circuit currents around the axon. As a result of such localized changes in membrane potential, adjacent resting channels in the axon are activated, and excitation of an adjacent portion of the axonal membrane occurs. This brings about propagation of the action potential without decrement along the axon. The region that has undergone depolarization remains momentarily in a refractory state. In myelinated fibers, permeability changes occur only at the nodes of Ranvier, thus causing a rapidly progressing type of jumping, or saltatory, conduction. The puffer fish poison *tetrodotoxin* and a close congener found in some shellfish, *saxitoxin*, selectively block axonal conduction; they do so by blocking the voltage-sensitive Na^+ channel and preventing the increase in Na^+ permeability associated with the rising phase of the action potential. In contrast, *batrachotoxin*, an extremely potent steroidal alkaloid secreted by a South American frog, produces paralysis through a selective increase in permeability of the Na^+ channel, which induces a persistent depolarization. Scorpion toxins are peptides that also cause persistent depolarization, but they do so by inhibiting the inactivation process (*see* Catterall, 2000). Na^+ and Ca^{2+} channels are discussed in more detail in Chapters 14, 31, and 34.

Junctional Transmission. The arrival of the action potential at the axonal terminals initiates a series of events that trigger transmission of an excitatory or inhibitory impulse across the synapse or neuroeffector junction. These events, diagrammed in Figure 6–2, are:

1. *Storage and release of the transmitter.* The non-peptide (small molecule) neurotransmitters are largely synthesized in the region of the axonal terminals and stored there in synaptic vesicles. Peptide neurotransmitters (or precursor peptides) are found in large dense-core vesicles that are transported down the axon from their site of synthesis in the cell body. During the resting state, there is a continual slow release of isolated quanta of the transmitter; this produces electrical responses at the postjunctional membrane [miniature end-plate potentials (*mepps*)] that are associated with the maintenance of physiological responsiveness of the effector organ. A low level of spontaneous activity within the motor units of skeletal muscle is particularly important because skeletal muscle lacks inherent tone. The action potential causes the synchronous release of several hundred quanta of neurotransmitter. Depolarization of the axonal terminal triggers this process; a critical step in most but not all nerve endings is the influx of Ca^{2+}, which enters the axonal cytoplasm and promotes fusion between the axoplasmic membrane and those vesicles in close proximity to it (*see* Meir *et al.*, 1999; Hille *et al.*, 1999). The contents of the vesicles, including enzymes and other proteins, then are discharged to the exterior by a process termed *exocytosis*. Synaptic vesicles may either fully exocytose with complete fusion and subsequent endocytosis or form a transient pore that closes after transmitter has escaped (Murthy and Stevens, 1998).

Synaptic vesicles are clustered in discrete areas underlying the presynaptic plasma membrane, termed *active zones;* they often are aligned with the tips of postsynaptic folds. Some 20 to 40 proteins, playing distinct roles as transporter or trafficking proteins, are found in the vesicle. Neurotransmitter transport into the vesicle is driven by an electrochemical gradient generated by the vacuolar proton pump.

The function of the trafficking proteins is less well understood, but the vesicle protein synaptobrevin (VAMP) assembles with the plasma membrane proteins SNAP-25 and syntaxin 1 to form a core complex that initiates or drives the vesicle–plasma membrane fusion process (Jahn *et al.*, 2003). The submillisecond triggering of exocytosis by Ca^{2+} appears to be mediated by a separate family of proteins, the synaptotagmins. GTP-binding proteins of the Rab 3 family regulate the fusion process and cycle on and off the vesicle through GTP hydrolysis. Several other regulatory proteins of less well-defined function—synapsin, synaptophysin, and synaptogyrin—also play a role in fusion and exocytosis, as do proteins such as RIM and neurexin that are found on the active zones of the plasma membrane. Many of the trafficking proteins are homologous to those used in vesicular transport in yeast.

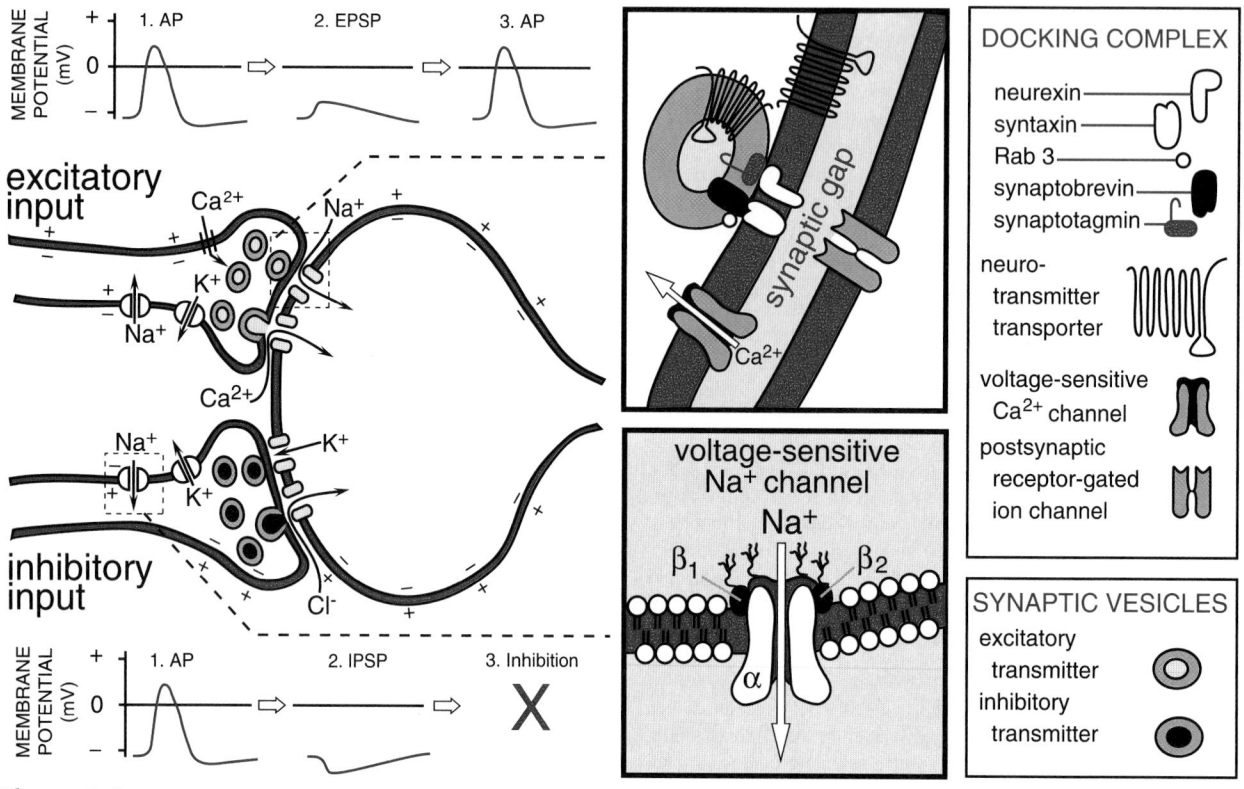

**Figure 6–2. *Steps involved in excitatory and inhibitory neurotransmission. 1.* The nerve action potential (AP) consists of a transient self-propagated reversal of charge on the axonal membrane. (The internal potential E_i goes from a negative value, through zero potential, to a slightly positive value primarily through increases in Na$^+$ permeability and then returns to resting values by an increase in K$^+$ permeability.) When the AP arrives at the presynaptic terminal, it initiates release of the excitatory or inhibitory transmitter. Depolarization at the nerve ending and entry of Ca^{2+} initiate docking and then fusion of the synaptic vesicle with the membrane of the nerve ending. Docked and fused vesicles are shown. *2.* Combination of the excitatory transmitter with postsynaptic receptors produces a localized depolarization, the excitatory postsynaptic potential (EPSP), through an increase in permeability to cations, most notably Na$^+$. The inhibitory transmitter causes a selective increase in permeability to K$^+$ or Cl$^-$, resulting in a localized hyperpolarization, the inhibitory postsynaptic potential (IPSP). *3.* The EPSP initiates a conducted AP in the postsynaptic neuron; this can be prevented, however, by the hyperpolarization induced by a concurrent IPSP. The transmitter is dissipated by enzymatic destruction, by reuptake into the presynaptic terminal or adjacent glial cells, or by diffusion. (Modified from Eccles, 1964, 1973; Katz, 1966; Catterall, 1992; Jahn and Südhof, 1994.)

Over the past 30 years an extensive variety of receptors has been identified on soma, dendrites, and axons of neurons, where they respond to neurotransmitters or modulators released from the same neuron or from adjacent neurons or cells (Langer, 1997, Miller, 1998, Westfall, 2004). Soma–dendritic receptors are those receptors located on or near the cell body and dendrites; when activated, they primarily modify functions of the soma–dendritic region such as protein synthesis and generation of action potentials. Presynaptic receptors are those presumed to be located on, in, or near axon terminals or varicosities; when activated, they modify functions of the terminal region such as synthesis and release of transmitters. Two main classes of presynaptic receptors have been identified on most neurons, including sympathetic and parasympathetic terminals. Heteroreceptors are presynaptic receptors that respond to neurotransmitters, neuromodulators, or neurohormones released from adjacent neurons or cells. For example, norepinephrine can influence the release of ACh from parasympathetic neurons by acting on α_{2A}, α_{2B}, and α_{2C} receptors, whereas ACh can influence the release of norepinephrine from sympathetic neurons by acting on M$_2$ and M$_4$ receptors (*see* below). The other class of presynaptic receptors consists of autoreceptors, which are receptors located on or close to those axon terminals of a neuron through which the neuron's own transmitter can modify transmitter synthesis and release. For example, norepinephrine released from sympathetic neurons may interact with α_{2A} and α_{2C} receptors to inhibit neurally released norepinephrine. Similarly, ACh released from parasympathetic neurons may interact with M$_2$ and M$_4$ receptors to inhibit neurally released ACh.

Presynaptic nicotinic receptors enhance transmitter release in motor neurons (Bowman *et al.*, 1990) and in a variety of other central and peripheral synapses (MacDermott *et al.*, 1999).

Adenosine, dopamine, *glutamate,* γ-aminobutyric acid (GABA), *prostaglandins,* and *enkephalins* have been shown to influence neurally mediated release of various neurotransmitters. The receptors for these agents exert their modulatory effects in part by altering the function of prejunctional ion channels (Tsien *et al.,* 1988; Miller, 1998). A number of ion channels that directly control transmitter release are found in presynaptic terminals (Meir *et al.,* 1999).

2. *Combination of the transmitter with postjunctional receptors and production of the postjunctional potential.* The transmitter diffuses across the synaptic or junctional cleft and combines with specialized receptors on the postjunctional membrane; this often results in a localized increase in the ionic permeability, or conductance, of the membrane. With certain exceptions (noted below), one of three types of permeability change can occur: (a) a generalized increase in the permeability to cations (notably Na^+ but occasionally Ca^{2+}), resulting in a localized depolarization of the membrane, *i.e.,* an excitatory postsynaptic potential (EPSP); (b) a selective increase in permeability to anions, usually Cl^-, resulting in stabilization or actual hyperpolarization of the membrane, which constitutes an inhibitory postsynaptic potential (IPSP); or (c) an increased permeability to K^+. Because the K^+ gradient is directed out of the cell, hyperpolarization and stabilization of the membrane potential occur (an IPSP).

It should be emphasized that the potential changes associated with the EPSP and IPSP at most sites are the results of passive fluxes of ions down their concentration gradients. The changes in channel permeability that cause these potential changes are specifically regulated by the specialized postjunctional receptors for the neurotransmitter that initiates the response (*see* Chapter 12 and below). These receptors may be clustered on the effector cell surface, as seen at the neuromuscular junctions of skeletal muscle and other discrete synapses, or distributed more uniformly, as observed in smooth muscle.

By using microelectrodes that form high-resistance seals on the surface of cells, electrical events associated with a single neurotransmitter-gated channel can be recorded (*see* Hille, 1992). In the presence of an appropriate neurotransmitter, the channel opens rapidly to a high-conductance state, remains open for about a millisecond, and then closes. A short squarewave pulse of current is observed as a result of the channel's opening and closing. The summation of these microscopic events gives rise to the EPSP. The graded response to a neurotransmitter usually is related to the frequency of opening events rather than to the extent of opening or the duration of opening. High-conductance ligand-gated ion channels usually permit passage of Na^+ or Cl^-; K^+ and Ca^{2+} are involved less frequently. The preceding ligand-gated channels belong to a large superfamily of ionotropic receptor proteins that includes the nicotinic, glutamate, and certain serotonin (5-HT_3) and purine receptors, which conduct primarily Na^+, cause depolarization, and are excitatory, and GABA and glycine receptors, which conduct Cl^-, cause hyperpolarization, and are inhibitory. The nicotinic, GABA, gly-

cine, and 5-HT_3 receptors are closely related, whereas the glutamate and purinergic ionotropic receptors have distinct structures (Karlin and Akabas, 1995). Neurotransmitters also can modulate the permeability of K^+ and Ca^{2+} channels indirectly. In these cases, the receptor and channel are separate proteins, and information is conveyed between them by G proteins (*see* Chapter 1). Other receptors for neurotransmitters act by influencing the synthesis of intracellular second messengers and do not necessarily cause a change in membrane potential. The most widely documented examples of receptor regulation of second-messenger systems are the activation or inhibition of adenylyl cyclase and the increase in intracellular concentrations of Ca^{2+} that results from release of the ion from internal stores by *inositol trisphosphate* (*see* Chapter 1).

3. *Initiation of postjunctional activity.* If an EPSP exceeds a certain threshold value, it initiates a propagated action potential in a postsynaptic neuron or a muscle action potential in skeletal or cardiac muscle by activating voltage-sensitive channels in the immediate vicinity. In certain smooth muscle types in which propagated impulses are minimal, an EPSP may increase the rate of spontaneous depolarization, cause Ca^{2+} release, and enhance muscle tone; in gland cells, the EPSP initiates secretion through Ca^{2+} mobilization. An IPSP, which is found in neurons and smooth muscle but not in skeletal muscle, will tend to oppose excitatory potentials simultaneously initiated by other neuronal sources. Whether a propagated impulse or other response ensues depends on the summation of all the potentials.

4. *Destruction or dissipation of the transmitter.* When impulses can be transmitted across junctions at frequencies up to several hundred per second, it is obvious that there should be an efficient means of disposing of the transmitter following each impulse. At cholinergic synapses involved in rapid neurotransmission, high and localized concentrations of *acetylcholinesterase* (AChE) are available for this purpose. On inhibition of AChE, removal of the transmitter is accomplished principally by diffusion. Under these circumstances, the effects of released ACh are potentiated and prolonged (see Chapter 8).

Rapid termination of norepinephrine occurs by a combination of simple diffusion and reuptake by the axonal terminals of most of the released norepinephrine. Termination of the action of amino acid transmitters results from their active transport into neurons and surrounding glia. Peptide neurotransmitters are hydrolyzed by various peptidases and dissipated by diffusion; specific uptake mechanisms have not been demonstrated for these substances.

5. *Nonelectrogenic functions.* The continual quantal release of neurotransmitters in amounts insufficient to elicit a postjunctional response probably is important in the transjunctional control of neurotransmitter action. The activity and turnover of enzymes involved in the synthesis and inactivation of neurotransmitters, the density of presynaptic and postsynaptic receptors, and other characteristics of synapses probably are controlled by trophic actions of neurotransmitters or other trophic factors released by the neuron or the target cells (Sanes and Lichtman, 1999).

Cholinergic Transmission

The synthesis, storage, and release of ACh follow a similar life cycle in all cholinergic synapses, including those at skeletal neuromuscular junctions, preganglionic sympathetic and parasympathetic terminals, postganglionic parasympathetic varicosities, postganglionic sympathetic varicosities innervating sweat glands in the skin, and in the CNS. The neurochemical events that underlie cholinergic neurotransmission are summarized in Figure 6–3 (*see* Whittaker, 1988, for review). Two enzymes, choline acetyltransferase and AChE, are involved in ACh synthesis and degradation, respectively.

Choline Acetyltransferase. Choline acetyltransferase catalyzes the final step in the synthesis of ACh—the acetylation of choline with acetyl coenzyme A (CoA) (*see* Wu and Hersh, 1994). The primary structure of choline acetyltransferase is known from molecular cloning, and its immunocytochemical localization has proven useful for identification of cholinergic axons and nerve cell bodies.

Acetyl CoA for this reaction is derived from pyruvate *via* the multistep pyruvate dehydrogenase reaction or is synthesized by acetate thiokinase, which catalyzes the reaction of acetate with ATP to form an enzyme-bound acyladenylate (acetyl AMP). In the presence of CoA, transacetylation and synthesis of acetyl CoA proceed.

Choline acetyltransferase, like other protein constituents of the neuron, is synthesized within the perikaryon and then is transported along the length of the axon to its terminal. Axonal terminals contain a large number of mitochondria, where acetyl CoA is synthesized. Choline is taken up from the extracellular fluid into the axoplasm by active transport. The final step in the synthesis occurs within the cytoplasm, following which most of the ACh is sequestered within synaptic vesicles. Although moderately potent inhibitors of choline acetyltransferase exist, they have no therapeutic utility in part because the uptake of choline is the rate-limiting step in ACh biosynthesis.

Choline Transport. Transport of choline from the plasma into neurons is accomplished by distinct high- and low-affinity transport systems. The high-affinity system (K_m = 1 to 5 μM) is unique to cholinergic neurons, is

dependent on extracellular Na^+, and is inhibited by *hemicholinium*. Plasma concentrations of choline approximate 10 μM; thus, the concentration of choline does not limit its availability to cholinergic neurons. Much of the choline formed from AChE-catalyzed hydrolysis of ACh is recycled into the nerve terminal. The cloning of the high-affinity choline transporter found in presynaptic terminals reveals a sequence and structure differing from those of other neurotransmitter transporters but similar to that of the Na^+-dependent glucose transporter family (Ferguson and Blakely, 2004).

Storage of ACh. After its synthesis from choline, ACh is taken up by the storage vesicles principally at the nerve terminals. The vesicles are transported anterogradely from the cell body *via* the microtubules, with little ACh incorporation taking place during this process.

There appear to be two types of vesicles in cholinergic terminals: electron-lucent vesicles (40 to 50 nm in diameter) and dense-cored vesicles (80 to 150 nm). The core of the vesicles contains both ACh and ATP, at an estimated ratio of 10:1, which are dissolved in the fluid phase with metal ions (Ca^{2+} and Mg^{2+}) and a proteoglycan called *vesiculin*. Vesiculin is negatively charged and is thought to sequester the Ca^{2+} or ACh. It is bound within the vesicle, with the protein moiety anchoring it to the vesicular membrane. In some cholinergic terminals there are peptides, such as VIP, that act as cotransmitters at some junctions. The peptides usually are located in the dense-cored vesicles. Vesicular membranes are rich in lipids, primarily cholesterol and phospholipids, as well as protein. The proteins include ATPase, which is ouabain-sensitive and thought to be involved in proton pumping and in vesicular inward transport of Ca^{2+}. Other proteins include protein kinase (involved in phosphorylation mechanisms of Ca^{2+} uptake), calmodulin, atractyloside-binding protein (which acts as an ATP carrier), and synapsin (which is thought to be involved with exocytosis).

The vesicular transporter allows for the uptake of ACh into the vesicle, has considerable concentrating power, is saturable, and is ATPase-dependent. The process is inhibited by vesamicol (Figure 6–3). Inhibition by *vesamicol* is noncompetitive and reversible and does not affect the vesicular ATPase. The gene for choline acetyltransferase and the vesicular transporter are found at the same locus, with the transporter gene positioned in the first intron of the transferase gene. Hence a common promoter regulates the expression of both genes (Eiden, 1998).

Estimates of the ACh content of synaptic vesicles range from 1000 to over 50,000 molecules per vesicle, and it has been calculated that a single motor nerve terminal contains 300,000 or more vesicles. In addition, an uncertain but possibly significant amount of ACh is present in the extravesicular cytoplasm. Recording the electrical events associated with the opening of single channels at the motor end plate during continuous application of ACh has permitted estimation of the potential change induced by a single molecule of ACh (3×10^{-7} V); from such calculations it is evident that even the lower estimate of the ACh content per vesicle (1000 molecules) is sufficient to account for the magnitude of the mepps.

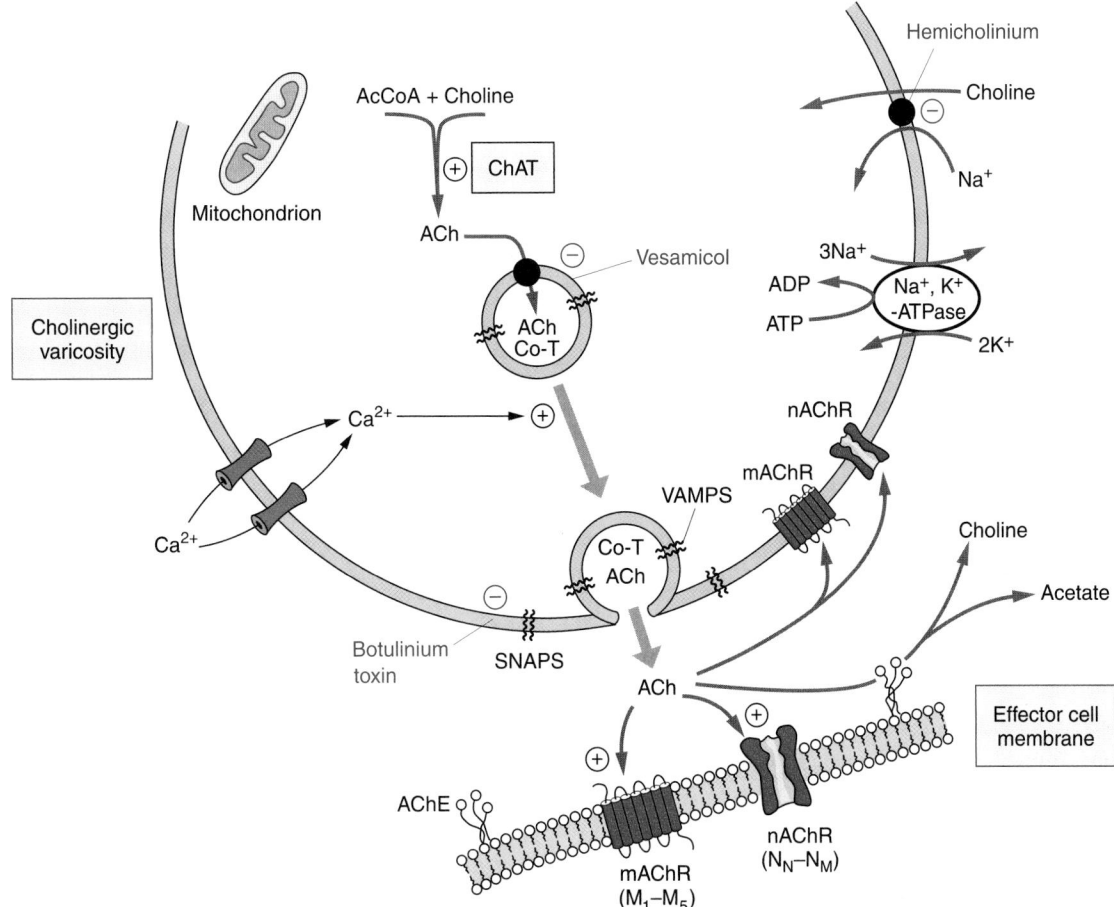

Figure 6–3. *Schematic representations of a cholinergic neuroeffector junction showing features of the synthesis, storage, and release of acetylcholine (ACh) and receptors on which ACh acts.* The synthesis of ACh in the varicosity depends on the uptake of choline *via* a sodium-dependent carrier. This uptake can be blocked by *hemicholinium*. Choline and the acetyl moiety of acetyl coenzyme A, derived from mitochondria, form ACh, a process catalyzed by the enzyme choline acetyltransferase (ChAT). ACh is transported into the storage vesicle by another carrier that can be inhibited by *vesamicol*. ACh is stored in vesicles along with other potential cotransmitters (Co-T) such as ATP and VIP at certain neuroeffector junctions. Release of ACh and the Co-T occurs on depolarization of the varicosity, which allows the entry of Ca^{2+} through voltage-dependent Ca^{2+} channels. Elevated $[Ca^{2+}]_{in}$ promotes fusion of the vesicular membrane with the cell membrane, and exocytosis of the transmitters occurs. This fusion process involves the interaction of specialized proteins associated with the vesicular membrane (VAMPs, vesicle-associated membrane proteins) and the membrane of the varicosity (SNAPs, synaptosome-associated proteins). The exocytotic release of ACh can be blocked by *botulinum toxin*. Once released, ACh can interact with the muscarinic receptors (mAChR), which are GPCRs, or nicotinic receptors (nAChR), which are ligand-gated ion channels, to produce the characteristic response of the effector. ACh also can act on presynaptic mAChRs or nAChRs to modify its own release. The action of ACh is terminated by metabolism to choline and acetate by acetylcholinesterase (AChE), which is associated with synaptic membranes.

Release of Acetylcholine. Fatt and Katz recorded at the motor end plate of skeletal muscle and observed the random occurrence of small (0.1 to 3.0 mV) spontaneous depolarizations at a frequency of approximately 1 Hz. The magnitude of these mepps is considerably below the threshold required to fire a muscle action potential (AP); that they are due to the release of ACh is indicated by their enhancement by *neostigmine* (an anti-ChE agent) and their block-

ade by D-*tubocurarine* (a competitive antagonist that acts at nicotinic receptors). These results led to the hypothesis that ACh is released from motor nerve endings in constant amounts, or quanta. The likely morphological counterpart of quantal release was discovered shortly thereafter in the form of synaptic vesicles by De Robertis and Bennett. Most of the storage and release properties of ACh originally investigated in motor end plates apply to other fast-responding synapses. When an AP arrives at the motor nerve terminal, there is a synchronous release of 100 or more quanta (or vesicles) of ACh.

The release of ACh and other neurotransmitters by exocytosis through the prejunctional membrane is inhibited by botulinum and tetanus toxins from *Clostridium*. The *Clostridium* toxins, consisting of disulfide-linked heavy and light chains, bind to an as-yet-unidentified receptor on the membrane of the cholinergic nerve terminal. Through endocytosis, they are transported into the cytosol. The light chain is a Zn^{2+}-dependent protease that becomes activated and hydrolyzes components of the core or SNARE complex involved in exocytosis. The various serotypes of botulinum toxin digest select proteins in the plasma membrane (syntaxin and SNAP-25) and the synaptic vesicle (synaptobrevin). Therapeutic uses of botulinum toxin are described in Chapters 9 and 63.

By contrast, tetanus toxin primarily has a central action because it is transported in retrograde fashion up the motor neuron to its soma in the spinal cord. From there the toxin migrates to inhibitory neurons that synapse with the motor neuron and blocks exocytosis in the inhibitory neuron. The block of release of inhibitory transmitter gives rise to tetanus or spastic paralysis. The toxin from the venom of black widow spiders (α-latrotoxin) binds to neurexins, transmembrane proteins that reside on the nerve terminal membrane, resulting in massive synaptic vesicle exocytosis (Schiavo *et al.*, 2000).

Acetylcholinesterase (AChE). For ACh to serve as a neurotransmitter in the motor system and at other neuronal synapses, it must be removed or inactivated within the time limits imposed by the response characteristics of the synapse. At the neuromuscular junction, immediate removal is required to prevent lateral diffusion and sequential activation of adjacent receptors. Modern biophysical methods have revealed that the time required for hydrolysis of ACh at the neuromuscular junction is less than a millisecond. The K_m of AChE for ACh is approximately 50 to 100 μM. Choline has only 10^{-3} to 10^{-5} the potency of ACh at the neuromuscular junction.

While AChE is found in cholinergic neurons (dendrites, perikarya, and axons), it is distributed more widely than cholinergic synapses. It is highly concentrated at the postsynaptic end plate of the neuromuscular junction. Butyrylcholinesterase (BuChE; also known as *pseudocholinesterase*) is present in low abundance in glial or satellite cells but is virtually absent in neuronal elements of the central and peripheral nervous systems. BuChE is synthesized primarily in the liver and is found in liver and plasma; its likely vestigial physiological function is the hydrolysis of ingested esters from plant sources. AChE and BuChE typically are distinguished by the relative rates of ACh and butyrylcholine hydrolysis and by effects of selective inhibitors (*see* Chapter 8). Almost all pharmacological effects of the anti-ChE agents are due to the inhibition of AChE, with the consequent accumulation of endogenous ACh in the vicinity of the nerve terminal. Distinct but single genes encode AChE and BuChE in mammals; the diversity

of molecular structure of AChE arises from alternative mRNA processing (Taylor *et al.*, 2000).

AChE also has been proposed to have multiple nonclassical biological functions that are not obvious and that remain controversial (Soreg and Seidman, 2001). These nonclassical functions include neuritogenesis, cell adhesion, synaptogenesis, amyloid fiber assembly, activation of dopamine receptors, hematopoiesis, and thrombopoiesis.

Characteristics of Cholinergic Transmission at Various Sites. There are marked differences among various sites of cholinergic transmission with respect to architecture and fine structure, the distributions of AChE and receptors, and the temporal factors involved in normal function. In skeletal muscle, for example, the junctional sites occupy a small, discrete portion of the surface of the individual fibers and are relatively isolated from those of adjacent fibers; in the superior cervical ganglion, approximately 100,000 ganglion cells are packed within a volume of a few cubic millimeters, and both the presynaptic and postsynaptic neuronal processes form complex networks.

Skeletal Muscle. Stimulation of a motor nerve results in the release of ACh from perfused muscle; close intra-arterial injection of ACh produces muscular contraction similar to that elicited by stimulation of the motor nerve. The amount of ACh (10^{-17} mol) required to elicit an end-plate potential (EPP) following its micro-iontophoretic application to the motor end plate of a rat diaphragm muscle fiber is equivalent to that recovered from each fiber following stimulation of the phrenic nerve.

The combination of ACh with nicotinic ACh receptors at the external surface of the postjunctional membrane induces an immediate, marked increase in cation permeability. On receptor activation by ACh, its intrinsic channel opens for about 1 ms; during this interval, about 50,000 Na^+ ions traverse the channel. The channel-opening process is the basis for the localized depolarizing EPP within the end plate, which triggers the muscle AP. The latter, in turn, leads to contraction.

Following section and degeneration of the motor nerve to skeletal muscle or of the postganglionic fibers to autonomic effectors, there is a marked reduction in the threshold doses of the transmitters and of certain other drugs required to elicit a response; *i.e.,* denervation supersensitivity occurs. In skeletal muscle, this change is accompanied by a spread of the receptor molecules from the end-plate region to the adjacent portions of the sarcoplasmic membrane, which eventually involves the entire muscle surface. Embryonic muscle also exhibits this uniform sensitivity to ACh prior to innervation. Hence, innervation represses the expression of the receptor gene by the nuclei that lie in extrajunctional regions of the muscle fiber and directs the subsynaptic nuclei to express the structural and functional proteins of the synapse (Sanes and Lichtman, 1999).

Autonomic Effectors. Stimulation or inhibition of autonomic effector cells occurs on activation of muscarinic acetylcholine receptors (*see* below). In this case, the effector is coupled to the receptor by a G protein (*see* Chapter 1). In contrast to skeletal muscle and neurons, smooth muscle and the cardiac conduction system [sinoatrial (SA) node, atrium, atrioventricular (AV) node, and the His–Purkinje system] normally exhibit intrinsic activity, both electrical and mechanical, that is modulated but not initiated by nerve impulses.

In the basal condition, unitary smooth muscle exhibits waves of depolarization and/or spikes that are propagated from cell to cell at rates considerably slower than the AP of axons or skeletal muscle. The spikes apparently are initiated by rhythmic fluctuations in the membrane resting potential. Application of ACh (0.1 to 1 μM) to isolated intestinal muscle causes a decrease in the resting potential (*i.e.*, the membrane potential becomes less negative) and an increase in the frequency of spike production, accompanied by a rise in tension. A primary action of ACh in initiating these effects through muscarinic receptors is probably partial depolarization of the cell membrane brought about by an increase in Na^+ and, in some instances, Ca^{2+} conductance. ACh also can produce contraction of some smooth muscles when the membrane has been depolarized completely by high concentrations of K^+, provided that Ca^{2+} is present. Hence, ACh stimulates ion fluxes across membranes and/or mobilizes intracellular Ca^{2+} to cause contraction.

In the heart, spontaneous depolarizations normally arise from the SA node. In the cardiac conduction system, particularly in the SA and AV nodes, stimulation of the cholinergic innervation or the direct application of ACh causes inhibition, associated with hyperpolarization of the membrane and a marked decrease in the rate of depolarization. These effects are due, at least in part, to a selective increase in permeability to K^+ (Hille, 1992).

Autonomic Ganglia. The primary pathway of cholinergic transmission in autonomic ganglia is similar to that at the neuromuscular junction of skeletal muscle. Ganglion cells can be discharged by injecting very small amounts of ACh into the ganglion. The initial depolarization is the result of activation of nicotinic ACh receptors, which are ligand-gated cation channels with properties similar to those found at the neuromuscular junction. Several secondary transmitters or modulators either enhance or diminish the sensitivity of the postganglionic cell to ACh. This sensitivity appears to be related to the membrane potential of the postsynaptic nerve cell body or its dendritic branches. Ganglionic transmission is discussed in more detail in Chapter 9.

Actions of Acetylcholine at Prejunctional Sites. As described earlier, both cholinergic and adrenergic nerve terminal varicosities contain autoreceptors and heteroreceptors. ACh release therefore is subject to complex regulation by mediators, including ACh itself acting on M_2 and M_4 autoreceptors, and other transmitters (*e.g.*, norepinephrine acting on α_{2A}- and α_{2C} adrenergic receptors) (Philipp and Hein, 2004; Wess, 2004) or substances produced locally in tissues (*e.g.*, NO). ACh-mediated inhibition of ACh release following activation of M_2 and M_4 autoreceptors is thought to represent a physiological negative-feedback control mechanism. At some neuroeffector junctions such as the myenteric plexus in the GI tract or the SA node in the heart, sympathetic and parasympathetic nerve terminals often lie juxtaposed to each other. The opposing effects of norepinephrine and ACh, therefore, result not only from the opposite effects of the two transmitters on the smooth muscle or cardiac cells but also from the inhibition of ACh release by norepinephrine or inhibition of norepinephrine release by ACh acting on heteroreceptors on para-

sympathetic or sympathetic terminals. The muscarinic autoreceptors and heteroreceptors also represent drug targets for both agonists and antagonists. Muscarinic agonists can inhibit the electrically induced release of ACh, whereas antagonists will enhance the evoked release of transmitter. The parasympathetic nerve terminal varicosities also may contain additional heteroreceptors that could respond by inhibition or enhancement of ACh release by locally formed autacoids, hormones, or administered drugs. In addition to α_{2A} and α_{2C} adrenergic receptors, other inhibitory heteroreceptors on parasympathetic terminals include adenosine A_1 receptors, histamine H_3 receptors, and opioid receptors. Evidence also exists for β_2-adrenoceptive facilitatory receptors (for review, *see* Broadly, 1996).

Extraneuronal Cholinergic Systems. ACh is present in the vast majority of human cells and organs, including epithelial cells (airways, alimentary tract, epidermis, glandular tissue), mesothelial and endothelial cells, circulating cells (platelets), and immune cells (mononuclear cells, macrophages). Although the exact function of non-neuronal ACh is not known precisely, proposed roles include the regulation of elementary cell functions such as mitosis, locomotion, automaticity, ciliary activity, cell–cell contact, barrier function, respiration and secretion, and regulation of lymphocyte function (Wessler *et al.*, 1998; Kawashima and Fujii, 2000).

Cholinergic Receptors and Signal Transduction. Sir Henry Dale noted that the various esters of choline elicited responses that were similar to those of either *nicotine* or muscarine depending on the pharmacological preparation. A similarity in response also was noted between muscarine and nerve stimulation in those organs innervated by the craniosacral divisions of the autonomic nervous system. Thus, Dale suggested that ACh or another ester of choline was a neurotransmitter in the autonomic nervous system; he also stated that the compound had dual actions, which he termed a "nicotine action" (*nicotinic*) and a "muscarine action" (*muscarinic*).

The capacities of *tubocurarine* and *atropine* to block nicotinic and muscarinic effects of ACh, respectively, provided further support for the proposal of two distinct types of cholinergic receptors. Although Dale had access only to crude plant alkaloids of then unknown structure from *Amanita muscaria* and *Nicotiana tabacum,* this classification remains as the primary subdivision of cholinergic receptors. Its utility has survived the discovery of several distinct subtypes of nicotinic and muscarinic receptors.

Although ACh and certain other compounds stimulate both muscarinic and nicotinic cholinergic receptors, several other agonists and antagonists are selective for one of the two major types of receptors. ACh is a flexible molecule, and indirect evidence suggests that the conformations of the neurotransmitter are distinct when it is bound to nicotinic or muscarinic cholinergic receptors.

Nicotinic receptors are ligand-gated ion channels whose activation always causes a rapid (millisecond) increase in cellular permeability to Na^+ and Ca^{2+}, depolarization, and excitation. By contrast, muscarinic receptors are G protein–coupled receptors (GPCRs). Responses to muscarinic agonists are slower; they may be either excitatory or inhibitory, and they are not necessarily linked to changes in ion permeability.

The primary structures of various species of nicotinic receptors (Numa *et al.*, 1983; Changeux and Edelstein, 1998) and muscarinic receptors (Bonner, 1989; Caulfield and Birdsall, 1998) have been deduced from the sequences of their respective genes. That these two types of receptors belong to distinct families of proteins is not surprising, retrospectively, in view of their distinct differences in chemical specificity and function.

Subtypes of Nicotinic Acetylcholine Receptors

The nicotinic ACh receptors (nAChRs) are members of a superfamily of ligand-gated ion channels. The receptors exist at the skeletal neuromuscular junction, autonomic ganglia, and adrenal medulla and in the CNS. They are the natural targets for ACh as well as pharmacologically administered drugs, including nicotine. The receptor forms a pentameric structure consisting of homomeric α and β subunits. In humans, eight α subunits (α_2 through α_7, α_9, and α_{10}) and three β subunits (β_2 through β_4) have been cloned. A further α_8 subunit has been cloned in chickens but is not present in mammals. Both the muscle and neuronal nAChRs share structural and functional properties with other ligand-gated channels such as the $GABA_A$, $5-HT_3$, and glycine receptors. The muscle nAChR is the best-characterized ligand-gated ion channel both because large quantities of receptors have been purified from *Torpedo* electrical organs and because of the existence of highly specific agonists and antagonists (Picciotto *et al.*, 2001).

The muscle nicotinic receptor contains four distinct subunits in a pentameric complex ($\alpha\beta\delta\gamma$ or $\alpha_2\beta\delta\varepsilon$). Receptors in embryonic or denervated muscle contain a γ subunit, whereas an ε subunit replaces the γ subunit in adult innervated muscle (Table 6–2). This change in expression of the genes encoding the γ and ε subunits gives rise to small differences in ligand selectivity but may be more important for dictating rates of turnover of the receptors or their tissue localization.

The muscle and neuronal subunits share the basic topography of a large extracellular N-terminal domain that contributes to agonist binding, four hydrophobic transmembrane domains (TM_1 through TM_4), a large

cytoplasmic loop between TM_3 and TM_4, and a short extracellular C terminus. The M_2 transmembrane region is thought to form the ion pore of the nAChR (Picciotto *et al.*, 2001).

Functional neuronal nAChRs also exist as pentamers composed of two α and three β subunits with "duplex" (α/β) or "triplex" (α_x, $\alpha_y\beta$, or $\alpha\beta_x\beta_y$) conformation (De Biasi, 2002). The *in vivo* composition and functional role of most of the nAChRs is unclear. Autonomic ganglia form homomeric α_7 and heteromeric α_3/β_4, with $(\alpha_3)_2(\beta_4)_3$ being the most prevalent.

The pentameric structure of the neuronal nAChR and the considerable molecular diversity of its subunits offer the possibility of a large number of nAChRs with different physiological properties. These receptors may subserve a variety of discrete functions and thus represent novel drug targets for a wide variety of therapeutic agents. The stoichiometry of most nAChRs in brain is still uncertain, although an abundant nAChR $\alpha_4\beta_3$ is proposed to have two α_4 and three β_3 subunits (Lindstrom, 2000). More complex combinations with three ($\alpha_3\beta_4\alpha_5$) or four ($\alpha_3\beta_2\beta_4\alpha_5$) different subunits have been identified. Until recently, few selective ligands were available that affect nAChR function, but the list of selective agents is expanding considerably (Loyd and Williams, 2000). For example, the neuronal nAChR subunits on presynaptic terminals of dopamine neurons projecting to the striatum have been fully defined (Luetje, 2004), as has the complete subunit composition of four major presynaptic nAChR subtypes in the striatum (Salminen *et al.*, 2004). The α conotoxin MII–sensitive class of receptors consists of $\alpha_6\beta_2\beta_3$ and $\alpha_3\alpha_6\beta_2\beta_3$, whereas the α conotoxin MII–resistant class consists of $\alpha_4\beta_2$ and $\alpha_4\alpha_5\beta_2$ subunits. It can be expected that similar advances soon will be made with other neuronal nAChRs.

Owing to the large number of permutations of α and β subunits, it is not possible to make a pharmacological classification of all the subtypes at this time. Distinctions between nAChRs are listed in Table 6–2. The structure, function, distribution, and subtypes of nicotinic receptors are described in more detail in Chapter 9.

Subtypes of Muscarinic Receptors. In mammals, five distinct subtypes of muscarinic ACh receptors (mAChRs) have been identified, each produced by a different gene. Like the different forms of nicotinic receptors, these variants have distinct anatomical locations in the periphery and CNS and differing chemical specificities. The mAChRs are GPCRs (see Table 6–3 for characteristics of the mAChRs).

Different experimental approaches including immunohistochemical and mRNA hybridization studies have shown that mAChRs are present in virtually all organs, tissues, and cell types (Table 6–3), although certain subtypes often predominate specific sites. For example, the M_2 receptor is the predominant subtype in the heart, whereas the M_3 receptor is the predominant subtype in the bladder (Dhein *et al.*, 2001; Fetscher *et al.*, 2002). In the periphery, mAChRs mediate the classical muscarinic actions of

Table 6–2
Characteristics of Subtypes of Nicotinic Acetylcholine Receptors (nAChRs)

RECEPTOR (PRIMARY RECEPTOR SUBTYPE)*	MAIN SYNAPTIC LOCATION	MEMBRANE RESPONSE	MOLECULAR MECHANISM	AGONISTS	ANTAGONISTS
Skeletal muscle (N_M) $(\alpha_1)_2\beta_1\varepsilon\delta$ adult $(\alpha_1)_2\beta_1\gamma\delta$ fetal	Skeletal neuro-muscular junction (postjunctional)	Excitatory; end-plate depolarization; skeletal muscle contraction	Increased cation permeability (Na^+; K^+)	ACh Nicotine Succinyl-choline	Atracurium Vecuronium *d*-Tubocurarine Pancuronium α-Conotoxin α-Bungarotoxin
Peripheral neuronal (N_N) $(\alpha_3)_2(\beta_4)_3$	Autonomic ganglia; adrenal medulla	Excitatory; depolarization; firing of postganglion neuron; depolarization and secretion of catecholamines	Increased cation permeability (Na^+; K^+)	ACh Nicotine Epibatidine Dimethylphenylpiperazinium	Trimethaphan Mecamylamine
Central neuronal (CNS) $(\alpha_4)_2(\beta_4)_3$ (α-btox-insensitive)	CNS; pre- and postjunctional	Pre- and postsynaptic excitation Prejunctional control of transmitter release	Increased cation permeability (Na^+; K^+)	Cytisine, epibatidine Anatoxin A	Mecamylamine Dihydro-β-erythrodine Erysodine Lophotoxin
$(\alpha_7)_5$ (α-btox-sensitive)	CNS; Pre- and postsynaptic	Pre- and postsynaptic excitation Prejunctional control of transmitter release	Increased permeability (Ca^{2+})	Anatoxin A	Methyllycaconitine α-Bungarotoxin α-Conotoxin IMI

*Nine individual subunits have been identified and cloned in human brain, which combine in various conformations to form individual receptor subtypes. The structure of individual receptors and the subtype composition are incompletely understood. Only a finite number of naturally occurring functional nAChR constructs have been identified. α-btox, α-bungarotoxin.

ACh in organs and tissues innervated by parasympathetic nerves, although receptors may be present at sites that lack parasympathetic innervation (*e.g.*, most blood vessels). In the CNS, mAChRs are involved in regulating a large number of cognitive, behavior, sensory, motor, and autonomic functions. Owing to the lack of specific muscarinic agonists and antagonists that demonstrate selectivity for individual mAChRs and the fact that most organs and tissues express multiple mAChRs, it has been a challenge to assign specific pharmacological functions to distinct mAChRs. The development of gene-targeting techniques in mice has been very helpful in defining specific functions (Table 6–3) (*see* Wess, 2004).

The basic functions of muscarinic cholinergic receptors are mediated by interactions with G proteins and thus by G protein–induced changes in the function of distinct member-bound effector molecules. The M_1, M_3, and M_5 subtypes couple through the pertussis toxin–insensitive G_{11} and G_{13} that are responsible for stimulation of phospholipase C activity. The immediate result is hydrolysis of

membrane phosphatidylinositol 4,5 diphosphate to form inositol polyphosphates. Inositol trisphosphate (IP_3) causes release of intracellular Ca^{2+} from the endoplasmic reticulum, with activation of Ca^{2+}-dependent phenomena such as contraction of smooth muscle and secretion (Berridge, 1993) (*see* Chapter 1). The second product of the phospholipase C reaction, diacylglycerol, activates protein kinase C (in conjunction with Ca^{2+}). This arm of the pathway plays a role in the phosphorylation of numerous proteins, leading to various physiological responses. Activation of M_1, M_3, and M_5 receptors can also cause the activation of phospholipase A_2, leading to the release of arachidonic acid and consequent eicosanoid synthesis, resulting in autocrine/paracrine stimulation of adenylyl cyclase and an increase in cyclic AMP.

Stimulation of M_2 and M_4 cholinergic receptors leads to interaction with other G proteins, (*e.g.*, G_i and G_o) with a resulting inhibition of adenylyl cyclase leading to a decrease in cyclic AMP, activation of inwardly rectifying K^+ channels, and inhibition of voltage-gated Ca^{2+} channels (van Koppen and Kaiser, 2003). The

Table 6-3

Characteristics of Muscarinic Acetylcholine Receptor Subtypes (mAChRs)

RECEPTOR	SIZE; CHROMOSOME LOCATION	CELLULAR AND TISSUE LOCATION*	CELLULAR RESPONSE†	FUNCTIONAL RESPONSE‡
M_1	460 aa 11q 12-13	CNS; Most abundant in cerebral cortex, hippocampus and striatum Autonomic ganglia Glands (gastric and salivary) Enteric nerves	Activation of PLC; ↑ IP_3 and ↑DAG → ↑Ca^{2+} and PKC Depolarization and excitation (↑ sEPSP) Activation of PLD_2, PLA_2; ↑ AA Couples *via* $G_{q/11}$	Increased cognitive function (learning and memory) Increased seizure activity Decrease in dopamine release and locomotion Increase in depolarization of autonomic ganglia Increase in secretions
M_2	466 aa 7 q 35-36	Widely expressed in CNS, heart, smooth muscle, autonomic nerve terminals	Inhibition of adenylyl cyclase, ↓cAMP Activation of inwardly rectifying K^+ channels Inhibition of voltage-gated Ca^{2+} channels Hyperpolarization and inhibition Couples *via* G_i/G_o (PTX-sensitive)	*Heart:* SA node: slowed spontaneous depolarization; hyperpolarization, ↓HR AV node: decrease in conduction velocity Atrium: ↓ refractory period, ↓ contraction Ventricle: slight ↓ contraction *Smooth muscle:* ↑ Contraction *Peripheral nerves:* Neural inhibition *via* autoreceptors and heteroreceptor ↓ Ganglionic transmission. *CNS:* Neural inhibition ↑ Tremors; hypothermia; analgesia
M_3	590 aa 1q 43-44	Widely expressed in CNS (< than other mAChRs) Abundant in smooth muscle and glands Heart	Activation of PLC; ↑ IP_3 and ↑DAG → ↑Ca^{2+} and PKC Depolarization and excitation (↑ sEPSP) Activation of PLD_2, PLA_2; ↑ AA Couples *via* $G_{q/11}$	*Smooth muscle* ↑ contraction (predominant in some, *e.g.* bladder) *Glands:* ↑ secretion (predominant in salivary gland) Increases food intake, body weight fat deposits Inhibition of dopamine release Synthesis of NO

(Continued)

Table 6–3

Characteristics of Muscarinic Acetylcholine Receptor Subtypes (mAChRs) (Continued)

RECEPTOR	SIZE; CHROMOSOME LOCATION	CELLULAR AND TISSUE LOCATION*	CELLULAR RESPONSE[†]	FUNCTIONAL RESPONSE[‡]
M_4	479 aa 11p 12-11.2	Preferentially expressed in CNS, particularly forebrain	Inhibition of adenylyl cyclase, $\downarrow$cAMP Activation of inwardly rectifying K^+ channels Inhibition of voltage-gated Ca^{2+} channels Hyperpolarization and inhibition Couples *via* Gi/G$_o$ (PTX-sensitive)	Autoreceptor- and heteroreceptor-mediated inhibition of transmitter release in CNS and periphery. Analgesia; cataleptic activity Facilitation of dopamine release
M_5	532 aa 15q 26	Expressed in low levels in CNS and periphery Predominant mAchR in dopamine neurons in VTA and substantia nigra	Activation of PLC; $\uparrow$ IP$_3$ and $\uparrow$DAG $\rightarrow$ $\uparrow$Ca^{2+} and PKC Depolarization and excitation ($\uparrow$ sEPSP) Activation of PLD$_2$, PLA$_2$; $\uparrow$ AA Couples *via* G$_{q/11}$	Mediator of dilation in cerebral arteries and arterioles (?) Facilitates dopamine release Augmentation of drug seeking behavior and reward (*e.g.,* opiates, cocaine)

*Most organs, tissues, and cells express multiple mAChRs. [†]M_1, M_3, and M_5 mAChRs appear to couple to the same G proteins and signal through similar pathways. Likewise, M_2 and M_4 mAChRs couple through similar G proteins and signal through similar pathways. [‡]Despite the fact that in many tissues, organs, and cells multiple subtypes of mAChRs coexist, one subtype may predominate in producing a particular function; in others, there may be equal predominance. ABBREVIATIONS: PLC, phospholipase C; IP$_3$, inositol-1,4,5-triphosphate; DAG, diacylglycerol; PLD$_2$, phospholipase D; AA, arachidonic acid; PLA, phospholipase A; cAMP, cyclic AMP; AV node, atrioventricular node; HR, heart rate; PTX, pertussis toxin; VTA, ventral tegmentum area.

157

functional consequences of these effects are hyperpolarization and inhibition of excitable membranes. These are most clear in myocardium, where inhibition of adenylyl cyclase and activation of K$^+$ conductances account for the negative chronotropic and inotropic effects of ACh.

Following activation by classical or allosteric agonists, mAChRs can be phosphorylated by a variety of receptor kinases and second-messenger regulated kinases; the phosphorylated mAChR subtypes then can interact with β-arrestin and presumably other adaptor proteins. As a result, the various mAChR signaling pathways may be differentially altered, leading to short- or long-term desensitization of a particular signaling pathway, receptor-mediated activation of the MAP kinase pathway downstream of mAChR phosphorylation, and long-term potentiation of mAChR-mediated phospholipase C stimulation. Agonist activation of mAChRs also may induce receptor internalization and down-regulation (van Koppen and Kaiser, 2003).

Adrenergic Transmission

Under this general heading are norepinephrine (NE), the principal transmitter of most sympathetic postganglionic fibers and of certain tracts in the CNS, dopamine, the predominant transmitter of the mammalian extrapyramidal system and of several mesocortical and mesolimbic neuronal pathways, and epinephrine, the major hormone of the adrenal medulla. Collectively, these three amines are called *catecholamines.*

A tremendous amount of information about catecholamines and related compounds has accumulated in recent years partly because of the importance of interactions between the endogenous catecholamines and many of the drugs used in the treatment of hypertension, mental disorders, and a variety of other conditions. The details of these interactions and of the pharmacology of the sympathomimetic amines themselves will be found in subsequent chapters. The basic physiological, biochemical, and pharmacological features are presented here.

Synthesis, Storage, and Release of Catecholamines. **Synthesis.** The steps in the synthesis of dopamine, norepinephrine (noradrenaline), and epinephrine (adrenaline) are shown in Figure 6–4. Tyrosine is sequentially 3-hydroxylated and decarboxylated to form dopamine. Dopamine is β-hydroxylated to yield norepinephrine, which is N-methylated in chromaffin tissue to give epinephrine. The enzymes involved have been identified, cloned, and characterized (Nagatsu, 1991). Table 6–4 summarizes some of the important characteristics of the four enzymes. These enzymes are not completely specific; consequently, other endogenous substances, as well as certain drugs, are also substrates. For example, 5-hydroxytryptamine (5-HT, sero-

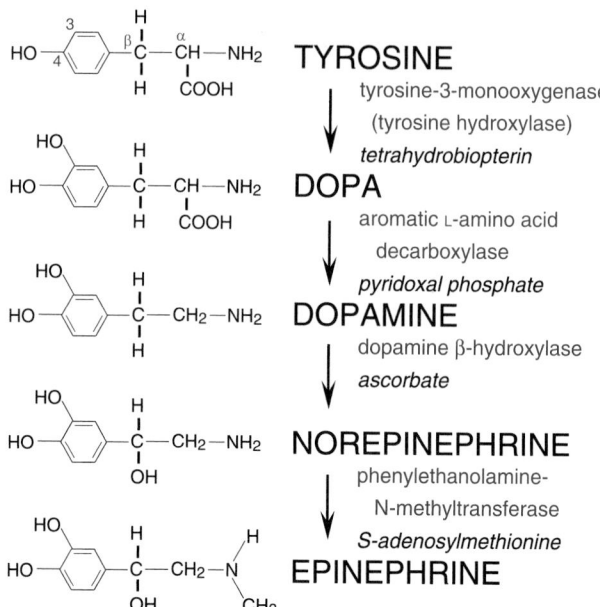

Figure 6–4. ***Steps in the enzymatic synthesis of dopamine, norepinephrine, and epinephrine.*** The enzymes involved are shown in blue; essential cofactors in italics. The final step occurs only in the adrenal medulla and in a few epinephrine-containing neuronal pathways in the brainstem.

tonin) can be produced from 5-hydroxy-L-tryptophan by aromatic L-amino acid decarboxylase (or dopa decarboxylase). Dopa decarboxylase also converts dopa into dopamine, and methyldopa to α-methyldopamine, which, in turn, is converted by dopamine β-hydroxylase (DβH) to methylnorepinephrine.

The hydroxylation of tyrosine by tyrosine hydroxylase generally is regarded as the rate-limiting step in the biosynthesis of catecholamines (Zigmond *et al.*, 1989); this enzyme is activated following stimulation of sympathetic nerves or the adrenal medulla. The enzyme is a substrate for PKA, PKC, and CaM kinase; kinase-catalyzed phosphorylation may be associated with increased hydroxylase activity (Zigmond *et al.*, 1989; Daubner *et al.*, 1992). This is an important acute mechanism for increasing catecholamine synthesis in response to elevated nerve stimulation. In addition, there is a delayed increase in tyrosine hydroxylase gene expression after nerve stimulation. This increased expression can occur at multiple levels of regulation, including transcription, RNA processing, regulation of RNA stability, translation, and enzyme stability (Kumer and Vrana, 1996). These mechanisms serve to maintain the content of catecholamines in response to increased transmitter release. In addition, tyrosine hydroxylase is subject to feedback

Table 6–4
Enzymes for Synthesis of Catecholamines

ENZYME	OCCURRENCE	SUBCELLULAR DISTRIBUTION	COFACTOR REQUIREMENT	SUBSTRATE SPECIFICITY	COMMENTS
Tyrosine hydroxylase	Widespread; sympathetic nerves	Cytoplasmic	Tetrahydro-biopterin, O_2, Fe^{2+}	Specific for L-tyrosine	Rate limiting step. Inhibition can lead to depletion of NE
Aromatic L-amino acid decarboxylase	Widespread; sympathetic nerves	Cytoplasmic	Pyridoxal phosphate	Nonspecific	Inhibition does not alter tissue NE and Epi appreciably
Dopamine β-hydrox-ylase	Widespread; sympathetic nerves	Synaptic vesicles	Ascorbic acid, O_2 (contains copper)	Nonspecific	Inhibition can decrease NE and Epi levels
Phenylethanolamine *N*-methyltrans-ferase	Largely in adrenal gland	Cytoplasmic	*S*-Adenosyl methionine (CH_3 donor)	Nonspecific	Inhibition leads to decrease in adrenal catecholamines; under control of glucocorticoids

inhibition by catechol compounds, which allosterically modulate enzyme activity.

Tyrosine hydroxylase deficiency has been reported in humans and is characterized by generalized rigidity, hypokinesia, and low cerebrospinal fluid (CSF) levels of norepinephrine and dopamine metabolites homovanillic acid and 3-methoxy-4-hydroxyphenylethylene glycol (Wevers *et al.*, 1999). Tyrosine hydroxylase knockout is embryonically lethal in mice, presumably because the loss of catecholamines results in altered cardiac function. Interestingly, residual levels of dopamine are present in these mice. It has been suggested that tyrosinase may be an alternate source for catecholamines, although tyrosinase-derived catecholamines are clearly not sufficient for survival (Carson and Robertson, 2002).

DβH deficiency in humans is characterized by orthostatic hypotension, ptosis of the eyelids, retrograde ejaculation, and elevated plasma levels of dopamine. In the case of DH-deficient mice, there is about 90% embryonic mortality (Carson and Robertson, 2002).

Our understanding of the cellular sites and mechanisms of synthesis, storage, and release of catecholamines derives from studies of sympathetically innervated organs and the adrenal medulla. Nearly all the norepinephrine content of the former is confined to the postganglionic sympathetic fibers; it disappears within a few days after section of the nerves. In the adrenal medulla, catecholamines are stored in chromaffin granules (Aunis, 1998). These vesicles contain extremely high concentrations of catecholamines (approximately 21% dry weight), ascorbic acid, and ATP, as well as specific proteins such as chromogranins, DβH, and peptides including enkephalin and neuropeptide Y. Interestingly, vasostatin-1, the N-terminal fragment of chromogranin A, has been found to have antibacterial and antifungal

activity (Lugardon *et al.*, 2000), as have other chromogranin A fragments such as chromofungin, vasostatin II, prochromacin, and chromacin I and II (Taupenot *et al.*, 2003). Two types of storage vesicles are found in sympathetic nerve terminals: large dense-core vesicles corresponding to chromaffin granules and small dense-core vesicles containing norepinephrine, ATP, and membrane-bound DβH.

The main features of the mechanisms of synthesis, storage, and release of catecholamines and their modifications by drugs are summarized in Figure 6–5. In the case of adrenergic neurons, the enzymes that participate in the formation of norepinephrine are synthesized in the cell bodies of the neurons and then are transported along the axons to their terminals. In the course of synthesis (Figure 6–5), the hydroxylation of tyrosine to dopa and the decarboxylation of dopa to dopamine take place in the cytoplasm. About half the dopamine formed in the cytoplasm then is actively transported into the DβH-containing storage vesicles, where it is converted to norepinephrine; the remainder, which escapes capture by the vesicles, is deaminated to 3,4-dihydroxyphenylacetic acid (DOPAC) and subsequently *O*-methylated to homovanillic acid (HVA). The adrenal medulla has two distinct catecholamine-containing cell types: those with norepinephrine and those with primarily epinephrine. The latter cell population contains the enzyme phenylethanolamine-*N*-methyltransferase (PNMT). In these cells, the norepinephrine formed in the granules leaves these structures, presumably by diffusion, and is methylated in the cytoplasm to epinephrine. Epinephrine then reenters the chromaffin granules, where it is stored until released. In adults, epinephrine accounts for approximately 80% of the catecholamines of the adrenal medulla, with norepinephrine making up most of the remainder (von Euler, 1972).

A major factor that controls the rate of synthesis of epinephrine, and hence the size of the store available for release from the adrenal medulla, is the level of glucocorticoids secreted by the

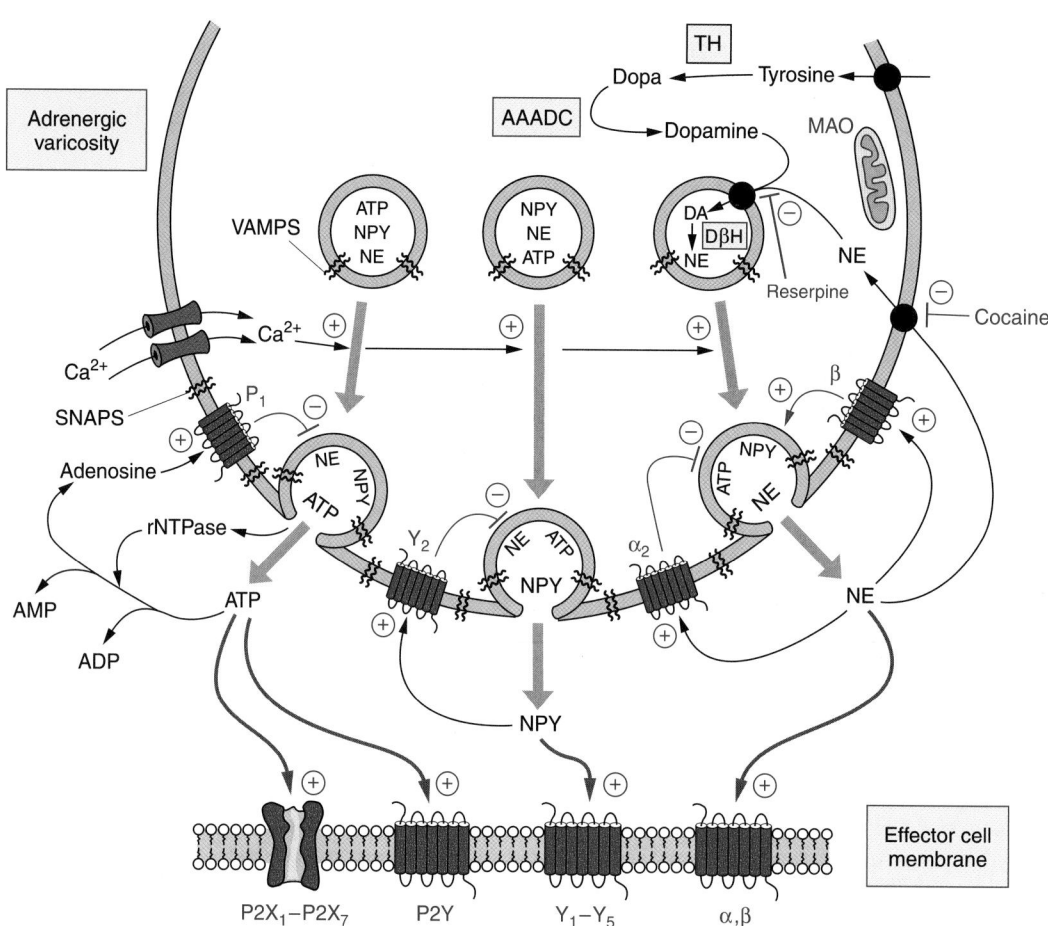

Figure 6–5. **Schematic representation of an adrenergic neuroeffector junction showing features of the synthesis, storage, release, and receptors for norepinephrine (NE), the cotransmitters neuropeptide Y (NPY), and ATP.** Tyrosine is transported into the varicosity and is converted to DOPA by tyrosine hydroxylase (TH) and DOPA to dopamine *via* the action of aromatic L-amino acid decarboxylase (AAADC). Dopamine is taken up into the vesicles of the varicosity by a transporter that can be blocked by reserpine. Cytoplasmic NE also can be taken up by this transporter. Dopamine is converted to NE within the vesicle *via* the action of dopamine-β-hydroxylase (DβH). NE is stored in vesicles along with other cotransmitters, NPY and ATP, depending on the particular neuroeffector junction. Release of the transmitters occurs upon depolarization of the varicosity, which allows entry of Ca^{2+} through voltage-dependent Ca^{2+} channels. Elevated levels of Ca^{2+} promote the fusion of the vesicular membrane with the membrane of the varicosity, with subsequent exocytosis of transmitters. This fusion process involves the interaction of specialized proteins associated with the vesicular membrane (VAMPs, vesicle-associated membrane proteins) and the membrane of the varicosity (SNAPs, synaptosome-associated proteins). In this schematic representation, NE, NPY, and ATP are stored in the same vesicles. Different populations of vesicles, however, may preferentially store different proportions of the cotransmitters. Once in the synapse, NE can interact with α and β adrenergic receptors to produce the characteristic response of the effector. The adrenergic receptors are GPCRs. α and β receptors also can be located presynaptically where NE can either diminish ($α_2$), or facilitate (β) its own release and that of the cotransmitters. The principal mechanism by which NE is cleared from the synapse is *via* a cocaine-sensitive neuronal uptake transporter. Once transported into the cytosol, NE can be restored in the vesicle or metabolized by monoamine oxidase (MAO). NPY produces its effects by activating NPY receptors, of which there are at least five types (Y_1 through Y_5). NPY receptors are GPCRs. NPY can modify its own release and that of the other transmitters *via* presynaptic receptors of the Y_2 type. NPY is removed from the synapse by metabolic breakdown by peptidases. ATP produces its effects by activating P2X receptors or P2Y receptors. P2X receptors are ligand-gated ion channels; P2Y receptors are GPCRs. There are multiple subtypes of both P2X and P2Y receptors. As with the other cotransmitters, ATP can act prejunctionally to modify its own release *via* receptors for ATP or *via* its metabolic breakdown to adenosine that acts on P1 (adenosine) receptors. ATP is cleared from the synapse primarily by releasable nucleotidases (rNTPase) and by cell-fixed ectonucleotidases.

adrenal cortex. The intra-adrenal portal vascular system carries the corticosteroids directly to the adrenal medullary chromaffin cells, where they induce the synthesis of PNMT (Figure 6–4). The activities of both tyrosine hydroxylase and DβH also are increased in the adrenal medulla when the secretion of glucocorticoids is stimulated (Carroll *et al.*, 1991; Viskupic *et al.*, 1994). Thus, any stress that persists sufficiently to evoke an enhanced secretion of corticotropin mobilizes the appropriate hormones of both the adrenal cortex (predominantly cortisol in humans) and medulla (epinephrine). This remarkable relationship is present only in certain mammals, including humans, in which the adrenal chromaffin cells are enveloped entirely by steroid-secreting cortical cells. In the dogfish, for example, where the chromaffin cells and steroid-secreting cells are located in independent, noncontiguous glands, epinephrine is not formed. Nonetheless, there is evidence indicating that PMNT is expressed in mammalian tissues such as brain, heart, and lung, leading to extra-adrenal epinephrine synthesis (Kennedy *et al.*, 1993).

In addition to its *de novo* synthesis, norepinephrine stores in the terminal portions of the adrenergic fibers are also replenished by active transport of norepinephrine previously released to the extracellular fluid by the norepinephrine transporter (NET, originally named *uptake 1*) (*see* below). To effect the reuptake of norepinephrine into adrenergic nerve terminals and to maintain the concentration gradient of norepinephrine within the vesicles, at least two distinct carrier-mediated transport systems are involved: one across the axoplasmic membrane from the extracellular fluid to the cytoplasm mentioned earlier and the other from the cytoplasm into the storage vesicles, the vesicular monoamine transporter (VMAT-2).

Uptake by the NET is more important than extraneuronal uptake and metabolism of norepinephrine released by neurons. It has been estimated that the sympathetic nerves as a whole remove approximately 87% of released norepinephrine by NET compared with 5% by extraneuronal uptake (ENT, *uptake 2*; *see* below) and 8% diffusion to the circulation. In contrast, clearance of circulating catecholamines is primarily by nonneuronal mechanisms, with liver and kidney accounting for over 60% of the clearance of circulating catecholamines. Because the VMAT-2 has a much higher affinity for norepinephrine than does monoamine oxidase (MAO), over 70% of recaptured norepinephrine is sequestered into storage vesicles (Eisenhofer, 2001).

Storage of Catecholamines. Catecholamines are stored in vesicles, ensuring their regulated release; this storage decreases intraneuronal metabolism of these transmitters and their leakage outside the cell. The vesicular amine transporter (VMAT-2) extensively appears to be driven by pH and potential gradients that are established by an ATP-dependent proton translocase. For every molecule of amine taken up, two H$^+$ ions are extruded (Brownstein and Hoffman, 1994). Monoamine transporters are relatively promiscuous and transport dopamine, norepinephrine, epinephrine, and serotonin, for example, as well as *meta-iodobenzylguanidine,* can be used to image chromaffin cell tumors (Schuldiner, 1994). *Reserpine* inhibits monoamine transport into storage vesicles and ultimately leads to depletion of catecholamine from sympathetic

nerve endings and in the brain. Several vesicular transport cDNAs have been cloned; these cDNAs reveal open reading frames predictive of proteins with 12 transmembrane domains (*see* Chapter 2). Regulation of the expression of these various transporters may be important in the regulation of synaptic transmission (Varoqui and Erickson, 1997).

There are two neuronal membrane transporters for catecholamines, the norepinephrine transporter (NET) mentioned earlier and the dopamine transporter (DAT); their characteristics are depicted in Table 6–5. The NET is also present in the adrenal medulla, the liver, and the placenta, whereas the DAT is present in the stomach, pancreas, and kidney (Eisenhofer, 2001).

NET is Na$^+$-dependent and is blocked selectively by a number of drugs, including *cocaine* and tricyclic antidepressants such as *imipramine*. This transporter has a high affinity for norepinephrine and a somewhat lower affinity for epinephrine (Table 6–5); the synthetic β adrenergic receptor agonist *isoproterenol* is not a substrate for this system. A number of highly specific neurotransmitter transporters have been identified. High-affinity transporters include those for dopamine, norepinephrine, serotonin, and a variety of amino acid transmitters (Amara and Kuhar, 1993; Brownstein and Hoffman, 1994; Masson *et al.*, 1999). These transporters are members of an extended family sharing common structural motifs, particularly the putative 12-transmembrane helices. These plasma membrane transporters appear to have greater substrate specificity than do vesicular transporters and may be viewed as targets ("receptors") for specific drugs such as cocaine (dopamine transporter) or *fluoxetine* (serotonin transporter).

Certain sympathomimetic drugs (*e.g., ephedrine* and *tyramine*) produce some of their effects indirectly by displacing norepinephrine from the nerve terminals to the extracellular fluid, where it then acts at receptor sites of the effector cells. The mechanisms by which these drugs release norepinephrine from nerve endings are complex. All such agents are substrates for NET. As a result of their transport across the neuronal membrane and release into the axoplasm, they make carrier available at the inner surface of the membrane for the outward transport of norepinephrine ("facilitated exchange diffusion"). In addition, these amines are able to mobilize norepinephrine stored in the vesicles by competing for the vesicular uptake process. Reserpine, which depletes vesicular stores of norepinephrine, also inhibits this uptake mechanism, but in contrast with the indirect-acting sympathomimetic amines, it enters the adrenergic nerve ending by passive diffusion across the axonal membrane.

Table 6–5
Characteristics of Transporters for Endogenous Catecholamines

TYPE OF TRANSPORTER	SUBSTRATE SPECIFICITY	TISSUE	REGION/CELL TYPE	INHIBITORS
Neuronal				
NET	DA > NE > Epi	All sympathetically innervated tissue	Sympathetic nerves	Desipramine, cocaine, nisoxetine
		Adrenal medulla	Chromaffin cells	
		Liver	Capillary endothelial cells	
		Placenta	Syncytiotrophoblast	
DAT	DA >> NE > Epi	Kidney	Endothelium	Cocaine, imazindol
		Stomach	Parietal and endothelial cells	
		Pancreas	Pancreatic duct	
Nonneuronal:				
OCT 1	DA ≈ Epi >> NE	Liver	Hepatocytes	Isocyanines; corticosterone
		Intestine	Epithelial cells	
		Kidney (not human)	Distal tubule	
OCT 2	DA >> NE > Epi	Kidney	Medullary proximal and distal tubules	Isocyanines; corticosterone
		Brain	Glial cells of DA-rich regions, some non-adrenergic neurons	
ENT (OCT 3)	Epi >> NE > DA	Liver	Hepatocytes	Isocyanines; corticosterone; *O*-methyl-isoproterenol
		Brain	Glial cells, others	
		Heart	Myocytes	
		Blood vessels	Endothelial cells	
		Kidney	Cortex, proximal and distal tubules	
		Placenta	Syncytiotrophoblasts (basal membrane)	
		Retina	Photoreceptors, ganglion amacrine cells	

ABBREVIATIONS: NET, norepinephrine transporter, originally known as uptake 1; DAT, dopamine transporter; ENT (OCT3), extraneuronal transporter, originally known as uptake 2; OCT 1, OCT 2, organic cation transporters; Epi, epinephrine; NE, norepinephrine; DA, dopamine.

The actions of indirect-acting sympathomimetic amines are subject to *tachyphylaxis*. For example, repeated administration of tyramine results in rapidly decreasing effectiveness, whereas repeated administration of norepinephrine does not reduce effectiveness and, in fact, reverses the tachyphylaxis to tyramine. Although these phenomena have not been explained fully, several hypotheses have been proposed. One possible explanation is that the pool of neurotransmitter available for displacement by these drugs is small relative to the total amount stored in the sympathetic nerve ending. This pool is presumed to reside in close proximity to the plasma membrane, and the norepinephrine of such vesicles may be replaced by the less potent amine following repeated administration of the latter substance. In any case, neurotransmitter release by displacement is not associated with the release of

DβH and does not require extracellular Ca^{2+}; thus, it is presumed not to involve exocytosis.

There are also three extraneuronal transporters that handle a wide range of endogenous and exogenous substrates. The extraneuronal amine transporter (ENT), originally named *uptake-2* and also designated *OCT3,* is an organic cation transporter. Relative to NET, ENT exhibits lower affinity for catecholamines, favors epinephrine over norepinephrine or dopamine, and shows a higher maximum rate of catecholamine uptake. The ENT is not Na^+-dependent and displays a completely different profile of pharmacological inhibition. Other members of this family are the organic cation transporters OCT1 and OCT2 (*see* Chapter 2). All three can transport catecholamines in addition to a wide variety of other organic acids, including serotonin, histamine, choline, spermine, guanidine, and creatinine (Eisenhofer, 2001). The characteristics and location of the nonneuronal transporters are summarized in Table 6–5.

Release of Catecholamines. The full sequence of steps by which the nerve impulse effects the release of norepinephrine from sympathetic neurons is not known. In the adrenal medulla, the triggering event is the liberation of ACh by the preganglionic fibers and its interaction with nicotinic receptors on chromaffin cells to produce a localized depolarization; a subsequent step is the entrance of Ca^{2+} into these cells, which results in the extrusion by exocytosis of the granular contents, including epinephrine, ATP, some neuroactive peptides or their precursors, chromogranins, and DβH. Influx of Ca^{2+} likewise plays an essential role in coupling the nerve impulse, membrane depolarization, and opening of voltage-gated Ca^{2+} channels with the release of norepinephrine at sympathetic nerve terminals. Blockade of N-type Ca^{2+} channels leads to hypotension likely owing to inhibition of norepinephrine release. Ca^{2+}-triggered secretion involves interaction of highly conserved molecular scaffolding proteins leading to docking of granules at the plasma membrane and ultimately leading to secretion (Aunis, 1998).

Reminiscent of the release of ACh at cholinergic terminals, various synaptic proteins, including the plasma membrane proteins syntaxin and synaptosomal protein 25kDa (SNAP-25), and the vesicle membrane protein synaptobrevin form a complex that interacts in an ATP-dependent manner with the soluble proteins *N*-ethylmaleimide-sensitive fusion protein (NSF) and soluble NSF attachment proteins (SNAPs). The ability of synaptobrevin, syntaxin, and SNAP-25 to bind SNAPs has led to their designation as *SNAP receptors* (SNAREs). It has been hypothesized that most, if not all, intracellular fusion events are mediated by SNARE interactions (Boehm and Kubista, 2002). As with cholinergic neurotransmission, important evidence supporting the involvement of SNARE proteins (*e.g.,* SNAP-25, syntaxin, and synaptobrevin) in transmitter release comes from the fact that botulinum neurotoxins and tetanus toxin, which potently block neurotransmitter release, proteolyze these proteins.

Enhanced activity of the sympathetic nervous system is accompanied by an increased concentration of both DβH and chromogranins in the circulation, supporting the argument that the process of release following adrenergic nerve stimulation also involves exocytosis.

Adrenergic fibers can sustain the output of norepinephrine during prolonged periods of stimulation without exhausting their reserve supply, provided that synthesis and uptake of the transmitter are unimpaired. To meet increased needs for norepinephrine, acute regulatory mechanisms are evoked involving activation of tyrosine hydroxylase and DβH (*see* above).

Prejunctional Regulation of Norepinephrine Release

The release of the three sympathetic cotransmitters can be modulated by prejunctional autoreceptors and heteroreceptors. Following their release from sympathetic terminals, all three cotransmitters—norepinephrine, neuropeptide Y (NPY), and ATP—can feedback on prejunctional receptors to inhibit the release of each other (Westfall, *et al.,* 2002; Westfall, 2004). The most thoroughly studied have been prejunctional α_2 adrenergic receptors. The α_{2A} and α_{2C} adrenergic receptors are the principal prejunctional receptors that inhibit sympathetic neurotransmitter release, whereas the α_{2B} adrenergic receptors also may inhibit transmitter release at selected sites. Antagonists of this receptor, in turn, can enhance the electrically evoked release of sympathetic neurotransmitter. NPY, acting on Y_2 receptors, and ATP-derived adenosine, acting on P1 receptors, also can inhibit sympathetic neurotransmitter release. Numerous heteroreceptors on sympathetic nerve varicosities also inhibit the release of sympathetic neurotransmitters; these include: M_2 and M_4 muscarinic, serotonin, PGE_2, histamine, enkephalin, and dopamine receptors. Enhancement of sympathetic neurotransmitter release can be produced by activation of β_2 adrenergic receptors, angiotensin II receptors, and nACh receptors. All these receptors can be targets for agonists and antagonists.

Termination of the Actions of Catecholamines. The actions of norepinephrine and epinephrine are terminated by (1) reuptake into nerve terminals by NET; (2) dilution by diffusion out of the junctional cleft and uptake at extraneuronal sites by ENT, OCT 1, and OCT 2; and (3) metabolic transformation. Two enzymes are important in the initial steps of metabolic transformation of catecholamines—monoamine oxidase (MAO) and catechol-*O*-methyltransferase (COMT). In addition, catecholamines are metabolized by sulfotransferases (Dooley, 1998) (*see* Chapter 3). However, termination of action by a powerful degradative enzymatic pathway, such as that provided by AChE at sites of cholinergic transmission, is absent from the adrenergic nervous system. The importance of neuronal reuptake of catecholamines is shown by observations that inhibitors of this process (*e.g.,* cocaine and imipramine) potentiate the effects of the neurotransmitter; inhibitors of MAO and COMT have relatively little effect. However, MAO metabolizes transmitter that is released within the nerve terminal. COMT, particularly in the liver, plays a major role in the metabolism of endogenous circulating and administered catecholamines.

Both MAO and COMT are distributed widely throughout the body, including the brain; the highest concentrations of each are in the liver and the kidney. However, little or no COMT is found in sympathetic neurons. In the brain, there is also no significant COMT in presynaptic terminals, but it is found in some postsynaptic neurons and glial cells. In the kidney, COMT is localized in proximal tubular epithelial cells, where dopamine is synthesized, and is thought to exert local diuretic and natriuretic effects. The physiological substrates for COMT include L-dopa, all three endogenous catecholamines (dopamine, norepinephrine, and epinephrine), their hydroxylated metabolites, catecholestrogens, ascorbic acid, and dihydroxyindolic intermediates of melanin (*see* review by Männistö and Kaakkola, 1999). There are distinct differences in the cytological locations of the two enzymes; MAO is associated chiefly with the outer surface of mitochondria, including those within the terminals of sympathetic or central noradrenergic neuronal fibers, whereas COMT is largely cytoplasmic. These factors are of importance both in determining the primary metabolic pathways followed by catecholamines in various circumstances and in explaining the effects of certain drugs. Two different isozymes of MAO (MAO-A and MAO-B) are found in widely varying proportions in different cells in the CNS and in peripheral tissues. In the periphery, MAO-A is located in the syncytiotrophoblast layer of term placenta and liver, whereas MAO-B is located in platelets, lymphocytes, and liver. In the brain, MAO-A is located in all regions containing catecholamines, with the highest abundance in the locus ceruleus. MAO-B, on the other hand, is found primarily in regions that are known to synthesize and store serotonin. MAO-B is most prominent in the nucleus raphe dorsalis but also in the posterior hypothalamus and in glial cells in regions known to contain nerve terminals. MAO-B is also present in osteocytes around blood vessels (Abell and Kwan, 2001). Selective inhibitors of these two isozymes are available (*see* Chapter 17). Irreversible antagonists of MAO-A (*e.g., phenelzine, tranylcypromine,* and *isocarboxazid*) enhance the bioavailability of tyramine contained in many foods; tyramine-induced norepinephrine release from sympathetic neurons may lead to markedly increased blood pressure (hypertensive crisis). Selective MAO-B inhibitors (*e.g., selegiline*) or reversible MAO-A–selective inhibitors (*e.g., moclobemide*) are less likely to cause this potential interaction (Volz and Geiter, 1998; Wouters, 1998). MAO inhibitors are useful in the treatment of Parkinson's disease and mental depression (*see* Chapters 17 and 20).

Most of the epinephrine and norepinephrine that enters the circulation—from the adrenal medulla or following administration or that is released by exocytosis from sympathetic fibers—is methylated by COMT to metanephrine or normetanephrine, respectively (Figure 6–6). Norepinephrine that is released intraneuronally by drugs such as reserpine is deaminated initially by MAO to 3,4-dihydroxyphenylglycolaldehyde (DOPGAL) (Figure 6–6). The aldehyde is reduced by aldehyde reductase to 3,4-dihydroxyphenylethylene glycol (DOPEG) or is oxidized by aldehyde dehydrogenase to form

3,4-dihydroxymandelic acid (DOMA). 3-Methoxy-4-hydroxymandelic acid [generally but incorrectly called *vanillylmandelic acid* (VMA)] is the major metabolite of catecholamines excreted in the urine. The corresponding product of the metabolic degradation of dopamine, which contains no hydroxyl group in the side chain, is homovanillic acid (HVA). Other metabolic reactions are described in Figure 6–6. Measurement of the concentrations of catecholamines and their metabolites in blood and urine is useful in the diagnosis of pheochromocytoma, a catecholamine-secreting tumor of the adrenal medulla.

Inhibitors of MAO (*e.g., pargyline* and *nialamide*) can cause an increase in the concentration of norepinephrine, dopamine, and 5-HT in the brain and other tissues accompanied by a variety of pharmacological effects. No striking pharmacological action in the periphery can be attributed to the inhibition of COMT. However, the COMT inhibitors *entacapone* and *tocapone* have been found to be efficacious in the therapy of Parkinson's disease (Chong and Mersfelder, 2000) (*see* Chapter 20).

Classification of Adrenergic Receptors. Crucial to understanding the remarkably diverse effects of the catecholamines and related sympathomimetic agents is an understanding of the classification and properties of the different types of adrenergic receptors (or adrenoceptors). Elucidation of the characteristics of these receptors and the biochemical and physiological pathways they regulate has increased our understanding of the seemingly contradictory and variable effects of catecholamines on various organ systems. Although structurally related (*see* below), different receptors regulate distinct physiological processes by controlling the synthesis or release of a variety of second messengers (Tables 6–6 and 6–7).

Based on studies of the abilities of epinephrine, norepinephrine, and other related agonists to regulate various physiological processes, Ahlquist first proposed the existence of more than one adrenergic receptor. It was known that these drugs could cause either contraction or relaxation of smooth muscle depending on the site, the dose, and the agent chosen. For example, norepinephrine was known to have potent excitatory effects on smooth muscle and correspondingly low activity as an inhibitor; isoproterenol displayed the opposite pattern of activity. Epinephrine could both excite and inhibit smooth muscle. Thus, Ahlquist proposed the designations α and β for receptors on smooth muscle where catecholamines produce excitatory and inhibitory responses, respectively. An exception is the gut, which generally is relaxed by activation of either α or β receptors. The rank order of potency of agonists is isoproterenol > epinephrine $\geq$ norepinephrine for β adrenergic receptors and epinephrine $\geq$ norepinephrine >> isoproterenol for α adrenergic receptors (Table 6–3). This initial classification was corroborated by the finding that certain antagonists produce selective blockade of the effects of adrenergic nerve impulses and sympathomimetic agents at α receptors (*e.g., phenoxybenzamine*), whereas others produce selective β receptor blockade (*e.g., propranolol*).

β Receptors later were subdivided into β_1 (*e.g.,* those in the myocardium) and β_2 (smooth muscle and most other sites) because

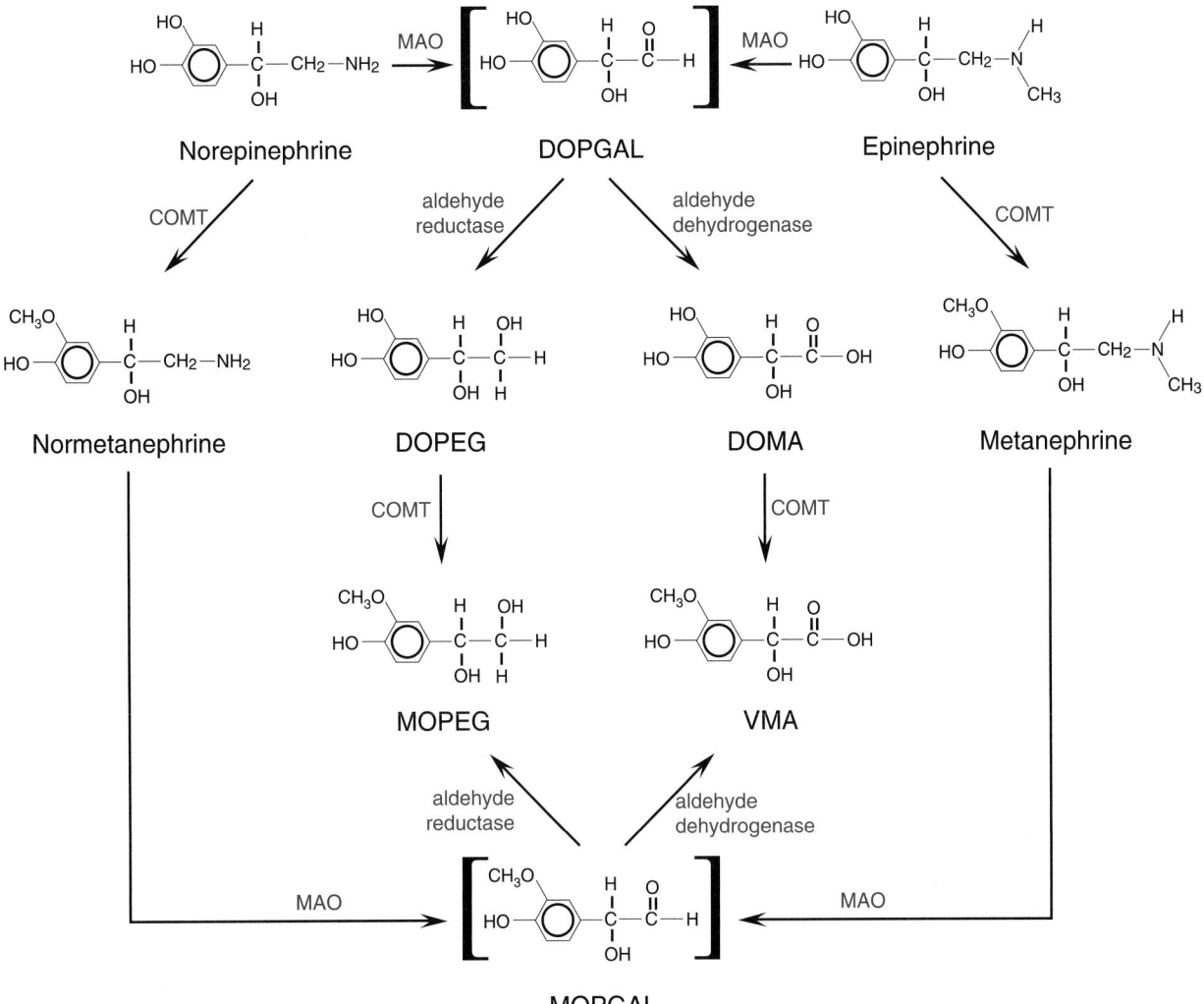

Figure 6–6. *Steps in the metabolic disposition of catecholamines.* Norepinephrine and epinephrine are first oxidatively deaminated by monoamine oxidase (MAO) to 3,4-dihydroxyphenylglycoaldehyde (DOPGAL) and then either reduced to 3,4-dihydroxyphenyl-ethylene glycol (DOPEG) or oxidized to 3,4-dihydroxymandelic acid (DOMA). Alternatively, they can be methylated initially by cate-chol-*O*-methyltransferase (COMT) to normetanephrine and metanephrine, respectively. Most of the products of either type of reaction then are metabolized by the other enzyme to form the major excretory products in blood and urine, 3-methoxy-4-hydroxyphenylethyl-ene glycol (MOPEG or MHPG) and 3-methoxy-4-hydroxymandelic acid (VMA). Free MOPEG is largely converted to VMA. The glycol and, to some extent, the *O*-methylated amines and the catecholamines may be conjugated to the corresponding sulfates or glu-curonides. (Modified from Axelrod, 1966, and others.)

epinephrine and norepinephrine essentially are equipotent at the former sites, whereas epinephrine is 10 to 50 times more potent than norepinephrine at the latter. Antagonists that discriminate between β_1 and β_2 receptors subsequently were developed (*see* Chapter 10). A human gene that encodes a third β receptor (designated β_3) has been isolated (Emorine *et al.*, 1989; Granneman *et al.*, 1993). Since the β_3 receptor is about tenfold more sensitive to norepinephrine than to epinephrine and is relatively resistant to blockade by antago-nists such as propranolol, it may mediate responses to catecho-la-mine at sites with "atypical" pharmacological characteristics (*e.g.*,

adipose tissue). Although the adipocytes are a major site of β_3 adre-nergic receptors, all three β adrenergic receptors are present in both white adipose tissue (WAT) and brown adipose tissue (BAT). Ani-mals treated with β_3 receptor agonists exhibit a vigorous thermogen-ic response as well as lipolysis (Robidoux *et al.*, 2004). Polymor-phisms in the β_3 receptor gene may be related to risk of obesity or type 2 diabetes in some populations (Arner and Hoffstedt, 1999). Also, there has been interest in the possibility that β_3-receptor–selective agonists may be beneficial in treating these disorders (Weyer *et al.*, 1999).

Table 6–6
Characteristics of Subtypes of Adrenergic Receptors*

RECEPTOR	AGONISTS	ANTAGONISTS	TISSUE	RESPONSES
α_1[†]	Epi ≥ NE >> Iso Phenylephrine	Prazosin	Vascular smooth muscle GU smooth muscle Liver[‡] Intestinal smooth muscle Heart	Contraction Contraction Glycogenolysis; gluconeogenesis Hyperpolarization and relaxation Increased contractile force; arrhythmias
α_2[†]	Epi ≥ NE >> Iso Clonidine	Yohimbine	Pancreatic islets (β cells) Platelets Nerve terminals Vascular smooth muscle	Decreased insulin secretion Aggregation Decreased release of NE Contraction
β_1	Iso > Epi = NE Dobutamine	Metoprolol CGP 20712A	Juxtaglomerular cells Heart	Increased renin secretion Increased force and rate of contraction and AV nodal conduction velocity
β_2	Iso > Epi >> NE Terbutaline	ICI 118551	Smooth muscle (vascular, bronchial, GI, and GU) Skeletal muscle Liver[‡]	Relaxation Glycogenolysis; uptake of K^+ Glycogenolysis; gluconeogenesis
β_3[§]	Iso = NE > Epi BRL 37344	ICI 118551 CGP 20712A	Adipose tissue	Lipolysis

ABBREVIATIONS: Epi, epinephrine; NE, norepinephrine; Iso, isoproterenol; GI, gastrointestinal; GU, genitourinary. *This table provides examples of drugs that act on adrenergic receptors and of the location of subtypes of adrenergic receptors. [†]At least three subtypes each of α_1 and α_2 adrenergic receptors are known, but distinctions in their mechanisms of action have not been clearly defined. [‡]In some species (*e.g.*, rat), metabolic responses in the liver are mediated by α_1 adrenergic receptors, whereas in others (*e.g.*, dog) β_2 adrenergic receptors are predominantly involved. Both types of receptors appear to contribute to responses in human beings. [§]Metabolic responses in adipocytes and certain other tissues with atypical pharmacological characteristics may be mediated by this subtype of receptor. Most β adrenergic receptor antagonists (including propranolol) do not block these responses.

The heterogeneity of α adrenergic receptors also is now appreciated. The initial distinction was based on functional and anatomical considerations when it was realized that norepinephrine and other α-adrenergic receptors could profoundly inhibit the release of norepinephrine from neurons (Westfall, 1977) (Figure 6–5). Indeed, when sympathetic nerves are stimulated in the presence of certain α receptor antagonists, the amount of norepinephrine liberated by each nerve impulse increases markedly. This feedback-inhibitory effect of norepinephrine on its release from nerve terminals is mediated by α receptors that are pharmacologically distinct from the classical postsynaptic α receptors. Accordingly, these presynaptic α adrenergic receptors were designated α_2, whereas the postsynaptic "excitatory" α receptors were designated α_1 (*see* Langer, 1997). Compounds such as *clonidine* are more potent agonists at α_2 than at α_1 receptors; by contrast, *phenylephrine* and *methoxamine* selectively activate postsynaptic α_1 receptors. Although there is little evidence to suggest that α_1 adrenergic receptors function presynaptically in the autonomic nervous system, it now is clear that α_2 receptors

also are present at postjunctional or nonjunctional sites in several tissues. For example, stimulation of postjunctional α_2 receptors in the brain is associated with reduced sympathetic outflow from the CNS and appears to be responsible for a significant component of the antihypertensive effect of drugs such as clonidine (*see* Chapter 10). Thus, the anatomical concept of prejunctional α_2 and postjunctional α_1 adrenergic receptors has been abandoned in favor of a pharmacological and functional classification (Table 6–6 and 6–8).

Cloning revealed additional heterogeneity of both α_1 and α_2 adrenergic receptors (Bylund, 1992). There are three pharmacologically defined α_1 receptors (α_{1A}, α_{1B}, and α_{1D}) with distinct sequences and tissue distributions (Tables 6–6 and 6–8). There are also three cloned subtypes of α_2 receptors (α_{2A}, α_{2B}, and α_{2C}) (Table 6–8). Distinct patterns of distribution of these subtypes exist.

Owing to the lack of sufficiently subtype-selective ligands, the precise physiological function and therapeutic potential of the subtypes of adrenergic receptors have not been elucidated fully. Great

Table 6–7
Adrenergic Receptors and Their Effector Systems

ADRENERGIC RECEPTOR	G PROTEIN	EXAMPLES OF SOME BIOCHEMICAL EFFECTORS
β_1	G_s	↑ adenylyl cyclase, ↑ L-type Ca^{2+} channels
β_2	G_s	↑ adenylyl cyclase
β_3	G_s	↑ adenylyl cyclase
α_1 Subtypes	G_q	↑ phospholipase C
	G_q	↑ phospholipase D
	G_q, G_i/G_o	↑ phospholipase A_2
	G_q	? ↑ Ca^{2+} channels
α_2 Subtypes	$G_{i\ 1,\ 2,\ or\ 3}$	↓ adenylyl cyclase
	G_i ($\beta\gamma$ subunits)	↑ K^+ channels
	G_o	↓ Ca^{2+} channels (L- and N-type)
	?	↑ PLC, PLA_2

advances in our understanding have been made through the use of genetic approaches using transgenic and receptor knockout experiments in mice (discussed below). These mouse models have been used to identify the particular receptor subtypes and pathophysiological relevance of individual adrenergic receptors subtypes (Steinberg, 2002; Tanoue *et al.*, 2002a, 2002b, 2002c; Hein and Schmitt, 2003; Philipp and Hein, 2004).

Molecular Basis of Adrenergic Receptor Function. All of the adrenergic receptors are GPCRs that link to heterotrimeric G proteins. Each major type shows preference for a particular class of G proteins, *i.e.*, α_1 to G_q, α_2 to G_i, and β to G_s (Table 6–7). The responses that follow activation of all types of adrenergic receptors result from G protein–mediated effects on the generation of second messengers and on the activity of ion channels. As discussed in Chapter 1, these systems involve three interacting proteins—the GPCR, the coupling G protein, and effector enzymes or ion channels. The pathways overlap broadly with those discussed for muscarinic acetylcholine receptors and are summarized in Table 6–7.

Structure of Adrenergic Receptors. Adrenergic receptors constitute a family of closely related proteins that are related both structurally and functionally to GPCRs for a wide variety of other hormones and neurotransmitters (Lefkowitz, 2000). The GPCR family includes the muscarinic ACh receptors and the visual "photon receptor"

rhodopsin (*see* Chapter 1). Ligand binding, site-directed labeling, and mutagenesis have revealed that the conserved membrane-spanning regions are crucially involved in ligand binding (Strader *et al.*, 1994; Hutchins, 1994). These regions appear to create a ligand-binding pocket analogous to that formed by the membrane-spanning regions of rhodopsin to accommodate the covalently attached chromophore, retinal, with molecular models placing catecholamines either horizontally (Strader *et al.*, 1994) or perpendicularly (Hutchins, 1994) in the bilayer. The crystal structure of mammalian rhodopsin confirms a number of predictions about the structure of GPCRs (Palczewski *et al.*, 2000).

β Adrenergic Receptors. The three β receptors share approximately 60% amino acid sequence identity within the presumed membrane-spanning domains where the ligand-binding pocket for epinephrine and norepinephrine is found. Based on results of site-directed mutagenesis, individual amino acids in the β_2 receptor that interact with each of the functional groups on the catecholamine agonist molecule have been identified.

β Receptors regulate numerous functional responses, including heart rate and contractility, smooth muscle relaxation, and multiple metabolic events (Table 6–1). All three of the β receptor subtypes (β_1, β_2, and β_3) couple to G_s and activate adenylyl cyclase (Table 6–7). However, recent data suggest differences in downstream signals and events activated by the three β receptors (Lefkowitz, 2000; Ma and Huang, 2002). Catecholamines promote β receptor feedback regulation, *i.e.*, desensitization and receptor down-regulation (Kohout and Lefkowitz, 2003). β Receptors differ in the extent to which they undergo such regulation, with the β_2 receptor being the most susceptible. Stimulation of β adrenergic receptors leads to the accumulation of cyclic AMP, activation of the PKA, and altered function of numerous cellular proteins as a result of their phosphorylation (*see* Chapter 1). In addition, G_s can enhance directly the activation of voltage-sensitive Ca^{2+} channels in the plasma membrane of skeletal and cardiac muscle.

Several reports demonstrate that β_1, β_2, and β_3 receptors differ in their intracellular signaling pathways and subcellular location. While the positive chronotropic effects of β_1 receptor activation are clearly mediated *via* G_s in myocytes, dual coupling of β_2 receptors to G_s and G_i occurs in myocytes from newborn mice. Stimulation of β_2 receptors caused a transient increase in heart rate that is followed by a prolonged decrease. Following pretreatment with pertussis toxin, which prevents activation of G_i, the negative chronotropic effect of β_2 activation is abolished. It is thought that these specific signaling properties of β receptor subtypes are linked to subtype-selective association with intracellular scaffolding and signaling proteins (Baillie and Houslay, 2005).

Table 6–8
Subtypes of Adrenergic Receptors

SUBTYPE	GENE LOCATION IN HUMAN CHROMOSOME	TISSUE LOCALIZATION	SUBTYPE DOMINANT EFFECTS
α_{1A}	8	Heart, liver, cerebellum cerebral cortex, prostate, lung, vas deferens, blood vessels	Predominant receptor causing contraction of smooth muscle including vasoconstriction in numerous arteries and veins. With α_{1B} promotes cardiac growth and structure
α_{1B}	5	Kidney, spleen, lung, cerebral cortex, blood vessels	Most abundant subtype in heart; with α_{1A} promotes cardiac growth and structure
α_{1D}	20	Platelets, cerebral cortex, prostate, hippocampus, aorta, coronary arteries	Predominant receptor causing vasoconstriction in the aorta and coronary arteries
α_{2A}	10	Platelets, cerebral cortex, locus ceruleus, spinal cord, sympathetic neurons; autonomic ganglia	Predominant inhibitory autoreceptor in sympathetic nerve varicosities. Predominant receptor mediating α_2 agonist–induced antinociception, sedation, hypotension, and hypothermia
α_{2B}	2	Liver, kidney, blood vessels	Predominant receptor mediating α_2-induced vasoconstriction
α_{2C}	4	Cerebral cortex	Predominant receptor modulating dopamine neurotransmission. Predominant inhibitory receptor on adrenal medulla
β_1	$10_{q240q26}$	Heart, kidney, adipocytes, other tissues	Predominant receptor in heart producing + inotropic and chronotropic effects
β_2	$5_{q32-q32}$	Heart; vascular, bronchial, and GI smooth muscle; glands; leukocytes; hepatocytes	Prominent receptor in smooth muscle producing relaxation; highly polymorphic
β_3	$8_{p12-p11.2}$	Adipose tissue, GI tract, other tissue	Prominent adrenergic receptor producing metabolic effects

β_2 Receptors normally are confined to caveolae in cardiac myocyte membranes. The activation of PKA by AMP and the importance of compartmentation of components of the cyclic AMP pathway are discussed in Chapter 1.

α Adrenergic Receptors. The deduced amino acid sequences from the three α_1 receptor genes (α_{1A}, α_{1B}, and α_{1D}) and three α_2 receptor genes (α_{2A}, α_{2B}, and α_{2C}) conform to the well-established GPCR paradigm (Zhong and Minneman, 1999; Bylund, 1992). While not as thoroughly investigated as β receptors, the general structural features and their relation to the functions of ligand binding and G protein activation appear to agree with those set forth in Chapter 1 and above for the β receptors. Within the membrane-spanning domains, the three α_1 adrenergic receptors share approximately 75% identity in amino acid residues, as do the three α_2 receptors, but the α_1 and α_2 subtypes are no more similar than are the α and β subtypes (approximately 30% to 40%).

α_2 Adrenergic Receptors. As shown in Table 6–7, α_2 receptors couple to a variety of effectors (Aantaa et al., 1995; Bylund, 1992). Inhibition of adenylyl cyclase activity was the first effect observed, but in some systems the enzyme actually is stimulated by α_2 adrenergic receptors, either by G_i $\beta\gamma$ subunits or by weak direct stimulation of G_s. The physiological significance of these latter processes is not currently clear. α_2 Receptors activate G protein–gated K^+ channels, resulting in membrane hyperpolarization.

In some cases (*e.g.*, cholinergic neurons in the myenteric plexus) this may be Ca^{2+}-dependent, whereas in others (*e.g.*, muscarinic ACh receptors in atrial myocytes) it results from direct interaction of $\beta\gamma$ subunits with K^+ channels. α_2 Receptors also can inhibit voltage-gated Ca^{2+} channels; this is mediated by G_o. Other second-messenger systems linked to α_2 receptor activation include acceleration of Na^+/H^+ exchange, stimulation of phospholipase $C_{\beta 2}$ activity and arachidonic acid mobilization, increased phosphoinositide hydrolysis, and increased intracellular availability of Ca^{2+}. The latter is involved in the smooth muscle–contracting effect of α_2 adrenergic receptor agonists. In addition, the α_2 receptors activate mitogen-activated protein kinases (MAPKs) likely *via* $\beta\gamma$ subunits released from pertussis toxin–sensitive G proteins (Della Rocca *et al.*, 1997; Richman and Regan, 1998). This and related pathways lead to activation of a variety of tyrosine kinase–mediated downstream events. These pathways are reminiscent of pathways activated by tyrosine kinase activities of growth factor receptors. Although α_2 receptors may activate several different signaling pathways, the exact contribution of each to many physiological processes is not clear. The α_{2A} receptor plays a major role in inhibiting norepinephrine release from sympathetic nerve endings and suppressing sympathetic outflow from the brain, leading to hypotension (MacMillan *et al.*, 1996; Docherty, 1998; Kable *et al.*, 2000).

In the CNS, α_{2A} receptors, which appear to be the most dominant adrenergic receptor, probably produce the antinociceptive effects, sedation, hypothermia, hypotension, and behavioral actions of α_2 agonists (Lakhlani *et al.*, 1997). The α_{2C} receptor occurs in the ventral and dorsal striatum and hippocampus. It appears to modulate dopamine neurotransmission and various behavioral responses. The α_{2B} receptor is the main receptor mediating α_2-induced vasoconstriction, whereas the α_{2C} receptor is the predominant receptor inhibiting the release of catecholamines from the adrenal medulla and modulating dopamine neurotransmission in the brain.

α_1 Adrenergic Receptors. Stimulation of α_1 receptors results in the regulation of multiple effector systems. A primary mode of signal transduction involves activation of the G_q-PLC_β-IP_3-Ca^{2+} pathway and the activation of other Ca^{2+} and calmodulin sensitive pathways such as CaM kinases (*see* Chapter 1). For example, α_1 receptors regulate hepatic glycogenolysis in some animal species; this effect results from the activation of phosphorylase kinase by the mobilized Ca^{2+}, aided by the inhibition of glycogen synthase caused by PKC-mediated phosphorylation. PKC phosphorylates many substrates, including membrane proteins such as channels, pumps, and ion-exchange proteins (*e.g.*, Ca^{2+}-transport ATPase). These effects presumably lead to regulation of various ion conductances.

α_1 Receptor stimulation of phospholipase A_2 leads to the release of free arachidonate, which is then metabolized *via* the cyclooxygenase and lipoxygenase pathways to the bioactive prostaglandins and leukotrienes, respectively (*see* Chapter 25). Stimulation of phospholipase A_2 activity by various agonists (including epinephrine acting at α_1 receptors) is found in many tissues and cell lines, suggesting that this effector is physiologically important. Phospholipase D hydrolyzes phosphatidylcholine to yield phosphatidic acid (PA). Although PA itself may act as a second messenger by releasing Ca^{2+} from intracellular stores, it also is metabolized to the second messenger DAG. Phospholipase D is an effector for ADP-ribosylating factor (ARF), suggesting that phospholipase D may play a role in membrane trafficking. Finally, some evidence in vascular

smooth muscle suggests that α_1 receptors are capable of regulating a Ca^{2+} channel *via* a G protein.

In most smooth muscles, the increased concentration of intracellular Ca^{2+} ultimately causes contraction as a result of activation of Ca^{2+}-sensitive protein kinases such as the calmodulin-dependent myosin light-chain kinase; phosphorylation of the light chain of myosin is associated with the development of tension (Stull *et al.*, 1990). In contrast, the increased concentration of intracellular Ca^{2+} that result from stimulation of α_1 receptors in gastrointestinal smooth muscle causes hyperpolarization and relaxation by activation of Ca^{2+}-dependent K^+ channels (McDonald *et al.*, 1994).

As with α_2 receptors, there is considerable evidence demonstrating that α_1 receptors activate MAPKs and other kinases such as PI3 kinase leading to important effects on cell growth and proliferation (Dorn and Brown, 1999; Gutkind, 1998). For example, prolonged stimulation of α_1 receptors promotes growth of cardiac myocytes and vascular smooth muscle cells. The α_{1A} receptor is the predominant receptor causing vasoconstriction in many vascular beds, including the following arteries: mammary, mesenteric, splenic, hepatic, omental, renal, pulmonary, and epicardial coronary. It is also the predominant subtype in the vena cava and the saphenous and pulmonary veins (Michelotti *et al.*, 2001). Together with the α_{1B} receptor subtype, it promotes cardiac growth and structure. The α_{1B} receptor subtype is the most abundant subtype in the heart, whereas the α_{1D} receptor subtype is the predominant receptor causing vasoconstriction in the aorta. There is evidence to support the idea that α_{1B} receptors mediate behaviors such as reaction to novelty and exploration and are involved in behavioral sensitizations and in the vulnerability to addiction (*see* Chapter 23).

Localization of Adrenergic Receptors. Presynaptically located α_2 and β_2 receptors fulfill important roles in the regulation of neurotransmitter release from sympathetic nerve endings. Presynaptic α_2 receptors also may mediate inhibition of release of neurotransmitters other than norepinephrine in the central and peripheral nervous systems. Both α_2 and β_2 receptors are located at postsynaptic sites, *e.g.*, on many types of neurons in the brain. In peripheral tissues, postsynaptic α_2 receptors are found in vascular and other smooth muscle cells (where they mediate contraction), adipocytes, and many types of secretory epithelial cells (intestinal, renal, endocrine). Postsynaptic β_2 receptors can be found in the myocardium (where they mediate contraction) as well as on vascular and other smooth muscle cells (where they mediate relaxation). Both α_2 and β_2 receptors may be situated at sites that are relatively remote from nerve terminals releasing norepinephrine. Such extrajunctional receptors typically are found on vascular smooth muscle cells and blood elements (platelets and leukocytes) and may be activated preferentially by circulating catecholamines, particularly epinephrine.

In contrast, α_1 and β_1 receptors appear to be located mainly in the immediate vicinity of sympathetic adrenergic nerve terminals in peripheral target organs, strategically placed to be activated during stimulation of these nerves. These receptors also are distributed widely in the mammalian brain.

The cellular distributions of the three α_1 and three α_2 receptor subtypes still are incompletely understood. *In situ* hybridization of receptor mRNA and receptor subtype-specific antibodies indicates that α_{2A} receptors in the brain may be both pre- and postsynaptic. These findings and other studies indicate that this receptor subtype functions as a presynaptic autoreceptor in central noradrenergic neurons (Aantaa *et al.,* 1995; Lakhlani *et al.,* 1997). Using similar approaches, α_{1A} mRNA was found to be the dominant subtype message expressed in prostatic smooth muscle (Walden *et al.,* 1997).

Refractoriness to Catecholamines. Exposure of catecholamine-sensitive cells and tissues to adrenergic agonists causes a progressive diminution in their capacity to respond to such agents. This phenomenon, variously termed *refractoriness, desensitization,* or *tachyphylaxis,* can limit the therapeutic efficacy and duration of action of catecholamines and other agents (*see* Chapter 1). Although descriptions of such adaptive changes are common, the mechanisms are incompletely understood. They have been studied most extensively in cells that synthesize cyclic AMP in response to β receptor agonists.

Multiple mechanisms are involved in desensitization, including rapid events such as receptor phosphorylation by both G-protein receptor kinases (GRKs) and by signaling kinases such as PKA and PKC and receptor sequestration and uncoupling from G proteins. More slowly occurring events also are seen, such as receptor endocytosis, which decreases receptor number. An understanding of the mechanisms involved in regulation of GPCR desensitization has developed over the last few years (Perry and Lefkowitz, 2002; Lefkowitz *et al.,* 2002, Kohout and Lefkowitz, 2003). Such regulation is very complex and exceeds the simplistic model of GPCR phosphorylation by GRKs followed by arrestin binding and uncoupling of G protein signaling. It is known that GRK activities are extensively regulated by numerous interactions with and modifications by other proteins. β-Arrestin, now recognized as a scaffolding protein, can physically interrupt signaling to the G proteins as well as to further enhance GPCR desensitization by causing translocation of cytosolic proteins to the receptor (*e.g.,* phosphodiesterase and c-Src). These, in turn, can turn off signaling at its source by degrading cyclic AMP or phosphorylating GRK2 to enhance its activity to the receptor.

RELATIONSHIP BETWEEN THE NERVOUS AND THE ENDOCRINE SYSTEMS

The theory of neurohumoral transmission by its very designation implies at least a superficial resemblance between the nervous and endocrine systems. It is now clear that the similarities extend considerably deeper, particularly with respect to the autonomic nervous system. In the regulation of homeostasis, the autonomic nervous system is responsible for rapid adjustments to changes in the environment, which it effects at both its ganglionic synapses and its postganglionic terminals by the liberation of chemical agents that act transiently at their immediate sites of release. The endocrine system, in contrast, regu-

lates slower, more generalized adaptations by releasing hormones into the systemic circulation to act at distant, widespread sites over periods of minutes to hours or days. Both systems have major central representations in the hypothalamus, where they are integrated with each other and with subcortical, cortical, and spinal influences. The neurohumoral theory provides a unitary concept of the functioning of the nervous and endocrine systems in which the differences largely relate to the distances over which the released mediators travel.

PHARMACOLOGICAL CONSIDERATIONS

The foregoing sections contain numerous references to the actions of drugs considered primarily as tools for the dissection and elucidation of physiological mechanisms. This section presents a classification of drugs that act on the peripheral nervous system and its effector organs at some stage of neurotransmission. In the subsequent four chapters, the systematic pharmacology of the important members of each of these classes is described.

Each step involved in neurotransmission (Figures 6–2, 6–3, and 6–5) represents a potential point of therapeutic intervention. This is depicted in the diagrams of the cholinergic and adrenergic terminals and their postjunctional sites (Figure 6–3 and 6–5). Drugs that affect processes involved in each step of transmission at both cholinergic and adrenergic junctions are summarized in Table 6–9, which lists representative agents that act *via* the mechanisms described below.

Interference with the Synthesis or Release of the Transmitter. **Cholinergic.** *Hemicholinium* (HC-3), a synthetic compound, blocks the transport system by which choline accumulates in the terminals of cholinergic fibers, thus limiting the synthesis of the ACh store available for release. *Vesamicol* blocks the transport of ACh into its storage vesicles, preventing its release. The site on the presynaptic nerve terminal for block of ACh release by botulinum toxin was discussed previously; death usually results from respiratory paralysis unless patients with respiratory failure receive artificial ventilation. Injected locally, *botulinum toxin type A* is used in the treatment of certain ophthalmological conditions associated with spasms of ocular muscles (*e.g.,* strabismus and blepharospasm) (*see* Chapter 63) and for a wide variety of unlabeled

Table 6–9

Representative Agents Acting at Peripheral Cholinergic and Adrenergic Neuroeffector Junctions

MECHANISM OF ACTION	SYSTEM	AGENTS	EFFECT
1. Interference with synthesis of transmitter	Cholinergic	Choline acetyl transferase inhibitors	Minimal depletion of ACh
	Adrenergic	α-Methyltyrosine (inhibition of tyrosine hydroxylase)	Depletion of NE
2. Metabolic transformation by same pathway as precursor of transmitter	Adrenergic	Methyldopa	Displacement of NE by α-methyl-NE, which is an α_2 agonist, similar to clonidine, that reduces sympathetic outflow from CNS.
3. Blockade of transport system at nerve terminal membrane	Cholinergic	Hemicholinium	Block of choline uptake with consequent depletion of ACh
	Adrenergic	Cocaine, imipramine	Accumulation of NE at receptors
4. Blockade of transport system of storage vesicle	Cholinergic	Vesamicol	Block of ACh storage
	Adrenergic	Reserpine	Destruction of NE by mitochondrial MAO, and depletion from adrenergic terminals
5. Promotion of exocytosis or displacement of transmitter from axonal terminal	Cholinergic	Latrotoxins	Cholinomimetic followed by anticholinergic
	Adrenergic	Amphetamine, tyramine	Adrenomimetic
6. Prevention of release of transmitter	Cholinergic	Botulinum toxin	Anticholinergic
	Adrenergic	Bretylium, guanadrel	Antiadrenergic
7. Mimicry of transmitter at postjunctional sites	Cholinergic		
	Muscarinic*	Methacholine, bethanachol	Cholinomimetic
	Nicotinic†	Nicotine, epibatidine, cytisine	Cholinomimetic
	Adrenergic		
	α_1	Phenylephrine	Selective α_1 adrenomimetic
	α_2	Clonidine	Adrenomimetic (periphery); reduced sympathetic outflow (CNS)
	α_1, α_2	Oxymetazoline	Non-selective α adrenomimetic
	β_1	Dobutamine	Selective cardiac stimulation (also activates α_1 receptors)
	β_2	Terbutaline, albuterol metaproterenol	Selective β_2 receptor agonist (selective inhibition of smooth muscle contraction)
	β_1, β_2	Isoproterenol	Nonselective β adrenomimetic

(Continued)

Table 6–9
Representative Agents Acting at Peripheral Cholinergic and Adrenergic Neuroeffector Junctions (Continued)

MECHANISM OF ACTION	SYSTEM	AGENTS	EFFECT
8. Blockade of postsynaptic receptor	Cholinergic		
	Muscarinic[*]	Atropine	Muscarinic blockade
	Nicotinic (N_M)[†]	*d*-tubucurarine, atracurium	Neuromuscular blockade
	Nicotinic (N_N)[†]	trimethaphan	Ganglionic blockade
	Adrenergic		
	α_1, α_2	Phenoxybenzamine	Nonselective α receptor blockade (irreversible)
	α_1, α_2	Phentolamine	Nonselective α receptor blockade (reversible)
	α_1	Prazosin, terazosin, doxasozin	Selective α_1 receptor blockade (reversible)
	α_2	Yohimbine	Selective α_2 receptor blockade
	β_1, β_2	Propranolol	Nonselective β receptor blockade
	β_1	Metoprolol, atenolol	Selective β_1 receptor blockade (cardiac)
	β_2	—	Selective β_2 receptor blockade (smooth muscle)
9. Inhibition of enzymatic breakdown of transmitter	Cholinergic	AChE inhibitors (edrophonium, neostigmine, pyridostigmine)	Cholinomimetic (muscarinic sites) Depolarization blockade (nicotinic sites)
	Adrenergic	Nonselective MAO inhibitors (paragyline, nialamide)	Little direct effect on NE or sympathetic response; potentiation of tyramine
		Selective MAO-B inhibitor (selegeline)	Adjunct in Parkinson's disease
		Peripheral COMT inhibitor (entacapone)	
		Peripheral and central COMT inhibitor (tolcapone)	Adjunct in Parkinson's disease

ABBREVIATIONS: ACh, acetylcholine; AChE, acetylcholine esterase; COMT, catechol-*O*-methyl transferase; MAO, monoamine oxidase; NE, norepinephrine. [*]At least five subtypes of muscarinic receptors exist. Agonists show little selectivity for subtypes whereas several antagonists show partial subtype selectivity (*see* Table 6–3). [†]Two subtypes of muscle acetylcholine nicotinic receptors and several subtypes of neuronal receptors have been identified (*see* Table 6–2).

uses ranging from treatment of muscle dystonias and palsy (*see* Chapter 9) to cosmetic erasure of facial lines and wrinkles (*see* Chapter 62).

Adrenergic. α-*Methyltyrosine* (*metyrosine*) blocks the synthesis of norepinephrine by inhibiting tyrosine hydroxylase, the enzyme that catalyzes the rate-limiting step in catecholamine synthesis. This drug occasionally may be useful in treating selected patients with pheochromocytoma. On the other hand, *methyldopa,* an inhibitor of aromatic L-amino acid decarboxylase, is—like dopa itself— successively decarboxylated and hydroxylated in its side chain to form the putative "false neurotransmitter" α-methylnorepinephrine. The use of methyldopa in the treatment of hypertension is discussed in Chapter 32. *Bretylium, guanadrel,* and *guanethidine* act by preventing the release of norepinephrine by the nerve impulse. However, such agents can transiently stimulate the release of norepinephrine because of their capacity to displace the amine from storage sites.

Promotion of the Release of the Transmitter. *Cholinergic.*

The ability of cholinergic agents to promote the release of ACh is limited presumably because ACh and other cholinomimetic agents are quaternary amines and do not readily cross the axonal membrane into the nerve ending. The *latrotoxins* from black widow spider venom and stonefish are known to promote neuroexocytosis by binding to receptors on the neuronal membrane.

Adrenergic. Several drugs that promote the release of the adrenergic mediator already have been discussed. On the basis of the rate and duration of the drug-induced release of norepinephrine from adrenergic terminals, one of two opposing effects can predominate. Thus tyramine, *ephedrine, amphetamine,* and related drugs cause a relatively rapid, brief liberation of the transmitter and produce a sympathomimetic effect. On the other hand, reserpine, by blocking the vesicular amine transporter (VAMT 2) uptake of amines, produces a slow, prolonged depletion of the adrenergic transmitter from adrenergic storage vesicles, where it is largely metabolized by intraneuronal MAO. The resulting depletion of transmitter produces the equivalent of adrenergic blockade. Reserpine also causes the depletion of serotonin, dopamine, and possibly other, unidentified amines from central and peripheral sites, and many of its major effects may be a consequence of the depletion of transmitters other than norepinephrine.

As discussed earlier, deficiencies of tyrosine hydroxylase in humans cause a neurologic disorder (Carson and Robertson, 2002) that can be treated by supplementation with the dopamine precursor *levodopa.*

A syndrome caused by congenital DβH deficiency has been described; this syndrome is characterized by the absence of norepinephrine and epinephrine, elevated concentrations of dopamine, intact baroreflex afferent fibers and cholinergic innervation, and undetectable concentrations of plasma DβH activity (Carson and Robertson, 2002). Patients have severe orthostatic hypotension, ptosis of the eyelids, and retrograde ejaculations. *Dihydroxyphenylserine* (L-DOPS) has been shown to improve postural hypotension in this rare disorder. This therapeutic approach cleverly takes advantage of the nonspecificity of aromatic L-amino acid decarboxylase, which synthesizes norepinephrine directly from this drug in the absence of DβH (Man in't Veld *et al.,* 1988; Robertson *et al.,* 1991). Despite the restoration of plasma norepinephrine in humans with L-DOPS, epinephrine levels are not restored, leading to speculations that PNMT may require DβH for appropriate functioning (Carson and Robertson, 2002).

Agonist and Antagonist Actions at Receptors. *Cholinergic.*

The nicotinic receptors of autonomic ganglia and skeletal muscle are not identical; they respond differently to certain stimulating and blocking agents, and their pentameric structures contain different combinations of homologous subunits (Table 6–2). *Dimethylphenylpiperazinium* (DMPP) and *phenyltrimethylammonium* (PTMA) show some selectivity for stimulation of autonomic ganglion cells and end plates of skeletal muscle, respectively. *Trimethaphan* and *hexamethonium* are relatively selective competitive and noncompetitive ganglionic blocking agents. Although tubocurarine effectively blocks transmission at both motor end plates and autonomic ganglia, its action at the former site predominates. *Succinylcholine,* a depolarizing agent, produces selective neuromuscular blockade. Transmission at autonomic ganglia and the adrenal medulla is complicated further by the presence of muscarinic receptors in addition to the principal nicotinic receptors (*see* Chapter 9).

Various toxins in snake venoms exhibit a high degree of specificity in the cholinergic nervous system. The α-neurotoxins from the Elapidae family interact with the agonist-binding site on the nicotinic receptor. α-*Bungarotoxin* is selective for the muscle receptor and interacts with only certain neuronal receptors, such as those containing α_7 through α_9 subunits. Neuronal bungarotoxin shows a wider range of inhibition of neuronal receptors. A second group of toxins, called the *fasciculins,* inhibits AChE. A third group of toxins, termed the *muscarinic toxins* (MT$_1$ through MT$_4$), includes partial agonists and antagonists for the muscarinic receptors. Venoms from the Viperidae family of snakes and the fish-hunting cone snails also have relatively selective toxins for nicotinic receptors.

Muscarinic ACh receptors, which mediate the effects of ACh at autonomic effector cells, now can be divided into five subclasses. Atropine blocks all the muscarinic responses to injected ACh and related cholinomimetic drugs whether they are excitatory, as in the intestine, or inhibitory, as in the heart. Newer muscarinic agonists, *pirenzepine* for M_1, *tripitramine* for M_2, and *darifenacin* for M_3, show selectivity as muscarinic blocking agents. Several muscarinic antagonists show sufficient selectivity in the clinical setting to minimize the bothersome side effects seen with the nonselective agents at therapeutic doses (*see* Chapter 7).

Adrenergic. A vast number of synthetic compounds that bear structural resemblance to the naturally occurring catecholamines can interact with α and β adrenergic receptors to produce sympathomimetic effects (*see* Chapter 10). Phenylephrine acts selectively at α_1 receptors, whereas clonidine is a selective α_2 adrenergic agonist. Isoproterenol exhibits agonist activity at both β_1 and β_2 receptors. Preferential stimulation of cardiac β_1 receptors follows the administration of *dobutamine*. *Terbutaline* is an example of a drug with relatively selective action on β_2 receptors; it produces effective bronchodilation with minimal effects on the heart. The main features of adrenergic blockade, including the selectivity of various blocking agents for α and β adrenergic receptors, have been mentioned (*see* Chapter 10). Again, partial dissociation of effects at β_1 and β_2 receptors has been achieved, as exemplified by the β_1 receptor antagonists *metoprolol* and *atenolol*, which antagonize the cardiac actions of catecholamines while causing somewhat less antagonism at bronchioles. *Prazosin* and *yohimbine* are representative of α_1 and α_2 receptor antagonists, respectively, although prazosin has a relatively high affinity at α_{2B} and α_{2C} subtypes compared with α_{2A} receptors. Several important drugs that promote the release of norepinephrine or deplete the transmitter resemble, in their effects, activators or blockers of postjunctional receptors (*e.g.,* tyramine and reserpine, respectively).

Interference with the Destruction of the Transmitter. **Cholinergic.** The anti-ChE agents (*see* Chapter 8) constitute a chemically diverse group of compounds, the primary action of which is inhibition of AChE, with the consequent accumulation of endogenous ACh. At the neuromuscular junction, accumulation of ACh produces depolarization of end plates and flaccid paralysis. At postganglionic muscarinic effector sites, the response is either excessive stimulation resulting in contraction and secretion or an inhibitory response mediated by hyperpolarization. At ganglia, depolarization and enhanced transmission are observed.

Adrenergic. The reuptake of norepinephrine by the adrenergic nerve terminals *via* NET is the major mechanism for terminating its transmitter action. Interference with this process is the basis of the potentiating effect of cocaine on responses to adrenergic impulses and injected catecholamines. It also has been suggested that the antidepressant actions and some of the adverse effects of imipramine and related drugs are due to a similar action at adrenergic synapses in the CNS (*see* Chapter 17).

Entacapone and *tolcapone* are nitro catechol-type COMT inhibitors. Entacapone is a peripherally acting COMT inhibitor, whereas tolcapone also inhibits COMT activity in the brain. COMT inhibition has been shown to attenuate levodopa toxicity on dopamine neurons and enhance dopamine action in the brain of patients with Parkinson's disease (*see* Chapter 20). On the other hand, nonselective MAO inhibitors, such as tranylcypromine, potentiate the effects of tyramine and may potentiate effects of neurotransmitters. While most MAO inhibitors used as antidepressants inhibit both MAO-A and MAO-B, selective MAO-A and MAO-B inhibitors are available. Selegiline is a selective and irreversible MAO-B inhibitor that also has been used as an adjunct in the treatment of Parkinson's disease.

OTHER AUTONOMIC NEUROTRANSMITTERS

The vast majority of neurons in both the central and peripheral nervous systems contain more than one substance with potential or demonstrated activity at relevant postjunctional sites (*see* Chapter 12). In some cases, especially in peripheral structures, it has been possible to demonstrate that two or more such substances are contained within individual nerve terminals and are released simultaneously on nerve stimulation. Although the anatomical separation of the parasympathetic and sympathetic components of the autonomic nervous system and the actions of ACh and norepinephrine (their primary neurotransmitters) still provides the essential framework for studying autonomic function, a host of other chemical messengers such as purines, eicosanoids, NO, and peptides modulate or mediate responses that follow stimulation of the autonomic nervous system. An expanded view of autonomic neurotransmission has evolved to include instances where substances other than ACh or norepinephrine are released and may function as cotransmitters, neuromodulators, or even primary transmitters.

The evidence for cotransmission in the autonomic nervous system usually encompasses the following considerations: (1) A portion of responses to stimulation of preganglionic or postganglionic nerves or to field stimulation of target structures persists in the presence of concentrations of muscarinic or adrenergic antagonists that completely block their respective agonists. (2) The candidate substance can be detected within nerve fibers that course through target tissues. (3) The substance can be recovered on microdialysis or in the venous or perfusion effluent following electrical stimulation; such release often can be blocked by tetrodotoxin. (4) Effects of electrical stimulation are mimicked by the application of the substance and are inhibited in the presence of specific antagonists. When such antagonists are not available, reliance often is placed on neutralizing antibodies or selective desensitization produced by prior exposure to the substance. A more recent approach to this challenging problem is the use of knockout mice that do not express the putative cotransmitter.

A number of problems confound interpretation of such evidence. It is particularly difficult to establish that substances that fulfill all the listed criteria originate within the autonomic nervous system. In some instances, their origin can be traced to sensory fibers, to intrinsic neurons, or to nerves innervating blood vessels. Also, there may be marked synergism between the candidate substance and known or unknown transmitters (Lundberg, 1996). In knockout mice, compensatory mechanisms or transmitter redundancy may disguise even well-defined actions (Hökfelt *et al.*, 2000). Finally, it should be recognized that the putative cotransmitter may have primarily a trophic function in maintaining synaptic connectivity or in expressing a particular receptor.

It long has been known that ATP and ACh coexist in cholinergic vesicles (Dowdall *et al.*, 1974) and that ATP, NPY, and catecholamines are found within storage granules in nerves and the adrenal medulla (*see* above). ATP is released along with the transmitters, and either it or its metabolites have a significant function in synaptic transmission in some circumstances (*see* below). Recently, attention has focused on the growing list of peptides that are found in the adrenal medulla, nerve fibers, or ganglia of the autonomic nervous system or in the structures that are innervated by the autonomic nervous system. This list includes the enkephalins, substance P and other tachykinins, somatostatin, gonadotropin-releasing hormone, cholecystokinin, calcitonin gene–related peptide, galanin, pituitary adenylyl cyclase–activating pep-

tide, VIP, chromogranins, and NPY (Darlison and Richter, 1999; Lundberg, 1996; Bennett, 1997, Hökfelt *et al.*, 2000). Some of the orphan GPCRs discovered in the course of genome-sequencing projects may represent receptors for undiscovered peptides or other cotransmitters. The evidence for widespread transmitter function in the autonomic nervous system is substantial for VIP and NPY, and further discussion is confined to these peptides. The possibility that abnormalities in function of neuropeptide cotransmitters, in type 2 diabetes, for example, contribute to disease pathogenesis remains of interest (Ahren, 2000).

Cotransmission in the Autonomic Nervous System. The evidence is substantial that ATP plays a role in sympathetic nerves as a cotransmitter with norepinephrine (Stjärne, 1989; Westfall *et al.*, 1991, 2002; Silinsky *et al.*, 1998; Burnstock, 1999). For example, the rodent vas deferens is supplied with a dense sympathetic innervation, and stimulation of the nerves results in a biphasic mechanical response that consists of an initial rapid twitch followed by a sustained contraction. The first phase of the response is mediated by ATP acting on postjunctional P2X receptors, whereas the second phase is mediated mainly by norepinephrine acting on α_1 receptors (Sneddon and Westfall, 1984). The cotransmitters apparently are released from the same types of nerves because pretreatment with *6-hydroxydopamine,* an agent that specifically destroys adrenergic nerves, abolished both phases of the neurogenically induced biphasic contraction. It has been assumed that the sympathetic nerves store ATP and norepinephrine in the same synaptic vesicles, and therefore, on release, the two cotransmitters are released together (Stjärne, 1989). This may not always be the case, and ATP and norepinephrine may be released from separate subsets of vesicles and subject to differential regulation.

While part of the metabolism of ATP, once released into the neuroeffector junction, is by extracellularly directed membrane-bound nucleotidases to ADP, AMP, and adenosine (Gordon, 1986), the majority of the metabolism occurs *via* the action of releasable nucleotidases. There is also evidence that ATP and its metabolites exert presynaptic modulatory effects on transmitter release *via* P2 receptors and receptors for adenosine. In addition to evidence showing that ATP is a cotransmitter with norepinephrine, there is also evidence that ATP may be a cotransmitter with ACh in certain postganglionic parasympathetic nerves, *e.g.*, in the urinary bladder.

The NPY family of peptides is distributed widely in the central and peripheral nervous systems and consists of three members: NPY, pancreatic polypeptide, and peptide YY. NPY has been shown to be colocalized and core-leased with norepinephrine and ATP in most sympathetic nerves in the peripheral nervous system, especially those innervating blood vessels (*see* Westfall, 2004). There is also convincing evidence that NPY exerts prejunctional modulatory effects on transmitter release and synthesis. Moreover, there are numerous examples of postjunctional interactions that are consistent with a cotransmitter role for NPY at various sympathetic neuroeffector junctions. Thus, it seems that NPY, together with norepinephrine and ATP, is the third sympathetic cotransmitter. The functions of NPY include (1) direct postjunctional contractile effects; (2) potentiation of the contractile effects of the other sympathetic cotransmitters; and (3) inhibitory modulation of the nerve stimulation–induced release of all three sympathetic cotransmitters.

Studies with selective NPY-Y_1 antagonists provide evidence that the principal postjunctional receptor is of the Y_1 subtype, although other receptors are also present at some sites and may exert physiological actions. Studies with selective NPY-Y_2 antagonists suggest that the principal prejunctional receptor is of the Y_2 subtype both in the periphery and in the CNS. Again, there is evidence for a role for other NPY receptors, and clarification awaits the further development of selective antagonists. NPY also can act prejunctionally to inhibit the release of ACh, CGRP, and substance P. In the CNS, NPY exists as a cotransmitter with catecholamines in some neurons and with peptides and mediators in others. A prominent action of NPY is the presynaptic inhibition of the release of various neurotransmitters, including norepinephrine, dopamine, GABA, glutamate, and serotonin, as well as inhibition or stimulation of various neurohormones such as gonadotropin-releasing hormone, vasopressin, and oxytocin. Evidence also exists for stimulation of norepinephrine and dopamine release. NPY also acts on autoreceptors to inhibit its own release. NPY may use several mechanisms to produce its presynaptic effects, including: inhibition of Ca^{2+} channels, activation of K^+ channels, and perhaps regulation of the vesicle release complex at some point distal to calcium entry. NPY also may play a role in several pathophysiological conditions. The further development of selective NPY agonists and antagonists should enhance understanding about the physiological and pathophysiological roles of NPY.

The pioneering studies of Hökfelt and coworkers, which demonstrated the existence of VIP and ACh in peripheral autonomic neurons, initiated interest in the possibility of peptidergic cotransmission in the autonomic nervous system. Subsequent work has confirmed the frequent association of these two substances in autonomic fibers, including parasympathetic fibers that innervate smooth muscle and exocrine glands and cholinergic sympathetic neurons that innervate sweat glands (Hökfelt *et al.*, 2000).

The role of VIP in parasympathetic transmission has been studied most extensively in the regulation of salivary secretion. The evidence for cotransmission includes the release of VIP following stimulation of the chorda lingual nerve and the incomplete blockade by

atropine of vasodilation when the frequency of stimulation is raised; the latter observation may indicate independent release of the two substances, which is consistent with histochemical evidence for storage of ACh and VIP in separate populations of vesicles. Synergism between ACh and VIP in stimulating vasodilation and secretion also has been described. VIP may be involved in parasympathetic responses in the GI tract, where it may facilitate sphincter relaxation, and the trachea.

Nonadrenergic, Noncholinergic Transmission by Purines. The smooth muscle of many tissues that are innervated by the autonomic nervous system shows inhibitory junction potentials following stimulation by field electrodes (Bennett, 1997). Since such responses frequently are undiminished in the presence of adrenergic and muscarinic cholinergic antagonists, these observations have been taken as evidence for the existence of nonadrenergic, noncholinergic (NANC) transmission in the autonomic nervous system.

Burnstock (1996) and his colleagues have compiled compelling evidence for the existence of purinergic neurotransmission in the gastrointestinal tract, genitourinary tract, and certain blood vessels; ATP has fulfilled all the criteria for a neurotransmitter listed earlier. However, in at least some circumstances, primary sensory axons may be an important source of ATP (Burnstock, 2000). Although adenosine is generated from the released ATP by ectoenzymes and releasable nucleotidases, its primary function appears to be modulatory by causing feedback inhibition of release of the transmitter.

Adenosine can be transported from the cell cytoplasm to activate extracellular receptors on adjacent cells. The efficient uptake of adenosine by cellular transporters and its rapid rate of metabolism to inosine or to adenine nucleotides contribute to its rapid turnover. Several inhibitors of adenosine transport and metabolism are known to influence extracellular adenosine and ATP concentrations (Sneddon *et al.*, 1999).

The purinergic receptors found on the cell surface may be divided into the adenosine (P1) receptors and the receptors for ATP (P2X and P2Y receptors) (Fredholm *et al.*, 2000). Both of the P1 and P2 receptors have various subtypes. Methylxanthines such as *caffeine* and *theophylline* preferentially block adenosine receptors (*see* Chapter 27). There are four adenosine receptors (A1, A2A, A2B, and A3) and multiple subtypes of P2X and P2Y receptors throughout the body. The adenosine receptors and the P2Y receptors mediate their responses *via* G proteins, whereas the P2X receptors are a subfamily of ligand-gated ion channels (Burnstock, 2000).

Modulation of Vascular Responses by Endothelium-Derived Factors. Furchgott and colleagues demonstrated that an intact endothelium was necessary to achieve vascular relaxation in response to ACh (Furchgott, 1999). This inner cellular layer of the blood vessel now is known to modulate autonomic and hormonal effects on the contractility of blood vessels. In response to a variety of vasoactive agents and even physical stimuli, the endothelial cells release a short-lived vasodilator called *endothelium-derived relaxing factor* (EDRF), now known to be NO. Less commonly, an endothelium-derived hyperpolarizing factor (EDHF) and endothelium-derived contracting factor (EDCF) of as yet undefined compositions are released (Vanhoutte, 1996). EDCF formation depends on cyclooxygenase activity.

Products of inflammation and platelet aggregation (*e.g.*, serotonin, histamine, bradykinin, purines, and thrombin) exert all or part of their action by stimulating the production of NO. Endothelial cell–dependent mechanisms of relaxation are important in a variety of vascular beds, including the coronary circulation (Hobbs *et al.*, 1999). Activation of specific GPCRs on endothelial cells promotes NO production. NO diffuses readily to the underlying smooth muscle and induces relaxation of vascular smooth muscle by activating the soluble form of guanylyl cyclase, which increases cyclic GMP concentrations. Nitrovasodilating drugs used to lower blood pressure or to treat ischemic heart disease probably act through conversion to or release of NO (*see* Chapter 31). NO also has been shown to be released from certain nerves (*nitrergic*) innervating blood vessels and smooth muscles of the gastrointestinal tract. NO has a negative inotropic action on the heart.

Alterations in the release or action of NO may affect a number of major clinical situations such as atherosclerosis (Hobbs *et al.*, 1999; Ignarro, 1999). Furthermore, there is evidence suggesting that the hypotension of endotoxemia or that induced by cytokines is mediated by induction of enhanced release of NO; consequently, increased release of NO may have pathological significance in septic shock. NO is synthesized from L-arginine and molecular oxygen by *nitric oxide synthase* (NOS). There are three known forms of this enzyme (Moncada *et al.*, 1997). One form (eNOS) is constitutive, residing in the endothelial cell and synthesizing NO over short periods in response to receptor-mediated increases in cellular Ca^{2+}. A second form (nNOS) is responsible for the Ca^{2+}-dependent NO synthesis neurons. The third form of NOS (iNOS) is induced after activation of cells by cytokines and bacterial endotoxins

and, once expressed, synthesizes NO for long periods of time. This Ca^{2+}-independent, high-output form is responsible for the above-mentioned toxic manifestations of NO. Glucocorticoids inhibit the expression of inducible, but not constitutive, forms of NOS in vascular endothelial cells. However, other endothelium-derived factors also may be involved in vasodilation and hyperpolarization of the smooth muscle cell. There has been considerable interest in the possibility that NOS inhibitors might have therapeutic benefit, for example, in septic shock and neurodegenerative diseases (Hobbs *et al.*, 1999). Conversely, diminished production of NO by the endothelial cell layer in atherosclerotic coronary arteries may contribute to the risk of myocardial infarction.

Full contractile responses of cerebral arteries also require an intact endothelium. A family of peptides, termed *endothelins,* is stored in vascular endothelial cells. Their release onto smooth muscle promotes contraction by stimulation of endothelin receptors. Endothelins contribute to the maintenance of vascular homostasis by acting *via* multiple endothelin receptors (Sokolovsky, 1995) to reverse the response to NO (Rubanyi and Polokoff, 1994). In isolated cell systems, several G-protein-linked responses to endothelins are quasi-irreversible (Hilal-Dandan *et al.*, 1997).

BIBLIOGRAPHY

Ahren, B. Autonomic regulation of islet hormone secretion: Implications for health and disease. *Diabetologia,* **2000,** *43*:393–410.

Altschuler, S.M., Bao, X.M., Bieger, D., Hopkins, D.A., and Miselis, R.R. Viscerotopic representation of the upper alimentary tract in the rat: sensory ganglia and nuclei of the solitary and spinal trigeminal tracts. *J. Comp. Neurol.* **1989,** *283*:248–268.

Arner, P., and Hoffstedt, J. Adrenoceptor genes in human obesity. *J. Intern. Med.,* **1999,** *245*:667–672.

Carroll, J.M., Evinger, M.J., Goodman, H.M., and Joh, T.H. Differential and coordinate regulation of TH and PNMT mRNAs in chromaffin cell cultures by second messenger system activation and steroid treatment. *J. Mol. Neurosci.,* **1991,** *3*:75–83.

Daubner, S.C., Lauriano, C., Haycock, J.W., and Fitzpatrick, P.F. Site-directed mutagenesis of serine 40 of rat tyrosine hydroxylase: Effects of dopamine and cAMP-dependent phosphorylation on enzyme activity. *J. Biol. Chem.,* **1992,** *267*:12639–12646.

Della Rocca, G.J., van Biesen, T., Daaka, Y., *et al.* Ras-dependent mitogen-activated protein kinase activation by G protein–coupled receptors: Convergence of G_i- and G_q-mediated pathways on calcium/calmodulin, Pyk2, and Src kinase. *J. Biol. Chem.,* **1997,** *272*:19125–19132.

Dowdall, M.J., Boyne, A.F., and Whittaker, V.P. Adenosine triphosphate, a constituent of cholinergic synaptic vesicles. *Biochem. J.,* **1974,** *140*:1–12.

Emorine, L.J., Marullo, S., Briend-Sutren, M.M., *et al.* Molecular characterization of the human β_3-adrenergic receptor. *Science,* **1989,** *245*:1118–1121.

Fetscher, C., Fleichman, M., Schmidt, M., Krege, S., and Michel, M.C. M_3 muscarinic receptors mediate contraction of human urinary bladder. *Br J Pharmacol.* **2002,** *136*:641–643.

Granneman, J.G., Lahners, K.N., and Chaudhry, A. Characterization of the human β_3-adrenergic receptor gene. *Mol. Pharmacol.,* **1993,** *44*:264–270.

Hilal-Dandan, R., Villegas, S., Gonzalez, A., and Brunton, L. The quasi-irreversible nature of endothelin binding and G protein-linked signaling in cardiac myocytes. *J. Pharmacol. Exp. Therap.,* **1997,** *281*:267–273.

Hille, B., Billiard, J., Babcock, D.F., Nguyen, T., and Koh, D.S. Stimulation of exocytosis without a calcium signal. *J. Physiol.,* **1999,** *520*:23–31.

Kable, J.W., Murrin, L.C., and Bylund, D.B. In vivo gene modification elucidates subtype-specific functions of $\alpha(2)$-adrenergic receptors. *J. Pharmacol. Exp. Ther.,* **2000,** *293*:1–7.

Kennedy, B., Elayan, H., and Ziegler, M.G. Glucocorticoid elevation of mRNA encoding epinephrine-forming enzyme in lung. *Am. J. Physiol.,* **1993,** *265*:L117–120.

Kumer, S.C., and Vrana, K.E. Intricate regulation of tyrosine hydroxylase activity and gene expression. *J. Neurochem.,* **1996,** *67*:443–462.

Lakhlani, P.P., MacMillan, L.B., Guo, T.Z., *et al.* Substitution of a mutant α_{2A}-adrenergic receptor via "hit and run" gene targeting reveals the role of this subtype in sedative, analgesic, and anesthetic-sparing responses in vivo. *Proc. Natl. Acad. Sci. U.S.A.,* **1997,** *94*:9950–9955.

Lugardon, K., Raffner, R., Goumon, Y., *et al.* Antibacterial and antifungal activities of vasostatin-1, the N-terminal fragment of chromogranin A. *J. Biol. Chem.,* **2000,** *275*:10745–10753.

MacMillan, L.B., Hein, L., Smith, M.S., Piascik, M.T., and Limbird, L.E. Central hypotensive effects of the α_{2A}-adrenergic receptor subtype. *Science,* **1996,** *9*:801–803.

Moncada, S., Higgs, A., and Furchgott, R. International Union of Pharmacology nomenclature in nitric oxide research. *Pharmacol. Rev.,* **1997,** *49*:137–142.

Murthy, V.N., and Stevens, C.F. Synaptic vesicles retain their identity through the endocytic cycle. *Nature,* **1998,** *392*:497–501.

Palczewski, K., Kumasaka, T., Hori, T., *et al.* Crystal structure of rhodopsin: A G protein–coupled receptor. *Science,* **2000,** *289*:739–745.

Richman, J.G., and Regan, J.W. α_2-Adrenergic receptors increase cell migration and decrease F-actin labeling in rat aortic smooth muscle cells. *Am. J. Physiol.,* **1998,** *274*:C654–662.

Salminen, O., Murphy, K.L., McIntosh, J.M., *et al.* Subunit composition and pharmacology of two classes of striatal presynaptic nicotinic acetylcholine receptors mediating dopamine release in mice. *Mol. Pharmacol.,* **2004,** *65*:1526–1535.

Sneddon, P., and Westfall, D.P. Pharmacological evidence that adenosine trisphosphate and noradrenaline are co-transmitters in the guinea-pig vas deferens. *J. Physiol.,* **1984,** *347*:561–580.

Sneddon, P., Westfall, T.D., Todorov, L.D., *et al.* Modulation of purinergic neurotransmission. *Prog. Brain Res.,* **1999,** *120*:11–20.

Tanoue, A., Koba, M., Miyawaki, S., *et al.* Role of the α_{1D}-adrenergic receptor in the development of salt-induced hypertension. *Hypertension,* **2002a,** *40*:101–106.

Tanoue, A., Koshimizu, T.A., and Tsujimoto, G. Transgenic studies of

α_1-adrenergic receptor subtype function. *Life Sci.,* **2002b,** *71*:2207–2215.

Tanoue, A., Nasa, Y., Koshimizu, T., *et al.* The α_{1D}-adrenergic receptor directly regulates arterial blood pressure via vasoconstriction. *J. Clin. Invest.,* **2002c,** *109*:765–775.

Varoqui, H., and Erickson, J.D. Vesicular neurotransmitter transporters: Potential sites for the regulation of synaptic function. *Mol. Neurobiol.,* **1997,** *15*:165–191.

Viskupic, E., Kvetnansky, R., Sabban, E.L., *et al.* Increase in rat adrenal phenylethanolamine *N*-methyltransferase mRNA level caused by immobilization stress depends on intact pituitary-adrenocortical axis. *J. Neurochem.,* **1994,** *63*:808–814.

Walden, P.D., Durkin, M.M., Lepor, H., *et al.* Localization of mRNA and receptor binding sites for the α_{1A}-adrenoceptor subtype in the rat, monkey, and human urinary bladder and prostate. *J. Urol.,* **1997,** *157*:1032–1038.

Wang, Z. Shi, H., and Wang, H. Functional M_3 muscarinic acetylcholine receptors in mammalian hearts. *Br. J. Pharmacol.,* **2004,** *142*:395–408.

Wevers, R.A., de Rijk-van Andel, J.F., Brautigam, C., *et al.* A review of biochemical and molecular genetic aspects of tyrosine hydroxylase deficiency including a novel mutation (291delC). *J. Inherit. Metab. Dis.,* **1999,** *22*:364–373.

MONOGRAPHS AND REVIEWS

Aantaa, R., Marjamaki, A., and Scheinin, M. Molecular pharmacology of α_2-adrenoceptor subtypes. *Ann. Med.,* **1995,** *27*:439–449.

Abell, C.W., and Kwan, S.W. Molecular characterization of monoamine oxidases A and B. *Prog. Nucleic Acid Res. Mol. Biol.,* **2001,** *65*:129–156.

Amara, S.G., and Kuhar, M.J. Neurotransmitter transporters: recent progress. *Annu. Rev. Neurosci.,* **1993,** *16*:73–93.

Andresen, M.C., and Kunze, D.L. Nucleus tractus solitarius: Gateway to neural circulatory control. *Annu. Rev. Physiol.,* **1994,** *56*:93–116.

Aunis, D. Exocytosis in chromaffin cells of the adrenal medulla. *Int. Rev. Cytol.,* **1998,** *181*:213–320.

Axelrod, J. Methylation reactions in the formation and metabolism of catecholamines and other biogenic amines. *Pharmacol. Rev.,* **1966,** *18*:95–113.

Baillie, G., and Houslay, M. Arrestin times for compartmentalized cAMP signalling and phosphodiesterase-4 enzymes. *Curr. Opin. Cell Biol.,* **2005,** *17*:129–134.

Boehm, S., and Kubista, H. Fine tuning of sympathetic transmitter release via ionotropic and metabotropic presynaptic receptors. *Pharmacol. Rev.,* **2002,** *54*:43–99.

Bonner, T.I. The molecular basis of muscarinic receptor diversity. *Trends Neurosci.,* **1989,** *12*:148–151.

Bowman, W.C., Prior, C., and Marshall, I.G. Presynaptic receptors in the neuromuscular junction. *Ann. N.Y. Acad. Sci.,* **1990,** *604*:69–81.

Broadley, K.J. *Autonomic Pharmacology.* Taylor and Francis, London, **1996.**

Brownstein, M.J., and Hoffman, B.J. Neurotransmitter transporters. *Recent Prog. Horm. Res.,* **1994,** *49*:27–42.

Burnstock, G. Purinergic neurotransmission. *Semin. Neurosci.,* **1996,** *8*:171–257.

Burnstock, G. Purinergic cotransmission. *Brain Res. Bull.* **1999,** *50*:355–357.

Burnstock, G. P2X receptors in sensory neurons. *Br. J. Anaesth.,* **2000,** *84:*476–488.

Bylund, D.B. Subtypes of α_1- and α_2-adrenergic receptors. *FASEB J.,* **1992,** 6:832–839.

Carson, R.P., and Robertson, D. Genetic manipulation of noradrenergic neurons. *J. Pharmacol. Exp. Ther.,* **2002,** *301:*410–407.

Catterall, W.A. Cellular and molecular biology of voltage-gated sodium channels. *Physiol. Rev.,* **1992,** *72:*S15–48.

Catterall, W.A. From ionic currents to molecular mechanisms: The structure and function of voltage-gated sodium channels. *Neuron,* **2000,** *26:*13–25.

Caulfield, M.P., and Birdsall, N.J. International Union of Pharmacology: XVII. Classification of muscarinic acetylcholine receptors. *Pharmacol. Rev.,* **1998,** *50:*279–290.

Changeux, J.P., and Edelstein, S.J. Allosteric receptors after 30 years. *Neuron,* **1998,** *21:*959–980.

Chong, B.S., and Mersfelder, T.L. Entacapone. *Ann. Pharmacother.,* **2000,** *34:*1056–1065.

Cooke, H.J. "Enteric tears": Chloride secretion and its neural regulation. *News Physiol. Sci.,* **1998,** *13:*269–274.

Costa, M., Brookes, S.J., Steele, P.A., *et al.* Neurochemical classification of myenteric neurons in the guinea-pig ileum. *Neuroscience,* **1996,** *75:*949–967.

Costa, M., Brookes, S.J., and Hennig, G.W. Anatomy and physiology of the enteric nervous system. *Gut,* **2000,** *47:*15–19.

Darlison, M.G., and Richter, D. Multiple genes for neuropeptides and their receptors: Co-evolution and physiology. *Trends Neurosci.,* **1999,** *22:*81–88.

DeBiasi, M. Nicotinic mechanisms in the autonomic control of organ systems. *J. Neurobiol.,* **2002,** *53:*568–579.

Dhein, S., van Koppen, C.J., and Brodde, O.E. Muscarinic receptors in the mammalian heart. *Pharmacol. Res.,* **2001,** *44:*161–182.

Docherty, J.R. Subtypes of functional α_1- and α_2-adrenoceptors. *Eur. J. Pharmacol.,* **1998,** *361:*1–15.

Dooley, T.P. Cloning of the human phenol sulfotransferase gene family: Three genes implicated in the metabolism of catecholamines, thyroid hormones and drugs. *Chem. Biol. Interact.,* **1998,** *109:*29–41.

Dorn, G.W., and Brown, J.H. G_q signaling in cardiac adaptation and maladaptation. *Trends Cardiovasc. Med.,* **1999,** *9:*26–34.

Eccles, J.C. *The Physiology of Synapses.* Springer-Verlag, Berlin, **1964.**

Eccles, J.C. *The Understanding of the Brain.* McGraw-Hill, New York, **1973.**

Eiden, L.E. The cholinergic gene locus. *J. Neurochem.,* **1998,** *70:*2227–2240.

Eisenhofer, G. The role of neuronal and extraneuronal plasma membrane transporters in the inactivation of peripheral catecholamines. *Pharmacol. Ther.,* **2001,** *91:*35–62.

Ferguson, S., and Blakely, R. The choline transporter resurfaces: New roles for synaptic vesicles? *Mol. Interv.,* **2004,** *4:*22–37.

Fredholm, B.B., Ijzerman, A.P., Jacobson, K.A., and Linden, J. Adenosine receptors. In, *The IUPHAR Compendium of Receptor Characterization and Classification.* **2000,** pp. 78–87.

Furchgott, R.F. Endothelium-derived relaxing factor: Discovery, early studies, and identification as nitric oxide. *Biosci. Rep.,* **1999,** *19:*235–251.

Galligan, J.J. Pharmacology of synaptic transmission in the enteric nervous system. *Curr. Opin. Pharmacol.,* **2002,** *2:*623–629.

Gordon, J.L. Extracellular ATP: Effects, sources and fate. *Biochem. J.,* **1986,** *233:*309–319.

Gutkind, J.S. The pathways connecting G protein–coupled receptors to the nucleus through divergent mitogen-activated protein kinase cascades. *J. Biol. Chem.,* **1998,** *273:*1839–1842.

Hall, Z.W., and Sanes, J.R. Synaptic structure and development: the neuromuscular junction. *Cell,* **1993,** *72:*99–121.

Hall, R.A., and Lefkowitz, R.J. Regulation of G protein–coupled receptor signaling by scaffold proteins. *Circ. Res.,* **2002,** *91:*672–680.

Hein, L., and Schmitt, J.P. α_1-Adrenoceptors in the heart: Friend or foe? *J. Mol. Cell. Cardiol.,* **2003,** *35:*1183–1185.

Hille, B. *Ionic Channels of Excitable Membranes,* 2d ed. Sinauer Associates, Sunderland, MA, **1992.**

Hobbs, A.J., Higgs, A., and Moncada, S. Inhibition of nitric oxide synthase as a potential therapeutic target. *Annu. Rev. Pharmacol. Toxicol.,* **1999,** *39:*191–220.

Hökfelt, T., Broberger, C., Xu, Z.Q., *et al.* Neuropeptides: An overview. *Neuropharmacology,* **2000,** *39:*1337–1356.

Horowitz, B., Ward, S.M., and Sanders, K.M. Cellular and molecular basis for electrical rhythmicity in gastrointestinal muscles. *Annu. Rev. Physiol.,* **1999,** *61:*19–43.

Hutchins, C. Three-dimensional models of the D1 and D2 dopamine receptors. *Endocr. J.,* **1994,** *2:*7–23.

Ignarro, L.J., Cirino, G., Casini, A., and Napoli, C. Nitric oxide as a signaling molecule in the vascular system: An overview. *J. Cardiovasc. Pharmacol.,* **1999,** *34:*879–886.

Jahn, R., Lang, T., and Südhof, T. Membrane fusion. *Cell,* **2003,** *112:*519–533.

Karlin, A., and Akabas, M.H. Toward a structural basis for the function of nicotinic acetylcholine receptors and their cousins. *Neuron,* **1995,** *15:*1231–1244.

Katz, B. *Nerve, Muscle, and Synapse.* McGraw-Hill, New York, **1966.**

Kawashima, K., and Fujii, T. Extraneuronal cholinergic system in lymphocytes. *Pharmacol. Ther.,* **2000,** *86:*29–48.

Kohout, T.A., and Lefkowitz, R.J. Regulation of G protein–coupled receptor kinases and arrestins during receptor desensitization. *Mol. Pharmacol.,* **2003,** *63:*9–18.

Kunze, W.A.A., and Furness, J.B. The enteric nervous system and regulation of intestinal motility. *Annu. Rev. Physiol.,* **1999,** *61:*117–142.

Langer, S.Z. 25 years since the discovery of presynaptic receptors: Present knowledge and future perspectives. *Trends Pharmacol. Sci.,* **1997,** *18:*95–99.

Lefkowitz, R.J. G protein–coupled receptors: III. New roles for receptor kinases and β-arrestins in receptor signaling and desensitization. *J. Biol. Chem.,* **1998,** *273:*18677–18680.

Lefkowitz, R.J. The superfamily of heptahelical receptors. *Nature Cell Biol.,* **2000,** *2:*E133–136.

Lefkowitz, R.J., Pierce, K.L., and Luttrell, L.M. Dancing with different partners: protein kinase A phosphorylation of seven membrane-spanning receptors regulates their G protein–coupling specificity. *Mol. Pharmacol.,* **2002,** *62:*971–974.

Lindstom, J.M. Acetylcholine receptors and myasthenia. *Muscle Nerve,* **2000,** *23:*453–477.

Lloyd, G.K., and Williams, M. Neuronal nicotinic acetylcholine receptors as novel drug targets. *J. Pharmacol. Exp. Ther.,* **2000,** *292:*461–467.

Luetje, C.W. Getting past the asterisk: The subunit composition of presynaptic nicotinic receptors that modulate striatal dopamine release. *Mol. Pharmacol.,* **2004,** *65:*1333–1335.

Ma, Y.C., and Huang, X.Y. Novel signaling pathways through the β-adrenergic receptors. *Trends Cardiovasc. Med.,* **2002,** *12:*46–49.

MacDermott, A.B., Role, L.W., and Siegelbaum, S.A. Presynaptic ionotropic receptors and the control of transmitter release. *Annu. Rev. Neurosci.,* **1999,** *22*:443–485.

Man in't Veld, A., Boomsma, F., Lenders, J., *et al.* Patients with congenital dopamine *β*-hydroxylase deficiency: A lesson in catecholamine physiology. *Am. J. Hypertens.,* **1988,** *1*:231–238.

Männistö, P.T., and Kaakkola, S. Catechol-*O*-methyltransferase (COMT): Biochemistry, molecular biology, pharmacology, and clinical efficacy of the new selective COMT inhibitors. *Pharmacol. Rev.* **1999,** *51*:593–628.

Masson, J., Sagne, C., Hamon, M., and Mestikawy, S.E. Neurotransmitter transporters in the central nervous system. *Pharmacol. Rev.,* **1999,** *51*:439–464.

McDonald, T.F., Pelzer, S., Trautwein, W., and Pelzer, D.J. Regulation and modulation of calcium channels in cardiac, skeletal, and smooth muscle cells. *Physiol. Rev.,* **1994,** *74*:365–507.

Meir, A., Ginsburg, S., Butkevich, A., *et al.* Ion channels in presynaptic nerve terminals and control of transmitter release. *Physiol. Rev.,* **1999,** *79*:1019–1088.

Michelotti, G.A., Price, D.T., and Schwinn, D.A. *α₁*-Adrenergic receptor regulation: Basic science and clinical implications. *Pharmacol. Ther.,* **2000,** *88*:281–309.

Miller, R.J. Presynaptic receptors. *Ann. Rev. Pharmacol. Toxicol.,* **1998,** *38*:201–227.

Nagatsu, T. Genes for human catecholamine-synthesizing enzymes. *Neurosci. Res.,* **1991,** *12*:315–345.

Numa, S., Noda, M., Takahashi, H., *et al.* Molecular structure of the nicotinic acetylcholine receptor. *Cold Spring Harbor Symp. Quant. Biol.,* **1983,** *48*:57–69.

Perry, S.J., and Lefkowitz, R.J. Arresting developments in heptahelical receptor signaling and regulation. *Trends Cell Biol.,* **2002,** *12*:130–138.

Philipp, M., and Hein, L. Adrenergic receptor knockout mice: Distinct functions of 9 receptor subtypes. *Pharmacol. Ther.,* **2004,** *101*:65–74.

Picciotto, M.R., Caldarone, B.J., Brunzell, D.H., *et al.* Neuronal nicotinic acetylcholine receptor subunit knockout mice: Physiological and behavioral phenotypes and possible clinical implications. *Pharmacol. Ther.,* **2001,** *92*:89–108.

Robertson, D., Haile, V., Perry, S.E., *et al.* Dopamine *β*-hydroxylase deficiency: A genetic disorder of cardiovascular regulation. *Hypertension,* **1991,** *18*:1–8.

Robidoux, J., Martin, T.L., and Collins, S. *β*-Adrenergic receptors and regulation of energy expenditure: A family affair. *Annu. Rev. Pharmacol. Toxicol.,* **2004,** *44*:297–323.

Rubanyi, G.M., and Polokoff, M.A. Endothelins: Molecular biology, biochemistry, pharmacology, physiology, and pathophysiology. *Pharmacol. Rev.,* **1994,** *46*:325–415.

Sanes, J.R., and Lichtman, J.W. Development of the vertebrate neuromuscular junction. *Annu. Rev. Neurosci.,* **1999,** *22*:389–442.

Saper, C.B. The central autonomic nervous system: Conscious visceral perception and autonomic pattern generation. *Annu. Rev. Neurosci.,* **2002,** *25*:433–469.

Saper, C.B. Pain as a visceral sensation. *Prog. Brain Res.,* **2000,** *122*:237–243.

Schiavo, G., Matteoli, M., and Montecucco, C. Neurotoxins affecting neuroexocytosis. *Physiol. Rev.,* **2000,** *80*:717–766.

Schuldiner, S. A molecular glimpse of vesicular monoamine transporters. *J. Neurochem.,* **1994,** *62*:2067–2078.

Silinsky, E.M., von Kügelgen, I., Smith, A., and Westfall, D.P. Functions of extracellular nucleotides in peripheral and central neuronal

tissues. In, *The P2 Nucleotide Receptors.* (Turner, J.T., Weisman, G.A. and Fedan, J.S., eds.) Humana Press, Totowa, NJ, **1998,** pp. 259–290.

Sneddon, P., Westfall, T.D., Todorov, L.D., *et al.* Modulation of purinergic neurotransmission. *Prog. Brain Res.,* **1999,** *120*:11–20.

Sokolovsky, M. Endothelin receptor subtypes and their role in transmembrane signaling mechanisms. *Pharmacol. Ther.,* **1995,** *68*:435–471.

Soreq, H., and Seidman, S. Acetylcholinesterase: New roles for an old actor. *Nature Rev. Neurosci.,* **2001,** *2*:294–302.

Steinberg, S.F. *α₁*-Adrenergic receptor subtype function in cardiomyocytes: Lessons from genetic models in mice. *J. Mol. Cell. Cardiol.,* **2002,** *34*:1141–1145.

Stjärne, L. Basic mechanisms and local modulation of nerve impulse-induced secretion of neurotransmitters from individual sympathetic nerve varicosities. *Rev. Physiol. Biochem. Pharmacol.,* **1989,** *112*:1–137.

Starke, K. Presynaptic *α*-autoreceptors. *Rev. Physiol. Biochem. Pharmacol.,* **1987,** *107*:73–146.

Starke, M.E., and Szurszewski, J.H. Role of nitric oxide in gastrointestinal and hepatic function and disease. *Gastroenterology,* **1992,** *103*:1928–1949.

Strader, C.D., Fong, T.M., Tota, M.R., Underwood, D., and Dixon, R.A. Structure and function of G protein–coupled receptors. *Annu. Rev. Biochem.,* **1994,** *63*:101–132.

Stull, J.T., Bowman, B.F., Gallagher, P.J., *et al.* Myosin phosphorylation in smooth and skeletal muscles: Regulation and function. *Prog. Clin. Biol. Res.,* **1990,** *327*:107–126.

Taupenot, L., Harper, K.L., and O'Connor, D.T. The chromogranin–secretogranin family. *New Eng. J. Med.,* **2003,** *348*:1134–1149.

Taylor, P., Luo, Z.D., and Camp, S. The genes encoding the cholinesterases: Structure, evolutionary relationships and regulation of their expression. In, *Cholinesterase and Cholinesterase Inhibitors.* (Giacobini, E., ed.) London, Martin Dunitz, **2000,** pp. 63–80.

Tsien, R.W., Lipscombe, D., Madison, D.V., Bley, K.R., and Fox, A.P. Multiple types of neuronal calcium channels and their selective modulation. *Trends Neurosci.,* **1988,** *11*:431–438.

van Koppen, C.J., and Kaiser, B. Regulation of muscarinic acetylcholine signaling. *Pharmacol. Ther.,* **2003,** *98*:197–220.

Vanhoutte, P.M. Endothelium-dependent responses in congestive heart failure. *J. Mol. Cell. Cardiol.,* **1996,** *28*:2233–2240.

Volz, H.P., and Gleiter, C.H. Monoamine oxidase inhibitors: A perspective on their use in the elderly. *Drugs Aging,* **1998,** *13*:341–355.

von Euler, U.S. Synthesis, uptake and storage of catecholamines in adrenergic nerves: The effects of drugs. In, *Catecholamines: Handbuch der Experimentellen Pharmakologie,* Vol. 33. (Blaschko, H., and Muscholl, E., eds.) Springer-Verlag, Berlin, **1972,** pp. 186–230.

Lagercrantz, H., and Wennmalm, A., eds.) Academic Press, London, **1981,** pp. 3–12.

Wess, J. Muscarinic acetylcholine receptor knockout mice: Novel phenotypes and clinical implication. *Annu. Rev. Pharmacol. Toxicol.,* **2004,** *44*:423–450.

Wessler, I., Kirkpatrick, J., and Racke, K. Non-neuronal acetylcholine, a locally acting molecule widely distributed in biological systems: Expression and function in humans. *Pharmacol. Ther.,* **1998,** *77*:59–79.

Westfall, D.P., Dalziel, H.H., and Forsyth, K.M. ATP as neurotransmitter, cotransmitter and neuromodulator. In, *Adenosine and Adenine Nucleotides as Regulators of Cellular Function.* (Phillis, Ted, ed.) CRC Press, Boca Raton, FL, **1991,** pp. 295–305.

Westfall, D.P., Todorov, L.D., and Mihaylova-Todorova, S.T. ATP as a cotransmitter in sympathetic nerves and its inactivation by releasable enzymes. *J. Pharmacol. Exp. Ther.,* **2002,** *303*:439–444.

Westfall, T.C. Local regulation of adrenergic neurotransmission. *Physiol. Rev.,* **1977,** *57*:659–728.

Westfall, T.C. Prejunctional effects of neuropeptide Y and its role as a cotransmitter. *Exp. Pharmacol.,* **2004,** *162*:138–183.

Weyer, C., Gautier, J.F., and Danforth, E. Development of β_3-adrenoceptor agonists for the treatment of obesity and diabetes: An update. *Diabetes Metab.,* **1999,** *25*:11–21.

Whittaker, V.P. (ed.). *The Cholinergic Synapse: Handbook of Experimental Pharmacology,* Vol. 86. Springer-Verlag, Berlin, **1988.**

Wouters, J. Structural aspects of monoamine oxidase and its reversible inhibition. *Curr. Med. Chem.,* **1998,** *5*:137–162.

Wu, D., and Hersh, L.B. Choline acetyltransferase: Celebrating its fiftieth year. *J. Neurochem.,* **1994,** *62*:1653–1663.

Zhong, H., and Minneman, K.P. α_1-Adrenoceptor subtypes. *Eur. J. Pharmacol.,* **1999,** *375*:261–276.

Zigmond, R.E., Schwarzschild, M.A., and Rittenhouse, A.R. Acute regulation of tyrosine hydroxylase by nerve activity and by neurotransmitters via phosphorylation. *Annu. Rev. Neurosci.,* **1989,** *12*:415–461.

MUSCARINIC RECEPTOR AGONISTS AND ANTAGONISTS

Joan Heller Brown and Palmer Taylor

ACETYLCHOLINE AND ITS MUSCARINIC RECEPTOR TARGET

Muscarinic acetylcholine receptors in the peripheral nervous system are found primarily on autonomic effector cells innervated by postganglionic parasympathetic nerves. Muscarinic receptors also are present in ganglia and on some cells, such as endothelial cells of blood vessels, that receive little or no cholinergic innervation. Within the central nervous system (CNS), the hippocampus, cortex, and thalamus have high densities of muscarinic receptors.

Acetylcholine (ACh), the naturally occurring neurotransmitter for these receptors, has virtually no systemic therapeutic applications because its actions are diffuse, and its hydrolysis, catalyzed by both acetylcholinesterase (AChE) and plasma butyrylcholinesterase, is rapid. Muscarinic agonists mimic the effects of ACh at these sites. These agonists typically are longer-acting congeners of ACh or natural alkaloids that display little selectivity for the various subtypes of muscarinic receptors. Several of these agents stimulate nicotinic as well as muscarinic receptors.

The mechanisms of action of endogenous ACh at the postjunctional membranes of the effector cells and neurons that correspond to the four classes of cholinergic synapses are discussed in Chapter 6. To recapitulate, these synapses are found at (1) autonomic effector sites, innervated by postganglionic parasympathetic fibers (and a small number of cholinergic sympathetic fibers); (2) sympathetic and parasympathetic ganglion cells and the adrenal medulla, innervated by preganglionic autonomic fibers; (3) motor endplates on skeletal muscle, innervated

by somatic motor nerves; and (4) certain synapses peripherally and within the CNS (Krnjević, 2004), where the actions can be either pre- or postsynaptic. When ACh is administered systemically, it potentially can act at all of these sites; however, as a quaternary ammonium compound, its CNS penetration is limited, and butyrylcholinesterase in the plasma reduces the concentrations of ACh that reach peripheral areas with low blood flow.

The actions of ACh and related drugs at autonomic effector sites are referred to as *muscarinic,* based on the original observation that muscarine acts selectively at those sites and produces the same qualitative effects as ACh. Accordingly, the muscarinic, or parasympathomimetic, actions of the drugs considered in this chapter are practically equivalent to the effects of postganglionic parasympathetic nerve impulses listed in Table 6–1; the differences between the actions of the classical muscarinic agonists are largely quantitative, as they show limited selectivity for one organ system or another. Muscarinic receptors also are present on autonomic ganglion cells and in the adrenal medulla. Muscarinic stimulation of ganglia and the adrenal medulla usually is thought to modulate nicotinic stimulation. All of the actions of ACh and its congeners at muscarinic receptors can be blocked by *atropine.* The *nicotinic* actions of cholinergic agonists refer to their initial stimulation, and often in high doses to subsequent blockade, of autonomic ganglion cells, the adrenal medulla, and the neuromuscular junction, actions comparable to those of nicotine.

Properties and Subtypes of Muscarinic Receptors

Muscarinic receptors were characterized initially by analysis of the responses of cells and tissues in the periphery and the CNS. Differential effects of two muscarinic agonists, *bethanechol* and McN-A-

343, on the tone of the lower esophageal sphincter led to the initial designation by Goyal and Rattan (1978) of muscarinic receptors as M_1 (ganglionic) and M_2 (effector cell) (*see* Chapter 6). The basis for the selectivity of these agonists is unclear, as there is limited evidence that agonists discriminate appreciably among the subtypes of muscarinic receptors (Eglen *et al.*, 1996; Caulfield and Birdsall, 1998). However, subsequent radioligand binding studies definitively revealed distinct populations of antagonist binding sites (Hammer *et al.*, 1980). In particular, the muscarinic antagonist *pirenzepine* was shown to bind with high affinity to sites in cerebral cortex and sympathetic ganglia (M_1) but to have lower affinity for sites in cardiac muscle, smooth muscle, and various glands. These data explain the ability of pirenzepine to block agonist-induced responses that are mediated by muscarinic receptors in sympathetic and myenteric ganglia at concentrations considerably lower than those required to block responses that result from direct stimulation of receptors in various effector organs. Antagonists that can further discriminate among various subtypes of muscarinic receptors are now available. For example, *tripitramine* displays selectivity for cardiac M_2 relative to M_3 muscarinic receptors, while *darifenacin* is relatively selective for antagonizing glandular and smooth muscle M_3 relative to M_2 receptors (Caulfield and Birdsall, 1998; Birdsall *et al.*, 1998; Levine *et al.*, 1999).

The cloning of the cDNAs that encode muscarinic receptors identified five distinct gene products (Bonner *et al.*, 1987), now designated as M_1 through M_5 (*see* Chapter 6). All of the known muscarinic receptor subtypes interact with members of a group of heterotrimeric guanine nucleotide-binding regulatory proteins (G proteins) that in turn are linked to various cellular effectors (*see* Chapter 1). Regions within the receptor responsible for the specificity of G protein coupling have been defined primarily by receptor mutants and chimeras formed between receptor subtypes. In particular, one region at the carboxyl-terminal end of the third intracellular loop of the receptor has been implicated in the specificity of G protein coupling and shows extensive homology within M_1, M_3, and M_5 receptors and between M_2 and M_4 receptors (Wess, 1996; Caulfield, 1993; Caulfield and Birdsall, 1998). Conserved regions in the second intracellular loop also confer specificity for proper G protein recognition. Although selectivity is not absolute, stimulation of M_1 or M_3 receptors causes hydrolysis of polyphosphoinositides and mobilization of intracellular Ca^{2+} as a consequence of activation of the G_q-PLC pathway (*see* Chapter 6); this effect in turn results in a variety of Ca^{2+}-mediated events, either directly or as a consequence of the phosphorylation of target proteins. In contrast, M_2 and M_4 muscarinic receptors inhibit adenylyl cyclase and regulate specific ion channels (*e.g.*, enhancement of K^+ conductance in cardiac atrial tissue) through subunits released from pertussis toxin–sensitive G proteins (G_i and G_0) that are distinct from the G proteins used by M_1 and M_3 receptors (*see* Chapter 1).

Studies using muscarinic receptor subtype–specific antibodies and ligands demonstrate discrete localization of the muscarinic receptor subtypes, for example within brain regions and in different populations of smooth muscle cells (Levey, 1993; Yasuda *et al.*, 1993; Eglen *et al.*, 1996; Caulfield and Birdsall, 1998). The M_1 through M_5 subtypes have been disrupted through gene targeting to create null alleles for each of these genes (Hamilton *et al.*, 1997; Gomeza *et al.*, 1999; Matsui *et al.*, 2000; Yamada *et al.*, 2001a; Yamada *et al.*, 2001b; Wess, 2004). All of the muscarinic receptor subtype deletions yield mice that are viable and fertile. Studies using these mice indicate that *pilocarpine*-induced seizures are mediated through M_1, *oxotremorine*-induced tremors through M_2,

analgesia through M_2 and M_4, and hypothermia through M_2 and other subtypes. *Carbachol* and vagally induced bradycardia are lost in M_2 receptor knockout mice, while mice lacking the M_3 receptor show loss of cholinergic bronchoconstriction and urinary bladder contraction (Fisher *et al.*, 2004; Wess, 2004). Full abolition of cholinergic bronchoconstriction, salivation, pupillary constriction, and bladder contraction generally requires deletion of more than a single receptor subtype. The minimal phenotypic alteration that accompanies deletion of a single receptor subtype suggests functional redundancy between receptor subtypes in various tissues.

Pharmacological Properties

Cardiovascular System. ACh has four primary effects on the cardiovascular system: vasodilation, a decrease in cardiac rate (the negative chronotropic effect), a decrease in the rate of conduction in the specialized tissues of the sinoatrial (SA) and atrioventricular (AV) nodes (the negative dromotropic effect), and a decrease in the force of cardiac contraction (the negative inotropic effect). The last effect is of lesser significance in ventricular than in atrial muscle. Certain of the above responses can be obscured by baroreceptor and other reflexes that dampen the direct responses to ACh.

Although ACh rarely is given systemically, its cardiac actions are important because of the involvement of cholinergic vagal impulses in the actions of the cardiac glycosides, antiarrhythmic agents, and many other drugs; afferent stimulation of the viscera during surgical interventions also stimulates vagal release of ACh.

The intravenous injection of a small dose of ACh produces a transient fall in blood pressure owing to generalized vasodilation, usually accompanied by reflex tachycardia. A considerably larger dose is required to elicit bradycardia or block of AV nodal conduction from a direct action of ACh on the heart. If large doses of ACh are injected after the administration of atropine, an increase in blood pressure is observed; the increase is caused by direct stimulation of the adrenal medulla and sympathetic ganglia to release catecholamines into the circulation and at postganglionic sympathetic nerve endings, respectively.

ACh produces dilation of essentially all vascular beds, including those of the pulmonary and coronary vasculature. Vasodilation of coronary beds is mediated by stimulation of local production of NO and may be elicited by baroreceptor or chemoreceptor reflexes or by direct electrical stimulation of the vagus (Feigl, 1998). However, neither parasympathetic vasodilator nor sympathetic vasoconstrictor tone plays a major role in the regulation of coronary blood flow relative to the effects of local oxygen tension and autoregulatory metabolic factors such as adenosine (Berne and Levy, 1997).

Dilation of vascular beds by exogenously administered ACh is due to muscarinic receptors, primarily of the M_3 subtype (Bruning *et al.*, 1994; Eglen *et al.*, 1996; Caulfield and Birdsall, 1998), despite the lack of apparent cholinergic innervation of most blood vessels. The muscarinic receptors responsible for relaxation are located on the endothelial cells of the vasculature; occupation of these receptors by agonist activates the G_q–PLC–IP_3 pathway of endothelial cells, leading to Ca^{2+}-calmodulin–dependent activation of endothelial NO synthase (eNOS) and production of NO (endothelium-derived relaxing factor) (Moncada and Higgs, 1995), which diffuses to adjacent smooth muscle cells and causes them to relax (Furchgott, 1999; Ignarro *et al.*, 1999) (*see* Chapters 1 and 6). Vasodilation also may arise indirectly due to inhibition of norepinephrine release from adrenergic nerve endings by ACh. If the endothelium is damaged, as occurs under various pathophysiological conditions, ACh can stimulate receptors on vascular smooth muscle cells and cause vasoconstriction by activation of the G_q–PLC–IP_3 pathway. There is also evidence of NO-based (nitrergic) neurotransmission in peripheral blood vessels (Toda and Okamura, 2003).

Cholinergic stimulation affects cardiac function both directly and by inhibiting the effects of adrenergic activation. The latter depends on the level of sympathetic drive to the heart and results in part from inhibition of cyclic AMP formation and reduction in L-type Ca^{2+} channel activity, mediated through M_2 receptors (Brodde and Michel, 1999). The functional role of M_3 receptors in the human heart is unknown (Willmy-Matthes *et al.*, 2003). Inhibition of adrenergic stimulation of the heart arises not only from the capacity of ACh to modulate or depress the myocardial response to catecholamines, but also from a capacity to inhibit the release of norepinephrine from sympathetic nerve endings. There are also inhibitory M_2 receptors that regulate ACh release in the human heart (Oberhauser *et al.*, 2001). Cholinergic innervation of the ventricular myocardium is less dense, and the parasympathetic fibers terminate largely on specialized conduction tissue such as the Purkinje fibers but also on ventricular myocytes (Kent *et al.*, 1976; Levy and Schwartz, 1994).

In the SA node, each normal cardiac impulse is initiated by the spontaneous depolarization of the pacemaker cells (*see* Chapter 34). At a critical level—the threshold potential—this depolarization initiates an action potential. The action potential is conducted through the atrial muscle fibers to the AV node and thence through the Purkinje system to the ventricular muscle. ACh slows the heart rate by decreasing the rate of spontaneous diastolic depolarization (the pacemaker current) and by increasing the repolarizing K^+ current at the SA node; attainment of the threshold potential and the succeeding events in the cardiac cycle are therefore delayed (DiFrancesco, 1993).

In atrial muscle, ACh decreases the strength of contraction. This occurs largely indirectly, as a result of decreasing cyclic AMP and Ca^{2+} channel activity. Direct inhibitory effects are seen at higher ACh concentrations and result from M_2 receptor–mediated activation of G protein–regulated K^+ channels (Wickman and Clapham, 1995). The rate of impulse conduction in the normal atrium is either unaffected or may increase in response to ACh. The increase is due to the activation of additional Na^+ channels, possibly in response to the ACh-induced hyperpolarization. The combination of these factors is the basis for the perpetuation or exacerbation by vagal impulses of atrial flutter or fibrillation arising at an ectopic focus. In contrast, primarily in the AV node and to a much lesser extent in the Purkinje conducting system, ACh slows conduction and increases the refractory period. The decrement in AV nodal conduction usually is responsible for the complete heart block that may be observed when large quantities of cholinergic agonists are administered systemically. With an increase in vagal tone, such as is produced by the *digitalis* glycosides, the increased refractory period can contribute to the reduction in the frequency with which aberrant atrial impulses are transmitted to the ventricle, and thus decrease the ventricular rate during atrial flutter or fibrillation.

In the ventricle, ACh, whether released by vagal stimulation or applied directly, also has a negative inotropic effect, although it is smaller than that observed in the atrium. In humans and most mammals, inhibition is most apparent when there is concomitant adrenergic stimulation or underlying sympathetic tone (Levy and Schwartz, 1994; Brodde and Michel, 1999; Lewis *et al.*, 2001). Automaticity of Purkinje fibers is suppressed, and the threshold for ventricular fibrillation is increased (Kent and Epstein, 1976). Sympathetic and vagal nerve terminals lie in close proximity, and muscarinic receptors are believed to exist at presynaptic as well as postsynaptic sites (Wellstein and Pitschner, 1988).

Gastrointestinal and Urinary Tracts. Although stimulation of vagal input to the gastrointestinal tract increases tone, amplitude of contraction, and secretory activity of the stomach and intestine, such responses are inconsistently seen with administered ACh. Poor perfusion of visceral organs and rapid hydrolysis by plasma butyrylcholinesterase limit access of systemically administered ACh to visceral muscarinic receptors. Parasympathetic sacral innervation causes detrusor muscle contraction, increased voiding pressure, and ureter peristalsis, but for similar reasons these responses are not evident with administered ACh.

Table 7–1
Some Pharmacological Properties of Choline Esters and Natural Alkaloids

MUSCARINIC AGONIST	SUSCEPTIBILITY TO CHOLINESTERASES	MUSCARINIC ACTIVITY					NICOTINIC ACTIVITY
		Cardio-vascular	*Gastro-intestinal*	*Urinary Bladder*	*Eye (Topical)*	*Antagonism by Atropine*	
Acetylcholine	+++	++	++	++	+	+++	++
Methacholine	+	+++	++	++	+	+++	+
Carbachol	−	+	+++	+++	++	+	+++
Bethanechol	−	±	+++	+++	++	+++	−
Muscarine	−	++	+++	+++	++	+++	−
Pilocarpine	−	+	+++	+++	++	+++	−

Miscellaneous Effects. The influence of ACh and parasympathetic innervation on various organs and tissues is discussed in detail in Chapter 6. ACh and its analogs stimulate secretion by all glands that receive parasympathetic innervation, including the lacrimal, tracheobronchial, salivary, and digestive glands. The effects on the respiratory system, in addition to increased tracheobronchial secretion, include bronchoconstriction and stimulation of the chemoreceptors of the carotid and aortic bodies. When instilled into the eye, muscarinic agonists produce miosis (*see* Chapter 63).

Synergisms and Antagonisms. The muscarinic actions of ACh and all the drugs of this class are blocked by atropine, primarily through competitive occupation of muscarinic receptor sites on the autonomic effector cells and secondarily on autonomic ganglion cells. The nicotinic actions of ACh and its derivatives at autonomic ganglia are blocked by *hexamethonium* and *trimethaphan*; nicotinic actions at the neuromuscular junction of skeletal muscle are antagonized by *d-tubocurarine* and other competitive blocking agents (*see* Chapter 9).

CHOLINOMIMETIC CHOLINE ESTERS AND NATURAL ALKALOIDS

Muscarinic cholinergic receptor agonists can be divided into two groups: (1) ACh and several synthetic choline esters, and (2) the naturally occurring cholinomimetic alkaloids (particularly pilocarpine, *muscarine*, and *arecoline*) and their synthetic congeners.

Methacholine (acetyl-β-methylcholine) differs from ACh chiefly in its greater duration and selectivity of action. Its action is more prolonged because the added methyl group increases its resistance to hydrolysis by cholinesterases. Its selectivity is manifested by slight nicotinic and a predominance of muscarinic actions, the

latter being manifest in the cardiovascular system (Table 7–1).

Carbachol and bethanechol, which are unsubstituted carbamoyl esters, are completely resistant to hydrolysis by cholinesterases; their half-lives are thus sufficiently long that they become distributed to areas of low blood flow. Bethanechol has mainly muscarinic actions, showing some selectivity on gastrointestinal tract and urinary bladder motility. Carbachol retains substantial nicotinic activity, particularly on autonomic ganglia. It is likely that both its peripheral and its ganglionic actions are due, at least in part, to the release of endogenous ACh from the terminals of cholinergic fibers.

The three major natural alkaloids in this group—pilocarpine, muscarine, and arecoline—have the same principal sites of action as the choline esters discussed above. Muscarine acts almost exclusively at muscarinic receptor sites, and the classification of the receptors as such is derived from this fact. Arecoline also acts at nicotinic receptors. Pilocarpine has a dominant muscarinic action, but it causes anomalous cardiovascular responses; the sweat glands are particularly sensitive to the drug. Although these naturally occurring alkaloids are of great value as pharmacological tools, present clinical use is restricted largely to the employment of pilocarpine as a sialagogue and miotic agent (*see* Chapter 63).

History and Sources. Of the several hundred synthetic choline derivatives investigated, only methacholine, carbachol, and bethanechol have had clinical applications. The structures of these compounds are shown in Figure 7–1. Methacholine, the β-methyl analog of ACh, was studied by Hunt and Taveau as early as 1911. Carbachol and bethanechol, its β-methyl analog, were synthesized and investigated in the 1930s. Pilocarpine is the chief alkaloid obtained from the leaflets of South American shrubs of the genus *Pilocarpus*. Although it was long known by the natives that the chewing of leaves of *Pilocarpus* plants caused salivation, the first experiments were apparently

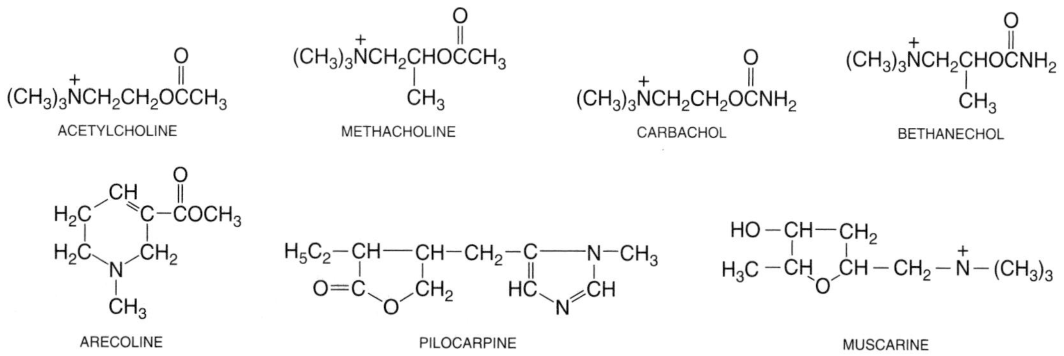

Figure 7–1. *Structural formulas of acetylcholine, choline esters, and natural alkaloids that stimulate muscarinic receptors.*

performed in 1874 by the Brazilian physician Coutinhou. The alkaloid was isolated in 1875, and shortly thereafter the actions of pilocarpine on the pupil and on the sweat and salivary glands were described by Weber.

The poisonous effects of certain species of mushrooms have been known since ancient times, but it was not until Schmiedeberg isolated the alkaloid muscarine from *Amanita muscaria* in 1869 that its properties could be systematically investigated. Arecoline is the chief alkaloid of areca or betel nuts, the seeds of *Areca catechu*. The red-staining betel nut is consumed as a euphoretic by the natives of the Indian subcontinent and East Indies in a masticatory mixture known as betel and composed of the nut, shell lime, and leaves of *Piper betle*, a climbing species of pepper.

Structure–Activity Relationships. The muscarinic alkaloids show marked differences as well as interesting relationships in structure when compared to the quaternary esters of choline (Figure 7–1). Arecoline and pilocarpine are tertiary amines. Muscarine, a quaternary ammonium compound, shows more limited absorption. McN-A-343 is an agonist that was originally proposed to stimulate M_1 receptors with some selectivity. While it is clear that McN-A-343 can stimulate sympathetic ganglia and inhibitory neurons in the myenteric plexus, this is a functional rather than a subtype-specific effect. Indeed, no therapeutically useful agonists with true M_1 or other subtype specificity are known (Caulfield and Birdsall, 1998; Eglen *et al.*, 2001).

Pharmacological Properties

Gastrointestinal Tract. All muscarinic agonists are capable of stimulating smooth muscle of the gastrointestinal tract, thereby increasing tone and motility; large doses will cause spasm and tenesmus. Unlike methacholine, carbachol, bethanechol, and pilocarpine stimulate the GI tract without significant cardiovascular effects.

Urinary Tract. The choline esters and pilocarpine contract the detrusor muscle of the bladder, increase voiding pressure, decrease bladder capacity, and increase ureteral peristalsis. In addition, the trigone and external sphincter muscles relax. Selectivity for bladder stimulation relative to cardiovascular activity is evident for bethanechol. In animals with experimental spinal cord lesions, muscarinic agonists promote evacuation of the bladder (Yoshimura *et al.*, 2000).

Exocrine Glands. The choline esters and muscarinic alkaloids stimulate secretion of glands that receive parasympathetic or sympathetic cholinergic innervation, including the lacrimal, salivary, digestive, tracheobronchial, and sweat glands. Pilocarpine in particular causes marked diaphoresis in human beings; 2 to 3 liters of sweat may be secreted. Salivation also is increased markedly. Oral administration of pilocarpine causes a more continuous production of saliva. Muscarine and arecoline also are potent diaphoretic agents. Accompanying side effects may include hiccough, salivation, nausea, vomiting, weakness, and occasionally collapse. These alkaloids also stimulate the lacrimal, gastric, pancreatic, and intestinal glands, and the mucous cells of the respiratory tract.

Respiratory System. In addition to tracheobronchial secretions, bronchial smooth muscle is stimulated by the muscarinic agonists. Asthmatic patients respond with intense bronchoconstriction, secretions, and a reduction in vital capacity. These actions form the basis of the methacholine challenge test used to diagnose airway hyperreactivity.

Cardiovascular System. Continuous intravenous infusion of methacholine elicits hypotension and bradycardia, just as ACh does but at 1/200 the dose. Muscarine, at small doses, also leads to a marked fall in blood pressure and a slowing or temporary cessation of the heartbeat. In contrast, carbachol and bethanechol generally cause only a transient fall in blood pressure at doses that affect the gastrointestinal and urinary tracts. Likewise, pilocarpine produces only a brief fall in blood pressure. However, if this is preceded by an appropriate dose of a nicotinic receptor antagonist, pilocarpine produces a marked rise in pressure. Both the vasodepressor and pressor responses are prevented by atropine; the latter effect also is abolished by α adrenergic receptor antagonists. These actions of pilocarpine have not been fully explained, but may arise from ganglionic and adrenomedullary stimulation.

Eye. Muscarinic agonists stimulate the pupillary constrictor and ciliary muscles when applied locally to the eye, causing pupil constriction and a loss of ability to accommodate to far vision.

Central Nervous System. The intravenous injection of relatively small doses of pilocarpine, muscarine, or arecoline evokes a characteristic cortical arousal or activation response in cats, similar to that produced by injection of anticholinesterase agents or by electrical stimulation of the brainstem reticular formation. The arousal response to all of these drugs is reduced or blocked by atropine and related agents (Krnjevíc, 1974). Being quaternary, the choline esters do not cross the blood–brain barrier.

Therapeutic Uses

Acetylcholine (MIOCHOL-E) is available as an ophthalmic surgical aid for the rapid production of miosis. *Bethanechol chloride* (carbamyl-β-methylcholine chloride; URECHOLINE, others) is available in tablets and as an injection and is used as a stimulant of the smooth muscle of the gastrointestinal tract, and in particular, the urinary bladder. *Pilocarpine hydrochloride* (SALAGEN) is available as 5- or 7.5-mg oral doses for treatment of xerostomia or as ophthalmic solutions (PILOCAR, others) of varying strength. *Methacholine chloride* (acetyl-β-methylcholine chloride; PROVOCHOLINE) may be administered for diagnosis of bronchial hyperreactivity. The unpredictability of absorption and intensity of response has precluded its use as a vasodilator or cardiac vagomimetic agent. *Cevimeline* (EVOXAC) is a newer muscarinic agonist available orally for use in treatment of xerostomia.

Gastrointestinal Disorders. Bethanechol can be of value in certain cases of postoperative abdominal distention and in gastric atony or gastroparesis. The oral route is preferred; the usual dosage is 10 to 20 mg, three or four times daily. Bethanechol is given by mouth before each main meal in cases without complete retention; when gastric retention is complete and nothing passes into the duodenum, the subcutaneous route is necessary because of poor stomach absorption. Bethanechol likewise has been used to advantage in certain patients with congenital megacolon and with adynamic ileus secondary to toxic states. Prokinetic agents with combined cholinergic-agonist and dopamine-antagonist activity (*e.g., metoclopramide*) or serotonin-antagonist activity (*see* Chapter 37) have largely replaced bethanechol in gastroparesis or esophageal reflux disorders.

Urinary Bladder Disorders. Bethanechol may be useful in treating urinary retention and inadequate emptying of the bladder when organic obstruction is absent, as in postoperative and postpartum urinary retention and in certain cases of chronic hypotonic, myogenic, or neurogenic bladder (Wein, 1991). α Adrenergic receptor antagonists are useful adjuncts in reducing outlet resistance of the internal sphincter (*see* Chapter 10). Bethanechol may enhance contractions of the detrusor muscle after spinal injury if the vesical reflex is intact, and some benefit has been noted in partial sensory or motor paralysis of the bladder. Catheterization thus can be avoided. For acute retention, multiple subcutaneous doses of 2.5 mg of bethanechol may be administered. The stomach should be empty at the time the drug is injected. In chronic cases, 10 to 50 mg of the drug may be given orally two to four times daily with meals to avoid nausea and vomiting. When voluntary or spontaneous voiding begins, bethanechol is then slowly withdrawn.

Xerostomia. Pilocarpine is administered orally in 5- to 10-mg doses given three times daily for the treatment of xerostomia that follows head and neck radiation treatments or that is associated with Sjögren's syndrome (Wiseman and Faulds, 1995; Porter *et al.*, 2004). The latter is an autoimmune disorder occurring primarily in women in whom secretions, particularly salivary and lacrimal, are compromised (Anaya and Talal, 1999; Nusair and Rubinow, 1999). Provided salivary parenchyma maintains residual function, enhanced salivary secretion, ease of swallowing, and subjective improvement in hydration of the oral cavity are achieved. Side effects typify cholinergic

stimulation, with sweating being the most common complaint. Bethanechol is an oral alternative that produces less diaphoresis (Epstein *et al.*, 1994). Cevimeline (EVOXAC) is a newer agonist with activity at M_3 muscarinic receptors. These receptors are found on lacrimal and salivary gland epithelia. Cevimeline has a long-lasting sialogogic action and may have fewer side effects than pilocarpine (Anaya and Talal, 1999). It also enhances lacrimal secretions in Sjögren's syndrome (Ono *et al.*, 2004).

Ophthalmological. Pilocarpine also is used in the treatment of glaucoma, where it is instilled into the eye usually as a 0.5% to 4% solution. An ocular insert (OCUSERT PILO-20) that releases 20 μg of pilocarpine per hour over 7 days also is marketed for the control of elevated intraocular pressure. Pilocarpine usually is better tolerated than are the anticholinesterases, and pilocarpine is the standard cholinergic agent in the treatment of open-angle glaucoma. Reduction of intraocular pressure occurs within a few minutes and lasts 4 to 8 hours. The ophthalmic use of pilocarpine alone and in combination with other agents is discussed in Chapter 63. The miotic action of pilocarpine is useful in reversing a narrow-angle glaucoma attack and overcoming the mydriasis produced by atropine; alternated with mydriatics, pilocarpine is employed to break adhesions between the iris and the lens.

CNS. Agonists that show functional selectivity for M_1 and M_2 receptors have been targets for drug development, and some have been in clinical trial for use in treating the cognitive impairment associated with Alzheimer's disease. The potential advantage of such agonists would arise from stimulating postsynaptic M_1 receptors in the CNS without concomitantly stimulating the presynaptic M_2 receptors that inhibit release of endogenous ACh. However, lack of efficacy in improvement of cognitive function has diminished enthusiasm for this approach (Eglen *et al.*, 1999).

Precautions, Toxicity, and Contraindications

Muscarinic agonists are administered subcutaneously to achieve an acute response and orally to treat more chronic conditions. Should serious toxic reactions to these drugs arise, *atropine sulfate* (0.5 to 1 mg in adults) should be given subcutaneously or intravenously. *Epinephrine* (0.3 to 1 mg, subcutaneously or intramuscularly) also is of value in overcoming severe cardiovascular or bronchoconstrictor responses.

Major contraindications to the use of the muscarinic agonists are asthma, hyperthyroidism, coronary insufficiency, and acid-peptic disease. Their bronchoconstrictor action is liable to precipitate an asthma attack, and hyperthyroid patients may develop atrial fibrillation. Hypotension induced by these agents can severely reduce coronary blood flow, especially if it is already compromised. Other possible undesirable effects of the cholinergic agents are flushing, sweating, abdominal cramps, belching, a sensation of tightness in the urinary bladder, difficulty in visual accommodation, headache, and salivation.

Toxicology

Poisoning from pilocarpine, muscarine, or arecoline is characterized chiefly by exaggeration of their various parasympathomimetic effects and resembles that produced by consumption of mushrooms of the genus *Inocybe* (*see* below). Treatment consists of the parenteral administration of atropine in doses sufficient to cross the blood–brain barrier and measures to support the respiratory and cardiovascular systems and to counteract pulmonary edema.

Mushroom Poisoning (Mycetism). Mushroom poisoning has been known for centuries. The Greek poet Euripides (fifth century B.C.) is said to have lost his wife and three children from this cause. In recent years the number of cases of mushroom poisoning has been increasing as the result of the current popularity of the consumption of wild mushrooms. Various species of mushrooms contain many toxins, and species within the same genus may contain distinct toxins.

Although *Amanita muscaria* is the source from which muscarine was isolated, its content of the alkaloid is so low (approximately 0.003%) that muscarine cannot be responsible for the major toxic effects. Much higher concentrations of muscarine are present in various species of *Inocybe* and *Clitocybe*. The symptoms of intoxication attributable to muscarine develop within 30 to 60 minutes of ingestion; they include salivation, lacrimation, nausea, vomiting, headache, visual disturbances, abdominal colic, diarrhea, bronchospasm, bradycardia, hypotension, and shock. Treatment with atropine (1 to 2 mg intramuscularly every 30 minutes) effectively blocks these effects (Köppel, 1993; Goldfrank, 1998).

Intoxication produced by *A. muscaria* and related *Amanita* species arises from the neurologic and hallucinogenic properties of muscimol, ibotenic acid, and other isoxazole derivatives. These agents stimulate excitatory and inhibitory amino acid receptors. Symptoms range from irritability, restlessness, ataxia, hallucinations, and delirium to drowsiness and sedation. Treatment is mainly supportive; benzodiazepines are indicated when excitation predominates, whereas atropine often exacerbates the delirium.

Mushrooms from *Psilocybe* and *Panaeolus* species contain psilocybin and related derivatives of tryptamine. They also cause short-lasting hallucinations. *Gyromitra* species (false morels) produce gastrointestinal disorders and a delayed hepatotoxicity. The toxic substance, acetaldehyde methylformylhydrazone, is converted in the body to reactive hydrazines. Although fatalities from liver and kidney failure have been reported, they are far less frequent than with amatoxin-containing mushrooms.

The most serious form of mycetism is produced by *Amanita phalloides,* other *Amanita* species, *Lepiota,* and *Galerina* species (Goldfrank, 1998). These species account for more than 90% of all fatal cases. Ingestion of as little as 50 g of *A. phalloides* (deadly nightcap) can be fatal. The principal toxins are the amatoxins (α- and β-amanitin), a group of cyclic octapeptides that inhibit RNA polymerase II and hence block mRNA synthesis. This causes cell death, manifested particularly in the gastrointestinal mucosa, liver, and kidneys. Initial symptoms, which often are unnoticed, or when present are due to other toxins, include diarrhea and abdominal cramps. A symptom-free period lasting up to 24 hours is followed by hepatic and renal malfunction. Death occurs in 4 to 7 days from renal and hepatic failure (Goldfrank, 1998). Treatment is largely supportive; *penicillin, thioctic acid,* and *silibinin* may be effective antidotes, but the evidence is based largely on anecdotal studies (Köppel, 1993).

Because the severity of toxicity and treatment strategies for mushroom poisoning depend on the species ingested, their identification should be sought. Often symptomatology is delayed, limiting the value of gastric lavage and administration of activated charcoal. Regional poison control centers in the United States maintain up-to-date information on the incidence of poisoning in the region and treatment procedures.

MUSCARINIC RECEPTOR ANTAGONISTS

The class of drugs referred to here as muscarinic receptor antagonists includes (1) the naturally occurring alkaloids, atropine and *scopolamine;* (2) semisynthetic derivatives of these alkaloids, which primarily differ from the parent compounds in their disposition in the body or their duration of action; and (3) synthetic congeners, some of which show selectivity for particular subtypes of muscarinic receptors. Noteworthy agents among the synthetic derivatives are *homatropine* and *tropicamide,* which have a shorter duration of action than atropine, and *methylatropine, ipratropium,* and *tiotropium,* which are quaternized and do not cross the blood–brain barrier or readily cross membranes. The latter two agents are given by inhalation in the treatment of chronic obstructive pulmonary disease and are pending approval for use in bronchial asthma. Ipratropium also has an FDA-approved indication for perennial- and common cold–associated rhinorrhea. The synthetic derivatives possessing partial receptor selectivity include pirenzepine, used in the treatment of acid-peptic disease in some countries, and *tolterodine, oxybutynin,* and several others, used in the treatment of urinary incontinence.

Muscarinic receptor antagonists prevent the effects of ACh by blocking its binding to muscarinic cholinergic receptors at neuroeffector sites on smooth muscle, cardiac muscle, and gland cells; in peripheral ganglia; and in the CNS. In general, muscarinic receptor antagonists cause little blockade at nicotinic receptor sites. However, the quaternary ammonium antagonists generally exhibit a greater degree of nicotinic blocking activity, and consequently are more likely to interfere with ganglionic or neuromuscular transmission.

Cholinergic transmission appears to be both muscarinic and nicotinic at spinal, subcortical, and cortical levels in the brain (*see* Chapter 12). At high or toxic doses, central effects of atropine and related drugs are observed, generally consisting of CNS stimulation followed by depression. Since quaternary compounds penetrate the blood–brain barrier poorly, they have little or no effect on the CNS.

Parasympathetic neuroeffector junctions in different organs vary in their sensitivity to muscarinic receptor antagonists (Table 7–2). Small doses of atropine depress salivary and bronchial secretion and sweating. With larger doses, the pupil dilates, accommodation of the lens to near vision is inhibited, and vagal effects on the heart are

Table 7–2
Effects of Atropine in Relation to Dose

DOSE	EFFECTS
0.5 mg	Slight cardiac slowing; some dryness of mouth; inhibition of sweating
1 mg	Definite dryness of mouth; thirst; acceleration of heart, sometimes preceded by slowing; mild dilation of pupils
2 mg	Rapid heart rate; palpitation; marked dryness of mouth; dilated pupils; some blurring of near vision
5 mg	All the above symptoms marked; difficulty in speaking and swallowing; restlessness and fatigue; headache; dry, hot skin; difficulty in micturition; reduced intestinal peristalsis
10 mg and more	Above symptoms more marked; pulse rapid and weak; iris practically obliterated; vision very blurred; skin flushed, hot, dry, and scarlet; ataxia, restlessness, and excitement; hallucinations and delirium; coma

blocked so that the heart rate is increased. Larger doses antagonize parasympathetic control of the urinary bladder and gastrointestinal tract, thereby inhibiting micturition and decreasing the tone and motility of the gut. Still larger doses are required to inhibit gastric motility and particularly secretion. Thus, doses of atropine and most related muscarinic receptor antagonists that depress gastric secretion also almost invariably affect salivary secretion, ocular accommodation, micturition, and gastrointestinal tone. This hierarchy of relative sensitivities is not a consequence of differences in the affinity of atropine for the muscarinic receptors at these sites because atropine lacks selectivity toward different muscarinic receptor subtypes. More likely determinants include the degree to which the functions of various end organs are regulated by parasympathetic tone and the involvement of intramural neurons and reflexes.

The actions of most clinically available muscarinic receptor antagonists differ only quantitatively from those of atropine, considered below as the prototype of the group. No antagonist in the receptor-selective category, including pirenzepine, is completely selective (*i.e.*, can be used to define a single receptor subtype relative to all other receptor subtypes). In fact, clinical efficacy of some

agents may arise from a balance of antagonistic actions on two or more receptor subtypes.

History. The naturally occurring muscarinic receptor antagonists atropine and scopolamine are alkaloids of the belladonna (Solanaceae) plants. Preparations of belladonna were known to the ancient Hindus and have been used by physicians for many centuries. During the time of the Roman Empire and in the Middle Ages, the deadly nightshade shrub was frequently used to produce obscure and often prolonged poisoning. This prompted Linnaeus to name the shrub *Atropa belladonna,* after Atropos, the oldest of the three Fates, who cuts the thread of life. The name *belladonna* derives from the alleged use of this preparation by Italian women to dilate their pupils; modern-day fashion models are known to use this same device for visual appeal. Atropine (*d,l-hyoscyamine*) also is found in *Datura stramonium,* also known as Jamestown or jimson weed. Scopolamine (*l-hyoscine*) is found chiefly in *Hyoscyamus niger* (henbane). In India, the root and leaves of the jimson weed plant were burned and the smoke inhaled to treat asthma. British colonists observed this ritual and introduced the belladonna alkaloids into western medicine in the early 1800s.

Accurate study of the actions of belladonna dates from the isolation of atropine in pure form by Mein in 1831. In 1867, Bezold and Bloebaum showed that atropine blocked the cardiac effects of vagal stimulation, and 5 years later Heidenhain found that it prevented salivary secretion produced by stimulation of the chorda tympani. Many semisynthetic congeners of the belladonna alkaloids and a large number of synthetic muscarinic receptor antagonists have been prepared, primarily with the objective of altering gastrointestinal or bladder activity without causing dry mouth or pupillary dilation.

Chemistry. Atropine and scopolamine are esters formed by combination of an aromatic acid, tropic acid, and complex organic bases, either tropine (tropanol) or scopine. Scopine differs from tropine only in having an oxygen bridge between the carbon atoms designated as 6 and 7 (Figure 7–2). Homatropine is a semisynthetic compound produced by combining the base tropine with mandelic acid. The corresponding quaternary ammonium derivatives, modified by the addition of a second methyl group to the nitrogen, are *methylatropine nitrate, methscopolamine bromide,* and *homatropine methylbromide.* Ipratropium and tiotropium also are quaternary tropine analogs esterified with synthetic aromatic acids.

Structure–Activity Relationships. An intact ester of tropine and tropic acid is essential for antimuscarinic action, since neither the free acid nor the basic alcohol exhibits significant antimuscarinic activity. The presence of a free OH group in the acyl portion of the ester also is important for activity. When given parenterally, quaternary ammonium derivatives of atropine and scopolamine are generally more potent than their parent compounds in both muscarinic receptor and ganglionic (nicotinic) blocking activities. The quaternary derivatives, when given orally, are poorly and unreliably absorbed.

Both tropic and mandelic acids have an enantiomeric center (boldface **C** in the formulas in Figure 7–2). Scopolamine is *l*-hyoscine and is much more active than *d*-hyoscine. Atropine is racemized during extraction and consists of *d,l*-hyoscyamine, but antimuscarinic activity is almost wholly due to the naturally occurring *l*

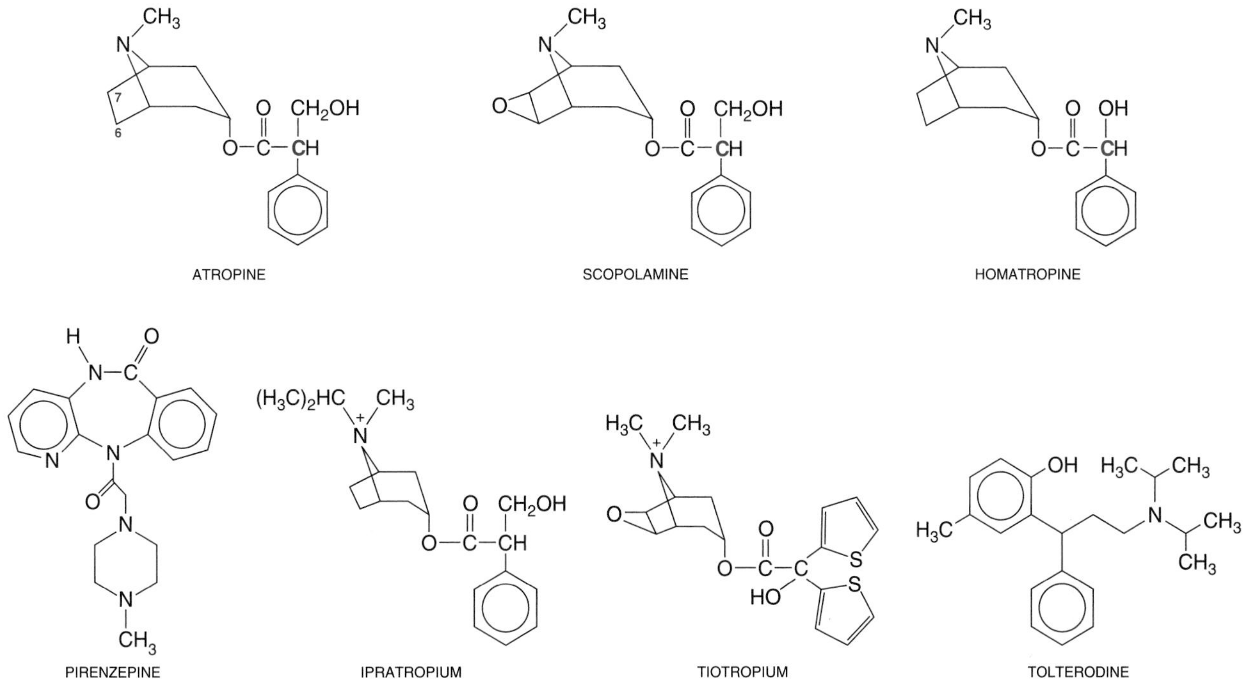

Figure 7–2. *Structural formulas of the belladonna alkaloids and semisynthetic and synthetic analogs.* The blue **C** identifies an asymmetric carbon atom.

isomer. Synthetic derivatives show a wide latitude of structures that spatially replicate the aromatic acid and the bridged nitrogen of the tropine.

Mechanism of Action. Atropine and related compounds compete with ACh and other muscarinic agonists for a common binding site on the muscarinic receptor. Based on the position of retinol in the mammalian rhodopsin structure (Palczewski *et al.*, 2000), the binding site for competitive antagonists and acetylcholine likely is in a cleft formed by several of the receptor's 7 transmembrane helices. An aspartic acid present in the *N*-terminal portion of the third transmembrane helix of all 5 muscarinic receptor subtypes is believed to form an ionic bond with the cationic quaternary nitrogen in acetylcholine and the tertiary or quaternary nitrogen of the antagonists (Wess, 1996; Caulfield and Birdsall, 1998).

Since antagonism by atropine is competitive, it can be overcome if the concentration of ACh at receptor sites of the effector organ is increased sufficiently. Muscarinic receptor antagonists inhibit responses to postganglionic cholinergic nerve stimulation less readily than they inhibit responses to injected choline esters. The difference may be due to release of ACh by cholinergic nerve terminals so close to receptors that very high concentrations of the transmitter gain access to the receptors in the neuroeffector junction.

Pharmacological Properties: The Prototypical Alkaloids Atropine and Scopolamine

Atropine and scopolamine differ quantitatively in antimuscarinic actions, particularly in their ability to affect the CNS. Atropine has almost no detectable effect on the CNS in doses that are used clinically. In contrast, scopolamine has prominent central effects at low therapeutic doses. The basis for this difference is probably the greater permeation of scopolamine across the blood–brain barrier. Because atropine has limited CNS effects, it is preferred to scopolamine for most purposes.

Central Nervous System. Atropine in therapeutic doses (0.5 to 1 mg) causes only mild vagal excitation as a result of stimulation of the medulla and higher cerebral centers. With toxic doses of atropine, central excitation becomes more prominent, leading to restlessness, irritability, disorientation, hallucinations, or delirium (*see* discussion of atropine poisoning, below). With still larger doses, stimulation is followed by depression, leading to circulatory collapse and respiratory failure after a period of paralysis and coma.

Scopolamine in therapeutic doses normally causes CNS depression manifested as drowsiness, amnesia, fatigue, and dreamless sleep, with a reduction in rapid eye movement (REM) sleep. It also causes euphoria and is therefore subject to some abuse. The depressant and amnesic effects formerly were sought when scopolamine was used as an adjunct to anesthetic agents or for preanesthetic medication. However, in the presence of severe pain, the same doses of scopolamine can occasionally cause excitement, restlessness, hallucinations, or delirium. These excitatory effects resemble those of toxic doses of atropine. Scopolamine also is effective in preventing motion sickness. This action is probably either on the cortex or the vestibular apparatus.

The belladonna alkaloids and related muscarinic receptor antagonists have long been used in parkinsonism. These agents can be effective adjuncts to treatment with *levodopa* (*see* Chapter 20). Muscarinic receptor antagonists also are used to treat the extrapyramidal symptoms that commonly occur as side effects of conventional antipsychotic drug therapy (*see* Chapter 18). Certain antipsychotic drugs are relatively potent muscarinic-receptor antagonists (Richelson, 1999), and these cause fewer extrapyramidal side effects.

Ganglia and Autonomic Nerves. Cholinergic neurotransmission in autonomic ganglia is mediated primarily by activation of nicotinic ACh receptors, resulting in the generation of action potentials (*see* Chapters 6 and 9). ACh and other cholinergic agonists also cause the generation of slow excitatory postsynaptic potentials that are mediated by ganglionic M_1 muscarinic receptors. This response is particularly sensitive to blockade by pirenzepine. The extent to which the slow excitatory response can alter impulse transmission through the different sympathetic and parasympathetic ganglia is difficult to assess, but the effects of pirenzepine on responses of end organs suggest a physiological modulatory function for the ganglionic M_1 receptor (Caulfield, 1993; Eglen *et al.*, 1996; Birdsall *et al.*, 1998; Caulfield and Birdsall, 1998).

Pirenzepine inhibits gastric acid secretion at doses that have little effect on salivation or heart rate. Since the muscarinic receptors on the parietal cells do not appear to have a high affinity for pirenzepine, the M_1 receptor responsible for alterations in gastric acid secretion is postulated to be localized in intramural ganglia (Eglen *et al.*, 1996). Blockade of ganglionic muscarinic receptors (rather than those at the neuroeffector junction) also appears to underlie the ability of pirenzepine to inhibit the relaxation of the lower esophageal sphincter. Likewise, blockade of parasympathetic ganglia may contribute to the response to muscarinic antagonists in lung and heart (Wellstein and Pitschner, 1988).

Presynaptic muscarinic receptors also are present on terminals of sympathetic and parasympathetic neurons. Blockade of these presynaptic receptors, which are of variable subtype, generally augments neurotransmitter release. Nonselective muscarinic blocking agents may thus augment ACh release, partially counteracting their effective postsynaptic receptor blockade.

Since muscarinic receptor antagonists can alter autonomic activity at the ganglion and postganglionic neuron, the ultimate response of end organs to blockade of muscarinic receptors is difficult to predict. Thus, while direct blockade at neuroeffector sites predictably reverses the usual effects of the parasympathetic nervous system, concomitant inhibition of ganglionic or presynaptic receptors may produce paradoxical responses.

Eye. Muscarinic receptor antagonists block the cholinergic responses of the pupillary sphincter muscle of the iris and the ciliary muscle controlling lens curvature (*see* Chapter 63). Thus, they dilate the pupil (mydriasis) and paralyze accommodation (cycloplegia). The wide pupillary dilation results in photophobia; the lens is fixed for far vision, near objects are blurred, and objects may appear smaller than they are. The normal pupillary reflex constriction to light or upon convergence of the eyes is abolished. These effects can occur after either local or systemic administration of the alkaloids. However, conventional systemic doses of atropine (0.6 mg) have little ocular effect, in contrast to equal doses of scopolamine, which cause definite mydriasis and loss of accommodation. Locally applied atropine or scopolamine produces ocular effects of considerable duration; accommodation and pupillary reflexes may not fully recover for 7 to 12 days. Other muscarinic receptor antagonists with shorter durations of action are therefore preferred as mydriatics in ophthalmological practice (*see* Chapter 63). Sympathomimetic agents also cause pupillary dilation but without loss of accommodation. Pilocarpine, choline esters, *physostigmine* (ophthalmic solution discontinued in the United States), and *isoflurophate* (DFP) in sufficient concentrations can partially or fully reverse the ocular effects of atropine.

Muscarinic receptor antagonists administered systemically have little effect on intraocular pressure except in patients predisposed to narrow-angle glaucoma, in whom the pressure may occasionally rise dangerously. The rise in pressure occurs when the anterior chamber is narrow and the iris obstructs outflow of aqueous humor into the trabeculae. Muscarinic antagonists may precipitate a first attack in unrecognized cases of this relatively rare condition. In patients with open-angle glaucoma, an acute rise in pressure is unusual. Atropinelike drugs generally can be used safely in this latter condition, particularly if the patient also is adequately treated with an appropriate miotic agent.

Cardiovascular System. **Heart.** The main effect of atropine on the heart is to alter the rate. Although the dominant response is tachycardia, the heart rate often decreases transiently with average clinical doses (0.4 to 0.6 mg). The slowing is rarely marked, about 4 to 8 beats per minute, and is usually absent after rapid intravenous injection. There are no accompanying changes in blood pressure or cardiac output. This unexpected effect once was thought to be due to central vagal stimulation; however, cardiac slowing also is seen with muscarinic receptor antagonists that do not readily enter the brain. Human studies show that pirenzepine is equipotent with atropine in decreasing heart rate and that its prior administration can prevent any further decrease by atropine (Wellstein and Pitschner, 1988).

Larger doses of atropine cause progressively increasing tachycardia by blocking vagal effects on M_2 receptors on the SA nodal pacemaker. The resting heart rate is increased by about 35 to 40 beats per minute in young men given 2 mg of atropine intramuscularly. The maximal heart rate (*e.g.*, in response to exercise) is not altered by atropine. The influence of atropine is most noticeable in healthy young adults, in whom vagal tone is considerable. In infancy and old age, even large doses of atropine may fail to accelerate the heart. Atropine often produces cardiac arrhythmias, but without significant cardiovascular symptoms.

With low doses of scopolamine (0.1 or 0.2 mg), the cardiac slowing is greater than with atropine. With higher doses, a transient cardioacceleration may be observed.

Adequate doses of atropine can abolish many types of reflex vagal cardiac slowing or asystole—for example, from inhalation of irritant vapors, stimulation of the carotid sinus, pressure on the eyeballs, peritoneal stimulation, or injection of contrast dye during cardiac catheterization. It also prevents or abruptly abolishes bradycardia or asystole caused by choline esters, acetylcholinesterase inhibitors, or other parasympathomimetic drugs, as well as cardiac arrest from electrical stimulation of the vagus.

The removal of vagal influence on the heart by atropine also may facilitate AV conduction. Atropine shortens the functional refractory period of the AV node and can increase ventricular rate in patients who have atrial fibrillation or flutter. In certain cases of second-degree heart block (*e.g.,* Wenckebach AV block), in which vagal activity is an etiological factor (such as with digitalis toxicity), atropine may lessen the degree of block. In some patients with complete heart block, the idioventricular rate may be accelerated by atropine; in others it is stabilized. Atropine may improve the clinical condition of patients with inferior or posterior wall myocardial infarction by relieving severe sinus or nodal bradycardia or AV block.

Circulation. Atropine, in clinical doses, completely counteracts the peripheral vasodilation and sharp fall in blood pressure caused by choline esters. In contrast, when given alone, its effect on blood vessels and blood pressure is neither striking nor constant. This result is expected because most vascular beds lack significant cholinergic innervation. The presence of cholinergic sympathetic vasodilator fibers to vessels supplying skeletal muscle is not well documented in humans; they do not appear to be involved in the normal regulation of tone.

Atropine in toxic, and occasionally therapeutic, doses can dilate cutaneous blood vessels, especially those in the blush area (atropine flush). This may be a compensatory reaction permitting the radiation of heat to offset the atropine-induced rise in temperature that can accompany inhibition of sweating.

Respiratory Tract. The parasympathetic nervous system plays a major role in regulating bronchomotor tone. A diverse set of stimuli cause a reflex increase in parasympathetic activity that contributes to bronchoconstriction. Vagal fibers synapse and activate nicotinic and M_1 muscarinic receptors in parasympathetic ganglia located in the airway wall; short postganglionic fibers release ACh, which acts on M_3 muscarinic receptors in airway smooth muscle. The submucosal glands also are innervated by parasympathetic neurons and also have predominantly M_3 receptors. Largely owing to the introduction of inhaled ipratropium and tiotropium, anticholinergic therapy of chronic obstructive pulmonary disease and asthma has been revived (Barnes and Hansel, 2004).

The belladonna alkaloids inhibit secretions of the nose, mouth, pharynx, and bronchi, and thus dry the mucous membranes of the respiratory tract. This action is especially marked if secretion is excessive and was the basis for the use of atropine and scopolamine to prevent irritating anesthetics such as diethyl ether from increasing bronchial secretion. Reduction of mucous secretion and mucociliary clearance resulting in mucus plugs are undesirable side effects of atropine in patients with airway disease.

Inhibition by atropine of bronchoconstriction caused by histamine, bradykinin, and the eicosanoids presumably reflects the participation of parasympathetic efferents in the bronchial reflexes elicited by these agents. The ability to block the indirect bronchoconstrictive effects of these mediators that are released during attacks of asthma forms the basis for the use of anticholinergic agents, along with β adrenergic receptor agonists, in the treatment of this disease (*see* Chapter 27).

Gastrointestinal Tract. Interest in the actions of muscarinic receptor antagonists on the stomach and intestine led to their use as antispasmodic agents for gastrointestinal disorders and in the treatment of peptic ulcer disease. Although atropine can completely abolish the effects of ACh (and other parasympathomimetic drugs) on the motility and secretions of the gastrointestinal tract, it inhibits only incompletely the effects of vagal impulses. This difference is particularly striking in the effects of atropine on gut motility. Preganglionic vagal fibers that innervate the GI synapse not only with postganglionic cholinergic fibers, but also with a network of noncholinergic intramural neurons. These neurons, which form the enteric plexus, utilize numerous neurotransmitters or neuromodulators including 5-hydroxytryptamine (5-HT), dopamine, and peptides. Since therapeutic doses of atropine do not block responses to gastrointestinal hormones or to noncholinergic neurohumoral transmitters, release of these substances from the intramural neurons can still effect changes in motility. Similarly, while vagal activity modulates gastrin-elicited histamine release and gastric acid secretion, the actions of gastrin can occur independent of vagal tone. Histamine H_2 receptor antagonists and proton pump inhibitors have replaced nonselective muscarinic antagonists as inhibitors of acid secretion (*see* Chapter 36).

Secretions. *Salivary secretion* appears to be mediated through M_3 receptors and is particularly sensitive to inhibition by muscarinic receptor antagonists, which can completely abolish the copious, watery, parasympathetically induced secretion. The mouth becomes dry, and swallowing and talking may become difficult. Gastric secretions during the cephalic and fasting phase are also reduced markedly by muscarinic receptor antagonists. In contrast, the intestinal phase of gastric secretion is only partially inhibited. The concentration of acid is not necessarily lowered because secretion of HCO_3^- as well as of H^+ is blocked. The gastric cells that secrete mucin and proteolytic enzymes are more directly under vagal influence than are the acid-secreting cells, and atropine decreases their secretory function.

Motility. The parasympathetic nerves enhance both tone and motility and relax sphincters, thereby favoring the passage of gastrointestinal contents. Both in normal subjects and in patients with gastrointestinal disease, muscarinic antagonists produce prolonged inhibitory effects on the motor activity of the stomach, duodenum, jejunum, ileum, and colon, characterized by a reduction in tone and in amplitude and frequency of peristaltic contractions. Relatively large doses are needed to produce such inhibition. The intestine has a complex system of intramural nerve plexuses that regulate motility independent of parasympathetic control; vagal impulses from the medulla serve to modulate the effects of the intrinsic reflexes (*see* Chapter 6).

Other Smooth Muscle. *Urinary Tract.* Muscarinic antagonists decrease the normal tone and amplitude of contractions of the ureter and bladder, and often eliminate drug-induced enhancement of ureteral tone. However, this inhibition is not achieved in the absence of inhibition of salivation and lacrimation and blurring of vision. Control of bladder contraction apparently is mediated by multiple muscarinic receptor subtypes. Receptors of the M_2 subtype appear most prevalent in the bladder, yet studies with selective antagonists suggest that the M_3 receptor mediates detrusor muscle contraction. The M_2 receptor may act to inhibit β adrenergic receptor–mediated relaxation of the bladder and may be involved primarily in the filling stages to diminish urge incontinence (Hegde and Eglen, 1999; Chapple, 2000). In addition, presynaptic M_1 receptors appear to facilitate the release of ACh from parasympathetic nerve terminals (Somogyi and de Groat, 1999).

Biliary Tract. Atropine exerts a mild antispasmodic action on the gallbladder and bile ducts in humans. However, this effect usually is not sufficient to overcome or prevent the marked spasm and increase in biliary duct pressure induced by opioids. The nitrites (*see* Chapter 31) are more effective than atropine in this respect.

Sweat Glands and Temperature. Small doses of atropine or scopolamine inhibit the activity of sweat glands innervated by sympathetic cholinergic fibers, and the skin becomes hot and dry. Sweating may be depressed enough to raise the body temperature, but only notably so after large doses or at high environmental temperatures.

Pharmacologic Properties: The Quaternary Derivatives Ipratropium and Tiotropium

Ipratropium bromide (ATROVENT, others) is a quaternary ammonium compound formed by the introduction of an isopropyl group to the N atom of atropine. A similar agent, *oxitropium bromide,* an *N*-ethyl-substituted, quaternary derivative of scopolamine, is available in Europe. The most recently developed and bronchoselective member of this family is tiotropium bromide (SPIRIVA), which has a longer duration of action. Ipratropium appears to block all subtypes of muscarinic receptors and thus blocks presynaptic muscarinic inhibition of ACh release, whereas tiotropium shows some selectivity for M_1 and M_3 receptors. Tiotropium has a lower affinity for M_2 receptors, minimizing its presynaptic effect on ACh release.

Ipratropium produces bronchodilation, tachycardia, and inhibition of secretion similar to that of atropine when it is administered parenterally. Although somewhat more potent than atropine, ipratropium and tiotropium lack appreciable action on the CNS but have greater inhibitory effects on ganglionic transmission. An unexpected and therapeutically important property of ipratropium and tiotropium, evident upon either local or parenteral administration, is their minimal inhibitory effect on mucociliary clearance relative to atropine. Hence, the use of these agents in patients with airway disease minimizes the increased accumulation of lower airway secretions encountered with atropine.

When ipratropium or tiotropium is inhaled, its action is confined almost exclusively to the mouth and airways. Dry mouth is the only side effect reported frequently. Selectivity results from the very inefficient absorption of the drug from the lungs or the gastrointestinal tract. The degree of bronchodilation achieved by these agents is thought to reflect the level of basal parasympathetic tone, supplemented by reflex activation of cholinergic pathways brought about by various stimuli. In normal individuals, inhalation of the drugs can provide virtually complete protection against the bronchoconstriction produced by the subsequent inhalation of such irritants as sulfur dioxide, ozone, or cigarette smoke. However, atopic patients with asthma or patients with demonstrable bronchial hyperresponsiveness are less well protected. Although these drugs cause a marked reduction in sensitivity to methacholine in asthmatic subjects, more modest inhibition of responses to challenge with histamine, bradykinin, or $PGF_{2\alpha}$ is achieved, and little protection is afforded against the bronchoconstriction induced by serotonin or the leukotrienes.

The principal clinical use of ipratropium and tiotropium is in the treatment of chronic obstructive pulmonary disease; they are less effective in most asthmatic patients (Barnes and Hansel, 2004; Gross, 2004). Ipratropium is FDA approved for the treatment of perennial and common cold–associated rhinorrhea. The therapeutic use of ipratropium and tiotropium is discussed further in Chapter 27.

Absorption, Fate, and Excretion of Muscarinic Antagonists. The belladonna alkaloids and the tertiary synthetic and semisynthetic derivatives are absorbed rapidly from the gastrointestinal tract. They also enter the circulation when applied locally to the mucosal surfaces of the body. Absorption from intact skin is limited, although efficient absorption does occur in the postauricular region for some agents, allowing delivery *via* transdermal patch. Systemic absorption of inhaled or orally ingested quaternary muscarinic receptor antagonists is minimal. The quaternary ammonium derivatives of the belladonna alkaloids also penetrate the conjunctiva of the eye less readily. Central effects are also lacking, because the quaternary agents do not cross the blood–brain barrier. Atropine has a half-life of ~4 hours; hepatic metabolism accounts for the elimination of about half of a dose; the remainder is excreted unchanged in the urine.

Ipratropium is administered as an aerosol or solution for inhalation whereas tiotropium is administered as a dry powder. As with most drugs administered by inhalation, about 90% of the dose is swallowed. Most of the swallowed drug appears in the feces. After inhalation, maximal responses usually develop over 30 to 90 minutes, with tiotropium having the slower onset. The effects of ipratropium last for 4 to 6 hours, while tiotropium's effects persist for 24 hours, and the drug is amenable to once-daily dosing (Barnes and Hansel, 2004).

THERAPEUTIC USES OF MUSCARINIC RECEPTOR ANTAGONISTS

Muscarinic receptor antagonists have been employed in a wide variety of clinical conditions, predominantly to inhibit effects of parasympathetic nervous system activity. The major limitation in the use of the nonselective drugs is often failure to obtain desired therapeutic responses without concomitant side effects. The latter usually are not serious but are sufficiently disturbing to decrease patient compliance, particularly during long-term administration. Selectivity has been achieved by local administration, either by pulmonary inhalation or instillation in the eye. Minimal systemic absorption and dilution from the site of action minimize systemic effects. Subtype-selective muscarinic receptor antagonists hold the most promise for treating specific clinical symptoms, but few show absolute selectivity.

Respiratory Tract. Atropine, related belladonna alkaloids, and synthetic analogs reduce secretion in both the upper and lower respiratory tracts. This effect in the nasopharynx may provide some symptomatic relief of acute rhinitis associated with coryza or hay fever, although such therapy does not affect the natural course of the condition. It is probable that the contribution of antihistamines employed in "cold" mixtures is due primarily to their antimuscarinic properties, except in conditions with an allergic basis.

Systemic administration of belladonna alkaloids or their derivatives for bronchial asthma or chronic obstructive pulmonary disease carries the disadvantage of reducing bronchial secretions and inspissation of the residual secretions. This viscid material is difficult to remove from the respiratory tree, and its presence can dangerously obstruct airflow and predispose to infection.

Ipratropium and tiotropium, administered by inhalation, do not produce adverse effects on mucociliary clearance, in contrast to atropine and other muscarinic antagonists. Thus, their anticholinergic properties can be exploited safely in the treatment of airway disease. These agents often are used with inhalation of long-acting β adrenergic receptor agonists, although there is little evidence of true synergism. The muscarinic antagonists are more effective in chronic obstructive pulmonary disease, particularly when cholinergic tone is evident. β adrenergic receptor agonists control best the intermittent exacerbations of asthma (*see* Chapter 27).

Genitourinary Tract. Overactive urinary bladder disease can be successfully treated with muscarinic receptor antagonists. These agents can include synthetic substitutes of atropine, such as tolterodine and *trospium chloride*, which lower intravesicular pressure, increase capacity, and reduce the frequency of contractions by antagonizing parasympathetic control of the bladder. There is renewed interest in muscarinic antagonists as a modality for treating this increasingly common disorder, as well as for treating enuresis in children, particularly when a progressive increase in bladder capacity is the objective. These agents also are used to reduce urinary frequency in spastic paraplegia and to increase the capacity of the bladder (Chapple, 2000; Goessl *et al.*, 2000).

Oxybutynin (DITROPAN, others) and its more active enantiomer, (S)-oxybutynin, tolterodine (DETROL), trospium chloride (SANCTURA), darifenacin (ENABLEX), *solifenacin* (VESICARE), and *flavoxate* (URIS-PAS) are indicated for overactive bladder. Side effects of dry mouth and eyes limit the tolerability of these drugs with continued use, and patient acceptance declines. In an attempt to overcome this limitation, oxybutynin is marketed as a transdermal system (OXYTROL) that delivers 3.9 mg/day and is associated with a lower incidence of side effects than the oral immediate- or extended-release formulations. Tolterodine (DETROL) is a potent muscarinic antagonist that shows selectivity for the urinary bladder in animal models and in clinical studies. Its selectivity and greater patient acceptance is surprising, because studies on isolated receptors do not reveal a unique subtype selectivity (Chapple, 2000; Abrams *et al.*, 1998; Abrams *et al.*, 1999). Inhibition of a particular complement of receptors in the bladder may give rise to synergism and clinical efficacy. Tolterodine is metabolized by CYP2D6 to a 5-hydroxymethyl metabolite. Since this metabolite possesses similar activity to the parent drug, variations in CYP2D6 levels do not affect the duration of action of the drug.

Trospium is a quaternary amine long used in Europe and approved recently for use in the United States for treatment of overactive bladder. It has been shown to be as effective as oxybutynin (*see* below) with better tolerability. Solifenacin is newly approved for overactive bladder with a favorable efficacy:side effect ratio (Chapple *et al.*, 2004). Stress urinary incontinence has been treated with some success with *duloxetine* (YENTREVE), that acts centrally to influence serotonin and norepinephrine levels (Millard *et al.*, 2004).

Tripitramine and darifenacin are selective antagonists for M_2 and M_3 muscarinic receptors, respectively. They are of potential utility in blocking cholinergic bradycardia (M_2) and smooth muscle activity or epithelial secretions (M_3).

Gastrointestinal Tract. Muscarinic receptor antagonists were once the most widely used drugs for the management of peptic ulcer. Although they can reduce gastric motility and the secretion of gastric acid, antisecretory doses produce pronounced side effects, such as dry mouth, loss of visual accommodation, photophobia, and difficulty in urination. As a consequence, patient compliance in the long-term management of symptoms of acid-peptic disease with these drugs is poor.

Pirenzepine is a tricyclic drug, similar in structure to *imipramine*. Pirenzepine has selectivity for M_1 over M_2 and M_3 receptors (Caulfield, 1993; Caulfield and Birdsall, 1998). However, pirenzepine's affinities for M_1 and M_4 receptors are comparable, so it does not possess total M_1 selectivity.

Telenzepine is an analog of pirenzepine that has higher potency and similar selectivity for M_1 muscarinic receptors. Both drugs are used in the treatment of acid-peptic disease in Europe, Japan, and Canada, but not currently in the United States. At therapeutic doses of pirenzepine, the incidence of dry mouth, blurred vision, and central muscarinic disturbances are relatively low. Central effects are not seen because of the drug's limited penetration into the CNS. Because of pirenzepine's relative selectivity for M_1 receptors, it clearly offers a marked improvement over atropine.

Most studies indicate that pirenzepine (100 to 150 mg per day) produces about the same rate of healing of duodenal and gastric ulcers as the H_2-receptor antagonists *cimetidine* or *ranitidine*; it also may be effective in preventing the recurrence of ulcers (Carmine and Brogden, 1985; Tryba and Cook, 1997). Side effects necessitate drug withdrawal in <1% of patients. Studies in human

subjects have shown pirenzepine to be more potent in inhibiting gastric acid secretion produced by neural stimuli than by muscarinic agonists, supporting the postulated localization of M_1 receptors at ganglionic sites. H_2-receptor antagonists and proton pump inhibitors generally are considered to be the current drugs of choice to reduce gastric acid secretion (*see* Chapter 36).

The belladonna alkaloids (atropine, *belladonna tincture*, l-hyoscyamine sulfate [ANASPAZ, LEVSIN, others], and scopolamine), and combinations with sedatives (*e.g.*, *phenobarbital* [DONNATAL, others] or *butabarbital* [BUTIBEL]), antianxiety agents (*e.g.*, *chlordiazepoxide* [LIBRAX, others], or *ergotamine* [BELLAMINE]) also have been used in a wide variety of conditions known or supposed to involve irritable bowel and increased tone (spasticity) or motility of the gastrointestinal tract. The belladonna alkaloids and their synthetic substitutes can reduce tone and motility when administered in maximal tolerated doses, and they might be expected to be efficacious if the condition simply involves excessive smooth muscle contraction, a point that is often in doubt. M_3-selective antagonists might achieve more selectivity, but M_3 receptors also exert a dominant influence on salivation, bronchiolar secretion and contraction, and bladder motility. Alternative agents for treatment of irritable bowel syndrome and its associated diarrhea are discussed in Chapter 38. Diarrhea sometimes associated with irritative conditions of the lower bowel, such as mild dysenteries and diverticulitis, may respond to atropine-like drugs. However, more severe conditions such as *Salmonella* dysentery, ulcerative colitis, and Crohn's disease respond poorly. The belladonna alkaloids and synthetic substitutes are very effective in reducing excessive salivation, such as drug-induced salivation and that associated with heavy-metal poisoning and parkinsonism.

Uses in Ophthalmology. Effects limited to the eye are obtained by local administration of muscarinic receptor antagonists to produce mydriasis and cycloplegia. Cycloplegia is not attainable without mydriasis and requires higher concentrations or more prolonged application of a given agent. Mydriasis often is necessary for thorough examination of the retina and optic disc and in the therapy of iridocyclitis and keratitis. The belladonna mydriatics may be alternated with miotics for breaking or preventing the development of adhesions between the iris and the lens. Complete cycloplegia may be necessary in the treatment of iridocyclitis and choroiditis and for accurate measurement of refractive errors. In instances in which complete cycloplegia is required, more effective agents such as atropine or scopolamine are preferred to drugs such as *cyclopentolate* and tropicamide.

Homatropine hydrobromide (ISOPTO HOMATROPINE, others), a semisynthetic derivative of atropine (Figure 7–2), *cyclopentolate hydrochloride* (CYCLOGYL, others), and tropicamide (MYDRIACYL, others) are agents used in ophthalmological practice. These agents are preferred to topical atropine or scopolamine because of their shorter duration of action. Additional information on the ophthalmological properties and preparations of these and other drugs is provided in Chapter 63.

Cardiovascular System. The cardiovascular effects of muscarinic receptor antagonists are of limited clinical application. Generally, these agents are used in coronary care units for short-term interventions or in surgical settings.

Atropine may be considered in the initial treatment of patients with acute myocardial infarction in whom excessive vagal tone causes sinus or nodal bradycardia. Sinus bradycardia is the most common arrhythmia seen during acute myocardial infarction of the inferior or posterior wall. Atropine may prevent further clinical deterioration in cases of high vagal tone or AV block by restoring heart rate to a level sufficient to maintain adequate hemodynamic status and to eliminate AV nodal block. Dosing must be judicious; doses that are too low can cause a paradoxical bradycardia (*see* above), while excessive doses will cause tachycardia that may extend the infarct by increasing the demand for oxygen.

Atropine occasionally is useful in reducing the severe bradycardia and syncope associated with a hyperactive carotid sinus reflex. It has little effect on most ventricular rhythms. In some patients, atropine may eliminate premature ventricular contractions associated with a very slow atrial rate. It also may reduce the degree of AV block when increased vagal tone is a major factor in the conduction defect, such as the second-degree AV block that can be produced by digitalis.

Central Nervous System. For many years, the belladonna alkaloids and subsequently synthetic substitutes were the only agents helpful in the treatment of parkinsonism. Levodopa or levodopa along with *carbidopa* now is the treatment of choice, but alternative or concurrent therapy with muscarinic receptor antagonists may be required in some patients (*see* Chapter 20). Centrally acting agents such as benztropine have been shown to be efficacious in preventing dystonias or parkinsonian symptoms in patients treated with antipsychotic drugs (Arana *et al.*, 1988) (*see* Chapter 20).

The belladonna alkaloids were among the first drugs to be used in the prevention of motion sickness. Scopolamine is the most effective prophylactic agent for short (4- to 6-hour) exposures to severe motion, and probably for exposures of up to several days. All agents used to combat motion sickness should be given prophylactically; they are much less effective after severe nausea or vomiting has developed. A transdermal preparation of scopolamine (TRANSDERM SCOP) has been shown to be highly effective when used prophylactically for the prevention of motion sickness. The drug, incorporated into a multilayered adhesive unit, is applied to the postauricular mastoid region, an area where transdermal absorption of the drug is especially efficient, and over a period of about 72 hours, approximately 0.5 mg of scopolamine is delivered. Dry mouth is common, drowsiness is not infrequent, and blurred vision occurs in some individuals. Mydriasis and cycloplegia can occur by inadvertent transfer of the drug to the eye from the fingers after handling the patch. Rare but severe psychotic episodes have been reported. The use of scopolamine to produce tranquilization and amnesia in a variety of circumstances, including labor, is declining and of questionable value. Given alone in the presence of pain or severe anxiety, scopolamine may induce outbursts of uncontrolled behavior.

Benztropine mesylate (COGENTIN, others), *biperiden* (AKINETON), *procyclidine* (KEMADRIN), and *trihexyphenidyl hydrochloride* (ARTANE, others) are tertiary-amine muscarinic receptor antagonists (together with the ethanolamine antihistamine *diphenhydramine* [BENADRYL, others]) that gain access to the CNS and can therefore be used when anticholinergics are indicated to treat parkinsonism and the extrapyramidal side effects of antipsychotic drugs. These drugs are discussed in Chapter 20.

Uses in Anesthesia. The use of anesthetics that are relatively nonirritating to the bronchi has virtually eliminated the need for prophylactic use of muscarinic receptor antagonists. Atropine commonly is given to block responses to vagal reflexes induced by surgical manipulation of visceral organs. Atropine or glycopyrrolate is used with *neostigmine* to block its parasympathomimetic effects when the latter agent is used to reverse skeletal muscle relaxation after surgery (*see* Chapter 9). Serious cardiac arrhythmias have occasionally occurred, perhaps because of the initial bradycardia produced by atropine combined with the cholinomimetic effects of neostigmine.

Anticholinesterase Poisoning. The use of atropine in large doses for the treatment of poisoning by anticholinesterase organophosphorus insecticides is discussed in Chapter 8. Atropine also may be used to antagonize the parasympathomimetic effects of *pyridostigmine* or other anticholinesterase agents administered in the treatment of myasthenia gravis. It does not interfere with the salutary effects at the skeletal neuromuscular junction. It is most useful early in therapy, before tolerance to muscarinic side effects has developed.

Other Muscarinic Antagonists. **Methscopolamine.** Methscopolamine bromide (PAMINE) is a quaternary ammonium derivative of scopolamine and therefore lacks the central actions of scopolamine. Its use has been limited chiefly to gastrointestinal diseases. It is less potent than atropine and is poorly absorbed; however, its action is more prolonged, the usual oral dose (2.5 mg) acting for 6 to 8 hours.

Homatropine Methylbromide. Homatropine methylbromide is the quaternary derivative of homatropine. It is less potent than atropine in antimuscarinic activity, but it is four times more potent as a ganglionic blocking agent. It is available in combination with *hydrocodone* as an antitussive combination (HYCODAN) and has been used for relief of gastrointestinal spasms and as an adjunct in peptic ulcer disease.

Glycopyrrolate. *Glycopyrrolate* (ROBINUL, others) is employed orally to inhibit gastrointestinal motility and also is used parenterally to block the effects of vagal stimulation during anesthesia and surgery.

Dicyclomine hydrochloride (BENTYL, others), *flavoxate hydrochloride* (URISPAS, others), *oxybutynin chloride* (DITROPAN, others), and *tolterodine tartrate* (DETROL) are tertiary amines and *trospium chloride* (SANCTURA) is a quaternary amine; all are used for their antispasmodic properties. These agents appear to exert some nonspecific direct relaxant effect on smooth muscle. In therapeutic doses they decrease spasm of the gastrointestinal tract, biliary tract, ureter, and uterus.

Mepenzolate Bromide. *Mepenzolate bromide* (CENTIL) is a quaternary amine with peripheral actions similar to those of atropine. It is indicated for adjunctive therapy of peptic ulcer disease and has been used as an antispasmodic for the relief of GI disorders.

Propantheline. *Propantheline bromide* (PRO-BANTHINE) is one of the more widely used of the synthetic nonselective muscarinic receptor antagonists. High doses produce the symptoms of ganglionic blockade, and toxic doses block the skeletal neuromuscular junction. Its duration of action is comparable to that of atropine.

POISONING BY MUSCARINIC RECEPTOR ANTAGONISTS AND OTHER DRUGS WITH ANTICHOLINERGIC PROPERTIES

The deliberate or accidental ingestion of natural belladonna alkaloids is a major cause of poisonings. Many histamine H$_1$-receptor antagonists, phenothiazines, and tricyclic antidepressants also block muscarinic receptors, and in sufficient dosage, produce syndromes that include features of atropine intoxication.

Among the tricyclic antidepressants, *protriptyline* and *amitriptyline* are the most potent muscarinic receptor antagonists, with an affinity for the receptor that is approximately one-tenth that reported for atropine. Since these drugs are administered in therapeutic doses considerably higher than the effective dose of atropine, antimuscarinic effects often are observed clinically (*see* Chapter 17). In addition, overdose with suicidal intent is a danger in the population using antidepressants. Fortunately, most of the newer antidepressants and selective serotonin reuptake inhibitors are far less anticholinergic (Cusack *et al.*, 1994). In contrast, the newer antipsychotic drugs, classified as "atypical" and characterized by their low propensity for inducing extrapyramidal side effects, include agents that are potent muscarinic receptor antagonists. In particular, *clozapine* binds to human brain muscarinic receptors with one fifth the affinity of atropine; *olanzapine* also is a potent muscarinic receptor antagonist (Richelson, 1999). Accordingly, dry mouth is a prominent side effect of these drugs. A paradoxical side effect of clozapine is increased salivation and drooling, possibly the result of partial agonist properties of this drug (Richelson, 1999).

Infants and young children are especially susceptible to the toxic effects of muscarinic antagonists. Indeed, cases of intoxication in children have resulted from conjunctival instillation for ophthalmic refraction and other ocular effects. Systemic absorption occurs either from the nasal mucosa after the drug has traversed the nasolacrimal duct or from the GI tract if the drug is swallowed. Poisoning with *diphenoxylate*-atropine (LOMOTIL, others), used to treat diarrhea, has been extensively reported in the pediatric literature. Transdermal preparations of scopolamine used for motion sickness have been noted to cause toxic psychoses, especially in children and in the elderly. Serious intoxication may occur in children who ingest berries or seeds containing belladonna alkaloids. Poisoning from ingestion and smoking of jimson weed, or thorn apple, is seen with some frequency today.

Table 7–2 shows the oral doses of atropine causing undesirable responses or symptoms of overdosage. These symptoms are predictable results of blockade of parasympathetic innervation. In cases of full-blown atropine poisoning, the syndrome may last 48 hours or longer. Intravenous injection of the anticholinesterase agent physostigmine may be used for confirmation. If physostigmine does not elicit the expected salivation, sweating, bradycardia, and intestinal hyperactivity, intoxication with atropine or a related agent is almost certain. Depression and circulatory collapse are evident only in cases of severe intoxication; the blood pressure declines, convulsions may ensue, respiration becomes inadequate, and death due to respiratory failure may follow after a period of paralysis and coma.

Measures to limit intestinal absorption should be initiated without delay if the poison has been taken orally (*see* Chapter 64). For symptomatic treatment, slow intravenous injection of physostigmine rapidly abolishes the delirium and coma caused by large doses of atropine, but carries some risk of overdose in mild atropine intoxication. Since physostigmine is metabolized rapidly, the patient may again lapse into coma within 1 to 2 hours, and repeated doses may be needed (*see* Chapter 8). If marked excitement is present and more specific treatment is not available, a benzodiazepine is the most suitable agent for sedation and for control of convulsions. Phenothiazines or agents with antimuscarinic activity should not be used, because their antimuscarinic action is likely to intensify toxicity. Support of respiration and control of hyperthermia may be necessary. Ice bags and alcohol sponges help to reduce fever, especially in children.

CLINICAL SUMMARY

The availability of cDNAs encoding five distinct muscarinic receptor subtypes has facilitated the development of subtype-selective agonists and antagonists. This approach has been more successful with antagonists; even here, a high degree of receptor subtype selectivity that eliminates unwanted side effects has been difficult to achieve. Subtype-selective muscarinic receptor antagonists show promise in certain therapeutic settings, for example, in the treatment of urinary incontinence and for management of irritable bowel syndrome. Therapeutic efficacy can be enhanced by targeting unique subsets of receptors that control muscarinic responses within a particular end organ. Local application by inhalation or instillation into the eye has resulted in organ selectivity of selected antagonists. Inhalation with quaternary antagonists has proved useful in the treatment of pulmonary conditions, particularly chronic obstructive pulmonary disease.

BIBLIOGRAPHY

Abrams, P., Freeman, R., Anderstrom, C., and Mattiasson, A. Tolterodine, a new antimuscarinic agent: as effective but better tolerated than oxybutynin in patients with an overactive bladder. *Br. J. Urol.,* **1998,** *81:*801–810.

Arana, G.W., Goff, D.C., Baldessarini, R.J., and Keepers, G.A. Efficacy of anticholinergic prophylaxis for neuroleptic-induced acute dystonia. *Am. J. Psychiatry,* **1988,** *145:*993–996.

Bonner, T.I., Buckley, N.J., Young, A.C., and Brann, M.R. Identification of a family of muscarinic acetylcholine receptor genes. *Science,* **1987,** *237:*527–532.

Bruning, T.A., Hendriks, M.G., Chang, P.C., Kuypers, E.A., and van Zwieten, P.A. *In vivo* characterization of vasodilating muscarinic-receptor subtypes in humans. *Circ. Res.,* **1994,** *74:*912–919.

Chapple, R.R., Rechberger, T., Al-Shukri, S., *et al.* Randomized, double-blind placebo- and tolterodine-controlled trial of the once-daily antimuscarinic agent solifenacin in patients with symptomatic overactive bladder. *BJU International,* **2004,** *93:*303–310.

Cusack, B., Nelson, A., and Richelson, E. Binding of antidepressants to human brain receptors: focus on newer generation compounds. *Psychopharmacology (Berl.),* **1994,** *114:*559–565.

Epstein, J.B., Burchell, J.L., Emerton, S., Le, N.D., and Silverman, S. Jr. A clinical trial of bethanechol in patients with xerostomia after radiation therapy. A pilot study. *Oral Surg. Oral Med. Oral Pathol.,* **1994,** *77:*610–614.

Feigl, E.O. Neural control of coronary blood flow. *J. Vasc. Res.,* **1998,** *35:*85–92.

Fisher, J.T., Vincent, S.G., Gomeza, J., Yamada, M., and Wess, J. Loss of vagally mediated bradycardia and bronchoconstriction in mice lacking M_2 or M_3 muscarinic acetylcholine receptors. *FASEB J.,* **2004,** *18:*711–713.

Goessl, C., Sauter, T., Michael, T., *et al.* Efficacy and tolerability of tolterodine in children with detrusor hyperreflexia. *Urology,* **2000,** *55:*414–418.

Gomeza, J., Shannon, H., Kostenis, E., *et al.* Pronounced pharmacologic deficits in M_2 muscarinic acetylcholine receptor knockout mice. *Proc. Natl. Acad. Sci. U.S.A.,* **1999,** *96:*1692–1697.

Hamilton, S.E., Loose, M.D., Qi, M., *et al.* Disruption of the M_1 receptor gene ablates muscarinic receptor-dependent M current regulation and seizure activity in mice. *Proc. Natl. Acad. Sci. U.S.A.,* **1997,** *94:*13311–13316.

Hammer, R., Berrie, C.P., Birdsall, N.J., Burgen, A.S., and Hulme, E.C. Pirenzepine distinguishes between different subclasses of muscarinic receptors. *Nature,* **1980,** *283:*90–92.

Kent, K.M., and Epstein, S.E. Neural basis for the genesis and control of arrhythmias associated with myocardial infarction. *Cardiology,* **1976,** *61:*61–74.

Levey, A.I. Immunological localization of m1–m5 muscarinic acetylcholine receptors in peripheral tissues and brain. *Life Sci.,* **1993,** *52:*441–448.

Lewis, M.E., Al-Khalidi, A.H., Bonser, R.S., *et al.* Vagus nerve stimulation decreases left ventricular contractility in vivo in the human and pig heart. *J Physiol.,* **2001,** *534:*547–552.

Matsui, M., Motomura, D., Karasawa, H., *et al.* Multiple functional defects in peripheral autonomic organs in mice lacking muscarinic acetylcholine receptor gene for the M_3 subtype. *Proc. Natl. Acad. Sci. U.S.A.,* **2000,** *97:*9579–9584.

Millard, R.J., Moore, K., Rencken, R., Yalcin, I., and Bump, R.C. Duloxetine *vs.* placebo in the treatment of stress urinary incontinence:

A four-continent randomized clinical trial. *BJU International,* **2004,** *93:*311–318.

Oberhauser, V., Schwertfeger, E., Rutz, T., Beyersdorf, F., and Rump, L.C. Acetylcholine release in human heart atrium: influence of muscarinic autoreceptors, diabetes, and age. *Circulation,* **2001,** *103:*1638–1643.

Ono, M., Takamura, E., Shinozaki, K., *et al.* Therapeutic effect of cevimeline on dry eye in patients with Sjögren's syndrome: a randomized, double-blind clinical study. *Am. J. Ophthalmology,* **2004,** *138:*6–17.

Palczewski, K., Kumasaka, T., Hori, T., *et al.* Crystal structure of rhodopsin: A G protein–coupled receptor. *Science,* **2000,** *289:*739–745.

Porter, S.R., Scully, C., and Hegarty, A.M. An update of the etiology and management of xerostomia. *Oral Surg. Oral Med. Oral Pathol. Oral Radiol. Endod.,* **2004,** *97:*28–46.

Richelson, E. Receptor pharmacology of neuroleptics: relation to clinical effects. *J. Clin. Psychiatry,* **1999,** *10*(suppl):5–14.

Wellstein, A., and Pitschner, H.F. Complex dose-response curves of atropine in man explained by different functions of M_1- and M_2-cholinoceptors. *Naunyn Schmiedebergs Arch. Pharmacol.,* **1988,** *338:*19–27.

Willmy-Matthes, P., Leineweber, K., Wangemann, T., Silber, R.E., and Brodde, O.E. Existence of functional M_3-muscarinic receptors in the human heart. *Naunyn Schmiedebergs Arch. Pharmacol.,* **2003,** *368:*316–319.

Yamada, M., Lamping, K.G., Duttaroy, A., *et al.* Cholinergic dilation of cerebral blood vessels is abolished in M_5 muscarinic acetylcholine receptor knockout mice. *Proc. Natl. Acad. Sci. U.S.A.,* **2001b,** *98:*14096–14101.

Yamada, M., Miyakawa, T., Duttaroy, A., *et al.* Mice lacking the M_3 muscarinic acetylcholine receptor are hypophagic and lean. *Nature,* **2001a,** *410:*207–212.

Yasuda, R.P., Ciesla, W., Flores, L.R., *et al.* Development of antisera selective for M_4 and M_5 muscarinic cholinergic receptors: distribution of M_4 and M_5 receptors in rat brain. *Mol. Pharmacol.,* **1993,** *43:*149–157.

MONOGRAPHS AND REVIEWS

Abrams, P., Larsson, G., Chapple, C., and Wein, A.J. Factors involved in the success of antimuscarinic treatment. *B.J.U. Int.,* **1999,** *83*(suppl 2):42–47.

Anaya, J.M., and Talal, N. Sjögren's syndrome comes of age. *Semin. Arthritis Rheum.,* **1999,** *28:*355–359.

Barnes, P.J., and Hansel, T.T. Prospects for new drugs for chronic obstructive pulmonary disease. *Lancet,* **2004,** *364:*985–996.

Berne, R.M., and Levy, M.N. In, *Cardiovascular Physiology,* 8th ed. Mosby, St. Louis, **2001.**

Birdsall, N.J.M., Buckley, N.J., Caulfield, M.P., *et al.* Muscarinic acetylcholine receptors. In, *The IUPHAR Compendium of Receptor Characterization and Classification.* IUPHAR Media, London, **1998,** pp. 36–45.

Brodde, O.E., and Michel, M.C. Adrenergic and muscarinic receptors in the human heart. *Pharmacol. Rev.,* **1999,** *51:*651–690.

Carmine, A.A., and Brogden, R.N. Pirenzepine. A review of its pharmacodynamic and pharmacokinetic properties and therapeutic efficacy in peptic ulcer disease and other allied diseases. *Drugs,* **1985,** *30:*85–126.

Caulfield, M.P., and Birdsall, N.J. International Union of Pharmacology, XVII. Classification of muscarinic acetylcholine receptors. *Pharmacol. Rev.,* **1998,** *50:*279–290.

Caulfield, M.P. Muscarinic receptors—characterization, coupling and function. *Pharmacol. Ther.,* **1993,** *58:*319–379.

Chapple, C.R., Yamanishi, T., and Chess-Williams, R. Muscarinic receptor subtypes and management of the overactive bladder. *Urology,* **2002,** *60:*82–89.

DiFrancesco, D. Pacemaker mechanisms in cardiac tissue. *Annu. Rev. Physiol.,* **1993,** *55:*455–472.

Eglen, R.M., Choppin, A., and Watson, N. Therapeutic opportunities from muscarinic receptor research. *Trends Pharmacol. Sci.,* **2001,** *22:*409–414.

Eglen, R.M., Choppin, A., Dillon, M.P., and Hegde, S. Muscarinic receptor ligands and their therapeutic potential. *Curr. Opin. Chem. Biol.,* **1999,** *3:*426–432.

Eglen, R.M., Hedge, S.S., and Watson, N. Muscarinic receptor subtypes and smooth muscle function. *Pharmacol. Rev.,* **1996,** *48:*531–565.

Furchgott, R.F. Endothelium-derived relaxing factor: discovery, early studies, and identification as nitric oxide. *Biosci. Rep.,* **1999,** *19:*235–251.

Goldfrank, L.R. Mushrooms: toxic and hallucinogenic. In, *Goldfrank's Toxicologic Emergencies,* 6th ed. (Goldfrank, L.R., Flomenbaum, N.E., Lewin, N.A., *et al.,* eds.) Appleton & Lange, Stamford, CT, **1998,** pp. 1207–1220.

Goyal, R.K., and Rattan, S. Neurohumoral, hormonal, and drug receptors for the lower esophageal sphincter. *Gastroenterology,* **1978,** *74:*598–619.

Gross, N.J. Tiotropium bromide. *Chest,* **2004,** *126:*1946–1953.

Hegde, S.S., and Eglen, R.M. Muscarinic receptor subtypes modulating smooth muscle contractility in the urinary bladder. *Life Sci.,* **1999,** *64:*419–428.

Ignarro, L.J., Cirino, G., Casini, A., and Napoli, C. Nitric oxide as a signaling molecule in the vascular system: an overview. *J. Cardiovasc. Pharmacol.,* **1999,** *34:*879–886.

Köppel, C. Clinical symptomatology and management of mushroom poisoning. *Toxicon,* **1993,** *31:*1513–1540.

Krnjević, K. Chemical nature of synaptic transmission in vertebrates. *Physiol. Rev.,* **1974,** *54:*418–540.

Krnjević, K. Synaptic mechanisms modulated by acetylcholine in cerebral cortex. *Prog. Brain Res.,* **2004,** *145:*81–93.

Levine, R., Birdsall, N.M.J., and Nathanson, N.M., eds. Proceedings of the 8th International Symposium on Subtypes of Muscarinic Receptors. *Life Sci.,* **1999,** *64:*355–596.

Levy, M.N., and Schwartz, P.J., eds. *Vagal Control of the Heart: Experimental Basis and Clinical Implications.* Futura, Armonk, NY, **1994.**

Moncada, S., and Higgs, E.A. Molecular mechanisms and therapeutic strategies related to nitric oxide. *FASEB J.,* **1995,** *9:*1319–1330.

Nusair, S., and Rubinow, A. The use of oral pilocarpine in xerostomia and Sjögren's syndrome. *Semin. Arthritis Rheum.,* **1999,** *28:*360–367.

Somogyi, G.T., and de Groat, W.C. Function, signal transduction mechanisms and plasticity of presynaptic muscarinic receptors in the urinary bladder. *Life Sci.,* **1999,** *64:*411–418.

Toda, N., and Okamura, T. The pharmacology of nitric oxide in the peripheral nervous system of blood vessels. *Pharmacol. Rev.* **2003,** *55:*271–324.

Tryba, M., and Cook, D. Current guidelines on stress ulcer prophylaxis. *Drugs,* **1997,** *54:*581–596.

Wein, A.J. Practical uropharmacology. *Urol. Clin. North Am.,* **1991,** *18:*269–281.

Wess, J. Molecular biology of muscarinic acetylcholine receptors. *Crit. Rev. Neurobiol.,* **1996,** *10:*69–99.

Wess, J. Muscarinic acetylcholine receptor knockout mice: novel phenotypes and clinical implications. *Annu. Rev. Pharmacol. Toxicol.,* **2004,** *44:*423–450.

Wickman, K., and Clapham, D.E. Ion channel regulation by G proteins. *Physiol. Rev.,* **1995,** *75:*868–885.

Wiseman, L.R., and Faulds, D. Oral pilocarpine: a review of its pharmacological properties and clinical potential in xerostomia. *Drugs,* **1995,** *49:*143–155.

Yoshimura, N., Smith, C.P., Chancellor, M.B., and de Groat, W.C. Pharmacologic and potential biologic interventions to restore bladder function after spinal cord injury. *Curr. Opin. Neurol.,* **2000,** *13:*677–681.

ANTICHOLINESTERASE AGENTS

Palmer Taylor

The function of acetylcholinesterase (AChE) in terminating the action of acetylcholine (ACh) at the junctions of the various cholinergic nerve endings with their effector organs or postsynaptic sites is considered in Chapter 6. Drugs that inhibit AChE are called *anticholinesterase* (anti-ChE) *agents.* They cause ACh to accumulate in the vicinity of cholinergic nerve terminals and thus are potentially capable of producing effects equivalent to excessive stimulation of cholinergic receptors throughout the central and peripheral nervous systems. In view of the widespread distribution of cholinergic neurons across animal species, it is not surprising that the anti-ChE agents have received extensive application as toxic agents, in the form of agricultural insecticides, pesticides, and potential chemical warfare "nerve gases." Nevertheless, several compounds of this class are widely used therapeutically; others that cross the blood–brain barrier have been approved or are in clinical trials for the treatment of Alzheimer's disease.

Prior to World War II, only the "reversible" anti-ChE agents were generally known, of which *physostigmine* is the prototype. Shortly before and during World War II, a new class of highly toxic chemicals, the organophosphates, was developed chiefly by Schrader at I.G. Farbenindustrie, first as agricultural insecticides and later as potential chemical warfare agents. The extreme toxicity of these compounds was found to be due to their "irreversible" inactivation of AChE, which resulted in prolonged enzyme inhibition. Since the pharmacological actions of both classes of anti-ChE agents are qualitatively similar, they are discussed here as a group. Interactions of anti-ChE agents with other drugs acting at peripheral autonomic synapses and the neuromuscular junction are described in Chapters 7 and 9.

History. Physostigmine, also called *eserine,* is an alkaloid obtained from the Calabar or ordeal bean, the dried, ripe seed of *Physostigma*

venenosum, Balfour, a perennial plant found in tropical West Africa. The Calabar bean once was used by native tribes of West Africa as an "ordeal poison" in trials for witchcraft. A pure alkaloid was isolated by Jobst and Hesse in 1864 and named physostigmine. The first therapeutic use of the drug was in 1877 by Laqueur, in the treatment of glaucoma, one of its clinical uses today. Interesting accounts of the history of physostigmine have been presented by Karczmar (1970) and Holmstedt (2000).

As a result of the basic research of Stedman and associates in elucidating the chemical basis of the activity of physostigmine, others began systematic investigations of a series of substituted aromatic esters of alkyl carbamic acids. *Neostigmine* was introduced into therapeutics in 1931 for its stimulant action on the GI tract and subsequently was reported to be effective in the symptomatic treatment of myasthenia gravis.

Remarkably, the first account of the synthesis of a highly potent organophosphorus anti-ChE, *tetraethyl pyrophosphate* (TEPP), was published by Clermont in 1854. It is even more remarkable that the investigator survived to report on the compound's taste; a few drops should have been lethal. Modern investigations of the organophosphorus compounds date from the 1932 publication of Lange and Krueger on the synthesis of dimethyl and diethyl phosphorofluoridates. The authors' statement that inhalation of these compounds caused a persistent choking sensation and blurred vision apparently was instrumental in leading Schrader to explore this class for insecticidal activity.

Upon synthesizing approximately 2000 compounds, Schrader defined the structural requirements for insecticidal (and, as learned subsequently, for anti-ChE) activity (*see* below) (Gallo and Lawryk, 1991). One compound in this early series, *parathion* (a phosphorothioate), later became the most widely used insecticide of this class. *Malathion,* which currently is used extensively, also contains the thionophosphorus bond found in parathion. Prior to and during World War II, the efforts of Schrader's group were directed toward the development of chemical warfare agents. The synthesis of several compounds of much greater toxicity than parathion, such as *sarin, soman,* and *tabun,* were kept secret by the German government. Investigators in the Allied countries also followed Lange and Krueger's lead in the search for potentially toxic compounds; diisopropyl phosphorofluoridate (*diisopropyl fluorophosphate;* DFP), synthesized by McCombie and Saunders, was studied most extensively by British and American scientists.

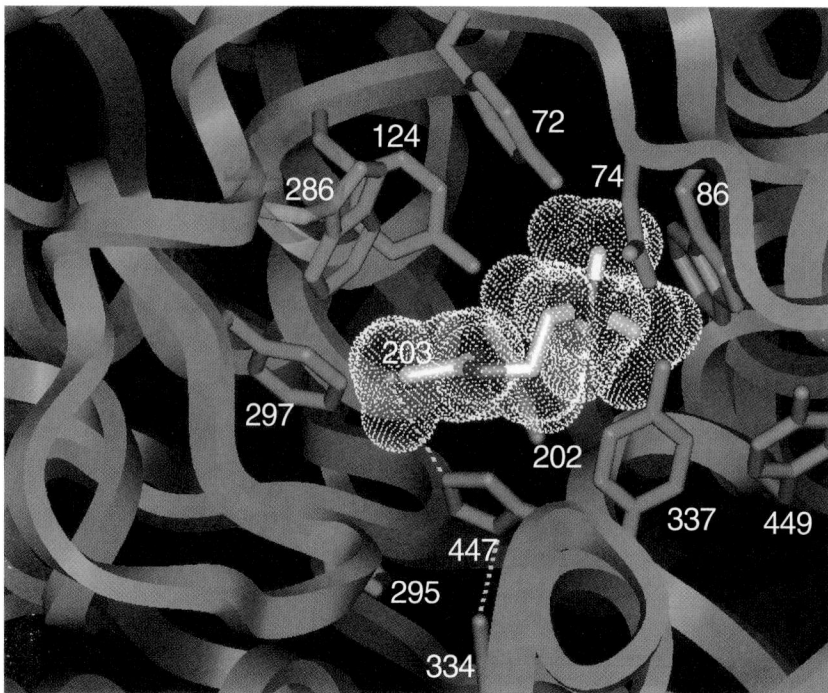

Figure 8–1. ***The active center gorge of mammalian acetylcholinesterase.*** Bound acetylcholine is shown by the dotted structure depicting its van der Waals radii. The crystal structure of mouse cholinesterase active center, which is virtually identical to human AChE, is shown (Bourne *et al.*, 1995). Included are the side chains of (a) the catalytic triad, Glu_{334}, His_{447}, Ser_{203} (hydrogen bonds are denoted by the dotted lines); (b) acyl pocket, Phe_{295} and Phe_{297}; (c) choline subsite, Trp_{86}, Glu_{202}, and Tyr_{337}; and (d) the peripheral site: Trp_{286}, Tyr_{72}, Tyr_{124}, and Asp_{74}. Tyrosines 337 and 449 are further removed from the active center but likely contribute to stabilization of certain ligands. The catalytic triad, choline subsite, and acyl pocket are located at the base of the gorge, while the peripheral site is at the lip of the gorge. The gorge is 18 to 20 Å deep, with its base centrosymmetric to the subunit.

In the 1950s, a series of aromatic carbamates was synthesized and found to have substantial selective toxicity against insects and to be potent anti-ChE agents (Ecobichon, 2000).

Structure of Acetylcholinesterase. AChE exists in two general classes of molecular forms: simple homomeric oligomers of catalytic subunits (*i.e.*, monomers, dimers, and tetramers) and heteromeric associations of catalytic subunits with structural subunits (Massoulié, 2000; Taylor *et al.*, 2000). The homomeric forms are found as soluble species in the cell, presumably destined for export or for association with the outer membrane of the cell, typically through an attached glycophospholipid. One heteromeric form, largely found in neuronal synapses, is a tetramer of catalytic subunits disulfide-linked to a 20,000-dalton lipid-linked subunit. Similar to the glycophospholipid-attached form, it is found in the outer surface of the cell membrane. The other heteromeric form consists of tetramers of catalytic subunits, disulfide linked to each of three strands of a collagen-like structural subunit. This molecular species, whose molecular mass approaches 10^6 daltons, is associated with the basal lamina of junctional areas of skeletal muscle.

Molecular cloning revealed that a single gene encodes vertebrate AChEs (Schumacher *et al.*, 1986; Taylor *et al.*, 2000). However, multiple gene products arise from alternative processing of the mRNA that differ only in their carboxyl-termini; the portion of the gene encoding the catalytic core of the enzyme is invariant. Hence, the individual AChE species can be expected to show identical substrate and inhibitor specificities.

A separate, structurally related gene encodes butyrylcholinesterase, which is synthesized in the liver and is primarily found in plasma (Lockridge *et al.*, 1987). The cholinesterases define a superfamily of proteins whose structural motif is the α, β hydrolase–fold (Cygler *et al.*, 1993). The family includes several esterases, other hydrolases not found in the nervous system, and surprisingly, proteins without hydrolase activity such as thyroglobulin and members of the tactin and neuroligin families of proteins (Taylor *et al.*, 2000).

The three-dimensional structures of AChEs show the active center to be nearly centrosymmetric to each subunit, residing at the base of a narrow gorge about 20 Å in depth (Sussman *et al.*, 1991; Bourne *et al.*, 1995). At the base of the gorge lie the residues of the catalytic triad: serine 203, histidine 447, and glutamate 334 in mammals (Figure 8–1). The catalytic mechanism resembles that of other hydrolases; the serine hydroxyl group is rendered highly nucleophilic through a charge-relay system involving the carboxylate anion from glutamate, the imidazole of histidine, and the hydroxyl of serine (Figure 8–2A).

During enzymatic attack of ACh, an ester with trigonal geometry, a tetrahedral intermediate between enzyme and substrate is

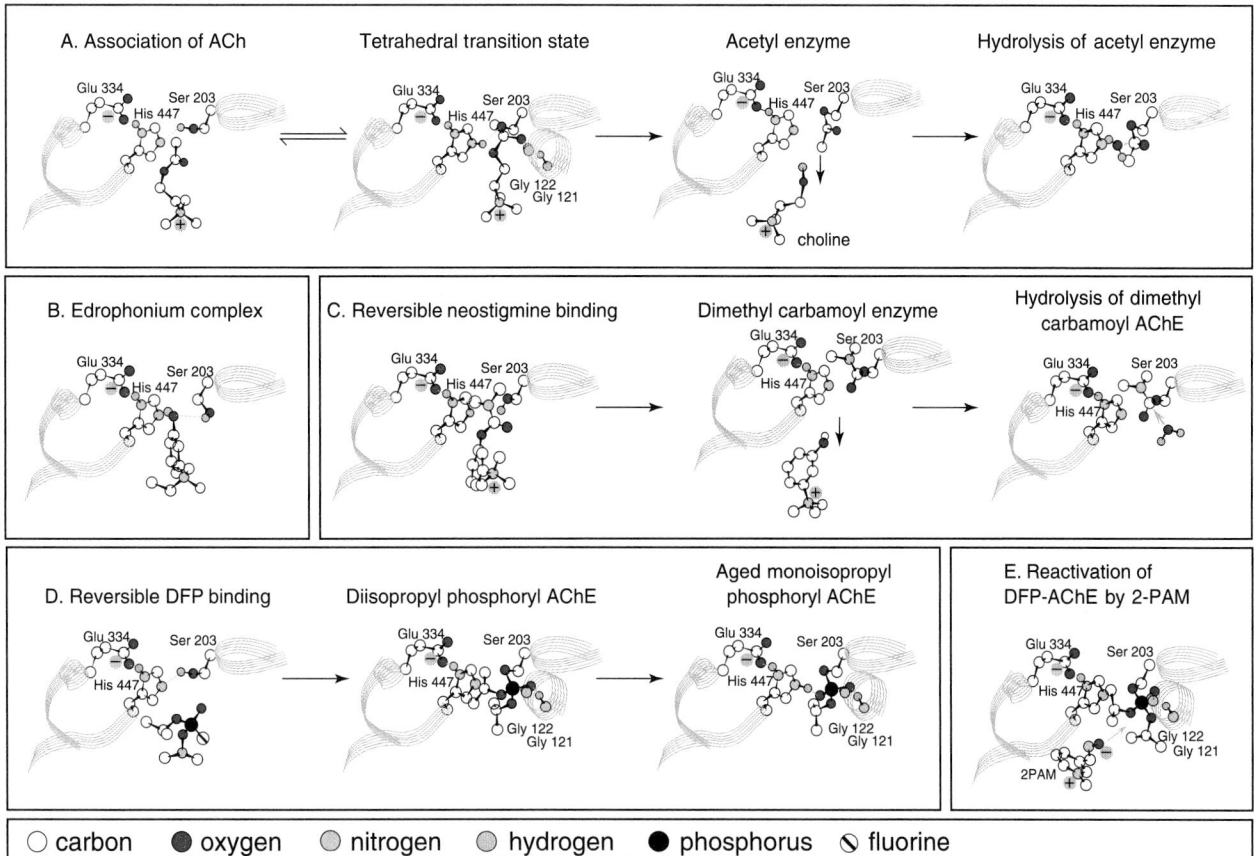

Figure 8–2. *Steps involved in the hydrolysis of acetylcholine by acetylcholinesterase and in the inhibition and reactivation of the enzyme.* Only the three residues of the catalytic triad shown in Figure 8–1 are depicted. The associations and reactions shown are: **A.** Acetylcholine (ACh) catalysis: binding of ACh, formation of a tetrahedral transition state, formation of the acetyl enzyme with liberation of choline, rapid hydrolysis of the acetyl enzyme with return to the original state. **B.** Reversible binding and inhibition by edrophonium. **C.** Neostigmine reaction with and inhibition of AChE: reversible binding of neostigmine, formation of the dimethyl carbamoyl enzyme, slow hydrolysis of the dimethyl carbamoyl enzyme. **D.** Diisopropyl fluorophosphate (DFP) reaction and inhibition of AChE: reversible binding of DFP, formation of the diisopropyl phosphoryl enzyme, formation of the aged monoisopropyl phosphoryl enzyme. Hydrolysis of the diisopropyl enzyme is very slow and is not shown. The aged monoisopropyl phosphoryl enzyme is virtually resistant to hydrolysis and reactivation. The tetrahedral transition state of ACh hydrolysis resembles the conjugates formed by the tetrahedral phosphate inhibitors and accounts for their potency. Amide bond hydrogens from Gly 121 and 122 stabilize the carbonyl and phorphoryl oxygens. **E.** Reactivation of the diisopropyl phosphoryl enzyme by pralidoxime (2-PAM). 2-PAM attack of the phosphorus on the phosphorylated enzyme will form a phospho-oxime with regeneration of active enzyme. The individual steps of phosphorylation reaction and oxime reaction have been characterized by mass spectrometry (Jennings *et al.*, 2004).

formed (Figure 8–2A) that collapses to an acetyl enzyme conjugate with the concomitant release of choline. The acetyl enzyme is very labile to hydrolysis, which results in the formation of acetate and active enzyme (Froede and Wilson, 1971; Rosenberry, 1975). AChE is one of the most efficient enzymes known: one molecule of AChE can hydrolyze 6×10^5 ACh molecules per minute; this yields a turnover time of 150 microseconds.

Mechanism of Action of AChE Inhibitors. The mechanisms of the action of compounds that typify the three classes of anti-ChE agents are also shown in Figure 8–2.

Three distinct domains on AChE constitute binding sites for inhibitory ligands and form the basis for specificity differences between AChE and butyrylcholinesterase: the acyl pocket of the active center, the choline subsite of the active center, and the peripheral anionic site (Taylor and Radic', 1994; Reiner and Radic', 2000). Reversible inhibitors, such as *edrophonium* and *tacrine*, bind to the choline subsite in the vicinity of tryptophan 86 and glutamate 202 (Silman and Sussman, 2000) (Figure 8–2B). Edrophonium has a brief duration of action because its quaternary structure facilitates renal elimination and it binds reversibly to the AChE active center. Additional reversible inhibitors, such as *donepezil,* bind with higher affinity to the active center.

Other reversible inhibitors, such as *propidium* and the snake peptidic toxin *fasciculin,* bind to the peripheral anionic site on AChE. This site resides at the rim of the gorge and is defined by tryptophan 286 and tyrosines 72 and 124 (Figure 8–1).

Drugs that have a carbamoyl ester linkage, such as physostigmine and neostigmine, are hydrolyzed by AChE, but much more slowly than is ACh. The quaternary amine neostigmine and the tertiary amine physostigmine exist as cations at physiological pH. By serving as alternate substrates to ACh (Figure 8–2C), attack by the active center serine generates the carbamoylated enzyme. The carbamoyl moiety resides in the acyl pocket outlined by phenylalanines 295 and 297. In contrast to the acetyl enzyme, methylcarbamoyl AChE and dimethylcarbamoyl AChE are far more stable (the half-life for hydrolysis of the dimethylcarbamoyl enzyme is 15 to 30 minutes). Sequestration of the enzyme in its carbamoylated form thus precludes the enzyme-catalyzed hydrolysis of ACh for extended periods of time. *In vivo,* the duration of inhibition by the carbamoylating agents is 3 to 4 hours.

The organophosphorus inhibitors, such as diisopropyl fluorophosphate (DFP), serve as true hemisubstrates, since the resultant conjugate with the active center serine phosphorylated or phosphonylated is extremely stable (Figure 8–2D). The organophosphorus inhibitors are tetrahedral in configuration, a configuration that resembles the transition state formed in carboxyl ester hydrolysis. Similar to the carboxyl esters, the phosphoryl oxygen binds within the oxyanion hole of the active center. If the alkyl groups in the phosphorylated enzyme are ethyl or methyl, spontaneous regeneration of active enzyme requires several hours. Secondary (as in DFP) or tertiary alkyl groups further enhance the stability of the phosphorylated enzyme, and significant regeneration of active enzyme usually is not observed. Hence, the return of AChE activity depends on synthesis of a new enzyme. The stability of the phosphorylated enzyme is enhanced through "aging," which results from the loss of one of the alkyl groups.

From the foregoing account, it is apparent that the terms *reversible* and *irreversible* as applied to the carbamoyl ester and organophosphorate anti-ChE agents, respectively, reflect only quantitative differences in rates of decarbamoylation or dephosphorylation of the conjugated enzyme. Both chemical classes react covalently with the enzyme serine in essentially the same manner as does ACh.

Action at Effector Organs. The characteristic pharmacological effects of the anti-ChE agents are due primarily to the prevention of hydrolysis of ACh by AChE at sites of cholinergic transmission. Transmitter thus accumulates, enhancing the response to ACh that is liberated by cholinergic impulses or that is spontaneously released from the nerve ending. Virtually all acute effects of moderate doses of organophosphates are attributable to this action. For example, the characteristic miosis that follows local application of DFP to the eye is not observed after chronic postganglionic denervation of the eye because there is no source from which to release endogenous ACh. The consequences of enhanced concentrations of ACh at motor endplates are unique to these sites and are discussed below.

The tertiary amine and particularly the quaternary ammonium anti-ChE compounds may have additional direct actions at certain cholinergic receptor sites. For example, the effects of neostigmine on the spinal cord and neuromuscular junction are based on a combination of its anti-ChE activity and direct cholinergic stimulation.

Chemistry and Structure–Activity Relationships. The structure–activity relationships of anti-ChE agents are reviewed in previous editions of this book. Only agents of general therapeutic or toxicological interest are considered here.

Noncovalent Inhibitors. While these agents interact by reversible and noncovalent association with the active site in AChE, they differ in their disposition in the body and their affinity for the enzyme. Edrophonium, a quaternary drug whose activity is limited to peripheral nervous system synapses, has a moderate affinity for AChE. Its volume of distribution is limited and renal elimination is rapid, accounting for its short duration of action. By contrast, tacrine and donepezil (Figure 8–3) have higher affinities for AChE, are more hydrophobic, and readily cross the blood–brain barrier to inhibit AChE in the central nervous system (CNS). Their partitioning into lipid and their higher affinities for AChE account for their longer durations of action.

"Reversible" Carbamate Inhibitors. Drugs of this class that are of therapeutic interest are shown in Figure 8–3. Early studies showed that the essential moiety of the physostigmine molecule was the methylcarbmate of an amine-substituted phenol. The quaternary ammonium derivative neostigmine is a compound of equal or greater potency. *Pyridostigmine* is a close congener that also is used to treat myasthenia gravis.

An increase in anti-ChE potency and duration of action can result from the linking of two quaternary ammonium moieties. One such example is the miotic agent *demecarium,* which consists of two neostigmine molecules connected by a series of ten methylene groups. The second quaternary group confers additional stability to the interaction by associating with a negatively charged amino side chain, Asp74, near the rim of the gorge. Carbamoylating inhibitors with high lipid solubilities (*e.g.,* rivastigmine), which readily cross the blood–brain barrier and have longer durations of action, are approved or in clinical trial for the treatment of Alzheimer's disease (Giacobini, 2000; Cummings, 2004) (*see* Chapter 20).

The carbamate insecticides *carbaryl* (SEVIN), *propoxur* (BAYGON), and *aldicarb* (TEMIK), which are used extensively as garden insecticides, inhibit ChE in a fashion identical with other carbamoylating inhibitors. The symptoms of poisoning closely resemble those of the organophosphates (Baron, 1991; Ecobichon, 2000). Carbaryl has a particularly low toxicity from dermal absorption. It is used topically for control of head lice in some countries. Not all carbamates in garden formulations are ChE inhibitors; the dithiocarbamates are fungicidal.

Organophosphorus Compounds. The general formula for this class of ChE inhibitors is presented in Table 8–1. A great variety of substituents is possible: R_1 and R_2 may be alkyl, alkoxy, aryloxy, amido, mercaptan, or other groups, and X, the leaving group, typically a conjugate base of a weak acid, is a halide, cyanide, thiocyanate, phenoxy, thiophenoxy, phosphate, thiocholine, or carboxylate group. For a compilation of the organophosphorus compounds and their toxicity, *see* Gallo and Lawryk (1991).

DFP produces virtually irreversible inactivation of AChE and other esterases by alkylphosphorylation. Its high lipid solubility, low molecular weight, and volatility facilitate inhalation, transdermal absorption, and penetration into the CNS. After desulfuration, the insecticides in current use form the dimethoxy or diethoxyphosphoryl enzyme.

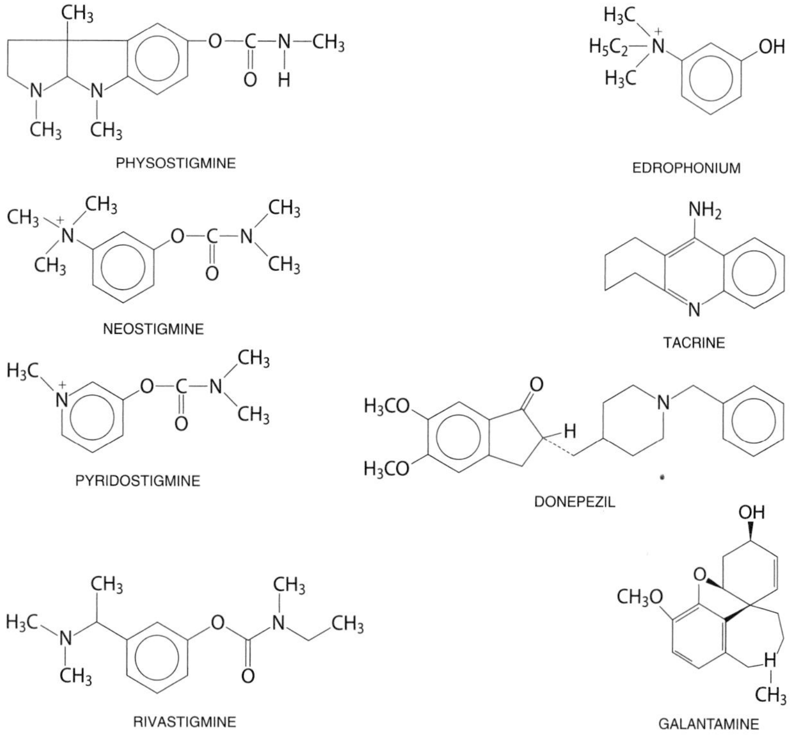

Figure 8–3. *Representative "reversible" anticholinesterase agents employed clinically.*

The "nerve gases"—tabun, sarin, and soman—are among the most potent synthetic toxins known; they are lethal to laboratory animals in nanogram doses. Insidious employment of these agents has occurred in warfare and terrorism attacks (Nozaki and Aikawa, 1995).

Because of their low volatility and stability in aqueous solution, parathion and *methylparathion* were widely used as insecticides. Acute and chronic toxicity has limited their use, and potentially less hazardous compounds have replaced them for home and garden use. These compounds are inactive in inhibiting AChE *in vitro; paraoxon* is the active metabolite. The phosphoryl oxygen for sulfur substitution is carried out predominantly by hepatic CYPs. This reaction also occurs in the insect, typically with more efficiency. Other insecticides possessing the phosphorothioate structure have been widely employed for home, garden, and agricultural use. These include *diazinon* (SPECTRACIDE, others) and *chlorpyrifos* (DURSBAN, LORSBAN). Chlorpyrifos recently has been placed under restricted use because of evidence of chronic toxicity in the newborn animal. For the same reason, diazinon was banned for indoor use in the United States in 2001 and will be phased out of all outdoor residential use by 2005.

Malathion (CHEMATHION, MALA-SPRAY) also requires replacement of a sulfur atom with oxygen *in vivo,* conferring resistance to mammalian species. Also, this insecticide can be detoxified by hydrolysis of the carboxyl ester linkage by plasma carboxylesterases, and plasma carboxylesterase activity dictates species resistance to malathion. The detoxification reaction is much more rapid in mammals and birds than in insects (Costa *et al.,* 1987). In recent years, malathion has been employed in aerial spraying of relatively populous areas for control of citrus orchard-destructive Mediterranean fruit flies and mosquitoes that harbor and transmit viruses harmful to human beings, such as the West Nile encephalitis virus.

Evidence of acute toxicity from malathion arises only with suicide attempts or deliberate poisoning (Bardin *et al.,* 1994). The lethal dose in mammals is about 1 g/kg. Exposure to the skin results in a small fraction (<10%) of systemic absorption. Malathion is used topically in the treatment of pediculosis (lice) infestations.

Among the quaternary ammonium organophosphorus compounds (group E in Table 8–1), only *echothiophate* is useful clinically and is limited to ophthalmic administration. Being positively charged, it is not volatile and does not readily penetrate the skin.

Metrifonate is a low-molecular-weight organophosphate that is spontaneously converted to the active phosphoryl ester, *dimethyl 2,2-dichlorovinyl phosphate* (DDVP, *dichlorvos*). Both metrifonate and DDVP readily cross the blood–brain barrier to inhibit AChE in the CNS. Metrifonate originally was developed for the treatment of schistosomiasis (*see* Chapter 41). Its capacity to inhibit AChE in the CNS and its reported low toxicity led to its clinical trial in treatment of Alzheimer's disease (Cummings *et al.,* 1999; Cummings, 2004); a low incidence of skeletal muscle paralysis may limit its acceptance.

PHARMACOLOGICAL PROPERTIES

Generally, the pharmacological properties of anti-ChE agents can be predicted by knowing those loci where ACh is released physiologically by nerve impulses, the degree of nerve impulse activity, and the responses of the corresponding effector organs to ACh (*see* Chapter 6). The

Table 8–1
Chemical Classification of Representative Organophosphorus Compounds of Particular Pharmacological or Toxicological Interest

General formula

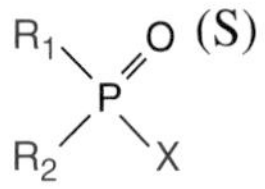

Group A, X = halogen, cyanide, or thiocyanate leaving group; group B, X = alkylthio, arylthio, alkoxy, or aryloxy leaving group; group C, thionophosphorus or thio-thionophosphorus compounds; group D, pyrophosphates and similar compounds; group E, quaternary ammonium leaving group. R_1 can be an alkyl (phosphonates), alkoxy (phosphorates) or an alkylamino (phosphoramidates) group.

GROUP	STRUCTURAL FORMULA	COMMON, CHEMICAL, AND OTHER NAMES	COMMENTS
A	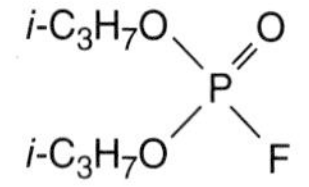	DFP; Isoflurophate; diisopropyl fluorophosphate	Potent, irreversible inactivator
	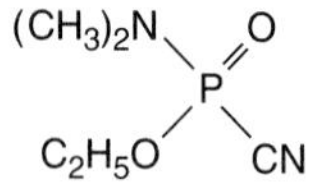	Tabun Ethyl *N*-dimethylphosphoramidocyanidate	Extremely toxic "nerve gas"
	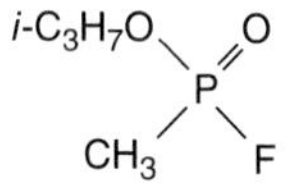	Sarin (GB) Isopropyl methylphosphonofluoridate	Extremely toxic "nerve gas"
	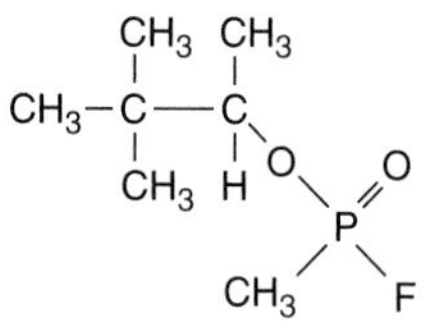	Soman (GD) Pinacolyl methylphosphonofluoridate	Extremely toxic "nerve gas"
B	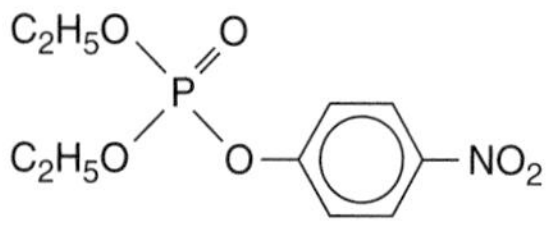	Paraoxon (MINTACOL), E 600 *O,O*-Diethyl *O*-(4-nitrophenyl)-phosphate	Active metabolite of parathion
	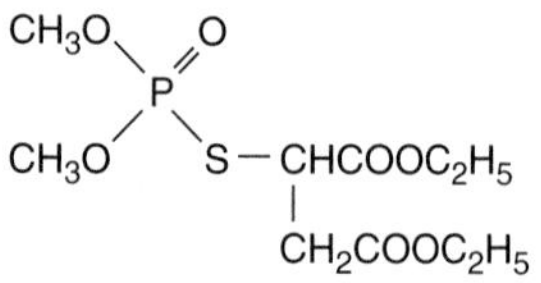	Malaoxon *O,O*-Dimethyl *S*-(1,2-dicarboxyethyl)-phosphorothioate	Active metabolite of malathion
C	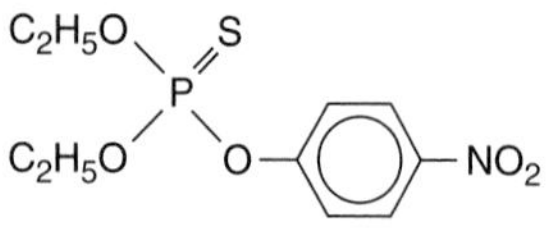	Parathion *O,O*-Diethyl *O*-(4-nitrophenyl)-phosphorothioate	Employed as agricultural insecticide, resulting in numerous cases of accidental poisoning; phased out of agricultural use in 2003.
	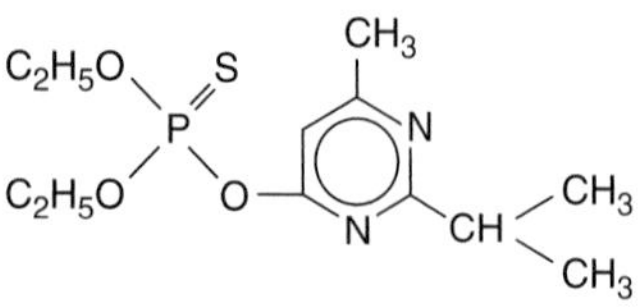	Diazinon, Dimpylate *O,O*-Diethyl *O*-(2-isopropyl-6-methyl-4-pyrimidinyl) phosphorothioate	Insecticide in wide use for gardening and agriculture; now banned for indoor use and being phased out of all outdoor use in 2005

(Continued)

Table 8–1
Chemical Classification of Representative Organophosphorus Compounds of Particular Pharmacological or Toxicological Interest (Continued)

GROUP	STRUCTURAL FORMULA	COMMON, CHEMICAL, AND OTHER NAMES	COMMENTS
		Chlorpyrifos O,O-Diethyl O-(3,5,6-trichloro-2-pyridyl) phosphorothioate	Insecticide with restricted use in consumer products and limited to nonresidential settings
		Malathion O,O-Dimethyl S-(1,2-dicarbethoxyethyl) phosphorodithioate	Widely employed insecticide of greater safety than parathion or other agents because of rapid detoxification by higher organisms
D		TEPP Tetraethyl pyrophosphate	Early insecticide
E		Echothiophate (PHOSPHOLINE IODIDE), MI-217 Diethoxyphosphinylthiocholine iodide	Extremely potent choline derivative; employed in treatment of glaucoma; relatively stable in aqueous solution

anti-ChE agents potentially can produce all the following effects: (1) stimulation of muscarinic receptor responses at autonomic effector organs; (2) stimulation, followed by depression or paralysis, of all autonomic ganglia and skeletal muscle (nicotinic actions); and (3) stimulation, with occasional subsequent depression, of cholinergic receptor sites in the CNS. Following toxic or lethal doses of anti-ChE agents, most of these effects can be noted (*see* below). However, with smaller doses, particularly those used therapeutically, several modifying factors are significant. In general, compounds containing a quaternary ammonium group do not penetrate cell membranes readily; hence, anti-ChE agents in this category are absorbed poorly from the GI tract or across the skin and are excluded from the CNS by the blood–brain barrier after moderate doses. On the other hand, such compounds act preferentially at the neuromuscular junctions of skeletal muscle, exerting their action both as anti-ChE agents and as direct agonists. They have comparatively less effect at autonomic effector sites and ganglia. In contrast, the more lipid-soluble agents are well absorbed after oral administration, have ubiquitous effects at both peripheral and central cholinergic sites, and may be sequestered in lipids for long periods of time. Lipid-soluble organophosphorus agents

also are well absorbed through the skin, and the volatile agents are transferred readily across the alveolar membrane (Storm *et al.*, 2000).

The actions of anti-ChE agents on autonomic effector cells and on cortical and subcortical sites in the CNS, where the receptors are largely of the muscarinic type, are blocked by *atropine*. Likewise, atropine blocks some of the excitatory actions of anti-ChE agents on autonomic ganglia, since both nicotinic and muscarinic receptors are involved in ganglionic neurotransmission (*see* Chapter 9).

The sites of action of anti-ChE agents of therapeutic importance are the CNS, eye, intestine, and the neuromuscular junction of skeletal muscle; other actions are of toxicological consequence.

Eye. When applied locally to the conjunctiva, anti-ChE agents cause conjunctival hyperemia and constriction of the pupillary sphincter muscle around the pupillary margin of the iris (miosis) and the ciliary muscle (block of accommodation reflex with resultant focusing to near vision). Miosis is apparent in a few minutes and can last several hours to days. Although the pupil may be "pinpoint" in size, it generally contracts further when exposed to light. The block of accommodation is more transient and generally disappears before termination of miosis. Intraocular pressure, when elevated, usually falls as the result of facilitation of outflow of the aqueous humor (*see* Chapter 63).

Gastrointestinal Tract. In humans, neostigmine enhances gastric contractions and increases the secretion of gastric acid. After bilateral vagotomy, the effects of neostigmine on gastric motility are greatly reduced. The lower portion of the esophagus is stimulated by neostigmine; in patients with marked achalasia and dilation of the esophagus, the drug can cause a salutary increase in tone and peristalsis.

Neostigmine also augments motor activity of the small and large bowel; the colon is particularly stimulated. Atony produced by muscarinic-receptor antagonists or prior surgical intervention may be overcome, propulsive waves are increased in amplitude and frequency, and movement of intestinal contents is thus promoted. The total effect of anti-ChE agents on intestinal motility probably represents a combination of actions at the ganglion cells of Auerbach's plexus and at the smooth muscle fibers, as a result of the preservation of ACh released by the cholinergic preganglionic and postganglionic fibers, respectively (*see* Chapter 37).

Neuromuscular Junction. Most of the effects of potent anti-ChE drugs on skeletal muscle can be explained adequately on the basis of their inhibition of AChE at neuromuscular junctions. However, there is good evidence for an accessory direct action of neostigmine and other quaternary ammonium anti-ChE agents on skeletal muscle. For example, the intra-arterial injection of neostigmine into chronically denervated muscle, or muscle in which AChE has been inactivated by prior administration of DFP, evokes an immediate contraction, whereas physostigmine does not.

Normally, a single nerve impulse in a terminal motor-axon branch liberates enough ACh to produce a localized depolarization (endplate potential) of sufficient magnitude to initiate a propagated muscle action potential. The ACh released is rapidly hydrolyzed by AChE, such that the lifetime of free ACh within the nerve-muscle synapse (~200 microseconds) is shorter than the decay of the endplate potential or the refractory period of the muscle. Therefore, each nerve impulse gives rise to a single wave of depolarization. After inhibition of AChE, the residence time of ACh in the synapse increases, allowing for lateral diffusion and rebinding of the transmitter to multiple receptors. Successive stimulation of neighboring receptors to the release site in the endplate results in a prolongation of the decay time of the endplate potential. Quanta

released by individual nerve impulses are no longer isolated. This action destroys the synchrony between endplate depolarizations and the development of the action potentials. Consequently, asynchronous excitation and fasciculations of muscle fibers occur. With sufficient inhibition of AChE, depolarization of the endplate predominates, and blockade owing to depolarization ensues (*see* Chapter 9). When ACh persists in the synapse, it also may depolarize the axon terminal, resulting in antidromic firing of the motoneuron; this effect contributes to fasciculations that involve the entire motor unit.

The anti-ChE agents will reverse the antagonism caused by competitive neuromuscular blocking agents (*see* Chapter 9). Neostigmine is not effective against the skeletal muscle paralysis caused by *succinylcholine;* this agent also produces neuromuscular blockade by depolarization, and depolarization will be enhanced by neostigmine.

Actions at Other Sites. Secretory glands that are innervated by postganglionic cholinergic fibers include the bronchial, lacrimal, sweat, salivary, gastric (antral G cells and parietal cells), intestinal, and pancreatic acinar glands. Low doses of anti-ChE agents augment secretory responses to nerve stimulation, and higher doses actually produce an increase in the resting rate of secretion.

Anti-ChE agents increase contraction of smooth muscle fibers of the bronchioles and ureters, and the ureters may show increased peristaltic activity.

The cardiovascular actions of anti-ChE agents are complex, since they reflect both ganglionic and postganglionic effects of accumulated ACh on the heart and blood vessels and actions in the CNS. The predominant effect on the heart from the peripheral action of accumulated ACh is bradycardia, resulting in a fall in cardiac output. Higher doses usually cause a fall in blood pressure, often as a consequence of effects of anti-ChE agents on the medullary vasomotor centers of the CNS.

Anti-ChE agents augment vagal influences on the heart. This shortens the effective refractory period of atrial muscle fibers and increases the refractory period and conduction time at the SA and AV nodes. At the ganglionic level, accumulating ACh initially is excitatory on nicotinic receptors, but at higher concentrations, ganglionic blockade ensues as a result of persistent depolarization of the cell membrane. The excitatory action on the parasympathetic ganglion cells would tend to reinforce the diminished cardiac output, whereas the opposite sequence would result from the action of ACh on sympathetic ganglion cells. Excitation followed by inhibition also is elicited by ACh at the central medullary vasomotor and cardiac centers. All of these effects are complicated further by the hypoxemia resulting from the bronchoconstrictor and secretory actions of increased ACh on the respiratory system; hypoxemia, in turn, can reinforce both sympathetic tone and ACh-induced discharge of epinephrine from the adrenal medulla. Hence, it is not surprising that an increase in heart rate is seen with severe ChE inhibitor poisoning. Hypoxemia probably is a major factor in the CNS depression that appears after large doses of anti-ChE agents. The CNS-stimulant effects are antagonized by atropine, although not as completely as are the muscarinic effects at peripheral autonomic effector sites.

Absorption, Fate, and Excretion. Physostigmine is absorbed readily from the GI tract, subcutaneous tissues, and mucous membranes. The conjunctival instillation of solutions of the drug may result in systemic effects if measures (*e.g.,* pressure on the inner canthus) are not taken to prevent absorption from the nasal mucosa. Parenterally administered physostigmine is largely destroyed within 2 hours, mainly by hydrolytic cleavage by plasma esterases; renal excretion plays only a minor role in its elimination.

Neostigmine and pyridostigmine are absorbed poorly after oral administration, such that much larger doses are needed than by the parenteral route. Whereas the effective parenteral dose of neostigmine is 0.5 to 2 mg, the equivalent oral dose may be 15 to 30 mg or more. Neostigmine and pyridostigmine are destroyed by plasma esterases, and the quaternary aromatic alcohols and parent compounds are excreted in the urine; the half-lives of these drugs are only 1 to 2 hours (Cohan *et al.,* 1976).

Organophosphorus anti-ChE agents with the highest risk of toxicity are highly lipid-soluble liquids; many have high vapor pressures. The less volatile agents that are commonly used as agricultural insecticides (*e.g.,* diazinon, malathion) generally are dispersed as aerosols or as dusts adsorbed to an inert, finely particulate material. Consequently, the compounds are absorbed rapidly through the skin and mucous membranes following contact with moisture, by the lungs after inhalation, and by the GI tract after ingestion (Storm *et al.,* 2000).

Following their absorption, most organophosphorus compounds are excreted almost entirely as hydrolysis products in the urine. Plasma and liver esterases are responsible for hydrolysis to the corresponding phosphoric and phosphonic acids. However, the CYPs are responsible for converting the inactive phosphorothioates containing a phosphorus-sulfur (thiono) bond to phosphorates with a phosphorus-oxygen bond, resulting in their activation. These enzymes also play a role in the inactivation of certain organophosphorus agents.

The organophosphorus anti-ChE agents are hydrolyzed by two families of enzymes: the carboxylesterases and the paraoxonases (A-esterases). These enzymes are found in the plasma and liver and scavenge or hydrolyze a large number of organophosphorus compounds by cleaving the phosphoester, anhydride, PF, or PCN bonds. The paraoxonases are low-molecular-weight enzymes, requiring Ca^{2+} for catalysis, whose natural substrate is unclear. Some of the isozymes are associated with high density lipoproteins, and in addition to their capacity to hydrolyze organophosphates, they may control low density lipoprotein oxidation, thereby exerting a protective effect in athero-

sclerosis (Harel *et al.,* 2004; Mackness *et al.,* 2004). Genetic polymorphisms that govern organophosphate substrate specificity and possible susceptibility to atherosclerosis have been found (Costa *et al.,* 2003; Mackness *et al.,* 2004). Wide variations in paraoxonase activity exist among animal species. Young animals are deficient in carboxylesterases and paraoxonases, which may account for age-related toxicities seen in newborn animals and suspected to be a basis for toxicity in human beings (Padilla *et al.,* 2004).

Plasma and hepatic carboxylesterases (aliesterases) and plasma butyrylcholinesterase are inhibited irreversibly by organophosphorus compounds (Lockridge and Masson, 2000); their scavenging capacity for organophosphates can afford partial protection against inhibition of AChE in the nervous system. The carboxylesterases also catalyze hydrolysis of malathion and other organophosphorus compounds that contain carboxyl-ester linkages, rendering them less active or inactive. Since carboxylesterases are inhibited by organophosphates, toxicity from exposure to two organophosphorus insecticides can be synergistic.

TOXICOLOGY

The toxicological aspects of the anti-ChE agents are of practical importance to clinicians. In addition to numerous cases of accidental intoxication from the use and manufacture of organophosphorus compounds as agricultural insecticides (over 40 have been approved for use in the United States), these agents have been used frequently for homicidal and suicidal purposes, largely because of their accessibility. Organophosphorus agents account for as much as 80% of pesticide-related hospital admissions. The World Health Organization documents pesticide toxicity as a widespread global problem; most poisonings occur in developing countries (Bardin *et al.,* 1994; Landrigan *et al.,* 2000). Occupational exposure occurs most commonly by the dermal and pulmonary routes, while oral ingestion is most common in cases of nonoccupational poisoning.

In the United States, the Environmental Protection Agency (EPA), by virtue of revised risk assessments and the Food Quality Protection Act of 1996, has placed several organophosphate insecticides on restricted use or phase-out status in consumer products for home and garden use. A primary concern relates to children, since the developing nervous system may be particularly susceptible to certain of these agents. The Office of Pesticide Programs of the EPA provides continuous reviews of the status of organophosphate pesticides, their tolerance reassessments, and revisions of risk assessments through their Web site (www.epa.gov/pesticides/op/). Public comment is sought prior to decisions on revisions.

Acute Intoxication. The effects of acute intoxication by anti-ChE agents are manifested by muscarinic and nicotinic signs and symptoms, and, except for compounds of extremely low lipid solubility, by signs referable to the CNS. Systemic effects appear within minutes after inhalation of vapors or aerosols. In contrast, the onset of symptoms is delayed after gastrointestinal and percutaneous absorption. The duration of effects is determined largely by the properties of the compound: its lipid solubility, whether it must be activated to form the oxon, the stability of the organophosphorus-AChE bond, and whether "aging" of the phosphorylated enzyme has occurred.

After local exposure to vapors or aerosols or after their inhalation, ocular and respiratory effects generally appear first. Ocular manifestations include marked miosis, ocular pain, conjunctival congestion, diminished vision, ciliary spasm, and brow ache. With acute systemic absorption, miosis may not be evident due to sympathetic discharge in response to hypotension. In addition to rhinorrhea and hyperemia of the upper respiratory tract, respiratory effects consist of tightness in the chest and wheezing respiration, caused by the combination of bronchoconstriction and increased bronchial secretion. Gastrointestinal symptoms occur earliest after ingestion and include anorexia, nausea and vomiting, abdominal cramps, and diarrhea. With percutaneous absorption of liquid, localized sweating and muscle fasciculations in the immediate vicinity are generally the earliest symptoms. Severe intoxication is manifested by extreme salivation, involuntary defecation and urination, sweating, lacrimation, penile erection, bradycardia, and hypotension.

Nicotinic actions at the neuromuscular junctions of skeletal muscle usually consist of fatigability and generalized weakness, involuntary twitchings, scattered fasciculations, and eventually severe weakness and paralysis. The most serious consequence is paralysis of the respiratory muscles. Knockout mice lacking AChE can survive under highly supportive conditions and with a special diet, but they exhibit continuous tremors and are stunted in growth (Xie *et al.*, 2000). Mice that selectively lack AChE in skeletal muscle but have normal or near normal expression in brain and organs innervated by the autonomic nervous system grow normally and can reproduce, but have continuous tremors (Camp *et al.*, 2004). These studies show that cholinergic systems can partially adapt to chronically diminished hydrolytic capacity for AChE.

The broad spectrum of effects of acute AChE inhibition on the CNS includes confusion, ataxia, slurred speech, loss of reflexes, Cheyne-Stokes respiration, generalized convulsions, coma, and central respiratory paralysis. Actions on the vasomotor and other cardiovascular centers in the medulla oblongata lead to hypotension.

The time of death after a single acute exposure may range from less than 5 minutes to nearly 24 hours, depending on the dose, route, agent, and other factors. The cause of death primarily is respiratory failure, usually accompanied by a secondary cardiovascular component. Peripheral muscarinic and nicotinic as well as central actions all contribute to respiratory compromise; effects include laryngospasm, bronchoconstriction, increased tracheobronchial and salivary secretions, compromised voluntary control of the diaphragm and intercostal muscles, and central respiratory depression. Blood pressure may fall to alarmingly low levels and cardiac arrhythmias intervene. These effects usually result from hypoxemia and often are reversed by assisted pulmonary ventilation.

Delayed symptoms appearing after 1 to 4 days and marked by persistent low blood ChE and severe muscle weakness are termed the *intermediate syndrome* (Marrs, 1993; De Bleecker *et al.*, 1992; Lotti, 2002). A delayed neurotoxicity also may be evident after severe intoxication (*see* below).

Diagnosis and Treatment. The diagnosis of severe, acute anti-ChE intoxication is made readily from the history of exposure and the characteristic signs and symptoms. In suspected cases of milder acute or chronic intoxication, determination of the ChE activities in erythrocytes and plasma generally will establish the diagnosis (Storm *et al.*, 2000). Although these values vary considerably in the normal population, they usually are depressed well below the normal range before symptoms are evident.

Atropine in sufficient dosage (*see* below) effectively antagonizes the actions at muscarinic receptor sites, including increased tracheobronchial and salivary secretion, bronchoconstriction, bradycardia, and to a moderate extent, peripheral ganglionic and central actions. Larger doses are required to get appreciable concentrations of atropine into the CNS. Atropine is virtually without effect against the peripheral neuromuscular compromise, which can be reversed by *pralidoxime* (2-PAM), a cholinesterase reactivator.

In moderate or severe intoxication with an organophosphorus anti-ChE agent, the recommended adult dose of pralidoxime is 1 to 2 g, infused intravenously over not less than 5 minutes. If weakness is not relieved or if it recurs after 20 to 60 minutes, the dose should be repeated. Early treatment is very important to assure that the oxime reaches the phosphorylated AChE while the latter still can be reactivated. Many of the alkylphosphates are extremely lipid soluble, and if extensive partitioning into body fat has occurred and desulfuration is required for inhibition of AChE, toxicity will persist and symptoms may recur after initial treatment. With severe toxicities from the lipid-soluble agents, it is necessary to continue treatment with atropine and pralidoxime for a week or longer.

General supportive measures also are important, including: (1) termination of exposure, by removal of the patient or application of a gas mask if the atmosphere remains contaminated, removal and destruction of contaminated clothing, copious washing of contaminated skin or mucous membranes with water, or gastric lavage; (2) maintenance of a patent airway, including endobronchial aspiration; (3) artificial respiration, if required; (4) administration of oxygen; (5) alleviation of persistent convulsions with *diazepam* (5 to 10 mg, intravenously); and (6) treatment of shock (Marrs, 1993; Bardin *et al.*, 1994).

Atropine should be given in doses sufficient to cross the blood–brain barrier. Following an initial injection of 2 to 4 mg, given intravenously if possible, otherwise intramuscularly, 2 mg should be given every 5 to 10 minutes until muscarinic symptoms disappear, if they reappear, or until signs of atropine toxicity appear. More than 200 mg may be required on the first day. A mild degree of atropine block then should be maintained for as long as symptoms are evident. Whereas the AChE reactivators can be of great benefit in the therapy of anti-ChE intoxication (*see* below), their use must be regarded as a supplement to the administration of atropine.

Cholinesterase Reactivators. Although the phosphorylated esteratic site of AChE undergoes hydrolytic regeneration at a slow or negligible rate, Wilson found that nucleophilic agents, such as hydroxylamine (NH_2OH), hydroxamic acids (RCONH—OH), and oximes (RCH=NOH), reactivate the enzyme more rapidly than does spontaneous hydrolysis. He reasoned that selective reactivation could be achieved by a site-directed nucleophile, wherein interaction of a quaternary nitrogen with the negative subsite of the active center would place the nucleophile in close apposition to the phosphorus. This goal was achieved to a remarkable degree by Wilson and Ginsburg with pyridine-2-aldoxime methyl chloride (pralidoxime) (Figure 8–2E);

reactivation with this compound occurs at a million times the rate of that with hydroxylamine. The oxime is oriented proximally to exert a nucleophilic attack on the phosphorus; a phosphoryloxime is formed, leaving the regenerated enzyme.

Several *bis*-quaternary oximes are even more potent as reactivators for insecticide and nerve gas poisoning (*see* below); an example is HI-6, which is used in Europe as an antidote. The structures of pralidoxime and HI-6 are:

PRALIDOXIME (2-PAM)

HI-6

The velocity of reactivation of phosphorylated AChE by oximes depends on their accessibility to the active center serine (Wong *et al.*, 2000). Furthermore, certain phosphorylated AChEs can undergo a fairly rapid process of "aging," so that within the course of minutes or hours they become completely resistant to the reactivators. "Aging" is due to the loss of one alkoxy group, leaving a much more stable monoalkyl- or monoalkoxy-phosphoryl-AChE (Figure 8–2D and E). Organophosphorus compounds containing tertiary alkoxy groups are more prone to "aging" than are congeners containing the secondary or primary alkoxy groups. The oximes are not effective in antagonizing the toxicity of the more rapidly hydrolyzing carbamoyl ester inhibitors; since pralidoxime itself has weak anti-ChE activity, it is not recommended for the treatment of overdosage with neostigmine or physostigmine or poisoning with carbamoylating insecticides such as carbaryl.

Pharmacology, Toxicology, and Disposition. The reactivating action of oximes *in vivo* is most marked at the skeletal neuromuscular junction. Following a dose of an organophosphorus compound that produces total blockade of transmission, the intravenous injection of an oxime can restore the response to stimulation of the motor nerve within a few minutes. Antidotal effects are less striking at autonomic effector sites, and the quaternary ammonium group restricts entry into the CNS.

Although high doses or accumulation of oximes can inhibit AChE and cause neuromuscular blockade, they should be given until one can be assured of clearance of the offending organophosphate. Many organophosphates partition into lipid and are released slowly as the active entity.

Current antidotal therapy for organophosphate exposure resulting from warfare or terrorism includes parenteral atropine, an oxime (2-PAM or HI-6), and a benzodiaz-

epine as an anticonvulsant. Parenterally administered human butyrylcholinesterase is under development as an antidote, to scavenge the inhibitor in the plasma before it reaches peripheral and central tissue sites (Doctor, 2003). Because this effect of butyrylcholinesterase is stoichiometric rather than catalytic, large quantities are required.

The oximes and their metabolites are readily eliminated by the kidney.

Delayed Neurotoxicity of Organophosphorus Compounds. Certain fluorine-containing organophosphorus anti-ChE agents (*e.g.,* DFP, *mipafox*) have in common with the triarylphosphates, of which *tri-orthocresylphosphate* (TOCP) is the classical example, the property of inducing delayed neurotoxicity. This syndrome first received widespread attention following the demonstration that TOCP, an adulterant of Jamaica ginger, was responsible for an outbreak of thousands of cases of paralysis that occurred in the United States during Prohibition.

The clinical picture is that of a severe polyneuropathy manifested initially by mild sensory disturbances, ataxia, weakness, muscle fatigue and twitching, reduced tendon reflexes, and tenderness to palpation. In severe cases, the weakness may progress to flaccid paralysis and muscle wasting. Recovery may require several years and may be incomplete.

Toxicity from this organophosphate-induced delayed polyneuropathy is not dependent upon inhibition of cholinesterases; instead a distinct esterase, termed *neurotoxic esterase*, is linked to the lesions (Johnson, 1993). This enzyme has a substrate specificity for hydrophobic esters, but its natural substrate and function remain unknown (Glynn, 2000). Myopathies that result in generalized necrotic lesions and changes in endplate cytostructure also are found in experimental animals after long-term exposure to organophosphates (Dettbarn, 1984; De Bleecker *et al.*, 1992).

THERAPEUTIC USES

Current use of anti-AChE agents is limited to four conditions in the periphery: atony of the smooth muscle of the intestinal tract and urinary bladder, glaucoma, myasthenia gravis, and reversal of the paralysis of competitive neuromuscular blocking drugs (*see* Chapter 9). Long-acting and hydrophobic ChE inhibitors are the only inhibitors with well-documented efficacy, albeit limited, in the treatment of dementia symptoms of Alzheimer's disease. Physostigmine, with its shorter duration of action, is useful in the treatment of intoxication by atropine and several drugs with anticholinergic side effects (*see* below); it also is indicated for the treatment of Friedreich's or other inherited ataxias. Edrophonium has been used for terminating attacks of paroxysmal supraventricular tachycardia.

Available Therapeutic Agents. The compounds described here are those commonly used as anti-ChE drugs and ChE reactivators in the United States. Preparations used solely for ophthalmic purposes are described in Chapter 63. Conventional dosages and routes of administration are given in the discussion of therapeutic applications (*see* below).

Physostigmine salicylate (ANTILIRIUM) is available for injection. *Physostigmine sulfate ophthalmic ointment* and *physostigmine salicylate ophthalmic solution* also are available. *Pyridostigmine bromide* is available for oral (MESTINON) or parenteral (REGONOL, MESTINON) use. *Neostigmine bromide* (PROSTIGMIN) is available for oral use. *Neostigmine methylsulfate* (PROSTIGMIN) is marketed for parenteral injection. *Ambenonium chloride* (MYTELASE) is available for oral use. Tacrine (COGNEX), donepezil (ARICEPT), rivastigmine (EXELON), and *galantamine* (REMINYL) have been approved for the treatment of Alzheimer's disease.

Pralidoxime chloride (PROTOPAM CHLORIDE) is the only AChE reactivator currently available in the United States and can be obtained in a parenteral formulation. HI-6 is available in several European and Near Eastern countries.

Paralytic Ileus and Atony of the Urinary Bladder. In the treatment of both these conditions, neostigmine generally is preferred among the anti-ChE agents. The direct parasympathomimetic agents (Chapter 7) are employed for the same purposes.

Neostigmine is used for the relief of abdominal distension and acute colonic pseudo-obstruction from a variety of medical and surgical causes (Ponec *et al.*, 1999). The usual subcutaneous dose of neostigmine methylsulfate for postoperative paralytic ileus is 0.5 mg, given as needed. Peristaltic activity commences 10 to 30 minutes after parenteral administration, whereas 2 to 4 hours are required after oral administration of neostigmine bromide (15 to 30 mg). It may be necessary to assist evacuation with a small low enema or gas with a rectal tube.

When neostigmine is used for the treatment of atony of the detrusor muscle of the urinary bladder, postoperative dysuria is relieved, and the time interval between operation and spontaneous urination is shortened. The drug is used in a similar dose and manner as in the management of paralytic ileus. Neostigmine should not be used when the intestine or urinary bladder is obstructed, when peritonitis is present, when the viability of the bowel is doubtful, or when bowel dysfunction results from inflammatory bowel disease.

Glaucoma and Other Ophthalmologic Indications. Glaucoma is a complex disease characterized by an increase in intraocular pressure that, if sufficiently high and persistent, leads to damage to the optic disc at the juncture of the optic nerve and the retina; irreversible blindness can result. Of the three types of glaucoma—primary, secondary, and congenital—anti-AChE agents are of value in the management of the primary as well as of certain categories of the secondary type (*e.g.*, aphakic glaucoma, following cataract extraction); congenital glaucoma rarely responds to any therapy other than surgery. Primary glaucoma is subdivided into narrow-angle (acute congestive) and wide-angle (chronic simple) types, based on the configuration of the angle of the anterior chamber where the aqueous humor is reabsorbed.

Narrow-angle glaucoma is nearly always a medical emergency in which drugs are essential in controlling the acute attack, but the long-range management is often surgical (*e.g.*, peripheral or complete iridectomy). Wide-angle glaucoma, on the other hand, has a gradual, insidious onset and is not generally amenable to surgical improvement; in this type, control of intraocular pressure usually is dependent upon continuous drug therapy.

Since the cholinergic agonists and ChE inhibitors also block accommodation and induce myopia, these agents produce transient blurring of far vision, limited visual acuity in low light, and loss of vision at the margin when instilled in the eye. With long-term administration of the cholinergic agonists and anti-ChE agents, the compromise of vision diminishes. Nevertheless, other agents without these side effects, such as β adrenergic receptor antagonists, prostaglandin analogs, or carbonic anhydrase inhibitors, have become the primary topical therapies for open-angle glaucoma (Alward, 1998) (*see* Chapter 63), with AChE inhibitors held in reserve for the chronic conditions when patients become refractory to the above agents. Topical treatment with long-acting ChE inhibitors such as echothiophate gives rise to symptoms characteristic of systemic ChE inhibition. Echothiophate treatment in advanced glaucoma may be associated with the production of cataracts (Alward, 1998).

Anti-ChE agents have been employed locally in the treatment of a variety of other less common ophthalmologic conditions, including accommodative esotropia and myasthenia gravis confined to the extraocular and eyelid muscles. Adie (or tonic pupil) syndrome results from dysfunction of the ciliary body, perhaps because of local nerve degeneration. Low concentrations of physostigmine are reported to decrease the blurred vision and pain associated with this condition. In alternation with a mydriatic drug such as atropine, short-acting anti-ChE agents have proven useful for breaking adhesions between the iris and the lens or cornea. (For a complete account of the use of anti-ChE agents in ocular therapy, *see* Chapter 63.)

Myasthenia Gravis. Myasthenia gravis is a neuromuscular disease characterized by weakness and marked fatigability of skeletal muscle (Drachman, 1994); exacerbations and partial remissions occur frequently. Jolly noted the similarity between the symptoms of myasthenia gravis and curare poisoning in animals and suggested that physostigmine, an agent then known to antagonize curare, might be of therapeutic value. Forty years elapsed before his suggestion was given systematic trial.

The defect in myasthenia gravis is in synaptic transmission at the neuromuscular junction. When a motor nerve of a normal subject is stimulated at 25 Hz, electrical and mechanical responses are well sustained. A suitable margin of safety exists for maintenance of neuromuscular transmission. Initial responses in the myasthenic patient may be normal, but they diminish rapidly, which explains the difficulty in maintaining voluntary muscle activity for more than brief periods.

The relative importance of prejunctional and postjunctional defects in myasthenia gravis was a matter of considerable debate until Patrick and Lindstrom found that rabbits immunized with the nicotinic receptor purified from electric eels slowly developed muscular weakness and respiratory difficulties that resembled the symptoms of myasthenia gravis. The rabbits also exhibited decremental responses following repetitive nerve stimulation, enhanced sensitivity to curare, and following the administration of anti-AChE agents, symptomatic and electrophysiological improvement of neuromuscular transmission. Although this experimental allergic myasthenia gravis and the naturally occurring disease differ somewhat, this animal model prompted intense investigation into whether the natural disease represented an autoimmune response directed toward the ACh receptor. Antireceptor antibodies are detectable in sera of 90% of patients with the disease, although the clinical status of the patient does not correlate precisely with the antibody titer (Drachman *et al.*, 1982; Drachman, 1994; Lindstrom, 2000).

The picture that emerges is that myasthenia gravis is caused by an autoimmune response primarily to the ACh receptor at the postjunctional endplate. These antibodies reduce the number of receptors detectable either by snake α-neurotoxin-binding assays (Fambrough *et al.*, 1973) or by electrophysiological measurements of ACh sensitivity (Drachman, 1994). The autoimmune reaction enhances receptor degradation (Drachman *et al.*, 1982). Immune complexes along with marked ultrastructural abnormalities appear in the synaptic cleft and enhance receptor degradation. These events appear to be a consequence of complement-mediated lysis of junctional folds in the endplate. A related disease that also compromises neuromuscular transmission is Lambert-Eaton syndrome. Here, antibodies are directed against Ca^{2+} channels that are necessary for presynaptic release of ACh (Lang *et al.*, 1998).

In a subset of approximately 10% of patients presenting with a myasthenic syndrome, muscle weakness has a congenital rather than an autoimmune basis. Characterization of biochemical and genetic bases of the congenital condition has shown mutations to occur in the acetylcholine receptor which affect ligand-binding and channel-opening kinetics (Engel *et al.*, 2003). Other mutations occur as a deficiency in the form of AChE that contains the collagen-like tail unit (Ohno *et al.*, 2000). As expected, following administration of anti-ChE agents (*see* below), subjective improvement is not seen in most congenital myasthenic patients.

Diagnosis. Although the diagnosis of autoimmune myasthenia gravis usually can be made from the history, signs, and symptoms, its differentiation from certain neurasthenic, infectious, endocrine, congenital, neoplastic, and degenerative neuromuscular diseases can be challenging. However, myasthenia gravis is the only condition in which the aforementioned deficiencies can be improved dramatically by anti-ChE medication. The edrophonium test for evaluation of possible myasthenia gravis is performed by rapid intravenous injection of 2 mg of *edrophonium chloride*, followed 45 seconds later by an additional 8 mg if the first dose is without effect; a positive response consists of brief improvement in strength, unaccompanied by lingual fasciculation (which generally occurs in nonmyasthenic patients).

An excessive dose of an anti-ChE drug results in a *cholinergic crisis*. The condition is characterized by weakness resulting from generalized depolarization of the motor endplate; other features result from overstimulation of muscarinic receptors. The weakness resulting from depolarization block may resemble myasthenic weakness, which is manifest when anti-ChE medication is insufficient. The distinction is of obvious practical importance, since the former is treated by withholding, and the latter by administering, the anti-ChE agent. When the edrophonium test is performed cautiously, limiting the dose to 2 mg and with facilities for respiratory resuscitation available, a further decrease in strength indicates cholinergic crisis, while improvement signifies myasthenic weakness. *Atropine sulfate*, 0.4 to 0.6 mg or more intravenously, should be given immediately if a severe muscarinic reaction ensues (for complete details, *see* Osserman *et al.*, 1972; Drachman, 1994). Detection of anti-receptor antibodies in muscle biopsies or plasma is now widely employed to establish the diagnosis.

Treatment. Pyridostigmine, neostigmine, and ambenonium are the standard anti-ChE drugs used in the symptomatic treatment of myasthenia gravis. All can increase the response of myasthenic muscle to repetitive nerve impulses, primarily by the preservation of endogenous ACh. Following AChE inhibition, receptors over a greater cross-sectional area of the endplate presumably are exposed to concentrations of ACh that are sufficient for channel opening and production of a postsynaptic endplate potential.

When the diagnosis of myasthenia gravis has been established, the optimal single oral dose of an anti-ChE agent can be determined empirically. Baseline recordings are made for grip strength, vital capacity, and a number of signs and symptoms that reflect the strength of various muscle groups. The patient then is given an oral dose of pyridostigmine (30 to 60 mg), neostigmine (7.5 to 15 mg), or ambenonium (2.5 to 5 mg). The improvement in muscle strength and changes in other signs and symptoms are noted at frequent intervals until there is a return to the basal state. After an hour or longer in the basal state, the drug is given again, with the dose increased to one and one-half times the initial amount, and the same observations are repeated. This sequence is continued, with increasing increments of one-half the initial dose, until an optimal response is obtained.

The duration of action of these drugs is such that the interval between oral doses required to maintain a reasonably even level of strength usually is 2 to 4 hours for neostigmine, 3 to 6 hours for pyridostigmine, or 3 to 8 hours for ambenonium. However, the dose required may vary from day to day, and physical or emotional stress, intercurrent infections, and menstruation usually necessitate an increase in the frequency or size of the dose. In addition, unpredictable exacerbations and remissions of the myasthenic state may require adjustment of dosage. Although myasthenia gravis requires physician care at regular intervals, most patients can be taught to modify their dosage regimens according to their changing requirements. Pyridostigmine is available in sustained-release tablets containing a total of 180 mg, of which 60 mg is released immediately and 120 mg over several hours; this preparation is of value in maintaining patients for 6- to 8-hour periods, but should be limited to use at bedtime. Muscarinic cardiovascular and gastrointestinal side effects of anti-ChE agents generally can be controlled by atropine or other anticholinergic drugs (*see* Chapter 7). However, these anticholinergic drugs mask many side effects of an excessive dose of an anti-ChE agent. In most patients, tolerance develops eventually to the muscarinic effects, so that anticholinergic medication is not necessary. A number of drugs, including curariform agents and certain antibiotics and general anesthetics, interfere with neuromuscular transmission (*see* Chapter 9); their administration to patients with myasthenia gravis is hazardous without proper adjustment of anti-ChE dosage and other appropriate precautions.

Other therapeutic measures should be considered as essential elements in the management of this disease. Controlled studies reveal that glucocorticoids promote clinical improvement in a high percentage of patients. However, when treatment with steroids is continued over prolonged periods, a high incidence of side effects may result (*see* Chapter 59). Gradual lowering of maintenance doses and alternate-day regimens of short-acting steroids are used to minimize side effects. Initiation of steroid treatment augments muscle weakness; however, as the patient improves with continued administration of steroids, doses of anti-ChE drugs can be reduced (Drachman, 1994). Other immunosuppressive agents such as *azathioprine* and *cyclosporine* also have been beneficial in more advanced cases (*see* Chapter 52).

Thymectomy should be considered in myasthenia associated with a thymoma or when the disease is not controlled adequately by anti-ChE agents and steroids. The relative risks and benefits of the surgical procedure *versus* anti-ChE and glucocorticoid treatment require careful assessment in each case. Since the thymus contains myoid cells with nicotinic receptors (Schluep *et al.*, 1987), and a predominance of patients have thymic abnormalities, the thymus may be responsible for the initial pathogenesis. It also is the source of autoreactive T-helper cells. However, the thymus is not required for perpetuation of the condition.

In keeping with the presumed autoimmune etiology of myasthenia gravis, plasmapheresis and immune therapy have produced beneficial results in patients who have remained disabled despite thymectomy and treatment with steroids and anti-ChE agents (Drachman, 1994; Drachman, 1996). Improvement in muscle strength correlates with the reduction of the titer of antibody directed against the nicotinic ACh receptor.

Prophylaxis in Cholinesterase Inhibitor Poisoning. Studies in experimental animals have shown that pretreatment with pyridostigmine reduces the incapacitation and mortality associated with nerve agent poisoning, particularly for agents such as soman that show rapid aging. The first large-scale administration of pyridostigmine to humans occurred in 1990 in anticipation of nerve-agent attack in the first Persian Gulf War. At an oral dose of 30 mg every 8 hours, the incidence of side effects was around 1%, but fewer than 0.1% of the subjects had responses sufficient to warrant discontinuing the drug in the setting of military action (Keeler *et al.*, 1991). Long-term follow-up indicates that veterans of the Persian Gulf War who received pyridostigmine showed a low incidence of a neurologic syndrome, now termed the *Persian Gulf War syndrome*. It is characterized by impaired cognition, ataxia, confusion, myoneuropathy, adenopathy, weakness, and incontinence (Haley *et al.*, 1997; Institute of Medicine, 2003). While pyridostigmine has been implicated by some as the causative agent, the absence of similar neuropathies in pyridostigmine-treated myasthenic patients makes it far more likely that a combination of agents, including combusted organophosphates and insect repellents in addition to pyridostigmine, contributed to this persisting syndrome. It also is difficult to distinguish residual chemical toxicity from posttraumatic stress experienced after combat action. Pyridostigmine has recently been approved by the FDA for prophylaxis against soman, an organophosphate that rapidly ages following inhibition of cholinesterases.

Intoxication by Anticholinergic Drugs. In addition to atropine and other muscarinic agents, many other drugs, such as the phenothiazines, antihistamines, and tricyclic antidepressants, have central and peripheral anticholinergic activity. Physostigmine is potentially useful in reversing the central anticholinergic syndrome produced by overdosage or an unusual reaction to these drugs (Nilsson, 1982). The effectiveness of physostigmine in reversing the anticholinergic effects of these agents has been clearly documented. However, other toxic effects of the tricyclic antidepressants and phenothiazines (*see* Chapters 17 and 18), such as intraventricular conduction deficits and ventricular arrhythmias, are not reversed by physostigmine. In addition, physostigmine may precipitate seizures; hence, its usually small potential benefit must be weighed against this risk. The initial intravenous or intramuscular dose of physostigmine is 2 mg, with additional doses given as necessary. Physostigmine, a tertiary amine, crosses the blood–brain barrier, in contrast to the quaternary anti-AChE drugs. The use of anti-ChE agents to reverse the effects of competitive neuromuscular blocking agents is discussed in Chapter 9.

Alzheimer's Disease. A deficiency of intact cholinergic neurons, particularly those extending from subcortical areas such as the nucleus basalis of Meynert, has been observed in patients with progressive dementia of the Alzheimer type (Markesbery, 1998). Using a rationale similar to that in other CNS degenerative diseases (*see* Chapter 20), therapy for enhancing concentrations of cholinergic

neurotransmitters in the CNS was investigated (Mayeux and Sano, 1999). In 1993, the FDA approved tacrine (tetrahydroaminoacridine) for use in mild to moderate Alzheimer's disease, but a high incidence of hepatotoxicity limits the utility of this drug. About 30% of the patients receiving low doses of tacrine within 3 months have alanine aminotransferase values three times normal; upon discontinuing the drug, liver function values return to normal in 90% of the patients. Other side effects are typical of AChE inhibitors.

More recently, donepezil was approved for clinical use. At 5- and 10-mg daily oral doses, improved cognition and global clinical function were seen in the 21- to 81-week intervals studied (Dooley and Lamb, 2000). In long-term studies, the drug delayed symptomatic progression of the disease for periods up to 55 weeks. Side effects are largely attributable to excessive cholinergic stimulation, with nausea, diarrhea, and vomiting being most frequently reported. The drug is well tolerated in single daily doses. Usually, 5-mg doses are administered at night for 4 to 6 weeks; if this dose is well tolerated, the dose can be increased to 10 mg daily.

Rivastigmine, a long-acting carbamoylating inhibitor, recently has been approved for use in the United States and Europe. Although fewer studies have been conducted, its efficacy, tolerability, and side effects are similar to those of donepezil (Corey-Bloom *et al.*, 1998; Giacobini, 2000). *Eptastigmine*, another carbamoylating inhibitor, was associated with adverse hematologic effects in two studies, resulting in suspension of clinical trials. Galantamine is another AChE inhibitor recently approved by the FDA. It has a side-effect profile similar to those of donepezil and rivastigmine.

Therapeutic strategies with new compounds are directed at maximizing the ratio of central to peripheral ChE inhibition and the use of ChE inhibitors in conjunction with selective cholinergic agonists and antagonists. Combination therapy and other therapeutic strategies are presented in Chapter 20.

BIBLIOGRAPHY

Bourne, Y., Marchot, P., and Taylor, P. Acetylcholinesterase inhibition by fasciculin: crystal structure of the complex. *Cell,* **1995,** *83:*493–506.

Burkhart, C.G. Relationship of treatment resistant head lice to the safety and efficacy of pediculicides. *Mayo Clinic Proceedings,* **2004,** *79:*661–666.

Cohan, S.L., Pohlmann, J.L.W., Mikszewski, J., and O'Doherty, D.S. The pharmacokinetics of pyridostigmine. *Neurology,* **1976,** *26:*536–539.

Corey-Bloom, J., Anand, R., and Veach, J. A randomized trial evaluating the efficacy and safety of ENA 713 (rivastigmine tartrate), a new acetylcholinesterase inhibitor, in patients with mild to moderately severe Alzheimer's disease. *Int. J. Psychopharmacol.,* **1998,** *1:*55–65.

Costa, L.G., Cole, T.B., and Furlong, C.E. Polymorphisms of paroxonase and their significance in clinical toxicology of organophosphates. *J Toxicol Clin Toxicol,* **2003,** *41:*37–45.

Cummings, J.L., Cyrus, P.A., and Bieber, F. Metrifonate treatment of cognitive deficits in Alzheimer's disease. *Neurology,* **1999,** *50:*1214–1221.

Cygler, M., Schrag, J., Sussman, J.L., *et al.* Relationship between sequence conservation and three dimensional structure in a large family of esterases, lipases and related proteins. *Protein Sci.,* **1993,** *2:*366–382.

Drachman, D.B., Adams, R.N., Josifek, L.F., and Self, S.G. Functional activities of autoantibodies to acetylcholine receptors and the clinical severity of myasthenia gravis. *N. Engl. J. Med.,* **1982,** *307:*769–775.

Fambrough, D.M., Drachman, D.B., and Satyamurti, S. Neuromuscular junction in myasthenia gravis: decreased acetylcholine receptors. *Science,* **1973,** *182:*293–295.

Haley, R.W., Kurt, T.L., and Hom, J. Is there a Gulf War syndrome? *JAMA,* **1997,** *277:*215–222.

Harel, M., Aharoni, A., Gaidukov, L., *et al.* Structure and evolution of the serum paraoxonase family of detoxifying and anti-atherosclerotic enzymes. *Nat. Struct. Mol. Biol.,* **2004,** *11:*412–419.

Jennings, L.L., Malecki, M., Komives, E.A., and Taylor, P. Direct analysis of the kinetic profiles of organophosphate-acetylcholinesterase adducts by MALDI-TOF mass spectrometry. *Biochemistry,* **2003,** *42(37):*11083–11091.

Keeler, J.R., Hurst, C.G., and Dunn, M.A. Pyridostigmine used as a nerve agent pretreatment under wartime conditions. *JAMA,* **1991,** *266:*693–695.

Lockridge, O., Bartels, C.F., Vaughan, T.A., *et al.* Complete amino acid sequence of human serum cholinesterase. *J. Biol. Chem.,* **1987,** *262:*549–557.

Lockridge, O., and Masson, P. Pesticides and susceptible populations: People with butyrylcholinesterase genetic variants may be at risk. *Neurotoxicology,* **2000,** *21:*113–126.

Nilsson, E. Physostigmine treatment in various drug-induced intoxications. *Ann. Clin. Res.,* **1982,** *14:*165–172.

Nozaki, H., and Aikawa, N. Sarin poisoning in Tokyo subway. *Lancet,* **1995,** *346:*1446–1447.

Padilla, S., Sung, H.-J., and Moser, V.C. Further assessment of an in vitro screen that may help identify organophosphate insecticides that are more acutely toxic to the young. *J. Toxicol. & Environ. Health,* **2004,** *67:*1477–1489.

Patrick, J., and Lindstrom, J. Autoimmune response to acetylcholine receptor. *Science,* **1973,** *180:*871–872.

Ponec, R.J., Saunders, M.D., and Kimmey, M.B. Neostigmine for the treatment of acute colonic pseudoobstruction. *N. Engl. J. Med.,* **1999,** *341:*137–141.

Schluep, M., Wilcox, N., Vincent, A., Dhoot, G.K., and Newson-Davis, J. Acetylcholine receptors in human thymic myoid cells in situ: an immunohistological study. *Ann. Neurol.,* **1987,** *22:*212–222.

Schumacher, M., Camp, S., Maulet, Y., *et al.* Primary structure of *Torpedo californica* acetylcholinesterase deduced from its cDNA sequence. *Nature,* **1986,** *319:*407–409.

Sussman, J.L., Harel, M., Frolow, F., *et al.* Atomic structure of acetylcholinesterase from *Torpedo californica:* a prototypic acetylcholine-binding protein. *Science,* **1991,** *253:*872–879.

Wong, L., Radic, Z., Bruggemann, R.J., *et al.* Mechanism of oxime reactivation of acetylcholinesterase analyzed by chirality and mutagenesis. *Biochemistry,* **2000,** *39:*5750–5757.

Xie, W., Stribley, J.A., Chatonnet, A., *et al.* Postnatal development delay and supersensitivity to organophosphate in gene-targeted mice lacking acetylcholinesterase. *J. Pharmacol. Exp. Ther.,* **2000,** *293:*892–902.

MONOGRAPHS AND REVIEWS

Alward, W.L.M. Medical management of glaucoma. *N. Engl. J. Med.,* **1998,** *339:*1298–1307.

Bardin, P.G., van Eeden, S.F., Moolman, J.A., Foden, A.P., and Joubert, J.R. Organophosphate and carbamate poisoning. *Arch. Intern. Med.,* **1994,** *154:*1433–1441.

Baron, R.L. Carbamate insecticides. In, *Handbook of Pesticide Toxicology,* Vol. 3. (Hayes, W.J., Jr., and Laws, E.R., Jr., eds.) Academic Press, San Diego, CA, **1991,** pp. 1125–1190.

Camp, S., Zhang, L., Marquez, M., de la Torre, B., Long, J.M., Bucht, G., and Taylor, P. Acetylcholinesterase gene modification in transgenic animals: functional consequences of selected exon and regulatory region deletion. In: *Chemico-Biological Interactions,* **2005,** in press.

Costa, L.G., Galli, C.L., and Murphy, S.D. (eds.) *Toxicology of Pesticides: Experimental, Clinical, and Regulatory Perspectives. NATO Advanced Study Institute Series H,* Vol. 13. Springer-Verlag, Berlin, **1987.**

Cummings, J.L. Alzheimer's Disease. *N. Engl. J. Med.,* **2004,** *351:*56–67.

De Bleecker, J.L., De Reuck, J.L., and Willems, J.L. Neurological aspects of organophosphate poisoning. *Clin. Neurol. Neurosurg.,* **1992,** *94:*93–103.

Dettbarn, W.D. Pesticide induced muscle necrosis: mechanisms and prevention. *Fundam. Appl. Toxicol.,* **1984,** *4:*S18–S26.

Dooley, M., and Lamb, H.M. Donepezil: a review of its use in Alzheimer's disease. *Drugs Aging,* **2000,** *16:*199–226.

Doctor, B.P. Butyrylcholinesterase: its use for prophylaxis of organophosphate exposure. In, *Butyrylcholinesterase: Its Function and Inhibitors.* (E. Giacobini, ed.) Martin Dunitz, London, **2003,** pp. 163-177.

Drachman, D.B. Myasthenia gravis. *N. Engl. J. Med.,* **1994,** *330:*1797–1810.

Drachman, D.B. Immunotherapy in neuromuscular disorders: current and future strategies. *Muscle Nerve,* **1996,** *19:*1239–1251.

Ecobichon, D.J. Carbamates. In, *Experimental and Clinical Neurotoxicology,* 2nd ed. (Spencer, P.S., and Schauburg, H.H., eds.) Oxford University Press, New York, **2000.**

Engel, A.G., Ohno, K., and Sine, S.M. Sleuthing molecular targets for neurological diseases at the neuromuscular junction. *Nature Reviews (Neuroscience),* **2003,** *4:*339–352.

Froede, H.C., and Wilson, I.B. Acetylcholinesterase. In, *The Enzymes,* Vol. 5. (Boyer, P.D., ed.) Academic Press, New York, **1971,** pp. 87–114.

Gallo, M.A., and Lawryk, N.J. Organic phosphorus pesticides. In, *Handbook of Pesticide Toxicology,* Vol. 2. (Hayes, W.J., Jr., and Laws, E.R., Jr., eds.) Academic Press, San Diego, CA, **1991,** pp. 917–1123.

Giacobini, E. Cholinesterase inhibitors: from the Calabar bean to Alzheimer's therapy. In, *Cholinesterases and Cholinesterase Inhibitors.* (Giacobini, E., ed.) Martin Dubitz, London, **2000,** pp. 181–227.

Glynn, P. Neural development and neurodegeneration: two faces of neuropathy target esterase. *Prog. Neurobiol.,* **2000,** *61:*61–74.

Holmstedt, B., Cholinesterase inhibitors: an introduction. In, *Cholinesterases and Cholinesterase Inhibitors.* (Giacobini, E., ed.) Martin Dunitz, London, **2000,** pp. 1–8.

Institute of Medicine (National Academy of Science-USA). *Gulf War and Health Volume 2,* National Academies Press, Washington, D.C., **2003,** 600pp.

Johnson, M.K. Symposium introduction: retrospect and prospects for neuropathy target esterase (NTE) and the delayed polyneuropathy (OPIDP) induced by some organophosphorus esters. *Chem. Biol. Interact.,* **1993,** *87:*339–346.

Karczmar, A.G. History of the research with anticholinesterase agents. In, *Anticholinesterase Agents,* Vol. 1, *International Encyclopedia of Pharmacology and Therapeutics,* Sect. 13. (Karczmar, A.G., ed.) Pergamon Press, Oxford, **1970,** pp. 1–44.

Landrigan, P.J., Claudio, L., and McConnell, R. Pesticides. In, *Environmental Toxicants: Human Exposures and Their Health Effects.* (Lippman, M., ed.) Wiley, New York, **2000,** pp. 725–739.

Lang, B., Waterman, S., Pinto, A., *et al.* The role of autoantibodies in Lambert-Eaton myasthenic syndrome. *Ann. N.Y. Acad. Sci.,* **1998,** *841:*596–605.

Lindstrom, J.M. Acetylcholine receptors and myasthenia. *Muscle Nerve,* **2000,** *23:*453–477.

Lotti, M. Low-level exposures to organophosphorus esters and peripheral nerve function. *Muscle Nerve,* **2002,** *25:*492–504.

Mackness, M., Durrington, P., and Mackness, B. Paraoxonase 1 activity, concentration and genotype in cardiovascular disease. *Curr. Opin. Lipidol.,* **2004,** *15:*399–404.

Markesbery, W.R. (ed.) *Neuropathology of Dementing Disorders.* Arnold, London, **1998.**

Marrs, T.C. Organophosphate poisoning. *Pharmacol. Ther.,* **1993,** *58:*51–66.

Massoulié, J. Molecular forms and anchoring of acetylcholinesterase. In, *Cholinesterases and Cholinesterase Inhibitors.* (Giacobini, E., ed.) Martin Dunitz, London, **2000,** pp. 81–103.

Mayeux, R., and Sano, M. Treatment of Alzheimer's disease. *N. Engl. J. Med.,* **1999,** *341:*1670–1679.

Ohno, K., Engle, A.G., Brengman, B.S., *et al.* The spectrum of mutations causing end plate acetylcholinesterase deficiency. *Ann. Neurol.,* **2000,** *47:*162–170.

Osserman, K.E., Foldes, F.F., and Genkins, G. Myasthenia gravis. In, *Neuromuscular Blocking and Stimulating Agents,* Vol. 11, *International Encyclopedia of Pharmacology and Therapeutics,* Sect. 14. (Cheymol, J., ed.) Pergamon Press, Oxford, **1972,** pp. 561–618.

Reiner, E., and Radic', Z. Mechanism of action of cholinesterase inhibitors. In, *Cholinesterases and Cholinesterase Inhibitors.* (Giacobini, E., ed.) Martin Dunitz, London, **2000,** pp. 103–120.

Rosenberry, T.L. Acetylcholinesterase. *Adv. Enzymol. Relat. Areas Mol. Biol.,* **1975,** *43:*103–218.

Silman, I., and Sussman, J.L. Structural studies on acetylcholinesterase. In, *Cholinesterases and Cholinesterase Inhibitors.* (Giacobini, E., ed.) Martin Dunitz, London, **2000,** pp. 9–26.

Storm, J.E., Rozman, K.K., and Doull, J. Occupational exposure limits for 30 organophosphate pesticides based on inhibition of red blood cell acetylcholinesterase. *Toxicology,* **2000,** *150:*1–29.

Taylor, P., Luo, Z.D., and Camp, S. The genes encoding the cholinesterases: structure, evolutionary relationships and regulation of their expression. In, *Cholinesterases and Cholinesterase Inhibitors.* (Giacobini, E., ed.) Martin Dunitz, London, **2000,** pp. 63–80.

Taylor, P., and Radic', Z. The cholinesterases: from genes to proteins. *Annu. Rev. Pharmacol. Toxicol.,* **1994,** *34:*281–320.

AGENTS ACTING AT THE NEUROMUSCULAR JUNCTION AND AUTONOMIC GANGLIA

Palmer Taylor

The nicotinic acetylcholine (ACh) receptor mediates neurotransmission postsynaptically at the neuromuscular junction and peripheral autonomic ganglia; in the CNS, it largely controls release of neurotransmitters from presynaptic sites. The receptor is called *nicotinic acetylcholine receptor* because it is stimulated by both the neurotransmitter ACh and the alkaloid *nicotine*. Distinct subtypes of nicotinic receptors exist at the neuromuscular junction and the ganglia, and several pharmacological agents that act at these receptors discriminate between them. Neuromuscular blocking agents are distinguished by whether they cause depolarization of the motor end plate and thus are classified either as *competitive* (*stabilizing*) agents, of which *curare* is the classical example, or as *depolarizing* agents, such as *succinylcholine*. The competitive and depolarizing agents are used widely to achieve muscle relaxation during anesthesia. Ganglionic agents act by stimulating or blocking nicotinic receptors on the postganglionic neuron.

THE NICOTINIC ACETYLCHOLINE RECEPTOR

The concept of the nicotinic ACh receptor, with which ACh combines to initiate the end-plate potential (EPP) in muscle or an excitatory postsynaptic potential (EPSP) in peripheral ganglia, was introduced in Chapter 6. Classical studies of the actions of curare and nicotine made this the prototypical pharmacological receptor over a century ago. By taking advantage of specialized structures that have evolved to mediate cholinergic neurotransmission and natural toxins that block motor

activity, peripheral and then central nicotinic receptors were isolated and characterized. These accomplishments represent landmarks in the development of molecular pharmacology.

The electrical organs from the aquatic species of *Electrophorus* and, especially, *Torpedo* provide rich sources of nicotinic receptor. The electrical organ is derived embryologically from myoid tissue; however, in contrast to skeletal muscle, up to 40% of the surface of the membrane is excitable and contains cholinergic receptors. In vertebrate skeletal muscle, motor end plates occupy 0.1% or less of the cell surface. The discovery of seemingly irreversible antagonism of neuromuscular transmission by α toxins from venoms of the krait, *Bungarus multicinctus*, or varieties of the cobra, *Naja naja,* offered suitable markers for identification of the receptor. The *a* toxins are peptides of about 7000 daltons. Radioisotope-labeled toxins were used by Changeux and colleagues in 1970 to assay the isolated cholinergic receptor *in vitro* (*see* Changeux and Edelstein, 1998). The *a* toxins have extremely high affinities and slow rates of dissociation from the receptor, yet the interaction is noncovalent. *In situ* and *in vitro,* their behavior resembles that expected for a high-affinity antagonist. Since cholinergic neurotransmission mediates motor activity in marine vertebrates and mammals, a large number of peptide, terpinoid, and alkaloid toxins that block the nicotinic receptors have evolved to enhance predation or protect plant and animal species from predation (Taylor *et al.*, 2000).

Purification of the receptor from *Torpedo* ultimately led to isolation of complementary DNAs (cDNAs) that encode each of the subunits. These cDNAs, in turn, permitted the cloning of genes encoding the multiple receptor subunits from mammalian neurons and muscle (Numa *et al.*, 1983). By simultaneously expressing the genes that encode the individual subunits in cellular systems in various permutations and by measuring binding and the electrophysiological events that result from activation by agonists, researchers have been able to correlate functional properties with details of primary structures of the receptor subtypes (Lindstrom, 2000; Karlin, 2002).

Nicotinic Receptor Structure. The nicotinic receptor of the electrical organ and vertebrate skeletal muscle is a pentamer composed of four distinct subunits (α, β, γ, and δ) in the stoichiometric ratio of 2:1:1:1, respectively. In mature, innervated muscle end plates, the γ subunit is replaced by ε, a closely related subunit. The individual subunits are about 40% identical in their amino acid sequences, arising from a common primordial gene.

The nicotinic receptor became the prototype for other pentameric ligand-gated ion channels, which include the receptors for the inhibitory amino acids (γ-aminobutyric acid and glycine) and certain serotonin (5-HT$_3$) receptors. Each of the subunits in the pentameric receptor has a molecular mass of 40,000 to 60,000 daltons. The amino-terminal 210 residues constitute virtually all the extracellular domain. This is followed by four transmembrane-spanning (TM) domains; the region between the third and fourth domains forms most of the cytoplasmic component (Figure 9–1).

Each of the subunits within the nicotinic ACh receptor has an extracellular and an intracellular exposure on the postsynaptic membrane. The five subunits are arranged around a pseudo–axis of symmetry to circumscribe an internally located channel (Changeux and Edelstein, 1998; Karlin, 2000). The receptor is an asymmetrical molecule (14 × 8 nm) of 250,000 daltons, with the bulk of the non-membrane-spanning domain on the extracellular surface. In junctional areas (*i.e.*, the motor end plate in skeletal muscle and the ventral surface of the electrical organ), the receptor is present at high densities (10,000/μm^2) in a regular packing order. This ordering of the receptors has allowed electron microscopic image reconstruction of its molecular structure (Figure 9–2).

An ACh-binding protein homologous to only the extracellular domain of the nicotinic receptor has been identified in fresh- and saltwater snails and characterized structurally and pharmacologically (Brejc *et al.*, 2001). This protein assembles as a homomeric pentamer and binds nicotinic receptor ligands with the expected selec-

tivity; its crystal structure reveals an atomic organization expected of the nicotinic receptor. Moreover, fusion of the ACh-binding protein and the transmembrane spans of the receptor yields a functional protein that exhibits the channel gating and changes in state expected of the receptor (Bouzat *et al.*, 2004). This binding protein serves as both a structural and functional surrogate of the receptor and has provided a detailed understanding of the determinants governing ligand specificity of the nicotinic receptor.

The agonist-binding sites are found at the subunit interfaces, but in muscle, only two of the five subunit interfaces, αγ and αδ, have evolved to bind ligands. The binding of agonists, reversible competitive antagonists, and the elapid α toxin is mutually exclusive and involves overlapping surfaces on the receptor. Both subunits forming the subunit interface contribute to ligand specificity.

Measurements of membrane conductances demonstrate that rates of ion translocation are sufficiently rapid (5 × 10^7 ions per second) to require ion translocation through an open channel rather than by a rotating carrier of ions. Moreover, agonist-mediated changes in ion permeability (typically an inward movement of primarily Na$^+$ and secondarily Ca^{2+}) occur through a cation channel intrinsic to the receptor structure. The second transmembrane-spanning region on each of the five subunits forms the internal perimeter of the channel. The agonist-binding site is intimately coupled with an ion channel; in the muscle receptor, simultaneous binding of two agonist molecules results in a rapid conformational change that opens the channel. Both the binding and gating response show positive cooperativity. Details on the kinetics of channel opening have evolved from electrophysiological patch-clamp techniques that distinguish the individual opening and closing events of a single receptor molecule (Sakmann, 1992).

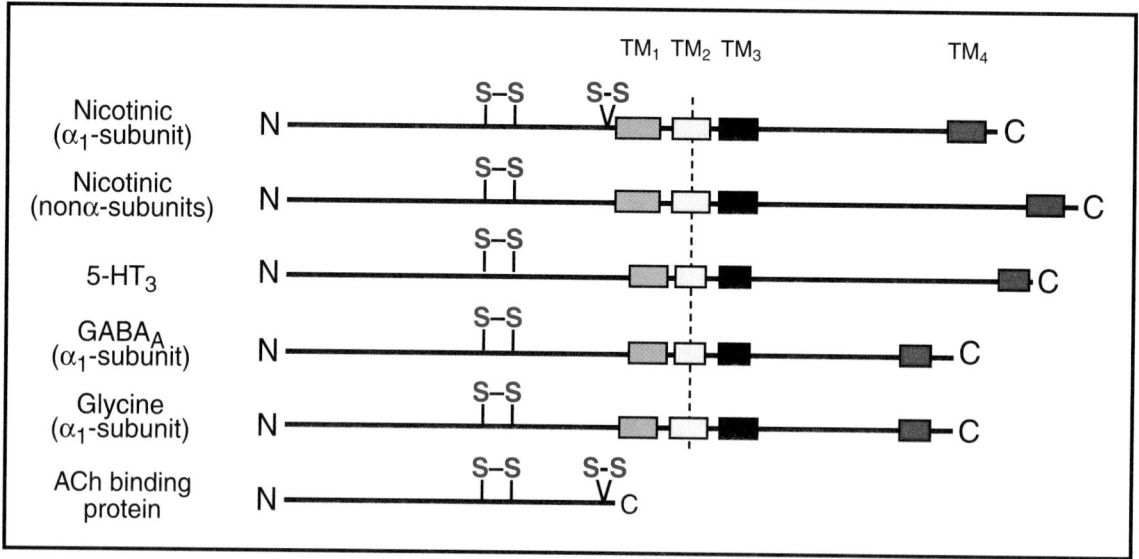

Figure 9–1. *Subunit organization of pentameric ligand-gated ion channels and the ACh binding protein.* For each receptor, the amino terminal region of about 210 amino acids is found in the extracellular surface. It is then followed by four hydrophobic regions that span the membrane (TM$_1$–TM$_4$), leaving the small carboxyl terminus on the extracellular surface. The TM$_2$ region is α-helical, and TM$_2$ regions from each subunit of the pentameric receptor line the internal pore of the receptor. Two disulfide loops at positions 128–142 and 192–193 are found in the α-subunit of the nicotinic receptor. The 128–142 motif is conserved in the family of receptors, whereas the vicinal cysteines at 192 and 193 distinguish α-subunits and the acetylcholine binding protein from β, γ, δ, and ε in the nicotinic receptor.

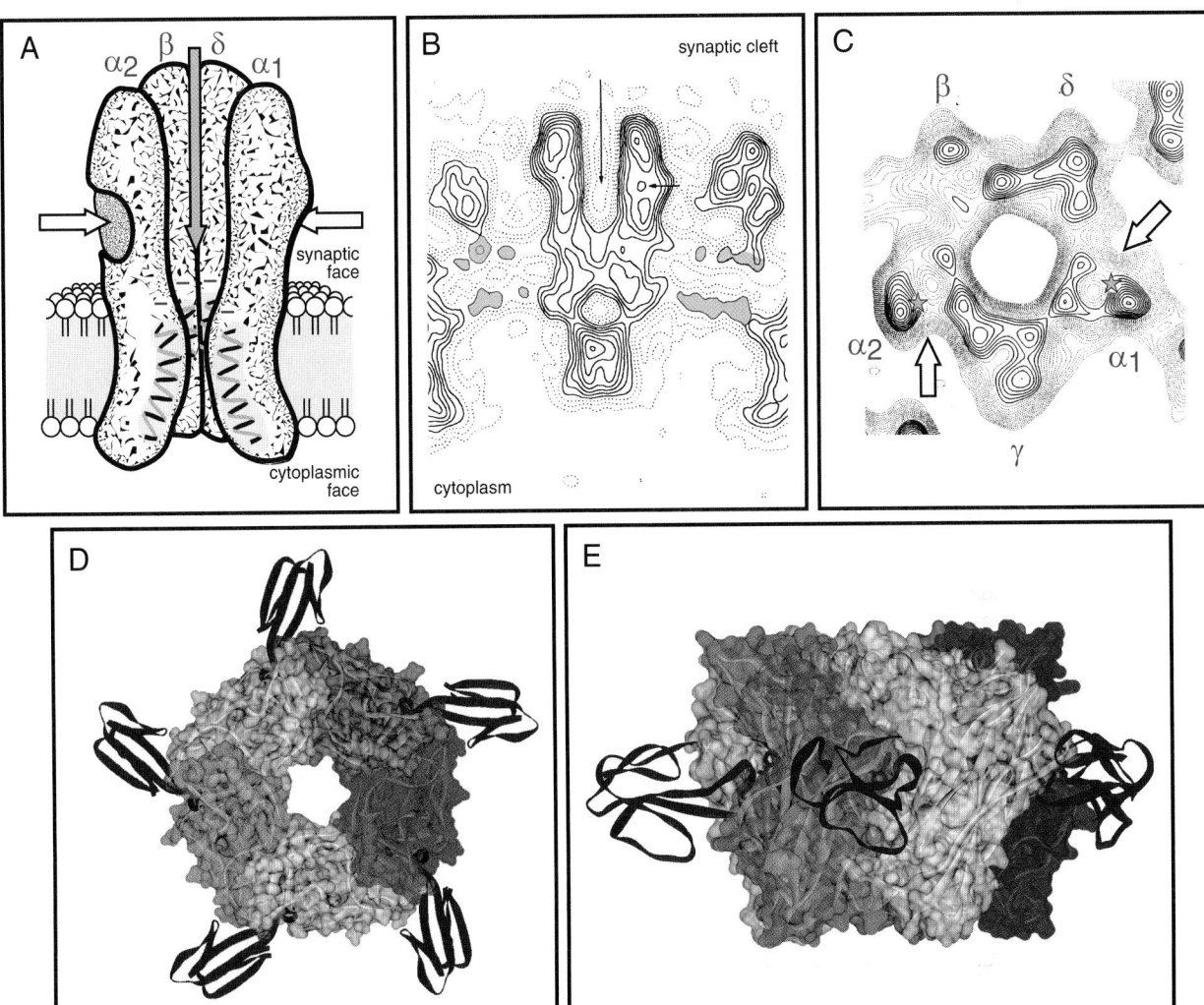

Figure 9–2. Molecular structure of the nicotinic acetylcholine receptor. A. Longitudinal view with the γ subunit removed. The remaining subunits, two copies of α, one of β, and one of δ, are shown to surround an internal channel with an outer vestibule and its constriction located deep in the membrane bilayer region. Spans of α-helices with slightly bowed structures form the perimeter of the channel and come from the TM_2 region of the linear sequence (*see* Figure 9–1). Acetylcholine (ACh)–binding sites, indicated by arrows, are found at the $\alpha\gamma$ and $\alpha\delta$ (not visible) interfaces. Panels ***B*** and ***C*** show data on which the structure is based. ***B.*** Longitudinal view of the electron density of receptor molecules packed in a tubular membrane. Arrows indicate the synaptic surface entry to the pore and agonist site. The additional density in the cytoplasmic region below the receptor arises from an anchoring protein attached to the receptor. ***C.*** Cross-sectional view of the image-reconstructed electron density taken 30 Å above the plane of the membrane. Pseudofivefold symmetry is evident. The arrows denote the presumed route of entry of the ligand (ACh) to the binding site (shown by the star). $\alpha1$ and $\alpha2$ in this panel are identical in sequence; the numeric designations show that there are two copies of the α-subunit in the pentamer (*see* Unwin, 1993 and 2005). The ACh binding protein (panels ***D*** and ***E***) is homologous to the extracellular domain of the nicotinic receptor (*see* Figure 9–1). The protein is a homopentamer that binds nicotinic receptor ligands with the expected selectivity and, when fused with the TM portions of the receptor, yields a functional ligand-gated channel. The subunit structure of the ACh binding protein is clear from the top view (panel ***D***) and side view (panel ***E***).

NEURONAL ACETYLCHOLINE RECEPTOR COMPOSITION AND STRUCTURE

Cloning by sequence homology identified the genes encoding the vertebrate nicotinic receptor. Neuronal nicotinic receptors found in ganglia and the CNS also exist as pentamers of one, two, or more subunits. Although only a single subunit of the α-type sequence (denoted as $\alpha 1$) is found in abundance in muscle, along with β, δ, and γ or ε, at least eight subtypes of α ($\alpha 2$ through $\alpha 9$) and three of the non-α type (designated as $\beta 2$ through $\beta 4$) are found in neuronal tissues. Although not all permutations of α and β subunits lead to functional receptors, the diversity in subunit composition is large and exceeds the capacity of ligands to distinguish subtypes on the basis of their selectivity. Studies of neuronal receptor subunit abundance and associations in brain and the periphery have enabled investigators to identify subunit combinations that confer function. For example, the $\alpha 3/\beta 4$ and $\alpha 3/\beta 2$ subtypes are prevalent in peripheral ganglia, whereas the $\alpha 4/\beta 2$ subtype is most prevalent in brain. The subtypes $\alpha 2$ through $\alpha 6$ and $\beta 2$ through $\beta 4$ associate as heteromeric pentamers composed of two or three distinct subtypes, whereas $\alpha 7$ through $\alpha 9$ often are seen as homomeric associations. Distinctive selectivities of the receptor subtypes for Na^+ and Ca^{2+} suggest that certain subtypes may possess functions other than rapid trans-synaptic signaling.

NEUROMUSCULAR BLOCKING AGENTS

History, Sources, and Chemistry. *Curare* is a generic term for various South American arrow poisons. The drug has a long and romantic history. It has been used for centuries by the Indians along the Amazon and Orinoco Rivers for immobilizing and paralyzing wild animals used for food; death results from paralysis of skeletal muscles. The preparation of curare was long shrouded in mystery and was entrusted only to tribal witch doctors. Soon after the discovery of the American continent, Sir Walter Raleigh and other early explorers and botanists became interested in curare, and late in the sixteenth century, samples of the native preparations were brought to Europe. Following the pioneering work of the scientist/explorer von Humboldt in 1805, the botanical sources of curare became the object of much field research. The curares from eastern Amazonia come from *Strychnos* species. These and other South American species of *Strychnos* contain chiefly quaternary neuromuscular-blocking alkaloids, whereas the Asiatic, African, and Australian species nearly all contain tertiary strychnine-like alkaloids.

Curare was the important tool that Claude Bernard used to demonstrate a locus of drug action at or near the nerve terminations of muscle. The modern clinical use of curare apparently dates from 1932, when West employed highly purified fractions in patients with tetanus and spastic disorders. Research on curare was accel-

ated greatly by the work of Gill, who, after prolonged and intimate study of the native methods of preparing curare, brought to the United States a sufficient amount of the authentic drug to permit chemical and pharmacological investigations. Griffith and Johnson reported the first trial of curare for promoting muscular relaxation in general anesthesia in 1942. Details of the fascinating history of curare, its nomenclature, and the chemical identification of the curare alkaloids are presented in previous editions of this book.

King established the essential structure of *tubocurarine* in 1935 (Figure 9–3). A synthetic derivative, *metocurine* (formerly called *dimethyl tubocurarine*), contains three additional methyl groups, one of which quaternizes the second nitrogen; the other two form methyl ethers at the phenolic hydroxyl groups. This compound possesses two to three times the potency of tubocurarine in human beings. The most potent curare alkaloids are the toxiferines, obtained from *Strychnos toxifera*. A semisynthetic derivative, *alcuronium chloride* (*N,N'*-diallylnortoxiferinium dichloride), was widely used clinically in Europe and elsewhere. The seeds of the trees and shrubs of the genus *Erythrina*, widely distributed in tropical and subtropical areas, contain erythroidines that possess curare-like activity.

Gallamine is one of a series of synthetic substitutes for curare described by Bovet and coworkers in 1949. Early structure–activity studies led to the development of the polymethylene *bis*-trimethylammonium series (referred to as the *methonium compounds*). The most potent agent at the neuromuscular junction was found when the chain contained 10 carbon atoms—*decamethonium* (C10) (Figure 9–3). The member of the series containing 6 carbon atoms in the chain— hexamethonium (C6)—was found to be essentially devoid of neuromuscular blocking activity but is particularly effective as a ganglionic blocking agent (*see* below).

Classification and Chemical Properties of Neuromuscular Blocking Agents

At present, only a single depolarizing agent, succinylcholine, is in general clinical use, whereas multiple competitive or nondepolarizing agents are available (Figure 9–3). Therapeutic selection should be based on achieving a pharmacokinetic profile consistent with the duration of the interventional procedure and minimizing cardiovascular compromise or other side effects (Table 9–1). Two general classifications are useful because they are helpful in distinguishing side effects and pharmacokinetic behavior. The first relates to the duration of drug action, and these agents are categorized as long-, intermediate-, and short-acting. The persistent blockade and difficulty in complete reversal after surgery with D-tubocurarine, metocurine, *pancuronium*, and *doxacurium* led to the development of *vecuronium* and *atracurium*, agents of intermediate duration. This was followed by the development of a short-acting agent, *mivacurium*. Often the long-acting agents are the more potent, requiring the use of low concentrations. The necessity of administering potent agents in low concentrations delays their onset. *Rocuronium* is an agent of intermediate duration but of rapid onset and lower potency. Its rapid onsets allows it

Competitive Agents

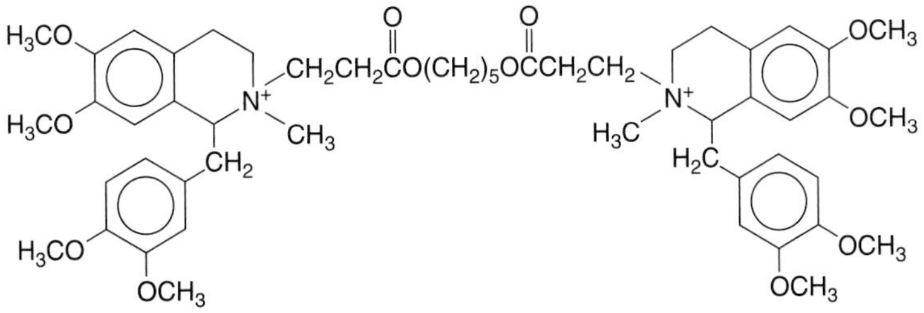

ATRACURIUM

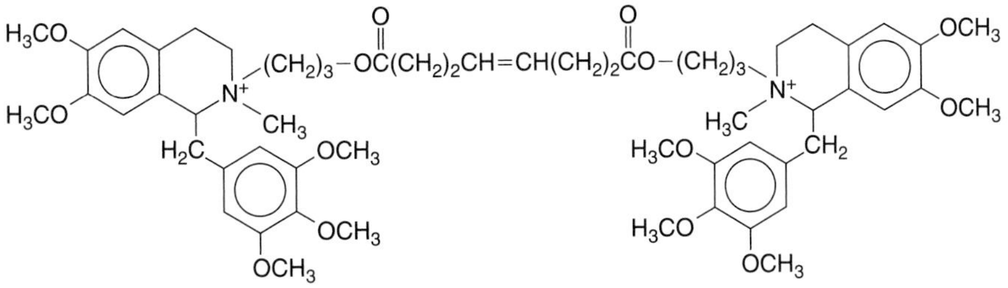

MIVACURIUM

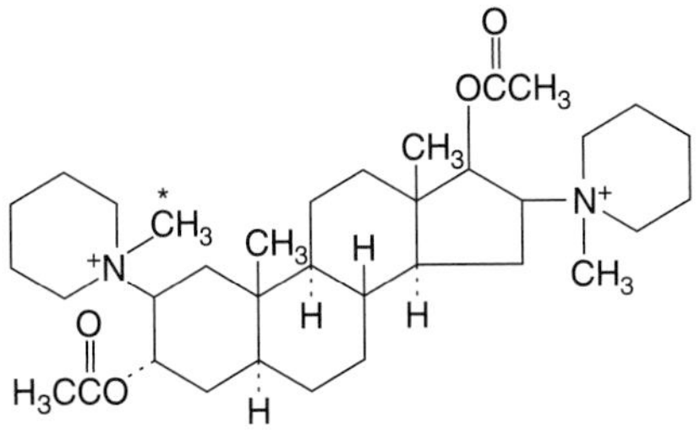

PANCURONIUM

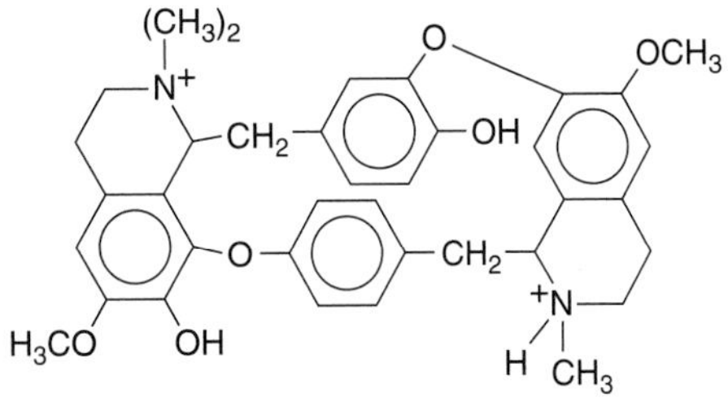

TUBOCURARINE

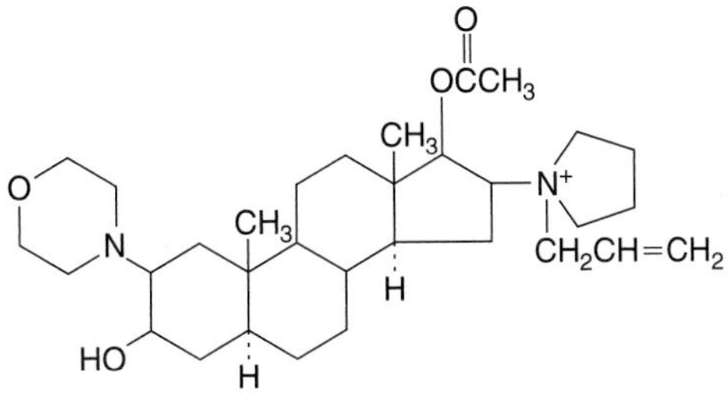

ROCURONIUM

Depolarizing Agents

$(CH_3)_3\overset{+}{N}{-}(CH_2)_{10}{-}\overset{+}{N}(CH_3)_3$

DECAMETHONIUM

$(H_3C)_3{-}\overset{+}{N}CH_2CH_2O\overset{O}{\overset{\|}{C}}CH_2CH_2\overset{O}{\overset{\|}{C}}OCH_2CH_2\overset{+}{N}{-}(CH_3)_3$

SUCCINYLCHOLINE

Figure 9–3. ***Structural formulas of major neuromuscular blocking agents.*** (*The methyl group is absent in vecuronium.)

Table 9–1
Classification of Neuromuscular Blocking Agents

AGENT	CHEMICAL CLASS	PHARMACOLOGICAL PROPERTIES	TIME OF ONSET, MIN	CLINICAL DURATION, MIN	MODE OF ELIMINATION
Succinylcholine (ANECTINE, others)	Dicholine ester	Ultrashort duration; depolarizing	1–1.5	5–8	Hydrolysis by plasma cholinesterases
D-Tubocurarine	Natural alkaloid (cyclic benzyl-isoquinoline)	Long duration; competitive	4–6	80–120	Renal elimination; liver clearance
Atracurium (TRACRIUM)	Benzylisoquinoline	Intermediate duration; competitive	2–4	30–60	Hofmann degradation; hydrolysis by plasma esterases; renal elimination
Doxacurium (NUROMAX)	Benzylisoquinoline	Long duration; competitive	4–6	90–120	Renal elimination
Mivacurium (MIVACRON)	Benzylisoquinoline	Short duration; competitive	2–4	12–18	Hydrolysis by plasma cholinesterases
Pancuronium (PAVULON)	Ammonio steroid	Long duration; competitive	4–6	120–180	Renal elimination
Pipecuronium (ARDUAN)	Ammonio steroid	Long duration; competitive	2–4	80–100	Renal elimination; liver metabolism and clearance
Rocuronium (ZEMURON)	Ammonio steroid	Intermediate duration; competitive	1–2	30–60	Liver metabolism
Vecuronium (NORCURON)	Ammonio steroid	Intermediate duration; competitive	2–4	60–90	Liver metabolism and clearance; renal elimination

to be used as an alternative to succinylcholine in rapid-induction anesthesia and in relaxing the laryngeal and jaw muscles to facilitate tracheal intubation (Bevan, 1994; Savarese *et al.*, 2000).

The second useful classification is derived from the chemical nature of the agents and includes the natural alkaloids or their congeners, the ammonio steroids, and the benzylisoquinolines (Table 9–1). The natural alkaloid D-tubocurarine and the semisynthetic alkaloid alcuronium seldom are used. Apart from a shorter duration of action, the newer agents exhibit greatly diminished frequency of side effects, chief of which are ganglionic blockade, block of vagal responses, and histamine release. The prototype ammonio steroid, pancuronium, induces virtually no histamine release; however, it blocks muscarinic receptors, and this antagonism is manifested primarily in vagal blockade and tachycardia. Tachycardia is eliminated in the newer ammonio steroids, vecuronium and rocuronium.

The benzylisoquinolines appear to be devoid of vagolytic and ganglionic blocking actions but show a slight propensity for histamine release. The unusual metabolism of the prototype compound atracurium and its newer congener mivacurium confers special indications for use of these compounds. For example, atracurium's disappearance from the body depends on hydrolysis of the ester moiety by plasma esterases and by a spontaneous or Hofmann degradation (cleavage of the *N*-alkyl portion in the benzylisoquinoline). Hence two routes for degradation are available, both of which remain functional in renal failure. Mivacurium is extremely sensitive to catalysis by cholinesterase or other plasma hydrolases, therein accounting for its short duration of action.

Structure–Activity Relationships. Several structural features distinguish competitive and depolarizing neuromuscular blocking agents. The competitive agents (*e.g.*, tubocurarine, the benzylisoquinolines, and the ammonio steroids) are relatively bulky, rigid molecules, whereas the depolarizing agents [*e.g., decamethonium* (no longer marketed in the United States) and succinylcholine] generally have more flexible structures that enable free bond rotations (Figure 9–3). While the distance between quaternary groups in the flexible depolarizing agents can vary up to the limit of the maximal bond distance (1.45 nm for decamethonium), the distance for the rigid competitive blockers is typically 1.0 ± 0.1 nm. L-Tubocurarine is considerably less potent than D-tubocurarine, perhaps because the D-isomer has all the hydrophilic groups localized uniquely to one surface.

Pharmacological Properties

Skeletal Muscle. A localized paralytic action of curare was first described by Claude Bernard in the 1850s. That the site of action of D-tubocurarine and other competitive blocking agents was the motor end plate (a thickened region of postjunctional membrane) subsequently was established by fluorescence and electron microscopy, microiontophoretic application of drugs, patch-clamp analysis of single channels, and intracellular recording. Competitive antagonists combine with the nicotinic ACh receptor at the end plate and thereby competitively block the binding of ACh. When the drug is applied directly to the end plate of a single isolated muscle fiber, the muscle cell becomes insensitive to motor-nerve impulses and to directly applied ACh; however, the end-plate region and the remainder of the muscle fiber membrane retain their normal sensitivity to K^+ depolarization, and the muscle fiber still responds to direct electrical stimulation.

To analyze further the action of antagonists at the neuromuscular junction, consider certain details of receptor activation by ACh. The steps involved in ACh release by the nerve action potential, the development of miniature end-plate potentials (MEPPs), their summation to form a postjunctional end-plate potential (EPP), the triggering of the muscle action potential, and contraction were described in Chapter 6. Biophysical studies with patch electrodes revealed that the fundamental event elicited by ACh or other agonists is an "all or none" opening and closing of the individual receptor channels, which gives rise to a squarewave pulse with an average open-channel conductance of 20 to 30 ps and a duration that is exponentially distributed around a time of about 1 ms. The *duration* of channel opening is far more dependent on the nature of the agonist than is the magnitude of the open-channel conductance (*see* Sakmann, 1992).

Increasing concentrations of the competitive antagonist tubocurarine diminish progressively the amplitude of the excitatory postjunctional EPP. The amplitude of this potential may fall to below 70% of its initial value before it is insufficient to initiate the propagated muscle action potential; this provides a safety factor in neuromuscular transmission. Analysis of the antagonism of tubocurarine on single-channel events shows that, as expected for a competitive antagonist, tubocurarine reduces the frequency of channel-opening events but does not affect the conductance or duration of opening for a single channel (Katz and Miledi, 1978). At higher concentrations, curare and other competitive antagonists block the channel directly in a fashion that is noncompetitive with agonists and dependent on membrane potential (Colquhoun *et al.*, 1979).

The decay time of the MEPP is of the same duration as the average lifetime of channel opening (1 to 2 ms). Since the MEPPs are a consequence of the spontaneous release of one or more quanta of ACh ($\sim 10^5$ molecules), individual molecules of ACh released into the synapse have only a transient opportunity to activate the receptor and do not rebind successively to receptors to activate multiple channels before being hydrolyzed by acetylcholinesterase. The concentration of unbound ACh in the synapse from nerve-released ACh diminishes more rapidly than does the decay of the EPP (or current).

If anticholinesterase (anti-ChE) drugs are present, the EPP is prolonged up to 25 to 30 ms, which is indicative of the rebinding of transmitter to neighboring receptors before diffusion from the synapse. It is therefore not surprising that anti-ChE agents and tubocurarine act in opposing directions, since increasing the duration of ACh retention in the synapse should favor occupation of the receptor by transmitter and displace tubocurarine.

Simultaneous binding by two agonist molecules at the respective $\alpha\gamma$ and $\alpha\delta$ subunit interfaces of the receptor is required for activation. Activation shows positive cooperativity and thus occurs over a narrow range of concentrations (Sine and Claudio, 1991; Changeux and Edelstein, 1998). Although two competitive antagonist or snake *a*-toxin molecules can bind to each receptor molecule at the agonist sites, the binding of one molecule of antagonist to each receptor is sufficient to render it nonfunctional (Taylor *et al.*, 1983).

The depolarizing agents, such as succinylcholine, act by a different mechanism. Their initial action is to depolarize the membrane by opening channels in the same manner as ACh. However, they persist for longer durations at the neuromuscular junction primarily because of their resistance to acetylcholinesterase. The depolarization is thus longer-lasting, resulting in a brief period of repetitive excitation that may elicit transient muscle fasciculations. The initial phase is followed by block of neuromuscular transmission and flaccid paralysis. This arises because released ACh binds to receptors on an already depolarized end plate. It is the *change* in EPP elicited by the transient increases in ACh that triggers action potentials. An end plate depolarized from −80 to −55 mV by a depolarizing blocking agent is resistant to further depolarization by ACh. In humans, a sequence of repetitive excitation (fasciculations) followed by block of transmission and neuromuscular paralysis is elicited by depolarizing agents; however, this sequence is influenced by such factors as the anesthetic agent used concurrently, the type of muscle, and the rate of drug administration. The characteristics of depolarization and competitive blockade are contrasted in Table 9–2.

In other animal species and occasionally in humans, decamethonium and succinylcholine produce a blockade that has unique features, some of which combine those of the depolarizing and the competitive agents; thus this type of action is termed a *dual mechanism*. In such cases, the depolarizing agents produce initially the characteristic fasciculations and potentiation of the maximal twitch, followed by the rapid onset of neuromuscular block; this block is potentiated by anti-ChE agents. However, following the onset of blockade, there is a poorly sustained response to tetanic stimulation

Table 9–2

Comparison of Competitive (D-Tubocurarine) and Depolarizing (Decamethonium) Blocking Agents

	D-TUBOCURARINE	DECAMETHONIUM
Effect of D-tubocurarine administered previously	Additive	Antagonistic
Effect of decamethonium administered previously	No effect, or antagonistic	Some tachyphylaxis; but may be additive
Effect of anticholinesterase agents on block	Reversal of block	No reversal
Effect on motor end plate	Elevated threshold to acetylcholine; no depolarization	Partial, persisting depolarization
Initial excitatory effect on striated muscle	None	Transient fasciculations
Character of muscle response to indirect tetanic stimulation during *partial* block	Poorly sustained contraction	Well-sustained contraction

SOURCE: Based on data in Paton and Zaimis, 1952; Zaimis, 1976.

of the motor nerve, intensification of the block by tubocurarine, and lack of potentiation by anti-ChE agents. The dual action of the depolarizing blocking agents also is seen in intracellular recordings of membrane potential; when agonist is applied continuously, the initial depolarization is followed by a gradual repolarization. The second phase, repolarization, in many respects resembles receptor desensitization.

Under clinical conditions, with increasing concentrations of succinylcholine and over time, the block may convert slowly from a depolarizing to a nondepolarizing type, termed *phase I* and *phase II blocks* (Durant and Katz, 1982). The pattern of neuromuscular blockade produced by depolarizing drugs in anesthetized patients appears to depend, in part, on the anesthetic; fluorinated hydrocarbons may be more apt to predispose the motor end plate to nondepolarization blockade after prolonged use of succinylcholine or decamethonium (*see* Fogdall and Miller, 1975). The characteristics of phase I and phase II blocks are shown in Table 9–3.

During the initial phase of application, depolarizing agents produce channel opening, which can be measured by the statistical analysis of fluctuation of muscle EPPs. The probability of channel opening associated with the binding of drug to the receptor is less with decamethonium than with ACh (Katz and Miledi, 1978) and also may result from decamethonium block of the receptor channel (Adams and Sakmann, 1978).

Although the observed fasciculations also may be a consequence of stimulation of the prejunctional nerve terminal by the depolarizing agent, giving rise to stimulation of the motor unit in an antidromic fashion, the primary site of action of both competitive and depolarizing blocking agents is the postjunctional membrane. Presynaptic actions of the competitive agents may become significant on repetitive high-frequency stimulation because prejunctional nicotinic receptors may be involved in the mobilization of ACh for release from the nerve terminal (Bowman *et al.*, 1990; Van der Kloot and Molgo, 1994).

Many drugs and toxins block neuromuscular transmission by other mechanisms, such as interference with the synthesis or release of ACh (Van der Kloot and Molgo, 1994; Ferguson and Blakely, 2004) (*see* Chapter 6), but most of these agents are not

Table 9–3

Clinical Responses and Monitoring of Phase I and Phase II Neuromuscular Blockade by Succinylcholine Infusion

RESPONSE	PHASE I	PHASE II
End-plate membrane potential	Depolarized to −55mV	Repolarization toward −80 mV
Onset	Immediate	Slow transition
Dose-dependence	Lower	Ususally higher or follows prolonged infusion
Recovery	Rapid	More prolonged
Train of four and tetanic stimulation	No fade	Fade*
Acetylcholinesterase inhibition	Augments	Reverses or antagonizes
Muscle response	Fasciculations → flaccid paralysis	Flaccid paralysis

*Post-tetanic potentiation follows fade.

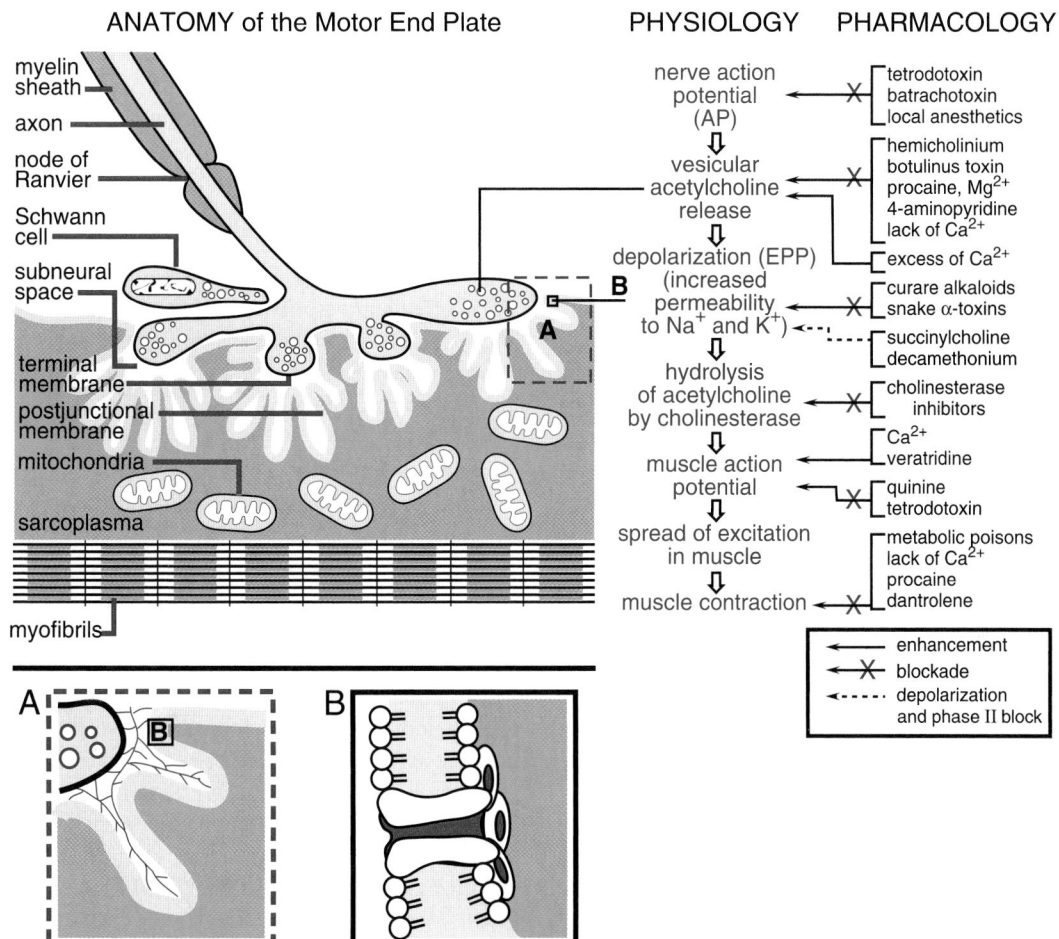

Figure 9–4. *Sites of action of agents at the neuromuscular junction and adjacent structures.* The anatomy of the motor end plate, shown at the left, and the sequence of events from liberation of acetylcholine (ACh) by the nerve action potential (AP) to contraction of the muscle fiber, indicated by the middle column, are described in Chapter 6. The modification of these processes by various agents is shown on the right; an arrow marked with an X indicates inhibition or block; an unmarked arrow indicates enhancement or activation. The insets are enlargements of the indicated structures. The highest magnification depicts the receptor in the bilayer of the postsynaptic membrane. A more detailed view of the receptor is shown in Figure 9–2.

employed clinically for this purpose. One exception is *botulinum toxin,* which has been administered locally into muscles of the orbit in the management of ocular blepharospasm and strabismus and has been used to control other muscle spasms and to facilitate facial muscle relaxation (*see* Chapters 6 and 63). This toxin also has been injected into the lower esophageal sphincter to treat achalasia (*see* Chapter 38). *Dantrolene* blocks release of Ca^{2+} from the sarcoplasmic reticulum and is used in the treatment of malignant hyperthermia (*see* below). The sites of action and interrelationship of several agents that serve as pharmacological tools are shown in Figure 9–4.

Sequence and Characteristics of Paralysis. When an appropriate dose of a competitive blocking agent is injected intravenously in human beings, motor weakness progresses to a total flaccid paralysis. Small, rapidly moving muscles

such as those of the eyes, jaw, and larynx relax before those of the limbs and trunk. Ultimately, the intercostal muscles and finally the diaphragm are paralyzed, and respiration then ceases. Recovery of muscles usually occurs in the reverse order to that of their paralysis, and thus the diaphragm ordinarily is the first muscle to regain function (Feldman and Fauvel, 1994; Savarese *et al.,* 2000).

After a single intravenous dose of 10 to 30 mg of a depolarizing agent such as succinylcholine, muscle fasciculations, particularly over the chest and abdomen, occur briefly; then relaxation occurs within 1 minute, becomes maximal within 2 minutes, and disappears as a rule within 5 minutes. Transient apnea usually occurs at the time of maximal effect.

Muscle relaxation of longer duration is achieved by continuous intravenous infusion. After infusion is discontinued, the effects of the drug usually disappear rapidly because of its rapid hydrolysis by plasma and hepatic butyrylcholinesterase. Muscle soreness may follow the administration of succinylcholine. Small prior doses of competitive blocking agents have been employed to minimize fasciculations and muscle pain caused by succinylcholine. However, this procedure is controversial because it increases the requirement for the depolarizing drug.

During prolonged depolarization, muscle cells may lose significant quantities of K^+ and gain Na^+, Cl^-, and Ca^{2+}. In patients in whom there has been extensive injury to soft tissues, the efflux of K^+ following continued administration of succinylcholine can be life-threatening. The life-threatening complications of succinylcholine-induced hyperkalemia are discussed below, but it is important to stress that there are many conditions for which succinylcholine administration is contraindicated or should be undertaken with great caution. The change in the nature of the blockade produced by succinylcholine (from phase I to phase II) presents an additional complication with long-term infusions.

Central Nervous System. Tubocurarine and other quaternary neuromuscular blocking agents are virtually devoid of central effects following ordinary clinical doses because of their inability to penetrate the blood–brain barrier. The most decisive experiment performed to resolve whether or not curare significantly affects central functions in the dose range used clinically was that of Smith and associates. Smith (an anesthesiologist) permitted himself to receive intravenously two and one-half times the amount of tubocurarine necessary for paralysis of all skeletal muscles. Adequate respiratory exchange was maintained by artificial respiration. At no time was there any evidence of lapse of consciousness, clouding of sensorium, analgesia, or disturbance of special senses. Despite adequate artificially controlled respiration, Smith experienced "shortness of breath" and the sensation of choking due to the accumulation of unswallowed saliva in the pharynx. The experience was decidedly unpleasant. It was concluded that tubocurarine given intravenously even in large doses has no significant central stimulant, depressant, or analgesic effects and that its sole action in anesthesia is the peripheral paralytic effect on skeletal muscle.

Autonomic Ganglia and Muscarinic Sites.
Neuromuscular blocking agents show variable potencies in producing ganglionic blockade. Just as at the motor end plate, ganglionic blockade by tubocurarine and other stabilizing drugs is reversed or antagonized by anti-ChE agents.

At the doses of tubocurarine once used clinically, partial blockade probably is produced both at autonomic ganglia and at the adrenal medulla, which results in a fall in blood pressure and tachycardia. Pancuronium shows less ganglionic blockade at common clinical doses. Atracurium, vecuronium, doxacurium, *pipecuronium* (no longer

marketed in the United States), mivacurium, and rocuronium are even more selective (Pollard, 1994; Savarese *et al.*, 2000). The maintenance of cardiovascular reflex responses usually is desired during anesthesia. Pancuronium has a vagolytic action, presumably from blockade of muscarinic receptors, that leads to tachycardia.

Of the depolarizing agents, succinylcholine at doses producing neuromuscular relaxation rarely causes effects attributable to ganglionic blockade. However, cardiovascular effects are sometimes observed, probably owing to the successive stimulation of vagal ganglia (manifested by bradycardia) and sympathetic ganglia (resulting in hypertension and tachycardia).

Histamine Release.
Tubocurarine produces typical histamine-like wheals when injected intracutaneously or intraarterially in humans, and some clinical responses to neuromuscular blocking agents (*e.g.*, bronchospasm, hypotension, excessive bronchial and salivary secretion) appear to be caused by the release of histamine. Succinylcholine, mivacurium, doxacurium, and atracurium also cause histamine release, but to a lesser extent unless administered rapidly. The ammonio steroids, pancuronium, vecuronium, pipecuronium, and rocuronium, have even less tendency to release histamine after intradermal or systemic injection (Basta, 1992; Watkins, 1994). Histamine release typically is a direct action of the muscle relaxant on the mast cell rather than IgE-mediated anaphylaxis (Watkins, 1994).

Actions of Neuromuscular Blocking Agents with Life-Threatening Implications.
The depolarizing agents can release K^+ rapidly from intracellular sites; this may be a factor in production of the prolonged apnea in patients who receive these drugs while in electrolyte imbalance. Succinylcholine-induced hyperkalemia is a life-threatening complication of that drug. For example, such alterations in the distribution of K^+ are of particular concern in patients with congestive heart failure who are receiving digoxin or diuretics. For the same reason, caution should be used or depolarizing blocking agents should be avoided in patients with extensive soft tissue trauma or burns. A higher dose of a competitive blocking agent often is indicated in these patients. In addition, succinylcholine administration is contraindicated or should be given with great caution in patients with nontraumatic rhabdomyolysis, ocular lacerations, spinal cord injuries with paraplegia or quadriplegia, or muscular dystrophies. Succinylcholine no longer is indicated for children 8 years of age and younger unless emergency intubation or securing an airway is necessary. Hyperkalemia, rhabdomyolysis, and cardiac arrest have been reported. A subclinical dystrophy frequently is associated

with these adverse responses (Savarese *et al.*, 2000). Neonates also may have an enhanced sensitivity to competitive neuromuscular blocking agents.

Synergisms and Antagonisms. Interactions between competitive and depolarizing neuromuscular blocking agents already have been considered (Table 9–2). From a clinical viewpoint, important pharmacological interactions of these drugs are with certain general anesthetics, certain antibiotics, Ca^{2+} channel blockers, and anti-ChE compounds.

Since the anti-ChE agents *neostigmine, pyridostigmine,* and *edrophonium* preserve endogenous ACh and also act directly on the neuromuscular junction, they can be used in the treatment of overdosage with competitive blocking agents. Similarly, on completion of the surgical procedure, many anesthesiologists employ neostigmine or edrophonium to reverse and decrease the duration of competitive neuromuscular blockade. Succinylcholine should never be administered after reversal of competitive blockade with neostigmine; in this circumstance, a prolonged and intense blockade often results. A muscarinic antagonist (*atropine* or *glycopyrrolate*) is used concomitantly to prevent stimulation of muscarinic receptors and thereby to avoid slowing of the heart rate. The anti-ChE agents, however, are synergistic with the depolarizing blocking agents, particularly in their initial phase of action. Since they will not reverse depolarizing neuromuscular blockade and, in fact, can enhance it, the distinction in the type of neuromuscular blocking agent must be clear.

Many inhalational anesthetics (*e.g., halothane, isoflurane,* and *enflurane*) exert a stabilizing effect on the postjunctional membrane and therefore act synergistically with the competitive blocking agents. Consequently, when such blocking drugs are used for muscle relaxation as adjuncts to these anesthetics, their doses should be reduced (*see* Fogdall and Miller, 1975).

Aminoglycoside antibiotics produce neuromuscular blockade by inhibiting ACh release from the preganglionic terminal (through competition with Ca^{2+}) and to a lesser extent by noncompetitively blocking the receptor. The blockade is antagonized by Ca^{2+} salts but only inconsistently by anti-ChE agents (*see* Chapter 45). The *tetracyclines* also can produce neuromuscular blockade, possibly by chelation of Ca^{2+}. Additional antibiotics that have neuromuscular blocking action, through both presynaptic and postsynaptic actions, include *polymyxin B, colistin, clindamycin,* and *lincomycin* (*see* Pollard, 1994). Ca^{2+} *channel blockers* enhance neuromuscular blockade produced by both competitive and depolarizing antagonists. It is not clear whether this is a result of a diminution of Ca^{2+}-dependent release of transmitter from the nerve ending or is a postsynaptic action. When neuromuscular blocking agents are administered to patients receiving these agents, dose adjustments should be considered; if recovery of spontaneous respiration is delayed, Ca^{2+} salts may facilitate recovery.

Miscellaneous drugs that may have significant interactions with either competitive or depolarizing neuromuscular blocking agents include *trimethaphan* (no longer marketed in the United States),

opioid analgesics, procaine, lidocaine, quinidine, phenelzine, phenytoin, propranolol, magnesium salts, corticosteroids, digitalis glycosides, chloroquine, catecholamines, and *diuretics* (*see* Pollard, 1994; Savarese *et al.*, 2000).

Toxicology. The important untoward responses of the neuromuscular blocking agents include prolonged apnea, cardiovascular collapse, those resulting from histamine release, and, rarely, anaphylaxis. Failure of respiration to become adequate in the postoperative period may not always be due directly to excessive muscle paralysis from the drug. An obstruction of the airway, decreased arterial P_{CO_2} secondary to hyperventilation during the operative procedure, or the neuromuscular depressant effect of excessive amounts of neostigmine used to reverse the action of the competitive blocking drugs also may be implicated. Directly related factors may include alterations in body temperature; electrolyte imbalance, particularly of K^+ (discussed earlier); low plasma butyrylcholinesterase levels, resulting in a reduction in the rate of destruction of succinylcholine; the presence of latent myasthenia gravis or of malignant disease such as small cell carcinoma of the lung (Eaton-Lambert myasthenic syndrome); reduced blood flow to skeletal muscles, causing delayed removal of the blocking drugs; and decreased elimination of the muscle relaxants secondary to reduced renal function. Great care should be taken when administering these agents to dehydrated or severely ill patients.

Malignant Hyperthermia. Malignant hyperthermia is a potentially life-threatening event triggered by the administration of certain anesthetics and neuromuscular blocking agents. The clinical features include contracture, rigidity, and heat production from skeletal muscle resulting in severe hyperthermia, accelerated muscle metabolism, metabolic acidosis, and tachycardia. Uncontrolled release of Ca^{2+} from the sarcoplasmic reticulum of skeletal muscle is the initiating event. Although the halogenated hydrocarbon anesthetics (*e.g.,* halothane, isoflurane, and *sevoflurane*) and succinylcholine alone have been reported to precipitate the response, most of the incidents arise from the combination of depolarizing blocking agent and anesthetic. Susceptibility to malignant hyperthermia, an autosomal dominant trait, is associated with certain congenital myopathies such as *central core disease*. In the majority of cases, however, no clinical signs are visible in the absence of anesthetic intervention.

Determination of susceptibility is made with an *in vitro* contracture test on a fresh biopsy of skeletal muscle, where contractures in the presence of halothane and caffeine are measured. In over 50% of the families, a linkage is found between the phenotype as measured by the contracture test and a mutation in the gene (*RyR-1*) encoding the skeletal muscle ryanodine receptor (RYR-1). Over 20 mutations in a region of the gene that encodes the cytoplasmic face of the receptor have been described. Other loci have been identified on the L-type Ca^{2+} channel (voltage-gated dihydropyridine receptor) and on other associated proteins or channel subunits. The large size of *RyR-1* and the genetic heterogeneity of the condition have precluded random genotypic determination for malignant hyperthermia (Hopkins, 2000; Jurkat-Rott *et al.*, 2000).

Treatment entails intravenous administration of *dantrolene* (DANTRIUM), which blocks Ca^{2+} release and the metabolic sequelae. Dantrolene inhibits Ca^{2+} release from the sarcoplasmic reticulum of skeletal muscle by limiting the capacity of Ca^{2+} and calmodulin to activate RYR-1 (Fruen *et al.*, 1997). RYR-1 and the L-type Ca^{2+} channel are juxtaposed to associate at a triadic junction formed between the T-tubule and the sarcoplasmic reticulum. The L-type channel with its T-tubular location serves as the voltage sensor receiving the depolarizing activation signal. The intimate coupling of the two proteins at the triad, along with a host of modulatory proteins in the two organelles and the surrounding cytoplasm, regulates the release of and response to Ca^{2+} (Lehmann-Horn and Jurkat-Rott, 1999).

Rapid cooling, inhalation of 100% oxygen, and control of acidosis should be considered adjunct therapy in malignant hyperthermia. Declining fatality rates for malignant hyperthermia relate to anesthesiologists' awareness of the condition and the efficacy of dantrolene.

Patients with central core disease, so named because of the presence of myofibrillar cores seen on biopsy of slow-twitch muscle fibers, show muscle weakness in infancy and delayed motor development. These individuals are highly susceptible to malignant hyperthermia with the combination of an anesthetic and a depolarizing neuromuscular blocker. Central core disease has five allelic variants of *RyR-1* in common with malignant hyperthermia. Patients with other muscle syndromes or dystonias also have an increased frequency of contracture and hyperthermia in the anesthesia setting. Succinylcholine in susceptible individuals also induces *masseter muscle rigidity,* which may complicate endotracheal tube insertion and airway management. This condition has been correlated with a mutation in the gene encoding the α subunit of the voltage-sensitive Na^{+} channel (Vita *et al.*, 1995). Masseter muscle rigidity can be an early sign of the onset of malignant hyperthermia if the anesthetic combination is continued (Hopkins, 2000).

Respiratory Paralysis. Treatment of respiratory paralysis arising from an adverse reaction or overdose of a neuromuscular blocking agent should be by positive-pressure artificial respiration with oxygen and maintenance of a patent airway until recovery of normal respiration is ensured. With the competitive blocking agents, this may be hastened by the administration of neostigmine methylsulfate (0.5 to 2 mg intravenously) or edrophonium (10 mg intravenously, repeated as required) (Watkins, 1994).

Interventional Strategies for Other Toxic Effects. Neostigmine effectively antagonizes only the skeletal muscular blocking action of the competitive blocking agents and may aggravate such side effects as hypotension or induce bronchospasm. In such circumstances, *sympathomimetic amines* may be given to support the blood pressure. Atropine or glycopyrrolate is administered to counteract muscarinic stimulation. *Antihistamines* are definitely beneficial to counteract the responses that follow the release of histamine, particularly when administered before the neuromuscular blocking agent.

Absorption, Fate, and Excretion. Quaternary ammonium neuromuscular blocking agents are very poorly and irregularly absorbed from the gastrointestinal tract. This fact was well known to the South American Indians, who ate with impunity the flesh of game killed with curare-poisoned arrows. Absorption is quite adequate from intramuscular sites. Rapid onset is achieved with intravenous administration. The more potent agents, of course, must be given in lower concentrations, and diffusional requirements slow their rate of onset.

When long-acting competitive blocking agents such as D-tubocurarine and pancuronium are administered, blockade may diminish after 30 minutes owing to redistribution of the drug, yet residual blockade and plasma levels of the drug persist. Subsequent doses show diminished redistribution. Long-acting agents may accumulate with multiple doses.

The ammonio steroids contain ester groups that are hydrolyzed in the liver. Typically, the metabolites have about one-half the activity of the parent compound and contribute to the total relaxation profile. Ammonio steroids of intermediate duration of action, such as vecuronium, and rocuronium (Table 9–1), are cleared more rapidly by the liver than is pancuronium. The more rapid decay of neuromuscular blockade with compounds of intermediate duration argues for sequential dosing of these agents rather than administering a single dose of a long-duration neuromuscular blocking agent (Savarese *et al.*, 2000).

Atracurium is converted to less active metabolites by plasma esterases and spontaneous degradation. Because of these alternative routes of metabolism, atracurium does not exhibit an increased half-life in patients with impaired renal function and therefore is the agent of choice in this setting

(Hunter, 1994). Mivacurium shows an even greater susceptibility to butyrylcholinesterase catalysis, and thus has the shortest duration among the nondepolarizing blockers.

The extremely brief duration of action of succinylcholine also is due largely to its rapid hydrolysis by the butyrylcholinesterase of liver and plasma. Among the occasional patients who exhibit prolonged apnea following the administration of succinylcholine or mivacurium, most have an atypical plasma cholinesterase or a deficiency of the enzyme owing to allelic variations (Pantuck, 1993; Primo-Parmo *et al.*, 1996), hepatic or renal disease, or a nutritional disturbance; however, in some, the enzymatic activity in plasma is normal (Whittaker, 1986).

Therapeutic Uses

The main clinical use of the neuromuscular blocking agents is as an adjuvant in surgical anesthesia to obtain relaxation of skeletal muscle, particularly of the abdominal wall, to facilitate operative manipulations. With muscle relaxation no longer dependent on the depth of general anesthesia, a much lighter level of anesthesia suffices. Thus, the risk of respiratory and cardiovascular depression is minimized, and postanesthetic recovery is shortened. These considerations notwithstanding, neuromuscular blocking agents cannot be used to substitute for inadequate depth of anesthesia. Otherwise, a risk of reflex responses to painful stimuli and conscious recall may occur.

Muscle relaxation is also of value in various orthopedic procedures, such as the correction of dislocations and the alignment of fractures. Neuromuscular blocking agents of short duration often are used to facilitate intubation with an endotracheal tube and have been used to facilitate laryngoscopy, bronchoscopy, and esophagoscopy in combination with a general anesthetic agent.

Neuromuscular blocking agents are administered parenterally, nearly always intravenously. As potentially hazardous drugs, they should be administered to patients only by anesthesiologists and other clinicians who have had extensive training in their use and in a setting where facilities for respiratory and cardiovascular resuscitation are immediately at hand. Detailed information on dosage and monitoring the extent of muscle relaxation can be found in anesthesiology textbooks (Pollard, 1994; Savarese *et al.*, 2000).

Measurement of Neuromuscular Blockade in Humans. Assessment of neuromuscular block usually is performed by stimulation of the ulnar nerve. Responses are monitored from compound action potentials or muscle tension developed in the adductor pollicis (thumb) muscle. Responses to repetitive or tetanic stimuli are most useful for evaluation of blockade of transmission because individual measurements of twitch tension must be related to control values obtained prior to the adminis-

tration of drugs. Thus, stimulus schedules such as the "train of four" and the "double burst" or responses to tetanic stimulation are preferred procedures (Waud and Waud, 1972; Drenck *et al.*, 1989). Rates of onset of blockade and recovery are more rapid in the airway musculature (jaw, larynx, and diaphragm) than in the thumb. Hence, tracheal intubation can be performed before onset of complete block at the adductor pollicis, whereas partial recovery of function of this muscle allows sufficient recovery of respiration for extubation (Savarese *et al.*, 2000). Differences in rates of onset of blockade, recovery from blockade, and intrinsic sensitivity between the stimulated muscle and those of the larynx, abdomen, and diaphragm should be considered.

Use to Prevent Trauma during Electroshock Therapy. Electroconvulsive therapy (ECT) of psychiatric disorders occasionally is complicated by trauma to the patient; the seizures induced may cause dislocations or fractures. Inasmuch as the muscular component of the convulsion is not essential for benefit from the procedure, neuromuscular blocking agents and *thiopental* are employed. The combination of the blocking drug, the anesthetic agent, and postictal depression usually results in respiratory depression or temporary apnea. An endotracheal tube and oxygen always should be available. An oropharyngeal airway should be inserted as soon as the jaw muscles relax (after the seizure) and provision made to prevent aspiration of mucus and saliva. Succinylcholine or mivacurium is used most often because of the brevity of relaxation. A cuff may be applied to one extremity to prevent the effects of the drug in that limb; evidence of an effective electroshock is provided by contraction of the group of protected muscles. These agents are also used in capital punishment by electrocution. Although a convulsive response is blocked, ethical concerns have been raised because all motor function is blocked.

Control of Muscle Spasms. Several agents, many of limited efficacy, have been used to treat spasticity involving the α-motor neuron with the objective of increasing functional capacity and relieving discomfort. Agents that act in the CNS at either higher centers or the spinal cord to block spasms are considered in Chapter 20. These include *baclofen*, the *benzodiazepines*, and *tizanidine*. Botulinum toxin and dantrolene act peripherally.

The anaerobic bacterium *Clostridium botulinum* produces a family of toxins targeted to presynaptic proteins and that block the release of ACh (*see* Chapter 6). *Botulinum toxin A* (BOTOX), by blocking ACh release, produces flaccid paralysis of skeletal muscle and diminished activity of parasympathetic and sympathetic cholinergic synapses. Inhibition lasts from several weeks to 3 to 4 months, and restoration of function requires nerve sprouting. Immunoresistance may develop with continued use (Davis and Barnes, 2000). Originally approved for the treatment of the ocular conditions of strabismus and blepharospasm and for hemifacial spasms, botulinum toxin has been used to treat spasms and dystonias such as adductor spasmodic dysphonia, oromandibular dystonia, cervical dystonia and spasms associated with the lower esophageal sphincter and anal fissures. Its dermatological uses include treatment of hyperhidrosis of the palms and axillae that is

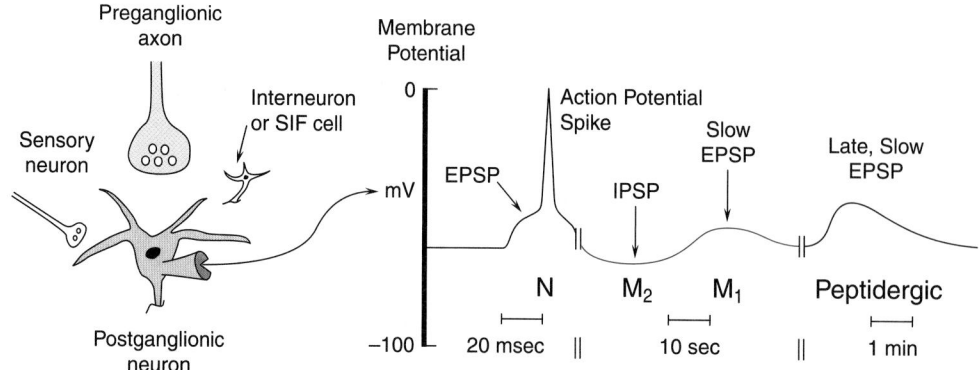

Figure 9–5. *Autonomic ganglion cells and the excitatory and inhibitory postsynaptic potentials (EPSP and IPSP) recorded from the postganglionic nerve cell body after stimulation of the preganglionic nerve fiber.* The initial EPSP, if of sufficient magnitude, triggers an action potential spike, which is followed by a slow IPSP, a slow EPSP, and a late, slow EPSP. The slow IPSP and slow EPSP are not seen in all ganglia. The subsequent electrical events are thought not to trigger spikes directly but rather to increase or decrease the probability of a subsequent EPSP reaching a threshold to trigger a spike. Other interneurons, such as catecholamine-containing, small, intensely fluorescent (SIF) cells, and axon terminals from sensory, afferent neurons also release transmitters and are thought to influence the slow potentials of the postganglionic neuron. A number of cholinergic, peptidergic, adrenergic, and amino acid receptors are found on the dendrites and soma of the postganglionic neuron and the interneurons. The preganglionic terminal releases acetylcholine and peptides; the interneurons store and release catecholamines, amino acids, and peptides; and the sensory afferent nerve terminals release peptides. The initial EPSP is mediated through nicotinic (N) receptors, the slow IPSP and EPSP through M_2 and M_1 muscarinic receptors, and the late, slow EPSP through several types of peptidergic receptors, as detailed in the text (Weight *et al.*, 1979; Jan and Jan, 1983; Elfvin *et al.*, 1993).

resistant to topical and iontophoretic remedies and removal of facial lines associated with excessive nerve stimulation and muscle activity. Treatment involves local intramuscular or intradermal injections (Boni *et al.*, 2000). Botox treatments also have become a popular cosmetic procedure for those seeking a wrinkle-free face. The effect is temporary.

In addition to its use in managing an acute attack of malignant hyperthermia (*see* above), dantrolene also has been explored in the treatment of spasticity and hyperreflexia. With its peripheral action, it causes a generalized weakness. Thus, its use should be reserved to nonambulatory patients with severe spasticity. Hepatotoxicity has been reported with continued use, requiring liver function tests (Kita and Goodkin, 2000).

GANGLIONIC NEUROTRANSMISSION

Neurotransmission in autonomic ganglia has long been recognized to be a far more complex process than that described by a single neurotransmitter–receptor system; intracellular recordings reveal at least four different changes in potential that can be elicited by stimulation of the preganglionic nerve (Weight *et al.*, 1979) (Figure 9–5). The primary event involves a rapid depolarization of postsynaptic sites by ACh. The receptors are nicotinic, and the path-

way is sensitive to classical blocking agents such as *hexamethonium* and trimethaphan. Activation of this primary pathway gives rise to an initial excitatory postsynaptic potential (EPSP). This rapid depolarization is due primarily to an inward Na^+ and perhaps Ca^{2+} current through a neuronal type of nicotinic-receptor channel. Multiple nicotinic-receptor subunits (*e.g.*, $\alpha3$, $\alpha5$, $\alpha7$, $\beta2$, and $\beta4$) have been identified in ganglia, with $\alpha3$ and $\beta2$ being most abundant.

An action potential is generated in the postganglionic neuron when the initial EPSP attains a critical amplitude. In mammalian sympathetic ganglia *in vivo*, it may be necessary for multiple synapses to be activated before transmission is effective. Discrete end plates with focal localization of receptors do not exist in ganglia; rather, the dendrites and nerve cell bodies contain the receptors.

Iontophoretic application of ACh to the ganglion results in a depolarization with a latency of less than 1 ms; this decays over a period of 10 to 50 ms (Ascher *et al.*, 1979). Measurements of single-channel conductances indicate that the characteristics of nicotinic-receptor channels of the ganglia and the neuromuscular junction are quite similar.

The secondary events that follow the initial depolarization are insensitive to hexamethonium or other nicotinic antagonists. They include the slow EPSP, the late slow EPSP, and an inhibitory postsynaptic potential (IPSP). ACh action on muscarinic receptors generates the slow EPSP, which is blocked by atropine or antagonists that are selective for M_1 muscarinic receptors (*see* Chapter 7). The slow EPSP has a longer latency and a duration of 30 to 60 seconds. In contrast, the late slow EPSP lasts for several minutes and is initiated by the action of peptides released from presynaptic nerve endings or interneurons in specific ganglia (Dun, 1983). The peptides and ACh may be released from the same nerve ending, but the enhanced stability of the peptide in the ganglion extends its sphere of influence to postsynaptic sites beyond those in immediate proximity to the nerve ending. The slow EPSPs result from decreased K^+ conductance (Weight *et al.*, 1979). The K^+ conductance has been called an *M current,* and it regulates the sensitivity of the cell to repetitive fast-depolarizing events (Adams *et al.*, 1982).

Like the slow EPSP, the IPSP is unaffected by the classical nicotinic-receptor blocking agents. Electrophysiological and neurochemical evidence suggests that catecholamines participate in the generation of the IPSP. *Dopamine* and *norepinephrine* cause hyperpolarization of ganglia, and both the IPSP and catecholamine-induced hyperpolarization are blocked by α adrenergic receptor antagonists. Since the IPSP is sensitive in most systems to blockade by both atropine and α adrenergic receptor antagonists, ACh that is released at the preganglionic terminal may act on catecholamine-containing interneurons to stimulate the release of dopamine or norepinephrine; the catecholamine, in turn, produces hyperpolarization (an IPSP) of ganglion cells. At least in some ganglia, a muscarinic link in the IPSP is mediated through M_2 muscarinic receptors (*see* Chapter 7). Histochemical studies indicate that dopamine- or norepinephrine-containing small, intensely fluorescent (SIF) cells and adrenergic nerve terminals are present in ganglia. Details of the functional linkage between the SIF cells and the electrogenic mechanism of the IPSP remain to be resolved (Prud'homme *et al.*, 1999; Slavikova *et al.*, 2003).

The relative importance of the secondary pathways and even the nature of the modulating transmitters appear to differ among individual ganglia and between parasympathetic and sympathetic ganglia. A variety of peptides, including gonadotropin-releasing hormone, substance P, angiotensin, calcitonin gene–related peptide, vasoactive intestinal polypeptide, neuropeptide Y, and enkephalins, have been identified in ganglia by immunofluorescence. They appear localized to particular cell bodies, nerve fibers, or SIF cells, are released on nerve stimulation, and are presumed to mediate the late slow EPSP (Elfvin *et al.*, 1993). Other neurotransmitter substances, such as 5-hydroxytryptamine and γ-aminobutyric acid, are known to modify ganglionic transmission. Precise details of their modulatory actions are not understood, but they appear to be most closely associated with the late slow EPSP and inhibition of the M current in various ganglia. It should be emphasized that the secondary synaptic events only modulate the initial EPSP. Conventional ganglionic blocking agents can inhibit ganglionic transmission completely; the same cannot be said for muscarinic antagonists or α adrenergic receptor agonists (Volle, 1980).

Drugs that stimulate cholinergic receptor sites on autonomic ganglia can be grouped into two categories. The first group consists of drugs with nicotinic specificity, including nicotine itself. Their excitatory effects on ganglia are rapid in onset, are blocked by ganglionic nicotinic-receptor antagonists, and mimic the initial EPSP. The second group is composed of agents such as *muscarine, McN-A-343*, and *methacholine*. Their excitatory effects on ganglia are delayed in onset, blocked by atropine-like drugs, and mimic the slow EPSP.

Ganglionic blocking agents acting on the nicotinic receptor may be classified into two groups. The first

group includes drugs that initially stimulate the ganglia by an ACh-like action and then block them because of a persistent depolarization (*e.g.,* nicotine); prolonged application of nicotine results in desensitization of the cholinergic receptor site and continued blockade (Volle, 1980). The blockade of autonomic ganglia produced by the second group of blocking drugs, of which hexamethonium and trimethaphan are prototypes, does not involve prior ganglionic stimulation or changes in ganglionic potentials. These agents impair transmission either by competing with ACh for ganglionic nicotinic-receptor sites or by blocking the channel. Trimethaphan acts by competition with ACh, analogous to the mechanism of action of curare at the neuromuscular junction. Hexamethonium appears to block the channel after it opens. This action shortens the duration of current flow because the open channel either becomes occluded or closes (Gurney and Rang, 1984). Regardless of the mechanism, the initial EPSP is blocked, and ganglionic transmission is inhibited.

GANGLIONIC STIMULATING DRUGS

History. Two natural alkaloids, nicotine and *lobeline*, exhibit peripheral actions by stimulating autonomic ganglia. Nicotine (Figure 9–6) was first isolated from leaves of tobacco, *Nicotiana tabacum,* by Posselt and Reiman in 1828, and Orfila initiated the first pharmacological studies of the alkaloid in 1843. Langley and Dickinson painted the superior cervical ganglion of rabbits with nicotine and demonstrated that its site of action was the ganglion rather than the preganglionic or postganglionic nerve fiber. Lobeline, from *Lobelia inflata,* has many of the same actions as nicotine but is less potent.

A number of synthetic compounds also have prominent actions at ganglionic receptor sites. The actions of the "onium" compounds, of which *tetramethylammonium* (TMA) is the simplest prototype, were explored in considerable detail in the last half of the nineteenth century and the early twentieth century.

Nicotine

Nicotine is of considerable medical significance because of its toxicity, presence in tobacco, and propensity for conferring a dependence on its users. The chronic effects of nicotine and the untoward effects of the chronic use of tobacco are considered in Chapter 23.

Nicotine is one of the few natural liquid alkaloids. It is a colorless, volatile base ($pK_a = 8.5$) that turns brown and acquires the odor of tobacco on exposure to air.

Pharmacological Actions. The complex and often unpredictable changes that occur in the body after administration of nicotine are due not only to its actions on a variety of neuroeffector and chemosensitive sites but also to the fact that the alkaloid can stimulate and desensitize receptors. The ultimate response of any one system represents the summation of stimulatory and inhibitory effects of nicotine. For example, the drug can increase heart rate by excitation of sympathetic

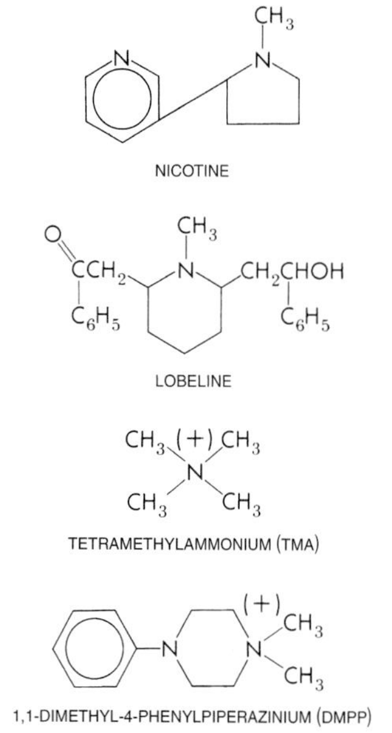

Figure 9–6. *Ganglionic stimulants.*

or paralysis of parasympathetic cardiac ganglia, and it can slow heart rate by paralysis of sympathetic or stimulation of parasympathetic cardiac ganglia. In addition, the effects of the drug on the chemoreceptors of the carotid and aortic bodies and on brain centers influence heart rate, as do also the cardiovascular compensatory reflexes resulting from changes in blood pressure caused by nicotine. Finally, nicotine elicits a discharge of epinephrine from the adrenal medulla, which accelerates heart rate and raises blood pressure.

Peripheral Nervous System. The major action of nicotine consists initially of transient stimulation and subsequently of a more persistent depression of all autonomic ganglia. Small doses of nicotine stimulate the ganglion cells directly and may facilitate impulse transmission. When larger doses of the drug are applied, the initial stimulation is followed very quickly by a blockade of transmission. Whereas stimulation of the ganglion cells coincides with their depolarization, depression of transmission by adequate doses of nicotine occurs both during the depolarization and after it has subsided. Nicotine also possesses a biphasic action on the adrenal medulla; small doses evoke the discharge of catecholamines, and larger doses prevent their release in response to splanchnic nerve stimulation.

The effects of nicotine on the neuromuscular junction are similar to those on ganglia. However, with the exception of avian and de-nervated mammalian muscle, the stimulant phase is obscured largely by the rapidly developing paralysis. In the latter stage, nicotine also produces neuromuscular blockade by receptor desensitization.

Nicotine, like ACh, is known to stimulate a number of sensory receptors. These include mechanoreceptors that respond to stretch or pressure of the skin, mesentery, tongue, lung, and stomach; chemoreceptors of the carotid body; thermal receptors of the skin and tongue; and pain receptors. Prior administration of hexamethonium prevents stimulation of the sensory receptors by nicotine but has little, if any, effect on the activation of sensory receptors by physiological stimuli.

Central Nervous System. Nicotine markedly stimulates the CNS. Low doses produce weak analgesia; with higher doses, tremors leading to convulsions at toxic doses are evident. The excitation of respiration is a prominent action of nicotine; although large doses act directly on the medulla oblongata, smaller doses augment respiration reflexly by excitation of the chemoreceptors of the carotid and aortic bodies. Stimulation of the CNS with large doses is followed by depression, and death results from failure of respiration owing to both central paralysis and peripheral blockade of muscles of respiration.

Nicotine induces vomiting by both central and peripheral actions. The central component of the vomiting response is due to stimulation of the emetic chemoreceptor trigger zone in the area postrema of the medulla oblongata. In addition, nicotine activates vagal and spinal afferent nerves that form the sensory input of the reflex pathways involved in the act of vomiting. Studies in isolated higher centers of the brain and spinal cord reveal that the primary sites of action of nicotine in the CNS are prejunctional, causing the release of other transmitters. Accordingly, the stimulatory and pleasure–reward actions of nicotine appear to result from release of excitatory amino acids, dopamine, and other biogenic amines from various CNS centers (MacDermott *et al.*, 1999). Release of excitatory amino acids may account for much of nicotine's stimulatory action.

Chronic exposure to nicotine in several systems causes a marked increase in the density or number of nicotinic receptors (Di Chiara *et al.*, 2000; Stitzel *et al.*, 2000). While the details of the mechanism are not yet understood, the response may be compensatory to the desensitization of receptor function by nicotine.

Cardiovascular System. When administered intravenously to dogs, nicotine characteristically produces an increase in heart rate and blood pressure. The latter is usually more sustained. In general, the cardiovascular responses to nicotine are due to stimulation of sympathetic ganglia and the adrenal medulla, together with the discharge of catecholamines from sympathetic nerve endings. Also contributing to the sympathomimetic response to nicotine is the activation of chemoreceptors of the aortic and carotid bodies, which reflexly results in vasoconstriction, tachycardia, and elevated blood pressure.

Gastrointestinal Tract. The combined activation of parasympathetic ganglia and cholinergic nerve endings by nicotine results in increased tone and motor activity of the bowel. Nausea, vomiting, and occasionally diarrhea are observed following systemic absorption of nicotine in an individual who has not been exposed to nicotine previously.

Exocrine Glands. Nicotine causes an initial stimulation of salivary and bronchial secretions that is followed by inhibition.

Absorption, Fate, and Excretion. Nicotine is readily absorbed from the respiratory tract, buccal membranes, and skin. Severe poisoning has resulted from percutaneous absorption. Being a relatively strong base, its absorption from the stomach is limited. Intestinal absorption is far more efficient. Nicotine in chewing tobacco, because it is absorbed more slowly than inhaled nicotine, has a longer duration of effect. The average cigarette contains 6 to 11 mg nicotine and delivers about 1 to 3 mg nicotine systemically to the smoker; bioavailability can increase as much as threefold with intensity of puffing and technique of the smoker (Henningfield, 1995; Benowitz, 1998). Nicotine is available in several dosage forms to help achieve abstinence from tobacco use. Efficacy results primarily from preventing a withdrawal or abstinence syndrome. Nicotine may be administered orally as a gum (*nicotine polacrilex*, NICORETTE), transdermal patch (NICODERM, HABITROL, others), a nasal spray (NICOTROL NS), and a vapor inhaler (NICOTROL INHALER). The first two are used most widely, and the objective is to obtain a sustained plasma nicotine concentration lower than venous blood concentrations after smoking. Arterial blood concentrations immediately following inhalation can be as much as tenfold higher than venous concentrations. The efficacy of the preceding dosage forms in producing abstinence from smoking is enhanced when linked to counseling and motivational therapy (Henningfield, 1995; Fant *et al.*, 1999; Benowitz, 1999) (*see* Chapter 23).

Approximately 80% to 90% of nicotine is altered in the body, mainly in the liver but also in the kidney and lung. Cotinine is the major metabolite, with nicotine-1'-*N*-oxide and 3-hydroxycotinine and conjugated metabolites found in lesser quantities (Benowitz, 1998). The profile of metabolites and the rate of metabolism appear to be similar in smokers and nonsmokers. The half-life of nicotine following inhalation or parenteral administration is about 2 hours. Nicotine and its metabolites are eliminated rapidly by the kidney. The rate of urinary excretion of nicotine diminishes when the urine is alkaline. Nicotine also is excreted in the milk of lactating women who smoke; the milk of heavy smokers may contain 0.5 mg/L.

Acute Nicotine Poisoning. Poisoning from nicotine may occur from accidental ingestion of nicotine-containing insecticide sprays or in children from ingestion of tobacco products. The acutely fatal dose of nicotine for an adult is probably about 60 mg of the base. Smoking tobacco usually contains 1% to 2% nicotine. Apparently, the gastric absorption of nicotine from tobacco taken by mouth is delayed because of slowed gastric emptying, so vomiting caused by the central effect of the initially absorbed fraction may remove much of the tobacco remaining in the GI tract.

The onset of symptoms of acute, severe nicotine poisoning is rapid; they include nausea, salivation, abdominal pain, vomiting, diarrhea, cold sweat, headache, dizziness, disturbed hearing and vision, mental confusion, and marked weakness. Faintness and prostration ensue; the blood pressure falls; breathing is difficult; the pulse is weak, rapid, and irregular; and collapse may be followed by terminal convulsions. Death may result within a few minutes from respiratory failure.

Therapy. Vomiting may be induced, or gastric lavage should be performed. Alkaline solutions should be avoided. A slurry of activated charcoal is then passed through the tube and left in the stomach. Respiratory assistance and treatment of shock may be necessary.

Other Ganglionic Stimulants

Stimulation of ganglia by tetramethylammonium (TMA) or *1,1-dimethyl-4-phenylpiperazinium iodide* (DMPP) differs from that produced by nicotine in that the initial stimulation is not followed by a dominant blocking action. DMPP is about three times more potent and slightly more ganglion-selective than nicotine. Although parasympathomimetic drugs stimulate ganglia, their effects usually are obscured by stimulation of other neuroeffector sites. McN-A-343 represents an exception to this; in certain tissues its primary action appears to occur at muscarinic M_1 receptors in ganglia.

GANGLIONIC BLOCKING DRUGS

The chemical diversity of compounds that block autonomic ganglia without causing prior stimulation is shown in Figure 9–7.

History and Structure–Activity Relationship. Although Marshall first described the "nicotine-paralyzing" action of *tetraethylammonium* (TEA) on ganglia in 1913, TEA was largely overlooked until Acheson and Moe published their definitive analyses of the effects of the ion on the cardiovascular system and autonomic ganglia. The *bis*-quaternary ammonium salts were developed and studied independently by Barlow and Ing and Paton and Zaimis. The prototypical ganglionic blocking drug in this series, hexamethonium (C6), has a bridge of six methylene groups between the two quaternary

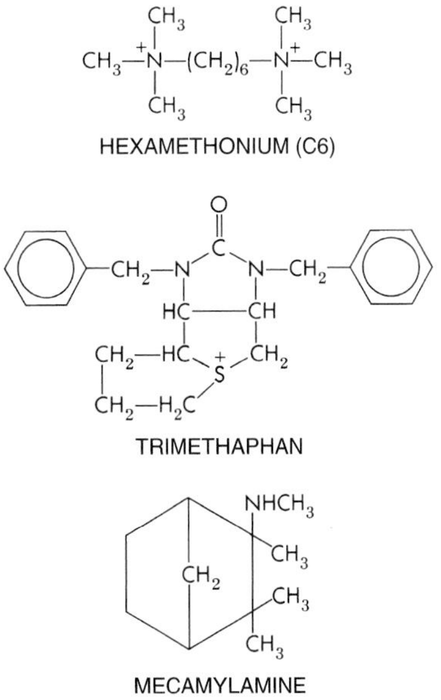

Figure 9–7. *Ganglionic blocking agents.*

nitrogen atoms (Figure 9–7). It has minimal neuromuscular and muscarinic blocking activities.

Triethylsulfoniums, like the quaternary and *bis*-quaternary ammonium ions, possess ganglionic blocking actions. This knowledge led to the development of sulfonium ganglionic blocking agents such as trimethaphan (Figure 9–7). *Mecamylamine,* a secondary amine, was introduced into therapy for hypertension in the mid-1950s.

Pharmacological Properties. Nearly all the physiological alterations observed after the administration of ganglionic blocking agents can be anticipated with reasonable accuracy by a careful inspection of Figure 6–1 and by knowing which division of the autonomic nervous system exercises dominant control of various organs (Table 9–4). For example, blockade of sympathetic ganglia interrupts adrenergic control of arterioles and results in vasodilation, improved peripheral blood flow in some vascular beds, and a fall in blood pressure.

Generalized ganglionic blockade also may result in atony of the bladder and gastrointestinal tract, cycloplegia, xerostomia, diminished perspiration, and by abolishing circulatory reflex pathways, postural hypotension. These changes represent the generally undesirable features of ganglionic blockade, which severely limit the therapeutic efficacy of ganglionic blocking agents.

Cardiovascular System. Existing sympathetic tone is critical in determining the degree to which blood pressure is lowered by ganglionic blockade; thus blood pressure may be decreased only minimally in recumbent normotensive subjects but may fall markedly in sitting or standing subjects. Postural hypotension was a major limitation in ambulatory patients receiving ganglionic blocking drugs.

Changes in heart rate following ganglionic blockade depend largely on existing vagal tone. In humans, mild tachycardia usually accompanies the hypotension, a sign that indicates fairly complete ganglionic blockade. However, a decrease may occur if the heart rate is high initially.

Cardiac output often is reduced by ganglionic blocking drugs in patients with normal cardiac function as a consequence of diminished venous return resulting from venous dilation and peripheral

Table 9–4
Usual Predominance of Sympathetic or Parasympathetic Tone at Various Effector Sites, and Consequences of Autonomic Ganglionic Blockade

SITE	PREDOMINANT TONE	EFFECT OF GANGLIONIC BLOCKADE
Arterioles	Sympathetic (adrenergic)	Vasodilation; increased peripheral blood flow; hypotension
Veins	Sympathetic (adrenergic)	Dilation: peripheral pooling of blood; decreased venous return; decreased cardiac output
Heart	Parasympathetic (cholinergic)	Tachycardia
Iris	Parasympathetic (cholinergic)	Mydriasis
Ciliary muscle	Parasympathetic (cholinergic)	Cycloplegia—focus to far vision
Gastrointestinal tract	Parasympathetic (cholinergic)	Reduced tone and motility; constipation; decreased gastric and pancreatic secretions
Urinary bladder	Parasympathetic (cholinergic)	Urinary retention
Salivary glands	Parasympathetic (cholinergic)	Xerostomia
Sweat glands	Sympathetic (cholinergic)	Anhidrosis
Genital tract	Sympathetic and parasympathetic	Decreased stimulation

pooling of blood. In patients with cardiac failure, ganglionic blockade frequently results in increased cardiac output owing to a reduction in peripheral resistance. In hypertensive subjects, cardiac output, stroke volume, and left ventricular work are diminished.

Although total systemic vascular resistance is decreased in patients who receive ganglionic blocking agents, changes in blood flow and vascular resistance of individual vascular beds are variable. Reduction of cerebral blood flow is small unless mean systemic blood pressure falls below 50 to 60 mmHg. Skeletal muscle blood flow is unaltered, but splanchnic and renal blood flow decrease following the administration of a ganglionic blocking agent.

Absorption, Fate, and Excretion. The absorption of quaternary ammonium and sulfonium compounds from the enteric tract is incomplete and unpredictable. This is due both to the limited ability of these ionized substances to penetrate cell membranes and to the depression of propulsive movements of the small intestine and gastric emptying. Although the absorption of mecamylamine is less erratic, a danger exists of reduced bowel activity leading to frank paralytic ileus.

After absorption, the quaternary ammonium- and sulfonium-blocking agents are confined primarily to the extracellular space and are excreted mostly unchanged by the kidney. Mecamylamine concentrates in the liver and kidney and is excreted slowly in an unchanged form.

Untoward Responses and Severe Reactions. Among the milder untoward responses observed are visual disturbances, dry mouth, conjunctival suffusion, urinary hesitancy, decreased potency, subjective chilliness, moderate constipation, occasional diarrhea, abdominal discomfort, anorexia, heartburn, nausea, eructation, and bitter taste and the signs and symptoms of syncope caused by postural hypotension. More severe reactions include marked hypotension, constipation, syncope, paralytic ileus, urinary retention, and cycloplegia.

Therapeutic Uses. Of the ganglionic blocking agents that have appeared on the therapeutic scene, only mecamylamine (INVER-

SINE) is currently available in the United States. Ganglionic blocking agents have been supplanted by superior agents for the treatment of chronic hypertension (*see* Chapter 32). Alternative agents also are available for management of acute hypertensive crises.

The therapeutic use of the ganglionic blocking agents in the production of controlled hypotension [*e.g.*, reduction in blood pressure during surgery to minimize hemorrhage in the operative field, to reduce blood loss in various orthopedic procedures, and to facilitate surgery on blood vessels (Fukusaki *et al.*, 1999)] has been supplanted largely by *nitroprusside* or depressor sedatives.

BIBLIOGRAPHY

Adams, P.R., and Sakmann, B. Decamethonium both opens and blocks endplate channels. *Proc. Natl. Acad. Sci. U.S.A.*, **1978,** *75:*2994–2998.

Adams, P.R., Brown, D.A., and Constanti, A. Pharmacological inhibition of the M-current. *J. Physiol.*, **1982,** *332:*223–262.

Ascher, P., Large, W.A., and Rang, H.P. Studies on the mechanism of action of acetylcholine antagonists on rat parasympathetic ganglion cells. *J. Physiol.*, **1979,** *295:*139–170.

Bouzat, C., Gumilar, F., Spitzmaul, G., *et al.* Coupling of agonist binding to channel gating in an ACh-binding protein linked to an ion channel. *Nature*, **2004,** *430:*896–900.

Brejc, K., van Dijk, W.J., Klaassen, R.V., *et al.* Crystal structure of an ACh-binding protein reveals the ligand-binding domain of nicotinc receptors. *Nature*, **2001,** *411:*269–276.

Colquhoun, D., Dreyer, F., and Sheridan, R.E. The actions of tubocurarine at the frog neuromuscular junction. *J. Physiol.*, **1979,** *293:*247–284.

Drenck, N.E., Ueda, N., Olsen, N.V., *et al.* Manual evaluation of residual curarization using double-burst stimulation: A comparison with train-of-four. *Anesthesiology,* **1989,** *70:*578–581.

Fogdall, R.P., and Miller, R.D. Neuromuscular effects of enflurane, alone and combined with D-tubocurarine, pancuronium, and succinylcholine, in man. *Anesthesiology,* **1975,** *42*:173–178.

Fruen, B.R., Mickelson, J.R., and Louis, C.F. Dantrolene inhibition of sarcoplasmic reticulum Ca^{2+} release by direct and specific action at skeletal muscle ryanodine receptors. *J. Biol. Chem.,* **1997,** *272*:26965–26971.

Fukusaki, M., Miyako, M., Hara, T., *et al.* Effects of controlled hypotension with sevoflurane anesthesia on hepatic function of surgical patients. *Eur. J. Anaesthesiol.,* **1999,** *16*:111–116.

Gurney, A.M., and Rang, H.P. The channel-blocking action of methonium compounds on rat submandibular ganglion cells. *Br. J. Pharmacol.,* **1984,** *82*:623–642.

Jan, Y.N., and Jan, L.Y. A LHRH-like peptidergic neurotransmitter capable of action at a distance in autonomic ganglia. *Trends Neurosci.,* **1983,** *6*:320–325.

Katz, B., and Miledi, R. A re-examination of curare action at the motor end plate. *Proc. R. Soc. Lond. [Biol.],* **1978,** *203*:119–133.

Pantuck, E.J. Plasma cholinesterase: gene and variations. *Anesth. Analg.,* **1993,** *77*:380–386.

Primo-Parmo, S.L., Bartels, C.F., Wiersema, B., *et al.* Characterization of 12 silent alleles of the human butyrylcholinesterase (*BCHE*) gene. *Am. J. Hum. Genet.,* **1996,** *58*:52–64.

Prud'homme, M., Houdeau, E., Serghini, R., Tillet, Y., Schemann, M., and Rousseau, J. Small intensely fluorescent cells of the rat paracervical ganglion. *Brain Res.,* **1999,** *821*:141–149.

Sine, S.M., and Claudio, T. γ- and δ-subunits regulate the affinity and cooperativity of ligand binding to the acetylcholine receptor. *J. Biol. Chem.,* **1991,** *266*:19369–19377.

Slavikova, J., Kuncova, J., Reischig, J., and Dvorakova, M. Catecholaminergic neurons in the rat intrinsic cardiac nervous system. *Neurochem. Res.,* **2003,** *28*:593–598.

Unwin, N. Nicotinic acetylcholine receptor at 9 Å resolution. *J. Mol. Biol.,* **1993,** *229*:1101–1124.

Unwin, N. Refined structure of the nicotinic acetylcholine receptor at 4Å resolution. *J. Mol. Biol.,* **2005,** *346*:967–989.

Vita, G.M., Olckers, A., Jedlicka, A.E., *et al.* Masseter muscle rigidity associated with glycine 1306-to-alanine mutation in the adult muscle sodium channel α-subunit gene. *Anesthesiology,* **1995,** *82*:1097–1103.

Waud, B.E., and Waud, D.R. The relation between the response to "train-of-four" stimulation and receptor occlusion during competitive neuromuscular block. *Anesthesiology,* **1972,** *37*:413–416.

MONOGRAPHS AND REVIEWS

Basta, S.J. Modulation of histamine release by neuromolecular blocking drugs. *Curr. Opin. Anaesthesiol.,* **1992,** *5*:512–566.

Benowitz, N.L. In, *Nicotine Safety and Toxicity.* (Benowitz, N.L., ed.) Oxford University Press, New York, **1998,** pp. 3–28.

Benowitz, N.L. Nicotine addiction. *Primary Care,* **1999,** *26*:611–653.

Bevan, D.R. Newer neuromuscular blocking agents. *Pharmacol. Toxicol.,* **1994,** *74*:3–9.

Boni, R., Kryden, O.P., and Burg, G. Revival of the use of botulinum toxin: Application in dermatology. *Dermatology,* **2000,** *200*:287–291.

Bowman, W.C., Prior, C., and Marshall, I.G. Presynaptic receptors in the neuromuscular junction. *Ann. N.Y. Acad. Sci.,* **1990,** *604*:69–81.

Changeux, J.P., and Edelstein, S.J. Allosteric receptors after 30 years. *Neuron,* **1998,** *21*:959–980.

Davis, E., and Barnes, M.P. Botulinum toxin and spasticity. *J. Neurol. Neurosurg. Psychiatry,* **2000,** *68*:141–147.

Di Chiara, G. Behavioral pharmacology and neurobiology of nicotine reward and dependence. In, *Neuronal Nicotinic Receptors.* (Clementi, F., Fornasari, D., and Gotti, C., eds.) Springer-Verlag, Berlin, **2000,** pp. 603–750.

Durant, N.N., and Katz, R.L. Suxamethonium. *Br. J. Anaesth.,* **1982,** *54*:195–208.

Elfvin, L.G., Lindh, B., and Hokfelt, T. The chemical neuroanatomy of sympathetic ganglia. *Annu. Rev. Neurosci.,* **1993,** *16*:471–507.

Engel, A., Ohno, K., and Sine, S. Sleuthing molecular targets for neurological diseases at the neuromuscular junction. *Nat. Rev. Neurosci.,* **2003,** *4*:339–352.

Fant, R.V., Owen, L.L., and Henningfield, J.E. Nicotine replacement therapy. *Primary Care,* **1999,** *26*:633–652.

Feldman, S.A., and Fauvel, N. Onset of neuromuscular block. In, *Applied Neuromuscular Pharmacology.* (Pollard, B.J., ed.) Oxford University Press, Oxford, England, **1994,** pp. 69–84.

Ferguson, S., and Blakely, R. The choline transporter resurfaces: New roles for synaptic vesicles? *Mol. Interv.,* **2004,** *4*:22–37.

Henningfield, J.E. Nicotine medications for smoking cessation. *New Engl. J. Med.,* **1995,** *333*:1196–1203.

Hopkins, P.M. Malignant hyperthermia: Advances in clinical management and diagnosis. *Br. J. Anaesth.,* **2000,** *85*:118–128.

Hunter, J.M. Muscle relaxants in renal disease. *Acta Anaesthesiol. Scand. Suppl.,* **1994,** *102*:2–5.

Jurkat-Rott, K., McCarthy, T., and Lehmann-Horn, F. Genetics and pathogenesis of malignant hyperthermia. *Muscle Nerve,* **2000,** *23*:4–17.

Karlin, A. Emerging structures of nicotinic acetylcholine receptors. *Nature Rev. Neurosci.,* **2002,** *3*:102–114.

Kita, M., and Goodkin, D.E. Drugs used to treat spasticity. *Drugs,* **2000,** *59*:487–495.

Lehmann-Horn, F., and Jurkat-Rott, K. Voltage-gated ion channels and hereditary disease. *Physiol. Rev.,* **1999,** *79*:1317–1372.

Lindstrom, J.M. The structures of neuronal nicotinic receptors. In, *Neuronal Nicotinic Receptors.* (Clementi, F., Fornasari, D., and Gotti, C., eds.) Springer-Verlag, Berlin, **2000,** pp. 101–162.

MacDermott, A.B., Role, L.W., and Siegelbaum, S.A. Presynaptic ionotropic receptors and the control of transmitter release. *Annu. Rev. Neurosci.,* **1999,** *22*:443–485.

Numa, S., Noda, M., Takahashi, H., *et al.* Molecular structure of the nicotinic acetylcholine receptor. *Cold Spring Harbor Symp. Quant. Biol.,* **1983,** *48*:57–69.

Pollard, B.J. Interactions involving relaxants. In, *Applied Neuromuscular Pharmacology.* (Pollard, B.J., ed.) Oxford University Press, Oxford, England, **1994,** pp. 202–248.

Sakmann, B. Elementary steps in synaptic transmission revealed by currents through single ion channels. *Science,* **1992,** *256*:503–512.

Savarese, J.J., Caldwell, J.E., Lein, C.A., and Miller, R.D. Pharmacology of muscle relaxants and their antagonists. In, *Anesthesia,* 5th ed. (Miller, R.D., ed.) Churchill-Livingstone, Philadelphia, **2000,** pp. 412–490.

Stitzel, J.A., Leonard, S.S., and Collins, A.C. Genetic regulation of nicotine-related behaviors and brain nicotinic receptors. In, *Neuronal Nicotinic Receptors.* (Clementi, F., Fornasari, D., and Gotti, C., eds.) Springer-Verlag, Berlin, **2000,** pp. 563–586.

Taylor, P., Brown, R.D., and Johnson, D.A. The linkage between ligand occupation and response of the nicotinic acetylcholine receptor. In, *Current Topics in Membranes and Transport,* vol. 18. (Kleinzeller, A., and Martin, B.R., eds.) Academic Press, New York, **1983,** pp. 407–444.

Taylor, P., Osaka, H., Molles, B., Keller, S.H., and Malany, S. Contributions of studies of the nicotinic receptor from muscle to defining structural and functional properties of ligand-gated ion channels. In, *Neuronal Nicotinic Receptors*. (Clementi, F., Fornasari, D., and Gotti, C., eds.) Springer-Verlag, Berlin, **2000,** pp. 79–100.

Van der Kloot, W., and Molgo, J. Quantal acetylcholine release at the vertebrate neuromuscular junction. *Physiol. Rev.,* **1994,** *74*:899–991.

Volle, R.L. Nicotinic ganglion-stimulating agents. In, *Pharmacology of Ganglionic Transmission*. (Kharkevich, D.A., ed.) Springer-Verlag, Berlin, **1980,** pp. 281–312.

Watkins, J. Adverse reaction to neuromuscular blockers: Frequency, investigation, and epidemiology. *Acta Anaesthesiol. Scand. Suppl.,* **1994,** *102*:6–10.

Whittaker, M. Cholinesterase. In, *Monographs in Human Genetics,* vol. 11. (Beckman, L., ed.) S. Karger, Basel, **1986,** p. 231.

ADRENERGIC AGONISTS AND ANTAGONISTS

Thomas C. Westfall and David P. Westfall

I. CATECHOLAMINES AND SYMPATHOMIMETIC DRUGS

Most of the actions of catecholamines and sympathomimetic agents can be classified into seven broad types: (1) a peripheral excitatory action on certain types of smooth muscle, such as those in blood vessels supplying skin, kidney, and mucous membranes, and on gland cells, such as those in salivary and sweat glands; (2) a peripheral inhibitory action on certain other types of smooth muscle, such as those in the wall of the gut, in the bronchial tree, and in blood vessels supplying skeletal muscle; (3) a cardiac excitatory action that increases heart rate and force of contraction; (4) metabolic actions, such as an increase in the rate of glycogenolysis in liver and muscle and liberation of free fatty acids from adipose tissue; (5) endocrine actions, such as modulation (increasing or decreasing) of the secretion of insulin, renin, and pituitary hormones; (6) actions in the central nervous system (CNS), such as respiratory stimulation, an increase in wakefulness and psychomotor activity, and a reduction in appetite; and (7) prejunctional actions that either inhibit or facilitate the release of neurotransmitters, the inhibitory action being physiologically more important. Many of these actions and the receptors that mediate them are summarized in Tables 6–1 and 6–8. Not all sympathomimetic drugs show each of the above types of action to the same degree. However, many of the differences in their effects are only quantitative; therefore, the pharmacological properties of these drugs as a class are described in detail for the prototypical agent, *epinephrine*.

Appriation of the pharmacological properties of the drugs described in this chapter depends on an understanding of the classification, distribution, and mechanism of action of α and β adrenergic receptors (*see* Figure 10–1 and Chapter 6).

CLASSIFICATION OF SYMPATHOMIMETIC DRUGS

Catecholamines and sympathomimetic drugs are classified as direct acting, indirect acting, or mixed acting sympathomimetics (Figure 10–2). Direct-acting sympathomimetic drugs act directly on one or more of the adrenergic receptors. These agents may exhibit considerable selectivity for a specific receptor subtype (*e.g., phenylephrine* for α_1, *terbutaline* for β_2) or may have no or minimal selectivity and act on several receptor types (*e.g.,* epinephrine for α_1, α_2, β_1, β_2, β_3 receptors; *norepinephrine* for α_1, α_2, β_1 receptors). Indirect-acting drugs increase the availability of norepinephrine or epinephrine to stimulate adrenergic receptors. This can be accomplished in several ways: (1) by releasing or displacing norepinephrine from sympathetic nerve varicosities; (2) by blocking the transport of norepinephrine into sympathetic neurons (*e.g.,* cocaine); or (3) by blocking the metabolizing enzymes, monoamine oxidase (MAO) (*e.g., pargyline*) or catechol-*O*-methyltransferase (COMT) (*e.g., entacapone*). Drugs that indirectly release norepinephrine and also directly activate receptors are referred to as mixed-acting sympathomimetic drugs (*e.g., ephedrine, dopamine*).

Prototypical drugs for these various mechanisms are listed in Figure 10–2. Although this classification is convenient, there probably is a continuum of activity from predominantly direct-acting to predominantly indirect-acting drugs. Thus, this classification is relative rather than absolute.

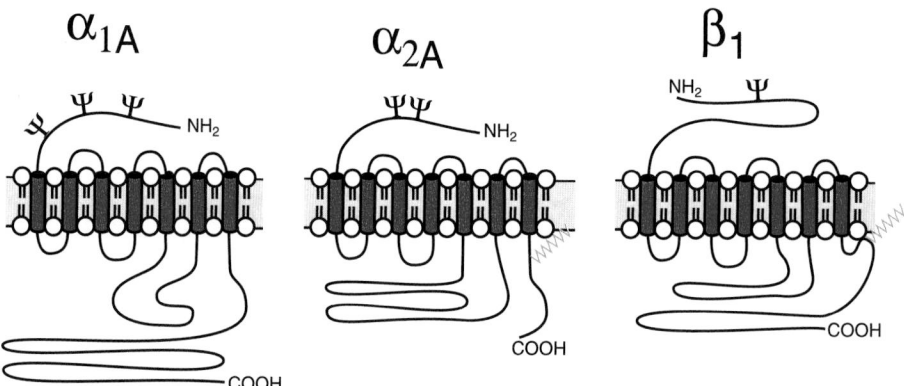

Figure 10–1. *Subtypes of adrenergic receptors.* All of the adrenergic receptors are heptaspanning GPCRs. A representative of each type is shown; each type has three subtypes: $\alpha_{1A, 1B, and 1D}$, $\alpha_{2A, 2B, and 2C}$, and $\beta_{1, 2, and 3}$. All β receptor subtypes are coupled to stimulation of adenylyl cyclase activity; similarly, all α_2 adrenergic receptor subtypes affect the same effector systems (*i.e.,* inhibition of adenylyl cyclase, activation of receptor-operated K^+ channels, and inhibition of Ca^{2+} channels). In contrast, there is evidence that different α_1 adrenergic receptor subpopulations couple to different effector systems, the G_q-PLC-IP$_3$ pathway being a major effector. ψ indicates a site for *N*-glycosylation. ᔕᔕᔕᔕ indicates a site for thio-acetylation.

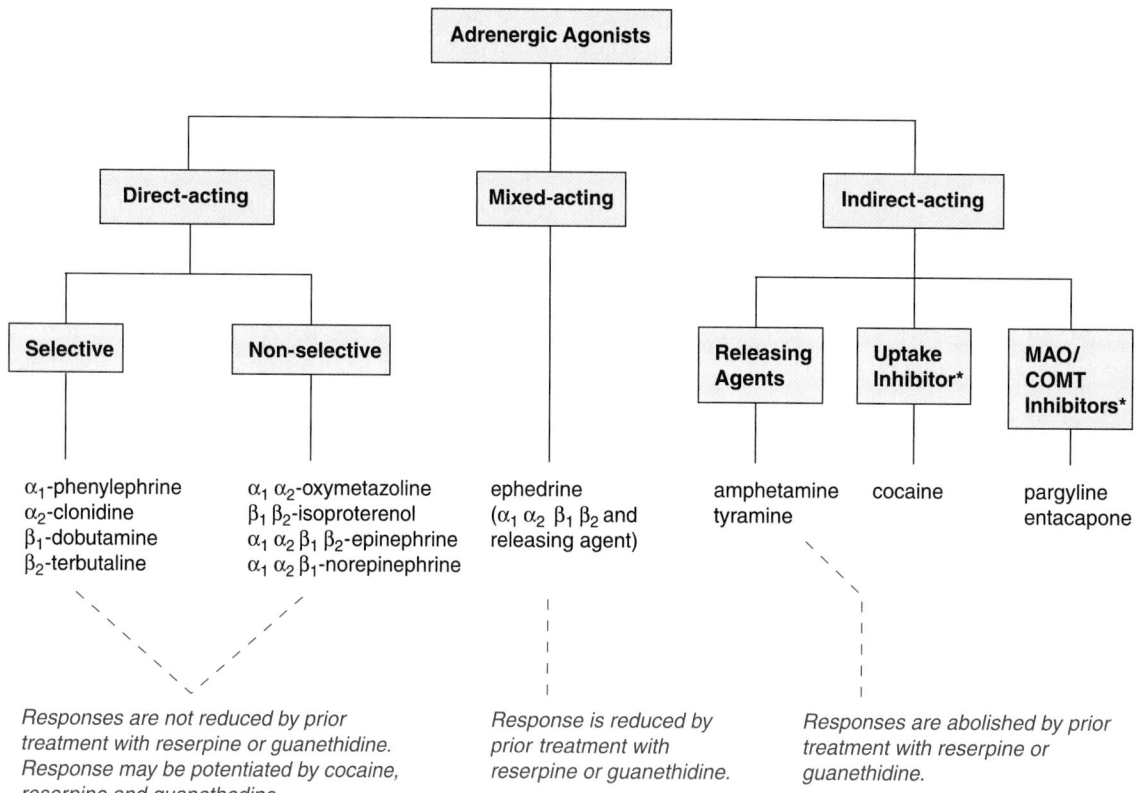

Figure 10–2. *Classification of adrenergic receptor agonists (sympathomimetic amines) or drugs that produce sympathomimetic-like effects.* For each category, a prototypical drug is shown. *Not actually sympathetic drugs but produce sympathomimetic-like effects.

A feature of direct-acting sympathomimetic drugs is that their responses are not reduced by prior treatment with *reserpine* or *guanethidine*, which deplete norepinephrine from sympathetic neurons. After transmitter depletion, the actions of direct-acting sympathomimetic drugs actually may increase because the loss of the neurotransmitter induces compensatory changes that upregulate receptors or enhance the signaling pathway. In contrast, the responses of indirect-acting sympathomimetic drugs (*e.g.*, *amphetamine*, *tyramine*) are abolished by prior treatment with reserpine or guanethidine. The cardinal feature of mixed-acting sympathomimetic drugs is that their effects are blunted, but not abolished, by prior treatment with reserpine or guanethidine.

Since the actions of norepinephrine are more pronounced on α and β_1 receptors than on β_2 receptors, many noncatecholamines that release norepinephrine have predominantly α receptor–mediated and cardiac effects. However, certain noncatecholamines with both direct and indirect effects on adrenergic receptors show significant β_2 activity and are used clinically for these effects. Thus, ephedrine, although dependent on release of norepinephrine for some of its effects, relieves bronchospasm by its action on β_2 receptors in bronchial smooth muscle, an effect not seen with norepinephrine. Moreover, some noncatecholamines (*e.g.*, *phenylephrine*) act primarily and directly on target cells. It therefore is impossible to predict precisely the effects of noncatecholamines solely on their ability to provoke norepinephrine release.

Chemistry and Structure–Activity Relationship of Sympathomimetic Amines. *β-Phenylethylamine* (Table 10–1) can be viewed as the parent compound of the sympathomimetic amines, consisting of a benzene ring and an ethylamine side chain. The structure permits substitutions to be made on the aromatic ring, the α- and β-carbon atoms, and the terminal amino group to yield a variety of compounds with sympathomimetic activity. Norepinephrine, epinephrine, dopamine, *isoproterenol*, and a few other agents have hydroxyl groups substituted at positions 3 and 4 of the benzene ring. Since *o*-dihydroxybenzene is also known as *catechol*, sympathomimetic amines with these hydroxyl substitutions in the aromatic ring are termed *catecholamines*.

Many directly acting sympathomimetic drugs influence both α and β receptors, but the ratio of activities varies among drugs in a continuous spectrum from predominantly α activity (phenylephrine) to predominantly β activity (isoproterenol). Despite the multiplicity of the sites of action of sympathomimetic amines, several generalizations can be made (Table 10–1).

Separation of Aromatic Ring and Amino Group. By far the greatest sympathomimetic activity occurs when two carbon atoms separate the ring from the amino group. This rule applies with few exceptions to all types of action.

Substitution on the Amino Group. The effects of amino substitution are most readily seen in the actions of catecholamines on α

and β receptors. Increase in the size of the alkyl substituent increases β receptor activity (*e.g.*, isoproterenol). Norepinephrine has, in general, rather feeble β_2 activity; this activity is greatly increased in epinephrine by the addition of a methyl group. A notable exception is phenylephrine, which has an *N*-methyl substituent but is an α-selective agonist. β_2-Selective compounds require a large amino substituent, but depend on other substitutions to define selectivity for β_2 rather than for β_1 adrenergic receptors. In general, the smaller the substitution on the amino group, the greater the selectivity for α activity, although *N*-methylation increases the potency of primary amines. Thus, α activity is maximal in epinephrine, less in norepinephrine, and almost absent in isoproterenol.

Substitution on the Aromatic Nucleus. Maximal α and β activity depends on the presence of hydroxyl groups on positions 3 and 4. When one or both of these groups are absent, with no other aromatic substitution, the overall potency is reduced. Phenylephrine is thus less potent than epinephrine at both α and β receptors, with β_2 activity almost completely absent. Studies of the β adrenergic receptor suggest that the hydroxyl groups on serine residues 204 and 207 probably form hydrogen bonds with the catechol hydroxyl groups at positions 3 and 4, respectively (Strader *et al.*, 1989). It also appears that aspartate 113 is a point of electrostatic interaction with the amine group on the ligand. Since the serines are in the fifth membrane-spanning region and the aspartate is in the third (*see* Chapter 6), it is likely that catecholamines bind parallel to the plane of the membrane, forming a bridge between the two membrane spans. However, models involving dopamine receptors suggest alternative possibilities (Hutchins, 1994).

Hydroxyl groups in positions 3 and 5 confer β_2 receptor selectivity on compounds with large amino substituents. Thus, *metaproterenol*, terbutaline, and other similar compounds relax the bronchial musculature in patients with asthma, but cause less direct cardiac stimulation than do the nonselective drugs. The response to noncatecholamines is partly determined by their capacity to release norepinephrine from storage sites. These agents thus cause effects that are mostly mediated by α and β_1 receptors, since norepinephrine is a weak β_2 agonist. Phenylethylamines that lack hydroxyl groups on the ring and the β-hydroxyl group on the side chain act almost exclusively by causing the release of norepinephrine from sympathetic nerve terminals.

Since substitution of polar groups on the phenylethylamine structure makes the resultant compounds less lipophilic, unsubstituted or alkyl-substituted compounds cross the blood–brain barrier more readily and have more central activity. Thus, ephedrine, amphetamine, and *methamphetamine* exhibit considerable CNS activity. In addition, as noted above, the absence of polar hydroxyl groups results in a loss of direct sympathomimetic activity.

Catecholamines have only a brief duration of action and are ineffective when administered orally, because they are rapidly inactivated in the intestinal mucosa and in the liver before reaching the systemic circulation (*see* Chapter 6). Compounds without one or both hydroxyl substituents are not acted upon by COMT, and their oral effectiveness and duration of action are enhanced.

Groups other than hydroxyls have been substituted on the aromatic ring. In general, potency at α receptors is reduced and β receptor activity is minimal; the compounds may even block β receptors. For example, *methoxamine*, with methoxy substituents at positions 2 and 5, has highly selective α-stimulating activity,

Table 10–1
Chemical Structures and Main Clinical Uses of Important Sympathomimetic Drugs†

Structural template: benzene ring (positions 1–6) attached to β-CH — α-CH — NH

Drug	Ring substituent	β (CH)	α (CH)	NH	α Receptor A	α Receptor N	α Receptor P	α Receptor V	β Receptor B	β Receptor C	β Receptor U	CNS, 0
Phenylethylamine		H	H	H								
Epinephrine	3-OH,4-OH	OH	H	CH_3	A		P	V	B	C		
Norepinephrine	3-OH,4-OH	OH	H	H			P		B			
Dopamine	3-OH,4-OH	H	H	H			P			C		
Dobutamine	3-OH,4-OH	H	H	1*								
Colterol	3-OH,4-OH	OH	H	$C(CH_3)_3$					B			
Ethylnorepinephrine	3-OH,4-OH	OH	CH_2CH_3	H					B			
Isoproterenol	3-OH,4-OH	OH	H	$CH(CH_3)_2$					B	C		
Isoetharine	3-OH,4-OH	OH	CH_2CH_3	$CH(CH_3)_2$					B			
Metaproterenol	3-OH,5-OH	OH	H	$CH(CH_3)_2$					B			
Terbutaline	3-OH,5-OH	OH	H	$C(CH_3)_3$					B		U	
Metaraminol	3-OH	OH	CH_3	H		N	P					
Phenylephrine	3-OH	OH	H	CH_3			P					
Tyramine	4-OH	H	H	H								
Hydroxyamphetamine	4-OH	H	CH_3	H								
Ritodrine	4-OH	OH	CH_3	2*						C		
Prenalterol	4-OH	OH‡	H	$-CH(CH_3)_2$							U	
Methoxamine	2-OCH_3,5-OCH_3	OH	CH_3	H			P					
Albuterol	3-CH_2OH,4-OH	OH	H	$C(CH_3)_3$					B		U	
Amphetamine		H	CH_3	H								CNS, 0
Methamphetamine		H	CH_3	CH_3								CNS, 0
Benzphetamine		H	CH_3	3*								0
Ephedrine		OH	CH_3	CH_3		N	P		B	C		
Phenylpropanolamine		OH	CH_3	H		N	P					
Mephentermine		H	4*	CH_3		N	P					0
Phentermine		H	4*	H		N						0
Propylhexedrine	5*	H	CH_3	CH_3		N						
Diethylpropion			6*									0
Phenmetrazine			7*									0
Phendimetrazine			8*									0

240

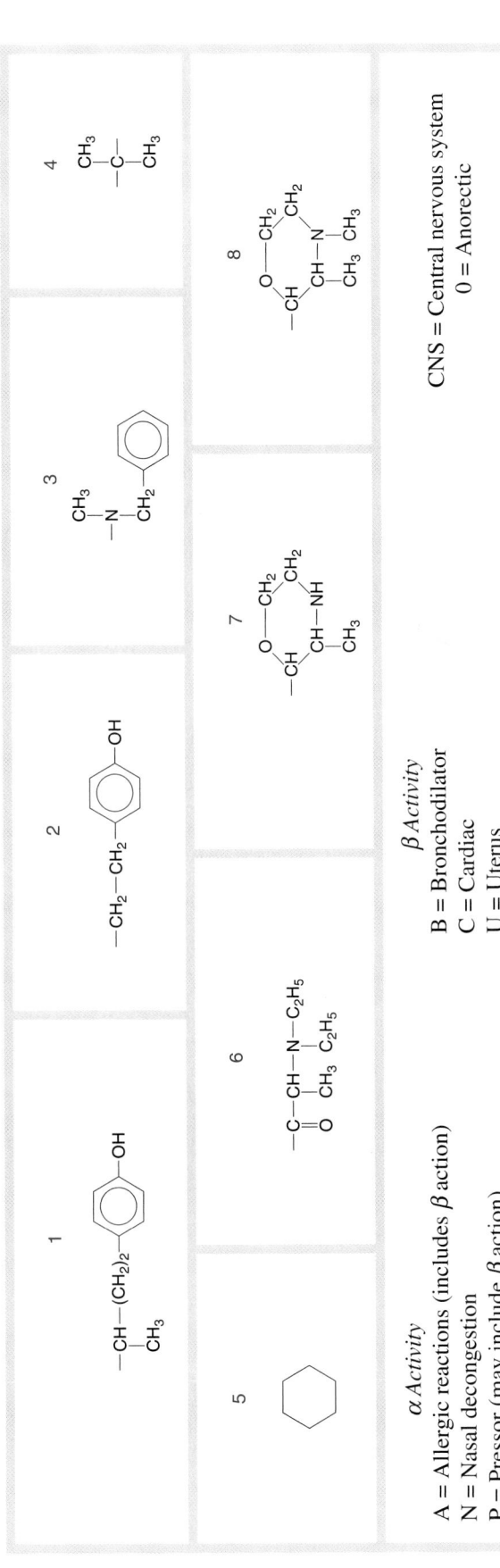

α *Activity*

A = Allergic reactions (includes β action)
N = Nasal decongestion
P = Pressor (may include β action)
V = Other local vasoconstriction
     (*e.g.*, in local anesthesia)

β *Activity*

B = Bronchodilator
C = Cardiac
U = Uterus

CNS = Central nervous system
0 = Anorectic

*Numbers bearing an asterisk refer to the substituents numbered in the bottom rows of the table; substituent 3 replaces the N atom, substituent 5 replaces the phenyl ring, and 6, 7, and 8 are attached directly to the phenyl ring, replacing the ethylamine side chain. †The α and β in the prototypical formula refer to positions of the C atoms in the ethylamine side chain. ‡Prenalterol has — OCH₂— between the aromatic ring and the carbon atom designated as β in the prototypical formula.

241

and in large doses blocks β receptors. *Albuterol*, a β_2-selective agonist, has a substituent at position 3 and is an important exception to the general rule of low β receptor activity. The structure of albuterol is:

$$\text{CH}_2\text{OH}$$
$$\text{HO} - \bigcirc - \text{CHOHCH}_2\text{NHC(CH}_3)_3$$

ALBUTEROL

Substitution on the α-Carbon Atom. This substitution blocks oxidation by MAO, greatly prolonging the duration of action of noncatecholamines because their degradation depends largely on the action of this enzyme. The duration of action of drugs such as ephedrine or amphetamine is thus measured in hours rather than in minutes. Similarly, compounds with an α-methyl substituent persist in the nerve terminals and are more likely to release norepinephrine from storage sites. Agents such as *metaraminol* exhibit a greater degree of indirect sympathomimetic activity.

Substitution on the β-Carbon Atom. Substitution of a hydroxyl group on the β carbon generally decreases actions within the CNS, largely because it lowers lipid solubility. However, such substitution greatly enhances agonist activity at both α and β adrenergic receptors. Although ephedrine is less potent than methamphetamine as a central stimulant, it is more powerful in dilating bronchioles and increasing blood pressure and heart rate.

Optical Isomerism. Substitution on either α- or β-carbon yields optical isomers. Levorotatory substitution on the β-carbon confers the greater peripheral activity, so that the naturally occurring *l*-epinephrine and *l*-norepinephrine are at least 10 times as potent as their unnatural *d*-isomers. Dextrorotatory substitution on the α carbon generally results in a more potent compound. *d*-Amphetamine is more potent than *l*-amphetamine in central but not peripheral activity.

Physiological Basis of Adrenergic Receptor Function.
An important factor in the response of any cell or organ to sympathomimetic amines is the density and proportion of α and β adrenergic receptors. For example, norepinephrine has relatively little capacity to increase bronchial airflow, since the receptors in bronchial smooth muscle are largely of the β_2 subtype. In contrast, isoproterenol and epinephrine are potent bronchodilators. Cutaneous blood vessels physiologically express almost exclusively α receptors; thus, norepinephrine and epinephrine cause constriction of such vessels, whereas isoproterenol has little effect. The smooth muscle of blood vessels that supply skeletal muscles has both β_2 and α receptors; activation of β_2 receptors causes vasodilation, and stimulation of α receptors constricts these vessels. In such vessels, the threshold concentration for activation of β_2 receptors by epinephrine is lower than that for α receptors, but when both types of receptors are activated at high concentrations of epinephrine, the response to α receptors predominates. Physiological concentrations of epinephrine primarily cause vasodilation.

The ultimate response of a target organ to sympathomimetic amines is dictated not only by the direct effects of the agents, but also by the reflex homeostatic adjustments of the organism. One of the most striking effects of many sympathomimetic amines is a rise in arterial blood pressure caused by stimulation of vascular α adrenergic receptors. This stimulation elicits compensatory reflexes that are mediated by the carotid–aortic baroreceptor system. As a result, sympathetic tone is diminished and vagal tone is enhanced; each of these responses leads to slowing of the heart rate. Conversely, when a drug (*e.g.*, a β_2 agonist) lowers mean blood pressure at the mechano-receptors of the carotid sinus and aortic arch, the baroreceptor reflex works to restore pressure by reducing parasympathetic (vagal) outflow from the CNS to the heart, and increasing sympathetic outflow to the heart and vessels. The baroreceptor reflex effect is of special importance for drugs that have little capacity to activate β receptors directly. With diseases such as atherosclerosis, which may impair baroreceptor mechanisms, the effects of sympathomimetic drugs may be magnified (Chapleau *et al.*, 1995).

False-Transmitter Concept. Indirectly acting amines are taken up into sympathetic nerve terminals and storage vesicles, where they replace norepinephrine in the storage complex. Phenylethylamines that lack a β-hydroxyl group are retained there poorly, but β-hydroxylated phenylethylamines and compounds that subsequently become hydroxylated in the synaptic vesicle by dopamine β-hydroxylase are retained in the synaptic vesicle for relatively long periods of time. Such substances can produce a persistent diminution in the content of norepinephrine at functionally critical sites. When the nerve is stimulated, the contents of a relatively constant number of synaptic vesicles are apparently released by exocytosis. If these vesicles contain phenylethylamines that are much less potent than norepinephrine, activation of postsynaptic α and β receptors will be diminished.

This hypothesis, known as the *false-transmitter concept,* is a possible explanation for some of the effects of MAO inhibitors. Phenylethylamines normally are synthesized in the GI tract as a result of the action of bacterial tyrosine decarboxylase. The tyramine formed in this fashion usually is oxidatively deaminated in the GI tract and the liver, and the amine does not reach the systemic circulation in significant concentrations. However, when an MAO inhibitor is administered, tyramine may be absorbed systemically and transported into sympathetic nerve terminals, where its catabolism again is prevented because of the inhibition of MAO at this site; the tyramine then is β-hydroxylated to octopamine and stored in the vesicles in this form. As a consequence, norepinephrine gradually is displaced, and stimulation of the nerve terminal results in the release of a relatively small amount of norepinephrine along with a fraction of octopamine. The latter amine has relatively little ability to activate either α or β receptors. Thus, a functional impairment of sympathetic transmission parallels long-term administration of MAO inhibitors.

Despite such functional impairment, patients who have received MAO inhibitors may experience severe hypertensive crises if they ingest cheese, beer, or red wine. These and related foods, which are produced by fermentation, contain a large quantity of tyramine, and to a lesser degree, other phenylethylamines. When gastrointestinal and hepatic MAO are inhibited, the large quantity of tyramine that is ingested is absorbed rapidly and reaches the systemic circulation in high concentration. A massive and precipitous release of norepinephrine can result, with consequent hypertension that can be severe enough to cause myocardial infarction or a stroke. The properties of various MAO inhibitors (reversible or irreversible; selective or nonselective at MAO-A and MAO-B) are discussed in Chapter 17.

ENDOGENOUS CATECHOLAMINES

Epinephrine

Epinephrine (adrenaline) is a potent stimulant of both α and β adrenergic receptors, and its effects on target organs are thus complex. Most of the responses listed in Table 6–1 are seen after injection of epinephrine, although the occurrence of sweating, piloerection, and mydriasis depends on the physiological state of the subject. Particularly prominent are the actions on the heart and on vascular and other smooth muscle.

Blood Pressure. Epinephrine is one of the most potent vasopressor drugs known. If a pharmacological dose is given rapidly by an intravenous route, it evokes a characteristic effect on blood pressure, which rises rapidly to a peak that is proportional to the dose. The increase in systolic pressure is greater than the increase in diastolic pres-

sure, so that the pulse pressure increases. As the response wanes, the mean pressure may fall below normal before returning to control levels.

The mechanism of the rise in blood pressure due to epinephrine is threefold: (1) a direct myocardial stimulation that increases the strength of ventricular contraction (positive inotropic action); (2) an increased heart rate (positive chronotropic action); and (3) vasoconstriction in many vascular beds—especially in the precapillary resistance vessels of skin, mucosa, and kidney—along with marked constriction of the veins. The pulse rate, at first accelerated, may be slowed markedly at the height of the rise of blood pressure by compensatory vagal discharge. Small doses of epinephrine (0.1 $\mu g/kg$) may cause the blood pressure to fall. The depressor effect of small doses and the biphasic response to larger doses are due to greater sensitivity to epinephrine of vasodilator β_2 receptors than of constrictor α receptors.

The effects are somewhat different when the drug is given by slow intravenous infusion or by subcutaneous injection. Absorption of epinephrine after subcutaneous injection is slow due to local vasoconstrictor action; the effects of doses as large as 0.5 to 1.5 mg can be duplicated by intravenous infusion at a rate of 10 to 30 μg per minute. There is a moderate increase in systolic pressure due to increased cardiac contractile force and a rise in cardiac output (Figure 10–3). Peripheral resistance decreases, owing to a dominant action on β_2 receptors of vessels in skeletal muscle, where blood flow is enhanced; as a consequence, diastolic pressure usually falls. Since the mean blood pressure is not, as a rule, greatly elevat-

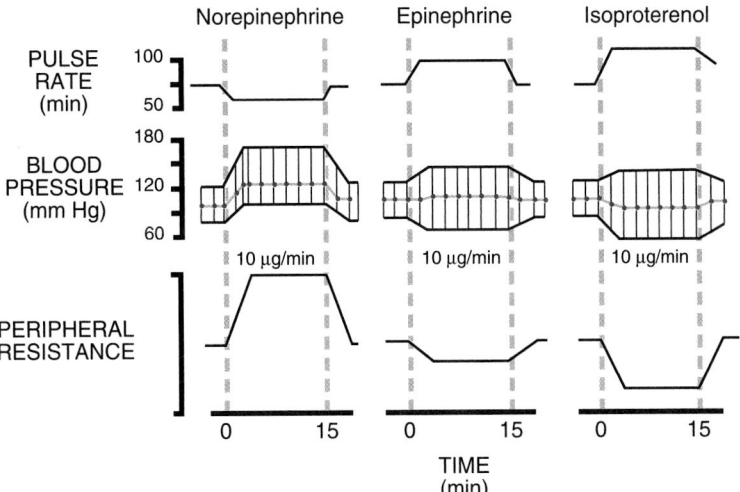

Figure 10–3. **Effects of intravenous infusion of norepinephrine, epinephrine, or isoproterenol in humans.** (Modified from Allwood *et al.*, 1963, with permission.)

ed, compensatory baroreceptor reflexes do not appreciably antagonize the direct cardiac actions. Heart rate, cardiac output, stroke volume, and left ventricular work per beat are increased as a result of direct cardiac stimulation and increased venous return to the heart, which is reflected by an increase in right atrial pressure. At slightly higher rates of infusion, there may be no change or a slight rise in peripheral resistance and diastolic pressure, depending on the dose and the resultant ratio of α to β responses in the various vascular beds; compensatory reflexes also may come into play. The details of the effects of intravenous infusion of epinephrine, norepinephrine, and isoproterenol in humans are compared in Table 10–2 and Figure 10–3.

Vascular Effects. The chief vascular action of epinephrine is exerted on the smaller arterioles and precapillary sphincters, although veins and large arteries also respond to the drug. Various vascular beds react differently, which results in a substantial redistribution of blood flow.

Injected epinephrine markedly decreases cutaneous blood flow, constricting precapillary vessels and small venules. Cutaneous vasoconstriction accounts for a marked decrease in blood flow in the hands and feet. The "after congestion" of mucosa following the vasoconstriction from locally applied epinephrine probably is due to changes in vascular reactivity as a result of tissue hypoxia rather than to β agonist activity of the drug on mucosal vessels.

Blood flow to skeletal muscles is increased by therapeutic doses in humans. This is due in part to a powerful β_2-mediated vasodilator action that is only partially counterbalanced by a vasoconstrictor action on the α receptors that also are present in the vascular bed. If an α receptor antagonist is given, the vasodilation in muscle is more pronounced, the total peripheral resistance is decreased, and the mean blood pressure falls (epinephrine reversal). After the administration of a nonselective β receptor antagonist, only vasoconstriction occurs, and the administration of epinephrine is associated with a considerable pressor effect.

The effect of epinephrine on cerebral circulation is related to systemic blood pressure. In usual therapeutic doses, the drug has relatively little constrictor action on cerebral arterioles. It is physiologically advantageous that the cerebral circulation does not constrict in response to activation of the sympathetic nervous system by stressful stimuli. Indeed, autoregulatory mechanisms tend to limit the increase in cerebral blood flow caused by increased blood pressure.

Doses of epinephrine that have little effect on mean arterial pressure consistently increase renal vascular resistance and reduce

Table 10–2
Comparison of the Effects of Intravenous Infusion of Epinephrine and Norepinephrine in Human Beings*

EFFECT	EPI	NE
Cardiac		
Heart rate	+	−[†]
Stroke volume	++	++
Cardiac output	+++	0,−
Arrhythmias	++++	++++
Coronary blood flow	++	++
Blood pressure		
Systolic arterial	+++	+++
Mean arterial	+	++
Diastolic arterial	+,0,−	++
Mean pulmonary	++	++
Peripheral circulation		
Total peripheral resistance	−	++
Cerebral blood flow	+	0,−
Muscle blood flow	+++	0,−
Cutaneous blood flow	−−	−−
Renal blood flow	−	−
Splanchnic blood flow	+++	0,+
Metabolic effects		
Oxygen consumption	++	0,+
Blood glucose	+++	0,+
Blood lactic acid	+++	0,+
Eosinopenic response	+	0
Central nervous system		
Respiration	+	+
Subjective sensations	+	+

*0.1 to 0.4 µg/kg per minute. [2]*Abbreviations:* Epi, epinephrine; NE, norepinephrine; +, increase; 0, no change; −, decrease; †, after atropine, +. After Goldenberg *et al.,* 1950.

renal blood flow by as much as 40%. All segments of the renal vascular bed contribute to the increased resistance. Since the glomerular filtration rate is only slightly and variably altered, the filtration fraction is consistently increased. Excretion of Na^+, K^+, and Cl^- is decreased; urine volume may be increased, decreased, or unchanged. Maximal tubular reabsorptive and excretory capacities are unchanged. The secretion of renin is increased as a consequence of a direct action of epinephrine on β_1 receptors in the juxtaglomerular apparatus.

Arterial and venous pulmonary pressures are raised. Although direct pulmonary vasoconstriction occurs, redistribution of blood from the systemic to the pulmonary circulation, due to constriction of the more powerful musculature in the systemic great veins, doubtless plays an important part in the increase in pulmonary pressure. Very high concentrations of epinephrine may cause pulmonary edema precipitated by elevated pulmonary capillary filtration pressure and possibly by "leaky" capillaries.

Coronary blood flow is enhanced by epinephrine or by cardiac sympathetic stimulation under physiological conditions. The increased flow, which occurs even with doses that do not increase the aortic blood pressure, is the result of two factors. The first is the increased relative duration of diastole at higher heart rates (*see* below); this is partially offset by decreased blood flow during systole because of more forceful contraction of the surrounding myocardium and an increase in mechanical compression of the coronary vessels. The increased flow during diastole is further enhanced if aortic blood pressure is elevated by epinephrine; as a consequence, total coronary flow may be increased. The second factor is a metabolic dilator effect that results from the increased strength of contraction and myocardial oxygen consumption due to the direct effects of epinephrine on cardiac myocytes. This vasodilation is mediated in part by adenosine released from cardiac myocytes, which tends to override a direct vasoconstrictor effect of epinephrine that results from activation of α receptors in coronary vessels.

Cardiac Effects.

Epinephrine is a powerful cardiac stimulant. It acts directly on the predominant β_1 receptors of the myocardium and of the cells of the pacemaker and conducting tissues; β_2, β_3, and α receptors also are present in the heart, although there are considerable species differences. Considerable recent interest has focused on the role of β_1 and β_2 receptors in the human heart, especially in heart failure. The heart rate increases, and the rhythm often is altered. Cardiac systole is shorter and more powerful, cardiac output is enhanced, and the work of the heart and its oxygen consumption are markedly increased. Cardiac efficiency (work done relative to oxygen consumption) is lessened. Direct responses to epinephrine include increases in contractile force, accelerated rate of rise of isometric tension, enhanced rate of relaxation, decreased time to peak tension, increased excitability, acceleration of the rate of spontaneous beating, and induction of automaticity in specialized regions of the heart.

In accelerating the heart, epinephrine preferentially shortens systole so that the duration of diastole usually is not reduced. Indeed, activation of β receptors increases the rate of relaxation of ventricular muscle. Epinephrine speeds the heart by accelerating the slow depolarization of sinoatrial (SA) nodal cells that takes place during diastole, *i.e.,* during phase 4 of the action potential (*see* Chapter 34). Consequently, the transmembrane potential of the pacemaker cells rises more rapidly to the threshold level of action potential initiation. The amplitude of the action potential and the maximal rate of depolarization (phase 0) also are increased. A shift in the location of the pacemaker within the SA node often occurs, owing to activation of latent pacemaker cells. In Purkinje fibers, epinephrine also accelerates diastolic depolarization and may activate latent pacemaker cells. These changes do not occur in atrial and ventricular muscle fibers, where epinephrine has little effect on the stable, phase 4 membrane potential after repolarization. If large doses of epinephrine

are given, premature ventricular contractions occur and may herald more serious ventricular arrhythmias. This rarely is seen with conventional doses in humans, but ventricular extrasystoles, tachycardia, or even fibrillation may be precipitated by release of endogenous epinephrine when the heart has been sensitized to this action of epinephrine by certain anesthetics or by myocardial ischemia. The mechanism of induction of these cardiac arrhythmias is not clear.

Some effects of epinephrine on cardiac tissues are largely secondary to the increase in heart rate and are small or inconsistent when the heart rate is kept constant. For example, the effect of epinephrine on repolarization of atrial muscle, Purkinje fibers, or ventricular muscle is small if the heart rate is unchanged. When the heart rate is increased, the duration of the action potential is consistently shortened, and the refractory period is correspondingly decreased.

Conduction through the Purkinje system depends on the level of membrane potential at the time of excitation. Excessive reduction of this potential results in conduction disturbances, ranging from slowed conduction to complete block. Epinephrine often increases the membrane potential and improves conduction in Purkinje fibers that have been excessively depolarized.

Epinephrine normally shortens the refractory period of the human atrioventricular (AV) node by direct effects on the heart, although doses of epinephrine that slow the heart through reflex vagal discharge may indirectly tend to prolong it. Epinephrine also decreases the grade of AV block that occurs as a result of disease, drugs, or vagal stimulation. Supraventricular arrhythmias are apt to occur from the combination of epinephrine and cholinergic stimulation. Depression of sinus rate and AV conduction by vagal discharge probably plays a part in epinephrine-induced ventricular arrhythmias, since various drugs that block the vagal effect confer some protection. The actions of epinephrine in enhancing cardiac automaticity and in causing arrhythmias are effectively antagonized by β receptor antagonists such as propranolol. However, α_1 receptors exist in most regions of the heart, and their activation prolongs the refractory period and strengthens myocardial contractions.

Cardiac arrhythmias have been seen in patients after inadvertent intravenous administration of conventional subcutaneous doses of epinephrine. Premature ventricular contractions can appear, which may be followed by multifocal ventricular tachycardia or ventricular fibrillation. Pulmonary edema also may occur.

Epinephrine decreases the amplitude of the T wave of the electrocardiogram (ECG) in normal persons. In animals given relatively larger doses, additional effects are seen on the T wave and the ST segment. After decreasing in amplitude, the T wave may become biphasic, and the ST segment can deviate either above or below the isoelectric line. Such ST-segment changes are similar to those seen in patients with angina pectoris during spontaneous or epinephrine-induced attacks of pain. These electrical changes therefore have been attributed to myocardial ischemia. Also, epinephrine as well as other catecholamines may cause myocardial cell death, particularly after intravenous infusions. Acute toxicity is associated with contraction band necrosis and other pathological changes. Recent interest has focused on the possibility that prolonged sympathetic stimulation of the heart, such as in congestive cardiomyopathy, may promote apoptosis of cardiomyocytes.

Effects on Smooth Muscles.

The effects of epinephrine on the smooth muscles of different organs and systems depend on the type of adrenergic receptor in the muscle (*see* Table 6–1). The effects on vascular smooth muscle are of major physiological importance, whereas those on gastrointestinal smooth muscle are relatively minor. Gastrointestinal smooth muscle is, in general, relaxed by epinephrine. This effect is due to activation of both α and β receptors. Intestinal tone and the frequency and amplitude of spontaneous contractions are reduced. The stomach usually is relaxed and the pyloric and ileocecal sphincters are contracted, but these effects depend on the preexisting tone of the muscle. If tone already is high, epinephrine causes relaxation; if low, contraction.

The responses of uterine muscle to epinephrine vary with species, phase of the sexual cycle, state of gestation, and dose given. Epinephrine contracts strips of pregnant or nonpregnant human uterus *in vitro* by interaction with α receptors. The effects of epinephrine on the human uterus *in situ,* however, differ. During the last month of pregnancy and at parturition, epinephrine inhibits uterine tone and contractions. β_2-Selective agonists, such as *ritodrine* or terbutaline, have been used to delay premature labor, although their efficacy is limited. Effects of these and other drugs on the uterus are discussed below.

Epinephrine relaxes the detrusor muscle of the bladder as a result of activation of β receptors and contracts the trigone and sphincter muscles owing to its α agonist activity. This can result in hesitancy in urination and may contribute to retention of urine in the bladder. Activation of smooth muscle contraction in the prostate promotes urinary retention.

Respiratory Effects. Epinephrine affects respiration primarily by relaxing bronchial muscle. It has a powerful bronchodilator action, most evident when bronchial muscle is contracted because of disease, as in bronchial asthma, or in response to drugs or various autacoids. In such situations, epinephrine has a striking therapeutic effect as a physiological antagonist to substances that cause bronchoconstriction.

The beneficial effects of epinephrine in asthma also may arise from inhibition of antigen-induced release of inflammatory mediators from mast cells, and to a lesser extent from diminution of bronchial secretions and congestion within the mucosa. Inhibition of mast cell secretion is mediated by β_2 receptors, while the effects on the mucosa are mediated by α receptors; however, other drugs, such as glucocorticoids and leukotriene-receptor antagonists, have much more profound antiinflammatory effects in asthma (*see* Chapter 27).

Effects on the Central Nervous System. Because of the inability of this rather polar compound to enter the CNS, epinephrine in conventional therapeutic doses is not a powerful CNS stimulant. While the drug may cause restlessness, apprehension, headache, and tremor in many persons, these effects in part may be secondary to the effects of epinephrine on the cardiovascular system, skeletal muscles, and intermediary metabolism; that is,

they may be the result of somatic manifestations of anxiety. Some other sympathomimetic drugs more readily cross the blood–brain barrier.

Metabolic Effects. Epinephrine has a number of important influences on metabolic processes. It elevates the concentrations of glucose and lactate in blood by mechanisms described in Chapter 6. Insulin secretion is inhibited through an interaction with α_2 receptors and is enhanced by activation of β_2 receptors; the predominant effect seen with epinephrine is inhibition. Glucagon secretion is enhanced by an action on the β receptors of the α cells of pancreatic islets. Epinephrine also decreases the uptake of glucose by peripheral tissues, at least in part because of its effects on the secretion of insulin, but also possibly due to direct effects on skeletal muscle. Glycosuria rarely occurs. The effect of epinephrine to stimulate glycogenolysis in most tissues and in most species involves β receptors (*see* Chapter 6).

Epinephrine raises the concentration of free fatty acids in blood by stimulating β receptors in adipocytes. The result is activation of triglyceride lipase, which accelerates the triglyceride breakdown to free fatty acids and glycerol. The calorigenic action of epinephrine (increase in metabolism) is reflected in humans by an increase of 20% to 30% in oxygen consumption after conventional doses. This effect mainly is due to enhanced breakdown of triglycerides in brown adipose tissue, providing an increase in oxidizable substrate (*see* Chapter 6).

Miscellaneous Effects. Epinephrine reduces circulating plasma volume by loss of protein-free fluid to the extracellular space, thereby increasing hematocrit and plasma protein concentration. However, conventional doses of epinephrine do not significantly alter plasma volume or packed red cell volume under normal conditions, although such doses are reported to have variable effects in the presence of shock, hemorrhage, hypotension, or anesthesia. Epinephrine rapidly increases the number of circulating polymorphonuclear leukocytes, likely due to β receptor–mediated demargination of these cells. Epinephrine accelerates blood coagulation in laboratory animals and humans and promotes fibrinolysis.

The effects of epinephrine on secretory glands are not marked; in most glands secretion usually is inhibited, partly owing to the reduced blood flow caused by vasoconstriction. Epinephrine stimulates lacrimation and a scanty mucus secretion from salivary glands. Sweating and pilomotor activity are minimal after systemic administration of epinephrine, but occur after intradermal injection of very dilute solutions of either epinephrine or norepinephrine. Such effects are inhibited by α receptor antagonists.

Mydriasis is readily seen during physiological sympathetic stimulation but not when epinephrine is instilled into the conjunctival sac of normal eyes. However, epinephrine usually lowers intraocular pressure; the mechanism of this effect is not clear but probably reflects reduced production of aqueous humor due to vasoconstriction and enhanced outflow (*see* Chapter 63).

Although epinephrine does not directly excite skeletal muscle, it facilitates neuromuscular transmission, particularly that following prolonged rapid stimulation of motor nerves. In apparent contrast to the effects of α receptor activation at presynaptic nerve terminals in the autonomic nervous system (α_2 receptors), stimulation of α receptors causes a more rapid increase in transmitter release from the somatic motor neuron, perhaps as a result of enhanced influx of Ca^{2+}. These responses likely are mediated by α_1 receptors. These actions may explain in part the ability of epinephrine (given intra-arterially) to briefly increase strength of the injected limb of patients with myasthenia gravis. Epinephrine also acts directly on white, fast-twitch muscle fibers to prolong the active state, thereby increasing peak tension. Of greater physiological and clinical importance is the capacity of epinephrine and selective β_2 agonists to increase physiological tremor, at least in part due to β receptor–mediated enhancement of discharge of muscle spindles.

Epinephrine promotes a fall in plasma K^+, largely due to stimulation of K^+ uptake into cells, particularly skeletal muscle, due to activation of β_2 receptors. This is associated with decreased renal K^+ excretion. These receptors have been exploited in the management of hyperkalemic familial periodic paralysis, which is characterized by episodic flaccid paralysis, hyperkalemia, and depolarization of skeletal muscle. The β_2-selective agonist albuterol apparently is able to ameliorate the impairment in the ability of the muscle to accumulate and retain K^+.

The administration of large or repeated doses of epinephrine or other sympathomimetic amines to experimental animals damages arterial walls and myocardium, even inducing necrosis in the heart indistinguishable from myocardial infarction. The mechanism of this injury is not yet clear, but α and β receptor antagonists and Ca^{2+} channel blockers may afford substantial protection against the damage. Similar lesions occur in many patients with pheochromocytoma or after prolonged infusions of norepinephrine.

Absorption, Fate, and Excretion. As indicated above, epinephrine is not effective after oral administration because it is rapidly conjugated and oxidized in the GI mucosa and liver. Absorption from subcutaneous tissues occurs relatively slowly because of local vasoconstriction and the rate may be further decreased by systemic hypotension, for example in a patient with shock. Absorption is more rapid after intramuscular injection. In emergencies, it may be necessary to administer epinephrine intravenously. When relatively concentrated solutions (1%) are nebulized and inhaled, the actions of the drug largely are restricted to the respiratory tract; however, systemic reactions such as arrhythmias may occur, particularly if larger amounts are used.

Epinephrine is rapidly inactivated in the body. The liver, which is rich in both of the enzymes responsible for destroying circulating epinephrine (COMT and MAO), is particularly important in this regard (*see* Figure 6–6 and Table 6–5). Although only small amounts appear in the urine of normal persons, the urine of patients with pheochromocytoma may contain relatively large amounts of epinephrine, norepinephrine, and their metabolites.

Epinephrine is available in a variety of formulations geared for different clinical indications and routes of administration, such as by injection (usually subcutaneously but sometimes intravenously), by inhalation, or topically. Several practical points are worth noting. First, epinephrine is unstable in alkaline solution; when exposed to air or light, it turns pink from oxidation to adrenochrome and then brown from formation of polymers. Epinephrine injection is available in 1 mg/ml (1:1000), 0.1 mg/ml (1:10,000), and 0.5 mg/ml (1:2,000) solutions. The usual adult dose given subcutaneously ranges from 0.3 to 0.5 mg. The intravenous route is used cautiously if an immediate and reliable effect is mandatory. If the solution is given by vein, it must be adequately diluted and injected very slowly. The dose is seldom as much as 0.25 mg, except for cardiac arrest, when larger doses may be required. Epinephrine suspensions are used to slow subcutaneous absorption and must never be injected intravenously. *Also, a 1% (10 mg/ml; 1:100) formulation is available for administration via inhalation; every precaution must be taken not to confuse this 1:100 solution with the 1:1000 solution designed for parenteral administration, because inadvertent injection of the 1:100 solution can be fatal.*

Toxicity, Adverse Effects, and Contraindications. Epinephrine may cause disturbing reactions, such as restlessness, throbbing headache, tremor, and palpitations. The effects rapidly subside with rest, quiet, recumbency, and reassurance.

More serious reactions include cerebral hemorrhage and cardiac arrhythmias. The use of large doses or the accidental, rapid intravenous injection of epinephrine may result in cerebral hemorrhage from the sharp rise in blood pressure. Ventricular arrhythmias may follow the administration of epinephrine. Angina may be induced by epinephrine in patients with coronary artery disease.

The use of epinephrine generally is contraindicated in patients who are receiving nonselective β receptor blocking drugs, since its unopposed actions on vascular α_1 receptors may lead to severe hypertension and cerebral hemorrhage.

Therapeutic Uses. The clinical uses of epinephrine are based on its actions on blood vessels, heart, and bronchial muscle. In the past, the most common use of epinephrine was to relieve respiratory distress due to bronchospasm; however, β_2-selective agonists now are preferred. A major use is to provide rapid relief of hypersensitivity reactions, including anaphylaxis, to drugs and other allergens. Epinephrine also is used to prolong the action of local anesthetics, presumably by decreasing local blood flow (*see* Chapter 14). Its cardiac effects may be of use in restoring cardiac rhythm in patients with cardiac arrest due to various causes. It also is used as a topical hemostatic agent on bleeding surfaces such as in the mouth or in bleeding peptic ulcers during endoscopy of the stomach and duodenum. Systemic absorption of the drug can occur with dental application. In addition, inhalation of epinephrine may be useful in the treatment of postintubation and infectious croup. The therapeutic uses of epinephrine, in relation to other sympathomimetic drugs, are discussed later in this chapter.

Norepinephrine

Norepinephrine (levarterenol, *l*-noradrenaline, *l*-β-[3,4-dihydroxyphenyl]-α-aminoethanol) is a major chemical mediator liberated by mammalian postganglionic sympathetic nerves. It differs from epinephrine only by lacking the methyl substitution in the amino group (Table 10–1). Norepinephrine constitutes 10% to 20% of the catecholamine content of human adrenal medulla and as much as 97% in some pheochromocytomas, which may not express the enzyme phenylethanolamine-*N*-methyltransferase. The history of its discovery and its role as a neurohumoral mediator are discussed in Chapter 6.

Pharmacological Properties. The pharmacological actions of norepinephrine and epinephrine have been extensively compared *in vivo* and *in vitro* (Table 10–2). Both drugs are direct agonists on effector cells, and their actions differ mainly in the ratio of their effectiveness in stimulating α and β_2 receptors. They are approximately equipotent in stimulating β_1 receptors. Norepinephrine is a potent α agonist and has relatively little action on β_2 receptors; however, it is somewhat less potent than epinephrine on the α receptors of most organs.

Cardiovascular Effects. The cardiovascular effects of an intravenous infusion of 10 μg of norepinephrine per minute in humans are shown in Figure 10–3. Systolic and diastolic pressures, and usually pulse pressure, are increased. Cardiac output is unchanged or decreased, and total peripheral resistance is raised. Compensatory vagal reflex activity slows the heart, overcoming a direct cardioaccelerator action, and stroke volume is increased. The peripheral vascular resistance increases in most vascular beds, and renal blood flow is reduced. Norepinephrine constricts mesenteric vessels and reduces splanchnic and hepatic blood flow. Coronary flow usually is increased, probably owing both to indirectly induced coronary dilation, as with epinephrine, and to elevated blood pressure. Although generally a poor β_2 receptor agonist, norepinephrine may increase coronary blood flow directly by stimulating β_2 receptors on coronary vessels (Sun *et al.*, 2002). The physiological significance of this is not yet established. Patients with Prinzmetal's variant angina may be supersensitive to the α adrenergic vasoconstrictor effects of norepinephrine.

Unlike epinephrine, small doses of norepinephrine do not cause vasodilation or lower blood pressure, since the blood vessels of skeletal muscle constrict rather than dilate; α adrenergic receptor antagonists therefore abolish the pressor effects but do not cause significant reversal (*i.e.*, hypotension).

Other Effects. Other responses to norepinephrine are not prominent in humans. The drug causes hyperglycemia and other metabolic effects similar to those produced by epinephrine, but these are observed only when large doses are given because norepinephrine is not as effective a "hormone" as epinephrine. Intradermal injection of suitable doses causes sweating that is not blocked by atropine.

Absorption, Fate, and Excretion. Norepinephrine, like epinephrine, is ineffective when given orally and is absorbed poorly from sites of subcutaneous injection. It is rapidly inactivated in the body by the same enzymes that methylate and oxidatively deaminate epinephrine (*see* above). Small amounts normally are found in the urine. The excretion rate may be greatly increased in patients with pheochromocytoma.

Toxicity, Adverse Effects, and Precautions. The untoward effects of norepinephrine are similar to those of epinephrine, although there typically is greater elevation of blood pressure with norepinephrine. Excessive doses can cause severe hypertension, so careful blood pressure monitoring generally is indicated during systemic administration of this agent.

Care must be taken that necrosis and sloughing do not occur at the site of intravenous injection owing to extravasation of the drug. The infusion should be made high in the limb, preferably through a long plastic cannula extending centrally. Impaired circulation at injection sites, with or without extravasation of norepinephrine, may be relieved by infiltrating the area with *phentolamine*, an α receptor antagonist. Blood pressure must be determined frequently during the infusion and particularly during adjustment of the rate of the infusion. Reduced blood flow to organs such as kidney and intestines is a constant danger with the use of norepinephrine.

Therapeutic Uses and Status. Norepinephrine (LEVOPHED, others) has only limited therapeutic value. The use of it and other sympathomimetic amines in shock is discussed later in this chapter. In the treatment of low blood pressure, the dose is titrated to the desired pressor response.

Dopamine

Dopamine (3,4-dihydroxyphenylethylamine) (Table 10–1) is the immediate metabolic precursor of norepinephrine and epinephrine; it is a central neurotransmitter particularly important in the regulation of movement (*see* Chapters 12, 18, and 20) and possesses important intrinsic pharmacological properties. In the periphery, it is synthesized in epithelial cells of the proximal tubule and is thought to exert local diuretic and natriuretic effects. Dopamine is a substrate for both MAO and COMT and thus is ineffective when administered orally. Classification of dopamine receptors is described in Chapters 12 and 20.

Pharmacological Properties. ***Cardiovascular Effects.*** The cardiovascular effects of dopamine are mediated by several distinct types of receptors that vary in their affinity for dopamine. At low concentrations, the primary interaction of dopamine is with vascular D_1 receptors, especially in the renal, mesenteric, and coronary beds. By activating adenylyl cyclase and raising intracellular concentrations of cyclic AMP, D_1 receptor stimulation leads to vasodilation (Missale *et al.*, 1998). Infusion of low doses of dopamine causes an increase in glomerular filtration rate, renal blood flow, and Na^+ excretion. Activation of D_1 receptors on renal tubular cells decreases sodium transport by cAMP-dependent and cAMP-independent mechanisms. Increasing cAMP production in the proximal tubular cells and the medullary part of the thick ascending limb of the loop of Henle inhibits the Na^+-H^+ exchanger and the Na^+,K^+-ATPase pump. The renal tubular actions of dopamine that cause natriuresis may be augmented by the increase in renal blood flow and the small increase in the glomerular filtration rate that follow its administration. The resulting increase in hydrostatic pressure in the peritubular capillaries and reduction in oncotic pressure may contribute to diminished reabsorption of sodium by the proximal tubular cells. As a consequence, dopamine has pharmacologically appropriate effects in the management of states of low cardiac output associated with compromised renal function, such as severe congestive heart failure.

At somewhat higher concentrations, dopamine exerts a positive inotropic effect on the myocardium, acting on β_1 adrenergic receptors. Dopamine also causes the release of norepinephrine from nerve terminals, which contributes to its effects on the heart. Tachycardia is less prominent during infusion of dopamine than of isoproterenol (*see* below). Dopamine usually increases systolic blood pressure and pulse pressure and either has no effect on diastolic blood pressure or increases it slightly. Total peripheral resistance usually is unchanged when low or intermediate doses of dopamine are given, probably because of the ability of dopamine to reduce regional arterial resistance in some vascular beds, such as mesenteric and renal, while causing only minor increases in others. At high concentrations, dopamine activates vascular α_1 receptors, leading to more general vasoconstriction.

Other Effects. Although there are specific dopamine receptors in the CNS, injected dopamine usually has no central effects because it does not readily cross the blood–brain barrier.

Precautions, Adverse Reactions, and Contraindications. Before dopamine is administered to patients in shock, hypovolemia should be corrected by transfusion of whole blood, plasma, or other appropriate fluid. Untoward effects due to overdosage generally are attributable to excessive sympathomimetic activity (although this also

may be the response to worsening shock). Nausea, vomiting, tachycardia, anginal pain, arrhythmias, headache, hypertension, and peripheral vasoconstriction may be encountered during dopamine infusion. Extravasation of large amounts of dopamine during infusion may cause ischemic necrosis and sloughing. Rarely, gangrene of the fingers or toes has followed prolonged infusion of the drug.

Dopamine should be avoided or used at a much reduced dosage (one-tenth or less) if the patient has received a MAO inhibitor. Careful adjustment of dosage also is necessary in patients who are taking tricyclic antidepressants.

Therapeutic Uses. Dopamine (INTROPIN, others) is used in the treatment of severe congestive failure, particularly in patients with oliguria and low or normal peripheral vascular resistance. The drug also may improve physiological parameters in the treatment of cardiogenic and septic shock. While dopamine may acutely improve cardiac and renal function in severely ill patients with chronic heart disease or renal failure, there is relatively little evidence supporting long-term benefit in clinical outcome (Marik and Iglesias, 1999). The management of shock is discussed below.

Dopamine hydrochloride is used only intravenously. The drug initially is administered at a rate of 2 to 5 $\mu g/kg$ per minute; this rate may be increased gradually up to 20 to 50 $\mu g/kg$ per minute or more as the clinical situation dictates. During the infusion, patients require clinical assessment of myocardial function, perfusion of vital organs such as the brain, and the production of urine. Most patients should receive intensive care, with monitoring of arterial and venous pressures and the ECG. Reduction in urine flow, tachycardia, or the development of arrhythmias may be indications to slow or terminate the infusion. The duration of action of dopamine is brief, and hence the rate of administration can be used to control the intensity of effect.

Related drugs include *fenoldopam* and *dopexamine*. Fenoldopam (CORLOPAM), a benzazepine derivative, is a rapidly acting vasodilator used for control of severe hypertension (*e.g.*, malignant hypertension with end-organ damage) in hospitalized patients for not more than 48 hours. Fenoldopam is an agonist for D_1 peripheral dopamine receptors and binds with moderate affinity to α_2 adrenergic receptors; it has no significant affinity for D_2 receptors or α_1 or β adrenergic receptors. Fenoldopam is a racemic mixture; the R-isomer is the active component. It dilates a variety of blood vessels, including coronary arteries, afferent and efferent arterioles in the kidney, and mesenteric arteries (Murphy *et al.*, 2001).

Less than 6% of an orally administered dose is absorbed because of extensive first-pass formation of sulfate, methyl, and glucuronide conjugates. The elimination half-life of intravenously infused fenoldopam, estimated from the decline in plasma concentration in hypertensive patients after the cessation of a 2-hour infusion, is 10 minutes. Adverse effects are related to the vasodilation and include headache, flushing, dizziness, and tachycardia or bradycardia.

Dopexamine (DOPACARD) is a synthetic analog related to dopamine with intrinsic activity at dopamine D_1 and D_2 receptors as well as at β_2 receptors; it may have other effects such as inhibition of catecholamine uptake (Fitton and Benfield, 1990). It appears to have favorable hemodynamic actions in patients with severe congestive heart failure, sepsis, and shock. In patients with low cardiac output, dopexamine infusion significantly increases stroke volume with a decrease in systemic vascular resistance. Tachycardia and hypotension can occur, but usually only at high infusion rates. Dopexamine is not currently available in the United States.

β ADRENERGIC RECEPTOR AGONISTS

β Adrenergic receptor agonists have been utilized in many clinical settings but now play a major role only in the treatment of bronchoconstriction in patients with asthma (reversible airway obstruction) or chronic obstructive pulmonary disease (COPD). Minor uses include management of preterm labor, treatment of complete heart block in shock, and short-term treatment of cardiac decompensation after surgery or in patients with congestive heart failure or myocardial infarction.

Epinephrine first was used as a bronchodilator at the beginning of the past century, and ephedrine was introduced into western medicine in 1924, although it had been used in China for thousands of years. The next major advance was the development in the 1940s of isoproterenol, a β receptor–selective agonist; this provided a drug for asthma that lacked α receptor activity. The recent development of β_2-selective agonists has resulted in drugs with even more valuable characteristics, including adequate oral bioavailability, lack of α adrenergic activity, and diminished likelihood of some adverse cardiovascular effects.

β Receptor agonists may be used to stimulate the rate and force of cardiac contraction. The chronotropic effect is useful in the emergency treatment of arrhythmias such as *torsades de pointes,* bradycardia, or heart block (*see* Chapter 34), whereas the inotropic effect is useful when it is desirable to augment myocardial contractility. The therapeutic uses of β receptor agonists are discussed later in the chapter.

Isoproterenol

Isoproterenol (isopropylarterenol, isopropyl norepinephrine, isoprenaline, isopropyl noradrenaline, d,l-β-[3,4-dihydroxyphenyl]-α-isopropylaminoethanol) (Table 10–1) is a potent, nonselective β receptor agonist with very low affinity for α receptors. Consequently, isoproterenol has powerful effects on all β receptors and almost no action at α receptors.

Pharmacological Actions. The major cardiovascular effects of isoproterenol (compared with epinephrine

and norepinephrine) are illustrated in Figure 10–3. Intravenous infusion of isoproterenol lowers peripheral vascular resistance, primarily in skeletal muscle but also in renal and mesenteric vascular beds. Diastolic pressure falls. Systolic blood pressure may remain unchanged or rise, although mean arterial pressure typically falls. Cardiac output is increased because of the positive inotropic and chronotropic effects of the drug in the face of diminished peripheral vascular resistance. The cardiac effects of isoproterenol may lead to palpitations, sinus tachycardia, and more serious arrhythmias; large doses of isoproterenol may cause myocardial necrosis in animals.

Isoproterenol relaxes almost all varieties of smooth muscle when the tone is high, but this action is most pronounced on bronchial and GI smooth muscle. It prevents or relieves bronchoconstriction. Its effect in asthma may be due in part to an additional action to inhibit antigen-induced release of histamine and other mediators of inflammation; this action is shared by β_2 receptor–selective stimulants.

Absorption, Fate, and Excretion. Isoproterenol is readily absorbed when given parenterally or as an aerosol. It is metabolized primarily in the liver and other tissues by COMT. Isoproterenol is a relatively poor substrate for MAO and is not taken up by sympathetic neurons to the same extent as are epinephrine and norepinephrine. The duration of action of isoproterenol therefore may be longer than that of epinephrine, but it still is brief.

Toxicity and Adverse Effects. Palpitations, tachycardia, headache, and flushing are common. Cardiac ischemia and arrhythmias may occur, particularly in patients with underlying coronary artery disease.

Therapeutic Uses. Isoproterenol (ISUPREL, others) may be used in emergencies to stimulate heart rate in patients with bradycardia or heart block, particularly in anticipation of inserting an artificial cardiac pacemaker or in patients with the ventricular arrhythmia *torsades de pointes.* In disorders such as asthma and shock, isoproterenol largely has been replaced by other sympathomimetic drugs (*see* below and Chapter 27).

Dobutamine

Dobutamine resembles dopamine structurally but possesses a bulky aromatic substituent on the amino group (Table 10–1). The pharmacological effects of dobutamine are due to direct interactions with α and β receptors; its actions do not appear to result from release of norepinephrine from sympathetic nerve endings, nor are they exerted *via* dopaminergic receptors. Although dobutamine originally was thought to be a relatively selective β_1 receptor agonist, it now is clear that its pharmacological effects are complex. Dobutamine possesses a center of asymmetry; both enantiomeric forms are present in the racemic mixture used clinically. The (−) isomer of dobutamine is a potent agonist at α_1 receptors and is capable of causing marked pressor responses. In contrast, (+)-dobutamine is a potent α_1 receptor antagonist, which can block the effects of (−)-dobutamine. The effects of these two isomers are mediated *via* β receptors. The (+) isomer is a more potent β receptor agonist than the (−) isomer (approximately tenfold). Both isomers appear to be full agonists.

Cardiovascular Effects. The cardiovascular effects of racemic dobutamine represent a composite of the distinct pharmacological properties of the (−) and (+) stereoisomers. Dobutamine has relatively more prominent inotropic than chronotropic effects on the heart compared to isoproterenol. Although not completely understood, this useful selectivity may arise because peripheral resistance is relatively unchanged. Alternatively, cardiac α_1 receptors may contribute to the inotropic effect. At equivalent inotropic doses, dobutamine enhances automaticity of the sinus node to a lesser extent than does isoproterenol; however, enhancement of atrioventricular and intraventricular conduction is similar for both drugs.

In animals, administration of dobutamine at a rate of 2.5 to 15 μg/kg per minute increases cardiac contractility and cardiac output. Total peripheral resistance is not greatly affected. The relatively constant peripheral resistance presumably reflects counterbalancing of α_1 receptor–mediated vasoconstriction and β_2 receptor–mediated vasodilation (Ruffolo, 1987). Heart rate increases only modestly when the rate of administration of dobutamine is maintained at less than 20 μg/kg per minute. After administration of β receptor antagonists, infusion of dobutamine fails to increase cardiac output, but total peripheral resistance increases, confirming that dobutamine has modest direct effects on α adrenergic receptors in the vasculature.

Adverse Effects. In some patients, blood pressure and heart rate increase significantly during dobutamine administration; this may require reduction of the rate of infusion. Patients with a history of hypertension may exhibit such an exaggerated pressor response more frequently. Since dobutamine facilitates atrioventricular conduction, patients with atrial fibrillation are at risk of marked increases in ventricular response rates; digoxin or other measures may be required to prevent this from occurring. Some patients may develop ventricular ectopic activity. As with any inotropic agent, dobutamine potentially may increase the size of a myocardial infarct by increasing myocardial oxygen demand. This risk must be balanced against the patient's overall clinical status. The efficacy of dobutamine over a period of more than a few days is uncertain; there is evidence for the development of tolerance.

Therapeutic Uses. Dobutamine (DOBUTREX, others) is indicated for the short-term treatment of cardiac decompensation that may occur after cardiac surgery or in patients with congestive heart failure or acute myocardial infarction. Dobutamine increases cardiac output and stroke volume in such patients, usually without a marked increase in heart rate. Alterations in blood pressure or peripheral resistance usually are minor, although some patients may have marked increases in blood pressure or heart rate. Clinical evidence of longer-term efficacy remains uncertain. An infusion of dobutamine in combination with echocardiography is useful in the noninvasive assessment of patients with coronary artery disease (Madu *et al.*, 1994). Stressing of the heart with dobutamine may reveal cardiac abnormalities in carefully selected patients.

Dobutamine has a half-life of about 2 minutes; the major metabolites are conjugates of dobutamine and 3-*O*-methyldobutamine. The onset of effect is rapid. Consequently, a loading dose is not required, and steady-state concentrations generally are achieved within 10 minutes of initiation of the infusion. The rate of infusion required to increase cardiac output typically is between 2.5 and 10 μg/kg per minute, although higher infusion rates occasionally are required. The rate and duration of the infusion are determined by the clinical and hemodynamic responses of the patient.

β_2-Selective Adrenergic Receptor Agonists

Some of the major adverse effects of β receptor agonists in the treatment of asthma are caused by stimulation of β_1 receptors in the heart. Accordingly, drugs with preferential affinity for β_2 receptors compared with β_1 receptors have been developed. However, this selectivity is not absolute and is lost at high concentrations of these drugs.

A second strategy that has increased the usefulness of several β_2-selective agonists in the treatment of asthma has been structural modification that results in lower rates of metabolism and enhanced oral bioavailability (compared with catecholamines). Modifications have included placing the hydroxyl groups at positions 3 and 5 of the phenyl ring or substituting another moiety for the hydroxyl group at position 3. This has yielded drugs such as metaproterenol, terbutaline, and albuterol, that are not substrates for COMT. Bulky substituents on the amino group of catecholamines contribute to potency at β receptors with decreased activity at α receptors and decreased metabolism by MAO. A final strategy to enhance preferential activation of pulmonary β_2 receptors is the administration by inhalation of small doses of the drug in aerosol form. This approach typically leads to effective activation of β_2 receptors in the bronchi but very low systemic drug concentrations. Consequently, there is less potential to activate cardiac β_1 receptors or to stimulate β_2 receptors in skeletal muscle, which can cause tremor and thereby limit oral therapy.

Administration of β receptor agonists by aerosol (*see* Chapter 27) typically leads to a very rapid therapeutic response, generally within minutes, although some agonists such as *salmeterol* have a delayed onset of action (*see* below). While subcutaneous injection also causes prompt bronchodilation, the peak effect of a drug given orally may be delayed for several hours. Aerosol therapy depends on the delivery of drug to the distal airways. This, in turn, depends on the size of the particles in the aerosol and respiratory parameters such as inspiratory flow rate, tidal volume, breath-holding time, and airway diameter. Only about 10% of an inhaled dose actually enters the lungs; much of the remainder is swallowed and ultimately may be absorbed. Successful aerosol therapy requires that each patient master the technique of drug administration. Many patients, particularly children and the elderly, do not use optimal techniques, often because of inadequate instructions or incoordination. In these patients, spacer devices may enhance the efficacy of inhalation therapy (*see* Chapter 27).

In the treatment of asthma, β receptor agonists are used to activate pulmonary receptors that relax bronchial smooth muscle and decrease airway resistance. Although this action appears to be a major therapeutic effect of these drugs in patients with asthma, evidence suggests that β receptor agonists also may suppress the release of leukotrienes and histamine from mast cells in lung tissue, enhance mucociliary function, decrease microvascular permeability, and possibly inhibit phospholipase A_2 (Seale, 1988). The relative importance of these actions in the treatment of human asthma remains to be determined. However, it is becoming increasingly clear that airway inflammation is directly involved in airway hyperresponsiveness; consequently, the use of antiinflammatory drugs such as inhaled steroids may have primary importance (*see* Chapter 27). The use of β agonists for the treatment of asthma is discussed in Chapter 27.

Metaproterenol. Metaproterenol (called *orciprenaline* in Europe), along with terbutaline and *fenoterol*, belongs to the structural class of resorcinol bronchodilators that have hydroxyl groups at positions 3 and 5 of the phenyl ring (rather than at positions 3 and 4 as in catechols) (Table 10–1). Consequently, metaproterenol is resistant to methylation by COMT, and a substantial fraction (40%) is absorbed in active form after oral administration. It is excreted primarily as glucuronic acid conjugates. Metaproterenol is considered to be β_2 selective, although it probably is less selective than albuterol or terbutaline and hence is more prone to cause cardiac stimulation.

Effects occur within minutes of inhalation and persist for several hours. After oral administration, onset of action is slower, but effects last 3 to 4 hours. Metaproterenol (ALUPENT, others) is used for the long-term treatment of obstructive airway diseases, asthma, and for treatment of acute bronchospasm (*see* Chapter 27). Side effects are similar to the short- and intermediate-acting sympathomimetic bronchodilators.

Terbutaline. Terbutaline is a β_2-selective bronchodilator. It contains a resorcinol ring and thus is not a substrate for COMT methylation. It is effective when taken orally, subcutaneously, or by inhalation.

Effects are observed rapidly after inhalation or parenteral administration; after inhalation its action may persist for 3 to 6 hours. With oral administration, the onset of effect may be delayed for 1 to 2 hours. Terbutaline (BRETHINE, others) is used for the long-term treatment of obstructive airway diseases and for treatment of acute bronchospasm, and also is available for parenteral use for the emergency treatment of status asthmaticus (*see* Chapter 27).

Albuterol. Albuterol (VENTOLIN, PROVENTIL, others) is a selective β_2 receptor agonist with pharmacological properties and therapeutic indications similar to those of terbutaline. It is administered either by inhalation or orally for the symptomatic relief of bronchospasm.

When administered by inhalation, it produces significant bronchodilation within 15 minutes, and effects persist for 3 to 4 hours. The cardiovascular effects of albuterol are considerably weaker than those of isoproterenol when doses that produce comparable bronchodilation are administered by inhalation. Oral albuterol has the potential to delay preterm labor. Although rare, CNS and respiratory side effects are sometimes observed.

Isoetharine. *Isoetharine* was the first β_2-selective drug widely used for the treatment of airway obstruction. However, its degree of selectivity for β_2 receptors may not approach that of some of the other agents. Although resistant to metabolism by MAO, it is a catecholamine and thus is a good substrate for COMT (Table 10–1). Consequently, it is used only by inhalation for the treatment of acute episodes of bronchoconstriction.

Pirbuterol. *Pirbuterol* is a relatively selective β_2 agonist. Its structure is identical to albuterol except for the substitution of a pyridine ring for the benzene ring. Pirbuterol acetate (MAXAIR) is available for inhalation therapy; dosing is typically every 4 to 6 hours.

Bitolterol. *Bitolterol* (TORNALATE) is a novel β_2 agonist in which the hydroxyl groups in the catechol moiety are protected by esterification with 4-methylbenzoate. Esterases in the lung and other tissues hydrolyze this prodrug to the active form, colterol, or terbutyl-norepinephrine (Table 10–1). Animal studies suggest that these esterases are present in higher concentrations in lung than in tissues such as the heart. The duration of effect of bitolterol after inhalation ranges from 3 to 6 hours.

Fenoterol. Fenoterol (BEROTEC) is a β_2-selective receptor agonist. After inhalation, it has a prompt onset of action, and its effect typically is sustained for 4 to 6 hours. Fenoterol is under investigation for use in the United States. The possible association of fenoterol use with increased deaths from asthma in New Zealand is controversial (Pearce *et al.*, 1995; Suissa and Ernst, 1997).

Formoterol. *Formoterol* (FORADIL) is a long-acting β_2-selective receptor agonist. Significant bronchodilation occurs within minutes of inhalation of a therapeutic dose, which may persist for up to 12 hours (Faulds *et al.*, 1991). It is highly lipophilic and has high affinity for β_2 receptors. Its major advantage over many other β_2-selective agonists is this prolonged duration of action, which may be particularly advantageous in settings such as nocturnal asthma. Formoterol's sustained action is due to its insertion into the lipid bilayer of the plasma membrane, from which it gradually diffuses to provide prolonged stimulation of β_2 receptors (Nelson, 1995). It is FDA approved for treatment of asthma, bronchospasm, prophylaxis of exercise-induced bronchospasm, and chronic obstructive pulmonary disease (COPD). It can be used concomitantly with short-acting β_2 agonists, glucocorticoids (inhaled or systemic), and theophylline (Goldsmith and Keating, 2004).

Procaterol. *Procaterol* (MASCACIN, others) is a β_2-selective receptor agonist. After inhalation, it has a prompt onset of action that is sustained for about 5 hours. Procaterol is not available in the United States.

Salmeterol. Salmeterol (SEREVENT) is a selective β_2 receptor agonist with a prolonged duration of action (>12 hours); it has at least fiftyfold greater selectivity for β_2 receptors than albuterol. It provides symptomatic relief and improves lung function and quality of life in patients with COPD; in this setting, it is as effective as the cholinergic antagonist *ipratropium* and more effective than oral *theophylline*. It has additive effects when used in combination with inhaled ipratropium or oral theophylline. Like formoterol, it is highly lipophilic and has a sustained duration of action; for salmeterol, this long action reflects binding to a specific site within the β_2 receptor that allows for its prolonged activation. It also may have antiinflammatory activity. Salmeterol is metabolized by CYP3A4 to α-hydroxy-salmeterol, which is eliminated primarily in the feces. Since the onset of action of inhaled salmeterol is relatively slow, it is not suitable monotherapy for acute breakthrough attacks of bronchospasm. Salmeterol or formoterol are the agents of choice for nocturnal asthma in patients who remain symptomatic despite antiinflammatory agents and other standard management.

Like formoterol, salmeterol generally is well tolerated but has the potential to increase heart rate and plasma glucose concentration, to produce tremors, and to decrease plasma potassium concentration through effects on extrapulmonary β_2 receptors. Salmeterol should not be used more than twice daily (morning and evening) and should not be used to treat acute asthma symptoms, which should be treated with a short-acting β_2 agonist (*e.g.*, albuterol) when breakthrough symptoms occur despite twice-daily use of salmeterol (Redington, 2001).

Ritodrine.
Ritodrine is a selective β_2 receptor agonist that was developed specifically for use as a uterine relaxant. Nevertheless, its pharmacological properties closely resemble those of the other agents in this group.

Ritodrine is rapidly but incompletely (30%) absorbed following oral administration, and 90% of the drug is excreted in the urine as inactive conjugates; about 50% of ritodrine is excreted unchanged after intravenous administration. The pharmacokinetic properties of ritodrine are complex and incompletely defined, especially in pregnant women.

Therapeutic Uses. Ritodrine may be administered intravenously to selected patients to arrest premature labor. Ritodrine and related drugs can prolong pregnancy. However, β_2-selective agonists may not have clinically significant benefits on perinatal mortality and may actually increase maternal morbidity. Given modern improvements in the care of premature babies, it is possible that existing clinical trials may not have had sufficient statistical power to demonstrate subtle, but potentially important, clinical effects. In a multicenter trial comparing *nifedipine* with ritodrine in managing preterm labor, nifedipine was associated with a longer postponement of delivery, fewer maternal side effects, and fewer admissions to the neonatal intensive care unit (Papatsonis *et al.*, 1997).

Adverse Effects of β_2-Selective Agonists.
The major adverse effects of β receptor agonists occur as a result of excessive activation of β receptors. Patients with underlying cardiovascular disease are particularly at risk for significant reactions. However, the likelihood of adverse effects can be greatly decreased in patients with lung disease by administering the drug by inhalation rather than orally or parenterally.

Tremor is a relatively common adverse effect of the β_2-selective receptor agonists. Tolerance generally develops to this effect; it is not clear whether tolerance reflects desensitization of the β_2 receptors of skeletal muscle or adaptation within the CNS. This adverse effect can be minimized by starting oral therapy with a low dose of drug and progressively increasing the dose as tolerance to the tremor develops. Feelings of restlessness, apprehension, and anxiety may limit therapy with these drugs, particularly oral or parenteral administration.

Tachycardia is a common adverse effect of systemically administered β receptor agonists. Stimulation of heart rate occurs primarily *via* β_1 receptors. It is uncertain to what extent the increase in heart rate also is due to activation of cardiac β_2 receptors or to reflex effects that stem from β_2 receptor–mediated peripheral vasodilation. However, during a severe asthma attack, heart rate actually may decrease during therapy with a β agonist, presumably because of improvement in pulmonary function with consequent reduction in endogenous cardiac sympathetic stimulation. In patients without cardiac disease, β agonists rarely cause significant arrhythmias or myocardial ischemia; however, patients with underlying coronary artery disease or preexisting arrhythmias are at greater risk. The risk of adverse cardiovascular effects also is increased in patients who are receiving MAO inhibitors. In general, at least 2 weeks should elapse between the use of MAO inhibitors and administration of β_2 receptor agonists or other sympathomimetics.

Arterial O_2 tension may fall when treatment of patients with acute exacerbations of asthma is begun; this may be due to drug-induced pulmonary vascular dilation, which leads to increased ventilation:perfusion mismatch. This effect usually is small and transient. Supplemental oxygen should be given if necessary. Severe pulmonary edema has been reported in women receiving ritodrine or terbutaline for premature labor.

The results of a number of epidemiologic studies have suggested a possible connection between prolonged use of β receptor agonists and death or near-death from asthma (Suissa *et al.*, 1994). While exact interpretation of these results is difficult, these studies have raised questions about the role of β agonists in the treatment of chronic asthma. Tolerance to effects of β agonists has been studied extensively, both *in vitro* and *in vivo* (*see* Chapter 6). Their long-term systemic administration leads to downregulation of β receptors in some tissues and decreased pharmacological responses. However, it appears likely that tolerance to the pulmonary effects of these drugs is not a major clinical problem for the majority of asthmatics, who do not exceed recommended dosages of β receptor agonists over prolonged periods.

There is some evidence suggesting that regular use of β_2-selective agonists may cause increased bronchial hyperreactivity and deterioration in disease control (Hancox *et al.*, 1999). To what extent this potential adverse association may be even more unfavorable for very long-acting β agonists or excess doses of medication is not yet known (Beasley *et al.*, 1999). However, for patients requiring regular use of these drugs over prolonged periods, strong consideration should be given to additional or alternative therapy, such as the use of inhaled glucocorticoids.

Large doses of β receptor agonists cause myocardial necrosis in laboratory animals. When given parenterally, these drugs also may increase the concentrations of glucose, lactate, and free fatty acids in plasma and decrease the concentration of K^+. The decrease in K^+ concentration may be especially important in patients with cardiac disease, particularly those taking *digoxin* and diuretics. In some diabetic patients, hyperglycemia may be worsened by these drugs, and higher doses of insulin may be required. All these adverse effects are far less likely with inhalation therapy than with parenteral or oral therapy.

α_1-SELECTIVE ADRENERGIC RECEPTOR AGONISTS

The major clinical effects of a number of sympathomimetic drugs are due to activation of α adrenergic receptors in vascular smooth muscle. As a result, peripheral vascular resistance is increased and blood pressure is maintained or elevated. Although the clinical utility of these drugs is limited, they may be useful in the treatment of some patients with hypotension, including orthostatic hypotension, or shock. Phenylephrine and methoxamine (discontinued in the United States) are direct-acting vasoconstrictors and are selective activators of α_1 receptors. *Mephentermine* and metaraminol act both directly and indirectly. *Midodrine* is a prodrug that is converted, after oral administration, to desglymidodrine, a direct-acting α_1 agonist.

Phenylephrine

Phenylephrine is a selective α_1 receptor agonist; it activates β receptors only at much higher concentrations.

Chemically, phenylephrine differs from epinephrine only in lacking a hydroxyl group at position 4 on the benzene ring (Table 10–1). The pharmacological effects of phenylephrine are similar to those of methoxamine. The drug causes marked arterial vasoconstriction during intravenous infusion. Phenylephrine (NEO-SYNEPHRINE, others) also is used as a nasal decongestant and as a mydriatic in various nasal and ophthalmic formulations (*see* Chapter 63 for ophthalmic uses).

Mephentermine

Mephentermine (Table 10–1) is a sympathomimetic drug that acts both directly and indirectly; it has many similarities to ephedrine (*see* below). After an intramuscular injection, the onset of action is prompt (within 5 to 15 minutes), and effects may last for several hours. Since the drug releases norepinephrine, cardiac contraction is enhanced, and cardiac output and systolic and diastolic pressures usually are increased. The change in heart rate is variable, depending on the degree of vagal tone. Adverse effects are related to CNS stimulation, excessive rises in blood pressure, and arrhythmias. Mephentermine (WYAMINE SULFATE) is used to prevent hypotension, which frequently accompanies spinal anesthesia.

Metaraminol

Metaraminol (ARAMINE) (Table 10–1) is a sympathomimetic drug with prominent direct effects on vascular α adrenergic receptors. Metaraminol also is an indirectly acting agent that stimulates the release of norepinephrine. The drug has been used in the treatment of hypotensive states or off-label to relieve attacks of paroxysmal atrial tachycardia, particularly those associated with hypotension (*see* Chapter 34 for preferable treatments of this arrhythmia).

Midodrine

Midodrine (PROAMATINE) is an orally effective α_1 receptor agonist. It is a prodrug; its activity is due to its conversion to an active metabolite, desglymidodrine, which achieves peak concentrations about 1 hour after a dose of midodrine. The half-life of desglymidodrine is about 3 hours. Consequently, the duration of action is about 4 to 6 hours. Midodrine-induced rises in blood pressure are associated with both arterial and venous smooth muscle contraction. This is advantageous in the treatment of patients with autonomic insufficiency and postural hypotension (McClellan *et al.*, 1998). A frequent complication in these patients is supine hypertension. This can be minimized by avoiding dosing prior to bedtime and elevating the head of the bed. Very cautious use of a short-acting antihypertensive drug at bedtime may be useful in some patients. Typical dosing, achieved by careful titration of blood pressure responses, varies between 2.5 and 10 mg three times daily.

α_2-SELECTIVE ADRENERGIC RECEPTOR AGONISTS

α_2-Selective adrenergic agonists are used primarily for the treatment of systemic hypertension. Their efficacy as antihypertensive agents is somewhat surprising, since many blood vessels contain postsynaptic α_2 adrenergic receptors that promote vasoconstriction (*see* Chapter 6). Indeed, *clonidine*, the prototypic α_2 agonist, was initially developed as a vasoconstricting nasal decongestant. Its capacity to lower blood pressure results from activation of α_2 receptors in the cardiovascular control centers of the CNS; such activation suppresses the outflow of sympathetic nervous system activity from the brain.

In addition, α_2 agonists reduce intraocular pressure by decreasing the production of aqueous humor. This action first was reported for clonidine and suggested a potential role for α_2 receptor agonists in the management of ocular hypertension and glaucoma. Unfortunately, clonidine lowered systemic blood pressure even if applied topically to the eye (Alward, 1998). Two derivatives of clonidine, *apraclonidine* and *brimonidine*, have been developed that retain the ability to decrease intraocular pressure with little or no effect on systemic blood pressure.

Clonidine

Clonidine, an imidazoline, was synthesized in the early 1960s and found to produce vasoconstriction that was mediated by α receptors. During clinical testing of the drug as a topical nasal decongestant, clonidine was found to cause hypotension, sedation, and bradycardia. The structural formula of clonidine is:

CLONIDINE

Pharmacological Effects. The major pharmacological effects of clonidine involve changes in blood pressure and heart rate, although the drug has a variety of other important actions. Intravenous infusion of clonidine causes an acute rise in blood pressure, apparently because of activation of postsynaptic α_2 receptors in vascular smooth muscle. The affinity of clonidine for these receptors is high, although the drug is a partial agonist with relatively low efficacy at these sites. The hypertensive response that follows parenteral administration of clonidine generally is not seen when the drug is given orally. However, even after intravenous administration, the transient vasoconstriction is followed by a more prolonged hypotensive response that results from decreased sympathetic outflow from the CNS. The exact mechanism by which clonidine lowers blood pressure is

not completely understood. The effect appears to result, at least in part, from activation of α_2 receptors in the lower brainstem region. This central action has been demonstrated by infusing small amounts of the drug into the vertebral arteries or by injecting it directly into the cisterna magna.

Questions remain about whether the sympatho-inhibitory action of clonidine results solely from its α_2 receptor agonism or whether part or all of its actions are mediated by imidazoline receptors. Imidazoline receptors include three subtypes (I_1, I_2, and I_3) and are widely distributed in the body, including the CNS. Clonidine, as an imidazoline, binds to these imidazoline receptors, in addition to its well-described binding to α_2 receptors. Two newer antihypertensive imidazolines, *rilmenidine* and *moxonidine*, have profiles of action similar to clonidine, suggesting a role for I_1 receptors. However, the lack of an antihypertensive effect of clonidine in knockout mice lacking α_{2A} receptors supports a key role for these receptors in blood pressure regulation (MacMillan *et al.*, 1996; Zhu *et al.*, 1999). Others argue that, while the action of clonidine may be mediated by α_2 receptors, the I_1 receptor mediates the effects of moxonidine and rilmenidine. Finally, the α_2 receptor and the imidazoline receptors may cooperatively regulate vasomotor tone and may jointly mediate the hypotensive actions of centrally acting drugs with affinity for both receptor types.

Clonidine decreases discharges in sympathetic preganglionic fibers in the splanchnic nerve and in postganglionic fibers of cardiac nerves. These effects are blocked by α_2-selective antagonists such as *yohimbine*. Clonidine also stimulates parasympathetic outflow, which may contribute to the slowing of heart rate as a consequence of increased vagal tone and diminished sympathetic drive. In addition, some of the antihypertensive effects of clonidine may be mediated by activation of presynaptic α_2 receptors that suppress the release of norepinephrine, ATP, and NPY from postganglionic sympathetic nerves. Clonidine decreases the plasma concentration of norepinephrine and reduces its excretion in the urine.

Absorption, Fate, and Excretion. Clonidine is well absorbed after oral administration, and its bioavailability is nearly 100%. The peak concentration in plasma and the maximal hypotensive effect are observed 1 to 3 hours after an oral dose. The elimination half-life of the drug ranges from 6 to 24 hours, with a mean of about 12 hours. About half of an administered dose can be recovered unchanged in the urine, and the half-life of the drug may increase with renal failure. There is good correlation between plasma concentrations of clonidine and its pharmacological effects. A transdermal delivery patch permits continuous administration of clonidine as an alternative to oral therapy. The drug is released at an approximately constant rate for a week; 3 or 4 days are required to reach steady-state concentrations in plasma. When the patch is removed, plasma concentrations remain stable for about 8 hours and then decline gradually over a period of several days; this decrease is associated with a rise in blood pressure.

Adverse Effects. The major adverse effects of clonidine are dry mouth and sedation. These responses occur in at least 50% of patients and may require drug discontinuation. However, they may diminish in intensity after several weeks of therapy. Sexual dysfunction also may occur. Marked bradycardia is observed in some patients. These and some of the other adverse effects of clonidine frequently are related to dose, and their incidence may be lower with transdermal administration of clonidine, since antihypertensive efficacy may be achieved while avoiding the relatively high peak concentrations that occur after oral administration of the drug. About 15% to 20% of patients develop contact dermatitis when using clonidine in the transdermal system. Withdrawal reactions follow abrupt discontinuation of long-term therapy with clonidine in some hypertensive patients.

Therapeutic Uses. The major therapeutic use of clonidine (CATAPRES, others) is in the treatment of hypertension (*see* Chapter 32). Clonidine also has apparent efficacy in the off-label treatment of a range of other disorders. Stimulation of α_2 receptors in the GI tract may increase absorption of sodium chloride and fluid and inhibit secretion of bicarbonate. This may explain why clonidine has been found to be useful in reducing diarrhea in some diabetic patients with autonomic neuropathy. Clonidine also is useful in treating and preparing addicted subjects for withdrawal from narcotics, alcohol, and tobacco (*see* Chapter 23). Clonidine may help ameliorate some of the adverse sympathetic nervous activity associated with withdrawal from these agents, as well as decrease craving for the drug. The long-term benefits of clonidine in these settings and in neuropsychiatric disorders remain to be determined. Clonidine may be useful in selected patients receiving anesthesia because it may decrease the requirement for anesthetic and increase hemodynamic stability (Hayashi and Maze, 1993; *see* Chapter 13). Other potential benefits of clonidine and related drugs such as *dexmedetomidine* (PRECEDEX; a relatively selective α_2 receptor agonist with sedative properties) in anesthesia include preoperative sedation and anxiolysis, drying of secretions, and analgesia. Transdermal administration of clonidine (CATAPRES-TTS) may be useful in reducing the incidence of menopausal hot flashes.

Acute administration of clonidine has been used in the differential diagnosis of patients with hypertension and suspected pheochromocytoma. In patients with primary hypertension, plasma concentrations of norepinephrine are markedly suppressed after a single dose of clonidine; this response is not observed in many patients with pheochromocytoma. The capacity of clonidine to activate postsynaptic α_2 receptors in vascular smooth muscle has been exploited in a limited number of patients whose autonomic failure is so severe that reflex sympathetic responses on standing are absent; postural hypotension is thus marked. Since the central effect of clonidine on blood pressure is unimportant in these patients, the drug can elevate blood pressure and improve the symptoms of postural hypotension. Among the other off-label uses of clonidine are atrial fibrillation, attention-deficit/hyperactivity disorder, constitutional growth delay in children, *cyclosporine*-associated nephrotoxicity, Tourette's syndrome, hyperhidrosis, mania, posthepatic neuralgia, psychosis, restless leg syndrome, ulcerative colitis, and allergy-induced inflammatory reactions in patients with extrinsic asthma.

Apraclonidine

Apraclonidine (IOPIDINE) is a relatively selective α_2 receptor agonist that is used topically to reduce intraocular pressure. It can reduce elevated as well as normal intraocular pressure whether accompanied by glaucoma or not. The reduction in intraocular pressure occurs with minimal or no effects on systemic cardiovascular parameters; thus, apraclonidine

is more useful than clonidine for ophthalmic therapy. Apparently apraclonidine does not cross the blood–brain barrier. The mechanism of action of apraclonidine is related to α_2 receptor–mediated reduction in the formation of aqueous humor.

The clinical utility of apraclonidine is most apparent as short-term adjunctive therapy in glaucoma patients whose intraocular pressure is not well controlled by other pharmacological agents such as β receptor antagonists, parasympathomimetics, or carbonic anhydrase inhibitors. The drug also is used to control or prevent elevations in intraocular pressure that occur in patients after laser trabeculoplasty or iridotomy (*see* Chapter 63).

Brimonidine

Brimonidine (ALPHAGAN), is another clonidine derivative that is administered ocularly to lower intraocular pressure in patients with ocular hypertension or open-angle glaucoma. Brimonidine is a α_2-selective agonist that reduces intraocular pressure both by decreasing aqueous humor production and by increasing outflow (*see* Chapter 63). The efficacy of brimonidine in reducing intraocular pressure is similar to that of the β receptor antagonist *timolol*. Unlike apraclonidine, brimonidine can cross the blood–brain barrier and can produce hypotension and sedation, although these CNS effects are slight compared to those of clonidine. As with all α_2 receptor agonists, this drug should be used with caution in patients with cardiovascular disease.

Guanfacine

Guanfacine is a phenylacetylguanidine derivative. Its structural formula is:

GUANFACINE

Guanfacine (TENEX) is an α_2 receptor agonist that is more selective for α_2 receptors than is clonidine. Like clonidine, guanfacine lowers blood pressure by activation of brainstem receptors with resultant suppression of sympathetic activity. The drug is well absorbed after oral administration and has a large volume of distribution (4 to 6 liters/kg). About 50% of guanfacine appears unchanged in the urine; the rest is metabolized. The half-time for elimination ranges from 12 to 24 hours. Guanfacine and clonidine appear to have similar efficacy for the treatment of hypertension. The pattern of adverse effects also is similar for the two drugs, although it has been suggested that some of these effects may be milder and occur less frequently with guanfacine (Sorkin and Heel, 1986). A withdrawal syndrome may occur after the abrupt discontinuation of guanfacine, but it appears to be less frequent and milder than the syndrome that follows clonidine withdrawal. Part of this difference may relate to the longer half-life of guanfacine.

Guanabenz

Guanabenz and guanfacine are closely related chemically and pharmacologically. The structural formula of guanabenz is:

GUANABENZ

Guanabenz (WYTENSIN, others) is a centrally acting α_2 agonist that decreases blood pressure by a mechanism similar to those of clonidine and guanfacine. Guanabenz has a half-life of 4 to 6 hours and is extensively metabolized by the liver. Dosage adjustment may be necessary in patients with hepatic cirrhosis. The adverse effects caused by guanabenz (*e.g.,* dry mouth and sedation) are similar to those seen with clonidine.

Methyldopa

Methyldopa (α-methyl-3,4-dihydroxyphenylalanine) is a centrally acting antihypertensive agent. It is metabolized to α-methylnorepinephrine in the brain, and this compound is thought to activate central α_2 receptors and lower blood pressure in a manner similar to that of clonidine. Methyldopa is discussed in more detail in Chapter 32.

Tizanidine

Tizanidine (ZANAFLEX, others) is a muscle relaxant used for the treatment of spasticity associated with cerebral and spinal disorders. It also is an α_2 receptor agonist with some properties similar to those of clonidine (Wagstaff and Bryson, 1997).

MISCELLANEOUS SYMPATHOMIMETIC AGONISTS

Amphetamine

Amphetamine, racemic β-phenylisopropylamine (Table 10–1), has powerful CNS stimulant actions in addition to the peripheral α and β actions common to indirect-acting sympathomimetic drugs. Unlike epinephrine, it is effective after oral administration and its effects last for several hours.

Cardiovascular Responses. Amphetamine given orally raises both systolic and diastolic blood pressure. Heart rate often is reflexly slowed; with large doses, cardiac arrhythmias may occur. Cardiac output is not enhanced by therapeutic doses, and cerebral blood flow does not change much. The *l*-isomer is slightly more potent than the *d*-isomer in its cardiovascular actions.

Other Smooth Muscles. In general, smooth muscles respond to amphetamine as they do to other sympathomimetic amines. The contractile effect on the sphincter of the urinary bladder is particularly marked, and for this reason amphetamine has been used in treating enuresis and incontinence. Pain and difficulty in micturition occasionally occur. The gastrointestinal effects of amphetamine are

unpredictable. If enteric activity is pronounced, amphetamine may cause relaxation and delay the movement of intestinal contents; if the gut already is relaxed, the opposite effect may occur. The response of the human uterus varies, but there usually is an increase in tone.

Central Nervous System. Amphetamine is one of the most potent sympathomimetic amines in stimulating the CNS. It stimulates the medullary respiratory center, lessens the degree of central depression caused by various drugs, and produces other signs of CNS stimulation. These effects are thought to be due to cortical stimulation and possibly to stimulation of the reticular activating system. In contrast, the drug can obtund the maximal electroshock seizure discharge and prolong the ensuing period of depression. In elicitation of CNS excitatory effects, the *d*-isomer (*dextroamphetamine*) is three to four times more potent than the *l*-isomer.

The psychic effects depend on the dose and the mental state and personality of the individual. The main results of an oral dose of 10 to 30 mg include wakefulness, alertness, and a decreased sense of fatigue; elevation of mood, with increased initiative, self-confidence, and ability to concentrate; often, elation and euphoria; and increase in motor and speech activities. Performance of simple mental tasks is improved, but, although more work may be accomplished, the number of errors may increase. Physical performance—in athletes, for example—is improved, and the drug often is abused for this purpose. These effects are not invariable and may be reversed by overdosage or repeated usage. Prolonged use or large doses are nearly always followed by depression and fatigue. Many individuals given amphetamine experience headache, palpitation, dizziness, vasomotor disturbances, agitation, confusion, dysphoria, apprehension, delirium, or fatigue (*see* Chapter 23).

Fatigue and Sleep. Prevention and reversal of fatigue by amphetamine have been studied extensively in the laboratory, in military field studies, and in athletics. In general, the duration of adequate performance is prolonged before fatigue appears, and the effects of fatigue are at least partly reversed. The most striking improvement appears to occur when performance has been reduced by fatigue and lack of sleep. Such improvement may be partly due to alteration of unfavorable attitudes toward the task. However, amphetamine reduces the frequency of attention lapses that impair performance after prolonged sleep deprivation and thus improves execution of tasks requiring sustained attention. The need for sleep may be postponed, but it cannot be avoided indefinitely. When the drug is discontinued after long use, the pattern of sleep may take as long as 2 months to return to normal.

Analgesia. Amphetamine and some other sympathomimetic amines have a small analgesic effect, but it is not sufficiently pronounced to be therapeutically useful. However, amphetamine can enhance the analgesia produced by opiates.

Respiration. Amphetamine stimulates the respiratory center, increasing the rate and depth of respiration. In normal individuals, usual doses of the drug do not appreciably increase respiratory rate or minute volume. Nevertheless, when respiration is depressed by centrally-acting drugs, amphetamine may stimulate respiration.

Depression of Appetite. Amphetamine and similar drugs have been used for the treatment of obesity, although the wisdom of this use is at best questionable. Weight loss in obese humans treated with amphetamine is almost entirely due to reduced food intake and only in small measure to increased metabolism. The site of action probably is in the lateral hypothalamic feeding center; injection of amphetamine into this area, but not into the ventromedial region, suppresses food intake. Neurochemical mechanisms of action are unclear but may involve increased release of norepinephrine and/or dopamine (Samanin and Garattini, 1993). In humans, tolerance to the appetite suppression develops rapidly. Hence, continuous weight reduction usually is not observed in obese individuals without dietary restriction (Bray, 1993).

Mechanisms of Action in the CNS. Amphetamine appears to exert most or all of its effects in the CNS by releasing biogenic amines from their storage sites in nerve terminals. The alerting effect of amphetamine, its anorectic effect, and at least a component of its locomotor-stimulating action presumably are mediated by release of norepinephrine from central noradrenergic neurons. These effects can be prevented in experimental animals by treatment with α-methyltyrosine, an inhibitor of tyrosine hydroxylase, and therefore of catecholamine synthesis. Some aspects of locomotor activity and the stereotyped behavior induced by amphetamine probably are a consequence of the release of dopamine from dopaminergic nerve terminals, particularly in the neostriatum. Higher doses are required to produce these behavioral effects, and this correlates with the higher concentrations of amphetamine required to release dopamine from brain slices or synaptosomes *in vitro*. With still higher doses of amphetamine, disturbances of perception and overt psychotic behavior occur. These effects may be due to release of 5-hydroxytryptamine (serotonin, 5-HT) from serotonergic neurons and of dopamine in the mesolimbic system. In addition, amphetamine may exert direct effects on central receptors for 5-HT (*see* Chapter 11).

Toxicity and Adverse Effects. The acute toxic effects of amphetamine usually are extensions of its therapeutic actions, and as a rule result from overdosage. CNS effects commonly include restlessness, dizziness, tremor, hyperactive reflexes, talkativeness, tenseness, irritability, weakness, insomnia, fever, and sometimes euphoria. Confusion, aggressiveness, changes in libido, anxiety, delirium, paranoid hallucinations, panic states, and suicidal or homicidal tendencies occur, especially in mentally ill patients. However, these psychotic effects can be elicited in any individual if sufficient quantities of amphetamine are ingested for a prolonged period. Fatigue and depression usually follow central stimulation. Cardiovascular effects are common and include headache, chilliness, pallor or flushing, palpitation, cardiac arrhythmias, anginal pain, hypertension or hypotension, and circulatory collapse. Excessive sweating occurs. Gastrointestinal symptoms include dry mouth, metallic taste, anorexia, nausea, vomiting, diarrhea, and abdominal cramps. Fatal poisoning usually terminates in convulsions and coma, and cerebral hemorrhages are the main pathological findings.

The toxic dose of amphetamine varies widely. Toxic manifestations occasionally occur as an idiosyncratic reaction after as little as

2 mg, but are rare with doses of less than 15 mg. Severe reactions have occurred with 30 mg, yet doses of 400 to 500 mg are not uniformly fatal. Larger doses can be tolerated after chronic use of the drug.

Treatment of acute amphetamine intoxication may include acidification of the urine by administration of ammonium chloride; this enhances the rate of elimination. Sedatives may be required for the CNS symptoms. Severe hypertension may require administration of *sodium nitroprusside* or an α adrenergic receptor antagonist.

Chronic intoxication with amphetamine causes symptoms similar to those of acute overdosage, but abnormal mental conditions are more common. Weight loss may be marked. A psychotic reaction with vivid hallucinations and paranoid delusions, often mistaken for schizophrenia, is the most common serious effect. Recovery usually is rapid after withdrawal of the drug, but occasionally the condition becomes chronic. In these persons, amphetamine may act as a precipitating factor hastening the onset of incipient schizophrenia.

The abuse of amphetamine as a means of overcoming sleepiness and of increasing energy and alertness should be discouraged. The drug should be used only under medical supervision. The amphetamines are schedule II drugs under federal regulations. The additional contraindications and precautions for the use of amphetamine generally are similar to those described above for epinephrine. Its use is inadvisable in patients with anorexia, insomnia, asthenia, psychopathic personality, or a history of homicidal or suicidal tendencies.

Dependence and Tolerance. Psychological dependence often occurs when amphetamine or dextroamphetamine is used chronically, as discussed in Chapter 23. Tolerance almost invariably develops to the anorexigenic effect of amphetamines, and often is seen also in the need for increasing doses to maintain improvement of mood in psychiatric patients. Tolerance is striking in individuals who are dependent on the drug, and a daily intake of 1.7 g without apparent ill effects has been reported. Development of tolerance is not invariable, and cases of narcolepsy have been treated for years without requiring an increase in the initially effective dose.

Therapeutic Uses. Amphetamine is used chiefly for its CNS effects. Dextroamphetamine (DEXEDRINE, others), with greater CNS action and less peripheral action, was used off-label for obesity (but no longer is approved for this purpose because of the risk of abuse) and is FDA approved for the treatment of narcolepsy and attention-deficit/hyperactivity disorder. Their uses are discussed below.

Methamphetamine

Methamphetamine (DESOXYN) is closely related chemically to amphetamine and ephedrine (Table 10–1). In the brain, methamphetamine releases dopamine and other biogenic amines, and inhibits neuronal and vesicular monoamine transporters as well as MAO.

Small doses have prominent central stimulant effects without significant peripheral actions; somewhat larger doses produce a sustained rise in systolic and diastolic blood pressures, due mainly to cardiac stimulation. Cardiac output is increased, although the heart rate may be reflexly slowed. Venous constriction causes peripheral venous pressure to increase. These factors tend to increase the venous return, and thus cardiac output. Pulmonary arterial pressure is raised, probably owing to increased cardiac output. Methamphetamine is a schedule II drug under federal regulations and has high potential for abuse (*see* Chapter 23). It is widely used as a cheap, accessible recreational drug and methamphetamine abuse is a widespread phenomenon. Its illegal production in clandestine laboratories throughout the United States is common. It is used principally for its central effects, which are more pronounced than those of amphetamine and are accompanied by less prominent peripheral actions. These uses are discussed below.

Methylphenidate

Methylphenidate is a piperidine derivative that is structurally related to amphetamine and has the following formula:

METHYLPHENIDATE

Methylphenidate (RITALIN, others) is a mild CNS stimulant with more prominent effects on mental than on motor activities. However, large doses produce signs of generalized CNS stimulation that may lead to convulsions. Its pharmacological properties are essentially the same as those of the amphetamines. Methylphenidate also shares the abuse potential of the amphetamines and is listed as a schedule II controlled substance in the United States. Methylphenidate is effective in the treatment of narcolepsy and attention-deficit/hyperactivity disorder, as described below.

Methylphenidate is readily absorbed after oral administration and reaches peak concentrations in plasma in about 2 hours. The drug is a racemate; its more potent (+) enantiomer has a half-life of about 6 hours, and the less potent (−) enantiomer has a half-life of about 4 hours. Concentrations in the brain exceed those in plasma. The main urinary metabolite is a deesterified product, ritalinic acid, which accounts for 80% of the dose. The use of methylphenidate is contraindicated in patients with glaucoma.

Dexmethylphenidate

Dexmethylphenidate (FOCALIN) is the *d*-threo enantiomer of racemic methylphenidate. It is FDA approved for the treatment of attention-deficit/hyperactivity disorder and is listed as a schedule II controlled substance in the United States.

Pemoline

Pemoline (CYLERT, others) is structurally dissimilar to methylphenidate but elicits similar changes in CNS function with minimal effects on the cardiovascular system. It is a schedule IV controlled substance in the United States and is employed in treating attention-deficit/hyperactivity disorder. It can be given once daily because of its long half-life. Clinical improvement may require treatment for 3 to 4 weeks. Use of pemoline has been associated with severe hepatic failure.

Ephedrine

Ephedrine is both an α and a β receptor agonist; in addition, it enhances release of norepinephrine from sympathetic neurons and therefore is a mixed-acting sympathomimetic drug. Ephedrine contains two asymmetrical carbon atoms (Table 10–1); only *l*-ephedrine and racemic ephedrine are used clinically.

Pharmacological Actions. Ephedrine does not contain a catechol moiety and is effective after oral administration. The drug stimulates heart rate and cardiac output and variably increases peripheral resistance; as a result, ephedrine usually increases blood pressure. Stimulation of the α receptors of smooth muscle cells in the bladder base may increase the resistance to the outflow of urine. Activation of β receptors in the lungs promotes bronchodilation. Ephedrine is a potent CNS stimulant. After oral administration, effects of the drug may persist for several hours. Ephedrine is eliminated in the urine largely as unchanged drug, with a half-life of about 3 to 6 hours.

Therapeutic Uses and Toxicity. In the past, ephedrine was used to treat Stokes-Adams attacks with complete heart block and as a CNS stimulant in narcolepsy and depressive states. It has been replaced by alternate treatments in each of these disorders. In addition, its use as a bronchodilator in patients with asthma has become much less extensive with the development of β_2-selective agonists. Ephedrine has been used to promote urinary continence, although its efficacy is not clear. Indeed, the drug may cause urinary retention, particularly in men with benign prostatic hyperplasia. Ephedrine also has been used to treat the hypotension that may occur with spinal anesthesia.

Untoward effects of ephedrine include hypertension, particularly after parenteral administration or with higher-than-recommended oral dosing. Insomnia is a common CNS adverse effect. Tachyphylaxis may occur with repetitive dosing. Concerns have been raised about the safety of ephedrine. Usual or higher-than-recommended doses may cause important adverse effects in susceptible individuals and are especially of concern in patients with underlying cardiovascular disease that might be unrecognized. Of potentially greater cause for concern, large amounts of herbal preparations containing ephedrine (ma huang, *ephedra*) are utilized around the world. There can be considerable variability in the content of ephedrine in these preparations, which may lead to inadvertent consumption of higher-than-usual doses of ephedrine and its isomers. Because of this, the FDA has banned the sale of dietary supplements containing ephedra effective April, 2004.

Other Sympathomimetic Agents

Several sympathomimetic drugs are used primarily as vasoconstrictors for local application to the nasal mucous membrane or the

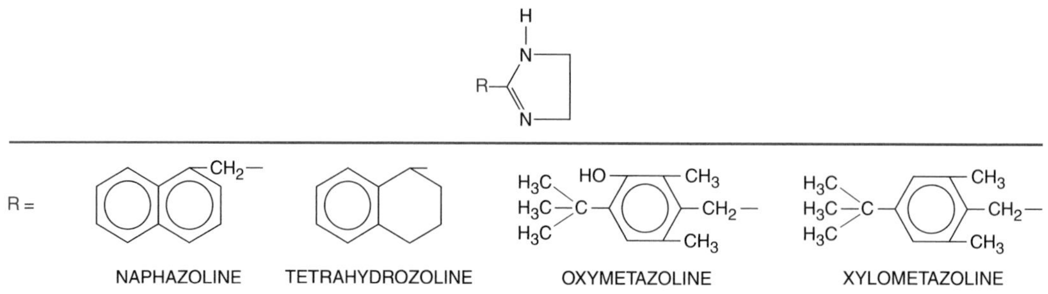

Figure 10–4. *Chemical structures of imidazoline derivatives.*

eye. The structures of *propylhexedrine* (BENZEDREX, others), *naphazoline* (PRIVINE, NAPHCON, others), *oxymetazoline* (AFRIN, OCU-CLEAR, others), and *xylometazoline* (OTRIVIN, others) are depicted in Table 10–1 and Figure 10–4. *Ethylnorepinephrine* (BRONKEPH-RINE) (Table 10–1) is a β receptor agonist that is used as a bronchodilator. The drug also has α receptor agonist activity; this effect may cause local vasoconstriction and thereby reduce bronchial congestion.

Phenylephrine (*see* above), *pseudoephedrine* (SUDAFED, others) (a stereoisomer of ephedrine), and *phenylpropanolamine* are the sympathomimetic drugs that have been used most commonly in oral preparations for the relief of nasal congestion. Pseudoephedrine is available without a prescription in a variety of solid and liquid dosage forms. Phenylpropanolamine shares the pharmacological properties of ephedrine and is approximately equal in potency except that it causes less CNS stimulation. The drug has been available without prescription in tablets and capsules. In addition, numerous proprietary mixtures marketed for the oral treatment of nasal and sinus congestion contain one of these sympathomimetic amines, usually in combination with an H_1-histamine receptor antagonist. Also, phenylpropanolamine suppresses appetite by mechanisms possibly different from those of amphetamines. Concern about the possibility that phenylpropanolamine increases the risk of hemorrhagic stroke led the FDA in 2000 to issue a public warning about the risk. In response to this warning, most manufacturers have voluntarily stopped marketing products containing phenylpropanolamine in the United States and the FDA is in the process of withdrawing approval for the drug.

THERAPEUTIC USES OF SYMPATHOMIMETIC DRUGS

The variety of vital functions that are regulated by the sympathetic nervous system and the success that has attended efforts to develop therapeutic agents that can influence adrenergic receptors selectively have resulted in a class of drugs with a large number of important therapeutic uses.

Shock. Shock is a clinical syndrome characterized by inadequate perfusion of tissues; it usually is associated with hypotension and ultimately with the failure of organ systems (Hollenberg *et al.*, 1999). Shock is an immediately life-threatening impairment of delivery of oxygen and nutrients to the organs of the body. Causes of shock include hypovolemia (due to dehydration or blood loss), cardiac failure (extensive myocardial infarction, severe arrhythmia, or cardiac mechanical defects such as ventricular septal defect), obstruction to cardiac output (due to pulmonary embolism, pericardial tamponade, or aortic dissection), and peripheral circulatory dysfunction (sepsis or anaphylaxis). Recent research on shock has focused on the accompanying increased permeability of the GI mucosa to pancreatic proteases, and on the role of these degradative enzymes on microvascular inflammation and multiorgan failure (Scmid-Schonbein and Hugli, 2005). The treatment of shock consists of specific efforts to reverse the underlying pathogenesis as well as nonspecific measures aimed at correcting hemodynamic abnormalities. Regardless of etiology, the accompanying fall in blood pressure generally leads to marked activation of the sympathetic nervous system. This, in turn, causes peripheral vasoconstriction and an increase in the rate and force of cardiac contraction. In the initial stages of shock these mechanisms may maintain blood pressure and cerebral blood flow, although blood flow to the kidneys, skin, and other organs may be decreased, leading to impaired production of urine and metabolic acidosis (Ruffolo, 1992).

The initial therapy of shock involves basic life-support measures. It is essential to maintain blood volume, which often requires monitoring of hemodynamic parameters. Specific therapy (*e.g.,* antibiotics for patients in septic shock) should be initiated immediately. If these measures do not lead to an adequate therapeutic response, it may be necessary to use vasoactive drugs in an effort to improve abnormalities in blood pressure and flow. This therapy generally is empirically based on response to hemodynamic measurements. Many of these pharmacological approaches, while apparently clinically reasonable, are of uncertain efficacy. Adrenergic receptor agonists may be used in an attempt to increase myocardial contractility or to modify peripheral vascular resistance. In general terms, β receptor agonists increase heart rate and force of contraction, α receptor agonists increase peripheral vascular resistance, and dopamine promotes dilation of renal and splanchnic vascular beds, in addition to activating β and α receptors (Breslow and Ligier, 1991).

Cardiogenic shock due to myocardial infarction has a poor prognosis; therapy is aimed at improving peripheral blood flow. Definitive therapy, such as emergency cardiac catheterization followed by surgical revascularization or angioplasty, may be very important. Mechanical left ventricular assist devices also may help to maintain cardiac output and coronary perfusion in critically ill patients. In the setting of severely impaired cardiac output, falling blood pressure leads to intense sympathetic outflow and vasoconstriction. This may further decrease cardiac output as the damaged heart pumps against a higher peripheral resistance. Medical intervention is designed to optimize cardiac filling pressure (preload), myocardial contractility, and peripheral resistance (afterload). Preload may be increased by administration of intravenous fluids or reduced with drugs such as diuretics and nitrates. A number of sympathomimetic amines have been used to increase the force of contraction of the heart. Some of these drugs have disadvantages: isoproterenol is a powerful chronotropic agent and can greatly increase myocardial oxygen demand; norepinephrine intensifies peripheral vasoconstriction; and epinephrine increases heart rate and may predispose the heart to dangerous arrhythmias. Dopamine is an effective inotropic agent that causes less increase in heart rate than does isoproterenol. Dopamine also promotes renal arterial dilation; this may be useful in preserving renal function. When given in high doses (greater than 10 to 20 μg/kg per minute), dopamine activates α receptors, causing peripheral and renal vasoconstriction. Dobutamine has complex pharmacological actions that are mediated by its stereoisomers; the clinical effects of the drug are to increase myocardial contractility with little increase in heart rate or peripheral resistance.

In some patients in shock, hypotension is so severe that vasoconstricting drugs are required to maintain a blood pressure that is adequate for CNS perfusion (Kulka and Tryba, 1993). Alpha agonists such as norepinephrine, phenylephrine, metaraminol, mephentermine, midodrine, ephedrine, epinephrine, dopamine, and methoxamine all have been used for this purpose. This approach may be advantageous in patients with hypotension due to failure of the sympathetic nervous system (*e.g.,* after spinal anesthesia or injury). However, in patients with other forms of shock, such as cardiogenic shock, reflex vasoconstriction generally is intense, and α receptor agonists may further compromise blood flow to organs such as the kidneys and gut and adversely increase the work of the heart. Indeed, vasodilating drugs such as *nitroprusside* are more likely to improve blood flow and decrease cardiac work in such patients by decreasing afterload if a minimally adequate blood pressure can be maintained.

The hemodynamic abnormalities in septic shock are complex and poorly understood. Most patients with septic shock initially have low or barely normal peripheral vascular resistance, possibly owing to excessive effects of endogenously produced nitric oxide as well as normal or increased cardiac output. If the syndrome progresses, myocardial depression, increased peripheral resistance, and impaired tissue oxygenation occur. The primary treatment of septic shock is antibiotics. Data on the comparative value of various adrenergic agents in the treatment of septic shock are limited. Therapy with drugs such as dopamine or dobutamine is guided by hemodynamic monitoring, with individualization of therapy depending on the patient's overall clinical condition.

Hypotension. Drugs with predominantly α agonist activity can be used to raise blood pressure in patients with decreased peripheral resistance in conditions such as spinal anesthesia or intoxication with antihypertensive medications. However, hypotension *per se* is not an indication for treatment with these agents unless there is inadequate perfusion of organs such as the brain, heart, or kidneys. Furthermore, adequate replacement of fluid or blood may be more appropriate than drug therapy for many patients with hypotension. In patients with spinal anesthesia that interrupts sympathetic activation of the heart, injections of ephedrine increase heart rate as well as peripheral vascular resistance; tachyphylaxis may occur with repetitive injections, necessitating the use of a directly acting drug.

Patients with orthostatic hypotension (excessive fall in blood pressure with standing) often represent a pharmacological challenge. There are diverse causes for this disorder, including the Shy-Drager syndrome and idiopathic autonomic failure. Therapeutic approaches include physical maneuvers and a variety of drugs (*fludrocortisone*, prostaglandin synthesis inhibitors, somatostatin analogs, *caffeine*, vasopressin analogs, and dopamine antagonists). A number of sympathomimetic drugs also have been used in treating this disorder. The ideal agent would enhance venous constriction prominently and produce relatively little arterial constriction so as to avoid supine hypertension. No such agent currently is available. Drugs used in this disorder to activate α_1 receptors include both direct- and indirect-acting agents. Midodrine shows promise in treating this challenging disorder.

Hypertension. Centrally acting α_2 receptor agonists such as clonidine are useful in the treatment of hypertension. Drug therapy of hypertension is discussed in Chapter 32.

Cardiac Arrhythmias. Cardiopulmonary resuscitation in patients with cardiac arrest due to ventricular fibrillation, electromechanical dissociation, or asystole may be facilitated by drug treatment. Epinephrine is an important therapeutic agent in patients with cardiac arrest; epinephrine and other α agonists increase diastolic pressure and improve coronary blood flow. Alpha agonists also help to preserve cerebral blood flow during resuscitation. Cerebral blood vessels are relatively insensitive to the vasoconstricting effects of catecholamines, and perfusion pressure is increased. Consequently, during external cardiac massage, epinephrine facilitates distribution of the limited cardiac output to the cerebral and coronary circulations. Although it had been thought that the β adrenergic effects of epinephrine on the heart made ventricular fibrillation more susceptible to conversion with electrical countershock, tests in animal models have not confirmed this hypothesis. The optimal dose of epinephrine in patients with cardiac arrest is unclear. Once a cardiac rhythm has been restored, it may be necessary to treat arrhythmias, hypotension, or shock.

In patients with paroxysmal supraventricular tachycardias, particularly those associated with mild hypotension, careful infusion of an α agonist such as phenylephrine or methoxamine to raise blood pressure to about 160 mm Hg may end the arrhythmia by increasing vagal tone. However, this method of treatment has been replaced largely by Ca^{2+} channel blockers with clinically significant effects on the AV node, β receptor antagonists, *adenosine*, and electrical cardioversion (*see* Chapter 34). Beta agonists such as isoproterenol may be used as adjunctive or temporizing therapy with atropine in patients with marked bradycardia who are compromised hemodynamically; if long-term therapy is required, a cardiac pacemaker usually is the treatment of choice.

Congestive Heart Failure. Sympathetic stimulation of β receptors in the heart is an important compensatory mechanism for maintenance of cardiac function in patients with congestive heart failure (Francis and Cohn, 1986). Responses mediated by β receptors are blunted in the failing human heart. While β agonists may increase cardiac output in acute emergency settings such as shock, long-term therapy with β agonists as inotropic agents is not efficacious. Indeed, interest has grown in the use of β receptor antagonists in the treatment of patients with congestive heart failure (*see* Chapter 33).

Local Vascular Effects of α Adrenergic Receptor Agonists. Epinephrine is used in many surgical procedures in the nose, throat, and larynx to shrink the mucosa and improve visualization by limiting hemorrhage. Simultaneous injection of epinephrine with local anesthetics retards the absorption of the anesthetic and increases the duration of anesthesia (*see* Chapter 14). Injection of α agonists into the penis may be useful in reversing priapism, a complication of the use of α receptor antagonists or PDE5 inhibitors (*e.g.*, sildenafil) in the treatment of erectile dysfunction. Both phenylephrine and oxymetazoline are efficacious vasoconstrictors when applied locally during sinus surgery.

Nasal Decongestion. α Receptor agonists are used extensively as nasal decongestants in patients with allergic or vasomotor rhinitis and in acute rhinitis in patients with upper respiratory infections. These drugs probably decrease resistance to airflow by decreasing the volume of the nasal mucosa; this may occur by activation of α receptors in venous capacitance vessels in nasal tissues that have erectile characteristics. The receptors that mediate this effect appear to be α_1 receptors. Interestingly, α_2 receptors may mediate contraction of arterioles that supply nutrition to the nasal mucosa. Intense constriction of these vessels may cause structural damage to the mucosa. A major limitation of therapy with nasal decongestants is that loss of efficacy, "rebound" hyperemia, and worsening of symptoms often occur with chronic use or when the drug is stopped. Although mechanisms are uncertain, possibilities include receptor desensitization and damage to the mucosa. Agonists that are selective for α_1 receptors may be less likely to induce mucosal damage (DeBernardis *et al.*, 1987).

For decongestion, α agonists may be administered either orally or topically. Oral ephedrine often causes CNS adverse effects. Pseudoephedrine is a stereoisomer of ephedrine that is less potent than ephedrine in producing tachycardia, increased blood pressure, and CNS stimulation. Sympathomimetic decongestants should be used with great caution in patients with hypertension and in men with prostatic enlargement, and they are contraindicated in patients who are taking MAO inhibitors. A variety of compounds (*see* above) are available for topical use in patients with rhinitis. Topical decongestants are particularly useful in acute rhinitis because of their more selective site of action, but they are apt to be used excessively by patients, leading to rebound congestion. Oral decongestants are much less likely to cause rebound congestion but carry a greater risk of inducing adverse systemic effects. Indeed, patients with uncontrolled hypertension or ischemic heart disease generally should carefully avoid the oral consumption of over-the-counter products or herbal preparations containing sympathomimetic drugs.

Asthma. Use of β adrenergic agonists in the treatment of asthma is discussed in Chapter 27.

Allergic Reactions. Epinephrine is the drug of choice to reverse the manifestations of serious acute hypersensitivity reactions (*e.g.*, from food, bee sting, or drug allergy). A subcutaneous injection of epinephrine rapidly relieves itching, hives, and swelling of lips, eyelids, and tongue. In some patients, careful intravenous infusion of epinephrine may be required to ensure prompt pharmacological effects. This treatment may be life-saving when edema of the glottis threatens airway patency or when there is hypotension or shock in patients with anaphylaxis. In addition to its cardiovascular effects, epinephrine is thought to activate β receptors that suppress the release from mast cells of mediators such as histamine and leukotrienes. Although glucocorticoids and antihistamines frequently are administered to patients with severe hypersensitivity reactions, epinephrine remains the mainstay.

Ophthalmic Uses. Application of various sympathomimetic amines for diagnostic and therapeutic ophthalmic use is discussed in Chapter 63.

Narcolepsy. Narcolepsy is characterized by hypersomnia, including attacks of sleep that may occur suddenly under conditions that are not normally conducive to sleep. Some patients respond to treatment with tricyclic antidepressants or MAO inhibitors. Alternatively, CNS stimulants such as amphetamine, dextroamphetamine, or methamphetamine may be useful (Mitler *et al.*, 1993). *Modafinil* (PROVIGIL), a CNS stimulant, may have benefit in narcolepsy (Fry, 1998). In the United States, it is a schedule IV controlled substance. Its mechanism of action in narcolepsy is unclear and may not involve adrenergic receptors. Therapy with amphetamines is complicated by the risk of abuse and the likelihood of the development of tolerance. Depression, irritability, and paranoia also may occur. Amphetamines may disturb nocturnal sleep, which increases the difficulty of avoiding daytime attacks of sleep in these patients.

Narcolepsy in rare individuals is caused by mutations in the related orexin neuropeptides (also called hypocretins), which are expressed in the lateral hypothalamus, or in their G protein–coupled receptors (Mignot, 2004). Although such mutations are not present in most subjects with narcolepsy, the levels of orexins in the CSF are markedly diminished, suggesting that deficient orexin signaling may play a pathogenic role. The association of these neuropeptides and their cognate GPCRs with narcolepsy provides an attractive target for the development of novel pharmacotherapies for this disorder.

Weight Reduction. Obesity arises as a consequence of positive caloric balance. Optimally, weight loss is achieved by a gradual increase in energy expenditure from exercise combined with dieting to decrease the caloric intake. However, this obvious approach has a relatively low success rate. Consequently, alternative forms of treatment, including surgery or medications, have been developed in an effort to increase the likelihood of achieving and maintaining weight loss. Amphetamine was found to produce weight loss in early studies of patients with narcolepsy and was subsequently used in the treatment of obesity. The drug promotes weight loss by suppressing appetite rather than by increasing energy expenditure. Other anorexic drugs include methamphetamine, dextroamphetamine, *phentermine, benzphetamine, phendimetrazine, phenmetrazine, diethylpropion, mazindol,* phenylpropanolamine, and *sibutramine* (a mixed adrenergic/serotonergic drug). In short-term (up to 20 weeks), double-blind controlled studies, amphetamine-like drugs have been shown to be more effective than placebo in promoting weight loss; the rate of weight loss typically is increased by about 0.5 pound per week with these drugs. There is little to choose among these drugs in terms of efficacy. However, long-term weight loss has not been demonstrated unless these drugs are taken continuously (Bray, 1993). In addition, other important issues have not yet been resolved, including the selection of patients who might benefit from these drugs, whether the drugs should be administered continuously or intermittently, and the duration of treatment. Adverse effects of treatment include the potential for drug abuse and habituation, serious worsening of hypertension (although in some patients blood pressure actually may fall, presumably as a consequence of weight loss), sleep disturbances, palpitations, and dry mouth. These agents may be effective adjuncts in the treatment of obesity. However, available evidence does not support the isolated use of these drugs in the absence of a more comprehensive program that stresses exercise and modification of diet. β_3 Receptor agonists were found to have remarkable antiobesity and antidiabetic effects in rodents. However, pharmaceutical companies have not yet succeeded in developing β_3 receptor agonists for the treatment of these conditions in humans, perhaps because of important differences in β_3 receptors between humans and rodents. With the cloning of the human β_3 receptor, compounds with favorable metabolic effects have been developed. The use of β_3 agonists in the treatment of obesity remains a possibility for the future (Robidoux *et al.*, 2004; Fernandez-Lopez *et al.*, 2002).

Attention-Deficit/Hyperactivity Disorder (ADHD). This syndrome, usually first evident in childhood, is characterized by excessive motor activity, difficulty in sustaining attention, and impulsiveness. Children with this disorder frequently are troubled by difficulties in school, impaired interpersonal relationships, and excitability. Academic underachievement is an important characteristic. A substantial number of children with this syndrome have characteristics that persist into adulthood, although in modified form. Behavioral therapy may be helpful in some patients. Catecholamines may be involved in the control of attention at the level of the cerebral cortex. A variety of stimulant drugs have been utilized in the treatment of ADHD, and they are particularly indicated in moderate-to-severe cases. Dextroamphetamine has been demonstrated to be more effective than placebo. Methylphenidate is effective in children with ADHD and is the most common intervention (Swanson and Volkow, 2003). Treatment may start with a dose of 5 mg of methylphenidate in the morning and at lunch; the dose is increased gradually over a period of weeks depending on the response as judged by parents, teachers, and the clinician. The total daily dose generally should not exceed 60 mg; because of its short duration of action, most children require two or three doses of methylphenidate each day. The timing of doses is adjusted individually in accordance with rapidity of onset of effect and duration of action. Methylphenidate, dextroamphetamine, and amphetamine probably have similar efficacy in ADHD and are the preferred drugs in this disorder (Elia *et al.*, 1999). Pemoline appears to be less effective, although like sustained-release preparations of methylphenidate (RITALIN SR, CONCERTA, METADATE) and amphetamine (ADDERAL XR), it may be used once daily in children and adults. Potential adverse effects of these medications include insomnia, abdominal pain, anorexia, and weight loss that may be associated with suppression of growth in children. Minor symptoms may be transient or may respond to adjustment of dosage or administration of the drug with meals. Other drugs that have been utilized include tricyclic antidepressants, antipsychotic agents, and clonidine (Fox and Rieder, 1993).

II. ADRENERGIC RECEPTOR ANTAGONISTS

Many types of drugs interfere with the function of the sympathetic nervous system and thus have profound effects on the physiology of sympathetically innervated organs. Several of these drugs are important in clinical medicine, particularly for the treatment of cardiovascular diseases. Drugs that decrease the amount of norepinephrine released as a consequence of sympathetic nerve stimulation or that inhibit sympathetic nervous activity by suppressing sympathetic outflow from the brain are discussed in Chapter 32.

The remainder of this chapter focuses on drugs termed adrenergic receptor *antagonists,* which inhibit the interaction of norepinephrine, epinephrine, and other sympathomimetic drugs with α and β receptors (*see* Figure 10–5). Almost all of these agents are competitive antagonists; an important exception is *phenoxybenzamine*, an irreversible antagonist that binds covalently to α receptors. There are important structural differences among the various types of adrenergic receptors (*see* Chapter 6). Since compounds have been developed that have different affinities for the various receptors, it is possible to interfere selectively with responses that result from stimulation of the sympathetic nervous system. For example, selective antagonists of β_1 receptors block most actions of epinephrine and norepinephrine on the heart, while having less effect on β_2 receptors in bronchial smooth muscle and no effect on responses mediated by α_1 or α_2 receptors. Detailed knowledge of the autonomic nervous system and the sites of action of drugs that act on adrenergic receptors is essential for understanding the pharmacological properties and therapeutic uses of this important class of drugs. Additional background material is presented in Chapter 6. Because of their unique antipsychotic activity in the CNS, drugs that block dopamine receptors are considered in Chapter 18.

α ADRENERGIC RECEPTOR ANTAGONISTS

The α adrenergic receptors mediate many of the important actions of endogenous catecholamines. Responses of particular clinical relevance include α_1 receptor–

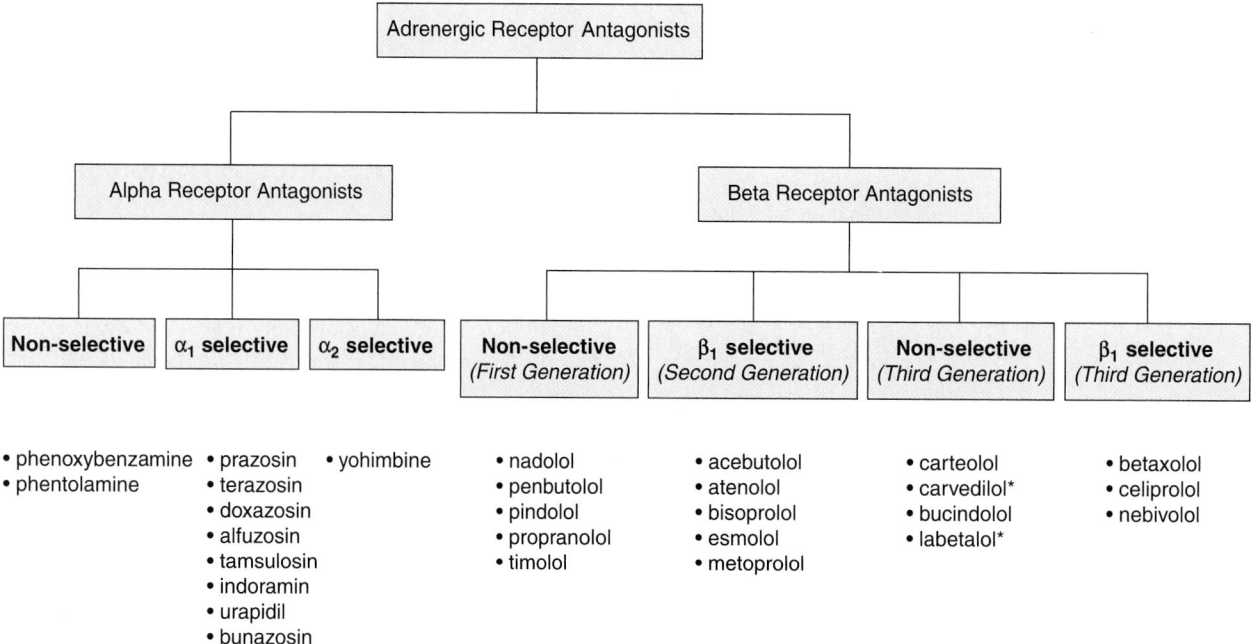

Figure 10–5. ***Classification of adrenergic receptor antagonists.*** Drugs marked by an asterisk (*) also block α_1 receptors.

mediated contraction of arterial and venous smooth muscle. The α_2 receptors are involved in suppressing sympathetic output, increasing vagal tone, facilitating platelet aggregation, inhibiting the release of norepinephrine and acetylcholine from nerve endings, and regulating metabolic effects. These effects include suppression of insulin secretion and inhibition of lipolysis. The α_2 receptors also mediate contraction of some arteries and veins.

Alpha receptor antagonists have a wide spectrum of pharmacological specificities (Table 10–3) and are chemically heterogeneous (Figure 10–6). Some of these drugs have markedly different affinities for α_1 and α_2 receptors. For example, *prazosin* is much more potent in blocking α_1 than α_2 receptors (*i.e.*, α_1 selective), whereas yohimbine is α_2 selective; *phentolamine* has similar affinities for both of these receptor subtypes. More recently, agents that discriminate among the various subtypes of a particular receptor have become available; for example *tamsulosin* has higher potency at α_{1A} than at α_{1B} receptors.

Chemistry. The structural formulas of a number of α receptor antagonists are shown in Figure 10–6. These structurally diverse drugs can be divided into a number of major groups including β-haloethylamine alkylating agents, imidazoline analogs, piperazinyl quinazolines, and indole derivatives. Table 10–3 summarizes the pharmacological properties of drugs in three of these groups.

Pharmacological Properties

Cardiovascular System. Some of the most important effects of α receptor antagonists observed clinically are on the cardiovascular system. Actions in both the CNS and the periphery are involved; the outcome depends on the cardiovascular status of the patient at the time of drug administration and the relative selectivity of the agent for α_1 and α_2 receptors.

α_1 Receptor Antagonists. Blockade of α_1 adrenergic receptors inhibits vasoconstriction induced by endogenous catecholamines; vasodilation may occur in both arteriolar resistance vessels and veins. The result is a fall in blood pressure due to decreased peripheral resistance. The magnitude of such effects depends on the activity of the sympathetic nervous system at the time the antagonist is administered and thus is less in supine than in upright subjects and is particularly marked if there is hypovolemia. For most α receptor antagonists, the fall in blood pressure is opposed by baroreceptor reflexes that cause increases in heart rate and cardiac output, as well as fluid retention. These reflexes are exaggerated if the antagonist also blocks α_2 receptors on peripheral sympathetic nerve endings, leading to enhanced release of norepinephrine and increased stimulation of postsynaptic β_1 receptors in the heart and on juxtaglomerular cells (Starke *et al.*, 1989) (*see* Chapter 6). Although stimula-

Table 10–3

*Comparative Information About α Adrenergic Receptor Antagonists**

	HALOALKYLAMINES	IMIDAZOLINES	QUINAZOLINES
Prototype	Phenoxybenzamine (DIBENZYLINE) (PBZ)	Phentolamine (REGITINE)	Prazosin (MINIPRESS)
Others		Tolazoline (PRISCOLINE)	Terazosin (HYTRIN) Doxazosin (CARDURA) Trimazosin (CARDOVAR) Alfuzosin (UROXATRAL)
Antagonism	Irreversible	Competitive	Competitive
Selectivity	α_1 with some α_2	Nonselective between α_1 and α_2	Selective for α_1; does not distinguish among α_1 subtypes
Hemodynamic effects	Decreased PVR and blood pressure Venodilation is prominent Cardiac stimulation (cardiovascular reflexes and enhanced NE release due to α_2 antagonism)	Similar to PBZ	Decreased PVR and blood pressure Veins less susceptible than arteries; thus, postural hypotension less of a problem Cardiac stimulation is less (NE release is not enhanced due to α_1 selectivity)
Actions other than α blockade	Some antagonism of ACh, 5-HT, and histamine Blockade of neuronal and extraneuronal uptake	Cholinomimetic; adrenomimetic; histamine-like actions Antagonism of 5-HT	At high doses some direct vasodilator action, probably due to PDE inhibition
Routes of administration	Intravenous and oral; oral absorption incomplete and erratic	Similar to PZB	Oral
Adverse reactions	Postural hypotension, tachycardia, miosis, nasal stuffiness, failure of ejaculation	Same as PBZ, plus GI disturbances due to cholinomimetic and histamine-like actions	Some postural hypotension, especially with the first dose; less of a problem overall than with PBZ or phentolamine
Therapeutic uses	Conditions of catecholamine excess (*e.g.*, pheochromocytoma) Peripheral vascular disease	Same as PBZ	Primary hypertension Benign prostatic hypertrophy

*Adapted from Westfall, 2004. *Abbreviations:* ACh, acetylcholine; 5-HT, 5-hydroxytryptamine; PBZ, phenoxybenzamine; NE, norepinephrine; PVR, peripheral vascular resistance.

Alkylating agent

PHENOXYBENZAMINE

Benzenesulfonamide

TAMSULOSIN

Imidazolines

PHENTOLAMINE

TOLAZOLINE

Piperazinyl quinazolines

PRAZOSIN

TERAZOSIN

DOXAZOSIN

Indoles

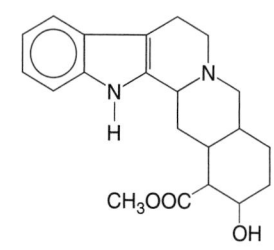

YOHIMBINE

INDORAMIN

Figure 10–6. *Structural formulas of some α adrenergic receptor antagonists.*

tion of α_1 receptors in the heart may cause an increased force of contraction, the importance of blockade at this site in humans is uncertain.

Blockade of α_1 receptors also inhibits vasoconstriction and the increase in blood pressure produced by the administration of a sympathomimetic amine. The pattern of effects depends on the adrenergic agonist that is administered: pressor responses to phenylephrine can be completely suppressed; those to norepinephrine are only incompletely blocked because of residual stimulation of cardiac β_1 receptors; and pressor responses to epinephrine may be transformed to vasodepressor effects because of residual stimulation of β_2 receptors in the vasculature with resultant vasodilation.

α_2 *Adrenergic Receptor Antagonists.* The α_2 receptors have an important role in regulation of the activity of the sympathetic nervous system, both peripherally and centrally. As mentioned above, activation of presynaptic α_2 receptors inhibits the release of norepinephrine and other cotransmitters from peripheral sympathetic nerve endings. Activation of α_2 receptors in the pontomedullary region of the CNS inhibits sympathetic nervous system activity and leads to a fall in blood pressure; these receptors are a site of action for drugs such as clonidine. Blockade of α_2 receptors with selective antagonists such as yohimbine thus can increase sympathetic outflow and potentiate the release of norepinephrine from nerve endings, leading to activation of α_1 and β_1 receptors in the heart and peripheral vasculature with a consequent rise in blood pressure. Antagonists that also block α_1 receptors give rise to similar effects on sympathetic outflow and release of norepinephrine, but the net increase in blood pressure is prevented by inhibition of vasoconstriction.

Although certain vascular beds contain α_2 receptors that promote contraction of smooth muscle, it is thought that these receptors are preferentially stimulated by circulating catecholamines, whereas α_1 receptors are activated by norepinephrine released from sympathetic nerve fibers. In other vascular beds, α_2 receptors reportedly promote vasodilation by stimulating the release of NO from endothelial cells. The physiological role of vascular α_2 receptors in the regulation of blood flow within various vascular beds is uncertain. The α_2 receptors contribute to smooth muscle contraction in the human saphenous vein, whereas α_1 receptors are more prominent in dorsal hand veins. The effects of α_2 receptor antagonists on the cardiovascular system are dominated by actions in the CNS and on sympathetic nerve endings.

Other Actions of α *Adrenergic Receptor Antagonists.* Catecholamines increase the output of glucose from the liver; in humans this effect is mediated predominantly by β receptors, although α receptors may contribute (Rosen *et al.*, 1983). Alpha

receptor antagonists therefore may reduce glucose release. Receptors of the α_{2A} subtype facilitate platelet aggregation; the effect of blockade of platelet α_2 receptors *in vivo* is not clear. Activation of α_2 receptors in the pancreatic islets suppresses insulin secretion; conversely, blockade of pancreatic α_2 receptors may facilitate insulin release (*see* Chapter 60). Alpha receptor antagonists reduce smooth muscle tone in the prostate and neck of the bladder, thereby decreasing resistance to urine outflow in benign prostatic hypertrophy (*see* below).

Phenoxybenzamine and Related Haloalkylamines

Phenoxybenzamine is a haloalkylamine that blocks α_1 and α_2 receptors irreversibly. Although phenoxybenzamine may have slight selectivity for α_1 receptors, it is not clear whether this has any significance in humans.

Chemistry. The haloalkylamine adrenergic blocking drugs are closely related chemically to the nitrogen mustards; as in the latter, the tertiary amine cyclizes with the loss of chlorine to form a reactive etheniminium or aziridinium ion (*see* Chapter 51). The molecular configuration directly responsible for blockade probably is a highly reactive carbonium ion formed upon cleavage of the three-membered ring. It is presumed that the arylalkyl amine moiety of the molecule is responsible for the relative specificity of action of these agents, since the reactive intermediate probably reacts with sulfhydryl, amino, and carboxyl groups in many proteins. Because of these chemical reactions, phenoxybenzamine is covalently conjugated with α receptors. Consequently, receptor blockade is irreversible, and restoration of cellular responsiveness to α receptor agonists probably requires the synthesis of new receptors.

Pharmacological Properties. The major effects of phenoxybenzamine result from blockade of α receptors in smooth muscle. Phenoxybenzamine causes a progressive decrease in peripheral resistance and an increase in cardiac output that is due, in part, to reflex sympathetic nerve stimulation. Tachycardia may be accentuated by enhanced release of norepinephrine (because of α_2 blockade) and decreased inactivation of the amine because of inhibition of neuronal and extraneuronal uptake mechanisms (*see* below and Chapter 6). Pressor responses to exogenously administered catecholamines are impaired. Indeed, hypotensive responses to epinephrine occur because of unopposed β receptor–mediated vasodilation. Although phenoxybenzamine has relatively little effect on supine blood pressure in normotensive subjects, there is a marked fall in blood pressure on standing because of antagonism of compensatory vasoconstriction. In addition, the ability to respond to hypovolemia and anesthetic-induced vasodilation is impaired.

Phenoxybenzamine inhibits the uptake of catecholamines into both sympathetic nerve terminals and extraneuronal tissues. In addition to blockade of α receptors, substituted β haloalkylamines irreversibly inhibit responses to 5-HT, histamine, and ACh. However, somewhat higher doses of phenoxybenzamine are required to produce these effects than to produce blockade of α receptors. More detailed discussion can be found in earlier editions of this textbook.

The pharmacokinetic properties of phenoxybenzamine are not well understood. The half-life of phenoxybenzamine probably is less than 24 hours. However, since the drug irreversibly inactivates α receptors, the duration of its effect is dependent not only on the presence of the drug, but also on the rate of synthesis of α receptors. Many days may be required before the number of functional α receptors on the surface of target cells returns to normal. Blunted maximal responses to catecholamines may not be as persistent, since there are "spare" α_1 receptors in vascular smooth muscle.

Therapeutic Uses. A major use of phenoxybenzamine (DIBEN-ZYLINE) is in the treatment of pheochromocytoma. Pheochromocytomas are tumors of the adrenal medulla and sympathetic neurons that secrete enormous quantities of catecholamines into the circulation. The usual result is hypertension, which may be episodic and severe. The vast majority of pheochromocytomas are treated surgically; however, phenoxybenzamine is almost always used to treat the patient in preparation for surgery. The drug controls episodes of severe hypertension and minimizes other adverse effects of catecholamines, such as contraction of plasma volume and injury of the myocardium. A conservative approach is to initiate treatment with phenoxybenzamine (at a dosage of 10 mg twice daily) 1 to 3 weeks before the operation. The dose is increased every other day until the desired effect on blood pressure is achieved. Therapy may be limited by postural hypotension; nasal stuffiness is another frequent adverse effect. The usual daily dose of phenoxybenzamine in patients with pheochromocytoma is 40 to 120 mg given in two or three divided portions. Prolonged treatment with phenoxybenzamine may be necessary in patients with inoperable or malignant pheochromocytoma. In some patients, particularly those with malignant disease, administration of *metyrosine* may be a useful adjuvant (Perry *et al.*, 1990). Metyrosine is a competitive inhibitor of tyrosine hydroxylase, the rate-limiting enzyme in the synthesis of catecholamines (*see* Chapter 6). Beta receptor antagonists also are used to treat pheochromocytoma, but only after the administration of an α receptor antagonist (*see* below).

Albeit off-label, phenoxybenzamine was the first α receptor antagonist used in the medical therapy of benign prostatic hyperplasia (BPH); blockade of α adrenergic receptors in smooth muscle of the prostate and bladder base may decrease both obstructive symptoms and the need to urinate at night. While the results were promising, significant adverse effects occurred and as a result, phenoxybenzamine is not used to treat BPH. Alpha receptor antagonists such as *doxazosin* and *terazosin* are preferred for this disorder (*see* below). Phenoxybenzamine has been used off-label to control the manifestations of autonomic hyperreflexia in patients with spinal cord transection.

Toxicity and Adverse Effects. The major adverse effect of phenoxybenzamine is postural hypotension. This often is accompanied by reflex tachycardia and other arrhythmias. Hypotension can be par-

ticularly severe in hypovolemic patients or under conditions that promote vasodilation (administration of vasodilator drugs, exercise, ingestion of alcohol or large quantities of food). Reversible inhibition of ejaculation may occur because of impaired smooth muscle contraction in the vas deferens and ejaculatory ducts. Phenoxybenzamine is mutagenic in the Ames test, and repeated administration of this drug to experimental animals causes peritoneal sarcomas and lung tumors. The clinical significance of these findings is not known.

Phentolamine and Tolazoline

Phentolamine, an imidazoline, is a competitive α receptor antagonist that has similar affinities for α_1 and α_2 receptors. Its effects on the cardiovascular system are very similar to those of phenoxybenzamine.

Phenoxybenzamine and phentolamine have played an important role in the establishment of the importance of α receptors in cardiovascular regulation. They sometimes are referred to as "classical" α blockers to distinguish them from more recently developed compounds such as prazosin and its derivatives. Phentolamine also can block receptors for 5-HT, and it causes release of histamine from mast cells; phentolamine also blocks K^+ channels (McPherson, 1993). *Tolazoline* is a related but somewhat less potent compound; it is no longer marketed in the United States. Tolazoline and phentolamine stimulate GI smooth muscle, an effect that is antagonized by *atropine*, and they also enhance gastric acid secretion. Tolazoline stimulates secretion by salivary, lacrimal, and sweat glands as well.

The pharmacokinetic properties of phentolamine are not known, although the drug is extensively metabolized.

Therapeutic Uses. Phentolamine (REGITINE) can be used in short-term control of hypertension in patients with pheochromocytoma. Rapid infusions of phentolamine may cause severe hypotension, so the drug should be administered cautiously. Phentolamine also may be useful to relieve pseudo-obstruction of the bowel in patients with pheochromocytoma; this condition may result from the inhibitory effects of catecholamines on intestinal smooth muscle. Phentolamine has been used locally to prevent dermal necrosis after the inadvertent extravasation of an α receptor agonist. The drug also may be useful for the treatment of hypertensive crises that follow the abrupt withdrawal of clonidine or that may result from the ingestion of tyramine-containing foods during the use of nonselective MAO inhibitors. Although excessive activation of α receptors is important in the development of severe hypertension in these settings, there is little information about the safety and efficacy of phentolamine compared with those of other antihypertensive agents in the treatment of such patients. Direct intracavernous injection of phentolamine (in combination with *papaverine*) has been proposed as a treatment for male sexual dysfunction. The long-term efficacy of this treatment is not known. Intracavernous injection of phentolamine may cause orthostatic hypotension and priapism; pharmacological reversal of drug-induced erections can be achieved with an α receptor agonist such as phenylephrine. Repetitive intrapenile injections may cause fibrotic reactions. Buccally or orally administered phentolamine may have efficacy in some men with sexual dysfunction (Becker *et al.*, 1998).

Toxicity and Adverse Effects. Hypotension is the major adverse effect of phentolamine. In addition, reflex cardiac stimulation may cause alarming tachycardia, cardiac arrhythmias, and ischemic cardiac events, including myocardial infarction. GI stimulation may result in abdominal pain, nausea, and exacerbation of peptic ulcer. Phentolamine should be used with particular caution in patients with coronary artery disease or a history of peptic ulcer.

Prazosin and Related Drugs

Prazosin, the prototype of a family of agents that contain a piperazinyl quinazoline nucleus, is a potent and selective α_1 receptor antagonist. Due in part to its greater α_1 receptor selectivity, the quinazoline class of α receptor antagonists exhibits greater clinical utility and has largely replaced the nonselective haloalkylamine (*e.g.,* phenoxybenzamine) and imidazoline (*e.g.,* phentolamine) α receptor antagonists. The affinity of prazosin for α_1 adrenergic receptors is about one thousandfold greater than that for α_2 adrenergic receptors. Prazosin has similar potencies at α_{1A}, α_{1B}, and α_{1D} subtypes. Interestingly, the drug also is a relatively potent inhibitor of cyclic nucleotide phosphodiesterases, and it originally was synthesized for this purpose. The pharmacological properties of prazosin have been characterized extensively, and the drug frequently is used for the treatment of hypertension (*see* Chapter 32).

Pharmacological Properties. Prazosin. The major effects of prazosin result from its blockade of α_1 receptors in arterioles and veins. This leads to a fall in peripheral vascular resistance and in venous return to the heart. Unlike other vasodilating drugs, administration of prazosin usually does not increase heart rate. Since prazosin has little or no α_2 receptor–blocking effect at concentrations achieved clinically, it probably does not promote the release of norepinephrine from sympathetic nerve endings in the heart. In addition, prazosin decreases cardiac preload and thus has little tendency to increase cardiac output and rate, in contrast to vasodilators such as hydralazine that have minimal dilatory effects on veins. Although the combination of reduced preload and selective α_1 receptor blockade might be sufficient to account for the relative absence of reflex tachycardia, prazosin also may act in the CNS to suppress sympathetic outflow. Prazosin appears to depress baroreflex function in hypertensive patients. Prazosin and related drugs in this class tend to have favorable effects on serum lipids in humans, decreasing low-density lipoproteins (LDL) and triglycerides while increasing concentrations of high-density lipoproteins (HDL). Prazosin and related drugs may have effects on cell

growth unrelated to antagonism of α_1 receptors (Yang *et al.*, 1997; Hu *et al.*, 1998).

Prazosin (MINIPRESS, others) is well absorbed after oral administration, and bioavailability is about 50% to 70%. Peak concentrations of prazosin in plasma generally are reached 1 to 3 hours after an oral dose. The drug is tightly bound to plasma proteins (primarily α_1-acid glycoprotein), and only 5% of the drug is free in the circulation; diseases that modify the concentration of this protein (*e.g.,* inflammatory processes) may change the free fraction. Prazosin is extensively metabolized in the liver, and little unchanged drug is excreted by the kidneys. The plasma half-life is approximately 2 to 3 hours (this may be prolonged to 6 to 8 hours in congestive heart failure). The duration of action of the drug typically is 7 to 10 hours in the treatment of hypertension.

The initial dose should be 1 mg, usually given at bedtime so that the patient will remain recumbent for at least several hours to reduce the risk of syncopal reactions that may follow the first dose of prazosin. Therapy is begun with 1 mg given two or three times daily, and the dose is titrated upward depending on the blood pressure. A maximal effect generally is observed with a total daily dose of 20 mg in patients with hypertension. In the treatment of benign prostatic hyperplasia (BPH), doses from 1 to 5 mg twice daily typically are used. The twice-daily dosing requirement for prazosin is a disadvantage compared with newer α_1 receptor antagonists.

Terazosin. Terazosin (HYTRIN, others) is a close structural analog of prazosin (Kyncl, 1993; Wilde *et al.,* 1993). It is less potent than prazosin but retains high specificity for α_1 receptors; terazosin does not discriminate among α_{1A}, α_{1B}, and α_{1D} receptors. The major distinction between the two drugs is in their pharmacokinetic properties.

Terazosin is more soluble in water than is prazosin, and its bioavailability is high (>90%). The half-time of elimination of terazosin is approximately 12 hours, and its duration of action usually extends beyond 18 hours. Consequently, the drug may be taken once daily to treat hypertension and BPH in most patients. Terazosin has been found more effective than finasteride in treatment of BPH (Lepor *et al.,* 1996). An interesting aspect of the action of terazosin and doxazosin in the treatment of lower urinary tract problems in men with BPH is the induction of apoptosis in prostate smooth muscle cells. This apoptosis may lessen the symptoms associated with chronic BPH by limiting cell proliferation. The apoptotic effect of terazosin and doxazosin appears to be related to the quinazoline moiety rather than α_1 receptor antagonism; tamsulosin, a nonquinazoline α_1 receptor antagonist, does not produce apoptosis (Kyprianou, 2003). Only about 10% of terazosin is excreted unchanged in the urine. An initial first dose of 1 mg is recommended. Doses are titrated upward depending on the therapeutic response. Doses of 10 mg/day may be required for maximal effect in BPH.

Doxazosin. Doxazosin (CARDURA, others) is another structural analog of prazosin. It also is a highly selective antagonist at α_1 receptors, although nonselective among

α_1 receptor subtypes, but it differs in its pharmacokinetic profile (Babamoto and Hirokawa, 1992).

The half-life of doxazosin is approximately 20 hours, and its duration of action may extend to 36 hours. The bioavailability and extent of metabolism of doxazosin and prazosin are similar. Most doxazosin metabolites are eliminated in the feces. The hemodynamic effects of doxazosin appear to be similar to those of prazosin. Doxazosin should be given initially as a 1-mg dose in the treatment of hypertension or BPH. Similarly to terazosin, doxazosin may have beneficial actions in the long-term management of BPH related to apoptosis that are independent of α_1 receptor antagonism.

Alfuzosin.

Alfuzosin (UROXATRAL) is a quinazoline-based α_1 receptor antagonist with similar affinity at all of the α_1 receptor subtypes (Foglar *et al.*, 1995; Kenny *et al.*, 1996). It has been used extensively in treating BPH. Its bioavailability is about 64%; it has a half-life of 3 to 5 hours. The recommended dosage is one 10-mg extended-release tablet daily to be taken after the same meal each day.

Tamsulosin.

Tamsulosin (FLOMAX), a benzenesulfonamide, is an α_1 receptor antagonist with some selectivity for α_{1A} (and α_{1D}) subtypes compared to α_{1B} subtype (Kenny *et al.*, 1996). This selectivity may favor blockade of α_{1A} receptors in prostate. Tamsulosin is efficacious in the treatment of BPH with little effect on blood pressure (Wilde and McTavish, 1996; Beduschi *et al.*, 1998). Tamsulosin is well absorbed and has a half-life of 5 to 10 hours. It is extensively metabolized by CYPs. Tamsulosin may be administered at a 0.4-mg starting dose; a dose of 0.8 mg ultimately will be more efficacious in some patients. Abnormal ejaculation is an adverse effect of tamsulosin.

Adverse Effects.

A major potential adverse effect of prazosin and its congeners is the first-dose effect; marked postural hypotension and syncope sometimes are seen 30 to 90 minutes after a patient takes an initial dose.

Syncopal episodes also have occurred with a rapid increase in dosage or with the addition of a second antihypertensive drug to the regimen of a patient who already is taking a large dose of prazosin. The mechanisms responsible for such exaggerated hypotensive responses or for the development of tolerance to these effects are not clear. An action in the CNS to reduce sympathetic outflow may contribute (*see* above). The risk of the first-dose phenomenon is minimized by limiting the initial dose (*e.g.*, 1 mg at bedtime), by increasing the dosage slowly, and by introducing additional antihypertensive drugs cautiously.

Since orthostatic hypotension may be a problem during long-term treatment with prazosin or its congeners, it is essential to check standing as well as recumbent blood pressure. Nonspecific adverse effects such as headache, dizziness, and asthenia rarely limit treatment with prazosin. The nonspecific complaint of dizziness generally is not due to orthostatic hypotension. Although not extensively documented, the adverse effects of the structural analogs of prazosin appear to be similar to those of the parent compound. For tamsu-

losin, at a dose of 0.4 mg daily, effects on blood pressure are not expected, although impaired ejaculation may occur.

Therapeutic Uses.

Prazosin and its congeners have been used successfully in the treatment of essential hypertension (*see* Chapter 32). Considerable interest has focused on the use of α_1 receptor antagonists in the treatment of hypertension, predicted by the tendency of these drugs to improve rather than worsen lipid profiles and glucose-insulin metabolism in patients with hypertension who are at risk for atherosclerotic disease (Grimm, 1991). Also, catecholamines are powerful stimulators of vascular smooth muscle hypertrophy, acting *via* α_1 receptors (Okazaki *et al.*, 1994). To what extent these effects of α_1 antagonists have clinical significance in diminishing the risk of atherosclerosis is not known.

Additional uses for α antagonists, covered below, are in congestive heart failure and in the management of lower urinary tract problems secondary to benign prostatic hypertrophy.

Congestive Heart Failure. Alpha receptor antagonists have been used in the treatment of congestive heart failure, as have other vasodilating drugs. The short-term effects of prazosin in these patients are due to dilation of both arteries and veins, resulting in a reduction of preload and afterload, which increases cardiac output and reduces pulmonary congestion. In contrast to results obtained with inhibitors of angiotensin-converting enzyme or a combination of *hydralazine* and an organic nitrate, prazosin has not been found to prolong life in patients with congestive heart failure (Cohn *et al.*, 1986).

Benign Prostatic Hyperplasia (BPH). BPH produces symptomatic urethral obstruction in a significant percentage of older men that leads to weak stream, urinary frequency, and nocturia. These symptoms are due to a combination of mechanical pressure on the urethra due to the increase in smooth muscle mass and the α_1 receptor–mediated increase in smooth muscle tone in the prostate and neck of the bladder (Kyprianou, 2003). Alpha$_1$ receptors in the trigone muscle of the bladder and urethra contribute to the resistance to outflow of urine. Prazosin reduces this resistance in some patients with impaired bladder emptying caused by prostatic obstruction or parasympathetic decentralization from spinal injury (Kirby *et al.*, 1987; Andersson, 1988). The efficacy and importance of α receptor antagonists in the medical treatment of benign prostatic hyperplasia have been demonstrated in multiple controlled clinical trials. Transurethral resection of the prostate is the accepted surgical treatment for symptoms of urinary obstruction in men with BPH; however, there are some serious potential complications (*e.g.*, risk of impotence), and improvement may not be permanent. Other, less invasive procedures also are available. Medical therapy has utilized α receptor antagonists for many years. Finasteride, (PROPECIA) and *dutasteride* (AVODART), two drugs that inhibit conversion of testosterone to dihydrotestosterone (*see* Chapter 58), and can reduce prostate volume in some patients, are approved for this indication. However, the overall efficacy appears less than that observed with α_1 receptor antagonists (Lepor *et al.*, 1996). Selective α_1 receptor antagonists have efficacy in BPH owing to relaxation of smooth muscle in the bladder neck, prostate capsule, and prostatic urethra. These drugs rapidly improve urinary flow, whereas the actions of finasteride are typically delayed for months. Recent studies show that combination therapy with doxazosin and finasteride reduces the risk of overall clinical progression of BPH significantly more than treatment with either drug alone (McConnell *et al.*, 2003). Prazosin, terazosin, doxazosin, tamsulosin, and alfuzosin have been studied extensively and used widely in patients with benign prostatic hyperplasia (Cooper *et al.*, 1999). With the exception of tamsulosin, the comparative efficacies of each of these drugs, especially in comparison with relative adverse effects such as postural hypotension, appear similar, although direct comparisons are limited. Tamsulosin at the recommended dose of 0.4 mg daily is less likely to cause orthostatic hypotension than are the other drugs. There is growing evidence that the predominant α_1 receptor subtype expressed in the human prostate is the α_{1A} receptor (Forray *et al.*, 1994; Ruffulo and Hieble, 1999). Developments in this area will provide the basis for the selection of α receptor antagonists with specificity for the relevant subtype of α_1 receptor. However, the possibility remains that some of the symptoms of BPH are due to α_1 receptors in other sites, such as bladder, spinal cord, or brain.

Other Disorders. Although anecdotal evidence suggested that prazosin might be useful in the treatment of patients with variant angina (Prinzmetal's angina) due to coronary vasospasm, several small controlled trials have failed to demonstrate a clear benefit. Some studies have indicated that prazosin can decrease the incidence of digital vasospasm in patients with Raynaud's disease; however, its relative efficacy as compared with other vasodilators (*e.g.*, Ca^{2+} channel blockers) is not known. Prazosin may have some benefit in patients with other vasospastic disorders (Spittell and Spittell, 1992). Prazosin decreases ventricular arrhythmias induced by coronary artery ligation or reperfusion in laboratory animals; the therapeutic potential for this use in humans is not known. Prazosin also may be useful for the treatment of patients with mitral or aortic valvular insufficiency, presumably because of reduction of afterload.

Additional α Adrenergic Receptor Antagonists

Ergot Alkaloids. The ergot alkaloids were the first adrenergic receptor antagonists to be discovered, and most aspects of their general pharmacology were disclosed in the classic studies of Dale. Ergot alkaloids exhibit a complex variety of pharmacological properties. To varying degrees, these agents act as partial agonists or antagonists at α receptors, dopamine receptors, and serotonin receptors. Additional information about the ergot alkaloids is in Chapter 11 and in previous editions of this book.

Indoramin. *Indoramin* is a selective, competitive α_1 receptor antagonist that has been used for the treatment of hypertension. Competitive antagonism of histamine H_1 and 5-HT receptors also is evident. As an α_1-selective antagonist, indoramin lowers blood pressure with minimal tachycardia. The drug also decreases the incidence of attacks of Raynaud's phenomenon.

The bioavailability of indoramin generally is less than 30% (with considerable variability), and it undergoes extensive first-pass metabolism. Little unchanged drug is excreted in the urine, and some of the metabolites may be biologically active. The elimination half-life is about 5 hours. Some of the adverse effects of indoramin

include sedation, dry mouth, and failure of ejaculation. Although indoramin is an effective antihypertensive agent, it has complex pharmacokinetics and lacks a well-defined place in current therapy. Indoramin currently is not available in the United States.

Ketanserin. Although developed as a 5-HT-receptor antagonist, *ketanserin* also blocks α_1 receptors. Ketanserin is discussed in Chapter 11.

Urapidil. *Urapidil* is a novel, selective α_1 receptor antagonist that has a chemical structure distinct from those of prazosin and related compounds. Blockade of peripheral α_1 receptors appears to be primarily responsible for the hypotension produced by urapidil, although it has actions in the CNS as well. The drug is extensively metabolized and has a half-life of 3 hours. The role of urapidil in the treatment of hypertension remains to be determined. Urapidil is not currently available for clinical use in the United States.

Bunazosin. *Bunazosin* is an α_1-selective antagonist of the quinazoline class that has been shown to lower blood pressure in patients with hypertension (Harder and Thurmann, 1994). Bunazosin is not currently available in the United States.

Yohimbine. Yohimbine (YOCON) is a competitive antagonist that is selective for α_2 receptors. The compound is an indolealkylamine alkaloid and is found in the bark of the tree *Pausinystalia yohimbe* and in *Rauwolfia* root; its structure resembles that of reserpine. Yohimbine readily enters the CNS, where it acts to increase blood pressure and heart rate; it also enhances motor activity and produces tremors. These actions are opposite to those of clonidine, an α_2 agonist (Grossman *et al.*, 1993). Yohimbine also is an antagonist of 5-HT. In the past, it was used extensively to treat male sexual dysfunction. Although efficacy never was clearly demonstrated, there is renewed interest in the use of yohimbine in the treatment of male sexual dysfunction. The drug enhances sexual activity in male rats and may benefit some patients with psychogenic erectile dysfunction (Reid *et al.*, 1987). However, the efficacies of PDE5 inhibitors (*e.g.*, *sildenafil*, *vardenafil*, and *tadalafil*) and *apomorphine* have been much more conclusively demonstrated in oral treatment of erectile dysfunction. Several small studies suggest that yohimbine also may be useful for diabetic neuropathy and in the treatment of postural hypotension.

Neuroleptic Agents. Natural and synthetic compounds of several other chemical classes developed primarily because they are antagonists of D_2 dopamine receptors also exhibit α receptor blocking activity. *Chlorpromazine*, *haloperidol*, and other neuroleptic drugs of the phenothiazine and butyrophenone types produce significant α receptor blockade in both laboratory animals and humans.

β ADRENERGIC RECEPTOR ANTAGONISTS

Competitive antagonists of β adrenergic receptors, or β blockers, have received enormous clinical attention because of their efficacy in the treatment of hypertension, ischemic heart disease, congestive heart failure, and certain arrhythmias.

History. Ahlquist's hypothesis that the effects of catecholamines were mediated by activation of distinct α and β receptors provided the initial impetus for the synthesis and pharmacological evaluation of β receptor blocking agents (*see* Chapter 6). The first such selective agent was *dichloroisoproterenol*. However, this compound is a partial agonist, and this property was thought to preclude its safe clinical use. Sir James Black and his colleagues initiated a program in the late 1950s to develop additional agents of this type. Although the usefulness of their first antagonist, *pronethalol*, was limited by the production of thymic tumors in mice, *propranolol* soon followed.

Chemistry. The structural formulas of some β receptor antagonists in general use are shown in Figure 10–7. The structural similarities between agonists and antagonists that act on β receptors are closer than those between α receptor agonists and antagonists. Substitution of an isopropyl group or other bulky substituent on the amino nitrogen favors interaction with β receptors. There is a rather wide tolerance for the nature of the aromatic moiety in the nonselective β receptor antagonists; however, the structural tolerance for β_1-selective antagonists is far more constrained.

Overview. Propranolol is a competitive β receptor antagonist and remains the prototype to which other β antagonists are compared. Additional β antagonists can be distinguished by the following properties: relative affinity for β_1 and β_2 receptors, intrinsic sympathomimetic activity, blockade of α receptors, differences in lipid solubility, capacity to induce vasodilation, and pharmacokinetic properties. Some of these distinguishing characteristics have clinical significance, and they help guide the appropriate choice of a β receptor antagonist for an individual patient.

Propranolol has equal affinity for β_1 and β_2 adrenergic receptors; thus, it is a nonselective β adrenergic receptor antagonist. Agents such as *metoprolol, atenolol, acebutolol, bisoprolol,* and *esmolol* have somewhat greater affinity for β_1 than for β_2 receptors; these are examples of β_1-selective antagonists, even though the selectivity is not absolute. Propranolol is a pure antagonist, and it has no capacity to activate β receptors. Several β blockers (*e.g.,* pindolol and acebutolol) activate β receptors partially in the absence of catecholamines; however, the intrinsic activities of these drugs are less than that of a full agonist such as isoproterenol. These partial agonists are said to have intrinsic sympathomimetic activity. Substantial sympathomimetic activity would be counterproductive to the response desired from a β antagonist; however, slight residual activity may, for example, prevent profound bradycardia or neg-

ative inotropy in a resting heart. The potential clinical advantage of this property, however, is unclear and may be disadvantageous in the context of secondary prevention of myocardial infarction (*see* below). In addition, other β receptor antagonists have been found to have the property of inverse agonism (*see* Chapter 1). These drugs can decrease basal activity of β receptor signaling by shifting the equilibrium of spontaneously active receptors toward the inactive state (Chidiac *et al.,* 1994). Several β receptor antagonists also have local anesthetic or membrane stabilizing activity, similar to lidocaine, that is independent of β blockade. Such drugs include propranolol, acebutolol, and *carvedilol*. Pindolol, metoprolol, *betaxolol*, and *labetalol* have slight membrane stabilizing effects. Although most β receptor antagonists do not block α adrenergic receptors, labetalol, carvedilol, and *bucindolol* are examples of agents that block both α_1 and β adrenergic receptors. In addition to carvedilol, labetalol, and bucindolol, many other β receptor antagonists have vasodilating properties due to various mechanisms discussed below. These include *celiprolol, nebivolol, nipradilol, carteolol,* betaxolol, *bopindolol,* and *bevantolol* (Toda, 2003).

Pharmacological Properties

As in the case of α receptor blocking agents, the pharmacological properties of β receptor antagonists can be explained largely from knowledge of the responses elicited by the receptors in the various tissues and the activity of the sympathetic nerves that innervate these tissues (*see* Table 6–1). For example, β receptor blockade has relatively little effect on the normal heart of an individual at rest, but has profound effects when sympathetic control of the heart is dominant, as during exercise or stress.

In this chapter, β-adrenergic receptor antagonists are classified as Non-Subtype Selective β Receptor Antagonists ("First Generation"), β_1-Selective Receptor Antagonists ("Second Generation"), and Non-Subtype or Subtype Selective β Receptor Antagonists *with additional cardiovascular actions* ("Third Generation"). These latter drugs have additional cardiovascular properties (especially vasodilation) that seem unrelated to β blockade. Table 10–4 summarizes important pharmacological and pharmacokinetic properties of β receptor antagonists.

Cardiovascular System. The major therapeutic effects of β receptor antagonists are on the cardiovascular system. It is important to distinguish these effects in normal subjects from those in subjects with cardiovascular disease such as hypertension or myocardial ischemia.

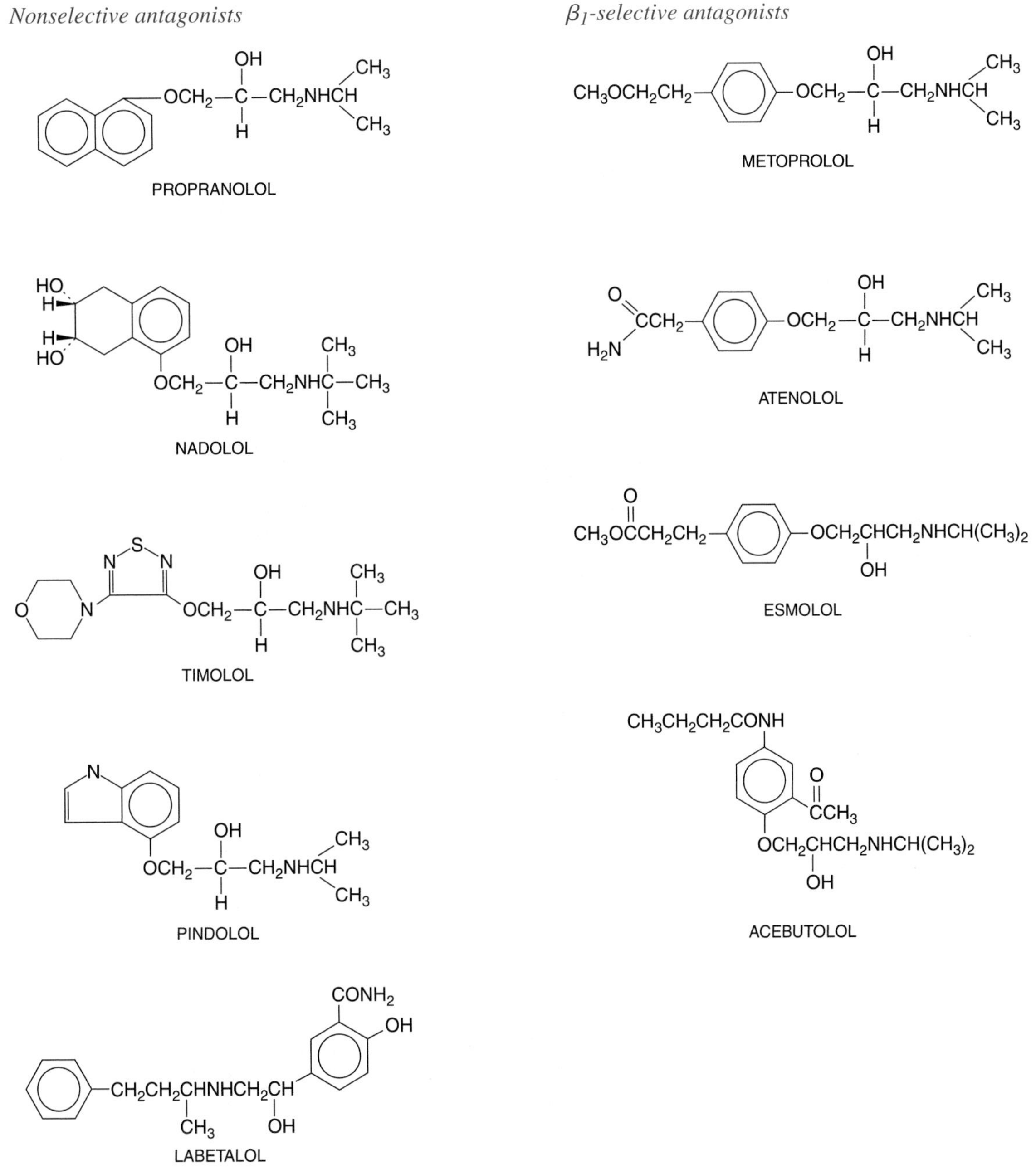

Nonselective antagonists

β₁-selective antagonists

PROPRANOLOL

NADOLOL

TIMOLOL

PINDOLOL

LABETALOL

METOPROLOL

ATENOLOL

ESMOLOL

ACEBUTOLOL

Figure 10–7. *Structural formulas of some β adrenergic receptor antagonists.*

Since catecholamines have positive chronotropic and inotropic actions, β receptor antagonists slow the heart rate and decrease myocardial contractility. When tonic stimulation of β receptors is low, this effect is correspondingly modest. However, when the sympathetic nervous system is activated, as during exercise or stress, β receptor antagonists attenuate the expected rise in heart rate. Short-term administration of β receptor antagonists such as propranolol decreases cardiac output; peripheral resistance increases in proportion to maintain blood pressure as a result of blockade of vascular β_2 receptors and compensatory reflexes, such as increased sympathetic nervous system activity, leading to activation of vascular α receptors. However, with long-term use of β receptor antagonists,

Table 10–4
Pharmacological/Pharmacokinetic Properties of β Receptor Blocking Agents

DRUG	MEMBRANE STABILIZING ACTIVITY	INTRINSIC AGONIST ACTIVITY	LIPID SOLUBILITY	EXTENT OF ABSORPTION (%)	ORAL BIOAVAILABILITY (%)	PLASMA $t_{\frac{1}{2}}$ (hours)	PROTEIN BINDING (%)
Classical non-selective β blockers: First generation							
Nadolol	0	0	Low	30	30–50	20–24	30
Penbutolol	0	+	High	≈100	~100	~5	80–98
Pindolol	+	+++	Low	>95	~100	3–4	40
Propranolol	++	0	High	<90	30	3–5	90
Timolol	0	0	Low to Moderate	90	75	4	<10
$β_1$-Selective β blockers: Second generation							
Acebutolol	+	+	Low	90	20–60	3–4	26
Atenolol	0	0	Low	90	50–60	6–7	6–16
Bisoprolol	0	0	Low	≤90	80	9–12	~30
Esmolol	0	0	Low	NA	NA	0.15	55
Metoprolol	+*	0	Moderate	~100	40–50	3–7	12
Non-selective β blockers with additional actions: Third generation							
Carteolol	0	++	Low	85	85	6	23–30
Carvedilol	++	0	Moderate	>90	~30	7–10	98
Labetalol	+	+	Low	>90	~33	3–4	~50
$β_1$-selective β blockers with additional actions: Third generation							
Betaxolol	+	0	Moderate	>90	~80	15	50
Celiprolol	0	+	Low	~74	30–70	5	4–5

*Detectable only at doses much greater than required for β blockade.

total peripheral resistance returns to initial values (Mimran and Ducailar, 1988) or decreases in patients with hypertension (Man in't Veld *et al.*, 1988). With β antagonists that also are $α_1$ receptor antagonists, such as labetalol, carvedilol, and bucindolol, cardiac output is maintained with a greater fall in peripheral resistance. This also is seen with β receptor antagonists that are direct vasodilators.

β Receptor antagonists have significant effects on cardiac rhythm and automaticity. Although it had been thought that these effects were due exclusively to blockade of $β_1$ receptors, $β_2$ receptors likely also regulate heart rate in humans (Brodde and Michel, 1999; Altschuld and Billman, 2000). $β_3$ Receptors also have been identified in normal myocardial tissue in several species, including humans (Moniotte *et al.*, 2001). In con-

trast to $β_1$ and $β_2$ receptors, $β_3$ receptors are linked to G_i and their stimulation inhibits cardiac contraction and relaxation. The physiological role of $β_3$ receptors in the heart remains to be established (Morimoto *et al.*, 2004). β Receptor antagonists reduce sinus rate, decrease the spontaneous rate of depolarization of ectopic pacemakers, slow conduction in the atria and in the AV node, and increase the functional refractory period of the AV node.

Although high concentrations of many β blockers produce quinidine-like effects (membrane-stabilizing activity), it is doubtful that this is significant at usual doses of these agents. However, this effect may be important when there is overdosage. Interestingly, there is some evidence suggesting that *d*-propranolol may suppress ventricular arrhythmias independently of β receptor blockade (Murray *et al.*, 1990).

The cardiovascular effects of β receptor antagonists are most evident during dynamic exercise. In the presence of β receptor blockade, exercise-induced increases in heart rate and myocardial contractility are attenuated. However, the exercise-induced increase in cardiac output is less affected because of an increase in stroke volume (Shephard, 1982). The effects of β receptor antagonists on exercise are somewhat analogous to the changes that occur with normal aging. In healthy elderly persons, catecholamine-induced increases in heart rate are smaller than in younger individuals; however, the increase in cardiac output in older people may be preserved because of an increase in stroke volume during exercise. β Blockers tend to decrease work capacity, as assessed by their effects on intense short-term or more prolonged steady-state exertion (Kaiser *et al.*, 1986). Exercise performance may be impaired to a lesser extent by β_1-selective agents than by nonselective antagonists. Blockade of β_2 receptors tends to blunt the increase in blood flow to active skeletal muscle during submaximal exercise (Van Baak, 1988). Blockade of β receptors also may attenuate catecholamine-induced activation of glucose metabolism and lipolysis.

Coronary artery blood flow increases during exercise or stress to meet the metabolic demands of the heart. By increasing heart rate, contractility, and systolic pressure, catecholamines increase myocardial oxygen demand. However, in patients with coronary artery disease, fixed narrowing of these vessels attenuates the expected increase in flow, leading to myocardial ischemia. β Receptor antagonists decrease the effects of catecholamines on the determinants of myocardial oxygen consumption. However, these agents may tend to increase the requirement for oxygen by increasing end-diastolic pressure and systolic ejection period. Usually, the net effect is to improve the relationship between cardiac oxygen supply and demand; exercise tolerance generally is improved in patients with angina, whose capacity to exercise is limited by the development of chest pain (*see* Chapter 31).

Activity as Antihypertensive Agents. β Receptor antagonists generally do not reduce blood pressure in patients with normal blood pressure. However, these drugs lower blood pressure in patients with hypertension. Despite their widespread use, the mechanisms responsible for this important clinical effect are not well understood. The release of renin from the juxtaglomerular apparatus is stimulated by the sympathetic nervous system *via* β_1 receptors, and this effect is blocked by β receptor antagonists (*see* Chapter 30). However, the relationship between this phenomenon and the fall in blood pressure is not clear. Some investigators have found that the antihypertensive effect of propranolol is most marked in patients with elevated concentrations of plasma renin, as compared with patients with low or normal concentrations of renin. However, β receptor antagonists are effective even in patients with low plasma renin, and pindolol is an effective antihypertensive agent that has little or no effect on plasma renin activity.

Presynaptic β receptors enhance the release of norepinephrine from sympathetic neurons, but the importance of diminished release of norepinephrine to the antihypertensive effects of β antagonists is unclear. Although β blockers would not be expected to decrease the contractility of vascular smooth muscle, long-term administration of these drugs to hypertensive patients ultimately leads to a fall in peripheral vascular resistance (Man in't Veld *et al.*, 1988). The mechanism for this important effect is not known, but this delayed fall in peripheral vascular resistance in the face of a persistent reduction of cardiac output appears to account for much of the antihypertensive effect of these drugs. Although it has been hypothesized that central actions of β blockers also may contribute to their antihypertensive effects, there is relatively little evidence to support this possibility, and drugs that poorly penetrate the blood–brain barrier are effective antihypertensive agents.

As indicated above, some β receptor antagonists have additional effects that may contribute to their capacity to lower blood pressure. These drugs all produce peripheral vasodilation; at least six properties have been proposed to contribute to this effect, including production of nitric oxide, activation of β_2 receptors, blockade of α_1 receptors, blockade of Ca^{2+} entry, opening of K^+ channels, and antioxidant activity. The ability of vasodilating β receptor antagonists to act through one or more of these mechanisms is depicted in Table 10–5 and Figure 10–8. These mechanisms appear to contribute to the antihypertensive effects by enhancing hypotension, increasing peripheral blood flow, and decreasing afterload. Two of these agents (*e.g.*, celiprolol and nebivolol) also have been observed to produce vasodilation and thereby reduce preload.

Although further clinical trials are needed, these agents may be associated with a lower incidence of bronchospasm, impaired lipid metabolism, impotence, reduced regional blood flow, increased vascular resistance, and withdrawal symptoms. A lower incidence of these adverse effects would be particularly beneficial in patients who have insulin resistance and diabetes mellitus in addition to hypertension (Toda, 2003). The clinical significance in humans of some of these relatively subtle differences in pharmacological properties still is unclear. Particular interest has focused on patients with congestive heart failure or peripheral arterial occlusive disease.

Propranolol and other nonselective β receptor antagonists inhibit the vasodilation caused by isoproterenol and augment the pressor response to epinephrine. This is particularly significant in patients with a pheochromocytoma, in whom β receptor antagonists should be used only after adequate α receptor blockade has been established. This

Table 10–5
Third-Generation β Receptor Antagonists with Additional Cardiovascular Actions: Proposed Mechanisms Contributing to Vasodilation

NITRIC OXIDE PRODUCTION	β₂ RECEPTOR AGONISM	α₁ RECEPTOR ANTAGONISM	Ca²⁺ ENTRY BLOCKADE	K⁺ CHANNEL OPENING	ANTIOXIDANT ACTIVITY
Celiprolol*	Celiprolol*	Carvedilol	Carvedilol	Tilisolol*	Carvedilol
Nebivolol*	Carteolol	Bucindolol*	Betaxolol		
Carteolol	Bopindolol*	Bevantolol*	Bevantolol*		
Bopindolol*		Nipradilol*			
Nipradilol*		Labetalol			

*Not currently available in the United States, where most are under investigation for use.

avoids uncompensated α receptor–mediated vasoconstriction caused by epinephrine secreted from the tumor.

Pulmonary System. Nonselective β receptor antagonists such as propranolol block β₂ receptors in bronchial smooth muscle. This usually has little effect on pulmonary function in normal individuals. However, in patients with COPD, such blockade can lead to life-threatening bronchoconstriction. Although β₁-selective antagonists or antagonists with intrinsic sympathomimetic activity are less likely than propranolol to increase airway resistance in patients with asthma, these drugs should be used only with great caution, if at all, in patients with bronchospastic diseases. Drugs such as celiprolol, with β₁ receptor

selectivity and β₂ receptor partial agonism, are of potential promise, although clinical experience is limited (Pujet *et al.*, 1992).

Metabolic Effects. β Receptor antagonists modify the metabolism of carbohydrates and lipids. Catecholamines promote glycogenolysis and mobilize glucose in response to hypoglycemia. Nonselective β blockers may delay recovery from hypoglycemia in type 1 (insulin-dependent) diabetes mellitus, but infrequently in type 2 diabetes mellitus. In addition to blocking glycogenolysis, β receptor antagonists can interfere with the counterregulatory effects of catecholamines secreted during hypoglycemia by blunting the perception of symptoms such as tremor,

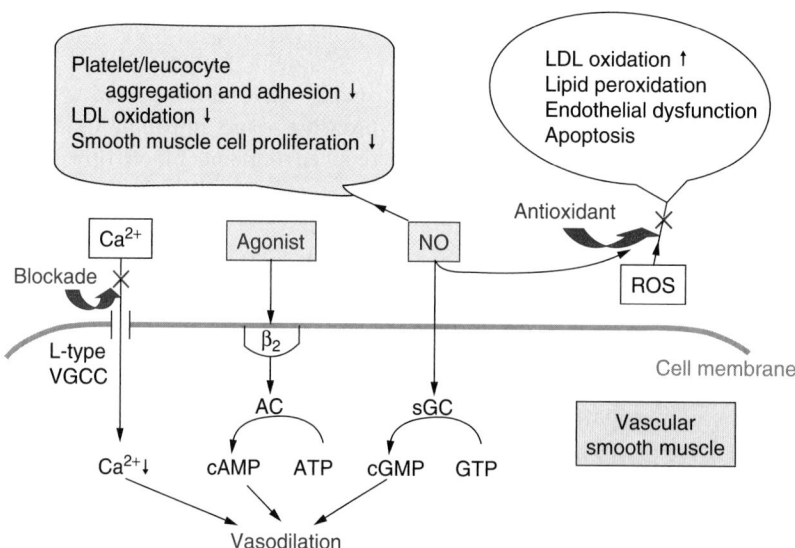

Figure 10–8. *Mechanisms underlying actions of vasodilating β blockers in blood vessels.* ROS, reactive oxygen species; sGC, soluble guanylyl cyclase; AC, adenylyl cyclase; L-type VGCC, L-type voltage gated Ca²⁺ channel. (Reproduced with permission from Toda, 2003.)

tachycardia, and nervousness. Thus, β adrenergic receptor antagonists should be used with great caution in patients with labile diabetes and frequent hypoglycemic reactions. If such a drug is indicated, a β_1-selective antagonist is preferred, since these drugs are less likely to delay recovery from hypoglycemia (Dunne *et al.*, 2001; DiBari *et al.*, 2003).

The β receptors mediate activation of hormone-sensitive lipase in fat cells, leading to release of free fatty acids into the circulation (*see* Chapter 6). This increased flux of fatty acids is an important source of energy for exercising muscle. β Receptor antagonists can attenuate the release of free fatty acids from adipose tissue. Nonselective β receptor antagonists consistently reduce HDL cholesterol, increase LDL cholesterol, and increase triglycerides. In contrast, β_1-selective antagonists, including celiprolol, carteolol, nebivolol, carvedilol, and bevantolol, reportedly improve the serum lipid profile of dyslipidemic patients. While drugs such as propranolol and atenolol increase triglycerides, plasma triglycerides are reduced with chronic celiprolol, carvedilol, and carteolol (Toda, 2003).

In contrast to classical β blockers, which decrease insulin sensitivity, the vasodilating β receptor antagonists (*e.g.,* celiprolol, nipradilol, carteolol, carvedilol, and *dilevalol*) increase insulin sensitivity in patients with insulin resistance. Together with their cardioprotective effects, improvement in insulin sensitivity from vasodilating β receptor antagonists may partially counterbalance the hazard from worsened lipid abnormalities associated with diabetes. If β blockers are to be used, β_1-selective or vasodilating β receptor antagonists are preferred. In addition, it may be necessary to use β receptor antagonists in conjunction with other drugs, (*e.g.,* HMG-CoA reductase inhibitors) to ameliorate adverse metabolic effects (Dunne *et al.*, 2001).

β Receptor agonists decrease the plasma concentration of K^+ by promoting the uptake of the ion, predominantly into skeletal muscle. At rest, an infusion of epinephrine causes a decrease in the plasma concentration of K^+. The marked increase in the concentration of epinephrine that occurs with stress (such as myocardial infarction) may cause hypokalemia, which could predispose to cardiac arrhythmias. The hypokalemic effect of epinephrine is blocked by an experimental antagonist, ICI 118551, which has a high affinity for β_2 and β_3 receptors. Exercise causes an increase in the efflux of K^+ from skeletal muscle. Catecholamines tend to buffer the rise in K^+ by increasing its influx into muscle. β blockers negate this buffering effect.

Other Effects. β Receptor antagonists block catecholamine-induced tremor. They also block inhibition of mast-cell degranulation by catecholamines.

NON-SUBTYPE-SELECTIVE β ADRENERGIC RECEPTOR ANTAGONISTS

Propranolol

In view of the extensive experience with propranolol (INDERAL, others), it is a useful prototype (Table 10–4).

Propranolol interacts with β_1 and β_2 receptors with equal affinity, lacks intrinsic sympathomimetic activity, and does not block α receptors.

Absorption, Fate, and Excretion. Propranolol is highly lipophilic and is almost completely absorbed after oral administration. However, much of the drug is metabolized by the liver during its first passage through the portal circulation; on average, only about 25% reaches the systemic circulation. In addition, there is great interindividual variation in the presystemic clearance of propranolol by the liver; this contributes to enormous variability in plasma concentrations (approximately twentyfold) after oral administration of the drug and contributes to the wide range of doses in terms of clinical efficacy. A clinical disadvantage of propranolol is that multiple, increasing steps in drug dose may be required over time. The degree of hepatic extraction of propranolol declines as the dose is increased. The bioavailability of propranolol may be increased by the concomitant ingestion of food and during long-term administration of the drug.

Propranolol has a large volume of distribution (4 liters/kg) and readily enters the CNS. Approximately 90% of the drug in the circulation is bound to plasma proteins. It is extensively metabolized, with most metabolites appearing in the urine. One product of hepatic metabolism is 4-hydroxypropranolol, which has some β adrenergic antagonist activity.

Analysis of the distribution of propranolol, its clearance by the liver, and its activity is complicated by the stereospecificity of these processes (Walle *et al.*, 1988). The (–)-enantiomers of propranolol and other β blockers are the active forms of the drug. The (–)-enantiomer of propranolol appears to be cleared more slowly from the body than is the inactive enantiomer. The clearance of propranolol may vary with hepatic blood flow and liver disease and also may change during the administration of other drugs that affect hepatic metabolism. Monitoring of plasma concentrations of propranolol has found little application, since the clinical endpoints (reduction of blood pressure and heart rate) are readily determined. The relationships between the plasma concentrations of propranolol and its pharmacodynamic effects are complex; for example, despite its short half-life in plasma (about 4 hours), its antihypertensive effect is sufficiently long-lived to permit administration twice daily. Some of the (–)-enantiomer of propranolol and other β blockers is taken up into sympathetic nerve endings and is released upon sympathetic nerve stimulation (Walle *et al.*, 1988).

A sustained-release formulation of propranolol (INDERAL LA) has been developed to maintain therapeutic concentrations of propranolol in plasma throughout a 24-hour period. Suppression of exercise-induced tachycardia is maintained throughout the dosing interval, and patient compliance may be improved.

Therapeutic Uses. For the treatment of hypertension and angina, the initial oral dose of propranolol generally is 40 to 80 mg per day. The dose may then be titrated upward until the optimal response is obtained. For the treatment of angina, the dose may be increased at intervals of less than 1 week, as indicated clinically. In hypertension, the full blood-pressure response may not develop for several weeks. Typically, doses are less than 320 mg per day. If propranolol is taken twice daily for hypertension, blood pressure should be measured just prior to a dose to ensure that the duration of effect is sufficiently prolonged. Adequacy of β adrenergic blockade can be assessed by measuring suppression of exercise-induced tachycardia. Propranolol also is used to treat supraventricular arrhythmias/tachycardias, ventricular arrhythmias/tachycardias, premature ventricular contractions, digitalis-induced tachyarrhythmias, myocardial infarction, pheochromocytoma, and the prophylaxis of migraine. It also has been used for several off-label indications including parkinsonian tremors (sustained-release only), akathisia induced by antipsychotic drugs, variceal bleeding in portal hypertension, and generalized anxiety disorder (Table 10–6). Propranolol may be administered intravenously for the management of life-threatening arrhythmias or to patients under anesthesia. Under these circumstances, the usual dose is 1 to 3 mg, administered slowly (less than 1 mg per minute) with careful and frequent monitoring of blood pressure, ECG, and cardiac function. If an adequate response is not obtained, a second dose may be given after several minutes. If bradycardia is excessive, atropine should be administered to increase heart rate. Change to oral therapy should be initiated as soon as possible.

Nadolol

Nadolol (CORGARD, others) is a long-acting antagonist with equal affinity for β_1 and β_2 receptors. It is devoid of both membrane-stabilizing and intrinsic sympathomimetic activity. A distinguishing characteristic of nadolol is its relatively long half-life of 12 to 24 hours. It can be used to treat both hypertension and angina pectoris. Unlabeled uses have included migraine prophylaxis, parkinsonian tremors, and variceal bleeding in portal hypertension.

Absorption, Fate, and Excretion. Nadolol is very soluble in water and is incompletely absorbed from the gut; its bioavailability is about 35%. Interindividual variability is less than with propranolol. The low lipid solubility of nadolol may result in lower concentrations of the drug in the brain as compared with more lipid-soluble β receptor antagonists. Although it frequently has been suggested that the incidence of CNS adverse effects is lower with hydrophilic β receptor antagonists, data from controlled trials to support this contention are limited. Nadolol is not extensively metabolized and is largely excreted intact in the urine. The half-life of the drug in plasma is approximately 20 hours; consequently, it generally is administered once daily. Nadolol may accumulate in patients with renal failure, and dosage should be reduced in such individuals.

Timolol

Timolol (BLOCADREN, others) is a potent, non-subtype-selective β receptor antagonist. It has no intrinsic sympathomimetic or membrane-stabilizing activity. It is used

to treat hypertension, congestive heart failure, migraine prophylaxis, and has been widely used in the treatment of open-angle glaucoma and intraocular hypertension.

Absorption, Fate, and Excretion. Timolol is well absorbed from the gastrointestinal tract. It is metabolized extensively by CYP2D6 in the liver and undergoes first-pass metabolism. Only a small amount of unchanged drug appears in the urine. The half-life in plasma is about 4 hours. Interestingly, the ocular formulation of timolol (TIMOPTIC, others), used for the treatment of glaucoma, may be extensively absorbed systemically (*see* Chapter 63); adverse effects can occur in susceptible patients, such as those with asthma or congestive heart failure. The systemic administration of *cimetidine* with topical ocular timolol increases the degree of β blockade, resulting in a reduction of resting heart rate, intraocular pressure, and exercise tolerance (Ishii *et al.*, 2000).

Pindolol

Pindolol (VISKEN, others) is a non-subtype-selective β receptor antagonist with intrinsic sympathomimetic activity. It has low membrane-stabilizing activity and low lipid solubility.

Although only limited data are available, β blockers with slight partial agonist activity may produce smaller reductions in resting heart rate and blood pressure. Hence, such drugs may be preferred as antihypertensive agents in individuals with diminished cardiac reserve or a propensity for bradycardia. Nonetheless, the clinical significance of partial agonism has not been substantially demonstrated in controlled trials but may be of importance in individual patients (Fitzgerald, 1993). Agents such as pindolol block exercise-induced increases in heart rate and cardiac output.

Absorption, Fate, and Excretion. Pindolol is almost completely absorbed after oral administration and has moderately high bioavailability. These properties tend to minimize interindividual variation in the plasma concentrations of the drug that are achieved after its oral administration. Approximately 50% of pindolol ultimately is metabolized in the liver. The principal metabolites are hydroxylated derivatives that subsequently are conjugated with either glucuronide or sulfate before renal excretion. The remainder of the drug is excreted unchanged in the urine. The plasma half-life of pindolol is about 4 hours; clearance is reduced in patients with renal failure.

β_1-SELECTIVE ADRENERGIC RECEPTOR ANTAGONISTS

Metoprolol

Metoprolol (LOPRESSOR, others) is a β_1-selective receptor antagonist that is devoid of intrinsic sympathomimetic activity and membrane-stabilizing activity.

Table 10-6
Summary of Adrenergic Agonists and Antagonists

CLASS	DRUGS	PROMINENT PHARMACOLOGICAL ACTIONS	PRINCIPAL THERAPEUTIC APPLICATIONS	UNTOWARD EFFECTS	COMMENTS
Direct-acting non-selective agonists	Epinephrine ($\alpha_1, \alpha_2, \beta_1, \beta_2, \beta_3$)	Increase in heart rate Increase in blood pressure Increased contractility Slight decrease in PVR Increase in cardiac output Vasoconstriction (viscera) Vasodilation (skeletal muscle) Increase in blood glucose and lactic acid	Open-angle glaucoma With local anesthetics to prolong action Anaphylactic shock Complete heart block or cardiac arrest Bronchodilator in asthma	Palpitation Cardiac arrhythmias Cerebral hemorrhage Headache Tremor Restlessness	Not given orally Life saving in anaphylaxis or cardiac arrest
	Norepinephrine ($\alpha_1, \alpha_2, \beta_1, >> \beta_2$)	Increase in systolic and diastolic blood pressure Vasoconstriction Increase in PVR Direct increase in heart rate and contraction Reflex decrease in heart rate	Hypotension	Similar to Epi Hypertension	Not absorbed orally
β Receptor Agonists Non-selective ($\beta_1 + \beta_2$)	Isoproterenol	IV administration Decrease in PVR Increase in cardiac output Tachyarrhythmias Bronchodilation	Bronchodilator in asthma Complete heart block or cardiac arrest Shock	Palpitations Tachycardia Headache Flushed skin Cardiac ischemia in patients with CAD	Administered by inhalation in asthma

(Continued)

Table 10-6
Summary of Adrenergic Agonists and Antagonists (Continued)

CLASS	DRUGS	PROMINENT PHARMACOLOGICAL ACTIONS	PRINCIPAL THERAPEUTIC APPLICATIONS	UNTOWARD EFFECTS	COMMENTS
β_1-selective	Dobutamine	Increase in contractility Some increase in heart rate Increase in AV conduction	Short-term treatment of cardiac decompensation after surgery, or patients with CHF or MI	Increase in blood pressure and heart rate.	Use with caution in patients with hypertension or cardiac arrhythmias Used only IV
β_2-selective (intermediate acting)	Albuterol Bitolterol Fenoterol Isoetharine Metaproterenol Procaterol Terbutaline Ritodrine	Relaxation of bronchial smooth muscle Relaxation of uterine smooth muscle Activation of other β_2 receptors after systemic administration	Bronchodilators for treatment of asthma and COPD Short/intermediate-acting drugs for acute bronchospasm Ritodrine, to stop premature labor	Skeletal muscle tremor Tachycardia and other cardiac effects seen after systemic administration (much less with inhalational use)	Use with caution in patients with CV disease (reduced by inhalational administration) Minimal side effects
(Long acting)	Formoterol Salmeterol		Best choice for prophylaxis due to long action		Long action favored for prophylaxis
α Receptor agonists					
α_1-selective	Methoxamine Phenylephrine Mephentermine Metaraminol Midodrine	Vasoconstriction	Nasal congestion (used topically) Postural hypotension	Hypertension Reflex bradycardia Dry mouth, sedation, rebound hypertension upon abrupt withdrawal	Mephentermine and metaraminol also act indirectly to release NE Midodrine is a prodrug converted *in vivo* to an active compound

α_2-selective	Clonidine Apraclonidine Guanfacine Guanabenz Brimonidine α-methyldopa	Decrease sympathetic outflow from brain to periphery resulting in decreased PVR and blood pressure Decrease nerve-evoked release of sympathetic transmitters Decrease production of aqueous humor	Adjunctive therapy in shock Hypertension To reduce sympathetic response to withdrawal from narcotics, alcohol, and tobacco Glaucoma		Apraclonidine and brimonidine used topically for glaucoma and ocular hypertension Methyldopa is converted in CNS to α-methyl NE, an effective α_2 agonist
Indirect-acting	Amphetamine Methamphetamine Methylphenidate (releases NE peripherally; NE, DA, 5-HT centrally)	CNS stimulation Increase in blood pressure Myocardial stimulation	Treatment of ADHD Narcolepsy Obesity (rarely)	Restlessness Tremor Insomnia Anxiety Tachycardia Hypertension Cardiac arrhythmias	Schedule II drugs Marked tolerance occurs Chronic use leads to dependence Can result in hemorrhagic stroke in patients with underlying disease Long-term use can cause paranoid schizophrenia
Mixed-acting	Dopamine (α_1, α_2, β_1, D_1; releases NE)	Vasodilation (coronary, renal mesenteric beds) Increase in glomerular filtration rate and natriuresis Increase in heart rate and contractility Increase in systolic blood pressure	Cardiogenic shock Congestive heart failure Treatment of acute renal failure	High doses lead to vasoconstriction	Important for its ability to maintain renal blood flow Administered IV
	Ephedrine (α_1, α_2, β_1, β_2; releases NE)	Similar to epinephrine but longer lasting CNS stimulation	Bronchodilator for treatment of asthma Nasal congestion Treatment of hypotension and shock	Restlessness Tremor Insomnia Anxiety Tachycardia Hypertension	Administered by all routes Not commonly used

(Continued)

Table 10-6
Summary of Adrenergic Agonists and Antagonists (Continued)

CLASS	DRUGS	PROMINENT PHARMACOLOGICAL ACTIONS	PRINCIPAL THERAPEUTIC APPLICATIONS	UNTOWARD EFFECTS	COMMENTS
α Blockers Non-selective (classical α blockers)	Phenoxybenzamine Phentolamine Tolazoline	Decrease in PVR and blood pressure Venodilation	Treatment of catecholamine excess (*e.g.*, pheochromocytoma)	Postural hypotension Failure of ejaculation	Cardiac stimulation due to initiation of reflexes and to enhanced release of NE via α_2 receptor blockade. Phenoxybenzamine produces long-lasting α-receptor blockade and at high doses can block neuronal and extraneuronal uptake of amines
α_1-selective	Prazosin Terazosin Doxazosin Trimazosin Alfuzosin Tamsulosin	Decrease in PVR and blood pressure Relax smooth muscles in neck of urinary bladder and in prostate	Primary hypertension Increase urine flow in BPH	Postural hypotension when therapy instituted	Prazosin and related quinazolines are selective for α_1 receptors but not among α_1 subtypes Tamsulosin exhibits some selectivity for α_{1A} receptors
β Blockers Non-selective (1st generation)	Nadolol Penbutolol Pindolol Propranolol Timolol	Decrease in heart rate Decrease in contractility Decrease in cardiac output Slow conduction in atria and AV node Increase refractory period, AV node Bronchoconstriction Prolonged hypoglycemia Decrease in plasma FFA	Angina pectoris Hypertension Cardiac arrhythmias CHF Pheochromocytoma Glaucoma Hypertropic obstructive cardiomyopathy Hyperthyroidism Migraine prophylaxis	Bradycardia Negative inotropic effect Decrease in cardiac output Bradyarrhythmias Reduction in AV conduction Bronchoconstriction Fatigue	Pharmacological effects depend largely on degree of sympathoadrenal tone Bronchoconstriction (of concern in asthmatics and COPD) Hypoglycemia (concern in hypoglycemics and diabetics)

282

Class	Drugs		Adverse effects	Properties
Non-selective (1st generation) *(continued)*		Reduction in HDL cholesterol Increase in LDL cholesterol and triglycerides Hypokalemia	Acute panic symptoms Substance abuse with-drawal Variceal bleeding in portal hypertension	Sleep disturbances (insomnia, night-mares) Prolongation of hypoglycemia Sexual dysfunction in men Drug interactions	Membrane stabilizing effect (propranolol, acebutolol, carvedilol, and betaxolol only) ISA (strong for pindolol; weak for penbutolol, carteolol, labetalol, and betaxolol)
β_1-selective (2nd generation)	Acebutolol Atenolol Bisoprolol Esmolol Metoprolol				
Non-selective (3rd generation) vasodilators	Carteolol Carvedilol Bucindolol Labetalol	(Membrane stabilizing effect) (ISA) (Vasodilation)			Vasodilation seen in 3rd generation drugs; multiple mechanisms (α_1 antagonism; β_2 agonism; release of NO; Ca^{2+} channel blockade; opening of K^+ channels; others)
β_1-selective (3rd generation) vasodilators	Betaxolol Celiprolol Nebivolol				

ADHD, attention-deficit/hyperactivity disorder; AV, atrioventricular; BPH, benign prostatic hypertrophy; CAD, coronary artery disease; CHF, congestive heart failure; COPD, chronic obstructive pulmonary disease; CV, cardiovascular; DA, dopamine; D_1, subtype 1 dopamine receptor; Epi, epinephrine; FFA, free fatty acids; 5-HT, serotonin; ISA, intrinsic sympathomimetic activity; MI, myocardial infarction; NE, norepinephrine; NO, nitric oxide; PVR, peripheral vascular resistance.

Absorption, Fate, and Excretion. Metoprolol is almost completely absorbed after oral administration, but bioavailability is relatively low (about 40%) because of first-pass metabolism. Plasma concentrations of the drug vary widely (up to seventeenfold), perhaps because of genetically determined differences in the rate of metabolism. Metoprolol is extensively metabolized in the liver, with CYP2D6 the major enzyme involved, and only 10% of the administered drug is recovered unchanged in the urine. The half-life of metoprolol is 3 to 4 hours, but can increase to 7 to 8 hours in CYP2D6 poor metabolizers. It recently has been reported that CYP2D6 poor metabolizers have a fivefold higher risk for developing adverse effects during metoprolol treatment than patients who are not poor metabolizers (Wuttke *et al.*, 2002). An extended-release formulation (TOPROL XL) is available for once-daily administration.

Therapeutic Uses. For the treatment of hypertension, the usual initial dose is 100 mg per day. The drug sometimes is effective when given once daily, although it frequently is used in two divided doses. Dosage may be increased at weekly intervals until optimal reduction of blood pressure is achieved. If the drug is taken only once daily, it is important to confirm that blood pressure is controlled for the entire 24-hour period. Metoprolol generally is used in two divided doses for the treatment of stable angina. For the initial treatment of patients with acute myocardial infarction, an intravenous formulation of metoprolol tartrate is available. Oral dosing is initiated as soon as the clinical situation permits. Metoprolol generally is contraindicated for the treatment of acute myocardial infarction in patients with heart rates of less than 45 beats per minute, heart block greater than first-degree (PR interval ≥0.24 second), systolic blood pressure <100 mm Hg, or moderate-to-severe heart failure. Metoprolol also has been proven to be effective in chronic heart failure. It has been shown in randomized trials to be associated with a striking reduction in all-cause mortality and hospitalization for worsening heart failure and a modest reduction in all-cause hospitalization (MERIT-HF Study Group, 1999; Prakash and Markham, 2000).

Atenolol

Atenolol (TENORMIN, others) is a β_1-selective antagonist that is devoid of intrinsic sympathomimetic and membrane stabilizing activity (Wadworth *et al.*, 1991). Atenolol is very hydrophilic and appears to penetrate the CNS only to a limited extent. Its half-life is somewhat longer than that of metoprolol.

Absorption, Fate, and Excretion. Atenolol is incompletely absorbed (about 50%), but most of the absorbed dose reaches the systemic circulation. There is relatively little interindividual variation in the plasma concentrations of atenolol; peak concentrations in different patients vary over only a fourfold range. The drug is excreted largely unchanged in the urine, and the elimination half-life is about 5 to 8 hours. The drug accumulates in patients with renal failure, and dosage should be adjusted for patients whose creatinine clearance is less than 35 ml/minute.

Therapeutic Uses. The initial dose of atenolol for the treatment of hypertension usually is 50 mg per day, given once daily. If an ade-

quate therapeutic response is not evident within several weeks, the daily dose may be increased to 100 mg; higher doses are unlikely to provide any greater antihypertensive effect. Atenolol has been shown to be efficacious, in combination with a diuretic, in elderly patients with isolated systolic hypertension.

Esmolol

Esmolol (BREVIBLOC, others) is a β_1-selective antagonist with a very short duration of action. It has little if any intrinsic sympathomimetic activity, and it lacks membrane-stabilizing actions. Esmolol is administered intravenously and is used when β blockade of short duration is desired or in critically ill patients in whom adverse effects of bradycardia, heart failure, or hypotension may necessitate rapid withdrawal of the drug.

Absorption, Fate, and Excretion. Esmolol has a half-life of about 8 minutes and an apparent volume of distribution of approximately 2 liters/kg. The drug contains an ester linkage, and it is hydrolyzed rapidly by esterases in erythrocytes. The half-life of the carboxylic acid metabolite of esmolol is far longer (4 hours), and it accumulates during prolonged infusion of esmolol. However, this metabolite has very low potency as a β receptor antagonist (1/500 of the potency of esmolol); it is excreted in the urine.

The onset and cessation of β receptor blockade with esmolol are rapid; peak hemodynamic effects occur within 6 to 10 minutes of administration of a loading dose, and there is substantial attenuation of β blockade within 20 minutes of stopping an infusion. Esmolol may have striking hypotensive effects in normal subjects, although the mechanism of this effect is unclear.

Because esmolol is used in urgent settings where immediate onset of β blockade is warranted, a partial loading dose typically is administered, followed by a continuous infusion of the drug. If an adequate therapeutic effect is not observed within 5 minutes, the same loading dose is repeated, followed by a maintenance infusion at a higher rate. This process, including progressively greater infusion rates, may need to be repeated until the desired endpoint (*e.g.*, lowered heart rate or blood pressure) is approached.

Acebutolol

Acebutolol (SECTRAL, others) is a selective β_1 adrenergic receptor antagonist with some intrinsic sympathomimetic and membrane-stabilizing activity.

Absorption, Fate, and Excretion. Acebutolol is well absorbed, and undergoes significant first-pass metabolism to an active metabolite, diacetolol, which accounts for most of the drug's activity. The elimination half-life of acebutolol typically is about 3 hours, but the half-life of diacetolol is 8 to 12 hours; it is excreted in the urine.

Therapeutic Uses. The initial dose of acebutolol in hypertension usually is 400 mg per day; it may be given as a single dose, but two divided doses may be required for adequate control of blood pressure. Optimal responses usually occur with doses of 400 to 800 mg per day (range 200 to 1200 mg). For treatment of ventricular arrhythmias, the drug should be given twice daily.

Bisoprolol

Bisoprolol (ZEBETA) is a highly selective β_1 receptor antagonist that does not have intrinsic sympathomimetic or membrane-stabilizing activity (McGavin and Keating, 2002). It is approved for the treatment of hypertension and has been investigated in randomized, double-blind multicenter trials in combination with ACE inhibitors and diuretics in patients with moderate-to-severe chronic heart failure (Simon *et al.*, 2003). All-case mortality was significantly lower with bisoprolol than placebo.

Bisoprolol generally is well tolerated and side effects include dizziness, bradycardia, hypotension, and fatigue. Bisoprolol is well absorbed following oral administration with bioavailability of ~90%. It is eliminated by renal excretion (50%) and liver metabolism to pharmacologically inactive metabolites (50%). Bisoprolol has a plasma half-life of 11 to 17 hours. Bisoprolol can be considered a standard treatment option when selecting a β blocker for use in combination with ACE inhibitors and diuretics in patients with stable, moderate-to-severe chronic heart failure and in treating hypertension (McGavin and Keating, 2002; Owen, 2002; Simon *et al.*, 2003).

β Receptor Antagonists with Additional Cardiovascular Effects ("Third Generation" β Blockers)

In addition to the classical non-subtype selective and β_1-selective adrenergic receptor antagonists, there also are a series of drugs that possess vasodilatory actions. These effects are produced through a variety of mechanisms including α_1 adrenergic receptor blockade (labetalol, carvedilol, bucindolol, bevantolol, nipradilol), increased production of NO (celiprolol, nebivolol, carteolol, bopindolol, and nipradolol), β_2-agonist properties (celiprolol, carteolol, and bopindolol), Ca^{2+} entry blockade (carvedilol, betaxolol, and bevantolol), opening of K^+ channels (*tilisolol*), or antioxidant action (carvedilol) (Toda, 2003). These actions are summarized in Table 10–5 and Figure 10–8. Many third generation β receptor antagonists are not yet available in the United States but have undergone clinical trials and are on the market in other countries.

Labetalol

Labetalol (NORMODYNE, TRANDATE, others) is representative of a class of drugs that act as competitive antagonists at both α_1 and β receptors. Labetalol has two optical centers, and the formulation used clinically contains equal amounts of the four diastereomers. The pharmacological properties of the drug are complex, because each isomer displays different relative activities. The properties of the mixture include selective blockade of α_1 receptors (as compared with the α_2 subtype), blockade of β_1 and β_2 receptors, partial agonist activity at β_2 receptors, and inhibition of neuronal uptake of norepinephrine (cocaine-like effect) (*see* Chapter 6). The potency of the mixture for β receptor blockade is fivefold to tenfold that for α_1 receptor blockade.

The pharmacological effects of labetalol have become clearer since the four isomers were separated and tested individually. The R,R isomer is about four times more potent as a β receptor antagonist than is racemic labetalol, and it accounts for much of the β blockade produced by the mixture of isomers, although it no longer is in development as a separate drug (dilevalol). As an α_1 antagonist, this isomer is less than 20% as potent as the racemic mixture. The R,S isomer is almost devoid of both α and β blocking effects. The S,R isomer has almost no β blocking activity, yet is about five times more potent as an α_1 blocker than is racemic labetalol. The S,S isomer is devoid of β blocking activity and has a potency similar to that of racemic labetalol as an α_1 receptor antagonist. The R,R isomer has some intrinsic sympathomimetic activity at β_2 adrenergic receptors; this may contribute to vasodilation. Labetalol also may have some direct vasodilating capacity.

The actions of labetalol on both α_1 and β receptors contribute to the fall in blood pressure observed in patients with hypertension. α_1 Receptor blockade leads to relaxation of arterial smooth muscle and vasodilation, particularly in the upright position. The β_1 blockade also contributes to a fall in blood pressure, in part by blocking reflex sympathetic stimulation of the heart. In addition, the intrinsic sympathomimetic activity of labetalol at β_2 receptors may contribute to vasodilation.

Labetalol is available in oral form for therapy of chronic hypertension and as an intravenous formulation for use in hypertensive emergencies. Labetalol has been associated with hepatic injury in a limited number of patients (Clark *et al.*, 1990).

Absorption, Fate, and Excretion. Although labetalol is completely absorbed from the gut, there is extensive first-pass clearance; bioavailability is only about 20% to 40% and is highly variable. Bioavailability may be increased by food intake. The drug is rapidly and extensively metabolized in the liver by oxidative biotransformation and glucuronidation; very little unchanged drug is found in the urine. The rate of metabolism of labetalol is sensitive to changes in hepatic blood flow. The elimination half-life of the drug is about 8 hours. The half-life of the R,R isomer of labetalol (dilevalol) is about 15 hours. Labetalol provides an interesting and challenging example of pharmacokinetic-pharmacodynamic modeling applied to a drug that is a racemic mixture of isomers with different kinetics and pharmacological actions (Donnelly and Macphee, 1991).

Carvedilol

Carvedilol (COREG) is a third-generation β receptor antagonist that has a unique pharmacological profile. It blocks

β_1, β_2, and α_1 receptors similarly to labetalol, but also has antioxidant and antiproliferative effects. It has membrane-stabilizing activity but it lacks intrinsic sympathomimetic activity. Carvedilol produces vasodilation. It is thought that the additional properties (e.g., antioxidant and anti-proliferative effects) contribute to the beneficial effects seen in treating congestive heart failure. Carvedilol does not increase β receptor density and is not associated with high levels of inverse agonist activity (Keating and Jarvis, 2003; Cheng et al., 2001).

Carvedilol has been tested in numerous double-blind, random-ized studies including the following: U.S. Carvedilol Heart Failure Trials Program, Carvedilol or Metoprolol European Trial (COMET) (Poole-Wilson et al., 2003), Carvedilol Prospective Randomised Cumulative Survival (COPERNICUS) trial, and the Carvedilol Post Infarct Survival Control in LV Dysfunction (CAPRICORN) trial (Cleland, 2003). These trials showed that carvedilol improves ven-tricular function and reduces mortality and morbidity in patients with mild-to-severe congestive heart failure. Several experts recom-mend it as the standard treatment option in this setting. In addition, carvedilol combined with conventional therapy reduces mortality and attenuates myocardial infarction. In patients with chronic heart failure, carvedilol reduces cardiac sympathetic drive, but it is not clear if α_1 receptor–mediated vasodilation is maintained over long periods of time.

Absorption, Fate, Excretion. Carvedilol is rapidly absorbed fol-lowing oral administration, with peak plasma concentrations occurring in 1 to 2 hours. It is highly lipophilic and thus is exten-sively distributed into extravascular tissues. It is >95% protein bound and is extensively metabolized in the liver, predominantly by CYP2D6 and CYP2C9. The half life is 7 to 10 hours. Stereose-lective first-pass metabolism results in more rapid clearance of S(−)-carvedilol than R(+)-carvedilol. No significant changes in the pharmacokinetics of carvedilol were seen in elderly patients with hypertension, and no change in dosage is needed in patients with moderate-to-severe renal insufficiency (Cleland, 2003; Keating and Jarvis, 2003).

Bucindolol

Bucindolol (SANDONORM) is a third-generation non-selective β receptor antagonist with some α_1 receptor blocking as well as β_2 and β_3 agonistic properties. Although not precisely understood, it appears to be a vasodilator via its β_2 agonistic action as well as ancil-lary mechanisms (Andreka et al., 2002; Maack et al., 2000).

Bucindolol increases left ventricular systolic ejection fraction and decreases peripheral resistance, thereby reducing afterload. It increases plasma HDL cholesterol, but does not affect plasma tri-glycerides. In contrast to other β receptor antagonists used in large multicenter trials (e.g., carvedilol), bucindolol was not asso-ciated with improved survival compared with placebo (The β-

Blocker Evaluation of Survival Trial Investigators, 2001). Although the reasons for a lack of benefit in mortality in the BEST trial are not clear, bucindolol has intrinsic sympathomimet-ic activity that may be detrimental in the long-term treatment of heart failure (Andreka et al., 2002). Bucindolol is not currently on the U.S. market.

Celiprolol

Celiprolol (SELECTOR) is a third-generation cardioselec-tive, β receptor antagonist. It has low lipid solubility and possesses weak vasodilating and bronchodilating effects attributed to partial selective β_2 agonist activity and possibly papaverine-like relaxant effects on smooth muscle (including bronchial). It also has been reported to have peripheral α_2-adrenergic receptor inhibitory activity and to promote NO release. There is evidence for intrinsic sympathomimetic activity at the β_2 recep-tor. Celiprol is devoid of membrane-stabilizing activity. Weak α_2 antagonistic properties are present, but are not considered clinically significant at therapeutic doses (Toda, 2003).

Celiprolol reduces heart rate and blood pressure and can increase the functional refractory period of the atrioventricular node. Oral bioavailability ranges from 30% to 70%, and peak plasma levels are seen at 2 to 4 hours. It is largely unmetabolized and is excreted unchanged in the urine and feces. Celiprolol does not undergo first-pass metabolism. The predominant mode of excretion is renal. Celiprolol is a safe and effective drug for treat-ment of hypertension and angina (Witchitz et al., 2000; Felix et al., 2001).

Nebivolol

Nebivolol has a hemodynamic profile different from classic β receptor antagonists such as atenolol, pro-pranolol, and pindolol. It acutely lowers arterial blood pressure without depressing left ventricular function, and reduces systemic vascular resistance. This reduc-tion in systemic vascular resistance is due to a direct vasorelaxant effect that is mediated at least in part by NO (Ignarro et al., 2002). Nebivolol appears to be the most selective β_1 receptor antagonist available clinical-ly and is devoid of intrinsic sympathomimetic activity, inverse agonist activity, and α_1 receptor blocking properties (de Groot et al., 2004; Brixius et al., 2001). It does not alter exercise capacity in healthy individu-als but does inhibit both ADP and collagen-induced platelet aggregation.

Nebivolol is a racemate containing equal amounts of the d- and l-enantiomers. The d-isomer is the active β-blocking compo-nent, while the l-isomer is responsible for the release of nitric oxide. Nebivolol was effective in treating hypertension and diastolic heart failure in several well-controlled clinical trials (Czuriga *et al.*, 2003; Rosei *et al.*, 2003; Nodari *et al.*, 2003). Although not yet on the market in the United States, a New Drug Application has been submitted to the FDA for use in the management of hypertension.

Other β Receptor Antagonists

Many other β receptor antagonists have been synthesized and evaluated to varying extents. *Oxprenolol* (no longer marketed in the United States), and *penbutolol* (LEVATOL) are non–subtype-selective β blockers with intrinsic sympathomimetic activity. *Medroxalol* is a nonselective β blocker with α_1 receptor–blocking activity (Rosendorff, 1993). *Levobunolol* (BETAGAN LIQUIFILM, others) is a non–subtype-selective β antagonist used as a topical agent in the treatment of glaucoma (Brooks and Gillies, 1992). Betaxolol (BETOP-TIC), a β_1-selective antagonist, is available as an ophthalmic preparation for glaucoma and an oral formulation for systemic hypertension. Betaxolol may be less likely to induce bronchospasm than are the ophthalmic preparations of the nonselective β blockers timolol and levobunolol. Similarly, ocular administration of carteolol (OCUPRESS) may be less likely than timolol to have systemic effects, possibly because of its intrinsic sympathomimetic activity; cautious monitoring is required nonetheless. *Sotalol* (BETAPACE, BETAPACE AF, others) is a nonselective β antagonist that is devoid of membrane-stabilizing actions. However, it has antiarrhythmic actions independent of its ability to block β adrenergic receptors (Fitton and Sorkin, 1993) (*see* Chapter 34). *Propafenone* (RYTH-MOL) is a Na^+-channel blocking drug that also is a β adrenergic receptor antagonist.

ADVERSE EFFECTS AND PRECAUTIONS

The most common adverse effects of β receptor antagonists arise as pharmacological consequences of blockade of β receptors; serious adverse effects unrelated to β receptor blockade are rare.

Cardiovascular System. Because the sympathetic nervous system provides critical support for cardiac performance in many individuals with impaired myocardial function, β receptor antagonists may induce congestive heart failure in susceptible patients. Thus, β receptor blockade may cause or exacerbate heart failure in patients with compensated heart failure, acute myocardial infarction, or cardiomegaly. It is not known whether β receptor antagonists that possess intrinsic sympathomimetic activity or peripheral vasodilating properties are safer in these settings. Nonetheless, there is convincing evidence that chronic administration of β receptor antagonists is efficacious in prolonging life in the therapy of heart failure in selected patients (*see* below and Chapter 33).

Bradycardia is a normal response to β receptor blockade; however, in patients with partial or complete atrioventricular conduction defects, β antagonists may cause life-threatening bradyarrhythmias. Particular caution is indicated in patients who are taking other drugs, such as *verapamil* or various antiarrhythmic agents, which may impair sinus-node function or AV conduction.

Some patients complain of cold extremities while taking β receptor antagonists. Symptoms of peripheral vascular disease may worsen, although this is uncommon, or Raynaud's phenomenon may develop. The risk of worsening intermittent claudication probably is very small with this class of drugs, and the clinical benefits of β antagonists in patients with peripheral vascular disease and coexisting coronary artery disease may be very important.

Abrupt discontinuation of β receptor antagonists after long-term treatment can exacerbate angina and may increase the risk of sudden death. The underlying mechanism is unclear, but it is well established that there is enhanced sensitivity to β adrenergic receptor agonists in patients who have undergone long-term treatment with certain β receptor antagonists after the blocker is withdrawn abruptly. For example, chronotropic responses to isoproterenol are blunted in patients who are receiving β receptor antagonists; however, abrupt discontinuation of propranolol leads to greater-than-normal sensitivity to isoproterenol. This increased sensitivity is evident several days after stopping propranolol and may persist for at least 1 week. Such enhanced sensitivity can be attenuated by tapering the dose of the β blocker for several weeks before discontinuation. Supersensitivity to isoproterenol also has been observed after abrupt discontinuation of metoprolol, but not of pindolol. This enhanced β responsiveness may result from up-regulation of β receptors. The number of β receptors on circulating lymphocytes is increased in subjects who have received propranolol for long periods; pindolol has the opposite effect. Optimal strategies for discontinuation of β blockers are not known, but it is prudent to decrease the dose gradually and to restrict exercise during this period.

Pulmonary Function. A major adverse effect of β receptor antagonists is caused by blockade of β_2 receptors in bronchial smooth muscle. These receptors are particularly important for promoting bronchodilation in patients with bronchospastic disease, and β blockers may cause a life-threatening increase in airway resistance in such patients. Drugs with selectivity for β_1 adrenergic receptors or those with intrinsic sympathomimetic activity at β_2 adrenergic receptors may be somewhat less likely to induce bronchospasm. Since the selectivity of current β blockers for β_1 receptors is modest, these drugs should be avoided if at all possible in patients with asthma. However, in some patients with chronic obstructive pulmonary disease, the potential advantage of using β receptor antagonists after myocardial infarction may outweigh the risk of worsening pulmonary function (Gottlieb *et al.*, 1998).

Central Nervous System. The adverse effects of β receptor antagonists that are referable to the CNS may include fatigue, sleep disturbances (including insomnia and nightmares), and depression. The previously ascribed association between these drugs and depression (Thiessen *et al.*, 1990) may not be substantiated by more recent clinical studies (Gerstman *et al.*, 1996; Ried *et al.*, 1998). Interest has focused on the relationship between the incidence of the adverse effects of β receptor antagonists and their lipophilicity; however, no clear correlation has emerged.

Metabolism. As described above, β adrenergic blockade may blunt recognition of hypoglycemia by patients; it also may delay recovery from insulin-induced hypoglycemia. β Receptor antagonists should be used with great caution in patients with diabetes who are prone to hypoglycemic reactions; β_1-selective agents may be preferable for these patients. The benefits of β receptor antagonists in type 1 diabetes with myocardial infarction may outweigh the risk in selected patients (Gottlieb *et al.*, 1998).

Miscellaneous. The incidence of sexual dysfunction in men with hypertension who are treated with β receptor antagonists is not clearly defined. Although experience with the use of β adrenergic receptor antagonists in pregnancy is increasing, information about the safety of these drugs during pregnancy still is limited.

Overdosage. The manifestations of poisoning with β receptor antagonists depend on the pharmacological properties of the ingested drug, particularly its β_1 selectivity, intrinsic sympathomimetic activity, and membrane-stabilizing properties (Frishman, 1983). Hypotension, bradycardia, prolonged AV conduction times, and widened QRS complexes are common manifestations of overdosage. Seizures and depression may occur. Hypoglycemia is rare, and bronchospasm is uncommon in the absence of pulmonary disease. Significant bradycardia should be treated initially with atropine, but a cardiac pacemaker often is required. Large doses of isoproterenol or an α receptor agonist may be necessary to treat hypotension. Glucagon has positive chronotropic and inotropic effects on the heart that are independent of interactions with β adrenergic receptors, and the drug has been useful in some patients.

Drug Interactions. Both pharmacokinetic and pharmacodynamic interactions have been noted between β receptor antagonists and other drugs. Aluminum salts, *cholestyramine*, and *colestipol* may decrease the absorption of β blockers. Drugs such as *phenytoin*, *rifampin*, and *phenobarbital*, as well as smoking, induce hepatic biotransformation enzymes and may decrease plasma concentrations of β receptor antagonists that are metabolized extensively (*e.g.*, propranolol). Cimetidine and hydralazine may increase the bioavailability of agents such as propranolol and metoprolol by affecting hepatic blood flow. β Receptor antagonists can impair the clearance of *lidocaine*.

Other drug interactions have pharmacodynamic explanations. For example, β antagonists and Ca^{2+} channel blockers have additive effects on the cardiac conducting system. Additive effects on blood pressure between β blockers and other antihypertensive agents often are employed to clinical advantage. However, the antihypertensive effects of β receptor antagonists can be opposed by *indomethacin* and other nonsteroidal antiinflammatory drugs (*see* Chapter 26).

THERAPEUTIC USES

Cardiovascular Diseases

β Receptor antagonists are used extensively in the treatment of hypertension (*see* Chapter 32), angina and acute coronary syndromes (*see* Chapter 31), and congestive heart failure (*see* Chapter 33). These drugs also are used frequently in the treatment of supraventricular and ventricular arrhythmias (*see* Chapter 34).

Myocardial Infarction. A great deal of interest has focused on the use of β receptor antagonists in the treatment of acute myocardial infarction and in the prevention of recurrences for those who have survived an initial attack. Numerous trials have shown that β receptor antagonists administered during the early phases of acute myocardial infarction and continued long-term may decrease mortality by about 25% (Freemantle *et al.*, 1999). The precise mechanism is not known, but the favorable effects of β receptor antagonists may stem from decreased myocardial oxygen demand, redistribution of myocardial blood flow, and antiarrhythmic actions. There is likely much less benefit if β adrenergic receptor antagonists are administered for only a short time. In studies of secondary prevention, the most extensive, favorable clinical trial data are available for propranolol, metoprolol, and timolol. In spite of these proven benefits, many patients with myocardial infarction do not receive a β adrenergic receptor antagonist.

Congestive Heart Failure. It is a common clinical observation that acute administration of β receptor antagonists can worsen markedly or even precipitate congestive heart failure in compensated patients with multiple forms of heart disease, such as ischemic or congestive cardiomyopathy. Consequently, the hypothesis that β receptor antagonists might be efficacious in the long-term treatment of heart failure originally seemed counterintuitive to many physicians. However, the reflex sympathetic responses to heart failure may stress the failing heart and exacerbate the progression of the disease, and blocking those responses could be beneficial. A number of well-designed randomized clinical trials involving numerous patients have demonstrated that certain β receptor antagonists are highly effective treatment for patients with all grades of heart failure secondary to left ventricular systolic dysfunction. The drugs have been shown to improve myocardial function, to improve life quality, and to prolong life. From the point of view of the history of therapeutic advances in the treatment of congestive heart failure, it is interesting to note how this drug class has moved from being completely contraindicated to being the standard of care in many settings.

Large trials have been conducted with carvedilol, bisoprolol, metoprolol, *xamoterol*, bucindolol, betaxol, nebivolol, and *talinolol* (Cleland, 2003). Carvedilol, metoprolol, and bisoprolol all have been shown to reduce the mortality rate in large cohorts of patients with stable chronic heart failure regardless of severity (Bolger and Al-Nasser, 2003; Cleland, 2003). In the initial use of β blockers for treating heart failure, the beginning effects often are neutral or even adverse. Benefits accumulate gradually over a period of weeks to months, although benefits from the third-generation vasodilator β blocker carvedilol may be seen within days in patients with severe heart failure. There also is a reduction in the hospitalization of patients along with a reduction in mortality with fewer sudden deaths and deaths caused by progressive heart failure. These benefits extend to patients with asthma and with diabetes mellitus (Dunne *et al.*, 2001; Self *et al.*, 2003; Cruickshank, 2002; Salpeter, 2003). Patients in atrial fibrillation and heart failure can also benefit from β blockade (Kühlkamp *et al.*, 2002). On the other hand, patients with heart failure and atrial fibrillation are associated with a higher mortality, and the benefit derived from β blockers may not be comparable to those in sinus rhythm (Fung *et al.*, 2003). Long-term β blockade reduces cardiac volume, myocardial hypertrophy, and filling pressure, and increases ejection fraction (*e.g.*, ventricular remodeling). β Receptor antagonists impact mortality even before beneficial effects on ventricular function are observed, possibly due to prevention of arrhythmias or a reduction in acute vascular events.

Some patients are unable to tolerate β blockers. Hopefully, ongoing trials will identify the common characteristics that define this population so that β blockers can be avoided in these patients (Bolger and Al-Nasser, 2003). Because of the real possibility of acutely worsening cardiac function, β receptor antagonists should be initiated only by clinicians experienced in patients with congestive heart failure. As might be anticipated, starting with very low doses of drug and advancing doses slowly over time, depending on each patient's response, are critical for the safe use of these drugs in patients with congestive heart failure.

It is unknown whether it is necessary to block only the β_1 adrenergic receptor or whether nonselective agents would be more desirable in the management of heart failure. Blockade of β_2 adrenergic receptors can enhance peripheral vasoconstriction and bronchoconstriction and therefore have a deleterious effect. On the

other hand, blocking β_2 adrenergic receptors might be advantageous due to more effectively protecting cardiac cells from catecholamine excess and hypokalemia. Some propose that nonselective β antagonists that block both β_1 and β_2 receptors and also have peripheral vasodilatory actions (third-generation β blockers) may offer the best myocardial, metabolic, and hemodynamic benefit (Cleland, 2003) (*see* Chapter 33). Some experts have recommended that β blockers be considered as part of the standard treatment regimen for all patients with mild-to-moderate heart failure (Goldstein, 2002; Maggioni *et al.*, 2003).

β **Adrenergic Receptor Signaling in Heart Failure and its Treatment.** The underlying cellular or subcellular mechanisms leading to the beneficial effects of β blockers are unclear. Sympathetic nervous system activity is increased in patients with congestive heart failure (Bristow *et al.*, 1985). Infusions of β agonists are toxic to the heart in several animal models. Also, overexpression of β receptors in transgenic mice leads to a dilated cardiomyopathy (Engelhardt *et al.*, 1999). A number of changes in β receptor signaling occur in the myocardium of patients with heart failure and in a variety of animal models (Post *et al.*, 1999). Decreased numbers and functioning of β_1 receptors consistently have been found in heart failure, leading to attenuation of β receptor–mediated stimulation of positive inotropic responses in the failing heart. These changes may be due in part to increased expression of β adrenergic receptor kinase-1 (βARK-1, GRK2) (Lefkowitz *et al.*, 2000) (*see* Chapter 6).

It is of potential interest that β_2 receptor expression is relatively maintained in these settings of heart failure. While both β_1 and β_2 receptors activate adenylyl cyclase *via* G_s, there is evidence suggesting that β_2 receptors also stimulate G_i, which may attenuate contractile responses and lead to activation of other effector pathways downstream of G_i (Lefkowitz *et al.*, 2000). Overexpression of β_2 adrenergic receptors in mouse heart is associated with increased cardiac force without the development of cardiomyopathy (Liggett *et al.*, 2000). The stimulation of β_3 adrenergic receptors inhibits contraction and relaxation (Gauthier *et al.*, 2000). In contrast to β_1 and β_2 receptors, β_3 receptors are upregulated in heart failure (Moniotte *et al.*, 2001). This has led to the hypothesis that in severe congestive heart failure, as β_1 and β_2 receptor pathways *via* G_s become less responsive, the inhibitory effects of the β_3 receptor pathway may contribute to the detrimental effects of sympathetic stimulation in congestive heart failure (Morimoto *et al.*, 2004). Thus, the blockade of β_3 receptors by β receptor antagonists (*e.g.*, carvedilol) could improve the acute tolerability and benefit of β_1 and β_2 receptor antagonists (Moniotte *et al.*, 2001; Morimoto *et al.*, 2004).

The mechanisms by which β receptor antagonists decrease mortality in patients with congestive heart failure are still unclear. Perhaps this is not surprising, given that the mechanism by which this class of drugs lowers blood pressure in patients with hypertension remains elusive despite years of investigation (*see* Chapter 32). This is much more than an academic undertaking; a deeper understanding of involved pathways could lead to selection of the most appropriate drugs available as well as the development of novel compounds with especially desirable properties. The potential differences among β_1, β_2, and β_3 receptor function in heart failure is one example of the complexity of adrenergic pharmacology of this syndrome. Recent research provides evidence for multiple affinity states of the β_1 receptor, for cell-type specific coupling of β receptor subtypes to signalling pathways other than

G_s-adenylyl cyclase–cyclic AMP, and for altered receptor properties when β_2 and β_3 receptors for hetero-oligomers (Rozec *et al.*, 2003; Breit *et al.*, 2004). Such findings suggest opportunities for the development of more focused β antagonist therapy in the future.

A number of mechanisms have been proposed to play a role in the beneficial effects of β receptor antagonists in heart failure. Since excess effects of catecholamines may be toxic to the heart, especially *via* activation of β_1 receptors, inhibition of the pathway may help preserve myocardial function. Also, antagonism of β receptors in the heart may attenuate cardiac remodeling, which ordinarily might have deleterious effects on cardiac function. Interestingly, activation of β receptors may promote myocardial cell death *via* apoptosis (Singh *et al.*, 2000). In addition, properties of certain β receptor antagonists that are due to other, unrelated properties of these drugs may be potentially important. For example, afterload reduction by drugs such as carvedilol may be relevant. The potential importance of the α_1 antagonistic and antioxidant properties of carvedilol in its beneficial effects in patients with heart failure is not clear (Ma *et al.*, 1996).

Use of β Antagonists in Other Cardiovascular Diseases. β Receptor antagonists, particularly propranolol, are used in the treatment of hypertrophic obstructive cardiomyopathy. Propranolol is useful for relieving angina, palpitations, and syncope in patients with this disorder. Efficacy probably is related to partial relief of the pressure gradient along the outflow tract. β Blockers also may attenuate catecholamine-induced cardiomyopathy in pheochromocytoma.

β Blockers are used frequently in the medical management of acute dissecting aortic aneurysm; their usefulness comes from reduction in the force of myocardial contraction and the rate of development of such force. Nitroprusside is an alternative, but when given in the absence of β receptor blockade, it causes an undesirable tachycardia. Patients with Marfan's syndrome may develop progressive dilation of the aorta, which may lead to aortic dissection and regurgitation, a major cause of death in these patients. Chronic treatment with propranolol may be efficacious in slowing the progression of aortic dilation and its complications in patients with Marfan's syndrome (Shores *et al.*, 1994).

Glaucoma

β Receptor antagonists are very useful in the treatment of chronic open-angle glaucoma. Six drugs currently are available: carteolol (OCUPRESS, others), betaxolol (BETAOPTIC, others), levobunolol (BETAGAN, others), *metipranolol* (OPTIPRANOLOL, others), timolol (TIMOPTIC, others), and *levobetaxolol* (BETAXON). Timolol, levobunolol, carteolol, and metipranolol are nonselective, while betaxolol and levobetaxolol are β_1 selective. None of the agents has significant membrane-stabilizing or intrinsic sympathomimetic activities. Topically administered β blockers have little or no effect on pupil size or accommodation and are devoid of blurred vision and night blindness often seen with miotics. These agents decrease the production of aqueous

humor, which appears to be the mechanism for their clinical effectiveness.

The drugs generally are administered as eye drops and have an onset in approximately 30 minutes with a duration of 12 to 24 hours. While topically administered β blockers usually are well tolerated, systemic absorption can lead to adverse cardiovascular and pulmonary effects in susceptible patients. They therefore should be used with great caution in glaucoma patients at risk for adverse systemic effects of β receptor antagonists (*e.g.*, patients with bronchial asthma, severe COPD, or those with bradyarrhythmias. The use of topically administered β blockers for treatment of glaucoma is discussed further in Chapter 63. Recently three β blockers (betaxolol, metipranolol, and timolol) also have been observed to confer protection to retinal neurons, apparently related to their ability to attenuate neuronal Ca^{2+} and Na^+ influx (Wood *et al.*, 2003). Betaxolol is the most effective antiglaucoma drug at reducing Na^+/Ca^{2+} influx. It is thought that β blockers may be able to blunt ganglion cell death in glaucoma and that levobetaxolol may be a more important neuroprotectant than timolol because of its greater capacity to block Na^+ and Ca^{2+} influx (Osborne *et al.*, 2004).

Other Uses

Many of the signs and symptoms of hyperthyroidism are reminiscent of the manifestations of increased sympathetic nervous system activity. Indeed, excess thyroid hormone increases the expression of β receptors in some types of cells. β Receptor antagonists control many of the cardiovascular signs and symptoms of hyperthyroidism and are useful adjuvants to more definitive therapy. In addition, propranolol inhibits the peripheral conversion of thyroxine to triiodothyronine, an effect that may be independent of β receptor blockade. However, caution is advised in treating patients with cardiac enlargement, since the use of β receptor antagonists may precipitate congestive heart failure (*see* Chapter 56 for further discussion of the treatment of hyperthyroidism).

Propranolol, timolol, and metoprolol are effective for the prophylaxis of migraine (Tfelt-Hansen, 1986); the mechanism of this effect is not known, and these drugs are not useful for treatment of acute attacks of migraine.

Propranolol and other β blockers are effective in controlling acute panic symptoms in individuals who are required to perform in public or in other anxiety-provoking situations. Public speakers may be calmed by the prophylactic administration of the drug, and the performance of musicians may be improved. Tachycardia, muscle tremors, and other evidence of increased sympathetic activity are reduced. Propranolol also may be useful in the treatment of essential tremor.

β Blockers may be of some value in the treatment of patients undergoing withdrawal from alcohol or those with akathisia. Propranolol and nadolol are efficacious in the primary prevention of variceal bleeding in patients with portal hypertension caused by cirrhosis of the liver (Villanueva *et al.*, 1996; Bosch, 1998). *Isosorbide mononitrate* may augment the fall in portal pressure seen in some patients treated with β receptor antagonists. These drugs also may be beneficial in reducing the risk of recurrent variceal bleeding.

Selection of a β Receptor Antagonist

The various β receptor antagonists that are used for the treatment of hypertension and angina appear to have similar efficacies. Selection of the most appropriate drug for an individual patient should be based on pharmacokinetic and pharmacodynamic differences among the drugs, cost, and whether there are concurrent medical problems. For some diseases (*e.g.,* myocardial infarction, migraine, cirrhosis with varices, and congestive heart failure), it should not be assumed that all members of this class of drugs are interchangeable; the appropriate drug should be selected from those that have documented efficacy for the disease. β_1-Selective antagonists are preferable in patients with bronchospasm, diabetes, peripheral vascular disease, or Raynaud's phenomenon. Although no clinical advantage of β receptor antagonists with intrinsic sympathomimetic activity has been clearly established, such drugs may be preferable in patients with bradycardia. In addition, third generation β antagonists that block α_1 receptors, stimulate β_2 receptors, enhance NO production, block Ca^{2+} entry, open K^+ channels, or possess antioxidant properties may offer therapeutic advantages.

BIBLIOGRAPHY

Allwood, M.J., Cobbold, A.F., and Ginsberg, J. Peripheral vascular effects of noradrenaline, isopropylnoradrenaline, and dopamine. *Br. Med. Bull.,* **1963,** *19:*132–136.

Andreka, P., Aiyar, N., Olson, L.C., *et al.* Bucinolol displays intrinsic sympathomimetic activity in human myocardium. *Circulation,* **2002,** *105:*2429–2434.

Becker, A.J., Stief, C.G., Machtens, S., *et al.* Oral phentolamine as treatment for erectile dysfunction. *J. Urol.,* **1998,** *159:*1214–1216.

Breit, A., Lagace, M., and Bouvier, M. Hetero-oligomerization between β_2 and β_3 receptors generates a β-adrenergic signaling unit with distinct funtional properties. *J. Biol. Chem.,* **2004,** *279:*28756–28765.

Brixius, K., Bundkirchen, A., Bölck, B., Mehlhorn, U., and Schwinger, R.H. Nebivolol, bucindolol, metoprolol and carvedilol are devoid of intrinsic sympathomimetic activity in human myocardium. *Br. J. Pharmacol.,* **2001,** *133:*1330–1338.

Chapleau, M.W., Cunningham, J.T., Sullivan, M.J., Wachtel, R.E., and Abboud, F.M. Structural versus functional modulation of the arterial baroreflex. *Hypertension,* **1995,** *26:*341–347.

Chidiac, P., Hebert, T.E., Valiquette, M., Dennis, M., and Bouvier, M. Inverse agonist activity of β-adrenergic antagonists. *Mol. Pharmacol.,* **1994,** *45:*490–499.

Clark, J.A., Zimmerman, H.J., and Tanner, L.A. Labetalol hepatotoxicity. *Ann. Intern. Med.,* **1990,** *113:*210–213.

Cohn, J.N., Archibald, D.G., Ziesche, S., *et al.* Effect of vasodilator therapy on mortality in chronic congestive heart failure. Results of a Veterans Administration Cooperative Study. *N. Engl. J. Med.,* **1986,** *314:*1547–1552.

Czuriga, I., Riecansky, I., Bodnar, J., *et al.* for the NEBIS investigators, NEBIS Investigators Group. Comparison of the new cardioselective β-blocker nebivolol with bisoprolol in hypertension: The nebivolol, bisoprolol multicenter study (NEBIS). *Cardiovasc. Drugs Ther.,* **2003,** *17:*257–263.

DeBernardis, J.F., Winn, M., Kerkman, D.J., *et al.* A new nasal decongestant, A-57219: a comparison with oxymetazoline. *J. Pharm. Pharmacol.,* **1987,** *39:*760–763.

Engelhardt, S., Hein, L., Wiesmann, F., and Lohse, M.J. Progressive hypertrophy and heart failure in β_1-adrenergic receptor transgenic mice. *Proc. Natl. Acad. Sci. U.S.A.,* **1999,** *96:*7059–7064.

Felix, S.B., Stangl, V., Kieback, A., *et al.* Acute hemodynamic effects of β-blockers in patients with severe congestive heart failure: Comparison of celiprolol and esmolol. *J. Cardiovasc. Pharmacol.,* **2001,** *38:*666–671.

Foglar, R., Shibata, K., Horie, K., Hirasawa, A., and Tsujimoto, G. Use of recombinant α_1-adrenoceptors to characterize subtype selectivity of drugs for the treatment of prostatic hypertrophy. *Eur. J. Pharmacol.,* **1995,** *288:*201–207.

Forray, C., Bard, J.A., Wetzel, J.M., *et al.* The α_1-adrenergic receptor that mediates smooth muscle contraction in human prostate has the pharmacological properties of the cloned human α 1c subtype. *Mol. Pharmacol.,* **1994,** *45:*703–708.

Gottlieb, S.S., McCarter, R.J., and Vogel, R.A. Effect of β-blockade on mortality among high-risk and low-risk patients after myocardial infarction. *N. Engl. J. Med.,* **1998,** *339:*489–497.

de Groot, A.A., Mathy, M.J., van Zwieten, P.A., and Peters, S.L. Antioxidant activity of nebivolol in the rat aorta. *J. Cardiovasc. Pharmacol.,* **2004,** *43:*148–153.

Grossman, E., Rosenthal, T., Peleg, E., Holmes, C., and Goldstein, D.S. Oral yohimbine increases blood pressure and sympathetic nervous outflow in hypertensive patients. *J. Cardiovasc. Pharmacol.,* **1993,** *22:*22–26.

Hancox, R.J., Aldridge, R.E., Cowan, J.O., *et al.* Tolerance to β-agonists during acute bronchoconstriction. *Eur. Respir. J.,* **1999,** *14:*283–287.

Harder, S., and Thurmann, P. Concentration/effect relationship of bunazosin, a selective α_1-adrenoceptor antagonist in hypertensive patients after single and multiple oral doses. *Int. J. Clin. Pharmacol. Ther.,* **1994,** *32:*38–43.

Hu, Z.W., Shi, X.Y., and Hoffman, B.B. Doxazosin inhibits proliferation and migration of human vascular smooth-muscle cells independent of α_1-adrenergic receptor antagonism. *J. Cardiovasc. Pharmacol.,* **1998,** *31:*833–839.

Ignarro, L.J., Byrns, R.E., Trinh, K. Sisodia, M., and Buga, G.M. Nebivolol: a selective β_1 adrenergic receptor antagonist that relaxes vascular smooth muscle by nitric-oxide and cyclic GMP-dependent mechanisms. *Nitric Oxide,* **2002,** *7:*75–82.

Ishii, Y., Nakamura, K., Tsutsumi, K., *et al.* Drug interaction between cimetidine and timolol ophthalmic solution: effect on heart rate and intraocular pressure in healthy Japanese volunteers. *J. Clin. Pharmacol.,* **2000,** *40:*193–199.

Kaiser, P., Tesch, P.A., Frisk-Holmberg, M., Juhlin-Dannfelt, A., and Kaijser, L. Effect of β_1-selective and nonselective β-blockade on work capacity and muscle metabolism. *Clin. Physiol.,* **1986,** *6:*197–207.

Kenny, B.A., Miller, A.M., Williamson, I.J., *et al.* Evaluation of the pharmacological selectivity profile of α_1 adrenoceptor antagonists at prostatic α_1 adrenoceptors: binding, functional and in vivo studies. *Br. J. Pharmacol.*, **1996**, *118:*871–878.

Kirby, R.S., Coppinger, S.W., Corcoran, M.O., *et al.* Prazosin in the treatment of prostatic obstruction. A placebo-controlled study. *Br. J. Urol.*, **1987**, *60:*136–142.

Lepor, H., Williford, W.O., Barry, M.J., *et al.* The efficacy of terazosin, finasteride, or both in benign prostatic hyperplasia. Veterans Affairs Cooperative Studies Benign Prostatic Hyperplasia Study Group. *N. Engl. J. Med.*, **1996**, *335:*533–539.

Liggett, S.B., Tepe, N.M., Lorenz, J.N., *et al.* Early and delayed consequences of β_2-adrenergic receptor overexpression in mouse hearts: critical role for expression level. *Circulation,* **2000**, *101:*1707–1714.

Ma, X.L., Yue, T.L., Lopez, B.L., *et al.* Carvedilol, a new β adrenoreceptor blocker and free radical scavenger, attenuates myocardial ischemia–reperfusion injury in hypercholesterolemic rabbits. *J. Pharmacol. Exp. Ther.*, **1996**, *277:*128–136.

Maack, C., Cremers, B., Flesch, M., *et al.* Different intrinsic activities of bucindolol, carvedilol and metoprolol in human failing myocardium. *Br. J. Pharmacol.*, **2000**, *130:*1131–1139.

MacMillan, L.B., Hein, L., Smith, M.S., Piascik, M.T., and Limbird, L.E. Central hypotensive effects of the α_{2A}-adrenergic receptor subtype. *Science,* **1996**, *273:*801–803.

Maggioni, A.P., Sinagra, G., Opasich, C., *et al.* β Blockers in patients with congestive heart failure: guided use in clinical practice investigators. Treatment of chronic heart failure with β adrenergic blockade beyond controlled clinical trials: The BRING-UP experience. *Heart,* **2003**, *89:*299–305.

Marik, P.E., and Iglesias, J. Low-dose dopamine does not prevent acute renal failure in patients with septic shock and oliguria. NORASEPT II Study Investigators. *Am. J. Med.,* **1999**, *107:*387–390.

MERIT-HF Study Group. Effect of metoprolol CR/XL in chronic heart failure: Metoprolol CR/XL Randomised Intervention Trial in Congestive Heart Failure (MERIT-HF). *Lancet,* **1999**, *353:*2001–2007.

Mignot, E. Sleep, sleep disorders, and hypocretin (orexin). *Sleep Med.,* **2004**, *5:*S2–S8.

Moniotte, S., Kobzik, L., Feron O., *et al.* Upregulation of β_3-adrenoceptors and altered contractile response to inotropic amines in human failing myocardium. *Circulation,* **2001**, *103:*1649–1655.

Morimoto, A., Hasegawa, H., Cheng, H-J., Little, W.C., and Cheng, C.P. Endogenous β_3-adrenoceptor activation contributes to left ventricular and cardiomyocyte dysfunction in heart failure. *Am. J. Physiol. Heart Circ. Physiol.,* **2004**, *286:*H2425–H2433.

Murray, K.T., Reilly, C., Koshakji, R.P., *et al.* Suppression of ventricular arrhythmias in man by *d*-propranolol independent of β-adrenergic receptor blockade. *J. Clin. Invest.,* **1990**, *85:*836–842.

Nodari, S., Metra, M., Dei Cas, L. β-Blocker treatment of patients with diastolic heart failure and atrial hypertension. A prospective, randomized comparison of the long-term effects of atenolol vs. nebivolol. *Eur. J. Heart Failure,* **2003**, *5:*621–627.

Okazaki, M., Hu, Z-W., Fujinaga, M., and Hoffman, B.B. α_1 Adrenergic receptor-induced c-*fos* gene expression in rat aorta and cultured vascular smooth muscle cells. *J. Clin. Invest.,* **1994**, *94:*210–218.

Osborne, N.N., Wood, J.P., Chidlow, G., *et al.* Effectiveness of levobetaxolol and timolol at blunting retinal ischaemia is related to their calcium and sodium blocking activities: relevance to glaucoma. *Brain Res. Bull.,* **2004**, *62:*525–528.

Papatsonis, D.N., van Geijn, H.P., *et al.* Nifedipine and ritodrine in the management of preterm labor: a randomized multicenter trial. *Obstet. Gynecol.,* **1997**, *90:*230–234.

Pearce, N., Beasley, R., Crane, J., Burgess, C., and Jackson, R. End of the New Zealand asthma mortality epidemic. *Lancet,* **1995**, *345:*41–44.

Perry, R.R., Keiser, H.R., Norton, J.A., *et al.* Surgical management of pheochromocytoma with the use of metyrosine. *Ann. Surg.,* **1990**, *212:*621–628.

Pujet, J.C., Dubreuil, C., Fleury, B., Provendier, O., and Abella, M.L. Effects of celiprolol, a cardioselective β-blocker, on respiratory function in asthmatic patients. *Eur. Respir. J.,* **1992**, *5:*196–200.

Reid, K., Surridge, D.H., Morales, A., *et al.* Double-blind trial of yohimbine in treatment of psychogenic impotence. *Lancet,* **1987**, *2:*421–423.

Rosei, E.A., Rizzoni, D., Comini, S., and Boari, G., Nebivolol-Lisinopril Study Group. Evaluation of the efficacy and tolerability of nebivolol versus lisinopril in the treatment of essential arterial hypertension: A randomized, multicentre, double blind study. *Blood Press. Suppl.,* **2003**, *1:*30–35.

Rosen, S.G., Clutter, W.E., Shah, S.D., *et al.* Direct α-adrenergic stimulation of hepatic glucose production in human subjects. *Am. J. Physiol.,* **1983**, *245:*E616–E626.

Rozec, B., Noireaud, J., Trochu, J., and Gauthier, C. Place of β_3-adrenoceptors among other β-adrenoceptor sub-types in the regulation of the cardiovascular system. *Arch. Mal Coeur Vaiss.,* **2003**, *96:*905–913.

Shmid-Schonbein, G., and Hugli, T. A new hypothesis for microvascular inflammation in shock and multiorgan failure: self-digestion by pancreatic enzymes. *Microcirc.,* **2005**, *12:*71–82.

Shores, J., Berger, K.R., Murphy, E.A., and Pyeritz, R.E. Progression of aortic dilatation and the benefit of long-term β-adrenergic blockade in Marfan's syndrome. *N. Engl. J. Med.,* **1994**, *330:*1335–1341.

Simon, T., Mary-Krause, M., Funck-Brentano, C., Lechat, P., and Jaillon, P. Bisoprolol dose-response relationship in patients with congestive heart failure: a subgroups analysis in the cardiac insufficiency bisoprolol study (CIBIS II). *Eur. Heart J.,* **2003**, *24:*552–559.

Spittell, J.A. Jr., and Spittell, P.C. Chronic pernio: another cause of blue toes. *Int. Angiol.,* **1992**, *11:*46–50.

Strader, C.D., Candelore, M.R., Hill, W.S., Sigal, I.S., and Dixon, R.A. Identification of two serine residues involved in agonist activation of the β-adrenergic receptor. *J. Biol. Chem.,* **1989**, *264:*13572–13578.

Suissa, S., and Ernst, P. Optical illusions from visual data analysis: example of the New Zealand asthma mortality epidemic. *J. Clin. Epidemiol.,* **1997**, *50:*1079–1088.

Suissa, S., Ernst, P., Boivin, J.F., *et al.* A cohort analysis of excess mortality in asthma and the use of inhaled β-agonists. *Am. J. Respir. Crit. Care. Med.,* **1994**, *149:*604–610.

Sun, D., Huang, A., Mital, S., *et al.* Norepinephrine elicits β_2-receptor-mediated dilation of isolated human coronary arterioles. *Circulation,* **2002**, *106:*550–555.

The β-Blocker Evaluation of Survival Trial Investigators. A trial of the β-blocker bucindolol in patients with advanced chronic heart failure. *N. Engl. J. Med.,* **2001**, *344:*1659–1667.

Thiessen, B.Q., Wallace, S.M., Blackburn, J.L., Wilson, T.W., and Bergman, U. Increased prescribing of antidepressants subsequent to β-blocker therapy. *Arch. Intern. Med.,* **1990,** *150:*2286–2290.

Villanueva, C., Balanzo, J., Novella, M.T., *et al.* Nadolol plus isosorbide mononitrate compared with sclerotherapy for the prevention of variceal rebleeding. *N. Engl. J. Med.,* **1996,** *334:*1624–1629.

Witchitz, S., Cohen-Solal, A., Dartois, N., *et al.* Treatment of heart failure with celiprolol, a cardioselective β blocker with β-2 agonist vasodilator properties. The CELICARD Group. *Am. J. Cardiol.,* **2000,** *85:*1467–1471.

Wood, J.P., Schmidt, K.G., Melena, J., *et al.* The β-adrenoceptor antagonists metipranolol and timolol are retinal neuroprotectants: comparison with betaxolol. *Exp. Eye Res.,* **2003,** *76:*505–516.

Wuttke, H., Rau, T., Heide, R., *et al.* Increased frequency of cytochrome P450 2D6 poor metabolizers among patients with metoprolol-associated adverse effects. *Clin. Pharmacol. Ther.,* **2002,** *72:*429–437.

Yang, G., Timme, T.L., Park, S.H., *et al.* Transforming growth factor β 1 transduced mouse prostate reconstitutions: II. Induction of apoptosis by doxazosin. *Prostate,* **1997,** *33:*157–163.

Zhu, Q.-M., Lesnick, J.D., Jasper, J.R., *et al.* Cardiovascular effects of rilmedidine, moxonidine and clonidine in conscious wild-type and D79N α_{2A}-adrenoceptor transgenic mice. *Br. J. Pharmacol.,* **1999,** *126:*1522–1530.

MONOGRAPHS AND REVIEWS

Altschuld, R.A., and Billman, G.E. β_2-Adrenoceptors and ventricular fibrillation. *Pharmacol. Ther.,* **2000,** *88:*1–14.

Alward, W.L. Medical management of glaucoma. *N. Engl. J. Med.,* **1998,** *339:*1298–1307.

Andersson, K.E. Current concepts in the treatment of disorders of micturition. *Drugs,* **1988,** *35:*477–494.

Babamoto, K.S., and Hirokawa, W.T. Doxazosin: a new α_1-adrenergic antagonist. *Clin. Pharm.,* **1992,** *11:*415–427.

Beasley, R., Pearce, N., Crane, J., and Burgess, C. β-Agonists: what is the evidence that their use increases the risk of asthma morbidity and mortality? *J. Allergy Clin. Immunol.,* **1999,** *104:*S18–S30.

Beduschi, M.C., Beduschi, R., and Oesterling, J.E. α-Blockade therapy for benign prostatic hyperplasia: from a nonselective to a more selective α_{1A}-adrenergic antagonist. *Urology,* **1998,** *51:*861–872.

Bolger, A.P., and Al-Nasser, F. β-Blockers for chronic heart failure: surviving longer but feeling better? *Int. J. Cardiol.,* **2003,** *92:*1–8.

Bosch, J. Medical treatment of portal hypertension. *Digestion,* **1998,** *59:*547–555.

Bray, G.A. Use and abuse of appetite-suppressant drugs in the treatment of obesity. *Ann. Intern. Med.,* **1993,** *119:*707–713.

Breslow, M.J., and Ligier, B. Hyperadrenergic states. *Crit. Care Med.,* **1991,** *19:*1566–1579.

Bristow, M.R., Kantrowitz, N.E., Ginsburg, R., and Fowler, M.B. β-Adrenergic functions in heart muscle disease and heart failure. *J. Mol. Cell Cardiol.,* **1985,** *17*(suppl 2):41–52.

Brodde, O.E., and Michel, M.C. Adrenergic and muscarinic receptors in the human heart. *Pharmacol. Rev.,* **1999,** *51:*651–690.

Brooks, A.M., and Gillies, W.E. Ocular β-blockers in glaucoma management. Clinical pharmacological aspects. *Drugs Aging,* **1992,** *2:*208–221.

Cheng, J., Kamiya, K., and Kodama, I. Carvedilol: Molecular and cellular basis for its multifaceted therapeutic potential. *Cardiovasc. Drug Rev.,* **2001,** *19:*152–171.

Cleland, J.G. β-Blockers for heart failure: why, which, when, and where. *Med. Clin. North Am.,* **2003,** *87:*339–371.

Cooper, K.L., McKiernan, J.M., and Kaplan, S.A. α-Adrenoceptor antagonists in the treatment of benign prostatic hyperplasia. *Drugs,* **1999,** *57:*9–17.

Cruickshank, J.M. β-Blockers and diabetes. The bad guys come good. *Cardiovasc. Drugs Ther.,* **2002,** *16:*457–470.

DiBari, M., Marchionni, N., and Pahor, M. β-blockers after acute myocardial infarction in elderly patients with diabetes mellitus: time to reassess. *Drugs Aging,* **2003,** *20:*13–22.

Donnelly, R., and Macphee, G.J. Clinical pharmacokinetics and kinetic-dynamic relationships of dilevalol and labetalol. *Clin. Pharmacokinet.,* **1991,** *21:*95–109.

Dunne, F., Kendall, M.J., and Martin, U. β-Blockers in the management of hypertension in patients with type 2 diabetes mellitus: Is there a role? *Drugs,* **2001,** *61:*428–435.

Elia, J., Ambrosini, P.J., and Rapoport, J.L. Treatment of attention-deficit-hyperactivity disorder. *N. Engl. J. Med.,* **1999,** *340:*780–788.

Faulds, D., Hollingshead, L.M., and Goa, K.L. Formoterol. A review of its pharmacological properties and therapeutic potential in reversible obstructive airways disease. *Drugs,* **1991,** *42:*115–137.

Fernandez-Lopez, J.A., Remesar, X., Foz, M., and Alemany, M. Pharmacological approaches for the treatment of obesity. *Drugs,* **2002,** *62:*915–944.

Fitton, A., and Benfield, P. Dopexamine hydrochloride. A review of its pharmacodynamic and pharmacokinetic properties and therapeutic potential in acute cardiac insufficiency. *Drugs,* **1990,** *39:*308–330.

Fitton, A., and Sorkin, E.M. Sotalol. An updated review of its pharmacological properties and therapeutic use in cardiac arrhythmias. *Drugs,* **1993,** *46:*678–719.

Fitzgerald, J.D. Do partial agonist β-blockers have improved clinical utility? *Cardiovasc. Drugs Ther.,* **1993,** *7:*303–310.

Fox, A.M., and Rieder, M.J. Risks and benefits of drugs used in the management of the hyperactive child. *Drug Saf.,* **1993,** *9:*38–50.

Francis, G.S., and Cohn, J.N. The autonomic nervous system in congestive heart failure. *Annu. Rev. Med.,* **1986,** *37:*235–247.

Freemantle, N., Cleland, J., Young, P., Mason, J., and Harrison, J. β Blockade after myocardial infarction: systematic review and meta regression analysis. *BMJ,* **1999,** *318:*1730–1737.

Frishman, W.H. Pindolol: a new β-adrenoceptor antagonist with partial agonist activity. *N. Engl. J. Med.,* **1983,** *308:*940–944.

Fry, J.M. Treatment modalities for narcolepsy. *Neurology,* **1998,** *50*(2 suppl 1):S43–S48.

Fung, J.W., Yu, C.M., Kum, L.C., Yip, G.W., and Sanderson, J.E. Role of β-blocker therapy in heart failure and atrial fibrillation. *Cardiac Electrophysiol. Rev.,* **2003,** *7:*236–242.

Gauthier, C., Langin, D., and Balligand, J.L. β_3 adrenoceptors in the cardiovascular system. *Trends Pharmacol. Sci.,* **2000,** *21:*426–431.

Gerstman, B.B., Jolson, H.M., Bauer, M., *et al.* The incidence of depression in new users of β-blockers and selected antihypertensives. *J. Clin. Epidemiol.,* **1996,** *49:*809–815.

Goldenberg, M., Aranow, H., Jr., Smith, A.A., and Faber, M. Pheochromocytoma and essential hypertensive vascular disease. *Arch. Intern. Med.,* **1950,** *86:*823–836.

Goldsmith, D.R., and Keating, G.M. Budesonide/fomoterol: A review of its use in asthma. *Drugs,* **2004,** *64:*1597–1618.

Goldstein, S. Benefits of β-blocker therapy for heart failure. *Arch. Int. Med.,* **2002,** *162:*641–648.

Grimm, R.H., Jr. Antihypertensive therapy: taking lipids into consideration. *Am. Heart J.,* **1991,** *122:*910–918.

Hayashi, Y., and Maze, M. α_2 Adrenoceptor agonists and anaesthesia. *Br. J. Anaesth.,* **1993,** *71:*108–118.

Hollenberg, S.M., Kavinsky, C.J., and Parrillo, J.E. Cardiogenic shock. *Ann. Intern. Med.,* **1999,** *131:*47–59.

Hutchins, C. Three-dimensional models of the D1 and D2 dopamine receptors. *Endocr. J.,* **1994,** *2:*7–23.

Keating, G.M., and Jarvis, B. Carvedilol: A review of its use in chronic heart failure. *Drugs,* **2003,** *63:*1697–1741.

Kühlkamp, V., Bosch, R., Mewis, C., and Seipel, L. Use of β-blockers in atrial fibrillation. *Am. J. Cardiovasc. Drugs,* **2002,** *2:*37–42.

Kulka, P.J., and Tryba, M. Inotropic support of the critically ill patient. A review of the agents. *Drugs,* **1993,** *45:*654–667.

Kyncl, J.J. Pharmacology of terazosin: an α_1-selective blocker. *J. Clin. Pharmacol.,* **1993,** *33:*878–883.

Kyprianou, N. Doxazosin and terazosin suppress prostate growth by inducing apoptosis. Clinical significance. *J. Urol.,* **2003,** *169:*1520–1525.

Lefkowitz, R.J., Rockman, H.A., and Koch, W.J. Catecholamines, cardiac β-adrenergic receptors, and heart failure. *Circulation,* **2000,** *101:*1634–1637.

McClellan, K.J., Wiseman, L.R., and Wilde, M.I. Midodrine. A review of its therapeutic use in the management of orthostatic hypotension. *Drugs Aging,* **1998,** *12:*76–86.

McConnell, J.D., Roehrborn, C.G., Bautista, O.M., *et al.* The long-term effect of doxazosin, finasteride, and combination therapy on the clinical progression of benign prostatic hyperplasia. *N. Engl. J. Med.,* **2003,** *349:*2387–2398.

McGavin, J.K., and Keating, G.M. Bisoprolol. A review of its use in chronic heart failure. *Drugs,* **2002,** *62:*2677–2696.

McPherson, G.A. Current trends in the study of potassium channel openers. *Gen. Pharmacol.,* **1993,** *24:*275–281.

Madu, E.C., Ahmar, W., Arthur, J., and Fraker, T.D., Jr. Clinical utility of digital dobutamine stress echocardiography in the noninvasive evaluation of coronary artery disease. *Arch. Intern. Med.,* **1994,** *154:*1065–1072.

Man in't Veld, A.J., Van den Meiracker, A.H., and Schalekamp, M.A. Do β blockers really increase peripheral vascular resistance? Review of the literature and new observations under basal conditions. *Am. J. Hypertens.,* **1988,** *1:*91–96.

Mimran, A., and Ducailar, G. Systemic and regional haemodynamic profile of diuretics and α- and β-blockers. A review comparing acute and chronic effects. *Drugs,* **1988,** *35*(suppl 6):60–69.

Missale, C., Nash, S.R., Robinson, S.W., Jaber, M., and Caron, M.G. Dopamine receptors: from structure to function. *Physiol. Rev.,* **1998,** *78:*189–225.

Mitler, M.M., Erman, M., and Hajdukovic, R. The treatment of excessive somnolence with stimulant drugs. *Sleep,* **1993,** *16:*203–206.

Murphy, M.B., Murray, C., and Shorten, G.D. Fenoldopam: a selective peripheral dopamine receptor agonist for the treatment of severe hypertension. *N. Engl. J. Med.,* **2001,** *345:*1548–1557.

Nelson, H.S. β-Adrenergic bronchodilators. *N. Engl. J. Med.,* **1995,** *333:*499–506.

Owen, A. Optimising the use of β-blockers in older patients with heart failure. *Drugs Aging,* **2002,** *19:*671–684.

Poole-Wilson P.A., Swedberg K., Cleland J.G., *et al.* Comparison of carvedilol and metoprolol on clinical outcomes in patients with chronic heart failure in the Carvedilol Or Metoprolol European Trial (COMET): randomised controlled trial. *Lancet,* **2003,** *362:*7–13.

Post, S.R., Hammond, H.K., and Insel, P.A. β-Adrenergic receptors and receptor signaling in heart failure. *Annu. Rev. Pharmacol. Toxicol.,* **1999,** *39:*343–360.

Prakash, A., and Markham, A. Metoprolol: a review of its use in chronic heart failure. *Drugs,* **2000,** *60:*647–678.

Redington, A.E. Step one for asthma treatment: β_2-agonists or inhaled corticosteroids? *Drugs,* **2001,** *61:*1231–1238.

Ried, L.D., McFarland, B.H., Johnson, R.E., and Brody, K.K. β-Blockers and depression: the more the murkier? *Ann. Pharmacother.,* **1998,** *32:*699–708.

Robidoux, J., Martin, T.L., and Collins, S. β-Adrenergic receptors and regulation of energy expenditure: a family affair. *Annu. Rev. Pharmacol. Toxicol.,* **2004,** *44:*297–323.

Rosendorff, C. β-Blocking agents with vasodilator activity. *J. Hypertens. Suppl.,* **1993,** *11:*S37–S40.

Ruffolo, R.R., Jr. Fundamentals of receptor theory: basics for shock research. *Circ. Shock,* **1992,** *37:*176–184.

Ruffolo, R.R., Jr. The pharmacology of dobutamine. *Am. J. Med. Sci.,* **1987,** *294:*244–248.

Ruffolo, R.R., Jr., and Hieble, J.P. Adrenoceptor pharmacology: urogenital applications. *Eur. Urol.,* **1999,** *36*(suppl 1):17–22.

Salpeter, S.R. Cardioselective β blocker use in patients with asthma and chronic obstructive pulmonary disease: an evidence-based approach to standard of care. *Respir. Med.,* **2003,** *24:*564–572.

Samanin, R., and Garattini, S. Neurochemical mechanism of action of anorectic drugs. *Pharmacol. Toxicol.,* **1993,** *73:*63–68.

Seale, J.P. Whither β-adrenoceptor agonists in the treatment of asthma? *Prog. Clin. Biol. Res.,* **1988,** *263:*367–377.

Self, T., Soberman, J.E., Bubla, J.M., and Chafen, C.C. Cardioselective β-blockers in patients with asthma and concomitant heart failure or history of myocardial infarction: when do benefits outweigh risks? *J. Asthma,* **2003,** *40:*839–845.

Shephard, R.J. *Physiology and Biochemistry of Exercise.* Praeger, New York, 1982, pp. 228–229.

Singh, K., Communal, C., Sawyer, D.B., and Colucci, W.S. Adrenergic regulation of myocardial apoptosis. *Cardiovasc. Res.,* **2000,** *45:*713–719.

Sorkin, E.M., and Heel, R.C. Guanfacine. A review of its pharmacodynamic and pharmacokinetic properties and therapeutic efficacy in the treatment of hypertension. *Drugs,* **1986,** *31:*301–336.

Starke, K., Gothert, M., and Kilbinger, H. Modulation of neurotransmitter release by presynaptic autoreceptors. *Physiol. Rev.,* **1989,** *69:*864–989.

Swanson, J.M., and Volkow, N.D. Serum and brain concentrations of methylphenidate: implications for use and abuse. *Neurosci. Biobehav. Rev.,* **2003,** *27:*615–621.

Tfelt-Hansen, P. Efficacy of β-blockers in migraine. A critical review. *Cephalalgia,* **1986,** *6*(suppl 5):15–24.

Toda, N. Vasodilating β-adrenoceptor blockers as cardiovascular therapeutics. *Pharmacol. Ther.,* **2003,** *100:*215–234.

Van Baak, M.A. β-Adrenoceptor blockade and exercise. An update. *Sports Med.,* **1988,** *5:*209–225.

Wadworth, A.N., Murdoch, D., and Brogden, R.N. Atenolol. A reappraisal of its pharmacological properties and therapeutic use in cardiovascular disorders. *Drugs,* **1991,** *42:*468–510.

Wagstaff, A.J., and Bryson, H.M. Tizanidine. A review of its pharmacology, clinical efficacy and tolerability in the management of spasticity associated with cerebral and spinal disorders. *Drugs,* **1997,** *53:*435–452.

Walle, T., Webb, J.G., Bagwell, E.E., *et al.* Stereoselective delivery and actions of β receptor antagonists. *Biochem. Pharmacol.,* **1988,** *37:*115–124.

Westfall, D.P. Adrenoceptor antagonists. In, (Craig, C.R., and Stitzel, R.E., eds.) *Modern Pharmacology.* Baltimore, Lippincott Williams & Wilkins, **2004,** pp. 109–120.

Wilde, M.I., and McTavish, D. Tamsulosin. A review of its pharmacological properties and therapeutic potential in the management of symptomatic benign prostatic hyperplasia. *Drugs,* **1996,** *52:*883–898.

Wilde, M.I., Fitton, A., and Sorkin, E.M. Terazosin. A review of its pharmacodynamic and pharmacokinetic properties, and therapeutic potential in benign prostatic hyperplasia. *Drugs Aging,* **1993,** *3:*258–277.

5-HYDROXYTRYPTAMINE (SEROTONIN): RECEPTOR AGONISTS AND ANTAGONISTS

Elaine Sanders-Bush and Steven E. Mayer

5-Hydroxytryptamine (5-HT, serotonin) is a regulator of smooth muscle in the cardiovascular system and the gastrointestinal tract, an enhancer of platelet aggregation, and a neurotransmitter in the central nervous system (CNS). 5-HT is found in high concentrations in enterochromaffin cells throughout the gastrointestinal tract, in storage granules in platelets, and broadly throughout the CNS. Although 5-HT is implicated in the regulation of a number of physiological processes and their malfunction, the exact sites and modes of its action are still being defined. Fourteen 5-HT-receptor subtypes have been delineated by pharmacological analyses and cDNA cloning. The availability of cloned receptors has allowed the development of subtype-selective drugs and the elucidation of actions of 5-HT at a molecular level. Increasingly, therapeutic goals are being achieved by drugs that target selectively one or more of the subtypes of 5-HT receptors.

History. In the 1930s, Erspamer began to study the distribution of enterochromaffin cells, which stained with a reagent for indoles. The highest concentrations were found in gastrointestinal mucosa, followed by platelets and the CNS. Page and colleagues were the first to isolate and chemically characterize a vasoconstrictor substance released from platelets in clotting blood. This substance, named *serotonin*, was shown to be identical to the indole isolated by Erspamer. The discovery of biosynthetic and degradative pathways for 5-HT and clinical interest in the pressor effects of 5-HT led to the hypothesis that the symptoms of patients with tumors of intestinal enterochromaffin cells (carcinoid syndrome) result from abnormally high production of 5-HT. Several hundred milligrams of 5-HT and its metabolites may be excreted daily in patients with carcinoid tumors. The gross effects of 5-HT, produced in excess in malignant carcinoid, gave some indication of the physiologic and pharmacologic actions of 5-HT. For example, these patients often display psychotic behaviors similar to those produced by lysergic acid diethylamide (LSD). Several naturally occurring hallucinogenic tryptaminelike substances were identified from animal and plant sources, suggest-

ing that these substances or congeners might be formed *in vivo* and could explain the abnormal behavior of carcinoid patients. In the mid-1950s, 5-HT was proposed as a neurotransmitter in the mammalian CNS. For additional details about the discovery and effects of 5-HT, *see* Sjoerdsma and Palfreyman, 1990.

Source and Chemistry. 5-HT, 3-(β-aminoethyl)-5-hydroxyindole, is widely distributed in the animal and plant kingdoms (*see* Figure 11–1 for chemical structures). It occurs in vertebrates; in tunicates, mollusks, arthropods, and coelenterates; and in fruits and nuts. It also is present in venoms, including those of the common stinging nettle and of wasps and scorpions. Numerous synthetic or naturally occurring congeners of 5-HT have pharmacological activity. Many of the *N*- and *O*-methylated indoleamines, such as *N,N*-dimethyltryptamine, are hallucinogens. Because these compounds are behaviorally active and might be synthesized *via* known metabolic pathways, they have long been considered candidates for endogenous psychotomimetic substances, potentially responsible for some psychotic behaviors. Another close relative of 5-HT, *melatonin* (5-methoxy-*N*-acetyltryptamine), is formed by sequential *N*-acetylation and *O*-methylation (Figure 11–2). Melatonin is the principal indoleamine in the pineal gland, where it may be said to constitute a pigment of the imagination. Its synthesis is controlled by external factors including environmental light. Melatonin induces pigment lightening in skin cells and suppresses ovarian functions; it also serves a role in regulating biological rhythms and shows promise in the treatment of jet lag and other sleep disturbances (Cajochen *et al.*, 2003).

Synthesis and Metabolism. 5-HT is synthesized by a two-step pathway from the essential amino acid *tryptophan* (Figure 11–2). Tryptophan is actively transported into the brain by a carrier protein that also transports other large neutral and branched-chain amino acids. The levels of tryptophan in the brain are influenced not only by its plasma concentration, but also by the plasma concentrations of other amino acids that compete for the brain uptake carrier. *Tryptophan hydroxylase*, a mixed-function oxidase that requires molecular oxygen and a reduced pteridine cofactor for activity, is the rate-limiting enzyme in the synthetic pathway. A second, brain-specific isoform of tryptophan hydroxylase has been cloned (Walther *et al.*, 2003); although its distribution differs markedly from that of the classical

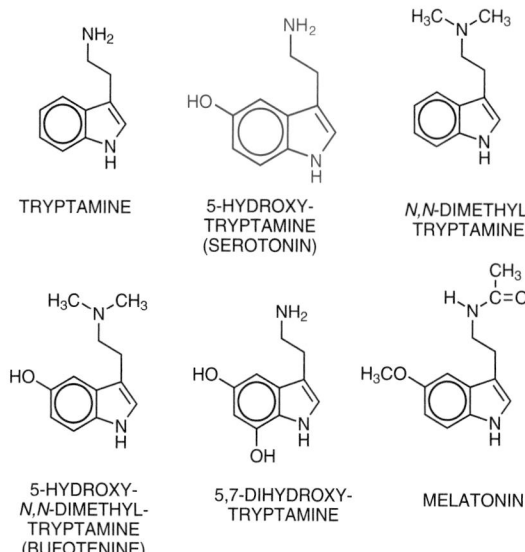

Figure 11–1. *Structures of representative indolealkylamines.*

enzyme, it is not clear whether this translates into differences in function and regulation. Unlike tyrosine hydroxylase, tryptophan hydroxylase is not regulated by end-product inhibition, although regulation by phosphorylation is common to both enzymes. Brain tryptophan hydroxylase is not generally saturated with substrate; consequently the concentration of tryptophan in the brain influences the synthesis of 5-HT.

The enzyme that converts L-5-hydroxytryptophan to 5-HT, aromatic L-amino acid decarboxylase, is widely distributed and has a broad substrate specificity. A long-standing debate about whether L-5-hydroxytryptophan decarboxylase and L-dopa decarboxylase are identical enzymes was clarified when cDNA cloning confirmed that a single gene product decarboxylates both amino acids. 5-Hydroxytryptophan is not detected in the brain because it is rapidly decarboxylated. The synthesized product, 5-HT, is stored in secretory granules by a vesicular transporter; stored 5-HT is released by exocytosis from serotonergic neurons. In the nervous system, the action of released 5-HT is terminated by neuronal uptake mediated by a specific transporter. The 5-HT transporter is localized in the membrane of serotonergic axon terminals (where it terminates the action of 5-HT in the synapse) and in the membrane of platelets (where it takes up 5-HT from the blood). This uptake system is the only way that platelets acquire 5-HT, as they lack the enzymes required to synthesize 5-HT. The 5-HT transporter, as well as other monoamine transporters, has been cloned (*see* Chapters 2 and 12). The deduced amino-acid sequence and predicted membrane topology place the amine transporters in a family clearly distinct from the transport proteins that concentrate amines in intracellular storage vesicles. Furthermore, the vesicular transporter is a nonspecific amine carrier, while the 5-HT transporter and the other amine transporters are highly specific. Neither pharmacological studies nor cDNA cloning has provided evidence to support the existence of multiple 5-HT transporters. Studies have found that the 5-HT transporter is regulated by phosphorylation with subsequent internalization (Ramamoorthy and Blakely, 1999), providing a mechanism for dynamic regulation of serotonergic transmission.

Figure 11–2. *Synthesis and inactivation of serotonin.* Synthetic enzymes are identified in blue lettering, and cofactors are shown in black lowercase letters.

The principal route of metabolism of 5-HT involves oxidative deamination by monoamine oxidase (MAO), forming an acetaldehyde intermediate; the aldehyde is converted to 5-hydroxyindole acetic acid (5-HIAA) by a ubiquitous enzyme, aldehyde dehydrogenase (Figure 11–2). An alternative route, reduction of the acetaldehyde to an alcohol, 5-hydroxytryptophol, is normally insignificant. 5-HIAA is actively transported out of the brain by a process that is sensitive to the nonspecific transport inhibitor probenecid. Since 5-HIAA formation accounts for nearly 100% of the metabolism of 5-HT in brain, the turnover rate of brain 5-HT is estimated by measuring the rate of rise of 5-HIAA after administration of probenecid. 5-HIAA from brain and peripheral sites of 5-HT storage and metabolism is excreted in the urine along with small amounts of 5-hydroxytryptophol sulfate or glucuronide conjugates. The usual range of urinary excretion of 5-HIAA by a normal adult is 2 to 10 mg daily. Larger amounts are excreted by patients with malignant carcinoid, providing a reliable diagnostic test for the disease. Ingestion of ethyl alcohol results in elevated amounts of reduced nicotinamide adenine dinucleotide (NADH), which diverts 5-hydroxyindole acetaldehyde from the oxidative route to the reductive pathway (Figure 11–2), and tends to increase the excretion of 5-hydroxytryptophol and correspondingly reduces the excretion of 5-HIAA.

Two isoforms of monoamine oxidase (MAO-A and -B) were distinguished initially on the basis of substrate and inhibitor specificities. Both isoforms have been cloned, and the properties of the cloned enzymes are consistent with the pharmacological profiles established previously (Shih, 1991; *see* Chapters 10 and 17). MAO-A preferentially metabolizes 5-HT and norepinephrine; *clorgyline* is a specific inhibitor of this enzyme. MAO-B prefers β-phenylethylamine and benzylamine as substrates; low dose *selegiline* is a relatively selective inhibitor of MAO-B. Dopamine and tryptamine are metabolized equally well by both isoforms. Neurons contain both isoforms of MAO, localized primarily in the outer membrane of mitochondria. MAO-B is the principal isoform in platelets, which contain large amounts of 5-HT.

Other minor pathways of metabolism of 5-HT, such as sulfation and *O*- or *N*-methylation, have been suggested. The latter reaction could lead to formation of an endogenous psychotropic substance, 5-hydroxy-*N,N*-dimethyltryptamine (*bufotenine;* Figure 11–1). However, other methylated indoleamines such as *N,N*-dimethyltryptamine and 5-methoxy-*N,N*-dimethyltryptamine are far more active hallucinogens and are more likely candidates to be endogenous psychotomimetics.

PHYSIOLOGICAL FUNCTIONS OF SEROTONIN

Multiple 5-HT Receptors

Based on data from early studies of 5-HT's actions in peripheral tissues, researchers hypothesized that the multiple actions of 5-HT involved interaction with multiple 5-HT-receptor subtypes. Extensive pharmacological characterization and the cloning of receptor cDNAs have confirmed this hypothesis (for an extensive review *see* Barnes and Sharp, 1999). The multiple 5-HT-receptor subtypes cloned comprise the largest known neurotransmitter-receptor family. The 5-HT-receptor subtypes are expressed in distinct but often overlapping patterns (Palacios *et al.*, 1990) and are coupled to

different transmembrane-signaling mechanisms (Table 11–1). Four 5-HT-receptor families with defined functions currently are recognized: $5-HT_1$ through $5-HT_4$. The $5-HT_1$, $5-HT_2$, and $5-HT_{4-7}$ receptor families are members of the superfamily of GPCRs (*see* Chapter 1). The $5-HT_3$ receptor, on the other hand, is a ligand-gated ion channel that gates Na^+ and K^+ and has a predicted membrane topology akin to that of the nicotinic cholinergic receptor (*see* Chapter 9).

History of 5-HT Receptor Subtypes. Gaddum and Picarelli (1957) proposed the existence of two 5-HT-receptor subtypes, which they termed *M* and *D receptors*. M receptors were believed to be located on parasympathetic nerve endings, controlling the release of acetylcholine, whereas D receptors were thought to be located on smooth muscle. Although subsequent studies in both the periphery and brain were consistent with the notion of multiple subtypes of 5-HT receptor, the radioligand-binding studies of Peroutka and Snyder (1979) provided the first definitive evidence for 2 distinct recognition sites for 5-HT. $5-HT_1$ receptors had a high affinity for [^{3}H]5-HT, while $5-HT_2$ receptors had a low affinity for [^{3}H]5-HT and a high affinity for [^{3}H]spiperone. Subsequently, high affinity for 5-HT was used as a primary criterion for classifying a receptor subtype as a member of the $5-HT_1$ receptor family. This classification strategy proved to be invalid; for example, a receptor expressed in the choroid plexus was named the $5-HT_{1C}$ receptor because it was the third receptor shown to have a high affinity for 5-HT. However, based on its pharmacological properties, second-messenger function, and deduced amino acid sequence, the $5-HT_{1C}$ receptor clearly belonged to the $5-HT_2$ receptor family and was subsequently renamed the $5-HT_{2C}$ receptor. The current classification scheme (Hoyer *et al.*, 1994) proposes 7 subfamilies of 5-HT receptors (Table 11–1). It is likely that further modifications of this scheme will be required. Convincing evidence suggests that the $5-HT_{1D\beta}$ receptor is the human homolog of the $5-HT_{1B}$ receptor originally characterized and subsequently cloned from rodent brain. The current designation for species homologs of the same receptor protein is confusing and requires resolution. Although the rat $5-HT_{1B}$ receptor and the human $5-HT_{1D}$ receptor show greater than 95% amino-acid sequence homology, they have distinct pharmacological properties. The rat $5-HT_{1B}$ receptor has an affinity for β adrenergic antagonists, such as pindolol and propranolol, that is 2 to 3 orders of magnitude higher than that of the human $5-HT_{1D}$ receptor. This difference appears to be due to a single amino acid difference in the seventh transmembrane span (threonine in the human $5-HT_{1D}$ receptor *versus* asparagine in the rodent $5-HT_{1B}$ receptor).

$5-HT_1$ Receptors. All 5 members of the $5-HT_1$-receptor subfamily inhibit adenylyl cyclase. At least one $5-HT_1$-receptor subtype, the $5-HT_{1A}$ receptor, also activates a receptor-operated K^+ channel and inhibits a voltage-gated Ca^{2+} channel, a common property of receptors coupled to the pertussis toxin–sensitive G_i/G_o family of G proteins. The $5-HT_{1A}$ receptor is found in the raphe nuclei of the brainstem, where it functions as an inhibitory, somatodendritic autoreceptor on cell bodies of serotonergic neurons

Table 11–1
Serotonin Receptor Subtypes

	STRUCTURAL FAMILIES					
	5-HT$_1$, 5-HT$_2$, 5-HT$_{4-7}$ G protein–coupled receptor				5-HT$_3$ 5-HT–gated ion channel	
SUBTYPE	GENE STRUCTURE	SIGNAL TRANSDUCTION	LOCALIZATION	FUNCTION	SELECTIVE AGONIST	SELECTIVE ANTAGONIST
5-HT$_{1A}$	Intronless	Inhibition of AC	Raphe nuclei Hippocampus	Autoreceptor	8-OH-DPAT	WAY 100135
5-HT$_{1B}$*	Intronless	Inhibition of AC	Subiculum Substantia nigra	Autoreceptor	—	—
5-HT$_{1D}$	Intronless	Inhibition of AC	Cranial blood vessels	Vasoconstriction	Sumatriptan	—
5-HT$_{1E}$	Intronless	Inhibition of AC	Cortex Striatum	—	—	—
5-HT$_{1F}$†‡	Intronless	Inhibition of AC	Brain and periphery	—	—	—
5-HT$_{2A}$ (D receptor)	Introns	Activation of PLC	Platelets Smooth muscle Cerebral cortex	Platelet aggregation Contraction Neuronal excitation	α-Methyl-5-HT, DOI	Ketanserin LY53857 MDL 100,907
5-HT$_{2B}$	Introns	Activation of PLC	Stomach fundus	Contraction	α-Methyl-5-HT, DOI	LY53857
5-HT$_{2C}$	Introns	Activation of PLC	Choroid plexus	—	α-Methyl-5-HT, DOI	LY53857 Mesulergine
5-HT$_3$ (M receptor)	Introns	Ligand-operated ion channel	Peripheral nerves Area postrema Hippocampus	Neuronal excitation	2-Methyl-5-HT	Ondansetron Tropisetron
5-HT$_4$	Introns	Activation of AC	Hippocampus GI tract	Neuronal excitation	Renzapride	GR 113808
5-HT$_{5A}$	Introns	Inhibition of AC	Hippocampus	Unknown	—	—
5-HT$_{5B}$	Introns	Unknown			—	—
5-HT$_6$	Introns	Activation of AC	Striatum	Unknown	—	—
5-HT$_7$	Introns	Activation of AC	Hypothalamus Intestine	Unknown	—	—

*Also referred to as 5-HT$_{1D\beta}$. †Also referred to as 5-HT$_{1E\beta}$. ABBREVIATIONS: AC, adenylyl cyclase; PLC, phospholipase C; 8-OH-DPAT, 8-hydroxy-(2-N,N-dipropylamino)-tetraline; DOI, 1-(2,5-dimethoxy-4-iodophenyl)isopropylamine.

(Figure 11–3). Another subtype, the 5-HT_{1D} receptor, functions as an autoreceptor on axon terminals, inhibiting 5-HT release as does its rat homolog, 5-HT_{1B}. 5-HT_{1D} receptors, abundantly expressed in the substantia nigra and basal ganglia, may regulate the firing rate of dopamine-containing cells and the release of dopamine at axonal terminals.

5-HT₂ Receptors.

The 3 subtypes of 5-HT_2 receptors are linked to phospholipase C with the generation of two second messengers, *diacylglycerol* (a cofactor in the activation of protein kinase C) and *inositol trisphosphate* (which mobilizes intracellular stores of Ca^{2+}). The 5-HT_2-receptor subtypes couple to pertussis toxin–insensitive G proteins, such as G_q and G_{11}. 5-HT_{2A} receptors are broadly distributed in the CNS, primarily in serotonergic terminal areas. High densities of 5-HT_{2A} receptors are found in prefrontal, parietal, and somatosensory cortex, claustrum, and in platelets. 5-HT_{2A} receptors in the GI tract are thought to correspond to the D subtype of 5-HT receptor originally described by Gaddum and Picarelli. 5-HT_{2B} receptors originally were described in stomach fundus. The expression of 5-HT_{2B} receptor mRNA is highly restricted in the CNS. 5-HT_{2C} receptors have a very high density in the choroid plexus, an epithelial tissue that is the primary site of cerebrospinal fluid production. The 5-HT_{2C} receptor has been implicated in feeding behavior and susceptibility to seizure (Tecott *et al.*, 1995). The 5-HT_{2C} receptor is regulated by RNA editing, a posttranscriptional event that alters expression of the genetic code at the level of RNA (Burns *et al.*, 1997). Multiple receptor isoforms with alterations of as many as 3 amino acids within the second intracellular loop are predicted, and these edited isoforms have modified G protein–coupling efficiencies (Sanders-Bush *et al.*, 2003).

5-HT₃ Receptors.

The 5-HT_3 receptor is unique, being the only monoamine neurotransmitter receptor that is known to function as a ligand-operated ion channel. The 5-HT_3 receptor corresponds to Gaddum and Picarelli's M receptor. Activation of 5-HT_3 receptors elicits a rapidly desensitizing depolarization, mediated by the gating of cations. These receptors are located on parasympathetic terminals in the GI tract, including vagal and splanchnic afferents. In the CNS, a high density of 5-HT_3 receptors is found in the solitary tract nucleus and in the area postrema. 5-HT_3 receptors in both the gastrointestinal tract and the CNS participate in the emetic response, providing an anatomical basis for the antiemetic property of 5-HT_3-receptor antagonists. Most ligand-operated ion channels are composed of multiple subunits; however, the original, cloned 5-HT_3-receptor subunit forms functional channels that gate cations when expressed in *Xenopus* oocytes or in cultured cells (Maricq *et al.*, 1991). Nevertheless, extensive pharmacological and physiological data obtained in tissues and in intact animals clearly suggest the existence of multiple components of 5-HT_3 receptors. Recently, splice variants of the 5-HT_3 receptor have been identified, perhaps explaining the observed functional diversity.

5-HT₄ Receptors.

5-HT_4 receptors are widely distributed throughout the body. In the CNS, the receptors are found on neurons of the superior and inferior colliculi and in the hippocampus. In the GI tract, 5-HT_4 receptors are located on neurons of the myenteric plexus and on smooth muscle and secretory cells. The 5-HT_4 receptor is thought to evoke secretion in the alimentary tract and to facilitate the peristaltic reflex. 5-HT_4 receptors couple to G_s to activate adenylyl cyclase, leading to a rise in intracellular levels of cyclic AMP (cAMP) (Hegde and Eglen, 1996). The latter effect may explain the utility of prokinetic benzamides in gastrointestinal disorders (*see* Chapter 37).

Additional Cloned 5-HT Receptors. Two other cloned receptors, 5-HT_6 and 5-HT_7, are linked to activation of adenylyl cyclase. Multiple splice variants of the 5-HT_7 receptor have been found, although functional distinctions are not clear. The absence of selective agonists and antagonists has foiled definitive studies of the role of the 5-HT_6 and 5-HT_7 receptors. Circumstantial evidence suggests that 5-HT_7 receptors play a role in smooth-muscle relaxation in the GI

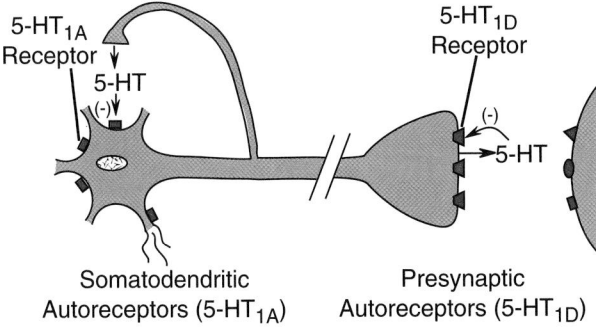

Figure 11–3. Two classes of 5-HT autoreceptors with differential localizations. Somatodendritic 5-HT_{1A} autoreceptors decrease raphe cell firing when activated by 5-HT released from axon collaterals of the same or adjacent neurons. The receptor subtype of the presynaptic autoreceptor on axon terminals in the forebrain has different pharmacological properties and has been classified as 5-HT_{1D} (in human beings) or 5-HT_{1B} (in rodents). This receptor modulates the release of 5-HT. Postsynaptic 5-HT_1 receptors are also indicated.

tract and the vasculature. The atypical antipsychotic drug clozapine has a high affinity for 5-HT_6 and 5-HT_7 receptors; whether this property is related to the broader effectiveness of clozapine compared to conventional antipsychotic drugs is not known. Clozapine appears to be effective in many patients who do not respond to conventional antipsychotic drugs (*see* Chapter 18). Two subtypes of the 5-HT_5 receptor have been cloned; although the 5-HT_{5A} receptor has been shown to inhibit adenylyl cyclase, functional coupling of the cloned 5-HT_{5B} receptor has not yet been described.

Sites of 5-HT Action

Enterochromaffin Cells. Enterochromaffin cells, identified histologically, are located in the GI mucosa, with the highest density found in the duodenum. These cells synthesize 5-HT from tryptophan and store 5-HT and other autacoids, such as the vasodilator peptide substance P and other kinins. Basal release of enteric 5-HT is augmented by mechanical stretching, such as that caused by food or the administration of hypertonic saline, and also by efferent vagal stimulation. 5-HT probably has an additional role in stimulating motility *via* the myenteric network of neurons, located between the layers of smooth muscle (Gershon, 2003; *see also* Chapter 37). The greatly enhanced secretion of 5-HT and other autacoids in malignant carcinoid leads to a multitude of cardiovascular, gastrointestinal, and CNS abnormalities. In addition, the synthesis of large amounts of 5-HT by carcinoid tumors may result in tryptophan and niacin deficiencies (pellagra).

Platelets. Platelets differ from other formed elements of blood in expressing mechanisms for uptake, storage, and endocytotic release of 5-HT. 5-HT is not synthesized in platelets, but is taken up from the circulation and stored in secretory granules by active transport, similar to the uptake and storage of norepinephrine by sympathetic nerve terminals (*see* Chapters 6 and 12). Thus, Na^+-dependent transport across the surface membrane of platelets is followed by uptake into dense core granules *via* an electrochemical gradient generated by an H^+-translocating ATPase. A gradient of 5-HT as high as 1000:1 with an internal concentration of 0.6 M in the dense core storage vesicles can be maintained by platelets. Measuring the rate of Na^+-dependent 5-HT uptake by platelets provides a sensitive assay for 5-HT-uptake inhibitors.

Main functions of platelets include adhesion, aggregation, and thrombus formation to plug holes in the endothelium; conversely, the functional integrity of the endothelium is critical for platelet action. A complex local interplay of multiple factors, including 5-HT, regulates thrombosis and hemostasis (*see* Chapters 25 and 54). When platelets make contact with injured endothelium, they release substances that promote platelet aggregation, and secondarily, they release 5-HT (Figure 11–4). 5-HT binds to platelet 5-HT_{2A} receptors and elicits a weak aggregation response that is markedly augmented by the presence of collagen. If the damaged blood vessel is injured to a depth where vascular smooth muscle is exposed, 5-HT exerts a direct vasoconstrictor effect, thereby contributing to hemostasis, which is enhanced by locally released autacoids (thromboxane A_2, kinins, and vasoactive peptides). Conversely, 5-HT may stimulate production of nitric oxide and antagonize its own vasoconstrictor action, as well as the vasoconstriction produced by other locally released agents.

Cardiovascular System. The classical response of blood vessels to 5-HT is contraction, particularly in the splanchnic, renal, pulmonary, and cerebral vasculatures. This response also occurs in bronchial

smooth muscle. 5-HT also induces a variety of responses by the heart that are the result of activation of multiple 5-HT-receptor subtypes, stimulation or inhibition of autonomic nerve activity, or dominance of reflex responses to 5-HT (Saxena and Villalón, 1990). Thus 5-HT has positive inotropic and chronotropic actions on the heart that may be blunted by simultaneous stimulation of afferent nerves from baroreceptors and chemoreceptors. An effect on vagus nerve endings elicits the Bezold-Jarisch reflex, causing extreme bradycardia and hypotension. The local response of arterial blood vessels to 5-HT also may be inhibitory, the result of stimulated nitric oxide (NO) and prostaglandin synthesis and blockade of norepinephrine release from sympathetic nerves. On the other hand, 5-HT amplifies the local constrictor actions of norepinephrine, angiotensin II, and histamine, which reinforce the hemostatic response to 5-HT.

Gastrointestinal Tract. Enterochromaffin cells in the mucosa appear to be the location of the synthesis and most of the storage of 5-HT in the body and are the source of circulating 5-HT. 5-HT released from these cells enters the portal vein and is subsequently metabolized by MAO-A in the liver. 5-HT that survives hepatic oxidation is rapidly removed by the endothelium of lung capillaries and then inactivated by MAO. 5-HT released by mechanical or vagal stimulation also acts locally to regulate GI function. Motility of gastric and intestinal smooth muscle may be either enhanced or inhibited *via* at least 6 subtypes of 5-HT receptors (Table 11–2). The stimulatory response occurs at nerve endings on longitudinal and circular enteric muscle (5-HT_4), at postsynaptic cells of the enteric ganglia (5-HT_3 and 5-HT_{1P}), and by direct effects of 5-HT on the smooth-muscle cells (5-HT_{2A} in intestine and 5-HT_{2B} in stomach fundus). In esophagus, 5-HT acting at 5-HT_4

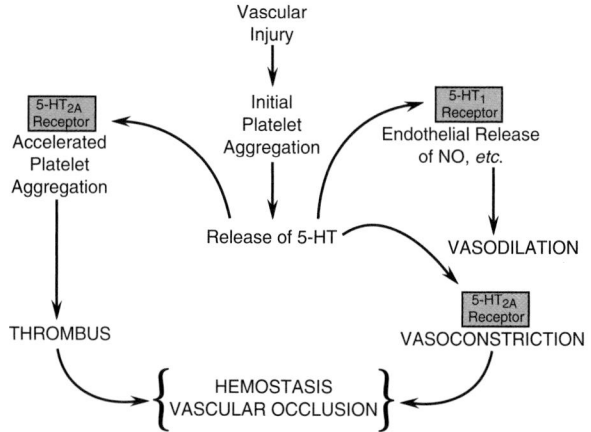

Figure 11–4. Schematic representation of the local influences of platelet 5-HT. The release of 5-HT stored in platelets is triggered by aggregation. The local actions of 5-HT include feedback actions on platelets (shape change and accelerated aggregation) mediated by interaction with platelet 5-HT_{2A} receptors, stimulation of NO production mediated by 5-HT_1-like receptors on vascular endothelium, and contraction of vascular smooth muscle mediated by 5-HT_{2A} receptors. These influences act in concert with many other mediators that are not shown to promote thrombus formation and hemostasis. *See* Chapter 54 for details of adhesion and aggregation of platelets and factors contributing to thrombus formation and blood clotting.

Table 11–2
Some Actions of 5-HT in the Gastrointestinal Tract

SITE	RESPONSE	RECEPTOR
Enterochromaffin cells	Release of 5-HT	5-HT_3
	Inhibition of 5-HT release	5-HT_4
Enteric ganglion cells	Release of ACh	5-HT_4
(presynaptic)	Inhibition of ACh release	5-HT_{1P}, 5-HT_{1A}
Enteric ganglion cells	Fast depolarization	5-HT_3
(postsynaptic)	Slow depolarization	5-HT_{1P}
Smooth muscle, intestinal	Contraction	5-HT_{2A}
Smooth muscle, stomach fundus	Contraction	5-HT_{2B}
Smooth muscle, esophagus	Contraction	5-HT_4

ABBREVIATION: ACh, acetylcholine.

receptors causes either relaxation or contraction, depending on the species. Abundant 5-HT_3 receptors on vagal and other afferent neurons and on enterochromaffin cells play a pivotal role in emesis (*see* Chapter 37). Serotonergic terminals have been described in the myenteric plexus. Enteric 5-HT is released in response to acetylcholine, sympathetic nerve stimulation, increases in intraluminal pressure, and lowered pH (Gershon, 2003), triggering peristaltic contraction.

Central Nervous System. A multitude of brain functions are influenced by 5-HT, including sleep, cognition, sensory perception, motor activity, temperature regulation, nociception, mood, appetite, sexual behavior, and hormone secretion. All of the cloned 5-HT receptors are expressed in the brain, often in overlapping domains. Although patterns of 5-HT receptor expression in individual neurons have not been defined, it is likely that multiple 5-HT receptor subtypes with similar or opposing actions are expressed in individual neurons, leading to a tremendous diversity of actions.

The principal cell bodies of 5-HT neurons are located in raphe nuclei of the brainstem and project throughout the brain and spinal cord (*see* Chapter 12). In addition to being released at discrete synapses, release of serotonin also seems to occur at sites of axonal swelling, termed *varicosities,* which do not form distinct synaptic contacts (Descarries *et al.,* 1990). 5-HT released at nonsynaptic varicosities is thought to diffuse to outlying targets, rather than acting on discrete synaptic targets. Such nonsynaptic release with an ensuing widespread influence of 5-HT is consistent with the idea that 5-HT acts as a neuromodulator as well as a neurotransmitter (*see* Chapter 12).

Serotonergic nerve terminals contain all of the proteins needed to synthesize 5-HT from L-tryptophan (Figure 11–2). Newly formed 5-HT is rapidly accumulated in synaptic vesicles, where it is protected from MAO. 5-HT released by nerve-impulse flow is reaccumulated into the pre-synaptic terminal by an Na^+-dependent carrier, the 5-HT transporter. Pre-synaptic re-uptake is a highly efficient mechanism for terminating the action of 5-HT released by nerve-impulse flow. MAO localized in postsynaptic elements and surrounding cells rapidly inactivates 5-HT that escapes neuronal re-uptake and storage.

Electrophysiology. The physiological consequences of 5-HT release vary with the brain area and the neuronal element involved, as well as with the population of 5-HT receptor subtype(s) expressed

(Aghajanian and Sanders-Bush, 2002). 5-HT has direct excitatory and inhibitory actions (Table 11–3), which may occur in the same preparation, but with distinct temporal patterns. For example, in hippocampal neurons, 5-HT elicits hyperpolarization mediated by 5-HT_{1A} receptors followed by a slow depolarization mediated by 5-HT_4 receptors.

5-HT_{1A} receptor–induced membrane hyperpolarization and reduction in input resistance results from an increase in K^+ conductance. These ionic effects, which are blocked by pertussis toxin, are independent of cAMP, suggesting that 5-HT_{1A} receptors couple directly, *via* subunits of G_i- or G_o-like G proteins, to receptor-operated K^+ channels (Andrade *et al.,* 1986). Somatodendritic 5-HT_{1A} receptors on raphe cells also elicit a K^+-dependent hyperpolarization. The G protein involved is pertussis toxin–sensitive, but the K^+ current apparently is different from the current elicited at postsynaptic 5-HT_{1A} receptors in the hippocampus. The precise signaling mechanism involved in inhibition of 5-HT release by the 5-HT_{1D} autoreceptor at the synaptic terminal is not known, although inhibition of voltage-gated calcium channels likely contributes.

Slow depolarization induced by 5-HT_{2A}-receptor activation in areas such as the prefrontal cortex, nucleus accumbens, and facial motor nucleus involves a decrease in K^+ conductance. A second, distinct mechanism involving Ca^{2+}-activated membrane currents

Table 11–3
Electrophysiological Effects of 5-HT Receptors

SUBTYPE	RESPONSE
$5\text{-HT}_{1A,B}$	Increase K^+ conductance
	Hyperpolarization
5-HT_{2A}	Decrease K^+ conductance
	Slow depolarization
5-HT_3	Gating of Na^+, K^+
	Fast depolarization
5-HT_4	Decrease K^+ conductance
	Slow depolarization

enhances neuronal excitability and potentiates the response to excitatory signals such as glutamate. The role of the phosphoinositide signaling cascade in these physiological actions of $5\text{-}HT_{2A}$ receptors has not been clearly defined. In areas where $5\text{-}HT_1$ and $5\text{-}HT_{2A}$ receptors coexist, the effect of 5-HT may reflect a combination of the two opposing responses: a prominent $5\text{-}HT_1$ receptor–mediated hyperpolarization and an opposing $5\text{-}HT_{2A}$ receptor–mediated depolarization. When $5\text{-}HT_{2A}$ receptors are blocked, hyperpolarization is enhanced. In many cortical areas, $5\text{-}HT_{2A}$ receptors are localized on both GABAergic interneurons and pyramidal cells. Activation of interneurons enhances GABA (γ-aminobutyric acid) release, which secondarily slows the firing rate of pyramidal cells. Thus there is the potential for the $5\text{-}HT_{2A}$ receptor to differentially regulate cortical pyramidal cells, depending on the specific target cells (interneurons *versus* pyramidal cells). $5\text{-}HT_{2C}$ receptors have been shown to depress a K^+ current in *Xenopus* oocytes expressing the cloned receptor mRNA; a similar action has not been definitively identified in the brain. The $5\text{-}HT_4$ receptor, which is coupled to activation of adenylyl cyclase, also elicits a slow neuronal depolarization mediated by a decrease in K^+ conductance. It is not clear why two distinct 5-HT receptor families linked to different signaling pathways can elicit a common neurophysiological action. Yet another receptor, the $5\text{-}HT_{1P}$ receptor, elicits a slow depolarization. This receptor, which couples to activation of adenylyl cyclase, is restricted to the enteric nervous system and has a unique pharmacological profile (Gershon, 2003).

The fast depolarization elicited by $5\text{-}HT_3$ receptors reflects direct gating of an ion channel intrinsic to the receptor structure itself. The $5\text{-}HT_3$ receptor–induced inward current has the characteristics of a cation-selective, ligand-operated channel. Membrane depolarization is mediated by simultaneous increases in Na^+ and K^+ conductance. Patch–clamp analyses confirm that the $5\text{-}HT_3$ receptor functions as a receptor–ion channel complex, comparable to the nicotinic cholinergic receptor. $5\text{-}HT_3$ receptors have been characterized in the CNS and in sympathetic ganglia, primary afferent parasympathetic and sympathetic nerves, enteric neurons, and neuronally derived clonal cell lines such as NG108-15 cells. The pharmacological properties of $5\text{-}HT_3$ receptors, which are different from those of other 5-HT receptors, suggest that multiple $5\text{-}HT_3$ receptor subtypes may exist and may correspond to different combinations of subunits (*see* Chapter 12).

Behavior. The behavioral alterations elicited by drugs that interact with 5-HT receptors are extremely diverse. Many animal behavioral models for initial assessment of agonist and antagonist properties of drugs depend on aberrant motor or reflex responses, such as startle reflexes, hind-limb abduction, head twitches, and other stereotypical behaviors. Operant behavioral paradigms, such as drug discrimination, provide models of specific 5-HT receptor activation and are useful for exploring the action of CNS-active drugs, including agents that interact with 5-HT. For example, investigations of the mechanism of action of hallucinogenic drugs have relied heavily on drug discrimination (as discussed below). The following discussion focuses on animal models that may relate to pathological conditions in human beings and will not attempt to cover the voluminous literature dealing with 5-HT and behavior. *See* Lucki, 1998; Bonasera and Tecott, 2000; and Swerdlow *et al.*, 2000, for excellent reviews on this topic.

Sleep-Wake Cycle. Control of the sleep-wake cycle is one of the first behaviors in which a role for 5-HT was identified. Following pioneering work in cats (for review *see* Jouvet, 1999), many studies showed that depletion of 5-HT with *p*-chlorophenylalanine, a tryptophan hydroxylase inhibitor, elicited insomnia that was reversed by the 5-HT precursor, 5-hydroxytryptophan. Conversely, treatment with L-tryptophan or with nonselective 5-HT agonists accelerated sleep onset and prolonged total sleep time. 5-HT antagonists reportedly can increase and decrease slow-wave sleep, probably reflecting interacting or opposing roles for subtypes of 5-HT receptors. One relatively consistent finding in humans and in laboratory animals is an increase in slow-wave sleep following administration of a selective $5\text{-}HT_{2A/2C}$-receptor antagonist such as ritanserin.

Aggression and Impulsivity. Studies in laboratory animals and in human beings suggest that 5-HT serves a critical role in aggression and impulsivity. Many human studies reveal a correlation between low cerebrospinal fluid 5-HIAA and violent impulsivity and aggression. As an example, low 5-HIAA is associated with violent suicidal acts, but not with suicidal ideation *per se*. As with many effects of 5-HT, pharmacological studies of aggressive behavior in laboratory animals are not definitive, but suggest a role for 5-HT. Two genetic studies have reinforced and amplified this notion. The $5\text{-}HT_{1B}$ receptor was the first 5-HT receptor whose function was investigated in knockout mice. Knockout mice lacking this receptor exhibited extreme aggression (Saudou *et al.*, 1994), suggesting either a role for $5\text{-}HT_{1B}$ receptors in the development of neuronal pathways important in aggression or a direct role in the mediation of aggressive behavior. A human genetic study identified a point mutation in the gene encoding MAO-A, which was associated with extreme aggressiveness and mental retardation (Brunner *et al.*, 1993), and this has been confirmed in knockout mice lacking MAO-A (Cases *et al.*, 1995). These genetic studies add credence to the proposition that abnormalities in 5-HT are related to aggressive behaviors.

Anxiety and Depression. The effects of 5-HT-active drugs, like the selective serotonin reuptake inhibitors (SSRIs), in anxiety and depressive disorders strongly suggest an effect of 5-HT in the neurochemical mediation of these disorders. However, 5-HT-related drugs with clinical effects in anxiety and depression have varied effects in classical animal models of these disorders, depending on the experimental paradigm, species, and strain. For example, the effective anxiolytic *buspirone* (BUSPAR, *see* Chapter 17), a $5\text{-}HT_{1A}$-receptor partial agonist, does not reduce anxiety in classical approach-avoidance paradigms that were instrumental in development of anxiolytic benzodiazepines. However, buspirone and other $5\text{-}HT_{1A}$-receptor agonists are effective in other animal behavioral tests used to predict anxiolytic effects. Furthermore, studies in $5\text{-}HT_{1A}$-receptor knockout mice suggest a role for this receptor in anxiety, and possibly depression. Agonists of certain 5-HT receptors, including $5\text{-}HT_{2A}$ and $5\text{-}HT_{2C}$ receptors (*e.g.,* *m*-chlorophenylpiperazine [mCPP]), have been shown to have anxiogenic properties in laboratory animal and human studies. Similarly, these receptors have been implicated in the animal models of depression, such as learned helplessness.

An impressive finding in human beings with depression is the abrupt reversal of the antidepressant effects of drugs such as SSRIs by manipulations that rapidly reduce the amount of 5-HT in the brain. These approaches include administration of *p*-chlorophenylalanine or a tryptophan-free drink containing large quantities of neutral amino acids (Delgado *et al.*, 1990). Curiously, this kind of 5-HT depletion has not been shown to worsen or to induce depression in nondepressed subjects, suggesting that the continued presence of 5-HT is required to maintain the effects of these drugs. This clinical finding adds credence to somewhat less convincing neurochemical findings that suggest a role for 5-HT in the pathogenesis of depression.

Pharmacological Manipulation of the Amount of 5-HT in Tissues

Experimental strategies for evaluating the role of 5-HT depend on techniques that manipulate tissue levels of 5-HT or block 5-HT receptors. Until recently, manipulation of the levels of endogenous 5-HT was the more commonly used strategy, because the actions of 5-HT antagonists were poorly understood.

Tryptophan hydroxylase, the rate-limiting enzyme in 5-HT synthesis, is a vulnerable site. A diet low in tryptophan reduces the concentration of brain 5-HT; conversely, ingestion of a tryptophan load increases levels of 5-HT in the brain. In addition, administration of a tryptophan hydroxylase inhibitor causes a profound depletion of 5-HT. The most widely used selective tryptophan hydroxylase inhibitor is *p*-chlorophenylalanine, which acts irreversibly. *p*-Chlorophenylalanine produces profound, long-lasting depletion of 5-HT levels with no change in levels of catecholamines.

p-Chloroamphetamine and other halogenated amphetamines promote 5-HT release from platelets and neurons. A rapid release of 5-HT is followed by a prolonged and selective depletion of 5-HT in brain. The halogenated amphetamines are valuable experimental tools and two of them, *fenfluramine* and *dexfenfluramine,* were used clinically to reduce appetite; these drugs were withdrawn from the United States market in 1998 after reports of cardiac toxicity associated with their use. The mechanism of action of this class of drugs is controversial. A profound reduction in levels of 5-HT in the brain lasts for weeks and is accompanied by an equivalent loss of proteins selectively localized in 5-HT neurons (5-HT transporter and tryptophan hydroxylase), suggesting that the halogenated amphetamines have a neurotoxic action. Despite these long-lasting biochemical deficits, neuroanatomical signs of neuronal death are not readily apparent. Another class of compounds, ring-substituted tryptamine derivatives such as 5,7-dihydroxytryptamine (*see* Figure 11–1) leads to unequivocal degeneration of 5-HT neurons. In adult animals, 5,7-dihydroxytryptamine selectively destroys serotonergic axon terminals; the remaining intact cell bodies allow eventual regeneration of axon terminals. In newborn animals, degeneration is permanent because 5,7-dihydroxytryptamine destroys serotonergic cell bodies as well as axon terminals.

Another highly specific mechanism for altering synaptic availability of 5-HT is inhibition of presynaptic reaccumulation of neuronally released 5-HT. SSRIs, such as *fluoxetine* (PROZAC), potentiate and prolong the action of 5-HT released by neuronal activity. When coadministered with L-5-hydroxytryptophan, SSRIs elicit a profound activation of serotonergic responses. SSRIs are the most widely used treatment for endogenous depression (*see* Chapter 17). *Sibutramine* (MERIDIA), an inhibitor of the reuptake of 5-HT, norepinephrine, and dopamine, is used as an appetite suppressant in the management of obesity. The drug is converted to two active metabolites that probably account for its therapeutic effects. Whether effects on a single neurotransmitter are primarily responsible for sibutramine's effects in obese patients is unclear.

Nonselective treatments that alter 5-HT levels include MAO inhibitors and reserpine. MAO inhibitors block the principal route of degradation, thereby increasing levels of 5-HT, whereas reserpine releases intraneuronal stores with subsequent depletion of 5-HT. These treatments profoundly alter levels of 5-HT throughout the body. However, because comparable changes occur in the levels of catecholamines, reserpine and MAO inhibitors are of limited utility as research tools. At one time or another, both have been used in the treatment of mental diseases: reserpine as an antipsychotic drug (*see* Chapter 18) and MAO inhibitors as antidepressants (*see* Chapter 17).

5-HT-RECEPTOR AGONISTS AND ANTAGONISTS

5-HT-Receptor Agonists

Direct-acting 5-HT-receptor agonists have widely different chemical structures, as well as diverse pharmacological properties (Table 11–4). This diversity is not surprising in light of the number of 5-HT-receptor subtypes. $5-HT_{1A}$ receptor–selective agonists have helped elucidate the functions of this receptor in the brain and have resulted in a new class of antianxiety drugs including buspirone, *gepirone,* and *ipsapirone* (*see* Chapter 17). $5-HT_{1D}$ receptor–selective agonists, such as *sumatriptan,* have unique properties that result in constriction of intracranial blood vessels. Sumatriptan was first in a series of new serotonin-receptor agonists available for treatment of acute migraine attacks (*see* below). Other such agents now FDA approved in the United States for the acute treatment of migraine include *zolmitriptan* (ZOMIG), *naratriptan* (AMERGE), and *rizatriptan* (MAXALT), all of which are selective for $5-HT_{1D}$ and $5-HT_{1B}$ receptors. A number of $5-HT_4$ receptor–selective agonists have been developed or are being developed for the treatment of disorders of the GI tract (*see* Chapter 37). These classes of selective 5-HT-receptor agonists are discussed in more detail in the chapters that deal directly with treatment of the relevant pathological conditions.

Table 11–4
Serotonergic Drugs: Primary Actions and Clinical Uses

RECEPTOR	ACTION	DRUG EXAMPLES	CLINICAL DISORDER
5-HT$_{1A}$	Partial agonist	Buspirone, ipsaperone	Anxiety, depression
5-HT$_{1D}$	Agonist	Sumatriptan	Migraine
5-HT$_{2A/2C}$	Antagonist	Methysergide, trazodone, risperidone, ketanserin	Migraine, depression, schizophrenia
5-HT$_3$	Antagonist	Ondansetron	Chemotherapy-induced emesis
5-HT$_4$	Agonist	Cisapride	Gastrointestinal disorders
5-HT transporter	Inhibitor	Fluoxetine, sertraline	Depression, obsessive-compulsive disorder, panic disorder, social phobia, posttraumatic stress disorder

5-HT-Receptor Agonists and Migraine. Migraine headache afflicts 10% to 20% of the population, producing a morbidity estimated at 64 million missed workdays per year in the United States. Although migraine is a specific neurological syndrome, the manifestations vary widely. The principal types are: migraine without aura (common migraine); migraine with aura (classic migraine), which includes subclasses of migraine with typical aura, migraine with prolonged aura, migraine without headache, and migraine with acute-onset aura; and several other rarer types. Auras also may appear without a subsequent headache. Premonitory aura may begin as long as 24 hours before the onset of pain and often is accompanied by photophobia, hyperacusis, polyuria, and diarrhea, and by disturbances of mood and appetite. A migraine attack may last for hours or days and be followed by prolonged pain-free intervals. The frequency of migraine attacks is extremely variable, but usually ranges from 1 to 2 a year to 1 to 4 per month.

The therapy of migraine headaches is complicated by the variable responses among and within individual patients and by the lack of a firm understanding of the pathophysiology of the syndrome. The efficacy of antimigraine drugs varies with the absence or presence of aura, duration of the headache, its severity and intensity, and as yet undefined environmental and genetic factors (Deleu *et al.*, 1998). A rather vague and inconsistent pathophysiological characteristic of migraine is the spreading depression of neural impulses from a focal point of vasoconstriction followed by vasodilation. However, it is unlikely that vasoconstriction followed by vasodilation (spreading depression) or vasodilation alone accounts for the local edema and focal tenderness often observed in migraine patients.

Consistent with the hypothesis that 5-HT is a key mediator in the pathogenesis of migraine, 5-HT-receptor agonists have become the mainstay for acute treatment of migraine headaches. This hypothesis is based on evidence obtained in laboratory experiments and on the following evidence obtained in human beings: (1) Plasma and platelet concentrations of 5-HT vary with the different phases of the migraine attack. (2) Urinary concentrations of 5-HT and its metabolites are elevated during most migraine attacks. (3) Migraine may be precipitated by agents such as reserpine and fenfluramine that release biogenic amines, including serotonin, from intracellular storage sites. New treatments for the prevention of migraines, such as botulinum toxin and newer antiepileptic drugs, have unique mechanisms of action, presumably unrelated to 5-HT (Ashkenazi and Silberstein, 2004).

5-HT$_1$-Receptor Agonists: The Triptans. The introduction of sumatriptan (IMITREX), zolmitriptan (ZOMIG), naratriptan (AMERGE), and rizatriptan (MAXALT and MAXALT-MLT) in the therapy of migraine has led to significant progress in preclinical and clinical research on migraine. The selective pharmacological effects of these agents, dubbed the *triptans,* at 5-HT$_1$ receptors have led to insights into the pathophysiology of migraine. Clinically, the drugs are effective, acute antimigraine agents. Their ability to decrease, rather than exacerbate, the nausea and vomiting of migraine is an important advance in the treatment of the condition.

History. Sumatriptan emerged from the first experimentally based approach to identify and develop a novel therapy for migraine. In 1972, Humphrey and colleagues initiated a project aimed at identifying novel therapeutic agents in the treatment of migraine (Humphrey *et al.*, 1990). The goal of this project was to develop selective vasoconstrictors of the extracranial circulation based on the theories of the etiology of migraine prevalent in the early 1970s. Humphrey and colleagues focused on the identification of 5-HT receptors in the carotid vasculature based on the evidence that the efficacy of traditional antimigraine drugs such as ergota-

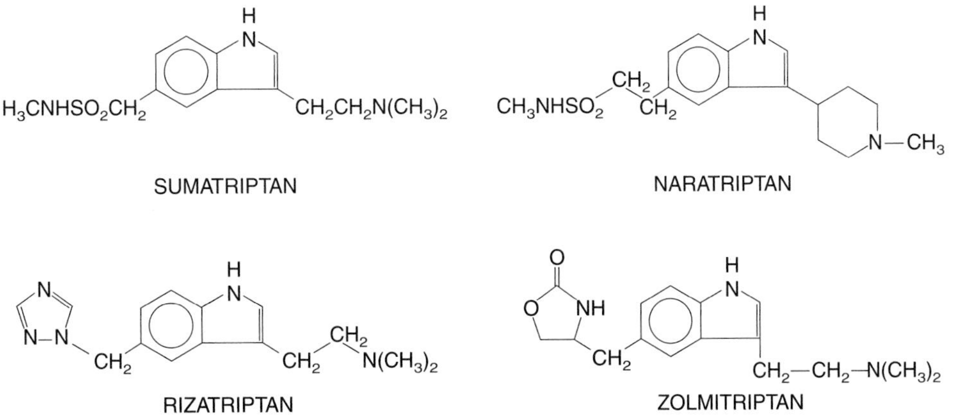

Figure 11–5. *Structures of the triptans (selective 5-HT$_1$-receptor agonists).*

mine derived from their capacity to induce vasoconstriction of the carotid arteriovenous anastomoses, presumably *via* their effects on 5-HT receptors. The synthesis of many novel tryptamine analogs was followed by determination of their actions on *in vitro* vascular preparations and in intact animals. Sumatriptan, first synthesized in 1984, potently contracted the dog isolated saphenous vein, a vessel believed to contain the novel 5-HT receptor located in the carotid circulation. Sumatriptan became available for clinical use in the United States in 1992; since then, several other triptans have been approved for clinical use (Gladstone and Gawel, 2003).

Chemistry. The triptans are indole derivatives, with substituents on the 3 and 5 positions. Their structures are given in Figure 11–5.

Pharmacological Properties. In contrast to ergot alkaloids (*see* below), the pharmacological effects of the triptans appear to be limited to the 5-HT$_1$ family of receptors, providing evidence that this receptor subclass plays an important role in the acute relief of a migraine attack. The triptans are much more selective agents than are ergot alkaloids in that they interact potently with 5-HT$_{1D}$ and 5-HT$_{1B}$ receptors and have a low or no affinity for other subtypes of 5-HT receptors. The triptans are essentially inactive at α_1 and α_2 adrenergic, β adrenergic, dopaminergic, muscarinic cholinergic, and benzodiazepine receptors. Clinically effective doses of the triptans do not correlate well with their affinity for either 5-HT$_{1A}$ or 5-HT$_{1E}$ receptors, but do correlate well with their affinities for both 5-HT$_{1B}$ and 5-HT$_{1D}$ receptors. Current data are thus consistent with the hypothesis that 5-HT$_{1B}$ and/or 5-HT$_{1D}$ receptors are the most likely receptors involved in the mechanism of action of acute antimigraine drugs.

Mechanism of Action. Two hypotheses have been proposed to explain the efficacy of 5-HT$_{1B/1D}$-receptor agonists in migraine. One hypothesis implicates the capacity of these receptors to cause constriction of intracranial blood vessels including arteriovenous anastomoses. According to a prominent pathophysiological model of migraine, unknown events lead to the abnormal dilation of carotid arteriovenous anastomoses in the head. As much as 80% of carotid arterial blood flow has been reported to be "shunted" *via* these anastomoses, located mainly in the cranial skin and ears, diverting blood from the capillary beds and thereby producing cerebral ischemia and hypoxia. Based on this model, an effective antimigraine agent would close the shunts and restore blood flow to the brain. Indeed, ergotamine, dihydroergotamine, and sumatriptan share the capacity to produce this vascular effect with a pharmacological specificity that mirrors the effects of these agents on 5-HT$_{1B}$- and 5-HT$_{1D}$-receptor subtypes.

An alternative hypothesis concerning the significance of one or more 5-HT$_1$ receptors in migraine pathophysiology relates to the observation that both 5-HT$_{1B}$ and 5-HT$_{1D}$ receptors serve as presynaptic autoreceptors, modulating neurotransmitter release from neuronal terminals (Figure 11–3). 5-HT$_1$ agonists may block the release of proinflammatory neuropeptides at the level of the nerve terminal in the perivascular space. Indeed, ergotamine, dihydroergotamine, and sumatriptan can block the development of neurogenic plasma extravasation in dura mater associated with depolarization of perivascular axons following capsaicin injection or unilateral electrical stimulation of the trigeminal nerve (Moskowitz, 1992). The ability of potent 5-HT$_1$-receptor agonists to inhibit endogenous neurotransmitter release in the perivascular space could account for their efficacy in the acute treatment of migraine.

Absorption, Fate, and Excretion. When given subcutaneously, sumatriptan reaches its peak plasma concentration in approximately 12 minutes. Following oral administration, peak plasma concentrations occur within 1 to 2 hours. Bioavailability following the subcutaneous route of administration is approximately 97%; after oral administration or nasal spray, bioavailability is only 14% to 17%. The elimination half-life is approximately 1 to 2 hours. Sumatriptan is metabolized predominantly by MAO-A, and its metabolites are excreted in the urine.

Zolmitriptan reaches its peak plasma concentration 1.5 to 2 hours after oral administration. Its bioavailability is about 40% following oral ingestion. Zolmitriptan is converted to an active *N*-desmethyl metabolite, which has severalfold higher affinity for 5-HT$_{1B}$ and 5-HT$_{1D}$ receptors than does the parent drug. Both the metabolite and the parent drug have half-lives of 2 to 3 hours.

Naratriptan, administered orally, reaches its peak plasma concentration in 2 to 3 hours and has an absolute bioavailability of about 70%. It is the longest acting of the triptans, having a half-life of about 6 hours. Fifty percent of an administered dose of naratriptan is excreted unchanged in the urine, and about 30% is excreted as products of oxidation by CYPs.

Rizatriptan has an oral bioavailability of about 45% and reaches peak plasma levels within 1 to 1.5 hours after oral ingestion of tablets of the drug. An orally disintegrating dosage form has a somewhat slower rate of absorption, yielding peak plasma levels of the drug 1.6 to 2.5 hours after administration. The principal route of metabolism of rizatriptan is *via* oxidative deamination by MAO-A.

Plasma protein-binding of the triptans ranges from about 14% (sumatriptan and rizatriptan) to 30% (naratriptan).

Adverse Effects and Contraindications. Rare but serious cardiac events have been associated with the administration of 5-HT$_1$ agonists, including coronary artery vasospasm, transient myocardial ischemia, atrial and ventricular arrhythmias, and myocardial infarction, predominantly in patients with risk factors for coronary artery disease. In general, however, only minor side effects are seen with the triptans in the acute treatment of migraine. As much as 83% of patients experience at least one side effect after subcutaneous injection of sumatriptan. Most patients report transient mild pain, stinging, or burning sensations at the site of injection. The most common side effect of sumatriptan nasal spray is a bitter taste. Orally administered triptans can cause paresthesias; asthenia and fatigue; flushing; feelings of pressure, tightness, or pain in the chest, neck, and jaw; drowsiness; dizziness; nausea; and sweating.

The triptans are contraindicated in patients who have a history of ischemic or vasospastic coronary artery disease, cerebrovascular or peripheral vascular disease, or other significant cardiovascular diseases. Because triptans may cause an acute, usually small, increase in blood pressure, they also are contraindicated in patients with uncontrolled hypertension. Naratriptan is contraindicated in patients with severe renal or hepatic impairment. Rizatriptan should be used with caution in patients with renal or hepatic disease but is not contraindicated in such patients. Sumatriptan, rizatriptan, and zolmitriptan are contraindicated in patients who are taking monoamine oxidase inhibitors.

Use in Treatment of Migraine. The triptans are effective in the acute treatment of migraine (with or without aura), but are not intended for use in prophylaxis of migraine. Treatment with these agents should begin as soon as possible after onset of a migraine attack. Oral dosage forms of the triptans are the most convenient to use, but they may not be practical in patients experiencing

migraine-associated nausea and vomiting. Approximately 70% of individuals report significant headache relief from a 6-mg subcutaneous dose of sumatriptan. This dose may be repeated once within a 24-hour period if the first dose does not relieve the headache. An oral formulation and a nasal spray of sumatriptan also are available. The onset of action is as early as 15 minutes with the nasal spray. The recommended oral dose of sumatriptan is 25 to 100 mg, which may be repeated after 2 hours up to a total dose of 200 mg over a 24-hour period. When administered by nasal spray, from 5 to 20 mg of sumatriptan is recommended. The dose can be repeated after 2 hours up to a maximum dose of 40 mg over a 24-hour period. Zolmitriptan is given orally in a 1.25- to 2.5-mg dose, which can be repeated after 2 hours, up to a maximum dose of 10 mg over 24 hours, if the migraine attack persists. Naratriptan is given orally in a 1- to 2.5-mg dose, which should not be repeated until 4 hours after the previous dose. The maximum dose over a 24-hour period should not exceed 5 mg. The recommended oral dose of rizatriptan is 5 to 10 mg. The dose can be repeated after 2 hours up to a maximum dose of 30 mg over a 24-hour period. The safety of treating more than 3 or 4 headaches over a 30-day period with triptans has not been established. Triptans should not be used concurrently with (or within 24 hours of) an ergot derivative (*see* below), nor should one triptan be used concurrently or within 24 hours of another.

Ergot and the Ergot Alkaloids. The dramatic abortive effect of ergot ingested during pregnancy has been recognized for more than 2000 years. The active principles of ergot were isolated and chemically identified in the early 20th century. The elucidation of the constituents of ergot and their complex actions was an important chapter in the evolution of modern pharmacology, even though the very complexity of their actions limits their therapeutic uses (Table 11–5). The pharmacological effects of the ergot alkaloids are varied and complex; in general, the effects result from their actions as partial agonists or antagonists at adrenergic, dopaminergic, and serotonergic receptors (*see also* Chapter 10). The spectrum of effects depends on the agent, dosage, species, tissue, physiological and endocrinological state, and experimental conditions.

History. Ergot is the product of a fungus (*Claviceps purpurea*) that grows on rye and other grains. The contamination of an edible grain by a poisonous, parasitic fungus spread death for centuries. As early as 600 B.C., an Assyrian tablet alluded to a "noxious pustule in the ear of grain." Written descriptions of ergot poisoning first appeared in the Middle Ages. Strange epidemics were described in which the characteristic symptom was gangrene of the feet, legs, hands, and arms. In severe cases, the tissue became dry and black, and mummified limbs separated off without loss of blood. Limbs were said to be consumed by the holy fire, blackened like charcoal with agonizing burning sensa-

Table 11–5
Pharmacological Actions of Selected Ergot Alkaloids

COMPOUND	Pharmacological Actions		
	INTERACTIONS WITH TRYPTAMINERGIC RECEPTORS	INTERACTIONS WITH DOPAMINERGIC RECEPTORS	INTERACTIONS WITH α ADRENERGIC RECEPTORS
Ergotamine	Partial agonist in certain blood vessels; antagonist in various smooth muscles; poor agonist/antagonist in CNS	No notable actions on central or peripheral structures; high emetic potency	Partial agonist and antagonist in blood vessels and various smooth muscles; mainly antagonist in CNS
Dihydroergotamine	Partial agonist and antagonist in a few smooth muscles	Nonselective antagonist in sympathetic ganglia; low emetic potency	Partial agonist; antagonist in blood vessels, various smooth muscles, peripheral nervous system, and CNS
Bromocriptine	Only a few weak antagonistic actions reported	Partial agonist/antagonist in CNS; presumed agonist in inhibiting secretion of prolactin; less emetic potency than ergotamine	No agonistic effects; less potent antagonist than dihydroergotamine
Ergonovine, methyl ergonovine	Partial agonists in human umbilical and placental blood vessels; selective and fairly potent antagonists in various smooth muscles; partial agonists/antagonists in CNS	Weak antagonists in certain blood vessels; partial agonists/antagonists in CNS; less potent than bromocriptine in producing emesis or inhibiting secretion of prolactin	Partial agonists in blood vessels (less than ergotamine); little antagonistic action
Methysergide	Partial agonist in blood vessels and areas of CNS; selective and very potent antagonist in many tissues and areas of CNS	Little evidence for agonistic or antagonistic activity; no emetic activity	Little or no agonistic or antagonistic action

tions. The disease was called holy fire or St. Anthony's fire in honor of the saint at whose shrine relief was said to be obtained. The relief that followed migration to the shrine of St. Anthony was probably real, for the sufferers received a diet free of contaminated grain during their sojourn at the shrine. The symptoms of ergot poisoning were not restricted to limbs. A frequent complication of ergot poisoning was abortion. Indeed, ergot was known as an obstetrical herb before it was identified as the cause of St. Anthony's fire.

Chemistry. The ergot alkaloids can all be considered to be derivatives of the tetracyclic compound 6-methylergoline (Table 11–6). The naturally occurring alkaloids contain a substituent in the beta configurations at position 8 and a double bond in ring D. The natural alkaloids of therapeutic interest are amide derivatives of *d*-lysergic acid. The first pure ergot alkaloid, ergotamine, was obtained in 1920, followed by the isolation of ergonovine in 1932. Numerous semisynthetic derivatives of the ergot alkaloids have been prepared by catalytic hydrogenation of the natural alkaloids, *e.g.,* dihydroergotamine. Another synthetic derivative, *bromocriptine* (2-bromo-α-ergocriptine), is used to control the secretion of prolactin (*see*

Chapter 55), a property derived from its dopamine agonist effect. Other products of this series include lysergic acid diethylamide (LSD), a potent hallucinogenic drug, and methysergide, a serotonin antagonist. These drugs are discussed later in this chapter.

Absorption, Fate, and Excretion. The oral administration of ergotamine by itself generally results in low or undetectable systemic drug concentrations, because of extensive first-pass metabolism. Bioavailability after sublingual administration probably is less than 1% and is inadequate for therapeutic purposes. The bioavailability after administration of rectal suppositories is greater. Ergotamine is metabolized in the liver by largely undefined pathways, and 90% of the metabolites are excreted in the bile. Only traces of unmetabolized drug are found in urine and feces. Despite a plasma half-life of approximately 2 hours, ergotamine produces vasoconstriction that lasts for 24 hours or longer. Dihydroergotamine is eliminated more rapidly than ergotamine, presumably due to its rapid hepatic clearance.

Ergonovine and methylergonovine are rapidly absorbed after oral administration and reach peak concentrations in plasma within 60 to 90 minutes that are more than tenfold those achieved with an

Table 11–6
Natural and Semisynthetic Ergot Alkaloids

| A. AMINE ALKALOIDS AND CONGENERS | | | | B. AMINO ACID ALKALOIDS | | |

Alkaloid	X	Y	Alkaloid§	R(2')	R'(5')
d-Lysergic acid	—COOH	—H	Ergotamine	—CH₃	—CH₂—phenyl
d-Isolysergic acid	—H	—COOH	Ergosine	—CH₃	—CH₂CH(CH₃)₂
d-Lysergic acid diethylamide (LSD)	—C—N(CH₂CH₃)₂ ‖ O	—H	Ergostine	—CH₂CH₃	—CH₂—phenyl
Ergonovine (ergometrine)	—C—NH—CHCH₂OH ‖ | O CH₃	—H	Ergotoxine group: Ergocornine Ergocristine α-Ergocryptine β-Ergocryptine	—CH(CH₃)₂ —CH(CH₃)₂ —CH(CH₃)₂ —CH(CH₃)₂	—CH(CH₃)₂ —CH₂—phenyl —CH₂CH(CH₃)₂ —CHCH₂CH₃ | CH₃
Methylergonovine	CH₂CH₃ | —C—NH—CH ‖ \ O CH₂OH	—H	Bromocriptine¶	—CH(CH₃)₂	—CH₂CH(CH₃)₂
Methysergide*	CH₂CH₃ | —C—NH—CH ‖ \ O CH₂OH	—H			
Lisuride	—H	O ‖ —NH—C—N(CH₂CH₃)₂			
Lysergol	—CH₂OH	—H			
Lergotrile†,‡	—CH₂CN	—H			
Metergoline*,†	O ‖ —CH₂—NH—C—O—CH₂—phenyl	—H			

*Contains methyl substitution at N1. †Contains hydrogen atoms at C9 and C10. ‡Contains chlorine atom at C2. §Dihydro derivatives contain hydrogen atoms at C9 and C10. ¶Contains bromine atom at C2.

equivalent dose of ergotamine. An uterotonic effect in postpartum women can be observed within 10 minutes after oral administration of 0.2 mg of ergonovine. Judging from the relative durations of action, ergonovine is metabolized and/or eliminated more rapidly than is ergotamine. The half-life of methylergonovine in plasma ranges between 0.5 and 2 hours.

Use in the Treatment of Migraine. The multiple pharmacological effects of ergot alkaloids have complicated the determination of their precise mechanism of action in the acute treatment of migraine. Based on the mechanism of action of sumatriptan and other 5-HT$_{1B/1D}$-receptor agonists (discussed above), the actions of ergot alkaloids at 5-HT$_{1B/1D}$ receptors likely mediate their *acute* antimigraine effects. The ergot derivative methysergide, which acts more commonly as a 5-HT-receptor *antagonist,* has been used for the prophylactic treatment of migraine headaches and is discussed below, in the section on 5-HT-receptor antagonists.

The use of ergot alkaloids for migraine should be restricted to patients having frequent, moderate migraine or infrequent, severe migraine attacks. As with other medications used to abort an attack, the patient should be advised to take ergot preparations as soon as possible after the onset of a headache. Gastrointestinal absorption of ergot alkaloids is erratic, perhaps contributing to the large variation in

patient response to these drugs. Accordingly, available preparations currently in the United States include sublingual tablets of *ergotamine tartrate* (ERGOMAR) and a nasal spray and solution for injection of *dihydroergotamine mesylate* (MIGRANAL and D.H.E. 45, respectively). The recommended dose for ergotamine tartrate is 2 mg sublingually, which can be repeated at 30-minute intervals if necessary up to a total dose of 6 mg in a 24-hour period or 10 mg a week. Dihydroergotamine mesylate injections can be given intravenously, subcutaneously, or intramuscularly. The recommended dose is 1 mg, which can be repeated after 1 hour if necessary up to a total dose of 2 mg (intravenously) or 3 mg (subcutaneously or intramuscularly) in a 24-hour period or 6 mg in a week. The dose of dihydroergotamine mesylate administered as a nasal spray is 0.5 mg (one spray) in each nostril, repeated after 15 minutes for a total dose of 2 mg (4 sprays). The safety of more than 3 mg over 24 hours or 4 mg over 7 days has not been established.

Adverse Effects and Contraindications. Nausea and vomiting, due to a direct effect on CNS emetic centers, occur in approximately 10% of patients after oral administration of ergotamine, and in about twice that number after parenteral administration. This side effect is problematic, since nausea and sometimes vomiting are part of the symptomatology of a migraine headache. Leg weakness is common, and muscle pains that occasionally are severe may occur in the extremities. Numbness and tingling of fingers and toes are other reminders of the ergotism that this alkaloid may cause. Precordial distress and pain suggestive of angina pectoris, as well as transient tachycardia or bradycardia, also have been noted, presumably as a result of coronary vasospasm induced by ergotamine. Localized edema and itching may occur in an occasional hypersensitive patient, but usually do not necessitate interruption of ergotamine therapy. In the event of acute or chronic poisoning (ergotism), treatment consists of complete withdrawal of the offending drug and symptomatic measures. The latter include attempts to maintain adequate circulation by agents such as anticoagulants, low-molecular-weight dextran, and potent vasodilator drugs, such as intravenous sodium nitroprusside. Dihydroergotamine has lower potency than does ergotamine as an emetic and as a vasoconstrictor and oxytocic.

Ergot alkaloids are contraindicated in women who are or may become pregnant, because the drugs may cause fetal distress and miscarriage. Ergot alkaloids also are contraindicated in patients with peripheral vascular disease, coronary artery disease, hypertension, impaired hepatic or renal function, and sepsis. Ergot alkaloids should not be taken within 24 hours of the use of the triptans, and should not be used concurrently with other drugs that can cause vasoconstriction.

Use of Ergot Alkaloids in Postpartum Hemorrhage. All of the natural ergot alkaloids markedly increase the motor activity of the uterus. After small doses, contractions are increased in force or frequency, or both, but are followed by a normal degree of relaxation. As the dose is increased, contractions become more forceful and prolonged, resting tone is dramatically increased, and sustained contracture can result. Although this characteristic precludes their use for induction or facilitation of labor, it is quite compatible with their use postpartum or after abortion to control bleeding and maintain uterine contraction. The gravid uterus is very sensitive, and small doses of ergot alkaloids can be given immediately postpartum to obtain a marked uterine response, usually without significant side effects. In current obstetric practice, ergot alkaloids are used primarily to prevent postpartum hemorrhage. Although all natural ergot alkaloids have qualitatively the same effect on the uterus, *ergonovine* is the most active and also is less toxic than ergotamine. For these reasons ergonovine and its semisynthetic derivative *methylergonovine* have replaced other ergot preparations as uterine-stimulating agents in obstetrics.

D-Lysergic Acid Diethylamide (LSD). Of the many drugs that are nonselective 5-HT agonists, LSD is the most remarkable. This ergot derivative profoundly alters human behavior, eliciting perception disturbances such as sensory distortion (especially visual and auditory) and hallucinations at doses as low as 1 μg/kg. The potent, mind-altering effects of LSD explain its abuse by human beings (*see* Chapter 23), as well as the fascination of scientists with the mechanism of action of LSD. The chemical structure of LSD is shown in Table 11–6.

LSD was synthesized in 1943 by Albert Hoffman, who discovered its unique properties when he accidentally ingested the drug. The chemical precursor, lysergic acid, occurs naturally in a fungus that grows on wheat and rye, but it is devoid of hallucinogenic actions. LSD contains an indolealkylamine moiety embedded within its structure, and early investigators postulated that it would interact with 5-HT receptors. Extensive studies have shown that LSD interacts with brain 5-HT receptors as an agonist/partial agonist. LSD mimics 5-HT at 5-HT$_{1A}$

autoreceptors on raphe cell bodies, producing a marked slowing of the firing rate of serotonergic neurons. In the raphe, LSD and 5-HT are equi-effective; however, in areas of serotonergic axonal projections (such as visual relay centers), LSD is far less effective than is 5-HT. Current theories focus on the ability of hallucinogens such as LSD to promote glutamate release in thalamocortical terminals, thus causing a dissociation between sensory relay centers and cortical output (Aghajanian and Marek, 1999). In drug discrimination, an animal behavioral model thought to reflect the subjective effects of abused drugs, the discriminative stimulus effects of LSD and other hallucinogenic drugs appear to be mediated by activation of 5-HT$_{2A}$ receptors (Glennon, 1990). Consistent with these behavioral results, analyses of receptor-linked phosphoinositide hydrolysis show that LSD and other hallucinogenic drugs act as partial or full agonists at 5-HT$_{2A}$ and 5-HT$_{2C}$ receptors. An important unanswered question is whether the agonist property of hallucinogenic drugs at 5-HT$_{2C}$ receptors contributes to the behavioral alterations. LSD also interacts potently with many other 5-HT receptors, including cloned receptors whose functions have not yet been determined. On the other hand, the hallucinogenic phenethylamine derivatives such as 1-(4-bromo-2,5-dimethoxyphenyl)-2-aminopropane are selective 5-HT$_{2A/2C}$-receptor agonists. Promising signs of progress in understanding the actions of hallucinogens are arising from clinical investigations of hallucinogens. It is now possible to test in human beings the hypotheses developed in animal models. For example, positron emission tomography (PET) imaging studies (Vollenweider *et al.*, 1997) revealed that administration of the hallucinogen psilocybin mimics the pattern of brain activation found in schizophrenic patients experiencing hallucinations. Consistent with animal studies, this action of psilocybin is blocked by pretreatment with 5-HT$_{2A/2C}$ antagonists (for a review, *see* Vollenweider and Geyer, 2001).

8-Hydroxy-(2-N,N-Dipropylamino)-Tetraline (8-OH-DPAT). This prototypic 5-HT$_{1A}$-selective receptor agonist is a valuable experimental tool. The structure of 8-OH-DPAT is:

8-OH-DPAT

8-OH-DPAT does not interact with other members of the 5-HT$_1$-receptor subfamily or with 5-HT$_2$, 5-HT$_3$, or 5-HT$_4$ receptors. 8-OH-DPAT reduces the firing rate of raphe cells by activating 5-HT$_{1A}$ autoreceptors and inhibits neuronal firing in terminal fields (*e.g.*, hippocampus) by direct interaction with postsynaptic 5-HT$_{1A}$ receptors. A series of long-chain arylpiperazines, such as buspirone, gepirone, and ipsapirone, are selective partial agonists at 5-HT$_{1A}$ receptors. Other closely related arylpiperazines act as 5-HT$_{1A}$-receptor antagonists. Buspirone, the first clinically available drug in this series, has been effective in the treatment of anxiety (*see* Chapter 17). The sedative properties of the benzodiazepines, which buspirone does not have, may explain why patients usually prefer the benzodiazepines to relieve anxiety. Other arylpiperazines are being developed for treatment of depression as well as anxiety.

m-Chlorophenylpiperazine (mCPP). The actions of mCPP *in vivo* primarily reflect activation of 5-HT$_{1B}$ and/or 5-HT$_{2A/2C}$ receptors, although this agent is not subtype-

selective in radioligand-binding studies *in vitro*. mCPP (structure below) is an active metabolite of the antidepressant drug *trazodone* (DESYREL).

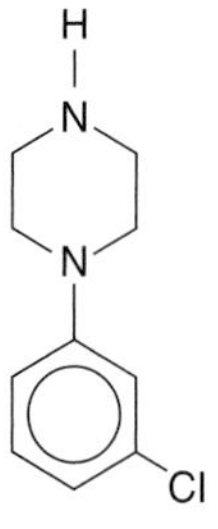

mCPP

mCPP has been employed to probe brain 5-HT function in human beings. The drug alters a number of neuroendocrine parameters and elicits profound behavioral effects, with anxiety as a prominent symptom (Murphy, 1990). mCPP elevates cortisol and prolactin secretion, probably *via* a combination of 5-HT$_1$- and 5-HT$_{2A/2C}$-receptor activation. It also increases growth hormone secretion, apparently by a 5-HT-independent mechanism. 5-HT$_{2A/2C}$ receptors appear to mediate at least part of the anxiogenic effects of mCPP, as 5-HT$_{2A/2C}$-receptor antagonists attenuate mCPP-induced anxiety. Animal studies suggest a greater involvement of the 5-HT$_{2C}$ receptor in anxiogenic actions of mCPP.

5-HT-Receptor Antagonists

The properties of 5-HT-receptor antagonists also vary widely. Ergot alkaloids and related compounds tend to be nonspecific 5-HT-receptor antagonists; however, a few ergot derivatives such as *metergoline* bind preferentially to members of the 5-HT$_2$-receptor family. A number of selective antagonists for 5-HT$_{2A/2C}$ and 5-HT$_3$ receptors are currently available. Members of these drug classes have widely different chemical structures, with no common structural motif predictably conveying high affinity. Ketanserin is the prototypic 5-HT$_{2A}$-receptor antagonist (*see* below). A large series of 5-HT$_3$-receptor antagonists are being explored for treatment of various gastrointestinal disturbances. *Ondansetron* (ZOFRAN), *dolasetron* (ANZEMET), and *granisetron* (KYTRIL), all 5-HT$_3$-receptor antagonists, have proven to be highly efficacious in the treatment of chemotherapy-induced nausea (*see* Chapter 37).

Clinical effects of 5-HT-related drugs often exhibit a significant delay in onset. This is particularly the case with drugs used to treat affective disorders such as anxiety and depression (*see* Chapter 17). This delayed onset has generated considerable interest in potential adaptive changes in

5-HT-receptor density and sensitivity after chronic drug treatments. Laboratory studies have documented agonist-promoted receptor subsensitivity and down-regulation of 5-HT-receptor subtypes, a compensatory response common to many neurotransmitter systems. However, an unusual adaptive process, *antagonist*-induced down-regulation of 5-HT$_{2C}$ receptors, takes place in rats and mice after chronic treatment with receptor antagonists (Gray and Roth, 2001). The mechanism of this paradoxical regulation of 5-HT$_{2A/2C}$ receptors has generated considerable interest, since many clinically effective drugs, including clozapine, ketanserin, and amitriptyline, exhibit this unusual property. These drugs, as well as several other 5-HT$_{2A/2C}$-receptor antagonists, possess negative intrinsic activity, reducing constitutive (spontaneous) receptor activity as well as blocking agonist occupancy (Barker *et al.*, 1994). This property of negative intrinsic activity or inverse agonism is frequently observed when constitutive (agonist-independent) activity can be measured; in the absence of constitutive activity, inverse agonists behave as competitive antagonists (for reviews *see* Milligan, 2003; and Kenakin, 2004). Another group of 5-HT$_{2A/2C}$-receptor antagonists was found to act in the classical manner, simply blocking receptor occupancy by agonists. Even though there is only scant evidence for constitutive activity *in vivo*, drug development has been further refined by focusing on reduction of preexisting constitutive neuronal activity as opposed to blockade of excess neurotransmitter action.

Ketanserin. Ketanserin (SUFREXAL) (structure below) opened a new era in 5-HT-receptor pharmacology. Ketanserin potently blocks 5-HT$_{2A}$ receptors, less potently blocks 5-HT$_{2C}$ receptors, and has no significant effect on 5-HT$_3$ or 5-HT$_4$ receptors or any members of the 5-HT$_1$-receptor family. Notably, ketanserin also has high affinity for α adrenergic receptors and histamine H$_1$ receptors (Janssen, 1983).

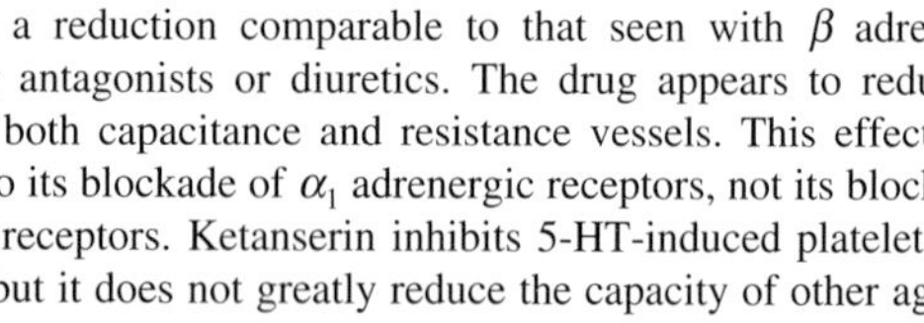

KETANSERIN

Ketanserin lowers blood pressure in patients with hypertension, causing a reduction comparable to that seen with β adrenergic-receptor antagonists or diuretics. The drug appears to reduce the tone of both capacitance and resistance vessels. This effect likely relates to its blockade of α_1 adrenergic receptors, not its blockade of 5-HT$_{2A}$ receptors. Ketanserin inhibits 5-HT-induced platelet aggregation, but it does not greatly reduce the capacity of other agents to cause aggregation. Ketanserin is not yet marketed in the United States but is available in Europe. Severe side effects after treatment with ketanserin have not been reported. Its oral bioavailability is about 50%, and its plasma half-life is 12 to 25 hours. The primary mechanism of inactivation is hepatic metabolism.

Chemical relatives of ketanserin such as *ritanserin* are more selective 5-HT$_{2A}$-receptor antagonists with low affinity for α_1 adrenergic receptors. However, ritanserin, as well as most other 5-HT$_{2A}$-receptor antagonists, also potently antagonize 5-HT$_{2C}$ receptors. The physiological significance of 5-HT$_{2C}$-receptor blockade is unknown. MDL 100,907 is the prototype of a new series of potent 5-HT$_{2A}$-receptor antagonists, with high selectivity for 5-HT$_{2A}$ *versus* 5-HT$_{2C}$ receptors. Clinical trials of MDL 100,907 in the treatment of schizophrenia have been inconclusive.

Atypical Antipsychotic Drugs. *Clozapine* (CLOZARIL), a 5-HT$_{2A/2C}$-receptor antagonist, represents a class of atypical antipsychotic drugs with reduced incidence of extrapyramidal side effects compared to the classical neuroleptics, and possibly a greater efficacy for reducing negative symptoms of schizophrenia (*see* Chapter 18). Clozapine also has a high affinity for subtypes of dopamine receptors.

One of the newest strategies for the design of additional atypical antipsychotic drugs is to combine 5-HT$_{2A/2C}$ and dopamine D$_2$-receptor–blocking actions in the same molecule (Meltzer, 1999). *Risperidone* (RISPERDAL), for example, is a potent 5-HT$_{2A}$- and D$_2$-receptor antagonist. Low doses of risperidone have been reported to attenuate negative symptoms of schizophrenia with a low incidence of extrapyramidal side effects. Extrapyramidal effects are commonly seen, however, with doses of risperidone in excess of 6 mg/day. Other atypical antipsychotic agents— *quetiapine* (SEROQUEL) and *olanzapine* (ZYPREXA)—act on multiple receptors, but their antipsychotic properties are thought to be due to antagonism of dopamine and serotonin.

Methysergide. *Methysergide* (SANSERT; 1-methyl-*d*-lysergic acid butanolamide) is a congener of methylergonovine (Table 11–6).

Methysergide blocks 5-HT$_{2A}$ and 5-HT$_{2C}$ receptors, but appears to have partial agonist activity in some preparations. Methysergide inhibits the vasoconstrictor and pressor effects of 5-HT, as well as the actions of 5-HT on various types of extravascular smooth muscle. It has been found to both block and mimic the central effects of 5-HT. Methysergide is not selective: it also interacts with 5-HT$_1$ receptors, but its therapeutic effects appear primarily to reflect blockade of 5-HT$_2$ receptors. Although methysergide is an ergot derivative, it has only weak vasoconstrictor and oxytocic activity.

Methysergide has been used for the prophylactic treatment of migraine and other vascular headaches, including Horton's syndrome. It is without benefit when given during an acute migraine attack. The protective effect takes 1 to 2 days to develop and disappears slowly when treatment is terminated. This might be due to the accumulation of an active metabolite of methysergide, methylergometrine, which is more potent than the parent drug. Methysergide

also has been used to combat diarrhea and malabsorption in patients with carcinoid tumors, and may be beneficial in the postgastrectomy dumping syndrome; both of these conditions have a 5-HT–mediated component. However, methysergide is ineffective against other substances (*e.g.*, kinins) that also are released by carcinoid tumors. For this reason, the preferred agent to treat malabsorption in carcinoid patients is a somatostatin analog, *octreotide acetate* (SANDOSTATIN), which inhibits the secretion of all the mediators released by the carcinoid tumors (*see* Chapter 55).

Side effects of methysergide are usually mild and transient, although drug withdrawal is infrequently required to reverse more severe reactions. Common side effects include gastrointestinal disturbances (heartburn, diarrhea, cramps, nausea, and vomiting), and symptoms related to vasospasm-induced ischemia (numbness and tingling of extremities, pain in the extremities, and low back and abdominal pain). Effects attributable to central actions include unsteadiness, drowsiness, weakness, lightheadedness, nervousness, insomnia, confusion, excitement, hallucinations, and even frank psychotic episodes. Reactions suggestive of vascular insufficiency and exacerbation of angina pectoris have been observed in a few patients. A potentially serious complication of prolonged treatment is inflammatory fibrosis, giving rise to various syndromes that include retroperitoneal fibrosis, pleuropulmonary fibrosis, and coronary and endocardial fibrosis. Usually the fibrosis regresses after drug withdrawal, although persistent cardiac valvular damage has been reported. Because of this danger, other drugs are preferred for the prophylactic treatment of migraine (*see* earlier discussion of migraine therapy). If methysergide is used chronically, treatment should be interrupted for 3 weeks or more every 6 months.

Cyproheptadine. The structure of *cyproheptadine* (PERIACTIN; *see* below) resembles that of the phenothiazine histamine H$_1$-receptor antagonists, and indeed, it is an effective H$_1$-receptor antagonist. Cyproheptadine also has prominent 5-HT blocking activity on smooth muscle by virtue of its binding to 5-HT$_{2A}$ receptors. In addition, it has weak anticholinergic activity and possesses mild CNS depressant properties.

CYPROHEPTADINE

Cyproheptadine shares the properties and uses of other H$_1$-receptor antagonists (*see* Chapter 24). It is effective in controlling skin allergies, particularly the accompanying pruritus. In allergic conditions, the action of cyproheptadine as a 5-HT-receptor antagonist is irrelevant, since 5-HT$_{2A}$ receptors are not involved in human allergic responses. Some physicians recommend cyproheptadine to counteract the sexual side effects of selective 5-HT-reuptake inhibitors such as fluoxetine and sertraline (*see* Chapter 17). The 5-HT blocking actions of cyproheptadine explain its value in the postgastrectomy dumping syndrome, intestinal hypermotility of carcinoid, and migraine prophylaxis. Cyproheptadine is not, however, a preferred treatment for these conditions.

Side effects of cyproheptadine include those common to other H$_1$-receptor antagonists, such as drowsiness. Weight gain and increased growth in children have been observed and attributed to impaired regulation of growth-hormone secretion.

BIBLIOGRAPHY

Andrade, R., Malenka, R.C., and Nicoll, R.A. A G protein couples serotonin and GABA-B receptors to the same channels in hippocampus. *Science*, **1986**, *234*:1261–1265.

Barker, E.L., Westphal, R.S., Schmidt, D., and Sanders-Bush, E. Constitutively active 5HT$_{2C}$ receptors reveal novel inverse agonist activity of receptor ligands. *J. Biol. Chem.*, **1994**, *269*:11687–11690.

Brunner, H.C., Nelen, M., Breakefield, X.O., *et al.* Abnormal behavior associated with a point mutation in the structural gene for monoamine oxidase A. *Science,* **1993**, *262*:578–580.

Burns, C.M., Chu, H., Rueter, S.M., *et al.* Regulation of serotonin-2C receptor G-protein coupling by RNA editing. *Nature*, **1997**, *387*:303–308.

Cases, O., Seif, I., Grimsby, J., *et al.* Aggressive behavior and altered amounts of brain serotonin and norepinephrine in mice lacking MAOA. *Science*, **1995**, *268*:1763–1766.

Delgado, P.L., Charney, D.S., Price, L.H., *et al.* Serotonin function and the mechanism of antidepressant action. Reversal of antidepressant-induced remission by rapid depletion of plasma tryptophan. *Arch. Gen. Psychiatry*, **1990**, *47*:411–418.

Gaddum, J.H., and Picarelli, Z.P. Two kinds of tryptamine receptors. *Br. J. Pharmacol.*, **1957**, *12*:323–328.

Maricq, A.V., Peterson, A.S., Brake, A.J., *et al.* Primary structure and functional expression of the 5HT3 receptor, a serotonin-gated ion channel. *Science*, **1991**, *254*:432–437.

Peroutka, S.J., and Snyder, S.H. Multiple serotonin receptors: differential binding of [³H]5-hydroxytryptamine, [³H]lysergic acid diethylamide and [³H]spiroperidol. *Mol. Pharmacol.*, **1979**, *16*:687–699.

Ramamoorthy, S., and Blakely, R.D. Phosphorylation and sequestration of serotonin transporters differentially modulated by psychostimulants. *Science*, **1999**, *285*:763–766.

Saudou, F., Amara, D.A., Dierich, A., *et al.* Enhanced aggressive behavior in mice lacking 5-HT$_{1B}$ receptor. *Science*, **1994**, *265*:1875–1878.

Tecott, L.H., Sun, L.M., Akana, S.F., *et al.* Eating disorder and epilepsy in mice lacking 5-HT$_{2C}$ serotonin receptors. *Nature*, **1995**, *374*:542–546.

Vollenweider, F.X., Leenders, K.L., Scharfetter, C., *et al.* Positron emission tomography and fluorodeoxyglucose studies of metabolic hyperfrontality and psychopathology in the psilocybin model of psychosis. *Neuropsychopharmacology,* **1997**, *16*:357–372.

MONOGRAPHS AND REVIEWS

Aghajanian, G.K., and Marek, G.J. Serotonin and hallucinogens. *Neuropsychopharmacology*, **1999**, *21*(suppl 1):S16–S23.

Aghajanian, G.K., and Sanders-Bush, E. Serotonin. In, *Psychopharmacology: The Fifth Generation of Progress.* (Davis, K.L., Charney, D., Coyle J.T., and Nemeroff, C., eds.) Lippincott Williams & Wilkins, Baltimore, **2002**, pp. 15–35.

Ashkenazi, A., and Silberstein, S.D. Botulinum toxin and other new approaches to migraine therapy. *Annu. Rev. Med.*, **2004**, *55*:505–518.

Barnes, N.M., and Sharp, T. A review of central 5-HT receptors and their function. *Neuropharmacology*, **1999**, *38*:1083–1152.

Bonasera, S.J., and Tecott, L.H. Mouse models of serotonin receptor function: toward a genetic dissection of serotonin systems. *Pharmacol. Ther.*, **2000**, *88*:133–142.

Cajochen, C., Krauchi, K., and Wirz-Justice A. Role of melatonin in the regulation of human circadian rhythms and sleep. *J. Neuroendocrinol.*, **2003**, *15*:432–437.

Deleu, D., Hanssens, Y., and Worthing, E.A. Symptomatic and prophylactic treatment of migraine: a critical reappraisal. *Clin. Neuropharmacol.*, **1998**, *21*:267–279.

Descarries, L., Audet, M.A., Doucet, G., *et al.* Morphology of central serotonin neurons. Brief review of quantified aspects of their distribution and ultrastructural relationships. *Ann. N.Y. Acad. Sci.,* **1990**, *600*:81–92.

Gershon, M.D. Serotonin and its implication for the management of irritable bowel syndrome. *Rev. Gastroenterol. Disord.*, **2003**, *3*(suppl 2):S25–S34.

Gladstone, J.P., and Gawel, M. Newer formulations of the triptans: advances in migraine management. *Drugs*, **2003**, *63*:2285–2305.

Glennon, R.A. Do classical hallucinogens act as 5-HT$_2$ agonists or antagonists? *Neuropsychopharmacology*, **1990**, *3*:509–517.

Gray, J.A., and Roth, B.L. Paradoxical trafficking and regulation of 5-HT$_{2A}$ receptors by agonists and antagonists. *Brain Res. Bull.*, **2001**, *56*:441–451.

Hegde, S.S., and Eglen, R.M. Peripheral 5-HT$_4$ receptors. *FASEB J.*, **1996**, *10*:1398–1407.

Hoyer, D., Clarke, D.E., Fozard, J.R., *et al.* International Union of Pharmacology classification of receptors for 5-hydroxytryptamine (serotonin). *Pharmacol. Rev.*, **1994**, *46*:157–203.

Humphrey, P.P., Aperley, E., Feniuk, W., and Perren, M.J. A rational approach to identifying a fundamentally new drug for the treatment of migraine. In, *Cardiovascular Pharmacology of 5-Hydroxytryptamine: Prospective Therapeutic Applications.* (Saxena, P.R., Wallis, D.I., Wouters, W., and Bevan, P., eds.) Kluwer Academic Publishers, Dordrecht, Netherlands, **1990**, pp. 417–431.

Janssen, P.A.J. 5-HT$_2$ receptor blockade to study serotonin-induced pathology. *Trends Pharmacol. Sci.*, **1983**, *4*:198–206.

Jouvet, M. Sleep and serotonin: an unfinished story. *Neuropsychopharmacology*, **1999**, *21*(suppl 2):24S–27S.

Kenakin, T. Efficacy as a vector: the relative prevalence and paucity of inverse agonism. *Mol. Pharmacol.*, **2004**, *65*:2–11.

Lucki, I. The spectrum of behaviors influenced by serotonin. *Biol. Psychiatry*, **1998**, *44*:151–162.

Meltzer, H.Y. The role of serotonin in antipsychotic drug action. *Neuropsychopharmacology*, **1999**, *21*(suppl 2):106S–115S.

Milligan, G. Constitutive activity and inverse agonists of G protein-coupled receptors: a current perspective. *Mol. Pharmacol.*, **2003**, *64*:1271–1276.

Moskowitz, M.A. Neurogenic *versus* vascular mechanisms of sumatriptan and ergot alkaloids in migraine. *Trends Pharmacol. Sci.*, **1992**, *13*:307–311.

Murphy, D.L. Neuropsychiatric disorders and the multiple human brain serotonin receptor subtypes and subsystems. *Neuropsychopharmacology*, **1990**, *3*:457–471.

Palacios, J.M., Waeber, C., Hoyer, D., and Mengod, G. Distribution of serotonin receptors. *Ann. N.Y. Acad. Sci.*, **1990**, *600*:36–52.

Sanders-Bush, E., Fentress, H., and Hazelwood, L. Serotonin 5-HT$_2$ receptors: molecular and genomic diversity. *Mol. Interv.*, **2003**, *3*:319–330.

Saxena, P.R., and Villalón, C.M. Cardiovascular effects of serotonin agonists and antagonists. *J. Cardiovasc. Pharmacol.*, **1990**, *15*(suppl 7):S17–S34.

Shih, J.C. Molecular basis of human MAO A and B. *Neuropsychopharmacology*, **1991**, *4*:1–7.

Sjoerdsma, A., and Palfreyman, M.G. History of serotonin and serotonin disorders. *Ann. N.Y. Acad. Sci.*, **1990**, *600*:1–8.

Swerdlow, N.R., Braff, D.L., and Geyer, M.A. Animal models of deficient sensorimotor gating: what we know, what we think we know, and what we hope to know soon. *Behav. Pharmacol.*, **2000**, *11*:185–204.

Vollenweider, F.X., and Geyer, M.A. A systems model of altered consciousness: integrating natural and drug-induced psychoses. *Brain Res. Bull.*, **2001**, *56*:495–507.

Walther, D.J., Peter, J.U., Bashammakh, S., *et al.* Synthesis of serotonin by a second tryptophan hydroxylase isoform. *Science*, **2003**, *299*:76.

SECTION III
Drugs Acting on the Central Nervous System

NEUROTRANSMISSION AND THE CENTRAL NERVOUS SYSTEM

Floyd E. Bloom

Drugs that act upon the central nervous system (CNS) influence the daily lives of everyone. These agents are invaluable therapeutically because they can produce specific physiological and psychological effects. Without general anesthetics, modern surgery would be impossible. Drugs that affect the CNS can selectively relieve pain, reduce fever, suppress disordered movement, induce sleep or arousal, reduce appetite, and allay the tendency to vomit. Selectively acting drugs can be used to treat anxiety, depression, mania, or schizophrenia and do so without altering consciousness (*see* Chapters 17 and 18).

The nonmedical self-administration of CNS-active drugs is a widespread practice. Socially acceptable stimulants and antianxiety agents produce stability, relief, and even pleasure. However, the excessive use of such drugs can affect lives adversely when their uncontrolled, compulsive use leads to physical dependence on the drug or to toxic side effects, including lethal overdosage (*see* Chapters 22 and 23).

The quality of drugs that affect the nervous system and behavior presents extraordinary scientific challenge—the attempt to understand the cellular and molecular basis for the enormously complex and varied functions of the human brain. In this effort, pharmacologists have two major goals: to use drugs to elucidate the mechanisms that operate in the normal CNS and to develop appropriate drugs to correct pathophysiological events in the abnormal CNS.

Elucidating the sites and mechanisms of action of CNS drugs demands an understanding of the cellular and molecular biology of the brain. Although knowledge of the anatomy, physiology, and chemistry of the nervous system is far from complete, the acceleration of interdisciplinary research on the CNS has led to remarkable progress. This chapter introduces guidelines and fundamental principles for the comprehensive analysis of drugs that affect the CNS. Specific therapeutic approaches to neurological and psychiatric disorders are discussed in Chapters 13 through 23.

ORGANIZATIONAL PRINCIPLES OF THE BRAIN

The brain is an assembly of interrelated neural systems that regulate their own and each other's activity in a dynamic, complex fashion largely through intercellular chemical neurotransmission (for additional references, *see* Bloom, 1996; Nestler *et al.*, 2001; Cooper *et al.*, 2003).

Macrofunctions of the Brain Regions

The large anatomical divisions provide a superficial classification of the distribution of brain functions.

Cerebral Cortex. The two cerebral hemispheres constitute the largest division of the brain. Regions of the cortex are classified in several ways: (1) by the modality of information processed (*e.g.,* sensory, including somatosensory, visual, auditory, and olfactory, as well as motor and associational); (2) by anatomical position (frontal, temporal, parietal, and occipital); and (3) by the geometric relationship between cell types in the major cortical layers ("cytoarchitectonic" classifications). The specialized functions of a cortical region arise from the interplay between connections from other regions of the cortex (corticocortical systems) and noncortical areas of the brain (subcortical systems) and a basic intracortical processing module of approximately 100 vertically connected cortical columns (Mountcastle, 1997). Varying numbers of adjacent columnar modules may be functionally, but transiently, linked into larger information-processing ensembles. The pathology of Alzheimer's disease, for example, destroys the integrity of the columnar modules and the corticocortical connections (*see* Chapter 20).

Cortical areas termed association areas process information from primary cortical sensory regions to produce higher cortical functions such as abstract thought, memory, and consciousness. The cerebral cortices also provide supervisory integration of the autonomic nervous system and integrate somatic and vegetative functions, including those of the cardiovascular and gastrointestinal systems.

Limbic System. The "limbic system" is an archaic term for an assembly of brain regions (hippocampal formation, amygdaloid complex, septum, olfactory nuclei, basal ganglia, and selected nuclei of the diencephalon) grouped around the subcortical borders of the underlying brain core to which a variety of complex emotional and motivational functions have been attributed. Modern neuroscience avoids this term because those ill-defined regions of the "limbic system" do not function consistently as a system. Parts of these limbic regions also participate individually in functions that can be more precisely defined. Thus, the basal ganglia or neostriatum (the *caudate nucleus, putamen, globus pallidus,* and *lentiform nucleus*) form an essential regulatory segment of the *extrapyramidal motor system.* This system complements the function of the pyramidal (or voluntary) motor system. Damage to the extrapyramidal system depresses the ability to initiate voluntary movements and causes disorders characterized by involuntary movements, such as the tremors and rigidity of Parkinson's disease or the uncontrollable limb movements of Huntington's chorea (*see* Chapter 20). Similarly, the hippocampus may be crucial to the formation of recent memory, since this function is lost in patients with extensive bilateral damage to the hippocampus. Memory also is disrupted by Alzheimer's disease, which destroys the intrinsic structure of the hippocampus as well as parts of the frontal cortex.

Diencephalon. The *thalamus* lies in the center of the brain, beneath the cortex and basal ganglia and above the hypothalamus. The neurons of the thalamus are arranged into distinct clusters, or nuclei, which are either paired or midline structures. These nuclei act as relays between the incoming sensory pathways and the cortex, between the discrete regions of the thalamus and the hypothalamus, and between the basal ganglia and the association regions of the cerebral cortex. The thalamic nuclei and the basal ganglia also exert regulatory control over visceral functions; aphagia and adipsia, as well as general sensory neglect, follow damage to the corpus striatum or to selected circuits ending there. The *hypothalamus* is the

principal integrating region for the entire autonomic nervous system and regulates body temperature, water balance, intermediary metabolism, blood pressure, sexual and circadian cycles, secretion of the adenohypophysis, sleep, and emotion. Recent advances in the cytophysiological and chemical dissection of the hypothalamus have clarified the connections and possible functions of individual hypothalamic nuclei.

Midbrain and Brainstem. The *mesencephalon, pons,* and *medulla oblongata* connect the cerebral hemispheres and thalamus-hypothalamus to the spinal cord. These "bridge portions" of the CNS contain most of the nuclei of the cranial nerves, as well as the major inflow and outflow tracts from the cortices and spinal cord. These regions contain the *reticular activating system,* an important but incompletely characterized region of gray matter linking peripheral sensory and motor events with higher levels of nervous integration. The major monoamine-containing neurons of the brain (*see* below) are found here. Together, these regions represent the points of central integration for coordination of essential reflexive acts, such as swallowing and vomiting, and those that involve the cardiovascular and respiratory systems; these areas also include the primary receptive regions for most visceral afferent sensory information. The reticular activating system is essential for the regulation of sleep, wakefulness, and level of arousal, as well as for coordination of eye movements. The fiber systems projecting from the reticular formation have been called "nonspecific" because the targets to which they project are relatively more diffuse in distribution than those of many other neurons (*e.g.,* specific thalamocortical projections). However, the chemically homogeneous components of the reticular system innervate targets in a coherent and functional manner despite their broad distribution.

Cerebellum. The cerebellum arises from the posterior pons behind the cerebral hemispheres. It also is highly laminated and redundant in its detailed cytological organization. The lobules and folia of the cerebellum project onto specific deep cerebellar nuclei, which in turn make relatively selective projections to the motor cortex (by way of the thalamus) and to the brainstem nuclei concerned with vestibular (position-stabilization) function. In addition to maintaining the proper tone of antigravity musculature and providing continuous feedback during volitional movements of the trunk and extremities, the cerebellum also may regulate visceral function (*e.g.,* heart rate, so as to maintain blood flow despite changes in posture). In addition, the cerebellum plays a significant role in learning and memory.

Spinal Cord. The spinal cord extends from the caudal end of the medulla oblongata to the lower lumbar vertebrae. Within this mass of nerve cells and tracts, the sensory information from skin, muscles, joints, and viscera is locally coordinated with motoneurons and with primary sensory relay cells that project to and receive signals from higher levels. The spinal cord is divided into anatomical segments (cervical, thoracic, lumbar, and sacral) that correspond to divisions of the peripheral nerves and spinal column (*see* Figure 6–1). Ascending and descending tracts of the spinal cord are located within the white matter at the perimeter of the cord, while intersegmental connections and synaptic contacts are concentrated within the H-shaped internal mass of gray matter. Sensory information flows into the dorsal cord, and motor commands exit *via* the ventral portion. The preganglionic neurons of the autonomic nervous system (*see* Chapter 6) are found in the intermediolateral columns of the gray matter. Autonomic reflexes (*e.g.*, changes in skin vasculature with alteration of temperature) can be elicited within local segments of the spinal cord, as shown by the maintenance of these reflexes after the cord is severed.

Microanatomy of the Brain

Neurons operate either within layered structures (such as the olfactory bulb, cerebral cortex, hippocampal formation, and cerebellum) or in clustered groupings (the defined collections of central neurons which aggregate into nuclei). The specific connections between neurons within or across the macro-divisions of the brain are essential to the brain's functions. It is through their patterns of neuronal circuitry that individual neurons form functional ensembles to regulate the flow of information within and between the regions of the brain.

Cellular Organization of the Brain. Present understanding of the cellular organization of the CNS can be viewed from the perspective of the size, shape, location, and interconnections between neurons (*see* Cooper *et al.*, 2003; Shepherd, 2003, for additional references).

Cell Biology of Neurons. Neurons are classified according to function (sensory, motor, or interneuron), location, or identity of the transmitter they synthesize and release. Microscopic analysis of a neuron focuses on its general shape, and in particular the complexity of the afferent receptive surfaces on the dendrites and cell body that receive synaptic contacts from other neurons. Neurons exhibit the cytological characteristics of highly active secretory cells with large nuclei: large amounts of smooth and rough endoplasmic reticulum; and frequent clusters of specialized smooth endoplasmic reticulum (Golgi complex), in which secretory products of the cell are packaged into membrane-bound organelles for transport from the cell body proper to the axon or dendrites (Figure 12–1). Neurons and their cellular extensions are rich in microtubules, which support the complex cellular structure and assist in the reciprocal transport of essential macromolecules and organelles between the cell body and the distant axon or dendrites. The sites of interneuronal communication in the CNS are termed *synapses* (*see* below). Although synapses are functionally analogous to "junctions" in the somatic motor and autonomic nervous systems, the central junctions contain an array of specific proteins presumed to be the active zone for transmitter release and response (Husi *et al.*, 2000). Like peripheral "junctions," central synapses also are denoted by accumulations of tiny (500 to 1500 Å) organelles, termed *synaptic vesicles*. The proteins of these vesicles have been shown to have specific roles in transmitter storage, vesicle docking onto presynaptic membranes, voltage- and Ca^{2+}-dependent secretion (*see* Chapter 6), and recycling and restorage of released transmitter (Murthy *et al.*, 2003; Jahn, 2004).

Supportive Cells. Neurons are not the only cells in the CNS. According to most estimates, neurons are outnumbered, perhaps by an order of magnitude, by the various supportive cells: the macroglia, the microglia, the cells of the vascular elements comprising

the intracerebral vasculature as well as the cerebrospinal fluid–forming cells of the choroid plexus found within the intracerebral ventricular system, and the meninges, which cover the surface of the brain and comprise the cerebrospinal fluid–containing envelope. Macroglia are the most abundant supportive cells; some are categorized as *astrocytes* (cells interposed between the vasculature and the neurons, often surrounding individual compartments of synaptic complexes). Astrocytes play a variety of metabolic support roles including furnishing energy intermediates and supplementary removal of extracellular neurotransmitter secretions (Pellerin *et al.*, 2003). The *oligodendroglia*, a second prominent category of macroglia, are the myelin-producing cells. Myelin, made up of multiple layers of their compacted membranes, insulates segments of long axons bioelectrically and accelerates action potential conduction velocity. Microglia are relatively uncharacterized supportive cells believed to be of mesodermal origin and related to the macrophage/monocyte lineage (Carson *et al.*, 1998; Carson, 2002). Some microglia reside within the brain, while additional cells of this class may be recruited to the brain during periods of inflammation following either microbial infection or other brain injury. The response of the brain to inflammation differs strikingly from that of other tissues and presents a therapeutic response that may transcend specific diseases (Ransohoff, 2002; Rosenberg, 2002; Raber *et al.*, 1998).

Blood–Brain Barrier. Apart from the exceptional instances in which drugs are introduced directly into the CNS, the concentration of the agent in the blood after oral or parenteral administration differs substantially from its concentration in the brain. The *blood–brain barrier* (BBB) is an important boundary between the periphery and the CNS that forms a permeability barrier to the passive diffusion of substances from the bloodstream into various regions of the CNS. Evidence of the barrier is provided by the greatly diminished rate of access of chemicals from plasma to the brain (*see* Chapter 1). This barrier is nonexistent in the peripheral nervous system, and is much less prominent in the hypothalamus and in several small, specialized organs (the circumventricular organs) lining the third and fourth ventricles of the brain: the median eminence, area postrema, pineal gland, subfornical organ, and subcommissural organ. While the BBB imposes severe limitations on the diffusion of macromolecules from the bloodstream into the brain, selective barriers to permeation into and out of the brain also exist for small, charged molecules such as neurotransmitters, their precursors and metabolites, and some drugs. These diffusional barriers are viewed as a combination of the partition of solute across the vasculature (which governs passage by definable properties such as molecular weight, charge, and lipophilicity) and the presence or absence of energy-dependent transport systems (*see* Chapter 2). The brain clears metabolites of transmitters into the cerebrospinal fluid by excretion *via* the acid transport system of the choroid plexus. Substances that rarely gain access to the brain from the bloodstream often can reach the brain when injected directly into the cerebrospinal fluid. Under certain conditions, it may be possible to open the BBB, at least transiently, to permit the entry of chemotherapeutic agents. Cerebral ischemia and inflammation also modify the BBB, increasing access to substances that ordinarily would not affect the brain.

Response to Damage: Repair and Plasticity in the CNS

Because the neurons of the CNS are terminally differentiated cells, they do not undergo proliferative responses to damage, although

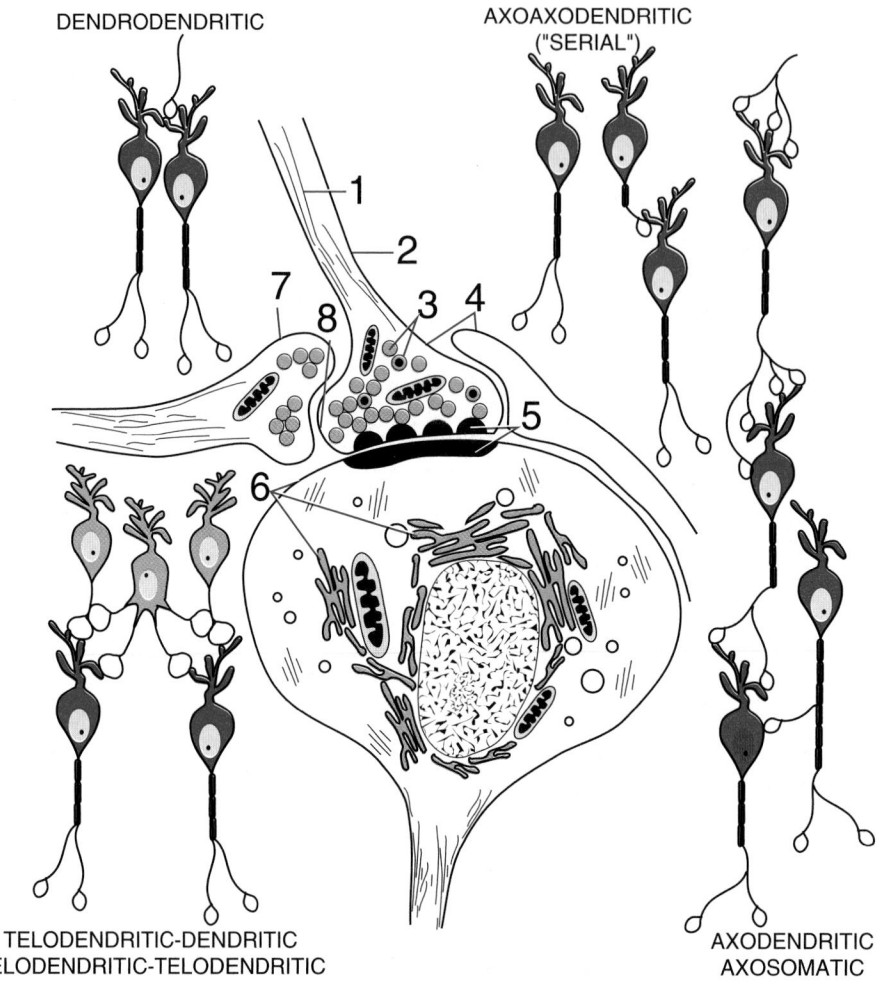

DENDRODENDRITIC

AXOAXODENDRITIC ("SERIAL")

TELODENDRITIC-DENDRITIC
TELODENDRITIC-TELODENDRITIC

AXODENDRITIC
AXOSOMATIC

Figure 12–1. ***Schematic view of the drug-sensitive sites in prototypical synaptic complexes.*** In the center, a postsynaptic neuron receives a somatic synapse (shown greatly oversized) from an axonic terminal; an axoaxonic terminal is shown in contact with this presynaptic nerve terminal. Drug-sensitive sites include: (1) microtubules and molecular motors responsible for bidirectional transport of macromolecules between the neuronal cell body and distal processes; (2) electrically conductive membranes; (3) sites for the synthesis and storage of transmitters; (4) sites for the active uptake of transmitters by nerve terminals or glia; (5) sites for the release of transmitter; (6) postsynaptic receptors, cytoplasmic organelles, and postsynaptic proteins for expression of synaptic activity and for long-term mediation of altered physiological states; and (7) presynaptic receptors on adjacent presynaptic processes and (8) on nerve terminals (autoreceptors). Around the central neuron are schematic illustrations of the more common synaptic relationships in the CNS. (Modified from Bodian, 1972, and Cooper *et al.*, 2003.)

recent evidence suggests the possibility of neural stem cell proliferation as a natural means for replacement of neurons in selected areas of the CNS (Gage, 2002); this may provide a future means of repair (Steindler *et al.*, 2002). As a result, neurons have evolved other adaptive mechanisms to maintain function following injury. These adaptive mechanisms endow the brain with considerable capacity for structural and functional modification well into adulthood, including some of the phenomena of memory and learning (Linden, 2003).

INTEGRATIVE CHEMICAL COMMUNICATION IN THE CENTRAL NERVOUS SYSTEM

The cardinal role of the CNS is to integrate information from a variety of external and internal sources, to optimize the needs of the organism within the demands of the environment. These integrative concepts transcend individual transmitter systems and emphasize the means by which neuronal activity is normally coordinated. Only through a detailed understanding of these integrative functions, and their failure in certain pathophysiological conditions, can effective and specific therapeutic approaches be developed for neurological and psychiatric disorders. The molecular and cellular mechanisms of neural integration are linked to clinical therapeutics because untreatable diseases and unexpected nontherapeutic side effects of drugs often reveal previously unrecognized mechanisms of pathophysiology. The capacity to link molecular processes to normal and pathological behavior provides an exciting aspect of modern neuropharmacological research. *A central underlying concept of neuropsychopharmacology is that drugs that influence behavior and improve the functional status of patients with neurological or psychiatric diseases act by enhancing or blunting the effectiveness of specific combinations of synaptic transmitter actions.*

Four research strategies provide the neuroscientific substrates of neuropsychological phenomena: molecular (or biochemical), cellular, multicellular (or systems), and behavioral. The intensively exploited molecular and biochemical levels have been the traditional focus for characterizing drugs that alter behavior. Molecular discoveries provide biochemical probes for identifying the appropriate neuronal sites and their mediative mechanisms. Such mechanisms include: (1) ion channels, which provide for changes in excitability induced by neurotransmitters; (2) neurotransmitter receptors; (3) auxiliary intramembranous and cytoplasmic transductive molecules that couple these receptors to intracellular effectors for short-term changes in excitability and for longer-term regulation through alterations in gene expression (Sofroniew *et al.*, 2001); and (4) transporters for the conservation of released transmitter molecules by reaccumulation into nerve terminals, and then into synaptic vesicles (*see* Chapter 6). Vesicular transporters are distinct from the plasma membrane proteins involved in transmitter uptake into nerve terminals (Figure 12–2) (Nestler *et al.*, 2001; Cooper *et al.*, 2003). Thus, the most basic cellular phenomena of neurons are now understood in terms of such discrete molecular entities. It has long been known that electrical excitability of neurons is achieved through modifications of the ion channels that all neurons express in abundance in their plasma membranes. However, we now understand in considerable detail how the three major cations, Na^+, K^+ and Ca^{2+}, and the Cl^- anions are regulated in their flow through highly discriminative ion channels (Figures 12–3 and 12–4). In addition to these ion channels, two other families of channels have been recognized: cyclic nucleotide-modulated channels, and transient receptor potential (TRP) channels.

Voltage-dependent ion channels (Figure 12–3) provide for rapid changes in ion permeability along axons and within dendrites and for the excitation-secretion coupling that releases neurotransmitters from presynaptic sites (Catterall and Epstein, 1992; Catterall, 1993). The major cation channels have been defined by functional assessment of recombinant proteins with and without constrained molecular modifications (Figure 12–3A). The intrinsic membrane-embedded domains of the Na^+ and Ca^{2+} channels are

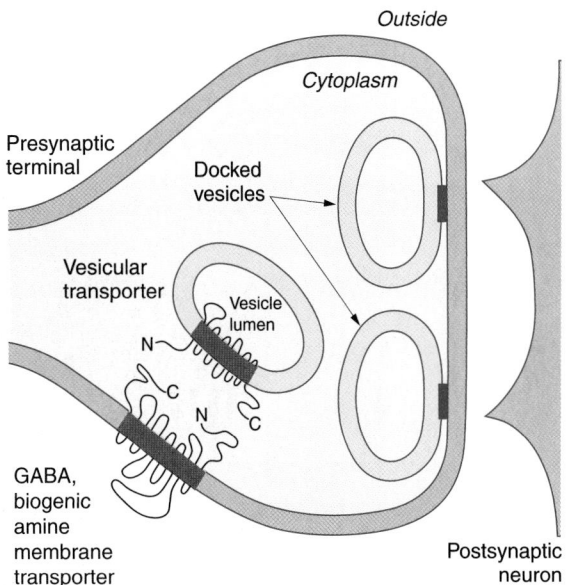

Figure 12–2. ***Predicted structural motif for neurotransmitter transporters.*** Transporters for the conservation of released amino acid or amine transmitters all share a 12-transmembrane domain structure, although the exact orientation of the amino terminus is not clear. Transporters for amine transmitters found on synaptic vesicles also share a 12-transmembrane domain structure, but one that is distinct from the transporters of the plasma membrane. *See* Chapter 2 for structural details of pharmacologically important transport proteins.

envisioned as four tandem repeats of a putative six-transmembrane domain, while the K^+ channel family contains greater molecular diversity. One structural form of voltage-regulated K^+ channels consists of subunits composed of a single putative six-transmembrane domain (Figure 12–3C). The inward rectifier K^+ channel structure, in contrast, retains the general configuration corresponding to transmembrane spans 5 and 6 with the interposed "pore region" that penetrates only the exofacial surface membrane. These two structural categories of K^+ channels can form hetero-oligomers, giving rise to multiple possibilities for regulation by voltage, neurotransmitters, assembly with intracellular auxiliary proteins, or posttranslational modifications. X-ray crystallography confirms these configurations for the K^+ channel (MacKinnon, 2003).

Ligand-gated ion channels, regulated by the binding of neurotransmitters, form a distinct group of ion channels (Figure 12–4). The structurally defined channel molecules now can be examined to determine how drugs, toxins, and imposed voltages alter neuronal excitability (Table 12–1). Within the CNS, variants of the K^+ channels (the delayed rectifier, the Ca^{2+}-activated K^+ channel, and the after-hyperpolarizing K^+ channel) regulated by intracellular second messengers repeatedly have been shown to underlie complex forms of synaptic modulation (Greengard, 2001).

Cyclic nucleotide–modulated channels consist of two groups: the cyclic nucleotide–gated (CNG) channels, which play key roles in sensory transduction for olfactory and photoreceptors, and the hyperpolarization-activated, cyclic nucleotide–gated (HCN) chan-

Ion channels

A

α₁ subunits for Ca²⁺, Na⁺ channels

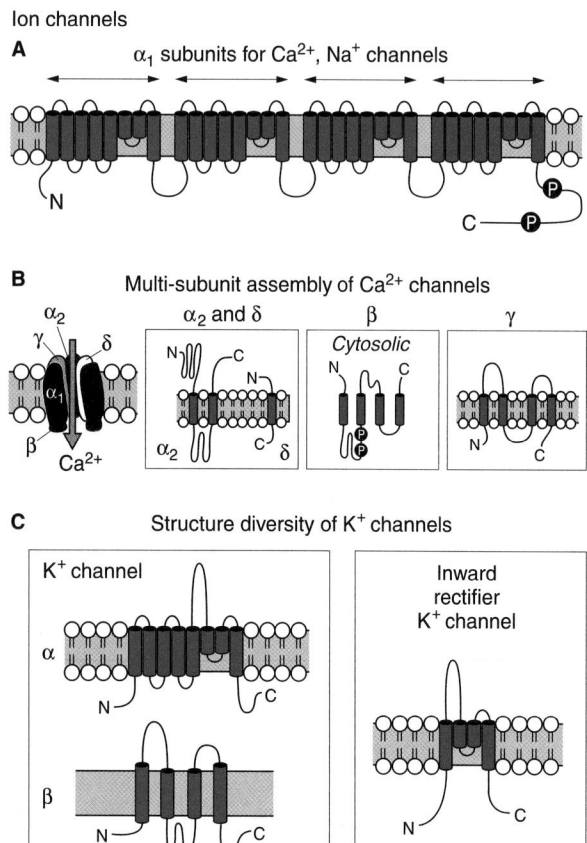

B   Multi-subunit assembly of Ca²⁺ channels

C   Structure diversity of K⁺ channels

Figure 12–3. The major molecular motifs of ion channels that establish and regulate neuronal excitability in the central nervous system. A. The α subunits of the Ca²⁺ and Na⁺ channels share a similar presumptive six-transmembrane structure, repeated four times, in which an intramembranous segment separates transmembrane segments 5 and 6. *B.* The Ca²⁺ channel also requires several auxiliary small proteins (α_2, β, γ, and δ). The α_2 and δ subunits are linked by a disulfide bond (*not shown*). Regulatory subunits also exist for Na⁺ channels. *C.* Voltage-sensitive K⁺ channels (K$_v$) and the rapidly activating K⁺ channel (K$_a$) share a similar presumptive six-transmembrane domain similar in overall configuration to one repeat unit within the Na⁺ and Ca²⁺ channel structure, while the inwardly rectifying K⁺ channel protein (K$_{ir}$) retains the general configuration of just loops 5 and 6. Regulatory β subunits (cystosolic) can alter K$_v$ channel functions. Channels of these two overall motifs can form heteromultimers (Krapivinsky *et al.*, 1995).

nels. The latter channels are unique cation channels that open with hyperpolarization and close with depolarization; upon direct binding of cyclic AMP or cyclic GMP, the activation curves for the channels are shifted to more hyperpolarized potentials. These channels play essential roles in cardiac pacemaker cells and presumably in rhythmically discharging neurons (Hofmann *et al.*, 2004).

Transient receptor potential (TRP) channels, named for their role in *Drosophila* phototransduction, are a family of hexaspanning receptors with a pore domain between the fifth and sixth transmembrane segments, and a common 25-amino acid TRP "box" C-terminal of the sixth transmembrane domain; these channels are found across the phylogenetic scale from bacteria to mammals. Members of the TRPV subfamily serve as the receptors for endogenous cannabinoids, such as anadamide (*see* section on diffusible mediators, *below*) and the hot pepper toxin, capsaicin (Clapham *et al.*, 2004).

Research at the cellular level identifies specific neurons and their most proximate synaptic connections that may mediate a behavior or the behavioral effects of a given drug. For example, research into the basis of emotion exploits both molecular and behavioral leads to the most likely brain sites at which behavioral changes pertinent to emotion can be analyzed. Such research provides clues as to the nature of the interactions in terms of interneuronal communication (*i.e.*, excitation, inhibition, or the more complex forms of synaptic interaction).

An understanding at the systems level is required to assemble the descriptive structural and functional properties of specific central transmitter systems, linking the neurons that make and release a given neurotransmitter to its behavioral effects. While many such transmitter-to-behavior linkages have been postulated, it has proven difficult to validate the essential involvement of specific transmitter-defined neurons in mediating specific mammalian behavior.

Research at the behavioral level often can illuminate the integrative phenomena that link populations of neurons (often through operationally or empirically defined ways) into extended specialized circuits, ensembles, or "systems" that integrate the physiological expression of a learned, reflexive, or spontaneously generated behavioral response. The entire concept of "animal models" of human psychiatric diseases rests on the assumption that scientists can appropriately infer from observations of behavior and physiology (heart rate, respiration, locomotion, etc.) that the states experienced by animals are equivalent to the emotional states experienced by human beings

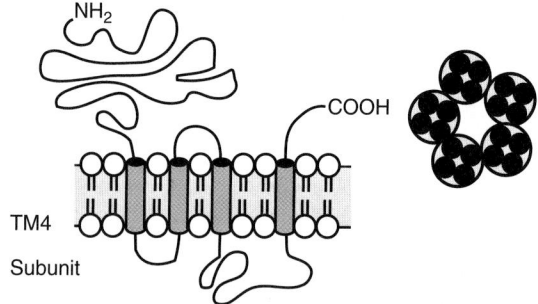

Figure 12–4. Ionophore receptors for neurotransmitters are composed of subunits with four transmembrane domains and are assembled as tetramers or pentamers (at right). The predicted motif shown likely describes nicotinic cholinergic receptors for ACh, GABA$_A$ receptors for gamma-aminobutyric acid, and receptors for glycine. Ionophore receptors for glutamate, however, probably are not accurately represented by this schematic motif.

Table 12–1

Overview of Transmitter Pharmacology in the Central Nervous System

TRANSMITTER	TRANSPORTER BLOCKER*	RECEPTOR SUBTYPE	AGONISTS	RECEPTOR-EFFECTOR COUPLING MOTIF (IR/GPCR)	SELECTIVE ANTAGONISTS
GABA	Guvacine, nipecotic acid	GABA$_A$ α, β, γ, δ, σ isoforms	Muscimol Isoguvacine THIP	IR: classical fast inhibitory transmission via Cl$^-$ channels	Bicuculline Picrotoxin SR 95531
	(β-Alanine for glia)	GABA$_B$	Baclofen 3-Aminopropyl-phosphinic acid	IR: pre- and post-synaptic effects	2-hydroxy-*s*-Saclofen CGP35348 CGP55845
		GABA$_C$		IR: slow, sustained responses via Cl$^-$ channels	
Glycine	? Sarcosine	α and β subunits	β-Alanine; taurine	IR: classical fast inhibitory transmission via Cl$^-$ channels (insensitive to bicuculline and picrotoxin)	Strychnine
Glutamate	—	AMPA	Quisqualate	IR: classical fast excitatory transmission via cation channels	NBQX
Aspartate	—	GLU 1-4	Kainate AMPA		CNQX GYK153665
		KA GLU 5-7; KA 1,2	Domoic acid Kainate		CNQX LY294486
		NMDA NMDA 1,2$_{A-D}$	NMDA GLU, ASP	IR: depolarization Mg^{2+}-gated slow excitatory transmission	MK801 AP5 Ketamine, PCP
		mGLU 1,5 (Group I mGluRs)	3,5-DHPG	GPCRs: modulatory; regulate ion channels, second messenger production, and protein phosphorylation *In vitro* coupling; Group I, G$_q$; Groups II and III, G$_i$	
		mGLU 2,3 (Group II mGluRs)	APDC LY354740		
		mGLU 4,6,7,8 (Group III mGluRs)	L-AP4		

(Continued)

Table 12-1
Overview of Transmitter Pharmacology in the Central Nervous System (Continued)

TRANSMITTER	TRANSPORTER BLOCKER*	RECEPTOR SUBTYPE	AGONISTS	RECEPTOR-EFFECTOR COUPLING MOTIF (IR/GPCR)	SELECTIVE ANTAGONISTS
Acetylcholine	—	Nicotinic		IR: classical fast excitatory transmission *via* cation channels	α-Bungarotoxin
		$\alpha 2$–4 and $\beta 2$–4 isoforms $\alpha 7$			Me-Lyaconitine
		Muscarinic M_{1-4}		GPCR: modulatory M_1, M_3; G_q, $\uparrow IP_3/Ca^{2+}$ M_2, M_4; G_i; $\downarrow cAMP$	M_1: Pirenzepine M_2: Methoctramine M_3: Hexahydrosiladifenidol M_4: Tropicamide
Dopamine	Cocaine; mazindol; GBR12-395; nomifensine	D_{1-5}	D_1: SKF38393 D_2: Bromocriptine D_3: 7-OH-DPAT	GPCR: D_1 D_5; G_s coupled; $D_{2,3,4}$: G_i coupled	D_1: SCH23390 D_2: Sulpiride, domperidone
Norepinephrine	Desmethyl-imipramine; mazindol, cocaine	α_{1A-D} α_{2A-C}	α_{1A}: NE > EPI α_{2A}: Oxymetazoline	GCPR: $G_{q/11}$ coupled GCPR: $G_{i/o}$ coupled	WB4101 α_{2A-C}: Yohimbine α_{2B}, α_{2C}: Prazosin
		β_{1-3}	β_1: EPI = NE β_2: EPI >> NE β_3: NE > EPI	GPCR: G_s coupled GPCR: $G_s/G_{i/o}$ coupled	β_1: Atenolol β_2: Butoxamine β_3: BRL 37344
Serotonin	Clomipramine; sertraline; fluoxetine	$5-HT_{1A-F}$	$5-HT_{1A}$: 8-OH-DPAT $5-HT_{1B}$: CP93129 $5-HT_{1D}$: LY694247	GPCR: $G_{i/o}$ coupled	$5-HT_{1A}$: WAY101135 $5-HT_{1D}$ GR127935
		$5-HT_{2A-C}$	α-Me-5-HT, DOB	GPCR: $G_{q/11}$ coupled	LY53857; ritanserin; mesulergine; ketanserin
		$5-HT_3$	2-Me-5-HT; m-CPG	IR: classical fast excitatory transmission *via* cation channels	Tropisetron: ondansetron; granisetron
		$5-HT_{4-7}$	$5-HT_4$: BIMU8; RS67506; renzapride	GPCR: $5-HT_{4,6,7}$; G_s coupled $5-HT_5$; G_s coupled?	$5-HT_4$: GR113808; SB204070

Ligand	Receptor	Agonist	Signal Transduction	Antagonist
Histamine	H_1	2-Pyridylethylamine 2-Me-histamine	GPCR: $G_{q/11}$ coupled	Mepyramine
	H_2	Methylhistamine; dimaprit, impromadine	GPCR: G_s coupled	Ranitidine, famotidine, cimetidine
	H_3	H_3: R-α-Me-histamine	GPCR: $G_{i/o}$? Autoreceptor function: inhibits transmitter release	H_3: Thioperamide
	H_4	Imetit, clobenpropit	GPCR: G_q, G_i?	JNJ777120
Vasopressin	$V_{1A,B}$	—	GPCR: $G_{q/11}$ coupled; modulatory; regulates ion channels, second messenger production, and protein phosphorylation	V_{1A}: SR 49059
	V_2	DDAVP	GPCR: G_s coupled	$d(CH_2)_5$ [dIle^{2}Ile^4]AVP
Oxytocin		[Thr^4,Gly^7]OT	GPCR: $G_{q/11}$ coupled	$d(CH_2)_5$ [Tyr(Me)^2, Thr^4, Orn^8]OT$_{1-8}$
Tachykinins	NK_1 (SP > NKA > NKB)	Substance P Me ester	GPCR: $G_{q/11}$ coupled; modulatory; regulates ion channels, second messenger production, and protein phosphorylation	SR140333 LY303870 CP99994 GR94800 GR159897 SR142802 SR223412 [Pro^7]NKB
	NK_2 (NKA > NKB > SP)	β-[Ala^8]NKA$_{4-10}$		
	NK_3 (NKB > NKA > SP)	GR138676		
CCK	CCK_A	CCK8 >> gastrin 5 = CCK4	GPCR: $G_{q/11}$ and G_s coupled	Devazepide; lorglumide
	CCK_B	CCK8 > gastrin 5 = CCK4	GPCR: $G_{q/11}$ coupled	CI988; L365260; YM022
NPY	Y_1 Y_2 Y_{4-6}	[Pro^{34}]NPY NPY$_{13-36}$; NPY$_{18-36}$ NPY$_{13-36}$; NPY$_{18-36}$	GPCR: $G_{i/o}$ coupled	—

(Continued)

Table 12–1
Overview of Transmitter Pharmacology in the Central Nervous System (Continued)

TRANSMITTER	TRANSPORTER BLOCKER*	RECEPTOR SUBTYPE	RECEPTOR-EFFECTOR COUPLING MOTIF (IR/GPCR)	AGONISTS	SELECTIVE ANTAGONISTS
Neurotensin	—	NTS1 NTS2	GPCR: $G_{q/11}$ coupled	—	SR48692
Opioid peptides	—	μ (β-endorphin)	GPCR: $G_{i/o}$ coupled	DAMGO, sufentanil; DALDA	CTAP; CTOP; β-FNA
		δ (Met^5-Enk)		DPDPE; DSBULET; SNC-80	Naltrindole; DALCE; ICI174864; SB205588
		κ (Dyn A)		U69593; CI977; ICI174864	Nor-binaltorphimine; 7-[3-(1-piperidinyl) propanamido] morphan
Somatostatin	—	sst$_{1A-C}$ sst$_{2A,B}$	GPCR: $G_{i/o}$ coupled	SRIF1A; seglitide Octreotide; seglitide, BIM23027	— Cyanamid 154806
		sst$_{3,4}$ sst$_5$		BIM23052, NNC269100 L362855	BIM23056
Purines	—	P1 (A$_{1,2a,2b,3}$)	A$_1$; GPCR: $G_{i/o}$ coupled	A$_1$: N6-cyclopentyladeno-sine	8-Cyclopentyltheophylline; DPCPX
			A$_{2a}$: GPCR: G_s coupled	A$_{2a}$: CGS21680; APEC; HENECA	CO66713; SCH58261; ZM241385
		P2X	IR: transductive effects not yet determined	α,β-methylene ATP	Suramin (nonselective)
		P2Y	GPCR: $G_{i/o}$ and $G_{q/11}$ coupled	ADP βF	Suramin

*In some instances (*e.g.*, acetylcholine, purines), agents that inhibit metabolism of the transmitter(s) have effects that are analogous to those of inhibitors of transport of other transmitters. Receptor-effector coupling consists of ion channel mechanisms for ionotropic receptors (IR) or coupling to G proteins for GPCRs. All GPCRs modulate neuronal activity by affecting second messenger production, protein phosphorylation, and ion channel function by mechanisms described in Chapter 1. In general, G_s couples to adenylyl cyclase to activate cyclic AMP production, while coupling to G_i inhibits adenylyl cyclase; coupling to G_q activates the PLC-IP$_3$-Ca^{2+} pathway; $\beta\gamma$ subunits of G proteins may modulate ion channels directly. ABBREVIATIONS: 7-OH-DPAT, 7-hydroxy-2 (di-n-propyl-amino) tetralin; 5-HT, 5-hydroxytryptamine (serotonin); L-AP4, L-amino-4-phosphonobutyrate; APDC, 1S, 4R-4-aminopyrrolidine2-4-dicarboxylate; AVP, arginine vasopressin; CCK, cholecystokinin; CTAP, DPhe-Cys-Tyr-DTrp-Arg-Thr-Pen-Thr-NH$_2$; CTOP, DPhe-Cys-Tyr-DTrp-Orn-Thr-Pen-Thr-NH$_2$; DALCE, [DAla^2, Leu^5, Cys^6]enkephalin; DAMGO, [D-Ala^2,N-Me-Phe^4,Gly^5-ol]-enkephalin; DDAVP, 1-desamino-8-D-arginine vasopressin; DHPG, dihydroxyphenylglycine; DPDPE, [d-Pen^2, d-Pen^5] enkephalin; DSBULET, Tyr-d-Ser-o-butyl-Gly-Phe-Leu-Thr; EPI, epinephrine; NE, norepinephrine; NK, neurokinin; NPY, neuropeptide Y; OT, oxytocin; PCP, phencyclidine; SP, substance P; SRIF, somatotropin release-inhibiting factor; THIP, 4,5,6,7-tetrahydroisoxazolo [5,4-c]-pyridone; VP, vasopressin. All other abbreviations represent experimental drugs coded by their manufacturers.

326

expressing similar physiological changes (Cowan *et al.*, 2000 and 2002; *see* Chapter 17).

Identification of Central Transmitters

An essential step in understanding the functional properties of neurotransmitters within the context of the circuitry of the brain is to identify which substances are the transmitters for specific interneuronal connections. The criteria for the rigorous identification of central transmitters require the same data used to establish the transmitters of the autonomic nervous system (*see* Chapter 6).

1. *The transmitter must be shown to be present in the presynaptic terminals of the synapse and in the neurons from which those presynaptic terminals arise.* Extensions of this criterion involve the demonstration that the presynaptic neuron synthesizes the transmitter substance, rather than simply storing it after accumulation from a nonneural source. Microscopic cytochemistry with antibodies or *in situ* hybridization, subcellular fractionation, and biochemical analysis of brain tissue are particularly suited to satisfy this criterion. These techniques often are combined in experimental animals with the production of surgical or chemical lesions of presynaptic neurons or their tracts to demonstrate that the lesion eliminates the proposed transmitter from the target region. Detection of the mRNA for specific neurotransmitter receptors within postsynaptic neurons using molecular biological methods can identify candidate postsynaptic cells.

2. *The transmitter must be released from the presynaptic nerve concomitantly with presynaptic nerve activity.* This criterion is best satisfied by electrical stimulation of the nerve pathway *in vivo* and collection of the transmitter in an enriched extracellular fluid within the synaptic target area. Demonstrating release of a transmitter formerly required sampling for prolonged intervals, but modern approaches employ minute microdialysis tubing or microvoltametric electrodes capable of sensitive detection of amine and amino acid transmitters within spatially and temporally meaningful dimensions (Bourne and Nicoll, 1993). Release of transmitter also can be studied *in vitro* by ionic or electrical activation of thin brain slices or subcellular fractions that are enriched in nerve terminals. The release of all transmitter substances so far studied, including presumptive transmitter release from dendrites, is voltage-dependent and requires the influx of Ca^{2+} into the presynaptic terminal. However, transmitter release is relatively insensitive to extracellular Na^+ or to tetrodotoxin, which blocks transmembrane movement of Na^+.

3. *When applied experimentally to the target cells, the effects of the putative transmitter must be identical to the effects of stimulating the presynaptic pathway.* This criterion can be met loosely by qualitative comparisons (*e.g.*, both the substance and the pathway inhibit or excite the target cell). More convincing is the demonstration that the ionic conductances activated by the pathway are the same as those activated by the candidate transmitter. Alternatively, the criterion can be satisfied less rigorously by demonstration of the pharmacological identity of receptors (order of potency of agonists and antagonists). In general, pharmacological antagonism of the actions of the pathway and those of the candidate transmitter should be achieved by similar concentrations of antagonist. To be convincing, the antagonistic drug should not affect responses of the target neurons to other unrelated pathways or to chemically distinct transmitter candidates. Actions that are qualitatively identical to those that follow stimulation of the pathway also should be observed with synthetic agonists that mimic the actions of the transmitter.

Other studies, especially those implicating peptides as neurotransmitters, suggest that many brain and spinal-cord synapses contain more than one transmitter substance (Hökfelt *et al.*, 2003). Substances that coexist in a given synapse are presumed to be released together, but in a frequency-dependent fashion, with higher-frequency bursts mediating peptide release. Coexisting substances may either act jointly on the postsynaptic membrane, or affect release of transmitter from the presynaptic terminal. Clearly, if more than one substance transmits information, no single agonist or antagonist would faithfully mimic or fully antagonize activation of a given presynaptic element. Costorage and corelease of ATP and norepinephrine are an example (Burnstock, 1995).

CNS Transmitter Discovery Strategies

The earliest transmitters considered for central roles were acetylcholine and norepinephrine, largely because of their established roles in the somatic motor and autonomic nervous systems. In the 1960s, serotonin, epinephrine, and dopamine also were investigated as potential CNS transmitters; although histochemical, biochemical, and pharmacological data yielded results consistent with their roles as neurotransmitters, not all criteria were satisfied. In the early 1970s, the availability of selective and potent antagonists of gamma-aminobutyric acid (GABA), glycine, and glutamate, all known to be enriched in brain, led to their general acceptance as transmitter substances. Also at this time, a search for hypothalamic-hypophyseal factors led to an improvement in the technology to isolate, purify, sequence, and synthetically replicate a growing family of neuropeptides (Hökfelt *et al.*, 2003). This advance, coupled with the widespread application of immunohistochemistry, strongly supported the view that neuropeptides act as transmitters. Adaptation of bioassay technology from studies of pituitary secretions to other effectors (such as smooth-muscle contractility), and later, competitive binding assays with radioactive ligands, gave rise to the discovery of endogenous peptide ligands for drugs acting at opiate receptors (*see* Chapter 21). The search for endogenous factors whose receptors constituted the drug binding sites later was extended to the benzodiazepine receptors and to a series of endogenous lipid amides as the natural ligands for the cannabinoid receptors, termed the endocannabinoids (Piomelli, 2003).

Assessment of Receptor Properties. Until the 1990s, central synaptic receptors were characterized either by examination of their capacity to bind radiolabeled agonists or antagonists (and on the ability of other unlabeled compounds to compete for such binding sites) or by electrophysiological or biochemical consequences of receptor activation of neurons *in vivo* or *in vitro*. Radioligand-binding assays can quantify binding sites within a region, track their appearance throughout the phylogenetic scale and during brain development, and evaluate how physiologic or pharmacologic manipulation regulates receptor number or affinity (Nestler *et al.*, 2001; Cooper *et al.*, 2003).

The properties of the cellular response to the transmitter can be studied electrophysiologically by the use of microiontophoresis (involving recording from single cells and highly localized drug administration). The patch-clamp technique can be used to study the electrical properties of single ion channels and their regulation by neurotransmitters. These direct electrophysiological tests of neuronal responsiveness can provide qualitative and quantitative information on the receptor-specific effects of a putative transmitter substance (*see* Neubig *et al.*, 2003, for a comprehensive receptor database). Receptor properties also can be studied biochemically when the activated receptor is coupled to an enzymatic reaction, such as the synthesis of a second messenger and its biochemical sequelae.

Molecular biological techniques have led to the identification of mRNAs (or cDNAs) for the receptors for virtually every natural ligand considered as a neurotransmitter. A common practice is to introduce these coding sequences into test cells (frog oocytes or mammalian cells) and to assess the relative effects of ligands on second-messenger production in such cells. Molecular cloning studies have revealed two major motifs (Figures 12–4 and 12–5) and one minor motif of transmitter receptors. Oligomeric ion channel receptors composed of multiple subunits usually have four transmembrane domains (Figure 12–4). The ion channel receptors (ionotropic receptors, or IRs) for neurotransmitters contain sites for reversible phosphorylation by protein kinases and phosphoprotein phosphatases and for voltage-gating. Receptors with this structure include nicotinic cholinergic receptors; the receptors for the amino acids GABA, glycine, glutamate, and aspartate; and the 5-HT$_3$ receptor.

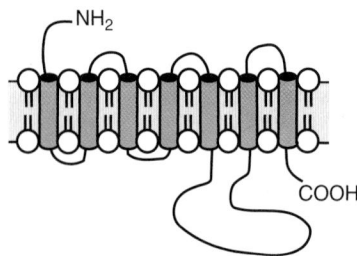

Figure 12–5. *G protein–coupled receptors are composed of a single subunit, with seven transmembrane domains.* For small neurotransmitters, the binding pocket is buried within the bilayer; sequences in the second cytoplasmic loop and projecting out of the bilayer at the base of transmembrane spans 5 and 6 have been implicated in agonist-facilitated G protein coupling (*see* Chapter 1).

The second major motif comprises the G protein–coupled receptors (GPCRs), a large family of heptahelical receptors with varying cytoplasmic loop lengths connecting the transmembrane domains (Figure 12–5). Multiple mutagenesis strategies have defined how the activated receptors (themselves subject to reversible phosphorylation at one or more functionally distinct sites) can interact with the heterotrimeric GTP-binding protein complex. Such protein-protein interactions can activate, inhibit, or otherwise regulate effector systems such as adenylate cyclase or phospholipase C, and ion channels, such as voltage-gated Ca^{2+} channels or receptor-operated K^+ channels (*see* Chapter 1). GPCRs are employed by muscarinic cholinergic receptors, one subtype each of GABA and glutamate receptors, and all other aminergic and peptidergic receptors. Transfecting cells lacking GPCRs with mRNAs for GPCRs with no known ligands has led to the identification of novel neuropeptide ligands for these "orphan" receptors (Robas *et al.*, 2003). A third receptor motif is that of a growth factor receptor (GFR), a monospanning membrane protein that has an extracellular binding domain that regulates an intracellular catalytic activity, such as the atrial natriuretic peptide–binding domain that regulates the activity of the membrane-bound guanylyl cyclase (*see* Figure 1–7). Dimerization of GPCRs and GFRs apparently contributes to their activities, as does localization within or outside of caveolae in the membrane (Milligan, 2004) (*see* Chapter 1).

An additional ligand-binding motif expressed within the CNS involves the transporters that conserve transmitters after secretion by an ion-dependent reuptake process (Figure 12–2). These neurotransmitter transporters share a molecular motif with 12 transmembrane domains, similar to glucose transporters and adenylyl cyclase (*see* Chapter 2) (Nestler *et al.*, 2001).

Postsynaptic receptivity of CNS neurons is regulated continuously in terms of the number of receptor sites and the threshold required to generate a response. Receptor number often depends on the concentration of agonist to which the target cell is exposed. Thus, chronic excess of agonist can lead to a reduced number of receptors (desensitization or down-regulation) and consequently to subsensitivity or tolerance to the transmitter. For many GPCRs, short-term down-regulation is achieved by the actions of G protein–linked receptor kinases (GRKs) and internalization of the receptors (*see* Chapter 1). Conversely, deficit of agonist or prolonged pharmacologic blockade of receptors can lead to increased numbers of receptors and supersensitivity of the system. These adaptive processes become especially important when drugs are used to treat chronic illness of the CNS. After prolonged exposure to drug, the actual mechanisms underlying the therapeutic effect may differ strikingly from those that operate when the agent is first introduced. Similar adaptive modifications of neuronal systems also can occur at presynaptic sites, such as those concerned with transmitter synthesis, storage, and release (Murthy and Camilli, 2003).

NEUROTRANSMITTERS, HORMONES, AND MODULATORS: CONTRASTING PRINCIPLES OF NEURONAL REGULATION

Neurotransmitters. Given a definite effect of a neuron on a target cell, a substance found in or secreted by the neuron and producing the effect operationally would be the transmitter from the neuron to the target cell. In some cases, transmitters may produce minimal effects on bioelectric properties, yet activate or inactivate biochemical mechanisms necessary for responses to other circuits. Alternatively, the action of a transmitter may vary with the context of ongoing synaptic events—enhancing excitation or inhibition, rather than operating to impose direct excitation or inhibition (Cooper *et al.*, 2003). Each chemical substance that fits within the broad definition of a transmitter may therefore require operational definition within the spatial and temporal domains in which a specific cell-cell circuit is defined. Those same properties may or may not be generalized to other cells that are contacted by the same presynaptic neurons, with the differences in operation related to differences in postsynaptic receptors and the mechanisms by which the activated receptor produces its effect.

Classically, electrophysiological signs of the action of a *bona fide* transmitter fall into two major categories: (1) *excitation*, in which ion channels are opened to permit net influx of positively charged ions, leading to depolarization with a reduction in the electrical resistance of the membrane; and (2) *inhibition*, in which selective ion movements lead to hyperpolarization, also with decreased membrane resistance. There also may be many "nonclassical" transmitter mechanisms operating in the CNS. In some cases, either depolarization or hyperpolarization is accompanied by a *decreased* ionic conductance (increased membrane resistance) as actions of the transmitter lead to the closure of ion channels (so-called leak channels) that normally are open in some resting neurons (Shepherd, 2003). For transmitters such as monoamines and certain peptides, a "conditional" action may be involved, *i.e.*, a transmitter substance may enhance or suppress the response of the target neuron to classical excitatory or inhibitory transmitters while producing little or no change in membrane potential or ionic conductance when applied alone. Such conditional responses are termed *modulatory*, and specific categories of modulation have been hypothesized (Burnstock, 1995; Aston-Jones *et al.*, 2001). Regardless of the mechanisms that underlie such synaptic operations, their temporal and biophysical characteristics differ substantially from the rapid onset-offset effects previously thought to describe all synaptic events. These differences have thus raised the issue of whether substances that produce slow synaptic effects should be described as neurotransmitters. Some of the alternative terms and the relevant molecules are described below.

Neurohormones. Peptide-secreting cells of the hypothalamicohypophyseal circuits originally were described as neurosecretory cells, receiving synaptic information from other central neurons, yet secreting transmitters in a hormone-like fashion into the circulation. The transmitter released from such neurons was termed a *neurohormone*, *i.e.,* a substance secreted into the blood by a neuron. This term has lost much of its original meaning, because these hypothalamic neurons also may form traditional synapses with central neurons. Cytochemical evidence indicates that the same substances that are secreted as hormones from the posterior pituitary (oxytocin, arginine-vasopressin; *see* Chapters 29 and 55), mediate transmission at these sites. Thus the designation *hormone* relates to the site of release at the posterior pituitary and does not necessarily describe all the actions of the peptide.

Neuromodulators. The distinctive feature of a modulator is that it originates from nonsynaptic sites, yet influences the excitability of nerve cells. Florey (1967) specifically designated substances such as CO_2 and ammonia, arising from active neurons or glia, as potential modulators through nonsynaptic actions. Similarly, circulating steroid hormones, steroids produced in the nervous system (*i.e.*, neurosteroids), locally released adenosine, and other purines, eicosanoids, and nitric oxide (NO) are all now regarded as modulators (*see* below).

Neuromediators. Substances that participate in eliciting the postsynaptic response to a transmitter fall under this heading. The clearest examples of such effects are provided by the involvement of cyclic AMP, cyclic GMP, and inositol phosphates as second messengers at specific sites of synaptic transmission (*see* Chapters 1, 6, 7, 10, and 11). However, it is technically difficult to demonstrate in brain that a change in the concentration of cyclic nucleotides occurs prior to the generation of the synaptic potential and that this change in concentration is both necessary and sufficient for its generation. It is possible that changes in the concentration of second messengers can occur and enhance the generation of synaptic potentials. Second messenger–dependent protein phosphorylation can initiate a complex cascade of molecular events that regulate the properties of membrane and cytoplasmic proteins central to neuronal excitability (Greengard, 2001). These possibilities are particularly pertinent to the action of drugs that augment or reduce transmitter effects (*see* below).

Neurotrophic Factors. Neurotrophic factors are substances produced within the CNS by neurons, astrocytes, microglia, or transiently invading peripheral inflammatory or immune cells that assist neurons in their attempts to repair damage. Seven categories of neurotrophic peptides are recognized: (1) the classic neurotrophins (nerve growth factor, brain-derived neurotrophic factor, and the related neurotrophins); (2) the neuropoietic factors, which have effects both in brain and in myeloid cells (*e.g.*, cholinergic differentiation factor [also called leukemia inhibitory factor], ciliary neurotrophic factor, and some interleukins); (3) growth factor peptides, such as epidermal growth factor, transforming growth factors α and β, glial cell–derived neurotrophic factor, and activin A; (4) the fibroblast growth factors; (5) insulin-like growth factors; (6) platelet-derived growth factors; and (7) axon guidance molecules, some of which are also capable of affecting cells of the immune system. Drugs designed to elicit the formation and secretion of these products or to emulate their actions may ultimately provide useful adjuncts to rehabilitative treatments (Huang and Reichardt, 2001).

CENTRAL NEUROTRANSMITTERS

The view that synapses are drug-modifiable control points within neuronal networks requires explicit delineation of the sites at which given neurotransmitters may operate and the degree of specificity with which such sites may be affected. One principle that underlies the following summaries of individual transmitter substances is the chemical-specificity hypothesis of Dale: A given neuron releases the same transmitter substance at each of its synaptic terminals. Because of the growing indications that some neurons contain more than one transmitter substance (Hökfelt *et al.*, 2000), Dale's hypothesis has been modified to indicate that a given neuron secretes the same set of transmitters from all its terminals. Even this theory may require revision. For example, it is not clear whether a neuron that secretes a given peptide will process the precursor peptide to the same end product at all of its synaptic terminals. Table 12–1 summarizes the pharmacological properties of the transmitters in the CNS that have been studied extensively. Neurotransmitters are discussed below as groups of substances within given chemical categories: amino acids, amines, and neuropeptides. Other substances that may participate in central synaptic transmission include purines (such as adenosine and ATP), nitric oxide (Boehning and Snyder, 2003), and arachidonic acid derivatives (Piomelli, 2003).

Amino Acids. The CNS contains uniquely high concentrations of certain amino acids, notably glutamate and gamma-aminobutyric acid (GABA) (Figure 12–6). Although these amino acids potently alter neuronal discharge, physiologists initially were reluctant to accept them as central neurotransmitters. Their ubiquitous distribution within the brain and the consistent observation that they produced prompt, powerful, and readily reversible but redundant effects on every neuron tested seemed out of keeping with the extreme heterogeneity of distribution and responsivity seen for other putative transmitters. The dicarboxylic amino acids (*e.g.*, glutamate and aspartate) produced near universal excitation, while the monocarboxylic ω-amino acids (*e.g.*, GABA, glycine, β-alanine, and taurine) produced qualitatively similar, consistent inhibitions. Following the emergence of selective antagonists to the amino acids, identification of selective receptors and receptor subtypes became possible. These data, together with the development of methods for mapping the ligands and their receptors, led to widespread acceptance that the amino acids GABA, glycine, and glutamate are central transmitters. The structures of glycine, glutamate, GABA, and some related compounds are shown in Figure 12–6.

GABA. GABA, the major inhibitory neurotransmitter in the mammalian CNS, was identified as a unique chemical constituent of brain in 1950, but its potency as a CNS depressant was not immediately recognized. GABA initially was identified as the only inhibitory amino acid found exclusively in nerves that inhibit the crustacean

stretch receptor; moreover, the GABA content accounted for the inhibitory potency of extracts from these nerves. Finally, GABA release correlated with the frequency of nerve stimulation and identical increases in muscle Cl^- conductance accompanied GABA application and stimulation of the inhibitory nerve (for further historical references, *see* the ninth edition of this book).

These same physiological and pharmacological properties helped to establish a role for GABA in the mammalian CNS. Substantial data support the idea that GABA mediates the inhibitory actions of local interneurons in the brain and may also mediate presynaptic inhibition within the spinal cord. Presumptive GABA-containing inhibitory synapses have been demonstrated most clearly between cerebellar Purkinje neurons and their targets in Deiter's nucleus; between small interneurons and the major output cells of the cerebellar cortex, olfactory bulb, cuneate nucleus, hippocampus, and lateral septal nucleus; and between the vestibular nucleus and the trochlear motoneurons. GABA also mediates inhibition within the cerebral cortex and between the caudate nucleus and the substantia nigra. GABA-containing neurons and nerve terminals have been localized with immunocytochemical methods that visualize glutamic acid decarboxylase, the enzyme that catalyzes the synthesis of GABA from glutamic acid, or by *in situ* hybridization of the mRNA for this protein. GABA-containing neurons frequently coexpress one or more neuropeptides (*see* below). The most useful compounds for confirmation of GABA-mediated effects have been bicuculline and picrotoxin (Figure 12–6); however, many convulsants whose actions previously were unexplained (including penicillin and pentylenetetrazol) also may act as relatively selective antagonists of the action of GABA. Useful therapeutic effects have not yet been obtained through the use of agents that mimic GABA (such as muscimol), inhibit its active reuptake (such as 2,4-diaminobutyrate, nipecotic acid, and guvacine), or alter its turnover (such as aminooxyacetic acid).

GABA receptors have been divided into three main types: A, B, and C. The most prominent GABA-receptor subtype, the $GABA_A$ receptor, is a ligand-gated Cl^- ion channel, an "ionotropic receptor" that is opened after release of GABA from presynaptic neurons. The $GABA_B$ receptor is a GPCR. The $GABA_C$ receptor is a transmitter-gated Cl^- channel. The $GABA_A$ receptor subunit proteins have been well characterized due to their abundance. The receptor also has been extensively characterized as the site of action of many neuroactive drugs (*see* Chapters 16 and 22), notably benzodiazepines, barbiturates, ethanol, anesthetic steroids, and volatile anesthetics. Based on sequence homology to the first reported $GABA_A$ subunit cDNAs, more than 15 other subunits have been cloned and appear to be expressed in multiple multimeric, pharmacologically distinctive combinations. In addition to these subunits, which are products of separate genes, splice variants for several subunits have been described. The $GABA_A$ receptor, by analogy with the nicotinic cholinergic receptor, may be either a pentameric or tetrameric protein in which the subunits assemble together around a central ion pore typical for all ionotropic receptors (*see* below). The major form of the $GABA_A$ receptor contains at least three different subunits—α, β, and γ—but their stoichiometry is not known (Whiting, 2003). All three subunits are required to interact with benzodiazepines with the profile expected of the native $GABA_A$ receptor, and inclusion of variant α, β, or γ subunits alters the pharmacological profiles. The $GABA_B$ or metabotropic GABA receptor interacts with G_i to inhibit adenylyl cyclase, activate K^+ channels, and reduce Ca^{2+} conductance. Presynaptic $GABA_B$ receptors function as autoreceptors, inhibiting GABA release, and may play the same role on neurons releasing other transmitters. There are two subtypes of $GABA_B$ receptors, 1a and 1b. The $GABA_C$ recep-

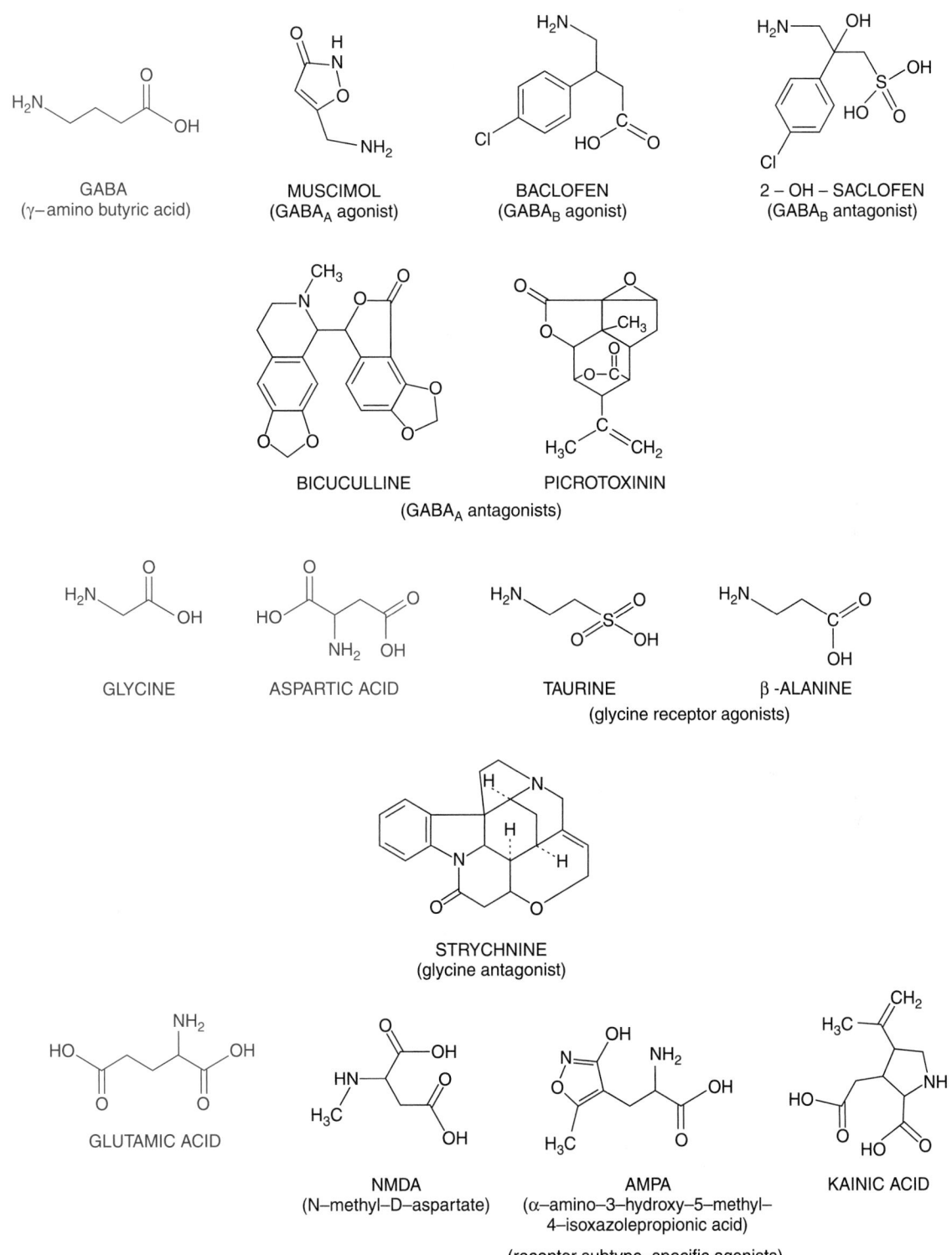

Figure 12–6. *Amino acid transmitters and congeners.*

tor is less widely distributed than the A and B subtypes and is pharmacologically distinct: GABA is more potent by an order of magnitude at $GABA_C$ than at $GABA_A$ receptors, and a number of $GABA_A$ agonists (*e.g.*, baclofen) and modulators (*e.g.*, benzodiazepines and barbiturates) seem not to interact with $GABA_C$ receptors. $GABA_C$ receptors are found in the retina, spinal cord, superior colliculus, and pituitary (Johnston, 2002; Johnston *et al.*, 2003).

Glycine. Many of the features described for the $GABA_A$ receptor family also apply to the inhibitory glycine receptor that is prominent in the brainstem and spinal cord. Multiple subunits assemble into a variety of glycine receptor subtypes (*see* ninth edition of this volume for earlier references). These pharmacological subtypes are detected in brain tissue with particular neuroanatomical and neurodevelopmental profiles. However, as with the $GABA_A$ receptor, the complete functional significance of the glycine receptor subtypes is not known. There is evidence for clustering of glycine receptors by the anchoring protein gephyrin (Sola *et al.*, 2004).

Glutamate and Aspartate. Glutamate and aspartate are found in very high concentrations in brain, and both amino acids have powerful excitatory effects on neurons in virtually every region of the CNS. Their widespread distribution initially obscured their roles as transmitters, but there now is broad acceptance that glutamate and possibly aspartate are the principal fast ("classical") excitatory transmitters throughout the CNS (Bleich *et al.*, 2003; Conn, 2003). Over the past decade, multiple subtypes of receptors for excitatory amino acids have been cloned, expressed, and characterized pharmacologically, based on the relative potencies of synthetic agonists and the discovery of potent and selective antagonists (Kotecha and MacDonald, 2003).

Glutamate receptors are classed functionally either as ligand-gated ion channel ("ionotropic") receptors or as "metabotropic" (G protein–coupled) receptors. Neither the precise number of subunits that assembles to generate a functional glutamate ionotropic receptor ion channel *in vivo* nor the intramembranous topography of each subunit has been established unequivocally. The ligand-gated ion channels are further classified according to the identity of agonists that selectively activate each receptor subtype, and are broadly divided into *N*-methyl-D-aspartate (NMDA) receptors and "non-NMDA" receptors. The non-NMDA receptors include the α-amino-3-hydroxy-5-methyl-4-isoxazole propionic acid (AMPA), and kainic acid (KA) receptors (Figure 12–6). Selective antagonists for these receptors now are available (Herrling, 1997). In the case of NMDA receptors, agonists include open-channel blockers such as phencyclidine (PCP or "angel dust"), antagonists such as 5,7-dichlorokynurenic acid, which act at an allosteric glycine-binding site, and the novel antagonist ifenprodil, which may act as a closed-channel blocker. In addition, the activity of NMDA receptors is sensitive to pH and also can be modulated by a variety of endogenous modulators including Zn^{2+}, some neurosteroids, arachidonic acid, redox reagents, and polyamines such as spermine. Additional diversity of glutamate receptors arises by alternative splicing or by single-base editing of mRNAs encoding the receptors or receptor subunits. Alternative splicing has been described for metabotropic receptors and for subunits of NMDA, AMPA, and kainate receptors. For some subunits of AMPA and kainate receptors, the RNA sequence differs from the genomic sequence in a single codon of the receptor subunit and determines the Ca^{2+} permeability of the receptor channel (Seeburg *et al.*, 2001; Schmauss and Howe, 2002). AMPA and kainate receptors mediate fast depolarization at most glutamatergic synapses in the brain and spinal cord. NMDA receptors also are involved in normal synaptic transmission, but activation of NMDA receptors is associated more closely with the induction of various forms of synaptic plasticity rather than with fast point-to-point signaling in the brain. AMPA or kainate receptors and

NMDA receptors may be co-localized at many glutamatergic synapses. A well-characterized phenomenon involving NMDA receptors is the induction of long-term potentiation (LTP). LTP refers to a prolonged (hours to days) increase in the size of a postsynaptic response to a presynaptic stimulus of given strength. Activation of NMDA receptors is obligatory for the induction of one type of LTP that occurs in the hippocampus. NMDA receptors normally are blocked by Mg^{2+} at resting membrane potentials. Thus, activation of NMDA receptors requires not only binding of synaptically released glutamate, but simultaneous depolarization of the postsynaptic membrane. This is achieved by activation of AMPA/kainate receptors at nearby synapses by inputs from different neurons. AMPA receptors also are dynamically regulated to affect their sensitivity to the synergism with NMDA. Thus, NMDA receptors may function as coincidence detectors, being activated only when there is simultaneous firing of two or more neurons. Interestingly, NMDA receptors also can induce long-term depression (LTD; the converse of LTP) at CNS synapses. Apparently the frequency and pattern of synaptic stimulation dictates whether a synapse undergoes LTP or LTD (Nestler *et al.*, 2001; Cooper *et al.*, 2003).

Glutamate Excitotoxicity. High concentrations of glutamate produce neuronal cell death by mechanisms that have only recently begun to be clarified. Initially, the cascade of events leading to neuronal death was thought to be triggered exclusively by excessive activation of NMDA or AMPA/kainate receptors, allowing significant influx of Ca^{2+} into the neurons. Such glutamate neurotoxicity was thought to underlie the damage that occurs after ischemia or hypoglycemia in the brain, during which a massive release and impaired reuptake of glutamate in the synapse would lead to excess stimulation of glutamate receptors and subsequent cell death. Although NMDA receptor antagonists can attenuate neuronal cell death induced by activation of these receptors (Herrling, 1997), even the most potent antagonists cannot prevent all such damage, causing additional efforts to salvage the therapeutic potential for glutamate antagonists as neuroprotectants. More recent studies (Gillessen *et al.*, 2002; Frandsen and Schousboe, 2003) implicate both local depletion of Na^+ and K^+, as well as small but significant elevations of extracellular Zn^{2+} as factors that can activate both necrotic and pro-apoptotic cascades, leading to neuronal death.

Because of the widespread distribution of glutamate receptors in the CNS, they have become targets for diverse therapeutic interventions. For example, a role for disordered glutamatergic transmission in the etiology of chronic neurodegenerative diseases and in schizophrenia has been postulated (*see* Chapters 18 and 20).

Acetylcholine. After acetylcholine (ACh) was identified as the transmitter at neuromuscular and parasympathetic neuroeffector junctions, and at the major synapse of autonomic ganglia (*see* Chapter 6), the amine began to receive considerable attention as a potential central neurotransmitter. Based on its irregular distribution within the CNS and the observation that peripheral cholinergic drugs could produce marked behavioral effects after central administration, many investigators addressed the possibility that ACh also might be a central neurotransmitter. In the late 1950s, Eccles and colleagues satisfied the experimental criteria to identify ACh as a neurotransmitter for the excitation of spinal cord Renshaw interneurons by the recurrent axon collaterals of spinal motoneurons. Subsequently, the capacity of ACh to elicit neuronal discharge has been replicated on scores of CNS cells (*see* Shepherd, 2003, for more recent references).

In most regions of the CNS, the effects of ACh, assessed either by iontophoresis or by radioligand binding assays, appear to be generated by interaction with a mixture of nicotinic and muscarinic receptors. Several presumptive cholinergic pathways have been proposed in addition to that of the motoneuron-Renshaw cell. By a combination of immunocytochemistry of choline acetyltransferase (ChAT; the enzyme that synthesizes ACh) and ligand binding, or *in situ* hybridization studies for the detection of neurons expressing subunits of nicotinic and muscarinic receptors, eight major clusters of ACh neurons and their pathways have been characterized (Nestler *et al.*, 2001; Cooper *et al.*, 2003; Shepherd, 2003).

Catecholamines. The brain contains separate neuronal systems that utilize three different catecholamines—dopamine, norepinephrine, and epinephrine. Each system is anatomically distinct and serves separate, but similar, functional roles within its field of innervation (*see* Nestler *et al.*, 2001; Cooper *et al.*, 2003; Shepherd, 2003, for additional details).

Dopamine. Although dopamine (DA) originally was regarded only as a precursor of norepinephrine, assays of distinct regions of the CNS revealed that the distributions of dopamine and norepinephrine are markedly different. In fact, more than half the CNS content of catecholamine is dopamine, and extremely large amounts are found in the basal ganglia (especially the caudate nucleus), the nucleus accumbens, the olfactory tubercle, the central nucleus of the amygdala, the median eminence, and restricted fields of the frontal cortex. Of these myriad connections, most attention has been directed to the long projections between the major dopamine-containing nuclei in the substantia nigra and ventral tegmentum and their targets in the striatum, in the limbic zones of the cerebral cortex, and in other major limbic regions (but in general not to the hippocampus). At the cellular level, the actions of dopamine depend on receptor subtype expression and the contingent convergent actions of other transmitters to the same target neurons.

Initial pharmacological studies discriminated between two subtypes of dopamine receptors: D_1 (which couples to G_S and adenylyl cyclase) and D_2 (which couples to G_i to inhibit adenylyl cyclase). Subsequent cloning studies identified three additional genes encoding subtypes of dopamine receptors: one resembling the D_1 receptor, D_5; and two resembling the D_2 receptor, D_3 and D_4, as well as two isoforms of the D_2 receptor that differ in the predicted length of their third intracellular loops, D_2 short (D_{2S}) and D_2 long (D_{2L}) (Nestler *et al.*, 2001; Cooper *et al.*, 2003). The D_1 and D_5 receptors activate adenylyl cyclase. The D_2 receptors couple to multiple effector systems, including the inhibition of adenylyl cyclase activity, suppression of Ca^{2+} currents, and activation of K^+ currents. The effector systems to which the D_3 and D_4 receptors couple have not been unequivocally defined (Greengard, 2001). Dopamine receptors have been implicated in the pathophysiology of schizophrenia and Parkinson's disease (*see* Chapters 18 and 20).

Norepinephrine. There are relatively large amounts of norepinephrine within the hypothalamus and in certain zones of the limbic system, such as the central nucleus of the amygdala and the dentate gyrus of the hippocampus. However, this catecholamine also is present in significant, although lower, amounts in most brain regions. Detailed mapping studies indicate that noradrenergic neurons of the locus ceruleus innervate specific target cells in a large

number of cortical, subcortical, and spinomedullary fields (Nestler *et al.*, 2001; Cooper *et al.*, 2003). Although norepinephrine has been firmly established as the transmitter at synapses between presumptive noradrenergic pathways and a wide variety of target neurons, a number of features of the mode of action of this biogenic amine have complicated the acquisition of convincing evidence. These problems largely reflect its "nonclassical" electrophysiological synaptic actions, which result in "state-dependent" or "enabling" effects. For example, stimulation of the locus ceruleus depresses the spontaneous activity of target neurons in the cerebellum; this is associated with a slowly developing hyperpolarization and a decrease in membrane conductance. However, activation of the locus ceruleus enhances the higher firing rates produced by stimulation of excitatory inputs to these neurons to a lesser degree, and excitatory postsynaptic potentials are enhanced. All consequences of activation of the locus ceruleus are mimicked by iontophoretic application of norepinephrine and are effectively blocked by α adrenergic antagonists. Although the mechanisms underlying these effects are obscure, there is convincing evidence for intracellular mediation by cyclic AMP (for additional references, *see* Aston-Jones *et al.*, 2001; Nestler *et al.*, 2001; Cooper *et al.*, 2003).

Three types of adrenergic receptors (α_1, α_2, and β) and their subtypes have been described in the CNS; all are GPCRs. As in the periphery, these central subtypes can be similarly distinguished in terms of their pharmacological properties and their distribution (*see* Chapter 10 for details). The β adrenergic receptors are coupled to stimulation of adenylyl cyclase activity. The α_1 adrenergic receptors are associated predominantly with neurons, while α_2 adrenergic receptors are more characteristic of glial and vascular elements. The α_1 receptors couple to G_q to stimulate phospholipase C. The α_1 receptors on noradrenergic target neurons of the neocortex and thalamus respond to norepinephrine with prazosin-sensitive, depolarizing responses due to decreases in K^+ conductances (both voltage-sensitive and voltage-insensitive). However, stimulation of α_1 receptors also can augment cyclic AMP accumulation in neocortical slices in response to vasoactive intestinal polypeptide, possibly an example of G_q-G_S cross-talk involving Ca^{2+}/calmodulin and/or PKC (Ostrom *et al.*, 2003). α_2 Adrenergic receptors are prominent on noradrenergic neurons, where they presumably couple to G_i, inhibit adenylyl cyclase, and mediate a hyperpolarizing response due to enhancement of an inwardly rectifying K^+ channel. In cortical projection fields, α_2 receptors may help restore functional declines of senescence. Until functional roles are better defined among these receptor subtypes, studies of knockout mice lacking these receptors may be revealing (MacMillan *et al.*, 1998).

Epinephrine. Neurons in the CNS that contain epinephrine were recognized only after the development of sensitive enzymatic assays and immunocytochemical staining techniques for phenylethanolamine-*N*-methyltransferase. Epinephrine-containing neurons are found in the medullary reticular formation and make restricted connections to a few pontine and diencephalic nuclei, eventually coursing as far rostrally as the paraventricular nucleus of the dorsal midline thalamus. Their physiological properties have not been identified.

5-Hydroxytryptamine. Following the chemical determination that a biogenic substance found both in serum ("serotonin") and in gut ("enteramine") was 5-hydroxytryptamine (5-HT), assays for this substance revealed its presence in brain (*see* Chapter 11). Subsequent studies of 5-HT have provided pivotal advances in our understanding of the neuropharmacology of the CNS. In mammals, 5-hydroxytryptaminergic neurons are found in nine nuclei lying in or adjacent to the midline (raphe) regions of the pons and upper brainstem.

In the mammalian CNS, cells receiving cytochemically demonstrable 5-HT input, such as the suprachiasmatic nucleus, ventrolateral geniculate body, amygdala, and hippocampus, exhibit a uniform and dense investment of reactive terminals.

Molecular biological approaches have led to identification of 14 distinct mammalian 5-HT receptor subtypes (*see* Chapter 11 for details). These subtypes exhibit characteristic ligand-binding profiles, couple to different intracellular signaling systems, exhibit subtype-specific distributions within the CNS, and mediate distinct behavioral effects of 5-HT. The 5-HT receptors fall into four broad classes: the $5-HT_1$ and $5-HT_2$ classes both are GPCRs and include multiple isoforms within each class; the $5-HT_3$ receptor is a ligand-gated ion channel with structural similarity to the α subunit of the nicotinic acetylcholine receptor. Similarly to some glutamate receptors, mRNA editing has also been observed for the $5-HT_{2C}$ subtype (Niswender *et al.*, 2001). Members of the $5-HT_4$, $5-HT_5$, $5-HT_6$, and $5-HT_7$ classes all are GPCRs, but have not yet been fully studied electrophysiologically or operationally in the CNS.

The $5-HT_1$ receptor subset is composed of at least five receptor subtypes ($5-HT_{1A}$, $5-HT_{1B}$, $5-HT_{1D}$, $5-HT_{1E}$, and $5-HT_{1F}$) that are linked to inhibition of adenylyl cyclase activity or to regulation of K^+ or Ca^{2+} channels. As an example of the potency and complexity of serotonergic neurotransmission, the $5-HT_{1A}$ receptors are abundantly expressed on 5-HT neurons of the dorsal raphe nucleus, where they are thought to be involved in temperature regulation. They also are found in regions of the CNS associated with mood and anxiety such as the hippocampus and amygdala. Activation of $5-HT_{1A}$ receptors opens an inwardly rectifying K^+ conductance, which leads to hyperpolarization and neuronal inhibition. These receptors can be activated by the drugs buspirone and ipsapirone, which are used to treat anxiety and panic disorders (*see* Chapter 17). In contrast, $5-HT_{1D}$ receptors are potently activated by the drug sumatriptan, which is currently prescribed for acute management of migraine headaches (*see* Chapters 11 and 21).

The $5-HT_2$ receptor class has three subtypes: $5-HT_{2A}$, $5-HT_{2B}$, and $5-HT_{2C}$; these receptors couple to pertussis toxin–insensitive G proteins (*e.g.*, G_q and G_{11}) and link to activation of phospholipase C. Based on ligand binding and mRNA *in situ* hybridization patterns, $5-HT_{2A}$ receptors are enriched in forebrain regions such as the neocortex and olfactory tubercle, as well as in several nuclei arising from the brainstem. The $5-HT_{2C}$ receptor, which is very similar in sequence and pharmacology to the $5-HT_{2A}$ receptor, is expressed abundantly in the choroid plexus, where it may modulate cerebrospinal fluid production (*see* Chapter 11).

The $5-HT_3$ receptors function as ligand-gated ion channels; these receptors were first recognized in the peripheral autonomic nervous system. Within the CNS, they are expressed in the area postrema and solitary tract nucleus, where they couple to potent depolarizing responses that show rapid desensitization to continued 5-HT exposure. Actions of 5-HT at central $5-HT_3$ receptors can lead to emesis and antinociceptive actions, and $5-HT_3$ antagonists are beneficial in the management of chemotherapy-induced emesis (*see* Chapter 37).

Within the CNS, $5-HT_4$ receptors occur on neurons within the inferior and superior colliculi and in the hippocampus. Activation of $5-HT_4$ receptors stimulates the G_s-adenylyl cyclase–cyclic AMP pathway. Other 5-HT receptors are less well studied in the CNS.

The $5-HT_6$ and $5-HT_7$ receptors also couple to G_s-adenylyl cyclase; their affinity for clozapine may relate to its antipsychotic efficacy (*see* Chapters 11 and 18). Of the two subtypes of $5-HT_5$ receptors, the $5-HT_{5A}$ receptor seems to inhibit cyclic AMP synthesis, while $5-HT_{5B}$ receptor-effector coupling has not been described.

The hallucinogen lysergic acid diethylamide (LSD) interacts with 5-HT, primarily through $5-HT_2$ receptors. When applied iontophoretically, LSD and 5-HT both potently inhibit the firing of raphe (5-HT) neurons, whereas LSD and other hallucinogens are far more potent excitants on facial motoneurons that receive innervation from the raphe. The inhibitory effect of LSD on raphe neurons offers a plausible explanation for its hallucinogenic effects, namely that these effects result from depression of activity in a system that tonically inhibits visual and other sensory inputs. However, typical LSD-induced behavior is still seen in animals with destroyed raphe nuclei or after blockade of the synthesis of 5-HT by *p*-chlorophenylalanine (Aghajanian and Marek, 1999).

Histamine. For many years, histamine and antihistamines that are active in the periphery have been known to produce significant effects on animal behavior. Recent evidence suggests that histamine also may be a central neurotransmitter. Biochemical detection of histamine synthesis by neurons and direct cytochemical localization of these neurons have defined a histaminergic system in the CNS. Most of these neurons are located in the ventral posterior hypothalamus; they give rise to long ascending and descending tracts to the entire CNS that are typical of the patterns characteristic of other aminergic systems. Based on the presumptive central effects of histamine antagonists, the histaminergic system is thought to regulate arousal, body temperature, and vascular dynamics.

Four subtypes of histamine receptors have been described; all are GPCRs. H_1 receptors, the most prominent, are located on glia and vessels as well as on neurons and act to mobilize Ca^{2+} in receptive cells through the G_q-PLC pathway. H_2 receptors couple *via* G_S to the activation of adenylyl cyclase, perhaps in concert with H_1 receptors in certain circumstances. H_3 receptors, which have the greatest sensitivity to histamine, are localized selectively in basal ganglia and olfactory regions in the rat; consequences of H_3 receptor activation remain unresolved but may include reduced Ca^{2+} influx and feedback inhibition of transmitter synthesis and release (*see* Chapter 24). The expression of H_4 receptors is confined to cells of hematopoietic origin: eosinophils, T cells, mast cells, basophils, and dendritic cells. H_4 receptors appear to couple to $G_{i/o}$ and G_q, and are postulated to play a role in inflammation and chemotaxis (*see* Chapter 24 and Thurmond *et al.*, 2004). Unlike the monoamines and amino acid transmitters, there does not appear to be an active process for histamine after its release. In addition, no direct evidence had been obtained for release of histamine from neurons either *in vivo* or *in vitro* (Schwartz *et al.*, 1994) until recently (Yoshitake *et al.*, 2003).

Peptides. The discovery during the 1980s of numerous novel peptides in the CNS, each capable of regulating neural function, produced considerable excitement and an imposing catalog of entities as well as potential medications based upon their receptors (Darlison and Richter, 1999; Hökfelt *et al.*, 2003). In addition, certain peptides previously thought to be restricted to the gut or to endocrine glands also have been found in the CNS. Relatively detailed neuronal maps are available that show immunoreactivity to peptide-specific antisera. While some CNS peptides may function on their own, most are now thought to act mainly in concert with coexisting transmitters, both amines and amino acids. As noted above, some neurons may contain two or more transmitters, and their release can be independently regulated. Listed below are several approaches that have utility in analyzing the expanding systems of peptidergic neurons.

Organization by Peptide Families. Because of significant homology in amino acid sequences, families of related molecules can be defined as either *ancestral* or *concurrent*. The ancestral relationship is illustrated by peptides such as the tachykinin or the vasotocin (vasopressin/oxytocin) family, in which species' differences can be correlated with modest variations in peptide structure. The concurrent relationship is best exemplified by the endorphins and by the glucagonsecretin family. In the endorphin superfamily, three major systems of endorphin peptides (pro-opiomelanocortin, proenkephalin, and prodynorphin) and at least two populations of minor opioid peptides (the endomorphins and the orphanin/nociceptin peptide) exist in independent neuronal circuits (Cooper *et al.*, 2003, for review). These natural opioid peptides arise from independent but homologous genes. The peptides all share some actions at receptors once classified generally as "opioid," but now are undergoing progressive refinement (*see* Chapter 21). In the glucagon family, multiple and somewhat homologous peptides are found simultaneously in different cells of separate organ systems: glucagon and vasoactive intestinal polypeptide (VIP) in pancreatic islets; secretin in duodenal mucosa; VIP and related peptides in enteric, autonomic, and central neurons (Magistretti *et al.*, 1999); and growth hormone–releasing hormone only in central neurons (Guillemin *et al.*, 1984). The general metabolic effects produced by this family can be viewed as leading to increased blood glucose. To some degree, ancestral and concurrent relationships are not mutually exclusive. For example, multiple members of the tachykinin/substance P family within mammalian brains and intestines may account for the apparent existence of subsets of receptors for these peptides. The mammalian terminus of the vasotocin family also shows two concurrent products, vasopressin and oxytocin, each having evolved to perform separate functions once executed by single vasotocin-related peptides in lower phyla.

Organization by Anatomic Pattern. Some peptide systems follow rather consistent anatomical organizations. Thus, the hypothalamic peptides oxytocin, vasopressin, pro-opiomelanocortin, gonadotropin-releasing hormone, and growth hormone-releasing hormone all tend to be synthesized by single large clusters of neurons that give off multibranched axons to several distant targets. Other peptides, such as somatostatin, cholecystokinin, and enkephalin, can have patterns varying from moderately long hierarchical connections to short-axon, local-circuit neurons that are widely distributed throughout the brain (*see* 10th edition of this volume for earlier references).

Organization by Function. Since almost all peptides were identified initially on the basis of bioassays, their names reflect these biologically assayed functions (*e.g.*, thyrotropin-releasing hormone and vasoactive intestinal polypeptide). These names become trivial if more ubiquitous distributions and additional functions are discovered.

Some general integrative role might be hypothesized for widely separated neurons (and other cells) that make the same peptide. However, a more parsimonious view is that each peptide has unique messenger roles at the cellular level that are used repeatedly in functionally similar pathways within functionally distinct systems. The cloning of the major members of the opioid-peptide receptors revealed unexpected, and as yet unexplained, homology with receptors for somatostatin, angiotensin, and other peptides. For example, open-system methods of peptide-encoding brain mRNAs have yielded unexpected members of the somatostatin and secretin families (Sutcliffe, 2001).

Comparison with Other Transmitters. Peptides differ in several important respects from the monoamine and amino acid transmitters considered earlier. Peptide synthesis is performed in the rough endoplasmic reticulum. The propeptide is cleaved (processed) to the secreted form as secretory vesicles are transported from the perinuclear cytoplasm to the nerve terminals. Furthermore, no active mechanisms for peptides have been described. This increases the dependency of peptidergic nerve terminals on distant sites of synthesis. Perhaps most importantly, linear chains of amino acids can assume many conformations at their receptors, making it difficult to define the sequences and their steric relationships that are critical for activity.

Until recently, it has been difficult to develop nonpeptidic synthetic agonists or antagonists that interact with specific peptide receptors. Such agents now are being developed for many neuropeptides (Hökfelt *et al.*, 2003). Nature also has had limited success in this regard, since only one plant alkaloid, morphine, has been found to act selectively at peptidergic synapses. Fortunately for pharmacologists, morphine was discovered before the endorphins, or rigid molecules capable of acting at peptide receptors might have been deemed impossible to develop.

Other Regulatory Substances.

In addition to these major families of neurotransmitters, other endogenous substances also may participate in the regulated flow of signals between neurons, but in sequences of events that differ somewhat from the conventional concepts of neurotransmitter function. These substances have significant potential as regulatory factors and as targets for future drug development.

Purines. Adenosine and *uridine di-* and *triphosphates* have roles as extracellular signaling molecules (Edwards and Robertson, 1999; Robertson *et al.*, 2001). ATP is a component of the adrenergic storage vesicle and is released with catecholamines. Intracellular nucleotides may also reach the cell surface by other means (Lazarowski *et al.*, 2003a), and extracellular adenosine can result from cellular release or extracellular production from adenine nucleotides (Jackson and Raghvendra, 2004). These extracellular nucleotides and adenosine act on a family of purinergic receptors that is divided into two classes, P1 and P2. The P1 receptors are GPCRs that interact with adenosine; two of these receptors (A_1 and A_3) couple to G_i and two (A_{2a} and A_{2b}) couple to G_s; methylxanthines antagonize A_1 and A_3 receptors (*see* Chapter 27). Activation of A_1 receptors is associated with inhibition of adenylyl cyclase, activation of K^+ currents, and in some instances, with activation of PLC; stimulation of A_2 receptors activates adenylyl cyclase. The P2 class consists of a large number of P2X receptors that are ligand-gated ion channels, and of the P2Y receptors, a large subclass of GPCRs that couple to G_q or G_s and their associated effectors. The $P2Y_{14}$ receptor is expressed in the CNS; it interacts with UDP-glucose and may couple to G_q (Chambers *et al.*, 2000; Lazarowski *et al.*, 2003b). The co-storage of ATP and catecholamines in adrenergic storage vesicles and their co-release from adrenergic nerves suggests that P2Y receptors in the synaptic region will be stimulated whenever a nerve releases catecholamine. There is *in vitro* evidence for synergistic $G_q \rightarrow G_s$ crosstalk (enhanced β adrenergic response) when β_2 receptors and G_q-linked P2Y receptors are activated simultaneously (Meszaros *et al.*, 2000).

Although many of these receptors can be detected in brain, most of the current interest stems from pharmacological rather than physiological observations. Adenosine can act presynaptically throughout the cortex and hippocampal formation to inhibit the release of amine and amino acid transmitters. ATP-regulated responses have been linked pharmacologically to a variety of supracellular functions, including anxiety, stroke, and epilepsy.

Diffusible Mediators. Certain physiological regulators in systems throughout the body recently have been examined for their roles within the CNS.

Arachidonic acid, normally stored within the cell membrane as a glycerol ester, can be liberated during phospholipid hydrolysis (by pathways involving phospholipases A_2, C, and D). Phospholipases are activated by a variety of receptors (*see* Chapter 1). Arachidonic acid can be converted to highly reactive regulators by three major enzymatic pathways (*see* Chapter 25): cyclooxygenases (leading to *prostaglandins* and *thromboxanes*), lipoxygenases (leading to the *leukotrienes* and other transient catabolites of eicosatetraenoic acid), and CYPs (which are inducible and also expressed at low levels in brain). Arachidonic acid metabolites have been implicated as diffusible modulators in the CNS, particularly for LTP and other forms of plasticity (De Petrocellis *et al.*, 2004).

Nitric oxide (NO) has been recognized as an important regulator of vascular and inflammatory mediation for more than a decade, but came into focus with respect to roles in the CNS after successful efforts to characterize brain nitric oxide synthases (NOS; *see* Boehning and Snyder, 2003). Both constitutive and inducible forms of NOS are expressed in the brain. The availability of potent inhibitors of NOS (such as methyl arginine and nitroarginine) and of NO donors (such as nitroprusside) has led to reports of the presumptive involvement of nitric oxide in a host of CNS phenomena, including LTP, activation of the soluble guanylyl cyclase, neurotransmitter release, and enhancement of glutamate (NMDA)-mediated neurotoxicity. Subsequently, rational analysis based on proposed mechanisms of NO action through binding to the iron in the active site of target enzymes led to the idea that carbon monoxide (CO) may be a second gaseous, labile, diffusible intercellular regulator, at least in the regulation of the soluble guanylyl cyclase in cultured neurons.

Cytokines. The term *cytokines* encompasses a large and diverse family of polypeptide regulators that are produced widely throughout the body by cells of diverse embryological origin. The effects of cytokines are known to be regulated by the conditions imposed by other cytokines, interacting as a network with variable effects leading to synergistic, additive, or opposing actions. Tissue-produced peptidic factors termed *chemokines* serve to attract cells of the immune and inflammatory lines into interstitial spaces. These special cytokines have received much attention as potential regulators in nervous system inflammation (as in early stages of dementia, following infection with human immunodeficiency virus, and during recovery from traumatic injury). The more conventional neuronal- and glial-derived growth-enhancing and growth-retardant factors were mentioned above. The fact that neurons and astrocytes may be induced under some pathophysiological conditions to express cytokines or other growth factors further blurs the dividing line between neurons and glia (Wang *et al.*, 2002; Campbell, 2004).

ACTIONS OF DRUGS IN THE CNS

Specificity and Nonspecificity of CNS Drug Actions. The effect of a drug is considered to be specific in the CNS when it affects an identifiable molecular mechanism unique to target cells that bear receptors for that drug. Conversely, a drug is regarded as nonspecific when it produces effects on many different target cells and acts by diverse molecular mechanisms. This distinction often is a property of the dose-response relationship of the drug and the cell or mechanisms under scrutiny (*see* Chapters 1 and 5). Even a drug that is highly specific when tested at a low concentration may exhibit nonspecific actions at higher doses. Conversely, even generally acting drugs may not act equally on all levels of the CNS. For example, sedatives, hypnotics, and general anesthetics would have very limited utility if central neurons that control the respiratory and cardiovascular systems were especially sensitive to their actions. Drugs with specific actions may produce nonspecific effects if the dose and route of administration produce high tissue concentrations.

Drugs whose mechanisms currently appear to be primarily general or nonspecific are classed according to whether they produce behavioral depression or stimulation. Specifically acting CNS drugs can be classed more definitively according to their locus of action or specific therapeutic usefulness. The absence of overt behavioral effects does not rule out the existence of important central actions for a given drug. For example, the impact of muscarinic cholinergic antagonists on the behavior of normal animals may be subtle, but these agents are used extensively in the treatment of movement disorders and motion sickness (*see* Chapter 7).

General (Nonspecific) CNS Depressants. This category includes the anesthetic gases and vapors, the aliphatic alcohols, and some hypnotic-sedative drugs. These agents share the capacity to depress excitable tissue at all levels of the CNS, leading to a decrease in the amount of transmitter released by the nerve impulse, as well as to general depression of postsynaptic responsiveness and ion movement. At subanesthetic concentrations, these agents (*e.g.*, ethanol) can exert relatively specific effects on certain groups of neurons, which may account for differences in their behavioral effects, especially the propensity to produce dependence (*see* Chapters 13, 16, and 22).

General (Nonspecific) CNS Stimulants. The drugs in this category include pentylenetetrazol and related agents that are capable of powerful excitation of the CNS, and the methylxanthines, which have a much weaker stimulant action. Stimulation may be accomplished by one of two general mechanisms: (1) by blockade of inhibition or (2) by direct neuronal excitation (which may involve increased transmitter release, more prolonged transmitter action, labilization of the postsynaptic membrane, or decreased synaptic recovery time).

Drugs That Selectively Modify CNS Function. The agents in this group may cause either depression or excitation. In some instances, a drug may produce both effects simultaneously on different systems. Some agents in this category have little effect on the level of excitability in doses that are used therapeutically. The principal classes of these CNS drugs are: anticonvulsants, drugs used in treating Parkinson's disease, opioid and nonopioid analgesics, appetite suppressants, antiemetics, analgesic-antipyretics, certain stimulants, neuroleptics (antidepressants and antimanic and antipsychotic agents), tranquilizers, sedatives, and hypnotics. Although not yet a broad class, medications employed in the treatment of Alzheimer's disease (cholinesterase inhibitors and antiglutamate neuroprotectants) and compounds promising in the symptomatic treatment of Huntington's disease (tetrabenazine for the depletion of monoamines and reduction in tremor) also may be included.

Although selectivity of action may be remarkable, a drug usually affects several CNS functions to varying degrees. When only one constellation of effects is wanted in a therapeutic situation, the remaining effects of the drug are regarded as limitations in selectivity (*i.e.,* unwanted side effects). The specificity of a drug's action frequently is overestimated. This is partly due to the fact that the drug is identified with the effect that is implied by the class name.

General Characteristics of CNS Drugs.

Combinations of centrally acting drugs frequently are administered to therapeutic advantage (*e.g.,* an anticholinergic drug and levodopa for Parkinson's disease). However, other combinations of drugs may be detrimental because of potentially dangerous additive or mutually antagonistic effects.

The effect of a CNS drug is additive with the physiological state and with the effects of other depressant and stimulant drugs. For example, anesthetics are less effective in a hyperexcitable subject than in a normal patient; the converse is true for stimulants. In general, the depressant effects of drugs from all categories are additive (*e.g.,* the fatal combination of barbiturates or benzodiazepines with ethanol), as are the effects of stimulants. Therefore, respiration depressed by morphine is further impaired by depressant drugs, while stimulant drugs can augment the excitatory effects of morphine to produce vomiting and convulsions.

Antagonism between depressants and stimulants is variable. Some instances of true pharmacological antagonism among CNS drugs are known; for example, opioid antagonists are very selective in blocking the effects of opioid analgesics. However, the antagonism exhibited between two CNS drugs is usually physiological in nature. For example, an individual whose CNS is depressed by an opiate cannot be returned entirely to normal by stimulation by caffeine.

The selective effects of drugs on specific neurotransmitter systems may be additive or competitive. This potential for drug interaction must be considered whenever such drugs are administered concurrently. To minimize such interactions, a drug-free period may be required when modifying therapy, and development of desensitized and supersensitive states with prolonged therapy may limit the speed with which one drug may be halted and another started. An excitatory effect is commonly observed with low concentrations of certain depressant drugs due either to depression of inhibitory systems or to a transient increase in the release of excitatory transmitters. Examples are the stage of excitement during induction of general anesthesia and the stimulant effects of alcohol. The excitatory phase occurs only with low concentrations of the depressant; uniform depression ensues with increasing drug concentration. The excitatory effects can be minimized, when appropriate, by pretreatment with a depressant drug that is devoid of such effects (*e.g.,* benzodiazepines in preanesthetic medication). Acute, excessive stimulation of the cerebrospinal axis normally is followed by depression, which is in part a consequence of neuronal fatigue and exhaustion of stores of transmitters. Postictal depression is additive with the effects of depressant drugs. Acute, drug-induced depression generally is not followed by stimulation. However, chronic drug-induced sedation or depression may be followed by prolonged hyperexcitability upon abrupt withdrawal of the medication (barbiturates or alcohol). This type of hyperexcitability can be controlled effectively by the same or another depressant drug (*see* Chapters 16, 17, and 18).

Organization of CNS–Drug Interactions.

The structural and functional properties of neurons provide a means to specify the possible sites at which drugs could interact, specifically or generally, in the CNS (Figure 12–1). In this scheme, drugs that affect neuronal energy metabolism, membrane integrity, or transmembrane ionic equilibria would be generally acting compounds. Similarly general in action would be drugs (*e.g.,* colchicine) that affect the two-way intracellular transport systems. These general effects still can exhibit different dose–response or time–response relationships, based, for example, on such neuronal properties as rate of firing, dependence of discharge on external stimuli or internal pacemakers, resting ionic fluxes, or axon length. In contrast, when drug actions can be related to specific aspects of the metabolism, release, or function of a neurotransmitter, the site, specificity, and mechanism of action of a drug can be defined by systematic studies of dose–response and time–response relationships. From such data, the most sensitive, rapid, or persistent neuronal event can be identified.

Transmitter-dependent actions of drugs can be grouped into presynaptic and postsynaptic categories. The presynaptic category includes all of the events in the perikaryon and nerve terminal that regulate transmitter synthesis (including the acquisition of adequate substrates and cofactors), storage, release, and metabolism. Transmitter concentrations can be lowered by blockade of synthesis, storage, or both. The amount of transmitter released per impulse generally is stable but also can be regulated. The effective concentration of transmitter may be increased by inhibition of or by blockade of metabolic enzymes. The transmitter that is released at a synapse also can exert actions on the terminal from which it was released by interacting with receptors at these sites (termed *autoreceptors*; *see* above). Activation of presynaptic autoreceptors can slow the rate of discharge of transmitter and thereby provide a feedback mechanism that controls the concentration of transmitter in the synaptic cleft.

The postsynaptic category includes all the events that follow release of the transmitter in the vicinity of the postsynaptic receptor. Examples include the molecular mechanisms by which receptor occupancy alters the properties of the membrane of the postsynaptic cell (shifts in membrane potential), as well as more enduring biochemical actions (*e.g.*, changes in second messenger concentrations, protein kinase and phosphatase activities, and phosphoprotein formation). Direct postsynaptic effects of drugs generally require relatively high affinity for the receptors or resistance to metabolic degradation. Each of these presynaptic or postsynaptic actions potentially is highly specific and can be envisioned as restricted to a single, chemically defined subset of CNS cells.

Convergence, Synergism, and Antagonism Result from Transmitter Interactions. Although the power of the reductionist approach to clone cDNAs for receptors or receptor subunits and to determine their properties by expression in cells that do not normally express the receptor or subunit cannot be underestimated, *the simplicity of cell culture models of this type may divert attention from the complexity of the intact CNS.* A given neurotransmitter may interact simultaneously with all of the various isoforms of its receptor on neurons that also are under the influence of multiple other afferent pathways and their transmitters. Thus, attempts to predict the behavioral or therapeutic consequences of drugs designed to elicit precise and restricted receptor actions in simple model systems may fail as a consequence of the complexity of the interactions possible, including differences between normal and diseased tissue.

BIBLIOGRAPHY

Aston-Jones, G., Chen, S., Zhu, Y., and Oshinsky, M.L. A neural circuit for circadian regulation of arousal. *Nat. Neurosci.*, **2001,** *4:*732–738.

Bodian, D. Neuron junctions: a revolutionary decade. *Anat. Rec.,* **1972,** *174:*73–82.

Carson, M.J., *et al.* Mature microglia resemble immature antigen-presenting cell. *Glia.*, **1998,** *22:*72-85.

Carson, M.J. Microglia as liaisons between the immune and central nervous systems: functional implications for multiple sclerosis. *Glia,* **2002,** *40:*218–231.

Chambers, J.K., Macdonald, L.E., *et al.* A G-protein-coupled receptor for UDP-glucose. *J. Biol. Chem.*, **2000,** *275:*10767–10771.

Florey, E. Neurotransmitters and modulators in the animal kingdom. *Fed. Proc.,* **1967,** *26:*1164–1176.

Frandsen, A., and Schousboe, A. AMPA receptor-mediated neurotoxicity: role of Ca^{2+} and desensitization. *Neurochem. Res.,* **2003,** *28:*1495–1499.

Gage, F.H. Neurogenesis in the adult brain. *J. Neurosci.,* **2002,** *22:*612–613.

Guillemin, R., Zeytin, F., Ling, N., *et al.* Growth hormone-releasing factor: chemistry and physiology. *Proc. Soc. Exp. Biol. Med.,* **1984,** *175:*407–413.

Husi, H., *et al.* Proteomic analysis of NMDA receptor-adhesion protein signaling complexes. *Nat. Neurosci.,* **2000,** *3:*661–669.

Jahn, R. Principles of exocytosis and membrane fusion. *Ann. N.Y. Acad. Sci.,* **2004,** *1014:*170–178.

Johnston, G.A., Chebib, M., Hanrahan, J.R., and Mewett K.N. $GABA_C$ receptors as drug targets. *Curr. Drug Targets CNS Neurol. Disord.,* **2003,** *2:*260–268.

Johnston, G.A. Medicinal chemistry and molecular pharmacology of $GABA_C$ receptors. *Curr. Top. Med. Chem.,* **2002,** *2:*903–913.

Krapivinsky, G., Gordon, E.A., Wickman, K., *et al.* The G-protein-gated atrial K^+ channel I_{KACh} is a heteromultimer of two inwardly rectifying K^+-channel proteins. *Nature,* **1995,** *374:*135–141.

Lazarowski, E.R., Shea, D.A., Boucher, R.C. and Harden, T.K. Release of cellular UDP-glucose as a potential extracellular signaling molecule. *Mol. Pharmacol.,* **2003a,** *63:*1190–1197.

MacKinnon, R. Potassium channels. *FEBS Lett.,* **2003,** *555:*62–65.

MacMillan, L.B., Lakhlani, P.P., Hein, L., *et al.* In vivo mutation of the α_{2A}-adrenergic receptor by homologous recombination reveals the role of this receptor subtype in multiple physiological processes. *Adv. Pharmacol.,* **1998,** *42:*493–496.

Meszaros, J.G., Gonzalez, A.M., Endo-Mochizuki, Y., *et al.* Identification of G protein-coupled signaling pathways in cardiac fibroblasts: crosstalk between G_q and G_s. *Am. J. Physiol. Cell Physiol.,* **2000,** *278:*C154–C162.

Niswender, C.M., Herrick-Davis, K., Dilley, G.E., *et al.* RNA editing of the human serotonin $5-HT_{2C}$ receptor, alterations in suicide and implications for serotonergic pharmacotherapy. *Neuropsychopharmacology,* **2001,** *24:*478–491.

Ostrom, R.S., Naugle, J.E., Hase, M., *et al.* Angiotensin II enhances adenylyl cyclase signaling via Ca^{2+}/Calmodulin. G_q-G_s cross-talk regulates collagen production in cardiac fibroblasts. *J. Biol. Chem.,* **2003,** *278:*24461–24468.

Pellerin, L., and Magistretti, P.J. How to balance the brain energy budget while spending glucose differently. *J. Physiol.,* **2003,** *546*(Pt 2):325.

Raber, J., *et al.* Inflammatory cytokines: putative regulators of neuronal and neuro-endocrine function. *Brain Res. Brain Res. Rev.,* **1998,** *26:*320–326.

Ransohoff, R.M. The chemokine system in neuroinflammation: an update. *J. Infect. Dis.,* **2002,** *186*(Suppl 2):S152–S156.

Rosenberg, G.A. Matrix metalloproteinases in neuroinflammation. *Glia,* **2002,** *39:*279–291.

Sola, M., Bavro, V.N., Timmins, J., *et al.* Structural basis of dynamic glycine receptor clustering by gephyrin. *EMBO. J.,* **2004,** *23:*2510–2519.

Steindler, D.A., and Pincus, D.W. Stem cells and neuropoiesis in the adult human brain. *Lancet,* **2002,** *359:*1047–1054.

Thurmond, R.L., Desai, P.J., Dunford, P.J., *et al.* A potent and selective histamine H_4 receptor antagonist with antiinflammatory properties. *J. Pharmacol. Exp. Ther.,* **2004,** *309:*404–413.

Yoshitake, T., Yamaguchi, M., Nohta, H., *et al.* Determination of histamine in microdialysis samples from rat brain by microbore column liquid chromatography following intramolecular excimer-forming derivatization with pyrene-labeling reagent. *J. Neurosci. Methods,* **2003,** *127:*11–17.

MONOGRAPHS AND REVIEWS

Aghajanian, G.K., and Marek, G.J. Serotonin and hallucinogens. *Neuropsychopharmacology,* **1999,** *21*(2 Suppl):16S–23S.

Bleich, S., Romer, K., Wiltfang J., and Kornhuber, J. Glutamate and the glutamate receptor system: a target for drug action. *Int. J. Geriatr. Psychiatry,* **2003,** *18*(Suppl 1):S33–S40.

Bloom, F.E. Neurotransmission and the central nervous system. In, *Goodman and Gilman's The Pharmacological Basis of Therapeutics,* 9ᵗʰ ed. (Hardman, J.G. and Limbird, L.E., eds.) McGraw-Hill, New York, **1996,** pp. 267–293.

Boehning, D., and Snyder, S.H. Novel neural modulators. *Annu. Rev. Neurosci.,* **2003,** *26:*105–131.

Bourne, H.R., and Nicoll, R. Molecular machines integrate coincident synaptic signals. *Cell,* **1993,** *72:*65–75.

Burnstock, G. Noradrenaline and ATP: co-transmitters and neuromodulators. *J. Physiol. Pharmacol.,* **1995,** *46*(4):365–384.

Campbell, I.L. Chemokines as plurifunctional mediators in the CNS: implications for the pathogenesis of stroke. *Ernst Schering Res. Found. Workshop,* **2004,** *45:*31–51.

Catterall, W., and Epstein, P.N. Ion channels. *Diabetologia,* **1992,** *2:*S23–S33.

Catterall, W.A. Structure and function of voltage-gated ion channels. *Trends Neurosci.,* **1993,** *16:*500–506.

Clapham, D.E., Julius, D., Montell, C., and Schultz, G. Transient Receptor Channels. Available at: http://www.iuphar-db.org/iuphar-ic/TRPC.html. Accessed March 26, 2004.

Conn, P.J. Physiological roles and therapeutic potential of metabotropic glutamate receptors. *Ann. N.Y. Acad. Sci.,* **2003,** *1003:*12–21.

Cooper, J., Bloom, F., and Roth, R. *The Biochemical Basis of Neuropharmacology.* Oxford University Press, New York, **2003.**

Cowan, W.M., Harter, D.H., and Kandel, E.R. The emergence of modern neuroscience: some implications for neurology and psychiatry. *Annu. Rev. Neurosci.,* **2000,** *23:*343–391.

Cowan, W.M., Kopnisky, K.L., and Hyman, S.E. The Human Genome Project and its impact on psychiatry. *Annu. Rev. Neurosci.,* **2002,** *25:*1–50.

Darlison, M.G., and Richter, D. Multiple genes for neuropeptides and their receptors: co-evolution and physiology. *Trends Neurosci.,* **1999,** *22:*81–88.

De Petrocellis, L., Cascio, M.G., Di Marzo, V., *et al.* The endocannabinoid system: a general view and latest additions. Cannabinoids and memory: animal studies. *Br. J. Pharmacol.,* **2004,** *141:*765–774.

Edwards, F.A., and Robertson, S.J. The function of A₂ adenosine receptors in the mammalian brain: evidence for inhibition vs. enhancement of voltage gated calcium channels and neurotransmitter release. *Prog. Brain Res.,* **1999,** *120:*265–273.

Gillessen, T., Budd, S.L., and Lipton, S.A. Excitatory amino acid neurotoxicity. *Adv. Exp. Med. Biol.,* **2002,** *513:*3–40.

Greengard, P. The neurobiology of dopamine signaling. *Biosci. Rep.,* **2001,** *21:*247–269.

Herrling, P. Excitatory amino acids. In, *Clinical Results with Antagonists.* Academic Press, San Diego, **1997.**

Hofmann, F., Biel, M., and Kaupp, U.B. Cyclic Nucleotide-modulated Channels. Available at: http://www.iuphar-db.org/iuphar-ic/CNGA.html. Accessed March 26, 2004.

Hökfelt, T., Bartfai, T., and Bloom, F. Neuropeptides: opportunities for drug discovery. *Lancet. Neurol.,* **2003,** *2:*463–472.

Hökfelt, T., Broberger, C., Xu, Z.-Q.D., *et al.* Neuropeptides—an Overview. *Neuropharmacology,* **2000,** *39:*1337–1356.

Huang, E.J., and Reichardt, L.F. Neurotrophins: Roles in neuronal development and function. *Annu. Rev. Neurosci.,* **2001,** *24:*677–736.

Jackson, E.K., and Raghvendra, D.K. The extracellular cyclic AMP-adenosine pathway in renal physiology. *Annu. Rev. Physiol.,* **2004,** *66:*571–599.

Kotecha, S.A., and MacDonald, J.F. Signaling molecules and receptor transduction cascades that regulate NMDA receptor-mediated synaptic transmission. *Int. Rev. Neurobiol.,* **2003,** *54:*51–106.

Lazarowski, E.R., Boucher, R.C., and Harden, T.K. Mechanisms of release of nucleotides and integration of the action as P2X- and P2Y-receptor activating molecules. *Mol. Pharmacol.,* **2003b,** *64:*785–795.

Linden, D.J. Neuroscience. From molecules to memory in the cerebellum. *Science,* **2003,** *301:*1682–1685.

Magistretti, P., Cardinaux, J., and Martin, J.L. VIP and PACAP in the CNS: regulators of glial energy metabolism and modulators of glutamatergic signaling. *Ann. N.Y. Acad. Sci.,* **1999,** *865:*213–225.

Milligan, G. G protein-coupled receptor dimerization: function and ligand pharmacology. *Mol. Pharmacol.,* **2004,** *66:*1–7.

Mountcastle, V.B. The columnar organization of the neocortex. *Brain,* **1997,** *120:*701–722.

Murthy, V.N., and Camilli, P.D. Cell biology of the presynaptic terminal. *Annu. Rev. Neurosci.,* **2003,** *26:*701–728.

Nestler, E.J., Hyman, S.E., and Malenka, R.C. *Molecular Neuropharmacology.* McGraw-Hill, New York, **2001.**

Neubig, R., Spedding, M., Kenakin, T., and Christopoulos, A. International Union of Pharmacology Committee on Receptor Nomenclature and Drug Classification. XXXVIII. Update on Terms and Symbols in Quantitative Pharmacology. *Pharmacol. Rev.,* **2003,** *55:*597–606.

Piomelli, D. The molecular logic of endocannabinoid signaling. *Nat. Rev. Neurosci.,* **2003,** *4:*873–884.

Robas, N., O'Reilly, M., Katugampola, S., and Fidock, M. Maximizing serendipity: strategies for identifying ligands for orphan G-protein-coupled receptors. *Curr. Opin. Pharmacol.,* **2003,** *3:*121–126.

Robertson, S.J., Ennion, S.J., Evans, R.J., and Edwards, F.A. Synaptic P2X receptors. *Curr. Opin. Neurobiol.,* **2001,** *11:*378–386.

Schmauss, C., and Howe, J.R. RNA editing of neurotransmitter receptors in the mammalian brain. *Sci. STKE.,* **2002,** *2002:*PE26.

Schwartz, J.-C., Arrang, J.-M., Garbarg, M., and Traiffort, E. Histamine. In, *Psychopharmacology: The Fourth Generation of Progress.* (Bloom, F.E. and Kupfer, D.J., eds.) Raven Press, New York, **1994,** pp. 397–406.

Seeburg, P.H., Single, F., Kuner, T., Higuchi, M., and Sprengel, R. Genetic manipulation of key determinants of ion flow in glutamate receptor channels in the mouse. *Brain Res.,* **2001,** *907:*233–243.

Shepherd, G.M. *The Synaptic Organization of the Brain.* Oxford University Press, New York, **2003.**

Sofroniew, M.V., Howe, C.L., and Mobley, W.C. Nerve growth factor signaling, neuroprotection, and neural repair. *Annu. Rev. Neurosci.,* **2001,** *24:*1217–1281.

Sutcliffe, J.G. Open-system approaches to gene expression in the CNS. *J. Neurosci.,* **2001,** *21:*8306–8309.

Wang, J., Asensio, V.C., and Campbell, I.L. Cytokines and chemokines as mediators of protection and injury in the central nervous system assessed in transgenic mice. *Curr. Top. Microbiol. Immunol.,* **2002,** *265:*23–48.

Whiting, P.J. The GABAₐ receptor gene family: new opportunities for drug development. *Curr. Opin. Drug Discov. Devel.,* **2003,** *6:*648–657.

GENERAL ANESTHETICS

Alex S. Evers, C. Michael Crowder, and Jeffrey R. Balser

General anesthetics depress the central nervous system to a sufficient degree to permit the performance of surgery and other noxious or unpleasant procedures. Not surprisingly, general anesthetics have low therapeutic indices and thus require great care in administration. While all general anesthetics produce a relatively similar anesthetic state, they are quite dissimilar in their secondary actions (side effects) on other organ systems. The selection of specific drugs and routes of administration to produce general anesthesia is based on their pharmacokinetic properties and on the secondary effects of the various drugs, in the context of the proposed diagnostic or surgical procedure and with the consideration of the individual patient's age, associated medical condition, and medication use. Anesthesiologists also employ sedatives (*see* Chapter 16), neuromuscular blocking agents (*see* Chapter 9), and local anesthetics (*see* Chapter 14) as the situation requires.

Before describing the general features of anesthesia, the basic principles that underlie anesthetic actions, and the specific properties of inhalational and intravenous anesthetics and the practical aspects of their use, it is sobering to recall the time, not so very long ago, when surgical anesthesia did not exist, and to be reminded of the development of this field since 1846.

Historical Perspectives. Although Crawford Long, a physician in rural Georgia, first used *ether* anesthesia in 1842, not until the first public demonstration in 1846 by William T.G. Morton, a Boston dentist and medical student, did general anesthesia achieve worldwide discovery, spawning a revolution in medical care. The operating room, now known as "the ether dome" where Gilbert Abbott underwent surgery in an unconscious state at the Massachusetts General Hospital, remains a memorial to this day. Although no longer used in modern practice,

ether was the ideal "first" anesthetic. Chemically, it is readily made in pure form and is relatively nontoxic to vital organs. A liquid at room temperature, it readily vaporizes, and as such is easy to administer. Unlike *nitrous oxide,* ether is potent, so it can produce anesthesia without diluting the oxygen in room air to hypoxic levels. Finally, ether does not greatly compromise respiration or circulation, crucial properties at a time when our understanding of human physiology and technical prowess did not allow for assisted respiration and circulation.

Chloroform was the next anesthetic to receive wide use. Introduced by the Scottish obstetrician James Simpson in 1847, it became quite popular, perhaps because its odor is more pleasant than that of ether. Other than this and its nonflammability, there was little to recommend it; the drug is a hepatotoxin and a severe cardiovascular depressant. Despite the relatively high incidence of intraoperative and postoperative death associated with the use of chloroform, it was championed, especially in Great Britain, for nearly 100 years.

It was at a stage show that Horace Wells, a dentist, noted that while under the influence of nitrous oxide, one of the participants injured himself yet felt no pain. The next day Wells, while breathing nitrous oxide, had one of his own teeth extracted painlessly by a colleague. Shortly thereafter, in 1845, Wells attempted to demonstrate his discovery at the Massachusetts General Hospital in Boston. Unfortunately the patient cried out during the operation, the demonstration was deemed a failure, and nitrous oxide fell into disuse until 1863 when Gardner Q. Colton, a showman, entrepreneur, and partially trained physician reintroduced the drug into American dental and surgical practice. In 1868, the coadministration of nitrous oxide and oxygen was described by Edmond Andrews, a Chicago surgeon, and soon thereafter the two gases became available in steel cylinders, greatly increasing their practical use.

The anesthetic properties of *cyclopropane* were accidentally discovered in 1929 when chemists were analyzing impurities in an isomer, propylene. After extensive clinical trials at the University of Wisconsin, the drug was introduced into practice; cyclopropane was perhaps the most widely used general anesthetic for the next 30 years. However, cyclopropane was flammable, indeed explosive, and with the increasing use of electronic equipment and electrocautery, the need for a safe, nonflammable anesthetic was clear. Efforts by the British Research Council and by chemists at Imperial Chemical Industries were rewarded by the development of *halothane*, a nonflammable anesthetic agent that was introduced into clinical practice in 1956 and quickly became the dominant anesthetic. Most of the newer agents, which are halogenated alkanes and ethers, are modeled after halothane.

Although the desirability of an intravenous anesthetic agent must have been apparent to physicians early in the 20th century, the drugs at hand were few and unsatisfactory. The situation changed dramatically in 1935, when Lundy demonstrated the clinical usefulness of *thiopental*, a rapidly-acting thiobarbiturate. It originally was considered useful as a sole anesthetic agent, but the doses required resulted in serious depression of the circulatory, respiratory, and nervous systems. However, thiopental and other intravenous anesthetics now have become the most common agents for induction of general anesthesia.

GENERAL PRINCIPLES OF SURGICAL ANESTHESIA

Unlike the practice of every other branch of medicine, anesthesia is usually neither therapeutic nor diagnostic. The exceptions to this, such as treatment of status asthmaticus with halothane and intractable angina with epidural local anesthetics, should not obscure this critical point that permeates the training and practice of the specialty. Hence, administration of general anesthesia, as well as the development of new anesthetic agents and physiologic monitoring technology, has been driven by three general objectives:

1. *Minimizing the potentially deleterious direct and indirect effects of anesthetic agents and techniques.*
2. *Sustaining physiologic homeostasis during surgical procedures* that may involve major blood loss, tissue ischemia, reperfusion of ischemic tissue, fluid shifts, exposure to a cold environment, and impaired coagulation.
3. *Improving postoperative outcomes* by choosing techniques that block or treat components of the *surgical stress response,* which may lead to short- or long-term sequelae (Mangano *et al.*, 1996; Balser *et al.*, 1998).

Hemodynamic Effects of General Anesthesia. The most prominent physiological effect of anesthesia induction, associated with the majority of both intravenous and inhalational agents, is a decrease in systemic arterial blood pressure. The causes include direct vasodilation, myocardial depression or both, a blunting of baroreceptor control, and a generalized decrease in central sympathetic tone (Sellgren *et al.*, 1990). Agents vary in the magnitude of their specific effects (*see* below), but in all cases the hypotensive response is enhanced by underlying volume

depletion or preexisting myocardial dysfunction. Even anesthetics that show minimal hypotensive tendencies under normal conditions (*e.g., etomidate* and *ketamine*) must be used with caution in trauma victims, in whom intravascular volume depletion is being compensated by intense sympathetic discharge. Smaller-than-normal anesthetic dosages are employed in patients presumed to be sensitive to hemodynamic effects of anesthetics.

Respiratory Effects of General Anesthesia. Airway maintenance is essential following induction of anesthesia, as nearly all general anesthetics reduce or eliminate both ventilatory drive and the reflexes that maintain airway patency. Therefore, ventilation generally must be assisted or controlled for at least some period during surgery. The gag reflex is lost, and the stimulus to cough is blunted. Lower esophageal sphincter tone also is reduced, so both passive and active regurgitation may occur. Endotracheal intubation was introduced by Kuhn in the early 1900s and has been a major reason for a decline in the number of aspiration deaths during general anesthesia. Muscle relaxation is valuable during the induction of general anesthesia where it facilitates management of the airway, including endotracheal intubation. Neuromuscular blocking agents commonly are used to effect such relaxation (*see* Chapter 9), reducing the risk of coughing or gagging during laryngoscopic-assisted instrumentation of the airway, and thus reducing the risk of aspiration prior to secure placement of an endotracheal tube. Alternatives to an endotracheal tube include a facemask and a laryngeal mask, an inflatable mask placed in the oropharynx forming a seal around the glottis. The choice of airway management is based on the type of procedure and characteristics of the patient.

Hypothermia. Patients commonly develop hypothermia (body temperature <36°C) during surgery. The reasons for the hypothermia include low ambient temperature, exposed body cavities, cold intravenous fluids, altered thermoregulatory control, and reduced metabolic rate. General anesthetics lower the core temperature set point at which thermoregulatory vasoconstriction is activated to defend against heat loss. Furthermore, vasodilation produced by both general and regional anesthesia offsets cold-induced peripheral vasoconstriction, thereby redistributing heat from central to peripheral body compartments, leading to a decline in core temperature (Sessler, 2000). Metabolic rate and total body oxygen consumption decrease with general anesthesia by about 30%, reducing heat generation.

Even small drops in body temperatures may lead to an increase in perioperative morbidity, including cardiac complications (Frank *et al.*, 1997), wound infections

(Kurz *et al.*, 1996), and impaired coagulation. Prevention of hypothermia has emerged as a major goal of anesthetic care. Modalities to maintain normothermia include using warm intravenous fluids, heat exchangers in the anesthesia circuit, forced-warm-air covers, and new technology involving water-filled garments with microprocessor feedback control to a core temperature set point.

Nausea and Vomiting. Nausea and vomiting in the postoperative period continue to be significant problems following general anesthesia and are caused by an action of anesthetics on the chemoreceptor trigger zone and the brainstem vomiting center, which are modulated by serotonin (5-HT), histamine, acetylcholine, and dopamine. The 5-HT$_3$-receptor antagonist *ondansetron* (*see* Chapter 37) is very effective in suppressing nausea and vomiting. Common treatments also include *droperidol, metoclopramide, dexamethasone,* and avoidance of N$_2$O. The use of *propofol* as an induction agent and the nonsteroidal antiinflammatory drug *ketorolac* as a substitute for opioids may decrease the incidence and severity of postoperative nausea and vomiting.

Other Emergence and Postoperative Phenomena. The physiological changes accompanying emergence from general anesthesia can be profound. Hypertension and tachycardia are common as the sympathetic nervous system regains its tone and is enhanced by pain. Myocardial ischemia can appear or markedly worsen during emergence in patients with coronary artery disease. Emergence excitement occurs in 5% to 30% of patients and is characterized by tachycardia, restlessness, crying, moaning and thrashing, and various neurological signs. Postanesthesia shivering occurs frequently because of core hypothermia. A small dose of *meperidine* (12.5 mg) lowers the shivering trigger temperature and effectively stops the activity. The incidence of all of these emergence phenomena is greatly reduced when opioids are employed as part of the intraoperative regimen.

Airway obstruction may occur during the postoperative period because residual anesthetic effects continue to partially obtund consciousness and reflexes (especially in patients who normally snore or who have sleep apnea). Strong inspiratory efforts against a closed glottis can lead to negative-pressure pulmonary edema. Pulmonary function is reduced postoperatively following all types of anesthesia and surgery, and hypoxemia may occur. Hypertension can be prodigious, often requiring aggressive treatment.

Pain control can be complicated in the immediate postoperative period. The respiratory suppression associated with opioids can be problematic among postoperative patients who still have a substantial residual anesthetic effect. Patients can alternate between screaming in apparent agony and being deeply somnolent with airway obstruction, all in a matter of moments. The nonsteroidal antiinflammatory agent ketorolac (30 to 60 mg intravenously) frequently is effective, and the development of injectable cyclooxygenase-2 inhibitors (*see* Chapter 26) holds promise for analgesia without respiratory depression. In addition, regional anesthetic techniques are an important part of a perioperative multimodal approach that employs local anesthetic wound infiltration; epidural, spinal, and plexus blocks; and nonsteroidal antiinflammatory drugs, opioids, α_2 adrenergic-receptor agonists, and NMDA-receptor antagonists. Patient-controlled administration of intravenous and epidural analgesics makes use of small, computerized pumps activated on demand but programmed with safety limits to prevent overdose. The agents used are opioids (frequently *morphine*) by the intravenous route, and opioid, local anesthetic, or both, by the epidural route. These techniques have revolutionized postoperative pain management, can be continued for hours or days, and promote ambulation and improved bowel function until oral pain medications are initiated.

ACTIONS AND MECHANISMS OF GENERAL ANESTHETICS

The Anesthetic State

General anesthetics are a structurally diverse class of drugs that produce a common end point—a behavioral state referred to as *general anesthesia*. In the broadest sense, general anesthesia can be defined as a global but reversible depression of central nervous system (CNS) function resulting in the loss of response to and perception of all external stimuli. While this definition is appealing in its simplicity, it is not useful for two reasons: First, it is inadequate because anesthesia is not simply a deafferented state; for example, amnesia is an important aspect of the anesthetic state. Second, not all general anesthetics produce identical patterns of deafferentation. Barbiturates, for example, are very effective at producing amnesia and loss of consciousness, but are not effective as analgesics.

An alternative way of defining the anesthetic state is to consider it as a collection of "component" changes in behavior or perception. The components of the anesthetic state include *amnesia, immobility* in response to noxious stimulation, *attenuation of autonomic responses* to noxious stimulation, *analgesia,* and *unconsciousness*. It is important to remember that general anesthesia is useful

Table 13-1
Properties of Inhalational Anesthetic Agents

ANESTHETIC AGENT	MAC* (vol %)	MAC$_{AWAKE}$[†] (vol %)	EC$_{50}$[‡] FOR SUPPRESSION OF MEMORY (vol %)	VAPOR PRESSURE (mm Hg at 20°C)	PARTITION COEFFICIENT AT 37°C			RECOVERED AS METABOLITES (%)
					Blood:Gas	*Brain:Blood*	*Fat:Blood*	
Halothane	0.75	0.41	—	243	2.3	2.9	51	20
Isoflurane	1.2	0.4	0.24	250	1.4	2.6	45	0.2
Enflurane	1.6	0.4	—	175	1.8	1.4	36	2.4
Sevoflurane	2	0.6	—	160	0.65	1.7	48	3
Desflurane	6	2.4	—	664	0.45	1.3	27	0.02
Nitrous oxide	105	60.0	52.5	Gas	0.47	1.1	2.3	0.004
Xenon	71	32.6	—	Gas	0.12	—	—	0

*MAC (minimum alveolar concentration) values are expressed as vol %, the percentage of the atmosphere that is anesthetic. A value of MAC greater than 100% means that hyperbaric conditions would be required. †MAC$_{awake}$ is the concentration at which appropriate responses to commands are lost. ‡EC$_{50}$ is the concentration that produces memory suppression in 50% of patients. —, Not available.

only insofar as it facilitates the performance of surgery or other noxious procedures. The performance of surgery usually requires an immobilized patient who does not have an excessive autonomic response to surgery (blood pressure and heart rate) and who has amnesia for the procedure. Thus, the essential components of the anesthetic state are immobilization, amnesia, and attenuation of autonomic responses to noxious stimulation. Indeed, if an anesthetic produces profound amnesia, it can be difficult in principle to determine if it also produces either analgesia or unconsciousness.

Measurement of Anesthetic Potency

Given the essential requirement that a general anesthetic agent provide an immobilized patient, the potency of general anesthetic agents usually is measured by determining the concentration of general anesthetic that prevents movement in response to surgical stimulation. For inhalational anesthetics, anesthetic potency is measured in MAC units, with 1 MAC defined as the *minimum alveolar concentration* that prevents movement in response to surgical stimulation in 50% of subjects. The strengths of MAC as a measurement are that (1) alveolar concentrations can be monitored continuously by measuring end-tidal anesthetic concentration using infrared spectroscopy or mass spectrometry; (2) it provides a direct correlate of the free concentration of the anesthetic at its site(s) of action in the CNS; (3) it is a simple-to-measure end point that reflects an important clinical goal. End points other than immobilization also can be used to measure anesthetic potency.

For example, the ability to respond to verbal commands (MAC$_{awake}$) (Stoelting *et al.*, 1970) and the ability to form memories (Dwyer *et al.*, 1992) also have been correlated with alveolar anesthetic concentration. Interestingly, verbal response and memory formation both are suppressed at a fraction of MAC. Furthermore, the ratio of the anesthetic concentrations required to produce amnesia and immobility vary significantly among different inhalational anesthetic agents (nitrous oxide *vs.* isoflurane) (Table 13-1), suggesting that anesthetic agents may produce these behavioral end points *via* different cellular and molecular mechanisms. The potency of intravenous anesthetic agents is somewhat more difficult to measure because there is not an available method to measure blood or plasma anesthetic concentration continuously, and because the free concentration of the drug at its site of action cannot be determined. Generally, the potency of intravenous agents is defined as the free plasma concentration (at equilibrium) that produces loss of response to surgical incision (or other end points) in 50% of subjects.

Mechanisms of Anesthesia

The molecular and cellular mechanisms by which general anesthetics produce their effects have remained one of the great mysteries of pharmacology. For most of the 20th century, it was theorized that all anesthetics act by a common mechanism (*the unitary theory of anesthesia*). The leading unitary theory was that anesthesia is produced by perturbation of the physical properties of cell membranes. This thinking was based largely on the observation that the anesthetic potency of a gas correlated with its solubility in olive oil. This correlation, referred to as the *Meyer-Overton rule,* was interpreted as implicating the lipid bilayer as the likely target of anesthetic action. Clear exceptions to the Meyer-Overton rule have now been noted (Koblin *et al.,* 1994). For example, inhalational and intravenous anesthetics can be enantioselective in their action as anesthetics (etomidate, steroids, *isoflurane*) (Tomlin *et al.,* 1998; Lysko *et al.,* 1994; Wittmer *et al.,* 1996). The fact that enantiomers have unique actions but identical physical properties indicates that properties other than bulk solubility are important in determining anesthetic action. This realization has focused thinking on identification of specific protein binding sites for anesthetics.

One impediment to understanding the mechanisms of anesthesia has been the difficulty in precisely defining anesthesia. A substantial body of work indicates that an anesthetic agent produces different components of the anesthetic state *via* actions at different anatomic loci in the nervous system and may produce these component effects *via* different cellular and molecular actions. Moreover, increasing evidence supports the hypothesis that different anesthetic agents produce specific components of anesthesia *via* actions at different molecular targets. Given these insights, the unitary theory of anesthesia has been largely discarded.

Anatomic Sites of Anesthetic Action. In principle, general anesthetics could interrupt nervous system function at myriad levels, including peripheral sensory neurons, the spinal cord, the brainstem, and the cerebral cortex. Delineation of the precise anatomic sites of action is difficult because many anesthetics diffusely inhibit electrical activity in the CNS. For example, isoflurane at 2 MAC can cause electrical silence in the brain (Newberg *et al.,* 1983). Despite this, *in vitro* studies have shown that specific cortical pathways exhibit markedly different sensitivities to both inhalational and intravenous anesthetics (MacIver and Roth, 1988; Nicoll, 1972). This suggests that anesthetics may produce specific components of the anesthetic state *via* actions at specific sites in the CNS. Consistent with this possibility, studies show that inhalational anesthetics produce immobilization in response to a surgical incision (the end point used in determining MAC) by action on the spinal cord (Rampil, 1994; Antognini and Schwartz, 1993). Given that amnesia or unconsciousness cannot result from anesthetic actions in the spinal cord, different components of anesthesia are produced at different sites in the CNS. Indeed, recent studies show that the sedative effects of *pentobarbital* and propofol (GABAergic anesthetics) are mediated by GABA$_A$ receptors in the tuberomammillary nucleus (Nelson *et al.,* 2002), and the sedative effects of the intravenous anesthetic *dexmedetomidine* (an α_2 adrenergic-receptor agonist) are produced *via* actions in the locus ceruleus (Mizobe *et al.,* 1996). These findings suggest that the sedative actions of some anesthetics share the neuronal pathways involved in endogenous sleep. While the sites at which other intravenous and inhalational anesthetics produce unconsciousness have not been identified, inhalational anesthetics depress the excitability of thalamic neurons (Ries and Puil,

1999). This suggests the thalamus as a potential locus for the sedative effects of inhalational anesthetics, since blockade of thalamocortical communication would produce unconsciousness. Finally, both intravenous and inhalational anesthetics depress hippocampal neurotransmission (Kendig *et al.,* 1991), a probable locus for their amnestic effects.

Cellular Mechanisms of Anesthesia. General anesthetics produce two important physiologic effects at the cellular level. First, the inhalational anesthetics can hyperpolarize neurons (Nicoll and Madison, 1982). This may be an important effect on neurons serving a pacemaker role and on pattern-generating circuits. It also may be important in synaptic communication, since reduced excitability in a postsynaptic neuron may diminish the likelihood that an action potential will be initiated in response to neurotransmitter release. Second, at anesthetizing concentrations, both inhalational and intravenous anesthetics have substantial effects on synaptic transmission and much smaller effects on action-potential generation or propagation (Larrabee and Posternak, 1952). The inhalational anesthetics inhibit excitatory synapses and enhance inhibitory synapses in various preparations. It seems likely that these effects are produced by both pre- and postsynaptic actions of the inhalational anesthetics. The inhalational anesthetic isoflurane clearly can inhibit neurotransmitter release (Perouansky *et al.,* 1995; MacIver *et al.,* 1996), while the small reduction in presynaptic action potential amplitude produced by isoflurane (3% reduction at MAC concentration) substantially inhibits neurotransmitter release (Wu *et al.,* 2004b). The latter effect occurs because the reduction in the presynaptic action potential is amplified into a much larger reduction in presynaptic Ca^{2+} influx, which in turn is amplified into an even greater reduction in transmitter release. This effect may account for the majority of the reduction in transmitter release by inhalational anesthetics at some excitatory synapses. Inhalational anesthetics also can act postsynaptically, altering the response to released neurotransmitter. These actions are thought to be due to specific interactions of anesthetic agents with neurotransmitter receptors.

The intravenous anesthetics produce a narrower range of physiological effects. Their predominant actions are at the synapse, where they have profound and relatively specific effects on the postsynaptic response to released neurotransmitter. Most of the intravenous agents act predominantly by enhancing inhibitory neurotransmission, whereas ketamine predominantly inhibits excitatory neurotransmission at glutamatergic synapses.

Molecular Actions of General Anesthetics. The electrophysiological effects of general anesthetics at the cellular level suggest several potential molecular targets for anesthetic action. There is strong evidence that ligand-gated ion channels are important targets for anesthetic action. Chloride channels gated by the inhibitory GABA$_A$ receptors (*see* Chapters 12 and 16) are sensitive to clinical concentrations of a wide variety of anesthetics, including the halogenated inhalational agents and many intravenous agents (propofol, barbiturates, etomidate, and neurosteroids) (Krasowski and Harrison, 1999). At clinical concentrations, general anesthetics increase the sensitivity of the GABA$_A$ receptor to GABA, thus enhancing inhibitory neurotransmission and depressing nervous system activity. The action of anesthetics on the GABA$_A$ receptor probably is mediated by binding of the anesthetics to specific sites on the GABA$_A$-receptor protein, since point mutations of the receptor can eliminate the effects of the anesthetic on ion channel function (Mihic *et al.,* 1997). There likely are specific binding sites for at least several classes of anesthetics, as mutations in various regions (and subunits) of the GABA$_A$ receptor selectively affect the actions of various anesthetics (Belelli *et al.*, 1997; Krasowski and Harrison, 1999). Notably, none of the general anesthetics competes with GABA for its binding site on the receptor. The capacity of propofol and etomidate to inhibit the response to noxious stimuli is mediated by a specific site on the β_3 subunit of the GABA$_A$ receptor (Jurd *et al.*, 2003), whereas the sedative effects of these anesthetics are mediated by the same site on the β_2 subunit (Reynolds *et al.*, 2003). These results indicate that two components of anesthesia *can* be mediated by GABA$_A$ receptors; for anesthetics other than propofol and etomidate, which components of anesthesia *are* produced by actions on GABA$_A$ receptors remains a matter of conjecture.

Structurally closely related to the GABA$_A$ receptors are other ligand-gated ion channels including glycine receptors and neuronal nicotinic acetylcholine receptors. Glycine receptors may play a role in mediating inhibition by anesthetics of responses to noxious stimuli. Clinical concentrations of inhalational anesthetics enhance the capacity of glycine to activate glycine-gated chloride channels (glycine receptors), which play an important role in inhibitory neurotransmission in the spinal cord and brainstem. Propofol (Hales and Lambert, 1988), neurosteroids, and barbiturates also potentiate glycine-activated currents, whereas etomidate and ketamine do not (Mascia *et al.*, 1996). Subanesthetic concentrations of the inhalational anesthetics inhibit some classes of neuronal nicotinic acetylcholine receptors (Violet *et al.*, 1997; Flood *et al.*, 1997). However, these actions do not appear to mediate anesthetic immobilization (Eger *et al.*, 2002); rather, neuronal nicotinic receptors could mediate other components of anesthesia such as analgesia or amnesia.

The only general anesthetics that do not have significant effects on GABA$_A$ or glycine receptors are ketamine, nitrous oxide, cyclopropane, and *xenon*. These agents inhibit a different type of ligand-gated ion channel, the *N*-methyl-D-aspartate (NMDA) receptor (*see* Chapter 12). NMDA receptors are glutamate-gated cation channels that are somewhat selective for calcium and are involved in long-term modulation of synaptic responses (long-term potentiation) and glutamate-mediated neurotoxicity. Ketamine inhibits NMDA receptors by binding to the *phencyclidine* site on the NMDA-receptor protein (Anis *et al.*, 1983), and the NMDA receptor is thought to be the principal molecular target for ketamine's anesthetic actions. Nitrous oxide (Mennerick *et al.*, 1998; Jevtovic-Todorovic *et al.*, 1998), cyclopropane (Raines *et al.*, 2001), and xenon (Franks *et al.*, 1998; de Sousa *et al.*, 2000) are potent and selective inhibitors of NMDA-activated currents, suggesting that these agents also may produce unconsciousness *via* actions on NMDA receptors.

Inhalational anesthetics have two other known molecular targets that may mediate some of their actions. Halogenated inhalational anesthetics activate some members of a class of K$^+$ channels known as two-pore domain channels (Gray *et al.*, 1998; Patel *et al.*, 1999); other two-pore domain channel family members are activated by xenon, nitrous oxide, and cyclopropane (Gruss *et al.*, 2004). These channels are important in setting the resting membrane potential of neurons and may be the molecular locus through which these agents hyperpolarize neurons. A second target is the molecular machinery involved in neurotransmitter release. In *Caenorhabditis elegans,* the action of inhalational anesthetics requires a protein complex (syntaxin, SNAP-25, synaptobrevin) involved in synaptic neurotransmitter release (van Swinderen *et al.*, 1999). These molecular interactions may explain in part the capacity of inhalational anesthetics to cause presynaptic inhibition in the hippocampus and could contribute to the amnesic effect of inhalational anesthetics.

Summary. Current evidence supports the view that most intravenous general anesthetics act predominantly through GABA$_A$ receptors and perhaps through some interactions with other ligand-gated ion channels. The halogenated inhalational agents have a variety of molecular targets, consistent with their status as complete (all components) anesthetics. Nitrous oxide, ketamine, and xenon constitute a third category of general anesthetics that are likely to produce unconsciousness *via* inhibition of the NMDA receptor and/or activation of two-pore-domain K$^+$ channels. The molecular mechanisms of general anesthetics are reviewed by Rudolph and Antkowiak (2004).

PARENTERAL ANESTHETICS

Pharmacokinetic Principles

Parenteral anesthetics are small, hydrophobic, substituted aromatic or heterocyclic compounds (Figure 13–1). Hydrophobicity is the key factor governing their pharmacokinetics (Shafer and Stanski, 1992). After a single intravenous bolus, these drugs preferentially partition into the highly perfused and lipophilic tissues of the brain and spinal cord where they produce anesthesia within a single circulation time. Subsequently blood levels fall rapidly, resulting in drug redistribution out of the CNS back into the blood. The anesthetic then diffuses into less perfused

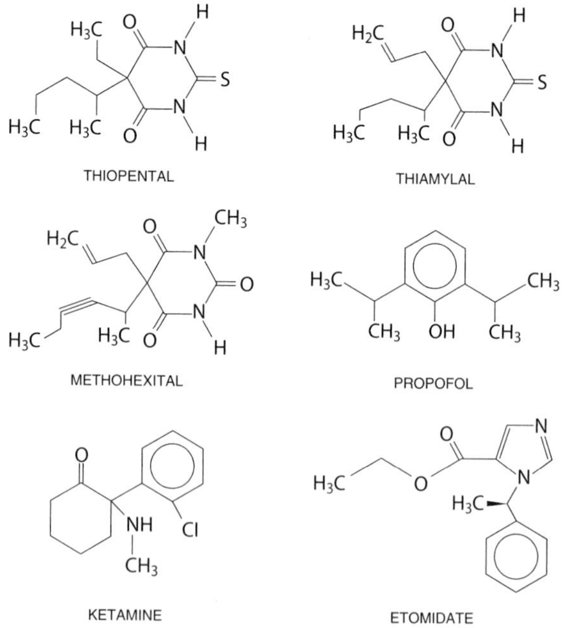

Figure 13–1. Structures of parenteral anesthetics.

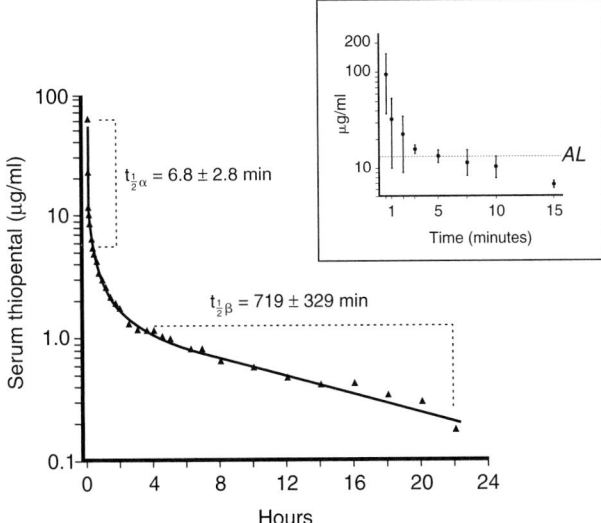

Figure 13–2. Thiopental serum levels after a single intravenous induction dose. Thiopental serum levels after a bolus can be described by two time constants, $t_{\frac{1}{2}}\alpha$ and $t_{\frac{1}{2}}\beta$. The initial fall is rapid ($t_{\frac{1}{2}}\alpha$ <10 min) and is due to redistribution of drug from the plasma and the highly perfused brain and spinal cord into less well-perfused tissues such as muscle and fat. During this redistribution phase, serum thiopental concentration falls to levels at which patients awaken (AL, awakening level; *see* inset—the average thiopental serum concentration in 12 patients after a 6-mg/kg intravenous bolus of thiopental). Subsequent metabolism and elimination is much slower and is characterized by a half-life ($t_{\frac{1}{2}}\beta$) of more than 10 hours. (Adapted with permission from Burch and Stanski, 1983.)

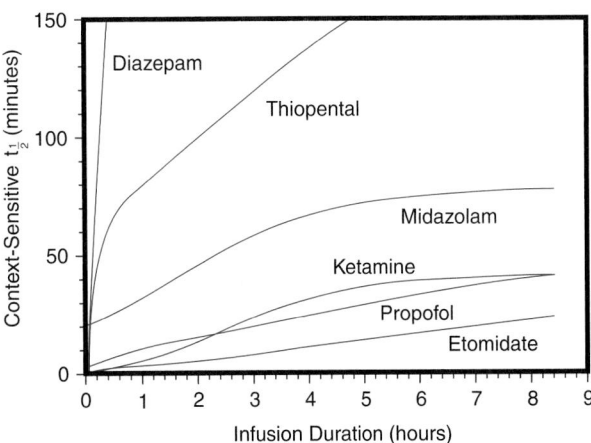

Figure 13–3. Context-sensitive half-time of general anesthetics. The duration of action of single intravenous doses of anesthetic/hypnotic drugs is similarly short for all and is determined by redistribution of the drugs away from their active sites (*see* Figure 13–2). However, after prolonged infusions, drug half-lives and durations of action are dependent on a complex interaction between the rate of redistribution of the drug, the amount of drug accumulated in fat, and the drug's metabolic rate. This phenomenon has been termed the *context-sensitive half-time*; that is, the half-time of a drug can be estimated only if one knows the context—the total dose and over what time period it has been given. Note that the half-times of some drugs such as etomidate, propofol, and ketamine increase only modestly with prolonged infusions; others (*e.g.,* diazepam and thiopental) increase dramatically. (Reproduced with permission from Reves *et al.,* 1994.)

tissues such as muscle and viscera, and at a slower rate into the poorly perfused but very hydrophobic adipose tissue. Termination of anesthesia after single boluses of parenteral anesthetics primarily reflects redistribution out of the CNS rather than metabolism (Figure 13–2). After redistribution, anesthetic blood levels fall according to a complex interaction between the metabolic rate and the amount and lipophilicity of the drug stored in the peripheral compartments (Hughes *et al.,* 1992; Shafer and Stanski, 1992). Thus, parenteral anesthetic half-lives are "context-sensitive," and the degree to which a half-life is contextual varies greatly from drug to drug, as might be predicted based on their differing hydrophobicities and metabolic clearances (Table 13–2 and Figure 13–3). For example, after a single bolus of thiopental, patients usually emerge from anesthesia within 10 minutes; however, a patient may require more than a day to awaken from a prolonged thiopental infusion. Most individual variability in sensitivity to parenteral anesthetics can be accounted for by pharmacokinetic factors (Wada *et al.,* 1997). For

example, in patients with lower cardiac output, the relative perfusion of and fraction of anesthetic dose delivered to the brain is higher; thus, patients in septic shock or with cardiomyopathy usually require lower doses of anesthetic. The elderly also typically require a smaller anesthetic dose, primarily because of a smaller initial volume of distribution (Homer and Stanski, 1985). As described below, similar principles govern the pharmacokinetics of the hydrophobic inhalational anesthetics, with the added complexity of drug uptake by inhalation.

SPECIFIC PARENTERAL AGENTS

Barbiturates

Chemistry and Formulations. Anesthetic barbiturates are derivatives of barbituric acid (2,4,6-trioxohexahydropyrimidine), with either an oxygen or sulfur at the 2-position (Figure 13–1). The three barbiturates used for clinical anesthesia are *sodium thiopental, thia-*

Table 13–2
Pharmacological Properties of Parenteral Anesthetics

DRUG	FORMULATION	IV INDUCTION DOSE (mg/kg)	MINIMAL HYPNOTIC LEVEL (μg/ml)	INDUCTION DOSE DURATION (min)	$T_{\frac{1}{2}\beta}$ (hours)	CL (ml·min⁻¹·kg⁻¹)	PROTEIN BINDING (%)	V_{SS} (L/kg)
Thiopental	25 mg/ml in aqueous solution + 1.5 mg/ml Na_2CO_3; pH = 10–11	3–5	15.6	5–8	12.1	3.4	85	2.3
Methohexital	10 mg/ml in aqueous solution + 1.5 mg/ml Na_2CO_3; pH = 10–11	1–2	10	4–7	3.9	10.9	85	2.2
Propofol	10 mg/ml in 10% soybean oil, 2.25% glycerol, 1.2% egg PL, 0.005% EDTA or 0.025% Na-MBS; pH = 4.5–7	1.5–2.5	1.1	4–8	1.8	30	98	2.3
Etomidate	2 mg/ml in 35% PG; pH = 6.9	0.2–0.4	0.3	4–8	2.9	17.9	76	2.5
Ketamine	10, 50, or 100 mg/ml in aqueous solution; pH = 3.5–5.5	0.5–1.5	1	10–15	3.0	19.1	27	3.1

SOURCES: Thiopental: Clarke *et al.*, 1968; Burch and Stanski, 1983; Hudson *et al.*, 1983; Hung *et al.*, 1992; methohexital: Brand *et al.*, 1963; Clarke *et al.*, 1968; Kay and Stephenson, 1981; Hudson *et al.*, 1983; McMurray *et al.*, 1986; propofol: Kirkpatrick *et al.*, 1988; Langley and Heel, 1988; Shafer *et al.*, 1988; etomidate: Doenicke, 1974; Meuldermans and Heykants, 1976; Fragen *et al.*, 1983; ketamine: Hebron *et al.*, 1983; Chang and Glazko, 1974; Clements and Nimmo, 1981; White *et al.*, 1982; Dayton *et al.*, 1983. ABBREVIATIONS: $t_{\frac{1}{2}\beta}$, β phase half-life; *CL*, clearance; *Vss*, volume of distribution at steady state; EDTA, ethylenediaminetetraacetic acid; Na-MBS, Na-metabisulfite; PG, propylene glycol; PL, phospholipid.

mylal, and *methohexital.* Sodium thiopental (PENTOTHAL) has been used most frequently for inducing anesthesia. The barbiturate anesthetics are supplied as racemic mixtures despite enantioselectivity in their anesthetic potency (Andrews and Mark, 1982). Barbiturates are formulated as the sodium salts with 6% sodium carbonate and reconstituted in water or isotonic saline to produce 1% (methohexital), 2% (thiamylal), or 2.5% (thiopental) alkaline solutions with pHs of 10 to 11. Once reconstituted, thiobarbiturates are stable in solution for up to 1 week, methohexital for up to 6 weeks if refrigerated. *Mixing with more acidic drugs commonly used during anesthetic induction can result in precipitation of the barbiturate as the free acid; thus, standard practice is to delay the administration of other drugs until the barbiturate has cleared the intravenous tubing.*

Dosages and Clinical Use.
Recommended intravenous dosing for parenteral anesthetics in a healthy young adult is given in Table 13–2.

The typical induction dose (3 to 5 mg/kg) of thiopental produces unconsciousness in 10 to 30 seconds with a peak effect in 1 minute and duration of anesthesia of 5 to 8 minutes. Neonates and infants usually require a higher induction dose (5 to 8 mg/kg), whereas elderly and pregnant patients require less (1 to 3 mg/kg) (Homer and Stanski 1985; Jonmarker *et al.*, 1987; Gin *et al.*, 1997). Dosage calculation based on lean body mass reduces individual variation in dosage requirements. Doses can be reduced by 10% to 50% after premedication with benzodiazepines, opiates, or α_2 adrenergic agonists, because of their additive hypnotic effect (Short *et al.*, 1991; Nishina *et al.*, 1994; Wang *et al.*, 1996). Thiamylal is approximately equipotent with and in all aspects similar to thiopental. Methohexital (BREVITAL) is threefold more potent but otherwise similar to thiopental in onset and duration of action. Thiopental and thiamylal produce little to no pain on injection; methohexital elicits mild pain. Veno-irritation can be reduced by injection into larger non-hand veins and by prior intravenous injection of lidocaine (0.5 to 1 mg/kg). Intra-arterial injection of thiobarbiturates can induce a severe inflammatory and potentially necrotic reaction and should be avoided. Thiopental often evokes the taste of garlic just prior to inducing anesthesia. Methohexital and to a lesser degree the other barbiturates can produce excitement phenomena such as muscle tremor, hypertonus, and hiccups. For induction of pediatric patients without IV access, all three drugs can be given per rectum at approximately tenfold the IV dose.

Pharmacokinetics and Metabolism.
Pharmacokinetic parameters for parenteral anesthetics are given in Table 13–2. As discussed above, the principal mechanism limiting anesthetic duration after single doses is redistribution of these hydrophobic drugs from the brain to other tissues. However, after multiple doses or infusions, the duration of action of the barbiturates varies considerably depending on their clearances.

Methohexital differs from the other two intravenous barbiturates in its much more rapid clearance; thus, it accumulates less during prolonged infusions (Schwilden and Stoeckel, 1990). Because of their slow elimination and large volumes of distribution, prolonged infusions or very large doses of thiopental and thiamylal can produce unconsciousness lasting several days. Even single induction doses of thiopental and to a lesser degree methohexital can produce psychomotor impairment lasting up to 8 hours (Korttila *et al.*, 1975; Beskow *et al.*, 1995). Methohexital had been used frequently for outpatient procedures for which rapid return to an alert state is particularly desirable, but for this use it now has been largely replaced by propofol (*see* below). All three barbiturates are primarily eliminated by hepatic metabolism and renal excretion of inactive metabolites; a small fraction of thiopental undergoes desulfuration to the longer-acting hypnotic pentobarbital (Chan *et al.*, 1985). Each drug is highly protein bound (Table 13–2). Hepatic disease or other conditions that reduce serum protein concentration will decrease the volume of distribution and thereby increase the initial free concentration and hypnotic effect of an induction dose.

Side Effects. *Nervous System.*
Besides producing a general anesthesia, barbiturates reduce the cerebral metabolic rate, as measured by cerebral oxygen consumption ($CMRO_2$), in a dose-dependent manner. Induction doses of thiopental reduce $CMRO_2$ by 25% to 30% with a maximal decrease of 55% occurring at two to five times that dose (Stullken *et al.*, 1977). As a consequence of the decrease in $CMRO_2$, cerebral blood flow and intracranial pressure are similarly reduced (Shapiro *et al.*, 1973).

Because it markedly lowers cerebral metabolism, thiopental has been used as a protectant against cerebral ischemia. At least one human study suggests that thiopental may be efficacious in ameliorating ischemic damage in the perioperative setting (Nussmeier *et al.*, 1986). Thiopental also reduces intraocular pressure (Joshi and Bruce, 1975). Presumably in part due to their CNS depressant activity, barbiturates are effective anticonvulsants. Thiopental in particular is a proven medication in the treatment of status epilepticus (Modica *et al.*, 1990).

Cardiovascular.
The anesthetic barbiturates produce dose-dependent decreases in blood pressure. The effect is due primarily to vasodilation, particularly venodilation, and to a lesser degree to a direct decrease in cardiac contractility. Typically, heart rate increases as a compensatory response to a lower blood pressure, although barbiturates also blunt the baroreceptor reflex.

Hypotension can be severe in patients with an impaired ability to compensate for venodilation such as those with hypovolemia, cardiomyopathy, valvular heart disease, coronary artery disease, cardiac tamponade, or β adrenergic blockade. Thiopental is not contraindicated in patients with coronary artery disease because the ratio of myocardial oxygen supply to demand appears to be adequately maintained within a patient's normal blood pressure range (Reiz *et al.*, 1981). None of the barbiturates has been shown to be arrhythmogenic.

Respiratory.
Barbiturates are respiratory depressants. Induction doses of thiopental decrease minute ventilation and tidal volume with a smaller and inconsistent decrease in respiratory rate (Grounds *et al.*, 1987); reflex responses

to hypercarbia and hypoxia are diminished by anesthetic barbiturates (Hirshman *et al.*, 1975), and at higher doses or in the presence of other respiratory depressants such as opiates, apnea can result. With the exception of uncommon anaphylactoid reactions, these drugs have little effect on bronchomotor tone and can be used safely in asthmatics (Kingston and Hirshman, 1984).

Other Side Effects. Short-term administration of barbiturates has no clinically significant effect on the hepatic, renal, or endocrine systems. A single induction dose of thiopental does not alter tone of the gravid uterus, but may produce mild transient depression of newborn activity (Kosaka *et al.*, 1969). True allergies to barbiturates are rare (Baldo *et al.*, 1991); however, direct drug-induced histamine release is occasionally seen (Sprung *et al.*, 1997). Barbiturates can induce fatal attacks of porphyria in patients with acute intermittent or variegate porphyria and are contraindicated in such patients. Unlike inhalational anesthetics and succinylcholine, barbiturates and all other parenteral anesthetics apparently do not trigger malignant hyperthermia (Rosenberg *et al.*, 1997).

Propofol

Chemistry and Formulations. Propofol now is the most commonly used parenteral anesthetic in the United States. The active ingredient in propofol, 2,6-diisopropylphenol, is essentially insoluble in aqueous solutions and is formulated only for IV administration as a 1% (10 mg/ml) emulsion in 10% soybean oil, 2.25% glycerol, and 1.2% purified egg phosphatide. In the United States, disodium EDTA (0.05 mg/ml) or sodium metabisulfite (0.25 mg/ml) is added to inhibit bacterial growth. Nevertheless, significant bacterial contamination of open containers has been associated with serious patient infection; propofol should be either administered or discarded shortly after removal from sterile packaging.

Dosage and Clinical Use. The induction dose of propofol (DIPRIVAN) in a healthy adult is 1.5 to 2.5 mg/kg and it has an onset and duration of anesthesia similar to thiopental (Table 13–2). As with barbiturates, dosages should be reduced in the elderly and in the presence of other sedatives and increased in young children. Because of its reasonably short elimination half-life, propofol often is used for maintenance of anesthesia as well as for induction. For short procedures, small boluses (10% to 50% of the induction dose) every 5 minutes or as needed are effective. An infusion of propofol produces a more stable drug level (100 to 300 μg/kg per minute) and is better suited for longer-term anesthetic maintenance. Infusion rates should be tailored to patient response and the levels of other hypnotics. Sedating doses of propofol are 20% to 50% of those required for general anesthesia. However, even at these lower doses, caregivers should be vigilant and prepared for all of the side effects of propofol discussed below, particularly airway obstruction and apnea. Propofol elicits pain on injection that can be reduced with

lidocaine and the use of larger arm and antecubital veins. Excitatory phenomena during induction with propofol occur at about the same frequency as with thiopental, but much less frequently than with methohexital (Langley and Heel, 1988).

Pharmacokinetics and Metabolism. The pharmacokinetics of propofol are governed by the same principles that apply to barbiturates. Onset and duration of anesthesia after a single bolus are similar to thiopental (Langley and Heel, 1988). Recovery after multiple doses or infusion has been shown to be much faster after propofol than after thiopental or even methohexital (Doze *et al.*, 1986; Langley and Heel, 1988).

Propofol's shorter duration after infusion can be explained by its very high clearance, coupled with the slow diffusion of drug from the peripheral to the central compartment (Figure 13–3). The rapid clearance of propofol explains its less severe hangover compared with barbiturates, and may allow for a more rapid discharge from the recovery room. Propofol is metabolized in the liver to less active metabolites that are renally excreted (Simons *et al.*, 1988); however, its clearance exceeds hepatic blood flow, and anhepatic metabolism has been demonstrated (Veroli *et al.*, 1992). Propofol is highly protein bound, and its pharmacokinetics, like those of the barbiturates, may be affected by conditions that alter serum protein levels (Kirkpatrick *et al.*, 1988).

Side Effects. Nervous System. The CNS effects of propofol are similar to those of barbiturates.

Propofol decreases $CMRO_2$, cerebral blood flow, and intracranial and intraocular pressures by about the same amount as thiopental (Langley and Heel, 1988). Like thiopental, propofol has been used in patients at risk for cerebral ischemia (Ravussin and de Tribolet, 1993); however, no human outcome studies have been performed to determine its efficacy as a neuroprotectant. Results from studies on the anticonvulsant effects of propofol have been mixed; some data even suggest it has proconvulsant activity when combined with other drugs (Modica *et al.*, 1990). Thus, unlike thiopental, propofol is not a proven acute intervention for seizures.

Cardiovascular. Propofol produces a dose-dependent decrease in blood pressure that is significantly greater than that produced by thiopental (Grounds *et al.*, 1985; Langley and Heel 1988). The fall in blood pressure can be explained by both vasodilation and mild depression of myocardial contractility (Grounds *et al.*, 1985). Propofol appears to blunt the baroreceptor reflex or is directly vagotonic because smaller increases in heart rate are seen for any given drop in blood pressure after doses of propofol (Langley and Heel, 1988). As with thiopental, propofol should be used with caution in patients at risk for or intolerant of decreases in blood pressure.

Respiratory and Other Side Effects. At equipotent doses, propofol produces a slightly greater degree of respiratory depression than thiopental (Blouin *et al.*, 1991). Patients given propofol should be monitored to ensure adequate oxygenation and ventilation. Propofol appears to be less likely than barbiturates to provoke bronchospasm (Pizov *et al.*, 1995). It has no clinically significant effects on hepatic, renal, or endocrine organ systems. Unlike thiopental, propofol appears to have significant anti-emetic action and is a good choice for sedation or anesthesia of patients at high risk for nausea and vomiting (McCollum *et al.*, 1988). Propofol provokes anaphylactoid reactions and histamine release at about the same low frequency as thiopental (Laxenaire *et al.*, 1992). Although propofol does cross placental membranes, it is considered safe for use in pregnant women, and like thiopental, only transiently depresses activity in the newborn (Abboud *et al.*, 1995).

Etomidate

Chemistry and Formulation. Etomidate is a substituted imidazole that is supplied as the active D-isomer (Figure 13–1). Etomidate is poorly soluble in water and is formulated as a 2 mg/ml solution in 35% propylene glycol. Unlike thiopental, etomidate does not induce precipitation of neuromuscular blockers or other drugs frequently given during anesthetic induction.

Dosage and Clinical Use. Etomidate (AMIDATE) is primarily used for anesthetic induction of patients at risk for hypotension.

Induction doses of etomidate (0.2 to 0.4 mg/kg) have a rapid onset and short duration of action (Table 13–2) and are accompanied by a high incidence of pain on injection and myoclonic movements. Lidocaine effectively reduces the pain of injection (Galloway *et al.*, 1982), while myoclonic movements can be reduced by premedication with either benzodiazepines or opiates. Etomidate is pharmacokinetically suitable for infusion for anesthetic maintenance (10 µg/kg per minute) or sedation (5 µg/kg per minute); however, long-term infusions are not recommended for reasons discussed below. Etomidate also may be given rectally (6.5 mg/kg) with an onset of about 5 minutes.

Pharmacokinetics and Metabolism. An induction dose of etomidate has a rapid onset; redistribution limits the duration of action (Table 13–2). Metabolism occurs in the liver, primarily to inactive compounds (Heykants *et al.*, 1975; Gooding and Corssen, 1976). Elimination is both renal (78%) and biliary (22%). Compared to thiopental, the duration of action of etomidate increases less with repeated doses (Figure 13–3). The plasma protein binding of etomidate is high but less than that of barbiturates and propofol (Table 13–2).

Side Effects. Nervous System. The effects of etomidate on cerebral blood flow, metabolism, and intracranial and intraocular pressures are similar to those of thiopental

(Modica *et al.*, 1992). Etomidate has been used as a protectant against cerebral ischemia; however, animal studies have failed to show a consistent beneficial effect (Drummond *et al.*, 1995), and no controlled human trials have been performed. Etomidate has been shown in some studies to be a proconvulsant and is not a proven treatment for seizures (Modica *et al.*, 1990).

Cardiovascular. Cardiovascular stability after induction is a major advantage of etomidate over either barbiturates or propofol. Induction doses of etomidate typically produce a small increase in heart rate and little or no decrease in blood pressure or cardiac output (Criado *et al.*, 1980). Etomidate has little effect on coronary perfusion pressure while reducing myocardial oxygen consumption (Kettler *et al.*, 1974). Thus, of all induction agents, etomidate is best suited to maintain cardiovascular stability in patients with coronary artery disease, cardiomyopathy, cerebral vascular disease, or hypovolemia.

Respiratory and Other Side Effects. The degree of respiratory depression due to etomidate appears to be less than that due to thiopental (Morgan *et al.*, 1977). Like methohexital, etomidate may induce hiccups but does not significantly stimulate histamine release. Despite minimal cardiac and respiratory effects, etomidate does have two major drawbacks. First, etomidate has been associated with nausea and vomiting (Fragen *et al.*, 1979). Second, etomidate inhibits adrenal biosynthetic enzymes required for the production of cortisol and some other steroids, possibly inhibiting the adrenocortical stress response (Ledingham *et al.*, 1983). Even single induction doses of etomidate may mildly and transiently reduce cortisol levels (Wagner *et al.*, 1984), but no significant differences in outcome after short-term administration have been found, even for variables specifically known to be associated with adrenocortical suppression (Wagner *et al.*, 1984). Thus, while etomidate is not recommended for long-term infusion, it appears safe for anesthetic induction and has some unique advantages in patients prone to hemodynamic instability.

Ketamine

Chemistry and Formulation. Ketamine is an arylcyclohexylamine, a congener of phencyclidine (Figure 13–1). It is supplied as a racemic mixture even though the S-isomer is more potent with fewer side effects (White *et al.*, 1982). Although more lipophilic than thiopental, ketamine is water soluble and available as 10-, 50-, and 100-mg/ml solutions in sodium chloride plus the preservative benzethonium chloride.

Dosage and Clinical Use. Ketamine (KETALAR, others) has unique properties that make it useful for anesthetizing patients at risk for hypotension and bronchospasm and for certain pediatric procedures. However, significant side effects limit its routine use. Ketamine rapidly produces a hypnotic state quite distinct from that of other anesthetics. Patients have profound analgesia, unresponsiveness to commands, and amnesia, but may have their eyes open, move their limbs involuntarily, and breathe spontaneously. This cataleptic state has been termed *dissociative anesthesia.*

Ketamine typically is administered intravenously but also is effective by intramuscular, oral, and rectal routes. The induction doses are 0.5 to 1.5 mg/kg IV, 4 to 6 mg/kg IM, and 8 to 10 mg/kg PR (White *et al.*, 1982). Onset of action after an intravenous dose is similar to that of the other parenteral anesthetics, but the duration of anesthesia of a single dose is longer (Table 13–2). For anesthetic maintenance, ketamine occasionally is continued as an infusion (25 to 100 μg/kg per minute) (White *et al.*, 1982). Ketamine does not elicit pain on injection or true excitatory behavior as described for methohexital, although involuntary movements produced by ketamine can be mistaken for anesthetic excitement.

Pharmacokinetics and Metabolism. The onset and duration of an induction dose of ketamine are determined by the same distribution/redistribution mechanism operant for all the other parenteral anesthetics.

Ketamine is hepatically metabolized to norketamine, which has reduced CNS activity; norketamine is further metabolized and excreted in urine and bile (Chang *et al.*, 1974). Ketamine has a large volume of distribution and rapid clearance that make it suitable for continuous infusion without the drastic lengthening in duration of action seen with thiopental (Table 13–2 and Figure 13–3). Protein binding is much lower with ketamine than with the other parenteral anesthetics (Table 13–2).

Side Effects. Nervous System. Ketamine has indirect sympathomimetic activity (White *et al.*, 1992). Ketamine's behavioral effects are distinct from those of other anesthetics. The ketamine-induced cataleptic state is accompanied by nystagmus with pupillary dilation, salivation, lacrimation, and spontaneous limb movements with increased overall muscle tone. Although ketamine does not produce the classic anesthetic state, patients are amnestic and unresponsive to painful stimuli. Ketamine produces profound analgesia, a distinct advantage over other parenteral anesthetics (White *et al.*, 1982).

Unlike other parenteral anesthetics, ketamine increases cerebral blood flow and intracranial pressure (ICP) with minimal alteration of cerebral metabolism. These effects can be attenuated by concurrent administration of thiopental and/or benzodiazepines along with hyperventilation (Belopavlovic and Buchthal, 1982; Mayberg *et al.*, 1995). However, given that other anesthetics actually reduce ICP and cerebral metabolism, ketamine is relatively contraindicated for patients with increased intracranial pressure or those at risk for cerebral ischemia. In some

studies, ketamine increased intraocular pressure, and its use for induction of patients with open eye injuries is controversial (Whitacre and Ellis, 1984). The effects of ketamine on seizure activity appear mixed, without either strong pro- or anticonvulsant activity (Modica *et al.*, 1990). Emergence delirium characterized by hallucinations, vivid dreams, and illusions is a frequent complication of ketamine that can result in serious patient dissatisfaction and can complicate postoperative management (White *et al.*, 1982). Delirium symptoms are most frequent in the first hour after emergence and appear to occur less frequently in children (Sussman, 1974). Benzodiazepines reduce the incidence of emergence delirium (Dundee and Lilburn, 1978).

Cardiovascular. Unlike other anesthetics, induction doses of ketamine typically increase blood pressure, heart rate, and cardiac output. The cardiovascular effects are indirect and are most likely mediated by inhibition of both central and peripheral catecholamine reuptake (White *et al.*, 1982). Ketamine has direct negative inotropic and vasodilating activity, but these effects usually are overwhelmed by the indirect sympathomimetic action (Pagel *et al.*, 1992). Thus, ketamine is a useful drug, along with etomidate, for patients at risk for hypotension during anesthesia. While not arrhythmogenic, ketamine increases myocardial oxygen consumption and is not an ideal drug for patients at risk for myocardial ischemia (Reves *et al.*, 1978).

Respiratory. The respiratory effects of ketamine are perhaps the best indication for its use. Induction doses of ketamine produce small and transient decreases in minute ventilation, but respiratory depression is less severe than with other general anesthetics (White *et al.*, 1982). Ketamine is a potent bronchodilator due to its indirect sympathomimetic activity and perhaps some direct bronchodilating activity (Hirshman *et al.*, 1979). Thus, ketamine is particularly well-suited for anesthetizing patients at high risk for bronchospasm.

Summary of Parenteral Anesthetics

Parenteral anesthetics are the most common drugs used for anesthetic induction of adults. Their lipophilicity, coupled with the relatively high perfusion of the brain and spinal cord, results in rapid onset and short duration after a single bolus dose. However, these drugs ultimately accumulate in fatty tissue, prolonging recovery if multiple doses are given, particularly for drugs with lower rates of clearance. Each anesthetic has its own unique set of properties and side effects (summarized in Table 13–3). Thiopental and propofol are the two most commonly used

Table 13–3
Some Pharmacological Effects of Parenteral Anesthetics*

DRUG	CBF	CMRO$_2$	ICP	MAP	HR	CO	RR	$\dot{V}_E$
Thiopental	---	---	---	-	+	-	-	--
Etomidate	---	---	---	0	0	0	-	-
Ketamine	++	0	++	+	++	+	0	0
Propofol	---	---	---	--	+	-	--	---

ABBREVIATIONS: CBF, cerebral blood flow; CMRO$_2$, cerebral oxygen consumption; ICP, intracranial pressure; MAP, mean arterial pressure; HR, heart rate; CO, cardiac output; RR, respiratory rate; $\dot{V}_E$, minute ventilation. *Typical effects of a single induction dose in human beings; *see* text for references. Qualitative scale from --- to +++ = slight, moderate, or large decrease or increase, respectively; 0 indicates no significant change.

parenteral agents. Thiopental has a long-established track record of safety. Propofol is advantageous for procedures where rapid return to a preoperative mental status is desirable. Etomidate usually is reserved for patients at risk for hypotension and/or myocardial ischemia. Ketamine is best suited for patients with asthma or for children undergoing short, painful procedures.

INHALATIONAL ANESTHETICS

Introduction

A wide variety of gases and volatile liquids can produce anesthesia. The structures of the currently used inhalational anesthetics are shown in Figure 13–4. One of the troublesome properties of the inhalational anesthetics is their low safety margin. The inhalational anesthetics have therapeutic indices (LD$_{50}$/ED$_{50}$) that range from 2 to 4, making these among the most dangerous drugs in clinical use. The toxicity of these drugs is largely a function of their side effects, and each of the inhalational anesthetics has a unique side-effect profile. Hence, the selection of an inhalational anesthetic often is based on matching a patient's pathophysiology with drug side-effect profiles. The specific adverse effects of each of the inhalational anesthetics are emphasized in the following sections. The inhalational anesthetics also vary widely in their physical properties. Table 13–1 lists the important physical properties of the inhalational agents in clinical use. These properties are important because they govern the pharmacokinetics of the inhalational agents. Ideally, an inhalational agent would produce a rapid induction of anesthesia and a rapid recovery following discontinuation. The pharmacokinetics of the inhalational agents are reviewed in the following section.

Pharmacokinetic Principles

The inhalational agents are some of the very few pharmacological agents administered as gases. The fact that these agents behave as gases rather than as liquids requires that different pharmacokinetic constructs be used in analyzing their uptake and distribution. It is essential to understand that inhalational anesthetics distribute between tissues (or between blood and gas) such that equilibrium is achieved when the partial pressure of anesthetic gas is equal in the two tissues. When a person has breathed an inhalational anesthetic for a sufficiently long time that all tissues are

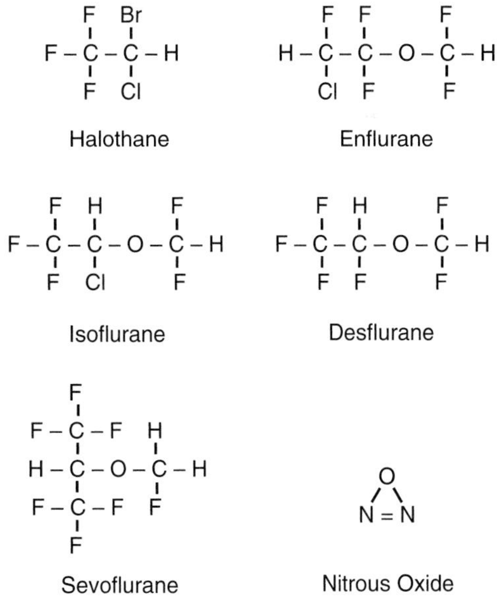

Figure 13–4. Structures of inhalational general anesthetics. Note that all inhalational general anesthetic agents except nitrous oxide and halothane are ethers and that fluorine progressively replaces other halogens in the development of the halogenated agents. All structural differences are associated with important differences in pharmacological properties.

equilibrated with the anesthetic, the partial pressure of the anesthetic in all tissues will be equal to the partial pressure of the anesthetic in inspired gas. It is important to note that while the partial pressure of the anesthetic may be equal in all tissues, the concentration of anesthetic in each tissue will be different. Indeed, anesthetic partition coefficients are defined as the ratio of anesthetic concentration in two tissues when the partial pressures of anesthetic are equal in the two tissues. Blood:gas, brain:blood, and fat:blood partition coefficients for the various inhalational agents are listed in Table 13–1. These partition coefficients show that inhalational anesthetics are more soluble in some tissues (*e.g.,* fat) than they are in others (*e.g.,* blood), and that there is significant range in the solubility of the various inhalational agents in such tissues.

In clinical practice, one can monitor the equilibration of a patient with anesthetic gas. Equilibrium is achieved when the partial pressure in inspired gas is equal to the partial pressure in end-tidal (alveolar) gas. This defines equilibrium because it is the point at which there is no net uptake of anesthetic from the alveoli into the blood. For inhalational agents that are not very soluble in blood or any other tissue, equilibrium is achieved quickly, as illustrated for nitrous oxide in Figure 13–5. If an agent is more soluble in a tissue such as fat, equilibrium may take many hours to reach. This occurs because fat represents a huge anesthetic reservoir that will be filled slowly because of the modest blood flow to fat. This is illustrated by the slow approach of halothane alveolar partial pressure to inspired partial pressure of halothane in Figure 13–5.

In considering the pharmacokinetics of anesthetics, one important parameter is the speed of anesthetic induction. Anesthesia is produced when anesthetic partial pressure in brain is equal to or greater than MAC. Because the brain is well perfused, anesthetic partial pressure in brain becomes equal to the partial pressure in alveolar gas (and in blood) over the course of several minutes. Therefore, anesthesia is achieved shortly after alveolar partial pressure reaches MAC. While the rate of rise of alveolar partial pressure will be slower for anesthetics that are highly soluble in blood and other tissues, this limitation on speed of induction can be overcome largely by delivering higher inspired partial pressures of the anesthetic.

Elimination of inhalational anesthetics is largely the reverse process of uptake. For agents with low blood and tissue solubility, recovery from anesthesia should mirror anesthetic induction, regardless of the duration of anesthetic administration. For inhalational agents with high blood and tissue solubility, recovery will be a function of the duration of anesthetic administration. This occurs because the accumulated amounts of anesthetic in the fat

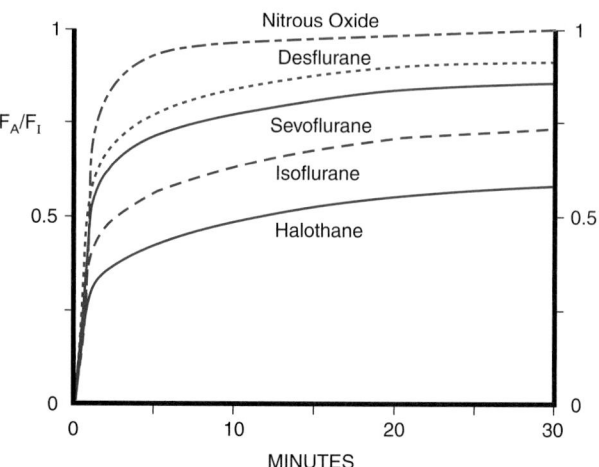

Figure 13–5. Uptake of inhalational general anesthetics. The rise in end-tidal alveolar (F_A) anesthetic concentration toward the inspired (F_I) concentration is most rapid with the least soluble anesthetics, nitrous oxide and desflurane, and slowest with the most soluble anesthetic, halothane. All data are from human studies. (Reproduced with permission from Eger, 2000.)

reservoir will prevent blood (and therefore alveolar) partial pressures from falling rapidly. Patients will be arousable when alveolar partial pressure reaches MAC_{awake}, a partial pressure somewhat lower than MAC (Table 13–1).

Halothane

Chemistry and Formulation. Halothane (FLUOTHANE) is 2-bromo-2-chloro-1,1,1-trifluoroethane (Figure 13–4). Halothane is a volatile liquid at room temperature and must be stored in a sealed container. Because halothane is a light-sensitive compound that also is subject to spontaneous breakdown, it is marketed in amber bottles with thymol added as a preservative. Mixtures of halothane with oxygen or air are neither flammable nor explosive.

Pharmacokinetics. Halothane has a relatively high blood:gas partition coefficient and high fat:blood partition coefficient (Table 13–1). Induction with halothane therefore is relatively slow, and the alveolar halothane concentration remains substantially lower than the inspired halothane concentration for many hours of administration. Because halothane is soluble in fat and other body tissues, it will accumulate during prolonged administration. Therefore, the speed of recovery from halothane is lengthened as a function of duration of administration.

Approximately 60% to 80% of halothane taken up by the body is eliminated unchanged *via* the lungs in the first 24 hours after its administration. A substantial amount of the halothane not eliminated in exhaled gas is biotransformed by hepatic CYPs. The major metabolite of halothane is trifluoroacetic acid, which is formed by removal of bromine and chlorine ions (Gruenke *et al.*, 1988). Trifluoroacetic acid, bromine, and chlorine all can be detected in the urine. Trifluoroacetylchloride, an intermediate in oxidative metabolism of halothane, can trifluoroacetylate several proteins in the liver. An immune reaction to these altered proteins may be responsible for the rare cases of fulminant halothane-induced hepatic necrosis (Kenna *et al.*, 1988). A minor reductive pathway accounts for approximately 1% of halothane metabolism that generally is observed only under hypoxic conditions (Van Dyke *et al.*, 1988).

Clinical Use. Halothane, introduced in 1956, was the first of the modern, halogenated inhalational anesthetics used in clinical practice. It is a potent agent that usually is used for maintenance of anesthesia. It is not pungent and is therefore well tolerated for inhalation induction of anesthesia. This is most commonly done in children, in whom preoperative placement of an intravenous catheter can be difficult. Anesthesia is produced by halothane at end-tidal concentrations of 0.7% to 1%. The use of halothane in the United States has diminished substantially in the past decade because of the introduction of newer inhalational agents with better pharmacokinetic and side-effect profiles. Halothane continues to be extensively used in children because it is well tolerated for inhalation induction and because the serious side effects appear to be diminished in children. Halothane has a low cost and therefore still is widely used in developing countries.

Side Effects. Cardiovascular System. The most predictable side effect of halothane is a dose-dependent reduction in arterial blood pressure. Mean arterial pressure typically decreases about 20% to 25% at MAC concentrations of halothane. This reduction in blood pressure primarily is the result of direct myocardial depression leading to reduced cardiac output (Figure 13–6). Myocardial depression is thought to result from attenuation of depolarization-induced intracellular calcium transients (Lynch, 1997). Halothane-induced hypotension usually is accompanied by either bradycardia or a normal heart rate. This absence of a tachycardic (or contractile) response to reduced blood pressure is thought to be due to an inability of the heart to respond to the effector arm of the baroreceptor reflex. Heart rate can be increased during halothane anesthesia by exogenous catecholamine or by sympathoadrenal stimulation. Halothane-induced reductions in blood pressure and heart rate generally disappear after several hours of constant halothane administration, presumably because of progressive sympathetic stimulation.

Halothane does not cause a significant change in systemic vascular resistance. Nonetheless, it does alter the resistance and autoregulation of specific vascular beds, leading to redistribution of blood flow. The vascular beds of the skin and brain are dilated directly by halothane, leading to increased cerebral blood flow and skin perfusion. Conversely, autoregulation of renal, splanchnic, and

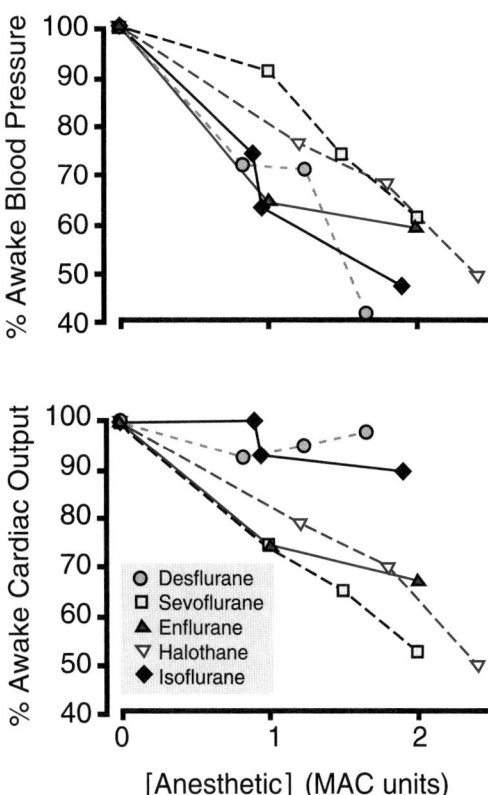

Figure 13–6. *Influence of inhalational general anesthetics on the systemic circulation.* While all of the inhalational anesthetics reduce systemic blood pressure in a dose-related manner (*top*), the lower figure shows that cardiac output is well preserved with isoflurane and desflurane, and therefore that the causes of hypotension vary with the agent. (Data are from human studies except for sevoflurane, where data are from swine; Bahlman *et al.*, 1972; Cromwell *et al.*, 1971; Weiskopf *et al.*, 1991; Calverley *et al.*, 1978; Stevens *et al.*, 1971; Eger *et al.*, 1970; Weiskopf *et al.*, 1988.)

cerebral blood flow is inhibited by halothane, leading to reduced perfusion of these organs in the face of reduced blood pressure. Coronary autoregulation is largely preserved during halothane anesthesia. Finally, halothane inhibits hypoxic pulmonary vasoconstriction, leading to increased perfusion to poorly ventilated regions of the lung and an increased alveolar:arterial oxygen gradient.

Halothane also has significant effects on cardiac rhythm. Sinus bradycardia and atrioventricular rhythms occur frequently during halothane anesthesia but usually are benign. These rhythms result mainly from a direct depressive effect of halothane on sinoatrial node discharge. Halothane also can sensitize the myocardium to the arrhythmogenic effects of epinephrine (Sumikawa *et al.*, 1983). Premature ventricular contractions and sustained ventricular tachycardia can be observed during halothane anesthesia when exogenous administration or endogenous adrenal production elevates plasma epinephrine levels. Epinephrine-induced arrhythmias during halothane anesthesia are thought to be mediated by a synergistic effect on α_1 and β_1 adrenergic receptors (Hayashi *et al.*, 1988).

Respiratory System. Spontaneous respiration is rapid and shallow during halothane anesthesia. The decreased alveolar ventilation results in an elevation in arterial CO_2 tension from 40 mm Hg to >50 mm Hg at 1 MAC (Figure 13–7). The elevated CO_2 does not provoke a compensatory increase in ventilation, because halothane causes a concentration-dependent inhibition of the ventilatory response to CO_2 (Knill and Gelb, 1978). This action of halothane is thought to be mediated by depression of central chemoceptor mechanisms. Halothane also inhibits peripheral chemoceptor responses to arterial hypoxemia. Thus, neither hemodynamic (tachycardia and hypertension) nor ventilatory responses to hypoxemia are observed during halothane anesthesia, making it prudent to monitor arterial oxygenation directly. Halothane also is an effective bronchodilator (Yamakage, 1992) and has been effectively used as a treatment of last resort in patients with status asthmaticus (Gold and Helrich, 1970).

Nervous System. Halothane dilates the cerebral vasculature, increasing cerebral blood flow under most conditions. This increase in blood flow can increase intracranial pressure in patients with space-occupying intracranial masses, brain edema, or preexisting intracranial hypertension. For this reason, halothane is relatively contraindicated in patients at risk for elevated intracranial pressure. Halothane also attenuates autoregulation of cerebral blood flow. For this reason, cerebral blood flow can decrease when arterial blood pressure is markedly decreased. Modest decreases in cerebral blood flow generally are well tolerated because halothane also reduces cerebral metabolic consumption of O_2.

Muscle. Halothane causes some relaxation of skeletal muscle *via* its central depressant effects. Halothane also potentiates the actions of nondepolarizing muscle relaxants (curariform drugs; *see* Chapter 9), increasing both their duration of action and the magnitude of their effect. Halothane and the other halogenated inhalational anesthetics can trigger malignant hyperthermia, a syndrome characterized by severe muscle contraction, rapid development of hyperthermia, and a massive increase in metabolic rate in genetically susceptible patients. This syndrome frequently is fatal and is treated by immediate discontinuation of the anesthetic and administration of dantrolene.

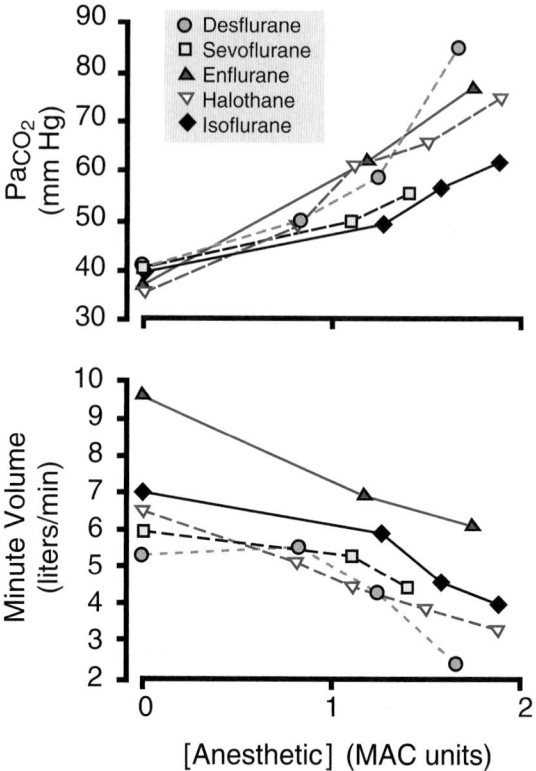

Figure 13–7. Respiratory effects of inhalational anesthetics. Spontaneous ventilation with all of the halogenated inhalational anesthetics reduces minute volume of ventilation in a dose-dependent manner (*lower panel*). This results in an increased arterial carbon dioxide tension (*top panel*). Differences among agents are modest. (Data from Doi and Ikada, 1987; Lockhart *et al.*, 1991; Munson *et al.*, 1966; Calverley *et al.*, 1978; Fourcade *et al.*, 1971.)

Uterine smooth muscle is relaxed by halothane. This is a useful property for manipulation of the fetus (version) in the prenatal period and for delivery of retained placenta postnatally. Halothane, however, inhibits uterine contractions during parturition, prolonging labor and increasing blood loss, and therefore is not used as an analgesic or anesthetic for labor and vaginal delivery.

Kidney. Patients anesthetized with halothane usually produce a small volume of concentrated urine. This is the consequence of halothane-induced reduction of renal blood flow and glomerular filtration rate, which may be reduced by 40% to 50% at 1 MAC. Halothane-induced changes in renal function are fully reversible and are not associated with long-term nephrotoxicity.

Liver and Gastrointestinal Tract. Halothane reduces splanchnic and hepatic blood flow as a consequence of reduced perfusion pressure, as discussed above. This reduced blood flow has not been shown to produce detrimental effects on hepatic or GI function.

Halothane can produce fulminant hepatic necrosis in a small number of patients. This syndrome generally is characterized by fever, anorexia, nausea, and vomiting, developing several days after anesthesia and can be accompanied by a rash and peripheral eosinophilia. There is a rapid progression to hepatic failure, with a fatality rate of approximately 50%. This syndrome occurs in about 1 in 10,000 patients receiving halothane and is referred to as *halothane hepatitis* (Subcommittee on the National Halothane Study, 1966). Current thinking is that halothane hepatitis is the result of an immune response to hepatic proteins that become trifluoroacetylated as a consequence of halothane metabolism (*see* Pharmacokinetics, above).

Isoflurane

Chemistry and Physical Properties. Isoflurane (FORANE, others) is 1-chloro-2,2,2-trifluoroethyl difluoromethyl ether (Figure 13–4). It is a volatile liquid at room temperature and is neither flammable nor explosive in mixtures of air or oxygen.

Pharmacokinetics. Isoflurane has a blood:gas partition coefficient substantially lower than that of halothane or *enflurane* (Table 13–1). Consequently, induction with isoflurane and recovery from isoflurane are relatively rapid. Changes in anesthetic depth also can be achieved more rapidly with isoflurane than with halothane or enflurane. More than 99% of inhaled isoflurane is excreted unchanged *via* the lungs. Approximately 0.2% of absorbed isoflurane is oxidatively metabolized by CYP2E1 (Kharasch and Thummel, 1993). The small amount of isoflurane degradation products produced is insufficient to produce any renal, hepatic, or other organ toxicity. Isoflurane does not appear to be a mutagen, teratogen, or carcinogen (Eger *et al.*, 1978).

Clinical Use. Isoflurane is a commonly used inhalational anesthetic worldwide. It is typically used for maintenance of anesthesia *after induction* with other agents because of its pungent odor, but induction of anesthesia can be achieved in less than 10 minutes with an inhaled concentration of 3% isoflurane in O_2; this concentration is reduced to 1% to 2% for maintenance of anesthesia. The use of other drugs such as opioids or nitrous oxide reduces the concentration of isoflurane required for surgical anesthesia.

Side Effects. Cardiovascular System. Isoflurane produces a concentration-dependent decrease in arterial blood pressure. Unlike halothane, cardiac output is well maintained with isoflurane, and hypotension is the result of decreased systemic vascular resistance (Figure 13–6). Isoflurane produces vasodilation in most vascular beds, with particularly pronounced effects in skin and muscle.

Isoflurane is a potent coronary vasodilator, simultaneously producing increased coronary blood flow and decreased myocardial O_2 consumption. In theory, this makes isoflurane a particularly safe anesthetic to use for patients with ischemic heart disease. However, concern has been raised that isoflurane may produce myocardial ischemia by inducing "coronary steal" (*i.e.,* the diversion of blood flow from poorly perfused to well perfused areas) (Buffington *et al.*, 1988). This concern has not been substantiated in subsequent animal and human studies. Patients anesthetized with isoflurane generally have mildly elevated heart rates as a compensatory response to reduced blood pressure; however, rapid changes in isoflurane concentration can produce both transient tachycardia and hypertension due to isoflurane-induced sympathetic stimulation.

Respiratory System. Isoflurane produces concentration-dependent depression of ventilation. Patients spontaneously breathing isoflurane have a normal respiration rate but a reduced tidal volume, resulting in a marked reduction in alveolar ventilation and an increase in arterial CO_2 tension (Figure 13–7). Isoflurane is particularly effective at depressing the ventilatory response to hypercapnia and hypoxia (Hirshman *et al.*, 1977). While isoflurane is an effective bronchodilator, it also is an airway irritant and can stimulate airway reflexes during induction of anesthesia, producing coughing and laryngospasm.

Nervous System. Isoflurane, like halothane, dilates the cerebral vasculature, producing increased cerebral blood flow and the risk of increased intracranial pressure. Isoflurane also reduces cerebral metabolic O_2 consumption. Isoflurane causes less cerebral vasodilation than do either enflurane or halothane, making it a preferred agent for neurosurgical procedures (Drummond *et al.*, 1983). The modest effects of isoflurane on cerebral blood flow can be reversed readily by hyperventilation (McPherson *et al.*, 1989).

Muscle. Isoflurane produces some relaxation of skeletal muscle *via* its central effects. It also enhances the effects of both depolarizing and nondepolarizing muscle relaxants. Isoflurane is more potent than halothane in its potentiation of neuromuscular blocking agents. Like other halogenated inhalational anesthetics, isoflurane relaxes uterine smooth muscle and is not recommended for analgesia or anesthesia for labor and vaginal delivery.

Kidney. Isoflurane reduces renal blood flow and glomerular filtration rate, resulting in a small volume of concentrated urine. Changes in renal function observed during isoflurane anesthesia are rapidly reversed, with no long-term renal sequelae or toxicities.

Liver and Gastrointestinal Tract. Splanchnic and hepatic blood flows are reduced with increasing doses of isoflurane as systemic arterial pressure decreases. Liver function tests are minimally affected by isoflurane, with no reported incidence of hepatic toxicity.

Enflurane

Chemical and Physical Properties. Enflurane (ETHRANE, others) is 2-chloro-1,1,2-trifluoroethyl difluoromethyl ether (Figure 13–4). It is a clear, colorless liquid at room temperature with a mild, sweet odor. Like other inhalational anesthetics, it is volatile and must be stored in a sealed bottle. It is nonflammable and nonexplosive in mixtures of air or oxygen.

Pharmacokinetics. Because of its relatively high blood:gas partition coefficient, induction of anesthesia and recovery from enflurane are relatively slow (Table 13–1). Enflurane is metabolized to a modest extent, with 2% to 8% of absorbed enflurane undergoing oxidative metabolism in the liver by CYP2E1 (Kharasch *et al.*, 1994). Fluoride ions are a by-product of enflurane metabolism, but plasma fluoride levels are low and nontoxic. Patients taking isoniazid exhibit enhanced metabolism of enflurane with significantly elevated serum fluoride concentrations (Mazze *et al.*, 1982).

Clinical Use. As with isoflurane, enflurane is primarily utilized for maintenance rather than induction of anesthesia.

Surgical anesthesia can be induced with enflurane in less than 10 minutes with an inhaled concentration of 4% in oxygen. Anesthesia can be maintained with concentrations from 1.5% to 3%. As with other anesthetics, the enflurane concentrations required to produce anesthesia are reduced when it is coadministered with nitrous oxide or opioids. Use of enflurane has decreased substantially in recent years with the introduction of newer inhalational agents with preferable pharmacokinetic and side-effect profiles.

Side Effects. **Cardiovascular System.** Enflurane causes a concentration-dependent decrease in arterial blood pressure. Hypotension is due, in part, to depression of myocardial contractility, with some contribution from peripheral vasodilation (Figure 13–6). Enflurane has minimal effects on heart rate and produces neither the bradycardia seen with halothane nor the tachycardia seen with isoflurane.

Respiratory System. The respiratory effects of enflurane are similar to those of halothane. Spontaneous ventilation with enflurane produces a pattern of rapid, shallow breathing. Minute ventilation is markedly decreased, and a Pa_{CO_2} of 60 mm Hg can be seen with 1 MAC of enflurane (Figure 13–7). Enflurane produces a greater depression of the ventilatory responses to hypoxia and hypercarbia than do either halothane or isoflurane (Hirshman *et al.*, 1977). Enflurane, like other inhalational anesthetics, is an effective bronchodilator.

Nervous System. Enflurane is a cerebral vasodilator and thus can increase intracranial pressure in some patients. Like other inhalational anesthetics, enflurane reduces cerebral metabolic O_2 consumption. Enflurane has an unusual property of producing electrical seizure activity. High concentrations of enflurane or profound hypocarbia during enflurane anesthesia result in a characteristic high-voltage, high-frequency electroencephalographic (EEG) pattern that progresses to spike-and-dome complexes. The spike-and-dome pattern can be punctuated by frank seizure activity that may or may not be accompanied by peripheral motor manifestations of seizure activity. The seizures are self-limited and are not thought to produce permanent damage. Epileptic patients are not particularly susceptible to enflurane-induced seizures. Nonetheless, enflurane generally is not used in patients with seizure disorders.

Muscle. Enflurane produces significant skeletal muscle relaxation in the absence of muscle relaxants. It also significantly enhances the effects of nondepolarizing muscle relaxants. As with other inhalational agents, enflurane relaxes uterine smooth muscle. It is not widely used for obstetric anesthesia.

Kidney. Like other inhalational anesthetics, enflurane reduces renal blood flow, glomerular filtration rate, and urinary output. These effects are rapidly reversed upon drug discontinuation. Enflurane metabolism produces significant plasma levels of fluoride ions (20 to 40 μmol) and can produce transient urinary-concentrating defects following prolonged administration (Mazze *et al.*, 1977). There is scant evidence of long-term nephrotoxicity following enflurane use, and it is safe to use in patients with renal impairment, provided that the depth of enflurane anesthesia and the duration of administration are not excessive.

Liver and Gastrointestinal Tract. Enflurane reduces splanchnic and hepatic blood flow in proportion to reduced arterial blood pressure. Enflurane does not appear to alter liver function or to be hepatotoxic.

Desflurane

Chemistry and Physical Properties. *Desflurane* (SUPRANE) is difluoromethyl 1-fluoro-2,2,2-trifluoromethyl ether (Figure 13–4). It is a highly volatile liquid at room temperature (vapor pressure = 681 mm Hg) and thus must be stored in tightly sealed bottles. Delivery of a precise concentration of desflurane requires the use of a specially heated vaporizer that delivers pure vapor that then is diluted appropriately with other gases (O_2, air, or N_2O). Desflurane is nonflammable and nonexplosive in mixtures of air or oxygen.

Pharmacokinetics. Desflurane has a very low blood:gas partition coefficient (0.42) and also is not very soluble in fat or other peripheral tissues (Table 13–1). For this reason, the alveolar (and blood) concentration rapidly rises to the level of inspired concentration. Indeed, within five minutes of administration, the alveolar concentration reaches 80% of the inspired concentration. This provides for a very rapid induction of anesthesia and for rapid changes in depth of anesthesia following changes in the inspired concentration. Emergence from anesthesia also is very rapid with desflurane. The time to awakening following desflurane is half as long as with halothane or *sevoflurane* and usually does not exceed 5 to 10 minutes in the absence of other sedative agents (Smiley *et al.*, 1991).

Desflurane is metabolized to a minimal extent, and more than 99% of absorbed desflurane is eliminated unchanged *via* the lungs. A small amount of absorbed desflurane is oxidatively metabolized by hepatic CYPs. Virtually no serum fluoride ions are detectable in serum after desflurane administration, but low concentrations of trifluoroacetic acid are detectable in serum and urine (Koblin *et al.*, 1988).

Clinical Use. Desflurane is a widely used anesthetic for outpatient surgery because of its rapid onset of action and rapid recovery. The drug is irritating to the airway in awake patients and can provoke coughing, salivation, and bronchospasm. Anesthesia therefore usually is induced with an intravenous agent, with desflurane subsequently administered for maintenance of anesthesia. Maintenance of anesthesia usually requires inhaled concentrations of 6% to 8%. Lower concentrations of desflurane are required if it is coadministered with nitrous oxide or opioids.

Side Effects. **Cardiovascular System.** Desflurane, like all inhalational anesthetics, causes a concentration-dependent decrease in blood pressure. Desflurane has a very modest negative inotropic effect and produces hypotension primarily by decreasing systemic vascular resistance (Eger, 1994) (Figure 13–6). Cardiac output thus is well preserved during desflurane anesthesia, as is blood flow to the major organ beds (splanchnic, renal, cerebral, and coronary). Marked increases in heart rate often are noted during induction of desflurane anesthesia and during abrupt increases in the delivered concentration of desflurane. This transient tachycardia results from desflurane-induced stimulation of the sympathetic nervous system (Ebert and Muzi, 1993). Unlike some inhalational anesthetics, the hypotensive effects of desflurane do not wane with increasing duration of administration.

Respiratory System. Similarly to halothane and enflurane, desflurane causes a concentration-dependent increase in respiratory rate and a decrease in tidal volume. At low concentrations (less than 1 MAC) the net effect is to preserve minute ventilation. At desflurane concentrations greater than 1 MAC, minute ventilation is markedly depressed, resulting in elevated arterial CO_2 tension (Pa_{CO_2}) (Figure 13–7) (Lockhart *et al.*, 1991). Patients spontaneously breathing desflurane at concentrations greater than 1.5 MAC will have extreme elevations of Pa_{CO_2} and may become apneic. Desflurane, like other inhalational agents, is a bronchodilator. However, it also is a strong airway irritant, and can cause coughing, breath-holding, laryngospasm, and excessive respiratory secretions. Because of its irritant properties, desflurane is not used for induction of anesthesia.

Nervous System. Desflurane decreases cerebral vascular resistance and cerebral metabolic O_2 consumption. Under conditions of normocapnia and normotension, desflurane produces an increase in cerebral blood flow and can increase intracranial pressure in patients with poor intracranial compliance. The vasoconstrictive response to hypocapnia is preserved during desflurane anesthesia, and increases in intracranial pressure thus can be prevented by hyperventilation.

Muscle. Desflurane produces direct skeletal muscle relaxation as well as enhancing the effects of nondepolarizing and depolarizing neuromuscular blocking agents (Caldwell *et al.*, 1991).

Kidney. Desflurane has no reported nephrotoxicity. This is consistent with its minimal metabolic degradation.

Liver and Gastrointestinal Tract. Desflurane is not known to affect liver function tests or to cause hepatotoxicity.

Sevoflurane

Chemistry and Physical Properties. Sevoflurane (ULTANE) is fluoromethyl 2,2,2-trifluoro-1-[trifluoromethyl]ethyl ether (Figure 13–4). It is a clear, colorless, volatile liquid at room temperature and must be stored in a sealed bottle. It is nonflammable and nonexplosive in mixtures of air or oxygen. Sevoflurane can undergo an exothermic reaction with desiccated CO_2 absorbent (BARALYME) to produce airway burns (Fatheree and Leighton, 2004) or spontaneous ignition, explosion and fire (Wu *et al.*, 2004a). *Care must be taken to ensure that sevoflurane is not used with an anesthesia machine in which the CO_2 absorbent has been dried by prolonged gas flow through the absorbent. Sevoflurane reaction with desiccated CO_2 absorbent also can produce CO, which can result in serious patient injury.*

Pharmacokinetics. The low solubility of sevoflurane in blood and other tissues provides for rapid induction of anesthesia, rapid changes in anesthetic depth following changes in delivered concentration, and rapid emergence following discontinuation of administration (Table 13–1).

Approximately 3% of absorbed sevoflurane is biotransformed. Sevoflurane is metabolized in the liver by CYP2E1, with the predominant product being hexafluoroisopropanol (Kharasch *et al.*, 1995). Hepatic metabolism of sevoflurane also produces inorganic fluoride. Serum fluoride concentrations peak shortly after surgery and decline rapidly. Interaction of sevoflurane with soda lime also produces decomposition products. The major product of interest is referred to as compound A and is pentafluoroisopropenyl fluoromethyl ether (*see* Side Effects: Kidney, below) (Hanaki *et al.*, 1987).

Clinical Use. Sevoflurane is widely used, particularly for outpatient anesthesia, because of its rapid recovery profile. It is well-suited for inhalation induction of anesthesia (particularly in children) because it is not irritating to the airway. Induction of anesthesia is rapidly achieved using inhaled concentrations of 2% to 4% sevoflurane.

Side Effects. **Cardiovascular System.** Sevoflurane, like all other halogenated inhalational anesthetics, produces a concentration-dependent decrease in arterial blood pressure. This hypotensive effect primarily is due to systemic vasodilation, although sevoflurane also produces a concentration-dependent decrease in cardiac output (Figure 13–6). Unlike isoflurane or desflurane, sevoflurane does not produce tachycardia and thus may be a preferable agent in patients prone to myocardial ischemia.

Respiratory System. Sevoflurane produces a concentration-dependent reduction in tidal volume and increase in respiratory rate in spontaneously breathing patients. The increased respiratory frequency does not compensate for reduced tidal volume, with the net effect being a reduction in minute ventilation and an increase in Pa_{CO_2} (Doi and Ikeda, 1987) (Figure 13–7). Sevoflurane is not irritating to the airway and is a potent bronchodilator. Because of this combination of properties, sevoflurane is the most effective clinical bronchodilator of the inhalational anesthetics (Rooke *et al.*, 1997).

Nervous System. Sevoflurane produces effects on cerebral vascular resistance, cerebral metabolic O_2 consumption, and cerebral blood flow that are very similar to those produced by isoflurane and desflurane. While sevoflurane can increase intracranial pressure in patients with poor intracranial compliance, the response to hypocapnia is preserved during sevoflurane anesthesia, and increases in intracranial pressure can be prevented by hyperventilation.

Muscle. Sevoflurane produces skeletal muscle relaxation and enhances the effects of nondepolarizing and depolarizing neuromuscular blocking agents. Its effects are similar to those of other halogenated inhalational anesthetics.

Kidney. Controversy has surrounded the potential nephrotoxicity of sevoflurane with the degradation product produced by interaction of sevoflurane with the CO_2 absorbent soda lime. Biochemical evidence of transient renal injury has been reported in human volunteers (Eger *et al.*, 1997). Large clinical studies have shown no evidence of increased serum creatinine, blood urea nitrogen, or any other evidence of renal impairment following sevoflurane administration (Mazze *et al.*, 2000). *The current recommendation of the FDA is that sevoflurane be administered with fresh gas flows of at least 2 L/min to minimize accumulation of compound A.*

Liver and Gastrointestinal Tract. Sevoflurane is not known to cause hepatotoxicity or alterations of hepatic function tests.

Nitrous Oxide

Chemical and Physical Properties. Nitrous oxide (dinitrogen monoxide; N_2O) is a colorless, odorless gas at room temperature (Figure 13–4). It is sold in steel cylinders and must be delivered through calibrated flow meters provided on all anesthesia machines. Nitrous oxide is neither flammable nor explosive, but it does support com-

bustion as actively as oxygen does when it is present in proper concentration with a flammable anesthetic or material.

Pharmacokinetics. Nitrous oxide is very insoluble in blood and other tissues (Table 13–1). This results in rapid equilibration between delivered and alveolar anesthetic concentrations and provides for rapid induction of anesthesia and rapid emergence following discontinuation of administration. The rapid uptake of N_2O from alveolar gas serves to concentrate coadministered halogenated anesthetics; this effect (the "second gas effect") speeds induction of anesthesia. On discontinuation of N_2O administration, nitrous oxide gas can diffuse from blood to the alveoli, diluting O_2 in the lung. This can produce an effect called *diffusional hypoxia. To avoid hypoxia, 100% O_2 rather than air should be administered when N_2O is discontinued.*

Nitrous oxide is almost completely eliminated by the lungs, with some minimal diffusion through the skin. Nitrous oxide is not biotransformed by enzymatic action in human tissue, and 99.9% of absorbed nitrous oxide is eliminated unchanged. Nitrous oxide can be degraded by interaction with vitamin B_{12} in intestinal bacteria. This results in inactivation of methionine synthesis and can produce signs of vitamin B_{12} deficiency (megaloblastic anemia and peripheral neuropathy) following long-term nitrous oxide administration (O'Sullivan *et al.*, 1981). For this reason, N_2O is not used as a chronic analgesic or as a sedative in critical care settings.

Clinical Use. Nitrous oxide is a weak anesthetic agent and produces reliable surgical anesthesia only under hyperbaric conditions. It does produce significant analgesia at concentrations as low as 20% and usually produces sedation in concentrations between 30% and 80%. It frequently is used in concentrations of approximately 50% to provide analgesia and sedation in outpatient dentistry. Nitrous oxide cannot be used at concentrations above 80% because this limits the delivery of an adequate amount of oxygen. Because of this limitation, nitrous oxide is used primarily as an adjunct to other inhalational or intravenous anesthetics. Nitrous oxide substantially reduces the requirement for inhalational anesthetics. For example, at 70% nitrous oxide, the MAC for other inhalational agents is reduced by about 60%, allowing for lower concentrations of halogenated anesthetics and a lesser degree of side effects.

One major problem with N_2O is that it will exchange with N_2 in any air-containing cavity in the body. Moreover, because of their differential blood:gas partition coefficients, nitrous oxide will enter the cavity faster than nitrogen escapes, thereby increasing the volume and/or pressure in this cavity. Examples of air collections that can be expanded by nitrous oxide include a pneumothorax, an obstructed middle ear, an air embolus, an obstructed loop of bowel, an intraocular air bubble, a pulmonary bulla, and intracranial air. Nitrous oxide should be avoided in these clinical settings.

Side Effects. **Cardiovascular System.** Although N_2O produces a negative inotropic effect on heart muscle *in vitro,* depressant effects on cardiac function generally are not observed in patients because of the stimulatory effects of nitrous oxide on the sympathetic nervous system. The cardiovascular effects of nitrous oxide also are heavily influenced by the concomitant administration of other anesthetic agents. When nitrous oxide is coadministered with halogenated inhalational anesthetics, it generally produces an increase in heart rate, arterial blood pressure, and cardiac output. In contrast, when nitrous oxide is coadministered with an opioid, it generally decreases arterial blood pressure and cardiac output. Nitrous oxide also increases venous tone in both the peripheral and pulmonary vasculature. The effects of N_2O on pulmonary vascular resistance can be exaggerated in patients with pre-existing pulmonary hypertension (Schulte-Sasse *et al.*, 1982) and the drug generally is not used in these patients.

Respiratory System. Nitrous oxide causes modest increases in respiratory rate and decreases in tidal volume in spontaneously breathing patients. The net effect is that minute ventilation is not significantly changed and Pa_{CO_2} remains normal. However, even modest concentrations of nitrous oxide markedly depress the ventilatory response to hypoxia. Thus, it is prudent to monitor arterial O_2 saturation directly in patients receiving or recovering from nitrous oxide.

Nervous System. When administered alone, nitrous oxide can significantly increase cerebral blood flow and intracranial pressure. When nitrous oxide is coadministered with intravenous anesthetic agents, increases in cerebral blood flow are attenuated or abolished. When nitrous oxide is added to a halogenated inhalational anesthetic, its vasodilatory effect on the cerebral vasculature is slightly reduced.

Muscle. Nitrous oxide does not relax skeletal muscle and does not enhance the effects of neuromuscular blocking drugs. Unlike the halogenated anesthetics, nitrous oxide does not trigger malignant hyperthermia.

Kidney, Liver, and Gastrointestinal Tract. Nitrous oxide is not known to produce any changes in renal or hepatic function and is neither nephrotoxic nor hepatotoxic.

Xenon

Xenon is an inert gas that first was identified as an anesthetic agent in 1951. It is not approved for use in the United States and is unlikely to enjoy widespread use because it is a rare gas that cannot be manufactured and must be extracted from air. This limits the quantities of available xenon gas and renders xenon very expensive. Despite these shortcomings, xenon has properties that make it a virtually ideal anesthetic gas that ultimately may be used in critical situations (Lynch *et al.*, 2000).

Xenon is extremely insoluble in blood and other tissues, providing for rapid induction and emergence from anesthesia (Table 13–1). It is sufficiently potent to produce surgical anesthesia when administered with 30% oxygen. Most importantly, xenon has minimal side effects. It has no effects on cardiac output or cardiac rhythm and is not thought to have a significant effect on systemic vascular resistance. It also does not affect pulmonary function and is not known to have any hepatic or renal toxicity. Finally, xenon is not metabolized in the human body. Xenon is an anesthetic that may be available in the future if limitations on its availability and its high cost can be overcome.

ANESTHETIC ADJUNCTS

A general anesthetic is rarely given as the sole agent. Rather, anesthetic adjuncts usually are used to augment specific components of anesthesia, permitting lower doses of general anesthetics with fewer side effects. Because they are such an integral part of general anesthetic drug regimens, their use as anesthetic adjuncts is described briefly here. The detailed pharmacology of each drug is covered in other chapters.

Benzodiazepines

While benzodiazepines (*see* Chapter 16) can produce anesthesia similar to that of barbiturates, they are more commonly used for sedation rather than general anesthesia because prolonged amnesia and sedation may result from anesthetizing doses. As adjuncts, benzodiazepines are used for anxiolysis, amnesia, and sedation prior to induction of anesthesia or for sedation during procedures not requiring general anesthesia. The benzodiazepine most frequently used in the perioperative period is *midazolam* (VERSED) followed distantly by *diazepam* (VALIUM), and *lorazepam* (ATIVAN). Midazolam is water soluble and typically is administered intravenously but also can be given orally, intramuscularly, or rectally; oral midazolam is particularly useful for sedation of young children. Midazolam produces minimal venous irritation as opposed to diazepam and lorazepam, which are formulated in propylene glycol and are painful on injection, sometimes producing thrombophlebitis. Midazolam has the pharmacokinetic advantage, particularly over lorazepam, of being more rapid in onset and shorter in duration of effect. Sedative doses of midazolam (0.01 to 0.07 mg/kg intravenously) reach peak effect in about 2 minutes and provide sedation for about 30 minutes (Reves *et al.*, 1985). Elderly patients tend to be more sensitive to and have a slower recovery from benzodiazepines (Jacobs *et al.*, 1995); thus, titration to the desired effect of smaller doses in this age group is prudent. Midazolam is hepatically metabolized with a clearance (6 to 11 ml/min per kg), similar to that of methohexital and about 20 and 7 times higher than those of diazepam and lorazepam, respectively (Reves *et al.*, 1985). Either for prolonged sedation or for general anesthetic maintenance, midazolam is more suitable for infusion than are other benzodiazepines, although its duration of action does significantly increase with prolonged infusions (Figure 13–3). Benzodiazepines reduce both cerebral blood flow and metabolism, but at equi-anesthetic doses are less potent in this respect than are barbiturates. They are effective anticonvulsants and sometimes are given to treat status epilepticus (Modica *et al.*, 1990). Benzodiazepines modestly decrease blood pressure and respiratory drive, occasionally resulting in apnea (Reves *et al.*, 1985). Thus, blood pressure and respiratory rate should be monitored in patients sedated with intravenous benzodiazepines.

α₂ Adrenergic Agonists. In 1999 the FDA approved the α_2 adrenergic agonist dexmedetomidine (PRECEDEX) for short-term sedation of critically ill adults. Dexmedetomidine is now widely used in the intensive care unit setting and is beginning to be administered off-label in other clinical scenarios including as an anesthetic adjunct. Dexmedetomidine is an imidazole derivative that is highly selective for the α_2 adrenergic receptor (Kamibayashi *et al.*, 2000). Activation of the α_{2A} adrenergic receptor by dexmedetomidine produces both sedation and analgesia, but does not reliably provide general anesthesia, even at maximal doses (Aho *et al.*, 1992; Lakhlani *et al.*, 1997).

The most common side effects of dexmedetomidine include hypotension and bradycardia, both of which are attributed to decreased catecholamine release by activation peripherally and in the CNS of the α_{2A}-receptor (Lakhlani *et al.*, 1997). Nausea and dry mouth also are common untoward reactions. At higher drug concentrations, the α_{2B}-subtype is activated, resulting in hypertension and a further decrease in heart rate and cardiac output. Dexmedetomidine has the very useful property of producing sedation and analgesia with minimal respiratory depression (Belleville *et al.*, 1992); thus, it is particularly valuable in sedation of patients who are not endotracheally intubated and mechanically ventilated. The sedation produced by dexmedetomidine has been noted to be more akin to natural sleep, with patients relatively easy to arouse (Hall *et al.*, 2000). However, dexmedetomidine does not appear to provide reliable amnesia and additional agents may need to be employed if lack of recall is desirable (Coursin and Maccioli, 2001).

Dexmedetomidine is supplied as an aqueous solution of the hydrochloride salt and should be diluted in normal saline to a final concentration of 4 μg/ml for intravenous delivery, the only approved route of administration. The recommended loading dose is 1 μg/kg given over 10 minutes, followed by infusion at a rate of 0.2 to 0.7 μg/kg per hour. Infusions for longer than 24 hours are not recommended because of a potential for rebound hypertension. Reduced

doses should be considered in patients with risk factors for severe hypotension. The distribution and terminal half-lives are 6 minutes and 2 hours, respectively (Khan *et al.*, 1999). Dexmedetomidine is highly protein bound and is primarily hepatically metabolized; the glucuronide and methyl conjugates are renally excreted (Bhana *et al.*, 2000).

In summary, dexmedetomidine is a relatively new sedative-hypnotic that provides analgesia with little respiratory depression and in most patients a tolerable decrease in blood pressure and heart rate. Dexmedetomidine is likely to be increasingly used for sedation and as an anesthetic adjunct.

Analgesics

With the exception of ketamine, neither parenteral nor currently available inhalational anesthetics are effective analgesics. Thus, analgesics typically are administered with general anesthetics to reduce anesthetic requirement and minimize hemodynamic changes produced by painful stimuli. Nonsteroidal antiinflammatory drugs, cyclooxygenase-2 inhibitors, or acetaminophen sometimes provide adequate analgesia for minor surgical procedures. However, because of the rapid and profound analgesia produced, opioids are the primary analgesics used during the perioperative period.

Fentanyl (SUBLIMAZE), *sufentanil* (SUFENTA), *alfentanil* (ALFENTA), *remifentanil* (ULTIVA), meperidine (DEMEROL), and morphine are the major parenteral opioids used in the perioperative period. The primary analgesic activity of each of these drugs is produced by agonist activity at μ-opioid receptors (Pasternak, 1993). Their order of potency (relative to morphine) is: sufentanil (1000x) > remifentanil (300x) > fentanyl (100x) > alfentanil (15x) > morphine (1x) > meperidine (0.1x) (Clotz and Nahata, 1991; Glass *et al.*, 1993; Martin, 1983). Pharmacological properties of these agents are discussed in more detail in Chapter 21.

The choice of a perioperative opioid is based primarily on duration of action, given that at appropriate doses, all produce similar analgesia and side effects. Remifentanil has an ultrashort duration of action (~10 minutes) and accumulates minimally with repeated doses or infusion (Glass *et al.*, 1993); it is particularly well suited for procedures that are briefly painful, but for which little analgesia is required postoperatively. Single doses of fentanyl, alfentanil, and sufentanil all have similar intermediate durations of action (30, 20, and 15 minutes, respectively), but recovery after prolonged administration varies considerably (Shafer *et al.*, 1991). Fentanyl's duration of action lengthens most with infusion, sufentanil's much less so, and alfentanil's the least. Except for remifentanil, all of the above-mentioned opioids are metabolized in the liver followed by renal and biliary excretion of the metabolites (Tegeder *et al.*, 1999). Remifentanil is hydrolyzed by tissue and plasma esterases (Westmoreland *et al.*, 1993). After prolonged administration, morphine metabolites have significant analgesic and hypnotic activity (Christrup, 1997).

During the perioperative period, opioids often are given at induction to preempt responses to predictable painful stimuli (*e.g.*, endotracheal intubation and surgical incision). Subsequent doses either by bolus or infusion are titrated to the surgical stimulus and the patient's hemodynamic response. Marked decreases in respiratory rate and heart rate with much smaller reductions in blood pressure are seen to varying degrees with all opioids (Bowdle, 1998). Muscle rigidity that can impair ventilation sometimes accompanies larger doses of opioids. The incidence of sphincter of Oddi spasm is increased with all opioids, although morphine appears to be more potent in this regard (Hahn *et al.*, 1988). The frequency and severity of nausea, vomiting, and pruritus after emergence from anesthesia are increased by all opioids to about the same degree (Watcha *et al.*, 1992). A useful side effect of meperidine is its capacity to reduce shivering, a common problem during emergence from anesthesia (Pauca *et al.*, 1984); other opioids are not as efficacious against shivering, perhaps due to less κ-receptor agonist activity. Finally, opioids often are administered intrathecally and epidurally for management of acute and chronic pain. Neuraxial opioids with or without local anesthetics can provide profound analgesia for many surgical procedures; however, respiratory depression and pruritus usually limit their use to major operations.

Neuromuscular Blocking Agents

The practical aspects of the use of neuromuscular blockers as anesthetic adjuncts are briefly described here. The detailed pharmacology of this drug class is presented in Chapter 9.

Depolarizing (*e.g., succinylcholine*) and nondepolarizing muscle relaxants (*e.g., pancuronium*) often are administered during the induction of anesthesia to relax muscles of the jaw, neck, and airway and thereby facilitate laryngoscopy and endotracheal intubation. Barbiturates will precipitate when mixed with muscle relaxants and should be allowed to clear from the intravenous line prior to injection of a muscle relaxant. Following induction, continued muscle relaxation is desirable for many procedures to aid surgical exposure and to provide additional insurance of immobility. Of course, muscle relaxants are not by themselves anesthetics and should not be used in lieu of adequate anesthetic depth. The action of nondepolarizing muscle relaxants usually is antagonized, once muscle paralysis is no longer desired, with an acetylcholinesterase inhibitor such as *neostigmine* or *edrophonium* (*see* Chapter 8) combined with a muscarinic receptor antagonist (*e.g., glycopyrolate* or *atropine*) (*see* Chapter 7) to offset the muscarinic activation resulting from esterase inhibition. Other than histamine release by some agents, nondepolarizing muscle relaxants used in this manner have few side effects. However, succinylcholine has multiple serious side effects (bradycardia, hyperkalemia, and severe myalgia) including induction of malignant hyperthermia in susceptible individuals.

BIBLIOGRAPHY

Abboud, T.K., Zhu, J., Richardson, M., Peres Da Silva, E., and Donovan, M. Intravenous propofol vs thiamylal-isoflurane for caesarean section, comparative maternal and neonatal effects. *Acta. Anaesthesiol. Scand.*, **1995**, *39:*205–209.

Aho, M., Erkola, O., Kallio, A., Scheinin, H., and Korttila, K. Dexmedetomidine infusion for maintenance of anesthesia in patients undergoing abdominal hysterectomy. *Anesth. Analg.*, **1992**, *75:*940–946.

Andrews, P.R., and Mark, L.C. Structural specificity of barbiturates and related drugs. *Anesthesiology*, **1982**, *57:*314–320.

Antognini, J.F., and Schwartz, K. Exaggerated anesthetic requirements in the preferentially anesthetized brain. *Anesthesiology*, **1993**, *79:*1244–1249.

Bahlman, S.H., Eger, E.I. II, Halsey, M.J., *et al.* The cardiovascular effects of halothane in man during spontaneous ventilation. *Anesthesiology*, **1972**, *36:*494–502.

Baldo, B.A., Fisher, M.M., and Harle, D.G. Allergy to thiopentone. *Clin. Rev. Allergy*, **1991**, *9:*295–308.

Balser, J.R., Martinez, E.A., Winters, B., *et al.* Beta-adrenergic blockade accelerates conversion of postoperative supraventricular tachyarrhythmias. *Anesthesiology*, **1998**, *89:*1052–1059.

Belelli, D., Lambert, J.J., Peters, J.A., Wafford, K., and Whiting, P.J. The interaction of the general anesthetic etomidate with the gamma-aminobutyric acid type A receptor is influenced by a single amino acid. *Proc. Natl. Acad. Sci. U.S.A.*, **1997**, *94:*11031–11036.

Belleville, J.P., Ward, D.S., Bloor, B.C., and Maze, M. Effects of intravenous dexmedetomidine in humans. I. Sedation, ventilation, and metabolic rate. *Anesthesiology*, **1992**, *77:*1125–1133.

Belopavlovic, M., and Buchthal, A. Modification of ketamine-induced intracranial hypertension in neurosurgical patients by pretreatment with midazolam. *Acta. Anaesthesiol. Scand.*, **1982**, *26:*458–462.

Beskow, A., Werner, O., and Westrin, P. Faster recovery after anesthesia in infants after intravenous induction with methohexital instead of thiopental. *Anesthesiology*, **1995**, *83:*976–979.

Bhana, N., Goa, K.L., and McClellan, K.J. Dexmedetomidine. *Drugs*, **2000**, *59:*263–268; discussion 269–270.

Blouin, R.T., Conard, P.F., and Gross, J.B. Time course of ventilatory depression following induction doses of propofol and thiopental. *Anesthesiology*, **1991**, *75:*940–944.

Bowdle, T.A. Adverse effects of opioid agonists and agonist-antagonists in anaesthesia. *Drug Saf.*, **1998**, *19:*173–189.

Brand, L., Mark, L.C., Snell, M.M., Vrindten, P., and Dayton, P.G. Physiologic disposition of methohexital in man. *Anesthesiology*, **1963**, *24:*331–335.

Buffington, C.W., Davis, K.B., Gillespie, S., and Pettinger, M. The prevalence of steal-prone coronary anatomy in patients with coronary artery disease: an analysis of the Coronary Artery Surgery Studio Registry. *Anesthesiology*, **1988**, *69:*721–727.

Burch, P.G., and Stanski, D.R. The role of metabolism and protein binding in thiopental anesthesia. *Anesthesiology*, **1983**, *58:*146–152.

Caldwell, J.E., Laster, M.J., Magorian, T., *et al.* The neuromuscular effects of desflurane, alone and combined with pancuronium or succinylcholine in humans. *Anesthesiology*, **1991**, *74:*412–418.

Calverley, R.K., Smith, N.T., Jones, C.W., Prys-Roberts, C., and Eger, E.I. II. Ventilatory and cardiovascular effects of enflurane anesthesia during spontaneous ventilation in man. *Anesth. Analg.*, **1978**, *57:*610–618.

Chan, H.N., Morgan, D.J., Crankshaw, D.P., and Boyd, M.D. Pentobarbitone formation during thiopentone infusion. *Anaesthesia*, **1985**, *40:*1155–1159.

Christrup, L.L. Morphine metabolites. *Acta Anaesthesiol. Scand.*, **1997**, *41:*116–122.

Clarke, R.S., Dundee, J.W., Barron, D.W., and McArdle, L. Clinical studies of induction agents. XVXVI. The relative potencies of thiopentone, methohexitone and propanidid. *Br. J. Anesth.*, **1968**, *40:*593–601.

Clements, J.A., and Nimmo, W.S. Pharmacokinetics and analgesic effect of ketamine in man. *Br. J. Anaesth.,* **1981,** *53:*27–30.

Coursin, D.B., and Maccioli, G.A. Dexmedetomidine. *Curr. Opin. Crit. Care,* **2001,** *7:*221–226.

Criado, A., Maseda, J., Navarro, E., Escarpa, A., and Avello, F. Induction of anaesthesia with etomidate: haemodynamic study of 36 patients. *Br. J. Anaesth.,* **1980,** *52:*803–806.

Cromwell, T.H., Stevens, W.C., Eger, E.I., *et al.* The cardiovascular effects of compound 469 (Forane) during spontaneous ventilation and CO_2 challenge in man. *Anesthesiology,* **1971,** *35:*17–25.

Dayton, P.G., Stiller, R.L., Cook, D.R., and Perel, J.M. The binding of ketamine to plasma proteins: emphasis on human plasma. *Eur. J. Clin. Pharmacol.,* **1983,** *24:*825–831.

Doenicke, A. Etomidate, a new intravenous hypnotic. *Acta. Anaesthesiol. Belg.,* **1974,** *25:*307–315.

Doi, M., and Ikeda, K. Respiratory effects of sevoflurane. *Anesth. Analg.,* **1987,** *66:*241–244.

Doze, V.A., Westphal, L.M., and White, P.F. Comparison of propofol with methohexital for outpatient anesthesia. *Anesth. Analg.,* **1986,** *65:*1189–1195.

Drummond, J.C., Cole, D.J., Patel, P.M., and Reynolds, L.W. Focal cerebral ischemia during anesthesia with etomidate, isoflurane, or thiopental: a comparison of the extent of cerebral injury. *Neurosurgery,* **1995,** *37:*742–748; discussion 748–749.

Drummond, J.C., Todd, M.M., Toutant, S.M., and Shapiro, H.M. Brain surface protrusion during enflurane, halothane, and isoflurane anesthesia in cats. *Anesthesiology,* **1983,** *59:*288–293.

Dundee, J.W., and Lilburn, J.K. Ketamine-lorazepam. Attenuation of psychic sequelae of ketamine by lorazepam. *Anaesthesia,* **1978,** *33:*312–314.

Dwyer, R., Bennett, H.L., Eger, E.I. II, and Peterson, N. Isoflurane anesthesia prevents unconscious learning. *Anesth. Analg.,* **1992,** *75:*107–112.

Ebert, T.J., and Muzi, M. Sympathetic hyperactivity during desflurane anesthesia in healthy volunteers. A comparison with isoflurane. *Anesthesiology,* **1993,** *79:*444–453.

Eger, E.I. II, Koblin, D.D., Bowland, T., *et al.* Nephrotoxicity of sevoflurane versus desflurane anesthesia in volunteers. *Anesth. Analg.,* **1997,** *84:*160–168.

Eger, E.I. II, Smith, N.T., Stoelting, R.K., *et al.* Cardiovascular effects of halothane in man. *Anesthesiology,* **1970,** *2:*396–409.

Eger, E.I. II, White, A.E., Brown, C.L., *et al.* A test of the carcinogenicity of enflurane, isoflurane, halothane, methoxyflurane, and nitrous oxide in mice. *Anesth. Analg.,* **1978,** *57:*678–694.

Eger, E.I. II, Zhang, Y., Laster, M., *et al.* Acetylcholine receptors do not mediate the immobilization produced by inhaled anesthetics. *Anesth. Analg.,* **2002,** *94:*1500–1504.

Flood, P., Ramirez-Latorre, J., and Role, L. $\alpha 4\beta 2$ Neuronal nicotinic acetylcholine receptors in the central nervous system are inhibited by isoflurane and propofol, but α7-type nicotinic acetylcholine receptors are unaffected. *Anesthesiology,* **1997,** *86:*859–865.

Fourcade, H.E., Stevens, W.C., Larson, C.P. Jr., *et al.* The ventilatory effects of Forane, a new inhaled anesthetic. *Anesthesiology,* **1971,** *35:*26–31.

Fragen, R.J., Avram, M.J., Henthorn, T.K., and Caldwell, N.J. A pharmacokinetically designed etomidate infusion regimen for hypnosis. *Anesth. Analg.,* **1983,** *62:*654–660.

Fragen, R.J., and Caldwell, N. Comparison of a new formulation of etomidate with thiopental—side effects and awakening times. *Anesthesiology,* **1979,** *50:*242–244.

Frank, S.M., Fleisher, L.A., Breslow, M.J., *et al.* Perioperative maintenance of normothermia reduces the incidence of morbid cardiac events. A randomized clinical trial. *JAMA,* **1997,** *277:*1127–1134.

Franks, N.P., Dickinson, R., de Sousa, S.L., Hall, A.C., and Lieb, W.R. How does xenon produce anaesthesia? *Nature,* **1998,** *396:*324.

Galloway, P.A., Nicoll, J.M., and Leiman, B.C. Pain reduction with etomidate injection. *Anaesthesia,* **1982,** *37:*352–353.

Gin, T., Mainland, P., Chan, M.T., and Short, T.G. Decreased thiopental requirements in early pregnancy. *Anesthesiology,* **1997,** *86:*73–78.

Glass, P.S., Hardman, D., Kamiyama, Y., *et al.* Preliminary pharmacokinetics and pharmacodynamics of an ultra-short-acting opioid: remifentanil (GI87084B). *Anesth. Analg.,* **1993,** *77:*1031–1040.

Gold, M.I., and Helrich, M. Pulmonary mechanics during general anesthesia: V. status asthmaticus. *Anesthesiology,* **1970,** *32:*422–428.

Gooding, J.M., and Corssen, G. Etomidate: an ultrashort-acting nonbarbiturate agent for anesthesia induction. *Anesth. Analg.,* **1976,** *55:*286–289.

Gray, A.T., Winegar, B.D., Leonoudakis, D.J., *et al.* TOK1 is a volatile anesthetic stimulated K^+ channel. *Anesthesiology,* **1998,** *88:*1076–1084.

Grounds, R.M., Maxwell, D.L., Taylor, M.B., Aber, V., and Royston, D. Acute ventilatory changes during i.v. induction of anaesthesia with thiopentone or propofol in man. Studies using inductance plethysmography. *Br. J. Anaesth.,* **1987,** *59:*1098–1102.

Grounds, R.M., Twigley, A.J., Carli, F., Whitwam, J.G., and Morgan, M. The haemodynamic effects of intravenous induction. Comparison of the effects of thiopentone and propofol. *Anaesthesia,* **1985,** *40:*735–740.

Gruenke, L.D., Konopka, K., Koop, D.R., and Waskell, L.A. Characterization of halothane oxidation by hepatic microsomes and purified cytochromes P-450 using a gas chromatographic mass spectrometric assay. *J. Pharmacol. Exp. Ther.,* **1988,** *246:*454–459.

Gruss, M., Bushell, T.J., Bright, D.P., *et al.* Two-pore-domain K^+ channels are a novel target for the anesthetic gases xenon, nitrous oxide and cyclopropane. *Mol. Pharmacol.,* **2004,** *65:*443–452.

Hahn, M., Baker, R., and Sullivan, S. The effect of four narcotics on cholecystokinin octapeptide stimulated gallbladder contraction. *Aliment. Pharmacol. Ther.,* **1988,** *2:*129–134.

Hales, T.G., and Lambert, J.J. Modulation of the $GABA_A$ receptor by propofol. *Br. J. Pharmacol.,* **1988,** *93:*84P.

Hall, J.E., Uhrich, T.D., Barney, J.A., Arain, S.R., and Ebert, T.J. Sedative, amnestic, and analgesic properties of small-dose dexmedetomidine infusions. *Anesth. Analg.,* **2000,** *90:*699–705.

Hanaki, C., Fujii, K., Morio, M., and Tashima, T. Decomposition of sevoflurane by soda lime. *Hiroshima J. Med. Sci.,* **1987,** *36:*61–67.

Hayashi, Y., Sumikawa, K., Tashiro, C., Yamatodani, A., and Yoshiya, I. Arrhythmogenic threshold of epinephrine during sevoflurane, enflurane, and isoflurane anesthesia in dogs. *Anesthesiology,* **1988,** *69:*145–147.

Hebron, B.S., Edbrooke, D.L., Newby, D.M., and Mather, S.J. Pharmacodynamics of etomidate associated with prolonged i.v. infusion. *Br. J. Anaesth.,* **1983,** *55:*281–287.

Heykants, J.J., Meuldermans, W.E., Michiels, L.J., Lewi, P.J., and Janssen, P.A. Distribution, metabolism and excretion of etomidate, a short-acting hypnotic drug, in the rat. Comparative study of *(R)*-(+)-(–)-Etomidate. *Arch. Int. Pharmacodyn. Ther.,* **1975,** *216:*113–129.

Hirshman, C.A., Downes, H., Farbood, A., and Bergman, N.A. Ketamine block of bronchospasm in experimental canine asthma. *Br. J. Anaesth.,* **1979,** *51:*713–718.

Hirshman, C.A., McCullough, R.E., Cohen, P.J., and Weil, J.V. Depression of hypoxic ventilatory response by halothane, enflurane and isoflurane in dogs. *Br. J. Anaesth.,* **1977,** *49:*957–963.

Hirshman, C.A., McCullough, R.E., Cohen, P.J., and Weil, J.V. Hypoxic ventilatory drive in dogs during thiopental, ketamine, or pentobarbital anesthesia. *Anesthesiology,* **1975,** *43:*628–634.

Homer, T.D., and Stanski, D.R. The effect of increasing age on thiopental disposition and anesthetic requirement. *Anesthesiology,* **1985,** *62:*714–724.

Hudson, R.J., Stanski, D.R., and Burch, P.G. Pharmacokinetics of methohexital and thiopental in surgical patients. *Anesthesiology,* **1983,** *59:*215–219.

Hughes, M.A., Glass, P.S., and Jacobs, J.R. Context-sensitive half-time in multicompartment pharmacokinetic models for intravenous anesthetic drugs. *Anesthesiology,* 1992, *76:*334–341.

Hung, O.R., Varvel, J.R., Shafer, S.L., and Stanski, D.R. Thiopental pharmacodynamics. II. Quantitation of clinical and electroencephalographic depth of anesthesia. *Anesthesiology,* **1992,** *77:*237–244.

Jacobs, J.R., Reves, J.G., Marty, J., White, W.D., Bai, S.A., *et al.* Aging increases pharmacodynamic sensitivity to the hypnotic effects of midazolam. *Anesth. Analg.,* **1995,** *80:*143–148.

Jevtovic-Todorovic, V., Todorovic, S.M., Mennerick, S., *et al.* Nitrous oxide (laughing gas) is an NMDA antagonist, neuroprotectant and neurotoxin. *Nat. Med.,* **1998,** *4:*460–463.

Jonmarker, C., Westrin, P., Larsson, S., and Werner, O. Thiopental requirements for induction of anesthesia in children. *Anesthesiology,* **1987,** *67:*104–107.

Joshi, C., and Bruce, D.L. Thiopental and succinylcholine: action on intraocular pressure. *Anesth. Analg.,* **1975,** *54:*471–475.

Jurd, R., Arras, M., Lambert, S., *et al.* General anesthetic actions in vivo strongly attenuated by a point mutation in the GABA$_A$ receptor β3 subunit. *FASEB J.,* **2003,** *17:*250–252.

Kamibayashi, T., and Maze, M. Clinical uses of α_2-adrenergic agonists. *Anesthesiology,* **2000,** *93:*1345–1349.

Kay, B., and Stephenson, D.K. Dose-response relationship for disoprofol (ICI 35868; Diprivan). Comparison with methohexitone. *Anaesthesia,* **1981,** *36:*863–867.

Kenna, J.G., Satoh, H., Christ, D.D., and Pohl, L.R. Metabolic basis of a drug hypersensitivity: antibodies in sera from patients with halothane hepatitis recognize liver neoantigens that contain the trifluoroacetyl group derived from halothane. *J. Pharmacol. Exp. Ther.,* **1988,** *2435:*1103–1109.

Kettler, D., Sonntag, H., Donath, U., Regensburger, D., and Schenk, H.D. Haemodynamics, myocardial mechanics, oxygen requirement and oxygenation of the human heart during induction of anaesthesia with etomidate. *Anaesthesist,* **1974,** *23:*116–121.

Khan, Z.P., Munday, I.T., Jones, R.M., *et al.* Effects of dexmedetomidine on isoflurane requirements in healthy volunteers. 1: Pharmacodynamic and pharmacokinetic interactions. *Br. J. Anaesth.,* **1999,** *83:*372–380.

Kharasch, E.D., Armstrong, A.S., Gunn, K., *et al.* Clinical sevoflurane metabolism and disposition. II. The role of cytochrome P450 2E1 in fluoride and hexafluoroisopropanol formation. *Anesthesiology,* **1995,** *82:*1379–1388.

Kharasch, E.D., and Thummel, K.E. Identification of cytochrome P450 2E1 as the predominant enzyme catalyzing human liver microsomal defluorination of sevoflurane, isoflurane, and methoxyflurane. *Anesthesiology,* **1993,** *79:*795–807.

Kharasch, E.D., Thummel, K.E., Mautz, D., and Bosse, S. Clinical enflurane metabolism by cytochrome P450 2E1. *Clin. Pharmacol. Ther.,* **1994,** *55:*434–440.

Kingston, H.G., and Hirshman, C.A. Perioperative management of the patient with asthma. *Anesth. Analg.,* **1984,** *63:*844–855.

Kirkpatrick, T., Cockshott, I.D., Douglas, E.J., and Nimmo, W.S. Pharmacokinetics of propofol (diprivan) in elderly patients. *Br. J. Anaesth.,* **1988,** *60:*146–150.

Knill, R.L., and Gelb, A.W. Ventilatory responses to hypoxia and hypercapnia during halothane sedation and anesthesia in man. *Anesthesiology,* **1978,** *49:*244–251.

Koblin, D.D., Chortkoff, B.S., Laster, M.J., *et al.* Polyhalogenated and perfluorinated compounds that disobey the Meyer-Overton hypothesis. *Anesth. Analg.,* **1994,** *79:*1043–1048.

Koblin, D.D., Eger, E.I. II, Johnson, B.H., Konopka, K., and Waskell, L. I-653 resists degradation in rats. *Anesth. Analg.,* **1988,** *67:*534–538.

Korttila, K., Linnoila, M., Ertama, P., and Hakkinen, S. Recovery and simulated driving after intravenous anesthesia with thiopental, methohexital, propanidid, or alphadione. *Anesthesiology,* **1975,** *43:*291–299.

Kosaka, Y., Takahashi, T., and Mark, L.C. Intravenous thiobarbiturate anesthesia for cesarean section. *Anesthesiology,* **1969,** *31:*489–506.

Kurz, A., Sessler, D.I., and Lenhardt, R. Perioperative normothermia to reduce the incidence of surgical-wound infection and shorten hospitalization. Study of Wound Infection and Temperature Group. *N. Engl. J. Med.,* **1996,** *334:*1209–1215.

Lakhlani, P.P., MacMillan, L.B., Guo, T.Z., *et al.* Substitution of a mutant α_{2a}-adrenergic receptor via "hit and run" gene targeting reveals the role of this subtype in sedative, analgesic, and anesthetic-sparing responses in vivo. *Proc. Natl. Acad. Sci. USA,* **1997,** *94:*9950–9955.

Langley, M.S., and Heel, R.C. Propofol. A review of its pharmacodynamic and pharmacokinetic properties and use as an intravenous anaesthetic. *Drugs,* **1988,** *35:*334–372.

Larrabee, M.G., and Posternak, J.M. Selective action of anesthetics on synapses and axons in mammalian sympathetic ganglia. *J. Neurophysiol.,* **1952,** *15:*91–114.

Laxenaire, M.C., Mata-Bermejo, E., Moneret-Vautrin, D.A., and Gueant, J.L. Life-threatening anaphylactoid reactions to propofol. *Anesthesiology,* **1992,** *77:*275–280.

Ledingham, I.M., and Watt, I. Influence of sedation on mortality in critically ill multiple trauma patients. *Lancet,* **1983,** *1:*1270.

Lockhart, S.H., Rampil, I.J., Yasuda, N., Eger, E.I. II, and Weiskopf, R.B. Depression of ventilation by desflurane in humans. *Anesthesiology,* **1991,** *74:*484–488.

Lysko, G.S., Robinson, J.L., Casto, R., and Ferrone, R.A. The stereospecific effects of isoflurane isomers *in vivo. Eur. J. Pharmacol.,* **1994,** *263:*25–29.

McCollum, J.S., Milligan, K.R., and Dundee, J.W. The antiemetic action of propofol. *Anaesthesia,* **1988,** *43:*239–240.

MacIver, M.B., Mikulec, A.A., Amagasu, S.M., and Monroe, F.A. Volatile anesthetics depress glutamate transmission *via* presynaptic actions. *Anesthesiology,* **1996,** *85:*823–834.

McMurray, T.J., Robinson, F.P., Dundee, J.W., Riddell, J.G., and McClean, E. A method for producing constant plasma concentration of drugs. Application to methohexitone. *Br. J. Anaesth.,* **1986,** *58:*1085–1090.

MacIver, M.B., and Roth, S.H. Inhalational anaesthetics exhibit pathway-specific and differential actions on hippocampal synaptic responses *in vitro. Br. J. Anaesth.,* **1988,** *60:*680–691.

McPherson, R.W., Briar, J.E., and Traystman, R.J. Cerebrovascular responsiveness to carbon dioxide in dogs with 1.4% and 2.8% isoflurane. *Anesthesiology,* **1989,** *70:*843–850.

Mangano, D.T., Layug, E.L., Wallace, A., and Tateo, I. Effect of atenolol on mortality and cardiovascular morbidity after noncardiac surgery. Multicenter Study of Perioperative Ischemia Research Group. *N. Engl. J. Med.,* **1996,** *335:*1713–1720.

Martin, W.R. Pharmacology of opioids. *Pharmacol. Rev.,* **1983,** *35:*283–323.

Mascia, M.P., Machu, T.K., and Harris, R.A. Enhancement of homomeric glycine receptor function by long-chain alcohols and anaesthetics. *Br. J. Pharmacol.,* **1996,** *119:*1331–1336.

Mayberg, T.S., Lam, A.M., Matta, B.F., Domino, K.B., and Winn, H.R. Ketamine does not increase cerebral blood flow velocity or intracranial pressure during isoflurane/nitrous oxide anesthesia in patients undergoing craniotomy. *Anesth. Analg.,* **1995,** *81:*84–89.

Mazze, R.I., Callan, C.M., Galvez, S.T., Delgado-Herrera, L., and Mayer, D.B. The effects of sevoflurane on serum creatinine and blood urea nitrogen concentrations: a retrospective, twenty-two-center, comparative evaluation of renal function in adult surgical patients. *Anesth. Analg.,* **2000,** *90:*683–688.

Mazze, R.I., Calverley, R.K., and Smith, N.T. Inorganic fluoride nephrotoxicity: prolonged enflurane and halothane anesthesia in volunteers. *Anesthesiology,* **1977,** *46:*265–271.

Mazze, R.I., Woodruff, R.E., and Heerdt, M.E. Isoniazid-induced enflurane defluorination in humans. *Anesthesiology,* **1982,** *57:*5–8.

Mennerick, S., Jevtovic-Todorovic, V., Todorovic, S.M., *et al.* Effect of nitrous oxide on excitatory and inhibitory synaptic transmission in hippocampal cultures. *J. Neurosci.,* **1998,** *18:*9716–9726.

Meuldermans, W.E., and Heykants, J.J. The plasma protein binding and distribution of etomidate in dog, rat and human blood. *Arch. Int. Pharmacodyn. Ther.,* **1976,** *221:*150–162.

Mihic, S.J., Ye, Q., Wick, M.J., *et al.* Sites of alcohol and volatile anaesthetic action on $GABA_A$ and glycine receptors. *Nature,* **1997,** *389:*385–389.

Mizobe, T., Maghsoudi, K., Sitwala, K., *et al.* Antisense technology reveals the α_{2A} adrenergic receptor to be the subtype mediating the hypnotic response to the highly selective agonist, dexmedetomidine, in the locus coeruleus of the rat. *J. Clin. Invest.,* **1996,** *98:*1076–1080.

Modica, P.A., and Tempelhoff, R. Intracranial pressure during induction of anaesthesia and tracheal intubation with etomidate-induced EEG burst suppression. *Can. J. Anaesth.,* **1992,** *39:*236–241.

Morgan, M., Lumley, J., and Whitwam, J.G. Respiratory effects of etomidate. *Br. J. Anaesth.,* **1977,** *49:*233–236.

Munson, E.S., Larson, C.P. Jr., Bahbad, A.A., *et al.* The effects of halothane, fluroxene and cyclopropane on ventilation: a comparative study in man. *Anesthesiology,* **1966,** *27:*716–728.

Nelson, L.E., Guo, T.Z., Lu, J., *et al.* The sedative component of anesthesia is mediated by $GABA_A$ receptors in an endogenous sleep pathway. *Nat. Neurosci.,* **2002,** *5:*979–984.

Newberg, L.A., Milde, J.J., and Michenfelder, J.D. The cerebral metabolic effects of isoflurane at and above concentrations that suppress cortical electrical activity. *Anesthesiology,* **1983,** *59:*23–28.

Nicoll, R.A. The effects of anaesthetics on synaptic excitation and inhibition in the olfactory bulb. *J. Physiol.,* **1972,** *223:*803–814.

Nicoll, R.A., and Madison, D.V. General anesthetics hyperpolarize neurons in the vertebrate central nervous system. *Science,* **1982,** *217:*1055–1057.

Nishina, K., Mikawa, K., Maekawa, N., Takao, Y., and Obara, H. Clonidine decreases the dose of thiamylal required to induce anesthesia in children. *Anesth. Analg.,* **1994,** *79:*766–768.

Nussmeier, N.A., Arlund, C., and Slogoff, S. Neuropsychiatric complications after cardiopulmonary bypass: cerebral protection by a barbiturate. *Anesthesiology,* **1986,** *64:*165–170.

O'Sullivan, H., Jennings, F., Ward, K., *et al.* Human bone marrow biochemical function and megaloblastic hematopoiesis after nitrous oxide anesthesia. *Anesthesiology,* **1981,** *55:*645–649.

Pagel, P.S., Kampine, J.P., Schmeling, W.T., and Warltier, D.C. Ketamine depresses myocardial contractility as evaluated by the preload recruitable stroke work relationship in chronically instrumented dogs

with autonomic nervous system blockade. *Anesthesiology,* **1992,** *76:*564–572.

Pasternak, G.W. Pharmacological mechanisms of opioid analgesics. *Clin Neuropharmacol,* **1993,** *16:*1–18.

Patel, A.J., Honore, E., Lesage, F., *et al.* Inhalational anesthetics activate two-pore-domain background K^+ channels. *Nat. Neurosci.,* **1999,** *2:*422–426.

Pauca, A.L., Savage, R.T., Simpson, S., and Roy, R.C. Effect of pethidine, fentanyl and morphine on post-operative shivering in man. *Acta. Anaesthesiol. Scand.,* **1984,** *28:*138–143.

Perouansky, M., Barnaov, D., Salman, M., and Yaari, Y. Effects of halothane on glutamate receptor–mediated excitatory postsynaptic currents. A patch-clamp study in adult mouse hippocampal slices. *Anesthesiology,* **1995,** *83:*109–119.

Pizov, R., Brown, R.H., Weiss, Y.S., *et al.* Wheezing during induction of general anesthesia in patients with and without asthma. A randomized, blinded trial. *Anesthesiology,* **1995,** *82:*1111–1116.

Raines, D.E., Claycomb, R.J., Scheller, M., and Forman, S.A. Nonhalogenated alkane anesthetics fail to potentiate agonist actions on two ligand-gated ion channels. *Anesthesiology,* **2001,** *95:*470–477.

Rampil, I.J. Anesthetic potency is not altered after hypothermic spinal cord transection in rats. *Anesthesiology,* **1994,** *80:*606–610.

Ravussin, P., and de Tribolet, N. Total intravenous anesthesia with propofol for burst suppression in cerebral aneurysm surgery: preliminary report of 42 patients. *Neurosurgery,* **1993,** *32:*236–240.

Reiz, S., Balfors, E., Friedman, A., Haggmark, S., and Peter, T. Effects of thiopentone on cardiac performance, coronary hemodynamics and myocardial oxygen consumption in chronic ischemic heart disease. *Acta. Anaesthesiol. Scand.,* **1981,** *25:*103–110.

Reves, J.G., Lell, W.A., McCracken, L.E. Jr., Kravetz, R.A., and Prough, D.S. Comparison of morphine and ketamine anesthetic technics for coronary surgery: a randomized study. *South. Med. J.,* **1978,** *71:*33–36.

Reynolds, D.S., Rosahl, T.W., Cirone, J., *et al.* Sedation and anesthesia mediated by distinct $GABA_A$ receptor isoforms. *J. Neurosci.,* **2003,** 23:8608–8617.

Ries, C.R., and Puil, E. Mechanism of anesthesia revealed by shunting actions of isoflurane on thalamocortical neurons. *J. Neurophysiol.,* **1999,** *81:*1795–1801.

Rooke, G.A., Choi, J.H., and Bishop, M.J. The effect of isoflurane, halothane, sevoflurane and thiopental/nitrous oxide on respiratory resistance after tracheal intubation. *Anesthesiology,* **1997,** *86:*1294–1299.

Rosenberg, H., Fletcher, J.E., and Seitman, D. Pharmacogenetics. In, *Clinical Anesthesia,* 3rd ed. (Barash, P.G., Cullen, B.F., Stoelting, R.K., eds., translator). Lippincott-Raven, Philadelphia, **1997,** pp. 489–517.

Schulte-Sasse, U., Hess, W., and Tarnow, J. Pulmonary vascular responses to nitrous oxide in patients with normal and high pulmonary vascular resistance. *Anesthesiology,* **1982,** *57:*9–13.

Schwilden, H., and Stoeckel, H. Effective therapeutic infusions produced by closed-loop feedback control of methohexital administration during total intravenous anesthesia with fentanyl. *Anesthesiology,* **1990,** *73:*225–229.

Sellgren, J., Ponten, J., and Wallin, B.G. Percutaneous recording of muscle nerve sympathetic activity during propofol, nitrous oxide, and isoflurane anesthesia in humans. *Anesthesiology,* **1990,** *73:*20–27.

Sessler, D.I. Perioperative heat balance. *Anesthesiology,* **2000,** *92:*578–596.

Shafer, A., Doze., V.A., Shafer, S.L., and White, P.F. Pharmacokinetics and pharmacodynamics of propofol infusions during general anesthesia. *Anesthesiology,* **1988,** *69:*348–356.

Shafer, S.L., and Stanski, D.R. Improving the clinical utility of anesthetic drug pharmacokinetics. *Anesthesiology,* **1992,** *76:*327–330.

Shafer, S.L., and Varvel, J.R. Pharmacokinetics, pharmacodynamics, and rational opioid selection. *Anesthesiology,* **1991,** *74:*53–63.

Shapiro, H.M., Galindo, A., Wyte, S.R., and Harris, A.B. Rapid intraoperative reduction of intracranial pressure with thiopentone. *Br. J. Anaesth.,* **1973,** *45:*1057–1062.

Short, T.G., Galletly, D.C., and Plummer, J.L. Hypnotic and anaesthetic action of thiopentone and midazolam alone and in combination. *Br. J. Anaesth.,* **1991,** *66:*13–19.

Simons, P.J., Cockshott, I.D., Douglas, E.J., *et al.* Disposition in male volunteers of a subanaesthetic intravenous dose of an oil in water emulsion of 14C-propofol. *Xenobiotica,* **1988,** *18:*429–440.

Smiley, R.M., Ornstein, E., Matteo, R.S., Pantuck, E.J., and Pantuck, C.B. Desflurane and isoflurane in surgical patients: comparison of emergence time. *Anesthesiology,* **1991,** *74:*425–428.

de Sousa, S.L., Dickinson, R., Lieb, W.R., and Franks, N.P. Contrasting synaptic actions of the inhalational general anesthetics isoflurane and xenon. *Anesthesiology,* **2000,** *92:*1055–1066.

Sprung, J., Schoenwald, P.K., and Schwartz, L.B. Cardiovascular collapse resulting from thiopental-induced histamine release. *Anesthesiology,* **1997,** *86:*1006–1007.

Stevens, W.C., Cromwell, T.H., Halsey, M.J., *et al.* The cardiovascular effects of a new inhalational anesthetic, Forane, in human volunteers at constant arterial carbon dioxide tension. *Anesthesiology,* **1971,** *35:*8–16.

Stoelting, R.K., Longnecker, D.E., and Eger, E.I. II. Minimum alveolar concentration in man on awakening from methoxyflurane, halothane, ether and fluroxene anesthesia: MAC$_{awake}$. *Anesthesiology,* **1970,** *33:*5–9.

Stullken, E.H. Jr., Milde, J.H., Michenfelder, J.D., and Tinker, J.H. The nonlinear responses of cerebral metabolism to low concentrations of halothane, enflurane, isoflurane, and thiopental. *Anesthesiology,* **1977,** *46:*28–34.

Subcommittee on the National Halothane Study of the Committee on Anesthesia, National Academy of Sciences–National Research Council. Summary of the National Halothane Study. Possible association between halothane anesthesia and postoperative hepatic necrosis. *JAMA,* **1966,** *197:*775–788.

Sumikawa, K., Ishizaka, N., and Suzaki, M. Arrhythmogenic plasma levels of epinephrine during halothane, enflurane, and pentobarbital anesthesia in the dog. *Anesthesiology,* **1983,** *58:*322–325.

Sussman, D.R. A comparative evaluation of ketamine anesthesia in children and adults. *Anesthesiology,* **1974,** *40:*459–464.

van Swinderen, B., Saifee, O., Shebester, L., *et al.* A neomorphic syntaxin mutation blocks volatile-anesthetic action in *Caenorhabditis elegans. Proc. Natl. Acad. Sci. USA,* **1999,** *96:*2479–2484.

Tegeder, I., Lotsch, J., and Geisslinger, G. Pharmacokinetics of opioids in liver disease. *Clin Pharmacokinet.,* **1999,** *37:*17–40.

Tomlin, S.L., Jenkins, A., Lieb, W.R., and Franks, N.P. Stereoselective effects of etomidate optical isomers on gamma-aminobutyric acid type A receptors and animals. *Anesthesiology,* **1998,** *88:*708–717.

Van Dyke, R.A., Baker, M.T., Jansson, I., and Schenkman, J. Reductive metabolism of halothane by purified cytochrome P-450. *Biochem. Pharmacol.,* **1988,** *37:*2357–2361.

Veroli, P., O'Kelly, B., Bertrand, F., *et al.* Extrahepatic metabolism of propofol in man during the anhepatic phase of orthotopic liver transplantation. *Br. J. Anaesth.,* **1992,** *68:*183–186.

Violet, J.M., Downie, D.L., Nakisa, R.C., Lieb, W.R., and Franks, N.P. Differential sensitivities of mammalian neuronal and muscle nicotinic acetylcholine receptors to general anesthetics. *Anesthesiology,* **1997,** *86:*866–874.

Wada, D.R., Bjorkman, S., Ebling, W.F., *et al.* Computer simulation of the effects of alterations in blood flows and body composition on thiopental pharmacokinetics in humans. *Anesthesiology,* **1997,** *87:*884–899.

Wagner, R.L., White, P.F., Kan, P.B., Rosenthal, M.H., and Feldman, D. Inhibition of adrenal steroidogenesis by the anesthetic etomidate. *N. Engl. J. Med.,* **1984,** *310:*1415–1421.

Wang, L.P., Hermann, C., and Westrin, P. Thiopentone requirements in adults after varying pre-induction doses of fentanyl. *Anaesthesia,* **1996,** *51:*831–835.

Weiskopf, R.B., Cahalan, M.K., Eger, E.I., *et al.* Cardiovascular actions of desflurane in normocarbic volunteers. *Anesth. Analg.,* **1991,** *73:*143–156.

Weiskopf, R.B., Holmes, M.A., Eger, E.I. II, *et al.* Cardiovascular effects of 1653 in swine. *Anesthesiology,* **1988,** *69:*303–309.

Westmoreland, C.L., Hoke, J.F., Sebel, P.S., Hug, C.C. Jr., and Muir, K.T. Pharmacokinetics of remifentanil (GI87084B) and its major metabolite (GI90291) in patients undergoing elective inpatient surgery. *Anesthesiology,* **1993,** *79:*893–903.

Whitacre, M.M., and Ellis, P.P. Outpatient sedation for ocular examination. *Surv. Ophthalmol.,* **1984,** *28:*643–652.

Wittmer, L.L., Hu, Y., Kalkbrenner, M., Evers, A.S., Zorumski, C.F., *et al.* Enantioselectivity of steroid-induced gamma-aminobutyric acidA receptor modulation and anesthesia. *Mol. Pharmacol.,* **1996,** *50:*1581–1586.

Yacoub, O., Doell, D., Kryger, M.H., and Anthonisen, N.R. Depression of hypoxic ventilatory response by nitrous oxide. *Anesthesiology,* **1976,** *45:*385–389.

Yamakage, M. Direct inhibitory mechanisms of halothane on canine tracheal smooth muscle contraction. *Anesthesiology,* **1992,** *77:*546–553.

MONOGRAPHS AND REVIEWS

Andrews, P.R., and Mark, L.C. Structural specificity of barbiturates and related drugs. *Anesthesiology,* **1982,** *57:*314–320.

Baldo, B.A., Fisher, M.M., and Harle, D.G. Allergy to thiopentone. *Clin. Rev. Allergy,* **1991,** *9:*295–308.

Bowdle, T.A. Adverse effects of opioid agonists and agonist-antagonists in anaesthesia. *Drug Saf.,* **1998,** *19:*173–189.

Chang, T., and Glazko, A.J. Biotransformation and disposition of ketamine. *Int. Anesthesiol. Clin.,* **1974,** *12:*157–177.

Christrup, L.L. Morphine metabolites. *Acta. Anaesthesiol. Scand.,* **1997,** *41:*116–122.

Clotz, M.A., and Nahata, M.C. Clinical uses of fentanyl, sufentanil, and alfentanil. *Clin. Pharm.,* **1991,** *10:*581–593.

Eger, E.I. II. New inhaled anesthetics. *Anesthesiology,* **1994,** *80:*906–922.

Eger, E.I. II. Uptake and distribution. In, *Anesthesia,* 5th ed. (Miller, R.D., ed.) Churchill Livingstone, Philadelphia, **2000,** pp. 74–95.

Fatheree, R.S., and Leighton, B.L. Acute respiratory distress syndrome after an exothermic Baralyme®-sevoflurane reaction. *Anesthesiology,* **2004,** *101:*531–533.

Kendig, J.J., MacIver, M.B., and Roth, S.H. Anesthetic actions in the hippocampal formation. *Ann. N.Y. Acad. Sci.,* **1991,** *625:*37–53.

Kingston, H.G., and Hirshman, C.A. Perioperative management of the patient with asthma. *Anesth. Analg.,* **1984,** *63:*844–855.

Krasowski, M.D., and Harrison, N.L. General anaesthetic actions on ligand-gated ion channels. *Cell. Mol. Life Sci.,* **1999,** *55:*1278–1303.

Langley, M.S., and Heel, R.C. Propofol. A review of its pharmacodynamic and pharmacokinetic properties and use as an intravenous anaesthetic. *Drugs,* **1988,** *35:*334–372.

Lynch, C. III. Myocardial excitation-contraction coupling. In, *Anesthesia: Biologic Foundations.* (Yaksh, T.L., Lynch, C. III, and Zapol, W.M., eds.) Lippincott-Raven, Philadelphia, **1997,** pp. 1047–1079.

Lynch, C. III, Baum, J., and Tenbrinck, R. Xenon anesthesia. *Anesthesiology,* **2000,** *92:*865–868.

Martin, W.R. Pharmacology of opioids. *Pharmacol. Rev.,* **1983,** *35:*283–323.

Modica, P.A., Tempelhoff, R., and White, P.F. Pro- and anticonvulsant effects of anesthetics. *Anesth. Analg.,* **1990,** *70:*433–444.

Pasternak, G.W. Pharmacological mechanisms of opioid analgesics. *Clin. Neuropharmacol.,* **1993,** *16:*1–18.

Reves, J.G., Fragen, R.J., Vinik, H.R., and Greenblatt, D.J. Midazolam: pharmacology and uses. *Anesthesiology,* **1985,** *62:*310–324.

Reves, J.G., Glass, P.S.A., and Lubarsky, D.A. Nonbarbiturate intravenous anesthetics. In, *Anesthesia,* 4th ed. (Miller, R.D., ed.) Churchill Livingstone, New York, **1994,** pp. 228–272.

Rosenberg, H., Fletcher, J.E., and Seitman, D. Pharmacogenetics. In, *Clinical Anesthesia,* 3rd ed. (Barash, P.G., Cullen, B.F., and Stoelting, R.K., eds.) Lippincott-Raven, Philadelphia, **1997,** pp. 489–517.

Rudolph, U., and Antkowiak, B. Molecular and neuronal substrates for general anaesthetics. *Nat. Rev. Neurosci.,* **2004,** *5:*709–720.

Tegeder, I., Lotsch, J., and Geisslinger, G. Pharmacokinetics of opioids in liver disease. *Clin. Pharmacokinet.,* **1999,** *37:*17–40.

Watcha, M.F., and White, P.F. Postoperative nausea and vomiting. Its etiology, treatment, and prevention. *Anesthesiology,* **1992,** *77:*162–184.

White, P.F., Way, W.L., and Trevor, A.J. Ketamine—its pharmacology and therapeutic uses. *Anesthesiology,* **1982,** *56:*119–136.

Wu, J., Previte, J.P., Adler, E., Myers, T., Ball, J., *et al.* Spontaneous ignition, explosion and fire with sevoflurane and barium hydroxide lime. *Anesthesiology,* **2004a,** *101:*534–537.

Wu, X-S., Sun, J-Y., Evers, A.S., Crowder, M., and Wu, L-G. Isoflurane inhibits transmitter release and the presynaptic action potential. *Anesthesiology,* **2004b,** *100:*663–670.

LOCAL ANESTHETICS

William A. Catterall and Kenneth Mackie

Local anesthetics bind reversibly to a specific receptor site within the pore of the Na^+ channels in nerves and block ion movement through this pore. When applied locally to nerve tissue in appropriate concentrations, local anesthetics can act on any part of the nervous system and on every type of nerve fiber, reversibly blocking the action potentials responsible for nerve conduction. Thus, a local anesthetic in contact with a nerve trunk can cause both sensory and motor paralysis in the area innervated. These effects of clinically relevant concentrations of local anesthetics are reversible with recovery of nerve function and no evidence of damage to nerve fibers or cells in most clinical applications.

History. The first local anesthetic, *cocaine*, was serendipitously discovered to have anesthetic properties in the late 19th century. Cocaine occurs in abundance in the leaves of the coca shrub (*Erythroxylon coca*). For centuries, Andean natives have chewed an alkali extract of these leaves for its stimulatory and euphoric actions. Cocaine was first isolated in 1860 by Albert Niemann. He, like many chemists of that era, tasted his newly isolated compound and noted that it caused a numbing of the tongue. Sigmund Freud studied cocaine's physiological actions, and Carl Koller introduced cocaine into clinical practice in 1884 as a topical anesthetic for ophthalmological surgery. Shortly thereafter, Halstead popularized its use in infiltration and conduction block anesthesia.

Chemistry and Structure–Activity Relationship. Cocaine is an ester of benzoic acid and the complex alcohol 2-carbomethoxy, 3-hydroxy-tropane (Figure 14–1). Because of its toxicity and addictive properties (*see* Chapter 23), a search for synthetic substitutes for cocaine began in 1892 with the work of Einhorn and colleagues, resulting in the synthesis of *procaine*, which became the prototype for local anesthetics for nearly half a century. The most widely used agents today are procaine, *lidocaine, bupivacaine,* and *tetracaine*.

The typical local anesthetics contain hydrophilic and hydrophobic moieties that are separated by an intermediate ester or amide linkage (Figure 14–1). A broad range of compounds containing these minimal structural features can satisfy the requirements for action as local anesthetics. The hydrophilic group usually is a tertiary amine but also may be a secondary amine; the hydrophobic moiety must be aromatic. The nature of the linking group determines some of the pharmacological properties of these agents. For example, local anesthetics with an ester link are hydrolyzed readily by plasma esterases.

The structure–activity relationship and the physicochemical properties of local anesthetics have been reviewed by Courtney and Strichartz (1987). Hydrophobicity increases both the potency and the duration of action of the local anesthetics. This arises because association of the drug at hydrophobic sites enhances the partitioning of the drug to its sites of action and decreases the rate of metabolism by plasma esterases and hepatic enzymes. In addition, the receptor site for these drugs on Na^+ channels is thought to be hydrophobic (*see* below), so that receptor affinity for anesthetic agents is greater for more hydrophobic drugs. Hydrophobicity also increases toxicity, so that the therapeutic index is decreased for more hydrophobic drugs.

Molecular size influences the rate of dissociation of local anesthetics from their receptor sites. Smaller drug molecules can escape from the receptor site more rapidly. This characteristic is important in rapidly firing cells, in which local anesthetics bind during action potentials and dissociate during the period of membrane repolarization. Rapid binding of local anesthetics during action potentials causes the frequency- and voltage-dependence of their action (*see* below).

Mechanism of Action.
Local anesthetics act at the cell membrane to prevent the generation and the conduction of nerve impulses. Conduction block can be demonstrated in squid giant axons from which the axoplasm has been removed.

Local anesthetics block conduction by decreasing or preventing the large transient increase in the permeability of excitable membranes to Na^+ that normally is produced by a slight depolarization of the membrane (*see* Chapter 12) (Strichartz and Ritchie, 1987). This action of local anesthetics is due to their direct interaction with voltage-gated Na^+ channels. As the anesthetic action progressively develops in a nerve, the threshold for electrical excitability gradually increases, the rate of rise of the action poten-

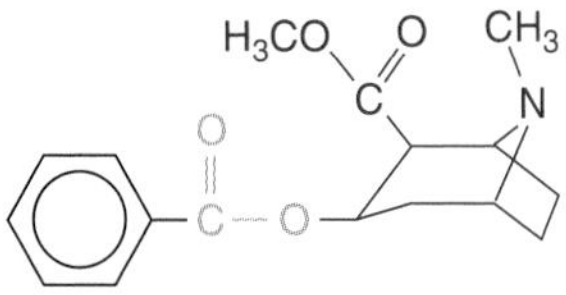

COCAINE

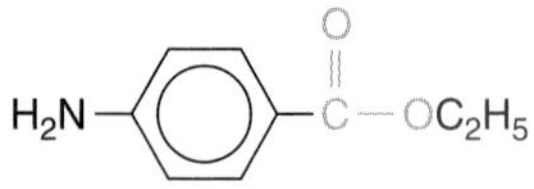

BENZOCAINE

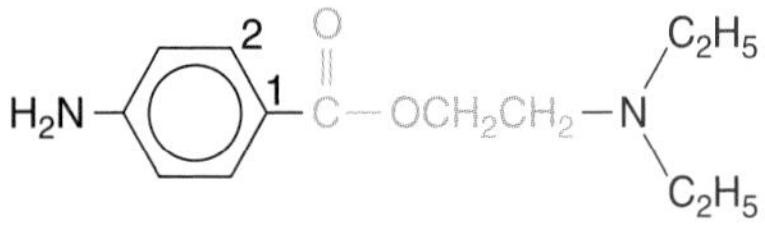

PROCAINE

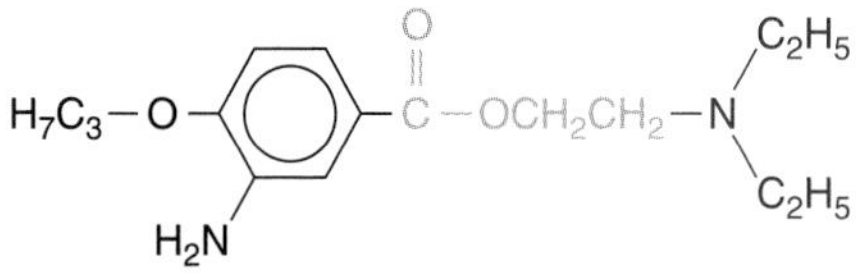

PROPARACAINE

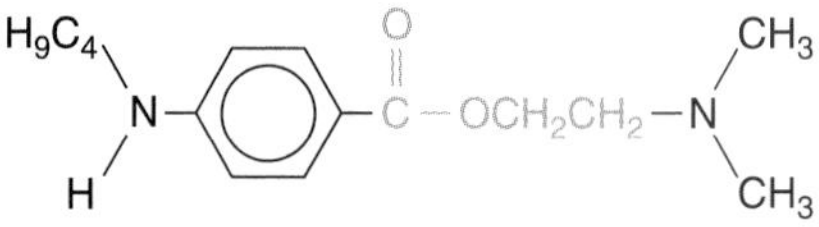

TETRACAINE

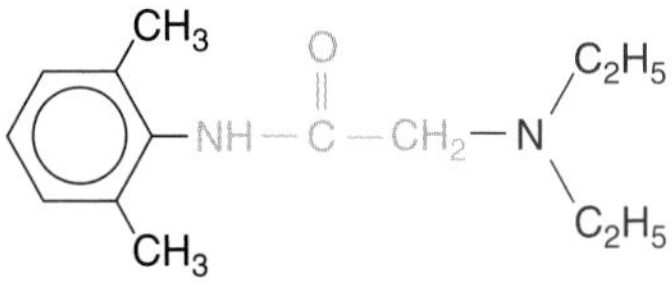

LIDOCAINE

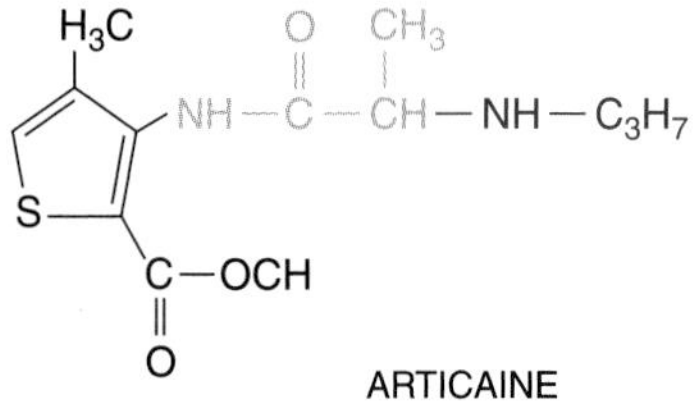

ARTICAINE

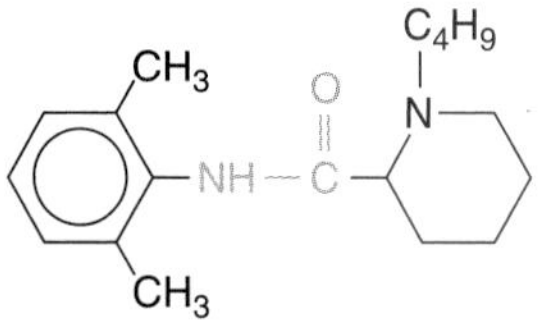

BUPIVACAINE

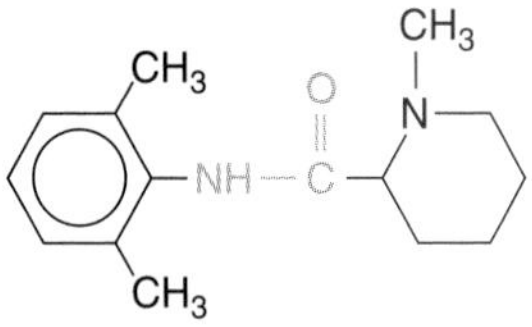

MEPIVACAINE

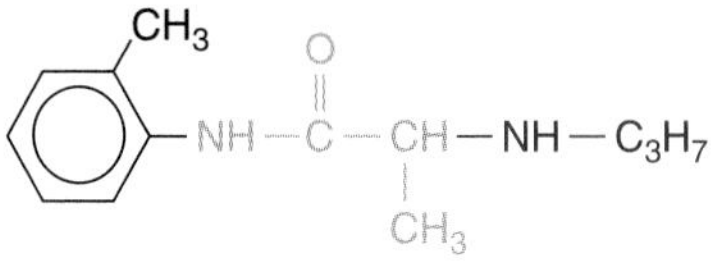

PRILOCAINE

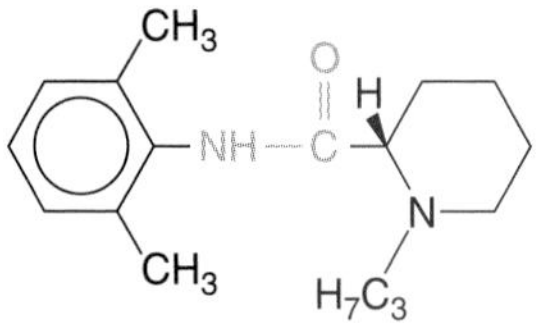

ROPIVACAINE

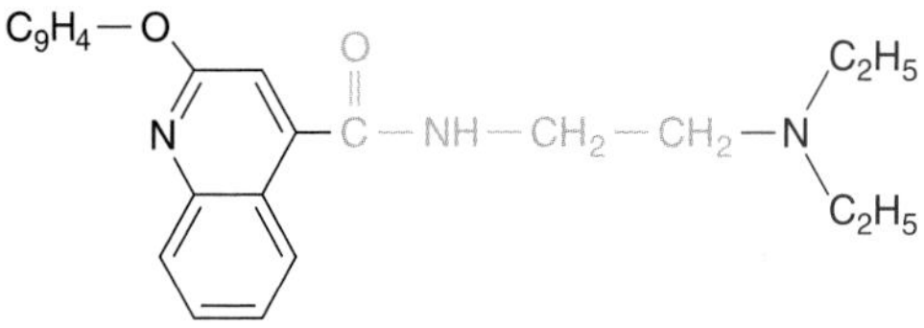

DIBUCAINE

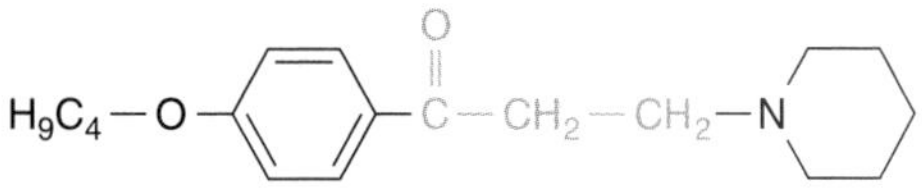

DYCLORINE

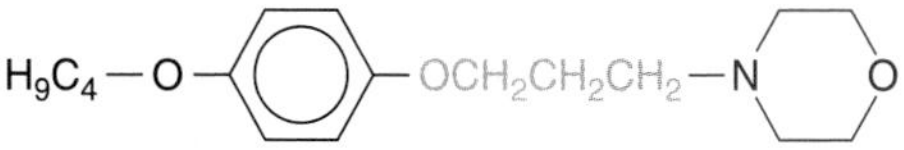

PRAMOXINE

tial declines, impulse conduction slows, and the safety factor for conduction decreases. These factors decrease the probability of propagation of the action potential, and nerve conduction eventually fails.

Local anesthetics can bind to other membrane proteins (Butterworth and Strichartz, 1990). In particular, they can block K^+ channels (Strichartz and Ritchie, 1987). However, since the interaction of local anesthetics with K^+ channels requires higher concentrations of drug, blockade of conduction is not accompanied by any large or consistent change in resting membrane potential.

Quaternary analogs of local anesthetics block conduction when applied internally to perfused giant axons of squid but are relatively ineffective when applied externally. These observations suggest that the site at which local anesthetics act, at least in their charged form, is accessible only from the inner surface of the membrane (Narahashi and Frazier, 1971; Strichartz and Ritchie, 1987). Therefore, local anesthetics applied externally first must cross the membrane before they can exert a blocking action.

Although a variety of physicochemical models have been proposed to explain how local anesthetics achieve conduction block (Courtney and Strichartz, 1987), it now is generally accepted that the major mechanism of action of these drugs involves their interaction with one or more specific binding sites within the Na^+ channel (Butterworth and Strichartz, 1990). The Na^+ channels of the mammalian brain are complexes of glycosylated proteins with an aggregate molecular size in excess of 300,000 daltons; the individual subunits are designated α (260,000 daltons) and β_1 to β_4 (33,000 to 38,000 daltons). The large α subunit of the Na^+ channel contains four homologous domains (I to IV); each domain is thought to consist of six transmembrane segments in α-helical conformation (S1 to S6; Figure 14–2) and an additional, membrane-reentrant pore (P) loop. The Na^+-selective transmembrane pore of the channel presumably resides in the center of a nearly symmetrical structure formed by the four homologous domains. The voltage dependence of channel opening is hypothesized to reflect conformational changes that result from the movement of "gating charges" (voltage sensors) in response to changes in the transmembrane potential. The gating charges are located in the S4 transmembrane helix; the S4 helices are both hydrophobic and positively charged, containing lysine or arginine residues at every third position. It is postulated that these residues move perpendicular to the plane of the membrane under the influence of the transmembrane potential, initiating a series of conformational changes in all four domains, which leads to the open state of the channel (Catterall, 2000; Figure 14–2).

The transmembrane pore of the Na^+ channel is thought to be surrounded by the S5 and S6 transmembrane helices and the short membrane-associated segments between them that form the P loop. Amino acid residues in these short segments are the most critical determinants of the ion conductance and selectivity of the channel.

After it opens, the Na^+ channel inactivates within a few milliseconds due to closure of an inactivation gate. This functional gate is formed by the short intracellular loop of protein that connects homologous domains III and IV (Figure 14–2). The loop folds over the intracellular mouth of the transmembrane pore during the process of inactivation and also binds to an inactivation gate "receptor" formed by the intracellular mouth of the pore.

Amino acid residues important for local anesthetic binding are found in the S6 segment in domains I, III, and IV (Ragsdale *et al.*, 1994; Yarov-Yarovoy *et al.*, 2002). Hydrophobic amino acid residues near the center and the intracellular end of the S6 segment may interact directly with bound local anesthetics (Figure 14–3). Experimental mutation of a large hydrophobic amino acid residue (isoleucine) to a smaller one (alanine) near the extracellular end of this segment creates a pathway for access of charged local anesthetic drugs from the extracellular solution to the receptor site. These findings place the local anesthetic receptor site within the intracellular half of the transmembrane pore of the Na^+ channel, with part of its structure contributed by amino acids in the S6 segments of domains I, III, and IV.

Frequency- and Voltage-Dependence of Local Anesthetic Action. The degree of block produced by a given concentration of local anesthetic depends on how the nerve has been stimulated and on its resting membrane

---

Figure 14–1. *Structural formulas of selected local anesthetics.* Most local anesthetics consist of a hydrophobic (aromatic) moiety (black), a linker region (light blue), and a substituted amine (hydrophilic region, in dark blue). The structures above are grouped by the nature of the linker region. Procaine is a prototypic ester-type local anesthetic; esters generally are well hydrolyzed by plasma esterases, contributing to the relatively short duration of action of drugs in this group. Lidocaine is a prototypic amide-type local anesthetic; these structures generally are more resistant to clearance and have longer durations of action. There are exceptions, including benzocaine (poorly water soluble; used only topically) and the structures with a ketone, an amidine, and an ether linkage. *Chloroprocaine has a chlorine atom on C2 of the aromatic ring of procaine.

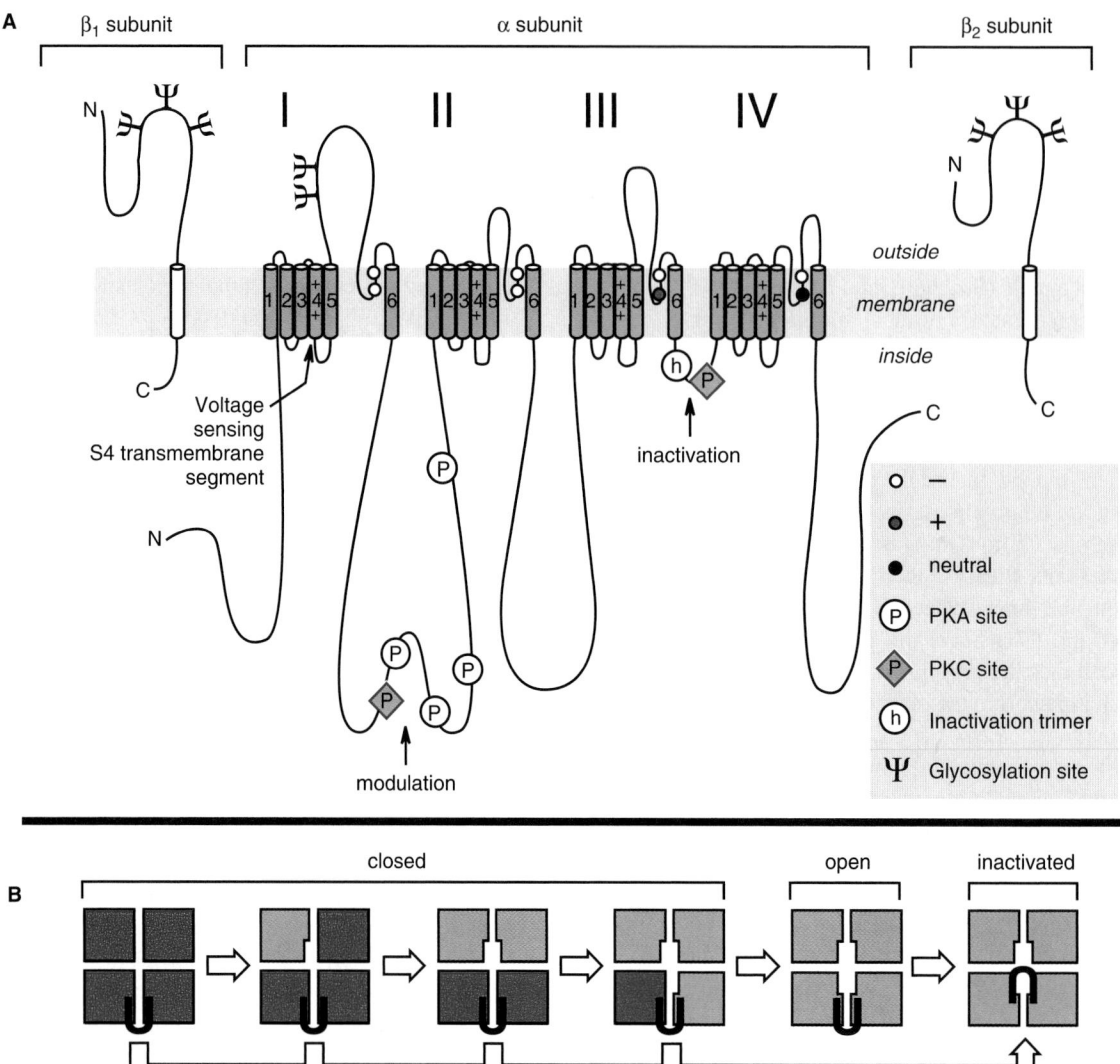

Figure 14–2. *Structure and function of voltage-gated Na⁺ channels.* ***A.*** A two-dimensional representation of the α (center), β_1 (left), and β_2 (right) subunits of the voltage-gated Na⁺ channel from mammalian brain. The polypeptide chains are represented by continuous lines with length approximately proportional to the actual length of each segment of the channel protein. Cylinders represent regions of transmembrane α helices. Ψ indicates sites of demonstrated N-linked glycosylation. Note the repeated structure of the four homologous domains (I through IV) of the α subunit. **Voltage Sensing.** The S4 transmembrane segments in each homologous domain of the α subunit serve as voltage sensors. (+) represents the positively charged amino acid residues at every third position within these segments. Electrical field (negative inside) exerts a force on these charged amino acid residues, pulling them toward the intracellular side of the membrane; depolarization allows them to move outward. **Pore.** The S5 and S6 transmembrane segments and the short membrane-associated loop between them (P loop) form the walls of the pore in the center of an approximately symmetrical square array of the four homologous domains (*see* Panel ***B***). The amino acid residues indicated by circles in the P loop are critical for determining the conductance and ion selectivity of the Na⁺ channel and its ability to bind the extracellular pore-blocking toxins tetrodotoxin and saxitoxin. **Inactivation.** The short intracellular loop connecting homologous domains III and IV serves as the inactivation gate of the Na⁺ channel. It is thought to fold into the intracellular mouth of the pore and occlude it within a few milliseconds after the channel opens. Three hydrophobic residues (isoleucine–phenylalanine–methionine; IFM) at the position marked **h** appear to serve as an inactivation particle, entering the intracellular mouth of the pore and binding therein to an inactivation gate receptor there. **Modulation.** The gating of the Na⁺ channel can be modulated by protein phosphorylation. Phosphorylation of the inactivation gate between homologous domains III and IV by protein kinase C slows inactivation. Phosphorylation of sites in the intracellular loop between homologous domains I and II by either protein kinase C (⬥) or cyclic AMP–dependent protein kinase (Ⓟ) reduces Na⁺ channel activation. ***B.*** The four homologous domains of the Na⁺ channel α subunit are illustrated as a square array, as viewed looking down on the membrane. The sequence of conformational changes that the Na⁺ channel undergoes during activation and inactivation is diagrammed. Upon depolarization, each of the four homologous domains sequentially undergoes a conformational change to an activated state. After all four domains have activated, the Na⁺ channel can open. Within a few milliseconds after opening, the inactivation gate between domains III and IV closes over the intracellular mouth of the channel and occludes it, preventing further ion conductance. (*Adapted from* Catterall, 2000, *with permission.*)

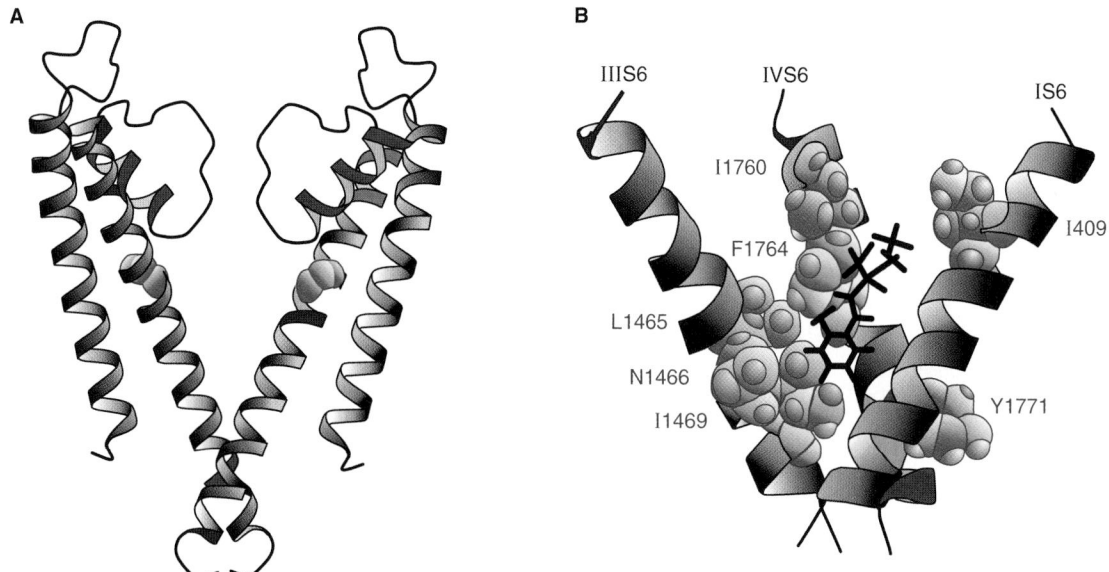

Figure 14–3. *The local anesthetic receptor site.* *A*. A drawing of the pore structure of a bacterial K⁺ channel (KcsA), which is related to the sodium channel. The KcsA channel has two transmembrane segments, analogous to the S5 and S6 segments of sodium channels. The S6-like segment forms the walls of the inner pore while the *P* loop forms the narrow ion selectivity filter at its extracellular (top) end. Four separate KcsA subunits form the pore in their center; only two of the subunits are shown here. *B*. A structural model of the local anesthetic receptor site. The S6 segments from domains I, III, and IV of the sodium channel α subunit are illustrated, based on the structure of the KcsA channel (panel *A*). The amino acid residues in these three transmembrane segments that contribute to the local anesthetic receptor site are indicated in single letter code and are presented in space-filling representation (light blue). An etidocaine molecule (black) is illustrated bound in the receptor site. Substitutions of the light blue residues with alanine reduce the affinity for local anesthetic block of sodium channels. It therefore is likely that the side chains of these amino acid residues contact bound local anesthetics in their receptor site. I1760 and I409 likely form the outer boundary of the local anesthetic receptor site. Mutations of I1760 allow drug access to the receptor site from the extracellular side (Ragsdale *et al.*, 1994; Yarov-Yarovoy *et al.*, 2002).

potential. Thus, a resting nerve is much less sensitive to a local anesthetic than one that is repetitively stimulated; higher frequency of stimulation and more positive membrane potential cause a greater degree of anesthetic block. These frequency- and voltage-dependent effects of local anesthetics occur because the local anesthetic molecule in its charged form gains access to its binding site within the pore only when the Na⁺ channel is in an open state and because the local anesthetic binds more tightly to and stabilizes the inactivated state of the Na⁺ channel (Courtney and Strichartz, 1987; Butterworth and Strichartz, 1990). Local anesthetics exhibit these properties to different extents depending on their pK_a, lipid solubility and molecular size. In general, the frequency dependence of local anesthetic action depends critically on the rate of dissociation from the receptor site in the pore of the Na⁺ channel. A high frequency of stimulation is required for rapidly dissociating drugs so that drug binding during the action potential exceeds drug dissociation between action potentials. Dissociation of smaller and more hydrophobic drugs is more rapid, so a higher frequency of stimulation is

required to yield frequency-dependent block. Frequency-dependent block of ion channels is most important for the actions of antiarrhythmic drugs (*see* Chapter 34).

Differential Sensitivity of Nerve Fibers to Local Anesthetics. Although there is great individual variation, for most patients treatment with local anesthetics causes the sensation of pain to disappear first, followed by loss of the sensations of temperature, touch, deep pressure, and finally motor function (Table 14–1). Classical experiments with intact nerves showed that the δ wave in the compound action potential, which represents slowly conducting, small-diameter myelinated fibers, was reduced more rapidly and at lower concentrations of cocaine than was the α wave, which represents rapidly conducting, large-diameter fibers (Gasser and Erlanger, 1929). In general, autonomic fibers, small unmyelinated C fibers (mediating pain sensations), and small myelinated Aδ fibers (mediating pain and temperature sensations) are blocked before the larger myelinated Aγ, Aβ, and Aα fibers (mediating postural, touch, pressure, and motor

Table 14-1
Susceptibility to Block of Types of Nerve Fibers

CONDUCTION BIOPHYSICAL CLASSIFICATION	ANATOMIC LOCATION	MYELIN	DIAMETER, μM	CONDUCTION VELOCITY, M·SEC^{-1}	FUNCTION	CLINICAL SENSITIVITY TO BLOCK
A fibers						
A α	Afferent to and efferent	Yes	6–22	10–85	Motor and	+
A β	from muscles and joints				proprioception	++
A γ	Efferent to muscle spindles	Yes	3–6	15–35	Muscle tone	++
A δ	Sensory roots and afferent peripheral nerves	Yes	1–4	5–25	Pain, temperature, touch	+++
B fibers	Preganglionic sympathetic	Yes	<3	3–15	Vasomotor, visceromotor, sudomotor, pilomotor	++++
C fibers						
Sympathetic	Postganglionic sympathetic	No	0.3–1.3	0.7–1.3	Vasomotor, visceromotor, sudomotor, pilomotor	++++
Dorsal root	Sensory roots and afferent peripheral nerves	No	0.4–1.2	0.1–2	Pain, temperature, touch	++++

SOURCE: Adapted from Carpenter and Mackey, 1992, with permission.

information; reviewed in Raymond and Gissen, 1987). The differential rate of block exhibited by fibers mediating different sensations is of considerable practical importance in the use of local anesthetics.

The precise mechanisms responsible for this apparent specificity of local-anesthetic action on pain fibers are not known, but several factors may contribute. The initial hypothesis from the classical work on intact nerves was that sensitivity to local-anesthetic block increases with decreasing fiber size, consistent with high sensitivity for pain sensation mediated by small fibers and low sensitivity for motor function mediated by large fibers (Gasser and Erlanger, 1929). However, when nerve fibers are dissected from nerves to allow direct measurement of action potential generation, no clear correlation of the concentration dependence of local anesthetic block with fiber diameter is observed (Franz and Perry, 1974; Fink and Cairns, 1984; Huang *et al.*, 1997). Therefore, it is unlikely that the fiber size *per se* determines the sensitivity to local anesthetic block under steady-state conditions. However, the spacing of nodes of Ranvier increases with the size of nerve fibers. Because a fixed number of nodes must be blocked to prevent conduction, small fibers with closely

spaced nodes of Ranvier may be blocked more rapidly during treatment of intact nerves, because the local anesthetic reaches a critical length of nerve more rapidly (Franz and Perry, 1974). Differences in tissue barriers and location of smaller C fibers and Aδ fibers in nerves also may influence the rate of local anesthetic action.

Effect of pH. Local anesthetics tend to be only slightly soluble as unprotonated amines. Therefore, they generally are marketed as water-soluble salts, usually hydrochlorides. Inasmuch as the local anesthetics are weak bases (typical pK_a values range from 8 to 9), their hydrochloride salts are mildly acidic. This property increases the stability of the local anesthetic esters and catecholamines added as vasoconstrictors. Under usual conditions of administration, the pH of the local anesthetic solution rapidly equilibrates to that of the extracellular fluids.

Although the unprotonated species of the local anesthetic is necessary for diffusion across cellular membranes, it is the cationic species that interacts preferentially with Na$^+$ channels. The results of experiments on anesthetized mammalian nonmyelinated fibers support this conclusion (Ritchie and Greengard, 1966). In these experiments, conduction could be blocked or unblocked merely by adjusting the pH of the bathing medium to 7.2 or 9.6, respectively, without altering the amount of anesthetic present. The primary role of the cationic form also was demonstrated by Narahashi and Frazier, who perfused the extracellular and axoplasmic surface of the giant squid axon with tertiary and quaternary amine local anesthetics (Narahashi and Frazier, 1971). However, the unprotonated molecular forms also possess some anesthetic activity (Butterworth and Strichartz, 1990).

Prolongation of Action by Vasoconstrictors. The duration of action of a local anesthetic is proportional to the time of contact with nerve. Consequently, maneuvers that keep the drug at the nerve prolong the period of anesthesia. For instance, cocaine inhibits the neuronal membrane transporters for catecholamines, thereby potentiating the effect of norepinephrine at α adrenergic receptors in the vasculature, resulting in vasoconstriction and reduced cocaine absorption in vascular beds where α adrenergic effects predominate (*see* Chapters 6 and 10). *Ropivacaine* and bupivacaine also cause vasoconstriction. In clinical practice, a vasoconstrictor, usually epinephrine, is often added to local anesthetics. The vasoconstrictor performs a dual service. By decreasing the rate of absorption, it not only localizes the anesthetic at the desired site, but also allows the rate at which it is destroyed in the body to keep pace with the rate at which it is absorbed into the circulation. This reduces its systemic toxicity. It should be noted, however, that epinephrine also dilates skeletal muscle vascular beds through actions at β_2 adrenergic receptors, and therefore has the potential to increase systemic toxicity of anesthetic deposited in muscle tissue.

Some of the vasoconstrictor agent may be absorbed systemically, occasionally to an extent sufficient to cause untoward reactions (*see* below). There also may be delayed wound healing, tissue edema, or necrosis after local anesthesia. These effects seem to occur partly because sympathomimetic amines increase the oxygen consumption of the tissue; this, together with the vasoconstriction, leads to hypoxia and local tissue damage. The use of vasoconstrictors in local-anesthetic preparations for anatomical regions with limited collateral circulation could produce irreversible hypoxic damage, tissue necrosis, and gangrene, and therefore is contraindicated.

Undesired Effects of Local Anesthetics. In addition to blocking conduction in nerve axons in the peripheral nervous system, local anesthetics interfere with the function of all organs in which conduction or transmission of impulses occurs. Thus, they have important effects on the central nervous system (CNS), the autonomic ganglia, the neuromuscular junction, and all forms of muscle (for review *see* Covino, 1987; Garfield and Gugino, 1987; Gintant and Hoffman, 1987). The danger of such adverse reactions is proportional to the concentration of local anesthetic achieved in the circulation. In general, in local anesthetics with chiral centers, the *S*-enantiomer is less toxic than the R-enantiomer (McClure, 1996).

Central Nervous System. Following absorption, local anesthetics may cause CNS stimulation, producing restlessness and tremor that may progress to clonic convulsions. In general, the more potent the anesthetic, the more readily convulsions may be produced. Alterations of CNS activity are thus predictable from the local anesthetic agent in question and the blood concentration achieved. Central stimulation is followed by depression; death usually is caused by respiratory failure.

The apparent stimulation and subsequent depression produced by applying local anesthetics to the CNS presumably is due solely to depression of neuronal activity; a selective depression of inhibitory neurons is thought to account for the excitatory phase *in vivo*. Rapid systemic administration of local anesthetics may produce death with no or only transient signs of CNS stimulation. Under these conditions, the concentration of the drug probably rises so rapidly that all neurons are depressed simultaneously. Airway control and ventilatory support are essential features of treatment in the late stage of intoxication. Benzodiazepines or rapidly acting barbiturates administered intravenously are the drugs of choice for both the prevention and arrest of convulsions (*see* Chapter 16).

Although drowsiness is the most frequent complaint that results from the CNS actions of local anesthetics, lidocaine may produce dysphoria or euphoria and muscle twitching. Moreover, both lidocaine and procaine may produce a loss of consciousness that is preceded only by symptoms of sedation (Covino, 1987). Whereas other local anesthetics also show the effect, cocaine has a particularly prominent effect on mood and behavior. These effects of cocaine and its potential for abuse are discussed in Chapter 23.

Cardiovascular System. Following systemic absorption, local anesthetics act on the cardiovascular system (Covino, 1987). The primary site of action is the myocardium, where decreases in electrical excitability, conduction rate, and force of contraction occur. In addition, most local anesthetics cause arteriolar dilation. Untoward cardiovascular effects usually are seen only after high systemic concentrations are attained and effects on the CNS are produced. However, on rare occasions, lower doses of some local anesthetics will cause cardiovascular collapse and death, probably due to either an action on the pacemaker or the sudden onset of ventricular fibrillation. It should be noted that ventricular tachycardia and fibrillation are relatively uncommon consequences of local anesthetics other than bupivacaine. The effects of local anesthetics such as lidocaine and *procainamide*, which also are used as antiarrhythmic drugs, are discussed in Chapter 34. Finally, it should be stressed that untoward cardiovascular effects of local anesthetic agents may result from their inadvertent intravascular administration, especially if epinephrine also is present.

Smooth Muscle. Local anesthetics depress contractions in the intact bowel and in strips of isolated intestine (Zipf and Dittmann, 1971). They also relax vascular and bronchial smooth muscle, although low concentrations initially may produce contraction (Covino, 1987). Spinal and epidural anesthesia, as well as instillation of local anesthetics into the peritoneal cavity, cause sympathetic nervous system paralysis, which can result in increased tone of gastrointestinal musculature (*see* below). Local anesthetics may increase the resting tone and decrease the contractions of isolated human uterine muscle; however, uterine contractions seldom are depressed directly during intrapartum regional anesthesia.

Neuromuscular Junction and Ganglionic Synapse. Local anesthetics also affect transmission at the neuromuscular junction. Procaine, for example, can block the response of skeletal muscle to maximal motor-nerve volleys and to acetylcholine at concentrations at which the muscle responds normally to direct electrical stimulation. Similar effects occur at autonomic ganglia. These effects are due to block of the ion channel of the acetylcholine receptor by high concentrations of the local anesthetics (Neher and Steinbach, 1978; Charnet *et al.*, 1990).

Hypersensitivity to Local Anesthetics.

Rare individuals are hypersensitive to local anesthetics. The reaction may manifest itself as an allergic dermatitis or a typical asthmatic attack (Covino, 1987). It is important to distinguish allergic reactions from toxic side effects and from the effects of co-administered vasoconstrictors. Hypersensitivity seems to occur more frequently with local anesthetics of the ester type and frequently extends to chemically related compounds. For example, individuals sensitive to procaine also may react to structurally similar compounds (*e.g.,* tetracaine) through reaction to a common metabolite. Although allergic responses to agents of the amide type are uncommon, solutions of such agents may contain preservatives such as methylparaben that may provoke an allergic reaction (Covino, 1987). Local anesthetic preparations containing a vasoconstrictor also may elicit allergic responses due to the sulfite added as an antioxidant for the catecholamine/vasoconstrictor.

Metabolism of Local Anesthetics.

The metabolic fate of local anesthetics is of great practical importance, because their toxicity depends largely on the balance between their rates of absorption and elimination. As noted above, the rate of absorption of many anesthetics can be reduced considerably by the incorporation of a vasoconstrictor agent in the anesthetic solution. However, the rate of degradation of local anesthetics varies greatly, and this is a major factor in determining the safety of a particular agent. Since toxicity is related to the free concentration of drug, binding of the anesthetic to proteins in the serum and to tissues reduces the concentration of free drug in the systemic circulation, and consequently reduces toxicity. For example, in intravenous regional anesthesia of an extremity, about half of the original anesthetic dose still is tissue bound 30 minutes after the restoration of normal blood flow (Arthur, 1987).

Some of the common local anesthetics (*e.g.,* tetracaine) are esters. They are hydrolyzed and inactivated primarily by a plasma esterase, probably plasma cholinesterase. The liver also participates in hydrolysis of local anesthetics. Since spinal fluid contains little or no esterase, anesthesia produced by the intrathecal injection of an anesthetic agent will persist until the local anesthetic agent has been absorbed into the circulation.

The amide-linked local anesthetics are, in general, degraded by the hepatic CYPs (cytochrome P450 enzymes), the initial reactions involving *N*-dealkylation and subsequent hydrolysis (Arthur, 1987). However, with *prilocaine*, the initial step is hydrolytic, forming *o*-toluidine metabolites that can cause methemoglobinemia. The extensive use of amide-linked local anesthetics in patients with severe hepatic disease requires caution. The amide-linked local anesthetics are extensively (55% to 95%) bound to plasma proteins, particularly α_1-acid glycoprotein. Many factors increase (*e.g.*, cancer, surgery, trauma, myocardial infarction, smoking, and uremia) or decrease (*e.g.*, oral contraceptives) the level of this glycoprotein, thereby changing the amount of anesthetic delivered to the liver for metabolism and thus influencing systemic toxicity. Age-related changes in protein binding of local anesthetics also occur. The neonate is relatively deficient in plasma proteins that bind local anesthetics and thereby is more susceptible to toxicity. Plasma proteins are not the sole determinant of local anesthetic availability. Uptake by the lung also may play an important role in the distribution of amide-linked local anesthetics in the body (Arthur, 1987). Reduced cardiac output slows delivery of the amide compounds to the liver, reducing their metabolism and prolonging their plasma half-lives (*see* Chapter 34).

COCAINE

Chemistry. Cocaine, an ester of benzoic acid and methylecgonine, occurs in abundance in the leaves of the coca shrub. Egconine is an amino alcohol base closely related to tropine, the amino alcohol in atropine. It has the same fundamental structure as the synthetic local anesthetics (Figure 14–1).

Pharmacological Actions and Preparations. The clinically desired actions of cocaine are the blockade of nerve impulses, as a consequence of its local anesthetic properties, and local vasoconstriction, secondary to inhibition of local norepinephrine reuptake. Toxicity and its potential for abuse have steadily decreased the clinical uses of cocaine. Its high toxicity is due to reduced catecholamine uptake in both the central and peripheral nervous systems. Its euphoric properties are due primarily to inhibition of catecholamine uptake, particularly in the CNS. Other local anesthetics do not block the uptake of norepinephrine and do not produce the sensitization to catecholamines, vasoconstriction, or mydriasis characteristic of cocaine. Currently, cocaine is used primarily for topical anesthesia of the upper respiratory tract, where its combination of both vasoconstrictor and local anesthetic properties provide anesthesia and shrinking of the mucosa. Cocaine hydrochloride is provided as a 1%, 4%, or 10% solution for topical application. For most applications, the 1% or 4% preparation is preferred to reduce toxicity. Because of its abuse potential, cocaine is listed as a schedule II drug by the U.S. Drug Enforcement Agency.

LIDOCAINE

Lidocaine (XYLOCAINE, others), an aminoethylamide (Figure 14–1), is the prototypical amide local anesthetic.

Pharmacological Actions. Lidocaine produces faster, more intense, longer lasting, and more extensive anesthesia than does an equal concentration of procaine. Lidocaine is an alternative choice for individuals sensitive to ester-type local anesthetics.

Absorption, Fate, and Excretion. Lidocaine is absorbed rapidly after parenteral administration and from the gastrointestinal and respiratory tracts. Although it is effective when used without any vasoconstrictor, epinephrine decreases the rate of absorption, such that the toxicity is decreased and the duration of action usually is prolonged. In addition to preparations for injection, an iontophoretic, needle-free drug-delivery system for a solution of lidocaine and epinephrine (IONTOCAINE) is available. This system generally is used for dermal procedures and provides anesthesia to a depth of up to 10 mm.

A lidocaine transdermal patch (LIDODERM) is used for relief of pain associated with postherpetic neuralgia. The combination of lidocaine (2.59%) and prilocaine (2.5%) in an occlusive dressing (EMLA ANESTHETIC DISC) is used as an anesthetic prior to venipuncture, skin graft harvesting, and infiltration of anesthetics into genitalia.

Lidocaine is dealkylated in the liver by CYPs to monoethylglycine xylidide and glycine xylidide, which can be metabolized further to monoethylglycine and xylidide. Both monoethylglycine xylidide and glycine xylidide retain local anesthetic activity. In humans, about 75% of the xylidide is excreted in the urine as the further metabolite 4-hydroxy-2, 6-dimethylaniline (Arthur, 1987).

Toxicity. The side effects of lidocaine seen with increasing dose include drowsiness, tinnitus, dysgeusia, dizziness, and twitching. As the dose increases, seizures, coma, and respiratory depression and arrest will occur. Clinically significant cardiovascular depression usually occurs at serum lidocaine levels that produce marked CNS effects. The metabolites monoethylglycine xylidide and glycine xylidide may contribute to some of these side effects.

Clinical Uses. Lidocaine has a wide range of clinical uses as a local anesthetic; it has utility in almost any application where a local anesthetic of intermediate duration is needed. Lidocaine also is used as an antiarrhythmic agent (*see* Chapter 34).

BUPIVACAINE

Pharmacological Actions. Bupivacaine (MARCAINE, SENSORCAINE), is a widely used amide local anesthetic; its structure is similar to that of lidocaine except that the amine-containing group is a butyl piperidine (Figure 14–1). *Levobupivacaine* (CHIROCAINE), the *S*-enantiomer of bupivacaine, also is available. Bupivacaine is a potent agent capable of producing prolonged anesthesia. Its long duration of action plus its tendency to provide more sensory than motor block has made it a popular drug for providing prolonged analgesia during labor or the postoperative period. By taking advantage of indwelling catheters and continuous infusions, bupivacaine can be used to provide several days of effective analgesia.

Toxicity. Bupivacaine and *etidocaine*, below, are more cardiotoxic than equi-effective doses of lidocaine. Clinically, this is manifested by severe ventricular arrhythmias and myocardial depression after inadvertent intravascular administration of large doses of bupivacaine. Although lidocaine and bupivacaine both rapidly block cardiac Na^+ channels during systole, bupivacaine dissociates much more slowly than does lidocaine during diastole, so a significant fraction of Na^+ channels at physiological heart rates remains blocked with bupivacaine at the end of diastole (Clarkson and Hondeghem, 1985). Thus, the block by bupivacaine is cumulative and substantially more than would be predicted by its local anesthetic potency. At least a portion of the cardiac toxicity of bupivacaine may be mediated centrally, as direct injection of small quantities of bupivacaine into the medulla can produce malignant ventricular arrhythmias (Thomas *et al.*, 1986). Bupivacaine-induced cardiac toxicity can be very difficult to treat, and its severity is enhanced by coexisting acidosis, hypercarbia, and hypoxemia. The *S*-enantiomer and the racemate are equally efficacious and potent; however, both animal studies (Groban *et al.*, 2001) and experience in humans (Foster and Markham, 2000) suggest that levobupivacaine is less cardiotoxic.

OTHER SYNTHETIC LOCAL ANESTHETICS

The number of synthetic local anesthetics is so large that it is impractical to consider them all here. Some local anesthetic agents are too toxic to be given by injection. Their use is restricted to topical application to the eye (*see* Chapter 63), the mucous membranes, or the skin (*see* Chapter 62). Many local anesthetics are suitable, however, for infiltration or injection to produce nerve block; some of them also are useful for topical application. The main categories of local anesthetics are given below; agents are listed alphabetically. (*See* Figure 14–1 for structures.)

Local Anesthetics Suitable for Injection

Articaine. *Articaine* (SEPTOCAINE) is a recently introduced amino amide, approved in the United States for dental and periodontal procedures. It exhibits a rapid onset (1 to 6 minutes) and duration of action of approximately 1 hour.

Chloroprocaine. *Chloroprocaine* (NESACAINE), an ester local anesthetic introduced in 1952, is a chlorinated derivative of procaine. Its major assets are its rapid onset and short duration of action and its reduced acute toxicity due to its rapid metabolism (plasma half-life approximately 25 seconds). Enthusiasm for its use has been tempered by reports of prolonged sensory and motor block after epidural or subarachnoid administration of large doses. This toxicity appears to have been a consequence of low pH and the use of sodium metabisulfite as a preservative in earlier formulations. There are no reports of neurotoxicity with newer preparations of chloroprocaine, which contain calcium EDTA as the preservative, although these preparations also are not recommended for intrathecal administration. A higher-than-expected incidence of muscular back pain following epidural anesthesia with 2-chloroprocaine also has been reported (Stevens *et al.*, 1993). This back pain is thought to be due to tetany in the paraspinus muscles, which may be a consequence of Ca^{2+} binding by the EDTA included as a preservative; the incidence of back pain appears to be related to the volume of drug injected and its use for skin infiltration.

Etidocaine. *Etidocaine* (DURANEST), is a long-acting amino amide with an onset of action faster than that of bupivacaine and comparable to that of lidocaine, and a duration of action similar to that of bupivacaine. Compared to bupivacaine, etidocaine produces preferential motor blockade. Thus, while it is useful for surgery requiring intense skeletal muscle relaxation, its utility in labor or postoperative analgesia is limited. Its cardiac toxicity is similar to that of bupivacaine. Etidocaine no longer is marketed in the United States.

Mepivacaine. *Mepivacaine* (CARBOCAINE, POLOCAINE) is an intermediate-acting amino amide. Its pharmacological properties are similar to those of lidocaine. Mepivacaine, however, is more toxic to the neonate and thus is not used in obstetrical anesthesia. The increased toxicity of mepivacaine in the neonate is related to ion trapping of this agent because of the lower pH of neonatal blood and the pK_a of mepivacaine rather than to its slower metabolism in the neonate. It appears to have a slightly higher therapeutic index in adults than does lidocaine. Its onset of action is similar to that of lidocaine and its duration slightly longer (about 20%) than that of lidocaine in the absence of a coadministered vasoconstrictor. Mepivacaine is not effective as a topical anesthetic.

Prilocaine. *Prilocaine* (CITANEST) is an intermediate-acting amino amide. It has a pharmacological profile similar to that of lidocaine. The primary differences are that it causes little vasodilation and thus can be used without a vasoconstrictor if desired, and its increased volume of distribution reduces its CNS toxicity, making it suitable for intravenous regional blocks (*see* below). It is unique among the local anesthetics in its propensity to cause methemoglobinemia. This effect is a consequence of the metabolism of the aromatic ring to *o*-toluidine. Development of methemoglobinemia is dependent on the total dose administered, usually appearing after a dose of 8 mg/kg. In healthy persons, methemoglobinemia usually is not a problem. If necessary, it can be treated by the

intravenous administration of methylene blue (1 to 2 mg/kg). Methemoglobinemia following prilocaine has limited its use in obstetrical anesthesia, because it complicates evaluation of the newborn. Also, methemoglobinemia is more common in neonates due to decreased resistance of fetal hemoglobin to oxidant stresses and the immaturity of enzymes in the neonate that convert methemoglobin back to the ferrous state.

Ropivacaine. The cardiac toxicity of bupivacaine stimulated interest in developing a less toxic, long-lasting local anesthetic. One result of that search was the development of the amino ethylamide ropivacaine (NAROPIN), the *S*-enantiomer of 1-propyl-2′,6′-pipecoloxylidide. The *S*-enantiomer was chosen because it has a lower toxicity than the *R*-isomer (McClure, 1996). Ropivacaine is slightly less potent than bupivacaine in producing anesthesia. In several animal models, it appears to be less cardiotoxic than equi-effective doses of bupivacaine. In clinical studies, ropivacaine appears to be suitable for both epidural and regional anesthesia, with a duration of action similar to that of bupivacaine. Interestingly, it seems to be even more motor-sparing than bupivacaine.

Procaine. Procaine (NOVOCAIN), introduced in 1905, was the first synthetic local anesthetic and is an amino ester. It has been supplanted by newer agents, and its use now is confined to infiltration anesthesia and occasionally for diagnostic nerve blocks. This is because of its low potency, slow onset, and short duration of action. While its toxicity is fairly low, it is hydrolyzed *in vivo* to produce para-aminobenzoic acid, which inhibits the action of sulfonamides. Thus, large doses should not be administered to patients taking sulfonamide drugs.

Tetracaine. *Tetracaine* (PONTOCAINE), is a long-acting amino ester. It is significantly more potent and has a longer duration of action than procaine. Tetracaine may exhibit increased systemic toxicity because it is more slowly metabolized than the other commonly used ester local anesthetics. Currently, it is widely used in spinal anesthesia when a drug of long duration is needed. Tetracaine also is incorporated into several topical anesthetic preparations. With the introduction of bupivacaine, tetracaine is rarely used in peripheral nerve blocks because of the large doses often necessary, its slow onset, and its potential for toxicity.

Local Anesthetics Used Primarily to Anesthetize Mucous Membranes and Skin

Some anesthetics are either too irritating or too ineffective to be applied to the eye. However, they are useful as topical anesthetic agents on the skin and/or mucous membranes. These preparations are effective in the symptomatic relief of anal and genital pruritus, poison ivy rashes, and numerous other acute and chronic dermatoses. They sometimes are combined with a glucocorticoid or antihistamine and are available in a number of proprietary formulations (*see* Figure 14–1 for structures).

Dibucaine (NUPERCAINAL) is a quinoline derivative. Its toxicity resulted in its removal from the United States market as an injectable preparation; however, it retains wide popularity outside the United States as a spinal anesthetic. It currently is available as a cream and an ointment for use on the skin.

Dyclonine hydrochloride (DYCLONE) has a rapid onset of action and duration of effect comparable to that of procaine. It is absorbed through the skin and mucous membranes. The compound has been used as 0.5% or 1% solution for topical anesthesia during endoscopy, for oral mucositis pain following radiation or chemotherapy, and for anogenital procedures; however, marketing of these solutions has been discontinued in the United States. Dyclonine is an active ingredient in a number of over-the-counter medications including sore throat lozenges (SUCRETS, others), a gel for cold sores (TANAC), and a 0.75% solution (SKIN SHIELD) to protect against contact dermatitis.

Pramoxine hydrochloride (ANUSOL, TRONOTHANE, others) is a surface anesthetic agent that is not a benzoate ester. Its distinct chemical structure may help minimize the danger of cross-sensitivity reactions in patients allergic to other local anesthetics. Pramoxine produces satisfactory surface anesthesia and is reasonably well tolerated on the skin and mucous membranes. It is too irritating to be used on the eye or in the nose. Various preparations, usually containing 1% pramoxine, are available for topical application.

Anesthetics of Low Solubility

Some local anesthetics are poorly soluble in water, and consequently are too slowly absorbed to be toxic. They can be applied directly to wounds and ulcerated surfaces, where they remain localized for long periods of time, producing a sustained anesthetic action. Chemically, they are esters of para-aminobenzoic acid lacking the terminal amino group possessed by the previously described local anesthetics. The most important member of the series is benzocaine (ethyl aminobenzoate; AMERICAINE ANESTHETIC, others). Benzocaine is structurally similar to procaine, but lacks the terminal diethylamino group (Figure 14–1). It is incorporated into a large number of topical preparations. Benzocaine can cause methemoglobinemia (*see* text concerning methemoglobinemia caused by prilocaine, above); consequently, dosing recommendations must be followed carefully.

Local Anesthetics Largely Restricted to Ophthalmological Use

Anesthesia of the cornea and conjunctiva can be obtained readily by topical application of local anesthetics. However, most of the local anesthetics described above are too irritating for ophthalmological use. The first local anesthetic used in ophthalmology, cocaine, has the severe disadvantages of producing mydriasis and corneal sloughing and has fallen out of favor. The two compounds used most frequently today are *proparacaine* (ALCAINE, OPHTHAINE, others) and tetracaine (Figure 14–1). In addition to being less irritating during administration, proparacaine has the added advantage of bearing little antigenic similarity to the other benzoate local anesthetics. Thus, it sometimes can be used in individuals sensitive to the amino ester local anesthetics.

For use in ophthalmology, these local anesthetics are instilled a single drop at a time. If anesthesia is incomplete, successive drops are applied until satisfactory conditions are obtained. The duration of anesthesia is determined chiefly by the vascularity of the tissue; thus it is longest in normal cornea and shortest in inflamed conjunctiva. In the latter case repeated instillations may be necessary to maintain adequate anesthesia for the duration of the procedure. Long-term administration of topical anesthesia to the eye has been associated with retarded healing, pitting and sloughing of the corneal epithelium, and predisposition of the eye to inadvertent injury. Thus, these drugs should not be prescribed for self-administration. For drug delivery, pharmacokinetic, and toxicity issues unique to drugs for ophthalmic use, *see* Chapter 63.

Tetrodotoxin and Saxitoxin

These two biological toxins also block the pore of the Na^+ channel. *Tetrodotoxin* is found in the gonads and other visceral tissues of some fish of the order Tetraodontiformes (to which the Japanese *fugu*, or puffer fish, belongs); it also occurs in the skin of some newts of the family Salamandridae and of the Costa Rican frog *Atelopus*. *Saxitoxin*, and possibly some related toxins, are elaborated by the dinoflagellates *Gonyaulax catenella* and *Gonyaulax tamarensis* and are retained in the tissues of clams and other shellfish that eat these organisms. Given the right conditions of temperature and light, the *Gonyaulax* may multiply so rapidly as to discolor the ocean, causing the condition known as *red tide*. Shellfish feeding on *Gonyaulax* at this time become extremely toxic to human beings and are responsible for periodic outbreaks of paralytic shellfish poisoning (Stommel and Watters, 2004). Although the toxins are chemically different from each other, their mechanisms of action are similar (Ritchie, 1980). Both toxins, in nanomolar concentrations, specifically block the outer mouth of the pore of Na^+ channels in the membranes of excitable cells. As a result, the action potential is blocked. The receptor site for these toxins is formed by amino acid residues in the *P* loop of the Na^+ channel α subunit (Figure 14–2) in all four domains (Terlau *et al.*, 1991; Catterall, 2000). Not all Na^+ channels are equally sensitive to tetrodotoxin; some Na^+ channels in cardiac myocytes and dorsal root ganglion neurons are resistant, and a tetrodotoxin-resistant Na^+ channel is expressed when skeletal muscle is denervated. Tetrodotoxin and saxitoxin are two of the most potent poisons known; the minimal lethal dose of each in the mouse is about 8 μg/kg. Both toxins have caused fatal poisoning in humans due to paralysis of the respiratory muscles. Therefore the treatment of severe cases of poisoning requires support of respiration. Blockade of vasomotor nerves, together with a relaxation of vascular smooth muscle, seems to be responsible for the hypotension that is characteristic of tetrodotoxin poisoning. Early gastric lavage and pressor support also are indicated. If the patient survives paralytic shellfish poisoning for 24 hours, the prognosis is good.

CLINICAL USES OF LOCAL ANESTHETICS

Local anesthesia is the loss of sensation in a body part without the loss of consciousness or the impairment of central control of vital functions. It offers two major advantages. First, physiological perturbations associated with general anesthesia are avoided; second, neurophysiological responses to pain and stress can be modified beneficially. As discussed above, local anesthetics potentially can produce deleterious side effects. Proper choice of a local anesthetic and care in its use are the primary determinants in avoiding toxicity. There is a poor relationship between the amount of local anesthetic injected and peak plasma levels in adults. Furthermore, peak plasma levels vary widely depending on the area of injection. They are highest with interpleural or intercostal blocks and lowest with subcutaneous infiltration. Thus, recommended maximum doses serve only as general guidelines.

The following discussion summarizes the pharmacological and physiological consequences of the use of local anesthetics categorized by method of administration. A more comprehensive discussion of their use and administration is presented in textbooks on regional anesthesia (*e.g.*, Cousins and Bridenbaugh, 1998).

Topical Anesthesia

Anesthesia of mucous membranes of the nose, mouth, throat, tracheobronchial tree, esophagus, and genitourinary tract can be produced by direct application of aqueous solutions of salts of many local anesthetics or by suspension of the poorly soluble local anesthetics. Tetracaine (2%), lidocaine (2% to 10%), and cocaine (1% to 4%) typically are used. Cocaine is used only in the nose, nasopharynx, mouth, throat, and ear, where it uniquely produces vasoconstriction as well as anesthesia. The shrinking of mucous membranes decreases operative bleeding while improving surgical visualization. Comparable vasoconstriction can be achieved with other local anesthetics by the addition of a low concentration of a vasoconstrictor such as phenylephrine (0.005%). Epinephrine, topically applied, has no significant local effect and does not prolong the duration of action of local anesthetics applied to mucous membranes because of poor penetration. *Maximal* safe total dosages for topical anesthesia in a healthy 70-kg adult are 300 mg for lidocaine, 150 mg for cocaine, and 50 mg for tetracaine.

Peak anesthetic effect following topical application of cocaine or lidocaine occurs within 2 to 5 minutes (3 to 8 minutes with tetracaine), and anesthesia lasts for 30 to 45 minutes (30 to 60 minutes with tetracaine). Anesthesia is entirely superficial; it does not extend to submucosal structures. This technique does not alleviate joint pain or discomfort from subdermal inflammation or injury.

Local anesthetics are absorbed rapidly into the circulation following topical application to mucous membranes or denuded skin. Thus, topical anesthesia always carries the risk of systemic toxic reactions. Systemic toxicity has occurred even following the use of local anesthetics to control discomfort associated with severe diaper rash in infants. Absorption is particularly rapid when local anesthetics are applied to the tracheobronchial tree. Concentrations in blood after instillation of local anesthetics into the airway are nearly the same as those following intravenous injection. Surface anesthetics for the skin and cornea have been described above.

The introduction of an eutectic mixture of lidocaine (2.5%) and prilocaine (2.5%) (EMLA) bridges the gap between topical and infiltration anesthesia. The efficacy of this combination lies in the fact that the mixture of prilocaine and lidocaine has a melting point less than that of either compound alone, existing at room temperature as an oil that can penetrate intact skin. EMLA cream produces anesthesia to a maximum depth of 5 mm and is applied as a cream on intact skin under an occlusive dressing, which must be left in place for at least 1 hour. It is effective for procedures involving skin and superficial subcutaneous structures (*e.g.*, venipuncture and skin graft harvesting). The component local anesthetics will be absorbed into the systemic circulation, potentially producing toxic effects (*see* above). Guidelines are available to calculate the maximum amount of cream that can be applied and area of skin covered. It must not be used on mucous membranes or abraded skin, as rapid absorption across these surfaces may result in systemic toxicity.

Infiltration Anesthesia

Infiltration anesthesia is the injection of local anesthetic directly into tissue without taking into consideration the course of cutaneous nerves. Infiltration anesthesia can be so superficial as to include only the skin. It also can include deeper structures, including intra-abdominal organs, when these too are infiltrated.

The duration of infiltration anesthesia can be approximately doubled by the addition of epinephrine (5 μg/ml) to the injection solution; epinephrine also decreases peak concentrations of local anesthetics in blood. *Epinephrine-containing solutions should not, however, be injected into tissues supplied by end arteries—for example, fingers and toes, ears, the nose, and the penis. The resulting vasoconstriction may cause gangrene.* For the same reason, epinephrine should be avoided in solutions injected intracutaneously. Since epinephrine also is absorbed into the circulation, its use should be avoided in those for whom adrenergic stimulation is undesirable.

The local anesthetics used most frequently for infiltration anesthesia are lidocaine (0.5% to 1%), procaine (0.5% to 1%), and bupivacaine (0.125% to 0.25%). When used without epinephrine, up to 4.5 mg/kg of lidocaine, 7 mg/kg of procaine, or 2 mg/kg of bupivacaine can be employed in adults. When epinephrine is added, these amounts can be increased by one-third.

The advantage of infiltration anesthesia and other regional anesthetic techniques is that it can provide satisfactory anesthesia without disrupting normal bodily functions. The chief disadvantage of infiltration anesthesia is that relatively large amounts of drug must be used to anesthetize relatively small areas. This is no problem with minor surgery. When major surgery is performed, however, the amount of local anesthetic that is required makes systemic toxic reactions likely. The amount of anesthetic required to anesthetize an area can be reduced significantly and the duration of anesthesia increased markedly by specifically blocking the nerves that innervate the area of interest. This can be done at one of several levels: subcutaneously, at major nerves, or at the level of the spinal roots.

Field Block Anesthesia

Field block anesthesia is produced by subcutaneous injection of a solution of local anesthetic in order to anesthetize the region distal to the injection. For example, subcutaneous infiltration of the proximal portion of the volar surface of the forearm results in an extensive area of cutaneous anesthesia that starts 2 to 3 cm distal to the site of injection. The same principle can be applied with particular benefit to the scalp, the anterior abdominal wall, and the lower extremity.

The drugs, concentrations, and doses recommended are the same as for infiltration anesthesia. The advantage of field block anesthesia is that less drug can be used to provide a greater area of anesthesia than when infiltration anesthesia is used. Knowledge of the relevant neuroanatomy obviously is essential for successful field block anesthesia.

Nerve Block Anesthesia

Injection of a solution of a local anesthetic into or about individual peripheral nerves or nerve plexuses produces even greater areas of anesthesia than do the techniques described above. Blockade of mixed peripheral nerves and nerve plexuses also usually anesthetizes somatic motor nerves, producing skeletal muscle relaxation, which is essential for some surgical procedures. The areas of sensory and motor block usually start several centimeters distal to the site of injection. Brachial plexus blocks are particularly useful for procedures on the upper extremity and shoulder. Intercostal nerve blocks are effective for anesthesia and relaxation of the anterior abdominal wall. Cervical plexus block is appropriate for surgery of the neck.

Sciatic and femoral nerve blocks are useful for surgery distal to the knee. Other useful nerve blocks prior to surgical procedures include blocks of individual nerves at the wrist and at the ankle, blocks of individual nerves such as the median or ulnar at the elbow, and blocks of sensory cranial nerves.

There are four major determinants of the onset of sensory anesthesia following injection near a nerve. These are the proximity of the injection to the nerve, concentration and volume of drug, the degree of ionization of the drug, and time. Local anesthetic is never intentionally injected into the nerve, as this would be painful and could cause nerve damage. Instead, the anesthetic agent is deposited as close to the nerve as possible. Thus the local anesthetic must diffuse from the site of injection into the nerve, where it acts. The rate of diffusion is determined chiefly by the concentration of the drug, its degree of ionization (ionized local anesthetic diffuses more slowly), its hydrophobicity, and the physical characteristics of the tissue surrounding the nerve. Higher concentrations of local anesthetic will provide a more rapid onset of peripheral nerve block. The utility of higher concentrations, however, is limited by systemic toxicity and by direct neural toxicity of concentrated local anesthetic solutions. For a given concentration, local anesthetics with lower pK_a values tend to have a more rapid onset of action because more drug is uncharged at neutral pH. For example, the onset of action of lidocaine occurs in about 3 minutes; 35% of lidocaine is in the basic form at pH 7.4. In contrast, the onset of action of bupivacaine requires about 15 minutes; only 5% to 10% of bupivacaine is uncharged at this pH. Increased hydrophobicity might be expected to speed onset by increased penetration into nerve tissue. However, it also will increase binding in tissue lipids. Furthermore, the more hydrophobic local anesthetics also are more potent (and toxic) and thus must be used at lower concentrations, decreasing the concentration gradient for diffusion. Tissue factors also play a role in determining the rate of onset of anesthetic effects. The amount of connective tissue that must be penetrated can be significant in a nerve plexus compared to isolated nerves and can slow or even prevent adequate diffusion of local anesthetic to the nerve fibers.

Duration of nerve block anesthesia depends on the physical characteristics of the local anesthetic used and the presence or absence of vasoconstrictors. Especially important physical characteristics are lipid solubility and protein binding. Local anesthetics can be broadly divided into three categories: those with a short (20 to 45 minutes) duration of action in mixed peripheral nerves, such as procaine; those with an intermediate (60 to 120 minutes) duration of action, such as lidocaine and mepivacaine; and those with a long (400 to 450 minutes) duration of action, such as bupivacaine, ropivacaine, and tetracaine. Block duration of the intermediate-acting local anesthetics such as lidocaine can be prolonged by the addition of epinephrine (5 μg/ml). The degree of block prolongation in peripheral nerves following the addition of epinephrine appears to be related to the intrinsic vasodilatory properties of the local anesthetic and thus is most pronounced with lidocaine.

The types of nerve fibers that are blocked when a local anesthetic is injected about a mixed peripheral nerve depend on the concentration of drug used, nerve-fiber size, internodal distance, and frequency and pattern of nerve-impulse transmission (*see* above). Anatomical factors are similarly important. A mixed peripheral nerve or nerve trunk consists of individual nerves surrounded by an investing epineurium. The vascular supply usually is centrally located. When a local anesthetic is deposited about a peripheral nerve, it diffuses from the outer surface toward the core along a concentration gradient (DeJong, 1994; Winnie *et al.*, 1977). Consequently, nerves in the outer mantle of the mixed nerve are blocked first. These fibers usually are distributed to more proximal anatomical structures than are those situated near the core of the mixed nerve and often are motor. If the volume and concentration of local anesthetic solution deposited about the nerve are adequate, the local anesthetic eventually will diffuse inward in amounts adequate to block even the most centrally located fibers. Lesser amounts of drug will block only nerves in the mantle and the smaller and more sensitive central fibers. Furthermore, since removal of local anesthetics occurs primarily in the core of a mixed nerve or nerve trunk, where the vascular supply is located, the duration of blockade of centrally located nerves is shorter than that of more peripherally situated fibers.

The choice of local anesthetic and the amount and concentration administered are determined by the nerves and the types of fibers to be blocked, the required duration of anesthesia, and the size and health of the patient. For blocks of 2 to 4 hours, lidocaine (1% to 1.5%) can be used in the amounts recommended above (*see* "Infiltration Anesthesia"). Mepivacaine (up to 7 mg/kg of a 1% to 2% solution) provides anesthesia that lasts about as long as that from lidocaine. Bupivacaine (2 to 3 mg/kg of a 0.25% to 0.375% solution) can be used when a longer duration of action is required. Addition of 5 μg/ml epinephrine slows systemic absorption and therefore prolongs duration and lowers the plasma concentration of the intermediate-acting local anesthetics.

Peak plasma concentrations of local anesthetics depend on the amount injected, the physical characteristics of the local anesthetic, whether epinephrine is used, the rate of blood flow to the site of injection, and the surface area exposed to local anesthetic. This is of particular importance in the safe application of nerve block anesthesia, since the potential for systemic reactions is related to peak free serum concentrations. For example, peak concentrations of lidocaine in blood following injection of 400 mg without epinephrine for intercostal nerve blocks average 7 μg/ml; the same amount of lidocaine used for block of the brachial plexus results in peak concentrations in blood of approximately 3 μg/ml (Covino and Vassallo, 1976). Therefore, the amount of local anesthetic that can be injected must be adjusted according to the anatomical site of the nerve(s) to be blocked to minimize untoward effects. Addition of epinephrine can decrease peak plasma concentrations by 20% to 30%. Multiple nerve blocks (*e.g.,* intercostal block) or blocks performed in vascular regions require reduction in the amount of anesthetic that can be given safely, because the surface area for absorption or the rate of absorption is increased.

Intravenous Regional Anesthesia (Bier's Block)

This technique relies on using the vasculature to bring the local anesthetic solution to the nerve trunks and endings. In this technique, an extremity is exsanguinated with an Esmarch (elastic) bandage, and a proximally located tourniquet is inflated to 100 to 150 mm Hg above the systolic blood pressure. The Esmarch bandage is removed, and the local anesthetic is injected into a previously cannulated vein. Typically, complete anesthesia of the limb ensues within 5 to 10 minutes. Pain from the tourniquet and the potential for ischemic nerve injury limits tourniquet inflation to 2 hours or less. However, the tourniquet should remain inflated for at least 15 to 30 minutes to prevent toxic amounts of local anesthetic from entering the circulation following deflation. Lidocaine, 40 to 50 ml (0.5 ml/kg in children) of a 0.5% solution without epinephrine is the drug of choice for this technique. For intravenous regional anesthesia in adults using a 0.5% solution without epinephrine, the dose administered should not exceed 4 mg/kg. A few clinicians prefer prilocaine (0.5%) over lidocaine because of its higher therapeutic index. The attractiveness of this technique lies in its simplicity. Its primary disadvantages are that it can be used only for a few anatomical regions, sensation (*i.e.*, pain) returns quickly after tourniquet deflation, and premature release or failure of the tourniquet can produce toxic levels of local anesthetic (*e.g.*, 50 ml of 0.5% lidocaine contains 250 mg of lidocaine). For the last reason and because their longer durations of action offer no advantages, the more cardiotoxic local anesthetics, bupivacaine and etidocaine, are not recommended for this technique. Intravenous regional anesthesia is used most often for surgery of the forearm and hand, but can be adapted for the foot and distal leg.

Spinal Anesthesia

Spinal anesthesia follows the injection of local anesthetic into the cerebrospinal fluid (CSF) in the lumbar space. For a number of reasons, including the ability to produce anesthesia of a considerable fraction of the body with a dose of local anesthetic that produces negligible plasma levels, spinal anesthesia remains one of the most popular forms of anesthesia. In most adults, the spinal cord terminates above the second lumbar vertebra; between that point and the termination of the thecal sac in the sacrum, the lumbar and sacral roots are bathed in CSF. Thus, in this region there is a relatively large volume of CSF within which to inject drug, thereby minimizing the potential for direct nerve trauma.

A brief discussion of the physiological effects of spinal anesthesia relating to the pharmacology of the local anesthetics used is presented here. See more specialized texts (*e.g.*, Cousins and Bridenbaugh, 1998) for additional details.

Physiological Effects of Spinal Anesthesia. Most of the physiological side effects of spinal anesthesia are a consequence of the sympathetic blockade produced by local anesthetic block of the sympathetic fibers in the spinal nerve roots. A thorough understanding of these physiological effects is necessary for the safe and successful application of spinal anesthesia. Although some of them may be deleterious and require treatment, others can be beneficial for the patient or can improve operating conditions. Most sympathetic fibers leave the spinal cord between T1 and L2 (*see* Chapter 6, Figure 6–1). Although local anesthetic is injected below these levels in the lumbar portion of the dural sac, cephalad spread of the local anesthetic occurs with all but the smallest volumes injected. This cephalad spread is of considerable importance in the practice of spinal anesthesia and potentially is under the control of numerous variables, of which patient position and baricity (density of the drug relative to the density of the CSF) are the most important (Greene, 1983). The degree of sympathetic block is related to the height of sensory anesthesia; often the level of sympathetic blockade is several spinal segments higher, since the preganglionic sympathetic fibers are more sensitive to low concentrations of local anesthetic. The effects of sympathetic blockade involve both the actions (now partially unopposed) of the parasympathetic nervous system and the response of the unblocked portion of the sympathetic nervous system. Thus, as the level of sympathetic block ascends, the actions of the parasympathetic nervous system are increasingly dominant, and the compensatory mechanisms of the unblocked sympathetic nervous system are diminished. As most sympathetic nerve fibers leave the cord at T1 or below, few additional effects of sympathetic blockade are seen with cervical levels of spinal anesthesia. The con-

sequences of sympathetic blockade will vary among patients as a function of age, physical conditioning, and disease state. Interestingly, sympathetic blockade during spinal anesthesia appears to be inconsequential in healthy children.

Clinically, the most important effects of sympathetic blockade during spinal anesthesia are on the cardiovascular system. At all but the lowest levels of spinal blockade, some vasodilation will occur. Vasodilation is more marked on the venous than on the arterial side of the circulation, resulting in blood pooling in the venous capacitance vessels. This reduction in circulating blood volume is well tolerated at low levels of spinal anesthesia in healthy patients. With an increasing level of block, this effect becomes more marked and venous return becomes gravity-dependent. If venous return decreases too much, cardiac output and organ perfusion decline precipitously. Venous return can be increased by a modest (10° to 15°) head-down tilt or by elevating the legs. At high levels of spinal blockade, the cardiac accelerator fibers, which exit the spinal cord at T1 to T4, will be blocked. This is detrimental in patients dependent on elevated sympathetic tone to maintain cardiac output (*e.g.*, during congestive heart failure or hypovolemia), and it also removes one of the compensatory mechanisms available to maintain organ perfusion during vasodilation. Thus, as the level of spinal block ascends, the rate of cardiovascular compromise can accelerate if not carefully observed and treated. Sudden asystole also can occur, presumably because of loss of sympathetic innervation in the continued presence of parasympathetic activity at the sinoatrial node (Caplan, *et al.*, 1988). In the usual clinical situation, blood pressure serves as a surrogate marker for cardiac output and organ perfusion. Treatment of hypotension usually is warranted when the blood pressure decreases to about 30% of *resting* values. Therapy is aimed at maintaining brain and cardiac perfusion and oxygenation. To achieve these goals, administration of oxygen, fluid infusion, manipulation of patient position, and the administration of vasoactive drugs are all options. In particular, patients typically are administered a bolus (500 to 1000 ml) of fluid prior to the administration of spinal anesthesia in an attempt to prevent some of the deleterious effects of spinal blockade. Since the usual cause of hypotension is decreased venous return, possibly complicated by decreased heart rate, drugs with preferential venoconstrictive and chronotropic properties are preferred. For this reason, ephedrine, 5 to 10 mg intravenously, often is the drug of choice. In addition to the use of ephedrine to treat deleterious effects of sympathetic blockade, direct-acting α_1 adrenergic receptor agonists such as phenylephrine (*see* Chapter 10) can be administered either by bolus or continuous infusion.

A beneficial effect of spinal anesthesia partially mediated by the sympathetic nervous system is on the intestine. Sympathetic fibers originating from T5 to L1 inhibit peristalsis; thus, their blockade produces a small, contracted intestine. This, together with a flaccid abdominal musculature, produces excellent operating conditions for some types of bowel surgery. The effects of spinal anesthesia on the respiratory system mostly are mediated by effects on the skeletal musculature. Paralysis of the intercostal muscles will reduce a patient's ability to cough and clear secretions, which may produce dyspnea in patients with bronchitis or emphysema. It should be noted that respiratory arrest during spinal anesthesia is seldom due to paralysis of the phrenic nerves or to toxic levels of local anesthetic in the CSF of the fourth ventricle. It is much more likely to be due to medullary ischemia secondary to hypotension.

Pharmacology of Spinal Anesthesia. Currently in the United States, the drugs most commonly used in spinal anesthesia are lidocaine, tetracaine, and bupivacaine. Procaine occasionally is used for diagnostic blocks when a short duration of action is desired. The choice of local anesthetic is primarily determined by the desired duration of anesthesia. General guidelines are to use lidocaine for short procedures, bupivacaine for intermediate to long procedures, and tetracaine for long procedures. As mentioned above, the factors contributing to the distribution of local anesthetics in the CSF have received much attention because of their importance in determining the height of block. The most important pharmacological factors include the amount, and possibly the volume, of drug injected and its baricity. The speed of injection of the local anesthesia solution also may affect the height of the block, just as the position of the patient can influence the rate of distribution of the anesthetic agent and the height of blockade achieved (*see* below). For a given preparation of local anesthetic, administration of increasing amounts leads to a fairly predictable increase in the level of block attained. For example, 100 mg of lidocaine, 20 mg of bupivacaine, or 12 mg of tetracaine usually will result in a T4 sensory block. More complete tables of these relationships can be found in standard anesthesiology texts. Epinephrine often is added to spinal anesthetics to increase the duration or intensity of block. Epinephrine's effect on duration of block is dependent on the technique used to measure duration. A commonly used measure of block duration is the length of time it takes for the block to recede by two dermatomes from the maximum height of the block, while a second is the duration of block at some specified level, typically L1. In most studies, addition of 200 μg of epinephrine to tetracaine solutions prolongs the duration of block by both measures. However, addition of epinephrine to lidocaine or bupivacaine does not affect the first measure of duration, but does prolong the block at lower levels. In different clinical situations, one or the other measure of anesthesia duration may be more relevant, and this must be kept in mind when deciding whether to add epinephrine to spinal local anesthetics. The mechanism of action of vasoconstrictors in prolonging spinal anesthesia is uncertain. It has been hypothesized that these agents decrease spinal cord blood flow, decreasing clearance of local anesthetic from the CSF, but this has not been convincingly demonstrated. Epinephrine and other α adrenergic agonists have been shown to decrease nociceptive transmission in the spinal cord, and studies in genetically modified mice suggest that α_{2A} adrenergic receptors play a principal role in this response (Stone *et al.*, 1997). It is possible that these actions contribute to the effects of epinephrine.

Drug Baricity and Patient Position. The baricity of the local anesthetic injected will determine the direction of migration within the dural sac. Hyperbaric solutions will tend to settle in the dependent portions of the sac, while hypobaric solutions will tend to migrate in the opposite direction. Isobaric solutions usually will stay in the vicinity where they were injected, diffusing slowly in all directions. Consideration of the patient position during and after the performance of the block and the choice of a local anesthetic of the appropriate baricity is crucial for a successful block during some surgical procedures. For example, a saddle (perineal) block is best performed with a hyperbaric anesthetic in the sitting position, with the patient remaining in that position until the anesthetic level has become "fixed." On the other hand, for a saddle block in the prone, jackknife position, a hypobaric local anesthetic is appropriate. Lidocaine and bupivacaine are marketed in both isobaric and hyperbaric preparations, and if desired, can be diluted with sterile, preservative-free water to make them hypobaric.

Complications of Spinal Anesthesia. Persistent neurological deficits following spinal anesthesia are extremely rare. Thorough evaluation of a suspected deficit should be performed in collaboration with a neurologist. Neurological sequelae can be both immediate and late. Possible causes include introduction of foreign substances (such as disinfectants or talc) into the subarachnoid space, infection, hematoma, or direct mechanical trauma. Aside from drainage of an abscess or hematoma, treatment usually is ineffective; thus, avoidance and careful attention to detail while performing spinal anesthesia are necessary. High concentrations of local anesthetic can cause irreversible block. After administration, local anesthetic solutions are diluted rapidly, quickly reaching nontoxic concentrations. However, there are several reports of transient or longer-lasting neurological deficits following lidocaine spinal anesthesia, particularly with 5% lidocaine (*i.e.,* 180 mmol) in 7.5% glucose (Hodgson *et al.*, 1999). Spinal anesthesia sometimes is regarded as contraindicated in patients with preexisting disease of the spinal cord. No experimental evidence exists to support this hypothesis. Nonetheless, it is prudent to avoid spinal anesthesia in patients with progressive diseases of the spinal cord. However, spinal anesthesia may be very useful in patients with fixed, chronic spinal cord injury.

A more common sequela following any lumbar puncture, including spinal anesthesia, is a postural headache with classic features. The incidence of headache decreases with increasing age of the patient and decreasing needle diameter. Headache following lumbar puncture must be thoroughly evaluated to exclude serious complications such as meningitis. Treatment usually is conservative, with bed rest and analgesics. If this approach fails, an epidural blood patch with the injection of autologous blood can be performed; this procedure usually is successful in alleviating post–dural puncture headaches, although a second blood patch may be necessary. If two epidural blood patches are ineffective in relieving the headache, the diagnosis of post–dural puncture headache should be reconsidered. Intravenous caffeine (500 mg as the benzoate salt administered over 4 hours) also has been advocated for the treatment of post–dural puncture headache. However, the efficacy of caffeine is less than that of a blood patch, and relief usually is transient.

Evaluation of Spinal Anesthesia. Spinal anesthesia is a safe and effective technique, especially during surgery involving the lower abdomen, the lower extremities, and the perineum. It often is combined with intravenous medication to provide sedation and amnesia. The physiological perturbations associated with low spinal anesthesia often have less potential harm than those associated with general anesthesia. The same does not apply for high spinal anesthesia. The sympathetic blockade that accompanies levels of spinal anesthesia adequate for mid- or upper-abdominal surgery, coupled with the difficulty in achieving visceral analgesia, is such that equally satisfactory and safer operating conditions can be realized by combining the spinal anesthetic with a "light" general anesthetic or by the administration of a general anesthetic and a neuromuscular blocking agent.

Epidural Anesthesia

Epidural anesthesia is administered by injecting local anesthetic into the epidural space—the space bounded by the ligamentum flavum posteriorly, the spinal periosteum laterally, and the dura anteriorly. Epidural anesthesia can be performed in the sacral hiatus (caudal anesthesia) or in the lumbar, thoracic, or cervical regions of the spine. Its current popularity arises from the development of catheters that can be placed into the epidural space, allowing either continuous infusions or repeated bolus administration of local anesthetics. The primary site of action of epidurally administered local anesthetics is on the spinal nerve roots. However, epidurally administered local anesthetics also may act on the spinal cord and on the paravertebral nerves.

The selection of drugs available for epidural anesthesia is similar to that for major nerve blocks. As for spinal anesthesia, the choice of drugs to be used during epidural anesthesia is dictated primarily by the duration of anesthesia desired. However, when an epidural catheter is placed, short-acting drugs can be administered repeatedly, providing more control over the duration of block. Bupivacaine, 0.5% to 0.75%, is used when a long duration of surgical block is desired. Due to enhanced cardiotoxicity in pregnant patients, the 0.75% solution is not approved for obstetrical use. Lower concentrations—0.25%, 0.125%, or 0.0625%—of bupivacaine, often with 2 μg/ml of fentanyl added, frequently are used to provide analgesia during labor. They also are useful preparations for providing postoperative analgesia in certain clinical situations. Lidocaine 2% is the most frequently used intermediate-acting epidural local anesthetic. Chloroprocaine, 2% or 3%, provides rapid onset and a very short duration of anesthetic action. However, its use in epidural anesthesia has been clouded by controversy regarding its potential ability to cause neurological complications if the drug is accidentally injected into the subarachnoid space (*see* above). The duration of action of epidurally administered local anesthetics frequently is prolonged, and systemic toxicity decreased, by addition of epinephrine. Addition of epinephrine also makes inadvertent intravascular injection easier to detect and modifies the effect of sympathetic blockade during epidural anesthesia.

For each anesthetic agent, a relationship exists between the volume of local anesthetic injected epidurally and the segmental level of anesthesia achieved. For example, in 20- to 40-year-old, healthy, nonpregnant patients, each 1 to 1.5 ml of 2% lidocaine will give an additional segment of anesthesia. The amount needed decreases with increasing age and also decreases during pregnancy and in children.

The concentration of local anesthetic used determines the type of nerve fibers blocked. The highest concentrations are used when sympathetic, somatic sensory, and somatic motor blockade are required. Intermediate concentrations allow somatic sensory anesthesia without muscle relaxation. Low concentrations will block only preganglionic sympathetic fibers. As an example, with bupivacaine these effects might be achieved with concentrations of 0.5%, 0.25%, and 0.0625%, respectively. The total amounts of drug that can be injected with safety at one time are approximately those mentioned above under "Nerve Block Anesthesia" and "Infiltration Anesthesia." Performance of epidural anesthesia requires a greater degree of skill than does spinal anesthesia. The technique of epidural anesthesia and the volumes, concentrations, and types of drugs used are described in detail in standard texts on regional anesthesia (*e.g.*, Cousins and Bridenbaugh, 1998).

A significant difference between epidural and spinal anesthesia is that the dose of local anesthetic used can produce high concentrations in blood following absorption from the epidural space. Peak concentrations of lidocaine in blood following injection of 400 mg (without epinephrine) into the lumbar epidural space average 3 to 4 μg/ml; peak concentrations of bupivacaine in blood average 1 μg/ml after the lumbar epidural injection of 150 mg. Addition of epinephrine (5 μg/ml) decreases peak plasma concentrations by about 25%. Peak blood concentrations are a function of the total dose of drug administered rather than the concentration or volume of solution following epidural injection (Covino and Vassallo, 1976). The risk of inadvertent intravascular injection is increased in epidural anesthesia, as the epidural space contains a rich venous plexus.

Another major difference between epidural and spinal anesthesia is that there is no zone of differential sympathetic blockade with epidural anesthesia; thus, the level of sympathetic block is close to the level of sensory block. Because epidural anesthesia does not result in the zones of differential sympathetic blockade observed during spinal anesthesia, cardiovascular responses to epidural anesthesia might be expected to be less prominent. In practice this is not the case; the potential advantage of epidural anesthesia is offset by the cardiovascular responses to the high concentration of anesthetic in blood that occurs during epidural anesthesia. This is most apparent when, as is often the case, epinephrine is added to the epidural injection. The resulting concentration of epinephrine in blood is sufficient to produce significant β_2 adrenergic receptor-mediated vasodilation. As a consequence, blood pressure decreases, even though cardiac output increases due to the positive inotropic and chronotropic effects of epinephrine (*see* Chapter 10). The result is peripheral hyperperfusion and hypotension. Differences in cardiovascular responses to equal levels of spinal and epidural anesthesia also are observed when a local anesthetic such as lidocaine is used without epinephrine. This may be a consequence of the direct effects of high concentrations of lidocaine on vascular smooth muscle and the heart. The magnitude of the differences in responses to equal sensory levels of spinal and epidural anesthesia varies, however, with the local anesthetic used for the epidural injection (assuming no epinephrine is used). For example, local anesthetics such as bupivacaine, which are highly lipid soluble, are distributed less into the circulation than are less lipid-soluble agents such as lidocaine.

High concentrations of local anesthetics in blood during epidural anesthesia are especially important when this technique is used to control pain during labor and delivery. Local anesthetics cross the placenta, enter the fetal circulation, and at high concentrations may cause depression of the neonate. The extent to which they do so is determined by dosage, acid–base status, the level of protein binding in both maternal and fetal blood, placental blood flow, and solubility of the agent in fetal tissue. These concerns have been lessened by the trend toward using more dilute solutions of bupivacaine for labor analgesia.

Epidural and Intrathecal Opiate Analgesia. Small quantities of opioid injected intrathecally or epidurally produce segmental analgesia (Yaksh and Rudy, 1976). This observation led to the clinical use of spinal and epidural opioids during surgical procedures and for the relief of postoperative and chronic pain (Cousins and Mather, 1984). As with local anesthesia, analgesia is confined to sensory nerves that enter the spinal cord dorsal horn in the vicinity of the injection. Presynaptic opioid receptors inhibit the release of substance P and other neurotransmitters from primary afferents, while postsynaptic opioid receptors decrease the activity of certain dorsal horn neurons in the spinothalamic tracts (Willcockson, *et al.*, 1986; *see* also Chapters 6 and 21). Since conduction in autonomic, sensory, and motor nerves is not affected by the opioids, blood pressure, motor function, and non-nociceptive sensory perception typically are not influenced by spinal opioids. The volume-evoked micturition reflex is inhibited, as manifested by urinary retention. Other side effects include pruritus and nausea and vomiting in susceptible individuals. Delayed respiratory depression and sedation, presumably from cephalad spread of opioid within the CSF, occurs infrequently with the doses of opioids currently used.

Spinally administered opioids by themselves do not provide satisfactory anesthesia for surgical procedures. Thus, opioids have found the greatest use in the treatment of postoperative and chronic pain. In selected patients, spinal or epidural opioids can provide excellent analgesia following thoracic, abdominal, pelvic, or lower extremity surgery without the side effects associated with high doses of systemically administered opioids. For postoperative analgesia, spinally administered morphine, 0.2 to 0.5 mg, usually will provide 8 to 16 hours of analgesia. Placement of an epidural catheter and repeated boluses or an infusion of opioid permits an increased duration of analgesia. Many opioids have been used epidurally. Morphine, 2 to 6 mg, every 6 hours, commonly is used for bolus injections, while fentanyl, 20 to 50 μg/hour, often combined with bupivacaine, 5 to 20 mg/hour, is used for infusions. For cancer pain, repeated doses of epidural opioids can provide analgesia of several months' duration. The dose of epidural morphine, for example, is far less than the dose of systemically administered morphine that would be required to provide similar analgesia. This reduces the complications that usually accompany the administration of high doses of systemic opioids, particularly sedation and constipation. Unfortunately, as with systemic opioids, tolerance will develop to the analgesic effects of epidural opioids, but this usually can be managed by increasing the dose.

BIBLIOGRAPHY

Caplan, R.A., Ward, R.J., Posner, K., and Cheney, F.W. Unexpected cardiac arrest during spinal anesthesia: a closed claims analysis of predisposing factors. *Anesthesiology,* **1988,** *68:*5–11.

Charnet, P., Labarca, C., Leonard, R.J., *et al.* An open-channel blocker interacts with adjacent turns of α-helices in the nicotinic acetylcholine receptor. *Neuron,* **1990,** *4:*87–95.

Clarkson, C.W., and Hondeghem, L.M. Mechanism for bupivacaine depression of cardiac conduction: fast block of sodium channels during the action potential with slow recovery from block during diastole. *Anesthesiology,* **1985,** *62:*396–405.

Cousins, M.J., and Mather, L.E. Intrathecal and epidural administration of opioids. *Anesthesiology,* **1984,** *61:*276–310.

Fink, B.R., and Cairns, A.M. Differential slowing and block of conduction by lidocaine in individual afferent myelinated and unmyelinated axons. *Anesthesiology,* **1984,** *60:*111–120.

Foster, R.H., and Markham, A. Levobupivacaine: a review of its pharmacology and use as a local anesthetic. *Drugs,* **2000,** *59:*551–579.

Franz, D.N., and Perry, R.S. Mechanisms for differential block among single myelinated and nonmyelinated axons by procaine. *J. Physiol.,* **1974,** *236:*193–210.

Gasser, H.S., and Erlanger, J. The role of fiber size in the establishment of a nerve block by pressure or cocaine. *Am. J. Physiol.,* **1929,** *88:*581–591.

Hodgson, P.S., Neal, J.M., Pollock, J.E., and Liu, S.S. The neurotoxicity of drugs given intrathecally. *Anesth. Analg.,* **1999,** *88:*797–809.

Huang, J.H., Thalhammer, J.G., Raymond, S.A., and Strichartz, G.R. Susceptibility to lidocaine of impulses in different somatosensory fibers of rat sciatic nerve. *J. Pharmacol. Exp. Ther.,* **1997,** *292:*802–811.

Narahashi, T., and Frazier, D.T. Site of action and active form of local anesthetics. *Neurosci. Res. (N.Y.),* **1971,** *4:*65–99.

Neher, E., and Steinbach, J.H. Local anesthetics transiently block currents through single acetylcholine-receptor channels. *J. Physiol.,* **1978,** *277:*153–176.

Ragsdale, D.R., McPhee, J.C., Scheuer, T., and Catterall, W.A. Molecular determinants of state-dependent block of Na$^+$ channels by local anesthetics. *Science,* **1994,** *265:*1724–1728.

Stevens, R.A., Urmey, W.F., Urquhart, B.L., and Kao, T.C. Back pain after epidural anesthesia with chloroprocaine. *Anesthesiology,* **1993,** *78:*492–497.

Stommel, E.W., and Watters, M.R. Marine neurotoxins: ingestible toxins. *Curr. Treat. Options Neurol.,* **2004,** *6:*105–114.

Stone, L.S., MacMillan, L.B., Kitto, K.F., *et al.* The α_{2a} adrenergic receptor subtype mediates spinal analgesia evoked by α_2 agonists and is necessary for spinal adrenergic-opioid synergy. *J. Neurosci.,* **1997,** *17:*7157–7165.

Terlau, H., Heinemann, S.H., Stühmer, W., *et al.* Mapping the site of block by tetrodotoxin and saxitoxin of sodium channel II. *FEBS Lett.,* **1991,** *293:*93–96.

Thomas, R.D., Behbehani, M.M., Coyle, D.E., and Denson, D.D. Cardiovascular toxicity of local anesthetics: an alternative hypothesis. *Anesth. Analg.,* **1986,** *65:*444–450.

Willcockson, W.S., Kim, J., Shin, H.K., *et al.* Actions of opioid on primate spinothalamic tract neurons. *J. Neurosci.,* **1986,** *6:*2509–2520.

Winnie, A.P., Tay, C.H., Patel, K.P., *et al.* Pharmacokinetics of local anesthetics during plexus blocks. *Anesth. Analg.,* **1977,** *56:*852–861.

Yaksh, T.L., and Rudy, T.A. Analgesia mediated by a direct spinal action of narcotics. *Science,* **1976,** *192:*1357–1358.

Yarov-Yarovoy, V., McPhee, J.C., Idsvoog, D., *et al.* Role of amino acid residues in transmembrane segments IS6 and IIS6 of the sodium channel α subunit in voltage-dependent gating and drug block. *J. Biol. Chem.,* **2002,** *277:*35393–35401.

MONOGRAPHS AND REVIEWS

Arthur, G.R. Pharmacokinetics. In, *Local Anesthetics.* (Strichartz, G.R., ed.) *Handbook of Experimental Pharmacology,* Vol. 81. Springer-Verlag, Berlin, **1987,** pp. 165–186.

Butterworth, J.F. IV, and Strichartz, G.R. Molecular mechanisms of local anesthesia: a review. *Anesthesiology,* **1990,** *72:*711–734.

Carpenter, R.L., and Mackey, D.C. Local anesthetics. In, *Clinical Anesthesia,* 2nd ed. (Barash, P.G., Cullen, B.F., and Stoelting, R.K., eds.) Lippincott, Philadelphia, **1992,** pp. 509–541.

Catterall, W.A. From ionic currents to molecular mechanisms: the structure and function of voltage-gated sodium channels. *Neuron,* **2000,** *26:*13–25.

Courtney, K.R., and Strichartz, G.R. Structural elements which determine local anesthetic activity. In, *Local Anesthetics.* (Strichartz, G.R., ed.) *Handbook of Experimental Pharmacology,* Vol. 81. Springer-Verlag, Berlin, **1987,** pp. 53–94.

Cousins, M.J., and Bridenbaugh, P.O., eds. *Neural Blockade in Clinical Anesthesia and Management of Pain,* 3rd ed. Lippincott-Raven, Philadelphia, **1998.**

Covino, B.G. Toxicity and systemic effects of local anesthetic agents. In, *Local Anesthetics.* (Strichartz, G.R., ed.) *Handbook of Experimental Pharmacology,* Vol. 81. Springer-Verlag, Berlin, **1987,** pp. 187–212.

Covino, B.G., and Vassallo, H.G. *Local Anesthetics: Mechanisms of Action and Clinical Use.* Grune & Stratton, New York, **1976.**

DeJong, R.H. *Local Anesthetics.* Mosby, St. Louis, MO, **1994.**

Garfield, J.M., and Gugino, L. Central effects of local anesthetics. In, *Local Anesthetics.* (Strichartz, G.R., ed.) *Handbook of Experimental Pharmacology,* Vol. 81. Springer-Verlag, Berlin, **1987,** pp. 253–284.

Gintant, G.A., and Hoffman, B.F. The role of local anesthetic effects in the actions of antiarrhythmic drugs. In, *Local Anesthetics.* (Strichartz,

G.R., ed.) *Handbook of Experimental Pharmacology,* Vol. 81. Springer-Verlag, Berlin, **1987,** pp. 213–251.

Greene, N.M. Uptake and elimination of local anesthetics during spinal anesthesia. *Anesth. Analg.,* **1983,** *62:*1013–1024.

Groban, L., Deal, D.D., Vernon, J.C., *et al.* Cardiac resuscitation after incremental overdosage with lidocaine, bupivacaine, levobupivacaine, and ropivacaine in anesthetized dogs. *Anesth. Analg.,* **2001,** *92:*37–43.

McClure, J.H. Ropivacaine. *Br. J. Anaesth.,* **1996,** *76:*300–307.

Raymond, S.A., and Gissen, A.J. Mechanism of differential nerve block. In, *Local Anesthetics.* (Strichartz, G.R., ed.) *Handbook of Experimental Pharmacology,* Vol. 81. Springer-Verlag, Berlin, **1987,** pp. 95–164.

Ritchie, J.M., and Greengard, P. On the mode of action of local anesthetics. *Annu. Rev. Pharmacol.,* **1966,** *6:*405–430.

Ritchie, J.M. Tetrodotoxin and saxitoxin and the sodium channels of excitable tissues. *Trends Pharmacol. Sci.,* **1980,** *1:*275–279.

Strichartz, G.R., and Ritchie, J.M. The action of local anesthetics on ion channels of excitable tissues. In, *Local Anesthetics.* (Strichartz, G.R., ed.) *Handbook of Experimental Pharmacology,* Vol. 81. Springer-Verlag, Berlin, **1987,** pp. 21–53.

Zipf, H.F., and Dittmann, E.C. General pharmacological effects of local anesthetics. In, *Local Anesthetics,* Vol. 1. *International Encyclopedia of Pharmacology and Therapeutics,* Sect. 8. (Lechat, P., ed.) Pergamon Press, Oxford, **1971,** pp. 191–238.

THERAPEUTIC GASES
Oxygen, Carbon Dioxide, Nitric Oxide, and Helium

Brett A. Simon, Eric J. Moody, and Roger A. Johns

OXYGEN

Oxygen (O_2) is essential for animal existence. Hypoxia is a life-threatening condition in which oxygen delivery is inadequate to meet the metabolic demands of the tissues. Since oxygen delivery is the product of blood flow and oxygen content, hypoxia may result from alterations in tissue perfusion, decreased oxygen tension in the blood, or decreased oxygen-carrying capacity. In addition, hypoxia may result from restricted oxygen transport from the microvasculature to cells or impaired utilization within the cell. Irrespective of cause, an inadequate supply of oxygen ultimately results in the cessation of aerobic metabolism and oxidative phosphorylation, depletion of high-energy compounds, cellular dysfunction, and death.

History. Soon after Priestley's discovery of oxygen in 1772 and Lavoisier's elucidation of its role in respiration, Beddoes introduced oxygen therapy with his 1794 publication entitled "Considerations on the Medicinal Use and Production of Factitious Airs." Beddoes, overcome with enthusiasm for his project, treated all kinds of diseases with oxygen, including such diverse conditions as scrofula, leprosy, and paralysis. Such indiscriminate therapeutic applications naturally led to many failures, and Beddoes died a disconsolate man. The pioneer investigations of Haldane, Hill, Barcroft, Krogh, L. J. Henderson, and Y. Henderson provided a sound physiological basis for oxygen therapy (Sackner, 1974). Although Paul Bert had studied therapeutic aspects of hyperbaric oxygen in 1870 and identified oxygen toxicity, the use of oxygen at pressures above one atmosphere for therapeutic purposes did not begin until the 1950s.

Normal Oxygenation

Oxygen makes up 21% of air, which at sea level represents a partial pressure of 21 kPa (158 mmHg). While the fraction (percentage) of oxygen remains constant regardless of atmospheric pressure, the partial pressure of oxygen (PO_2) decreases with lower atmospheric pressure. Since the partial pressure drives the diffusion of oxygen, ascent to elevated altitude reduces the uptake and delivery of oxygen to the tissues. Conversely, increases in atmospheric pressure (*e.g.*, hyperbaric therapy or breathing at depth) raise the PO_2 in inspired air and increase gas uptake. As the air is delivered to the distal airways and alveoli, the PO_2 decreases by dilution with carbon dioxide and water vapor and by uptake into the blood. Under ideal conditions, when ventilation and perfusion are well matched, the alveolar PO_2 will be approximately 14.6 kPa (110 mmHg). The corresponding alveolar partial pressures of water and carbon dioxide are 6.2 kPa (47 mmHg) and 5.3 kPa (40 mmHg), respectively. Under normal conditions, there is complete equilibration of alveolar gas and capillary blood, and the PO_2 in end-capillary blood is typically within a fraction of a kilopascal of that in the alveoli. In some diseases, the diffusion barrier for gas transport may be increased, or, during exercise, when high cardiac output reduces capillary transit time, full equilibration may not occur, and the alveolar–end-capillary PO_2 gradient may be increased.

The PO_2 in arterial blood, however, is further reduced by venous admixture (shunt), the addition of mixed venous blood from the pulmonary artery, which has a PO_2 of approximately 5.3 kPa (40 mmHg). Together, the diffusional barrier, ventilation–perfusion mismatches, and the shunt fraction are the major causes of the alveolar-to-arterial oxygen gradient, which is normally 1.3 to 1.6 kPa (10 to 12 mmHg) when air is breathed and 4.0 to 6.6 kPa (30 to 50 mmHg) when 100% oxygen is breathed.

Oxygen is delivered to the tissue capillary beds by the circulation and again follows a gradient out of the blood and into cells. Tissue extraction of oxygen typically reduces the PO_2 of venous blood by an additional 7.3 kPa (55 mmHg). Although the PO_2 at the site of cellular oxygen utilization—the mitochondria—is not known, oxidative phosphorylation can continue at a PO_2 of only a few millimeters of mercury (Robiolio *et al.*, 1989).

In the blood, oxygen is carried primarily in chemical combination with hemoglobin and is to a small extent dissolved in solution. The quantity of oxygen combined with hemoglobin depends on the PO_2, as illustrated by the sigmoidal oxyhemoglobin dissociation curve (Figure 15–1). Hemoglobin is about 98% saturated with oxygen when air is breathed under normal circumstances, and it binds 1.3 ml of oxygen per gram when fully saturated. The steep slope of this curve with falling PO_2 facilitates unloading of oxygen from

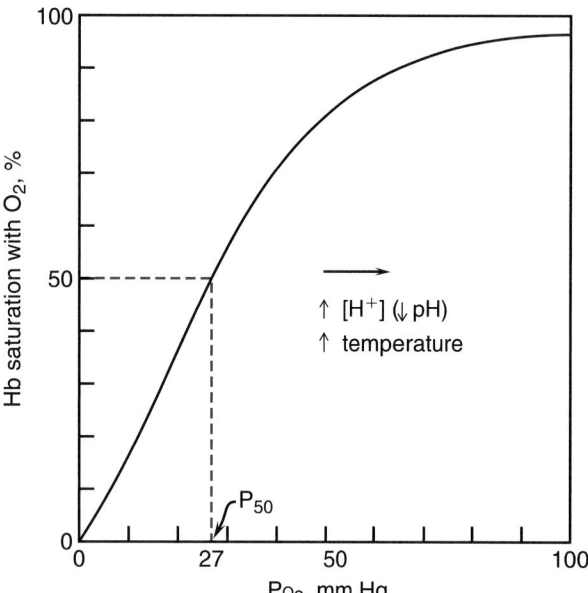

Figure 15–1. *Oxyhemoglobin dissociation curve for whole blood.* The relationship between P_{O_2} and hemoglobin (Hb) saturation is shown. The P_{50}, or the P_{O_2} resulting in 50% saturation, is indicated as well. An increase in temperature or a decrease in pH (as in working muscle) shifts this relationship to the right, reducing the hemoglobin saturation at the same P_{O_2} and thus aiding in the delivery of oxygen to the tissues.

hemoglobin at the tissue level and reloading when desaturated mixed venous blood arrives at the lung. Shifting of the curve to the right with increasing temperature, increasing P_{CO_2}, and decreasing pH, as is found in metabolically active tissues, lowers the oxygen saturation for the same P_{O_2} and thus delivers additional oxygen where and when it is most needed. However, the flattening of the curve with higher P_{O_2} indicates that increasing blood P_{O_2} by inspiring oxygen-enriched mixtures can increase the amount of oxygen carried by hemoglobin only minimally. Further increases in blood oxygen content can occur only by increasing the amount of oxygen dissolved in plasma. Because of the low solubility of oxygen (0.226 ml/L per kilopascal or 0.03 ml/L per millimeter of mercury at 37°C), breathing 100% oxygen can increase the amount of oxygen dissolved in blood by only 15 ml/L, less than one-third of normal metabolic demands. However, if the inspired P_{O_2} is increased to 3 atm (304 kPa) in a hyperbaric chamber, the amount of dissolved oxygen is sufficient to meet normal metabolic demands even in the absence of hemoglobin (Table 15–1).

Oxygen Deprivation

An understanding of the causes and effects of oxygen deficiency is necessary for the rational therapeutic use of the gas. *Hypoxia* is the term used to denote insufficient oxygenation of the tissues. *Hypoxemia* generally implies a failure of the respiratory system to oxygenate arterial blood.

Pulmonary Mechanisms of Hypoxemia. Classically, there are five causes of hypoxemia: low inspired oxygen fraction ($F_{I_{O_2}}$), increased diffusion barrier, hypoventilation, ventilation–perfusion ($\dot{V}/\dot{Q}$) mismatch, and shunt or venous admixture.

Low $F_{I_{O_2}}$ is a cause of hypoxemia only at high altitude or in the event of equipment failure, such as a gas blender malfunction or a mislabeled compressed-gas tank. An increase in the barrier to diffusion of oxygen within the lung is rarely a cause of hypoxemia in a resting subject, except in end-stage parenchymal lung disease. Both these problems may be alleviated with administration of supplemental oxygen, the former by definition and the latter by increasing the gradient driving diffusion.

Hypoventilation causes hypoxemia by reducing the alveolar P_{O_2} in proportion to the buildup of carbon dioxide in the alveoli. During hypoventilation, there is decreased delivery of oxygen to the alveoli, whereas its removal by the blood remains the same, causing its alveolar concentration to fall. The opposite occurs with carbon dioxide. This is described by the alveolar gas equation: $PA_{O_2} = PI_{O_2} - (PA_{CO_2}/R)$, where PA_{O_2} and PA_{CO_2} are the alveolar partial pressures of oxygen and carbon dioxide, PI_{O_2} is the partial pressure of oxygen in the inspired gas, and R the respiratory quotient. Under normal conditions, breathing room air at sea level (corrected for the partial pressure of water vapor), the PI_{O_2} is about 20 kPa (150 mmHg), the PA_{CO_2} about 5.3 kPa (40 mmHg), R is 0.8, and thus the PA_{O_2} is normally around 13.3 kPa (100 mmHg). It would require substantial hypoventilation, with the PA_{CO_2} rising to over 9.8 kPa (72 mmHg), to cause the PA_{O_2} to fall below 7.8 kPa (60 mmHg). This cause of hypoxemia is readily prevented by administration of even small amounts of supplemental O_2.

Shunt and $\dot{V}/\dot{Q}$ mismatch are related causes of hypoxemia but with an important distinction in their responses to supplemental oxygen. Optimal gas exchange occurs when blood flow ($\dot{Q}$) and ventilation ($\dot{V}$) are matched quantitatively. However, regional variations in $\dot{V}/\dot{Q}$ matching typically exist within the lung, particularly in the presence of lung disease. As ventilation increases relative to blood flow, the alveolar P_{O_2} (PA_{O_2}) increases; because of the flat shape of the oxyhemoglobin dissociation curve at high P_{O_2} (Figure 15–1), this increased PA_{O_2} does not contribute much to the oxygen content of the blood. Conversely, as the $\dot{V}/\dot{Q}$ ratio falls and perfusion increases relative to ventilation, the PA_{O_2} of the blood leaving these regions falls relative to regions with better matched ventilation and perfusion. Since the oxyhemoglobin dissociation curve is steep at these lower P_{O_2} values, the oxygen saturation and content of the pulmonary

Table 15–1
The Carriage of Oxygen in Blood*

ARTERIAL PO$_2$, kPa (mmHg)	Arterial O$_2$ Content (ml O$_2$/liter)			MIXED VENOUS PO$_2$, kPa (mmHg)	Mixed Venous O$_2$ Content (ml O$_2$/liter)			EXAMPLES
	DISSOLVED	BOUND TO HEMOGLOBIN	TOTAL		DISSOLVED	BOUND TO HEMOGLOBIN	TOTAL	
4.0 (30)	0.9	109	109.9	2.7 (20)	0.6	59	59.6	High altitude; respiratory failure breathing air
12.0 (90)	2.7	192	194.7	5.5 (41)	1.2	144	145.2	Normal person breathing air
40.0 (300)	9.0	195	204	5.9 (44)	1.3	153	154.3	Normal person breathing 50% O$_2$
79.7 (600)	18	196	214	6.5 (49)	1.5	163	164.5	Normal person breathing 100% O$_2$
239 (1800)	54	196	250	20.0 (150)	4.5	196	200.5	Normal person breathing hyperbaric O$_2$

*This table illustrates the carriage of oxygen in the blood under a variety of circumstances. As arterial O$_2$ tension increases, the amount of dissolved O$_2$ increases in direct proportion to the PO$_2$, but the amount of oxygen bound to hemoglobin reaches a maximum of 196 ml O$_2$/liter (100% saturation of hemoglobin at 15 g/dl). Further increases in O$_2$ content require increases in dissolved oxygen. At 100% inspired O$_2$, dissolved O$_2$ still provides only a small fraction of total demand. Hyperbaric oxygen therapy is required to increase the amount of dissolved oxygen to supply all or a large part of metabolic requirements. Note that, during hyperbaric oxygen therapy, the hemoglobin in the mixed venous blood remains fully saturated with O$_2$. The figures in this table are approximate and are based on the assumptions of 15 g/dl hemoglobin, 50 ml O$_2$/liter whole-body oxygen extraction, and constant cardiac output. When severe anemia is present, arterial PO$_2$ remains the same, but arterial content is lower; oxygen extraction continues, resulting in lower O$_2$ content and tension in mixed venous blood. Similarly, as cardiac output falls significantly, the same oxygen extraction occurs from a smaller volume of blood and results in lower mixed venous oxygen content and tension.

389

venous blood falls significantly. At the extreme of low $\dot{V}/\dot{Q}$ ratios, there is no ventilation to a perfused region, and a pure shunt results; thus the blood leaving the region has the same low P_{O_2} and high $P_{A_{CO_2}}$ as mixed venous blood.

The deleterious effect of $\dot{V}/\dot{Q}$ mismatch on arterial oxygenation is a direct result of the asymmetry of the oxyhemoglobin dissociation curve. Adding supplemental oxygen generally will make up for the fall in $P_{A_{O_2}}$ in low $\dot{V}/\dot{Q}$ units and thereby improve arterial oxygenation. However, since there is no ventilation to units with pure shunt, supplemental oxygen will not be effective in reversing hypoxemia from this cause. Because of the steep oxyhemoglobin dissociation curve at low P_{O_2}, even moderate amounts of pure shunt will cause significant hypoxemia despite oxygen therapy (Figure 15–2). For the same reason, factors that decrease mixed venous P_{O_2}, such as decreased cardiac output or increased oxygen consumption, enhance the hypoxemic effects of $\dot{V}/\dot{Q}$ mismatch and shunt.

Nonpulmonary Causes of Hypoxia. In addition to failure of the respiratory system to oxygenate the blood adequately, a number of other factors can contribute to hypoxia at the tissue level. These may be divided into categories of oxygen delivery and oxygen utilization. Oxygen delivery decreases globally when cardiac output falls or locally when regional blood flow is compromised, such as from a vascular occlusion (*e.g.,* stenosis, thrombosis, or microvascular occlusion) or increased downstream pressure (*e.g.,* compartment syndrome, venous stasis, or venous hypertension). Decreased oxygen-carrying capacity of the blood likewise will reduce oxygen delivery, such as occurs with anemia, carbon monoxide poisoning, or hemoglobinopathy. Finally, hypoxia may occur when transport of oxygen from the capillaries to the tissues is decreased (edema) or utilization of the oxygen by the cells is impaired (cyanide toxicity).

Effects of Hypoxia. There has been a considerable increase in our understanding of the cellular and biochemical changes that occur after acute and chronic hypoxia. Regardless of the cause, hypoxia produces a marked alteration in gene expression, mediated in part by hypoxia-inducible factor-1α (Semenza, 2003). Ultimately, hypoxia results in the cessation of aerobic metabolism, exhaustion of high-energy intracellular stores, cellular dysfunction, and death. The time course of cellular demise depends on the tissue's relative metabolic requirements, oxygen and energy stores, and anaerobic capacity. Survival times (the time from the onset of circulatory arrest to significant organ dysfunction) range from 1 minute in the cerebral cortex to around 5 minutes in the heart and 10 minutes in the kidneys and liver, with the potential for some degree of recovery if reperfused. Revival times (the duration of hypoxia beyond which recovery is no longer possible) are approximately four to five times longer. Less severe degrees of hypoxia have progressive physiological effects on different organ systems (Nunn, 2000b).

Respiratory System. Hypoxia stimulates the carotid and aortic baroreceptors to cause increases in both the rate and depth of ventilation. Minute volume almost doubles when normal individuals inspire gas with a P_{O_2} of 6.6 kPa (50 mmHg). Dyspnea is not always experienced with simple hypoxia but occurs when the respiratory minute volume approaches half the maximal breathing capacity; this may occur with minimum exertion in patients in whom maximal breathing capacity is reduced by lung disease. In general, little warning precedes the loss of consciousness resulting from hypoxia.

Cardiovascular System. Hypoxia causes reflex activation of the sympathetic nervous system *via* both autonomic and humoral mechanisms, resulting in tachycardia and increased cardiac output. Peripheral vascular resistance, however, decreases primarily *via* local autoregulatory

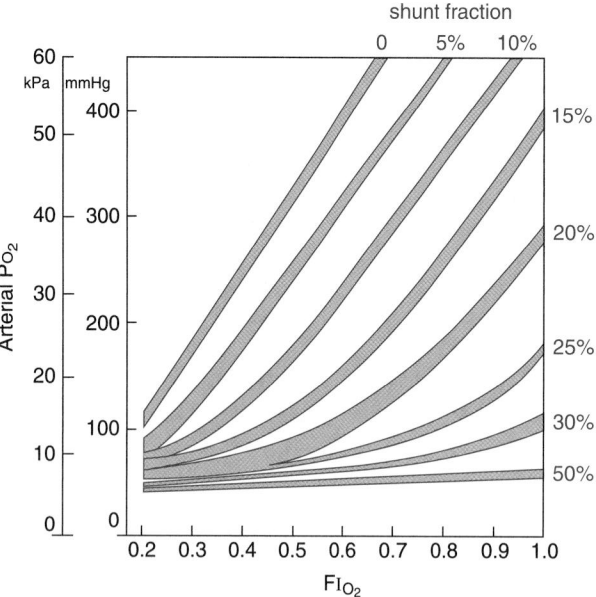

Figure 15–2. *Effect of shunt on arterial oxygenation.* The iso-shunt diagram shows the effect of changing inspired oxygen concentration on arterial oxygenation in the presence of different amounts of pure shunt. As shunt fraction increases, even an inspired oxygen fraction (FI_{O_2}) of 1.0 is ineffective at increasing the arterial P_{O_2}. This estimation assumes hemoglobin (Hb) from 10 to 14 g/dl, arterial P_{CO_2} of 3.3 to 5.3 kPa (25 to 40 mmHg), and an arterial–venous (a–v) O_2 content difference of 5 ml/100 ml. Redrawn from Benatar *et al.,* 1973, with permission.

mechanisms, with the net result that blood pressure generally is maintained unless hypoxia is prolonged or severe. In contrast to the systemic circulation, hypoxia causes pulmonary vasoconstriction and hypertension, an extension of the normal regional vascular response that matches perfusion with ventilation to optimize gas exchange in the lung (hypoxic pulmonary vasoconstriction).

Central Nervous System (CNS). The CNS is least able to tolerate hypoxia. Hypoxia is manifest initially by decreased intellectual capacity and impaired judgment and psychomotor ability. This state progresses to confusion and restlessness and ultimately to stupor, coma, and death as the arterial PO_2 decreases below 4 to 5.3 kPa (30 to 40 mmHg). Victims often are unaware of this progression.

Cellular and Metabolic Effects. When the mitochondrial PO_2 falls below about 0.13 kPa (1 mmHg), aerobic metabolism stops, and the less efficient anaerobic pathways of glycolysis become responsible for the production of cellular energy. End products of anaerobic metabolism, such as lactic acid, are released into the circulation in measurable quantities. Energy-dependent ion pumps slow, and transmembrane ion gradients dissipate. Intracellular concentrations of Na^+, Ca^{2+}, and H^+ increase, finally leading to cell death. The time course of cellular demise depends on the relative metabolic demands, oxygen storage capacity, and anaerobic capacity of the individual organs. Restoration of perfusion and oxygenation prior to hypoxic cell death paradoxically can result in an accelerated form of cell injury (ischemia–reperfusion syndrome), which is thought to result from the generation of highly reactive oxygen free radicals (McCord, 1985).

Adaptation to Hypoxia. Long-term hypoxia results in adaptive physiological changes; these have been studied most thoroughly in persons exposed to high altitude. Adaptations include increased numbers of pulmonary alveoli, increased concentrations of hemoglobin in blood and myoglobin in muscle, and a decreased ventilatory response to hypoxia. Short-term exposure to high altitude produces similar adaptive changes. In susceptible individuals, however, acute exposure to high altitude may produce *acute mountain sickness,* a syndrome characterized by headache, nausea, dyspnea, sleep disturbances, and impaired judgment progressing to pulmonary and cerebral edema (Johnson and Rock, 1988). Mountain sickness is treated with supplemental oxygen, descent to lower altitude, or an increase in ambient pressure. Diuretics (*carbonic anhydrase inhibitors*) and steroids also may be helpful. The syndrome usually can be avoided by a slow ascent to altitude, permitting time for adaptation to occur.

Certain aspects of fetal and newborn physiology are strongly reminiscent of adaptation mechanisms found in hypoxia-tolerant animals (Mortola, 1999; Singer, 1999), including shifts in the oxyhemoglobin dissociation curve (fetal hemoglobin), reductions in metabolic rate and body temperature (hibernation-like mode), reductions in heart rate and circulatory redistribution (as in diving mammals), and redirection of energy utilization from growth to mainte-

nance metabolism. These adaptations probably account for the relative tolerance of the fetus and neonate to both chronic (uterine insufficiency) and short-term hypoxia.

Oxygen Inhalation

Physiological Effects of Oxygen Inhalation. Oxygen inhalation is used primarily to reverse or prevent the development of hypoxia; other consequences usually are minor. However, when oxygen is breathed in excessive amounts or for prolonged periods, secondary physiological changes and toxic effects can occur.

Respiratory System. Inhalation of oxygen at 1 atm or above causes a small degree of respiratory depression in normal subjects, presumably as a result of loss of tonic chemoreceptor activity. However, ventilation typically increases within a few minutes of oxygen inhalation because of a paradoxical increase in the tension of carbon dioxide in tissues. This increase results from the increased concentration of oxyhemoglobin in venous blood, which causes less efficient removal of carbon dioxide from the tissues (Plewes and Farhi, 1983).

In a small number of patients whose respiratory center is depressed by long-term retention of carbon dioxide, injury, or drugs, ventilation is maintained largely by stimulation of carotid and aortic chemoreceptors, commonly referred to as the *hypoxic drive.* The provision of too much oxygen can depress this drive, resulting in respiratory acidosis. In these cases, supplemental oxygen should be titrated carefully to ensure adequate arterial saturation. If hypoventilation results, then mechanical ventilatory support with or without tracheal intubation should be provided.

Expansion of poorly ventilated alveoli is maintained in part by the nitrogen content of alveolar gas; nitrogen is poorly soluble and thus remains in the airspaces while oxygen is absorbed. High oxygen concentrations delivered to poorly ventilated lung regions dilute the nitrogen content and can promote absorption atelectasis, occasionally resulting in an increase in shunt and a paradoxical worsening of hypoxemia after a period of oxygen administration.

Cardiovascular System. Aside from reversing the effects of hypoxia, the physiological consequences of oxygen inhalation on the cardiovascular system are of little significance. Heart rate and cardiac output are slightly reduced when 100% oxygen is breathed; blood pressure changes little. While pulmonary arterial pressure changes little in normal subjects with oxygen inhalation, elevated pulmonary artery pressures in patients living at high altitude who have chronic hypoxic pulmonary hypertension may reverse with oxygen therapy or return to sea level. In particular, in neonates with congenital heart disease and left-to-right shunting of cardiac output, oxygen supplementation must be regulated carefully because of the risk of further reducing pulmonary vascular resistance and increasing pulmonary blood flow.

Metabolism. Inhalation of 100% oxygen does not produce detectable changes in oxygen consumption, carbon dioxide production, respiratory quotient, or glucose utilization.

Oxygen Administration

Oxygen is supplied as a compressed gas in steel cylinders, and a purity of 99% is referred to as *medical grade.* Most hospitals have oxygen piped from insulated liquid oxygen containers to areas of frequent use. For safety, oxygen cylinders and piping are color-coded (green in the United States), and some form of mechanical indexing of valve connections is used to prevent the connection of other gases to oxygen systems. Oxygen concentrators, which employ molecular sieve, membrane, or electrochemical technologies, are available for low-flow home use. Such systems produce 30% to 95% oxygen depending on the flow rate.

Oxygen is delivered by inhalation except during extracorporeal circulation, when it is dissolved directly into the circulating blood. Only a closed delivery system with an airtight seal to the patient's airway and complete separation of inspired from expired gases can precisely control $F_{I_{O_2}}$. In all other systems, the actual delivered $F_{I_{O_2}}$ will depend on the ventilatory pattern (*i.e.,* rate, tidal volume, inspiratory–expiratory time ratio, and inspiratory flow) and delivery system characteristics.

Low-Flow Systems. Low-flow systems, in which the oxygen flow is lower than the inspiratory flow rate, have a limited ability to raise the $F_{I_{O_2}}$ because they depend on entrained room air to make up the balance of the inspired gas. The $F_{I_{O_2}}$ of these systems is extremely sensitive to small changes in the ventilatory pattern. Devices such as face tents are used primarily for delivering humidified gases to patients and cannot be relied on to provide predictable amounts of supplemental oxygen. Nasal cannulae—small, flexible prongs that sit just inside each naris—deliver oxygen at 1 to 6 L/min. The nasopharynx acts as a reservoir for storing the oxygen, and patients may breathe through either the mouth or nose as long as the nasal passages remain patent. These devices typically deliver 24% to 28% $F_{I_{O_2}}$ at 2 to 3 L/min. Up to 40% $F_{I_{O_2}}$ is possible at higher flow rates, although this is poorly tolerated for more than brief periods because of mucosal drying. The simple facemask, a clear plastic mask with side holes for clearance of expiratory gas and inspiratory air entrainment, is used when higher concentrations of oxygen delivered without tight control are desired. The maximum $F_{I_{O_2}}$ of a facemask can be increased from around 60% at 6 to 15 L/min to greater than 85% by adding a 600- to 1000-ml reservoir bag. With this partial rebreathing mask, most of the inspired volume is drawn from the reservoir, avoiding dilution by entrainment of room air.

High-Flow Systems. The most commonly used high-flow oxygen delivery device is the Venturi mask, which uses a specially designed mask insert to entrain room air reliably in a fixed ratio and thus provides a relatively constant $F_{I_{O_2}}$ at relatively high flow rates. Typically, each insert is designed to operate at a specific oxygen flow rate, and different inserts are required to change the $F_{I_{O_2}}$. Lower delivered $F_{I_{O_2}}$ values use greater entrainment ratios, resulting in higher total (oxygen plus entrained air) flows to the patient, ranging from 80 L/min for 24% $F_{I_{O_2}}$ to 40 L/min at 50% $F_{I_{O_2}}$. While these flow rates are much higher than those obtained with low-flow devices, they still may be lower than the peak inspiratory flows for patients in respiratory distress, and thus the actual delivered oxygen concentration may be lower than the nominal value. Oxygen nebulizers, another type of Venturi device, provide patients with humidified oxygen at 35% to 100% $F_{I_{O_2}}$ at high flow rates. Finally, oxygen blenders provide high inspired oxygen concentrations at very high flow rates. These devices mix high-pressure compressed air and oxygen to achieve any concentration of oxygen from 21% to 100% at flow rates of up to 100 L/min. These same blenders are used to provide control of $F_{I_{O_2}}$ for ventilators, CPAP/BiPAP machines, oxygenators, and other devices with similar requirements. Again, despite the high flows, the delivery of high $F_{I_{O_2}}$ to an individual patient also depends on maintaining a tight-fitting seal to the airway and/or the use of reservoirs to minimize entrainment of diluting room air.

Monitoring of Oxygenation. Monitoring and titration are required to meet the therapeutic goal of oxygen therapy and to avoid complications and side effects. Although cyanosis is a physical finding of substantial clinical importance, it is not an early, sensitive, or reliable index of oxygenation. Cyanosis appears when about 5 g/dl of deoxyhemoglobin is present in arterial blood, representing an oxygen saturation of about 67% when a normal amount of hemoglobin (15 g/dl) is present. However, when anemia lowers the hemoglobin to 10 g/dl, then cyanosis does not appear until the arterial blood saturation has decreased to 50%. Invasive approaches for monitoring oxygenation include intermittent laboratory analysis of arterial or mixed venous blood gases and placement of intravascular cannulae capable of continuous measurement of oxygen tension. The latter method, which relies on fiberoptic oximetry, is used frequently for the continuous measurement of mixed venous hemoglobin saturation as an index of tissue extraction of oxygen, usually in critically ill patients.

Noninvasive monitoring of arterial oxygen saturation now is widely available from transcutaneous pulse oximetry, in which oxygen saturation is measured from the differential absorption of light by oxyhemoglobin and deoxyhemoglobin and the arterial saturation determined from the pulsatile component of this signal. Application is simple, and calibration is not required. Because pulse oximetry measures hemoglobin saturation and not P_{O_2}, it is not sensitive to increases in P_{O_2} that exceed levels required to saturate the blood fully. However, pulse oximetry is very useful for monitoring the adequacy of oxygenation during procedures requiring sedation or anesthesia, rapid evaluation and monitoring of potentially compromised patients, and titrating oxygen therapy in situations where toxicity from oxygen or side effects of excess oxygen are of concern.

Complications of Oxygen Therapy. Administration of supplemental oxygen is not without potential complications. In addition to the potential to promote absorption atelectasis and depress ventilation (discussed earlier), high flows of dry oxygen can dry out and irritate mucosal surfaces of the airway and the eyes, as well as decrease mucociliary transport and clearance of secretions. Humidified oxygen thus should be used when prolonged therapy (>1 hour) is required. Finally, any oxygen-enriched atmosphere constitutes a fire hazard, and appropriate precautions must be taken both in the operating room and for patients on oxygen at home.

It is important to realize that hypoxemia still can occur despite the administration of supplemental oxygen. Furthermore, when supplemental oxygen is administered, desaturation occurs at a later time after airway obstruction or hypoventilation, potentially delaying the detection of these critical events. Therefore, whether or not oxygen is administered to a patient at risk for these problems, it is essential that both oxygen saturation and adequacy of ventilation be assessed frequently.

Therapeutic Uses of Oxygen

Correction of Hypoxia. As stated earlier, the primary therapeutic use of oxygen is to correct hypoxia. However, hypoxia is most commonly a manifestation of an underlying disease, and administration of oxygen thus should be viewed as a symptomatic or temporizing therapy. Efforts must be directed at correcting the cause of the hypoxia. For example, airway obstruction is unlikely to respond to an increase in inspired oxygen tension without relief of the obstruction. More important, while hypoxemia owing to hypoventilation after a narcotic overdose can be improved with supplemental oxygen administration, the patient remains at risk for respiratory failure if ventilation is not increased through stimulation, narcotic reversal, or mechanical ventilation. The hypoxia that results from most pulmonary diseases can be alleviated at least partially by administration of oxygen, thereby allowing time for definitive therapy to reverse the primary process. Thus, administration of oxygen is a basic and important treatment to be used in all forms of hypoxia, with the understanding that the response will vary in a way that generally is predictable from knowledge of the underlying pathophysiological processes.

Reduction of Partial Pressure of an Inert Gas. Since nitrogen constitutes some 79% of ambient air, it also is the predominant gas in most gas-filled spaces in the body. In certain situations, such as bowel distension from obstruction or ileus, intravascular air embolism, or pneumothorax, it is desirable to reduce the volume of these air-filled spaces. Since nitrogen is relatively insoluble, inhalation of high concentrations of oxygen (and thus low concentrations of nitrogen) rapidly lowers the total-body partial pressure of nitrogen and provides a substantial gradient for the removal of nitrogen from gas spaces. Administration of oxygen for air embolism is additionally beneficial because it also helps to relieve the localized hypoxia distal to the embolic vascular obstruction. In the case of *decompression sickness*, or *bends*, lowering of inert gas tension in blood and tissues by oxygen inhalation prior to or during a barometric decompression can reduce the degree of supersaturation that occurs after decompression so that bubbles do not form. If bubbles do form in either tissues or the vasculature, administration of oxygen is based on the same rationale as that described for gas embolism.

Hyperbaric Oxygen Therapy. Oxygen is administered at greater than atmospheric pressure for a number of conditions when 100% oxygen at 1 atm is insufficient (Buras, 2000; Shank and Muth, 2000; Myers, 2000). To achieve concentrations of greater than 1 atm, a hyperbaric chamber must be used. These chambers range from small, single-person units to multiroom establishments that may include complex medical equipment. Smaller, one-person chambers typically are pressurized with oxygen, whereas larger ones are pres-

surized with air, and a patient must wear a mask to receive the oxygen at the increased pressure. The larger chambers are more suitable for critically ill patients who require ventilation, monitoring, and constant attendance. Any chamber must be built to withstand pressures that may range from 200 to 600 kPa (2 to 6 atm), although inhaled oxygen tension that exceeds 300 kPa (3 atm) rarely is used (*see* Oxygen Toxicity, below).

Hyperbaric oxygen therapy has two components: increased hydrostatic pressure and increased oxygen pressure. Both factors are necessary for the treatment of decompression sickness and air embolism. The hydrostatic pressure reduces bubble volume, and the absence of inspired nitrogen increases the gradient for elimination of nitrogen and reduces hypoxia in downstream tissues. Increased oxygen pressure at the tissue level is the primary therapeutic goal for most of the other indications for hyperbaric oxygen. For example, even a small increase in PO_2 in previously ischemic areas may enhance the bactericidal activity of leukocytes and increase angiogenesis. Thus, repetitive brief exposures to hyperbaric oxygen are a useful adjunct in the treatment of chronic refractory osteomyelitis, osteoradionecrosis, or crush injury or for the recovery of compromised skin, tissue grafts, or flaps. Furthermore, increased oxygen tension itself can be bacteriostatic; the spread of infection with *Clostridium perfringens* and production of toxin by the bacteria are slowed when oxygen tensions exceed 33 kPa (250 mmHg), justifying the early use of hyperbaric oxygen in clostridial myonecrosis (gas gangrene).

Hyperbaric oxygen also is useful in selected instances of generalized hypoxia. In CO poisoning, hemoglobin (Hb) and myoglobin become unavailable for O_2 binding because of the high affinity of these proteins for CO. This affinity is ~250 times greater than the affinity for O_2; thus, an alveolar concentration of CO = 0.4 mm Hg (1/250th that of alveolar O_2, which is ~100 mm Hg), will compete equally with O_2 for binding sites on Hb. A high PO_2 facilitates competition of O_2 for Hb binding sites as CO is exchanged in the alveoli; i.e., the high PO_2 increases the probability that O_2 rather than CO will bind to Hb once CO dissociates. In addition, hyperbaric O_2 will increase the availability of dissolved O_2 in the blood (*see* Table 15–1). In a randomized clinical trial (Weaver *et al.*, 2002), hyperbaric oxygen decreased the incidence of long- and short-term neurological sequelae after CO intoxication. The occasional use of hyperbaric oxygen in cyanide poisoning has a similar rationale. Hyperbaric oxygen also may be useful in severe short-term anemia because sufficient oxygen can be dissolved in the plasma at 3 atm to meet metabolic needs. However, such treatment must be limited because oxygen toxicity depends on increased PO_2, not on the oxygen content of the blood.

Hyperbaric oxygen therapy has been used in such diverse conditions as multiple sclerosis, traumatic spinal cord injury, cerebrovascular accidents, bone grafts and fractures, and leprosy; however, data from well-controlled clinical trials are not sufficient to justify these uses.

Oxygen Toxicity

Oxygen is used in cellular energy production and is crucial for cellular metabolism. However, oxygen also may have deleterious actions at the cellular level. Oxygen toxicity probably results from increased production of hydrogen peroxide and reactive agents such as superoxide anion, singlet oxygen, and hydroxyl radicals (Carraway and Piantadosi, 1999) that attack and damage lipids, proteins, and other macromolecules, especially those in biological membranes. A number of factors limit the toxicity of oxygen-derived reactive agents, including enzymes such as superoxide dismutase, glutathione peroxidase, and catalase, which scavenge toxic oxygen by-products, and reducing agents such as iron, glutathione, and ascorbate. These factors, however, are insufficient to limit the destructive actions of oxygen when patients are exposed to high concentrations over an extended time period. Tissues show differential sensitivity to oxygen toxicity, which is likely the result of differences in both their production of reactive compounds and their protective mechanisms.

Respiratory Tract. The pulmonary system is usually the first to exhibit toxicity, a function of its continuous exposure to the highest oxygen tensions in the body. Subtle changes in pulmonary function can occur within 8 to 12 hours of exposure to 100% oxygen (Sackner *et al.*, 1975). Increases in capillary permeability, which will increase the alveolar/arterial oxygen gradient and ultimately lead to further hypoxemia, and decreased pulmonary function can be seen after only 18 hours of exposure (Davis *et al.*, 1983; Clark, 1988). Serious injury and death, however, require much longer exposures. Pulmonary damage is directly related to the inspired oxygen tension, and concentrations of less than 0.5 atm appear to be safe over long time periods. The capillary endothelium is the most sensitive tissue of the lung. Endothelial injury results in loss of surface area from interstitial edema and leaks into the alveoli (Crapo *et al.*, 1980).

Decreases of inspired oxygen concentrations remain the cornerstone of therapy for oxygen toxicity. Modest decreases in toxicity also have been observed in animals treated with antioxidant enzymes (White *et al.*, 1989). Tolerance also may play a role in protection from oxygen toxicity; animals exposed briefly to high oxygen tensions are subsequently more resistant to toxicity (Kravetz *et al.*, 1980; Coursin *et al.*, 1987). Sensitivity in human beings also can be altered by preexposure to both high and low oxygen concentrations (Hendricks *et al.*, 1977; Clark, 1988). These studies strongly suggest that changes in alveolar surfactant and cellular levels of antioxidant enzymes play a role in protection from oxygen toxicity.

Retina. Retrolental fibroplasia can occur when neonates are exposed to increased oxygen tensions (Betts *et al.*, 1977). These changes can progress to blindness and are likely caused by angiogenesis (Kushner *et al.*, 1977; Ashton, 1979). The incidence of this disorder has decreased with an improved appreciation of the issues and avoidance of excessive inspired oxygen concentrations. Adults do not seem to develop the disease.

Central Nervous System. CNS problems are rare, and toxicity occurs only under hyperbaric conditions where exposure exceeds 200 kPa (2 atm). Symptoms include seizures and visual changes, which resolve when oxygen tension is returned to normal. These problems are a further reason to replace oxygen with helium under hyperbaric conditions (*see* below).

CARBON DIOXIDE

Transfer and Elimination of Carbon Dioxide

Carbon dioxide (CO_2) is produced by the body's metabolism at approximately the same rate as oxygen consumption. At rest, this value is about 3 ml/kg per minute, but it may increase dramatically with heavy exercise. Carbon dioxide diffuses readily from the cells into the bloodstream, where it is carried partly as bicarbonate ion (HCO_3^-), partly in chemical combination with hemoglobin and plasma proteins, and partly in solution at a partial pressure of about 6 kPa (46 mmHg) in mixed venous blood. Carbon dioxide is transported to the lung, where it is normally exhaled at the same rate at which it is produced, leaving a partial pressure of about 5.2 kPa (40 mmHg) in the alveoli and in arterial blood. An increase in PCO_2 results in a respiratory acidosis and may be due to decreased ventilation or the inhalation of carbon dioxide, whereas an increase in ventilation results in decreased PCO_2 and a respiratory alkalosis. Since carbon dioxide is freely diffusible, the changes in blood PCO_2 and pH soon are reflected by intracellular changes in PCO_2 and pH.

Effects of Carbon Dioxide

Alterations in PCO_2 and pH have widespread effects in the body, particularly on respiration, circulation, and the CNS. More complete discussions of these and other effects are found in textbooks of physiology (*see* Nunn, 2000a).

Respiration. Carbon dioxide is a rapid, potent stimulus to ventilation in direct proportion to the inspired carbon dioxide. Inhalation of 10% carbon dioxide can produce minute volumes of 75 L/min in normal individuals. Carbon dioxide acts at multiple sites to stimulate ventilation. Respiratory integration areas in the brainstem are acted on by impulses from medullary and peripheral arterial chemoreceptors. The mechanism by which carbon dioxide acts on these receptors probably involves changes in pH (Nattie, 1999). Elevated PCO_2 causes bronchodilation, whereas hypocarbia causes constriction of airway smooth muscle; these responses may play a role in matching pulmonary ventilation and perfusion (Duane *et al.*, 1979).

Circulation. The circulatory effects of carbon dioxide result from the combination of its direct local effects and its centrally mediated effects on the autonomic nervous system. The direct effect of carbon dioxide on the heart, diminished contractility, results from pH changes (van den Bos *et al.*, 1979). The direct effect on systemic blood vessels results in vasodilation. Carbon dioxide causes widespread activation of the sympathetic nervous system and an increase in the plasma concentrations of epinephrine, norepinephrine, angiotensin, and other vasoactive peptides (Staszewska-Barczak and Dusting, 1981). The results of sympathetic nervous system activation generally are opposite to the local effects of carbon dioxide. The sympathetic effects consist of increases in cardiac contractility, heart rate, and vasoconstriction (*see* Chapter 10).

The balance of opposing local and sympathetic effects, therefore, determines the total circulatory response to carbon dioxide. The net effect of carbon dioxide inhalation is an increase in cardiac output, heart rate, and blood pressure. In blood vessels, however, the direct vasodilating actions of carbon dioxide appear more important, and total peripheral resistance decreases when the PCO_2 is increased. Carbon dioxide also is a potent coronary vasodilator. Cardiac arrhythmias associated with increased PCO_2 are due to the release of catecholamines.

Hypocarbia results in opposite effects: decreased blood pressure and vasoconstriction in skin, intestine, brain, kidney, and heart. These actions are exploited clinically in the use of hyperventilation to diminish intracranial hypertension.

Central Nervous System. Hypercarbia depresses the excitability of the cerebral cortex and increases the cutaneous pain threshold through a central action. This central depression has therapeutic importance. For example, in patients who are hypoventilating from narcotics or anesthetics, increasing PCO_2 may result in further CNS depression, which in turn may worsen the respiratory depression. This positive-feedback cycle can be deadly. The inhalation of high concentrations of carbon dioxide (about 50%) produces marked cortical and subcortical depression of a type similar to that produced by anesthetic agents. Under certain circumstances, inspired carbon dioxide (25% to 30%) can result in subcortical activation and seizures.

Methods of Administration

Carbon dioxide is marketed in gray metal cylinders as the pure gas or as carbon dioxide mixed with oxygen. It usually is administered at a concentration of 5% to 10% in combination with oxygen by means of a facemask. Another method for the temporary administration of carbon dioxide is by rebreathing, *e.g.,* from an anesthesia breathing circuit when the soda lime canister is bypassed or from something as simple as a paper bag. A potential safety issue exists in that tanks containing carbon dioxide plus oxygen are the same color as those containing 100% carbon dioxide. When tanks containing carbon dioxide and oxygen have been used inadvertently where a fire hazard exists (*e.g.,* in the presence of electrocautery during laparoscopic surgery), explosions and fires have resulted.

Therapeutic Uses

Inhalation of carbon dioxide is used less commonly today than in the past because there are now more effective treatments for most indications. Inhalation of carbon dioxide has been used during anesthesia to increase the speed of induction and emergence from inhalational anesthesia by increasing minute ventilation and cerebral blood flow. However, this technique results in some degree of respiratory acidosis. Hypocarbia, with its attendant respiratory alkalosis, still has some uses in anesthesia. It constricts cerebral vessels, decreasing brain size slightly, and thus may facilitate the performance of neurosurgical operations. Although carbon dioxide stimulates respiration, it is not useful in situations where respiratory depression has resulted in hypercarbia or acidosis because further depression results.

A common use of carbon dioxide is for insufflation during endoscopic procedures (*e.g.,* laparoscopic surgery) because it is highly soluble and does not support combustion. Any inadvertent gas emboli thus are dissolved and eliminated more easily *via* the respiratory system.

Recently, carbon dioxide has been shown to be helpful during open cardiac surgery, where it is used to flood the surgical field. Because of its density, carbon dioxide displaces the air surrounding the open heart so that any gas bubbles trapped in the heart are carbon dioxide rather than insoluble nitrogen (Nadolny and Svensson, 2000). For the same reasons, CO_2 is used to de-bubble cardiopulmonary bypass and extracorporeal membrane oxygenation (ECMO) circuits. It also can be used to adjust pH during bypass procedures when a patient is cooled.

NITRIC OXIDE

Nitric oxide (NO), a free-radical gas long known as an air pollutant and a potential toxin, is an endogenous cell-signaling molecule of great physiological importance. As knowledge of the important actions of NO has evolved, interest in the use of NO as a therapeutic agent has grown.

Endogenous NO is produced from L-arginine by a family of enzymes called *NO synthases.* NO is both an intracellular and a cell–cell messenger implicated in a wide range of physiological and pathophysiological events in numerous cell types, including the cardiovascular, immune, and nervous systems. NO activates the soluble guanyl cyclase, increasing cellular cyclic GMP (*see* Chapter 1). In the vasculature, basal release of NO produced by endothelial cells is a primary determinant of resting vascular tone; NO causes vasodilation when synthesized in response to shear stress or a variety of vasodilating agents (*see* Chapter 32). It also inhibits platelet aggregation and adhesion. Impaired NO production has been implicated in diseases such as atherosclerosis, hypertension, cerebral and coronary vasospasm, and ischemia–reperfusion injury. In the immune system, NO serves as an effector of macrophage-induced cytotoxicity, and overproduction of NO is a mediator of inflammation. In neurons, NO acts as a mediator of long-term potentiation, cytotoxicity resulting from *N*-methyl-D-aspartate (NMDA), and non-adrenergic noncholinergic neurotransmission; NO has been implicated in mediating central nociceptive pathways (*see* Chapter 6).

The physiology and pathophysiology of endogenous NO have been reviewed extensively (Nathan, 2004; Ignarro and Napoli, 2005).

Therapeutic Use of NO

Inhalation of NO gas has received considerable therapeutic attention owing to its ability to dilate selectively the pulmonary vasculature with minimal systemic cardiovascular effects (Steudel *et al.*, 1999). The lack of effect of inhaled NO on the systemic circulation is due to its strong binding to and inactivation by oxyhemoglobin on exposure to the pulmonary circulation. Ventilation–perfusion matching is preserved or improved by NO because inhaled NO is distributed only to ventilated areas of the lung and dilates only those vessels directly adjacent to the ventilated alveoli. Thus, inhaled NO will decrease elevated pulmonary artery pressure and pulmonary vascular resistance and often improve oxygenation (Steudel *et al.*, 1999; Haddad *et al.*, 2000).

Owing to its selective pulmonary vasodilating action, inhaled NO is being studied as a potential therapeutic agent for numerous diseases associated with increased pulmonary vascular resistance. Therapeutic trials of inhaled NO in a wide range of such conditions have confirmed its ability to decrease pulmonary vascular resistance and often increase oxygenation, but in all but a few cases these trials have yet to demonstrate long-term improvement in terms of morbidity or mortality (Dellinger, 1999; Cheifetz, 2000). Inhaled NO has been approved by the FDA only for use in newborns with persistent pulmonary hypertension and has become the first-line therapy for this disease (Hwang *et al.*, 2004; Mourani *et al.*, 2004). In this disease state, NO inhalation has been shown to reduce significantly the necessity for extracorporeal membrane oxygenation, although overall mortality has been unchanged (Kinsella *et al.*, 1997; Roberts *et al.*, 1997). Notably, numerous trials of inhaled NO in adult and pediatric acute respiratory distress syndrome, as well as a recent meta-analysis, have failed to demonstrate an impact on outcome (Dellinger, 1999; Cheifetz, 2000; Sokol *et al.*, 2003). Several small studies and case reports have suggested potential benefits of inhaled NO in a variety of conditions, including weaning from cardiopulmonary bypass in adult and congenital heart disease patients, primary pulmonary hypertension, pulmonary embolism, acute chest syndrome in sickle-cell patients, congenital diaphragmatic hernia, high-altitude pulmonary edema, and lung transplantation (Steudel *et al.*, 1999; Haddad *et al.*, 2000; Tanus-Santos and Theodorakis, 2002). Larger prospective, randomized studies either have not yet been performed or have failed to confirm any

changes in outcome. Outside of clinical investigation, therapeutic use and benefit of inhaled NO presently are limited to newborns with persistent pulmonary hypertension.

Diagnostic Uses of NO

Inhaled NO also is used in several diagnostic applications. Inhaled NO can be used during cardiac catheterization to evaluate safely and selectively the pulmonary vasodilating capacity of patients with heart failure and infants with congenital heart disease. Inhaled NO also is used to determine the diffusion capacity (DL) across the alveolar–capillary unit. NO is more effective than carbon dioxide in this regard because of its greater affinity for hemoglobin and its higher water solubility at body temperature (Steudel *et al.*, 1999; Haddad *et al.*, 2000).

NO is produced from the nasal passages and from the lungs of normal human subjects and can be detected in exhaled gas. The measurement of exhaled NO has been investigated for its utility in assessment of respiratory tract diseases. Measurement of exhaled NO may prove to be useful in diagnosis and assessment of severity of asthma and in respiratory tract infections (Haddad *et al.*, 2000; Zeidler *et al.*, 2003).

Toxicity of NO

Administered at low concentrations (0.1 to 50 ppm), inhaled NO appears to be safe and without significant side effects. Pulmonary toxicity can occur with levels higher than 50 to 100 ppm. In the context of NO as an atmospheric pollutant, the Occupational Safety and Health Administration places the 7-hour exposure limit at 50 ppm. Part of the toxicity of NO may be related to its further oxidation to nitrogen dioxide (NO_2) in the presence of high concentrations of oxygen. Even low concentrations of NO_2 (2 ppm) have been shown to be highly toxic in animal models, with observed changes in lung histopathology, including loss of cilia, hypertrophy, and focal hyperplasia in the epithelium of terminal bronchioles. It is important, therefore, to keep NO_2 formation during NO therapy at a low level. This can be achieved through appropriate filters and scavengers and the use of high-quality gas mixtures. Laboratory studies have suggested potential additional toxic effects of chronic low doses of inhaled NO, including surfactant inactivation and the formation of peroxynitrite by interaction with superoxide. The ability of NO to inhibit or alter the function of a number of iron- and heme-containing proteins—including cyclooxygenase, lipoxygenases, and oxidative cytochromes—as well as its interactions with ADP-ribosylation, suggests a need for further investigation of the toxic potential of NO under therapeutic conditions (Steudel *et al.*, 1999; Haddad *et al.*, 2000).

The development of methemoglobinemia is a significant complication of inhaled NO at higher concentrations, and rare deaths have been reported with overdoses of NO. The blood content of methemoglobin, however, generally will not increase to toxic levels with appropriate use of inhaled NO. Methemoglobin concentrations should be monitored intermittently during NO inhalation (Steudel *et al.*, 1999; Haddad *et al.*, 2000).

Inhaled NO can inhibit platelet function and has been shown to increase bleeding time in some clinical studies, although bleeding complications have not been reported.

In patients with impaired function of the left ventricle, NO has a potential to further impair left ventricular performance by dilating the pulmonary circulation and increasing the blood flow to the left ventricle, thereby increasing left atrial pressure and promoting pulmonary edema formation. Careful monitoring of cardiac output, left atrial pressure, or pulmonary capillary wedge pressure is important in this situation (Steudel *et al.*, 1999).

Despite these concerns, there are limited reports of inhaled NO-related toxicity in humans. The most important requirements for safe NO inhalation therapy include (1) continuous measurement of NO and NO_2 concentrations using either chemiluminescence or electrochemical analyzers; (2) frequent calibration of monitoring equipment; (3) intermittent analysis of blood methemoglobin levels; (4) the use of certified tanks of NO; and (5) administration of the lowest NO concentration required for therapeutic effect (Steudel *et al.*, 1999).

Methods of Administration

Courses of treatment of patients with inhaled NO are highly varied, extending from 0.1 to 40 ppm in dose and for periods of a few hours to several weeks in duration. The minimum effective inhaled NO concentration should be determined for each patient to minimize the chance for toxicity. Commercial NO systems are available that will accurately deliver inspired NO concentrations between 0.1 and 80 ppm and simultaneously measure NO and NO_2 concentrations. A constant inspired concentration of NO is obtained by administering NO in nitrogen to the inspiratory limb of the ventilator circuit in either a pulse or continuous mode. While inhaled NO may be administered to spontaneously breathing patients *via* a closely fitting mask, it usually is delivered during mechanical ventilation. Nasal prong administration is being employed in therapeutic trials of home administration for treatment of primary pulmonary hypertension (Steudel *et al.*, 1999; Haddad *et al.*, 2000).

Acute discontinuation of NO inhalation can lead to a rebound pulmonary artery hypertension with an increase in right-to-left intrapulmonary shunting and a decrease in oxygenation. To avoid this phenomenon, a graded decrease of inhaled NO concentration is important in the process of weaning a patient from inhaled NO (Steudel *et al.*, 1999; Haddad *et al.*, 2000).

HELIUM

Helium is an inert gas whose low density, low solubility, and high thermal conductivity provide the basis for its medical and diagnostic uses. Helium is produced by separation from liquefied natural gas and is supplied in brown cylinders. Helium can be mixed with oxygen and administered by mask or tracheal tube. Under hyperbaric conditions, it can be substituted for the bulk of other gases, resulting in a mixture of much lower density that is easier to breathe.

The primary uses of helium are in pulmonary function testing, the treatment of respiratory obstruction, during laser airway surgery, for diving at depth, and most recently, as a label in imaging studies. The determinations of residual lung volume, functional residual capacity, and related lung volumes require a highly diffusible nontoxic gas that is insoluble (and thus does not leave the lung *via* the bloodstream) so that, by dilution, the lung volume can be measured. Helium is well suited to these needs and is much cheaper than alternatives. In these tests, a breath of a known concentration of helium is given, and the concentration of helium then is measured in the mixed expired gas, allowing calculation of the other pulmonary volumes.

Pulmonary gas flow is normally laminar, but with increased flow rate or narrowed flow pathway, a component becomes turbulent. Helium can be added to oxygen to treat the turbulence due to airway obstruction: the density of helium is substantially less than that of air and the viscosity of helium is greater than that of air; addition of helium reduces the Reynolds number of the mixture (the Reynolds number is proportional to density and inversely proportional to viscosity), thereby reducing turbulence. Indeed, flow rates are increased with lower density gases. Thus, with mixtures of helium and oxygen, the work of breathing is less. Several factors limit the utility of this approach, however. Oxygenation is often the principal problem in airway obstruction, and the practical need for increased inspired O_2 concentration may limit the fraction of helium that can be used. Furthermore, even though helium reduces the Reynolds number of the gas mixture, the viscosity of helium is higher than that of air, and the increased viscosity increases the resistance to flow according to Poiseuille's law, whereby flow is inversely proportional to viscosity.

Helium has high thermal conductivity, which makes it useful during laser surgery on the airway. This more rapid conduction of heat away from the point of contact of the laser beam reduces the spread of tissue damage and the likelihood that the ignition point of flammable materials in the airway will be reached. Its low density improves the flow through the small endotracheal tubes typically used in such procedures.

Recently, laser-polarized helium has been used as an inhalational contrast agent for pulmonary magnetic resonance imaging. Optical pumping of nonradioactive helium increases the signal from the gas in the lung sufficiently to permit detailed imaging of the airways and inspired airflow patterns (Kauczor *et al.*, 1998).

Hyperbaric Applications. The depth and duration of diving activity are limited by oxygen toxicity, inert gas (nitrogen) narcosis, and nitrogen supersaturation when decompressing. Oxygen toxicity is a problem with prolonged exposure to compressed air at 500 kPa (5 atm) or more. This problem can be minimized by dilution of oxygen with helium, which lacks narcotic potential even at very high pressures and is quite insoluble in body tissues. This low solubility reduces the likelihood of bubble formation after decompression, which therefore can be achieved more rapidly. The low density of helium also reduces the work of breathing in the otherwise dense hyperbaric atmosphere. The lower heat capacity of helium also decreases respiratory heat loss, which can be significant when diving at depth.

BIBLIOGRAPHY

Ashton, N. The pathogenesis of retrolental fibroplasia. *Ophthalmology,* **1979,** *86*:1695–1699.

Benatar, S.R., Hewlett, A.M., and Nunn, J.F. The use of iso-shunt lines for control of oxygen therapy. *Br. J. Anaesth.,* **1973,** *45*:711–718.

Betts, E.K., Downes, J.J., Schaffer, D.B., and Johns, R. Retrolental fibroplasia and oxygen administration during general anesthesia. *Anesthesiology,* **1977,** *47*:518–520.

Cheifetz, I.M. Inhaled nitric oxide: plenty of data, no consensus. *Crit. Care Med.,* **2000,** *28*:902–903.

Clark, J.M. Pulmonary limits of oxygen tolerance in man. *Exp. Lung Res.,* **1988,** *14*:897–910.

Coursin, D.B., Cihla, H.P., Will, J.A., and McCreary, J.L. Adaptation to chronic hyperoxia: Biochemical effects and the response to subsequent lethal hyperoxia. *Am. Rev. Respir. Dis.,* **1987,** *135*:1002–1006.

Crapo, J.D., Barry, B.E., Foscue, H.A., and Shelburne, J. Structural and biochemical changes in rat lungs occurring during exposures to lethal and adaptive doses of oxygen. *Am. Rev. Respir. Dis.,* **1980,** *122*:123–143.

Davis, W.B., Rennard, S.I., Bitterman, P.B., and Crystal, R.G. Pulmonary oxygen toxicity: Early reversible changes in human alveolar structures induced by hyperoxia. *New Engl. J. Med.,* **1983,** *309*:878–883.

Dellinger, R.P. Inhaled nitric oxide in acute lung injury and acute respiratory distress syndrome: Inability to translate physiologic benefit to clinical outcome benefit in adult clinical trials. *Intensive Care Med.,* **1999,** *25*:881–883.

Duane, S.F., Weir, E.K., Stewart, R.M., and Niewoehner, D.E. Distal airway responses to changes in oxygen and carbon dioxide tensions. *Respir. Physiol.,* **1979,** *38*:303–311.

Hendricks, P.L., Hall, D.A., Hunter, W.L., Jr., and Haley, P.J. Extension of pulmonary O_2 tolerance in man at 2 ATA by intermittent O_2 exposure. *J. Appl. Physiol.,* **1977,** *42*:593–599.

Hwang, S.J., Lee, K.H., Hwang, J.H., *et al.* Factors affecting the response to inhaled nitric oxide therapy in persistent pulmonary hypertension of the newborn infants. *Yonsei Med. J.,* **2004,** *45*:49–55.

Johnson, T.S., and Rock, P.B. Current concepts: Acute mountain sickness. *New Engl. J. Med.,* **1988,** *319*:841–845.

Kauczor, H., Surkau, R., and Roberts, T. MRI using hyperpolarized noble gases. *Eur. Radiol.,* **1998,** *8*:820–827.

Kinsella, J.P., Truog, W.E., Walsh, W.F., *et al.* Randomized, multicenter trail of inhaled nitric oxide and high-frequency oscillatory ventilation in severe, persistent pulmonary hypertension of the newborn. *J. Pediatr.,* **1997,** *131*:55–62.

Kravetz, G., Fisher, A.B., and Forman, H.J. The oxygen-adapted rat model: Tolerance to oxygen at 1.5 and 2 ATA. *Aviat. Space Environ. Med.,* **1980,** *51*:775–777.

Kushner, B.J., Essner, D., Cohen, I.J., and Flynn, J.T. Retrolental fibroplasias: II. Pathologic correlation. *Arch. Ophthalmol.,* **1977,** *95*:29–38.

McCord, J.M. Oxygen-derived free radicals in postischemic tissue injury. *New Engl. J. Med.,* **1985,** *312*:159–163.

Mortola, J.P. How newborn mammals cope with hypoxia. *Respir. Physiol.,* **1999,** *116*:95–103.

Mourani, P.M., Ivy, D.D., Gao, D., and Abman, S.H. Pulmonary vascular effects of inhaled nitric oxide and oxygen tension in bronchopul-

monary dysplasia. *Am. J. Respir. Crit. Care Med.,* **2004,** *107*:1006–1013.

Nadolny, E.M., and Svensson, L.G. Carbon dioxide field flooding techniques for open-heart surgery: monitoring and minimizing potential adverse effects. *Perfusion,* **2000,** *15*:151–153.

Plewes, J.L., and Farhi, L.E. Peripheral circulatory responses to acute hyperoxia. *Undersea Biomed. Res.,* **1983,** *10*:123–129.

Roberts, J.D., Jr., Fineman, J.R., Morin, F.C., 3rd, *et al.* Inhaled nitric oxide and persistent pulmonary hypertension of the newborn. The Inhaled Nitric Oxide Study Group. *New Engl. J. Med.,* **1997,** *336*:605–610.

Robiolio, M., Rumsey, W.L., and Wilson, D.F. Oxygen diffusion and mitochondrial respiration in neuroblastoma cells. *Am. J. Physiol.,* **1989,** *256*:C1207–C1213.

Sackner, M.A., Landa, J., Hirsch, J., and Zapata, A. Pulmonary effects of oxygen breathing: A 6-hour study in normal men. *Ann. Intern. Med.,* **1975,** *82*:40–43.

Singer, D. Neonatal tolerance to hypoxia: A comparative-physiological approach. *Comp. Biochem. Physiol. A. Mol. Integr. Physiol.,* **1999,** *123*:221–234.

Sokol, J., Jacobs, S.E., and Bohn, D. Inhaled nitric oxide for acute hypoxic respiratory failure in children and adults: A meta-analysis. *Anesth. Analg.,* **2003,** *97*:989–998.

Staszewska-Barczak, J., and Dusting, G.J. Importance of circulating angiotensin II for elevation of arterial pressure during acute hypercapnia in anaesthetized dogs. *Clin. Exp. Pharmacol. Physiol.,* **1981,** *8*:189–201.

Tanus-Santos, J.E., and Theodorakis, M.J. Is there a place for inhaled nitric oxide in the therapy of acute pulmonary embolism? *Am. J. Respir. Med.,* **2002,** *1*:167–176.

van den Bos, G.C., Drake, A.J., and Noble, M.I. The effect of carbon dioxide upon myocardial contractile performance, blood flow and oxygen consumption. *J. Physiol.,* **1979,** *287*:149–161.

Weaver, L.K., Hopkins, R.O., Chan, K.J., *et al.* Hyperbaric oxygen for acute carbon monoxide poisoning. *New Engl. J. Med.,* **2002,** *347*:1057–1067.

White, C.W., Jackson, J.H., Abuchowski, A., *et al.* Polyethylene glycol-attached antioxidant enzymes decrease pulmonary oxygen toxicity in rats. *J. Appl. Physiol.,* **1989,** *66*:584–590.

Zeidler, M.R., Kleerup, E.C., and Tashkin, D.P. Exhaled nitric oxide in the assessment of asthma. *Curr. Opin. Pulm. Med.,* **2004,** *10*:31–36.

MONOGRAPHS AND REVIEWS

Buras, J. Basic mechanisms of hyperbaric oxygen in the treatment of ischemia–reperfusion injury. *Int. Anesthesiol. Clin.,* **2000,** *38*:91–109.

Carraway, M.S., and Piantadosi, C.A. Oxygen toxicity. *Respir. Care Clin. North Am.,* **1999,** *5*:265–295.

Haddad, E., Millatt, L.J., and Johns, R.A. Clinical applications of inhaled NO. In, *Lung Physiology* (Kadowitz, P., ed.) Marcel Dekker, New York, **2000.**

Ignarro, L.J., and Napoli, C. Novel features of nitric oxide, endothelial nitric oxide synthase, and atherosclerosis. *Curr. Diab. Rep.,* **2005,** *5*:17–23.

Myers, R.A. Hyperbaric oxygen therapy for trauma: Crush injury, compartment syndrome, and other acute traumatic peripheral ischemias. *Int. Anesthesiol. Clin.,* **2000,** *38*:139–151.

Nathan, C. The moving frontier in nitric oxide-dependent signaling. *Sci. STKE,* **2004,** *257*:pp. 52.

Nattie, E. CO$_2$, brainstem chemoreceptors and breathing. *Prog. Neurobiol.,* **1999,** *59*:299–331.

Nunn, J.F. Carbon dioxide. In, *Nunn's Applied Respiratory Physiology*, 5th ed. (Lumb, A.B., ed.) Butterworth-Heineman, Oxford, England, **2000a,** pp. 222–248.

Nunn, J.F. Hypoxia. In, *Nunn's Applied Respiratory Physiology*, 5th ed. (Lumb, A.B., ed.) Butterworth-Heineman, Oxford, England, **2000b,** pp. 472–479.

Sackner, M.A. A history of oxygen usage in chronic obstructive pulmonary disease. *Am. Rev. Respir. Dis.,* **1974,** *110*:25–34.

Semenza, G.L. Angiogenesis in ischemia and neoplastic disorders. *Annu. Rev. Med.,* **2003,** *54*:17–28.

Shank, E.S., and Muth, C.M. Decompression illness, iatrogenic gas embolism, and carbon monoxide poisoning: The role of hyperbaric oxygen therapy. *Int. Anesthesiol. Clin.,* **2000,** *38*:111–138.

Steudel, W., Hurford, W.E., and Zapol, W.M. Inhaled nitric oxide: Basic biology and clinical applications. *Anesthesiology,* **1999,** *91*:1090–1121.

Travadi, J.N., and Patole, S.K. Phosphodiesterase inhibitors for persistent pulmonary hypertension of the newborn: A review. *Pediatr. Pulmonol.,* **2003,** *36*:529–535.

HYPNOTICS AND SEDATIVES

Dennis S. Charney, S. John Mihic, and R. Adron Harris

A great variety of agents have the capacity to depress the function of the central nervous system (CNS) such that calming or drowsiness (sedation) is produced. Older sedative-hypnotic drugs depress the CNS in a dose-dependent fashion, progressively producing sedation, sleep, unconsciousness, surgical anesthesia, coma, and ultimately, fatal depression of respiration and cardiovascular regulation. The CNS depressants discussed in this chapter include benzodiazepines, barbiturates, and sedative-hypnotic agents of diverse chemical structure (*e.g., paraldehyde* and *chloral hydrate*).

A *sedative* drug decreases activity, moderates excitement, and calms the recipient, whereas a *hypnotic* drug produces drowsiness and facilitates the onset and maintenance of a state of sleep that resembles natural sleep in its electroencephalographic characteristics and from which the recipient can be aroused easily. The latter effect sometimes is called *hypnosis,* but the sleep induced by hypnotic drugs does not resemble the artificially induced passive state of suggestibility also called *hypnosis.*

The nonbenzodiazepine sedative-hypnotic drugs belong to a group of agents that depress the CNS in a dose-dependent fashion, progressively producing calming or drowsiness (sedation), sleep (pharmacological hypnosis), unconsciousness, coma, surgical anesthesia, and fatal depression of respiration and cardiovascular regulation. They share these properties with a large number of chemicals, including general anesthetics (*see* Chapter 13) and aliphatic alcohols, most notably ethanol (*see* Chapter 22). Only two landmarks on the continuum of CNS depression produced by increasing concentrations of these agents can be defined with a reasonable degree of precision: surgical anesthesia, a state in which painful stimuli elicit no behavioral or autonomic response (*see* Chapter 13), and death,

resulting from sufficient depression of medullary neurons to disrupt coordination of cardiovascular function and respiration. The "end points" at lower concentrations of CNS depressants are defined with less precision—in terms of deficits in cognitive function (including attention to environmental stimuli) or motor skills (*e.g.,* ataxia) or of the intensity of sensory stimuli needed to elicit some reflex or behavioral response. Other important indices of decreased CNS activity, such as analgesia and seizure suppression, do not necessarily fall along this continuum; they may not be present at subanesthetic concentrations of a CNS-depressant drug (*e.g.,* a barbiturate), or they may be achieved with minimal sedation or other evidence of CNS depression (*e.g.,* with low doses of opioids, *phenytoin,* or *ethosuximide*).

Sedation is a side effect of many drugs that are not general CNS depressants (*e.g.,* antihistamines and neuroleptics). Although such agents can intensify the effects of CNS depressants, they usually produce more specific therapeutic effects at concentrations far lower than those causing substantial CNS depression. For example, they cannot induce surgical anesthesia in the absence of other agents. The benzodiazepine sedative-hypnotics resemble such agents; although coma may occur at very high doses, neither surgical anesthesia nor fatal intoxication is produced by benzodiazepines in the absence of other drugs with CNS-depressant actions; an important exception is *midazolam,* which has been associated with decreased tidal volume and respiratory rate. Moreover, specific antagonists of benzodiazepines exist. This constellation of properties sets the benzodiazepines apart from other sedative-hypnotic drugs and imparts a measure of safety that has resulted in benzodiazepines largely displacing older agents for the treatment of insomnia and anxiety.

History. Since antiquity, alcoholic beverages and potions containing *laudanum* and various herbals have been used to induce sleep. In the middle of the nineteenth century, *bromide* was the first agent to be introduced specifically as a sedative-hypnotic. Chloral hydrate, paraldehyde, *urethane,* and *sulfonal* came into use before the introduction of *barbital* in 1903 and *phenobarbital* in 1912. Their success spawned the synthesis and testing of more than 2500 barbiturates, of which approximately 50 were distributed commercially. The barbiturates were so dominant that less than a dozen other sedative-hypnotics were marketed successfully before 1960.

The partial separation of sedative-hypnotic-anesthetic from anticonvulsant properties embodied in phenobarbital led to searches for agents with more selective effects on CNS functions. As a result, relatively nonsedating anticonvulsants, notably phenytoin and *trimethadione*, were developed in the late 1930s and early 1940s (*see* Chapter 19). The advent of *chlorpromazine* and *meprobamate* in the early 1950s, with their taming effects in animals, and the development of increasingly sophisticated methods for evaluating the behavioral effects of drugs set the stage in the 1950s for the synthesis of *chlordiazepoxide* by Sternbach and the discovery of its unique pattern of actions by Randall. The introduction of chlordiazepoxide into clinical medicine in 1961 ushered in the era of benzodiazepines. Most of the benzodiazepines that have reached the marketplace were selected for high anxiolytic potency in relation to their depression of CNS function. However, all benzodiazepines possess sedative-hypnotic properties to varying degrees; these properties are exploited extensively clinically, especially to facilitate sleep. Mainly because of their remarkably low capacity to produce fatal CNS depression, the benzodiazepines have displaced the barbiturates as sedative-hypnotic agents.

BENZODIAZEPINES

All benzodiazepines in clinical use have the capacity to promote the binding of the major inhibitory neurotransmitter γ-aminobutyric acid (GABA) to the GABA$_A$ subtype of GABA receptors, which exist as multisubunit, ligand-gated chloride channels, thereby enhancing the GABA-induced ionic currents through these channels (*see* Chapter 12). Pharmacological investigations have provided evidence for heterogeneity among sites of binding and action of benzodiazepines, whereas biochemical and molecular biological investigations have revealed the numerous varieties of subunits that make up the GABA-gated chloride channels expressed in different neurons. Since receptor subunit composition appears to govern the interaction of various allosteric modulators with these channels, there has been a surge in efforts to find agents displaying different combinations of benzodiazepinelike properties that may reflect selective actions on one or more subtypes of GABA receptors.

These efforts led to the development of *zolpidem*, an imidazopyridine, and the pyrazolopyrimidines *zaleplon* and *indiplon* (under review by the Food and Drug Administration); these compounds all apparently exert sedative-hypnotic effects by interacting with a subset of benzodiazepine binding sites.

Although the benzodiazepines exert qualitatively similar clinical effects, important quantitative differences in their pharmacodynamic spectra and pharmacokinetic properties have led to varying patterns of therapeutic application. A number of distinct mechanisms of action are thought to contribute to the sedative-hypnotic, muscle-relaxant, anxiolytic, and anticonvulsant effects of the benzodiazepines, and specific subunits of the GABA$_A$ receptor are responsible for specific pharmacological properties of benzodiazepines. While only the benzodiazepines used primarily for hypnosis are discussed in detail, this chapter describes the general properties of the group and important differences among individual agents (*see* Chapters 17 and 19).

Chemistry. The structures of the benzodiazepines in use in the United States are shown in Table 16–1, as are those of a few related compounds discussed below. The term *benzodiazepine* refers to the portion of the structure composed of a benzene ring (A) fused to a seven-membered diazepine ring (B). Since all the important benzodiazepines contain a 5-aryl substituent (ring C) and a 1,4-diazepine ring, the term has come to mean the 5-aryl-1,4-benzodiazepines. Various modifications in the structure of the ring systems have yielded compounds with similar activities, including 1,5-benzodiazepines (*e.g.*, *clobazam*) and compounds in which the fused benzene ring is replaced with heteroaromatic systems such as thieno (*e.g.*, *brotizolam*). The chemical nature of substituents at positions 1 to 3 can vary widely and can include triazolo or imidazolo rings fused at positions 1 and 2. Replacement of ring C with a keto function at position 5 and a methyl substituent at position 4 is an important structural feature of the benzodiazepine antagonist *flumazenil* (ROMAZICON).

In addition to various benzodiazepine or imidazobenzodiazepine derivatives, a large number of nonbenzodiazepine compounds compete with classic benzodiazepines or flumazenil for binding at specific sites in the CNS. These include representatives from the β-carbolines (containing an indole nucleus fused to a pyridine ring), imidazopyridines (*e.g.*, *zolpidem*; *see* below), imidazopyrimidines, imidazoquinolones, and cyclopyrrolones (*e.g.*, *zopiclone*).

Pharmacological Properties

Virtually all effects of the benzodiazepines result from their actions on the CNS. The most prominent of these effects are sedation, hypnosis, decreased anxiety, muscle relaxation, anterograde amnesia, and anticonvulsant activity. Only two effects of these drugs result from peripheral actions: coronary vasodilation, seen after

Table 16–1
Benzodiazepines: Names and Structures*

BENZODIAZEPINE	R_1	R_2	R_3	R_7	R_2'
Alprazolam	[Fused triazolo ring][b]		—H	—Cl	—H
Brotizolam†	[Fused triazolo ring][b]		—H	[Thieno ring A][c]	—Cl
Chlordiazepoxide[a]	(—)	—NHCH$_3$	—H	—Cl	—H
Clobazam[a],†	—CH$_3$	=O	—H	—Cl	—H
Clonazepam	—H	=O	—H	—NO$_2$	—Cl
Clorazepate	—H	=O	—COO$^-$	—Cl	—H
Demoxepam[a],†,‡	—H	=O	—H	—Cl	—H
Diazepam	—CH$_3$	=O	—H	—Cl	—H
Estazolam	[Fused triazolo ring][d]		—H	—Cl	—H
Flumazenil[a]	[Fused imidazo ring][e]		—H	—F	[=O at C$_5$][g]
Flurazepam	—CH$_2$CH$_2$N(C$_2$H$_5$)$_2$	=O	—H	—Cl	—F
Lorazepam	—H	=O	—OH	—Cl	—Cl
Midazolam	[Fused imadazo ring][f]		—H	—Cl	—F
Nitrazepam†	—H	=O	—H	—NO$_2$	—H
Nordazepam†,§	—H	=O	—H	—Cl	—H
Oxazepam	—H	=O	—OH	—Cl	—H
Prazepam†	$-CH_2-CH\overset{CH_2}{\underset{CH_2}{<}}$	=O	—H	—Cl	—H
Quazepam	—CH$_2$CF$_3$	=O	—H	—Cl	—F
Temazepam	—CH$_3$	=O	—OH	—Cl	—H
Triazolam	[Fused triazolo ring][b]		—H	—Cl	—Cl

*Alphabetical footnotes refer to alterations of the general formula; symbolic footnotes are used for other comments. †Not available for clinical use in the United States. ‡Major metabolite of chlordiazepoxide. §Major metabolite of diazepam and others; also referred to as nordiazepam and desmethyldiazepam. [a]No substituent at position 4, except for chlordiazepoxide and demoxepam, which are N-oxides; R_4 is —CH$_3$ in flumazenil, in which there is no double bond between positions 4 and 5; R_4 is =O in clobazam, in which position 4 is C and position 5 is N.

[g]No ring C.

intravenous administration of therapeutic doses of certain benzodiazepines, and neuromuscular blockade, seen only with very high doses.

A number of benzodiazepinelike effects have been observed *in vivo* and *in vitro* and have been classified as *full agonistic effects* (*i.e.,* faithfully mimicking agents such as *diazepam* with relatively low fractional occupancy of binding sites) or *partial agonistic effects* (*i.e.,* producing less intense maximal effects and/or requiring relatively high fractional occupancy compared with agents such as diazepam). Some compounds produce effects opposite to those of diazepam in the absence of benzodiazepinelike agonists and have been termed *inverse agonists; partial inverse agonists* also have been recognized. The vast majority of effects of agonists and inverse agonists can be reversed or prevented by the benzodiazepine antagonist *flumazenil*, which competes with agonists and inverse agonists for binding to the GABA$_A$ receptor. In addition, compounds from other chemical classes can act to block only the effects of agonists or inverse agonists.

Central Nervous System. While benzodiazepines affect activity at all levels of the neuraxis, some structures are affected preferentially. The benzodiazepines do not produce the same degrees of neuronal depression as do barbiturates and volatile anesthetics. All the benzodiazepines have similar pharmacological profiles. Nevertheless, the drugs differ in selectivity, and the clinical usefulness of individual benzodiazepines thus varies considerably.

As the dose of a benzodiazepine is increased, sedation progresses to hypnosis and then to stupor. The clinical literature often refers to the "anesthetic" effects and uses of certain benzodiazepines, but the drugs do not cause a true general anesthesia because awareness usually persists, and relaxation sufficient to allow surgery cannot be achieved. However, at "preanesthetic" doses, there is amnesia for events subsequent to administration of the drug; this may create the illusion of previous anesthesia.

Although considerable attempts have been made to separate the anxiolytic actions of benzodiazepines from their sedative-hypnotic effects, distinguishing between these behaviors still is problematic. Measurements of anxiety and sedation are difficult in human beings, and the validity of animal models for anxiety and sedation is uncertain. The existence of multiple benzodiazepine receptors may explain in part the diversity of pharmacological responses in different species.

Animal Models of Anxiety. In animal models of anxiety, most attention has focused on the ability of benzodiazepines to increase locomotor, feeding, or drinking behavior that has been suppressed by novel or aversive stimuli. In one paradigm, animal behaviors that previously had been rewarded by food or water are punished periodically by an electric shock. The time during which shocks are delivered is signaled by some auditory or visual cue, and untreated animals stop performing almost completely when the cue is perceived. The difference in behavioral responses during the punished and unpunished periods is eliminated by benzodiazepine agonists, usually at doses that do not reduce the rate of unpunished responses or produce other signs of impaired motor function. Similarly, rats placed in an unfamiliar environment exhibit markedly reduced exploratory behavior (neophobia), whereas animals treated with benzodiazepines do not. Opioid analgesics and neuroleptic (antipsychotic) drugs do not increase suppressed behaviors, and phenobarbital and meprobamate usually do so only at doses that also reduce spontaneous or unpunished behaviors or produce ataxia.

The difference between the dose required to impair motor function and that necessary to increase punished behavior varies widely among the benzodiazepines and depends on the species and experimental protocol. Although such differences may have encouraged the marketing of some benzodiazepines as selective sedative-hypnotic agents, they have not predicted with any accuracy the magnitude of sedative effects among those benzodiazepines marketed as anxiolytic agents.

Tolerance to Benzodiazepines. Studies on tolerance in laboratory animals often are cited to support the belief that disinhibitory effects of benzodiazepines are distinct from their sedative-ataxic effects. For example, tolerance to the depressant effects on rewarded or neutral behavior occurs after several days of treatment with benzodiazepines; the disinhibitory effects of the drugs on punished behavior are augmented initially and decline after 3 to 4 weeks (*see* File, 1985). Although most patients who ingest benzodiazepines chronically report that drowsiness wanes over a few days, tolerance to the impairment of some measures of psychomotor performance (*e.g.,* visual tracking) usually is not observed. The development of tolerance to the anxiolytic effects of benzodiazepines is a subject of debate (Lader and File, 1987). However, many patients can maintain themselves on a fairly constant dose; increases or decreases in dosage appear to correspond with changes in problems or stresses. Nevertheless, some patients either do not reduce their dosage when stress is relieved or steadily escalate dosage. Such behavior may be associated with the development of drug dependence (*see* Chapter 23).

Some benzodiazepines induce muscle hypotonia without interfering with normal locomotion and can decrease rigidity in patients with cerebral palsy. In contrast to effects in animals, there is only a limited degree of selectivity in human beings. *Clonazepam* in nonsedative doses does cause muscle relaxation, but diazepam and most other benzodiazepines do not. Tolerance occurs to the muscle relaxant and ataxic effects of these drugs.

Experimentally, benzodiazepines inhibit seizure activity induced by either *pentylenetetrazol* or *picrotoxin,* but *strychnine-* and maximal electroshock-induced seizures are suppressed only at doses that also severely impair locomotor activity. Clonazepam, *nitrazepam,* and *nordazepam* have more selective anticonvulsant activity than most other benzodiazepines. Benzodiazepines also suppress photic seizures in baboons and ethanol-withdrawal seizures in human beings. However, the development of tolerance to the anticonvulsant effects has limited the usefulness of benzodiazepines in the treatment of recurrent seizure disorders in human beings (*see* Chapter 19).

Although analgesic effects of benzodiazepines have been observed in experimental animals, only transient analgesia is apparent in humans after intravenous administration. Such effects actually may involve the production of amnesia. However, unlike the barbiturates, the benzodiazepines do not cause hyperalgesia.

Effects on the Electroencephalogram (EEG) and Sleep Stages. The effects of benzodiazepines on the waking EEG resemble those of other sedative-hypnotic drugs. Alpha activity is decreased, but there is an increase in low-voltage fast activity. Tolerance occurs to these effects.

Most benzodiazepines decrease sleep latency, especially when first used, and diminish the number of awakenings and the time spent in stage 0 (a stage of wakefulness). Time in stage 1 (descending drowsiness) usually is decreased, and there is a prominent decrease in the time spent in slow-wave sleep (stages 3 and 4). Most benzodiazepines increase the time from onset of spindle sleep to the first burst of rapid-eye-movement (REM) sleep, and the time spent in REM sleep usually is shortened. However, the number of cycles of REM sleep usually is increased, mostly late in the sleep time. *Zolpidem* and *zaleplon* suppress REM sleep to a lesser extent than do benzodiazepines and thus may be superior to benzodiazepines for use as hypnotics (Dujardin *et al.*, 1998).

Despite the shortening of stage 4 and REM sleep, benzodiazepine administration typically increases total sleep time largely because of increased time spent in stage 2 (which is the major fraction of non-REM sleep). The effect is greatest in subjects with the shortest baseline total sleep time. In addition, despite the increased number of REM cycles, the number of shifts to lighter sleep stages (1 and 0) and the amount of body movement are diminished. Nocturnal peaks in the secretion of growth hormone, prolactin, and luteinizing hormone are not affected. During chronic nocturnal use of benzodiazepines, the effects on the various stages of sleep usually decline within a few nights. When such use is discontinued, the pattern of drug-induced changes in sleep parameters may "rebound," and an increase in the amount and density of REM sleep may be especially prominent. If the dosage has not been excessive, patients usually will note only a shortening of sleep time rather than an exacerbation of insomnia.

Although some differences in the patterns of effects exerted by the various benzodiazepines have been noted, their use usually imparts a sense of deep or refreshing sleep. It is uncertain to which effect on sleep parameters this feeling can be attributed. As a result, variations in the pharmacokinetic properties of individual benzodiazepines appear to be much more important determinants of their effects on sleep than are any potential differences in their pharmacodynamic properties.

Molecular Targets for Benzodiazepine Actions in the CNS.

Benzodiazepines are believed to exert most of their effects by interacting with inhibitory neurotransmitter receptors directly activated by GABA. GABA receptors are membrane-bound proteins that can be divided into two major subtypes: $GABA_A$ and $GABA_B$ receptors. The ionotropic $GABA_A$ receptors are composed of five subunits that coassemble to form an integral chloride channel. $GABA_A$ receptors are responsible for most inhibitory neurotransmission in the CNS. In

contrast, the metabotropic $GABA_B$ receptors are G protein–coupled receptors. Benzodiazepines act at $GABA_A$ but not $GABA_B$ receptors by binding directly to a specific site that is distinct from that of GABA binding. Unlike barbiturates, benzodiazepines do not activate $GABA_A$ receptors directly but rather require GABA to express their effects; *i.e.,* they only modulate the effects of GABA. Benzodiazepines and GABA analogs bind to their respective sites on brain membranes with nanomolar affinity. Benzodiazepines modulate GABA binding, and GABA alters benzodiazepine binding in an allosteric fashion.

Benzodiazepines and related compounds can act as agonists, antagonists, or inverse agonists at the benzodiazepine-binding site on $GABA_A$ receptors. Agonists at the binding site increase and inverse agonists decrease the amount of chloride current generated by $GABA_A$-receptor activation. Agonists at the benzodiazepine binding site shift the GABA concentration–response curve to the left, whereas inverse agonists shift the curve to the right. Both these effects are blocked by antagonists at the benzodiazepine binding site. In the absence of an agonist or inverse agonist for the benzodiazepine binding site, an antagonist for this binding site does not affect $GABA_A$-receptor function. One such antagonist, flumazenil, is used clinically to reverse the effects of high doses of benzodiazepines. The behavioral and electrophysiological effects of benzodiazepines also can be reduced or prevented by prior treatment with antagonists at the GABA-binding site (*e.g., bicuculline*).

The strongest evidence that benzodiazepines act directly on $GABA_A$ receptors comes from recombinant expression of cDNAs encoding subunits of the receptor complex, which resulted in high-affinity benzodiazepine binding sites and GABA-activated chloride conductances that were enhanced by benzodiazepine receptor agonists (Burt, 2003). The properties of the expressed receptors generally resemble those of $GABA_A$ receptors found in most CNS neurons. Each $GABA_A$ receptor is believed to consist of a pentamer of homologous subunits. Thus far 16 different subunits have been identified and classified into seven subunit families: six α, three β, three γ, and single δ, ε, π, and θ subunits. Additional complexity arises from RNA splice variants of some of these subunits (*e.g., $\gamma 2$* and $\alpha 6$). The exact subunit structures of native $GABA_A$ receptors still are unknown, but it is thought that most GABA receptors are composed of α, β, and γ subunits that coassemble with some uncertain stoichiometry. The multiplicity of subunits generates heterogeneity in $GABA_A$ receptors and is responsible, at least in part, for the pharmacological diversity in benzodiazepine effects in behavioral, biochemical, and functional studies. Studies of cloned $GABA_A$ receptors have shown that the coassembly of a γ subunit with α and β subunits confers benzodiazepine sensitivity to $GABA_A$ receptors (Burt, 2003). Receptors composed solely of α and β subunits produce functional $GABA_A$ receptors that also respond to barbiturates, but they neither bind nor are affected by benzodiazepines. Benzodiazepines are believed to bind at the interface between α and γ subunits, and both subunits determine the pharmacology of the benzodiazepine binding site (Burt, 2003). For example, receptors containing the $\alpha 1$ subunit are pharmacologically distinct from receptors containing $\alpha 2$, $\alpha 3$, or $\alpha 5$ subunits (Pritchett and Seeburg, 1990), reminiscent of the pharmacological heterogeneity detected with radioligand-binding studies using brain membranes. Receptors containing the $\alpha 6$ subunit do not display high-affinity binding of diazepam and appear to be selective for the benzodiazepine receptor inverse agonist RO 15-4513, which has been tested as an alcohol antagonist (Lüddens *et al.*, 1990). The subtype of γ subunit also modulates benzodiazepine pharmacology, with lower-affinity binding observed in receptors containing the $\gamma 1$ subunit. Although theoretically approximately a million different GABA$_A$ receptors could be assembled from all these different subunits, constraints for the assembly of these receptors apparently limit their numbers (Sieghart *et al.*, 1999).

An understanding of which GABA$_A$ receptor subunits are responsible for particular effects of benzodiazepines *in vivo* is emerging. The mutation to arginine of a histidine residue at position 101 of the GABA$_A$ receptor $\alpha 1$ subunit renders receptors containing that subunit insensitive to the GABA-enhancing effects of diazepam (Kleingoor *et al.*, 1993). Mice bearing these mutated subunits fail to exhibit the sedative, the amnestic, and, in part, the anticonvulsant effects of diazepam while retaining sensitivity to the anxiolytic, muscle-relaxant, and ethanol-enhancing effects. Conversely, mice bearing the equivalent mutation in the $\alpha 2$ subunit of the GABA$_A$ receptor are insensitive to the anxiolytic effects of diazepam (Burt, 2003). The attribution of specific behavioral effects of benzodiazepines to individual receptor subunits will aid in the development of new compounds exhibiting fewer undesired side effects. For example, the experimental compound L838,417 enhances the effects of GABA on receptors composed of $\alpha 2$, $\alpha 3$, or $\alpha 5$ subunits but lacks efficacy on receptors containing the $\alpha 1$ subunit; it is thus anxiolytic but not sedating (Burt, 2003).

GABA$_A$ receptor subunits also may play roles in the targeting of assembled receptors to their proper locations in synapses. In knockout mice lacking the $\gamma 2$ subunit, GABA$_A$ receptors did not localize to synapses, although they were formed and translocated to the cell surface (Essrich *et al.*, 1998). The synaptic clustering molecule gephyrin also plays a role in receptor localization.

GABA$_A$ Receptor-Mediated Electrical Events: In Vivo Properties. The remarkable safety of the benzodiazepines is likely related to the fact that their effects *in vivo* depend on the presynaptic release of GABA; in the absence of GABA, benzodiazepines have no effects on GABA$_A$ receptor function. Although barbiturates also enhance the effects of GABA at low concentrations, they directly activate GABA receptors at higher concentrations, which can lead to profound CNS depression (*see* below). Further, the behavioral and sedative effects of benzodiazepines can be ascribed in part to potentiation of GABA-ergic pathways that serve to regulate the firing of neurons containing various monoamines (*see* Chapter 12). These neurons are known to promote behavioral arousal and are important mediators of the inhibitory effects of fear and punishment on behavior. Finally, inhibitory effects on muscular hypertonia or the spread of seizure activity can be rationalized by potentiation of inhibitory GABA-ergic circuits at various levels of the neuraxis. In most studies conducted *in vivo* or *in situ,* the local or systemic administration of benzodiazepines reduces spontaneous or evoked electrical activity of major (large) neurons in all regions of the brain and spinal cord. The activity of these neurons is regulated in part by small inhibitory interneurons (predominantly GABA-ergic) arranged in feedback and feedforward types of circuits. The magnitude of the effects produced by benzodiazepines varies widely depending on such factors as the types of inhibitory circuits that are operating, the sources and intensity of excitatory input, and the manner in which experimental manipulations are performed and assessed. For example, feedback circuits often involve powerful inhibitory synapses on the neuronal soma near the axon hillock, which are supplied predominantly by recurrent pathways. The synaptic or exogenous application of GABA to this region increases chloride conductance and can prevent neuronal discharge by shunting electric currents that otherwise would depolarize the membrane of the initial segment. Accordingly, benzodiazepines markedly prolong the period after brief activation of recurrent GABA-ergic pathways during which neither spontaneous nor applied excitatory stimuli can evoke neuronal discharge; this effect is reversed by the GABA$_A$-receptor antagonist *bicuculline.*

Molecular Basis for Benzodiazepine Regulation of GABA$_A$ Receptor-Mediated Electrical Events. Electrophysiological studies *in vitro* have shown that the enhancement of GABA-induced chloride currents by benzodiazepines results primarily from an increase in the frequency of bursts of chloride channel opening produced by submaximal amounts of GABA (Twyman *et al.*, 1989). Inhibitory synaptic transmission measured after stimulation of afferent fibers is potentiated by benzodiazepines at therapeutically relevant concentrations. Prolongation of spontaneous miniature inhibitory postsynaptic currents (IPSCs) by benzodiazepines also has been observed. Although sedative barbiturates also enhance such chloride currents, they do so by prolonging the duration of individual channel-opening events. Macroscopic measurements of GABA$_A$ receptor-mediated currents indicate that benzodiazepines shift the GABA concentration–response curve to the left without increasing the maximum current evoked with GABA. These findings collectively are consistent with a model in which benzodiazepines exert their major actions by increasing the gain of inhibitory neurotransmission mediated by GABA$_A$ receptors. As noted earlier, certain experimental benzodiazepines and other structurally related compounds act as inverse agonists to reduce GABA-induced chloride currents, promote convulsions, and produce other *in vivo* effects opposite to those induced by the benzodiazepines in clinical use (*see* Gardner *et al.*, 1993). A few compounds, most notably flumazenil, can block the effects of clinically used benzodiazepines and inverse agonists *in vitro* and *in vivo*, but they have no detectable actions by themselves. Although benzodiazepines appear to act mainly at GABA$_A$ receptors, some observations are difficult to reconcile with the hypothesis that all benzodiazepines effects are mediated *via* GABA$_A$ receptors. Low concentrations of benzodiazepines that are not blocked by bicuculline or picrotoxin induce depressant effects on hippocampal neurons (Polc, 1988). The induction of sleep in rats by benzodiazepines also is insensitive to bicuculline or picrotoxin but is prevented by flumazenil (*see* Mendelson, 1992). At higher concentrations, corresponding to those producing hypnosis and amnesia during preanesthetic medication (*see* Chapter 13) or those achieved during the treatment of status epilepticus (*see* Chapter 19), the actions of the benzodiazepines may involve a number of other mechanisms. These include inhibition of the uptake of adenosine and the resulting potentiation of the actions of this endogenous neuronal depressant (*see* Phillis and O'Regan, 1988), as well as the GABA-independent inhibition of Ca^{2+} currents, Ca^{2+}-dependent release of neurotransmitter, and *tetrodotoxin*-sensitive Na^+ channels (*see* Macdonald and McLean, 1986).

The macromolecular complex containing GABA-regulated chloride channels also may be a site of action of general anesthetics, ethanol, inhaled drugs of abuse, and certain metabolites of endogenous steroids (Whiting, 2003). Among the latter, *allopregnanolone* (3α-hydroxy, 5α-dihydroprogesterone) is of particular interest. This compound, a metabolite of progesterone that can be formed in the brain from precursors in the circulation, as well as from those synthesized by glial cells, produces barbituratelike effects, including promotion of GABA-induced chloride currents and enhanced binding of benzodiazepines and GABA-receptor agonists. As with the barbiturates, higher concentrations of the steroid activate chloride currents in the absence of GABA, and its effects do not require the presence of a γ subunit in GABA$_A$ receptors expressed in transfected cells. Unlike the barbiturates, however, the steroid cannot reduce excitatory responses to glutamate (*see* below). These effects are produced very rapidly and apparently are mediated by interactions at sites on the cell surface. A congener of allopregnanolone (*alfaxalone*) was used previously outside the United States for the induction of anesthesia.

Respiration. Hypnotic doses of benzodiazepines are without effect on respiration in normal subjects, but special care must be taken in the treatment of children (Kriel *et al.*, 2000) and individuals with impaired hepatic function, such as alcoholics (Guglielminotti *et al.*, 1999). At higher doses, such as those used for preanesthetic medication or for endoscopy, benzodiazepines slightly depress alveolar ventilation and cause respiratory acidosis as the result of a decrease in hypoxic rather than hypercapnic drive; these effects are exaggerated in patients with chronic obstructive pulmonary disease (COPD), and alveolar hypoxia and/or CO_2 narcosis may result. These drugs can cause apnea during anesthesia or when given with opioids. Patients severely intoxicated with benzodiazepines only require respiratory assistance when they also have ingested another CNS-depressant drug, most commonly ethanol.

In contrast, hypnotic doses of benzodiazepines may worsen sleep-related breathing disorders by adversely affecting control of the upper airway muscles or by decreasing the ventilatory response to CO_2 (*see* Guilleminault, in Symposium, 1990). The latter effect may cause hypoventilation and hypoxemia in some patients with severe COPD, although benzodiazepines may improve sleep and sleep structure in some instances. In patients with obstructive sleep apnea (OSA), hypnotic doses of benzodiazepines may decrease muscle tone in the upper airway and exaggerate the impact of apneic episodes on alveolar hypoxia, pulmonary hypertension, and cardiac ventricular load. Many clinicians consider the presence of OSA to be a contraindication to the use of alcohol or any sedative-hypnotic agent, including a benzodiazepine; caution also should be exercised with patients who snore regularly, because partial airway obstruction may be converted to OSA under the influence of these drugs. In addition, benzodiazepines may promote the appearance of episodes of apnea during REM sleep (associated with decreases in oxygen saturation) in patients recovering from a myocardial infarction (Guilleminault, in Symposium, 1990); however, no impact of these drugs on survival of patients with cardiac disease has been reported.

Cardiovascular System. The cardiovascular effects of benzodiazepines are minor in normal subjects except in severe intoxication; the adverse effects in patients with obstructive sleep disorders or cardiac disease were noted above. In preanesthetic doses, all benzodiazepines decrease blood pressure and increase heart rate. With midazolam, the effects appear to be secondary to a decrease in peripheral resistance, but with diazepam, they are secondary to a decrease in left ventricular work and cardiac output. Diazepam increases coronary flow, possibly by an action to increase interstitial concentrations of adenosine, and the accumulation of this cardiodepressant metabolite also may explain the negative inotropic effects of the drug. In large doses, midazolam decreases cerebral blood flow and oxygen assimilation considerably (Nugent *et al.*, 1982).

Gastrointestinal Tract. Benzodiazepines are thought by some gastroenterologists to improve a variety of "anxiety related" gastrointestinal disorders. There is a paucity of evidence for direct actions. Benzodiazepines partially protect against stress ulcers in rats, and diazepam markedly decreases nocturnal gastric secretion in human beings. Other agents are considerably more effective in acid-peptic disorders (*see* Chapter 36).

Absorption, Fate, and Excretion. The physicochemical and pharmacokinetic properties of the benzodiazepines greatly affect their clinical utility. They all have high lipid–water distribution coefficients in the nonionized form; nevertheless, lipophilicity varies more than fiftyfold according to the polarity and electronegativity of various substituents.

All the benzodiazepines are absorbed completely, with the exception of *clorazepate;* this drug is decarboxylated rapidly in gastric juice to *N*-desmethyldiazepam (nordazepam), which subsequently is absorbed completely. Some benzodiazepines (*e.g.*, *prazepam* and *flurazepam*) reach the systemic circulation only in the form of active metabolites.

Drugs active at the benzodiazepine receptor may be divided into four categories based on their elimination half-lives: (1) ultra-short-acting benzodiazepines, (2) short-acting agents, with half-lives less than 6 hours, including *triazolam,* the nonbenzodiazepine *zolpidem* (half-life approximately 2 hours), and zopiclone (half-life 5 to 6 hours), (3) intermediate-acting agents, with half-lives of 6 to 24 hours, including *estazolam* and *temazepam,* and (4) long-acting agents, with half-lives of greater than 24 hours, including flurazepam, diazepam, and *quazepam.*

The benzodiazepines and their active metabolites bind to plasma proteins. The extent of binding correlates strongly with lipid solubility and ranges from about 70% for *alprazolam* to nearly 99% for diazepam. The concentration in the cerebrospinal fluid is approximately equal to the concentration of free drug in plasma. While competition with other protein-bound drugs may occur, no clinically significant examples have been reported.

The plasma concentrations of most benzodiazepines exhibit patterns that are consistent with two-compartment models (*see* Chapter 1), but three-compartment models appear to be more appropriate for the compounds with the highest lipid solubility. Accordingly, there is rapid uptake of benzodiazepines into the brain and other highly perfused organs after intravenous administration (or oral administration of a rapidly absorbed compound); rapid uptake is followed by a phase of redistribution into tissues that are less well perfused, especially muscle and fat. Redistribution is most rapid for drugs with the highest lipid solubility. In the regimens used for nighttime sedation, the rate of redistribution sometimes can have a greater influence than the rate of biotransformation on the duration of CNS effects (Dettli, in Symposium, 1986a). The kinetics of redistribution of diazepam and other lipophilic benzodiazepines are complicated by enterohepatic circulation. The volumes of distribution of the benzodiazepines are large and in many cases are increased in elderly patients. These drugs cross the placental barrier and are secreted into breast milk.

The benzodiazepines are metabolized extensively by cytochrome P450 enzymes, particularly CYP3A4 and CYP2C19. Some benzodiazepines, such as *oxazepam,* are conjugated directly and are not metabolized by these enzymes (*see* Tanaka, 1999). *Erythromycin, clarithromycin, ritonavir, itraconazole, ketoconazole, nefazodone,* and grapefruit juice are inhibitors of CYP3A4 and can affect the metabolism of benzodiazepines (Dresser *et al.,* 2000). Because active metabolites of some benzodiazepines are biotransformed more slowly than are the parent compounds, the duration of action of many benzodiazepines bears little relationship to the half-life of elimination of the drug that has been administered. For example, the half-life of flurazepam in plasma is 2 to 3 hours, but that of a major active metabolite (*N*-desalkylflurazepam) is 50 hours or more. Conversely, the rate of biotransformation of agents that are inactivated by the initial reaction is an important determinant of their duration of action; these agents include oxazepam, *lorazepam,* temazepam, triazolam, and midazolam. Metabolism of the benzodiazepines occurs in three major stages. These and the relationships between the drugs and their metabolites are shown in Table 16–2.

For benzodiazepines that bear a substituent at position 1 (or 2) of the diazepine ring, the initial and most rapid phase of metabolism involves modification and/or removal of the substituent. With the exception of triazolam, alprazolam, estazolam, and midazolam, which contain either a fused triazolo or imidazolo ring, the eventual products are *N*-desalkylated compounds that are biologically active. One such compound, nordazepam, is a major metabolite common to the biotransformation of diazepam, clorazepate, and prazepam; it also is formed from demoxepam, an important metabolite of chlordiazepoxide.

The second phase of metabolism involves hydroxylation at position 3 and also usually yields an active derivative (*e.g.,* oxazepam from nordazepam). The rates of these reactions are usually very much slower than the first stage (half-lives > 40 to 50 hours) such that appreciable accumulation of hydroxylated products with intact substituents at position 1 does not occur. There are two significant exceptions to this rule: (1) Small amounts of temazepine accumulate during the chronic administration of diazepam (not shown in Table 16–2), and (2) following the replacement of sulfur with oxygen in quazepam, most of the resulting 2-oxoquazepam is hydroxylated slowly at position 3 without removal of the *N*-alkyl group. However, only small amounts of the 3-hydroxyl derivative accumulate during the chronic administration of quazepam because this compound is conjugated at an unusually rapid rate. In contrast, the *N*-desalkylflurazepam that is formed by the "minor" metabolic pathway does accumulate during quazepam administration, and it contributes significantly to the overall clinical effect.

The third major phase of metabolism is the conjugation of the 3-hydroxyl compounds, principally with glucuronic acid; the half-lives of these reactions usually are between 6 and 12 hours, and the products invariably are inactive. Conjugation is the only major route of metabolism for oxazepam and lorazepam and is the preferred pathway for temazepam because of the slower conversion of this compound to oxazepam. Triazolam and alprazolam are metabolized principally by initial hydroxylation of the methyl group on the fused triazolo ring; the absence of a chlorine residue in ring C of alprazolam slows this reaction significantly. The products, sometimes referred to as α-*hydroxylated compounds,* are quite active but are metabolized very rapidly, primarily by conjugation with glucuronic acid, such that there is no appreciable accumulation of active metabolites. The fused triazolo ring in estazolam lacks a methyl group and is hydroxylated to only a limited extent; the major route of metabolism involves the formation of the 3-hydroxyl derivative. The corresponding hydroxyl derivatives of triazolam and alprazolam also are formed to a significant extent. Compared with compounds without the triazolo ring, the rate of this reaction for all three drugs is unusually swift, and the 3-hydroxyl compounds are rapidly conjugated or oxidized further to benzophenone derivatives before excretion.

Midazolam is metabolized rapidly, primarily by hydroxylation of the methyl group on the fused imidazo ring; only small amounts

Table 16–2

Major Metabolic Relationships among Some of the Benzodiazepines

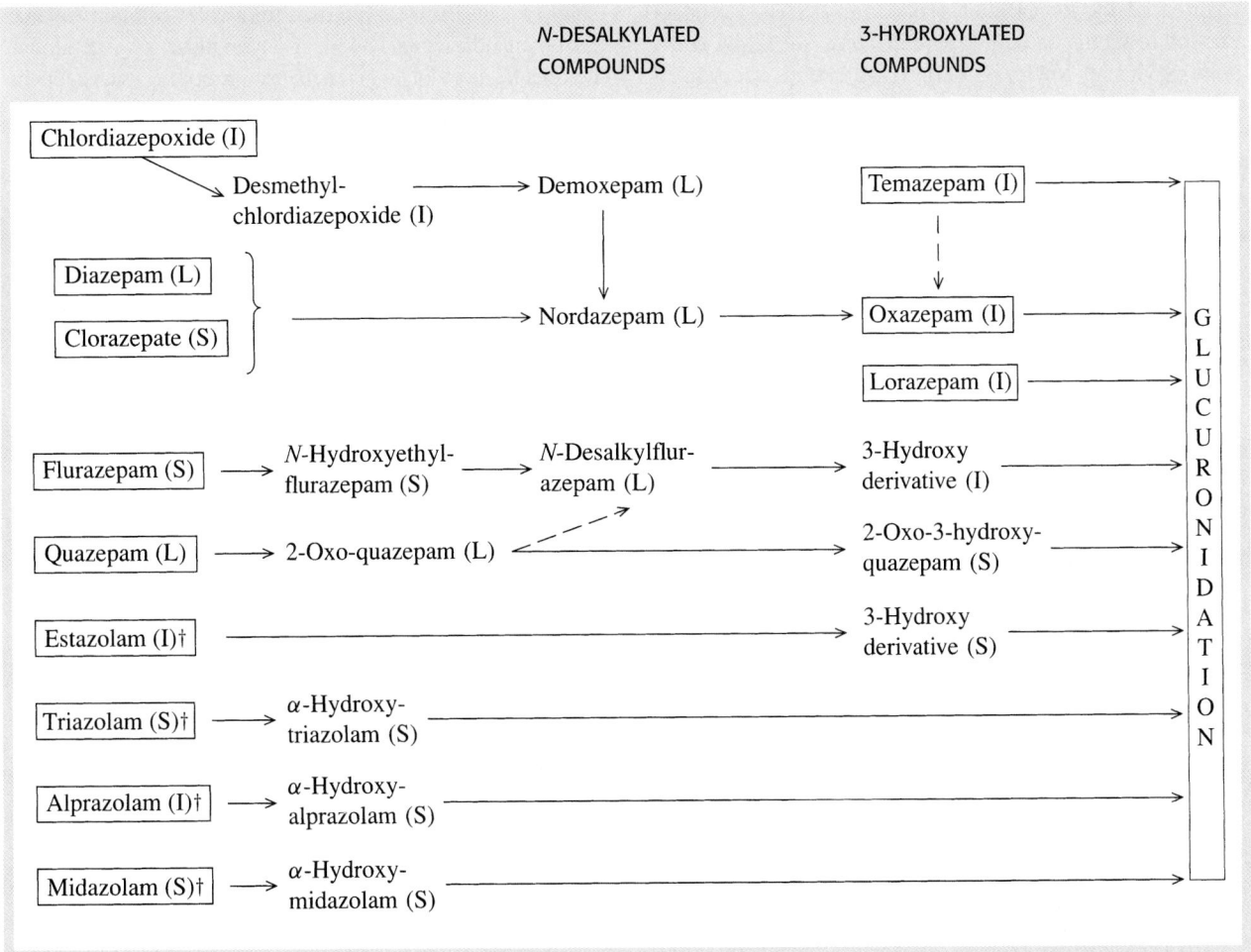

*Compounds enclosed in boxes are marketed in the United States. The approximate half-lives of the various compounds are denoted in parentheses; S (short-acting), $t_{\frac{1}{2}} < 6$ hours; I (intermediate-acting), $t_{\frac{1}{2}} = 6$ to 24 hours; L (long-acting), $t_{\frac{1}{2}} = >24$ hours. All compounds except clorazepate are biological-ly active; the activity of 3-hydroxydesalkylflurazepam has not been determined. Clonazepam (not shown) is an *N*-desalkyl compound, and it is metabo-lized primarily by reduction of the 7-NO$_2$ group to the corresponding amine (inactive), followed by acetylation; its half-life is 20 to 40 hours. †*See* text for discussion of other pathways of metabolism.

of 3-hydroxyl compounds are formed. The α-hydroxylated com-pound, which has appreciable biological activity, is eliminated with a half-life of 1 hour after conjugation with glucuronic acid. Variable and sometimes substantial accumulation of this metabolite has been noted during intravenous infusion (Oldenhof *et al.*, 1988).

The aromatic rings (A and C) of the benzodiazepines are hydroxylated only to a small extent. The only important metabolism at these sites is reduction of the 7-nitro substituents of clonazepam, nitrazepam, and *flunitrazepam*; the half-lives of these reactions are usually 20 to 40 hours. The resulting amines are inactive and are acetylated to varying degrees before excretion.

Because the benzodiazepines apparently do not significantly induce the synthesis of hepatic cytochrome P450 enzymes, their chronic administration usually does not result in the accelerated metabolism of other substances or of the benzodiazepines. *Cimeti-dine* and oral contraceptives inhibit *N*-dealkylation and 3-hydroxyla-

tion of benzodiazepines. Ethanol, isoniazid, and phenytoin are less effective in this regard. These reactions usually are reduced to a greater extent in elderly patients and in patients with chronic liver disease than are those involving conjugation.

An ideal hypnotic agent would have a rapid onset of action when taken at bedtime, a sufficiently sustained action to facilitate sleep throughout the night, and no residual action by the following morning. Among the benzodiaz-epines that are used commonly as hypnotic agents, triaz-olam theoretically fits this description most closely. Because of the slow rate of elimination of *desalkylflurazepam,* flu-razepam (or quazepam) might seem to be unsuitable for this purpose. In practice, there appear to be some disadvantages to the use of agents that have a relatively rapid rate of disappearance, including the early-morning insomnia that is experienced by some patients and a greater likelihood of rebound insomnia on drug discontinuation (*see* Gillin *et al.*, 1989; Roth and Roehrs, 1992). With careful selection of dosage, flurazepam and other benzodiazepines with slower rates of elimination than triazolam can be used effectively. The biotransformation and pharmacokinetic properties of the benzodiazepines have been reviewed (Greenblatt, 1991; Laurijssens and Greenblatt, 1996).

Therapeutic Uses

The therapeutic uses and routes of administration of individual benzodiazepines that are marketed in the United States are summarized in Table 16–3. It should be emphasized that most benzodiazepines can be used interchangeably. For example, diazepam can be used for alcohol withdrawal, and most benzodiazepines work as hypnotics. In general, the therapeutic uses of a given benzodiazepine depend on its half-life and may not match the Food and Drug Administration (FDA) approved indications. Benzodiazepines that are useful as anticonvulsants have a long half-life, and rapid entry into the brain is required for efficacy in treatment of status epilepticus. A short elimination half-life is desirable for hypnotics, although this carries the drawback of increased abuse liability and severity of withdrawal after drug discontinuation. Antianxiety agents, in contrast, should have a long half-life despite the drawback of the risk of neuropsychological deficits caused by drug accumulation.

Table 16–3
Trade Names, Routes of Administration, and Therapeutic Uses of Benzodiazepines

COMPOUND (TRADE NAME)	ROUTES OF ADMINISTRATION*	EXAMPLES OF THERAPEUTIC USES†	COMMENTS	$t_{\frac{1}{2}}$, HOURS‡	USUAL SEDATIVE-HYPNOTIC DOSAGE, MG¶
Alprazolam (XANAX)	Oral	Anxiety disorders, agoraphobia	Withdrawal symptoms may be especially severe	12±2	—
Chlordiazepoxide (LIBRIUM, others)	Oral, IM, IV	Anxiety disorders, management of alcohol withdrawal, anesthetic premedication	Long-acting and self-tapering because of active metabolites	10±3.4	50–100, qd–qid§
Clonazepam (KLONOPIN)	Oral	Seizure disorders, adjunctive treatment in acute mania and certain movement disorders	Tolerance develops to anticonvulsant effects	23±5	—
Clorazepate (TRANXENE, others)	Oral	Anxiety disorders, seizure disorders	Prodrug; activity due to formation of nordazepam during absorption	2.0±0.9	3.75–20, bid–qid§
Diazepam (VALIUM, others)	Oral, IM, IV, rectal	Anxiety disorders, status epilepticus, skeletal muscle relaxation, anesthetic premedication	Prototypical benzodiazepine	43±13	5–10, tid–qid§
Estazolam (PROSOM)	Oral	Insomnia	Contains triazolo ring; adverse effects may be similar to those of triazolam	10–24	1–2

(Continued)

Table 16–3
Trade Names, Routes of Administration, and Therapeutic Uses of Benzodiazepines (Continued)

COMPOUND (TRADE NAME)	ROUTES OF ADMINISTRATION*	EXAMPLES OF THERAPEUTIC USES†	COMMENTS	$t_{\frac{1}{2}}$, HOURS‡	USUAL SEDATIVE-HYPNOTIC DOSAGE, MG¶
Flurazepam (DALMANE)	Oral	Insomnia	Active metabolites accumulate with chronic use	74±24	15–30
Lorazepam (ATIVAN)	Oral, IM, IV	Anxiety disorders, pre-anesthetic medication	Metabolized solely by conjugation	14±5	2–4
Midazolam (VERSED)	IV, IM	Preanesthetic and intraoperative medication	Rapidly inactivated	1.9±0.6	—#
Oxazepam (SERAX)	Oral	Anxiety disorders	Metabolized solely by conjugation	8.0±2.4	15–30, tid–qid§
Quazepam (DORAL)	Oral	Insomnia	Active metabolites accumulate with chronic use	39	7.5–15
Temazepam (RESTORIL)	Oral	Insomnia	Metabolized mainly by conjugation	11±6	7.5–30
Triazolam (HALCION)	Oral	Insomnia	Rapidly inactivated; may cause disturbing daytime side effects	2.9±1.0	0.125–0.25

*IM, intramuscular injection; IV, intravenous administration; qd, once a day; bid, twice a day; tid, three times a day; qid, four times a day. †The therapeutic uses are identified as examples to emphasize that most benzodiazepines can be used interchangeably. In general, the therapeutic uses of a given benzodiazepine are related to its half-life and may not match the marketed indications. The issue is addressed more extensively in the text. ‡Half-life of active metabolite may differ. See Appendix II for additional information. ¶For additional dosage information, see Chapter 13 (anesthesia), Chapter 17 (anxiety), and Chapter 19 (seizure disorders). §Approved as a sedative-hypnotic only for management of alcohol withdrawal; doses in a nontolerant individual would be smaller. #Recommended doses vary considerably depending on specific use, condition of patient, and concomitant administration of other drugs.

Untoward Effects. At the time of peak concentration in plasma, hypnotic doses of benzodiazepines can be expected to cause varying degrees of lightheadedness, lassitude, increased reaction time, motor incoordination, impairment of mental and motor functions, confusion, and anterograde amnesia. Cognition appears to be affected less than motor performance. *All these effects can greatly impair driving and other psychomotor skills, especially if combined with ethanol.* When the drug is given at the intended time of sleep, the persistence of these effects during the waking hours is adverse. These dose-related residual effects can be insidious because most subjects underestimate the degree of their impair-ment. Residual daytime sleepiness also may occur, even though successful drug therapy can reduce the daytime sleepiness resulting from chronic insomnia (*see* Dement, 1991). The intensity and incidence of CNS toxicity generally increase with age; both pharmacokinetic and pharmacodynamic factors are involved (*see* Meyer, 1982; Monane, 1992).

Other relatively common side effects of benzodiazepines are weakness, headache, blurred vision, vertigo, nausea and vomiting, epigastric distress, and diarrhea; joint pains, chest pains, and incontinence are much more rare. Anticonvulsant benzodiazepines sometimes actually increase the frequency of seizures in patients with epilepsy. The possible adverse effects of alterations in the sleep pattern are discussed below.

Adverse Psychological Effects. Benzodiazepines may cause paradoxical effects. Flurazepam occasionally increases the incidence of nightmares—especially during the first week of use—and sometimes causes garrulousness, anxiety, irritability, tachycardia, and sweating. Amnesia, euphoria, restlessness, hallucinations, and hypomanic behavior have been reported to occur during use of various benzodiazepines. The release of bizarre uninhibited behavior has been noted in some users, whereas hostility and rage may occur in others; collectively, these are sometimes referred to as *disinhibition* or *dyscontrol reactions.* Paranoia, depression, and suicidal ideation also occasionally may accompany the use of these agents. Such paradoxical or disinhibition reactions are rare and appear to be dose-related. Because of reports of an increased incidence of confusion and abnormal behaviors, triazolam has been banned in the United Kingdom, although the FDA declared triazolam to be safe and effective in low doses of 0.125 to 0.25 mg. Surveys in the United Kingdom after the ban found that patients did not have fewer side effects with replacement treatments (Hindmarch *et al.,* 1993), which is consonant with controlled studies that do not support the conclusion that such reactions occur more frequently with any one benzodiazepine than with others (*see* Jonas *et al.,* 1992; Rothschild, 1992).

Chronic benzodiazepine use poses a risk for development of dependence and abuse (Woods *et al.,* 1992), but not to the same extent as seen with older sedatives and other recognized drugs of abuse (Ulenhuth *et al.,* 1999). Abuse of benzodiazepines includes the use of flunitrazepam (ROHYPNOL) as a "date-rape drug" (Woods and Winger, 1997). Mild dependence may develop in many patients who have taken therapeutic doses of benzodiazepines on a regular basis for prolonged periods. Withdrawal symptoms may include temporary intensification of the problems that originally prompted their use (*e.g.,* insomnia or anxiety). Dysphoria, irritability, sweating, unpleasant dreams, tremors, anorexia, and faintness or dizziness also may occur, especially when withdrawal of the benzodiazepine occurs abruptly (Petursson, 1994). Hence, it is prudent to taper the dosage gradually when therapy is to be discontinued. Despite their adverse effects, benzodiazepines are relatively safe drugs. Even huge doses are rarely fatal unless other drugs are taken concomitantly. Ethanol is a common contributor to deaths involving benzodiazepines, and true coma is uncommon in the absence of another CNS depressant. Although overdosage with a benzodiazepine rarely causes severe cardiovascular or respiratory depression, therapeutic doses can further compromise respiration in patients with COPD or obstructive sleep apnea (*see* discussion of effects on respiration, above).

A wide variety of allergic, hepatotoxic, and hematologic reactions to the benzodiazepines may occur, but the incidence is quite low; these reactions have been associated with the use of flurazepam and triazolam but not with temazepam. Large doses taken just before or during labor may cause hypothermia, hypotonia, and mild respiratory depression in the neonate. Abuse by the pregnant mother can result in a withdrawal syndrome in the newborn.

Except for additive effects with other sedative or hypnotic drugs, reports of clinically important pharmacodynamic interactions between benzodiazepines and other drugs have been infrequent. Ethanol increases both the rate of absorption of benzodiazepines and the associated CNS depression. *Valproate* and benzodiazepines in combination may cause psychotic episodes. Pharmacokinetic interactions were discussed earlier.

Novel Benzodiazepine-Receptor Agonists

Hypnotics in this class include *zolpicone* (not available in the United States), zolpidem (AMBIEN), zaleplon (SONATA), and indiplon (under review by the FDA). Although the chemical structures of these compounds do not resemble those of benzodiazepines, it is assumed that their therapeutic efficacies are due to agonist effects on the benzodiazepine site of the GABA$_A$ receptor.

Zaleplon and zolpidem are effective in relieving sleep-onset insomnia. Both drugs have been approved by the FDA for use for up to 7 to 10 days at a time. Zaleplon and zolpidem have sustained hypnotic efficacy without occurrence of rebound insomnia on abrupt discontinuation (Mitler, 2000; Walsh *et al.,* 2000). Zaleplon and zolpidem have similar degrees of efficacy. Zolpidem has a half-life of about 2 hours, which is sufficient to cover most of a typical 8-hour sleep period, and is presently approved for bedtime use only. Zaleplon has a shorter half-life, about 1 hour, which offers the possibility for safe dosing later in the night, within 4 hours of the anticipated rising time. As a result, zaleplon is approved for use immediately at bedtime or when the patient has difficulty falling asleep after bedtime. Because of its short half-life, zaleplon has not been shown to be different from placebo in measures of duration of sleep and number of awakenings. Zaleplon and zolpidem may differ in residual side effects; late-night administration of zolpidem has been associated with morning sedation, delayed reaction time, and anterograde amnesia, whereas zaleplon has no more side effects than placebo.

Zaleplon. Zaleplon (SONATA) is a nonbenzodiazepine and is a member of the pyrazolopyrimidine class of compounds. The structural formula is:

ZALEPLON

Zaleplon preferentially binds to the benzodiazepine-binding site on GABA$_A$ receptors containing the α1 receptor subunit. Zaleplon is absorbed rapidly and reaches peak plasma concentrations in about

1 hour. Its half-life is approximately 1 hour. Its bioavailability is approximately 30% because of presystemic metabolism. Zaleplon has a volume of distribution of approximately 1.4 L/kg and plasma-protein binding of approximately 60%. Zaleplon is metabolized largely by aldehyde oxidase and to a lesser extent by CYP3A4. Its oxidative metabolites are converted to glucuronides and eliminated in urine. Less than 1% of zaleplon is excreted unchanged in urine. None of zaleplon's metabolites is pharmacologically active.

Zaleplon (usually administered in 5-, 10-, or 20-mg doses) has been studied in clinical trials of patients with chronic or transient insomnia (for a review, *see* Dooley and Plosker, 2000). Studies have focused on its effects in decreasing sleep latency. Zaleplon-treated subjects with either chronic or transient insomnia have experienced shorter periods of sleep latency than have placebo-treated subjects. Tolerance to zaleplon does not appear to occur, nor do rebound insomnia or withdrawal symptoms after stopping treatment.

Zolpidem. Zolpidem (AMBIEN) is a nonbenzodiazepine sedative-hypnotic drug that became available in the United States in 1993 after 5 years of use in Europe (Holm and Goa, 2000). It is classified as an imidazopyridine and has the following chemical structure:

ZOLPIDEM

Although the actions of zolpidem are due to agonist effects on $GABA_A$ receptors and generally resemble those of benzodiazepines, it produces only weak anticonvulsant effects in experimental animals, and its relatively strong sedative actions appear to mask anxiolytic effects in various animal models of anxiety (*see* Langtry and Benfield, 1990). Although chronic administration of zolpidem to rodents produces neither tolerance to its sedative effects nor signs of withdrawal when the drug is discontinued and flumazenil is injected (Perrault *et al.*, 1992), tolerance and physical dependence have been observed with chronic administration of zolpidem to baboons (Griffiths *et al.*, 1992).

Unlike the benzodiazepines, zolpidem has little effect on the stages of sleep in normal human subjects. The drug is as effective as benzodiazepines in shortening sleep latency and prolonging total sleep time in patients with insomnia. After discontinuation of zolpidem, the beneficial effects on sleep reportedly persist for up to 1 week (Herrmann *et al.*, 1993), but mild rebound insomnia on the first night also has occurred (Anonymous, 1993). Tolerance and physical dependence develop only rarely and under unusual circumstances (Cavallaro *et al.*, 1993; Morselli, 1993). Indeed, zolpidem-induced improvement in sleep time of chronic insomniacs was sustained during as much as 6 months of treatment without signs of withdrawal or rebound after stopping the drug (Kummer *et al.*, 1993). Nevertheless, zolpidem is approved only for the short-term treatment of insomnia. At therapeutic doses (5 to 10 mg), zolpidem infrequently produces residual daytime sedation or amnesia, and the incidence of other adverse effects (*e.g.*, gastrointestinal complaints or dizziness) also is low. As with the benzodiazepines, large overdoses of zolpidem do not produce severe respiratory depression unless other agents (*e.g.*, ethanol) also are ingested (Garnier *et al.*,

1994). Hypnotic doses increase the hypoxia and hypercarbia of patients with obstructive sleep apnea.

Zolpidem is absorbed readily from the gastrointestinal tract; first-pass hepatic metabolism results in an oral bioavailability of about 70%, but this value is lower when the drug is ingested with food because of slowed absorption and increased hepatic blood flow. Zolpidem is eliminated almost entirely by conversion to inactive products in the liver, largely through oxidation of the methyl groups on the phenyl and imidazopyridine rings to the corresponding carboxylic acids. Its plasma half-life is approximately 2 hours in individuals with normal hepatic blood flow or function. This value may be increased twofold or more in those with cirrhosis and also tends to be greater in older patients; adjustment of dosage often is necessary in both categories of patients. Although little or no unchanged zolpidem is found in the urine, elimination of the drug is slower in patients with chronic renal insufficiency largely owing to an increase in its apparent volume of distribution.

Flumazenil: A Benzodiazepine-Receptor Antagonist

Flumazenil (ROMAZICON) is an imidazobenzodiazepine (Table 16–1) that behaves as a specific benzodiazepine antagonist (Hoffman and Warren, 1993). Flumazenil binds with high affinity to specific sites on the $GABA_A$ receptor, where it competitively antagonizes the binding and allosteric effects of benzodiazepines and other ligands. Both the electrophysiological and behavioral effects of agonist or inverse-agonist benzodiazepines and β-carbolines also are antagonized. In animal models, the intrinsic pharmacological actions of flumazenil have been subtle; effects resembling those of inverse agonists sometimes have been detected at low doses, whereas slight benzodiazepinelike effects often have been evident at high doses. The evidence for intrinsic activity in human subjects is even more vague, except for modest anticonvulsant effects at high doses. However, anticonvulsant effects cannot be relied on for therapeutic utility because the administration of flumazenil may precipitate seizures under certain circumstances (*see* below).

Flumazenil is available only for intravenous administration. Although absorbed rapidly after oral administration, less than 25% of the drug reaches the systemic circulation owing to extensive first-pass hepatic metabolism; effective oral doses are apt to cause headache and dizziness (Roncari *et al.*, 1993). On intravenous administration, flumazenil is eliminated almost entirely by hepatic metabolism to inactive products with a half-life of about 1 hour; the duration of clinical effects usually is only 30 to 60 minutes.

The primary indications for the use of flumazenil are the management of suspected benzodiazepine overdose and the reversal of sedative effects produced by benzodiazepines administered during either general anesthesia or diagnostic and/or therapeutic procedures.

The administration of a series of small injections is preferred to a single bolus injection. A total of 1 mg flumazenil given over 1 to 3 minutes usually is sufficient to abolish the effects of therapeutic doses of benzodiazepines; patients with suspected benzodiazepine overdose should respond adequately to a cumulative dose of 1 to 5 mg given over 2 to 10 minutes; a lack of response to 5 mg flumazenil strongly suggests that a benzodiazepine is not the major cause of sedation. Additional courses of treatment with flumazenil may be needed within 20 to 30 minutes should sedation reappear. Flumazenil is not effective in single-drug overdoses with either barbiturates or tricyclic antidepressants. To the contrary, the administration of flumazenil in these settings may be associated with the onset of seizures, especially in patients poisoned with tricyclic antidepressants

(Spivey, 1992). Seizures or other withdrawal symptoms also may be precipitated in patients who had been taking benzodiazepines for protracted periods and in whom tolerance and/or dependence may have developed.

BARBITURATES

The barbiturates were used extensively as sedative-hypnotic drugs. Except for a few specialized uses, they have been replaced largely by the much safer benzodiazepines.

Chemistry. Barbituric acid is 2,4,6-trioxohexahydropyrimidine. This compound lacks central depressant activity, but the presence of alkyl or aryl groups at position 5 confers sedative-hypnotic and sometimes other activities. The general structural formula for the barbiturates and the structures of selected compounds are included in Table 16–4.

The carbonyl group at position 2 takes on acidic character because of lactam–lactim ("keto"–"enol") tautomerization, which is favored by its location between the two electronegative amido nitrogens. The lactim form is favored in alkaline solution, and salts result. Barbiturates in which the oxygen at C2 is replaced by sulfur sometimes are called *thiobarbiturates*. These compounds are more lipid-soluble than the corresponding *oxybarbiturates*. In general, structural changes that increase lipid solubility decrease duration of action, decrease latency to onset of activity, accelerate metabolic degradation, and increase hypnotic potency.

Pharmacological Properties

The barbiturates reversibly depress the activity of all excitable tissues. The CNS is exquisitely sensitive, and even when barbiturates are given in anesthetic concentrations, direct effects on peripheral excitable tissues are weak. However, serious deficits in cardiovascular and other peripheral functions occur in acute barbiturate intoxication.

Central Nervous System. *Sites and Mechanisms of Action on the CNS.* Barbiturates act throughout the CNS; non-anesthetic doses preferentially suppress polysynaptic responses. Facilitation is diminished, and inhibition usually is enhanced. The site of inhibition is either postsynaptic, as at cortical and cerebellar pyramidal cells and in the cuneate nucleus, substantia nigra, and thalamic relay neurons, or presynaptic, as in the spinal cord. Enhancement of inhibition occurs primarily at synapses where neurotransmission is mediated by GABA acting at $GABA_A$ receptors.

The barbiturates exert several distinct effects on excitatory and inhibitory synaptic transmission. For example, *(–)-pentobarbital* potentiates GABA-induced increases in chloride conductance and depresses voltage-activated Ca^{2+} currents at similar concentrations (below 10 μM) in isolated hippocampal neurons; above 100 μM, chloride conductance is increased in the absence of GABA (ffrench-Mullen *et al.*, 1993). Phenobarbital is less efficacious and much less potent in producing these effects, whereas *(+)-pentobarbital* has

only weak activity. Thus the more selective anticonvulsant properties of phenobarbital and its higher therapeutic index may be explained by its lower capacity to depress neuronal function as compared with the anesthetic barbiturates.

As noted earlier, the mechanisms underlying the actions of barbiturates on $GABA_A$ receptors appear to be distinct from those of either GABA or the benzodiazepines for reasons that include the following: (1) Although barbiturates also enhance the binding of GABA to $GABA_A$ receptors in a chloride-dependent and picrotoxin-sensitive fashion, they promote (rather than displace) the binding of benzodiazepines; (2) barbiturates potentiate GABA-induced chloride currents by prolonging periods during which bursts of channel opening occur rather than by increasing the frequency of these bursts, as benzodiazepines do; (3) only α and β (not γ) subunits are required for barbiturate action; and (4) barbiturate-induced increases in chloride conductance are not affected by the deletion of the tyrosine and threonine residues in the β subunit that govern the sensitivity of $GABA_A$ receptors to activation by agonists (Amin and Weiss, 1993).

Sub-anesthetic concentrations of barbiturates also can reduce glutamate-induced depolarizations (Macdonald and McLean, 1982) (*see also* Chapter 12); only the AMPA subtypes of glutamate receptors sensitive to kainate or quisqualate appear to be affected (Marszalec and Narahashi, 1993). At higher concentrations that produce anesthesia, pentobarbital suppresses high-frequency repetitive firing of neurons, apparently as a result of inhibiting the function of voltage-dependent, tetrodotoxin-sensitive Na^+ channels; in this case, however, both stereoisomers are about equally effective (Frenkel *et al.*, 1990). At still higher concentrations, voltage-dependent K^+ conductances are reduced. Taken together, the findings that barbiturates activate inhibitory $GABA_A$ receptors and inhibit excitatory AMPA receptors can explain their CNS-depressant effects (Saunders and Ho, 1990).

The barbiturates can produce all degrees of depression of the CNS, ranging from mild sedation to general anesthesia. The use of barbiturates for general anesthesia is discussed in Chapter 13. Certain barbiturates, particularly those containing a 5-phenyl substituent (*e.g.,* phenobarbital and *mephobarbital*), have selective anticonvulsant activity (*see* Chapter 19). The anti-anxiety properties of the barbiturates are inferior to those exerted by the benzodiazepines.

Except for the anticonvulsant activities of phenobarbital and its congeners, the barbiturates possess a low degree of selectivity and therapeutic index. Thus, it is not possible to achieve a desired effect without evidence of general depression of the CNS. Pain perception and reaction are relatively unimpaired until the moment of unconsciousness, and in small doses, the barbiturates increase the reaction to painful stimuli. Hence they cannot be relied on to produce sedation or sleep in the presence of even moderate pain.

Effects on Stages of Sleep. Hypnotic doses of barbiturates increase the total sleep time and alter the stages of sleep in a dose-dependent manner. Like the benzodiazepines, these drugs decrease sleep latency, the number of awakenings, and the durations of REM and slow-wave sleep. During repetitive nightly administration, some tolerance to the effects on sleep occurs within a few days, and the effect on total sleep time may be reduced by as much as 50% after 2 weeks of use. Discontinuation leads to rebound increases in all the parameters reported to be decreased by barbiturates.

Tolerance. Pharmacodynamic (functional) and pharmacokinetic tolerance to barbiturates can occur. The former contributes more to the decreased effect than does the latter. With chronic administration of gradually increasing doses, pharmacodynamic tolerance continues to develop over a period of weeks to months, depending on the dosage schedule, whereas pharmacokinetic tolerance reaches its

Table 16–4
Structures, Trade Names, and Major Pharmacological Properties of Selected Barbiturates

GENERAL FORMULA:

$$R_3-N-C_2-N-H$$
$$O=C_2^3-C_{5}^{5}(R_{5a})(R_{5b})$$
(or S=)*

COMPOUND (TRADE NAMES)	R_3	R_{5a}	R_{5b}	ROUTES OF ADMINISTRATION†	HALF-LIFE, HOURS	THERAPEUTIC USES	COMMENTS
Amobarbital (AMYTAL)	—H	—C_2H_5	—$CH_2CH_2CH(CH_3)_2$	IM, IV	10–40	Insomnia, preoperative sedation, emergency management of seizures	Only sodium salt administered parenterally
Butabarbital (BUTISOL, others)	—H	—C_2H_5	—$CH(CH_3)CH_2CH_3$	Oral	35–50	Insomnia, preoperative sedation	Redistribution shortens duration of action of single dose to 8 hours
Butalbital	—H	—$CH_2CH=CH_2$	$CH_2CH(CH_3)_2$	Oral	35–88	Marketed in combination with analgesics	Therapeutic efficacy questionable.
Mephobarbital (MEBARAL)	—CH_3	—C_2H_5	(phenyl ring)	Oral	10–70	Seizure disorders, daytime sedation	Second-line anticonvulsant
Methohexital (BREVITAL)	—CH_3	—$CH_2CH=CH_2$	—$CH(CH_3)C\equiv CCH_2CH_3$	IV	3–5‡	Induction and maintenance of anesthesia	Only sodium salt is available; single injection provides 5 to 7 minutes of anesthesia‡
Pentobarbital (NEMBUTAL)	—H	—C_2H_5	—$CH(CH_3)CH_2CH_2CH_3$	Oral, IM, IV, rectal	15–50	Insomnia, preoperative sedation, emergency management of seizures	Only sodium salt administered parenterally

(Continued)

Table 16-4

Structures, Trade Names, and Major Pharmacological Properties of Selected Barbiturates (Continued)

GENERAL FORMULA:

COMPOUND (TRADE NAMES)	R_3	R_{5a}	R_{5b}	ROUTES OF ADMINISTRATION†	HALF-LIFE, HOURS	THERAPEUTIC USES	COMMENTS
Phenobarbital (LUMINAL, others)	—H	—C_2H_5	(phenyl ring)	Oral, IM, IV	80–120	Seizure disorders, status epilepticus, daytime sedation	First-line anti-convulsant; only sodium salt administered parenterally
Secobarbital (SECONAL)	—H	—$CH_2CH=CH_2$	—$CH(CH_3)CH_2CH_2CH_3$	Oral	15–40	Insomnia, preoperative sedation	Only sodium salt is available
Thiopental (PENTOTHAL)	—H	—C_2H_5	—$CH(CH_3)CH_2CH_2CH_3$	IV	8–10‡	Induction and/or maintenance of anesthesia, preoperative sedation, emergency management of seizures	Only sodium salt is available; single injections provide short periods of anesthesia‡

*O except in thiopental, where it is replaced by S. †IM, intramuscular injection; IV, intravenous administration. ‡Value represents terminal half-life due to metabolism by the liver; redistribution following parenteral administration produces effects lasting only a few minutes.

peak in a few days to a week. Tolerance to the effects on mood, sedation, and hypnosis occurs more readily and is greater than that to the anticonvulsant and lethal effects; thus, as tolerance increases, the therapeutic index decreases. Pharmacodynamic tolerance to barbiturates confers tolerance to all general CNS-depressant drugs, including ethanol.

Abuse and Dependence. Like other CNS-depressant drugs, barbiturates are abused, and some individuals develop a dependence on them. Moreover, the barbiturates may have euphoriant effects. These topics are discussed in Chapter 23.

Peripheral Nervous Structures. Barbiturates selectively depress transmission in autonomic ganglia and reduce nicotinic excitation by choline esters. This effect may account, at least in part, for the fall in blood pressure produced by intravenous oxybarbiturates and by severe barbiturate intoxication. At skeletal neuromuscular junctions, the blocking effects of both *tubocurarine* and *decamethonium* are enhanced during barbiturate anesthesia. These actions probably result from the capacity of barbiturates at hypnotic or anesthetic concentrations to inhibit the passage of current through nicotinic cholinergic receptors. Several distinct mechanisms appear to be involved, and little stereoselectivity is evident.

Respiration. Barbiturates depress both the respiratory drive and the mechanisms responsible for the rhythmic character of respiration. The neurogenic drive is diminished by hypnotic doses but usually no more so than during natural sleep. However, neurogenic drive is essentially eliminated by a dose three times greater than that used normally to induce sleep. Such doses also suppress the hypoxic drive and, to a lesser extent, the chemoreceptor drive. At still higher doses, the powerful hypoxic drive also fails. However, the margin between the lighter planes of surgical anesthesia and dangerous respiratory depression is sufficient to permit the ultra-short-acting barbiturates to be used, with suitable precautions, as anesthetic agents.

The barbiturates only slightly depress protective reflexes until the degree of intoxication is sufficient to produce severe respiratory depression. Coughing, sneezing, hiccoughing, and laryngospasm may occur when barbiturates are employed as intravenous anesthetic agents. Indeed, laryngospasm is one of the chief complications of barbiturate anesthesia.

Cardiovascular System. When given orally in sedative or hypnotic doses, the barbiturates do not produce significant overt cardiovascular effects except for a slight decrease in blood pressure and heart rate such as occurs in normal sleep. In general, the effects of *thiopental* anesthesia on the cardiovascular system are benign in comparison with those of the volatile anesthetic agents; there usually is either no change or a fall in mean arterial pressure (*see* Chapter 13). Apparently, a decrease in cardiac output usually is sufficient to offset an increase in total calculated peripheral resistance, which sometimes is accompanied by an increase in heart rate. Cardiovascular reflexes are obtunded by partial inhibition of ganglionic transmission. This is most evident in patients with congestive heart failure or hypovolemic shock, whose reflexes already are operating maximally and in whom barbiturates can cause an exaggerated fall in blood pressure. Because barbiturates also impair reflex cardiovascular adjustments to inflation of the lung, positive-pressure respiration should be used cautiously and only when necessary to maintain adequate pulmonary ventilation in patients who are anesthetized or intoxicated with a barbiturate.

Other cardiovascular changes often noted when thiopental and other intravenous thiobarbiturates are administered after conventional preanesthetic medication include decreased renal and cerebral blood flow with a marked fall in CSF pressure. Although cardiac arrhythmias are observed only infrequently, intravenous anesthesia with barbiturates can increase the incidence of ventricular arrhythmias, especially when *epinephrine* and *halothane* also are present. Anesthetic concentrations of barbiturates have direct electrophysiological effects on the heart; in addition to depressing Na^+ channels, they reduce the function of at least two types of K^+ channels (Nattel *et al.*, 1990; Pancrazio *et al.*, 1993). However, direct depression of cardiac contractility occurs only when doses several times those required to cause anesthesia are administered, which probably contributes to the cardiovascular depression that accompanies acute barbiturate poisoning.

Gastrointestinal Tract. The oxybarbiturates tend to decrease the tone of the gastrointestinal musculature and the amplitude of rhythmic contractions. The locus of action is partly peripheral and partly central, depending on the dose. A hypnotic dose does not significantly delay gastric emptying in human beings. The relief of various GI symptoms by sedative doses is probably largely due to the central-depressant action.

Liver. The best known effects of barbiturates on the liver are those on the microsomal drug-metabolizing system (*see* Chapter 3). Acutely, the barbiturates combine with several CYPs and inhibit the biotransformation of a number of other drugs and endogenous substrates, such as steroids; other substrates may reciprocally inhibit barbiturate biotransformations. Drug interactions may result even when the other substances and barbiturates are oxidized by different microsomal enzyme systems.

Chronic administration of barbiturates markedly increases the protein and lipid content of the hepatic smooth endoplasmic reticulum, as well as the activities of glucuronyl transferase and CYPs 1A2, 2C9, 2C19, and 3A4. The induction of these enzymes increases the metabolism of a number of drugs and endogenous substances, including steroid hormones, cholesterol, bile salts, and vitamins K and D. This also results in an increased rate of barbiturate metabolism, which partly accounts for tolerance to barbiturates. Many sedative-hypnotics, various anesthetics, and ethanol also are metabolized by and/or induce the microsomal enzymes, and some degree of cross-tolerance therefore can occur. Not all microsomal biotransformations of drugs and endogenous substrates are affected equally, but a convenient rule of thumb is that at maximal induction in human beings, the rates are approximately doubled. The inducing effect is not limited to the microsomal enzymes; *e.g.*, there are increases in δ-aminolevulinic acid (ALA) synthetase, a mitochondrial enzyme, and aldehyde dehydrogenase, a cytosolic enzyme. The effect of barbiturates on ALA synthetase can cause dangerous disease exacerbations in persons with intermittent porphyria.

Kidney. Severe oliguria or anuria may occur in acute barbiturate poisoning largely as a result of the marked hypotension.

Absorption, Fate, and Excretion. For sedative-hypnotic use, the barbiturates usually are administered orally (Table 16–4). Such doses are absorbed rapidly and probably completely; sodium salts are absorbed more rapidly than the corresponding free acids, especially from liquid formulations. The onset of action varies from 10 to 60 minutes, depending on the agent and the formulation, and is delayed by the presence of food in the stomach. When necessary, intramuscular injections of solutions of the sodium salts should be placed deeply into large muscles to avoid the pain and possible necrosis that can result at more superficial sites. With some agents, special preparations are available for rectal administration. The intravenous route usually is reserved for the management of status epilepticus (phenobarbital sodium) or for the induction and/or maintenance of general anesthesia (*e.g., thiopental* or *methohexital*).

Barbiturates are distributed widely, and they readily cross the placenta. The highly lipid-soluble barbiturates, led by those used to induce anesthesia, undergo redistribution after intravenous injection. Uptake into less vascular tissues, especially muscle and fat, leads to a decline in the concentration of barbiturate in the plasma and brain. With thiopental and methohexital, this results in the awakening of patients within 5 to 15 minutes of the injection of the usual anesthetic doses (*see* Chapter 13).

Except for the less lipid-soluble *aprobarbital* and phenobarbital, nearly complete metabolism and/or conjugation of barbiturates in the liver precedes their renal excretion. The oxidation of radicals at C5 is the most important biotransformation that terminates biological activity. Oxidation results in the formation of alcohols, ketones, phenols, or carboxylic acids, which may appear in the urine as such or as glucuronic acid conjugates. In some instances (*e.g.,* phenobarbital), *N*-glycosylation is an important metabolic pathway. Other biotransformations include *N*-hydroxylation, desulfuration of thiobarbiturates to oxybarbiturates, opening of the barbituric acid ring, and *N*-dealkylation of *N*-alkylbarbiturates to active metabolites (*e.g.,* mephobarbital to phenobarbital). About 25% of phenobarbital and nearly all of aprobarbital are excreted unchanged in the urine. Their renal excretion can be increased greatly by osmotic diuresis and/or alkalinization of the urine.

The metabolic elimination of barbiturates is more rapid in young people than in the elderly and infants, and half-lives are increased during pregnancy partly because of the expanded volume of distribution. Chronic liver disease, especially cirrhosis, often increases the half-life of the biotransformable barbiturates. Repeated administration, especially of phenobarbital, shortens the half-life of barbiturates that are metabolized as a result of the induction of microsomal enzymes (*see* above).

None of the barbiturates used for hypnosis in the United States appears to have an elimination half-life that is short enough for elimination to be virtually complete in 24 hours (Table 16-4). However, the relationship between duration of action and half-time of elimination is complicated by the fact that enantiomers of optically active barbiturates often differ in both biological potencies and rates of biotransformation. Nevertheless, all these barbiturates will accumulate during repetitive administration unless appropriate adjustments in dosage are made. Furthermore, the persistence of the drug in plasma during the day favors the development of tolerance and abuse.

Therapeutic Uses

The major uses of individual barbiturates are listed in Table 16–4. As with the benzodiazepines, selection of particular barbiturates for a given therapeutic indication is based primarily on pharmacokinetic considerations.

CNS Uses. Although barbiturates largely have been replaced by benzodiazepines and other compounds for sedation, phenobarbital and *butabarbital* are still available as "sedatives" in a host of combinations of questionable efficacy for the treatment of functional gastrointestinal disorders and asthma. They also are included in analgesic combinations, possibly counterproductively. Barbiturates, especially butabarbital and phenobarbital, are used sometimes to antagonize unwanted CNS-stimulant effects of various drugs, such as *ephedrine, dextroamphetamine,* and *theophylline,* although a preferred approach is adjustment of dosage or substitution of alternative therapy for the primary agents. Phenobarbital still is used to treat hypnosedative withdrawal (Martin *et al.,* 1979).

Barbiturates are employed in the emergency treatment of convulsions, such as occur in tetanus, eclampsia, status epilepticus, cerebral hemorrhage, and poisoning by convulsant drugs; however, benzodiazepines generally are superior in these uses. Phenobarbital sodium is used most frequently because of its anticonvulsant efficacy; however, even when administered intravenously, 15 minutes or more may be required for it to attain peak concentrations in the brain. The ultra-short- and short-acting barbiturates have a low ratio of anticonvulsant to hypnotic action, and these drugs or inhalational anesthetic agents are employed only when general anesthesia must be used to control seizures refractory to other measures. Diazepam usually is chosen for the emergency treatment of seizures. The use of barbiturates in the symptomatic therapy of epilepsy is discussed in Chapter 19.

Ultra-short-acting agents such as thiopental or methohexital continue to be employed as intravenous anesthetics (*see* Chapter 13). In children, the rectal administration of methohexital sometimes is used for the induction of anesthesia or for sedation during imaging procedures. Short- and ultra-short-acting barbiturates occasionally are used as adjuncts to other agents for obstetrical anesthesia. Although studies have failed to affirm gross depression of respiration in full-term infants, premature infants clearly are more susceptible. Since evaluation of the effects on the fetus and neonate is difficult, it therefore is prudent to avoid the use of barbiturates in this setting.

The barbiturates are employed as diagnostic and therapeutic aids in psychiatry; these uses sometimes are referred to as *narcoanalysis* and *narcotherapy,* respectively. In low concentrations, *amobarbital* has been administered directly into the carotid artery before neurosurgery as a means of identifying the dominant cerebral hemisphere for speech. Use of this procedure has been expanded to include a more extensive neuropsychological evaluation of patients with medically intractable seizure disorders who may benefit from surgical therapy (*see* Smith and Riskin, 1991).

Anesthetic doses of barbiturates attenuate cerebral edema resulting from surgery, head injury, or cerebral ischemia, and they may decrease infarct size and increase survival. General anesthetics do not provide protection. The procedure is not without serious danger, however, and the ultimate benefit to the patient has been questioned (*see* Shapiro, 1985; Smith and Riskin, 1991).

Hepatic Metabolic Uses.   Because hepatic glucuronyl transferase and the bilirubin-binding Y protein are increased by the barbiturates, phenobarbital has been used successfully to treat hyperbilirubinemia and kernicterus in the neonate. The nondepressant barbiturate *phetharbital* (*N*-phenylbarbital) works equally well. Phenobarbital may improve the hepatic transport of bilirubin in patients with hemolytic jaundice.

Untoward Effects.   *After-Effects.*   Drowsiness may last for only a few hours after a hypnotic dose of barbiturate, but residual CNS depression sometimes is evident the following day, and subtle distortions of mood and impairment of judgment and fine motor skills may be demonstrable. For example, a 200-mg dose of *secobarbital* has been shown to impair performance of driving or flying skills for 10 to 22 hours. Residual effects also may take the form of vertigo, nausea, vomiting, or diarrhea or sometimes may be manifested as overt excitement. The user may awaken slightly intoxicated and feel euphoric and energetic; later, as the demands of daytime activities challenge possibly impaired faculties, the user may display irritability and temper.

Paradoxical Excitement.   In some persons, barbiturates produce excitement rather than depression, and the patient may appear to be inebriated. This type of idiosyncrasy is relatively common among geriatric and debilitated patients and occurs most frequently with phenobarbital and *N*-methylbarbiturates. Barbiturates may cause restlessness, excitement, and even delirium when given in the presence of pain and may worsen a patient's perception of pain.

Hypersensitivity.   Allergic reactions occur, especially in persons with asthma, urticaria, angioedema, or similar conditions. Hypersensitivity reactions include localized swellings, particularly of the eyelids, cheeks, or lips, and erythematous dermatitis. Rarely, exfoliative dermatitis may be caused by phenobarbital and can prove fatal; the skin eruption may be associated with fever, delirium, and marked degenerative changes in the liver and other parenchymatous organs.

Drug Interactions.   Barbiturates combine with other CNS depressants to cause severe depression; ethanol is the most frequent offender, and interactions with first-generation antihistamines also are common. Isoniazid, methylphenidate, and monoamine oxidase inhibitors also increase the CNS-depressant effects.

Barbiturates competitively inhibit the metabolism of certain other drugs; however, the greatest number of drug interactions results from induction of hepatic CYPs and the accelerated disappearance of many drugs and endogenous substances. The metabolism of vitamins D and K is accelerated, which may hamper bone mineralization and lower Ca^{2+} absorption in patients taking phenobarbital and may be responsible for the reported coagulation defects in neonates whose mothers had been taking phenobarbital. Hepatic enzyme induction enhances metabolism of endogenous steroid hormones, which may cause endocrine disturbances, as well as of oral contraceptives, which may result in unwanted pregnancy. Barbiturates also induce the hepatic generation of toxic metabolites of chlorocarbon anesthetics and carbon tetrachloride and consequently promote lipid peroxidation, which facilitates the periportal necrosis of the liver caused by these agents.

Other Untoward Effects.   Because barbiturates enhance porphyrin synthesis, they are absolutely contraindicated in patients with acute intermittent porphyria or porphyria variegata. In hypnotic doses, the effects of barbiturates on the control of respiration are minor; however, in the presence of pulmonary insufficiency, serious respiratory depression may occur, and the drugs thus are contraindicated. Rapid intravenous injection of a barbiturate may cause cardiovascular collapse before anesthesia ensues, so the CNS signs of depth of anesthesia may fail to give an adequate warning of impending toxicity. Blood pressure can fall to shock levels; even slow intravenous injection of barbiturates often produces apnea and occasionally laryngospasm, coughing, and other respiratory difficulties.

Barbiturate Poisoning. The incidence of barbiturate poisoning has declined markedly, largely as a result of their decreased use as sedative-hypnotic agents. Nevertheless, poisoning with barbiturates is a significant clinical problem, and death occurs in a few percent of cases (Gary and Tresznewsky, 1983). Most of the cases are the result of deliberate attempts at suicide, but some are from accidental poisonings in children or in drug abusers. The lethal dose of barbiturate varies, but severe poisoning is likely to occur when more than 10 times the full hypnotic dose has been ingested at once. If alcohol or other depressant drugs also are present, the concentrations that can cause death are lower.

In severe intoxication, the patient is comatose; respiration is affected early. Breathing may be either slow or rapid and shallow. Superficial observation of respiration may be misleading with regard to actual minute volume and to the degree of respiratory acidosis and cerebral hypoxia. Eventually, blood pressure falls because the effect of the drug and of hypoxia on medullary vasomotor centers; depression of cardiac contractility and sympathetic ganglia also contributes. Pulmonary complications (*e.g.,* atelectasis, edema, and bronchopneumonia) and renal failure are likely to be the fatal complications of severe barbiturate poisoning.

The treatment of acute barbiturate intoxication is based on general supportive measures, which are applicable in most respects to poisoning by any CNS depressant. Hemodialysis or hemoperfusion is necessary only rarely, and the use of CNS stimulants is contraindicated because they increase the mortality rate.

Constant attention must be paid to the maintenance of a patent airway and adequate ventilation and to the prevention of pneumonia; oxygen should be administered. After precautions to avoid aspiration, gastric lavage should be considered if fewer than 24 hours have elapsed since ingestion, because the barbiturate can reduce GI motility. After lavage, the administration of activated charcoal and a cathartic such as *sorbitol* may shorten the half-life of the less lipid-soluble agents such as phenobarbital. If renal and cardiac functions are satisfactory, and the patient is hydrated, forced diuresis and alkalinization of the urine will hasten the excretion of aprobarbital and phenobarbital. Measures to prevent or treat atelectasis should be taken, and mechanical ventilation should be initiated when indicated.

In severe acute barbiturate intoxication, circulatory collapse is a major threat. Often the patient is admitted to the hospital with severe hypotension or shock, and dehydration frequently is severe. Hypovolemia must be corrected, and if necessary, the blood pressure can be supported with *dopamine.* Acute renal failure consequent to shock and hypoxia accounts for perhaps one-sixth of the deaths. In the event of renal failure, hemodialysis should be instituted.

MISCELLANEOUS SEDATIVE-HYPNOTIC DRUGS

Many drugs with diverse structures have been used for their sedative-hypnotic properties, including *paraldehyde* (introduced before the barbiturates), *chloral hydrate, ethchlorvynol, glutethimide, methyprylon, ethinamate,* and *meprobamate* (introduced just before the benzodiazepines).

With the exception of meprobamate, the pharmacological actions of these drugs generally resemble those of the barbiturates: they all are general CNS depressants that can produce profound hypnosis with little or no analgesia; their effects on the stages of sleep are similar to those of the barbiturates; their therapeutic index is limited, and acute intoxication, which produces respiratory depression and hypotension, is managed similarly to barbiturate poisoning; their chronic use can result in tolerance and physical dependence; and the syndrome after chronic use can be severe and life-threatening. The properties of meprobamate bear some resemblance to those of the benzodiazepines, but the drug has a distinctly higher potential for abuse and has less selective anti-anxiety effects. The clinical use of these agents has decreased markedly, and deservedly so. Nevertheless, some of them are useful in certain settings, particularly in hospitalized patients.

The chemical structures and major pharmacological properties of paraldehyde, ethchlorvynol (PLACIDYL, others), chloral hydrate (NOCTEC, others), and meprobamate are presented in Table 16–5. Further information on glutethimide, methyprylon, and ethinamate can be found in previous editions of this book.

Paraldehyde. Paraldehyde is a polymer of acetaldehyde, but it perhaps is best regarded as a cyclic polyether. It has a strong odor and a disagreeable taste. Orally, it is irritating to the throat and stomach, and it is not administered parenterally because of its injurious effects on tissues. When given rectally as a retention enema, the drug is diluted with olive oil.

Oral paraldehyde is absorbed rapidly and distributed widely; sleep usually ensues in 10 to 15 minutes after hypnotic doses. About 70% to 80% of a dose is metabolized in the liver, probably by depolymerization to acetaldehyde and subsequent oxidation to acetic acid, which ultimately is converted to carbon dioxide and water; most of the remainder is exhaled, producing a strong characteristic smell to the breath. Commonly observed consequences of poisoning with the drug include acidosis, gastritis, and fatty changes in the liver and kidney with toxic hepatitis and nephrosis.

The clinical uses of paraldehyde include the treatment of withdrawal reactions (especially delirium tremens in hospitalized patients) and other psychiatric states characterized by excitement. Paraldehyde also has been used for the treatment of convulsions (including status epilepticus) in children. Individuals who become addicted to paraldehyde may have become acquainted with the drug during treatment of their alcoholism and then, despite its disagreeable taste and odor, prefer it to alcohol.

Chloral Hydrate. Chloral hydrate is formed by adding one molecule of water to the carbonyl group of chloral (2,2,2-trichloroacetaldehyde). In addition to its hypnotic use, the drug has been employed in the past for the production of sedation in children undergoing diagnostic, dental, or other potentially uncomfortable procedures.

Chloral hydrate is reduced rapidly to the active compound, trichloroethanol (CCl_3CH_2OH), largely by alcohol dehydrogenase in the liver; significant amounts of chloral hydrate are not found in the blood after its oral administration. Therefore, its pharmacological effects probably are caused by trichloroethanol. Indeed, the latter compound can exert barbiturate-like effects on $GABA_A$-receptor channels *in vitro* (Lovinger *et al.,* 1993). Trichloroethanol is conjugated mainly with glucuronic acid, and the product (urochloralic acid) is excreted mostly into the urine.

Chloral hydrate is irritating to the skin and mucous membranes. These irritant actions give rise to an unpleasant taste, epigastric distress, nausea, and occasional vomiting, all of which are particularly likely to

Table 16–5
Structures, Trade Names, and Major Pharmacological Properties of Miscellaneous Sedative-Hypnotic Drugs

COMPOUND (TRADE NAMES)	STRUCTURE	ROUTES OF ADMINISTRATION	HALF-LIFE, HOURS	COMMENTS
Paraldehyde (PARAL)		Oral, rectal	4–10	Used to treat delirium tremens in hospitalized patients; eliminated by hepatic metabolism (75%) and exhalation (25%), toxicities include acidosis, hepatitis, and nephrosis
Chloral hydrate	$CCl_3CH(OH)_2$	Oral, rectal	5–10*	Rapidly converted by hepatic alcohol dehydrogenase to trichloroethanol, which is largely responsible for the effects of chloral hydrate; chronic use may cause hepatic damage; withdrawal syndrome is severe
Ethchlorvynol‡ (PLACIDYL)		Oral	10–20†	Redistribution shortens duration of action of single doses to 4 to 5 hours, which may result in early morning awakening; idiosyncratic responses include marked excitement, especially in the presence of pain
Meprobamate (MILTOWN, others)		Oral	6–17	Approved only for treatment of anxiety disorders, but widely used as a nighttime sedative; overdosage can cause severe hypotension, respiratory depression, and death

*Value is for elimination of trichloroethanol, to which effects can be attributed. †Value represents terminal half-life due to metabolism by the liver; redistribution shortens duration of action to less than 5 hours. ‡Not available for use in the United States.

occur if the drug is insufficiently diluted or taken on an empty stomach. Undesirable CNS effects include lightheadedness, malaise, ataxia, and nightmares. Rarely, patients may exhibit idiosyncratic reactions to chloral hydrate and may be disoriented and incoherent and show paranoid behavior. Acute poisoning by chloral hydrate may cause jaundice. Individuals using chloral hydrate chronically may exhibit sudden, acute intoxication, which can be fatal; this situation results either from an overdose or from a failure of the detoxification mechanism owing to hepatic damage; parenchymatous renal injury also may occur. Sudden withdrawal from the habitual use of chloral hydrate may result in delirium and seizures, with a high frequency of death when untreated.

Ethchlorvynol. In addition to pharmacological actions that are very similar to those of barbiturates, ethchlorvynol has anticonvulsant and muscle-relaxant properties. Ethchlorvynol is absorbed rapidly and distributed widely after oral administration. Two-compartment kinetics are manifest, with a distribution half-life of about 1 to 3 hours and an elimination half-life of 10 to 20 hours. As a result, the duration of action of the drug is relatively short, and early-morning awakening may occur after its administration at bedtime. Approximately 90% of the drug eventually is metabolized in the liver. Ethchlorvynol is used as a short-term hypnotic for the management of insomnia.

The most common side effects caused by ethchlorvynol are a mintlike aftertaste, dizziness, nausea, vomiting, hypotension, and facial numbness. Mild "hangover" also is relatively common. An occasional patient responds with profound hypnosis, muscular weakness, and syncope unrelated to marked hypotension. Idiosyncratic responses range from mild stimulation to marked excitement and hysteria. Hypersensitivity reactions include urticaria, rare but sometimes fatal thrombocytopenia, and occasionally, cholestatic jaundice. Acute intoxication resembles that produced by barbiturates, except for more severe respiratory depression and a relative bradycardia. Ethchlorvynol may enhance the hepatic metabolism of other drugs such as oral anticoagulants, and it is contraindicated in patients with intermittent porphyria.

Meprobamate. Meprobamate is a *bis*-carbamate ester; it was introduced as an antianxiety agent in 1955, and this remains its only approved use in the United States. However, it also became popular as a sedative-hypnotic drug, and it is discussed here mainly because of its continued use for such purposes. The question of whether the sedative and antianxiety actions of meprobamate differ is unanswered, and clinical proof for the efficacy of meprobamate as a selective antianxiety agent in human beings is lacking.

The pharmacological properties of meprobamate resemble those of the benzodiazepines in a number of ways. Meprobamate can release suppressed behaviors in experimental animals at doses that cause little impairment of locomotor activity, and although it can cause widespread depression of the CNS, it cannot produce anesthesia. However, ingestion of large doses of meprobamate alone can cause severe or even fatal respiratory depression, hypotension, shock, and heart failure. Meprobamate appears to have a mild analgesic effect in patients with musculoskeletal pain, and it enhances the analgesic effects of other drugs.

Meprobamate is well absorbed when administered orally. Nevertheless, an important aspect of intoxication with meprobamate is the formation of gastric bezoars consisting of undissolved meprobamate tablets; hence treatment may require endoscopy, with mechanical removal of the bezoar. Most of the drug is metabolized in the liver, mainly to a side-chain hydroxy derivative and a glucuronide; the kinetics of elimination may depend on the dose. The half-life of meprobamate may be prolonged during its chronic administration, even though the drug can induce some hepatic CYPs.

The major unwanted effects of the usual sedative doses of meprobamate are drowsiness and ataxia; larger doses produce considerable impairment of learning and motor coordination and prolongation of reaction time. Like the benzodiazepines, meprobamate enhances the CNS depression produced by other drugs.

The abuse of meprobamate has continued despite a substantial decrease in the clinical use of the drug. *Carisoprodol* (SOMA), a skeletal muscle relaxant whose active metabolite is meprobamate, also has abuse potential and has become a popular "street drug" (Reeves *et al.*, 1999). Meprobamate is preferred to the benzodiazepines by subjects with a history of drug abuse. After long-term medication, abrupt discontinuation evokes a withdrawal syndrome usually characterized by anxiety, insomnia, tremors, and, frequently, hallucinations; generalized seizures occur in about 10% of cases. The intensity of symptoms depends on the dosage ingested.

Others. *Etomidate* (AMIDATE) is used in the United States and other countries as an intravenous anesthetic, often in combination with *fentanyl*. It is advantageous because it lacks pulmonary and vascular depressant activity, although it has a negative inotropic effect on the heart. Its pharmacology and anesthetic uses are described in Chapter 13. It also is used in some countries as a sedative-hypnotic drug in intensive care units, during intermittent positive-pressure breathing, in epidural anesthesia, and in other situations. Because it is administered only intravenously, its use is limited to hospital settings. The myoclonus commonly seen after anesthetic doses is not seen after sedative-hypnotic doses.

Clomethiazole has sedative, muscle relaxant, and anticonvulsant properties. It is used outside the United States for hypnosis in elderly and institutionalized patients, for preanesthetic sedation, and especially in the management of withdrawal from ethanol (*see* Symposium, 1986b). Given alone, its effects on respiration are slight, and the therapeutic index is high. However, deaths from adverse interactions with ethanol are relatively frequent.

Propofol (DIPRIVAN) is a rapidly acting and highly lipophilic diisopropylphenol used in the induction and maintenance of general anesthesia (*see* Chapter 13), as well as in the maintenance of long-term sedation. Propofol sedation is of a similar quality to that produced by midazolam. Emergence from sedation occurs quickly owing to its rapid clearance (McKeage and Perry, 2003). Propofol has found use in intensive care sedation in adults (McKeage and Perry, 2003), as well as for sedation during gastrointestinal endoscopy procedures (Heuss and Inauen, 2004) and transvaginal oocyte retrieval (Dell and Cloote, 1998). Although its mechanism of action is not understood completely, propofol is believed to act primarily through enhancement of GABA$_A$-receptor function. Effects on other ligand-gated and G protein–coupled receptors, however, also have been reported (Trapani *et al.*, 2000).

Nonprescription Hypnotic Drugs. As part of the ongoing systematic review of over-the-counter (OTC) drug products, the FDA has ruled that *diphenhydramine* is the only ingredient that is recognized as generally safe and effective for use in nonprescription sleep aids. Despite the prominent sedative side effects encountered during the use of antihistamines previously included in OTC sleep aids (*e.g.*, *doxylamine* and *pyrilamine*), these agents have been eliminated as ingredients in the OTC nighttime sleep aids marketed in the United States. With an elimination half-life of about 9 hours, the nighttime use of diphenhydramine can be associated with prominent residual daytime sleepiness.

MANAGEMENT OF INSOMNIA

Insomnia is one of the most common complaints in general medical practice, and its treatment is predicated on proper diagnosis. Although the precise function of sleep is not known, adequate sleep improves the quality of daytime wakefulness, and hypnotics should be used judiciously to avoid its impairment.

A number of pharmacological agents are available for the treatment of insomnia. The "perfect" hypnotic would allow sleep to occur with normal sleep architecture rather than produce a pharmacologically altered sleep pattern. It would not cause next-day effects, either of rebound anxiety or of continued sedation. It would not interact with other medications. It could be used chronically without causing dependence or rebound insomnia on discontinuation. Regular moderate exercise meets these criteria but often is not effective by itself, and many patients may not be able to exercise. However, even small amounts of exercise often are effective in promoting sleep.

Controversy in the management of insomnia revolves around two issues: pharmacological *versus* nonpharmacological treatment and the use of short-acting *versus* long-acting hypnotics. The side effects of hypnotic medications must be weighed against the sequelae of chronic insomnia, which include a fourfold increase in serious accidents (Balter and Uhlenhuth, 1992). Two aspects of the management of insomnia traditionally have been underappreciated: a search for specific medical causes and the use of nonpharmacological treatments. In addition to appropriate pharmacological treatment, the management of insomnia should correct identifiable causes, address inadequate sleep hygiene, eliminate performance anxiety related to falling asleep, provide entrainment of the biological clock so that maximum sleepiness occurs at the hour of attempted sleep, and suppress the use of alcohol and OTC sleep medications (Nino-Murcia, 1992).

Categories of Insomnia. The National Institute of Mental Health Consensus Development Conference (1984) divided insomnia into three categories:

1. *Transient insomnia* lasts less than 3 days and usually is caused by a brief environmental or situational stressor. It may respond to attention to sleep hygiene rules. If hypnotics are prescribed, they should be used at the lowest dose and for only 2 to 3 nights. However, benzodiazepines given acutely before important life events, such as examinations, may result in impaired performance (James and Savage, 1984).
2. *Short-term insomnia* lasts from 3 days to 3 weeks and usually is caused by a personal stressor such as illness, grief, or job problems. Again, sleep hygiene education is the first step. Hypnotics may be used adjunctively for 7 to 10 nights. Hypnotics are best used intermittently during this time, with the patient skipping a dose after 1 to 2 nights of good sleep.
3. *Long-term insomnia* is insomnia that has lasted for more than 3 weeks; no specific stressor may be identifiable. A more complete medical evaluation is necessary in these patients, but most do not need an all-night sleep study.

Insomnia Accompanying Major Psychiatric Illnesses. The insomnia caused by major psychiatric illnesses often responds to specific pharmacological treatment for that illness. In major depressive episodes with insomnia, for example, the selective serotonin reuptake inhibitors, which may cause insomnia as a side effect, usually will result in *improved* sleep because they treat the depressive syndrome. In patients whose depression is responding to the serotonin reuptake inhibitor but who have persistent insomnia as a side effect of the medication, judicious use of evening *trazodone* may improve sleep (Nierenberg *et al.*, 1994), as well as augment the antidepressant effect of the reuptake inhibitor. However, the patient should be monitored for priapism, orthostatic hypotension, and arrhythmias.

Adequate control of anxiety in patients with anxiety disorders often produces adequate resolution of the accompanying insomnia. Sedative use in the anxiety disorders is decreasing because of a growing appreciation of the effectiveness of other agents, such as β adrenergic receptor antagonists (*see* Chapter 10) for performance anxiety and serotonin reuptake inhibitors for obsessive-compulsive disorder and perhaps generalized anxiety disorder. The profound insomnia of patients with acute psychosis owing to schizophrenia or mania usually responds to dopamine-receptor antagonists (*see* Chapter 18). Benzodiazepines often are used adjunctively in this situation to reduce agitation; their use also will result in improved sleep.

Insomnia Accompanying Other Medical Illnesses. For long-term insomnia owing to other medical illnesses, adequate treatment of the underlying disorder, such as congestive heart failure, asthma, or COPD, may resolve the insomnia.

Adequate pain management in conditions of chronic pain, including terminal cancer pain, will treat both the pain and the insomnia and may make hypnotics unnecessary.

Many patients simply manage their sleep poorly. *Adequate attention to sleep hygiene, including reduced caffeine intake, avoidance of alcohol, adequate exercise, and regular sleep and wake times, often will reduce the insomnia.*

Conditioned (Learned) Insomnia. In those who have no major psychiatric or other medical illness and in whom attention to sleep hygiene is ineffective, attention should be directed to conditioned (learned) insomnia. These patients have associated the bedroom with activities consistent with wakefulness rather than sleep. In such patients, the bed should be used only for sex and sleep. All other activities associated with waking, even such quiescent activities as reading and watching television, should be done outside the bedroom.

Sleep-State Misperception. Some patients complain of poor sleep but have been shown to have no objective polysomnographic evidence of insomnia. They are difficult to treat.

Long-Term Insomnia. Nonpharmacological treatments are important for all patients with long-term insomnia. These include education about sleep hygiene, adequate exercise (where possible), relaxation training, and behavioral-modification approaches, such as sleep-restriction and stimulus-control therapies. In sleep-restriction therapy, the patient keeps a diary of the amount of time spent in bed and then chooses a time in bed of 30 to 60 minutes less than this time. This induces a mild sleep debt, which aids sleep onset. In stimulus-control therapy, the patient is instructed to go to bed only when sleepy, to use the bedroom only for sleep and sex, to get up and leave the bedroom if sleep does not occur within 15 to 20 minutes, to return to bed again only when sleepy, to arise at the same time each morning regardless of sleep quality the preceding night, and to avoid daytime naps. Nonpharmacological treatments for insomnia have been found to be particularly effective in reducing sleep-onset latency and time awake after sleep onset (Morin *et al.*, 1994).

Side effects of hypnotic agents may limit their usefulness for insomnia management. The use of hypnotics for long-term insomnia is problematic for many reasons. Long-term hypnotic use leads to a decrease in effectiveness and may produce rebound insomnia on discontinuance. Almost all hypnotics change sleep architecture. The barbiturates reduce REM sleep; the benzodiazepines reduce slow-wave non-REM sleep and, to a lesser extent, REM sleep. While the significance of these findings is not clear, there is an emerging consensus that slow-wave sleep is particularly important for physical restorative processes. REM sleep may aid in the consolidation of learning. The blockade of slow-wave sleep by benzodiazepines may partly account for their diminishing effectiveness over the long term, and it also may explain their effectiveness in blocking sleep terrors, a disorder of arousal from slow-wave sleep.

Long-acting benzodiazepines can cause next-day confusion, with a concomitant increase in falls, whereas shorter-acting agents can produce rebound next-day anxiety. Paradoxically, the acute amnestic effects of benzodiazepines may be responsible for the patient's subsequent report of restful sleep. Triazolam has been postulated to induce cognitive changes that blur the subjective distinction between waking and sleeping (Mendelson, 1993). Anterograde amnesia may be more common with triazolam. While the performance-disruptive effects of alcohol and diphenhydramine are reduced after napping, those of triazolam are not (Roehrs *et al.*, 1993).

Benzodiazepines may worsen sleep apnea. Some hypersomnia patients do not feel refreshed after a night's sleep and so may ask for sleeping pills to improve the quality of their sleep. The consensus is that hypnotics should not be given to patients with sleep apnea, especially of the obstructive type, because these agents decrease upper airway muscle tone while also decreasing the arousal response to hypoxia (Robinson and Zwillich, 1989). These individuals benefit from all-night sleep studies to guide treatment.

Insomnia in Older Patients.

The elderly, like the very young, tend to sleep in a *polyphasic* (multiple sleep episodes per day) pattern rather than the *monophasic* pattern characteristic of younger adults. They may have single or multiple daytime naps in addition to nighttime sleep. This pattern makes assessment of adequate sleep time difficult. Anyone who naps regularly will have shortened nighttime sleep without evidence of impaired daytime wakefulness, regardless of age. This pattern is exemplified in "siesta" cultures and probably is adaptive.

Changes in the pharmacokinetic profiles of hypnotic agents occur in the elderly because of reduced body water, reduced renal function, and increased body fat, leading to a longer half-life for benzodiazepines. A dose that produces pleasant sleep and adequate daytime wakefulness during week 1 of administration may produce daytime confusion and amnesia by week 3 as the level continues to rise, particularly with long-acting hypnotics. For example, the benzodiazepine diazepam is highly lipid soluble and is excreted by the kidney. Because of the increase in body fat and the decrease in

renal excretion that typically occur from age 20 to 80, the half-life of the drug may increase fourfold over this span.

Elderly people who are living full lives with relatively unimpaired daytime wakefulness may complain of insomnia because they are not sleeping as long as they did when they were younger. Injudicious use of hypnotics in these individuals can produce daytime cognitive impairment and so impair overall quality of life.

Once an older patient has been taking benzodiazepines for an extended period, whether for daytime anxiety or for nighttime sedation, terminating the drug can be a long, involved process. Since attempts at drug withdrawal may not be successful, it may be necessary to leave the patient on the medication, with adequate attention to daytime side effects.

Management of Patients after Long-Term Treatment with Hypnotic Agents.

Patients who have been taking hypnotics for many months or even years pose a special problem (Fleming, 1993). If a benzodiazepine has been used regularly for more than 2 weeks, it should be tapered rather than discontinued abruptly. In some patients on hypnotics with a short half-life, it is easier to switch first to a hypnotic with a long half-life and then to taper. In a study in which the nonbenzodiazepine agent zopiclone was abruptly substituted for a benzodiazepine agent for 1 month and then itself abruptly terminated, improved sleep was reported during the zopiclone treatment, and withdrawal effects were absent on discontinuation of zopiclone (Shapiro *et al.*, 1993).

The onset of withdrawal symptoms from medications with a long half-life may be delayed. Consequently, the patient should be warned about the symptoms associated with withdrawal effects.

Prescribing Guidelines for the Management of Insomnia.

Hypnotics that act at $GABA_A$ receptors, including the benzodiazepine hypnotics and the newer agents zolpidem, zopiclone, and zaleplon, are preferred to barbiturates because they have a greater therapeutic index, are less toxic in overdose, have smaller effects on sleep architecture, and have less abuse potential. Compounds with a shorter half-life are favored in patients with sleep-onset insomnia but without significant daytime anxiety who need to function at full effectiveness all day. These compounds also are appropriate for the elderly because of a decreased risk of falls and respiratory depression. However, the patient and physician should be aware that early-morning awakening, rebound daytime anxiety, and amnestic episodes also may occur.

These undesirable side effects are more common at higher doses of the benzodiazepines.

Benzodiazepines with longer half-lives are favored for patients who have significant daytime anxiety and who may be able to tolerate next-day sedation but would be impaired further by rebound daytime anxiety. These benzodiazepines also are appropriate for patients receiving treatment for major depressive episodes because the short-acting agents can worsen early-morning awakening. However, longer-acting benzodiazepines can be associated with next-day cognitive impairment or delayed daytime cognitive impairment (after 2 to 4 weeks of treatment) as a result of drug accumulation with repeated administration.

Older agents such as barbiturates, glutethimide, and meprobamate should be avoided for the management of insomnia. They have high abuse potential and are dangerous in overdose.

BIBLIOGRAPHY

Amin, J., and Weiss, D.S. GABA$_A$ receptor needs two homologous domains of the β-subunit for activation by GABA but not by pentobarbital. *Nature,* **1993,** *366*:565–569.

Balter, M.B., and Uhlenhuth, E.H. New epidemiologic findings about insomnia and its treatment. *J. Clin. Psychiatry,* **1992,** *53*(suppl):34–39.

Cavallaro, R., Regazzetti, M.G., Covelli, G., and Smeraldi, E. Tolerance and withdrawal with zolpidem. *Lancet,* **1993,** *342*:374–375.

Dell, R.G. and Cloote, A.H. Patient-controlled sedation during transvaginal oocyte retrieval: An assessment of patient acceptance of patient-controlled sedation using a mixture of propofol and alfentanil. *Eur. J. Anaesthesiol.,* **1998,** *15*:210–215.

Dresser, G.K., Spence, J.D., and Bailey, D.G. Pharmacokinetic–pharmacodynamic consequences and clinical relevance of cytochrome P450 3A4 inhibition. *Clin. Pharmacokinet.,* **2000,** *38*:41–57.

Dujardin, K., Guieu, J.D., Leconte-Lambert, C., *et al.* Comparison of the effects of zolpidem and flunitrazepam on sleep structure and daytime cognitive functions: A study of untreated insomniacs. *Pharmacopsychiatry,* **1998,** *31*:14–18.

Fleming, J.A. The difficult to treat insomniac patient. *J. Psychosom. Res.,* **1993,** *37*(suppl 1):45–54.

ffrench-Mullen, J.M., Barker, J.L., and Rogawski, M.A. Calcium current block by (–)-pentobarbital, phenobarbital, and CHEB but not (+)-pentobarbital in acutely isolated hippocampal CA1 neurons: Comparison with effects on GABA-activated Cl⁻ current. *J. Neurosci.,* **1993,** *13*:3211–3221.

Frenkel, C., Duch, D.S., and Urban, B.W. Molecular actions of pentobarbital isomers on sodium channels from human brain cortex. *Anesthesiology,* **1990,** *72*:640–649.

Griffiths, R.R., Sannerud, C.A., Ator, N.A., and Brady, J.V. Zolpidem behavioral pharmacology in baboons: Self-injection, discrimination, tolerance and withdrawal. *J. Pharmacol. Exp. Ther.,* **1992,** *260*:1199–1208.

Guglielminotti, J., Maury, E., Alzieu, M., *et al.* Prolonged sedation requiring mechanical ventilation and continuous flumazenil infusion after routine doses of clonazepam for alcohol withdrawal syndrome. *Intensive Care Med.,* **1999,** *25*:1435–1436.

Herrmann, W.M., Kubicki, S.T., Boden, S., *et al.* Pilot controlled, double-blind study of the hypnotic effects of zolpidem in patients with chronic "learned" insomnia: Psychometric and polysomnographic evaluation. *J. Int. Med. Res.,* **1993,** *21*:306–322.

Hindmarch, I., Fairweather, D.B., and Rombaut, N. Adverse events after triazolam substitution. *Lancet,* **1993,** *341*:55.

James, I. and Savage, I. Beneficial effect of nadolol on anxiety-induced disturbances of performance in musicians: A comparison with diazepam and placebo. *Am. Heart J.,* **1984,** *108*:1150–1155.

Kriel, R.L., Cloyd, J.C., and Pellock, J.M. Respiratory depression in children receiving diazepam for acute seizures: A prospective study. *Dev. Med. Child Neurol.,* **2000,** *42*:429–430.

Kummer, J., Guendel, L., Linden, J., *et al.* Long-term polysomnographic study of the efficacy and safety of zolpidem in elderly psychiatric inpatients with insomnia. *J. Int. Med. Res.,* **1993,** *21*:171–184.

Lader, M., and File, S. The biological basis of benzodiazepine dependence. *Psychol. Med.,* **1987,** *17*:539–547.

Lovinger, D.M., Zimmerman, S.A., Levitin, M., *et al.* Trichloroethanol potentiates synaptic transmission mediated by γ-aminobutyric acid$_A$ receptors in hippocampal neurons. *J. Pharmacol. Exp. Ther.,* **1993,** *264*:1097–1103.

Lüddens, H., Pritchett, D.B., Köhler, M., *et al.* Cerebellar GABA$_A$ receptor selective for a behavioural alcohol antagonist. *Nature,* **1990,** *346*:648–651.

Macdonald, R.L., and McLean, M.J. Cellular bases of barbiturate and phenytoin anticonvulsant drug action. *Epilepsia,* **1982,** *23*(suppl 1):S7–S18.

Marszalec, W., and Narahashi, T. Use-dependent pentobarbital block of kainate and quisqualate currents. *Brain Res.,* **1993,** *608*:7–15.

Martin, P.R., Bhushan, C.M., Kapur, B.M., *et al.* Intravenous phenobarbital therapy in barbiturate and other hypnosedative withdrawal reactions: A kinetic approach. *Clin. Pharmacol. Ther.* **1979,** *26*:256–264.

Mendelson, W.B. Pharmacologic alteration of the perception of being awake or asleep. *Sleep,* **1993,** *16*:641–646.

Meyer, B.R. Benzodiazepines in the elderly. *Med. Clin. North Am.,* **1982,** *66*:1017–1035.

Monane, M. Insomnia in the elderly. *J. Clin. Psychiatry,* **1992,** *53*(suppl):23–28.

Morin, C.M., Culbert, J.P., and Schwartz, S.M. Nonpharmacological interventions for insomnia: A meta-analysis of treatment efficacy. *Am. J. Psychiatry,* **1994,** *151*:1172–1180.

Morselli, P.L. Zolpidem side effects. *Lancet,* **1993,** *342*:868–869.

Nattel, S., Wang, Z.G., and Matthews, C. Direct electrophysiological actions of pentobarbital at concentrations achieved during general anesthesia. *Am. J. Physiol.,* **1990,** *259*:H1743–H1751.

Nierenberg, A.A., Adler, L.A., Peselow, E., *et al.* Trazodone for antidepressant-associated insomnia. *Am. J. Psychiatry,* **1994,** *151*:1069–1072.

Nugent, M., Artru, A.A., and Michenfelder, J.D. Cerebral metabolic, vascular and protective effects of midazolam maleate: Comparison to diazepam. *Anesthesiology,* **1982,** *56*:172–176.

Oldenhof, H., de Jong, M., Steenhoek, A., and Janknegt, R. Clinical pharmacokinetics of midazolam in intensive care patients, a wide interpatient variability? *Clin. Pharmacol. Ther.,* **1988,** *43*:263–269.

Pancrazio, J.J., Frazer, M.J., and Lynch, C., III. Barbiturate anesthetics depress the resting K⁺ conductance of myocardium. *J. Pharmacol. Exp. Ther.,* **1993,** *265*:358–365.

Perrault, G., Morel, E., Sanger, D.J., and Zivkovic, B. Lack of tolerance and physical dependence upon repeated treatment with the novel hypnotic zolpidem. *J. Pharmacol. Exp. Ther.,* **1992,** *263:*298–303.

Polc, P. Electrophysiology of benzodiazepine receptor ligands: Multiple mechanisms and sites of action. *Prog. Neurobiol.,* **1988,** *31:*349–423.

Reeves, R.R., Carter, O.S., Pinkofsky, H.B., *et al.* Carisoprodol (SOMA): Abuse potential and physician unawareness. *J. Addict. Dis.,* **1999,** *18:*51–56.

Roehrs, T., Claiborue, D., Knox, M., and Roth, T. Effects of ethanol, diphenhydramine, and triazolam after a nap. *Neuropsychopharmacology,* **1993,** *9:*239–245.

Roncari, G., Timm, U., Zell, M., *et al.* Flumazenil kinetics in the elderly. *Eur. J. Clin. Pharmacol.,* **1993,** *45:*585–587.

Roth, T., and Roehrs, T.A. Issues in the use of benzodiazepine therapy. *J. Clin. Psychiatry,* **1992,** *53*(suppl):14–18.

Shapiro, C.M., MacFarlane, J.G., and MacLean, A.W. Alleviating sleep-related discontinuance symptoms associated with benzodiazepine withdrawal: A new approach. *J. Psychosom. Res.,* **1993,** *37*(suppl 1):55–57.

Spivey, W.H. Flumazenil and seizures: An analysis of 43 cases. *Clin. Ther.,* **1992,** *14:*292–305.

Trapani, G., Altomare, C., Liso, G., *et al.* Propofol in anesthesia: Mechanism of action, structure–activity relationships, and drug delivery. *Curr. Med. Chem.,* **2000,** *7:*249–271.

Twyman, R.E., Rogers, C.J., and Macdonald, R.L. Differential regulation of -aminobutyric acid receptor channels by diazepam and phenobarbital. *Ann. Neurol.,* **1989,** *25:*213–220.

Uhlenhuth, E.H., Balter, M.B., Ban, T.A., and Yang, K. International study of expert judgment on therapeutic use of benzodiazepines and other psychotherapeutic medications: IV. Therapeutic dose dependence and abuse liability of benzodiazepines in the long-term treatment of anxiety disorders. *J. Clin Psychopharmacol.,* **1999,** *19*(6 suppl 2):23S–29S.

Walsh, J.K., Vogel, G.W., Schart, M., *et al.* A five-week polysomnographic assessment of zaleplon 10 mg for the treatment of primary insomnia. *Sleep Med.,* **2000,** *1:*41–49.

MONOGRAPHS AND REVIEWS

Anonymous. Zolpidem for insomnia. *Med. Lett. Drugs Ther.,* **1993,** *35:*35–36.

Burt, D.R. Reducing GABA receptors. *Life Sci.,* **2003,** *73:*1741–1758.

Dement, W.C. Objective measurements of daytime sleepiness and performance comparing quazepam with flurazepam in two adult populations using the Multiple Sleep Latency Test. *J. Clin. Psychiatry,* **1991,** *52*(suppl):31–37.

Dooley, M., and Plosker, G.L. Zaleplon: A review of its use in the treatment of insomnia. *Drugs,* **2000,** *60:*413–445.

Essrich, C., Lorez, M., Benson, J.A., *et al.* Postsynaptic clustering of major $GABA_A$ receptor subtypes requires the $\gamma 2$ subunit and gephyrin. *Nature Neurosci.,* **1998,** *1:*563–571.

File, S.E. Tolerance to the behavioral actions of benzodiazepines. *Neurosci. Biobehav. Rev.,* **1985,** *9:*113–121.

Gardner, C.R., Tully, W.R., and Hedgecock, C.J. The rapidly expanding range of neuronal benzodiazepine receptor ligands. *Prog. Neurobiol.,* **1993,** *40:*1–61.

Garnier, R., Guerault, E., Muzard, D., *et al.* Acute zolpidem poisoning—analysis of 344 cases. *J. Toxicol. Clin. Toxicol.,* **1994,** *32:*391–404.

Gary, N.E., and Tresznewsky, O. Clinical aspects of drug intoxication: Barbiturates and a potpourri of other sedatives, hypnotics, and tranquilizers. *Heart Lung,* **1983,** *12:*122–127.

Gillin, J.C., Spinweber, C.L., and Johnson, L.C. Rebound insomnia: A critical review. *J. Clin. Psychopharmacol.,* **1989,** *9:*161–172.

Greenblatt, D.J. Benzodiazepine hypnotics: Sorting the pharmacokinetic facts. *J. Clin. Psychiatry,* **1991,** *52*(suppl):4–10.

Heuss, L.T., and Inauen, W. The dawning of a new sedative: Propofol in gastrointestinal endoscopy. *Digestion,* **2004,** *69:*20–26.

Hoffman, E.J., and Warren, E.W. Flumazenil: A benzodiazepine antagonist. *Clin. Pharm.,* **1993,** *12:*641–656.

Holm, K.J., and Goa, K.L. Zolpidem: An update of its pharmacology, therapeutic efficacy and tolerability in the treatment of insomnia. *Drugs,* **2000,** *59:*865–889.

Jonas, J.M., Coleman, B.S., Sheridan, A.Q., and Kalinske, R.W. Comparative clinical profiles of triazolam versus other shorter-acting hypnotics. *J. Clin. Psychiatry,* **1992,** *53*(suppl):19–31.

Kleingoor, C., Wieland, H.A., Korpi, E.R., *et al.* Current potentiation by diazepam but not GABA sensitivity is determined by a single histidine residue. *Neuroreport,* **1993,** *4:*187–190.

Langtry, H.D., and Benfield, P. Zolpidem: A review of its pharmacodynamic and pharmacokinetic properties and therapeutic potential. *Drugs,* **1990,** *40:*291–313.

Laurijssens, B.E., and Greenblatt, D.J. Pharmacokinetic–pharmacodynamic relationships for benzodiazepines (review). *Clin. Pharmacokinet.,* **1996,** *30:*52–76.

Macdonald, R.L., and McLean, M.J. Anticonvulsant drugs: mechanisms of action. *Adv. Neurol.,* **1986,** *44:*713–736.

McKeage, K., and Perry, C.M. Propofol: A review of its use in intensive care sedation of adults. *CNS Drugs,* **2003,** *17:*235–272.

Mendelson, W.B. Neuropharmacology of sleep induction by benzodiazepines. *Crit. Rev. Neurobiol.,* **1992,** *6:*221–232.

Mitler, M.M. Nonselective and selective benzodiazepine receptor agonists—where are we today? *Sleep,* **2000,** *23*(suppl 1):S39–S47.

National Institute of Mental Health Consensus Development Conference. Drugs and insomnia: The use of medications to promote sleep. *JAMA,* **1984,** *251:*2410–2414.

Nino-Murcia, G. Diagnosis and treatment of insomnia and risks associated with lack of treatment. *J. Clin. Psychiatry,* **1992,** *53*(suppl):43–47.

Petursson, H. The benzodiazepine withdrawal syndrome. *Addiction,* **1994,** *89:*1455–1459.

Phillis, J.W., and O'Regan, M.H. The role of adenosine in the central actions of the benzodiazepines. *Prog. Neuropsychopharmacol. Biol. Psychiatry,* **1988,** *12:*389–404.

Pritchett, D.B., and Seeburg, P.H. γ-Aminobutyric acid A receptor $\alpha 5$-subunit creates novel type II benzodiazepine receptor pharmacology. *J. Neurochem.,* **1990,** *54:*1802–1804.

Robinson, R.W., and Zwillich, C.W. The effect of drugs on breathing during sleep. In, *Principles and Practice of Sleep Medicine.* (Kryger, M.H., Roth, T., and Dement, W.C., eds.) Saunders, Philadelphia, **1989.**

Rothschild, A.J. Disinhibition, amnestic reactions, and other adverse reactions secondary to triazolam: A review of the literature. *J. Clin. Psychiatry,* **1992,** *53*(suppl):69–79.

Saunders, P.A., and Ho, I.K. Barbiturates and the $GABA_A$ receptor complex. *Prog. Drug Res.,* **1990,** *34:*261–286.

Shapiro, H.M. Barbiturates in brain ischaemia. *Br. J. Anaesth.,* **1985,** *57:*82–95.

Sieghart, W., Fuchs, K., Tretter, V., *et al.* Structure and subunit composition of $GABA_A$ receptors. *Neurochem Int.,* **1999,** *34:*379–385.

Smith, M.C., and Riskin, B.J. The clinical use of barbiturates in neurological disorders. *Drugs,* **1991,** *42*:365–378.

Symposium (various authors). Modern hypnotics and performance. (Nicholson, A., Hippius, H., Rüther, E., and Dunbar, G., eds.) *Acta Psychiatr. Scand. Suppl.,* **1986a,** *332*:3–174.

Symposium (various authors). Chlormethiazole 25 years: Recent developments and historical perspectives. (Evans, J.G., Feuerlein, W., Glatt, M.M., Kanowski, S., and Scott, D.B., eds.) *Acta Psychiatr. Scand. Suppl.,* **1986b,** *329*:1–198.

Symposium (various authors). Critical issues in the management of insomnia: Investigators report on estazolam. (Roth. T., ed.) *Am. J. Med.,* **1990,** *88*(suppl):1S–48S.

Tanaka, E. Clinically significant pharmacokinetic drug interactions with benzodiazepines. *J. Clin. Pharm. Ther.,* **1999,** *24*:347–355.

Whiting, P.J. The GABA$_A$ receptor gene family: New opportunities for drug development. *Curr. Opin. Drug. Discov. Dev.,* **2003,** 6:648–657.

Woods, J.H., Katz, J.L., and Winger, G. Benzodiazepines: Use, abuse, and consequences. *Pharmacol. Rev.,* **1992,** *44*:151–347.

Woods, J.H., and Winger, G. Abuse liability of flunitrazepam. *J. Clin. Psychopharmacol.,* **1997,** *17*:1S–57S.

DRUG THERAPY OF DEPRESSION AND ANXIETY DISORDERS

Ross J. Baldessarini

The availability and use of drugs with demonstrable efficacy in psychiatric disorders has grown since the late 1950s to the point that 10% to 15% of prescriptions written in the U.S. are for medications intended to affect mental processes—to sedate, stimulate or otherwise modify mood, thinking or behavior. The optimal use of psychotropic drugs requires familiarity with the differential diagnosis of psychiatric conditions (American Psychiatric Association, 2000; and Sadock and Sadock, 2000).

The development of psychotropic agents has occurred in conjunction with studies of receptor-effector systems and bio-synthetic and degradative pathways of monoamine neurotransmitters (e.g., catecholamines and serotonin [5-HT], as described in Chapters 6, 11 and 12). Mechanistic interpretations of the efficacy of psychotropic drugs in the CNS have propelled investigations into the causes of mental illness (Baldessarini, 2000). The antipsychotic, mood-stabilizing, and antidepressant agents used to treat the most severe mental illnesses have had a remarkable impact on psychiatric practice and theory—an impact that legitimately can be called revolutionary and one that is experiencing continued innovation.

Although the rational development and assessment of efficacy of any drug is imperfect, the psychoactive drugs are particularly challenging. We do not understand the underlying pathogenesis of these disorders. Moreover, the essential characteristics of human mental disorders cannot be reproduced in animal models, just as affective states, communication, and social relationships in animals are difficult to compare with corresponding human conditions. Thus, screening procedures in animals for the discovery of novel psychotherapeutic agents have been of limited utility. Finally, clinical evaluation of new drugs is hampered by the lack of homogeneity within diagnostic groups and difficulty in applying valid and sensitive measurements of therapeutic effect. As a consequence, clinical trials of psychotropic agents often have yielded equivocal or inconsistent results. However, contemporary pharmacology provides many techniques for characterizing the actions of known psychotropic and other CNS-active agents at the cellular and molecular levels (*see* Chapters 1 and 12). Strategies that define the affinity of compounds for specific receptors or transporters can identify new agents and hopefully provide novel drugs for the therapy of psychiatric disorders (Kent, 2000).

Biological Hypotheses in Mental Illness. The introduction of relatively effective and selective drugs for the management of patients with schizophrenia and bipolar disorder encouraged the formulation of biological concepts for the pathogenesis of these major mental illnesses. In addition, other agents have been shown to mimic some of the symptoms of severe mental illness. These include LSD, which induces hallucinations and altered emotional states; antihypertensive agents such as reserpine, which can induce depression; and stimulants, which can induce manic or psychotic states when taken in excess. A leading hypothesis that arose from such considerations was that antidepressants enhance the biological activity of monoamine neurotransmitters in the CNS and that anti-adrenergic compounds may induce depression. These observations led to speculation that a deficiency of aminergic transmission in the CNS might cause depression, whereas an excess may result in mania. Further, antipsychotic-antimanic agents antagonize the neurotransmitter actions of dopamine in the forebrain, suggesting a possible state of functional overactivity of dopamine in the limbic system or cerebral cortex in schizophrenia or mania. Alternatively, an endogenous psychotomimetic compound might be produced either uniquely or in excessive quantities in psychotic patients. This "pharmacocentric" approach to the construction of hypotheses was appealing and gained strong encouragement from studies of the actions of antipsychotic and antidepressant drugs while further encouraging development of similar agents. In turn, the plausibility of such biological hypotheses has generated interest in genetic and clinical biochemical studies. Despite extensive efforts, attempts to document metabolic changes in human subjects predicted by these hypotheses have not provided consistent or compelling corroboration (Baldessarini, 2000; Musselman *et al.*, 1998). Moreover, results of genetic studies have demonstrated that inheritance accounts for only a portion of the causation of mental illnesses, leaving room for environmental and psychological hypotheses.

The antipsychotic, antianxiety, antimanic, and antidepressant drugs have effects on cortical, limbic, hypothalamic, and brainstem mechanisms that are of fundamental importance in the regulation of arousal, consciousness, affect, and autonomic functions. Physiological and pharmacological modifications of these brain regions may have important behavioral consequences and useful clinical effects regardless of the underlying cause of any mental disorder. The lack of diagnostic or even syndromal specificity of most psychotropic drugs tends to reduce the chances of finding a discrete metabolic correlate for a specific disease conceived simply on the actions of therapeutic agents. Finally, technical problems in studying changes in brain metabolism *in vivo* or the postmortem chemistry of the human brain are formidable. Among these are artifacts introduced by drug treatment itself.

In summary, there is no definitive link between discrete biological lesions and the pathogenesis of the most severe mental illnesses (other than delirium and the dementias). Even without such a link, we can provide effective medical treatment for psychiatric patients. It would be clinical folly to underestimate the importance of psychological and social factors in the manifestations of mental illnesses or to overlook psychological aspects of the conduct of biological therapies (Baldessarini, 2000).

CHARACTERIZATION OF DEPRESSIVE AND ANXIETY DISORDERS

The primary clinical manifestations of major depression are significant depression of mood and impairment of function. Some features of depressive disorders overlap those of the anxiety disorders, including *panic-agoraphobia* syndrome, severe *phobias, generalized anxiety disorder, social anxiety disorder, posttraumatic stress disorder,* and *obsessive-compulsive disorder.* Extremes of mood also may be associated with psychosis, as manifested by disordered or delusional thinking and perceptions that often are congruent with the predominant mood. Conversely, secondary changes in mood may be associated with psychotic disorders. This overlap of disorders can lead to errors in diagnosis and suboptimal treatment (American Psychiatric Association, 2000). Mood and anxiety disorders are the most common mental illnesses, each affecting up to 10% of the general population at some time in their lives (Kessler *et al.*, 1994).

Clinical depression must be distinguished from normal grief, sadness, disappointment, and the dysphoria or demoralization often associated with medical illness. The condition is underdiagnosed and frequently undertreated (McCombs *et al.*, 1990; Suominen *et al.*, 1998). Major depression is characterized by feelings of intense sadness and despair, mental slowing and loss of concentration, pessimistic worry, lack of pleasure, self-deprecation, and variable agitation or hostility. Physical changes also occur, particularly in severe, vital, or "melancholic" depression. These include insomnia or hypersomnia; altered eating patterns, with anorexia and weight loss or sometimes overeating; decreased energy and libido; and disruption of the normal circadian and ultradian rhythms of activity, body temperature, and many endocrine functions. As many as 10% to 15% of individuals with severe clinical depression, and up to 25% of those with bipolar disorder, display suicidal behavior at some time (Tondo *et al.*, 2003). Depressed patients usually respond to antidepressant drugs, or, in severe or treatment-resistant cases, to electroconvulsive therapy (ECT). This method remains the most rapid and effective treatment for severe acute depression and sometimes is life-saving for acutely suicidal patients (Rudorfer *et al.*, 1997). Efficacy of other forms of biological treatment of depression (*e.g.*, magnetic stimulation of the brain, or electrical stimulation of the vagus nerve) has not been well established. The decision to treat with an antidepressant is guided by the presenting clinical syndrome, its severity, and by the patient's personal and family history.

The major disorders of mood or affect include the syndromes of *major depression* (formerly termed *melancholia*) and *bipolar disorder* (formerly termed *manic-depressive disorder*). The lifetime prevalence of bipolar disorder is 1% to 2% for type I (with *mania*). It is about twice that rate if cases of recurrent depression with milder upswings of mood (*hypomania*) are included (type II bipolar disorder). Lifetime risk for major depression is considerably higher, at 5% to 10%, and approximately twice the risk in women than in men. These disorders commonly include disordered autonomic functioning (*e.g.*, altered rhythms of activity, sleep, and appetite) and behavior, as well as persistent abnormalities of mood. These disorders are associated with increased risk of self-harm or suicide as well as increased mortality from stress-sensitive general medical conditions, medical complications of comorbid abuse of alcohol or illicit drugs, or from accidents. Bipolar disorder is marked by a high likelihood of recurrences of severe depression and manic excitement, often with psychotic features.

The less pervasive psychiatric disorders include conditions formerly termed *psychoneuroses,* which currently are viewed as anxiety-associated disorders. The ability to comprehend reality is retained, but suffering and disability sometimes are severe. Anxiety disorders may be acute and transient, or more commonly, recurrent or persistent. Their symptoms may include mood changes (fear, panic, or dysphoria) or limited abnormalities of thought (obsessions, irrational fears, or phobias) or of behavior (avoidance, rituals or compulsions, pseudoneurological or "hysterical" conversion signs, or fixation on imagined or exaggerated physical symptoms). In such disorders drugs can have beneficial effects, particularly by modifying associated anxiety and depression to facilitate a more comprehensive program of treatment and rehabilitation. Antidepressants and sedative-antianxiety agents are commonly used to treat anxiety disorder.

Antidepressants

Most antidepressants exert important actions on the metabolism of monoamine neurotransmitters and their receptors, particularly norepinephrine and serotonin (Buckley and Waddington, 2000; Owens *et al.*, 1997) (Table 17–1).

History. *Monoamine Oxidase Inhibitors.* In 1951 *isoniazid* and its isopropyl derivative, ipronazid, were developed for the treatment of tuberculosis. Ipronazid, a hydrazine derivative, was observed to have mood-elevating effects in patients with tuberculosis, but owing to hepatotoxicity was abandoned for this use. In 1952 Zeller and coworkers found that ipronazid, in contrast to isoniazid, inhibited monoamine oxidase (MAO). Following investigations by Kline and by Crane in the mid-1950s, ipronazid (MARSILID) was used to treat depressed patients; historically, it was the first antidepressant to be used clinically (Healy, 1997). Two other hydrazine-derivative inhibitors of MAO, *phenelzine* (the structural analog of phenethylamine, an endogenous amine) and *isocarboxazid*, subsequently were introduced into clinical practice. *Tranylcypromine,* structurally related to amphetamine, was the first MAO inhibitor unrelated to hydrazine to be discovered and brought to the market. The development of reversible, selective MAO inhibitors with potentially broad applications (e.g., selegiline [eldepryl] for Parkinson's disease) was stimulated by the understanding that the early MAO inhibitors result in irreversible and nonselective blockade of both MAO-A and MAO-B, which were responsible for the metabolic breakdown of dopamine, norepinephrine, and serotonin in neuronal tissues. Three other MAO inhibitors that are used for purposes unrelated to MAO inhibition are *furazolidone* (FUROXONE, an anti-infective); *procarbazine* (MATULANE; N-methylhydrazine, indicated for the treatment of Hodgkin's disease); and *linezolid* (ZYVOX, an antibiotic used for serious infections).

Tricyclic Antidepressants and Selective Serotonin Reuptake Inhibitors. Häfliger and Schindler in the late 1940s synthesized a series of more than 40 iminodibenzyl derivatives for possible use as antihistamines, sedatives, analgesics, and antiparkinsonism drugs. One of these was imipramine, a dibenzazepine compound, which differs from the phenothiazines by replacement of the sulfur with an ethylene bridge to produce a seven-membered central ring analogous to the benzazepine antipsychotic agents (*see* Chapter 18). Following screening in animals, a few compounds, including imipramine, were selected for therapeutic trial on the basis of sedative or hypnotic properties. During clinical investigation of these putative phenothiazine analogs, Kuhn (1958) fortuitously found that unlike the phenothiazines, imipramine was relatively ineffective in quieting agitated psychotic patients, but it had a remarkable effect on depressed patients. Since then, indisputable evidence of its effectiveness in major depression has accumulated (Potter *et al.*, 1998; Thase and Nolen, 2000).

Older tricyclic antidepressants with a tertiary-amine side chain (including amitriptyline, doxepin, and imipramine) block neuronal uptake of both serotonin and norepinephrine, whereas clomipramine is relatively selective against serotonin (Table 17–2). Following this lead, even more selective serotonin reuptake inhibitors were developed in the early 1970s, arising from observations by Carlsson that antihistamines, including chlorpheniramine and diphenhydramine inhibited the transport of serotonin or norepinephrine. Chemical modifications led to the earliest selective serotonin reuptake inhibitor, *zimelidine,* soon followed by development of *fluoxetine* and *fluvoxamine* (Table 17–2) (Carlsson and Wong, 1997; Fuller, 1992; Masand and Gupta, 1999; Tollefson and Rosenbaum, 1998; Wong and Bymaster, 1995). Although first to market, zimelidine was withdrawn due to an association with febrile illness and Guillain-Barré ascending paralysis. Thus, fluoxetine and fluvoxamine were the first widely used selective serotonin reuptake inhibitors (often abbreviated as SSRIs or SRIs). Development of these agents was paralleled by the identification of compounds with selectivity for norepinephrine reuptake, along with others effective against both serotonin and norepinephrine reuptake—again with potential for applications beyond depression and/or anxiety (*e.g., atomoxetine* [STRATTERA]).

Chemistry and Structure-Activity Relationships. *Tricyclic Antidepressants.* The search for compounds related chemically to imipramine yielded multiple analogs. In addition to the dibenzazepines, imipramine and its secondary-amine congener and major active metabolite *desipramine,* and its 3-chloro derivative *clomipramine,* there are *amitriptyline* and its *N*-demethylated metabolite *nortriptyline* (dibenzocycloheptadienes), as well as *doxepin* (a dibenzoxepine) and *protriptyline* (a dibenzocycloheptatriene). Other structurally related agents are *trimipramine* (a dibenzazepine, with only weak effects on amine transport); *maprotiline* (a "tetracyclic" containing an additional ethylene bridge across the central six-carbon ring); and *amoxapine* (a piperazinyldibenzoxazepine with mixed antidepressant and neuroleptic properties). Since these agents all have a three-ring molecular core and most share pharmacological (norepinephrine-reuptake inhibition) and clinical (antidepressant and anxiolytic) properties, the name "tricyclic antidepressants" is used for this group. Structures and other features of antidepressant compounds are given in Table 17–1.

Selective Serotonin Reuptake Inhibitors. Citalopram and fluoxetine are racemates; *sertraline* and *paroxetine* are separate enantiomers. Escitalopram is the (*S*)-enantiomer of citalopram. Fluoxetine and its major metabolite norfluoxetine are highly active against serotonin transport and also may have antimigraine effects not found with the (*R*)-enantiomer of fluoxetine. The (*R*)-enantiomer of fluoxetine also is active against serotonin transport and is shorter acting than the (*S*)-enantiomer, but its clinical development was halted due to adverse electrocardiographic effects. (*R*)-Norfluoxetine is virtually inactive (Wong *et al.*, 1993). Structure-activity relationships are not well established for the SSRIs. However, it is known that the *para*-location of the CF_3 substituent of fluoxetine (Table 17–1) is critical for serotonin transporter potency. Its removal and substitution at the *ortho*-position with a methoxy group yields *nisoxetine,* a highly selective norepinephrine-uptake inhibitor.

Table 17-1
Antidepressants: Chemical Structures, Dose and Dosage Forms, and Side Effects

NONPROPRIETARY NAME (TRADE NAME)	DOSE AND DOSAGE FORMS			AMINE EFFECTS	SIDE EFFECTS								
	Usual Dose, mg/day	Extreme Dose, mg/day	Dosage Form		Agitation	Seizures	Sedation	Hypotension	Anticholinergic Effects	Gastrointestinal Effects	Weight Gain	Sexual Effects	Cardiac Effects
Norepinephrine Reuptake Inhibitors: Tertiary Amine Tricyclics													
Amitriptyline (ELAVIL and others) — C, H, C=CH(CH₂)₂N(CH₃)₂	100–200	25–300	O, I	NE, 5-HT	0	2+	3+	3+	3+	0/+	2+	2+	3+
Clomipramine (ANAFRANIL) — C, Cl, N—(CH₂)₃N(CH₃)₂	100–200	25–250	O	NE, 5-HT	0	3+	2+	2+	3+	+	2+	3+	3+
Doxepin (ADAPIN, SINEQUAN) — O, H, C=CH(CH₂)₂N(CH₃)₂	100–200	25–300	O	NE, 5-HT	0	2+	3+	2+	2+	0-+	2+	2+	3+
Imipramine (TOFRANIL and others) — C, H, N—(CH₂)₃N(CH₃)₂	100–200	25–300	O, I	NE, 5-HT	0/+	2+	2+	2+	2+	0/+	2+	2+	3+
(+)-Trimipramine (SURMONTIL) — C, H, N—CH₂CHCH₂N(CH₃)₂	75–200	25–300	O	NE, 5-HT	0	2+	3+	2+	3+	0/+	2+	2+	3+
Norepinephrine Reuptake Inhibitors: Secondary Amine Tricyclics													
Amoxapine (ASENDIN)	200–300	50–600	O	NE, DA	0	2+	+	2+	+	0/+	+	2+	2+
Desipramine (NORPRAMIN)	100–200	25–300	O	NE	+	+	0/+	+	+	0/+	+	2+	2+

432

Selective Serotonin Reuptake Inhibitors

Drug													
Maprotiline (LUDIOMIL) — CH₂CH₂CH₂NHCH₃	100–150	25–225	O	NE	0/+	3+	2+	2+	2+	0/+	+	2+	2+
Nortriptyline (PAMELOR) — CH₂CH₂CH₂NHCH₃	75–150	25–250	O	NE	0	+	+	+	+	0/+	+	2+	2+
Protriptyline (VIVACTIL) — CH₂CH₂CH₂NHCH₃	15–40	10–60	O	NE	2+	2+	0/+	+	+	2+	0/+	+	2+	3+
(±)-Citalopram (CELEXA)	20–40	10–60	O	5-HT	0/+	0	0/+	0	0	3+	0	3+	0
(+)-Escitalopram (LEXAPRO)	20–40	10–60	O	5-HT	0/+	0	0/+	0	0	3+	0	3+	0
(±)-Fluoxetine (PROZAC) — O–CHCH₂CH₂NHCH₃	20–40	5–50	O	5-HT	+	0/+	0/+	0	0	3+	0/+	3+	0/+

Maprotiline (LUDIOMIL): CH₂CH₂CH₂NHCH₃

Nortriptyline (PAMELOR): CH₂CH₂CH₂NHCH₃

Protriptyline (VIVACTIL): CH₂CH₂CH₂NHCH₃

(±)-Citalopram (CELEXA): F ... N≡C ... (CH₂)₃N(CH₃)₂

(+)-Escitalopram (LEXAPRO): NC ... (S) ... NMe₂ ... F

(±)-Fluoxetine (PROZAC): F₃C ... O–CHCH₂CH₂NHCH₃

(Continued)

Table 17–1

Antidepressants: Chemical Structures, Dose and Dosage Forms, and Side Effects (Continued)

NONPROPRIETARY NAME (TRADE NAME)	DOSE AND DOSAGE FORMS			AMINE EFFECTS	SIDE EFFECTS								
	Usual Dose, mg/day	Extreme Dose, mg/day	Dosage Form		Agitation	Seizures	Sedation	Hypotension	Anticholinergic Effects	Gastrointestinal Effects	Weight Gain	Sexual Effects	Cardiac Effects
Selective Serotonin Reuptake Inhibitors (*cont.*)													
Fluvoxamine (LUVOX)	100–200	50–300	O	5-HT	0	0	0/+	0	0	3+	0	3+	0
(–)-Paroxetine (PAXIL)	20–40	10–50	O	5-HT	+	0	0/+	0	0/+	3+	0	3+	0
(+)-Sertraline (ZOLOFT)	100–150	50–200	O	5-HT	+	0	0/+	0	0	3+	0	3+	0
(±)-Venlafaxine (EFFEXOR)	75–225	25–375	O	5-HT, NE	0/+	0	0	0	0	3+	0	3+	0/+

434

Atypical Antidepressants

Compound														
(−)-Atomoxetine (STRATTERA)	40–80 (children: 1.0–1.4 mg/kg)	20–150	O	NE	0	0	0	0	0	0/+	0	0	0
Bupropion (WELLBUTRIN)	200–300	100–450	O	DA, ?NE	3+	4+	0	0	0	2+	0	0	0
(+)-Duloxetine (CYMBALTA)	80–100	40–120	O	NE, 5-HT	+	0	0/+	0/+	0	0/+	0/+	0/+	0/+
(±)-Mirtazapine (REMERON)	15–45	7.5–45	O	5-HT, NE	0	0	4+	0/+	0	0/+	0/+	0	0
Nefazodone* (SERZONE)	200–400	100–600	O	5-HT	0	0	3+	0	0	2+	0/+	0/+	0/+

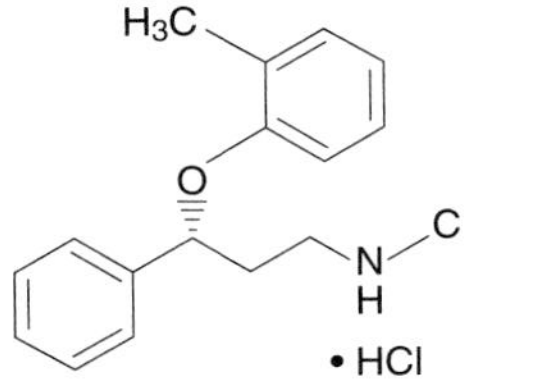

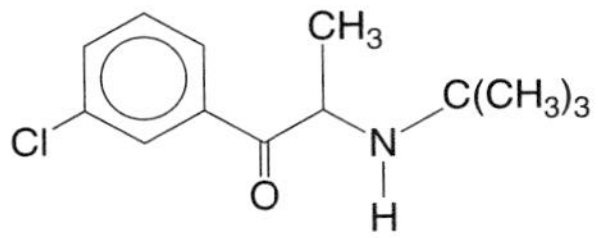

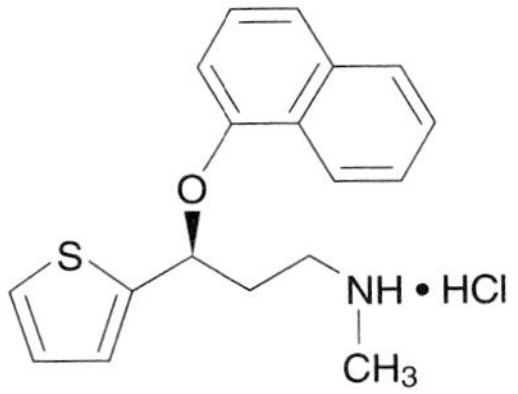

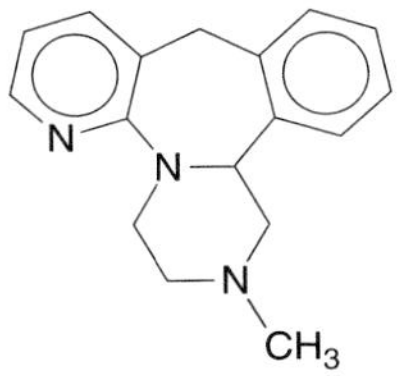

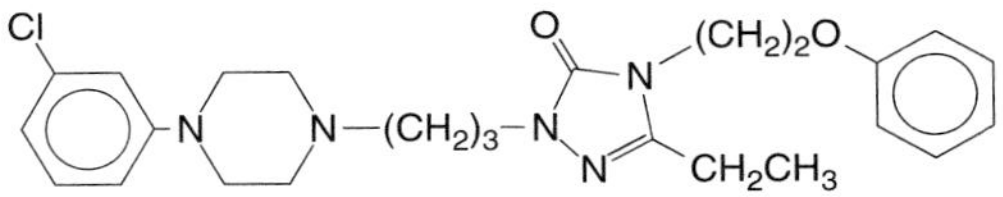

(−)-Atomoxetine (STRATTERA): H₃C–O–, •HCl, with N–H, C substituents

Bupropion (WELLBUTRIN): CH₃, C(CH₃)₃, N–H, O, Cl

(+)-Duloxetine (CYMBALTA): NH•HCl, CH₃, O, S

(±)-Mirtazapine (REMERON): N–CH₃, N

Nefazodone* (SERZONE): –(CH₂)₂O–, CH₂CH₃, O, N–(CH₂)₃–N, Cl

(Continued)

435

Table 17-1
Antidepressants: Chemical Structures, Dose and Dosage Forms, and Side Effects (Continued)

NONPROPRIETARY NAME (TRADE NAME)	DOSE AND DOSAGE FORMS			AMINE EFFECTS	SIDE EFFECTS								
	Usual Dose, mg/day	Extreme Dose, mg/day	Dosage Form		Agitation	Seizures	Sedation	Hypotension	Anticholinergic Effects	Gastrointestinal Effects	Weight Gain	Sexual Effects	Cardiac Effects
Atypical Antidepressants (cont.)													
Trazodone† (DESYREL)	150–200	50–600	O	5-HT	0	0	3+	0	0	2+	+	+	0/+
Monoamine Oxidase Inhibitors													
Phenelzine (NARDIL)	30–60	15–90	O	NE, 5-HT, DA	0/+	0	+	+	0	0/+	+	3+	0
Tranylcypromine (PARNATE)	20–30	10–60	O	NE, 5-HT, DA	2+	0	0	+	0	0/+	+	2+	0
(−)-Selegiline (ELDEPRYL)	10	5–20	O	DA, ?NE, ?5-HT	0	0	0	0	0	0	0	+	0

Note: Most of the drugs are hydrochloride salts, but SURMONTIL and LUVOX are maleates; CELEXA is a hydrobromide, and REMERON is a free-base. Selegiline is approved for early Parkinson's disease, but may have antidepressant effects, especially at daily doses ≥20 mg, and is under investigation for administration by transdermal patch. ABBREVIATIONS: O, oral tablet or capsule; I, injectable; NE, norepinephrine; DA, dopamine; 5-HT, 5-hydroxytryptamine, serotonin; 0, negligible; 0/+, minimal; +, mild; 2+, moderate; 3+, moderately severe; 4+, severe. *Nefazodone: additional side effect of impotence (+) and some risk of hepatic toxicity. †Trazodone: additional side effect of priapism (+).

436

Table 17–2

Potencies of Antidepressants at Human Transporters for Monoamine Neurotransmitters

DRUG	NET	SERT	DAT	SELECTIVITY FOR NE OR 5-HT
NE-selective agents				
Desipramine	0.83	17.5	3,200	21.1
Protriptyline	1.40	19.6	2,130	14
Norclomipramine	2.50	41	—	16.4
Atomoxetine	3.52	43	1,270	12.2
Nortriptyline	4.35	18.5	1,140	4.25
Oxaprotiline	5	4,000	4,350	800
Lofepramine	5.30	71.4	18,500	13.5
Reboxetine	7.14	58.8	11,500	8.24
Maprotiline	11.1	5,900	1,000	532
Nomifensine	15.6	1,000	55.6	64.1
Amoxapine	16.1	58.5	4,350	3.63
Doxepin	29.4	66.7	12,200	2.27
Mianserin	71.4	4,000	9,100	56
Viloxazine	156	17,000	100,000	109
Mirtazapine	4,760	100,000	100,000	21.0
5-HT–selective agents				
Paroxetine	40	0.125	500	320
Clomipramine	37	0.280	2,200	132
Sertraline	417	0.293	25	1,423
Fluoxetine	244	0.810	3,600	301
S-Citalopram	7,840	1.10	>10,000	7,127
R,S-Citalopram	5,100	1.38	28,000	3,696
Imipramine	37	1.41	8,300	26.2
Duloxetine	11.2	1.55	—	7.23
Fluvoxamine	1,300	2.22	9,100	586
Amitriptyline	34.5	4.33	3,200	7.97
Nor$_1$-citalopram	780	7.40	—	105
Dothiepin	45.5	8.33	5,300	5.46
Venlafaxine	1,060	9.10	9,100	116
Milnacipran	83.3	9.10	71,400	9.15
Nor$_2$-citalopram	1,500	24	—	62.5
Norfluoxetine	410	25	1,100	16.4
Norsertraline	420	76	440	55
Zimelidine	9,100	152	12,000	59.9
Trazodone	8,300	160	7,140	51.9
Nefazodone	60	200	360	1.80
Trimipramine	2,400	1,500	10,000	264
Bupropion	52,600	9,100	526	5.78

Note: Potency is expressed as inhibition constant (K_i) in nanomoles, based on radioactive ligand transport competition assays with membranes from cell lines transfected with human genes for specific transporter proteins (T). Agents are ranked in descending order of potency (increasing K_i) for the norepinephrine-transporter (NET) or serotonin transporter (SERT). Selectivity is based on the ratio of K_i values. Some drugs listed are not available for clinical use in the United States. Note that the most potent NET-selective agent is desipramine; the least potent is mirtazapine, and the most selective for NET over the SERT are oxaprotiline and its congener maprotiline. For SERT, the most potent agents are paroxetine and clomipramine; the least potent is bupropion, and citalopram is the most selective over NET. Bupropion is the only agent with some selectivity for the dopamine transporter (DAT) over NET and SERT.

SOURCES: Data adapted from Frazer, 1997; Owens *et al.*, 1997; and Leonard and Richelson, 2000.

Monoamine Oxidase Inhibitors. The nonselective MAO inhibitors in clinical use are reactive hydrazines (phenelzine and isocarboxazid) or amphetamine derivatives (tranylcypromine). Selegiline, a propargylamine, contains a reactive acetylenic bond and is relatively specific for MAO-B (Cesura and Pletscher, 1992). Following their oxidation to reactive intermediates by MAO, each of these "suicide" substrates interacts irreversibly to inactivate the flavin prosthetic group of the MAO enzyme (Krishnan, 1998). Cyclization of the side chain of amphetamine resulted in tranylcypromine. After formation of a reactive imine intermediate by MAO, inhibition of MAO by this cyclopropylamine derivative may involve the reaction of a sulfhydryl group in the active site of MAO. Due to the irreversible inactivation of MAO, these compounds produce long-acting inhibition that may persist for up to 2 weeks after drug discontinuation. Short-acting, reversible inhibitors of MAO-A (RIMAs) with antidepressant activity are being investigated. These include a piperidylbenzofuran (*brofaromine*), a morpholinobenzamide (*moclobemide*; [AURORIX, MANERIX]) and an oxazolidinone (toloxatone) (Danish University Antidepressant Group, 1993; Delini-Stula *et al.*, 1988).

Pharmacological Properties. Tricyclic Antidepressants and Other Norepinephrine-Reuptake Inhibitors.

Knowledge of the pharmacological properties of antidepressant drugs remains incomplete, and coherent interpretation is limited by a lack of a compelling psychobiological theory of mood disorders. The actions of imipramine-like tricyclic antidepressants include a range of complex, secondary adaptations to their initial and sustained actions as inhibitors of norepinephrine neuronal transport (reuptake) and variable blockade of serotonin transport (Table 17–2) (Barker and Blakely, 1995; Beasley *et al.*, 1992; Leonard and Richelson, 2000; Potter *et al.*, 1998; Wamsley *et al.*, 1987). Tricyclic-type antidepressants with secondary-amine side chains or the *N*-demethylated (*nor*) metabolites of agents with tertiary-amine moieties (*e.g.*, amoxapine, desipramine, maprotiline, *norclomipramine*, *nordoxepin*, and nortriptyline) are relatively selective inhibitors of norepinephrine transport. Most tertiary-amine tricyclic antidepressants also inhibit the reuptake of serotonin.

It is likely that relatively selective inhibitors of norepinephrine reuptake, including atomoxetine and *reboxetine*, share many of the actions of older inhibitors of norepinephrine transport (Kent, 2000; Kratochvil *et al.*, 2003) such as desipramine (Delgado and Michaels, 1999). Among the tricyclic antidepressants, trimipramine is exceptional in that it lacks prominent inhibitory effects at monoamine transport (Table 17–2), and its clinical actions remain unexplained.

The tricyclic and other norepinephrine-active antidepressants do not block dopamine transport (Table 17–2), thereby differing from CNS stimulants, including cocaine, methylphenidate, and amphetamines (*see* Chapter 10). Nevertheless, they may facilitate effects of dopamine indirectly by inhibiting the nonspecific transport of dopamine into noradrenergic terminals in cerebral cortex. Tricyclic antidepressants also can desensitize D_2 dopamine autoreceptors, through uncertain mechanisms and with uncertain behavioral contributions (Potter *et al.*, 1998).

In addition to their transport-inhibiting effects, tricyclic antidepressants variably interact with adrenergic receptors (Table 17–3). The presence or absence of such receptor interactions appears to be critical for responses to increased availability of extracellular norepinephrine in or near synapses. Most tricyclic antidepressants have at least moderate and selective affinity for α_1 adrenergic receptors, much less for α_2, and virtually none for β receptors. The α_2 receptors include presynaptic autoreceptors that limit the neurophysiological activity of noradrenergic neurons ascending from the locus ceruleus in brainstem to supply mid- and forebrain projections. The same noradrenergic neurons provide descending projections to the spinal cord preganglionic cholinergic efferents to the peripheral autonomic ganglia (*see* Chapters 6 and 10). Autoreceptor mechanisms also reduce the synthesis of norepinephrine through the rate-limiting enzyme tyrosine hydroxylase, presumably through α_2 adrenergic receptor attenuation of cyclic AMP–mediated phosphorylation-activation of the enzyme. Activation of these receptors inhibits transmitter release by incompletely defined molecular and cellular actions that likely include suppression of voltage-gated Ca^{2+} currents and activation of G protein–coupled, receptor-operated K^+ currents (Foote and Aston-Jones, 1995).

The α_2 receptor–mediated, presynaptic, negative-feedback mechanisms are rapidly activated after administration of tricyclic antidepressants. By limiting synaptic availability of norepinephrine, such mechanisms normally tend to maintain functional homeostasis. However, with repeated drug exposure, α_2-receptor responses eventually are diminished. This loss may result from desensitization secondary to increased exposure to the endogenous agonist ligand norepinephrine, or alternatively from prolonged occupation of the norepinephrine transporter itself *via* an allosteric effect, as suggested for inhibitors of serotonin transporters on serotonergic neurons (Chaput *et al.*, 1991). Over a period of days to weeks, this adaptation allows the presynaptic production and release of norepinephrine to return to, or even exceed, baseline levels (Foote and Aston-Jones, 1995; Heninger and Charney, 1987; Potter *et al.*, 1998). However, long-term treatment eventually can reduce the expression of tyrosine hydroxylase as well as the norepinephrine transporter (NET) protein (Nestler *et al.*, 1990; Zhu *et al.*, 2002; Zhu *et al.*, 2004).

Table 17–3
Potencies of Selected Antidepressants at Muscarinic, Histamine H_1, and α_1 Adrenergic Receptors

	Receptor Type		
DRUG	M*	H_1	α_1
Amitriptyline	17.9	1.10	27.0
Amoxapine	1000	25.0	50.0
Atomoxetine	≥1000	≥1000	≥1000
Bupropion	40,000	6700	4550
R,S-Citalopram	1800	380	1550
S-Citalopram	1240	1970	3870
Clomipramine	37.0	31.2	38.5
Desipramine	196	110	130
Doxepin	83.3	0.24	23.8
Duloxetine	3000	2300	8300
Fluoxetine	2000	6250	5900
Fluvoxamine	24,000	>100,000	7700
Imipramine	90.9	11.0	90.9
Maprotiline	560	2.00	90.9
Mirtazapine	670	0.14	500
Nefazodone	11,000	21.3	25.6
Nortriptyline	149	10.0	58.8
Paroxetine	108	22,000	>100,000
Protriptyline	25.0	25.0	130
Reboxetine	6700	312	11,900
Sertraline	625	24,000	370
Trazodone	>100,000	345	35.7
Trimipramine	58.8	0.27	23.8
Venlafaxine	>100,000	>100,000	>100,000

Note: Data (K_i values in nM) are adapted from Leonard and Richelson, 2000, and reflect the ability of the antidepressant drug to compete with radioligands selective for muscarinic cholinergic receptors (M), histamine H_1-receptors (H_1), and α_1 adrenergic receptors (α_1). Note that anticholinergic potency is particularly high with amitriptyline, protriptyline, clomipramine, trimipramine, doxepin, and imipramine; relatively high with paroxetine among selective serotonin reuptake inhibitors; and lowest with venlafaxine, trazodone, bupropion, fluvoxamine, and nefazodone. This effect contributes to many diverse autonomic effects. Antihistaminic potency is highest with the relatively sedating agents mirtazapine, doxepin, trimipramine, and amitriptyline, and lowest with venlafaxine, fluvoxamine, sertraline, and paroxetine. Anti–α_1 adrenergic potency is highest with doxepin, trimipramine, nefazodone, amitriptyline, trazodone, clomipramine, amoxapine, nortriptyline, imipramine, and maptrotiline and particularly low with paroxetine, venlafaxine, reboxetine, fluvoxamine and fluoxetine. *Data were obtained with a radioligand that is nonselective for muscarinic receptor subtypes.

The density of functional postsynaptic β adrenergic receptors also gradually down-regulates over several weeks of repeated treatment with various types of antidepressants, including tricyclics, some SSRIs, MAO inhibitors, and electroshock (a model of ECT) in animals (Sulser and Mobley, 1980). Combinations of a serotonin transport inhibitor with a tricyclic antidepressant may have a more rapid β adrenergic receptor–desensitizing effect. The pharmacologic basis of this interaction is not clear, nor is its potential for superior clinical efficacy proven (Nelson *et al.*, 1991). It is unlikely that diminished β-receptor signaling contributes directly to the mood-elevating effects of antidepressant treatment, since β-blockers tend to induce or worsen depression in vulnerable persons. Nevertheless, loss of inhibitory β adrenergic influences on serotonergic neurons may enhance release of serotonin and thus contribute indirectly to antidepressant effects (Leonard and Richelson, 2000; Wamsley *et al.*, 1987) (*see* Chapter 10).

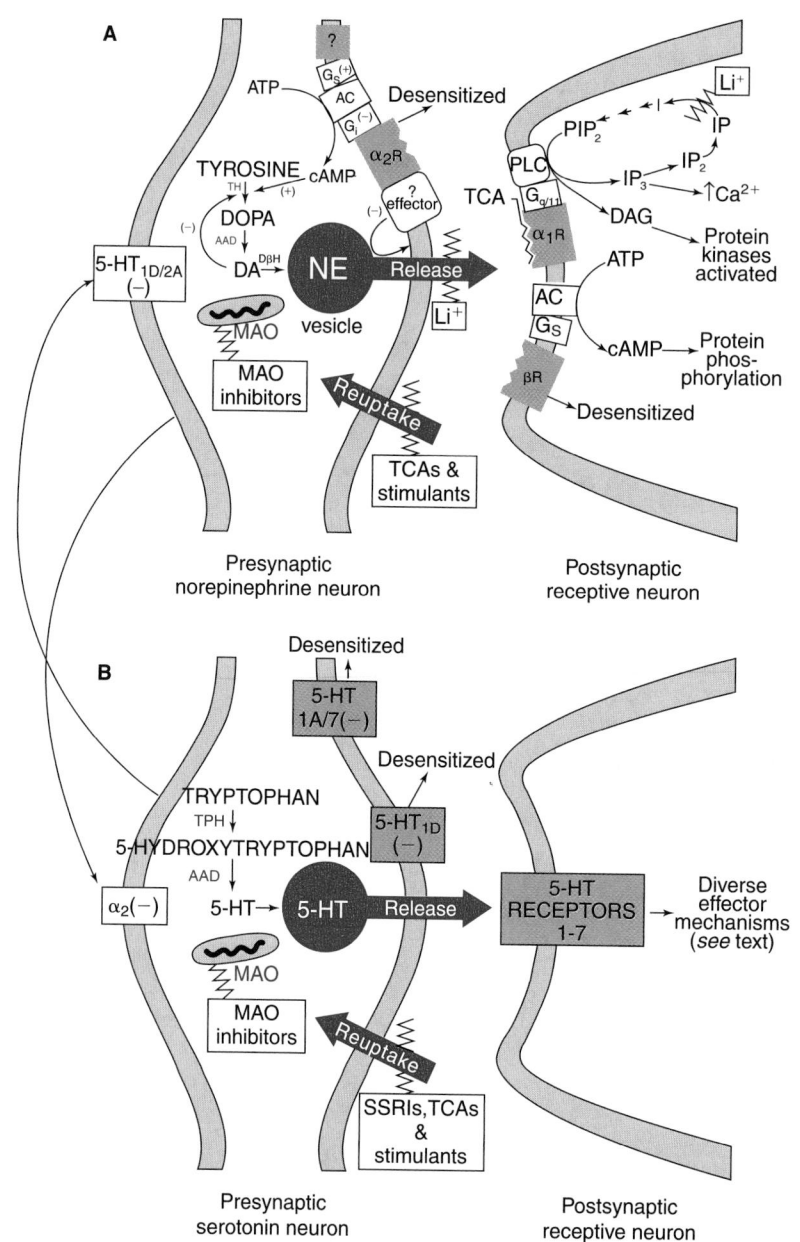

Figure 17–1.* *Sites of action of antidepressants. A. In varicosities ("terminals") along terminal arborizations of norepinephrine (NE) neurons projecting from brainstem to forebrain, L-tyrosine is oxidized to dihydroxyphenylalanine (L-DOPA) by tyrosine hydroxylase (TH), then decarboxylated to dopamine (DA) by aromatic L-amino acid decarboxylase (AAD) and stored in vesicles, where sidechain oxidation by dopamine β-hydroxylase (DβH) converts DA to NE. Following exocytotic release by depolarization in the presence of Ca^{2+} (inhibited by lithium), NE interacts with postsynaptic α and β adrenergic receptor (R) subtypes as well as presynaptic α_2 autoreceptors. Regulation of NE release by α_2 receptors is principally through attenuation of Ca^{2+} currents and activation of K^+ currents. Inactivation of trans-synaptic communication occurs primarily by active transport ("reuptake") into presynaptic terminals (inhibited by most tricyclic antidepressants [TCAs] and stimulants), with secondary deamination (by mitochondrial monoamine oxidase [MAO], blocked by MAO inhibitors). Blockade of inactivation of NE by TCAs initially leads to α_2 receptor–mediated inhibition of firing rates, metabolic activity, and transmitter release from NE neurons; gradually, however, α_2 autoreceptor response diminishes and presynaptic activity returns. Postsynaptically, β adrenergic receptors activate the G_S-adenylyl cyclase (AC) to cyclic AMP (cAMP) pathway. Adrenergic α_1 (and other) receptors activate the phospholipase C–G_q–IP_3 pathway with secondary modulation of intracellular Ca^{2+} and protein kinases. Postsynaptic β receptors also desensitize, but α_1 receptors do not. (*Continued*)

With tricyclic antidepressant therapy, postsynaptic α_1 adrenergic receptors may be partially blocked initially, probably contributing to early hypotensive effects of many tricyclics. Over weeks of treatment, α_1 receptors remain available and may even become more sensitive to norepinephrine as clinical mood-elevating effects gradually emerge. Therefore, as antidepressant treatment gradually becomes clinically effective, inactivation of transmitter reuptake continues to be blocked, presynaptic production and release of norepinephrine returns to or may exceed baseline levels, and a postsynaptic α_1 adrenergic mechanism is in place to provide a critical functional output.

Additional neuropharmacological changes that may contribute to the clinical effects of tricyclic antidepressants include indirect facilitation of serotonin (and perhaps dopamine) neurotransmission through excitatory α_1 "heteroceptors" on other monoaminergic neurons, or desensitized, inhibitory α_2 autoreceptors, as well as D_2 dopamine autoreceptors. Activated release of serotonin and dopamine may, in turn, lead to secondary down-regulation of serotonin 5-HT$_1$ autoreceptors, postsynaptic 5-HT$_2$ receptors, and perhaps dopamine D_2 autoreceptors and postsynaptic D_2 receptors (Leonard and Richelson, 2000).

Other adaptive changes have been observed in response to long-term treatment with tricyclic antidepressants. These include altered sensitivity of muscarinic acetylcholine receptors as well as decreases in gamma-aminobutyric acid (GABA$_B$) receptors and possibly N-methyl-D-aspartate (NMDA) glutamate receptors (Kitamura *et al.*, 1991; Leonard and Richelson, 2000). In addition, cyclic AMP production is increased and the activities of protein kinases altered in some cells, including those acting on cytoskeletal and other structural proteins that may alter neuronal growth and sprouting (Racagni *et al.*, 1991; Wong *et al.*, 1991). Transcription and neurotrophic factors also are affected, including the cyclic AMP–response-element binding protein (CREB) and brain-derived neurotrophic factor (BDNF) (Duman *et al.*, 1997; Siuciak *et al.*, 1997). Additional changes may be indirect effects of antidepres-

sant treatment or may reflect recovery from depressive illness. These include normalization of glucocorticoid release and glucocorticoid receptor sensitivity, as well as shifts in the production of prostaglandins and cytokines and in lymphocyte functions (Kitayama *et al.*, 1988; Leonard and Richelson, 2000).

The complex molecular and cellular changes induced by repeated antidepressant administration remain incompletely understood. Nevertheless, their occurrence underscores the important concept that repeated administration of neuroactive or psychotropic agents triggers a cascade of adaptive processes. The neuropharmacology of tricyclic antidepressants, in particular, is not accounted for simply by blockade of the transport-mediated removal of norepinephrine, even though this effect is no doubt a crucial initiating event that induces a series of important secondary adaptations (Duman *et al.*, 1997; Hyman and Nestler, 1996; Leonard and Richelson, 2000). Interactions of antidepressants with monoaminergic synaptic transmission are illustrated in Figure 17–1.

Selective Serotonin Reuptake Inhibitors (SSRIs). The late and indirect actions of these antidepressant and antianxiety agents remain less well understood than are those of tricyclic antidepressants. However, there are striking parallels between responses in the noradrenergic and serotonergic systems. Like tricyclic antidepressants, which block norepinephrine reuptake, the SSRIs block neuronal transport of serotonin both immediately and chronically, leading to complex secondary responses (Table 17–2).

Increased synaptic availability of serotonin stimulates a large number of postsynaptic 5-HT receptor types (Azmitia and Whitaker-Azmitia, 1995) (*see* Chapter 11). Stimulation of 5-HT$_3$ receptors is suspected to contribute to common adverse effects haracteristic of this class of drugs, including gastrointestinal (nausea and vomiting) and sexual effects (delayed or impaired orgasm). Stimulation of 5-HT$_{2C}$ receptors may contribute to the agitation or restlessness sometimes induced by serotonin reuptake inhibitors.

Figure 17–1. (Continued) Sites of action of antidepressants. B. Selective serotonin reuptake inhibitors (SSRIs) have analogous actions to TCAs at serotonin-containing neurons, and TCAs can interact with serotonergic neurons and receptors (*see* text and Chapters 11 and 12). Serotonin is synthesized from L-tryptophan by a relatively rate-limiting tryptophan hydroxylase (TPH), and the resulting 5-hydroxytryptophan is deaminated by AAD to 5-hydroxytryptamine (5-HT, serotonin). Following release, 5-HT interacts with a large number of postsynaptic 5-HT receptors that exert their effects through a variety of PLG and AC-mediated mechanisms. Inhibitory autoreceptors include types 5-HT$_{1A}$ and perhaps 5-HT$_7$ receptor subtypes at serotonin cell bodies and dendrites, as well as 5-HT$_{1D}$ receptors at the nerve terminals; these receptors probably become desensitized following prolonged treatment with a SSRI antidepressant that blocks 5-HT transporters. The adrenergic and serotonergic systems also influence each other, in part through complementary heteroceptor mechanisms (inhibitory α_2 receptors on 5-HT neurons, and inhibitory 5-HT$_{1D}$ and 5-HT$_{2A}$ receptors on noradrenergic neurons).

An important parallel in responses of serotonin and norepinephrine neurons is that negative feedback mechanisms rapidly emerge to restore homeostasis (Azmitia and Whitaker-Azmitia, 1995). In the serotonin system, 5-HT_1–subtype autoreceptors (types 1A and 7 at raphe cell bodies and dendrites, type 1D at terminals) suppress serotonin neurons in the raphe nuclei of the brainstem, inhibiting both tryptophan hydroxylase (probably through reduced phosphorylation-activation) and neuronal release of serotonin. Repeated treatment leads to gradual down-regulation and desensitization of autoreceptor mechanisms over several weeks (particularly of 5-HT_{1D} receptors at nerve terminals), with a return or increase of presynaptic activity, production, and release of serotonin (Blier *et al.*, 1990; Chaput *et al.*, 1991; Tome *et al.*, 1997). Additional secondary changes include gradual down-regulation of postsynaptic 5-HT_{2A} receptors that may contribute to antidepressant effects directly, as well as by influencing the function of noradrenergic and other neurons *via* serotonergic heteroceptors. Many other postsynaptic 5-HT receptors presumably remain available to mediate increased serotonergic transmission and contribute to the mood-elevating and anxiolytic effects of this class of drugs.

As in responses to norepinephrine-transport inhibitors, complex late adaptations occur upon repeated treatment with serotonin reuptake inhibitors. These may include indirect enhancement of norepinephrine output by reduction of tonic inhibitory effects of 5-HT_{2A} heteroceptors. Finally, similar nuclear and cellular adaptations occur as with the tricyclic antidepressants, including increased intraneuronal cyclic AMP, activation/phosphorylation or transcription factors (*e.g.*, CREB), and increased production of BDNF (Azmitia and Whitaker-Azmitia, 1995; Hyman and Nestler, 1996).

Other Drugs Affecting Monoamine Neurotransmitters. Drugs that significantly inhibit dopamine uptake include the older psychostimulants (*see* Chapter 10) (Fawcett and Busch, 1998). These agents provide only limited benefit in major depression and may worsen agitation, psychosis, insomnia, and anorexia associated with severe depressive illness. *Nomifensine* is a structurally distinct antidepressant that inhibits the transport of both norepinephrine and dopamine; it was withdrawn from clinical use in 1996 owing to risk of hemolytic anemia and intravascular hemolysis. The aromatic aminoketone *bupropion* and its amphetaminelike active metabolites also inhibit dopamine and norepinephrine transport (Ascher *et al.*, 1995). The MAO inhibitor tranylcypromine is amphetaminelike in structure but interacts only weakly at dopamine transporters.

The phenylpiperazine *nefazodone,* and to a lesser extent, the structurally related *trazodone* have at least weak inhibitory actions on serotonin transport, and nefazodone also may have a minor effect on norepinephrine transport. This agent also has a prominent direct antagonistic effect at 5-HT_{2A} receptors that may contribute to antidepressant and anxiolytic activity. Both drugs also may inhibit presynaptic 5-HT_1 subtype autoreceptors to enhance neuronal release of serotonin, though they probably also exert at least partial-agonist effects on postsynaptic 5-HT_1 receptors (Table 17–3) (Golden *et al.*, 1998). Trazodone also blocks cerebral α_1 adrenergic and H_1-histamine receptors (Table 17–3), possibly contributing to its tendency to induce priapism and sedation, respectively.

Finally, the atypical antidepressants *mirtazapine* and *mianserin* are structural analogs of serotonin with potent antagonistic effects at several postsynaptic serotonin receptor types (including 5-HT_{2A}, 5-HT_{2C}, and 5-HT_3 receptors) and can produce gradual down-regulation of 5-HT_{2A} receptors (Golden *et al.*, 1998). Mirtazapine also limits the effectiveness of inhibitory α_2 adrenergic heteroceptors on serotonergic neurons as well as inhibitory α_2 autoreceptors and 5-HT_{2A} heteroceptors on noradrenergic neurons. These effects may enhance release of amines and contribute to the antidepressant effects of these drugs. Mirtazapine also is a potent histamine H_1-receptor antagonist and is relatively sedating. Mianserin is not used in the United States owing largely to an association with bone marrow suppression.

Monoamine Oxidase Inhibitors. The MAOs comprise two structurally related flavin-containing enzymes, designated MAO-A and MAO-B, that share approximately 70% of their amino acids but are encoded by distinct genes (Abell and Kwan, 2000). They are localized in mitochondrial membranes and widely distributed throughout the body in nerve terminals, the liver, intestinal mucosa, platelets, and other organs. Within the CNS, MAO-A is expressed predominantly in noradrenergic neurons, while MAO-B is expressed in serotonergic and histaminergic neurons. MAO activity is closely linked functionally with an aldehyde reductase and an aldehyde dehydrogenase, depending on the substrate and tissue.

MAO regulates the metabolic degradation of catecholamines, serotonin, and other endogenous amines in the CNS and peripheral tissues. Hepatic MAO has a crucial defensive role in inactivating circulating monoamines or compounds, such as the indirect-acting sympathomimetic tyramine, that are ingested or originate in the gut and get absorbed into the portal circulation. Inhibition of this enzyme system by MAO inhibitors causes a reduction in metabolism and a subsequent increase in the concentrations of biogenic amines. Of the two major molecular species of MAO, MAO-A preferentially deaminates epinephrine, norepinephrine, and serotonin, and is selectively inhibited by clorgyline. MAO-B metabolizes phenethylamine and is inhibited by selegiline. Dopamine and tyramine are metabolized by both MAO isozymes and both types are inhibited by phenelzine, tranylcypromine, and isocarboxazid.

Experimentally, selective MAO-A inhibitors are thought to be more effective in treating major depression than type B inhibitors (Krishnan, 1998). The MAO-B inhibitor selegiline is approved for treatment of early Parkinson's disease and acts by potentiating remaining dopamine in degenerating nigrostriatal neurons and possibly by reducing neuronal damage due to reactive products of the oxidative metabolism of dopamine or other potential neurotoxins (*see* Chapter 20). Selegiline also has antidepressant effects, particularly at doses higher than 10 mg that also inhibit MAO-A or yield amphetamine-like metabolites. Administered experimentally in a transdermal dosage form, selegiline has a limited effect on MAO-A in the gut, possibly allowing liberalization of the tyramine-restricted diet that otherwise is necessary to avoid potentially fatal hypertensive crises (Wecker *et al.*, 2003). Several short-acting selective inhibitors of MAO-A (*e.g.*, brofaromine and moclobemide) and *toloxatone* have at least moderate antidepressant effects and are less likely to potentiate the pressor actions of tyramine and other indirect-acting sympathomimetic amines than are the nonselective, irreversible MAO inhibitors (Delini-Stula *et al.*, 1988; Kuhn and Muller, 1996; Lotufo-Neto *et al.*, 1999; Mann *et al.*, 1989).

In the clinical setting MAO inhibition occurs rapidly, and is usually maximal within a few days. As with other antidepressants, clinical benefits usually are delayed for several weeks. This delay remains unexplained but may reflect secondary adaptations, including downregulation of serotonergic and adrenergic receptors. Evaluation of MAO activity in human subjects taking an MAO inhibitor has led to the impression that favorable clinical responses are likely to occur when human platelet MAO-B is inhibited by at least 85%. This relationship is best established for the nonselective MAO-A and MAO-B inhibitor phenelzine, and it suggests the need to use aggressive dosages to achieve the maximal therapeutic potential of MAO inhibitors. Finally, despite long-lasting inhibition of MAO by the irreversible inhibitors of MAO, optimal therapeutic benefit appears to require daily dosing.

Absorption and Bioavailability. Most antidepressants are fairly well absorbed after oral administration. A notable exception is that the bioavailability of nefazodone is only about 20%. The MAO inhibitors are absorbed readily when given by mouth. High doses of the strongly anticholinergic tricyclic antidepressants (Table 17–1) can slow gastrointestinal activity and gastric emptying time, resulting in slower or erratic drug absorption and complicating management of acute overdosages. Serum concentrations of most tricyclic antidepressants peak within several hours. Intravenous administration of some tricyclic antidepressants (notably clomipramine) or intramuscular injection (amitriptyline) was used at one time, particularly with severely depressed, anorexic patients who refused oral medication (DeBattista and Schatzberg, 1999), but injectable formulations are no longer commercially available in the United States.

Distribution and Serum Level Monitoring. Once absorbed, tricyclic antidepressants are widely distributed. They are relatively lipophilic and strongly bind to plasma proteins and constituents of tissues, leading to apparent volumes of distribution that can be as high as 10 to 50 L/kg. The tendency of tricyclic antidepressants and their relatively cardiotoxic, ring-hydroxy metabolites to accumulate in cardiac tissue adds to their cardiotoxic risks (Pollock and Perel, 1989; Prouty and Anderson, 1990; Wilens *et al.*, 1992). Serum concentrations of antidepressants that correlate meaningfully with clinical effects are not securely established except for a few tricyclic antidepressants (particularly amitriptyline, desipramine, imipramine, and nortriptyline), typically at concentrations of approximately 100 to 250 ng/ml (Perry *et al.*, 1994) (Table 17–4). Toxic effects of tricyclic antidepressants can be expected at serum concentrations above 500 ng/ml, while levels above 1 μg/ml can be fatal (Burke and Preskorn, 1995; Catterson *et al.*, 1997; Preskorn, 1997; van Harten, 1993).

The utility of therapeutic drug monitoring in the routine clinical use of antidepressants is limited, and the relative safety of modern antidepressants has led to a diminished interest in this approach to guiding clinical dosing. Individual variance in tricyclic antidepressant levels in response to a given dose is as high as ten- to thirtyfold and is due largely to genetic control of hepatic cytochrome P450 isoenzymes (CYPs) (DeVane and Nemeroff, 2000). Predictable relationships between initial disposition of a relatively small test dose of nortriptyline or desipramine and doses required to achieve theoretically optimal serum concentrations have been proposed as a guide to clinical dosing of individual patients. Serum concentrations of antidepressants can be misleading when obtained postmortem for forensic purposes (Prouty and Anderson, 1990).

Metabolism, Half-Lives, and Duration of Action. Tricyclic antidepressants are oxidized by hepatic microsomal enzymes, followed by conjugation with glucuronic acid. The major metabolite of imipramine is desipramine; biotransformation of imiprimine or desipramine occurs largely by oxidation to 2-hydroxy metabolites, which retain some ability to block the transport of amines and have particularly prominent cardiac depressant actions. In contrast, amitriptyline and its major demethylated byproduct, nortriptyline, undergo preferential oxidation at the 10 position. The 10-hydroxy metabolites may have some biological activity, and may be less cardiotoxic than the 2-hydroxy metabolites of imipramine or desipramine (Pollock and Perel, 1989). Conjugation of ring-hydroxylated metabolites with glucuronic acid extinguishes any remaining biological activity. The *N*-demethylated metabolites of several tricyclic antidepressants are pharmacologically active and may accumulate in concentrations approaching or exceeding those of the parent drug, to contribute variably to overall pharmacodynamic activity.

Amoxapine is oxidized predominantly to the 8-hydroxy metabolite and less of the 7-hydroxy metabolite. The 8-hydroxy metabolite is pharmacologically active, including antagonistic interactions with D_2 dopamine receptors. Amoxapine has some risk of extrapyramidal side effects, including tardive dyskinesia, reminiscent of those of the *N*-methylated congener loxapine, a typical neuroleptic (*see* Chapter 18).

Mirtazapine is also *N*-demethylated and undergoes aromatic hydroxylation. Trazodone and nefazodone both are *N*-dealkylated to yield *meta*-chlorophenylpiperazine (mCPP), an active metabolite with serotonergic activity. Bupropion yields active metabolites that include amphetaminelike compounds. Clomipramine, fluoxetine, sertraline, and *venlafaxine* are *N*-demethylated to norclomipramine,

Table 17–4
Disposition of Antidepressants

DRUG	ELIMINATION HALF-LIFE,* HOURS, PARENT (ACTIVE METABOLITE)	TYPICAL SERUM CONCENTRATIONS, ng/ml	PREFERRED CYP ISOZYMES‡
Tertiary-amine tricyclic antidepressants			2D6, 2C19, 3A3/4
Amitriptyline	16 (30)	100–250	
Clomipramine	32 (70)	150–500	
Doxepin	16 (30)	150–250	
Imipramine	12 (30)	175–300	
Trimipramine	16 (30)	100–300	
Secondary-amine tricyclic antidepressants			2D6, 2C19, 3A3/4
Amoxapine	8 (30)	200–500	
Desipramine	30	125–300	
Maprotiline	48	200–400	
Nortriptyline	30	60–150	
Protriptyline	80	100–250	
Selective serotonin reuptake inhibitors			
R,S-Citalopram	36	75–150	3A4, 2C19
S-Citalopram	30	40–80	3A4, 2C19
Fluoxetine	50 (240)	100–500	2D6, 2C9
Fluvoxamine	18	100–200	2D6, 1A2, 3A4, 2C9
Paroxetine	22	30–100	2D6
Sertraline	24 (66)	25–50	2D6
Venlafaxine†	5 (11)	—	2D6, 3A4
Atypical agents			
Atomoxetine	5 (child: 3)	—	2D6, 3A3/4
Bupropion†	14	75–100	2B6
Duloxetine	11	—	2D6
Mirtazapine	16–30	—	2D6
Nefazodone	3	—	3A3/4
Reboxetine	12	—	—
Trazodone	6	800–1600	2D6

*Half-life is the approximate elimination (β) half-life (limited data for newer agents). Half-life values given in parentheses are those of active metabolites (commonly *N*-demethylated) that contribute to overall duration of action. †Agents available in slow-release forms that delay absorption but not elimination half-life; venlafaxine also inhibits norepinephrine transport at higher doses. ‡Some serotonin reuptake inhibitors inhibit the hepatic oxidation of other agents: potent inhibition is produced by fluoxetine (2D6 and other CYP isozymes), fluvoxamine (1A2, 2C8, and 3A3/4), paroxetine (2D6), and nefazodone (3A3/4); sertraline produces moderate effects at high doses (2D6 and others); citalopram (2C19) and venlafaxine have weak interactions. Serum concentrations are levels encountered at typical clinical doses and not intended as guidelines to optimal dosing. Information was obtained from manufacturers' product information summaries.

norfluoxetine, norsertraline, and desmethylvenlafaxine, respectively (DeVane and Nemeroff, 2000; van Harten, 1993). As occurs with the tertiary-amine tricyclic antidepressants, the *N*-demethylated metabolites of serotonin reuptake inhibitors also are eliminated more slowly, and some are pharmacologically active. Norclomipramine contributes noradrenergic activity. Norfluoxetine is a very long-acting inhibitor of serotonin transport (elimination half-life approximately 10 days) (Table 17–4) that requires several weeks for elimination (Wong *et al.*, 1993). Norfluoxetine also competes for hepatic CYPs and thereby elevates blood levels of other agents, including tricyclic antidepressants. These effects can persist for days after administration of the parent drug has been stopped. Norsertraline, though also eliminated relatively slowly (half-life of 60 to 70 hours), appears to contribute limited pharmacological activity or risk of drug interactions. Nornefazodone contributes little to the biological activity or duration of action of nefazodone.

With some notable exceptions, inactivation and elimination of most antidepressants occurs over a period of several days. Generally, secondary-amine tricyclic antidepressants and the *N*-demethylated derivatives of serotonin reuptake inhibitors have elimination half-lives about twice those of the parent drugs (van Harten, 1993). Nevertheless, most tricyclics are almost completely eliminated within 7 to 10 days. An exceptionally long-acting tricyclic antidepressant is protriptyline (half-life of about 80 hours). Most MAO inhibitors are long acting, because recovery from their effects requires the synthesis of new enzyme over a period of 1 to 2 weeks.

At the other extreme, trazodone, nefazodone, and venlafaxine have short half-lives (about 3 to 6 hours), as does the active 4-hydroxy metabolite of venlafaxine (half-life of about 11 hours). The half-life of bupropion is about 14 hours. Owing to rapid aromatic hydroxylation, the half-life of nefazodone is very short (about 3 hours). The shorter duration of action of these agents usually implies the need for multiple daily doses. Some short-acting antidepressants have been prepared in slow-release preparations (notably bupropion and venlafaxine), to allow less frequent dosing and potentially to temper side effects related to agitation and GI disturbance.

Antidepressants are metabolized more rapidly by children and more slowly by patients over 60 years of age as compared with young adults (Wilens *et al.*, 1992). Dosages are adjusted accordingly, sometimes to daily doses in children that far exceed those typically given to adults (Wilens *et al.*, 1992).

The hydrazide MAO inhibitors are thought to be cleaved to liberate pharmacologically active products (*e.g.,* hydrazines). They are inactivated primarily by acetylation. About one-half the population of the United States and Europe (and more in certain Asian and Arctic regions) are "slow acetylators" of hydrazine-type drugs, including phenelzine, and this genetic trait may contribute to exaggerated effects observed in some patients given standard doses of phenelzine (*see* Chapters 3 and 4).

Interactions with Cytochrome P450 Isoenzymes. The metabolism of most antidepressants is greatly dependent on the activity of hepatic CYPs (*see* Chapter 3). Most tricyclic antidepressants are extensively oxidized by CYP1A2. *Citalopram,* imipramine, and the *meta*-chlorophenylpiperidine metabolite of trazodone and nefazodone are substrates for CYP2C19, while atomoxetine,

duloxetine, mirtazapine, paroxetine, trazodone, and some tricyclics are substrates for CYP2D6. Nefazodone and some tricyclic and SSRI antidepressants are oxidized by CYP3A3/4 (DeVane and Nemeroff, 2000; Lantz *et al.,* 2003; Sauer *et al.,* 2003; Skinner *et al.,* 2003; van Harten, 1993). In general, CYP1A2 and CYP2D6 mediate aromatic hydroxylation, and CYP3A3/4 mediate *N*-dealkylation and *N*-oxidation reactions in the metabolism of antidepressants.

Some antidepressants not only are substrates for metabolism by CYPs but also can inhibit the metabolic clearance of other drugs, sometimes producing clinically significant drug-drug interactions (*see* below). Notable inhibitory interactions include fluvoxamine with CYP1A2; fluoxetine and fluvoxamine with CYP2C9, and fluvoxamine with CYP1A2 and CYP2C19; paroxetine, fluoxetine, and less actively, sertraline with CYP2D6; norfluoxetine with CYP3A4; and fluvoxamine and nefazodone with CYP3A3/4. Citalopram or *S*-citalopram and venlafaxine interact much less with CYPs (Caccia, 2004; DeVane and Nemeroff, 2000; Hansten and Horn, 2000; Hemeryck and Belpaire, 2002; Preskorn, 1997; Spina *et al.,* 2003; Weber, 1999). Atomoxetine has weak effects on the metabolism of most other agents, but its clearance is inhibited by some SSRIs including paroxetine (Sauer *et al.,* 2003). Duloxetine can inhibit the metabolism of agents such as desipramine that are metabolized extensively through CYP2D6, and its own metabolism is inhibited by some SSRIs including paroxetine (Lantz *et al.,* 2003; Skinner *et al.,* 2003).

Potentially clinically significant interactions include the tendency for fluvoxamine to increase circulating concentrations of oxidatively metabolized benzodiazepines, clozapine, theophylline, and warfarin. Sertraline and fluoxetine can increase levels of benzodiazepines, clozapine, and warfarin. Paroxetine increases levels of clozapine, theophylline, and warfarin. Fluoxetine also potentiates tricyclic antidepressants and some class IC antiarrhythmics with a narrow therapeutic index (including *encainide, flecainide,* and *propafenone; see* Chapter 34). Nefazodone potentiates benzodiazepines other than *lorazepam* and *oxazepam.*

Tolerance and Physical Dependence. Some tolerance to the sedative and autonomic effects of tricyclic antidepressants and to the initial nausea commonly associated with serotonin reuptake inhibitors tends to develop with continued drug use. The medical literature contains case reports of possible "tolerance" to the therapeutic effects of antidepressants after continued use. However, it is important to emphasize that various antidepressants have been used for months or years by patients with severe recurring depression without obvious loss of efficacy, though such therapeutic tolerance may occur more often with serotonin reuptake inhibitors than with older agents (Viguera *et al.*, 1998). Sometimes this loss of benefit may be overcome by increasing the dose of antidepressant, by temporary addition of lithium or perhaps a small dose of an antipsychotic agent, or by changing to an antidepressant in a different class (Byrne and Rothschild, 1998). To avoid toxicity and precipitation of "serotonin syndrome" (*see* Drug Interactions, below), extreme caution is advised when these strategies are employed.

Occasionally, patients show physical dependence on the tricyclic antidepressants, with malaise, chills, coryza, muscle aches, and sleep disturbance following abrupt discontinuation, particularly of high doses. Similar reactions, along with gastrointestinal and sensory symptoms (paresthesias) and irritability, also occur with abrupt discontinuation of serotonin reuptake inhibitors, particularly with paroxetine and venlafaxine (Schatzberg *et al.*, 1997; Tollefson and Rosenbaum, 1998). Withdrawal reactions from MAO inhibitors may be severe, commencing 24 to 72 hours after drug discontinuation. MAO inhibitor withdrawal reactions are more common in patients using tranylcypromine and isocarboxazid at doses significantly in excess of the usual therapeutic range. Symptoms range from nausea, vomiting, and malaise to nightmares, agitation, psychosis, and convulsions.

Some withdrawal effects may reflect increased cholinergic activity following its inhibition by such agents as amitriptyline, imipramine, and paroxetine, but serotonergic mechanisms may contribute to the effects of abrupt discontinuation of serotonin reuptake inhibitors. Some of these reactions can be confused with clinical worsening of depressive symptoms. Emergence of agitated or manic reactions also has been observed after abrupt discontinuation of tricyclics. Such reactions to antidepressant discontinuation indicate that it is wise to discontinue antidepressants gradually over at least a week, or longer when feasible.

Another reaction to treatment discontinuation is suspected with several psychotropic agents, involving a period of risk of recurrence of morbidity that is greater than would be predicted by the natural history of untreated illness, particularly if long-term maintenance medication is withdrawn rapidly (Baldessarini *et al.*, 1999; Viguera *et al.*, 1998). This risk probably extends over several months. Evidence for the occurrence of this phenomenon is particularly strong with lithium in bipolar disorder, is likely with some antipsychotics, and may occur with anti-

depressants (Baldessarini *et al.*, 1999; Viguera *et al.*, 1998). Such risk may be reduced by gradual discontinuation of long-term medication over at least several weeks (*see* Chapter 18).

Adverse Effects. Significant adverse effects of antidepressants are common. Tricyclic antidepressants routinely produce adverse autonomic responses, in part related to their relatively potent antimuscarinic effects. These include dry mouth and a sour or metallic taste, epigastric distress, constipation, dizziness, tachycardia, palpitations, blurred vision (poor accommodation with increased risk of glaucoma), and urinary retention. Cardiovascular effects include orthostatic hypotension, sinus tachycardia, and variable prolongation of cardiac conduction times with the potential for arrhythmias, particularly with overdoses.

In the absence of cardiac disease, the principal problem associated with imipraminelike agents is postural hypotension, probably related to anti–α_1 adrenergic actions. Hypotension can be severe, with falls and injuries (Ray *et al.*, 1987; Roose, 1992). Among tricyclics, nortriptyline may have a relatively low risk of inducing postural blood pressure changes. Tricyclic antidepressants are avoided following an acute myocardial infarction; in the presence of defects in bundle-branch conduction or slowed repolarization; or when other cardiac depressants (including other psychotropic agents such as thioridazine) are being administered. They have direct cardiac-depressing actions like those of class I antiarrhythmics, related to actions at fast Na^+ channels (*see* Chapter 34). Mild congestive heart failure and the presence of some cardiac arrhythmias are not absolute contraindications to the short-term use of a tricyclic antidepressant when depression and its associated medical risks are severe, safer alternatives fail, and appropriate medical care is provided (Glassman *et al.*, 1993). Nevertheless, modern nontricyclic antidepressants—notably the SSRIs—have less risk and are a prudent choice for cardiac patients. ECT also can be an option.

Weakness and fatigue are attributable to central effects of tricyclic antidepressants, particularly tertiary amines (Table 17–1) and mirtazapine, all of which have potent central antihistaminic effects. Trazodone and nefazodone also are relatively sedating. Other CNS effects include variable risk of confusion or delirium, in large part owing to atropine-like effects of tricyclic antidepressants. Epileptic seizures can occur; this is especially likely with daily doses of bupropion above 450 mg, maprotiline above 250 mg, or acute overdoses of amoxapine or tricyclics (Johnston *et al.*, 1991). The risk of cerebral or cardiac intoxication can increase if such agents are given in relatively high doses, particularly when combined with

SSRIs that inhibit their metabolism (Table 17–4). MAO inhibitors can induce sedation or behavioral excitation and have a high risk of inducing postural hypotension, sometimes with sustained mild elevations of diastolic blood pressure.

Miscellaneous toxic effects of tricyclic antidepressants include jaundice, leukopenia, and rashes, but these are very infrequent. Weight gain is a common adverse effect of many antidepressants, but is less likely with the SSRIs, and is rare with bupropion (Table 17–1). Excessive sweating also is common, but its pathophysiology is not known.

Newer antidepressants generally present fewer or different side effects and toxic risks than older tricyclics and MAO inhibitors. As a group, the SSRIs have a high risk of nausea and vomiting, headache, and sexual dysfunction, including inhibited ejaculation in men and impaired orgasm in women. Adverse sexual effects also occur with tricyclic antidepressants but are less common with bupropion, nefazodone, and mirtazapine. Trazodone can produce priapism in men, presumably due to antiadrenergic actions. Some SSRIs, and perhaps fluoxetine in particular, have been associated with agitation and restlessness that resembles akathisia (see Chapter 18) (Hamilton and Opler, 1992). Bupropion can act as a stimulant, with agitation, anorexia, and insomnia. SSRIs, while generally less likely to produce adverse cardiovascular effects than older antidepressants, can elicit electrophysiological changes in cardiac tissue, including interference with Na^+ and Ca^{2+} channels (Pacher et al., 1999). SSRIs can also induce the syndrome of inappropriate secretion of antidiuretic hormone with hyponatremia (see Chapter 29) (Fisher et al., 2002). Nefazodone has been associated with apparently increased risk of hepatic toxicity that has led to its removal in some countries. Such reactions are not unknown with tricyclic and MAO inhibitor antidepressants, but rarely are associated with the SSRIs (Lucena et al., 2003).

Another risk of antidepressants in vulnerable patients (particularly those with unrecognized bipolar depression) is switching, sometimes suddenly, from depression to hypomanic or manic excitement, or mixed, dysphoric-agitated, manic-depressive states. To some extent this effect is dose-related, and is somewhat more likely in adults treated with tricyclic antidepressants than with serotonin reuptake inhibitors, bupropion, and perhaps with MAO inhibitors. Risk of mania with newer sedating antidepressants, including nefazodone and mirtazapine, also may be relatively low, but some risk of inducing mania can be expected with any treatment that elevates mood (Sachs et al., 1994), including in children with unsuspected bipolar disorder (Faedda et al., 2004).

Safety through the Life Cycle. Most antidepressants appear to be generally safe during pregnancy, in that pro-posed teratogenic associations in newborns exposed to several tricyclic antidepressants and some newer antidepressants (particularly fluoxetine) are not convincing (McGrath et al., 1999; Wisner et al., 1999). Most antidepressants and lithium are secreted in breast milk, at least in small quantities, and their safety in nursing infants is neither established nor safely assumed (Birnbaum et al., 1999). For severe depression during pregnancy and lactation, ECT can be a relatively safe and effective alternative.

Major affective disorders are being recognized more often in children, and antidepressants increasingly are used in this age group. Children are vulnerable to the cardiotoxic and seizure-inducing effects of high doses of tricyclic antidepressants (Kutcher, 1997). Deaths have occurred in children after accidental or deliberate overdosage with only a few hundred milligrams of drug, and several cases of unexplained sudden death have been reported in preadolescent children treated with desipramine (Biederman et al., 1995). Most children are relatively protected by vigorous hepatic metabolic clearing mechanisms that eliminate many drugs rapidly. Indeed, attaining serum concentrations of desipramine like those encountered in adults (Table 17–4) may require doses of 5 mg/kg of body weight (or more in some school-age children) compared to only 2 to 3 mg/kg in adults (Wilens et al., 1992). Risk-benefit considerations of antidepressants in pediatric populations remain uncertain, particularly since many trials of tricyclic antidepressants in children have failed to show substantial superiority to placebo. The efficacy of modern agents, including SSRIs, is not securely established other than for fluoxetine (Kutcher, 1997; Milin et al., 2003; Ryan, 2003; Wagner et al., 2003; Williams and Miller, 2003) and sertraline; both have shown efficacy in depressed children in placebo-controlled trials (Emslie et al., 2002; Wagner et al., 2003). Other antidepressants have received little assessment in juveniles with various disorders (Emslie et al., 1999; Kutcher, 1997; Steingard et al., 1995; Milin et al., 2003; Ryan, 2003). Antidepressants appear to be more effective in adolescents. In children, they risk inducing agitated states that may represent mania in undiagnosed juvenile bipolar disorder (Faedda et al., 2004). The possibility that suicidal risk may increase in some juveniles treated with SSRIs also has been suggested, with proposed restrictions on their use (Whittington et al., 2004).

Among geriatric patients, dizziness, postural hypotension, constipation, delayed micturition, edema, and tremor are found commonly with tricyclic antidepressants. These patients are much more likely to tolerate SSRIs and other modern antidepressants (Catterson et al., 1997; Flint, 1998; Newman and Hassan, 1999; Oshima and Higuchi,

1999; Small, 1998). Risks in geriatric patients are higher due to decreased metabolic clearance of antidepressants and less ability to tolerate them.

Toxic Effects of Acute Overdoses. Acute poisoning with tricyclic antidepressants or MAO inhibitors is potentially life-threatening. Fatalities are much less common since modern antidepressants have widely replaced these drugs; however, suicide rates have not declined consistently as clinical usage of modern antidepressants has increased (Tondo *et al.*, 2003; Helgason *et al.*, 2004). Deaths have been reported with acute doses of approximately 2 g of imipramine, and severe intoxication can be expected at doses above 1 g, or about a week's supply. If a patient is severely depressed, potentially suicidal, impulsive, or has a history of substance abuse, prescribing a relatively safe antidepressant agent with close clinical follow-up is appropriate. If a potentially lethal agent is prescribed, it is best dispensed in small, sublethal quantities, with the risk that sustained adherence to recommended treatment may be compromised.

Acute poisoning with a tricyclic antidepressant often is clinically complex (Nicotra *et al.*, 1981). A typical pattern is brief excitement and restlessness, sometimes with myoclonus, tonic-clonic seizures, or dystonia, followed by rapid development of coma, often with depressed respiration, hypoxia, depressed reflexes, hypothermia, and hypotension. Antidepressants that have relatively strong antimuscarinic potency commonly induce an atropine-like syndrome of mydriasis, flushed dry skin and dry mucosae, absent bowel sounds, urinary retention, and tachycardia or other cardiac arrhythmias. A tricyclic antidepressant–intoxicated patient must be treated early, ideally in an intensive care unit. Gastric lavage with activated charcoal sometimes is useful, but dialysis and diuresis are ineffective. Coma abates gradually over 1 to 3 days, and excitement and delirium may reappear. Risk of life-threatening cardiac arrhythmias continues for at least several days, requiring close medical supervision (Settle, 1998; Buckley and Faunce, 2003; Cheeta *et al.*, 2004).

Cardiac toxicity and hypotension can be especially difficult to manage in patients with overdoses of tricyclic antidepressants. The most common cardiac effect is sinus tachycardia, due both to anticholinergic effects and diminished uptake of norepinephrine. Delayed depolarization due to inhibition of the sodium current may be evidenced by a prolonged QT interval or widened QRS complex. Intravenous administration of sodium bicarbonate can improve hypotension and cardiac arrhythmias, although the precise roles of alkalinization versus increased sodium have not been established. Cardiac glycosides and type I antiarrhythmic drugs such as quinidine, procainamide, and disopyramide are contraindicated, but phenytoin and lidocaine can be used for ventricular arrhythmias. If the prolonged QT interval results in *torsades de pointes*, magnesium, isoproterenol, and atrial pacing may be employed. Hypotension that does not respond to alkalinization should be treated with norepinephrine and intravenous fluids.

Effects of MAO inhibitor overdosage include agitation, hallucinations, hyperreflexia, fever, and convulsions. Both hypotension and hypertension can occur. Treatment of such intoxication is problematic, but conservative treatment often is successful.

Drug Interactions. Antidepressants are associated with several clinically important drug interactions (Hansten and Horn, 2000; Leipzig and Mendelowitz, 1992). Binding of tricyclic antidepressants to plasma albumin can be reduced by competition with a number of drugs, including phenytoin, aspirin, aminopyrine, scopolamine, and phenothiazines. Barbiturates and many anticonvulsant agents (particularly carbamazepine), as well as cigarette smoking, can increase the hepatic metabolism of antidepressants by inducing CYPs.

Conversely, the tendency for several SSRIs to compete for the metabolism of other drugs can lead to significant and potentially dangerous drug interactions. For example, during the use of combinations of SSRIs with tricyclic antidepressants, as is sometimes done to achieve more rapid therapeutic effect or to manage otherwise treatment resistant depressed patients, serum concentrations of the tricyclic drug may rise to toxic levels. Such an interaction can persist for days after discontinuing fluoxetine, due to the prolonged elimination half-life of norfluoxetine (Nelson *et al.*, 1991). As discussed above, several serotonin reuptake inhibitors are potent inhibitors of human hepatic CYPs (Crewe *et al.*, 1992). Venlafaxine, citalopram, and sertraline appear to have relatively low risk of such interactions (Caccia, 1998; Ereshefsky *et al.*, 1996; Preskorn, 1997; Preskorn, 1998). Significant interactions may be most likely in persons who are relatively rapid metabolizers through the microsomal oxidase system, including children (DeVane and Nemeroff, 2000; Preskorn, 1997; Preskorn, 1998).

Examples of drug interactions with SSRIs include potentiation of agents metabolized prominently by CYP1A2 (*e.g.,* β adrenergic receptor antagonists, caffeine, several antipsychotic agents, and most tricyclic antidepressants); CYP2C9 (carbamazepine); CYP2C19 (barbiturates, imipramine, propranolol, and phenytoin); CYP2D6 (β adrenergic receptor antagonists, some antipsychotics, and many antidepressants); and CYP3A3/4 (benzodiazepines, carbamazepine, many antidepressants, and several antibiotics). This specialized topic is reviewed elsewhere (DeVane and Nemeroff, 2000; Hansten and Horn, 2000; Preskorn, 1997; Weber, 1999) (*see* Chapter 3).

Antidepressants potentiate the effects of alcohol and probably other sedatives. The anticholinergic activity of tricyclic antidepressants can add to that of antiparkinsonism agents, antipsychotic drugs of low potency (especially clozapine and thioridazine), or other compounds with antimuscarinic activity to produce toxic effects. Tricyclic antidepressants have prominent and potentially dangerous potentiative interactions with biogenic amines such as norepinephrine, which normally are removed from their site of action by neuronal reuptake. However, these inhibitors of norepinephrine transport block the effects of indirectly acting amines such as tyramine, which must be taken up by sympathetic neurons to release norepinephrine. Presumably by a similar mechanism, tricyclic antidepressants prevent the antihypertensive action of adrenergic neuron blocking agents such as guanadrel. Tricyclic agents and trazodone also can block the centrally mediated antihypertensive action of clonidine.

Selective serotonin reuptake inhibitors and virtually any agent with serotonin-potentiating activity can interact dangerously or even fatally with MAO inhibitors (particularly long-acting MAO inhibitors). Other agents also have been implicated in dangerous interactions with MAO inhibitors, including meperidine and perhaps other phenylpiperidine analgesics, as well as pentazocine, dextromethorphan, fenfluramine, and infrequently, tricyclic antidepressants (Ener *et al.*, 2003). The resulting reactions are referred to as "serotonin syndrome." Serotonin syndrome most commonly occurs in patients receiving combination therapy with 2 or more serotonergic agents. Besides the combination of MAO inhibitors with SSRIs, other drug combinations or conditions that increase serotonin synthesis (*e.g.*, L-tryptophan) or release (*e.g.*, amphetamines and cocaine), that act as serotonin agonists (*e.g.*, buspirone, dihydroergotamine, and sumatriptan), or that otherwise increase serotonin activity (*e.g.*, ECT and lithium) all have been implicated in the development of serotonin syndrome. This syndrome typically includes akathisia-like restlessness, muscle twitches and myoclonus, hyperreflexia, sweating, penile erection, shivering, and tremor as a prelude to more severe intoxication, with seizures and coma. The reaction often is self-limiting if the diagnosis is made quickly and the offending agents are discontinued. The precise pathophysiological mechanisms underlying these toxic syndromes remain ill-defined. Newer MAO inhibitors (*e.g.*, selegiline, moclobemide, and perhaps St. John's wort preparations) also should be considered to have some risk of such interactions (Mason *et al.* 2000; Ener *et al.* 2003).

To avoid drug toxicity and prevent the precipitation of serotonin syndrome, duration of effect should be considered when switching between antidepressants. For example, an MAO inhibitor should not be started for 5 weeks after discontinuing fluoxetine, and 2 to 3 weeks should elapse between stopping a nonselective MAO inhibitor and initiating therapy with a tricyclic antidepressant.

The cerebral intoxication reactions associated with MAO inhibitors are distinguished from the hypertensive interaction of MAO inhibitors with indirectly acting pressor phenethylamines (*see* Chapter 10) such as tyramine. This interaction requires scrupulous avoidance of many agents, such as over-the-counter cold remedies containing indirect-acting sympathomimetic drugs (*see* Chapter 10) (Gardner *et al.*, 1996; Healy, 1997; Leipzig and Mendelowitz, 1992). Fatal intracranial bleeding has occurred in such hypertensive reactions. Headache is a common symptom, and fever frequently accompanies the hypertensive episode. Meperidine should never be used for such headaches (it could prove to be fatal), and blood pressure should be evaluated immediately when a patient taking an MAO inhibitor reports a severe throbbing headache or a feeling of pressure in the head. MAO inhibitors also can potentiate the effects of stimulants and bupropion (Weber, 1999; Hansten and Horn, 2000).

Therapeutic Uses. In addition to their use in adult major depression syndrome (*see* Drug Treatment of Mood Disorders, below), the various antidepressant agents have found broad utility in other disorders that may or may not be related psychobiologically to the mood disorders. Encouragement to find new indications has increased with the advent of newer agents that are less toxic, simpler to use, and often better accepted by both physicians and patients (Edwards, 1995; Edwards *et al.*, 1997; Tollefson and Rosenbaum, 1998). Current applications include rapid but temporary suppression of enuresis with low (*e.g.*, 25 mg) pre-bedtime doses of tricyclic antidepressants, including imipramine and nortriptyline, by uncertain mechanisms in children and in geriatric patients, as well as a beneficial effect of duloxetine on urinary stress incontinence (Moore, 2004).

Antidepressants have a growing role in other disorders, including *attention-deficit/hyperactivity disorder* in children and adults, for which imipramine, desipramine, and nortriptyline appear to be effective, even in patients responding poorly to or who are intolerant of the stimulants (*e.g.*, methylphenidate) that have been the standard agents for this disorder. Newer norepinephrine selective reuptake inhibitors also may be useful in this disorder; atomoxetine is approved for this application (Biederman *et al.*, 2004; Kratochvil *et al.*, 2003; Simpson and Plosker, 2004). Utility of SSRIs in this syndrome is not established, and bupropion, despite its similarity to stimulants, appears to have limited efficacy (Kutcher, 1997; Spencer *et al.*, 1993; Wilens *et al.*, 1992). Antidepressants tend to provide a more sustained and continuous improvement of the symptoms of attention-deficit/hyperactivity disorder than do the stimulants, and they do not induce tics or other abnormal movements sometimes associated with the use of stimulants. Indeed, desipramine and nortriptyline may effectively treat tic disorders, either in association with the use of stimulants or in patients with both attention deficit disorder and Tourette's syndrome (Spencer *et al.*, 1993). Antidepressants also are leading choices in the treatment of severe anxiety disorders, including panic disorder with agoraphobia, generalized anxiety disorder, social phobia, and obsessive-compulsive disorder (Feighner, 1999; Geller *et al.*, 2003; Masand and Gupta, 1999; Pigott and Seay, 1999; Pollack *et al.*, 2003; Rickels and Rynn, 2002; Sheehan, 2002; Waugh and Goa, 2003), as well as for the common comorbidity of anxiety in depressive illness (Boerner and Moller, 1999; Hoehn-Saric *et al.*, 2000). Antidepressants, especially SSRIs, also are employed in the management of posttraumatic stress disorder, which is marked by anxiety, startle, painful recollection of the traumatic events, and disturbed sleep (Asnis *et al.*, 2004). Initially, nonsedating antidepressants (Table 17–1) often are tolerated poorly by anxious patients, requiring slowly increased doses. Their beneficial actions typically are delayed for several weeks in anxiety disorders, just as they are in major depression.

For panic disorder, tricyclic antidepressants and MAO inhibitors, as well as high-potency benzodiazepines (notably alprazolam, clonazepam, and lorazepam) (*see* Chapter 16) are effective in blocking the autonomic expression of panic itself, thus facilitating a comprehensive rehabilitation program (Argyropoulos and Nutt, 1999; Sheehan, 2002). Imipramine and phenelzine are well-studied antidepressants for panic disorder. SSRIs also may be effective (Sheehan, 2002), but β adrenergic receptor antagonists, buspirone, and low-potency benzodiazepines usually are not, and bupropion can worsen anxiety (Taylor, 1998).

The SSRIs are agents of choice in obsessive-compulsive disorder, as well as in possibly related syndromes of impulse dyscontrol or obsessive preoccupations, including compulsive gambling, trichotillomania, bulimia (but usually not anorexia) nervosa, and body dysmorphic disorder (Agras, 1998; Geller *et al.*, 1998; Hoehn-Saric *et al.*, 2000; Pigott and Seay, 1999; Sadock and Sadock, 2000). Although their benefits may be limited, SSRIs offer an important advance in the medical treatment of these often chronic and sometimes incapacitating disorders for which no other medical treatment by itself has been consistently effective. The effectiveness of pharmacological treatment for these disorders is greatly enhanced by use of behavioral treatments (Miguel *et al.*, 1997).

In addition to the wide use of modern antidepressants to treat depression associated with general medical illnesses (Schwartz *et al.*, 1989), several psychosomatic disorders may respond at least partly to treatment with tricyclic antidepressants, MAO inhibitors, or SSRIs. These include chronic pain disorders, including diabetic and other peripheral neuropathic syndromes (for which tertiary-amine tricyclics probably are superior to fluoxetine, and both duloxetine and venlafaxine also may be effective); fibromyalgia; peptic ulcer and irritable bowel syndrome; hot flashes of menopause; chronic fatigue; cataplexy; tics; migraine; and sleep apnea (Bradley *et al.*, 2003; Goldstein *et al.*, 2004; Gruber *et al.*, 1996; Guttuso, 2004; Masand and Gupta, 1999; Nemeroff *et al.*, 2002; Spencer *et al.*, 1993; Vu, 2004). These disorders may have some psychobiological relationship to mood or anxiety disorders (Hudson and Pope, 1990).

Drug Treatment of Mood Disorders

Disorders of mood (*affective disorders*) are very common, both in general medical practice and in psychiatry. The

severity of these conditions covers an extraordinarily broad range, from normal grief reactions and dysthymia to severe, incapacitating psychotic and melancholic illnesses that may result in death. The lifetime risk of suicide in severe forms of major affective disorders requiring hospitalization is 10% to 15%, but as low at 3% to 5% in less severely ill outpatients. These statistics do not begin to represent the morbidity and cost of these frequently underdiagnosed and undertreated illnesses. Perhaps 30% to 40% of cases of clinical depression are diagnosed, and a much smaller proportion of those diagnosed are adequately treated (Isacsson *et al.*, 1992; Katon *et al.*, 1992; Kind and Sorensen, 1993; McCombs *et al.*, 1990; Suominen *et al.*, 1998).

Clearly, not all types of human grief and misery call for medical treatment, and even severe mood disorders have a high rate of spontaneous remission provided that sufficient time (often a matter of months) passes. Antidepressants generally are reserved for the more severe and incapacitating depressive disorders. The most satisfactory results tend to occur in patients who have moderately severe illnesses with "endogenous" or "melancholic" characteristics without psychotic features (American Psychiatric Association, 2000; Montgomery, 1995; Peselow *et al.*, 1992; Sadock and Sadock, 2000). The data from clinical research in support of the efficacy of antidepressant agents for adult major depression generally are convincing (Burke and Preskorn, 1995; Keller *et al.*, 1998; Kasper *et al.*, 1994; Montgomery and Roberts, 1994; Workman and Short, 1993). Nevertheless, a number of shortcomings continue to be associated with all drugs used to treat affective disorders.

A major problem with antidepressants is that because placebo response rates tend to be as high as 30% to 40% among research subjects diagnosed with major depression (Healy, 1997), and possibly even higher in some anxiety disorders, statistical and clinical distinctions between active drug and placebo are difficult to prove (Fairchild *et al.*, 1986; Kahn *et al.*, 2000). Assessment-based changes in clinical ratings of depressive symptoms, rather than categorization as "treatment responsive," often yields small average differences between active antidepressants and placebo in contemporary outpatient trials involving adult patients with depressive illness of only moderate severity, and even smaller and less consistent effects in juvenile depression (Healy, 1997; Kahn *et al.*, 2000; Moncrieff *et al.*, 2004; Storosum *et al.*, 2004; Whittington *et al.*, 2004). Separation of response rates to active antidepressants from placebo improves when patients are selected for moderate but not extreme severity, presence and persistence of classic melancholic or endogenous symptoms, and absence of psychotic features or of mixed bipolar states. Various metabolic, endocrinological, or other physiological testing procedures only marginally predict responses to antidepressant treatment and clinical utility (Baldessarini, 2000). These circumstances highlight the importance of continued reliance on placebo-controlled studies in the development of new agents, since comparisons against standard agents yielding no difference can risk an erroneous inference of equal efficacy.

Information on special depressed populations (pediatric, geriatric, medically ill, hospitalized, recurrently or chronically ill, and bipolar depressed patients) continues to be limited, despite the long-standing medical need for such information. Pediatric studies often have failed to show superiority of antidepressant drugs over placebo, particularly with older antidepressants, but also with most serotonin reuptake inhibitors, and the future of tricyclic antidepressant use in children is uncertain (Hazell *et al.*, 2002; Milin *et al.*, 2003; Whittington *et al.*, 2004). Geriatric depression includes an excess of chronic and psychotic illnesses, which tend to respond less well to antidepressant treatment alone, but may do better with ECT or when an antipsychotic agent is added (Schatzberg, 2003). Despite lack of consistency and convincingly demonstrated efficacy, the modern antidepressants have largely replaced the tricyclics as first-line options in children, adolescents, and the elderly, largely owing to their relative safety (*see* Safety Through the Life Cycle, above) (Montano, 1999). Finally, evidence concerning clinical dose-response and dose-risk relationships is especially limited with this class of drugs.

Choice of Antidepressant Medication and Dosing. The usual dosages and dose ranges of antidepressant medications are listed in Table 17–1, along with the severity of common side effects. Although they usually are used initially in divided doses, the relatively long half-lives and wide range of tolerated concentrations of most antidepressants permit gradual transition to a single daily dose. With the tricyclic antidepressants, dosing is most safely done with single doses up to the equivalent of 150 mg of imipramine.

Tricyclic and Selective Serotonin Reuptake Inhibitors. The imipramine-like tricyclics have been largely supplanted by the newer, less-toxic SSRIs and other atypical modern agents, which now are accepted broadly as drugs of first choice, particularly for medically ill or potentially suicidal patients and in the elderly and young (Brown and Khan, 1994; Flint, 1998; Oshima and Higuchi, 1999; Small, 1998; Whittington *et al.*, 2004). MAO inhibitors commonly are reserved for patients who fail to respond to vigorous trials of at least one of the newer agents and a standard tricyclic antidepressant, administered alone or with lithium or low doses of triiodothyronine to enhance overall therapeutic effectiveness (Bauer and Döpfmer, 1999; Lasser and Baldessarini, 1997; Yamada and Yashuhara,

2004). The somewhat less anticholinergic secondary-amine tricyclics, particularly nortriptyline and desipramine, can be considered as an alternative or a second choice for elderly or medically ill patients, particularly if administered in moderate, divided doses (Table 17–1). Despite their potential for less favorable responses to simple antidepressant therapy, patients with severe, prolonged, disabling, psychotic, suicidal, or bipolar depression require vigorous and prompt medical intervention. Underdiagnosis of depressive illnesses arises in part from the sometimes misleading clinical presentation of many depressed patients with nonspecific somatic complaints, anxiety, or insomnia. In the past, undertreatment arose from the reluctance of physicians to prescribe potentially toxic or pharmacologically complicated tricyclic or MAO inhibitor antidepressants, especially to medically ill or elderly patients. This pattern is changing with the wide acceptance of less-toxic and better-accepted antidepressants among the serotonin reuptake inhibitors and atypical agents (Anderson, 2001; Montano, 1999).

MAO Inhibitors. Indications for the MAO inhibitors are limited and must be weighed against their potential toxicity and their complex interactions with other drugs. The MAO inhibitors generally are considered drugs of late choice for the treatment of severe depression, even though the evidence for the efficacy of adequate doses of tranylcypromine or phenelzine is convincing. Despite the favorable results obtained with tranylcypromine and with doses of phenelzine above 45 mg per day (Davis *et al.*, 1987; Krishnan, 1998), the possibility of toxic reactions has limited their acceptance by many clinicians and patients (Yamada and Yasuhara, 2004). Nevertheless, MAO inhibitors sometimes are used when vigorous trials of several standard antidepressants have been unsatisfactory and when ECT is refused. In addition, MAO inhibitors may have selective benefits for conditions other than typical major depression, including illnesses marked by phobias and anxiety or panic as well as dysphoria, and possibly in chronic dysthymic conditions (Liebowitz, 1993; Versiani, 1998). Similar benefits, however, may be found with imipramine-like agents or SSRIs.

Stimulants and Experimental Treatment Modalities. Stimulants, with or without added sedatives, are an outmoded and ineffective treatment for severe depression. Stimulants such as methylphenidate or amphetamines demonstrate well-established effectiveness for the treatment of pediatric and adult attention disorder (Zhang and Baldessarini, 2004), and some clinicians continue to use them in the short-term treatment of other selected patients (Fawcett and Busch, 1998), including some geriatric patients and those with mild dysphoria, temporary demoralization, or lack of energy associated with medical illnesses. However, none of these possible indications has been investigated systematically (Chiarello and Cole, 1987).

Experimental treatments for psychotic forms of severe depression include use of the glucocorticoid/progesterone receptor antagonist–abortifacient mifepristone (RU-486) (Belanoff *et al.*, 2002; Schatzberg, 2003).

Bipolar Forms of Depression. A particularly difficult clinical challenge is the safe and effective treatment of bipolar depression (*see* Chapter 18). This condition sometimes is misdiagnosed in patients with bipolar disorder who present with mixed dysphoric-agitated moods, who then are inappropriately treated with an antidepressant without a mood stabilizing agent to protect against worsening agitation or mania (Wehr and Goodwin, 1987; Ghaemi *et al.*, 2004; Faedda *et al.*, 2004). For this reason the management of manic, mixed, and depressive mood states in bipolar disorder best relies on lithium or other mood-stabilizing agents, notably the anticonvulsant lamotrigine, as the primary treatment (*see* Chapter

18). An antidepressant can be added cautiously and temporarily to treat bipolar depression, but the additional benefit and safety of sustained combinations of an antidepressant with a mood stabilizer are unproven (Ghaemi *et al.*, 2003; Ghaemi *et al.*, 2004; Hadjipavlou *et al.*, 2004; Post *et al.*, 2003). The choice of antidepressant in bipolar depression remains uncertain. Moderate doses of desipramine or nortriptyline have been used in the past; currently, the short-acting SSRIs, bupropion, nefazodone, or mirtazapine often are employed despite a lack of data regarding rational choice of agent, dose, or timing (Zornberg and Pope, 1993; Ghaemi *et al.*, 2003; Martin *et al.*, 2004). Bupropion and SSRIs in moderate doses may have a reduced tendency to induce mania or mood destabilization. The first combination SSRI/atypical antipsychotic (fluoxetine/olanzapine; SYMBYAX) recently was FDA approved for treatment of depressive episodes associated with bipolar disorder (Ketter *et al.*, 2004).

Duration of Treatment. The natural history of major depression (either as unipolar depression or depressive phases of bipolar disorder) is that individual episodes tend to remit spontaneously over 6 to 12 months; however, there is a high risk of relapse of depression for at least several months following discontinuation of a successful trial of antidepressant treatment. This risk is estimated at 50% within 6 months and 65% to 70% at 1 year of follow-up, rising to 85% by 3 years (Baldessarini and Tohen, 1988; Viguera *et al.*, 1998). To minimize this risk, it is best to continue antidepressant medication for not less than 6 months following apparent clinical recovery. Continued use of initially therapeutic doses is recommended, although tolerability and acceptance by patients may require flexibility in this regard at later times.

Many depressed patients follow a recurring course of episodic illness, often with lesser levels of symptoms and disability between major episodes, and therefore merit consideration of long-term maintenance medication to reduce the risk of recurrence, particularly in patients with 3 or more relatively severe episodes or chronic depressive or dysthymic disorders (Keller *et al.*, 1998; Viguera *et al.*, 1998). Such treatment has been tested for as long as 5 years, using relatively high doses of imipramine, with evidence that early dose reduction led to a higher risk of relapse (Frank *et al.*, 1993; Kupfer *et al.*, 1992). Long-term supplementation of an antidepressant with lithium may enhance the result (Baldessarini and Tohen, 1988). Prolonged maintenance treatment of patients with recurring major depression for more than a year has rarely been evaluated with modern antidepressants, and long-term dose-response data with any antidepressant are very limited (Frank *et al.*, 1993; Hirschfeld, 2000; Keller *et al.*, 1998; Viguera *et al.*, 1998). The decision to recommend indefinitely prolonged maintenance treatment with an antidepressant is guided by the past history of multiple, and especially severe or life-threatening, recurrences and the impression that recurrence risk is greater in older patients. Due to evidence that rapid discontinuation or even a sharp reduction in doses of antidepressants and lithium may contribute to excess early recurrence of illness, gradual reduction and close clinical follow-up over at least several weeks are recommended when maintenance treatment is to be discontinued, and ideally, even when stopping continuation therapy within the months following recovery from an acute episode of depression (Greden, 1998; Viguera *et al.*, 1998; Baldessarini *et al.*, 1999).

Other short-acting, reversible inhibitors of MAO-A (*e.g.*, brofaromine or moclobemide) appear to be moderately effective antidepressants with reduced risk of inducing hypertension when combined with indirectly acting sympathomimetic pressor amines (*see* Chapter 10).

PHARMACOTHERAPY OF ANXIETY

Anxiety is a cardinal symptom of many psychiatric disorders and an almost inevitable component of many medical and surgical conditions. Indeed, it is a universal human emotion, closely allied with appropriate fear and presumably serving psychobiologically adaptive purposes. A most important clinical generalization is that anxiety is rather infrequently a "disease" in itself. Anxiety that is typically associated with the former "psychoneurotic" disorders is not readily explained in biological or psychological terms; contemporary hypotheses implicate overactivity of adrenergic systems or dysregulation of serotonergic systems in the CNS (Stein and Uhde, 1998). In addition, symptoms of anxiety commonly are associated with depression and especially with dysthymic disorder (chronic depression of moderate severity), panic disorder, agoraphobia and other specific phobias, obsessive-compulsive disorder, eating disorders, and many personality disorders (Boerner and Moller, 1999; Liebowitz, 1993). Sometimes, despite a thoughtful evaluation of a patient, no treatable primary illness is found, or if one is found and treated, it may be desirable to deal directly with the anxiety at the same time. In such situations antianxiety medications are frequently and appropriately used (Taylor, 1998).

Currently, the benzodiazepines and the SSRIs are the most commonly employed medicinal treatments for the common clinical anxiety disorders (*see* Chapter 16). Some high-potency benzodiazepines (alprazolam, clonazepam, and lorazepam) are effective in severe anxiety with strong autonomic overactivity (panic disorder), as are several antidepressants, as discussed above. For generalized or nonspecific anxiety, the benzodiazepine selected seems to make little difference (Rickels and Rynn, 2002). In the elderly or in patients with impaired hepatic function, oxazepam in small, divided doses sometimes is favored due to its brief action and direct conjugation and elimination. The latter property is shared by lorazepam, but not by alprazolam (*see* Chapter 16). Benzodiazepines sometimes are given to patients presenting with anxiety mixed with symptoms of depression, although the efficacy of these agents in altering the core features of severe major depression has not been demonstrated (Argyropoulos and Nutt, 1999; Boerner and Moller, 1999; Liebowitz, 1993).

The most favorable responses to the benzodiazepines are obtained in situations that involve relatively acute anxiety reactions in medical or psychiatric patients who have either modifiable primary illnesses or primary anxiety disorders. However, this group of anxious patients also has a high response rate to placebo and is likely to undergo spontaneous improvement. Antianxiety drugs also are used in the management of more persistent or recurrent primary anxiety disorders; guidelines for their appropriate long-term use for such disorders are less clear (Hollister *et al.*, 1993; Zohar, 2003).

Although there has been concern about the potential for habituation and abuse of benzodiazepines, some studies suggest that physicians tend to be conservative and may even undertreat patients with anxiety. They may either withhold drug unless symptoms or dysfunction are severe, or cease treatment within a few weeks, with a high proportion of relapses. Patients with personality disorders or a past history of abuse of sedatives or alcohol may be particularly at risk of dose escalation and dependence on benzodiazepines. Benzodiazepines carry some risk of impairing cognition and skilled motor functions, particularly in the elderly, in whom they are a common cause of confusion, delirium (sometimes mistaken for primary dementia), and falls with fractures (Ray *et al.*, 1987; Lawlor *et al.*, 2003). Risk of fatality on acute overdose of benzodiazepines is limited in the absence of other cerebrotoxins, including alcohol.

A particularly controversial aspect of the use of benzodiazepines, especially those of high potency, is in long-term management of patients with sustained or recurring symptoms of anxiety (Argyropoulos and Nutt, 1999; Hollister *et al.*, 1993; Soumerai *et al.*, 2003). Clinical benefit has been found for at least several months in such cases, but it is unclear to what extent the long-term benefits can be distinguished from nonspecific ("placebo") effects following development of tolerance on the one hand, or prevention of related withdrawal-emergent anxiety on the other.

In the past, other classes of CNS-active drugs were used for daytime sedation and to treat anxiety. Such drugs included the *propanediol carbamates* (notably meprobamate), and the barbiturates (*see* Chapter 16). Their use for anxiety is now obsolete due primarily to their tendency to cause unwanted degrees of sedation or frank intoxication at doses required to alleviate anxiety. Meprobamate and the barbiturates also can induce tolerance, physical dependence, severe withdrawal reactions, and life-threatening toxicity with overdosage.

The antihistamine *hydroxyzine* is an effective antianxiety agent, but only at doses (about 400 mg per day) that produce marked sedation (*see* Chapter 24). *Propranolol* and *metoprolol*, lipophilic β adrenergic receptor antagonists that enter the CNS, can reduce the autonomic symptoms (nervousness and muscle tremor) associated with specific situational or social phobias, but do not appear to be effective in generalized anxiety or panic disorder (*see* Chapter 10). Similarly, other antiadrenergic agents, including *clonidine*, may modify autonomic expression of anxiety, but have not been demonstrated convincingly to be clinically useful in the treatment of severe anxiety disorders (*see* Chapters 10 and 32).

Another class of agents with beneficial effects in disorders marked by anxiety or dysphoria of moderate intensity are the azapirones (azaspirodecanediones), currently represented clinically by buspirone (BUSPAR) (Ninan *et al.*, 1998). The azapirones have limited antidopaminergic actions *in vivo* and do not induce clinical extrapyramidal side effects. Also, they do not interact with binding sites for benzodiazepines or facilitate the action of GABA. They are not anticonvulsant (and may even lower seizure threshold slightly), do not appear to cause tolerance or withdrawal reactions, and do not show cross-tolerance with benzodiazepines or other sedatives. Buspirone and several experimental congeners (*e.g.*, *gepirone*, *ipsapirone*, and *tiospirone*) have selective affinity for serotonin receptors of the 5-HT$_{1A}$ type, for which they appear to be partial agonists (*see* Chapter 11).

Buspirone has beneficial actions in anxious patients, particularly those with generalized anxiety of mild or moderate severity (Ninan *et al.*, 1998; Taylor, 1998). Unlike potent benzodiazepines and antidepressants, buspirone lacks beneficial actions in severe anxiety with panic attacks. It is not efficacious as a monotherapy in obsessive-compulsive disorder, although it may have useful anti-obsessional activity when added to SSRIs (which are efficacious as monotherapy). A lack of cross-tolerance is consistent with a lack of clinical protection against withdrawal-emergent anxiety when changing abruptly from treatment with a benzodiazepine to buspirone; a gradual transition between these classes of antianxiety agents is more likely to be tolerated (Lader, 1987). Of note, the risk of suicide with buspirone is very low.

CLINICAL SUMMARY

Major affective and anxiety disorders continue to represent the most common psychiatric illnesses, and are those most often encountered by primary-care clinicians. Major depression may well represent a spectrum of disorders, varying in severity from mild and self-limited conditions that approach everyday human distress to extraordinarily severe, psychotic, incapacitating, and deadly diseases. Rates of diagnosis and appropriate treatment of major mood disorders have improved somewhat in recent years with the advent of better-accepted and safer mood-altering medicines. Nevertheless, the majority of patients with depression or bipolar disorder are diagnosed after years of delay, if at all, and many remain inadequately treated or studied, especially children, the elderly, those with bipolar depression, and those with severe, chronic, or psychotic forms of depression.

The major limitation to developing new antidepressant and antianxiety drugs is a fundamental lack of a coherent pathophysiology and etiology for major depression, bipolar disorder, and common anxiety disorders. Current medications (SSRIs and tricyclic antidepressants) focus on blockade of norepinephrine and serotonin uptake, thereby prolonging their synaptic effects. The relative success of these agents creates a conceptual impasse that limits identification of novel therapeutic targets for these disorders (Murphy *et al.*, 1995; Healy, 1997). Nevertheless, a number of novel products aimed at the treatment of depression or anxiety disorders are in development (NDA Pipeline, 2004). These include other inhibitors of neuronal transport of one or more monoamines, including norepinephrine or dopamine, as well as serotonin (*e.g.*, BTS-74398, DOV-216303, MCI-225; *milnacipran*, [DALCIPRAN, IXEL]); serotonin agonists (e.g., sunepitron, PRX-0002), largely for anxiety; serotonin antagonists (e.g., AR-A2, deramciclane, SB-243213), mainly for depression; agents with partial-agonist effects at dopamine and serotonin receptors, much like some atypical antipsychotics (*e.g.*, SLV-308, SLV-318); inhibitors of MAO-A (moclobemide, selegiline); inhibitors of phosphodiesterase 4 (e.g., MEM-1414); glutamate α-amino-3-hydroxy-5-methyl-4-isoxazole propionic acid (AMPA) receptor modulators (*ampakines*; *e.g.*, CX-516); glutamate metabotropic receptor agonists for anxiety (e.g., LY-544344); GABA$_A$ receptor agonists for anxiety (*e.g.,* CP-615003, DOV-51892; *ocinaplon, pagoclone*); inhibitors of neurokinin-1 (substance-P) receptors (e.g., CP-122721, GB-823296, GW-597599, R-673, SB-823296); ligands for cerebral sigma-2 sites (e.g., LU-28179); corticotropin (CRF-1) receptor antagonists (e.g., AG-561, AVE-4579, DPC-368, NBI-30775, SB-733620); and the metabolic methyl donor S-adenosyl-L-methionine.

BIBLIOGRAPHY

Abell, C.W., and Kwan, S.W. Molecular characterization of monoamine oxidases A and B. *Prog. Nucl. Acid Res. Mol. Biol.,* **2000,** *65:*129–156.

Anderson, I.M. Meta-analytical studies on new antidepressants. *Br. Med. Bull.,* **2001,** *57:*161–178.

Argyropoulos, S.V., and Nutt, D.J. The use of benzodiazepines in anxiety and other disorders. *Eur. Neuropsychopharmacol.,* **1999,** *9*(suppl 6):S407–S412.

Ascher, J.A., Cole, J.O., Colin, J.N., *et al.* Bupropion: a review of its mechanism of antidepressant activity. *J. Clin. Psychiatry,* **1995,** *56:*395–401.

Asnis, G.M., Kohn, S.R., Henderson, M., and Brown, N.L. SSRIs vs. non-SSRIs in post-traumatic stress disorder: update with recommendations. *Drugs,* **2004,** *64:*383–404.

Azmitia, E.C., and Whitaker-Azmitia, P.M. Anatomy, cell biology, and plasticity of the seronergic system. In, *Psychopharmacology: The Fourth Generation of Progress.* (Bloom, F.E., and Kupfer, D.L., eds.) Raven Press, New York, **1995,** pp. 443–449.

Baldessarini, R.J., and Jamison, J.R. Effects of medical interventions on suicidal behavior. Summary and conclusions. *J. Clin. Psychiatry,* **1999,** *60*(suppl 2):117–122.

Baldessarini, R.J., and Tohen, M. Is there a long-term protective effect of mood-altering agents in unipolar depressive disorder? In, *Psycho-*

pharmacology: Current Trends. (Casey, D.E., and Christensen, A.V., eds.) Springer-Verlag, Berlin, **1988,** pp. 130–139.

Baldessarini, R.J., Tondo, L., and Viguera, A.C. Discontinuing psychotropic agents. *J. Psychopharmacology,* **1999,** *13:*292–293.

Barker, E.L., and Blakely, R.D. Norepinephrine and serotonin transporters: molecular targets of antidepressant drugs. In, *Psychopharmacology: The Fourth Generation of Progress.* (Bloom, F.E., and Kupfer, D.L., eds.) Raven Press, New York, **1995,** pp. 321–333.

Bauer, M., and Döpfmer, S. Lithium augmentation in treatment-resistant depression: meta-analysis of placebo-controlled studies. *J. Clin. Psychopharmacol.,* **1999,** *19:*427–434.

Beasley, C.M., Masica, D.N., and Potvin, J.H. Fluoxetine: a review of receptor and functional effects and their clinical implications. *Psychopharmacology (Berl.),* **1992,** *107:*1–10.

Belanoff, J.K., Rothschild, A.J., Cassidy, F., *et al.* Open-label trial of C-1073 (mifepristone) for psychotic major depression. *Biol. Psychiatry,* **2002,** *52:*386–392.

Berger, F.M. The pharmacological properties of 2-methyl-2-n-propyl-1,3 propanediol dicarbamate (MILTOWN), a new interneuronal blocking agent. *J. Pharmacol. Exp. Ther.,* **1954,** *112:*413–423.

Biederman, J., Spencer, T., and Wilens, T. Evidence-based pharmacotherapy for attention-deficit hyperactivity disorder. *Int. J. Neuropsychopharmacol.,* **2004,** *7:*77–97.

Biederman, J., Thisted, R.A., Greenhill, L.L., and Ryan, N.D. Estimation of the association between desipramine and the risk for sudden death in 5- to 14-year-old children. *J. Clin. Psychiatry,* **1995,** *56:*87–93.

Birnbaum, C.S., Cohen, L.S., Bailey, J.W., *et al.* Serum concentrations of antidepressants and benzodiazepines in nursing infants: a case series. *Pediatrics,* **1999,** *104:*1–11.

Blier, P., de Montigny C., and Chaput, Y. A role for the serotonin system in the mechanism of action of antidepressant treatments: preclinical evidence. *J. Clin. Psychiatry,* **1990,** *51*(suppl):14–20.

Boerner, R.J., and Moller, H.J. The importance of new antidepressants in the treatment of anxiety/depressive disorders. *Pharmacopsychiatry,* **1999,** *32:*119–126.

Bradley, R.H., Barkin, R.L., Jerome, J., DeYoung, K., and Dodge, C.W. Efficacy of venlafaxine for the long term treatment of chronic pain with associated major depressive disorder. *Am. J. Ther.,* **2003,** *10:*318–323.

Brown, W.A., and Khan, A. Which depressed patients should receive antidepressants? *CNS Drugs,* **1994,** *1:*341–347.

Buckley, N.A., and Faunce, T.A. 'Atypical' antidepressants in overdose: clinical considerations with respect to safety. *Drug Saf.,* **2003,** *26:*539–551.

Burke, M.J., and Preskorn, S.H. Short-term treatment of mood disorders with standard antidepressants. In, *Psychopharmacology: The Fourth Generation of Progress.* (Bloom, F.E., and Kupfer, D.L., eds.) Raven Press, New York, **1995,** pp. 1053–1065.

Byrne, S.E., and Rothschild, A.J. Loss of antidepressant efficacy during maintenance therapy: possible mechanisms and treatments. *J. Clin. Psychiatry,* **1998,** *59:*279–288.

Caccia, S. Metabolism of the newer antidepressants. An overview of the pharmacological and pharmacokinetic implications. *Clin. Pharmacokinet.,* **1998,** *34:*281–302.

Caccia S. Metabolism of the newest antidepressants: comparisons with related predecessors. *Drugs,* **2004,** *7:*143–150.

Carlsson A., and Wong, D.T. Correction: a note on the discovery of selective serotonin reuptake inhibitors. *Life Sci.,* **1997,** *61:*1203.

Catterson, M.L., Preskorn, S.H., and Martin, R.L. Pharmacodynamic and pharmacokinetic considerations in geriatric psychopharmacology. *Psychiatr. Clin. North Am.,* **1997,** *20:*205–218.

Cesura, A.M., and Pletscher, A. The new generation of monoamine oxidase inhibitors. *Prog. Drug Res.*, **1992,** *38:*171–297.

Chaput, Y., de Montigny, C., and Blier, P. Presynaptic and postsynaptic modifications of the serotonin system by long-term administration of antidepressant treatments. An *in vivo* electrophysiologic study in the rat. *Neuropsychopharmacology*, **1991,** *5:*219–229.

Cheeta, S., Schifano, F., Oyefeso, A., Webb, L., and Ghodse, A.H. Antidepressant-related deaths and antidepressant prescriptions in England and Wales, 1998–2000. *Br. J. Psychiatry*, **2004,** *184:*41–47.

Chiarello, R.J., and Cole, J.O. The use of psychostimulants in general psychiatry. A reconsideration. *Arch. Gen. Psychiatry*, **1987,** *44:*286–295.

Crewe, H.K., Lennard, M.S., Tucker, G.T., Woods, F.R., and Haddock, R.E. The effect of selective serotonin reuptake inhibitors on cytochrome P450 2D6 (CYP2D6) activity in human liver microsomes. *Br. J. Clin. Pharmacol.*, **1992,** *34:*262–265.

Danish University Antidepressant Group. Moclobemide: a reversible MAO-A inhibitor showing weaker antidepressant effect than clomipramine in a controlled multicenter study. *J. Affect. Disord.*, **1993,** *28:*105–116.

Davis, J.M., Janicak, P.G., and Bruninga, K. The efficacy of MAO inhibitors in depression; a meta-analysis. *Psychiatric Ann.*, **1987,** *17:*825–831.

Delgado, P.L., and Michaels, T. Reboxetine: a review of efficacy and tolerability. *Drugs Today*, **1999,** *35:*725–737.

Delini-Stula, A., Radeke, E., and Waldmeier, P.S. Basic and clinical aspects of the new monoamine oxidase inhibitors. In, *Psychopharmacology: Current Trends.* (Casey, D.E., and Christensen, A.V., eds.) Springer-Verlag, Berlin, **1988,** pp. 147–158.

Ditto, K.E. SSRI discontinuation syndrome. *Postgrad. Med.*, **2003,** *114:*79–84.

Duman, R.S., Heninger, G.R., and Nestler, E.J. A molecular and cellular theory of depression. *Arch. Gen. Psychiatry*, **1997,** *54:*597–606.

Edwards, J.G. Drug choice in depression: selective serotonin reuptake inhibitors or tricyclic antidepressants? *CNS Drugs*, **1995,** *4:*141–159.

Edwards, J.G., Inman, W.H.W., Wilton, L., Pearce, G.L., and Kubota, K. Drug safety monitoring of 12,692 patients treated with fluoxetine. *Hum. Psychopharmacol. Clin. Exp.*, **1997,** *12:*127–137.

Emslie, G.J., Heiligenstein, J.H., Wagner, K.D., *et al.* Fluoxetine for acute treatment of depression in children and adolescents: a placebo-controlled, randomized clinical trial. *J. Am. Acad. Child Adolesc. Psychiatry*, **2002,** *41:*1205–1215.

Emslie, G.J., Walkup, J.T., Pliszka, S.R., and Ernst, M. Nontricyclic antidepressants: current trends in children and adolescents. *J. Am. Acad. Child Adolesc. Psychiatry*, **1999,** *38:*517–528.

Ener, R.A., Meglathery, S.B., Van Decker, W.A., and Gallagher, R.M. Serotonin syndrome and other serotonergic disorders. *Pain Med.*, **2003,** *4:*63–74.

Ereshefsky, L., Riesenman, C., and Lam, Y.W. Serotonin selective reuptake inhibitor drug interactions and the cytochrome P450 system. *J. Clin. Psychiatry*, **1996,** *57*(suppl 8):17–24.

Faedda, G.L., Baldessarini, R.J., Glovinsky, I.P., and Austin, N.B. Mania with antidepressant and stimulant treatment in pediatric manic-depressive illness. *J. Affect. Disord.*, **2004,** 82:149–158.

Fairchild, C.J., Rush, A.J., Vasavada, N., Giles, D.E., and Khatami, M. Which depressions respond to placebo? *Psychiatry Res.*, **1986,** *18:*217–226.

Fisher, A., Davis, M., Croft-Baker, J., Purcell, P., and McLean, A. Citalopram-induced severe hyponatraemia with coma and seizure. *Adverse Drug React., Toxicol. Rev.*, **2002,** *21:*179–187.

Flint, A.J. Choosing appropriate antidepressant therapy in the elderly. A risk-benefit assessment of available agents. *Drugs Aging*, **1998,** *13:*269–280.

Foote, S.L., and Aston-Jones, G.S. Pharmacology and physiology of central noradrenergic systems. In, *Psychopharmacology: The Fourth Generation of Progress.* (Bloom, F.E., and Kupfer, D.L., eds.) Raven Press, New York, **1995,** pp. 335–345.

Frank, E., Kupfer, D.J., Perel, J.M., *et al.* Comparison of full-dose versus half-dose pharmacotherapy in the maintenance treatment of recurrent depression. *J. Affect. Disord.*, **1993,** *27:*139–145.

Gardner, D.M., Shulman, K.I., Walker, S.E., and Tailor, S.A. The making of a user-friendly MAOI diet. *J. Clin. Psychiatry*, **1996,** *57:*99–104.

Geller, D.A., Biederman, J., Stewart, S.E., *et al.* Which SSRI? A meta-analysis of pharmacotherapy trials in pediatric obsessive-compulsive disorder. *Am. J. Psychiatry*, **2003,** *160:*1919–1928.

Ghaemi, S.N., Hsu, D.J., Soldani, F., and Goodwin, F.K. Antidepressants in bipolar disorder: the case for caution. *Bipolar Disord.*, **2003,** *5:*421–433.

Ghaemi, S.N., Rosenquist, K.J., Ko, J.Y., *et al.* Antidepressant treatment in bipolar vs. unipolar depression. *Am. J. Psychiatry*, **2004,** *161:*163–165.

Glassman, A.H., Roose, S.P., and Bigger, J.T. Jr. The safety of tricyclic antidepressants in cardiac patients. Risk-benefit reconsidered. *J.A.M.A.*, **1993,** *269:*2673–2675.

Goldstein, D.J., Lu, Y., Detke, M.J., *et al.* Effects of duloxetine on painful physical symptoms associated with depression. *Psychosomatics*, **2004,** *45:*17–28.

Greden, J.F. Do long-term treatments alter lifetime course? *J. Psychiatr. Res.*, **1998,** *32:*197–199.

Gruber, A.J., Hudson, J.I., and Pope, H.G. Jr. The management of treatment-resistant depression in disorders on the interface of psychiatry and medicine. Fibromyalgia, chronic fatigue syndrome, migraine, irritable bowel syndrome, atypical facial pain, and premenstrual dysphoric disorder. *Psychiatr. Clin. North Am.*, **1996,** *19:*351–369.

Guttuso, T. Jr. Hot flashes refractory to HRT and SSRI therapy but responsive to gabapentin therapy. *J. Pain Symptom Manage.*, **2004,** 27:274–276.

Hadjipavlou, G., Mok, H., and Yatham, L.N. Pharmacotherapy of bipolar II disorder: a critical review of current evidence. *Bipolar Disord.*, **2004,** *6:*14–25.

Hamilton, M.S., and Opler, L.A. Akathisia, suicidality, and fluoxetine. *J. Clin. Psychiatry*, **1992,** *53:*401–406.

van Harten, J. Clinical pharmacokinetics of selective serotonin reuptake inhibitors. *Clin. Pharmacokinet.*, **1993,** *24:*203–220.

Hazell, P., O'Connell, D., Heathcote, D., and Henry, D. Tricyclic drugs for depression in children and adolescents. *Cochrane Database Syst. Rev.*, **2002,** *2:*CD002317.

Helgason, T., Tómasson, H., and Zoëga, T. Antidepressants and public health in Iceland: time series analysis of national data. *Br. J. Psychiatry*, **2004,** *184:*157–162.

Hemeryck, A., and Belpaire, F.M. Selective serotonin reuptake inhibitors and cytochrome P-450 mediated drug-drug interactions: an update. *Curr. Drug Metab.*, **2002,** *3:*13–37.

Heninger, G.R., and Charney, D.S. Mechanisms of action of antidepressant treatments: implications for the etiology and treatment of depressive disorders. In, *Psycopharmacology: The Third Generation of Progress.* (Meltzer, H.Y., ed.) New York, Raven Press, **1987,** pp. 535–544.

Hoehn-Saric, R., Ninan, P., Black, D.W., *et al.* Multicenter double-blind comparison of sertraline and desipramine for concurrent obsessive-compulsive and major depressive disorders. *Arch. Gen. Psychiatry,* **2000,** *57:*76–82.

Hirschfeld, R.M. Antidepressants in long-term therapy: review of tricyclic antidepressants and selective serotonin reuptake inhibitors. *Acta Psychiatr. Scand. Suppl.,* **2000,** *403:*35–38.

Hudson, J.I., and Pope, H.G. Jr. Affective spectrum disorder: does antidepressant response identify a family of disorders with a common pathophysiology? *Am. J. Psychiatry,* **1990,** *147:*552–564.

Hyman, S.E., and Nestler, E.J. Initiation and adaptation: a paradigm for understanding psychotropic drug action. *Am. J. Psychiatry,* **1996,** *153:*151–162.

Isacsson, G., Boëthius, G., and Bergman, U. Low level of antidepressant prescription for people who later commit suicide: 15 years of experience from a population-based drug database in Sweden. *Acta Psychiatr. Scand.,* **1992,** *85:*444–448.

Johnston, J.A., Lineberry, C.G., Ascher, J.A., *et al.* A 102-center prospective study of seizure in association with bupropion. *J. Clin. Psychiatry,* **1991,** *52:*450–456.

Kahn, A., Warner, H.A., and Brown, W.A. Symptom reduction and suicide risk in patients treated with placebo in antidepressant clinical trials: an analysis of the Food and Drug Administration database. *Arch. Gen. Psychiatry,* **2000,** *57:*311–317.

Kasper, S., Höflich, G., Scholl, H.-P., and Möller, H.-J. Safety and antidepressant efficacy of selective serotonin re-uptake inhibitors. *Hum. Psychopharmacol.,* **1994,** *9:*1–12.

Katon, W., von Korff M., Lin, E., Bush, T., and Ormel, J. Adequacy and duration of antidepressant treatment in primary care. *Med. Care,* **1992,** *30:*67–76.

Keller, M.B., Kocsis, J.K., Thase, M.E., *et al.* Maintenance phase efficacy of sertraline for chronic depression: a randomized controlled trial. *J.A.M.A.,* **1998,** *280:*1665–1672.

Kessler, R.C., McGonagle, K.A., Zhao, S., *et al.* Lifetime and 12-month prevalence of DSM-III-R psychiatric disorders in the United States. Results from the National Comorbidity Study. *Arch. Gen. Psychiatry,* **1994,** *51:*8–19.

Ketter, T.A., Wang, P.W., Nowakowska, C., Marsh, W.K. New medication treatment options for bipolar disorders. *Acta Psychiatr. Scand. Suppl.,* **2004,** (suppl. 422):18–33.

Kind, P., and Sorensen, J. The costs of depression. *Int. Clin. Psychopharmacol.,* **1993,** *7:*191–195.

Kitamura, Y., Zhao, X.H., Takei, M., and Nomura, Y. Effects of antidepressants on the glutamatergic system in mouse brain. *Neurochem. Int.,* **1991,** *19:*247–253.

Kitayama, I., Janson, A.M., Cintra, A., *et al.* Effects of chronic imipramine treatment on glucocorticoid receptor immunoreactivity in various regions of the rat brain. Evidence for selective increases of glucocorticoid receptor immunoreactivity in the locus coeruleus and 5-hydroxytryptamine nerve cell groups of the rostral ventromedial medulla. *J. Neural Transm.,* **1988,** *73:*191–203.

Kline, N.S. Clinical experience with iproniazid (marsilid). *J. Clin. Exp. Psychopathol.,* **1958,** *19*(suppl):72–78.

Knapp, M.J., Knopman, D.S., Solomon, P.R., *et al.* A 30-week randomized controlled trial of high-dose tacrine in patients with Alzheimer's disease. The Tacrine Study Group. *JAMA,* **1994,** *271:*985–991.

Kuhn, R. The treatment of depressive states with G22355 (imipramine hydrochloride). *Am. J. Psychiatry,* **1958,** *115:*459–464.

Kratochvil, C.J., Vaughan, B.S., Harrington, M.J., and Burke, W.J. Atomoxetine: a selective noradrenaline reuptake inhibitor for the treatment of attention-deficit/hyperactivity disorder. *Expert Opin. Pharmacother.,* **2003,** *4:*1165–1174.

Kuhn, W., and Muller, T. The clinical potential of deprenyl in neurologic and psychiatric disorders. *J. Neural Transm. Suppl.,* **1996,** *48:*85–93.

Kupfer, D.J., Frank, E., Perel, J.M., *et al.* Five-year outcome for maintenance therapies in recurrent depression. *Arch. Gen. Psychiatry,* **1992,** *49:*769–773.

Lader, M. Long-term anxiolytic therapy: the issue of drug withdrawal. *J. Clin. Psychiatry,* **1987,** *48*(suppl 12):12–16.

Lasser, R.A., and Baldessarini, R.J. Thyroid hormones in depressive disorders: a reappraisal of clinical utility. *Harv. Rev. Psychiatry,* **1997,** *4:*291–305.

Lawlor, D.A., Patel, R., and Ebrahim, S. Association between falls in elderly women and chronic diseases and drug use: cross sectional study. *B.M.J.,* **2003,** *327:*712–717.

Liebowitz, M.R. Depression with anxiety and atypical depression. *J. Clin. Psychiatry,* **1993,** *54*(suppl):10–14.

Lotufo-Neto, F., Trivedi, M., and Thase, M.E. Meta-analysis of the reversible inhibitors of monoamine oxidase type A moclobemide and brofaromine in the treatment of depression. *Neuropsychopharmacology,* **1999,** *20:*226–247.

Lucena, M.I., Carvajal, A., Andrade, R.J., and Velasco, A. Antidepressant-induced hepatotoxicity. *Expert Opin. Drug Safety,* **2003,** *2:*249–262.

McCombs, J.S., Nichol, M.B., Stimmel, G.L., *et al.* The cost of antidepressant drug therapy failure: a study of antidepressant use patterns in a Medicaid population. *J. Clin. Psychiatry,* **1990,** *51*(suppl):60–69.

McGrath, C., Buist, A., and Norman, T.R. Treatment of anxiety during pregnancy: effects of psychotropic drug treatment on the developing fetus. *Drug Saf.,* **1999,** *20:*171–186.

Mann, J.J., Aarons, S.F., Wilner, P.J., *et al.* A controlled study of the antidepressant efficacy and side effects of (–)-deprenyl. A selective monoamine oxidase inhibitor. *Arch. Gen. Psychiatry,* **1989,** *46:*45–50.

Martin, A., Young, C., Leckman, J.F., *et al.* Age effects on antidepressant-induced manic conversion. *Arch. Pediatr. Adolesc. Med.,* **2004,** *158:*773–780.

Mason, P.J., Morris, V.A., and Balcezak, T.J. Serotonin syndrome. Presentation of 2 cases and review of the literature. *Medicine (Baltimore),* **2000,** *79:*201–209.

Miguel, E.C., Rauch, S.L., and Jenicke, M.A. Obsessive-compulsive disorder. *Psychiatr. Clin. North Am.,* **1997,** *20:*863–883.

Milin, R., Walker, S., and Chow, J. Major depressive disorder in adolescence: a brief review of the recent treatment literature. *Can. J. Psychiatry,* **2003,** *48:*600–606.

Moncrieff, J., Wessely, S., and Hardy, R. Active placebos vs. antidepressants for depression. *Cochrane Database Syst. Rev.,* **2004,** *1:*CD003012.

Montano, C.B. Primary care issues related to the treatment of depression in elderly patients. *J. Clin. Psychiatry,* **1999,** *60*(suppl 20):45–51.

Montgomery, S.A., and Roberts, A. SSRIs: well tolerated treatment for depression. *Hum. Psychopharmacol.,* **1994,** *9*(suppl 1):S7–S10.

Montgomery, S.A. Selective serotonin reuptake inhibitors in the acute treatment of depression. In, *Psychopharmacology: The Fourth Generation of Progress.* (Bloom, F.E., and Kupfer, D.L., eds.) Raven Press, New York, **1995,** pp. 1043–1051.

Moore K. Duloxetine: New approach for treating stress urinary incontinence. *Int. J. Gynaecol. Obstet.,* **2004,** *86*(suppl. 1):S53–S62.

NDA Pipeline. Available at: http://www.ndapipeline.com. Accessed Dec. 2004.

Nelson, J.C., Mazure, C.M., Bowers, M.B. Jr., and Jatlow, P.I. A preliminary, open study of the combination of fluoxetine and desipramine for rapid treatment of major depression. *Arch. Gen. Psychiatry*, **1991**, *48:*303–307.

Nemeroff, C.B., Schatzberg, A.F., Goldstein, D.J., *et al.* Duloxetine for the treatment of major depressive disorder. *Psychopharmacol. Bull.,* **2002**, *36:*106–132.

Nestler, E.J., McMahohn, A., Sabban, E.L., Tallman, J.F., and Duman, R.S. Chronic antidepressant administration decreases the expression of tyrosine hydroxylase in the rat locus coeruleus. *Proc. Natl. Acad. Sci. U.S.A.*, **1990**, *87:*7522–7526.

Newman, S.C., and Hassan, A.I. Antidepressant use in the elderly population in Canada: results from a national survey. *J. Gerontol. A. Biol. Sci. Med. Sci.*, **1999**, *54:*M527–M530.

Nicotra, M.B., Rivera, M., Pool, J.L., and Noall, M.W. Tricyclic antidepressant overdose: clinical and pharmacologic observations. *Clin. Toxicol.*, **1981**, *18:*599–613.

Oshima, A., and Higuchi, T. Treatment guidelines for geriatric mood disorders. *Psychiatry Clin. Neurosci.*, **1999**, *53*(suppl):S55–S59.

Owens, M.J., Morgan, W.N., Plott, S.J., and Nemeroff, C.B. Neurotransmitter receptor and transporter binding profile of antidepressants and their metabolites. *J. Pharmacol. Exp. Ther.*, **1997**, *283:*1305–1322.

Pacher, P., Ungvari, Z., Nanasi, P.P., Furst, S., and Kecskemeti, V. Speculations on difference between tricyclic and selective serotonin reuptake inhibitor antidepressants on their cardiac effects. Is there any? *Curr. Med. Chem.*, **1999**, *6:*469–480.

Perry, P.J., Zeilman, C., and Arndt, S. Tricyclic antidepressant concentrations in plasma: an estimate of their sensitivity and specificity as a predictor of response. *J. Clin. Psychopharmacol.*, **1994**, *14:*230–240.

Peselow, E.D., Sanfilipo, M.P., Difiglia, C., and Fieve, R.R. Melancholic/endogenous depression and response to somatic treatment and placebo. *Am. J. Psychiatry*, **1992**, *149:*1324–1334.

Pigott, T.A., and Seay, S.M. A review of the efficacy of selective serotonin reuptake inhibitors in obsessive-compulsive disorder. *J. Clin. Psychiatry*, **1999**, *60:*101–106.

Pollock, B.G., and Perel, J.M. Hydroxy metabolites of tricyclic antidepressants: evaluation of relative cardiotoxicity. In, *Clinical Pharmacology in Psychiatry: From Molecular Studies to Clinical Reality.* (Dahl, S.G., and Gram, L.F., eds.) Springer-Verlag, Berlin, **1989**, pp. 232–236.

Pollack, M.H., Allgulander, C., Bandelow, B., *et al.* WCA recommendations for the long-term treatment of panic disorder. *CNS Spectrums*, **2003**, *8*(8 suppl 1):17–30.

Post, R.M., Baldassano, C.F., Perlis, R.H., and Ginsberg, D.L. Treatment of bipolar depression. *CNS Spectrums*, **2003**, *8:*1–10.

Preskorn, S.H. Debate resolved: there are differential effects of serotonin selective reuptake inhibitors on cytochrome P450 enzymes. *J. Psychopharmacol.*, **1998**, *12:*S89–S97.

Prouty, R.W., and Anderson, W.H. The forensic science implications of site and temporal influences on postmortem blood-drug concentrations. *J. Forensic Sci.*, **1990**, *35:*243–270.

Racagni, G., Tinelli, D., and Bianchi, E. cAMP-dependent binding proteins and endogenous phosphorylation after antidepressant treatment. In, *5-Hydroxytryptamine in Psychiatry: A Spectrum of Ideas.* (Sandler, M., Coppen, A., and Hartnet, S., eds.) Oxford University Press, New York, **1991**, pp. 116–123.

Raskin, J., Goldstein, D.J., Mallinckrodt, C.H., and Ferguson, M.B. Duloxetine in the long-term treatment of major depressive disorder. *J. Clin. Psychiatry*, **2003**, *64:*1237–1244.

Ray, W.A., Griffin, M.R., Schaffner, W., Baugh, D.K., and Melton, L.J. III. Psychotropic drug use and the risk of hip fracture. *N. Engl. J. Med.*, **1987**, *316:*363–369.

Rickels, K., and Rynn, M. Pharmacotherapy of generalized anxiety disorder. *J. Clin. Psychiatry*, **2002**, *63*(suppl 14):9–16.

Roose, S.P., Glassman, A.H., Attia, E., and Woodring, S. Comparative efficacy of selective serotonin reuptake inhibitors and tricyclics in the treatment of melancholia. *Am. J. Psychiatry*, **1994**, *151:*1735–1739.

Roose, S.P. Modern cardiovascular standards for psychotropic drugs. *Psychopharmacol. Bull.*, **1992**, *28:*35–43.

Ryan, N.D. Child and adolescent depression: short-term treatment effectiveness and long-term opportunities. *Int. J. Methods Psychiatr. Res.*, **2003**, *12:*44–53.

Sachs, G.S., Lafer, B., Stoll, A.L., *et al.* A double-blind trial of bupropion versus desipramine for bipolar depression. *J. Clin. Psychiatry*, **1994**, *55:*391–393.

Sauer, J.M., Ponsler, G.D., Mattiuz, E.L., *et al.* Disposition and metabolic fate of atomoxetine hydrochloride. *Drug Metab. Dispos.*, **2003**, *31:*98–107.

Schatzberg, A.F., Haddad, P., Kaplan, E.M., *et al.* Serotonin reuptake discontinuation syndrome: a hypothetical definition. Discontinuation Consensus panel. *J. Clin. Psychiatry*, **1997**, *58*(suppl 7):5–10.

Schatzberg, A.F. New approaches to managing psychotic depression. *J. Clin. Psychiatry*, **2003**, *64*(suppl 1):19–23.

Schwartz, J.A., Speed, N., and Bereford, T.P. Antidepressants in the medically ill: prediction of benefits. *Int. J. Psychiatry Med.*, **1989**, *19:*363–369.

Settle, E.C. Jr. Antidepressant drugs: disturbing and potentially dangerous adverse effects. *J. Clin. Psychiatry*, **1998**, *59*(suppl 16):25–30.

Sheehan, D.V. The management of panic disorder. *J. Clin. Psychiatry*, **2002**, *63*(suppl 14):17–21.

Simpson D., and Plosker, G.L. Atomoxetine: a review of its use in adults with attention deficit hyperactivity disorder. *Drugs*, **2004**, *64:*205–222.

Siuciak, J.A., Lewis, D.R., Wiegand, S.J., and Lindsay, R.M. Antidepressant-like effect of brain-derived neurotrophic factor (BDNF). *Pharmacol. Biochem. Behav.*, **1997**, *56:*131–137.

Skinner, M.H., Kuan, H.Y., Pan, A., *et al.* Duloxetine is both an inhibitor and a substrate of cytochrome P450-2D6 in healthy volunteers. *Clin. Pharmacol. Ther.*, **2003**, *73:*170–177.

Small, G.W. Treatment of geriatric depression. *Depression Anxiety*, **1998**, *8*(suppl 1):32–42.

Soumerai, S.B., Simoni-Wastila, L., Singer, C., *et al.* Lack of relationship between long-term use of benzodiazepines and escalation to high dosages. *Psychiatr. Serv.*, **2003**, *54:*1006–1011.

Spencer, T., Biederman, J., Wilens, T., Steingard, R., and Geist, D. Nortriptyline treatment of children with attention-deficit hyperactivity disorder and tic disorder or Tourette's syndrome. *J. Am. Acad. Child Adolesc. Psychiatry*, **1993**, *32:*205–210.

Spina, E., Scordo, M.G., and D'Arrigo, C. Metabolic drug interactions with new psychotropic agents. *Fundament. Clin. Pharmacol.*, **2003**, *17:*517–538.

Steingard, R.J., DeMaso, D.R., Goldman, S.J., Shorrock, K.L., and Bucci, J.P. Current perspectives on the pharmacotherapy of depressive disorders in children and adolescents. *Harv. Rev. Psychiatry*, **1995**, *2:*313–326.

Storosum, J.G., Elferink, A.J., van Zwieten, B.J., van den Brink, W., and Huyser, J. Natural course and placebo response in short-term, placebo-controlled studies in major depression: a meta-analysis of published and non-published studies. *Pharmacopsychiatry*, **2004**, *37:*32–36.

Suominen K.H., Isometsä, E.T., Hendriksson, M.M., Ostamo, A.I., and Lönnqvist, J.K. Inadequate treatment for major depression both before and after attempted suicide. *Am. J. Psychiatry*, **1998**, *155:*1778–1780.

Thase, M.E., and Nolen, W. Tricyclic antidepressants and classical monoamine oxidase inhibitors: contemporary clinical use. In, *Schizo-*

phrenia and Mood Disorders: The New Drug Therapies in Clinical Practice. (Buckley, P.F., and Waddington, J.L., eds.) Butterworth-Heinemann, Boston, **2000,** pp. 85–99.

Tome, M.B., Isaac, M.T., Harte, R., and Holland, C. Paroxetine and pindolol: a randomized trial of serotonergic autoreceptor blockade in the reduction of antidepressant latency. *Int. Clin. Psychopharmacol.,* **1997,** *12:*81–89.

Tondo, L., Isacsson, L., and Baldessarini, R.J. Suicidal behavior in bipolar disorder: Risk and prevention. *CNS Drugs,* **2003,** *17:*491–511.

Versiani, M. Pharmacotherapy of dysthymic and chronic depressive disorders: overview with focus on moclobemide. *J. Affect. Disord.,* **1998,** *51:*323–332.

Viguera, A.C., Baldessarini, R.J., and Friedberg, J. Discontinuing antidepressant treatment in major depression. *Harv. Rev. Psychiatry,* **1998,** *5:*293–306.

Vu, T.N. Current pharmacologic approaches to treating neuropathic pain. *Curr. Pain Headache Report,* **2004,** *8:*15–18.

Wagner, K.D., Ambrosini, P., Rynn, M., *et al.* Efficacy of sertraline in the treatment of children and adolescents with major depressive disorder: two randomized controlled trials. *J.A.M.A.,* **2003,** *290:*1033–1041.

Wamsley, J.K., Byerley, W.F., McCabe, R.T., *et al.* Receptor alterations associated with serotonergic agents: an autoradiographic analysis. *J. Clin. Psychiatry,* **1987,** *48*(suppl):19–25.

Waugh, J., and Goa, K.L. Escitalopram: a review of its use in the management of major depressive and anxiety disorders. *CNS Drugs,* **2003,** *17:*343–362.

Wecker, L., James, S., Copeland, N., and Pacheco, M.A. Transdermal selegiline: targeted effects on monoamine oxidases in the brain. *Biol. Psychiatry,* **2003,** *54:*1099–1104.

Wehr, T.A., and Goodwin, F.K. Can antidepressants cause mania and worsen the course of affective illness? *Am. J. Psychiatry,* **1987,** *144:*1403–1411.

Whittington, C.J., Kendall, T., Fonagy, P., *et al.* Selective serotonin reuptake inhibitors in childhood depression: Systematic review of published versus unpublished data. *Lancet,* **2004,** *363:*1341–1345.

Wilens, T.E., Biederman, J., Baldessarini, R.J., Puopolo, P.R., and Flood, J.G. Developmental changes in serum concentrations of desipramine and 2-hydroxydesipramine during treatment with desipramine. *J. Am. Acad. Child Adolesc. Psychiatry,* **1992,** *31:*691–698.

Williams, T.P., and Miller, B.D. Pharmacologic management of anxiety disorders in children and adolescents. *Curr. Opin. Pediatr.,* **2003,** *15:*483–490.

Wisner, K.L., Gelenberg, A.J., Leonard, H., Zarin, D., and Frank, E. Pharmacologic treatment of depression during pregnancy. *J.A.M.A.,* **1999,** *282:*1264–1269.

Wong, D.T., and Bymaster, F.P. Development of antidepressant drugs. Fluoxetine (PROZAC) and other selective serotonin reuptake inhibitors. *Adv. Exp. Med. Biol.,* **1995,** *363:*77–95.

Wong, D.T., Bymaster, F.P., Reid, L.R., *et al.* Norfluoxetine enantiomers as inhibitors of serotonin uptake in rat brain. *Neuropsychopharmacology,* **1993,** *8:*337–344.

Wong, K.L., Bruch, R.C., and Farbman, A.I. Amitriptyline-mediated inhibition of neurite outgrowth from chick embryonic cerebral explants involves a reduction in adenylate cyclase activity. *J. Neurochem.,* **1991,** *57:*1223–1230.

Workman, E.A., and Short, D.D. Atypical antidepressants versus imipramine in the treatment of major depression: a meta-analysis. *J. Clin. Psychiatry,* **1993,** *54:*5–12.

Yamada, M., and Yasuhara, H. Clinical pharmacology of MAO inhibitors: safety and future. *Neurotoxicology,* **2004,** *25:*215–221.

Zhang, K., and Baldessarini, R.J. Attention-deficit/hyperactivity disorder (ADHD). In, *Manual of Neurological and Psychiatric Disorders.* (Tarazi, F.I., and Schatz, J.A., eds). Humana Press, Totawa, N.J., **2004,** in press.

Zhu, M.-Y., Kim, C.-H., Hwang, D.-Y., Baldessarini, R.J., and Kim, K.-S. Effects of desipramine treatment on norepinephrine transporter gene expression in cultured SK-N-BE(2)M17 cells and rat brain tissue. *J. Neurochem.,* **2002,** *82:*146–153.

Zhu, M.-Y., Wang, W.-P., Baldessarini, R.J., Kim, K.-S. Effects of desipramine treatment on tyrosine hydroxylase gene expression in cultured SK-N-BE(2)M17 cells and rat brain tissue. *J. Neurochem.,* **2004,** in press.

Zornberg, G.L., and Pope, H.G. Jr. Treatment of depression in bipolar disorder: new directions for research. *J. Clin. Psychopharmacol.,* **1993,** *13:*397–408.

MONOGRAPHS AND REVIEWS

Agras, W.S. Treatment of eating disorders. In, *The American Psychiatric Press Textbook of Psychopharmacology,* 2nd ed. (Schatzberg, A.F., and Nemeroff, C.B., eds.) American Psychiatric Press, Washington, D.C., **1998,** pp. 869–879.

American Psychiatric Association. *Diagnostic and Statistical Manual of Mental Disorders: DSM-IV,* 4th ed., text revision. APA Press, Washington, D.C., **2000.**

Baldessarini, R.J. Fifty years of biomedical psychiatry and psychopharmacology in America. In, *American Psychiatry After World War II: (1944–1994).* (Menninger R., and Nemiah, J., eds.) American Psychiatric Press, Washington, D.C., **2000,** pp. 371–412.

Buckley, P.F., and Waddington, J.L., eds. *Schizophrenia and Mood Disorders: The New Drug Therapies in Clinical Practice.* Butterworth-Heinemann, Boston, **2000.**

Caldwell, A.E. History of psychopharmacology. In, *Principles of Psychopharmacology,* 2nd ed. (Clark, W.G., and del Giudice, J., eds.) Academic Press, New York, **1978,** pp. 9–40.

Cornish, J.W., McNicholas, L.F., and O'Brien, C.P. Treatment of substance-related disorders. In, *The American Psychiatric Press Textbook of Psychopharmacology,* 2nd ed. (Schatzberg, A.F., and Nemeroff, C.B., eds.) American Psychiatric Press, Washington, D.C., **1998,** pp. 851–867.

DeBattista, C., and Schatzberg, A.F. Universal psychotropic dosing and monitoring guidelines. *The Economics of Neuroscience (TEN),* **1999,** *1:*75–84.

DeVane, C.L., and Nemeroff, C.B. Psychotropic drug interactions. *The Economics of Neuroscience (TEN),* **2000,** *2:*55–75.

Fawcett, J., and Busch, K.A. Stimulants in psychiatry. In, *The American Psychiatric Press Textbook of Psychopharmacology,* 2nd ed. (Schatzberg, A.F., and Nemeroff, C.B., eds.) American Psychiatric Press, Washington, D.C., **1998,** pp. 503–522.

Feighner, J.P. Overview of antidepressants currently used to treat anxiety disorders. *J. Clin. Psychiatry,* **1999,** *60*(suppl 22):18–22.

Frazer, A. Antidepressants. *J. Clin. Psychiatry,* **1997,** *58*(supp. 6):9–25.

Fuller, R.W. Basic advances in serotonin pharmacology. *J. Clin. Psychiatry,* **1992,** *53*(suppl):36–45.

Geller, D.A., Biederman, J., Jones, J., *et al.* Obsessive-compulsive disorder in children and adolescents: a review. *Harv. Rev. Psychiatry,* **1998,** *5:*260–273.

Golden, R.N., Dawkins, K., Nicholas, L., and Bebchuk, J.M. Trazodone, nefazodone, bupropion, and mirtazapine. In, *The American Psychiatric Press Textbook of Psychopharmacology,* 2nd ed. (Schatzberg, A.F., and Nemeroff, C.B., eds.) American Psychiatric Press, Washington, D.C., **1998,** pp. 251–269.

Grossberg, G.T., Corey-Bloom, J., Small, G.W., and Tariot, P.N. Emerging therapeutic strategies in Alzheimer's disease. *J. Clin. Psychiatry*, **2004**, *65:*255–266.

Hansten, P.D., and Horn, J.R. *Drug Interactions Analysis and Management Quarterly.* Applied Therapeutics, Vancouver, Wa., **2000.**

Healy, D. *The Antidepressant Era.* Harvard University Press, Cambridge, Ma., **1997.**

Hollister, L.E., Müller-Oerlinghausen, B., Rickels, K., and Shader, R.I. Clinical uses of benzodiazepines. *J. Clin. Psychopharmacol.*, **1993,** *13:*1S–169S.

Kent, J.M. SNaRIs, NaSSAs, and NaRIs: new agents for the treatment of depression. *Lancet*, **2000,** *355:*911–918.

Krishnan, K.R.R. Monoamine oxidase inhibitors. In, *The American Psychiatric Press Textbook of Psychopharmacology,* 2nd ed. (Schatzberg, A.F., and Nemeroff, C.B., eds.) American Psychiatric Press, Washington, D.C., **1998,** pp. 239–249.

Kutcher, S.P. *Child & Adolescent Psychopharmacology.* Saunders, Philadelphia, **1997.**

Leipzig, R.M., and Mendelowitz, A. Adverse psychotropic drug interactions. In, *Adverse Effects of Psychotropic Drugs.* (Kane, J.M., and Lieberman, J.A., eds.) Guilford Press, New York, **1992,** pp. 13–76.

Leonard, B.E., and Richelson, E. Synaptic effects of antidepressants. In, *Schizophrenia and Mood Disorders: The New Drug Therapies in Clinical Practice.* (Buckley, P.F., and Waddington, J.L., eds.) Butterworth-Heinemann, Boston, **2000,** pp. 67–84.

Marin, D.B., and Davis, K.L. Cognitive enhancers. In, *The American Psychiatric Press Textbook of Psychopharmacology,* 2nd ed. (Schatzberg, A.F., and Nemeroff, C.B., eds.) American Psychiatric Press, Washington, D.C., **1998,** pp. 473–486.

Masand, P.S., and Gupta, S. Selective serotonin-reuptake inhibitors: an update. *Harv. Rev. Psychiatry*, **1999,** *7:*69–84.

Murphy, D.L., Mitchell, P.B., and Potter, W.Z. Novel pharmacological approaches to the treatment of depression. In, *Psychopharmacology: The Fourth Generation of Progress.* (Bloom, F.E., and Kupfer, D.L., eds.) Raven Press, New York, **1995,** pp. 1143–1153.

Musselman, D.L., DeBattista, C., Nathan, K.I., *et al.* Biology of mood disorders. In, *The American Psychiatric Press Textbook of Psychopharmacology,* 2nd ed. (Schatzberg, A.F., and Nemeroff, C.B., eds.) American Psychiatric Press, Washington, D.C., **1998,** pp. 549–588.

Ninan, P.T., Cole, J.O., and Yonkers, K.A. Nonbenzodiazepine anxiolytics. In, *The American Psychiatric Press Textbook of Psychopharmacology,* 2nd ed. (Schatzberg, A.F., and Nemeroff, C.B., eds.) American Psychiatric Press, Washington, D.C., **1998,** pp. 287–300.

Potter, W.Z., Manji, H.K., and Rudorfer, M.V. Tricyclics and tetracyclics. In, *The American Psychiatric Press Textbook of Psychopharmacology,* 2nd ed. (Schatzberg, A.F., and Nemeroff, C.B., eds.) American Psychiatric Press, Washington, D.C., **1998,** pp. 199–218.

Preskorn, S.H. Clinically relevant pharmacology of selective serotonin reuptake inhibitors: an overview with emphasis on pharmacokinetics and effects on oxidative drug metabolism. *Clin. Pharmacokinet.*, **1997,** *32*(suppl 1):1–21.

Rudorfer, M.V., Henry, M.E., and Sackein, H.A. Electroconvulsive therapy. In, *Psychiatry,* Vol. 1. (Tasman, A., Kay, J., and Lieberman, J.A., eds.) Saunders, Philadelphia, **1997,** pp. 1535–1551.

Sadock, B.J., and Sadock, V.A., eds. *Kaplan & Sadock's Comprehensive Textbook of Psychiatry,* 7th ed. Lippincott Williams & Wilkins, Philadelphia, **2000.**

Singer, T.P., Von Korff, R.W., and Murphy, D., eds. *Monoamine Oxidase: Structure, Function, and Altered Functions.* Academic Press, New York, **1979.**

Stein, M.B., and Uhde, T.W. Biology of anxiety disorders. In, *The American Psychiatric Press Textbook of Psychopharmacology,* 2nd ed. (Schatzberg, A.F., and Nemeroff, C.B., eds.) American Psychiatric Press, Washington, D.C., **1998,** pp. 609–628.

Sulser, F., and Mobley, P.L. Biochemical effects of antidepressants in animals. In, *Psychotropic Agents. Handbook of Experimental Pharmacology,* Vol. 55, Pt. I. (Hoffmeister, F. and Stille, G., eds.) Springer-Verlag, Berlin, **1980,** pp. 471–490.

Taylor, C.B. Treatment of anxiety disorders. In, *The American Psychiatric Press Textbook of Psychopharmacology,* 2nd ed. (Schatzberg, A.F., and Nemeroff, C.B., eds.) American Psychiatric Press, Washington, D.C., **1998,** pp. 775–789.

Tollefson, G.D., and Rosenbaum, J.F. Selective serotonin-reuptake inhibitors. In, *The American Psychiatric Press Textbook of Psychopharmacology,* 2nd ed. (Schatzberg, A.F., and Nemeroff, C.B., eds.) American Psychiatric Press, Washington, D.C., **1998,** pp. 219–237.

Weber, S.S. Drug interactions with antidepressants. *CNS Special Edition,* **1999,** *1:*47–55.

Zohar, J. (ed.) WCA recommendations for the long-term treatment of anxiety disorders. *CNS Spectrums,* **2003,** *8*(suppl 1):1–52.

CHAPTER
18

PHARMACOTHERAPY OF PSYCHOSIS AND MANIA

Ross J. Baldessarini and Frank I. Tarazi

I. Drugs Used in the Treatment of Psychoses

The psychotic disorders include schizophrenia, the manic phase of bipolar (manic-depressive) illness, acute idiopathic psychotic illnesses, and other conditions marked by severe agitation. All exhibit major disturbances in reasoning, often with delusions and hallucinations. Several classes of drugs are effective for symptomatic treatment. Antipsychotic agents also are useful alternatives to electroconvulsive therapy (ECT) in severe depression with psychotic features, and sometimes are used in the management of patients with psychotic disorders associated with delirium or dementia, or induced by other agents (*e.g.*, stimulants or L-dopa).

Effective and clinically employed antipsychotic agents include *phenothiazines,* structurally similar *thioxanthenes, benzepines, butyrophenones* (phenylbutylpiperidines), *diphenylbutylpiperidines, indolones,* and other heterocyclic compounds. Because these chemically dissimilar drugs share many properties, information about their pharmacology and clinical uses is grouped. Particular attention is paid to *chlorpromazine,* the prototype of the phenothiazine–thioxanthene group of antipsychotic agents, and to *haloperidol,* the original butyrophenone and representative of several related classes of aromatic butylpiperidine derivatives. Contrasts to chemically dissimilar modern agents are highlighted.

The term *neuroleptic* is often applied to drugs that have relatively prominent experimental and clinical evidence of antagonism of D_2-dopamine receptor activity, with substantial risk of adverse extrapyramidal neurological effects (*see* Chapter 12) and increased release of prolactin. The term *atypical antipsychotic* is applied to agents that are associat-

ed with substantially lower risks of such extrapyramidal effects. Representative examples include *aripiprazole, clozapine, quetiapine, ziprasidone,* and low doses of *olanzapine* and *risperidone* (Blin, 1999; Markowitz *et al.*, 1999).

Although the antipsychotic drugs have had a revolutionary, beneficial impact on medical and psychiatric practice, their liabilities, especially the adverse effects of the older typical or neuroleptic agents, must be emphasized. Newer antipsychotics are atypical in having less risk of extrapyramidal side effects, but these agents present their own spectrum of adverse effects, including hypotension, seizures, weight gain, and increased risk of type II diabetes mellitus and hyperlipidemia.

The psychoses are among the most severe psychiatric disorders, in which there is not only marked impairment of behavior, but also a serious inability to think coherently, to comprehend reality, or to gain insight into the presence of these abnormalities. These common disorders (affecting perhaps 1% of the population at some age) typically include symptoms of false beliefs (*delusions*) and abnormal sensations (*hallucinations*). Their etiological basis remains unknown, although genetic, neurodevelopmental, and environmental causative factors have all been proposed. Representative syndromes in this category include schizophrenia, brief psychoses, and delusional disorders. Psychotic features also occur in major mood disorders, particularly mania and severe melancholic depression. Psychotic illnesses are characterized by disordered thought processes (as inferred from illogical or highly idiosyncratic communications) with disorganized or irrational behavior and varying degrees of altered mood that can range from excited agitation to severe emotional withdrawal. Idiopathic psychoses characterized by chronically disordered thinking and emotional withdrawal, and often associated with delusions and auditory hallucinations, are called *schizophrenia.* Acute and recurrent idiopathic psychoses that bear an uncertain relationship to schizophrenia or the major affective disorders also occur. Delusions that are more or less isolated are characteristic of *delusional disorder* or *paranoia.*

The beneficial effects of antipsychotic drugs are not limited to schizophrenia. They also are employed in disorders ranging from postsurgical delirium and amphetamine intoxication to paranoia, mania, psychotic depression, and the agitation of Alzheimer's dementia. They are especially useful in severe depression and possibly in other conditions marked by severe turmoil or agitation.

TRICYCLIC ANTIPSYCHOTIC AGENTS

Several dozen phenothiazine antipsychotic drugs and chemically related agents are used worldwide. Other phenothiazines are marketed primarily for their antiemetic, antihistaminic, or anticholinergic effects.

History. The early development of the antipsychotic agents is well summarized by Swazey (1974) and Caldwell (1978), and is recounted in the personal observations of Tuillier (1999). In the early 1950s, some antipsychotic effects were obtained with extracts of the *Rauwolfia* plant, then with large doses of its purified active alkaloid *reserpine*, which Woodward later chemically synthesized. Although reserpine and related alkaloids that also deplete monoamines from their vesicular storage sites in nerve terminals exert antipsychotic effects, these are relatively weak and are associated with severe side effects, including sedation, hypotension, diarrhea, anergy, and depressed mood. Thus the clinical utility of reserpine primarily was to treat hypertension.

Phenothiazines were synthesized initially in Europe in the late nineteenth century as a consequence of the development of aniline dyes such as methylene blue. In the late 1930s a phenothiazine derivative, *promethazine*, was found to have antihistaminic and sedative effects. This discovery led to relatively unsuccessful attempts to use promethazine and other antihistamines to treat agitation in psychiatric patients. Promethazine was noted to prolong barbiturate sleeping time in rodents, and the drug was introduced into clinical anesthesia as a potentiating and autonomic stabilizing agent. This work prompted a search for phenothiazine derivatives with similar effects, and led in 1949–1950, to Charpentier's synthesis of chlorpromazine. Soon thereafter, Laborit and his colleagues described the ability of this compound to potentiate anesthetics and produce "artificial hibernation." Chlorpromazine by itself did not cause a loss of consciousness, but diminished arousal and motility, with some tendency to promote sleep. These central actions soon became known as *ataractic* or *neuroleptic*.

The first attempts to treat mental illness with chlorpromazine were made in Paris in 1951 and early 1952 by Paraire and Sigwald (Swazey, 1974). In 1952 Delay and Deniker became convinced that chlorpromazine achieved more than symptomatic relief of agitation or anxiety and that it had an ameliorative effect upon psychotic processes in diverse disorders, including mania and schizophrenia. In 1954 Lehmann and Hanrahan as well as Winkelman reported the initial use of chlorpromazine in North America for the treatment of psychomotor excitement and manic states as well as schizophrenia (Swazey, 1974). Clinical studies soon revealed that chlorpromazine was effective in the treatment of psychotic disorders of various types.

Chemistry and Structure–Activity Relationships. Phenothiazines have a tricyclic structure in which two benzene rings are linked by a sulfur and a nitrogen atom (Table 18–1). The chemically related thioxanthenes have a carbon in place of the nitrogen at position 10 with the R_1 moiety linked through a double bond. Substitution of an electron-withdrawing group at position 2 increases the antipsychotic efficacy of phenothiazines and other tricyclic congeners (*e.g.*, chlorpromazine *vs. promazine*). The nature of the substituent at position 10 also influences pharmacological activity. As can be seen in Table 18–1, the phenothiazines and thioxanthenes can be divided into three groups on the basis of substitution at this site. Those with an aliphatic side chain include chlorpromazine and *triflupromazine*. These compounds are relatively low in potency but not in clinical efficacy. Those with a *piperidine* ring in the side chain include *thioridazine* and *mesoridazine*; they have a somewhat lower incidence of adverse extrapyramidal effects, possibly due to increased central antimuscarinic activity, but have depressant effects on cardiac conduction and repolarization. Several potent phenothiazine antipsychotic compounds have a *piperazine* group in the side chain; *fluphenazine, perphenazine,* and *trifluoperazine* are examples. Most of these compounds have relatively weak antimuscarinic activity; their use at standard doses entails a greater risk of inducing adverse extrapyramidal effects, but a lower tendency to produce sedation or autonomic side effects, such as hypotension. Several piperazine phenothiazines are esterified at a free hydroxyl with long-chain fatty acids to produce long-acting, highly lipophilic prodrugs. The *decanoates* of fluphenazine and haloperidol are used commonly in the United States; several others (including esters of *pipotiazine* and perphenazine) are available elsewhere.

Thioxanthenes also have aliphatic or piperazine side-chain substituents. The analog of chlorpromazine among the thioxanthenes is *chlorprothixene*. Piperazine-substituted thioxanthenes include *clopenthixol, cis-flupentixol, piflutixol,* and *thiothixene*. They are all potent and effective antipsychotic agents, although only thiothixene (NAVANE) is available in the United States. Since thioxanthenes have an olefinic double bond between the central-ring carbon atom at position 10 and the side chain, geometric isomers exist. The *cis* isomers are more active. A series of experimental antipsychotic agents (*acridanes*) retain the sulfur and replace the nitrogen of the phenothiazine central ring with a carbon atom.

The antipsychotic phenothiazines and thioxanthenes have three carbon atoms interposed between position 10 of the central ring and the first amino nitrogen atom of the side chain at this position; the amine is always tertiary. Antihistaminic phenothiazines (*e.g.*, promethazine) or strongly anticholinergic phenothiazines (*e.g.*, ethopropazine, diethazine) have only two carbon atoms separating the amino group from position 10 of the central ring. Metabolic *N*-dealkylation of the side chain or increasing the size of amino *N*-alkyl substituents reduces antidopaminergic and antipsychotic activity.

Additional tricyclic antipsychotic agents are the benzepines, containing a 7-member central ring, of which *lox-*

Table 18–1
Selected Antipsychotic Drugs: Chemical Structures, Doses and Dosage Forms, and Side Effects*

NONPROPRIETARY NAME/TRADE NAME		DOSE AND DOSAGE FORMS			SIDE EFFECTS		
Phenothiazines		*Adult Antipsychotic Oral Dose Range (Daily)*		*Single IM Dose‡*	*Sedative*	*Extra-pyramidal*	*Hypotensive*
R_1	R_2	Usual, mg	Extreme,§ mg	Usual, mg			
Chloropromazine hydrochloride (THORAZINE) —$(CH_2)_3$—$N(CH_3)_2$	—Cl	200–800	30–2000 O, SR, L, I, S	25–50	+++	++	IM+++ Oral++
Mesoridazine besylate (SERENTIL)	—SCH_3 $\overset{\|}{O}$	75–300	30–400 O, L, I	25	+++	+	++
Thioridazine hydrochloride (MELLARIL)	—SCH_3	150–600	20–800 O, L		+++	+	+++
Fluphenazine hydrochloride Fluphenazine enanthate Fluphenazine decanoate (PERMITIL and PROLIXIN) (PROLIXIN) —$(CH_2)_3$—N◯N—$(CH_2)_2$— OH	—CF_3	2–20	0.5–30 O, L, I	1.25–2.5 (decanoate or enanthate: 12.5–50 every 1–4 weeks)	+	++++	+
Perphenazine (TRILAFON) $(CH_2)_3$— N◯N—$(CH_2)_2$— OH	—Cl	8–32	4–64 O, L, I	5–10	++	++	+
Trifluoperazine hydrochloride (STELAZINE) —$(CH_2)_3$— N◯N— CH_3	—CF_3	5–20	2–30 O, L, I	1–2	+	+++	+

(Continued)

Table 18–1
Selected Antipsychotic Drugs: Chemical Structures, Doses and Dosage Forms, and Side Effects* (Continued)

NONPROPRIETARY NAME/TRADE NAME		DOSE AND DOSAGE FORMS			SIDE EFFECTS		
Thioxanthenes		*Adult Antipsychotic Oral Dose Range (Daily)*		*Single IM Dose‡*	*Sedative*	*Extra-pyramidal*	*Hypotensive*
R_1	R_2	Usual, mg	Extreme,§ mg	Usual, mg			
Chlorprothixene (TARACTAN)	—Cl	50–400	30–600	25–50 O, L, I	+++	++	++
Thiothixene hydrochloride (NAVANE)	—SO₂ | N(CH₃)₂	5–30	2–30	2–4 O, L, I	+ to ++	+++	++
Other Heterocyclic Compounds Aripiprazole (ABILIFY)		10–15	5–30	O	0/+	0	0/+
Clozapine (CLOZARIL)		150–450	12.5–900	O	+++	0	+++
Haloperidol; haloperidol decanoate (HALDOL)		2–20	1–100	2–5 (haloperidol decanoate: 25–250 every 2–4 weeks) O, L, I	+	++++	+

(Continued)

Table 18–1

Selected Antipsychotic Drugs: Chemical Structures, Doses and Dosage Forms, and Side Effects* (Continued)

NONPROPRIETARY NAME/TRADE NAME	DOSE AND DOSAGE FORMS			SIDE EFFECTS		
Other Heterocyclic Compounds (cont.)	*Adult Antipsychotic Oral Dose Range (Daily)*		*Single IM Dose‡*	*Sedative*	*Extra-pyramidal*	*Hypotensive*
R_1	Usual, mg	Extreme,§ mg	Usual, mg			
Loxapine succinate (LOXITANE) 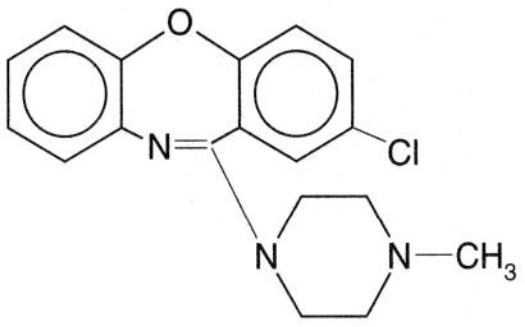	60–100	20–250	12.5–50	+	++	+
			O, L, I			
Molindone hydrochloride (MOBAN) 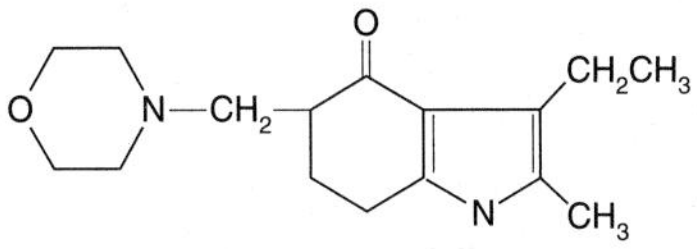	50–225	15–225		++	++	+
			O, L			
Olanzapine (ZYPREXA) 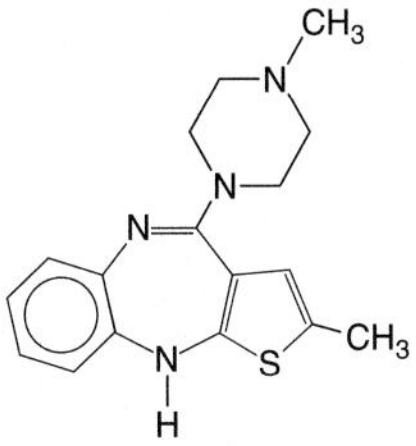	5–10	2.5–20		+	+	++
			O, I			
Pimozide (ORAP) 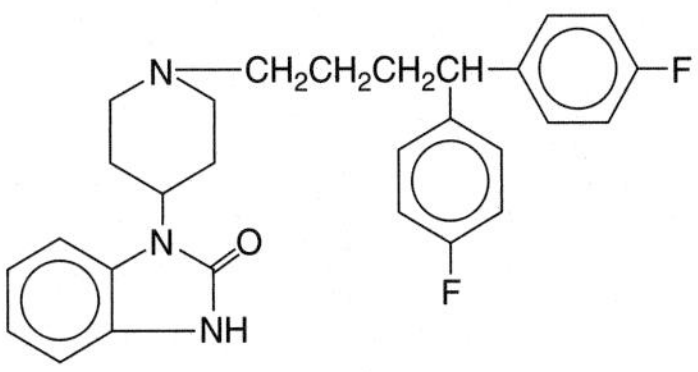	2–6	1–10		+	+++	+
			O			
Quetiapine fumarate (SEROQUEL) 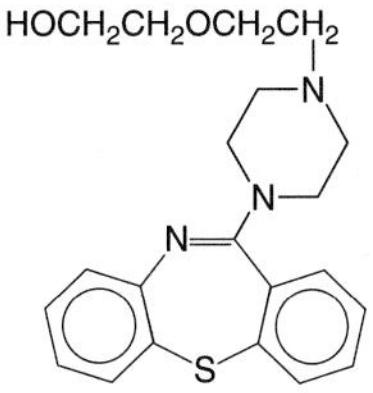	300–500	50–750		+++	0	++
			O			

(Continued)

Table 18–1
Selected Antipsychotic Drugs: Chemical Structures, Doses and Dosage Forms, and Side Effects* (Continued)

NONPROPRIETARY NAME/TRADE NAME	DOSE AND DOSAGE FORMS			SIDE EFFECTS		
Other Heterocyclic Compounds (cont.)	*Adult Antipsychotic Oral Dose Range (Daily)*		*Single IM Dose‡*	*Sedative*	*Extra-pyramidal*	*Hypotensive*
R_1	Usual, mg	Extreme,§ mg	Usual, mg			
Risperidone (RISPERDAL)	2–8	0.25–16		++	++	+++
			O, I (long-acting)			
Ziprasidone (GEODON)	80–160	20–160		+/++	0/+	+
			O, I [hydrochloride (O), mesylate (I)]			

*Antipsychotic agents for use in children under age 12 years include chlorpromazine, chlorprothixene (>6 years), thioridazine, and triflupromazine (among agents of low potency); and prochlorperazine and trifluoperazine (>6 years) (among agents of high potency). Haloperidol (orally) has also been used extensively in children. †Dosage forms are indicated as follows: I, regular or long-acting injection; L, oral liquid or oral liquid concentrate; O, oral solid; S, suppository; SR, oral, sustained-release ‡Except for the enanthate and decanoate forms of fluphenazine and haloperidol decanoate, dosage can be given intramuscularly up to every 6 hours for agitated patients. Haloperidol lactate has been given intravenously; this is experimental. §Extreme dosage ranges are occasionally exceeded cautiously and only when other appropriate measures have failed. Side effects: 0, absent; +, low; ++, moderate; +++, moderately high; ++++, high The indicated salts are not shown in the formulas but are commercially available forms of the drugs.

apine (a dibenzoxazepine; Table 18–1) and clozapine (a dibenzodiazepine) are available in the United States. Loxapine-like agents include potent and typical neuroleptics with prominent antidopaminergic activity (*e.g., clothiapine, metiapine, zotepine,* and others). They have an electron-withdrawing moiety at position 2, relatively close to the side-chain nitrogen atoms. Clozapine-like, atypical antipsychotic agents may lack a substituent on the aromatic ring (*e.g.,* quetiapine, a dibenzothiazepine), have an analogous methyl substituent (notably olanzapine; Table 18–1), or have an electron-donating substituent at position 8 (*e.g.,* clozapine, *fluperlapine,* and others). In addition to their moderate potencies at dopamine receptors, clozapinelike agents interact with varying affinities at several other classes of receptors (α_1 and α_2 adrenergic, 5-HT$_{1A}$, 5-HT$_{2A}$, 5-HT$_{2C}$, muscarinic cholinergic, histamine H$_1$, and others). Some are highly effective antipsychotic agents; clozapine

in particular has proved effective even in chronically ill patients who respond poorly to standard neuroleptics (Baldessarini and Frankenburg, 1991).

The introduction of clozapine strongly stimulated searches for additional, safer agents with antipsychotic activity and an atypically low risk of adverse extrapyramidal neurological effects. This search led to a series of atypical antipsychotic agents (Table 18–1) with some pharmacological similarities to clozapine: the structurally similar olanzapine and quetiapine, the mixed antidopaminergic-antiserotonergic agent risperidone (a benzisoxazole) (Owens and Risch, 1998; Waddington and Casey, 2000), and the newer agents ziprasidone (a benzisothiazolpiprazinylindolone derivative) (Seeger *et al.,* 1995) and aripiprazole (a quinolinone derivative) (Inoue *et al.,* 1996).

The butyrophenone (phenylbutylpiperidine) neuroleptics include haloperidol, originally developed as a substituted derivative of the phenylpiperidine analgesic meperidine (Janssen, 1974). Other experimental heterocyclic-substituted phenylbutylpiperidines include the *spiperones*. An analogous compound, *droperidol,* is a very short-acting, highly sedating neuroleptic that today is used almost exclusively in anesthesia (*see* Chapter 13). Additional analogs in the diphenylbutylpiperidine series include *fluspirilene, penfluridol,* and *pimozide* (Neumeyer and Booth, 2002). These are potent neuroleptics with prolonged action. In the United States, pimozide is indicated for the treatment of Tourette's syndrome and other tic disorders, although it also is an effective antipsychotic.

Several other classes of heterocyclic compounds have antipsychotic effects, but too few are available or sufficiently well characterized to permit conclusions regarding structure–activity relationships (Abraham, 2003; Neumeyer and Booth, 2002). These include several indole compounds (notably *molindone* and *oxypertine*) and structurally related compounds (including *sertindole* and ziprasidone). Another experimental compound, *butaclamol,* is a potent antidopaminergic agent that has a pentacyclic structure with a dibenzepine core and structural and pharmacological similarity to loxapine-like rather than clozapine-like dibenzepines. Its active (dextrorotatory) and inactive enantiomeric forms have been useful in characterizing the stereochemistry of sites of action of neuroleptics at dopamine receptors.

Risperidone has prominent antiserotonergic (5-HT$_{2A}$), antidopaminergic (D$_2$-like), antiadrenergic (α_1), and antihistaminic (H$_1$) activity, as well as very low antimuscarinic activity. Although risperidone and clozapine share relatively high serotonin 5-HT$_{2A}$ and lower dopamine D$_2$-receptor affinities, risperidone has much more potent antidopaminergic and much less potent antimuscarinic activity. Unlike clozapine, it can induce extrapyramidal symptoms and prominent hyperprolactinemia. Nevertheless, risperidone can be considered an "atypical" antipsychotic in that its adverse extrapyramidal neurological effects are limited at low daily doses (*i.e.,* 6 mg or less), usually with adequate antipsychotic effects.

A growing series of heterocyclic antipsychotic agents are the enantiomeric, substituted *benzamides*. These include the gastroenterological agents *metoclopramide* and *cisapride,* which have antiserotonergic as well as peripheral anti–D$_2$-dopaminergic actions. In addition, several benzamides, like the butyrophenones and their congeners, are relatively selective antagonists at central D$_2$ dopamine receptors, and many have neuroleptic-antipsychotic activity. Experimental examples include *epidepride, eticlopride, nemonapride, raclopride, remoxipride,* and *sultopride. Sulpiride* is employed clinically as a sedative outside the United States; and its congener, *amisulpride,* is an effective antipsychotic that is not available in the United States.

The search for novel compounds that share the antidopaminergic and potent antiserotonergic actions of risperidone and clozapine led to the development of the indole-like heterocyclic agent ziprasidone. Ziprasidone (GEODON) is in clinical use, although it is associated with prolongation of the QTc interval. Ziprasidone is a combined dopamine D$_2$/5-HT$_{2A,2C,1D}$ receptor antagonist and 5-HT$_{1A}$ agonist (Gunasekara *et al.*, 2002; Stimmel *et al.*, 2002). In addition, ziprasidone has an antidepressant-like pharmacological feature: It inhibits 5-HT and norepinephrine reuptake with moderate potency. The combination of 5-HT$_{1D}$ antagonism, 5-HT$_{1A}$ agonism, and inhibition of monoamine reuptake by ziprasidone is consistent with potential for antidepressant or anxiolytic activity in patients with psychotic disorders. Ziprasidone also is indicated for the treatment of schizophrenia and mania (Stimmel *et al.*, 2002).

Efforts to develop dopamine D$_2$ receptor partial agonists as potential atypical antipsychotics produced *aripiprazole* (ABILIFY). In addition to its partial-agonist activity at D$_2$ receptors, aripiprazole has partial-agonist effects at serotonin 5-HT$_{1A}$ receptors, as well as antagonistic activity at 5-HT$_{2A}$ receptors (Potkin *et al.*, 2003). Other similar agents, including *bifeprunox,* are currently in clinical testing.

Pharmacological Properties

Antipsychotic drugs share many pharmacological effects and therapeutic applications (Davis *et al.*, 2003; Lehman *et al.*, 2003; Leucht *et al.*, 2003a; Leucht *et al.*, 2003b; Owens and Risch, 1998). Chlorpromazine and haloperidol are prototypic of the older, standard neuroleptic-type agents against which newer agents are compared and contrasted. Many antipsychotic drugs, especially chlorpromazine and other agents of low potency, have a prominent sedative effect. This is particularly conspicuous early in treatment, although some tolerance typically develops. Sedation can be of added value when very agitated psychotic patients are treated. Despite their sedative effects, neuroleptic drugs generally are not used to treat anxiety disorders or insomnia, largely because of their adverse autonomic and neurologic effects, which paradoxically can include severe anxiety and restlessness (akathisia). The risk of developing adverse extrapyramidal effects, including tardive dyskinesia, following long-term administration of neuroleptic drugs makes them less desirable than several alternative treatments for anxiety disorders (*see* Chapter 17).

The term *neuroleptic*—introduced to denote the effects of chlorpromazine and reserpine on the behavior of laboratory animals and in psychiatric patients—was intended to contrast their effects to those of sedatives and other CNS depressants. The neuroleptic syndrome involves suppression of spontaneous movements and complex behaviors, whereas spinal reflexes and unconditioned nociceptive-avoidance behaviors remain intact. In humans, neuroleptic drugs reduce initiative and interest in the environment as well as manifestations of emotion. Such effects led to their being considered "tranquilizers" before their unique antipsychotic and antimanic effects were well established. In clinical use, there may be some initial drowsiness and slowness in response to external stimuli. However, subjects are easily aroused, can answer questions, and retain intact cognition. Ataxia, incoordination, or dysarthria do not occur at ordinary doses. Typically, psychotic patients soon become less agitated, withdrawn or autistic patients sometimes become more responsive and communicative, and aggressive and impulsive behavior diminishes. Gradually (usually over a period of days), psychotic symptoms of hallucinations, delusions, and disorganized or incoherent thinking ameliorate. Neuroleptic agents also exert characteristic neurological effects—including bradykinesia, mild rigidity, tremor, and subjective restlessness (akathisia)—that resemble the signs of Parkinson's disease.

Although the term *neuroleptic* initially encompassed this whole unique syndrome and is still used as a synonym for *antipsychotic,* it now is used to emphasize the more neurological aspects of the syndrome (*i.e.,* the parkinsonian and other extrapyramidal effects). Except for clozapine, aripiprazole, quetiapine, ziprasidone, and low doses of olanzapine and risperidone, antipsychotic drugs available in the United States also have effects on movement and posture and so can be called neuroleptic. However, the more general term *antipsychotic* is preferable, and the growing number of modern atypical antipsychotic drugs with little extrapyramidal action has reinforced this trend.

Behavioral Effects.   Several animal behavioral models that mimic different aspects of psychotic disorders and predict the efficacy or potential adverse effects of antipsychotic agents have been proposed (Arnt and Skarsfeld, 1998; Geyer and Ellenbroek, 2003). Among the oldest of these is *conditioned avoidance* in response to an aversive stimulus, such as a foot-shock, following a warning stimulus. Escape or avoidance responses in such circumstances are selectively inhibited by most antipsychotics, whereas unconditioned escape or avoidance responses are not. Since correlations between antipsychotic effectiveness and conditioned avoidance tests are effective for many types of antipsychotics, they have been important in pharmaceutical screening procedures. Nevertheless, despite their empirical utility and quantitative characteristics, effects on conditioned avoidance have not provided important insights into the basis of clinical antipsychotic effects. For example, the effects of antipsychotic drugs on conditioned avoidance, but not their clinical actions, are subject to tolerance and are blocked by anticholinergic agents. Moreover, close correlation between the potencies of drugs in conditioned avoidance tests and their ability to block the behavioral effects of dopaminergic agonists suggests that such avoidance tests may select for antidopaminergic agents with extrapyramidal and other neurological effects (Fielding and Lal, 1978; Janssen and Van Bever, 1978; Arnt and Skarsfeldt, 1998).

Another classical animal model is the effect of antipsychotics on *motor activity*. Nearly all antipsychotics, including newer agents, diminish spontaneous motor activity and reverse increases in motor activity induced by apomorphine, amphetamine, or phencyclidine (PCP) (Ellenbroek, 1993). Antipsychotics also block apomorphine-induced climbing in mice, which is believed to reflect D_2-like receptor activation.

A third model is *latent inhibition*—the retarding effects of prior stimulus exposure on subsequent stimulus-response learning (Feldon and Weiner, 1992). Most antipsychotics reverse amphetamine-induced reduction in latent inhibition. A related model is *prepulse inhibition* (PPI) of startle, which mimics deficits in sensory gating and information processing documented in many psychotic patients (Perry *et al.*, 1999). PPI is the reduction in startle response following presentation of a low-intensity, nonstartling stimulus (the prepulse) shortly before a stronger startle stimulus (Swerdlow *et al.*, 1994). PPI can be disrupted by administration of agonists and releasers of dopamine (apomorphine and amphetamine, respectively), serotonin (2,5-dimethoxy-4-iodoamphetamine [DOI]), and 3,4-methylenedioxymethamphetamine (MDMA), as well as glutamate N-methyl-D-aspartate (NMDA) receptor antagonists (PCP, ketamine). As expected, virtually all typical and atypical antipsychotics with appreciable affinity for D_2 receptors block apomorphine-induced disruption of PPI. In contrast, only atypical antipsychotics, and not typical neuroleptics, reverse the PPI disruption induced by serotonin agonists or releasers, or by NMDA antagonists.

Auditory sensory gating (ASG) involves the response to two identical stimuli. It is reduced in many psychotic patients and disrupted in animals given amphetamine or PCP (Ellenbroek *et al.*, 1999). Typical neuroleptics such as haloperidol can normalize amphetamine- and PCP-induced deficits in this behavior, but effects of newer atypical agents are less well studied.

So-called "negative" social and cognitive symptoms of schizophrenia, particularly social withdrawal and isolation, can be mimicked in at least two animal models: amphetamine-induced social isolation in monkeys, and PCP-induced social withdrawal in rats. In both models, drug-treated animals avoid interactions with other animals. These social deficits are partially reversed by newer antipsychotics but not older neuroleptics (Ellenbroek *et al.*, 1999).

Extrapyramidal Effects of Antipsychotics. The acute adverse clinical effects of antipsychotic agents are best mimicked in animals by assessing catalepsy in rats (immobility that allows an animal to be placed in abnormal postures that persist) or dystonia in monkeys. Late dyskinetic effects of antipsychotics are represented by the development of vacuous chewing movements in rats (Casey, 1996; Ellenbroek *et al.*, 1999).

A particularly disturbing adverse effect of most antipsychotics is restless activity, termed *akathisia*, which is not readily mimicked by animal behavior. The cataleptic immobility of animals treated with classical antipsychotics resembles the catatonia seen in some psychotic patients and in a variety of metabolic and neurological disorders affecting the CNS. In patients, catatonic signs, along with other features of psychotic illnesses, are sometimes relieved by antipsychotic agents. However, rigidity and bradykinesia, which mimic catatonia, can be induced by administering large doses of potent traditional neuroleptics, and reversed by their removal or by addition of an antimuscarinic-antiparkinson agent (Fielding and Lal, 1978; Janssen and Van Bever, 1978). Theories concerning mechanisms underlying these extrapyramidal reactions and descriptions of their clinical presentations and management are provided below.

Effects on Cognitive Functions. Several cognitive functions, including auditory processing and attention, spatial organization, verbal learning, semantic and verbal memory, and executive functions, are impaired in schizophrenia patients and are a major source of social and occupational dysfunction and disability (Saykin *et al.*, 1991). Potent D_2-antagonist neuroleptics have very limited beneficial effects on such functions. Some atypical antipsychotic agents with mixed $D_2/5$-HT_{2A} activity (including clozapine, quetiapine, olanzapine, and risperidone), as well as the D_2 partial agonist aripiprazole, seem to improve cognitive functioning in psychotic patients (Kasper and Resinger, 2003; Purdon, 2000). Nevertheless, significant long-term gains in social and occupational function during long-term treatment of chronically psychotic patients with these drugs are not well documented.

Effects on Sleep. Antipsychotic drugs have inconsistent effects on sleep patterns but tend to normalize sleep disturbances characteristic of many psychoses and mania. The ability to prolong and enhance the effect of opioid and hypnotic drugs appears to parallel the sedative, rather than the neuroleptic, potency of a particular agent, so that potent, less-sedating antipsychotics do not enhance sleep.

Effects on Specific Areas of the Nervous System. The antipsychotic drugs affect all levels of the central nervous system. Although knowledge of the actions underlying the antipsychotic and many of the neurological effects of antipsychotic drugs remains incomplete, theories based on their ability to antagonize the actions of dopamine as a neurotransmitter in the basal ganglia and limbic portions of the forebrain are most prominent. Although supported by a large body of data, these theories reflect a degree of circularity in the consideration of antipsychotic drug candidates for development after identifying their antidopaminergic activity (Baldessarini, 2000).

Cerebral Cortex. Since psychosis involves disordered thought processes, cortical effects of antipsychotic drugs are of particular interest. Antipsychotic drugs interact with dopaminergic projections to the prefrontal and deep-temporal (limbic) regions of the cerebral cortex, with relative sparing of these areas from adaptive changes in dopamine metabolism that would suggest tolerance to the actions of neuroleptics (Bunney *et al.*, 1987).

Seizure Threshold. Many neuroleptic drugs can lower the seizure threshold and induce discharge patterns in the electroencephalogram (EEG)—effects associated with epileptic seizure disorders. Clozapine, olanzapine, and aliphatic phenothiazines with low potency (such as chlorpromazine) seem particularly able to do this, while the more potent piperazine phenothiazines and thioxanthenes (notably fluphenazine and thiothixene), risperidone, and quetiapine are much less likely to have this effect (Baldessarini and Frankenburg, 1991; Centorrino *et al.*, 2002). The butyrophenones and molindone variably and unpredictably rarely cause seizures. Clozapine has a clearly dose-related risk of inducing EEG abnormalities and seizures in nonepileptic patients (Baldessarini and Frankenburg, 1991; Centorrino *et al.*, 2002). Antipsychotic agents, especially clozapine, olanzapine, and low-potency phenothiazines and thioxanthenes, should be used with *extreme caution,* if at all, in untreated epileptic patients and in patients undergoing withdrawal from CNS depressants such as alcohol, barbiturates, or benzodiazepines. Most antipsychotic drugs, especially the piperazines as well as the newer atypical agents aripiprazole, quetiapine, risperidone, and ziprasidone, can be used safely in epileptic patients if moderate doses are attained gradually and if concomitant anticonvulsant drug therapy is maintained (*see* Chapter 19).

Basal Ganglia. Because the extrapyramidal effects of many antipsychotic drugs are prominent, a great deal of interest has centered on their actions in the basal ganglia, notably the caudate nucleus, putamen, globus pallidus, and allied nuclei, which play a crucial role in the control of posture and the extrapyramidal aspects of movement. The critical pathogenic role of dopamine deficiency in this region in Parkinson's disease, the potent activity of neuroleptics as dopamine receptor antagonists, and the striking resemblance between clinical manifestations of Parkinson's disease and some of the neurological effects of neuroleptic drugs have all focused attention on the role of deficient dopaminergic activity in some of the neuroleptic-induced extrapyramidal effects (Carlsson, 1992).

The hypothesis that interference with dopamine signaling in the mammalian forebrain might contribute to the neurological and possibly the antipsychotic effects of the neuroleptic drugs arose from the observation that they consistently increased cerebral tissue concentrations of dopamine metabolites, but variably affected the metabolism of other neurotransmitters. The importance of dopamine also was supported by histochemical studies, which indicated a preferential distribution of dopamine-containing fibers between midbrain and the basal ganglia (notably the nigrostriatal tract) and in the hypothalamus (*see* Chapter 12) (Neumeyer *et al.*, 2003). Other dopamine-containing neurons project from midbrain tegmental nuclei to forebrain regions associated with the limbic system and to temporal and prefrontal cerebral cortical areas closely related functionally to the limbic system. Thus a simplistic but attractive concept arose: many adverse extrapyramidal neurological and neuroendocrinological effects of the neuroleptics are mediated by anti-dopaminergic effects in the basal ganglia and hypothalamic systems, whereas their antipsychotic effects are mediated by modification of dopaminergic neurotransmission in the limbic and mesocortical systems.

Antagonism of dopamine-mediated synaptic neurotransmission is an important action of many antipsychotics (Carlsson, 1992). Thus, neuroleptic drugs (but not their inactive congeners) initially increase the rate of production of dopamine metabolites, the rate of conversion of the precursor amino acid L-tyrosine to L-dihydroxy-phenylalanine (L-dopa) and its metabolites, and initially increase the rate of firing of dopamine-containing cells in the midbrain. These effects presumably represent adaptive responses of neuronal systems aimed at reducing the impact of impaired synaptic transmission at dopaminergic terminals in the forebrain.

Evidence supporting this interpretation includes the observation that small doses of neuroleptics block behavioral or neuroendocrine effects of systemically administered or intracerebrally injected dopaminergic agonists. Examples include apomorphine-induced stereotyped gnawing behavior and release of growth hormone in the rat. Many antipsychotic drugs also block the effects of agonists on dopamine-sensitive adenylyl cyclase associated with D_1/D_5-dopamine receptors in forebrain tissue (Figure 18–1). Atypical antipsychotic drugs such as clozapine and quetiapine are characterized by low affinity or weak actions in such tests (Campbell *et al.*, 1991). Initially, the standard antipsychotics increase firing and metabolic activity in dopaminergic neurons. These responses eventually are replaced by diminished presynaptic activity ("depolarization inactivation") with reduced firing and production of dopamine, particularly in the extrapyramidal basal ganglia (Bunney *et al.*, 1987). The timing of these adaptive changes following the administration of neuroleptics correlates well with the gradual evolution of parkinsonian brady-kinesia over several days (Tarsy *et al.*, 2002).

Radioligand-binding and autoradiographic assays for dopamine receptor subtypes have been used to define more precisely the mechanism of action of antipsychotic agents (Baldessarini and Tarazi, 1996; Civelli *et al.*, 1993; Neve and Neve, 1997; Tarazi *et al.*, 1997, 2001) (Table 18–2 and Figure 18–1). Estimated clinical potencies of most antipsychotic drugs correlate well with their relative potencies *in vitro* to inhibit binding of radioligands to D_2-dopamine receptors. This correlation with drug potency is partly obscured by the tendency of antipsychotics to accumulate in brain tissue to different degrees (Tsuneizumi *et al.*, 1992; Cohen *et al.*, 1992). Nevertheless, almost all clinically effective antipsychotic agents (with the notable exception of clozapine and quetiapine) have high or moderate affinity for D_2 receptors. Although some antipsychotics (especially thioxanthenes, phenothiazines, and clozapine) bind with relatively high affinity to D_1 receptors, they also block D_2 receptors and other D_2-like receptors, including the D_3 and D_4 subtypes (Sokoloff *et al.*, 1990; Van Tol *et al.*, 1991; Baldessarini and Tarazi, 1996; Tarazi and Baldessarini, 1999; Tarazi *et al.*, 1997, 2001). Butyrophenones and congeners (*e.g.,* haloperidol, pimozide, *N*-methylspiperone) and experimental benzamide neuroleptics are relatively selective antagonists of D_2 and D_3

dopamine receptors, with either high (nemonapride) or low (eticlopride, raclopride, remoxipride) D_4 affinity. The physiological and clinical consequences of selectively blocking D_1/D_5 receptors remain obscure, although experimental benzazepines (*e.g.,* SCH-23390 or SCH-39166 [ecopipam]) with such properties, but apparently with weak antipsychotic effects, are known (Daly and Waddington, 1992; Karlsson *et al.*, 1995; Kebabian *et al.*, 1997).

Many other antipsychotic agents are active α_1 adrenergic antagonists (Baldessarini *et al.*, 1992; Richelson, 1999). This action may contribute to sedative and hypotensive side effects or may underlie useful psychotropic effects, although assessment of the psychotropic potential of centrally active antiadrenergic agents is limited.

Many antipsychotic agents also have affinity for forebrain 5-HT_{2A}-serotonin receptors, including aripiprazole, clozapine, olanzapine, quetiapine, risperidone, and ziprasidone (Chouinard *et al.*, 1993; Leysen *et al.*, 1994) (*see* Chapter 11). This mixture of moderate affinities for several CNS receptor types (including muscarinic acetylcholine and H_1-histamine receptors) may contribute to the distinct pharmacological profiles of the atypical antipsychotic agent clozapine (Baldessarini and Frankenburg, 1991) and other newer atypical antipsychotics (Ichikawa and Meltzer, 1999; Meltzer and Nash, 1991).

Limbic System. Dopaminergic projections from the midbrain terminate on septal nuclei, the olfactory tubercle and basal forebrain, the amygdala, and other structures within the temporal and prefrontal cerebral lobes and the hippocampus. The dopamine hypothesis has focused considerable attention on the mesolimbic and mesocortical systems as possible sites where antipsychotic effects are mediated. Speculations about the pathophysiology of idiopathic psychoses such as schizophrenia have long centered on dopaminergic functions in the limbic system (Baldessarini, 2000). Such speculation has been given indirect encouragement by repeated "natural experiments" that have associated psychotic mental phenomena with lesions of the temporal lobe and other portions of the limbic system, as well as by psychotic syndromes produced by excessive exposure to psychostimulants.

Certain important effects of antipsychotic drugs are similar in extrapyramidal and limbic regions, including effects on ligand-binding assays for dopaminergic receptors. However, the extrapyramidal and antipsychotic actions of these drugs differ in several ways. For example, while some acute extrapyramidal effects of neuroleptics tend to diminish or disappear with time or with concurrent administration of anticholinergic drugs, antipsychotic effects do not. Dopaminergic subsystems in the forebrain differ functionally and in their physiological responses to drugs (Bunney *et al.*, 1987; Moore, 1987; Wolf and Roth, 1987). For example, anticholinergic agents block the increased turnover of dopamine in the basal ganglia induced by neuroleptic agents, but not in limbic areas containing dopaminergic terminals. Further, tolerance to the enhanced dopamine metabolism by antipsychotics is much less prominent in cortical and limbic areas than in extrapyramidal areas (Carlsson, 1992).

Newer Dopaminergic Receptors in Basal Ganglia and Limbic System. The discovery that D_3 and D_4 receptors are preferentially expressed in limbic areas has led to efforts to identify selective inhibitors for these receptors that might have antipsychotic efficacy and low

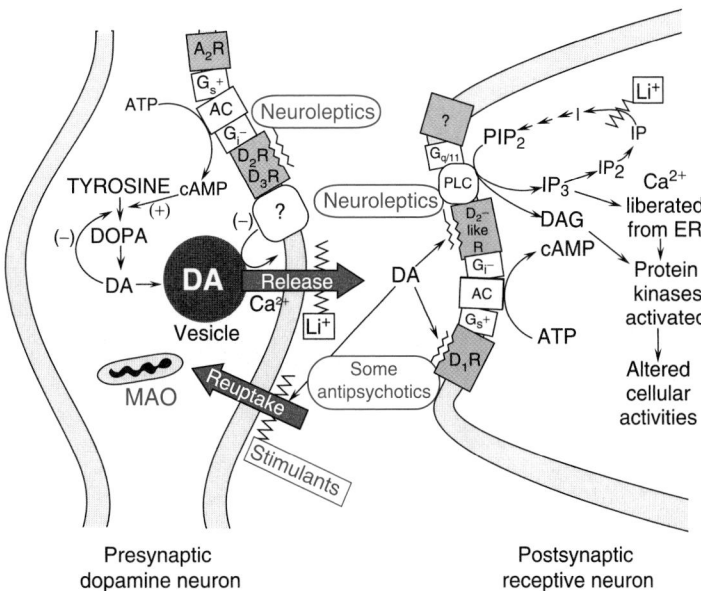

Figure 18–1. *Sites of action of neuroleptics and lithium.* In varicosities ("terminals") along terminal arborizations of dopamine (DA) neurons projecting from midbrain to forebrain, tyrosine is oxidized to dihydroxyphenylalanine (DOPA) by tyrosine hydroxylase (TH), the rate-limiting step in catecholamine biosynthesis, then decarboxylated to DA by aromatic L-amino acid decarboxylase (AAD) and stored in vesicles. Following exocytotic release (inhibited by Li^+) by depolarization in the presence of Ca^{2+}, DA interacts with postsynaptic receptors (R) of D_1 and D_2 types (and structurally similar but less prevalent D_1-like and D_2-like receptors), as well as with presynaptic D_2 and D_3 autoreceptors. Inactivation of transsynaptic communication occurs primarily by active transport ("reuptake") of DA into presynaptic terminals (inhibited by many stimulants), with secondary deamination by mitochondrial monoamine oxidase (MAO). Postsynaptic D_1 receptors, through G_s, activate adenylyl cyclase (AC) to increase cyclic AMP (cAMP), whereas D_2 receptors inhibit AC through G_i. D_2 receptors also activate receptor-operated K^+ channels, suppress voltage-gated Ca^{2+} currents, and stimulate phospholipase C (PLC), perhaps *via* the $\beta\gamma$ subunits liberated from activated G_i (*see* Chapter 1), activating the IP_3-Ca^{2+} pathway, thereby modulating a variety of Ca^{2+}-dependent activities including protein kinases. Lithium inhibits the phosphatase that liberates inositol (I) from inositol phosphate (IP). Both Li^+ and valproate can modify the abundance or function of G proteins and effectors, as well as protein kinases and several cell and nuclear regulatory factors. D_2-like autoreceptors suppress synthesis of DA by diminishing phosphorylation of rate-limiting TH, and by limiting DA release (possibly through modulation of Ca^{2+} or K^+ currents). In contrast, presynaptic A_2 adenosine receptors (A_2R) activate AC and, *via* cyclic AMP production, TH activity. Nearly all antipsychotic agents block D_2 receptors and autoreceptors; some also block D_1 receptors (Table 18–2). Initially in antipsychotic treatment, DA neurons activate and release more DA, but following repeated treatment, they enter a state of physiological depolarization inactivation, with diminished production and release of DA, in addition to continued receptor blockade. ER, endoplasmic reticulum.

risk of extrapyramidal effects. Clozapine has modest selectivity for dopamine D_4 receptors over other dopamine-receptor types. D_4 receptors, preferentially localized in cortical and limbic brain regions in relatively low abundance (Tarazi and Baldessarini, 1999; Van Tol *et al.*, 1991), are upregulated after repeated administration of most typical and atypical antipsychotic drugs (Tarazi *et al.*, 1997, 2001). These receptors may contribute to clinical antipsychotic actions, but agents that are D_4 selective (*e.g.*, L-745,870, sonepiprazole) or mixed D_4/5-HT_{2A} antagonists (*e.g.*, fananserin) have not proved effective in the treatment of psychotic patients (Baldessarini, 1997; Corrigan *et al.*, 2004; Kebabian *et al.*, 1997; Kramer *et al.*, 1997; Lahti *et al.*, 1998; Tarazi and Baldessarini, 1999; Truffinet *et al.*, 1999). Other D_4-selective compounds may emerge as novel treatments for other neuropsychiatric disorders, including attention-deficit/hyperactivity disorder or cognitive symptoms of psychotic disorders (Tarazi and Baldessarini, 1999; Zhang *et al.*, 2004).

In contrast to effects on D_2 and D_4 receptors, long-term administration of typical and atypical antipsychotic drugs does not alter D_3 receptor levels in rat forebrain regions (Tarazi *et al.*, 1997, 2001). These findings suggest that D_3 receptors are unlikely to play a pivotal role in antipsychotic drug actions, perhaps because their avid affinity for endogenous dopamine prevents their interaction with antipsychotics (Levant, 1997). Agents partially selective for the D_3-dopamine receptor include several hydroxyaminotetralins (particularly R[+]-7-hydroxy-*N,N*-dipropylaminotetralin; the tricyclic analog PD-128,907); the hexahydrobenzophenanthridines, *nafadotride* and BP-897; and others in development (Baldessarini *et al.*, 1993; Sautel *et al.*, 1995; Kebabian *et al.*, 1997; Pilla *et al.*, 1999). The subtle and atypical functional activities of cerebral D_3 receptors suggest that D_3 agonists rather than antagonists may have useful psychotropic effects, particularly in antagonizing stimulant-reward and dependence behaviors (Shafer and Levant, 1998; Pilla *et al.*, 1999).

Table 18–2
Potencies of Standard and Experimental Antipsychotic Agents at Neurotransmitter Receptors[*][‡]

RECEPTOR	DOPAMINE D_2	SEROTONIN $5\text{-}HT_2$	$5\text{-}HT_{2A}/D_2$ RATIO	DOPAMINE D_1	DOPAMINE D_4	MUSCARINIC CHOLINERGIC	ADRENERGIC α_1	ADRENERGIC α_2	HISTAMINE H_1
Drugs									
Ziprasidone	0.42	0.42	1	525	32	≥1000	10	260	47
cis-Thiothixene	0.45	130	289	340	77	2500	11	200	6
Sertindole	0.45	0.38	0.84	28	21	≥10,000	0.77	1700	500
Fluphenazine	0.80	19	24	15	9.30	2000	9	1600	21
Zotepine	1	0.63	0.63	84	5.80	550	3.40	960	3.40
Perphenazine	1.40	5.60	4	—	—	1500	10	510	—
Thioridazine	2.30	41	17.8	22	12	10	1.10	—	—
Pimozide	2.50	13	5.20	—	30	—	—	—	—
Risperidone	3.30	0.16	0.05	750	17	>10,000	2	56	59
Aripiprazole	3.40	3.40	1	265	44	>10,000	57	—	61
Haloperidol	4	36	9	45	10	>20,000	6.20	3800	1890
Ziprasidone	4.79	0.42	0.09	339	39	≥10,000	10	—	47
Mesoridazine	5.00	6.30	1.26	—	13	—	—	—	—
Sulpiride	7.40	≥1000	135	≥1000	52	≥1000	≥1000	—	—
Olanzapine	11	4	0.36	31	9.60	1.89	19	230	7.14
Chlorpromazine	19	1.40	0.07	56	12	60	0.60	750	9.10
Loxapine	71	1.69	0.02	—	12	62	28	2400	5
Pipamperone	93	1.20	0.01	2450	—	≥5000	66	680	≥5000
Molindone	125	5000	40	—	—	—	2500	625	>10,000
Amperozide	140	20	0.14	260	1164	1700	130	590	730
Quetiapine	160	294	1.84	455	9.6	120	62	2500	11
Clozapine	180	1.60	0.01	38	9.6	7.50	9	160	2.75
Melperone	199	32	0.16	—	230	—	—	—	—
Remoxipride	275	≥10,000	36	≥10,000	3690	≥10,000	≥10,000	2900	≥10,000

[*]Data are Ki values (nM) determined by competition with radioligands for binding to the indicated receptors. [†]Compounds are in rank-order of dopamine D_2-receptor affinity; $5\text{-}HT_{2A}/D_2$ ratio indicates relative preference for D_2 *vs.* serotonin $5\text{-}HT_{2A}$ receptors. Compounds include clinically used and experimental agents. [‡]Muscarinic-cholinergic-receptor Ki values are pooled results obtained with radioligands that are nonselective for muscarinic-receptor subtypes or that are selective for the M_1 subtype.

SOURCES: Data are averaged from Roth *et al.*, 1995; Seeger *et al.*, 1995; Schotte *et al.*, 1996; Richelson, 1999; and a personal written communication from E. Richelson 1/26/00.

In Vivo *Occupation of Cerebral Neurotransmitter Receptors.* Levels of occupation of dopamine receptors and other receptors in human brain can be estimated with positron emission tomography (PET) brain imaging in patients treated with antipsychotic drugs. Such analyses not only support conclusions arising from laboratory studies of receptor occupancy (Table 18–2) but also assist in predicting clinical efficacy, extrapyramidal side effects, and clinical dosing, even in advance of controlled clinical trials (Farde *et al.*, 1995; Kasper *et al.*, 2002; Kapur and Seeman, 2001; Waddington and Casey, 2000). For example, occupation of more than 75% of D_2 receptors in the basal ganglia is associated with risk of acute extrapyramidal dysfunctions and is commonly found with clinical doses of typical neuroleptics (Farde *et al.*, 1995). In contrast, therapeutic doses of clozapine usually are associated with lower levels of occupation of D_2 receptors (averaging 40% to 50%), but higher levels of occupation (70% to 90%) of cortical $5\text{-}HT_{2A}$ receptors (Kapur *et al.*, 1999; Kapur and Seeman, 2001; Nordstrom *et al.*, 1995). Of the novel atypical antipsychotics, quetiapine has a notable clozapinelike *in vivo* receptor-occupancy profile, resembling clozapine's levels of occupation of both D_2 (40% to 50%) and $5\text{-}HT_{2A}$ receptors (50% to 70%; Gefvert *et al.*, 2001). Olanzapine and risperidone also block cortical $5\text{-}HT_{2A}$ receptors at high levels (80% to 100%), with greater occupancy at D_2 sites (typically 50% to 90%) than either clozapine or quetiapine (Farde *et al.*, 1995; Nordstrom *et al.*, 1998; Kapur *et al.*, 1999). In addition to its relatively high levels of D_2-receptor occupation, olanzapine is more antimuscarinic than is risperidone, perhaps contributing to its lower risk of acute extrapyramidal effects (Tables 18–1 and 18–2).

Clinical PET studies also indicate that ziprasidone occupies both D_2 and $5\text{-}HT_{2A}$ receptors. At conventional clinical doses, ziprasidone occupied 77% of striatal D_2 receptors and over 98% of cortical $5\text{-}HT_{2A}$ receptors (Bench *et al.*, 1996). Aripiprazole (10 to 30 mg) resulted in dose-dependent D_2 receptor occupancy (up to 84% to 94%; Yokoi *et al.*, 2002). Despite such high levels of D_2 receptor occupation, acute extrapyramidal side effects are virtually unknown with aripiprazole, consistent with evidence that it acts as a D_2 partial agonist.

Hypothalamus and Endocrine Systems. Endocrine changes occur because of effects of antipsychotic drugs on the hypothalamus or pituitary, including their antidopaminergic actions. Most older antipsychotics, reserpine, and risperidone increase prolactin secretion.

This effect on prolactin secretion probably is due to a blockade of the pituitary actions of the tuberoinfundibular dopaminergic neurons; these neurons project from the arcuate nucleus of the hypothalamus to the median eminence, where they deliver dopamine to the anterior pituitary *via* the hypophyseoportal blood vessels. D_2-dopaminergic receptors on lactotropes in the anterior pituitary mediate the tonic prolactin-inhibiting action of dopamine (Ben-Jonathan, 1985) (*see* Chapter 55).

Correlations between the potencies of antipsychotic drugs in stimulating prolactin secretion and causing behavioral effects are excellent for many types of agents (Sachar, 1978). Aripiprazole, clozapine, olanzapine, quetiapine, and ziprasidone are exceptional in having minimal or transient effects on prolactin (Argo *et al.*, 2004; Arvanitis and Miller, 1997; Compton and Miller, 2002), while olanzapine produces only minor, transient increases in prolactin levels (Tollefson and Kuntz, 1999). Risperidone has an unusually potent prolactin-elevating effect, even at doses with little extrapyramidal impact (Grant and Fitton, 1994). Effects of neuroleptics on prolactin secretion generally occur at lower doses than do their antipsychotic effects. This may reflect their action outside the blood–brain barrier in the adenohypophysis, or differences in the regulation of pituitary and cerebral D_2 receptors. Little tolerance develops to the effect of antipsychotic drugs on prolactin secretion, even after years of treatment, correlating with a relative lack of up- or down-regulation of pituitary D_2 receptors and their relative sensitivity to dopamine partial agonists such as bromocriptine (Baldessarini *et al.*, 1994; Campbell *et al.*, 1989). However, the hyperprolactinemia effect of antipsychotics is rapidly reversible when the drugs are discontinued (Bitton and Schneider, 1992). This activity is presumed to be responsible for the breast engorgement and galactorrhea that occasionally are associated with their use, sometimes even in male patients given high doses of neuroleptics.

Because antipsychotic drugs are used chronically and thus cause sustained hyperprolactinemia, there has been concern about their possible contribution to risk of carcinoma of the breast, although supportive clinical evidence is lacking (Dickson and Glazer, 1999; Mortensen, 1994). Nevertheless, antipsychotic and other agents that stimulate secretion of prolactin should be avoided in patients with established carcinoma of the breast, particularly with metastases. Perhaps due to the effects of hyperprolactinemia, some antipsychotic drugs reduce the secretion of gonadotropins and sex steroids, which can cause amenorrhea in women and sexual dysfunction or infertility in men.

The effects of standard antipsychotics on other hypothalamic neuroendocrine functions are less well characterized, although these agents inhibit the release of growth hormone and may reduce stress-induced secretion of corticotropin-releasing hormone (CRH). Despite their capacity to interfere with secretion of pituitary growth hormone, classical antipsychotics are poor therapy for acromegaly, and there is no evidence that they retard growth or development of children. In addition, some antipsychotics can decrease secretion of neurohypophyseal hormones.

In addition to neuroendocrine effects, it is likely that other autonomic effects of antipsychotic drugs are mediated by the hypothalamus. An important example is the poikilothermic effect of chlorpromazine and other neuroleptic agents, which impairs the body's ability to regulate temperature such that hypo- or hyperthermia may result, depending on the ambient temperature. Clozapine can induce moderate elevations of body temperature that can be confusing clinically. Central effects on temperature regulation and cardiovascular and respiratory functioning probably contribute to the features of *neuroleptic malignant syndrome* (*see* below).

Brainstem. Clinical doses of antipsychotic agents usually have little effect on respiration. However, vasomotor reflexes mediated by either the hypothalamus or the brainstem are depressed by some antipsychotics, which may lead to hypotension. This risk is associated particularly with older low-potency antipsychotics and with risperidone. Even in cases of acute overdose with suicidal intent, the antipsychotic drugs usually do not cause life-threatening coma or suppress vital functions. Haloperidol has been administered intravenously in doses exceeding 500 mg/24 hours to control agitation in delirious patients (Tesar *et al.*, 1985), although such aggressive dosing increased the risks of potentially life-threatening cardiac depressant effects (Hassaballa and Balk, 2003).

Chemoreceptor Trigger Zone (CTZ). Most antipsychotics protect against the nausea- and emesis-inducing effects of apomorphine and certain ergot alkaloids, all of which can interact with central dopaminergic receptors in the CTZ of the medulla. The antiemetic effect of most neuroleptics occurs with low doses. It can contribute to toxicity of acute overdoses of mixed agents by preventing their elimination by vomiting. Drugs or other stimuli that cause emesis by an action on the nodose ganglion or locally on the gastrointestinal tract are not antagonized by antipsychotic drugs, but potent piperazines and butyrophenones are sometimes effective against nausea caused by vestibular stimulation.

Autonomic Nervous System. Since various antipsychotic agents have antagonistic interactions at peripheral, α adrenergic, serotonin (5-HT$_{2A/2C}$), and histamine (H$_1$) receptors, their effects on the autonomic nervous system are complex and unpredictable. Chlorpromazine, clozapine, and thioridazine have particularly significant α adrenergic antagonistic activity. The potent piperazine tricyclic neuroleptics (*e.g.*, fluphenazine, trifluoperazine), haloperidol, and risperidone, have antipsychotic effects even when used in low doses, and show little antiadrenergic activity in patients.

The muscarinic-cholinergic blocking effects of most antipsychotic drugs are relatively weak, but the blurred vision commonly associated with chlorpromazine may be due to an anticholinergic action on the ciliary muscle. Chlorpromazine regularly produces miosis, which can be due to α adrenergic blockade. Other phenothiazines can cause mydriasis. This is especially likely to occur with clozapine or thioridazine, which are potent muscarinic antagonists. Chlorpromazine can cause constipation and decreased gastric secretion and motility; clozapine can decrease the efficiency of clearing saliva and severely impair intestinal motility (Rabinowitz *et al.*, 1996; Theret *et al.*, 1995). Decreased sweating and salivation also result from the anticholinergic effects of such drugs. Acute urinary retention is uncommon but can occur in males with prostatism. Anticholinergic effects are least frequently caused by the potent antipsychotics such as haloperidol and risperidone. However, olanzapine has substantial anticholinergic activity that may tend to offset its considerable D$_2$ antidopamine effects on the extrapyramidal system (Tarazi *et al.*, 2001). Clozapine is sufficiently anticholinergic as to induce an atropinelike poisoning on overdose (Schuster *et al.*, 1977). Its prominent, pharmacologically active metabolite, norclozapine, has allosteric agonist effects at the acetylcholine M$_1$ receptor and may potentiate the function of NMDA glutamate receptors (Sur

et al., 2003). The phenothiazines inhibit ejaculation without interfering with erection. Thioridazine produces this effect with some regularity, sometimes limiting its acceptance by men.

Kidney and Electrolyte Balance. Chlorpromazine may have weak diuretic effects in animals and human beings because of a depressant action on the secretion of vasopressin (also called antidiuretic hormone or ADH), inhibition of reabsorption of water and electrolytes by a direct action on the renal tubule, or both. The syndrome of idiopathic polydipsia and hyponatremia sometimes associated with psychotic illness has responded to clozapine, presumably *via* CNS actions (Siegel *et al.*, 1998).

Cardiovascular System. Chlorpromazine has complex actions on the cardiovascular system, directly affecting the heart and blood vessels and indirectly acting through CNS and autonomic reflexes. Chlorpromazine and less potent antipsychotic agents, as well as reserpine, risperidone, and olanzapine, can cause orthostatic hypotension, usually with rapid development of tolerance (Ray *et al.*, 1987).

Thioridazine, mesoridazine, and other phenothiazines with low potency, as well as ziprasidone, droperidol, and perhaps high doses of haloperidol have a potentially clinically significant direct negative inotropic action and a quinidinelike effect on the heart. Electrocardiographic (ECG) changes include prolongation of the QTc and PR intervals, blunting of T waves, and depression of the ST segment. Thioridazine in particular causes a high incidence of QTc- and T-wave changes and may rarely produce ventricular arrhythmias and sudden death (Zareba and Lin, 2003). These effects are less common with potent antipsychotic agents. Ziprasidone also has the propensity to prolong QTc, and prudent practice calls for extra caution when this agent, thioridazine, or mesoridazine are used in combination with other agents that depress cardiac conduction (*see* Chapter 34) (Daniel, 2003; Taylor, 2003).

Miscellaneous Pharmacological Effects. Interactions of antipsychotic drugs with central neurotransmitters other than dopamine may contribute to their antipsychotic effects or other actions. For example, many antipsychotics enhance the turnover of acetylcholine, especially in the basal ganglia, perhaps secondary to the blockade of inhibitory dopaminergic heteroceptors on cholinergic neurons. In addition, there is an inverse relationship between antimuscarinic potency of antipsychotic drugs in the brain and the likelihood of extrapyramidal effects (Snyder and Yamamura, 1977). Chlorpromazine and low-potency antipsychotic agents, including clozapine and quetiapine, have antagonistic actions at histamine receptors that probably contribute to their sedative effects.

Absorption, Distribution, Fate, and Excretion. Some antipsychotic drugs have erratic and unpredictable patterns of absorption after oral administration. Parenteral (intramuscular) administration increases the bioavailability of active drug four- to tenfold. Most antipsychotic drugs are highly lipophilic, highly membrane- or protein-bound, and accumulate in the brain, lung, and other tissues with a rich blood supply. They also enter the fetal circulation and breast milk. It is virtually impossible and usually not necessary to remove these agents by dialysis.

The stated elimination half-lives with respect to total concentrations in plasma are typically 20 to 40 hours. However, complex patterns of delayed elimination may occur with some agents, particularly the butyrophenones and their congeners (Cohen *et al.*, 1992). Biological effects of single doses of most antipsychotics usually persist for at least 24 hours, permitting once-daily dosing once the patient has adjusted to initial side effects. Elimination from the plasma may be more rapid than from sites of high lipid content and binding, notably in the CNS, but direct pharmacokinetic studies on this issue are few and inconclusive (Sedvall, 1992). Metabolites of some agents have been detected in the urine several months after drug administration was discontinued. Slow removal of drug may contribute to the typically delayed exacerbation of psychosis after stopping drug treatment. Repository ("depot") preparations of esters of neuroleptic drugs, as well of risperidone, incorporated into carbohydrate microspheres, are absorbed and eliminated much more slowly than are oral preparations. For example, half of an oral dose of fluphenazine hydrochloride is eliminated in about 20 hours, while the decanoate ester injected intramuscularly has a nominal half-life of 7 to 10 days. Clearance of fluphenazine decanoate and normalization of hyperprolactinemia following repeated dosing can require 6 to 8 months (Sampath *et al.*, 1992). Effects of long-acting risperidone (RISPERIDAL CONSTA) are delayed for 2 to 3 weeks because of slow biodegradation of the microspheres and persist for at least 2 weeks after the injections are discontinued (Harrison and Goa, 2004).

The antipsychotic drugs are metabolized by oxidative processes mediated largely by hepatic cytochrome P450 isozymes (CYPs) and by glucuronidation, sulfation, and other conjugation processes. Hydrophilic metabolites of these drugs are excreted in the urine and to some extent in the bile. Most oxidized metabolites of antipsychotic drugs are biologically inactive; a few (*e.g.*, 7-hydroxychlorpromazine, mesoridazine, several *N*-demethylated metabolites of phenothiazines, the labile hydroxy metabolite of haloperidol, 9-hydroxyrisperidone, and dehydroaripiprazole) are not. These active metabolites may contribute to biological activity of the parent compound and complicate correlating blood drug levels with clinical effects (Baldessarini *et al.*, 1988). Less potent antipsychotic drugs like chlorpromazine may weakly induce their own hepatic metabolism, since their concentrations in blood are lower after several weeks of treatment at the same dosage. Alterations of gastrointestinal motility also may contribute. The fetus, the infant, and the elderly have diminished capacity to metabolize and eliminate antipsychotic agents, while young children tend to metabolize these drugs more rapidly than do adults (Kowatch and DelBello, 2003; Kutcher, 1997; Frazier *et al.*, 2003).

With several antipsychotic agents, bioavailability and drug acceptance by hospitalized patients is somewhat increased with liquid concentrates and rapidly disintegrating tablets that yield peak serum concentrations of chlorpromazine and other phenothiazines within 2 to 4 hours. Intramuscular administration avoids much of the first-pass enteric metabolism and provides measurable concentrations in plasma within 15 to 30 minutes. Bioavailability of chlorpromazine may be increased up to tenfold with injections, but the clinical dose usually is decreased by only three- to fourfold. Gastrointestinal absorption of chlorpromazine is modified unpredictably by food and probably is decreased by antacids. Concurrent administration of anticholinergic antiparkinsonian agents does not appreciably diminish intestinal absorption of neuroleptic agents (Simpson *et al.*, 1980). Chlorpromazine and other antipsychotic agents bind significantly to membranes and to plasma proteins. Typically, more than 85% of the drug in plasma is bound to albumin. Concentrations of some neuroleptics (*e.g.*, haloperidol) in brain can be more than 10 times those in the blood (Tsuneizumi *et al.*, 1992). Their apparent volume of distribution may be as high as 20 liters per kilogram.

Disappearance of chlorpromazine from plasma varies widely and includes a rapid distribution phase (half-life about 2 hours) and a slower elimination phase (half-life about 30 hours). The half-life of elimination from human brain is not known but may be estimated using modern brain-scanning technologies (Sedvall, 1992). Approximate elimination half-lives of clinically employed antipsychotic agents are provided in Table 18–3.

Table 18–3
Elimination Half-Lives of Antipsychotic Drugs

DRUG	HALF-LIFE (HOURS)[*]
Aripiprazole	75
Chlorpromazine	24 (8–35)
Clozapine	12 (4–66)
Fluphenazine	18 (14–24)
Haloperidol	24 (12–36)[†]
Loxapine	8 (3–12)
Mesoridazine	30 (24–48)
Molindone	12 (6–24)
Olanzapine	30 (20–54)
Perphenazine	12 (8–21)
Pimozide	55 (29–111)[†]
Quetiapine	6
Risperidone	20–24[‡]
Thioridazine	24 (6–40)
Thiothixene	34
Trifluoperazine	18 (14–24)[§]
Ziprasidone	7.5

[*]Average and range. [†]May have multiphasic elimination with much longer terminal half-life. [‡]Half-life of the main active metabolite (parent drug half-life ca. 3–4 hours). [§]Estimated, assuming similarity to fluphenazine. SOURCES: Data from Ereshefsky (1996) and United States Pharmacopoeia, 2004.

Attempts to correlate plasma concentrations of chlorpromazine or its metabolites with clinical responses have been unsuccessful (Baldessarini *et al.*, 1988; Cooper *et al.*, 1976). Studies have revealed wide variations (at least tenfold) in plasma concentrations among individuals. Although plasma concentrations of chlorpromazine below 30 ng/ml are not likely to produce an adequate antipsychotic response, and levels above 750 ng/ml are likely to be poorly tolerated (Rivera-Calimlim and Hershey, 1984), the plasma concentrations that are associated with optimal clinical responses are not known. Again, modern brain-imaging techniques with radioligands for relevant cerebral receptors should provide correlations of receptor occupancy and plasma concentrations of specific drugs, as has been reported for haloperidol (Wolkin *et al.*, 1989), but few other agents (Gefvert *et al.*, 2001; Tauscher *et al.*, 2002).

At least 10 chlorpromazine metabolites occur in appreciable quantities in humans (Morselli, 1977). Quantitatively, the most important of these are nor$_2$-chlorpromazine (bis-demethylated), chlorophenothiazine (dealkylation), methoxy and hydroxy products, and glucuronide conjugates of the hydroxylated compounds. In the urine, 7-hydroxylated and *N*-dealkylated (nor and nor$_2$) metabolites and their conjugates predominate. Chlorpromazine and other phenothiazines are metabolized extensively by CYP2D6.

The pharmacokinetics and metabolism of thioridazine and fluphenazine are similar to those of chlorpromazine, but the strong anticholinergic action of thioridazine on the gut may modify its own absorption. Major metabolites of thioridazine and fluphenazine include *N*-demethylated, ring-hydroxylated, and *S*-oxidized products (Neumeyer and Booth, 2002). Concentrations of thioridazine in plasma are relatively high (hundreds of nanograms per milliliter), possibly because of its relative hydrophilicity. Thioridazine is prominently converted to the active product mesoridazine, which probably contributes to the antipsychotic activity of thioridazine.

The biotransformation of the thioxanthenes is similar to that of the phenothiazines, except that metabolism to sulfoxides is common and ring-hydroxylated products are uncommon. Piperazine derivatives of the phenothiazines and thioxanthenes also are handled much like chlorpromazine, although metabolism of the piperidine ring itself occurs.

Elimination of haloperidol and chemically related agents from human plasma is not a log-linear function, and the apparent half-life increases with observation time to a very prolonged terminal half-life of approximately 1 week (Cohen *et al.*, 1992). Haloperidol and other butyrophenones are metabolized primarily by an *N*-dealkylation reaction and the resultant inactive fragments can be conjugated with glucuronic acid. The metabolites of haloperidol are inactive, with the possible exception of a hydroxylated product formed by reduction of the keto moiety that may be reoxidized to haloperidol (Korpi *et al.*, 1983). A potentially neurotoxic derivative of haloperidol, a substituted phenylpiperidine analogous to the parkinsonism-inducing agent methylphenyltetrahydropyridine (MPTP), has been described and found in nanomolar quantities in postmortem brain tissue of persons who had been treated with haloperidol (Castagnoli *et al.*, 1999). Its pathophysiological significance is unknown. Typical plasma concentrations of haloperidol encountered clinically are about 5 to 20 ng/ml. These correspond to 80% to 90% occupancy of D$_2$-dopamine receptors in human basal ganglia, as demonstrated by PET brain scanning (Wolkin *et al.*, 1989).

For clozapine, typical peak serum concentrations after a single oral dose of 200 mg (100 to 770 ng/ml) are reached at 2.5 hours after administration, and serum levels during treatment are about 300 to 500 ng/ml. Clozapine is metabolized preferentially by

CYP3A4 into demethylated, hydroxylated, and *N*-oxide derivatives that are excreted in urine and feces. The elimination half-life of clozapine varies with dose and dosing frequency but averages about 12 hours (Table 18–3; Baldessarini and Frankenburg, 1991).

The clozapine analog olanzapine also is well absorbed, but about 40% of an oral dose is metabolized before reaching the systemic circulation. Plasma concentrations of olanzapine peak at about 6 hours after oral administration, and its elimination half-life ranges from 20 to 54 hours (Table 18–3). Major, readily excreted metabolites of olanzapine are the inactive 10-*N*-glucuronide and 4′-nor derivatives, formed mainly by the action of CYP1A2, with CYP2D6 as a minor alternative pathway (United States Pharmacopoeia, 2004).

The clozapine analog quetiapine is readily absorbed after oral administration. It reaches peak plasma levels after 1.5 hours, with a mean elimination half-life of 6 hours (Table 18–3). It is highly metabolized by hepatic CYP3A4 to inactive and readily excreted sulfoxide and acidic derivatives (United States Pharmacopoeia, 2004).

Risperidone is well absorbed and is metabolized in the liver by CYP2D6 to an active metabolite, 9-hydroxyrisperidone. Since this metabolite and risperidone are nearly equipotent, the clinical efficacy of the drug reflects both compounds. Following oral administration, peak plasma concentrations of risperidone and of its 9-hydroxy metabolite occur at 1 and 3 hours, respectively. The mean elimination half-life of both compounds is about 22 hours (Table 18–3).

The oral absorption of ziprasidone is increased up to twofold by food, and its elimination half-life is 6 to 7 hours (Beedham *et al.*, 2003; Stimmel *et al.*, 2002). Ziprasidone is highly metabolized to four major metabolites, only one of which, S-methyldihydroziprasidone, likely contributes to its clinical activity. In humans, less than 5% of the dose is excreted unchanged. Reduction by aldehyde oxidase accounts for about 66% of ziprasidone metabolism; two oxidative pathways involving hepatic CYP3A4 account for the remainder.

Bioavailability of aripiprazole is around 87%, with peak plasma concentrations attained at 3 to 5 hours after dosing. It is metabolized by dehydrogenation, oxidative hydroxylation, and N-dealkylation, largely mediated by hepatic CYPs 3A4 and 2D6 (Winans, 2003). Elimination half-life is approximately 75 hours, and the active metabolite, dehydroaripiprazole, has an elimination half-life of about 94 hours (Table 18–3).

Tolerance and Physical Dependence. As defined in Chapter 23, the antipsychotic drugs are not addicting. However, some degree of physical dependence may occur, with malaise and difficulty in sleeping developing several days after an abrupt drug discontinuation following prolonged use.

Some tolerance to sedative effects of antipsychotics usually develops over days or weeks. Loss of efficacy with prolonged treatment is not known to occur with antipsychotic agents. However, tolerance to antipsychotic drugs and cross-tolerance among the agents are demonstrable in behavioral and biochemical experiments in animals, particularly those directed toward evaluation of the blockade of dopaminergic receptors in the basal ganglia (Baldessarini and Tarsy, 1979). This form of tolerance may be less prominent in limbic and cortical areas of the forebrain. One correlate of tolerance in forebrain dopaminergic systems is the development of supersensitivity of those systems, which probably is mediated by upregulation and sensitization of dopamine receptors, particularly D$_2$ receptors. These changes may underlie the clinical phenomenon of withdrawal-emergent dyskinesias (*e.g.*, choreoathetosis on abrupt discontinuation of antipsychotic agents, especially following prolonged use of high doses of potent agents) and may contribute to the pathophysiology of tardive dyskinesias (Baldessarini *et al.*, 1980).

Although cross-tolerance may occur among antipsychotic drugs, clinical problems occur in making rapid changes from high doses of one type of agent to another. Sedation, hypotension, and other autonomic effects or acute extrapyramidal reactions can result. Worsening of the clinical condition that routinely follows discontinuation of maintenance treatment with antipsychotic agents appears to depend on the rate of drug discontinuation (Viguera *et al.*, 1997). Clinical worsening of psychotic symptoms is particularly likely after rapid discontinuation of clozapine and is difficult to control with alternative antipsychotics (Baldessarini *et al.*, 1997).

Preparations and Dosage. The number of clinically employed agents with known antipsychotic effects is large. Table 18–1 summarizes those currently marketed in the United States for the treatment of psychotic disorders or mania.

Prochlorperazine (COMPAZINE) has questionable utility as an antipsychotic agent and frequently produces acute extrapyramidal reactions. It is rarely employed in psychiatry, although it is used as an antiemetic.

Thiethylperazine (TORECAN), marketed only as an antiemetic, is a potent dopaminergic antagonist with many neurolepticlike properties. At high doses, it may be an efficacious antipsychotic agent (Rotrosen *et al.*, 1978). Long-acting repository preparations of several antipsychotic agents, including phenothiazines, thioxanthenes, butyrophenones, diphenylbutylpiperidines, and benzamides are available in other countries. However, in the United States only the decanoates of fluphenazine and haloperidol and an injected carbohydrate microsphere preparation of risperidone are commonly employed as long-acting repository preparations.

Toxic Reactions and Adverse Effects.

Antipsychotic drugs have a high therapeutic index and are generally safe agents. Furthermore, most phenothiazines, haloperidol, clozapine, and quetiapine have relatively flat dose–response curves and can be used over a wide range of dosages (Table 18–1). Although occasional deaths from overdoses have been reported, fatalities are rare in patients given medical care unless the overdose is complicated by concurrent ingestion of alcohol or other drugs. Based on animal data, the therapeutic index is lower for thioridazine and chlorpromazine than for the more potent phenothiazines (Janssen and Van Bever, 1978). Adults have survived doses of chlorpromazine up to 10 grams, and deaths from an overdose of haloperidol alone appear to be unknown, although the neuroleptic malignant syndrome and dystonic reactions that compromise respiration can be lethal.

Adverse effects often are extensions of the many pharmacological actions of these drugs. The most important are those on the cardiovascular, central and autonomic nervous, and endocrine systems. Other dangerous effects are seizures, agranulocytosis, cardiac toxicity, and pigmentary degeneration of the retina, all of which are rare (*see* below).

Therapeutic doses of phenothiazines may cause faintness, palpitations, and anticholinergic effects including nasal stuffiness, dry mouth, blurred vision, constipation, worsening of glaucoma, and urinary retention in males with prostatism.

Adverse Cardiovascular and Cerebrovascular Effects. The most common adverse cardiovascular effect is orthostatic hypotension, which may result in syncope, falls, and injuries. Hypotension is most likely to occur with administration of the phenothiazines with aliphatic side chains or atypical antipsychotics. Potent neuroleptics generally produce less hypotension.

Some antipsychotic agents depress cardiac repolarization, as reflected in the QT interval corrected for heart rate (QTc). Prolongations above 500 msec can be dangerous clinically, particularly by increasing the risk of *torsades de pointes*, which often is a precursor of fatal cardiac arrest (*see* Chapter 34). Such cardiac depressant effects are especially prominent with thioridazine and its active metabolite, mesoridazine, as well as pimozide and perhaps high doses of haloperidol, and to some extent with ziprasidone (Daniel, 2003; Hassaballa and Balk, 2003; Taylor, 2003). These drugs are used cautiously, if at all, in combination with other agents with known cardiac-depressant effects, including tricyclic antidepressants (*see* Chapter 17), certain antiarrhythmic agents (*see* Chapter 34), other antipsychotics with similar actions (such as pimozide and thioridazine), or specific dopamine antagonists (cisapride and metoclopramide; *see* Chapter 37).

Clozapine has rarely been associated with myocarditis and cardiomyopathy (La Grenade, *et al.*, 2001). Some clinical observations have suggested increased risk of stroke among elderly patients treated with risperidone and perhaps olanzapine (Wooltorton, 2002). The clinical significance of these uncommon cardiac and cerebrovascular events remains uncertain.

Adverse Neurological Effects. Many neurological syndromes, particularly involving the extrapyramidal motor system, occur following the use of most antipsychotic drugs. These reactions are particularly prominent with the high-potency D_2 dopamine receptor antagonists (tricyclic piperazines and butyrophenones). Acute adverse extrapyramidal effects are less likely with aripiprazole, clozapine, quetiapine, thioridazine, and ziprasidone, or low doses of olanzapine or risperidone. The neurological effects associated with antipsychotic drugs have been reviewed in detail (Baldessarini and Tarsy, 1979; Baldessarini *et al.*, 1980; Baldessarini, 1984; Baldessarini *et al.*, 1990; Kane *et al.*, 1992; Tarsy *et al.*, 2002).

Six distinct neurological syndromes are characteristic of older neuroleptic-antipsychotic drugs. Four of these

Table 18–4
Neurological Side Effects of Neuroleptic Drugs

REACTION	FEATURES	TIME OF MAXIMAL RISK	PROPOSED MECHANISM	TREATMENT
Acute dystonia	Spasm of muscles of tongue, face, neck, back; may mimic seizures; *not* hysteria	1 to 5 days	Unknown	Antiparkinsonian agents are diagnostic and curative[*]
Akathisia	Motor restlessness; *not* anxiety or "agitation"	5 to 60 days	Unknown	Reduce dose or change drug; antiparkinsonian agents,[†] benzodiazepines or propranolol[‡] may help
Parkinsonism	Bradykinesia, rigidity, variable tremor, mask facies, shuffling gait	5 to 30 days; can recur even after a single dose	Antagonism of dopamine	Antiparkinsonian agents helpful[†]
Neuroleptic malignant syndrome	Catatonia, stupor, fever, unstable blood pressure, myoglobinemia; can be fatal	Weeks; can persist for days after stopping neuroleptic	Antagonism of dopamine may contribute	Stop neuroleptic immediately; dantrolene or bromocriptine[§] may help; antiparkinsonian agents not effective
Perioral tremor ("rabbit syndrome")	Perioral tremor (may be a late variant of parkinsonism)	After months or years of treatment	Unknown	Antiparkinsonian agents often help[†]
Tardive dyskinesia	Oral-facial dyskinesia; widespread choreoathetosis or dystonia	After months or years of treatment (worse on withdrawal)	Excess function of dopamine hypothesized	Prevention crucial; treatment unsatisfactory

[*]Many drugs have been claimed to be helpful for acute dystonia. Among the most commonly employed treatments are diphenhydramine hydrochloride, 25 or 50 mg intramuscularly, or benztropine mesylate, 1 or 2 mg intramuscularly or slowly intravenously, followed by oral medication with the same agent for a period of days to perhaps several weeks thereafter. [†]For details regarding the use of oral antiparkinsonian agents, *see* the text and Chapter 20: Treatment of Central Nervous System Degenerative Disorders. [‡]Propranolol often is effective in relatively low doses (20–80 mg per day). Selective β_1 adrenergic receptor antagonists are less effective. [§]Despite the response to dantrolene, there is no evidence of an abnormality of Ca^{2+} transport in skeletal muscle; with lingering neuroleptic effects, bromocriptine may be tolerated in large doses (10–40 mg per day).

(acute dystonia, akathisia, parkinsonism, and the rare neuroleptic malignant syndrome) usually appear soon after administration of the drug. Two (tardive dyskinesias or dystonias, and rare perioral tremor) are late-appearing syndromes that evolve during prolonged treatment. The clinical features of these syndromes and guidelines for their management are summarized in Table 18–4.

Acute dystonic reactions commonly occur with the initiation of neuroleptic therapy, particularly with agents of high potency, and may include facial grimacing, torticollis, oculogyric crisis, and abnormal contraction of spinal muscles (including opisthotonos) and of muscles involved

in breathing. These syndromes may be mistaken for hysterical reactions or epileptic seizures, but respond dramatically to parenteral administration of anticholinergic antiparkinson drugs. Oral administration of anticholinergic agents also can prevent dystonia, particularly in young male patients given a high-potency neuroleptic (Arana *et al.*, 1988). Although readily treated, acute dystonic reactions are terrifying to patients. Sudden death has occurred, probably due to impaired respiration caused by dystonia of pharyngeal, laryngeal, and other muscles. Dystonia is especially common in young men. It usually is not immediate but occurs within the first 24 to 48 hours of treatment, with diminishing risk thereafter except with repeated injections of long-acting agents. This timing, in association with the gradual emergence of bradykinesia, parallels the presynaptic adaptations that occur in dopaminergic neurons within the first week of exposure to neuroleptic agents.

Akathisia refers to strong subjective feelings of anxious distress or discomfort and a compelling need to be in constant movement rather than to follow any specific movement pattern. Patients typically feel that they must get up and walk or continuously move about and may be unable to control this tendency. Akathisia may be mistaken for agitation in psychotic patients, and the distinction is critical, since agitation might be treated with an increase in dosage. Because akathisia often responds poorly to antiparkinson drugs, treatment typically requires reduction of dosage or a change of the antipsychotic drug. Antianxiety agents or moderate doses of a relatively lipophilic β adrenergic receptor antagonist such as propranolol may be beneficial (Lipinski *et al.*, 1984; Reiter *et al.*, 1987). This common syndrome often interferes with patient adherence to neuroleptic treatment but frequently is not diagnosed. Akathisia occurs with newer antipsychotic agents, including risperidone, olanzapine, and even occasionally with clozapine (Tarsy *et al.*, 2002). This pattern adds to the impression that the underlying pathophysiology differs from that of the more clearly extrapyramidal reactions, such as dystonia and bradykinesia.

A *parkinsonian syndrome* that can be indistinguishable from idiopathic Parkinson's disease (*paralysis agitans*) commonly develops gradually during administration of antipsychotic drugs. This adverse effect, which almost certainly reflects deficient dopaminergic function in the extrapyramidal basal ganglia, varies in incidence with different agents (Tables 18–1 and 18–4). Clinically, there is a generalized slowing and impoverishment of volitional movement (bradykinesia or akinesia) with masked facies and reduced arm movements during walking. The syndrome characteristically evolves gradually over days to weeks as the risk of acute dystonia diminishes. The most noticeable signs are slowing of movements, and sometimes rigidity and variable tremor at rest, especially involving the upper extremities. "Pill-rolling" movements and other types of resting tremor (at a frequency of 3 to 5 Hz, as in Parkinson's disease) may be seen, although they are less prominent in neuroleptic-induced than in idiopathic parkinsonism. Bradykinesia and masked facies may be mistaken for clinical depression. This reaction usually is managed by use of either antiparkinson agents with anticholinergic properties, or amantadine (*see* Chapter 20). The use of levodopa or a directly acting dopamine

agonist incurs the risk of inducing agitation and worsening the psychotic illness. Antipsychotic agents sometimes are required in the clinical management of patients with idiopathic Parkinson's disease with spontaneous psychotic illness or psychotic reactions to dopaminergic therapy (*see* Chapter 20). Clozapine and perhaps quetiapine are least likely to worsen the neurological disorder (Menza *et al.*, 1999; Parkinson Study Group, 1999). Risperidone, olanzapine, and typical neuroleptics are relatively poorly tolerated by patients with Parkinson's disease, and aripiprazole and ziprasidone have not been adequately investigated in this setting (Tarsy *et al.*, 2002).

The rare *neuroleptic malignant syndrome* (NMS) resembles a very severe form of parkinsonism, with coarse tremor and catatonia, fluctuating in intensity. It includes signs of autonomic instability (hyperthermia and labile pulse, blood pressure, and respiration rate), stupor, elevation of creatine kinase in serum, and sometimes myoglobinemia with potential nephrotoxicity. In its most severe form, this syndrome may persist for more than a week after the offending agent is discontinued. Mortality exceeds 10%, mandating immediate medical attention. This reaction has been associated with various types of antipsychotics, but its prevalence may be greater when relatively high doses of potent agents are used, especially when they are administered parenterally. Aside from cessation of antipsychotic treatment and provision of supportive care, specific treatment is unsatisfactory; administration of *dantrolene* or the dopaminergic agonist *bromocriptine* may be helpful (Addonizio *et al.*, 1987; Pearlman, 1986). Although dantrolene also is used to manage the syndrome of malignant hyperthermia induced by general anesthetics, the neuroleptic-induced form of catatonia and hyperthermia probably is not associated with a defect in Ca^{2+} metabolism in skeletal muscle. Atypical antipsychotic agents including clozapine, olanzapine, and risperidone are associated with an atypical, but potentially lethal, neuroleptic malignant–like syndrome that is marked by fever and delirium without muscle rigidity (Farver, 2003).

Tardive dyskinesia is a late-appearing neurological syndrome (or syndromes) associated with neuroleptic drugs. It occurs more frequently in older patients, and risk may be somewhat greater in patients with mood disorders than in those with schizophrenia. Its prevalence averages 15% to 25% in young adults treated with older antipsychotics for more than a year. There is an annual incidence of 3% to 5% and a somewhat smaller annual rate of spontaneous remission, even with continued neuroleptic treatment. The risk is much lower with clozapine; lower with aripiprazole, olanzapine, and ziprasidone; and intermediate with risperidone (Correll *et al.*, 2004; Tarsy *et al.*, 2002). Tardive dyskinesia is characterized by stereotyped, repetitive, painless, involuntary, quick choreiform (tic-like) movements of the face, eyelids (blinks or spasm), mouth (grimaces), tongue, extremities, or trunk. There are varying degrees of slower athetosis (twisting movements) and sustained dystonic postures, which are more common in young men and may be disabling. Late (tardive) emergence of disorders marked mainly by dystonia or akathisia (restlessness) also are seen. These movements all disappear in sleep (as do many other extrapyramidal syndromes), vary in intensity over time, and are dependent on the level of arousal or emotional distress, sometimes reappearing during acute psychiatric illnesses following prolonged disappearance.

Tardive dyskinetic movements can be suppressed partially by use of a potent neuroleptic, and perhaps with a dopamine-depleting agent such as reserpine or tetrabenazine, but such interventions are reserved for severe dyskinesia, particularly with continuing psychosis. Some dyskinetic patients, typically those with dystonic features, benefit from use of clozapine, which has a very low risk of tardive dyskinesia. Symptoms sometimes persist indefinitely after discontinuation of neuroleptic medication. More often, they diminish or disappear gradually over months of follow-up, especially in younger patients (Gardos *et al.*, 1994; Morgenstern and Glazer, 1993; Smith and Baldessarini, 1980). Antiparkinson agents typically have little effect on, or may even exacerbate, tardive dyskinesia and other forms of choreoathetosis, such as in Huntington's disease. No adequate treatment of these conditions has been established (Adler *et al.*, 1999; Soares and McGrath, 1999; Tarsy *et al.*, 2002).

There is no established neuropathology in tardive dyskinesia, and its pathophysiological basis remains obscure. Compensatory increases in the function of dopamine as a neurotransmitter in the basal ganglia could be involved, including increased abundance and sensitivity of dopamine D_2-like receptors resulting from long-term administration of different classes of antipsychotic drugs (Baldessarini and Tarsy, 1979; Tarazi *et al.* 1997, 2001). This hypothesis is supported by the dissimilarities of therapeutic responses in patients with Parkinson's disease and those with tardive dyskinesia, and by the similar responses of patients with other choreoathetotic dyskinesias such as Huntington's disease (*see* Chapter 20). Thus antidopaminergic drugs tend to suppress manifestations of tardive dyskinesia and Huntington's disease, whereas dopaminergic agonists worsen them. In contrast to parkinsonism, antimuscarinic agents tend to worsen tardive dyskinesia, while cholinergic agents usually are ineffective. In laboratory animals, supersensitivity to dopaminergic agonists usually lasts only for a few weeks after withdrawal of dopamine antagonists. This phenomenon most likely plays a role in variants of tardive dyskinesia that resolve rapidly, usually referred to as *withdrawal-emergent dyskinesias*. The theoretical and clinical

aspects of this problem have been reviewed in detail (Baldessarini and Tarsy, 1979; Baldessarini *et al.*, 1980; Kane *et al.*, 1992).

A rare movement disorder that can appear late in chronic treatment with antipsychotic agents is *perioral tremor,* often referred to as the "rabbit syndrome" (Schwartz and Hocherman, 2004) because of the peculiar movements that characterize it. Rabbit syndrome shares many features with parkinsonism, because the tremor has a frequency of about 3 to 5 Hz, and often responds favorably to anticholinergic agents and removal of the offending agent.

Certain therapeutic guidelines should be followed to minimize the neurological syndromes that complicate the use of antipsychotic drugs. Routine use of antiparkinson agents in an attempt to avoid early extrapyramidal reactions usually is unnecessary; it adds complexity, side effects, and expense to the regimen. Antiparkinson agents are best reserved for cases of overt extrapyramidal reactions that respond favorably to such intervention. The need for such agents for the treatment of acute dystonic reactions ordinarily diminishes with time, but parkinsonism and akathisia typically persist. The thoughtful and conservative use of antipsychotic drugs, particularly modern atypical agents, in patients with chronic or frequently recurrent psychotic disorders almost certainly can reduce the risk of tardive dyskinesia. Although reduction of the dose of an antipsychotic agent is the best way to minimize its adverse neurological effects, this may not be practical in a patient with uncontrollable psychotic illness. The best preventive practice is to use the minimum dose of an antipsychotic drug that is effective. The growing number of modern atypical antipsychotic agents with a low risk of inducing extrapyramidal side effects provides an alternative for many patients, particularly those with continuing psychotic symptoms plus dyskinesia (Baldessarini and Frankenburg, 1991; Tarsy *et al.*, 2002).

Weight Gain and Metabolic Effects. Weight gain and its associated long-term complications can occur with extended treatment with most antipsychotic and antimanic drugs. Weight gain is especially prominent with clozapine and olanzapine; somewhat less with quetiapine; even less with fluphenazine, haloperidol, and risperidone; and is very low with aripiprazole, molindone, and ziprasidone (Allison *et al.*, 1999). Adverse effects of weight gain likely include increased risk of new-onset or worsening of type 2 diabetes mellitus, hypertension, and hyperlipidemia. Only some of these consequences are explained by risk factors associated with major psychiatric disorders themselves. The anticipated long-term public health impact of these emerging problems is not yet well defined (Cohen, 2004; Gaulin *et al.*, 1999; Henderson *et al.*, 2000; McIntyre *et al.*, 2003; Wirshing *et al.*, 1998). In some patients with morbid increases in weight, the airway may be compromised (*Pickwickian syndrome*), especially during sleep (including *sleep apnea*).

Blood Dyscrasias. Mild leukocytosis, leukopenia, and eosinophilia occasionally occur with antipsychotic treatment, particularly with clozapine and less often with phenothiazines of low potency. It is difficult to determine whether leukopenia that develops during the administration of such agents is a forewarning of impending agranulocytosis. This serious complication occurs in not more than 1 in 10,000 patients receiving chlorpromazine or other low-potency agents (other than clozapine); it usually appears within the first 8 to 12 weeks of treatment (Alvir *et al.*, 1993).

Bone marrow suppression, or less commonly agranulocytosis, has been associated with the use of clozapine. The incidence approaches 1% within several months of treatment, independent of dose, without regular monitoring of white blood cell counts. Because blood dyscrasia may develop suddenly, the appearance of fever, malaise, or apparent respiratory infection in a patient being treated with an antipsychotic drug should be followed immediately by a complete blood count. Risk of agranulocytosis is greatly reduced, though not eliminated, by frequent white blood cell counts in patients being treated with clozapine, as is required in the United States (weekly for 6 months and biweekly thereafter). The safety of resuming even low doses of clozapine or other antipsychotics following recovery from agranulocytosis should not be assumed (Iqbal *et al.*, 2003).

Skin Reactions. Dermatological reactions to the phenothiazines, including urticaria or dermatitis, occur in about 5% of patients receiving chlorpromazine. Contact dermatitis may occur in personnel who handle chlorpromazine, and there may be a degree of cross-sensitivity to other phenothiazines. Sunburn and photosensitivity resembling severe sunburn occur and require use of an effective sunscreen preparation. Epithelial keratopathy often is observed in patients on long-term therapy with chlorpromazine, and opacities in the cornea and in the lens of the eye have been noted. Pigmentary retinopathy has been reported, particularly following doses of thioridazine in excess of 1000 mg per day. A maximum daily dose of 800 mg currently is recommended. Dermatological reactions to modern atypical antipsychotic agents are uncommon.

Gastrointestinal and Hepatic Effects. A mild jaundice, typically occurring early in therapy, may be observed in some patients receiving chlorpromazine. Pruritus is rare. The reaction probably is a manifestation of hypersensitivity because eosinophilia and eosinophilic infiltration of the liver occur unrelated to dose. Desensitization to chlorpromazine may occur with repeated administration, and jaundice may or may not recur if the same drug is given again. When the psychiatric disorder calls for uninterrupted drug therapy for a patient with neuroleptic-induced jaundice, it probably is safest to use low doses of a potent, dissimilar agent. Hepatic dysfunction with other antipsychotic agents is uncommon.

Clozapine specifically has two important risks of intestinal dysfunction: potentially severe ileus (Theret *et al.*, 1995) and sialor-

rhea, which may be related to deficient pharyngeal-esophageal clearing mechanisms most noticeable during sleep (Rabinowitz *et al.*, 1996).

Interactions with Other Drugs. The phenothiazines and thioxanthenes, especially those of lower potency, affect the actions of a number of other drugs, sometimes with important clinical consequences (DeVane and Nemeroff, 2000; Goff and Baldessarini, 1993). Antipsychotic drugs can strongly potentiate the effect of medically prescribed sedatives and analgesics, alcohol, nonprescription sedatives and hypnotics, antihistamines, and cold remedies. Chlorpromazine increases the miotic and sedative effects of morphine and may increase its analgesic actions. The drug markedly increases the respiratory depression produced by meperidine and can be expected to have similar effects when administered concurrently with other opioids. Obviously, neuroleptic drugs inhibit the actions of dopaminergic agonists and levodopa and worsen the neurological symptoms of Parkinson's disease (Tarsy *et al.*, 2002).

Other interactions involve the cardiovascular system. Chlorpromazine, some other antipsychotic drugs, and their *N*-demethylated metabolites may block the antihypertensive effects of guanethidine, probably by blocking its uptake into sympathetic nerves. Molindone and the more potent antipsychotic agents are less likely to cause this effect. Low-potency phenothiazines can promote postural hypotension, possibly due to their α adrenergic blocking properties. Thus interactions between phenothiazines and antihypertensive agents are unpredictable.

The antimuscarinic action of clozapine and thioridazine can cause tachycardia and enhance the peripheral and central effects (confusion, delirium) of other anticholinergic agents, such as the tricyclic antidepressants and antiparkinson agents.

Sedatives or anticonvulsants (*e.g., carbamazepine, oxcarbazepine, phenobarbital,* and *phenytoin,* but not *valproate*) that induce CYPs (*see* Chapter 3) can enhance the metabolism of antipsychotic and many other agents (including anticoagulants and oral contraceptives), sometimes with significant clinical consequences. Conversely, selective serotonin reuptake inhibitors including *fluvoxamine, fluoxetine, paroxetine, venlafaxine, sertraline,* and *nefazodone* (*see* Chapter 17) compete for these enzymes and can elevate circulating levels of neuroleptics (Goff and Baldessarini, 1993).

DRUG TREATMENT OF PSYCHOSES

Short-Term Treatment. The antipsychotic drugs are not specific to the type of illness being treated. They clearly are effective in acute psychoses of unknown etiology, including mania, acute idiopathic psychoses, and acute exacerbations of schizophrenia. The best studied indications are for the acute and chronic phases of schizophrenia and in acute mania. Antipsychotic drugs also are used empirically in many other neuromedical and idiopathic disorders with prominent psychotic symptoms or severe agitation.

Acceptance that neuroleptic agents are indeed antipsychotics came slowly. However, many clinical trials and five decades of clinical experience have established that they are effective and superior to sedatives, such as the barbiturates and benzodiazepines, or alternatives, such as electroconvulsive shock or other medical or psychological therapies (Baldessarini *et al.*, 1990). The "target" symptoms for which antipsychotic agents are especially effective include agitation, combativeness, hostility, hallucinations, acute delusions, insomnia, anorexia, poor self-care, negativism, and sometimes withdrawal and seclusiveness. More variable or delayed are improvements in motivation and cognition, including insight, judgment, memory, orientation, and functional recovery. The most favorable prognosis is for patients with acute illnesses of brief duration who had functioned relatively well prior to the illness.

No one drug or combination of drugs selectively affects a particular symptom complex in groups of psychotic patients. Although individual patients may apparently respond better with one agent than another, this can be determined only by trial and error. It is sometimes claimed that certain agents (particularly newer antipsychotic drugs) are specifically effective against "negative" symptoms in psychotic disorders (*e.g.,* abulia, social withdrawal, and lack of motivation). However, evidence supporting this proposal remains inconsistent, and such benefits usually are limited (Moller, 1999; Arango *et al.*, 2004). Generally, "positive" (irrational thinking, delusions, agitated turmoil, hallucinations) and "negative" symptoms tend to respond or not respond together with overall clinical improvement. This tendency is well documented with typical neuroleptics as well as modern atypical antipsychotic agents. It is clear that aripiprazole, clozapine, quetiapine, and ziprasidone induce less bradykinesia and other parkinsonian effects than do typical neuroleptics. In addition, aripiprazole and ziprasidone are minimally sedating. Minimizing such side effects is sometimes interpreted clinically as specific improvement in impoverished affective responsiveness and energy level.

The short-term clinical superiority of modern antipsychotic agents over older neuroleptics has been particularly hard to prove, and some comparison trials involve nonequivalent dosing of novel and older agents. Moreover, comparisons among modern agents are even less numerous, and their findings remain largely inconclusive (Gardner *et al.*, 2005). Nevertheless, at least in the United States, the modern atypical agents have come to dominate clinical practice, owing mainly to their perceived superior tolerability and acceptability.

It is important to simplify the treatment regimen and to ensure that the patient is receiving the drug. In cases of suspected severe and dangerous noncompliance or with failure of oral treatment, the patient can be treated with injections of fluphenazine decanoate, haloperidol decanoate, or other long-acting preparations, including risperidone microspheres.

Because the choice of an antipsychotic drug cannot be made reliably on the basis of anticipated therapeutic effect, drug selection often depends on likely tolerability of specific side effects, the need for sedation, or on a previous favorable response. If the patient has a history of cardiovascular disease or stroke and the threat from hypotension is serious, a modern atypical agent or a potent older neuroleptic should be used in the smallest dose that is effective (Table 18–1; DeBattista and Schatzberg, 1999). If it seems important to minimize the risk of acute extrapyramidal symptoms, aripiprazole, clozapine, quetiapine, ziprasidone, or a low dose of olanzapine or risperidone should be considered. If the patient would be seriously discomfited by interference with ejaculation or if there are serious risks of cardiovascular or other autonomic toxicity, low doses of a potent neuroleptic might be preferred. If sedative effects are undesirable, a potent agent (aripiprazole or ziprasidone) is preferable. Small doses of antipsychotic drugs of high or moderate potency may be safest in the elderly, in whom the possible risk of stroke with risperidone and olanzapine must be considered. If hepatic function is compromised or there is a potential threat of jaundice, low doses of a high-potency agent may be used. The physician's experience with a particular drug may outweigh other considerations. *Skill in the use of antipsychotic drugs depends on selection of an adequate but not excessive dose, knowledge of what to expect, and judgment as to when to stop therapy or change drugs.*

Some patients do not respond satisfactorily to antipsychotic drug treatment, and many chronically ill schizophrenia patients, while helped during periods of acute exacerbation of illness, may show unsatisfactory responses during less acute intervals. Individual nonresponders cannot be identified beforehand with certainty, but a substantial minority of psychotic patients do poorly with any antipsychotic medicine, including clozapine. If a patient does not improve after a course of seemingly adequate treatment and fails to respond to another drug given in adequate dosage, the diagnosis should be reevaluated.

Usually 2 to 3 weeks or more are required to demonstrate obvious beneficial effects in schizophrenia patients. Maximum benefit in chronically ill patients may require several months. In contrast, improvement of some acutely psychotic or manic patients can be seen within 48 hours. Aggressive dosing with high doses of an antipsychotic drug at the start of an acute episode of psychosis has not been found to increase either the magnitude or the rate of therapeutic responses (Baldessarini *et al.*, 1988). However, parenteral agents in moderate doses can bring about rapid sedation and may be useful in acute behavioral control. Sedatives, such as the potent benzodiazepines, can be used briefly during the initiation of antipsychotic therapy, but are not effective in the long-term treatment of chronically psychotic, and especially, schizophrenic patients (Bradwejn *et al.*, 1990). After the initial response, drugs usually are used in conjunction with psychological, supportive, and rehabilitative treatments.

There is no convincing evidence that combinations of antipsychotic drugs offer clear or consistent advantages. A combination of an antipsychotic drug and an antidepressant may be useful in some cases, especially in depressed psychotic patients or in cases of agitated major depression with psychotic features. The first combination antipsychotic/antidepressant (olanzapine/fluoxetine; SYMBYAX) was recently FDA approved in the United States for treatment of depressive episodes associated with bipolar disorder. However, antidepressants and stimulants are unlikely to reduce apathy and withdrawal in schizophrenia, and they may induce clinical worsening in some cases. Adjunctive addition of lithium or an antimanic anticonvulsant may add benefit in some psychotic patients with prominent affective, aggressive, or resistant symptoms (Hosak and Libiger,

2002), and may produce earlier improvements in psychotic symptoms of acute schizophrenia patients (Casey *et al.*, 2003).

Optimal dosage of antipsychotic drugs requires individualization to determine doses that are effective, well tolerated, and accepted by the patient. Dose–response relationships for antipsychotic and adverse effects overlap, and it can be difficult to determine an end-point of a desired therapeutic response (DeBattista and Schatzberg, 1999). Typical effective daily doses are approximately 300 to 500 mg of chlorpromazine, 5 to 15 mg of haloperidol, 200 to 500 mg of clozapine, 5 to 15 mg of olanzapine, 4 to 6 mg of risperidone, 400 to 800 mg of quetiapine, 80 to 160 mg of ziprasidone, 5 to 30 mg of aripiprazole, or their equivalent. Doses of as little as 50 to 200 mg of chlorpromazine per day (or 2 to 6 mg of haloperidol or fluphenazine, 2 mg of risperidone, or 5 mg of olanzapine) may be effective and be better tolerated by many patients, especially after the initial improvement of acute symptoms (Baldessarini *et al.*, 1988, 1990). Careful observation of the patient's changing response is the best guide to dosage.

To achieve control of symptoms in the treatment of acute psychoses, the dose of antipsychotic drug is increased as tolerated during the first few days. The dose is then adjusted during the next several weeks as the patient's condition warrants. Parenteral short-acting medication sometimes is indicated for acutely agitated patients; 5 mg of haloperidol or fluphenazine, or a comparable dose of another agent, is given intramuscularly. Short-acting injectable preparations of both olanzapine and ziprasidone also have been developed (Altamura *et al.*, 2003; Wright *et al.*, 2003; Zimbroff, 2003). Desired clinical effects usually can be obtained by administering additional doses at intervals of 4 to 8 hours for the first 24 to 72 hours, because the appearance of effects may be delayed for several hours. Rarely is it necessary to administer a total daily dose of more than 20 to 30 mg of fluphenazine or haloperidol, 600 to 900 mg of clozapine, 6 to 8 mg of risperidone, 15 to 20 mg of olanzapine, 120 to 160 mg of ziprasidone (or up to 40 mg intramuscularly), or 20 to 30 mg of aripiprazole (or an equivalent amount of another agent). Severe and poorly controlled agitation usually can be managed safely by use of adjunctive sedation (*e.g.,* with a benzodiazepine such as lorazepam) and close supervision in a secure setting.

One must remain alert for acute dystonic reactions, which are especially likely to appear early with aggressive use of potent neuroleptics. Hypotension is most likely to occur if an agent of low potency, such as chlorpromazine, is given in a high dose or by injection and may occur early in treatment with atypical antipsychotic agents. Some antipsychotic drugs, including fluphenazine, other piperazines, and haloperidol, have been given in doses of several hundred milligrams a day without serious adverse effects. However, such high doses of potent agents do not yield significantly or consistently superior results in the treatment of acute or chronic psychosis, and may even yield inferior antipsychotic effects with increased risk of neurological, cardiovascular, and other adverse effects (Baldessarini *et al.*, 1988, 1990). After an initial period of stabilization, regimens based on a single daily dose (typically 5 to 10 mg per day of haloperidol or fluphenazine, 2 to 4 mg of risperidone, 5 to 15 mg of olanzapine, or their equivalent) often are effective and safe. The time of administration may be varied to minimize adverse effects.

Table 18–1 gives the usual and extreme ranges of dosage for antipsychotic drugs used in the United States (DeBattista and Schatzberg, 1999; United States Pharmacopoeia, 2004). The ranges have been established for the most part in the treatment of young and middle-aged adult patients diagnosed with schizophrenia or mania. Acutely disturbed hospitalized patients often require higher

doses of an antipsychotic drug than do more stable outpatients. However, the concept that a low or flexible maintenance dose often will suffice during follow-up care of a partially recovered or chronic psychotic patient is supported by several appropriately controlled trials (Baldessarini *et al.*, 1988, 1990; Herz *et al.*, 1991).

Despite the great success of the antipsychotic drugs, their use alone does not constitute optimal care of psychotic or manic patients. The acute care, protection, and support of such patients, as well as their long-term care and rehabilitation, also are critically important. Detailed reviews of the clinical use of antipsychotic drugs are available (Baldessarini *et al.*, 1990; Marder, 1998; Worrel *et al.*, 2000).

Long-Term Treatment. In reviews of nearly 30 controlled prospective studies involving several thousand schizophrenic patients, the mean overall relapse rate was 58% for patients withdrawn from antipsychotic drugs and given a placebo *versus* only 16% of those who continued on drug therapy (Baldessarini *et al.*, 1990; Gilbert *et al.*, 1995; Viguera *et al.*, 1997). Daily dosage in chronic cases often can be lowered to 50 to 200 mg of chlorpromazine or its equivalent without signs of relapse (Baldessarini *et al.*, 1988), but rapid dose reduction or discontinuation appears to increase risk of exacerbation or relapse (Viguera *et al.*, 1997). Flexible therapy in which dosage is adjusted to changing current requirements can be useful and can reduce the incidence of adverse effects.

If the modern or atypical antipsychotic agents have superiority to older neuroleptics, this advantage is most important in the long-term treatment of chronic or recurrent psychotic illnesses, where it is standard practice to continue maintenance treatment with moderate and well-tolerated doses of an antipsychotic agent indefinitely, as long as the clinical indications, benefits, and tolerability remain clear. The only agent with securely proven superiority, not only to older neuroleptics but also to some modern antipsychotics, is clozapine (Baldessarini and Frankenburg, 1991; Bagnall *et al.*, 2003; Davis *et al.*, 2003; Kane *et al.*, 1988; Leucht *et al.*, 2003a, 2003b; Tuunainen *et al.*, 2004; Wahlbeck *et al.*, 1999). Nevertheless, there is some evidence that modern atypical antipsychotics may yield superior results in long-term treatment, if only due to superior tolerability and adherence to treatment (Bagnall *et al.*, 2003; Czernansky *et al.*, 2003). Currently, the cost-benefit analysis does not always favor the more expensive modern agents (Rosenheck *et al.*, 2003; Gardner *et al.*, 2005).

Maintenance with injections of the decanoate ester of fluphenazine or haloperidol every 2 to 4 weeks, or with long-acting risperidone microspheres every 2 or 3 weeks, can be very effective (Kane *et al.*, 1983; Harrison and Goa, 2004; Lasser *et al.*, 2005). However, an expectation of superiority of long-acting injected antipsychotics is not well supported by available studies, most of which involve randomization of patients who already are largely cooperative with long-term oral treatment (Adams *et al.*, 2001; Bhanji *et al.*, 2004; Schooler, 2003). Further studies are required, ideally among difficult, complex, and poorly treatment-adherent populations of chronically psychotic patients.

Special Populations. The treatment of some symptoms and behaviors associated with delirium or dementia is another accepted use for the antipsychotic drugs. They may be administered temporarily while a specific and correctable structural, infectious, metabolic, or toxic cause is vigorously sought. They sometimes are used for prolonged periods when no correctable cause can be found. There are no drugs of choice or clearly established dosage guidelines for such indications, although older neuroleptics of high potency are preferred (Prien, 1973). Modern atypical agents have not established their place in the management of delirium or dementia (Ely *et al.*, 2004). In patients with delirium without likelihood of seizures, frequent small doses (*e.g.,* 2 to 6 mg) of haloperidol or another potent antipsychotic may be effective in controlling agitation. Agents with low potency should be avoided because of their greater tendency to produce sedation, hypotension, and seizures, and those with central anticholinergic effects may worsen confusion and agitation.

A challenging special population are Parkinson's disease patients with psychotic symptoms related to dopaminergic therapy (Neumeyer *et al.*, 2003) (*see* Chapter 20). Standard neuroleptics, risperidone (even in small doses), and olanzapine often produce unacceptable worsening of bradykinesia-akinesia. Clozapine is relatively well tolerated and effective, though more complicated to use. Use of moderate doses of newer agents with very low risk of parkinsonism (aripiprazole, quetiapine, ziprasidone) requires further study (Tarsy *et al.*, 2002).

Most antipsychotics are rapidly effective in the treatment of mania and often are used concomitantly with the institution of lithium or anticonvulsant therapy (*see* below). Adequate studies of possible long-term preventive effects of antipsychotic drugs in manic-depressive illness are starting to emerge (Tohen *et al.*, 2003; Yatham, 2003).

Antipsychotic drugs also may have a limited role in the treatment of severe depression. Controlled studies have demonstrated the efficacy of several antipsychotic drugs in some depressed patients, especially those with striking agitation or psychotic features, and addition of an antipsychotic to an antidepressant in psychotic depression may yield results approaching those obtained with ECT (Brotman *et al.*, 1987; Chan *et al.*, 1987). Antipsychotic agents ordinarily are not used for the treatment of anxiety disorders. The use of clozapine in patients with schizophrenia and a high risk of suicidal behavior may reduce the risk of suicide attempts. Clozapine is the first drug to be FDA approved for an antisuicide indication (Meltzer *et al.*, 2003; Hennen and Baldessarini, 2004).

Drug treatment of childhood psychosis and other behavioral disorders of children is confused by diagnostic inconsistencies and a paucity of controlled trials. Antipsychotics can benefit children with disorders characterized by features that occur in adult psychoses, mania, autism, or Tourette's syndrome. Low doses of the more potent or modern atypical agents usually are preferred in an attempt to avoid interference with daytime activities or performance in school (Kutcher, 1997; Findling *et al.*, 1998). Attention deficit disorder, with or without hyperactivity, responds poorly to antipsychotic agents, but often if the condition is not comorbid with bipolar disorder, responds very well to stimulants and some antidepressants (Faedda *et al.*, 2004; Kutcher, 1997). Information on dosages of antipsychotic drugs for children is limited, as is the number of drugs currently approved in the United States for use in preadolescents. The recommended doses of antipsychotic agents for school-aged children with moderate degrees of agitation are lower than those for acutely psychotic children, who may require daily doses similar to those used in adults (Kutcher, 1997; Table 18–1).

Most relevant experience with pediatric patients is with chlorpromazine, for which the recommended dose is approximately 0.5 mg/kg of body weight given at intervals of 4 to 6 hours orally or 6 to 8 hours intramuscularly. Suggested dosage limits are 200 mg per day (orally) for preadolescents, 75 mg per day (intramuscularly) for children aged 5 to 12 years or weighing 23 to 45 kg, and 40 mg per day (intramuscularly) for children under 5 years of age or weighing

less than 23 kg. Usual single doses for other agents of relatively low potency are thioridazine, 0.25 to 0.5 mg/kg, and chlorprothixene, 0.5 to 1 mg/kg, to a total of 100 mg/day (over the age of 6). For neuroleptics of high potency, daily doses are trifluoperazine, 1 to 15 mg (6 to 12 years of age) and 1 to 30 mg (over 12 years of age); fluphenazine, 0.05 to 0.10 mg/kg, up to 10 mg (over 5 years of age); and perphenazine, 0.05 to 0.10 mg/kg, up to 6 mg (over 1 year of age). Haloperidol and pimozide have been used in children, especially for Tourette's syndrome; haloperidol is recommended for use in a dosage of 2 to 16 mg per day in children over 12 years of age. Doses of modern atypical antipsychotic agents for children and adolescents with psychotic or manic illness usually are started at the lower end of the range prescribed for adults (Findling, 2002; King *et al.*, 2003; Sikich *et al.*, 2004; Stigler *et al.*, 2001).

Poor tolerance of the adverse effects of the antipsychotic drugs often limits the dose in elderly patients. One should proceed cautiously, using small, divided doses of agents with moderate or high potency, with the expectation that elderly patients will require doses that are one-half or less of those needed for young adults (Eastham and Jeste, 1997; Jeste *et al.*, 1999a, 1999b; Zubenko and Sunderland, 2000). As previously mentioned, the potential risk of stroke associated with risperidone and olanzapine in elderly patients should be considered (Wooltorton, 2002).

MISCELLANEOUS MEDICAL USES FOR ANTIPSYCHOTIC DRUGS

Antipsychotic drugs have a variety of uses in addition to the treatment of psychotic or manic patients. Predominant among these are the treatment of nausea and vomiting, alcoholic hallucinosis, certain neuropsychiatric diseases such as autism and others marked by movement disorders (notably Tourette's syndrome and Huntington's disease), and occasionally, pruritus and intractable hiccough.

Nausea and Vomiting. Many antipsychotic agents can prevent vomiting due to specific etiologies when given in relatively low, nonsedative doses. This use is discussed in Chapter 37.

Other Neuropsychiatric Disorders. Antipsychotic drugs are useful in the management of several syndromes with psychiatric features that also are characterized by movement disorders. These include *Gilles de la Tourette's syndrome* (marked by tics, other involuntary movements, aggressive outbursts, grunts, and vocalizations that frequently are obscene) and Huntington's disease (marked by severe and progressive choreoathetosis, psychiatric symptoms, and dementia, with a well-characterized genetic basis; *see* Chapter 20). Haloperidol currently is regarded as a drug of choice for these conditions, although it probably is not unique in its antidyskinetic actions. Pimozide also is used (typically in daily doses of 2 to 10 mg). Pimozide carries some risk of impairing cardiac repolarization, and it should be discontinued if the QTc interval exceeds 500 msec. Clonidine and tricyclic antidepressants such as nortriptyline also may be effective in Tourette's syndrome (Spencer *et al.*, 1993).

Withdrawal Syndromes. Antipsychotic drugs are *not* useful in the management of withdrawal from opioids, and their use in the management of withdrawal from barbiturates, other sedatives, or alcohol is contraindicated because of the high risk of seizures. They can be used safely and effectively in psychoses associated with chronic alcoholism—especially the syndrome known as *alcoholic hallucinosis* (Sadock and Sadock, 2000).

II. TREATMENT OF MANIA

ANTIMANIC MOOD-STABILIZING AGENTS: LITHIUM

Lithium carbonate was introduced into psychiatry in 1949 for the treatment of mania (Cade, 1949; Mitchell *et al.*, 1999). However, it was not FDA approved for this purpose in the United States until 1970, in part due to concerns of American physicians about its safety following reports of severe intoxication with lithium chloride from its uncontrolled use as a substitute for sodium chloride in patients with cardiac disease. Evidence for both the safety and the efficacy of lithium salts in the treatment of mania and the prevention of recurrent attacks of bipolar manic-depressive illness is both abundant and convincing (Baldessarini *et al.*, 2002; Davis *et al.*, 1999; Geddes *et al.*, 2004; Mitchell *et al.*, 1999). In recent years the limitations and adverse effects of lithium salts have become increasingly well appreciated, and efforts to find alternative antimanic or mood-stabilizing agents have intensified (Davis *et al.*, 1999; Goodwin and Jamison, 1990). The most successful alternatives or adjuncts to lithium to date are the anticonvulsants carbamazepine, *lamotrigine*, and valproic acid. Atypical antipsychotic agents also appear to be useful (Baldessarini *et al.*, 2003b; Goldsmith *et al.*, 2004; Post, 2000; Tohen *et al.*, 2003).

History. Lithium urate is very water soluble, and lithium salts were used in the nineteenth century as a treatment of gout. Lithium bromide was employed in that era as a sedative (including in manic patients) and as a putative anticonvulsant. Thereafter, lithium salts were unpopular until the late 1940s, when lithium chloride was employed as a salt substitute for cardiac and other chronically ill patients. This ill-advised use led to several reports of severe intoxication and death and to considerable notoriety concerning lithium salts within the medical profession. Cade, in Australia, while look-

ing for toxic nitrogenous substances in the urine of mental patients for testing in guinea pigs, administered lithium salts to the animals in an attempt to increase the solubility of urates. Lithium carbonate made the animals lethargic, and in an inductive leap, Cade gave lithium carbonate to several agitated or manic psychiatric patients, reporting that this treatment seemed to have a specific effect in mania (Cade, 1949; Mitchell *et al.*, 1999).

Chemistry. Lithium is the lightest of the alkali metals (group Ia); the salts of this monovalent cation share some characteristics with those of Na^+ and K^+. Li^+ is readily assayed in biological fluids and can be detected in brain tissue by magnetic resonance spectroscopy (Riedl *et al.*, 1997). Traces of the ion occur normally in animal tissues, but it has no known physiological role. Lithium carbonate and lithium citrate currently are used therapeutically in the United States.

Pharmacological Properties

Therapeutic concentrations of lithium ion (Li^+) have almost no discernible psychotropic effects in normal individuals. It is not a sedative, depressant, or euphoriant, and this characteristic differentiates Li^+ from other psychotropic agents. The general biology and pharmacology of Li^+ have been reviewed in detail (Jefferson *et al.*, 1983). The precise mechanism of action of Li^+ as a mood-stabilizing agent remains unknown, although many molecular and cellular actions of Li^+, as well as similarities of actions of other mood-stabilizing agents, including valproate, have been described (Manji *et al.*, 1999b, 2003; Manji and Zarate, 2002).

An important characteristic of Li^+ is that, unlike Na^+ and K^+, it has a relatively small gradient of distribution across biological membranes. Although it can replace Na^+ in supporting a single action potential in a nerve cell, it is not a "substrate" for the Na^+ pump and therefore cannot maintain membrane potentials. It is uncertain whether therapeutic concentrations of Li^+ (about 0.5 to 1 mEq per liter) affect the transport of other monovalent or divalent cations by nerve cells.

Central Nervous System. In addition to possibly altering cation distribution in the CNS, much attention has centered on the effects of therapeutic concentrations of Li^+ on the metabolism of the biogenic monoamines that have been implicated in the pathophysiology of mood disorders and on second-messenger and other intracellular molecular mechanisms involved in signal transduction, gene regulation, and cell survival (Jope, 1999; Lenox and Manji, 1998; Manji *et al.*, 1999a, 1999b, 2003; Manji and Zarate, 2002).

In animal brain tissue, Li^+ at concentrations of 1 to 10 mEq per liter inhibits the depolarization-provoked and Ca^{2+}-dependent release of norepinephrine and dopamine, but *not* serotonin, from nerve terminals (Baldessarini and Vogt, 1988). Li^+ may even transiently enhance release of serotonin, especially in the limbic system (Treiser *et al.*, 1981; Manji *et al.*, 1999a, 1999b; Wang and Friedman, 1989). The ion has limited effects on catecholamine-sensitive adenylyl cyclase activity or on the binding of ligands to monoamine receptors in brain tissue (Manji *et al.*, 1999b; Turkka *et al.*, 1992). However, Li$^+$ can modify some hormonal responses mediated by adenylyl cyclase or phospholipase C in other tissues, including the actions of vasopressin and thyroid-stimulating hormone on their peripheral target tissues (Manji *et al.*, 1999b; Urabe *et al.*, 1991). There is some evidence that Li$^+$ can inhibit the effects of receptor-blocking agents that cause supersensitivity in such systems (Bloom *et al.*, 1983). In part, the actions of Li$^+$ may reflect its ability to interfere with the activity of both stimulatory and inhibitory G proteins (G$_s$ and G$_i$) by keeping them in their less active $\alpha\beta\gamma$ trimeric state (Jope, 1999; Manji *et al.*, 1999b).

A consistently reported, selective action of Li$^+$ is to inhibit inositol monophosphatase (Berridge *et al.*, 1989) and thus interfere with the phosphatidylinositol pathway (Figure 18–1). This effect can lead to decreases in cerebral inositol concentrations, which can be detected with magnetic resonance spectroscopy in human brain tissue (Manji *et al.*, 1999a, 1999b). Physiological consequences of this effect may include interference with neurotransmission mechanisms by affecting the phosphatidylinositol pathway (Lenox and Manji, 1998; Manji *et al.*, 1999b).

Lithium treatment also leads to consistent decreases in the functioning of protein kinases in brain tissue, including PKC (Jope, 1999; Lenox and Manji, 1998), particularly subtypes α and β (Manji *et al.*, 1999b). Among other proposed antimanic or mood-stabilizing agents, this effect also is shared with valproic acid (particularly for PKC) but not carbamazepine (Manji *et al.*, 1993). In turn, these effects may alter the release of amine neurotransmitters and hormones (Wang and Friedman, 1989; Zatz and Reisine, 1985) as well as the activity of tyrosine hydroxylase (Chen *et al.*, 1998). A major substrate for cerebral PKC is the myristolated alanine-rich PKC-kinase substrate (MARCKS) protein, which has been implicated in synaptic and neuronal plasticity. The expression of MARCKS protein is reduced by treatment with both Li$^+$ and valproate, but not by carbamazepine or antipsychotic, antidepressant, or sedative drugs (Watson and Lenox, 1996; Watson *et al.*, 1998). Both Li$^+$ and valproate treatment inhibit glycogen synthase kinase-3β (GSK-3β), which is involved in neuronal and nuclear regulatory processes, including limiting expression of the regulatory protein β-catenin (Chen *et al.*, 1999b; Manji *et al.*, 1999b). Li$^+$ and valproic acid both interact with nuclear regulatory factors that affect gene expression. Such effects include increasing DNA binding of the transcription factor activator protein-1 (AP-1), as well as altered expression of other transcription factors, including AMI-1β or PEBP-2β (Chen *et al.*, 1999a, 1999c).

Treatment with Li$^+$ and valproate has been associated with increased expression of the regulatory protein B-cell lymphocyte protein-2 (bcl-2), which is associated with protection against neuronal degeneration (Chen *et al.*, 1999c; Manji *et al.*, 1999c). The significance of interactions of mood-stabilizing agents with cell-regulatory factors, and their potential utility in preventing cell loss or other pathological changes in brain tissue in various neuropsychiatric disorders remains to be clarified (Bauer *et al.*, 2003; Manji *et al.*, 2003; Manji and Zarate, 2002).

Absorption, Distribution, and Excretion.   Li$^+$ is absorbed readily and almost completely from the gastrointestinal tract. Complete absorption occurs in about 8 hours, with

peak plasma concentrations occurring 2 to 4 hours after an oral dose. Slow-release preparations of lithium carbonate provide a slower rate of absorption and thereby minimize early peaks in plasma concentrations of the ion, but absorption can be variable, lower gastrointestinal tract symptoms may be increased, and elimination rate is not altered with such preparations. Li$^+$ initially is distributed in the extracellular fluid, then gradually accumulates in various tissues; it does not bind appreciably to plasma proteins. The concentration gradient across plasma membranes is much smaller than those for Na$^+$ and K$^+$. The final volume of distribution (0.7 to 0.9 liter per kilogram) approaches that of total body water and is much lower than that of most other psychotropic agents, which are lipophilic and protein bound. Passage through the blood–brain barrier is slow, and when a steady state is achieved, the concentration of Li$^+$ in the cerebrospinal fluid and in brain tissue is about 40% to 50% of the concentration in plasma. The kinetics of Li$^+$ can be monitored in human brain with magnetic resonance spectroscopy (Plenge *et al.*, 1994; Riedl *et al.*, 1997).

Approximately 95% of a single dose of Li$^+$ is eliminated in the urine. From one- to two-thirds of an acute dose is excreted during a 6- to 12-hour initial phase of excretion, followed by slow excretion over the next 10 to 14 days. The elimination half-life averages 20 to 24 hours. With repeated administration, Li$^+$ excretion increases during the first 5 to 6 days until a steady state is reached between ingestion and excretion. When therapy with Li$^+$ is stopped, there is a rapid phase of renal excretion followed by a slow 10- to 14-day phase. Since 80% of the filtered Li$^+$ is reabsorbed by the proximal renal tubules, clearance of Li$^+$ by the kidney is about 20% of that for creatinine, ranging between 15 and 30 ml per minute. This rate is somewhat lower in elderly patients (10 to 15 ml per minute). Loading with Na$^+$ produces a small enhancement of Li$^+$ excretion, but Na$^+$ depletion promotes a clinically important degree of retention of Li$^+$.

Although the pharmacokinetics of Li$^+$ vary considerably among subjects, the volume of distribution and clearance are relatively stable in an individual patient. However, a well-established regimen can be complicated by occasional periods of Na$^+$ loss, as may occur with an intercurrent febrile, diarrheal, or other medical illness, with losses or restrictions of fluids and electrolytes, or during treatment with a diuretic. Heavy sweating may be an exception due to a preferential secretion of Li$^+$ over Na$^+$ in sweat (Jefferson *et al.*, 1982).

Most of the renal tubular reabsorption of Li$^+$ occurs in the proximal tubule. Nevertheless, Li$^+$ retention can be increased by any diuretic that leads to depletion of Na$^+$, particularly the thiazides (*see* Chapter 28) (Siegel *et al.*, 1998). Renal excretion can be increased by administration of osmotic diuretics, acetazolamide, or aminophylline, although they are of little help in the management of Li$^+$

intoxication. Triamterene may increase excretion of Li$^+$, suggesting that some reabsorption of the ion may occur in the distal nephron. However, spironolactone does not increase the excretion of Li$^+$. Some nonsteroidal antiinflammatory agents can facilitate renal proximal tubular resorption of Li$^+$ and thereby increase concentrations in plasma to toxic levels. This interaction appears to be particularly prominent with indomethacin, but also may occur with *ibuprofen*, *naproxen*, and cyclooxygenase-2 (COX-2) inhibitors, and possibly less so with *sulindac* and *aspirin* (Siegel *et al.*, 1998; Phelan *et al.*, 2003). A potential drug–drug interaction can occur with angiotensin-converting enzyme inhibitors, causing lithium retention (*see* Chapter 29).

Less than 1% of ingested Li$^+$ leaves the human body in the feces, and 4% to 5% is secreted in sweat. Li$^+$ is secreted in saliva in concentrations about twice those in plasma, while its concentration in tears is about equal to that in plasma. Since the ion also is secreted in human milk, women receiving Li$^+$ should not breast-feed infants.

Serum Level Monitoring and Dose. Because of the low therapeutic index for Li$^+$, periodic determination of serum concentrations is crucial. Li$^+$ cannot be used with adequate safety in patients who cannot be tested regularly. Concentrations considered to be effective and acceptably safe are between 0.6 and 1.25 mEq per liter. The range of 0.9 to 1.1 mEq per liter is favored for treatment of acutely manic or hypomanic patients. Somewhat lower values (0.6 to 0.75 mEq per liter) are considered adequate and are safer for long-term use for prevention of recurrent manic-depressive illness. Some patients may not relapse at concentrations as low as 0.5 to 0.6 mEq per liter, and lower levels usually are better tolerated (Maj *et al.*, 1986; Tondo *et al.*, 1998, 2001a). The recommended concentration usually is attained by doses of 900 to 1500 mg of lithium carbonate per day in outpatients and 1200 to 2400 mg per day in hospitalized manic patients. The optimal dose tends to be larger in younger and heavier individuals.

Serum concentrations of Li$^+$ have been found to follow a clear dose-effect relationship between 0.4 and 0.9 mEq per liter, with a corresponding dose-dependent rise in polyuria and tremor as indices of adverse effects, and little gain in benefit at levels above 0.75 mEq per liter (Maj *et al.*, 1986). This pattern indicates the need for individualization of serum levels to obtain a favorable risk-benefit relationship. The concentration of Li$^+$ in blood usually is measured at a trough of the daily oscillations that result from repetitive administration (*i.e.,* from samples obtained 10 to 12 hours after the last oral dose of the day). Peaks can be two or three times higher at a steady state. When the peaks are reached, intoxication may result, even when concentrations in morning samples of plasma at the daily nadir are in the acceptable range of 0.6 to 1 mEq per liter. Single daily doses, with relatively large oscillations of the plasma concentration of Li$^+$, may reduce the polyuria sometimes associated with this treatment, but the average

reduction is quite small (Baldessarini *et al.*, 1996b; Hetmar *et al.*, 1991). Nevertheless, because of the low margin of safety of Li$^+$ and because of its short half-life during initial distribution, divided daily doses are usually indicated even with slow-release formulations.

Toxic Reactions and Side Effects. The occurrence of toxicity is related to the serum concentration of Li$^+$ and its rate of rise following administration. Acute intoxication is characterized by vomiting, profuse diarrhea, coarse tremor, ataxia, coma, and convulsions. Symptoms of milder toxicity are most likely to occur at the absorptive peak of Li$^+$ and include nausea, vomiting, abdominal pain, diarrhea, sedation, and fine tremor. The more serious effects involve the nervous system and include mental confusion, hyperreflexia, gross tremor, dysarthria, seizures, and cranial nerve and focal neurological signs, progressing to coma and death. Sometimes both cognitive and motor neurological damage may be irreversible. Other toxic effects are cardiac arrhythmias, hypotension, and albuminuria. Other adverse effects common even in therapeutic dose ranges include nausea, diarrhea, daytime drowsiness, polyuria, polydipsia, weight gain, fine hand tremor, and dermatological reactions including acne (Baldessarini *et al.*, 1996b).

Therapy with Li$^+$ is associated initially with a transient increase in the excretion of 17-hydroxycorticosteroids, Na$^+$, K$^+$, and water. This effect usually is not sustained beyond 24 hours. In the subsequent 4 to 5 days, the excretion of K$^+$ becomes normal, Na$^+$ is retained, and in some cases dependent edema forms. Na$^+$ retention has been associated with increased aldosterone secretion and responds to administration of spironolactone. However, this maneuver incurs the risk of promoting the retention of Li$^+$ and increasing its concentration in plasma (*see* Chapter 28). Edema and Na$^+$ retention frequently disappear spontaneously after several days.

A small number of patients treated with Li$^+$ develop a benign, diffuse, nontender thyroid enlargement suggestive of compromised thyroid function. This effect may be associated with previous thyroiditis, particularly in middle-aged women. In patients treated with Li$^+$, thyroid uptake of iodine is increased, plasma protein–bound iodine and free thyroxine tend to be slightly low, and thyroid-stimulating hormone (TSH) secretion may be moderately elevated. These effects appear to result from interference with the iodination of tyrosine, and therefore the synthesis of thyroxine. However, patients usually remain euthyroid, and overt hypothyroidism is rare. In patients who do develop goiter, discontinuation of Li$^+$ or treatment with thyroid hormone results in shrinkage of the gland. Adding supplemental thyroid hormones to bipolar disorder patients with low-normal thyroid hormone levels and continued depression or anergy may be useful clinically, although this is an area of considerable controversy. Moreover, proposed use of high doses of thyroxine (T$_4$) to control rapid-cycling bipolar disorder is not established as a safe practice (Bauer and Whybrow, 1990; Baumgartner *et al.*, 1994; Lasser and Baldessarini, 1997).

The kidneys' ability to concentrate urine decreases during Li$^+$ therapy. Polydipsia and polyuria occur in patients treated with Li$^+$, occasionally to a disturbing degree. Acquired nephrogenic diabetes insipidus can occur in patients maintained at therapeutic plasma concentrations of the ion (*see* Chapter 29) (Siegel *et al.*, 1998). Typically, mild polyuria appears early in treatment and then disappears. Late-developing polyuria is an indication to evaluate renal function, lower the dose of Li$^+$, or consider adding a potassium-sparing agent such as amiloride (preferred to potassium-wasting thiazides) to counteract the polyuria (*see* Chapter 28) (Batlle *et al.*, 1985; Kosten and Forrest, 1986). Polyuria disappears with cessation of Li$^+$ therapy. The mechanism of polyuria may involve inhibition of the action of vasopressin on renal adenylyl cyclase as reflected in elevated circulating vasopressin and lack of responsiveness to exogenous vasopressin or synthetic analogs (Boton *et al.*, 1987; Siegel *et al.*, 1998). The result is decreased vasopressin stimulation of renal reabsorption of water. However, Li$^+$ also may alter renal function at steps beyond cyclic AMP synthesis. The effect of Li$^+$ on water metabolism is not sufficiently predictable to be therapeutically useful in treatment of the syndrome of inappropriate secretion of antidiuretic hormone. Evidence of chronic inflammatory changes in biopsied renal tissue has been found in a minority of patients given Li$^+$ for prolonged periods. Since progressive, clinically significant impairment of renal function is rare, these are considered incidental findings by most experts. Nevertheless, plasma creatinine and urine volume should be monitored during long-term use of Li$^+$ (Boton *et al.*, 1987; Hetmar *et al.*, 1991).

Li$^+$ also has a weak action on carbohydrate metabolism, causing an increase in skeletal muscle glycogen accompanied by depletion of glycogen from the liver.

The prolonged use of Li$^+$ causes a benign and reversible depression of the T wave of the ECG, an effect not related to depletion of Na$^+$ or K$^+$.

Li$^+$ routinely causes EEG changes characterized by diffuse slowing, widened frequency spectrum, and potentiation with disorganization of background rhythm. Seizures have been reported in nonepileptic patients with therapeutic plasma concentrations of Li$^+$. Myasthenia gravis may worsen during treatment with Li$^+$ (Neil *et al.*, 1976).

A benign, sustained increase in circulating polymorphonuclear leukocytes occurs during the chronic use of Li$^+$ and is reversed within a week after termination of treatment.

Allergic reactions such as dermatitis and vasculitis can occur with Li$^+$ administration. Worsening of acne vulgaris is a common problem, and some patients may experience mild alopecia.

In pregnancy, maternal polyuria may be exacerbated by lithium. Concomitant use of lithium with natriuretics and a low-Na$^+$ diet during pregnancy can contribute to maternal and neonatal Li$^+$ intoxication. During postpartum diuresis one can anticipate potentially toxic retention of Li$^+$ by the mother. Lithium freely crosses the placenta, and fetal or neonatal lithium toxicity may develop when maternal blood levels are within the therapeutic range. Lithium also is secreted in breast milk of nursing mothers. The use of Li$^+$ in pregnancy has been associated with neonatal goiter, CNS depression, hypotonia ("floppy baby" syndrome), and cardiac murmur. All of these conditions reverse with time, and no long-term neurobehavioral sequelae have been observed (Committee on Drugs. American Academy of Pediatrics, 2000; Iqbal *et al.*, 2001; Pinelli *et al.*, 2002).

The use of Li$^+$ in early pregnancy may be associated with an increase in the incidence of cardiovascular anomalies of the newborn, especially Ebstein's malformation (Cohen *et al.*, 1994). The basal risk of Ebstein's anomaly (malformed tricuspid valve, usually with a septal defect) of about 1 per 20,000 live births may rise severalfold, but probably not above 1 per 2500. Moreover, the defect typically is

detectable *in utero* by ultrasonography and often is surgically correctable after birth. In contrast, the antimanic anticonvulsants valproic acid and probably carbamazepine have an associated risk of irreversible spina bifida that may exceed 1 per 100, and so do not represent a rational alternative for pregnant women (Viguera *et al.*, 2000, 2002). In balancing the risk *vs.* benefit of using Li$^+$ in pregnancy, it is important to evaluate the risk of untreated manic-depressive disorder and to consider conservative measures, such as deferring intervention until symptoms arise or using a safer treatment, such as a neuroleptic or ECT (Cohen *et al.*, 1994; Viguera *et al.*, 2000, 2002).

Treatment of Lithium Intoxication. There is no specific antidote for Li$^+$ intoxication, and treatment is supportive. Vomiting induced by rapidly rising plasma Li$^+$ may tend to limit absorption, but fatalities have occurred. Care must be taken to assure that the patient is not Na$^+$- and water-depleted. Dialysis is the most effective means of removing the ion from the body and is necessary in severe poisonings, *i.e.,* in patients exhibiting symptoms of toxicity or patients with serum Li$^+$ concentrations greater than 4 mEq/L in acute overdoses or greater than 1.5 mEq/L in chronic overdoses.

Interactions with Other Drugs. Interactions between Li$^+$ and diuretics (especially spironolactone and amiloride) and nonsteroidal anti-inflammatory agents have been discussed above (*see* Absorption, Distribution, and Excretion and Toxic Reactions and Side Effects; Siegel *et al.*, 1998). Relative to thiazides and other diuretics that deplete Na$^+$, retention of Li$^+$ may be limited during administration of the weakly natriuretic agent amiloride as well as the loop diuretic furosemide. Amiloride and other diuretic agents (sometimes with reduced doses of Li$^+$) have been used safely to reverse the syndrome of diabetes insipidus occasionally associated with Li$^+$ therapy (Batlle *et al.*, 1985; Boton *et al.*, 1987) (*see* Chapter 29).

Li$^+$ often is used in conjunction with antipsychotic, sedative, antidepressant, and anticonvulsant drugs. A few case reports have suggested a risk of increased CNS toxicity when Li$^+$ was combined with haloperidol; however, this finding is at variance with many years of experience with this combination. Antipsychotic drugs may prevent nausea, which can be an early sign of Li$^+$ toxicity. There is, however, no absolute contraindication to the concurrent use of Li$^+$ and psychotropic drugs. Finally, anticholinergic and other agents that alter gastrointestinal motility also may alter Li$^+$ concentrations in blood over time.

Therapeutic Uses

Drug Treatment of Bipolar Disorder. Treatment with Li$^+$ ideally is conducted in cooperative patients with normal Na$^+$ intake and with normal cardiac and renal function. Occasionally, patients with severe systemic illnesses are treated with Li$^+$, provided that the indications are compelling. Treatment of acute mania and the prevention of recurrences of bipolar illness in otherwise healthy adults or adolescents currently are the only uses approved by the FDA, even though the primary indication for Li$^+$

treatment is for long-term prevention of recurrences of major affective illness, particularly both mania and depression in bipolar I or II disorders (Baldessarini *et al.*, 1996b, 2002; Goodwin and Jamison, 1990; Shulman *et al.*, 1996; Tondo *et al.*, 1998).

In addition, on the basis of compelling evidence of efficacy, Li⁺ sometimes is used as an alternative or adjunct to antidepressants in severe, especially melancholic, recurrent depression, as a supplement to antidepressant treatment in acute major depression, including in patients who present clinically with only mild mood elevations or hypomania (bipolar II disorder), or as an adjunct when later response to an antidepressant alone is unsatisfactory (Austin *et al.*, 1991; Bauer and Döpfmer, 1999). In major affective disorders, lithium is associated with stronger evidence of reduction of suicide risk than any other treatment (Baldessarini *et al.*, 2003a; Tondo *et al.*, 2001b).

The beneficial effects of Li⁺ in major depression may be associated with the presence of clinical or biological features also found in bipolar affective disorder (Goodwin and Jamison, 1990; Baldessarini *et al.*, 1996b). Growing clinical experience also suggests the utility of Li⁺ in the management of childhood disorders that are marked by adultlike manic depression or by severe changes in mood and behavior, which are probable precursors to bipolar disorder in adults (Baldessarini *et al.*, 1996b; Faedda *et al.*, 1995, 2004).

Li⁺ has been evaluated in many additional disorders marked by an episodic course, including premenstrual dysphoria, episodic alcohol abuse, and episodic violence (Baldessarini *et al.*, 1996b, 2002). Evidence of efficacy in most of these conditions has been unconvincing. The side effects of the Li⁺ ion have been exploited in the management of hyperthyroidism and the syndrome of inappropriate antidiuretic hormone secretion, as well as in the reversal of spontaneous or drug-induced leukopenias, but usually with limited benefit.

Formulations.   Most preparations currently used in the United States are tablets or capsules of lithium carbonate. Slow-release preparations of lithium carbonate also are available, as is a liquid preparation of lithium citrate (with 8 mEq of Li⁺, equivalent to 300 mg of carbonate salt, per 5 ml or 1 teaspoonful of citrate liquid). Salts other than the carbonate have been used, but the carbonate salt is favored for tablets and capsules because it is relatively less hygroscopic and less irritating to the gut than other salts, especially the chloride.

Drug Treatment of Mania and Prophylactic Treatment of Bipolar Disorder.   The modern treatment of the manic, depressive, and mixed-mood phases of bipolar disorder was revolutionized by the introduction of lithium in 1949, its gradual acceptance worldwide by the 1960s, and late official acceptance in the United States in 1970, initially for acute mania only, and later primarily for prevention of recurrences of mania. Lithium is effective in acute mania, but is rarely employed as a sole treatment due to its slow onset of action, need for monitoring blood Li⁺ concentrations, and the difficulties associated with adherence to the therapeutic regimen by highly agitated and uncooperative manic patients. Rather, an antipsychotic or potent sedative benzodiazepine (such as *lorazepam* or *clonazepam*) commonly is used to attain a degree of control of acute agitation (Licht, 1998; Tohen and Zarate, 1998). Alternatively, the anticonvulsant sodium valproate can provide rapid antimanic effects (Pope *et al.*, 1991; Bowden *et al.*, 1994), particularly when doses as high as 30 mg/kg and later 20 mg/kg daily are used to rapidly obtain serum concentrations of 90 to 120 μg/ml (Grunze *et al.*, 1999; Hirschfeld *et al.*, 1999). Once patients are stabilized and cooperative, Li⁺ then can be introduced for longer-term mood stabilization, or the anticonvulsant may be continued alone (*see* below).

Li⁺ or an alternative antimanic agent usually is continued for at least several months after full recovery from a manic episode, due to a high risk of relapse or of cycling into depression within 12 months (Goodwin and Jamison, 1990). The clinical decision to recommend more prolonged maintenance treatment is based on balancing the frequency and severity of past episodes of manic-depressive illness, the age and estimated reliability of the patient, and the risk of adverse effects (Baldessarini *et al.*, 1996b; Zarin and Pass, 1987). Regardless of the number of previous episodes of mania or depression, or delay in initiating maintenance treatment, Li⁺ remains by far the best established long-term treatment to prevent recurrences of mania (and bipolar depression) (Baethge *et al.*, 2003; Baldessarini *et al.*, 2002; Bratti *et al.*, 2003; Davis *et al.*, 1999; Geddes *et al.*, 2004; Goodwin and Jamison, 1990). There is compelling evidence of substantial lowering of risk of suicide and suicide attempts during treatment with lithium but not with either carbamazepine or *divalproex* (Baldessarini *et al.*, 2003a; Goodwin *et al.*, 2003; Thies-Flechtner *et al.*, 1996; Tondo *et al.*, 2001).

Owing to the limited tolerability of Li⁺ and its imperfect protection from recurrences of bipolar illness, antimanic anticonvulsants, particularly sodium valproate and carbamazepine, also have been employed prophylactically in bipolar disorder. However, research supporting their long-term use remains limited (Calabrese *et al.*, 1992, 2002; Davis *et al.*, 1999; Bowden *et al.*, 2000; Davis *et al.*, 2000). There is growing evidence for the inferiority of carbamazepine compared to lithium (Dardennes *et al.*,

1995; Davis *et al.*, 1999; Denicoff *et al.*, 1997; Greil *et al.*, 1997; Post *et al.*, 1998; Post, 2000) and carbamazepine is not FDA approved for bipolar disorder. Divalproex, the sodium salt of valproic acid, is FDA approved for mania and is extensively used off-label for long-term prophylactic treatment of bipolar disorder patients. In addition, lamotrigine is the first agent given FDA approval for long-term prophylactic treatment in bipolar disorder without an indication for acute mania; it is particularly effective against bipolar depression with minimal risk of inducing mania (Bowden *et al.*, 2004; Calabrese *et al.*, 2002; Goldsmith *et al.*, 2004). Other anticonvulsants that may have utility in bipolar disorder (*topiramate, zonisamide,* and the carbamazepine congener *oxcarbazepine*) remain under investigation (Centorrino *et al.*, 2003; Evins, 2003).

Relevant pharmacology and dosing guidelines for the anticonvulsants are provided in Chapter 19. Doses established for their anticonvulsant effects are assumed to be appropriate for the treatment of manic-depressive patients, although formal dose–response studies in psychiatric patients are lacking. Thus, dosing usually is adjusted to provide plasma concentrations of 6 to 12 μg/ml for carbamazepine and 60 to 120 μg/ml for valproic acid. It also is common to combine Li^+ with an anticonvulsant, particularly valproate, when patients fail to be fully protected from recurrences of bipolar illness by monotherapy (Freeman and Stoll, 1998).

Antipsychotic drugs commonly have been employed empirically to manage manic and psychotic illness in bipolar disorder patients. Indeed, standard neuroleptics have been a mainstay of the treatment of acute mania (only chlorpromazine is FDA approved for this indication, although haloperidol has also been widely used) and for manic episodes that break through prophylactic treatment with Li^+ or an anticonvulsant (Segal *et al.*, 1998; Sernyak *et al.*, 1994; Tohen and Zarate, 1998). However, the older antipsychotics are not used routinely for long-term prophylactic treatment in bipolar disorder because their effectiveness is untested, some may worsen depression, and the risk of tardive dyskinesia in these syndromes may be higher than in schizophrenia (Kane, 1999).

Several modern, better-tolerated antipsychotic agents have recently received FDA approval for use in acute mania (olanzapine, quetiapine, and risperidone) (Baldessarini *et al.*, 2003b; Keck and Licht, 2001; Tohen *et al.*, 1999, 2003; Vieta *et al.*, 2004). There is also evidence of antimanic efficacy of others (aripiprazole, ziprasidone) (Keck *et al.*, 2003; Yatham, 2003). There also is evidence of long-term effectiveness of olanzapine in bipolar I disorder (Tohen *et al.*, 2003), for which olanzapine has

received an FDA approved indication. Other atypical antipsychotic drugs are under investigation for long-term prophylactic treatment of bipolar disorder. The risks and benefits of the atypical antipsychotic agents aripiprazole and ziprasidone for treatment of bipolar disorder require further study. Ziprasidone can have stimulating or apparent mood-elevating actions with an uncertain risk of inducing mania (Baldassano *et al.*, 2003).

Other alternatives to Li^+ (*e.g.*, calcium channel blockers, long-chain unsaturated fatty acids) have been less well evaluated and are not established options for bipolar disorder (Dubovsky, 1998; Pazzaglia *et al.*, 1998; Stoll *et al.*, 1999).

Discontinuation of maintenance treatment with Li^+ carries a high risk of early recurrence and of suicidal behavior over a period of several months, even if the treatment had been successful for several years. Recurrence is much more rapid than is predicted by the natural history of untreated bipolar disorder, in which cycle lengths average about 1 year (Baldessarini *et al.*, 1996b, 1999; Tondo *et al.*, 1998). This risk probably can be moderated by slowing the gradual removal of Li^+ when that is medically feasible (Faedda *et al.*, 1993; Baldessarini *et al.*, 1999). Significant risk also is suspected after rapid discontinuation or even sharp dosage reduction during maintenance treatment with other agents, including antipsychotic, antidepressant, and antianxiety drugs (Baldessarini *et al.*, 1996a, 1999). This phenomenon hinders clinical researchers from employing and interpreting results from common study designs in which an ongoing maintenance treatment is interrupted to compare continued treatment to a placebo, to an alternative treatment, or to compare higher *vs.* lower doses (Baldessarini *et al.*, 1996a). As a result, direct comparisons between different maintenance options are limited.

Novel Treatments for Psychotic Disorders

Acceptance of clozapine for general use, and growing evidence that no alternative has proved superior in antipsychotic efficacy to clozapine, have stimulated interest in discovering other antipsychotic agents with a low risk of extrapyramidal neurological side effects and high efficacy, and without the need to monitor for the hematologic toxicity of clozapine (Baldessarini and Frankenburg, 1991). Not surprisingly, a substantial number of potential new antipsychotic agents with effects on dopaminergic systems are in development (NDA Pipeline, 2004). They include additional mixed *dopamine D_2/serotonin 5-HT$_{2A}$ antagonists* (*e.g., AD-5423, asenapine, blonanserin, clothiapine, DHA-clozapine, GSK-773812, iloperidone, mazapertine, terguride*). Others are D_2 *partial agonists* like aripiprazole (*e.g., bifeprunox*, CI-1007, DAB-452, *roxindole*). A few combine D_2 antagonist activity with *muscarinic agonist* or *antagonist* activity (*e.g.*, BuTAC, AC-42, AC-90222). Several are D_3-*receptor antagonists* (*e.g.*, AVE-5997, DTA-201, S-33138) whose behavioral effects remain to be determined. Several D_4 antagonists also have been brought to clinical trial, but have proved ineffective for the treatment of typical symptoms of schizophrenia.

Treatments that involve even more novel principles of antipsychotic action have remained elusive, but some have been proposed. Several involve targets other than the dopamine receptors that have dominated antipsychotic drug development for a half-century. Compounds that enhance glutamatergic neurotransmission have provided some interesting leads. Some act by stimulating the *glycine modulatory site* of the NMDA receptor (*e.g.*, L-glycine, serine, D-cycloserine, S-18841). Others are *ampakines* that stimulate AMPA receptors (CX-516, ORG-23430, ORG-24448). Both types of glutamate enhancers may augment the beneficial therapeutic effects of atypical antipsychotic agents, particularly by improving cognition, but may not be effective or well tolerated when given alone (Goff *et al.*, 1999, 2001). In addition, preclinical studies suggest that novel compounds targeting selective G protein-coupled *metabotropic glutamate receptors,* GluR2/3 (LY354740, LY379268), mGluR3 (*N*-acetylaspartyl-glutamate [NAAG]), or mGlu5 (2-methyl-6-[phenylethy-nyl]-pyridine [MPEP]) may improve cognitive deficits in schizophrenia (Moghaddam, 2004). Finally, the active metabolite *norclozapine* appears to potentiate NMDA glutamatergic and M_1 cholinergic receptor activity (Sur *et al.*, 2003).

The development of antipsychotic agents that effect serotonergic neurotransmission, and recent advances in characterizing 5-HT receptor types have encouraged development of drugs selective for various serotonin receptors (*see* Chapter 11). Such potential novel antipsychotic agents include 5-HT_{2A}-receptor inverse agonists (AC-90179, ACP-103, AR-116081), 5-HT_6-receptor antagonists (SB-271046, SB-742457), and 5-HT_7-receptor antagonists (SB-269970). The clinical utility of such agents remains to be proved.

Additional novel products that target different molecular elements and cellular pathways and are aimed at improving particular symptoms of schizophrenia also are under development. They include α_4-β_2 nicotinic receptor agonists (*e.g.*, S1B-1553A), a cannabinoid CB_1 antagonist (SR141716), neurokinin-3 antagonists (SB-223412, SR-142801), neurotensin modulators (AC-7954, NT-69L, SR-48692), a somatostatin stimulator (FK-960), a urotensin-2 agonist (AC-7954), adenosine receptor agonist/modula-tors (allopurinol, dipyridamole), a PLA_2 inhibitor (SC-111), a PDE5 inhibitor (T-0156), a PDE10A inhibitor (*papaverine*), sigma-1 site modulators (E-5842, NE-100), COX-2 inhibitors (celecoxib, GSK-644784), and neuros-teroids [*dehydroepiandrosterone* (DHEA) and its sulfate derivative (DHEA-S)] (Miyamoto *et al.*, 2004; NDA Pipeline, 2004).

Novel Treatments for Bipolar Disorder

The clinical successes of valproate and carbamazepine as antimanic agents, and of lamotrigine as a mood-stabilizing agent, have strongly encouraged exploration of the growing number of other anticonvulsants being introduced into neurological practice (*see* Chapter 19). Several anticonvulsants are currently being tested in clinical trials (Ferrier and Calabrese, 2000; Keck and McElroy, 1998; Manji *et al.*, 2000; Post *et al.*, 1998; Post, 2000). Aside from extensions of the known principles of applying anticonvulsants and antipsychotics for the treatment of bipolar disorder, some highly innovative concepts have emerged. Given the overlapping actions of lithium and valproate, it may be possible to develop novel antimanic agents that act directly on effector mechanisms that mediate the actions of adrenergic and other neurotransmitter receptors (Manji *et al.*, 1999b). Under experimental development are drugs that affect PKC, such as the antiestrogen *tamoxifen* (Beb-chuk *et al.*, 2000) and other novel kinase-inhibiting agents. For bipolar disorder, a critical challenge is to develop safe and effective antidepressants that do not induce mania and mood-stabilizing agents that consistently outperform lithium in broad effectiveness, with improved safety (*see* Baldessarini *et al.*, 1996b, 2002; Stoll *et al.*, 1994).

CLINICAL SUMMARY

Clinically effective antipsychotic agents include tricyclic phenothiazines, thioxanthenes, and benzepines, as well as butyrophenones and congeners, other heterocyclics, and experimental benzamides. Virtually all of these drugs block D_2-dopamine receptors and reduce dopaminergic neurotransmission in the forebrain; some also interact with D_1, D_3, D_4, 5-HT_{2A}, 5-HT_{2C}, α, and H_1 receptors. Antipsychotic drugs are relatively lipophilic and are metabolized mainly by hepatic oxidative enzymes; some have complex elimination kinetics. These drugs offer effective symptomatic treatment of both organic and idiopathic psychotic disorders with acceptable safety and practicality. Highly potent antipsychotic agents tend to have more adverse extrapyramidal neurological effects; less potent agents have more sedative, hypotensive, and autonomic adverse effects. For older typical or "neuroleptic" antipsychotic agents, characteristic neurological adverse effects include dystonia, akathisia, bradykinesia, tremor, and acute as well as late dyskinesias. Other antipsychotic agents (e.g., aripiprazole, clozapine, quetiapine, ziprasidone, low doses of olanzapine and risperidone) have limited extrapyramidal effects and therefore are considered "atypical." Treatment of acute psychotic illness typically involves daily doses up to the equivalent of 10 to 20 mg of fluphenazine or haloperidol (at serum concentrations of about 5 to 20 ng/ml), 300 to 600 mg of chlorpromazine, 200 to 500 mg of clozapine, 10 to 20 mg of olanzapine, 4 to 6 mg of risperidone, or the equivalent dose of another modern agent. Higher doses usually are not more effective but they increase risks of adverse effects. Long-term maintenance treatment usually requires relatively low doses, and late loss of efficacy (tolerance) is virtually unknown.

The treatment of mania and recurrences of mania and depression in bipolar disorder have long relied on the use of lithium. Lithium has a low therapeutic index and its safe use requires close control of serum concentrations. Antipsychotic agents commonly are used to control acute mania, with or without psychotic features; some agents (e.g., olanzapine) appear to have long-term mood-stabilizing effects. Potent sedative-anticonvulsant benzodiazepines, notably clonazepam and lorazepam (see Chapter 16) are used adjunctively for rapid sedation in acute mania. Additional alternative or adjunctive treatments for mania include the anticonvulsants sodium divalproex and carbamazepine. Lamotrigine has long-term protective effects in bipolar disorder, particularly for depression. Other anticonvulsants with preliminary support for efficacy in bipolar disorder include *levetiracetam*, oxcarbazepine, *topiramate*, and *zonisamide* (see Chapter 19).

BIBLIOGRAPHY

Adams, C.E., Fenton, M.K., Quraishi, S., and David, A.S. Systematic meta-review of depot antipsychotic drugs for people with schizophrenia. *Br. J. Psychiatry*, **2001**, *179:*290–299.

Addonizio, G., Susman, V.L., and Roth, S.D. Neuroleptic malignant syndrome: review and analysis of 115 cases. *Biol. Psychiatry*, **1987**, *22:*1004–1020.

Adler, L.A., Rotrosen, J., Edson, R., *et al.* Vitamin E treatment for tardive dyskinesia. *Arch. Gen. Psychiatry*, **1999**, *56:*836–841.

Allison, D.B., Mentore, J.L., Heo, M., *et al.* Antipsychotic-induced weight gain: a comprehensive research synthesis. *Am. J. Psychiatry*, **1999**, *156:*1686–1696.

Altamura, A.C., Sassella, F., Santini, A., *et al.* Intramuscular preparations of antipsychotics: uses and relevance in clinical practice. *Drugs*, **2003**, *63:*493–512.

Alvir, J.M., Lieberman, J.A., Safferman, A.Z., Schwimmer, J.L., and Schaaf, J.A. Clozapine-induced agranulocytosis. Incidence and risk factors in the United States. *N. Engl. J. Med.*, **1993**, *329:*162–167.

Arana, G.W., Goff, D.C., Baldessarini, R.J., and Keepers, G.A. Efficacy for anticholinergic prophylaxis of neuroleptic-induced acute dystonia. *Am. J. Psychiatry*, **1988**, *145:*993–996.

Arango, C., Buchanan, R.W., Kirkpatrick, B., and Carpenter, W.T. The deficit syndrome in schizophrenia: implications for the treatment of negative symptoms. *Eur. Psychiatry*, **2004**, *19:*21–26.

Argo, T.R., Carnahan, R.M., and Perry, P.J. Aripiprazole, a novel atypical antipsychotic drug. *Pharmacotherapy*, **2004**, *24:*212–228.

Arnt, J., and Skarsfeldt, T. Do novel antipsychotics have similar pharmacological characteristics? A review of the evidence. *Neuropsychopharmacology*, **1998**, *18:*63–101.

Arvanitis, L.A., and Miller, B.G. Multiple fixed doses of "Seroquel" (quetiapine) in patients with acute exacerbation of schizophrenia: a comparison with haloperidol and placebo. The Seroquel Trial 13 Study Group. *Biol. Psychiatry*, **1997**, *42:*233–246.

Austin, M.P., Souza, F.G., and Goodwin, G.M. Lithium augmentation in antidepressant-resistant patients. A quantitative analysis. *Br. J. Psychiatry*, **1991**, *159:*510–514.

Baethge, C., Baldessarini, R.J., Bratti, I.M., and Tondo, L. Effect of treatment-latency on outcome in bipolar disorder. *Can. J. Psychiatry*, **2003**, *48:*449–457.

Baldassano, C.F., Ballas, C., Datto, S.M., *et al.* Ziprasidone-associated mania: case series and review of the mechanism. *Bipolar Disord.*, **2003**, *5:*72–75.

Baldessarini, R.J., Campbell A., Ben-Jonathan N., *et al.* Effects of aporphine isomers on rat prolactin. *Neurosci. Lett.*, **1994**, *176:*269–271.

Baldessarini, R.J., Cohen, B.M., and Teicher, M.H. Significance of neuroleptic dose and plasma level in the pharmacological treatment of psychoses. *Arch. Gen. Psychiatry*, **1988**, *45:*79–91.

Baldessarini, R.J., Hennen, J., Wilson, M., *et al.* Olanzapine vs. placebo in acute mania: Treatment responses in subgroups. *J. Clin. Psychopharmacol.*, **2003b**, *23:*370–376.

Baldessarini, R.J., Huston-Lyons, D., Campbell, A., *et al.* Do central antiadrenergic actions contribute to the atypical properties of clozapine? *Br. J. Psychiatry Suppl.*, **1992**, *17:*12–16.

Baldessarini, R.J., Kula, N.S., McGrath, C.R., *et al.* Isomeric selectivity at dopamine D_3 receptors. *Eur. J. Pharmacol.*, **1993**, *239:*269–270.

Baldessarini, R.J., Suppes, T., and Tondo, L. Lithium withdrawal in bipolar disorder: implications for clinical practice and experimental therapeutics research. *Am. J. Therapeutics*, **1996a**, *3:*492–496.

Baldessarini, R.J., Tarazi, F.I., Kula, N.S., and Gardner, D.M. Clozapine withdrawal: serotonergic or dopaminergic mechanisms? *Arch. Gen. Psychiatry*, **1997**, *45:*761–762.

Baldessarini, R.J., Tondo, L., and Hennen, J. Treatment-latency and previous episodes: relationships to pretreatment morbidity and response to maintenance treatment in bipolar I and II disorders. *Bipolar Disord.*, **2003c**, *5:*169–179.

Baldessarini, R.J., Tondo, L., Hennen, J., and Viguera, A.C. Is lithium still worth using? An update of selected recent research. *Harv. Rev. Psychiatry*, **2002**, *10:*59–75.

Baldessarini RJ, Tondo L, Hennen J: Lithium treatment and suicide risk in major affective disorders: Update and new findings. *J. Clin. Psychiatry*, **2003a**, *64*(suppl 5):44–52.

Baldessarini, R.J., Tondo, L., and Viguera, A.C. Effects of discontinuing lithium maintenance treatment. *Bipolar Disord.*, **1999**, *1:*17–24.

Baldessarini, R.J., and Vogt, M. Release of [³H]dopamine and analogous monoamines from rat striatal tissue. *Cell. Mol. Neurobiol.*, **1988**, *8:*205–216.

Batlle, D.C., von Riotte, A.B., Gaviria, M., and Grupp, M. Amelioration of polyuria by amiloride in patients receiving long-term lithium therapy. *N. Engl. J. Med.*, **1985**, *312:*408–414.

Bauer, M., Alda, M., Priller, J., and Young, L.T. Implications of the neuroprotective effects of lithium for the treatment of bipolar and neurodegenerative disorders. *Pharmacopsychiatry,* **2003**, *36*(suppl 3):S250–S254.

Bauer, M., and Döpfmer, S. Lithium augmentation in treatment-resistant depression: meta-analysis of placebo-controlled studies. *J. Clin. Psychopharmacol.*, **1999**, *19:*427–434.

Bauer, M.E., and Whybrow, P.C. Rapid cycling bipolar affective disorder II. Treatment of refractory rapid cycling with high-dose levothyroxine: a preliminary study. *Arch. Gen. Psychiatry,* **1990**, *47:*435–440.

Baumgartner, A., Bauer, M., and Hellweg, R. Treatment of intractable non–rapid cycling bipolar affective disorder with high-dose thyroxine: an open clinical trial. *Neuropsychopharmacology,* **1994**, *10:*183–189.

Bebchuk, J.M., Arfken, C.L., Dolan-Manji, S., et al. A preliminary investigation of a protein kinase C inhibitor in the treatment of acute mania. *Arch. Gen. Psychiatry,* **2000**, *57:*95–97.

Beedham, C., Miceli, J.J., and Obach, R.S. Ziprasidone metabolism, aldehyde oxidase, and clinical implications. *J. Clin. Psychopharmacol.*, **2003**, *23:*229–232.

Bench, C.J., Lammertsma, A.A., Grasby, P.M., et al. The time course of binding to striatal dopamine D₂ receptors by the neuroleptic ziprasidone (CP-88,059-01) determined by positron emission tomography. *Psychopharmacology (Berl.)*, **1996**, *124:*141–147.

Berridge, M.J., Downes, C.P., and Hanley, M.R. Neural and developmental actions of lithium: a unifying hypothesis. *Cell,* **1989**, *59:*411–419.

Bhanji, N.H., Chouinard, G., and Margolese, H.C. Review of compliance, depot intramuscular antipsychotics and the new long-acting injectable atypical antipsychotic risperidone in schizophrenia. *Eur. Neuropsychopharmacol.*, **2004**, *14:*87–92.

Bitton, R., and Schneider, B. Endocrine, metabolic, and nutritional effects of psychotropic drugs. In, *Adverse Effects of Psychotropic Drugs.* (Kane, J.M., and Leiberman, J.A., eds.) Guilford Press, New York, **1992**, pp. 341–355.

Blin, O. A comparative review of new antipsychotics. *Can. J. Psychiatry,* **1999**, *44:*235–244.

Bloom, F.E., Baetge, G., Deyo, S., et al. Chemical and physiological aspects of the actions of lithium and antidepressant drugs. *Neuropharmacology,* **1983**, *22*(3 Spec. No.):359–365.

Boton, R., Gaviria, M., and Batlle, D.C. Prevalence, pathogenesis, and treatment of renal dysfunction associated with chronic lithium therapy. *Am. J. Kidney Dis.*, **1987**, *10:*329–345.

Bowden, C.L., Asnis, G.M., Ginsberg, L.D., et al. Safety and tolerability of lamotrigine for bipolar disorder. *Drug Saf.*, **2004**, *27:*173–184.

Bowden, C.L., Brugger, A.M., Swann, A.C., et al. Efficacy of divalproex vs. lithium and placebo in the treatment of mania. The Depakote Mania Study Group. *J.A.M.A.*, **1994**, *271:*918–924.

Bowden, C.L., Calabrese, J.R., McElroy, S.L., et al. A randomized, placebo-controlled 12-month trial of divalproex and lithium in the treatment of outpatients with bipolar I disorder. Divalproex Bipolar Study Group. *Arch. Gen. Psychiatry,* **2000**, *57:*481–489.

Bradwejn, J., Shriqui, C., Koszycki, D., and Meterissian, G. Double-blind comparison of the effects of clonazepam and lorazepam in acute mania. *J. Clin. Psychopharmacol.*, **1990**, *10:*403–408.

Bratti, I.M., Baldessarini, R.J., Baethge, C., and Tondo, L. Pretreatment episode count and response to lithium treatment in manic-depressive illness. *Harvard Rev. Psychiatry,* **2003**, *11:*245–256.

Brotman, A.W., Falk, W.E., and Gelenberg, A.J. Pharmacologic treatment of acute depressive subtypes. In, *Psychopharmacology: The Third Generation of Progress.* (Meltzer, H.Y., ed.) Raven Press, New York, **1987**, pp. 1031–1040.

Bunney, B.S., Sesack, S.R., and Silva, N.L. Midbrain dopaminergic systems: neurophysiology and electrophysiological pharmacology. In, *Psychopharmacology: The Third Generation of Progress.* (Meltzer, H.Y., ed.) Raven Press, New York, **1987**, pp. 113–126.

Cade, J.F.J. Lithium salts in the treatment of psychotic excitement. *Med. J. Austral.,* **1949**, *2:*349–352.

Calabrese, J.R., Markovitz, P.J., Kimmel, S.E., and Wagner, S.C. Spectrum of efficacy of valproate in 78 rapid-cycling bipolar patients. *J. Clin. Psychopharmacol.*, **1992**, *12:*53S–56S.

Calabrese, J.R., Shelton, M.D., Rapport, D.J., Kimmel, S.E., and Elhaj, O. Long-term treatment of bipolar disorder with lamotrigine. *J. Clin. Psychiatry,* **2002**, *63*(suppl 10):18–22.

Campbell, A., Baldessarini, R.J., Cremens, C., et al. Bromocriptine antagonizes behavioral effects of cocaine in the rat. *Neuropsychopharmacology,* **1989**, *2:*209–224.

Campbell, A., Yeghiayan, S., Baldessarini, R.J., and Neumeyer, J.L. Selective antidopaminergic effects of S(+)N-*n*-propylnoraporphines in limbic versus extrapyramidal sites in rat brain: comparisons with typical and atypical antipsychotic agents. *Psychopharmacology,* **1991**, *103:*323–329.

Casey, D.E., Daniel, D.G., Wassef, A.A., et al. Effect of divalproex combined with olanzapine or risperidone in patients with an acute exacerbation of schizophrenia. *Neuropsychopharmacology,* **2003**, *28:*182–192.

Casey, D.E. Side effect profiles of new antipsychotic agents. *J. Clin. Psychiatry,* **1996**, *57*(suppl 11):40–45.

Castagnoli, N. Jr., Castagnoli, K.P., Van der Schyf, C.J., et al. Enzyme-catalyzed bioactivation of cyclic tertiary amines to form potential neurotoxins. *Pol. J. Pharmacol.*, **1999**, *51:*31–38.

Centorrino, F., Albert, M.J., Berry, J.M., et al. Oxcarbazepine: clinical experience with hospitalized psychiatric patients. *Bipolar Disord.*, **2003**, *5:*370–374.

Centorrino, F., Price, B.H., Tuttle, M., et al. Electroencephalographic abnormalities during treatment with typical and atypical antipsychotics. *Am. J. Psychiatry,* **2002**, *159:*109–115.

Chan, C.H., Janicak, P.G., Davis, J.M., et al. Response of psychotic and nonpsychotic depressed patients to tricyclic antidepressants. *J. Clin. Psychiatry,* **1987**, *48:*197–200.

Chen, G., Huang, L.D., Jiang, Y.M., and Manji, H.K. The mood-stabilizing agent valproate inhibits the activity of glycogen synthase kinase-3. *J. Neurochem.*, **1999b**, *72:*1327–1330.

Chen, G., Yuan, P.X., Jiang, Y.M., et al. Lithium increases tyrosine hydroxylase levels both *in vivo* and *in vitro. J. Neurochem.*, **1998**, *70:*1768–1771.

Chen, G., Yuan, P.X., Jiang, Y.M., et al. Valproate robustly enhances AP-1 mediated gene expression. *Brain Res. Mol. Brain Res.*, **1999a**, *64:*52–58.

Chen, G., Zeng, W.Z., Yuan, P.X., et al. The mood-stabilizing agents lithium and valproate robustly increase the levels of the neuroprotective protein bcl-2 in the CNS. *J. Neurochem.*, **1999c**, *72:*879–882.

Chouinard, G., Jones, B., Remington, G., et al. A Canadian multicenter placebo-controlled study of fixed doses of risperidone and haloperidol in the treatment of chronic schizophrenic patients. *J. Clin. Psychopharmacol.*, **1993**, *13:*25–40.

Cohen, D. Atypical antipsychotics and new onset diabetes mellitus. An overview of the literature. *Pharmacopsychiatry*, **2004**, *37:*1–11.

Cohen, L.S., Friedman, J.M., Jefferson, J.W., *et al.* A reevaluation of risk of *in utero* exposure to lithium. *J.A.M.A.*, **1994**, *271:*146–150.

Cohen, B.M., Tsuneizumi, T., Baldessarini, R.J., *et al.* Differences between antipsychotic drugs in persistence of brain levels and behavioral effects. *Psychopharmacology (Berl.)*, **1992**, *108:*338–344.

Committee on Drugs. American Academy of Pediatrics. Use of psychoactive medication during pregnancy and possible side effects on the fetus and newborn. *Pediatrics*, **2000**, *105:*880.

Compton, M.T., and Miller, A.H. Antipsychotic-induced hyperprolactinemia and sexual dysfunction. *Psychopharmacol. Bull.*, **2002**, *36:*143–164.

Correll, C.U., Leucht, S., and Kane, J.M. Lower risk for tardive dyskinesia associated with second-generation antipsychotics: systematic review of 1-year studies. *Am. J. Psychiatry*, **2004**, *161:*414–425.

Corrigan, M.H., Gallen, C.C., Bonura, M.L., and Merchant, K.M., for the Sonepiprazole Study Group. Effectiveness of the selective D4 antagonist sonepiprazole in schizophrenia: A placebo-controlled study. *Biol. Psychiatry*, **2004**, *55:*445–451.

Csernansky, J.G., Mahmoud, R., and Brenner, R. Comparison of risperidone and haloperidol for the prevention of relapse in patients with schizophrenia. *N. Engl. J. Med.*, **2002**, *346:*16–22.

Daly, S.A., and Waddington, J.L. Two directions of dopamine D1/D2 receptor interaction in studies of behavioural regulation: a finding generic to four new, selective dopamine D1 receptor antagonists. *Eur. J. Pharmacol.*, **1992**, *213:*251–258.

Daniel, D.G. Tolerability of ziprasidone: an expanding perspective. *J. Clin. Psychiatry*, **2003**, *64*(suppl 19):40–49.

Dardennes, R., Even, C., Bange, F., and Heim, A. Comparison of carbamazepine and lithium in the prophylaxis of bipolar disorders. A meta-analysis. *Br. J. Psychiatry*, **1995**, *166:*378–381.

Davis, J.M., Chen, N., and Glick, I.D. A meta-analysis of the efficacy of second-generation antipsychotics. *Arch. Gen. Psychiatry*, **2003**, *60:*553–564.

Davis, J.M., Janicak, P.G., and Hogan, D.M. Mood stabilizers in the prevention of recurrent affective disorders: a meta-analysis. *Acta. Psychiatr. Scand.*, **1999**, *100:*406–417.

Denicoff, K.D., Smith-Jackson, E.E., Bryan, A.L., *et al.* Valproate prophylaxis in a prospective clinical trial of refractory bipolar disorder. *Am. J. Psychiatry*, **1997**, *154:*1456–1458.

Denicoff, K.D., Smith-Jackson, E.E., Disney, E.R., *et al.* Comparative prophylactic efficacy of lithium, carbamazepine, and the combination in bipolar disorder. *J. Clin. Psychiatry*, **1997**, *58:*470–478.

Dickson, R.A., and Glazer, W.M. Neuroleptic-induced hyperprolactinemia. *Schizophr. Res.*, **1999**, *35*(suppl):S75–S86.

Eastham, J.H., and Jeste, D.V. Treatment of schizophrenia and delusional disorder in the elderly. *Eur. Arch. Psychiatry Clin. Neurosci.*, **1997**, *247:*209–218.

Ellenbroek, B.A., Sams Dodd, F., and Cools, A.R. Simulation models for schizophrenia. In, *Atypical Antipsychotics.* (Ellenbroek, B.A., and Cools, A.R., eds.) Birkhauser Verlag, Basel, **1999**, pp. 121–142.

Ellenbroek, B.A. Treatment of schizophrenia: clinical and preclinical evaluation of neuroleptic drugs. *Pharmacol. Ther.*, **1993**, *57:*1–78.

Ely, E.W., Stephens, R.K, Jackson, J.C., *et al.* Current opinions regarding the importance, diagnosis, and management of delirium in the intensive care unit: a survey of 912 healthcare professionals. *Crit. Care Med.*, **2004**, *32:*106–112.

Ereshefsky, L. Pharmacokinetics and drug interactions: update for new antipsychotics. *J. Clin. Psychiatry*, **1996**, *57*(suppl 11):12–25.

Evins, A.E. Efficacy of newer anticonvulsant medications in bipolar spectrum mood disorders. *J. Clin. Psychiatry*, **2003**, *64*(suppl 8):9–14.

Faedda, G.L., Baldessarini, R.J., Glovinsky, I.P., and Austin, N.B. Mania with antidepressant and stimulant treatment in pediatric manic-depressive illness. *J. Affect. Disord.*, **2004**, *82:*149–158.

Faedda, G.L., Baldessarini, R.J., Suppes, T., *et al.* Pediatric-onset bipolar disorder: a neglected clinical and public health problem. *Harv. Rev. Psychiatry*, **1995**, *3:*171–195.

Faedda, G.L., Tondo, L., Baldessarini, R.J., Suppes, T., and Tohen, M. Outcome after rapid *vs.* gradual discontinuation of lithium treatment in bipolar disorders. *Arch. Gen. Psychiatry*, **1993**, *50:*448–455.

Farde, L., Nyberg, S., Oxenstierna, G., *et al.* Positron emission tomography studies on D_2 and $5HT_2$ receptor binding in risperidone-treated schizophrenic patients. *J. Clin. Psychopharmacol.*, **1995**, *15:*19S–23S.

Farver, D.K. Neuroleptic malignant syndrome induced by atypical antipsychotics. *Expert Opin. Drug Saf.*, **2003**, *2:*21–35.

Feldon. J., and Weiner I. From an animal model of an attentional deficit towards new insights into the pathophysiology of schizophrenia. *J. Psychiatr. Res.*, **1992**, *26:*345–366.

Findling, R.L. Use of quetiapine in children and adolescents. *J. Clin. Psychiatry*, **2002**, *63*(suppl 13):27–31.

Frazier, J.A., Cohen, L.G., Jacobsen, L., *et al.* Clozapine pharmacokinetics in children and adolescents with childhood-onset schizophrenia. *J. Clin. Psychopharmacol.*, **2003**, *23:*87–91.

Freeman, M.P., and Stoll, A.L. Mood stabilizer combinations: a review of safety and efficacy. *Am. J. Psychiatry*, **1998**, *155:*12–21.

Gardner, D., Baldessarini, R.J., and Waraich, P. Modern antipsychotic agents: A brief overview. *Can. Med. Assoc. J.*, **2005**, in press.

Gardos, G., Casey, D.E., Cole, J.O., *et al.* Ten-year outcome of tardive dyskinesia. *Am. J. Psychiatry*, **1994**, *151:*836–841.

Gaulin, B.D., Markowitz, J.S., Caley, C.F., *et al.* Clozapine-associated elevation of serum triglycerides. *Am. J. Psychiatry*, **1999**, *156:*1270–1272.

Geddes, J.R., Burgess, S., Hawton, K., *et al.* Long-term lithium therapy for bipolar disorder: systematic review and meta-analysis of randomized controlled trials. *Am. J. Psychiatry*, **2004**, *161:*217–222.

Gefvert O., Lundberg T., Wieselgren I.M., *et al.* D(2) and 5HT(2A) receptor occupancy of different doses of quetiapine in schizophrenia: PET study. *Eur. Neuropsychopharmacol.*, **2001**, *11:*105–110.

Geyer M.A., and Ellenbroek, B. Animal behavior models of the mechanisms underlying antipsychotic atypicality. *Prog. Neuropsychopharmacol. Biol. Psychiatry*, **2003**, *27:*1071–1079.

Gilbert, P.L., Harris, M.J., McAdams, L.A., and Jeste, D.V. Neuroleptic withdrawal in schizophrenic patients. A review of the literature. *Arch. Gen. Psychiatry*, **1995**, *52:*173–188.

Goff, D.C., and Baldessarini, R.J. Drug interactions with antipsychotic agents. *J. Clin. Psychopharmacol.*, **1993**, *13:*57–67.

Goff, D.C., Leahy, L., Berman, I., *et al.* A placebo-controlled pilot study of the ampakine CX516 added to clozapine in schizophrenia. *J. Clin. Psychopharmacol.*, **2001**, *21:*484–487.

Goff, D.C., Tsai, G., Levitt, J., *et al.* A placebo-controlled trial of D-cycloserine added to conventional neuroleptics in patients with schizophrenia. *Arch. Gen. Psychiatry*, **1999**, *56:*21–27.

Goldsmith, D.R., Wagstaff, A.J., Ibbotson, T., and Perry, C.M. Spotlight on lamotrigine in bipolar disorder. *CNS Drugs*, **2004**, *18:*63–67.

Goodwin, F.K., Fireman, B., Simon, G.E., *et al.* Suicide risk in bipolar disorder during treatment with lithium and divalproex. *J.A.M.A.*, **2003**, *290:*1467–1473.

Grant, S., and Fitton, A. Risperidone. A review of its pharmacology and therapeutic potential in the treatment of schizophrenia. *Drugs*, **1994**, *48:*253–273.

Greil, W., Ludwig-Mayerhofer, W., Erazo, N., *et al.* Lithium versus carbamazepine in the maintenance treatment of bipolar disorders—a randomised study. *J. Affect. Disord.,* **1997,** *43:*151–161.

Grunze, H., Erfurth, A., Amann, B., *et al.* Intravenous valproate loading in acutely manic and depressed bipolar I patients. *J. Clin. Psychopharmacol.,* **1999,** *19:*303–309.

Harrison, T.S., and Goa, K.L. Long-acting risperidone: review of its use in schizophrenia. *CNS Drugs,* **2004,** *18:*113–132.

Hassaballa, H.A., and Balk, R.A. *Torsade de pointes* associated with the administration of intravenous haloperidol: review of the literature and practical guidelines for use. *Expert Opin. Drug Saf.,* **2003,** *2:*543–547.

Henderson, D.C., Cagliero, E., Gray, C., *et al.* Clozapine, diabetes mellitus, weight gain, and lipid abnormalities: A five-year naturalistic study. *Am. J. Psychiatry,* **2000,** *157:*975–981.

Hennen, J., and Baldessarini, R.J. Reduced suicidal risk during treatment with clozapine: A meta-analysis. *Schizophrenia Res.,* **2004,** in press.

Herz, M.I., Glazer, W.M., Mostert, M.A., *et al.* Intermittent *vs.* maintenance medication in schizophrenia. Two-year results. *Arch. Gen. Psychiatry,* **1991,** *48:*333–339.

Hetmar, O., Povlsen, U.J., Ladefoged, J., and Bolwig, T.G. Lithium: long-term effects on the kidney. A prospective follow-up study ten years after kidney biopsy. *Br. J. Psychiatry,* **1991,** *158:*53–58.

Hirschfeld, R.M., Allen, M.H., McEvoy, J.P., *et al.* Safety and tolerability of oral loading divalproex sodium in acutely manic bipolar patients. *J. Clin. Psychiatry,* **1999,** *60:*815–818.

Ichikawa, J., and Meltzer, H.Y. Relationship between dopaminergic and serotonergic neuronal activity in the frontal cortex and the action of typical and atypical antipsychotic drugs. *Eur. Arch. Psychiatry Clin. Neurosci.,* **1999,** *249*(suppl 4):90–98.

Inoue, T., Domae, M., Yamada, K., and Furukawa, T. Effects of the novel antipsychotic agent 7-(4-[4-(2,3-dichlorophenyl)-1-piperazinyl]butyloxy)-3,4-dihydro-2(1H)-quinolinone (OPC-14597) on prolactin release from the rat anterior pituitary gland. *J. Pharmacol. Exp. Ther.,* **1996,** *277:*137–143.

Iqbal, M.M., Gundlapalli, S.P., Ryan, W.G., *et al.* Effects of antimanic mood-stabilizing drugs on fetuses, neonates, and nursing infants. *South. Med. J.,* **2001,** *94:*304.

Iqbal, M.M., Rahman, A., Husain, Z., *et al.* Clozapine: clinical review of adverse effects and management. *Ann. Clin. Psychiatry,* **2003,** *15:*33–48.

Jefferson, J.W., Greist, J.H., Clagnaz, P.J., *et al.* Effect of strenuous exercise on serum lithium level in man. *Am. J. Psychiatry,* **1982,** *139:*1593–1595.

Jeste, D.V., Lacro, J.P., Bailey, A., *et al.* Lower incidence of tardive dyskinesia with risperidone compared with haloperidol in older patients. *J. Am. Geriatr. Soc.,* **1999a,** *47:*716–719.

Jeste, D.V., Rockwell, E., Harris, M.J., *et al.* Conventional *vs.* newer antipsychotics in elderly patients. *Am. J. Geriatr. Psychiatry,* **1999b,** *7:*70–76.

Jope, R.S. A bimodal model of the mechanism of action of lithium. *Mol. Psychiatry,* **1999,** *4:*21–25.

Kane, J.M., Honigfeld, G., Singer, J., and Meltzer, H.Y. Clozapine for the treatment resistant schizophrenic: A double-blind comparison with chlorpromazine. *Arch. Gen. Psychiatry,* **1988,** *45:*789–796.

Kane, J.M., Rifkin, A., Woerner, M., *et al.* Low-dose neuroleptic treatment of outpatient schizophrenics. I. Preliminary results for relapse rates. *Arch. Gen. Psychiatry,* **1983,** *40:*893–896.

Kane, J.M. Tardive dyskinesia in affective disorders. *J. Clin. Psychiatry,* **1999,** *60*(suppl 5):43–47.

Kapur, S., and Seeman, P. Does fast dissociation from the dopamine D_2 receptor explain the action of atypical antipsychotics?: new hypothesis. *Am. J. Psychiatry,* **2001,** *158:*360–369.

Kapur, S., Zipursky, R.B., and Remington, G. Clinical and theoretical implications of 5-HT_2 and D_2 receptor occupancy of clozapine, risperidone, and olanzapine in schizophrenia. *Am. J. Psychiatry,* **1999,** *156:*286–293.

Karlsson, P., Smith, L., Farde, L., *et al.* Lack of apparent antipsychotic effect of the D_1-dopamine receptor antagonist SCH-39166 in acutely ill schizophrenic patients. *Psychopharmacology (Berl.),* **1995,** *121:*309–316.

Kasper, S., and Resinger, E. Cognitive effects and antipsychotic treatment. *Psychoneuroendocrinology,* **2003,** *28*(suppl 1):27–38.

Kasper, S., Tauscher, J., Willeit, M., *et al.* Receptor and transporter imaging studies in schizophrenia, depression, bulimia and Tourette's disorder: implications for psychopharmacology. *World J. Biol. Psychiatry,* **2002,** *3:*133–146.

Keck, P.E., Jr., Marcus, R., Tourkodimitris, S., *et al.* Placebo-controlled, double-blind study of the efficacy and safety of aripiprazole in patients with acute bipolar mania. *Am. J. Psychiatry,* **2003,** *160:*1651–1658.

Korpi, E.R., Phelps, B.H., Granger, H., *et al.* Simultaneous determination of haloperidol and its reduced metabolite in serum and plasma by isocratic liquid chromatography with electrochemical detection. *Clin. Chem.,* **1983,** *29:*624–628.

Kosten, T.R., and Forrest, J.N. Treatment of severe lithium-induced polyuria with amiloride. *Am. J. Psychiatry,* **1986,** *143:*1563–1568.

Kowatch, R.A., and DelBello, M.P. Use of mood stabilizers and atypical antipsychotics in children and adolescents with bipolar disorders. *CNS Spectrums,* **2003,** *8:*273–280.

Kramer, M.S., Last, B., Getson, A., and Reines, S.A. The effects of a selective D_4 dopamine receptor antagonist (L-745,870) in acutely psychotic inpatients with schizophrenia. D_4 Dopamine Antagonist Group. *Arch. Gen. Psychiatry,* **1997,** *54:*567–572.

La Grenade, L., Graham, D., and Trontell, A. Myocarditis and cardiomyopathy associated with clozapine use in the United States. *N. Engl. J. Med.,* **2001,** *345:*224–225.

Lahti, A.C., Weiler, M., Carlsson, A., and Tamminga, C.A. Effects of the D_3 and autoreceptor-preferring dopamine antagonist (+)-UH232 in schizophrenia. *J. Neural Transm.,* **1998,** *105:*719–734.

Lasser, R.A., and Baldessarini, R.J. Thyroid hormones in depressive disorders: a reappraisal of clinical utility. *Harv. Rev. Psychiatry,* **1997,** *4:*291–305.

Lasser, R.A., Bossie, C., Gharabawi, G.M., and Baldessarini, R.J. Clinical improvements in 336 stable, chronically psychotic patients changed form oral to long-acting risperidone: a 12-month open trial. *J. Clin. Psychiatry,* **2005,** in press.

Lehman, A.F., Buchanan, R.W., Dickerson, F.B., *et al.* Evidence-based treatment for schizophrenia. *Psychiatr. Clin. North Am.,* **2003,** *26:*939–954.

Leucht, S., Barnes, T.R.E., Kissling, W., *et al.* Relapse prevention in schizophrenia with new-generation antipsychotics: a systematic review and exploratory meta-analysis of randomized, controlled trials. *Am J Psychiatry* **2003a,** *160:*1209–1222.

Leucht, S., Wahlbeck, K., Hamann, J., and Kissling, W. New generation antipsychotics *vs.* low-potency conventional antipsychotics: a systematic review and meta-analysis. *Lancet,* **2003b,** *361:*1582–1589.

Leysen, J.E., Janssen, P.M., Megens, A.A., and Schotte, A. Risperidone: a novel antipsychotic with balanced serotonin-dopamine antagonism, receptor occupancy profile, and pharmacologic activity. *J. Clin. Psychiatry,* **1994,** *55*(suppl):5–12.

Licht, R.W. Drug treatment of mania: a critical review. *Acta. Psychiatr. Scand.,* **1998,** *97:*387–397.

Lipinski, J.F. Jr., Zubenko, G.S., Cohen, B.M., and Barreira, P.J. Propranolol in the treatment of neuroleptic-induced akathisia. *Am. J. Psychiatry,* **1984,** *141:*412–415.

McIntyre, R.S., Trakas, K., Lin, D., *et al.* Risk of weight gain associated with antipsychotic treatment. *Can. J. Psychiatry,* **2003,** *48:*689–694.

Maj, M., Starace, F., Nolfe, G., and Kemali, D. Minimum plasma lithium levels required for effective prophylaxis in DSM III bipolar disorder: a prospective study. *Pharmacopsychiatry,* **1986,** *19:*420–423.

Manji, H.K., Etcheberrigaray, G., Chen, R., and Olds, J.L. Lithium decreases membrane-associated protein kinase C in hippocampus: selectivity for the alpha isozyme. *J. Neurochem.,* **1993,** *61:*2303–2310.

Markowitz, J.S., Brown, C.S., and Moore, T.R. Atypical antipsychotics. Part I: Pharmacology, pharmacokinetics, and efficacy. *Ann. Pharmacother.,* **1999,** *33:*73–85.

Meltzer, H.Y., Alphs, L., Green, A.I., *et al.* Clozapine treatment for suicidality in schizophrenia. *Arch. Gen. Psychiatry,* **2003,** *60:*82–91.

Meltzer, H.Y., and Nash, J.F. Effects of antipsychotic drugs on serotonin receptors. *Pharmacol. Rev.,* **1991,** *43:*587–604.

Menza, M.M., Palermo, B., and Mark, M. Quetiapine as an alternative to clozapine in the treatment of dopamimetic psychosis in patients with Parkinson's disease. *Ann. Clin. Psychiatry,* **1999,** *11:*141–144.

Moghaddam, B. Targeting metabotropic glutamate receptors for treatment of the cognitive symptoms of schizophrenia. *Psychopharmacology (Berl.),* **2004,** *174:*39–44.

Moller, H.J. Atypical neuroleptics: a new approach in the treatment of negative symptoms. *Eur. Arch. Psychiatry Clin. Neurosci.,* **1999,** *249*(suppl 4):99–107.

Moore, K.E. Hypothalamic dopaminergic neuronal systems. In, *Psychopharmacology: The Third Generation of Progress.* (Meltzer, H.Y., ed.) Raven Press, New York, **1987,** pp. 127–139.

Morgenstern, H., and Glazer, W.M. Identifying risk factors for tardive dyskinesia among long-term outpatients maintained with neuroleptic medications. Results of the Yale Tardive Dyskinesia Study. *Arch. Gen. Psychiatry,* **1993,** *50:*723–733.

Mortensen, P.B. The occurrence of cancer in first admitted schizophrenic patients. *Schizophr. Res.,* **1994,** *12:*185–194.

NDA Pipeline. Available at: http://www.ndapipeline.com. Accessed Dec., **2004.**

Neil, J.F., Himmelhoch, J.M., and Licata, S.M. Emergence of myasthenia gravis during treatment with lithium carbonate. *Arch. Gen. Psychiatry,* **1976,** *33:*1090–1092.

Nordstrom, A.L., Farde, L., Nyberg, S., *et al.* D_1, D_2, and 5-HT_2 receptor occupancy in relation to clozapine serum concentration: a PET study of schizophrenic patients. *Am. J. Psychiatry,* **1995,** *152:*1444–1449.

Nordstrom, A.L., Nyberg, S., Olsson, H., and Farde, L. Positron emission tomography finding of a high striatal D_2 receptor occupancy in olanzapine-treated patients. *Arch. Gen. Psychiatry,* **1998,** *55:*283–284.

Parkinson Study Group. Low-dose clozapine for the treatment of drug-induced psychosis in Parkinson's disease. *N. Engl. J. Med.,* **1999,** *340:*757–763.

Pazzaglia, P.J., Post, R.M., Ketter, T.A., *et al.* Nimodipine monotherapy and carbamazepine augmentation in patients with refractory recurrent affective illness. *J. Clin. Psychopharmacol.,* **1998,** *18:*404–413.

Pearlman, C.A. Neuroleptic malignant syndrome: a review of the literature. *J. Clin. Psychopharmacology,* **1986,** *6:*257–273.

Perry, W., Geyer M.A., and Braff, D.L. Sensorimotor gating and thought disturbance measured in close temporal proximity in schizophrenic patients. *Arch. Gen. Psychiatry,* **1999,** *56:*277–281.

Phelan, K.M., Mosholder, A.D., and Lu, S. Lithium interaction with the cyclooxygenase-2 inhibitors rofecoxib and celecoxib and other nonsteroidal anti-inflammatory drugs. *J. Clin. Psychiatry,* **2003,** *64:*1328–1334.

Pilla, M., Perachon, S., Sautel, F., *et al.* Selective inhibition of cocaine-seeking behaviour by a partial D_3 receptor agonist. *Nature,* **1999,** *400:*371–375.

Pinelli, J.M., Symington, A.J., Cunningham, K.A., and Paes, B.A. Case report and review of the perinatal implications of maternal lithium use. *Am. J. Obstet. Gynecol.,* **2002,** *187:*245.

Plenge, P., Stensgaard, A., Jensen, H.V., *et al.* 24-hour lithium concentration in human brain studied by ^7Li magnetic resonance spectroscopy. *Biol. Psychiatry,* **1994,** *36:*511–516.

Pope, H.G. Jr., McElroy, S.L., Keck, P.E. Jr., and Hudson, J.I. Valproate in the treatment of acute mania. A placebo-controlled study. *Arch. Gen. Psychiatry,* **1991,** *48:*62–68.

Post, R.M., Denicoff, K.D., Frye, M.A., *et al.* A history of the use of anticonvulsants as mood stabilizers in the last two decades of the 20th century. *Neuropsychobiology,* **1998,** *38:*152–166.

Potkin, S.G., Saha, A.R., Kujawa, M.J., *et al.* Aripiprazole, an antipsychotic with a novel mechanism of action, and risperidone *vs.* placebo in patients with schizophrenia and schizoaffective disorder. *Arch. Gen. Psychiatry,* **2003,** *60:*681–690.

Purdon, S.E. Measuring neuropsychological change in schizophrenia with novel antipsychotic medications. *J. Psychiatry Neurosci.,* **2000,** *25:*108–116.

Rabinowitz, T., Frankenburg, F.R., Centorrino, F., and Kando, J. The effect of clozapine on saliva flow rate: a pilot study. *Biol. Psychiatry,* **1996,** *40:*1132–1134.

Ray, W.A., Griffin, M.R., Schaffner, W., *et al.* Psychotropic drug use and the risk of hip fracture. *N. Engl. J. Med.,* **1987,** *316:*363–369.

Reiter, S., Adler, L., Angrist, B., Corwin, J., and Rotrosen, J. Atenolol and propranolol in neuroleptic-induced akathisia. *J. Clin. Psychopharmacol.,* **1987,** *7:*279–280.

Richelson, E. Receptor pharmacology of neuroleptics: relation to clinical effects. *J. Clin. Psychiatry,* **1999,** *60*(suppl 10):5–14.

Riedl, U., Barocka, A., Kolem, H., *et al.* Duration of lithium treatment and brain lithium concentration in patients with unipolar and schizoaffective disorder: a study with magnetic resonance spectroscopy. *Biol. Psychiatry,* **1997,** *41:*844–850.

Rosenheck, R., Perlick, D., Bingham, S., *et al.* Effectiveness and cost of olanzapine and haloperidol in the treatment of schizophrenia: a randomized controlled trial. *J.A.M.A.,* **2003,** *290:*2693–2702.

Roth, B.L., Tandra, S., Burgess, L.H., *et al.* D_4 dopamine receptor affinity does not distinguish between typical and atypical antipsychotic drugs. *Psychopharmacology (Berl.),* **1995,** *120:*365–368.

Rotrosen, J., Angrist, B.M., Gershon, S., *et al.* Thiethylperazine: clinical antipsychotic efficacy and correlation with potency in predictive systems. *Arch. Gen. Psychiatry,* **1978,** *35:*1112–1118.

Sampath, G., Shah, A., Krska, J., and Soni, S.D. Neuroleptic discontinuation in the very stable schizophrenic patient: relapse rates and serum neuroleptic levels. *Hum. Psychopharmacol.,* **1992,** *7:*255–264.

Sautel, F., Griffon, N., Sokoloff, P., *et al.* Nafadotide, a potent preferential dopamine D_3 receptor antagonist, activates locomotion in rodents. *J. Pharmacol. Exp. Ther.,* **1995,** *275:*1239–1246.

Saykin, A.J., Gur, R.C., Gur, R.E., *et al.* Neuropsychological function in schizophrenia. Selective impairment in memory and learning. *Arch. Gen. Psychiatry,* **1991,** *48:*618–624.

Schooler, N.R. Relapse and rehospitalization: comparing oral and depot antipsychotics. *J. Clin. Psychiatry,* **2003,** *64*(suppl 16):14–17.

Schotte, A., Janssen, P.F., Gommeren, W., *et al.* Risperidone compared with new and reference antipsychotic drugs: *in vitro* and *in vivo* receptor binding. *Psychopharmacology (Berl.),* **1996,** *124:*57–73.

Schuster, P., Gabriel, E., Kufferle, B., *et al.* Reversal by physostigmine of clozapine-induced delirium. *Clin. Toxicol.,* **1977,** *10:*437–441.

Schwartz, M., and Hocherman, S. Antipsychotic-induced rabbit syndrome: epidemiology, management and pathophysiology. *CNS Drugs*, **2004**, *18:*213–220.

Sedvall, G. The current status of PET scanning with respect to schizophrenia. *Neuropsychopharmacology*, **1992**, *7:*41–54.

Seeger, T.F., Seymour, P.A., Schmidt, A.W., *et al.* Ziprasidone (CP-88,059): a new antipsychotic with combined dopamine and serotonin receptor antagonists activity. *J. Pharmacol. Exp. Ther.*, **1995**, *275:*101–113.

Segal, J., Berk, M., and Brook, S. Risperidone compared with both lithium and haloperidol in mania: a double-blind randomized controlled trial. *Clin. Neuropharmacol.*, **1998**, *21:*176–180.

Sernyak, M.J., Griffin, R.A., Johnson, R.M., *et al.* Neuroleptic exposure following inpatient treatment of acute mania with lithium and neuroleptic. *Am. J. Psychiatry*, **1994**, *151:*133–135.

Shafer, R.A., and Levant, B. The D_3 dopamine receptor in cellular and organismal function. *Psychopharmacology (Berl.)*, **1998**, *135:*1–16.

Siegel, A.J., Baldessarini, R.J., Klepser, M.B., and McDonald, J.C. Primary and drug-induced disorders of water homeostasis in psychiatric patients: principles of diagnosis and management. *Harv. Rev. Psychiatry*, **1998**, *6:*190–200.

Sikich, L., Hamer, R.M., Bashford, R.A., *et al.* Pilot study of risperidone, olanzapine, and haloperidol in psychotic youth. *Neuropsychopharmacology*, **2004**, *29:*133–145.

Simpson, G.M., Cooper, T.B., Bark, N., *et al.* Effect of antiparkinsonian medication on plasma levels of chlorpromazine. *Arch. Gen. Psychiatry*, **1980**, *37:*205–208.

Smith, J.M., and Baldessarini, R.J. Changes in prevalence, severity, and recovery in tardive dyskinesia with age. *Arch. Gen. Psychiatry*, **1980**, *37:*1368–1373.

Snyder, S.H., and Yamamura, H.I. Antidepressants and the muscarinic acetylcholine receptor. *Arch. Gen. Psychiatry*, **1977**, *34:*236–239.

Soares, K.V., and McGrath, J.J. The treatment of tardive dyskinesia: a systematic review and meta-analysis. *Schizophr. Res.*, **1999**, *39:*1–16.

Sokoloff, P., Giros, B., Martres, M.P., *et al.* Molecular cloning and characterization of a novel dopamine receptor (D_3) as a target for neuroleptics. *Nature*, **1990**, *347:*146–151.

Spencer, T., Biederman, J., Wilens, T., *et al.* Nortriptyline treatment of children with attention-deficit hyperactivity disorder and tic disorder or Tourette's syndrome. *J. Am. Acad. Child Adolesc. Psychiatry*, **1993**, *32:*205–210.

Stigler, K.A., Potenza, M.N., and McDougle, C.J. Tolerability profile of atypical antipsychotics in children and adolescents. *Paediatr. Drugs*, **2001**, *3:*927–942.

Stimmel, G.L., Gutierrez, M.A., and Lee, V. Ziprasidone: An atypical antipsychotic drug for the treatment of schizophrenia. *Clin. Ther.*, **2002**, *24:*24–37.

Stoll, A.L., Mayer, P.V., Kolbrener, M., *et al.* Antidepressant-associated mania: a controlled comparison with spontaneous mania. *Am. J. Psychiatry*, **1994**, *151:*1642–1645.

Stoll, A.L., Severus, W.E., Freeman, M.P., *et al.* Omega 3 fatty acids in bipolar disorder: a preliminary double-blind, placebo-controlled trial. *Arch. Gen. Psychiatry*, **1999**, *56:*407–412.

Sur, C., Mallorga, P.J., Wittmann, M., *et al.* N-desmethyclozapine, an allosteric agonist at muscarinic-1 receptor, potentiates N-methyl-D-aspartate receptor activity. *Proc. Natl. Acad. Sci. U.S.A.*, **2003**, *100:*13674–13679.

Swerdlow, N.R., Braff, D.L., Taaid, N., and Geyer, M.A. Assessing the validity of an animal model of deficient sensorimotor gating in schizophrenic patients. *Arch. Gen. Psychiatry*, **1994**, *51:*139–154.

Tarazi, F.I., Yeghiayan, S.K., Baldessarini, R.J., *et al.* Long-term effects of S(+)N-*n*-propylnorapomorphine compared with typical and atypical antipsychotics: differential increases of cerebrocortical D_2-like and striatolimbic D_4-like dopamine receptors. *Neuropsychopharmacology*, **1997**, *17:*186–196.

Tarazi, F.I., Zhang, K., and Baldessarini, R.J. Long-term effects of olanzapine, risperidone, and quetiapine on dopamine receptor subtypes: Implications for antipsychotic drug treatment. *J. Pharmacol. Exp. Ther.*, **2001**, *297:*711–717.

Tarsy, D., Baldessarini, R.J., and Tarazi, F.I. Extrapyramidal dysfunction associated with modern antipsychotic drugs. *CNS Drugs*, **2002**, *16:*23–45.

Tauscher, J., Jones, C., Remington, G., *et al.* Significant dissociation of brain and plasma kinetics with antipsychotics. *Mol. Psychiatry*, **2002**, *7:*317–321.

Tesar, G.E., Murray, G.B., and Cassem, N.H. Use of high-dose intravenous haloperidol in the treatment of agitated cardiac patients. *J. Clin. Psychopharmacol.*, **1985**, *5:*344–347.

Taylor, D. Ziprasidone in the management of schizophrenia: the QT interval issue in context. *CNS Drugs*, **2003**, *17:*423–430.

Theret, L., Germain, M.L., and Burde, A. Current aspects of the use of clozapine in the Chalons-sur-Marne Psychiatric Hospital: intestinal occlusion with clozapine. *Ann. Med. Psychol. (Paris)*, **1995**, *153:*474–477.

Thies-Flechtner, K., Müller-Oerlinghausen, B., Seibert, W., *et al.* Effect of prophylactic treatment on suicide risk in patients with major affective disorders: Data from a randomized prospective trial. *Pharmacopsychiatry*, **1996**, *29:*103–107.

Tohen, M., Ketter, T.A, Zarate, C.A., *et al.* Olanzapine versus divalproex sodium for the treatment of acute mania and maintenance of remission: 47-week study. *Am. J. Psychiatry*, **2003**, *160:*1263–1271.

Tohen, M., Sanger, T.M., McElroy, S.L., *et al.* Olanzapine versus placebo in the treatment of acute mania. Olanzapine Study Group. *Am. J. Psychiatry*, **1999**, *156:*702–709.

Tohen, M., and Zarate, C.A. Jr. Antipsychotic agents and bipolar disorder. *J. Clin. Psychiatry*, **1998**, *59*(suppl 1):38–48.

Tollefson, G.D., and Kuntz, A.J. Review of recent clinical studies with olanzapine. *Br. J. Psychiatry Suppl.*, **1999**, 30–35.

Tondo, L., Baldessarini, R.J., and Floris, G. Long-term effectiveness of lithium maintenance treatment in types I and II bipolar disorders. *Br. J. Psychiatry*, **2001a**, *178*(suppl 40):184–190.

Tondo, L., Baldessarini, R.J., Hennen, J., and Floris, G. Lithium maintenance treatment of depression and mania in bipolar I and II bipolar disorders. *Am. J. Psychiatry*, **1998**, *155:*638–645.

Tondo, L., Hennen, J., and Baldessarini, R.J. Reduced suicide risk with long-term lithium treatment in major affective illness: A meta-analysis. *Acta. Psychiatr. Scand.*, **2001b**, *104:*163–172.

Turkka, J., Bitram, J.A., Manji, H.K., *et al.* Effects of chronic lithium on agonist and antagonist binding to β-adrenergic receptors of rat brain. *Lithium*, **1992**, *3:*43–47.

Treiser, S.L., Cascio, C.S., O'Donohue, T.L., *et al.* Lithium increases serotonin release and decreases serotonin receptors in the hippocampus. *Science*, **1981**, *213:*1529–1531.

Truffinet, P., Tamminga, C.A., Fabre, L.F., *et al.* Placebo-controlled study of the D_4/5-HT$_{2A}$ antagonist fananserin in the treatment of schizophrenia. *Am. J. Psychiatry*, **1999**, *156:*419–425.

Tsuneizumi, T., Babb, S.M., and Cohen, B.M. Drug distribution between blood and brain as a determinant of antipsychotic drug effects. *Biol. Psychiatry*, **1992**, *32:*817–824.

Urabe, M., Hershmann, J.M., Pang, X.P., *et al.* Effect of lithium on function and growth of thyroid cells *in vitro*. *Endocrinology*, **1991**, *129:*807–814.

Van Tol, H.H., Bunzow, J.R., Guan, H.C., *et al.* Cloning of the gene for a human dopamine D_4 receptor with high affinity for the antipsychotic clozapine. *Nature,* **1991,** *350:*610–614.

Vieta, E., Brugue, E., Goikolea, J.M., *et al.* Acute and continuation risperidone monotherapy in mania. *Hum. Psychopharmacol.,* **2004,** *19:*41–45.

Viguera, A.C., Baldessarini, R.J., Hegarty, J.M., *et al.* Clinical risk following abrupt and gradual withdrawal of maintenance neuroleptic treatment. *Arch. Gen. Psychiatry,* **1997,** *54:*49–55.

Viguera, A.C., Cohen, L.S., Baldessarini, R.J., and Nonacs, R. Managing bipolar disorder in pregnancy: Weighing the risks and benefits. *Can. J. Psychiatry,* **2002,** *47:*426–436.

Viguera, A.C., Nonacs, R., Cohen, L.S., *et al.* Risk of recurrence of bipolar disorder in pregnant and nonpregnant women after discontinuing lithium maintenance. *Am. J. Psychiatry,* **2000,** *157:*179–184.

Wahlbeck, K., Cheine, M., Essali, A., and Adams, C. Evidence of clozapine's effectiveness in schizophrenia: a systematic review and meta-analysis of randomized trials. *Am. J. Psychiatry,* **1999,** *156:*990–999.

Wang, H.Y., and Friedman, E. Lithium inhibition of protein kinase C activation–induced serotonin release. *Psychopharmacology (Berl.),* **1989,** *99:*213–218.

Watson, D.G., and Lenox, R.H. Chronic lithium-induced down-regulation of MARCKS in immortalized hippocampal cells: potentiation by muscarinic receptor activation. *J. Neurochem.,* **1996,** *67:*767–777.

Watson, D.G., Watterson, J.M., and Lenox, R.H. Sodium valproate down-regulates the myristoylated alanine-rich C kinase substrate (MARCKS) in immortalized hippocampal cells: a property of protein kinase C–mediated mood stabilizers. *J. Pharmacol. Exp. Ther.,* **1998,** *285:*307–316.

Wirshing, D.A., Spellberg, B.J., Erhard, S.M., *et al.* Novel antipsychotics and new onset diabetes. *Biol. Psychiatry,* **1998,** *44:*778–783.

Wolkin, A., Brodie, J.D., Barouche, F., *et al.* Dopamine receptor occupancy and plasma haloperidol levels. *Arch. Gen. Psychiatry,* **1989,** *46:*482–484.

Wooltorton, E. Risperidone (Risperdal): increased rate of cerebrovascular events in dementia trials. *C.M.A.J.,* **2002,** *26:*1269–1270.

Wright, P., Lindborg, S.R., Birkett, M., *et al.* Intramuscular olanzapine and intramuscular haloperidol in acute schizophrenia: antipsychotic efficacy and extrapyramidal safety during the first 24 hours of treatment. *Can. J. Psychiatry,* **2003,** *48:*716–721.

Yatham, L.N. Efficacy of atypical antipsychotics in mood disorders. *J. Clin. Psychopharmacol.,* **2003,** *23*(3 suppl 1):S9–S14.

Yokoi, F., Grunder, G., Biziere, K., *et al.* Dopamine D2 and D3 receptor occupancy in normal humans treated with the antipsychotic drug aripiprazole (OPC 14597): a study using positron emission tomography and [^{11}C]raclopride. *Neuropsychopharmacology,* **2002,** *27:*248–259.

Zareba, W., and Lin, D.A. Antipsychotic drugs and QT interval prolongation. *Psychiatr. Quart.,* **2003,** *74:*291–306.

Zarin, D.A., and Pass, T.M. Lithium and the single episode. When to begin long-term prophylaxis for bipolar disorder. *Med. Care,* **1987,** *25:*S76–S84.

Zatz, M., and Reisine, T.D. Lithium induces corticotropin secretion and desensitization in cultured anterior pituitary cells. *Proc. Natl. Acad. Sci. U.S.A.,* **1985,** *82:*1286–1290.

Zhang, K., Grady, C.J., Tsapakis, E.M., *et al.* Regulation of working memory by dopamine D_4 receptor in rats. *Neuropsychopharmacology,* **2004,** *29:*1648–1655.

Zimbroff, D.L. Management of acute psychosis: from emergency to stabilization. *CNS Spectrums,* **2003,** *8*(11 suppl 2):10–15.

Zubenko, G.S., and Sunderland, T. Geriatric psychopharmacology: why does age matter? *Harv. Rev. Psychiatry,* **2000,** *7:*311–333.

MONOGRAPHS AND REVIEWS

Abraham, D. (ed.) *Burger's Medicinal Chemistry and Drug Discovery,* 6th ed. Wiley, New York, **2003.**

Bagnall, A.M., Jones, L., Ginnelly, L., *et al.* A systematic review of atypical antipsychotic drugs in schizophrenia. *Health Technol. Assess.,* **2003,** *7:*1–193.

Baldessarini, R.J. American biological psychiatry and psychopharmacology 1944–1994. Chapter 16. In, *American Psychiatry After World War II 1944–1994.* (Menninger, R.W. and Nemiah, J.C., eds.) APA Press, Washington, D.C., **2000,** pp. 371–412.

Baldessarini, R.J., and Frankenburg, F.R. Clozapine. A novel antipsychotic agent. *N. Engl. J. Med.,* **1991,** *324:*746–754.

Baldessarini, R.J., and Tarazi, F.I. Brain dopamine receptors: a primer on their current status, basic and clinical. *Harv. Rev. Psychiatry,* **1996,** *3:*301–325.

Baldessarini, R.J., Cohen, B.M., and Teicher, M.H. Pharmacological treatment. In, *Schizophrenia: Treatment of Acute Psychotic Episodes.* (Levy, S.T., and Ninan, P.T., eds.) American Psychiatric Press, Washington, D.C., **1990,** pp. 61–118.

Baldessarini, R.J., Cole, J.O., Davis, J.M., *et al.* Tardive Dyskinesia: A Task Force Report of the American Psychiatric Association. Task Force Report No. 18. American Psychiatric Association, Washington, D.C., **1980.**

Baldessarini, R.J. Dopamine receptors and clinical medicine. In, *The Dopamine Receptors.* (Neve, K.A., and Neve, R.L., eds.) Humana Press, Totowa, N.J., **1997,** pp. 457–498.

Baldessarini, R.J., Faedda, G.L., and Suppes, T. Treatment response in pediatric, adult, and geriatric bipolar disorder patients. In, *Mood Disorders Across the Life Span.* (Shulman, K., Tohen, M., and Kutcher, S.P., eds.) Wiley-Liss, New York, **1996b,** pp. 299–338.

Baldessarini, R.J., and Tarsy, D. Relationship of the actions of neuroleptic drugs to the pathophysiology of tardive dyskinesia. *Int. Rev. Neurobiol.,* **1979,** *21:*1–45.

Ben-Jonathan, N. Dopamine: a prolactin-inhibiting hormone. *Endocr. Rev.,* **1985,** *6:*564–589.

Caldwell, A.E. History of psychopharmacology. In, *Principles of Psychopharmacology,* 2nd ed. (Clark, W.G., and del Giudice, J., eds.) Academic Press, New York, **1978,** pp. 9–40.

Carlsson, A. Fifteen years of continued research in psychopharmacology. *Pharmacopsychiatry,* **1992,** *25:*22–24.

Civelli, O., Bunzow, J.R., and Grandy, D.K. Molecular diversity of the dopamine receptors. *Annu. Rev. Pharmacol. Toxicol.,* **1993,** *33:*281–307.

Cooper, T.B., Simpson, G.M., and Lee, J.H. Thymoleptic and neuroleptic drug plasma levels in psychiatry: current status. *Int. Rev. Neurobiol.,* **1976,** *19:*269–309.

Davis, J.M., Janicak, P.G., and Hogan, D.M. Mood stabilizers in the prevention of recurrent affective disorders: a meta-analysis. *Acta. Psychiatr. Scand.,* **1999,** *100:*406–417.

Davis, L.L., Ryan, W., Adinoff, B., and Petty, F. Comprehensive review of the psychiatric uses of valproate. *J. Clin. Psychopharmacol.,* **2000,** *20:*1S–17S.

DeBattista, C., and Schatzberg, A.F. Universal psychotropic dosing and monitoring guidelines. *The Economics of Neuroscience (TEN),* **1999,** *1:*75–84.

DeVane, C.L., and Nemeroff, C.B. Psychotropic drug interactions. *The Economics of Neuroscience (TEN),* **2000,** *2:*55–75.

Dubovsky, S.L. Calcium channel antagonists as novel agents for the treatment of bipolar disorder. In, *Textbook of Psychopharmacology* (Schatzberg, A.F., and Nemeroff, C.B., eds.) American Psychiatric Press, Washington, D.C., **1998,** pp. 455–469.

Ferrier, N., and Calabrese, J. Lamotrigine, gabapentin, and the new anticonvulsants: efficacy in mood disorders. In, *Schizophrenia and Mood Disorders: The New Drug Therapies in Clinical Practice.* (Buckley, P.F., and Waddington, J.L., eds.) Butterworth-Heinemann, Boston, **2000,** pp. 190–198.

Fielding, S., and Lal, H. Behavioral actions of neuroleptics. In, *Handbook of Psychopharmacology,* Vol. 10. (Iversen, L.L., Iversen, S.D., and Snyder, S.H., eds.) Plenum Press, New York, **1978,** pp. 91–128.

Findling, R.L., Schulz, S.C., Reed, M.D., and Blumer, J.L. The antipsychotics. A pediatric perspective. *Pediatr. Clin. North Am.,* **1998,** *45:*1205–1232.

Goodwin, F.K., and Jamison, K.R. *Manic-Depressive Illness.* Oxford University Press, New York, **1990.**

Gunasekara, N.S., Spencer, C.M., and Keating, G.M. Ziprasidone: A review of its use in schizophrenia and schizoaffective disorder. *Drugs,* **2002,** *62:*1217–1251.

Hosak, L., and Libiger, J. Antiepileptic drugs in schizophrenia: a review. *Eur. Psychiatry,* **2002,** *17:*371–378.

Janssen, P.A.J., and Van Bever, W.F. Preclinical psychopharmacology of neuroleptics. In, *Principles of Psychopharmacology,* 2nd ed. (Clark, W.G., and del Giudice, J., eds.) Academic Press, New York, **1978,** pp. 279–295.

Janssen, P.A.J. Butyrophenones and diphenylbutylpiperidines. In, *Psychopharmacological Agents,* Vol. 3. (Gordon, M., ed.) Academic Press, New York, **1974,** pp. 128–158.

Jefferson, J.W., Greist, J.H., and Ackerman, D.L. *Lithium Encyclopedia for Clinical Practice.* American Psychiatric Press, Washington, D.C., **1983.**

Kane, J.M., Jeste, D.V., Barnes, T.R.E., *et al. Tardive Dyskinesia: A Task Force Report of the American Psychiatric Association.* American Psychiatric Association, Washington, D.C., **1992.**

Kebabian, J.W., Tarazi, F.I., Kula, N.S., and Baldessarini, R.J. Compounds selective for dopamine receptor subtypes. *Drug Discov. Today,* **1997,** *2:*333–340.

Keck, P., and Licht, R. Antipsychotic medications in the treatment of mood disorders. In, *Schizophrenia and Mood Disorders: The New Drug Therapies in Clinical Practice.* (Buckley, P.F., and Waddington, J.L., eds.) Butterworth-Heinemann, Boston, **2000,** pp. 199–211.

Keck, P., and McElroy, S.L. Antiepileptic drugs. In, *The American Psychiatric Press Textbook of Psychopharmacology.* (Schatzberg, A.F., and Nemeroff, C.B., eds.) American Psychiatric Press, Washington, D.C., **1998,** pp. 431–454.

King, B., Zwi, K., Nunn, K., *et al.* Use of risperidone in a paediatric population. *J. Paediatr. Child Health,* **2003,** *39:*523–527.

Kutcher, S.P. *Child & Adolescent Psychopharmacology.* Saunders, Philadelphia, **1997.**

Lenox, R.H., and Manji, H.K. In, *The American Psychiatric Press Textbook of Psychopharmacology.* (Schatzberg, A.F., and Nemeroff, C.B., eds.) American Psychiatric Press, Washington, D.C., **1998,** pp. 379–429.

Levant, B. The D_3 dopamine receptor: neurobiology and potential clinical relevance. *Pharmacol. Rev.,* **1997,** *49:*231–252.

Manji, H.K., Bebchuck, J.M., Moore, G.J., *et al.* Modulation of CNS signal transduction pathways and gene expression by mood-stabilizing agents: therapeutic implications. *J. Clin. Psychiatry,* **1999a,** *60*(suppl 2):27–39.

Manji, H.K., Bowden, C.L., and Belmaker, R.H., eds. *Bipolar Medications: Mechanisms of Action.* American Psychiatric Press, Washington, D.C., **2000.**

Manji, H.K., McNamara, R., Chen, G., and Lenox, R.H. Signalling pathways in the brain: cellular transduction of mood stabilization in the treatment of manic-depressive illness. *Aust. N.Z. J. Psychiatry,* **1999b,** *33*(suppl):S65–S83.

Manji, H.K., Moore, G.J., and Chen, G. Lithium at 50: have the neuroprotective effects of this unique cation been overlooked? *Biol. Psychiatry,* **1999c,** *46:*929–940.

Manji, H.K., Quiroz, J.A., Payne, J.L., *et al.* The underlying neurobiology of bipolar disorder. *World Psychiatry,* **2003,** *2:*137–146.

Manji, H.K., and Zarate, C.A. Molecular and cellular mechanisms underlying mood stabilization in bipolar disorder: implications for the development of improved therapeutics. *Mol. Psychiatry,* **2002,** *7*(suppl 1):S1–S7.

Marder, S.R. Antipsychotic medications. In, *The American Psychiatric Press Textbook of Psychopharmacology.* (Schatzberg, A.F., and Nemeroff, C.B., eds.) American Psychiatric Press, Washington, D.C., **1998,** pp. 309–321.

Mitchell, P.B., Hadzi-Pavlovic, D., and Manji, H.K., eds. Fifty years of treatment for bipolar disorder: a celebration of John Cade's discovery. *Aust. N.Z. J. Psychiatry,* **1999,** *33*(suppl):S1–S122.

Miyamoto, S., Duncan, G.E., Marx, C.E., and Lieberman, J.A. Treatments for schizophrenia: a critical review of pharmacology and mechanisms of action of antipsychotic drugs. *Mol. Psychiatry,* **2005,** *10:*79–104.

Morselli, P.L. Psychotropic drugs. In, *Drug Disposition During Development.* (Morselli, P.L., ed.) Halsted Press, New York, **1977,** pp. 431–474.

Neumeyer, J.L., and Booth, R.G. Neuroleptics and anxiolytic agents. In, *Principles of Medicinal Chemistry,* 4th ed. (Foye, W.O., Williams, D.A., and Lemke, T.L., eds.) Lippincott Williams & Wilkins, Philadelphia, **2002,** pp. 408–433.

Neumeyer, J.L., Booth, R.G., and Baldessarini, R.J. Therapeutic and diagnostic agents for Parkinson's disease. Chapter 12 in Vol. 6. (Abraham, D. ed.) *Burger's Medicinal Chemistry and Drug Discovery,* 6th ed. Wiley, New York, **2003,** pp. 711–741.

Neve, K.A., and Neve, R.L., eds. *The Dopamine Receptors.* Humana Press, Totowa, N.J., **1997.**

Owens, M.J., and Risch, S.C. Atypical antipsychotics. In, *The American Psychiatric Press Textbook of Psychopharmacology* (Schatzberg, A.F., and Nemeroff, C.B., eds.) American Psychiatric Press, Washington, D.C., **1998,** pp. 323–348.

Post, R.M. Psychopharmacology of mood-stabilizers. In, *Schizophrenia and Mood Disorders: The New Drug Therapies in Clinical Practice.* (Buckley, P.F., and Waddington, J.L., eds.) Butterworth-Heinemann, Boston, **2000,** pp. 127–154.

Prien, R.F. Chemotherapy in chronic organic brain syndrome: a review of the literature. *Psychopharmacol. Bull.,* **1973,** *9:*5–20.

Rivera-Calimlim, L., and Hershey, L. Neuroleptic concentrations and clinical response. *Annu. Rev. Pharmacol. Toxicol.,* **1984,** *24:*361–386.

Sachar, E.J. Neuroendocrine responses to psychotropic drugs. In, *Psychopharmacology: A Generation of Progress.* (Lipton, M.A., DiMascio, A., and Killam, K.F., eds.) Raven Press, New York, **1978,** pp. 499–507.

Sadock, B.J., and Sadock, V.A., eds. *Kaplan and Sadock's Comprehensive Textbook of Psychiatry,* 7th ed. Lippincott Williams & Wilkins, Philadelphia, **2000.**

Shulman, K., Tohen, M., and Kutcher, S.P., eds. *Mood Disorders Across the Life Span.* Wiley, New York, **1996.**

Swazey, J.P. *Chlorpromazine in Psychiatry: A Study in Therapeutic Innovation.* M.I.T. Press, Cambridge, MA, **1974.**

Tarazi, F.I., and Baldessarini, R.J. Dopamine D$_4$ receptors: significance for molecular psychiatry at the millennium. *Mol. Psychiatry,* **1999,** *4:*529–538.

Thuillier, J. *The Ten Years That Changed the Face of Mental Illness* (Healy, D., translator). Martin Dunitz, London, **1999.**

Tuunainen, A., Wahlbeck, K., and Gilbody, S.M. Newer atypical antipsychotic medication *vs.* clozapine for schizophrenia (Cochrane Review). In, *The Cochrane Library,* John Wiley & Sons, Chichester, UK, Issue 2, **2004.**

United States Pharmacopoeia. *USP DI. Drug Information for the Health Care Provider.* Micromedex, Englewood, CO, **2004.**

Waddington, J., and Casey, D. Comparative pharmacology of classical and novel (second-generation) antipsychotics. In, *Schizophrenia and Mood Disorders: The New Drug Therapies in Clinical Practice.*

(Buckley, P.F., and Waddington, J.L., eds.) Butterworth-Heinemann, Boston, **2000,** pp. 1–13.

Wagstaff, A.J., and Bryson, H.M. Clozapine: a review of its pharmacological properties and therapeutic use. *CNS Drugs,* **1995,** *4:*370–400.

Winans E. Aripiprazole. *Am. J. Health Syst. Pharmacy,* **2003,** *60:*2437–2445.

Wolf, M.E., and Roth, R.H. Dopamine autoreceptors. In, *Dopamine Receptors.* (Creese, I., and Fraser, C.M., eds.) A.R. Liss, New York, **1987,** pp. 45–96.

Worrel, J.A., Marken, P.A., Beckman, S.E., and Ruehter, V.L. The atypical antipsychotic agents: a critical review. *Am. J. Health Syst. Pharm.,* **2000,** *57:*238–255.

Zhang, K., Davids, E., and Baldessarini, R.J. Attention-deficit/hyperactivity disorder (ADHD). In, *Neurological and Psychiatric Disorders: From Bench to Bedside* (Tarazi, F.I., and Schatz, J.A., eds). Humana Press, Totawa, N.J., **2005.**

PHARMACOTHERAPY OF THE EPILEPSIES

James O. McNamara

The epilepsies are common and frequently devastating disorders, affecting approximately 2.5 million people in the United States alone. More than 40 distinct forms of epilepsy have been identified. Epileptic seizures often cause transient impairment of consciousness, leaving the individual at risk of bodily harm and often interfering with education and employment. Therapy is symptomatic in that available drugs inhibit seizures, but neither effective prophylaxis nor cure is available. Compliance with medication is a major problem because of the need for long-term therapy together with unwanted effects of many drugs.

The mechanisms of action of antiseizure drugs fall into three major categories. Drugs effective against the most common forms of epileptic seizures, partial and secondarily generalized tonic-clonic seizures, appear to work by one of two mechanisms. One is to limit the sustained, repetitive firing of neurons, an effect mediated by promoting the inactivated state of voltage-activated Na^+ channels. A second mechanism appears to involve enhanced γ-aminobutyric acid (GABA)–mediated synaptic inhibition, an effect mediated either by a presynaptic or postsynaptic action. Drugs effective against absence seizure, a less common form of epileptic seizure, limit activation of a particular voltage-activated Ca^{2+} channel known as the T current.

Although many treatments are available, much effort is being devoted to novel approaches. Many of these approaches center on elucidating the genetic causes and the cellular and molecular mechanisms by which a normal brain becomes epileptic, insights that promise to provide molecular targets for both symptomatic and preventive therapies.

TERMINOLOGY AND EPILEPTIC SEIZURE CLASSIFICATION

The term *seizure* refers to a transient alteration of behavior due to the disordered, synchronous, and rhythmic firing of populations of brain neurons. The term *epilepsy* refers to a disorder of brain function characterized by the periodic and unpredictable occurrence of seizures. Seizures can be "nonepileptic" when evoked in a normal brain by treatments such as electroshock or chemical convulsants or "epileptic" when occurring without evident provocation. Pharmacological agents in current clinical use inhibit seizures, and thus are referred to as antiseizure drugs. Whether any of these prevent the development of epilepsy (epileptogenesis) is uncertain.

Seizures are thought to arise from the cerebral cortex, and not from other central nervous system (CNS) structures such as the thalamus, brainstem, or cerebellum. Epileptic seizures have been classified into *partial* seizures, those beginning focally in a cortical site, and *generalized* seizures, those that involve both hemispheres widely from the outset (Commission on Classification and Terminology, 1981). The behavioral manifestations of a seizure are determined by the functions normally served by the cortical site at which the seizure arises. For example, a seizure involving motor cortex is associated with clonic jerking of the body part controlled by this region of cortex. A *simple* partial seizure is associated with preservation of consciousness. A *complex* partial seizure is associated with impairment of consciousness. The majority of complex partial seizures originate from the temporal lobe. Examples of generalized seizures include absence, myoclonic, and tonic-clonic. The type of epileptic seizure is one determinant of the drug selected for therapy. More detailed information is presented in Table 19–1.

Table 19–1
Classification of Epileptic Seizures

SEIZURE TYPE	FEATURES	CONVENTIONAL ANTISEIZURE DRUGS	RECENTLY DEVELOPED ANTISEIZURE DRUGS
Partial seizures:			
Simple partial	Diverse manifestations determined by the region of cortex activated by the seizure (*e.g.*, if motor cortex representing left thumb, clonic jerking of left thumb results; if somatosensory cortex representing left thumb, paresthesia of left thumb results), lasting approximating 20 to 60 seconds. *Key feature is preservation of consciousness.*	Carbamazepine, phenytoin, valproate	Gabapentin, lamotrigine, levetiracetam, tiagabine, topiramate, zonisamide
Complex partial	Impaired consciousness lasting 30 seconds to 2 minutes, often associated with purposeless movements such as lip smacking or hand wringing.	Carbamazepine, phenytoin, valproate	Gabapentin, lamotrigine, levetiracetam, tiagabine, topiramate, zonisamide
Partial with secondarily generalized tonic-clonic seizure	Simple or complex partial seizure evolves into a tonic-clonic seizure with loss of consciousness and sustained contractions (tonic) of muscles throughout the body followed by periods of muscle contraction alternating with periods of relaxation (clonic), typically lasting 1 to 2 minutes.	Carbamazepine, phenobarbital, phenytoin, primidone, valproate	Gabapentin, lamotrigine, levetiracetam, tiagabine, topiramate, zonisamide
Generalized seizures:			
Absence seizure	Abrupt onset of impaired consciousness associated with staring and cessation of ongoing activities typically lasting less than 30 seconds.	Ethosuximide, valproate	Lamotrigine
Myoclonic seizure	A brief (perhaps a second), shocklike contraction of muscles which may be restricted to part of one extremity or may be generalized.	Valproate	Lamotrigine, topiramate
Tonic-clonic seizure	As described above for partial with secondarily generalized tonic-clonic seizures except that it is not preceded by a partial seizure.	Carbamazepine, phenobarbital, phenytoin, primidone, valproate	Lamotrigine, topiramate

Apart from this epileptic seizure classification, an additional classification specifies *epileptic syndromes,* which refer to a cluster of symptoms frequently occurring together and include seizure types, etiology, age of onset, and other factors (Commission on Classification and Terminology, 1989). More than 40 distinct epileptic syndromes have been identified and categorized into partial *versus* generalized epilepsies. The partial epilepsies may consist of any of the partial seizure types (Table 19–1) and account for roughly 60% of all epilepsies. The etiology commonly consists of a lesion in some part of the cortex, such as a tumor, developmental malformation, damage due to trauma or stroke, etc. Such lesions often are evident on brain magnetic resonance imaging (MRI). Alternatively, the etiology may be genetic. The generalized epilepsies are characterized most commonly by one or more of the generalized seizure types listed in Table 19–1 and account for approximately 40% of all epilepsies. The etiology is usually genetic. The most common generalized epilepsy is referred to as juvenile myoclonic epilepsy, accounting for approximately 10% of all epileptic syndromes. The age of onset is in the early teens, and the condition is characterized by myoclonic, tonic-clonic, and often absence seizures. Like most of the generalized-onset epilepsies, juvenile myoclonic epilepsy is a complex genetic disorder that is probably due to inheritance of multiple susceptibility genes; there is a familial clustering of cases, but the pattern of inheritance is not mendelian. The classification of epileptic syndromes guides clinical assessment and management, and in some instances, selection of antiseizure drugs.

NATURE AND MECHANISMS OF SEIZURES AND ANTISEIZURE DRUGS

Partial Epilepsies. More than a century ago, John Hughlings Jackson, the father of modern concepts of epilepsy, proposed that seizures were caused by "occasional, sudden, excessive, rapid and local discharges of gray matter," and that a generalized convulsion resulted when normal brain tissue was invaded by the seizure activity initiated in the abnormal focus. This insightful proposal provided a valuable framework for thinking about mechanisms of partial epilepsy. The advent of the electroencephalogram (EEG) in the 1930s permitted the recording of electrical activity from the scalp of humans with epilepsy and demonstrated that the epilepsies are disorders of neuronal excitability.

The pivotal role of synapses in mediating communication among neurons in the mammalian brain suggested that defective synaptic function might lead to a seizure. That is, a reduction of inhibitory synaptic activity or enhancement of excitatory synaptic activity might be expected to trigger a seizure; pharmacological studies of seizures supported this notion. The neurotransmitters mediating the bulk of synaptic transmission in the mammalian brain are amino acids, with γ-aminobutyric acid (GABA) and glutamate being the principal inhibitory and excitatory neurotransmitters, respectively (*see* Chapter 12). Pharmacological studies disclosed that *antagonists* of the $GABA_A$ receptor or *agonists* of different glutamate-receptor subtypes (NMDA, AMPA, or *kainic acid*) (*see* Chapter 12) trigger seizures in experimental animals *in vivo*. Conversely, pharmacological agents that enhance GABA-mediated synaptic inhibition suppress seizures in diverse models. Glutamate-receptor antagonists also inhibit seizures in diverse models, including seizures evoked by electroshock and chemical convulsants such as pentylenetetrazol.

Such studies support the idea that pharmacological regulation of synaptic function can regulate the propensity for seizures and

provide a framework for electrophysiological analyses aimed at elucidating the role of both synaptic and nonsynaptic mechanisms in expression of seizures and epilepsy. Progress in techniques of electrophysiology has fostered the progressive refinement of the level of analysis of seizure mechanisms from the EEG to populations of neurons (field potentials) to individual neurons to individual synapses and individual ion channels on individual neurons. Cellular electrophysiological studies of epilepsy over roughly two decades beginning in the mid-1960s were focused on elucidating the mechanisms underlying the *depolarization shift* (DS), the intracellular correlate of the "interictal spike" (Figure 19–1). The interictal (or between-seizures) spike is a sharp waveform recorded in the EEG of patients with epilepsy; it is asymptomatic in that it is accompanied by no detectable change in the patient's behavior. The location of the interictal spike helps localize the brain region from which seizures originate in a given patient. The DS consists of a large depolarization of the neuronal membrane associated with a burst of action potentials. In most cortical neurons, the DS is generated by a large excitatory synaptic current that can be enhanced by activation of voltage-regulated intrinsic membrane currents. Although the mechanisms generating the DS are increasingly understood, it remains unclear whether the interictal spike triggers a seizure, inhibits a seizure, or is an epiphenomenon with respect to seizure occurrence in an epileptic brain. While these questions remain unanswered, study of the mechanisms of DS generation set the stage for inquiry into the cellular mechanisms of a seizure.

During the 1980s, a diversity of *in vitro* models of seizures were developed in isolated brain slice preparations, in which many synaptic connections are preserved. Electrographic events with features similar to those recorded during seizures *in vivo* have been produced in hippocampal slices by multiple methods, including altering ionic constituents of media bathing the brain slices (McNamara, 1994) such as low Ca^{2+}, zero Mg^{2+}, or elevated K^+. The accessibility and experimental control provided by these preparations has permitted mechanistic investigations into the induction of seizures. Analyses of multiple *in vitro* models confirmed the importance of synaptic function in initiation of a seizure, demonstrating that subtle (*e.g.*, 20%) reductions of inhibitory synaptic function could lead to epileptiform activity and that activation of excitatory synapses could be pivotal in seizure initiation. Many other important factors were identified, including the volume of the extracellular space as well as intrinsic properties of a neuron, such as voltage-regulated ion channels including those gating K^+, Na^+, and Ca^{2+} ions (Traynelis and Dingledine, 1988). Identification of these diverse synaptic and nonsynaptic factors controlling seizures *in vitro* provides potential pharmacological targets for regulating seizure susceptibility *in vivo*.

Additional studies have centered on understanding the mechanisms by which a normal brain is transformed into an epileptic brain. Some common forms of partial epilepsy arise months to years after cortical injury sustained as a consequence of stroke, trauma, or other factors. An effective prophylaxis administered to patients at high risk would be highly desirable. The drugs described in this chapter provide symptomatic therapy; that is, the drugs inhibit seizures in patients with epilepsy. No effective antiepileptogenic agent has been identified.

Understanding the mechanisms of epileptogenesis in cellular and molecular terms should provide a framework for development of novel therapeutic approaches. The availability of animal models provides an opportunity to investigate the underlying mechanisms.

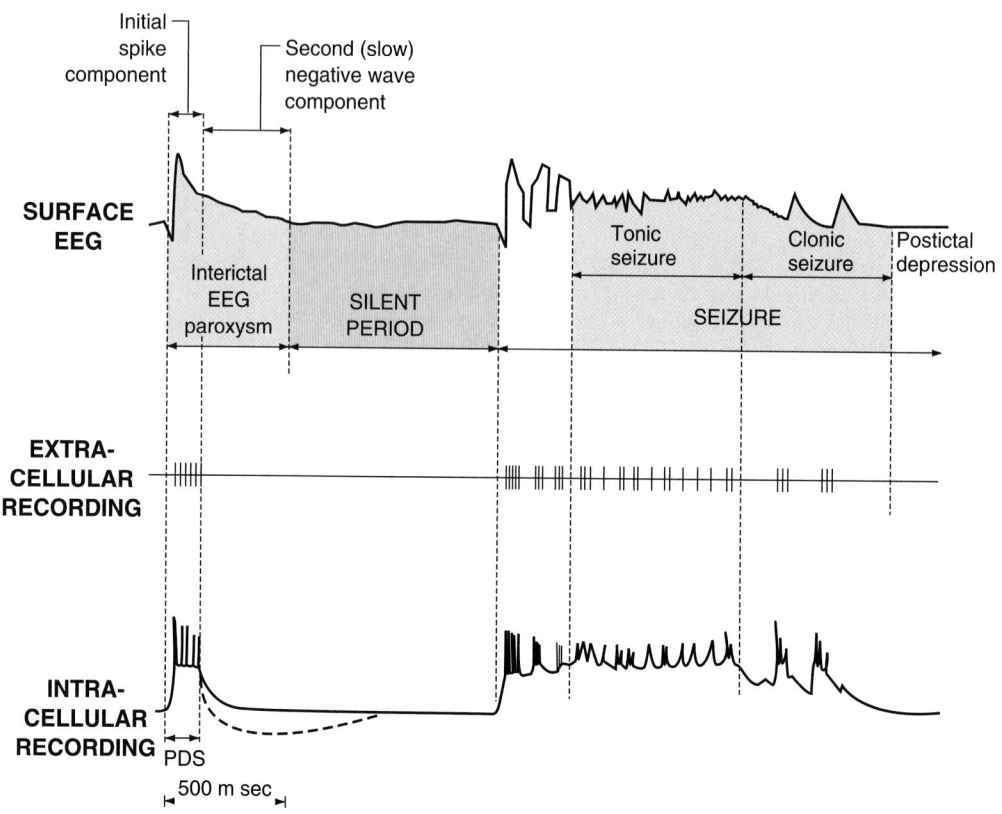

Figure 19–1. *Relations among cortical EEG, extracellular, and intracellular recordings in a seizure focus induced by local application of a convulsant agent to mammalian cortex.* The extracellular recording was made through a high-pass filter. Note the high-frequency firing of the neuron evident in both extracellular and intracellular recording during the paroxysmal depolarization shift (PDS). (Modified with permission from Ayala *et al.*, 1973.)

One model, termed "kindling," is induced by periodic administration of brief, low-intensity electrical stimulation of the amygdala or other limbic structures. Initial stimulations evoke a brief electrical seizure recorded on the EEG without behavioral change, but repeated (*e.g.,* 10 to 20) stimulations result in progressive intensification of seizures, culminating in tonic-clonic seizures. Once established, the enhanced sensitivity to electrical stimulation persists for the life of the animal. Despite the exquisite propensity to intense seizures, spontaneous seizures or a truly epileptic condition do not occur until 100 to 200 stimulations have been administered. The ease of control of kindling induction (*i.e.,* stimulations administered at the investigator's convenience), its graded onset, and the ease of quantitating epileptogenesis (number of stimulations required to evoke tonic-clonic seizures) simplify experimental study. In mice, deletion of the gene encoding the receptor tyrosine kinase, TrkB, prevents epileptogenesis in the kindling model (He *et al.*, 2004), which advances TrkB and its downstream signaling pathways as attractive targets for developing small molecule inhibitors for prevention of epilepsy in individuals at high risk.

Additional models are produced by induction of continuous seizures for hours ("status epilepticus"), with the inciting agent being a chemoconvulsant, such as kainic acid or *pilocarpine*, or sustained electrical stimulation. The fleeting episode of status epilepticus is followed weeks later by the onset of spontaneous seizures, an intriguing parallel to the scenario of complicated febrile seizures in

young children preceding the emergence of spontaneous seizures years later. In contrast to the limited or absent neuronal loss characteristic of the kindling model, overt destruction of hippocampal neurons occurs in the status epilepticus models, reflecting aspects of hippocampal sclerosis observed in humans with severe limbic seizures. Indeed, the recent discovery that complicated febrile seizures precede and presumably are the cause of hippocampal sclerosis in young children (VanLandingham *et al.*, 1998) establishes yet another commonality between these models and the human condition.

Several questions arise with respect to these models. What transpires during the latent period between status epilepticus and emergence of spontaneous seizures that causes the epilepsy? Might similar mechanisms be operative in kindling development and during the latent period following status epilepticus? Might an antiepileptogenic agent that was effective in one of these models be effective in other models?

Important insights into the mechanisms of action of drugs that are effective against partial seizures have emerged in the past two decades (Macdonald and Greenfield, 1997). These insights largely have emerged from electrophysiological studies of relatively simple *in vitro* models, such as neurons isolated from the mammalian CNS and maintained in primary culture. The experimental control and accessibility provided by these models—together with careful attention to clinically relevant concentrations of the drugs—led to clarification of their mechanisms. Although it is difficult to prove unequivocally that a given drug effect observed *in vitro* is both necessary and sufficient to inhibit a seizure in an animal or human being *in vivo*, there is an excellent likelihood that the putative mechanisms identified do in fact underlie the clinically relevant antiseizure effects.

Electrophysiological analyses of individual neurons during a partial seizure demonstrate that the neurons undergo depolarization and fire action potentials at high frequencies (Figure 19–1). This pattern of neuronal firing is characteristic of a seizure and is uncommon during physiological neuronal activity. Thus, selective inhibition of this pattern of firing would be expected to reduce seizures with minimal unwanted effects. *Carbamazepine, lamotrigine, phenytoin,* and *valproic acid* inhibit high-frequency firing at concentrations known to be effective at limiting seizures in humans (Macdonald and Greenfield, 1997). Inhibition of the high-frequency firing is thought to be mediated by reducing the ability of Na$^+$ channels to recover from inactivation (Figure 19–2). That is, depolarization-triggered opening of the Na$^+$ channels in the axonal membrane of a neuron is required for an action potential; after opening, the channels spontaneously close, a process termed *inactivation*. This inactivation is thought to cause the refractory period, a short time after an action potential during which it is not possible to evoke another action potential. Upon recovery from inactivation, the Na$^+$ channels are again poised to participate in another action potential. Because firing at a slow rate permits sufficient time for Na$^+$ channels to recover from inactivation, inactivation has little or no effect on low-frequency firing. However, reducing the rate of recovery of Na$^+$ channels from inactivation would limit the ability of a neuron to fire at high frequencies, an effect that likely underlies the effects of carbamazepine, lamotrigine, phenytoin, *topiramate,* valproic acid, and *zonisamide* against partial seizures.

Insights into mechanisms of seizures suggest that enhancing GABA-mediated synaptic inhibition would reduce neuronal excitability and raise the seizure threshold. Several drugs are thought to inhibit seizures by regulating GABA-mediated synaptic inhibition through an action at distinct sites of the synapse (Macdonald and

Greenfield, 1997). The principal postsynaptic receptor of synaptically released GABA is termed the GABA$_A$ receptor (*see* Chapter 16). Activation of the GABA$_A$ receptor inhibits the postsynaptic cell by increasing the inflow of Cl$^-$ ions into the cell, which tends to hyperpolarize the neuron. Clinically relevant concentrations of both benzodiazepines and barbiturates enhance GABA$_A$ receptor–mediated inhibition through distinct actions on the GABA$_A$ receptor (Figure 19–3), and this enhanced inhibition probably underlies the effectiveness of these compounds against partial and tonic-clonic seizures in humans. At higher concentrations, such as might be used for status epilepticus, these drugs also can inhibit high-frequency firing of action potentials. A second mechanism of enhancing GABA-mediated synaptic inhibition is thought to underlie the antiseizure mechanism of *tiagabine*; tiagabine inhibits the GABA transporter, GAT-1, and reduces neuronal and glial uptake of GABA (Suzdak and Jansen, 1995) (Figure 19–3).

Generalized-Onset Epilepsies: Absence Seizures.
In contrast to partial seizures, which arise from localized regions of the cerebral cortex, generalized-onset seizures arise from the reciprocal firing of the thalamus and cerebral cortex (Huguenard, 1999). Among the diverse forms of generalized seizures, absence seizures have been studied most intensively. The striking synchrony in appearance of generalized seizure discharges in widespread areas of neocortex led to the idea that a structure in the thalamus and/or brainstem (the "centrencephalon") synchronized these seizure discharges. Focus on the thalamus in particular emerged from the demonstration that low-frequency stimulation of midline thalamic structures triggered EEG rhythms in the cortex similar to spike-and-wave discharges characteristic of absence seizures. Intracerebral electrode recordings from humans subsequently demonstrated the presence of thalamic and neocortical involvement in the spike-and-wave discharge of absence seizures.

Many of the structural and functional properties of the thalamus and neocortex that lead to the generalized spike-and-wave discharges have been elucidated (Huguenard, 1999). The EEG hallmark of an absence seizure is generalized spike-and-wave discharges at a frequency of 3 per second (3 Hz). These bilaterally synchronous spike-and-wave discharges, recorded locally from electrodes in both the thalamus and the neocortex, represent oscillations between the thalamus and neocortex. A comparison of EEG and intracellular recordings reveals that the EEG spikes are associated with the firing of action potentials and the following slow wave with prolonged inhibition. These reverberatory, low-frequency rhythms are made possible by a combination of factors, including reciprocal excitatory synaptic connections between the neocortex and thalamus as well as intrinsic properties of neurons in the thalamus (Huguenard, 1999). One intrinsic property of thalamic neurons that is pivotally involved in the generation of the 3-Hz spike-and-wave discharges is a particular form of voltage-regulated Ca^{2+} current, the low threshold ("T") current. In contrast to its small size in most neurons, the T current in many neurons throughout the thalamus has a large amplitude. Indeed, bursts of action potentials in thalamic neurons are mediated

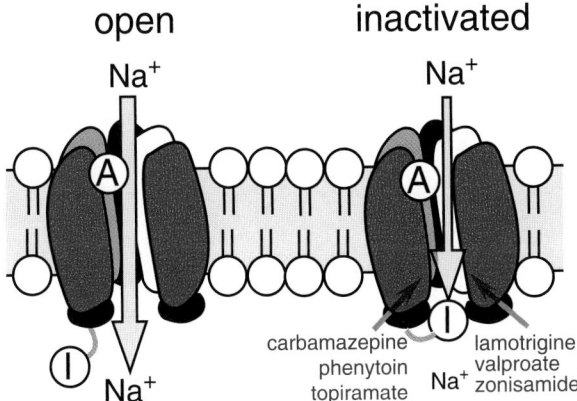

open   **inactivated**

carbamazepine   lamotrigine
phenytoin   valproate
topiramate   zonisamide

Figure 19–2. *Antiseizure drug–enhanced Na$^+$ channel inactivation.* Some antiseizure drugs (shown in blue text) prolong the inactivation of the Na$^+$ channels, thereby reducing the ability of neurons to fire at high frequencies. Note that the inactivated channel itself appears to remain open, but is blocked by the inactivation gate (I). A, activation gate.

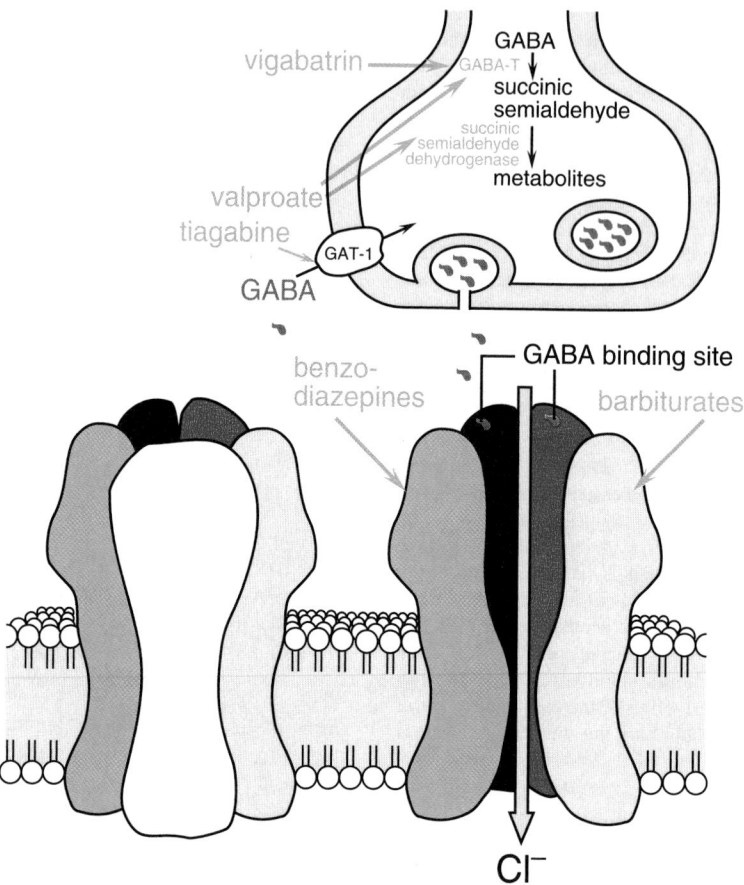

Figure 19–3. Enhanced GABA synaptic transmission. In the presence of GABA, the $GABA_A$ receptor (structure on left) is opened, allowing an influx of Cl⁻, which in turn increases membrane polarization (*see* Chapter 16). Some antiseizure drugs (shown in larger blue text) act by reducing the metabolism of GABA. Others act at the $GABA_A$ receptor, enhancing Cl⁻ influx in response to GABA. As outlined in the text, gabapentin acts presynaptically to promote GABA release; its molecular target is currently under investigation. GABA-T, GABA transaminase; GAT-1, GABA transporter.

by activation of the T current. The T current plays an amplifying role in thalamic oscillations, with one oscillation being the 3-Hz spike-and-wave discharge of the absence seizure. Importantly, the principal mechanism by which anti–absence-seizure drugs (*ethosuximide*, valproic acid) are thought to act is by inhibition of the T current (Figure 19–4) (Macdonald and Kelly, 1993). Thus, inhibiting voltage-regulated ion channels is a common mechanism of action of antiseizure drugs, with anti–partial-seizure drugs inhibiting voltage-activated Na⁺ channels and anti–absence-seizure drugs inhibiting voltage-activated Ca^{2+} channels.

Genetic Approaches to the Epilepsies. Genetic caus-es contribute to a wide diversity of human epilepsies. Genetic causes are solely responsible for some rare forms inherited in an autosomal dominant or autosomal reces-sive manner. Genetic causes also are mainly responsible for some more common forms such as juvenile myoclonic epilepsy (JME) or childhood absence epilepsy (CAE), the majority of which are likely due to inheritance of two or

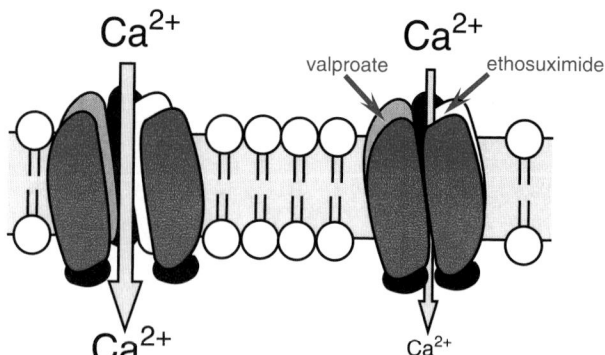

Figure 19–4. Antiseizure drug–induced reduction of cur-rent through T-type Ca^{2+} channels. Some antiseizure drugs (shown in blue text) reduce the flow of Ca^{2+} through T-type Ca^{2+} channels (*see* Chapter 12), thus reducing the pacemaker current that underlies the thalamic rhythm in spikes and waves seen in generalized absence seizures.

more susceptibility genes. Genetic determinants also may contribute some degree of risk to epilepsies caused by injury of the cerebral cortex.

Enormous progress has been made in understanding the genetics of mammalian epilepsy. Mutant genes have been identified for a number of symptomatic epilepsies, in which the epilepsy seems to be a manifestation of some profound neurodegenerative disease. Because most patients with epilepsy are neurologically normal, elucidating the mutant genes underlying familial epilepsy in otherwise normal individuals is of particular interest; this led to the successful identification of 11 distinct genes implicated in distinct, albeit rare idiopathic epilepsy syndromes that account for less than 1% of all of the human epilepsies. Interestingly, almost all of the mutant genes encode ion channels that are gated by voltage or ligands (Scheffer and Berkovic, 2003). Mutations have been identified in voltage-gated sodium and potassium channels and in channels gated by GABA and acetylcholine. The genotype-phenotype correlations of these genetic syndromes are complex; the same mutation in one channel can be associated with divergent clinical syndromes ranging from simple febrile seizures to intractable seizures with intellectual decline. Conversely, clinically indistinguishable epilepsy syndromes have been associated with mutation of distinct genes. The implication of genes encoding ion channels in familial epilepsy is particularly interesting because episodic disorders involving other organs also result from mutations of these genes. For example, episodic disorders of the heart (cardiac arrhythmias), skeletal muscle (periodic paralyses), cerebellum (episodic ataxia), vasculature (familial hemiplegic migraine), and other organs all have been linked to mutations in genes encoding components of voltage-gated ion channels (Ptacek, 1997).

The cellular electrophysiological consequences of some of these mutations exhibit an intriguing relationship to mechanisms of seizures and antiseizure drugs. For example, generalized epilepsy with febrile seizures (GEFS+) is caused by a point mutation in the β subunit of a voltage-gated Na^+ channel ($SCN1B$). As described previously, several antiseizure drugs act on Na^+ channels to promote their inactivation; the phenotype of the mutated Na^+ channel appears to involve defective inactivation (Wallace et al., 1998).

In no instance is it clear how a genotype leads to the epileptic phenotype, but the generation of mice with mutations in candidate genes should provide powerful tools with which to elucidate how the genotype produces the phenotype. The known human mutated channels, however, suggest some intriguing molecular targets for development of antiseizure drugs acting by novel mechanisms. Moreover, it seems likely that many additional epilepsy genes will be identified.

ANTISEIZURE DRUGS: GENERAL CONSIDERATIONS

History. The first antiepileptic drug was *bromide*, which was used in the late nineteenth century. *Phenobarbital* was the first synthetic organic agent recognized as having antiseizure activity. Its usefulness, however, was limited to generalized tonic clonic seizures, and to a lesser degree, simple and complex partial seizures. It had no effect on absence seizures. Merritt and Putnam developed the electroshock seizure test in experimental animals to screen chemical agents for antiseizure effectiveness; in the course of screening a variety of drugs, they discovered that *diphenylhydantoin* (later renamed phenytoin) suppressed seizures in the absence of sedative effects. The electroshock seizure test is extremely valuable, because drugs that are effective against tonic hindlimb extension induced by electroshock generally have proven to be effective against partial and tonic-clonic seizures in humans. Another screening test, seizures induced by the chemoconvulsant pentylenetetrazol, is most useful in identifying drugs that are effective against myoclonic seizures in humans. These screening tests are still used. The chemical structures of most of the drugs introduced before 1965 were closely related to phenobarbital. These included the hydantoins and the succinimides. Between 1965 and 1990, the chemically distinct structures of the benzodiazepines, an iminostilbene (carbamazepine), and a branched-chain carboxylic acid (valproic acid) were introduced, followed in the 1990s by a phenyltriazine (lamotrigine), a cyclic analog of GABA (*gabapentin*), a sulfamate-substituted monosaccharide (*topiramate*), a nipecotic acid derivative (*tiagabine*), and a pyrrolidine derivative (*levetiracetam*).

Therapeutic Aspects. The ideal antiseizure drug would suppress all seizures without causing any unwanted effects. Unfortunately, the drugs used currently not only fail to control seizure activity in some patients, but frequently cause unwanted effects that range in severity from minimal impairment of the CNS to death from aplastic anemia or hepatic failure. The clinician who treats patients with epilepsy is thus faced with the task of selecting the appropriate drug or combination of drugs that best controls seizures in an individual patient at an acceptable level of untoward effects. As a general rule, complete control of seizures can be achieved in up to 50% of patients, while another 25% can be improved significantly. The degree of success varies as a function of seizure type, cause, and other factors.

To minimize toxicity, treatment with a single drug is preferred. If seizures are not controlled with the initial agent at adequate plasma concentrations, substitution of a second drug is preferred to the concurrent administration of another agent. However, multiple-drug therapy may be required, especially when two or more types of seizure occur in the same patient.

Measurement of drug concentrations in plasma facilitates optimizing antiseizure medication, especially when therapy is initiated, after dosage adjustments, in the event of therapeutic failure, when toxic effects appear, or when multiple-drug therapy is instituted. However, clinical effects of some drugs do not correlate well with their concentrations in plasma, and recommended concentrations are only guidelines for therapy. The ultimate therapeutic regimen must be determined by clinical assessment of effect and toxicity.

The general principles of the drug therapy of the epilepsies are summarized below, following discussion of the individual agents.

HYDANTOINS

Phenytoin

Phenytoin (diphenylhydantoin, DILANTIN) is effective against all types of partial and tonic-clonic seizures but not absence seizures. Properties of other hydantoins (*ethotoin*, PEGANONE) are described in previous editions of this book.

History. Phenytoin was first synthesized in 1908 by Biltz, but its anticonvulsant activity was not discovered until 1938. In contrast to the earlier accidental discovery of the antiseizure properties of bromide and phenobarbital, phenytoin was the product of a search among nonsedative structural relatives of phenobarbital for agents capable of suppressing electroshock convulsions in laboratory animals. It was introduced for the treatment of epilepsy in the same year. Since this agent is not a sedative in ordinary doses, it established that antiseizure drugs need not induce drowsiness and encouraged the search for drugs with selective antiseizure action.

Structure–Activity Relationship. Phenytoin has the following structural formula:

PHENYTOIN

A 5-phenyl or other aromatic substituent appears essential for activity against generalized tonic-clonic seizures. Alkyl substituents in position 5 contribute to sedation, a property absent in phenytoin. The carbon 5 position permits asymmetry, but there appears to be little difference in activity between isomers.

Pharmacological Effects. Central Nervous System.
Phenytoin exerts antiseizure activity without causing general depression of the CNS. In toxic doses, it may produce excitatory signs and at lethal levels a type of decerebrate rigidity.

The most significant effect of phenytoin is its ability to modify the pattern of maximal electroshock seizures. The characteristic tonic phase can be abolished completely, but the residual clonic seizure may be exaggerated and prolonged. This seizure-modifying action is observed with many other antiseizure drugs that are effective against generalized tonic-clonic seizures. By contrast, phenytoin does not inhibit clonic seizures evoked by pentylenetetrazol.

Mechanism of Action. Phenytoin limits the repetitive firing of action potentials evoked by a sustained depolarization of mouse spinal cord neurons maintained *in vitro* (McLean and Macdonald, 1986b). This effect is mediated by a slowing of the rate of recovery of voltage-activated Na^+ channels from inactivation, an action that is both voltage- (greater effect if membrane is depolarized) and use-dependent. These effects of phenytoin are evident at concentrations in the range of therapeutic drug levels in cerebrospinal fluid (CSF) in humans, which correlate with the free (or unbound) concentration of phenytoin in the serum. At these concentrations, the effects on Na^+ channels are selective, and no changes of spontaneous activity or responses to iontophoretically applied GABA or glutamate are detected. At concentrations five- to tenfold higher, multiple effects of phenytoin are evident, including reduction of spontaneous activity and enhancement of responses to GABA; these effects may underlie some of the unwanted toxicity associated with high levels of phenytoin.

Pharmacokinetic Properties. Phenytoin is available in two types of oral formulations that differ in their pharmacokinetics: rapid-release and extended-release forms. Once-daily dosing is possible only with the extended-release formulations, and due to differences in dissolution and other formulation-dependent factors, the plasma phenytoin level may change when converting from one formulation to another. Confusion also can arise because different formulations can include either phenytoin or phenytoin sodium. Therefore, comparable doses can be approximated by considering "phenytoin equivalents," but serum level monitoring is also necessary to assure therapeutic safety.

The pharmacokinetic characteristics of phenytoin are influenced markedly by its binding to serum proteins, by the nonlinearity of its elimination kinetics, and by its metabolism by CYPs. Phenytoin is extensively bound (about 90%) to serum proteins, mainly albumin. Small variations in the percentage of phenytoin that is bound dramatically affect the absolute amount of free (active) drug; increased proportions of free drug are evident in the neonate, in patients with hypoalbuminemia, and in uremic patients. Some agents, such as *valproate*, can compete with phenytoin for binding sites on plasma proteins; when combined with valproate-mediated inhibition of phenytoin metabolism, marked increases in free phenytoin can

Table 19–2
Interactions of Antiseizure Drugs with Hepatic Microsomal Enzymes[*]

DRUG	INDUCES CYP	INDUCES UGT	INHIBITS CYP	INHIBITS UGT	METABOLIZED BY CYP	METABOLIZED BY UGT
Carbamazepine	2C9;3A families	Yes			1A2;2C8;2C9;3A4	No
Ethosuximide	No	No	No	No	Uncertain	Uncertain
Gabapentin	No	No	No	No	No	No
Lamotrigine	No	Yes	No	No	No	Yes
Levetiracetam	No	No	No	No	No	No
Oxcarbazepine	3A4/5	Yes	2C19	Weak	No	Yes
Phenobarbital	2C;3A families	Yes	Yes	No	2C9;2C19	No
Phenytoin	2C;3A families	Yes	Yes	No	2C9;2C19	No
Primidone	2C;3A families	Yes	Yes	No	C9;2C19	No
Tiagabine	No	No	No	No	3A4	No
Topiramate	No	No	2C19	No		
Valproate	No	No	2C9	Yes	2C9;2C19	Yes
Zonisamide	No	No	No	No	3A4	Yes

[*]CYP, cytochrome P450; UGT, uridine diphosphate-glucuronosyltransferase. SOURCE: Based on Anderson, 1998.

result. Measurement of free rather than total phenytoin permits direct assessment of this potential problem in patient management.

Phenytoin is one of the few drugs for which the rate of elimination varies as a function of its concentration (*i.e.,* the rate is nonlinear). The plasma half-life of phenytoin ranges between 6 and 24 hours at plasma concentrations below 10 μg/ml but increases with higher concentrations; as a result, plasma drug concentration increases disproportionately as dosage is increased, even with small adjustments for levels near the therapeutic range.

The majority (95%) of phenytoin is metabolized principally in the hepatic endoplasmic reticulum by CYP2C9/10 and to a lesser extent CYP2C19 (Table 19–2). The principal metabolite, a parahydroxyphenyl derivative, is inactive. Because its metabolism is saturable, other drugs that are metabolized by these enzymes can inhibit the metabolism of phenytoin and increase its plasma concentration. Conversely, the degradation rate of other drugs that are substrates for these enzymes can be inhibited by phenytoin; one such drug is *warfarin*, and addition of phenytoin to a patient receiving warfarin can lead to bleeding disorders (*see* Chapter 54). An alternative mechanism of drug interactions arises from phenytoin's ability to induce diverse CYPs (*see* Chapter 3); coadministration of phenytoin and medications metabolized by these enzymes can lead to an increased degradation of such medications. Of particular note in this regard are oral contraceptives, which are metabolized by CYP3A4; treatment with phenytoin could enhance the metabolism of oral contraceptives and lead to unplanned pregnancy. The potential teratogenic effects of phenytoin underscore the importance of attention to this interaction. Carbamazepine, *oxcarbazepine*, phenobarbital, and *primidone* also can induce CYP3A4 and likewise might increase degradation of oral contraceptives.

The low aqueous solubility of phenytoin hindered its intravenous use and led to production of *fosphenytoin,* a water-soluble prodrug. Fosphenytoin (CEREBYX) is converted into phenytoin by phosphatases in liver and red blood cells with a half-life of 8 to 15 minutes. Fosphenytoin is extensively bound (95% to 99%) to human plasma proteins, primarily albumin. This binding is saturable and fosphenytoin displaces phenytoin from protein binding sites. Fosphenytoin is useful for adults with partial or generalized seizures when intravenous or intramuscular administration is indicated.

Toxicity. The toxic effects of phenytoin depend on the route of administration, the duration of exposure, and the dosage.

When fosphenytoin, the water-soluble prodrug, is administered intravenously at an excessive rate in the emergency treatment of status epilepticus, the most notable toxic signs are cardiac arrhythmias, with or without hypotension, and/or CNS depression. Although cardiac toxicity occurs more frequently in older patients and in those with known cardiac disease, it also can develop in young, healthy patients. These complications can be minimized by administering fosphenytoin at a rate of less than 150 mg of phenytoin sodium equivalents per minute, a rate that therefore should not be exceeded. Acute oral overdosage results primarily in signs referable to the cerebellum and vestibular system; high doses have been associated with marked cerebellar atrophy. Toxic effects associated with chronic treatment also are primarily dose-related cerebellar-vestibular effects but also include other CNS effects, behavioral changes, increased frequency of seizures, gastrointestinal symptoms, gingival hyperplasia, osteomalacia, and megaloblastic anemia. Hirsutism is an annoying untoward effect in young females. Usually, these phenomena can be diminished by proper adjustment of dosage. Serious adverse effects, including those on the skin, bone marrow, and liver, probably are manifestations of drug allergy. Although rare, they necessitate withdrawal of the drug. Moderate elevation of the plasma concentrations of hepatic transaminases sometimes are observed; since these changes are transient and may result in part from induced synthesis of the enzymes, they do not necessitate withdrawal of the drug.

Gingival hyperplasia occurs in about 20% of all patients during chronic therapy and is probably the most common manifestation of phenytoin toxicity in children and young adolescents. It may be more frequent in those individuals who also develop coarsened facial features. The overgrowth of tissue appears to involve altered collagen metabolism. Toothless portions of the gums are not affected. The condition does not necessarily require withdrawal of medication and can be minimized by good oral hygiene.

A variety of endocrine effects have been reported. Inhibition of release of antidiuretic hormone (ADH) has been observed in patients with inappropriate ADH secretion. Hyperglycemia and glycosuria appear to be due to inhibition of insulin secretion. Osteomalacia, with hypocalcemia and elevated alkaline phosphatase activity, has been attributed to both altered metabolism of vitamin D and the attendant inhibition of intestinal absorption of Ca^{2+}. Phenytoin also increases the metabolism of vitamin K and reduces the concentration of vitamin K–dependent proteins that are important for normal Ca^{2+} metabolism in bone. This may explain why the osteomalacia is not always ameliorated by the administration of vitamin D.

Hypersensitivity reactions include morbilliform rash in 2% to 5% of patients and occasionally more serious skin reactions, including Stevens-Johnson syndrome. Systemic lupus erythematosus and potentially fatal hepatic necrosis have been reported rarely. Hematological reactions include neutropenia and leukopenia. A few instances of red-cell aplasia, agranulocytosis, and mild thrombocytopenia also have been reported. Lymphadenopathy, resembling Hodgkin's disease and malignant lymphoma, is associated with reduced immunoglobulin A (IgA) production. Hypoprothrombinemia and hemorrhage have occurred in the newborns of mothers who received phenytoin during pregnancy; vitamin K is effective treatment or prophylaxis.

Plasma Drug Concentrations. A good correlation usually is observed between the total concentration of phenytoin in plasma and its clinical effect. Thus, control of seizures generally is obtained with con-

centrations above 10 μg/ml, while toxic effects such as nystagmus develop at concentrations around 20 μg/ml.

Drug Interactions. Concurrent administration of any drug metabolized by CYP2C9 or CYP2C10 can increase the plasma concentration of phenytoin by decreasing its rate of metabolism. Carbamazepine, which may enhance the metabolism of phenytoin, causes a well-documented *decrease* in phenytoin concentration. Conversely, phenytoin reduces the concentration of carbamazepine. Interaction between phenytoin and phenobarbital is variable.

Therapeutic Uses. *Epilepsy.* Phenytoin is one of the more widely used antiseizure agents, and it is effective against partial and tonic-clonic but not absence seizures. The use of phenytoin and other agents in the therapy of epilepsies is discussed further at the end of this chapter. Phenytoin preparations differ significantly in bioavailability and rate of absorption. In general, patients should consistently be treated with the same drug from a single manufacturer. However, if it becomes necessary to temporarily switch between products, care should be taken to select a therapeutically equivalent product and patients should be monitored for loss of seizure control or onset of new toxicities.

Other Uses. Some cases of trigeminal and related neuralgias appear to respond to phenytoin, but carbamazepine may be preferable. The use of phenytoin in the treatment of cardiac arrhythmias is discussed in Chapter 34.

ANTISEIZURE BARBITURATES

The pharmacology of the barbiturates as a class is considered in Chapter 16; discussion in this chapter is limited to the two barbiturates used for therapy of the epilepsies.

Phenobarbital

Phenobarbital (LUMINAL, others) was the first effective organic antiseizure agent. It has relatively low toxicity, is inexpensive, and is still one of the more effective and widely used drugs for this purpose.

Structure–Activity Relationship. The structural formula of phenobarbital (5-phenyl-5-ethylbarbituric acid) is shown in Chapter 16. The structure–activity relationships of the barbiturates have been studied extensively. Maximal antiseizure activity is obtained when one substituent at carbon 5 position is a phenyl group. The 5,5-diphenyl derivative has less antiseizure potency than does phenobarbital, but it is virtually devoid of hypnotic activity. By contrast, 5,5-dibenzyl barbituric acid causes convulsions.

Antiseizure Properties. Most barbiturates have antiseizure properties. However, only some of these agents, such as phenobarbital, exert maximal antiseizure action at doses below those required for hypnosis, which determines their clinical utility as antiseizure agents. Phenobarbital is active in most antiseizure tests in animals but is relatively nonselective. It inhibits tonic hindlimb extension in the maximal electroshock model, clonic seizures evoked by pentylenetetrazol, and kindled seizures.

Mechanism of Action. The mechanism by which phenobarbital inhibits seizures likely involves potentiation of synaptic inhibition through an action on the $GABA_A$ receptor. Intracellular recordings of mouse cortical or spinal cord neurons demonstrated that phenobarbital enhances responses to iontophoretically applied GABA. These effects have been observed at therapeutically relevant concentrations of phenobarbital. Analyses of single channels in outside-out patches isolated from mouse spinal cord neurons demonstrated that phenobarbital increased the $GABA_A$ receptor–mediated current by increasing the duration of bursts of $GABA_A$ receptor–mediated currents without changing the frequency of bursts (Twyman *et al.*, 1989). At levels exceeding therapeutic concentrations, phenobarbital also limits sustained repetitive firing; this may underlie some of the antiseizure effects of higher concentrations of phenobarbital achieved during therapy of status epilepticus.

Pharmacokinetic Properties. Oral absorption of phenobarbital is complete but somewhat slow; peak concentrations in plasma occur several hours after a single dose. It is 40% to 60% bound to plasma proteins and bound to a similar extent in tissues, including brain. Up to 25% of a dose is eliminated by pH-dependent renal excretion of the unchanged drug; the remainder is inactivated by hepatic microsomal enzymes, principally CYP2C9, with minor metabolism by CYP2C19 and CYP2E1. Phenobarbital induces uridine diphosphate-glucuronosyltransferase (UGT) enzymes as well as the CYP2C and CYP3A subfamilies. Drugs metabolized by these enzymes can be more rapidly degraded when coadministered with phenobarbital; importantly, oral contraceptives are metabolized by CYP3A4.

Toxicity. Sedation, the most frequent undesired effect of phenobarbital, is apparent to some extent in all patients upon initiation of therapy, but tolerance develops during chronic medication. Nystagmus and ataxia occur at excessive dosage. Phenobarbital sometimes produces irritability and hyperactivity in children, and agitation and confusion in the elderly.

Scarlatiniform or morbilliform rash, possibly with other manifestations of drug allergy, occurs in 1% to 2% of patients. Exfoliative dermatitis is rare. Hypoprothrombinemia with hemorrhage has been observed in the newborns of mothers who have received phenobarbital during pregnancy; vitamin K is effective for treatment or prophylaxis. As with phenytoin, megaloblastic anemia that responds to folate and osteomalacia that responds to high doses of vitamin D occur during chronic phenobarbital therapy of epilepsy. Other adverse effects of phenobarbital are discussed in Chapter 16.

Plasma Drug Concentrations. During long-term therapy in adults, the plasma concentration of phenobarbital averages 10 μg/ml per daily dose of 1 mg/kg; in children, the value is 5 to 7 μg/ml per 1 mg/kg. Although a precise relationship between therapeutic results and concentration of drug in plasma does not exist, plasma concentrations of 10 to 35 μg/ml are usually recommended for control of seizures.

The relationship between plasma concentration of phenobarbital and adverse effects varies with the development of tolerance. Sedation, nystagmus, and ataxia usually are absent at concentrations below 30 μg/ml during long-term therapy, but adverse effects may be apparent for several days at lower concentrations when therapy is initiated or whenever the dosage is increased. Concentrations greater than 60 μg/ml may be associated with marked intoxication in the nontolerant individual.

Since significant behavioral toxicity may be present despite the absence of overt signs of toxicity, the tendency to maintain patients, particularly children, on excessively high doses of phenobarbital should be resisted. The plasma phenobarbital concentration should be increased above 30 to 40 μg/ml only if the increment is adequately tolerated and only if it contributes significantly to control of seizures.

Drug Interactions. Interactions between phenobarbital and other drugs usually involve induction of the hepatic CYPs by phenobarbital (*see* Chapters 3 and 16). The variable interaction with phenytoin has been discussed above. Concentrations of phenobarbital in plasma may be elevated by as much as 40% during concurrent administration of valproic acid (*see* below).

Therapeutic Uses. Phenobarbital is an effective agent for generalized tonic-clonic and partial seizures. Its efficacy, low toxicity, and low cost make it an important agent for these types of epilepsy. However, its sedative effects and its tendency to disturb behavior in children have reduced its use as a primary agent.

Mephobarbital (MEBARAL) is *N*-methylphenobarbital. It is *N*-demethylated in the hepatic endoplasmic reticulum, and most of its activity during long-term therapy can be attributed to the accumulation of phenobarbital. Consequently, the pharmacological properties, toxicity, and clinical uses of mephobarbital are the same as those for phenobarbital.

IMINOSTILBENES

Carbamazepine

Carbamazepine (TEGRETOL, CARBATROL, others) was initially approved in the United States for use as an antiseizure agent in 1974. It has been employed since the 1960s for the treatment of trigeminal neuralgia. It is now considered to be a primary drug for the treatment of partial and tonic-clonic seizures.

Chemistry. Carbamazepine is related chemically to the tricyclic antidepressants. It is a derivative of iminostilbene with a carbamyl group at the 5 position; this moiety is essential for potent antiseizure activity. The structural formula of carbamazepine is:

CARBAMAZEPINE

Pharmacological Effects. Although the effects of carbamazepine in animals and humans resemble those of phenytoin in many ways, the two drugs exhibit important differences. Carbamazepine has been found to produce therapeutic responses in manic-depressive patients, including some in whom lithium carbonate is not effective. Further, carbamazepine has antidiuretic effects that are sometimes associated with reduced concentrations of antidiuretic hormone (ADH) in plasma. The mechanisms responsible for these effects of carbamazepine are not clearly understood.

Mechanism of Action. Like phenytoin, carbamazepine limits the repetitive firing of action potentials evoked by a sustained depolarization of mouse spinal cord or cortical neurons maintained *in vitro* (McLean and Macdonald, 1986b). This appears to be mediated by a slowing of the rate of recovery of voltage-activated Na^+ channels from inactivation. These effects of carbamazepine are evident at concentrations in the range of therapeutic drug levels in CSF in humans. The effects of carbamazepine are selective at these concentrations, in that there are no effects on spontaneous activity or on responses to iontophoretically applied GABA or glutamate. The carbamazepine metabolite, 10,11-epoxycarbamazepine, also limits sustained repetitive firing at therapeutically relevant concentrations, suggesting that this metabolite may contribute to the antiseizure efficacy of carbamazepine.

Pharmacokinetic Properties.

The pharmacokinetics of carbamazepine are complex. They are influenced by its limited aqueous solubility and by the ability of many antiseizure drugs, including carbamazepine itself, to increase their conversion to active metabolites by hepatic oxidative enzymes.

Carbamazepine is absorbed slowly and erratically after oral administration. Peak concentrations in plasma usually are observed 4 to 8 hours after oral ingestion, but may be delayed by as much as 24 hours, especially following the administration of a large dose. The drug distributes rapidly into all tissues. Approximately 75% of carbamazepine binds to plasma proteins and concentrations in the CSF appear to correspond to the concentration of free drug in plasma.

The predominant pathway of metabolism in humans involves conversion to the 10,11-epoxide. This metabolite is as active as the parent compound in various animals, and its concentrations in plasma and brain may reach 50% of those of carbamazepine, especially during the concurrent administration of phenytoin or phenobarbital. The 10,11-epoxide is metabolized further to inactive compounds, which are excreted in the urine principally as glucuronides. Carbamazepine also is inactivated by conjugation and hydroxylation. Hepatic CYP3A4 is primarily responsible for biotransformation of carbamazepine. Carbamazepine induces CYP2C, CYP3A, and UGT, thus enhancing the metabolism of drugs degraded by these enzymes. Of particular importance in this regard are oral contraceptives, which are also metabolized by CYP3A4.

Toxicity. Acute intoxication with carbamazepine can result in stupor or coma, hyperirritability, convulsions, and respiratory depression. During long-term therapy, the more frequent untoward effects of the drug include drowsiness, vertigo, ataxia, diplopia, and blurred vision. The frequency of seizures may increase, especially with overdosage. Other adverse effects include nausea, vomiting, serious hematological toxicity (aplastic anemia, agranulocytosis), and hypersensitivity reactions (dermatitis, eosinophilia, lymphadenopathy, splenomegaly). A late complication of therapy with carbamazepine is retention of water, with decreased osmolality and concentration of Na^+ in plasma, especially in elderly patients with cardiac disease.

Some tolerance develops to the neurotoxic effects of carbamazepine, and they can be minimized by gradual increase in dosage or adjustment of maintenance dosage. Various hepatic or pancreatic abnormalities have been reported during therapy with carbamazepine, most commonly a transient elevation of hepatic transaminases in plasma in 5% to 10% of patients. A transient, mild leukopenia occurs in about 10% of patients during initiation of therapy and usually resolves within the first 4 months of continued treatment; transient thrombocytopenia also has been noted. In about 2% of patients, a persistent leukopenia may develop that requires withdrawal of the drug. The initial concern that aplastic anemia might be a frequent complication of long-term therapy with carbamazepine has not materialized. In most cases, the administration of multiple drugs or the presence of another underlying disease has made it difficult to establish a causal relationship. In any event, the prevalence of aplastic anemia appears to be about 1 in 200,000 patients who are treated with the drug. It is not clear whether monitoring of hematological function can avert the development of irreversible aplastic anemia. Although carbamazepine is carcinogenic in rats, it is not known to be carcinogenic in humans. The induction of fetal malformations during the treatment of pregnant women is discussed below.

Plasma Drug Concentrations. There is no simple relationship between the dose of carbamazepine and concentrations of the drug in plasma. Therapeutic concentrations are reported to be 6 to 12 μg/ml, although considerable variation occurs. Side effects referable to the CNS are frequent at concentrations above 9 μg/ml.

Drug Interactions. Phenobarbital, phenytoin, and valproate may increase the metabolism of carbamazepine by inducing CYP3A4; carbamazepine may enhance the biotransformation of phenytoin. Concurrent administration of carbamazepine may lower concentrations of valproate, lamotrigine, tiagabine, and topiramate. Carbamazepine reduces both the plasma concentration and therapeutic effect of *haloperidol*. The metabolism of carbamazepine may be inhibited by *propoxyphene, erythromycin, cimetidine, fluoxetine,* and *isoniazid.*

Therapeutic Uses. Carbamazepine is useful in patients with generalized tonic-clonic and both simple and complex partial seizures. When it is used, renal and hepatic function and hematological parameters should be monitored. The therapeutic use of carbamazepine is discussed further at the end of this chapter.

Carbamazepine was introduced by Blom in the early 1960s and is now the primary agent for treatment of trigeminal and glossopharyngeal neuralgias. It is also effective for lightning tabetic pain associated with bodily wasting. Most patients with neuralgia benefit initially, but only 70% obtain continuing relief. Adverse effects have required discontinuation of medication in 5% to 20% of patients. The therapeutic range of plasma concentrations for antiseizure therapy serves as a guideline for its use in neuralgia. Carbamazepine also has found use in the treatment of bipolar affective disorders, as discussed further in Chapter 18.

Oxcarbazepine

Oxcarbazepine (TRILEPTAL) (10,11-dihydro-10-oxocarbamazepine) is a keto analog of carbamazepine. Oxcarbazepine functions as a prodrug, in that it is almost immediately converted to its main active metabolite, a 10-monohydroxy derivative, which is inactivated by glucuronide conjugation and eliminated by renal excretion. Its mechanism of action is similar to that of carbamazepine. Oxcarbazepine is a less potent enzyme inducer than is carbamazepine, and substitution of oxcarbazepine for carbamazepine is associated with increased levels of phenytoin and valproic acid, presumably because of reduced induction of hepatic enzymes. Oxcarbazepine does not induce the hepatic enzymes involved in its own degradation. Although oxcarbazepine does not appear to reduce the anticoagulant effect of warfarin, it does induce CYP3A and thus reduces plasma levels of steroid oral contraceptives. It has been approved for monotherapy or adjunct therapy for partial seizures in adults and as adjunctive therapy for partial seizures in children ages 4 to 16.

SUCCINIMIDES

Ethosuximide

Ethosuximide (ZARONTIN) is a primary agent for the treatment of absence seizures.

Structure–Activity Relationship. Ethosuximide has the following structural formula:

ETHOSUXIMIDE

The structure–activity relationship of the succinimides is in accord with that for other antiseizure classes. *Methsuximide* (CELONTIN) has phenyl substituents and is more active against maximal electroshock seizures. It is no longer in common use. Discussion of its properties can be found in previous editions of this book. Ethosuximide, with alkyl substituents, is the most active of the succinimides against seizures induced by pentylenetetrazol and is the most selective for absence seizures.

Pharmacological Effects. The most prominent characteristic of ethosuximide at nontoxic doses is protection against clonic motor seizures induced by pentylenetetrazol. By contrast, at nontoxic doses ethosuximide does not inhibit tonic hindlimb extension of electroshock seizures or kindled seizures. This profile correlates with efficacy against absence seizures in humans.

Mechanism of Action. Ethosuximide reduces low threshold Ca^{2+} currents (T currents) in thalamic neurons (Coulter *et al.*, 1989). The thalamus plays an important role in generation of 3-Hz spike-and-wave rhythms typical of absence seizures (Coulter, 1998). Neurons in the thalamus exhibit a large-amplitude T-current spike that underlies bursts of action potentials and likely plays an important role in thalamic oscillatory activity such as 3-

Hz spike-and-wave activity. At clinically relevant concentrations, ethosuximide inhibits the T current, as is evident in voltage-clamp recordings of acutely isolated, ventrobasal thalamic neurons from rats and guinea pigs. Ethosuximide reduces this current without modifying the voltage dependence of steady-state inactivation or the time course of recovery from inactivation. By contrast, succinimide derivatives with convulsant properties do not inhibit this current. Ethosuximide does not inhibit sustained repetitive firing or enhance GABA responses at clinically relevant concentrations. Current data are consistent with the idea that inhibition of T currents is the mechanism by which ethosuximide inhibits absence seizures.

Pharmacokinetic Properties. Absorption of ethosuximide appears to be complete, with peak concentrations in plasma within about 3 hours after a single oral dose. Ethosuximide is not significantly bound to plasma proteins; during long-term therapy, its concentration in the CSF is similar to that in plasma. The apparent volume of distribution averages 0.7 L/kg.

Approximately 25% of the drug is excreted unchanged in the urine. The remainder is metabolized by hepatic microsomal enzymes, but whether CYPs are responsible is unknown. The major metabolite, the hydroxyethyl derivative, accounts for about 40% of administered drug, is inactive, and is excreted as such and as the glucuronide in the urine. The plasma half-life of ethosuximide averages between 40 and 50 hours in adults and approximately 30 hours in children.

Toxicity. The most common dose-related side effects are gastrointestinal complaints (nausea, vomiting, and anorexia) and CNS effects (drowsiness, lethargy, euphoria, dizziness, headache, and hiccough). Some tolerance to these effects develops. Parkinsonlike symptoms and photophobia also have been reported. Restlessness, agitation, anxiety, aggressiveness, inability to concentrate, and other behavioral effects have occurred primarily in patients with a prior history of psychiatric disturbance.

Urticaria and other skin reactions, including Stevens-Johnson syndrome, as well as systemic lupus erythematosus, eosinophilia, leukopenia, thrombocytopenia, pancytopenia, and aplastic anemia also have been attributed to the drug. The leukopenia may be transient despite continuation of the drug, but several deaths have resulted from bone marrow depression. Renal or hepatic toxicity has not been reported.

Plasma Drug Concentrations. During long-term therapy, the plasma concentration of ethosuximide averages

about 2 μg/ml per daily dose of 1 mg/kg. A plasma concentration of 40 to 100 μg/ml usually is required for satisfactory control of absence seizures.

Therapeutic Uses. Ethosuximide is effective against absence seizures but not tonic-clonic seizures.

An initial daily dose of 250 mg in children (3 to 6 years old) and 500 mg in older children and adults is increased by 250-mg increments at weekly intervals until seizures are adequately controlled or toxicity intervenes. Divided dosage is required occasionally to prevent nausea or drowsiness associated with once-daily dosing. The usual maintenance dose is 20 mg/kg per day. Increased caution is required if the daily dose exceeds 1500 mg in adults or 750 to 1000 mg in children. The use of ethosuximide and the other antiseizure agents is discussed further at the end of the chapter.

VALPROIC ACID

The antiseizure properties of valproic acid (DEPAKENE, others) were discovered serendipitously when it was employed as a vehicle for other compounds that were being screened for antiseizure activity.

Chemistry. Valproic acid (*n*-dipropylacetic acid) is a simple branched-chain carboxylic acid; its structural formula is:

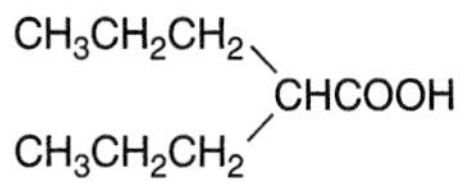

$$CH_3CH_2CH_2\diagdown$$
$$CHCOOH$$
$$CH_3CH_2CH_2\diagup$$

VALPROIC ACID

Certain other branched-chain carboxylic acids have potencies similar to that of valproic acid in antagonizing pentylenetetrazol-induced convulsions. However, increasing the number of carbon atoms to nine introduces marked sedative properties. Straight-chain acids have little or no activity.

Pharmacological Effects. Valproic acid is strikingly different from phenytoin or ethosuximide in that it is effective in inhibiting seizures in a variety of models. Like phenytoin and carbamazepine, valproate inhibits tonic hindlimb extension in maximal electroshock seizures and kindled seizures at nontoxic doses. Like ethosuximide, valproic acid at subtoxic doses inhibits clonic motor seizures induced by pentylenetetrazol. Its efficacy in diverse models parallels its efficacy against absence as well as partial and generalized tonic-clonic seizures in humans.

Mechanism of Action. Valproic acid produces effects on isolated neurons similar to those of phenytoin and ethosuximide. At therapeutically relevant concentrations, valproate inhibits sustained repetitive firing induced by depolarization of mouse cortical or spinal cord neurons (McLean and Macdonald, 1986a). The action is similar to that of both phenytoin and carbamazepine and appears to be mediated by a prolonged recovery of voltage-activated Na^+ channels from inactivation. Valproic acid does not modify neuronal responses to iontophoretically applied GABA. In neurons isolated from the nodose ganglion, valproate also produces small reductions of the low-threshold (T) Ca^{2+} current (Kelly *et al.*, 1990) at clinically relevant but slightly higher concentrations than those that limit sustained repetitive firing; this effect on T currents is similar to that of ethosuximide in thalamic neurons (Coulter *et al.*, 1989). Together, these actions of limiting sustained repetitive firing and reducing T currents may contribute to the effectiveness of valproic acid against partial and tonic-clonic seizures and absence seizures, respectively.

Another potential mechanism that may contribute to valproate's antiseizure actions involves metabolism of GABA. Although valproate has no effect on responses to GABA, it does increase the amount of GABA that can be recovered from the brain after the drug is administered to animals. *In vitro,* valproate can stimulate the activity of the GABA synthetic enzyme, glutamic acid decarboxylase, and inhibit GABA degradative enzymes, GABA transaminase and succinic semialdehyde dehydrogenase. Thus far it has been difficult to relate the increased GABA levels to the antiseizure activity of valproate.

Pharmacokinetic Properties. Valproic acid is absorbed rapidly and completely after oral administration. Peak concentration in plasma is observed in 1 to 4 hours, although this can be delayed for several hours if the drug is administered in enteric-coated tablets or is ingested with meals. The apparent volume of distribution for valproate is about 0.2 L/kg. Its extent of binding to plasma proteins is usually about 90%, but the fraction bound is reduced as the total concentration of valproate is increased through the therapeutic range. Although concentrations of valproate in CSF suggest equilibration with free drug in the blood, there is evidence for carrier-mediated transport of valproate both into and out of the CSF.

The vast majority of valproate (95%) undergoes hepatic metabolism, with less than 5% excreted unchanged in urine. Its hepatic metabolism occurs mainly by UGT enzymes and β-oxidation. Valproate is a substrate for CYP2C9 and CYP2C19, but metabolism by these enzymes accounts for a relatively minor portion of its elimination. Some of the drug's metabolites, notably 2-propyl-2-pentenoic acid and 2-propyl-4-pentenoic acid, are nearly as potent antiseizure agents as the parent compound; however, only the former (2-en-valproic acid) accumulates in plasma and brain to a potentially significant extent. The half-life of valproate is approximately 15 hours but is reduced in patients taking other antiepileptic drugs.

Toxicity. The most common side effects are transient gastrointestinal symptoms, including anorexia, nausea, and vomiting in about 16% of patients. Effects on the CNS include sedation, ataxia, and tremor; these symptoms occur infrequently and usually respond to a decrease in dosage. Rash, alopecia, and stimulation of appetite have been observed occasionally and weight gain has been seen with chronic valproic acid treatment in some patients. Valproic acid has several effects on hepatic function. Elevation of hepatic transaminases in plasma is observed in up to 40% of patients and often occurs asymptomatically during the first several months of therapy.

A rare complication is a fulminant hepatitis that is frequently fatal (Dreifuss *et al.*, 1989). Pathological examination reveals a microvesicular steatosis without evidence of inflammation or hypersensitivity reaction. Children below 2 years of age with other medical conditions who were given multiple antiseizure agents were especially likely to suffer fatal hepatic injury. At the other extreme, there were no deaths reported for patients over the age of 10 years who received only valproate. Acute pancreatitis and hyperammonemia also have been frequently associated with the use of valproic acid. Valproic acid can also produce teratogenic effects such as neural tube defects.

Plasma Drug Concentrations. The concentration of valproate in plasma that is associated with therapeutic effects is approximately 30 to 100 μg/ml. However, there is a poor correlation between the plasma concentration and efficacy. There appears to be a threshold at about 30 to 50 μg/ml; this is the concentration at which binding sites on plasma albumin begin to become saturated.

Drug Interactions. Valproate primarily inhibits the metabolism of drugs that are substrates for CYP2C9, including phenytoin and phenobarbital. Valproate also inhibits UGT and thus inhibits the metabolism of lamotrigine and lorazepam. A high proportion of valproate is bound to albumin, and the high molar concentrations of valproate in the clinical setting result in valproate's displacing phenytoin and other drugs from albumin. With respect to phenytoin in particular, valproate's inhibition of the drug's metabolism is exacerbated by displacement of phenytoin from albumin. The concurrent administration of valproate and *clonazepam* has been associated with the development of absence status epilepticus; however, this complication appears to be rare.

Therapeutic Uses. Valproate is effective in the treatment of absence, myoclonic, partial, and tonic-clonic seizures. The initial daily dose usually is 15 mg/kg, increased at weekly intervals by 5 to 10 mg/kg per day to a maximum daily dose of 60 mg/kg. Divided doses should be given when the total daily dose exceeds 250 mg. The therapeutic uses of valproate in epilepsy are discussed further at the end of this chapter.

BENZODIAZEPINES

The benzodiazepines are employed clinically primarily as sedative-antianxiety drugs; their pharmacology is described in Chapters 16 and 17. Discussion here is limited to consideration of their usefulness in the therapy of the epilepsies. A large number of benzodiazepines have broad antiseizure properties, but only clonazepam (KLONOPIN) and *clorazepate* (TRANXENE-SD, others) have been approved in the United States for the long-term treatment of certain types of seizures. *Diazepam* (VALIUM, DIASTAT; others) and *lorazepam* (ATIVAN) have well-defined roles in the management of status epilepticus. The structures of the benzodiazepines are shown in Chapter 16.

Antiseizure Properties. In animals, prevention of pentylenetetrazol-induced seizures by the benzodiazepines is much more prominent than is their modification of the maximal electroshock seizure pattern. Clonazepam is unusually potent in antagonizing the effects of pentylenetetrazol, but it is almost without action on seizures induced by maximal electroshock. Benzodiazepines, including clonazepam, suppress the spread of kindled seizures and generalized convulsions produced by stimulation of the amygdala, but do not abolish the abnormal discharge at the site of stimulation.

Mechanism of Action. The antiseizure actions of the benzodiazepines, as well as other effects that occur at nonsedating doses, result in large part from their ability to enhance GABA-mediated synaptic inhibition. Molecular cloning and study of recombinant receptors have demonstrated that the benzodiazepine receptor is an integral part of the $GABA_A$ receptor (*see* Chapter 16). At therapeutically relevant concentrations, benzodiazepines act at subsets of $GABA_A$ receptors and increase the frequency, but not duration, of openings at GABA-activated Cl^- channels (Twyman *et al.*, 1989). At higher concentrations, diazepam and many other benzodiazepines can reduce sustained high-frequency firing of neurons, similar to the effects of phenytoin, carbamazepine, and valproate. Although these concentrations correspond to concentrations achieved in patients during treatment of status epilepticus with diazepam, they are considerably higher than those associated with antiseizure or anxiolytic effects in ambulatory patients.

Pharmacokinetic Properties. Benzodiazepines are well absorbed after oral administration, and concentrations in plasma are usually maximal within 1 to 4 hours. After intravenous administration, they are redistributed in a manner typical of that for highly lipid-soluble agents (*see* Chapter 1). Central effects develop promptly, but wane rapidly as the drugs move to other tissues. Diazepam is redistributed especially rapidly, with a half-life of redistribution of about 1 hour. The extent of

binding of benzodiazepines to plasma proteins correlates with lipid solubility, ranging from approximately 99% for diazepam to about 85% for clonazepam (*see* Appendix II).

The major metabolite of diazepam, *N*-desmethyl-diazepam, is somewhat less active than the parent drug and may behave as a partial agonist. This metabolite also is produced by the rapid decarboxylation of clorazepate following its ingestion. Both diazepam and *N*-desmethyl-diazepam are slowly hydroxylated to other active metabolites, such as *oxazepam*. The half-life of diazepam in plasma is between 1 and 2 days, while that of *N*-desmethyl-diazepam is about 60 hours. Clonazepam is metabolized principally by reduction of the nitro group to produce inactive 7-amino derivatives. Less than 1% of the drug is recovered unchanged in the urine. The half-life of clonazepam in plasma is about 1 day. Lorazepam is metabolized chiefly by conjugation with glucuronic acid; its half-life in plasma is about 14 hours.

Toxicity. The principal side effects of long-term oral therapy with clonazepam are drowsiness and lethargy. These occur in about 50% of patients initially, but tolerance often develops with continued administration. Muscular incoordination and ataxia are less frequent. Although these symptoms usually can be kept to tolerable levels by reducing the dosage or the rate at which it is increased, they sometimes force drug discontinuation. Other side effects include hypotonia, dysarthria, and dizziness. Behavioral disturbances, especially in children, can be very troublesome; these include aggression, hyperactivity, irritability, and difficulty in concentration. Both anorexia and hyperphagia have been reported. Increased salivary and bronchial secretions may cause difficulties in children. Seizures are sometimes exacerbated, and status epilepticus may be precipitated if the drug is discontinued abruptly. Other aspects of the toxicity of the benzodiazepines are discussed in Chapter 16. Cardiovascular and respiratory depression may occur after the intravenous administration of diazepam, clonazepam, or lorazepam, particularly if other antiseizure agents or central depressants have been administered previously.

Plasma Drug Concentrations. Because tolerance affects the relationship between drug concentration and drug antiseizure effect, plasma concentrations of benzodiazepines are of limited value.

Therapeutic Uses. Clonazepam is useful in the therapy of absence seizures as well as myoclonic seizures in children. However, tolerance to its antiseizure effects usually develops after 1 to 6 months of administration, after which some patients will no longer respond to clonazepam at any dosage. The initial dose of clonazepam for adults should not exceed 1.5 mg per day and for children 0.01 to 0.03 mg/kg per day. The dose-dependent side effects are reduced if two or three divided doses are given each day. The dose may be increased every 3 days in amounts of 0.25 to 0.5 mg per day in children and 0.5 to 1 mg per day in adults. The maximal recommended dose is 20 mg per day for adults and 0.2 mg/kg per day for children.

While diazepam is an effective agent for treatment of status epilepticus, its short duration of action is a disadvantage, leading to the more frequent use of lorazepam. Although diazepam is not useful as an oral agent for the treatment of seizure disorders, clorazepate is effective in combination with certain other drugs in the treatment of partial seizures. The maximal initial dose of clorazepate is 22.5 mg per day in three portions for adults and 15 mg per day in two doses in children. Clorazepate is not recommended for children under the age of 9.

OTHER ANTISEIZURE DRUGS

Gabapentin

Gabapentin (NEURONTIN) is an antiseizure drug that consists of a GABA molecule covalently bound to a lipophilic cyclohexane ring. Gabapentin was designed to be a centrally active GABA agonist, with its high lipid solubility aimed at facilitating its transfer across the blood–brain barrier. The structure of gabapentin is:

$$H_2N \qquad COOH$$

GABAPENTIN

Pharmacological Effects and Mechanisms of Action. Gabapentin inhibits tonic hindlimb extension in the electroshock seizure model. Interestingly, gabapentin also inhibits clonic seizures induced by pentylenetetrazol. Its efficacy in both these tests parallels that of valproic acid and distinguishes it from phenytoin and carbamazepine. The anticonvulsant mechanism of action of gabapentin is unknown. Despite its design as a GABA agonist, gabapentin does not mimic GABA when iontophoretically applied to neurons in primary culture. Gabapentin may promote nonvesicular release of GABA through a poorly understood mechanism (Honmou *et al.*, 1995). Gabapentin binds a protein in cortical membranes with an amino acid sequence identical to that of the $\alpha2\delta$ subunit of the L type of voltage-sensitive Ca^{2+} channel, yet gabapentin does not affect Ca^{2+} currents of the T, N, or L types of Ca^{2+} channels in dorsal root ganglion cells (Macdonald and Greenfield, 1997). Gabapentin has not been found consistently to reduce sustained repetitive firing of action potentials (Macdonald and Kelly, 1993).

Pharmacokinetics. Gabapentin is absorbed after oral administration and is not metabolized in humans. It is not bound to plasma proteins. It is excreted unchanged, mainly in the urine. Its half-life, when it is used as monotherapy, is 4 to 6 hours. It has no known interactions with other antiseizure drugs.

Therapeutic Uses. Gabapentin is effective for partial seizures, with and without secondary generalization, when used in addition to other antiseizure drugs.

Double-blind placebo-controlled trials of adults with refractory partial seizures demonstrated that addition of gabapentin to other antiseizure drugs was superior to placebo (Sivenius *et al.*, 1991). A double-blind study of gabapentin (900 or 1800 mg/day) monotherapy disclosed that gabapentin was equivalent to carbamazepine (600 mg/day) for newly diagnosed partial or generalized epilepsy (Chadwick *et al.*, 1998). Gabapentin also is being used for the treatment of migraine, chronic pain, and bipolar disorder.

Gabapentin usually is effective in doses of 900 to 1800 mg daily in three doses, although 3600 mg may be required in some patients to achieve reasonable seizure control. Therapy usually is begun with a low dose (300 mg once on the first day), which is increased in daily increments of 300 mg until an effective dose is reached.

Toxicity. Overall, gabapentin is well tolerated with the most common adverse effects of somnolence, dizziness, ataxia, and fatigue. These effects usually are mild to moderate in severity but resolve within 2 weeks of onset during continued treatment.

Lamotrigine

Lamotrigine (LAMICTAL) is a phenyltriazine derivative initially developed as an antifolate agent based on the incorrect idea that reducing folate would effectively combat seizures. Structure–activity studies indicate that its effectiveness as an antiseizure drug is unrelated to its antifolate properties (Macdonald and Greenfield, 1997). Approved by the FDA in 1994, its chemical structure is:

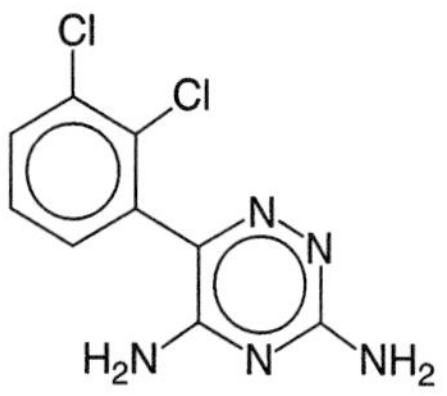

LAMOTRIGINE

Pharmacological Effects and Mechanisms of Action. Lamotrigine suppresses tonic hindlimb extension in the maximal electroshock model and partial and secondarily generalized seizures in the kindling model, but does not inhibit clonic motor seizures induced by pentylenetetrazol. Lamotrigine blocks sustained repetitive firing of mouse spinal cord neurons and delays the recovery from inactivation of recombinant Na^+ channels, mechanisms similar to those of phenytoin and carbamazepine (Xie *et al.*, 1995). This may well explain lamotrigine's actions on partial and secondarily generalized seizures. However, as mentioned below, lamotrigine is effective against a broader spectrum of seizures than phenytoin and carbamazepine, suggesting that lamotrigine may have actions in addition to regulating recovery from inactivation of Na^+ channels. The mechanisms underlying its broad spectrum of actions are incompletely understood. One possibility involves lamotrigine's inhibition of glutamate release in rat cortical slices treated with veratridine, a Na^+ channel activator, raising the possibility that lamotrigine inhibits synaptic release of glutamate by acting at Na^+ channels themselves.

Pharmacokinetics. Lamotrigine is completely absorbed from the gastrointestinal tract and is metabolized primarily by glucuronidation. The plasma half-life of a single dose is 15 to 30 hours. Administration of phenytoin, carbamazepine, or phenobarbital reduces the half-life and plasma concentrations of lamotrigine. Conversely, addition of valproate markedly increases plasma concentrations of lamotrigine, likely by inhibiting glucuronidation. Addition of lamotrigine to valproic acid produces a reduction of valproate concentrations by approximately 25% over a few weeks. Concurrent use of lamotrigine and carbamazepine is associated with increases of the 10,11-epoxide of carbamazepine and clinical toxicity in some patients.

Therapeutic Use. Lamotrigine is useful for monotherapy and add-on therapy of partial and secondarily generalized

tonic-clonic seizures in adults and Lennox-Gastaut syndrome in both children and adults. Lennox-Gastaut syndrome is a disorder of childhood characterized by multiple seizure types, mental retardation, and refractoriness to antiseizure medication.

A double-blind comparison of lamotrigine and carbamazepine monotherapy and also of lamotrigine and phenytoin monotherapy in newly diagnosed partial or generalized tonic-clonic seizures revealed lamotrigine to be equivalent to carbamazepine and phenytoin, respectively (Brodie *et al.*, 1995; Steiner *et al.*, 1999). A double-blind, placebo-controlled trial of addition of lamotrigine to existing antiseizure drugs further demonstrated effectiveness of lamotrigine against tonic-clonic seizures and drop attacks in children with the Lennox-Gastaut syndrome (Motte *et al.*, 1997). Lamotrigine was also found to be superior to placebo in a double-blind study of children with newly diagnosed absence epilepsy (Frank *et al.*, 1999).

Patients who are already taking a hepatic enzyme–inducing antiseizure drug (such as carbamazepine, phenytoin, phenobarbital, or primidone, but not valproate) should be given lamotrigine initially at 50 mg per day for 2 weeks. The dose is increased to 50 mg twice per day for 2 weeks and then increased in increments of 100 mg/day each week up to a maintenance dose of 300 to 500 mg/day divided into two doses. For patients taking valproate in addition to an enzyme-inducing antiseizure drug, the initial dose should be 25 mg every other day for 2 weeks, followed by an increase to 25 mg/day for 2 weeks; the dose then can be increased by 25 to 50 mg/day every 1 to 2 weeks up to a maintenance dose of 100 to 150 mg/day divided into two doses.

Toxicity. The most common adverse effects are dizziness, ataxia, blurred or double vision, nausea, vomiting, and rash when lamotrigine was added to another antiseizure drug. A few cases of Stevens-Johnson syndrome and disseminated intravascular coagulation have been reported. The incidence of serious rash in pediatric patients (approximately 0.8%) is higher than in the adult population (0.3%).

Levetiracetam

Levetiracetam (KEPPRA) is a pyrrolidine, the racemically pure S-enantiomer of α-ethyl-2-oxo-1-pyrrolidineacetamide. Its structure is:

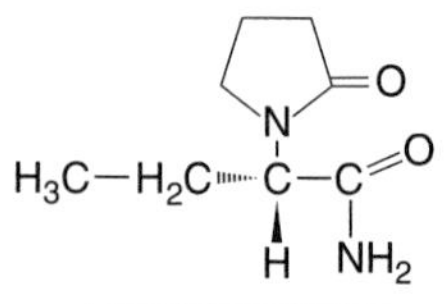

LEVETIRACETAM

Pharmacological Effects and Mechanism of Action. Levetiracetam exhibits a novel pharmacological profile insofar as it inhibits partial and secondarily generalized tonic-clonic seizures in the kindling model, yet is ineffective against maximum electroshock- and pentylene-tetrazol-induced seizures, findings consistent with clinical effectiveness against partial and secondarily generalized tonic-clonic seizures. The mechanism by which levetiracetam exerts these antiseizure effects is unknown. No evidence for an action on voltage-gated Na+ channels or either GABA- or glutamate-mediated synaptic transmission has emerged. A stereoselective binding site has been identified in rat brain membranes and the synaptic vesicle protein SVZA has been shown to be a brain-binding target of levetiracetam (Lynch *et al.*, 2004).

Pharmacokinetics. Levetiracetam is rapidly and almost completely absorbed after oral administration and is not bound to plasma proteins. Ninety-five percent of the drug and its inactive metabolite are excreted in the urine, 65% of which is unchanged drug; 24% of the drug is metabolized by hydrolysis of the acetamide group. It neither induces nor is a high-affinity substrate for CYP isoforms or glucuronidation enzymes and thus is devoid of known interactions with other antiseizure drugs, oral contraceptives, or anticoagulants.

Therapeutic Use. A double-blind, placebo-controlled trial of adults with refractory partial seizures demonstrated that addition of levetiracetam to other antiseizure medications was superior to placebo. Insufficient evidence is available with respect to use of levetiracetam as monotherapy for partial or generalized epilepsy.

Toxicity. The drug is well tolerated. The most frequently reported adverse effects are somnolence, asthenia, and dizziness.

Tiagabine

Tiagabine (GABITRIL) is a derivative of nipecotic acid and was approved by the FDA in 1998 for treating partial seizures in adults when used in addition to other drugs. Its structure is:

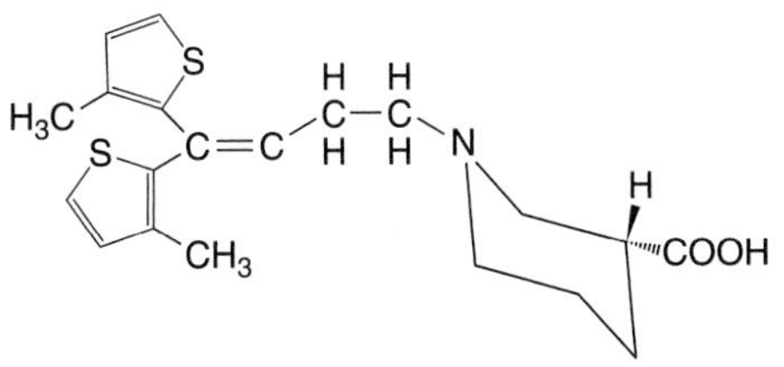

TIAGABINE

Pharmacological Effects and Mechanism of Action. Tiagabine inhibits the GABA transporter, GAT-1, and thereby reduces GABA uptake into neurons and glia. In CA1 neurons of the hippocampus, tiagabine increases the duration of inhibitory synaptic currents, findings consistent with prolonging the effect of GABA at inhibitory synapses through reducing its reuptake by GAT-1. Tiagabine inhibits maximum electroshock seizures and both limbic and secondarily generalized tonic-clonic seizures in the kindling model, results suggestive of clinical efficacy against partial and tonic-clonic seizures.

Pharmacokinetics. Tiagabine is rapidly absorbed after oral administration, extensively bound to serum or plasma proteins, and metabolized mainly in the liver, predominantly by CYP3A. Its half-life of about 8 hours is shortened by 2 to 3 hours when coadministered with hepatic enzyme–inducing drugs such as phenobarbital, phenytoin, or carbamazepine.

Therapeutic Use. Double-blind, placebo-controlled trials have established tiagabine's efficacy as add-on therapy of refractory partial seizures with or without secondary generalization. Its efficacy for monotherapy for newly diagnosed or refractory partial and generalized epilepsy has not been established.

Toxicity. The principal adverse effects include dizziness, somnolence, and tremor; they appear to be mild to moderate in severity and appear shortly after initiation of therapy. The fact that tiagabine and other drugs thought to enhance effects of synaptically released GABA can facilitate spike-and-wave discharges in animal models of absence seizures raises the possibility that tiagabine may be contraindicated in patients with generalized absence epilepsy. Patients with a history of spike-and-wave discharges have been reported to have exacerbations of their EEG abnormalities.

Topiramate

Topiramate (TOPAMAX) is a sulfamate-substituted monosaccharide. Its structure is:

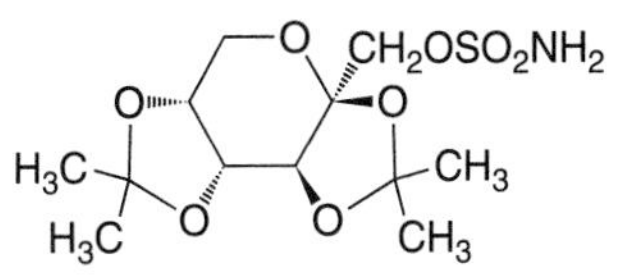

TOPIRAMATE

Pharmacological Effects and Mechanisms of Action. Topiramate reduces voltage-gated Na+ currents in cerebellar granule cells and may act on the inactivated state of the channel in a manner similar to that of phenytoin. In addition, topiramate activates a hyperpolarizing K^+ current, enhances postsynaptic $GABA_A$-receptor currents, and also limits activation of the AMPA-kainate-subtype(s) of glutamate receptor. Topiramate also is a weak carbonic anhydrase inhibitor. Topiramate inhibits maximal electroshock and pentylenetetrazol-induced seizures as well as partial and secondarily generalized tonic-clonic seizures in the kindling model, findings predictive of a broad spectrum of antiseizure actions clinically.

Pharmacokinetics. Topiramate is rapidly absorbed after oral administration, exhibits little (10% to 20%) binding to plasma proteins, and is mainly excreted unchanged in the urine. The remainder undergoes metabolism by hydroxylation, hydrolysis, and glucuronidation with no single metabolite accounting for more than 5% of an oral dose. Its half-life is about 1 day. Reduced estradiol plasma concentrations occur with concurrent topiramate, suggesting the need for higher doses of oral contraceptives when coadministered with topiramate.

Therapeutic Use. A double-blind study revealed topiramate to be equivalent to valproate and carbamazepine in children and adults with newly diagnosed partial and primary generalized epilepsy (Privitera *et al.*, 2003). Additional studies disclosed topiramate to be effective as monotherapy for refractory partial epilepsy (Sachdeo *et al.*, 1997) and refractory generalized tonic-clonic seizures (Biton *et al.*, 1999). Topiramate also was found to be significantly more effective than placebo against both drop attacks and tonic-clonic seizures in patients with Lennox-Gastaut syndrome (Sachdeo *et al.*, 1999).

Toxicity. Topiramate is well tolerated. The most common adverse effects are somnolence, fatigue, weight loss, and nervousness. It can precipitate renal calculi, which is most likely due to inhibition of carbonic anhydrase. Topiramate has been associated with cognitive impairment and patients may complain about a change in the taste of carbonated beverages.

Felbamate

Felbamate (FELBATOL) is a dicarbamate which was approved by the FDA for partial seizures in 1993. An association between felbamate and aplastic anemia in at least 10 cases resulted in a recommendation by the FDA and the manufacturer for the immediate withdrawal

of most patients from treatment with this drug. The structure of felbamate is:

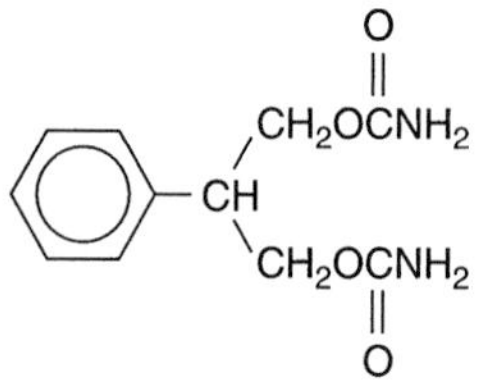

FELBAMATE

Felbamate is effective in both the maximal electroshock and pentylenetetrazol seizure models. Clinically relevant concentrations of felbamate inhibit NMDA-evoked responses and potentiate GABA-evoked responses in whole-cell, voltage-clamp recordings of cultured rat hippocampal neurons (Rho *et al.*, 1994). This dual action on excitatory and inhibitory transmitter responses may contribute to the wide spectrum of action of the drug in seizure models.

An active control, randomized, double-blind protocol demonstrated the efficacy of felbamate in patients with poorly controlled partial and secondarily generalized seizures (Sachdeo *et al.*, 1992). Felbamate also was found to be efficacious against seizures in patients with Lennox-Gastaut syndrome (The Felbamate Study Group in Lennox-Gastaut Syndrome, 1993). The clinical efficacy of this compound, which inhibited responses to NMDA and potentiated those to GABA, underscores the potential value of additional antiseizure agents with similar mechanisms of action.

Zonisamide

Zonisamide (ZONEGRAN) is a sulfonamide derivative with the following chemical structure:

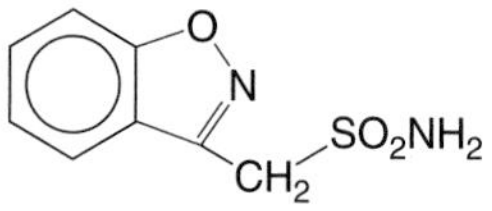

ZONISAMIDE

Pharmacological Effects and Mechanism of Action. Zonisamide inhibits the T-type Ca^{2+} currents. In addition, zonisamide inhibits the sustained, repetitive firing of spinal cord neurons, presumably by prolonging the inactivated state of voltage-gated Na^+ channels in a manner similar to actions of phenytoin and carbamazepine. Zonisamide inhibits tonic hindlimb extension evoked by maximal electroshock and inhibits both partial and secondarily generalized seizures in the kindling model, results predictive of clinical effectiveness against partial and secondarily generalized tonic-clonic seizures. Zonisamide does not inhibit minimal clonic seizures induced by pentylenetetrazol, suggesting that the drug will not be effective clinically against myoclonic seizures.

Pharmacokinetics. Zonisamide is almost completely absorbed after oral administration, has a long half-life (about 63 hours), and is about 40% bound to plasma protein. Approximately 85% of an oral dose is excreted in the urine, principally as unmetabolized zonisamide and a glucuronide of sulfamoylacetyl phenol, which is a product of metabolism by CYP3A4. Phenobarbital, phenytoin, and carbamazepine decrease the plasma concentration/dose ratio of zonisamide, whereas lamotrigine increases this ratio. Conversely, zonisamide has little effect on the plasma concentrations of other antiseizure drugs.

Therapeutic Use. Double-blind, placebo-controlled studies of patients with refractory partial seizures demonstrated that addition of zonisamide to other drugs was superior to placebo. There is insufficient evidence for its efficacy as monotherapy for newly diagnosed or refractory epilepsy.

Toxicity. Overall, zonisamide is well tolerated. The most common adverse effects include somnolence, ataxia, anorexia, nervousness, and fatigue. Approximately 1% of individuals develop renal calculi during treatment with zonisamide, which may relate to its ability to inhibit carbonic anhydrase.

Acetazolamide

Acetazolamide, the prototype for the carbonic anhydrase inhibitors, is discussed in Chapter 28. Its antiseizure actions are discussed in previous editions of this textbook. Although it is sometimes effective against absence seizures, its usefulness is limited by the rapid development of tolerance. Adverse effects are minimal when it is used in moderate dosage for limited periods.

GENERAL PRINCIPLES AND CHOICE OF DRUGS FOR THE THERAPY OF THE EPILEPSIES

Early diagnosis and treatment of seizure disorders with a single appropriate agent offers the best prospect of achieving prolonged seizure-free periods with the lowest risk of toxicity. An attempt should be made to determine the cause of the epilepsy with the hope of discovering a correctable lesion, either structural or metabolic. The drugs commonly used for distinct seizure types are listed in Table 19–1. The efficacy combined with the unwanted effects of a given drug determine which particular drug is optimal for a given patient.

The first issue that arises is whether and when to initiate treatment. For example, it may not be necessary to initiate antiseizure therapy after an isolated tonic-clonic seizure in a healthy young adult who lacks a family history of epilepsy and who has a normal neurological exam, a normal EEG, and a normal brain MRI scan. That is, the odds of seizure recurrence in the next year (15%) approximate the risk of a drug reaction sufficiently severe to warrant discontinuation of medication (Bazil and Pedley, 1998). Alternatively, a similar seizure occurring in an individual with a positive family history of epilepsy, an abnormal neurological exam, an abnormal EEG, and an abnormal MRI carries a risk of recurrence approximating 60%, odds that favor initiation of therapy.

Unless extenuating circumstances such as status epilepticus exist, only monotherapy should be initiated. Initial dosage usually is that expected to provide a plasma drug concentration during the plateau state at least in the lower portion of the range associated with clinical efficacy. To minimize dose-related adverse effects, therapy with many drugs is initiated at reduced dosage. Dosage is increased at appropriate intervals, as required for control of seizures or as limited by toxicity, and such adjustment is preferably assisted by monitoring of drug concentrations in plasma. Compliance with a properly selected, single drug in maximal tolerated dosage results in complete control of seizures in approximately 50% of patients. If a seizure occurs despite optimal drug levels, the physician should assess the presence of potential precipitating factors such as sleep deprivation, a concurrent febrile illness, or drugs; drugs might consist of large amounts of caffeine or even over-the-counter medications, which can include drugs that can lower the seizure threshold.

If compliance has been confirmed yet seizures persist, another drug should be substituted. Unless serious adverse effects of the drug dictate otherwise, dosage always should be reduced gradually when a drug is being discontinued to minimize risk of seizure recurrence. In the case of partial seizures in adults, the diversity of available drugs permits selection of a second drug that acts by a distinct mechanism. Among previously untreated patients, 47% became seizure free with the first drug and an additional 14% became seizure free with a second or third drug (Kwan and Brodie, 2000).

In the event that therapy with a second single drug also is inadequate, many physicians resort to treatment with two drugs simultaneously. This decision should not be taken lightly, because most patients obtain optimal seizure control with fewest unwanted effects when taking a single drug. Nonetheless, some patients will not be controlled adequately without the simultaneous use of two or more antiseizure agents. No properly controlled studies have systematically compared one particular drug combination with another. The chances of complete control with this approach are not high, as evidenced by Kwan and Brodie (2000), who found that epilepsy was controlled by treatment with two drugs in only 3% of patients. It seems wise to select two drugs that act by distinct mechanisms (*e.g.*, one that promotes Na$^+$ channel inactivation and another that enhances GABA-mediated synaptic inhibition). Additional issues that warrant careful consideration are the unwanted effects of each drug and the potential drug interactions. As specified in Table 19–2, many of these drugs induce expression of CYPs and thereby impact the metabolism of themselves and/or other drugs. Overall, drugs introduced after 1990 present fewer problems with respect to drug interactions.

Essential to optimal management of epilepsy is the filling out of a seizure chart by the patient or a relative. Frequent visits to the physician or seizure clinic may be necessary early in the period of treatment, since hematological and other possible side effects may require consideration of a change in medication. Long-term follow-up with neurological examinations and possibly EEG and neuroimaging studies is appropriate. Most crucial for successful management is regularity of medication, since faulty compliance is the most frequent cause for failure of therapy with antiseizure drugs.

Measurement of plasma drug concentration at appropriate intervals greatly facilitates the initial adjustment of dosage for individual differences in drug elimination and the subsequent adjustment of dosage to minimize dose-related adverse effects without sacrifice of seizure control. Periodic monitoring during maintenance therapy can detect failure of the patient to take the medication as prescribed. Knowledge of plasma drug concentration can be especially helpful during multiple-drug therapy. If toxicity occurs, monitoring helps to identify the particular drug(s) responsible, and if pharmacokinetic drug interaction occurs, monitoring can guide readjustment of dosage.

Duration of Therapy. Once initiated, antiseizure drugs are typically continued for at least 2 years. If the patient is seizure free after 2 years, consideration should be given to tapering and discontinuing therapy. Factors associated with high risk for recurrent seizures following discontinuation of therapy include EEG abnormalities, a known structural lesion, abnormalities on neurological exam, and history of frequent seizures or medically refractory seizures prior to control. Conversely, factors associated with low risk for recurrent seizures include idiopathic epilepsy, normal EEG, onset in childhood, and seizures easily controlled with a single drug. The risk of recurrent seizures approximates 25% in low-risk individuals and exceeds 50% in high-risk individuals (Anonymous, 1996). Typically 80% of recurrences will occur within 4 months of discontinuing therapy. The clinician and patient must weigh the risk of recurrent seizure and the associated potential deleterious consequences (*e.g.*, loss of driving privileges) against the various implications of continuing medication including cost, unwanted effects, implications of diagnosis of epi-

lepsy, etc. Any taper ideally is performed slowly over a period of several months.

Simple and Complex Partial and Secondarily Generalized Tonic-Clonic Seizures. The efficacy and toxicity of carbamazepine, phenobarbital, and phenytoin for treatment of partial and secondarily generalized tonic-clonic seizures in adults have been examined in a double-blind prospective study (Mattson *et al.*, 1985). A subsequent double-blind prospective study compared carbamazepine with valproate (Mattson *et al.*, 1992). Carbamazepine and phenytoin were the most effective overall for single-drug therapy of partial or generalized tonic-clonic seizures. The choice between carbamazepine and phenytoin required assessment of toxic effects of each drug. Decreased libido and impotence were associated with all three drugs (carbamazepine 13%, phenobarbital 16%, and phenytoin 11%). The study comparing carbamazepine with valproate revealed that carbamazepine provided superior control of complex partial seizures. With respect to adverse effects, carbamazepine was more commonly associated with skin rash, but valproate was more commonly associated with tremor and weight gain. Overall, the data demonstrated that carbamazepine and phenytoin are preferable for treatment of partial seizures, but phenobarbital and valproic acid are also efficacious.

Control of secondarily generalized tonic-clonic seizures did not differ significantly with carbamazepine, phenobarbital, or phenytoin (Mattson *et al.*, 1985). Valproate was as effective as carbamazepine for control of secondarily generalized tonic-clonic seizures (Mattson *et al.*, 1992). Since secondarily generalized tonic-clonic seizures usually coexist with partial seizures, these data indicate that among drugs introduced before 1990, carbamazepine and phenytoin are the first-line drugs for these conditions.

One key issue confronting the treating physician is the optimal drug for initiating treatment in the patient newly diagnosed with partial or generalized onset epilepsy. At first glance, this issue may appear unimportant because approximately 50% of newly diagnosed patients become seizure free with the first drug, whether old or new drugs are used (Kwan and Brodie, 2000). However, responsive patients typically receive the initial drug for several years, underscoring the importance of proper drug selection. Among the drugs available before 1990, phenytoin, carbamazepine, and phenobarbital induce hepatic CYPs, thereby complicating use of multiple antiseizure drugs as well as impacting metabolism of oral contraceptives, warfarin, and many other drugs. These drugs also enhance metabolism of endogenous compounds including gonadal steroids and vitamin D, potentially impacting reproductive function and bone density. By contrast, most of the newer drugs have little if any effect on the CYPs. Factors arguing against use of recently introduced drugs include higher costs and less clinical experience with the compounds.

Ideally, a prospective study would systematically compare newly introduced antiseizure drugs with drugs available before 1990 in a study design adjusting dose as needed and observing responses for extended periods of time (*e.g.*, 2 years or more), in much the same manner as that used when comparing the older antiseizure drugs with one another as described above (Mattson *et al.*, 1985).

Unfortunately, such a study has not been performed. Many of the studies referenced in description of newer drugs did compare a new with an older antiseizure drug, but study design did not permit declaring a clearly superior drug; moreover, differences in study design and patient populations preclude comparing a new drug with multiple older drugs or with other new drugs. The use of recently introduced antiseizure drugs for newly diagnosed epilepsy was thoughtfully considered following a comprehensive analysis of scientific literature conducted jointly by subcommittees of the American Academy of Neurology and the American Epilepsy Society (French *et al.*, 2004a; French *et al.*, 2004b); these authors concluded that available evidence supported the use of gabapentin, lamotrigine, and topiramate for newly diagnosed partial or mixed seizure disorders. None of these drugs, however, has been approved by the FDA for either of these indications. Insufficient evidence was available on the remaining newly introduced drugs to permit meaningful assessment of their effectiveness for this indication.

Absence Seizures. The best data indicate that ethosuximide and valproate are equally effective in the treatment of absence seizures (Mikati and Browne, 1988). Between 50% and 75% of newly diagnosed patients can be rendered free of seizures following therapy with either drug. In the event that tonic-clonic seizures are present or emerge during therapy, valproate is the agent of first choice. French and others concluded that available evidence indicates that lamotrigine is also effective for newly diagnosed absence epilepsy despite the fact that lamotrigine is not approved for this indication by the FDA.

Myoclonic Seizures. Valproic acid is the drug of choice for myoclonic seizures in the syndrome of juvenile myoclonic epilepsy, in which myoclonic seizures often coexist with tonic-clonic and also absence seizures. No trials have been conducted examining any of the newly introduced drugs for patients with juvenile myoclonic epilepsy or other idiopathic generalized epilepsy syndromes.

Febrile Convulsions. Two to four percent of children experience a convulsion associated with a febrile illness. From 25% to 33% of these children will have another febrile convulsion. Only 2% to 3% become epileptic in later years, a sixfold increase in risk compared with the general population. Several factors are associated with an increased risk of developing epilepsy: preexisting neurological disorder or developmental delay, a family history of epilepsy, or a complicated febrile seizure (*i.e.*, the febrile seizure lasted more than 15 minutes, was one-sided, or was followed by a second seizure in the same day). If all of these risk factors are present, the risk of developing epilepsy is approximately 10%.

Concern regarding the increased risk of developing epilepsy or other neurological sequelae led many physicians to prescribe antiseizure drugs prophylactically after a febrile seizure. Uncertainties regarding the efficacy of prophylaxis for reducing epilepsy combined with substantial side effects of phenobarbital prophylaxis (Farwell *et al.*, 1990) argue against the use of chronic therapy for prophylactic purposes (Freeman, 1992). For children at high risk of developing recurrent febrile seizures and epilepsy, rectally administered diazepam at the time of fever may prevent recurrent seizures and avoid side effects of chronic therapy.

Seizures in Infants and Young Children. Infantile spasms with hypsarrhythmia are refractory to the usual antiseizure agents; *corticotropin* or the glucocorticoids are commonly used. A randomized study found *vigabatrin* (γ-vinyl GABA) to be efficacious in comparison to placebo (Appleton *et al.*, 1999). Constriction of visual fields has been reported in some adults treated with vigabatrin (Miller *et al.*, 1999). The drug received orphan drug status for the treatment of infantile spasms in the United States in 2000 and also is available in other countries.

The Lennox-Gastaut syndrome is a severe form of epilepsy which usually begins in childhood and is characterized by cognitive impairments and multiple types of seizures including tonic-clonic, tonic, atonic, myoclonic, and atypical absence seizures. Addition of lamotrigine to other antiseizure drugs resulted in improved seizure control in comparison to placebo in a double-blind trial (Motte *et al.*, 1997), demonstrating lamotrigine to be an effective and well-tolerated drug for this treatment-resistant form of epilepsy. Felbamate also was found to be effective for seizures in this syndrome, but the occasional occurrence of aplastic anemia has limited its use (French *et al.*, 1999). Topiramate has also been demonstrated to be effective for Lennox-Gastaut syndrome (Sachdeo *et al.*, 1999).

Status Epilepticus and Other Convulsive Emergencies. Status epilepticus is a neurological emergency. Mortality for adults approximates 20% (Lowenstein and Alldredge, 1998). The goal of treatment is rapid termination of behavioral and electrical seizure activity; the longer the episode of status epilepticus is untreated, the more difficult it is to control and the greater the risk of permanent brain damage. Critical to the management is a clear plan, prompt treatment with effective drugs in adequate doses, and attention to hypoventilation and hypotension. Since hypoventilation may result from high doses of drugs used for treatment, it may be necessary to assist respiration temporarily. Drugs should be administered by the intravenous route only. Because of slow and unreliable absorption, the intramuscular route has no place in treatment of status epilepticus. To assess the optimal initial drug regimen, a double-blind, multicenter trial compared four intravenous treatments: diazepam followed by phenytoin; lorazepam; phenobarbital; and phenytoin alone (Treiman *et al.*, 1998). The treatments were shown to have similar efficacies, in that success rates ranged from 44% to 65%, but lorazepam alone was significantly better than phenytoin alone. No significant differences were found with respect to recurrences or adverse reactions.

Antiseizure Therapy and Pregnancy. Use of antiseizure drugs has diverse implications of great importance for the health of women, issues considered in guidelines articulated by the American Academy of Neurology (Morrell, 1998). These issues include interactions with oral contraceptives, potential teratogenic effects, and effects on vitamin K metabolism in pregnant women.

The effectiveness of oral contraceptives appears to be reduced by concomitant use of antiseizure drugs. The failure rate of oral contraceptives is 3.1/100 years in women receiving antiseizure drugs compared to a rate of 0.7/100 years in nonepileptic women. One attractive explanation of the increased failure rate is the increased rate of oral contraceptive metabolism caused by antiseizure drugs that induce hepatic enzymes (Table 19–2); particular caution is needed with antiseizure drugs that induce CYP3A4.

Epidemiological evidence suggests that antiseizure drugs have teratogenic effects. These teratogenic effects add to the deleterious consequences of oral contraceptive failure. Infants of epileptic mothers are at twofold greater risk of major congenital malformations than offspring of nonepileptic mothers (4% to 8% compared to 2% to 4%). These malformations include congenital heart defects, neural tube defects, and others. Inferring causality from the associations found in large epidemiological studies with many uncontrolled variables can be hazardous, but a causal role for antiseizure drugs is suggested by association of congenital defects with higher concentrations of a drug or with polytherapy compared to monotherapy. Phenytoin, carbamazepine, valproate, and phenobarbital all have been associated with teratogenic effects. The antiseizure drugs introduced after 1990 have teratogenic effects in animals but whether such effects occur in humans is yet uncertain. One consideration for a woman with epilepsy who wishes to become pregnant is a trial free of antiseizure drug; monotherapy with careful attention to drug levels is another alternative. Polytherapy with toxic levels should be avoided. Folate supplementation (0.4 mg/day) has been recommended by the U.S. Public Health Service for all women of childbearing age to reduce the likelihood of neural tube defects, and this is appropriate for epileptic women as well.

Antiseizure drugs that induce CYPs have been associated with vitamin K deficiency in the newborn, which can result in a coagulopathy and intracerebral hemorrhage. Treatment with vitamin K_1, 10 mg/day during the last month of gestation, has been recommended for prophylaxis.

BIBLIOGRAPHY

Anderson, G.D. A mechanistic approach to antiepileptic drug interactions. *Ann. Pharmacother.*, **1998**, *32:*554–563.

Appleton, R.E., Peters, A.C., Mumford, J.P., and Shaw, D.E. Randomised, placebo-controlled study of vigabatrin as first-line treatment of infantile spasms. *Epilepsia*, **1999**, *40:*1627–1633.

Ayala, G.F., Dichter, M., Gumnit, R.J., Matsumoto, H., and Spencer, W.A. Genesis of epileptic interictal spikes. New knowledge of cortical feedback systems suggests a neurophysiological explanation of brief paroxysms. *Brain Res.*, **1973**, *52:*1–17.

Biton, V., Montouris, G.D., Ritter, F., *et al.* A randomized, placebo-controlled study of topiramate in primary generalized tonic-clonic seizures: Topiramate YTC Study Group. *Neurology*, **1999**, *52:*1330–1337.

Brodie, M.J., Richens, A., and Yuen, A.W. Double-blind comparison of lamotrigine and carbamazepine in newly diagnosed epilepsy. UK Lamotrigine/Carbamazepine Monotherapy Trial Group. *Lancet*, **1995**, *345:*476–479.

Chadwick, D.W., Anhut, H., Grenier, M.J., *et al.* A double-blind trial of gabapentin monotherapy for newly diagnosed partial seizures: International Gabapentin Monotherapy Study Group 945-77. *Neurology*, **1998**, *51:*1282–1288.

Commission on Classification and Terminology of the International League Against Epilepsy. Proposal for revised clinical and electroencephalographic classification of epileptic seizures. *Epilepsia*, **1981**, *22:*489–501.

Commission on Classification and Terminology of the International League Against Epilepsy. Proposal for revised classification of epilepsies and epileptic syndromes. *Epilepsia*, **1989**, *30:*389–399.

Coulter, D.A., Huguenard, J.R., and Prince, D.A. Characterization of ethosuximide reduction of low-threshold calcium current in thalamic neurons. *Ann. Neurol.*, **1989**, *25:*582–593.

Dreifuss, F.E., Langer, D.H., Moline, K.A., and Maxwell, J.E. Valproic acid hepatic fatalities. II. U.S. experience since 1984. *Neurology*, **1989**, *39:*201–207.

Farwell, J.R., Lee, Y.J., Hirtz, D.G., *et al.* Phenobarbital for febrile seizures—effects on intelligence and on seizure recurrence. *N. Engl. J. Med.*, **1990**, *322:*364–369.

The Felbamate Study Group in Lennox-Gastaut Syndrome. Efficacy of felbamate in childhood epileptic encephalopathy (Lennox-Gastaut syndrome). *N. Engl. J. Med.*, **1993**, *328:*29–33.

Frank, L.M., Enlow, T., Holmes, G.L., *et al.* Lamictal (lamotrigine) monotherapy for typical absence seizure in children. *Epilepsia*, **1999**, *40:*973–979.

He, X.P., Kotloski, R., Nef, S., *et al.* Conditional deletion of TrkB but not BDNF prevents epileptogenesis in the kindling model. *Neuron*, **2004**, *43:*31–42.

Honmou, O., Kocsis, J.D., and Richerson, G.B. Gabapentin potentiates the conductance increase induced by nipecotic acid in CA1 pyramidal neurons *in vitro*. *Epilepsy Res.*, **1995**, *20:*193–202.

Kelly, K.M., Gross, R.A., and Macdonald, R.L. Valproic acid selectively reduces the low-threshold (T) calcium current in rat nodose neurons. *Neurosci. Lett.*, **1990**, *116:*233–238.

Kwan, P., and Brodie, M.J. Early identification of refractory epilepsy. *N. Engl. J. Med.*, **2000**, *342:*314–319.

Lynch, B.A., Lambeng, N., Nocka, K., *et al.* The synaptic vesicle protein SV2A is the binding site for the antiepileptic drug levetiracetam. *Proc. Natl. Acad. Sci. USA.*, **2004**, *101:*9861–9866.

McLean, M.J., and Macdonald, R.L. Carbamazepine and 10,11-epoxycarbamazepine produce use- and voltage-dependent limitation of rapidly firing action potentials of mouse central neurons in cell culture. *J. Pharmacol. Exp. Ther.*, **1986b**, *238:*727–738.

McLean, M.J., and Macdonald, R.L. Sodium valproate, but not ethosuximide, produces use- and voltage-dependent limitation of high-frequency repetitive firing of action potentials of mouse central neurons in cell culture. *J. Pharmacol. Exp. Ther.*, **1986a**, *237:*1001–1011.

Mattson, R.H., Cramer, J.A., and Collins, J.F. A comparison of valproate with carbamazepine for the treatment of complex partial seizures and secondarily generalized tonic-clonic seizures in adults. The Department of Veterans Affairs Epilepsy Cooperative Study No. 264 Group. *N. Engl. J. Med.*, **1992**, *327:*765–771.

Mattson, R.H., Cramer, J.A., Collins, J.F., *et al.* Comparison of carbamazepine, phenobarbital, phenytoin, and primidone in partial and secondarily generalized tonic-clonic seizures. *N. Engl. J. Med.*, **1985**, *313:*145–151.

Miller, N.R., Johnson, M.A., Paul, S.R., *et al.* Visual dysfunction in patients receiving vigabatrin: clinical and electrophysiologic findings. *Neurology*, **1999**, *53:*2082–2087.

Morrell, M.J. Guidelines for the care of women with epilepsy. *Neurology*, **1998**, *51:*S21–S27.

Motte, J., Trevathan, E., Arvidsson, J.F., *et al.* Lamotrigine for generalized seizures associated with the Lennox-Gastaut syndrome. Lamictal Lennox-Gastaut Study Group. *N. Engl. J. Med.*, **1997**, *337:*1807–1812.

Privitera, M.D., Brodie, M.J., Mattson, R.H., *et al.* Topiramate, carbamazepine and valproate monotherapy: double-blind comparison in newly diagnosed epilepsy. *Acta Neurol. Scand.*, **2003**, *107:*165–175.

Ptacek, L.J. Channelopathies: ion channel disorders of muscle as a paradigm for paroxysmal disorders of the nervous system. *Neuromuscul. Disord.*, **1997**, *7:*250–255.

Rho, J.M., Donevan, S.D., and Rogawski, M.A. Mechanism of action of the anticonvulsant felbamate: opposing effects on *N*-methyl-D-aspartate and GABA$_A$ receptors. *Ann. Neurol.*, **1994**, *35:*229–234.

Sachdeo, R.C., Glauser, T.A., Ritter, F., *et al.* A double-blind, randomized trial of topiramate in Lennox-Gastaut syndrome: Topiramate YL Study Group. *Neurology*, **1999**, *52:*1882–1887.

Sachdeo R., Kramer, L.D., Rosenberg, A., and Sachdeo, S. Felbamate monotherapy: controlled trial in patients with partial onset seizures. *Ann. Neurol.*, **1992**, *32:*386–392.

Sachdeo, R.C., Leroy, R.F., Krauss, G.L., *et al.* Tiagabine therapy for complex partial seizures: a dose-frequency study: the Tiagabine Study Group. *Arch. Neurol.*, **1997**, *54:*595–601.

Sivenius, J., Kalviainen, R., Ylinen, A., *et al.* Double-blind study of gabapentin in the treatment of partial seizures. *Epilepsia,* **1991,** *32:*539–542.

Steiner, T.J., Dellaportas, C.I., Findley, L.S., *et al.* Lamotrigine monotherapy in newly diagnosed untreated epilepsy: a double-blind comparison with phenytoin. *Epilepsia,* **1999,** *40:*601–607.

Suzdak, P.D., and Jansen, J.A. A review of the preclinical pharmacology of tiagabine: a potent and selective anticonvulsant GABA uptake inhibitor. *Epilepsia,* **1995,** *36:*612–626.

Traynelis, S.F., and Dingledine, R. Potassium-induced spontaneous electrographic seizures in the rat hippocampal slice. *J. Neurophysiol.,* **1988,** *59:*259–276.

Treiman, D.M., Meyers, P.D., Walton, N.Y., *et al.* A comparison of four treatments for generalized convulsive status epilepticus. Veterans Affairs Status Epilepticus Cooperative Study Group. *N. Engl. J. Med.,* **1998,** *339:*792–798.

Twyman, R.E., Rogers, C.J., and Macdonald, R.L. Differential regulation of γ-aminobutyric acid receptor channels by diazepam and phenobarbital. *Ann. Neurol.,* **1989,** *25:*213–220.

VanLandingham, K.E., Heinz, E.R., Cavazos, J.E., and Lewis, D.V. Magnetic resonance imaging evidence of hippocampal injury after prolonged focal febrile convulsions. *Ann. Neurol.,* **1998,** *43:*413–426.

Wallace, R.H., Wang, D.W., Singh, R., *et al.* Febrile seizures and generalized epilepsy associated with a mutation in the Na$^+$-channel β1 subunit gene *SCN1B. Nat. Genet.,* **1998,** *19:*366–370.

Xie, X., Lancaster, B., Peakman, T., and Garthwaite, J. Interaction of the antiepileptic drug lamotrigine with recombinant rat brain type IIA Na$^+$ channels and with native Na$^+$ channels in rat hippocampal neurones. *Pflugers Arch.,* **1995,** *430:*437–446.

MONOGRAPHS AND REVIEWS

Anonymous. Practice parameter: a guideline for discontinuing antiepileptic drugs in seizure-free patients—summary statement. Report of the Quality Standards Subcommittee of the American Academy of Neurology. *Neurology,* **1996,** *47:*600–602.

Bazil, C.W., and Pedley, T.A. Advances in the medical treatment of epilepsy. *Annu. Rev. Med.,* **1998,** *49:*135–162.

Coulter, D.A. Thalamocortical anatomy and physiology. In, *Epilepsy: A Comprehensive Textbook,* Vol. 1. (Engel, J. Jr., and Pedley, T.A., eds.) Lippincott-Raven, Philadelphia, **1998,** pp. 341–353.

Freeman, J.M. The best medicine for febrile seizures. *N. Engl. J. Med.,* **1992,** *327:*1161–1163.

French, J.A., Kanner, A.M., Bautista, J., *et al.* Efficacy and tolerability of the new antiepileptic drugs. I: Treatment of new-onset epilepsy: Report of the TTA and QSS subcommittees of the American Academy of Neurology and American Epilepsy Society. *Neurology,* **2004a,** *62:*1252–1260.

French, J.A., Kanner, A.M., Bautista, J., *et al.* Efficacy and tolerability of the new antiepileptic drugs. II: Treatment of refractory epilepsy: Report of the TTA and QSS subcommittees of the American Academy of Neurology and the American Epilepsy Society. *Neurology,* **2004b,** *62:*1261–1273.

French, J., Smith, M., Faught, E., and Brown, L. Practice advisory: The use of felbamate in the treatment of patients with intractable epilepsy: Report of the Quality Standards Subcommittee of the American Academy of Neurology and the American Epilepsy Society. *Neurology,* **1999,** *52:*1540–1545.

Huguenard, J.R. Neuronal circuitry of thalamocortical epilepsy and mechanisms of antiabsence drug action. *Adv. Neurol.,* **1999,** *79:*991–999.

Lowenstein, D.H., and Alldredge, B.K. Status epilepticus. *N. Engl. J. Med.,* **1998,** *338:*970–976.

Macdonald, R.L., and Greenfield, L.J. Jr. Mechanisms of action of new antiepileptic drugs. *Curr. Opin. Neurol.,* **1997,** *10:*121–128.

Macdonald, R.L., and Kelly, K.M. Antiepileptive drug mechanisms of action. *Epilepsia,* **1993,** *34*(suppl 5):51–58.

McNamara, J.O. Cellular and molecular basis of epilepsy. *J. Neurosci.,* **1994,** *14:*3413–3425.

Mikati, M.A., and Browne, T.R. Comparative efficacy of antiepileptic drugs. *Clin. Neuropharmacol.,* **1988,** *11:*130–140.

Scheffer, I.E., and Berkovic, S.F. The genetics of human epilepsy. *Trends. Pharm. Sci.,* **2003,** *24:*428-433.

TREATMENT OF CENTRAL NERVOUS SYSTEM DEGENERATIVE DISORDERS

David G. Standaert and Anne B. Young

Neurodegenerative disorders are characterized by progressive and irreversible loss of neurons from specific regions of the brain. Prototypical neurodegenerative disorders include Parkinson's disease (PD) and Huntington's disease (HD), where loss of neurons from structures of the basal ganglia results in abnormalities in the control of movement; Alzheimer's disease (AD), where the loss of hippocampal and cortical neurons leads to impairment of memory and cognitive ability; and amyotrophic lateral sclerosis (ALS), where muscular weakness results from the degeneration of spinal, bulbar, and cortical motor neurons. As a group, these disorders are relatively common and represent a substantial medical and societal problem. They are primarily disorders of later life, developing in individuals who are neurologically normal, although childhood-onset forms of each of the disorders are recognized. PD is observed in more than 1% of individuals over the age of 65 (Tanner, 1992), whereas AD affects as many as 10% of the same population (Evans *et al.*, 1989). HD, which is a genetically determined autosomal dominant disorder, is less frequent in the population as a whole but affects, on average, 50% of each generation in families carrying the gene. ALS also is relatively rare but often leads rapidly to disability and death (Kurtzke, 1982).

At present, the pharmacological therapy of neurodegenerative disorders is limited mostly to symptomatic treatments that do not alter the course of the underlying disease. Symptomatic treatment for PD, where the neurochemical deficit produced by the disease is well defined, is, in general, relatively successful, and a number of effective agents are available. The available treatments for AD, HD, and ALS are much more limited in effectiveness, and the need for new strategies is particularly acute.

SELECTIVE VULNERABILITY AND NEUROPROTECTIVE STRATEGIES

Selective Vulnerability. The most striking feature of this group of disorders is the exquisite specificity of the disease processes for particular types of neurons. For example, in PD there is extensive destruction of the dopaminergic neurons of the substantia nigra, whereas neurons in the cortex and many other areas of the brain are unaffected (Gibb, 1992; Fearnley and Lees, 1994). In contrast, neural injury in AD is most severe in the hippocampus and neocortex, and even within the cortex, the loss of neurons is not uniform but varies dramatically in different functional regions (Arnold *et al.*, 1991). Even more striking is the observation that in HD the mutant gene responsible for the disorder is expressed throughout the brain and in many other organs, yet the pathological changes are most prominent in the neostriatum (Vonsattel *et al.*, 1985; Landwehrmeyer *et al.*, 1995). In ALS, there is loss of spinal motor neurons and the cortical neurons that provide their descending input (Tandan and Bradley, 1985). The diversity of these patterns of neural degeneration has led to the proposal that the process of neural injury must be viewed as the interaction of genetic and environmental influences with the intrinsic physiological characteristics of the affected populations of neurons. These intrinsic factors may include susceptibility to excitotoxic injury, regional variation in capacity for oxidative metabolism, and the production of toxic free radicals as by-products of cellular metabolism (Figure 20–1). The factors that convey selective vulnerability may prove to be important targets for neuroprotective agents to slow the progression of neurodegenerative disorders.

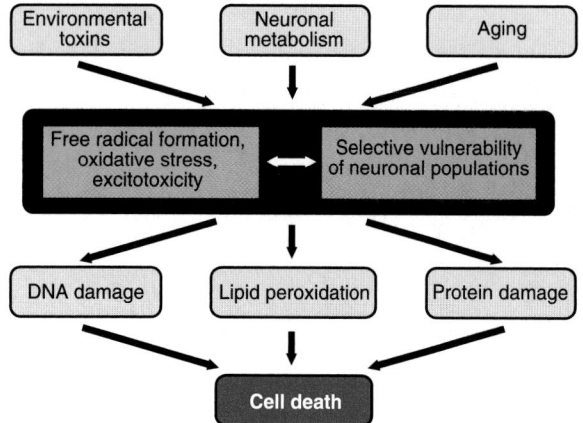

Figure 20–1. *Mechanisms of selective neuronal vulnerability in neurodegenerative diseases.*

Genetics. It has long been suspected that genetic predisposition plays an important role in the etiology of neurodegenerative disorders, and some of the responsible mechanisms have now been discovered. HD is transmitted by autosomal dominant inheritance, and the molecular nature of the genetic defect has been defined (*discussed below*). Most cases of PD, AD, or ALS are sporadic, but families with a high incidence of each of these diseases have been identified, and these studies have begun to yield important clues to the pathogenesis of the disorders. In the case of PD, mutations in four different proteins can lead to genetically determined forms of the disease: α-synuclein, an abundant synaptic protein; parkin, a ubiquitin hydrolase; UCHL1, which also participates in ubiquitin-mediated degradation of proteins in the brain; and DJ-1, a protein thought to be involved in the neuronal response to stress (Gwinn-Hardy, 2002). In AD, mutations in the genes coding for the amyloid precursor protein (APP) and proteins known as the presenilins, which may be involved in APP processing, lead to inherited forms of the disease (Selkoe, 2002). Mutations in the gene coding for copper-zinc superoxide dismutase (*SOD1*) account for about 2% of the cases of adult-onset ALS (Cudkowicz and Brown, 1996). Although these mutations are rare, their importance extends beyond the families that carry them because they point to pathways and mechanisms that also may underlie the more common, sporadic cases of these diseases.

Genetically determined cases of PD, AD, and ALS are infrequent, but it is likely that an individual's genetic background has an important role in determining the probability of acquiring these diseases. Apolipoprotein E (apo E) has been identified as the first of what are likely to be many genetic risk factors for AD. Four distinct isoforms of this protein, which is well known to be involved in transport of cholesterol and lipids in blood, exist. Although all the isoforms carry out their primary role in lipid metabolism equally well, individuals who are homozygous for the apo E 4 allele ("4/4") have a much higher lifetime risk of AD than do those homozygous for the apo E 2 allele ("2/2"). The mechanism by which the apo E 4 protein increases the risk of AD is not known, but a secondary function of the protein in β-amyloid aggregation or processing of APP has been suggested (Roses, 1997).

Environmental Triggers. Infectious agents, environmental toxins, and acquired brain injury have been proposed to have a role in the etiology of neurodegenerative disorders. The role of infection is best documented in the numerous cases of PD that developed following the epidemic of encephalitis lethargica (Von Economo's encephalitis) in the early part of the 20th century. Most contemporary cases of PD are not preceded by encephalitis, and there is no convincing evidence for an infectious contribution to HD, AD, or ALS. Traumatic brain injury has been suggested as a trigger for neurodegenerative disorders, and in the case of AD there is some evidence to support this view (Cummings *et al.*, 1998). At least one toxin, *N*-methyl-4-phenyl-1,2,3,6-tetrahydropyridine (MPTP; *discussed below*), can induce a condition closely resembling PD. More recently, the widely used agricultural pesticide rotenone has been shown to induce a parkinsonian condition in rodents, but sustained parenteral treatment was required (Betarbet, 2002). Whether environmental exposure to these or similar agents may contribute to human PD is unknown.

Excitotoxicity. The term *excitotoxicity* was coined by Olney (1969) to describe the neural injury that results from the presence of excess glutamate in the brain. Glutamate is used as a neurotransmitter by many different neural systems and is believed to mediate most excitatory synaptic transmission in the mammalian brain (*see* Chapter 12). Although glutamate is required for normal brain function, the presence of excessive amounts of glutamate can lead to excitotoxic cell death (Lipton and Rosenberg, 1994). The destructive effects of glutamate are mediated by glutamate receptors, particularly those of the *N*-methyl-D-aspartate (NMDA) type. Unlike other glutamate-gated ion channels, which primarily regulate the flow of Na^+, activated NMDA-receptor channels allow an influx of Ca^{2+}, which in excess can activate a variety of potentially destructive processes. The activity of NMDA-receptor channels is regulated not only by the concentration of glutamate in the synaptic space but also by a voltage-dependent blockade of the channel by Mg^{2+}; thus entry of Ca^{2+} into neurons through NMDA-receptor channels requires binding of glutamate to NMDA receptors as well as depolarization of the neuron (*e.g.,* by the activity of glutamate at non-NMDA receptors), which relieves the blockade of NMDA-receptor channels by extracellular Mg^{2+}. Excitotoxic injury is thought to make an important contribution to the neural death that occurs in acute processes such as stroke and head trauma (Choi and Rothman, 1990). In the chronic neurodegenerative disorders, the role of excitotoxicity is less certain; regional and cellular differences in susceptibility to excitotoxic injury, conveyed, for example, by differences in types of glutamate receptors, may contribute to selective vulnerability.

Energy Metabolism and Aging. The excitotoxic hypothesis provides a link between selective patterns of neuronal injury, the effects of aging, and observations on the metabolic capacities of neurons (Beal *et al.,* 1993). Since blockade of the NMDA-receptor channel by Mg^{2+} depends on the membrane potential, disturbances that impair the metabolic capacity of neurons will tend to relieve Mg^{2+} blockade and predispose to excitotoxic injury. The capacity of neurons for oxidative metabolism declines progressively with age perhaps in part because of a progressive accumulation of mutations in the mitochondrial genome (Wallace, 1992). Patients with PD exhibit several defects in energy metabolism that are even greater than expected for their age, most notably a reduction in the function of complex I of the mitochondrial electron-transport chain (Schapira *et al.,* 1990). Additional evidence for the role of metabolic defects in the etiology of neural degeneration comes from the study of patients who inadvertently self-administered MPTP, a "designer drug" that resulted in symptoms of severe and irreversible parkinsonism (Ballard *et al.,* 1985). Subsequent studies have shown that a metabolite of MPTP induces degeneration of neurons similar to that observed in idiopathic PD and that its mechanism of action appears to be related to an ability to impair mitochondrial energy metabolism in dopaminergic neurons (Przedborski and Jackson-Lewis, 1998). The pesticide rotenone, which also can induce dopaminergic injury, has a similar mechanism of action (Beterbet *et al.,* 2002). In rodents, neural degeneration similar to that observed in HD can be produced either by direct administration of large doses of NMDA-receptor agonists or by more chronic administration of inhibitors of mitochondrial oxidative metabolism, suggesting that disturbances of energy metabolism may underlie the selective pathology of HD as well (Beal *et al.,* 1986, 1993).

Oxidative Stress. Although neurons depend on oxidative metabolism for survival, a consequence of this process is the production of reactive compounds such as hydrogen peroxide and oxyradicals (Cohen and Werner, 1994). Unchecked, these reactive species can lead to DNA damage, peroxidation of membrane lipids, and neuronal death. Several mechanisms serve to limit this *oxidative stress,* including the presence of reducing compounds such as ascorbate and glutathione and enzymatic mechanisms such as superoxide dismutase, which catalyzes the reduction of superoxide radicals. Oxidative stress also may be relieved by aminosteroid agents that serve as free radical scavengers. In PD, attention has focused on the possibility that oxidative stress induced by the metabolism of dopamine may underlie the selective vulnerability of dopaminergic neurons (Jenner, 1998). The primary catabolic pathway of dopamine to 3,4-dihydroxyphenylacetic acid (DOPAC) is catalyzed by monoamine oxidase (MAO) and generates hydrogen peroxide. Hydrogen peroxide, in the presence of ferrous ion, which is relatively abundant in the basal ganglia, can generate hydroxyl free radicals (the Fenton reaction) (Figure 20–2). If the protective mechanisms are inadequate because of inherited or acquired deficiency, the oxyradicals could cause degeneration of dopaminergic neurons. This hypothesis has led to several proposals for therapeutic agents to retard neuronal loss in PD. Two candidates, the free radical scavenger *tocopherol* (vitamin E) and the MAO inhibitor *selegiline* (*discussed below*), have been tested in a large-scale clinical trial, but neither was shown to have a substantial neuroprotective effect (Parkinson Study Group, 1993).

PARKINSON'S DISEASE (PD)

Clinical Overview. Parkinsonism is a clinical syndrome consisting of four cardinal features: bradykinesia (slowness and poverty of movement), muscular rigidity, resting tremor (which usually abates during voluntary movement), and an impairment of postural balance leading to disturbances of gait and falling (Lang, 1998). The most common cause of parkinsonism is idiopathic PD, first described by James Parkinson in 1817 as *paralysis agitans,* or the "shaking palsy." The pathological hallmark of PD is a loss of the pigmented, dopaminergic neurons of the substantia nigra pars compacta, with the appearance of intracellular inclusions known as *Lewy bodies* (Gibb, 1992; Fearnley and Less, 1994). Progressive loss of dopamine-containing neurons is a feature of normal aging; however, most people do not lose the 70% to 80% of dopaminergic neurons required to cause symptomatic PD. Without treatment, PD progresses over 5 to 10 years to a

The reaction of dopamine metabolism producing free radicals is shown below:

$$\text{DOPAMINE} + O_2 + H_2O \xrightarrow[\text{AD}]{\text{MAO}} \text{DOPAC} + NH_3 + H_2O_2$$

$$H_2O_2 + Fe^{2+} \xrightarrow[\text{Reaction}]{\text{Fenton}} {}^{\bullet}OH + OH^- + Fe^{3+}$$

Figure 20–2. Production of free radicals by the metabolism of dopamine. Dopamine is converted by monamine oxidase (MAO) and aldehyde dehydrogenase (AD) to 3,4-dihydroxyphenylacetic acid (DOPAC), producing hydrogen peroxide (H_2O_2). In the presence of ferrous iron, H_2O_2 undergoes spontaneous conversion, forming a hydroxyl free radical (the Fenton reaction).

rigid, akinetic state in which patients are incapable of caring for themselves. Death frequently results from complications of immobility, including aspiration pneumonia or pulmonary embolism. The availability of effective pharmacological treatment has altered radically the prognosis of PD; in most cases, good functional mobility can be maintained for many years, and the life expectancy of adequately treated patients is increased substantially. It is important to recognize that several disorders other than PD also may produce parkinsonism, including some relatively rare neurodegenerative disorders, stroke, and intoxication with dopamine-receptor antagonists. Drugs in common clinical use that may cause parkinsonism include antipsychotics such as *haloperidol* and *thorazine* (*see* Chapter 18) and antiemetics such as *prochloperazine* and *metoclopramide* (*see* Chapter 37). Although a complete discussion of the clinical diagnostic approach to parkinsonism exceeds the scope of this chapter, the distinction between PD and other causes of parkinsonism is important because parkinsonism arising from other causes usually is refractory to all forms of treatment.

Pathophysiology. The primary deficit in PD is a loss of the neurons in the substantia nigra pars compacta that provide dopaminergic innervation to the striatum (caudate and putamen). The current understanding of the pathophysiology of PD can be traced to neurochemical investigations that demonstrated a reduction in the striatal dopamine content in excess of 80%. This paralleled the loss of neurons from the substantia nigra, suggesting that replacement of dopamine could restore function (Cotzias *et al.*, 1969; Hornykiewicz, 1973). These fundamental observations led to an extensive investigative effort to understand the metabolism and actions of dopamine and to learn how a deficit in dopamine gives rise to the clinical features of PD. We now have a model of the function of the basal ganglia that, while incomplete, is still useful.

Dopamine Synthesis and Metabolism. Dopamine, a catecholamine, is synthesized in the terminals of dopaminergic neurons from

tyrosine and stored, released, and metabolized by processes described in Chapter 6 and summarized in Figures 20–3 and 20–4.

Dopamine Receptors. The actions of dopamine in the brain are mediated by a family of dopamine-receptor proteins (Figure 20–5).

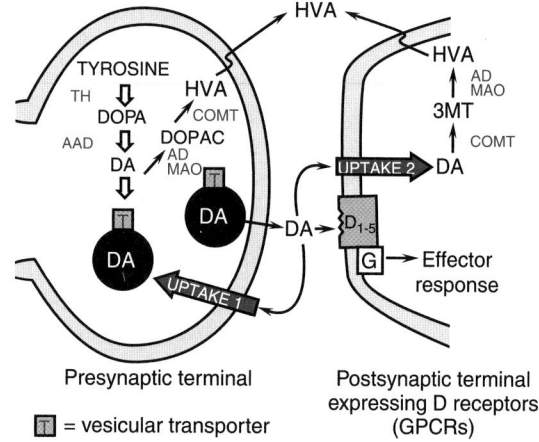

= vesicular transporter

Figure 20–3. Dopaminergic terminal. Dopamine (DA) is synthesized in neuronal terminals from tyrosine by the sequential actions of tyrosine hydroxylase (TH), producing the intermediary L-dihydroxyphenylalanine (L-DOPA), and aromatic L-amino acid decarboxylase (AAD). In the terminal, DA is transported into storage vesicles by a vesicular membrane transporter (T). Release, triggered by depolarization and entry of Ca^{2+}, allows dopamine to act on a variety of postsynaptic GPCRs for DA. The D_1 and D_2 receptors are important in brain regions involved in PD. The differential actions of DA on postsynaptic targets bearing different types of DA receptors have important implications for the function of neural circuits. The actions of DA are terminated by reuptake into the nerve terminal (where DA may be restored or metabolized) or uptake into the postsynaptic cell (where DA is metabolized). Metabolism occurs by the sequential actions of the enzymes catechol-*O*-methyltransferase (COMT), monoamine oxidase (MAO), and aldehyde dehydrogenase (AD). 3MT, 3-methoxytyramine; DOPAC, 3,4-dihydroxyphenylacetic acid; HVA, 3-methoxy-4-hydroxy-phenylacetic acid (*see* Figure 20–4). In humans, HVA is the principal metabolite of DA. (From Cooper *et al.*, 1996, with permission.)

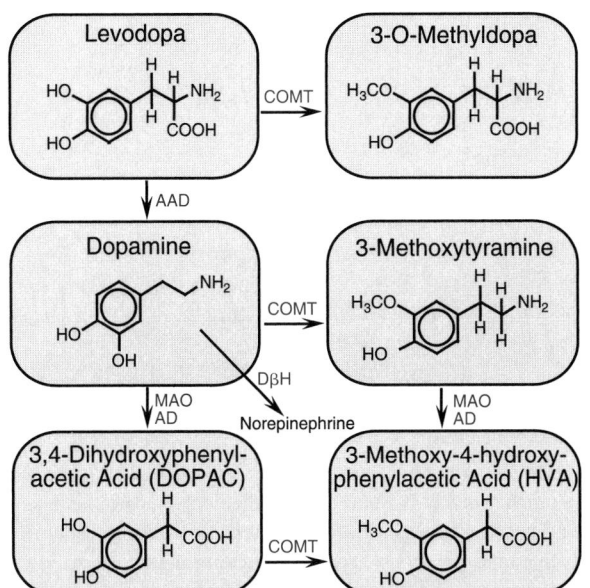

Figure 20–4. Metabolism of levodopa (L-DOPA). AD, aldehyde dehydrogenase; COMT, catechol-*O*-methyltransferase; DβH, dopamine β-hydroxylase; AAD, aromatic L-amino acid decarboxylase; MAO, monoamine oxidase.

Two types of dopamine receptors were identified in the mammalian brain using pharmacological techniques: D_1 receptors, which stimulate the synthesis of the intracellular second messenger cyclic AMP, and D_2 receptors, which inhibit cyclic AMP synthesis as well as suppress Ca^{2+} currents and activate receptor-operated K^+ currents. Application of molecular genetics to the study of dopamine receptors has revealed a more complex receptor situation than envisioned

originally. At present, five distinct dopamine receptors are known (*see* Missale *et al.*, 1998, and Chapter 12). All the dopamine receptors are heptahelical G protein–coupled receptors (GPCRs) (*see* Chapter 1).

The five dopamine receptors can be divided into two groups on the basis of their pharmacological and structural properties (Figure 20–5). The D_1 and D_5 proteins have a long intracellular carboxy-terminal tail and are members of the class defined pharmacologically as D_1; they stimulate the formation of cyclic AMP and phosphatidyl inositol hydrolysis. The D_2, D_3, and D_4 receptors share a large third intracellular loop and are of the D_2 class. They decrease cyclic AMP formation and modulate K^+ and Ca^{2+} currents. Each of the five dopamine receptor proteins has a distinct anatomical pattern of expression in the brain. The D_1 and D_2 proteins are abundant in the striatum and are the most important receptor sites with regard to the causes and treatment of PD. The D_4 and D_5 proteins are largely extrastriatal, whereas D_3 expression is low in the caudate and putamen but more abundant in the nucleus accumbens and olfactory tubercle.

Neural Mechanism of Parkinsonism. Considerable effort has been devoted to understanding how the loss of dopaminergic input to the neurons of the neostriatum gives rise to the clinical features of PD (for review, *see* Albin *et al.*, 1989; Mink and Thach, 1993; and Wichmann and DeLong, 1993). The basal ganglia can be viewed as a modulatory side loop that regulates the flow of information from the cerebral cortex to the motor neurons of the spinal cord (Figure 20–6). The neostriatum is the principal input structure of the basal ganglia and receives excitatory glutamatergic input from many areas of the cortex. Most neurons within the striatum are projection neurons that innervate other basal ganglia structures. A small but important subgroup of striatal neurons consists of interneurons that connect neurons within the striatum but do not project beyond its borders. Acetylcholine and neuropeptides are used as transmitters by these striatal interneurons.

The outflow of the striatum proceeds along two distinct routes, termed the *direct* and *indirect pathways.* The direct pathway is

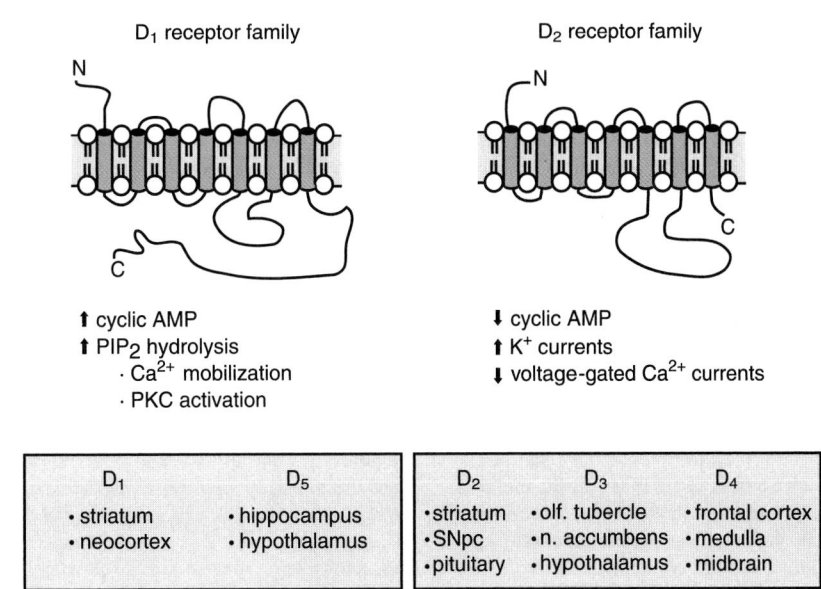

Figure 20–5. Distribution and characteristics of dopamine receptors in the ceontral nervous system. SNpc, substantia nigra pars compacta.

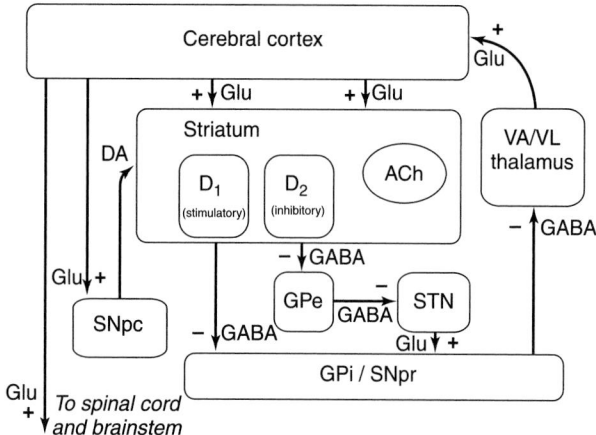

Figure 20–6. *Schematic wiring diagram of the basal ganglia.* The striatum is the principal input structure of the basal ganglia and receives excitatory glutamatergic input from many areas of cerebral cortex. The striatum contains projection neurons expressing predominantly D_1 or D_2 dopamine receptors, as well as interneurons that use acetylcholine (ACh) as a neurotransmitter. Outflow from the striatum proceeds along two routes. The direct pathway, from the striatum to the substantia nigra pars reticulata (SNpr) and globus pallidus interna (GPi), uses the inhibitory transmitter GABA. The indirect pathway, from the striatum through the globus pallidus externa (GPe) and the subthalamic nucleus (STN) to the SNpr and GPi consists of two inhibitory GABAergic links and one excitatory glutamatergic projection (Glu). The substantia nigra pars compacta (SNpc) provides dopaminergic innervation to the striatal neurons, giving rise to both the direct and indirect pathways, and regulates the relative activity of these two paths. The SNpr and GPi are the output structures of the basal ganglia and provide feedback to the cerebral cortex through the ventroanterior and ventrolateral nuclei of the thalamus (VA/VL).

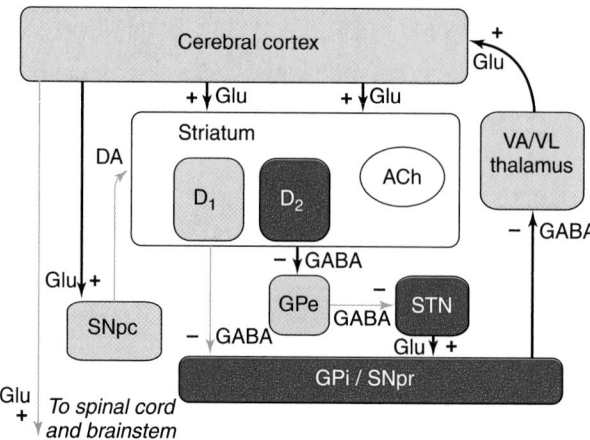

Figure 20–7. *The basal ganglia in Parkinson's disease.* The primary defect is destruction of the dopaminergic neurons of the SNpc. The striatal neurons that form the direct pathway from the striatum to the SNpr and GPi express primarily the *excitatory* D_1 dopamine receptor, whereas the striatal neurons that project to the GPe and form the indirect pathway express the *inhibitory* D_2 dopamine receptor. Thus, loss of the dopaminergic input to the striatum has a differential effect on the two outflow pathways; the direct pathway to the SNpr and GPi is less active (*structures in light blue*), whereas the activity in the indirect pathway is increased (*structures in dark blue*). The net effect is that neurons in the SNpr and GPi become more active. This leads to increased inhibition of the VA/VL thalamus and reduced excitatory input to the cortex. (*See* legend to Figure 20–6 for definitions of anatomical abbreviations.)

formed by neurons in the striatum that project directly to the output stages of the basal ganglia, the substantia nigra pars reticulata (SNpr) and the globus pallidus interna (GPi); these, in turn, relay to the ventroanterior and ventrolateral thalamus, which provides excitatory input to the cortex. The neurotransmitter of both links of the direct pathway is γ-aminobutyric acid (GABA), which is inhibitory, so that the net effect of stimulation of the direct pathway at the level of the striatum is to increase the excitatory outflow from the thalamus to the cortex. The indirect pathway is composed of striatal neurons that project to the globus pallidus externa (GPe). This structure, in turn, innervates the subthalamic nucleus (STN), which provides outflow to the SNpr and GPi output stage. As in the direct pathway, the first two links—the projections from striatum to GPe and GPe to STN—use the inhibitory transmitter GABA; however, the final link—the projection from STN to SNpr and GPi—is an excitatory glutamatergic pathway. Thus the net effect of stimulating the indirect pathway at the level of the striatum is to reduce the excitatory outflow from the thalamus to the cerebral cortex.

The key feature of this model of basal ganglia function, which accounts for the symptoms observed in PD as a result of loss of

dopaminergic neurons, is the differential effect of dopamine on the direct and indirect pathways (Figure 20–7). The dopaminergic neurons of the substantia nigra pars compacta (SNpc) innervate all parts of the striatum; however, the target striatal neurons express distinct types of dopamine receptors. The striatal neurons giving rise to the direct pathway express primarily the *excitatory* D_1 dopamine receptor protein, whereas the striatal neurons forming the indirect pathway express primarily the *inhibitory* D_2 type. Thus dopamine released in the striatum tends to increase the activity of the direct pathway and reduce the activity of the indirect pathway, whereas the depletion that occurs in PD has the opposite effect. The net effect of the reduced dopaminergic input in PD is to increase markedly the inhibitory outflow from the SNpr and GPi to the thalamus and reduce excitation of the motor cortex.

There are several limitations of this model of basal ganglia function (Parent and Ciccetti, 1998). In particular, recent work has shown that the anatomical connections are considerably more complex than envisioned originally. In addition, many of the pathways involved use not just one but several neurotransmitters. For example, the neuropeptides substance P and dynorphin are found predominantly in striatal neurons making up the direct pathway, whereas most of the indirect pathway neurons express enkephalin. These transmitters are expected to have slow modulatory effects on signaling, in contrast to the rapid effects of glutamate and GABA, but the functional significance of these modulatory effects remains unclear. Nevertheless, the model is useful and has important implications for

Table 20-1
Commonly Used Medications for the Treatment of Parkinson's Disease

AGENT	TYPICAL INITIAL DOSE	TOTAL DAILY DOSE– USEFUL RANGE	COMMENTS
Carbidopa/levodopa	25 mg carbidopa + 100 mg levodopa ("25/100" tablet), twice or three times a day	200–1200 mg levodopa	
Carbidopa/levodopa sustained release	50 mg carbidopa + 200 mg levodopa ("50/200 sustained release" tablet) twice a day	200–1200 mg levodopa	Bioavailability 75% of immediate release form
Bromocriptine	1.25 mg twice a day	3.75–40 mg	Titrate slowly
Pergolide	0.05 mg once a day	0.75–5 mg	Titrate slowly
Ropinirole	0.25 mg three times a day	1.5–24 mg	
Pramipexole	0.125 mg three times a day	1.5–4.5 mg	
Entacapone	200 mg with each dose of levodopa/carbidopa	600–2000 mg	
Tolcapone	100 mg twice a day or three times a day	200–600 mg	May be hepatotoxic; requires monitoring of liver enzymes
Selegiline	5 mg twice a day	2.5–10 mg	
Amantadine	100 mg twice a day	100–200 mg	
Trihexyphenidyl HCl	1 mg twice a day	2–15 mg	

the rational design and use of pharmacological agents in PD. First, it suggests that to restore the balance of the system through stimulation of dopamine receptors, the complementary effect of actions at both D_1 and D_2 receptors, as well as the possibility of adverse effects that may be mediated by D_3, D_4, or D_5 receptors, must be considered. Second, it explains why replacement of dopamine is not the only approach to the treatment of PD. Drugs that inhibit cholinergic receptors have long been used for treatment of parkinsonism. Although their mechanisms of action are not completely understood, it seems likely that their effect is mediated at the level of the striatal projection neurons, which normally receive cholinergic input from striatal cholinergic interneurons. Few clinically useful drugs for parkinsonism are presently available based on actions through GABA and glutamate receptors, even though both have crucial roles in the circuitry of the basal ganglia. However, they represent a promising avenue for drug development (Hallet and Standaert, 2004).

TREATMENT OF PARKINSON'S DISEASE

Commonly used medications for the treatment of PD are summarized in Table 20–1.

Levodopa

Levodopa (L-DOPA, LARODOPA, L-3,4-dihydroxyphenylalanine), the metabolic precursor of dopamine, is the single most effective agent in the treatment of PD.

Levodopa is itself largely inert; both its therapeutic and adverse effects result from the decarboxylation of levodopa to dopamine. When administered orally, levodopa is absorbed rapidly from the small bowel by the transport system for aromatic amino acids. Concentrations of the drug in plasma usually peak between 0.5 and 2 hours after an oral dose. The half-life in plasma is short (1 to 3 hours). The rate and extent of absorption of levodopa depends on the rate of gastric emptying, the pH of gastric juice, and the length of time the drug is exposed to the degradative enzymes of the gastric and intestinal mucosa. Competition for absorption sites in the small bowel from dietary amino acids also may have a marked effect on the absorption of levodopa; administration of levodopa with meals delays absorption and reduces peak plasma concentrations. Entry of the drug into the central nervous system (CNS) across the blood–brain barrier also is mediated by a membrane transporter for aromatic amino acids, and competition between dietary protein and levodopa may occur at this level. In the brain, levodopa is converted to dopamine by decarboxylation primarily within the presynaptic terminals of dopaminergic neurons in the stratium. The dopamine produced is responsible for the therapeutic effectiveness of the drug in PD; after release, it is either transported back into dopaminergic terminals by the presynaptic uptake mechanism or metabolized by the actions of MAO and catechol-*O*-methyltransferase (COMT) (Figure 20–4).

In practice, levodopa is almost always administered in combination with a peripherally acting inhibitor of aromatic L-amino acid decarboxylase, such as *carbidopa* or *benserazide* (available outside the United States), that do not penetrate well into the CNS. If levodopa is administered alone, the drug is largely decarboxylated by enzymes in the intestinal mucosa and other peripheral sites so that relatively little unchanged drug reaches the cerebral circulation and probably less than 1% penetrates the CNS. In addition, dopamine release into the circulation by peripheral conversion of levodopa produces undesirable effects, particularly nausea. Inhibition of peripheral decarboxylase markedly increases the fraction of administered levodopa that remains unmetabolized and available to cross the blood–brain barrier (*see* Figure 20–9) and reduces the incidence of gastrointestinal side effects. In most individuals, a daily dose of 75 mg carbidopa is sufficient to prevent the development of nausea. For this reason, the most commonly prescribed form of carbidopa/levodopa (SINEMET, ATAMET) is the *25/100* form, containing 25 mg carbidopa and 100 mg levodopa. With this formulation, dosage schedules of three or more tablets daily provide acceptable inhibition of decarboxylase in most individuals. Occasionally, individuals will require larger doses of carbidopa to minimize gastrointestinal side effects, and administration of supplemental carbidopa (LODOSYN) alone may be beneficial.

Levodopa therapy can have a dramatic effect on all the signs and symptoms of PD. Early in the course of the disease, the degree of improvement in tremor, rigidity, and bradykinesia may be nearly complete. In early PD, the duration of the beneficial effects of levodopa may exceed the plasma lifetime of the drug, suggesting that the nigrostriatal dopamine system retains some capacity to store and release dopamine. A principal limitation of the long-term use of levodopa therapy is that with time this apparent "buffering" capacity is lost, and the patient's motor state may fluctuate dramatically with each dose of levodopa. A common problem is the development of the "wearing off" phenomenon: each dose of levodopa effectively improves mobility for a period of time, perhaps 1 to 2 hours, but rigidity and akinesia return rapidly at the end of the dosing interval. Increasing the dose and frequency of administration can improve this situation, but this often is limited by the development of *dyskinesias,* excessive and abnormal involuntary movements. Dyskinesias are observed most often when the plasma levodopa concentration is high, although in some individuals dyskinesias or dystonia may be triggered when the level is rising or falling. These movements can be as uncomfortable and disabling

as the rigidity and akinesia of PD. In the later stages of PD, patients may fluctuate rapidly between being "off," having no beneficial effects from their medications, and being "on" but with disabling dyskinesias, a situation called the *on/off phenomenon.*

Recent evidence has indicated that induction of the on/off phenomena and dyskinesias may be the result of an active process of adaptation to variations in brain and plasma levodopa levels. This process of adaptation is apparently complex, involving not only alterations in the function of dopamine receptors but also downstream changes in the postsynaptic striatal neurons, including modification of NMDA glutamate receptors (Mouradian and Chase, 1994; Chase, 1998, Hallett and Standaert, 2004). When levodopa levels are maintained constant by intravenous infusion, dyskinesias and fluctuations are greatly reduced, and the clinical improvement is maintained for up to several days after returning to oral levodopa dosing (Mouradian *et al.*, 1990). A sustained-release formulation consisting of carbidopa/levodopa in an erodable wax matrix (SINEMET CR) has been marketed in an attempt to produce more stable plasma levodopa levels than can be obtained with oral administration of standard carbidopa/levodopa formulations. This formulation is helpful in some cases, but absorption of the sustained-release formulation is not entirely predictable. Another technique used to overcome the on/off phenomenon is to sum the total daily dose of carbidopa/levodopa and give equal amounts every 2 hours rather than every 4 or 6 hours.

An important unanswered question regarding the use of levodopa in PD is whether this medication alters the course of the underlying disease or merely modifies the symptoms. Two aspects of levodopa treatment and the outcome of PD are of concern. First, if the production of free radicals as a result of dopamine metabolism contributes to the death of nigrostriatal neurons, then the addition of levodopa actually might accelerate the process, although no convincing evidence for such an effect has yet been obtained. Second, it is well established that the undesirable on/off fluctuations and wearing off phenomena are observed almost exclusively in patients treated with levodopa, but it is not known if delaying treatment with levodopa will delay the appearance of these effects. In view of these uncertainties, most practitioners have adopted a pragmatic approach, using levodopa only when the symptoms of PD cause functional impairment.

In addition to motor fluctuations and nausea, several other adverse effects may be observed with levodopa treatment. A common and troubling adverse effect is the induction of hallucinations and confusion; these effects are particularly common in the elderly and in those with pre-existing cognitive dysfunction and often limit the ability to treat parkinsonian symptoms adequately. Conventional antipsychotic agents, such as the phenothiazines, are effective against levodopa-induced psychosis but may cause marked worsening of parkinsonism, probably through actions at the D_2 dopamine receptor. A recent approach has been to use the "atypical" antipsychotic agents, which are effective in the treatment of psychosis but do not cause or worsen parkinsonism (*see* Chapter 18). The most effective of these are *clozapine* and *quetiapine* (Friedman and Factor, 2000).

Peripheral decarboxylation of levodopa and release of dopamine into the circulation may activate vascular dopamine receptors and produce orthostatic hypotension. The actions of dopamine at α and β adrenergic receptors may induce cardiac arrhythmias, especially in patients with pre-existing conduction disturbances. Administration of levodopa with nonspecific inhibitors of MAO, such as *phenelzine* and *tranylcypromine,* markedly accentuates the actions of levodopa and may precipitate life-threatening hypertensive crisis and hyperpyrexia; nonspecific MAO inhibitors always should be discontinued at least 14 days before levodopa is administered (note that this prohibition does not include the MAO-B subtype-specific inhibitor *selegiline,* which, as discussed below, often is administered safely in combination with levodopa). Abrupt withdrawal of levodopa or other dopaminergic medications may precipitate the *neuroleptic malignant syndrome* more commonly observed after treatment with dopamine antagonists.

Dopamine-Receptor Agonists. An alternative to levodopa is the use of drugs that are direct agonists of striatal dopamine receptors, an approach that offers several potential advantages. Since enzymatic conversion of these drugs is not required for activity, they do not depend on the functional capacities of the nigrostriatal neurons. Most dopamine-receptor agonists in clinical use have durations of action substantially longer than that of levodopa and often are useful in the management of dose-related fluctuations in motor state. Finally, if the hypothesis that free radical formation as a result of dopamine metabolism contributes to neuronal death is correct, then dopamine-receptor agonists may have the potential to modify the course of the disease by reducing endogenous release of dopamine as well as the need for exogenous levodopa.

Four orally administered dopamine-receptor agonists are available for treatment of PD: two older agents, *bromocriptine* (PARLODEL) and *pergolide* (PERMAX); and two newer, more selective compounds, *ropinirole* (REQUIP) and *pramipexole* (MIRPEX). Bromocriptine and pergolide both are ergot derivatives and share a similar spectrum of therapeutic actions and adverse effects. Bromocriptine is a strong agonist of the D_2 class of dopamine receptors and a partial antagonist of the D_1 receptors, whereas pergolide is an agonist of both classes. Ropinirole and pramipexole (Figure 20–8) have selective activity at D_2 class sites (specifically at the D_2 and D_3 receptor proteins) and little or no activity at D_1 class sites. All four of the drugs are well absorbed orally and have similar therapeutic actions. Like levodopa, they can relieve the clinical symptoms of PD. The duration of action of the dopamine agonists (8 to 24 hours) often is longer than that of levodopa (6 to 8 hours), and they are particularly effective in the treatment of patients who have developed on/off phenomena. All four also may produce hallucinosis or confusion, similar to that observed with levodopa, and may worsen orthostatic hypotension.

The principal distinction between the newer, more selective agents and the older ergot derivatives is in their tolerability and speed of titration. Initial treatment with bro-

Figure 20–8. Structures of selective dopamine D_2-receptor agonists.

mocriptine or pergolide may cause profound hypotension, so they should be initiated at low dosage. The ergot derivatives also often induce nausea and fatigue with initial treatment. Symptoms usually are transient, but they require slow upward adjustment of the dose over a period of weeks to months. Ropinirole and pramipexole can be initiated more quickly, achieving therapeutically useful doses in a week or less. They generally cause less gastrointestinal disturbance than do the ergot derivatives, but they can produce nausea and somnolence. The somnolence in some cases may be quite severe, and several instances of sudden attacks of irresistible sleepiness leading to motor vehicle accidents have been reported (Frucht *et al.*, 1999). This effect seems to be uncommon, but it is prudent to advise patients of this possibility and to switch to another treatment if sleepiness interferes with the activities of daily life. Recent reports have associated long-term use of pergolide with significant cardiac valvular disease. If these reports are confirmed, this may be another important factor favoring the use of the nonergot agents.

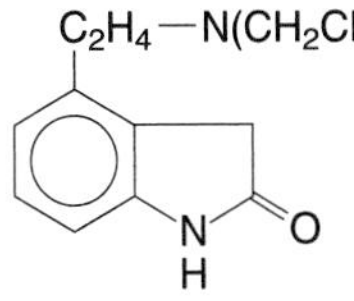

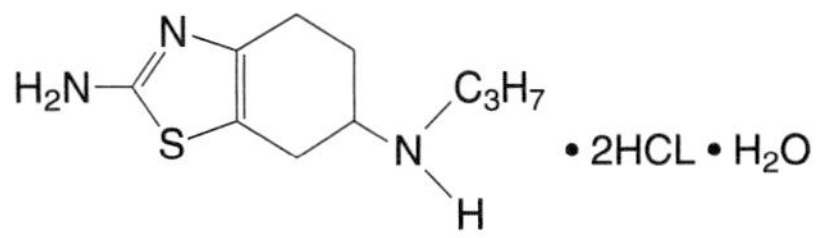

The introduction of pramipexole and ropinirole has led to a substantial change in the clinical use of dopamine agonists in PD. Because these selective agonists are well tolerated, they are used increasingly as initial treatment for PD rather than as adjuncts to levodopa. This change has been driven by two factors: (1) the belief that because of their longer duration of action, dopamine agonists may be less likely than levodopa to induce on/off effects and dyskinesias and (2) the concern that levodopa may contribute to oxidative stress, thereby accelerating loss of dopaminergic neurons. Two large controlled clinical trials comparing levodopa with pramipexole or ropinirole as initial treatment of PD have provided convincing evidence for a reduced rate of motor fluctuation in patients treated with these agonists. This benefit was accompanied by an increased rate of adverse effects in both studies, especially somnolence and hallucinations (Parkinson Study Group, 2000; Rascol *et al.*, 2000). At present, many experts favor dopamine agonists as initial therapy in younger patients with PD and levodopa as the initial treatment in older patients who may be more vulnerable to the adverse cognitive effects of the agonists.

Apomorphine (APOKYN) is a dopaminergic agonist that can be administered by subcutaneous injection. It has high affinity for D_4 receptors; moderate affinity for D_2, D_3, D_5, and adrenergic $\alpha 1D$, $\alpha 2B$, and $\alpha 2C$ receptors; and low affinity for D_1 receptors. Apomorphine has been used in Europe for many years and was approved recently by the U.S. Food and Drug Administration (FDA) as a "rescue therapy" for the acute intermittent treatment of "off" episodes in patients with a fluctuating response to dopaminergic therapy. In addition to being associated with the side effects discussed earlier for the oral dopamine agonists, apomorphine also is highly emetogenic and requires pre- and post-treatment antiemetic therapy. It is recommended that oral trimethobenzamide (TIGAN), at a dose of 300 mg three times daily, be started three days prior to the initial dose of apomorphine and continued at least during the first 2 months of therapy. Based on reports of profound hypotension and loss of consciousness when apomorphine was administered with ondansetron, the concomitant use of apomorphine with antiemetic drugs of the $5\text{-}HT_3$ antagonist class is contraindicated. Other potentially serious side effects of apomorphine include QT prolongation, injection-site reactions, and the development of a pattern of abuse characterized by increasingly frequent dosing leading to hallucinations, dyskinesia, and abnormal behavior. Because of these potential adverse effects, use of apomorphine is appropriate only when other measures, such as oral dopamine agonists or COMT inhibitors, have failed to control the "off" episodes. Apomorphine therapy should be initiated in a setting where the patient can be monitored carefully, beginning with a 2-mg test dose. If this is tolerated, it can be titrated slowly up to a maximum dosage of 6 mg. For effective control of symptoms, patients may require three or more injections daily.

Catechol-O-Methyltransferase (COMT) Inhibitors.
A recently developed class of drugs for the treatment of PD consists of inhibitors of COMT. COMT and MAO are responsible for the catabolism of levodopa as well as dopamine. COMT transfers a methyl group from the donor *S*-adenosyl-L-methionine, producing the pharmacologically inactive compounds 3-*O*-methyl DOPA (from levodopa) and 3-methoxytyramine (from dopamine) (Figure 20–9). When levodopa is administered orally, nearly 99% of the drug is catabolized and does not reach the brain. Most is

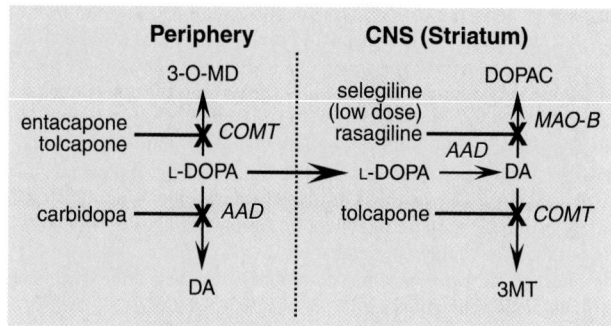

Figure 20–9. Pharmacological preservation of L-DOPA and striatal dopamine. The principal site of action of inhibitors of catechol-*O*-methyltransferase (COMT) (such as tolcapone and entacapone) is in the peripheral circulation. They block the *O*-methylation of levodopa (L-DOPA) and increase the fraction of the drug available for delivery to the brain. Tolcapone also has effects in the CNS. Inhibitors of MAO-B, such as low-dose selegiline and rasagiline, will act within the CNS to reduce oxidative deamination of DA, thereby enhancing vesicular stores. AAD, aromatic L-amino acid decarboxylase; DA, dopamine; DOPAC, 3,4-dihydroxyphenylacetic acid; MAO, monoamine oxidase; 3MT, 3-methoxyltyramine; 3-O-MD, 3-*O*-methyl DOPA.

converted by aromatic L-amino acid decarboxylase (AAD) to dopamine, which causes nausea and hypotension. Addition of an AAD inhibitor such as carbidopa reduces the formation of dopamine but increases the fraction of levodopa that is methylated by COMT. The principal therapeutic action of the COMT inhibitors is to block this peripheral conversion of levodopa to 3-*O*-methyl DOPA, increasing both the plasma half-life of levodopa as well as the fraction of each dose that reaches the CNS.

Two COMT inhibitors presently are available for this use in the United States, *tolcapone* (TASMAR) and *entacapone* (COMTAN). Both these agents have been shown in double-blind trials to reduce the clinical symptoms of "wearing off" in patients treated with levodopa/carbidopa (Parkinson Study Group, 1997; Kurth *et al.*, 1997). Although the magnitude of their clinical effects and mechanisms of action are similar, they differ with respect to pharmacokinetic properties and adverse effects. Tolcapone has a relatively long duration of action, allowing for administration two to three times a day, and appears to act by both central and peripheral inhibition of COMT. The duration of action of entacapone is short, around 2 hours, so it usually is administered simultaneously with each dose of levodopa/carbidopa. The action of entacapone is attributable principally to peripheral inhibition of COMT. The common adverse effects of these agents are similar to those observed in patients treated with levodopa/carbidopa alone and include nausea, orthostatic hypotension, vivid dreams, confusion, and hallucinations. An important adverse effect associated with tolcapone is hepatotoxicity. In clinical trials, up to 2% of the patients treated had increases in serum alanine aminotransferase and aspartate transaminase; after marketing, three fatal cases of fulminant hepatic failure in patients taking tolcapone were observed, leading to addition of a warning to the label. At present, tolcapone should be used only in patients who have not responded to other therapies and with appropriate monitoring for hepatic injury. Entacapone has not been associated with hepatotoxicity and requires no special monitoring. Entacapone also is available in fixed-dose combinations with levodopa/carbidopa (STALEVO).

Selective MAO-B Inhibitors. Two isoenzymes of MAO oxidize monoamines. While both isoenzymes (MAO-A and MAO-B) are present in the periphery and inactivate monoamines of intestinal origin, the isoenzyme MAO-B is the predominant form in the striatum and is responsible for most of the oxidative metabolism of dopamine in the brain. At low to moderate doses (10 mg/day or less), *selegiline* (ELDEPRYL) is a selective inhibitor of MAO-B, leading to irreversible inhibition of the enzyme (Olanow, 1993). Unlike nonspecific inhibitors of MAO (such as phenelzine, tranylcypromine, and isocarboxazid), selegiline does not inhibit peripheral metabolism of catecholamines; thus it can be taken safely with levodopa. Selegiline also does not cause the lethal potentiation of catecholamine action observed when patients taking nonspecific MAO inhibitors ingest indirectly acting sympathomimetic amines such as the tyramine found in certain cheeses and wine. Doses of selegiline higher than 10 mg daily can produce inhibition of MAO-A and should be avoided.

Selegiline has been used for several years as a symptomatic treatment for PD, although its benefit is modest. The basis of the efficacy of selegiline is presumed to be its capacity to retard the breakdown of dopamine in the striatum. With the recent emergence of interest in the potential role of free radicals and oxidative stress in the pathogenesis of PD, it has been proposed that the ability of selegiline to retard the metabolism of dopamine might confer neuroprotective properties. In support of this idea, selegiline can protect animals from MPTP-induced parkinsonism by blocking the conversion of MPTP to its toxic metabolite (1-methyl-4-phenylpyridium ion), a transformation mediated by MAO-B. The potential protective role of selegiline in idiopathic PD was evaluated in multicenter randomized trials; these studies showed a symptomatic effect of selegiline in PD, but longer follow-up failed to provide any definite evidence of ability to retard the loss of dopaminergic neurons (Parkinson Study Group, 1993).

Selegiline is generally well tolerated in patients with early or mild PD. In patients with more advanced PD or underlying cognitive impairment, selegiline may accentuate the adverse motor and cognitive effects of levodopa therapy. Metabolites of selegiline include amphetamine and methamphetamine, which may cause anxiety, insomnia, and other adverse symptoms. A related compound, rasagiline, also acts through inhibition of MAO-B but does not form these undesirable metabolites. Rasagiline has shown efficacy in both early and advanced PD but is not yet approved for use in the United States. Interestingly, selegiline, like the nonspecific MAO inhibitors, can lead to the development of stupor, rigidity, agitation, and hyperthermia after administration of the analgesic meperidine; the basis of this interaction is uncertain. There also have been case reports of adverse effects resulting from interactions between selegiline and tricyclic antidepressants and between selegiline and serotonin-reuptake inhibitors. The combination of selegiline and serotonin-reuptake inhibitors seems well tolerated in patients with PD, and many patients do take these combinations of medications without apparent adverse interaction; nonetheless, concomitant administration of selegiline and serotonergic drugs should be done with caution.

Muscarinic Receptor Antagonists. Antagonists of muscarinic acetylcholine receptors were used widely for the treatment of PD before the discovery of levodopa. The biological basis for the therapeutic actions of anticholinergics is not completely understood. It seems likely that they act within the neostriatum through the receptors that normally mediate the response to intrinsic cholinergic innervation of this structure, which arises primarily from cholinergic striatal interneurons. Several muscarinic cholinergic receptors have been cloned (*see* Chapters 7 and 12); like the dopamine receptors, these are GPCRs. Five subtypes of muscarinic receptors have been identified; at least four and probably all five subtypes are present in the striatum, although each has a distinct distribution (Hersch *et al.*, 1994). Several drugs with anticholinergic properties currently are used in the treatment of PD, including *trihexyphenidyl* (ARTANE, 2 to 4 mg three times per day), *benztropine mesylate* (COGENTIN, 1 to 4 mg two times per day), and *diphenhydramine hydrochloride* (BENADRYL, 25 to 50 mg three to four times per day). *Diphenhydramine* also is a histamine H_1 antagonist (*see* Chapter 24). All have modest antiparkinsonian activity that is useful in the treatment of early PD or as an adjunct to dopamimetic therapy. The adverse effects of these drugs are a result of their anticholinergic properties. Most troublesome are sedation and mental confusion. They also may produce constipation, urinary retention, and blurred vision through cycloplegia; they must be used with caution in patients with narrow-angle glaucoma.

Amantadine. Amantadine (SYMMETREL), an antiviral agent used for the prophylaxis and treatment of influenza A (*see* Chapter 49), has antiparkinsonian activity. Amantadine has several pharmacological effects; it is not clear which properties are responsible for its antiparkinsonian actions. Amantadine appears to alter dopamine release in the striatum and also has anticholinergic properties. The most significant action of amantadine may be its ability to block NMDA glutamate receptors (Hallett and Standaert, 2004). In any case, the effects of amantadine in PD are modest. It is used as initial therapy of mild PD. It also may be helpful as an adjunct in patients on levodopa with dose-related fluctuations and dyskinesias. The antidyskinetic properties of amantadine have been attributed to actions at NMDA receptors, although the closely related NMDA receptor antagonist *memantine* (discussed below) does not seem to have this effect. Amantadine usually is administered in a dose of 100 mg twice a day and is well tolerated. Dizziness, lethargy, anticholinergic effects, and sleep disturbance, as well as nausea and vomiting, have been observed occasionally, but even when present, these effects are mild and reversible.

Neuroprotective Treatments for Parkinson's Disease. It would be desirable to identify a treatment that modifies the progressive degeneration that underlies PD rather than simply controlling the symptoms. Current research strategies are based on the mechanistic approaches described earlier (*e.g.,* energy metabolism, oxidative stress, environmental triggers, and excitotoxicity) and on discoveries related to the genetics of PD (Cantuti-Castelvetri and Standaert, 2004). Some of the strongest evidence for a neuroprotective action has emerged from long-term studies of the effects of the dopamine agonists pramipexole and ropinerole. The therapeutic effects of these are related to actions at postsynaptic dopamine receptors, but they also can activate presynaptic autoreceptors found on dopamine terminals, which are principally of the D_2 class. By stimulating presynaptic receptors, pramipexole and ropinerole may reduce endogenous dopamine production and release and thereby diminish oxidative stress. Two trials have attempted to examine the effect of pramipexole or ropinirole on neurodegeneration in PD (Whone *et al.,* 2003; Parkinson Study Group, 2002). Both trials observed that in patients treated with one of these agonists, there

was a reduced rate of loss of markers of dopaminergic neurotransmission measured by brain imaging compared with a similar group of patients treated with levodopa. These intriguing data should be viewed cautiously, particularly because there is considerable uncertainty about the relationship of the imaging techniques used and the true rate of neurodegeneration (Albin and Frey, 2003). Another strategy under study is the use of compounds that augment cellular energy metabolism such coenzyme Q10, a cofactor required for the mitochondrial electron-transport chain. A small study has demonstrated that this drug is well tolerated in PD and has suggested that coenzyme Q10 may slow the course of the disease (Shults *et al.,* 2002).

ALZHEIMER'S DISEASE (AD)

Clinical Overview. AD produces an impairment of cognitive abilities that is gradual in onset but relentless in progression. Impairment of short-term memory usually is the first clinical feature, whereas retrieval of distant memories is preserved relatively well into the course of the disease. As the condition progresses, additional cognitive abilities are impaired, among them the ability to calculate, exercise visuospatial skills, and use common objects and tools (ideomotor apraxia). The level of arousal or alertness of the patient is not affected until the condition is very advanced, nor is there motor weakness, although muscular contractures are an almost universal feature of advanced stages of the disease. Death, most often from a complication of immobility such as pneumonia or pulmonary embolism, usually ensues within 6 to 12 years of onset. The diagnosis of AD is based on careful clinical assessment of the patient and appropriate laboratory tests to exclude other disorders that may mimic AD; at present, no direct antemortem confirmatory test exists.

Pathophysiology. AD is characterized by marked atrophy of the cerebral cortex and loss of cortical and subcortical neurons. The pathological hallmarks of AD are senile plaques, which are spherical accumulations of the protein β-amyloid accompanied by degenerating neuronal processes, and neurofibrillary tangles, composed of paired helical filaments and other proteins (Arnold *et al.,* 1991; Braak and Braak, 1994). Although small numbers of senile plaques and neurofibrillary tangles can be observed in intellectually normal individuals, they are far more abundant in patients with AD, and the abundance of tangles is roughly proportional to the severity of cognitive impairment. In advanced AD, senile plaques and neurofibrillary tangles are numerous and most abundant in the hippocampus and associative regions of the cortex, whereas areas such as the visual and motor cortices are relatively spared. This corresponds to the clinical features of marked impairment of memory and abstract reasoning, with preservation of vision and movement. The factors underlying the selective vulnerability of particular cortical neurons to the pathological effects of AD are not known.

Neurochemistry. The neurochemical disturbances that arise in AD have been studied intensively (Johnston, 1992). Direct analysis of neurotransmitter content in the cerebral cortex shows a reduction of many transmitter substances that parallels neuronal loss; there is a striking and disproportionate deficiency of acetylcholine. The anatomical basis of the cholinergic deficit is the atrophy and degeneration of subcortical cholinergic neurons, particularly those in the basal forebrain (nucleus basalis of Meynert), that provide cholinergic innervation to the whole cerebral cortex. The selective deficiency of acetylcholine in AD, as well as the observation that central cholinergic antagonists such as atropine can induce a confusional state that bears some resemblance to the dementia of AD, has given rise to the "cholinergic hypothesis," which proposes that a deficiency of acetylcholine is critical in the genesis of the symptoms of AD (Perry, 1986). Although the conceptualization of AD as a "cholinergic deficiency syndrome" in parallel with the "dopaminergic deficiency syndrome" of PD provides a useful framework, it is important to note that the deficit in AD is far more complex, involving multiple neurotransmitter systems, including serotonin, glutamate, and neuropeptides, and that in AD there is destruction of not only cholinergic neurons but also the cortical and hippocampal targets that receive cholinergic input.

Role of β-Amyloid. The presence of aggregates of β-amyloid is a constant feature of AD. Until recently, it was not clear whether the amyloid protein was causally linked to the disease process or merely a by-product of neuronal death. The application of molecular genetics has shed some light on this question. β-amyloid from affected brains and found to be a short polypeptide of 42 to 43 amino acids. This information led to cloning of amyloid precursor protein (APP), a much larger protein of more than 700 amino acids, which is expressed widely by neurons throughout the brain in normal individuals as well as in those with AD. The function of APP is unknown, although the structural features of the protein suggest that it may serve as a cell surface receptor for an as-yet-unidentified ligand. The production of β-amyloid from APP appears to result from abnormal proteolytic cleavage of APP by the β-site APP-cleaving enzyme BACE. This may be an important target of future therapies (Vassar *et al.*, 1999).

Analysis of APP gene structure in pedigrees exhibiting autosomal dominant inheritance of AD has shown that in some families, mutations of the β-amyloid-forming region of APP are present, whereas in others, mutations of proteins involved in the processing of APP are implicated (Selkoe, 2002). These results suggest that it is possible for abnormalities in APP or its processing to cause AD. The vast majority of cases of AD, however, are not familial, and structural abnormality of APP or related proteins has not been observed consistently in these sporadic cases of AD. As noted earlier, common alleles of the apo E protein have been found to influence the probability of developing AD. Many investigators believe that modifying the metabolism of APP might alter the course of AD in both familial and sporadic cases, but no clinically practical strategies have been developed.

Treatment of Alzheimer's Disease. A major approach to the treatment of AD has involved attempts to augment the cholinergic function of the brain (Johnston, 1992). An early approach was the use of precursors of acetylcholine

synthesis, such as *choline chloride* and *phosphatidyl choline (lecithin)*. Although these supplements generally are well tolerated, randomized trials have failed to demonstrate any clinically significant efficacy.

A somewhat more successful strategy has been the use of inhibitors of acetylcholinesterase (AChE), the catabolic enzyme for acetylcholine (*see* Chapter 8). *Physostigmine,* a rapidly acting, reversible AChE inhibitor, produces improved responses in animal models of learning, and some studies have demonstrated mild transitory improvement in memory following physostigmine treatment in patients with AD. The use of physostigmine has been limited because of its short half-life and tendency to produce symptoms of systemic cholinergic excess at therapeutic doses.

Four inhibitors of AChE currently are approved by the FDA for treatment of Alzheimer's disease: *tacrine* (1,2,3,4-tetrahydro-9-aminoacridine; COGNEX), *donepezil* (ARICEPT), *rivastigmine* (EXCELON), and *galantamine* (RAZADYNE) (Mayeux and Sano, 1999). Tacrine is a potent centrally acting inhibitor of AChE (Freeman and Dawson, 1991). Studies of oral tacrine in combination with lecithin have confirmed that there is indeed an effect of tacrine on some measures of memory performance, but the magnitude of improvement observed with the combination of lecithin and tacrine is modest at best (Chatellier and Lacomblez, 1990). The side effects of tacrine often are significant and dose-limiting; abdominal cramping, anorexia, nausea, vomiting, and diarrhea are observed in up to one-third of patients receiving therapeutic doses, and elevations of serum transaminases are observed in up to 50% of those treated. Because of significant side effects, tacrine is not used widely clinically. Donepezil is a selective inhibitor of AChE in the CNS with little effect on AChE in peripheral tissues. It produces modest improvements in cognitive scores in Alzheimer's disease patients (Rogers and Friedhoff, 1998) and has a long half-life (*see* Appendix II), allowing once-daily dosing. Rivastigmine and galantamine are dosed twice daily and produce a similar degree of cognitive improvement. Adverse effects associated with donepezil, rivastigmine, and galantamine are similar in character but generally less frequent and less severe than those observed with tacrine; they include nausea, diarrhea, vomiting, and insomnia. Donepezil, rivastigmine, and galantamine are not associated with the hepatotoxicity that limits the use of tacrine.

An alternative strategy for the treatment of AD is the use of the NMDA glutamate-receptor antagonist memantine (NAMENDA). Memantine produces a use-dependent blockade of NMDA receptors. In patients with moderate to severe AD, use of memantine is associated with a reduced rate of clinical deterioration (Reisberg *et al.*, 2003). Whether this is due to a true disease-modifying effect, possibly reduced excitotoxicity, or is a symptomatic effect of the drug is unclear. Adverse effects of memantine usually are mild and reversible and may include headache or dizziness.

HUNTINGTON'S DISEASE

Clinical Features. HD is a dominantly inherited disorder characterized by the gradual onset of motor incoordination and cognitive decline in midlife. Symptoms develop insidiously, either as a movement disorder manifest by brief, jerklike movements of the extremities, trunk, face, and neck (chorea) or as personality changes or both. Fine motor incoordination and impairment of rapid eye movements are early features. Occasionally, especially when the onset of symptoms occurs before age 20, choreic movements are less prominent; instead, bradykinesia and dystonia predominate. As the disorder progresses, the involuntary movements become more severe, dysarthria and dysphagia develop, and balance is impaired. The cognitive disorder manifests first as slowness of mental processing and difficulty in organizing complex tasks. Memory is affected, but affected persons rarely lose their memory of family, friends, and the immediate situation. Such persons often become irritable, anxious, and depressed. Less frequently, paranoia and delusional states are manifest. The outcome of HD is invariably fatal; over a course of 15 to 30 years, the affected person becomes totally disabled and unable to communicate, requiring full-time care; death ensues from the complications of immobility (Hayden, 1981; Harper, 1991).

Pathology and Pathophysiology. HD is characterized by prominent neuronal loss in the striatum (caudate/putamen) of the brain (Vonsattel *et al.*, 1985). Atrophy of these structures proceeds in an orderly fashion, first affecting the tail of the caudate nucleus and then proceeding anteriorly from mediodorsal to ventrolateral. Other areas of the brain also are affected, although much less severely; morphometric analyses indicate that there are fewer neurons in cerebral cortex, hypothalamus, and thalamus. Even within the striatum, the neuronal degeneration of HD is selective. Interneurons and afferent terminals are largely spared, whereas the striatal projection neurons (the medium spiny neurons) are severely affected. This leads to large decreases in striatal GABA concentrations, whereas somatostatin and dopamine concentrations are relatively preserved (Ferrante *et al.*, 1987).

Selective vulnerability also appears to underlie the most conspicuous clinical feature of HD, the development of chorea. In most adult-onset cases, the medium spiny neurons that project to the GPi and SNpr (the indirect pathway) appear to be affected earlier than

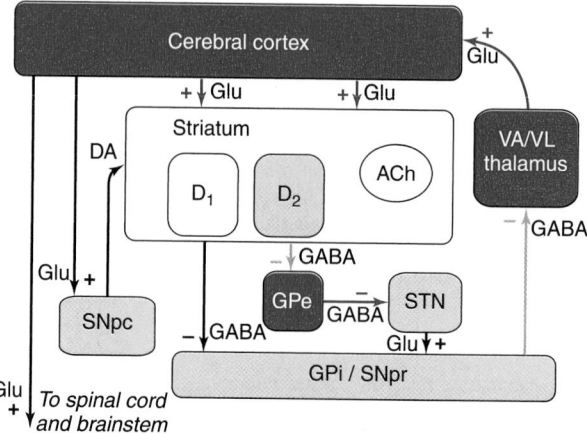

Figure 20–10. *The basal ganglia in Huntington's disease.* HD is characterized by loss of neurons from the striatum. The neurons that project from the striatum to the GPe and form the indirect pathway are affected earlier in the course of the disease than those which project to the GPi. This leads to a loss of inhibition of the GPe. The increased activity in this structure, in turn, inhibits the STN, SNpr, and GPi, resulting in a loss of inhibition to the VA/VL thalamus and increased thalamocortical excitatory drive. Structures in light blue have reduced activity in HD, whereas structures in dark blue have increased activity. (*See* legend to Figure 20–6 for definitions of anatomical abbreviations.)

those projecting to the GPe (the direct pathway) (Albin *et al.*, 1992). The disproportionate impairment of the indirect pathway increases excitatory drive to the neocortex, producing involuntary choreiform movements (Figure 20–10). In some individuals, rigidity rather than chorea is the predominant clinical feature; this is especially common in juvenile-onset cases. In these cases the striatal neurons giving rise to both the direct and indirect pathways are impaired to a comparable degree.

Genetics. HD is an autosomal dominant disorder with nearly complete penetrance. The average age of onset is between 35 and 45 years, but the range varies from as early as age 2 to as late as the middle 80s. Although the disease is inherited equally from mother and father, more than 80% of those developing symptoms before age 20 inherit the defect from the father. This is an example of *anticipation*, or the tendency for the age of onset of a disease to decline with each succeeding generation, which also is observed in other neurodegenerative diseases with similar genetic mechanisms. Known homozygotes for HD show clinical characteristics identical to the typical HD heterozygote, indicating that the unaffected chromosome does not attenuate the disease symptomatology. Until the discovery of the genetic defect responsible for HD, *de novo* mutations causing HD were thought to be unusual; but it is now clear that the disease can arise from unaffected parents, especially when one carries an "intermediate allele," as described below.

The discovery of the genetic mutation responsible for Huntington's disease was the product of an arduous 10-year, multi-investigator collaborative effort. In 1993, a region near the end of the short arm of chromosome 4 was found to contain a polymorphic $(CAG)_n$ trinucleotide repeat that was significantly expanded in all individuals with HD (Huntington's Disease Collaborative Research Group, 1993). The expansion of this trinucleotide repeat is the genetic alteration responsible for HD. The range of CAG repeat length in normal individuals is between 9 and 34 triplets, with a median repeat length on normal chromosomes of 19. The repeat length in HD varies from 40 to over 100. Repeat lengths of 35 to 39 represent intermediate alleles; some of these individuals develop HD late in life, whereas others are not affected. Repeat length is correlated inversely with age of onset. The younger the age of onset, the higher is the probability of a large repeat number. This correlation is most powerful in individuals with onset before age 30; with onset above age 30, the correlation is weaker. Thus, repeat length cannot serve as an adequate predictor of age of onset in most individuals. Several other neurodegenerative diseases also arise through expansion of a CAG repeat, including hereditary spinocerebellar ataxias and Kennedy's disease, a rare inherited disorder of motor neurons.

Selective Vulnerability. The mechanism by which the expanded trinucleotide repeat leads to the clinical and pathological features of HD is unknown. The HD mutation lies within a gene designated *IT15*. The *IT15* gene is very large (10 kilobases) and encodes a protein of approximately 348,000 daltons or 3144 amino acids. The trinucleotide repeat, which encodes the amino acid glutamine, occurs at the 5 end of *IT15* and is followed directly by a second, shorter repeat of $(CCG)_n$ that encodes proline. The protein, named *huntingtin,* does not resemble any other known protein, and the normal function of the protein has not been identified. Mice with a genetic knockout of huntingtin die early in embryonic life, so it must have an essential cellular function. It is thought that the mutation results in a *gain of function; i.e.,* the mutant protein acquires a new function or property not found in the normal protein.

The HD gene is expressed widely throughout the body. High levels of expression are present in brain, pancreas, intestine, muscle, liver, adrenals, and testes. In brain, expression of *IT15* does not correlate with neuron vulnerability: Although the striatum is most severely affected, neurons in all regions of the brain express similar levels of *IT15* mRNA (Landwehrmeyer *et al.,* 1995).

The ability of the HD mutation to produce selective neural degeneration despite nearly universal expression of the gene among neurons may be related to metabolic or excitotoxic mechanisms. For many years it has been noted that HD patients are thin, suggesting the presence of a systemic disturbance of energy metabolism. In animal models, agonists for the NMDA subtype of excitatory amino acid receptor can cause pathology similar to that seen in HD when they are injected into the striatum (Beal *et al.,* 1986). Interestingly, inhibitors of complex II of the mitochondrial respiratory chain also can produce HD-like striatal lesions—even when given systemically (Beal *et al.,* 1993). Furthermore, this pathology can be diminished by NMDA-receptor antagonists, suggesting that this is an example of a metabolic impairment giving rise to excitotoxic neuronal injury. Thus the link between the widespread expression of the gene for the abnormal *IT15* protein in HD and the selective vulnerability of neurons in the disease may arise from the interaction of a widespread defect in energy metabolism with the intrinsic properties of striatal neurons, including their capacity and need for oxidative metabolism, as well as the types of glutamate receptors present.

An alternative mechanism for the neurodegeneration observed in HD has arisen from studies of effects of the disease on gene expression. In both the human disease and animal models there are striking and selective alterations in patterns of gene expression. This has led to the "transcriptional hypothesis" that suggests that the abnormal function of mutant huntingtin may be an ability to alter or interfere with mechanisms of gene transcription (Cha, 2000).

These two hypotheses have given rise to trials of several different types of therapies in animal models and patients with HD, addressing on the one hand, metabolic defects and energy defects through treatment with agents such as coenzyme Q10 and, on the other hand, drugs that alter gene transcription. None of these approaches is yet established to be effective in altering the course of the disease.

Symptomatic Treatment of Huntington's Disease. Practical treatment for symptomatic HD emphasizes the selective use of medications (Shoulson, 1992). No current medication slows the progression of the disease, and many medications can impair function because of side effects. Treatment is needed for patients who are depressed, irritable, paranoid, excessively anxious, or psychotic. Depression can be treated effectively with standard antidepressant drugs with the caveat that drugs with substantial anticholinergic profiles can exacerbate chorea. *Fluoxetine (see* Chapter 17) is effective treatment for both the depression and the irritability manifest in symptomatic HD. *Carbamazepine (see* Chapter 19) also has been found to be effective for depression. Paranoia, delusional states, and psychosis usually require treatment with antipsychotic drugs, but the doses required often are lower than those usually used in primary psychiatric disorders. These agents also reduce cognitive function and impair mobility and thus should be used in the lowest doses possible and should be discontinued when the psychiatric symptoms resolve. In individuals with predominantly rigid HD, *clozapine, quetiapine (see* Chapter 18), or carbamazepine may be more effective for treatment of paranoia and psychosis.

The movement disorder of HD *per se* only rarely justifies pharmacological therapy. For those with large-amplitude chorea causing frequent falls and injury, dopamine-depleting agents such as *tetrabenazine* and *reserpine (see* Chapter 32) can be tried, although patients must be monitored for hypotension and depression. Antipsychotic agents also can be used, but these often do not improve overall function because they decrease fine motor coordination and increase rigidity. Many HD patients exhibit worsening of involuntary movements as a result of anxiety or stress. In these situations, judicious use of sedative or anxiolytic benzodiazepines can be very helpful. In juvenile-onset cases where rigidity rather than chorea predominates, dopamine agonists have had variable success in the improvement of rigidity. These individuals also occasionally develop myoclonus and seizures that can be responsive to *clonazepam, valproic acid,* and other anticonvulsants.

AMYOTROPHIC LATERAL SCLEROSIS (ALS)

Clinical Features and Pathology. ALS is a disorder of the motor neurons of the ventral horn of the spinal cord and the cortical neurons that provide their afferent input. The ratio of males to females affected is approximately 1.5:1 (Kurtzke, 1982). The disorder is characterized by rapidly progressive weakness, muscle atrophy and fasciculations, spasticity, dysarthria, dysphagia, and respiratory compromise. Sensory function generally is spared, as is cognitive, autonomic, and oculomotor activity. ALS usually is progressive and fatal, with most affected patients dying of respiratory compromise and pneumonia after 2 to 3 years, although occasional individuals have a more indolent course and survive for many years. The pathology of ALS corresponds closely to the clinical features: There is prominent loss of the spinal and brainstem motor neurons that project to striated muscles (although the oculomotor neurons are spared), as well as loss of the large pyramidal motor neurons in layer V of motor cortex, which are the origin of the descending corticospinal tracts. In familial cases, Clarke's column and the dorsal horns sometimes are affected (Rowland, 1994).

Etiology. About 10% of ALS cases are familial (FALS), usually with an autosomal dominant pattern of inheritance. Most of the mutations responsible have not been identified, but an important subset of FALS patients are families with a mutation in the gene for the enzyme SOD1 (Rosen *et al.*, 1993). Mutations in this protein account for about 20% of cases of FALS. Most of the mutations are alterations of single amino acids, but more than 30 different alleles have been found in different kindreds. Transgenic mice expressing mutant human *SOD1* develop a progressive degeneration of motor neurons that closely mimics the human disease, providing an important animal model for research and pharmaceutical trials. Interestingly, many of the mutations of *SOD1* that can cause disease do not reduce the capacity of the enzyme to perform its primary function, the catabolism of superoxide radicals. Thus, as may be the case in HD, mutations in *SOD1* may confer a toxic "gain of function," the precise nature of which is unclear.

More than 90% of ALS cases are sporadic and are not associated with abnormalities of *SOD1* or any other known gene. The cause of the motor neuron loss in sporadic ALS is unknown, but theories include autoimmunity, excitotoxicity, free radical toxicity, and viral infection (Rowland, 1994; Cleveland, 1999). Most of these ideas are not well supported by available data, but there is evidence that glutamate reuptake may be abnormal in the disease, leading to accumulation of glutamate and excitotoxic injury (Rothstein *et al.*, 1992). The only currently approved therapy for ALS, *riluzole,* is based on these observations.

Treatment of ALS with Riluzole. *Riluzole* (2-amino-6-[trifluoromethoxy]benzothiazole; RILUTEK) is an agent with complex actions in the nervous system (Bryson *et al.*, 1996). Its structure is as follows:

RILUZOLE

Riluzole is absorbed orally and is highly protein bound. It undergoes extensive metabolism in the liver by both cytochrome P450–mediated hydroxylation and glucuronidation. Its half-life is about 12 hours. *In vitro* studies have shown that riluzole has both presynaptic and postsynaptic effects. It inhibits glutamate release, but it also blocks postsynaptic NMDA- and kainate-type glutamate receptors and inhibits voltage-dependent sodium channels. Some of the effects of riluzole *in vitro* are blocked by pertussis toxin, implicating the drug's interaction with an as-yet-unidentified GPCR. In clinical trials riluzole has modest but genuine effects on the survival of patients with ALS. In the largest trial conducted to date, with nearly 1000 patients, the median duration of survival was extended by about 60 days (Lacomblez *et al.*, 1996). The recommended dose is 50 mg every 12 hours, taken 1 hour before or 2 hours after a meal. Riluzole usually is well tolerated, although nausea or diarrhea may occur. Rarely, riluzole may produce hepatic injury with elevations of serum transaminases, and periodic monitoring of these is recommended. Although the magnitude of the effect of riluzole on ALS is small, it represents a significant therapeutic milestone in the treatment of a disease refractory to all previous treatments.

Symptomatic Therapy of ALS: Spasticity. Spasticity is an important component of the clinical features of ALS in that the presence of spasticity often leads to considerable pain and discomfort and reduces mobility, which already is compromised by weakness. Furthermore, spasticity is the feature of ALS that is most amenable to present forms of treatment. *Spasticity* is defined as an increase in muscle tone characterized by an initial resistance to passive displacement of a limb at a joint, followed by a sudden relaxation (the so-called clasped-knife phenomenon). Spasticity is the result of the loss of descending inputs to the spinal motor neurons, and the character of the spasticity depends on which nervous system pathways are affected (Davidoff, 1990). Whole repertoires of movement can be generated directly at the spinal cord level; it is beyond the scope of this chapter to describe these in detail. The monosynaptic tendon-stretch reflex is the simplest of the spinal mechanisms contributing to spasticity. Primary Ia afferents from muscle spindles, activated when the muscle is stretched rapidly, synapse directly on motor neurons going to the stretched muscle, causing it to contract and resist the movement. A collateral of the primary Ia afferent synapses on a "Ia-coupled interneuron" that inhibits the motor neurons innervating the antagonist of the stretched muscle, allowing contraction of the muscle to be unopposed. Upper motor neurons from the cerebral cortex (the pyramidal neurons) suppress spinal reflexes and the lower motor neurons indirectly by activating the spinal cord inhibitory interneuron pools. The pyramidal neurons use glutamate as a neurotransmitter. When the pyramidal influences are removed, the reflexes are released from inhibition and become more active, leading to hyperreflexia. Other descending pathways from the brainstem, including the rubro-, reticulo-, and vestibulospinal pathways and the descending catecholamine pathways, also influence spinal reflex activity. When just the pyramidal pathway is affected, extensor tone in the legs and flexor tone in the arms are increased. When the vestibulospinal and catecholamine pathways are impaired, increased flexion of all extremities is observed, and light cutaneous stimulation can lead to disabling whole-body spasms. In ALS, pyramidal pathways are impaired with relative preservation of the other descending pathways, resulting in hyperactive deep-tendon reflexes, impaired fine motor coordination, increased extensor tone in the legs, and increased flexor tone in the arms. The gag reflex often is overactive as well.

The most useful agent for the symptomatic treatment of spasticity in ALS is *baclofen* (LIORESAL), a GABA$_B$-receptor agonist. Initial doses of 5 to 10 mg/day are recommended, but the dose can be increased to as much as 200 mg/day if necessary. If weakness occurs, the dose should be lowered. In addition to oral administration, baclofen also can be delivered directly into the space around the spinal cord by use of a surgically implanted pump and an intrathecal catheter. This approach minimizes the adverse effects of the drug, especially sedation, but it carries the risk of potentially life-threatening CNS depression and should be only used by physicians trained in delivering chronic intrathecal therapy. *Tizanidine* (ZANFLEX) is an agonist of α_2 adrenergic receptors in the CNS. It reduces muscle spasticity and is assumed to act by increasing presynaptic inhibition of motor neurons. Tizanidine is used most widely in the treatment of spasticity in multiple sclerosis or after stroke, but it also may be effective in patients with ALS. Treatment should be initiated at a low dose of 2 to 4 mg at bedtime and titrated upward gradually. Drowsiness, asthenia, and dizziness may limit

the dose that can be administered. *Benzodiazepines* (*see* Chapter 16) such as *clonazepam* (KLONIPIN) are effective antispasmodics, but they may contribute to respiratory depression in patients with advanced ALS. *Dantrolene* (DANTRIUM) also is approved in the United States for the treatment of muscle spasm. In contrast to the other agents discussed, dantrolene acts directly on skeletal muscle fibers, impairing calcium ion flux across the sarcoplasmic reticulum. Because it can exacerbate muscular weakness, it is not used in ALS but is effective in treating spasticity associated with stroke or spinal cord injury and in treating malignant hyperthermia (*see* Chapter 9). Dantrolene may cause hepatotoxicity, so it is important to perform liver function tests before and during therapy with the drug.

CLINICAL SUMMARY

The shared characteristic of all neurodegenerative disorders is the selective and progressive loss of neurons in specific brain structures. At the present time there are effective symptomatic therapies for several of the disorders, but few treatments that can substantially slow the underlying degenerative processes.

PD is characterized by the progressive loss of dopaminergic neurons in the substantia nigra pars compacta, producing abnormalities in the control of movement. The symptomatic therapy of PD is often very successful, producing effective control of many of the signs and symptoms. The single most effective therapy is levodopa, but long-term use of this agent is associated with undesirable side effects, wearing off, and dyskinesias. There also is uncertainty about the impact of levodopa on progression of the disease. An alternative to treatment with levodopa is the use of dopamine agonists such as pramipexole or ropinirole. There are also useful adjunctive therapies for PD, including inhibitors of the enzyme COMT, that prolong the action of levodopa, as well as drugs acting at acetylcholine receptors and other sites.

AD is associated with accumulation of abnormal aggregates of the protein β-amyloid, as well as neuronal degeneration with neurofibrillary tangles, and leads to progressive impairment of memory and cognition. Many different brain regions are affected, but there is particularly severe degeneration of cholinergic neurons in the basal forebrain. Most current therapies are based on augmenting cholinergic transmission through inhibition of acetylcholinesterase. This approach is modestly effective, producing partial improvement in memory and behavioral symptoms that may improve the quality of life of affected patients significantly.

HD is an autosomal dominant disorder caused by a mutation in the protein huntingtin. The defect leads to progressive motor and cognitive symptoms. At present there is no effective treatment for the primary disorder, although antidepressant and antipsychotic medications may be useful to control specific symptoms.

ALS (or Lou Gehrig's disease) is a progressive degenerative disease of spinal motor neurons leading to weakness and eventually paralysis. It is the most rapidly progressive of the common neurodegenerative disorders and often is fatal within 2 to 3 years of onset. The only therapy established to alter the course of ALS is the drug riluzole, which acts through inhibition of glutamate release as well as other mechanisms. The effect of this treatment is modest, prolonging survival by about 3 months.

An important goal of much current research in the pharmacology of neurodegenerative disorders is identification of drugs that can slow the underlying degenerative process. A number of candidate mechanisms have been identified that are shared among these disease, and there are clinical trials currently in progress seeking evidence of efficacy.

BIBLIOGRAPHY

Albin, R.L., Reiner, A., Anderson, K.D., *et al.* Preferential loss of striato–external pallidal projection neurons in presymptomatic Huntington's disease. *Ann. Neurol.*, **1992**, *31*:425–430.

Arnold, S.E., Hyman, B.T., Flory, J., Damasio, A.R., and Van Hoesen, G.W. The topographical and neuroanatomical distribution of neurofibrillary tangles and neuritic plaques in the cerebral cortex of patients with Alzheimer's disease. *Cereb. Cortex*, **1991**, *1*:103–116.

Ballard, P.A., Tetrud, J.W., and Lanston, J.W. Permanent human parkinsonism due to *N*-methyl-4-phenyl-1,2,3,6-tetrahydropyridine (MPTP): Seven cases. *Neurology*, **1985**, *35*:949–956.

Beal, M.F., Kowall, N.W., Ellison, D.W., *et al.* Replication of the neurochemical characteristics of Huntington's disease by quinolinic acid. *Nature*, **1986**, *321*:168–172.

Chase, T.N. Levodopa therapy: Consequences of nonphysiologic replacement of dopamine. *Neurology*, **1998**, *50*:S17–S25.

Chatellier, G., and Lacomblez, L. Tacrine (tetrahydroaminoacridine; THA) and lecithin in senile dementia of the Alzheimer type: A multicentre trial. Groupe Français d'Etude de la Tetrahydromaminoacridine. *BMJ*, **1990**, *300*:495–499.

Cohen, G., and Werner, P. Free radicals, oxidative stress and neurodegeneration. In, *Neurodegenerative Diseases*. (Calne, D.B., ed.) Saunders, Philadelphia, **1994**, pp. 139–161.

Cotzias, G.C., Papavasiliou, P.S., and Gellene, R. Modification of Parkinsonism: Chronic treatment with L-DOPA. *New Engl. J. Med.*, **1969**, *280*:337–345.

Cudkowicz, M.E., and Brown, R.H., Jr. An update on superoxide dismutase 1 in familial amyotrophic lateral sclerosis. *J. Neurol. Sci.*, **1996**, *139*(suppl):10–15.

Evans, D.A., Funkenstein, H.H., Albert, M.S., *et al.* Prevalence of

Alzheimer's disease in a community population of older persons: Higher than previously reported. *JAMA*, **1989**, *262*:2551–2556.

Ferrante, R.J., Kowall, N.W., Beal, M.F., *et al.* Morphologic and histochemical characteristics of a spared subset of striatal neurons in Huntington's disease. *J. Neuropathol. Exp. Neurol.*, **1987**, *46*:12–27.

Friedman, J.H., and Factor, S.A. Atypical antipsychotics in the treatment of drug-induced psychosis in Parkinson's disease. *Mov. Disord.*, **2000**, *15*:201–211.

Frucht, S., Rogers, J.G., Greene, P.E., Gordon, M.F., and Fahn, S. Falling asleep at the wheel: Motor vehicle mishaps in persons taking pramipexole and ropinirole. *Neurology*, **1999**, *52*:1908–1910.

Gibb, W.R. Neuropathology of Parkinson's disease and related syndromes. *Neurol. Clin.*, **1992**, *10*:361–376.

Hersch, S.M., Gutekunst, C.A., Rees, H.D., Heilman, C.J., and Levey, A.I. Distribution of m1-m4 muscarinic receptor proteins in the rat striatum: Light and electron microscopic immunocytochemistry using subtype-specific antibodies. *J. Neurosci.*, **1994**, *14*:3351–3363.

Hornykiewicz, O. Dopamine in the basal ganglia: Its role and therapeutic indications (including the clinical use of L-DOPA). *Br. Med. Bull.*, **1973**, *29*:172–178.

Huntington's Disease Collaborative Research Group. A novel gene containing a trinucleotide repeat that is expanded and unstable on Huntington's disease chromosomes. *Cell*, **1993**, *72*:971–983.

Jenkins, B.G., Koroshetz, W.J., Beal, M.F., and Rosen, B.R. Evidence for impairment of energy metabolism *in vivo* in Huntington's disease using localized ^{1}H NMR spectroscopy. *Neurology*, **1993**, *43*:2689–2695.

Jenner, P. Oxidative mechanisms in nigral cell death in Parkinson's disease. *Mov. Disord.*, **1998**, *13*(suppl 1):24–34.

Kurth, M.C., Adler, C.H., Hilaire, M.S., *et al.* Tolcapone improves motor function and reduces levodopa requirement in patients with Parkinson's disease experiencing motor fluctuations: A multicenter, double-blind, randomized, placebo-controlled trial. Tolcapone Fluctuator Study Group I. *Neurology*, **1997**, *48*:81–87.

Lacomblez, L., Bensimon, G., Leigh, P.N., Guillet, P., and Meininger, V. Dose-ranging study of riluzole in amyotrophic lateral sclerosis. *Lancet*, **1996**, *347*:1425–1431.

Landwehrmeyer, G.B., McNeil, S.M., Dure, L.S., *et al.* Huntington's disease gene: Regional and cellular expression in brain of normal and affected individuals. *Ann. Neurol.*, **1995**, *37*:218–230.

Lipton, S.A., and Rosenberg, P.A. Excitatory amino acids as a final common pathway for neurologic disorders. *New Engl. J. Med.*, **1994**, *330*:613–622.

Mouradian, M.M., Heuser, I.J., Baronti, F., and Chase, T.N. Modification of central dopaminergic mechanisms by continuous levodopa therapy for advanced Parkinson's disease. *Ann. Neurol.*, **1990**, *27*:18–23.

Olanow, C.W. MAO-B inhibitors in Parkinson's disease. *Adv. Neurol.*, **1993**, *60*:666–671.

Olney, J.W. Brain lesions, obesity, and other disturbances in mice treated with monosodium glutamate. *Science*, **1969**, *164*:719–721.

Parkinson Study Group. Effects of tocopherol and deprenyl on the progression of disability in early Parkinson's disease. *New Engl. J. Med.*, **1993**, *328*:176–183.

Parkinson Study Group. Entacapone improves motor fluctuations in levodopa-treated Parkinson's disease patients. *Ann. Neurol.*, **1997**, *42*: 747–755 (published erratum appears in *Ann. Neurol.*, **1998**, *44*:292).

Parkinson Study Group. Pramipexole vs. levodopa as initial treatment for Parkinson's disease: A randomized, controlled trial. *JAMA*, **2000**, *284*:1931–1938.

Parkinson Study Group. Dopamine transporter imaging to asses the effects of pramipexole vs levodopa on Parkinson disease progression. JAMA, **2002**, *287*:1653–1661.

Przedborski, S., and Jackson-Lewis, V. Mechanisms of MPTP toxicity. *Mov. Disord.,* **1998**, *13*(suppl 1):35–38.

Rascol, O., Brooks, D.J., Korczyn, A.D., *et al.* A five-year study of the incidence of dyskinesia in patients with early Parkinson's disease who were treated with ropinirole or levodopa. 056 Study Group. *New Engl. J. Med.,* **2000**, *342*:1484–1491.

Reisberg, B., Doody, R., Stoffler, A., *et al.* Memantine in moderate to severe Alzheimer's disease. *New Engl. J. Med.,* **2003**, *348:*1333-1341.

Rogers, S.L., and Friedhoff, L.T. Long-term efficacy and safety of done-pezil in the treatment of Alzheimer's disease: An interim analysis of the results of a U.S. multicentre open label extension study. *Eur. Neuropsychopharmacol.,* **1998**, *8*:67–75.

Rosen, D.R., Siddique, T., Patterson, D., *et al.* Mutations in Cu/Zn superoxide dismutase gene are associated with familial amyotrophic lateral sclerosis. *Nature,* **1993**, *362*:59–62 (published erratum appears in *Nature,* **1993**, *364*:362).

Roses, A.D. Apolipoprotein E, a gene with complex biological interactions in the aging brain. *Neurobiol. Dis.,* **1997**, *4*:170–185.

Rothstein, J.D., Marin, L.J., and Kuncl, R.W. Decreased glutamate transport by the brain and spinal cord in amyotrophic lateral sclerosis. *New Engl. J. Med.,* **1992**, *326*:1464–1468.

Schapira, A.H., Mann, V.M., Cooper, J.M., *et al.* Anatomic and disease specificity of NADH CoQ1 reductase (complex I) deficiency in Parkinson's disease. *J. Neurochem.,* **1990**, *55*:2142–2145.

Shults, C.W., Oakes, D., Kieburtz, K., *et al.* Effects of coenzyme Q10 in early Parkinson disease: Evidence of slowing of the functional decline. *Arch. Neurol.,* **2002**, *59*:1541–1550.

Tandan, R., and Bradley, W.G. Amyotrophic lateral sclerosis: 2. Etio-pathogenesis. *Ann. Neurol.,* **1985**, *18*:419–431.

Vassar, R., Bennett, B.D., Babu-Kahn, S., *et al.* β-Secretase cleavage of Alzheimer's amyloid precursor protein by the transmembrane aspartic protease BACE. *Science,* **1999**, *286*:735–741.

Vonsattel, J.P., Myers, R.H., Stevens, T.J., *et al.* Neuropathological classification of Huntington's disease. *J. Neuropathol. Exp. Neurol.,* **1985**, *44*:559–577.

Wallace, D.C. Mitochondrial genetics: A paradigm of aging and degenerative diseases? *Science,* **1992**, *256*:628–632.

Whone, A.L., Watts, R.L., Stoessl, A.J., *et al.* Slower progression of Parkinson's disease with ropinirole versus levodopa: The REAL-PET study. *Ann. Neurol.,* **2003**, *54*:93-101.

MONOGRAPHS AND REVIEWS

Albin, R.L., Young, A.B., and Penney, J.B. The functional anatomy of basal ganglia disorders. *Trends Neurosci.,* **1989**, *12*:366–375.

Albin, R.L., and Frey, K.A. Initial agonist treatment of Parkinson's disease: A critique. *Neurology,* **2003**, *60*:390–394.

Beal, M.F., Hyman, B.T., and Koroshetz, W. Do defects in mitochondrial energy metabolism underlie the pathology of neurodegenerative diseases? *Trends Neurosci.,* **1993**, *16*:125–131.

Betarbet, R., Sherer, T.B., Di Monte, D.A., and Greenamyre, J.T. Mechanistic approaches to Parkinson's disease. *Brain Pathology,* **2002**, *12*:499–510.

Braak, H., and Braak, E. Pathology of Alzheimer's disease. In, *Neurodegenerative Diseases.* (Calne, D.B., ed.) Saunders, Philadelphia, **1994**, pp. 585–614.

Bryson, H.M., Fulton, B., and Benfield, P. Riluzole: A review of its pharmacodynamic and pharmacokinetic properties and therapeutic potential in amyotrophic lateral sclerosis. *Drugs,* **1996**, *52*:549–563.

Cantuti-Castelvetri, I., and Standaert, D.G., Neuroprotective strategies for Parkinson's disease. *Curr. Neuropharm.,* **2004**, *2*:153–168.

Cha, J.H. Transcriptional dysregulation in Huntington's disease. *Trends Neurosci* **2000**, *23*:387–392.

Choi, D.W., and Rothman, S.M. The role of glutamate neurotoxicity in hypoxic-ischemic neuronal death. *Annu. Rev. Neurosci.,* **1990**, *13*:171–182.

Cleveland, D.W. From Charcot to SOD1: Mechanisms of selective motor neuron death in ALS. *Neuron,* **1999**, *24*:515–520.

Cooper, J.R., Bloom, F.E., and Roth, H.R., eds. *The Biochemical Basis of Neuropharmacology,* 7th ed. Oxford University Press, New York, **1996.**

Cummings, J.L., Vinters, H.V., Cole, G.M., and Khachaturian, Z.S. Alzheimer's disease: Etiologies, pathophysiology, cognitive reserve, and treatment opportunities. *Neurology,* **1998**, *51*:S2–S17.

Davidoff, R.A. Spinal neurotransmitters and the mode of action of antispasticity drugs. In, *The Origin and Treatment of Spasticity.* (Benecke, R., Emre, M., and Davidoff, R.A., eds.) Parthenon Publishing Group, Carnforth, England, **1990**, pp. 63–92.

Fearnley, J., and Lees, A. Pathology of Parkinson's disease. In, *Neurodegenerative Diseases.* (Calne, D.B., ed.) Saunders, Philadelphia, **1994**, pp. 545–554.

Freeman, S.E., and Dawson, R.M. Tacrine: A pharmacological review. *Prog. Neurobiol.,* **1991**, *36*:257–277.

Gwinn-Hardy, K. Genetics of parkinsonism. *Mov. Disord.,* **2002**, *17*:645-656.

Hallett, P.J, and Standaert, D.G. Rationale for and use of NMDA receptor antagonists in Parkinson's disease. *Pharmacol. Ther.,* **2004**, *102*:155–174.

Harper, P.S., ed. *Huntington's Disease.* Saunders, London, **1991.**

Hayden, M.R. *Huntington's Chorea.* Springer-Verlag, Berlin, **1981.**

Johnston, M.V. Cognitive disorders. In, *Principles of Drug Therapy in Neurology.* (Johnston, M.V., MacDonald, R.L., and Young, A.B., eds.) Davis, Philadelphia, **1992**, pp. 226–267.

Kurtzke, J.F. Epidemiology of amyotrophic lateral sclerosis. In, *Human Motor Neuron Diseases.* (Rowland, L.P., ed.) *Advances in Neurology,* Vol. 36. Raven Press, New York, **1982**, pp. 281–302.

Lang, A.E., and Lozano, A.M. Parkinson's disease. First of two parts. *New Engl. J. Med.,* **1998**, *339*:1044–1053.

Mayeux, R., and Sano, M. Treatment of Alzheimer's disease. *New Engl. J. Med.,* **1999**, *341*:1670–1679.

Mink, J.W., and Thach, W.T. Basal ganglia intrinsic circuits and their role in behavior. *Curr. Opin. Neurobiol.,* **1993**, *3*:950–957.

Missale, C., Nash, S.R., Robinson, S.W., Jaber, M., and Caron, M.G. Dopamine receptors: from structure to function. *Physiol. Rev.,* **1998**, *78*:189-225.

Mouradian, M.M., and Chase, T.N. Improved dopaminergic therapy of Parkinson's disease. In, *Movement Disorders 3.* (Marsden, C.D., and Fahn, S., eds.) Butterworth-Heinemann, Oxford, **1994**, pp. 181–199.

Parent, A., and Cicchetti, F. The current model of basal ganglia organization under scrutiny. *Mov. Disord.,* **1998**, *13*:199–202.

Perry, E.K. The cholinergic hypothesis—ten years on. *Br. Med. Bull.,* **1986**, *42*:63–69.

Rowland, L.P. Amyotrophic lateral sclerosis: theories and therapies. *Ann. Neurol.,* **1994**, *35*:129–130.

Selkoe, D.J., and Podlisny, M.B. Deciphering the genetic basis of Alzheimer's disease. *Annu. Rev. Genomics Hum. Genet.,* **2002**, *3*:67–99.

Shoulson, I. Huntington's disease. In, *Diseases of the Nervous System: Clinical Neurobiology.* (Asbury, A.K., McKhann, G.M., and McDonald, W.I., eds.) Saunders, Philadelphia, **1992**, pp. 1159–1168.

Tanner, C.M. Epidemiology of Parkinson's disease. *Neurol. Clin.,* **1992**, *10*:317–329.

Wichmann, T., and DeLong, M.R. Pathophysiology of parkinsonian motor abnormalities. *Adv. Neurol.,* **1993**, *60*:53–61.

OPIOID ANALGESICS

Howard B. Gutstein and Huda Akil

OVERVIEW

Opioids have been the mainstay of pain treatment for thousands of years, and they remain so today. Opioids such as *heroin* and *morphine* exert their effects by mimicking naturally occurring substances, called *endogenous opioid peptides* or *endorphins*. Much now is known about the basic biology of the endogenous opioid system and its molecular and biochemical complexity, widespread anatomy, and diversity. The diverse functions of this system include the best known sensory role, prominent in inhibiting responses to painful stimuli; a modulatory role in gastrointestinal, endocrine, and autonomic functions; an emotional role, evident in the powerful rewarding and addicting properties of opioids; and a cognitive role in the modulation of learning and memory. The endogenous opioid system is complex and subtle, with a great diversity in endogenous ligands (more than a dozen) yet with only four major receptor types. This chapter presents key facts about the biochemical and functional nature of the opioid system that then are used to understand the actions of clinically used opioid drugs and strategies for pain treatment.

Terminology. The term *opioid* refers broadly to all compounds related to opium. The word *opium* is derived from *opos*, the Greek word for "juice," the drug being derived from the juice of the opium poppy, *Papaver somniferum. Opiates* are drugs derived from opium, and they include the natural products *morphine, codeine,* and *thebaine,* and many semisynthetic derivatives. *Endogenous opioid peptides* are the naturally occurring ligands for opioid receptors. The term *endorphin* is used synonymously with endogenous opioid peptides but also refers to a specific endogenous opioid, β-endorphin. The term *narcotic* was derived from the Greek word for "stupor." At one time, the term referred to any drug that induced sleep, but then it became associated with opioids. It often is used in a legal context to refer to a variety of substances with abuse or addictive potential.

History. The first undisputed reference to opium is found in the writings of Theophrastus in the third century B.C. Arab physicians were well versed in the uses of opium; Arab traders introduced the drug to the Orient, where it was employed mainly for the control of dysenteries. During the Middle Ages, many of the uses of opium were appreciated. In 1680, Sydenham wrote: "Among the remedies which it has pleased Almighty God to give to man to relieve his sufferings, none is so universal and so efficacious as opium."

Opium contains more than 20 distinct alkaloids. In 1806, Sertürner reported the isolation of a pure substance in opium that he named *morphine,* after Morpheus, the Greek god of dreams. The discovery of other alkaloids in opium quickly followed—codeine by Robiquet in 1832 and *papaverine* by Merck in 1848. By the middle of the nineteenth century, the use of pure alkaloids in place of crude opium preparations began to spread throughout the medical world.

In addition to the remarkable beneficial effects of opioids, the toxic side effects and addictive potential of these drugs also have been known for centuries. These problems stimulated a search for potent synthetic opioid analgesics free of addictive potential and other side effects. Unfortunately, all synthetic compounds that have been introduced into clinical use share the liabilities of classical opioids. However, the search for new opioid agonists led to the synthesis of opioid antagonists and compounds with mixed agonist–antagonist properties, which expanded therapeutic options and provided important tools for exploring mechanisms of opioid actions.

Until the early 1970s, the endogenous opioid system was totally unknown. The actions of morphine, heroin, and other opioids as antinociceptive and addictive agents, while well described, typically were studied in the context of interactions with other neurotransmitter systems, such as monoaminergic and cholinergic. Some investigators suggested the existence of a specific opioid receptor because of the unique structural requirements of opiate ligands, but the presence of an opiate-like system in the brain remained unproven. A particularly misleading observation was that the administration of the opioid antagonist *naloxone* to a normal animal produced little effect, although the drug was effective in reversing or preventing the effects of exogenous opiates. The first physiological evidence suggesting an endogenous opioid system was the demonstration that analgesia produced by electrical stimulation of certain brain regions was reversed by naloxone (Akil *et al.,* 1972, 1976). Pharmacological evidence for an opiate receptor also was building. In 1973, investigators in three laboratories demonstrated opiate-binding sites in the brain (Pert and Snyder, 1973; Simon *et al.,* 1973; Terenius, 1973). This was the first use of radioligand-binding assays to demonstrate the presence of membrane-associated neurotransmitter receptors in the brain.

Stimulation-produced analgesia, its naloxone reversibility, and the discovery of opioid receptors strongly pointed to the existence of endogenous opioids. In 1975, Hughes and associates identified an endogenous opiate-like factor that they called *enkephalin* (from the head). Soon after, two more classes of endogenous opioid peptides were isolated, the *dynorphins* and *endorphins*. Details of these discoveries and the unique properties of the opioid peptides have been reviewed (Akil *et al.*, 1984).

Given the large number of endogenous ligands, it was not surprising that multiple classes of opioid receptors also were found. The concept of opioid receptor multiplicity arose shortly after the initial demonstration of opiate-binding sites. Based on *in vivo* studies in dogs, Martin and colleagues postulated the existence of multiple types of opiate receptors (Martin *et al.*, 1976). Receptor-binding studies and subsequent cloning confirmed the existence of three main receptor types: μ, δ, and κ. A fourth member of the opioid peptide receptor family, the *nociceptin/orphanin FQ* (N/OFQ) receptor, was cloned in 1994. This latter receptor is not, strictly speaking, opioid in its function, in that it does not interact with any of the classical opiate ligands, but it is part of the opioid family based on extensive sequence homology. In addition to these four major receptor classes, a number of subtypes have been proposed, such as ε, often based on bioassays from different species (Schulz *et al.*, 1979), ι (Oka, 1980), λ (Grevel and Sadee, 1983), and ζ (Zagon *et al.*, 1989). In 2000, the Committee on Receptor Nomenclature and Drug Classification of the International Union of Pharmacology adopted the terms *MOP, DOP,* and *KOP* to indicate μ, δ, and κ opioid peptide receptors, respectively. The original Greek letter designations are used in this and other chapters. The committee also recommended the term *NOP* for the N/OFQ receptor.

ENDOGENOUS OPIOID PEPTIDES

Three distinct families of classical opioid peptides have been identified: the *enkephalins, endorphins,* and *dynorphins*. Each family derives from a distinct precursor protein and has a characteristic anatomical distribution. These precursors, prepro-opiomelanocortin (POMC), preproenkephalin, and preprodynorphin, respectively, are encoded by three corresponding genes. Each precursor is subject to complex cleavages and post-translational modifications resulting in the synthesis of multiple active peptides. The opioid peptides share the common amino-terminal sequence of Tyr-Gly-Gly-Phe-(Met or Leu), which has been called the *opioid motif*. This motif is followed by various C-terminal extensions yielding peptides ranging from 5 to 31 residues (Table 21–1).

The major opioid peptide derived from POMC is β-endorphin. Although β-endorphin contains the sequence for met-enkephalin at its amino terminus, it is not converted to this peptide; met-enkephalin is derived from the processing of preproenkephalin. In addition to β-endorphin, the POMC precursor also is processed into the nonopioid peptides adrenocorticotropic hormone (ACTH),

melanocyte-stimulating hormone (α-MSH), and β-lipotropin (β-LPH). Previous biochemical work had suggested a common precursor for the stress hormone ACTH and the opioid peptide β-endorphin. This association implied a close physiological linkage between the stress axis and opioid systems, which was validated by many studies of the phenomenon of stress-induced analgesia (Akil *et al.*, 1986). Proenkephalin contains multiple copies of met-enkephalin, as well as a single copy of leu-enkephalin. Prodynorphin contains three peptides of differing lengths that all begin with the leu-enkephalin sequence: dynorphin A, dynorphin B, and neoendorphin (Figure 21–1). The anatomical distribution of these peptides in the CNS has been reviewed (Mansour *et al.*, 1988).

A novel endogenous opioid peptide was cloned in 1995 (Meunier *et al.*, 1995; Reinscheid *et al.*, 1995). This peptide has a significant sequence homology to dynorphin A, with an identical length of 17 amino acids, identical carboxy-terminal residues, and a slight modification of the amino-terminal opioid core (Phe-Gly-Gly-Phe instead of Tyr-Gly-Gly-Phe) (Table 21–1). The removal of this single hydroxyl group is sufficient to abolish interactions with the three classical opioid peptide receptors. This peptide was called *orphanin FQ* (OFQ) by one group of investigators and *nociceptin* (N) by another because it lowered pain threshold under certain conditions. Like the opioid precursors, the structure of the N/OFQ precursor (Figure 21–2) suggests that it may encode other biologically active peptides (Nothacker *et al.*, 1996). Immediately downstream of N/OFQ is a 17-amino-acid peptide (orphanin-2), which also starts with phenylalanine and ends with glutamine but is otherwise distinct from N/OFQ, as well as a putative peptide upstream from N/OFQ, which may be liberated on post-translational processing (*nocistatin*). The N/OFQ system represents a new neuropeptide system with a high degree of sequence identity to the opioid peptides. Indeed, it appears to be derived from a common opioid precursor that contains OFQ and enkephalin-like structures (Danielson *et al.*, 2001). However, the slight structural changes profoundly alter function. The common precursor apparently diverged through evolution to give rise to the opioid and the nonopioid branches of this family (Danielson *et al.*, 2001). Thus, N/OFQ has behavioral and pain modulatory properties distinct from those of the three classical opioid peptides (*see* below).

The anatomical distribution of POMC-producing cells is relatively limited within the CNS, occurring mainly in the arcuate nucleus and nucleus tractus solitarius. These neurons project widely

Table 21–1
Endogenous and Synthetic Opioid Peptides

<table>
<tr><th colspan="2" align="center">Selected Endogenous Opioid Peptides</th></tr>
<tr><td>[Leu⁵]enkephalin</td><td>**Tyr-Gly-Gly-Phe-Leu**</td></tr>
<tr><td>[Met⁵]enkephalin</td><td>**Tyr-Gly-Gly-Phe-Met**</td></tr>
<tr><td>Dynorphin A</td><td>**Tyr-Gly-Gly-Phe-Leu**-Arg-Arg-Ile-Arg-Pro-Lys-Leu-Lys-Trp-Asp-Asn-Gln</td></tr>
<tr><td>Dynorphin B</td><td>**Tyr-Gly-Gly-Phe-Leu**-Arg-Arg-Gln-Phe-Lys-Val-Val-Thr</td></tr>
<tr><td>α-Neoendorphin</td><td>**Tyr-Gly-Gly-Phe-Leu**-Arg-Lys-Tyr-Pro-Lys</td></tr>
<tr><td>β-Neoendorphin</td><td>**Tyr-Gly-Gly-Phe-Leu**-Arg-Lys-Tyr-Pro</td></tr>
<tr><td>β_h-Endorphin</td><td>**Tyr-Gly-Gly-Phe-Met**-Thr-Ser-Glu-Lys-Ser-Gln-Thr-Pro-Leu-Val-Thr-Leu-Phe-Lys-
Asn-Ala-Ile-Ile-Lys-Asn-Ala-Tyr-Lys-Lys-Gly-Glu</td></tr>
<tr><th colspan="2" align="center">Novel Endogenous Opioid-Related Peptides</th></tr>
<tr><td>Orphanin FQ/Nociceptin</td><td>Phe-**Gly-Gly-Phe-**Thr-Gly-Ala-Arg-Lys-Ser-Ala-Arg-Lys-Leu-Ala-Asn-Gln</td></tr>
<tr><th colspan="2" align="center">Selected Synthetic Opioid Peptides</th></tr>
<tr><td>DAMGO</td><td>[D-Ala²,MePhe⁴,Gly(ol)⁵]enkephalin</td></tr>
<tr><td>DPDPE</td><td>[D-Pen²,D-Pen⁵]enkephalin</td></tr>
<tr><td>DSLET</td><td>[D-Ser²,Leu⁵]enkephalin-Thr⁶</td></tr>
<tr><td>DADL</td><td>[D-Ala²,D-Leu⁵]enkephalin</td></tr>
<tr><td>CTOP</td><td>D-Phe-Cys-Tyr-D-Trp-Orn-Thr-Pen-Thr-NH₂</td></tr>
<tr><td>FK-33824</td><td>[D-Ala²,N-MePhe⁴,Met(O)⁵-ol]enkephalin</td></tr>
<tr><td>[D-Ala²]Deltorphin I</td><td>Tyr-D-Ala-Phe-Asp-Val-Val-Gly-NH₂</td></tr>
<tr><td>[D-Ala²,Glu⁴]Deltorphin
(Deltorphin II)</td><td>Tyr-D-Ala-Phe-Glu-Val-Val-Gly-NH₂</td></tr>
<tr><td>Morphiceptin</td><td>Tyr-Pro-Phe-Pro-NH₂</td></tr>
<tr><td>PL-017</td><td>Tyr-Pro-MePhe-D-Pro-NH₂</td></tr>
<tr><td>DALCE</td><td>[D-Ala²,Leu⁵,Cys⁶]enkephalin</td></tr>
</table>

to limbic and brainstem areas and to the spinal cord (Lewis *et al.*, 1987). There also is evidence of POMC production in the spinal cord (Gutstein *et al.*, 1992). The distribution of POMC corresponds to areas of the human brain where electrical stimulation can relieve pain (Pilcher *et al.*, 1988). Peptides from POMC occur in the anterior and intermediate lobes of the pituitary and also are contained in pancreatic islet cells. The peptides from prodynorphin and proenkephalin are distributed widely throughout the CNS and frequently are found together. Although each family of peptides typically is located in different groups of neurons, occasionally more than one family is expressed within the same neuron (Weihe *et al.*, 1988). Of particular note, proenkephalin peptides are present in areas of the CNS that are presumed to be related to the perception of pain (*e.g.*, laminae I and II of the spinal cord, the spinal trigeminal nucleus, and the periaqueductal gray), to the modulation of affective behavior (*e.g.*, amygdala, hippocampus, locus ceruleus, and the frontal cerebral cortex), to the modulation of motor control (*e.g.*, caudate nucleus and globus pallidus), to the regulation of the autonomic nervous system (*e.g.*, medulla oblongata), and to neuroendocrinological functions (*e.g.*, median eminence). Although there are a few long

enkephalinergic fiber tracts, these peptides are contained primarily in interneurons with short axons. The peptides from proenkephalin also are found in the adrenal medulla and in nerve plexuses and exocrine glands of the stomach and intestine.

The N/OFQ precursor has a unique anatomical distribution (Neal *et al.*, 1999b) that suggests important roles in hippocampus, cortex, and numerous sensory sites. N/OFQ produces a complex behavioral profile, including effects on drug reward and reinforcement (Bertorelli *et al.*, 2000), stress responsiveness (Devine *et al.*, 2001; Koster *et al.*, 1999), feeding behavior (Olszewski and Levine, 2004) and interplay with the stress system (Nicholson *et al.*, 2002), and learning and memory processes (Koster *et al.*, 1999). Studies of the effect of N/OFQ on pain sensitivity have produced conflicting results, perhaps because the effects of N/OFQ on pain sensitivity depend on the underlying behavioral state of the animal (Pan *et al.*, 2000) (*see* below). Analogous mechanisms also could explain some of the conflicting results with other physiological processes. However, more studies are needed before a general role can be ascribed to the N/OFQ system, including the investigation of other active peptides that may be derived from the precursor (Figure 21–2). For example, nocistatin

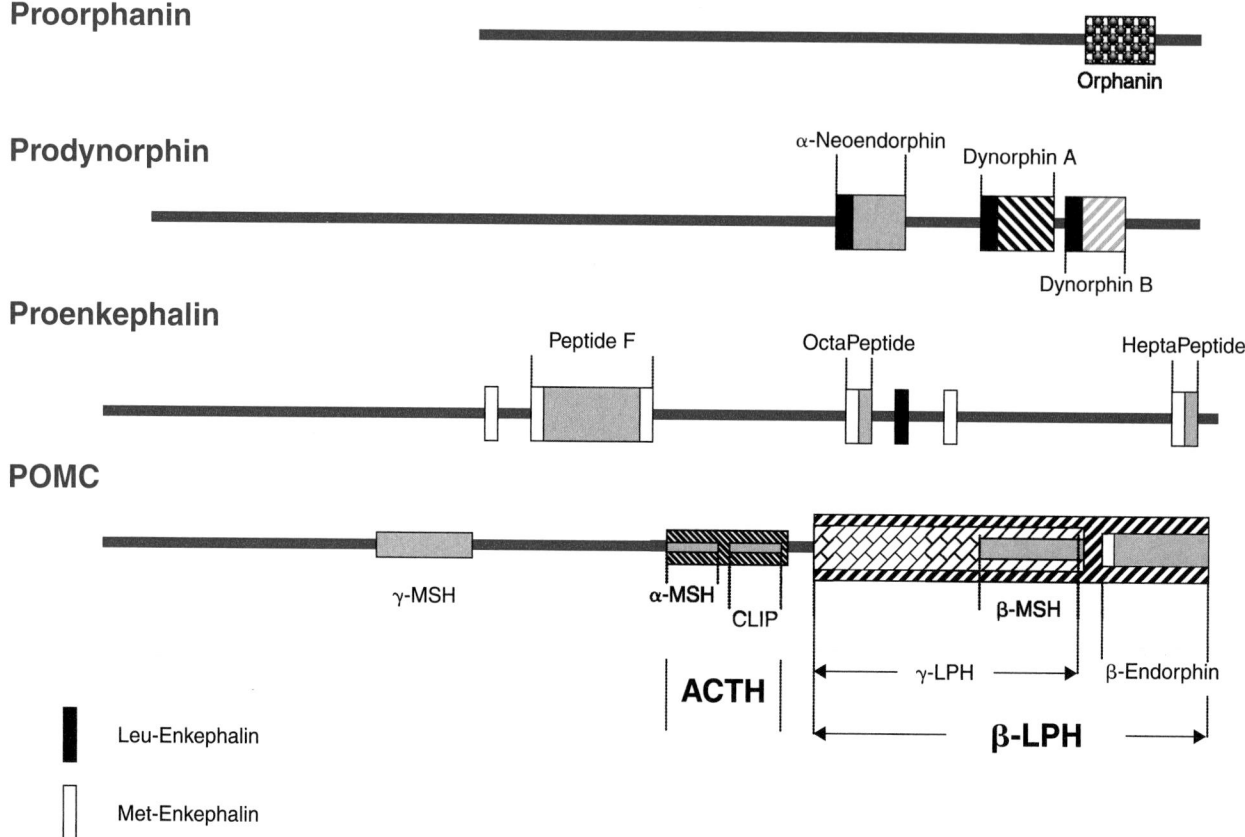

Figure 21–1. *Peptide precursors.* POMC, pro-opiomelanocortin; ACTH, adrenocorticotropic hormone; β-LPH, β-lipotropin. (From Akil *et al.*, 1998.)

has been tested behaviorally and found to produce effects opposite to those of N/OFQ (Okuda-Ashitaka *et al.*, 1998). These findings, coupled with the extensive anatomy of the system, suggest that the N/OFQ precursor plays a complex role in the brain and that it interacts with many of the functions of the classical endogenous opioids, sometimes in a complementary but often in an opposing fashion. Not all cells that make a given precursor polypeptide store and release the same mixture of active opioid peptides because of differential processing secondary to variations in the cellular complement of pepti-

dases that produce and degrade the active opioid fragments (Akil *et al.*, 1984). In addition, processing of these peptides is altered by physiological demands, leading to a different mix of peptides being released by the same cell under different conditions. For example, chronic morphine treatment (Bronstein *et al.*, 1990) or stress (Akil *et al.*, 1985) can alter the forms of β-endorphin released by cells, which could underlie some observed physiological adaptations. Although the endogenous opioid peptides appear to function as neurotransmitters, modulators of neurotransmission, or neurohormones, the full extent of their physiological role is not completely understood (Akil *et al.*, 1988). The elucidation of the physiological roles of the opioid peptides has been made more difficult by their frequent coexistence with other putative neurotransmitters within a given neuron.

110-127 Nocistatin	MPRVRSLFQEQEEPEPGMEEAGEMEQKQLQ
130-146 Orphanin	FQFGGFTGARKSARKLANQ
149-165 Orphanin-2	FSEFMRQYLVLSMQSSQ

Figure 21–2. *Human pro-orphanin-derived peptides.*

OPIOID RECEPTORS

Three classical opioid receptor types, μ, δ, and κ, have been studied extensively (Waldhoer *et al.*, 2004). The more recently discovered N/OFQ receptor, initially called the *opioid-receptor-like 1* (ORL-1) receptor or "orphan" opioid receptor, has added a dimension to the study of opioids.

Table 21–2
Classification of Opioid Receptor Subtypes and Actions from Animal Models

	RECEPTOR SUBTYPE	ACTIONS OF:	
		Agonist	*Antagonist*
Analgesia			
Supraspinal	μ, κ, δ	Analgesic	No effect
Spinal	μ, κ, δ	Analgesic	No effect
Respiratory function	μ	Decrease	No effect
Gastrointestinal tract	μ, κ	Decrease transit	No effect
Psychotomimesis	κ	Increase	No effect
Feeding	μ, κ, δ	Increase feeding	Decrease feeding
Sedation	μ, κ	Increase	No effect
Diuresis	κ	Increase	
Hormone regulation			
Prolactin	μ	Increase release	Decrease release
Growth hormone	μ and/or δ	Increase release	Decrease release
Neurotransmitter release			
Acetylcholine	μ	Inhibit	
Dopamine	μ, δ	Inhibit	
Isolated organ bioassays			
Guinea pig ileum	μ	Decrease contraction	No effect
Mouse vas deferens	d	Decrease contraction	No effect

The actions listed for antagonists are seen with the antagonist alone. All the correlations in this table are based on studies in rats and mice, which occasionally show species differences. Thus, any extensions of these associations to humans are tentative. Clinical studies do indicate that μ receptors elicit analgesia spinally and supraspinally. Preliminary work with a synthetic opioid peptide, [D-Ala^2,D-Leu^5]enkephalin, suggests that intrathecal δ agonists are analgesic in humans. Modified from Pasternak (1993).

Highly selective ligands that allowed for type-specific labeling of the three classical opioid receptors (*e.g.*, DAMGO for μ, DPDPE for δ, and U-50,488 and U-69,593 for κ) (Handa *et al.*, 1981; Mosberg *et al.*, 1983; Vonvoightlander *et al.*, 1983) became available in the early 1980s. These tools made possible the definition of ligand-binding characteristics of each of the receptor types and the determination of anatomical distribution of the receptors using autoradiographic techniques. Each major opioid receptor has a unique anatomical distribution in brain, spinal cord, and the periphery (Mansour *et al.*, 1988; Neal *et al.*, 1999b). These distinctive localization patterns suggested possible functions that subsequently have been investigated in pharmacological and behavioral studies.

The study of the biological functions of opioid receptors *in vivo* was aided by the synthesis of selective antagonists and agonists. Among the most commonly used antagonists are cyclic analogs of *somatostatin* such as CTOP as μ-receptor antagonists, a derivative of naloxone called *naltrindole* as a δ-receptor antagonist, and a bivalent derivative of *naltrexone* called *binaltorphimine* (nor-BNI) as a κ-receptor antagonist (Gulya *et al.*, 1986; Portoghese *et al.*, 1987, 1988). In general, functional studies using selective agonists and antagonists have revealed substantial parallels between μ and δ receptors and dramatic contrasts between μ/δ and κ receptors. *In vivo* infusions of selective antagonists and agonists also were used to establish the receptor types involved in mediating various opioid effects (Table 21–2).

Most of the clinically used opioids are relatively selective for μ receptors, reflecting their similarity to morphine (Tables 21–3 and 21–4). However, it is important to note that drugs that are relatively selective at standard doses will interact with additional receptor subtypes when given at sufficiently high doses, leading to possible changes in their pharmacological profile. This is especially true as doses are escalated to overcome tolerance. Some drugs, particularly mixed agonist–antagonist agents, interact with more than one receptor class at usual clinical doses. The actions of these drugs are particularly interesting because they may act as an agonist at one receptor and an antagonist at another.

Table 21–3

Actions and Selectivities of Some Opioids at the Various Opioid Receptor Classes

	RECEPTOR TYPES		
	μ	δ	κ
Drugs			
Morphine	+++		+
Methadone	+++		
Etorphine	+++	+++	+++
Levorphanol	+++		
Fentanyl	+++		
Sufentanil	+++	+	+
DAMGO	+++		
Butorphanol	P		+++
Buprenorphine	P		––
Naloxone	–––	–	––
Naltrexone	–––	–	–––
CTOP	–––		
Diprenorphine	–––	––	–––
β-Funaltrexamine	–––	–	++
Naloxonazine	–––	–	–
Nalorphine	–––		+
Pentazocine	P		++
Nalbuphine	––		++
Naloxone benzoylhydrazone	–––	–	–
Bremazocine	+++	++	+++
Ethylketocyclazocine	P	+	+++
U50,488			+++
U69,593			+++
Spiradoline	+		+++
nor-Binaltorphimine	–	–	–––
Naltrindole	–	–––	–
DPDPE		++	
[D-Ala^2,Glu^4]deltorphin		++	
DSLET	+	++	
Endogenous Peptides			
Met-enkephalin	++	+++	
Leu-enkephalin	++	+++	
β-Endorphin	+++	+++	
Dynorphin A	++		+++
Dynorphin B	+	+	+++
α-Neoendorphin	+	+	+++

Activities of drugs are given at the receptors for which the agent has reasonable affinity. +, agonist; –, antagonist; P, partial agonist; DAMGO, CTOP, DPDPE, DSLET, *see* Table 21–1. The number of symbols is an indication of potency; the ratio for a given drug denotes selectivity. These values were obtained primarily from animal studies and should be extrapolated to human beings with caution. Both β-funaltrexamine and naloxonazine are irreversible μ antagonists, but β-funaltrexamine also has reversible κ agonist activity.

There is little agreement regarding the exact classification of opioid receptor subtypes. Pharmacological studies have suggested the existence of multiple subtypes of each receptor. The complex literature on κ-opioid receptor subtypes (Akil and Watson, 1994) strongly suggests the presence of at least one additional subtype with high affinity for the benzomorphan class of opiate alkaloids. The data for δ-opioid receptor subtypes are intriguing. While early support for the possibility of multiple δ receptors came from radioligand-binding studies, the strongest evidence derives from behavioral studies (Jiang *et al.*, 1991), which led to the proposal that two δ-receptor sites exist, δ_1 and δ_2. In the case of the μ receptor, behavioral and pharmacological studies led to the proposal of μ_1 and μ_2 subtypes (Pasternak, 1986). The μ_1 site is proposed to be a very high affinity receptor with little discrimination between μ and δ ligands. A parallel hypothesis (Rothman *et al.*, 1988) holds that there is a high-affinity μ/δ complex rather than a distinct μ site. Although molecular cloning studies have not readily supported the existence of these subtypes as distinct molecules, recent findings (*see* below) regarding modified specificity for opioid ligands owing to heterodimerization of receptors may explain the observed pharmacological diversity.

Molecular Studies of Opioid Receptors and Their Ligands

For many years, the study of multiple opioid receptors greatly profited from the availability of a rich array of natural and synthetic ligands but was limited by the absence of opioid receptor clones. In 1992, the mouse δ receptor was cloned from the NG-108 cell line (Evans *et al.*, 1992). Subsequently, the other two major types of classical opioid receptors were cloned from various rodent species (Meng *et al.*, 1993; Thompson *et al.*, 1993). The N/OFQ receptor was cloned as a result of searches for novel types or subtypes of opioid receptors. The coding regions for the opioid peptide receptors subsequently were isolated and chromosomally assigned. In the case of μ, the cloned sequence is the classical morphine-like receptor rather than the proposed μ_1. With δ, no differentiation between the two proposed types by binding appears possible, and the cloned receptor recognizes all δ-selective ligands regardless of their behavioral assignment as δ_1 or δ_2. For κ, the cloned receptor is the classical receptor rather than the proposed benzomorphan-binding site. All four opioid receptors belong to the GPCR family (*see* Chapter 1) and share extensive sequence homologies (Figure 21–3). The N/OFQ receptor has high structural homology with the classical opioid receptors, but it has very low or no affinity for binding conventional opioid ligands. The structural similarities of the N/OFQ receptor and the three classical opioid receptors are highest in the transmembrane regions and cytoplasmic domains and lowest in the extracellular domains critical for ligand selectivity (Meng *et al.*, 1998) (Figure 21–3B).

Further cloning experiments may identify unique genes encoding opioid receptor subtypes; if multiple opioid receptor subtypes exist, however, they may derive from a single gene, and multiple mechanisms may provide distinct pharmacological profiles. Two potential pathways to opioid receptor diversity are alternative splicing of receptor RNA and dimerization of receptor proteins.

Alternative splicing of receptor heteronuclear RNA (*e.g.*, exon skipping and intron retention) is thought to play an important role in producing *in vivo* diversity within many members of the GPCR superfamily (Kilpatrick *et al.*, 1999). Splice variants may exist within each of the three opioid receptor families, and this alternative splicing of receptor transcripts may be crucial for the diversity of opioid receptors. A technique used widely to identify potential sites of alternative splicing is antisense oligodeoxynucleotide (ODN)

Table 21–4
Properties of the Cloned Opioid Receptors

RECEPTOR SUBTYPE	SELECTIVE LIGANDS		NONSELECTIVE LIGANDS		PUTATIVE ENDOGENOUS LIGANDS
	Agonists	Antagonists	Agonists	Antagonists	
μ	DAMGO Morphine Methadone Fentanyl Dermorphin	CTOP	Levorphanol Etorphine	Naloxone Naltrexone β-funaltrexamine	Enkephalin Endorphin
κ	Spiradoline U50,488 Dynorphin A	Nor-BNI	Levorphanol Etorphine EKC	Naloxone Naltrexone	Dynorphin A
δ	DPDPE Deltorphin DSLET	Naltrindole NTB BNTX	Levorphanol Etorphine	Naloxone Naltrexone	Enkephalin

ABBREVIATIONS: BNTX, 7 benzylidenenaltroxone; EKC, ethylketocyclazosine; NTB, benzofuran analog of naltrindole; nor-BNI, nor-binaltorphimine. DAMGO, CTOR, DPDPE, DSLET, *see* Table 21–1. SOURCE: Modified from Raynor *et al.* (1994).

mapping. The ability of antisense ODNs to target specific regions of cDNA permits the systematic evaluation of the contribution of individual exons to observed receptor properties. Use of this approach has demonstrated that antisense ODNs targeting of exon 1 of μ-opioid receptors blocks morphine analgesia, whereas administration of antisense ODNs targeting exon 2 does not block morphine analgesia but prevents the analgesia produced by heroin, *fentanyl,* and the morphine metabolite morphine-6-glucuronide (Pasternak, 2001). These results, which imply that unique μ-receptor mechanisms mediate the analgesic effects of a variety of opioids, are consistent with the proposal that unique receptor mechanisms are achieved through alternative splicing. The use of antisense ODNs and real-time polymerase chain reaction techniques also has led to the identification of potential sites for splice variation in the κ- and δ-opioid receptors (Wei *et al.*, 2004). Central to the claim that these results reflect the existence of splice variants is the *in vivo* isolation of such variants. A μ opioid receptor splice variant has been identified that differs considerably from the native receptor within its C terminus (Zimprich *et al.*, 1995). This variant exhibits a binding profile similar to that of the cloned μ opioid receptor but does not readily undergo the desensitization frequently observed after exposure to agonist. Thus, the existence of this splice variant cannot explain the differential analgesic sensitivities described earlier. Studies are investigating the *in vivo* relevance of putative splice variants.

The interaction of two receptors to form a unique structure (dimerization) also has been accorded an important role in regulating receptor function (Agnati *et al.*, 2003, Milligan, 2004). κ and δ opioid receptors have been shown to exist as homodimers (Levac *et al.*, 2002). However, the most interesting findings have been generated by studies showing dimerization between different opioid receptor types. κ and δ opioid receptors, as well as μ and δ opioid receptors, can exist as heterodimers in heterologous expression systems and *in vivo* (Devi, 2001). The dimerization of these receptors profoundly alters their pharmacological properties. The affinity of the heterodimers for highly selective agonists and antagonists is

reduced greatly. Instead, the heterodimers show greatest affinity for partially selective agonists such as *bremazocine* and some endogenous opioid peptides (Levac *et al.*, 2002). *In vivo* responses to morphine also may be altered (Gomes *et al.*, 2004), suggesting novel strategies for pain treatment. Receptor heterodimerization may explain, at least in part, the discrepancies between molecular and pharmacological properties of opioid receptors. Heterodimerization also may occur between opioid receptors and other types of GPCRs (Pfeiffer *et al.*, 2003), but the physiological significance of these interactions is not clear.

Given the existence of four families of endogenous ligands and cloned receptors, it seems reasonable to ask if there is a one-to-one correspondence among them. Previous studies using brain homogenates demonstrated that an orderly pattern of association between a set of opioid gene products and a given receptor does not exist. Although proenkephalin products generally are associated with δ receptors and prodynorphin products with κ receptors, much "crosstalk" is present (Mansour *et al.*, 1995). The cloning of the opioid receptors allowed this question to be addressed more systematically because each receptor could be expressed separately and then compared under identical conditions (Mansour *et al.*, 1997). The κ receptor exhibits the most selectivity across endogenous ligands, with affinities ranging from 0.1 nM for dynorphin A to approximately 100 nM for leu-enkephalin. In contrast, μ and δ receptors show only a tenfold difference between the most and least preferred ligand, with a majority of endogenous ligands exhibiting greater affinity for δ than for μ receptors. The limited selectivity of μ and δ receptors suggests that the μ and δ receptors recognize principally the Tyr-Gly-Gly-Phe core of the endogenous peptide, whereas the κ receptor requires this core *and* the arginine in position 6 of dynorphin A and other prodynorphin products (Table 21–1). Interestingly, proenkephalin products with arginine in position 6 (*i.e.,* met-enkephalin-Arg-Phe and met-enkephalin-Arg-Gly-Leu) are equally good κ-receptor ligands, arguing against the idea of a unique association between a given receptor and a given opioid precursor family.

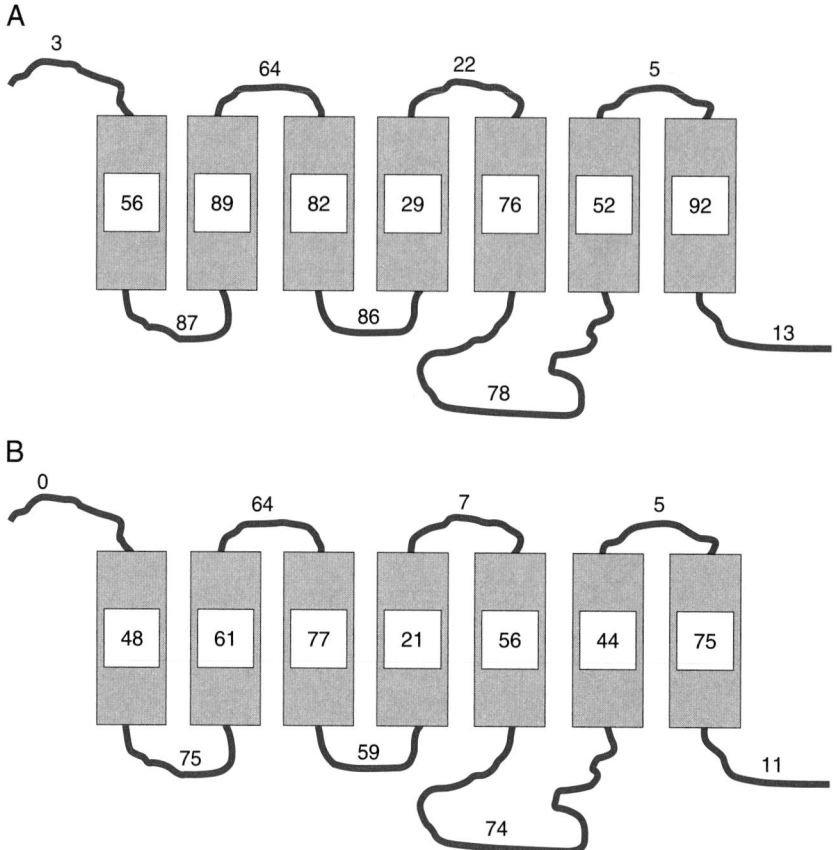

Figure 21–3. *A. Structural homology among the three opioid receptors. B. Structural homology among the three opioid receptors and the N/OFQ receptor.* Numbers indicate the percent of identical amino acids in the segment. (From Akil *et al.*, 1998, with permission.)

In sum, high-affinity interactions are possible between each of the peptide precursor families and each of the three receptor types, the only exception being the lack of high-affinity interaction between POMC-derived peptides and opioid receptors. Otherwise, at least one peptide product from each of the families exhibits high affinity (low nanomolar or subnanomolar) for each receptor. The relatively unimpressive affinity of the μ receptor toward all known endogenous ligands suggests that its most avid and selective ligand has not been identified, a notion being tested (*see* below).

Molecular Basis for Opioid Receptor Selectivity and Affinity. Previous studies of other peptide receptors suggested that peptides and small molecules may bind to GPCRs differently. Mutagenesis studies of small-ligand receptors (*e.g.,* adrenergic and dopamine receptors) showed that charged amino acid residues in the transmembrane domains were important in receptor binding and activation (Mansour *et al.*, 1992). This observation places the bound ligands within the receptor core formed by the transmembrane helices. On the other hand, studies with peptidergic receptors have demonstrated a critical role for extracellular loops in ligand recognition (Xie *et al.*, 1990). All three classical opioid receptors appear to combine both properties: Charged residues in transmembrane domains have been implicated in the high-affinity binding of most opioid ligands, whether alkaloid or peptide (Mansour *et al.*, 1997). However, critical interactions of opioid peptides with the extracellular domains also have been shown.

The opioid peptide Tyr-Gly-Gly-Phe core, sometimes called the *message,* appears to be necessary for interaction with the receptor-binding pocket; however, peptide *selectivity* resides in the carboxy-terminal extension beyond the tetrapeptide core, providing the *address* (Schwyzer, 1986). When the carboxy-terminal domain is long, it may interact with extracellular loops of the receptors, contributing to selectivity in a way that cannot be achieved by the much smaller alkaloids. Indeed, dynorphin A selectivity depends on the second extracellular loop of the κ receptor (Meng *et al.*, 1995), whereas δ- and μ-selective ligands have more complex mechanisms of selectivity that depend on multiple extracellular loops. These findings have led to the proposal that high selectivity is achieved by attraction to the most favored receptor and repulsion by the less favored receptor (Meng *et al.*, 1995). For example, the N/OFQ receptor does not bind any of the classical endogenous opioid peptides. However, mutating as few as four amino acids endows the N/OFQ receptor with the ability to recognize prodynorphin-derived peptides while retaining recognition of N/OFQ (Meng *et al.*, 1996), suggesting that unique mechanisms have evolved to ensure selectivity of the N/OFQ receptor for N/OFQ and against classical opioid peptides. Mechanisms involved in selectivity can be difficult to separate from mechanisms involved in affinity because the extracellular domains not only may allow interactions with the peptide ligands but also may be important in stabilizing these interactions.

Results of the research discussed above imply that the alkaloids are small enough to fit completely inside or near the mouth of the receptor core, whereas peptides bind to the extracellular loops and simultaneously extend to the receptor core to activate the common binding site. That one can truly separate the binding of peptides and alkaloids is demonstrated most clearly by a genetically engineered κ receptor (Coward *et al.*, 1998) that does not recognize endogenous peptide ligands yet retains full affinity and efficacy for small synthetic κ-receptor ligands, such as *spiradoline*. Given these differences in binding interactions with the receptor, it is possible that unique classes of ligands may activate the opioid receptor differently, leading to conformational changes of distinct quality or duration that may result in varying magnitudes and possibly different second-messenger events (Kenakin, 2002). This hypothesis is being tested (Quillan *et al.*, 2002; Alvarez *et al.*, 2002) and, if validated, may lead to novel strategies for differentially altering the interactions between the opioid receptors and signal-transduction cascades. The likely presence of receptor heterodimers that may have unique profiles and signaling properties provides a number of new directions for discovery of drugs that may target receptors in particular states (Bouvier, 2001; Wang *et al.*, 2005).

Opioid Receptor Signaling and Consequent Intracellular Events

Coupling of Opioid Receptors to Second Messengers. The μ, δ, and κ receptors in endogenous neuronal settings are coupled, *via* pertussis toxin–sensitive G proteins, to inhibition of adenylyl cyclase activity (Herz, 1993), activation of receptor-linked K^+ currents, and suppression of voltage-gated Ca^{2+} currents (Duggan and North, 1983). The hyperpolarization of the membrane potential by K^+-current activation and the limiting of Ca^{2+} entry by suppression of Ca^{2+} currents are tenable but unproven mechanisms for explaining blockade by opioids of neurotransmitter release and pain transmission in varying neuronal pathways. Studies with cloned receptors have shown that opioid receptors may couple to an array of other second-messenger systems, including activation of the MAP kinases and the phospholipase C (PLC)–mediated cascade leading to the formation of inositol triphosphate and diacylglycerol (Akil *et al.*, 1997). Prolonged exposure to opioids results in adaptations at multiple levels within these signaling cascades. The significance of these cellular-level adaptations lies in the causal relationship that may exist between them and adaptations seen at the organismic level, such as tolerance, sensitization, and withdrawal (Waldhoer *et al.*, 2004).

Receptor Desensitization, Internalization, and Sequestration after Chronic Exposure to Opioids. Transient administration of opioids leads to a phenomenon called *acute tolerance,* whereas sustained administration leads to the development of *classical* or *chronic tolerance. Tolerance* simply refers to a decrease in effectiveness of a drug with its repeated administration (*see* Chapter 23). Several studies have focused on putative cellular mechanisms of acute tolerance. Short-term receptor desensitization, which may underlie the development of tolerance, probably involves phosphorylation of the μ and δ receptors by PKC (Mestek *et al.*, 1995). A number of other kinases have been implicated in receptor desensitization, including PKA and β adrenergic receptor kinase (βARK) (Pei *et al.*, 1995; Wang *et al.*, 1994) (*see* below).

Like other GPCRs, μ and δ receptors can undergo rapid agonist-mediated internalization *via* a classic endocytic pathway (Gaudriault *et al.*, 1997), whereas κ receptors do not internalize after prolonged agonist exposure (Chu *et al.*, 1997). Interestingly, internalization of the μ and δ receptors apparently occurs *via* partially distinct endocytic pathways, suggesting *receptor*-specific interactions with different mediators of intracellular trafficking (Gaudriault *et al.*, 1997). It also is intriguing that these processes may be induced differentially as a function of the structure of the *ligand*. For example, certain agonists, such as *etorphine* and *enkephalins,* cause rapid internalization of the μ receptor, whereas morphine does not cause μ-receptor internalization, even though it decreases adenylyl cyclase activity equally well (Keith *et al.*, 1996). In addition, a truncated μ receptor with normal G protein coupling was shown to recycle constitutively from the membrane to cytosol (Segredo *et al.*, 1997), further indicating that activation of signal transduction and internalization are controlled by distinct molecular mechanisms. These studies also support the hypothesis that different ligands induce different conformational changes in the receptor that result in divergent intracellular events, and they may provide an explanation for differences in the efficacy and abuse potential of various opioids. One of the most interesting studies to evaluate the relevance of these alterations in signaling to the adaptations seen in response to opioid exposure *in vivo* was the demonstration that acute morphine-induced analgesia was enhanced in mice lacking β-arrestin 2 (Bohn *et al.*, 1999). Opioid-receptor internalization is mediated, at least in part, by the actions of GPCR kinases (GRKs). GRKs selectively phosphorylate agonist-bound receptors, thereby promoting interactions with β-arrestins, which interfere with G protein coupling and promote receptor internalization (Bohn *et al.*, 1999). Enhanced analgesia in mice lacking β-arrestin 2 is consistent with a role for the GRKs and arrestins in regulating responsivity to opioids *in vivo*. This result is even more intriguing given the inability of morphine to support arrestin translocation and receptor internalization *in vitro* (Whistler and von Zastrow, 1998) (*see* below).

Traditionally, long-term tolerance has been thought to be associated with increases in adenylyl cyclase activity—a counter-regulation to the decrease in cyclic AMP levels seen after acute opioid administration (Sharma *et al.*, 1977). Chronic treatment with μ-receptor opioids causes superactivation of adenylyl cyclase (Avidor-Reiss *et al.*, 1996). This effect is prevented by pretreatment with *pertussis toxin,* demonstrating involvement of $G_{i/o}$ proteins, and also by cotransfection with scavengers of G protein–$\beta\gamma$ dimers, indicating a role for this complex in superactivation. Alterations in levels of cyclic AMP clearly bring about numerous secondary changes (Nestler and Aghajanian, 1997).

Exciting recent findings suggest that the classic hypothesis of opioid tolerance development may need to be modified. For example, it appears that morphine does not efficiently promote μ-receptor internalization or receptor phosphorylation and desensitization (von Zastrow *et al.*, 2003; Koch *et al.*, 2005). When other μ agonists are subjected to similar analyses, widely divergent biochemical responses are observed. Unlike morphine, some opioids are very effective at cellular desensitization (Kovoor *et al.*, 1998). Some opioids rapidly induce receptor internalization, whereas morphine and other low-efficacy agonists do not (Whistler *et al.*, 1999). These studies collectively suggest that μ receptor desensitization and down-regulation are agonist-dependent, and they imply that different active receptor conformations caused by differing ligands produce a range of signaling responses (Kenakin, 2002). Concurrent studies of other GPCRs also have revealed that endocytosis and sequestration of receptors do not invariably lead to receptor degradation but also can result in receptor dephosphorylation and recycling to the surface of the cell (Krupnick and Benovic, 1998). Thus, receptor internalization may have divergent consequences, either reducing signaling by receptor inactivation and degradation or enhancing signaling by reactivating desensitized receptors.

Taken together, these findings suggest a novel hypothesis, namely, that opioid tolerance may not be related to receptor desensitization but rather to a lack of desensitization. Agonists that rapidly internalize opioid receptors also would rapidly desensitize signaling, but this desensitization would be at least partially reset by recycling of "reactivated" opioid receptors. It has been proposed that the lack of desensitization caused by morphine may result in prolonged receptor signaling, which, even though less efficient than that observed with other agonists, would lead to further downstream cellular adaptations that increase tolerance development (Borgland, 2001). Whistler and colleagues (1999) also have suggested that the measurement of relative agonist signaling *versus* endocytosis (RAVE) for opioid agonists could be predictive of the potential for tolerance development (Waldhoer *et al.*, 2004). A study by He and colleagues (2002) provides additional support for this concept, demonstrating that *DAMGO*, a μ agonist that alone causes receptor internalization, also will cause internalization of μ receptors in the presence of morphine, even when administered in concentrations that normally do not cause receptor internalization. In addition, these low concentrations of DAMGO inhibited the development of adenylyl cyclase supersensitivity by morphine. These intriguing *in vitro* findings were supported further by *in vivo* data demonstrating that coadministration of subthreshold amounts of DAMGO with morphine intraspinally in rats induced μ receptor endocytosis in the presence of morphine and markedly inhibited the development of morphine tolerance (He *et al.*, 2002). However, recent findings evaluating various aspects of this hypothesis *in vitro* have not confirmed these findings (Contet *et al.*, 2004). Further studies are needed to evaluate this new hypothesis.

An "Apparent Paradox." A paradox in evaluating the function of endogenous opioid systems is that a large number of endogenous ligands activate a small number of opioid receptors. This pattern is different from that of many other neurotransmitter systems, where a single ligand interacts with a large number of receptors having different structures and second messengers. Is this richness and complexity at the presynaptic level lost as multiple opioid ligands derived from different genes converge on only three receptors, or is this richness preserved through means yet to be discovered? One possibility is that molecular cloning has not revealed all opioid receptors. The complete sequence of the human and mouse genomes makes this less likely. Other options include splice variants, dimerization, and post-translational modification, as discussed previously. Even assuming that other receptors and variants will be found, the binding of many endogenous ligands to the three cloned classical receptors suggests a great deal of convergence. However, this convergence may be only apparent, since multiple mechanisms for achieving distinctive responses in the context of the biology described earlier may exist. Some issues to consider are:

1. The *duration of action* of endogenous ligands may be a crucial variable that has been overlooked and that may have clinical relevance.
2. The *pattern or profile of activation of multiple receptors by a ligand*, rather than activation of a single receptor, may be a crucial determinant of effect.

3. *Opioid genes may give rise to multiple active peptides with unique profiles of activity.* This patterning may be very complex and regulated by various stimuli.
4. *Differences in patterns and/or efficacy of intracellular signaling* produced by endogenous ligands at opioid receptors are under investigation. This issue may be particularly relevant for understanding physiological alterations after chronic administration of exogenous opioids.
5. *Intracellular trafficking of the receptors* may vary as a function of the receptor and of the ligand. This could have interesting implications for long-term adaptations during sustained treatment with opioids and after their withdrawal.

Understanding the complexity of endogenous opioid peptides and their patterns of interaction with multiple opioid receptors may help to define the similarities and differences between the endogenous modulation of these systems and their activation by drugs. These insights could be important in devising treatment strategies that maximize beneficial properties of opioids (*e.g.*, pain relief) while limiting their undesirable side effects, such as tolerance, dependence, and addiction.

EFFECTS OF CLINICALLY USED OPIOIDS

Morphine and most other clinically used opioid agonists exert their effects through μ opioid receptors. These drugs affect a wide range of physiological systems. They produce analgesia, affect mood and rewarding behavior (*see* Chapter 23), and alter respiratory, cardiovascular, gastrointestinal, and neuroendocrine function. δ Opioid receptor agonists also are potent analgesics in animals, and in some cases they have proved useful in humans (Moulin *et al.*, 1985). Agonists selective for κ receptors produce analgesia that has been shown in animals to be mediated primarily at spinal sites. Respiratory depression and miosis may be less severe with κ agonists. Instead of euphoria, κ receptor agonists produce dysphoric and psychotomimetic effects (Pfeiffer *et al.*, 1986). In neural circuitry mediating reward and analgesia, μ and κ agonists have been shown to have antagonistic effects (*see* below).

Mixed agonist–antagonist compounds were developed with the hope that they would have less addictive potential and less respiratory depression than morphine and related drugs. In practice, however, it has turned out that for the same degree of analgesia, the same intensity of side effects will occur. A "ceiling effect," limiting the amount of analgesia attainable, often is seen with these drugs. Some mixed agonist–antagonist drugs, such as *pentazocine* and *nalorphine,* can produce severe psychotomimetic effects that are not reversible with naloxone (suggesting that these undesirable side effects are not mediated through classical opioid receptors). Also, pentazocine and nalorphine can precipitate withdrawal in opioid-tolerant patients. For these reasons, the clinical use of these mixed agonist–antagonist drugs is limited.

Analgesia

In humans, morphine-like drugs produce analgesia, drowsiness, changes in mood, and mental clouding. A significant feature of the analgesia is that it occurs without loss of consciousness. When therapeutic doses of morphine are given to patients with pain, they report that the pain is less intense, less discomforting, or entirely gone; drowsiness commonly occurs. In addition to relief of distress, some patients experience euphoria.

When morphine in the same dose is given to a normal, pain-free individual, the experience may be unpleasant. Nausea is common, and vomiting may occur. There may be feelings of drowsiness, difficulty in mentation, apathy, and lessened physical activity. As the dose is increased, the subjective, analgesic, and toxic effects, including respiratory depression, become more pronounced. Morphine does not have anticonvulsant activity and usually does not cause slurred speech, emotional lability, or significant motor incoordination.

The relief of pain by morphine-like opioids is relatively selective, in that other sensory modalities are not affected. Patients frequently report that the pain is still present but that they feel more comfortable (*see* Therapeutic Uses of Opioid Analgesics, below). Continuous dull pain is relieved more effectively than sharp intermittent pain, but with sufficient amounts of opioid it is possible to relieve even the severe pain associated with renal or biliary colic.

Any meaningful discussion of the action of analgesic agents must include some distinction between *pain as a specific sensation,* subserved by distinct neurophysiological structures, and *pain as suffering* (the original sensation plus the reactions evoked by the sensation). It generally is agreed that all types of painful experiences, whether produced experimentally or occurring clinically as a result of pathology, include the original sensation and the reaction to that sensation. It also is important to distinguish between pain caused by stimulation of nociceptive receptors and transmitted over intact neural pathways (*nociceptive* pain) and pain that is caused by damage to neural structures, often involving neural supersensitivity (*neuropathic* pain). Although nociceptive pain usually is responsive to opioid analgesics, neuropathic pain typically responds poorly to opioid analgesics and may require higher doses of drug (McQuay, 1988).

In clinical situations, pain cannot be terminated at will, and the meaning of the sensation and the distress it engenders are markedly affected by the individual's previous experiences and current expectations. In experimentally produced pain, measurements of the effects of morphine on pain threshold have not always been consistent; some workers find that opioids reliably elevate the threshold, whereas many others do not obtain consistent changes. In contrast, moderate doses of morphine-like analgesics are effective in relieving clinical pain and increasing the capacity to tolerate experimentally induced pain. Not only is the sensation of pain altered by opioid analgesics, but the affective response is changed as well. This latter effect is best assessed by asking patients with clinical pain about the degree of relief produced by the drug administered. When pain does not evoke its usual responses (anxiety, fear, panic, and suffering), a patient's ability to tolerate the pain may be markedly increased even when the capacity to perceive the sensation is relatively unaltered. It is clear, however, that alteration of the emotional reaction to painful stimuli is not the sole mechanism of analgesia. Intrathecal administration of opioids can produce profound segmental analgesia without causing significant alteration of motor or sensory function or subjective effects (Yaksh, 1988).

Mechanisms and Sites of Opioid-Induced Analgesia. While cellular and molecular studies of opioid receptors are invaluable in understanding their function, it is crucial to place them in their anatomical and physiological context to fully understand the opioid system. Pain control by opioids must be considered in the context of brain circuits modulating analgesia and the functions of the various receptor types in these circuits (Fields *et al.*, 1991).

It is well established that the analgesic effects of opioids arise from their ability to directly inhibit the ascending transmission of nociceptive information from the spinal cord dorsal horn and to activate pain control circuits that descend from the midbrain *via* the rostral ventromedial medulla to the spinal cord dorsal horn. Opioid peptides and their receptors are found throughout these descending pain control circuits (Mansour *et al.*, 1995; Gutstein *et al.*, 1998). μ-Opioid receptor mRNA and/or ligand binding is seen throughout the periaqueductal gray (PAG), pontine reticular formation, median raphe, nucleus raphe magnus, and adjacent gigantocellular reticular nucleus in the rostral ventromedial medulla (RVM) and spinal cord. Evaluation of discrepancies between levels of ligand binding and mRNA expression provides important insights into the mechanisms of μ-opioid receptor–mediated analgesia. For instance, the presence of significant μ-opioid receptor ligand binding in the superficial dorsal horn but scarcity of mRNA expression (Mansour *et al.*, 1995) suggests that the majority of these spinal μ-receptor ligand-binding sites are located presynaptically on the terminals of primary afferent nociceptors. This conclusion is consistent with the high levels of μ-opioid receptor mRNA observed in dorsal root ganglia (DRG). A similar mismatch between μ-receptor ligand binding and mRNA expression is seen in the dorsolateral PAG (a high level of binding and sparse mRNA) (Gutstein *et al.*, 1998). δ-Opioid receptor mRNA and ligand binding have been demonstrated in the ventral and ventrolateral quadrants of the PAG, the pontine reticular formation, and the gigantocellular reticular nucleus, but only low levels are seen in the median raphe and nucleus raphe magnus. As with the μ-opioid receptor, there are significant numbers of δ-opioid receptor–binding sites in the dorsal horn but no detectable mRNA expression, suggesting an important role for presynaptic actions of the δ-opioid receptor in spinal analgesia. κ-Opioid receptor mRNA and ligand binding are widespread throughout the PAG, pontine reticular formation, median raphe, nucleus raphe magnus, and adjacent gigantocellular reticular nucleus. Again, κ-receptor ligand binding but minimal mRNA have been found in the dorsal horn. Although all three receptor mRNAs are found in the DRG, they are localized on different types of primary afferent cells. μ-Opioid receptor mRNA is present in medium- and large-diameter DRG cells, δ-opioid receptor mRNA in large-diameter cells, and κ-opioid receptor mRNA in small- and medium-diameter cells (Mansour *et al.*, 1995). This differential localization may be linked to functional differences in pain modulation.

The distribution of opioid receptors in descending pain control circuits indicates substantial overlap between μ and κ receptors. μ Receptors and κ receptors are most anatomically distinct from the δ-opioid receptor in the PAG, median raphe, and nucleus raphe magnus (Gutstein *et al.*, 1998). A similar differentiation of μ and κ receptors from δ is seen in the thalamus, suggesting that interactions between the κ and μ receptors may be important for modulating nociceptive transmission from higher nociceptive centers, as well as in the spinal cord dorsal horn. The actions of μ-receptor agonists are invariably analgesic, whereas those of κ-receptor agonists can be either analgesic or antianalgesic. Consistent with the anatomical overlap between the μ and κ receptors, the antianalgesic actions of the κ-receptor agonists appear to be mediated by functional antagonism of the actions of μ receptor agonists. The μ receptor produces analgesia within descending pain control circuits, at least in part, by the removal of γ-aminobutyric acid (GABA)–mediated inhibition of RVM-projecting neurons in the PAG and spinally projecting neurons in the RVM (Fields *et al.*, 1991). The pain-modulating effects of the κ receptor agonists in the brainstem appear to oppose those of μ receptor agonists. Application of a κ opioid agonist hyperpolarizes the same RVM neurons that are depolarized by a μ opioid agonist, and microinjections of a κ receptor agonist into the RVM antagonize the analgesia produced by microinjections of μ agonists into this region (Pan *et al.*, 1997). This is the strongest evidence to date demonstrating that opioids can have antianalgesic and analgesic effects, which may explain behavioral evidence for the reduction in hyperalgesia that follows injections of naloxone under certain circumstances.

As mentioned earlier, there is significant opioid-receptor ligand binding and little detectable receptor mRNA expression in the spinal cord dorsal horn but high levels of opioid-receptor mRNA in DRG. This distribution may suggest that the actions of opioid-receptor agonists relevant to analgesia at the spinal level are predominantly presynaptic. At least one presynaptic mechanism with potential clinical significance is inhibition of spinal tachykinin signaling. It is well known that opioids decrease the pain-evoked release of tachykinins from primary afferent nociceptors. Recently, the significance of this effect has been questioned. Trafton and colleagues (1999) have demonstrated that at least 80% of tachykinin signaling in response to noxious stimulation remains intact after the intrathecal administration of large doses of opioids. These results suggest that while opioid administration may reduce tachykinin release from primary afferent nociceptors, this reduction has little functional impact on the actions of tachykinins on postsynaptic pain-transmitting neurons. This implies either that tachykinins are not central to pain signaling and/or opioid-induced analgesia at the spinal level or that, contrary to the conclusions suggested by anatomical studies, presynaptic opioid actions may be of little analgesic significance.

Paralleling the important insights into mechanisms of opioid-induced analgesia at the brainstem and spinal levels, progress also has been made in understanding forebrain mechanisms. The actions of opioids in bulbospinal pathways are crucial in their analgesic efficacy, but the precise role of forebrain actions of opioids and whether these actions are independent of those in bulbospinal pathways are less well defined. Opioid actions in the forebrain clearly contribute to analgesia because decerebration prevents analgesia when rats are tested for pain sensitivity using the formalin test (Matthies and Franklin, 1992), and microinjection of opioids into several forebrain regions is analgesic in this test (Manning *et al.*, 1994). However, because these manipulations frequently do not change the analgesic efficacy of opioids in measures of acute-phasic nocicep-

tion, such as the tailflick test, a distinction has been made between forebrain-dependent mechanisms for morphine-induced analgesia in the presence of tissue injury and bulbospinal mechanisms for this analgesia in the absence of tissue injury. Manning and Mayer (1995a, 1995b) have shown that this distinction is not absolute. Analgesia induced by systemic administration of morphine in both the tailflick and formalin tests was disrupted either by lesioning or by reversibly inactivating the central nucleus of the amygdala, demonstrating that opioid actions in the forebrain contribute to analgesia in measures of tissue damage, as well as acute-phasic nociception.

Simultaneous administration of morphine at spinal and supraspinal sites results in synergy in analgesic response, with a tenfold reduction in the total dose of morphine necessary to produce equivalent analgesia at either site alone. The mechanisms responsible for spinal/supraspinal synergy are readily distinguished from those involved with supraspinal analgesia (Pick *et al.*, 1992). In addition to the well-described spinal/supraspinal synergy, synergistic μ/μ- and μ/δ-agonist interactions also have been observed within the brainstem between the PAG, locus coeruleus, and nucleus raphe magnus (Rossi *et al.*, 1993).

Opioids also can produce analgesia when administered peripherally. Opioid receptors are present on peripheral nerves and will respond to peripherally applied opioids and locally released endogenous opioid compounds when up-regulated during inflammatory pain states (Stein, 1993). During inflammation, immune cells capable of releasing endogenous opioids are present near sensory nerves, and a perineural defect allows opioids access to the nerves (Stein, 1993). This also may occur in neuropathic pain models (Kayser *et al.*, 1995), perhaps because of the presence of immune cells near damaged nerves (Monaco *et al.*, 1992) and perineural defects extant in these conditions.

The Role of N/OFQ and Its Receptor in Pain Modulation. N/OFQ mRNA and peptides are present throughout descending pain control circuits. For instance, N/OFQ-containing neurons are present in the PAG, the median raphe, throughout the RVM, and in the superficial dorsal horn (Neal *et al.*, 1999b). This distribution overlaps with that of opioid peptides, but the extent of colocalization is unclear. N/OFQ-receptor ligand binding and mRNA are seen in the PAG, median raphe, and RVM (Neal *et al.*, 1999a). Spinally, there is stronger N/OFQ-receptor mRNA expression in the ventral horn than in the dorsal horn but higher levels of ligand binding in the dorsal horn. There also are high N/OFQ-receptor mRNA levels in the DRG.

Despite clear anatomical evidence for a role of the N/OFQ system in pain modulation, its function is unclear. Targeted disruption of the N/OFQ receptor in mice had little effect on basal pain sensitivity in several measures, whereas targeted disruption of the N/OFQ precursor consistently elevated basal responses in the tailflick test, suggesting an important role for N/OFQ in regulating basal pain sensitivity (Koster *et al.*, 1999). Intrathecal injections of N/OFQ are analgesic (Xu *et al.*, 1996); however, supraspinal administration has produced either hyperalgesia, antiopioid effects, or a biphasic hyperalgesic/analgesic response (Mogil and Pasternak, 2001). These conflicting findings may be explained in part by a study in which it was shown that N/OFQ inhibits pain-facilitating and analgesia-facilitating neurons in the RVM (Pan *et al.*, 2000). Activation of endogenous analgesic circuitry was blocked by administration of N/OFQ. If the animal was hyperalgesic, the enhanced pain sensitivity also was blocked by N/OFQ. Thus, the effects of N/OFQ on pain responses appear to depend on the preexisting state of pain in the animal and the specific neural circuitry inhibited by N/OFQ (Heinricher, 2003).

Mood Alterations and Rewarding Properties

The mechanisms by which opioids produce euphoria, tranquility, and other alterations of mood (including rewarding properties) are not entirely clear. However, the neural systems that mediate opioid reinforcement are distinct from those involved in physical dependence and analgesia (Koob and Bloom, 1988). Behavioral and pharmacological data point to the role of dopaminergic pathways, particularly involving the nucleus accumbens (NAcc), in drug-induced reward. There is ample evidence for interactions between opioids and *dopamine* in mediating opioid-induced reward (*see* Chapter 23).

A full appreciation of mechanisms of drug-induced reward requires a more complete understanding of the NAcc and related structures at the anatomical level, as well as a careful examination of the interface between the opioid system and dopamine receptors. The NAcc, portions of the olfactory tubercle, and the ventral and medial portions of the caudate putamen constitute an area referred to as the *ventral striatum* (Heimer *et al.*, 1982). The ventral striatum is implicated in motivation and affect (limbic functions), whereas the dorsal striatum is involved in sensorimotor and cognitive functions (Willner *et al.*, 1991). The dorsal and ventral striata are heterogeneous structures that can be subdivided into distinct compartments. In the middle and caudal third of the NAcc, the characteristic distribution of neuroactive substances results in two unique compartments called the *core* and the *shell* (Heimer *et al.*, 1991). It is important to note that other reward-relevant brain regions (*e.g.*, the lateral hypothalamus and the medial prefrontal cortex) implicated with a variety of abused drugs are connected reciprocally to the shell of the NAcc. Thus the *shell of the NAcc* is the site that may be involved directly in the emotional and motivational aspects of drug-induced reward.

Prodynorphin- and proenkephalin-derived opioid peptides are expressed primarily in *output neurons* of the striatum and NAcc. All three opioid receptor types are present in the NAcc (Mansour *et al.*, 1988) and are thought to mediate, at least in part, the motivational effects of opiate drugs. Selective μ and δ receptor agonists are rewarding when defined by place preference (Shippenberg *et al.*, 1992) and intracranial self-administration (Devine and Wise, 1994) paradigms. Conversely, selective κ receptor agonists produce aversive effects (Cooper, 1991; Shippenberg *et al.*, 1992). Naloxone and selective μ antagonists also produce aversive effects (Cooper, 1991). Positive motivational effects of opioids are mediated partially by dopamine release at the level of the NAcc. Thus κ-receptor activation in these circuits inhibits dopamine release (Mulder and Schoffelmeer, 1993), whereas μ and δ receptor activation increases dopamine release (Devine *et al.*, 1993). Distinctive cell clusters in the shell of the NAcc contain proenkephalin, prodynorphin, μ receptors, and κ receptors, as well as dopamine receptors. These clusters may constitute a region where the motivational properties of dopaminergic and opioid drugs are processed.

The locus ceruleus (LC) contains noradrenergic neurons and high concentrations of opioid receptors and is postulated to play a crucial role in feelings of alarm, panic, fear, and anxiety. Neural activity in the LC is inhibited by exogenous opioids and endogenous opioidlike peptides.

Other CNS Effects

Whereas opioids are used clinically primarily for their pain-relieving properties, they produce a host of other effects. This is not surprising in view of the wide distribution of opioids and their receptors in the brain and the periphery. A brief summary of some of these effects is presented below. High doses of opioids can produce muscular rigidity in humans. Chest wall rigidity severe enough to compromise respiration is not uncommon during anesthesia with fentanyl, *alfentanil, remifentanil,* and *sufentanil* (Monk *et al.*, 1988). Opioids and endogenous peptides cause catalepsy, circling, and stereotypical behavior in rats and other animals.

Effects on the Hypothalamus. Opioids alter the equilibrium point of the hypothalamic heat-regulatory mechanisms such that body temperature usually falls slightly. However, chronic high dosage may increase body temperature (Martin, 1983).

Neuroendocrine Effects. Morphine acts in the hypothalamus to inhibit the release of gonadotropin-releasing hormone (GnRH) and corticotropin-releasing hormone (CRH), thus decreasing circulating concentrations of luteinizing hormone (LH), follicle-stimulating hormone (FSH), ACTH, and β-endorphin; the last two peptides usually are released simultaneously from corticotropes in the pituitary. As a result of the decreased concentrations of pituitary trophic hormones, the plasma concentrations of testosterone and cortisol decline. Secretion of thyrotropin is relatively unaffected.

The administration of μ agonists increases the concentration of prolactin in plasma probably by reducing the dopaminergic inhibition of its secretion. Although some opioids enhance the secretion of growth hormone, the administration of morphine or β-endorphin has little effect on the concentration of the hormone in plasma. With chronic administration, tolerance develops to the effects of morphine on hypothalamic-releasing factors. Patients maintained on *methadone* reflect this phenomenon; in women, menstrual cycles that had been disrupted by intermittent use of heroin return to normal; in men, circulating concentrations of LH and testosterone usually are within the normal range.

Although κ-receptor agonists inhibit the release of antidiuretic hormone and cause diuresis, the administration of μ-opioid receptor agonists tends to produce antidiuretic effects in humans.

Miosis. Morphine and most μ and κ agonists cause constriction of the pupil by an excitatory action on the parasympathetic nerve innervating the pupil. After toxic doses of μ agonists, *the miosis is marked, and pinpoint pupils are pathognomonic;* however, marked mydriasis occurs when asphyxia intervenes. Some tolerance to the miotic effect develops, but addicts with high circulating concentrations of opioids continue to have constricted pupils.

Therapeutic doses of morphine increase accommodative power and lower intraocular tension in normal and glaucomatous eyes.

Convulsions. In animals, high doses of morphine and related opioids produce convulsions. Several mechanisms appear to be involved, and different types of opioids produce seizures with different characteristics. Morphine-like drugs excite certain groups of neurons, especially hippocampal pyramidal cells; these excitatory effects probably result from inhibition of the release of GABA by interneurons (McGinty and Friedman, 1988). Selective δ agonists produce similar effects. These actions may contribute to the seizures that are produced by some agents at doses only moderately higher than those required for analgesia, especially in children. However, with most opioids, convulsions occur only at doses far in excess of those required to produce profound analgesia, and seizures are not seen when potent μ agonists are used to produce anesthesia. Naloxone is more potent in antagonizing convulsions produced by some opioids (*e.g.,* morphine, methadone, and *propoxyphene*) than those produced by others (*e.g., meperidine*). The production of convulsant metabolites of the latter agent may be partially responsible (*see* below). Anticonvulsant agents may not always be effective in suppressing opioid-induced seizures (*see* Chapter 19).

Respiration. Morphine-like opioids depress respiration at least in part by virtue of a direct effect on the brainstem respiratory centers. The respiratory depression is discernible even with doses too small to disturb consciousness and increases progressively as the dose is increased. In humans, death from morphine poisoning is nearly always due to respiratory arrest. Therapeutic doses of morphine in humans depress all phases of respiratory activity (rate, minute volume, and tidal exchange) and also may produce irregular and periodic breathing. The diminished respiratory volume is due primarily to a slower rate of breathing, and with toxic amounts, the rate may fall to three or four breaths per minute. Although effects on respiration are readily demonstrated, clinically significant respiratory depression rarely occurs with standard morphine doses in the absence of underlying pulmonary dysfunction. One important exception is when opioids are administered parenterally to women within 2 to 4 hours of delivery, which can lead to transient respiratory depression in the neonate because of transplacental passage of opioids. However, the combination of opioids with other medications, such as general anesthetics, tranquilizers, alcohol, or sedative-hypnotics, may present a greater risk of respiratory depression. Maximal respiratory depression occurs within 5 to 10 minutes of intravenous administration of morphine or within 30 or 90 minutes of intramuscular or subcutaneous administration, respectively.

Maximal respiratory depressant effects occur more rapidly with more lipid-soluble agents. After therapeutic doses, respiratory minute volume may be reduced for as long as 4 to 5 hours. The primary mechanism of respiratory depression by opioids involves a reduction in the responsiveness of the brainstem respiratory centers to carbon dioxide. Opioids also depress the pontine and medullary centers involved in regulating respiratory rhythmicity and the responsiveness of medullary respiratory centers to electrical stimulation (Martin, 1983).

Hypoxic stimulation of chemoreceptors still may be effective when opioids have decreased the responsiveness to CO_2, and the inhalation of O_2 thus may produce apnea. After large doses of morphine or other μ agonists, patients will breathe if instructed to do so, but without such instruction, they may remain relatively apneic.

Because of the accumulation of CO_2, respiratory rate and sometimes even minute volume can be unreliable indicators of the degree of respiratory depression that has been produced by morphine. Natural sleep also produces a decrease in the sensitivity of the medullary center to CO_2, and the effects of morphine and sleep are additive.

Numerous studies have compared morphine and morphine-like opioids with respect to their ratios of analgesic to respiratory-depressant activities, and most have found that when equianalgesic doses are used, there is no significant difference. Severe respiratory depression is less likely after the administration of large doses of selective κ agonists. High concentrations of opioid receptors and endogenous peptides are found in the medullary areas believed to be important in ventilatory control.

Cough. Morphine and related opioids also depress the cough reflex at least in part by a direct effect on a cough center in the medulla. There is, however, no obligatory relationship between depression of respiration and depression of coughing, and effective antitussive agents are available that do not depress respiration (*see* below). Suppression of cough by such agents appears to involve receptors in the medulla that are less sensitive to naloxone than those responsible for analgesia.

Nauseant and Emetic Effects. Nausea and vomiting produced by morphine-like drugs are side effects caused by direct stimulation of the chemoreceptor trigger zone for emesis in the area postrema of the medulla. Certain individuals never vomit after morphine, whereas others do so each time the drug is administered.

Nausea and vomiting are relatively uncommon in recumbent patients given therapeutic doses of morphine, but nausea occurs in approximately 40% and vomiting in 15% of ambulatory patients given 15 mg of the drug subcutaneously. This suggests that a vestibular component also is operative. Indeed, the nauseant and emetic effects of morphine are markedly enhanced by vestibular stimulation, and morphine and related synthetic analgesics produce an increase in vestibular sensitivity. All clinically useful μ agonists produce some degree of nausea and vomiting. Careful, controlled clinical studies usually demonstrate that, in equianalgesic dosage, the incidence of such side effects is not significantly lower than that seen with morphine. Antagonists to the 5-HT$_3$ serotonin receptor have supplanted phenothiazines and drugs used for motion sickness as the drugs of choice for the treatment of opioid-induced nausea and vomiting. Gastric prokinetic agents such as *metoclopramide* also are useful antinausea and antiemetic drugs (*see* Chapter 37).

Cardiovascular System. In the supine patient, therapeutic doses of morphinelike opioids have no major effect on blood pressure or cardiac rate and rhythm. Such doses do produce peripheral vasodilation, reduced peripheral resistance, and an inhibition of baroreceptor reflexes. Therefore, when supine patients assume the head-up position, orthostatic hypotension and fainting may occur. The peripheral arteriolar and venous dilation produced by morphine involves several mechanisms. Morphine and some other opioids provoke release of histamine, which sometimes plays a large role in the hypotension. However, vasodilation usually is only partially blocked by H$_1$ antagonists, but it is effectively reversed by naloxone. Morphine also blunts the reflex vasoconstriction caused by increased PCO$_2$ (*see* Chapter 15).

Effects on the myocardium are not significant in normal individuals. In patients with coronary artery disease but no acute medical problems, 8 to 15 mg morphine administered intravenously produces a decrease in oxygen consumption, left ventricular end-diastolic pressure, and cardiac work; effects on cardiac index usually are slight. In patients with acute myocardial infarction, the cardiovascular responses to morphine may be more variable than in normal subjects, and the magnitude of changes (*e.g.,* the decrease in blood pressure) may be more pronounced (Roth *et al.*, 1988).

Morphine may exert its well-known therapeutic effect in the treatment of angina pectoris and acute myocardial infarction by decreasing preload, inotropy, and chronotropy, thus favorably altering determinants of myocardial oxygen consumption and helping to relieve ischemia. It is not clear whether the analgesic properties of morphine in this situation are due to the reversal of acidosis that may stimulate local acid-sensing ion channels (McCleskey and Gold, 1999) or to a direct analgesic effect on nociceptive afferents from the heart.

When administered before experimental ischemia, morphine has been shown to produce cardioprotective effects. Morphine can mimic the phenomenon of ischemic preconditioning, where a short ischemic episode paradoxically protects the heart against further ischemia. This effect appears to be mediated through δ receptors signaling through a mitochondrial ATP-sensitive potassium channel in cardiac myocytes; the effect also is produced by other GPCRs signaling through G$_i$ (Fryer *et al.*, 2000). It also has been suggested recently that δ opioids can be antiarrhythmic and antifibrillatory during and after periods of ischemia (Fryer *et al.*, 2000), although other data suggest that δ opioids can be arrhythmogenic (McIntosh *et al.*, 1992).

Very large doses of morphine can be used to produce anesthesia; however, decreased peripheral resistance and blood pressure are troublesome. Fentanyl and sufentanil, which are potent and selective μ agonists, are less likely to cause hemodynamic instability during surgery in part because they do not cause the release of histamine (Monk *et al.*, 1988).

Morphine-like opioids should be used with caution in patients who have a decreased blood volume because these agents can aggravate hypovolemic shock. Morphine should be used with great care in patients with cor pulmonale because deaths after ordinary therapeutic doses have been reported. The concurrent use of certain phenothiazines may increase the risk of morphine-induced hypotension.

Cerebral circulation is not affected directly by therapeutic doses of morphine. However, opioid-induced respiratory depression and CO$_2$ retention can result in cerebral vasodilation and an increase in cerebrospinal fluid pressure; the pressure increase does not occur when PCO$_2$ is maintained at normal levels by artificial ventilation.

Gastrointestinal Tract. **Stomach.** Morphine and other μ agonists usually decrease the secretion of hydrochloric acid, although stimulation sometimes is evident. Activation of opioid receptors on parietal cells enhances secretion, but indirect effects, including increased secretion of somatostatin from the pancreas and reduced release of acetylcholine, appear to be dominant in most circumstances (Kromer, 1988). Relatively low doses of morphine decrease gastric motility, thereby prolonging gastric emptying time; this can increase the likelihood of esophageal reflux. The tone of the antral portion of the stomach and of the first part of the duodenum is increased, which often makes therapeutic intubation of the duodenum more difficult. Passage of the gastric contents through the duodenum may be delayed by as much as 12 hours, and the absorption of orally administered drugs is retarded.

Small Intestine. Morphine diminishes biliary, pancreatic, and intestinal secretions (De Luca and Coupar, 1996) and delays digestion of food in the small intestine. Resting tone is increased, and periodic spasms are observed. The amplitude of the nonpropulsive type of rhythmic, segmental contractions usually is enhanced, but propulsive contractions are decreased markedly. The upper part of the small intestine, particularly the duodenum, is affected more than the ileum. A period of relative atony may follow the hypertonicity. Water is absorbed more completely because of the delayed passage of bowel contents, and intestinal secretion is decreased; this increases the viscosity of the bowel contents.

In the presence of intestinal hypersecretion that may be associated with diarrhea, morphine-like drugs inhibit the transfer of fluid and electrolytes into the lumen by naloxone-sensitive actions on the intestinal mucosa and within the CNS (De Luca and Coupar, 1996; Kromer, 1988). Enteric muscle cells also may possess opioid receptors (Holzer, 2004). However, it is clear that opioids exert important effects on the submucosal plexus that lead to a decrease in the basal secretion by enterocytes and inhibition of the stimulatory effects of acetylcholine, prostaglandin E_2, and vasoactive intestinal peptide. The effects of opioids initiated either in the CNS or in the submucosal plexus may be mediated in large part by the release of norepinephrine and stimulation of α_2 adrenergic receptors on enterocytes.

Large Intestine. Propulsive peristaltic waves in the colon are diminished or abolished after administration of morphine, and tone is increased to the point of spasm. The resulting delay in the passage of bowel contents causes considerable desiccation of the feces, which, in turn, retards their advance through the colon. The amplitude of the nonpropulsive type of rhythmic contractions of the colon usually is enhanced. The tone of the anal sphincter is augmented greatly, and reflex relaxation in response to rectal distension is reduced. These actions, combined with inattention to the normal sensory stimuli for defecation reflex owing to the central actions of the drug, contribute to morphine-induced constipation.

Mechanism of Action on the Bowel. The usual gastrointestinal effects of morphine primarily are mediated by μ and δ opioid receptors in the bowel. However, injection of opioids into the cerebral ventricles or in the vicinity of the spinal cord can inhibit gastrointestinal propulsive activity as long as the extrinsic innervation to the bowel is intact. The relatively poor penetration of morphine into the CNS may explain how preparations such as *paregoric* can produce constipation at less than analgesic doses and may account for troublesome gastrointestinal side effects during the use of oral morphine for the treatment of cancer pain. Although some tolerance develops to the effects of opioids on gastrointestinal motility, patients who take opioids chronically remain constipated.

Biliary Tract. After the subcutaneous injection of 10 mg *morphine sulfate,* the sphincter of Oddi constricts, and the pressure in the common bile duct may rise more than tenfold within 15 minutes; this effect may persist for 2 hours or more. Fluid pressure also may increase in the gallbladder and produce symptoms that may vary from epigastric distress to typical biliary colic.

Some patients with biliary colic experience exacerbation rather than relief of pain when given opioids. Spasm of the sphincter of Oddi probably is responsible for elevations of plasma amylase and lipase that occur sometimes after morphine administration. All opioids can cause biliary spasm. *Atropine* only partially prevents morphine-induced biliary spasm, but opioid antagonists prevent or relieve it. *Nitroglycerin* (0.6 to 1.2 mg) administered sublingually also decreases the elevated intrabiliary pressure (Staritz, 1988).

Other Smooth Muscle. *Ureter and Urinary Bladder.* Therapeutic doses of morphine may increase the tone and amplitude of contractions of the ureter, although the response is variable. When the antidiuretic effects of the drug are prominent and urine flow decreases, the ureter may become quiescent.

Morphine inhibits the urinary voiding reflex and increases the tone of the external sphincter and the volume of the bladder; cath-

eterization sometimes is required after therapeutic doses of morphine. Stimulation of either μ or δ receptors in the brain or in the spinal cord exerts similar actions on bladder motility (Dray and Nunan, 1987). Tolerance develops to these effects of opioids on the bladder.

Uterus. If the uterus has been made hyperactive by oxytocics, morphine tends to restore the tone, frequency, and amplitude of contractions to normal.

Skin. Therapeutic doses of morphine cause dilation of cutaneous blood vessels. The skin of the face, neck, and upper thorax frequently becomes flushed. These changes may be due in part to the release of histamine and may be responsible for the sweating and some of the pruritus that occasionally follow the systemic administration of morphine (*see* below). Histamine release probably accounts for the urticaria commonly seen at the site of injection, which is not mediated by opioid receptors and is not blocked by naloxone. It is seen with morphine and meperidine but not with *oxymorphone,* methadone, fentanyl, or sufentanil.

Pruritus is a common and potentially disabling complication of opioid use. It can be caused by intraspinal and systemic injections of opioids, but it appears to be more intense after intraspinal administration (Ballantyne *et al.*, 1988). The effect appears to be mediated largely by dorsal horn neurons and is reversed by naloxone (Thomas *et al.*, 1992).

Immune System. The effects of opioids on the immune system are complex. Opioids modulate immune function by direct effects on cells of the immune system and indirectly *via* centrally mediated neuronal mechanisms (Sharp and Yaksh, 1997). The acute central immunomodulatory effects of opioids may be mediated by activation of the sympathetic nervous system, whereas the chronic effects of opioids may involve modulation of the hypothalamic–pituitary–adrenal (HPA) axis (Mellon and Bayer, 1998). Direct effects on immune cells may involve unique, incompletely characterized variants of the classical neuronal opioid receptors, with δ-receptor variants being most prominent (Sharp and Yaksh, 1997). Atypical receptors could account for the fact that it has been very difficult to demonstrate significant opioid binding on immune cells despite the observance of robust functional effects. In contrast, morphine-induced immune suppression largely is abolished in knockout mice lacking the μ receptor gene, suggesting that the μ receptor is a major target of morphine's actions on the immune system (Gaveriaux-Ruff *et al.*, 1998). A proposed mechanism for the immune suppressive effects of morphine on neutrophils is through a nitric oxide–dependent inhibition of NF-κB activation (Welters *et al.*, 2000). Others have proposed that the induction and activation of MAP kinase also may play a role (Chuang *et al.*, 1997).

The overall effects of opioids appear to be immunosuppressive, and increased susceptibility to infection and tumor spread have been observed. Infusion of the μ-receptor antagonist naloxone has been shown to improve survival after experimentally induced sepsis (Risdahl *et al.*, 1998). Such effects have been inconsistent in clinical situations possibly because of the use of confounding therapies and necessary opioid analgesics. In some situations, immune effects appear more prominent with acute administration than with chronic administration, which could have important implications for the care of the critically ill (Sharp and Yaksh, 1997). In contrast, opioids have been shown to reverse pain-induced immunosuppression and increase tumor metastatic potential in animal models (Page and Ben-Eliyahu, 1997). Therefore, opioids may either inhibit or augment immune function depending on the context in which they are used. These studies also indicate that withholding opioids in the presence of pain in immunocompromised patients actually could worsen immune function. An intriguing paper indicated that the partial μ-receptor agonist *buprenorphine* (*see* below) did not alter immune function when injected centrally into the mesencephalic PAG, whereas morphine did (Gomez-Flores and Weber, 2000). Taken together, these studies indicate that opioid-induced immune suppression may be clinically relevant both to the treatment of severe pain and in the susceptibility of opioid addicts to infection [*e.g.,* human immunodeficiency virus (HIV) infection and tuberculosis]. Different opioid agonists also may have unique immunomodulatory properties. Better understanding of these properties eventually should help to guide the rational use of opioids in patients with cancer or at risk for infection or immune compromise.

Tolerance and Physical Dependence

The development of tolerance and physical dependence with repeated use is a characteristic feature of all the opioid drugs. *Tolerance* to the effect of opioids or other drugs simply means that, over time, the drug loses its effectiveness and an increased dose is required to produce the same physiological response. *Dependence* refers to a complex and poorly understood set of changes in the homeostasis of an organism that causes a disturbance of the homeostatic set point of the organism if the drug is stopped. This disturbance often is revealed when administration of an opioid is stopped abruptly, resulting in *withdrawal. Addiction* is a behavioral pattern characterized by compulsive use of a drug and overwhelming involvement with its procurement and use. Tolerance and dependence are physiological responses seen in all patients and are not predictors of addiction (*see* Chapter 23). These processes appear to be quite distinct. For example, cancer pain often requires prolonged treatment with high doses of opioids, leading to tolerance and dependence. Yet abuse in this setting is very unusual (Foley, 1993). Neither the presence of tolerance and dependence nor the fear that they may develop should *ever* interfere with the appropriate use of opioids. Opioids can be discontinued in dependent patients once the need for analgesics is gone without subjecting them to withdrawal (*see* Chapter 23). Clinically, the dose can be decreased by 10% to 20% every other day and eventually stopped without signs and symptoms of withdrawal.

In vivo studies in animal models demonstrate the importance of neurotransmitters and their interactions with opioid pathways in the development of tolerance to morphine. Blockade of glutamate actions by NMDA (*N*-methyl-D-aspartate)–receptor antagonists blocks morphine tolerance (Trujillo and Akil, 1991). Since NMDA antagonists have no effect on the potency of morphine in naive animals, their effect cannot be attributed to poten-

tiation of opioid actions. Interestingly, the antitussive *dextromethorphan* (*see* below) has been shown to function as an NMDA antagonist. In animals, it can attenuate opioid tolerance development and reverse established tolerance (Elliott *et al.,* 1994). Nitric oxide production, possibly induced by NMDA-receptor activation, also has been implicated in tolerance because inhibition of nitric oxide synthase (NOS) also blocks morphine tolerance development (Kolesnikov *et al.,* 1993). Administering NOS inhibitors to morphine-tolerant animals also may reverse tolerance in certain circumstances. Although NMDA antagonists and nitric oxide synthase inhibitors are effective against tolerance to morphine and δ agonists such as DPDPE, they have little effect against tolerance to the κ agonists. Morphine dependence was thought to be closely related to tolerance because some treatments that block tolerance to morphine also block dependence. Nonetheless, it now is believed that distinct mechanisms underlie these two effects. The deletion of β-arrestin-2 inhibits the development of tolerance to morphine but does not inhibit the development of physical dependence (Bohn *et al.,* 2000). Deletion of GRK3 inhibits the development of tolerance to fentanyl but has no effect on the development of morphine tolerance (Terman *et al.,* 2004). GRK3 deletion also did not affect physical dependence. Taken together, these findings suggest that the signaling mechanisms underlying the development of opioid tolerance and physical dependence also may be agonist-dependent.

MORPHINE AND RELATED OPIOID AGONISTS

There are now many compounds with pharmacological properties similar to those of morphine, yet morphine remains the standard against which new analgesics are measured. However, responses of an individual patient may vary dramatically with different μ-opioid receptor agonists. For example, some patients unable to tolerate morphine may have no problems with an equianalgesic dose of methadone, whereas others can tolerate morphine and not methadone. If problems are encountered with one drug, another should be tried. Mechanisms underlying variations in individual responses to morphine-like agonists are poorly understood.

Source and Composition of Opium. Because the synthesis of morphine is difficult, the drug still is obtained from opium or extracted from poppy straw. Opium is obtained from the unripe seed capsules of the poppy plant, *Papaver somniferum.* The milky juice is dried and powdered to make powdered opium, which contains a number of alkaloids. Only a few—morphine, codeine, and papaverine—have clinical usefulness. These alkaloids can be divided into two distinct chemical classes, *phenanthrenes* and *benzylisoquinolines.* The principal phenanthrenes are morphine (10% of opium), codeine (0.5%), and thebaine (0.2%). The principal benzylisoquinolines are papaverine (1%), which is a smooth muscle relaxant (*see* the seventh and earlier editions of this book), and *noscapine* (6%).

Chemistry of Morphine and Related Opioids. The structure of morphine is shown in Table 21–5. Many semisynthetic derivatives are made by relatively simple modifications of morphine or thebaine. Codeine is methylmorphine, the methyl substitution being on the phenolic hydroxyl group. Thebaine differs from morphine only in that both hydroxyl groups are methylated and that the ring has two double bonds ($\Delta^{6,7}$, $\Delta^{8,14}$). Thebaine has little analgesic action but is a precursor of several important 14-OH compounds, such as *oxycodone* and naloxone. Certain derivatives of thebaine are more than 1000 times as potent as morphine (*e.g., etorphine*). *Diacetylmorphine*, or heroin, is made from morphine by acetylation at the 3 and 6 positions. *Apomorphine*, which also can be prepared from morphine, is a potent emetic and dopaminergic agonist (*see* Chapter 20). *Hydromorphone*, oxymorphone, *hydrocodone*, and oxycodone also are made by modifying the morphine molecule. The structural relationships between morphine and some of its surrogates and antagonists are shown in Table 21–5.

Structure–Activity Relationship of the Morphine-like Opioids. In addition to morphine, codeine, and the semisynthetic derivatives of the natural opium alkaloids, a number of other structurally distinct chemical classes of drugs have pharmacological actions similar to those of morphine. Clinically useful compounds include the morphinans, benzomorphans, methadones, phenylpiperidines, and propionanilides. Although the two-dimensional representations of these chemically diverse compounds appear to be quite different, molecular models show certain common characteristics, as indicated by the heavy lines in the structure of morphine shown in Table 21–5. Among the important properties of the opioids that can be altered by structural modification are their affinities for various species of opioid receptors, their activities as agonists *versus* antagonists, their lipid solubilities, and their resistance to metabolic breakdown. For example, blockade of the phenolic hydroxyl at position 3, as in codeine and heroin, drastically reduces binding to μ receptors; these compounds are converted *in vivo* to the potent analgesics morphine and 6-acetyl morphine, respectively.

Absorption, Distribution, Fate, and Excretion. *Absorption.*

In general, the opioids are absorbed readily from the gastrointestinal tract; absorption through the rectal mucosa is adequate, and a few agents (*e.g.,* morphine, hydromorphone) are available in suppositories. The more lipophilic opioids also are absorbed readily through the nasal or buccal mucosa (Weinberg *et al.,* 1988). Those with the greatest lipid solubility also can be absorbed transdermally (Portenoy *et al.,* 1993). Opioids are absorbed readily after subcutaneous or intramuscular injection and can penetrate the spinal cord adequately after epidural or intrathecal administration. Small amounts of morphine introduced epidurally or intrathecally into the spinal canal can produce profound analgesia that may last 12 to 24 hours. However, because of the hydrophilic nature of morphine, there is rostral spread of the drug in spinal fluid, and side effects, especially respiratory depression, can emerge up to 24 hours later as the opioid reaches supraspinal respiratory control centers. With highly lipophilic agents such as hydromorphone or fen-

tanyl, rapid absorption by spinal neural tissues produces very localized effects and segmental analgesia. The duration of action is shorter because of distribution of the drug in the systemic circulation, and the severity of respiratory depression may be more directly proportional to its concentration in plasma owing to a lesser degree of rostral spread (Gustafsson and Wiesenfeld-Hallin, 1988). However, patients receiving epidural or intrathecal fentanyl still should be monitored for respiratory depression.

With most opioids, including morphine, the effect of a given dose is less after oral than after parenteral administration because of variable but significant first-pass metabolism in the liver. For example, the bioavailability of oral preparations of morphine is only about 25%. The shape of the time–effect curve also varies with the route of administration, so the duration of action often is somewhat longer with the oral route. If adjustment is made for variability of first-pass metabolism and clearance, adequate relief of pain can be achieved with oral administration of morphine. Satisfactory analgesia in cancer patients is associated with a very broad range of steady-state concentrations of morphine in plasma (16 to 364 ng/ml) (Neumann *et al.,* 1982).

When morphine and most opioids are given intravenously, they act promptly. However, the more lipid-soluble compounds act more rapidly than morphine after subcutaneous administration because of differences in the rates of absorption and entry into the CNS. Compared with more lipid-soluble opioids such as codeine, heroin, and methadone, morphine crosses the blood–brain barrier at a considerably lower rate.

Distribution and Fate. About one-third of morphine in the plasma is protein-bound after a therapeutic dose. Morphine itself does not persist in tissues, and 24 hours after the last dose, tissue concentrations are low.

The major pathway for the metabolism of morphine is conjugation with glucuronic acid. The two major metabolites formed are *morphine-6-glucuronide* and *morphine-3-glucuronide*. Small amounts of morphine-3,6-diglucuronide also may be formed. Although the 3- and 6-glucuronides are quite polar, both still can cross the blood–brain barrier to exert significant clinical effects (Christup, 1997). Morphine-6-glucuronide has pharmacological actions indistinguishable from those of morphine. Morphine-6-glucuronide given systemically is approximately twice as potent as morphine in animal models (Paul *et al.,* 1989) and in humans (Osborne *et al.,* 1988). With chronic administration, it accounts for a significant portion of morphine's analgesic actions (Osborne *et al.,* 1988). Indeed, with chronic oral dosing, the blood levels

Table 21–5
Structures of Opioids and Opioid Antagonists Chemically Related to Morphine

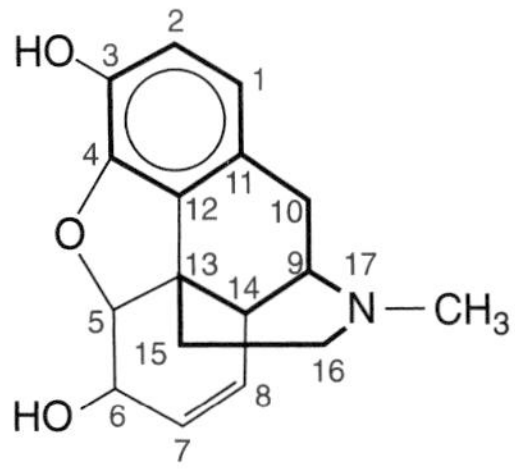

MORPHINE

NONPROPRIETARY NAME	CHEMICAL RADICALS AND POSITION*			OTHER CHANGES†
	3	*6*	*17*	
Morphine	—OH	—OH	—CH$_3$	—
Heroin	—OCOCH$_3$	—OCOCH$_3$	—CH$_3$	—
Hydromorphone	—OH	=O	—CH$_3$	(1)
Oxymorphone	—OH	=O	—CH$_3$	(1), (2)
Levorphanol	—OH	—H	—CH$_3$	(1), (3)
Levallorphan	—OH	—H	—CH$_2$CH=CH$_2$	(1), (3)
Codeine	—OCH$_3$	—OH	—CH$_3$	—
Hydrocodone	—OCH$_3$	=O	—CH$_3$	(1)
Oxycodone	—OCH$_3$	=O	—CH$_3$	(1), (2)
Nalmefene	—OH	=CH$_2$	—CH$_2$—◁ 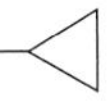	(1), (2)
Nalorphine	—OH	—OH	—CH$_2$CH=CH$_2$	—
Naloxone	—OH	=O	—CH$_2$CH=CH$_2$	(1), (2)
Naltrexone	—OH	=O	—CH$_2$—◁ 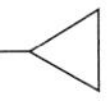	(1), (2)
Buprenorphine	—OH	—OCH$_3$	—CH$_2$—◁ 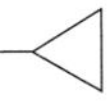	(1), (4)
Butorphanol	—OH	—H	—CH$_2$—◇ 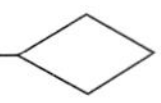	(1), (2), (3)
Nalbuphine	—OH	—OH	—CH$_2$—◇ 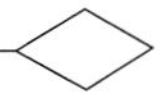	(1), (2)

*The numbers 3, 6, and 17 refer to positions in the morphine molecule, as shown above. †Other changes in the morphine molecule are: (1) Single instead of double bond between C7 and C8; (2) OH added to C14; (3) No oxygen between C4 and C5; (4) *Endo*etheno bridge between C6 and C14; 1-hydroxy-1,2,2-trimethylpropyl substitution on C7.

of morphine-6-glucuronide typically exceed those of morphine. Given its greater potency and its higher concentration, morphine-6-glucuronide may be responsible for most of morphine's analgesic activity in patients receiving chronic oral morphine. Morphine-6-glucuronide is excreted by the kidney. In renal failure, the levels of morphine-6-glucuronide can accumulate, perhaps explaining

morphine's potency and long duration in patients with compromised renal function. In adults, the half-life of morphine is about 2 hours; the half-life of morphine-6-glucuronide is somewhat longer. Children achieve adult renal function values by 6 months of age. In elderly patients, lower doses of morphine are recommended based on its smaller volume of distribution (Owen *et al.*,

1983) and the general decline in renal function in the elderly. Morphine-3-glucuronide, another important metabolite (Milne *et al.*, 1996), has little affinity for opioid receptors but may contribute to excitatory effects of morphine (Smith, 2000). Some investigators have shown that morphine-3-glucuronide can antagonize morphine-induced analgesia (Smith *et al.*, 1990), but this finding is not universal (Christup, 1997). *N*-Demethylation of morphine to normorphine is a minor metabolic pathway in humans but is more prominent in rodents (Yeh *et al.*, 1977). *N*-Dealkylation also is important in the metabolism of some congeners of morphine.

Excretion. Very little morphine is excreted unchanged. It is eliminated by glomerular filtration, primarily as morphine-3-glucuronide; 90% of the total excretion takes place during the first day. Enterohepatic circulation of morphine and its glucuronides occurs, which accounts for the presence of small amounts of morphine in the feces and in the urine for several days after the last dose.

Codeine.

In contrast to morphine, codeine is approximately 60% as effective orally as parenterally as an analgesic and as a respiratory depressant. Codeine analogs such as *levorphanol*, oxycodone, and methadone have a high ratio of oral-to-parenteral potency. The greater oral efficacy of these drugs reflects lower first-pass metabolism in the liver. Once absorbed, codeine is metabolized by the liver, and its metabolites are excreted chiefly as inactive forms in the urine. A small fraction (approximately 10%) of administered codeine is *O*-demethylated to morphine, and free and conjugated morphine can be found in the urine after therapeutic doses of codeine. Codeine has an exceptionally low affinity for opioid receptors, and the analgesic effect of codeine is due to its conversion to morphine. However, its antitussive actions may involve distinct receptors that bind codeine itself. The half-life of codeine in plasma is 2 to 4 hours.

The conversion of codeine to morphine is effected by the CYP2D6. Well-characterized genetic polymorphisms in CYP2D6 lead to the inability to convert codeine to morphine, thus making codeine ineffective as an analgesic for about 10% of the Caucasian population (Eichelbaum and Evert, 1996). Other polymorphisms can lead to enhanced metabolism and thus increased sensitivity to codeine's effects (Eichelbaum and Evert, 1996). Interestingly, there appears to be variation in metabolic efficiency among ethnic groups. For example, Chinese produce less morphine from codeine than do Caucasians and also are less sensitive to morphine's effects. The reduced sensitivity to morphine may be due to decreased production of morphine-6-glucuronide (Caraco *et al.*, 1999). Thus, it is important to consider the possibility of metabolic enzyme polymorphism in any patient who does not receive adequate analgesia from

codeine or an adequate response to other administered opioid prodrugs.

Tramadol.

Tramadol (ULTRAM) is a synthetic codeine analog that is a weak μ-opioid receptor agonist. Part of its analgesic effect is produced by inhibition of uptake of norepinephrine and serotonin. In the treatment of mild-to-moderate pain, tramadol is as effective as morphine or meperidine. However, for the treatment of severe or chronic pain, tramadol is less effective. Tramadol is as effective as meperidine in the treatment of labor pain and may cause less neonatal respiratory depression.

Tramadol is 68% bioavailable after a single oral dose and 100% available when administered intramuscularly. Its affinity for the μ-opioid receptor is only 1/6000 that of morphine. However, the primary *O*-demethylated metabolite of tramadol is two to four times as potent as the parent drug and may account for part of the analgesic effect. Tramadol is supplied as a racemic mixture, which is more effective than either enantiomer alone. The (+)-enantiomer binds to the μ receptor and inhibits serotonin uptake. The (−)-enantiomer inhibits norepinephrine uptake and stimulates α_2 adrenergic receptors (Lewis and Han, 1997). The compound undergoes hepatic metabolism and renal excretion, with an elimination half-life of 6 hours for tramadol and 7.5 hours for its active metabolite. Analgesia begins within an hour of oral dosing and peaks within 2 to 3 hours. The duration of analgesia is about 6 hours. The maximum recommended daily dose is 400 mg.

Common side effects of tramadol include nausea, vomiting, dizziness, dry mouth, sedation, and headache. Respiratory depression appears to be less than with equianalgesic doses of morphine, and the degree of constipation is less than that seen after equivalent doses of codeine (Duthie, 1998). Tramadol can cause seizures and possibly exacerbate seizures in patients with predisposing factors. While tramadol-induced analgesia is not entirely reversible by naloxone, tramadol-induced respiratory depression can be reversed by naloxone. However, the use of naloxone increases the risk of seizure. Physical dependence on and abuse of tramadol have been reported. Although its abuse potential is unclear, tramadol probably should be avoided in patients with a history of addiction. Because of its inhibitory effect on serotonin uptake, tramadol should not be used in patients taking monoamine oxidase (MAO) inhibitors (Lewis and Han, 1997) (*see* section on interaction of meperidine with other drugs below).

Heroin.

Heroin (diacetylmorphine) is rapidly hydrolyzed to 6-monoacetylmorphine (6-MAM), which, in turn, is hydrolyzed to morphine. Heroin and 6-MAM are more lipid soluble than morphine and enter the brain more readily. Evidence suggests that morphine and 6-MAM are responsible for the pharmacological actions of heroin. Heroin is excreted mainly in the urine largely as free and conjugated morphine.

Untoward Effects and Precautions.

Morphine and related opioids produce a wide spectrum of unwanted effects, including respiratory depression, nausea, vomiting, dizziness, mental clouding, dysphoria, pruritus, constipation, increased pressure in the biliary tract, urinary retention, and hypotension. The bases of these effects were described earlier. Rarely, a patient may develop delirium. Increased sensitivity to pain after analgesia has worn off also may occur.

A number of factors may alter a patient's sensitivity to opioid analgesics, including the integrity of the blood–brain barrier. For example, when morphine is administered to a newborn infant in weight-appropriate doses extrapolated from adults, unexpectedly profound analgesia and respiratory depression may be observed. This is due to the immaturity of the blood–brain barrier in neonates. As mentioned previously, morphine is hydrophilic, so proportionately less morphine normally crosses into the CNS than with more lipophilic opioids. In neonates or when the blood–brain barrier is compromised, lipophilic opioids may give more predictable clinical results than morphine. In adults, the *duration* of the analgesia produced by morphine increases progressively with age; however, the *degree* of analgesia that is obtained with a given dose changes little. Changes in pharmacokinetic parameters only partially explain these observations. The patient with severe pain may tolerate larger doses of morphine. However, as the pain subsides, the patient may exhibit sedation and even respiratory depression as the stimulatory effects of pain are diminished. The reasons for this effect are unclear.

All opioid analgesics are metabolized by the liver and should be used with caution in patients with hepatic disease because increased bioavailability after oral administration or cumulative effects may occur. Renal disease also significantly alters the pharmacokinetics of morphine, codeine, *dihydrocodeine,* meperidine, and propoxyphene. Although single doses of morphine are well tolerated, the active metabolite, morphine-6-glucuronide, may accumulate with continued dosing, and symptoms of opioid overdose may result (Chan and Matzke, 1987). This metabolite also may accumulate during repeated administration of codeine to patients with impaired renal function. When repeated doses of meperidine are given to such patients, the accumulation of normeperidine may cause tremor and seizures (Kaiko *et al.*, 1983). Similarly, the repeated administration of propoxyphene may lead to naloxone-insensitive cardiac toxicity caused by the accumulation of norpropoxyphene (Chan and Matzke, 1987).

Morphine and related opioids must be used cautiously in patients with compromised respiratory function (*e.g.*, emphysema, kyphoscoliosis, or severe obesi-

ty). In patients with cor pulmonale, death has occurred after therapeutic doses of morphine. Although many patients with such conditions seem to be functioning within normal limits, they are already using compensatory mechanisms, such as increased respiratory rate. Many have chronically elevated levels of plasma CO_2 and may be less sensitive to the stimulating actions of CO_2. The further imposition of the depressant effects of opioids can be disastrous. The respiratory-depressant effects of opioids and the related capacity to elevate intracranial pressure must be considered in the presence of head injury or an already elevated intracranial pressure. While head injury *per se* does not constitute an absolute contraindication to the use of opioids, the possibility of exaggerated depression of respiration and the potential need to control ventilation of the patient must be considered. Finally, since opioids may produce mental clouding and side effects such as miosis and vomiting, which are important signs in following the clinical course of patients with head injuries, the advisability of their use must be weighed carefully against these risks.

Morphine causes histamine release, which can cause bronchoconstriction and vasodilation. Morphine has the potential to precipitate or exacerbate asthmatic attacks and should be avoided in patients with a history of asthma. Other μ receptor agonists that do not release histamine, such as the fentanyl derivatives, may be better choices for such patients.

Patients with reduced blood volume are considerably more susceptible to the vasodilatory effects of morphine and related drugs, and these agents must be used cautiously in patients with hypotension from any cause.

Allergic phenomena occur with opioid analgesics but are uncommon. They usually are manifested as urticaria and other types of skin rashes such as fixed eruptions; contact dermatitis in nurses and pharmaceutical workers also occurs. Wheals at the site of injection of morphine, codeine, and related drugs are probably secondary to histamine release. Anaphylactoid reactions have been reported after intravenous administration of codeine and morphine, but such reactions are rare. Such reactions may be responsible for some of the sudden deaths, episodes of pulmonary edema, and other complications that occur among addicts who use heroin intravenously (*see* Chapter 23).

Interactions with Other Drugs. The depressant effects of some opioids may be exaggerated and prolonged by phenothiazines, MOA inhibitors, and tricyclic antidepressants; the mechanisms of these supra-additive effects are not understood fully but may involve alterations in the rate of metabolic transformation of the opioid or alterations in neurotransmitters involved in the actions of opioids. Some, but not all, phenothiazines reduce the amount of opioid required to produce a given level of analgesia. Depending on the specific agent, the respiratory-depressant effects also seem to be enhanced, the degree of sedation is increased, and the hypotensive effects of phenothiazines become an additional complication. Some phenothiazine derivatives enhance the sedative effects but at the same time seem to be antianalgesic and increase the amount of opioid required to produce satisfactory relief from pain. Small doses of *amphetamine* substantially increase the analgesic and euphoriant effects of morphine and may decrease its sedative side effects. A number of antihistamines exhibit modest analgesic actions; some (*e.g., hydroxyzine*) enhance the analgesic effects of low doses of opioids (Rumore and Schlichting, 1986). Antidepressants such as *desipramine* and *amitriptyline* are used in the treatment of chronic neuropathic pain but have limited intrinsic analgesic actions in acute pain. However, antidepressants may enhance morphine-induced analgesia (Levine *et al.*, 1986). The analgesic synergism between opioids and aspirinlike drugs is discussed below and in Chapter 26.

OTHER μ RECEPTOR AGONISTS

Levorphanol

Levorphanol (LEVO-DROMORAN) is the only commercially available opioid agonist of the morphinan series. The D-isomer (dextrorphan) is relatively devoid of analgesic action but may have inhibitory effects at NMDA receptors. The structure of levorphanol is shown in Table 21–5.

The pharmacological effects of levorphanol closely parallel those of morphine. However, clinical reports suggest that it may produce less nausea and vomiting. Levorphanol is metabolized less rapidly than morphine and has a half-life of about 12 to 16 hours; repeated administration at short intervals may thus lead to accumulation of the drug in plasma.

Meperidine and Congeners

The structural formulas of meperidine, a *phenylpiperidine,* and some of its congeners are shown in Figure 21–4. Meperidine is predominantly a μ receptor agonist, and it exerts its chief pharmacological action on the CNS and the neural elements in the bowel. Meperidine is no longer recommended for the treatment of chronic pain because of concerns over metabolite toxicity. It should not be used for longer than 48 hours or in doses greater than 600 mg/day (Agency for Health Care Policy and Research, 1992a).

Pharmacological Properties. *Central Nervous System.* Meperidine produces a *pattern* of effects similar but not identical to that described for morphine.

Analgesia. The analgesic effects of meperidine are detectable about 15 minutes after oral administration, peak in about 1 to 2 hours, and subside gradually. The onset of analgesic effect is faster (within 10 minutes) after subcutaneous or intramuscular administration, and the effect reaches a peak in about 1 hour that corresponds closely to peak concentrations in plasma. In clinical use, the duration of effective analgesia is approximately 1.5 to 3 hours. In general, 75 to 100 mg meperidine hydrochloride (*pethidine,* DEMEROL) given parenterally is approximately equivalent to 10 mg morphine, and in equianalgesic doses, meperidine produces as much sedation, respiratory depression, and euphoria as does morphine. In terms of total analgesic effect, meperidine is about one-third as effective when given orally as when administered parenterally. A few patients may experience dysphoria.

Other CNS Actions. Peak respiratory depression is observed within 1 hour of intramuscular administration, and there is a return toward normal starting at about 2 hours. Like other opioids, meperidine causes pupillary constriction, increases the sensitivity of the labyrinthine apparatus, and has effects on the secretion of pituitary hormones similar to those of morphine. Meperidine sometimes causes CNS excitation, characterized by tremors, muscle twitches, and seizures; these effects are due largely to accumulation of a metabolite, *normeperidine* (*see* below). As with morphine, respiratory depression is responsible for an accumulation of CO_2, which, in turn, leads to cerebrovascular dilation, increased cerebral blood flow, and elevation of cerebrospinal fluid pressure.

Cardiovascular System. The effects of meperidine on the cardiovascular system generally resemble those of morphine, including the ability to release histamine on parenteral administration. Intramuscular administration of meperidine does not affect heart rate significantly, but intravenous administration frequently produces a marked increase in heart rate.

Smooth Muscle. Meperidine has effects on certain smooth muscles qualitatively similar to those observed with other opioids. Meperidine does not cause as much constipation as does morphine even when given over prolonged periods of time; this may be related to its greater ability to enter the CNS, thereby producing analgesia at lower systemic concentrations. As with other opioids, clinical doses of meperidine slow gastric emptying sufficiently to delay absorption of other drugs significantly.

The uterus of a nonpregnant woman usually is mildly stimulated by meperidine. Administered before an oxytocic, meperidine does not exert any antagonistic effect. Therapeutic doses given during active labor do not delay the birth process; in fact, the frequency, duration, and amplitude of uterine contraction sometimes may be increased (Zimmer *et al.*, 1988). The drug does not interfere with normal postpartum contraction or involution of the uterus, and it does not increase the incidence of postpartum hemorrhage.

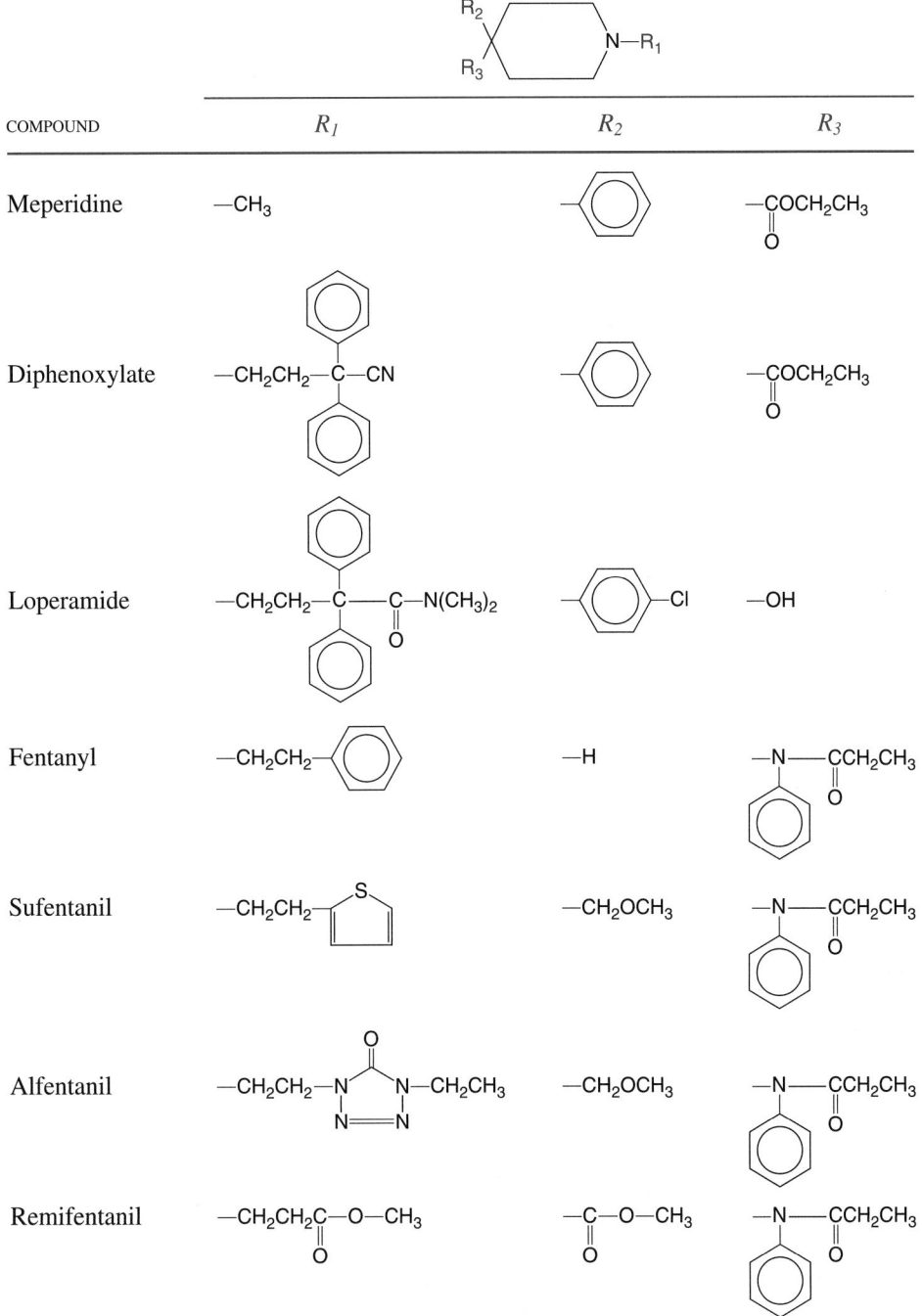

Figure 21–4. *Chemical structures of piperidine and phenylpiperidine analgesics.*

Absorption, Fate, and Excretion. Meperidine is absorbed by all routes of administration, but the rate of absorption may be erratic after intramuscular injection. The peak plasma concentration usually occurs at about 45 minutes, but the range is wide. After oral administration, only about 50% of the drug escapes first-pass metabolism to enter the circulation, and peak concentrations in plasma usually are observed in 1 to 2 hours.

In humans, meperidine is hydrolyzed to meperidinic acid, which, in turn, is partially conjugated. Meperidine also is *N*-demethylated to normeperidine, which then may be hydrolyzed to normeperidinic acid and subsequently conjugated. The clinical significance of the formation of normeperidine is discussed further below. Meperidine is metabolized chiefly in the liver, with a half-life of about 3 hours. In patients with cirrhosis, the bioavailability of meperidine is increased to as much as 80%, and the half-lives of both meperidine and normeperidine are prolonged. Approximately 60% of meperidine in plasma is protein-bound. Only a small amount of meperidine is excreted unchanged.

Untoward Effects, Precautions, and Contraindications.

The pattern and overall incidence of untoward effects that follow the use of meperidine are similar to those observed after equianalgesic doses of morphine, except that constipation and urinary retention may be less common. Patients who experience nausea and vomiting with morphine may not do so with meperidine; the converse also may be true. As with other opioids, tolerance develops to some of these effects. The contraindications generally are the same as for other opioids. In patients or addicts who are tolerant to the depressant effects of meperidine, large doses repeated at short intervals may produce an excitatory syndrome including hallucinations, tremors, muscle twitches, dilated pupils, hyperactive reflexes, and convulsions. These excitatory symptoms are due to the accumulation of normeperidine, which has a half-life of 15 to 20 hours compared with 3 hours for meperidine. Opioid antagonists can block the convulsant effect of normeperidine in the mouse. Since normeperidine is eliminated by the kidney and the liver, decreased renal or hepatic function increases the likelihood of such toxicity (Kaiko *et al.*, 1983).

Interactions with Other Drugs. Severe reactions may follow the administration of meperidine to patients being treated with MAO inhibitors. Two basic types of interactions can be observed. The most prominent is an excitatory reaction ("serotonin syndrome") with delirium, hyperthermia, headache, hyper- or hypotension, rigidity, convulsions, coma, and death. This reaction may be due to the ability of meperidine to block neuronal reuptake of serotonin and the resulting serotonergic overactivity (Stack *et al.*, 1988). Therefore, meperidine and its congeners should not be used in patients taking MAO inhibitors. Dextromethorphan also inhibits neuronal serotonin uptake and should be avoided in these patients. As discussed earlier, tramadol inhibits uptake of norepinephrine and serotonin and should not be used concomitantly with MAO inhibitors. Similar interactions with other opioids have not been observed clinically. Another type of interaction, a potentiation of opioid effect owing to inhibition of hepatic CYPs, also can be observed in patients taking MAO inhibitors, necessitating a reduction in the doses of opioids.

Chlorpromazine increases the respiratory-depressant effects of meperidine, as do tricyclic antidepressants; this is not true of *diazepam.* Concurrent administration of drugs such as *promethazine* or chlorpromazine also may greatly enhance meperidine-induced sedation without slowing clearance of the drug. Treatment with *phe-*

nobarbital or *phenytoin* increases systemic clearance and decreases oral bioavailability of meperidine; this is associated with an elevation of the concentration of normeperidine in plasma (Edwards *et al.*, 1982). As with morphine, concomitant administration of amphetamine has been reported to enhance the analgesic effects of meperidine and its congeners while counteracting sedation.

Therapeutic Uses. The major use of meperidine is for analgesia. Unlike morphine and its congeners, meperidine is not used for the treatment of cough or diarrhea. Single doses of meperidine also appear to be effective in the treatment of postanesthetic shivering. Meperidine, 25 to 50 mg, is used frequently with antihistamines, corticosteroids, *acetaminophen,* or nonsteroidal antiinflammatory drugs (NSAIDs) to prevent or ameliorate infusion-related rigors and shaking chills that accompany the intravenous administration of *amphotericin B, aldesleukin* (interleukin-2), *trastuzumab,* and *alemtuzumab.*

Meperidine crosses the placental barrier and even in reasonable analgesic doses causes a significant increase in the percentage of babies who show delayed respiration, decreased respiratory minute volume, or decreased oxygen saturation or who require resuscitation. Fetal and maternal respiratory depression induced by meperidine can be treated with naloxone. The fraction of drug that is bound to protein is lower in the fetus; concentrations of free drug thus may be considerably higher than in the mother. Nevertheless, meperidine produces less respiratory depression in the newborn than does an equianalgesic dose of morphine or methadone (Fishburne, 1982).

Congeners of Meperidine. *Diphenoxylate.* *Diphenoxylate* is a meperidine congener that has a definite constipating effect in humans. Its only approved use is in the treatment of diarrhea (*see* Chapter 37). Although single doses in the therapeutic range (*see* below) produce little or no morphine-like subjective effects, at high doses (40 to 60 mg) the drug shows typical opioid activity, including euphoria, suppression of morphine abstinence, and a morphine-like physical dependence after chronic administration. Diphenoxylate is unusual in that even its salts are virtually insoluble in aqueous solution, thus obviating the possibility of abuse by the parenteral route. *Diphenoxylate hydrochloride* is available only in combination with atropine sulfate (LOMOTIL, others). The recommended daily dosage of diphenoxylate for the treatment of diarrhea in adults is 20 mg in divided doses. *Difenoxin* (MOTOFEN), a metabolite of diphenoxylate, has actions similar to those of the parent compound.

Loperamide. Loperamide (IMODIUM, others), like diphenoxylate, is a piperidine derivative (Figure 21–3). It slows gastrointestinal motility by effects on the circular and longitudinal muscles of the intestine presumably as a result of its interactions with opioid receptors in the intestine. Some part of its antidiarrheal effect may be due to a reduction of gastrointestinal secretion (*see* above) (Kromer, 1988). In controlling chronic diarrhea, loperamide is as effective as diphenoxylate. In clinical studies, the most common side effect is abdominal cramps. Little tolerance develops to its constipating effect.

In human volunteers taking large doses of loperamide, concentrations of drug in plasma peak about 4 hours after ingestion; this long latency may be due to inhibition of gastrointestinal motility and to enterohepatic circulation of the drug. The apparent elimination half-life is 7 to 14 hours. Loperamide is poorly absorbed after oral administration and, in addition, apparently does not penetrate well into the brain because of P-glycoprotein transporter widely expressed in the brain endothelium (Sadeque *et al.*, 2000). Mice with deletions of one of the genes encoding the P-glycoprotein transporter have much higher brain levels and significant central effects after administration of loperamide (Schinkel *et al.*, 1996). Inhibition of P-glycoprotein by many clinically used drugs, such as *quinidine* and *verapamil,* possibly could lead to enhanced central effects of loperamide.

In general, loperamide is unlikely to be abused parenterally because of its low solubility; large doses of loperamide given to human volunteers do not elicit pleasurable effects typical of opioids. The usual dosage is 4 to 8 mg/day; the daily dose should not exceed 16 mg.

Fentanyl and Congeners

Fentanyl is a synthetic opioid related to the phenylpiperidines (Figure 21–3). The actions of fentanyl and its congeners, sufentanil, remifentanil, and alfentanil, are similar to those of other *μ*-receptor agonists. Alfentanil is seldom used now, and information concerning this drug can be found in the 10th edition of this text. Fentanyl is a popular drug in anesthetic practice because of its relatively shorter time to peak analgesic effect, rapid termination of effect after small bolus doses, and relative cardiovascular stability (*see* Chapter 13).

Pharmacological Properties. *Analgesia.* The analgesic effects of fentanyl and sufentanil are similar to those of morphine and other *μ* opioids. Fentanyl is approximately 100 times more potent than morphine, and sufentanil is approximately 1000 times more potent than morphine. These drugs are most commonly administered intravenously, although both also are commonly administered epidurally and intrathecally for acute postoperative and chronic pain management. Fentanyl and sufentanil are far more lipid soluble than morphine; thus the risk of delayed respiratory depression from rostral spread of intraspinally administered narcotic to respiratory centers is greatly reduced. The time to peak analgesic effect after intravenous administration of fentanyl and sufentanil is less than that for morphine and meperidine, with peak analgesia being reached after about 5 minutes, as opposed to approximately 15 minutes. Recovery from analgesic effects also occurs more quickly. However, with larger doses or prolonged infusions, the effects of these drugs become more lasting, with durations of action becoming similar to those of longer-acting opioids (*see* below).

Other CNS Effects. As with other *μ* opioids, nausea, vomiting, and itching can be observed with fentanyl. Muscle rigidity, while possible after all narcotics, appears to be more common after administration of bolus doses of fentanyl or its congeners. This effect is felt to be centrally mediated and may be due in part to their increased potency relative to morphine. Rigidity can be mitigated by avoiding bolus dosing, slower administration of boluses, and pretreatment with a nonopioid anesthetic induction agent. Rigidity can be treated with depolarizing or nondepolarizing neuromuscular blocking agents while controlling the patient's ventilation. Care must be taken to make sure that the patient is not simply immobilized but aware. Respiratory depression is similar to that observed with other *μ* receptor agonists, but the onset is more rapid. As with analgesia, respiratory depression after small doses is of shorter duration than with morphine but of similar duration after large doses or long infusions. As with morphine and meperidine, delayed respiratory depression also can be seen after the use of fentanyl or sufentanil, possibly owing to enterohepatic circulation. High doses of fentanyl can cause neuroexcitation and, rarely, seizure-like activity in humans (Bailey and Stanley, 1994). Fentanyl has minimal effects on intracranial pressure when ventilation is controlled and the arterial CO_2 concentration is not allowed to rise.

Cardiovascular System. Fentanyl and its derivatives decrease the heart rate and can mildly decrease blood pressure. However, these drugs do not release histamine and, in general, provide a marked degree of cardiovascular stability. Direct depressant effects on the myocardium are minimal. For this reason, high doses of fentanyl or sufentanil are commonly used as the primary anesthetic for patients undergoing cardiovascular surgery or for patients with poor cardiac function.

Absorption, Fate, and Excretion. These agents are highly lipid soluble and rapidly cross the blood–brain barrier. This is reflected in the half-life for equilibration between the plasma and cerebrospinal fluid of approximately 5 minutes for fentanyl and sufentanil. The levels in plasma and cerebrospinal fluid decline rapidly owing to redistribution of fentanyl from highly perfused tissue groups to other tissues, such as muscle and fat. As saturation of less well-perfused tissue occurs, the duration of effect of fentanyl and sufentanil approaches the length of their elimination half-lives of between 3 and 4 hours. Fentanyl and sufentanil undergo hepatic metabolism and renal excretion. Therefore, with the use of higher doses or prolonged infusions, fentanyl and sufentanil become longer acting.

Therapeutic Uses. *Fentanyl citrate* (SUBLIMAZE) and *sufentanil citrate* (SUFENTA) have gained widespread popularity as anesthetic adjuvants (*see* Chapter 13). They are used commonly either intravenously, epidurally, or intrathecally. Epidural use of fentanyl and sufentanil for postoperative or labor analgesia has gained increasing popularity. A combination of epidural opioids with local anesthetics permits reduction in the dosage of both components, minimizing the side effects of the local anesthetic (*i.e.,* motor blockade) and the opioid (*i.e.,* urinary retention, itching, and delayed respiratory depression in the case of morphine). Intravenous use of fentanyl and sufentanil for postoperative pain has been effective but limited by clinical concerns about muscle rigidity. However, the use of fentanyl and sufentanil in chronic pain treatment has become more widespread. Epidural and intrathecal infusions, both with and without local anesthetic, are used in the management of chronic malignant pain and selected cases of nonmalignant pain. Also, the development of novel, less invasive routes of administration for fentanyl has facilitated the use of these compounds in chronic pain management. Transdermal patches (DURAGESIC) that provide sustained release of fentanyl for 48 hours or more are available. However, factors promoting increased absorption (*e.g.,* fever) can lead to relative overdosage and increased side effects (*see* the section on alternative routes of administration, below). Also, the FENTANYL ORALET, a formulation that permits rapid absorption of fentanyl through the buccal mucosa (much like a lollipop), was tried as an anesthetic premedicant but did not gain wide acceptance owing to undesirable side effects in opioid-naive patients (nausea, vomiting, pruritus, and respiratory depression). This dosage form has been discontinued in the United States. A similar fentanyl product, ACTIQ, is available in higher strengths and is used for relief of breakthrough cancer pain (Ashburn *et al.*, 1989).

Remifentanil. This compound was developed in an effort to create an analgesic with a more rapid onset and predictable termination of effect. The potency of remifentanil is approximately equal to that of fentanyl. The pharmacological properties of remifentanil are similar to those of fentanyl and sufentanil. They have similar incidences of nausea, vomiting, and dose-dependent muscle rigidity. Nausea, vomiting, itching, and headaches have been reported when remifentanil has been used for conscious analgesia for painful procedures. Intracranial pressure changes are minimal when ventilation is controlled. Seizures after remifentanil administration have been reported.

Absorption, Fate, and Excretion. Remifentanil has a more rapid onset of analgesic action than fentanyl or sufentanil. Analgesic effects occur within 1 to 1.5 minutes. Remifentanil is unique in that it is metabolized by plasma esterases (Burkle *et al.*, 1996). Elimination is independent of hepatic metabolism or renal excretion, and the elimination half-life is 8 to 20 minutes. There is no prolongation of effect with repeated dosing or prolonged infusion. Age and weight can affect clearance of remifentanil, requiring that dosage be reduced in the elderly and based on lean body mass. However, neither of these conditions causes major changes in duration of effect. After 3- to 5-hour infusions of remifentanil, recovery of respiratory function can be seen within 3 to 5 minutes, whereas full recovery from all effects of remifentanil is observed within 15 minutes (Glass *et al.*, 1999). The primary metabolite, remifentanil acid, is 2000 to 4000 times less potent than remifentanil and is excreted renally. Peak respiratory depression after bolus doses of remifentanil occurs after 5 minutes (Patel and Spencer, 1996).

Therapeutic Uses. Remifentanil hydrochloride (ULTIVA) is useful for short, painful procedures that require intense analgesia and blunting of stress responses. The titratability of remifentanil and its consistent, rapid offset make it ideally suited for short surgical procedures where rapid recovery is desirable. Remifentanil also has been used successfully for longer neurosurgical procedures, where rapid emergence from anesthesia is important. However, in cases where postprocedural analgesia is required, remifentanil alone is a poor choice. In this situation, either a longer-acting opioid or another analgesic modality should be combined with remifentanil for prolonged analgesia, or another opioid should be used. Remifentanil is not used intraspinally because glycine in the drug vehicle can cause temporary motor paralysis. It generally is given by continuous intravenous infusion because its short duration of action makes bolus administration impractical.

Methadone and Congeners

Methadone is a long-acting μ-receptor agonist with pharmacological properties qualitatively similar to those of morphine.

Chemistry. Methadone has the following structural formula:

$$CH_3CH_2-\underset{\underset{O}{\|}}{C}-\overset{}{\underset{}{C}}-CH_2-\underset{\underset{CH_3}{}}{CH}-\underset{\underset{CH_3}{}}{N}\overset{CH_3}{}$$

METHADONE

The analgesic activity of the racemate is almost entirely the result of its content of L-methadone, which is 8 to 50 times more potent than the D isomer; D-methadone also lacks significant respiratory depressant action and addiction liability, but it does possess antitussive activity.

Pharmacological Actions. The outstanding properties of methadone are its analgesic activity, its efficacy by the oral route, its extended duration of action in suppressing withdrawal symptoms in physically dependent individuals, and its tendency to show persistent effects with repeated administration. Miotic and respiratory-depressant effects can be detected for more than 24 hours after a single dose, and on repeated administration, marked sedation is seen in some patients. Effects on cough, bowel motility, biliary tone, and the secretion of pituitary hormones are qualitatively similar to those of morphine.

Absorption, Fate, and Excretion. Methadone is absorbed well from the gastrointestinal tract and can be detected in plasma within 30 minutes of oral ingestion; it reaches peak concentrations at about 4 hours. After therapeutic doses, about 90% of methadone is bound to plasma proteins. Peak concentrations occur in the brain within 1 or 2 hours of subcutaneous or intramuscular administration, and this correlates well with the intensity and duration of analgesia. Methadone also can be absorbed from the buccal mucosa (Weinberg *et al.*, 1988).

Methadone undergoes extensive biotransformation in the liver. The major metabolites, the results of *N*-demethylation and cyclization to form pyrrolidines and pyrroline, are excreted in the urine and the bile along with small amounts of unchanged drug. The amount of methadone excreted in the urine is increased when the urine is acidified. The half-life of methadone is approximately 15 to 40 hours.

Methadone appears to be firmly bound to protein in various tissues, including brain. After repeated administration, there is gradual accumulation in tissues. When administration is discontinued, low concentrations are maintained in plasma by slow release from extravascular binding sites; this process probably accounts for the relatively mild but protracted withdrawal syndrome.

Side Effects, Toxicity, Drug Interactions, and Precautions. Side effects, toxicity, and conditions that alter sensitivity, as well as the treatment of acute intoxication, are similar to those described for morphine. During long-term administration, there may be excessive sweating, lymphocytosis, and increased concentrations of prolactin, albumin, and globulins in the plasma. *Rifampin* and phenytoin accelerate the metabolism of methadone and can precipitate withdrawal symptoms.

Tolerance and Physical Dependence. Volunteer postaddicts who receive subcutaneous or oral methadone daily develop partial tolerance to the nauseant, anorectic, miotic, sedative, respiratory-depressant, and cardiovascular effects of methadone. Tolerance develops more slowly to methadone than to morphine in some patients, especially with respect to the depressant effects; this may be related in part to cumulative effects of the drug or its metabolites. Tolerance to the constipating effect of methadone does not develop as fully as does tolerance to other effects. The behavior of addicts who use methadone parenterally is strikingly similar to that of morphine addicts, but many former heroin users treated with oral methadone show virtually no overt behavioral effects.

Development of physical dependence during the long-term administration of methadone can be demonstrated by drug withdrawal or by administration of an opioid antagonist. Subcutaneous administration of 10 to 20 mg methadone to former opioid addicts produces definite euphoria equal in duration to that caused by morphine, and its overall abuse potential is comparable with that of morphine.

Therapeutic Uses. The primary uses of *methadone hydrochloride* (DOLOPHINE, others) are relief of chronic pain, treatment of opioid abstinence syndromes, and treatment of heroin users. It is not used widely as an antiperistaltic agent. It should not be used in labor.

Analgesia. The onset of analgesia occurs 10 to 20 minutes after parenteral administration and 30 to 60 minutes after oral medication. The average minimal effective analgesic concentration in blood is about 30 ng/ml (Gourlay *et al.*, 1986). The typical oral dose is 2.5 to 15 mg depending on the severity of the pain and the response of the patient. The initial parenteral dose is usually 2.5 to 10 mg. Care must be taken when escalating the dosage because of the prolonged half-life of the drug and its tendency to accumulate over a period of several days with repeated dosing. Despite its longer plasma half-life, the duration of the analgesic action of single doses is essentially the same as that of morphine. With repeated use, cumulative effects are seen, so either lower dosages or longer intervals between doses become possible. In contrast to morphine, methadone and many of its congeners retain a considerable degree of their effectiveness when given orally. In terms of total analgesic effects, methadone given orally is about 50% as effective as the same dose administered intramuscularly; however, the oral–parenteral potency ratio is considerably lower when peak analgesic effect is considered. In equianalgesic doses, the pattern and incidence of untoward effects caused by methadone and morphine are similar.

Propoxyphene

Propoxyphene is structurally related to methadone (*see* below). Its analgesic effect resides in the D-isomer, D-propoxyphene (*dextropropoxyphene*). However, *levopropoxyphene* seems to have some antitussive activity. The structure of propoxyphene is as follows:

PROPOXYPHENE

Pharmacological Actions. Although slightly less selective than morphine, propoxyphene binds primarily to μ opioid receptors and produces analgesia and other CNS effects that are similar to those seen with morphine-like opioids. It is likely that at equianalgesic doses the incidence of side effects such as nausea, anorexia, constipation, abdominal pain, and drowsiness are similar to those of codeine.

As an analgesic, propoxyphene is about one-half to two-thirds as potent as codeine given orally. A dose of 90 to 120 mg of *propoxyphene hydrochloride* administered orally would equal the analgesic effects of 60 mg codeine, a dose that usually produces about as much analgesia as 600 mg *aspirin.* Combinations of propoxyphene and aspirin, like combinations of codeine and aspirin, afford a higher level of analgesia than does either agent given alone (Beaver, 1988).

Absorption, Fate, and Excretion. After oral administration, concentrations of propoxyphene in plasma reach their highest values at 1 to 2 hours. There is great variability between subjects in the rate of clearance and the plasma concentrations that are achieved. The average half-life of propoxyphene in plasma after a single dose is 6 to 12 hours, which is longer than that of codeine. In humans, the major route of metabolism is *N*-demethylation to yield *norpropoxyphene*. The half-life of norpropoxyphene is about 30 hours, and its accumulation with repeated doses may be responsible for some of the observed toxicity (Chan and Matzke, 1987).

Toxicity. Given orally, propoxyphene is approximately one-third as potent as orally administered codeine in depressing respiration. Moderately toxic doses usually produce CNS and respiratory depression, but with still larger doses the clinical picture may be complicated by convulsions in addition to respiratory depression. Delusions, hallucinations, confusion, cardiotoxicity, and pulmonary edema also have been noted. Respiratory-depressant effects are significantly enhanced when ethanol or sedative-hypnotics are ingested concurrently. Naloxone antagonizes the respiratory-depressant, convulsant, and some of the cardiotoxic effects of propoxyphene.

Tolerance and Dependence. Very large doses [800 mg propoxyphene hydrochloride (DARVON, others) or 1200 mg of the *napsylate* (DARVON-N) per day] reduce the intensity of the morphine withdrawal syndrome somewhat less effectively than do 1500-mg doses of codeine. Maximal tolerated doses are equivalent to daily doses of 20 to 25 mg morphine given subcutaneously. The use of higher doses of propoxyphene is prevented by untoward side effects and the occurrence of toxic psychoses. Very large doses produce some respiratory depression in morphine-tolerant addicts, suggesting that cross-tolerance between propoxyphene and morphine is incomplete. Abrupt discontinuation of chronically administered propoxyphene hydrochloride (up to 800 mg/day given for almost 2 months) results in mild abstinence phenomena, and large oral doses (300 to 600 mg) produce subjective effects that are considered pleasurable by postaddicts. The drug is quite irritating when administered either intravenously or subcutaneously, so abuse by these routes results in severe damage to veins and soft tissues.

Therapeutic Uses. Propoxyphene is recommended for the treatment of mild-to-moderate pain. Given acutely, the commonly prescribed combination of 32 mg propoxyphene with aspirin may not produce more analgesia than aspirin alone, and doses of 65 mg of the hydrochloride or 100 mg of the napsylate are suggested. Propoxyphene is given most often in combination with aspirin or *acetaminophen*.

The wide popularity of propoxyphene is largely a result of unrealistic overconcern about the addictive potential of codeine.

ACUTE OPIOID TOXICITY

Acute opioid toxicity may result from clinical overdosage, accidental overdosage in addicts, or attempts at suicide. Occasionally, a delayed type of toxicity may occur from the injection of an opioid into chilled skin areas or in patients with low blood pressure and shock. The drug is not fully absorbed, and therefore, a subsequent dose may be given. When normal circulation is restored, an excessive amount may be absorbed suddenly. It is difficult to define the exact amount of any opioid that is toxic or lethal to humans. Recent experiences with methadone indicate that in nontolerant individuals, serious toxicity may follow the oral ingestion of 40 to 60 mg. Older literature suggests that in the case of morphine, a normal, pain-free adult is not likely to die after oral doses of less than 120 mg or to have serious toxicity with less than 30 mg parenterally.

Symptoms and Diagnosis. The patient who has taken an overdose of an opioid usually is stuporous or, if a large overdose has been taken, may be in a profound coma. The respiratory rate will be very low, or the patient may be apneic, and cyanosis may be present. As respiratory exchange decreases, blood pressure, at first likely to be near normal, will fall progressively. If adequate oxygenation is restored early, the blood pressure will improve; if hypoxia persists untreated, there may be capillary damage, and measures to combat shock may be required. The pupils will be symmetrical and pinpoint in size; however, if hypoxia is severe, they may be dilated. Urine formation is depressed. Body temperature falls, and the skin becomes cold and clammy. The skeletal muscles are flaccid, the jaw is relaxed, and the tongue may fall back and block the airway. Frank convulsions occasionally may be noted in infants and children. When death occurs, it is nearly always from respiratory failure. Even if respiration is restored, death still may occur as a result of complications that develop during the period of coma, such as pneumonia or shock. Noncardiogenic pulmonary edema is seen commonly with opioid poisoning. It probably is not due to contaminants or to anaphylactoid reactions, and it has been observed after toxic doses of morphine, methadone, propoxyphene, and uncontaminated heroin.

The triad of coma, pinpoint pupils, and depressed respiration strongly suggests opioid poisoning. The finding of needle marks suggestive of addiction further supports the diagnosis. Mixed poisonings, however, are not uncommon. Examination of the urine and gastric contents for drugs may aid in diagnosis, but the results usually become available too late to influence treatment.

Treatment. The first step is to establish a patent airway and ventilate the patient. Opioid antagonists (*see* below)

can produce dramatic reversal of the severe respiratory depression, and the antagonist naloxone (*see* below) is the treatment of choice. However, care should be taken to avoid precipitating withdrawal in dependent patients, who may be extremely sensitive to antagonists. The safest approach is to dilute the standard naloxone dose (0.4 mg) and slowly administer it intravenously, monitoring arousal and respiratory function. With care, it usually is possible to reverse the respiratory depression without precipitating a major withdrawal syndrome. If no response is seen with the first dose, additional doses can be given. Patients should be observed for rebound increases in sympathetic nervous system activity, which may result in cardiac arrhythmias and pulmonary edema. For reversing opioid poisoning in children, the initial dose of naloxone is 0.01 mg/kg. If no effect is seen after a total dose of 10 mg, one can reasonably question the accuracy of the diagnosis. Pulmonary edema sometimes associated with opioid overdosage may be countered by positive-pressure respiration. Tonic-clonic seizures, occasionally seen as part of the toxic syndrome with meperidine and propoxyphene, are ameliorated by treatment with naloxone.

The presence of general CNS depressants does not prevent the salutary effect of naloxone, and in cases of mixed intoxications, the situation will be improved largely owing to antagonism of the respiratory-depressant effects of the opioid. However, some evidence indicates that naloxone and naltrexone also may antagonize some of the depressant actions of sedative-hypnotics (*see* below). One need not attempt to restore the patient to full consciousness. The duration of action of the available antagonists is shorter than that of many opioids; hence patients can slip back into coma. This is particularly important when the overdosage is due to methadone. The depressant effects of these drugs may persist for 24 to 72 hours, and fatalities have occurred as a result of premature discontinuation of naloxone. In cases of overdoses of these drugs, a continuous infusion of naloxone should be considered. Toxicity owing to overdose of pentazocine and other opioids with mixed actions may require higher doses of naloxone. The pharmacological actions of opioid antagonists are discussed in more detail below.

OPIOID AGONIST/ANTAGONISTS AND PARTIAL AGONISTS

The drugs described in this section differ from clinically used μ-opioid receptor agonists. Drugs such as *nalbuphine* and *butorphanol* are competitive μ-receptor antagonists but exert their analgesic actions by acting as agonists at κ receptors. Pentazocine qualitatively resembles these drugs, but it may be a weaker μ-receptor antagonist or partial agonist while retaining its κ-agonist activity. Buprenorphine, on the other hand, is a partial agonist at μ receptors.

The stimulus for the development of mixed agonist–antagonist drugs was a need for analgesics with less respiratory depression and addictive potential. The clinical use of these compounds is limited by undesirable side effects and limited analgesic effects.

Pentazocine

Pentazocine was synthesized as part of a deliberate effort to develop an effective analgesic with little or no abuse potential. It has agonistic actions and weak opioid antagonistic activity.

Pharmacological Actions. The pattern of CNS effects produced by pentazocine generally is similar to that of the morphine-like opioids, including analgesia, sedation, and respiratory depression. The analgesic effects of pentazocine are due to agonistic actions at κ opioid receptors. Higher doses of pentazocine (60 to 90 mg) elicit dysphoric and psychotomimetic effects. The mechanisms responsible for these side effects are not known but might involve activation of supraspinal κ receptors because it has been suggested that these untoward effects may be reversible by naloxone.

The cardiovascular responses to pentazocine differ from those seen with typical μ receptor agonists, in that high doses cause an increase in blood pressure and heart rate. Pentazocine acts as a weak antagonist or partial agonist at μ opioid receptors. Pentazocine does not antagonize the respiratory depression produced by morphine. However, when given to patients dependent on morphine or other μ-receptor agonists, pentazocine may precipitate withdrawal. Ceiling effects for analgesia and respiratory depression are observed above 50 to 100 mg pentazocine (Bailey and Stanley, 1994).

Tablets for oral use now contain *pentazocine hydrochloride* (equivalent to 50 mg of the base) and *naloxone hydrochloride* (equivalent to 0.5 mg of the base; TALWIN NX), which reduces the potential use of tablets as a source of injectable pentazocine. After oral ingestion, naloxone is destroyed rapidly by the liver; however, if the material is dissolved and injected, the naloxone produces aversive effects in subjects dependent on opioids. An oral dose of about 50 mg pentazocine results in analgesia equivalent to that produced by 60 mg codeine orally.

Nalbuphine

Nalbuphine is related structurally to naloxone and oxymorphone (Table 21–5). It is an agonist–antagonist opioid with a spectrum of effects that qualitatively resembles that of pentazocine; however, nalbuphine is a more potent antagonist at μ receptors and is less likely to produce dysphoric side effects than is pentazocine.

Pharmacological Actions and Side Effects. An intramuscular dose of 10 mg nalbuphine is equianalgesic to 10 mg morphine, with similar onset and duration of analgesic and subjective effects. Nalbuphine depresses respiration as much as do equianalgesic doses of morphine. However, nalbuphine exhibits a ceiling effect such that increases in dosage beyond 30 mg produce no further respiratory depression. However, a ceiling effect for analgesia also is reached at this point. In contrast to pentazocine and butorphanol, 10 mg nalbuphine given to patients with stable coronary artery disease does not produce an increase in cardiac index, pulmonary arterial pressure, or cardiac work, and systemic blood pressure is not significantly altered; these indices also are relatively stable when nalbuphine is given to patients with acute myocardial infarction (Roth *et al.*, 1988). Its gastrointestinal effects probably are similar to those of pentazocine. Nalbuphine produces few side effects at doses of 10 mg or less; sedation, sweating, and headache are the most common. At much higher doses (70 mg), psychotomimetic side effects (*e.g.*, dysphoria, racing thoughts, and distortions of body image) can occur. Nalbuphine is metabolized in the liver and has a half-life in plasma of 2 to 3 hours. Given orally, nalbuphine is 20% to 25% as potent as when given intramuscularly.

Tolerance and Physical Dependence. In subjects dependent on low doses of morphine (60 mg/day), nalbuphine precipitates an abstinence syndrome. Prolonged administration of nalbuphine can produce physical dependence. The withdrawal syndrome is similar in intensity to that seen with pentazocine. The potential for abuse of parenteral nalbuphine in subjects not dependent on μ receptor agonists probably is similar to that for parenteral pentazocine.

Therapeutic Uses. *Nalbuphine hydrochloride* (NUBAIN) is used to produce analgesia. Because it is an agonist–antagonist, administration to patients who have been receiving morphine-like opioids may create difficulties unless a brief drug-free interval is interposed. The usual adult dose is 10 mg parenterally every 3 to 6 hours; this may be increased to 20 mg in nontolerant individuals.

Butorphanol

Butorphanol is a morphinan congener with a profile of actions similar to those of pentazocine. The structural formula of butorphanol is shown in Table 21–5.

Pharmacological Actions and Side Effects. In postoperative patients, a parenteral dose of 2 to 3 mg butorphanol produces analgesia and respiratory depression approximately equal to that produced by 10 mg morphine or 80 to 100 mg meperidine; the onset, peak, and duration of action are similar to those that follow the administration of morphine. The plasma half-life of butorphanol is about 3 hours. Like pentazocine, analgesic doses of butorphanol produce an increase in pulmonary arterial pressure and in the work of the heart; systemic arterial pressure is slightly decreased (Popio *et al.*, 1978).

The major side effects of butorphanol are drowsiness, weakness, sweating, feelings of floating, and nausea. While the incidence of psychotomimetic side effects is lower than that with equianalgesic doses of pentazocine, they are qualitatively similar. Physical dependence on butorphanol can occur.

Therapeutic Uses. *Butorphanol tartrate* (STADOL) is better suited for the relief of acute pain than of chronic pain. Because of its side effects on the heart, it is less useful than morphine or meperidine in patients with congestive heart failure or myocardial infarction. The usual dose is between 1 and 4 mg of the tartrate given intramuscularly or 0.5 to 2 mg given intravenously every 3 to 4 hours. A nasal formulation (STADOL NS) is available and has proven to be effective. This formulation is particularly useful for patients with severe headaches who may be unresponsive to other forms of treatment.

Buprenorphine

Buprenorphine is a semisynthetic, highly lipophilic opioid derived from thebaine (Table 21–5). It is 25 to 50 times more potent than morphine.

Pharmacological Actions and Side Effects. Buprenorphine produces analgesia and other CNS effects that are qualitatively similar to those of morphine. About 0.4 mg buprenorphine is equianalgesic with 10 mg morphine given intramuscularly (Wallenstein *et al.*, 1986). Although variable, the duration of analgesia usually is longer than that of morphine. Some of the subjective and respiratory-depressant effects are unequivocally slower in onset and last longer than those of morphine. For example, peak miosis occurs about 6 hours after intramuscular injection, whereas maximal respiratory depression is observed at about 3 hours.

Buprenorphine appears to be a partial μ receptor agonist. Depending on the dose, buprenorphine may cause symptoms of abstinence in patients who have been receiving μ receptor agonists for several weeks. It antagonizes the respiratory depression produced by anesthetic doses of fentanyl about as well as does naloxone without completely reversing opioid pain relief (Boysen *et al.*, 1988). Although respiratory depression has not been a major problem, it is not clear whether there is a ceiling for this effect (as seen with nalbuphine and pentazocine). The respiratory depression and other effects of buprenorphine can be prevented by prior administration of naloxone, but they are not readily reversed by high doses of naloxone once the effects have been produced. This suggests that buprenorphine dissociates very slowly from opioid receptors. The half-life for dissociation from the μ receptor is 166 minutes for buprenorphine, as opposed to 7 minutes for fentanyl (Boas and Villiger, 1985). Therefore, plasma levels of buprenorphine may not parallel clinical effects. Cardiovascular and other side effects (*e.g.*, sedation, nausea, vomiting, dizziness, sweating, and headache) appear to be similar to those of morphine-like opioids.

Buprenorphine is relatively well absorbed by most routes. Administered sublingually, the drug (0.4 to 0.8 mg) produces satisfactory analgesia in postoperative patients. Concentrations in blood peak within 5 minutes of intramuscular injection and within 1 to 2 hours of oral or sublingual administration. While the half-life in plasma has been reported to be about 3 hours, this value bears little relationship to the rate of disappearance of effects (*see* above). Both *N*-dealkylated and conjugated metabolites are detected in the urine, but most of the drug is excreted unchanged in the feces. About 96% of the circulating drug is bound to protein.

Physical Dependence. When buprenorphine is discontinued, a withdrawal syndrome develops that is delayed in onset for 2 days to 2 weeks; this consists of typical but generally not very severe morphine-like withdrawal signs and symptoms, and it persists for about 1 to 2 weeks (Bickel *et al.*, 1988; Fudala *et al.*, 1989).

Therapeutic Uses. Buprenorphine (BUPRENEX; SUBUTEX) may be used as an analgesic and also has proven to be useful as a maintenance drug for opioid-dependent subjects (Johnson *et al.*, 2000). The usual intramuscular or intravenous dose for analgesia is 0.3 mg given every 6 hours. Sublingual doses of 0.4 to 0.8 mg also produce effective analgesia. Buprenorphine is metabolized to norbuprenorphine by CYP3A4. Thus care should be taken in treating patients who also are taking known inhibitors of CYP3A4 (*e.g.*, azole antifungals, macrolide antibiotics, and HIV protease inhibitors), as well as drugs that induce CYP3A4 activity (*e.g.*, anticonvulsants and *rifampin*).

Buprenorphine is approved by the Food and Drug Administration (FDA) for the treatment of opioid addiction. Treatment is initiated with buprenorphine alone administered sublingually, followed by maintenance therapy with a combination of buprenorphine and naloxone (SUBOXONE) to minimize abuse potential. The partial agonist properties of buprenorphine limit its usefulness for the treatment of addicts who require high maintenance doses of opioids. However, conversion to maintenance treatment with higher doses of methadone, a full agonist, is possible (Kreek *et al.*, 2002).

OPIOID ANTAGONISTS

Under ordinary circumstances, the drugs discussed in this section produce few effects unless opioids with agonistic actions have been administered previously. However, when the endogenous opioid systems are activated, as in shock or certain forms of stress, the administration of an opioid antagonist alone may have visible consequences. These agents have obvious therapeutic utility in the treatment of opioid overdose. As the understanding of the role of endogenous opioid systems in pathophysiological states increases, additional therapeutic indications for these antagonists may develop.

Chemistry. Relatively minor changes in the structure of an opioid can convert a drug that is primarily an agonist into one with antagonistic actions at one or more types of opioid receptors. The most common such substitution is that of a larger moiety (*e.g.*, an allyl or methylcyclopropyl group) for the *N*-methyl group that is typical of the μ-receptor agonists. Such substitutions transform morphine to *nalorphine, levorphanol* to *levallorphan,* and oxymorphone to naloxone or naltrexone (Table 21–5). In some cases, congeners are produced that are competitive antagonists at μ receptors but that also have agonistic actions at κ receptors. Nalorphine and levallorphan have such properties. Other congeners, especially naloxone and naltrexone, appear to be devoid of agonistic actions and probably interact with all types of opioid receptors, albeit with widely different affinities (Martin, 1983).

Nalmefene (REVIX) is a relatively pure μ-receptor antagonist that is more potent than naloxone (Dixon *et al.*, 1986). A number of other nonpeptide antagonists have been developed that are relatively selective for individual types of opioid receptors. These include *cypridime* and *β-funaltrexamine* (β-FNA) (*μ*), *naltrindole* (*δ*), and *norbinaltorphimine* (*κ*) (Portoghese, 1989).

Pharmacological Properties

If endogenous opioid systems have not been activated, the pharmacological actions of opioid antagonists depend on whether or not an opioid agonist has been administered previously, on the pharmacological profile of that opioid, and on the degree to which physical dependence on an opioid has developed.

Effects in the Absence of Opioid Drugs. Subcutaneous doses of naloxone (NARCAN) up to 12 mg produce no discernible subjective effects in humans, and 24 mg causes only slight drowsiness. Naltrexone (REVIA) also appears

to be a relatively pure antagonist but with higher oral efficacy and a longer duration of action. At doses in excess of 0.3 mg/kg naloxone, normal subjects show increased systolic blood pressure and decreased performance on tests of memory. High doses of naltrexone appeared to cause mild dysphoria in one study but almost no subjective effect in several others (Gonzalez and Brogden, 1988).

Although high doses of antagonists might be expected to alter the actions of endogenous opioid peptides, the detectable effects usually are both subtle and limited (Cannon and Liebeskind, 1987). Most likely this reflects the low levels of tonic activity of the opioid systems. In this regard, analgesic effects can be differentiated from endocrine effects, in which naloxone causes readily demonstrable changes in hormone levels (*see* below). It is interesting that naloxone appears to block the analgesic effects of placebo medications and acupuncture. In laboratory animals, the administration of naloxone will reverse or attenuate the hypotension associated with shock of diverse origins, including that caused by anaphylaxis, endotoxin, hypovolemia, and injury to the spinal cord; opioid agonists aggravate these conditions (Amir, 1988). Naloxone apparently acts to antagonize the actions of endogenous opioids that are mobilized by pain or stress and that are involved in the regulation of blood pressure by the CNS. Although neural damage that follows trauma to the spinal cord or cerebral ischemia also appears to involve endogenous opioids, it is not certain whether opioid antagonists can prevent damage to these or other organs and/or increase rates of survival. Nevertheless, opioid antagonists can reduce the extent of injury in some animal models, perhaps by blocking κ receptors (Faden, 1988).

As noted earlier, endogenous opioid peptides participate in the regulation of pituitary secretion apparently by exerting tonic inhibitory effects on the release of certain hypothalamic hormones (*see* Chapter 55). Thus, the administration of naloxone or naltrexone increases the secretion of gonadotropin-releasing hormone and corticotropin-releasing hormone and elevates the plasma concentrations of LH, FSH, and ACTH, as well as the steroid hormones produced by their target organs. Antagonists do not consistently alter basal or stress-induced concentrations of prolactin in plasma in men; paradoxically, naloxone *stimulates* the release of prolactin in women. Opioid antagonists augment the increases in plasma concentrations of cortisol and catecholamines that normally accompany stress or exercise. The neuroendocrine effects of opioid antagonists have been reviewed. Endogenous opioid peptides probably have some role in the regulation of feeding or energy metabolism because opioid antagonists increase energy expenditure and interrupt hibernation in appropriate species and induce weight loss in genetically obese rats. The antagonists also prevent stress-induced overeating and obesity in rats. These observations have led to the experimental use of opioid antagonists in the treatment of human obesity, especially that associated with stress-induced eating disorders. However, naltrexone does not accelerate weight loss in very obese subjects, even though short-term administration of opioid antagonists reduces food intake in lean and obese individuals (Atkinson, 1987).

Antagonistic Actions. Small doses (0.4 to 0.8 mg) of naloxone given intramuscularly or intravenously prevent or promptly reverse the effects of μ receptor agonists. In patients with respiratory depression, an increase in respiratory rate is seen within 1 or 2 minutes. Sedative effects are reversed, and blood pressure, if depressed, returns to normal. Higher doses of naloxone are required to antagonize the respiratory-depressant effects of buprenorphine; 1 mg naloxone intravenously completely blocks the effects of 25 mg heroin. Naloxone reverses the psychotomimetic and dysphoric effects of agonist–antagonist agents such as pentazocine, but much higher doses (10 to 15 mg) are required. The duration of antagonistic effects depends on the dose but usually is 1 to 4 hours. Antagonism of opioid effects by naloxone often is accompanied by "overshoot" phenomena. For example, respiratory rate depressed by opioids transiently becomes higher than that before the period of depression. Rebound release of catecholamines may cause hypertension, tachycardia, and ventricular arrhythmias. Pulmonary edema also has been reported after naloxone administration.

Effects in Physical Dependence. In subjects who are dependent on morphine-like opioids, small subcutaneous doses of naloxone (0.5 mg) precipitate a moderate-to-severe withdrawal syndrome that is very similar to that seen after abrupt withdrawal of opioids, except that the syndrome appears within minutes of administration and subsides in about 2 hours. The severity and duration of the syndrome are related to the dose of the antagonist and to the degree and type of dependence. Higher doses of naloxone will precipitate a withdrawal syndrome in patients dependent on pentazocine, butorphanol, or nalbuphine. Naloxone produces overshoot phenomena suggestive of early acute physical dependence 6 to 24 hours after a single dose of a μ agonist (Heishman *et al.*, 1989).

Tolerance and Physical Dependence. Even after prolonged administration of high doses, discontinuation of naloxone is not followed by any recognizable withdrawal syndrome, and the withdrawal of naltrexone, another relatively pure antagonist, produces very few signs and symptoms. However, long-term administration of antagonists increases the density of opioid receptors in the brain and causes a temporary exaggeration of responses to the subsequent administration of opioid agonists (Yoburn *et al.*, 1988). Naltrexone and naloxone have little or no potential for abuse.

Absorption, Fate, and Excretion. Although absorbed readily from the gastrointestinal tract, naloxone is almost completely metabolized by the liver before reaching the systemic circulation and thus must be administered parenterally. The drug is absorbed rapidly from parenteral sites of injection and is metabolized in the liver primarily by conjugation with glucuronic acid; other metabolites are produced in small amounts. The half-life of naloxone is about 1 hour, but its clinically effective duration of action can be even less.

Compared with naloxone, naltrexone retains much more of its efficacy by the oral route, and its duration of action approaches 24 hours after moderate oral doses. Peak concentrations in plasma are reached within 1 to 2 hours and then decline with an apparent half-life of approximately 3 hours; this value does not change with long-term use. Naltrexone is metabolized to 6-naltrexol, which is a weaker antagonist but has a longer half-life of about 13 hours. Naltrexone is much more potent than naloxone, and l00-mg oral doses given to patients addicted to opioids produce concentrations in tissues sufficient to block the euphorigenic effects of 25-mg intravenous doses of heroin for 48 hours (Gonzalez and Brogden, 1988).

Therapeutic Uses

Opioid antagonists have established uses in the treatment of opioid-induced toxicity, especially respiratory depression; in the diagnosis of physical dependence on opioids; and as therapeutic agents in the treatment of compulsive users of opioids, as discussed in Chapter 23. Their potential utility in the treatment of shock, stroke, spinal cord and brain trauma, and other disorders that may involve mobilization of endogenous opioid peptides remains to be established. Naltrexone is approved by the FDA for treatment of alcoholism (*see* Chapters 22 and 23).

Treatment of Opioid Overdosage. Naloxone hydrochloride is used to treat opioid overdose. As discussed earlier, it acts rapidly to reverse the respiratory depression associated with high doses of opioids. However, it should be used cautiously because it also can precipitate withdrawal in dependent subjects and cause undesirable cardiovascular side effects. By carefully titrating the dose of naloxone, it usually is possible to antagonize the respiratory-depressant actions without eliciting a full withdrawal syndrome. The duration of action of naloxone is relatively short, and it often must be given repeatedly or by continuous infusion. Opioid antagonists also have been employed effectively to decrease neonatal respiratory depression secondary to the intravenous or intramuscular administration of opioids to the mother. In the neonate, the initial dose is 10 μg/kg given intravenously, intramuscularly, or subcutaneously.

CENTRALLY ACTIVE ANTITUSSIVE AGENTS

Cough is a useful physiological mechanism that serves to clear the respiratory passages of foreign material and excess secretions. It should not be suppressed indiscriminately. There are, however, many situations in which cough does not serve any useful purpose but may, instead, only annoy the patient or prevent rest and sleep. Chronic cough can contribute to fatigue, especially in elderly patients. In such situations, the physician should use a drug that will reduce the frequency or intensity of the coughing. The cough reflex is complex, involving the central and peripheral nervous systems, as well as the smooth muscle of the bronchial tree. It has been suggested that irritation of the bronchial mucosa causes bronchoconstriction, which, in turn, stimulates cough receptors (which probably represent a specialized type of stretch receptor) located in tracheobronchial passages. Afferent conduction from these receptors is *via* fibers in the vagus nerve; central components of the reflex probably include several mechanisms or centers that are distinct from the mechanisms involved in the regulation of respiration.

The drugs that directly or indirectly can affect this complex mechanism are diverse. For example, cough may be the first or only symptom in bronchial asthma or allergy, and in such cases, bronchodilators (*e.g.*, β_2 adrenergic receptor agonists; *see* Chapter 10) have been shown to reduce cough without having any significant central effects; other drugs act primarily on the central or peripheral nervous system components of the cough reflex.

A number of drugs reduce cough as a result of their central actions, although the exact mechanisms still are not entirely clear. Included among them are the opioid analgesics discussed earlier (codeine and hydrocodone are the opioids most commonly used to suppress cough), as well as a number of nonopioid agents. Cough suppression often occurs with lower doses of opioids than those needed for analgesia. A 10- or 20-mg oral dose of codeine, although ineffective for analgesia, produces a demonstrable antitussive effect, and higher doses produce even more suppression of chronic cough.

In selecting a specific centrally active agent for a particular patient, the significant considerations are its antitussive efficacy against pathological cough and the incidence and type of side effects to be expected. In the majority of situations requiring a cough suppressant, liability for abuse need not be a major consideration. Most of the nonopioid agents now offered as antitussives are effective against cough induced by a variety of experimental techniques. However, the ability of these tests to predict clinical efficacy is limited.

Dextromethorphan. Dextromethorphan (D-3-methoxy-N-methylmorphinan) is the D-isomer of the codeine analog methorphan; however, unlike the L-isomer, it has no analgesic or addictive properties and does not act through opioid receptors. The drug acts centrally to elevate the threshold for coughing. Its effectiveness in patients with pathological cough has been demonstrated in controlled studies; its potency is nearly equal to that of codeine. Compared with codeine, dextromethorphan produces fewer subjective and gastrointestinal side effects (Matthys *et al.*, 1983). In therapeutic dosages, the drug does not inhibit ciliary activity, and its antitussive effects persist for 5 to 6 hours. Its toxicity is low, but extremely high doses may produce CNS depression.

Sites that bind dextromethorphan with high affinity have been identified in membranes from various regions of the brain (Craviso and Musacchio, 1983). Although dextromethorphan is known to function as an NMDA-receptor antagonist, the dextromethorphan-binding sites are not limited to the known distribution of NMDA receptors (Elliott *et al.*, 1994). Thus, the mechanism by which dextromethorphan exerts its antitussive effect still is not clear. Two other known antitussives, *carbetapentane* and *caramiphen,* also bind avidly to the dextromethorphan-binding sites, but codeine, levopropoxyphene, and other antitussive opioids (as well as naloxone) are not bound. Although *noscapine* (*see* below) enhances the affinity of dextromethorphan, it appears to interact with distinct binding sites (Karlsson *et al.,* 1988). The relationship of these binding sites to antitussive actions is not known; however, these observations, coupled with the ability of naloxone to antagonize the antitussive effects of codeine but not those of dextromethorphan, indicate that cough suppression can be achieved by a number of different mechanisms. The average adult dosage of *dextromethorphan hydrobromide* is 10 to 30 mg three to six times daily; however, as is the case with codeine, higher doses often are required. The drug generally is marketed for over-the-counter sale in numerous syrups and lozenges or in combinations with antihistamines and other agents.

Other Drugs. *Pholcodine* [3-*O*-(2-morpholinoethyl)morphine] is used clinically in many countries outside the United States. Although structurally related to the opioids, it has no opioid-like actions because the substitution at the 3-position is not removed by metabolism. Pholcodine is at least as effective as codeine as an antitussive; it has a long half-life and can be given once or twice daily.

Benzonatate (TESSALON) is a long-chain polyglycol derivative chemically related to *procaine* and believed to exert its antitussive action on stretch or cough receptors in the lung, as well as by a central mechanism. It has been administered by all routes; the oral dosage is 100 mg three times daily, but higher doses have been used.

THERAPEUTIC USES OF OPIOID ANALGESICS

Sir William Osler called morphine "God's own medicine." Opioids still are the mainstay of pain treatment. However, the development of new analgesic compounds and new routes of administration have increased the therapeutic options available to clinicians while at the same time helping to minimize undesirable side effects. This section provides guidelines for rational drug selection, discusses routes of administration other than the standard oral and parenteral methods, and outlines general principles for the use of opioids in acute and chronic pain states.

Extensive efforts by many individuals and organizations have resulted in the publication of many useful guidelines for the administration of opioids. These have been developed for a number of clinical situations, including treatment of acute pain, trauma, cancer, nonmalignant chronic pain, and pain in children (Agency for Health Care Policy and Research, 1992a, 1992b, 1994; International Association for the Study of Pain, 1992; American Pain Society, 2003; Grossman *et al.*, 1999; World Health Organization, 1998; Berde *et al.*, 1990). These guidelines provide comprehensive discussions of dosing regimens and drug selection and also provide protocols for the management of complex conditions. In the case of cancer pain, adherence to standardized protocols for cancer pain management (Agency for Health Care Policy and Research, 1994) has been shown to improve pain management significantly (Du Pen *et al.*, 1999). Guidelines for the oral and parenteral dosing of commonly used opioids are presented in Table 21–6.

These guidelines are for acute pain management in opioid-naive patients. Adjustments will need to be made for use in opioid-tolerant patients and in chronic pain states. For children younger than 6 months of age, especially those who are ill or premature, expert consultation should be obtained. The pharmacokinetics and potency of opioids can be altered substantially in these patients, and in some cases there is a significant risk of apnea. It also should be noted that there is substantial individual variability in responses to opioids. A standard intramuscular dose of 10 mg morphine sulfate will relieve severe pain adequately in only two of three patients. Adjustments will have to be made based on clinical response.

In general, it is recommended that opioids always be combined with other analgesic agents, such as NSAIDs or acetaminophen. In this way, one can take advantage of additive analgesic effects and minimize the dose of opioids and thus undesirable side effects. In some situations, NSAIDs can provide analgesia equal to that produced by 60 mg codeine. Potentiation of opioid action by NSAIDs may be due to increased conversion of arachidonic acid to 12-lipoxygenase products that facilitate effects of opioids on K^+ channels (Vaughan *et al.*, 1997). This "opioid sparing" strategy is the backbone of the "analgesic ladder" for pain management proposed by

Table 21-6
Dosing Data for Opioid Analgesics

DRUG	APPROXIMATE EQUIANALGESIC ORAL DOSE	APPROXIMATE EQUIANALGESIC PARENTERAL DOSE	RECOMMENDED STARTING DOSE (ADULTS MORE THAN 50 KG BODY WEIGHT)		RECOMMENDED STARTING DOSE (CHILDREN AND ADULTS LESS THAN 50 KG BODY WEIGHT)[1]	
			Oral	Parenteral	Oral	Parenteral
Opioid Agonist						
Morphine[2]	30 mg q3–4h (around-the-clock dosing) 60 mg q3–4h (single dose or intermittent dosing)	10 mg q3–4h	30 mg q3–4h	10 mg q3–4h	0.3 mg/kg q3–4h	0.1 mg/kg q3–4h
Codeine[3]	130 mg q3–4h	75 mg q3–4h	60 mg q3–4h	60 mg q2h (intramuscular/subcutaneous)	1 mg/kg q3–4h[4]	Not recommended
Hydromorphone[2] (DILAUDID)	7.5 mg q3–4h	1.5 mg q3–4h	6 mg q3–4h	1.5 mg q3–4h	0.06 mg/kg q3–4h	0.015 mg/kg q3–4h
Hydrocodone (in LORCET, LORTAB, VICODIN, others)	30 mg q3–4h	Not available	10 mg q3–4h	Not available	0.2 mg/kg q3–4h[4]	Not available
Levorphanol	4 mg q6–8h	2 mg q6–8h	4 mg q6–8h	2 mg q6–8h	0.04 mg/kg q6–8h	0.02 mg/kg q6–8h
Meperidine (DEMEROL)	300 mg q2–3h	100 mg q3h	Not recommended	100 mg q3h	Not recommended	0.75 mg/kg q2–3h
Methadone (DOLOPHINE, others)	20 mg q6–8h	10 mg q6–8h	20 mg q6–8h	10 mg q6–8h	0.2 mg/kg q6–8h	0.1 mg/kg q6–8h
Oxycodone (ROXICODONE, OXYCONTIN, also in PERCOCET, PERCODAN, TYLOX, others)[7]	30 mg q3–4h	Not available	10 mg q3–4h	Not available	0.2 mg/kg q3–4h[4]	Not available
Oxymorphone[2] (NUMORPHAN)	Not available	1 mg q3–4h	Not available	1 mg q3–4h	Not recommended	Not recommended
Propoxyphene (DARVON)	130 mg[5]	Not available	65 mg q4–6h[5]	Not available	Not recommended	Not recommended
Tramadol[6] (ULTRAM)	100 mg[5]	100 mg	50–100 mg q6h[5]	50–100 mg q6h[5]	Not recommended	Not recommended
Opioid Agonist–Antagonist or Partial Agonist						
Buprenorphine (BUPRENEX)	Not available	0.3–0.4 mg q6–8h	Not available	0.4 mg q6–8h	Not available	0.004 mg/kg q6–8h
Butorphanol (STADOL)	Not available	2 mg q3–4h	Not available	2 mg q3–4h	Not available	Not recommended
Nalbuphine (NUBAIN)	Not available	10 mg q3–4h	Not available	10 mg q3–4h	Not available	0.1 mg/kg q3–4h

NOTE: Published tables vary in the suggested doses that are equianalgesic to morphine. Clinical response is the criterion that must be applied for each patient; titration to clinical response is necessary. Because there is not complete cross tolerance among these drugs, it is usually necessary to use a lower than equianalgesic dose when changing drugs and to retitrate to response. *Caution:* Recommended doses do not apply to patients with renal or hepatic insufficiency or other conditions affecting drug metabolism and kinetics. [1]*Caution:* Doses listed for patients with body weight less than 50 kg cannot be used as initial starting doses in babies less than 6 months of age. Consult the *Clinical Practice Guideline for Acute Pain Management: Operative or Medical Procedures and Trauma* section on management of pain in neonates for recommendations. [2]For morphine, hydromorphone, and oxymorphone, rectal administration is an alternate route for patients unable to take oral medications, but equianalgesic doses may differ from oral and parenteral doses because of pharmacokinetic differences. [3]*Caution:* Codeine doses above 65 mg often are not appropriate due to diminishing incremental analgesia with increasing doses but con-tinually increasing constipation and other side effects. [4]*Caution:* Doses of aspirin and acetaminophen in combination opioid/NSAID preparations must also be adjusted to the patient's body weight. Maximum acetaminophen dose: 4 gm/day in adults, 90 mg/kg/day in children. [5]Doses for moderate pain not necessarily equivalent to 30 mg oral or 10 mg parenteral morphine. [6]Risk of seizures: parenteral formulation not available in the U.S. [7]OXYCONTIN is an extended-release preparation containing up to 160 mg of oxycodone per tablet and recommended for use every 12 hours. It has been subject to substantial abuse. ABBREVIATION: q, every. Modified from Agency for Healthcare Policy and Research, 1992a, with permission.

580

the World Health Organization (1990). Weaker opioids can be supplanted by stronger opioids in cases of moderate and severe pain. In addition, analgesics always should be dosed in a continuous or "around the clock" fashion rather than on an as-needed basis for chronic severe pain. This provides more consistent analgesic levels and avoids unnecessary suffering.

Factors guiding the selection of specific opioid compounds for pain treatment include potency, pharmacokinetic characteristics, and the routes of administration available. A more potent compound could be useful when high doses of opioid are required so that the medicine can be given in a smaller volume. Duration of action also is an important consideration. For example, a long-acting opioid such as methadone may be appropriate when less frequent dosing is desired. For short, painful procedures, a quick-acting, fast-dissipating compound such as remifentanil would be a useful choice. In special cases, where a lower addiction risk is required or in patients unable to tolerate other opioids, a partial agonist or mixed agonist–antagonist compound might be a rational choice. The properties of some commonly used orally administered opioids are discussed in more detail below.

Morphine is available for oral use in standard and controlled-release preparations. Owing to first-pass metabolism, morphine is two to six times less potent orally than it is parenterally. This is important to remember when converting a patient from parenteral to oral medication. There is wide variability in the first-pass metabolism, and the dose should be titrated to the patient's needs. In children who weigh less than 50 kg, morphine can be given at 0.1 mg/kg every 3 to 4 hours parenterally or at 0.3 mg/kg orally.

Codeine is used widely owing to its high oral/parenteral potency ratio. Orally, codeine at 30 mg is approximately equianalgesic to 325 to 600 mg aspirin. Combinations of codeine with aspirin or acetaminophen usually provide additive actions, and at these doses, analgesic efficacy can exceed that of 60 mg codeine (Beaver, 1988). Many drugs can be used instead of either morphine or codeine, as shown in Table 21–6. Oxycodone, with its high oral/parenteral potency ratio, is used widely in combination with aspirin (PERCODAN, others) or acetaminophen (PERCOCET 2.5/325, others), although it is available alone (ROXICODINE, others). Oxycodone also is available in a sustained-release formulation for chronic pain management (OXYCONTIN). Unfortunately, this formulation has been subject to widespread abuse leading to serious consequences, including death, and the FDA has strengthened warnings for this drug (*see* Chapter 23).

Heroin (diacetylmorphine) is not available for therapeutic use in the United States, although it has been used in the United Kingdom. Given intramuscularly, it is approximately twice as potent as morphine. Pharmacologically, heroin is very similar to morphine and does not appear to have any unique therapeutic advantages over the available opioids (Sawynok, 1986).

It also may be helpful to employ other agents (adjuvants) that enhance opioid analgesia and that may add beneficial effects of their own. For example, the combination of an opioid with a small dose of amphetamine may augment analgesia while reducing the sedative effects. Certain antidepressants, such as amitriptyline and desipramine, also may enhance opioid analgesia, and they may have analgesic actions in some types of neuropathic (deafferentation) pain (McQuay, 1988). Other potentially useful adjuvants include certain antihistamines, anticonvulsants such as *carbamazepine* and phenytoin, and glucocorticoids.

Alternative Routes of Administration

In addition to the traditional oral and parenteral formulations for opioids, many other methods of administration have been developed in an effort to improve therapeutic efficacy while minimizing side effects. These routes also improve the ease of use of opioids and increase patient satisfaction.

Patient-Controlled Analgesia (PCA). With this modality, the patient has limited control of the dosing of opioid from an infusion pump within tightly mandated parameters. PCA can be used for intravenous or epidural infusion. This technique avoids any delays in administration and permits greater dosing flexibility than other regimens, better adapting to individual differences in responsiveness to pain and to opioids. It also gives the patient a greater sense of control. With shorter-acting opioids, serious toxicity or excessive use rarely occurs. An early concern that self-administration of opioids would increase the probability of addiction has not materialized. PCA is suitable for adults and children, and it is preferred over intramuscular injections for postoperative pain control (Rodgers *et al.*, 1988).

Intraspinal Infusion. Administration of opioids into the epidural or intrathecal space provides more direct access to the first pain-processing synapse in the dorsal horn of the spinal cord. This permits the use of doses substantially lower than those required for oral or parenteral administration (Table 21–7). Systemic side effects thus are decreased. However, epidural opioids have their own dose-dependent side effects, such as itching, nausea, vomiting, respiratory depression, and urinary retention. The use of hydrophilic opioids such as preservative-free morphine (DURAMORPH, others) permits more rostral spread of the compound, allowing it to directly affect supraspinal sites. As a consequence, after intraspinal morphine, delayed respiratory depression can be observed for as long as 24 hours after a bolus dose. While the risk of delayed respiratory depression is reduced with more lipophilic opioids, it is not eliminated. Extreme vigilance and appropriate monitoring are required for all patients receiving intraspinal narcotics. Nausea and vomiting also are

Table 21–7
Intraspinal Opioids for the Treatment of Acute Pain

DRUG	SINGLE DOSE* (mg)	INFUSION RATE† (mg/h)	ONSET (MINUTES)	DURATION OF EFFECT OF A SINGLE DOSE‡ (HOURS)
Epidural				
Morphine	1–6	0.1–1.0	30	6–24
Meperidine	20–150	5–20	5	4–8
Methadone	1–10	0.3–0.5	10	6–10
Hydromorphone	1–2	0.1–0.2	15	10–16
Fentanyl	0.025–0.1	0.025–0.10	5	2–4
Sufentanil	0.01–0.06	0.01–0.05	5	2–4
Alfentanil	0.5–1	0.2	15	1–3
Subarachnoid				
Morphine	0.1–0.3		15	8–24+
Meperidine	10–30		?	10–24+
Fentanyl	0.005–0.025		5	3–6

*Low doses may be effective when administered to the elderly or when injected in the cervical or thoracic region. †If combining with a local anesthetic, consider using 0.0625% bupivacaine. ‡Duration of analgesia varies widely; higher doses produce longer duration. Adapted from International Association for the Study of Pain, 1992.

more prominent symptoms with intraspinal morphine. However, supraspinal analgesic centers also can be stimulated, possibly leading to synergistic analgesic effects.

Analogous to the relationship between systemic opioids and NSAIDs, intraspinal narcotics often are combined with local anesthetics. This permits the use of lower concentrations of both agents, minimizing local anesthetic–induced complications of motor blockade and the opioid-induced complications listed earlier. Epidural administration of opioids has become popular in the management of postoperative pain and for providing analgesia during labor and delivery. Lower systemic opioid levels are achieved with epidural opioids, leading to less placental transfer and less potential for respiratory depression of the newborn (Shnider and Levinson, 1987). Intrathecal administration of opioids as a single bolus ("spinal" anesthesia) also is popular for acute pain management. Chronic intrathecal infusions generally are reserved for use in chronic pain patients.

Peripheral Analgesia. As mentioned previously, opioid receptors on peripheral nerves have been shown to respond to locally applied opioids during inflammation (Stein, 1993). Peripheral analgesia permits the use of lower doses, applied locally, than those necessary to achieve a systemic effect. The effectiveness of this technique has been demonstrated in studies of postoperative pain (Stein, 1993). These studies also suggest that peripherally acting opioid compounds would be effective in other selected circumstances without entering the CNS to cause many undesirable side effects. Development of such compounds and expansion of clinical applications of this technique are active areas of research.

Rectal Administration. This route is an alternative for patients with difficulty swallowing or other oral pathology and who prefer a less invasive route than parenteral. This route is not well tolerated in most children. Onset of action is seen within 10 minutes. In the United States, morphine, hydromorphone, and oxymorphone are available in rectal suppository formulations.

Administration by Inhalation. Opioids delivered by nebulizer can be an effective means of analgesic drug delivery (Worsley et al., 1990). However, constant supervision is required when administering the drug, and variable delivery to the lungs can cause differences in therapeutic effect. In addition, possible environmental contamination is a concern.

Oral Transmucosal Administration. Opioids can be absorbed through the oral mucosa more rapidly than through the stomach. Bioavailability is greater owing to avoidance of first-pass metabolism, and lipophilic opioids are absorbed better by this route than are hydrophilic compounds such as morphine (Weinberg et al., 1988). A transmucosal delivery system that suspends fentanyl in a dissolvable matrix has been approved for clinical use (ACTIQ). Its primary indication is for treatment of breakthrough cancer pain (Ashburn et al., 1989). In this setting, transmucosal fentanyl relieves pain within 15 minutes, and patients easily can titrate the appropriate dose. Transmucosal fentanyl also has been studied as a premedicant for children. However, this technique has been largely abandoned owing to a substantial incidence of undesirable side effects such as respiratory depression, sedation, nausea, vomiting, and pruritus.

Transdermal or Iontophoretic Administration. Transdermal fentanyl patches are approved for use in sustained pain. The opioid permeates the skin, and a "depot" is established in the stratum corneum layer. Unlike other transdermal systems (i.e., transdermal *scopolamine*), anatomic position of the patch does not affect absorption. However, fever and external heat sources (heating pads, hot baths) can increase absorption of fentanyl and potentially lead to an overdose (Rose *et al.*, 1993). This modality is well suited for cancer pain treatment because of its ease of use, prolonged duration of action, and stable blood levels (Portenoy *et al.*, 1993). It may take up to 12 hours to develop analgesia and up to 16 hours to observe full clinical effect. Plasma levels stabilize after two sequential patch applications, and the kinetics do not appear to change with repeated applications (Portenoy *et al.*, 1993). However, there may be a great deal of variability in plasma levels after a given dose. The plasma half-life after patch removal is about 17 hours. Thus, if excessive sedation or respiratory depression is experienced, antagonist infusions may need to be maintained for an extended period. Dermatological side effects from the patches, such as rash and itching, usually are mild.

Iontophoresis is the transport of soluble ions through the skin by using a mild electric current. This technique has been employed with morphine (Ashburn *et al.*, 1992). Fentanyl and sufentanil have been chemically modified and applied by iontophoresis in rats (Thysman and Preat, 1993). Effective analgesia was achieved in less than 1 hour, suggesting that iontophoresis could be a promising modality for postoperative pain. It should be noted that increasing the applied current will increase drug delivery and could lead to overdose. However, unlike transdermal opioids, a drug reservoir does not build up in the skin, thus limiting the duration of both main and side effects.

Nonanalgesic Therapeutic Uses of Opioids. *Dyspnea.* Morphine is used to alleviate the dyspnea of acute left ventricular failure and pulmonary edema, and the response to intravenous morphine may be dramatic. The mechanism underlying this relief is not clear. It may involve an alteration of the patient's reaction to impaired respiratory function and an indirect reduction of the work of the heart owing to reduced fear and apprehension. However, it is more probable that the major benefit is due to cardiovascular effects, such as decreased peripheral resistance and an increased capacity of the peripheral and splanchnic vascular compartments (Vismara *et al.*, 1976). Nitroglycerin, which also causes vasodilation, may be superior to morphine in this condition (Hoffman and Reynolds, 1987). In patients with normal blood gases but severe breathlessness owing to chronic obstruction of airflow ("pink puffers"), dihydrocodeine, 15 mg orally before exercise, reduces the feeling of breathlessness and increases exercise tolerance (Johnson *et al.*, 1983). Nonetheless, opioids generally are contraindicated in pulmonary edema owing to respiratory irritants unless severe pain also is present; relative contraindications to the use of histamine-releasing opioids in asthma have been discussed.

Special Anesthesia. High doses of morphine or other opioids have been used as the primary anesthetic agents in certain surgical procedures. Although respiration is so depressed that physical assistance is required, patients can retain consciousness (*see* Chapter 13).

CLINICAL SUMMARY

Opioid analgesics provide symptomatic relief of pain, but the underlying disease remains. The clinician must weigh the benefits of this relief against any potential risk to the patient, which may be quite different in an acute compared with a chronic disease.

In acute problems, opioids will reduce the intensity of pain. However, physical signs (such as abdominal rigidity) generally will remain. Relief of pain also can facilitate history taking, examination, and the patient's ability to tolerate diagnostic procedures. Patients should not be evaluated inadequately because of the physician's unwillingness to prescribe analgesics, nor in most cases should analgesics be withheld for fear of obscuring the progression of underlying disease.

The problems that arise in the relief of pain associated with chronic conditions are more complex. Repeated daily administration of opioid analgesics eventually will produce tolerance and some degree of physical dependence. The degree will depend on the particular drug, the frequency of administration, and the quantity administered. The decision to control any chronic symptom, especially pain, by the repeated administration of an opioid must be made carefully. When pain is due to chronic nonmalignant disease, measures other than opioid drugs should be employed to relieve chronic pain if they are effective and available. Such measures include the use of NSAIDs, local nerve blocks, antidepressant drugs, electrical stimulation, acupuncture, hypnosis, or behavioral modification. However, highly selected subpopulations of chronic nonmalignant pain patients can be maintained adequately on opioids for extended periods of time (Portenoy, 1990).

In the usual doses, morphine-like drugs relieve suffering by altering the emotional component of the painful experience, as well as by producing analgesia. Control of pain, especially chronic pain, must include attention to both psychological factors and the social impact of the illness that sometimes play dominant roles in determining the suffering experienced by the patient. In addition to emotional support, the physician also must consider the substantial variability in the patient's capacity to tolerate pain and the response to opioids. As a result, some patients may require considerably more than the average dose of a drug to experience any relief from pain; others may require dosing at shorter intervals. Some clinicians, out of an exaggerated concern for the possibility of inducing addiction, tend to prescribe initial doses of opioids that are too small or given too infrequently to alleviate pain and then respond to the patient's continued complaints with an even more exaggerated concern about drug dependence despite the high probability that the request for more drug is only the expected consequence of the inadequate dosage initially prescribed (Sriwatanakul *et al.*, 1983). It also is important to note that infants and children probably are more apt to receive inadequate treatment for pain than are adults owing to communication difficulties, lack of familiarity with appropriate pain assessment methodologies, and inexperience with the use of strong opioids in children. If an illness or procedure causes pain for an adult, there is no reason to assume that it will produce less pain for a child (Yaster and Deshpande, 1988).

Pain of Terminal Illness and Cancer Pain. Opioids are not indicated in all cases of terminal illness, but the analgesia, tranquility, and even euphoria afforded by the use of opioids can make the final days far less distressing for the patient and family. Although physical dependence and tolerance may develop, this possibility should not in any way prevent physicians from fulfilling their primary obligation to ease the patient's discomfort. The physician should not wait until the pain becomes agonizing; *no patient should ever wish for death because of a physician's reluctance to use adequate amounts of effective opioids.* This sometimes may entail the regular use of opioid analgesics in substantial doses. Such patients, while they may be physically dependent, are not "addicts" even though they may need large doses on a regular basis. Physical dependence is not equivalent to addiction (*see* Chapter 23).

Most clinicians who are experienced in the management of chronic pain associated with malignant disease or terminal illness recommend that opioids be administered at sufficiently short, fixed intervals so that pain is continually under control and patients do not dread its return (Foley, 1993). Less drug is needed to prevent the recurrence of pain than to relieve it. Morphine remains the opioid of choice in most of these situations, and the route and dose should be adjusted to the needs of the individual patient. Many clinicians find that oral morphine is adequate in most situations. Sustained-release preparations of oral morphine and oxycodone are available that can be administered at 8-, 12- or 24-hour intervals (morphine) or 8- to 12-hour intervals (oxycodone). Superior control of pain often can be achieved with fewer side effects using the same daily dose; a decrease in the fluctuation of plasma concentrations of morphine may be partially responsible.

Constipation is an exceedingly common problem when opioids are used, and the use of stool softeners and laxatives should be initiated early. Amphetamines have demonstrable mood-elevating and analgesic effects and enhance opioid-induced analgesia. However, not all terminal patients require the euphoriant effects of amphetamine, and some experience side effects, such as anorexia. Controlled studies demonstrate no superiority of oral heroin over oral morphine. Similarly, after adjustment is made for potency, parenteral heroin is not superior to morphine in terms of analgesia, effects on mood, or side effects (Sawynok, 1986). Although tolerance does develop to oral opioids, many patients obtain relief from the same dosage for weeks or months. In cases where one opioid loses effectiveness, switching to another may provide better pain relief. "Cross-tolerance" among opioids exists, but clinically and experimentally, cross-tolerance among related μ receptor agonists is not complete. The reasons for this are not clear but may relate to differences between agonists in receptor-binding characteristics and subsequent cellular signaling interactions, as discussed earlier in this chapter.

When opioids and other analgesics are no longer satisfactory, nerve block, chordotomy, or other types of neurosurgical interventions such as neurostimulation may be required if the nature of the disease permits. Epidural or intrathecal administration of opioids may be useful when administration of opioids by usual routes no longer yields adequate relief of pain (*see* above). This technique has been used with ambulatory patients over periods of weeks or months (Gustafsson and Wiesenfeld-Hallin, 1988). Moreover, portable devices have been developed that permit the patient to control the parenteral administration of an opioid while remaining ambulatory (Kerr *et al.*, 1988). These devices use a pump that infuses the drug from a reservoir at a rate that can be tailored to the needs of the patient, and they include mechanisms to limit dosage and/or allow the patient to self-administer an additional "rescue" dose if there is a transient change in the intensity of pain.

BIBLIOGRAPHY

Akil, H., Mayer, D.J., and Liebeskind, J.C. Antagonism of stimulation-produced analgesia by naloxone, a narcotic antagonist. *Science,* **1976,** *191*:961–962.

Akil, H., Mayer, D.J., and Liebeskind, J.C. Comparison in the rat between analgesia induced by stimulation of periaqueductal gray matter and morphine analgesia. *C. R. Acad. Sci. Hebd. Seances Acad. Sci. Ser. D,* **1972,** *274*:3603–3605.

Akil, H., Shiomi, H., and Matthews, J. Induction of the intermediate pituitary by stress: Synthesis and release of a nonopioid form of β-endorphin. *Science,* **1985,** *227*:424–426.

Alvarez, V.A., Arttamangkul, S., Dang, V., *et al.,* μ-Opioid receptors: Ligand-dependent activation of potassium conductance, desensitization, and internalization. *J. Neurosci.,* **2002,** *22*:5769–5776.

Ashburn, M.A., Fine, P.G., and Stanley, T.H. Oral transmucosal fentanyl citrate for the treatment of breakthrough cancer pain: a case report. *Anesthesiology,* **1989,** *71*:615–617.

Ashburn, M.A., Stephen, R.L., Ackerman, E., *et al.* Iontophoretic delivery of morphine for postoperative analgesia. *J. Pain Symptom Manag.,* **1992,** *7*:27–33.

Atkinson, R.L. Opioid regulation of food intake and body weight in humans. *Fed. Proc.,* **1987,** *46*:178–182.

Avidor-Reiss, T., Nevo, I., Levy, R., Pfeuffer, T., and Vogel, Z. Chronic opioid treatment induces adenylyl cyclase V superactivation: Involvement of Gβγ. *J. Biol. Chem.,* **1996,** *271*:21309–21315.

Ballantyne, J.C., Loach, A.B., and Carr, D.B. Itching after epidural and spinal opiates. *Pain,* **1988,** *331*:149–160.

Beaver, W.T. Impact of nonnarcotic oral analgesics on pain management. *Am. J. Med.,* **1988,** *84*:3–15.

Bickel, W.K., Stitzer, M.L., Bigelow, G.E., *et al.* Buprenorphine: Dose-related blockade of opioid challenge effects in opioid dependent humans. *J. Pharmacol. Exp. Ther.,* **1988,** *247*:47–53.

Boas, R.A., and Villiger, J.W. Clinical actions of fentanyl and buprenorphine: The significance of receptor binding. *Br. J. Anaesth.,* **1985,** *57*:192–196.

Bohn, L.M., Lefkowitz, R.J., Gainetdinov, R.R., *et al.* Enhanced morphine analgesia in mice lacking β-arrestin 2. *Science,* **1999,** *286*:2495–2498.

Bohn, L.M., Gainetditov, R.R., Lin, F.T., Lefkowitz, R.J., and Caron, M.G. μ-Opioid desensitization by β-arrestin 2 determines morphine tolerance but not dependence. *Nature,* **2000,** *408*:720–723.

Boysen, K., Hertel, S., Chraemmer-Jorgensen, B., Risbo, A., and Poulsen, N.J. Buprenorphine antagonism of ventilatory depression following fentanyl anesthesia. *Acta Anaesthesiol. Scand.,* **1988,** *32*:490–492.

Bronstein, D.M., Przewlocki, R., and Akil, H. Effects of morphine treatment on pro-opiomelanocortin systems in rat brain. *Brain Res.,* **1990,** *519*:102–111.

Caraco, Y., Sheller, J., and Wood, A.J. Impact of ethnic origin and quinidine coadministration on codeine's disposition and pharmacokinetic effects. *J. Pharmacol. Exp. Ther.,* **1999,** *290*:413–422.

Chu, P., Murray, S., Lissin, D., and von Zastrow, M. δ and κ opioid receptors are differentially regulated by dynamin-dependent endocytosis when activated by the same alkaloid agonist. *J. Biol. Chem.,* **1997,** *272*:27124–27130.

Chuang, L.F., Killam, K.F., Jr., and Chuang, R.Y. Induction and activation of mitogen-activated protein kinases of human lymphocytes as one of the signaling pathways of the immunomodulatory effects of morphine sulfate. *J. Biol. Chem.,* **1997,** *272*:26815–26817.

Coward, P., Wada, H.G., Falk, M.S., *et al.* Controlling signaling with a specifically designed G$_i$-coupled receptor. *Proc. Natl. Acad. Sci. U.S.A.,* **1998,** *95*:352–357.

Craviso, G.L., and Musacchio, J.M. High-affinity dextromethorphan binding sites in guinea pig brain: II. Competition experiments. *Mol. Pharmacol.,* **1983,** *23*:629–640.

Danielson, P.B., Hoversten, M.T., Fitzpatrick, M., *et al.* Sturgeon orphanin, a molecular "fossil" that bridges the gap between the opioids and orphanin FQ/nociceptin. *J. Biol. Chem.,* **2001,** *276*:22114–22119.

Devine, D.P., Leone, P., Pocock, D., and Wise, R.A. Differential involvement of ventral tegmental *mu, delta,* and *kappa* opioid receptors in modulation of basal mesolimbic dopamine release: *in vivo* microdialysis studies. *J. Pharmacol. Exp. Ther.,* **1993,** *266*:1236–1246.

Devine, D.P., Watson, S., and Akil, H. Nociceptin/orphanin FQ regulates neuroendocrine function of the limbic hypothalamic pituitary adrenal axis. *Neuroscience,* **2001,** *102*:541–553.

Devine, D.P., and Wise, R.A. Self-administration of morphine, DAMGO, and DPDPE into the ventral tegmental area of rats. *J. Neurosci.,* **1994,** *14*:1978–1984.

Dixon, R., Howes, J., Gentile, J., *et al.* Nalmefene: Intravenous safety and kinetics of a new opioid antagonist. *Clin. Pharmacol. Ther.,* **1986,** *39*:49–53.

Dray, A., and Nunan, L. Supraspinal and spinal mechanisms in morphine-induced inhibition of reflex urinary bladder contractions in the rat. *Neuroscience,* **1987,** *22*:281–287.

Edwards, D.J., Svensson, C.K., Visco, J.P., and Lalka, D. Clinical pharmacokinetics of pethidine: 1982. *Clin. Pharmacokinet.,* **1982,** *7*:421–433.

Eichelbaum, M., and Evert, B. Influence of pharmacogenetics on drug disposition and response. *Clin. Exp. Pharmacol. Physiol.,* **1996,** *23*:983–985.

Elliott, K., Hynansky, A., and Inturrisi, C.E. Dextromethorphan attenuates and reverses analgesic tolerance to morphine. *Pain,* **1994,** *59*:361–368.

Evans, C.J., Keith, D.E., Jr., Morrison, H., Magendzo, K., and Edwards, R.H. Cloning of a delta opioid receptor by functional expression. *Science,* **1992,** *258*:1952–1955.

Fryer, R.M., Hsu, A.K., Nagase, H., and Gross, G.J. Opioid-induced cardioprotection against myocardial infarction and arrhythmias: mitochondrial versus sarcolemmal ATP-sensitive potassium channels. *J. Pharmacol. Exp. Ther.,* **2000,** *294*:451–457.

Fudala, P.J., and Bunker, E. Abrupt withdrawal of buprenorphine following chronic administration. *Clin. Pharmacol. Ther.,* **1989,** *45*:186.

Gaudriault, G., Nouel, D., Dal Farra, C., Beaudet, A., and Vincent, J.P. Receptor-induced internalization of selective peptidic mu and delta opioid ligands. *J. Biol. Chem.,* **1997,** *272*:2880–2888.

Gaveriaux-Ruff, C., Matthes, H.W., Peluso, J., and Kieffer, B.L. Abolition of morphine-immunosuppression in mice lacking the μ-opioid receptor gene. *Proc. Natl. Acad. Sci. U.S.A.,* **1998,** *95*:6326–6330.

Gomes, I., Gupta, A., Filipovska, J., *et al.* A role for heterodimerization of μ and δ opiate receptors in enhancing morphine analgesia. *Proc. Natl. Acad. Sci. U.S.A.* **2004,** *101*:5135–5139.

Gomez-Flores, R., and Weber, R.J. Differential effects of buprenorphine and morphine on immune and neuroendocrine functions following acute administration in the rat mesencephalon periaqueductal gray. *Immunopharmacology,* **2000,** *48*:145–156.

Gourlay, G.K., Cherry, D.A., and Cousins, M.J. A comparative study of the efficacy and pharmacokinetics of oral methadone and morphine in the treatment of severe pain in patients with cancer. *Pain,* **1986,** *25*:297–312.

Grevel, J., and Sadee, W. An opiate binding site in the rat brain is highly selective for 4,5-epoxymorphinans. *Science,* **1983,** *221*:1198–1201.

Gulya, K., Pelton, J.T., Hruby, V.J., and Yamamura, H.I. Cyclic somatostatin octapeptide analogues with high affinity and selectivity toward mu opioid receptors. *Life Sci.,* **1986,** *38*:2221–2229.

Gutstein, H.B., Bronstein, D.M., and Akil, H. β-Endorphin processing and cellular origins in rat spinal cord. *Pain,* **1992,** *51*:241–247.

Gutstein, H.B., Mansour, A., Watson, S.J., Akil, H., and Fields, H.L. Mu and kappa receptors in periaqueductal gray and rostral ventromedial medulla. *Neuroreport,* **1998,** *9*:1777–1781.

Handa, B.K., Land, A.C., Lord, J.A., *et al.* Analogues of β-LPH61-64 possessing selective agonist activity at μ-opiate receptors. *Eur. J. Pharmacol.,* **1981,** *70*:531–540.

He, L., Fong, J., von Zastrow, M., and Whistler, J.L. Regulation of opioid receptor trafficking and morphine tolerance by receptor oligomerization. *Cell,* **2002,** *108*:271–282.

Heimer, L., Zahm, D.S., Churchill, L., Kalivas, P.W., and Wohltmann, C. Specificity in the projection patterns of accumbal core and shell in the rat. *Neuroscience,* **1991,** *41*:89–125.

Heishman, S.J., Stitzer, M.L., Bigelow, G.E., and Liebson, I.A. Acute opioid physical dependence in postaddict humans: Naloxone dose effects after brief morphine exposure. *J. Pharmacol. Exp. Ther.,* **1989,** *248*:127–134.

Hoffman, J.R., and Reynolds, S. Comparison of nitroglycerin, morphine and furosemide in treatment of presumed prehospital pulmonary edema. *Chest, 1987, 92*:586–593.

Jiang, Q., Takemori, A.E., Sultana, M., *et al.* Differential antagonism of opioid delta antinociception by [D-Ala², Leu⁵, Cys⁶] enkephalin and naltrindole 5'-isothiocyanante: evidence for delta receptor subtypes. *J. Pharmacol. Exp. Ther., 1991, 257*:1069–1075.

Johnson, M.A., Woodcock, A.A., and Geddes, D.M. Dihydrocodeine for breathlessness in "pink puffers." *Br. Med. J. (Clin. Res. Ed.), 1983, 286*:675–677.

Johnson, R.E., Chutuape, M.A., Strain, E.C., *et al.* A comparison of levomethadyl acetate, buprenorphine, and methadone for opioid dependence. *New Engl. J. Med., 2000, 343*:1290–1297.

Kaiko, R.F., Foley, K.M., Grabinski, P.Y., *et al.* Central nervous system excitatory effects of meperidine in cancer patients. *Ann. Neurol., 1983, 13*:180–185.

Karlsson, M., Dahlstrom, B., and Neil, A. Characterization of high-affinity binding for the antitussive [³H]noscapine in guinea pig brain tissue. *Eur. J. Pharmacol., 1988, 145*:195–203.

Kayser, V., Lee, S.H., and Guilbaud, G. Evidence for a peripheral component in the enhanced antinociceptive effect of a low dose of systemic morphine in rats with peripheral mononeuropathy. *Neuroscience, 1995, 64*:537–545.

Keith, D.E., Murray, S.R., Zaki, P.A., *et al.* Morphine activates opioid receptors without causing their rapid internalization. *J. Biol. Chem., 1996, 271*:19021–19024.

Kerr, I.G., Sone, M., Deangelis, C., *et al.* Continuous narcotic infusion with patient-controlled analgesia for chronic cancer pain in outpatients. *Ann. Intern. Med., 1988, 108*:554–557.

Kolesnikov, Y.A., Pick, C.G., Ciszewska, G., and Pasternak, G.W. Blockade of tolerance to morphine but not to kappa opioids by a nitric oxide synthase inhibitor. *Proc. Natl. Acad. Sci. U.S.A., 1993, 90*:5162–5166.

Koster, A., Montkowski, A., Schulz, S., *et al.* Targeted disruption of the orphanin FQ/nociceptin gene increases stress susceptibility and impairs stress adaptation in mice. *Proc. Natl. Acad. Sci. U.S.A., 1999, 96*:10444–10449.

Kovoor, A., Celver, J.P., Wu, A. and Chavkin, C. Agonist induced homologous desensitization of mu-opioid receptors mediated by G protein–coupled receptor kinases is dependent on agonist efficacy. *Mol. Pharmacol., 1998, 54*:704–711.

Levine, J.D., Gordon, N.C., Smith, R., and McBryde, R. Desipramine enhances opiate postoperative analgesia. *Pain, 1986, 27*:45–49.

Manning, B.H., and Mayer, D.J. The central nucleus of the amygdala contributes to the production of morphine antinociception in the rat tail-flick test. *J. Neurosci., 1995a*, 8199–8213.

Manning, B.H., and Mayer, D.J. The central nucleus of the amygdala contributes to the production of morphine analgesia in the formalin test. *Pain, 1995b, 63*:141–152.

Manning, B.H., Morgan, M.J., and Franklin, K.B. Morphine analgesia in the formalin test: Evidence for forebrain and midbrain sites of action. *Neuroscience, 1994, 63*:289–294.

Mansour, A., Meng, F., Meador-Woodruff, J.H., *et al.* Site-directed mutagenesis of the human dopamine D2 receptor. *Eur. J. Pharmacol., 1992, 227*:205–214.

Mansour, A., Taylor, L.P, Fine, J.L., *et al.* Key residues defining the mu-opioid receptor binding pocket: A site-directed mutagenesis study. *J. Neurochem., 1997, 68*:344–353.

Martin, W.R., Eades, C.G., Thompson, J.A., Huppler, R.E., and Gilbert, P.E. The effects of morphine- and nalorphine-like drugs in nondependent and morphine-dependent chronic spinal dog, *J. Pharmacol. Exp. Ther., 1976, 197*:517–532.

Matthies, B.K., and Franklin, K.B. Formalin pain is expressed in decerebrate rats but not attenuated by morphine. *Pain, 1992, 51*:199–206.

Matthys, H., Bleicher, B., and Bleicher, U. Dextromethorphan and codeine: Objective assessment of antitussive activity in patients with chronic cough. *J. Int. Med. Res., 1983, 11*:92–100.

McIntosh, M., Kane, K., and Parratt, J. Effects of selective opioid receptor agonists and antagonists during myocardial ischaemia. *Eur. J. Pharmacol., 1992, 210*:37–44.

Mellon, R.D., and Bayer, B.M. Evidence for central opioid receptors in the immunomodulatory effects of morphine: Review of potential mechanism(s) of action. *J. Neuroimmunol., 1998, 83*:19–28.

Meng, F., Hoversten, M.T., Thompson, R.C., *et al.* A chimeric study of the molecular basis of affinity and selectivity of the kappa and the delta opioid receptors: Potential role of extracellular domains. *J. Biol. Chem., 1995, 270*:12730–12736.

Meng, F., Taylor, L.P., Hoversten, M.T., *et al.* Moving from the orphanin FQ receptor to an opioid receptor using four point mutations. *J. Biol. Chem., 1996, 271*:32016–32020.

Meng, F., Ueda, Y., Hoversten, M.T., *et al.* Creating a functional opioid alkaloid binding site in the orphanin FQ receptor through site-directed mutagenesis. *Mol Pharmacol., 1998, 53*:772–777.

Meng, F., Xie, G.X., Thompson, R.C., *et al.* Cloning and pharmacological characterization of a rat kappa opioid receptor. *Proc. Natl. Acad. Sci. U.S.A., 1993, 90*:9954–9958.

Mestek, A., Hurley, J.H., Bye, L.S., *et al.* The human μ opioid receptor: modulation of function desensitization by calcium/calmodulin-dependent protein kinase and protein kinase C. *J. Neurosci., 1995, 15*:2396–2406.

Meunier, J.-C., Mollereau, C., Toll, L., *et al.* Isolation and structure of the endogenous agonist of opioid receptor-like ORL₁ receptor. *Nature, 1995, 377*:532–535.

Monaco, S., Gehrmann, J., Raivich, G., and Kreutzberg, G.W. MHC-positive, ramified macrophages in the normal and injured rat peripheral nervous system. *J. Neurocytol., 1992, 21*:623–634.

Mosberg, H.I., Hurst, R., Hruby, V.J., *et al.* Bis-penicillamine enkephalins possess highly improved specificity toward delta opioid receptors. *Proc. Natl. Acad. Sci. U.S.A., 1983, 80*:5871–5874.

Moulin, D.E., Max, M.B., Kaiko, R.F., *et al.* The analgesic efficacy of intrathecal D-Ala²-D-Leu⁵-enkephalin in cancer patients with chronic pain. *Pain, 1985, 23*:213–221.

Neal, C.R., Jr., Mansour, A., Reinscheid, R., *et al.* Localization of orphanin FQ (nociceptin) peptide and messenger RNA in the central nervous system of the rat. *J. Comp. Neurol., 1999a, 406*:503–547.

Neal, C.R., Jr., Mansour, A., Reinscheid, R., *et al.* Opioid receptor-like (ORL1) receptor distribution in the rat central nervous system: Comparison of ORL1 receptor mRNA expression with ¹²⁵I-(¹⁴Tyr)-orphanin FQ binding. *J. Comp. Neurol., 1999b, 412*:563–605.

Neumann, P.B., Henriksen, H., Grosman, N., and Christensen, C.B. Plasma morphine concentrations during chronic oral administration in patients with cancer pain. *Pain, 1982, 13*:247–252.

Nicholson, J.R., Akil, H., and Watson, S.J. Orphanin FQ-induced hyperphagia is mediated by corticosterone and central glucocorticoid receptors. *Neuroscience, 2002, 115*:637–643.

Nothacker, H.P., Reinscheid, R.K., Mansour, A., *et al.* Primary structure and tissue distribution of the orphanin FQ precursor. *Proc. Natl. Acad. Sci. U.S.A., 1996, 93*:8677–8682.

Oka, T. Enkephalin receptor in the rabbit ileum. *Life Sci., 1980, 38*:1889–1898.

Okuda-Ashitaka, E., Minami, T., Tachibana, S., *et al.* Nocistatin, a peptide that blocks nociceptin action in pain transmission. *Nature, 1998, 392*:286–289.

Osborne, R.J., Joel, S.P., Trew, D., and Slevin, M.L. The analgesic activity of morphine-6-glucuronide. *Lancet,* **1988,** *1*:828.

Owen, J.A., Sitar, D.S., Berger, L., *et al.* Age-related morphine kinetics. *Clin. Pharmacol. Ther.,* **1983,** *34*:364–368.

Pan, Z.Z., Hirakawa, N., and Fields, H.L. A cellular mechanism for the bidirectional pain-modulating actions of orphanin FQ/nociceptin. *Neuron,* 2000, *26*:515–522.

Pan, Z.Z., Tershner, S.A., and Fields, H.L. Cellular mechanism for anti-analgesic action of agonists of the κ-opioid receptor. *Nature,* **1997,** *389*:382–385.

Paul, D., Standifer, K.M., Inturrisi, C.E., and Pasternak, G.W. Pharmacological characterization of morphine-6β-glucuronide, a very potent morphine metabolite. *J. Pharmacol. Exp. Ther.,* **1989,** *251*:477–483.

Pei, G., Kieffer, B.L., Lefkowitz, R.J., and Freedman, N.J. Agonist-dependent phosphorylation of the mouse delta-opioid receptor: involvement of G protein–coupled receptor kinases but not protein kinase C. *Mol. Pharmacol.,* **1995,** *48*:173–177.

Pert, C.B., and Snyder, S.H. Opiate receptor: demonstration in nervous tissue. *Science,* **1973,** *179*:1011–1014.

Pfeiffer, A., Brantl, V., Herz, A., and Emrich, H.M. Psychotomimesis mediated by kappa opiate receptors. *Science,* **1986,** *233*:774–776.

Pfeiffer, M., Kirsch, S., Stumm, R., *et al.* Heterodimerization of substance P and μ-opioid receptors regulates receptor trafficking and resensitization. *J. Biol. Chem.,* **2003,** *278*:51630–51637.

Pick, C.G., Roques, B., Gacel, G., and Pasternak, G.W. Supraspinal mu2-opioid receptors mediate spinal/supraspinal morphine synergy. *Eur. J. Pharmacol.,* **1992,** *220*:275–277.

Pilcher, W.H., Joseph, S.A., and McDonald, J.V. Immunocytochemical localization of pro-opiomelanocortin neurons in human brain areas subserving stimulation analgesia. *J. Neurosurg.,* **1988,** *68*:621–629.

Popio, K.A., Jackson, D.H., Ross, A.M., Schreiner, B.F., and Yu, P.N. Hemodynamic and respiratory effects of morphine and butorphanol. *Clin. Pharmacol. Ther.,* **1978,** *23*:281–287.

Portenoy, R.K., Southam, M.A., Gupta, S.K., *et al.* Transdermal fentanyl for cancer pain: Repeated dose pharmacokinetics. *Anesthesiology,* **1993,** *78*:36–43.

Portoghese, P.S., Lipowski, A.W., and Takemori, A.E. Binaltorphimine and nor-binaltorphimine, potent and selective kappa-opioid receptor antagonists. *Life Sci.,* **1987,** *40*:1287–1292.

Portoghese, P.S., Sultana, M., and Takemori, A.E. Naltrindole, a highly selective and potent nonpeptide delta opioid receptor antagonist. *Eur. J. Pharmacol.,* **1988,** *146*:185–186.

Quillan, J.M., Carlson, K.W., Song, C., Wang, D., and Sadée, W. Differential effects of μ-opioid receptor ligands on Ca²⁺ signaling. *J. Pharmcol. Exp. Ther.,* **2002,** *302*:1002–1012.

Reinscheid, R.K., Nothacker, H.P., Bourson, A., *et al.* Orphanin FQ: A neuropeptide that activates an opioid-like G protein–coupled receptor. *Science,* **1995,** *270*:792–794.

Rodgers, B.M., Webb, C.J., Stergios, D., and Newman, B.M. Patient-controlled analgesia in pediatric surgery. *J. Pediatr. Surg.,* **1988,** *23*:259–262.

Rose, P.G., Macfee, M.S., and Boswell, M.V. Fentanyl transdermal system overdose secondary to cutaneous hyperthermia. *Anesth. Analg.,* **1993,** *77*:390–391.

Rossi, G.C., Pasternak, G.W., and Bodnar, R.J. Synergistic brainstem interactions for morphine analgesia. *Brain Res.,* **1993,** *624*:171–180.

Roth, A., Keren, G., Gluck, A., Braun, S., and Laniado, S. Comparison of nalbuphine hydrochloride versus morphine sulfate for acute myocardial infarction with elevated pulmonary artery wedge pressure. *Am. J. Cardiol.,* **1988,** *62*:551–555.

Rothman, R.B., Long, J.B., Bykov, V., *et al.* β-FNA binds irreversibly to the opiate receptor complex: In vivo and in vitro evidence. *J. Pharmacol. Exp. Ther.,* **1988,** *247*:405–416.

Sadeque, A.J., Wandel, C., He, H., Shah, S., and Wood, A.J. Increased drug delivery to the brain by P-glycoprotein inhibition. *Clin. Pharmacol. Ther.,* **2000,** *68*:231–237.

Schinkel, A.H., Wagenaar, E., Mol, C.A., and van Deemter, L. P-glycoprotein in the blood–brain barrier of mice influences the brain penetration and pharmacological activity of many drugs. *J. Clin. Invest.,* **1996,** *97*:2517–2524.

Schulz, R., Faase, E., Wuster, M., and Herz, A. Selective receptors for β-endorphin on the rat vas deferens. *Life Sci.,* **1979,** *24*:843–849.

Schwyzer, R., Molecular mechanism of opioid receptor selection. *Biochemistry,* **1986,** *25*:6335–6342.

Segredo, V., Burford, N.T., Lameh, J., and Sadee, W. A constitutively internalizing and recycling mutant of the mu-opioid receptor. *J. Neurochem.,* **1997,** *68*:2395–2404.

Sharma, S.K., Klee, W.A., and Nirenberg, M. Opiate-dependent modulation of adenylate cyclase. *Proc. Natl. Acad. Sci. U.S.A.,* **1977,** *74*:3365–3369.

Simon, E.J., Hiller, J.M., and Edelman, I. Stereospecific binding of the potent narcotic analgesic ³H-etorphine to rat brain homogenate. *Proc. Natl. Acad. Sci. U.S.A.,* **1973,** *70*:1947–1949.

Smith, M.T. Neuroexcitatory effects of morphine and hydromorphone: evidence implicating the 3-glucuronide metabolites. *Clin. Exp. Pharmacol. Physiol.,* **2000,** *27*:524–528.

Smith, M.T., Watt, J.A., and Cramond, T. Morphine-3-glucuronide: A potent antagonist of morphine analgesia. *Life Sci.,* **1990,** *47*:579–585.

Sriwatanakul, K., Weis, O.F., Alloza, J.L., *et al.* Analysis of narcotic analgesic usage in the treatment of postoperative pain. *JAMA,* **1983,** *250*:926–929.

Terenius, L. Stereospecific interaction between narcotic analgesics and a synaptic plasma membrane fraction of rat brain cortex. *Acta Pharmacol. Toxicol. (Copenh.),* **1973,** *32*:317–320.

Terman, G.W., Jin, W., Cheong, Y.P., *et al.* G-protein receptor kinase 3 (GRK3) influences opioid analgesic tolerance but not opioid withdrawal. *Br. J. Pharmacol.,* **2004,** *141*:55–64.

Thomas, D.A., Williams, G.M., Iwata, K., Kenshalo, D.R., Jr., and Dubner, R. Effects of central administration of opioids on facial scratching in monkeys. *Brain Res.,* **1992,** *585*:315–317.

Thompson, R.C., Mansour, A., Akil, H., and Watson, S.J. Cloning and pharmacological characterization of a rat mu opioid receptor. *Neuron,* **1993,** *11*:903–913.

Thysman, S., and Preat, V. In vivo iontophoresis of fentanyl and sufentanil in rats: pharmacokinetics and acute antinociceptive effects. *Anesth. Analg.,* **1993,** *77*:61–66.

Trafton, J.A., Abbadie, C., Marchand, S., Mantyh, P.W., and Basbaum, A.I. Spinal opioid analgesia: how critical is the regulation of substance P signaling? *J. Neurosci.,* **1999,** *19*:9642–9653.

Trujillo, K.A., and Akil, H. Inhibition of morphine tolerance and dependence by the NMDA receptor antagonist MK-801. *Science,* **1991,** *251*:85–87.

Vaughan, C.W., Ingram, S.L., Connor, M.A., and Christie, M.J. How opioids inhibit GABA-mediated neurotransmission. *Nature,* **1997,** *390*:611–614.

Vismara, L.A., Leaman, D.M., and Zelis, R. The effects of morphine on venous tone in patients with acute pulmonary edema. *Circulation,* **1976,** *54*:335–337.

Vonvoigtlander, P.F., Lahti, R.A., and Ludens, J.H. U-50,488: A selective and structurally novel non-mu (kappa) opioid agonist. *J. Pharmacol. Exp. Ther.,* **1983,** *224*:7–12.

Wallenstein, S.L., Kaiko, R.F., Rogers, A.G., and Houde, R.W. Cross-over trials in clinical analgesic assays: Studies of buprenorphine and morphine. *Pharmacotherapy,* **1986,** *6*:228–235.

Wang, D., Xidochun, S., Bohn, L., Sadée, W. Opioid receptor homo- and heterodimerization in living cells by quantitative bioluminescence resonance energy transfer. *Mol. Pharmacol.,* **2005,** *67*:2173–2184.

Wang, J.B., Johnson, P.S., Persico, A.M., *et al.* Human mu opiate receptor. cDNA and genomic clones: Pharmacologic characterization and chromosomal assignment. *FEBS Lett.,* **1994,** *338*:217–222.

Weihe, E., Millan, M.J., Leibold, A., Nohr, D., and Herz, A. Co-localization of proenkephalin- and prodynorphin-derived opioid peptides in laminae IV/V spinal neurons revealed in arthritic rats. *Neurosci. Lett.,* **1988,** *29*:187–192.

Weinberg, D.S., Inturrisi, C.E., Reidenberg, B., *et al.* Sublingual absorption of selected opioid analgesics. *Clin. Pharmacol. Ther.,* **1988,** *44*:335–342.

Welters, I.D., Menzebach, A., Goumon, Y., *et al.* Morphine inhibits NF-κB nuclear binding in human neutrophils and monocytes by a nitric oxide-dependent mechanism. *Anesthesiology,* **2000,** *92*:1677–1684.

Whistler, J.L., and von Zastrow, M. Morphine-activated opioid receptors elude desensitization by β-arrestin. *Proc. Natl. Acad. Sci. U.S.A.,* **1998,** *95*:9914–9919.

Whistler, J.L., Chuang, H.H., Chu, P., Jan. L.Y., and von Zastrow, M. Functional dissociation of μ opioid receptor signaling and endocytosis: Implications for the biology of opiate tolerance and addiction. *Neuron,* **1999,** *23*:737–746.

Worsley, M.H., MacLeod, A.D., Brodie, M.J., Asbury, A.J., and Clark, C. Inhaled fentanyl as a method of analgesia. *Anaesthesia,* **1990,** *45*:449–451.

Xie, Y.B., Wang, H., and Segaloff, D.L. Extracellular domain of lutropin/choriogonadotropin receptor expressed in transfected cells binds choriogonadotropin with high affinity. *J. Biol. Chem.,* **1990,** *265*:21411–21414.

Xu, X.J., Hao, J.X., and Wiesenfeld-Hallin, Z. Nociceptin or antinociceptin: potent spinal antinociceptive effect of orphanin FQ/nociceptin in the rat. *Neuroreport,* **1996,** *7*:2092–2094.

Yeh, S.Y., Gorodetzky, C.W., and Krebs, H.A. Isolation and identification of morphine 3- and 6-glucuronides, morphine 3,6-diglucuronide, morphine 3-ethereal sulfate, normorphine, and normorphine 6-glucuronide as morphine metabolites in humans. *J. Pharm. Sci.,* **1977,** *66*:1288–1293.

Yoburn, B.C., Luke, M.C., Pasternak, G.W., and Inturrisi, C.E. Upregulation of opioid receptor subtypes correlates with potency changes of morphine and DADLE. *Life Sci.,* **1988,** *43*:1319–1324.

Zagon, I.S., Goodman, S.R., and McLaughlin, P.J. Characterization of zeta: A new opioid receptor involved in growth. *Brain Res.,* **1989,** *482*:297–305.

Zimmer, E.Z., Divon, M.Y., and Vadasz, A. Influence of meperidine on fetal movements and heart rate beat-to-beat variability in the active phase of labor. *Am. J. Perinatol.,* **1988,** *5*:197–200.

Zimprich, A., Simon, T., and Hollt, V. Cloning and expression of an isoform of the rat μ opioid receptor (rMOR1B) which differs in agonist induced desensitization from rMOR1. *FEBS Lett.,* **1995,** *359*:142–146.

MONOGRAPHS AND REVIEWS

Agency for Health Care Policy and Research. *Acute Pain Management in Infants, Children, and Adolescents: Operative and Medical Procedures.* No. 92-0020. U.S. Dept. of Health and Human Services, Rockville, MD, **1992a.**

Agency for Health Care Policy and Research. *Acute Pain Management: Operative or Medical Procedures and Trauma.* No. 92-0032. U.S. Dept. of Health and Human Services, Rockville, MD, **1992b.**

Agency for Health Care Policy and Research. *Management of Cancer Pain.* No. 94-0592. U.S. Dept. of Health and Human Services, Rockville, MD, **1994.**

Agnati, L. F., Ferre, S., Lluis, C., Franco, R., and Fuxe, K. Molecular mechanisms and therapeutical implications of intramembrane receptor/receptor interactions among heptahelical receptors with examples from the striatopallidal GABA neurons. *Pharmacol. Rev.,* **2003,** *55*:509–550.

Akil, H., Bronstein, D., and Mansour, A. Overview of the endogenous opioid systems: anatomical, biochemical, and functional issues. In, *Endorphins, Opiates and Behavioural Processes.* (Rodgers, R.J., and Cooper, S.J., eds.) Wiley, Chichester, England, **1988,** pp. 3–17.

Akil, H., Meng, F., Devine, D.P., and Watson, S.J. Molecular and neuroanatomical properties of the endogenous opioid system: Implications for treatment of opiate addiction. *Semin. Neurosci.,* **1997,** *9*:70–83.

Akil, H., Owens, C., Gutstein, H, *et al.* Endogenous opioids: Overview and current issues. *Drug Alcohol Depend.,* **1998,** *51*:127–140.

Akil, H., and Watson, S. Cloning of kappa opioid receptors: functional significance and future directions. In, *Neuroscience: From the Molecular to the Cognitive.* (Bloom, F.E., ed.) Elsevier, Amsterdam, **1994,** pp. 81–86.

Akil, H., Watson, S.J., Young, E., *et al.* Endogenous opioids: biology and function. *Annu. Rev. Neurosci.,* **1984,** *7*:223–255.

Akil, H., Young, E., Walker, J.M., and Watson, S.J. The many possible roles of opioids and related peptides in stress-induced analgesia. *Ann. N.Y. Acad. Sci.,* **1986,** *467*:140–153.

American Pain Society. *Principles of Analgesic Use in the Treatment of Acute Pain and Cancer Pain.* 5th ed. American Pain Society, Glenview, IL, **2003.**

Amir, S. Anaphylactic shock: Catecholamine actions in the response to opioid antagonists. *Prog. Clin. Biol. Res.,* **1988,** *264*:265–274.

Bailey, P.L., and Stanley, T.H. Intravenous opioid anesthetics. In, *Anesthesia,* 4th ed., vol. 1. (Miller, R.D., ed.) Churchill-Livingstone, New York, **1994,** pp. 291–387.

Berde, C., Ablin, A., Glazer, J., *et al.* American Academy of Pediatrics Report of the Subcommittee on Disease-Related Pain in Childhood Cancer. *Pediatrics,* **1990,** *86*:818–825.

Bertorelli, R., Calo, G., Ongini, E., and Regoli, D. Nociceptin/orphanin FQ and its receptor: A potential target for drug discovery. *Trends Pharmacol. Sci.,* **2000,** *21*:233–234.

Borgland, S.L. Acute opioid receptor desensitization and tolerance: is there a link? *Clin. Exp. Pharmacol. Physiol.,* **2001,** *28*:147–154.

Bouvier, M. Oligomerization of G protein–coupled transmitter receptors. *Nature Rev. Neurosci.,* **2001,** *2*:274–286.

Burkle, H., Dunbar, S., and Van Aken, H. Remifentanil: A novel, short-acting μ-opioid. *Anesth. Analg.,* **1996,** *83*:646–651.

Cannon, J., and Liebeskind, J. Analgesic effects of electrical brain stimulation and stress. In, *Neurotransmitters and Pain Control,* Vol. 9: *Pain and Headache.* (Akil, H., and Lewis, J.W., eds.) Karger, Basel, **1987,** pp. 283–294.

Chan, G.L., and Matzke, G.R. Effects of renal insufficiency on the pharmacokinetics and pharmacodynamics of opioid analgesics. *Drug Intell. Clin. Pharm.,* **1987,** *21*:773–783.

Christup, L.L. Morphine metabolites. *Acta Anaesthesiol. Scand.,* **1997,** *41*:116–122.

Contet, C., Kieffer, B.L., and Befort, K. Mu opioid receptor: A gateway to drug addiction. *Curr. Opin. Neurobiol.,* **2004,** *14*:370–378.

Cooper, S. Interactions between endogenous opioids and dopamine: Implications for reward and aversion. In, *The Mesolimbic Dopamine*

System: From Motivation to Action. (Willner, P., and Scheel-Kruger, J., eds.) Wiley, Chichester, England, **1991**, pp. 331–366.

De Luca, A., and Coupar, I.M. Insights into opioid action in the intestinal tract. *Pharmacol. Ther.,* **1996**, *2*:103–115.

Devi, L.A. Heterodimerization of G protein–coupled receptors: Pharmacology, signaling and trafficking. *Trends Pharmacol. Sci.,* **2001**, *22*:532–537.

Duggan, A.W., and North, R.A. Electrophysiology of opioids. *Pharmacol. Rev.,* **1983**, *35*:219–281.

Du Pen, S.L., Du Pen, A.R., Polissar, N., *et al.* Implementing guidelines for cancer pain management: Results of a randomized, controlled clinical trial. *J. Clin. Oncol.,* **1999**, *17*:361–370.

Duthie, D.J. Remifentanil and tramadol. *Br. J. Anaesth.,* **1998**, *81*:51–57.

Faden, A.I. Role of thyrotropin-releasing hormone and opiate receptor antagonists in limiting central nervous system injury. *Adv. Neurol.,* **1988**, *47*:531–546.

Fields, H.L., Heinricher, M.M., and Mason, P. Neurotransmitters in nociceptive modulatory circuits. *Annu. Rev. Neurosci.,* **1991**, *14*:219–245.

Fishburne, J.I. Systemic analgesia during labor. *Clin. Perinatol.,* **1982**, *9*:29–53.

Foley, K.M. Opioid analgesics in clinical pain management. In, *Handbook of Experimental Pharmacology,* Vol. 104: *Opioids II.* (Herz, A., ed.) Springer-Verlag, Berlin, **1993**, pp. 693–743.

Glass, P.S., Gan, T.J., and Howell, S. A review of the pharmacokinetics and pharmacodynamics of remifentanil. *Anesth. Analg.,* **1999**, *89*:S7–14.

Gonzalez, J.P., and Brogden, R.N. Naltrexone: A review of its pharmacodynamic and pharmacokinetic properties and therapeutic efficacy in the management of opioid dependence. *Drugs,* **1988**, *35*:192–213.

Grossman, S., Benedetti, C., Payne, R., and Syrjala, K. NCCN practice guidelines for cancer pain. *NCCN Proc.,* **1999**, *13*:33–44.

Gustafsson, L.L., and Wiesenfeld-Hallin, Z. Spinal opioid analgesia: A critical update. *Drugs,* **1988**, *35*:597–603.

Heimer, L., Switzer, R., and Hoesen, G.V. Ventral striatum and ventral pallidum: Components of the motor system? *Trends Neurosci.,* **1982**, *5*:83087.

Heinricher, M.M. Orphanin FQ/nociceptin: From neural circuitry to behavior. *Life Sci.,* **2003**, *73*:813–822.

Herz, A., ed. *Handbook of Experimental Pharmacology,* Vol. 104: *Opioids I.* Springer-Verlag, Berlin, **1993.**

Holzer, P. Opioids and opioid receptors in the enteric nervous system: From a problem in opioid analgesia to a possible new prokinetic therapy in humans. *Neurosci. Lett.,* **2004**, *361*:192–195.

International Association for the Study of Pain. *Management of Acute Pain: A Practical Guide.* IASP Publications, Seattle, WA, **1992.**

Kenakin, T. Drug efficacy at G protein–coupled receptors. *Annu. Rev. Pharmacol. Toxicol.,* **2002**, *42*:349–379.

Kilpatrick, G.J., Dautzenberg, F.M., Martin, G.R., and Eglen, R.M. 7TM receptors: The splicing on the cake. *Trends Pharmacol. Sci.,* **1999**, *20*:294–301.

Koch, T., Widera, A., Bartzsch, K. *et al.* Receptor endocytosis counteracts the development of opioid tolerance. *Mol. Pharmacol.,* **2005**, *67*:280–287.

Koob, G.F., and Bloom, F.E. Cellular and molecular mechanisms of drug dependence. *Science,* **1988**, *242*:715–723.

Kreek, M.J., LaForge, K.S., and Butelman, E. Pharmacotherapy of addictions. *Nature Rev. Drug Dis.,* **2002**, *1*:710–726.

Kromer, W. Endogenous and exogenous opioids in the control of gastrointestinal motility and secretion. *Pharmacol. Rev.,* **1988**, *40*:121–162.

Krupnick, J.G., and Benovic, J.L. The role of receptor kinases and arrestins in G protein–coupled receptor regulation. *Annu. Rev. Pharmacol. Toxicol.,* **1998**, *38*:289–319.

Levac, B.A.R., O'Dowd, B.F., and George, S.R. Oligomerization of opioid receptors: Generation of novel signaling units. *Curr. Opin. Pharmacol.,* **2002**, *2*:76–81.

Lewis, J., Mansour, A., Khachaturian, H., Watson, S., and Akil, H. Neurotransmitters and pain control. In, *Neurotransmitters and Pain Control,* Vol. 9: *Pain and Headache.* (Akil, H., and Lewis, J.W., eds.) Karger, Basil, **1987**, pp. 129–159.

Lewis, K.S., and Han, N.H. Tramadol: A new centrally acting analgesic. *Am. J. Health Syst. Pharm.,* **1997**, *54*:643–652.

Mansour, A., Fox, C.A., Akil, H., and Watson, S.J. Opioid-receptor mRNA expression in the rat CNS: Anatomical and functional implications. *Trends Neurosci.,* **1995**, *18*:22–29.

Mansour, A., Khachaturian, H., Lewis, M.E., Akil, H., and Watson, S.J. Anatomy of CNS opioid receptors. *Trends Neurosci.,* **1988**, *11*:308–314.

Martin, W.R. Pharmacology of opioids. *Pharmacol. Rev.,* **1983**, *35*:283–323.

McCleskey, E.W., and Gold, M.S. Ion channels of nociception. *Annu. Rev. Physiol.,* **1999**, *61*:835–856.

McGinty, J., and Friedman, D. Opioids in the hippocampus. *Natl. Inst. Drug Abuse Res. Monogr. Ser.,* **1988**, *82*:1–145.

McQuay, H.J. Pharmacological treatment of neuralgic and neuropathic pain. *Cancer Surv.,* **1988**, *7*:141–159.

Milligan, G. G protein–coupled receptor dimerization: function and ligand pharmacology. *Mol. Pharmacol.,* **2004**, *66*:1–7.

Milne, R.W., Nation, R.L., and Somogyi, A.A. The disposition of morphine and its 3- and 6-glucuronide metabolites in humans and animals, and the importance of the metabolites to the pharmacological effects of morphine. *Drug Metab. Rev.,* **1996**, *28*:345–472.

Mogil, J.S., and Pasternak, G.W. The molecular and behavioral pharmacology of the orphanin FQ/nociceptin peptide and receptor family. *Pharmacol. Rev.,* **2001**, *53*:381–415.

Monk, J.P., Beresford, R., and Ward, A. Sufentanil: A review of its pharmacological properties and therapeutic use. *Drugs,* **1988**, *36*:286–313.

Mulder, A., and Schoffelmeer, A. multiple opioid receptors and presynaptic modulation of neurotransmitter release in the brain. In, *Handbook of Experimental Pharmacology,* Vol. 104: *Opioids I.* (Herz, A., ed.) Springer-Verlag, Berlin, **1993**, pp. 125–144.

Nestler, E.J., and Aghajanian, G.K. Molecular and cellular basis of addiction. *Science,* **1997**, *278*:58–63.

Olszewski, P.K., and Levine, A.S. Characterization of influence of central nociceptin/orphanin FQ on consummatory behavior. *Endocrinology,* **2004**, *145*:2627–2632.

Page, G.G., and Ben-Eliyahu, S. The immune-suppressive nature of pain. *Semin. Oncol. Nurs.,* **1997**, *13*:10–15.

Pasternak, G.W. Multiple morphine and enkephalin receptors: Biochemical and pharmacological aspects. *Ann. N.Y. Acad. Sci.,* **1986**, *467*:130–139.

Pasternak, G.W. Insights into mu opioid pharmacology: The role of mu opioid receptor subtypes. *Life Sci.,* **2001**, *68*:2213–2219.

Pasternak, G.W. Pharmacological mechanisms of opioid analgesics. *Clin. Neuropharmacol.,* **1993**, *16*:1–8

Patel, S.S., and Spencer, C.M. Remifentanil. *Drugs,* **1996**, *52*:417–427.

Portenoy, R.K. Chronic opioid therapy in nonmalignant pain. *J. Pain Sympt. Manag.,* **1990**, *5*:S46–62.

Portoghese, P.S. Bivalent ligands and the message-address concept in the design of selective opioid receptor antagonists. *Trends Pharmacol. Sci.,* **1989**, *10*:230–235.

Risdahl, J.M., Khanna, K.V., Peterson, P.K., and Molitor, T.W. Opiates and infection. *J. Neuroimmunol.,* **1998,** *83*:4–18.

Rumore, M.M., and Schlichting, D.A. Clinical efficacy of antihistaminics as analgesics. *Pain,* **1986,** *25*:7–22.

Sawynok, J. The therapeutic use of heroin: a review of the pharmacological literature. *Can. J. Physiol. Pharmacol.,* **1986,** *64*:1–6.

Sharp, B., and Yaksh, T. Pain killers of the immune system. *Nature Med.,* **1997,** *3*:831–832.

Shippenberg, T.S., Herz, A., Spanagel, R., Bals-Kubik, R., and Stein, C. Conditioning of opioid reinforcement: Neuroanatomical and neurochemical substrates. *Ann. N.Y. Acad. Sci.,* **1992,** *654*:347–356.

Shnider, S.M., and Levinson, G. *Anesthesia for Obstetrics.* Williams & Wilkins, Baltimore, MD, **1987.**

Stack, C.G., Rogers, P., and Linter, S.P. Monoamine oxidase inhibitors and anesthesia: A review. *Br. J. Anaesth.,* **1988,** *60*:222–227.

Staritz, M. Pharmacology of the sphincter of Oddi. *Endoscopy,* **1988,** *20*(suppl.1):171–174.

Stein, C. Peripheral mechanisms of opioid analgesia. *Anesth. Analg.,* **1993,** *76*:182–191.

von Zastrow, M., Svingos, A., Haberstock-Debic, H., and Evans, C. Regulated endocytosis of opioid receptors: Cellular mechanisms and proposed roles in physiological adaptation to opiate drugs. *Curr. Opin. Neurobiol.,* **2003,** *13*:348–353.

Waldhoer, M., Bartlett, S., and WHistler, J. Opioid receptors. *Ann. Rev. Biochem.,* **2004,** *73*:953–990.

Wei, L.N., Law, P.Y., and Loh, H.H. Post-transcriptional regulation of opioid receptors in the nervous system. *Front. Biosci.,* **2004,** *9*:1665–1679.

Willner, P., Ahlenius, S., Muscat, R., and Scheel-Kruger, J. The mesolimbic dopamine system. In, *The Mesolimbic Dopamine System: From Motivation to Action.* (Willner, J., and Scheel-Kruger, J., eds.) Wiley, Chichester, England, **1991.**

World Health Organization. *Cancer Pain Relief and Palliative Care: Report of a WHO Expert Committee.* World Health Organization, Geneva, Switzerland, **1990.**

World Health Organization. *Cancer Pain Relief and Palliative Care in Children.* World Health Organization, Geneva, Switzerland, **1998.**

Yaksh, T.L. CNS mechanisms of pain and analgesia. *Cancer Surv.,* **1988,** *7*:5–28.

Yaster, M., and Deshpande, J.K. Management of pediatric pain with opioid analgesics. *J. Pediatr.,* **1988,** *113*:421–429.

ETHANOL

Michael Fleming, S. John Mihic, and R. Adron Harris

The two-carbon alcohol *ethanol*, CH$_3$CH$_2$OH, is a CNS depressant that is widely available to adults; its use is legal and accepted in many societies, and its abuse is a societal problem. The relevant pharmacological properties of ethanol include effects on the gastrointestinal, cardiovascular, and central nervous systems, effects on disease processes, and effects on prenatal development. Ethanol disturbs the fine balance between excitatory and inhibitory influences in the brain, producing disinhibition, ataxia, and sedation. Tolerance to ethanol develops after chronic use, and physical dependence is demonstrated on alcohol withdrawal (*see* Chapter 23). Understanding the cellular and molecular mechanisms of these myriad effects of ethanol *in vivo* requires an integration of knowledge from multiple biomedical sciences.

HISTORY AND OVERVIEW

Alcoholic beverages are so strongly associated with human society that fermentation is said to have developed in parallel with civilization. Indeed, there is speculation that human alcohol use is linked evolutionarily to a preference for fermenting fruit, where the presence of ethanol signals that the fruit is ripe but not yet rotten (Dudley, 2000) (the terms *ethanol* and *alcohol* are used interchangeably in this chapter).

The Arabs developed distillation about 800 C.E., and the word *alcohol* is derived from the Arabic for "something subtle." Alchemists of the Middle Ages were captivated by the invisible "spirit" that was distilled from wine and thought it to be a remedy for practically all diseases. The term *whiskey* is derived from *usquebaugh*, Gaelic for "water of life," and alcohol became the major ingredient of widely marketed "tonics" and "elixirs."

Although alcohol abuse and alcoholism are major health problems in many countries, the medical and social impacts of alcohol abuse have not always been appreciated. The economic burden to the U.S. economy is about $185 billion each year, and alcohol is responsible for more than 100,000 deaths annually. At least 14 million Americans meet the criteria for alcohol abuse or alcoholism, but medical diagnosis and treatment often are delayed until the disease is advanced and complicated by multiple social and health problems, making treatment difficult. Biological and genetic studies clearly place alcoholism among diseases with both genetic and environmental influences, but persistent stigmas and attribution to moral failure have impeded recognition and treatment of alcohol problems. A major challenge for physicians and researchers is to devise diagnostic and therapeutic approaches aimed at this major health problem.

Compared with other drugs, surprisingly large amounts of alcohol are required for physiological effects, resulting in its consumption more as a food than a drug. The alcohol content of beverages typically ranges from 4% to 6% (volume/volume) for beer, 10% to 15% for wine, and 40% and higher for distilled spirits (the "proof" of an alcoholic beverage is twice its percentage of alcohol; *e.g.*, 40% alcohol is 80 proof). A glass of beer or wine, a mixed drink, or a shot of spirits contains about 14 g alcohol, or about 0.3 mol ethanol. Consumption of 1 to 2 mol over a few hours is not uncommon. Thus, alcohol is consumed in gram quantities, whereas most other drugs are taken in milligram or microgram doses. Since the ratio of ethanol in end-expiratory alveolar air and ethanol in the blood is relatively consistent, blood alcohol levels (BALs) in human beings can be estimated readily by the measurement of alcohol levels in expired air; the partition coefficient for ethanol between blood and alveolar air is approximately 2000:1. Because of the causal relationship between excessive alcohol consumption and vehicular accidents, there has been a near-universal adoption of laws attempting to limit the operation of vehicles while under the influence of alcohol. Legally allowed BALs typically are set at or below 80 mg% (80 mg ethanol per

100 ml blood; 0.08% w/v), which is equivalent to a concentration of 17 mM ethanol in blood. A 12-oz bottle of beer, a 5-oz glass of wine, and a 1.5-oz "shot" of 40% liquor each contains approximately 14 g ethanol, and the consumption of one of these beverages by a 70-kg person would produce a BAL of approximately 30 mg%. However, it is important to note that this is approximate because the BAL is determined by a number of factors, including the rate of drinking, sex, body weight and water percentage, and the rates of metabolism and stomach emptying (*see* "Acute Alcohol Intoxication" below).

PHARMACOLOGICAL PROPERTIES

Absorption, Distribution, and Metabolism

After oral administration, ethanol is absorbed rapidly into the bloodstream from the stomach and small intestine and distributes into total-body water (0.5 to 0.7 L/kg). Peak blood levels occur about 30 minutes after ingestion of ethanol when the stomach is empty. Because absorption occurs more rapidly from the small intestine than from the stomach, delays in gastric emptying (owing, for example, to the presence of food) slow ethanol absorption. Because of first-pass metabolism by gastric and liver alcohol dehydrogenase (ADH), oral ingestion of ethanol leads to lower BALs than would be obtained if the same quantity were administered intravenously. Gastric metabolism of ethanol is lower in women than in men, which may contribute to the greater susceptibility of women to ethanol (Lieber, 2000). *Aspirin* increases ethanol bioavailability by inhibiting gastric ADH. Ethanol is metabolized largely by sequential hepatic oxidation, first to acetaldehyde by ADH and then to acetic acid by aldehyde dehydrogenase (ALDH) (Figure 22–1). Each metabolic step requires NAD^+; thus oxidation of 1 mol ethanol (46 g) to 1 mol acetic acid requires 2 mol NAD^+ (approximately 1.3 kg). This greatly exceeds the supply of NAD^+ in the liver; indeed, NAD^+ availability limits ethanol

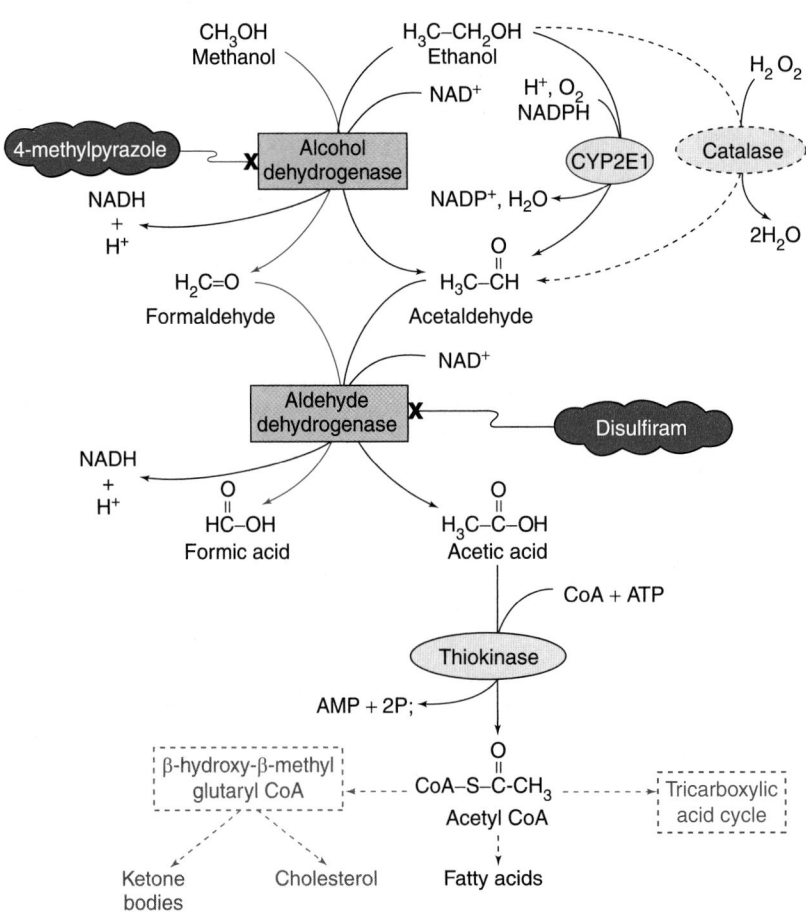

Figure 22–1. *Metabolism of ethanol and methanol.*

metabolism to about 8 g or 10 ml (approximately 170 mmol) per hour in a 70-kg adult, or approximately 120 mg/kg per hour. Thus, hepatic ethanol metabolism functionally saturates at relatively low blood levels compared with the high BALs achieved, and ethanol metabolism is a zero-order process (constant amount per unit time). Small amounts of ethanol are excreted in urine, sweat, and breath, but metabolism to acetate accounts for 90% to 98% of ingested ethanol, mostly owing to hepatic metabolism by ADH and ADLH. A hepatic cytochrome P450 enzyme, CYP2E1, also can contribute (Figure 22–1), especially at higher ethanol concentrations and under conditions such as alcoholism, where its activity may be induced. Catalase also can produce acetaldehyde from ethanol, but hepatic H_2O_2 availability usually is too low to support significant flux of ethanol through this pathway. Although CYP2E1 usually is not a major factor in ethanol metabolism, it can be an important site of interactions of ethanol with other drugs. CYP2E1 is induced by chronic consumption of ethanol, increasing the clearance of its substrates and activating certain toxins such as CCl_4. There can be decreased clearance of the same drugs, however, after acute consumption of ethanol because ethanol competes with them for oxidation by the enzyme system (*e.g., phenytoin* and *warfarin*). The large increase in the hepatic NADH:NAD$^+$ ratio during ethanol oxidation has profound consequences in addition to limiting the rate of ethanol metabolism. Enzymes requiring NAD$^+$ are inhibited; thus lactate accumulates, activity of the tricarboxylic acid cycle is reduced, and acetyl coenzyme A (acetyl CoA) accumulates (and it is produced in quantity from ethanol-derived acetic acid; Figure 22-1). The combination of increased NADH and elevated acetyl CoA supports fatty acid synthesis and the storage and accumulation of triacylglycerides. Ketone bodies accrue, exacerbating lactic acidosis. Ethanol metabolism by the CYP2E1 pathway produces elevated NADP$^+$, limiting the availability of NADPH for the regeneration of reduced glutathione (GSH), thereby enhancing oxidative stress.

The mechanisms underlying hepatic disease resulting from heavy ethanol use probably reflect a complex combination of these metabolic factors, CYP2E1 induction (and enhanced activation of toxins and production of H_2O_2 and oxygen radicals), and possibly enhanced release of endotoxin as a consequence of ethanol's effect on gram-negative flora in the gastrointestinal tract. Effects of heavy ethanol ingestion on various organs are summarized below; damage to tissues very likely reflects the poor nutritional status of alcoholics (malabsorption and lack of vitamins A and D and thiamine), suppression of immune function by ethanol, and a variety of other generalized effects.

The one-carbon alcohol *methanol* also is metabolized by ADH and ALDH, with damaging consequences (*see* below). Competition between methanol and ethanol for ADH forms the basis of the use of ethanol in methanol poisoning. Several drugs inhibit alcohol metabolism, including *4-methylprazole*, an ADH inhibitor useful in ethylene glycol poisoning, and *disulfiram,* an ALDH inhibitor used in treating alcoholism (*see* below). Ethanol also can competitively inhibit the metabolism of other substrates of ADH and CYP2E1, such as methanol and ethylene glycol, and therefore is an effective antidote.

EFFECTS OF ETHANOL ON PHYSIOLOGICAL SYSTEMS

William Shakespeare described the acute pharmacological effects of imbibing ethanol in the Porter scene (act 2, scene 3) of *Macbeth*. The Porter, awakened from an alcohol-induced sleep by Macduff, explains three effects of alcohol and then wrestles with a fourth effect that combines the contradictory aspects of soaring overconfidence with physical impairment:

> **Porter:** . . . and drink, sir, is a great provoker of three things.
> **Macduff:** What three things does drink especially provoke?
> **Porter:** Marry, sir, nose-painting [cutaneous vasodilation], sleep [CNS depression], and urine [a consequence of the inhibition of antidiuretic hormone (vasopressin) secretion, exacerbated by volume loading]. Lechery, sir, it provokes and unprovokes: it provokes the desire but it takes away the performance. Therefore much drink may be said to be an equivocator with lechery: it makes him and it mars him; it sets him on and it takes him off; it persuades him and disheartens him, makes him stand to and not stand to [the imagination desires what the corpus cavernosum cannot deliver]; in conclusion, equivocates him in a sleep, and, giving him the lie, leaves him.

More recent research has added details to Shakespeare's enumeration—*see* the bracketed additions to the Porter's words above and the section on organ systems below—but the most noticeable consequences of the recreational use of ethanol still are well summarized by the gregarious and garrulous Porter, whose delighted and devilish demeanor demonstrates a frequently observed influence of modest concentrations of ethanol on the CNS. The sections below detail ethanol's effects on physiological systems.

Central Nervous System

Although the public often views alcoholic drinks as stimulating, ethanol primarily is a CNS depressant. Ingestion of moderate amounts of ethanol, like that of other depressants such as barbiturates and benzodiazepines, can have anti-anxiety actions and produce behavioral disinhibition at a wide range of dosages. Individual signs of intoxication vary from expansive and vivacious affect to uncontrolled mood swings and emotional outbursts that may have violent components. With more severe intoxication, CNS function generally is impaired, and a condition of general anesthesia ultimately prevails. However, there is little margin between the anesthetic actions and lethal effects (usually owing to respiratory depression).

About 10% of alcohol drinkers progress to levels of consumption that are physically and socially detrimental. Chronic abuse is accompanied by tolerance, dependence, and craving for the drug (*see* below for a discussion of neuronal mechanisms; *see also* Chapter 23). Alcoholism is characterized by compulsive use despite clearly deleterious social and medical consequences. Alcoholism is a progressive illness, and brain damage from chronic alcohol abuse contributes to the deficits in cognitive functioning and judgment seen in alcoholics. Alcoholism is a leading cause of dementia in the United States (Oslin *et al.*, 1998). Chronic alcohol abuse results in shrinkage of the brain owing to loss of both white and gray matter (Kril and Halliday, 1999). The frontal lobes are particularly sensitive to damage by alcohol, and the extent of damage is determined by the amount and duration of alcohol consumption, with older alcoholics being more vulnerable than younger ones (Pfefferbaum *et al.*, 1998). It is important to note that ethanol itself is neurotoxic, and although malnutrition or vitamin deficiencies probably play roles in complications of alcoholism such as Wernicke's encephalopathy and Korsakoff's psychosis, most of the alcohol-induced brain damage in Western countries is due to alcohol itself. In addition to loss of brain tissue, alcohol abuse also reduces brain metabolism (as determined by positron-emission tomography), and this hypometabolic state rebounds to a level of increased metabolism during detoxification. The magnitude of decrease in metabolic state is determined by the number of years of alcohol use and the age of the patients (Volkow *et al.*, 1994; *see* "Mechanisms of CNS Actions" below).

Cardiovascular System

Serum Lipoproteins and Cardiovascular Effects. In most countries, the risk of mortality due to coronary heart disease (CHD) is correlated with a high dietary intake of saturated fat and elevated serum cholesterol levels. France is an exception to this rule, with relatively low mortality from CHD despite the consumption of high quantities of saturated fats by the French (the "French paradox"). Epidemiological studies suggest that widespread wine consumption (20 to 30 g ethanol per day) is one of the factors conferring a cardioprotective effect, with one to three drinks per day resulting in a 10% to 40% decreased risk of coronary heart disease compared with abstainers. In contrast, daily consumption of greater amounts of alcohol leads to an increased incidence of noncoronary causes of cardiovascular failure, such as arrhythmias, cardiomyopathy, and hemorrhagic stroke, offsetting the beneficial

effects of alcohol on coronary arteries; *i.e.,* alcohol has a J-shaped dose-mortality curve. Reduced risks for CHD are seen at intakes as low as one-half drink per day (Maclure, 1993). Young women and others at low risk for heart disease derive little benefit from light to moderate alcohol intake, whereas those of both sexes who are at high risk and who may have had a myocardial infarction clearly benefit. Data based on a number of prospective, cohort, cross-cultural, and case-control studies in diverse populations consistently reveal lower rates of angina pectoris, myocardial infarction, and peripheral artery disease in those consuming light (1 to 20 g/day) to moderate (21 to 40 g/day) amounts of alcohol.

One possible mechanism by which alcohol could reduce the risk of CHD is through its effects on blood lipids. Changes in plasma lipoprotein levels, particularly increases in high-density lipoprotein (HDL; *see* Chapter 35), have been associated with the protective effects of ethanol. HDL binds cholesterol and returns it to the liver for elimination or reprocessing, decreasing tissue cholesterol levels. Ethanol-induced increases in HDL-cholesterol thus could antagonize cholesterol accumulation in arterial walls, lessening the risk of infarction. Approximately half the risk reduction associated with ethanol consumption is explained by changes in total HDL levels (Langer *et al.*, 1992). HDL is found as two subfractions, named HDL_2 and HDL_3. Increased levels of HDL_2 (and possibly also HDL_3) are associated with reduced risk of myocardial infarction. Levels of both subfractions are increased following alcohol consumption (Gaziano *et al.*, 1993) and decrease when alcohol consumption ceases. Apolipoproteins A-I and A-II are constituents of HDL; some HDL particles contain only the former, whereas others are composed of both. Increased levels of both apolipoproteins A-I and A-II are associated with individuals who are daily heavy drinkers. In contrast, there are reports of decreased serum apolipoprotein(a) levels following acute alcohol consumption. Elevated apolipoprotein(a) levels have been associated with an increased risk for the development of atherosclerosis.

Although the cardioprotective effects of ethanol initially were noted in wine drinkers, all forms of alcoholic beverages confer cardioprotection. A variety of alcoholic beverages increase HDL levels while decreasing the risk of myocardial infarction. The flavonoids found in red wine (and purple grape juice) may have an additional antiatherogenic role by protecting low-density lipoprotein (LDL) from oxidative damage. Oxidized LDL has been implicated in several steps of atherogenesis (Hillbom *et al.*, 1998). Another way in which alcohol consumption conceivably could play a cardioprotective role is by altering factors involved in blood clotting. The formation of clots is an important step in the genesis of myocardial infarctions, and a number of factors maintain a balance between bleeding and clot dissolution. Alcohol consumption elevates the levels of tissue plasminogen activator, a clot-dissolving enzyme (Ridker *et al.*, 1994; *see* Chapter 54), decreasing the likelihood of clot formation. Decreased fibrinogen concentrations seen following ethanol consumption also could be cardioprotective (Rimm *et al.*, 1999), and epidemiological studies have linked the moderate consumption of ethanol to an inhibition of platelet activation (Rubin, 1999).

Should abstainers from alcohol be advised to consume ethanol in moderate amounts? The answer is *no*. There have been no randomized clinical trials to test the efficacy of daily alcohol use in reducing rates of coronary heart disease and mortality, and it is inappropriate for physicians to advocate alcohol ingestion solely to prevent heart disease. Many abstainers avoid alcohol because of a family history of alcoholism or for other health reasons, and it is imprudent to suggest that they begin drinking. Other lifestyle changes or medical treatments should be encouraged if patients are at risk for the development of CHD.

Hypertension. Heavy alcohol use can raise diastolic and systolic blood pressure (Klatsky, 1996). Studies indicate a positive, nonlinear association between alcohol use and hypertension that is unrelated to age, education, smoking status, or the use of oral contraceptives. Consumption above 30 g alcohol per day (more than two standard drinks) is associated with a 1.5 to 2.3 mm Hg rise in diastolic and systolic blood pressure. A time effect also has been demonstrated, with diastolic and systolic blood pressure elevation being greatest for persons who consumed alcohol within 24 hours of examination (Moreira *et al.*, 1998). Women may be at greater risk than men (Seppa *et al.*, 1996).

Several hypotheses have been proposed to explain the cause of alcohol-induced hypertension. One hypothesis holds that there is a direct pressor effect of alcohol caused by an unknown mechanism. Studies that have examined levels of renin, angiotensin, norepinephrine, antidiuretic hormone, cortisol, and other pressor mediators have been inconclusive. Newer hypotheses include increased intracellular Ca^{2+} levels with a subsequent increase in vascular reactivity, stimulation of the endothelium to release endothelin, and inhibition of endothelium-dependent NO production (Grogan and Kochar, 1994). Another hypothesis holds that there is an indirect effect. Some hypertensive alcoholic patients abstain before a physician visit (Iwase *et al.*, 1995), and as blood alcohol levels fall, acute withdrawal causes an elevation in blood pressure that is reflected in elevated blood pressure readings in the physician's office.

The prevalence of hypertension attributable to excess alcohol consumption is not known, but studies suggest a range of 5% to 11%. The prevalence probably is higher for men than for women because of higher alcohol consumption by men. A reduction in or cessation of alcohol use in heavy drinkers may reduce the need for antihypertensive medication or reduce the blood pressure to the normal range. A safe amount of alcohol consumption for hypertensive patients who are light drinkers (one to two drinks per occasion and less than 14 drinks per week) has not been determined. Factors to consider are a personal history of ischemic heart disease, a history of binge drinking, or a family history of alcoholism or of cerebrovascular accident. Hypertensive patients with any of these risk factors should abstain from alcohol use.

Cardiac Arrhythmias. Alcohol has a number of pharmacological effects on cardiac conduction, including prolongation of the QT interval, prolongation of ventricular repolarization, and sympathetic stimulation (Rossinen *et al.*, 1999; Kupari and Koskinen, 1998). Atrial arrhythmias associated with chronic alcohol use include supraventricular tachycardia, atrial fibrillation, and atrial flutter. Some 15% to 20% of idiopathic cases of atrial fibrillation may be induced by chronic ethanol use (Braunwald, 1997). Ventricular tachycardia may be responsible for the increased risk of unexplained sudden death that has been observed in persons who are alcohol-dependent (Kupari and Koskinen, 1998). During continued alcohol use, treatment of these arrhythmias may be more resistant to cardioversion, digoxin, or Ca^{2+} channel blocking agents (*see* Chapter 34). Patients with recurrent or refractory atrial arrhythmias should be questioned carefully about alcohol use.

Cardiomyopathy. Ethanol is known to have dose-related toxic effects on both skeletal and cardiac muscle. Numerous studies have shown that alcohol can depress cardiac contractility and lead to cardiomyopathy (Thomas *et al.*, 1994). Echocardiography demonstrates global hypokinesis. Fatty acid ethyl esters (formed from the enzymatic reaction of ethanol with free fatty acids) appear to play a role in the development of this disorder (Beckemeier and Bora, 1998). Approximately half of all patients with idiopathic cardiomyopathy are alcohol-dependent. Although the clinical signs and symptoms of idiopathic and alcohol-induced cardiomyopathy are similar, alcohol-induced cardiomyopathy has a better prognosis if patients are able to stop drinking. Women are at greater risk of alcohol-induced cardiomyopathy than are men (Urbano-Marquez *et al.*, 1995). Since 40% to 50% of persons with alcohol-induced cardiomyopathy who continue to drink die within 3 to 5 years, abstinence remains the primary treatment. Some patients respond to diuretics, angiotensin converting enzyme inhibitors, and vasodilators.

Stroke. Clinical studies indicate an increased incidence of hemorrhagic and ischemic stroke in persons who drink more than 40 to 60 g alcohol per day (Hansagi *et al.*, 1995). Many cases of stroke follow prolonged binge drinking, especially when stroke occurs in younger patients. Proposed etiological factors include alcohol-induced (1) cardiac arrhythmias and associated thrombus formation, (2) high blood pressure from chronic alcohol consumption and subsequent cerebral artery degeneration, (3) acute increases in systolic blood pressure and alterations in cerebral artery tone, and (4) head trauma. The effects on hemostasis, fibrinolysis, and blood clotting are variable and could prevent or precipitate acute stroke (Numminen *et al.*, 1996). The effects of alcohol on the formation of intracranial aneurysms are controversial, but the statistical association disappears when one controls for tobacco use and sex (Qureshi *et al.*, 1998).

Skeletal Muscle

Alcohol has a number of effects on skeletal muscle (Panzak *et al.*, 1998). Chronic, heavy, daily alcohol consumption is associated with decreased muscle strength, even when adjusted for other factors such as age, nicotine use, and chronic illness. Heavy doses of alcohol also can cause irreversible damage to muscle, reflected by a marked increase in the activity of creatine kinase in plasma. Muscle biopsies from heavy drinkers also reveal decreased glycogen stores and reduced pyruvate kinase activity (Vernet *et al.*, 1995). Approximately 50% of chronic heavy drinkers have evidence of type II fiber atrophy. These changes correlate with reductions in muscle protein synthesis and serum carnosinase activities (Wassif *et al.*, 1993). Most patients with chronic alcoholism show electromyographical changes, and many show evidence of a skeletal myopathy similar to alcoholic cardiomyopathy.

Body Temperature

Ingestion of ethanol causes a feeling of warmth because alcohol enhances cutaneous and gastric blood flow. Increased sweating also may occur. Heat, therefore, is lost more rapidly, and the internal body temperature falls. After consumption of large amounts of ethanol, the central temperature-regulating mechanism itself becomes depressed, and the fall in body temperature may become pronounced. The action of alcohol in lowering body temperature is greater and more dangerous when the ambient environmental temperature is low. Studies of deaths from hypothermia suggest that alcohol is a major risk factor in these events. Patients with ischemic limbs secondary to peripheral vascular disease are particularly susceptible to cold damage (Proano and Perbeck, 1994).

Diuresis

Alcohol inhibits the release of vasopressin (antidiuretic hormone; *see* Chapter 29) from the posterior pituitary gland, resulting in enhanced diuresis (Leppaluoto *et al.*, 1992). The volume loading that accompanies imbibing complements the diuresis that occurs as a result of reduced vasopressin secretion. Alcoholics have less urine output than do control subjects in response to a challenge dose with ethanol, suggesting that tolerance develops to the diuretic effects of ethanol (Collins *et al.*, 1992). Alcoholics withdrawing from alcohol exhibit increased vasopressin release and a consequent retention of water, as well as dilutional hyponatremia.

Gastrointestinal System

Esophagus. Alcohol frequently is either the primary etiologic factor or one of multiple causal factors associated with esophageal dysfunction. Ethanol also is associated with the development of esophageal reflux, Barrett's esophagus, traumatic rupture of the esophagus, Mallory-Weiss tears, and esophageal cancer. When compared with nonalcoholic nonsmokers, alcohol-dependent patients who smoke have a tenfold increased risk of developing cancer of the esophagus. There is little change in esophageal function at low blood alcohol concentrations, but at higher blood alcohol concentrations, a decrease in peristalsis and decreased lower esophageal sphincter pressure occur. Patients with chronic reflux esophagitis may respond to proton pump inhibitors (*see* Chapter 36) and abstinence from alcohol.

Stomach. Heavy alcohol use can disrupt the gastric mucosal barrier and cause acute and chronic gastritis. Ethanol appears to stimulate gastric secretions by exciting sensory nerves in the buccal and gastric mucosa and promoting the release of gastrin and histamine. Beverages containing more than 40% alcohol also have a direct toxic effect on gastric mucosa. While these effects are seen most often in chronic heavy drinkers, they can occur after moderate and short-term alcohol use. The diagnosis may not be clear because many patients have normal endoscopic examinations and upper gastrointestinal radiographs. Clinical symptoms include acute epigastric pain that is relieved with antacids or histamine H_2-receptor blockers (*see* Chapter 36).

Alcohol is not thought to play a role in the pathogenesis of peptic ulcer disease. Unlike acute and chronic gastritis, peptic ulcer disease is not more common in alcoholics. Nevertheless, alcohol exacerbates the clinical course and severity of ulcer symptoms. It appears to act synergistically with *Helicobacter pylori* to delay healing (Lieber, 1997a). Acute bleeding from the gastric mucosa, while uncommon, can be a life-threatening emergency. Upper gastrointestinal bleeding is associated more commonly with esophageal varices, traumatic rupture of the esophagus, and clotting abnormalities.

Intestines. Many alcoholics have chronic diarrhea as a result of malabsorption in the small intestine (Addolorato *et al.*, 1997). The major symptom is frequent loose stools. The rectal fissures and pruritus ani that frequently are associated with heavy drinking probably are related to chronic diarrhea. The diarrhea is caused by structural and functional changes in the small intestine (Papa *et al.*, 1998); the intestinal mucosa has flattened villi, and digestive enzyme levels often are decreased. These changes frequently are reversible after a period of abstinence. Treatment is based on replacing essential vitamins and electrolytes, slowing transit time with an agent such as loperamide (*see* Chapter 38), and abstaining from all alcoholic beverages. Patients with severe magnesium deficiencies (serum magnesium < 1 mEq/L) or symptomatic patients (a positive Chvostek's sign or asterixis) should receive 1 g magnesium sulfate intravenously or intramuscularly every 4 hours until the serum magnesium concentration is greater than 1 mEq/L (Sikkink and Fleming, 1992).

Pancreas. Heavy alcohol use is the most common cause of both acute and chronic pancreatitis in the United States. While pancreatitis has been known to occur after a single episode of heavy alcohol use, prolonged heavy drinking is common in most cases. Acute alcoholic pancreatitis is characterized by the abrupt onset of abdominal pain, nausea, vomiting, and increased levels of serum or urine pancreatic enzymes. Computed tomography is being used increasingly for diagnostic testing. While most attacks are not fatal, hemorrhagic pancreatitis can develop and lead to shock, renal failure, respiratory failure, and death. Management usually involves intravenous fluid replacement—often with nasogastric suction—and opioid pain medication. The etiology of acute pancreatitis probably is related to a direct toxic metabolic effect of alcohol on pancreatic acinar cells. Fatty acid esters and cytokines appear to play a major role (Schenker and Montalvo, 1998).

Two-thirds of patients with recurrent alcoholic pancreatitis will develop chronic pancreatitis. Chronic pancreatitis is treated by replacing the endocrine and exocrine deficiencies that result from pancreatic insufficiency. The development of hyperglycemia often requires insulin for control of blood-sugar levels. Pancreatic enzyme capsules containing lipase, amylase, and proteases may be necessary to treat malabsorption (*see* Chapter 37). The average lipase dose is 4000 to 24,000 units with each meal and snack. Many patients with chronic pancreatitis develop a chronic pain syndrome. While opioids may be helpful, non-narcotic methods for pain relief such as antiinflammatory drugs, tricyclic antidepressants, exercise, relaxation techniques, and self-hypnosis are preferred treatments for this population because cross-dependence to other drugs is common among alcoholics. In particular, for patients receiving chronic opioid therapy for chronic pancreatitis, treatment contracts and frequent assessments for signs of addiction are important.

Liver. Ethanol produces a constellation of dose-related deleterious effects in the liver (Fickert and Zatloukal, 2000). The primary effects are fatty infiltration of the liver, hepatitis, and cirrhosis. Because of its intrinsic toxicity, alcohol can injure the liver in the absence of dietary deficiencies (Lieber, 1994). The accumulation of fat in the liver is an early event and can occur in normal individuals after the ingestion of relatively small amounts of ethanol. This accumulation results from inhibition of both the tri-

carboxylic acid cycle and the oxidation of fat, in part, owing to the generation of excess NADH produced by the actions of ADH and ALDH (*see* Figure 22–1).

Fibrosis, resulting from tissue necrosis and chronic inflammation, is the underlying cause of alcoholic cirrhosis. Normal liver tissue is replaced by fibrous tissue. Alcohol can affect stellate cells in the liver directly; chronic alcohol use is associated with transformation of stellate cells into collagen-producing, myofibroblast-like cells (Lieber, 1998), resulting in deposition of collagen around terminal hepatic venules (Worner and Lieber, 1985). The histological hallmark of alcoholic cirrhosis is the formation of Mallory bodies, which are thought to be related to an altered cytokeratin intermediate cytoskeleton (Denk *et al.*, 2000).

A number of molecular mechanisms for alcoholic cirrhosis have been proposed. In nonhuman primate models, alcohol alters phospholipid peroxidation. Ethanol decreases phosphatidylcholine levels in hepatic mitochondria, a change associated with decreased oxidase activity and oxygen consumption (Lieber *et al.*, 1994a,b). Cytokines, such as transforming growth factor β and tumor necrosis factor α, can increase rates of fibrinogenesis and fibrosis in the liver (McClain *et al.*, 1993). Acetaldehyde is thought to have a number of adverse effects, including depletion of glutathione (Lieber, 2000), depletion of vitamins and trace metals, and decreased transport and secretion of proteins owing to inhibition of tubulin polymerization (Lieber, 1997b). *Acetaminophen*-induced hepatic toxicity (*see* Chapter 26) has been associated with alcoholic cirrhosis as a result of alcohol-induced increases in microsomal production of toxic acetaminophen metabolites (Whitcomb and Block, 1994). Liver failure secondary to cirrhosis and resulting in impaired clearance of toxins such as ammonia (*see* discussion of lactulose in Chapter 38) also may contribute to alcohol-induced hepatic encephalopathy. Ethanol also appears to increase intracellular free hydroxy-ethyl radical formation (Mantle and Preedy, 1999), and there is evidence that endotoxins may play a role in the initiation and exacerbation of alcohol-induced liver disease. Hepatitis C appears to be an important cofactor in the development of end-stage alcoholic liver disease (Regev and Jeffers, 1999).

Several strategies to treat alcoholic liver disease have been evaluated. *Prednisolone* may improve survival in patients with hepatic encephalopathy (Lieber, 1998). Nutrients such as *S-adenosylmethionine* and *polyunsaturated lecithin* have been found to have beneficial effects in nonhuman primates and are undergoing clinical trials. Other medications that have been tested include *oxandrolone, propylthiouracil* (Orrego *et al.*, 1987), and *colchicine* (Lieber, 1997b). At present, however, none of these drugs is approved for use in the United States for the treatment of alcoholic liver disease. The current primary treatment for liver failure is transplantation in conjunction with abstinence from ethanol. Long-term outcome studies suggest that patients who are alcohol-dependent have survival rates similar to those of patients with other types of liver disease. Alcoholics with hepatitis C may respond to interferon-2α (McCullough and O'Connor, 1998) (*see* Chapter 52).

Vitamins and Minerals

The almost complete lack of protein, vitamins, and most other nutrients in alcoholic beverages predisposes those who consume large quantities of alcohol to nutritional deficiencies. Alcoholics often present with these deficiencies owing to decreased intake, decreased absorption, or impaired utilization of nutrients. The peripheral neuropathy, Korsakoff's psychosis, and Wernicke's encephalopathy seen in alcoholics probably are caused by deficiencies of the B complex of vitamins (particularly thiamine), although direct toxicity produced by alcohol itself has not been ruled out (Harper, 1998). Chronic alcohol abuse decreases the dietary intake of retinoids and carotenoids and enhances the metabolism of retinol by the induction of degradative enzymes (Leo and Lieber, 1999). Retinol and ethanol compete for metabolism by ADH; vitamin A supplementation therefore should be monitored carefully in alcoholics when they are consuming alcohol to avoid retinol-induced hepatotoxicity. The chronic consumption of alcohol inflicts an oxidative stress on the liver owing to the generation of free radicals, contributing to ethanol-induced liver injury. The antioxidant effects of α-tocopherol (vitamin E) may ameliorate some of this ethanol-induced toxicity in the liver (Nordmann, 1994). Plasma levels of α-tocopherol often are reduced in myopathic alcoholics compared with alcoholic patients without myopathy.

Chronic alcohol consumption has been implicated in osteoporosis (*see* Chapter 61). The reasons for this decreased bone mass remain unclear, although impaired osteoblastic activity has been implicated. Acute administration of ethanol produces an initial reduction in serum parathyroid hormone (PTH) and Ca^{2+} levels, followed by a rebound increase in PTH that does not restore Ca^{2+} levels to normal. The hypocalcemia observed after chronic alcohol intake also appears to be unrelated to effects of alcohol on PTH levels, and alcohol likely inhibits bone remodeling by a mechanism independent of Ca^{2+}-regulating hormones (Sampson, 1997). Vitamin D also may play a role. Since vitamin D requires hydroxylation in the liver for activation, alcohol-induced liver damage can indirectly affect the role of vitamin D in the intestinal and renal absorption of Ca^{2+}.

Alcoholics tend to have lowered serum and brain levels of magnesium, which may contribute to their predisposition to brain injuries such as stroke (Altura and Altura, 1999). Deficits in intracellular magnesium levels may disturb cytoplasmic and mitochondrial bioenergetic pathways, potentially leading to calcium overload and ischemia. Although there is general agreement that total magnesium levels are decreased in alcoholics, it is less clear that this also applies to ionized Mg^{2+}, the physiologically active form (Hristova *et al.*, 1997). Magnesium sulfate sometimes is used in the treatment of alcohol with-

drawal, but its efficacy has been questioned (Erstad and Cotugno, 1995).

Sexual Function

Despite the widespread belief that alcohol can enhance sexual activities, the opposite effect is noted more often. Many drugs of abuse, including alcohol, have disinhibiting effects that may lead initially to increased libido. With excessive, long-term use, however, alcohol often leads to a deterioration of sexual function. While alcohol cessation may reverse many sexual problems, patients with significant gonadal atrophy are less likely to respond to discontinuation of alcohol consumption (Sikkink and Fleming, 1992).

Both acute and chronic alcohol use can lead to impotence in men. Increased blood alcohol concentrations lead to decreased sexual arousal, increased ejaculatory latency, and decreased orgasmic pleasure. The incidence of impotence may be as high as 50% in patients with chronic alcoholism. Additionally, many chronic alcoholics develop testicular atrophy and decreased fertility. The mechanism involved in this is complex and likely involves altered hypothalamic function and a direct toxic effect of alcohol on Leydig cells. Testosterone levels may be depressed, but many men who are alcohol-dependent have normal testosterone and estrogen levels. Gynecomastia is associated with alcoholic liver disease and is related to increased cellular response to estrogen and to accelerated metabolism of testosterone.

Sexual function in alcohol-dependent women is less clearly understood. Many female alcoholics complain of decreased libido, decreased vaginal lubrication, and menstrual cycle abnormalities. Their ovaries often are small and without follicular development. Some data suggest that fertility rates are lower for alcoholic women. The presence of comorbid disorders such as anorexia nervosa or bulimia can aggravate the problem. The prognosis for men and women who become abstinent is favorable in the absence of significant hepatic or gonadal failure (O'Farrell *et al.*, 1997).

Hematological and Immunological Effects

Chronic alcohol use is associated with a number of anemias. Microcytic anemia can occur because of chronic blood loss and iron deficiency. Macrocytic anemias and increases in mean corpuscular volume are common and may occur in the absence of vitamin deficiencies. Normochromic anemias also can occur owing to effects of chronic illness on hematopoiesis. In the presence of severe liver disease, morphological changes can include the development of burr cells, schistocytes, and ringed sideroblasts. Alcohol-induced sideroblastic anemia may respond to vitamin B_6 replacement (Wartenberg, 1998). Alcohol use also is associated with reversible thrombocytopenia, although platelet counts under 20,000/mm^3 are rare. Bleeding is uncommon unless there is an alteration in vitamin K_1–dependent clotting factors (*see* Chapter

Tolerance and Dependence

Tolerance is defined as a reduced behavioral or physiological response to the same dose of ethanol (*see* Chapter 23). There is a marked acute tolerance that is detectable soon after administration of ethanol. Acute tolerance can be demonstrated by measuring behavioral impairment at the same BALs on the ascending limb of the absorption phase of the BAL–time curve (minutes after ingestion of alcohol) and on the descending limb of the curve as BALs are lowered by metabolism (one or more hours after ingestion). Behavioral impairment and subjective feelings of intoxication are much greater at a given BAL on the ascending than on the descending limb. There also is a chronic tolerance that develops in the long-term heavy drinker. In contrast to acute tolerance, chronic tolerance often has a metabolic component owing to induction of alcohol-metabolizing enzymes.

Physical dependence is demonstrated by the elicitation of a withdrawal syndrome when alcohol consumption is terminated. The symptoms and severity are determined by the amount and duration of alcohol consumption and include sleep disruption, autonomic nervous system (sympathetic) activation, tremors, and in severe cases, seizures. In addition, two or more days after withdrawal, some individuals experience *delirium tremens,* characterized by hallucinations, delirium, fever, and tachycardia. Delirium tremens can be fatal. Another aspect of dependence is craving and drug-seeking behavior, often termed *psychological dependence.*

Ethanol tolerance and physical dependence are studied readily in animal models. Strains of mice with genetic differences in tolerance and dependence have been characterized, and a search for the relevant genes is under way (Crabbe, 2002). Neurobiological mechanisms of tolerance and dependence are not understood completely, but chronic alcohol consumption results in changes in synaptic and intracellular signaling likely owing to changes in gene expression. Most of the systems that are acutely affected by ethanol also are affected by chronic exposure, resulting in an adaptive or maladaptive response that can cause tolerance and dependence. In particular, chronic actions of ethanol likely require changes in signaling by glutamate and GABA receptors and intracellular systems such as PKC (Diamond and Gordon, 1997). There is an increase in NMDA-receptor function after chronic alcohol ingestion that may contribute to the CNS hyperexcitability and neurotoxicity seen during ethanol withdrawal (Chandler *et al.*, 1998). Arginine vasopressin, acting on V_1 receptors, maintains tolerance to ethanol in laboratory animals even after chronic ethanol administration has ceased (Hoffman *et al.*, 1990).

The neurobiological basis of the switch from controlled, volitional alcohol use to compulsive and uncontrolled addiction remains obscure. Impairment of the dopaminergic reward system and the resulting increase in alcohol consumption in an attempt to regain activation of the system is a possibility. In addition, the prefrontal cortex is particularly sensitive to damage from alcohol abuse and influences decision making and emotion, processes clearly compromised in the alcoholic (Pfefferbaum *et al.*, 1998). Thus, impairment of executive function in cortical regions by chronic alcohol consumption may be responsible for some of the lack of judgment and control that is expressed as obsessive alcohol consumption. The loss of brain volume and impairment of function seen in the chronic alcoholic is at least partially reversible by abstinence but will worsen with continued drinking (Pfefferbaum *et al.*, 1998). Early diagnosis and treatment of alcoholism are important in limiting the brain damage that promotes the progression to severe addiction.

Genetic Influences

The concept of alcoholism as a disease was first articulated by Jellinek in 1960; the subsequent acceptance of alcoholism and addiction as "brain diseases" led to a search for biological causes. Studies of rats and mice carried out in Chile, Finland, and the United States showed significant heritabilities (roughly 60%) for many behavioral actions of alcohol, including sedation, ataxia, and most notably, consumption (Crabbe, 2002). It has long been appreciated that alcoholism "runs in families"; a series of adoption (cross-fostering) and twin studies showed that human alcohol dependence does, indeed, have a genetic component. Although the genetic contribution varies among studies, it generally is in the range of 40% to 60%, which means that environmental variables also are critical for individual susceptibility to alcoholism.

The search for the genes and alleles responsible for alcoholism is complicated by the polygenetic nature of the disease and the general difficulty in defining multiple genes responsible for complex diseases. One fruitful area of research has been the study of why some populations (mainly Asian) are protected from alcoholism. This has been attributed to genetic differences in alcohol- and aldehyde-metabolizing enzymes. Specifically, genetic variants of ADH that exhibit high activity and variants of ALDH that exhibit low activity protect against heavy drinking. This is so because alcohol consumption by individuals who have these variants results in accumulation of acetaldehyde, which produces a variety of unpleasant effects (Li, 2000). These effects are similar to those of disulfiram therapy (*see* below), but the prophylactic, genetic form of inhibition of alcohol consumption is more effective than the pharmacotherapeutic approach, which is applied after alcoholism has developed.

In contrast to these protective genetic variants, there are little consistent data about genes responsible for increased risk for alcoholism. Several large-scale genetic studies of alcoholism currently are in progress, and these efforts, together with genetic studies in laboratory animals, may lead to identification of genes influencing susceptibility to alcoholism. These studies also may allow genetic classification of subtypes of alcoholism and thereby resolve some of the inconsistencies among study populations. For example, antisocial alcoholism is linked with a polymorphism in a serotonin receptor (5-HT$_{1B}$), but there is no association of this gene with non-antisocial alcoholism (Lappalainen *et al.*, 1998).

Another approach to understanding the inherited biology of alcoholism is to ask what behavioral or functional differences exist between individuals with high and low genetic risks for alcoholism.

This may be accomplished by studying young social drinkers with many or few alcoholic relatives [family history–positive (FHP) and family history–negative (FHN)]. Brain imaging by positron-emission tomography has been used in this context. A family history of alcoholism is linked to lower cerebellar metabolism and a blunted effect of a benzodiazepine (lorazepam) on cerebellar metabolism (Volkow *et al.*, 1995). Because GABA$_A$ receptors are the molecular site of benzodiazepine action, these results suggest that a genetic predisposition to alcoholism may be reflected in abnormal GABA$_A$ receptor function.

Schuckit and colleagues have studied actions of alcohol in FHP college students and have followed the study subjects for almost 20 years to determine which ones will develop alcoholism or alcohol abuse. Remarkably, a blunted behavioral and physiological response to alcohol in the original test is associated with a significantly greater risk for later development of alcohol-related problems (Schuckit and Smith, 2000). Studies with twins indicate a common genetic vulnerability for alcohol and nicotine dependence (True *et al.*, 1999), which is consistent with the high rate of smoking among alcoholics.

TERATOGENIC EFFECTS: FETAL ALCOHOL SYNDROME

In 1968, French researchers noted that children born to alcoholic mothers displayed a common pattern of distinct dysmorphology that later came to be known as *fetal alcohol syndrome* (FAS) (Lemoine *et al.*, 1968; Jones and Smith, 1973). The diagnosis of FAS typically is based on the observance of a triad of abnormalities in the newborn, including (1) a cluster of craniofacial abnormalities, (2) CNS dysfunction, and (3) pre- and/or postnatal stunting of growth. Hearing, language, and speech disorders also may become evident as the child ages (Church and Kaltenbach, 1997). Children who do not meet all the criteria for a diagnosis of FAS still may show physical and mental deficits consistent with a partial phenotype, termed *fetal alcohol effects* (FAEs) or *alcohol-related neurodevelopmental disorders*. The incidence of FAS is believed to be in the range of 0.5 to 1 per 1000 live births in the general U.S. population, with rates as high as 2 to 3 per 1000 in African-American and Native-American populations. A lower socioeconomic status of the mother rather than racial background *per se* appears to be primarily responsible for the higher incidence of FAS observed in those groups (Abel, 1995). The incidence of FAEs is likely higher than that of FAS, making alcohol consumption during pregnancy a major public health problem.

Craniofacial abnormalities commonly observed in the diagnosis of FAS consist of a pattern of microcephaly, a long and smooth philtrum, shortened palpebral fissures, a flat midface, and epicanthal folds. Magnetic resonance imaging studies demonstrate decreased volumes in the basal ganglia, corpus callosum, cerebrum, and cerebellum (Mattson *et*

al., 1992). The severity of alcohol effects can vary greatly and depends on the drinking patterns and amount of alcohol consumed by the mother. Maternal drinking in the first trimester has been associated with craniofacial abnormalities; facial dysmorphology also is seen in mice exposed to ethanol at the equivalent time in gestation.

CNS dysfunction following *in utero* exposure to alcohol manifests in the form of hyperactivity, attention deficits, mental retardation, and learning disabilities. FAS is the most common cause of preventable mental retardation in the Western world (Abel and Sokol, 1987), with afflicted children consistently scoring lower than their peers on a variety of IQ tests. It now is clear that FAS represents the severe end of a spectrum of alcohol effects. A number of studies have documented intellectual deficits, including mental retardation, in children not displaying the craniofacial deformities or retarded growth seen in FAS. Although cognitive improvements are seen with time, decreased IQ scores of FAS children tend to persist as they mature, indicating that the deleterious prenatal effects of alcohol are irreversible. Although a correlation exists between the amount of alcohol consumed by the mother and infant scores on mental and motor performance tests, there is considerable variation in performance on such tests among children of mothers consuming similar quantities of alcohol. The peak BAL reached may be a critical factor in determining the severity of deficits seen in the offspring. Although the evidence is not conclusive, there is a suggestion that even moderate alcohol consumption (two drinks per day) in the second trimester of pregnancy is correlated with impaired academic performance of offspring at age 6 (Goldschmidt *et al.*, 1996). Maternal age also may be a factor. Pregnant women over age 30 who drink alcohol create greater risks to their children than do younger women who consume similar amounts of alcohol (Jacobson *et al.*, 1996).

Children exposed prenatally to alcohol most frequently present with attentional deficits and hyperactivity, even in the absence of intellectual deficits or craniofacial abnormalities. Furthermore, attentional problems have been observed in the absence of hyperactivity, suggesting that the two phenomena are not necessarily related. Fetal alcohol exposure also has been identified as a risk factor for alcohol abuse by adolescents (Baer *et al.*, 1998). Apart from the risk of FAS or FAEs to the child, the intake of high amounts of alcohol by a pregnant woman, particularly during the first trimester, greatly increases the chances of spontaneous abortion.

Studies with laboratory animals have demonstrated many of the consequences of *in utero* exposure to ethanol observed in human beings, including hyperactivity, motor dysfunction, and learning deficits. In animals, *in utero* exposure to ethanol alters the expression patterns of a wide variety of proteins, changes neuronal migration patterns, and results in brain region–specific and cell type–specific alterations in neuronal numbers. Indeed, specific periods of vulnerability may exist for particular neuronal populations in the brain. Genetics also may play a role in determining vulnerability to ethanol: There are differences among strains of rats in susceptibility to the prenatal effects of ethanol. Finally, multidrug abuse, such as the concomitant administration of cocaine with ethanol, enhances fetal damage and mortality.

PHARMACOTHERAPY OF ALCOHOLISM

Currently, three drugs are approved in the United States for treatment of alcoholism: *disulfiram* (ANTABUSE), *nal-*

trexone (REVIA), and *acamprosate*. Disulfiram has a long history of use but has fallen into disfavor because of its side effects and problems with patient adherence to therapy. Naltrexone and acamprosate were introduced more recently. The goal of these medications is to assist the patient in maintaining abstinence.

Naltrexone

Naltrexone was approved by the FDA for treatment of alcoholism in 1994. It is chemically related to the highly selective opioid-receptor antagonist *naloxone* (NARCAN) but has higher oral bioavailability and a longer duration of action. Neither drug has appreciable opioid-receptor agonist effects. These drugs were used initially in the treatment of opioid overdose and dependence because of their ability to antagonize all the actions of opioids (*see* Chapters 21 and 23). Animal research and clinical experience suggested that naltrexone might reduce alcohol consumption and craving; this was confirmed in clinical trials (*see* O'Malley *et al.*, 2000; Johnson and Ait-Daoud, 2000). There is evidence that naltrexone blocks activation by alcohol of dopaminergic pathways in the brain that are thought to be critical to reward.

Naltrexone helps to maintain abstinence by reducing the urge to drink and increasing control when a "slip" occurs. It is not a "cure" for alcoholism and does not prevent relapse in all patients. Naltrexone works best when used in conjunction with some form of psychosocial therapy, such as cognitive behavioral therapy (Anton *et al.*, 1999). It typically is administered after detoxification and given at a dose of 50 mg/day for several months. Adherence to the regimen is important to ensure the therapeutic value of naltrexone and has proven to be a problem for some patients (Johnson and Ait-Daoud, 2000). The most common side effect of naltrexone is nausea, which is more common in women than in men and subsides if the patients abstain from alcohol (O'Malley *et al.*, 2000). When given in excessive doses, naltrexone can cause liver damage. It is contraindicated in patients with liver failure or acute hepatitis and should be used only after careful consideration in patients with active liver disease.

Nalmefene (REVEX) is another opioid antagonist that appears promising in preliminary clinical tests (Mason *et al.*, 1999). It has a number of advantages over naltrexone, including greater oral bioavailability, longer duration of action, and lack of dose-dependent liver toxicity.

Disulfiram

Disulfiram (tetraethylthiuram disulfide; ANTABUSE) was taken in the course of an investigation of its potential anthelminthic efficacy by two Danish physicians, who became ill at a cocktail party and were quick to realize that the compound had altered their responses to alcohol. They initiated a series of pharmacological and clinical studies that provided the basis for the use of disulfiram as an adjunct in the treatment of chronic alcoholism. Similar responses to alcohol ingestion are produced by various congeners of disulfiram, namely, *cyanamide,* the fungus *Coprinus atramentarius,* the hypoglycemic *sulfonylureas, metronidazole,* certain *cephalosporins,* and animal charcoal.

Disulfiram, given alone, is a relatively nontoxic substance, but it inhibits ALDH activity and causes the blood acetaldehyde concentration to rise to 5 to 10 times above the level achieved when ethanol is given to an individual not pretreated with disulfiram. Acetaldehyde, produced as a result of the oxidation of ethanol by ADH, ordinarily does not accumulate in the body because it is further oxidized almost as soon as it is formed primarily by ALDH. Following the administration of disulfiram, both cytosolic and mitochondrial forms of ALDH are irreversibly inactivated to varying degrees, and the concentration of acetaldehyde rises. It is unlikely that disulfiram itself is responsible for the enzyme inactivation *in vivo;* several active metabolites of the drug, especially diethylthiomethylcarbamate, behave as suicide-substrate inhibitors of ALDH *in vitro.* These metabolites reach significant concentrations in plasma following the administration of disulfiram (Johansson, 1992).

The ingestion of alcohol by individuals previously treated with disulfiram gives rise to marked signs and symptoms of acetaldehyde poisoning. Within 5 to 10 minutes, the face feels hot and soon afterward becomes flushed and scarlet in appearance. As the vasodilation spreads over the whole body, intense throbbing is felt in the head and neck, and a pulsating headache may develop. Respiratory difficulties, nausea, copious vomiting, sweating, thirst, chest pain, considerable hypotension, orthostatic syncope, marked uneasiness, weakness, vertigo, blurred vision, and confusion are observed. The facial flush is replaced by pallor, and the blood pressure may fall to shock levels.

Alarming reactions may result from the ingestion of even small amounts of alcohol in persons being treated with disulfiram. The use of disulfiram as a therapeutic agent thus is not without danger, and it should be attempted only under careful medical and nursing supervision. Patients must be warned that as long as they are taking disulfiram, the ingestion of alcohol in any form will make them sick and may endanger their lives. Patients must learn to avoid disguised forms of alcohol, as in sauces, fermented vinegar, cough syrups, and even after-shave lotions and back rubs.

The drug never should be administered until the patient has abstained from alcohol for at least 12 hours. In the initial phase of treatment, a maximal daily dose of 500 mg is given for 1 to 2 weeks. Maintenance dosage then ranges from 125 to 500 mg daily depending on tolerance to side effects. Unless sedation is prominent, the daily dose should be taken in the morning, the time when the resolve not to drink may be strongest. Sensitization to alcohol may last as long as 14 days after the last ingestion of disulfiram because of the slow rate of restoration of ALDH (Johansson, 1992).

Disulfiram and/or its metabolites can inhibit many enzymes with crucial sulfhydryl groups, and it thus has a wide spectrum of biological effects. It inhibits hepatic CYPs and thereby interferes with the metabolism of *phenytoin, chlordiazepoxide, barbiturates, warfarin,* and other drugs.

Disulfiram by itself usually is innocuous, but it may cause acneform eruptions, urticaria, lassitude, tremor, restlessness, headache, dizziness, a garlic-like or metallic taste, and mild GI disturbances. Peripheral neuropathies, psychosis, and ketosis also have been reported.

Acamprosate

Acamprosate (*N*-acetylhomotaurine, calcium salt), an analogue of GABA, is used widely in Europe for the treatment of alcoholism and was approved recently for use in the United States. A number of double-blind, placebo-controlled studies have demonstrated that acamprosate decreases drinking frequency and reduces relapse drinking in abstinent alcoholics. It acts in a dose-dependent manner (1.3 to 2 g/day) (Paille *et al.*, 1995) and appears to have efficacy similar to that of naltrexone. Studies in laboratory animals have shown that acamprosate decreases alcohol intake without affecting food or water consumption. Acamprosate generally is well tolerated by patients, with diarrhea being the main side effect (Garbutt *et al.*, 1999). No abuse liability has been noted. The drug undergoes minimal metabolism in the liver, is excreted primarily by the kidneys, and has an elimination half-life of 18 hours after oral administration (Wilde and Wagstaff, 1997). Concomitant use of disulfiram appears to increase the effectiveness of acamprosate, without any adverse drug interactions being noted (Besson *et al.*, 1998). The mechanism of action of acamprosate is obscure, although there is some evidence that it modulates the function of NMDA receptors in brain (Johnson and Ait-Daoud, 2000).

Other Agents

Ondansetron, a 5-HT$_3$-receptor antagonist and antiemetic drug (*see* Chapters 11 and 37), reduces alcohol consumption in laboratory animals and currently is being tested in humans. Preliminary findings suggest that ondansetron is effective in the treatment of early-onset alcoholics, who respond poorly to psychosocial treatment alone, although the drug does not appear to work well in other types of alcoholics (Johnson and Ait-Daoud, 2000). Ondansetron administration lowers the amount of alcohol consumed, particularly by drinkers who consume fewer than 10 drinks per day (Sellers *et al.*, 1994). It also decreases the subjective effects of ethanol on 6 of 10 scales measured, including the desire to drink (Johnson *et al.*, 1993), while at the same time not having any effect on the pharmacokinetics of ethanol.

Topiramate, a drug used for treating seizure disorders (*see* Chapter 19), appears useful for treating alcohol dependence. Compared with the placebo group, patients taking topiramate achieved more abstinent days and a lower craving for alcohol (Johnson *et al.*, 2003). The mechanism of action of topiramate is not well understood but is distinct from that of other drugs used for the treatment of dependence (*e.g.,* opioid antagonists), suggesting that it may provide a new and unique approach to pharmacotherapy of alcoholism.

BIBLIOGRAPHY

Addolorato, G., Montalto, M., Capristo, E., *et al.* Influence of alcohol on gastrointestinal motility: Lactulose breath hydrogen testing in orocecal transit time in chronic alcoholics, social drinkers, and teetotaler subjects. *Hepatogastroenterology,* **1997,** *44*:1076–1081.

Anders, D.L., Blevins, T., Sutton, G., *et al.* Fyn tyrosine kinase reduces the ethanol inhibition of recombinant NR1/NR2A but not NR1/NR2B NMDA receptors expressed in HEK 293 cells. *J. Neurochem.,* **1999,** *72*:1389–1393.

Anton, R.F., Moak, D.H., Waid, L.R., *et al.* Naltrexone and cognitive behavioral therapy for the treatment of outpatient alcoholics: Results of a placebo-controlled trial. *Am. J. Psychiatry,* **1999,** *156*:1758–1764.

Baer, J.S., Barr, H.M., Bookstein, F.L., *et al.* Prenatal alcohol exposure

and family history of alcoholism in the etiology of adolescent alcohol problems. *J. Stud. Alcohol.,* **1998,** *59*:533–543.

Beckemeier, M.E., and Bora, P.S. Fatty acid ethyl esters: Potentially toxic products of myocardial ethanol metabolism. *J. Mol. Cell. Cardiol.,* **1998,** *30*:2487–2494.

Besson, J., Aeby, F., Kasas, A., *et al.* Combined efficacy of acamprosate and disulfiram in the treatment of alcoholism: A controlled study. *Alcohol. Clin. Exp. Res.,* **1998,** *22*:573–579.

Carta, M., Ariwodola, O.J., Weiner, J.L., and Valenzuela, C.F. Alcohol potently inhibits the kainite receptor-dependent excitatory drive of hippocampal interneurons. *Proc. Natl. Acad. Sci. U.S.A.,* **2003,** *100*:6813–6818.

Collins, G.B., Brosnihan, K.B., Zuti, R.A., *et al.* Neuroendocrine, fluid balance, and thirst responses to alcohol in alcoholics. *Alcohol. Clin. Exp. Res.,* **1992,** *16*:228–233.

Constantinescu, A., Diamond, I., and Gordon, A.S. Ethanol-induced translocation of cAMP-dependent protein kinase to the nucleus: Mechanism and functional consequences. *J. Biol. Chem.,* **1999,** *274*:26985–26991.

Crabbe, J.C. Alcohol and genetics: New models. *Am. J. Med. Genet.,* **2002,** *114*:969–974.

Davies, A.G., Pierce-Shimomura, J.T., Kim, H., *et al.* A central role of the BK potassium channel in behavioral responses to ethanol in C. elegans. *Cell,* **2003,** 115:655–666.

Denk, H., Stumptner, C., and Zatloukal, K. Mallory bodies revisited. *J. Hepatol.,* **2000,** *32*:689–702.

Gaziano, J.M., Buring, J.E., Breslow, J.L., *et al.* Moderate alcohol intake, increased levels of high-density lipoprotein and its subfractions, and decreased risk of myocardial infarction. *New Engl. J. Med.,* **1993,** *329*:1829–1834.

Goldschmidt, L., Richardson, G.A., Stoffer, D.S., *et al.* Prenatal alcohol exposure and academic achievement at age six: A nonlinear fit. *Alcohol. Clin. Exp. Res.,* **1996,** *20*:763–770.

Hansagi, H., Romelsjo, A., Gerhardsson de Verdier, M., *et al.* Alcohol consumption and stroke mortality: 20-year follow-up of 15,077 men and women. *Stroke,* **1995,** *26*:1768–1773.

Harris, R.A., McQuilkin, S.J., Paylor, R., *et al.* Mutant mice lacking the γ isoform of protein kinase C show decreased behavioral actions of ethanol and altered function of γ-aminobutyrate type A receptors. *Proc. Natl. Acad. Sci. U.S.A.,* **1995,** *92*:3658–3662.

Hristova, E.N., Rehak, N.N., Cecco, S., *et al.* Serum ionized magnesium in chronic alcoholism: is it really decreased? *Clin. Chem.,* **1997,** *43*:394–399.

Iwase, S., Matsukawa, T., Ishihara, S., *et al.* Effect of oral ethanol intake on muscle sympathetic nerve activity and cardiovascular functions in humans. *J. Auton. Nerv. Syst.,* **1995,** *54*:206–214.

Jacobson, J.L., Jacobson, S.W., and Sokol, R.J. Increased vulnerability to alcohol-related birth defects in the offspring of mothers over 30. *Alcohol. Clin. Exp. Res.,* **1996,** *20*:359–363.

Johnson, B.A., and Ait-Daoud, N. Neuropharmacological treatments for alcoholism: Scientific basis and clinical findings. *Psychopharmacology (Berl.),* **2000,** *149*:327–344.

Johnson, B.A., Ait-Daoud, N., Bowden, C.L., *et al.* Oral topiramate for treatment of alcohol dependence: A randomized, controlled trial. *Lancet,* **2003,** *361*:1677–1685.

Johnson, B.A., Campling, G.M., Griffiths, P., and Cowen, P.J. Attenuation of some alcohol-induced mood changes and the desire to drink by 5-HT$_3$ receptor blockade: A preliminary study in healthy male volunteers. *Psychopharmacology (Berl.),* **1993,** *112*:142–144.

Jones, K.L., and Smith, D.W. Recognition of the fetal alcohol syndrome in early infancy. *Lancet,* **1973,** 2:999–1001.

Langer, R.D., Criqui, M.H., and Reed, D.M. Lipoproteins and blood pressure as biological pathways for effect of moderate alcohol consumption on coronary heart disease. *Circulation,* **1992,** *85*:910–915.

Lappalainen, J., Long, J.C., Eggert, M., *et al.* Linkage of antisocial alcoholism to the serotonin 5-HT$_{1B}$ receptor gene in two populations. *Arch. Gen. Psychiatry,* **1998,** *55*:989–994.

Lemoine, P., Harousseau, H., Borteyru, J.P., and Menuet, J.C. Les enfants de perents alcooliques: Anomalies observees. A propos de 127 cas. *Quest Medicale,* **1968,** *25*:476–482.

Leppaluoto, J., Vuolteenaho, O., Arjamaa, O., and Ruskoaho, H. Plasma immunoreactive atrial natriuretic peptide and vasopressin after ethanol intake in man. *Acta. Physiol. Scand.,* **1992,** *144*:121–127.

Lewohl, J.M., Wilson, W.R., Mayfield, R.D., *et al.* G protein–coupled inwardly rectifying potassium channels are targets of alcohol action. *Nature Neurosci.,* **1999,** *2*:1084–1090.

Lieber, C.S., Robins, S.J., and Leo, M.A. Hepatic phosphatidyl-ethanolamine methyltransferase activity is decreased by ethanol and increased by phosphatidylcholine. *Alcohol. Clin. Exp. Res.,* **1994a,** *18*:592–595.

Lieber, C.S., Robins, S.J., Li, J., *et al.* Phosphatidylcholine protects against fibrosis and cirrhosis in the baboon. *Gastroenterology,* **1994b,** *106*:152–159.

Mason, B.J., Salvato, F.R., Williams, L.D., *et al.* A double-blind, placebo-controlled study of oral nalmefene for alcohol dependence. *Arch. Gen. Psychiatry,* **1999,** *56*:719–724.

Mattson, S.N., Riley, E.P., Jernigan, T.L., *et al.* Fetal alcohol syndrome: A case report of neuropsychological, MRI, and EEG assessment of two children. *Alcohol. Clin. Exp. Res.,* **1992,** *16*:1001–1003.

McCullough, A.J., and O'Connor, J.F. Alcoholic liver disease: proposed recommendations for the American College of Gastroenterology. *Am. J. Gastroenterol.,* **1998,** *93*:2022–2036.

Menninger, J.A., Baron, A.E., and Tabakoff, B. Effects of abstinence and family history for alcoholism on platelet adenylyl cyclase activity. *Alcohol. Clin. Exp. Res.,* **1998,** *22*:1955–1961.

Moreira, L.B., Fuchs, F.D., Moraes, R.S., *et al.* Alcohol intake and blood pressure: The importance of time elapsed since last drink. *J. Hypertens.,* **1998,** *16*:175–180.

Numminen, H., Hillborn, M., and Juvela, S. Platelets, alcohol consumption, and onset of brain infarction. *J. Neurol. Neurosurg. Psychiatry,* **1996,** *61*:376–380.

O'Farrell, T.J., Choquette, K.A., Cutter, H.S., and Birchler, G.R. Sexual satisfaction and dysfunction in marriages of male alcoholics: Comparison with nonalcoholic maritally conflicted and nonconflicted couples. *J. Stud. Alcohol,* **1997,** *58*:91–99.

O'Malley, S.S., Krishnan-Sarin, S., Farren, C., and O'Connor, P.G. Naltrexone-induced nausea in patients treated for alcohol dependence: Clinical predictors and evidence for opioid-mediated effects. *J. Clin. Psychopharmacol.,* **2000,** *20*:69–76.

Orrego, H., Blake, J.E., Blendis, L.M., *et al.* Long-term treatment of alcoholic liver disease with propylthiouracil. *New Engl. J. Med.,* **1987,** *317*:1421–1427.

Paille, F.M., Guelfi, J.D., Perkins, A.C., *et al.* Double-blind, randomized multicentre trial of acamprosate in maintaining abstinence from alcohol. *Alcohol.,* **1995,** *30*:239–247.

Panzak, G., Tarter, R., Murali, S., *et al.* Isometric muscle strength in alcoholic and nonalcoholic liver-transplantation candidates. *Am. J. Drug Alcohol Abuse,* **1998,** *24*:449–512.

Papa, A., Tursi, A., Cammarota, G., *et al.* Effect of moderate and heavy alcohol consumption on intestinal transit time. *Panminerva Med.,* **1998,** *40*:183–185.

Pfefferbaum, A., Sullivan, E.V., Rosenbloom, M.J., *et al.* A controlled study of cortical gray matter and ventricular changes in alcoholic men over a 5-year interval. *Arch. Gen. Psychiatry,* **1998,** *55*:905–912.

Proano, E., and Perbeck, L. Effect of exposure to heat and intake of ethanol on the skin circulation and temperature in ischemic limbs. *Clin. Physiol.,* **1994,** *14*:305–310.

Qureshi, A.I., Suarez, J.I., Parekh, P.D., *et al.* Risk factors for multiple intracranial aneurysms. *Neurosurgery,* **1998,** *43*:22–26.

Ridker, P.M., Vaughan, D.E., Stampfer, M.J., *et al.* Association of moderate alcohol consumption and plasma concentration of endogenous tissue-type plasminogen activator. *JAMA,* **1994,** *272*:929–933.

Rimm, E.B., Williams, P., Fosher, K., *et al.* Moderate alcohol intake and lower risk of coronary heart disease: Meta-analysis of effects on lipids and haematostatic factors. *BMJ,* **1999,** *319*:1523–1528.

Rossinen, J., Sinisalo, J., Partanen, J., *et al.* Effects of acute alcohol infusion on duration and dispersion of QT interval in male patients with coronary artery disease and in healthy controls. *Clin. Cardiol.,* **1999,** *22*:591–594.

Schuckit, M.A. and Smith, T.L. The relationships of a family history of alcohol dependence, a low level of response to alcohol and six domains of life functioning to the development of alcohol use disorders. *J. Stud. Alcohol,* **2000,** *61*:827–835.

Sellers, E.M., Toneatto, T., Romach, M.K., *et al.* Clinical efficacy of the 5-HT$_3$ antagonist ondansetron in alcohol abuse and dependence. *Alcohol. Clin. Exp. Res.,* **1994,** *18*:879–885.

Seppa, K., Laippala, P., and Sillanaukee, P. High diastolic blood pressure: Common among women who are heavy drinkers. *Alcohol. Clin. Exp. Res.,* **1996,** *20*:47–51.

Smith, B.R., Horan, J.T., Gaskin, S., and Amit, Z. Exposure to nicotine enhances acquisition of ethanol drinking by laboratory rats in a limited access paradigm. *Psychopharmacology (Berl.),* **1999,** *142*:408–412.

Solem, M., McMahon, T., and Messing, R.O. Protein kinase A regulates inhibition of N- and P/Q-type calcium channels by ethanol in PC12 cells. *J. Pharmacol. Exp. Ther.,* **1997,** *282*:1487–1495.

Trudell, J.R., and Harris, R.A. Are sobriety and consciousness determined by water in protein cavities? *Alcohol Clin. Exp. Res.,* **2004,** *28*:1–3.

True, W.R., Xian, H., Scherrer, J.F., *et al.* Common genetic vulnerability for nicotine and alcohol dependence in men. *Arch. Gen. Psychiatry,* **1999,** *56*:655–661.

Urbano-Marquez, A., Estruch, R., Fernandez-Sola, J., *et al.* The greater risk of alcoholic cardiomyopathy and myopathy in women compared with men. *JAMA,* **1995,** *274*:149–154.

Vernet, M., Cadefau, J.A., Balaque, A., *et al.* Effect of chronic alcoholism on human muscle glycogen and glucose metabolism. *Alcohol. Clin. Exp. Res.,* **1995,** *19*:1295–1299.

Volkow, N.D., Wang, G.J., Begleiter, H., *et al.* Regional brain metabolic response to lorazepam in subjects at risk for alcoholism. *Alcohol. Clin. Exp. Res.,* **1995,** *19*:510–516.

Volkow, N.D., Wang, G.J., Hitzemann, R., *et al.* Recovery of brain glucose metabolism in detoxified alcoholics. *Am. J. Psychiatry,* **1994,** *151*:178–183.

Wallner, M., Hanchar, H.J., and Olsen, R.W. Ethanol enhances $a_4b_3\delta$ and $a_6b_3\delta$ γ-aminobutyric acid type A receptors at low concentrations known to affect humans. *Proc. Natl. Acad. Sci. U.S.A.,* **2003,** *100*:15218–15223.

Wassif, W.S., Preedy, V.R., Summers, B., *et al.* The relationship between muscle fibre atrophy factor, plasma carnosinase activities, and muscle RNA and protein composition in chronic alcoholic myopathy. *Alcohol Alcohol.,* **1993,** *28*:325–331.

Whitcomb, D.C., and Block, G.D. Association of acetaminophen hepatotoxicity with fasting and ethanol use. *JAMA,* **1994,** *272*:1845–1850.

Worner, T.M., and Lieber, C.S. Perivenular fibrosis as precursor lesion of cirrhosis. *JAMA,* **1985,** *254*:627–630.

MONOGRAPHS AND REVIEWS

Abel, E.L. An update on incidence of FAS: FAS is not an equal opportunity birth defect. *Neurotoxicol. Teratol.,* **1995,** *17*:437–443.

Abel, E.L., and Sokol, R.J. Incidence of fetal alcohol syndrome and economic impact of FAS-related anomalies. *Drug Alcohol Depend.,* **1987,** *19*:51–70.

Altura, B.M., and Altura, B.T. Association of alcohol in brain injury, headaches, and stroke with brain tissue and serum levels of ionized magnesium: A review of recent findings and mechanisms of action. *Alcohol,* **1999,** *19*:119–130.

Braunwald, E., ed. *Heart Disease: A Textbook of Cardiovascular Medicine,* 5th ed. Saunders, Philadelphia, **1997.**

Chandler, L.J., Harris, R.A., and Crews, F.T. Ethanol tolerance and synaptic plasticity. *Trends Pharmacol. Sci.,* **1998,** *19*:491–495.

Church, M.W., and Kaltenbach, J.A. Hearing, speech, language, and vestibular disorders in the fetal alcohol syndrome: A literature review. *Alcohol. Clin. Exp. Res.,* **1997,** *21*:495–512.

Diamond, I., and Gordon, A.S. Cellular and molecular neuroscience of alcoholism. *Physiol. Rev.,* **1997,** *77*:1–20.

Dopico, A.M., Chu, B., Lemos, J.R., and Treistman, S.N. Alcohol modulation of calcium-activated potassium channels. *Neurochem. Int.,* **1999,** *35*:103–106.

Dudley, R. Evolutionary origins of human alcoholism in primate frugivory. *Q. Rev. Biol.,* **2000,** *75*:3–15.

Erstad, B.L., and Cotugno, C.L. Management of alcohol withdrawal. *Am. J. Health Syst. Pharm.,* **1995,** *52*:697–709.

Fickert, P., and Zatloukal, K. Pathogenesis of alcoholic liver disease. In, *Handbook of Alcoholism.* (Zernig, G., Saria, A., Kurz, M., and O'Malley, S., eds.) CRC Press, Boca Raton, FL., **2000,** pp. 317–323.

Garbutt, J.C., West, S.L., Carey, T.S., *et al.* Pharmacological treatment of alcohol dependence: A review of the evidence. *JAMA,* **1999,** *281*:1318–1325.

Grogan, J.R., and Kochar, M.S. Alcohol and hypertension. *Arch. Fam. Med.,* **1994,** *3*:150–154.

Harper, C. The neuropathology of alcohol-specific brain damage, or does alcohol damage the brain? *J. Neuropathol. Exp. Neurol.,* **1998,** *57*:101–110.

Hillbom, M., Juvela, S., and Karttunen, V. Mechanisms of alcohol-related strokes, In, *Alcohol and Cardiovascular Diseases.* (Goode, J., ed.) Wiley, New York, **1998,** p. 193.

Hoffman, P.L., Ishizawa, H., Giri, P.R., *et al.* The role of arginine vasopressin in alcohol tolerance. *Ann. Med.,* **1990,** *22*:269–274.

Johansson, B. A review of the pharmacokinetics and pharmacodynamics of disulfiram and its metabolites. *Acta Psychiatr. Scand. Suppl.,* **1992,** *369*:15–26.

Klatsky, A.L. Alcohol, coronary disease, and hypertension. *Annu. Rev. Med.,* **1996,** *47*:149–160.

Kril, J.J., and Halliday, G.M. Brain shrinkage in alcoholics: A decade on and what have we learned? *Prog. Neurobiol.,* **1999,** *58*:381–387.

Kumar, S., Fleming, R.L., and Morrow, A.L. Ethanol regulation of aminobutyric acid$_A$ receptors: Genomic and nongenomic mechanisms. *Pharmacol. Ther.,* **2004,** *101*:211–226.

Kupari, M., and Koskinen, P. Alcohol, cardiac arrhythmias, and sudden death. In, *Alcohol and Cardiovascular Diseases.* (Goode, J., ed.) Wiley, New York, **1998,** p. 68.

Leo, M.A., and Lieber, C.S. Alcohol, vitamin A, and beta-carotene: Adverse interactions, including hepatotoxicity and carcinogenicity. *Am. J. Clin. Nutr.,* **1999,** *69*:1071–1085.

Li, T.K. Pharmacogenetics of responses to alcohol and genes that influence alcohol drinking. *J. Stud. Alcohol,* **2000,** *61*:5–12.

Lieber, C.S. Alcohol and the liver: Metabolism of alcohol and its role in hepatic and extrahepatic diseases. *Mt. Sinai J. Med.,* **2000,** *67*:84–94.

Lieber, C.S. Alcohol and the liver: 1994 update. *Gastroenterology,* **1994,** *106*:1085–1105.

Lieber, C.S. Gastric ethanol metabolism and gastritis: Interactions with other drugs, *Helicobacter pylori,* and antibiotic therapy (1957–1997): A review. *Alcohol. Clin. Exp. Res.,* **1997a,** *21*:1360–1366.

Lieber, C.S. Hepatic and other medical disorders of alcoholism: From pathogenesis to treatment. *J. Stud. Alcohol.,* **1998,** *59*:9–25.

Lieber, C.S. Pathogenesis and treatment of liver fibrosis in alcoholics: 1996 update. *Dig. Dis.,* **1997b,** *15*:42–66.

Maclure, M. Demonstration of deductive meta-analysis: Ethanol intake and risk of myocardial infarction. *Epidemiol Rev.,* **1993,** *15*:328–351.

Mantle, D., and Preedy, V.R. Free radicals as mediators of alcohol toxicity. *Adverse Drug React. Toxicol. Rev.,* **1999,** *18*:235–252.

McClain, C., Hill, D., Schmidt, J., and Diehl, A.M. Cytokines and alcoholic liver disease. *Semin. Liver Dis.,* **1993,** *13*:170–182.

Mehta, A.K., and Ticku, M.K. An update on GABA$_A$ receptors. *Brain Res. Brain Res. Rev.,* **1999,** *29*:196–217.

Mihic, S.J. Acute effects of ethanol on GABA$_A$ and glycine receptor function. *Neurochem. Int.,* **1999,** *35*:115–123.

Narahashi, T., Aistrup, G.L., Marszalec, W., and Nagata, K. Neuronal nicotinic acetylcholine receptors: A new target site of ethanol. *Neurochem. Int.,* **1999,** *35*:131–141.

Nordmann, R. Alcohol and antioxidant systems. *Alcohol.,* **1994,** *29*:513–522.

Oslin, D., Atkinson, R.M., Smith, D.M., and Hendrie, H. Alcohol-related dementia: Proposed clinical criteria. *Int. J. Geriatr. Psychiatry,* **1998,** *13*:203–212.

Regev, A., and Jeffers, L.J. Hepatitis C and alcohol. *Alcohol. Clin. Exp. Res.,* **1999,** *23*:1543–1551.

Rubin, R. Effect of ethanol on platelet function. *Alcohol. Clin. Exp. Res.,* **1999,** *23*:1114–1118.

Sampson, H.W. Alcohol, osteoporosis, and bone regulating hormones. *Alcohol. Clin. Exp. Res.,* **1997,** *21*:400–403.

Schenker, S., and Montalvo, R. Alcohol and the pancreas. *Recent Dev. Alcohol.,* **1998,** *14*:41–65.

Schirmer, M., Widerman, C., and Konwalinka, G. Immune system. In, *Handbook of Alcoholism.* (Zernig, G., Saria, A., Kurz, M., and O'Malley, S., eds.) CRC Press, Boca Raton, FL, **2000,** pp. 225–230.

Schuckit, M.A. *Drug and Alcohol Abuse: Clinical Guide to Diagnosis and Treatment,* 4th ed. Plenum Press, New York, **1995.**

Sikkink, J., and Fleming, M. Health effects of alcohol. In, *Addictive Disorders.* (Fleming, M.F., and Barry, K.L., eds.) Mosby–Year Book, St. Louis, **1992,** pp. 172–203.

Spies, C.D., and Rommelspacher, H. Alcohol withdrawal in the surgical patient: prevention and treatment. *Anesth. Analg.,* **1999,** *88*:946–954.

Tabakoff, B., and Hoffman, P.L. Adenylyl cyclases and alcohol. *Adv. Second Messenger Phosphoprotein Res.,* **1998,** *32*:173–193.

Thomas, A.P., Rozanski, D.J., Renard, D.C., and Rubin, E. Effects of ethanol on the contractile function of the heart: A review. *Alcohol. Clin. Exp. Res.,* **1994,** *18*:121–131.

Valenzuela, C.F., and Harris, R.A. Alcohol: Neurobiology. In, *Substance Abuse: A Comprehensive Textbook.* (Lowinson, J.H., Ruiz, P., Millman, R.B., Langrod, J.B., eds.) Williams & Wilkins, Baltimore, **1997,** pp. 119–142.

Wartenberg, A.A. Management of common medical problems. In, *Principles of Addiction Medicine,* 2d ed. (Graham, A.W. and Shultz, T.K., eds.) American Society of Addiction Medicine, Chevy Chase, MD, **1998,** pp. 731–740.

Wilde, M.I., and Wagstaff, A.J. Acamprosate: A review of its pharmacology and clinical potential in the management of alcohol dependence after detoxification. *Drugs,* **1997,** *53*:1038–1053.

DRUG ADDICTION AND DRUG ABUSE

Charles P. O'Brien

DRUG DEPENDENCE

There are many misunderstandings about the origins and even the definitions of drug abuse and addiction. Although many physicians are concerned about "creating addicts," relatively few individuals begin their drug addiction problems by misuse of prescription drugs. Confusion exists because the correct use of prescribed medications for pain, anxiety, and even hypertension commonly produces tolerance and physical dependence. These are *normal* physiological adaptations to repeated use of drugs from many different categories. Tolerance and physical dependence are explained in more detail later, but it must be emphasized that they *do not* imply abuse or addiction. This distinction is important because patients with pain sometimes are deprived of adequate opioid medication simply because they have shown evidence of tolerance or they exhibit withdrawal symptoms if the analgesic medication is stopped abruptly.

Definitions. Abuse and addiction have been defined and redefined by several organizations over the past 35 years. The reason for these revisions and disagreements is that abuse and addiction are behavioral syndromes that exist along a continuum from minimal use to abuse to addictive use. While tolerance and physical dependence are biological phenomena that can be defined precisely in the laboratory and diagnosed accurately in the clinic, there is an arbitrary aspect to the definitions of the overall behavioral syndromes of abuse and addiction. The most influential system of diagnosis for mental disorders is that published by the American Psychiatric Association (APA; *DSM IV*, 1994). The APA diagnostic system uses the term *substance dependence* instead of "addiction" for the overall behavioral syndrome. It also applies the same general criteria to all types of drugs regardless of their pharmacological class. Although accepted widely, this terminology can lead to confusion between *physical dependence* and *psychological dependence*. The term *addiction,* when used here, refers to compulsive drug use, the entire substance-dependence syndrome as defined in *DSM IV*. This should not be confused with physical dependence alone, a common error among physicians. *Addiction* is not used as a pejorative term but rather for clarity of communication.

The APA defines *substance dependence* (addiction) as a cluster of symptoms indicating that the individual continues use of the substance despite significant substance-related problems. Evidence of tolerance and withdrawal symptoms are included in the list of symptoms, but neither tolerance nor withdrawal is necessary or sufficient for a diagnosis of substance dependence. Dependence (addiction) requires three or more of the symptoms, whereas abuse can be diagnosed when only one or two symptoms are present. The chronic, relapsing nature of dependence (addiction) fulfills criteria for a chronic disease (McLellan *et al.*, 2000), but because of the voluntary component at initiation, the disease concept is controversial.

Origins of Substance Dependence. Many variables operate simultaneously to influence the likelihood that a given person will become a drug abuser or an addict. These variables can be organized into three categories: agent (drug), host (user), and environment (Table 23–1).

Agent (Drug) Variables. Drugs vary in their capacity to produce immediate good feelings in the user. Drugs that reliably produce intensely pleasant feelings (euphoria) are more likely to be taken repeatedly. *Reinforcement* refers to the capacity of drugs to produce effects that make the user wish to take them again. The more strongly reinforcing a drug is, the greater is the likelihood that the drug will be abused. Reinforcing properties of a drug can

Table 23–1
Multiple Simultaneous Variables Affecting Onset and Continuation of Drug Abuse and Addiction

---

Agent (drug)
Availability
Cost
Purity/potency
Mode of administration
  Chewing (absorption *via* oral mucous membranes)
  Gastrointestinal
  Intranasal
  Subcutaneous and intramuscular
  Intravenous
  Inhalation
  Speed of onset and termination of effects (pharmacokinetics: combination of agent and host)
Host (user)
Heredity
  Innate tolerance
  Speed of developing acquired tolerance
  Likelihood of experiencing intoxication as pleasure
Metabolism of the drug (nicotine and alcohol data already available)
Psychiatric symptoms
Prior experiences/expectations
Propensity for risk-taking behavior
Environment
Social setting
Community attitudes
  Peer influence, role models
Availability of other reinforcers (sources of pleasure or recreation)
Employment or educational opportunities
Conditioned stimuli: Environmental cues become associated with drugs after repeated use in the same environment

---

be measured reliably in animals. Generally, animals such as rats or monkeys equipped with intravenous catheters connected to lever-regulated pumps will work to obtain injections of the same drugs in roughly the same order of potency that human beings will. Thus, medications can be screened for their potential for abuse in human beings by the use of animal models.

Reinforcing properties of drugs are associated with their capacity to increase neuronal activity in critical brain areas (*see* Chapter 12). Cocaine, amphetamine, ethanol, opioids, cannabinoids, and nicotine all reliably increase extracellular fluid dopamine levels in the ventral striatum, specifically the nucleus accumbens region. In experimental animals, usually rats, brain microdialysis permits sampling of extracellular fluid while the animals are freely moving or receiving drugs. Smaller increases in dopamine in the nucleus accumbens also are observed when the rat is presented with sweet foods or a sexual partner. In contrast, drugs that block dopamine receptors generally produce bad feelings, *i.e.*, dysphoric effects. Neither animals nor human beings will take such drugs spontaneously. Despite strong correlative findings, a causal relationship between dopamine and euphoria/dysphoria has not been established, and other findings emphasize additional roles of serotonin, glutamine, norepinephrine, opiates, and γ-aminobutyric acid (GABA) in mediating the reinforcing effects of drugs.

The abuse liability of a drug is enhanced by rapidity of onset because effects that occur soon after administration are more likely to initiate the chain of events that leads to loss of control over drug taking. The pharmacokinetic variables that influence the time it takes the drug to reach critical receptor sites in the brain are explained in more detail in Chapter 1. The history of cocaine use illustrates the changes in abuse liability of the same compound, depending on the form and the route of administration.

When coca leaves are chewed, the cocaine is absorbed slowly through the buccal mucosa. This method produces low cocaine blood levels and correspondingly low levels in the brain. The mild stimulant effects produced by the chewing of coca leaves have a gradual onset, and this practice has produced little, if any, abuse or dependence despite use over thousands of years by natives of the Andes mountains. Beginning in the late 19th century, scientists isolated cocaine hydrochloride from coca leaves, and the extraction of pure cocaine became possible. Cocaine could be taken in higher doses by oral ingestion (GI absorption) or by absorption through the nasal mucosa, producing higher cocaine levels in the blood and a more rapid onset of stimulation. Subsequently, it was found that a solution of cocaine hydrochloride could be administered intravenously, giving a more rapid onset of stimulatory effects. Each newly available cocaine preparation that provided greater speed of onset and an increment in blood level was paralleled by a greater likelihood to produce addiction. In the 1980s, the availability of cocaine to the American public was increased further with the invention of crack cocaine. *Crack*, sold at a very low, albeit illegal, price ($1 to $3 per dose), is alkaloidal cocaine (free base), which can be readily vaporized by heating. Simply inhaling the vapors produces blood levels comparable with those resulting from intravenous cocaine owing to the large surface area for absorption into the pulmonary circulation following inhalation. The cocaine-containing blood then enters the left side of the heart and reaches the cerebral circulation without dilution by the systemic circulation. Inhalation of crack cocaine thus is much more likely to produce addiction than is chewing, drinking, or sniffing cocaine. This delivery method, with rapid drug brain levels, also is the preferred route for users of nicotine and cannabis.

Although the drug variables are important, they do not fully explain the development of abuse and addiction. Most people who experiment with drugs that have a high risk of producing addiction (addiction liability) do not intensify their drug use and lose control. The risk for

Table 23–2
Dependence among Users 1990–1992

AGENT	EVER USED* %	ADDICTION %	RISK OF ADDICTION %
Tobacco	75.6	24.1	31.9
Alcohol	91.5	14.1	15.4
Illicit drugs	51.0	7.5	14.7
Cannabis	46.3	4.2	9.1
Cocaine	16.2	2.7	16.7
Stimulants	15.3	1.7	11.2
Anxiolytics	12.7	1.2	9.2
Analgesics	9.7	0.7	7.5
Psychedelics	10.6	0.5	4.9
Heroin	1.5	0.4	23.1
Inhalants	6.8	0.3	3.7

*The ever-used and addiction percentages are those of the general population. The risk of addiction is specific to the drug indicated and refers to the percentage who met criteria for addiction among those who reported having used the agent at least once.
SOURCE: Anthony *et al.*, 1994, with permission.

developing addiction among those who try nicotine is about twice that for those who try cocaine (Table 23–2), but this does not imply that the pharmacological addiction liability of nicotine is twice that of cocaine. Rather, there are other variables listed in the categories of host factors and environmental conditions that influence the development of addiction.

Host (User) Variables. In general, effects of drugs vary among individuals. Even blood levels can show wide variation when the same dose of a drug on a milligram per kilogram basis is given to different people. Polymorphism of genes that encode enzymes involved in absorption, metabolism, and excretion and in receptor-mediated responses may contribute to the different degrees of reinforcement or euphoria observed among individuals (*see* Chapters 3 and 4).

Children of alcoholics show an increased likelihood of developing alcoholism, even when adopted at birth and raised by nonalcoholic parents. The studies of genetic influences in this disorder show only an *increased risk* for developing alcoholism, not a 100% determinism, consistent with a polygenic disorder that has multiple determinants. Even identical twins, who share the same genetic endowment, do not have 100% concordance when one twin is alcoholic. However, the concordance rate for identical twins is much higher than that for fraternal twins. The abuse of alcohol and other drugs tends to have some familial characteristics, suggesting that common mechanisms may be involved.

Innate tolerance to alcohol may represent a biological trait that contributes to the development of alcoholism. Data from a longitudinal study (Wilhelmsen *et al.*, 2003) show that sons of alcoholics have reduced sensitivity to alcohol when compared with other young men of the same age (22 years old) and drinking histories. Sensitivity to alcohol was measured as the effects of two different doses of ethanol in the laboratory on motor performance and subjective feelings of intoxication. When the men were re-examined 10 years later, those who had been most tolerant (insensitive) to alcohol at age 22 were the most likely to be diagnosed as alcohol dependent at age 32. The presence of tolerance predicted the development of alcoholism even in the group without a family history of alcoholism, but there were far fewer tolerant men in the negative-family-history group.

While innate tolerance increases vulnerability to alcoholism, impaired metabolism may *protect* against it. Ethanol is metabolized by sequential oxidation to acetaldehyde (by alcohol dehydrogenase) and then to acetic acid by aldehyde dehydrogenase (ALDH2) (*see* Figure 22–1). A common mutation in the ALDH2 gene results in a less effective enzyme. This allele has a high frequency in Asian populations and results in excess accumulation of acetaldehyde after the ingestion of alcohol. Those who are heterozygous for this allele experience a very unpleasant facial flushing reaction 5 to 10 minutes after ingesting alcohol; the reaction is more severe in individuals homozygous for the allele, and this genotype has not been found in alcoholics (Higuchi *et al.*, 1996). Similarly, individuals who inherit a gene associated with slow nicotine metabolism may experience unpleasant effects when beginning to smoke and reportedly have a lower probability of becoming nicotine dependent.

Psychiatric disorders constitute another category of host variables. Drugs may produce immediate, subjective effects that relieve preexisting symptoms. People with anxiety, depression, insomnia, or even subtle symptoms such as shyness may find, on experimentation or by accident, that certain drugs give them relief. However, the apparent beneficial effects are transient, and repeated use of the drug may lead to tolerance and eventually compulsive, uncontrolled drug use. While psychiatric symptoms are commonly seen in drug abusers presenting for treatment, most of these symptoms begin *after* the person starts abusing drugs. Thus, drugs of abuse appear to produce more psychiatric symptoms than they relieve.

Environmental Variables. Initiating and continuing illegal drug use appear to be influenced significantly by societal norms and peer pressure. Taking drugs may be seen initially as a form of rebellion against authority. In some communities, drug users and drug dealers are role models who seem to be successful and respected; thus, young people emulate them. There also may be a paucity of other options for pleasure, diversion, or income. These factors are particularly important in communities where educational levels are low and job opportunities scarce.

Pharmacological Phenomena. **Tolerance.** While abuse and addiction are complex conditions combining the many variables outlined earlier, there are a number of relevant pharmacological phenomena that occur independently of social and psychological dimensions. First are the changes in the way the body responds to a drug with repeated use. *Tolerance,* the most common response to

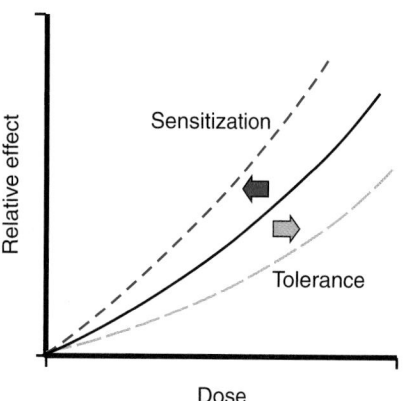

***Figure 23–1. Shifts in a dose–response curve with toler-
ance and sensitization.*** With tolerance, there is a shift of the
curve to the right such that doses higher than initial doses are
required to achieve the same effects. With sensitization, there is
a leftward shift of the dose–response curve such that for a given
dose, there is a greater effect than seen after the initial dose.

repetitive use of the same drug, can be defined as the
reduction in response to the drug after repeated administrations. Figure 23–1 shows an idealized dose–response
curve for an administered drug. As the dose of the drug
increases, the observed effect of the drug increases. With
repeated use of the drug, however, the curve shifts to the
right (tolerance). Thus a higher dose is required to produce the same effect that was once obtained at a lower
dose. *Diazepam,* for example, typically produces sedation
at doses of 5 to 10 mg in a first-time user, but those who
repeatedly use it to produce a kind of "high" may become
tolerant to doses of several hundreds of milligrams; some
abusers have had documented tolerance to more than
1000 mg/day. As outlined in Table 23–3, there are many
forms of tolerance likely arising *via* multiple mechanisms.

Table 23–3
Types of Tolerance

Innate (pre-existing sensitivity or insensitivity)
Acquired
  Pharmacokinetic (dispositional or metabolic)
  Pharmacodynamic
  Learned tolerance
    Behavioral
    Conditioned
  Acute tolerance
  Reverse tolerance (sensitization)
  Cross-tolerance

Tolerance develops to some drug effects much more rapidly than
to other effects of the same drug. For example, tolerance develops
rapidly to the euphoria produced by opioids such as heroin, and
addicts tend to increase their dose in order to re-experience that elusive "high." In contrast, tolerance to the gastrointestinal effects of
opiates develops more slowly. The discrepancy between tolerance to
euphorigenic effects (rapid) and tolerance to effects on vital functions (slow), such as respiration and blood pressure, can lead to
potentially fatal accidents in sedative abusers.

Innate tolerance refers to genetically determined sensitivity (or
lack of sensitivity) to a drug that is observed the first time that the
drug is administered. Innate tolerance was discussed earlier as a host
variable that influences the development of abuse or addiction.

Acquired tolerance can be divided into three major types: pharmacokinetic, pharmacodynamic, and learned tolerance, and includes
acute, reverse, and cross-tolerance (Table 23–3).

Pharmacokinetic, or dispositional, tolerance refers to changes in
the distribution or metabolism of a drug after repeated administrations such that a given dose produces a lower blood concentration
than the same dose did on initial exposure (*see* Chapter 1). The most
common mechanism is an increase in the rate of metabolism of the
drug. For example, *barbiturates* stimulate the production of higher
levels of hepatic CYPs, causing more rapid removal and breakdown
of barbiturates from the circulation. Since the same enzymes metabolize many other drugs, they too are metabolized more quickly. This
results in a decrease in their plasma levels as well and thus a reduction in their effects.

Pharmacodynamic tolerance refers to adaptive changes that have
taken place within systems affected by the drug so that response to a
given concentration of the drug is reduced. Examples include
drug-induced changes in receptor density or efficiency of receptor
coupling to signal-transduction pathways (*see* Chapters 1 and 12).

Learned tolerance refers to a reduction in the effects of a drug
owing to compensatory mechanisms that are acquired by past experiences. One type of learned tolerance is called *behavioral tolerance.* This simply describes the skills that can be developed through
repeated experiences with attempting to function despite a state of
mild to moderate intoxication. A common example is learning to
walk a straight line despite the motor impairment produced by alcohol intoxication. This probably involves both acquisition of motor
skills and the learned awareness of one's deficit, causing the person
to walk more carefully. At higher levels of intoxication, behavioral
tolerance is overcome, and the deficits are obvious.

Conditioned tolerance (situation-specific tolerance) develops
when environmental cues such as sights, smells, or situations consistently are paired with the administration of a drug. When a drug
affects homeostatic balance by producing sedation and changes in
blood pressure, pulse rate, gut activity, etc., there is usually a reflexive counteraction or adaptation in the direction of maintaining the
status quo. If a drug always is taken in the presence of specific environmental cues (*e.g.,* smell of drug preparation and sight of
syringe), these cues begin to predict the effects of the drug, and the
adaptations begin to occur even before the drug reaches its sites of
action. If the drug always is preceded by the same cues, the adaptive
response to the drug will be learned, and this will prevent the full
manifestation of the drug's effects (tolerance). This mechanism of
conditioned tolerance production follows classical (pavlovian) principles of learning and results in drug tolerance under circumstances
where the drug is "expected." When the drug is received under
novel or "unexpected" circumstances, conditioned tolerance does
not occur, and drug effects are enhanced.

The term *acute tolerance* refers to rapid tolerance developing with repeated use on a single occasion, such as in a "binge." For example, cocaine often is used in a binge, with repeated doses over one to several hours, sometimes longer, producing a decrease in response to subsequent doses of cocaine during the binge. This is the opposite of *sensitization,* observed with an intermittent dosing schedule, described below.

Sensitization. With stimulants such as cocaine or amphetamine, *reverse tolerance,* or *sensitization,* can occur. This refers to an increase in response with repetition of the same dose of the drug. Sensitization results in a shift to the left of the dose–response curve (Figure 23–1). For example, with repeated daily administration to rats of a dose of cocaine that produces increased motor activity, the effect increases over several days, even though the dose remains constant. A conditioned response also can be a part of sensitization to cocaine. Simply putting a rat into a cage where cocaine is expected or giving a placebo injection after several days of receiving cocaine under the same circumstances produces an increase in motor activity as though cocaine actually were given, *i.e.,* a conditioned response. Sensitization, in contrast to acute tolerance during a binge, requires a longer interval between doses, usually about 1 day.

Sensitization has been studied in rats equipped with microdialysis cannulas for monitoring extracellular dopamine (Kalivas and Duffy, 1990) (Figure 23–2). The initial response to 10 mg/kg of cocaine administered intraperitoneally is an increase in measured dopamine levels. After seven daily injections, the dopamine increase is significantly greater than on the first day, and the behavioral response also is greater. Figure 23–2 also provides an example of a conditioned response (learned drug effect) because injection of saline produced both an increase in dopamine levels and an increase in behavioral activity when administered 3 days after cocaine injections had stopped. Little research on sensitization has been conducted in human subjects, but the results suggest that the phenomenon can occur. It has been postulated that stimulant psychosis results from a sensitized response after long periods of use.

Cross-tolerance occurs when repeated use of a drug in a given category confers tolerance not only to that drug but also to other drugs in the same structural and mechanistic category. Understanding cross-tolerance is important in the medical management of persons dependent on any drug. *Detoxification* is a form of treatment for drug dependence that involves giving gradually decreasing doses of the drug to prevent withdrawal symptoms, thereby weaning the patient from the drug of dependence (*see* below). Detoxification can be accomplished with any medication in the same category as the initial drug of dependence. For example, users of heroin also are tolerant to other opioids. Thus, the detoxification of heroin-dependent patients can be accomplished with any medication that activates opiate receptors.

Physical Dependence

Physical dependence is a *state* that develops as a result of the adaptation (tolerance) produced by a resetting of homeostatic mechanisms in response to repeated drug use. Drugs can affect numerous systems that previously were in equilibrium; these systems find a new balance in the presence of inhibition or stimulation by a specific drug. A person in this adapted or physically dependent state

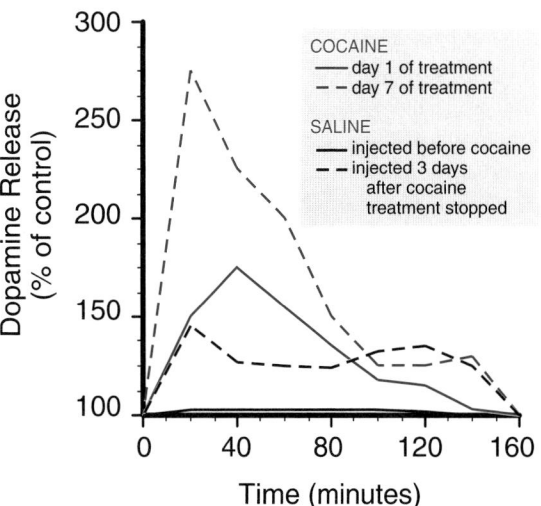

Figure 23–2. *Changes in dopamine detected in the extracellular fluid of the nucleus accumbens of rats after daily injections of cocaine (10 mg/kg, i.p.).* The first injection of cocaine produces a modest increase and the last, after 7 days, produces a much greater increase in dopamine release. The first saline injection produces no effect on dopamine levels, whereas the second, given 3 days after 7 days of cocaine injections, produces a significant rise in dopamine, presumably due to conditioning. (Adapted from Kalivas and Duffy, 1990, with permission.)

requires continued administration of the drug to maintain normal function. If administration of the drug is stopped abruptly, there is another imbalance, and the affected systems again must go through a process of readjusting to a new equilibrium without the drug.

Withdrawal Syndrome. The appearance of a withdrawal syndrome when administration of the drug is terminated is the only actual evidence of physical dependence. Withdrawal signs and symptoms occur when drug administration in a physically dependent person is terminated abruptly. Withdrawal symptoms have at least two origins: (1) removal of the drug of dependence and (2) CNS hyperarousal owing to readaptation to the absence of the drug of dependence. Pharmacokinetic variables are of considerable importance in the amplitude and duration of the withdrawal syndrome. Withdrawal symptoms are characteristic for a given category of drugs and tend to be *opposite* to the original effects produced by the drug before tolerance developed. Thus, abrupt termination of a drug (such as an opioid agonist) that produces miotic (constricted) pupils and slow heart rate will produce a withdrawal syndrome including dilated pupils and tachycardia. Tolerance, physical dependence, and withdrawal are all biological phenomena. They are the natural consequences of drug use and can be produced in experimental animals and in any human being who takes certain medications repeatedly. These symptoms in themselves do not imply that the individual is involved in abuse or addiction. *Patients who take medicine for appropriate medical indications and in correct dosages still may show tolerance, physical dependence, and withdrawal symptoms if the drug is stopped abruptly rather than gradually.* For example, a hypertensive patient receiving a β adrenergic receptor blocker such as *metoprolol* may have a good therapeutic response, but if the drug is stopped abruptly, the patient may experience a withdrawal syndrome consisting of rebound increased blood pressure temporarily higher than that prior to beginning the medication.

Medical addict is a term used to describe a patient in treatment for a medical disorder who has become "addicted" to the available prescribed drugs; the patient begins taking them in excessive doses, out of control. An example would be a patient with chronic pain, anxiety, or insomnia who begins using the prescribed medication more often than directed by the physician. If the physician restricts the prescriptions, the patient may begin seeing several doctors without the knowledge of the primary physician. Such patients also may visit emergency rooms for the purpose of obtaining additional medication. This scenario is very uncommon, considering the large number of patients who receive medications capable of producing tolerance and physical dependence. *Fear of producing such medical addicts results in needless suffering among patients with pain* because physicians needlessly limit appropriate medications. Tolerance and physical dependence are inevitable consequences of chronic treatment with opioids and certain other drugs, but tolerance and physical dependence by themselves do not imply "addiction."

CLINICAL ISSUES

The treatment of physically dependent individuals will be discussed with reference to the specific drug of abuse and dependence problems characteristic to each category: CNS depressants, including alcohol and other sedatives; nicotine and tobacco; opioids; psychostimulants, such as amphetamine and cocaine; cannabinoids; psychedelic drugs; and inhalants (volatile solvents, nitrous oxide, and ethyl ether). Abuse of combinations of drugs across these categories is common. Alcohol is so widely available that it is combined with practically all other categories. Some combinations reportedly are taken because of their interactive effects. An example is the combination of heroin and cocaine ("speedball"), which will be described with the opioid category. Alcohol and cocaine is another very common combination. When confronted with a patient exhibiting signs of overdose or withdrawal, the physician

must be aware of these possible combinations because each drug may require specific treatment.

CNS Depressants

Ethanol. Experimentation with ethanol is almost universal, and a high proportion of users finds the experience pleasant. More than 90% of American adults report experience with ethanol (commonly called *alcohol*), and approximately 70% report some level of current use. The lifetime prevalence of alcohol abuse and alcohol addiction (alcoholism) in this society is 5% to 10% for men and 3% to 5% for women.

Ethanol is classed as a depressant because it indeed produces sedation and sleep. However, the initial effects of alcohol, particularly at lower doses, often are perceived as stimulation owing to a suppression of inhibitory systems (*see* Chapter 22). Those who perceive only sedation from alcohol generally choose not to drink when evaluated in a test procedure (de Wit *et al.*, 1989).

Alcohol impairs recent memory and, in high doses, produces the phenomenon of "blackouts," after which the drinker has no memory of his or her behavior while intoxicated. The effects of alcohol on memory are unclear, but evidence suggests that reports from patients about their reasons for drinking and their behavior during a binge are not reliable. Alcohol-dependent persons often say that they drink to relieve anxiety or depression. When allowed to drink under observation, however, alcoholics typically become more dysphoric as drinking continues (Mendelson and Mello, 1979), thus not supporting the idea that alcoholics drink to relieve tension.

Tolerance, Physical Dependence, and Withdrawal. Mild intoxication by alcohol is familiar to almost everyone, but the symptoms vary among individuals. Some simply experience motor incoordination and sleepiness. Others initially become stimulated and garrulous. As the blood level increases, the sedating effects increase, with eventual coma and death occurring at high alcohol levels. The initial sensitivity (innate tolerance) to alcohol varies greatly among individuals and is related to family history of alcoholism (Wilhelmsen *et al.*, 2003). Experience with alcohol can produce greater tolerance (acquired tolerance) such that extremely high blood levels (300 to 400 mg/dl) can be found in alcoholics who do not appear grossly sedated. In these cases, the lethal dose does not increase proportionately to the sedating dose, and thus the margin of safety (therapeutic index) is decreased.

Heavy consumers of alcohol not only acquire tolerance but also inevitably develop a state of physical dependence. This often leads to drinking in the morning to restore blood alcohol levels diminished during the night. Eventually, they may awaken during the night and take a drink to avoid the restlessness produced by falling alcohol levels. The alcohol-withdrawal syndrome (Table 23–4)

Table 23–4
Alcohol Withdrawal Syndrome

Alcohol craving
Tremor, irritability
Nausea
Sleep disturbance
Tachycardia
Hypertension
Sweating
Perceptual distortion
Seizures (6 to 48 hours after last drink)
Visual (and occasionally auditory or tactile) hallucinations (12 to 48 hours after last drink)
Delirium tremens (48 to 96 hours after last drink; rare in uncomplicated withdrawal)
  Severe agitation
  Confusion
  Fever, profuse sweating
  Tachycardia
  Nausea, diarrhea
  Dilated pupils

generally depends on the size of the average daily dose and usually is "treated" by resumption of alcohol ingestion. Withdrawal symptoms are experienced frequently but usually are not severe or life-threatening until they occur in conjunction with other problems, such as infection, trauma, malnutrition, or electrolyte imbalance. In the setting of such complications, the syndrome of *delirium tremens* becomes likely (Table 23–4).

Alcohol produces cross-tolerance to other sedatives such as *benzodiazepines*. This tolerance is operative in abstinent alcoholics, but while the alcoholic is drinking, the sedating effects of alcohol add to those of other sedatives, making the combination more dangerous. This is particularly true for benzodiazepines, which are relatively safe in overdose when given alone but potentially are lethal in combination with alcohol.

The chronic use of alcohol and other sedatives is associated with the development of depression (McLellan *et al.*, 1979), and the risk of suicide among alcoholics is one of the highest of any diagnostic category. Cognitive deficits have been reported in alcoholics tested while sober. These deficits usually improve after weeks to months of abstinence. More severe recent memory impairment is associated with specific brain damage caused by nutritional deficiencies common in alcoholics, e.g., thiamine deficiency.

Alcohol is toxic to many organ systems. As a result, the medical complications of alcohol abuse and dependence include liver disease, cardiovascular disease, endocrine and gastrointestinal effects, and malnutrition, in addition to the CNS dysfunctions outlined earlier. Ethanol readily crosses the placental barrier, producing the *fetal alcohol syndrome*, a major cause of mental retardation (*see* Chapter 22).

Pharmacological Interventions. *Detoxification.* A patient who presents in a medical setting with an alcohol-withdrawal syndrome should be considered to have a potentially lethal condition. Although most mild cases of alcohol withdrawal never come to medical attention, severe cases require general evaluation; attention to hydration and electrolytes; vitamins, especially high-dose thiamine; and a sedating medication that has cross-tolerance with alcohol. To block or diminish the symptoms described in Table 23–4, a short-acting benzodiazepine such as *oxazepam* (SERAX) can be used at a dose of 15 to 30 mg every 4 to 6 hours according to the stage and severity of withdrawal; some authorities recommend a long-acting benzodiazepine unless there is demonstrated liver impairment. Anticonvulsants such as *carbamazepine* have been shown to be effective in alcohol withdrawal, although they appear not to relieve subjective symptoms as well as benzodiazepines. After medical evaluation, uncomplicated alcohol withdrawal can be treated effectively on an outpatient basis. When there are medical problems or a history of seizures, hospitalization is required.

Other Measures. Detoxification is only the first step of treatment. Complete abstinence is the objective of long-term treatment, and this is accomplished mainly by behavioral approaches. Medications that aid in the prevention of relapse are under development. *Disulfiram* (ANTABUSE; *see* Chapter 22) has been useful in some programs that focus behavioral efforts on ingestion of the medication. Disulfiram blocks aldehyde dehydrogenase, the second step in ethanol metabolism, resulting in the accumulation of acetaldehyde, which produces an unpleasant flushing reaction when alcohol is ingested. Knowledge of this unpleasant reaction helps the patient to resist taking a drink. Although quite effective pharmacologically, disulfiram has not been found to be effective in controlled clinical trials because so many patients failed to ingest the medication.

An FDA-approved medication used as an adjunct in the treatment of alcoholism is *naltrexone* (REVIA; *see* Chapter 22). This opiate-receptor antagonist has been shown to block some of the reinforcing properties of alcohol and has resulted in a decreased rate of relapse to alcohol drinking in the majority of published double-blind clinical trials. It works best in combination with behavioral treatment programs that encourage adherence to medication and to remaining abstinent from alcohol. A depot preparation with a duration of 30 days is currently under review by the FDA and would improve medication adherence, the major problem with the use of medications in alcoholism. One recent study linked abstinence in response to naltrexone therapy with a specific polymorphism in the gene encoding the μ opioid receptor (Oslin *et al.*, 2003), which has been linked to the reinforcing properties of alcohol and differential responses to μ-receptor antagonists. To the extent that these findings are confirmed, they may facilitate the identification of patients who are more likely to respond to pharmacotherapy with naltrexone.

Recently, the FDA approved another medication as an adjunct in the treatment of alcoholism. *Acamprosate* (Mason, 2003) is a competitive inhibitor of the *N*-methyl-D-aspartate (NMDA)–type glutamate receptor that is proposed to normalize the dysregulated neurotransmission associated with chronic ethanol intake and thereby to attenuate one of the mechanisms that lead to relapse. In several European studies, acamprosate has been shown to promote abstinence either alone or in combination with naltrexone.

Benzodiazepines. Benzodiazepines are among the most commonly prescribed drugs worldwide; they are used mainly for the treatment of anxiety disorders and insomnia (*see* Chapters 16 and 17). Considering their widespread use, intentional abuse of prescription benzodiazepines is relatively rare. When a benzodiazepine is taken for up to several weeks, there is little tolerance and no difficulty in stopping the medication when the condition no longer warrants its use. After several months, the proportion of patients who become tolerant increases, and reducing the dose or stopping the medication produces withdrawal symptoms (Table 23–5). It can be difficult to distinguish withdrawal symptoms from the reappearance of the anxiety symptoms for which the benzodiazepine was prescribed initially. Some patients may increase their dose over time because tolerance definitely develops to the sedative effects. Many patients and their physicians, however, contend that antianxiety benefits continue to occur long after tolerance to the sedating effects. Moreover, these patients continue to take the medication for years according to medical directions without increasing their dose and are able to function very effectively as long as they take the benzodiazepine. The degree to which tolerance develops to the anxiolytic effects of benzodiazepines is a subject of controversy. There is, however, good evidence that significant tolerance does not develop

Table 23–5
Benzodiazepine Withdrawal Symptoms

Following moderate dose usage
 Anxiety, agitation
 Increased sensitivity to light and sound
 Paresthesias, strange sensations
 Muscle cramps
 Myoclonic jerks
 Sleep disturbance
 Dizziness
Following high-dose usage
 Seizures
 Delirium

to all benzodiazepine actions because some effects of acute doses on memory persist in patients who have taken benzodiazepines for years. According to a task force that reviewed the issues and published guidelines on the proper medical use of benzodiazepines (American Psychiatric Association, 1990), intermittent use only when symptoms occur retards the development of tolerance and therefore is preferable to daily use. Patients with a history of alcohol- or other drug-abuse problems have an increased risk for the development of benzodiazepine abuse and should rarely, if ever, be treated with benzodiazepines on a chronic basis.

While relatively few patients who receive benzodiazepines for medical indications abuse their medication, there are individuals who specifically seek benzodiazepines for their ability to produce a "high." Among these abusers, there are differences in drug popularity; benzodiazepines that have a rapid onset, such as *diazepam* and *alprazolam,* tend to be the most desirable. The drugs may be obtained by simulating a medical condition and deceiving physicians or simply through illicit channels. Unsupervised use can lead to self-administration of large doses and therefore tolerance to the benzodiazepine's sedating effects. For example, while 5 to 20 mg/day of diazepam is a typical dose for a patient receiving prescribed medication, abusers may take over 1000 mg/day and not appear grossly sedated.

Abusers may combine benzodiazepines with other drugs to increase the effect. For example, it is part of the "street lore" that taking diazepam 30 minutes after an oral dose of *methadone* will produce an augmented high not obtainable with either drug alone.

While there is some illicit use of benzodiazepines as a primary drug of abuse, most of the unsupervised use seems to be by abusers of other drugs who are attempting to self-medicate the side effects or withdrawal effects of their primary drug of abuse. Thus, cocaine addicts often take diazepam to relieve the irritability and agitation produced by cocaine binges, and opioid addicts find that diazepam and other benzodiazepines relieve some of the anxiety symptoms of opioid withdrawal when they are unable to obtain their preferred drug.

Pharmacological Interventions. If patients receiving long-term benzodiazepine treatment by prescription wish to stop their medication, the process may take months of gradual dose reduction. Withdrawal symptoms (Table 23–5) may occur during this outpatient detoxification, but in most cases the symptoms are mild. If anxiety symptoms return, a nonbenzodiazepine such as *buspirone* may be prescribed, but this agent usually is less effective than benzodiazepines for treatment of anxiety in these patients. Some authorities recommend transferring the patient to a long-half-life benzodiazepine during detoxification; other recommended medications include the anticonvulsants *carbamazepine* and *phenobarbital*. Controlled studies comparing different treatment regimens are lacking. Since patients who have been on low doses of benzodiazepines for years usually have no adverse effects, the physician and patient should decide jointly whether detoxification and possible transfer to a new anxiolytic is worth the effort.

The specific benzodiazepine receptor antagonist *flumazenil* has been found useful in the treatment of overdose and in reversing the effects of long-acting benzodiazepines used in anesthesia (*see* Chapter 16). It has been tried in the treatment of persistent withdrawal symptoms after cessation of long-term benzodiazepine treatment.

Deliberate abusers of high doses of benzodiazepines usually require inpatient detoxification. Frequently, benzodiazepine abuse is part of a combined dependence involving alcohol, opioids, and cocaine. Detoxification can be a complex clinical pharmacological problem requiring knowledge of the pharmacokinetics of each drug. The patient's history may be unreliable not simply because of lying but also because the patient frequently does not *know* the true identity of drugs purchased on the street. Medication for detoxification should not be prescribed by the "cookbook" approach but by careful titration and patient observation. The withdrawal syndrome from diazepam, for example, may not become evident until the patient develops a seizure in the second week of hospitalization. One approach to complex detoxification is to focus on the CNS-depressant drug and temporarily hold the opioid component constant with a low dose of methadone. Opioid detoxification can begin later. A long-acting benzodiazepine such as diazepam or *clorazepate* (TRANXENE) or a long-acting barbiturate such as *phenobarbital* can be used to block the sedative withdrawal symptoms. The phenobarbital dose should be determined by a series of test doses and subsequent observations to determine the level of tolerance. Most complex detoxifications can be accomplished using this phenobarbital loading-dose strategy (*see* Robinson *et al.*, 1981).

After detoxification, the prevention of relapse requires a long-term outpatient rehabilitation program similar to the treatment of alcoholism. No specific medications have been found to be useful in the rehabilitation of sedative abusers, but, of course, specific psychiatric disorders such as depression or schizophrenia, if present, require appropriate medications.

Barbiturates and Nonbenzodiazepine Sedatives. The use of barbiturates and other nonbenzodiazepine sedating medications has declined greatly in recent years owing to

the increased safety and efficacy of newer medications (*see* Chapters 16 and 17). Abuse problems with barbiturates resemble those seen with benzodiazepines in many ways. Treatment of abuse and addiction should be handled similarly to interventions for the abuse of alcohol and benzodiazepines. Because drugs in this category frequently are prescribed as hypnotics for patients complaining of insomnia, physicians should be aware of the problems that can develop when the hypnotic agent is withdrawn. Insomnia rarely should be treated with medication as a primary disorder except when produced by short-term stressful situations. Insomnia often is a symptom of an underlying chronic problem, such as depression or respiratory dysfunction, or may be due simply to a change in sleep requirements with age. Prescription of sedative medications, however, can change the physiology of sleep with subsequent tolerance to these medication effects. When the sedative is stopped, there is a rebound effect with worsened insomnia. This medication-induced insomnia requires detoxification by gradual dose reduction.

Nicotine

The basic pharmacology of nicotine is discussed in Chapter 9. Because nicotine provides the reinforcement for cigarette smoking, the most common cause of preventable death and disease in the United States, it is arguably the most dangerous dependence-producing drug. The dependence produced by nicotine can be extremely durable, as exemplified by the high failure rate among smokers who try to quit. Although more than 80% of smokers express a desire to quit, only 35% try to stop each year, and fewer than 5% are successful in unaided attempts to quit (American Psychiatric Association, 1994).

Cigarette (nicotine) addiction is influenced by multiple variables. Nicotine itself produces reinforcement; users compare nicotine to stimulants such as cocaine or amphetamine, although its effects are of lower magnitude. While there are many casual users of alcohol and cocaine, few individuals who smoke cigarettes smoke a small enough quantity (5 cigarettes or fewer per day) to avoid dependence. Nicotine is absorbed readily through the skin, mucous membranes, and lungs. The pulmonary route produces discernible CNS effects in as little as 7 seconds. Thus each puff produces some discrete reinforcement. With 10 puffs per cigarette, the one-pack-per-day smoker reinforces the habit 200 times daily. The timing, setting, situation, and preparation all become associated repetitively with the effects of nicotine.

Nicotine has both stimulant and depressant actions. The smoker feels alert, yet there is some muscle relaxation. Nicotine activates the nucleus accumbens reward system in the brain, discussed earlier;

Table 23–6
Nicotine Withdrawal Symptoms

Irritability, impatience, hostility
Anxiety
Dysphoric or depressed mood
Difficulty concentrating
Restlessness
Decreased heart rate
Increased appetite or weight gain

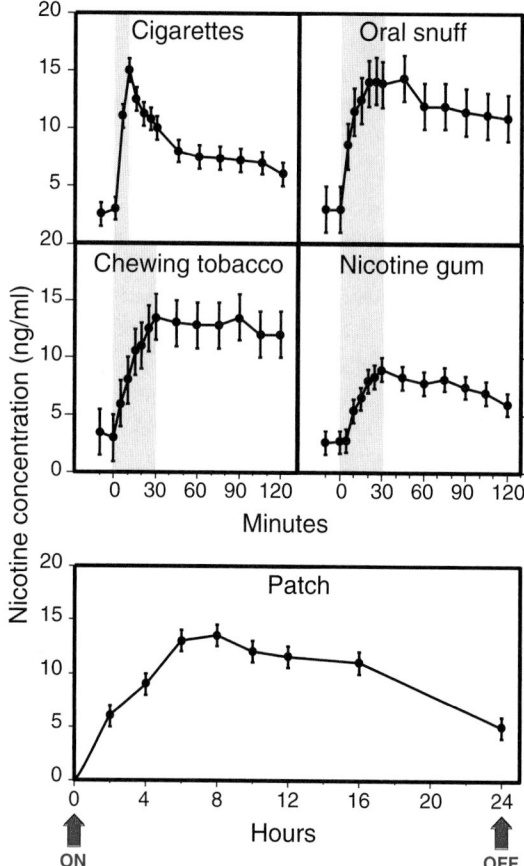

Figure 23–3. *Nicotine concentrations in blood resulting from five different nicotine delivery systems.* Shaded areas (upper panel) indicate the periods of exposure to nicotine. Arrows (lower panel) indicate when the nicotine patch was put on and taken off. (From Benowitz *et al.*, 1988, and Srivastava *et al.*, 1991, with permission.)

increased extracellular dopamine has been found in this region after nicotine injections in rats. Nicotine affects other systems as well, including the release of endogenous opioids and glucocorticoids.

There is evidence for tolerance to the subjective effects of nicotine. Smokers typically report that the first cigarette of the day after a night of abstinence gives the "best" feeling. Smokers who return to cigarettes after a period of abstinence may experience nausea if they return immediately to their previous dose. Persons naive to the effects of nicotine will experience nausea at low nicotine blood levels, and smokers will experience nausea if nicotine levels are raised above their accustomed levels.

Negative reinforcement refers to the benefits obtained from the termination of an unpleasant state. In dependent smokers, there is evidence that the urge to smoke correlates with a low blood nicotine level, as though smoking were a means to achieve a certain nicotine level and thus avoid withdrawal symptoms. Some smokers even awaken during the night to have a cigarette, which ameliorates the effect of low nicotine blood levels that could disrupt sleep. If the nicotine level is maintained artificially by a slow intravenous infusion, there is a decrease in the number of cigarettes smoked and in the number of puffs. Thus, smokers may be smoking to achieve the reward of nicotine effects, to avoid the pain of nicotine withdrawal, or most likely a combination of the two. Nicotine withdrawal symptoms are listed in Table 23–6.

Depressed mood (dysthymic disorder, affective disorder) is associated with nicotine dependence, but it is not known whether depression predisposes one to begin smoking or depression develops during the course of nicotine dependence. Depression increases significantly during smoking withdrawal, and this is cited as one reason for relapse.

Pharmacological Interventions. The nicotine withdrawal syndrome can be alleviated by nicotine-replacement therapy, available with (*e.g.,* NICOTROL INHALER and NICOTROL NASAL SPRAY) or without (*e.g.,* NICORETTE GUM and others and NICODERM TRANSDERMAL PATCH, NICOTROL TRANSDERMAL PATCH, and others) a prescription. Figure 23–3 shows the blood nicotine concentrations achieved by different methods of nicotine delivery. Because nicotine gum and a nicotine patch do not achieve the *peak levels* seen with cigarettes, they do not produce the same magnitude of subjective effects as nicotine. These methods do, however, suppress the symptoms of nicotine withdrawal. Thus smokers should be able to

transfer their dependence to the alternative delivery system and gradually reduce the daily nicotine dose with minimal symptoms. Although this results in more smokers achieving abstinence, most resume smoking over the ensuing weeks or months. Comparisons with placebo treatment show large benefits of nicotine replacement at 6 weeks, but the effect diminishes with time. The nicotine patch produces a steady blood level (Figure 23–3) and seems to have better patient compliance than that observed with nicotine gum. Verified abstinence rates at 12 months are reported to be in the range of 20%, which is worse than the success rate for any other addiction. The necessary goal of complete abstinence contributes to the poor success rate; when ex-smokers "slip" and begin smoking a little, they usually relapse quickly to their prior level of dependence. A sustained-release preparation of the antidepressant *bupropion* (*see* Chapter 17), improves abstinence rates among smokers. Newer agents such as the cannabinoid (CB-1) receptor antagonist *rimonabant* also have been reported to increase abstinence rates in clinical trials and are progressing through the FDA approval process. A combination of behavioral treatment with nicotine replacement to ease withdrawal and an anticraving medication to reduce relapse is currently considered the treatment of choice.

Opioids

Opioid drugs are used primarily for the treatment of pain (*see* Chapter 21). Some of the CNS mechanisms that reduce the perception of pain also produce a state of well-being or euphoria. Thus opioid drugs also are taken outside medical channels for the purpose of obtaining the effects on mood. This potential for abuse has generated much research on separating the mechanism of analgesia from that of euphoria in the hope of eventually developing a potent analgesic that does not activate brain reward systems. Although this research has led to advances in understanding the physiology of pain, the standard medications for severe pain remain the derivatives of the opium poppy (opiates) and synthetic drugs that activate the same receptors (opioids). Drugs modeled after the endogenous opioid peptides may one day provide more specific treatment, but none of these currently is available for clinical use. Medications that do not act at opiate receptors, such as the *nonsteroidal antiinflammatory drugs* (NSAIDs), have an important role in certain types of pain, especially chronic pain, but for acute pain and for severe chronic pain, the opioid drugs are most effective. Progress in pain control stems from a greater understanding of the mechanism of tolerance to μ opiate receptor–mediated analgesia, which involves NMDA receptors (Trujillo and Akil, 1991). By combining morphine with dextromethorphan, an NMDA-receptor antagonist, tolerance is impaired and analgesia is enhanced without an increase in the dose of opioid.

The subjective effects of opioid drugs are useful in the management of acute pain. This is particularly true in high-anxiety situations, such as the crushing chest pain of myocardial infarction, when the relaxing, anxiolytic effects complement the analgesia. Normal volunteers with no pain given opioids in the laboratory may report the effects as unpleasant because of side effects such as nausea, vomiting, and sedation. Patients with pain rarely develop abuse or addiction problems. Of course, patients receiving opioids over time develop tolerance routinely, and if the medication is stopped abruptly, they will show the signs of an opioid-withdrawal syndrome, the evidence for physical dependence.

Opioids never should be withheld from patients with cancer out of fear of producing addiction. If chronic opioid medication is indi-

cated, it is preferable to prescribe an orally active, slow-onset opioid with a long duration of action. These qualities reduce the likelihood of producing euphoria at onset and withdrawal symptoms as the medication wears off. *Methadone* is an excellent choice for the management of chronic severe pain. Controlled-release oral *morphine* (MS CONTIN, AVINZA) and controlled-release *oxycodone* (OXYCONTIN) are other possibilities. Rapid-onset, short-duration opioids are excellent for acute short-term use, such as during the postoperative period. As tolerance and physical dependence develop, however, the patient may experience the early symptoms of withdrawal between doses, and during withdrawal, the threshold for pain decreases. Thus, for chronic administration, the long-acting opioids are recommended. While methadone is long acting because of its metabolism to active metabolites, the long-acting version of oxycodone has been formulated to release slowly, thus changing a short-acting opioid into a long-acting one. Unfortunately, this mechanism can be subverted by breaking the tablet and making the full dose of oxycodone immediately available. This has led to diversion of oxycodone to illicit traffic because high-dose oxycodone produces euphoria that is sought by opiate abusers. The diversion of prescription opioids such as oxycodone and hydrocodone to illegal markets has become an important source of opiate abuse in the United States.

The major risk for abuse or addiction occurs in patients complaining of pain with no clear physical explanation or with evidence of a chronic disorder that is not life-threatening. Examples are chronic headaches, backaches, abdominal pain, or peripheral neuropathy. Even in these cases, an opioid may be considered as a brief emergency treatment, but long-term treatment with opioids should be used only after other alternatives have been exhausted. In the relatively rare patients who develop abuse, the transition from legitimate use to abuse often begins with patients returning to their physician earlier than scheduled to get a new prescription or visiting emergency rooms of different hospitals complaining of acute pain and asking for an opioid injection.

Heroin is the most important opiate that is abused. There is no legal supply of heroin for clinical use in the United States. Despite claims that heroin has unique analgesic properties for the treatment of severe pain, double-blind trials have found it to be no more effective than hydromorphone. However, heroin is widely available on the illicit market, and its price dropped sharply in the 1990s, continuing to the present, with purity increased tenfold. Previously, street heroin in the United States was highly diluted: Each 100-mg bag of powder had only about 4 mg heroin (range 0 to 8 mg), and the rest was filler such as quinine. In the mid-1990s, street heroin reached 45% to 75% purity in many large cities, with some samples testing as high as 90%. This means that the level of physical dependence among heroin addicts is relatively high and that users who interrupt regular dosing will develop more severe withdrawal symptoms. Whereas heroin previously required intravenous injection, the more potent supplies can be smoked or administered nasally (snorted), thus making the initiation of heroin use accessible to people who would not insert a needle into their veins. There is no accurate way to count the number of heroin addicts, but based on extrapolation from overdose deaths, number of applicants for treatment, and number of heroin addicts arrested, the estimates range from 800,000 to 1 million in the United States. Based on a stratified national sample of adults in the United States, approximately 1 in 4 individuals who report any use of heroin become addicted (Anthony *et al.*, 1994).

Tolerance, Dependence, and Withdrawal. Injection of a heroin solution produces a variety of sensations described as warmth, taste, or high and intense pleasure ("rush") often compared with sexual orgasm. There are some differences among the opioids in their acute effects, with *morphine* producing more of a histamine-releasing effect and *meperidine* producing more excitation or confusion. Even experienced opioid addicts, however, cannot distinguish between heroin and hydromorphone in double-blind tests. Thus, the popularity of heroin may be due to its availability on the illicit market and its rapid onset. After intravenous injection, the effects begin in less than a minute. Heroin has high lipid solubility, crosses the blood–brain barrier quickly, and is deacetylated to the active metabolites 6-monoacetyl morphine and morphine. After the intense euphoria, which lasts from 45 seconds to several minutes, there is a period of sedation and tranquility ("on the nod") lasting up to an hour. The effects of heroin wear off in 3 to 5 hours, depending on the dose. Experienced users may inject two to four times per day. Thus, the heroin addict is constantly oscillating between being "high" and feeling the sickness of early withdrawal (Figure 23–4). This produces many problems in the homeostatic systems regulated at least in part by endogenous opioids. For example, the hypothalamic–pituitary–gonadal axis and the hypothalamic–pituitary–adrenal axis are abnormal in heroin addicts. Women on heroin have irregular menses, and men have a variety of sexual performance problems. Mood also is affected. Heroin addicts are relatively docile and compliant after taking heroin, but during withdrawal, they become irritable and aggressive.

Based on patient reports, tolerance develops early to the euphoria-producing effects of opioids. There also is tolerance to the respiratory depressant, analgesic, sedative, and emetic properties. Heroin users tend to increase their daily dose, depending on their financial resources and the availability of the drug. If a supply is available, the dose can be increased progressively 100 times. Even in highly tolerant individuals, the possibility of overdose remains if tolerance is exceeded. Overdose is likely to occur when potency of the street sample is unexpectedly high or when the heroin is mixed with a far more potent opioid, such as *fentanyl* (SUBLIMAZE, others).

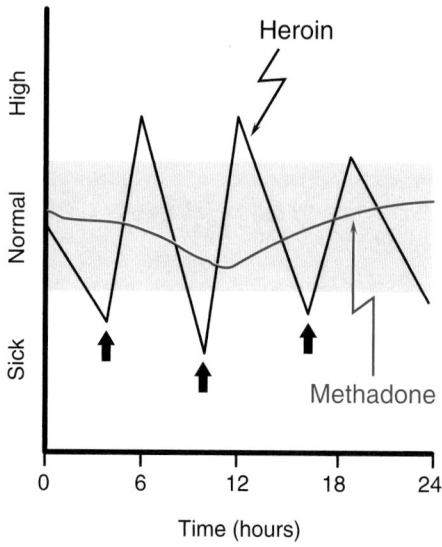

Figure 23–4. Differences in responses to heroin and methadone. A person who injects heroin (↑) several times per day oscillates between being sick and being high. In contrast, the typical methadone patient remains in the "normal" range (indicated in gray) with little fluctuation after dosing once per day. The ordinate values represent the subject's mental and physical state, not plasma levels of the drug.

Addiction to heroin or other short-acting opioids produces behavioral disruptions and usually becomes incompatible with a productive life. There is a significant risk for opioid abuse and dependence among physicians and other health care workers who have access to potent opioids, thus tempting them toward unsupervised experimentation. Physicians often begin by assuming that they can manage their own dose, and they may rationalize their behavior based on the beneficial effects of the drug. Over time, however, the typical unsupervised opioid user loses control, and behavioral changes are observed by family and coworkers. Apart from the behavioral changes and the risk of overdose, especially with very potent opioids, chronic use of opioids is relatively nontoxic.

Opioids frequently are used in combinations with other drugs. A common combination is heroin and cocaine ("speedball"). Users report an improved euphoria because of the combination, and there is evidence of an interaction, because cocaine reduces the signs of opiate withdrawal, and heroin may reduce the irritability seen in chronic cocaine users.

The mortality rate for street heroin users is very high. Early death comes from involvement in crime to support the habit; from uncertainty about the dose, the purity, and even the identity of what is purchased on the street; and from serious infections associated with nonsterile drugs and sharing of injection paraphernalia. Heroin users commonly

Table 23–7
Characteristics of Opioid Withdrawal

SYMPTOMS	SIGNS
Regular withdrawal	
Craving for opioids	Pupillary dilation
Restlessness, irritability	Sweating
Increased sensitivity to pain	Piloerection ("gooseflesh")
	Tachycardia
Nausea, cramps	Vomiting, diarrhea
Muscle aches	Increased blood pressure
Dysphoric mood	Yawning
Insomnia, anxiety	Fever
Protracted withdrawal	
Anxiety	Cyclic changes in weight,
Insomnia	pupil size, respiratory
Drug craving	center sensitivity

acquire bacterial infections producing skin abscesses; endocarditis; pulmonary infections, especially tuberculosis; and viral infections producing hepatitis C and acquired immune deficiency syndrome (AIDS).

As with other addictions, the first stage of treatment addresses physical dependence and consists of detoxification (Kosten and O'Conner, 2003). The opioid-withdrawal syndrome (Table 23–7) is very unpleasant but not life-threatening. It begins within 6 to 12 hours after the last dose of a short-acting opioid and as long as 72 to 84 hours after a very long-acting opioid medication. Heroin addicts go through early stages of this syndrome frequently when heroin is scarce or expensive. Some therapeutic communities as a matter of policy elect not to treat withdrawal so that the addict can experience the suffering while being given group support. The duration and intensity of the syndrome are related to the clearance of the individual drug. Heroin withdrawal is brief (5 to 10 days) and intense. *Methadone* withdrawal is slower in onset and lasts longer. Protracted withdrawal also is likely to be longer with methadone. (*See* more detailed discussions of protracted withdrawal under "Long-Term Management" below.)

Pharmacological Interventions. Opioid withdrawal signs and symptoms can be treated by three different approaches. The first and most commonly used approach depends on cross-tolerance and consists of transfer to a prescription opioid medication and then gradual dose reduction. The same principles of detoxification apply as for other types of physical dependence. It is convenient to change the patient from a short-acting opioid such as heroin to a long-acting one such as methadone. The initial dose of

methadone is typically 20 to 30 mg. This is a test dose to determine the level needed to reduce observed withdrawal symptoms. The first day's total dose then can be calculated depending on the response and then reduced by 20% per day during the course of detoxification.

A second approach to detoxification involves the use of oral *clonidine* (CATAPRES, others), a medication approved only for the treatment of hypertension (*see* Chapter 32). Clonidine is an α_2 adrenergic agonist that decreases adrenergic neurotransmission from the locus ceruleus. Many of the autonomic symptoms of opioid withdrawal such as nausea, vomiting, cramps, sweating, tachycardia, and hypertension result from the loss of opioid suppression of the locus ceruleus system during the abstinence syndrome. Clonidine, acting *via* distinct receptors but by cellular mechanisms that mimic opioid effects, can alleviate many of the symptoms of opioid withdrawal. However, clonidine does not alleviate generalized aches and opioid craving characteristic of opioid withdrawal. When using clonidine to treat withdrawal, the dose must be titrated according to the stage and severity of withdrawal, beginning with 0.2 mg orally. Postural hypotension commonly occurs when clonidine treatment is used for withdrawal. A similar drug, *lofexidine* (not yet available in the United States), has greater selectivity for α_{2A} adrenergic receptors and is associated with less of the hypotension that limits the usefulness of clonidine in this setting.

A third method of treating opioid withdrawal involves activation of the endogenous opioid system without medication. The techniques proposed include acupuncture and several methods of CNS activation using transcutaneous electrical stimulation. While attractive theoretically, this has not yet been found to be practical. Rapid antagonist-precipitated opioid detoxification under general anesthesia has received considerable publicity because it promises detoxification in several hours while the patient is unconscious and thus not experiencing withdrawal discomfort. A mixture of medications has been used, but morbidity and mortality as reported in the lay press are unacceptable, with no demonstrated advantage in long-term outcome.

Long-Term Management. If patients are simply discharged from the hospital after withdrawal from opioids, there is a high probability of a quick return to compulsive opioid use. Addiction is a chronic disorder that requires long-term treatment. Numerous factors influence relapse. One factor is that the withdrawal syndrome does not end in 5 to 7 days. There are subtle signs and symptoms often called the *protracted withdrawal syndrome* (Table 23–7) that persist for up to 6 months. Physiological measures tend to oscillate as though a new set point were being established; during this phase, outpatient drug-free treatment has a low probability of success, even when the patient has received intensive prior treatment while protected from relapse in a residential program.

The most successful treatment for heroin addiction consists of stabilization on methadone. Patients who relapse repeatedly during drug-free treatment can be transferred directly to methadone without requiring detoxification. The dose of methadone must be sufficient to prevent withdrawal symptoms for at least 24 hours. The introduction of *buprenorphine*, a partial agonist at μ opioid receptors (*see*

Chapter 21), represents a major change in the treatment of opiate addiction. This drug produces minimal withdrawal symptoms and has a low potential for overdose, a long duration of action, and the ability to block heroin effects. The laws governing the prescription of opioids for addicts were changed so that trained physicians could treat up to 30 patients with maintenance buprenorphine to prevent relapse to opiate addiction. Treatment can take place in the physician's private office rather than in a special center, as required for methadone. When taken sublingually, buprenorphine (SUBUTEX) is active, but it also has the potential to be dissolved and injected (abused). Thus, a buprenorphine-*naloxone* combination (SUBOXONE) is also available. When taken orally (sublingually), the naloxone moiety is not effective, but if the patient abuses the medication by injecting, the naloxone will block the mild subjective high that could be produced by buprenorphine alone.

Agonist or Partial-Agonist Maintenance. Patients receiving methadone or buprenorphine will not experience the ups and downs experienced while on heroin (Figure 23–4). Drug craving diminishes and may disappear. Neuroendocrine rhythms eventually are restored (Kreek *et al.*, 2002). Because of cross-tolerance (from methadone to heroin), patients who inject street heroin report a reduced effect from usual heroin doses. This cross-tolerance effect is dose-related, so higher methadone maintenance doses result in less illicit opioid use, as determined by random urine testing. Buprenorphine, as a partial agonist, has a ceiling effect at about 16 mg of the sublingual tablet equaling no more than 60 mg methadone. If the patient has a higher level of physical dependence, methadone, a full agonist, must be used. Patients become tolerant to the sedating effects of methadone and become able to attend school or function in a job. Opioids also have a persistent, mild, stimulating effect noticeable after tolerance to the sedating effect, such that reaction time is quicker and vigilance is increased while on a stable dose of methadone.

Antagonist Treatment. Another pharmacological option is opioid antagonist treatment. *Naltrexone* (REVIA; *see* Chapter 21) is an antagonist with a high affinity for the μ opioid receptor (MOR); it will competitively block the effects of heroin or other MOR agonists. Naltrexone has almost no agonist effects of its own and will not satisfy craving or relieve protracted withdrawal symptoms. For these reasons, naltrexone treatment does not appeal to the average heroin addict, but it can be used after detoxification for patients with high motivation to remain opioid-free. Physicians, nurses, and pharmacists who have frequent access to opioid drugs make excellent candidates for this treatment approach. A depot formulation of naltrexone that provides 30 days of medication after a single injection is in clinical trials. This formulation would eliminate the necessity of daily pill-taking and prevent relapse when the recently detoxified patient leaves a protected environment.

Cocaine and Other Psychostimulants

Cocaine. More than 23 million Americans are estimated to have used cocaine at some time, but the number of current users declined from an estimated 8.6 million occasional users and 5.8 million regular users to 3.6 million who are currently estimated to be chronic cocaine users. The number of frequent users (at least weekly) has remained steady since 1991 at about 640,000. Not all users become addicts, and the variables that influence this

risk are discussed at the beginning of this chapter. A key factor is the widespread availability of relatively inexpensive cocaine in the alkaloidal form (free base, "crack") suitable for smoking and the hydrochloride powder form suitable for nasal or intravenous use. Drug abuse in men occurs about twice as frequently as in women. However, smoked cocaine use is particularly common in young women of childbearing age, who may use cocaine in this manner as commonly as do men.

The reinforcing effects of cocaine and cocaine analogs correlate best with their effectiveness in blocking the transporter that recovers dopamine from the synapse. This leads to increased dopamine concentrations at critical brain sites (Ritz *et al.*, 1987). However, cocaine also blocks both norepinephrine (NE) and serotonin (5-HT) reuptake, and chronic use of cocaine produces changes in these neurotransmitter systems, as measured by reductions in the neurotransmitter metabolites 3-methoxy-4-hydroxyphenethyleneglycol (MOPEG or MHPG) and 5-hydroxyindoleacetic acid (5-HIAA).

The general pharmacology and legitimate use of cocaine are discussed in Chapter 14. Cocaine produces a dose-dependent increase in heart rate and blood pressure accompanied by increased arousal, improved performance on tasks of vigilance and alertness, and a sense of self-confidence and well-being. Higher doses produce euphoria, which has a brief duration and often is followed by a desire for more drug. Involuntary motor activity, stereotyped behavior, and paranoia may occur after repeated doses. Irritability and increased risk of violence are found among heavy chronic users. The half-life of cocaine in plasma is about 50 minutes, but inhalant (crack) users typically desire more cocaine after 10 to 30 minutes. Intranasal and intravenous uses also result in a high of shorter duration than would be predicted by plasma cocaine levels, suggesting that a declining plasma concentration is associated with termination of the high and resumption of cocaine seeking. This theory is supported by positron-emission tomographic imaging studies using ^{11}C-labeled cocaine, which show that the time course of subjective euphoria parallels the uptake and displacement of the drug in the corpus striatum (Volkow *et al.*, 1999). The major route for cocaine metabolism involves hydrolysis of each of its two ester groups. Benzoylecgonine, produced on loss of the methyl group, represents the major urinary metabolite and can be found in the urine for 2 to 5 days after a binge. As a result, benzoylecgonine tests are useful for detecting cocaine use; heavy users have detectable amounts of the metabolite in their urine for up to 10 days following a binge. Cocaine frequently is used in combination with other drugs. The cocaine–heroin combination was discussed earlier in the opioid section. Alcohol is another drug that cocaine users take to reduce the irritability experienced during heavy cocaine use. Some develop alcohol addiction in addition to their cocaine problem. An important metabolic interaction occurs when cocaine and alcohol are taken concurrently. Some cocaine is transesterified to cocaethylene, which is equipotent to cocaine in blocking dopamine reuptake (Hearn *et al.*, 1991).

Addiction is the most common complication of cocaine use. Some users, especially intranasal users, can continue intermittent use for years. Others become compulsive users despite elaborate methods to maintain control. Stimulants tend to be used much more irregularly than opioids, nicotine, and alcohol. Binge use is very common, and a binge may last hours to days, terminating only when supplies of the drug are exhausted.

Toxicity. Other risks of cocaine use, beyond the potential for addiction, involve cardiac arrhythmias, myocardial ischemia, myocarditis, aortic dissection, cerebral vasoconstriction, and seizures. Death from trauma also is associated with cocaine use. Pregnant cocaine users may experience premature labor and abruptio placentae (Chasnoff *et al.*, 1989). Attributing the developmental abnormalities reported in infants born to cocaine-using women simply to cocaine use is confounded by the infant's prematurity, multiple-drug exposure, and overall poor pre- and postnatal care.

Cocaine has been reported to produce a prolonged and intense orgasm if taken prior to intercourse, and its use is associated with compulsive and promiscuous sexual activity. Long-term cocaine use, however, usually results in reduced sexual drive; complaints of sexual problems are common among cocaine users presenting for treatment. Psychiatric disorders, including anxiety, depression, and psychosis, are common in cocaine users who request treatment. While some of these psychiatric disorders undoubtedly existed prior to the stimulant use, many develop during the course of the drug abuse (McLellan *et al.*, 1979).

Tolerance, Dependence, and Withdrawal. Sensitization is a consistent finding in animal studies of cocaine and other stimulants. Sensitization is produced by intermittent use and typically is measured by behavioral hyperactivity. In human cocaine users, sensitization for the euphoric effect typically is not seen. On the contrary, most experienced users report requiring more cocaine over time to obtain euphoria, *i.e.*, tolerance. In the laboratory, tachyphylaxis (rapid tolerance) has been observed with reduced effects when the same dose is given repeatedly in one session. Sensitization may involve conditioning (Figure 23–2). Cocaine users often report a strong response on seeing cocaine before it is administered, consisting of physiological arousal and increased drug craving with concomitant activation of brain limbic structures (Childress *et al.*, 1999). Sensitization in human beings has been linked to paranoid, psychotic manifestations of cocaine use based on the observation that cocaine-induced hallucinations and paranoia typically are seen after long-term exposure (mean 35 months) in vulnerable users (Satel *et al.*, 1991). Since cocaine typically is used intermittently, even heavy users go through frequent periods of withdrawal or "crash." The symptoms of withdrawal seen in users admitted to hospitals are listed in Table 23–8. Careful studies of cocaine users during withdrawal show gradual diminution of these symptoms over 1 to 3 weeks (Weddington *et al.*, 1990). Residual depression may be seen after cocaine withdrawal and should be treated with antidepressant agents if it persists (*see* Chapter 17).

Table 23–8
Cocaine Withdrawal Symptoms and Signs

Dysphoria, depression
Sleepiness, fatigue
Cocaine craving
Bradycardia

Pharmacological Interventions. Since cocaine withdrawal is generally mild, treatment of withdrawal symptoms usually is not required. The major problem in treatment is not detoxification but helping the patient to resist the urge to restart compulsive cocaine use. Rehabilitation programs involving individual and group psychotherapy based on the principles of Alcoholics Anonymous and behavioral treatments based on reinforcing cocaine-free urine tests result in significant improvement in the majority of cocaine users (Alterman *et al.*, 1994; Higgins *et al.*, 1994). Nonetheless, there is great interest in finding a medication that can aid in the rehabilitation of cocaine addicts.

Numerous medications have been tried in placebo-controlled clinical trials with cocaine addicts, but finding a medication that consistently improves the results of behavior therapy alone has been elusive. Animal models suggest that enhancing GABAergic inhibition can reduce reinstatement of cocaine self-administration. This finding prompted a controlled clinical trial of *topiramate* (TOPAMAX) that showed a significant improvement for this medication approved for use in epilepsy. Topiramate also was found to reduce the relapse rate in alcoholics, prompting current studies in patients dually dependent on cocaine and alcohol. *Baclofen* (LIORESAL, others), a GABA$_B$ agonist, was found in a single-site trial to reduce relapse in cocaine addicts and currently is being studied in a multiclinic trial. A different approach was taken using *modafinil* (PROVIGIL), a medication that increases alertness and is approved for the treatment of narcolepsy. This medication was found to reduce the euphoria produced by cocaine and to relieve cocaine withdrawal symptoms. After a single-site, double-blind study found it effective in reducing relapse, modafinil is being studied in a multisite trial among cocaine-dependent patients.

Two completely different approaches are also under study: a compound that competes with cocaine at the dopamine transporter and a vaccine that produces cocaine-binding antibodies. However, these should be regarded as innovative ideas that have yet to be shown to be useful clinically. The recent spate of positive findings from placebo-controlled trials suggests that an effective medication for cocaine addiction may be on the horizon. For now, the treatment of choice remains behavioral, with medication indicated for specific coexisting disorders such as depression.

Amphetamine and Related Agents. Subjective effects similar to those of cocaine are produced by *amphetamine, dextroamphetamine, methamphetamine, phenmetrazine, methylphenidate,* and *diethylpropion.* Amphetamines increase synaptic dopamine primarily by stimulating presynaptic release rather than by blockade of reuptake, as is the case with cocaine. Intravenous or smoked methamphetamine produces an abuse/dependence syndrome similar to that of cocaine, although clinical deterioration may progress more rapidly. In animal studies, methamphetamine in doses comparable with those used by human abusers produces neurotoxic effects in dopamine and serotonin neurons. Methamphetamine can be produced in small, clandestine laboratories starting with ephedrine, a widely available nonprescription stimulant. Oral stimulants, such as those prescribed in a weight-reduction program, have short-term efficacy because of tolerance development. Only a small proportion of patients introduced to these appetite suppressants subsequently exhibits dose escalation or drug seeking from various physicians; such patients may meet diagnostic criteria for abuse or addiction. *Fenfluramine* (no longer marketed in the United States) and *phenylpropanolamine* (no longer marketed in the United States) reduce appetite with no evidence of significant abuse potential. *Mazindol* (no longer marketed in the United States) also reduces appetite, with less stimulant properties than amphetamine.

Khat is a plant material widely chewed in East Africa and Yemen for its stimulant properties; these are due to the alkaloidal *cathinone,* a compound similar to amphetamine (Kalix, 1990). *Methcathinone,* a congener with similar effects, has been synthesized in clandestine laboratories, but widespread use in North America has not been reported. MDMA ("ecstasy") also has stimulant properties and will be discussed in the section on hallucinogens.

Caffeine. Caffeine, a mild stimulant, is the most widely used psychoactive drug in the world. It is present in soft drinks, coffee, tea, cocoa, chocolate, and numerous prescription and over-the-counter drugs. It mildly increases norepinephrine and dopamine release and enhances neural activity in numerous brain areas. Caffeine is absorbed from the digestive tract and is distributed rapidly throughout all tissues and easily crosses the placental barrier (*see* Chapter 27). Many of caffeine's effects are believed to occur by means of competitive antagonism at adenosine receptors. Adenosine is a neuromodulator that influences a number of functions in the CNS (*see* Chapters 12 and 27). The mild sedating effects that occur when adenosine activates particular adenosine-receptor subtypes can be antagonized by caffeine.

Tolerance occurs rapidly to the stimulating effects of caffeine. Thus a mild withdrawal syndrome has been produced in controlled studies by abrupt cessation of as little as one to two cups of coffee per day. Caffeine withdrawal consists of feelings of fatigue and sedation. With higher doses, headaches and nausea have been reported during withdrawal; vomiting is rare (Silverman *et al.,* 1992). Although a withdrawal syndrome can be demonstrated, few caffeine users report loss of control of caffeine intake or significant difficulty in reducing or stopping caffeine, if desired (Dews *et al.,* 1999). Thus, caffeine is not listed in the category of addicting stimulants (American Psychiatric Association, 1994).

Cannabinoids (Marijuana)

The cannabis plant has been cultivated for centuries both for the production of hemp fiber and for its presumed medicinal and psychoactive properties. The smoke from burning cannabis contains many chemicals, including 61 different cannabinoids that have been identified. One of these, Δ-9-tetrahydrocannabinol (Δ-9-THC), produces most of the characteristic pharmacological effects of smoked marijuana.

Surveys have shown that marijuana is the most commonly used illegal drug in the United States. Usage peaked during the late 1970s, when about 60% of high school seniors reported having used marijuana, and nearly 11% reported daily use. This declined steadily among high school seniors to about 40% reporting some use during their lifetime and 2% reporting daily use in the mid-1990s, followed by a gradual increase to 48% of 12th graders in 2002 reporting some use. Surveys among high school seniors tend to underestimate drug use because school dropouts are not surveyed.

Cannabinoid receptors CB-1 (mainly CNS) and CB-2 (peripheral) have been identified and cloned. An arachidonic acid derivative has been proposed as an endogenous ligand and named *anandamide.* While the physiological function of these receptors and their endogenous ligands are incompletely understood, they are likely to have important functions because they are dispersed widely with high densities in the cerebral cortex, hippocampus, striatum, and cerebellum (Iversen, 2003). Specific CB-1 antagonists have been developed and are in controlled clinical trials. One of these, *rimonabant,* has been reported to reduce relapse in cigarette smokers and to produce weight loss in obese patients.

The pharmacological effects of Δ-9-THC vary with the dose, route of administration, experience of the user, vulnerability to psychoactive effects, and setting of use. Intoxication with marijuana produces changes in mood, perception, and motivation, but the effect sought after by most users is the "high" and "mellowing out." This effect is described as different from the stimulant high and the opiate high. The effects vary with dose, but the typical marijuana smoker experiences a high that lasts about 2 hours. During this time, there is impairment of cognitive functions, perception, reaction time, learning, and memory. Impairments of coordination and tracking behavior have been reported to persist for several hours beyond the perception of the high. These impairments have obvious implications for the operation of a motor vehicle and performance in the workplace or at school.

Marijuana also produces complex behavioral changes such as giddiness and increased hunger. There are unsubstantiated claims of increased pleasure from sex and increased insight during a marijuana high. Unpleasant reactions such as panic or hallucinations and even acute psychosis may occur; several surveys indicate that 50% to 60% of marijuana users have reported at least one anxiety experience. These reactions are seen commonly with higher doses and with oral ingestion rather than smoked marijuana because smoking permits the regulation of dose according to the effects. While there is no convincing evidence that marijuana can produce a lasting schizophrenia-like syndrome, there are numerous clinical reports that marijuana use can precipitate a recurrence in people with a history of schizophrenia.

One of the most controversial of the reputed effects of marijuana is the production of an "amotivational syndrome." This syndrome is not an official diagnosis, but it has been used to describe young people who drop out of social activities and show little interest in school, work, or other goal-directed activity. When heavy marijuana use accompanies these symptoms, the drug often is cited as the cause, even though there are no data that demonstrate a causal relationship between marijuana smoking and these behavioral characteristics. There is no evidence that marijuana use damages brain cells or produces any permanent functional changes, although there are animal data indicating impairment of maze learning that persists for weeks after the last dose. These findings are consistent with clinical reports of gradual improvement in mental state after cessation of chronic high-dose marijuana use.

Several medicinal benefits of marijuana have been described. These include antinausea effects that have been applied to the relief of side effects of anticancer chemotherapy, muscle-relaxing effects, anticonvulsant effects, and reduction of intraocular pressure for the treatment of glaucoma. These medical benefits come at the cost of the psychoactive effects that often impair normal activities. Thus there is no clear advantage of marijuana over con-

Table 23–9
Marijuana Withdrawal Syndrome

Restlessness
Irritability
Mild agitation
Insomnia
Sleep EEG disturbance
Nausea, cramping

ventional treatments for any of these indications (Joy *et al.*, 1999). With the cloning of cannabinoid receptors, the discovery of endogenous ligands, and the synthesis of specific agonists and antagonists, it is likely that orally effective medications will be developed without the undesirable properties of smoked marijuana and without the deleterious effects of inhaling smoke particles and the chemical products of high-temperature combustion.

Tolerance, Dependence, and Withdrawal. Tolerance to most of the effects of marijuana can develop rapidly after only a few doses, but also disappears rapidly (Martin *et al.*, 2004). Tolerance to large doses has been found to persist in experimental animals for long periods after cessation of drug use. Withdrawal symptoms and signs typically are not seen in clinical populations. In fact, relative to the number of marijuana smokers, few patients ever seek treatment for marijuana addiction. A withdrawal syndrome in human subjects has been described following close observation of marijuana users given regular oral doses of the agent on a research ward (Table 23–9). This syndrome, however, is only seen clinically in persons who use marijuana on a daily basis and then suddenly stop. Compulsive or regular marijuana users do not appear to be motivated by fear of withdrawal symptoms, although this has not been studied systematically. A large study of psychotherapy for self-identified marijuana-dependent persons reported significant reductions in the use of marijuana after treatment, but there was no control group.

Pharmacological Interventions. Marijuana abuse and addiction have no specific treatments. Heavy users may suffer from accompanying depression and thus may respond to antidepressant medication, but this should be decided on an individual basis considering the severity of the affective symptoms after the marijuana effects have dissipated. The residual drug effects may continue for several weeks. The CB-1 receptor antagonist *rimonabant* has been reported to block the acute effects of smoked marijuana, but there have been no clinical trials of this medication in the treatment of marijuana dependence.

Psychedelic Agents

Perceptual distortions that include hallucinations, illusions, and disorders of thinking such as paranoia can be produced by toxic doses of many drugs. These phenomena also may be seen during toxic withdrawal from sedatives such as alcohol. There are, however, certain drugs that have as their primary effect the production of disturbances of perception, thought, or mood at low doses with minimal effects on memory and orientation. These are commonly called *hallucinogenic drugs,* but their use does not always result in frank hallucinations. In the late 1990s, the use of "club drugs" at all-night dance parties became popular. Such drugs include *methylenedioxymethamphetamine* (MDMA, "ecstasy"), *lysergic acid diethylamide* (LSD), *phencyclidine* (PCP), and *ketamine* (KETALAR). They often are used in association with illegal sedatives such as *flunitrazepam* (ROHYPNOL) or *γ-hydroxybutyrate* (GHB). The latter drug has the reputation of being particularly effective in preventing memory storage, so it has been implicated in "date rapes."

While psychedelic effects can be produced by a variety of different drugs, major psychedelic compounds come from two main categories. The indoleamine hallucinogens include LSD, *N,N-dimethyltryptamine* (DMT), and *psilocybin.* The phenethylamines include *mescaline, dimethoxymethylamphetamine* (DOM), *methylenedioxyamphetamine* (MDA), and MDMA. Both groups have a relatively high affinity for serotonin 5-HT$_2$ receptors (*see* Chapter 11), but they differ in their affinity for other subtypes of 5-HT receptors. There is a good correlation between the relative affinity of these compounds for 5-HT$_2$ receptors and their potency as hallucinogens in human beings (Titeler *et al.,* 1988). The 5-HT$_2$ receptor is further implicated in the mechanism of hallucinations by the observation that antagonists of that receptor, such as *ritanserin,* are effective in blocking the behavioral and electrophysiological effects of hallucinogenic drugs in animal models. However, LSD has been shown to interact with many receptor subtypes at nanomolar concentrations, and at present, it is not possible to attribute the psychedelic effects to any single 5-HT receptor subtype (Peroutka, 1994).

LSD. LSD is the most potent hallucinogenic drug and produces significant psychedelic effects with a total dose of as little as 25 to 50 μg. This drug is more than 3000 times more potent than mescaline. LSD is sold on the illicit market in a variety of forms. A popular contemporary system involves postage stamp-sized papers impregnated with varying doses of LSD (50 to 300 μg or more). Most street samples sold as LSD actually contain LSD. In contrast, the samples of mushrooms and other botanicals sold as sources of psilocybin and other psychedelics have a low probability of containing the advertised hallucinogen.

The effects of hallucinogenic drugs are variable, even in the same individual on different occasions. LSD is absorbed rapidly after oral administration, with effects beginning at 40 to 60 minutes, peaking at 2 to 4 hours, and gradually returning to baseline over 6 to 8 hours. At a dose of 100 μg, LSD produces perceptual distortions and sometimes hallucinations; mood changes, including elation, paranoia, or depression; intense arousal: and sometimes a feeling of panic. Signs of LSD ingestion include pupillary dilation, increased blood pressure and pulse, flushing, salivation, lacrimation, and hyperreflexia. Visual effects are prominent. Colors seem more intense, and shapes may appear altered. The subject may focus attention on unusual items such as the pattern of hairs on the back of the hand.

A "bad trip" usually consists of severe anxiety, although at times it is marked by intense depression and suicidal thoughts. Visual disturbances usually are prominent. The bad trip from LSD may be difficult to distinguish from reactions to anticholinergic drugs and phencyclidine. There are no documented toxic fatalities from LSD use, but fatal accidents and suicides have occurred during or shortly after intoxication. Prolonged psychotic reactions lasting 2 days or more may occur after the ingestion of a hallucinogen. Schizophrenic episodes may be precipitated in susceptible individuals, and there is some evidence that chronic use of these drugs is associated with the development of persistent psychotic disorders (McLellan *et al.,* 1979).

Claims about the potential of psychedelic drugs for enhancing psychotherapy and for treating addictions and other mental disorders have not been supported by controlled treatment outcome studies. Consequently, there is no current indication for these drugs as medications.

Tolerance, Physical Dependence, and Withdrawal. Frequent, repeated use of psychedelic drugs is unusual, and thus tolerance is not commonly seen. Tolerance does develop to the behavioral effects of LSD after three to four daily doses, but no withdrawal syndrome has been observed. Cross-tolerance among LSD, mescaline, and psilocybin has been demonstrated in animal models.

Pharmacological Intervention. Because of the unpredictability of psychedelic drug effects, any use carries some risk. Dependence and addiction do not occur, but users may require medical attention because of "bad trips." Severe agitation may require medication, and *diazepam* (20 mg orally) has been found to be effective. "Talking down" by reassurance also has been shown to be effective and is the management of first choice. Neuroleptic medications (*see* Chapter 18) may intensify the experience and thus are not indicated.

A particularly troubling after-effect of the use of LSD and similar drugs is the occurrence of episodic visual disturbances in a small proportion of former users. These originally were called "flashbacks" and resembled the experiences of prior LSD trips. There now is an official diagnostic category called the *hallucinogen persisting perception disorder* (HPPD; American Psychiatric Association,

1994). The symptoms include false fleeting perceptions in the peripheral fields, flashes of color, geometric pseudohallucinations, and positive afterimages (Abraham and Aldridge, 1993). The visual disorder appears stable in half the cases and represents an apparently permanent alteration of the visual system. Precipitants include stress, fatigue, emergence into a dark environment, marijuana, neuroleptics, and anxiety states.

MDMA ("Ecstasy") and MDA. MDMA and MDA are phenylethylamines that have stimulant as well as psychedelic effects. MDMA became popular during the 1980s on college campuses because of testimonials that it enhances insight and self-knowledge. It was recommended by some psychotherapists as an aid to the process of therapy, although no controlled data exist to support this contention. Acute effects are dose-dependent and include feelings of energy, altered sense of time, and pleasant sensory experiences with enhanced perception. Negative effects include tachycardia, dry mouth, jaw clenching, and muscle aches. At higher doses, visual hallucinations, agitation, hyperthermia, and panic attacks have been reported. A typical oral dose is one or two 100-mg tablets and lasts 3 to 6 hours, although dosage and potency of street samples are variable (approximately 100 mg per tablet).

MDA and MDMA produce degeneration of serotonergic nerve cells and axons in rats. While nerve degeneration has not been demonstrated in human beings, the cerebrospinal fluid of chronic MDMA users has been found to have low levels of serotonin metabolites (Ricaurte *et al.*, 2000). Thus, there is possible neurotoxicity with no evidence that the claimed benefits of MDMA actually occur.

Phencyclidine (PCP). PCP deserves special mention because of its widespread availability and because its pharmacological effects are different from those of the psychedelics such as LSD. PCP was developed originally as an anesthetic in the 1950s and later was abandoned because of a high frequency of postoperative delirium with hallucinations. It was classed as a dissociative anesthetic because, in the anesthetized state, the patient remains conscious with staring gaze, flat facies, and rigid muscles. PCP became a drug of abuse in the 1970s, first in an oral form and then in a smoked version enabling a better regulation of the dose. The effects of PCP have been observed in normal volunteers under controlled conditions. As little as 50 μg/kg produces emotional withdrawal, concrete thinking, and bizarre responses to projective testing. Catatonic posturing also is produced and resembles that of schizophrenia. Abusers taking higher doses may appear to be reacting to hallucinations and exhibit hostile or assaultive behavior. Anesthetic effects

increase with dosage; stupor or coma may occur with muscular rigidity, rhabdomyolysis, and hyperthermia. Intoxicated patients in the emergency room may progress from aggressive behavior to coma, with elevated blood pressure and enlarged nonreactive pupils.

PCP binds with high affinity to sites located in the cortex and limbic structures, resulting in blocking of *N*-methyl-D-aspartate (NMDA)–type glutamate receptors (*see* Chapter 12). LSD and other psychedelics do not bind to NMDA receptors. There is evidence that NMDA receptors are involved in ischemic neuronal death caused by high levels of excitatory amino acids; as a result, there is interest in PCP analogs that block NMDA receptors but with fewer psychoactive effects. Both PCP and ketamine ("Special K"), another "club drug," produce similar effects by altering the distribution of the neurotransmitter glutamate.

Tolerance, Dependence, and Withdrawal. PCP is reinforcing in monkeys, as evidenced by self-administration patterns that produce continuous intoxication. Human beings tend to use PCP intermittently, but some surveys report daily use in 7% of users queried. There is evidence for tolerance to the behavioral effects of PCP in animals, but this has not been studied systematically in human beings. Signs of a PCP withdrawal syndrome were observed in monkeys after interruption of daily access to the drug. These include somnolence, tremor, seizures, diarrhea, piloerection, bruxism, and vocalizations.

Pharmacological Intervention. Overdose must be treated by life support because there is no antagonist of PCP effects and no proven way to enhance excretion, although acidification of the urine has been proposed. PCP coma may last 7 to 10 days. The agitated or psychotic state produced by PCP can be treated with *diazepam*. Prolonged psychotic behavior requires neuroleptic medication (*see* Chapter 18). Because of the anticholinergic activity of PCP, neuroleptics with significant anticholinergic effects such as *chlorpromazine* should be avoided.

Inhalants

Abused inhalants consist of many different categories of chemicals that are volatile at room temperature and produce abrupt changes in mental state when inhaled. Examples include toluene (from model airplane glue), kerosene, gasoline, carbon tetrachloride, amyl nitrite, and nitrous oxide (*see* Chapter 64 for a discussion of the toxicology of such agents). There are characteristic patterns of response for each substance. Solvents such as toluene typically are used by children. The material usually is placed in a plastic bag and the vapors inhaled. After several minutes of inhalation, dizziness and intoxication occur. Aerosol sprays containing fluorocarbon propellants are another source of solvent intoxication. Prolonged exposure or daily use may result in damage to several organ systems. Clinical problems include cardiac arrhythmias, bone marrow depression, cerebral degeneration, and damage to liver, kidney, and peripheral nerves. Death occasionally has been attributed to inhalant abuse, probably *via* the mechanism of cardiac arrhythmias, especially accompanying exercise or upper airway obstruction.

Amyl nitrite produces dilation of smooth muscle and has been used in the past for the treatment of angina. It is a yellow, volatile, flammable liquid with a fruity odor. In recent years, amyl nitrite and *butyl nitrite* have been used to relax smooth muscle and enhance orgasm, particularly by male homosexuals. These agents are obtained in the form of room deodorizers and can produce a feeling of "rush," flushing, and dizziness. Adverse effects include palpitations, postural hypotension, and headache progressing to loss of consciousness.

Anesthetic gases such as *nitrous oxide* and *halothane* sometimes are used as intoxicants by medical personnel. Nitrous oxide also is abused by food-service employees because it is supplied for use as a propellant in disposable aluminum mini tanks for whipping cream canisters. Nitrous oxide produces euphoria and analgesia and then loss of consciousness. Compulsive use and chronic toxicity are reported rarely, but there are obvious risks of overdose associated with the abuse of this anesthetic. Chronic use has been reported to cause peripheral neuropathy.

CLINICAL SUMMARY

The management of drug abuse and addiction must be individualized according to the drugs involved and the associated psychosocial problems of the individual patient. An understanding of the pharmacology of the drug or combination of drugs ingested by the patient is essential to rational and effective treatment. This may be a matter of urgency for the treatment of overdose or for the detoxification of a patient who is experiencing withdrawal symptoms. It must be recognized, however, that the treatment of the underlying addictive disorder requires months or years of rehabilitation. The behavior patterns encoded in memory during thousands of prior drug ingestions do not disappear with detoxification from the drug, even after a typical 28-day inpatient rehabilitation program. Long periods of outpatient treatment are necessary. There probably will be periods of relapse and remission. While complete abstinence is the preferred goal, in reality, most patients are at risk to resume drug-seeking behavior and require a period of retreatment. Maintenance medication can be effective in some circumstances, such as methadone, buprenor-

phine, or naltrexone for opioid dependence and disulfiram, naltrexone, or acamprosate for alcoholism. The process can best be compared to the treatment of other chronic disorders such as diabetes, asthma, or hypertension. Long-term medication may be necessary, and cures are not likely. When viewed in the context of chronic disease, the available treatments for addiction are quite successful in that the majority of patients improve, but improvement does not necessarily persist after treatment has ceased (McLellan *et al.*, 2000; O'Brien, 1994).

Long-term treatment is accompanied by improvements in physical status as well as in mental, social, and occupational function. Unfortunately, there is general pessimism in the medical community about the benefits of treatment such that most of the therapeutic effort is directed at the complications of addiction, such as pulmonary, cardiac, and hepatic disorders. Prevention of these complications can be accomplished by addressing the underlying addictive disorder.

BIBLIOGRAPHY

Alterman, A.I., O'Brien, C.P., McLellan, A.T., *et al.* Effectiveness and costs of inpatient versus day hospital cocaine rehabilitation. *J. Nerv. Ment. Dis.,* **1994,** *182*:157–163.

Anthony, J.C., Warner, L.A., and Kessler, K.C. Comparative epidemiology of dependence on tobacco, alcohol, controlled substances and the inhalants: Basic findings from the national comorbidity survey. *Exp. Clin. Psychopharmacol.,* **1994,** 2:244–268.

Benowitz, N.L., Porchet, H., Sheiner, L., and Jacob, P. III. Nicotine absorption and cardiovascular effects with smokeless tobacco use: Comparison with cigarettes and nicotine gum. *Clin. Pharmacol. Ther.,* **1988,** *44*:23–28.

Chasnoff, I.J., Griffith, D.R., MacGregor, S., *et al.* Temporal patterns of cocaine use in pregnancy: Perinatal outcome. *JAMA,* **1989,** *261*:1741–1744.

Childress, A.R., Mozley, P.D., McElgin, W., *et al.* Limbic activation during cue-induced cocaine craving. *Am. J. Psychiatry,* **1999,** *156*:11–18.

de Wit, H., Pierri, J., and Johanson, C.E. Assessing individual differences in alcohol preference using a cumulative dosing procedure. *Psychopharmacology,* **1989,** 98:113–119.

Dews, P.B., Curtis, G.L., Hanford, K.J., and O'Brien, C.P. The frequency of caffeine withdrawal in a population-based survey and in a controlled, blinded pilot experiment. *J. Clin. Pharmacol.,* **1999,** *39*:1221–1232.

Hearn, W.L., Flynn, D.D., Hime, G.W., *et al.* Cocaethylene: A unique cocaine metabolite displays high affinity for the dopamine transporter. *J. Neurochem.,* **1991,** *56*:698–701.

Higgins, S.T., Budney, A.J., Bickel, W.K., *et al.* Outpatient behavioral treatment for cocaine dependence: One-year outcome. Presented at College on Problems of Drug Dependence 56th Annual Meeting, Palm Beach, FL, **1994.**

Higuchi S., Matsushita, S., Muramatsu, T., *et al.* Alcohol and aldehyde dehydrogenase genetypes and drinking behavior in Japanese. *Alcohol Clin. Exp. Res.*, **1996**, *20*:493–497.

Iversen, L. Cannabis and the brain. *Brain*, **2003**, *126*:1252–1270.

Kalivas, P.W., and Duffy, P. Effect of acute and daily cocaine treatment on extracellular dopamine in the nucleus accumbens. *Synapse*, **1990**, *5*:48–58.

Kosten, T.A. and O'Conner, P.G. Management of drug and alcohol withdrawal. *New Engl. J. Med.*, **2003**, *348*:1786–1795.

Kreek, M.J., LaForge, K.S., and Butelman, E. Pharmacotherapy of addictions. *Nature Rev. Drug Discov.*, **2002**, *1*:710–726.

Martin, B.R., Sim-Selley, L.J., and Selley, D.E. Signaling pathways involved in the development of cannabinoid tolerance. *Trends Pharmacol. Sci.*, **2004**, *25*:325–330.

McLellan, A.T., Woody, G.E., and O'Brien, C.P. Development of psychiatric illness in drug abusers: Possible role of drug preference. *New Engl. J. Med.*, **1979**, *301*:1310–1314.

Mason, B.J. Acamprosate and naltrexone treatment for alcohol dependence: An evidence-based risk benefits assessment. *Eur. Neuropsychopharmacol.*, **2003**, *13*:469–475.

Mendelson, J.H., and Mello, N.K. Medical progress: Biologic concomitants of alcoholism. *New Engl. J. Med.*, **1979**, *301*:912–921.

Oslin, D.W., Berrettini, W., Dranzler, H.R. *et al.* A functional polymorphism of the μ-opioid receptor gene is associated with naltrexone response in alcohol-dependent patients. *Neuropsychopharmacology*, **2003**, *28*:1546–1552.

Peroutka, S.J. 5-Hydroxytryptamine receptor interactions of *d*-lysergic acid diethylamide. In, *50 Years of LSD: Current status and Perspectives of Hallucinogens.* (Pletscher, A., and Ladewig, D., eds.) Parthenon Publishing, New York, **1994**, pp. 19–26.

Ricaurte, G.A., McCann, U.D., Szabo, Z., and Scheffel, U. Toxicodynamics and long-term toxicity of the recreational drug, 3,4-methylenedioxymethamphetamine (MDMA, "ecstasy"). *Toxicol. Lett.*, **2000**, *112–113*:143–146.

Ritz, M.C., Lamb, R.J., Goldberg, S.R., and Kuhar, M.J. Cocaine receptors on dopamine transporters are related to self-administration of cocaine. *Science*, **1987**, *237*:1219–1223.

Robinson G.M., Sellers, E.M., and Janecek, E. Barbiturate and hypnosedative withdrawal by a multiple oral phenobarbital loading dose technique. *Clin. Pharmacol. Ther.*, **1981**, *30*:71–76.

Satel, S.L., Southwick, S.M., and Gawin, F.H. Clinical features of cocaine-induced paranoia. *Am. J. Psychiatry*, **1991**, *148*:495–498.

Silverman, K., Evans, S.M., Strain, E.C., and Griffiths, R.R. Withdrawal syndrome after the double-blind cessation of caffeine consumption. *New Engl. J. Med.*, **1992**, *327*:1109–1114.

Srivastava, E.D., Russell, M.A., Feyerabend, C., *et al.* Sensitivity and tolerance to nicotine in smokers and nonsmokers. *Psychopharmacology*, **1991**, *105*:63–68.

Titeler, M., Lyon, R.A., and Glennon, R.A. Radioligand binding evidence implicates the brain 5-HT$_2$ receptor as a site of action for LSD and phenylisopropylamine hallucinogens. *Psychopharmacology*, **1988**, *94*:213–216.

Trujillo, K.A., and Akil, H. Inhibition of morphine tolerance and dependence by the NMDA receptor antagonist MK-801. *Science*, **1991**, *251*:85–87.

Volkow, N.D., Wang, G.J., Fowler, J.S., *et al.* Reinforcing effects of psychostimulants in humans are associated with increases in brain dopamine and occupancy of D$_2$ receptors. *J. Pharmacol. Exp. Ther.*, **1999**, *291*:409–415.

Weddington, W.W., Brown, B.S., Haertzen, C.A., *et al.* Changes in mood, craving, and sleep during short-term abstinence reported by male cocaine addicts. A controlled residential study. *Arch. Gen. Psychiatry*, **1990**, *47*:861–868.

MONOGRAPHS AND REVIEWS

Abraham, H.D., and Aldridge, A.M. Adverse consequences of lysergic acid diethylamide. *Addiction*, **1993**, *88*:1327–1334.

American Psychiatric Association. *Diagnostic and Statistical Manual of Mental Disorders*, 4th ed. (DSM IV). APA, Washington, **1994.**

American Psychiatric Association. *Benzodiazepine Dependence, Toxicity, and Abuse: A Task Force Report of the American Psychiatric Association.* APA, Washington, **1990.**

Joy, J.E., Watson, S.J., Benson, J.A., and Institute of Medicine. *Marijuana and Medicine: Assessing the Science Base.* National Academy Press, Washington, **1999.**

Kalix, P. Pharmacological properties of the stimulant khat. *Pharmacol. Ther.*, **1990**, *48*:397–416.

Kreek, M.J. Rationale for maintenance pharmacotherapy of opiate dependence. In, *Addictive States.* (O'Brien, C.P., and Jaffe, J.H., eds.) Raven Press, New York, **1992**, pp. 205–230.

McLellan, A.T., Lewis, D.C., O'Brien, C.P., and Kleber, H.D. Drug dependence, a chronic medical illness: Implications for treatment, insurance, and outcomes evaluation. *JAMA*, **2000**, *13*:1689–1695.

O'Brien, C.P. Treatment of alcoholism as a chronic disorder. In, *Toward a Molecular Basis of Alcohol Use and Abuse*, Experientia Supplementum, Vol. 71. (Jansson, B., Jörnvall, H., Rydberg, U., Terenius, L., and Vallee, B.L., eds.) Birkhäuser, Boston, **1994**, pp. 349–359.

Wilhelmsen, K.C., Schuckit, M. and Smith, T.L. The search for genes related to a low-level response to alcohol determined by alcohol challenges. *Alcohol Clin. Exp. Res.*, **2003**, *27*:1041–1047.

CHAPTER

24

HISTAMINE, BRADYKININ, AND THEIR ANTAGONISTS

Randal A. Skidgel and Ervin G. Erdös

HISTAMINE

History. The history of histamine (β-aminoethylimidazole) parallels that of acetylcholine (ACh). Both compounds were synthesized as chemical curiosities before their biological significance was recognized; they were first detected as uterine stimulants in extracts of ergot, from which they were subsequently isolated, and proved to be contaminants of ergot derived from bacterial action.

When Dale and Laidlaw subjected histamine to intensive pharmacological study, they discovered that it stimulated a host of smooth muscles and had an intense vasodepressor action. Remarkably, they observed that when a sensitized animal was injected with a normally inert protein, the immediate responses closely resembled those of poisoning by histamine. These observations anticipated by many years the discovery that endogenous histamine contributed to immediate hypersensitivity reactions and to responses to cellular injury. Best and colleagues (1927) isolated histamine from fresh samples of liver and lung, thereby establishing that this amine is a natural constituent of many mammalian tissues, hence the name *histamine* after the Greek word for tissue, *histos.*

Lewis and colleagues proposed that a substance with the properties of histamine ("H-substance") was liberated from the cells of the skin by injurious stimuli, including the reaction of antigen with antibody. We now know that endogenous histamine plays a role in the immediate allergic response and is an important regulator of gastric acid secretion. More recently, a role for histamine as a modulator of neurotransmitter release in the central and peripheral nervous systems

has emerged. The presence of histamine in tissue extracts delayed the acceptance of the discovery of some peptide and protein hormones (*e.g.,* gastrin) until the technology for separating the naturally occurring substances was sufficiently advanced (Grossman, 1966).

Early suspicions that histamine acts through more than one receptor have been borne out by the elucidation of four distinct classes of receptors for histamine, designated H_1 (Ash and Schild, 1966), H_2 (Black *et al.,* 1972), H_3 (Arrang *et al.,* 1987), and H_4 (Hough, 2001). H_1 receptors are blocked selectively by the classical "antihistamines" such as pyrilamine. Interest in the clinical use of H_1-receptor antagonists has been renewed owing to the development of second-generation antagonists collectively referred to as *nonsedating antihistamines.* The term *third generation* has been applied to some recently developed antihistamines, such as active metabolites of first- or second-generation antihistamines that are not further metabolized (*e.g.,* cetirizine derived from hydroxyzine or fexofenadine from terfenadine) or to antihistamines that have additional therapeutic effects. However, a review by the Consensus Group on New Generation Antihistamines concluded that none of the currently available antihistamines can be classified as true third-generation drugs, which they define as lacking in cardiotoxicity, drug–drug interactions, and central nervous system (CNS) effects with possible beneficial effects (*e.g.,* antiinflammatory) (Holgate *et al.,* 2003). The discovery of H_2 antagonists and their ability to inhibit gastric secretion has contributed greatly to the resurgence of interest in histamine in biology and clinical medicine (*see* Chapter 36). H_3 receptors were discovered as presynaptic autoreceptors on histamine-containing neurons that mediated feedback inhibition of the release and synthesis of histamine. The development of selective H_3-receptor agonists and antagonists has led to an increased understanding of the importance of H_3 receptors in histaminergic neurons *in vivo.* None of these H_3-receptor agonists or antagonists has yet emerged as a therapeutic agent. The H_4 receptor is more similar to the H_3 receptor

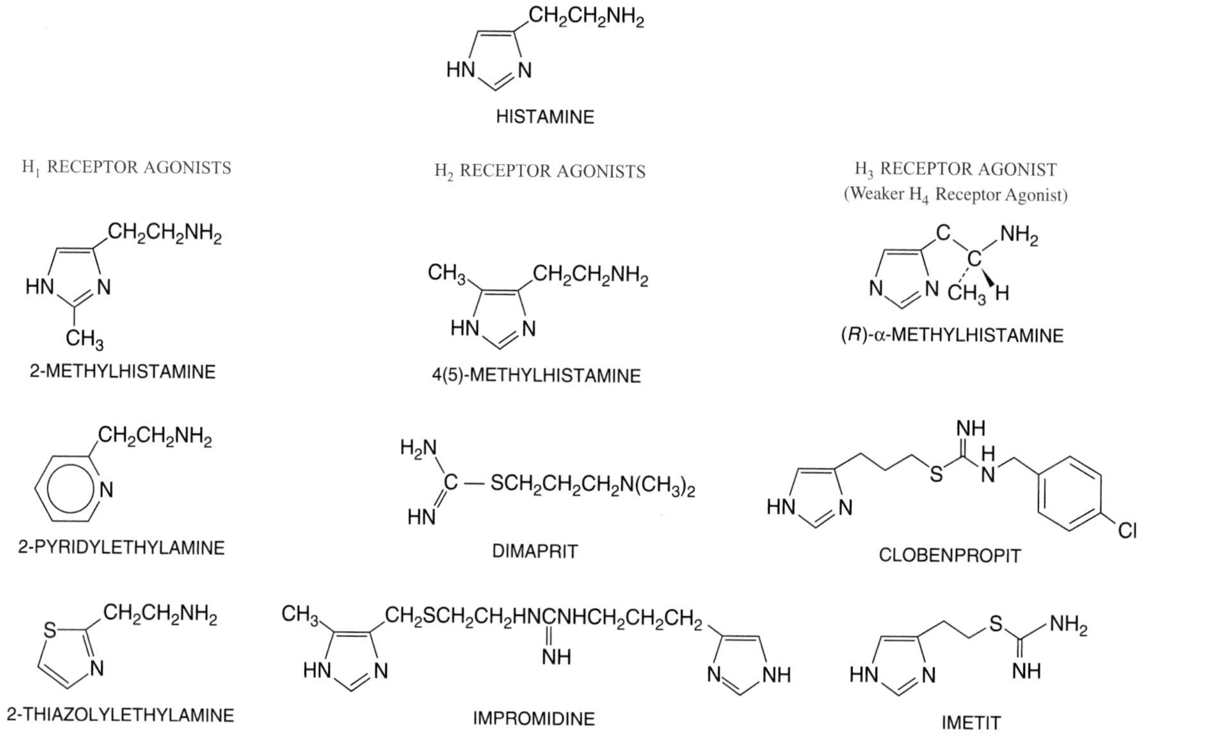

Figure 24–1. *Structure of histamine and some H₁, H₂, H₃, and H₄ agonists.* The H_3 agonists are weaker H_4 receptor agonists.

than to the other histamine receptors and is expressed in cells of hematopoietic lineage; the availability of an H_4-specific antagonist with antiinflammatory properties should help to define the biological roles of the H_4 receptor (Thurmond *et al.*, 2004).

Chemistry. Histamine is a hydrophilic molecule consisting of an imidazole ring and an amino group connected by two methylene groups. The pharmacologically active form at all histamine receptors is the monocationic Nγ—H tautomer, *i.e.*, the charged form of the species depicted in Figure 24–1, although different chemical

properties of this monocation may be involved in interactions with the H_1 and H_2 receptors (Ganellin and Parsons, 1982). The four classes of histamine receptors can be activated differently by analogs of histamine (Figure 24–1 and Table 24–1). Thus 2-methylhistamine preferentially elicits responses mediated by H_1 receptors, whereas 4(5)-methylhistamine has a preferential effect on H_2 receptors (Black *et al.*, 1972). A chiral analog of histamine with restricted conformational freedom, (R)-α-methylhistamine, is the preferred agonist at H_3-receptor sites, although it is a weak agonist of the H_4

Table 24–1
Characteristics of Histamine Receptors

	H_1	H_2	H_3	H_4
Size (amino acids)	487	359	373, 445, 365	390
G protein coupling (second messengers)	$G_{q/11}$ ($\uparrow Ca^{2+}$; $\uparrow cAMP$)	G_s ($\uparrow cAMP$)	$G_{i/o}$ ($\downarrow cAMP$)	$G_{i/o}$ ($\downarrow cAMP$; $\uparrow Ca^{2+}$)
Distribution	Smooth muscle, endothelial cells, CNS	Gastric parietal cells, cardiac muscle, mast cells, CNS	CNS: presynaptic, myenteric plexus	Cells of hematopoietic origin
Representative agonist	2-CH₃-histamine	Dimaprit	(R)-α-CH₃-histamine	Clobenpropit (partial?)
Representative antagonist	Chlorpheniramine	Ranitidine	Thioperamide Clobenpropit	JNJ7777120 Thioperamide

Compounds affecting the H_3 and H_4 receptors exhibit some lack of specificity, although JNJ7777120 seems to be a relatively specific H_4 antagonist. JNJ7777120 is 1-[(5-chloro-1H-indol-2-yl) carbonyl]-4-methylpiperazine (*see* Thurmond *et al.*, 2004).

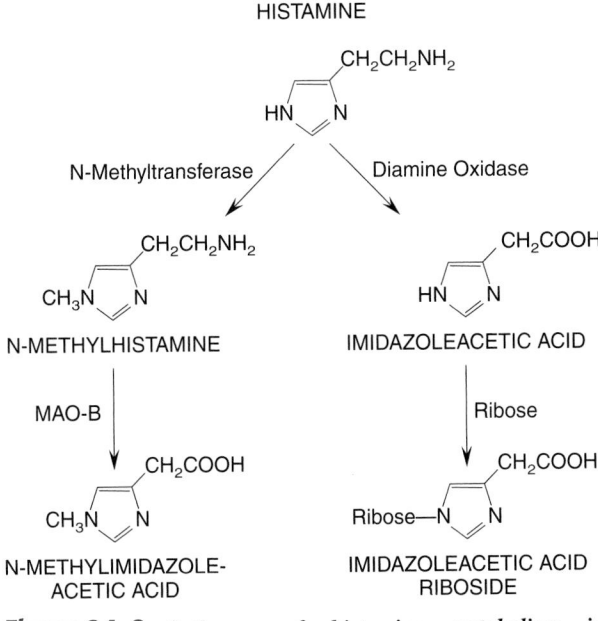

HISTAMINE

Figure 24–2. *Pathways of histamine metabolism in humans. See text for details.*

receptor as well (Hough, 2001). Indeed, a number of compounds have activity at both the H_3 and H_4 receptors.

Distribution and Biosynthesis of Histamine

Distribution. Histamine is widely, if unevenly, distributed throughout the animal kingdom and is present in many venoms, bacteria, and plants. Almost all mammalian tissues contain histamine in amounts ranging from less than 1 to more than 100 $\mu g/g$. Concentrations in plasma and other body fluids generally are very low, but human cerebrospinal fluid (CSF) contains significant amounts. The mast cell is the predominant storage site for histamine in most tissues (*see* below); the concentration of histamine is particularly high in tissues that contain large numbers of mast cells, such as skin, bronchial tree mucosa, and intestinal mucosa.

Synthesis, Storage, and Metabolism. Histamine is formed by the decarboxylation of the amino acid histidine by the enzyme L-histidine decarboxylase (Figure 24–2). Every mammalian tissue that contains histamine is capable of synthesizing it from histidine by virtue of its content of L-histidine decarboxylase. The chief site of histamine storage in most tissues is the mast cell; in the blood, it is the basophil. These cells synthesize histamine and store it in secretory granules. At the secretory granule pH of approximately 5.5, histamine is positively charged and ionically complexed with negatively charged acidic groups on other constituents of the secretory granule, primarily proteases and heparin or chondroitin sulfate proteoglycans (Serafin and Austen, 1987). The turnover rate of histamine in secretory granules is slow, and when tissues rich in mast cells are depleted of their histamine stores, it may take weeks before concentrations return to normal levels. Non–mast cell sites of histamine formation or storage include the epidermis, the gastric mucosa, neurons within the CNS, and cells in regenerating or rapidly growing tissues. Turnover is rapid at these non–mast cell sites because the histamine is released continuously

rather than stored. Non–mast cell sites of histamine production contribute significantly to the daily excretion of histamine metabolites in the urine. Since L-histidine decarboxylase is an inducible enzyme, the histamine-forming capacity at such sites is subject to regulation. Ingested histamine does not contribute to the body's store: Histamine, in the amounts normally ingested or formed by bacteria in the gastrointestinal tract, is metabolized rapidly and eliminated in the urine.

There are two major paths of histamine metabolism in humans (Figure 24–2). The more important of these involves ring methylation to form *N*-methylhistamine, catalyzed by histamine-*N*-methyltransferase, which is distributed widely. Most of the *N*-methylhistamine formed is then converted *N*-methylimidazoleacetic acid by monoamine oxidase (MAO), and this reaction can be blocked by monoamine oxidase (MAO) inhibitors (*see* Chapters 17 and 20). Alternatively, histamine may undergo oxidative deamination catalyzed mainly by the nonspecific enzyme diamine oxidase (DAO), yielding imidazoleacetic acid, which is then converted to imidazoleacetic acid riboside. These metabolites have little or no activity and are excreted in the urine. Measurement of *N*-methylhistamine in urine affords a more reliable index of histamine production than assessment of histamine itself. Artifactually elevated levels of histamine in urine arise from genitourinary tract bacteria that can decarboxylate histidine. In addition, the metabolism of histamine appears to be altered in patients with mastocytosis such that determination of histamine metabolites is a more sensitive diagnostic indicator of the disease than histamine.

Release and Functions of Endogenous Histamine

Histamine has important physiological roles. After its release from storage granules as a result of the interaction of antigen with immunoglobulin E (IgE) antibodies on the mast cell surface, histamine plays a central role in immediate hypersensitivity and allergic responses. The actions of histamine on bronchial smooth muscle and blood vessels account for many of the symptoms of the allergic response. In addition, certain clinically useful drugs can act directly on mast cells to release histamine, thereby explaining some of their untoward effects. Histamine has a major role in the regulation of gastric acid secretion and also modulates neurotransmitter release.

Role in Allergic Responses. The principal target cells of immediate hypersensitivity reactions are mast cells and basophils (Schwartz, 1994). As part of the allergic response to an antigen, reaginic (IgE) antibodies are generated and bind to the surfaces of mast cells and basophils *via* high-affinity F_c receptors that are specific for IgE. This receptor, FcεRI, consists of α, β, and two γ chains. The IgE molecules function as receptors for antigens and, *via* FcεRI, interact with signal-transduction systems in the membranes of sensitized cells (*see* Chapter 27). Atopic individuals develop IgE antibodies to commonly inhaled antigens. This is a heritable trait, and a candidate gene product has been identified as the β-chain of FcεRI. Antigen bridges the IgE molecules and activates signaling pathways in mast cells or basophils involving tyrosine kinases and subsequent phosphorylation of multiple protein substrates within 5 to 15 seconds of contact with antigen. Kinases implicated include the *Src*-related kinases Lyn and Syk. Prominent among the phosphorylated proteins are the β and γ subunits of FcεRI itself and phospholipases Cγl and

Cγ2 (with consequent production of IP$_3$ and mobilization of intra-cellular Ca^{2+}) (*see* Chapter 1). These events trigger the exocytosis of the contents of secretory granules (*see* Figure 6–2).

Release of Other Autacoids. The release of histamine only partially explains the biological effects that ensue from immediate hypersensitivity reactions. This is so because a broad spectrum of other inflammatory mediators is released on mast cell activation.

Stimulation of IgE receptors also activates phospholipase A$_2$ (PLA$_2$), leading to the production of a host of mediators, including platelet-activating factor (PAF) and metabolites of arachidonic acid. Leukotriene D$_4$, which is generated in this way, is a potent contractor of the smooth muscle of the bronchial tree (*see* Chapters 25 and 27). Kinins also are generated during some allergic responses. Thus the mast cell secretes a variety of inflammatory mediators in addition to histamine, each contributing to the major symptoms of the allergic response (*see* below).

Regulation of Mediator Release. The wide variety of mediators released during the allergic response explains the ineffectiveness of drug therapy focused on a single mediator. Considerable emphasis has been placed on the regulation of mediator release from mast cells and basophils, and these cells do contain receptors linked to signaling systems that can enhance or block the IgE-induced release of mediators.

Agents that act at muscarinic or α adrenergic receptors increase the release of mediators, although this effect is of little clinical significance. Epinephrine and related drugs that act through β_2 adrenergic receptors increase cellular cyclic AMP and thereby inhibit the secretory activities of mast cells. However, the beneficial effects of β adrenergic agonists in allergic states such as asthma are due mainly to their relaxant effect on bronchial smooth muscle (*see* Chapters 10 and 27). Cromolyn sodium is used clinically because it inhibits the release of mediators from mast and other cells in the lung (*see* Chapter 27).

Histamine Release by Drugs, Peptides, Venoms, and Other Agents. Many compounds, including a large number of therapeutic agents, stimulate the release of histamine from mast cells directly and without prior sensitization. Responses of this sort are most likely to occur following intravenous injections of certain categories of substances, particularly organic bases such as amides, amidines, quaternary ammonium compounds, pyridinium compounds, piperidines, and alkaloids (Rothschild, 1966). Tubocurarine, succinylcholine, morphine, some antibiotics, radiocontrast media, and certain carbohydrate plasma expanders also may elicit the response. The phenomenon is one of clinical concern, for it may account for unexpected anaphylactoid reactions. Vancomycin-induced "red-man syndrome" involving upper body and facial flushing and hypotension may be mediated through histamine release.

In addition to therapeutic agents, certain experimental compounds stimulate the release of histamine as their dominant pharmacological characteristic. The archetype is the polybasic substance known as *compound 48/80*. This is a mixture of low-molecular-weight polymers of *p*-methoxy-*N*-methylphenethylamine, of which the hexamer is most active.

Basic polypeptides often are effective histamine releasers, and over a limited range, their potency generally increases with the number of basic groups. For example, bradykinin is a poor histamine releaser, whereas kallidin (Lys-bradykinin) and substance P, with more positively charged amino acids, are more active. Some venoms, such as that of the wasp, contain potent histamine-releasing peptides (Johnson and Erdös, 1973). Polymyxin B is also very active. Since basic polypeptides are released on tissue injury, they constitute patho-

physiological stimuli to secretion for mast cells and basophils. Anaphylatoxins (C3a and C5a), which are low-molecular-weight peptides released during activation of complement, may act similarly.

Within seconds of the intravenous injection of a histamine liberator, human subjects experience a burning, itching sensation. This effect, most marked in the palms of the hand and in the face, scalp, and ears, is soon followed by a feeling of intense warmth. The skin reddens, and the color rapidly spreads over the trunk. Blood pressure falls, the heart rate accelerates, and the subject usually complains of headache. After a few minutes, blood pressure recovers, and crops of hives usually appear on the skin. Colic, nausea, hypersecretion of acid, and moderate bronchospasm also occur frequently. The effect becomes less intense with successive injections as the mast cell stores of histamine are depleted. Histamine liberators do not deplete tissues of non–mast cell histamine.

Mechanism of Histamine-Releasing Agents. Histamine-releasing substances activate the secretory responses of mast cells and basophils by causing a rise in intracellular Ca^{2+}. Some are ionophores and facilitate the entry of Ca^{2+} into the cell; others, such as neurotensin, act on specific G protein–coupled receptor. In contrast, basic secretogogues (*e.g.,* substance P, mastoparan, kallidin, compound 48/80, and polymyxin B) do not act *via* specific high-affinity receptors on mast cells. Their precise mechanism of action is still unclear but likely results from either interaction with a common cell surface binding site, such as a nonspecific G protein–coupled receptor, or by direct activation of G$_i$ proteins after being taken up by the cell (Ferry *et al.*, 2002). The downstream effectors appear to be $\beta\gamma$ subunits released from Gα_i, which activate the PLCβ–IP$_3$–Ca^{2+} pathway. Antigen–IgE complexes lead to mobilization of stored Ca^{2+} in phosphorylative activation of isoforms of PLCγ, as described earlier.

Histamine Release by Other Means. Clinical conditions in which release of histamine occurs in response to other stimuli include cold urticaria, cholinergic urticaria, and solar urticaria. Some of these involve specific secretory responses of the mast cells and cell-fixed IgE. However, histamine release also occurs whenever there is nonspecific cell damage from any cause. The redness and urticaria that follow scratching of the skin is a familiar example.

Increased Proliferation of Mast Cells and Basophils and Gastric Carcinoid Tumors. In urticaria pigmentosa (cutaneous mastocytosis), mast cells aggregate in the upper corium and give rise to pigmented cutaneous lesions that urticate (*i.e.,* sting) when stroked. In systemic mastocytosis, overproliferation of mast cells also is found in other organs. Patients with these syndromes suffer a constellation of signs and symptoms attributable to excessive histamine release, including urticaria, dermographism, pruritus, headache, weakness, hypotension, flushing of the face, and a variety of gastrointestinal effects such as peptic ulceration. Episodes of mast cell activation with attendant systemic histamine release are precipitated by a variety of stimuli, including exertion, emotional upset, exposure to heat, and exposure to drugs that release histamine directly or to which patients are allergic. In myelogenous leukemia, excessive numbers of basophils are present in the blood, raising its histamine content to high levels that may contribute to chronic pruritus. Gastric carcinoid tumors secrete histamine, which is responsible for episodes of vasodilation as part of the patchy "geographical" flush (Roberts *et al.*, 1979).

Gastric Acid Secretion. Acting at H$_2$ receptors, histamine is a powerful gastric secretagogue and evokes a copious secretion of acid from parietal cells (*see* Figure 36–1); it also increases the output of pepsin and intrinsic factor. Although the secretion of gastric acid also is evoked by stimulation of the vagus nerve and by the enteric hormone gastrin, presumably by activation of M_3 and CCK_2 receptors on the parietal cell, acetylcholine and gastrin also stimulate histamine release from the enterochromaffinlike cell. There is no doubt that histamine is the dominant physiological mediator of acid secretion: Blockade of H_2 receptors not only eliminates acid secretion in response to histamine but also causes nearly complete inhibition of responses to gastrin and vagal stimulation. The regulation of gastric acid secretion and the clinical utility of H_2 antagonists are discussed in Chapter 36.

Central Nervous System. There is substantial evidence that histamine functions as a neurotransmitter in the CNS. Histamine, histidine decarboxylase, and enzymes that catalyze the degradation of histamine are distributed nonuniformly in the CNS and are concentrated in synaptosomal fractions of brain homogenates. H_1 receptors are found throughout the CNS and are densely concentrated in the hypothalamus. Histamine increases wakefulness *via* H_1 receptors, explaining the potential for sedation by classical antihistamines. Histamine acting through H_1 receptors inhibits appetite (Ookuma *et al.*, 1993). Histamine-containing neurons may participate in the regulation of drinking, body temperature, and the secretion of antidiuretic hormone, as well as in the control of blood pressure and the perception of pain. Both H_1 and H_2 receptors seem to be involved in these responses (*see* Hough, 1988). Knockout of the H_1 receptor in mice by genetic engineering was associated with increased aggression, locomotion problems, and other neurological symptoms (Simons, 2003a). Central effects of histamine also may be mediated by presynaptic H_3 autoreceptors, which are found almost exclusively in the brain. This is consistent with changes in anxiety and cognition in animals treated with H_3-receptor antagonists or in mice in which the H_3 receptor was genetically deleted.

Pharmacological Effects

Receptor–Effector Coupling and Mechanisms of Action. Histamine receptors are GPCRs (Leurs *et al.*, 2001; Hough, 2001) (Table 24–1). The H_1 histamine receptors couple to $G_{q/11}$ and activate the $PLC–IP_3–Ca^{2+}$ pathway and its many possible sequelae, including activation of protein kinase C (PKC), Ca^{2+}–calmodulin–dependent enzymes (eNOS and various protein kinases), and PLA_2. H_2 receptors link to G_s to activate the adenylyl cyclase–cyclic AMP–protein kinase A (PKA) pathway, whereas H_3 and H_4 receptors couple to $G_{i/o}$ to inhibit adenylyl cyclase (Leurs *et al.*, 2001; Hough, 2001); activation of H_4 receptors also mobilizes stored Ca^{2+} in some cells. Armed with this information, with knowledge of the cellular expression of H-receptor subtypes, and with an understanding of the differentiated functions of a particular cell type, one can predict a cell's response to histamine. Of course, a cell in a physiological setting is exposed to a myriad of hormones simultaneously, and significant interactions may occur between signaling pathways, such as the $G_q \rightarrow G_s$ cross-talk described in a number of systems (Meszaros *et al.*, 2000). Furthermore, the differential expression of H-receptor subtypes on neigh-

boring cells and the unequal sensitivities of H-receptor–effector response pathways can cause parallel and opposing cellular responses to occur together, complicating interpretation of the overall response of a tissue. For example, activation of H_1 receptors on vascular endothelium stimulates the Ca^{2+}-mobilizing pathways (G_q–PLC–IP_3) and activates nitric oxide (NO) production by eNOS, relaxing nearby smooth muscle cells. Stimulation of H_1 receptors on smooth muscle similarly will mobilize Ca^{2+} but cause contraction, whereas activation of H_2 receptors on the same smooth muscle cell will link *via* G_s to enhanced cyclic AMP accumulation, activation of PKA, and then to relaxation (Leurs *et al.*, 2001; Toda, 1987).

The existence of multiple histamine receptors was predicted based on the studies of Ash and Schild and Black and colleagues a generation before the cloning of histamine receptors. Similarly, heterogeneity of H_3 receptors, predicted by kinetic and radioligand-binding studies, has been confirmed by cloning. This identified H_3 isoforms differing in the third intracellular loop TM6, TM7, and C-terminal tail and in their capacity to couple G_i, to inhibit adenylyl cyclase, and to activate mitogen-activated protein (MAP) kinase. Molecular cloning studies also have identified the H_4 receptor. H_1 and H_2 receptors are distributed widely in the periphery and in the CNS, but H_3 receptors are confined largely to the CNS. H_4 receptors, which also have been cloned, are mainly in cells of hematopoietic origin. In a species-dependent manner, adenosine receptors may interact with H_1 receptors. In the CNS of human beings, activation of adenosine A_1 receptors inhibits second-messenger generation *via* H_1 receptors. A possible mechanism for this is an interaction (cross-talk) between the G proteins to which the A_1 and H_1 receptors are functionally coupled, although multiple cell types and paracrine mediators also may be involved.

As Figures 24–1, 24–3, and 36–3 indicate, the pharmacologic definition of H_1, H_2, and H_3 receptors generally is clear: Relatively specific agonists and antagonists are available (Table 24–1). However, the H_4 receptor exhibits 35% to 40% homology to the H_3 receptor, and the two are harder to distinguish pharmacologically. High-affinity H_3 agonists interact with H_4 receptors as well, albeit with reduced potency, as do the H_3 antagonists *burimamide* and *clobenpropit*. Several nonimidazole compounds are selective H_3 antagonists. The atypical antipsychotic agent *clozapine* is an effective H_1-receptor antagonist, a weak H_3-receptor antagonist, but an H_4-receptor agonist in the rat. Many neuroleptics are H_1- and H_2-receptor antagonists, but it is unclear whether interactions with H receptors play a role in the effects of antipsychotic agents. The finding of high constitutive activity of the rat and human H_3 receptor has sparked a reexamination of the potential role of inverse agonists of H_3 recep-

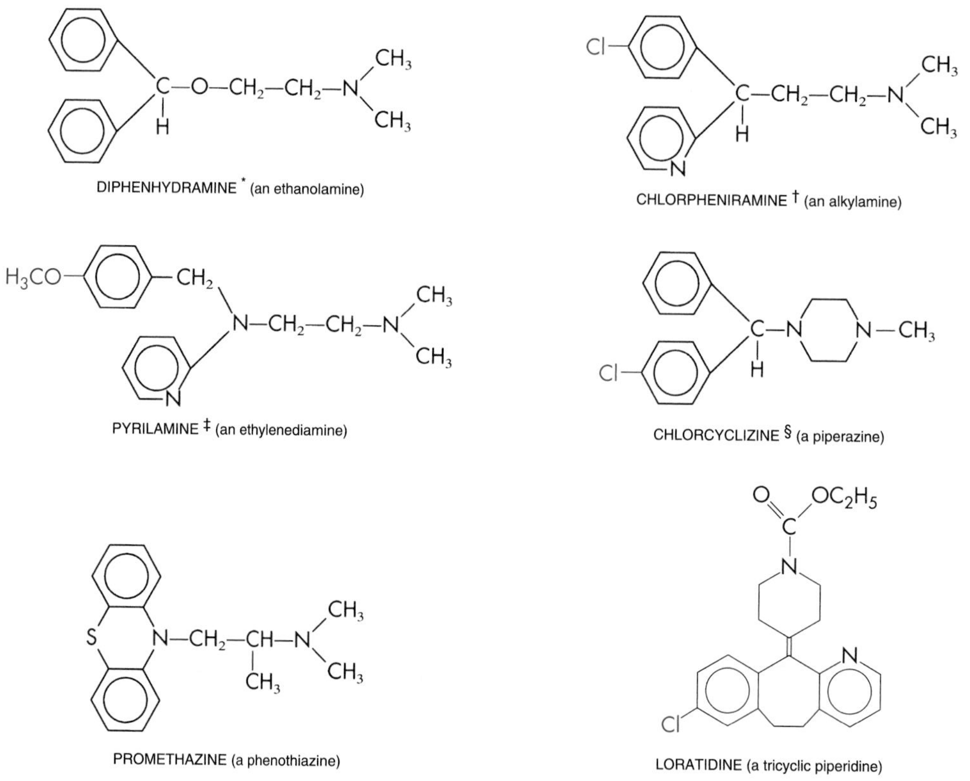

Figure 24–3. ***Representative H₁ antagonists.*** *Dimenhydrinate is a combination of diphenhydramine and 8-chlorotheophylline in equal molecular proportions. †Pheniramine is the same less Cl. ‡Tripelennamine is the same less H₃CO. §Cyclizine is the same less Cl.

tors as therapeutic modulators of H_3-receptor-mediated inhibition of histamine release from histaminergic neurons. H_1 receptors also are reported to express intrinsic or constitutive activity; thus many H_1 antagonists may function as inverse agonists (Leurs *et al.*, 2002). The synthesis of a selective H_4 antagonist (an indole–methylpiperazine derivative) with antiinflammatory properties was reported recently (*see* Thurmond *et al.*, 2004).

H₁ and H₂ Receptors. Once released, histamine can exert local or widespread effects on smooth muscles and glands. It contracts many smooth muscles, such as those of the bronchi and gut, but markedly relaxes others, including those in small blood vessels. Histamine also is a potent stimulus of gastric acid secretion (*see* above). Other, less prominent effects include formation of edema and stimulation of sensory nerve endings. Bronchoconstriction and contraction of the gut are mediated by H_1 receptors (Ash and Schild, 1966). Gastric secretion results from the activation of H_2 receptors and, accordingly, can be inhibited by H_2-receptor antagonists (*see* Chapter 36). Some responses, such as vascular dilation, are mediated by both H_1- and H_2-receptor stimulation.

H₃ and H₄ Receptors. H_3 receptors are expressed mainly in the CNS, especially in the basal ganglia, hippocampus, and cortex. H_3 receptors function as autoreceptors on histaminergic neurons, much like presynaptic α_2 receptors, inhibiting histamine release and modulating the release of other neurotransmitters. H_3 antagonists promote wakefulness; conversely, H_3 agonists promote sleep. H_3 receptors appear to have high constitutive activity; thus histamine release may be tonically inhibited, and inverse agonists may reduce receptor activation and increase histamine release from histaminergic neurons. H_4 receptors are on immune active cells such as eosinophils and neutrophils, as well as in the gastrointestinal (GI) tract and CNS. Activation of H_4 receptors on eosinophils induces a cellular shape change, chemotaxis, and up-regulation of adhesion molecules such as CD11b/CD18 and intercellular adhesion molecule (ICAM)-1 (*see* Ling *et al.*, 2004), suggesting that the histamine released from mast cells acts at H_4 receptors to recruit eosinophils. H_4 antagonists may be useful inhibitors of allergic and inflammatory responses.

Effects on Histamine Release. H_2-receptor stimulation increases cyclic AMP and leads to feedback inhibition of histamine release from mast cells and basophils. Activation of H_3 and H_4 receptors decreases cellular cyclic AMP (Oda *et al.*, 2000; Hough, 2001; Macglashan, 2003); H_3 receptors also may function as presynaptic autoinhibitory receptors on histaminergic neurons.

Histamine Toxicity from Ingestion. Histamine is the toxin in food poisoning from spoiled scombroid fish such as tuna (Morrow *et al.*, 1991), in which high histidine content combines with a large bacterial capacity to decarboxylate histidine to form large quantities of histamine. Ingestion of the fish causes severe nausea, vomiting, headache, flushing, and sweating. Histamine toxicity, manifested by headache and other symptoms, also can follow red wine consumption in persons who possibly have a diminished ability to degrade histamine. The symptoms of histamine poisoning can be suppressed by H_1-receptor antagonists.

Cardiovascular System. Histamine characteristically causes dilation of resistance vessels, an increase in capillary permeability, and an overall fall in systemic blood pressure. In some vascular beds, histamine will constrict veins, contributing to the extravasation of fluid and edema formation upstream of the capillaries and postcapillary venules.

Vasodilation. This is by far the most important vascular effect of histamine in human beings. Vasodilation involves both H_1 and H_2 receptors distributed throughout the resistance vessels in most vascular beds; however, quantitative differences are apparent in the degree of dilation that occurs in various beds. Activation of either the H_1 or H_2 receptor can elicit maximal vasodilation, but the responses differ. H_1 receptors have a higher affinity for histamine and mediate an endothelium–NO–dependent dilation that is relatively rapid in onset and short-lived. By contrast, activation of H_2 receptors (stimulating the cyclic AMP–PKA pathway in smooth muscle) causes dilation that develops more slowly and is more sustained. As a result, H_1 antagonists effectively counter small dilator responses to low concentrations of histamine but only blunt the initial phase of larger responses to higher concentrations of the amine. There seems to be a variable distribution of H_1 receptors on vascular smooth muscle as well, such that direct constrictor responses can be observed in vein, in skin and skeletal muscle, and in larger coronary arteries. Histamine causes hepatic venoconstriction in dogs (Chien and Krakoff, 1963).

Increased "Capillary" Permeability. This effect of histamine on small vessels results in outward passage of plasma protein and fluid into the extracellular spaces, an increase in the flow of lymph and its protein content, and edema formation. H_1 receptors on endothelial cells are the major mediators of this response; the role of H_2 receptors is uncertain.

Increased permeability results mainly from actions of histamine on postcapillary venules, where histamine causes the endothelial cells to contract and separate at their boundaries and thus to expose the basement membrane, which is freely permeable to plasma protein and fluid. The gaps between endothelial cells also may permit passage of circulating cells that are recruited to the tissues during the mast cell response. Recruitment of circulating leukocytes is promoted by H_1-receptor-mediated up-regulation of leukocyte adhesion. This process involves histamine-induced expression of the adhesion molecule P-selectin on the endothelial cells (Gaboury *et al.*, 1995).

Triple Response of Lewis. If histamine is injected intradermally, it elicits a characteristic phenomenon known as the *triple response* (Lewis, 1927). This consists of (1) a localized red spot extending for a few millimeters around the site of injection that appears within a few seconds and reaches a maximum in about a minute; (2) a brighter red flush, or "flare," extending about 1 cm or so beyond the original red spot and developing more slowly; and (3) a wheal that is discernible in 1 to 2 minutes and occupies the same area as the original small red spot at the injection site. The initial red spot results from the direct vasodilating effect of histamine (H_1-receptor-mediated NO production), the flare is due to histamine-induced stimulation of axon reflexes that cause vasodilation indirectly, and the wheal reflects histamine's capacity to increase capillary permeability (edema formation).

Constriction of Larger Vessels. Histamine tends to constrict larger blood vessels, in some species more than in others. In rodents, the effect extends to the level of the arterioles and may overshadow dilation of the finer blood vessels. A net increase in total peripheral resistance and an elevation in blood pressure can be observed. As noted earlier, H_1-receptor-mediated constriction may occur in some veins and in conduit coronary arteries (Toda, 1987).

Heart. Histamine affects both cardiac contractility and electrical events directly. It increases the force of contraction of both atrial and ventricular muscle by promoting the influx of Ca^{2+}, and it speeds heart rate by hastening diastolic depolarization in the sinoatrial (SA) node. It also acts directly to slow atrioventricular (AV) conduction, to increase automaticity, and in high doses especially, to elicit arrhythmias. With the exception of slowed AV conduction, which involves mainly H_1 receptors, all these effects are largely attributable to H_2 receptors and cyclic AMP accumulation. If histamine is given intravenously, direct cardiac effects of histamine are overshadowed by baroreceptor reflexes elicited by the reduced blood pressure.

Histamine Shock. Histamine given in large doses or released during systemic anaphylaxis causes a profound and progressive fall in blood pressure. As the small blood vessels dilate, they trap large amounts of blood, and as their permeability increases, plasma escapes from the circulation. Resembling surgical or traumatic shock, these effects diminish effective blood volume, reduce venous return, and greatly lower cardiac output.

Extravascular Smooth Muscle. Histamine stimulates or, more rarely, relaxes various smooth muscles. Contraction is due to activation of H_1 receptors, and relaxation (for the most part) is due to activation of H_2 receptors. Responses vary widely among species and even among humans (*see* Parsons, in Ganellin and Parsons, 1982). Bronchial muscle of guinea pigs is exquisitely sensitive. Minute doses of histamine also will evoke intense bronchoconstriction in patients with bronchial asthma and certain other pulmonary diseases; in normal human beings, the effect is much less pronounced. Although the spasmogenic influence of H_1 receptors is dominant in human bronchial muscle, H_2 receptors with dilator function also are present. Thus histamine-induced bronchospasm *in vitro* is potentiated slightly by H_2 blockade. In asthmatic subjects in particular, histamine-induced bronchospasm may involve an additional reflex component that arises from irritation of afferent vagal nerve endings (*see* Eyre and Chand, in Ganellin and Parsons, 1982; Nadel and Barnes, 1984).

The uterus of some species is contracted by histamine; in the human uterus, gravid or not, the response is negligible. Responses of intestinal muscle also vary with species and region, but the classical effect is contraction. Bladder, ureter, gallbladder, iris, and many other smooth muscle preparations are affected little or inconsistently by histamine.

Exocrine Glands. As mentioned earlier, histamine is an important physiological regulator of gastric acid secretion. This effect is mediated by H_2 receptors (*see* Chapter 36).

Peripheral Nerve Endings: Pain, Itch, and Indirect Effects. Histamine stimulates various nerve endings and sensory effects. Thus, when released in the epidermis, it causes itch; in the dermis, it evokes pain, sometimes accompanied by itching. Stimulant actions on one or another type of nerve ending, including autonomic afferents and efferents, were mentioned earlier as factors that contribute to the "flare" component of the triple response and to indirect effects of histamine on the bronchi and other organs. In the periphery, neuronal receptors for histamine are generally of the H_1 type (*see* Rocha e Silva, 1978; Ganellin and Parsons, 1982).

Clinical Uses

The practical applications of histamine are limited to uses as a diagnostic agent. Histamine (*histamine phosphate*) is used to assess nonspecific bronchial hyperreactivity in asthmatics and as a positive control injection during allergy skin testing.

H_1-RECEPTOR ANTAGONISTS

History. Antihistamine activity was first demonstrated by Bovet and Staub in 1937 with one of a series of amines with a phenolic ether moity. The substance 2-isopropyl-5-methylphenoxy-ethyldiethyl-amine protected guinea pigs against several lethal doses of histamine but was too toxic for clinical use. By 1944, Bovet and his colleagues had described *pyrilamine maleate,* an effective histamine antagonist of this category (*see* Bovet, 1950). The discovery of the highly effective diphenhydramine and *tripelennamine* soon followed (Ganellin and Parsons, 1982). In the 1980s, nonsedating H_1-histamine-receptor antagonists were developed for treatment of allergic diseases. Despite success in blocking allergic

responses to histamine, the antihistamines available in the early 1950s failed to inhibit a number of other responses to histamine, notably gastric acid secretion. The discovery of H_2 antagonists by Black and colleagues provided a new class of agents that antagonized histamine-induced acid secretion (Black *et al.*, 1972). The pharmacology of these drugs (*cimetidine, famotidine,* etc.) is described in Chapter 36.

Structure–Activity Relationship. All the available H_1-receptor antagonists are reversible competitive inhibitors of the interaction of histamine with H_1 receptors. Like histamine, many H_1 antagonists contain a substituted ethylamine moiety.

$$-\overset{|}{\underset{|}{C}}-\overset{|}{\underset{|}{C}}-N\diagdown^{\diagup}$$

Unlike histamine, which has a primary amino group and a single aromatic ring, most H_1 antagonists have a tertiary amino group linked by a two- or three-atom chain to two aromatic substituents and conform to the general formula

$$\overset{Ar_1}{\underset{Ar_2}{\diagdown}}X-\overset{|}{\underset{|}{C}}-\overset{|}{\underset{|}{C}}-N\diagdown^{\diagup}$$

where Ar is aryl and X is a nitrogen or carbon atom or a —C—O— ether linkage to the β-aminoethyl side chain. Sometimes the two aromatic rings are bridged, as in the tricyclic derivatives, or the ethylamine may be part of a ring structure (Figure 24–3) (Ganellin and Parsons, 1982).

Pharmacological Properties

Most H_1 antagonists have similar pharmacological actions and therapeutic applications. Their effects are largely predictable from knowledge of the consequences of the activation of H_1 receptors by histamines.

Smooth Muscle. H_1 antagonists inhibit most of the effects of histamine on smooth muscles, especially the constriction of respiratory smooth muscle. In guinea pigs, for example, death by asphyxia follows quite small doses of histamine, yet the animal may survive a hundred lethal doses of histamine if given an H_1 antagonist. In the same species, striking protection also is afforded against anaphylactic bronchospasm. This is not so in human beings, where allergic bronchoconstriction appears to be caused by a variety of mediators such as leukotrienes and PAF (*see* Chapter 25).

Within the vascular tree, the H_1 antagonists inhibit both the vasoconstrictor effects of histamine and, to a degree, the more rapid vasodilator effects that are mediated by activation of H_1 receptors on endothelial cells (synthesis/release of NO and other mediators). Residual vasodilation is due to H_2 receptors on smooth muscle and can be suppressed by administration of an H_2 antagonist. The efficacy of histamine antagonists on histamine-induced changes in systemic blood pressure parallels these vascular effects.

Capillary Permeability. H_1 antagonists strongly block the increased capillary permeability and formation of edema and wheal brought about by histamine.

Flare and Itch. The flare component of the triple response and the itching caused by intradermal injection of histamine are two different manifestations of the action of histamine on nerve endings. H_1 antagonists suppress both.

Exocrine Glands. H_1 antagonists do not suppress gastric secretion, but they do suppress histamine-evoked salivary, lacrimal, and other exocrine secretions with variable success. The antimuscarinic properties of many of these agents, however, may contribute to lessened secretion in cholinergically innervated glands and reduce ongoing secretion in, for example, the respiratory tree.

Immediate Hypersensitivity Reactions: Anaphylaxis and Allergy. During hypersensitivity reactions, histamine is one of the many potent autacoids released (*see* above), and its relative contribution to the ensuing symptoms varies widely with species and tissue. The protection afforded by histamine antagonists thus also varies accordingly. In humans, edema formation and itch are effectively suppressed. Other effects, such as hypotension, are less well antagonized. This may be explained by the participation of other types of H receptors and by effects of other mast cell mediators. These include those derived from arachidonic acid (released from membranes by PLA_2), which is converted by cyclooxygenases and lipoxygenases to prostaglandins, eicosatetratenoic acid derivatives, leukotrienes, and other mediators (Gelfand, *et al.*, 2004; Campbell and Harder, 1999) (*see* Chapter 25). Bronchoconstriction is reduced little, if at all.

Central Nervous System. The first-generation H_1 antagonists can both stimulate and depress the CNS. Stimulation occasionally is encountered in patients given conventional doses, who become restless, nervous, and unable to sleep. Central excitation also is a striking feature of overdose, which commonly results in convulsions, particularly in infants. Central depression, on the other hand, usually accompanies therapeutic doses of the older H_1 antagonists. Diminished alertness, slowed reaction times, and somnolence are common manifestations. Some of the H_1 antagonists are more likely to depress the CNS than others, and

patients vary in their susceptibility and responses to individual drugs. The ethanolamines (*e.g.*, diphenhydramine; Figure 24–3) are particularly prone to cause sedation.

The second-generation ("nonsedating") H_1 antagonists (*e.g., loratadine, cetirizine,* and *fexofenadine*) are largely excluded from the brain when given in therapeutic doses because they do not cross the blood–brain barrier appreciably. Their sedative effects are similar to those of placebo (Simons and Simons, 1994). Because of the sedation that occurs with first-generation antihistamines, these drugs cannot be tolerated or used safely by many patients unless given only at bedtime. Even then, patients may experience an antihistamine "hangover" in the morning, resulting in sedation with or without psychomotor impairment (Simons, 2003b). Thus the development of nonsedating antihistamines was an important advance that allowed the general use of these agents.

An interesting and useful property of certain H_1 antagonists is the capacity to counter motion sickness (*see* Chapters 7 and 37). This effect was first observed with *dimenhydrinate* and subsequently with diphenhydramine (the active moiety of dimenhydrinate), various piperazine derivatives, and *promethazine*.

Anticholinergic Effects. Many of the first-generation H_1 antagonists tend to inhibit responses to acetylcholine that are mediated by muscarinic receptors. These atropinelike actions are sufficiently prominent in some of the drugs to be manifest during clinical usage (*see* below). Promethazine has perhaps the strongest muscarinic-blocking activity among these agents and is among the most effective of the H_1 antagonists in combating motion sickness. Since *scopolamine* is a potent preventer of motion sickness (*see* Chapter 7), it is possible that the anticholinergic properties of H_1 antagonists are largely responsible for this effect. The second-generation H_1 antagonists have no effect on muscarinic receptors.

Local Anesthetic Effect. Some H_1 antagonists have local anesthetic activity, and a few are more potent than procaine. Promethazine (PHENERGAN) is especially active. However, the concentrations required for this effect are several orders of magnitude higher than those which antagonize histamine's interactions with its receptors.

Absorption, Fate, and Excretion. The H_1 antagonists are well absorbed from the GI tract. Following oral administration, peak plasma concentrations are achieved in 2 to 3 hours, and effects usually last 4 to 6 hours; however, some of the drugs are much longer acting (Table 24–2).

Extensive studies of the metabolic fate of the older H_1 antagonists are limited. Diphenhydramine, given orally, reaches a maximal concentration in the blood in about 2 hours, remains at about this level for another 2 hours, and then falls exponentially with a plasma elimination half-

Table 24–2

Preparations and Dosage of Representative H₁-Receptor Antagonists*

CLASS AND NONPROPRIETARY NAME	TRADE NAME	DURATION OF ACTION, HOURS	PREPARATIONS†	SINGLE DOSE (ADULT)
First-Generation Agents				
Tricyclic Dibenzoxepins				
Doxepin hydrochloride	SINEQUAN	6–24	O, L, T	10–150 mg
Ethanolamines				
Carbinoxamine maleate	RONDEC,¶ others	3–6	O, L	4–8 mg
Clemastine fumarate	TAVIST, others	12	O, L	1.34–2.68 mg
Diphenhydramine HCl	BENADRYL; others	12	O, L, I, T	25–50 mg
Dimenhydrinate	DRAMAMINE; others	4–6	O, L, I	50–100 mg
Ethylenediamines				
Pyrilamine maleate	POLY–HISTINE-D¶	4–6	O, L, T	25–50 mg
Tripelennamine HCl	PBZ	4–6	O	25–50 mg, 100 mg (sustained release)
Tripelennamine citrate	PBZ	4–6	L	37.5–75 mg
Alkylamines				
Chlorpheniramine maleate	CHLOR-TRIMETON; others	24	O, L, I	4 mg 8–12 mg (sustained release) 5–20 mg (injection)
Brompheniramine maleate	BROMPHEN; others	4–6	O, L, I	4 mg 8–12 mg (sustained release) 5–20 mg (injection)
Piperazines				
Hydroxyzine HCl	ATARAX; others	6–24	O, L, I	25–100 mg
Hydroxyzine pamoate	VISTARIL	6–24	O, L	25–100 mg
Cyclizine HCl	MAREZINE	4–6	O	50 mg
Cyclizine lactate	MAREZINE	4–6	I	50 mg
Meclizine HCl	ANTIVERT; others	12–24	O	12.5–50 mg
Phenothiazines				
Promethazine HCl	PHENERGAN; others	4–6	O, L, I, S	12.5–50 mg
Piperidines				
Cyproheptadine HCl§	PERIACTIN	4–6	O, L	4 mg
Phenindamine tartrate	NOLAHIST	4–6	O	25 mg
Second-Generation Agents				
Alkylamines				
Acrivastine‡	SEMPREX-D¶	6–8	O	8 mg
Piperazines				
Cetirizine hydrochloride‡	ZYRTEC	12–24	O	5–10 mg
Phthalazinones				
Azelastine hydrochloride‡	ASTELIN	12–24	T	2 sprays per nostril
Piperidines				
Levocabastine hydrochloride	LIVOSTIN	6–12	T	One drop
Loratadine	CLARITIN	24	O, L	10 mg
Desloratadine	CLARINEX, AERIUS	24	O	5 mg
Ebastine	EBASTEL	24	O	10–20 mg
Mizolastine	MIZOLLEN	24	O	10 mg
Fexofenadine	ALLEGRA, TELFAST	12–24	O	60 mg

HCl, hydrochloride. *For a discussion of phenothiazines, *see* Chapter 18. †Preparations are designated as follows: O, oral solids; L, oral liquids; I, Injection; S, suppository; T, topical. Many H₁-receptor antagonists also are available in preparations that contain multiple drugs. ‡Has mild sedating effects. ¶Trade name drug also contains other medications. §Also has antiserotonin properties.

time of about 4 to 8 hours. The drug is distributed widely throughout the body, including the CNS. Little, if any, is excreted unchanged in the urine; most appears there as metabolites. Other first-generation H_1 antagonists appear to be eliminated in much the same way (*see* Paton and Webster, 1985).

Peak concentrations of these drugs are achieved rapidly in the skin and persist after plasma levels have declined (Simons, 2003a). This is consistent with inhibition of "wheal and flare" responses to the intradermal injection of histamine or allergen, which last for 36 hours or more after treatment, even when concentrations in plasma are very low. Such results emphasize the need for flexibility in the interpretation of the recommended dosage schedules (Table 24–2); less frequent dosage may suffice. *Doxepin,* a tricyclic antidepressant (*see* Chapter 17), is one of the most potent antihistamines available; it is about 800 times more potent than diphenhydramine. This may account for the observation that doxepin can be effective in the treatment of chronic urticaria when other antihistamines have failed; it also is available as a topical preparation.

Like many other drugs that are metabolized extensively, H_1 antagonists are eliminated more rapidly by children than by adults and more slowly in those with severe liver disease. H_1-receptor antagonists also induce hepatic cytochrome P450 enzymes (CYPs) and thus may facilitate their own metabolism (*see* Paton and Webster, 1985).

The second-generation H_1 antagonist loratadine is absorbed rapidly from the GI tract and metabolized in the liver to an active metabolite by the hepatic CYPs (Simons and Simons, 1994) (*see* Chapter 3). Consequently, metabolism of loratadine can be affected by other drugs that compete for the P450 enzymes. Two other second-generation H_1 antagonists that were marketed previously, *astemizole* and *terfenadine,* also underwent metabolism by CYPs to active metabolites. Both these drugs were found in rare cases to induce a potentially fatal arrhythmia, *torsades de pointes,* when their metabolism was impaired, such as by liver disease or drugs that inhibit the CYP3A family (*see* Chapter 34). This led to the withdrawal of terfenadine and astemizole from the market in 1998 and 1999. The withdrawal of terfenadine prompted the development of its active metabolite, *fexofenadine,* as a replacement. This compound lacks the toxic side effects of terfenadine, is not sedating, and retains the antiallergic properties of the parent compound (Meeves and Appajosyula, 2003). Another antihistamine developed using this strategy is *desloratidine,* an active metabolite of loratidine. Cetirizine, loratadine, and fexofenadine are all well absorbed and are excreted mainly in the unmetabolized form. Cetirizine and loratadine are excreted primarily into the urine, whereas fexofenadine is excreted primarily in the feces.

Side Effects. Common Adverse Effects. The most frequent side effect in the first-generation H_1 antagonists is sedation. Although sedation may be a desirable adjunct in the treatment of some patients, it may interfere with the patient's daytime activities. Concurrent ingestion of alcohol or other CNS depressants produces an additive effect that impairs motor skills. Other untoward central actions include dizziness, tinnitus, lassitude, incoordination, fatigue, blurred vision, diplopia, euphoria, nervousness, insomnia, and tremors.

The next most frequent side effects involve the digestive tract and include loss of appetite, nausea, vomiting, epigastric distress, and constipation or diarrhea. Taking the drug with meals may reduce their incidence. H_1 antagonists appear to increase appetite and cause weight gain in rare patients. Other side effects apparently owing to the antimuscarinic actions of some of the first-generation H_1-receptor antagonists include dryness of the mouth and respiratory passages (sometimes inducing cough), urinary retention or frequency, and dysuria. These effects are not observed with second-generation H_1 antagonists.

Other Adverse Effects. Drug allergy may develop when H_1 antagonists are given orally but results more commonly from topical application. Allergic dermatitis is not uncommon; other hypersensitivity reactions include drug fever and photosensitization. Hematological complications such as leukopenia, agranulocytosis, and hemolytic anemia are very rare. Because H_1 antihistamines cross the placenta, caution must be used when they are taken by women who are or may become pregnant. Several antihistamines (*e.g., azelastine, hydroxyzine,* and fexofenadine) showed teratogenic effects in animal studies, whereas others (*e.g.,* chlorpheniramine, diphenhydramine, cetirizine, and loratadine) did not (*see* Simons, 2003b). Antihistamines can be excreted in small amounts in breast milk, and first-generation antihistamines taken by lactating mothers may cause symptoms in the nursing infant such as irritability, drowsiness, or respiratory depression (*see* Simons, 2003b). Since H_1 antagonists interfere with skin tests for allergy, they must be withdrawn well before such tests are performed.

In acute poisoning with H_1 antagonists, their central excitatory effects constitute the greatest danger. The syndrome includes hallucinations, excitement, ataxia, incoordination, athetosis, and convulsions. Fixed, dilated pupils with a flushed face, together with sinus tachycardia, urinary retention, dry mouth, and fever, lend the syndrome a remarkable similarity to that of *atropine* poisoning. Terminally, there is deepening coma with cardiorespiratory collapse and death usually within 2 to 18 hours. Treatment is along general symptomatic and supportive lines.

Available H₁ Antagonists. Summarized below are the therapeutic and side effects of a number of H₁ antagonists based on their chemical structures. Representative preparations are listed in Table 24-2.

Dibenzoxepin Tricyclics (Doxepin). Doxepin, the only drug in this class, is marketed as a tricyclic antidepressant (*see* Chapter 17). However, it also is a remarkably potent H₁ antagonist. It can cause drowsiness and is associated with anticholinergic effects. Doxepin is much better tolerated by patients who have depression than by those who do not. In nondepressed patients, sometimes even very small doses, *e.g.,* 20 mg, may be poorly tolerated because of disorientation and confusion.

Ethanolamines (Prototype: Diphenhydramine). These drugs possess significant antimuscarinic activity and have a pronounced tendency to sedation. About half of those treated with conventional doses experience somnolence. The incidence of GI side effects, however, is low with this group.

Ethylenediamines (Prototype: Pyrilamine). These include some of the most specific H₁ antagonists. Although their central effects are relatively feeble, somnolence occurs in a fair proportion of patients. GI side effects are quite common.

Alkylamines (Prototype: Chlorpheniramine). These are among the most potent H₁ antagonists. The drugs are less prone than some H₁ antagonists to produce drowsiness and are more suitable agents for daytime use, but again, a significant proportion of patients do experience sedation. Side effects involving CNS stimulation are more common than with other groups.

First-Generation Piperazines. The oldest member of this group, *chlorcyclizine,* has a more prolonged action and produces a comparatively low incidence of drowsiness. Hydroxyzine is a long-acting compound that is used widely for skin allergies; its considerable CNS-depressant activity may contribute to its prominent antipruritic action. *Cyclizine* and *meclizine* have been used primarily to counter motion sickness, although promethazine and diphenhydramine (dimenhydrinate) are more effective (as is scopolamine; *see* below).

Second-Generation Piperazines (Cetirizine). Cetirizine is the only drug in this class. It has minimal anticholinergic effects. It also has negligible penetration into the brain but is associated with a somewhat higher incidence of drowsiness than the other second-generation H₁ antagonists.

Phenothiazines (Prototype: Promethazine). Most drugs of this class are H₁ antagonists and also possess considerable anticholinergic activity. Promethazine, which has prominent sedative effects, and its many congeners are used primarily for their antiemetic effects (*see* Chapter 37).

First-Generation Piperidines (Cyproheptadine, Phenindamine). *Cyproheptadine* uniquely has both antihistamine and antiserotonin activity. Cyproheptadine and *phenindamine* cause drowsiness and also have significant anticholinergic effects.

Second-Generation Piperidines (Prototype: Terfenadine). Terfenadine and astemizole were withdrawn from the market. Current drugs in this class include loratadine, desloratadine, and fexofenadine. These agents are highly selective for H₁ receptors, lack significant anticholinergic actions, and penetrate poorly into the CNS. Taken together, these properties appear to account for the low incidence of side effects of piperidine antihistamines.

Therapeutic Uses

H₁ antagonists have an established and valued place in the symptomatic treatment of various immediate hypersensitivity reactions. In addition, the central properties of some of the series are of therapeutic value for suppressing motion sickness or for sedation.

Allergic Diseases. H₁ antagonists are most useful in acute types of allergy that present with symptoms of rhinitis, urticaria, and conjunctivitis. Their effect is confined to the suppression of symptoms attributable to the histamine released by the antigen–antibody reaction. In bronchial asthma, histamine antagonists have limited efficacy and are not used as sole therapy (*see* Chapter 27). In the treatment of systemic anaphylaxis, in which autacoids other than histamine play major roles, the mainstay of therapy is *epinephrine;* histamine antagonists have only a subordinate and adjuvant role. The same is true for severe angioedema, in which laryngeal swelling constitutes a threat to life.

Other allergies of the respiratory tract are more amenable to therapy with H₁ antagonists. The best results are obtained in seasonal rhinitis and conjunctivitis (hay fever, pollinosis), in which these drugs relieve the sneezing, rhinorrhea, and itching of eyes, nose, and throat. A gratifying response is obtained in most patients, especially at the beginning of the season when pollen counts are low; however, the drugs are less effective when the allergens are most abundant, when exposure to them is prolonged, and when nasal congestion is prominent. Topical preparations of antihistamines such as *levocabastine* (LIVOSTIN), *azelastine* (ASTELIN), *ketotifen* (ZADITOR), and *olopatadine* (PATANOL) have been shown to be effective in allergic conjunctivitis and rhinitis. Nasal sprays or topical ophthalmic preparations of these agents are available in the United States. Histamine causes the release of inflammatory cytokines and eicosanoids and increases expression of endothelial adhesion molecules (Holgate *et al.*, 2003; Gelfand *et al.*, 2004). In addition, H₁ receptors, either *via* constitutive activity or after stimulation by agonists, can activate the proinflammatory transcription factor NF-κB (Leurs *et al.*, 2002). Thus H₁ antihistamines have been investigated for potential antiinflammatory properties. Although H₁ antihistamines do exhibit a variety of antiinflammatory effects *in vitro* and in animal models, in many cases the doses required are higher than those normally achieved therapeutically, and clinical effectiveness has not yet been proven (Holgate *et al.*, 2003; Gelfand *et al.*, 2004).

Certain allergic dermatoses respond favorably to H₁ antagonists. Benefit is most striking in acute urticaria, although the itching in this condition is perhaps better controlled than are the edema and the erythema. Chronic urticaria is less responsive, but some benefit may occur in a fair proportion of patients. Furthermore, the combined use of H_1 and H_2 antagonists sometimes is effective when therapy with an H_1 antagonist alone has failed. As mentioned earlier, doxepin may be effective in the treatment of chronic urticaria that is refractory to other antihistamines. Angioedema also responds to treatment with H_1 antagonists, but the paramount importance of epinephrine in the severe attack must be re-emphasized, especially in life-threatening laryngeal edema (*see* Chapter 10). In this setting, it may be appropriate to also administer an H_1 antagonist by the intravenous route.

H_1 antagonists have a place in the treatment of pruritus. Some relief may be obtained in many patients suffering atopic dermatitis and contact dermatitis (although topical corticosteroids are more effective) and in such diverse conditions as insect bites and poison ivy. Various other pruritides without an allergic basis sometimes respond to antihistamine therapy, usually when the drugs are applied topically but occasionally when they are given orally. However, the possibility of producing allergic dermatitis with local application of H_1 antagonists must be recognized. Again, doxepin may be more effective in suppressing pruritus than are other antihistamines. Since these drugs inhibit allergic dermatoses, they should be withdrawn well before skin testing for allergies. The urticarial and edematous lesions of serum sickness respond to H_1 antagonists, but fever and arthralgia often do not.

Many drug reactions attributable to allergic phenomena respond to therapy with H_1 antagonists, particularly those characterized by itch, urticaria, and angioedema; serum-sickness reactions also respond to intensive treatment. However, explosive release of histamine generally calls for treatment with epinephrine, with H_1 antagonists being accorded a subsidiary role. Nevertheless, prophylactic treatment with an H_1 antagonist may reduce symptoms to a tolerable level when a drug known to be a histamine liberator is to be given.

Common Cold. Despite persistent popular belief, H_1 antagonists are without value in combating the common cold. The weak anticholinergic effects of the older agents may tend to lessen rhinorrhea, but this drying effect may do more harm than good, as may their tendency to induce somnolence.

Motion Sickness, Vertigo, and Sedation. Although scopolamine, given orally, parenterally, or transdermally, is the most effective of all drugs for the prophylaxis and treatment of motion sickness, some H_1 antagonists are useful in a broad range of milder conditions and offer the advantage of fewer adverse effects. These drugs include dimenhydrinate and the piperazines (*e.g.,* cyclizine and meclizine). Promethazine, a phenothiazine, is more potent and more effective; its additional antiemetic properties may be of value in reducing vomiting, but its pronounced sedative action usually is disadvantageous. Whenever possible, the various drugs should be administered an hour or so before the anticipated motion. Treatment after the onset of nausea and vomiting rarely is beneficial.

Some H_1 antagonists, notably dimenhydrinate and meclizine, often are of benefit in vestibular disturbances such as Meniere's disease and in other types of true vertigo. Only promethazine has usefulness in treating the nausea and vomiting subsequent to chemotherapy or radiation therapy for malignancies; however, other effective antiemetic drugs are available (*see* Chapter 37).

Diphenhydramine can reverse the extrapyramidal side effects caused by phenothiazines (*see* Chapter 18). The anticholinergic actions of this agent also can be used in the early stages of Parkinson's disease (*see* Chapter 20), but it is less effective than other agents.

The tendency of some H_1-receptor antagonists to produce somnolence has led to their use as hypnotics. H_1 antagonists, principally diphenhydramine, often are present in various proprietary remedies for insomnia that are sold over the counter. While these remedies generally are ineffective in the recommended doses, some sensitive individuals may derive benefit. The sedative and mild antianxiety activities of hydroxyzine and diphenhydramine have contributed to their use as weak anxiolytics.

H_2-Receptor Antagonists. The pharmacology and clinical utility of H_2 antagonists to inhibit gastric acid secretion are described in Chapter 36.

THE HISTAMINE H_3 RECEPTOR AND ITS LIGANDS

The H_3 receptor was characterized and localized in a variety of cells, including the cerebral histaminergic neurons using *(R)-α-methylhistamine,* a selective H_3 agonist, and *thioperamide,* an antagonist (Arrang *et al.,* 1987). The H_3 receptor was shown to couple to a pertussin toxin–sensitive G protein, and its cDNA was identified as an orphan heptahelical receptor (Lovenberg *et al.,* 1999). Further studies on the H_3 receptor uncovered a variety of isoforms resulting from alternative splicing, as well as interspecies differences, that can result in receptors with unique binding and signaling properties (Hancock *et al.,* 2003).

The H_3 receptors are localized on terminals as well as on cell bodies/dendrites in the hypothalamic tuberomammillary nucleus on histaminergic neurons. By inhibiting Ca^{2+} conductance, the activated H_3 receptor depresses neuronal firing at the level of cell bodies/dendrites and decreases histamine release from depolarized terminals. Thus H_3-receptor ligands are unique agents to modify histaminergic neurotransmission in brain; the agonists decrease it, and the antagonists increase it. H_3 receptors are also presynaptic heteroreceptors on a variety of neurons in brain and peripheral tissues, including noradrenergic, serotoninergic, GABAergic, and glutamatergic neurons, as well as on sensitive C-fibers. H_3 receptors in brain have significant constitutive activity in the absence of agonist both *in vitro* and *in vivo*; consequently, inverse agonists of high intrinsic activity (rather than neutral antagonists) will activate these neurons. H_3-receptor ligands currently are research tools to delineate the functional role of cerebral histamine and are drug candidates in neuropsychiatry (Schwartz and Arrang, 2002).

In the enterochromaffinlike cells of the stomach, H_3 receptors inhibit gastrin-induced release of histamine and, therefore, decrease HCl secretion mediated by H_2 receptors, but the effect is not large enough to warrant development of therapeutic agents. In contrast to histaminergic neurons, the H_3 receptors on other cell types may neither be tonically stimulated by endogenous histamine nor exhibit constitutive activity because inverse agonists/antagonists do not exert clear-cut effects. However, the receptors respond to agonists; *e.g.,* H_3 agonists decrease tachykinin release from capsaicin-sensitive C-fiber terminals and thereby reduce capsaicin-induced plasma extravasation and are antinociceptive. H_3 agonists also depress exaggerated catecholamine release in the heart, *e.g.,* during ischemia.

The H_3-receptor antagonists/inverse agonists that cross the blood–brain barrier have a range of central effects by activating histaminergic neurons, a consideration for therapeutic indications. In animal experiments, they induce a marked arousal at the expense of slow-wave sleep owing to the critical role of the posterior hypothalamic area in wakefulness. They also improve attention and learning, effects that are attributable to overstimulation of cortical H_1 receptors by endogenous histamine, which points to their possible application in pathological diurnal somnolence or minimal cognitive impairment.

The beneficial effects of these drugs in animal models of convulsions also suggest antiepileptic activity devoid of sedative side effects.

H_3 antagonists suppress food intake, increase locomotion, and increase anxiety (Leurs *et al.*, 1998), but recent H_3-receptor knockout mice unexpectedly exhibited obesity, reduced locomotion, and decreased anxiety (*see*, for example, Rizk *et al.*, 2004). This may reflect nonspecific actions of H_3-receptor antagonists or, more likely, the presence of compensatory mechanisms in the knockout mice.

Many early H_3 antagonists such as *impromidine* and burimamide had mixed effects because they also were agonists for the H_2 receptor. *Thioperamide* was the first specific H_3 antagonist available experimentally. A number of other imidazole derivatives have been developed as H_3 antagonists, including clobenpropit, *ciproxifan*, and *proxyfan*. Some H_3 antagonists can bind to α adrenergic receptors, H_4 receptors (*see* below), and CYPs, prompting an effort to develop more selective H_3-receptor antagonists using non-imidazole-based structures. For example, two piperazine amide antagonists (A-304121 and A-317920) were shown recently to have high affinity for the H_3 receptor without detectable binding to α_2 adrenergic, 5-HT$_3$, H_1, H_2, or H_4 receptors (Esbenshade *et al.*, 2003). Although none has yet been approved for clinical use, some H_3-receptor ligands are currently in phase II clinical trials. Their potential therapeutic indications derive from effects observed in animal models.

THE HISTAMINE H_4 RECEPTOR AND ITS LIGANDS

The discovery of a fourth histamine receptor with a unique pharmacology and distribution has opened new avenues of investigation (Hough, 2001). The H_4 receptor has the highest sequence similarity with the H_3 receptor and binds many H_3 agonists, although with lower affinity [*e.g.*, imetit and immepip have approximately 10 to 60 times lower and (*R*)-α-methylhistamine has approximately 200 to 500 times lower affinity for H_4] (Hough, 2001). The H_3 antagonist thioperamide also has significant H_4 antagonistic activity, whereas H_3 antagonists clobenpropit and burimamide are partial agonists of the H_4 receptor. The H_4 receptor couples through $G_{i/o}$ to decrease cyclic AMP accumulation and, presumably *via* the $\beta\gamma$ subunits, activates phospholipase Cβ and increases intracellular Ca^{2+} (Hough, 2001; Hofstra *et al.*, 2003).

Because the H_4 receptor is expressed primarily on cells of hematopoietic origin (notably mast cells, basophils, and eosinophils) and to a lesser extent in the intestine (Hough, 2001; Oda *et al.*, 2000; Hofstra *et al.*, 2003), there is great interest in the possible role of H_4 receptors in inflammatory processes. Indeed, the H_4 receptor can mediate histamine-induced chemotaxis of mast cells (Hofstra *et al.*, 2003), leukotriene B$_4$ production, and mast cell–dependent neutrophil recruitment induced by zymosan (Takeshita *et al.*, 2003). A potent and highly selective H_4-receptor antagonist (JNJ7777120) has been developed that can block all these H_4-mediated responses (Thurmond *et al.*, 2004). H_4 antagonists are promising drug candidates to treat inflammatory conditions involving mast cells and eosinophils, such as allergic rhinitis, asthma, and rheumatoid arthritis (Thurmond *et al.*, 2004).

CLINICAL SUMMARY OF THE HISTAMINE H_4 RECEPTOR AND ITS LIGANDS

H_1 Antihistamines. These medications are used widely in the treatment of allergic disorders. H_1 antihistamines are most effective in relieving the symptoms of seasonal rhinitis and conjunctivitis (*e.g.*, sneezing, rhinorrhea, and itching of the eyes, nose, and throat). In bronchial asthma, they have limited beneficial effects and are not useful as sole therapy. H_1-histamine antagonists are useful adjuncts to epinephrine in the treatment of systemic anaphylaxis or severe angioedema. Certain allergic dermatoses, such as acute urticaria, respond favorably to H_1 antagonists, which help to relieve the itch in atopic dermatitis or contact dermatitis but have no effect on the rash. Chronic urticaria is less responsive, but some benefit may occur, especially when combined with H_2 antagonists.

Side effects are most prominent with first-generation H_1 antihistamines (*e.g.*, diphenhydramine, chlorpheniramine, doxepin, and hydroxyzine), which cross the blood–brain barrier and cause sedation. Some of the first-generation H_1-receptor antagonists also have anticholinergic properties that can be responsible for symptoms such as dryness of the mouth and respiratory passages, urinary retention or frequency, and dysuria. The second-generation drugs (*e.g.*, cetirizine, loratadine, desloratadine, and fexofenadine) are largely devoid of these side effects because they do not penetrate the CNS and do not have antimuscarinic properties. Thus they are usually the drugs of choice for the treatment of allergic disorders.

The significant sedative effects of some first-generation antihistamines have led to their use in treating insomnia, although there are better drugs for this purpose. Hydroxyzine and diphenhydramine are used in some cases as weak anxiolytics. Some first-generation H_1 antagonists (*e.g.*, dimenhydrinate, cyclizine, meclizine, and promethazine) can prevent motion sickness, although scopolamine is more effective. Antiemetic effects of these H_1 antihistamines can be beneficial in treating vertigo or postoperative emesis.

Many H_1 antihistamines are metabolized by CYPs. Thus, inhibitors of CYP activity such as macrolide antibiotics (*e.g.*, erythromycin) or imidazole antifungals (*e.g.*, ketoconazole) can increase H_1 antihistamine levels, leading to toxicity. Some newer antihistamines, such as cetirizine, fexofenadine, levocabastine, and acrivastine, are not subject to these drug interactions.

Caution should be used in treating pregnant or lactating women with certain H_1 antihistamines, especially first-generations drugs, because of their possible teratogenic effects or symptomatic effects on infants owing to secretion into breast milk; cetirizine and loratadine are probably the best choices if H_1 antihistamines are required, but if they are not effective, diphenhydramine can be used safely in pregnant (but not breast-feeding) women.

H₂ Antihistamines. These drugs (*e.g.*, cimetidine and ranitidine) are used primarily to inhibit gastric acid secretion in the treatment of GI disorders and are discussed in detail in Chapter 36.

H₃ and H₄ Antihistamines. Although specific H₃- and H₄-receptor antagonists have been developed, no drugs have been approved for clinical use. Based on the functions of H₃ receptors in the CNS, H₃ antagonists have potential use in improving attention and learning, in stimulating arousal, and as antiepileptic agents. Because of the unique localization and function of H₄ receptors on cells of hematopoietic origin, H₄ antagonists are promising candidates to treat inflammatory conditions such as allergic rhinitis, asthma, and rheumatoid arthritis.

BRADYKININ, KALLIDIN, AND THEIR ANTAGONISTS

A number of factors, including tissue damage, allergic reactions, viral infections, and other inflammatory events, activate a series of proteolytic reactions that generate bradykinin and kallidin in the tissues. These peptides contribute to inflammatory responses as autacoids that act locally to produce pain, vasodilation, and increased vascular permeability. Much of their activity is due to stimulation of the release of potent mediators such as prostaglandins, NO, or endothelium-derived hyperpolarizing factor (EDHF).

A number of interesting discoveries have contributed to the elucidation of the functions of kinins. Kinin metabolites released by basic carboxypeptidases that were formally considered inactive degradation products are agonists of a receptor (B₁) that differs from that of intact kinins (B₂), whose expression is induced by tissue injury. Kinins and their des-Arg metabolites also release vasoactive agents and may be mediators of inflammation and pain. These findings may open novel avenues for therapeutic intervention in chronic inflammatory conditions.

History. In the 1920s and 1930s, Frey, Kraut, and Werle characterized a hypotensive substance in urine and found a similar material in saliva, plasma, and a variety of tissues (*see* Werle, 1970). The pancreas also was a rich source, so they named this material *kallikrein* after a Greek synonym for that organ, *kallikréas.* By 1937, Werle, Götze, and Keppler had established that kallikreins generate a pharmacologically active substance from an inactive precursor present in plasma. In 1948, Werle and Berek named the active substance *kallidin* and showed it to be a polypeptide cleaved from a plasma globulin that they termed *kallidinogen* (*see* Werle, 1970).

Interest in the field intensified when Rocha e Silva and associates reported that trypsin and certain snake venoms acted on plasma

globulin to produce a substance that lowered blood pressure and caused a slowly developing contraction of the gut (Rocha e Silva *et al.*, 1949; Beraldo and Andrade, 1997). Because of this slow response, they named the substance *bradykinin,* a term derived from the Greek words *bradys,* meaning "slow," and *kinein,* meaning "to move." In 1960, the nonapeptide bradykinin was isolated by Elliott and coworkers and synthesized by Boissonnas and associates. Shortly thereafter, kallidin was found to be a decapeptide—bradykinin with an additional lysine residue at the amino terminus (Beraldo and Andrade, 1997). These peptides have related chemical structures and pharmacological properties and are distributed widely in nature. For the whole group, the generic term *kinins* has been adopted, and kallidin and bradykinin are referred to as plasma kinins. The kinins had short half-lives because they were destroyed by plasma and tissue enzymes originally called *kininase I* and *kininase II.* The former released a single C-terminal amino acid; the latter, a dipeptide. Angiotensin converting enzyme (ACE) and kininase II later were shown to be the same enzyme (Yang *et al.*, 1970).

In 1970, Ferreira and colleagues reported the isolation of a bradykinin-potentiating factor from the venom of the Brazilian snake *Bothrops jararaca.* Ondetti and colleagues (1971) subsequently determined the structures of peptides from the venom that inhibited ACE. ACE inhibitors (*see* Chapter 30) are used widely in the treatment of hypertension, diabetic nephropathy, congestive heart failure, and post–myocardial infarction (Gavras *et al.*, 1974).

In 1980, Regoli and Barabé divided the kinin receptors into B₁ and B₂ classes based on the rank order of potency of kinin analogs, and this was validated at the molecular level by cloning of the B₁ and B₂ receptors (Bhoola *et al.*, 1992; Hess, 1997). A primary feature that distinguishes peptide ligands of the B₁ and B₂ receptors is the presence of a C-terminal Arg residue; intact kinins (bradykinin and kallidin) are agonists of the B₂ receptor, whereas their des-Arg forms ([des-Arg⁹]bradykinin and [des-Arg¹⁰]kallidin) are agonists for the B₁ receptor. First-generation kinin-receptor antagonists were developed in the mid-1980s (Vavrek and Stewart, 1985), and second-generation receptor-specific kinin antagonists were developed in the early 1990s. These antagonists have led to increasing acceptance of the importance of kinins. Studies involving B₁- and B₂-receptor knockout mice (Hess, 1997; Pesquero *et al.*, 2000) have furthered our understanding of the role of bradykinin in the regulation of cardiovascular homeostasis and inflammatory processes.

The Endogenous Kallikrein–Kininogen–Kinin System

Synthesis and Metabolism of Kinins. Bradykinin is a nonapeptide (Table 24–3). Kallidin has an additional lysine residue at the N-terminal position and is sometimes referred to as *lysyl-bradykinin.* The two peptides are cleaved from α₂ globulins termed *kininogens* (Figure 24–4). There are two kininogens, high-molecular-weight (HMW) and low-molecular-weight (LMW) kininogen. A number of serine proteases will generate kinins, but the highly specific proteases that release bradykinin and kallidin from the kininogens are termed *kallikreins* (*see* below).

Kallikreins. Bradykinin and kallidin are cleaved from HMW or LMW kininogens by plasma or tissue kallikrein, respectively (Figure 24–4). Plasma kallikrein and tissue kallikrein are distinct enzymes that are activated by different mechanisms (Bhoola *et al.*, 1992). Plasma prekallikrein is an inactive protein of about 88,000 daltons that complexes in a 1:1 ratio with its substrate, HMW kininogen. The ensuing proteolytic cascade is restrained by the protease inhibitors

Table 24–3
Structure of Kinin Agonists and Antagonists

NAME	STRUCTURE	FUNCTION
Bradykinin	Arg-Pro-Pro-Gly-Phe-Ser-Pro-Phe-Arg	Agonist, B_2
Kallidin	Lys-Arg-Pro-Pro-Gly-Phe-Ser-Pro-Phe-Arg	Agonist, B_2
[des-Arg^9]-bradykinin	Arg-Pro-Pro-Gly-Phe-Ser-Pro-Phe	Agonist, B_1
[des-Arg^{10}]-kallidin	Lys-Arg-Pro-Pro-Gly-Phe-Ser-Pro-Phe	Agonist, B_1
des-Arg^9-[Leu^8]-bradykinin	Arg-Pro-Pro-Gly-Phe-Ser-Pro-Leu	Antagonist, B_1
HOE 140	[D-Arg]-Arg-Pro-Hyp-Gly-Thi-Ser-Tic-Oic-Arg	Antagonist, B_2
CP 0127	B(D-Arg-Arg-Pro-Hyp-Gly-Phe-Cys-D-Phe-Leu-Arg)$_2$	Antagonist, B_2
FR 173657		Antagonist, B_2
FR 190997		Agonist, B_2

ABBREVIATIONS: Hyp, *trans*-4-hydroxy-Pro; Thi, β-(2-thienyl)-Ala; Tic, [D]-1,2,3,4-tetrahydroisoquinolin-3-yl-carbonyl; Oic, (3as,7as)-octahydroindol-2-yl-carbonyl. B, bissuccimidohexane.

present in plasma. Among the most important of these are the inhibitor of the activated first component of complement (C1-INH) and α_2-macroglobulin. Under experimental conditions, the kallikrein–kinin system is activated by the binding of factor XII, also known as *Hageman factor,* to negatively charged surfaces. Factor XII, a protease that is common to both the kinin and the intrinsic coagulation cascades (*see* Chapter 54), undergoes autoactivation and, in turn, activates kallikrein. Importantly, kallikrein further activates factor XII, thereby exerting a positive feedback on the system. *In vivo,* factor XII does not undergo autoactivation on binding to endothelial cells. Instead, the binding of a HMW kininogen–prekallikrein complex to a multiprotein receptor complex on endothelial cells leads to activation of prekallikrein by a lysosomal enzyme designated *prolylcarboxypeptidase,* which is also present on endothelial cell membranes (Schmaier, 2004). Kallikrein activates factor XII, cleaves HMW kininogen, and

activates prourokinase (Schmaier, 2004; Colman, 1999). Human tissue kallikrein is a member of a large multigene family of 15 members with high sequence identity that are clustered at chromosome 19q13.4 (Yousef and Diamandis, 2002). Only the classical (or "true") tissue kallikrein, hK1, generates kinins from kininogen. Another member, hK3, better known as the prostate-specific antigen (PSA), is an important marker in diagnosing prostate cancer.

Compared with plasma kallikrein, tissue kallikrein is a smaller protein (29,000 daltons). It is synthesized as a preproprotein in the epithelial cells or secretory cells of a number of tissues, including salivary glands, pancreas, prostate, and distal nephron. Tissue kallikrein is also expressed in human neutrophils. It acts locally near its sites of origin. The synthesis of tissue prokallikrein is controlled by a number of factors, including aldosterone in the kidney and salivary gland and androgens in certain other glands. The secretion of

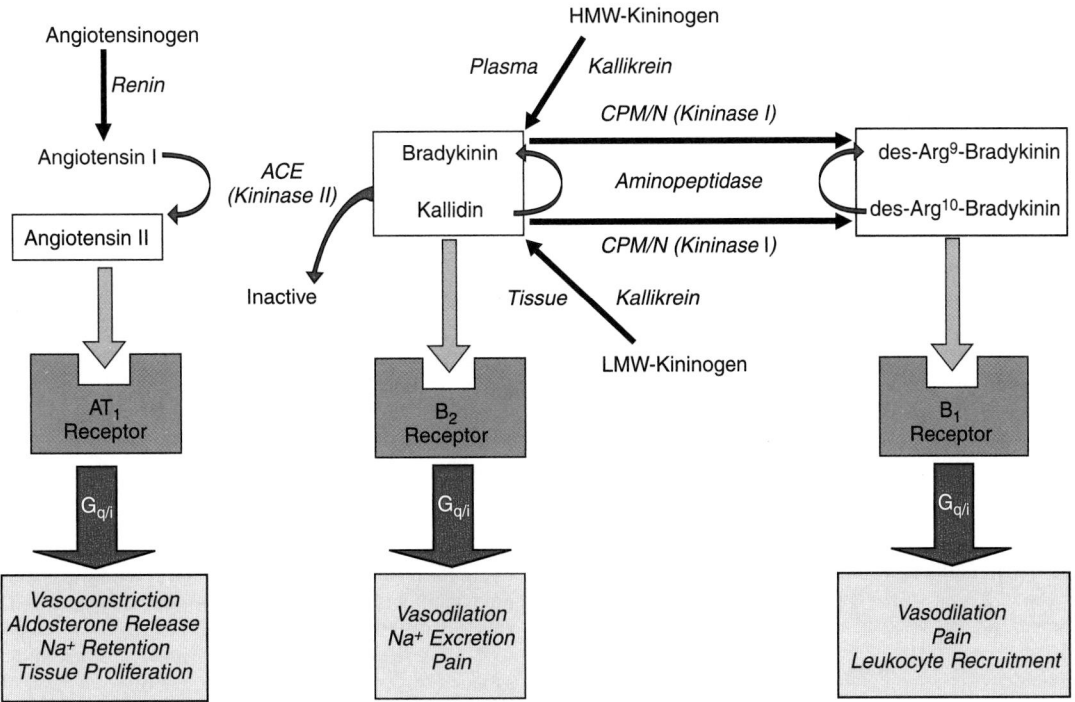

Figure 24–4. *Synthesis and receptor interactions of active peptides generated by the kallikrein–kinin and renin–angiotensin systems.* Bradykinin (BK) is generated by the action of *plasma* kallikrein on high-molecular-weight (HMW) kininogen, whereas kallidin (Lys-bradykinin) is synthesized by the hydrolysis of low-molecular-weight (LMW) kininogen by *tissue* kallikrein. Kallidin and BK are natural ligands of the B_2 receptor but can be converted to corresponding agonists of the B_1 receptor by removal of the C-terminal Arg by the action of kininase I–type enzymes: the plasma membrane–bound carboxypeptidase M (CPM) or soluble plasma carboxypeptidase N (CPN). Kallidin or [des-Arg^{10}]kallidin can be converted to the active peptides BK or [des-Arg^9]BK by aminopeptidase removal of the N-terminal Lys residue. In a parallel fashion, the inactive decapeptide angiotensin I (Ang I) is generated by the action of renin on the plasma substrate angiotensinogen. By removal of the C-terminal His–Leu dipeptide, angiotensin converting enzyme (ACE) generates the active peptide Ang II. These two systems have opposing effects. Whereas Ang II is a potent vasoconstrictor that also causes aldosterone release and Na$^+$ retention via activation of the AT$_1$ receptor, BK is a vasodilator that stimulates Na$^+$ excretion by activating the B_2 receptor. ACE generates active Ang II and at the same time inactivates BK and kallidin; thus its effects are prohypertensive, and ACE inhibitors are effective antihypertensive agents. The B_2 receptor mediates most of BK's effects under normal circumstances, whereas synthesis of the B_1 receptor is induced by inflammatory mediators and plays a major role in chronic inflammatory conditions. Both the B_1 and B_2 receptors couple through G_q to activate PLC and increase intracellular Ca^{2+}; the physiological response depends on receptor distribution on particular cell types and occupancy by agonist peptides. For instance, on endothelial cells, activation of B_2 receptors results in Ca^{2+}–calmodulin–dependent activation of eNOS and generation of NO, which causes cGMP accumulation and relaxation in neighboring smooth muscle cells. On smooth muscle cells, activation of kinin receptor coupling through the same pathway results in an increased [Ca^{2+}]$_i$ and contraction. B_1 and B_2 receptors also can couple through G_i to activate PLA$_2$, causing the release of arachidonic acid and the local generation of prostanoids and other metabolites. For further details, *see* text.

the tissue prokallikrein also may be regulated; *e.g.,* its secretion from the pancreas is enhanced by stimulation of the vagus nerve (*see* Margolius, 1989). The activation of tissue prokallikrein to kallikrein requires proteolytic cleavage to remove a 7–amino acid propeptide (Bhoola *et al.,* 1992).

Kininogens. The two substrates for the kallikreins, HMW kininogen and LMW kininogen, are derived from a single gene by alternative splicing. HMW kininogen and LMW kininogen have been divided into functional domains. The HMW kininogen contains 626 amino acid residues; the internal bradykinin sequence of 9 amino acid resi-

dues, domain 4, connects an N-terminal "heavy chain" sequence (362 amino acids). This consists of domains 1 through 3 and a C-terminal "light chain" sequence (255 amino acids) containing domains D5H and D6. LMW kininogen is identical to the larger form of the protein from the amino terminus through the bradykinin sequence; its short light chain differs (Takagaki *et al.,* 1985). HMW kininogen is cleaved by plasma and tissue kallikrein to yield bradykinin or kallidin, respectively. LMW kininogen is a substrate only of tissue kallikrein, and the product is kallidin. The kininogens also inhibit cysteine proteinases, inhibit thrombin binding, and exhibit antiadhesive and profibrinolytic properties.

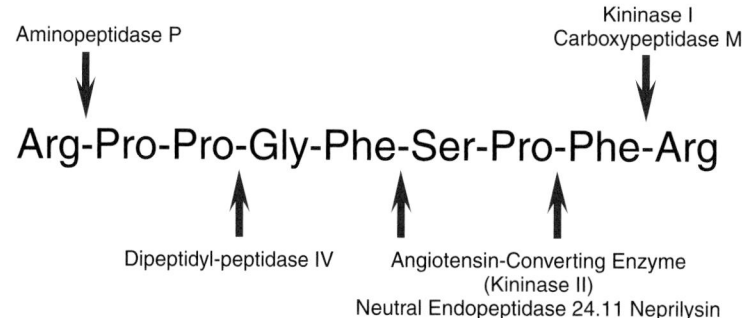

Figure 24–5. *Schematic diagram of the degradation of bradykinin.* Bradykinin and kallidin are inactivated primarily by kininase II [angiotensin converting enzyme (ACE)]. Neutral endopeptidase also cleaves bradykinin and kallidin at the Pro—Phe bond. In addition, aminopeptidase P inactivates bradykinin by hydrolyzing the N-terminal Arg^1—Pro^2 bond, leaving bradykinin susceptible to further degradation by dipeptidyl peptidase IV. Bradykinin and kallidin are converted to their respective des-Arg^9 or des-Arg^{10} metabolites by kininase I–type carboxypeptidases M and N. Unlike the parent compounds, these kinin metabolites are potent ligands for B_1-kinin receptors but not B_2-kinin receptors.

Metabolism. The decapeptide kallidin is about as active as the non-apeptide bradykinin even without conversion to bradykinin, which occurs when the N-terminal lysine residue is removed by a plasma aminopeptidase (Figure 24–4). The minimal effective structure required to elicit the classical responses on the B_2 receptor is that of the nonapeptide (Figure 24–5 and Table 24–3).

The kinins have an evanescent existence—their half-life in plasma is only about 15 seconds, and some 80% to 90% of the kinins may be destroyed in a single passage through the pulmonary vascular bed. Plasma concentrations of bradykinin are difficult to measure because inadequate inhibition of kininogenases or kininases in the blood can lead to artifactual formation or degradation of bradykinin during blood collection. Thus the reported physiological concentrations of bradykinin range from picomolar to femtomolar.

The principal catabolizing enzyme in the lung and other vascular beds is kininase II, or ACE (Figure 24–4) (*see* Chapter 30). Removal of the C-terminal dipeptide abolishes kininlike activity. Neutral endopeptidase 24.11 or neprilysin also inactivates kinins by cleaving off the C-terminal dipeptide (Skidgel and Erdös, 1998). A slower-acting enzyme, carboxypeptidase N (lysine carboxypeptidase, kininase I), releases the C-terminal arginine residue, producing [des-Arg^9]bradykinin and [des-Arg^{10}]kallidin (Table 24–3 and Figures 24–4 and 24–5), which are themselves potent B_1-kinin receptor agonists (Bhoola *et al.*, 1992; Skidgel and Erdös, 1998). Carboxypeptidase N is expressed constitutively in blood plasma, where its concentration is about 10^{-7} M (Skidgel and Erdös, 1998). Carboxypeptidase M, which also cleaves basic C-terminal amino acids, is a widely distributed plasma membrane–bound enzyme (Skidgel and Erdös, 1998) whose crystal structure was established recently. A familial carboxypeptidase N deficiency has been described in which affected individuals with low levels of this enzyme display angioedema or urticaria (*see* below; Skidgel and Erdös, 1998). Finally, aminopeptidase P can inactivate bradykinin by cleaving the N-terminal arginine, rendering bradykinin susceptible to further cleavage by dipeptidyl peptidase IV (Figure 24–5).

Bradykinin Receptors. There are at least two distinct receptors for kinins, which have been designated B_1 and B_2 (Bhoola *et al.*, 1992). Both are GPCRs, sharing 36% amino acid sequence identity (Hess, 1997). The classical bradykinin B_2 receptor is constitu-

tively expressed in most normal tissues, where it selectively binds bradykinin and kallidin (Table 24–3 and Figure 24–4) and mediates the majority of their effects. The B_1 receptor selectively binds to the C-terminal des-Arg metabolites of bradykinin and kallidin released by carboxypeptidase N or M (Table 24–3 and Figure 24–4) and is absent or expressed at low levels in most tissues. B_1-receptor expression is up-regulated by inflammation and by cytokines, endotoxins, and growth factors (Bhoola *et al.*, 1992; Dray and Perkins, 1993). Under these conditions, B_1-receptor effects may predominate.

The B_2 receptor activates PLA_2 and PLC *via* interaction with distinct G proteins. Kinin-induced PLC activation through G_q activates the IP_3–Ca^{2+} pathway, stimulating PKC activity and also enhancing NO synthesis and release. Bradykinin activates the proinflammatory transcription factor NF-κB through $G\alpha_q$ and $\beta\gamma$ subunits and also activates the MAP kinase pathway (Blaukat, 2003). Coupling of activated B_2 receptors to G_i leads to PLA_2 activation and the liberation of arachidonate from membrane-bound phospholipids, which is converted to a variety of potent inflammatory mediators and the vasodilator prostacyclin (*see* Chapter 25). Binding of bradykinin to the B_2 receptor leads to internalization of the agonist–receptor complex and thus to desensitization. In contrast, the B_1 receptor does not internalize after binding its ligand, [des-Arg]kinin, because it lacks the Ser/Thr-rich cluster present in the C-terminal tail of the B_2 receptor that mediates its sequestration after phosphorylation (Blaukat, 2003).

Because the bradykinin B_2 receptors are distributed widely and couple to several G proteins, receptor agonists are employed frequently as tools to activate and study signal transduction in a variety of cells. HOE-140 is the antagonist used most frequently to prove that cellular responses are mediated by B_2-receptor agonists. Nevertheless, increased signaling through the B_2 receptor does not necessarily require increased kinin generation because—at least in cultured cells—proteases such as kallikrein can activate the B_2 receptor directly, a response that is also blocked by HOE-140 (Hecquet *et al.*, 2000).

Some studies suggest that activation of the angiotensin AT_2 receptor has opposite effects to those of the angiotensin AT_1 receptor (*see* Chapter 30), effects that may be mediated in part through activation of the B_2 receptor (Widdop *et al.*, 2003).

Functions and Pharmacology of Kallikreins and Kinins

The availability of more specific bradykinin antagonists and the generation of bradykinin-receptor Knockout mice have advanced our understanding of the roles of the kinins significantly. These compounds currently are being investigated in diverse areas such as pain, inflammation and chronic inflammatory diseases, the cardiovascular system, and reproduction.

Pain. The kinins are powerful algesic agents that cause an intense burning pain when applied to the exposed base of a blister. Bradykinin excites primary sensory neurons and provokes the release of neuropeptides such as substance P, neurokinin A, and calcitonin gene–related peptide (Geppetti, 1993). Although there is overlap, B_2 receptors generally mediate acute bradykinin algesia, whereas the pain of chronic inflammation appears to involve increased numbers of B_1 receptors.

Inflammation. Kinins participate in a variety of inflammatory diseases. Plasma kinins increase permeability in the microcirculation. The effect, like that of histamine and serotonin in some species, is exerted on the small venules and involves separation of the junctions between endothelial cells. This, together with an increased hydrostatic pressure gradient, causes edema. Such edema, coupled with stimulation of nerve endings (*see* below), results in a "wheal and flare" response to intradermal injections in human beings.

In hereditary angioedema, bradykinin is formed, and there is depletion of the components of the kinin cascade during episodes of swelling, laryngeal edema, and abdominal pain. B_1 receptors on inflammatory cells such as macrophages can elicit production of the inflammatory mediators interleukin 1 (IL-1) and tumor necrosis factor α (TNF-α) (Dray and Perkins, 1993). Kinin levels are increased in a number of chronic inflammatory diseases, including rhinitis caused by inhalation of antigens and that associated with rhinoviral infection. Kinins may be significant in conditions such as gout, disseminated intravascular coagulation, inflammatory bowel disease, rheumatoid arthritis, and asthma. Kinins also may contribute to the skeletal changes seen in chronic inflammatory states. Kinins stimulate bone resorption through B_1 and possibly B_2 receptors, perhaps by osteoblast-mediated osteoclast activation (*see* Chapter 61).

Respiratory Disease. The kinins have been implicated in the pathophysiology of allergic airway disorders such as asthma and rhinitis. Inhalation or intravenous injection of kinins causes bronchospasm in asthmatic patients but not in normal individuals. This bradykinin-induced bronchoconstriction is blocked by anticholinergic agents but not by antihistamines or cyclooxygenase inhibitors. Similarly, nasal challenge with bradykinin is followed by sneezing and serious glandular secretions in patients with allergic rhinitis. A bradykinin B_2-receptor antagonist improved pulmonary function in patients with severe asthma.

Cardiovascular System. Urinary kallikrein concentrations are decreased in individuals with high blood pressure. In experimental animals and humans, infusion of bradykinin causes vasodilation and lowers blood pressure. Hypertensives also excrete less urinary kallikrein (Margolius, 1989, 1995). Bradykinin causes vasodilation by activating its B_2 receptor on endothelial cells. The endothelium-dependent dilation is mediated by NO, prostacyclin, and a hyperpolarizing epoxyeicosatrienoic acid that is a CYP-derived metabolite of arachidonic acid (Vanhoutte, 1989; Campbell *et al.*, 1996).

The availability of specific bradykinin antagonists and genetically altered animals has enhanced our understanding of the role of endogenous bradykinin in the regulation of blood pressure (Madeddu *et al.*, 1997). Basal blood pressure is normal in B_2-receptor antagonist–treated animals or B_2-receptor knockout mice. However, these animals exhibit an exaggerated blood pressure response to salt loading or activation of the renin–angiotensin system. These data suggest that the endogenous kallikrein–kinin system plays a minor role in the regulation of blood pressure under normal circumstances, but it may be important in hypertensive states.

The kallikrein–kinin system appears to be cardioprotective. Because part of the activity of the widely used ACE inhibitors is attributed to enhancement of bradykinin effects, much was learned about the function of kinins, such as their antiproliferative effects. Bradykinin contributes to the beneficial effect of preconditioning the heart against ischemia and reperfusion injury. In the presence of endothelial cells, bradykinin prevents vascular smooth muscle cell growth and proliferation. Bradykinin stimulates tissue plasminogen activator (tPA) release from the vascular endothelium (Brown *et al.*, 1999). In this way, bradykinin may contribute to the endogenous defense against cardiovascular events such as myocardial infarction and stroke.

Kinins also may increase sympathetic outflow *via* central and peripheral nervous mechanisms.

Kidney. Renal kinins act in a paracrine manner to regulate urine volume and composition (Saitoh *et al.*, 1995).

Kallikrein is synthesized and secreted by the connecting cells of the distal nephron. Tissue kininogen and kinin receptors are present in the cells of the collecting duct. Like other vasodilators, kinins increase renal blood flow. Bradykinin also causes natriuresis by inhibiting sodium reabsorption at the cortical collecting duct. Renal kallikreins are increased by treatment with mineralocorticoids, ACE inhibitors, and neutral endopeptidase (neprilysin) inhibitors.

Other Effects. The rat uterus in estrus is especially sensitive to contraction by kinins through the B_2 receptor. Kinins promote dilation of the fetal pulmonary artery, closure of the ductus arteriosus, and constriction of the umbilical vessels, all of which occur in the transition from fetal to neonatal circulation.

The kallikrein–kinin system also functions in many other areas in the body, serving to mediate edema formation and smooth muscle contraction. The slowly developing contraction of the isolated guinea pig ileum that the peptide induces first prompted the name *bradykinin*. The kinins also affect the CNS, in addition to their ability to disrupt the blood–brain barrier and allow increased CNS penetration. A bradykinin analog (RMP7) that is resistant to degradation by carboxypeptidase N and M and ACE has been tested in the laboratory and clinically to enhance the penetration of drugs to brain tumors through the blood–brain barrier (*see* Inamura *et al.*, 1994).

Potential Therapeutic Uses. Bradykinin contributes to many of the effects of the ACE inhibitors (Figure 24–4). *Aprotinin,* a kallikrein inhibitor, is administered to patients undergoing coronary bypass to minimize bleeding and blood requirements (*see* below). Kinin agonists potentially may increase the delivery of chemotherapeutic agents past the blood–brain barrier. Based on some of the actions outlined earlier, kinin antagonists are being tested in inflammatory conditions.

Kallikrein Inhibitors. Aprotinin (TRASYLOL) is a natural proteinase inhibitor obtained for commercial purposes from bovine lung, but it is identical with Kunitz's pancreatic trypsin inhibitor (Waxler and Rabito, 2003). Aprotinin inhibits mediators of the inflammatory response, fibrinolysis, and thrombin generation following cardiopulmonary bypass surgery, including kallikrein and plasmin. In several placebo-controlled, double-blind studies, administration of aprotinin reduced requirements for blood products in patients undergoing coronary artery bypass grafting. Depending on patient risk factors, aprotinin is given as a loading dose of either 1 or 2 million kallikrein inhibitor units (KIU), followed by continuous infusion of 250,000 or 500,000 KIU/h during surgery. Hypersensitivity reactions may occur with aprotinin, including anaphylactic or anaphylactoid reactions. The rate of such reactions is less than 1% in patients who have not been exposed previously to aprotinin and higher (1% to 9%) in patients who have been

exposed to aprotinin. A test dose of aprotinin (10,000 KIU) should be given prior to full dosing; however, this test is not risk-free. Aprotinin can interfere with an activated clotting time used to determine the effectiveness of heparin anticoagulation (*see* Chapter 54). For this reason, alternate methods must be used in patients treated with aprotinin. In one multicenter study, there was an increased closure rate of saphenous vein grafts in patients treated with aprotinin compared with placebo; there were no differences in rates of myocardial infarction or death (Waxler and Rabito, 2003).

Bradykinin and the Effects of ACE Inhibitors. ACE inhibitors are used widely in the treatment of hypertension, and they reduce mortality in patients with diabetic nephropathy, left ventricular dysfunction, previous myocardial infarction, or coronary artery disease. ACE inhibitors block the conversion of angiotensin I to angiotensin II, a potent vasoconstrictor and growth promoter (Figure 24–4) (*see* Chapter 30). Studies using the specific bradykinin B_2 antagonist HOE-140 demonstrate that bradykinin also contributes to many of the protective effects of ACE inhibitors. For example, administration of HOE-140 in animal models attenuates the favorable effects of ACE inhibitors on blood pressure, myocardial infarct size, and ischemic preconditioning (Linz *et al.*, 1995). Bradykinin-receptor antagonism also attenuates blood pressure lowering by acute ACE inhibition in human beings (Gainer *et al.*, 1998). The contribution of bradykinin to the effects of ACE inhibitors may result not only from decreased degradation of bradykinin but also from induction of enhanced receptor sensitivity (Marcic *et al.*, 1999).

Occasional patients receiving ACE inhibitors have experienced angioedema, which occurs most often shortly after initiating therapy. This is a class effect of ACE inhibitors and is thought to be connected to the inhibition of kinin metabolism by ACE (Slater *et al.*, 1988). ACE inhibitor–associated angioedema is more common in blacks than in Caucasians. A common side effect of ACE inhibitors (especially in women) is a chronic nonproductive cough that dissipates when the drug is stopped. The finding that angiotensin AT_1-receptor-subtype antagonists do not cause cough provides presumptive evidence for the role of bradykinin in this effect, but the mechanism and receptor subtype involved have not been clearly defined.

Preliminary data suggest that bradykinin also may contribute to the effects of the AT_1-receptor antagonists. During AT_1-receptor blockade, angiotensin II concentrations increase. Renal bradykinin concentrations also increase through the effects of angiotensin II on the unopposed AT_2-subtype receptor (Widdop *et al.*, 2003). Whether or not bradykinin contributes to the clinical effects of the

AT_1-receptor antagonists remains to be determined. In addition, a new class of antihypertensive agents, the combined ACE–neutral endopeptidase inhibitors, has been tested. These drugs inhibit two kinin-degrading enzymes; consequently, bradykinin may be expected to contribute more significantly to their clinical and side effects. In clinical trials, administration of the combination drug *omapatrilat* was associated with a threefold higher incidence of angioedema than was an ACE inhibitor alone, causing withdrawal of the combination and reduced enthusiasm for their further development.

Bradykinin Antagonists. The substitution of a D-aromatic amino acid for the proline residue at position seven conferred antagonist activity to bradykinin and blocked the action of ACE. The addition of an N-terminal D-arginine residue also increased the half-life of these antagonists. However, the early kinin antagonists were partial agonists and had short half-lives owing to enzymatic degradation by carboxypeptidase N *in vivo*. The longer-acting, more selective kinin antagonist HOE-140 was developed by substituting synthetic amino acids at positions seven [D-tetrahydroisoquinoline-3-carboxylic acid (Tic)] and eight [octahydroindole-2-carboxylic acid (Oic)] (Table 24–3). This compound has contributed to our understanding of the functions of bradykinin *in vitro* and *in vivo*.

The development of orally active nonpeptide-receptor antagonists promises to make bradykinin antagonism therapeutically feasible in the treatment of inflammatory disease. The first of these, WIN64338, suffered from having muscarinic cholinergic activity. More recently, the nonpeptide antagonist FR173657 (Table 24–3) has been shown to decrease bradykinin-induced edema and hypotension in animal models. On the other hand, synthetic B_2-receptor agonists (such as FR190997; Table 24–3) may be cardioprotective. Synthetic small-molecule bradykinin agonists or antagonists will not necessarily bind to the same extracellular domains of the B_2 receptor as the peptide but may interact with the hydrophobic transmembrane portion (Heitsch, 2003).

CLINICAL SUMMARY

Aprotinin (TRASYLOL), the potent inhibitor of kallikrein and other serine proteases, is employed clinically to reduce blood loss in patients undergoing coronary artery bypass surgery.

Because kinins and [des-Arg]kinins enhance pain and inflammation *via* activation of the two kinin receptors, B_2- and B_1-receptor antagonists may be useful in the future to treat inflammation. Although initial trials of peptide-based antagonists have not yet yielded convincingly positive effects, small synthetic nonpeptidic antagonists that absorb better and have more favorable pharmacokinetic profiles could be more promising therapeutic agents.

ACE inhibitors are widely used drugs in the treatment of hypertension, congestive heart failure, and diabetic nephropathy, and they reduce mortality in patients with a variety of cardiovascular risk factors (*see* Chapter 30). One effect of ACE inhibitors is to prevent the degradation of bradykinin. Because bradykinin, by activating its B_2 receptor, is responsible for many of the beneficial cardioprotective effects of ACE inhibitors, the search is on to find a suitable stable B_2 agonist for clinical evaluation. A major problem for such applications is to establish a safe therapeutic window between potentially protecting the heart and avoiding proinflammatory stimulation (Heitsch, 2003).

ACKNOWLEDGMENT

We are grateful for the helpful contributions of Dr. Jean-Charles Schwartz of INSERM U.109, Paris; Dr. Allen P. Kaplan of the Medical University of South Carolina, Charleston; Dr. Sara F. Rabito of Cook County Hospital, Chicago; and Dr. William B. Campbell of the Medical College of Wisconsin, Milwaukee.

BIBLIOGRAPHY

Arrang, J.-M., Garbarg, M., Lancelot, J.-C., *et al.* Highly potent and selective ligands for histamine H_3-receptors. *Nature,* **1987**, *327*:117–123.

Ash, A.S.F., and Schild, H.O. Receptors mediating some actions of histamine. *Br. J. Pharmacol.,* **1966**, *27*:427–439.

Best, C.H., Dale, H.H., Dudley, J.W., and Thorpe, W.V. The nature of the vasodilator constituents of certain tissue extract. *J. Physiol. (Lond.),* **1927**, *62*:397–417.

Black, J.W., Duncan, W.A., Durant, C.J., Ganellin, C.R., and Parsons, E.M. Definition and antagonism of histamine H_2-receptors. *Nature,* **1972**, *236*:385–390.

Brown, N.J., Gainer, J.V., Stein, C.M., and Vaughan, D.E. Bradykinin stimulates tissue plasminogen activator release in human vasculature. *Hypertension,* **1999**, *33*:1431–1435.

Campbell, W.B., Gebremedhin, D., Pratt, P.F., and Harder, D.R. Identification of epoxyeicosatrienoic acids as endothelium-derived hyperpolarizing factors. *Circ. Res.,* **1996**, *78*:415–423.

Chien, S., and Krakoff, L. Hemodynamics of dogs in histamine shock, with special reference to splanchnic blood volume and flow. *Circ. Res.,* **1963**, *12*:29–39.

Esbenshade, T.A., Krueger, K.M., Miller, T.R., *et al.* A. Two novel and selective nonimidazole histamine H_3 receptor antagonists A-304121 and A-317920: I. In Vitro Pharmacological Effects. *J. Pharmacol. Exp. Ther.,* **2003**, *305*:887–896.

Ferreira, S.H., Bartelt, D.C., and Greene, L.J. Isolation of bradykinin-potentiating peptides from *Bothrops jararaca* venom. *Biochemistry,* **1970**, *9*:2583–2593.

Gaboury, J.P., Johnston, B., Niu, X.-F., and Kubes, P. Mechanisms underlying acute mast cell–induced leukocyte rolling and adhesion *in vivo. J. Immunol.,* **1995**, *154*:804–813.

Gainer, J.V., Morrow, J.D., Loveland, A., King, D.J., and Brown, N.J. Effect of bradykinin-receptor blockade on the response to angiotensin-converting-enzyme inhibitor in normotensive and hypertensive subjects. *New Engl. J. Med.,* **1998**, *339*:1285–1292.

Gavras, H., Brunner, H.R., Laragh, J.H., *et al.* An angiotensin converting-enzyme inhibitor to identify and treat vasoconstrictor and volume factors in hypertensive patients. *New Engl. J. Med.,* **1974**, *291*:817–821.

Hecquet, C., Tan, F., Marcic, B.M., and Erdos, E.G. Human bradykinin B(2) receptor is activated by kallikrein and other serine proteases. *Mol. Pharmacol.,* **2000**, *58*:828–836.

Hofstra, C.L., Desai, P.J., Thurmond, R.L., and Fung-Leung, W.-P. Histamine H_4 receptor mediates chemotaxis and calcium mobilization of mast cells. *J. Pharmacol. Exp. Ther.,* **2003**, *305*:1212–1221.

Inamura, T., Nomura, T., Bartus, R.T., and Black K.L. Intracarotid infusion of RMP-7, a bradykinin analog: a method for selective drug delivery to brain tumors. *J. Neurosurg.,* **1994**, *81*:752–758.

Johnson, A.R., and Erdös, E.G. Release of histamine from mast cells by vasoactive peptides. *Proc. Soc. Exp. Biol. Med.,* **1973**, *142*:1252–1256.

Leurs, R., Wantanabe, T., and Timmerman, H. Histamine receptors are finally "coming out." *Trends Pharmacol. Sci.,* **2001**, *22*:337–339.

Ling, P., Ngo, K., Nguyen, S., *et al.* Histamine H_4 receptor mediates eosinophil chemotaxis with cell shape change and adhesion molecule up-regulation. *Brit. J. Pharmacol.,* **2004**, *142*:161–178.

Lovenberg, T.W., Roland, B.L., Wilson, S.J., *et al.* Cloning and functional expression of the human histamine H_3 receptor. *Mol. Pharmacol.,* **1999**, *55*:1101–1105.

Madeddu, P., Varoni, M.V., Palomba, D., *et al.* Cardiovascular phenotype of a mouse strain with disruption of bradykinin B_2-receptor gene. *Circulation,* **1997**, *96*:3570–3578.

Marcic, B., Deddish, P.A., Jackman, H.L., and Erdos, E.G. Enhancement of bradykinin and resensitization of its B_2 receptor. *Hypertension,* **1999**, *33*:835–843.

Meszaros, J.G., Gonzalez, A.M., Endo-Mochizuki, Y., *et al.* Identification of G protein–coupled pathways in cardiac fibroblasts: Cross-talk between G_q and G_s. *Am. J. Physiol.,* **2000**, *278*:C154–162.

Morrow, J.D., Margolies, G.R., Rowland, J., and Roberts, L.J., II. Evidence that histamine is the causative toxin of scombroid-fish poisoning. *New Engl. J. Med.,* **1991**, *324*:716–720.

Oda, T., Morikawa, N., Saito, Y., Masuho, Y., and Matsumoto, S.-I. Molecular cloning and characterization of a novel type of histamine receptor preferentially expressed in leukocytes. *J. Biol. Chem.,* **2000**, *275*:36781–36786.

Ondetti, M.A., Williams, N.J., Sabo, E.F., *et al.* Angiotensin-converting enzyme inhibitors from the venom of *Bothrops jararaca*: Isolation, elucidation of structure, and synthesis. *Biochemistry,* **1971**, *10*:4033–4039.

Ookuma, K., Sakata, T., Fukagawa, K., *et al.* Neuronal histamine in the hypothalamus suppresses food intake in rats. *Brain Res.,* **1993**, *628*:235–242.

Pesquero, J.B., Araujo, R.C., Heppenstall, P.A., *et al.* Hypoalgesia and altered inflammatory responses in mice lacking kinin B_1 receptors. *Proc. Natl. Acad. Sci. U.S.A.,* **2000**, *97*:8140–8145.

Rizk, A., Curley, J., Robertson, J., and Raber, J. Anxiety and cognition in histamine H_3 receptor–/– mice. *Eur. J. Neurosci.,* **2004**, *19*:1992–1996.

Roberts, L.J., II, Marney, S.R., Jr., and Oates, J.A. Blockade of the flush associated with metastatic gastric carcinoid syndrome by combined histamine H_1 and H_2 receptor antagonists: Evidence for an important role of H_2 receptors in human vasculature. *New Engl. J. Med.,* **1979**, *300*:236–238.

Rocha e Silva, M., Beraldo, W.T., and Rosenfeld, G. Bradykinin, a hypotensive and smooth muscle stimulating factor released from plasma globulin by snake venoms and by trypsin. *Am. J. Physiol.,* **1949**, *156*:261–273.

Saitoh, S., Scicli, A.G., Peterson, E., and Carretero, O.A. Effect of inhibiting renal kallikrein on prostaglandin E_2, water, and sodium excretion. *Hypertension,* **1995**, *25*:1008–1013.

Serafin, W.E., and Austen, K.F. Mediators of immediate hypersensitivity reactions. *New Engl. J. Med.,* **1987**, *317*:30–34.

Takagaki, Y., Kitamura, N., and Nakanishi, S. Cloning and sequence analysis of cDNAs for human high molecular weight and low molecular weight prekininogens: Primary structures of two human prekininogens. *J. Biol. Chem.,* **1985**, *260*:8601–8609.

Takeshita, K., Sakai, K., Bacon, K.B., and Gantner, F. Critical role of histamine H_4 receptor in leukotriene B_4 production and mast cell–dependent neutrophil recruitment induced by zymosan in vivo. *J. Pharmacol. Exp. Ther.,* **2003**, *307*:1072–1078.

Thurmond, R.L. Deais, P.J., Dunford, P.F., *et al.* A potent and selective histamine H_4 receptor antagonist with antiinflammatory properties. *J. Pharmacol. Exp. Ther.,* **2004**, *309*:404–413.

Toda, N. Is histamine a human coronary vasospastic substance? *Trends Pharmacol. Sci.,* **1987**, *8*:289–290.

Vavrek, R.J., and Stewart, J.M. Competitive antagonists of bradykinin. *Peptides,* **1985**, *6*:161–164.

Yang, H.Y.T., Erdös, E.G., and Levin, Y. A dipeptidyl carboxypeptidase that converts angiotensin I and inactivates bradykinin. *Biochim. Biophys. Acta,* **1970**, *214*:374–376.

MONOGRAPHS AND REVIEWS

Beraldo, W.T., and Andrade, S.P. Discovery of bradykinin and the kallikrein-kinin system. In, *The Kinin System.* (Farmer S. G., ed.) Academic Press, San Diego, **1997**, pp. 1–8.

Bhoola, K.D., Figueroa C.D., and Worthy, K. Bioregulation of kinins: Kallikreins, kininogens, and kininases. *Pharmacol. Rev.,* **1992**, *44*:1–80.

Blaukat, A. Structure and signalling pathways of kinin receptors. *Andrologia,* **2003**, *35*:17–23.

Bovet, D. Introduction to antihistamine agents and Antergan derivatives. *Ann. N.Y. Acad. Sci.,* **1950**, *50*:1089–1126.

Campbell, W.B., and Harder, D.R. Endothelium-derived hyperpolarizing factors and vascular cytochrome P450 metabolites of arachidonic acid in the regulation of tone. *Circ. Res.,* **1999**, *84*:484–488.

Colman, R.W. Biologic activities of the contact factors *in vivo*—potentiation of hypotension, inflammation, and fibrinolysis, and inhibition of cell adhesion, angiogenesis and thrombosis. *Thromb. Haemost.,* **1999**, *82*:1568–1577.

Dray, A., and Perkins, M. Bradykinin and inflammatory pain. *Trends Neurosci.,* **1993**, *16*:99–104.

Ferry, X., Brehin, S., Kamel, R., and Landry, Y. G protein–dependent activation of mast cell by peptides and basic secretagogues. *Peptides,* **2002**, *23*:1507–1515.

Ganellin, C.R., and Parsons, M.E., eds. *Pharmacology of Histamine Receptors.* PSG, Bristol, MA, **1982**.

Gelfand, E.W., Appajosyula, S., and Meeves, S. Antiinflammatory activity of H_1-receptor antagonists: Review of recent experimental research. *Curr. Med. Res. Opin.,* **2004**, *20*:73–81.

Geppetti, P. Sensory neuropeptide release by bradykinin: Mechanisms and pathophysiological implications. *Regul. Pept.,* **1993**, *47*:1–23.

Grossman, M.L. Some notes on the history of gastrin. In, *Gastrin.* (Grossman, M.L., ed.) University of California Press, Berkeley, **1966**, pp. 1–7.

Hancock, A.A., Esbenshade, T.A., Krueger, K.M., and Yao, B.B. Genetic and pharmacological aspects of histamine H_3 receptor heterogeneity. *Life Sci.,* **2003**, *73*:3043–3072.

Heitsch, H. The therapeutic potential of bradykinin B_2 receptor agonists in the treatment of cardiovascular disease. *Expert Opin. Invest. Drugs,* **2003,** *12*:759–770.

Hess, J.F. Molecular pharmacology of kinin receptors. In, *The Kinin System.* (Farmer, S.G., ed.) Academic Press, San Diego, **1997,** pp. 45–55.

Holgate, S.T., Canonica, G.W., Simons, F.E., *et al.* Consensus Group on New-Generation Antihistamines (CONGA): Present status and recommendations. *Clin. Exp. Allergy,* **2003,** *33*:1305–1324.

Hough, L.B. Genomics meets histamine receptors: New subtypes, new receptors. *Mol. Pharmacol.,* **2001,** *59*:415–419.

Hough, L.B. Cellular localization and possible functions for brain histamine: Recent progress. *Prog. Neurobiol.,* **1988,** *30*:469–505.

Leurs, R., Church, M.K., and Taglialatela, M. H_1 antihistamines: Inverse agonism, antiinflammatory actions and cardiac effects. *Clin. Exp. Allergy,* **2002,** *32*:489–498.

Leurs, R., Blandina, P., Tedford, C., and Timmerman, H. Therapeutic potential of histamine H_3 receptor agonists and antagonists. *Trends Pharmacol. Sci.,* **1998,** *19*:177–183.

Lewis, T. *The Blood Vessels of the Human Skin and Their Responses.* Shaw & Sons, London, **1927.**

Linz, W., Wiemer, G., Gohlke, P., Unger, T., and Schölkens, B. A. Contribution of kinins to the cardiovascular actions of angiotensin-converting enzyme inhibitors. *Pharmacol. Rev.,* **1995,** *47*:25–49.

Macglashan, D. Histamine: A mediator of inflammation. *J. Allergy Clin. Immunol.,* **2003,** *112*:S13–S19.

Madeddu, P. Receptor antagonists of bradykinin: A new tool to study the cardiovascular effects of endogenous kinins. *Pharmacol. Res.,* **1993,** *28*:107–128.

Margolius, H.S. Theodore Cooper Memorial Lecture. Kallikreins and kinins: Some unanswered questions about system characteristics and roles in human disease. *Hypertension,* **1995,** *26*:221–229.

Margolius, H.S. Tissue kallikreins and kinins: Regulation and roles in hypertensive and diabetic diseases. *Annu. Rev. Pharmacol. Toxicol.,* **1989,** *29*:343–364.

Meeves, S.G., and Appajosyula, S. Efficacy and safety profile of fexofenadine HCL: A unique therapeutic option in H_1-receptor antagonist treatment. *J. Allergy Clin. Immunol.,* **2003,** *112*:S29–S37.

Nadel, J.A., and Barnes, P.J. Autonomic regulation of the airways. *Annu. Rev. Med.,* **1984,** *35*:451–467.

Paton, D.M., and Webster, D.R. Clinical pharmacokinetics of H_1-receptor antagonists (the antihistamines). *Clin. Pharmacokinet.,* **1985,** *10*:477–497.

Rocha e Silva, M. ed., *Histamine II and Anti-Histaminics: Chemistry, Metabolism and Physiological and Pharmacological Actions [Hand-*buch der Experimentellen Pharmakologie],* Vol. 18, Pt. 2. Springer-Verlag, Berlin, **1978.**

Rothschild, A.M. Histamine release by basic compounds. In, *Histamine and Anti-Histamines. Handbook of Experimental Pharmacology,* Vol 18. (Rocha e Silva, M., ed.) Springer-Verlag, Berlin, **1966,** pp. 386–430.

Schmaier, A.H. The physiologic basis of assembly and activation of the plasma kallikrein/kinin system. *Thromb. Haemost.,* **2004,** *91*:1–3.

Schwartz, J.-C., and Arrang, J.M. Histamine. In, *Neuropsychopharmacology: The Fifth Generation of Progress.* (Davis, K.L., Charney, D., Coyle, J.T., and Nemeroff, C., eds.) Lippincott Williams & Wilkins, Philadelphia, **2002,** pp. 179–190.

Schwartz, L.B. Mast cells: Function and contents. *Curr. Opin. Immunol.,* **1994,** *6*:91–97.

Simons, F.E., and Simons, K.J. The pharmacology and use of H_1-receptor-antagonist drugs. *New Engl. J. Med.,* **1994,** *330*:1663–1670.

Simons, F.E. H_1-Antihistamines: More relevant than ever in the treatment of allergic disorders. *J. Allergy Clin. Immunol.,* **2003a,** *112*:S42–S52.

Simons, S.E.R. Antihistamines. In, *Middelton's Allergy: Principles and Practice,* 6th ed. (Adkinson, J., Franklin, N., Younginger, J.W., *et al.,* eds.) Mosby, Philadelphia, PA, **2003b,** pp. 834–869.

Skidgel, R.A., and Erdös, E.G. Enzymatic degradation of bradykinin. In, *Pro-inflammatory and Antiinflammatory Peptides.* (Said, S.I., ed.) Marcel Dekker, New York, **1998,** pp. 459–516.

Slater, E.E., Merrill, D.D., Guess, H.A., *et al.* Clinical profile of angioedema associated with angiotensin-converting enzyme inhibition. *JAMA,* **1988,** *260*:967–970.

Stark, H., Arrang, J.M., Ligneau, X., *et al.* The histamine H_3 receptor and its ligands. *Prog. Med. Chem.,* **2001,** *38*:279–308.

Vanhoutte, P.M. Endothelium and control of vascular function: State of the art lecture. *Hypertension,* **1989,** *13*:658–667.

Waxler, B., and Rabito, S.F. Aprotinin: A serine protease inhibitor with therapeutic actions: Its interaction with ACE inhibitors. *Curr. Pharm. Des.,* **2003,** *9*:777–787.

Werle, E. Discovery of the most important kallikreins and kallikrein inhibitors. In, *Bradykinin, Kallidin and Kallikrein [Handbuch der Experimentellen Pharmakologie],* Vol. 25. (Erdös, E.G., ed.) Springer-Verlag, Berlin, **1970,** pp. 1–6.

Widdop, R.E., Jones, E.S., Hannan, R.E., and Gaspari, T.A. Angiotensin AT_2 receptors: Cardiovascular hope or hype? *Br. J. Pharmacol.,* **2003,** *140*:809–824.

Yousef, G.M., and Diamandis, E.P. Human tissue kallikreins: A new enzymatic cascade pathway? *Biol. Chem.,* **2002,** *383*:1045–1057.

LIPID-DERIVED AUTACOIDS: EICOSANOIDS AND PLATELET-ACTIVATING FACTOR

Emer M. Smyth, Anne Burke, and Garret A. FitzGerald

Membrane lipids supply the substrate for the synthesis of eicosanoids and platelet-activating factor. Eicosanoids— arachidonate metabolites, including prostaglandins, prostacyclin, thromboxane A_2, leukotrienes, lipoxins and hepoxylins—are not stored but are produced by most cells when a variety of physical, chemical, and hormonal stimuli activate acyl hydrolases that make arachidonate available. Membrane glycerophosphocholine derivatives can be modified enzymatically to produce platelet-activating factor (PAF). PAF is formed by a smaller number of cell types, principally leukocytes, platelets, and endothelial cells. Eicosanoids and PAF lipids contribute to inflammation, smooth muscle tone, hemostasis, thrombosis, parturition, and gastrointestinal secretion. Several classes of drugs, most notably *aspirin,* the *traditional nonsteroidal antiinflammatory agents* (tNSAIDs), and the specific inhibitors of cyclooxygenase-2 (COX-2), such as the *coxibs,* owe their principal therapeutic effects to blockade of eicosanoid formation. In order to understand the therapeutic potential of selective inhibitors of eicosanoid synthesis and action, it is enlightening to first review the synthesis, metabolism, and mechanism of action of eicosanoids and PAF.

EICOSANOIDS

History. In 1930, Kurzrok and Lieb, two American gynecologists, observed that strips of uterine myometrium relax or contract when exposed to semen. Subsequentially, Goldblatt in England and von Euler in Sweden reported independently on smooth muscle–contracting and vasodepressor activities in seminal fluid and accessory reproductive glands. Von Euler identified the active material as a lipid-soluble acid, which he named *prostaglandin,* inferring its ori-

gin in the prostatic gland. Samuelsson, Bergström, and their colleagues elucidated the structures of prostaglandin E_1 (PGE_1) and prostaglandin $F_1\alpha$ ($PGF_1\alpha$) in 1962. In 1964, Bergström and coworkers and van Dorp and associates independently achieved the biosynthesis of PGE_2 from arachidonic acid using homogenates of sheep seminal vesicle. The discoveries of thromboxane A_2 (TxA_2), prostacyclin (PGI_2), and the leukotrienes followed in short order. Vane, Smith, and Willis reported that aspirin and NSAIDs act by inhibiting prostaglandin biosynthesis (Vane, 1971). This remarkable period of discovery culminated with the award of the Nobel Prize to Bergström, Samuelsson, and Vane in 1982. For his discovery of norepinephrine as the neurotransmitter in the sympathetic branch of the autonomic nervous system, von Euler shared the Nobel Prize in 1970 with Julius Axelrod and Bernard Katz.

Prostaglandins (PGs), leukotrienes (LTs), and related compounds are called *eicosanoids,* from the Greek *eikosi* ("twenty"). Precursor essential fatty acids contain 20 carbons and three, four, or five double bonds: 8,11,14-eicosatrienoic acid (dihomo-γ-linolenic acid), 5,8,11,14-eicosatetraenoic acid [arachidonic acid (AA); Figure 25–1], and 5,8,11,14,17-eicosapentaenoic acid (EPA). In humans, AA, the most abundant precursor, is either derived from dietary linoleic acid (9,12-octadecadienoic acid) or ingested directly as a dietary constituent. EPA is a major constituent of oils from fatty fish such as salmon.

Biosynthesis. Biosynthesis of eicosanoids is limited by the availability of substrate and depends primarily on the release of AA, esterified in the *sn*-2 domain of cell membrane phospholipids or other complex lipids, to the eicosanoid-synthesizing enzymes by acyl hydrolases, most notably phospholipase A_2. Chemical and physical stimuli activate the Ca^{2+}-dependent translocation of group IV cytosolic PLA_2 ($cPLA_2$), which has high affinity for AA, to the membrane, where it hydrolyzes the *sn*-2 ester bond of membrane phospholipids (particularly phosphatidylcholine and phosphatidylethanolamine), releasing arachidonate. Multiple additional PLA_2 isoforms [group IIA secretory ($sPLA_2$), group V ($sPLA_2$), group VI Ca^{2+} independent ($iPLA_2$), and group X ($sPLA_2$)] have been characterized. Under nonstimulated conditions, AA liberated by $iPLA_2$ is reincorporated into cell membranes, so there is negligible eicosanoid biosynthesis. While $cPLA_2$ dominates in the acute release of AA, the inducible $sPLA_2$ contributes under conditions

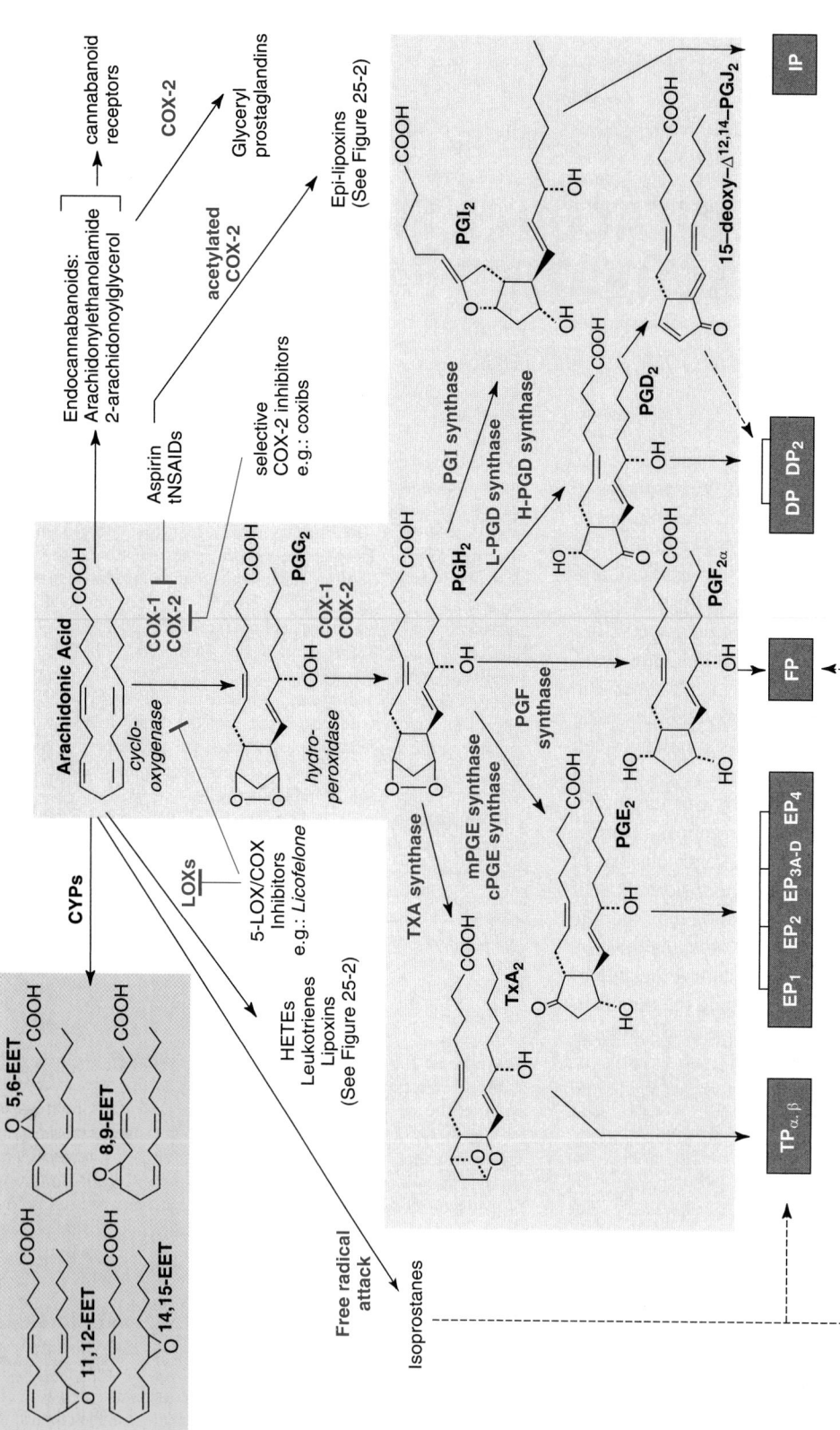

Figure 25–1. Metabolism of arachidonic acid. The cyclooxygenase (COX) pathway is highlighted in gray. The lipoxygenase (LOX) pathways are expanded in Figure 25–2. Major degradation pathways are shown in Figure 25–3. Cyclic endoperoxides (PGG$_2$ and PGH$_2$) arise from the sequential cyclooxygenase and hydroperoxidase actions of COX-1 or COX-2 on arachidonic acid released from membrane phospholipids. Subsequent products are generated by tissue-specific synthases and transduce their effects *via* membrane-bound receptors (*gray boxes*). Dashed lines indicate putative ligand–receptor interactions. EETs (*shaded in blue*) and isoprostanes are generated *via* CYP activity and nonenzymatic free radical attack, respectively. COX-2 can use modified arachidonoylglycerol, an endocannabinoid, to generate the glyceryl prostaglandins. Aspirin and tNSAIDs are nonselective inhibitors of COX-1 and COX-2 but do not affect LOX activity. Epilipoxins are generated by COX-2 following its acetylation by aspirin (Figure 25–2). Dual 5-LOX–COX inhibitors interfere with both pathways. *See text for other abbreviations.*

of sustained or intense stimulation of AA production. Once liberated, a portion of the AA is metabolized rapidly to oxygenated products by several distinct enzyme systems, including *cyclooxygenases, lipoxygenases,* and CYPs.

Products of Prostaglandin G/H Synthases. The prostaglandins prostacyclin and thromboxane, collectively termed *prostanoids,* can be considered analogs of unnatural compounds with the trivial names *prostanoic acid* and *thrombanoic acid,* with the structures shown below:

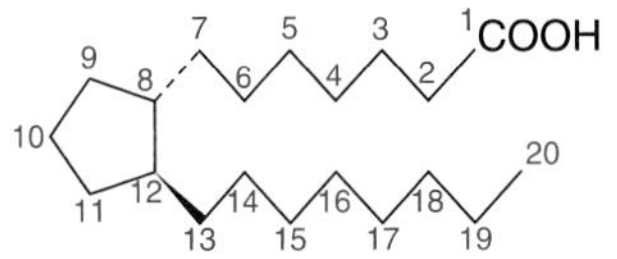

PROSTANOIC ACID

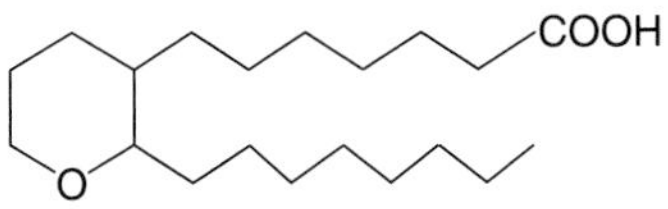

THROMBANOIC ACID

AA is metabolized successively to the cyclic endoperoxide prostaglandins G (PGG) and H (PGH) (Figure 25–1) by the cyclooxygenase (COX) and hydroperoxidase (HOX) activities of the prostaglandin G/H synthases. Isomerases and synthases effect the transformation of PGH_2 into terminal prostanoids distinguished by substitutions on their cyclopentane rings.

Prostaglandins of the E and D series are hydroxyketones, whereas the F_α prostaglandins are 1,3-diols (Figure 25–1). A, B, and C prostaglandins are unsaturated ketones that arise nonenzymatically from PGE during extraction procedures; it is unlikely that they occur biologically. PGJ_2 and related compounds result from the dehydration of PGD_2. Prostacyclin (PGI_2) has a double-ring structure; in addition to a cyclopentane ring, a second ring is formed by an oxygen bridge between carbons 6 and 9. Thromboxanes (Txs) contain a six-member oxirane ring instead of the cyclopentane ring of the prostaglandins. The main classes are further subdivided in accord with the number of double bonds in their side chains, as indicated by numerical subscripts. Dihomo-γ-linolenic acid is the precursor of the one series, AA for the two series, and EPA for the three series. Prostanoids derived from AA carry the subscript 2 and are the major series in mammals. There is little evidence that one- or three-series prostanoids are made in adequate amounts to be important under normal circumstances. However, the health benefits of dietary supplementation with ω-3 fatty acids remain a focus of investigation.

Synthesis of prostanoids is accomplished in a stepwise manner by a complex of microsomal enzymes. The first enzyme in this synthetic pathway is prostaglandin endoperoxide G/H synthase, which is colloquially called *cyclooxygenase,* or *COX.* There are two distinct COX isoforms, COX-1 and COX-2 (Smith *et al.,* 1996). COX-1 is expressed constitutively in most cells, whereas COX-2 is up-regulated by cytokines, shear stress, and growth factors. Thus COX-1 is considered to subserve housekeeping functions such as cytoprotection of the gastric epithelium (*see* Chapter 36). COX-2 is the major source of prostanoids formed in inflammation and cancer. This distinction is overly simplistic: There are physiological and pathophysiological processes in which each enzyme is uniquely involved and others in which they function coordinately (*see* Smith and Langenbach, 2001).

In addition to 61% amino acid identity, the crystal structures of COX-1 and COX-2 are remarkably similar (FitzGerald and Loll, 2001). Both isoforms are expressed as dimers homotypically inserted into the endoplasmic reticular membrane; their COX activity oxygenates and cyclizes unesterified AA to form PGG_2, whereas their HOX activity converts PGG_2 to PGH_2 (Smith and Langenbach, 2001). These chemically unstable intermediates are transformed enzymatically into the prostaglandins thromboxane and prostacyclin by isomerases and synthases that are expressed in a relatively cell-specific fashion such that most cells make one or two dominant prostanoids. For example, COX-1-derived TxA_2 is the dominant product in platelets, whereas COX-2-derived PGE_2 and TxA_2 dominate in activated macrophages. Two classes of PGE synthases have been cloned. Microsomal PGE synthases 1 and 2 colocalize with COX-2 in some, but not all, tissues and may be induced by cytokines and tumor promoters. Similarly, cytosolic PGE synthase colocalizes with COX-1 and may be important in constitutive formation of PGE_2. Two forms of PGD synthase and PGF synthase have been identified. In heterologous expression systems, COX-1 couples preferentially with TxA_2 and PGF synthase, whereas COX-2 prefers PGI_2 synthase (Smyth and FitzGerald, 2003).

Prostanoids are released from cells predominantly by facilitated transport through the prostaglandin transporter and possibly other transporters (*see* Schuster, 2002).

Products of Lipoxygenases. Lipoxygenases (LOXs) are a family of non-heme iron–containing enzymes that catalyze the oxygenation of polyenic fatty acids to corresponding lipid hydroperoxides (*see* Brash, 1999). The enzymes require a fatty acid substrate with two cis double bonds separated by a methylene group. AA, which contains several double bonds in this configuration, is metabolized to hydroperoxy eicosatetraenoic acids (HPETEs), which vary in the site of insertion of the hydroperoxy group. Analogous to PGG_2 and PGH_2, these unstable intermediates, normally with *S* chirality, are further metabolized by a variety of enzymes. HPETEs are converted to their corresponding hydroxy fatty acid (HETE) either nonenzymatically or by a peroxidase.

There are five active human lipoxygenases—5-LOX, 12(*S*)-LOX, 12(*R*)-LOX, 15-LOX-1, and 15-LOX-2—classified according to the site of hydroperoxy group insertion and, when necessary, the stereoconfiguration (*S* or *R*) of their products. Their expression is frequently cell-specific (Brash, 1999); platelets have only 12(*S*)-LOX, whereas leukocytes contain both 5(*S*)- and 12(*S*)-LOX (Figure 25–2). The epidermis contains a distinct subgroup of LOXs including epidermal 12(*S*)-, 12(*R*)- and 15-LOXs. A novel epidermal enzyme, lipoxygenase-3, has been reported to metabolize further the product of 12(*R*)-LOX in the skin (Yu *et al.,* 2003).

The 5-LOX pathway leads to the synthesis of the *leukotrienes* (LTs), which play a major role in the development and persistence of the inflammatory response (Brink *et al.,* 2003) (Figure 25–2). A nomenclature (LTB_4, LTB_5, etc.) similar to that of prostanoids applies to the subclassification of the LTs. When eosinophils, mast cells, polymorphonuclear leukocytes, or monocytes are activated, 5-LOX translocates to the nuclear membrane and associates with 5-LOX-activating protein (FLAP), an integral membrane protein essential for LT biosynthesis. FLAP may act as an AA transfer protein that presents the substrate to the 5-LOX (Brash, 1999). An experimental drug, MK-886, binds to FLAP and blocks LT production. A two-step reaction is catalyzed by 5-LOX: oxygenation of AA at C-5 to form 5-HPETE, followed by dehydration of 5-HPETE to an unstable 5,6-epoxide known as LTA_4. LTA_4 is transformed into bioactive eicosanoids by multiple pathways depending on the cellular

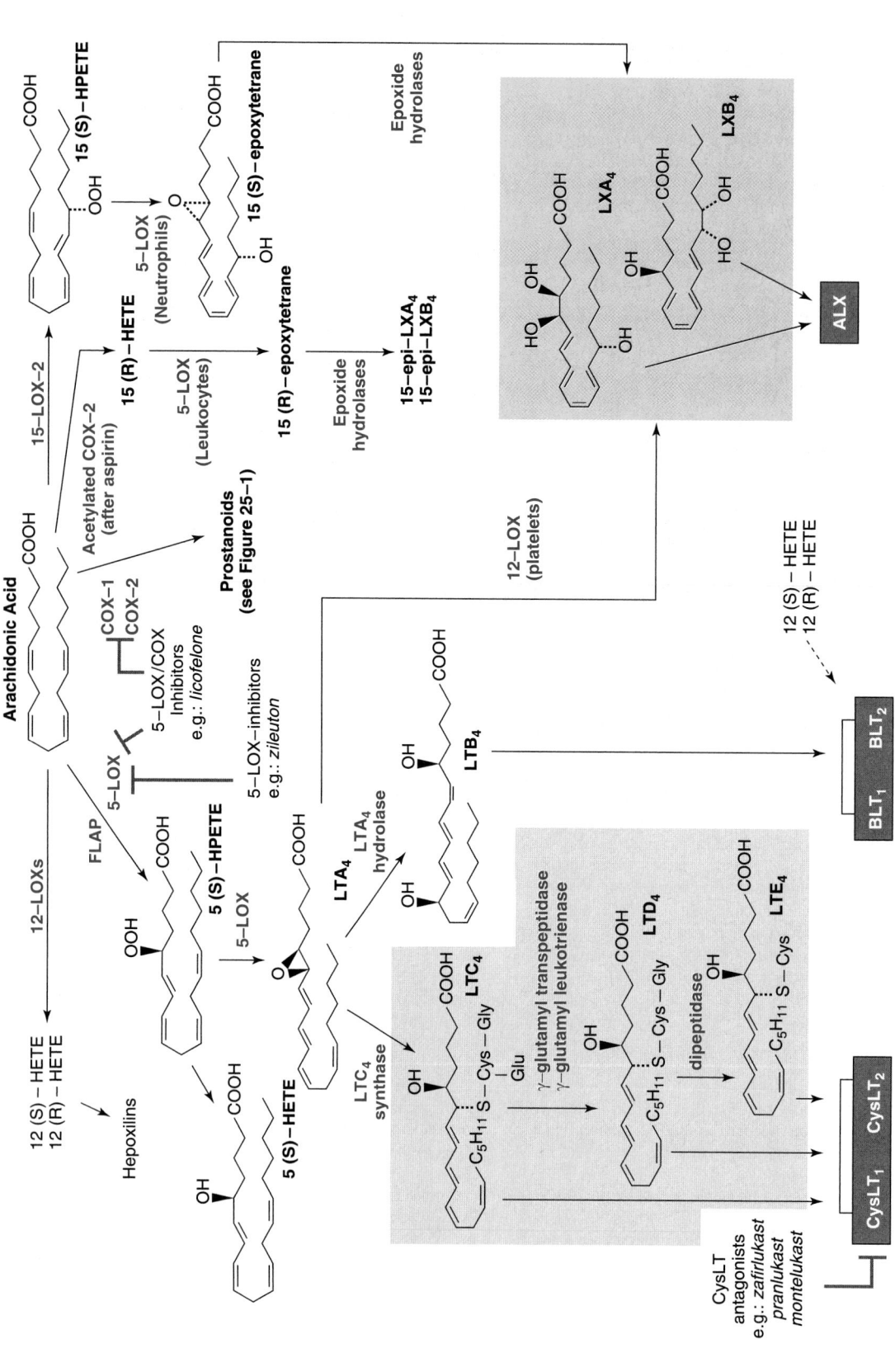

Figure 25–2. Lipoxygenase pathways of arachidonic acid metabolism. FLAP presents arachidonic acid to 5-LOX, leading to the generation of the LTs. Cysteinyl LTs are shaded in gray. Lipoxins (*shaded in blue*) are products of cellular interaction *via* a 5-LOX–12-LOX pathway or *via* a 15-LOX–5-LOX pathway. Biological effects are transduced *via* membrane-bound receptors (*dark gray boxes*). Dashed line indicates putative ligand–receptor interactions. Zileuton inhibits 5-LOX but not the COX pathways (expanded in Figure 25–1). Dual 5-LOX–COX inhibitors interfere with both pathways. CysLT antagonists prevent activation of the CysLT$_1$ receptor. *See text for abbreviations.*

context: transformation by LTA_4 hydrolase to a 5,12-dihydroxyeicosatetraenoic acid known as *LTB₄*; conjugation with reduced glutathione by LTC_4 synthase, in eosinophils, monocytes, and mast cells, to form LTC_4; and extracellular metabolism of the peptide moiety of LTC_4, leading to the removal of glutamic acid and subsequent cleavage of glycine, to generate LTD_4 and LTE_4, respectively (*see* Brash, 1999). LTC_4, LTD_4, and LTE_4, the *cysteinyl leukotrienes*, were known originally as the *slow-reacting substance of anaphylaxis* (SRS-A), first described more than 60 years ago (*see* Chapter 27). LTB_4 and LTC_4 are actively transported out of the cell.

15-LOX exists in at least two isoforms, 15-LOX-1 and 15-LOX-2. The former prefers linoleic acid as a substrate and forms 15(*S*)-hydroxyoctadecadienoic acid, whereas the latter uses AA to generate 15(*S*)-HETE. Platelet-type 12-LOX generates 12(*S*)-HETE from AA, whereas the leukocyte isozyme can synthesize both 12- and 15-HETE and often is referred to as *12/15-LOX*. 12-LOX can further metabolize LTA_4, the primary product of the 5-LOX pathway, to form the *lipoxins* LXA_4 and LXB_4. These mediators also can arise through 5-LOX metabolism of 15-HETE. 15(*R*)-HETE, derived from aspirin-acetylated COX-2, can be further transformed in leukocytes by 5-LOX to the *epilipoxins* 15-epi-LXA_4 or 15-epi-LXB_4, the so-called aspirin-triggered lipoxins (Brink *et al.*, 2003). 12-HETE also can undergo a catalyzed molecular rearrangement to epoxyhydroxyeicosatrienoic acids called *hepoxilins*.

The epidermal LOXs are distinct from "conventional" enzymes in their substrate preferences and products, and their roles in normal skin function are not clear. AA and linoleic acid apparently are not the natural substrates for the epidermal LOXs. Epidermal accumulation of 12(*R*)-HETE is a feature of psoriasis and icthyosis. Inhibitors of 12(*R*)-LOX are under investigation for the treatment of these proliferative skin disorders.

Products of Cytochrome P450. Multiple CYPs metabolize arachidonic acid (Capdevila and Falck, 2002). For instance, epoxyeicosatrienoic acids (EETs) can be formed by CYP epoxygenases, primarily CYP2C and CYP2J in humans. Four regioisomers (14,15-, 11,12-, 8,9-, and 5,6-EETs), each containing a mixture of the (*R,S*) and (*S,R*) enantiomers, are formed in a CYP isoform–specific manner. Their biosynthesis can be altered by pharmacological, nutritional, and genetic factors that affect CYP expression (*see* Chapter 3).

EETs are metabolized by numerous pathways. The corresponding dihydroxyeicosatrienoic acids (DHETs) are formed by epoxide hydrolases (EHs), whereas lysolipid acylation results in incorporation of EETs into cellular phospholipids. Glutathione conjugation and oxidation by COX and CYPs generate a series of glutathione conjugates, epoxyprostaglandins, diepoxides, tetrahydrofuran (THF) diols, and epoxyalcohols whose biological relevance is not known. Intracellular fatty acid–binding proteins (FABPs) may bind EETs and DHETs differentially, thus modulating their metabolism, activities, and targeting.

EETs are important modulators of cardiovascular and renal function. They are synthesized in endothelial cells and cause vasodilation in a number of vascular beds by activating the large conductance Ca^{2+}-activated K^+ channels of smooth muscle cells. This results in hyperpolarization of smooth muscle and thus relaxation, leading to reduced blood pressure. Substantial evidence indicates that EETs may function as endothelium-derived hyperpolarizing factors (EDHFs), particularly in the coronary circulation (Quilley and McGiff, 2000). Endogenous biosynthesis of EETs is increased in human syndromes of hypertension (Catella *et al.*, 1990). An analog of 11,12-EET abrogated the enhanced renal microvascular reactivity to angiotensin II (Ang II) associated with hypertension (Imig *et al.*, 2001), and blood pressure is lower in mice deficient in soluble EH (Sinal *et al.*, 2000);

these findings suggest that EH enzyme may be a potential pharmacological target for hypertension. Much evidence suggests the existence of EET receptors, although none has been cloned.

Other Pathways. The isoeicosanoids, a family of eicosanoid isomers, are formed nonenzymatically by direct free radical–based attack on AA and related lipid substrates (Lawson *et al.*, 1999; Fam and Morrow, 2003). Unlike eicosanoids, these compounds are generated initially on the esterified lipid in cell membranes, from which they are cleaved, presumably by phospholipases; the free isoeicosanoids circulate and are excreted in urine. Consequently, their production is not blocked *in vivo* by agents that suppress metabolism of free arachidonate, such as inhibitors of COX-1 or COX-2. The $PGF_{2\alpha}$ isomer F_2–I isoprostane 8-iso-$PGF_{2\alpha}$, also known as $iPF_{2\alpha}III$, was the first such compound to be identified. Unlike other isoprostanes studied to date, it may originate *via* a COX pathway or by a free radical–dependent mechanism. The former pathway does not contribute detectably to its levels in urine, although more abundant compounds, such as 8,12-iso-$PGF_{2\alpha}VI$, which are not formed *via* COXs, represent more attractive markers of lipid peroxidation *in vivo*. Since several isoprostanes can activate prostanoid receptors, it has been speculated that they may contribute to the pathophysiology of inflammatory responses in a manner insensitive to COX inhibitors.

In the brain, the endocannabinoids arachidonylethanolamide (anandamide) and 2-arachidonoylglycerol are endogenous ligands of cannabinoid receptors (Maccarrone and Finazzi-Agro, 2002). They mimic several pharmacological effects of Δ9-tetrahydrocannabinol, the active principle of *Cannabis sativa* preparations such as hashish and marijuana, including inhibition of adenylyl cyclase, inhibition of L-type Ca^{2+} channels, analgesia, and hypothermia. Glyceryl prostaglandins (PG-Gs) are generated by the oxygenation of 2-arachidonylglycerol by COX-2; their biological significance remains to be clarified.

Inhibitors of Eicosanoid Biosynthesis. A number of the biosynthetic steps just described can be inhibited by drugs. Inhibition of phospholipase A_2 decreases the release of the precursor fatty acid and thus the synthesis of all its metabolites. Since phospholipase A_2 is activated by Ca^{2+} and calmodulin, it may be inhibited by drugs that reduce the availability of Ca^{2+}. *Glucocorticoids* also inhibit phospholipase A_2, but they appear to do so indirectly by inducing the synthesis of a group of proteins termed *annexins* (formerly *lipocortins*) that modulate phospholipase A_2 activity (*see* Chapter 59). Glucocorticoids also down-regulate induced expression of COX-2 but not of COX-1 (Smith *et al.*, 1996). Aspirin and tNSAIDs were found originally to prevent the synthesis of prostaglandins from AA in tissue homogenates (Vane, 1971). It now is known that these drugs inhibit the COX but not the HOX moieties of the prostaglandin G/H synthases and thus the formation of their downstream prostanoid products. *These drugs do not inhibit LOXs and may result in increased formation of LTs by shunting of substrate to the lipoxygenase pathway.* Dual inhibitors of the COX and 5-LOX pathways are under investigation (Martel-Pelletier *et al.*, 2003). However, the interplay between these enzyme families remains to be defined by genetic and pharmacological approaches. Acetylated COX-2 generates 12(*R*)-HETE coincident with suppression of PG formation. The importance of this pathway remains to be established *in vivo.*

COX-1 and COX-2 differ in their sensitivity to inhibition by certain antiinflammatory drugs (Marnett *et al.,* 1999). This observation has led to the recent development of agents that selectively inhibit COX-2, including the coxibs (*see* Chapter 26). These drugs could have therapeutic advantages over NSAIDs because COX-2 is the predominant cyclooxygenase at sites of inflammation, whereas COX-1 is the major source of cytoprotective prostaglandins in the gastrointestinal tract. The matter is not settled, but the antiinflammatory actions of the coxibs were associated with improved gastrointestinal safety compared with their nonselective counterparts in at least one trial of clinical outcomes (Bombardier *et al.,* 2000; FitzGerald and Patrono, 2001). However, the theoretical disadvantage of unopposed COX-1 activity associated with these agents raises safety issues for renal function and thromboresistance of the vessel wall (FitzGerald, 2003). Indeed, a polymorphism of the COX-2 gene has been associated with a decreased risk of myocardial infarction and stroke (Cipollone *et al.,* 2004).

Since the metabolites of PGH_2 can produce a variety of biological effects (*see* below), there are theoretical advantages in compounds that preferentially and selectively inhibit the downstream enzymes that metabolize PGH_2. For example, agents that inhibit TxA_2 synthase might block platelet aggregation and induce vasodilation. Indeed, such drugs block TxA_2 production *in vitro* and *in vivo;* however, they have been disappointing in clinical development perhaps owing to activation of the TxA_2 receptor, the TP, by accumulated PGH_2 precursor. Their use in TP antagonists may circumvent this problem. Although some compounds with combined activities were evaluated, these agents did not have concordant potencies as enzyme inhibitors and receptor antagonists across the dosing range. Activation of the TP receptor by oxidized lipids could broaden the clinical indications for these compounds beyond their conventional targets in cardiovascular disease. More recently, mice lacking mPGE synthase-1 exhibited resistance to inflammatory stimuli similar to that observed after treatment with tNSAIDs. Inhibitors of PGE synthase-1 may retain the clinical efficacy of selective COX-2 inhibitors while avoiding cardiovascular complications attributable to suppression of COX-2-derived PGI_2.

Since leukotrienes mediate inflammation, efforts have focused on development of leukotriene-receptor antagonists and selective inhibitors of the LOXs. *Zileuton,* an inhibitor of 5-lipoxygenase, was marketed in the United States for the treatment of asthma but has been withdrawn. In addition, cysteinyl leukotriene-receptor antagonists, including *zafirlukast, pranlukast,* and *montelukast,* have established efficacy in the treatment of asthma (*see* Chapter 27). A common polymorphism in the gene for LTC_4 synthase that correlates with increased LTC_4 generation is associated with aspirin-intolerant asthma and with the efficacy of antileukotriene therapy (*see* Kanaoka and Boyce, 2004). Interestingly, while polymor-

phisms in the genes encoding 5-LOX or FLAP do not appear to be linked to asthma (Sayers *et al.,* 2003), studies have demonstrated an association of these genes with myocardial infarction, stroke (Helgadottir *et al.,* 2004), and atherosclerosis (Dwyer *et al.,* 2004); thus, inhibition of LT biosynthesis may be useful in the prevention of cardiovascular disease.

Eicosanoid Catabolism. Most eicosanoids are efficiently and rapidly inactivated. About 95% of infused PGE_2 (but not PGI_2) is inactivated during one passage through the pulmonary circulation. Broadly speaking, the enzymatic catabolic reactions are of two types: a relatively rapid initial step, catalyzed by widely distributed prostaglandin-specific enzymes, wherein prostaglandins lose most of their biological activity; and a second step in which these metabolites are oxidized, probably by enzymes identical to those responsible for the β and ω oxidation of fatty acids (Figure 25–3). The initial step is the oxidation of the 15-OH group to the corresponding ketone by prostaglandin 15-OH dehydrogenase (PGDH) (*see* Tai *et al.,* 2002). Two types of 15-PGDHs have been identified. Type I, an NAD^+-dependent enzyme, is the predominant form involved in eicosanoid catabolism. There is little circulating PGDH activity; thus, it is likely that metabolism first requires active transport to the intracellular space (*see* Schuster, 2002). The 15-keto compound then is reduced to the 13,14-dihydro derivative, a reaction catalyzed by prostaglandin Δ^{13}-reductase. This enzyme is identical to the LTB_4 12-hydroxydehydrogenase (*see* below). Subsequent steps consist of β and ω oxidation of the prostaglandin side chains, giving rise to polar dicarboxylic acids in the case of PGEs, which then are excreted in the urine as major metabolites (Figure 25–1); these reactions occur primarily in the liver.

Unlike PGE_2, PGD_2 initially is reduced *in vivo* to the F-ring prostaglandin $9\alpha11\beta$-PGF_2, which possesses significant biological activity. Subsequently, this compound undergoes metabolism similar to that of other eicosanoids (Figure 25–3). TxA_2 breaks down nonenzymatically ($t_{\frac{1}{2}} = 30$ seconds) into the chemically stable but biologically inactive TxB_2, which then is further metabolized by 11-hydroxy TxB_2 dehydrogenase to generate 11-dehydro-TxB_2 or by β-oxidation to form 2,3-dinor-TxB_2 (Figure 25–3).

The degradation of PGI_2 ($t_{\frac{1}{2}} = 3$ min) apparently begins with its spontaneous hydrolysis in blood to 6-keto-$PGF_1\alpha$. The metabolism of this compound in humans involves the same steps as those for PGE_2 and $PGF_{2\alpha}$.

The degradation of LTC_4 occurs in the lungs, kidney, and liver. The initial steps involve its conversion to LTE_4. LTC_4 also may be inactivated by oxidation of its cysteinyl sulfur to a sulfoxide. In leukocytes, LTB_4 is inactivated principally by oxidation by members of the CYP4F subfamily. Conversion to 12-oxo-LTB_4 by LTB 12-hydroxydehydrogenase (*see* above) is a key pathway in tissues other than leukocytes.

Pharmacological Properties of Eicosanoids

The eicosanoids show numerous and diverse effects in biological systems. This discussion highlights those that are thought to be the most important.

Cardiovascular System. In most vascular beds, PGE_2 elicits vasodilation and a drop in blood pressure (Narumiya *et al.,* 1999; Smyth and FitzGerald, 2003), although vasocon-

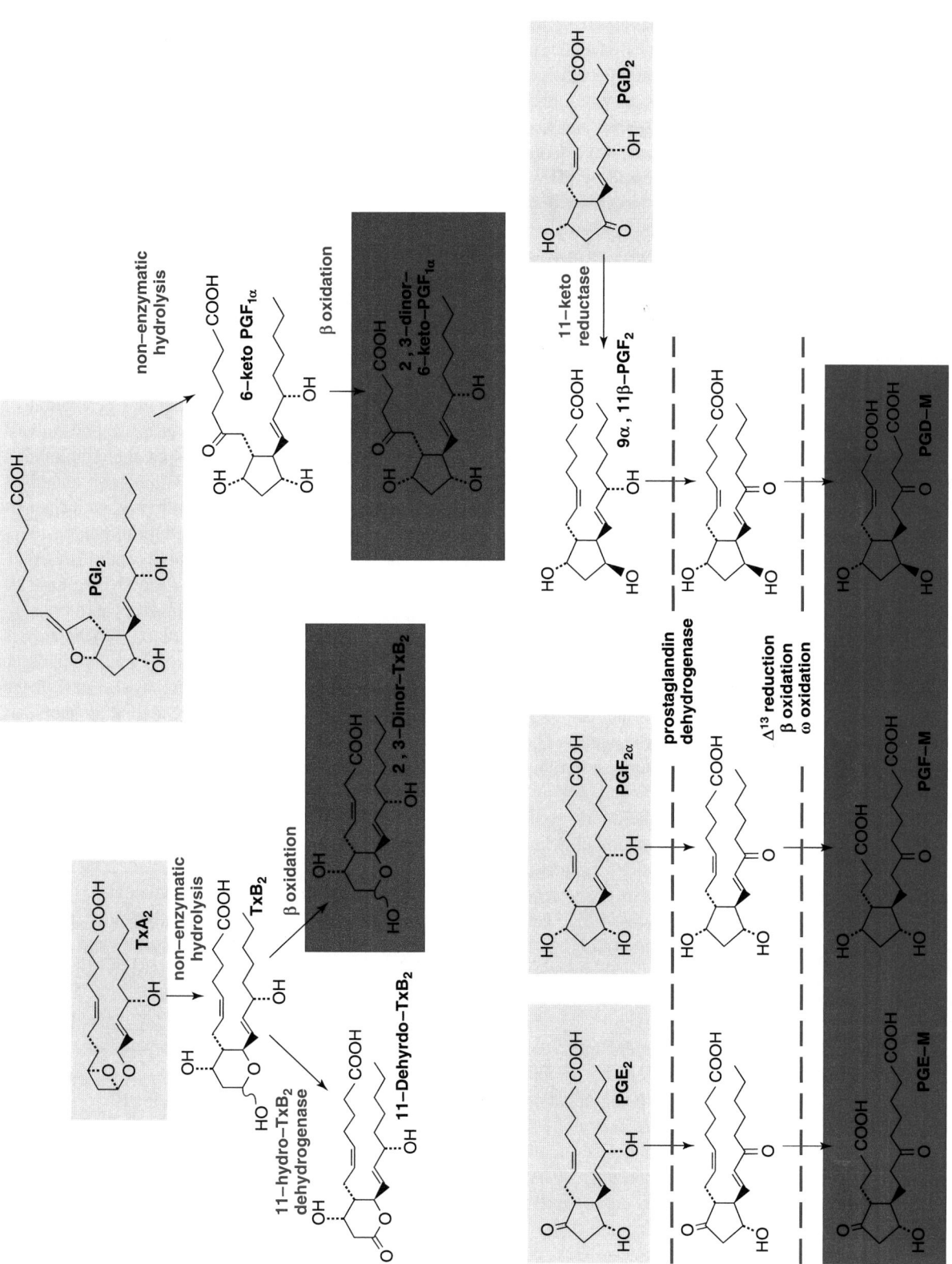

Figure 25–3. *Major pathways of prostanoid degradation.* Active metabolites are shaded in blue. Major urinary metabolites are shaded in gray. The blue dashed lines indicate reactions that use common enzymatic processes. M, metabolite. *See* text for other abbreviations.

strictor effects have been reported, depending on which PGE_2 receptor is activated (*see* below). Infusion of PGD_2 in humans results in flushing, nasal stuffiness, and hypotension; subsequent formation of F-ring metabolites may result in hypertension. Responses to $PGF_{2\alpha}$ vary with species and vascular bed; it is a potent constrictor of both pulmonary arteries and veins in humans. Blood pressure is increased by $PGF_{2\alpha}$ in some experimental animals owing to venoconstriction; however, in humans, $PGF_{2\alpha}$ does not alter blood pressure.

PGI_2 relaxes vascular smooth muscle, causing prominent hypotension and reflex tachycardia on intravenous administration. It is about five times more potent than PGE_2 in producing this effect. TxA_2 is a potent vasoconstrictor. It contracts vascular smooth muscle *in vitro* and is a vasoconstrictor in the whole animal and in isolated vascular beds.

Cardiac output generally is increased by prostaglandins of the E and F series. Weak, direct inotropic effects have been noted in various isolated preparations. In the intact animal, however, increased force of contraction and increased heart rate are in large measure a reflex consequence of a fall in total peripheral resistance.

LTC_4 and LTD_4 cause hypotension in humans (Brink *et al.*, 2003). This may result partly from a decrease in intravascular volume and also from decreased cardiac contractility secondary to a marked LT-induced reduction in coronary blood flow. Although LTC_4 and LTD_4 have little effect on most large arteries or veins, coronary arteries and distal segments of the pulmonary artery are contracted by nanomolar concentrations of these agents. The renal vasculature is resistant to this constrictor action, but the mesenteric vasculature is not.

The CysLTs have prominent effects on the microvasculature. LTC_4 and LTD_4 appear to act on the endothelial lining of postcapillary venules to cause exudation of plasma; they are more than a thousandfold more potent than histamine in this regard. At higher concentrations, LTC_4 and LTD_4 constrict arterioles and reduce exudation of plasma.

Isoprostanes usually are vasoconstrictors, although there are examples of vasodilation in preconstricted vessels.

Platelets. Low concentrations of PGE_2 enhance and higher concentrations inhibit platelet aggregation (Fabre *et al.*, 2001). Both PGI_2 and PGD_2 inhibit the aggregation of human platelets *in vitro*.

TxA_2, the major product of COX-1 in platelets, induces platelet aggregation. Perhaps more importantly, TxA_2 acts as an amplification signal for other, more potent platelet agonists such as thrombin and adenosine diphosphate (ADP) (FitzGerald, 1991). The actions of TxA_2 on platelets are restrained by PGI_2, which inhibits platelet aggregation by all recognized agonists. The biological

importance of 12-HETE formation is poorly understood, although deletion of the platelet 12-LOX augments ADP-induced platelet aggregation and AA-induced sudden death in mice. Some isoprostanes increase the response of platelets to pro-aggregatory agonists *in vitro*.

Inflammation and Immunity. Eicosanoids play a major role in the inflammatory and immune responses, as reflected by the clinical usefulness of the NSAIDs. While LTs generally are proinflammatory and lipoxins antiinflammatory, prostanoids can exert both kinds of activity.

LTB_4 is a potent chemotactic agent for polymorphonuclear leukocytes, eosinophils, and monocytes (Martel-Pelletier *et al.*, 2003). In higher concentrations, LTB_4 stimulates the aggregation of polymorphonuclear leukocytes and promotes degranulation and the generation of superoxide. LTB_4 promotes adhesion of neutrophils to vascular endothelial cells and their transendothelial migration and stimulates synthesis of proinflammatory cytokines from macrophages and lymphocytes. Prostaglandins generally inhibit lymphocyte function and proliferation, suppressing the immune response (Rocca and FitzGerald, 2002). PGE_2 depresses the humoral antibody response by inhibiting the differentiation of B-lymphocytes into antibody-secreting plasma cells. PGE_2 acts on T-lymphocytes to inhibit mitogen-stimulated proliferation and lymphokine release by sensitized cells. PGE_2 and TxA_2 also may play a role in T-lymphocyte development by regulating apoptosis of immature thymocytes (Tilley *et al.*, 2001). PGD_2, a major product of mast cells, is a potent chemoattractant for eosinophils and induces chemotaxis and migration of Th2 lymphocytes (Smyth and FitzGerald, 2003). The degradation product, 15d-PGJ_2, also may activate eosinophils *via* the DP2 (CRTH2) receptor (Monneret *et al.*, 2002).

Lipoxins have diverse effects on leukocytes, including activation of monocytes and macrophages and inhibition of the activation of neutrophils, eosinophils, and lymphocytes (McMahon and Godson, 2004).

Smooth Muscle. Prostaglandins contract or relax many smooth muscles besides those of the vasculature. The LTs contract most smooth muscles.

Bronchial and Tracheal Muscle. In general, $PGF_{2\alpha}$ and PGD_2 contract and PGE_2 and PGI_2 relax bronchial and tracheal muscle. Prostaglandin endoperoxides and TxA_2 constrict human bronchial smooth muscle. Although important in allergen-evoked bronchospasm in guinea pigs, these mediators, unlike PGD_2, do not appear relevant to this response in humans. Roughly 10% of people given aspirin or tNSAIDs develop bronchospasm (Szczeklik *et al.*, 2004). This appears attributable to a shift in AA metabolism to LT formation, as reflected by an increase in urinary LTE_4 in response to aspirin challenge in such individuals. This substrate diversion appears to involve COX-1; such patients do not develop bronchospasm when treated with selective inhibitors of COX-2. LTC_4 and its metabolites LTD_4 and LTE_4 are bronchoconstrictors in many species, including humans (Brink *et al.*, 2003). These LTs act principally on smooth muscle in the airways and are a thousand times more potent than histamine both *in vitro* and *in vivo*. They also stimulate bronchial mucus secretion and cause mucosal edema.

PGI_2 causes bronchodilation in most species; human bronchial tissue is particularly sensitive, and PGI_2 antagonizes bronchoconstriction induced by other agents.

Uterus. Strips of nonpregnant human uterus are contracted by $PGF_{2\alpha}$ and TxA_2 but are relaxed by E prostaglandins. Sensitivity to the contractile response is most prominent before menstruation, whereas relaxation is greatest at midcycle. Uterine strips obtained at hysterectomy from pregnant women are contracted by $PGF_{2\alpha}$ and by low concentrations of PGE_2. PGE_2, together with oxytocin, is essential for the onset of parturition. PGI_2 and high concentrations of PGE_2 produce relaxation. The intravenous infusion of PGE_2 or $PGF_{2\alpha}$ to pregnant women produces a dose-dependent increase in uterine tone and in the frequency and intensity of rhythmic uterine contractions. Uterine responsiveness to prostaglandins increases as pregnancy progresses but remains smaller than the response to oxytocin.

Gastrointestinal Muscle. The E and F prostaglandins stimulate contraction of the main longitudinal muscle from stomach to colon. Prostaglandin endoperoxides, TxA_2, and PGI_2 also produce contraction but are less active. Circular muscle generally relaxes in response to PGE_2 and contracts in response to $PGF_{2\alpha}$. The LTs have potent contractile effects. PGs reduce transit time in the small intestine and colon. Diarrhea, cramps, and reflux of bile have been noted in response to oral PGE; these are common side effects (along with nausea and vomiting) in patients given PGs for abortion. The E and F prostaglandins stimulate the movement of water and electrolytes into the intestinal lumen. Such effects may underlie the watery diarrhea that follows their oral or parenteral administration. By contrast, PGI_2 does not induce diarrhea; indeed, it prevents that provoked by other PGs.

PGE_2 appears to contribute to the water and electrolyte loss in cholera, a disease that is somewhat responsive to therapy with tNSAIDs.

Gastric and Intestinal Secretions. In the stomach, PGE_2 and PGI_2 contribute to increased mucus secretion (*cytoprotection*), reduced acid secretion, and reduced pepsin content. These effects result from their vasodilatory properties and probable direct effects on secretory cells. PGE_2 and its analogs also inhibit gastric damage caused by a variety of ulcerogenic agents and promote healing of duodenal and gastric ulcers (*see* Chapter 36). While COX-1 may be the dominant source of such cytoprotective PGs under physiological conditions, COX-2 predominates during ulcer healing. Selective inhibitors of COX-2 and deletion of the enzyme delay ulcer healing in rodents, but the impact of such drugs in humans is unclear. CysLTs, by constricting gastric blood vessels and enhancing production of pro-inflammatory cytokines, may contribute to the gastric damage.

Kidney and Urine Formation. PGs influence renal salt and water excretion by alterations in renal blood flow and by direct effects on renal tubules (Cheng and Harris, 2004). PGE_2 and PGI_2 infused directly into the renal arteries of dogs increase renal blood flow and provoke diuresis, natriuresis, and kaliuresis, with little change in glomerular filtration rate. TxA_2 decreases renal blood flow, decreases the rate of glomerular filtration, and participates in tubuloglo-

merular feedback. PGEs inhibit water reabsorption induced by antidiuretic hormone (ADH). PGE_2 also inhibits chloride reabsorption in the thick ascending limb of the loop of Henle in the rabbit. PGI_2, PGE_2, and PGD_2 stimulate renin secretion from the renal cortex apparently through a direct effect on the granular juxtaglomerular cells.

Eye. Although $PGF_{2\alpha}$ induces constriction of the iris sphincter muscle, its overall effect in the eye is to decrease intraocular pressure (IOP) by increasing the aqueous humor outflow of the eye *via* the uveoscleral and trabecular meshwork pathway. A variety of F prostaglandin-receptor agonists have proven effective in the treatment of open-angle glaucoma, a condition associated with the loss of COX-2 expression in the pigmented epithelium of the ciliary body (*see* Chapter 63).

Central Nervous System. While effects have been reported following injection of several PGs into discrete brain areas, the best established biologically active mediators are PGE_2 and PGD_2. The induction of fever by a range of endogenous and exogenous pyrogens appears to be mediated by PGE_2 (Smyth and FitzGerald, 2003). Exogenous $PGF_{2\alpha}$ and PGI_2 induce fever but do not contribute to the pyretic response. PGD_2 and TxA_2 do not induce fever. PGD_2 also appears to act on arachnoid trabecular cells in the basal forebrain to mediate an increase in extracellular adenosine that, in turn, facilitates induction of sleep.

PGs contribute to pain both peripherally and centrally. PLA_2 and COX-2 synthesis are increased at sites of local inflammation that are, in turn, associated with increased central PGE_2 biosynthesis (Samad *et al.*, 2002). PGE_2 and PGI_2 sensitize the peripheral nerve endings to painful stimuli by lowering the threshold of nociceptors. Centrally, PGE_2 can increase excitability in pain transmission neuronal pathways in the spinal cord. Hyperalgesia also is produced by LTB_4. The release of these eicosanoids during the inflammatory process thus serves as an amplification system for the pain mechanism (*see* below). The role of PGE_2 and PGI_2 in inflammation is discussed in Chapter 26. COX-2 has been implicated in several neurological diseases, and clinical trials of selective inhibitors of COX-2 are ongoing in the chemoprevention of Alzheimer's disease, Parkinson's disease, and epilepsy.

Endocrine System. A number of endocrine tissues respond to PGs. In a number of species, the systemic administration of PGE_2 increases circulating concentrations of adrenocorticotropic hormone (ACTH), growth hormone, prolactin, and gonadotropins. Other effects include stimulation of steroid production by the adrenals, stimulation of insulin release, and thyrotropin-like effects on the thyroid. The critical role of $PGF_{2\alpha}$ in parturition relies on its ability to induce an oxytocin-dependent decline in progesterone levels. PGE_2 works as part of a positive-feedback loop to induce oocyte maturation required for fertilization during and after ovulation.

LOX metabolites also have endocrine effects. 12-HETE stimulates the release of aldosterone from the adrenal cortex and mediates a portion of the aldosterone release stimulated by angiotensin II, but not that which occurs in response to ACTH.

Bone. PGs are strong modulators of bone metabolism. PGE_2 stimulates bone formation and resorption through osteoblastic and osteoclastic activities affecting bone strength and composition (Narumiya *et al.*, 1999; Smyth and FitzGerald, 2003).

Mechanism of Action of Eicosanoids. Many of the responses just described can be understood in light of the distribution of eicosanoid receptors and their coupling to second-messenger systems that modulate cellular activity.

Prostaglandin Receptors. PGs activate membrane receptors locally near their sites of formation. The diversity of their effects is explained to a large extent by their interaction with a diverse family of distinct receptors (Table 25–1). All eicosanoid receptors are G protein–coupled receptors that interact with G_s, G_i, and G_q to modulate the activities of adenylyl cyclase and phospholipase C (*see* Chapter 1). Single gene products have been identified for the receptors for prostacyclin (the IP receptor), $PGF_{2\alpha}$ (the FP receptor), and TxA_2 (the TP receptor). Four distinct

Table 25–1
Eicosanoid Receptors

RECEPTOR	PRIMARY LIGAND	SECONDARY LIGAND	PRIMARY COUPLING	MAJOR PHENOTYPE IN KNOCKOUT MICE
DP_1	PGD_2		$\uparrow$ cAMP (G_s)	$\downarrow$ Allergic asthma
DP_2/$CHRT_2$	PGD_2	15d-PGJ_2?	$\uparrow$ Ca^{2+}_i (G_i)	?
EP_1	PGE_2		G_q	Decreased response of colon to carcinogens
EP_2	PGE_2		$\uparrow$ cAMP	Impaired ovulation and fertilization; salt sensitive hypertension
EP_{3A-D}	PGE_2		$\downarrow$ cAMP (G_i) $\uparrow$ cAMP (G_s) $\uparrow$ PLC (G_q)	Resistance to pyrogens
EP_4	PGE_2		$\uparrow$ cAMP (G_s)	Patent ductus arteriosus
$FP_{A,B}$	$PGF_{2\alpha}$	IsoP?	G_q	Failure of parturition
IP	PGI_2	PGE_2	$\uparrow$ cAMP (G_s)	$\uparrow$ Thrombotic response, $\downarrow$ response to vascular injury
$TP_{\alpha,\beta}$	TxA_2	IsoPs	$\uparrow$ PLC (G_q, G_i, $G_{12/13}$, G_{16})	$\uparrow$ Bleeding time, $\uparrow$ response to vascular injury
BLT_1	LTB_4		G_{16}, G_i	Some suppression of inflammatory response
BLT_2	LTB_4	12(*S*)-HETE 12(*R*)-HETE	G_q-like, G_i-like, G_z-like	?
$CysLT_1$	LTD_4	LTC_4/LTE_4	$\uparrow$ PLC (G_q)	$\downarrow$ Innate and adaptive immune vascular permeability response, $\uparrow$ pulmonary inflammatory and fibrotic response
$CysLT_2$	LTC_4/LTD_4	LTE_4	$\uparrow$ PLC (G_q)	$\downarrow$ Pulmonary inflammatory and fibrotic response

This table lists the major classes of eicosanoid receptors and their signaling characteristics. Splice variants are indicated where appropriate. Major phenotypes in knockout mouse models are listed. ABBREVIATIONS: Ca^{2+}_i, cytosolic Ca^{2+}; cAMP, cyclic AMP; PLC, phospholipase C (activation leads to increased cellular inositol phosphate and diacyl glycerol generation and increased Ca^{2+}_i); IsoPs, isopostanes; DP_2 is a member of the fMLP receptor superfamily; fMLP, formyl-methionyl-leucyl-phenylalanine. *See* text for other abbreviations.

PGE_2 receptors (EP 1–4) and two PGD_2 receptors (DP$_1$ and DP$_2$) have been cloned. Additional isoforms of the TP (α and β), FP (A and B), and EP$_3$ (A–D) receptors can arise through differential mRNA splicing (Narumiya *et al.*, 1999; Smyth and FitzGerald, 2003).

Cell Signaling Pathways and Expression. The prostanoid receptors appear to derive from an ancestral EP receptor and share high homology. Phylogenetic comparison of this family reveals three subclusters: The first consists of the relaxant receptors EP$_2$, EP$_4$, IP, and DP$_1$, which increase cellular cyclic AMP generation; the second consists of the contractile receptors EP$_1$, FP, and TP, which increase cytosolic levels of Ca^{2+}; and a third, presently consisting only of EP$_3$, can couple to both elevation of intracellular calcium and a decrease in cyclic AMP. The DP$_2$ receptor is an exception and is unrelated to the other prostanoid receptors; rather, it is a member of the fMLP receptor superfamily (Table 25–1).

TP$_\alpha$ and TP$_\beta$ receptor isoforms couple *via* G$_q$ and several other G proteins to activate the PLC–IP$_3$–Ca^{2+} pathway. Activation of TP receptors also may activate or inhibit adenylyl cyclase *via* G$_s$ (TP$_\alpha$) or G$_i$ (TP$_\beta$), respectively, and signal *via* G$_q$ and related proteins to MAP kinase signaling pathways. TP is expressed in platelets, vasculature, lung, kidney, heart, thymus, and spleen.

The IP receptor couples with G$_s$ to stimulate adenylyl cyclase activity. It is expressed in many tissues and cells, including human kidney, lung, spine, liver, vasculature, and heart.

The DP$_1$ receptor also couples with adenylyl cyclase through G$_s$. It is the least abundant of the prostanoid receptors, with low levels of mRNA reported in mouse ileum, lung, stomach, and uterus. The DP$_1$ receptor is also expressed in the central nervous system (CNS), where it appears to be limited specifically to the leptomeninges. The DP$_2$ receptor couples with the G$_q$–PLC–IP$_3$ pathway to increase intracellular Ca^{2+}. It is found on T cells and eosinophils and at the fetal–maternal interface in human decidua.

The EP$_2$ and EP$_4$ receptors activate adenylate cyclase *via* G$_s$. The EP$_2$ receptor is expressed at much lower levels in most tissues and can be induced in response to inflammatory stimuli, suggesting distinct roles for these two G$_s$-coupled EP receptors. The EP$_1$ receptor, *via* an unclassified G protein, and the EP$_{3D}$ receptor, *via* G$_q$, activate the PLC–IP3–Ca^{2+} pathway. EP$_{3B}$/EP$_{3C}$ receptors couple with G$_s$-mediated activation of adenylyl cyclase; the EP$_{3D}$/EP$_{3A}$ isoforms inhibit adenylyl cyclase *via* G$_i$. EP$_1$ and EP$_2$ receptors have limited distribution compared with the distribution of EP$_3$ and EP$_4$ receptors.

The FP$_A$ and FP$_B$ receptors couple *via* G$_q$–PLC–IP$_3$ to mobilize cellular Ca^{2+} and activate protein kinase C (PKC). In addition, stimulation of FP activates Rho kinase, leading to the formation of actin stress fibers, phosphorylation of p125 focal adhesion kinase, and cell rounding. The FP receptor is expressed in kidney, heart, lung, stomach, and eye; it is most abundant in the corpus luteum, where its expression pattern varies during the estrus cycle.

Leukotriene and Lipoxin Receptors. Several receptors for the LTs and lipoxins have been identified (Brink *et al.*, 2003) (Table 25–1). Two receptors exist for both LTB$_4$ (BLT$_1$ and BLT$_2$) and the cysteinyl leukotrienes (CysLT$_1$ and CysLT$_2$). A single lipoxin receptor, ALX, is identical to the formyl peptide-1 (fMLP-1) receptor; the nomenclature now reflects LXA$_4$ as its natural and most potent ligand. A putative LXB$_4$ receptor has not yet been cloned. Receptors for the HETEs have been proposed but not yet isolated.

Cell Signaling Pathways and Expression. Phylogenetic comparison reveals two clusters of leukotriene/lipoxin receptors: the

chemoattractant receptors (BLT$_1$, BLT$_2$, and ALX), which also contain the DP$_2$ receptor for PGD$_2$, and the cysteinyl leukotriene receptors (CysLT$_1$ and CysLT$_2$). All are GPCRs and couple with G$_q$ and other G proteins (Table 25–1), depending on the cellular context. The BLT$_1$ receptor is expressed predominantly in leukocytes, thymus, and spleen, whereas BLT$_2$, the low-affinity receptor for LTB$_4$, is found in spleen, leukocytes, ovary, liver, and intestine. BLT$_2$ binds 12(*S*)- and 12(*R*)-HETE with reasonable affinity, although the biological relevance of this observation is not clear.

CysLT$_1$ receptors have been studied in greater detail than CysLT$_2$ receptors and mostly with LTD$_4$ as an agonist. Activation of G$_q$, leading to increased intracellular Ca^{2+}, is the primary signaling pathway reported. CysLT$_1$ is expressed in lung and intestinal smooth muscle, spleen, and peripheral blood leukocytes, whereas CysLT$_2$ is found in heart, spleen, peripheral blood leukocytes, adrenal medulla, and brain.

Responses to ALX receptor activation vary with cell type. In human neutrophils, AA release is stimulated, whereas Ca^{2+} mobilization is blocked; in monocytes, LXA$_4$ stimulates Ca^{2+} mobilization. The ALX receptor is expressed in lung, peripheral blood leukocytes, and spleen.

Other Agents. Other AA metabolites (*e.g.*, isoprostanes, epoxyeicosatrienoic acids, and hepoxilins) have potent biological activities, and there is evidence for distinct receptors for some of these substances. The isoprostanes appear to act as incidental ligands at the TP receptor (Audoly *et al.*, 2000), which may be important in the pathology of cardiovascular disease. Certain eicosanoids, most notably 15-deoxy-$\Delta^{12,14}$-PGJ$_2$ (15d-PGJ$_2$), a dehydration product of PGD$_2$, have been reported as endogenous ligands for a family of nuclear receptors called *peroxisome proliferator–activated receptors* (PPARs) that regulate lipid metabolism and cellular proliferation and differentiation. However, their affinities for PPARs are significantly lower than for cell surface receptors, raising doubt about the physiological relevance of the ligand–receptor interaction. 15d-PGJ$_2$ can bind PPARγ *in vitro*, but the quantities formed *in vivo* are orders of magnitude lower than those necessary for PPAR activation (Bell-Parikh *et al.*, 2003).

Endogenous Prostaglandins, Thromboxanes, and Leukotrienes: Functions in Physiological and Pathological Processes

The widespread biosynthesis and myriad of pharmacological actions of eicosanoids are reflected in their complex physiology and pathophysiology. The development of mice with targeted disruptions of genes regulating eicosanoid biosynthesis and ecosanoid receptors has revealed unexpected roles for these autacoids and has clarified hypotheses about their function (Austin and Funk, 1999; Narumiya and FitzGerald, 2001; Smyth and FitzGerald, 2003).

Platelets. Platelet aggregation leads to activation of membrane phospholipases, with the release of AA and consequent eicosanoid biosynthesis. In human platelets, TxA$_2$ and 12-HETE are the two major eicosanoids formed, although eicosanoids from other sources (*e.g.*, PGI$_2$ derived from vascular endothelium) also affect platelet function. A naturally occurring mutation in the first intracellular loop of the TP receptor is associated with a mild bleeding diathesis and resistance of platelet aggregability to TP agonists (Hirata *et al.*, 1994). The importance of the TxA_2 pathway is evident from the efficacy of low-dose aspirin in the secondary prevention of myocardial infarction and ischemic stroke. In addition, platelet thromboxane formation is augmented markedly in acute coronary artery syndromes (Fitzgerald *et al.*, 1986). Deletion of the TP receptor in the mouse prolongs bleeding time, renders platelets unresponsive to TP agonists, modifies their response to collagen but not to ADP, and blunts the response to vasopressors and the proliferative response to vascular injury.

PGI_2 inhibits platelet aggregation and disaggregates preformed clumps. Deficiency of the IP receptor in mice does not alter platelet aggregation significantly *ex vivo* (Yang *et al.*, 2002). However, PGI_2 does limit platelet activation by TxA_2 *in vivo*, reducing the thrombotic response to vascular injury (Cheng *et al.*, 2002). Deletion of the IP receptor augments the response to ischemia–reperfusion injury. High concentrations of PGE_2, released in response to major inflammatory mediators, also activate the IP receptor, inhibiting platelet aggregation. Low concentrations of PGE_2 activate the EP_3 receptor, leading to platelet aggregation (Fabre *et al.*, 2001).

Reproduction and Parturition. Studies with knockout mice confirm a role for PGs in reproduction and parturition (Austin and Funk, 1999; Narumiya and FitzGerald, 2001; Smyth and FitzGerald, 2003). COX-1-derived $PGF_{2\alpha}$ appears important for luteolysis, consistent with delayed parturition in mice deficient in COX-1. Subsequent up-regulation of COX-2 generates prostanoids, including $PGF_{2\alpha}$ and TxA_2, that are important in the final stages of parturition. Mice lacking both COX-1 and oxytocin undergo normal parturition, demonstrating the critical interplay between $PGF_{2\alpha}$ and oxytocin in onset of labor. EP_2-receptor-deficient mice demonstrate a preimplantation defect, which likely underlies some of the breeding difficulties seen in COX-2 knockouts.

Vasculature. Locally generated PGE_2 and PGI_2 modulate vascular tone. PGI_2, the major arachidonate metabolite released from the vascular endothelium, is derived primarily from COX-2 in humans (Catella-Lawson *et al.*, 1999; McAdam *et al.*, 1999) and is regulated by shear stress and by both vasoconstrictor and vasodilator autacoids. Knockout studies argue against a role for PGI_2 in the homeostatic maintenance of vascular tone; PGI synthase polymorphisms have been associated with essential hypertension and myocardial infarction (Smyth and FitzGerald, 2003). PGI_2 limits pulmonary hypertension induced by hypoxia and systemic hypertension induced by angiotensin II. Deficiency of EP_1 or EP_4 receptors reduces resting blood pressure in male mice; EP_1-receptor deficiency is associated with elevated renin–angiotensin activity. Both EP_2- and EP_4-receptor-deficient animals develop hypertension in response to a high-salt diet, reflecting the importance of PGE_2 in maintenance of renal blood flow and salt excretion (*see* below). PGI_2 and PGE_2 are implicated in the hypotension associated with septic shock. PGs also may play a role in the maintenance of placental blood flow.

COX-2-derived PGE_2, *via* the EP_4 receptor, maintains the ductus arteriosus patent until birth, when reduced PGE_2 levels (a consequence of increased PGE_2 metabolism) permit closure of the ductus arteriosus (Coggins *et al.*, 2002). The tNSAIDs induce closure of a patent ductus in neonates (*see* Chapter 26). Contrary to expectation, animals lacking the EP_4 receptor die with a patent ductus during the perinatal period (Table 25–1) because the mechanism for control of the ductus *in utero*, and its remodeling at birth, is absent. PGI_2 specifically limits TxA_2-induced smooth muscle proliferation in vascular injury, suggesting a role for these prostanoids in vascular remodeling (Cheng *et al.*, 2002).

Lung. A complex mixture of autacoids is released when sensitized lung tissue is challenged by the appropriate antigen. COX-derived bronchodilator (PGE_2) and bronchoconstrictor (*e.g.*, $PGF_{2\alpha}$, TxA_2, and PGD_2) substances are released. Polymorphisms in the genes for PGD_2 synthase and the TP receptor have been associated with asthma in humans, and deletion of DP_1 receptor in mice sharply reduces allergen-induced infiltration of lymphocytes and eosinophils and airway hyper-reactivity (Smyth and FitzGerald, 2003).

The CysLTs probably dominate during allergic constriction of the airway (Drazen, 1999). Deficiency of 5-LOX leads to reduced influx of eosinophils in airways and attenuates bronchoconstriction. Furthermore, unlike COX inhibitors and histaminergic antagonists, CysLT receptor antagonists and 5-LOX inhibitors are effective in the treatment of human asthma (*see* above). The relatively slow LT metabolism in lung contributes to the long-lasting bronchoconstriction that follows challenge with antigen and may be a factor in the high bronchial tone that is observed in asthmatics in periods between acute attacks (*see* Chapter 27).

Kidney. Long-term use of all COX inhibitors is limited by the development of hypertension, edema, and congestive heart failure in a significant number of patients. PGE_2, along with PGI_2, apparently derived from COX-2, plays a critical role in maintaining renal blood flow and salt excretion, whereas there is some evidence that the COX-1-derived vasoconstrictor TxA_2 may play a counterbalancing role. Biosynthesis of PGE_2 and PGI_2 is increased by factors that reduce renal blood flow (*e.g.*, stimulation of sympathetic nerves; angiotensin II).

Bartter's syndrome is an autosomal recessive trait that is manifested as hypokalemic metabolic alkalosis. The syndrome results from inappropriate renal salt absorption caused primarily by dysfunctional mutations in the Na^+–K^+–$2Cl^-$ cotransporter NKCC2, a target of loop diuretics in the ascending thick limb of the loop of Henle (Simon *et al.*, 1996) (*see* Chapter 28). The syndrome also can result from dysfunctional alterations in proteins whose activities can limit NKCC2 function: the K^+ channel ROMK2 (Kir1.1) that recycles K^+ into the tubular fluid; the basolateral membrane Cl^- channel, ClC–Kb; and Barttin, the integral membrane protein that forms the β-subunit of the ClC–Kb heteromer (O'Shaughnessy and Karet, 2004). The antenatal variant of Bartter's syndrome, owing to dysfunctional ROMK2, also is known as *hyperprostaglandin E syndrome*. The elevated PGE_2 may exacerbate the symptoms of salt and water loss. The relationship between dysfunctional ROMK2 and elevated PGE_2 synthesis is not clear. However, in patients with antenatal Bartter's syndrome, inhibition of COX-2 ameliorates many of the clinical symptoms (Nusing *et al.*, 2001).

Inflammatory and Immune Responses. PGs and LTs are synthesized in response to a host of stimuli that elicit inflammatory and immune responses, and eicosanoids contribute importantly to inflammation and immunity (Tilley *et al.*, 2001; Brink *et al.*, 2003). Prostanoid biosynthesis is increased significantly in inflamed tissue. Recruitment of leukocytes and the induction of COX-2 expression by inflammatory stimuli provided a rational basis for the development of COX-2-specific inhibitors for treatment of chronic inflammatory diseases (*see* Chapter 26). However, COX-1 also has a role in inflammation: It appears that COX-1 is responsible for acute and COX-2 for sustained prostanoid production following an inflammatory stimulus.

Prostanoids generally promote acute inflammation, although there are some exceptions, such as the inhibitory actions of PGE_2 on mast cell activation (Tilley *et al.*, 2001). Furthermore, deletion of COX-2 and, to a lesser extent, deletion of COX-1 are associated with greater severity of inflammatory colitis, consistent with the exacerbation of inflammatory bowel disease seen in patients receiving tNSAIDs. Both PGE_2 and PGI_2 markedly enhance edema formation and leukocyte infiltration by promoting blood flow in the inflamed region. Both have been associated with inflammatory pain, and both potentiate the pain-producing activity of bradykinin and other autacoids.

LTs are potent mediators of inflammation. Deletion of 5-LOX or FLAP reduces inflammatory responses (Austin and Funk, 1999). Generation of BLT_1-deficient mice confirms the role of LTB_4 in chemotaxis, adhesion, and recruitment of leukocytes to inflamed tissues (Toda *et al.*, 2002). Increased vascular permeability resulting from innate and adaptive immune challenges is offset in mice deficient in $CysLT_1$ or LTC_4 synthase (*see* Kanaoka and Boyce, 2004) (Table 25–1). Deletion either of LTC_4 synthase (and thus loss of CysLT biosynthesis) or $CysLT_2$ reduced chronic pulmonary inflammation and fibrosis in response to bleomycin. In contrast, absence of $CysLT_1$ led to an exaggerated response. These findings demonstrate a role for $CysLT_2$ in promoting, and an unexpected role for $CysLT_1$ in counteracting, chronic inflammation.

Cancer. There has been significant interest in the role of PGs and COX-2 in the development of malignancies. Angiogenesis, which is required for multistage carcinogenesis, is promoted by COX-2-derived TxA_2, PGE_2, and PGI_2. The role of COX-2 in colon cancer and breast cancer is an area of particular current interest. Various PGs induce proliferation of colon cancer cells, and COX inhibitors reduce colon tumor formation in experimental animals. Indeed, in large epidemiological studies, the incidental use of tNSAIDs is associated with a 40% to 50% reduction in relative risk of developing colon cancer. Furthermore, in patients with familial polyposis coli, cyclooxygenase inhibitors significantly decrease polyp formation (Williams *et al.*, 1999). A polymorphism in COX-2 has been associated with increased risk of colon cancer (Cox *et al.*, 2004). Several studies suggest that COX-2 expression is associated with markers of tumor progression in breast cancer. In mouse mammary tissue, COX-2 is pro-oncogenic (Liu *et al.*, 2001), whereas aspirin use is associated with a reduced risk of breast cancer in women, especially for hormone-receptor-positive tumors (Terry *et al.*, 2004).

Therapeutic Uses

Inhibitors and Antagonists. As a consequence of the important and diverse physiological roles of eicosanoids, mimicking their effects with stable agonists, inhibiting eicosanoid formation, and antagonizing eicosanoid receptors produce noticeable and therapeutically useful responses. As outlined earlier and in Chapter 26, the tNSAIDs and their subclass of selective COX-2 inhibitors are used widely as antiinflammatory drugs, whereas low-dose aspirin is employed frequently for cardioprotection. LT antagonists are useful clinically in the treatment of asthma, and FP agonists are used in the treatment of open-angle glau-

coma. EP agonists are used to induce labor and to ameliorate gastric irritation owing to tNSAIDs.

There are as yet no potent selective antagonists of prostanoid receptors in clinical use. TP antagonists are under evaluation in cardiovascular disease, whereas EP agonists and antagonists are under evaluation in the treatment of bone fracture and osteoporosis. Orally active antagonists of LTC_4 and D_4 have been approved for the treatment of asthma (*see* Chapter 27). These agents act by binding to the $CysLT_1$ receptor and include montelukast and zafirlukast. In patients with mild to moderately severe asthma, they cause bronchodilation, reduce the bronchoconstriction caused by exercise and exposure to antigen, and decrease the patient's requirement for the use of β_2 adrenergic agonists (Drazen, 1997). Their effectiveness in patients with aspirin-induced asthma also has been shown.

The use of eicosanoids or eicosanoid derivatives themselves as therapeutic agents is limited in part because systemic administration of prostanoids frequently is associated with significant adverse effects and because of their short half-lives in the circulation. Despite these limitations, however, several prostanoids are of clinical utility in the situations discussed below.

Therapeutic Abortion. There has been intense interest in the effects of the PGs on the female reproductive system. When given early in pregnancy, their action as *abortifacients* may be variable and often incomplete and accompanied by adverse effects. PGs appear, however, to be of value in missed abortion and molar gestation, and they have been used widely for the induction of midtrimester abortion. Several studies have shown that systemic or intravaginal administration of the PGE_1 analog *misoprostol* in combination with *mifepristone* (RU486) or *methotrexate* (Christin-Maitre *et al.*, 2000) is highly effective in the termination of early pregnancy.

PGE_2 or $PGF_{2\alpha}$ can induce labor at term. However, they may have more value when used to facilitate labor by promoting ripening and dilation of the cervix.

Gastric Cytoprotection. The capacity of several PG analogs to suppress gastric ulceration is a property of therapeutic importance. Of these, misoprostol (CYTOTEC), a PGE_1 analog, is approved by the Food and Drug Administration (FDA). Misoprostol appears to heal gastric ulcers about as effectively as the H_2-receptor antagonists (*see* Chapter 36); however, relief of ulcerogenic pain and healing of duodenal ulcers have not been achieved consistently with misoprostol. This drug currently is used primarily for the prevention of ulcers that often occur during long-term treatment with NSAIDs. In this setting, misoprostol appears to be as effective as the proton pump inhibitor *omeprazole*.

Impotence. PGE_1 (*alprostadil*) may be used in the treatment of impotence. Intracavernous injection of PGE_1 causes complete or partial erection in impotent patients who do not have disorders of the vascular system or cavernous body damage. The erection lasts for 1 to 3 hours and is sufficient for sexual intercourse. PGE_1 is more effective than papaverine. The agent is available as a sterile powder that is reconstituted with water for injections (CAVERJECT), although it has been superseded largely by the use of PDE5 inhibitors, such as *sildenafil, tadalafil,* and *vardenafil* (see Chapter 31).

Maintenance of Patent Ductus Arteriosus. The ductus arteriosus in neonates is highly sensitive to vasodilation by PGE$_1$. Maintenance of a patent ductus may be important hemodynamically in some neonates with congenital heart disease. PGE$_1$ (alprostadil, PROSTIN VR PEDIATRIC) is highly effective for palliative, but not definitive, therapy to maintain temporary patency until surgery can be performed. Apnea is observed in about 10% of neonates so treated, particularly those who weigh less than 2 kg at birth.

Pulmonary Hypertension. Primary pulmonary hypertension is a rare idiopathic disease that mainly affects young adults. It leads to right-sided heart failure and frequently is fatal. Long-term therapy with PGI$_2$ (*epoprostenol,* FLOLAN) has either delayed or precluded the need for lung or heart–lung transplantation in a number of patients. In addition, many affected individuals have had a marked improvement in symptoms after receiving treatment with PGI$_2$ (McLaughlin *et al.,* 1998). Epoprostenol also has been used successfully to treat portopulmonary hypertension that arises secondary to liver disease, again with a goal to facilitating ultimate transplantation (Krowka *et al.,* 1999).

PLATELET-ACTIVATING FACTOR

History. In 1971, Henson demonstrated that a soluble factor released from leukocytes caused platelets to aggregate. Benveniste and his coworkers characterized the factor as a polar lipid and named it *platelet-activating factor.* During this period, Muirhead described an antihypertensive polar renal lipid (APRL) produced by interstitial cells of the renal medulla that proved to be identical to PAF. Hanahan and coworkers then synthesized acetylglyceryletherphosphorylcholine (AGEPC) and determined that this phospholipid had chemical and biological properties identical with those of PAF. Independent determination of the structures of PAF and APRL showed them to be structurally identical to AGEPC. The commonly accepted name for this substance is platelet-activating factor (PAF); however, its actions extend far beyond platelets.

Chemistry and Biosynthesis. PAF is 1-*O*-alkyl-2-acetyl-*sn*-glycero-3-phosphocholine. Its structure is

$$^1CH_2-O-(CH_2)_n-CH_3$$
$$CH_3-C-O-^2C-H$$
$$\underset{O}{\|}$$
$$^3CH_2-O-\underset{\underset{O^-}{|}}{\overset{\overset{O}{\|}}{P}}-O-CH_2-CH_2-\overset{+}{N}(CH_3)_3$$

PLATELET-ACTIVATING FACTOR (*n* = 11 to 17)

PAF contains a long-chain alkyl group joined to the glycerol backbone in an ether linkage at position 1 and an acetyl group at position 2. PAF actually represents a family of phospholipids because the alkyl group at position 1 can vary in length from 12 to 18 carbon atoms. In human neutrophils, PAF consists predominantly of a mixture of the 16- and 18-carbon ethers, but its composition may change when cells are stimulated.

Like the eicosanoids, PAF is not stored in cells but is synthesized in response to stimulation. The major pathway by which PAF is generated involves the precursor 1-*O*-alkyl-2-acyl-glycerophosphocholine, a lipid found in high concentrations in the membranes of many

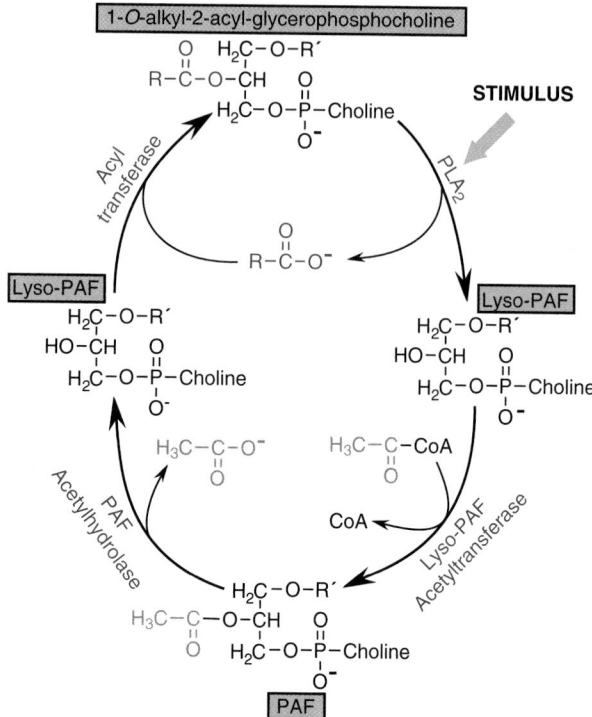

Figure 25–4. Synthesis and degradation of platelet-activating factor. RCOO$^-$ is a mixture of fatty acids but is enriched in arachidonic acid that may be metabolized to eicosanoids. CoA, coenzyme A.

types of cells. The 2-acyl substituents include AA. PAF is synthesized from this substrate in two steps (Figure 25–4). The first involves the action of phospholipase A$_2$, the initiating enzyme for eicosanoid biosynthesis, with the formation of 1-*O*-alkyl-2-lyso-glycerophosphocholine (lyso-PAF) and a free fatty acid (usually AA) (Prescott *et al.,* 2000). Eicosanoid and PAF biosynthesis thus is closely coupled, and deletion of cPLA$_2$ in mice leads to an almost complete loss of both prostanoid and PAF generation. The second, rate-limiting step is performed by the acetylcoenzyme-A-lyso-PAF acetyltransferase. PAF synthesis also can occur *de novo*; a phosphocholine substituent is transferred to alkyl acetyl glycerol by a distinct lysoglycerophosphate acetylcoenzyme-A transferase. This pathway may contribute to physiological levels of PAF for normal cellular functions. The synthesis of PAF may be stimulated during antigen–antibody reactions or by a variety of agents, including chemotactic peptides, thrombin, collagen, and other autacoids; PAF also can stimulate its own formation. Both the phospholipase and acetyltransferase are Ca^{2+}-dependent enzymes; thus, PAF synthesis is regulated by the availability of Ca^{2+}.

The inactivation of PAF also occurs in two steps (Stafforini *et al.,* 1997) (Figure 25–4). Initially, the acetyl group of PAF is removed by PAF acetylhydrolase to form lyso-PAF; this enzyme, a group VI phospholipase A$_2$, exists as secreted and intracellular isoforms and has marked specificity for phospholipids with short acyl chains at the *sn*-2 position. Lyso-PAF is then converted to a 1-*O*-alkyl-2-acyl-glycerophosphocholine by an acyltransferase.

PAF is synthesized by platelets, neutrophils, monocytes, mast cells, eosinophils, renal mesangial cells, renal medullary cells, and vascular endothelial cells. PAF is released from monocytes but retained by leukocytes and endothelial cells. In endothelial cells, it is displayed on the surface for juxtacrine signaling (Prescott *et al.*, 2000).

In addition to these enzymatic routes, PAF-like molecules can be formed from the oxidative fragmentation of membrane phospholipids (oxPLs) (Prescott *et al.*, 2002). These compounds are increased in settings of oxidant stress such as cigarette smoking and differ structurally from PAF in that they contain a fatty acid at the *sn*-1 position of glycerol joined through an ester bond and various short-chain acyl groups at the *sn*-2 position. OxPLs mimic the structure of PAF closely enough to bind to its receptor (*see below*) and elicit the same responses. Unlike the synthesis of PAF, which is highly controlled, oxPL production is unregulated; degradation by PAF acetylhydrolase, therefore, is necessary to suppress the toxicity of oxPLs. Levels of PAF acetylhydrolase (also known as *lipoprotein-associated phospholipase A_2*) are increased in colon cancer, cardiovascular disease, and stroke (Prescott *et al.*, 2002), and polymorphisms have been associated with altered risk of cardiovascular events (Ninio *et al.*, 2004). A common missense mutation in Japanese people is associated disproportionately with more severe asthma (Stafforini *et al.*, 1999).

Pharmacological Properties. *Cardiovascular System.* PAF is a potent dilator in most vascular beds; when administered intravenously, it causes hypotension in all species studied. PAF-induced vasodilation is independent of effects on sympathetic innervation, the renin–angiotensin system, or arachidonate, metabolism and likely results from a combination of direct and indirect actions. PAF induces vasoconstriction or vasodilation depending on the concentration, vascular bed, and involvement of platelets or leukocytes. For example, the intracoronary administration of very low concentrations of PAF increases coronary blood flow by a mechanism that involves the release of a platelet-derived vasodilator. Coronary blood flow is decreased at higher doses by the formation of intravascular aggregates of platelets and/or the formation of TxA_2. The pulmonary vasculature also is constricted by PAF, and a similar mechanism is thought to be involved.

Intradermal injection of PAF causes an initial vasoconstriction followed by a typical wheal and flare. PAF increases vascular permeability and edema in the same manner as histamine and bradykinin. The increase in permeability is due to contraction of venular endothelial cells, but PAF is more potent than histamine or bradykinin by three orders of magnitude.

Platelets. PAF potently stimulates platelet aggregation *in vitro*. While this is accompanied by the release of TxA_2 and the granular contents of the platelet, PAF does not require the presence of TxA_2 or other aggregating agents to produce this effect. The intravenous injection of PAF causes formation of intravascular platelet aggregates and thrombocytopenia.

Leukocytes. PAF stimulates polymorphonuclear leukocytes to aggregate, to release LTs and lysosomal enzymes, and to generate superoxide. Since LTB_4 is more potent in inducing leukocyte aggregation, it may mediate the aggregatory effects of PAF. PAF also promotes aggregation of monocytes and degranulation of eosinophils. It is chemotactic for eosinophils, neutrophils, and monocytes and promotes endothelial adherence and diapedesis of neutrophils. When given systemically, PAF causes leukocytopenia, with neutrophils showing the greatest decline. Intradermal injection causes the accumulation of neutrophils and mononuclear cells at the site of injection. Inhaled PAF increases the infiltration of eosinophils into the airways.

Smooth Muscle. PAF generally contracts gastrointestinal, uterine, and pulmonary smooth muscle. PAF enhances the amplitude of spontaneous uterine contractions; quiescent muscle contracts rapidly in a phasic fashion. These contractions are inhibited by inhibitors of PG synthesis. PAF does not affect tracheal smooth muscle but contracts airway smooth muscle. Most evidence suggests that another autacoid (*e.g.*, LTC_4 or TxA_2) mediates this effect of PAF. When given by aerosol, PAF increases airway resistance as well as the responsiveness to other bronchoconstrictors. PAF also increases mucus secretion and the permeability of pulmonary microvessels; this results in fluid accumulation in the mucosal and submucosal regions of the bronchi and trachea.

Stomach. In addition to contracting the fundus of the stomach, PAF is the most potent known ulcerogen. When given intravenously, it causes hemorrhagic erosions of the gastric mucosa that extend into the submucosa.

Kidney. When infused intrarenally in animals, PAF decreases renal blood flow, glomerular filtration rate, urine volume, and excretion of Na^+ without changes in systemic hemodynamics (Lopez-Novoa, 1999). These effects are the result of a direct action on the renal circulation. PAF exerts a receptor-mediated biphasic effect on afferent arterioles, dilating them at low concentrations and constricting them at higher concentrations. The vasoconstrictor effect appears to be mediated, at least in part, by COX products, whereas vasodilation is a consequence of the stimulation of NO production by endothelium.

Mechanism of Action of PAF. Extracellular PAF exerts its actions by stimulating a specific GPCR that is expressed in numerous cell types (Ishii *et al.*, 2002). The PAF receptor's strict recognition requirements, including a specific head group and specific atypical *sn*-2 residue, also are met by oxPLs. The PAF receptor couples with G_q to activate the PLC–IP_3–Ca^{2+} pathway and phospholipases A_2 and D such that AA is mobilized from diacylglycerol, resulting in the synthesis of PGs, TxA_2, or LTs, which may function as extracellular mediators of the effects of PAF. PAF also may exert actions without leaving its cell of origin. For example, PAF is synthesized in a regulated fashion by endothelial cells stimulated by inflammatory mediators. This PAF is presented on the surface of the endothelium, where it activates the PAF receptor on juxtaposed cells, including platelets, polymorphonuclear leukocytes, and monocytes, and acts cooperatively with P-selectin to promote adhesion (Prescott *et al.*, 2000). Endothelial cells under oxidant stress release oxPLs, which activate leukocytes and platelets and can spread tissue damage.

Receptor Antagonists. Many compounds have been described that are PAF-receptor antagonists that selectively inhibit the actions of PAF *in vivo* and *in vitro*. One would expect a PAF receptor antagonist to be a potent antiinflammatory agent that might be useful in the therapy of disorders such as asthma, sepsis, and other diseases in which PAF is postulated to play a role. However, trials in humans have been disappointing, and the clinical efficacy of PAF antagonists has yet to be realized.

Physiological and Pathological Functions of PAF. PAF generally is viewed as a mediator of pathological events. Dysregulation of PAF signaling or degradation has been associated with some human diseases, aided by data from genetically modified animals.

Platelets. Since PAF is synthesized by platelets and promotes aggregation, it was proposed as the mediator of cyclooxygenase inhibitor–resistant, thrombin-induced aggregation. However, PAF antagonists fail to block thrombin-induced aggregation, even though they prolong bleeding time and prevent thrombus formation in some experimental models. Thus, PAF does not function as an independent mediator of platelet aggregation but contributes to thrombus formation in a manner analogous to TxA_2 and ADP.

Reproduction and Parturition. A role for PAF in ovulation, implantation, and parturition has been suggested by numerous studies. However, PAF receptor–deficient mice are normal reproductively, indicating that PAF may not be essential for reproduction.

Inflammatory and Allergic Responses. The proinflammatory actions of PAF and its elaboration by endothelial cells, leukocytes, and mast cells under inflammatory conditions are well characterized. PAF and PAF-like molecules are thought to contribute to the pathophysiology of inflammatory disorders, including anaphylaxis, bronchial asthma, endotoxic shock, and skin diseases. The plasma concentration of PAF is increased in experimental anaphylactic shock, and the administration of PAF reproduces many of its signs and symptoms, suggesting a role for the autacoid in anaphylactic shock. In addition, mice overexpressing the PAF receptor exhibit bronchial hyperreactivity and increased lethality when treated with endotoxin (Ishii *et al.*, 2002). PAF receptor knockout mice display milder anaphylactic responses to exogenous antigen challenge, including less cardiac instability, airway constriction, and alveolar edema; they are, however, still susceptible to endotoxic shock. Deletion of the PAF receptor augments the lethality of infection with gram-negative bacteria while improving host defense against gram-positive pneumococcal pneumonia (Soares *et al.*, 2002; Rijneveld *et al.*, 2004).

Despite the broad implications of these observations, the effects of PAF antagonists in the treatment of inflammatory and allergic disorders have been disappointing. Although PAF antagonists reverse the bronchoconstriction of anaphylactic shock and improve survival in animal models, the impact of these agents on animal models of asthma and inflammation is marginal. Similarly, in patients with asthma, PAF antagonists partially inhibit the bronchoconstriction induced by antigen challenge but not by challenges by methacholine, exercise, or inhalation of cold air. These results may reflect the complexity of these pathological conditions and the likelihood that other mediators contribute to the inflammation associated with these disorders.

BIBLIOGRAPHY

Audoly, L.P., Rocca, B., Fabre, J.E., *et al.* Cardiovascular responses to the isoprostanes iPF2α-III and iPE₂-III are mediated via the thromboxane A₂ receptor *in vivo*. *Circulation*, **2000,** *101*:2833–2840.

Austin, S.C. and Funk, C.D. Insight into prostaglandin, leukotriene, and other eicosanoid functions using mice with targeted gene disruptions. *Prostaglandins Other Lipid Mediat.*, **1999,** *58*:231–252.

Bell-Parikh, L.C., Ide, T., Lawson, J.A., *et al.* Biosynthesis of 15-deoxy-δ12,14-PGJ₂ and the ligation of PPARγ. *J. Clin. Invest.*, **2003,** *112*:945–955.

Bombardier, C., Laine, L, Reicin, A., *et al.* Comparison of upper gastrointestinal toxicity of rofecoxib and naproxen in patients with rheumatoid arthritis. VIGOR Study Group. *New Engl. J. Med.*, **2000,** *343*:1520–1528.

Brash, A.R. Lipoxygenases: Occurrence, functions, catalysis, and acquisition of substrate. *J. Biol. Chem.*, **1999,** *274*:23679–23682.

Brink, C., Dahlen, S.E., Drazen, J., *et al.* International Union of Pharmacology: XXXVII. Nomenclature for leukotriene and lipoxin receptors. *Pharmacol. Rev.*, **2003,** *55*:195–227.

Capdevila, J.H., and Falck, J.R. Biochemical and molecular properties of the cytochrome P450 arachidonic acid monooxygenases. *Prostaglandins Other Lipid Mediat.*, **2002,** *68–69*:325–344.

Catella, F., Lawson, J.A., Fitzgerald, D.J., and FitzGerald, G.A. Endogenous biosynthesis of arachidonic acid epoxides in humans: Increased formation in pregnancy-induced hypertension. *Proc. Natl. Acad. Sci. U.S.A.*, **1990.** *87*:5893–5897.

Catella-Lawson, F., McAdams, B., Morrison, B.W., *et al.* Effects of specific inhibition of cyclooxygenase-2 on sodium balance, hemodynamics, and vasoactive eicosanoids. *J. Pharmacol. Exp. Ther.*, **1999,** *289*:735–741.

Cheng, H.F., and Harris, R.C. Cyclooxygenases, the kidney, and hypertension. *Hypertension*, **2004,** *43*:525–530.

Cheng, Y., Austin, S.C., Rocca, B., *et al.* Role of prostacyclin in the cardiovascular response to thromboxane A₂. *Science*, **2002,** *296*:539–541.

Christin-Maitre, S., Bouchard, P., and Spitz, I.M. Medical termination of pregnancy. *N. Engl. J. Med.*, **2000,** *342*:946–956.

Cipollone, F., Toniato, E. Martinotti, S., *et al.* A polymorphism in the cyclooxygenase 2 gene as an inherited protective factor against myocardial infarction and stroke. *JAMA*, **2004,** *291*:2221–2228.

Coggins, K.G., Latour, A., Nguyen, M.S., *et al.* Metabolism of PGE₂ by prostaglandin dehydrogenase is essential for remodeling the ductus arteriosus. *Nature Med.*, **2002,** *8*:91–92.

Cox, D.G., Pontes, C., Guino, E., *et al.* Polymorphisms in prostaglandin synthase 2/cyclooxygenase 2 (PTGS2/COX2) and risk of colorectal cancer. *Br. J. Cancer*, **2004,** *91*:339–343.

Drazen, J.M. Pharmacology of leukotriene receptor antagonists and 5-lipoxygenase inhibitors in the management of asthma. *Pharmacotherapy*, **1997,** *17*:22–30.

Drazen, J.M. Asthma therapy with agents preventing leukotriene synthesis or action. *Proc. Assoc. Am. Phys.*, **1999,** *111*:547–559.

Dwyer, J.H., Allayee, H., Dwyer, K.M., *et al.* Arachidonate 5-lipoxygenase promoter genotype, dietary arachidonic acid, and atherosclerosis. *New Engl. J. Med.*, **2004,** *350*:29–37.

Fabre, J.E., Nguyen, M., Athirakul, K., *et al.* Activation of the murine EP₃ receptor for PGE₂ inhibits cAMP production and promotes platelet aggregation. *J. Clin. Invest.*, **2001,** *107*:603–610.

Fam, S.S., and Morrow, J.D. The isoprostanes: Unique products of arachidonic acid oxidation—a review. *Curr. Med. Chem.*, **2003,** *10*:1723–1740.

Fitzgerald, D.J., Roy, L., Catella, F., and FitzGerald, G.A. Platelet activation in unstable coronary disease. *New Engl. J. Med.*, **1986,** *315*:983–989.

FitzGerald, G.A. Mechanisms of platelet activation: Thromboxane A₂ as an amplifying signal for other agonists. *Am. J. Cardiol.*, **1991,** *68*:11B–15B.

FitzGerald, G.A., and Loll, P. COX in a crystal ball: Current status and future promise of prostaglandin research. *J. Clin. Invest.*, **2001,** *107*:1335–1337.

FitzGerald, G.A., and Patrono, C. The coxibs, selective inhibitors of cyclooxygenase-2. *New Engl. J. Med.*, **2001,** *345*:433–442.

FitzGerald, G.A. COX-2 and beyond: Approaches to prostaglandin inhibitors in human disease. *Nat. Rev. Drug Discov.*, **2003,** 879–890.

Helgadottir, A., Manolescu, A., Thorleifssen, G., *et al.* The gene encoding 5-lipoxygenase activating protein confers risk of myocardial infarction and stroke. *Nature Genet.*, **2004,** *36*:233–239.

Hirata, T., Kakizuka, A., Ushikubi, F., et al. Arg60 to Leu mutation of the human thromboxane A_2 receptor in a dominantly inherited bleeding disorder. *J. Clin. Invest.*, **1994,** *94*:1662–1667.

Imig, J.D., Zhao, X., Falck, J.R., et al. Enhanced renal microvascular reactivity to angiotensin II in hypertension is ameliorated by the sulfonimide analog of 11,12-epoxyeicosatrienoic acid. *J. Hypertens.*, **2001,** *19*:983–992.

Ishii, S., Nagase, T., and Shimizu, T.. Platelet-activating factor receptor. *Prostaglandins Other Lipid Mediat.*, **2002,** *68–69*:599–609.

Kanaoka, Y., and Boyce, J.A. Cysteinyl leukotrienes and their receptors: Cellular distribution and function in immune and inflammatory responses. *J. Immunol.*, **2004,** *173*:1503–1510.

Krowka, M.J., Frantz, R.P., McGoon, M.D., et al. Improvement in pulmonary hemodynamics during intravenous epoprostenol (prostacyclin): A study of 15 patients with moderate to severe portopulmonary hypertension. *Hepatology*, **1999,** *30*:641–648.

Lawson, J.A., Rokach, J., and FitzGerald, G.A. Isoprostanes: Formation, analysis and use as indices of lipid peroxidation *in vivo*. *J. Biol. Chem.*, **1999,** *274*:24441–24444.

Liu, C.H., Chang, S.H., Narko, K., et al. Overexpression of cyclooxygenase-2 is sufficient to induce tumorigenesis in transgenic mice. *J. Biol. Chem.*, **2001,** *276*:18563–18569.

Lopez-Novoa, J.M. Potential role of platelet-activating factor in acute renal failure. *Kidney Int.*, **1999,** *55*:1672–1682.

Maccarrone, M., and Finazzi-Agro, A.. Endocannabinoids and their actions. *Vitam. Horm.*, **2002,** *65*:225–255.

Marnett, L.J., Rowlinson, S.W., Goodwin, D.C., et al. Arachidonic acid oxygenation by COX-1 and COX-2: Mechanisms of catalysis and inhibition. *J. Biol. Chem.*, **1999,** *274*:22903–22906.

Martel-Pelletier, J., Lajeunesse, D., Reboul, P., and Pelletier, J.P. Therapeutic role of dual inhibitors of 5-LOX and COX, selective and nonselective nonsteroidal antiinflammatory drugs. *Ann. Rheum. Dis.*, **2003,** *62*:501–509.

McAdam, B.F., Catella-Lawson, F., Mardini, I.A., et al. Systemic biosynthesis of prostacyclin by cyclooxygenase (COX)-2: the human pharmacology of a selective inhibitor of COX-2. *Proc. Natl. Acad. Sci. U.S.A.*, **1999,** *96*:272–277.

McLaughlin, V.V., Genthner, D.E., Panella, M.M., and Rich, S. Reduction in pulmonary vascular resistance with long-term epoprostenol (prostacyclin) therapy in primary pulmonary hypertension. *New Engl. J. Med.*, **1998,** *338*:273–277.

McMahon, B., and Godson, C. Lipoxins: Endogenous regulators of inflammation. *Am. J. Physiol. Renal Physiol.*, **2004,** *286*:F189–201.

Monneret, G., Li, H., Vasilescu, J., et al. 15-Deoxy-Δ12,14-prostaglandins D_2 and J_2 are potent activators of human eosinophils. *J. Immunol.*, **2002,** *168*:3563–3569.

Narumiya, S., and FitzGerald, G.A. Genetic and pharmacological analysis of prostanoid receptor function. *J. Clin. Invest.*, **2001,** *108*:25–30.

Narumiya, S., Sugimoto, Y., and Ushikubi, F. Prostanoid receptors: Structures, properties, and functions. *Physiol. Rev.*, **1999,** *79*:1193–1226.

Ninio, E., Tregouet, D., Carrier, J.I., et al. Platelet-activating factor-acetylhydrolase and PAF-receptor gene haplotypes in relation to future cardiovascular event in patients with coronary artery disease. *Hum. Mol. Genet.*, **2004,** *13*:1341–1351.

Nusing, R.M., Reinalter, S.C., Peters, M. Pathogenetic role of cyclooxygenase-2 in hyperprostaglandin E syndrome/antenatal Bartter syndrome: Therapeutic use of the cyclooxygenase-2 inhibitor nimesulide. *Clin. Pharmacol. Ther.*, **2001,** *70*:384–390.

O'Shaughnessy, K.M., and Karet, F.E. Salt handling and hypertension. *J. Clin. Invest.*, **2004,** *113*:1075–1081.

Prescott, S.M., McIntyre, T.M., Zimmerman, G.A., and Stafforini, D.M. Sol Sherry Lecture in Thrombosis: Molecular events in acute inflammation. *Arterioscler. Thromb. Vasc. Biol.*, **2002,** *22*:727–733.

Prescott, S.M., Zimmerman, G.A., Stafforini, D.M., and McIntyre, T.M. Platelet-activating factor and related lipid mediators. *Annu. Rev. Biochem.*, **2000,** *69*:419–445.

Quilley, J., and McGiff. J.C. Is EDHF an epoxyeicosatrienoic acid? *Trends Pharmacol. Sci.*, **2000,** *21*:121–124.

Rijneveld, A.W., Weijer, S., Florquin, S., et al. Improved host defense against pneumococcal pneumonia in platelet-activating factor receptor–deficient mice. *J. Infect. Dis.*, **2004,** *189*:711–716.

Rocca, B., and FitzGerald, G.A. Cyclooxygenases and prostaglandins: Shaping up the immune response. *Int. Immunopharmacol.*, **2002,** *2*:603–630.

Samad, T.A., Sapirstein, A., and Woolf, C.J. Prostanoids and pain: Unraveling mechanisms and revealing therapeutic targets. *Trends Mol. Med.*, **2002,** *8*:390–396.

Sayers, I., Barton, S., Rorke, S., et al. Promoter polymorphism in the 5-lipoxygenase (ALOX5) and 5-lipoxygenase-activating protein (ALOX5AP) genes and asthma susceptibility in a Caucasian population. *Clin. Exp. Allergy*, **2003,** *33*:1103–1110.

Schuster, V.L. Prostaglandin transport. *Prostaglandins Other Lipid Mediat.*, **2002,** *68–69*:633–647.

Simon, D.B., Karet, F.E., Hamdan, J.M. Bartter's syndrome, hypokalemic alkalosis with hypercalciuria, is caused by mutations in the Na^+–K^+–$2Cl^-$ co-transporter NKCC2. *Nature Genet.*, **1996,** *13*:183–188.

Sinal, C.J., Miyata, M., Tohkin, M, and Nagata, K., et al. Targeted disruption of soluble epoxide hydrolase reveals a role in blood pressure regulation. *J. Biol. Chem.*, **2000,** *275*:40504–40510.

Smith, W.L., Garavito, R.M., and DeWitt, D.L. Prostaglandin endoperoxide H synthases (cyclooxygenases)-1 and -2. *J. Biol. Chem.*, **1996,** *271*:33157–33160.

Smith, W.L., and Langenbach. R. Why there are two cyclooxygenase isozymes. *J. Clin. Invest.*, **2001,** *107*:1491–1495.

Smyth, E.M., and FitzGerald, G.A. Prostaglandin mediators. In, *Handbook of Cell Signaling*. (Bradshaw, R.D., ed) Academic Press, San Diego, **2003,** pp. 265–273.

Soares, A.C., Pinho, V.S., Souza, D.G., et al. Role of the platelet-activating factor (PAF) receptor during pulmonary infection with gram-negative bacteria. *Br. J. Pharmacol.*, **2002,** *137*:621–628.

Stafforini, D.M., McIntyre, T.M., Zimmerman, G.A., and Prescott, S.M. Platelet-activating factor acetylhydrolases. *J. Biol. Chem.*, **1997,** *272*:17895–17898.

Stafforini, D.M., Numao, T., Tsodikov, A., et al. Deficiency of platelet-activating factor acetylhydrolase is a severity factor for asthma. *J. Clin. Invest.*, **1999,** *103*:989–997.

Szczeklik, A., Sanak, M., Nizankowska-Mogilnicka, E., and Kielbasa, B. Aspirin intolerance and the cyclooxygenase–leukotriene pathways. *Curr. Opin. Pulm. Med.*, **2004,** *10*:51–56.

Tai, H.H., Ensor, C.M., Tong, M., et al. Prostaglandin catabolizing enzymes. *Prostaglandins Other Lipid Mediat.*, **2002,** *68–69*:483–493.

Terry, M.B., Gammon, M.D., Zhang, F.F., et al. Association of frequency and duration of aspirin use and hormone receptor status with breast cancer risk. *JAMA*, **2004,** *291*:2433–2440.

Tilley, S.L., Coffman, T.M., and Koller, B.H. Mixed messages: Modulation of inflammation and immune responses by prostaglandins and thromboxanes. *J. Clin. Invest.*, **2001,** *108*:15–23.

Toda, A., Yokomizo, T., and Shimizu, T. Leukotriene B_4 receptors. *Prostaglandins Other Lipid Mediat.*, **2002,** *68–69*:575–585.

Vane, J.R. Inhibition of prostaglandin synthesis as a mechanism of action for aspirin-like drugs. *Nature New Biol.*, **1971**, *231*:232–235.

Walt, R.P. Misoprostol for the treatment of peptic ulcer and antiinflammatory-drug-induced gastroduodenal ulceration. *New Engl. J. Med.*, **1992**, *327*:1575–1580.

Williams, C.S., Mann, M., and DuBois, R.N. The role of cyclooxygenases in inflammation, cancer, and development. *Oncogene*, **1999**, *18*:7908–7916.

Yang, J., Wu, J., Jiang, H., *et al.* Signaling through G_i family members in platelets: Redundancy and specificity in the regulation of adenylyl cyclase and other effectors. *J. Biol. Chem.*, **2002,** *277*:46035–46042.

Yu, Z., Schneider, C., Boeglin, W.E., *et al.* The lipoxygenase gene ALOXE3 implicated in skin differentiation encodes a hydroperoxide isomerase. *Proc. Natl. Acad. Sci. U.S.A.*, **2003,** *100*:9162–9167.

ANALGESIC-ANTIPYRETIC AGENTS; PHARMACOTHERAPY OF GOUT

Anne Burke, Emer Smyth, and Garret A. FitzGerald

This chapter describes *aspirin*, *acetaminophen*, the other non-narcotic nonsteroidal antiinflammatory drugs (NSAIDs) used to treat pain and inflammation, and the drugs used for hyperuricemia and gout.

Most currently available traditional NSAIDs (tNSAIDs) act by inhibiting the prostaglandin G/H synthase enzymes, colloquially known as the cyclooxygenases. The inhibition of cyclooxygenase-2 (COX-2) is thought to mediate, in large part, the antipyretic, analgesic, and antiinflammatory actions of tNSAIDs, while the simultaneous inhibition of cyclooxygenase-1 (COX-1) largely but not exclusively accounts for unwanted adverse effects in the gastrointestinal tract. Selective inhibitors of COX-2 are a subclass of NSAIDs that are also discussed. Aspirin, which irreversibly acetylates cyclooxygenase, is discussed, along with several structural subclasses of tNSAIDs, including propionic acid derivatives (*ibuprofen*, *naproxen*), acetic acid derivatives (*indomethacin*), and enolic acids (*piroxicam*), all of which compete in a reversible manner with the arachidonic acid (AA) substrate at the active site of COX-1 and COX-2. Acetaminophen is a very weak antiinflammatory drug; it is effective as an antipyretic and analgesic agent at typical doses that partly inhibit COXs, but appears to have fewer gastrointestinal side effects than the tNSAIDs.

Inflammation. The inflammatory process is the response to an injurious stimulus. It can be evoked by a wide variety of noxious agents (*e.g.*, infections, antibodies, or physical injuries). The ability to mount an inflammatory response is essential for survival in the face of environmental pathogens and injury; in some situations and diseases, the inflammatory response may be exaggerated and sustained without apparent benefit and even with severe adverse consequences. No matter what the initiating stimulus, the classic inflammatory response includes calor (warmth), dolor (pain), rubor (redness), and tumor (swelling).

Inflammatory responses occur in three distinct temporal phases, each apparently mediated by different mechanisms: (1) an acute phase, characterized by transient local vasodilation and increased capillary permeability; (2) a delayed, subacute phase characterized by infiltration of leukocytes and phagocytic cells; and (3) a chronic proliferative phase, in which tissue degeneration and fibrosis occur.

Many mechanisms are involved in the promotion and resolution of the inflammatory process (Serhan and Chiang, 2004; Kyriakis and Avruch, 2001). Although earlier studies emphasized the promotion of migration of cells out of the microvasculature, recent work has focused on adhesive interactions, including the E-, P-, and L-selectins, intercellular adhesion molecule-1 (ICAM-1), vascular cell adhesion molecule-1 (VCAM-1), and leukocyte integrins, in the adhesion of leukocytes and platelets to endothelium at sites of inflammation (Meager, 1999).

Activated endothelial cells play a key role in "targeting" circulating cells to inflammatory sites. Expression of the adhesion molecules varies among cell types involved in the inflammatory response. Cell adhesion occurs by recognition of cell-surface glycoproteins and carbohydrates on circulating cells due to the augmented expression of adhesion molecules on resident cells. Thus, endothelial activation results in leukocyte adhesion as the leukocytes recognize newly expressed L-selectin and P-selectin; other important interactions include those of endothelial-expressed E-selectin with sialylated Lewis X and other glycoproteins on the leukocyte surface and endothelial ICAM-1 with leukocyte integrins. It has been proposed that some, but not all, tNSAIDs may interfere with adhesion by inhibiting expression or activity of certain of these cell-adhesion molecules (Diaz-Gonzalez and Sanchez-Madrid, 1998). Novel classes of antiinflammatory drugs directed against cell-adhesion molecules are under active development but have not yet entered the clinical arena.

In addition to the cell-adhesion molecules outlined above, the recruitment of inflammatory cells to sites of injury involves the concerted interactions of several types of soluble mediators. These include the complement factor C5a, platelet-activating factor, and the eicosanoid LTB_4 (see Chapter 25). All can act as chemotactic agonists. Several cytokines also play essential roles in orchestrating the inflammatory process, especially interleukin-1 (IL-1) and tumor necrosis factor (TNF) (Dempsey et al., 2003). IL-1 and TNF are considered principal mediators of the biological responses to bacterial lipopolysaccharide (LPS, also called endotoxin). They are secreted by monocytes and macrophages, adipocytes, and other cells. Working in concert with each other and various cytokines and growth factors (including IL-8 and granulocyte-macrophage colony-stimulating factor; see Chapter 53), they induce gene expression and protein synthesis in a variety of cells to mediate and promote inflammation.

IL-1 comprises two distinct polypeptides (IL-1α and IL-1β) that bind to the same cell-surface receptors and produce similar biological responses. Plasma IL-1 levels are increased in patients with active inflammation. IL-1 can bind to two types of receptors, an 80-kd IL-1 receptor type 1 and a 68-kd IL-1 receptor type 2, which are present on different cell types.

TNF, originally termed "cachectin" because of its ability to produce a wasting syndrome, is composed of two closely related proteins: mature TNF (TNF-α) and lymphotoxin (TNF-β), both of which are recognized by the same cell-surface receptors. There are two types of TNF receptors, a 75-kd type 1 receptor and a 55-kd type 2 receptor. IL-1 and TNF produce many of the same proinflammatory responses.

A naturally occurring IL-1 receptor antagonist (IL-1ra), competes with IL-1 for receptor binding, blocks IL-1 activity in vitro and in vivo, and in experimental animals can prevent death induced by administration of bacteria or LPS. IL-1ra often is found in high levels in patients with various infections or inflammatory conditions. Thus, the balance between IL-1 and IL-1ra may contribute to the extent of an inflammatory response. Preliminary studies suggest that the administration of IL-1ra (designated anakinra)—by blocking IL-1 action on its receptor—may be beneficial in rheumatoid arthritis and other inflammatory conditions (Louie et al., 2003; Olson and Stein, 2004).

Other cytokines and growth factors [e.g., IL-2, IL-6, IL-8, and granulocyte/macrophage colony stimulating fac-

tor (GM-CSF)] contribute to manifestations of the inflammatory response. The concentrations of many of these factors are increased in the synovia of patients with inflammatory arthritis. Certain relevant peptides, such as substance P, which promotes firing of pain fibers, also are elevated and act in concert with cytokines at the site of inflammation. Other cytokines and growth factors counter the effects and initiate resolution of inflammation. These include transforming growth factor-β_1 (TGF-β_1), which increases extracellular matrix formation and acts as an immunosuppressant, IL-10, which decreases cytokine and prostaglandin E_2 formation by inhibiting monocytes, and interferon gamma, IFN-γ, which possesses myelosuppressive activity and inhibits collagen synthesis and collagenase production by macrophages.

Histamine was one of the first identified mediators of the inflammatory process. Although several H_1 histamine–receptor antagonists are available, they are useful only for the treatment of vascular events in the early transient phase of inflammation (see Chapter 24). Bradykinin and 5-hydroxytryptamine (serotonin, 5-HT) also may play a role in mediating inflammation, but their antagonists ameliorate only certain types of inflammatory response (see Chapter 24). Leukotriene (LT)-receptor antagonists (montelukast and zafirlukast) exert antiinflammatory actions and have been approved for the treatment of asthma (see Chapter 27). Another lipid autacoid, platelet-activating factor (PAF), has been implicated as an important mediator of inflammation; however, inhibitors of PAF synthesis and PAF-receptor antagonists have proven disappointing in the treatment of inflammation (see Chapter 25).

Intradermal, intravenous, or intra-arterial injections of small amounts of prostaglandins mimic many components of inflammation. Administration of prostaglandin E_2 (PGE$_2$) or prostacyclin (PGI$_2$) causes erythema and an increase in local blood flow. Such effects may persist for up to 10 hours with PGE$_2$ and include the capacity to counteract the vasoconstrictor effects of substances such as norepinephrine and angiotensin II, properties not generally shared by other inflammatory mediators. In contrast to their long-lasting effects on cutaneous vessels and superficial veins, prostaglandin-induced vasodilation in other vascular beds vanishes within a few minutes.

Although PGE$_1$ and PGE$_2$ (but not PGF$_{2\alpha}$) cause edema when injected into the hind paw of rats, it is not clear if they can increase vascular permeability in the postcapillary and collecting venules without the participation of other inflammatory mediators (e.g., bradykinin, histamine, and leukotriene C_4 [LTC$_4$]). Furthermore, PGE$_1$ is not produced in significant quantities in humans *in vivo*, except under rare circumstances such as essential fatty acid deficiency. Unlike LTs, prostaglandins are unlikely to be involved in chemotactic responses, even though they may promote the migration of leukocytes into an inflamed area by increasing blood flow.

Rheumatoid Arthritis. Although the detailed pathogenesis of rheumatoid arthritis is largely unknown, it appears to be an autoimmune disease driven primarily by activated T cells, giving rise to T cell–derived cytokines, such as IL-1 and TNF-α. Activation of B cells and the humoral response also are evident, although most of the antibodies generated are IgGs of unknown specificity, apparently elicited by polyclonal activation of B cells rather than from a response to a specific antigen.

Many cytokines, including IL-1 and TNF-α, have been found in the rheumatoid synovium. Glucocorticoids interfere with the synthesis and actions of cytokines, such as IL-1 or TNF-α (*see* Chapter 59). Although some of the actions of these cytokines are accompanied by the release of prostaglandins and thromboxane A_2 (TXA$_2$), COX inhibitors appear to block only their pyrogenic effects. In addition, many of the actions of the prostaglandins are inhibitory to the immune response, including suppression of the function of helper T cells and B cells and inhibition of the production of IL-1 (*see* Chapter 25). Thus, it has been suggested that COX-independent effects may contribute to the efficacy of NSAIDs in this setting. Besides an impact on adhesive interactions, salicylate and certain tNSAIDs can directly inhibit the activation and function of neutrophils, perhaps by blockade of integrin-mediated neutrophil responses by inhibiting downstream Erk signaling (Pillinger *et al.*, 1998).

NSAIDS: NONSTEROIDAL ANTIINFLAMMATORY DRUGS

All NSAIDs, including the subclass of selective COX-2 inhibitors, are antiinflammatory, analgesic, and antipyretic. NSAIDs are a chemically heterogeneous group of compounds, often chemically unrelated (although most of them are organic acids), which nevertheless share certain therapeutic actions and adverse effects. Aspirin also inhibits the COX enzymes but in a manner molecularly distinct from the competitive, reversible, active site inhibitors and is often distinguished from the NSAIDs. Similarly, acetaminophen, which is antipyretic and analgesic but largely devoid of antiinflammatory activity, also is conventionally segregated from the group despite its sharing NSAID activity with other actions relevant to its clinical action *in vivo*. General properties shared by aspirin, the NSAIDs, and acetaminophen as a class of COX inhibitors are considered first, followed by a discussion of important differences among representative drugs.

History. The history of aspirin provides an interesting example of the translation of a compound from the realm of herbal folklore to contemporary therapeutics. The use of willow bark and leaves to relieve fever has been attributed to Hippocrates, but was most clearly documented by the Rev. Edmund Stone in a 1763 letter to the president of the Royal Society. Similar properties were attributed to potions from Meadowsweet (*Spiraea ulmaria*), from which the name aspirin is derived. Salicin was crystalized in 1829 by Leroux, and Pina isolated salicylic acid in 1836. In 1859, Kolbe synthesized salicylic acid, and by 1874 it was being produced industrially. It soon was being used for rheumatic fever, gout, and as a general antipyretic. Its unpleasant taste and adverse gastrointestinal effects made it difficult to tolerate for more than short periods. In 1899, Hoffmann, a chemist at Bayer Laboratories, sought to improve the adverse-effect profile of salicylic acid (which his father was taking with difficulty for arthritis). He came across the earlier work of the French chemist, Gerhardt, who had acetylated salicylic acid in 1853, apparently ameliorating its adverse-effect profile but without improving its efficacy, and therefore abandoned the project. Hoffman resumed the quest, and Bayer began testing acetylsalicylic acid in animals by 1899—the first time that a drug was tested on animals in an industrial setting—and proceeded soon thereafter to human studies and the marketing of aspirin.

Mechanism of Action and Therapeutic Effects of NSAIDs

Although it had been used for almost a century, the mechanism of action of aspirin (and the tNSAIDs) was elucidated only in 1971, when John Vane and his associates demonstrated that low concentrations of aspirin and indomethacin inhibited the enzymatic production of prostaglandins (*see* Chapter 25). There was some evidence that prostaglandins participated in the pathogenesis of inflammation and fever at that time. Subsequent observations demonstrated that prostaglandins are released whenever cells are damaged and that aspirin and tNSAIDs inhibit their biosynthesis in all cell types. However, aspirin and tNSAIDs generally do not inhibit the formation of other inflammatory mediators, including other eicosanoids such as the LTs (*see* Chapter 25). While the clinical effects of these drugs are explicable in terms of inhibition of prostaglandin synthesis, substantial inter- and intraindividual differences in clinical response have been noted. At higher concentrations, NSAIDs also are known to reduce production of superoxide radicals, induce apoptosis, inhibit the expression of adhesion molecules, decrease nitric oxide synthase, decrease proinflammatory cytokines (*e.g.,* TNF-α, interleukin-1), modify lymphocyte activity, and alter cellular membrane functions. However, there are differing opinions as to whether these actions might contribute to the antiinflammatory activity of NSAIDs (Vane and Botting, 1998) at the concentrations attained during clinical dosing in people. The hypothesis that their antiinflammatory actions in humans derive from COX inhibition alone has not been rejected, based on current evidence.

Inhibition of Prostaglandin Biosynthesis by NSAIDs. The principal therapeutic effects of NSAIDs derive from their ability to inhibit prostaglandin production. The first enzyme in the prostaglandin synthetic pathway is prostaglandin G/H synthase, also known as cyclooxygenase or COX. This enzyme converts arachidonic acid (AA) to the unstable intermediates PGG$_2$ and PGH$_2$ and leads to the production of thromboxane A_2 (TXA$_2$) and a variety of prostaglandins (*see* Chapter 25) (Figures 25–1 and 25–2).

Therapeutic doses of aspirin and other NSAIDs reduce prostaglandin biosynthesis in humans, and there is a reasonably good correlation between the potency of these drugs as cyclooxygenase inhibitors and their antiinflammatory activity. Apparent discrepancies may be partially attributed to the experimental conditions, which do not always mimic the *in vivo* situation (*e.g.,* the effect of binding of the drugs to plasma proteins, or the effects of the drug on purified COX compared to intracellular COX). Further support linking cyclooxygenase inhibition to antiinflammatory activity is the high degree of stereoselectivity among several pairs of enantiomers of α-methyl arylacetic acids for inhibition of cyclooxygenase and suppression of inflammation; in each instance the *d* or (+) isomer is more potent in inhibiting cyclooxygenase and suppressing inflammation.

There are two forms of cyclooxygenase, cyclooxygenase-1 (COX-1) and cyclooxygenase-2 (COX-2). Splice variants of COX-1 that retain enzymatic activity have been described, one of which has been called "COX-3." It is not clear at present how relevant these splice variants are to prostaglandin synthesis and NSAID action in humans. COX-1 is a primarily constitutive isoform found in most normal cells and tissues, while cytokines and inflammatory mediators that accompany inflammation induce COX-2 production (Seibert *et al.,* 1997). However, COX-2 also is constitutively expressed in certain areas of kidney and brain (Breder *et al.,* 1995) and is induced in endothelial cells by laminar shear forces (Topper *et al.,* 1996). Importantly, COX-1, but not COX-2, is expressed as the dominant, constitutive isoform in gastric epithelial cells and is the major source of cytoprotective prostaglandin formation. Inhibition of COX-1 at this site is thought to account largely for the gastric adverse events that complicate therapy with tNSAIDs, thus providing the rationale for the development of NSAIDs specific for inhibition of COX-2 (FitzGerald and Patrono, 2001).

Aspirin and NSAIDs inhibit the COX enzymes and prostaglandin production; they do not inhibit the lipoxygenase pathways of AA metabolism and hence do not suppress LT formation (*see* Chapter 25). Glucocorticoids suppress the induced expression of COX-2, and thus COX-2–mediated prostaglandin production. They also inhibit the action of phospholipase A_2, which releases AA from the cell membrane. These effects contribute to the antiinflammatory actions of glucocorticoids, which are discussed in greater detail in Chapter 59. Table 26–1 provides a classification of NSAIDs and other analgesic and antipyretic agents based on their chemical structures.

Aspirin covalently modifies COX-1 and COX-2, irreversibly inhibiting cyclooxygenase activity. This is an important distinction from all the NSAIDs because the duration of aspirin's effects is related to the turnover rate of cyclooxygenases in different target tissues. The duration of effect of nonaspirin NSAIDs, which competitively inhibit the active sites of the COX enzymes, relates more directly to the time course of drug disposition. The importance of enzyme turnover in relief from aspirin action is most notable in platelets, which, being anucleate, have a markedly limited capacity for protein synthesis. Thus, the consequences of inhibition of platelet COX-1 (COX-2 is expressed only in megakaryocytes) last for the lifetime of the platelet. Inhibition of platelet COX-1–dependent TXA_2 formation therefore is cumulative with repeated doses of aspirin (at least as low as 30 mg/day) and takes roughly 8 to 12 days—the platelet turnover time—to recover once therapy has been stopped.

COXs are configured such that the active site is accessed by the AA substrate *via* a hydrophobic channel. Aspirin acetylates serine 530 of COX-1, located high up in the hydrophobic channel. Interposition of the bulky acetyl residue prevents the binding of AA to the active site of the enzyme and thus impedes the ability of the enzyme to make prostaglandins. Aspirin acetylates a homologous serine at position 516 in COX-2. Although covalent modification of COX-2 by aspirin also blocks the cyclooxygenase activity of this isoform, an interesting property not shared by COX-1 is that acetylated COX-2 synthesizes 15(*R*)-hydroxyeicosatetraenoic acid [15(*R*)-HETE]. This may be metabolized, at least *in vitro*, by 5-lipoxygenase to yield 15-epilipoxin A4, which has potent antiinflammatory properties (Serhan and Oliw, 2001). Due to these features, repeated doses of aspirin that acutely do not completely inhibit platelet COX-1–derived TXA_2 can exert a cumulative effect with complete blockade. This has been shown in randomized trials for doses as low as 30 mg per day. However, most of the clinical trials demonstrating cardioprotection from low-dose aspirin have used doses in the range of 75 to 81 mg/day.

The unique sensitivity of platelets to inhibition by such low doses of aspirin is related to their presystemic inhibition in the portal circulation before aspirin is deacetylated to salicylate on first pass through the liver (Pederson and FitzGerald, 1984). In contrast to aspirin, salicylic acid has no acetylating capacity. It is a weak, reversible competitive inhibitor of cyclooxygenase. High doses of salicylate inhibit the activation of NFκB *in vitro*, but the relevance of this property to the concentrations attained *in vivo* is not clear (Yin *et al.,* 1998).

The vast majority of NSAIDs listed in Table 26–1 are organic acids, and in contrast to aspirin, act as reversible, competitive inhibitors of cyclooxygenase activity. Even the nonacidic parent drug *nabumetone* is converted to an active acetic acid derivative *in vivo*. As organic acids, the compounds generally are well absorbed orally, highly bound to plasma proteins, and excreted either by glomerular filtration or by tubular secretion. They also accumulate in sites of inflammation, potentially confounding the relationship between plasma concentrations and duration of drug effect. The tNSAIDs include those with shorter (less than 6 hours) or longer (greater than 10 hours) half-lives.

Table 26-1

Classification and Comparison of Nonsteroidal Analgesics

CLASS/DRUG (substitution)	PHARMACOKINETICS		DOSING§		COMMENTS	COMPARED TO ASPIRIN
Salicylates						
Aspirin (acetyl ester)	Peak C_p*	1 hour	Antiplatelet	40–80 mg/d	Permanent platelet COX-1 inhibition (due to acetyl group)	
	Protein binding	80%–90%	Pain/fever	325–650 mg every 4–6 hours	Main side effects: GI, increased bleeding time, hypersensitivity reaction	
	Metabolites†	Salicyluric acid	Rheumatic fever	1 g every 4–6 hours		
	Half-life‡		Children	10 mg/kg every 4–6 hours	Avoid in children with acute febrile illness	
	Therapeutic	2–3 hours				
	High/toxic	15–30 hours				
Diflunisal (defluoro-phenyl)	Peak C_p	2–3 hours	250–500 mg every 8–12 hours		Not metabolized to salicylic acid	Analgesic and anti-inflammatory effects 4–5 times more potent
	Protein binding	99%			Competitive COX inhibitor	Antipyretic effect weaker
	Metabolites	Glucuronide			Excreted into breast milk	Fewer platelet and GI side effects
	Half-life	8–12 hours				
	Therapeutic					
Para-aminophenol derivative						
Acetaminophen	Peak C_p	30–60 min	10–15 mg/kg every 4 hours (maximum of 5 doses/24 hours)		Weak nonspecific inhibitor at common doses	Analgesic and anti-pyretic effects equivalent to aspirin
	Protein binding	20–50%			Potency may be modulated by peroxides	Antiinflammatory, GI, and platelet effects less than aspirin at 1000 mg/day
	Metabolites	Glucuronide conjugates (60%); sulfuric acid conjugates (35%)			Overdose leads to production of toxic metabolite and liver necrosis	
	Half-life	2 hours				
Acetic acid derivatives						
Indomethacin (methylated indole)	Peak C_p	1–2 hours	25 mg 2–3 times/day; 75–100 mg at night		Side effects (3%–50% of patients): frontal headache, neutropenia, thrombocytopenia; 20% discontinue therapy	10–40 times more potent; intolerance limits dose
	Protein binding	90%				
	Metabolites	O-demethylation (50%); unchanged (20%)				
	Half-life	$2^{1}/_{2}$ hours				

(Continued)

Table 26–1

Classification and Comparison of Nonsteroidal Analgesics (Continued)

CLASS/DRUG (substitution)	PHARMACOKINETICS		DOSING§	COMMENTS	COMPARED TO ASPIRIN
Sulindac (sulfoxide pro-drug)	Peak C_p	1–2 hours; 8 hours for sulfide metabolite; extensive enterohepatic circulation	150–200 mg twice/day	20% suffer GI side effects, 10% get CNS side effects	Efficacy comparable to aspirin
	Metabolites	Sulfone and conjugates (30%); sulindac and conjugates (25%)			
	Half-life	7 hours; 18 hours for metabolite			
Etodolac (pyranocarboxylic acid)	Peak C_p	1 hour	200–400 mg 3–4 times/day	Some COX-2 selectivity *in vitro*	100 mg etodolac, similar efficacy to aspirin 650 mg, but may be better tolerated
	Protein binding	99%			
	Metabolites	Hepatic metabolites			
	Half-life	7 hours			
Femanates (*N*-phenyl-anthranilates)				Isolated cases of hemolytic anemia reported	Efficacy similar to aspirin; GI side effects (25%)
Mefenamic acid	Peak C_p	2–4 hours	500-mg load, then 250 mg every 6 hours	May have some central action	
	Protein binding	High			
	Metabolites	Conjugates of 3-hydroxy and 3-carboxyl metabolites (20% recovered in feces)			
	Half-life	3–4 hours			
Meclofenamate	Peak C_p	0.5–2 hours	50–100 mg 4–6/day (maximum of 400 mg/day)		Efficacy similar to aspirin; 25% experience GI side effects
	Protein binding	99%			
	Metabolites	Hepatic metabolism; fecal and renal excretion			
	Half-life	2–3 hours			
Flufenamic acid	*Not available in United States*				

Drug	Parameter		Dose	Comments	
Tolmetin (heteroaryl acetate derivative)	Peak C_p Protein binding Metabolites Half-life	20–60 minutes 99% Oxidized to carboxylic acid/other derivatives, then conjugated 5 hours	400–600 mg 3 times/day Children (antiinflammatory): 20 mg/kg per day in 3–4 divided doses	Food delays and decreases peak absorption May persist longer in synovial fluid to give a biological efficacy longer than its plasma $t_{\frac{1}{2}}$	Efficacy similar 25%–40% develop side effects; 5%–10% discontinue drug
Ketorolac (pyrrolizine carboxylate)	Peak C_p Protein binding Metabolites Half-life	30–60 mins after IM route 99% Glucuronide conjugate (90%) 4–6 hours	<65 years: 20 mg (orally), then 10 mg every 4–6 hours (not to exceed 40 mg/24 hours); >65 years: 10 mg every 4–6 hours (not to exceed 40 mg/24 hours)	Commonly given parenterally (60 mg IM followed by 30 mg every 6 hours, or 30 mg IV every 6 hours) Also available as ocular preparation 0.25%, 1 drop every 6 hours	Potent analgesic, poor antiinflammatory
Diclofenac (phenylacetate derivatives)	Peak C_p Protein binding Metabolites Half-life	2–3 hours 99% Glucuronide and sulfide metabolites (renal 65%, bile 35%) 1–2 hours	50 mg 3 times/day or 75 mg 2 times/day	Also available as topical gel, ophthalmic solution, and oral tablets combined with misoprostol First-pass effect; oral bioavailability, 50%	More potent; 20% develop side effects, 2% discontinue use, 15% develop elevated liver enzymes
Proprionic acid derivatives				Intolerance of one does not preclude use of other proprionate derivative	Usually better tolerated
Ibuprofen	Peak C_p Protein binding Metabolites Half-life	15–30 minutes 99% Conjugates of hydroxyl and carboxyl metabolites 2–4 hours	Analgesia Antiinflammatory	200–400 mg every 4–6 hours 300 mg every 6–8 hours or 400–800 mg 3–4 times/day	10%–15% discontinue due to adverse effects Children's dosing Antipyretic: 5–10 mg/kg every 6 hours (maximum 40 mg/kg per day) Antiinflammatory: 20–40 mg/kg per day in 3–4 divided doses	Equipotent

(Continued)

Table 26–1
Classification and Comparison of Nonsteroidal Analgesics (Continued)

CLASS/DRUG (substitution)	PHARMACOKINETICS	DOSING§	COMMENTS	COMPARED TO ASPIRIN
Naproxen	Peak C_p 1 hour Protein binding 99% (less in elderly) Metabolites 6-demethyl and other metabolites Half-life 14 hours	250 mg 4 times/day or 500 mg 2 times/day Children Antiinflammatory— 5 mg/kg twice a day	Peak antiinflammatory effects may not be seen until 2–4 weeks of use Decreased protein binding and delayed excretion increase risk of toxicity in elderly	More potent *in vitro*; usually better tolerated; variably prolonged $t_{\frac{1}{2}}$ may afford cardioprotection in some individuals
Fenoprofen	Peak C_p 2 hours Protein binding 99% Metabolites Glucuronide, 4-OH metabolite Half-life 2 hours	200 mg 4–6 times/day; 300–600 mg 3–4 times/day		15% experience side effects; few discontinue use
Ketoprofen	Peak C_p 1–2 hours Protein binding 98% Metabolites Glucuronide conjugates Half-life 2 hours	Analgesia 25 mg 3–4 times/day; Antiinflammatory— 50–75 mg 3–4 times/day		30% develop side effects (usually GI, usually mild)
Flurbiprofen	Peak C_p 1–2 hours Protein binding 99% Metabolites Hydroxylates and conjugates Half-life 6 hours	200–300 mg/day in 2–4 divided doses	Available as a 0.03% ophthalmic solution	
Oxaprozin	Peak C_p 3–4 hours Protein binding 99% Major metabolites Oxidates and glucuronide conjugates Half-life 40–60 hours	600–1800 mg/day	Long $t_{\frac{1}{2}}$ allows for daily administration; slow onset of action; inappropriate for fever/acute analgesia	

Enolic acid derivatives

Drug		Dosage		
Piroxicam	Peak [drug]	3–5 hours	20 mg/day	May inhibit activation of neutrophils, activity of proteoglycanase, collagenases	Equipotent; perhaps better tolerated 20% develop side effects; 5% discontinue drug
	Protein binding	99%			
	Metabolites	Hydroxylates and then conjugated			
	Half-life	45–50 hours			Some COX-2 selectivity, especially at lower doses
Meloxicam	Peak [drug]	5–10 hours	7.5–15 mg/day		
	Protein binding	99%			
	Metabolites	Hydroxylation			Shows some COX-2 selectivity (active metabolite does not)
	Half-life	15–20 hours			
Nabumetone (naphthyl alkanone)	Peak [drug]	3–6 hours	500–1000 mg 1–2 times/day	A prodrug, rapidly metabolized to 6-methoxy-2-naphthyl-acetic acid; pharmacokinetics reflect active compound	Fewer GI side effects than many NSAIDs
	Protein binding	99%			
	Major metabolites	O-demethylation, then conjugation			
	Half-life	24 hours			

COX-2 selective inhibitors

					Marked decrease in gastrointestinal side effects and in platelet effects
				Evidence for cardiovascular adverse events	See text for overview of COX-2 inhibitors
Celecoxib [diaryl substituted pyrazone; (sulfonamide derivative)]	Peak [drug]	2–4 hours	100 mg 1–2 times/day	Substrate for CYP2C9; inhibitor of CYP2D6 Co-administration with inhibitors of CYP2C9 or substrates of CYP2D6 should be done with caution	
	Protein binding	97%			
	Metabolites	Carboxylic acid and glucuronide conjugates			
	Half-life	6–12 hours			
Valdecoxib (BEXTRA)	Peak [drug]	2–4 hours, delayed by food	20 mg twice daily 10 mg once daily Analgesia Primary dysmenorrhea	Substrate for CYP2C9 and CYP3A4; weak inhibitor of CYP2C9 and CYP2C19	Increased incidence of heart attack and stroke in patients undergoing bypass grafting
	Protein binding	98%			
	Metabolites	Hepatic metabolism to hydroxyl derivatives, then renal excretion			

(Continued)

Table 26–1
Classification and Comparison of Nonsteroidal Analgesics (Continued)

CLASS/DRUG (substitution)	PHARMACOKINETICS		DOSING§	COMMENTS	COMPARED TO ASPIRIN
	Half-life				
Valdecoxib (*cont.*)	7–8 hours			$t_{\frac{1}{2}}$ longer in elderly or with hepatic impairment	
Parecoxib Etoricoxib Lumaricoxib		*Not approved for use in the United States*			

*Time to peak plasma drug concentration (C_p) after a single dose. In general, food delays absorption but does not decrease peak concentration †The majority of NSAIDs undergo hepatic metabolism, and the metabolites are excreted in the urine. Major metabolites or disposal pathways are listed. ‡Typical half-life is listed for therapeutic doses; if much different with toxic dose, this is given also. §Limited dosing information given. For additional information, refer to text and product information literature. Additional references can be found in earlier editions of this textbook.

Most tNSAIDs inhibit both COX-1 and COX-2 with little selectivity, although some, conventionally thought of as tNSAIDs—*diclofenac, meloxicam,* and *nimesulide*—exhibit selectivity for COX-2 that is close to that of *celecoxib in vitro.* Indeed, meloxicam achieved approval in some countries as a selective inhibitor of COX-2. The hypothesis that the antiinflammatory effects of NSAIDs would be accompanied by a lower ulcerogenic potential propelled efforts to design drugs with greater selectivity for COX-2 *versus* COX-1 (FitzGerald and Patrono, 2001). These efforts led to the approval and marketing of *rofecoxib,* celecoxib, and *valdecoxib* as selective COX-2 inhibitors, known as the coxibs, and the development of others (*e.g., etoricoxib* and *lumiracoxib*). Based on whole blood assays, several previously marketed tNSAIDs also have selectivity ratios comparable to those of the least-selective of the novel COX-2 inhibitors, celecoxib. These include meloxicam, nimesulide, and diclofenac (Warner *et al.,* 1999; FitzGerald and Patrono, 2001).

Observational studies suggest that acetaminophen, which is a very weak antiinflammatory agent at the typical daily dose of 1000 mg, is associated with a reduced incidence of gastrointestinal adverse effects compared to tNSAIDs. At this dose, acetaminophen inhibits both cyclooxygenases by about 50%. The ability of acetaminophen to inhibit the enzyme is conditioned by the peroxide tone of the immediate environment (Boutaud *et al.,* 2002). This may partly explain the poor antiinflammatory activity of acetaminophen, since sites of inflammation usually contain increased concentrations of leukocyte-generated peroxides.

Pain. NSAIDs usually are classified as mild analgesics. However, consideration of the type of pain, as well as its intensity, is important in the assessment of analgesic efficacy. NSAIDs are particularly effective when inflammation has caused sensitization of pain receptors to normally painless mechanical or chemical stimuli. Pain that accompanies inflammation and tissue injury probably results from local stimulation of pain fibers and enhanced pain sensitivity (hyperalgesia), in part a consequence of increased excitability of central neurons in the spinal cord.

Bradykinin, released from plasma kininogen, and cytokines, such as TNF-α, IL-1, and IL-8, appear to be particularly important in eliciting the pain of inflammation. These agents liberate prostaglandins and probably other mediators that promote hyperalgesia. Neuropeptides, such as substance P and calcitonin gene-related peptide (CGRP), also may be involved in eliciting pain.

Large doses of PGE$_2$ or PGF$_{2\alpha}$, previously given to women by intramuscular or subcutaneous injection to induce abortion, cause intense local pain. Prostaglandins also can cause headache and vascular pain when infused intravenously. The capacity of prostaglandins to sensitize pain receptors to mechanical and chemical stimulation apparently results from a lowering of the threshold of the polymodal nociceptors of C fibers. In general, NSAIDs do not affect either hyperalgesia or pain caused by the direct action of prostaglandins, consistent with the notion that the analgesic effects of these agents are due to inhibition of prostaglandin synthesis. However, some data have suggested that relief of pain by these compounds may occur *via* mechanisms other than inhibition

of prostaglandin synthesis, including antinociceptive effects at peripheral or central neurons. Indeed, for all the use of NSAIDs in the relief of pain, we have a poor understanding of how the two COX enzymes interact in the mediation of the perception of pain, irrespective of any COX-independent actions of individual NSAIDs.

Fever. Regulation of body temperature requires a delicate balance between the production and loss of heat; the hypothalamus regulates the set point at which body temperature is maintained. This set point is elevated in fever, and NSAIDs promote its return to normal. These drugs do not influence body temperature when it is elevated by factors such as exercise or in response to ambient temperature.

Fever may reflect infection or result from tissue damage, inflammation, graft rejection, or malignancy. These conditions all enhance formation of cytokines such as IL-1β, IL-6, interferons, and TNF-α. The cytokines increase synthesis of PGE$_2$ in circumventricular organs in and adjacent to the preoptic hypothalamic area; PGE$_2$, in turn, increases cyclic AMP and triggers the hypothalamus to elevate body temperature by promoting an increase in heat generation and a decrease in heat loss. Aspirin and NSAIDs suppress this response by inhibiting PGE$_2$ synthesis. Prostaglandins, especially PGE$_2$, acting *via* its EP3 receptor, can produce fever when infused into the cerebral ventricles or when injected into the hypothalamus. As with pain, NSAIDs do not inhibit the fever caused by directly administered prostaglandins; rather they inhibit fever caused by agents that enhance the synthesis of IL-1 and other cytokines, which presumably cause fever, at least in part, by inducing the endogenous synthesis of prostaglandins.

Therapeutic Effects. All NSAIDs, including selective COX-2 inhibitors, are antipyretic, analgesic, and antiinflammatory, with the exception of acetaminophen, which is antipyretic and analgesic but is largely devoid of antiinflammatory activity.

When employed as analgesics, these drugs usually are effective only against pain of low-to-moderate intensity, such as dental pain. Although their maximal efficacy is generally much less than the opioids, NSAIDs lack the unwanted adverse effects of opiates in the CNS, including respiratory depression and the development of physical dependence. NSAIDs do not change the perception of sensory modalities other than pain. Chronic postoperative pain or pain arising from inflammation is controlled particularly well by NSAIDs, whereas pain arising from the hollow viscera usually is not relieved. An exception to this is menstrual pain. The release of prostaglandins by the endometrium during menstruation may cause severe cramps and other symptoms of primary dysmenorrhea; treatment of this condition with NSAIDs has met with considerable success (Marjoribanks *et al.,*

2003). Not surprisingly, the selective COX-2 inhibitors such as rofecoxib and etoricoxib are also efficacious in this condition.

NSAIDs reduce fever in most situations, but not the circadian variation in temperature or the rise in response to exercise or increased ambient temperature. Comparative analysis of the impact of tNSAIDs and selective COX-2 inhibitors suggests that COX-2 is the dominant source of prostaglandins that mediate the rise in temperature evoked by bacterial LPS administration (McAdam et al., 1999). This is consistent with the antipyretic clinical efficacy of both subclasses of NSAIDs.

It seems logical to select an NSAID with rapid onset for the management of fever associated with minor illness in adults. Due to the association with Reye's syndrome, aspirin and other salicylates are contraindicated in children and young adults less than 20 years old with fever associated with viral illness. Reye's syndrome is characterized by the acute onset of encephalopathy, liver dysfunction, and fatty infiltration of the liver and other viscera (Glasgow and Middleton, 2001). The etiology and pathophysiology are not clear. However, the epidemiologic evidence for an association between aspirin use in children and Reye's syndrome was sufficiently compelling that labeling of aspirin and aspirin-containing medications to indicate Reye's syndrome as a risk in children was mandated in 1986. Since then, the use of aspirin in children has declined dramatically, and Reye's syndrome has almost disappeared. Acetaminophen has not been implicated in Reye's syndrome and is the drug of choice for antipyresis in children and teens.

NSAIDs find their chief clinical application as anti-inflammatory agents in the treatment of musculoskeletal disorders, such as rheumatoid arthritis and osteoarthritis. In general, NSAIDs provide only symptomatic relief from pain and inflammation associated with the disease, do not arrest the progression of pathological injury to tissue, and are not considered to be "disease-modifying" anti-rheumatic drugs (see below). A number of NSAIDs are FDA approved for the treatment of ankylosing spondylitis and gout. The use of NSAIDs for mild arthropathies, together with rest and physical therapy, generally is effective. When the symptoms are limited either to trouble sleeping because of pain or significant morning stiffness, a single NSAID dose given at night may suffice. Patients with more debilitating disease may not respond adequately to full therapeutic doses of NSAIDs and may require aggressive therapy with second-line agents. The choice of drugs for children with juvenile rheumatoid arthritis commonly is restricted to those that have been specifically tested in children, such as aspirin (see discussion of Reye's syndrome, above, under "Fever"), naproxen, or tolmetin. Etoricoxib—not yet approved in the United States—also has been shown to be effective in the treatment of ankylosing spondylitis and gout.

Prostaglandins also have been implicated in the maintenance of patency of the ductus arteriosus, and indomethacin and other tNSAIDs have been used in neonates to close the inappropriately patent ductus. Both COX-1 and COX-2 appear to participate in maintaining patency of the ductus arteriosus in fetal lambs (Clyman et al., 1999), while in mice COX-2 appears to play the dominant role (Loftin et al., 2002). It is not known which isoform(s) is involved in maintaining patency of the fetal ductus in utero in humans.

Other Clinical Uses. *Systemic Mastocytosis.* Systemic mastocytosis is a condition in which there are excessive mast cells in the bone marrow, reticuloendothelial system, gastrointestinal system, bones, and skin. In patients with systemic mastocytosis, prostaglandin D_2, released from mast cells in large amounts, has been found to be the major mediator of severe episodes of vasodilation and hypotension; this PGD_2 effect is resistant to antihistamines. The addition of aspirin or ketoprofen has provided relief (Worobec, 2000). However, aspirin and tNSAIDs can cause degranulation of mast cells, so blockade with H_1 and H_2 histamine receptor antagonists should be established before NSAIDs are initiated.

Bartter's Syndrome. Bartter's syndrome includes a series of rare disorders (1-0.1/100,000) characterized by hypokalemic, hypochloremic metabolic alkalosis with normal blood pressure and hyperplasia of the juxtaglomerular apparatus. Fatigue, muscle weakness, diarrhea, and dehydration are the main symptoms. Distinct variants are caused by mutations in a $Na^+:K^+:2Cl^-$ cotransporter, an apical ATP-regulated K^+ channel, a basolateral Cl^- channel, a protein (barttin) involved in cotransporter trafficking, and the extracellular calcium-sensing receptor. Renal COX-2 is induced and biosynthesis of PGE_2 is increased. Treatment with indomethacin, combined with potassium repletion and spironolactone, is associated with improvement in the biochemical derangements and symptoms. Selective COX-2 inhibitors also have been used (Guay-Woodford, 1998).

Cancer Chemoprevention. Chemoprevention of cancer is an area where the potential use of aspirin and/or NSAIDs is under active investigation. Epidemiological studies suggested that frequent use of aspirin is associated with as much as a 50% decrease in the risk of colon cancer (Kune et al., 1998) and similar observations have been made with other cancers (Jacobs et al., 2004). NSAIDs have been used in patients with familial adenomatous polyposis (FAP), an inherited disorder characterized by multiple adenomatous colon polyps developing during adolescence and the inevitable occurrence of colon cancer by the sixth decade.

Studies in small numbers of patients over short periods of follow-up have shown a decrease in the polyp burden with the use of *sulindac*, celecoxib, or rofecoxib (Cruz-Correa *et al.*, 2002; Hallak *et al.*, 2003; Steinbach *et al.*, 2000). Celecoxib is approved as an adjunct to endoscopic surveillance and surgery in FAP based on superiority in a short-term placebo-controlled trial for polyp prevention/regression. However, more recent or longer-term studies have been somewhat disappointing with regard to the primary prevention of polyps (Giardiello *et al.*, 2002), and the prematurely terminated Adenoma Prevention with Celecoxib (APC) trial showed a 2.5 times increase in cardiovascular risk for patients taking 200 mg twice a day of celecoxib, and a 3.4 times increase in risk for patients taking 400 mg twice a day (Solomon *et al.*, 2005). Controlled evidence is not available to determine if selective COX-2 inhibitors differ from non-COX-2 selective tNSAIDs or aspirin in the extent of adenomatous colorectal polyp reduction in patients with FAP. Likewise, it is unknown whether there is even a clinical benefit from the reduction. Increased expression of COX-2 has been reported in multiple epithelial tumors, and in some cases the degree of expression has been related to prognosis. Deletion or inhibition of COX-2 dramatically inhibits polyp formation in mouse genetic models of polyposis coli. Although the phenotypes in these models do not completely recapitulate the human disease, deletion of COX-1 had a similar effect. Speculation as to how the two COXs might interact in tumorigenesis includes the possibility that products of COX-1 might induce expression of COX-2. However, the nature of this interaction is poorly understood, as are its therapeutic consequences. Meanwhile, large scale chemoprevention studies focused on aspirin, tNSAIDs, or specific inhibitors of COX-2 are underway (Rigas and Shiff, 2000).

Niacin Tolerability. Large doses of niacin (nicotinic acid) effectively lower serum cholesterol levels, reduce LDL, and raise HDL (*see* Chapter 35). However, niacin is tolerated poorly because it induces intense flushing. This flushing is mediated by a release of prostaglandin D_2 from the skin, which can be inhibited by treatment with aspirin (Jungnickel *et al.*, 1997) and would be susceptible to inhibition of PGD synthesis or antagonism of its DP receptors.

Adverse Effects of NSAID Therapy. Common adverse events that complicate therapy with aspirin and NSAIDs are outlined in Table 26–2. Age generally is correlated with an increased probability of developing serious adverse reactions to NSAIDs, and caution is warranted in choosing a lower starting dose for elderly patients.

Gastrointestinal. The most common symptoms associated with these drugs are gastrointestinal, including anorexia, nausea, dys-

Table 26–2
Common and Shared Side Effects of NSAIDs

SYSTEM	MANIFESTATIONS
GI (side effects decreased with COX-2–selective drugs)	Abdominal pain Nausea Anorexia Gastric erosions/ulcers Anemia GI hemorrhage Perforation Diarrhea
Renal	Salt and water retention Edema, worsening of renal function in renal/cardiac and cirrhotic patients Decreased effectiveness of antihypertensive medications Decreased effectiveness of diuretic medications Decreased urate excretion (especially with aspirin) Hyperkalemia
CNS	Headache Vertigo Dizziness Confusion Depression Lowering of seizure threshold Hyperventilation (salicylates)
Platelets (side effects decreased with COX-2–selective drugs)	Inhibited platelet activation Propensity for bruising Increased risk of hemorrhage
Uterus	Prolongation of gestation Inhibit labor
Hypersensitivity	Vasomotor rhinitis Angioneurotic edema Asthma Urticaria Flushing Hypotension Shock
Vascular	Closure of ductus arteriosus

pepsia, abdominal pain, and diarrhea. These symptoms may be related to the induction of gastric or intestinal ulcers, which is estimated to occur in 15% to 30% of regular users. Ulceration may range from small superficial erosions to full-thickness perforation of the muscularis mucosa. There may be single or multiple ulcers, and ulceration can be accompanied by gradual blood loss leading to anemia or by life-threatening hemorrhage. The risk is further increased in those with *Helicobacter pylori* infection, heavy alcohol consumption, or other risk factors for mucosal injury, including the concurrent use of glucocorticoids. Although there is a perception that tNSAIDs vary considerably in their tendency to cause such erosions and ulcers, this is based on overview analyses of small and heterogeneous studies, often at single doses of individual tNSAIDs. Large-scale comparative studies of tNSAIDs have not been performed, and there is no reliable information on which to assess the comparative likelihood of GI ulceration on antiinflammatory doses of aspirin *versus* tNSAIDs. Thus, most information is derived from the use of surrogate markers or from epidemiological datasets and suggests that the relative risk for serious adverse gastrointestinal events is elevated about threefold in tNSAID users compared to nonusers. Epidemiological studies suggest that combining low-dose aspirin (for cardioprotection) with other NSAIDs synergistically increases the likelihood of gastrointestinal adverse events (*see* section on drug interactions, below).

All of the selective COX-2 inhibitors have been shown to be less prone than equally efficacious doses of tNSAIDs to induce endoscopically visualized gastric ulcers (Deeks *et al.*, 2002), and this has provided the basis of FDA approval of valdecoxib and celecoxib. To date, three comparative studies of clinical outcome have been published, two of which reported a significant difference in serious gastrointestinal events. The VIGOR study showed that important gastrointestinal events—mainly bleeds—were reduced from 4% to 2% in subjects treated with rofecoxib (now withdrawn from the market worldwide), and the TARGET trial (which actually was two distinct comparative studies with naproxen and ibuprofen, respectively) showed a reduction in ulcer complications in patients taking lumiracoxib (Schnitzer *et al.*, 2004). In contrast, adverse events with celecoxib were not significantly decreased in the CLASS study (Silverstein *et al.*, 2000). While the outcome of the VIGOR study was consistent with the hypothesis that COX-2–selective inhibitors are associated with a decreased incidence of gastrointestinal adverse events, the results were tempered by a fivefold increase in the incidence of myocardial infarction, probably reflecting a cardiovascular hazard in predisposed individuals treated with selective COX-2 inhibitors together with a modest cardioprotective effect of naproxen (*see* cardiovascular section, below).

Gastric damage by NSAIDs can be brought about by at least two distinct mechanisms (*see* Chapter 36). Inhibition of COX-1 in gastric epithelial cells depresses mucosal cytoprotective prostaglandins, especially PGI_2 and PGE_2. These eicosanoids inhibit acid secretion by the stomach, enhance mucosal blood flow, and promote the secretion of cytoprotective mucus in the intestine. Inhibition of PGI_2 and PGE_2 synthesis may render the stomach more susceptible to damage and can occur with oral, parenteral, or transdermal administration of aspirin or NSAIDs. There is some evidence that COX-2 also contributes to constitutive formation of these prostaglandins by human gastric epithelium; products of COX-2 certainly contribute to ulcer healing in rodents (Mizuno *et al.*, 1997). This may partly reflect an impairment of angiogenesis by the inhibitors (Jones *et al.*, 1999). Indeed, coincidental deletion or inhibition of both COX-1 and COX-2 seems necessary to replicate NSAID-induced gastropathy in mice, and there is some evidence for gastric pathology in the face of prolonged inhibition

or deletion of COX-2 alone (Sigthorsson *et al.*, 2002). Another mechanism by which NSAIDs or aspirin may cause ulceration is by local irritation from contact of orally administered drug with the gastric mucosa. Local irritation allows backdiffusion of acid into the gastric mucosa and induces tissue damage. It also is possible that enhanced generation of lipoxygenase products (*e.g.,* LTs) contributes to ulcerogenicity in patients treated with NSAIDs.

Coadministration of the PGE_1 analog *misoprostol* or proton pump inhibitors (PPIs), which now are available over the counter in the United States, in conjunction with NSAIDs can be beneficial in the prevention of duodenal and gastric ulceration (Rostom *et al.*, 2002). While a combination of aspirin with a selective COX-2 inhibitor will undermine its distinction from a tNSAID with respect to serious GI complications, we do not know if the combination retains an advantage over aspirin plus a tNSAID.

Cardiovascular. Given their relatively short half-lives, tNSAIDs, unlike aspirin, are not thought to afford cardioprotection, and most epidemiological overviews are consistent with this likelihood (Garcia Rodriguez *et al.*, 2004). An exception in some individuals may be naproxen. Although there is considerable variation, a small study suggests that platelet inhibition might be anticipated throughout the dosing interval in some but not all individuals on naproxen (Capone *et al.*, 2004). Epidemiological evidence of cardioprotection is less impressive; it suggests about a 10% reduction in myocardial infarction, compared to 20% to 25% with low-dose aspirin. This would fit with heterogeneity of response to naproxen. Reliance on prescription databases may have constrained the ability of this approach to address the question with precision. Controlled evaluation of naproxen in cardioprotection has not been performed, and naproxen should not be used as a substitute for aspirin for this purpose. Several groups have attached nitric oxide–donating moieties to NSAIDs and to aspirin in the hope of reducing the incidence of adverse events. It seems likely that benefit may be attained by abrogation of the inhibition of angiogenesis by tNSAIDs during ulcer healing in rodents (Ma *et al.*, 2002). However, the clinical benefit of this strategy remains to be established. Similarly, LTs may accumulate in the presence of COX inhibition, and there is some evidence in rodents that combined lipoxygenase (LOX)-COX inhibition may be a useful strategy. Combined inhibitors are under clinical evaluation (Charlier and Michaux, 2003).

Selective inhibitors of COX-2 depress PGI_2 formation by endothelial cells without concomitant inhibition of platelet thromboxane. Experiments in mice suggest that PGI_2 restrains the cardiovascular effects of TXA_2, affording a mechanism by which selective inhibitors might increase the risk of thrombosis (McAdam *et al.*, 1999; Catella-Lawson *et al.*, 1999). This mechanism should pertain to individuals otherwise at risk of thrombosis, such as those with rheumatoid arthritis, as the relative risk of myocardial infarction is increased in these patients compared to patients with osteoarthritis or no arthritis. The incidence of myocardial infarction and stroke has diverged in such at-risk patients when COX-2 inhibitors are compared with tNSAIDs (FitzGerald, 2003). Placebo-controlled trials have now revealed an increased incidence of myocardial infarction and stroke in patients treated with rofecoxib (Bresalier *et al.*, 2005), valdecoxib (Nussmeier *et al.*, 2005), and celecoxib (Solomon *et al.*, 2005) consistent with a mechanism-based cardiovascular hazard for the class (FitzGerald, 2003). Regulatory agencies in the United States, Europe, and Australia have reviewed these studies and other available evidence and have concluded that all three drugs increase the risk of heart attack and stroke and will be labeled accordingly and restricted with respect to marketing directly to consumers. Patients at increased risk of cardiovascular disease or thrombosis are particularly prone to cardiovascular adverse events on these agents.

Blood Pressure, Renal, and Renovascular Adverse Events. tNSAIDs and COX-2 inhibitors have been associated with renal and renovascular adverse events (Cheng and Harris, 2004). NSAIDs have little effect on renal function or blood pressure in normal human subjects. However, in patients with congestive heart failure, hepatic cirrhosis, chronic kidney disease, hypovolemia, and other states of activation of the sympathoadrenal or renin-angiotensin systems, prostaglandin formation becomes crucial in model systems and in humans (Patrono and Dunn, 1987). NSAIDs are associated with loss of the prostaglandin-induced inhibition of both the reabsorption of Cl^- and the action of antidiuretic hormone, leading to the retention of salt and water. Experiments in mice that attribute the generation of vasodilator prostaglandins (PGE_2 and PGI_2) to COX-2 raise the likelihood that the incidence of hypertensive complications (either new onset or worsened control) induced by NSAIDs in patients may correlate with the degree of inhibition of COX-2 in the kidney and the selectivity with which it is attained (Qi *et al.*, 2002). Deletion of receptors for both PGI_2 and PGE_2 elevate blood pressure in mice, mechanistically integrating hypertension with a predisposition to thrombosis. Although this hypothesis has never been addressed directly, epidemiological studies suggest hypertensive complications occur more commonly in patients treated with coxibs than with tNSAIDs.

NSAIDs promote reabsorption of K^+ as a result of decreased availability of Na^+ at distal tubular sites and suppression of the prostaglandin-induced secretion of renin. The latter effect may account in part for the usefulness of NSAIDs in the treatment of Bartter's syndrome (*see above*).

Analgesic Nephropathy. Analgesic nephropathy is a condition of slowly progressive renal failure, decreased concentrating capacity of the renal tubule, and sterile pyuria. Risk factors are the chronic use of high doses of combinations of NSAIDs and frequent urinary tract infections. If recognized early, discontinuation of NSAIDs permits recovery of renal function.

Pregnancy and Lactation. In the hours before parturition, there is induction of myometrial COX-2 expression, and levels of prostaglandin E_2 and $F_{2\alpha}$ increase markedly in the myometrium during labor (Slater *et al.*, 2002). Prolongation of gestation by NSAIDs has been demonstrated in model systems and in humans. Some NSAIDs, particularly indomethacin, have been used off-label to terminate preterm labor. However, this use is associated with closure of the ductus arteriosus and impaired fetal circulation *in utero*, particularly in fetuses older than 32 weeks' gestation. COX-2–selective inhibitors have been used as tocolytic agents; this use has been associated with stenosis of the ductus arteriosus and oligohydramnios. Finally, the use of NSAIDs and aspirin late in pregnancy may increase the risk of postpartum hemorrhage. Therefore pregnancy, especially close to term, is a relative contraindication to the use of all NSAIDs, and their use must be weighed against potential fetal risk, even in cases of premature labor, and especially in cases of pregnancy-induced hypertension, where they have been used with questionable effect (Duley *et al.*, 2004).

Hypersensitivity. Certain individuals display hypersensitivity to aspirin and NSAIDs, as manifested by symptoms that range from vasomotor rhinitis with profuse watery secretions, angioede-

ma, generalized urticaria, and bronchial asthma to laryngeal edema, bronchoconstriction, flushing, hypotension, and shock. Aspirin intolerance is a contraindication to therapy with any other NSAID because cross-sensitivity can provoke a life-threatening reaction reminiscent of anaphylactic shock. Despite the resemblance to anaphylaxis, this reaction does not appear to be immunological in nature.

Although less common in children, this syndrome may occur in 10% to 25% of patients with asthma, nasal polyps, or chronic urticaria, and in 1% of apparently healthy individuals. It is provoked by even low doses (<80 mg) of aspirin and apparently involves COX inhibition. Cross-sensitivity extends to other salicylates, structurally dissimilar NSAIDs, and rarely acetaminophen (*see* below). Treatment of aspirin hypersensitivity is similar to that of other severe hypersensitivity reactions, with support of vital organ function and administration of epinephrine. Aspirin hypersensitivity is associated with an increase in biosynthesis of LTs, perhaps reflecting diversion of AA to lipoxygenase metabolism. Indeed, results in a small number of patients suggest that blockade of 5-lipoxygenase with the drug *zileuton* (no longer marketed in the United States) or use of the leukotriene receptor antagonists may ameliorate the symptoms and signs of aspirin intolerance, albeit incompletely.

Aspirin Resistance. All forms of treatment failure with aspirin have been collectively called "aspirin resistance." Although this has attracted much attention, there is little information concerning the prevalence of a stable, aspirin-specific resistance or the precise mechanisms that might convey this "resistance." Genetic variants of COX-1 that cosegregate with resistance have been described, but the relation to clinical outcome is not clear.

Drug Interactions

Concomitant NSAIDs and Low-Dose Aspirin. Many patients combine either tNSAIDs or COX-2 inhibitors with "cardioprotective" low-dose aspirin. Epidemiological studies suggest that this combination therapy increases significantly the likelihood of gastrointestinal adverse events over either class of NSAID alone.

Prior occupancy of the active site of platelet COX-1 by the commonly consumed tNSAID ibuprofen impedes access of aspirin to its target Ser 529 and prevents irreversible inhibition of platelet inhibition (Catella-Lawson *et al.*, 2001). Epidemiological studies have provided conflicting data as to whether this adversely impacts clinical outcomes, but they generally are constrained by the use of prescription databases to examine an interaction between two drug groups commonly obtained without prescription. Evidence in support of this interaction has been observed in comparing ibuprofen-treated patients with and without aspirin in two coxib outcome studies (CLASS and TARGET), but the trials were not powered to address this question definitively. In theory, this interaction should not occur with selective COX-2 inhibitors, because mature human platelets lack COX-2.

Other Drug Interactions. Angiotensin-converting enzyme (ACE) inhibitors act, at least partly, by preventing the breakdown of kinins that stimulate prostaglandin production. Thus, it is logical that NSAIDs might attenuate the effectiveness of ACE inhibitors by blocking the production of vasodilator and natriuretic prostaglandins. Due to hyperkalemia, the combination of NSAIDs and ACE inhibitors also can produce marked bradycardia leading to syncope, especially in the elderly and in patients with hypertension, diabetes mellitus, or ischemic heart disease. NSAIDs may increase the frequency or severity of gastrointestinal ulceration when combined with corticosteroids and augment the risk of bleeding in patients receiving *warfarin*. Many NSAIDs are highly bound to plasma proteins and thus may displace other drugs from their binding sites. Such interactions can occur in patients given salicylates or other NSAIDs together with warfarin, sulfonylurea hypoglycemic agents, or *methotrexate*; the dosage of such agents may require adjustment to prevent toxicity. The problem with warfarin is accentuated, both because almost all NSAIDs suppress normal platelet function and because some NSAIDs also increase warfarin levels by interfering with its metabolism; thus, concurrent administration should be avoided.

Pharmacokinetics and Pharmacodynamics. Most of the NSAIDs are rapidly and completely absorbed from the gastrointestinal tract, with peak concentrations occurring within 1 to 4 hours. Aspirin begins to acetylate platelets within minutes of reaching the presystemic circulation. The presence of food tends to delay absorption without affecting peak concentration. Most NSAIDs are extensively protein-bound (95% to 99%) and undergo hepatic metabolism and renal excretion. In general, NSAIDs are not recommended in the setting of advanced hepatic or renal disease due to their adverse pharmacodynamic effects (*see* below). Many NSAIDs metabolized by hepatic CYPs are subject to circadian variation in their metabolic disposition; however, the implications of this observation are not clear.

Other Clinical Considerations in the Rational Selection of Therapy. The choice of an agent for use as an antipyretic or analgesic is seldom a problem. Drugs with more rapid onset of action and shorter duration of action probably are preferable for simple fevers accompanying minor viral illnesses or pain after minor musculoskeletal injuries, whereas a longer duration of action may be preferable for postoperative pain management. Sometimes a loading dose of such NSAIDs may be required.

The choice among tNSAIDs for the treatment of chronic arthritic conditions such as rheumatoid arthritis largely is empirical. Substantial differences in response have been noted among individuals treated with the same tNSAID and within an individual treated with different tNSAIDs, even when the drugs are structurally related. It

is reasonable to give a drug for a week or two as a therapeutic trial and to continue it if the response is satisfactory. Initially, all patients should be asked about previous hypersensitivity to aspirin or any member of the NSAID class. Thereafter, low doses of the chosen agent should be prescribed to determine initial patient tolerance. Doses then may be adjusted to maximize efficacy or minimize adverse effects.

Adverse effects usually become manifest in the first weeks of therapy, although gastric ulceration and bleeding may present much later. If the patient does not achieve therapeutic benefit from one NSAID, another should be tried. It is best to avoid combination therapy with more than one NSAID. There is little evidence of extra benefit for the patient, and the risk of side effects is at least additive.

Placebo-controlled trials have now established that at least three selective inhibitors of COX-2—rofecoxib, valdecoxib, and celecoxib—confer an increased risk of heart attack and stroke. This would be expected to complicate treatment with newer, highly selective agents, such as lumiracoxib and etoricoxib, although definitive information is not yet available. However, of more immediate concern are some tNSAIDs, such as meloxicam and diclofenac, which resemble celecoxib in terms of their selectivity. Evidence for hazard with both drugs has been suggested from observational studies, but controlled trials to address this hypothesis have not been performed. The cardiovascular hazard from both celecoxib and rofecoxib—the two inhibitors for which data are available from placebo-controlled trials lasting more than 1 year—increased with chronicity of dosing. This is consistent with a mechanism-based acceleration of atherogenesis directly *via* inhibition of PGI_2 and indirectly due to the rise in blood pressure consequent to inhibition of COX-2 derived PGE_2 and PGI_2.

If COX-2 inhibitors are selected, they should be used at the lowest possible dose for the shortest period of time, and patients at risk of cardiovascular disease or prone to thrombosis should not be treated with these drugs. Small absolute risks of thrombosis attributable to these drugs may interact geometrically with small absolute risks from genetic variants like factor V Leiden or concomitant therapies, such as the anovulant pill.

A final important consideration in the selection of an NSAID is the cost of therapy, particularly since these agents frequently are used chronically.

Other forms of antiarthritic therapy should be considered for the seriously debilitated arthritis patient who cannot tolerate these drugs or in whom they are not adequately effective. Gold is discussed briefly in a separate section of this chapter. Other relevant drugs are discussed in separate chapters and include immunosuppressive agents, glucocorticoids, biologic agents including cytokine receptor inhibitors, antimalarials, and penicillamine.

For mild arthropathies, the scheme outlined above, together with rest and physical therapy, probably will be effective. When the patient has problems sleeping because of pain or morning stiffness, a larger single dose of the drug may be given at night. However, patients with more debilitating disease may not respond adequately, prompting the initiation of more aggressive therapy.

The choice of drugs for children is considerably restricted, and only drugs that have been extensively tested in children should be used. This commonly points towards naproxen and ibuprofen. The COX-2–selective inhibitor rofecoxib was approved by the FDA for juvenile rheumatoid arthritis but since has been withdrawn from the market worldwide.

Before 1986, aspirin was used extensively in children and found to be well tolerated, but concerns were raised about its role in Reye's syndrome. Aspirin still can be used in children as an analgesic or antirheumatism agent in the absence of a viral syndrome; however, its use for these purposes also has declined markedly.

THE SALICYLATES

Despite the introduction of many new drugs, aspirin is still the most widely consumed analgesic, antipyretic, and antiinflammatory agent and is the standard for the comparison and evaluation of the others. Prodigious amounts of the drug are consumed in the United States; some estimates place the quantity as high as 10,000 to 20,000 tons annually. Aspirin is the most common household analgesic; yet, because the drug is so generally available, the possibility of misuse and serious toxicity probably is underappreciated, and it remains a cause of fatal poisoning in children. The clinical pharmacology of the salicylates has been reviewed (Amann and Peskar, 2002).

Chemistry. Salicylic acid (orthohydroxybenzoic acid) is so irritating that it can only be used externally; therefore various derivatives of this acid have been synthesized for systemic use. These comprise two large classes, namely esters of salicylic acid obtained from substitutions within the carboxyl group and salicylate esters of organic acids, in which the carboxyl group is retained and substitution is made in the hydroxyl group. For example, aspirin is an ester of acetic acid. In addition, there are salts of salicylic acid. The chemical relationships can be seen from the structural formulas shown in Figure 26–1.

Structure–Activity Relationships. Salicylates generally act by virtue of their content of salicylic acid, although some of the unique effects of aspirin are caused by its capacity to acetylate proteins, as described above. Substitutions on the carboxyl or hydroxyl

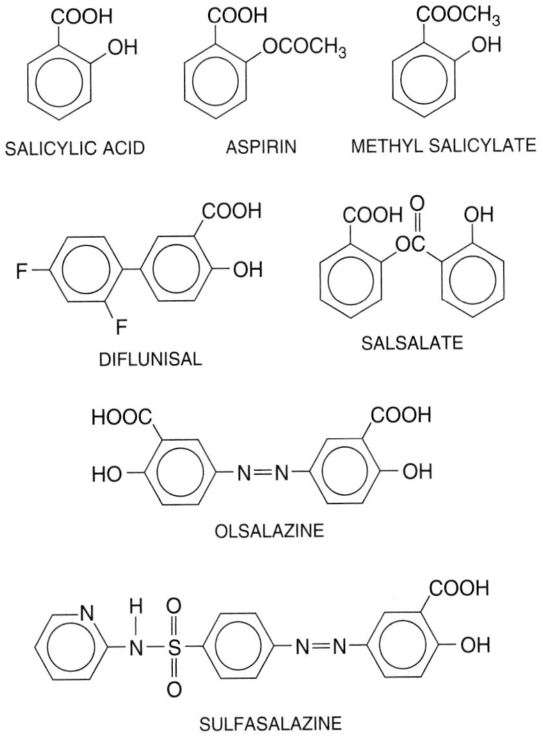

Figure 26–1. *Structural formulas of the salicylates.*

groups change the potency or toxicity of salicylates. The ortho position of the hydroxyl group is an important feature for the action of the salicylates. The effects of simple substitutions on the benzene ring have been studied extensively, and new salicylates are being synthesized. A difluorophenyl derivative, *diflunisal,* also is available for clinical use.

Pharmacological Properties of Therapeutic Doses

Analgesia. The types of pain usually relieved by salicylates are those of low intensity that arise from integumental structures rather than from viscera, especially headache, myalgia, and arthralgia. The salicylates are used more widely for pain relief than are any other classes of drugs. The salicylates alleviate pain by virtue of a peripheral action; direct effects on the CNS also may be involved.

Antipyresis. Salicylates usually lower elevated body temperatures rapidly and effectively. However, moderate doses that produce this effect also increase oxygen consumption and metabolic rate. These compounds have a pyretic effect at toxic doses, and sweating exacerbates the dehydration that occurs in salicylate intoxication (*see* below).

Respiration. Salicylates increase oxygen consumption and CO_2 production (especially in skeletal muscle) at full therapeutic doses; these effects are a result of uncoupling oxidative phosphorylation. The increased production of CO_2 stimulates respiration (mainly by an increase in depth of respiration with only a slight increase in rate). The increased alveolar ventilation balances the increased CO_2 production, and thus plasma CO_2 tension (P_{CO_2}) does not change or may decrease slightly.

Acid–Base and Electrolyte Balance and Renal Effects. Therapeutic doses of salicylate produce definite changes in the acid–base balance and electrolyte pattern. Compensation for the initial event, respiratory alkalosis (*see* above), is achieved by increased renal excretion of bicarbonate, which is accompanied by increased Na^+ and K^+ excretion; plasma bicarbonate is thus lowered, and blood pH returns toward normal. This is the stage of compensatory renal acidosis. This stage is seen most often in adults given intensive salicylate therapy and seldom proceeds further unless toxicity ensues (*see* below). Salicylates can cause retention of salt and water, as well as acute reduction of renal function in patients with congestive heart failure, renal disease, or hypovolemia. Although long-term use of salicylates alone rarely is associated with nephrotoxicity, the prolonged and excessive ingestion of analgesic mixtures containing salicylates in combination with other compounds can produce papillary necrosis and interstitial nephritis (*see* section on analgesic nephropathy, above).

Cardiovascular Effects. Low doses of aspirin (<100 mg daily) are used widely for their cardioprotective effects. At high therapeutic doses (>3 g daily), as might be given for acute rheumatic fever, salt and water retention can lead to an increase (up to 20%) in circulating plasma volume and decreased hematocrit (*via* a dilutional effect). There is a tendency for the peripheral vessels to dilate because of a direct effect on vascular smooth muscle. Cardiac output and work are increased. Those with carditis or compromised cardiac function may not have sufficient cardiac reserve to meet the increased demands, and congestive cardiac failure and pulmonary edema can occur. High doses of salicylates can produce noncardiogenic pulmonary edema, particularly in older patients who ingest salicylates regularly over a prolonged period.

Gastrointestinal Effects. The ingestion of salicylates may result in epigastric distress, nausea, and vomiting. Salicylates also may cause gastric ulceration, exacerbation of peptic ulcer symptoms (heartburn, dyspepsia), gastrointestinal hemorrhage, and erosive gastritis. These effects occur primarily with acetylated salicylates (*i.e.,* aspirin). Because nonacetylated salicylates lack the ability to acetylate cyclooxygenase and thereby irreversibly inhibit its activity, they are weaker inhibitors than aspirin.

Aspirin-induced gastric bleeding sometimes is painless, and if unrecognized may lead to iron-deficiency anemia (*see* Chapter 53). The daily ingestion of antiinflammatory doses of aspirin (4 or 5 g) results in an average fecal blood loss of between 3 and 8 ml per day, as compared with approximately 0.6 ml per day in untreated subjects. Gastroscopic examination of aspirin-treated subjects often reveals discrete ulcerative and hemorrhagic lesions of the gastric mucosa; in many cases, multiple hemorrhagic lesions with sharply demarcated areas of focal necrosis are observed. The incidence of bleeding may be higher with salicylates that dissolve slowly and deposit as particles in the gastric mucosal folds.

Hepatic Effects. Salicylates can cause hepatic injury, usually in patients treated with high doses of salicylates that result in plasma concentrations of more than 150 μg/ml. The injury is not an acute effect; rather, the onset characteristically occurs after several months of treatment. The majority of cases occur in patients with connective tissue disorders. There usually are no symptoms, simply an increase in serum levels of hepatic transaminases, but some patients note right upper quadrant abdominal discomfort and tenderness. Overt jaundice is uncommon. The injury usually is reversible upon discontinuation of salicylates. However, the use of salicylates is contraindicated in patients with chronic liver disease. Considerable evidence, as discussed above, implicates the use of salicylates as an important factor in the severe hepatic injury and encephalopathy observed in Reye's syndrome.

Uricosuric Effects. The effects of salicylates on uric acid excretion are markedly dependent on dose. Low doses (1 or 2 g per day) may decrease urate excretion and elevate plasma urate concentrations; intermediate doses (2 or 3 g per day) usually do not alter urate excretion; large doses (more than 5 g per day) induce uricosuria and lower plasma urate levels. However, such large doses are tolerated poorly. Even small doses of salicylate can block the effects of *probenecid* and other uricosuric agents that decrease tubular reabsorption of uric acid.

Effects on the Blood. Ingestion of aspirin by healthy individuals prolongs the bleeding time. For example, a single 325-mg dose of aspirin approximately doubles the mean bleeding time of normal persons for a period of 4 to 7 days. This effect is due to irreversible acetylation of platelet cyclooxygenase and the consequent reduced formation of TXA_2 until sufficient numbers of new, unmodified platelets are produced from megakaryocyte precursors.

Patients with severe hepatic damage, hypoprothrombinemia, vitamin K deficiency, or hemophilia should avoid aspirin because the inhibition of platelet hemostasis can result in hemorrhage. If possible, aspirin therapy should be stopped at least 1 week before surgery; care also should be exercised in the use of aspirin during long-term treatment with oral anticoagulant agents because of the combined danger of prolongation of bleeding time coupled with blood loss from the gastric mucosa. On the other hand, aspirin is used widely for the prophylaxis of thromboembolic disease, especially in the coronary and cerebral circulation, and is coupled frequently with oral anticoagulants in patients with bioprosthetic or mechanical heart valves (*see* Chapter 54).

Salicylates do not ordinarily alter the leukocyte or platelet count, the hematocrit, or the hemoglobin content. However, doses of 3 to 4 g per day markedly decrease plasma iron concentration and shorten erythrocyte survival time. Aspirin can cause a mild degree of hemolysis in individuals with a deficiency of glucose-6-phosphate dehydrogenase. As noted above (*Cardiovascular Effects*), high doses (>3 g daily) can expand plasma volume and decrease hematocrit by dilution.

Effects on Rheumatic, Inflammatory, and Immunological Processes and on Connective Tissue Metabolism. Although salicylates suppress clinical signs and even improve the histological picture in acute rheumatic fever, subsequent tissue damage, such as cardiac lesions and other visceral involvement, is unaffected by salicylate therapy. In addition to their effect on prostaglandin biosynthesis, the mechanism of action of the salicylates in rheumatic disease also may involve effects on other cellular and immunological processes in mesenchymal and connective tissues.

Because of the known relationship between rheumatic fever and immunological processes, attention has been directed to the capacity of salicylates to suppress a variety of antigen–antibody reactions. These include the inhibition of antibody production, of antigen–antibody aggregation, and of antigen-induced release of histamine. Salicylates also induce a nonspecific stabilization of capillary permeability during immunological insults. The concentrations of salicylates needed to produce these effects are high, and the relationship of these effects to the antirheumatic efficacy of salicylates is not clear.

Salicylates also can influence the metabolism of connective tissue, and these effects may be involved in their antiinflammatory action. For example, salicylates can affect the composition, biosynthesis, or metabolism of connective tissue mucopolysaccharides in the ground substance that provides barriers to the spread of infection and inflammation.

Metabolic Effects. *Oxidative Phosphorylation.* The uncoupling of oxidative phosphorylation by salicylates is similar to that induced by 2,4-dinitrophenol. The effect may occur with doses of salicylate used in the treatment of rheumatoid arthritis and can result in the inhibition of a number of ATP-dependent reactions. Other consequences include the salicylate-induced increase in O_2 uptake and CO_2 production (described above), the depletion of hepatic glycogen, and the pyretic effect of toxic doses of salicylate (*see* below). Salicylates in toxic doses may decrease aerobic metabolism and increase the production of strong organic acids.

Carbohydrate Metabolism. Large doses of salicylates may cause hyperglycemia and glycosuria and deplete liver and muscle glycogen.

Endocrine Effects. Long-term administration of salicylates decreases thyroidal uptake and clearance of iodine, but increases O_2 consumption and the rate of disappearance of thyroxine and triiodothyronine from the circulation. These effects probably are caused by the competitive displacement by salicylate of thyroxine and triiodothyronine from transthyretin and the thyroxine-binding globulin in plasma (*see* Chapter 56).

Salicylates and Pregnancy. There is no evidence that moderate therapeutic doses of salicylates are teratogenic in human beings; however, babies born to women who ingest salicylates for long periods may have significantly reduced birth weights. When administered during the third trimester there also is an increase in perinatal mortality, anemia, antepartum and postpartum hemorrhage, prolonged gestation, and complicated deliveries; thus, its use during this period should be avoided. As mentioned previously, administration of NSAIDs during the third trimester of pregnancy also can cause premature closure of the ductus arteriosus. The use of aspirin has been advocated for the treatment of women at high risk of preeclampsia, but it is estimated that treatment of 90 women is required to prevent one case of preeclampsia (Villar *et al.*, 2004).

Local Irritant Effects. Salicylic acid is irritating to skin and mucosa and destroys epithelial cells. The keratolytic action of the free acid is employed for the local treatment of warts, corns, fungal infections, and certain types of eczematous dermatitis. After treatment with salicylic acid, tissue cells swell, soften, and desquamate. *Methyl salicylate* (*oil of wintergreen*) is irritating to skin and gastric mucosa and is used as a counter-irritant for the relief of mild musculoskeletal pain.

Pharmacokinetics. *Absorption.* Orally ingested salicylates are absorbed rapidly, partly from the stomach but mostly from the upper small intestine. Appreciable concentrations are found in plasma in less than 30 minutes; after a single dose, a peak value is reached in about 1 hour and then declines gradually. The rate of absorption is determined by many factors, particularly the disintegration and dissolution rates of the tablets administered, the pH at the mucosal surface, and gastric emptying time.

Salicylate absorption occurs by passive diffusion primarily of nondissociated salicylic acid or acetylsalicylic acid across gastrointestinal membranes and hence is influenced by gastric pH. Even though salicylate is more ionized as the pH is increased, a rise in pH also increases the solubility of salicylate and thus dissolution of the tablets. The overall effect is to enhance absorption. As a result, there is little meaningful difference between the rates of absorption of sodium salicylate, aspirin, and the numerous buffered preparations of salicylates. The presence of food delays absorption of salicylates. Rectal absorption of salicylate usually is slower than oral absorption and is incomplete and inconsistent.

Salicylic acid is absorbed rapidly from the intact skin, especially when applied in oily liniments or ointments, and systemic poisoning has occurred from its application to large areas of skin. Methyl salicylate likewise is speedily absorbed when applied cutaneously; however, its gastrointestinal absorption may be delayed many hours, making gastric lavage effective for removal even in poisonings that present late after oral ingestion.

Distribution. After absorption, salicylates are distributed throughout most body tissues and transcellular fluids, primarily by pH-dependent passive processes. Salicylates are transported actively by a low-capacity, saturable system out of the CSF across the choroid plexus. The drugs readily cross the placental barrier.

The volume of distribution of usual doses of aspirin and sodium salicylate in normal subjects averages about 170 ml/kg of body weight; at high therapeutic doses, this volume increases to about 500 ml/kg because of saturation of binding sites on plasma proteins. Ingested aspirin mainly is absorbed as such, but some enters the systemic circulation as salicylic acid after hydrolysis by esterases in the gastrointestinal mucosa and liver. Aspirin can be detected in the plasma only for a short time as a result of hydrolysis in plasma, liver, and erythrocytes; for example, 30 minutes after a dose of 0.65 g, only 27% of the total plasma salicylate is in the acetylated form. Methyl salicylate also is hydrolyzed rapidly to salicylic acid, mainly in the liver.

Roughly 80% to 90% of the salicylate in plasma is bound to proteins, especially albumin, at concentrations encountered clinically; the proportion of the total that is bound declines as plasma concentrations increase. Hypoalbuminemia, as may occur in rheumatoid arthritis, is associated with a proportionately higher level of free salicylate in the plasma. Salicylate competes with a variety of compounds for plasma protein binding sites; these include *thyroxine, triiodothyronine, penicillin, phenytoin, sulfinpyrazone,* bilirubin, uric acid, and other NSAIDs such as naproxen. Aspirin is bound to a more limited extent; however, it acetylates human plasma albumin *in vivo* by reaction with the ε-amino group of lysine and may change the binding of other drugs to albumin. Aspirin also acetylates hormones, DNA, and hemoglobin and other proteins.

Biotransformation and Excretion. The biotransformation of salicylates takes place in many tissues, but particularly in the hepatic endoplasmic reticulum and mitochondria. The three chief metabolic products are salicyluric acid (the glycine conjugate), the ether or phenolic glucuronide, and the ester or acyl glucuronide. In addition, a small fraction is oxidized to gentisic acid (2,5-dihydroxybenzoic acid) and to 2,3-dihydroxybenzoic and 2,3,5-trihydroxybenzoic acids; gentisuric acid, the glycine conjugate of gentisic acid, also is formed.

Salicylates are excreted in the urine as free salicylic acid (10%), salicyluric acid (75%), salicylic phenolic (10%) and acyl glucuronides (5%), and gentisic acid (less than 1%). However, excretion of free salicylates is extremely variable and depends upon the dose and the urinary pH. In alkaline urine, more than 30% of the ingested drug may be eliminated as free salicylate, whereas in acidic urine this may be as low as 2%.

The plasma half-life for aspirin is about 20 minutes, and for salicylate 2 to 3 hours at antiplatelet doses, rising to 12 hours at usual antiinflammatory doses. The half-life of salicylate may be as long as 15 to 30 hours at high therapeutic doses or when there is intoxication. This dose-dependent elimination is the result of the limited capacity of the liver to form salicyluric acid and the phenolic glucuronide, resulting in a larger proportion of unchanged drug being excreted in the urine at higher doses.

Relationship of Plasma Salicylate Concentration to Therapeutic and Common Adverse Effects and Toxicity. Aspirin is one of the NSAIDs for which plasma salicylate can provide a means to monitor therapy and toxicity. Intermittent analgesic-antipyretic doses of aspirin typically produce plasma aspirin levels of less than 20 μg/ml and plasma salicylate levels of below 60 μg/ml. The daily ingestion of antiinflammatory doses of 4 to 5 g of aspirin produces plasma salicylate levels in the range of 120 to 350 μg/ml (Table 26–1). Optimal antiinflammatory effects for patients with rheumatic diseases require plasma salicylate concentrations of 150 to 300 μg/ml. Significant adverse effects can be seen at levels of more than 300 μg/ml. Hyperventilation generally occurs at concentrations greater than 350 μg/ml and other signs of intoxication, such as acidosis, at concentrations greater than 460 μg/ml. In the lower part of the range, the drug clearance is nearly constant (despite the fact that saturation of metabolic capacity is approached) because the fraction of drug that is free, and thus available for metabolism or excretion, increases as binding sites on plasma proteins are saturated. The total concentration of salicylate in plasma is thus a relatively linear function of dose at lower concentrations. At higher concentrations, however, as metabolic pathways of disposition become saturated, small increments in dose can disproportionately increase plasma salicylate concentration. Failure to anticipate this phenomenon can lead to toxicity. Since the range of plasma salicylate concentrations needed for optimal efficacy may overlap with those at which tinnitus (ringing of the ears) is noted, it is especially important to individualize antiinflammatory doses of aspirin. Tinnitus may be a reliable index of exceeding the acceptable plasma concentration in patients with normal hearing, but is not a reliable indicator in patients with preexisting hearing loss; thus, surveillance for this symptom is no substitute for periodic monitoring of serum salicylate levels.

The plasma concentration of salicylate is increased by conditions that decrease glomerular filtration rate or reduce proximal tubule secretion of salicylates, such as renal disease or the presence of inhibitors that compete for the transport system (*e.g.,* probenecid). Changes in urinary pH also have significant effects on salicylate excretion. For example, the clearance of salicylate is

about four times as great at pH 8 as at pH 6, and it is well above the glomerular filtration rate at pH 8. High rates of urine flow decrease tubular reabsorption, whereas the opposite is true in oliguria. The conjugates of salicylic acid with glycine and glucuronic acid do not readily back-diffuse across the renal tubular cells. Their excretion, therefore, is by glomerular filtration and proximal tubular secretion but is not pH dependent.

Therapeutic Uses

Systemic Uses. The two most commonly used preparations of salicylate for systemic effects are aspirin (acetylsalicylic acid) and sodium salicylate. The dose of salicylate depends on the condition being treated.

Other salicylates available for systemic use include *salsalate* (*salicylsalicylic acid;* DISALCID, others), which is hydrolyzed to salicylic acid during and after absorption, *sodium thiosalicylate* (injection; REXOLATE), *choline salicylate* (oral liquid; ARTHROPAN), and *magnesium salicylate* (tablets; MAGAN, MOMEMTUM, others). A combination of choline and magnesium salicylates (*choline magnesium, trisalicylate*, TRILISATE, others) also is available. Diflunisal (DOLOBID) is discussed below.

Antipyresis. Antipyretic therapy is reserved for patients in whom fever in itself may be deleterious and for those who experience considerable relief when fever is lowered. Little is known about the relationship between fever and the acceleration of inflammatory or immune processes; it may at times be a protective physiological mechanism. The course of the patient's illness may be obscured by the relief of symptoms and the reduction of fever by the use of antipyretic drugs. The antipyretic dose of salicylate for adults is 325 mg to 650 mg orally every 4 hours. Salicylates are contraindicated for fever associated with viral infection in children; for nonviral etiologies, 50 to 75 mg/kg per day has been given in four to six divided doses, not to exceed a total daily dose of 3.6 g. The route of administration nearly always is oral; parenteral administration (with sodium thiosalicylate) is rarely necessary. The rectal administration of aspirin suppositories may be necessary in infants or when the oral route is unavailable.

Analgesia. Salicylates are valuable for the nonspecific relief of minor aches and pain (*e.g.,* headache, arthritis, dysmenorrhea, neuralgia, and myalgia). For this purpose, they are prescribed in the same doses and manner as for antipyresis.

Rheumatoid Arthritis. Although aspirin is regarded as the standard against which other drugs should be compared for the treatment of rheumatoid arthritis, many clinicians favor the use of other NSAIDs perceived to have better gastrointestinal tolerability, even though this perception remains unproven by convincing clinical trials. As for NSAIDs, therapy with salicylates produces analgesia adequate to allow more effective movement and physical therapy in osteoarthritis and rheumatoid arthritis. In addition, aspirin therapy is associated with improvement in appetite, a feeling of well-being, and a reduction in the inflammation in joint tissues and surrounding structures. Patients with progressive or resistant disease require therapy with more toxic, second-line drugs, such as antimalarials, penicillamine, glucocorticoids, methotrexate, or immunosuppressive agents. In the United States, methotrexate is the second-line drug used most frequently, while in Europe, *sulfasalazine* is generally preferred.

Drug Interactions. The plasma concentration of salicylates generally is little affected by other drugs, but concurrent administration of aspirin lowers the concentrations of indomethacin, naproxen, keto-profen, and *fenoprofen*, at least in part by displacement from plasma proteins. Important adverse interactions of aspirin with warfarin, sulfonylureas, and methotrexate are mentioned above. Other interactions of aspirin include the antagonism of spironolactone-induced natriuresis and the blockade of the active transport of penicillin from CSF to blood.

Local Uses. *Inflammatory Bowel Disease. Mesalamine* (5-aminosal-icylic acid; ASACOL, others) is a salicylate that is used for its local effects in the treatment of inflammatory bowel disease (*see* Chapter 38). The drug is not effective orally because it is poorly absorbed and is inactivated before reaching the lower intestine. It currently is available as a suppository and rectal suspension enema (ROWASA) for treatment of mild to moderate proctosigmoiditis; a rectal suppository (CANASA, others) for the treatment of distal ulcerative colitis, proctosigmoiditis, or proctitis. Two oral formulations that deliver drug to the lower intestine, *olsalazine* (sodium azodisalicylate, a dimer of 5-aminosalicylate linked by an azo bond; DIPENTUM) and mesalamine formulated in a pH-sensitive polymer-coated oral preparation (ASACOL) and controlled-release capsule (PENTASA), are efficacious in treatment of inflammatory bowel disease, in particular ulcerative colitis. Sulfasalazine (salicylazosulfapyridine; AZULFIDINE) contains mesalamine linked covalently to sulfapyridine (*see* Chapter 38); it is absorbed poorly after oral administration, but it is cleaved to its active components by bacteria in the colon. The drug is of benefit in the treatment of inflammatory bowel disease, principally because of the local actions of mesalamine. Sulfasalazine and olsalazine also have been used in the treatment of rheumatoid arthritis and ankylosing spondylitis.

Salicylate Intoxication. Salicylate poisoning or serious intoxication often occurs in children and sometimes is fatal. The drugs should not be viewed as harmless household remedies, and salicylate intoxication should be seriously considered in any young child with coma, convulsions, or cardiovascular collapse. The fatal dose varies with the preparation of salicylate. Death has followed use of 10 to 30 g of sodium salicylate or aspirin in adults, but much larger amounts (130 g of aspirin in one case) have been ingested without a fatal outcome. The lethal dose of methyl salicylate (oil of wintergreen, sweet birch oil, gaultheria oil, betula oil) is considerably less than that of sodium salicylate. As little as 4 ml (4.7 g) of methyl salicylate may be fatal in children. Symptoms of poisoning by methyl salicylate differ little from those described below for aspirin. Central excitation, intense hyperpnea, and hyperpyrexia are prominent features. The odor of the drug can be detected easily on the breath and in the urine and vomitus. Poisoning by salicylic acid differs only in the increased prominence of GI symptoms due to the marked local irritation.

Salicylism. Mild chronic salicylate intoxication is called *salicylism*. When fully developed, the syndrome includes headache, dizziness, tinnitus, difficulty hearing, dimness of vision, mental confusion, lassitude, drowsiness, sweating, thirst, hyperventilation, nausea, vomiting, and occasionally diarrhea.

Neurological Effects. In high doses, salicylates have toxic effects on the CNS, consisting of stimulation (including convulsions) followed by depression. Confusion, dizziness, tinnitus, high-tone deafness,

delirium, psychosis, stupor, and coma may occur. The tinnitus and hearing loss of salicylate poisoning are caused by increased labyrinthine pressure or an effect on the hair cells of the cochlea, perhaps secondary to vasoconstriction in the auditory microvasculature. Tinnitus typically is observed at plasma salicylate concentrations of 200 to 450 $\mu g/ml$, and there is a close relationship between the extent of hearing loss and plasma salicylate concentration. An occasional patient may note tinnitus at lower plasma concentrations of salicylate. Tinnitus generally resolves within 2 or 3 days after withdrawal of the drug.

Salicylates induce nausea and vomiting, which result from stimulation of sites that are accessible from the CSF, probably in the medullary chemoreceptor trigger zone. In humans, centrally induced nausea and vomiting generally appear at plasma salicylate concentrations of about 270 $\mu g/ml$, but these same effects may occur at much lower plasma levels as a result of local gastric irritation.

Respiration. The respiratory effects of salicylates contribute to the serious acid–base balance disturbances that characterize poisoning by this class of compounds. Salicylates stimulate respiration directly and indirectly. Uncoupling of oxidative phosphorylation leads to increased peripheral CO_2 production and a compensatory increase in minute ventilation, usually with no overall change in PCO_2. Uncoupling of oxidative phosphorylation also leads to excessive heat production, and salicylate toxicity is associated with hyperthermia, particularly in children.

Salicylates directly stimulate the respiratory center in the medulla. This is characterized by an increase in depth and a pronounced increase in respiration rate. Patients with salicylate poisoning may have prominent increases in respiratory minute volume, and respiratory alkalosis ensues. This can be seen with plasma salicylate concentrations of 350 $\mu g/ml$, and marked hyperventilation occurs when the level approaches 500 $\mu g/ml$. However, should salicylate toxicity be associated with the coadministration of a barbiturate or opioid (*e.g.*, FIORINAL or DARVON COMPOUND 32), then central respiratory depression will prevent hyperventilation, and the salicylate-induced uncoupling of oxidative phosphorylation will be associated with a marked increase in plasma PCO_2 and respiratory acidosis.

Prolonged exposure to high doses of salicylates leads to depression of the medulla, with central respiratory depression and circulatory collapse, secondary to vasomotor depression. Because enhanced CO_2 production continues, respiratory acidosis ensues. Respiratory failure is the usual cause of death in fatal cases of salicylate poisoning.

Acid–Base Balance and Electrolytes. As described above, high therapeutic doses of salicylate are associated with a primary respiratory alkalosis and compensatory renal acidosis. Subsequent changes in acid–base status generally occur only when toxic doses of salicylates are ingested by infants and children or occasionally after large doses in adults.

The phase of primary respiratory alkalosis rarely is recognized in children with salicylate toxicity. They usually present in a state of mixed respiratory and renal acidosis, characterized by a decrease in blood pH, a low plasma bicarbonate concentration, and normal or nearly normal plasma PCO_2. Direct salicylate-induced depression of respiration prevents adequate respiratory hyperventilation to match the increased peripheral production of CO_2. Consequently, plasma PCO_2 increases and blood pH decreases. Because the concentration of bicarbonate in plasma already is low due to increased renal bicarbonate excretion, the acid–base status at this stage essentially is an uncompensated respiratory acidosis. Superimposed, however, is a true metabolic acidosis caused by accumulation of acids as a result of three processes. First, toxic concentrations of salicylates displace about 2 to 3 mEq per liter of plasma bicarbonate. Second, vasomotor depression caused by toxic doses of salicylates impairs renal function, with consequent accumulation of sulfuric and phosphoric acids. Third, salicylates in toxic doses may decrease aerobic metabolism as a result of inhibition of various enzymes. This derangement of carbohydrate metabolism leads to the accumulation of organic acids, especially pyruvic, lactic, and acetoacetic acids.

The same series of events also causes alterations of water and electrolyte balance. The low plasma P_{CO_2} leads to decreased renal tubular reabsorption of bicarbonate and increased renal excretion of Na^+, K^+, and water. Water also is lost by salicylate-induced sweating (especially in the presence of hyperthermia) and hyperventilation; dehydration, which can be profound, particularly in children, rapidly occurs. Because more water than electrolyte is lost through the lungs and by sweating, the dehydration is associated with hypernatremia. Prolonged exposure to high doses of salicylate also causes depletion of K^+ due to both renal and extrarenal factors.

Cardiovascular Effects. Toxic doses of salicylates lead to an exaggeration of the unfavorable cardiovascular responses seen at high therapeutic doses (*see* above), and central vasomotor paralysis occurs. Petechiae may be seen due to defective platelet function.

Metabolic Effects

Carbohydrate Metabolism. Large doses of salicylates may cause hyperglycemia and glycosuria and deplete liver and muscle glycogen; these effects are explained partly by the release of epinephrine. Such doses also reduce aerobic metabolism of glucose, increase glucose-6-phosphatase activity, and promote the secretion of glucocorticoids. There is a greater risk of hypoglycemia and subsequent permanent brain injury in children.

Nitrogen Metabolism. Salicylates in toxic doses cause a significant negative nitrogen balance, characterized by an aminoaciduria. Adrenocortical activation may contribute to the negative nitrogen balance by enhancing protein catabolism.

Fat Metabolism. Salicylates reduce lipogenesis by partially blocking incorporation of acetate into fatty acids; they also inhibit epinephrine-stimulated lipolysis in fat cells and displace long-chain fatty acids from binding sites on human plasma proteins. The combination of these effects leads to increased entry and enhanced oxidation of fatty acids in muscle, liver, and other tissues, and to decreased plasma concentrations of free fatty acids, phospholipid, and cholesterol; the oxidation of ketone bodies also is increased.

Endocrine Effects. Very large doses of salicylate stimulate steroid secretion by the adrenal cortex through an effect on the hypothalamus and transiently increase plasma concentrations of free corticosteroids by their displacement from plasma proteins. The therapeutic antiinflammatory effects of salicylate are independent of these effects.

Treatment. Salicylate poisoning represents an acute medical emergency, and death may result despite heroic efforts (Dargan *et al.*,

2002). Monitoring of salicylate levels is a useful guide to therapy but must be used in conjunction with an assessment of the patient's overall clinical condition, acid–base balance, formulation of salicylate ingested, timing, and dose.

There is no specific antidote for salicylate poisoning. Management begins with a rapid assessment (*see* Chapter 64) followed by the "A (airway), B (breathing), C (circulation), D (decontamination)" approach to medical emergencies.

Airway. Because of the need for respiratory alkalosis to compensate for the metabolic acidosis of salicylate toxicity, intubation should be avoided unless the patient demonstrates hypoventilation or obtundation.

Breathing. The use of paralytic agents and difficulty in achieving the very high minute volumes needed tend to induce respiratory acidosis in the patient. Aspirin ($pK_a = 3.5$) becomes non-ionized at an acidic pH and crosses the blood–brain barrier more readily, increasing its toxic central effects. It is the tissue rather than plasma levels that are dangerous to the patient. Noncardiogenic pulmonary edema interferes with oxygenation of the patient and high concentrations of inspired oxygen may be required.

Circulation. Aspirin poisoning leads to inappropriate vasodilation compounded by volume depletion and acidosis, which worsens vasodilation. Aggressive volume repletion with intravenous fluids should be instituted. The aim is to achieve large-volume diuresis to optimize salicylate elimination. If necessary, vasopressors (*e.g.*, norepinephrine, phenylephrine) are added.

Decontamination. Activated charcoal is used to prevent further absorption of aspirin from the GI tract. This is particularly important when enteric-coated aspirin, which has delayed absorption, has been ingested. Sodium bicarbonate should be administered to maintain the pH between 7.5 and 7.55, and if possible, the pH of the urine greater than 8. Forced alkaline diuresis maximizes salicylate elimination. Hemodialysis may be required if the above measures are inadequate, there is clinical deterioration despite therapy, or if plasma salicylate levels are greater than 1000 $\mu g/ml$. Plasma salicylate, glucose, pH, and potassium should be monitored frequently and therapy modified accordingly. Decreased CNS glucose levels may occur despite normal plasma glucose levels, and supplemental glucose should be given in cases of altered mental status, regardless of the plasma glucose levels.

Diflunisal

Diflunisal (DOLOBID) is a difluorophenyl derivative of salicylic acid (Figure 26–1).

It is almost completely absorbed after oral administration, and peak plasma concentrations occur within 2 to 3 hours. It is extensively bound to plasma albumin (99%). It is not converted to salicylic acid *in vivo*. About 90% of the drug is excreted as glucuronide conjugates, and its rate of elimination is dose-dependent. At the usual analgesic dose (500 to 750 mg per day), the plasma half-life averages between 8 and 12 hours (Davies, 1983). Diflunisal appears in the milk of lactating women.

Diflunisal is more potent than aspirin in antiinflammatory tests in animals and appears to be a competitive inhibitor of cyclooxygenase. However, it is largely devoid of antipyretic effects, perhaps because of poor penetration into the CNS. The drug has been used primarily as an analgesic in the treatment of osteoarthritis and musculoskeletal strains or sprains; in these circumstances it is about three to four times more potent than aspirin. The usual initial dose is 500 to 1000 mg, followed by 250 to 500 mg every 8 to 12 hours. For rheumatoid arthritis or osteoarthritis, 250 to 500 mg is administered twice daily; maintenance dosage should not exceed 1.5 g per day. Diflunisal does not produce auditory side effects and appears to cause fewer and less intense gastrointestinal and antiplatelet effects than does aspirin.

PARA-AMINOPHENOL DERIVATIVES: ACETAMINOPHEN

Acetaminophen (paracetamol; *N*-acetyl-*p*-aminophenol; TYLENOL, others) is the active metabolite of *phenacetin*, a so-called coal tar analgesic. (Due to its association with analgesic nephropathy, hemolytic anemia, and perhaps bladder cancer, phenacetin is no longer available for medicinal purposes.) Acetaminophen is an effective alternative to aspirin as an analgesic-antipyretic agent; however, its antiinflammatory effects are much weaker. While it is indicated for pain relief in patients with noninflammatory osteoarthritis, it is not a suitable substitute for aspirin or other NSAIDs in chronic inflammatory conditions such as rheumatoid arthritis. Acetaminophen is well tolerated and has a low incidence of gastrointestinal side effects. It is available without a prescription and is used as a common household analgesic. However, acute overdosage can cause severe hepatic damage, and the number of accidental or deliberate poisonings with acetaminophen continues to grow. Chronic use of less than 2 g/day is not typically associated with hepatic dysfunction.

History. *Acetanilide* is the parent member of this group of drugs. It was introduced into medicine in 1886 under the name antifebrin by Cahn and Hepp, who had discovered its antipyretic action accidentally. However, acetanilide proved to be excessively toxic. A number of chemical derivatives were developed and tested. One of the more satisfactory of these was phenacetin. It was introduced into therapy in 1887 and was extensively employed in analgesic mixtures until it was implicated in analgesic-abuse nephropathy and withdrawn in the 1980s. Discussion of its pharmacology can be found in earlier editions of this textbook.

Acetaminophen was first used in medicine by von Mering in 1893. However, it gained popularity only after 1949, when it was recognized as the major active metabolite of both acetanilide and phenacetin.

Pharmacological Properties. Acetaminophen has analgesic and antipyretic effects similar to those of aspirin. However, as mentioned above, it has only weak antiinflammatory effects and has been thought to have a generally poor ability to inhibit COX in the presence of high concentrations of peroxides, as are found at sites of inflammation. However, this aspect of its action has not been addressed rigorously. Certainly, the most commonly consumed daily dose, 1000 mg, results in roughly 50% inhibition of both COX-1 and COX-2 in whole blood assays *ex vivo* in healthy volunteers. It has been suggested that COX inhibition might be disproportionately pronounced in the brain, explaining its antipyretic efficacy (Boutaud *et al.*, 2002; Ouellet and Percival, 2001; Catella-Lawson *et al.*, 2001). A COX-1 splice variant identified in canine brain, termed COX-3, shows some susceptibility for inhibition by acetaminophen *in vitro* (Chandrasekharan *et al.*, 2002). However, it is presently unknown if this splice variant exists in human brain or if its inhibition relates to the efficacy of acetaminophen in humans. Minor metabolites contribute significantly to the toxic effects of acetaminophen (*see* below). The pharmacological properties of acetaminophen have been reviewed by Brune (1988).

Single or repeated therapeutic doses of acetaminophen have no effect on the cardiovascular and respiratory systems, on platelets, or on coagulation. Acid–base changes and uricosuric effects do not occur, nor does the drug produce the gastric irritation, erosion, or bleeding that may occur after salicylate administration.

Pharmacokinetics and Metabolism. Oral acetaminophen has excellent bioavailability. Peak plasma concentrations occur within 30 to 60 minutes and the half-life in plasma is about 2 hours after therapeutic doses. Acetaminophen is relatively uniformly distributed throughout most body fluids. Binding of the drug to plasma proteins is variable but less than with other NSAIDs; only 20% to 50% is bound at the concentrations encountered during acute intoxication. Some 90% to 100% of the drug may be recovered in the urine within the first day at therapeutic dosing, primarily after hepatic conjugation with glucuronic acid (about 60%), sulfuric acid (about 35%), or cysteine (about 3%); small amounts of hydroxylated and deacetylated metabolites also have been detected (Table 26–1). Children have less capacity for glucuronidation of the drug than do adults. A small proportion of acetaminophen undergoes CYP-mediated *N*-hydroxylation to form *N*-acetyl-*p*-benzoquinoneimine (NAPQI), a highly reactive intermediate. This metabolite normally reacts with sulfhydryl groups in glutathione (GSH) and thereby is rendered harmless. However, after ingestion of large doses of acetaminophen, the metabolite is formed in amounts sufficient to deplete hepatic GSH and contributes significantly to the toxic effects of overdose (*see* below).

Therapeutic Uses. Acetaminophen is a suitable substitute for aspirin for analgesic or antipyretic uses; it is particularly valuable for patients in whom aspirin is contraindicated (*e.g.*, those with peptic ulcer, aspirin hypersensitivity, children with a febrile illness). The conventional oral dose of acetaminophen is 325 to 1000 mg (650 mg rectally); total daily doses should not exceed 4000 mg (2000 mg/day for chronic alcoholics). The most common daily dose is 1000 mg, the dose at which epidemiological studies suggest that gastrointestinal adverse effects are less common than with therapeutic doses of tNSAIDs (Garcia Rodriguez *et al.*, 2004). Higher doses, which may accomplish complete inhibition of COXs, may approach the adverse effect profile of tNSAIDs. Single doses for children range from 40 mg to 480 mg, depending upon age and weight; no more than five doses should be administered in 24 hours. A dose of 10 mg/kg also may be used.

Toxicity and Common Adverse Effects. Acetaminophen usually is well tolerated at recommended therapeutic doses. Rash and other allergic reactions occur occasionally. The rash usually is erythematous or urticarial, but sometimes it is more serious and may be accompanied by drug fever and mucosal lesions. Patients who show hypersensitivity reactions to the salicylates only rarely exhibit sensitivity to acetaminophen. The use of acetaminophen has been associated anecdotally with neutropenia, thrombocytopenia, and pancytopenia.

The most serious acute adverse effect of overdosage of acetaminophen is a potentially fatal hepatic necrosis. Renal tubular necrosis and hypoglycemic coma also may occur. The mechanism by which overdosage with acetaminophen leads to hepatocellular injury and death involves its conversion to the toxic NAPQI metabolite (*see* Chapter 64). The glucuronide and sulfate conjugation pathways become saturated, and increasing amounts undergo CYP-mediated *N*-hydroxylation to form NAPQI. This is eliminated rapidly by conjugation with GSH and then further metabolized to a mercapturic acid and excreted into the urine. In the setting of acetaminophen overdose, hepatocellular levels of GSH become depleted. The highly reactive NAPQI metabolite binds covalently to cell macromolecules, leading to dysfunction of enzymatic systems and structural and metabolic disarray. Furthermore, depletion of intracellular GSH renders the hepatocytes highly susceptible to oxidative stress and apoptosis.

Hepatotoxicity. In adults, hepatotoxicity may occur after ingestion of a single dose of 10 to 15 g (150 to 250 mg/kg) of acetaminophen; doses of 20 to 25 g or more are potentially fatal. Conditions of CYP induction (*e.g.,* heavy alcohol consumption) or GSH depletion (*e.g.,* fasting or malnutrition) increase the susceptibility to hepatic injury, which has been documented, albeit uncommonly, with doses in the therapeutic range. Symptoms that occur during the first 2 days of acute poisoning by acetaminophen reflect gastric distress (nausea, abdominal pain, and anorexia) and belie the potential seriousness of the intoxication. Plasma transaminases become elevated, sometimes markedly so, beginning approximately 12 to 36 hours after ingestion. Clinical indications of hepatic damage are manifest within 2 to 4 days of ingestion of toxic doses, with right subcostal pain, tender hepatomegaly, jaundice, and coagulopathy. Renal impairment or frank renal failure may occur. Liver enzyme abnormalities typically peak 72 to 96 hours after ingestion. The onset of hepatic encephalopathy or worsening coagulopathy beyond this time indicates a poor prognosis. Biopsy of the liver reveals centrilobular necrosis with sparing of the periportal area. In nonfatal cases, the hepatic lesions are reversible over a period of weeks or months.

Management of Acetaminophen Overdose

Acetaminophen overdose constitutes a medical emergency. Severe liver damage occurs in 90% of patients with plasma concentrations of acetaminophen greater than 300 μg/ml at 4 hours or 45 μg/ml at 15 hours after the ingestion of the drug. Minimal hepatic damage can be anticipated when the drug concentration is less than 120 μg/ml at 4 hours or 30 μg/ml at 12 hours after ingestion. The nomogram provided in Figure 26–2 relates the plasma levels of acetaminophen and time after ingestion to the predicted severity of liver injury.

Early diagnosis and treatment of acetaminophen overdose is essential to optimize outcome. Perhaps 10% of poisoned patients

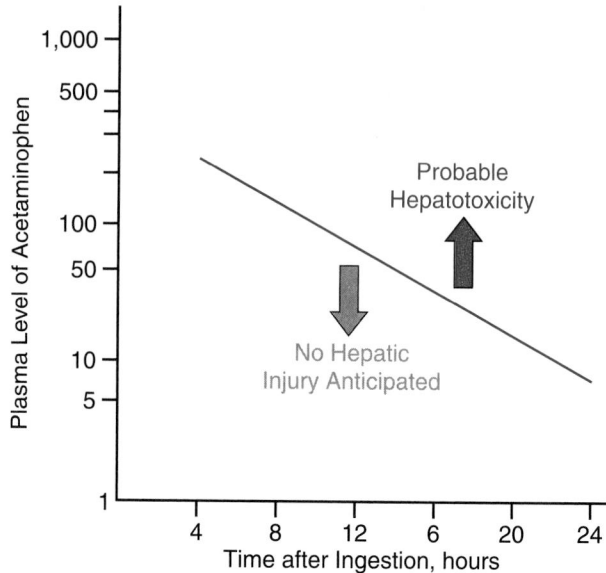

Figure 26–2. *Relationship of plasma levels of acetaminophen and time after acute ingestion to hepatic injury.* (Adapted with permission from Rumack *et al.*, 1981.)

who do not receive specific treatment develop severe liver damage; 10% to 20% of these eventually die of hepatic failure despite intensive supportive care. Activated charcoal, if given within 4 hours of ingestion, decreases acetaminophen absorption by 50% to 90% and is the preferred method of gastric decontamination. Gastric lavage generally is not recommended.

N-acetylcysteine (NAC) (MUCOMYST, MUCOSIL, PARVOLEX) is indicated for those at risk of hepatic injury. NAC therapy should be instituted in suspected cases of acetaminophen poisoning before blood levels become available, with treatment terminated if assay results subsequently indicate that the risk of hepatotoxicity is low.

NAC functions by detoxifying NAPQI. It both repletes GSH stores and may conjugate directly with NAPQI by serving as a GSH substitute. There is some evidence that in cases of established acetaminophen toxicity, NAC may protect against extrahepatic injury by its antioxidant and antiinflammatory properties (Keays *et al.*, 1991; Jones, 1998). Even in the presence of activated charcoal, there is ample absorption of NAC, and neither should activated charcoal be avoided nor NAC administration be delayed because of concerns of a charcoal-NAC interaction. Adverse reactions to NAC include rash (including urticaria, which does not require drug discontinuation), nausea, vomiting, diarrhea, and rare anaphylactoid reactions.

An oral loading dose of 140 mg/kg is given, followed by the administration of 70 mg/kg every 4 hours for 17 doses. Where available, the intravenous loading dose is 150 mg/kg by intravenous infusion in 100 ml of 5% dextrose over 15 minutes (for those weighing less than 20 kg), followed by 50 mg/kg by intravenous infusion in 250 ml of 5% dextrose over 4 hours, then 100 mg/kg by intravenous infusion in 500 ml of 5% dextrose over 16 hours.

Assistance in treatment of patients with acetaminophen overdose can be obtained from national poison centers: 1-800-222-1222 in the United States and 0870-600-6266 in the United Kingdom.

In addition to NAC therapy, aggressive supportive care is warranted. This includes management of hepatic and renal failure should they occur and intubation should the patient become obtunded. Hypoglycemia can result from liver failure, and plasma glucose should be monitored closely. Fulminant hepatic failure is an indication for liver transplantation, and a liver transplant center should be contacted early in the course of treatment of patients who develop severe liver injury despite NAC therapy.

ACETIC ACID DERIVATIVES: INDOMETHACIN, SULINDAC, AND ETODOLAC

Indomethacin was the product of a laboratory search for drugs with antiinflammatory properties. It was introduced in 1963 for the treatment of rheumatoid arthritis and related disorders. It is a nonselective COX inhibitor. Although indomethacin still is used clinically and is effective, toxicity and the availability of safer alternatives have limited its use. Sulindac was developed in an attempt to find a less toxic, but effective, congener of indomethacin and also is a nonselective COX inhibitor. The pharmacology of both drugs has been reviewed (Rainsford, 2003; Haanen, 2001). *Etodolac* is a structurally related tNSAID; it has been found to be a somewhat selective inhibitor of COX-2.

Indomethacin

Chemistry. The structural formula of indomethacin, a methylated indole derivative, is:

INDOMETHACIN

Pharmacological Properties. Indomethacin has prominent antiinflammatory and analgesic-antipyretic properties similar to those of the salicylates. Indomethacin is a more potent inhibitor of the cyclooxygenases than is aspirin, but patient intolerance generally limits its use to short-term dosing. Indomethacin has analgesic properties distinct from its antiinflammatory effects, and there is evidence for central and peripheral actions.

Indomethacin also inhibits the motility of polymorphonuclear leukocytes and depresses the biosynthesis of mucopolysaccharides. It also may have a direct, cyclooxygenase-independent vasoconstrictor effect (Edlund *et al.*, 1985). Observational studies have raised the possibility that indomethacin may increase the risk of myocardial infarction and stroke, but controlled clinical trials to address this hypothesis have not been performed.

Pharmacokinetics and Metabolism. Oral indomethacin has excellent bioavailability. Peak concentrations occur 1 to 2 hours after dosing (Table 26–1). Indomethacin is 90% bound to plasma proteins and tissues. The concentration of the drug in the CSF is low, but its concentration in synovial fluid is equal to that in plasma within 5 hours of administration.

Between 10% and 20% of indomethacin is excreted unchanged in the urine, partly by tubular secretion. The majority is converted to inactive metabolites, including those formed by *O*-demethylation (about 50%), conjugation with glucuronic acid (about 10%), and *N*-deacylation. Free and conjugated metabolites are eliminated in the urine, bile, and feces. There is enterohepatic cycling of the conjugates and probably of indomethacin itself. The half-life in plasma is variable, perhaps because of enterohepatic cycling, but averages about 2.5 hours.

Drug Interactions. The total plasma concentration of indomethacin plus its inactive metabolites is increased by concurrent administration of probenecid, but it is not clear if concomitant use requires dose adjustment. Indomethacin does not interfere with the uricosuric effect of probenecid.

Indomethacin does not directly modify the effect of warfarin, but platelet inhibition and gastric irritation increase the risk of bleeding; concurrent administration is not recommended. Indomethacin antagonizes the natriuretic and antihypertensive effects of *furosemide* and thiazide diuretics and blunts the antihypertensive effect of β receptor antagonists, AT_1 receptor antagonists, and ACE inhibitors.

Therapeutic Uses. A high rate of intolerance limits the long-term analgesic use of indomethacin (INDOCIN). Likewise, it is not used commonly as an analgesic or antipyretic unless the fever has been refractory to other agents (*e.g.,* Hodgkin's disease).

Indomethacin is effective for relieving joint pain, swelling, and tenderness, increasing grip strength, and decreasing the duration of morning stiffness. It is estimated to be approximately 20 times more potent than aspirin. Overall, about two-thirds of patients benefit from treatment with indomethacin, which typically is initiated at 25 mg two or three times daily. In some patients, 100 mg taken at night provides better nighttime analgesia and relief from morning stiffness. Failure to obtain adequate symptom relief with 100 mg within 7 to 10 days is an indication to try an alternative therapy.

When tolerated, indomethacin often is more effective than aspirin in the treatment of ankylosing spondylitis and osteoarthritis. It also is very effective in the treatment of acute gout, although it is not uricosuric.

Indomethacin is FDA approved for closure of persistent patent ductus arteriosus. A typical regimen involves the intravenous administration of 0.1 to 0.2 mg/kg every 12 hours for three doses. Successful closure can be expected in more than 70% of neonates treated with the drug. Such therapy is indicated primarily in premature infants who weigh between 500 and 1750 g, who have a hemodynamically significant patent ductus arteriosus, and in whom other supportive maneuvers have been attempted. Unexpectedly, treatment with indomethacin also may decrease the incidence and severity of intraventricular hemorrhage in low-birth-weight neonates (Ment *et al.*, 1994). The principal limitation of treating neonates is renal toxicity, and therapy is stopped if the output of urine falls to less than 0.6 ml/kg per hour. Renal failure, enterocolitis, thrombocytopenia, or hyperbilirubinemia are contraindications to the use of indomethacin.

Common Adverse Effects. A very high percentage (35% to 50%) of patients receiving usual therapeutic doses of indomethacin experience untoward symptoms, and about 20% must discontinue its use because of the side effects. Most adverse effects are dose-related.

Gastrointestinal complaints are common and can be serious. Diarrhea may occur and sometimes is associated with ulcerative lesions of the bowel. Underlying peptic ulcer disease is a contraindication to indomethacin use. Acute pancreatitis has been reported, as have rare, but potentially fatal, cases of hepatitis. The most frequent CNS effect (indeed, the most common side effect) is severe frontal headache, occurring in 25% to 50% of patients who take the drug for long periods. Dizziness, vertigo, light-headedness, and mental confusion may occur. Seizures have been reported, as have severe depression, psychosis, hallucinations, and suicide. Caution is advised when administering indomethacin to elderly patients or to those with underlying epilepsy, psychiatric disorders, or Parkinson's disease, because they are at greater risk for the development of serious CNS adverse effects.

Hematopoietic reactions include neutropenia, thrombocytopenia, and rarely aplastic anemia. As is common with other tNSAIDs, platelet function is impaired transiently during the dosing interval.

Sulindac

Chemistry. Sulindac is related closely to indomethacin; its structural formula is:

SULINDAC

Sulindac is a prodrug whose antiinflammatory activity resides in its sulfide metabolite.

Pharmacological Properties. Sulindac is less than half as potent as indomethacin. Because sulindac is a prodrug, it appears to be either inactive or relatively weak *in vitro* because it is not metabolized to its active sulfide metabolite. The sulfide metabolite is more than 500 times more potent than sulindac as an inhibitor of cyclooxygenase. The notion that gastric or intestinal mucosa is not directly exposed to high concentrations of active drug after oral administration of sulindac provides a rationale for the claim that there is a lower incidence of GI toxicity with sulindac as compared with indomethacin. This claim ignores the fact that the mucosa of the GI tract is directly exposed to circulating levels of active drug. Formal proof of the hypothetical advantage of sulindac is lacking, and the clinical experience in this regard has been disappointing. Similarly, early clinical studies suggesting that sulindac, in contrast to other NSAIDs, did not alter renal prostaglandin levels and therefore might avoid the association with hypertension in susceptible individuals, have been discredited (Kulling *et al.*, 1995). In short, the same precautions that apply to other NSAIDs regarding patients at risk for gastrointestinal toxicity or renal impairment also apply to sulindac.

Pharmacokinetics and Metabolism. The metabolism and pharmacokinetics of sulindac are complex. About 90% of the drug is absorbed in humans after oral administration (Table 26–1). Peak concentrations of sulindac in plasma are attained within 1 to 2 hours, while those of the sulfide metabolite occur about 8 hours after the oral administration of sulindac.

Sulindac undergoes two major biotransformations. It is oxidized to the sulfone and then reversibly reduced to the sulfide, the active metabolite. The sulfide is formed largely by the action of bowel microflora on sulindac excreted in the bile.

All three compounds are found in comparable concentrations in human plasma. The half-life of sulindac itself is about 7 hours, but the active sulfide has a half-life as long as 18 hours. Sulindac and its metabolites undergo extensive enterohepatic circulation, and all are bound extensively to plasma protein.

Little of the sulfide (or of its conjugates) is found in urine. The principal components excreted in the urine are the sulfone and its conjugates, which account for nearly 30% of an administered dose; sulindac and its conjugates account for about 20%. Up to 25% of an oral dose may appear as metabolites in the feces.

Therapeutic Uses. Sulindac (CLINORIL) has been used mainly for the treatment of rheumatoid arthritis, osteoarthritis, ankylosing spondylitis, and acute gout. Its analgesic and antiinflammatory effects are comparable to those achieved with aspirin. The most common dosage for adults is 150 to 200 mg twice a day. The drug usually is given with food to reduce gastric discomfort, although this may delay absorption and reduce its concentration in plasma. A use proposed for sulindac is to prevent colon cancer in patients with familial adenomatous polyposis (*see* above).

Common Adverse Effects. Although the incidence of toxicity is lower than with indomethacin, untoward reactions to sulindac are common. The typical gastrointestinal side effects are seen in nearly 20% of patients, but are thought to be less severe at common doses than with indomethacin. CNS side effects as described above for indomethacin are seen in up to 10% of patients. Rash and pruritus occur in 5% of patients. Transient elevations of hepatic transaminases in plasma are less common.

Etodolac

Etodolac is another acetic acid derivative with some degree of COX-2 selectivity. Thus, at antiinflammatory doses, the frequency of gastric irritation may be less than with other tNSAIDs (Warner *et al.*, 1999).

Pharmacokinetics and Metabolism. Etodolac is rapidly and well absorbed orally. It is highly bound to plasma protein and undergoes hepatic metabolism and renal excretion (Table 26–1). The drug may undergo enterohepatic circulation in humans; its half-life in plasma is about 7 hours.

Therapeutic Uses. A single oral dose (200 to 400 mg) of etodolac (LODINE) provides postoperative analgesia that typically lasts for 6 to 8 hours. Etodolac also is effective in the treatment of osteoarthritis and rheumatoid arthritis and the drug appears to be uricosuric. A sustained-release preparation (LODINE XL) is available, allowing once-a-day administration.

Common Adverse Effects. Etodolac appears to be relatively well tolerated. About 5% of patients who have taken the drug for up to 1 year discontinue treatment because of side effects, which include gastrointestinal intolerance, rashes, and CNS effects.

THE FENAMATES

The fenamates are a family of NSAIDs first discovered in the 1950s that are derivatives of *N*-phenylanthranilic acid. They include *mefenamic, meclofenamic,* and *flufenamic acids.*

Therapeutically, they have no clear advantages over several other tNSAIDs and frequently cause GI side effects.

Mefenamic acid (PONSTEL, PONSTAN [UK], DYSMAN [UK]) and *meclofenamate sodium* (MECLOMEN) have been used mostly in the short-term treatment of pain in soft-tissue injuries, dysmenorrhea, and in rheumatoid and osteoarthritis. These drugs are not recommended for use in children or pregnant women.

Mefenamic acid and meclofenamate, but not flufenamic acid, are available in the United States. All three are available in Europe. They are used rarely for chronic therapy of the arthritides.

Chemistry. Mefenamic acid and meclofenamate are *N*-substituted phenylanthranilic acids.

Pharmacological Properties. The fenamates are typical tNSAIDs. Mefenamic acid has central and peripheral actions, and meclofenamic acid (and perhaps other fenamates) may antagonize directly certain effects of prostaglandins, although it is not clear that receptor blockade is attained at therapeutic concentrations.

Pharmacokinetic Properties. These drugs are absorbed rapidly and have short durations of action. In humans, approximately 50% of a dose of mefenamic acid is excreted in the urine, primarily as the 3-hydroxymethyl and 3-carboxyl metabolites and their conjugates. Twenty percent of the drug is recovered in the feces, mainly as the unconjugated 3-carboxyl metabolite.

Common Adverse Effects and Precautions. Approximately 25% of users develop gastrointestinal side effects at therapeutic doses. Roughly 5% of patients develop a reversible elevation of hepatic transaminases. Diarrhea, which may be severe and associated with steatorrhea and inflammation of the bowel, also is relatively common. Autoimmune hemolytic anemia is a potentially serious but rare side effect.

The fenamates are contraindicated in patients with a history of gastrointestinal disease. If diarrhea or rash occur, these drugs should be stopped at once. Vigilance is required for signs or symptoms of hemolytic anemia.

TOLMETIN, KETOROLAC, AND DICLOFENAC

Tolmetin and *ketorolac* are structurally related heteroaryl acetic acid derivatives with different pharmacological fea-

tures. Diclofenac is a phenylacetic acid derivative that was developed specifically as an antiinflammatory agent.

Tolmetin

Tolmetin is an antiinflammatory, analgesic, and antipyretic agent introduced into clinical practice in the United States in 1976. Tolmetin, in recommended doses (200 to 600 mg three times a day), appears to be approximately equivalent in efficacy to moderate doses of aspirin. Tolmetin possesses typical tNSAID properties and side effects (Morley *et al.*, 1982).

Pharmacokinetics and Metabolism. Tolmetin demonstrates rapid and complete absorption, extensive plasma protein binding, and a short half-life (Table 26–1). It undergoes extensive hepatic metabolism, mostly by oxidation of the *para*-methyl group to a carboxylic acid. Metabolites are excreted in the urine. Accumulation of the drug in synovial fluid begins within 2 hours and persists for up to 8 hours after a single oral dose.

Therapeutic Uses. Tolmetin (*tolmetin sodium;* TOLECTIN) is approved in the United States for the treatment of osteoarthritis, rheumatoid arthritis, and juvenile rheumatoid arthritis; it also has been used in the treatment of ankylosing spondylitis. In general, tolmetin is thought to have similar therapeutic efficacy to aspirin. The maximum recommended dose is 2 g per day, typically given in divided doses with meals, milk, or antacids to lessen abdominal discomfort. However, peak plasma concentrations and bioavailability are reduced when the drug is taken with food.

Common Adverse Effects. Side effects occur in 25% to 40% of patients who take tolmetin, and 5% to 10% discontinue use of the drug. Gastrointestinal side effects are the most common (15%) and gastric ulceration has been observed. CNS side effects similar to those seen with indomethacin and aspirin occur, but they are less common and less severe.

Ketorolac

Ketorolac is a potent analgesic but only a moderately effective antiinflammatory drug. It is one of the few NSAIDs approved for parenteral administration. The structure of ketorolac is:

KETOROLAC

Pharmacological Properties. Ketorolac has greater systemic analgesic than antiinflammatory activity. Like other tNSAIDs, it inhibits platelet aggregation and promotes gastric ulceration. Ketorolac also has antiinflammatory activity when topically administered in the eye. The pharmacology of ketorolac has been reviewed (Buckley and Brogden, 1990).

Pharmacokinetics and Metabolism. Ketorolac has a rapid onset of action, extensive protein binding, and a short duration of action

(Table 26–1). Oral bioavailability is about 80%. Urinary excretion accounts for about 90% of eliminated drug, with about 10% excreted unchanged and the remainder as a glucuronidated conjugate. The rate of elimination is reduced in the elderly and in patients with renal failure.

Therapeutic Uses. Ketorolac (administered as the tromethamine salt TORADOL, ULTRAM) has been used as a short-term alternative (less than 5 days) to opioids for the treatment of moderate to severe pain and is administered intramuscularly, intravenously, or orally. Unlike opioids, tolerance, withdrawal, and respiratory depression do not occur. Like other NSAIDs, aspirin sensitivity is a contraindication to the use of ketorolac. Typical doses are 30 to 60 mg (intramuscular); 15 to 30 mg (intravenous); and 5 to 30 mg (oral). Ketorolac is used widely in postoperative patients, but it should not be used for routine obstetric analgesia. Topical (ophthalmic) ketorolac is FDA approved for the treatment of seasonal allergic conjunctivitis and postoperative ocular inflammation after cataract extraction.

Common Adverse Effects. Side effects at usual oral doses include somnolence, dizziness, headache, gastrointestinal pain, dyspepsia, nausea, and pain at the site of injection.

Diclofenac

Diclofenac is the most commonly used tNSAID in Europe (McNeely and Goa, 1999). The selective inhibitor of COX-2 lumiracoxib is an analog of diclofenac. The structure of diclofenac is:

DICLOFENAC

Pharmacological Properties. Diclofenac has analgesic, antipyretic, and antiinflammatory activities. Its potency against COX-2 is substantially greater than that of indomethacin, naproxen, or several other tNSAIDs. In addition, diclofenac appears to reduce intracellular concentrations of free AA in leukocytes, perhaps by altering its release or uptake. The selectivity of diclofenac for COX-2 resembles that of celecoxib. Indeed, the incidence of serious gastrointestinal adverse effects did not differ between celecoxib and diclofenac in the CLASS trial (Juni *et al.*, 2002). Furthermore, observational studies have raised the possibility of a cardiovascular hazard from chronic therapy with diclofenac. A large-scale randomized comparison of diclofenac and the selective COX-2 inhibitor etoricoxib is currently under way.

Pharmacokinetics. Diclofenac has rapid absorption, extensive protein binding, and a short half-life (Table 26–2). There is a substantial first-pass effect, such that only about 50% of diclofenac is available systemically. Diclofenac accumulates in synovial fluid after oral administration, which may explain why its duration of therapeutic effect is considerably longer than the plasma half-life. Diclofenac is metabolized in the liver by a

member of the CYP2C subfamily to 4-hydroxydiclofenac, the principal metabolite, and other hydroxylated forms; after glucuronidation and sulfation the metabolites are excreted in the urine (65%) and bile (35%).

Therapeutic Uses. Diclofenac is approved in the United States for the long-term symptomatic treatment of rheumatoid arthritis, osteoarthritis, and ankylosing spondylitis. Three formulations are available: an intermediate-release potassium salt (CATAFLAM), a delayed-release form (VOLTARIN, VOLTAROL [UK]), and an extended-release form (VOLTARIN-XR). The usual daily dosage for those indications is 100 to 200 mg, given in several divided doses. Diclofenac also is useful for short-term treatment of acute musculoskeletal pain, postoperative pain, and dysmenorrhea. Diclofenac is also available in combination with misoprostol, a PGE_1 analog (ARTHROTEC) (Davis *et al.*, 1995). This combination, which retains the efficacy of diclofenac while reducing the frequency of gastrointestinal ulcers and erosions, is cost-effective relative to the selective COX-2 inhibitors despite the cost of the added misoprostol (Morant *et al.*, 2002). In addition, an ophthalmic solution of diclofenac is available for treatment of postoperative inflammation following cataract extraction.

Common Adverse Effects. Diclofenac produces side effects (particularly gastrointestinal) in about 20% of patients, and approximately 2% of patients discontinue therapy as a result. Modest elevation of hepatic transaminases in plasma occurs in 5% to 15% of patients. Although usually moderate, transaminase values may increase more than threefold in a small percentage of patients. The elevations usually are reversible. Another member of this phenylacetic acid family of NSAIDs, *bromfenac*, was withdrawn from the market because of its association with severe, irreversible liver injury in some patients. Therefore, transaminases should be measured during the first 8 weeks of therapy with diclofenac, and the drug should be discontinued if abnormal values persist or if other signs or symptoms develop. Other untoward responses to diclofenac include CNS effects, rashes, allergic reactions, fluid retention, and edema, and rarely impairment of renal function. The drug is not recommended for children, nursing mothers, or pregnant women. Consistent with its preference for COX-2, and unlike ibuprofen, diclofenac does not interfere with the antiplatelet effect of aspirin (Catella-Lawson *et al.*, 2001). Given these observations, diclofenac is not a suitable alternative to a selective COX-2 inhibitor in individuals at risk of cardiovascular or cerebrovascular disease.

PROPIONIC ACID DERIVATIVES

Propionic acid derivatives are approved for use in the symptomatic treatment of rheumatoid arthritis, osteoarthritis, ankylosing spondylitis, and acute gouty arthritis; they also are used as analgesics, for acute tendinitis and bursitis, and for primary dysmenorrhea.

Ibuprofen, the most commonly used tNSAID in the United States, was the first member of the propionic acid class of NSAIDs to come into general use, and it is available without a prescription in the United States. Naprox-

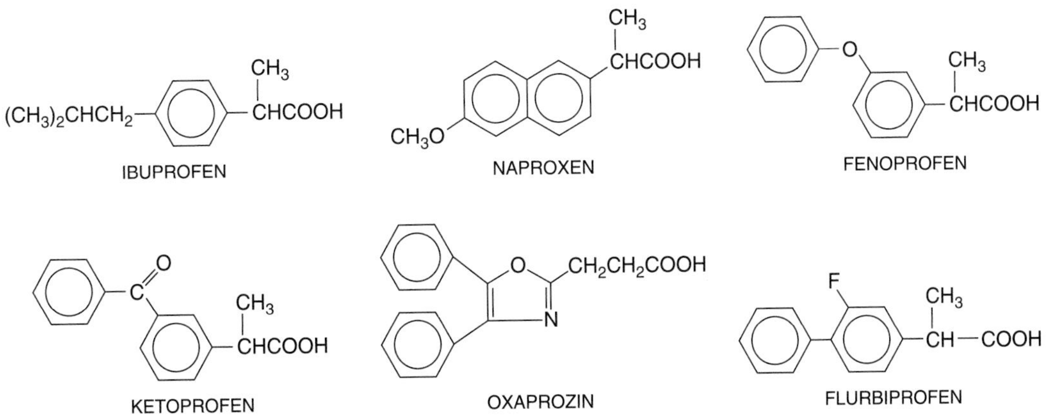

Figure 26–3. Chemical structures of the propionic acid derivatives.

en, also available without prescription, has a longer but variable half-life, making twice-daily administration feasible (and perhaps once daily in some individuals). Oxaprozin also has a long half-life and may possibly be given once daily. The structural formulas of these drugs are shown in Figure 26–3.

Small clinical studies suggest that the propionic acid derivatives are comparable in efficacy to aspirin for the control of the signs and symptoms of rheumatoid arthritis and osteoarthritis, perhaps with improved tolerability.

Ibuprofen, naproxen, *flurbiprofen,* fenoprofen, ketoprofen, and *oxaprozin*, which are available in the United States, are described individually below. Several additional agents in this class are in use or under study in other countries. These include *fenbufen, carprofen, pirprofen, indobufen,* and *tiaprofenic acid.*

Pharmacological Properties. The pharmacodynamic properties of the propionic acid derivatives do not differ significantly. All are nonselective cyclooxygenase inhibitors with the effects and side effects common to other tNSAIDs. Although there is considerable variation in their potency as COX inhibitors, this is not of obvious clinical consequence. Some of the propionic acid derivatives, particularly naproxen, have prominent inhibitory effects on leukocyte function, and some data suggest that naproxen may have slightly better efficacy with regard to analgesia and relief of morning stiffness (Hart and Huskisson, 1984). Epidemiological studies suggest that while the relative risk of myocardial infarction is unaltered by ibuprofen, it is reduced by around 10% by naproxen, compared to a reduction of 20% to 25% by aspirin. This suggestion of benefit accords with the clinical pharmacology of naproxen that suggests that some but not all individuals dosed with 500 mg twice daily sustain platelet inhibition throughout the dosing interval.

Drug Interactions. As do other NSAIDs, the propionic acid derivatives may interfere with the action of antihypertensive and diuretic agents, increase the risk of bleeding with warfarin, and increase the risk of bone marrow suppression with methotrexate. Ibuprofen also has been shown to interfere with the antiplatelet effects of aspirin (*see* above). There is also evidence for a similar interaction between aspirin and naproxen. In addition, propionic acid derivatives may interact with other drugs due to the high avidity for albumin. However, they have not been shown to alter the pharmacokinetics of the oral hypoglycemic drugs or warfarin.

Ibuprofen

Ibuprofen is supplied as tablets containing 200 to 800 mg; only the 200-mg tablets (ADVIL, MOTRIN, NUPRIN, BRUFEN [UK], ANADIN ULTRA [UK], others) are available without a prescription.

Doses of up to 800 mg four times daily can be used in the treatment of rheumatoid arthritis and osteoarthritis, but lower doses often are adequate. The usual dose for mild to moderate pain, such as that of primary dysmenorrhea, is 400 mg every 4 to 6 hours as needed. Ibuprofen has been reviewed (Davies, 1998a).

Pharmacokinetics. Ibuprofen is absorbed rapidly, bound avidly to protein, and undergoes hepatic metabolism (90% is metabolized to hydroxylate or carboxylate derivatives) and renal excretion of metabolites. The half-life is roughly 2 hours. Slow equilibration with the synovial space means that its antiarthritic effects may persist after plasma levels decline. In experimental animals, ibuprofen and its metabolites readily cross the placenta.

Common Adverse Effects. Ibuprofen is thought to be better tolerated than aspirin and indomethacin and has been used in patients with a history of gastrointestinal intolerance to other NSAIDs. Nevertheless, 5% to 15% of patients experience gastrointestinal side effects.

Other adverse effects of ibuprofen have been reported less frequently. They include thrombocytopenia, rashes, headache, dizziness, blurred vision, and in a few cases toxic amblyopia, fluid retention, and edema. Patients who develop ocular disturbances should discontinue the use of ibuprofen. Ibuprofen can be used occasionally by pregnant women; however, the concerns apply regarding third-trimester effects, including delay of parturition. Excretion into breast milk is thought to be minimal, so ibuprofen also can be used with caution by women who are breastfeeding.

Naproxen

The pharmacological properties and therapeutic uses of naproxen (ALEVE, NAPROSYN, others) have been reviewed (Davies and Anderson, 1997).

Pharmacokinetics. Naproxen is absorbed fully when administered orally. Food delays the rate but not the extent of absorption. Peak concentrations in plasma occur within 2 to 4 hours and are somewhat more rapid after the administration of naproxen sodium. Absorption is accelerated by the concurrent administration of sodium bicarbonate but delayed by magnesium oxide or aluminum hydroxide. Naproxen also is absorbed rectally, but more slowly than after oral administration. The half-life of naproxen in plasma is variable. About 14 hours in the young, it may increase about twofold in the elderly because of age-related decline in renal function (Table 26–1).

Metabolites of naproxen are excreted almost entirely in the urine. About 30% of the drug undergoes 6-demethylation, and most of this metabolite, as well as naproxen itself, is excreted as the glucuronide or other conjugates.

Naproxen is almost completely (99%) bound to plasma proteins after normal therapeutic doses. Naproxen crosses the placenta and appears in the milk of lactating women at approximately 1% of the maternal plasma concentration.

Common Adverse Effects. Typical gastrointestinal adverse effects with naproxen occur at approximately the same frequency as with indomethacin, but perhaps with less severity. CNS side effects range from drowsiness, headache, dizziness, and sweating, to fatigue, depression, and ototoxicity. Less common reactions include pruritus and a variety of dermatological problems. A few instances of jaundice, impairment of renal function, angioedema, thrombocytopenia, and agranulocytosis have been reported.

Fenoprofen

The pharmacological properties and therapeutic uses of fenoprofen (NALFON) have been reviewed (Brogden *et al.*, 1981).

Pharmacokinetics and Metabolism. Oral doses of fenoprofen are readily but incompletely (85%) absorbed. The presence of food in the stomach retards absorption and lowers peak concentrations in plasma, which usually are achieved within 2 hours. The concomitant administration of antacids does not seem to alter the concentrations that are achieved.

After absorption, fenoprofen binds avidly to protein, is extensively metabolized, and is excreted in the urine with a half-life of approximately 3 hours (Table 26–1).

Common Adverse Effects. The gastrointestinal side effects of fenoprofen are similar to those of ibuprofen or naproxen and occur in approximately 15% of patients.

Ketoprofen

Ketoprofen (ORUDIS, ORUVAIL) shares the pharmacological properties of other propionic acid derivatives (Veys, 1991) and is available for sale without a prescription in the United States. A more potent S-enantiomer is available in Europe (Barbanoj *et al.*, 2001). In addition to COX inhibition, ketoprofen may stabilize lysosomal membranes and antagonize the actions of bradykinin. It is unknown if these actions are relevant to its efficacy in humans.

Pharmacokinetics. Ketoprofen demonstrates a pharmacokinetic profile similar to fenoprofen (Table 26–1). It has a half-life in plasma of about 2 hours except in the elderly, in whom it is slightly prolonged. Ketoprofen is conjugated with glucuronic acid in the liver, and the conjugate is excreted in the urine. Patients with impaired renal function eliminate the drug more slowly.

Common Adverse Effects.
Approximately 30% of patients experience mild gastrointestinal side effects with ketoprofen, which are decreased if the drug is taken with food or antacids. Ketoprofen can cause fluid retention and increased plasma concentrations of creatinine. These effects generally are transient and asymptomatic and are more common in patients who are receiving diuretics or in those older than 60. Thus, renal function should be monitored in such patients.

Flurbiprofen

The pharmacological properties, therapeutic indications, and adverse effects of flurbiprofen (ANSAID) are similar to those of other antiinflammatory derivatives of propionic acid (Table 26–1) and have been reviewed (Davies, 1995). Flurbiprofen also has been investigated as an antiplatelet therapy; however, evidence that it offers an advantage over aspirin in this regard has not appeared.

Oxaprozin

Oxaprozin (DAYPRO) has similar pharmacological properties, adverse effects, and therapeutic uses to those of other propionic acid derivatives (Davies, 1998b). However, its pharmacokinetic properties differ considerably. Peak plasma levels are not achieved until 3 to 6 hours after an oral dose, while its half-life of 40 to 60 hours allows for once-daily administration.

ENOLIC ACIDS (OXICAMS)

The oxicam derivatives are enolic acids that inhibit COX-1 and COX-2 and have antiinflammatory, analgesic, and antipyretic activity. In general, they are nonselective COX inhibitors, although one member (meloxicam) shows modest COX-2 selectivity comparable to celecoxib in human blood *in vitro* and was approved as a selective COX-2 inhibitor in some countries (*see* below). They are similar in efficacy to aspirin, indomethacin, or naproxen for the long-term treatment of rheumatoid arthritis or osteoarthritis. Controlled trials comparing gastrointestinal tolerability with aspirin have not been performed. The main advantage suggested for these compounds is their long half-life, which permits once-a-day dosing.

Piroxicam

The pharmacological properties and therapeutic uses of piroxicam have been reviewed (Guttadauria, 1986).

Pharmacological Properties. Piroxicam is effective as an anti-inflammatory agent. It can inhibit activation of neutrophils, apparently independently of its ability to inhibit cyclooxygenase; hence, additional modes of antiinflammatory action have been proposed, including inhibition of proteoglycanase and collagenase in cartilage. Approximately 20% of patients experience side effects with piroxicam, and about 5% of patients discontinue use because of these effects.

Pharmacokinetics and Metabolism. Piroxicam is absorbed completely after oral administration and undergoes enterohepatic recirculation; peak concentrations in plasma occur within 2 to 4 hours (Table 26–1). Food may delay absorption. Estimates of the half-life in plasma have been variable; the average is roughly 50 hours.

After absorption, piroxicam is extensively (99%) bound to plasma proteins. Concentrations in plasma and synovial fluid are similar at steady state (*e.g.,* after 7 to 12 days). Less than 5% of the drug is excreted into the urine unchanged. The major metabolic transformation in humans is CYP-mediated hydroxylation of the pyridyl ring (predominantly by an isozyme of the CYP2C subfamily), and this inactive metabolite and its glucuronide conjugate account for about 60% of the drug excreted in the urine and feces.

Therapeutic Uses. Piroxicam (FELDENE) is approved in the United States for the treatment of rheumatoid arthritis and osteoarthritis. Due to its slow onset of action and delayed attainment of steady state, it is less suited for acute analgesia but has been used in acute gout. Caution is warranted in patients taking lithium because piroxicam can reduce the renal excretion of this drug to a clinically significant extent. The usual daily dose is 20 mg and because of the long half-life, steady-state blood levels are not reached for 7 to 12 days.

Meloxicam

Meloxicam (MOBIC) was approved recently by the FDA for use in osteoarthritis. It has been reviewed (Fleischmann *et al.*, 2002).

The recommended dose for meloxicam is 7.5 to 15 mg once daily for osteoarthritis and 15 mg once daily for rheumatoid arthritis.

Meloxicam demonstrates roughly tenfold COX-2 selectivity on average in *ex vivo* assays (Panara *et al.*, 1999). However, this is quite variable, and a clinical advantage or hazard has yet to be established. Indeed, even with surrogate markers, the relationship to dose is nonlinear. There is significantly less gastric injury compared to piroxicam (20 mg/day) in subjects treated with 7.5 mg/day of meloxicam, but the advantage is lost with 15 mg/day (Patoia *et al.*, 1996). Like diclofenac, meloxicam would not seem like a desirable alternative to prescribing celecoxib to patients at increased risk of myocardial infarction or stroke.

Other Oxicams

A number of other oxicam derivatives are under study or in use outside of the United States. These include several prodrugs of piroxicam (*ampiroxicam, droxicam,* and *pivoxicam*), which have been designed to reduce gastrointestinal irritation. However, as with sulindac, any theoretical diminution in gastric toxicity associated with administration of a prodrug is offset by gastric COX-1 inhibition from active drug circulating systemically. Other oxicams under study or in use outside the United States include *lornoxicam* (XEFO [UK]) (Balfour *et al.*, 1996), *cinnoxicam* (SINARTROL [ITALY]), *sudoxicam,* and *tenoxicam* (Nilsen, 1994). The efficacy and toxicity of these drugs are similar to those of piroxicam. Lornoxicam is unique among the enolic acid derivatives in that it has a rapid onset of action and a relatively short half-life (3 to 5 hours) (Skjodt and Davies, 1998).

Nabumetone

Nabumetone is an antiinflammatory agent approved in 1991 for use in the United States. It has been reviewed (Davies, 1997). The structure of nabumetone is:

NABUMETONE

Clinical trials with nabumetone (RELAFEN) have indicated substantial efficacy in the treatment of rheumatoid arthritis and osteoarthritis, with a relatively low incidence of side effects. The dose typically is 1000 mg given once daily. The drug also has off-label use in the short-term treatment of soft-tissue injuries.

Pharmacological Properties. Nabumetone is a prodrug; thus it is a weak inhibitor of COX *in vitro* but a potent COX inhibitor *in vivo*.

Pharmacokinetics and Metabolism. Nabumetone is absorbed rapidly and is converted in the liver to one or more active metabolites, principally 6-methoxy-2-naphthylacetic acid, a potent nonselective inhibitor of COX (Patrignani *et al.*, 1994). This metabolite, inactivated by *O*-demethylation in the liver, is then conjugated before excretion and is eliminated with a half-life of about 24 hours.

Side Effects. Nabumetone is associated with crampy lower abdominal pain and diarrhea, but the incidence of gastrointestinal ulceration appears to be lower than with other tNSAIDs (Scott *et al.*, 2000), although randomized, controlled studies directly comparing tolerability and clinical outcomes have not been performed. Other side effects include rash, headache, dizziness, heartburn, tinnitus, and pruritus.

PYRAZOLON DERIVATIVES

This group of drugs includes *phenylbutazone, oxyphenbutazone, antipyrine, aminopyrine,* and *dipyrone;* currently, only antipyrine otic drops are available in the United States. These drugs were used clinically for many years but have essentially been abandoned because of their propensity to cause irreversible agranulocytosis. Dipyrone was reintroduced in Europe approximately 10 years ago because epidemiological studies suggested that the risk of adverse effects was similar to that of acetaminophen and lower than that of aspirin. However, its use remains limited. The pyrazolone derivatives are discussed in previous editions of this book.

CYCLCOOXYGENASE-2 SELECTIVE NSAIDS

The therapeutic use of the tNSAIDs has been limited by poor tolerability. Chronic users are prone to experience gastrointestinal irritation in up to 20% of cases. However, the incidence of these adverse events had been falling sharply in the population prior to the introduction of the coxibs, perhaps reflecting a move away from use of high-dose aspirin as an antiinflammatory drug strategy. Studies of the immediate early genes induced by inflammation led to the discovery of a gene with significant homology to the original COX enzyme, now designated COX-2. Because expression of this second COX enzyme was regulated by cytokines and mitogens, it was proposed to be the dominant source of prostaglandin formation in inflammation and cancer. It further was proposed that the original, constitutively expressed COX was the predominant source of cytoprotective prostaglandins formed by the gastrointestinal epithelium. Thus, selective inhibition of COX-2 was postulated to afford efficacy similar to tNSAIDs but with better tolerability. Subsequent crystallization of COX-1 and COX-2 revealed remarkable conservation of tertiary structure. However, one difference was in the hydrophobic channel by which the AA substrate gains access to the COX active site, buried deep within the molecule. This channel is more accommodating in the COX-2 structure and consequently exhibits wider substrate specificity than in COX-1. It also contains a side pocket that in retrospect affords a structural explanation for the identification in screens of the two enzymes *in vitro* of small molecule inhibitors that are differentially specific for COX-2 (Smith *et al.*, 2000). Although there were differences in relative hierarchies, depending on whether screens were performed using recombinantly expressed enzymes, cells, or whole blood assays, most tNSAIDs expressed similar selectivity for inhibition of the two enzymes.

This section focuses on drugs that were developed specifically to favor inhibition of COX-2, of which the initial class are the coxibs. As discussed above, several older drugs (*e.g.,* nimesulide [not available in the United States], diclofenac, and meloxicam) exhibit relative selectivity for COX-2 inhibition in whole blood assays that resembles that of the first-approved specific inhibitor of COX-2, celecoxib (Brune and Hinz, 2004; FitzGerald and Patrono, 2001).

Three members of the initial class of COX-2 inhibitors, the coxibs, were approved for use in the United States and Europe. Both rofecoxib and valdecoxib have now been withdrawn from the market in view of their adverse event profile. Two others, *parecoxib* and etoricoxib, are approved in Europe but still under consideration in the United States. The newest drug in the class, lumiracoxib, is under consideration for approval in Europe and the United States. The relative degree of selectivity for COX-2 inhibition is lumiracoxib = etoricoxib > valdecoxib = rofecoxib >> celecoxib. However, there is considerable difference in response to the coxibs among individuals and it is not known how the degree of selectivity may relate to either efficacy or adverse effect profile, although it seems likely to be related to both. No controlled clinical trials comparing outcomes among the coxibs have been performed. The chemical structures of the coxibs are shown in Figure 26–4.

Pharmacokinetics. Most of the coxibs are distributed widely throughout the body. Celecoxib is particularly lipophilic, so it accumulates in fat and is readily transported into the CNS. Lumiracoxib is more acidic than the others, which may favor its accumulation at sites of inflammation. Despite these subtle differences, all of the coxibs achieve sufficient brain concentrations to have a central analgesic effect and all reduce prostaglandin formation in inflamed joints. All are well absorbed, but peak concentrations are achieved with lumiracoxib and etoricoxib in approximately 1 hour compared to 2 to 4 hours with the other agents (Table 26–1). All of the coxibs are extensively protein-bound (etoricoxib and rofecoxib approximately 90%, the others approximately 97% to 99%). Published estimates of the half-lives of these drugs vary (2 to 6 hours for lumiracoxib, 6 to 12 hours for celecoxib and valdecoxib, 15 to 18 hours for rofecoxib, and 20 to 26 hours for etoricoxib). However, peak plasma concentrations of lumiracoxib exceed considerably those necessary to inhibit COX-2, suggesting an extended pharmacodynamic half-life. Few data linking pharmacokinetics to pharmacodynamics for any of the coxibs are in the public domain. Likewise, there is little information on the

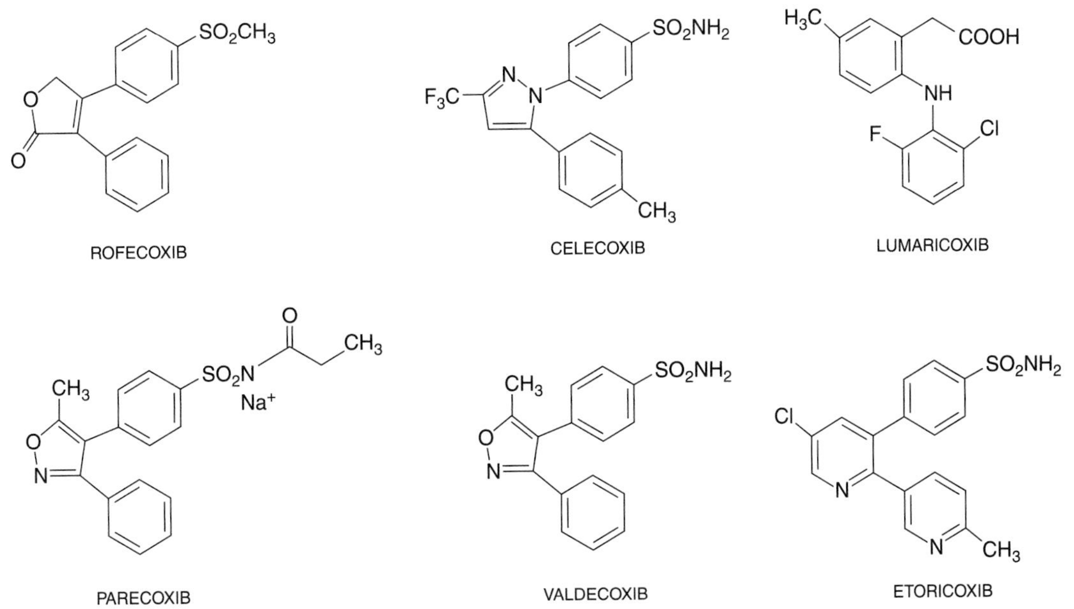

Figure 26–4. *Chemical structures of the coxibs.*

causes of inter- and intraindividual variability in drug response, which is considerable.

Drug–Drug Interactions. The coxibs are metabolized by a variety of CYPs, including CYP3A, CYP2C9, CYP2D6, and CYP1A2. Rofecoxib differs slightly in that the first step in its metabolism is catalyzed by cytosolic reductases. Celecoxib, valdecoxib, and the prodrug parecoxib all are metabolized predominantly by CYP2D6, which metabolizes approximately 20% of all drugs (*see* Chapter 3). Although it is poorly inducible, it has pharmacogenetic importance because polymorphic variants with very low activity differ in frequency among populations. The prevalence of homozygosity for these variants is approximately 10% in Caucasians, 5% in Indians, 2% to 3% in Africans, and 1% in Asians. Poor metabolizers are prone to develop high concentrations of relevant NSAIDs, while extensive metabolizers are prone to drug interactions involving competitive inhibition of the enzyme. For example, celecoxib inhibits the metabolism of *metoprolol* and results in its accumulation. Similar interactions have been observed with selective serotonin reuptake inhibitors, tricyclic antidepressants, some neuroleptic agents, and antiarrhythmic drugs. Valdecoxib (and parecoxib) are prone to similar interactions, while rofecoxib interacts with *theophylline.* Unlike tNSAIDs, specific inhibitors of COX-2 would not be expected to pharmacodynamically augment the bleeding risk on warfarin. However, both rofecoxib and valdecoxib may influence the disposition of warfarin, increasing measures of drug action such as the prothrombin times and amplifying the risk of bleeding. There are anecdotal suggestions of an interaction with methotrexate resulting in bone marrow depression. Specific COX-2 inhibitors, like tNSAIDs, may limit the effectiveness of several classes of antihypertensive drugs. Presently, the comparative incidence of renovascular complications on tNSAIDs *versus* COX-2 selective inhibitors is unknown. As with all NSAIDs, use of these drugs must be cau-

tious in patients with secondary hyperaldosteronism due to hepatic, cardiac, or renal decompensation.

Clinical Use. The first COX-2 inhibitors (*e.g.,* celecoxib, rofecoxib, and valdecoxib) gained FDA approval based on a superior side-effect profile in gastrointestinal endoscopy studies when compared to tNSAIDs. Subsequent to approval, clinical outcome studies against tNSAIDs were performed with celecoxib (the CLASS study; Silverstein *et al.,* 2000) and rofecoxib (the VIGOR study; Bombardier *et al.,* 2000). Only one of these, the VIGOR study, reported a significant difference in clinically significant gastrointestinal outcomes; these were halved from 4% on the tNSAID comparator, naproxen, to 2% on rofecoxib. Publication of the full dataset of the CLASS study revealed no difference between celecoxib and its comparators, ibuprofen and diclofenac (Juni *et al.,* 2002). While the results of these trials are reflected in the labeling of the coxibs, the data did not justify labeling the COX-2 selective inhibitors as a drug class distinct from the NSAIDs. All three of the FDA-approved coxibs have been shown to afford relief from postextraction dental pain and to afford dose-dependent relief from inflammation in osteoarthritis and rheumatoid arthritis. Celecoxib also is approved for the chemoprevention of polyposis coli; however, a placebo-controlled trial revealed a dose-dependent increase in myocardial infarction and stroke (Bresalier *et al.,* 2005).

Celecoxib

Celecoxib (CELEBREX) was approved for marketing in the United States in 1998. Details of its pharmacology have been reviewed (Davies *et al.*, 2000).

Pharmacokinetics. The bioavailability of oral celecoxib is not known, but peak plasma levels occur at 2 to 4 hours postdose. Celecoxib is bound extensively to plasma proteins. Little drug is excreted unchanged; most is excreted as carboxylic acid and glucuronide metabolites in the urine and feces. The elimination half-life is approximately 11 hours. The drug commonly is given once or twice per day during chronic treatment. Renal insufficiency is associated with a modest, clinically insignificant decrease in plasma concentration. Celecoxib has not been studied in patients with severe renal insufficiency. Plasma concentrations are increased by approximately 40% and 180% in patients with mild and moderate hepatic impairment, respectively, and dosages should be reduced by at least 50% in patients with moderate hepatic impairment. Significant interactions occur with *fluconazole* and *lithium* but not with *ketoconazole* or methotrexate. Celecoxib is metabolized predominantly by CYP2C9. Although not a substrate, celecoxib also is an inhibitor of CYP2D6. Clinical vigilance is necessary during coadministration of drugs that are known to inhibit CYP2C9 and drugs that are metabolized by CYP2D6.

Pharmacological Properties, Adverse Effects, and Therapeutic Uses. Effects attributed to inhibition of prostaglandin production in the kidney—hypertension and edema—occur with nonselective COX inhibitors and also with celecoxib. Studies in mice and some epidemiological evidence suggest that the likelihood of hypertension on NSAIDs reflects the degree of inhibition of COX-2 and the selectivity with which it is attained. Thus, the risk of thrombosis, hypertension, and accelerated atherogenesis are mechanistically integrated. The coxibs should be avoided in patients prone to cardiovascular or cerebrovascular disease. None of the coxibs has established clinical efficacy over tNSAIDs, while celecoxib has failed to establish superiority over tNSAIDs in reducing gastrointestinal adverse events. While selective COX-2 inhibitors do not interact to prevent the antiplatelet effect of aspirin, it now is thought that they lose their gastrointestinal advantage over a tNSAID alone when used in conjunction with aspirin. Experience with selective COX-2 inhibitors in patients who exhibit aspirin hypersensitivity is limited, and caution should be observed.

Celecoxib is approved in the United States for the treatment of osteoarthritis and rheumatoid arthritis. The recommended dose for treating osteoarthritis is 200 mg per day as a single dose or as two 100-mg doses. In the treatment of rheumatoid arthritis, the recommended dose is 100 to 200 mg twice per day. In the light of recent information on a potential cardiovascular hazard, physicians are advised to use the lowest possible dose for the shortest possible time. Current evidence does not support use of a coxib as a first choice among the tNSAIDs.

Valdecoxib

Pharmacokinetics. Valdecoxib (BEXTRA) is absorbed rapidly (1 to 2 hours), but peak serum concentrations are delayed by the presence of food (Table 26–1). It undergoes extensive hepatic metabolism by CYP3A4 and CYP2C9 and non–CYP-dependent glucu-

ronidation. Valdecoxib is a weak inhibitor of CYP2C9 and a weak to moderate inhibitor of CYP2C19. Concomitant administration of valdecoxib with known CYP3A4 and 2C9 inhibitors (*e.g.*, fluconazole and ketoconazole) increases plasma levels of valdecoxib. Coadministration of valdecoxib with warfarin (a CYP2C9 substrate) caused a small but significant increase in the plasma level and anticoagulation effect of warfarin. Interactions with *diazepam, glyburide, norethindrone, ethinyl estradiol, omeprazole,* and *dextromethorphan* also have been documented. The metabolites of valdecoxib are excreted in the urine. The half-life is approximately 7 to 8 hours but can be significantly prolonged in the elderly or those with hepatic impairment, with subsequent drug accumulation (Fenton *et al.*, 2004). Outside the United States, valdecoxib is available for injection.

Pharmacological Properties, Adverse Effects, and Therapeutic Uses. At therapeutic doses, valdecoxib has demonstrated significantly fewer endoscopically demonstrable lesions than tNSAIDs. Like other NSAIDs, valdecoxib can elevate blood pressure in predisposed individuals (Fenton *et al.*, 2004). Valdecoxib has received FDA approval for use in osteoarthritis, adult rheumatoid arthritis, and primary dysmenorrhea. It is also effective in moderate to severe acute pain, particularly if given preemptively (*e.g.*, before a dental procedure) and has been shown to decrease postoperative opioid requirements substantially (Fenton *et al.*, 2004). However, valdecoxib has been associated with a threefold increase in cardiovascular risk in two studies of patients undergoing cardiovascular bypass graft surgery (Furberg *et al.*, 2005). As with celecoxib, the FDA advisory committee reviewed the totality of the evidence and concluded that valdecoxib did indeed elevate the risk of heart attack and stroke and should be avoided in patients prone to these conditions. An additional concern was the causative link to Stevens-Johnson syndrome, a disfiguring skin condition that rarely complicates sulfonamides, like valdecoxib. Based on these considerations and the absence of established benefit compared to traditional NSAIDs, the FDA prompted withdrawal of valdecoxib from the market. No gastrointestinal outcome study with valdecoxib has been performed and there is no evidence that its clinical efficacy exceeds that of tNSAIDs. Thus, current evidence of benefit:risk would not support selection of valdecoxib as an NSAID of first choice, if at all. Finally, life-threatening skin reactions (including toxic epidermal necrolysis, Stevens-Johnson syndrome, and erythema multiforme) have been reported in association with valdecoxib. The drug must be discontinued at the first sign of rash, mucosal lesion, or any other sign of hypersensitivity. This additional hazard renders valdecoxib an unlikely therapeutic choice.

Rofecoxib

Rofecoxib (VIOXX) was introduced in 1999. Details of its pharmacodynamics, pharmacokinetics, therapeutic efficacy, and toxicity have been reviewed (Davies *et al.*, 2003). Based on interim analysis of data from the Adenomatous Polyp Prevention on Vioxx (APPROVe) study, which showed a significant (twofold) increase in the incidence of serious thromboembolic events in subjects receiving 25 mg of rofecoxib relative to placebo (Bresalier *et al.*, 2005), rofecoxib was withdrawn from the market worldwide (FitzGerald, 2004). The FDA advisory panel agreed that rofecoxib increased the risk of myocardial infarction and stroke and that the evidence accumulated was more substantial than for valdecoxib and appeared more convincing than for celecoxib. Only rofecoxib, however, has established superiority over tNSAIDs in terms of gastrointestinal outcomes, which adjusts the risk:benefit ratio. If reintroduced, it would only merit consideration in patients with severe gastrointestinal intolerance of tNSAIDs who were at demonstrably low risk of cardiovascular or cerebrovascular disease.

Other Coxibs

Clinical experience with other coxibs is limited. Parecoxib is a prodrug of valdecoxib and can be administered parenterally. Etoricoxib is given once a day and has been on the market in Europe. The European regulatory agency concluded that it, along with other coxibs, increased the risk of heart attack and stroke; they restricted specifically its use in patients with hypertension. Lumiracoxib is still under review in both Europe and the United States. Pharmacokinetic considerations are outlined in Table 26–1.

Parecoxib. **Pharmacokinetics.** Parecoxib is available outside of the United States for intravenous and intramuscular injection. It is absorbed rapidly (approximately 15 minutes) and converted (15 to 52 minutes) by deoxymethylation to valdecoxib, the active drug (Table 26–1) (Karim *et al.*, 2001).

Pharmacological Properties, Common Adverse Effects, and Therapeutic Uses. Parecoxib (DYNASTAT) is available in Germany and Australia, but not in the United Kingdom or United States. It is the only coxib available by injection and has been shown to be an effective analgesic for the perioperative period when patients are unable to take oral medication. However, it is not yet widely available, and clinical experience is limited. In general, the advantages and disadvantages pertaining to valdecoxib (*see* above) apply to parecoxib, including the risk of hypersensitivity or skin reactions.

Lumiracoxib. **Pharmacokinetics.** Lumiracoxib is unique among the coxibs in being a weak acid. It is rapidly and well absorbed, with peak plasma concentrations occurring in 1 to 3 hours. Its acidic nature allows it to penetrate well into areas of inflammation. The half-life in synovial fluid is considerably longer than in plasma. The concentration of lumiracoxib in synovial fluid 24 hours after administration of a single dose would be expected to result in substantial COX-2 inhibition. This may explain why once-daily dosing may suffice for some users despite its short plasma half-life. However, peak plasma concentrations greatly exceed those necessary to maximally inhibit COX-2, consistent with a longer pharmacodynamic half-life, reflected by sustained inhibition of prostacyclin metabolite excretion comparable to that observed with other coxibs. *In vitro*, lumiracoxib demonstrates greater COX-2 selectivity than any of the currently available coxibs (Tacconelli *et al.*, 2004).

Pharmacological Properties, Common Adverse Effects, and Therapeutic Uses. Lumiracoxib demonstrates potency similar to naproxen but with much greater COX-2 selectivity. Studies in small numbers of subjects showed little or no endoscopic evidence of gastric injury at high therapeutic doses (Kivitz *et al.*, 2004; Atherton *et al.*, 2004). It has been shown to be effective in the treatment of dysmenorrhea with efficacy similar to naproxen (Bitner *et al.*, 2004). It should be noted that these were not equivalence studies.

Further information regarding the safety of lumiracoxib has been provided by findings of the Therapeutic Arthritis Research and Gastrointestinal Event Trial (TARGET; Farkouh *et al.*, 2004; Schnitzer *et al.*, 2004). The trial actually consisted of two distinct studies comparing lumiracoxib to either ibuprofen or naproxen in more than 18,000 osteoarthritis patients in aggregate. Patients were aged 50 years or older and the trials were stratified on the basis of low-dose aspirin. Patients with significant preexisting coronary artery disease were excluded. TARGET detected an excess number of myocardial infarctions among patients taking lumiracoxib compared to naproxen and this difference was attenuated by aspirin. By contrast, ibuprofen appeared to undermine the beneficial effects of aspirin. The cardiovascular event rates on lumiracoxib differed considerably between the two studies, making their combined assessment complex. TARGET was grossly underpowered to assess the relative impact of lumiracoxib *versus* the tNSAIDs on vascular events. While lumiracoxib elevated blood pressure to a marginally lesser degree than the NSAIDs, these differences of a few millimeters of mercury on average were assessed retrospectively and are difficult to interpret. Lumiracoxib was associated with a significant decrease in the frequency of ulcer complications in patients not concurrently taking low-dose aspirin; the benefit disappeared, however, in patients taking aspirin. Finally, the frequency of greater than threefold elevation of hepatic transaminases was 2.6% for lumiracoxib *versus* 0.6% for the comparator tNSAIDs. Balanced against the tradeoffs of heightened risk for cardiovascular events and hepatotoxicity, the narrow gastrointestinal protective benefit of lumiracoxib makes its use difficult to justify, particularly in patients also taking low-dose aspirin.

Etoricoxib. **Pharmacokinetics.** Etoricoxib is incompletely (83%) absorbed and has a long half-life of approximately 20 to 26 hours (Table 26–1) (Rodrigues *et al.*, 2003). It is extensively metabolized before excretion. Small studies suggest that those with moderate hepatic impairment are prone to drug accumulation, and the dosing interval should be adjusted (Agrawal *et al.*, 2003). Renal insufficiency does not affect drug clearance (Agrawal *et al.*, 2004).

Pharmacological Properties, Common Adverse Effects, and Therapeutic Uses. Etoricoxib (ARCOXIA) is approved in the United Kingdom as a once-daily medicine for symptomatic relief in the treatment of osteoarthritis, rheumatoid arthritis, and acute gouty arthritis, as well as for the short-term treatment of musculoskeletal pain, postoperative pain, and primary dysmenorrhea (Patrignani *et al.*, 2003). Its COX-2 selectivity is second only to lumiracoxib, and in keeping with other coxibs, it shows decreased gastrointestinal injury as assessed endoscopically. A large randomized clinical outcome study of etoricoxib (MEDAL) is under way.

OTHER NONSTEROIDAL ANTIINFLAMMATORY DRUGS

Apazone (Azapropazone)

Apazone is a tNSAID that has antiinflammatory, analgesic, and antipyretic activity and is a potent uricosuric agent. It is available in

Europe but not the United States. Some of its function may arise from its ability to inhibit neutrophil migration, degranulation, and superoxide production.

Apazone has been used for the treatment of rheumatoid arthritis, osteoarthritis, ankylosing spondylitis, and gout, but usually is restricted to cases where other tNSAIDs have failed. Typical doses are 600 mg three times per day for acute gout. Once symptoms have abated, or for nongout indications, typical dosage is 300 mg three to four times per day. Clinical experience to date suggests that apazone is well tolerated. Mild gastrointestinal side effects (nausea, epigastric pain, dyspepsia) and rashes occur in about 3% of patients, while CNS effects (headache, vertigo) are reported less frequently. Precautions appropriate to other nonselective COX inhibitors also apply to apazone.

Nimesulide

Nimesulide is a sulfonanilide compound available in Europe that demonstrates COX-2 selectivity similar to celecoxib in whole blood assays. Additional effects include inhibition of neutrophil activation, decrease in cytokine production, decrease in degradative enzyme production, and possibly activation of glucocorticoid receptors (Bennet, 1999). Its structure is:

NIMESULIDE

Nimesulide is antiinflammatory, analgesic, and antipyretic and reportedly is associated with a low incidence of gastrointestinal adverse effects. Given its selectivity profile, it is not a logical alternative for patients switching from the coxibs because of the risk of cardiovascular and cerebrovascular events.

OTHER DRUGS FOR RHEUMATOID ARTHRITIS

Rheumatoid arthritis is an autoimmune disease that affects approximately 1% of the population. The pharmacological management of mild rheumatoid arthritis is geared towards symptomatic relief through the use of NSAIDs. Although they have antiinflammatory effects, they do not prevent or delay joint deformity. Thus, there now is a trend to use disease-modifying antirheumatic drugs earlier in the course of the disease (Olson and Stein, 2004; O'Dell, 2004). Most of these immunosuppressive and immune-modulatory agents have been discussed in other chapters (*see* Chapters 38 and 52) and will be mentioned only briefly here. The use of these agents early in the course of the disease must be weighed against their potentially serious adverse effects. Therapy is tailored to the individual patient, but short-term glucocorticoids often are used to bring the level of inflammation quickly under control. Glucocorticoids are not suitable for long-term use because of adrenal suppression, so methotrexate, sulfasalazine, or low-dose immunosuppressants commonly are used early in the course of the disease. Should these agents be

ineffective, TNF-receptor antagonists or IL-1–receptor antagonists may be administered. The combination of NSAIDs with these agents is increasingly common.

The older agents (gold, penicillamine, sulfasalazine, and *hydroxychloroquine*) have unclear mechanisms of action and with the exception of sulfasalazine, tend to have slight efficacy and significant side effects.

GOLD

Gold, in its elemental form, has been employed for centuries to relieve the itching palm. The more recent use of gold in the treatment of rheumatoid arthritis continues to wane as more effective and better-tolerated agents become available.

Gold is associated with serious adverse effects in the skin and mucous membranes (*e.g.,* erythema, glossitis, exfoliative dermatitis), kidneys (*e.g.,* proteinuria, membranous glomerulonephritis), and blood (*e.g.,* thrombocytopenia, leukopenia, agranulocytosis, aplastic anemia). These side effects tend to increase with cumulative dose. Gold therapy is reserved for patients with progressive disease who do not obtain satisfactory relief from therapy with NSAIDs and who cannot tolerate the more commonly used immunosuppressants or cytokine receptor antagonists. Gold should not be used if the disease is mild and usually is of little benefit in advanced disease.

The pharmacology of gold compounds is described in more detail in previous editions of this book.

PHARMACOTHERAPY OF GOUT

Gout results from the precipitation of urate crystals in the tissues and the subsequent inflammatory response. Acute gout usually causes an exquisitely painful distal monoarthritis, but it also can cause joint destruction, subcutaneous deposits (tophi), and renal calculi and damage. Gout affects approximately 0.5 to 1% of the population of Western countries.

The pathophysiology of gout is understood poorly. While a prerequisite, hyperuricemia does not inevitably lead to gout. Uric acid, the end product of purine metabolism, is relatively insoluble compared to its hypoxanthine and xanthine precursors, and normal serum urate levels approach the limit of solubility. In most patients with gout, hyperuricemia arises from underexcretion rather than overproduction of urate. Urate tends to crystallize in colder or more acidic conditions. Neutrophils ingesting urate crystals secrete inflammatory mediators that lower the local pH and lead to further urate precipitation.

The aims of treatment are to decrease the symptoms of an acute attack, decrease the risk of recurrent attacks, and lower serum urate levels. This section focuses on *colchicine, allopurinol,* and the uricosuric agents—probenecid, sulfinpyrazone, and *benzbromarone.*

Treatment of Acute Gout

Several tNSAIDs reportedly are effective in the treatment of acute gout. The specific COX-2 inhibitor etoricoxib has been shown to be effective in gout (Rubin *et al.,* 2004). When effective, NSAIDs should be given at relatively high doses for 3 to 4 days and then tapered for a total of 7 to 10 days. Indomethacin, naproxen, sulindac, and celecoxib all have been found to be effective, although the first three are the only NSAIDs that have received FDA approval for the treatment of gout. Aspirin is not used because it can inhibit urate excretion at low doses, and through its uricosuric actions increase the risk of renal calculi at higher doses. In addition, aspirin can inhibit the actions of uricosuric agents. Likewise, apazone should not be used in acute gout because of the concern that its uricosuric effects may promote nephrolithiasis.

Glucocorticoids and *corticotropin* (rarely used today) give rapid relief within hours of therapy. High doses are used initially and then tapered rapidly (*e.g.,* prednisone 30 to 60 mg/day for 3 days then tapered over 10 to 14 days), depending on the size and number of affected joints. Intra-articular glucocorticoids are useful if only a few joints are involved and septic arthritis has been ruled out. Further information on these agents is available in Chapter 59. Colchicine also is used in the treatment of acute gout (*see* below). There are anecdotal reports of the use of *ondansetron* in acute gout (*see* Chapter 11), but it is not used commonly for this purpose (Schworer and Ramadori, 1994).

Prevention of Recurrent Attacks

Recurrent attacks of gout can be prevented with the use of colchicine (*e.g.,* 0.6 mg daily or on alternate days). Indomethacin (25 mg/day) also has been used. These agents are used early in the course of uricosuric therapy when mobilization of urate is associated with a temporary increase in the risk of acute gouty arthritis.

Antihyperuricemic Therapy. Isolated hyperuricemia is not necessarily an indication for therapy, as not all of these patients develop gout. Persistently elevated uric acid levels, complicated by recurrent gouty arthritis, nephropathy, or subcutaneous tophi, can be lowered by allopurinol, which inhibits the formation of urate, or by uricosuric agents. Some physicians recommend measuring 24-hour urinary urate levels in patients who are on a low-purine diet to distinguish underexcretors from overproducers. However, tailored and empirical therapies have similar outcomes (Terkeltaub, 2003).

Certain drugs, particularly thiazide diuretics (*see* Chapter 28) and immunosuppressant agents (especially *cyclosporine*) may impair urate excretion and thereby increase the risk of gout.

Colchicine

Colchicine is one of the oldest available therapies for acute gout. Plant extracts containing colchicine were used for joint pain in the sixth century. Colchicine now is considered second-line therapy because it has a narrow thera-

peutic window and a high rate of side effects, particularly at higher doses.

Chemistry. The structural formula of colchicine is:

COLCHICINE

Its structure–activity relationship has been discussed (Levy *et al.,* 1991).

Mechanism of Action. Colchicine exerts a variety of pharmacological effects, but how these occur or how they relate to its activity in gout is not well understood. It has antimitotic effects, arresting cell division in G1 by interfering with microtubule and spindle formation (an effect shared with vinca alkaloids). This effect is greatest on cells with rapid turnover (*e.g.,* neutrophils and GI epithelium). Although somewhat controversial, colchicine may alter neutrophil motility in *ex vivo* assays (Levy *et al.,* 1991). Colchicine also renders cell membranes more rigid and decreases the secretion of chemotactic factors by activated neutrophils.

Colchicine inhibits the release of histamine-containing granules from mast cells, the secretion of insulin from pancreatic β cells, and the movement of melanin granules in melanophores. These processes also may involve interference with the microtubular system, but whether this occurs at clinically relevant concentrations is questionable.

Colchicine also exhibits a variety of other pharmacological effects. It lowers body temperature, increases the sensitivity to central depressants, depresses the respiratory center, enhances the response to sympathomimetic agents, constricts blood vessels, and induces hypertension by central vasomotor stimulation. It enhances gastrointestinal activity by neurogenic stimulation but depresses it by a direct effect, and alters neuromuscular function.

Pharmacokinetics and Metabolism. The absorption of colchicine is rapid but variable. Peak plasma concentrations occur 0.5 to 2 hours after dosing. In plasma, 50% of colchicine is protein-bound. There is significant enterohepatic circulation. The exact metabolism of colchicine is unknown but seems to involve deacetylation by the liver. Only 10% to 20% is excreted in the urine, although this increases in patients with liver disease. The kidney, liver, and spleen also contain high concentrations of colchicine, but it apparently is largely excluded from heart, skeletal muscle, and brain. The plasma half-life of colchicine is approximately 9 hours, but it can be detected in leukocytes and in the urine for at least 9 days after a single intravenous dose.

Toxic Effects. Exposure of the GI tract to large amounts of colchicine and its metabolites *via* enterohepatic circulation and the rapid rate of turnover of the gastrointestinal mucosa may explain why the GI tract is particularly susceptible to colchicine toxicity. Nausea, vomiting, diarrhea, and abdominal pain are the most common untoward effects of colchicine and the earliest signs of impending toxicity. Drug administration should be discontinued as soon as these symptoms occur. There is a latent period, which is not altered by dose or route of administration, of several hours or more between the administration of the drug and the onset of symptoms. For this reason, adverse effects are common during initial dosing for acute gout. However, since patients often remain relatively consistent in their response to a given dose of the drug, toxicity can be reduced or avoided during subsequent courses of therapy by reducing the dose. Acute intoxication causes hemorrhagic gastropathy. Intravenous colchicine sometimes is used to treat acute gouty arthritis when other medications are not effective, when the patient is unable to take oral medications, or when rapid therapeutic intervention is necessary. The narrow margin of safety for colchicine is even further diminished by intravenous administration because this route obviates early gastrointestinal side effects that can be a harbinger of serious systemic toxicity. Indiscriminate use of intravenous colchicine has been associated with preventable fatalities. Due to the high rate of serious bone marrow and renal complications (including death from sepsis), this route, although occasionally used, is not generally recommended.

Colchicine toxicity is associated with bone marrow suppression, particularly from the third to eighth days. There is a tendency toward leukocytosis with appearance of less mature forms. Chronic colchicine use may lead to agranulocytosis. Thrombocytopenia also can occur, and disseminated intravascular coagulation has been reported in cases of severe poisoning.

Chronic use is associated with a proximal myopathy. The associated weakness may go unrecognized, and creatine kinase levels should be monitored in those receiving chronic therapy. Ascending paralysis of the CNS has been reported with acute poisoning.

Proteinuria, hematuria, and acute tubular necrosis have been reported in severely intoxicated patients. Gouty nephropathy may occur in chronically treated patients. Azoospermia has been reported with chronic use.

There is no specific therapy for acute colchicine poisoning. Supportive measures should be used, particularly fluid repletion. Activated charcoal may decrease total colchicine exposure. Hemodialysis does not remove colchicine but may be required as part of supportive care. Colchicine antibodies and the use of granulocyte colony-stimulating factor to treat the leukopenia are under investigation.

Therapeutic Uses. *Acute Gout.* Colchicine dramatically relieves acute attacks of gout. It is effective in roughly two-thirds of patients if given within 24 hours of the onset of the attack. Pain, swelling, and redness abate within 12 hours and are completely gone within 48 to 72 hours. The typical oral dose is 0.6 mg each hour for a total of three doses. This dose should not be exceeded. Treatment with colchicine should not be repeated within 7 days to avoid cumulative toxicity.

Great care should be exercised in prescribing colchicine for elderly patients. For those with cardiac, renal, hepatic, or gastrointestinal disease, NSAIDs or glucocorticoids may be preferred.

Prevention of Acute Gout. The main indication for colchicine is in the prevention of recurrent gout, particularly in the early stages of antihyperuricemic therapy. The typical dose is 0.6 mg twice a day, which should be decreased for patients with impaired renal function. One suggestion is 0.6 mg/day for a creatinine clearance of 35 to 50 ml/minute, or in patients younger than 70 years of age, 0.6 mg every 2 to 3 days for creatinine clearances of 10 to 35 ml/minute, and avoidance in those with creatinine clearance of less than 10 ml/minute or with combined hepatic and renal disease (Terkeltaub, 2003).

Familial Mediterranean Fever. Daily administration of colchicine is useful for the prevention of attacks of familial Mediterranean fever and prevention of amyloidosis, which may complicate this disease (Zemer *et al.*, 1991).

There no longer is a role for colchicine in the treatment of primary biliary cirrhosis, psoriasis, or Behçet's disease.

Allopurinol

Allopurinol inhibits xanthine oxidase and prevents the synthesis of urate from hypoxanthine and xanthine. It is used to treat hyperuricemia in patients with gout and to prevent it in those with hematological malignancies about to undergo chemotherapy (acute tumor lysis syndrome). Even though underexcretion rather than overproduction is the underlying defect in most gout patients, allopurinol remains effective therapy.

History. Allopurinol initially was synthesized as a candidate antineoplastic agent but was found to lack antineoplastic activity. Subsequent testing showed it to be an inhibitor of xanthine oxidase that was useful clinically for the treatment of gout.

Chemistry and Pharmacological Properties. Allopurinol, an analog of hypoxanthine, has the following structural formula:

ALLOPURINOL

Both allopurinol and its primary metabolite, oxypurinol (alloxanthine), inhibit xanthine oxidase. Allopurinol competitively inhibits xanthine oxidase at low concentrations and is a noncompetitive inhibitor at high concentrations. Allopurinol also is a substrate for xanthine oxidase; the product of this reaction, oxypurinol, is also a noncompetitive inhibitor of the enzyme. The formation of oxypurinol, together with its long persistence in tissues, is responsible for much of the pharmacological activity of allopurinol.

In the absence of allopurinol, the dominant urinary purine is uric acid. During allopurinol treatment, the urinary purines include hypoxanthine, xanthine, and uric acid. Since each has its independent solubility, the concentration of uric acid in plasma is reduced and purine excretion increased, without exposing the urinary tract to an excessive load of uric acid. Despite their increased concentrations during allopurinol therapy, hypoxanthine and xanthine are efficiently excreted, and tissue deposition does not occur. There is a small risk of xanthine stones in patients with a very high urate load before allopurinol therapy, which can be minimized by liberal fluid intake and alkalization of the urine.

Allopurinol facilitates the dissolution of tophi and prevents the development or progression of chronic gouty arthritis by lowering the uric acid concentration in plasma below the limit of its solubility. The formation of uric acid stones virtually disappears with therapy, which prevents the development of nephropathy. Once significant renal injury has occurred, allopurinol cannot restore renal function but may delay disease progression. The incidence of acute attacks of gouty arthritis may increase during the early months of allopurinol therapy as a consequence of mobilization of tissue stores of uric acid.

Coadministration of colchicine helps suppress such acute attacks. After reduction of excess tissue stores of uric acid, the incidence of acute attacks decreases and colchicine can be discontinued.

In some patients, the allopurinol-induced increase in excretion of oxypurines is less than the reduction in uric acid excretion; this disparity primarily is a result of reutilization of oxypurines and feedback inhibition of *de novo* purine biosynthesis.

Pharmacokinetics. Allopurinol is absorbed relatively rapidly after oral ingestion, and peak plasma concentrations are reached within 60 to 90 minutes. About 20% is excreted in the feces in 48 to 72 hours, presumably as unabsorbed drug, and 10% to 30% is excreted unchanged in the urine. The remainder undergoes metabolism, mostly to oxypurinol. Oxypurinol is excreted slowly in the urine by glomerular filtration, counterbalanced by some tubular reabsorption. The plasma half-life of allopurinol is approximately 1 to 2 hours and of oxypurinol approximately 18 to 30 hours (longer in those with renal impairment). This allows for once-daily dosing and makes allopurinol the most commonly used antihyperuricemic agent.

Allopurinol and its active metabolite oxypurinol are distributed in total tissue water, with the exception of brain, where their concentrations are about one-third of those in other tissues. Neither compound is bound to plasma proteins. The plasma concentrations of the two compounds do not correlate well with therapeutic or toxic effects.

Drug Interactions. Allopurinol increases the half-life of probenecid and enhances its uricosuric effect, while probenecid increases the clearance of oxypurinol, thereby increasing dose requirements of allopurinol.

Allopurinol inhibits the enzymatic inactivation of *mercaptopurine* and its derivative *azathioprine* by xanthine oxidase. Thus, when allopurinol is used concomitantly with oral mercaptopurine or azathioprine, dosage of the antineoplastic agent must be reduced to one-fourth to one-third of the usual dose (*see* Chapters 38 and 51). This is of importance when treating gout in the transplant recipient. The risk of bone marrow suppression also is increased when allopurinol is administered with cytotoxic agents that are not metabolized by xanthine oxidase, particularly *cyclophosphamide*.

Allopurinol also may interfere with the hepatic inactivation of other drugs, including warfarin. Although the effect is variable, increased monitoring of prothrombin activity is recommended in patients receiving both medications.

It remains to be established whether the increased incidence of rash in patients receiving concurrent allopurinol and *ampicillin* should be ascribed to allopurinol or to hyperuricemia. Hypersensitivity reactions have been reported in patients with compromised renal function, especially those who are receiving a combination of allopurinol and a thiazide diuretic. The concomitant administration of allopurinol and theophylline leads to increased accumulation of an active metabolite of theophylline, 1-methylxanthine; the concentration of theophylline in plasma also may be increased (*see* Chapter 27).

Therapeutic Uses. Allopurinol (ZYLOPRIM, ALOPRIM, others) is available for oral use and provides effective therapy for the primary hyperuricemia of gout and the hyperuricemia secondary to polycy-

themia vera, myeloid metaplasia, other blood dyscrasias, or acute tumor lysis syndrome.

Allopurinol is contraindicated in patients who have exhibited serious adverse effects or hypersensitivity reactions to the medication, and in nursing mothers and children, except those with malignancy or certain inborn errors of purine metabolism (*e.g.,* Lesch-Nyhan syndrome). Allopurinol generally is used in complicated hyperuricemia (*see* above), to prevent acute tumor lysis syndrome, or in patients with hyperuricemia posttransplantation. If necessary, it can be used in conjunction with uricosuric agents.

The goal of therapy is to reduce the plasma uric acid concentration to less than 6 mg/dl (equivalent to 360 μmol). In the management of gout, it is customary to antecede allopurinol therapy with colchicine and to avoid starting allopurinol during an acute attack of gouty arthritis. Fluid intake should be sufficient to maintain daily urinary volume of more than 2 liters; slightly alkaline urine is preferred. An initial daily dose of 100 mg is increased by 100-mg increments at weekly intervals. Most patients can be maintained on 300 mg/day. Those with more severe gout may require 400 to 600 mg/day, and those with hematological malignancies may need up to 800 mg/day beginning 2 to 3 days before the start of chemotherapy. Daily doses in excess of 300 mg should be divided. Dosage must be reduced in patients in proportion to the reduction in glomerular filtration (*e.g.,* 300 mg/day if creatinine clearance is >90 ml/minute, 200 mg/day if creatinine clearance is between 60 and 90 ml/minute, 100 mg/day if creatinine clearance is 30 to 60 ml/minute, and 50 to 100 mg/day if creatinine clearance is <30 ml/minute) (Terkeltaub, 2003).

The usual daily dose in children with secondary hyperuricemia associated with malignancies is 150 to 300 mg, depending on age.

Allopurinol also is useful in lowering the high plasma concentrations of uric acid in patients with Lesch-Nyhan syndrome and thereby prevents the complications resulting from hyperuricemia; there is no evidence that it alters the progressive neurological and behavioral abnormalities that are characteristic of the disease.

Common Adverse Effects. Allopurinol is tolerated well by most patients. The most common adverse effects are hypersensitivity reactions that may occur after months or years of medication. The effects usually subside within a few days after medication is discontinued. Serious reactions preclude further use of the drug.

The cutaneous reaction caused by allopurinol is predominantly a pruritic, erythematous, or maculopapular eruption, but occasionally the lesion is urticarial or purpuric. Rarely, toxic epidermal necrolysis or Stevens-Johnson syndrome occurs, which can be fatal. The risk for Stevens-Johnson syndrome is limited primarily to the first 2 months of treatment (Roujeau *et al.*, 1995). Because the rash may precede severe hypersensitivity reactions, patients who develop a rash should discontinue allopurinol. If indicated, desensitization to allopurinol can be carried out starting at 10 to 25 μg per day, with the drug diluted in oral suspension and doubled every 3 to 14 days until the desired dose is reached. This is successful in approximately half of patients (Terkeltaub, 2003). Oxypurinol is available for compassionate use in the United States for patients intolerant of allopurinol. The safety of oxypurinol in patients with severe allopurinol hypersensitivity is unknown and not recommended.

Fever, malaise, and myalgias also may occur. Such effects are noted in about 3% of patients with normal renal function and more frequently in those with renal impairment. Transient leukopenia or leukocytosis and eosinophilia are rare reactions that may require cessation of therapy. Hepatomegaly and elevated levels of transaminases in plasma and progressive renal insufficiency also may occur.

Rasburicase

Rasburicase (ELITEK) is a recombinant urate-oxidase that catalyzes the enzymatic oxidation of uric acid into the soluble and inactive metabolite allantoin. It has been shown to lower urate levels more effectively than allopurinol (Bosly *et al.*, 2003). It is indicated for the initial management of elevated plasma uric acid levels in pediatric patients with leukemia, lymphoma, and solid tumor malignancies who are receiving anticancer therapy expected to result in tumor lysis and significant hyperuricemia.

Produced by a genetically modified *Saccharomyces cerevisiae* strain, the therapeutic efficacy may be hampered by the production of antibodies against the drug. Hemolysis in glucose-6-phosphate dehydrogenase (G6PD)-deficient patients, methemoglobinemia, acute renal failure, and anaphylaxis all have been associated with the use of rasburicase. Other frequently observed adverse reactions include vomiting, fever, nausea, headache, abdominal pain, constipation, diarrhea, and mucositis. Rasburicase causes enzymatic degradation of the uric acid in blood samples, and special handling is required to prevent spuriously low values for plasma uric acid in patients receiving the drug. The recommended dose of rasburicase is 0.15 mg/kg or 0.2 mg/kg as a single daily dose for 5 days, with chemotherapy initiated 4 to 24 hours after infusion of the first rasburicase dose.

URICOSURIC AGENTS

Uricosuric agents increase the rate of excretion of uric acid. In humans, urate is filtered, secreted, and reabsorbed by the kidneys. Reabsorption predominates, and the amount excreted usually is about 10% of that filtered. This process is mediated by a specific transporter, which can be inhibited.

The first step in urate reabsorption is its uptake from tubular fluid by a transporter that exchanges urate for either an organic or an inorganic anion. Uricosuric drugs compete with urate for the brush-border transporter, thereby inhibiting its reabsorption *via* the urate–anion exchanger system. However, transport is bidirectional, and depending on dosage, a drug may either decrease or increase the excretion of uric acid. Decreased excretion usually occurs at a low dosage, while increased excretion is observed at a higher dosage. Not all agents show this phenomenon, and one uricosuric drug may either add to or inhibit the action of another. The biphasic effect may be seen within the normal dosage range with some drugs such as salicylates.

Two mechanisms for a drug-induced decrease in urate excretion of urate have been advanced; they are not mutually exclusive. The first presumes that the small secretory movement of urate is inhibited by very low concentrations of the drug. Higher concentrations may inhibit urate reabsorption in the usual manner. The second proposal suggests that the urate-retaining anionic drug gains access to the intracellular fluid by an independent mechanism and promotes reabsorption of urate across the brush border by anion exchange.

There are two mechanisms by which one drug may nullify the uricosuric action of another. First, the drug may inhibit the secretion of the uricosuric agent, thereby denying it access to its site of action, the luminal aspect of the brush border. Second, the inhibition of urate secretion by one drug may counterbalance the inhibition of urate reabsorption by the other.

Many compounds have incidental uricosuric activity, probably by acting as exchangeable anions, but only probenecid is prescribed routinely for this purpose. Benzbromarone is an alternative uricosuric agent that is available in Europe. Conversely, a number of drugs and toxins cause retention of urate; these have been reviewed elsewhere (Maalouf *et al.*, 2004).

Probenecid

Chemistry. Probenecid is a highly lipid-soluble benzoic acid derivative (pK_a 3.4) with the following structural formula:

$$CH_3CH_2CH_2 \diagdown \atop CH_3CH_2CH_2 \diagup N-SO_2 - \bigcirc - COOH$$

PROBENECID

Pharmacological Actions. *Inhibition of Inorganic Acid Transport.* The actions of probenecid are confined largely to inhibition of the transport of organic acids across epithelial barriers. When tubular secretion of a substance is inhibited, its final concentration in the urine is determined by the degree of filtration, which in turn is a function of binding to plasma protein, and by the degree of reabsorption. The significance of each of these factors varies widely with different compounds. Usually, the end result is decreased tubular secretion of the compound, leading to decreased urinary and increased plasma concentration.

Uric acid is the only important endogenous compound whose excretion is known to be increased by probenecid. This results from inhibition of its reabsorption (*see* above). The uricosuric action of probenecid is blunted by the coadministration of salicylates.

Inhibition of Transport of Miscellaneous Substances. Probenecid inhibits the tubular secretion of a number of drugs, such as methotrexate and the active metabolite of *clofibrate*. It inhibits renal secretion of the inactive glucuronide metabolites of NSAIDs such as naproxen, ketoprofen, and indomethacin, and thereby can increase their plasma concentrations.

Inhibition of Monoamine Transport to CSF. Probenecid inhibits the transport of 5-hydroxyindoleacetic acid (5-HIAA) and other acidic metabolites of cerebral monoamines from the CSF to the plasma. The transport of drugs such as *penicillin G* also may be affected.

Inhibition of Biliary Excretion. Probenecid depresses the biliary secretion of certain compounds, including the diagnostic agents indocyanine green and bromosulphthalein (BSP). It also decreases the biliary secretion of *rifampin*, leading to higher plasma concentrations.

Absorption, Fate, and Excretion. Probenecid is absorbed completely after oral administration. Peak concentrations in plasma are reached in 2 to 4 hours. The half-life of the drug in plasma is dose-dependent and varies from less than 5 hours to more than 8 hours over the therapeutic range. Between 85% and 95% of the drug is bound to plasma albumin. The 5% to 15% of unbound drug is cleared by glomerular filtration. The majority of the drug is secreted actively by the proximal tubule. The high lipid solubility of the undissociated form results in virtually complete absorption by backdiffusion unless the urine is markedly alkaline. A small amount of probenecid glucuronide appears in the urine. It also is hydroxylated to metabolites that retain their carboxyl function and have uricosuric activity.

Common Adverse Effects. Probenecid is well tolerated. Approximately 2% of patients develop mild gastrointestinal irritation. The risk is increased at higher doses, and caution should be used in those with a history of peptic ulcer. It is ineffective in patients with renal insufficiency and should be avoided in those with creatinine clearance of <50 ml/minute. Hypersensitivity reactions usually are mild and occur in 2% to 4% of patients. Serious hypersensitivity is extremely rare. The appearance of a rash during the concurrent administration of probenecid and penicillin G presents the physician with an awkward diagnostic dilemma. Substantial overdosage with probenecid results in CNS stimulation, convulsions, and death from respiratory failure.

Therapeutic Use. *Gout.* Probenecid (BENEMID [US], BENURYL [UK]) is marketed for oral administration. The starting dose is 250 mg twice daily, increasing over 1 to 2 weeks to 500 to 1000 mg twice daily. Probenecid increases urinary urate levels. Liberal fluid intake therefore should be maintained throughout therapy to minimize the risk of renal stones. Probenecid should not be used in gouty patients with nephrolithiasis or with overproduction of uric acid. Concomitant colchicine or NSAIDs are indicated early in the course of therapy to avoid precipitating an attack of gout, which may occur in up to 20% of gouty patients treated with probenecid alone.

Combination with Penicillin. Probenecid was developed for the purpose of delaying the excretion of penicillin. Higher doses of probenecid are used as an adjuvant to prolong penicillin concentrations. This usually is confined to those being treated for gonorrhea or neurosyphilis infections or to cases where penicillin resistance may be an issue (*see* Chapter 44).

Sulfinpyrazone

History. Sulfinpyrazone was developed from phenylbutazone, an early NSAID whose toxicity precluded its continued use. Sulfinpyrazone lacks antiinflammatory and analgesic activity but has potent uricosuric effects. It rarely is used today.

Chemistry. Sulfinpyrazone is a strong organic acid ($pK_a = 2.8$) that readily forms soluble salts.

Pharmacological Actions. In sufficient doses, sulfinpyrazone potently inhibits the renal tubular reabsorption of uric acid. As with other uricosuric agents, small doses may reduce the excretion of uric acid. Like probenecid, sulfinpyrazone reduces the renal tubular secretion of many other organic anions. In addition, it may induce hypoglycemia by inhibiting the metabolism of the sulfonylurea oral hypoglycemic

agents. The hepatic metabolism of warfarin also is impaired. The uricosuric action of sulfinpyrazone is additive to that of probenecid, but it antagonizes that of salicylates. The inhibitory effect of sulfinpyrazone on platelet function is discussed in Chapter 54.

Absorption, Fate, and Excretion. Sulfinpyrazone is absorbed well after oral administration. It is bound strongly to plasma albumin (98% to 99%) and displaces other anionic drugs that have their highest affinity for the same binding site. Its plasma half-life is about 3 hours, but its uricosuric effect may persist for as long as 10 hours. Sulfinpyrazone is secreted by the proximal tubule and undergoes little passive backdiffusion. Approximately half of the orally administered dose appears in the urine within 24 hours, mostly (90%) as unchanged drug; the remaining 10% is eliminated as the N^1-*p*-hydroxyphenyl metabolite, which also is a potent uricosuric substance.

Common Adverse Effects. Gastrointestinal irritation occurs in roughly 10% to 15% of patients receiving sulfinpyrazone, and occasionally may lead patients to discontinue its use. Gastric distress is lessened when the drug is taken in divided doses with meals. Sulfinpyrazone should be given to patients with a history of peptic ulcer only with extreme caution. Hypersensitivity reactions, usually a rash with fever, do occur, but less frequently than with probenecid. Depression of hematopoiesis has been demonstrated, and periodic blood cell counts therefore are advised during prolonged therapy. Sulfinpyrazone should not be used by patients with underlying blood dyscrasias.

Therapeutic Use. Sulfinpyrazone (ANTURANE) is available for oral administration. The initial dosage for the treatment of chronic gout is 100 to 200 mg given twice daily. After the first week, the dosage may be gradually increased until a satisfactory lowering of plasma uric acid is achieved and maintained. This may require from 200 to 800 mg per day, divided in two to four doses and preferably given with meals or milk; a liberal fluid intake should be maintained. Larger doses are tolerated poorly and unlikely to produce a further uricosuric effect in resistant patients. Sulfinpyrazone is ineffective in patients with renal insufficiency and should be avoided in those with creatinine clearance of <50 ml/minute. As with probenecid, concomitant colchicine is indicated early in the course to avoid precipitating an attack of gout.

Benzbromarone

This is a potent uricosuric agent that is used in Europe. The drug is absorbed readily after oral ingestion, and peak concentrations in blood are achieved in about 4 hours. It is metabolized to monobromine and dehalogenated derivatives, both of which have uricosuric activity, and is excreted primarily in the bile. The uricosuric action is blunted by aspirin or sulfinpyrazone. No paradoxical retention of urate has been observed. It is a potent and reversible inhibitor of the urate–anion exchanger in the proximal tubule. As the micronized powder it is effective in a single daily dose of 40 mg to 80 mg, which makes it significantly more potent than other uricosuric drugs. It is effective in patients with renal insufficiency and may be useful clinically in patients who are either allergic or refractory to other drugs used for the treatment of gout. Preparations that combine allopurinol and benzbromarone are more effective than either drug alone in lowering serum uric acid levels, in spite of the fact that benzbromarone lowers plasma levels of oxypurinol, the active metabolite of allopurinol.

CONCLUSION

The emergence of clear evidence from placebo-controlled trials of a cardiovascular hazard for three coxibs has prompted a broad reappraisal of NSAID therapy. Selective inhibitors of COX-2 were developed to reduce gastrointestinal adverse effects and have never been shown to exhibit an efficacy advantage over tNSAIDs. The likelihood of hazard would be expected to be related to selectivity attained *in vivo*, dose, duration of action, and duration of dosing, as well as the underlying risk profile of an individual patient. It seems likely that some of the older drugs, specifically meloxicam and diclofenac, may closely resemble celecoxib, while naproxen may afford cardioprotection due to an extended half-life in some individuals, translating into a modest benefit when compared to aspirin.

BIBLIOGRAPHY

Agrawal, N.G., Matthews, C.Z., Mazenko, R.S., *et al.* Pharmacokinetics of etoricoxib in patients with renal impairment. *J. Clin. Pharmacol.,* **2004,** *44:*48–58.

Agrawal, N.G., Rose, M.J., Matthews, C.Z., *et al.* Pharmacokinetics of etoricoxib in patients with hepatic impairment. *J. Clin. Pharmacol.,* **2003,** *43:*1136–1148.

Atherton, C., Jones, J., McKaig, B., *et al.* Pharmacology and gastrointestinal safety of lumiracoxib, a novel cyclooxygenase-2 selective inhibitor: an integrated study. *Clin. Gastroenterol. Hepatol.,* **2004,** *2:*113–120.

Bennet, A. Overview of nimesulide. *Rheumatology,* **1999,** *38:*1–3.

Bitner, M., Kattenhorn, J., Hatfield, C., Gao, J., and Kellstein, D. Efficacy and tolerability of lumiracoxib in the treatment of primary dysmenorrhoea. *Int. J. Clin. Pract.,* **2004,** *58:*340–345.

Bombardier, C., Laine, L., Reicin, A., *et al.* Comparison of upper gastrointestinal toxicity of rofecoxib and naproxen in patients with rheumatoid arthritis. VIGOR Study Group. *N. Engl. J. Med.,* **2000,** *343:*1520–1528.

Bosly, A., Sonet, A., Pinkerton, C.R., *et al.* Rasburicase (recombinant urate oxidase) for the management of hyperuricemia in patients with cancer: report of an international compassionate use study. *Cancer,* **2003,** *98:*1048–1054.

Boutaud, O., Aronoff, D.M., Richardson, J.H., Marnett, L.J., and Oates, J.A. Determinants of the cellular specificity of acetaminophen as an inhibitor of prostaglandin H(2) synthases. *Proc. Natl. Acad. Sci. U.S.A.,* **2002,** *99:*7130–7135.

Breder, C.D., Dewitt, D., and Kraig, R.P. Characterization of inducible cyclooxygenase in rat brain. *J. Comp. Neurol.,* **1995,** *355:*296–315.

Bresalier, R.S., Sandler, R.S., Quan, H., *et al.* Cardiovascular events associated with rofecoxib in a colorectal adenoma chemoprevention trial. *N. Engl. J. Med.,* **2005,** *352:*1092–1102.

Capone, M.L., Tacconelli, S., Sciulli, M.G., *et al.* Clinical pharmacology of platelet, monocyte, and vascular cyclooxygenase inhibition by naproxen and low-dose aspirin in healthy subjects. *Circulation,* **2004,** *109:*1468–1471.

Catella-Lawson, F., McAdam, B., Morrison, B.W., *et al.* Effects of specific inhibition of cyclooxygenase-2 on sodium balance, hemodynamics, and vasoactive eicosanoids. *J. Pharmacol. Exp. Ther.,* **1999,** *289:*735–741.

Catella-Lawson, F., Reilly, M.P., Kapoor, S.C., *et al.* Cyclooxygenase inhibitors and the antiplatelet effects of aspirin. *N. Engl. J. Med.,* **2001,** *345:*1809–1817.

Chandrasekharan, N.V., Dai, H., Roos, K.L., *et al.* COX-3, a cyclooxygenase-1 variant inhibited by acetaminophen and other analgesic/antipyretic drugs: cloning, structure, and expression. *Proc. Natl. Acad. Sci. U.S.A.,* **2002,** *99:*13926–13931.

Charlier, C., and Michaux, C. Dual inhibition of cyclooxygenase-2 (COX-2) and 5-lipoxygenase (5-LOX) as a new strategy to provide safer non-steroidal anti-inflammatory drugs. *Eur. J. Med. Chem.,* **2003,** *38:*645–659.

Clyman, R.I., Hardy, P., Waleh, N., *et al.* Cyclooxygenase-2 plays a significant role in regulating the tone of the fetal lamb ductus arteriosus. *Am. J. Physiol.,* **1999,** *276:*R913–R921.

Cruz-Correa, M., Hylind, L.M., Romans, K.E., Booker, S.V., and Giardiello, F.M. Long-term treatment with sulindac in familial adenomatous polyposis: a prospective cohort study. *Gastroenterology,* **2002,** *122:*641–645.

Dargan, P.I., Wallace, C.I., and Jones, A.L. An evidence-based flowchart to guide the management of acute salicylate (aspirin) overdose. *Emerg. Med. J.,* **2002,** *19:*206–209.

Duley, L., Henderson-Smart, D.J., Knight, M., and King, J.F. Antiplatelet agents for preventing pre-eclampsia and its complications. *Cochrane Database Syst. Rev.,* **2004,** CD004659.

Edlund, A., Berglund, B., van Dorne, D., *et al.* Coronary flow regulation in patients with ischemic heart disease: release of purines and prostacyclin and the effect of inhibitors of prostaglandin formation. *Circulation,* **1985,** *71:*1113–1120.

Farkouh, M.E., Kirshner, H., Harrington, R.A., *et al.* Comparison of lumiracoxib with naproxen and ibuprofen in the Therapeutic Arthritis Research and Gastrointestinal Event Trial (TARGET), cardiovascular outcomes: randomised controlled trial. *Lancet,* **2004,** *364:*675–684.

Fenton, C., Keating, G.M., and Wagstaff, A.J. Valdecoxib: a review of its use in the management of osteoarthritis, rheumatoid arthritis, dysmenorrhoea and acute pain. *Drugs,* **2004,** *64:*1231–1261.

FitzGerald, G.A. COX-2 and beyond: Approaches to prostaglandin inhibition in human disease. *Nat. Rev. Drug Discov.,* **2003,** *2:*879–890.

FitzGerald, G.A. Coxibs and cardiovascular disease. *N. Engl. J. Med.,* **2004,** *351:*1709–1711.

Furberg, C.D., Psaty, B.M., and FitzGerald, G.A. Parecoxib, valdecoxib and cardiovascular risk. *Circulation,* **2005,** *111:*249.

Garcia Rodriguez, L.A., Varas-Lorenzo, C., Maguire, A., and Gonzalez-Perez, A. Nonsteroidal drugs and the risk of myocardial infarction in the general population. *Circulation,* **2004,** *109:*3000–3006.

Giardiello, F.M., Yang, V.W., Hylind, L.M., *et al.* Primary chemoprevention of familial adenomatous polyposis with sulindac. *N. Engl. J. Med.,* **2002,** *346:*1054–1059.

Hallak, A., Alon-Baron, L., Shamir, R., *et al.* Rofecoxib reduces polyp recurrence in familial polyposis. *Dig. Dis. Sci.,* **2003,** *48:*1998–2002.

Jacobs, E.J., Connell, C.J., Rodriguez, C., *et al.* Aspirin use and pancreatic cancer mortality in a large United States cohort. *J. Natl. Cancer Inst.,* **2004,** *96:*524–528.

Jones, M.K., Wang, H., Peskar, B.M., *et al*. Inhibition of angiogenesis by nonsteroidal anti-inflammatory drugs: insight into mechanisms and implications for cancer growth and ulcer healing. *Nat. Med.,* **1999,** *5:*1418–1423.

Jungnickel, P.W., Maloley, P.A., Vander Tuin, E.L., Peddicord, T.E., and Campbell, J.R. Effect of two aspirin pretreatment regimens on niacin-induced cutaneous reactions. *J. Gen. Intern. Med.,* **1997,** *12:*591–596.

Juni, P., Rutjes, A.W., and Dieppe, P.A. Are selective COX 2 inhibitors superior to traditional nonsteroidal antiinflammatory drugs? *BMJ,* **2002,** *324:*1287–1288.

Karim, A., Laurent, A., Slater, M.E., *et al*. A pharmacokinetic study of intramuscular (i.m.) parecoxib sodium in normal subjects. *J. Clin. Pharmacol.,* **2001,** *41:*1111–1119.

Keane, W.F. Merck announces voluntary worldwide withdrawal of Vioxx [Letter], Merck & Co. Inc., North Wales, PA, Sept. 30, 2004 http://www.vioxx.com/vioxx/documents/english/ hcp_notification_physicians.pdf.

Keays, R., Harrison, P.M., Wendon, J.A., *et al*. Intravenous acetylcysteine in paracetamol induced fulminant hepatic failure: a prospective controlled trial. *BMJ,* **1991,** *303:*1026–1029.

Kivitz, A.J., Nayiager, S., Schimansky, T., *et al*. Reduced incidence of gastroduodenal ulcers associated with lumiracoxib compared with ibuprofen in patients with rheumatoid arthritis. *Aliment. Pharmacol. Ther.,* **2004,** *19:*1189–1198.

Kulling, P.E., Backman, E.A., Skagius, A.S., and Beckman, E.A. Renal impairment after acute diclofenac, naproxen, and sulindac overdoses. *J. Toxicol. Clin. Toxicol.,* **1995,** *33:*173–177.

Kune, G.A., Kune, S., and Watson, L.F. Colorectal cancer risk, chronic illnesses, operations, and medications: case control results from the Melbourne Colorectal Cancer Study. *Cancer Res.,* **1998,** *48:*4399–4404.

Loftin, C.D., Trivedi, D.B., and Langenbach, R. Cyclooxygenase-1-selective inhibition prolongs gestation in mice without adverse effects on the ductus arteriosus. *J. Clin. Invest.,* **2002,** *110:*549–557.

Maalouf, N.M., Cameron, M.A., Moe, O.W., and Sakhaee, K. Novel insights into the pathogenesis of uric acid nephrolithiasis. *Curr. Opin. Nephrol. Hyperten.,* **2004,** *13:*181–189.

Ma, L., del Soldato, P., and Wallace, J.L. Divergent effects of new cyclooxygenase inhibitors on gastric ulcer healing: shifting the angiogenic balance. *Proc. Natl. Acad. Sci. U.S.A.,* **2002,** *99:*13243–13247.

McAdam, B.F., Catella-Lawson, F., Mardini, I.A., *et al*. Systemic biosynthesis of prostacyclin by cyclooxygenase (cox)-2: the human pharmacology of a selective inhibitor of COX-2. *Proc. Natl. Acad. Sci. U.S.A.,* **1999,** *96:*272–277.

Ment, L.R., Oh, W., Ehrenkranz, R.A., *et al*. Low-dose indomethacin and prevention of intraventricular hemorrhage: a multicenter randomized trial. *Pediatrics,* **1994,** *93:*543–550.

Mizuno, H., Sakamoto, C., Matsuda, K., *et al*. Induction of cyclooxygenase 2 in gastric mucosal lesions and its inhibition by the specific antagonist delays healing in mice. *Gastroenterology,* **1997,** *112:*387–397.

Morant, S.V., Shield, M.J., Davey, P.G., and MacDonald, T.M. A pharmacoeconomic comparison of misoprostol/diclofenac with diclofenac. *Pharmacoepidemiol. Drug Saf.,* **2002,** *11:*393–400.

Ouellet, M., and Percival, M.D. Mechanism of acetaminophen inhibition of cyclooxygenase isoforms. *Arch. Biochem. Biophys.,* **2001,** *38:*7273–7280.

Panara, M.R., Renda, G., Sciulli, M.G., *et al*. Dose-dependent inhibition of platelet cyclooxygenase-1 and monocyte cyclooxygenase-2 by

meloxicam in healthy subjects. *J. Pharmacol. Exp. Ther.,* **1999,** *290:*276–280.

Patoia, L., Santucci, L., Furno, P., *et al*. A 4-week, double-blind, parallel-group study to compare the gastrointestinal effects of meloxicam 7.5 mg, meloxicam 15 mg, piroxicam 20 mg and placebo by means of faecal blood loss, endoscopy and symptom evaluation in healthy volunteers. *B. Brit. J. Rheumatol.,* **1996,** *35:*61–67.

Patrignani, P., Capone, M.L., and Tacconelli, S. Clinical pharmacology of etoricoxib: a novel selective COX2 inhibitor. *Expert Opin. Pharmacother.,* **2003,** *4:*265–284.

Patrignani, P., Panara, M.R., Greco, A., *et al*. Biochemical and pharmacological characterization of the cyclooxygenase activity of human blood prostaglandin endoperoxide synthases. *J. Pharmacol. Exp. Ther.,* **1994,** *271:*1705–1712.

Pederson, A.K., and FitzGerald, G.A. Dose-related kinetics of aspirin: presystemic acetylation of platelet cyclooxygenase. *N. Engl. J. Med.,* **1984,** *311:*1206–1211.

Pillinger, M.H., Capodici, C., Rosenthal, P., *et al*. Modes of action of aspirin-like drugs: salicylates inhibit erk activation and integrin-dependent neutrophil adhesion. *Proc. Natl. Acad. Sci. U.S.A.,* **1998,** *95:*14540–14545.

Qi, Z., Hao, C.M., Langenbach, R.I., *et al*. Opposite effects of cyclooxygenase-1 and -2 activity on the pressor response to angiotensin II. *J. Clin. Invest.,* **2002,** *110:*61–69.

Rigas, B., and Shiff, S.J. Is inhibition of cyclooxygenase required for the chemopreventive effect of NSAIDs in colon cancer? A model reconciling the current contradiction. *Med. Hypotheses,* **2000,** *54:*210–215.

Rodrigues, A.D., Halpin, R.A., Geer, L.A., *et al*. Absorption, metabolism, and excretion of etoricoxib, a potent and selective cyclooxygenase-2 inhibitor, in healthy male volunteers. *Drug Metab. Dispos.,* **2003,** *31:*224–232.

Roujeau, J.C., Kelly, J.P., Naldi, L., *et al*. Medication use and the risk of Stevens-Johnson syndrome or toxic epidermal necrolysis. *N. Engl. J. Med.,* **1995,** *333:*1600–1607.

Rubin, B.R., Burton, R., Navarra, S., *et al*. Efficacy and safety profile of treatment with etoricoxib 120 mg once daily compared with indomethacin 50 mg three times daily in acute gout: a randomized controlled trial. *Arthritis Rheum.,* **2004,** *50:*598–606.

Rumack, B.H., Peterson, R.C., Koch, C.G., and Amara, I.A. Acetaminophen overdose. 662 cases with evaluation of oral acetylcysteine treatment. *Arch. Intern. Med.,* **1981,** *141:*380–385.

Schnitzer, T.J., Burmester, G.R., Mysler, E., *et al*. Comparison of lumiracoxib with naproxen and ibuprofen in the Therapeutic Arthritis Research and Gastrointestinal Event Trial (TARGET), reduction in ulcer complications: randomised controlled trial. *Lancet,* **2004,** *364:*665–674.

Schwörer, H., and Ramadori, G. Treatment of acute gouty arthritis with the 5-hydroxytryptamine antagonist ondansetron. *Clin. Investig.,* **1994,** *72:*811–813.

Scott, D.L., and Palmer, R.H. Safety and efficacy of nabumetone in osteoarthritis: emphasis on gastrointestinal safety. *Aliment. Pharmacol. Ther.,* **2000,** *14:*443–452.

Seibert, K., Zhang, Y., Leahy, K., *et al*. Distribution of COX-1 and COX-2 in normal and inflamed tissues. *Adv. Exp. Med. Biol.,* **1997,** *400A:*167–170.

Sigthorsson, G., Simpson, R.J., Walley, M., *et al*. COX-1 and 2, intestinal integrity, and pathogenesis of nonsteroidal anti-inflammatory drug enteropathy in mice. *Gastroenterology,* **2002,** *122:*1913–1923.

Silverstein, F.E., Faich, G., Goldstein, J.L., *et al*. Gastrointestinal toxicity with celecoxib vs. nonsteroidal antiinflammatory drugs for osteoarthritis and rheumatoid arthritis: the CLASS study: a randomized controlled trial. Celecoxib Long-term Arthritis Safety Study. *JAMA,* **2000,** *284:*1247–1255.

Smith, W.L., De Witt, D.L., and Garavito, R.M. Cyclooxygenases: structural, cellular, and molecular biology. *Annu. Rev. Biochem.,* **2000,** *29:*145–182.

Steinbach, G., Lynch, P.M., Phillips, R.K., *et al.* The effect of celecoxib, a cyclooxygenase-2 inhibitor, in familial adenomatous polyposis. *N. Engl. J. Med.,* **2000,** *342:*1946–1952.

Topper, J.N., Cai, J., Falb, D., and Gimbrone, M.A. Identification of vascular endothelial genes differentially responsive to fluid mechanical stimuli: cyclooxygenase-2, manganese superoxide dismutase, and endothelial cell nitric oxide synthase are selectively up-regulated by steady laminar shear stress. *Proc. Natl. Acad. Sci. U.S.A.,* **1996,** *93:*10417–10422.

Warner, T.D., Giuliano, F., Vojnovic, I., *et al.* Nonsteroid drug selectivities for cyclo-oxygenase-1 rather than cyclo-oxygenase-2 are associated with human gastrointestinal toxicity: a full in vitro analysis. *Proc. Natl. Acad. Sci. U.S.A.,* **1999,** *96:*7563–7568.

Yin, M.J., Yamamoto, Y., and Gaynor, R.B. The anti-inflammatory agents aspirin and salicylate inhibit the activity of I(kappa)B kinase-beta. *Nature,* **1998,** *396:*77–80.

Zemer, D., Livneh, A., Danon, Y.L., Pras, M., and Sohar, E. Long-term colchicine treatment in children with familial Mediterranean fever. *Arthritis. Rheum.,* **1991,** *34:*973–977.

MONOGRAPHS AND REVIEWS

Amann, R., and Peskar, B.A. Anti-inflammatory effects of aspirin and sodium salicylate. *Eur. J. Pharmacol.,* **2002,** *447:*1–9.

Balfour, J.A., Fitton, A., and Barradell, L.B. Lornoxicam. A review of its pharmacology and therapeutic potential in the management of painful and inflammatory conditions. *Drugs,* **1996,** *51:*639–657.

Barbanoj, M.J., Antonijoan, R.M., and Gich, I. Clinical pharmacokinetics of dexketoprofen. *Clin. Pharmacokin.,* **2001,** *40:*245–262.

Brogden, R.N., Heel, R.C., Speight, T.M., and Avery, G.S. Fenbufen: a review of its pharmacological properties and therapeutic use in rheumatic diseases and acute pain. *Drugs,* **1981,** *21:*1–22.

Brune, K., and Hinz, B. Selective cyclooxygenase-2 inhibitors: similarities and differences. *Scand. J. Rheumatol.,* **2004,** *33:*1–6.

Brune, K. The pharmacological profile of non-opioid (OTC) analgesics: aspirin, paracetamol (acetaminophen), ibuprofen, and phenazones. *Agents Actions Suppl* **1988,** *25:*9–19.

Buckley, M.M., and Brogden, R.N. Ketorolac. a review of its pharmacodynamic and pharmacokinetic properties, and therapeutic potential. *Drugs,* **1990,** *39:*86–109.

Cheng, H.F., and Harris, R.C. Cyclooxygenases, the kidney, and hypertension. *Hypertension,* **2004,** *43:*525–530.

Davies, N.M. Clinical pharmacokinetics of flurbiprofen and its enantiomers. *Clin. Pharmacokinet.,* **1995,** *28:*100–114.

Davies, N.M. Clinical pharmacokinetics of nabumetone. the dawn of selective cyclo-oxygenase-2 inhibition? *Clin. Pharmacokinet.,* **1997,** *33:*404–416.

Davies, N.M. Clinical pharmacokinetics of ibuprofen. The first 30 years. *Clin. Pharmacokinet.,* **1998a,** *34:*101–154.

Davies, N.M. Clinical pharmacokinetics of oxaprozin. *Clin. Pharmacokinet.,* **1998b,** *35:*425–436.

Davies, N.M., and Anderson, K.E. Clinical pharmacokinetics of naproxen. *Clin. Pharmacokinet.,* **1997,** *32:*268–293.

Davies, N.M., McLachlan, A.J., Day, R.O., and Williams, K.M. Clinical pharmacokinetics and pharmacodynamics of celecoxib: a selective cyclo-oxygenase-2 inhibitor. *Clin. Pharmacokinet.,* **2000,** *38:*225–242.

Davies, N.M., Teng, X.W., and Skjodt, N.M. Pharmacokinetics of rofecoxib: a specific cyclo-oxygenase-2 inhibitor. *Clin. Pharmacokinet.,* **2003,** *42:*545–556.

Davies, R.O. Review of the animal and clinical pharmacology of diflunisal. *Pharmacotherapy,* **1983,** *3:*9S–22S.

Davis, R., Yarker, Y.E., and Goa, K.L. Diclofenac/misoprostol. A review of its pharmacology and therapeutic efficacy in painful inflammatory conditions. *Drugs Aging,* **1995,** *7:*372–393.

Deeks, J.J., Smith, L.A., and Bradley, M.D. Efficacy, tolerability, and upper gastrointestinal safety of celecoxib for treatment of osteoarthritis and rheumatoid arthritis: systematic review of randomised controlled trials. *BMJ,* **2002,** *325:*619–626.

Dempsey, P.W., Doyle, S.E., He, J.Q., and Cheng, G. The signaling adaptors and pathways activated by TNF superfamily. *Cytokine Growth Factor Rev.,* **2003,** *14:*193–209.

Diaz-Gonzalez, F., and Sanchez-Madrid, F. Inhibition of leukocyte adhesion: an alternative mechanism of action for anti-inflammatory drugs. *Immunol. Today,* **1998,** *19:*169–172.

FitzGerald, G.A., and Patrono, C. The coxibs, selective inhibitors of cyclooxygenase-2. *N. Engl. J. Med.,* **2001,** *345:*433–442.

Fleischmann, R., Iqbal, I., and Slobodin, G. Meloxicam. *Expert Opin. Pharmacother.,* **2002,** *3:*1501–1512.

Glasgow, J.F., and Middleton, B. Reye syndrome—insights on causation and prognosis. *Arch. Dis. Child.,* **2001,** *85:*351–353.

Guay-Woodford, L.M. Bartter syndrome: unraveling the pathophysiologic enigma. *Am. J. Med.,* **1998,** *105:*151–161.

Guttadauria, M. The clinical pharmacology of piroxicam. *Acta Obstet. Gynecol. Scand. Suppl.,* **1986,** *138:*11–13.

Haanen, C. Sulindac and its derivatives: a novel class of anticancer agents. *Curr. Opin. Investig. Drugs,* **2001,** *2:*677–683.

Hart, F.D., and Huskisson, E.C. Nonsteroidal anti-inflammatory drugs. Current status and rational therapeutic use. *Drugs,* **1984,** *27:*232–255.

Jones, A.L. Mechanism of action and value of N-acetylcysteine in the treatment of early and late acetaminophen poisoning: a critical review. *J. Toxicol. Clin. Toxicol.,* **1998,** *36:*277–285.

Kyriakis, J.M., and Avruch, J. Mammalian mitogen-activated protein kinase signal transduction pathways activated by stress and inflammation. *Physiol. Rev.,* **2001,** *81:*807–869.

Levy, M., Spino, M., and Read, S.E. Colchicine: a state-of-the-art review. *Pharmacotherapy,* **1991,** *11:*196–211.

Louie, S.G., Park, B., and Yoon, H. Biological response modifiers in the management of rheumatoid arthritis. *Am. J. Health. Syst. Pharm.,* **2003,** *60:*346–355.

McNeely, W., and Goa, K.L. Diclofenac-potassium in migraine: a review. *Drugs,* **1999,** *57:*991–1003.

Marjoribanks, J., Proctor, M.L., and Farquhar, C. Nonsteroidal antiinflammatory drugs for primary dysmenorrhoea. *Cochrane Database Syst. Rev.,* **2003,** CD001751.

Meager, A. Cytokine regulation of cellular adhesion molecule expression in inflammation. *Cytokine Growth Factor Rev.,* **1999,** *10:*27–39.

Morley, P.A., Brogden, R.N., Carmine, A.A., *et al.* Zomepirac: a review of its pharmacological properties and analgesic efficacy. *Drugs,* **1982,** *23:*250–275.

Nilsen, O.G. Clinical pharmacokinetics of tenoxicam. *Clin. Pharmacokinet.,* **1994,** *26:*16–43.

Nussmeier, N.A., Whelton, A.A., Brown, M.T., *et al.* Complications of COX-2 inhibitors parecoxib and valdecoxib after cardiac surgery. *N. Engl. J. Med.,* **2005,** *352:*1081–1091.

O'Dell, J.R. Therapeutic strategies for rheumatoid arthritis. *N. Engl. J. Med.,* **2004,** *305:*2591–2602.

Olson, N.J., and Stein, C.M. New drugs for rheumatoid arthritis. *N. Engl. J. Med.,* **2004,** *350:*2167–2179.

Patrono, C., and Dunn, M.J. The clinical significance of inhibition of renal prostaglandin synthesis. *Kidney Int.,* **1987,** *32:*1–12.

Rainsford, K.D. Discovery, mechanisms of action and safety of ibuprofen. *Int. J. Clin. Pract. Suppl.,* **2003,** *135:*3–8.

Rostom, A., Dube, C., Wells, G., *et al.* Prevention of NSAID-induced gastroduodenal ulcers. *Cochrane Database Syst. Rev.,* **2002,** CD002296.

Serhan, C.N., and Chiang, N. Novel endogenous small molecules as the checkpoint controllers in inflammation and resolution: entree for resoleomics. *Rheum. Dis. Clin. North Am.,* **2004,** *30:*69–95.

Serhan, C.N., and Oliw, E. Unorthodox routes to prostanoid formation: new twists in cyclooxygenase-initiated pathways. *J. Clin. Invest.,* **2001,** *107:*1481–1489.

Skjodt, N.M., and Davies, N.M. Clinical pharmacokinetics of lornoxicam. A short half-life oxicam. *Clin. Pharmacokinet.,* **1998,** *34:*421–428.

Slater, D.M., Zervou, S., and Thornton, S. Prostaglandins and prostanoid receptors in human pregnancy and parturition. *J. Soc. Gynecol. Investig.,* **2002,** *9:*118–124.

Solomon, S.D., McMurray, J.V., Pfeffer, M.A., *et al.* Cardiovascular risk associated with celecoxib in a clinical trial for colorectal adenoma prevention. *N. Engl. J. Med.,* **2005,** *352:*1071–1080.

Tacconelli, S., Capone, M.L., and Patrignani, P. Clinical pharmacology of novel selective COX-2 inhibitors. *Curr. Pharm. Des.,* **2004,** *10:*589–601.

Terkeltaub, R.A. Clinical practice. Gout. *N. Engl. J. Med.,* **2003,** *349:*1647–1655.

Vane, J.R., and Botting, R.M. Mechanism of action of nonsteroidal antiinflammatory drugs. *Am. J. Med.,* **1998,** *104:*2S–8S.

Veys, E.M. 20 years' experience with ketoprofen. *Scand. J. Rheumat. Suppl.,* **1991,** *90:*1–44.

Villar, J., Abalos, E., Nardin, J.M., Merialdi, M., and Carroli, G. Strategies to prevent and treat preeclampsia: evidence from randomized controlled trials. *Semin. Nephrol.,* **2004,** *24:*607–615.

Worobec, A.S. Treatment of systemic mast cell disorders. *Hematol. Oncol. Clin. North Am.,* **2000,** *14:*659–687.

PHARMACOTHERAPY OF ASTHMA

Bradley J. Undem

Asthma is a common disorder, accounting in the United States for 1% to 3% of all office visits, 500,000 hospital admissions per year, more pediatric hospital admissions than any other single illness, and more than 5000 deaths annually.

The pharmacological therapy of asthma employs drugs aimed at reducing airway inflammation (*i.e.*, antiinflammatory agents) and drugs aimed more directly at decreasing bronchospasm (*i.e.*, bronchodilators). To these ends, six classes of therapeutic agents are presently indicated for asthma treatment: β adrenergic receptor agonists, glucocorticoids, leukotriene inhibitors, chromones, methylxanthines, and inhibitors of immunoglobulin E (IgE). Each of these classes is discussed below.

ASTHMA AS AN INFLAMMATORY ILLNESS

Asthma is associated with inflammation of the airway wall. Increased numbers of various types of inflammatory cells, most notably eosinophils but also basophils, mast cells, macrophages, and certain types of lymphocytes, can be found in airway wall biopsies and in bronchoalveolar lavage fluid from asthmatic patients. Inflammatory mediators and various cytokines also are increased in the airways of asthmatic subjects compared with healthy control subjects. How bronchial inflammation contributes to the asthmatic condition remains poorly understood. Even asthmatics with normal baseline lung function and no recent exacerbations of their asthma have increased numbers of inflammatory cells in their airways. Conversely, many individuals allergic to inhaled allergens have evidence of lower airway inflammation but suffer only from the symptoms of allergic rhinitis. The basis for this inflammation is not entirely clear. Many individuals with

asthma are atopic and have clearly defined allergen exposures that are partially or substantially responsible for their asthmatic inflammation. Epidemiological studies show a strong correlation between increasing IgE levels and the prevalence of asthma regardless of atopic status (Burrows *et al.*, 1989). Nonallergic individuals also can suffer from asthma, as is often seen in subjects in whom the onset of disease is later in life.

Although there are subtypes of asthma (allergic *versus* nonallergic), there are features of airway inflammation common to all asthmatic airways (Figure 27–1). Airway inflammation is thought to be triggered by innate and/or adapted immune responses. Although there may be multiple "triggers" for an inflammatory response (such as mast cell secretion), there is general agreement that a lymphocyte-directed eosinophilic bronchitis is a hallmark of asthma. The lymphocytes that participate in asthma pathology are biased toward the T-helper type 2 (Th2) phenotype, leading to increases in production of interleukin 4 (IL-4), IL-5, and IL-13. The IL-4 from Th2 cells (and basophils) provides help for IgE synthesis in B cells. The IL-5 provides support for eosinophil survival. The innate or adapted immune response triggers the production of additional cytokines and chemokines, resulting in trafficking of blood-borne cells (*i.e.*, eosinophils, basophils, neutrophils, and lymphocytes) into airway tissues, and these cells further generate a variety of autocoids and cytokines. The inflammatory cascade also leads to activation of resident cells within the airways that, in turn, can produce a panoply of cytokines, growth factors, chemokines, and autacoids. The chronic inflammatory response, over time, leads to epithelial shedding and reorganization, mucous hypersecretion, and airway wall remodeling most often exemplified by subepithelial fibrosis and smooth muscle hyperplasia. How these processes lead to attacks of asthma, which most often are induced or exacerbated by respiratory viral infections, remains unclear.

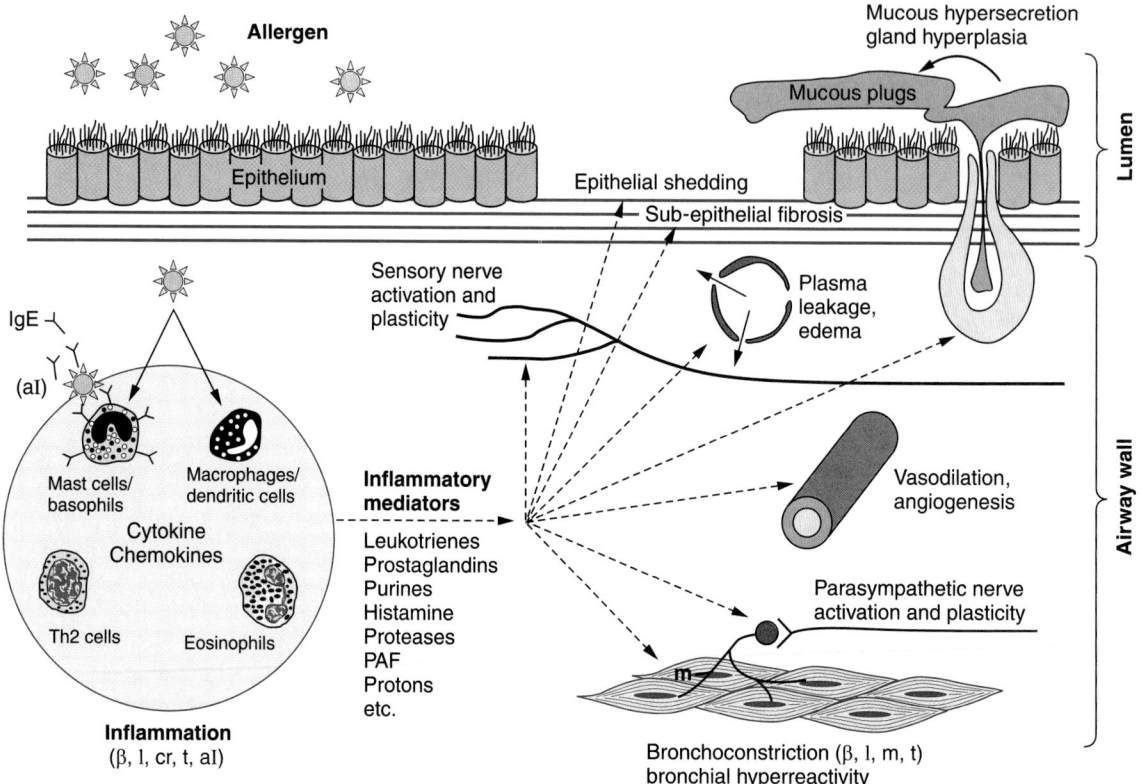

Figure 27–1. *Simplified view of allergic inflammation in the airways.* Asthma is an episodic narrowing of the bronchi thought to be caused by an underlying chronic inflammatory disorder. In allergic asthma, inhaled allergen initiates the inflammatory response by interacting with IgE bound to mast cells and basophils. This leads to a cascade of events involving other immune cells and resulting in the release of numerous inflammatory mediators into the interstitial space, where they influence the growth and function of cell types within the airway wall. The drugs available for the treatment of asthma are targeted at inhibiting the inflammatory responses and/or relaxing the bronchial smooth muscle. Letters denote the putative sites of action for the various classes of drugs used in treating asthma. β, β_2 adrenergic agonists; cs, corticosteroids; l, leukotriene modifiers; m, muscarinic receptor antagonists; cr, cromolyn; t, theophylline; aI, anti-IgE therapy. The sunburst (☼) symbolizes an allergen.

In addition to airway inflammation, asthmatics commonly exhibit bronchial hyperreactivity. Thus the concentration of a bronchial spasmogen, such as methacholine or histamine, needed to produce a 20% increase in airway resistance in asthmatics is often only 1% to 2% of the equally effective concentration in healthy control subjects. This bronchial hyperreactivity most often is nonspecific such that the airways are also inordinately reactive to stimuli such as strong odors, cold air, and pollutants. Little is known about specific mechanisms underlying this enigmatic hyperreactivity.

The pharmacotherapy of asthma centers on controlling the disease with drugs that inhibit airway inflammation. Other drugs that relax bronchial smooth muscle are used for more immediate and direct relief of the symptoms of asthma.

TREATMENT OF ASTHMA

Aerosol Delivery of Drugs

Topical application of drugs to the lungs can be accomplished by use of aerosols. In theory, this approach should produce a high local concentration in the lungs with a low systemic delivery, thereby significantly minimizing systemic side effects. The drugs used most commonly in the treatment of asthma, β_2 adrenergic receptor agonists and glucocorticoids, have potentially serious side effects when delivered systemically. Since the pathophysiology of asthma appears to involve the respiratory tract alone, the advantages of aerosol treatments with limited systemic effects are substantial. Indeed, in clinical practice, proba-

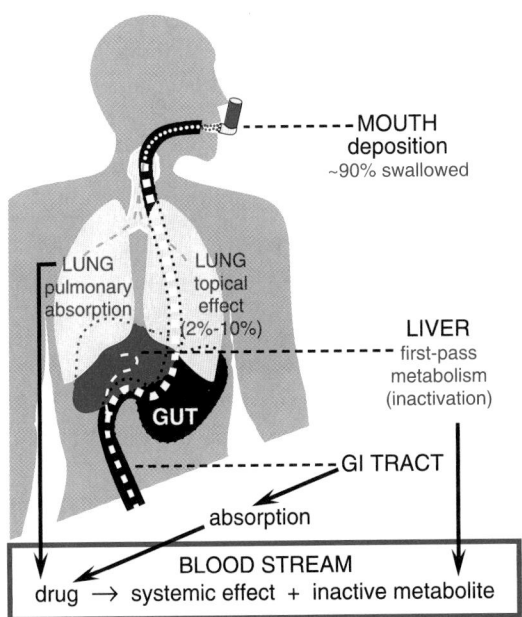

Figure 27–2. Schematic representations of the disposition of inhaled drugs. Inhalation therapy deposits asthma medications directly, but not exclusively, in the lungs. Distribution of inhaled drug between lungs and esophagus depends on particle size and efficiency of delivery to lungs. Most material, approximately 90%, will be swallowed and absorbed, entering the systemic circulation. Some drug also will be absorbed from the lungs. Optimal particle size for deposition in small airways is 1 to 5 μm.

bly more than 90% of asthmatic patients who are capable of manipulating inhaler devices can be managed by aerosol treatments alone. Because of the specialized nature of aerosol delivery and the substantial effects that these systems have on the therapeutic index, the principles of this delivery method are important to review.

The chemistry and physics of aerosol delivery systems have been reviewed (Taburet and Schmit, 1994). A schematic diagram of the fate of therapeutic agents delivered by this route is given in Figure 27-2. The critical determinant of the delivery of any particulate matter to the lungs is the size of the particles. Particles larger than 10 μm are deposited primarily in the mouth and oropharynx, whereas particles smaller than 0.5 μm are inhaled to the alveolae and subsequently exhaled without being deposited in the lungs. Particles with a diameter of 1 to 5 μm allow deposition of drugs in the small airways and therefore are the most effective. Unfortunately, no aerosol system in clinical use can produce uniform particles limited to the appropriate size range. A number of factors in addition to particle size determine effective deposition of drugs in the

bronchial tree, including the rate of breathing and breath-holding after inhalation. It is recommended that a slow, deep breath be taken and held for 5 to 10 seconds when administering drugs to the lungs.

As depicted in Figure 27–2, even under ideal circumstances only a small fraction of the aerosolized drug is deposited in the lungs, typically 2% to 10%. Most of the remainder is swallowed. Therefore, to minimize systemic effects, an aerosolized drug should be either poorly absorbed from the gastrointestinal system or rapidly inactivated *via* first-pass hepatic metabolism. Furthermore, any maneuvers that increase deposition in the lungs or decrease the percentage of drug reaching the gastrointestinal system should enhance the desired effects and reduce undesired systematic effects. For example, with metered-dose inhalers, a large-volume "spacer" can be attached to the inhaler. A spacer is a tube or expandable bellows that fits between the inhaler and the patient's mouth; the inhaler discharges into the spacer, and the patient inhales from it. A spacer can improve markedly the ratio of inhaled to swallowed drug by limiting the amount of larger particles (>10 μm) that reach the mouth and by reducing the need for the patient to coordinate accurately inhalation with inhaler activation (Bryant and Shimizu, 1988). This is not a trivial concern: More than 50% of patients using inhalers do not use proper technique and thus deposit too small a fraction of inhaled drug into the lungs.

The two types of devices used for aerosol therapy are *metered-dose inhalers* and *nebulizers*. Both devices provide a range of particle sizes that includes the desired 1- to 5-μm range. When used appropriately, they are equally effective in drug delivery to the lungs, even in the setting of fairly severe asthma exacerbations (Turner *et al.*, 1988; Benton *et al.*, 1989). Nevertheless, some clinicians and many patients prefer to use nebulizers for severe asthma exacerbations with poor inspiratory ability. Metered-dose inhalers offer the advantages of being cheaper and portable; nebulizers offer the advantage of not requiring hand-breathing coordination. In addition, nebulizer therapy can be delivered by facemask to young children or older patients who are confused. A substantial disadvantage of metered-dose inhalers is that most contain chlorofluorocarbons. Temporary exemptions have been given for these devices until safe alternative propellants can be developed. An albuterol metered-dose inhaler using hydrofluoroalkane as a propellant (PROVENTIL HFA) is available for clinical use in the United States.

An alternative to aerosolized delivery is the use of *dry-powder inhalers*. These typically use lactose or glucose powders to carry the drugs. One disadvantage of these devices is that a relatively high airflow is needed to suspend the powder properly. Young children, the elderly, and those suffering from a significant asthma exacerbation may be unable to generate such airflow rates. The dry powder can be irritating when inhaled. Storage of dry-powder inhalers in areas where there are wide temperature fluctuations or high humidity can impair their performance.

β_2 Adrenergic Receptor Agonists

The history, chemistry, pharmacological properties, and mechanisms of action of the β adrenergic agonists are discussed in Chapter 10. Their discussion here is restricted to their uses in asthma.

Mechanism of Action and Use in Asthma. The β adrenergic receptor agonists available for the treatment of asthma are selective for the β_2-receptor subtype. With few exceptions, they are delivered directly to the airways *via* inhalation. The agonists can be classified as short- or long-acting. This subclassification is useful from a pharmacological perspective: Short-acting agonists are used only for symptomatic relief of asthma, whereas long-acting agonists are used prophylactically in the treatment of the disease.

The mechanism of the antiasthmatic action of β adrenergic receptor agonists is undoubtedly linked to the direct relaxation of airway smooth muscle and consequent bronchodilation. Although human bronchial smooth muscle receives little or no sympathetic innervation, it nevertheless contains large numbers of β_2 adrenergic receptors. Stimulation of these receptors activates the G_s adenylyl cyclase–cyclic AMP pathway with a consequent reduction of in smooth muscle tone (Sylvester, 2004). β_2 Adrenergic receptor agonists also increase the conductance of large Ca^{2+}-sensitive K^+ channels in airway smooth muscle, leading to membrane hyperpolarization and relaxation. This occurs at least partly by mechanisms independent of adenylyl cyclase activity and cyclic AMP production and may involve the regulation of capacitative Ca^{2+} entry by small G proteins. (Kume *et al.*, 1994; Ostrom and Ehlert, 1998; Koike *et al.*, 2004; Sylvester, 2004).

There are β_2 adrenergic receptors on cell types in the airways other than bronchial smooth muscle. Of particular interest, stimulation of β_2 adrenergic receptors inhibits the function of numerous inflammatory cells, including mast cells, basophils, eosinophils, neutrophils, and lymphocytes. In general, stimulating β_2 adrenergic receptors in these cell types increases intracellular cyclic AMP, activating a signaling cascade that inhibits the release of inflammatory mediators and cytokines (Barnes, 1999).

As noted below, long-term exposure to β_2-agonists may desensitize some of these receptor-response pathways; thus there is little evidence that these drugs, used chronically, reduce airway inflammation.

Short-Acting β_2 Adrenergic Receptor Agonists. Drugs in this class include *albuterol* (PROVENTIL, VENTOLIN), *levalbuterol,* the (R)-enantiomer of albuterol (XOPENEX), *metaproterenol* (ALUPENT), *terbutaline* (BRETHAIRE), and

pirbuterol (MAXAIR). These drugs are used for acute inhalation treatment of bronchospasm. Terbutaline (BRETHINE, BRICANYL), albuterol, and metaproterenol also are available in oral dosage form. Each of the inhaled drugs has an onset of action within 1 to 5 minutes and produces bronchodilation that lasts for about 2 to 6 hours. When given in oral dosage forms, the duration of action is somewhat longer (oral terbutaline, for example, has a duration of action of 4 to 8 hours). Although there are slight differences in the relative β_2/β_1-receptor potency ratios among the drugs, all of them are selective for the β_2 subtype.

The most effective drugs in relaxing airway smooth muscle and reversing bronchoconstriction are short-acting β_2 adrenergic receptor agonists. They are the preferred treatment for rapid symptomatic relief of dyspnea associated with asthmatic bronchoconstriction (Fanta *et al.*, 1986; Nelson, 1995). Although these drugs are prescribed on an as-needed basis, it is imperative that guidelines be given to the patient so that reliance on relief of symptoms during times of deteriorating asthma does not occur. When the asthma symptoms become persistent, the patient should be reevaluated so that drugs aimed at controlling, in addition to reversing, the disease can be prescribed.

Long-Acting β Adrenergic Receptor Agonists. *Salmeterol xinafoate* (SEREVENT) and *formoterol* (FORADIL) are long-lasting adrenergic agents with very high selectivity for the β_2-receptor subtype (Cheung *et al.*, 1992; D'Alonzo *et al.*, 1994). Inhalation of salmeterol provides persistent bronchodilation lasting over 12 hours. The mechanism underlying the extended duration of action of salmeterol is not yet fully understood. The extended side chain on salmeterol renders it 10,000 times more lipophilic than albuterol (Brittain, 1990). The lipophilicity regulates the diffusion rate away from the receptor by determining the degree of partitioning in the lipid bilayer of the membrane. Subsequent to binding the receptor, the less lipophilic, short-acting agonists are removed rapidly from the receptor environment by diffusion in the aqueous phase. Unbound salmeterol, by contrast, persists in the membrane and only slowly dissociates from the receptor environment.

Long-acting β adrenergic receptor agonists relax airway smooth muscle and cause bronchodilation by the same mechanisms as short-duration agonists. Chronic treatment with a receptor agonist often leads to receptor desensitization and a diminution of effect. The rate and degree of β_2 adrenergic receptor desensitization depend on the cell type. For example, the β_2 receptors on human bronchial smooth muscle are relatively resistant to desensitization, whereas receptors on mast cells and lymphocytes are desensitized rapidly following agonist exposure (Chong and Peachell, 1999; Johnson and Coleman, 1995). This may help to explain why there is little evidence that these drugs are effective in inhibiting airway inflammation associated with asthma.

Several studies have evaluated the effect of adding a long-acting β_2 adrenergic agonist to inhaled glucocorticoid treatment in patients with persistent asthma (Jackson and Lipworth, 2004). Combinations examined include salmeterol–fluticasone and formoterol–budesonide. The data suggest that adding a long-acting β_2 adrenergic agonist to the inhaled steroid regimen is more effective than doubling the steroid dose. Thus, current management guidelines for asthma recommend that long-acting β_2 adrenergic agonists be added if symptoms persist in patients on low or medium doses of inhaled steroids. Because chronic treatment with long-lasting inhaled β_2 adrenergic agonists does not decrease airway inflammation significantly, most experts do not use them as sole agents for asthma treatment. A convenient fixed-dosage combination of salmeterol and fluticasone (ADVAIR) is marketed in the United States, and a fixed dosage combination of formoterol and budesonide is available in other countries.

Toxicity. Owing to their β_2-receptor selectivity and topical delivery, inhaled β adrenergic receptor agonists at recommended doses have relatively few side effects. A portion of inhaled drug is inevitably absorbed into the systemic circulation. At higher doses, therefore, these drugs may lead to increased heart rate, cardiac arrhythmias, and central nervous system (CNS) effects associated with β adrenergic receptor activation, as described in Chapter 10. This is of particular concern in patients with poorly controlled asthma, in whom there may be excessive and inappropriate reliance on symptomatic treatment with short-acting β receptor agonists.

Oral Therapy with β Adrenergic Receptor Agonists. The use of orally administered β adrenergic agonists for bronchodilation has not gained wide acceptance largely because of the greater risk of side effects, especially tremulousness, muscle cramps, cardiac tachyarrhythmias, and metabolic disturbances (*see* Chapter 10). There are two primary situations in which oral β adrenergic agonists are used. First, brief courses of oral therapy (albuterol or metaproterenol syrups) are well tolerated and effective in young children (<5 years old) who cannot manipulate metered-dose inhalers yet have occasional wheezing with viral upper respiratory infections. Second, in some patients with severe asthma exacerbations, any aerosol, whether delivered *via* a metered-dose inhaler or a nebulizer, can worsen cough and bronchospasm owing to local irritation. In this setting, oral therapy with β_2 adrenergic agonists (*e.g.,* albuterol, metaproterenol, or terbutaline tablets) can be effective. However, the frequency of adverse systemic side effects with orally administered agents is higher in adults than in children.

Even though stimulation of β adrenergic receptors inhibits the release of inflammatory mediators from mast cells, long-term administration of β_2-agonists, either orally or by inhalation, does not reduce bronchial hyperresponsiveness. Thus, other approaches are preferred for the treatment of chronic symptoms. As discussed below under "Pharmacogenetics," polymorphisms of the β_2 adrenergic receptor may correlate with response to therapy and adverse effects with β-agonists.

Glucocorticoids

The history, chemistry, pharmacological properties, and mechanisms of action of glucocorticoids are discussed in Chapter 59. The discussion here is restricted to their uses in asthma, as reviewed by Barnes and Pedersen (1993).

Systemic glucocorticoids long have been used to treat severe chronic asthma or severe acute exacerbations of asthma (McFadden, 1993; Greenberger, 1992). The development of aerosol formulations significantly improved the safety of glucocorticoid treatment, allowing it to be used for moderate asthma (Busse, 1993). Asthmatic subjects who require inhaled β_2 adrenergic agonists four or more times weekly are viewed as candidates for inhaled glucocorticoids (Anonymous, 1991; Israel and Drazen, 1994; Barnes, 1995).

Mechanism of Glucocorticoid Action in Asthma. Asthma is associated with airway inflammation, airway hyperreactivity, and acute bronchoconstriction. Glucocorticoids do not directly relax airway smooth muscle and thus have little effect on acute bronchoconstriction. By contrast, these agents are singularly effective in inhibiting airway inflammation. Very few mechanisms of inflammation escape the inhibitory effects of these drugs (*see* Chapter 59; Schleimer, 1998). The antiinflammatory effects of glucocorticoids in asthma include modulation of cytokine and chemokine production; inhibition of eicosanoid synthesis; marked inhibition of accumulation of basophils, eosinophils, and other leukocytes in lung tissue; and decreased vascular permeability (Schleimer, 1998). The profound and generalized antiinflammatory action of this class of drugs explains why they are currently the most effective drugs used in the treatment of asthma.

Inhaled Glucocorticoids. Although glucocorticoids are very effective in controlling asthma, treatment with systemic glucocorticoids comes at the cost of considerable adverse effects (*see* Chapter 59). A major advance in asthma therapy was the development of inhaled glucocorticoids that targeted the drug directly to the relevant site of inflammation. These formulations greatly enhance the therapeutic index of the drugs, substantially diminishing the number and degree of side effects without sacrificing clinical utility. There are currently five glucocorticoids available in the United States for inhalation therapy: *beclomethasone dipropionate* (BECLOVENT, VANCERIL), *triamcinolone acetonide* (AZMACORT), *flunisolide* (AEROBID), *budesonide* (PULMICORT), and *fluticasone propionate* (FLOVENT). While they differ markedly in their affinities for the glucocorticoid receptor, with fluticasone and budesonide having much higher affinities than beclomethasone, they are all effective in controlling asthma at the appropriate doses. Few studies have directly assessed the relative therapeutic index of the various formulations of inhaled steroids in the treatment of asthma, but available data indicate that none has a clearly superior therapeutic index (O'Byrne and Pedersen, 1998).

Inhaled glucocorticoids are used prophylactically to control asthma rather than acutely to reverse asthma symptoms. As with all prophylactic therapies, compliance is a significant concern. Issues relating to drug compliance, therefore, become relevant when choosing among the various steroid formulations. The newer, highly potent drugs (*e.g.*, fluticasone, flunisolide, and budesonide) can be effective with as little as one or two puffs administered twice or even once daily. This more convenient dosage regimen may be preferred by patients, providing improved compliance and better asthma control. The appropriate dose of steroid must be determined empirically. Important variables that influence the effective dose include the severity of disease, the particular steroid used, and the device used for drug delivery, which determines the actual quantity of drug delivered to the lungs (Smaldone, 1997). When determining the optimal dose, keep in mind that maximal improvement in lung function may not occur until after several weeks of treatment.

Asthmatic patients maintained on inhaled glucocorticoids show improvement in symptoms and lowered requirements for "rescue" with β_2 adrenergic agonists (Laitinen *et al.*, 1992; Haahtela *et al.*, 1994). Beneficial effects may be seen within 1 week; however, improvement, in terms of reduced bronchial hyperreactivity, may continue for several months (Juniper *et al.*, 1990). Inhaled glucocorticoids are superior to inhaled β_2-agonists for symptom control. In one study, improved bronchial hyperreactivity persisted throughout 2 years of treatment with inhaled budesonide (600 μg twice daily), and most patients were able to reduce their dose to 200 μg twice daily thereafter without worsened symptoms (Haahtela *et al.*, 1994). Complete discontinuation of budesonide generally was associated with increased bronchial hyperreactivity and worsened symptoms, although symptoms did not worsen in a third of patients. Thus a trial discontinuation of inhaled glucocorticoids should be considered in patients who are extremely well controlled.

Systemic Glucocorticoids. Systemic glucocorticoids are used for acute asthma exacerbations and chronic severe asthma. Substantial doses of glucocorticoids (*e.g.,* 40 to 60 mg prednisone or equivalent daily for 5 days; 1 to 2 mg/kg per day for children) often are used to treat acute exacerbations of asthma (Weinberger, 1987). Although an additional week at somewhat reduced dosage may be required, the steroids can be withdrawn abruptly once control of the symptoms by other medications has been restored; any suppression of adrenal function dissipates within 1 to 2 weeks. More protracted bouts of severe asthma may require longer treatment and slower tapering of the dose to avoid exacerbating asthma symptoms and suppressing pituitary/adrenal function. Previously, alternate-day therapy with oral prednisone was employed commonly in persistent asthma. Now most patients with asthma are better treated with inhaled glucocorticoids.

Toxicity. *Inhaled Glucocorticoids.* While there is a great deal of enthusiasm for inhaled glucocorticoids in asthma, local and systemic adverse effects remain a concern (Table 27–1). Some portion of any inhaled drug is swallowed. Therefore, inhaled drugs can reach the circulation by direct absorption from the lung or by absorption from the gas-

trointestinal tract. The newer glucocorticoids have extremely low oral bioavailability owing to extensive first-pass metabolism by the liver and reach the circulation almost exclusively by absorption from the lung (Brattsand and Axelsson, 1997). In contrast to the beneficial effects on asthma, which plateau at about 1600 μg/day, the probability of adverse effects continues to increase at higher doses. Oropharyngeal candidiasis and, more frequently, dysphonia can be encountered. The incidence of candidiasis can be reduced substantially by rinsing the mouth and throat with water after each use and by employing spacer or reservoir devices attached to the dispenser to decrease drug deposition in the oral cavity (Johnson, 1987). Appreciable suppression of the hypothalamic–pituitary–adrenal axis is difficult to document at doses below 800 μg/day and probably is rarely of physiologic importance even at doses up to 1600 μg/day. Modest but statistically significant decreases in bone mineral density do occur in female asthmatics receiving inhaled steroids, even when doses as low as 500 μg/day are employed (Ip *et al.*, 1994). Others have shown increases in markers for bone mineral turnover (serum osteocalcin and urine hydroxyproline levels) during treatment with inhaled glucocorticoids (Pavord and Knox, 1993; Israel and Drazen, 1994). While the clinical relevance of these bone metabolism findings remains to be determined, it is argued that inhaled glucocorticoid treatment should be reserved for moderate or severe asthma because such treatment is likely to last for many years (Israel and Drazen, 1994). Nonetheless, it has been suggested that the small risk of adverse effects at high doses of inhaled glucocorticoids is outweighed by the risks of inadequately controlling severe asthma (Barnes, 1995).

Systemic Glucocorticoids. The adverse effects of systemic administration of glucocorticoids are well known (*see* Chapter 59), but treatment for brief periods (5 to 10 days) causes relatively little dose-related toxicity. The most common adverse effects during a brief course are mood disturbances, increased appetite, impaired glucose control in diabetics, and candidiasis.

Leukotriene-Receptor Antagonists and Leukotriene-Synthesis Inhibitors

Zafirlukast (ACCOLATE) and *montelukast* (SINGULAIR) are leukotriene-receptor antagonists. *Zileuton* (ZYFLO) is an inhibitor of 5-lipoxygenase, which catalyzes the formation of leukotrienes from arachidonic acid.

History. The history of leukotrienes can be traced back to the classical pharmacological studies in the late 1930s by Kellaway and Trethewie. On investigating antigen-induced responses in guinea pigs sensitized to egg albumin, they discovered a slow-reacting smooth muscle–stimulating substance. They named the active ingredient *slow-reacting substance* (SRS) based on its pharmacological activity and concluded that it was a unique substance found only in immunologically sensitized tissues subsequently challenged with antigen. Decades later, SRS was renamed *slow-reacting substance of anaphylaxis* (SRS-A).

Two pivotal discoveries were required before the importance of SRS-A in allergic responses was proven. First was the discovery in 1973 by scientists at Fisons Pharmaceutical Company of an SRS-A antagonist called FPL 55712 (Augstein *et al.*, 1973), and second was the elucidation by Samuelsson and colleagues of the structure of SRS-A as a 5-lipoxygenase product of arachidonic acid, which they termed *cysteinyl leukotriene* (Murphy *et al.*, 1979; *see* Chapter 25). Soon thereafter, an enormous effort was undertaken by the pharmaceutical industry to discover novel inhibitors of leukotrienes as potential therapeutic

Table 27–1
Potential Adverse Effects Associated with Inhaled Glucocorticoids

ADVERSE EFFECT	RISK
Hypothalamic–pituitary–adrenal axis suppression	No significant risk until dosages of budesonide or beclomethasone increased to >1500 μg/day in adults or >400 μg/day in children
Bone resorption	Modest but significant effects at doses possibly as low as 500 μg/day
Carbohydrate and lipid metabolism	Minor, clinically insignificant changes occur with dosages of beclomethasone >1000 μg/day
Cataracts	Anecdotal reports, risk unproven
Skin thinning	Dosage-related effect with beclomethasone dipropionate over a range of 400 to 2000 μg/day
Purpura	Dosage-related increase in occurrence with beclomethasone over a range of 400 to 2000 μg/day
Dysphonia	Usually of little consequence
Candidiasis	Incidence <5%, reduced by use of spacer device
Growth retardation	Difficult to separate effect of disease from effect of treatment, but no discernible effects on growth when all studies are considered

SOURCE: Modified from Pavord and Knox (1993) and Barnes (1995).

agents for asthma. The strategies taken were either to reduce the synthesis of leukotrienes by inhibiting the 5-lipoxygenase enzyme or to antagonize the effects of leukotrienes at their receptors. These efforts bore fruit in the 1990s with the release of three new drugs for the treatment of asthma in the United States: the leukotriene-receptor antagonists zafirlukast (Krell *et al.*, 1990) and montelukast (Jones *et al.*, 1995) and the leukotriene-synthesis inhibitor zileuton (Carter *et al.*, 1991).

Chemistry. The chemical structures of zafirlukast, montelukast, and zileuton are shown below.

ZAFIRLUKAST

MONTELUKAST

ZILEUTON

Pharmacokinetics and Metabolism. The leukotriene-modifying drugs are administered orally. Zafirlukast is absorbed rapidly, with greater than 90% bioavailability. At therapeutic plasma concentrations, it is over 99% protein-bound. Zafirlukast is metabolized extensively by hepatic CYP2C9. The parent drug is responsible for its therapeutic activity, with metabolites being less than 10% as effective. The half-life of zafirlukast is approximately 10 hours.

Montelukast is absorbed rapidly, with about 60% to 70% bioavailability. At therapeutic concentrations, it is highly protein-bound (99%). It is metabolized extensively by CYP3A4 and CYP2C9. The half-life of montelukast is between 3 and 6 hours.

Zileuton is absorbed rapidly on oral administration and is metabolized extensively by CYPs and by UDP-glucuronosyltransferases. The parent molecule is responsible for its therapeutic action. Zileuton is a short-acting drug with a half-life of approximately 2.5 hours and also is highly protein-bound (93%).

Mechanism of Action in Asthma. Leukotriene-modifying drugs act either as competitive antagonists of leukotriene receptors or by inhibiting the synthesis of leukotrienes. The pharmacological properties of leukotrienes are discussed in detail in Chapter 25.

Leukotriene-Receptor Antagonists. Cysteinyl leukotrienes (cys-LTs) include leukotriene C4 (LTC4), leukotriene D4 (LTD4), and leukotriene E4 (LTE4). All the cys-LTs are potent constrictors of bronchial smooth muscle. On a molar basis, LTD4 is approximately 1000 times more potent than is histamine as a bronchoconstrictor (Dahlen *et al.*, 1980). The receptor responsible for the bronchoconstrictor effect of leukotrienes is the cys-LT1 receptor (Buckner *et al.*, 1986; Lynch *et al.*, 1999). Although each of the cys-LTs is an agonist at the cys-LT1 receptor, LTE4 is less potent than either LTC4 or LTD4. Zafirlukast and montelukast are selective high-affinity competitive antagonists for the cys-LT1 receptor (Krell *et al.*, 1990, Jones *et al.*, 1995). *Pranlukast* is another cys-LT1-receptor antagonist used in some countries in the treatment of asthma, but it is not approved for use in the United States. Inhibition of cys-LT-induced bronchial smooth muscle contraction likely is involved in the therapeutic effects of these agents to relieve the symptoms of asthma.

The effects of cys-LTs that are potentially relevant to bronchial asthma are not limited to bronchial smooth muscle contraction. Cys-LTs can increase microvascular leakage, increase mucous production, and enhance eosinophil and basophil influx into the airways (Hay *et al.*, 1995). The extent to which inhibiting these non–smooth muscle effects of leukotrienes contributes to the therapeutic effects of the drugs is not known. It may be noteworthy, however, that zafirlukast significantly inhibits the influx of basophils and lymphocytes entering the airways following experimental allergen challenge in asthmatic subjects (Calhoun *et al.*, 1998).

Leukotriene-Synthesis Inhibitors. The formation of leukotrienes depends on lipoxygenation of arachidonic acid by 5-lipoxygenase. Zileuton is a potent and selective inhibitor of 5-lipoxygenase activity and thus inhibits the formation of all 5-lipoxygenase products. Thus, in addition to inhibiting the formation of the cys-LTs, zileuton also inhibits the formation of leukotriene B4 (LTB4), a potent chemotactic autacoid, and other eicosanoids that depend on leukotriene A4 (LTA4) synthesis. In theory, the therapeutic effects of a 5-lipoxygenase inhibitor would include all those observed with the cys-LT1-receptor antagonists, as well as other effects that may result from inhibiting the formation of LTB4 and other 5-lipoxygenase products.

The pharmacological actions of cys-LTs are not fully accounted for by activation of the cys-LT1 receptor. For example, cys-LT-induced contraction of vascular smooth muscle (Gorenne *et al.*, 1995) and stimulation of expression of P-selectin by endothelial cells occur *via* cys-LT2 receptors (Pedersen *et al.*, 1997). This provides another theoretical advantage of zileuton over zafirlukast and montelukast because 5-lipoxygenase inhibitors would inhibit cys-LT effects regardless of the receptor subtypes involved. These theoretical advantages notwithstanding, studies to date do not prove that zileuton is significantly more efficacious than the cys-LT1-receptor antagonists in the treatment of asthma.

Toxicity. There are few adverse effects directly associated with inhibition of leukotriene synthesis or function. This likely is due to the fact that leukotriene production is limited predominantly to sites of inflammation.

Zafirlukast and Montelukast. In large clinical studies the adverse-effect profiles of these drugs were similar to that observed with placebo treatment. Very rarely, patients taking these drugs develop systemic eosinophilia and a vasculitis with features similar to Churg-Strauss syndrome. This problem, often associated with a reduction in glucocorticoid therapy, may represent the unmasking of a preexisting disease. Zafirlukast, but not montelukast, may interact with warfarin and increase prothrombin times, which should be monitored in patients subject to this interaction.

Zileuton. The adverse-effect profile in patients taking zileuton is similar to that in patients taking placebo. In about 4% to 5% of patients taking zileuton, however, there is an elevation in liver enzymes, generally within the first 2 months of therapy. Zileuton decreases the steady-state clearance of theophylline, substantially increasing its plasma concentrations. Zileuton also decreases warfarin clearance. Because of a variety of pharmacokinetic and safety issues, the drug is no longer used in the United States.

Use in Asthma. Although leukotriene inhibitors are effective prophylactic treatment for mild asthma, their role in asthma therapy is not clearly defined. Most clinical trials with these drugs have studied patients with mild asthma who were not taking glucocorticoids. In general, the studies show a modest but significant improvement in pulmonary function and a decrease in symptoms and asthma exacerbations. In a meta-analysis of clinical trials with zafirlukast, all studies showed some decrease in the rate of asthma exacerbations, with an average reduction of 50% (Barnes and Miller, 2000). When zafirlukast (Laitinen *et al.*, 1997) and montelukast (Malmstrom *et al.*, 1999) were compared with low-dose inhaled glucocorticoid therapy, the improvement in lung function and decreased dependence on short-acting β_2 adrenergic receptor agonist therapy was found to be greater in the glucocorticoid-treated subjects. There was little difference, however, between the steroid- and montelukast-treated subjects in the reduction in rate of asthma exacerbations. Clinical trials with antileukotriene drugs have revealed considerable heterogeneity in response to therapy, with patients falling into "responder" and "nonresponder" groups. For those who respond to antileukotriene therapy, the National Heart, Lung, and Blood Institute recognizes these drugs as alternatives to low-dose inhaled steroids for control of mild chronic asthma.

More studies are required to define the role of these drugs in moderate and severe asthma. Some clinical trials have demonstrated an ability of leukotriene antagonists to allow a reduction in the dose of inhaled steroid needed to control asthma exacerbations (Lofdahl *et al.*, 1999; Jarvis and Markham, 2000). If this is the case, it may be particularly relevant in children with more severe asthma. This class of drugs is not indicated for rapid bronchodilator therapy; thus patients are instructed to have short-acting β adrenergic receptor agonists available as rescue medication. Montelukast and zafirlukast are effective with once- or twice-daily treatment, respectively. In contrast, zileuton is taken four times a day. Liver enzymes should be monitored in patients beginning zileuton therapy to guard against the potential of liver toxicity.

Anti-IgE Therapy

Omalizumab (XOLAIR) is the first "biological drug" approved for the treatment of asthma. Omalizumab is a recombinant humanized monoclonal antibody targeted against IgE. IgE bound to omalizumab cannot bind to IgE receptors on mast cells and basophils, thereby preventing the allergic reaction at a very early step in the process (Figure 27–3).

History. In 1921, Prausnitz and Kustner provided conclusive evidence that a serum factor that they termed *reagin* was able to passively transfer allergic reactions from an allergic individuals to nonallergic subjects. It was some 45 years before the Ishizakas proved that reagin was a novel immunoglobulin termed E (IgE). IgE was found to bind with high affinity to receptors on mast cells and basophils, and the subsequent binding of antigen (allergen) to the bound IgE molecules resulted in cell activation and the release of various mediators of allergic inflammation (Tomioka and Ishizaka, 1971). It was recognized at once that a chemical that would prevent IgE from

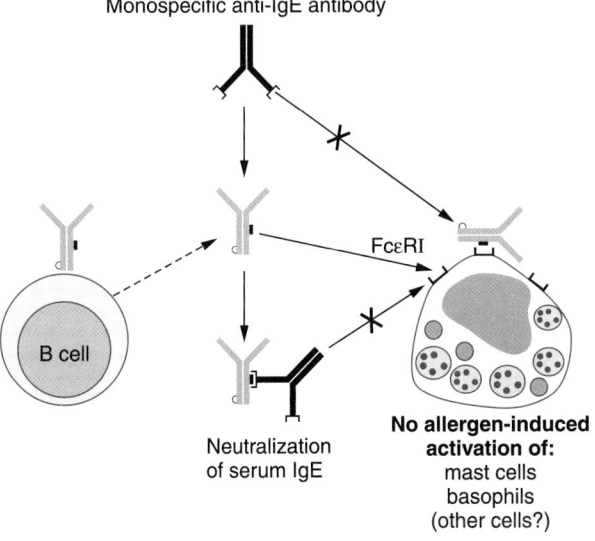

Monospecific anti-IgE antibody

B cell

FcεRI

Neutralization of serum IgE

No allergen-induced activation of:
mast cells
basophils
(other cells?)

Non-anaphylactic

Figure 27–3. Omalizumab is a monospecific anti-IgE antibody. Specific B-lymphocytes produce IgE antibodies. The Fc region of IgE heavy chains binds with high affinity to receptors (FcεRI) in the plasma membranes of mast cells and basophils (and other cells). Allergen interacts with the antigen-binding site of cell-bound IgE, causing FcεRI cross-linking and cell activation. Omalizumab neutralizes the free IgE in the serum by binding to the Fc regions of the heavy chains to form high-affinity IgE–anti-IgE complexes. This prevents the IgE from binding to FcεRI, thereby blocking allergen-induced cell activation.

binding to its receptor on mast cells and basophils would be a novel and powerful antiallergy drug. Various anti-IgE strategies met with little success until the discovery and development of "humanized" monoclonal antibodies. The rational idea of developing a monoclonal antibody targeted specifically against the receptor-binding site of IgE ultimately led to the discovery of omalizumab.

Chemistry. Omalizumab is a DNA-derived humanized monoclonal antibody of the IgG1κ subclass. It has a molecular weight of approximately 149,000. The antibody is produced in Chinese hamster ovary cells in cell culture. It is sold as a preservative-free powder. A vial of XOLAIR contains 202 mg omalizumab, as well as sucrose, L-histidine, and polysorbate 20.

Pharmacokinetics and Metabolism. Omalizumab is delivered as a single subcutaneous injection every 2 to 4 weeks. It has a bioavailability of about 60%, reaching peak serum levels after 7 to 8 days. The serum elimination half-life is 26 days, with a clearance rate of about 2.5 ml/kg per day. The elimination of omalizumab–IgE complexes occurs in the liver reticuloendothelial system at a rate somewhat faster than that of free IgG. Some intact omalizumab is also excreted in the bile. There is little evidence of specific uptake of omalizumab by any tissue.

Mechanism of Action. The Fc region of IgE binds with high affinity to the Fc epsilon receptor I (FcεRI). FcεRI is expressed on the surfaces of mast cells and basophils, as well as several other cell types. When an allergen interacts with the antigen-binding domains of IgE bound to FcεRI on mast cells and basophils, it cross-links the receptors and activates the cell. This, in turn, triggers the release of preformed granule-associated mediators such as histamine and tryptase. In addition, it results in the immediate production of eicosanoids, most notably LTC4 and prostaglandin D2 (PGD2) and, on a time scale of hours instead of minutes, the synthesis of various cytokines (Schroeder *et al.*, 2001; Krishnaswamy *et al.*, 2001). Omalizumab is an IgG antibody for which the antigen is the Fc region of the IgE antibody; thus it is an "anti-antibody antibody." Omalizumab binds tightly to free IgE in the circulation to form omalizumab–IgE complexes that have no affinity for FcεRI (Figure 27-3). At the recommended doses, omalizumab reduces free IgE by more than 95%, thereby limiting the amount of IgE bound to FcεR1-bearing cells. Omalizumab treatment also decreases the amount of FcεRI expressed on basophils and mast cells (MacGlashan *et al.*, 1997). For example, after treatment with omalizumab, the number of FcεRIs expressed on the surfaces of basophils decreased by more than 95% from a starting value of about 200,000 receptors per cell. This decrease in surface FcεRIs results from increased turnover of unbound receptors rather than decreased FcεRI synthesis (MacGlashan *et al.*, 2001; Borkowski *et al.*, 2001). Thus the effectiveness of omalizumab in reducing the amount of allergen-specific IgE bound to mast cells and basophils depends on the reduction of both free IgE and available FcεRIs on cell surfaces. Normally, IgE-mediated basophil activation is extremely efficacious, requiring antigen to interact with only a small fraction of the bound IgE to evoke a half-maximal response (MacGlashan, 1993). This predicts that drugs such as omalizumab will have little clinical effect until doses are given that reduce free IgE by greater than 90%.

Besides mast cells and basophils, monocytes, lymphocytes, certain antigen-presenting cells, and eosinophils express FcεRI. The effects of omalizumab on decreasing IgE binding and FcεRI expression on these cells also may contribute to the therapeutic effect of omalizumab (Prussin *et al.*, 2003).

Toxicity. The safety of omalizumab so far has been evaluated in only three large, randomized, placebo-controlled multicenter studies. Omalizumab generally was well tolerated in several large, placebo-controlled trials. The most frequent adverse effect was injection-site reactions (*e.g.*, redness, stinging, bruising, and induration), but these reactions also were seen at comparable frequencies with placebo. Low titers of antibodies against omalizumab developed in 1 of 1723 treated patients, whereas anaphylaxis was seen in 0.1% of treated patients. Malignancies of various types were observed in 20 of 4127 patients taking omalizumab, a higher frequency than the 5 malignancies in 2236 patients taking other asthma and allergy drugs. Additional studies are needed to determine if omalizumab does indeed cause cancers.

Use in Asthma. Omalizumab is indicated for adults and adolescents older than 12 years of age with allergies and moderate-to-severe persistent asthma. In this population, omalizumab has proven to be effective in reducing the dependency on inhaled and oral corticosteroids and in decreasing the frequency of asthma exacerbations (Soler *et al.*, 2001; Busse *et al.*, 2001). Omalizumab is not an acute bronchodilator and should not be used as a rescue medication or as a treatment of status asthmaticus.

Based on its mechanism of action, omalizumab has been used in the treatment of other allergic disorders, such as nasal allergy (Lin *et al.*, 2004) and food allergy (Leung *et al.*, 2003), but large-scale clinical trials are limited to asthma.

Cromolyn Sodium and Nedocromil Sodium

History and Chemistry. *Cromolyn* was synthesized in 1965 in an attempt to improve on the bronchodilator activity of khellin. This chromone, derived from the plant *Ammi visnaga*, had been used by the ancient Egyptians for its spasmolytic properties. Although devoid of the bronchodilating effect of the parent compound, cromolyn was found to inhibit antigen-induced bronchospasm as well as the release of histamine and other autacoids from sensitized rat mast cells. Cromolyn has been used in the United States for the treatment of asthma since 1973. The initial clinical results were disappointing, in retrospect largely owing to a misplaced hope that cromolyn would reduce or eliminate the need for systemic glucocorticoids in the treatment of patients with relatively severe asthma. However, its therapeutic role has been reevaluated in recent years, and cromolyn has emerged as one of the first-line agents in the treatment of mild to moderate asthma. *Nedocromil,* a compound with similar chemical and biological properties, became available in 1992 (Wasserman, 1993; Brogden and Sorkin, 1993). Cromolyn sodium (disodium cromoglycate) and nedocromil sodium have the following structures:

CROMOLYN SODIUM

NEDOCROMIL SODIUM

Mechanism of Action. Cromolyn and nedocromil have a variety of activities that may relate to their therapeutic efficacy in asthma. These include inhibiting mediator release from bronchial mast cells (Pearce *et al.*, 1989); reversing increased functional activation in leukocytes obtained from the blood of asthmatic patients (Murphy and Kelly, 1987); suppressing the activating effects of chemotactic peptides on human neutrophils, eosinophils, and monocytes (Kay *et al.*, 1987; Moqbel *et al.*, 1988); inhibiting parasympathetic and cough reflexes (Hargreaves and Benson, 1995; Fuller *et al.*, 1987); and inhibiting leukocyte trafficking in asthmatic airways (Hoshino and Nakamura, 1997). Suffice it to say that the mechanism of action of cromolyn and nedocromil in asthma is not known.

Pharmacokinetics. For asthma, cromolyn is given by inhalation using either solutions (delivered by aerosol spray or nebulizer) or, in some countries but not in the United States, powdered drug (mixed with lactose and delivered by a special turboinhaler). The pharmacological effects result from the topical deposition of the drug in the lung, since only about 1% of an oral dose of cromolyn is absorbed. Once absorbed, the drug is excreted unchanged in the urine and bile in about equal proportions. Peak concentrations in plasma occur within 15 minutes of inhalation, and excretion begins after some delay such that the biological half-life ranges from 45 to 100 minutes. The terminal half-time of elimination following intravenous administration is about 20 minutes. The pharmacokinetic properties of cromolyn have been reviewed (Murphy and Kelly, 1987).

Toxicity. Cromolyn and nedocromil generally are well tolerated by patients. Adverse reactions are infrequent and minor and include bronchospasm, cough or wheezing, laryngeal edema, joint swelling and pain, angioedema, headache, rash, and nausea. Such reactions have been reported at a frequency of less than 1 in 10,000 patients (*see* Murphy and Kelly, 1987). Very rare instances of anaphylaxis also have been documented. Nedocromil and cromolyn can cause a bad taste.

Use in Asthma. The main use of cromolyn (INTAL) and nedocromil (TILADE) is to prevent asthmatic attacks in individuals with mild to moderate bronchial asthma. These agents are ineffective in treating ongoing bronchoconstriction. When inhaled several times daily, cromolyn inhibits both the immediate and the late asthmatic responses to antigenic challenge or to exercise. With regular use for more than 2 to 3 months, bronchial hyperreactivity is reduced, as measured by response to challenge with histamine or methacholine (see Murphy and Kelly, 1987; Hoag and McFadden, 1991). Nedocromil generally is more effective than cromolyn in animal models and human beings (Brogden and Sorkin, 1993). Nedocromil is approved for use in asthmatic patients 12 years of age and older; cromolyn is approved for all ages.

Cromolyn and nedocromil generally are less effective than inhaled glucocorticoids in controlling asthma. Cromolyn (2 mg inhaled four times daily) was less effective than 200 μg twice daily of beclomethasone (Svendsen et al., 1987) or 4 mg four times daily of nedocromil (Brogden and Sorkin, 1993). Although necrodomil was roughly comparable with 200 μg beclomethasone inhaled twice daily, nedocromil was not as effective in controlling symptoms, reducing bronchodilator use, or improving bronchial hyperreactivity (Svendsen et al., 1989). In a second study, 4 mg nedocromil four times daily was as effective as 100 μg beclomethasone four times daily (Bel et al., 1990). In a thorough review, Brogden and Sorkin (1993) concluded that nedocromil is useful in patients with mild to moderate asthma as added therapy, as an alternative to regularly administered oral and inhaled β adrenergic agonists and oral methylxanthines, and possibly as an alternative to low-dose inhaled glucocorticoids.

The addition of cromolyn to inhaled glucocorticoid therapy yields no additional benefit in moderately severe asthma (Toogood et al., 1981). Nedocromil may allow a reduction of steroids in patients receiving high doses of inhaled steroids (Brogden and Sorkin, 1993). These studies were short term; whether or not long-term reduction in steroid dose is possible remains to be determined. In one study, the addition of nedocromil 4 mg four times daily for 8 weeks to high-dose inhaled glucocorticoid treatment resulted in modest improvements in patients with moderately severe asthma (Svendsen and Jorgensen, 1991). Because of its limited efficacy, the use of cromolyn for the treatment of asthma in the United States is decreasing.

In patients with systemic mastocytosis who have gastrointestinal symptoms owing to an excessive number of mast cells in the gastrointestinal mucosa, an oral preparation of cromolyn (GASTROCROM) is effective in reducing symptoms (Horan et al., 1990). The benefits reflect local action rather than systemic absorption; cromolyn is poorly absorbed, and only the gastrointestinal symptoms are improved in the treated patients.

Theophylline

Theophylline, a methylxanthine, is among the least expensive drugs used to treat asthma, and consequently, it remains a commonly used drug for this indication in many countries. In industrialized countries, the advent of inhaled glucocorticoids, β adrenergic receptor agonists,

and leukotriene-modifying drugs has diminished theophylline use significantly, and it has been relegated to a third- or fourth-line treatment in patients whose asthma is otherwise difficult to control.

Source and History. Theophylline, caffeine, and theobromine are three closely related plant alkaloids that are imbibed widely. At least half the population of the world consumes tea (containing caffeine and small amounts of theophylline and theobromine) prepared from the leaves of *Thea sinensis,* a bush native to southern China and now cultivated extensively in other countries. Cocoa and chocolate, from the seeds of *Theobroma cacao,* contain theobromine and some caffeine. Coffee, the most popular source of caffeine in the American diet, is extracted from the fruit of *Coffea arabica* and related species. Cola-flavored drinks usually contain considerable amounts of caffeine in part because of their content of extracts of the nuts of *Cola acuminata* and in part because caffeine is added during their production (see Graham, 1978).

The basis for the popularity of all caffeine-containing beverages is the ancient belief that they have stimulant and antisoporific actions that elevate mood, decrease fatigue, and increase capacity for work. Classical pharmacological studies principally of caffeine confirmed this belief and revealed that methylxanthines also possess other important pharmacological properties. These properties were exploited in a variety of therapeutic applications, in many of which caffeine now has been replaced by more effective agents. However, in recent years, there has been a resurgence of interest in the natural methylxanthines and their synthetic derivatives principally as a result of increased knowledge of their cellular basis of action.

Chemistry. Theophylline, caffeine, and theobromine are methylated xanthines. Caffeine is 1,3,7-trimethylxanthine; theophylline, 1,3-dimethylxanthine; and theobromine, 3,7-dimethylxanthine. The structural formulas of xanthine and the three naturally occurring xanthine derivatives are as follows:

XANTHINE

CAFFEINE

THEOPHYLLINE

THEOBROMINE

The solubility of the methylxanthines is low and is much enhanced by the formation of complexes (usually 1:1) with a wide variety of compounds. The most notable of these complexes is that between theophylline and ethylenediamine (to form *aminophylline*). The formation of complex double salts (e.g., caffeine and sodium benzoate) or true salts [e.g., *choline theophyllinate (oxtriphylline)*] also enhances aqueous solubility. These salts or complexes dissociate in aqueous solution to yield the parent methylxanthines and should not be confused with covalently modified derivatives such as *dyphylline* [1,3-dimethyl-7-(2, 3-dihydroxypropyl)xanthine].

A large number of derivatives of the methylxanthines have been prepared and examined for their ability to inhibit cyclic nucleotide phosphodiesterases (PDEs) (Beavo and Reifsnyder, 1990) and to antagonize receptor-mediated actions of adenosine (Daly, 1982; Linden, 1991), the two best characterized cellular actions of the methylxanthines. Although certain modifications dissociate these two activities to some degree, these compounds are not used therapeutically.

Mechanism of Action.   Theophylline inhibits cyclic nucleotide PDEs, thereby preventing breakdown of cyclic AMP and cyclic GMP to 5′-AMP and 5′-GMP, respectively. Inhibition of PDEs will lead to an accumulation of cyclic AMP and cyclic GMP, thereby increasing signal transduction through these pathways. The cyclic nucleotide PDEs are members of a superfamily of genetically distinct enzymes (Soderling and Beavo, 2000). Theophylline and related methylxanthines are relatively nonselective in the PDE subtypes they inhibit.

Cyclic nucleotide production is regulated by endogenous receptor–ligand interactions leading to activation of adenylyl cyclase and guanylyl cyclase. Inhibitors of PDEs therefore can be thought of as drugs that enhance the activity of endogenous autacoids, hormones, and neurotransmitters that signal *via* cyclic nucleotide messengers. This may explain why the *in vivo* potency often exceeds that observed *in vitro*.

Theophylline is a competitive antagonist at adenosine receptors (Fredholm and Persson, 1982). Adenosine can act as an autacoid and transmitter with myriad biological actions. Of particular relevance to asthma are the observations that adenosine can cause bronchoconstriction in asthmatics and potentiate immunologically induced mediator release from human lung mast cells (Cushley *et al.*, 1984; Peachell *et al.*, 1988). Inhibition of the actions of adenosine therefore also must be considered when attempting to explain the mechanism of action of theophylline (Feoktistov *et al.*, 1998).

Theophylline also may owe part of its antiinflammatory action to its ability to activate histone deacetylases in the nucleus (Ito *et al.*, 2002). In theory, the deacetylation of histones could decrease the transcription of several proinflammatory genes and potentiate the effect of corticosteroids.

Pulmonary System.   Theophylline effectively relaxes airway smooth muscle; this bronchodilation likely contributes to its acute therapeutic efficacy in asthma. Both adenosine receptor antagonism and PDE inhibition are likely involved in the bronchodilating effect of theophylline. Adenosine does not contract isolated human bronchial smooth muscle directly, but when it is inhaled, it acts as a potent bronchoconstrictor in asthmatic subjects (Cushley *et al.*,

1984). Therefore, inhibition of this function of adenosine may contribute to theophylline-induced bronchodilation in some asthmatic subjects. Inhibition of PDE4 and PDE5 effectively relaxes human isolated bronchial smooth muscle (Torphy *et al.*, 1993). It thus seems likely that inhibition of PDEs also contributes to the bronchodilating effect of theophylline. Studies with the related methylxanthine enprofylline (3-propylxanthine), which has been investigated extensively for treatment of asthma in Europe, also support a mechanistic role for PDE inhibition in the bronchodilator actions of theophylline. Enprofylline is more potent than theophylline as a bronchodilator but is much less potent in inhibiting most types of adenosine receptors (Pauwels *et al.*, 1985). The latter point, however, must be interpreted cautiously. Activation of the A_{2B} subtype of adenosine receptor causes several proinflammatory effects, and both theophylline and enprofylline are potent competitive antagonists of A_{2B} adenosine receptors (Feoktistov *et al.*, 1998).

Theophylline also inhibits synthesis and secretion of inflammatory mediators from numerous cell types, including mast cells and basophils (Page, 1999). This effect of theophylline likely is due to PDE inhibition and can be mimicked in large part with drugs that selectively inhibit PDE4 isozyme (Torphy and Undem, 1991). At therapeutic concentrations, the antiinflammatory effect of theophylline may be more relevant to the drug's therapeutic actions than direct bronchodilation, but this remains unproven (Page, 1999).

Consistent with an important role of PDE4 in obstructive lung disease, selective PDE4 inhibitors have been evaluated in clinical trials for the treatment of asthma and chronic obstructive pulmonary disease (COPD). In one study, cilomilast (ARIFLO; 15 mg twice daily for 10 weeks) decreased inflammatory cell infiltration significantly in bronchial biopsies of patients with COPD. Further studies are needed to define the role of PDE4 inhibitors in asthma and COPD, but these drugs are promising candidates for new approaches to asthma therapy.

Absorption, Fate, and Excretion.   The methylxanthines are absorbed readily after oral or parenteral administration. Absorption from rectal suppositories is slow and unreliable. Theophylline administered in liquids or uncoated tablets is absorbed rapidly and completely. Absorption also is complete from some, but not all, sustained-release formulations (*see* Hendeles and Weinberger, 1982). In the absence of food, solutions or uncoated tablets of theophylline produce maximal concentrations in plasma within 2 hours; caffeine is absorbed more rapidly, and maximal plasma concentrations are achieved within 1 hour. Numerous sustained-release preparations of theophylline are available, designed for dosing intervals of 8, 12, or 24 hours. There is marked interpatient variability with regard to the rate and extent of absorption and especially the effect of food and time of administration on these parameters (*see* Symposium, 1986a). Thus it is necessary to calibrate a given preparation in a given patient and to avoid substituting one apparently similar product for another.

Food ordinarily slows the rate of absorption of theophylline but does not limit its extent. With sustained-release preparations, food may decrease the bioavailability of theophylline with some products but may increase it with others. Recumbency or sleep also may reduce the rate or extent of absorption to an important degree. These factors make it difficult to maintain relatively constant concentrations of theophylline in plasma throughout the day. Concentrations required to alleviate asthmatic symptoms do not remain constant, and the emphasis has shifted toward designing dosing regimens that ensure peak concentrations in the early morning hours, when symptoms frequently worsen (*see* Symposium, 1988a).

Methylxanthines are distributed into all body compartments; they cross the placenta and pass into breast milk. The apparent volumes of distribution for caffeine and theophylline are between 0.4 and 0.6 L/kg. These values are considerably higher in premature infants. Theophylline is bound to plasma proteins to a greater extent than is caffeine, and the fraction bound declines as the concentration of methylxanthine increases. At therapeutic concentrations, the protein binding of theophylline averages about 60%, but it is decreased to about 40% in newborn infants and in adults with hepatic cirrhosis.

Methylxanthines are eliminated primarily by metabolism in the liver. Less than 15% and 5% of administered theophylline and caffeine, respectively, is recovered in the urine unchanged. Caffeine has a half-life in plasma of 3 to 7 hours; this increases by about two-fold in women during the later stages of pregnancy or with long-term use of oral contraceptives. In premature infants, the rate of elimination of both methylxanthines is quite slow; the average half-life for caffeine is more than 50 hours, whereas the mean values for theophylline obtained in various studies range between 20 and 36 hours. However, the latter values include the extensive conversion of theophylline to caffeine in these infants (see Symposium, 1981; Roberts, 1984).

There is marked individual variation in the rate of elimination of theophylline owing to both genetic and environmental factors; four-fold differences are not uncommon (see Lesko, in Symposium, 1986a). The half-life averages about 3.5 hours in young children, whereas values of 8 or 9 hours are more typical in adults. In most patients the drug obeys first-order elimination kinetics within the therapeutic range. At higher concentrations, zero-order kinetics become evident because of saturation of metabolic enzymes, prolonging the decline of theophylline concentrations to nontoxic levels.

Methylxanthine metabolism also is influenced by other diseases or drugs (Symposium, 1996a). Hepatic cirrhosis, congestive heart failure, and acute pulmonary edema all increase the half-life, as does concurrent therapy with cimetidine or erythromycin. In contrast, clearance is increased twofold by phenytoin or barbiturates, whereas cigarette smoking, rifampin, and oral contraceptives induce smaller changes.

Although scarcely detectable in adults, the conversion of theophylline to caffeine is significant in preterm infants (see Symposium, 1981; Roberts, 1984). In this setting, caffeine accumulates in plasma to a concentration approximately 25% that of theophylline. About 50% of the theophylline administered to such infants appears in the urine unchanged; the excretion of 1,3-dimethyluric acid, 1-methyluric acid, and caffeine derived from theophylline accounts for nearly all the remainder.

Toxicology. Fatal intoxications with theophylline have been much more frequent than with caffeine. Rapid intravenous administration of therapeutic doses of *aminophylline* (500 mg) sometimes results in sudden death that is probably due to cardiac arrhythmias, and the drug should be injected slowly over 20 to 40 minutes to avoid severe toxic symptoms. These include headache, palpitation, dizziness, nausea, hypotension, and precordial pain. Additional symptoms of toxicity include tachycardia, severe restlessness, agitation, and emesis; these effects are associated with plasma concentrations of more than 20 $\mu g/ml$. Focal and generalized seizures also can occur, sometimes without prior signs of toxicity.

Most toxicity results from repeated administration of theophylline by either oral or parenteral routes. Although convulsions and death have occurred at plasma concentrations as low as 25 $\mu g/ml$, seizures are relatively rare at concentrations below 40 $\mu g/ml$ (see Goldberg et al., in Symposium, 1986a). Patients with long-term theophylline intoxication appear to be much more prone to seizures than those who experience short-term overdoses. Such a dependence on the history of exposure to theophylline may contribute to the difficulty in establishing a relationship between the severity of toxic symptoms and the concentration of the drug in plasma (Aitken and Martin, 1987; Bertino and Walker, 1987), and greater caution is advised in treating intoxicated patients who have been ingesting theophylline regularly (see Paloucek and Rodvold, 1988). Treatment may include prophylactic administration of diazepam, perhaps in combination with phenytoin or phenobarbital; phenytoin also may be a useful alternative to lidocaine in the treatment of serious ventricular arrhythmias. Once seizures appear, they may be refractory to anticonvulsant therapy, sometimes necessitating general anesthesia or other measures used to treat status epilepticus (see Goldberg et al., in Symposium, 1986a).

The widespread use of sustained-release preparations of theophylline has renewed emphasis on measures to prevent continued absorption, particularly the use of oral activated charcoal and sorbitol as a cathartic (Goldberg et al., 1987). However, when plasma concentrations exceed 100 $\mu g/ml$, invasive measures usually are required, especially hemoperfusion through charcoal cartridges (see Paloucek and Rodvold, 1988).

Behavioral Toxicity. Moderate doses of caffeine can provoke intense feelings of anxiety, fear, or panic in some individuals. Even subjects with a history of light to moderate use of caffeine experience tension, anxiety, and dysphoria after ingesting 400 mg or more of the drug (see Griffiths and Woodson, in Symposium, 1988b). In infants who have received treatment for apnea of prematurity (see below), theophylline may produce persistent changes in sleep–wake patterns (Thoman et al., 1985), but long-term effects on behavior or cognitive development have yet to be identified (see Aranda et al., in Symposium, 1986a). There has been mounting concern that the treatment of asthmatic children with theophylline may produce depression, hyperactivity, or other behavioral toxicity. However, a study of academic performance of children treated or not with theophylline showed equal academic performance in asthmatic and non-asthmatic subjects (Lindgren et al., 1992). Even though it is difficult to factor out specific effects of theophylline from those caused by the illness or by other features of the treatment regimen, many investigators believe that most children will benefit from the use of alternative means of controlling their symptoms.

Use in Asthma. Theophylline has proven efficacy as a bronchodilator in asthma and formerly was considered first-line therapy. It now is relegated to a far less prominent role primarily because of the modest benefits it affords, its narrow therapeutic window, and the required monitoring of drug levels (Stoloff, 1994; Nasser and Rees, 1993). Nocturnal asthma can be improved with slow-release theophylline preparations (Self et al., 1992), but other interventions such as inhaled glucocorticoids or salmeterol probably are more effective (Meltzer et al., 1992).

Therapy usually is initiated by the administration of 12 to 16 mg/kg per day of theophylline (calculated as the free base) up to a maximum of 400 mg/day for at least 3 days (Weinberger, 1987). Children younger than 1 year of age require considerably less; the dose in milligrams per kilogram per day may be calculated as $0.2 \times$ (age in weeks) + 5. Starting with these low doses minimizes the early side effects of nausea, vomiting, nervousness, and insomnia that often subside with continued therapy and virtually eliminates the possibility of exceeding plasma concentrations of 20 μg/ml in patients older than age 1 year who do not have compromised hepatic or cardiac function. Thereafter, the dosage is increased in two successive stages to between 16 and 20 and, subsequently, 18 and 22 mg/kg per day (up to a maximum of 800 mg/day) depending on the age and clinical response of the patient and allowing at least 3 days between adjustments. The plasma concentration of theophylline is determined before a further adjustment in dosage is made. Although extended-release preparations of theophylline usually allow twice-daily dosing, variations in the rate and extent of absorption of such preparations require individualized calibration of dosing regimens for each patient and preparation.

Apnea of Preterm Infants. In premature infants, episodes of prolonged apnea lasting more than 15 seconds and accompanied by bradycardia pose the threat of recurrent hypoxemia and neurologic damage. Although they often are associated with serious systemic illness, in many instances no specific cause is found. Beginning with the work of Kuzemko and Paala (1973), methylxanthines have undergone numerous clinical trials for the treatment of apnea of undetermined origin. The oral or intravenous administration of methylxanthines can eliminate episodes of apnea that last more than 20 seconds and markedly reduces the number of episodes of shorter duration (*see* Symposium, 1981; Roberts, 1984; Aranda *et al.*, in Symposium, 1986a). Satisfactory responses may occur with plasma concentrations of theophylline of 4 to 8 μg/ml, but concentrations of nearly 13 μg/ml are required more frequently (Muttitt *et al.*, 1988). Still higher concentrations may produce a more regular pattern of respiration without further reduction in the frequency of episodes of apnea and bradycardia, and these usually are associated with a definite tachycardia. Therapeutic concentrations are achieved with loading doses of about 5 mg/kg of theophylline (calculated as the free base) and can be maintained with 2 mg/kg given every 12 or 24 hours (*see* Roberts, 1984). Although caffeine was used less frequently than theophylline initially, some physicians now prefer it because the dosing regimens are simpler and more predictable.

Anticholinergic Agents

There is a long history of the use of anticholinergic agents in the treatment of asthma. These agents are discussed in detail in Chapter 7. With the advent of inhaled β adrenergic agonists, use of anticholinergic agents declined. Renewed interest in anticholinergic agents paralleled the realization that parasympathetic pathways are important in bronchospasm in some asthmatics and the

availability of *ipratropium bromide* (ATROVENT), a quaternary muscarinic receptor antagonist that has better pharmacological properties than prior drugs. A particularly good response to ipratropium may be seen in the subgroup of asthmatic patients who experience psychogenic exacerbations (Neild and Cameron, 1985).

The cholinergic receptor subtype responsible for bronchial smooth muscle contraction is the muscarinic M_3 receptor. Although iprotropium and related compounds block all five muscarinic receptor subtypes with similar affinity, it is likely that M_3-receptor antagonism alone accounts for the bronchodilating effect. The bronchodilation produced by ipratropium in asthmatic subjects develops more slowly and usually is less intense than that produced by adrenergic agonists. Some asthmatic patients may experience a useful response lasting up to 6 hours. The variability in the response of asthmatic subjects to ipratropium presumably reflects differences in the strength of parasympathetic tone and in the degree to which reflex activation of cholinergic pathways participates in generating symptoms in individual patients. Hence the utility of ipratropium must be assessed on an individual basis by a therapeutic trial. The pharmacological properties and therapeutic uses of ipratropium have been reviewed (Gross,1988; *see also* Symposium, 1986b).

Combined treatment with ipratropium and β_2 adrenergic agonists results in slightly greater and more prolonged bronchodilation than with either agent alone in baseline asthma (Bryant and Rogers, 1992). In acute bronchoconstriction, the combination of a β_2 adrenergic agonist and ipratropium is more effective than either agent alone and more effective than simply giving more β_2 adrenergic agonist (Bryant, 1985; Bryant and Rogers, 1992). A large multicenter study showed that the asthmatic subjects with the worst initial lung function benefited most from combination therapy (Rebuck *et al.*, 1987). Thus the combination of a selective β_2 adrenergic agonist and ipratropium should be considered in acute treatment of severe asthma exacerbations. Ipratropium is available in metered-dose inhalers and as a nebulizer solution. A metered-dose inhaler containing a mixture of ipratropium and albuterol (COMBIVENT) also is available in the United States. In Europe, metered-dose inhalers containing a mixture of ipratropium and fenoterol are available (DUOVENT, BERODUAL).

Recently, tiotropium (SPIRIVA), a structural analogue of ipratropium, has been approved for the treatment of COPD and emphysema. Like ipratropium, tiotropium has high affinity for all muscarinic receptor subtypes, but it dissociates from the receptors much more slowly that ipratropium (Barnes, 2000). In particular, binding and functional studies indicate that tiotropium dissociates from muscarinic M_3 receptors more slowly than from muscarinic M_2 receptors. The high affinity of tiotropium for muscarinic receptors, combined with its very slow dissociation rate, permits once-daily dosing. The slow dissociation rate also provides a theoretical advantage in that it limits the capacity of large concentrations of the endogenous agonist acetylcholine to surmount the receptor blockade. Tiotropium is provided as a capsule containing a dry-powder formulation that is intended only for oral inhalation using the HandiHaler inhalation device.

Pharmacogenetics and Variability of Response to Asthma Medications. There is a wide degree of interindividual variability in the response of asthmatic subjects to pharmacotherapy. For example, some individuals benefit dramatically from treatment with leukotriene modifiers, whereas many others are essentially resistant to these treatments. Although more rare, the "steroid resistant" asthmatic receives relatively little benefit from treatment with inhaled corticosteroids. At present, it is impossible to predict who will benefit the most from a given treatment. This unpredictability of response largely reflects our limited understanding of the underlying pathophysiology of asthma. In addition, some component of this variability likely is explained by specific pharmacogenetic factors (Dewar and Hall, 2003).

Three functionally relevant mutations have been found in the promotor region of the gene encoding 5-lipoxygenase (In *et al.*, 1997). These mutations lead to a small decrease in promotor activity and leukotriene synthesis. About 35% of the population has at least one of these mutations in at least one allele. In one placebo-controlled clinical trial it was noted that individuals with mutations at both alleles responded less well to treatment with a 5-lipoxygenase inhibitor than did those with two wild-type alleles (Drazen *et al.*, 1999).

A variant of the β_2 adrenergic receptor in which glycine replaces arginine at position 16 (Gly 16) shows an increased rate of down-regulation in response to agonist exposure. This polymorphism occurs with equal frequency in asthmatic and nonasthmatic populations. There is some evidence that asthmatics who are homozygous for Gly 16 receptors are less responsive to β-agonist therapy than wild-type controls (Martinez *et al.*, 1997; Tan *et al.*, 1997). However, this was not noted in all studies (Hancox *et al.*, 1998).

There are several relatively rare genetic variants in the gene encoding the glucocorticoid receptor. Some of these variants produce receptors with a diminished affinity for glucocorticoid agonists. There is no evidence, however, that any glucocorticoid-receptor polymorphism is strongly associated with clinically relevant steroid resistance (Koper *et al.*, 1997). Consequently, attention is shifting away from polymorphisms in the receptor *per se* toward the numerous other candidate genes in the functional pathway of glucocorticoids as potential explanations for the unresponsiveness of some individuals to steroid therapy.

Use of Asthma Drugs in Rhinitis

Seasonal allergic rhinitis (hay fever) is caused by deposition of allergens on the nasal mucosa, resulting in an immediate hypersensitivity reaction. This reaction usually is not accompanied by asthma because the allergenic particles are too large to be inhaled into the lower airways (*e.g.*, pollens). Treatment for allergic rhinitis is similar to that for asthma. Topical glucocorticoids, including *beclomethasone* (BECONASE), *mometasone* (NASONEX), *budesonide* (RHINOCORT), *flunisolide* (NASAREL), *fluticasone* (FLONASE), and *triamcinolone* (NASACORT), can be highly effective with minimal side effects, particularly if treatment is instituted immediately prior to the allergy season. Topical glucocorticoids can be administered twice daily (beclomethasone and flunisolide) or even once daily (budesonide, mometasone, fluticasone, and triamcinolone). Cromolyn usually requires dosing three to six times daily for full effects. Rare instances of local candidiasis have been reported with glucocorticoids and probably can be avoided by rinsing the mouth after use. Unlike in asthma, antihistamines (*see* Chapter 24) afford considerable, though incomplete, symptom relief in allergic rhinitis. Nasal decongestants rely on β adrenergic agonists (*e.g.*, pseudoephedrine and phenylephrine) as vasoconstrictors and are discussed in Chapter 10. Anticholinergic agents such as ipratropium bromide (ATROVENT) are effective in inhibiting parasympathetic reflex–evoked secretions from serous glands lining the nasal mucosa.

Use of Asthma Drugs in COPD

Emphysema can be prevented or its progression slowed if the patient stops smoking (Ferguson and Cherniack, 1993). Pharmacological interventions can help patients to stop smoking. *Nicotine gum* (NICORETTE), *nicotine transdermal patches* (NICODERM), and the antidepressant agent *bupropion* (ZYBAN) are moderately useful when combined with other interventions such as support groups and physician encouragement. Clonidine may be helpful in reducing the craving for cigarettes. Treatment of nicotine addiction is discussed in Chapter 23.

The pharmacological treatment of established emphysema resembles that of asthma largely because the inflammatory/bronchospastic component of a patient's disease is the aspect amenable to therapy (Ferguson and Cherniack, 1993). For patients with emphysema who have a significant degree of active inflammation with bronchospasm and excessive mucus production, symptomatic use of inhaled ipratropium or a β_2 adrenergic agonist may be helpful. Ipratropium or tiotropium usually produces about the same modest degree of bronchodilation in patients with COPD as do maximal doses of β_2 adrenergic agonists. As in asthmatic patients, continuous use of bronchodilators is controversial, with some studies suggesting that it is associated with an unfavorable course of COPD (van Schayck et al., 1991). A subgroup of patients may respond favorably to short courses of oral glucocorticoids. Without a treatment trial, it is not possible to predict whether a particular patient will respond to glucocorticoids. Response to oral glucocorticoids may predict those patients who will respond to inhaled glucocorticoids. However, except for the treatment of acute bronchospastic episodes, glucocorticoids have given mixed results in the treatment of COPD (American Thoracic Society, 1987; Dompeling et al., 1993). In some patients, theophylline may be effective (Murciano et al., 1989); in others who have a profound response to β_2 adrenergic agonists, theophylline fails to produce additional bronchodilation beyond that achieved by maximal doses of the inhaled β adrenergic agonist.

In a minority of patients, emphysema results from a genetic deficiency of the plasma proteinase inhibitor α_1-antiproteinase (also called α_1-antitrypsin) (Crystal, 1990). Lung tissue destruction is caused by the unopposed action of neutrophil elastase and other proteinases. Purified α_1-antiproteinase (PROLASTIN) from human plasma is available for intravenous replacement.

CLINICAL SUMMARY

The principles underlying the therapy of asthma have remained unchanged over the past several decades. Bronchodilating drugs, exemplified by the *short-acting β_2 adrenergic receptor agonists,* are used acutely to reverse the bronchospasm of an asthma attack. Antiinflammatory drugs such as inhaled *glucocorticoids* are used to quell bronchial inflammation in an effort to reduce the severity and frequency of asthma attacks. In hospitalized patients, a short course of systemic steroids often is given, followed by a rapid taper. In patients who remain symptomatic despite inhaled glucocorticoid therapy, *long-acting β_2 adrenergic receptor agonists* may be added to the steroid regimen with good success. Once used widely, the *methylxanthines* now are used much less frequently owing to modest efficacy and narrow therapeutic window. Selective *PDE4 inhibitors,* which may provide similar efficacy with fewer adverse effects, are under evaluation in clinical trials. Other newer agents are directed at specific mechanisms underlying the initiation or progression of asthma. These include the *leukotriene-receptor antagonists* and the anti-IgE therapy *omalizumab.* Finally, the anticholinergic agent *tiotropium* was approved recently for the treatment of COPD in the United States.

BIBLIOGRAPHY

Aitken, M.L., and Martin, T.R. Life-threatening theophylline toxicity is not predictable by serum levels. *Chest,* **1987,** *91*:10–14.

Augstein, J., Farmer, J.B., Lee, T.B., et al. Selective inhibitor of slow reacting substance of anaphylaxis. *Nature New Biol.,* **1973,** *245*:215–217.

Barnes, N.C., and Miller, C.J. Effect of leukotriene receptor antagonist therapy on the risk of asthma exacerbations in patients with mild to moderate asthma: An integrated analysis of zafirlukast trials. *Thorax,* **2000,** *55*:478–483.

Barnes, P.J. Tiotropium bromide. *Exp. Opin. Invest. Drugs,* **2001,** *10*:733–740.

Bel, E.H., Timmers, M.C., Hermans, J., et al. The long-term effects of nedocromil sodium and beclomethasone dipropionate on bronchial responsiveness to methacholine in nonatopic asthmatic subjects. *Am. Rev. Respir. Dis.,* **1990,** *141*:21–28.

Benton, G., Thomas, R.C., Nickerson, B.G., et al. Experience with a metered-dose inhaler with a spacer in the pediatric emergency department. *Am. J. Dis. Child.,* **1989,** *143*:678–681.

Bertino, J.S., Jr., and Walker, J.W. Reassessment of theophylline toxicity: Serum concentrations, clinical course, and treatment. *Arch. Intern. Med.,* **1987,** *147*:757–760.

Borkowski, T.A., Jouvin, M.H., Lin, S.Y., and Kinet, J.P. Minimal requirements for IgE-mediated regulation of surface FcεRI. *J. Immunol.,* **2001,** *167*:1290–1296.

Brittain, R.T. Approaches to a long-acting, selective β_2-adrenoceptor stimulant. *Lung,* **1990,** *168*(suppl):111–114.

Bryant, D.H., and Rogers, P. Effects of ipratropium bromide nebulizer solution with and without preservatives in the treatment of acute and stable asthma. *Chest,* **1992,** *102*:742–747.

Bryant, E.E., and Shimizu, I. *Sample Design, Sampling Variance, and Estimation Procedures for the National Ambulatory Medical Care Survey.* DHHS Publication No. (PHS) 88-1382, U.S. Dept. of Health and Human Services, Hyattsville, MD., **1988.**

Buckner, C.K., Krell, R.D., Laravuso, R.B., et al. Pharmacological evidence that human intralobar airways do not contain different receptors that mediate contractions to leukotriene C4 and leukotriene D4. *J. Pharmacol. Exp. Ther.,* **1986,** *237*:558–562.

Burrows, B., Martinez, F.D., Halonen, M., et al. Association of asthma with serum IgE levels and skin-test reactivity to allergens. *New Engl. J. Med.,* **1989,** *320*:271–277.

Busse, W., Corren, J., Lanier, B.Q., *et al.* Omalizumab, anti-IgE recombinant humanized monoclonal antibody, for the treatment of severe allergic asthma. *J. Allergy Clin. Immunol.*, **2001**, *108*:184–190.

Calhoun, W.J., Lavins, B.J., Minkwitz, M.C., *et al.* Effect of zafirlukast (ACCOLATE) on cellular mediators of inflammation: Bronchoalveolar lavage fluid findings after segmental antigen challenge. *Am. J. Respir. Crit. Care Med.*, **1998**, *157*:1381–1389.

Carter, G.W., Young, P.R., Albert, D.H., *et al.* 5-Lipoxygenase inhibitory activity of zileuton. *J. Pharmacol. Exp. Ther.*, **1991**, *256*:929–937.

Cheung, D., Timmers, M.C., Zwinderman, A.H., *et al.* Long-term effects of a long-acting β_2-adrenoreceptor agonist, salmeterol, on airway hyperresponsiveness in patients with mild asthma. *New Engl. J. Med.*, **1992**, *327*:1198–1203.

Chong, L.K., and Peachell, P.T. β-Adrenoceptor reserve in human lung: A comparison between airway smooth muscle and mast cells. *Eur. J. Pharmacol.*, **1999**, *378*:115–122.

Cushley, M.J., Tattersfield, A.E., and Holgate, S.T. Adenosine-induced bronchoconstriction in asthma: Antagonism by inhaled theophylline. *Am. Rev. Respir. Dis.*, **1984**, *129*:380–384.

Dahlen, S.E., Hedqvist, P., Hammarstrom, S., and Samuelsson, B. Leukotrienes are potent constrictors of human bronchi. *Nature*, **1980**, *288*:484–486.

D'Alonzo, G.E., Nathan, R.A., Henochowicz, S., *et al.* Salmeterol xinafoate as maintenance therapy compared with albuterol in patients with asthma. *JAMA*, **1994**, *271*:1412–1416.

Drazen, J.M., Yandava, C.N., Dube, L., *et al.* Pharmacogenetic association between ALOX-5 promoter genotype and the response to anti-asthma treatment. *Nature Genet.*, **1999**, *22*:185–190.

Dompeling, E., van Schayck, C.P., van Grunsven, P.M., *et al.* Slowing the deterioration of asthma and chronic obstructive pulmonary disease observed during bronchodilator therapy by adding inhaled corticosteroids: A 4-year prospective study. *Ann. Intern. Med.*, **1993**, *118*:770–778.

Fanta, C.H., Rossing, T.H., and McFadden, E.R., Jr. Emergency room treatment of asthma: Relationships among therapeutic combinations, severity of obstruction and time course of response. *Am. J. Med.*, **1982**, *72*:416–422.

Fanta, C.H., Rossing, T.H., and McFadden, E.R., Jr. Treatment of acute asthma: Is combination therapy with sympathomimetics and methylxanthines indicated? *Am. J. Med.*, **1986**, *80*:5–10.

Feoktistov, I., Polosa, R., Holgate, S.T., and Biaggioni, I. Adenosine A2B receptors: A novel therapeutic target in asthma? *Trends Pharmacol. Sci.*, **1998**, *19*:148–153.

Fredholm, B.B., and Persson, C.G. Xanthine derivatives as adenosine receptor antagonists. *Eur. J. Pharmacol.*, **1982**, *81*:673–676.

Fuller, R.W., Dixon, C.M., Cuss, F.M., and Barnes, P.J. Bradykinin-induced bronchoconstriction in humans. Mode of action. *Am. Rev. Respir. Dis.*, **1987**, *135*:176–180.

Goldberg, M.J., Spector, R., Park, G.D., *et al.* The effect of sorbitol and activated charcoal on serum theophylline concentrations after slow-release theophylline. *Clin. Pharmacol. Ther.*, **1987**, *41*:108–111.

Gorenne, I., Ortiz, J.L., Labat, C., *et al.* Antagonism of leukotriene responses in human airways by BAY x7195. *Eur. J. Pharmacol.*, **1995**, *275*:207–212.

Greening, A.P., Ind, P.W., Northfield, M., and Shaw, G. Added salmeterol versus higher-dose corticosteroid in asthma patients with symptoms on existing inhaled corticosteroid. Allen and Hanbury's Limited UK Study. *Lancet*, **1994**, *344*:219–224.

Haahtela, T., Jarvinen, M., Kava, T., *et al.* Effects of reducing or discontinuing inhaled budesonide in patients with mild asthma. *New Engl. J. Med.*, **1994**, *331*:700–705.

Hancox, R.J., Sears, M.R., and Taylor, D.R. Polymorphism of the β_2-adrenoceptor and the response to long-term β_2-agonist therapy in asthma. *Eur. Respir. J.*, **1998**, *11*:589–593.

Hargreaves, M.R., and Benson, M.K. Inhaled sodium cromoglycate in angiotensin converting enzyme inhibitor cough. *Lancet*, **1995**, *345*:13–16.

Horan, R.F., Sheffer, A.L., and Austen, K.F. Cromolyn sodium in the management of systemic mastocytosis. *J. Allergy Clin. Immunol.*, **1990**, *85*:852–855.

Hoshino, M., and Nakamura, Y. The effect of inhaled sodium cromoglycate on cellular infiltration into the bronchial mucosa and the expression of adhesion molecules in asthmatics. *Eur. Respir. J.*, **1997**, *10*:858–865.

In, K.H., Asano K., Beier, D., *et al.* Naturally occurring mutations in the human 5-lipoxygenase gene promoter that modify transcription factor binding and reporter gene transcription. *J. Clin. Invest.*, **1997**, *99*:1130–1137.

Ip, M., Lam, K., Yam, L., *et al.* Decreased bone mineral density in premenopausal asthma patients receiving long-term inhaled steroids. *Chest*, **1994**, *105*:1722–1727.

Ito K., Lim S., Caramori G., *et al.* A molecular mechanism of action of theophylline: Induction of histone deacetylase activity to decrease inflammatory gene expression. *Proc. Natl. Acad. Sci. U.S.A.*, **2002**, *99*:8921–8926,.

Jones, T.R., Labelle, M., Belley, M., *et al.* Pharmacology of montelukast sodium (SINGULAIR), a potent and selective leukotriene D4 receptor antagonist. *Can. J. Physiol. Pharmacol.*, **1995**, *73*:191–201.

Juniper, E.F., Kline, P.A., Vanzeileghem, M.A., *et al.* Effect of long-term treatment with an inhaled corticosteroid (BUDESONIDE) on airway hyperresponsiveness and clinical asthma in nonsteroid-dependent asthmatics. *Am. Rev. Respir. Dis.*, **1990**, *142*:832–836.

Kay, A.B., Walsh, G.M., Moqbel, R., *et al.* Disodium cromoglycate inhibits activation of human inflammatory cells *in vitro*. *J. Allergy Clin. Immunol.*, **1987**, *80*:1–8.

Koike, K., Yamashita, Y., Horinouchi, T., Yamaki, F., and Tanak, Y. cAMP-independent mechanism is significantly involved in β_2-adrenoceptor-mediated tracheal relaxation. *Eur. J. Pharmacol.*, **2004**, *492*:65–70.

Koper, J.W., Stolk, R.P., de Lange, P., and Huizenga, N. Lack of association between five polymorphisms in the human glucocorticoid receptor gene and glucocorticoid resistance. *Hum. Gen.*, **1997**, *99*:663–668.

Krell, R.D., Aharony, D., Buckner, C.K., *et al.* The preclinical pharmacology of ICI 204,219: A peptide leukotriene antagonist. *Am. Rev. Respir. Dis.*, **1990**, *141*:978–987.

Kume, H., Hall, I.P., Washabau, R.J., *et al.* β-Adrenergic agonists regulate KCa channels in airway smooth muscle by cAMP-dependent and -independent mechanisms. *J. Clin. Invest.*, **1994**, *93*:371–379.

Kuzemko, J.A., and Paala, J. Apnoeic attacks in the newborn treated with aminophylline. *Arch. Dis. Child.*, **1973**, *48*:404–406.

Laitinen, L.A., Laitinen, A., and Haahtela, T. A comparative study of the effects of an inhaled corticosteroid, budesonide, and a β_2 agonist, terbutaline, on airway inflammation in newly diagnosed asthma: A randomized, double-blind, parallel-group controlled trial. *J. Allergy Clin. Immunol.*, **1992**, *90*:32–42.

Laitinen, L.A., Naya, I.P., Binks, S., Harris, A. Comparative efficacy of zafirlukast and low-dose steroids in asthmatics on pm β_2 agonists. *Eur. Respir. J.*, **1997**, *10*(suppl 4):4195–4205.

Leung, D.Y., Sampson, H.A., Yunginger, J.W., *et al.* Effect of anti-IgE therapy in patients with peanut allergy. *New Engl. J. Med.*, **2003**, *348*:986–993.

Li, X., Ward, C., Thien, F., *et al.* An anti-inflammatory effect of salmeterol, a long-acting β_2 agonist, assessed in airway biopsies and bronchoalveolar lavage in asthma. *Am. J. Respir. Crit. Care Med.,* **1999,** *160*:1493–1499.

Lin, H., Boesel, K.M., Griffith, D.T., *et al.* Omalizumab rapidly decreases nasal allergic response and FcRI on basophils. *J. Allergy Clin. Immunol.,* **2004,** *113*:297–302.

Lindgren, S., Lokshin, B., Stromquist, A., *et al.* Does asthma or treatment with theophylline limit children's academic performance? *New Engl. J. Med.,* **1992,** *327*:926–930.

Lofdahl, C.G., Reiss, T.F., Leff, J.A., *et al.* Randomized, placebo-controlled trial of effect of a leukotriene receptor antagonist, montelukast, on tapering inhaled corticosteroids in asthmatic patients. *BMJ,* **1999,** *319*:87–90.

Lynch, K.R., O'Neill, G.P., Liu, Q., *et al.* Characterization of the human cysteinyl leukotriene CysLT1 receptor. *Nature,* **1999,** *399*:789–793.

Macfarlane, J.T., and Lane, D.J. Irregularities in the use of regular aerosol inhalers. *Thorax,* **1980,** *35*:477–478.

MacGlashan, D.W., Jr. Releasability of human basophils: Cellular sensitivity and maximal histamine release are independent variables. *J. Allergy Clin. Immunol.,* **1993,** *91*:605–615.

MacGlashan, D.W., Jr., Bochner, B.S., Adelman, D.C., *et al.* Down-regulation of FcεRI expression on human basophils during in vivo treatment of atopic patients with anti-IgE antibody. *J. Immunol.,* **1997,** *158*:1438–1445.

MacGlashan, D., Jr., Xia, H.Z., Schwartz, L.B., and Gong, J. IgE-regulated loss, not IgE-regulated synthesis, controls expression of FcRI in human basophils. *J. Leukoc. Biol.,* **2001,** *70*:207–218.

Malmstrom, K., Rodriguez-Gomez, G., Guerra, J., *et al.* Oral montelukast, inhaled beclomethasone, and placebo for chronic asthma: A randomized, controlled trial. Montelukast/Beclomethasone Study Group. *Ann. Intern. Med.,* **1999,** *130*:487–495.

Martinez, F.D., Graves, P.E., Baldini, P.E., *et al.* Genetic polymorphisms of the β_2 adrenoceptor and response to albuterol in children with and without a history of wheezing. *J. Clin. Invest.,* **1997,** *100*:3184–3188.

Meltzer, E.O., Orgel, H.A., Ellis, E.F., *et al.* Long-term comparison of three combinations of albuterol, theophylline, and beclomethasone in children with chronic asthma. *J. Allergy Clin. Immunol.,* **1992,** *90*:2–11.

Moqbel, R., Cromwell, O., Walsh, G.M., *et al.* Effects of nedocromil sodium (TILADE) on the activation of human eosinophils and neutrophils and the release of histamine from mast cells. *Allergy,* **1988,** *43*:268–276.

Murciano, D., Auclair, M.H., Pariente, R., and Aubier, M. A randomized, controlled trial of theophylline in patients with severe chronic obstructive pulmonary disease. *New Engl. J. Med.,* **1989,** *320*:1521–1525.

Murphy, R.C., Hammarstrom, S., and Samuelsson, B. Leukotriene C: A slow-reacting substance from murine mastocytoma cells. *Proc. Natl. Acad. Sci. U.S.A.,* **1979,** *76*:4275–4279.

Murray, J.J., Tonnel, A.B., Brash, A.R., *et al.* Release of prostaglandin D₂ into human airways during acute antigen challenge. *New Engl. J. Med.,* **1986,** *315*:800–804.

Muttitt, S.C., Tierney, A.J., and Finer, N.N. The dose response of theophylline in the treatment of apnea of prematurity. *J. Pediatr.,* **1988,** *112*:115–121.

Neild, J.E., and Cameron, I.R. Bronchoconstriction in response to suggestion: Its prevention by an inhaled anticholinergic agent. *BMJ (Clin. Res. Ed.),* **1985,** *290*:674.

O'Byrne, P.M., and Pedersen, S. Measuring efficacy and safety of different inhaled corticosteroid preparations. *J. Allergy Clin. Immunol.,* **1998,** *102*:879–886.

Ostrom, R.S., and Ehlert F.J. M₂ muscarinic receptors inhibit forskolin—but not isoproterenol—mediated relaxation in bovine tracheal smooth muscle. *J. Pharmacol. Exp. Ther.,* **1998,** *287*:234–242.

Paloucek, F.P., and Rodvold, K.A. Evaluation of theophylline overdoses and toxicities. *Ann. Emerg. Med.,* **1988,** *17*:135–144.

Pauwels, R., Van Renterghem, D., Van der Straeten, M., *et al.* The effect of theophylline and enprofylline on allergen-induced bronchoconstriction. *J. Allergy Clin. Immunol.,* **1985,** *76*:583–590.

Peachell, P.T., Columbo, M., Kagey-Sobotka, A., *et al.* Adenosine potentiates mediator release from human lung mast cells. *Am. Rev. Respir. Dis.,* **1988,** *138*:1143–1151.

Pedersen, K.E., Bochner, B.S., and Undem, B.J. Cysteinyl leukotrienes induce P-selectin expression in human endothelial cells *via* a non-CysLT1 receptor-mediated mechanism. *J. Pharmacol. Exp. Ther.,* **1997,** *281*:655–662.

Prussin, C., Griffith, D.T., Boesel, K.M., *et al.* Omalizumab treatment down-regulates dendritic cell FcRI expression. *J. Allergy Clin. Immunol.,* **2003,** *112*:1147–1154.

Rebuck, A.S., Chapman, K.R., Abboud, R., *et al.* Nebulized anticholinergic and sympathomimetic treatment of asthma and chronic obstructive airways disease in the emergency room. *Am. J. Med.,* **1987,** *82*:59–64.

Saini, S.S., MacGlashan, D.W., Jr., Sterbinsky, S.A., *et al.* Down-regulation of human basophil IgE and FCεRIα surface densities and mediator release by anti-IgE-infusions is reversible *in vitro* and *in vivo. J. Immunol.,* **1999,** *162*:5624–5630.

Soler, M., Matz, J., Townley, R., *et al.* The anti-IgE antibody omalizumab reduces exacerbations and steroid requirement in allergic asthmatics. *Eur. Respir. J.,* **2001,** *18*:254–261.

Svendsen, U.G., Frolund, L., Madsen, F., and Nielsen, N.H. A comparison of the effects of nedocromil sodium and beclomethasone dipropionate on pulmonary function, symptoms, and bronchial responsiveness in patients with asthma. *J. Allergy Clin. Immunol.,* **1989,** *84*:224–231.

Svendsen, U.G., Frolund, L., Madsen, F., *et al.* A comparison of the effects of sodium cromoglycate and beclomethasone dipropionate on pulmonary function and bronchial hyperreactivity in subjects with asthma. *J. Allergy Clin. Immunol.,* **1987,** *80*:68–74.

Svendsen, U.G., and Jorgensen, H. Inhaled nedocromil sodium as additional treatment to high-dose inhaled corticosteroids in the management of bronchial asthma. *Eur. Respir. J.,* **1991,** *4*:992–999.

Sylvester, J.T. The tone of pulmonary smooth muscle: ROK and Rho music? *Am. J. Physiol. Lung Cell Mol. Physiol.,* **2004,** *287*:L624–630.

Tan, S., Hall, I.P., Dewar, J., *et al.* Association between β_2-adrenoceptor polymorphism and susceptibility to bronchodilator desensitization in moderately severe stable asthmatics. *Lancet,* **1997,** *350*:995–999.

Thoman, E.B., Davis, D.H., Raye, J.R., *et al.* Theophylline affects sleep–wake state development in premature infants. *Neuropediatrics,* **1985,** *16*:13–18.

Tomioka, H., and Ishizaka, K. Mechanisms of passive sensitization: II. Presence of receptors for IgE on monkey mast cells. *J. Immunol.,* **1971,** *107*:971–978.

Toogood, J.H., Jennings, B., and Lefcoe, N.M. A clinical trial of combined cromolyn/beclomethasone treatment for chronic asthma. *J. Allergy Clin. Immunol.,* **1981,** *67*:317–324.

Torphy, T.J., Undem, B.J., Cieslinski, L.B., *et al.* Identification, characterization, and functional role of phosphodiesterase isozymes in human airway smooth muscle. *J. Pharmacol. Exp. Ther.,* **1993,** *265*:1213–1223.

Turner, J.R., Corkery, K.J., Eckman, D., *et al.* Equivalence of continuous flow nebulizer and metered-dose inhaler with reservoir bag for treatment of acute airflow obstruction. *Chest,* **1988,** *93*:476–481.

van Schayck, C.P., Dompeling, E., van Herwaarden, C.L., *et al.* Bronchodilator treatment in moderate asthma or chronic bronchitis: continuous or on demand? A randomised, controlled study. *BMJ,* **1991,** *303*:1426–1431.

Woolcock, A., Lundback, B., Ringdal, N., and Jacques, L.A. Comparison of addition of salmeterol to inhaled steroids with doubling of the dose of inhaled steroids. *Am. J. Respir. Crit. Care Med.,* **1996,** *153*:1481–1488.

Wrenn, K., Slovis, C.M., Murphy, F., and Greenberg, R.S. Aminophylline therapy for acute bronchospastic disease in the emergency room. *Ann. Intern. Med.,* **1991,** *115*:241–247.

MONOGRAPHS AND REVIEWS

American Thoracic Society. Standards for the diagnosis and care of patients with chronic obstructive pulmonary disease (COPD) and asthma. *Am. Rev. Respir. Dis.,* **1987,** *136*:225–244.

Anonymous. *Executive Summary: Guidelines for the Diagnosis and Management of Asthma.* NIH Publication No. 91-3042A. NIH, Bethesda, MD, **1991,** pp. 1–44.

Barnes, P.J. Effect of β-agonists on inflammatory cells. *J. Allergy Clin. Immunol.,* **1999,** *104*:S10–S17.

Barnes, P.J. Inhaled glucocorticoids for asthma. *New Engl. J. Med.,* **1995,** *332*:868–875.

Barnes, P.J., and Pedersen, S. Efficacy and safety of inhaled corticosteroids in asthma. *Am. Rev. Respir. Dis.,* **1993,** *148*:S1–S26.

Beavo, J.A., and Reifsnyder, D.H. Primary sequence of cyclic nucleotide phosphodiesterase isozymes and the design of selective inhibitors. *Trends Pharmacol. Sci.,* **1990,** *11*:150–155.

Brattsand, R., and Axelsson, B.I. Basis of airway selectivity of inhaled glucocorticoids. In, *Inhaled Glucocorticoids in Asthma: Mechanisms and Clinical Actions.* (Schleimer, R.P., Busse, W.W., and O'Bryne, P., eds.) Marcel Dekker, New York, **1997,** pp. 351–379.

Brogden, R.N., and Sorkin, E.M. Nedocromil sodium: An updated review of its pharmacological properties and therapeutic efficacy in asthma. *Drugs,* **1993,** *45*:693–715.

Bryant, D.H. Nebulized ipratropium bromide in the treatment of acute asthma. *Chest,* **1985,** *88*:24–29.

Busse, W.W. What role for inhaled steroids in chronic asthma? *Chest,* **1993,** *104*:1565–1571.

Crystal, R.G. α_1-Antitrypsin deficiency, emphysema, and liver disease: Genetic basis and strategies for therapy. *J. Clin. Invest.,* **1990,** *85*:1343–1352.

Daly, J.W. Adenosine receptors: targets for future drugs. *J. Med. Chem.,* **1982,** *25*:197–207.

Dewar, J.C., and Hall, I.P. Personalised prescribing for asthma: Is pharmacogenetics the answer? *J. Pharm. Pharmacol.,* **2003,** *55*:279–289.

Ferguson, G.T., and Cherniack, R.M. Management of chronic obstructive pulmonary disease. *New Engl. J. Med.,* **1993,** *328*:1017–1022.

Graham, D.M. Caffeine—its identity, dietary sources, intake, and biological effects. *Nutr. Rev.,* **1978,** *36*:97–102.

Greenberger, P.A. Corticosteroids in asthma: Rationale, use, and problems. *Chest,* **1992,** *101*:418S–421S.

Gross, N.J. Ipratropium bromide. *New Engl. J. Med.,* **1988,** *319*:486–494.

Hay, D.W., Torphy, T.J., and Undem, B.J. Cysteinyl leukotrienes in asthma: Old mediators up to new tricks. *Trends Pharmacol. Sci.,* **1995,** *16*:304–309.

Hoag, J.E., and McFadden, E.R., Jr. Long-term effect of cromolyn sodium on nonspecific bronchial hyperresponsiveness: A review. *Ann. Allergy,* **1991,** *66*:53–63.

Holgate, S.T. Antihistamines in the treatment of asthma. *Clin. Rev. Allergy.,* **1994,** *12*:65–78.

Israel, E., and Drazen, J.M. Treating mild asthma: When are inhaled steroids indicated? *New Engl. J. Med.,* **1994,** *331*:737–739.

Jarvis, B., and Markham, A. Montelukast: A review of its therapeutic potential in persistent asthma. *Drugs,* **2000,** *59*:891–928.

Johnson, C.E. Aerosol corticosteroids for the treatment of asthma. *Drug Intell. Clin. Pharm.,* **1987,** *21*:784–790.

Johnson, M., and Coleman, R.A. Mechanisms of action of β_2-adrenoceptor agonists. In, *Asthma and Rhinitis.* (Busse, W.W., and Holgate, S.T., eds.) Blackwell Scientific Publications, Cambridge, MA, **1995,** pp. 1278–1295.

Krishnaswamy, G., Kelley, J., Johnson, D., *et al.* The human mast cell: functions in physiology and disease. *Front. Biosci.,* **2001,** *6*:D1109–1127.

McFadden, E.R., Jr. Dosages of corticosteroids in asthma. *Am. Rev. Respir. Dis.,* **1993,** *147*:1306–1310.

Murphy, S., and Kelly, H.W. Cromolyn sodium: A review of mechanisms and clinical use in asthma. *Drug Intell. Clin. Pharm.,* **1987,** *21*:22–35.

Nasser, S.S., and Rees, P.J. Theophylline: Current thoughts on the risks and benefits of its use in asthma. *Drug Saf.,* **1993,** *8*:12–18.

Nelson, H.S. β-Adrenergic bronchodilators. *New Engl. J. Med.,* **1995,** *333*:499–506.

Page, C.P. Recent advances in our understanding of the use of theophylline in the treatment of asthma. *J. Clin. Pharmacol.,* **1999,** *39*:237–240.

Pavord, I., and Knox, A. Pharmacokinetic optimisation of inhaled steroid therapy in asthma. *Clin. Pharmacokinet.,* **1993,** *25*:126–135.

Pearce, F.L., Al-Laith, M., Bosman, L., *et al.* Effects of sodium cromoglycate and nedocromil sodium on histamine secretion from mast cells from various locations. *Drugs,* **1989,** *37*(suppl 1):37–43.

Roberts, R.J. *Drug Therapy in Infants: Pharmacologic Principles and Clinical Experience.* Saunders, Philadelphia, **1984.**

Schleimer, R.P. Glucocorticosteroids: Their mechanisms of action and use in allergic diseases. In, *Allergy: Principles and Practice,* 5th ed. (Middleton, E., Jr., Ellis, E.F., Yuninger, J.W., *et al.,* eds.) Mosby, St. Louis, **1998,** pp. 638–660.

Schroeder, J.T., MacGlashan, D.W., Jr., and Lichtenstein, L.M. Human basophils: Mediator release and cytokine production. *Adv. Immunol.,* **2001,** *77*:93–122.

Self, T.H., Rumbak, M.J., Kelso, T.M., and Nicholas, R.A. Reassessment of the role of theophylline in the current therapy for nocturnal asthma. *J. Am. Board Fam. Pract.,* **1992,** *5*:281–288.

Smaldone, G.C. Determinants of dose and response to inhaled therapeutic agents in asthma. In, *Inhaled Glucocorticoids in Asthma: Mechanisms and Clinical Actions.* (Schleimer, R.P., Busse, W.W., and O'Bryne, P., eds.) Marcel Dekker, New York, **1997,** pp. 447–477.

Soderling, S.H., and Beavo, J.A. Regulation of cAMP and cGMP signaling: New phosphodiesterases and new functions. *Curr. Opin. Cell. Biol.,* **2000,** *12*:174–179.

Stoloff, S.W. The changing role of theophylline in pediatric asthma. *Am. Fam. Phys.,* **1994,** *49*:839–844.

Symposium. Asthma: A nocturnal disease. January 21–24, 1988, Laguna Niguel, California. Proceedings. (McFadden, E.R., Jr., ed.) *Am. J. Med.,* **1988a,** *85*:1–70.

Symposium. Cholinergic pathway in obstructive airways disease. (Bergofsky, E.H., ed.) *Am. J. Med.,* **1986b,** *81*:1–192.

Symposium. Developmental pharmacology of the methylxanthines. Introduction. (Soyka, L.F., ed.) *Semin. Perinatol.,* **1981,** *5*:303–304.

Symposium. Progress in understanding the relationship between the adenosine receptor system and actions of methylxanthines. (Carney, J.M., and Katz, J.L., eds.) *Pharmacol. Biochem. Behav.,* **1988b,** *29*:407–441.

Symposium. Update on theophylline. (Grant, J.A., and Ellis, E.F., eds.) *J. Allergy Clin. Immunol.,* **1986a,** *78*:669–824.

Taburet, A.M., and Schmit, B. Pharmacokinetic optimisation of asthma treatment. *Clin. Pharmacokinet.,* **1994,** *26*:396–418.

Torphy, T.J., and Undem, B.J. Phosphodiesterase inhibitors: New opportunities for the treatment of asthma. *Thorax,* **1991,** *46*:512–523.

Wasserman, S.I. A review of some recent clinical studies with nedocromil sodium. *J. Allergy Clin. Immunol.,* **1993,** *92*:210–215.

Weinberger, M. Pharmacologic management of asthma. *J. Adolesc. Health Care.,* **1987,** *8*:74–83.

CHAPTER

28

DIURETICS

Edwin K. Jackson

Diuretics increase the rate of urine flow and sodium excretion and are used to adjust the volume and/or composition of body fluids in a variety of clinical situations, including hypertension, heart failure, renal failure, nephrotic syndrome, and cirrhosis. This chapter first describes renal anatomy and physiology; then introduces diuretics with regard to chemistry, mechanism of action, site of action, effects on urinary composition, and effects on renal hemodynamics; and finally, integrates diuretic pharmacology with a discussion of mechanisms of edema formation and the role of diuretics in clinical medicine. Therapeutic applications of diuretics are expanded on in Chapters 32 (hypertension) and 33 (heart failure).

RENAL ANATOMY AND PHYSIOLOGY

Renal Anatomy. The main renal artery branches near the renal hilum into segmental arteries, which, in turn, subdivide to form interlobar arteries that pierce the renal parenchyma. The interlobar arteries curve at the border of the renal medulla and cortex to form arched vessels known as *arcuate arteries*. Arcuate arteries give rise to perpendicular branches, called *interlobular arteries,* that enter the renal cortex and supply blood to the afferent arterioles. A single afferent arteriole penetrates the glomerulus of each nephron and branches extensively to form the glomerular capillary nexus. These branches coalesce to form the efferent arteriole. Efferent arterioles of superficial glomeruli ascend toward the kidney surface before splitting into peritubular capillaries that service the tubular elements of the renal cortex. Efferent arterioles of juxtamedullary glomeruli descend into the medulla and divide to form the descending vasa recta, which supply blood to the

capillaries of the medulla. Blood returning from the medulla *via* the ascending vasa recta drains directly into the arcuate veins, and blood from the peritubular capillaries of the cortex enters the interlobular veins, which, in turn, connect with the arcuate veins. Arcuate veins drain into interlobar veins, which drain into segmental veins; blood leaves the kidney *via* the main renal vein.

The basic urine-forming unit of the kidney is the nephron, which consists of a filtering apparatus, the glomerulus, connected to a long tubular portion that reabsorbs and conditions the glomerular ultrafiltrate. Each human kidney is composed of approximately one million nephrons. The nomenclature for segments of the tubular portion of the nephron has become increasingly complex as renal physiologists have subdivided the nephron into shorter and shorter named segments. These subdivisions were based initially on the axial location of the segments but increasingly have been based on the morphology of the epithelial cells lining the various nephron segments. Figure 28–1 illustrates subdivisions of the nephron.

Glomerular Filtration. In the glomerular capillaries, a portion of the plasma water is forced through a filter that has three basic components: the fenestrated capillary endothelial cells, a basement membrane lying just beneath the endothelial cells, and the filtration slit diaphragms formed by the epithelial cells that cover the basement membrane on its urinary space side. Solutes of small size flow with filtered water (solvent drag) into the urinary (Bowman's) space, whereas formed elements and macromolecules are retained by the filtration barrier. For each nephron unit, the rate of filtration [single-nephron glomerular filtration rate (SNGFR)] is a function of the hydrostatic pressure in the glomerular capillaries (P_{GC}), the hydrostatic pressure in Bowman's space (which can be equated with pressure in the proximal tubule, P_T), the mean colloid osmotic pressure in the glomerular capillaries (Π_{GC}), the colloid osmotic pressure in the proximal tubule (Π_T), and the ultrafiltration coefficient (K_f), according to the equation

$$\text{SNGFR} = K_f[(P_{GC} - P_T) - (\Pi_{GC} - \Pi_T)] \qquad (28\text{–}1)$$

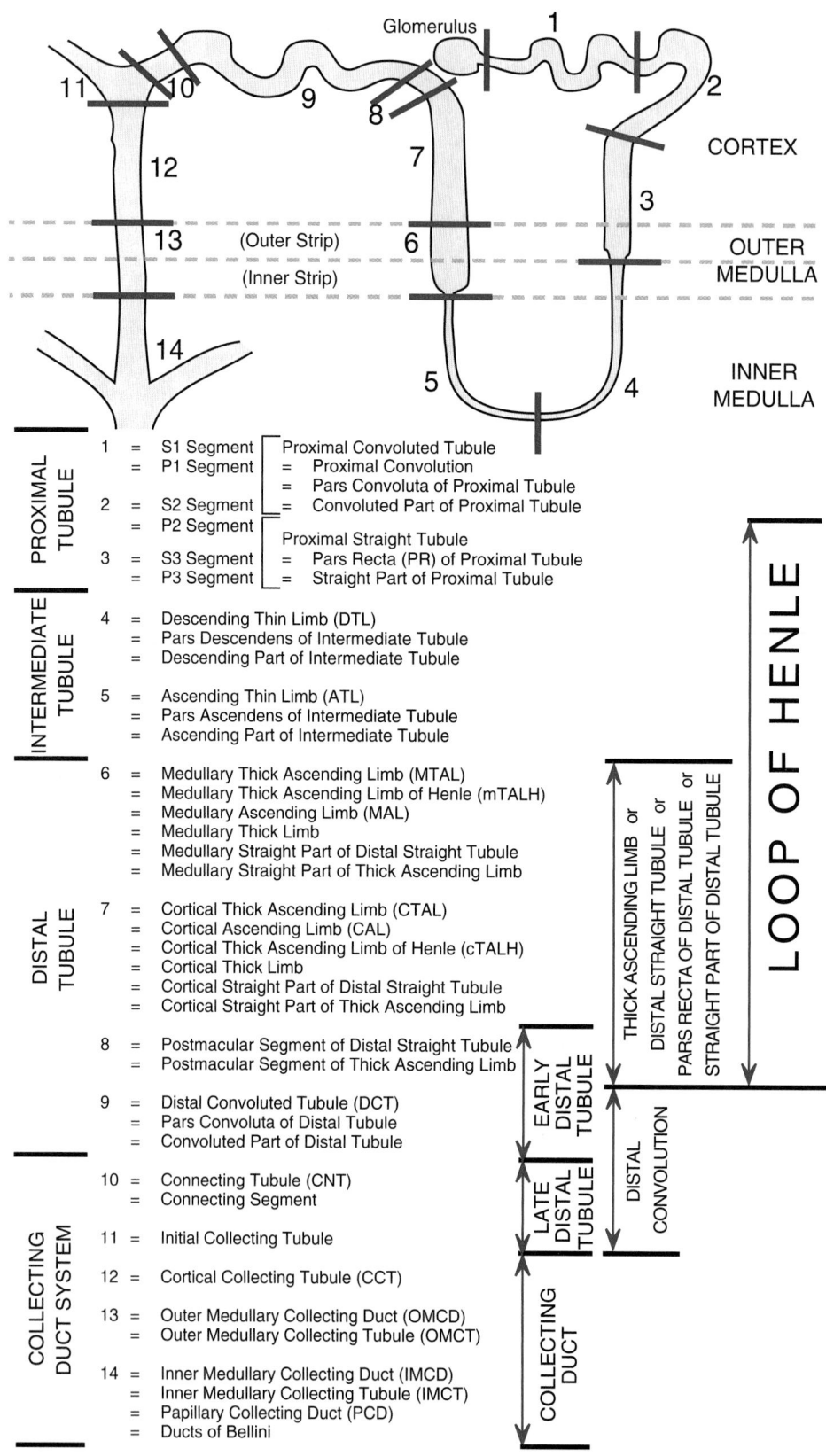

Figure 28–1. *Anatomy and nomenclature of the nephron.*

If $P_{GC} - P_T$ is defined as the transcapillary hydraulic pressure difference (ΔP), and if Π_T is negligible (as it usually is because little protein is filtered), then

$$\text{SNGFR} = K_f(\Delta P - \Pi_{GC}) \qquad (28\text{-}2)$$

This latter equation succinctly expresses the three major determinants of SNGFR. However, each of these three determinants can be influenced by a number of other variables. K_f is determined by the physicochemical properties of the filtering membrane and by the surface area available for filtration. ΔP is determined primarily by the arterial blood pressure and by the proportion of the arterial pressure that is transmitted to the glomerular capillaries. This is governed by the relative resistances of preglomerular and postglomerular vessels. Π_{GC} is determined by two variables, *i.e.*, the concentration of protein in the arterial blood entering the glomerulus and the single-nephron blood flow (Q_A). Q_A influences Π_{GC} because as blood transverses the glomerular capillary bed, filtration concentrates proteins in the capillaries, causing Π_{GC} to rise with distance along the glomerular bed. When Q_A is high, this effect is reduced; however, when Q_A is low, Π_{GC} may increase to the point that $\Pi_{GC} = \Delta P$, and filtration ceases (a condition known as *filtration equilibrium*).

Overview of Nephron Function. The kidney is designed to filter large quantities of plasma, reabsorb substances that the body must conserve, and leave behind and/or secrete substances that must be eliminated. The two kidneys in humans produce together approximately 120 ml of ultrafiltrate, yet only 1 ml/min of urine is produced. Therefore, greater than 99% of the glomerular ultrafiltrate is reabsorbed at a staggering energy cost. The kidneys consume 7% of total-body oxygen intake despite the fact that the kidneys make up only 0.5% of body weight.

The proximal tubule is contiguous with Bowman's capsule and takes a tortuous path until finally forming a straight portion that dives into the renal medulla. Based on the morphology of the epithelial cells lining the tubule, the proximal tubule has been subdivided into S1, S2, and S3 segments. Normally, approximately 65% of filtered Na^+ is reabsorbed in the proximal tubule, and since this part of the tubule is highly permeable to water, reabsorption is essentially isotonic.

Between the outer and inner strips of the outer medulla, the tubule abruptly changes morphology to become the descending thin limb (DTL), which penetrates the inner medulla, makes a hairpin turn, and then forms the ascending thin limb (ATL). At the juncture between the inner and outer medulla, the tubule once again changes morphology and becomes the thick ascending limb, which is made up of three segments: a medullary portion (MTAL), a cortical portion (CTAL), and a postmacular segment. Together the proximal straight tubule, DTL, ATL, MTAL, CTAL, and postmacular segment are known as the *loop of Henle*. The DTL is highly permeable to water, yet its permeability to NaCl and urea is low. In contrast, the ATL is permeable to NaCl and urea but is impermeable to water. The thick ascending limb actively reabsorbs NaCl but is impermeable to water and urea. Approximately 25% of filtered Na^+ is reabsorbed in the loop of Henle, mostly in the thick ascending limb, which has a large reabsorptive capacity.

The thick ascending limb passes between the afferent and efferent arterioles and makes contact with the afferent arteriole *via* a cluster of specialized columnar epithelial cells known as the *macula densa*. The macula densa is strategically located to sense concentrations of NaCl leaving the loop of Henle. If the concentration of NaCl is too high, the macula densa sends a chemical signal (perhaps adenosine or ATP) to the afferent arteriole of the same nephron, causing it to constrict. This, in turn, causes a reduction in P_{GC} and

Q_A and decreases SNGFR. This homeostatic mechanism, known as *tubuloglomerular feedback* (TGF), serves to protect the organism from salt and volume wasting. Besides mediating the TGF response, the macula densa also regulates renin release from the adjacent juxtaglomerular cells in the wall of the afferent arteriole.

Approximately 0.2 mm past the macula densa, the tubule changes morphology once again to become the distal convoluted tubule (DCT). The postmacular segment of the thick ascending limb and the distal convoluted tubule often are referred to as the *early distal tubule*. Like the thick ascending limb, the DCT actively transports NaCl and is impermeable to water. Since these characteristics impart the ability to produce a dilute urine, the thick ascending limb and the DCT are collectively called the *diluting segment of the nephron,* and the tubular fluid in the DCT is hypotonic regardless of hydration status. However, unlike the thick ascending limb, the DCT does not contribute to the countercurrent-induced hypertonicity of the medullary interstitium (*see* below).

The collecting duct system (connecting tubule + initial collecting tubule + cortical collecting duct + outer and inner medullary collecting ducts, *e.g.*, segments 10 to 14 in Figure 28–1) is an area of fine control of ultrafiltrate composition and volume. It is here that final adjustments in electrolyte composition are made, a process modulated by the adrenal steroid aldosterone. In addition, antidiuretic hormone (ADH; *see* Chapter 29) modulates permeability of this part of the nephron to water.

The more distal portions of the collecting duct pass through the renal medulla, where the interstitial fluid is markedly hypertonic. In the absence of ADH, the collecting duct system is impermeable to water, and a dilute urine is excreted. In the presence of ADH, the collecting duct system is permeable to water, so water is reabsorbed. The movement of water out of the tubule is driven by the steep concentration gradient that exists between the tubular fluid and the medullary interstitium.

The hypertonicity of the medullary interstitium plays a vital role in the ability of mammals and birds to concentrate urine and therefore is a key adaptation necessary for living in a terrestrial environment. This is accomplished *via* a combination of the unique topography of the loop of Henle and the specialized permeability features of the loop's subsegments. Although the precise mechanisms giving rise to the medullary hypertonicity have remained elusive, the "passive countercurrent multiplier hypothesis" is an intuitively attractive model that is qualitatively accurate (*see* Sands and Kokko, 1996). According to this hypothesis, the process begins with active transport in the thick ascending limb, which concentrates NaCl in the interstitium of the outer medulla. Since this segment of the nephron is impermeable to water, active transport in the ascending limb dilutes the tubular fluid. As the dilute fluid passes into the collecting-duct system, water is extracted if, and only if, ADH is present. Since the cortical and outer medullary collecting ducts have a low permeability to urea, urea is concentrated in the tubular fluid. The inner medullary collecting duct, however, is permeable to urea, so urea diffuses into the inner medulla, where it is trapped by countercurrent exchange in the vasa recta. Since the DTL is impermeable to salt and urea, the high urea concentration in the inner medulla extracts water from the DTL and concentrates NaCl in the tubular fluid of the DTL. As the tubular fluid enters the ATL, NaCl diffuses out of the salt-permeable ATL, thus contributing to the hypertonicity of the medullary interstitium.

General Mechanism of Renal Epithelial Transport. Figure 28–2 illustrates seven mechanisms by which solutes may cross renal epithelial cell membranes. If bulk water flow occurs across a membrane, solute molecules will be transferred by convection across the membrane, a process known as *solvent drag*. Solutes with sufficient lipid solubility

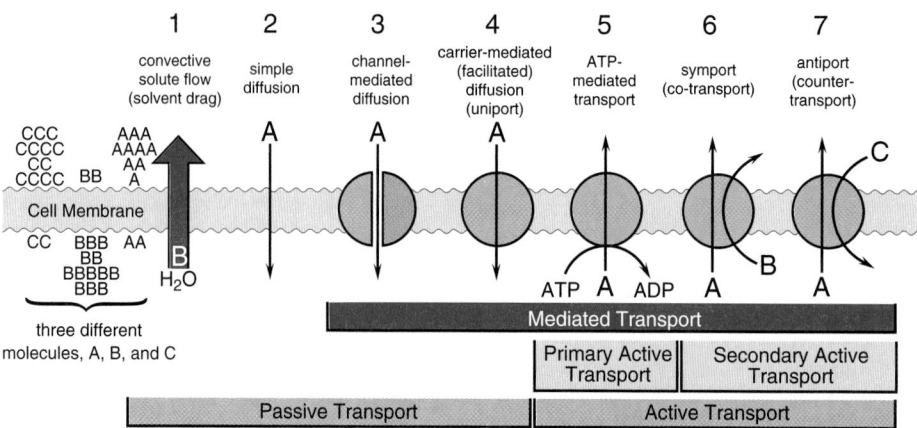

Figure 28–2. *Seven basic mechanisms for transmembrane transport of solutes.* 1, convective flow in which dissolved solutes are "dragged" by bulk water flow; 2, simple diffusion of lipophilic solute across membrane; 3, diffusion of solute through a pore; 4, transport of solute by carrier protein down electrochemical gradient; 5, transport of solute by carrier protein against electrochemical gradient with ATP hydrolysis providing driving force; 6 and 7, cotransport and countertransport, respectively, of solutes, with one solute traveling uphill against an electrochemical gradient and the other solute traveling down an electrochemical gradient.

also may dissolve in the membrane and diffuse across the membrane down their electrochemical gradients (simple diffusion). Many solutes, however, have limited lipid solubility, and transport must rely on integral proteins embedded in the cell membrane. In some cases the integral protein merely provides a conductive pathway (pore) through which the solute may diffuse passively (*channel-mediated diffusion*). In other cases the solute may bind to the integral protein and, owing to a conformational change in the protein, be transferred across the cell membrane down an electrochemical gradient (*carrier-mediated* or *facilitated diffusion,* also called *uniport*). However, this process will not result in net movement of solute against an electrochemical gradient. If solute must be moved "uphill" against an electrochemical gradient, then either primary active transport or secondary active transport is required. With primary active transport, ATP hydrolysis is coupled directly to conformational changes in the integral protein, thus providing the necessary free energy (*ATP-mediated transport*). Often, ATP-mediated transport is used to create an electrochemical gradient for a given solute, and the free energy of that solute gradient is then released to drive the "uphill" transport of other solutes. This process requires *symport* (cotransport of solute species in the same direction) or *antiport* (countertransport of solute species in opposite directions) and is known as *secondary active transport.*

The kinds of transport achieved in a particular nephron segment depend mainly on which transporters are present and whether they are embedded in the luminal or basolateral membrane. A general model of renal tubular transport is shown in Figure 28–3 and can be summarized as follows:

1. Na^+,K^+–ATPase (sodium pump) in the basolateral membrane hydrolyzes ATP, which results in the transport of Na^+ into the intercellular and interstitial spaces, the movement of K^+ into the cell, and the establishment and maintenance of an electrochemical gradient for Na^+ across the cell membrane directed inward. Although other ATPases exist in selected renal epithelial cells and participate in the transport of specific solutes (*e.g.,* Ca^{2+}–ATPase and H^+–ATPase), the bulk of all transport in the kidney is due to the abundant supply of Na^+,K^+–ATPase in the basolateral membranes of the renal epithelial cells and the separation of Na^+ and K^+ across the cell membrane.

2. Na^+ may diffuse across the luminal membrane *via* Na^+ channels into the epithelial cell down the electrochemical gradient for Na^+ that is established by the basolateral Na^+,K^+–ATPases. In addition, the free energy available in the electrochemical gradient for Na^+ is tapped by integral proteins in the luminal membrane, resulting in cotransport of various solutes against their electrochemical gradients by symporters (*e.g.,* Na^+–glucose, Na^+–$H_2PO_4^-$, and Na^+–amino acid). This process results in movement of Na^+ and cotransported solutes out of the tubular lumen into the cell. Also, antiporters (*e.g.,* Na^+–H^+) move Na^+ out of and some solutes into the tubular lumen.

3. Na^+ exits the basolateral membrane into the intercellular and interstitial spaces *via* the Na^+ pump or *via* symporters or antiporters in the basolateral membrane.

4. The action of Na^+-linked symporters in the luminal membrane causes the concentration of substrates for these symporters to rise in the epithelial cell. These electrochemical gradients then permit simple diffusion or mediated transport (*e.g.,* symporters, antiporters, uniporters, and channels) of solutes into the intercellular and interstitial spaces.

5. Accumulation of Na^+ and other solutes in the intercellular space creates a small osmotic pressure differential across the epithelial cell. In water-permeable epithelium, water moves into the intercellular spaces driven by the osmotic pressure differential. Water moves through aqueous pores in both the luminal and the basolateral cell membranes, as well as through the tight junctions (paracellular pathway). Bulk water flow carries some solutes into the intercellular space by solvent drag.

6. Movement of water into the intercellular space concentrates other solutes in the tubular fluid, resulting in an electrochemical gradient for these substances across the epithelium. Membrane-permeable solutes then move down their electrochemical gradients into the intercellular space *via* both the transcellular (*e.g.,* simple diffusion, symporters, antiporters, uniporters, and channels) and paracellular pathways. Membrane-impermeable solutes remain in the tubular lumen and are excreted in the urine with an obligatory amount of water.

7. As water and solutes accumulate in the intercellular space, the hydrostatic pressure increases, thus providing a driving force for bulk water flow. Bulk water flow carries solute (solute convection)

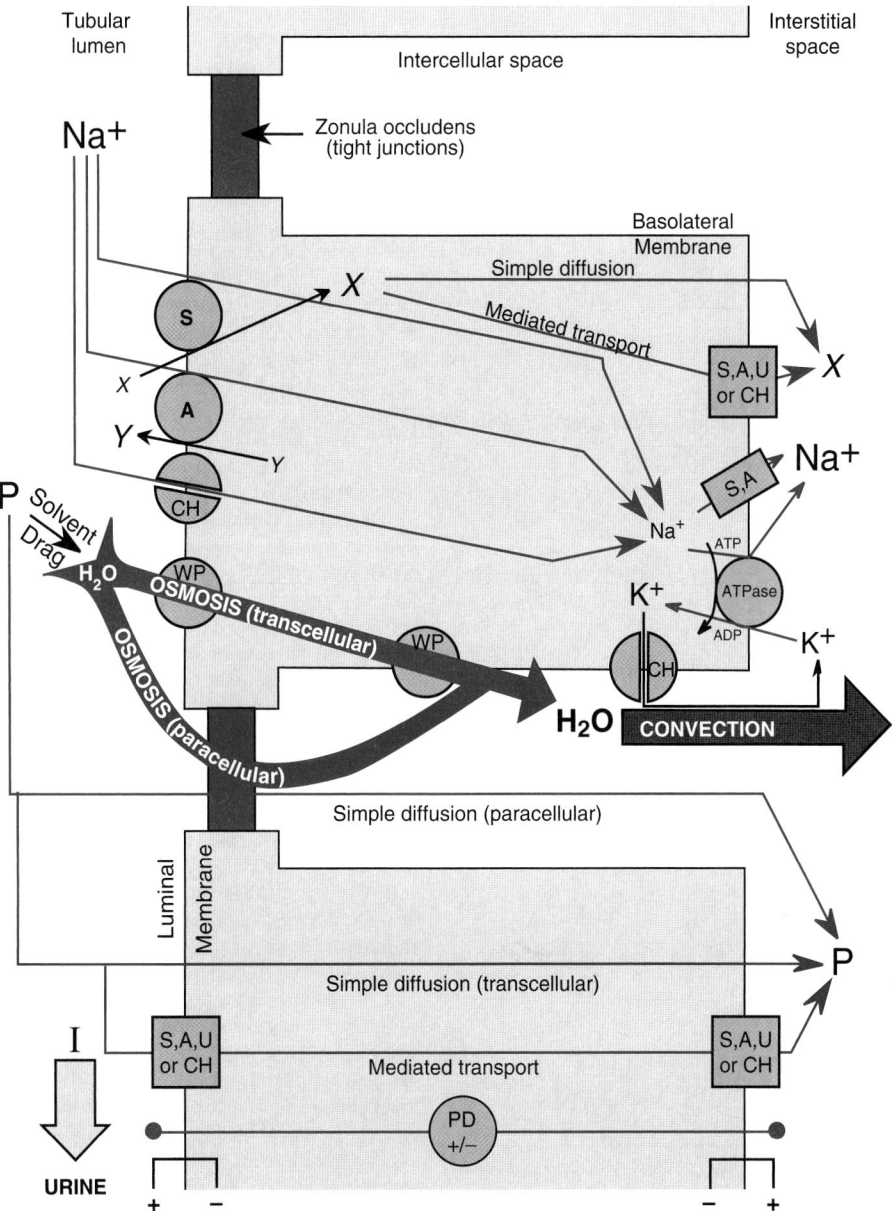

Figure 28–3. *Generic mechanism of renal epithelial cell transport (see text for details).* S, symporter; A, antiporter; CH, ion channel; WP, water pore; U, uniporter; ATPase, Na+,K+–ATPase (sodium pump); *X* and *Y,* transported solutes; *P,* membrane-permeable (reabsorbable) solutes; *I,* membrane-impermeable (nonreabsorbable) solutes; PD, potential difference across indicated membrane or cell.

out of the intercellular space into the interstitial space and, finally, into the peritubular capillaries. The movement of fluid into the peritubular capillaries is governed by the same Starling forces that determine transcapillary fluid movement for any capillary bed.

Mechanism of Organic Acid and Organic Base Secretion. The kidney is a major organ involved in the elimination of organic chemicals from the body. Organic molecules may enter the renal tubules by glomerular filtration of molecules not bound to plasma proteins or may be actively secreted directly into the tubules. The proximal tubule has

a highly efficient transport system for organic acids and an equally efficient but separate transport system for organic bases. Current models for these secretory systems are illustrated in Figure 28–4. Both systems are powered by the sodium pump in the basolateral membrane, involve secondary and tertiary active transport, and use a facilitated-diffusion step. There are at least nine different organic acid and five different organic base transporters; the precise roles that these transporters play in organic acid and base transport remain ill-defined (Dresser *et al.,* 2001). A family of organic anion transporters (OATs) countertransport organic anions with dicarboxylates (Figure

A Luminal space Epithelial cell Peritubular space

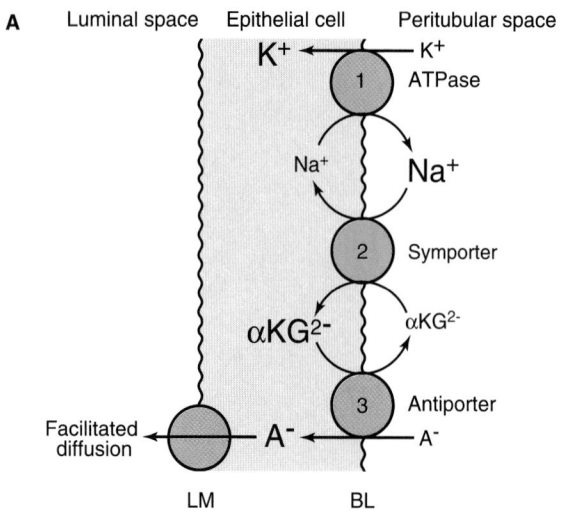

B Luminal space Epithelial cell Peritubular space

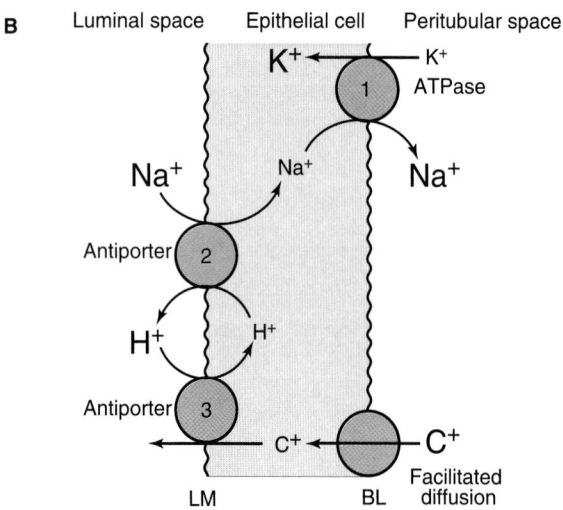

Figure 28–4. *Mechanisms of organic acid (A) and organic base (B) secretion in the proximal tubule.* The numbers 1, 2, and 3 refer to primary, secondary, and tertiary active transport. A^-, organic acid (anion); C^+, organic base (cation); αKG^{2-}, α-ketoglutarate but also other dicarboxylates. BL and LM indicate basolateral and luminal membranes, respectively.

28–4A). OATs most likely exist as α-helical dodecaspans connected by short segments of approximately 10 or fewer amino acids, except for large interconnecting stretches of amino acids between helices 1 and 2 and helices 6 and 7 (Eraly *et al.*, 2004).

Renal Handling of Specific Anions and Cations. Reabsorption of Cl^- generally follows reabsorption of Na^+. In segments of the tubule with low-resistance tight junctions (*i.e.*, "leaky" epithelium), such as the proximal tubule and thick ascending limb, Cl^- movement can

occur paracellularly. With regard to transcellular Cl^- flux, Cl^- crosses the luminal membrane *via* antiport with formate and oxalate (proximal tubule), symport with Na^+/K^+ (thick ascending limb), symport with Na^+ (DCT), and antiport with HCO_3^- (collecting-duct system). Cl^- crosses the basolateral membrane *via* symport with K^+ (proximal tubule and thick ascending limb), antiport with Na^+/HCO_3^- (proximal tubule), and Cl^- channels (thick ascending limb, DCT, collecting-duct system).

Eighty to ninety percent of filtered K^+ is reabsorbed in the proximal tubule (diffusion and solvent drag) and thick ascending limb (diffusion) largely *via* the paracellular pathway. In contrast, the DCT and collecting-duct system secrete variable amounts of K^+ *via* a conductive (channel-mediated) pathway. Modulation of the rate of K^+ secretion in the collecting-duct system, particularly by aldosterone, allows urinary excretion of K^+ to be matched with dietary intake. The transepithelial potential difference (V_T), lumen-positive in the thick ascending limb and lumen-negative in the collecting-duct system, provides an important driving force for K^+ reabsorption and secretion, respectively.

Most of the filtered Ca^{2+} (approximately 70%) is reabsorbed by the proximal tubule by passive diffusion *via* a paracellular route. Another 25% of filtered Ca^{2+} is reabsorbed by the thick ascending limb in part *via* a paracellular route driven by the lumen-positive V_T and in part by active transcellular Ca^{2+} reabsorption modulated by parathyroid hormone (PTH; *see* Chapter 61). Most of the remaining Ca^{2+} is reabsorbed in the DCT *via* a transcellular pathway. The transcellular pathway in the thick ascending limb and DCT involves passive influx of Ca^{2+} across the luminal membrane *via* Ca^{2+} channels, followed by extrusion of Ca^{2+} across the basolateral membrane by a Ca^{2+}–ATPase. Also, in the DCT, Ca^{2+} crosses the basolateral membrane *via* Na^+–Ca^{2+} antiport.

Inorganic phosphate (P_i) is largely reabsorbed (80% of filtered load) by the proximal tubule. An Na^+–P_i symporter uses the free energy of the Na^+ electrochemical gradient to transport P_i into the cell. The Na^+–P_i symporter is inhibited by PTH. P_i exits the basolateral membrane down its electrochemical gradient by a poorly understood transport system.

Only 20% to 25% of Mg^{2+} is reabsorbed in the proximal tubule, and only 5% is reabsorbed by the DCT and collecting-duct system. The bulk of Mg^{2+} is reabsorbed in the thick ascending limb *via* a paracellular pathway driven by the lumen-positive V_T. However, transcellular movement of Mg^{2+} also may occur with basolateral exit *via* Na^+–Mg^{2+} antiport or *via* a Mg^{2+}–ATPase.

The renal tubules play an extremely important role in the reabsorption of HCO_3^- and secretion of protons (tubular acidification) and thus participate critically in the maintenance of acid–base balance. These processes are described in the section on carbonic anhydrase inhibitors.

PRINCIPLES OF DIURETIC ACTION

By definition, diuretics are drugs that increase the rate of urine flow; however, clinically useful diuretics also increase the rate of excretion of Na^+ (natriuresis) and of an accompanying anion, usually Cl^-. NaCl in the body is the major determinant of extracellular fluid volume, and most clinical applications of diuretics are directed toward reducing extracellular fluid volume by decreasing total-body NaCl content. A sustained imbalance between dietary Na^+ intake and Na^+ loss is incompatible with life. A sustained positive Na^+ balance would result in volume overload with pulmonary edema, and a sustained negative Na^+ balance would result in volume depletion and cardiovascular collapse. Although continued administration of a diuretic causes a sustained net deficit in total-body Na^+, the time course of natriuresis is finite because renal compensatory mechanisms bring Na^+ excretion in line with Na^+ intake, a phenomenon known as *diuretic braking*. These compensatory, or braking, mechanisms include activation of the sympathetic nervous system, activation of the renin–angiotensin–aldosterone axis, decreased arterial blood pressure (which reduces pressure natriuresis), hypertrophy of renal epithelial cells, increased expression of renal epithelial transporters, and perhaps alterations in natriuretic hormones such as atrial natriuretic peptide (Ellison, 1999).

Historically, the classification of diuretics was based on a mosaic of ideas such as site of action (loop diuretics), efficacy (high-ceiling diuretics), chemical structure (thiazide diuretics), similarity of action with other diuretics (thiazidelike diuretics), effects on potassium excretion (potassium-sparing diuretics), etc. However, since the mechanism of action of each of the major classes of diuretics is now well understood, a classification scheme based on mechanism of action is used in this chapter.

Diuretics not only alter the excretion of Na^+ but also may modify renal handling of other cations (*e.g.*, K^+, H^+, Ca^{2+}, and Mg^{2+}), anions (*e.g.*, Cl^-, HCO_3^-, and $H_2PO_4^-$), and uric acid. In addition, diuretics may alter renal hemodynamics indirectly. Table 28–1 gives a comparison of the general effects of the major classes of diuretics.

INHIBITORS OF CARBONIC ANHYDRASE

Acetazolamide (DIAMOX) is the prototype of a class of agents that have limited usefulness as diuretics but have played a major role in the development of fundamental concepts of renal physiology and pharmacology.

Chemistry. When sulfanilamide was introduced as a chemotherapeutic agent, metabolic acidosis was recognized as a side effect. This observation led to the demonstration that sulfanilamide is an inhibitor of carbonic anhydrase. Subsequently, an enormous number of sulfonamides were synthesized and tested for the ability to inhibit carbonic anhydrase; of these compounds, acetazolamide has been studied most extensively. Table 28–2 lists the chemical structures of the three carbonic anhydrase inhibitors currently available in the United States—acetazolamide, *dichlorphenamide* (DARANIDE), and

methazolamide (GLAUCTABS). The common molecular motif of available carbonic anhydrase inhibitors is an unsubstituted sulfonamide moiety.

Mechanism and Site of Action. Proximal tubular epithelial cells are richly endowed with the zinc metalloenzyme carbonic anhydrase, which is found in the luminal and basolateral membranes (type IV carbonic anhydrase, an enzyme tethered to the membrane by a glycosylphosphatidylinositol linkage), as well as in the cytoplasm (type II carbonic anhydrase). Carbonic anhydrase plays a key role in $NaHCO_3$ reabsorption and acid secretion.

In the proximal tubule, the free energy in the Na^+ gradient established by the basolateral Na^+ pump is used by a Na^+–H^+ antiporter [also referred to as a Na^+–H^+ exchanger (NHE)] in the luminal membrane to transport H^+ into the tubular lumen in exchange for Na^+ (Figure 28–5). In the lumen, H^+ reacts with filtered HCO_3^- to form H_2CO_3, which decomposes rapidly to CO_2 and water in the presence of carbonic anhydrase in the brush border. Normally, the reaction between CO_2 and water occurs slowly, but carbonic anhydrase reversibly accelerates this reaction several thousand times. CO_2 is lipophilic and rapidly diffuses across the luminal membrane into the epithelial cell, where it reacts with water to form H_2CO_3, a reaction catalyzed by cytoplasmic carbonic anhydrase. (The actual reaction catalyzed by carbonic anhydrase is $OH^- + CO_2 \rightarrow HCO_3^-$; however, $H_2O \rightarrow OH^- + H^+$ and $HCO_3^- + H^+ \rightarrow H_2CO_3$, so the net reaction is $H_2O + CO_2 \rightarrow H_2CO_3$.) Continued operation of the Na^+–H^+ antiporter maintains a low proton concentration in the cell, so H_2CO_3 ionizes spontaneously to form H^+ and HCO_3, creating an electrochemical gradient for HCO_3^- across the basolateral membrane. The electrochemical gradient for HCO_3^- is used by a Na^+–HCO_3^- symporter [also referred to as the Na^+–HCO_3^- cotransporter (NBC)] in the basolateral membrane to transport $NaHCO_3$ into the interstitial space. The net effect of this process is transport of $NaHCO_3$ from the tubular lumen to the interstitial space, followed by movement of water (isotonic reabsorption). Removal of water concentrates Cl^- in the tubular lumen, and consequently, Cl^- diffuses down its concentration gradient into the interstitium *via* the paracellular pathway.

Carbonic anhydrase inhibitors potently inhibit (IC_{50} for acetazolamide is 10 nM) both the membrane-bound and cytoplasmic forms of carbonic anhydrase, resulting in nearly complete abolition of $NaHCO_3$ reabsorption in the proximal tubule. Studies with a high-molecular-weight carbonic anhydrase inhibitor that inhibits only luminal enzyme because of limited cellular permeability indicate that inhibition of both the membrane-bound and cytoplasmic pools of carbonic anhydrase contributes to the diuret-

Table 28–1
*Excretory and Renal Hemodynamic Effects of Diuretics**

	CATIONS					ANIONS			URIC ACID		RENAL HEMODYNAMICS			
	Na$^+$	K$^+$	H$^{+\dagger}$	Ca^{2+}	Mg^{2+}	Cl$^-$	HCO$_3^-$	H$_2$PO$_4^-$	Acute	Chronic	RBF	GFR	FF	TGF
Inhibitors of carbonic anhydrase (primary site of action is proximal tubule)	+	++	−	NC	V	(+)	++	++	I	−	−	−	NC	+
Osmotic diuretics (primary site of action is loop of Henle)	++	+	I	+	++	+	+	+	+	I	+	NC	−	I
Inhibitors of Na$^+$–K$^+$–2Cl$^-$ symport (primary site of action is thick ascending limb)	++	++	+	++	++	++	+‡	+‡	+	−	V(+)	NC	V(−)	−
Inhibitors of Na$^+$–Cl$^-$ symport (primary site of action is distal convoluted tubule)	+	++	+	V(−)	V(+)	+	+‡	+‡	+	−	NC	V(−)	V(−)	NC
Inhibitors of renal epithelial sodium channels (primary site of action is late distal tubule and collecting duct)	+	−	−	−	−	+	(+)	NC	I	I	NC	NC	NC	NC
Antagonists of mineralocorticoid receptors (primary site of action is late distal tubule and collecting duct)	+	−	−	I	−	+	(+)	I	I	−	NC	NC	NC	NC

*Except for uric acid, changes are for acute effects of diuretics in the absence of significant volume depletion, which would trigger complex physiological adjustments; ++, +, (+), −, NC, V, V(+), V(−) and I indicate marked increase, mild to moderate increase, slight increase, decrease, no change, variable effect, variable increase, variable decrease, and insufficient data, respectively. For cations and anions, the indicated effects refer to absolute changes in fractional excretion. RBF, renal blood flow; GFR, glomerular filtration rate; FF, filtration fraction; TGF, tubuloglomerular feedback. †H$^+$, titratable acid and NH4$^+$. ‡In general, these effects are restricted to those individual agents that inhibit carbonic anhydrase. However, there are notable exceptions in which symport inhibitors increase bicarbonate and phosphate (*e.g.,* metolazone, bumetanide) (*see* Puschett and Winaver, 1992).

744

Table 28–2
Inhibitors of Carbonic Anhydrase

DRUG	STRUCTURE	RELATIVE POTENCY	ORAL AVAILABILITY	$T_{\frac{1}{2}}$ (HOURS)	ROUTE OF ELIMINATION
Acetazolamide (DIAMOX)	CH$_3$CONH—S—SO$_2$NH$_2$ / N—N	1	~100%	6–9	R
Dichlorphenamide (DARAMIDE)	SO$_2$NH$_2$ / Cl / Cl / SO$_2$NH$_2$	30	ID	ID	ID
Methazolamide (GLAUCTABS)	CH$_3$CON—S—SO$_2$NH$_2$ / N—N / H$_3$C	>1; <10	~100%	~14	~25%, ~75% M

Abbreviations: R, renal excretion of intact drug; M, metabolism; ID, insufficient data.

ic activity of carbonic anhydrase inhibitors. Because of the large excess of carbonic anhydrase in proximal tubules, a high percentage of enzyme activity must be inhibited before an effect on electrolyte excretion is observed. Although the proximal tubule is the major site of action of carbonic anhydrase inhibitors, carbonic anhydrase also is involved in secretion of titratable acid in the collecting duct system (a process that involves a proton pump); therefore, the collecting duct system is a secondary site of action for this class of drugs.

Effects on Urinary Excretion. Inhibition of carbonic anhydrase is associated with a rapid rise in urinary HCO$_3^-$ excretion to approximately 35% of filtered load. This, along with inhibition of titratable acid and NH$_4^+$ secretion in the collecting-duct system, results in an increase in urinary pH to approximately 8 and development of a metabolic acidosis. However, even with a high degree of inhibition of carbonic anhydrase, 65% of HCO$_3^-$ is rescued from excretion by poorly understood mechanisms that may involve carbonic anhydrase-independent HCO$_3^-$ reabsorption at downstream sites. Inhibition of the transport mechanism described in the preceding section results in increased delivery of Na$^+$ and Cl$^-$ to the loop of Henle, which has a large reabsorptive capacity and captures most of the Cl$^-$ and a portion of the Na$^+$. Thus only a small increase in Cl$^-$

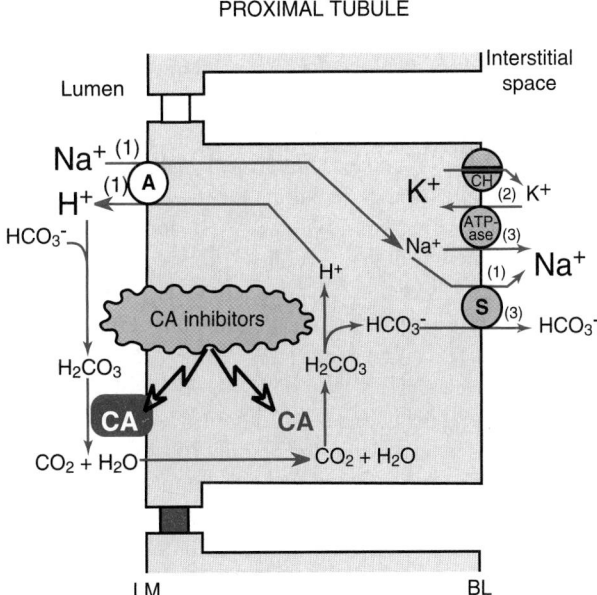

PROXIMAL TUBULE

Figure 28–5. *NaHCO$_3$ reabsorption in proximal tubule and mechanism of diuretic action of carbonic anhydrase inhibitors.* A, antiporter; S, symporter; CH, ion channel. (The actual reaction catalyzed by carbonic anhydrase is OH$^-$ + CO$_2$ → HCO$_3^-$; however, H$_2$O → OH$^-$ + H$^+$, and HCO$_3^-$ + H$^+$ → H$_2$CO$_3$, so the net reaction is H$_2$O + CO$_2$ → H$_2$CO$_3$.) Numbers in parentheses indicate stoichiometry. BL and LM indicate basolateral and luminal membranes, respectively.

excretion occurs, HCO_3^- being the major anion excreted along with the cations Na^+ and K^+. The fractional excretion of Na^+ may be as much as 5%, and the fractional excretion of K^+ can be as much as 70%. The increased excretion of K^+ is in part secondary to increased delivery of Na^+ to the distal nephron. The mechanism by which increased distal delivery of Na^+ enhances K^+ excretion is described in the section on inhibitors of sodium channels. Other mechanisms contributing to enhanced K^+ excretion include flow-dependent enhancement of K^+ secretion by the collecting duct, nonosmotic vasopressin release, and activation of the renin–angiotensin–aldosterone axis (Wilcox, 1999). Carbonic anhydrase inhibitors increase phosphate excretion (mechanism unknown) but have little or no effect on the excretion of Ca^{2+} or Mg^{2+}. The effects of carbonic anhydrase inhibitors on renal excretion are self-limiting probably because the resulting metabolic acidosis decreases the filtered load of HCO_3^- to the point that the uncatalyzed reaction between CO_2 and water is sufficient to achieve HCO_3^- reabsorption.

Effects on Renal Hemodynamics.
By inhibiting proximal reabsorption, carbonic anhydrase inhibitors increase delivery of solutes to the macula densa. This triggers TGF, which increases afferent arteriolar resistance and reduces renal blood flow (RBF) and glomerular filtration rate (GFR).

Other Actions.
Carbonic anhydrase is present in a number of extrarenal tissues, including the eye, gastric mucosa, pancreas, central nervous system (CNS), and erythrocytes. Carbonic anhydrase in the ciliary processes of the eye mediates the formation of large amounts of HCO_3^- in aqueous humor. Inhibition of carbonic anhydrase decreases the rate of formation of aqueous humor and consequently reduces intraocular pressure (IOP). Acetazolamide frequently causes paresthesias and somnolence, suggesting an action of carbonic anhydrase inhibitors in the CNS. The efficacy of acetazolamide in epilepsy is due in part to the production of metabolic acidosis; however, direct actions of acetazolamide in the CNS also contribute to its anticonvulsant action. Owing to interference with carbonic anhydrase activity in erythrocytes, carbonic anhydrase inhibitors increase CO_2 levels in peripheral tissues and decrease CO_2 levels in expired gas. Large doses of carbonic anhydrase inhibitors reduce gastric acid secretion, but this has no therapeutic applications. Acetazolamide causes vasodilation in human beings by opening vascular Ca^{2+}-activated K^+ channels (Pickkers *et al.*, 2001); however, the clinical significance of this effect is unclear.

Absorption and Elimination.
The oral bioavailability, plasma half-life, and route of elimination of the three currently available carbonic anhydrase inhibitors are listed in Table 28–2. Carbonic anhydrase inhibitors are avidly bound by carbonic anhydrase, and accordingly, tissues rich in this enzyme will have higher concentrations of carbonic anhydrase inhibitors following systemic administration.

Toxicity, Adverse Effects, Contraindications, Drug Interactions.
Serious toxic reactions to carbonic anhydrase inhibitors are infrequent; however, these drugs are sulfonamide derivatives and, like other sulfonamides, may cause bone marrow depression, skin toxicity, sulfonamidelike renal lesions, and allergic reactions in patients hypersensitive to sulfonamides (*see* Chapter 43). With large doses, many patients exhibit drowsiness and paresthesias. Most adverse effects, contraindications, and drug interactions are secondary to urinary alkalinization or metabolic acidosis, including (1) diversion of ammonia of renal origin from urine into the systemic circulation, a process that may induce or worsen hepatic encephalopathy (the drugs are contraindicated in patients with hepatic cirrhosis); (2) calculus formation and ureteral colic owing to precipitation of calcium phosphate salts in an alkaline urine; (3) worsening of metabolic or respiratory acidosis (the drugs are contraindicated in patients with hyperchloremic acidosis or severe chronic obstructive pulmonary disease); and (4) reduction of the urinary excretion rate of weak organic bases.

Therapeutic Uses.
Although *acetazolamide* is used for treatment of edema, the efficacy of carbonic anhydrase inhibitors as single agents is low, and carbonic anhydrase inhibitors are not employed widely in this regard. However, studies by Knauf and Mutschler (1997) indicate that the combination of acetazolamide with diuretics that block Na^+ reabsorption at more distal sites in the nephron causes a marked natriuretic response in patients with low basal fractional excretion of Na^+ (<0.2%) who are resistant to diuretic monotherapy. Even so, the long-term usefulness of carbonic anhydrase inhibitors often is compromised by the development of metabolic acidosis.

The major indication for carbonic anhydrase inhibitors is open-angle glaucoma. Carbonic anhydrase inhibitors also may be employed for secondary glaucoma and preoperatively in acute angle-closure glaucoma to lower IOP before surgery (*see* Chapter 63). Acetazolamide also is used for the treatment of epilepsy (*see* Chapter 19). The rapid development of tolerance, however, may limit the usefulness of carbonic anhydrase inhibitors for epilepsy. Acetazolamide may provide symptomatic relief

Table 28–3
Osmotic Diuretics

DRUG	STRUCTURE	ORAL AVAILABILITY	$T_{\frac{1}{2}}$ (HOURS)	ROUTE OF ELIMINATION
Glycerin (OSMOGLYN)	HO⌄OH / OH	Orally active	0.5–0.75	~80% M ~20% U
Isosorbide (ISMOTIC)	HO H H O / O H H OH	Orally active	5–9.5	R
Mannitol (OSMITROL)	OH OH OH OH / OH OH	Negligible	0.25–1.7*	~80% R ~20% M + B
Urea (UREAPHIL)	O / H_2N NH_2	Negligible	ID	R

*In renal failure, 6–36. *Abbreviations:* R, renal excretion of intact drug; M, metabolism; B, excretion of intact drug into bile; U, unknown pathway of elimination; ID, insufficient data.

in patients with altitude sickness; however, it is more appropriate to give acetazolamide as a prophylactic measure (Coote, 1991). Acetazolamide also is useful in patients with familial periodic paralysis (Links *et al.*, 1988). The mechanism for the beneficial effects of acetazolamide in altitude sickness and familial periodic paralysis is not clear, but it may be related to the induction of a metabolic acidosis. Finally, carbonic anhydrase inhibitors can be useful for correcting a metabolic alkalosis, especially an alkalosis caused by diuretic-induced increases in H⁺ excretion.

OSMOTIC DIURETICS

Osmotic diuretics are agents that are freely filtered at the glomerulus, undergo limited reabsorption by the renal tubule, and are relatively inert pharmacologically. Osmotic diuretics are administered in large enough doses to increase significantly the osmolality of plasma and tubular fluid. Table 28–3 gives the molecular structures of the four currently available osmotic diuretics— *glycerin* (OSMOGLYN), *isosorbide* (ISMOTIC), *mannitol* (OSMITROL), and *urea* (UREAPHIL).

Mechanism and Site of Action. For many years it was thought that osmotic diuretics act primarily in the proximal tubule. By acting as nonreabsorbable solutes, it was reasoned that osmotic diuretics limit the osmosis of water into the interstitial space and thereby reduce luminal Na⁺ concentration to the point that net Na⁺ reabsorption ceases. Although early micropuncture studies supported this concept, subsequent studies suggested that this mechanism, while operative, may be of only secondary importance and that the major site of action of osmotic diuretics is the loop of Henle.

By extracting water from intracellular compartments, osmotic diuretics expand the extracellular fluid volume, decrease blood viscosity, and inhibit renin release. These effects increase RBF, and the increase in renal medullary blood flow removes NaCl and urea from the renal medulla, thus reducing medullary tonicity. Under some circumstances, prostaglandins may contribute to the renal vasodilation and medullary washout induced by osmotic diuretics. A reduction in medullary tonicity causes a decrease in the extraction of water from the DTL, which, in turn, limits the concentration of NaCl in the tubular fluid entering the ATL. This latter effect diminishes the passive reabsorption of NaCl in the ATL. In addition, the marked ability of osmotic diuretics to inhibit reabsorption of Mg^{2+}, a cation that is reabsorbed mainly in the thick ascending limb, suggests that osmotic diuretics also interfere with transport processes in the thick ascending limb. The mechanism of this effect is unknown.

In summary, osmotic diuretics act both in the proximal tubule and the loop of Henle, with the latter being the primary site of action. Also, osmotic diuretics probably act by an osmotic effect in the tubules and by reducing medullary tonicity.

Effects on Urinary Excretion. Osmotic diuretics increase the urinary excretion of nearly all electrolytes, including Na^+, K^+, Ca^{2+}, Mg^{2+}, Cl^-, HCO_3^-, and phosphate.

Effects on Renal Hemodynamics. Osmotic diuretics increase RBF by a variety of mechanisms. Osmotic diuretics dilate the afferent arteriole, which increases P_{GC}, and dilute the plasma, which decreases Π_{GC}. These effects would increase GFR were it not for the fact that osmotic diuretics also increase P_T. In general, superficial SNGFR is increased, but total GFR is little changed.

Absorption and Elimination. The oral bioavailability, plasma half-life, and route of elimination of the four currently available osmotic diuretics are listed in Table 28–3. Glycerin and isosorbide can be given orally, whereas mannitol and urea must be administered intravenously.

Toxicity, Adverse Effects, Contraindications, Drug Interactions. Osmotic diuretics are distributed in the extracellular fluid and contribute to the extracellular osmolality. Thus water is extracted from intracellular compartments, and the extracellular fluid volume becomes expanded. In patients with heart failure or pulmonary congestion, this may cause frank pulmonary edema. Extraction of water also causes hyponatremia, which may explain the common adverse effects, including headache, nausea, and vomiting. On the other hand, loss of water in excess of electrolytes can cause hypernatremia and dehydration. In general, osmotic diuretics are contraindicated in patients who are anuric owing to severe renal disease or who are unresponsive to test doses of the drugs. Urea may cause thrombosis or pain if extravasation occurs, and it should not be administered to patients with impaired liver function because of the risk of elevation of blood ammonia levels. Both mannitol and urea are contraindicated in patients with active cranial bleeding. Glycerin is metabolized and can cause hyperglycemia.

Therapeutic Uses. A rapid decrease in GFR, *i.e.*, acute renal failure (ARF), is a serious medical condition that occurs in 5% of hospitalized patients and is associated with a significant mortality rate. ARF can be caused by diverse conditions both extrinsic (prerenal and postrenal failure) and intrinsic to the kidney. Acute tubular necrosis (ATN), *i.e.*, damage to tubular epithelial cells, accounts for most cases of intrinsic ARF. In animal models, mannitol is effective in attenuating the reduction in GFR associated with ATN when administered before the ischemic insult or offending nephrotoxin. The renal protection afforded by mannitol may be due to removal of obstructing tubular casts, dilution of nephrotoxic substances in the tubular fluid, and/or reduction of swelling of tubular elements *via* osmotic extraction of water. Although prophylactic mannitol is effective in animal models of ATN, the clinical efficacy of mannitol is less well established. Most published clinical studies have been uncontrolled, and controlled studies have not shown a benefit over hydration *per se* (*see* Kellum, 1998). In patients with mild to moderate renal insufficiency, hydration with 0.45% sodium chloride is as good as or better than either mannitol or furosemide in protection against decreases in GFR induced by radiocontrast agents (Soloman *et al.*, 1994). Studies of prophylactic mannitol indicate effectiveness in jaundiced patients undergoing surgery. However, in vascular and open-heart surgery, prophylactic mannitol maintains urine flow but not GFR. In established ATN, mannitol will increase urine volume in some patients, and patients converted from oliguric to nonoliguric ATN appear to recover more rapidly and require less dialysis compared with patients who do not respond to mannitol (Levinsky and Bernard, 1988). It is not clear whether these benefits are due to the diuretic or whether "responders" have lesser degrees of renal damage from the outset compared with "nonresponders." Repeated administration of mannitol to nonresponders is not recommended, and nowadays, loop diuretics are used more frequently to convert oliguric to nonoliguric ATN.

Another use for mannitol and urea is in the treatment of dialysis disequilibrium syndrome. Too rapid a removal of solutes from the extracellular fluid by hemodialysis or peritoneal dialysis results in a reduction in the osmolality of the extracellular fluid. Consequently, water moves from the extracellular compartment into the intracellular compartment, causing hypotension and CNS symptoms (*i.e.*, headache, nausea, muscle cramps, restlessness, CNS depression, and convulsions). Osmotic diuretics increase the osmolality of the extracellular fluid compartment and thereby shift water back into the extracellular compartment.

By increasing the osmotic pressure of the plasma, osmotic diuretics extract water from the eye and brain. All four osmotic diuretics are used to control IOP during acute attacks of glaucoma and for short-term reductions in IOP both preoperatively and postoperatively in patients who require ocular surgery. Also, mannitol and urea are used to reduce cerebral edema and brain mass before and after neurosurgery.

INHIBITORS OF NA$^+$–K$^+$–2CL$^-$ SYMPORT (LOOP DIURETICS, HIGH-CEILING DIURETICS)

Drugs in this group of diuretics inhibit the activity of the Na$^+$–K$^+$–2Cl$^-$ symporter in the thick ascending limb of the loop of Henle; hence these diuretics also are referred to as *loop diuretics*. Although the proximal tubule reabsorbs approximately 65% of the filtered Na$^+$, diuretics acting only in the proximal tubule have limited efficacy because the thick ascending limb has a great reabsorptive capacity and reabsorbs most of the rejectate from the proximal tubule. Diuretics acting predominantly at sites past the thick ascending limb also have limited efficacy because only a small percentage of the filtered Na$^+$ load reaches these more distal sites. In contrast, inhibitors of Na$^+$–K$^+$–2Cl$^-$ symport in the thick ascending limb are highly efficacious, and for this reason, they sometimes are called *high-ceiling diuretics*. The efficacy of inhibitors of Na$^+$–K$^+$–2Cl$^-$ symport in the thick ascending limb of the loop of Henle is due to a combination of two factors: (1) Approximately 25% of the filtered Na$^+$ load normally is reabsorbed by the thick ascending limb, and (2) nephron segments past the thick ascending limb do not possess the reabsorptive capacity to rescue the flood of rejectate exiting the thick ascending limb.

Chemistry. Inhibitors of Na$^+$–K$^+$–2Cl$^-$ symport are a chemically diverse group (Table 28–4). Only *furosemide* (LASIX), *bumetanide* (BUMEX), *ethacrynic acid* (EDECRIN), and *torsemide* (DEMADEX) are available currently in the United States. Furosemide and bumetanide contain a sulfonamide moiety. Ethacrynic acid is a phenoxyacetic acid derivative and torsemide is a sulfonylurea.

Mechanism and Site of Action. Inhibitors of Na$^+$–K$^+$–2Cl$^-$ symport act primarily in the thick ascending limb. Micropuncture of the DCT demonstrates that loop diuretics increase the delivery of solutes out of the loop of Henle. Also, *in situ* microperfusion of the loop of Henle and *in vitro* microperfusion of the CTAL indicate inhibition of transport by low concentrations of furosemide in the perfusate. Some inhibitors of Na$^+$–K$^+$–2Cl$^-$ symport may have additional effects in the proximal tubule; however, the significance of these effects is unclear.

It was thought initially that Cl$^-$ was transported by a primary active electrogenic transporter in the luminal membrane independent of Na$^+$. Discovery of furosemide-sensitive Na$^+$–K$^+$–2Cl$^-$ symport in other tissues prompted a more careful investigation of the Na$^+$ dependence of Cl$^-$ transport in the isolated perfused rabbit CTAL. Scrupulous removal of Na$^+$ from the luminal perfusate demonstrated the dependence of Cl$^-$ transport on Na$^+$.

It is now well accepted that flux of Na$^+$, K$^+$, and Cl$^-$ from the lumen into the epithelial cells in the thick ascending limb is mediated by a Na$^+$–K$^+$–2Cl$^-$ symporter (Hebert, 1999) (Figure 28–6). This symporter captures the free energy in the Na$^+$ electrochemical gradient established by the basolateral Na$^+$ pump and provides for "uphill" transport of K$^+$ and Cl$^-$ into the cell. K$^+$ channels in the luminal membrane (called *ROMK*) provide a conductive pathway for the apical recycling of this cation, and basolateral Cl$^-$ channels (called *CLC-Kb*) provide a basolateral exit mechanism for Cl$^-$. The luminal membranes of epithelial cells in the thick ascending limb have a large conductive pathway (channels) for K$^+$; therefore, the apical membrane voltage is determined by the equilibrium potential for K$^+$ (E_K) and is hyperpolarized. In contrast, the basolateral membrane has a large conductive pathway (channels) for Cl$^-$, so the basolateral membrane voltage is less negative than E_K; *i.e.*, conductance for Cl$^-$ depolarizes the basolateral membrane. Hyperpolarization of the luminal membrane and depolarization of the basolateral membrane result in a transepithelial potential difference of approximately 10 mV, with the lumen positive with respect to the interstitial space. This lumen-positive potential difference repels cations (Na$^+$, Ca^{2+}, and Mg^{2+}) and thereby provides an important driving force for the paracellular flux of these cations into the interstitial space.

As the name implies, inhibitors of Na$^+$–K$^+$–2Cl$^-$ symport bind to the Na$^+$–K$^+$–2Cl$^-$ symporter in the thick ascending limb and block its function, bringing salt transport in this segment of the nephron to a virtual standstill. The molecular mechanism by which this class of drugs blocks the Na$^+$–K$^+$–2Cl$^-$ symporter is unknown, but evidence suggests that these drugs attach to the Cl$^-$-binding site (Hannafin *et al.*, 1983) located in the symporter's transmembrane domain (Isenring and Forbush, 1997). Inhibitors of Na$^+$–K$^+$–2Cl$^-$ symport also inhibit Ca^{2+} and Mg^{2+} reabsorption in the thick ascending limb by abolishing the transepithelial potential difference that is the dominant driving force for reabsorption of these cations.

Na$^+$–K$^+$–2Cl$^-$ symporters are an important family of transport molecules found in many secretory and absorbing epithelia. The rectal gland of the dogfish shark is a particularly rich source of the protein,

Table 28–4
Inhibitors of Na⁺–K⁺–2Cl⁻ Symport (Loop Diuretics, High-Ceiling Diuretics)

DRUG	STRUCTURE	RELATIVE POTENCY	ORAL AVAILABILITY	$T_{\frac{1}{2}}$ (HOURS)	ROUTE OF ELIMINATION
Furosemide (LASIX)		1	~60%	~1.5	~65% R, ~35% M‡
Bumetanide (BUMEX)		40	~80%	~0.8	~62% R, ~38% M
Ethacrynic acid (EDECRIN)		0.7	~100%	~1	~67% R, ~33% M
Torsemide (DEMADEX)		3	~80%	~3.5	~20% R, ~80% M
Axosemide*		1	~12%	~2.5	~27% R, 63% M
Piretanide*		3	~80%	0.6–1.5	~50% R, ~50% M
Tripamide*		ID	ID	ID	ID

*Not available in the United States. ‡For furosemide, metabolism occurs predominantly in the kidney. *Abbreviations*: R, renal excretion of intact drug; M, metabolism; ID, insufficient data.

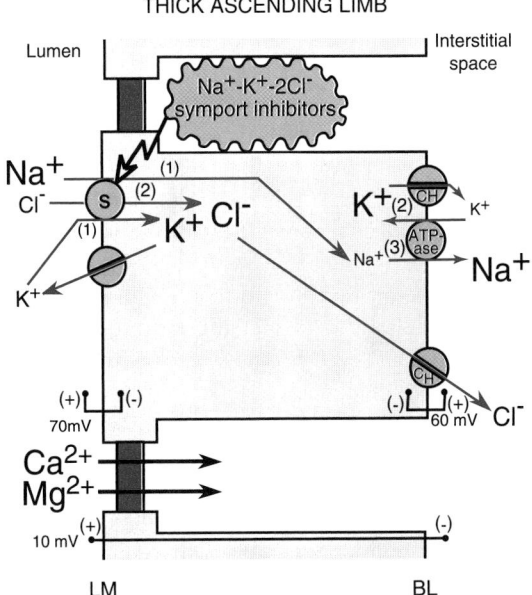

THICK ASCENDING LIMB

Figure 28–6. NaCl reabsorption in thick ascending limb and mechanism of diuretic action of Na⁺–K⁺–2Cl⁻ symport inhibitors. S, symporter; CH, ion channel. Numbers in parentheses indicate stoichiometry. Designated voltages are the potential differences across the indicated membrane or cell. The mechanisms illustrated here apply to the medullary, cortical, and postmacular segments of the thick ascending limb. BL and LM indicate basolateral and luminal membranes, respectively.

and a cDNA encoding a Na⁺–K⁺–2Cl⁻ symporter was isolated from a cDNA library obtained from the dogfish shark rectal gland by screening with antibodies to the shark symporter (Xu *et al.*, 1994). Molecular cloning revealed a deduced amino acid sequence of 1191 residues containing 12 putative membrane-spanning domains flanked by long N and C termini in the cytoplasm. Expression of this protein resulted in Na⁺–K⁺–2Cl⁻ symport that was sensitive to bumetanide. The shark rectal gland Na⁺–K⁺–2Cl⁻ symporter cDNA was used subsequently to screen a human colonic cDNA library, and this provided Na⁺–K⁺–2Cl⁻ symporter cDNA probes from this tissue. These latter probes were used to screen rabbit renal cortical and renal medullary libraries, which allowed cloning of the rabbit renal Na⁺–K⁺–2Cl⁻ symporter (Payne and Forbush, 1994). This symporter is 1099 amino acids in length, is 61% identical to the dogfish shark secretory Na⁺–K⁺–2Cl⁻ symporter, has 12 predicted transmembrane helices, and contains large N- and C-terminal cytoplasmic regions. Subsequent studies demonstrated that Na⁺–K⁺–2Cl⁻ symporters are of two varieties (*see* Kaplan *et al.*, 1996). The "absorptive" symporter (called *ENCC2, NKCC2,* or *BSC1*) is expressed only in the kidney, is localized to the apical membrane and subapical intracellular vesicles of the thick ascending limb, and is regulated by cyclic AMP/protein kinase A (Obermüller *et al.*, 1996; Kaplan *et al.*, 1996; Nielsen *et al.*, 1998; Plata *et al.*, 1999). At least six different isoforms of the absorptives symporter are generated by alternative mRNA splicing (Mount *et al.*, 1999), and alternative splicing of the absorptive symporter determines the dependency of transport on K⁺ (Plata *et al.*, 2001) The "secretory" symporter (called *ENCC3, NKCC1,* or *BSC2*) is a "housekeeping" protein that is expressed wide-

ly and, in epithelial cells, is localized to the basolateral membrane. The affinity of loop diuretics for the secretory symporter is somewhat less than for the absorptive symporter (*e.g.*, fourfold difference for bumetanide). A model of Na⁺–K⁺–2Cl⁻ symport has been proposed based on ordered binding of ions to the symporter (Lytle *et al.*, 1998). Mutations in the genes coding for the absorptive Na⁺–K⁺–2Cl⁻ symporter, the apical K⁺ channel, or the basolateral Cl⁻ channel are one cause of Bartter's syndrome (inherited hypokalemic alkalosis with salt wasting and hypotension) (*see* Simon and Lifton, 1998).

Effects on Urinary Excretion. Owing to blockade of the Na⁺–K⁺–2Cl⁻ symporter, loop diuretics increase in the urinary excretion of Na⁺ and Cl⁻ profoundly (*i.e.*, up to 25% of the filtered load of Na⁺). Abolition of the transepithelial potential difference also results in marked increases in the excretion of Ca²⁺ and Mg²⁺. Some (*e.g.*, furosemide) but not all (*e.g.*, bumetanide) sulfonamide-based loop diuretics have weak carbonic anhydrase–inhibiting activity. Drugs with carbonic anhydrase–inhibiting activity increase the urinary excretion of HCO₃⁻ and phosphate. The mechanism by which inhibition of carbonic anhydrase increases phosphate excretion is not known. All inhibitors of Na⁺–K⁺–2Cl⁻ symport increase the urinary excretion of K⁺ and titratable acid. This effect is due in part to increased delivery of Na⁺ to the distal tubule. The mechanism by which increased distal delivery of Na⁺ enhances excretion of K⁺ and H⁺ is discussed in the section on inhibitors of Na⁺ channels. Other mechanisms contributing to enhanced K⁺ and H⁺ excretion include flow-dependent enhancement of ion secretion by the collecting duct, nonosmotic vasopressin release, and activation of the renin–angiotensin–aldosterone axis (Wilcox, 1999). Acutely, loop diuretics increase the excretion of uric acid, whereas chronic administration of these drugs results in reduced excretion of uric acid. The chronic effects of loop diuretics on uric acid excretion may be due to enhanced transport in the proximal tubule secondary to volume depletion, leading to increased uric acid reabsorption, or to competition between the diuretic and uric acid for the organic acid secretory mechanism in the proximal tubule, leading to reduced uric acid secretion.

By blocking active NaCl reabsorption in the thick ascending limb, inhibitors of Na⁺–K⁺–2Cl⁻ symport interfere with a critical step in the mechanism that produces a hypertonic medullary interstitium. Therefore, loop diuretics block the kidney's ability to concentrate urine during hydropenia. Also, since the thick ascending limb is part of the diluting segment, inhibitors of Na⁺–K⁺–2Cl⁻ symport markedly impair the kidney's ability to excrete a dilute urine during water diuresis.

Effects on Renal Hemodynamics. If volume depletion is prevented by replacing fluid losses, inhibitors of Na⁺–

K^+–$2Cl^-$ symport generally increase total RBF and redistribute RBF to the midcortex. However, the effects on RBF are variable. The mechanism of the increase in RBF is not known but may involve prostaglandins. Nonsteroidal antiinflammatory drugs (NSAIDs) attenuate the diuretic response to loop diuretics in part by preventing prostaglandin-mediated increases in RBF. Loop diuretics block TGF by inhibiting salt transport into the macula densa so that the macula densa no longer can detect NaCl concentrations in the tubular fluid. Therefore, unlike carbonic anhydrase inhibitors, loop diuretics do not decrease GFR by activating TGF. Loop diuretics are powerful stimulators of renin release. This effect is due to interference with NaCl transport by the macula densa and, if volume depletion occurs, to reflex activation of the sympathetic nervous system and to stimulation of the intrarenal baroreceptor mechanism. Prostaglandins, particularly prostacyclin, may play an important role in mediating the renin-release response to loop diuretics.

Other Actions. Loop diuretics may cause direct vascular effects (Dormans *et al.*, 1996). Loop diuretics, particularly furosemide, acutely increase systemic venous capacitance and thereby decrease left ventricular filling pressure. This effect, which may be mediated by prostaglandins and requires intact kidneys, benefits patients with pulmonary edema even before diuresis ensues. Furosemide and ethacrynic acid can inhibit Na^+,K^+–ATPase, glycolysis, mitochondrial respiration, the microsomal Ca^{2+} pump, adenylyl cyclase, phosphodiesterase, and prostaglandin dehydrogenase; however, these effects do not have therapeutic implications. *In vitro,* high doses of inhibitors of Na^+–K^+–$2Cl^-$ symport can inhibit electrolyte transport in many tissues. Only in the inner ear, where alterations in the electrolyte composition of endolymph may contribute to drug-induced ototoxicity, is this effect important clinically.

Absorption and Elimination. The oral bioavailabilities, plasma half-lives, and routes of elimination of inhibitors of Na^+–K^+–$2Cl^-$ symport are listed in Table 28–4. Because furosemide, bumetanide, ethacrynic acid, and torsemide are bound extensively to plasma proteins, delivery of these drugs to the tubules by filtration is limited. However, they are secreted efficiently by the organic acid transport system in the proximal tubule and thereby gain access to their binding sites on the Na^+–K^+–$2Cl^-$ symport in the luminal membrane of the thick ascending limb. Probenecid shifts the plasma concentration–response curve to furosemide to the right by competitively inhibiting furosemide secretion by the organic acid transport system (Brater, 1983).

Approximately 65% of furosemide is excreted unchanged in the urine, and the remainder is conjugated to glucuronic acid in the kidney. Accordingly, in patients with renal, but not liver, disease, the elimination half-life of furosemide is prolonged. In contrast, bumetanide and torsemide have significant hepatic metabolism, so the elimination half-lives of these loop diuretics are prolonged by liver, but not renal, disease (Shankar and Brater, 2003).

Although the average oral availability of furosemide is approximately 60%, oral availability of furosemide varies from 10% to 100%. In contrast, oral availabilities of bumetanide and torsemide are reliably high. Heart failure patients have fewer hospitalizations and better quality of life with torsemide than with furosemide perhaps because of the more reliable absorption of torsemide (Shankar and Brater, 2003).

As a class, loop diuretics have short elimination half-lives, and prolonged-release preparations are not available. Consequently, often the dosing interval is too short to maintain adequate levels of loop diuretics in the tubular lumen. Note that torsemide has a longer $t_{\frac{1}{2}}$ than other agents available in the United States (Table 28–4). As the concentration of loop diuretic in the tubular lumen declines, nephrons begin to avidly reabsorb Na^+, which often nullifies the overall effect of the loop diuretic on total-body Na^+. This phenomenon of "postdiuretic Na^+ retention" can be overcome by restricting dietary Na^+ intake or by more frequent administration of the loop diuretic (Ellison, 1999).

Toxicity, Adverse Effects, Contraindications, Drug Interactions. Adverse effects unrelated to the diuretic efficacy are rare, and most adverse effects are due to abnormalities of fluid and electrolyte balance. Overzealous use of loop diuretics can cause serious depletion of total-body Na^+. This may be manifest as hyponatremia and/or extracellular fluid volume depletion associated with hypotension, reduced GFR, circulatory collapse, thromboembolic episodes, and in patients with liver disease, hepatic encephalopathy. Increased delivery of Na^+ to the distal tubule, particularly when combined with activation of the renin–angiotensin system, leads to increased urinary excretion of K^+ and H^+, causing a hypochloremic alkalosis. If dietary K^+ intake is not sufficient, hypokalemia may develop, and this may induce cardiac arrhythmias, particularly in patients taking cardiac glycosides. Increased Mg^{2+} and Ca^{2+} excretion may result in hypomagnesemia (a risk factor for cardiac arrhythmias) and hypocalcemia (rarely leading to tetany). Recent evidence suggests that loop diuretics should be avoided in postmenopausal osteopenic women, in whom increased Ca^{2+} excretion may have deleterious effects on bone metabolism (Rejnmark *et al.*, 2003).

Loop diuretics can cause ototoxicity that manifests as tinnitus, hearing impairment, deafness, vertigo, and a sense of fullness in the ears. Hearing impairment and deafness are usually, but not always, reversible. Ototoxicity occurs most frequently with rapid intravenous administration and least frequently with oral administration. Ethacrynic acid appears to induce ototoxicity more often than do other loop diuretics and should be used only in patients who cannot tolerate the other loop diuretics. Loop diuretics also can cause hyperuricemia (occasionally leading to gout) and hyperglycemia (infrequently precipitating diabetes mellitus) and can increase plasma levels of low-density lipoprotein (LDL) cholesterol and triglycerides while decreasing plasma levels of high-density lipoprotein (HDL) cholesterol. Other adverse effects include skin rashes, photosensitivity, paresthesias, bone marrow depression, and gastrointestinal disturbances.

Contraindications to the use of loop diuretics include severe Na^+ and volume depletion, hypersensitivity to sulfonamides (for sulfonamide-based loop diuretics), and anuria unresponsive to a trial dose of loop diuretic.

Drug interactions may occur when loop diuretics are coadministered with (1) aminoglycosides (synergism of ototoxicity caused by both drugs), (2) anticoagulants (increased anticoagulant activity), (3) digitalis glycosides (increased digitalis-induced arrhythmias), (4) lithium (increased plasma levels of lithium), (5) propranolol (increased plasma levels of propranolol), (6) sulfonylureas (hyperglycemia), (7) cisplatin (increased risk of diuretic-induced ototoxicity), (8) NSAIDs (blunted diuretic response and salicylate toxicity when given with high doses of salicylates), (9) probenecid (blunted diuretic response), (10) thiazide diuretics (synergism of diuretic activity of both drugs leading to profound diuresis), and (11) amphotericin B (increased potential for nephrotoxicity and toxicity and intensification of electrolyte imbalance).

Therapeutic Uses. A major use of loop diuretics is in the treatment of acute pulmonary edema. A rapid increase in venous capacitance in conjunction with a brisk natriuresis reduces left ventricular filling pressures and thereby rapidly relieves pulmonary edema. Loop diuretics also are used widely for the treatment of chronic congestive heart failure when diminution of extracellular fluid volume is desirable to minimize venous and pulmonary congestion (*see* Chapter 33). In this regard, a meta-analysis of randomized clinical trials demonstrates that diuretics cause a significant reduction in mortality and the risk of worsening heart failure, as well as an improvement in exercise capacity (Faris *et al.*, 2002).

Diuretics are used widely for the treatment of hypertension (*see* Chapter 32), and controlled clinical trials demonstrating reduced morbidity and mortality have been conducted with Na^+–Cl^- symport (thiazides and thiazidelike diuretics) but not Na^+–K^+–$2Cl^-$ symport inhibitors. Nonetheless, Na^+–K^+–$2Cl^-$ symport inhibitors appear to lower blood pressure as effectively as Na^+–Cl^- symport inhibitors while causing smaller perturbations in the lipid profile (van der Heijden *et al.*, 1998). However, the short elimination half-lives of loop diuretics render them less useful for hypertension than thiazide-type diuretics. The edema of nephrotic syndrome often is refractory to other classes of diuretics, and loop diuretics often are the only drugs capable of reducing the massive edema associated with this renal disease. Loop diuretics also are employed in the treatment of edema and ascites of liver cirrhosis; however, care must be taken not to induce encephalopathy or hepatorenal syndrome. In patients with a drug overdose, loop diuretics can be used to induce a forced diuresis to facilitate more rapid renal elimination of the offending drug. Loop diuretics, combined with isotonic saline administration to prevent volume depletion, are used to treat hypercalcemia. Loop diuretics interfere with the kidney's capacity to produce a concentrated urine. Consequently, loop diuretics combined with hypertonic saline are useful for the treatment of life-threatening hyponatremia. Loop diuretics also are used to treat edema associated with chronic renal insufficiency. However, animal studies have demonstrated that loop diuretics increase P_{GC} by activating the renin–angiotensin system, an effect that could accelerate renal injury (Lane *et al.*, 1998). Most patients with ARF receive a trial dose of a loop diuretic in an attempt to convert oliguric ARF to nonoliguric ARF. However, there is no evidence that loop diuretics prevent ATN or improve outcome in patients with ARF (Kellum, 1998).

INHIBITORS OF NA$^+$–CL$^-$ SYMPORT (THIAZIDE AND THIAZIDELIKE DIURETICS)

The benzothiadiazides were synthesized in an effort to enhance the potency of inhibitors of carbonic anhydrase. However, unlike carbonic anhydrase inhibitors, which primarily increase $NaHCO_3$ excretion, benzothiadiazides were found predominantly to increase NaCl excretion, an effect shown to be independent of carbonic anhydrase inhibition.

Chemistry. Inhibitors of Na^+–Cl^- symport are sulfonamides (Table 28–5), and many are analogues of 1,2,4-benzothiadiazine-1,1-dioxide. Because the original inhibitors of Na^+–Cl^- symport were benzothiadi-

Table 28–5
Inhibitors of Na⁺–K⁺ Symport (Thiazide and Thiazidelike Diuretics)

DRUG	STRUCTURE	RELATIVE POTENCY	ORAL AVAILABILITY	$T_{\frac{1}{2}}$ (HOURS)	ROUTE OF ELIMINATION
Bendroflumethiazide (NATURETIN)	$R_2 = H, R_3 = CH_2$ ⟨phenyl⟩, $R_6 = CF_3$	10	~100%	3–3.9	~30% R, ~70% M
Chlorothiazide (DIURIL)	$R_2 = H, R_3 = H, R_6 = Cl$ (Unsaturated between C3 and N4)	0.1	9–56% (dose-dependent)	~1.5	R
Hydrochlorothiazide (HYDRODIURIL)	$R_2 = H, R_3 = H, R_6 = Cl$	1	~70%	~2.5	R
Hydroflumethiazide (SALURON)	$R_2 = H, R_3 = H, R_6 = CF_3$	1	~50%	~17	40–80% R, 20–60% M
Methyclothiazide (ENDURON)	$R_2 = CH_3, R_3 = CH_2Cl, R_6 = Cl$	10	ID	ID	M
Polythiazide (RENESE)	$R_2 = CH_3, R_3 = CH_2SCH_2CF_3, R_6 = Cl$	25	~100%	~25	~25% R, ~75% U
Trichlormethiazide (NAQUA)	$R_2 = H, R_3 = CHCl_2, R_6 = Cl$	25	ID	2.3–7.3	R
Chlorthalidone (HYGROTON)		1	~65%	~47	~65% R, ~10% B, ~25% U
Indapamide (LOZOL)		20	~93%	~14	M
Metolazone (MYKROX, ZAROXOLYN)		10	~65%	ID	~80% R, ~10% B, ~10% M
Quinethazone (HYDROMOX)		1	ID	ID	ID

Abbreviations: R, renal excretion of intact drug; M, metabolism; B, excretion of intact drug into bile; U, unknown pathway of elimination; ID, insufficient data.

azine derivatives, this class of diuretics became known as *thiazide diuretics.* Subsequently, drugs that are pharmacologically similar to thiazide diuretics but are not thiazides were developed and are called *thiazidelike diuretics.* The term *thiazide diuretics* is used here to refer to all members of the class of inhibitors of Na⁺–Cl⁻ symport.

Mechanism and Site of Action. Some studies using split-droplet and stationary-microperfusion techniques have described reductions in proximal tubule reabsorption by thiazide diuretics; however, free-flow micropuncture studies have not consistently demonstrated increased solute delivery out of the proximal tubule following administration of thiazides. In contrast, micropuncture and *in situ* microperfusion studies clearly indicate that thiazide diuretics inhibit NaCl transport in the DCT. The DCT expresses thiazide binding sites and is accepted as the primary site of action of thiazide diuretics; the proximal tubule may represent a secondary site of action.

Figure 28–7 illustrates the current model of electrolyte transport in the DCT. As with other nephron segments, transport is powered by an Na⁺ pump in the basolateral membrane. The free energy in the electrochemical gradient for Na⁺ is harnessed by a Na⁺–Cl⁻ symporter in the luminal membrane that moves Cl⁻ into the epithelial cell against its electrochemical gradient. Cl⁻ then exits the basolateral membrane passively *via* a Cl⁻ channel. Thiazide diuretics inhibit the Na⁺–Cl⁻ symporter. In this regard, Na⁺ or Cl⁻ binding to the Na⁺–Cl⁻ symporter modifies thiazide-induced inhibition of the symporter, suggesting that the thiazide-binding site is shared or altered by both Na⁺ and Cl⁻ (Monroy, *et al.*, 2000).

DISTAL CONVOLUTED TUBULE

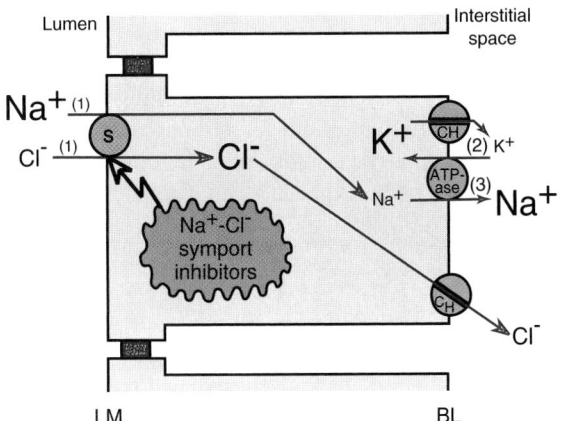

Figure 28–7. *NaCl reabsorption in distal convoluted tubule and mechanism of diuretic action of Na⁺–Cl⁻ symport inhibitors.* S, symporter; CH, ion channel. Numbers in parentheses indicate stoichiometry. BL and LM indicate basolateral and luminal membranes, respectively.

Using a functional expression strategy (Cl⁻-dependent Na⁺ uptake in *Xenopus* oocytes), Gamba *et al.* (1993) isolated a cDNA clone from the urinary bladder of the winter flounder that codes for a Na⁺–Cl⁻ symporter. This Na⁺–Cl⁻ symporter is inhibited by a number of thiazide diuretics (but not by furosemide, acetazolamide, or an amiloride derivative) and has 12 putative membrane-spanning domains, and its sequence is 47% identical to the cloned dogfish shark rectal gland Na⁺–K⁺–2Cl⁻ symporter. Subsequently, Gamba *et al.* (1994) cloned the rat and Mastroianni *et al.* (1996) cloned the human Na⁺–Cl⁻ symporter. The human Na⁺–Cl⁻ symporter has a predicted sequence of 1021 amino acids, 12 transmembrane domains, and 2 intracellular hydrophilic amino and carboxyl termini and maps to chromosome 16q13. The Na⁺–Cl⁻ symporter (called *ENCC1* or *TSC*) is expressed predominantly in the kidney (Chang *et al.*, 1996) and is localized to the apical membrane of DCT epithelial cells (Bachmann *et al.*, 1995; Obermüller *et al.*, 1995; Plotkin *et al.*, 1996). Expression of the Na⁺–Cl⁻ symporter is regulated by aldosterone (Velázquez *et al.*, 1996; Kim *et al.*, 1998; Bostonjoglo *et al.*, 1998). Mutations in the Na⁺–Cl⁻ symporter cause a form of inherited hypokalemic alkalosis called *Gitelman's syndrome* (Simon and Lifton, 1998).

Effects on Urinary Excretion. As would be expected from their mechanism of action, inhibitors of Na⁺–Cl⁻ symport increase Na⁺ and Cl⁻ excretion. However, thiazides are only moderately efficacious (*i.e.,* maximum excretion of filtered load of Na⁺ is only 5%) because approximately 90% of the filtered Na⁺ load is reabsorbed before reaching the DCT. Some thiazide diuretics also are weak inhibitors of carbonic anhydrase, an effect that increases HCO₃⁻ and phosphate excretion and probably accounts for their weak proximal tubular effects. Like inhibitors of Na⁺–K⁺–2Cl⁻ symport, inhibitors of Na⁺–Cl⁻ symport increase the excretion of K⁺ and titratable acid by the same mechanisms discussed for loop diuresis. Acute administration of thiazides increases the excretion of uric acid. However, uric acid excretion is reduced following chronic administration by the same mechanisms discussed for loop diuretics. The acute effects of inhibitors of Na⁺–Cl⁻ symport on Ca²⁺ excretion are variable; when administered chronically, thiazide diuretics decrease Ca²⁺ excretion (*see* Chapter 61). The mechanism involves increased proximal reabsorption owing to volume depletion, as well as direct effects of thiazides to increase Ca²⁺ reabsorption in the DCT. In this regard, inhibition of the Na⁺-Cl⁻ symporter in the luminal membrane decreases intracellular Na⁺ levels, thereby increasing the basolateral exit of Ca²⁺ *via* enhanced Na⁺–Ca²⁺ exchange (Friedman and Bushinsky, 1999). Thiazide diuretics may cause a mild magnesuria by a poorly understood mechanism, and there is increasing awareness that long-term use of thiazide diuretics may cause magnesium deficiency, particularly in the elderly (Wilcox, 1999). Since inhibitors of Na⁺–Cl⁻ symport inhibit transport in the cortical diluting segment, thiazide diuretics attenuate the ability of the kidney to excrete a dilute urine during water diuresis. However, since the DCT is not involved in the mechanism that generates a hypertonic medullary interstitium, thiazide diuretics do not alter the kidney's ability to concentrate urine during hydropenia.

Effects on Renal Hemodynamics. In general, inhibitors of Na^+–Cl^- symport do not affect RBF and only variably reduce GFR owing to increases in intratubular pressure. Since thiazides act at a point past the macula densa, they have little or no influence on TGF.

Other Actions. Thiazide diuretics may inhibit cyclic nucleotide phosphodiesterases, mitochondrial oxygen consumption, and renal uptake of fatty acids; however, these effects are not of clinical significance.

Absorption and Elimination. The relative potency, oral bioavailability, plasma half-life, and route of elimination of inhibitors of Na^+–Cl^- symport are listed in Table 28–5. Of special note is the wide range of half-lives for this class of drugs. Sulfonamides are organic acids and therefore are secreted into the proximal tubule by the organic acid secretory pathway. Since thiazides must gain access to the tubular lumen to inhibit the Na^+–Cl^- symporter, drugs such as probenecid can attenuate the diuretic response to thiazides by competing for transport into the proximal tubule. However, plasma protein binding varies considerably among thiazide diuretics, and this parameter determines the contribution that filtration makes to tubular delivery of a specific thiazide.

Toxicity, Adverse Effects, Contraindications, Drug Interactions. Thiazide diuretics rarely cause CNS (*e.g.,* vertigo, headache, paresthesias, xanthopsia, and weakness), gastrointestinal (*e.g.,* anorexia, nausea, vomiting, cramping, diarrhea, constipation, cholecystitis, and pancreatitis), hematological (*e.g.,* blood dyscrasias), and dermatological (*e.g.,* photosensitivity and skin rashes) disorders. The incidence of erectile dysfunction is greater with Na^+–Cl^- symport inhibitors than with several other antihypertensive agents (*e.g.,* β adrenergic receptor antagonists, Ca^{2+} channel blockers, angiotensin converting enzyme inhibitors, and α_1-receptor antagonists) (Grimm *et al.,* 1997) but usually is tolerable. As with loop diuretics, most serious adverse effects of thiazides are related to abnormalities of fluid and electrolyte balance. These adverse effects include extracellular volume depletion, hypotension, hypokalemia, hyponatremia, hypochloremia, metabolic alkalosis, hypomagnesemia, hypercalcemia, and hyperuricemia. Thiazide diuretics have caused

fatal or near-fatal hyponatremia, and some patients are at recurrent risk of hyponatremia when rechallenged with thiazides.

Thiazide diuretics also decrease glucose tolerance, and latent diabetes mellitus may be unmasked during therapy. The mechanism of the impaired glucose tolerance is not completely understood but appears to involve reduced insulin secretion and alterations in glucose metabolism. Hyperglycemia may be related in some way to K^+ depletion, in that hyperglycemia is reduced when K^+ is given along with the diuretic (Wilcox, 1999). In addition to contributing to hyperglycemia, thiazide-induced hypokalemia compromises the antihypertensive effect (Wilcox, 1999) and cardiovascular protection (Franse *et al.,* 2000) afforded by thiazides in patients with hypertension.

Thiazide diuretics also may increase plasma levels of LDL cholesterol, total cholesterol, and total triglycerides. Thiazide diuretics are contraindicated in individuals who are hypersensitive to sulfonamides.

With regard to drug interactions, thiazide diuretics may diminish the effects of anticoagulants, uricosuric agents used to treat gout, sulfonylureas, and insulin and may increase the effects of anesthetics, diazoxide, digitalis glycosides, lithium, loop diuretics, and vitamin D. The effectiveness of thiazide diuretics may be reduced by NSAIDs, whether nonselective or selective COX-2 inhibitors, and bile acid sequestrants (reduced absorption of thiazides). Amphotericin B and corticosteroids increase the risk of hypokalemia induced by thiazide diuretics.

A potentially lethal drug interaction warranting special emphasis is that involving thiazide diuretics and quinidine (Roden, 1993). Prolongation of the QT interval by quinidine can lead to the development of polymorphic ventricular tachycardia (*torsades de pointes*) owing to triggered activity originating from early after-depolarizations (*see* Chapter 34). Although usually self-limiting, *torsades de pointes* may deteriorate into fatal ventricular fibrillation. Hypokalemia increases the risk of quinidine-induced *torsades de pointes*, and thiazide diuretics cause hypokalemia. Thiazide diuretic–induced K^+ depletion may account for many cases of quinidine-induced *torsades de pointes.*

Therapeutic Uses. Thiazide diuretics are used for the treatment of the edema associated with heart (congestive heart failure), liver (hepatic cirrhosis), and renal (nephrotic syndrome, chronic renal failure, and acute glomerulonephritis) disease. With the possible exceptions of metolazone and indapamide, most thiazide diuretics are ineffective when the GFR is less than 30 to 40 ml/min.

Thiazide diuretics decrease blood pressure in hypertensive patients by increasing the slope of the renal pressure–natriuresis relationship (Saito and Kimura, 1996), and thiazide diuretics are used widely for the treatment of hypertension either alone or in combination with other antihypertensive drugs (*see* Chapter 32). In this regard, thiazide diuretics are inexpensive, as efficacious as other classes of antihypertensive agents, and well tolerated. Thiazides can be administered once daily, do not require dose titration, and have few contraindications. Moreover, thiazides have additive or synergistic effects when combined with other classes of antihypertensive agents. Although thiazides may increase the risk of sudden death (Hoes and Grobbee, 1996) and renal cell carcinoma marginally (Grossman *et al.*, 1999), in general, these agents are safe and reduce cardiovascular morbidity and mortality in hypertensive patients. Because the adverse effects of thiazides increase progressively in severity at doses higher than maximally effective antihypertensive doses, only low doses should be prescribed for hypertension (Kaplan, 1999). A common dose for hypertension is 25 mg/day of hydrochlorothiazide or the dose equivalent of another thiazide. The ALLHAT study (ALLHAT Officers and Coordinators for the ALLHAT Collaborative Research Group, 2002) provides strong evidence that thiazide diuretics are the best initial therapy for uncomplicated hypertension, a conclusion endorsed by the Joint National Committee on Prevention, Detection, Evaluation, and Treatment of High Blood Pressure (Chobanian *et al.*, 2003). Concern regarding the risk of diabetes should not cause physicians to avoid thiazides in nondiabetic hypertensives (Gress *et al.*, 2000). Recent studies suggest that

the antihypertensive response to thiazides is influenced by polymorphisms in the angiotensin-converting enzyme and α-adducin genes (Sciarrone *et al.*, 2003).

Thiazide diuretics, which reduce urinary excretion of Ca^{2+}, sometimes are employed to treat calcium nephrolithiasis and may be useful for the treatment of osteoporosis (*see* Chapter 61). Thiazide diuretics also are the mainstay for treatment of nephrogenic diabetes insipidus, reducing urine volume by up to 50%. The mechanism of this paradoxical effect remains unknown (Grønbeck *et al.*, 1998). Since other halides are excreted by renal processes similar to those for Cl^-, thiazide diuretics may be useful for the management of Br^- intoxication.

INHIBITORS OF RENAL EPITHELIAL NA+ CHANNELS (K+-SPARING DIURETICS)

Triamterene (DYRENIUM, MAXZIDE) and *amiloride* (MIDAMOR) are the only two drugs of this class in clinical use. Both drugs cause small increases in NaCl excretion and usually are employed for their antikaliuretic actions to offset the effects of other diuretics that increase K+ excretion. Consequently, triamterene and amiloride, along with spironolactone (*see* next section), often are classified as *potassium (K+)-sparing diuretics*.

Chemistry. Amiloride is a pyrazinoylguanidine derivative, and triamterene is a pteridine (Table 28–6). Both drugs are organic bases and are transported by the organic base secretory mechanism in the proximal tubule.

Table 28–6
Inhibitors of Renal Epithelial Na+ Channels (K+–Sparing Diuretics)

DRUG	STRUCTURE	RELATIVE POTENCY	ORAL AVAILABILITY	$T_{\frac{1}{2}}$ (HOURS)	ROUTE OF ELIMINATION
Amiloride (DYRENIUM)		1	15–25%	~21	R
Triamterene (MIDAMOR)		0.1	~50%	~4.2	M

Abbreviations: R, renal excretion of intact drug; M, metabolism; however, triamterene is transformed into an active metabolite that is excreted in the urine.

Mechanism and Site of Action. Available data suggest that triamterene and amiloride have similar mechanisms of action. Of the two, amiloride has been studied much more extensively, so its mechanism of action is known with a higher degree of certainty. As illustrated in Figure 28–8, principal cells in the late distal tubule and collecting duct have, in their luminal membranes, epithelial Na^+ channels that provide a conductive pathway for the entry of Na^+ into the cell down the electrochemical gradient created by the basolateral Na^+ pump. The higher permeability of the luminal membrane for Na^+ depolarizes the luminal membrane but not the basolateral membrane, creating a lumen-negative transepithelial potential difference. This transepithelial voltage provides an important driving force for the secretion of K^+ into the lumen *via* K^+ channels (ROMK) in the luminal membrane. Carbonic anhydrase inhibitors, loop diuretics, and thiazide diuretics increase the delivery of Na^+ to the late distal tubule and collecting duct, a situation that often is associated with increased K^+ and H^+ excretion. It is likely that the elevation in luminal Na^+ concentration in the distal nephron induced by such diuretics augments depolarization of the luminal membrane and thereby enhances the lumen-negative V_T, which facilitates K^+ excretion. In addition to principal cells, the collecting duct also contains type A intercalated cells that mediate the secretion of H^+ into the tubular lumen. Tubular acidification is driven by a luminal H^+–ATPase (proton pump), and this pump is aided by the partial depolarization of the luminal membrane. The luminal H^+–ATPase is of the vacuolar-type and is distinct from the gastric H^+–K^+–ATPase that is inhibited by drugs such as omeprazole. However, increased distal delivery of Na^+ is not the only mechanism by which diuretics increase K^+ and H^+ excretion. Activation of the renin–angiotensin–aldosterone axis by diuretics also contributes to diuretic-induced K^+ and H^+ excretion, as discussed in the section on mineralocorticoid antagonists.

Considerable evidence indicates that amiloride blocks epithelial Na^+ channels in the luminal membrane of principal cells in the late distal tubule and collecting duct perhaps by competing with Na^+ for negatively charged areas within the pore of the Na^+ channel. This evidence includes data from epithelia of nonrenal origin (amphibian skin and toad bladder), electrophysiological studies in isolated mammalian collecting ducts, and molecular studies that reconstitute channel subunits in lipid bilayers or express channel subunits in *Xenopus* oocytes. The renal epithelial Na^+ channels inhibited by this class of diuretics are not the same as voltage-gated Na^+ channels found in many electrically active cell types (*e.g.,* neurons and myocytes).

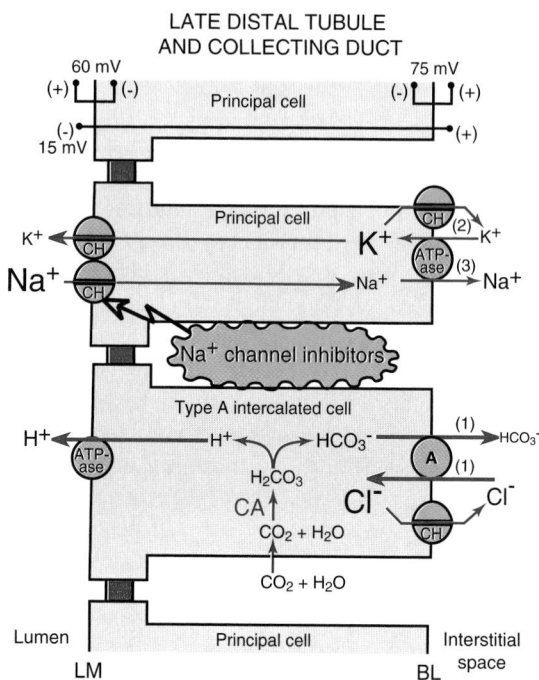

Figure 28–8. *Na^+ reabsorption in late distal tubule and collecting duct and mechanism of diuretic action of epithelial Na^+-channel inhibitors.* Cl^- reabsorption (*not shown*) occurs both paracellularly and transcellularly, and the precise mechanism of Cl^- transport appears to be species-specific. A, antiporter; CH, ion channel; CA, carbonic anhydrase. Numbers in parentheses indicate stoichiometry. Designated voltages are the potential differences across the indicated membrane or cell. BL and LM indicate basolateral and luminal membranes, respectively.

The amiloride-sensitive Na^+ channel (called *ENaC*) consists of three subunits (α, β, and γ) (Kleyman *et al.*, 1999). Although the α subunit is sufficient for channel activity, maximal Na^+ permeability is induced when all three subunits are coexpressed in the same cell, probably forming a tetrameric structure consisting of two α subunits, one β subunit, and one γ subunit. Studies in *Xenopus* oocytes expressing ENaC suggest that triamterene and amiloride bind to ENaC by similar mechanisms (Busch *et al.*, 1996). The K_i of amiloride for ENaC is submicromolar, and molecular studies have identified critical domains in ENaC that participate in amiloride binding (Kleyman *et al.*, 1999). Liddle's syndrome (pseudohyperaldosteronism) is an autosomal dominant form of low-renin, volume-expanded hypertension that is due to mutations in the β or γ subunits, leading to increased basal activity of ENaC (Ismailov *et al.*, 1999).

Effects on Urinary Excretion. Since the late distal tubule and collecting duct have a limited capacity to reabsorb solutes, blockade of Na^+ channels in this part of the nephron only mildly increases the excretion rates of Na^+ and Cl^- (approximately 2% of filtered load). Blockade of Na^+ channels hyperpolarizes the luminal membrane, reducing the lumen-negative transepithelial voltage. Since the lumen-negative potential difference normally opposes cation reabsorption and facilitates cation secretion, attenuation of the lumen-negative voltage decreases the excretion rates of K^+, H^+, Ca^{2+}, and Mg^{2+}. Volume contraction may increase reabsorption of uric acid in the proximal tubule; hence chronic administration of amiloride and triamterene may decrease uric acid excretion.

Effects on Renal Hemodynamics. Amiloride and triamterene have little or no effect on renal hemodynamics and do not alter TGF.

Other Actions. Amiloride, at concentrations higher than needed to elicit therapeutic effects, also blocks the Na^+–H^+ and Na^+–Ca^{2+} antiporters and inhibits Na^+,K^+–ATPase.

Absorption and Elimination. The relative potency, oral bioavailability, plasma half-life, and route of elimination for amiloride and triamterene are listed in Table 28–6. Amiloride is eliminated predominantly by urinary excretion of intact drug. Triamterene is metabolized extensively to an active metabolite, 4-hydroxytriamterene sulfate, and this metabolite is excreted in the urine. The pharmacological activity of 4-hydroxytriamterene sulfate is comparable with that of the parent drug. Therefore, the toxicity of triamterene may be enhanced in both hepatic disease (decreased metabolism of triamterene) and renal failure (decreased urinary excretion of active metabolite).

Toxicity, Adverse Effects, Contraindications, Drug Interactions. The most dangerous adverse effect of Na^+-channel inhibitors is hyperkalemia, which can be life-threatening. Consequently, amiloride and triamterene are contraindicated in patients with hyperkalemia, as well as in patients at increased risk of developing hyperkalemia (*e.g.*, patients with renal failure, patients receiving other K^+-sparing diuretics, patients taking angiotensin-converting enzyme inhibitors, or patients taking K^+ supplements). Even NSAIDs can increase the likelihood of hyperkalemia in patients receiving Na^+-channel inhibitors. Pentamidine and high-dose trimethoprim are used often to treat *Pneumocystis carinii* pneumonia in patients with acquired immune deficiency syndrome (AIDS). Because these compounds are weak inhibitors of ENaC, they too may cause hyperkalemia, and this may explain the frequent occurrence of hyperkalemia in AIDS patients (Kleyman *et al.*, 1999). Cirrhotic patients are prone to megaloblastosis because of folic acid deficiency, and triamterene, a weak folic acid antagonist, may increase the likelihood of this adverse event. Triamterene also can reduce glucose tolerance and induce photosensitization and has been associated with interstitial nephritis and renal stones. Both drugs can cause CNS, gastrointestinal, musculoskeletal, dermatological, and hematological adverse effects. The most common adverse effects of amiloride are nausea, vomiting, diarrhea, and headache; those of triamterene are nausea, vomiting, leg cramps, and dizziness.

Therapeutic Uses. Because of the mild natriuresis induced by Na^+-channel inhibitors, these drugs seldom are used as sole agents in the treatment of edema or hypertension. Rather, their major utility is in *combination* with other diuretics. Coadministration of a Na^+-channel inhibitor augments the diuretic and antihypertensive response to thiazide and loop diuretics. More important, the ability of Na^+-channel inhibitors to reduce K^+ excretion tends to offset the kaliuretic effects of thiazide and loop diuretics; consequently, the combination of a Na^+-channel inhibitor with a thiazide or loop diuretic tends to result in normal values of plasma K^+ (Hollenberg and Mickiewicz, 1989). Liddle's syndrome can be treated effectively with Na^+-channel inhibitors. Approximately 5% of people of African origin carry a *T594M* polymorphism in the β subunit of ENaC, and amiloride is particularly effective in lowering blood pressure in patients with hypertension who carry this polymorphism (Baker *et al.*, 2002). Aerosolized amiloride has been shown to improve mucociliary clearance in patients with cystic fibrosis. By inhibiting Na^+ absorption from the surfaces of airway epithelial cells, amiloride augments hydration of respiratory secretions and thereby improves mucociliary clearance. Amiloride also is useful for lithium-induced nephrogenic diabetes insipidus because it blocks Li^+ transport into the cells of the collecting tubules.

ANTAGONISTS OF MINERALOCORTICOID RECEPTORS (ALDOSTERONE ANTAGONISTS, K^+-SPARING DIURETICS)

Mineralocorticoids cause retention of salt and water and increase the excretion of K^+ and H^+ by binding to specific mineralocorticoid receptors. Early studies indicated that some spirolactones block the effects of mineralocorti-

Table 28–7
Mineralocorticoid Receptor Antagonists (Aldosterone Antagonists, Potassium-Sparing Diuretics)

DRUG	STRUCTURE	ORAL AVAILABILITY	$T_{\frac{1}{2}}$ (HOURS)	ROUTE OF ELIMINATION
Spironolactone (ALDACTONE)		~65%	~1.6	M
Canrenone*		ID	~16.5	M
Potassium canrenoate*		ID	ID	M
Eplerenone (INSPRA)		ID	~5	M

*Not available in United States. *Abbreviations*: M, metabolism; ID, insufficient data.

coids; this finding led to the synthesis of specific antagonists for the mineralocorticoid receptor (MR). Currently, two MR antagonists are available in the United States, *spironolactone* (a 17-spirolactone) and *eplerenone;* two others are available elsewhere (Table 28–7).

Mechanism and Site of Action. Epithelial cells in the late distal tubule and collecting duct contain cytosolic MRs that have a high affinity for aldosterone. This receptor is a member of the superfamily of receptors for steroid hormones, thyroid hormones, vitamin D, and retinoids (*see* Chapter 1). Aldosterone enters the epithelial cell from the basolateral membrane and binds to MRs; the MR–aldosterone complex translocates to the nucleus, where it binds to specific sequences of DNA (hormone-responsive elements) and thereby regulates the expression of multiple gene products called *aldosterone-induced proteins* (AIPs). Figure 28–9 illustrates some of the proposed effects of AIPs, including activation of "silent" Na+ channels and "silent" Na+ pumps that pre-exist in the cell

LATE DISTAL TUBULE
AND COLLECTING DUCT

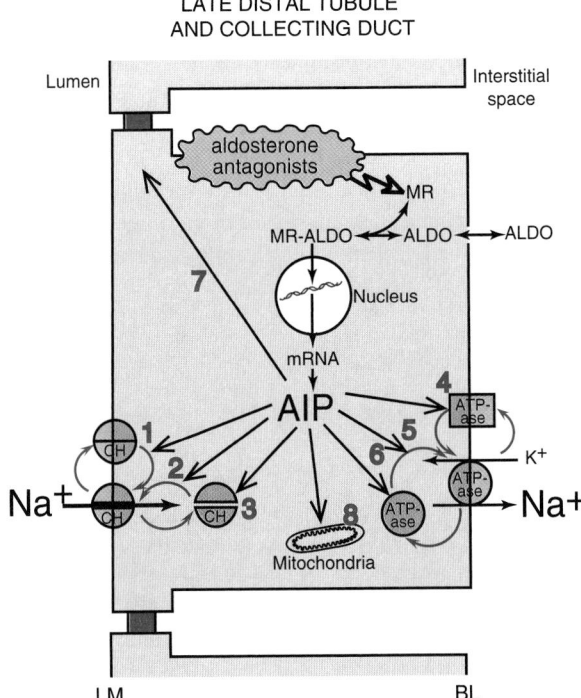

Figure 28–9. Effects of aldosterone on late distal tubule and collecting duct and diuretic mechanism of aldosterone antagonists. AIP, aldosterone-induced proteins; ALDO, aldosterone; MR, mineralocorticoid receptor; CH, ion channel; 1, activation of membrane-bound Na$^+$ channels; 2, redistribution of Na$^+$ channels from cytosol to membrane; 3, *de novo* synthesis of Na$^+$ channels; 4, activation of membrane-bound Na$^+$,K$^+$–ATPase; 5, redistribution of Na$^+$,K$^+$–ATPase from cytosol to membrane; 6, *de novo* synthesis of Na$^+$,K$^+$–ATPase; 7, changes in permeability of tight junctions; 8, increased mitochondrial production of ATP. BL and LM indicate basolateral and luminal membranes, respectively.

membrane, alterations in the cycling of Na$^+$ channels and Na$^+$ pumps between the cytosol and cell membrane such that more channels and pumps are located in the membrane, increased expression of Na$^+$ channels and Na$^+$ pumps, changes in permeability of the tight junctions, and increased activity of enzymes in the mitochondria that are involved in ATP production. The precise mechanisms by which AIPs alter transport are incompletely understood. However, the net effect of AIPs is to increase Na$^+$ conductance of the luminal membrane and sodium pump activity of the basolateral membrane. Consequently, transepithelial NaCl transport is enhanced, and the lumen-negative transepithelial voltage is increased. The latter effect increases the driving force for secretion of K$^+$ and H$^+$ into the tubular lumen.

Drugs such as spironolactone and eplerenone competitively inhibit the binding of aldosterone to the MR. Unlike the MR–aldosterone complex, the MR–spironolactone complex is not able to induce the synthesis of AIPs. Since spironolactone and eplerenone block the biological effects of aldosterone, these agents also are referred to as *aldosterone antagonists*. MR antagonists are the only diuretics that do not require access to the tubular lumen to induce diuresis.

Effects on Urinary Excretion. The effects of MR antagonists on urinary excretion are very similar to those induced by renal epithelial Na$^+$-channel inhibitors. However, unlike that of the Na$^+$-channel inhibitors, the clinical efficacy of MR antagonists is a function of endogenous levels of aldosterone. The higher the levels of endogenous aldosterone, the greater are the effects of MR antagonists on urinary excretion.

Effects on Renal Hemodynamics. MR antagonists have little or no effect on renal hemodynamics and do not alter TGF.

Other Actions. Spironolactone has some affinity toward progesterone and androgen receptors and thereby induces side effects such as gynecomastia, impotence, and menstrual irregularities. Owing to the 9,11-epoxide group, eplerenone has very low affinity for progesterone and androgen receptors (<1% and <0.1%, respectively) compared with spironolactone. Therapeutic concentrations of spironolactone block *ether-a-go-go*-related gene channels, and this may account for the antiarrythmic effects of spironolactone in heart failure (Caballero *et al.*, 2003). High concentrations of spironolactone have been reported to interfere with steroid biosynthesis by inhibiting cytochrome P450 steroid hydroxylases (*e.g.,* CYP11A1, CYP11B1, CYP11B2, CYP17, and CYP21). These effects have limited clinical relevance (*see* Chapter 59).

Absorption and Elimination. Spironolactone is absorbed partially (approximately 65%), is metabolized extensively (even during its first passage through the liver), undergoes enterohepatic recirculation, is highly protein-bound, and has a short half-life (approximately 1.6 hours). However, an active metabolite of spironolactone, canrenone, has a half-life of approximately 16.5 hours, which prolongs the biological effects of spironolactone. Although not available in the United States, canrenone and the K$^+$ salt of canrenoate also are in clinical use. Canrenoate is not active *per se* but is converted to canrenone in the body. Eplerenone has good oral availability and is eliminated primarily by metabolism (mediated by the hepatic cytochrome P450 isozyme CYP3A4) to inactive metabolites, with a $t_{\frac{1}{2}}$ of approximately 5 hours.

Toxicity, Adverse Effects, Contraindications, Drug Interactions. As with other K⁺-sparing diuretics, MR antagonists may cause life-threatening hyperkalemia. Indeed, hyperkalemia is the principal risk of MR antagonists. Therefore, these drugs are contraindicated in patients with hyperkalemia and in those at increased risk of developing hyperkalemia either because of disease or because of administration of other medications. MR antagonists also can induce metabolic acidosis in cirrhotic patients.

Salicylates may reduce the tubular secretion of canrenone and decrease the diuretic efficacy of spironolactone, and spironolactone may alter the clearance of digitalis glycosides. Owing to its affinity for other steroid receptors, spironolactone may cause gynecomastia, impotence, decreased libido, hirsutism, deepening of the voice, and menstrual irregularities. Spironolactone also may induce diarrhea, gastritis, gastric bleeding, and peptic ulcers (the drug is contraindicated in patients with peptic ulcers). CNS adverse effects include drowsiness, lethargy, ataxia, confusion, and headache. Spironolactone may cause skin rashes and, rarely, blood dyscrasias. Breast cancer has occurred in patients taking spironolactone chronically (cause and effect not established), and high doses of spironolactone have been associated with malignant tumors in rats. Whether or not therapeutic doses of spironolactone can induce malignancies remains an open question. Strong inhibitors of CYP3A4 (*see* Chapter 3) may increase plasma levels of eplerenone, and such drugs should not be administered to patients taking eplerenone, and vice versa. Other than hyperkalemia and gastrointestinal disorders, the rate of adverse events for eplerenone is similar to that of placebo (Pitt *et al.*, 2003).

Therapeutic Uses. As with other K⁺-sparing diuretics, spironolactone often is coadministered with thiazide or loop diuretics in the treatment of edema and hypertension. Such combinations result in increased mobilization of edema fluid while causing lesser perturbations of K⁺ homeostasis. Spironolactone is particularly useful in the treatment of primary hyperaldosteronism (adrenal adenomas or bilateral adrenal hyperplasia) and of refractory edema associated with secondary aldosteronism (cardiac failure, hepatic cirrhosis, nephrotic syndrome, and severe ascites). Spironolactone is considered the diuretic of choice in patients with hepatic cirrhosis. Spironolactone, added to standard therapy, substantially reduces morbidity and mortality (Pitt *et al.*, 1999) and ventricular arrhyth-

mias (Ramires *et al.*, 2000) in patients with heart failure (*see* Chapter 34).

Clinical experience with eplerenone is limited. Nonetheless, eplerenone appears to be a safe and effective antihypertensive drug (Ouzan *et al.*, 2002; Krum *et al.*, 2002; White *et al.*, 2003; Weinberger *et al.*, 2002). In patients with acute myocardial infarction complicated by left ventricular systolic dysfunction, addition of eplerenone to optimal medical therapy significantly reduces morbidity and mortality (Pitt *et al.*, 2003).

CLINICAL SUMMARY

Site and Mechanism of Action of Diuretics. An understanding of the site and mechanism of action of diuretics enhances comprehension of the clinically salient aspects of diuretic pharmacology. Figure 28–10 provides an overview of the many sites and mechanisms of actions of diuretics. Much of the pharmacology of diuretics can be deduced from this figure.

Mechanism of Edema Formation. A complex set of interrelationships (Figure 28–11) exists among the cardiovascular system, the kidneys, the CNS (Na⁺ appetite, thirst regulation), and the tissue capillary beds [distribution of extracellular fluid volume (ECFV)], so perturbations at one of these sites can affect all the remaining sites. A primary law of the kidney is that Na⁺ excretion is a steep function of mean arterial blood pressure (MABP) such that small increases in MABP cause marked increases in Na⁺ excretion (Guyton, 1991). Over any given time interval, the net change in total-body Na⁺ (either positive or negative) is simply the dietary Na⁺ intake minus the urinary excretion rate minus other losses (*e.g.*, sweating, fecal losses, and vomiting). When a net positive Na⁺ balance occurs, the concentration of Na⁺ in the extracellular fluid (ECF) will increase, stimulating water intake (thirst) and reducing urinary water output (*via* ADH release). Opposite changes occur during a net negative Na⁺ balance. Changes in water intake and output adjust ECFV concentration toward normal, thereby expanding or contracting total ECFV. Total ECFV is distributed among many body compartments; however, since the volume of ECF on the arterial side of the circulation pressurizes the arterial tree, it is this fraction of ECFV that determines MABP, and it is this fraction of ECFV that is "sensed" by the cardiovascular system and kidneys. Since MABP is a major determinant of Na⁺ output, a closed loop is established (Figure 28–11). This loop cycles until net Na⁺

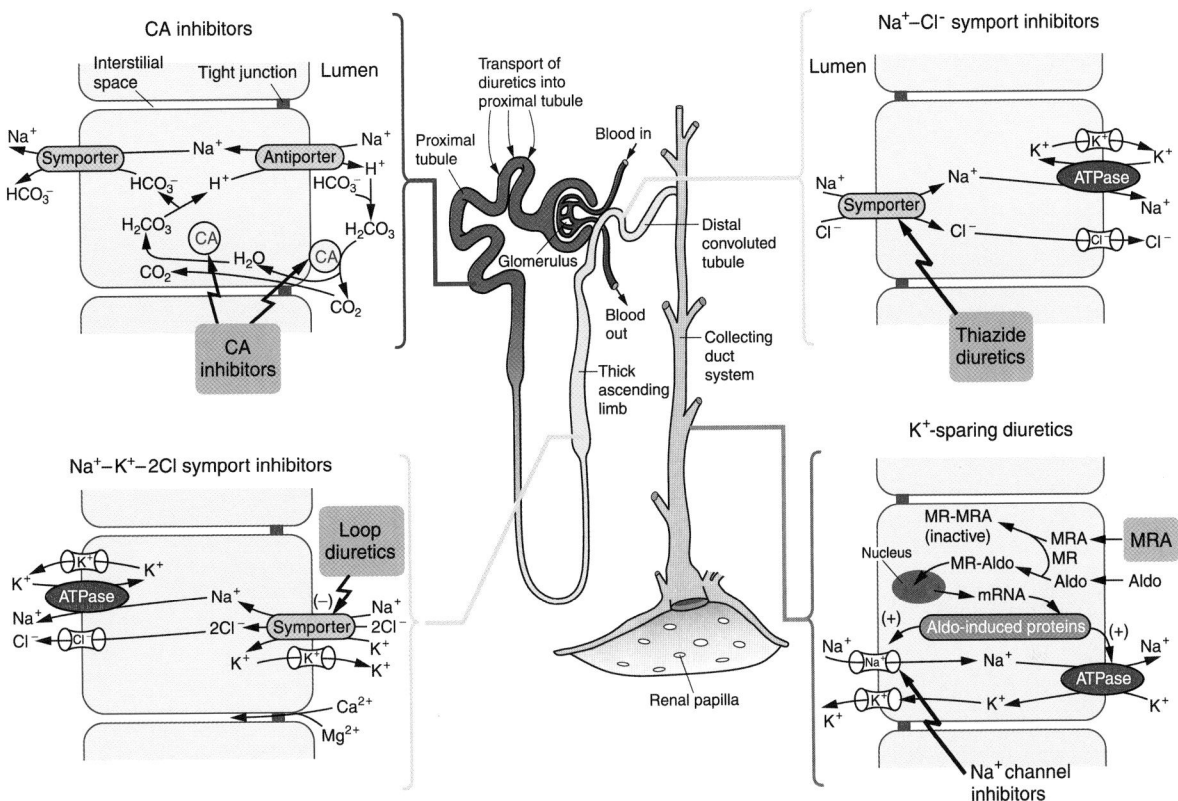

Figure 28–10. *Summary of the site and mechanism of action of diuretics.* Three important features of this summary figure are worth special note: (1) Transport of solute across epithelial cells in all nephron segments involves highly specialized proteins, which, for the most part, are apical and basolateral membrane integral proteins, (2) diuretics target and block the action of epithelial proteins involved in solute transport, and (3) the site and mechanism of action of a given class of diuretics are determined by the specific protein inhibited by the diuretic. CA, carbonic anhydrase; MR, mineralocorticoid receptor; MRA, mineralocorticoid receptor antagonist; Aldo, aldosterone.

accumulation is zero; *i.e.,* in the long run, Na$^+$ intake must equal Na$^+$ loss.

The preceding discussion implies that three fundamental types of perturbations contribute to venous congestion and/or edema formation:

1. A shift to the right in the renal pressure–natriuresis relationship (*e.g.,* chronic renal failure) causes reduced Na$^+$ excretion for any level of MABP. If all other factors remain constant, this would increase total-body Na$^+$, ECFV, and MABP. The additional ECFV would be distributed throughout various body compartments according to the state of cardiac function and prevailing Starling forces and would predispose toward venous congestion and/or edema. Even so, in the absence of any other predisposing factors for venous congestion and/or edema, a rightward shift in the renal pressure–natriuresis curve generally causes hypertension with only a slight (usually immeasurable) increase

in ECFV. As elucidated by Guyton and coworkers (Guyton, 1991), ECFV expansion triggers the following series of events: expanded ECFV → augmented cardiac output → enhanced vascular tone (*i.e.,* total-body autoregulation) → increased total peripheral resistance → elevated MABP → pressure natriuresis → reduction of ECFV and cardiac output toward normal. Most likely, a sustained rightward shift in the renal pressure–natriuresis curve is a necessary and sufficient condition for long-term hypertension but is only a predisposing factor for venous congestion and/or edema.

2. An increase in dietary Na$^+$ intake would have the same effects as a rightward shift in the renal pressure–natriuresis relationship (*i.e.,* increased MABP and predisposition to venous congestion/edema). However, changes in salt intake may have minimal or large effects depending on the shape of the patient's renal pressure–natriuresis curve.

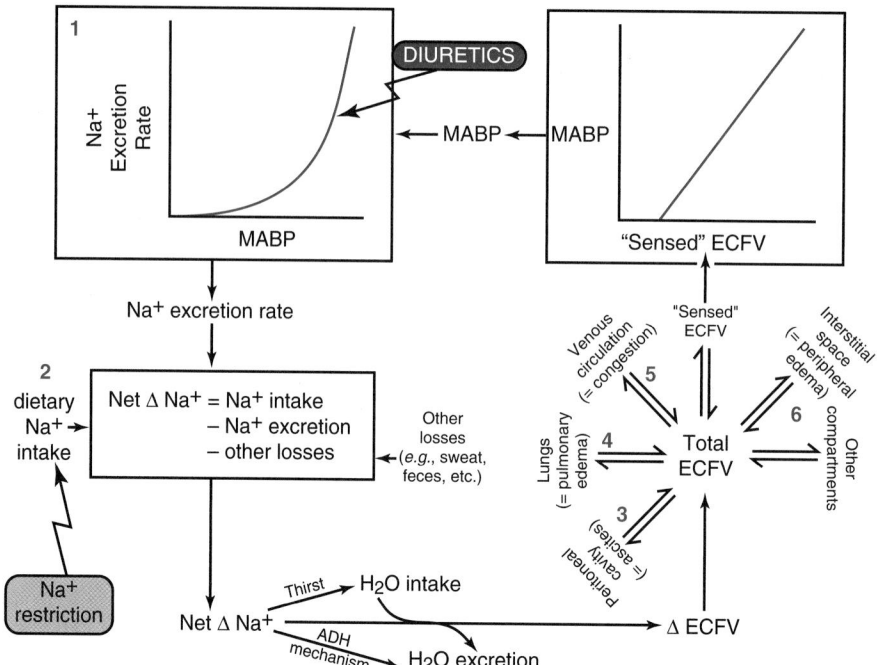

Figure 28–11. *Interrelationships among renal function, Na⁺ intake, water homeostasis, distribution of extracellular fluid volume, and mean arterial blood pressure.* Pathophysiological mechanisms of edema formation: 1, rightward shift of renal pressure natriuresis curve; 2, excessive dietary Na⁺ intake; 3, increased distribution of extracellular fluid volume (ECFV) to peritoneal cavity (*e.g.,* liver cirrhosis with increased hepatic sinusoidal hydrostatic pressure) leading to ascites formation; 4, increased distribution of ECFV to lungs (*e.g.,* left-sided heart failure with increased pulmonary capillary hydrostatic pressure) leading to pulmonary edema; 5, increased distribution of ECFV to venous circulation (*e.g.,* right-sided heart failure) leading to venous congestion; 6, peripheral edema caused by altered Starling forces causing increased distribution of ECFV to interstitial space (*e.g.,* diminished plasma proteins in nephrotic syndrome, severe burns, and liver disease).

3. Any pathophysiological alterations in the forces that govern the distribution of ECFV among the various body compartments would cause abnormal amounts of ECFV to be trapped at the site of altered forces. This would deplete the "sensed" ECFV, which would be restored back to normal by the mechanisms described earlier. ECFV may be trapped at several sites by different mechanisms. For instance, cirrhosis of the liver increases lymph in the space of Disse, leading to spillover *via* the glissonian wall into the peritoneal cavity (ascites). Left-sided heart failure, both acute and chronic, increases hydrostatic pressure in the lung capillaries, leading to pulmonary edema. Chronic right-sided heart failure redistributes ECFV from the arterial to the venous circulation, resulting in venous, hepatic, and splenic congestion and peripheral tissue edema. Decreased levels of plasma protein, particularly albumin (*e.g.,* in nephrotic syndrome, severe burns, and hepatic disease), increase the distribution of ECFV into the interstitial spaces, causing generalized peripheral edema. Peripheral edema also may be "idiopathic"

owing to unknown alterations in the Starling forces at the capillary bed.

The Role of Diuretics in Clinical Medicine. Another implication of the mechanisms illustrated in Figure 28–11 is that three fundamental strategies exist for mobilizing edema fluid: Correct the underlying disease, restrict Na⁺ intake, or administer diuretics. The most desirable course of action would be to correct the primary disease; however, this often is impossible. For instance, the increased hepatic sinusoidal pressure in cirrhosis of the liver and the urinary loss of protein in nephrotic syndrome are due to structural alterations in the portal circulation and glomeruli, respectively, that may not be remediable. Restriction of Na⁺ intake is the favored nonpharmacologic approach to the treatment of edema and hypertension and should be attempted; however, compliance is a major obstacle. Diuretics, therefore, remain the cornerstone for the treatment of edema or volume overload, particularly that owing to congestive heart failure, ascites, chronic renal failure, and nephrotic syndrome.

Whether a patient should receive diuretics and, if so, what therapeutic regimen should be used (*i.e.,* type of diuretic, dose, route of administration, and speed of mobilization of edema fluid) depend on the clinical situation. Massive pulmonary edema in patients with acute left-sided heart failure is a medical emergency requiring rapid, aggressive therapy including intravenous administration of a loop diuretic. In this setting, use of oral diuretics or diuretics with lesser efficacy is inappropriate. On the other hand, mild pulmonary and venous congestion associated with chronic heart failure is best treated with an oral loop or thiazide diuretic, the dosage of which should be titrated carefully to maximize the benefit-to-risk ratio. As mentioned previously, meta-analysis indicates that loop and thiazide diuretics decrease morbidity and mortality in heart failure patients (Faris *et al.*, 2002), and two randomized clinical trials with MR antagonists also demonstrate reduced morbidity and mortality in heart failure patients receiving optimal therapy with other drugs (Pitt *et al.*, 1999, 2003). Periodic administration of diuretics to cirrhotic patients with ascites may eliminate the necessity for or reduce the interval between paracenteses, adding to patient comfort and sparing protein reserves that are lost during the paracenteses. Although diuretics can reduce edema associated with chronic renal failure, increased doses of the more powerful loop diuretics usually are required. In the nephrotic syndrome, the response to diuretics often is disappointing. In chronic renal failure and cirrhosis, edema will not pose an immediate health risk. Even so, uncomfortable, oppressive, and/or disfiguring edema can greatly reduce quality of life, and the decision to treat will be based in part on quality-of-life issues. In such cases, only partial removal of edema fluid should be attempted, and the fluid should be mobilized slowly using a diuretic regimen that accomplishes the task with minimal perturbation of normal physiology. Brater (1998) provides a logically compelling algorithm for diuretic therapy (specific recommendations for drug, dose, route, and drug combinations) in patients with edema caused by renal, hepatic, or cardiac disorders. The basic features of "Brater's algorithm" are summarized in Figure 28-12.

In many clinical situations, edema is not caused by an abnormal intake of Na^+ or by an altered renal handling of Na^+. Rather, edema is the result of altered Starling forces at the capillary beds, *i.e.,* a "Starling trap." Use of diuretics in these clinical settings represents a judicious compromise between the edematous state and the hypovolumic state. In such conditions, reducing total ECFV with diuretics will decrease edema but also will cause depletion of "sensed" ECFV, possibly leading to hypotension, malaise, and asthenia.

Diuretic resistance refers to edema that is or has become refractory to a given diuretic. If diuretic resistance develops against a less efficacious diuretic, a more efficacious diuretic should be substituted, *e.g.,* a loop diuretic for a thiazide. However, resistance to loop diuretics is not uncommon and can be due to several causes. NSAIDs block prostaglandin-mediated increases in RBF and increase the expression of the Na^+–K^+–$2Cl^-$ symporter in the thick ascending limb (Fernández-Llama *et al.*, 1999), resulting in resistance to loop diuretics. Diuretic resistance induced by NSAIDs also occurs with selective COX-2 inhibitors (Kammerl *et al.*, 2001). In chronic renal failure, a reduction in RBF decreases the delivery of diuretics to the kidney, and accumulation of endogenous organic acids competes with loop diuretics for transport at the proximal tubule. Consequently, the concentration of diuretic at the active site in the tubular lumen is diminished. In nephrotic syndrome, the binding of diuretics has been postulated to limit response to the drugs; however, a recent study challenges the validity of this concept (Agarwal *et al.*, 2000). In hepatic cirrhosis, nephrotic syndrome, or heart failure, nephrons may have a diminished responsiveness to diuretics because of increased proximal tubular Na^+ reabsorption, leading to diminished delivery of Na^+ to the distal nephron segments (Knauf and Mutschler, 1997).

Faced with resistance to loop diuretics, the clinician has several options:

1. Bed rest may restore drug responsiveness by improving the renal circulation.
2. An increase in the dose of loop diuretic may restore responsiveness; however, nothing is gained by increasing the dose above that which causes a near-maximal effect (*i.e.,* the ceiling dose) of the diuretic.
3. Administration of smaller doses more frequently or a continuous intravenous infusion of a loop diuretic (Rudy *et al.*, 1991; Dormans *et al.*, 1996; Ferguson *et al.*, 1997) will increase the length of time that an effective concentration of the diuretic is at the active site.
4. Use of combination therapy to sequentially block more than one site in the nephron may result in a synergistic interaction between two diuretics. For instance, a combination of a loop diuretic with a K^+-sparing or a thiazide diuretic may improve therapeutic response; however, nothing is gained by the administration of two drugs of the same type. Thiazide diuretics with significant proximal tubular effects, *e.g.,* metolazone, are particularly well suited for sequential blockade when coadministered with a loop diuretic.
5. Reducing salt intake will diminish postdiuretic Na^+ retention that can nullify previous increases in Na^+ excretion.

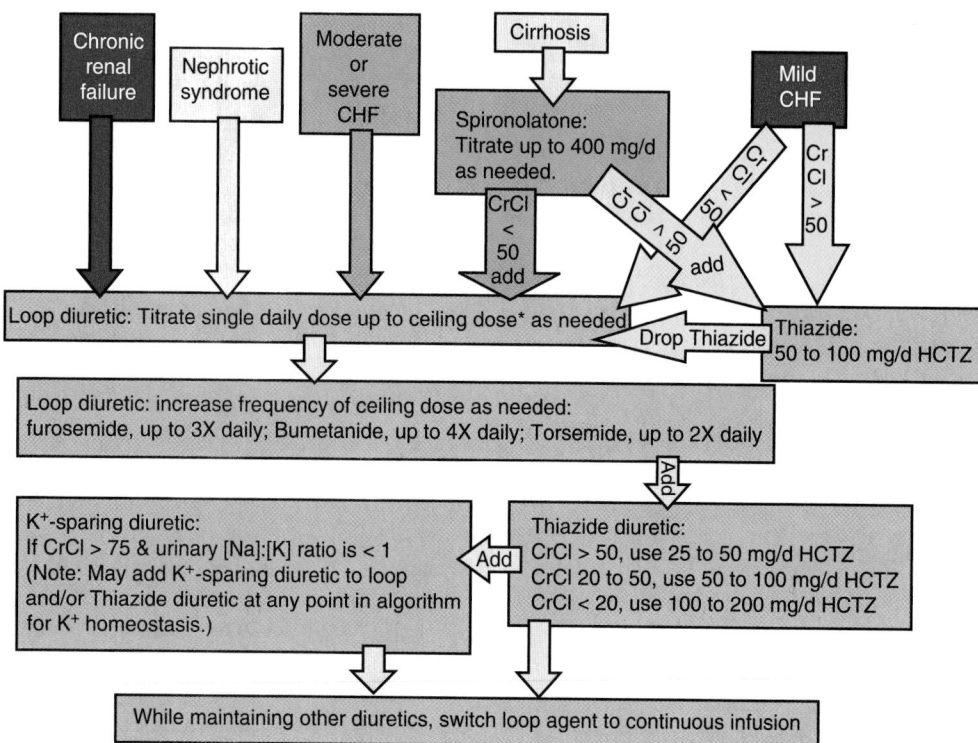

Figure 28–12. *"Brater's algorithm" for diuretic therapy of chronic renal failure, nephrotic syndrome, congestive heart failure, and cirrhosis.* Follow algorithm until adequate response is achieved. If adequate response is not obtained, advance to the next step. For illustrative purposes, the thiazide diuretic used in Brater's algorithm is hydrochlorothiazide (HCTZ). An alternative thiazide-type diuretic may be substituted with appropriate dosage adjustment so as to be pharmacologically equivalent to the recommended dose of HCTZ. *Do not combine two K$^+$-sparing diuretics because of the risk of hyperkalemia.* CrCl indicates creatinine clearance in milliliters per minute, and ceiling dose refers to the smallest dose of diuretic that produces a near-maximal effect. Ceiling doses of loop diuretics and dosing regimens for continuous intravenous infusions of loop diuretics are disease-state-specific. In this regard, *see* Brater (1998) for recommended dosages. Doses are for adults only.

6. Scheduling of diuretic administration shortly before food intake will provide effective concentrations of diuretic in the tubular lumen when the salt load is highest.

All currently available diuretics perturb K$^+$ homeostasis. However, studies in animals have established that blockade of adenosine A$_1$ receptors induces a brisk natriuresis without significantly increasing urinary K$^+$ excretion (Kuan *et al.*, 1993). Two clinical studies with FK453, a highly selective A$_1$-receptor antagonist, confirm that blockade of A$_1$ receptors induces natriuresis in human beings with minimal effects on K$^+$ excretion (Balakrishnan *et al.*, 1993; van Buren *et al.*, 1993). The natriuretic mechanism of this novel class of diuretics has been partially elucidated (Takeda *et al.*, 1993). Elevated intracellular cyclic AMP reduces basolateral Na$^+$–HCO$_3^-$ symport in proximal tubular cells. Endogenous adenosine normally acts on A$_1$ receptors in these cells to inhibit adenylyl cyclase and reduce cyclic AMP accumulation. Blockade of A$_1$ receptors removes this inhibition, permits cellular cyclic AMP to rise, and results in reduced activity of the Na$^+$–HCO$_3^-$ symporter. Because A$_1$ receptors are involved in TGF, A$_1$-receptor antagonists uncouple increased distal delivery of Na$^+$ from activation of TGF (Wilcox, 1999). Other mechanisms, including an effect in the collecting tubules, contribute to the natriuretic response to A$_1$-receptor antagonists; however, it is not known why this class of diuretics has little effect on K$^+$ excretion. In some patients, loop diuretics may compromise renal hemodynamics and actually reduce GFR, a phenomenon known as *diuretic intolerance*. Importantly, A$_1$-receptor antagonists tend to improve GFR in the setting of diuretic intolerance. A$_1$-receptor antagonists are in clinical trials as "renal friendly" diuretics for the treatment of edema owing to heart failure (Gottlieb *et al.*, 2002; Jackson, 2002).

BIBLIOGRAPHY

Agarwal, R., Gorski, J.C., Sundblad, K, and Brater, D.C. Urinary protein binding does not affect response to furosemide in patients with nephrotic syndrome. *J. Am. Soc. Nephrol.,* 2000, *11*:1100–1105.

Bachmann, S., Vel·zquez, H., Obermˌller, N., *et al.* Expression of the thiazide-sensitive Na–Cl cotransporter by rabbit distal convoluted tubule cells. *J. Clin. Invest.,* 1995, *96*:2510–2514.

Baker, E.H., Duggal, A., Dong, Y., *et al.* Amiloride, a specific drug for hypertension in black people with *T594M* variant? *Hypertension,* 2002, *40*:13–17.

Balakrishnan, V.S., Coles, G.A., and Williams, J.D. A potential role for endogenous adenosine in control of human glomerular and tubular function. *Am. J. Physiol.,* 1993, *265*:F504–F510.

Bostanjoglo, M., Reeves, W.B., Reilly, R.F., *et al.* 11β-Hydroxysteroid dehydrogenase, mineralocorticoid receptor, and thiazide-sensitive Na–Cl cotransporter expression by distal tubules. *J. Am. Soc. Nephrol.,* 1998, *9*:1347–1358.

Busch, A.E., Suessbrich, H., Kunzelmann, K. *et al.* Blockade of epithelial Na$^+$ channels by triamterenes: Underlying mechanisms and molecular basis. *Pflügers Arch.,* 1996, *432*:760–766.

Caballero, R., Morena, I., Gonzalez, T., *et al.* Spironolactone and its main metabolite, canrenoic acid, block human ether-a-go-go-related gene channels. *Circulation,* 2003, *107*:889–895.

Canessa, C.M., Schild, L., Buell, G., *et al.* Amiloride-sensitive epithelial Na$^+$ channel is made of three homologous subunits. *Nature,* 1994, *367*:463–467.

Chang, H., Tashiro, K., Hirai, M., *et al.* Identification of a cDNA encoding a thiazide-sensitive sodium–chloride cotransporter from the human and its mRNA expression in various tissues. *Biochem. Biophys. Res. Commun.,* 1996, *223*:324–328.

Dormans, T.P., van Meyel, J.J., Gerlag, P.G., *et al.* Diuretic efficacy of high-dose furosemide in severe heart failure: Bolus injection versus continuous infusion. *J. Am. Coll. Cardiol.,* 1996, *28*:376–382.

Faris, R., Flather, M., Purcell, H., *et al.* Current evidence supporting the role of diuretics in heart failure: A meta-analysis of randomised, controlled trials. *Int. J. Cardiol.,* 2002, *82*:149–158.

Ferguson, J.A., Sundblad, K.J., Becker, P.K., *et al.* Role of duration of diuretic effect in preventing sodium retention. *Clin. Pharmacol. Ther.,* 1997, *62*:203–208.

Fernandez-Llama, P., Ecelbarger, C.A., Ware, J.A., *et al.* Cyclooxygenase inhibitors increase Na–K–2Cl cotransporter abundance in thick ascending limb of Henle's loop. *Am. J. Physiol.,* 1999, *277*:F219–F226.

Franse, L.V., Pahor, M., Di Bari, M., *et al.* Hypokalemia associated with diuretic use and cardiovascular events in the Systolic Hypertension in the Elderly Program. *Hypertension,* 2000, *35*:1025–1030.

Gamba, G., Miyanoshita, A., Lombardi, M., *et al.* Molecular cloning, primary structure and characterization of two members of the mammalian electroneutral sodium–(potassium)–chloride cotransporter family expressed in kidney. *J. Biol. Chem.,* 1994, *269*:17713–17722.

Gamba, G., Saltzberg, S.N., Lombardi, M., *et al.* Primary structure and functional expression of a cDNA encoding the thiazide-sensitive, electroneutral sodium–chloride cotransporter. *Proc. Natl. Acad. Sci. USA,* 1993, *90*:2749–2753.

Gottlieb, S.S., Brater, D.C., Thomas, I., *et al.* BG9719 (CVT-124), an A$_1$ adenosine receptor antagonist, protects against the decline in renal function observed with diuretic therapy. *Circulation,* 2002, *105*:1348–1353.

Gress, T.W., Nieto, F.J., Shahar, E., Wofford, M.R., Brancati, F.L., Hypertension and antihypertensive therapy as risk factors for type 2 diabetes mellitus. Atherosclerosis Risk in Communities Study. *New Engl. J. Med.,* 2000, *342*:905–912.

Grimm, R.H., Jr., Grandits, G.A., Prineas, R.J., *et al.* Long-term effects on sexual function of five antihypertensive drugs and nutritional hygienic treatment in hypertensive men and women. Treatment of Mild Hypertension Study (TOMHS). *Hypertension,* 1997, *29*:8–14.

Grˉnbeck, L., Marples, D., Nielsen, S., and Christensen, S. Mechanism of antidiuresis caused by bendroflumethiazide in conscious rats with diabetes insipidus. *Br. J. Pharmacol.,* 1998, *123*:737–745.

Grossman, E., Messerli, F.H., and Goldbourt, U. Does diuretic therapy increase the risk of renal cell carcinoma? *Am. J. Cardiol.,* 1999, *83*:1090–1093.

Hollenberg, N.K., and Mickiewicz, C.W. Postmarketing surveillance in 70,898 patients treated with a triamterene/hydrochlorothiazide combination (MAXIDE). *Am. J. Cardiol.,* 1989, *63*:37B–41B.

Isenring, P., and Forbush, B., III. Ion and bumetanide binding by the Na–K–Cl cotransporter: Importance of transmembrane domains. *J. Biol. Chem.,* 1997, *272*:24556–24562.

Ismailov, I.I., Shlyonsky, V.G., Serpersu, E.H. *et al.* Peptide inhibition of ENaC. *Biochemistry,* 1999, *38*:354–363.

Kammerl, M.C., Nusing, R.M. Richthammer, W., Kramer, B.K., and Kurtz, A. Inhibition of COX-2 counteracts the effects of diuretics in rats. *Kidney Int.,* 2001, 60:1684–1691.

Kaplan, M.R., Plotkin, M.D., Lee, W.S., *et al.* Apical localization of the Na–K–Cl cotransporter *rBSC1* on rat thick ascending limbs. *Kidney Int.,* 1996, *49*:40–47.

Kim, G.H., Masilamani, S., Turner, R., *et al.* The thiazide-sensitive Na–Cl cotransporter is an aldosterone-induced protein. *Proc. Natl. Acad. Sci. USA,* 1998, *95*:14552–14557.

Knauf, H., and Mutschler, E. Sequential nephron blockade breaks resistance to diuretics in edematous states. *J. Cardiovasc. Pharmacol.,* 1997, *29*:367–372.

Krum, H., Nolly, H., Workman, D., *et al.* Efficacy of eplerenone added to renin–angiotensin blockade in hypertensive patients. *Hypertension,* 2002, *40*:117–123.

Kuan, C.J., Herzer, W.A., and Jackson, E.K. Cardiovascular and renal effects of blocking A$_1$ adenosine receptors. *J. Cardiovasc. Pharmacol.,* 1993, *21*:822–828.

Lane, P.H., Tyler, L.D., and Schmitz, P.G. Chronic administration of furosemide augments renal weight and glomerular capillary pressure in normal rats. *Am. J. Physiol.,* 1998, *275*:F230–F234.

Links, T.P., Zwarts, M.J., and Oosterhuis, H.J. Improvement of muscle strength in familial hypokalaemic periodic paralysis with acetazolamide. *J. Neurol. Neurosurg. Psychiatry,* 1988, *51*:1142–1145.

Lytle, C., McManus, T.J., and Haas, M. A model of Na–K–2Cl cotransport based on ordered ion binding and glide symmetry. *Am. J. Physiol.,* 1998, *274*:C299–C309.

Mastroianni, N., De Fusco, M., Zollo, M., *et al.* Molecular cloning, expression pattern, and chromosomal localization of the human Na–Cl thiazide-sensitive cotransporter (SLC12A3). *Genomics,* 1996, *35*:486–493.

Monroy, A., Plata, C., Hebert, S.C., and Gamba, G. Characterization of the thiazide-sensitive Na$^+$-Cl$^-$ cotransporter: A new model for ions and diuretics interaction. *Am. J. Physiol. Renal Physiol.,* 2000, *279*:F161–F169.

Mount, D.B., Baekgaard, A., Hall, A.E., *et al.* Isoforms of the Na$^+$-K$^+$-2Cl$^-$ cotransporter in murine TAL: I. Molecular characterization and intrarenal localization. *Am. J. Physiol.,* 1999, *276*:F347–F358.

Nielsen, S., Maunsbach, A.B., Ecelbarger, C.A., and Knepper, M.A. Ultrastructural localization of the Na–K–2Cl cotransporter in thick ascending limb and macula densa of rat kidney. *Am. J. Physiol.,* **1998,** *275:*F885–F893.

Oberm̧ller, N., Bernstein, P., Vel·zquez, H., *et al.* Expression of the thiazide-sensitive Na–Cl cotransporter in rat and human kidney. *Am. J. Physiol.,* **1995,** *269:*F900–F910.

Oberm̧ller, N., Kunchaparty, S., Ellison, D.H., and Bachmann, S. Expression of the Na–K–2Cl cotransporter by macula densa and thick ascending limb cells of rat and rabbit nephron. *J. Clin. Invest.,* **1996,** *98:*635–640.

Ouzan, J., Perault, C., Lincoff, A.M., Carre, E., and Mertes, M. The role of spironolactone in the treatment of patients with refractory hypertension. *Am. J. Hypertens.,* **2002,** *15:*333–339.

Payne, J.A., and Forbush, B., III. Alternatively spliced isoforms of the putative renal Na–K–Cl cotransporter are differentially distributed within the rabbit kidney. *Proc. Natl. Acad. Sci. USA,* **1994,** *91:*4544–4548.

Pickkers, P., Hughes, A.D., Russel, F.G., Thien, T., and Smits, P. *In vivo* evidence for K_{Ca} channel opening properties of acetazolamide in the human vasculature. *Br. J. Pharmacol.,* **2001,** *132:*443–450.

Pitt, B., Remme, W., Zannad, F., *et al.,* for the Eplerenone Post-Acute Myocardial Infarction Heart Failure Efficacy and Survival Study Investigators. Eplerenone, a selective aldosterone blocker, in patients with left ventricular dysfunction after myocardial infarction. *New Engl. J. Med.,* **2003,** *348:*1309–1321.

Pitt, B., Zannad, F., Remme, W., *et al.,* for the Randomized Aldactone Evaluation Study Investigators. The effect of spironolactone on morbidity and mortality in patients with severe heart failure. Randomized Aldactone Evaluation Study Investigators. *New Engl. J. Med.,* **1999,** *341:*709–717.

Plata, C., Meade, P., Hall, A., *et al.* Alternatively spliced isoform of apical Na⁺–K⁺–Cl⁻ cotransporter gene encodes a furosemide-sensitive Na⁺–Cl⁻ cotransporter. *Am. J. Physiol. Renal Physiol.,* **2001,** *280:*F574–F582.

Plata, C., Mount, D.B., Rubio, V., Hebert, S.C., and Gamba, G. Isoforms of the Na–K–2Cl cotransporter in murine TAL: II. Functional characterization and activation by cAMP. *Am. J. Physiol.,* **1999,** *276:*F359–F366.

Plotkin, M.D., Kaplan, M.R., Verlander, J.W., *et al.* Localization of the thiazide-sensitive Na–Cl cotransporter *rTSC1* in the rat kidney. *Kidney Int.,* **1996,** *50:*174–183.

Ramires, F.J., Mansur, A., Coelho, O., *et al.* Effect of spironolactone on ventricular arrhythmias in congestive heart failure secondary to idiopathic dilated or to ischemic cardiomyopathy. *Am. J. Cardiol.,* **2000,** *85:*1207–1211.

Rejnmark, L, Vestergaard, P., Pedersen, A.R., *et al.* Dose-effect relations of loop and thiazide diuretics on calcium homeostasis: A randomized, double-blinded, Latin-square, multiple cross-over study in postmenopausal osteopenic women. *Eur. J. Clin. Invest.,* **2003,** *33:*41–50.

Rudy, D.W., Voelker, J.R., Greene, P.K., Esparza, F.A., and Brater, D.C. Loop diuretics for chronic renal insufficiency: A continuous infusion is more efficacious than bolus therapy. *Ann. Intern. Med.,* **1991,** *115:*360–366.

Saito, F., and Kimura, G. Antihypertensive mechanism of diuretics based on pressure–natriuresis relationship. *Hypertension,* **1996,** *27:*914–918.

Sciarrone, M.T., Stella, P., Barlassina, C., *et al.* ACE and α-adducin polymorphism as markers of individual response to diuretic therapy. *Hypertension.* **2003,** *41:*398–403.

Solomon, R., Werner, C., Mann, D., DíElia, J., and Silva, P. Effects of saline, mannitol, and furosemide to prevent acute decreases in renal function induced by radiocontrast agents. *New Engl. J. Med.,* **1994,** *331:*1416–1420.

Takeda, M., Yoshitomi, K., and Imai, M. Regulation of Na⁺–3HCO₃⁻ cotransport in rabbit convoluted tubule via adenosine A_1 receptor. *Am. J. Physiol.,* **1993,** *265:*F511–F519.

The ALLHAT Officers and Coordinators for the ALLHAT Collaborative Research Group. The Antihypertensive and Lipid-Lowering Treatment to Prevent Heart Attack Trial. Major outcomes in high-risk hypertensive patients randomized to angiotensin-converting enzyme inhibitor or calcium channel blocker vs. diuretic: The Antihypertensive and Lipid-Lowering Treatment to Prevent Heart Attack Trial (ALLHAT). *JAMA,* **2002,** *288:*2981–2997.

van Buren, M., Bijlsma, J.A., Boer, P., van Rijn, H.J., and Koomans, H.A. Natriuretic and hypotensive effect of adenosine-1 blockade in essential hypertension. *Hypertension,* **1993,** *22:*728–734.

van der Heijden, M., Donders, S.H., Cleophas, T.J., *et al.* A randomized, placebo-controlled study of loop diuretics in patients with essential hypertension: The Bumetanide and Furosemide on Lipid Profile (BUFUL) Clinical Study report. *J. Clin. Pharmacol.,* **1998,** *38:*630–635.

Velazquez, H., Bartiss, A., Bernstein, P., and Ellison, D. H. Adrenal steroids stimulate thiazide-sensitive NaCl transport by rat renal distal tubules. *Am. J. Physiol.,* **1996,** *270:*F211–F219.

Weinberger, M.H., Roniker, B., Krause, S.L., and Weiss, R.J. Eplerenone, a selective aldosterone blocker, in mild to moderate hypertension. *Am. J. Hypertens.,* **2002,** *15:*709–716.

White, W.B., Carr, A.A., Krause, S., *et al.* Assessment of the novel selective aldosterone blocker eplerenone using ambulatory and clinical blood pressure in patients with systemic hypertension. *Am. J. Cardiol.,* **2003,** *92:*38–42.

Wilcox, C.S., Welch, W.J., Schreiner, G.F., and Belardinelli, L. Natriuretic and diuretic actions of a highly selective A_1 receptor antagonist. *J. Am. Soc. Nephrol.,* **1999,** *10:*714–720.

Xu, J.C., Lytle, C., Zhu, T.T., *et al.* Molecular cloning and functional expression of the bumetanide-sensitive Na–K–Cl cotransporter. *Proc. Natl. Acad. Sci. USA,* **1994,** *91:*2201–2205.

MONOGRAPHS AND REVIEWS

Brater, D.C. Clinical pharmacology of loop diuretics. *Drugs,* **1991,** *41:*14–22.

Brater, D.C. Diuretic therapy. *New Engl. J. Med.,* **1998,** *339:*387–395.

Chobanian, A., Bakris, G., Black, R., *et al.,* and National High Blood Pressure Education Program Coordinating Committee. Seventh report of the Joint National Committee on Prevention, Detection, Evaluation and Treatment of High Blood Pressure. *Hypertension,* **2003,** *42:*1206–1252.

Coote, J.H. Pharmacological control of altitude sickness. *Trends Pharmacol. Sci.,* **1991,** *12:*450–455.

Dormans, T.P., Pickkers, P., Russel, F.G., and Smits, P. Vascular effects of loop diuretics. *Cardiovasc. Res.,* **1996,** *32:*988–997.

Dresser, M.J., Leabman, M.K., and Giacomini, K.M. Transporters involved in the elimination of drugs in the kidney: Organic anion transporters and organic cation transporters. *J. Pharm. Sci.,* **2001,** *90:*397–421.

Ellison, D.H. Diuretic resistance: Physiology and therapeutics. *Semin. Nephrol.,* **1999,** *19:*581–597.

Eraly, S.A., Bush, K.T., Sampogna, R.V., Bhatnagar, V., and Nigam, S.K. The molecular pharmacology of organic anion transporters: From DNA to FDA? *Mol. Pharmacol.,* **2004,** *65:*479–487.

Friedman, P.A., and Bushinsky, D.A. Diuretic effects on calcium metabolism. *Semin. Nephrol.,* **1999,** *19*:551–556.

Guyton, A.C. Blood pressure control: Special role of the kidneys and body fluids. *Science,* **1991,** *252*:1813–1816.

Hebert, S.C. Molecular mechanisms. *Semin. Nephrol.,* **1999,** *19*:504–523.

Hoes, A.W., and Grobbee, D.E. Diuretics and risk of sudden death in hypertension: Evidence and potential implications. *Clin. Exp. Hypertens.,* **1996,** *18*:523–535.

Jackson, E.K. A$_1$ receptor antagonists as diuretic/natriuretic agents. *Drug Future,* **2002,** *27*:1057–1069.

Kaplan, M.R., Mount, D.B., and Delpire, E. Molecular mechanisms of NaCl cotransport. *Annu. Rev. Physiol.,* **1996,** *58*:649–668.

Kaplan, N.M. Diuretics: correct use in hypertension. *Semin. Nephrol.,* **1999,** *19*:569–574.

Kellum, J.A. Use of diuretics in the acute care setting. *Kidney Int. Suppl.,* **1998,** *66*:S67–S70.

Kleyman, T.R., Sheng, S., Kosari, F., and Kieber-Emmons, T. Mechanisms of action of amiloride: A molecular prospective. *Semin. Nephrol.,* **1999,** *19*:524–532.

Knauf, H., and Mutschler, E. Clinical pharmacokinetics and pharmacodynamics of torsemide. *Clin. Pharmacokinet.,* **1998,** *34*:1–24.

Levinsky, N.G., and Bernard, D.B. Mannitol and loop diuretics in acute renal failure. In, *Acute Renal Failure,* 2d ed. (Brenner, B.M., and Lazarus, J.M. eds.) Churchill-Livingstone, New York, 1988, pp. 841–856.

Puschett, J.B., and Winaver, J. Effects of diuretics on renal function. In, *Handbook of Physiology.* Sec. 8, Vol. 2. (Windhager, E.E. ed.) Oxford University Press, New York, 1992, pp. 2335–2404.

Roden, D.M. Torsade de pointes. *Clin. Cardiol.,* **1993,** *16*:683–686.

Sands, J.M., and Kokko, J.P. Current concepts of the countercurrent multiplication system. *Kidney Int. Suppl.,* **1996,** *57*:S93–S99.

Shankar, S.S., and Brater, D.C. Loop diuretics: from the Na–K–2Cl transporter to clinical use. *Am. J. Physiol. Renal Physiol.,* **2003,** *284*:F11–F21.

Simon, D.B., and Lifton, R.P. Mutations in Na(K)Cl transporters in Gitleman's and Bartter's syndromes. *Curr. Opin. Cell Biol.,* **1998,** *10*:450–454.

Wilcox, C.S. Metabolic and adverse effects of diuretics. *Semin. Nephrol.,* **1999,** *19*:557–568.

VASOPRESSIN AND OTHER AGENTS AFFECTING THE RENAL CONSERVATION OF WATER

Edwin K. Jackson

Precise regulation of body fluid osmolality is essential. It is controlled by a finely tuned, intricate homeostatic mechanism that operates by adjusting both the rate of water intake and the rate of solute-free water excretion by the kidneys—*i.e.,* water balance. Abnormalities in this homeostatic system can result from genetic diseases, acquired diseases, or drugs and may cause serious and potentially life-threatening deviations in plasma osmolality. This chapter describes the physiological mechanisms that regulate plasma osmolality, discusses the diseases that perturb those mechanisms, and examines pharmacological approaches for treating disorders of water balance.

Arginine vasopressin (the antidiuretic hormone in human beings) is the main hormone that regulates body fluid osmolality. Many diseases of water homeostasis and many pharmacological strategies for correcting such disorders pertain to vasopressin. Accordingly, this chapter focuses on vasopressin, including (1) chemistry (including the chemistry of vasopressin agonists and antagonists), (2) physiology (including anatomical considerations; the synthesis, transport, and storage of vasopressin; and the regulation of vasopressin secretion), (3) basic pharmacology (including vasopressin receptors and their signal-transduction pathways, renal actions of vasopressin, pharmacological modification of the antidiuretic response to vasopressin, and nonrenal actions of vasopressin), (4) diseases affecting the vasopressin system (diabetes insipidus, syndrome of inappropriate secretion of antidiuretic hormone, and other water-retaining states), and (5) clinical pharmacology of vasopressin peptides (therapeutic uses, pharmacokinetics, toxicities, adverse effects, contraindications, and drug interactions). A small number of other drugs can be used to treat abnormalities of water balance; a discussion of these agents is integrated into the section on diseases affecting the vasopressin system.

INTRODUCTION TO VASOPRESSIN

Immunoreactive vasopressin occurs in neurons from organisms belonging to the first animal phylum with a nervous system (*e.g., Hydra attenuata*), and vasopressinlike peptides have been isolated and characterized from both mammalian and nonmammalian vertebrates, as well as from invertebrates (Table 29–1). Genes encoding vasopressinlike peptides probably evolved more than 700 million years ago.

With the emergence of life on land, vasopressin became the mediator of a remarkable regulatory system for the conservation of water. The hormone is released by the posterior pituitary whenever water deprivation causes an increased plasma osmolality or whenever the cardiovascular system is challenged by hypovolemia and/or hypotension. In amphibians, the target organs for vasopressin are skin and the urinary bladder, whereas in other vertebrates, including humans, vasopressin acts primarily in the renal collecting duct. In each of these target tissues, vasopressin increases the permeability of the cell membrane to water, thus permitting water to move passively down an osmotic gradient across skin, bladder, or collecting duct into the extracellular compartment.

In view of the long evolutionary history of vasopressin, it is not surprising that vasopressin acts at sites in the nephron other than the collecting duct and on tissues other than the kidney. Vasopressin is a potent vasopressor; indeed, its name was chosen originally in recognition of this vasoconstrictor action. Vasopressin is a neurotransmitter; among its

Table 29–1
Vasopressin Receptor Agonists

I. NATURALLY OCCURRING VASOPRESSIN-LIKE PEPTIDES

	A	W	X	Y	Z
A. *Vertebrates*					
1. Mammals					
Arginine vasopressin* (AVP) (human beings and other mammals)	NH_2	Tyr	Phe	Gln	Arg
Lypressin* (pigs, marsupials)	NH_2	Tyr	Phe	Gln	Lys
Phenypressin (macropodids)	NH_2	Phe	Phe	Gln	Arg
2. Nonmammalian vertebrates					
Vasotocin	NH_2	Tyr	Ile	Gln	Arg
B. *Invertebrates*					
1. Arginine conopressin (*Conus striatus*)	NH_2	Ile	Ile	Arg	Arg
2. Lysine conopressin (*Conus geographicus*)	NH_2	Phe	Ile	Arg	Lys
3. Locust subesophageal ganglia peptide	NH_2	Leu	Ile	Thr	Arg

II. SYNTHETIC VASOPRESSIN PEPTIDES

	A	W	X	Y	Z
A. *V_1-selective agonists*					
1. V_{1a}-Selective Agonist [Phe², Ile³, Orn⁸]AVP	NH_2	Phe	Ile	Gln	Orn
2. V_{1b}-Selective Agonist Deamino [D-3-(3′-pyridyl)-Ala²]AVP	H	D-3-(3′-pyridyl)-Ala²	Phe	Gln	Arg
B. *V_2-selective agonists*					
1. Desmopressin* (DDAVP)	H	Tyr	Phe	Gln	D-Arg
2. Deamino[Val⁴, D-Arg⁸]AVP	H	Tyr	Phe	Val	D-Arg

III. NONPEPTIDE AGONIST

A. *OPC-51803*

*Available for clinical use.

actions in the central nervous system (CNS) are apparent roles in the secretion of adrenocorticotropic hormone (ACTH) and in the regulation of the cardiovascular system, temperature, and other visceral functions. Vasopressin also promotes the release of coagulation factors by the vascular endothelium and increases platelet aggregability; therefore, it may play a role in hemostasis.

PHYSIOLOGY OF VASOPRESSIN

Anatomy. The antidiuretic mechanism in mammals involves two anatomical components: a CNS component for the synthesis, transport, storage, and release of vasopressin and a renal collecting-duct system composed of epithelial cells that respond to vasopressin by increasing their permeability to water. The CNS component of the

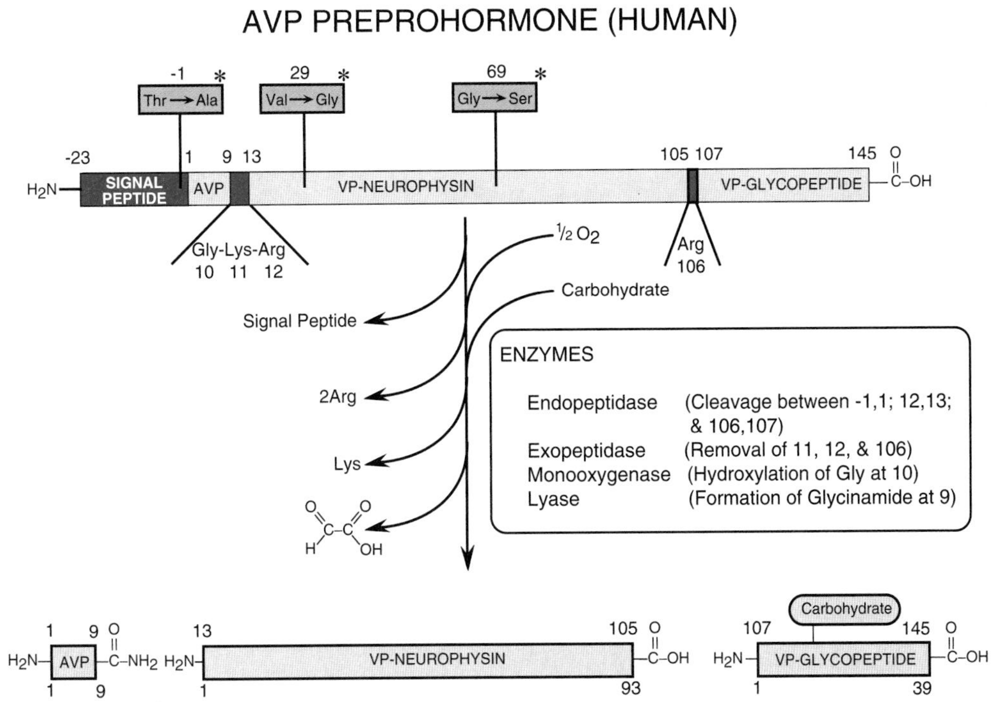

Figure 29–1. *Processing of the 168–amino acid human 8-arginine vasopressin (AVP) preprohormone to AVP, vasopressin (VP)–neurophysin, and VP–glycopeptide.* At least 40 mutations in the single gene on chromosome 20 that encodes AVP preprohormone give rise to central diabetes insipidus. *Boxes indicate mutations leading to central diabetes insipidus.

antidiuretic mechanism is called the *hypothalamiconeurohypophyseal system* and consists of neurosecretory neurons with perikarya located predominantly in two specific hypothalamic nuclei, the supraoptic nucleus (SON) and the paraventricular nucleus (PVN). The long axons of magnocellular neurons in the SON and PVN transverse the external zone of the median eminence to terminate in the neural lobe of the posterior pituitary (neurohypophysis), where they release vasopressin and oxytocin. In addition, axons of parvicellular neurons project to the external zone of the median eminence and release vasopressin directly into the pituitary portal circulation. The relevant anatomy of the renal collecting-duct system is described in Chapter 28.

Synthesis. Vasopressin and oxytocin are synthesized mainly in the perikarya of magnocellular neurons in the SON and PVN; the two hormones are synthesized predominantly in separate neurons. Parvicellular neurons in the PVN also synthesize vasopressin. Vasopressin synthesis appears to be regulated solely at the transcriptional level. In human beings, a 168–amino acid preprohormone (Figure 29–1) is synthesized, and a signal peptide (residues −23 to −1) ensures incorporation of the nascent polypeptide into ribosomes. During synthesis, the signal peptide is removed to form the vasopressin prohormone, which then is processed and incorporated into the Golgi compartment and then into membrane-associated granules. The prohormone contains three domains: vasopressin (residues 1 to 9), vasopressin (VP)–neurophysin (residues 13 to 105), and VP–glycopeptide (residues 107 to 145). The vasopressin domain is linked to the VP–neurophysin domain through a glycine–lysine–arginine–processing signal, and the VP–neurophysin is linked to the VP–glycopeptide domain by an arginine-processing signal. In the secretory granules, an endopeptidase, exopeptidase, monooxygenase,

and lyase act sequentially on the prohormone to produce vasopressin, VP–neurophysin (sometimes referred to as *neurophysin II* or *MSEL–neurophysin*), and VP–glycopeptide (sometimes called *copeptin*). The synthesis and transport of vasopressin depend on the conformation of the preprohormone. In particular, VP–neurophysin binds vasopressin and is critical to the correct processing, transport, and storage of vasopressin. Genetic mutations in either the signal peptide or VP–neurophysin give rise to central diabetes insipidus.

Transport and Storage. The process of axonal transport of vasopressin- and oxytocin-containing granules is rapid, and these hormone-laden granules arrive at their destinations within 30 minutes, ready for release by exocytosis when the magnocellular or parvicellular neurons are stimulated appropriately.

Maximal release of vasopressin occurs when impulse frequency is approximately 12 spikes per second for 20 seconds. Higher frequencies or longer periods of stimulation lead to diminished hormone release (fatigue). Appropriately, vasopressin-releasing cells demonstrate an atypical pattern of spike activity characterized by rapid phasic bursts (5 to 12 spikes per second for 15 to 60 seconds) separated by quiescent periods (15 to 60 seconds in duration). This pattern is orchestrated by activation and inactivation of ion channels in the magnocellular neurons and provides for optimal release of vasopressin.

Vasopressin Synthesis Outside the CNS. Vasopressin also is synthesized by the heart (Hupf *et al.*, 1999) and adrenal gland (Guillon *et al.*, 1998). In the heart, elevated wall stress increases vasopressin synthesis severalfold. Cardiac synthesis of vasopressin is predominantly vascular and perivascular and may contribute to impaired ventricular relaxation and coronary vasoconstriction. Vasopressin

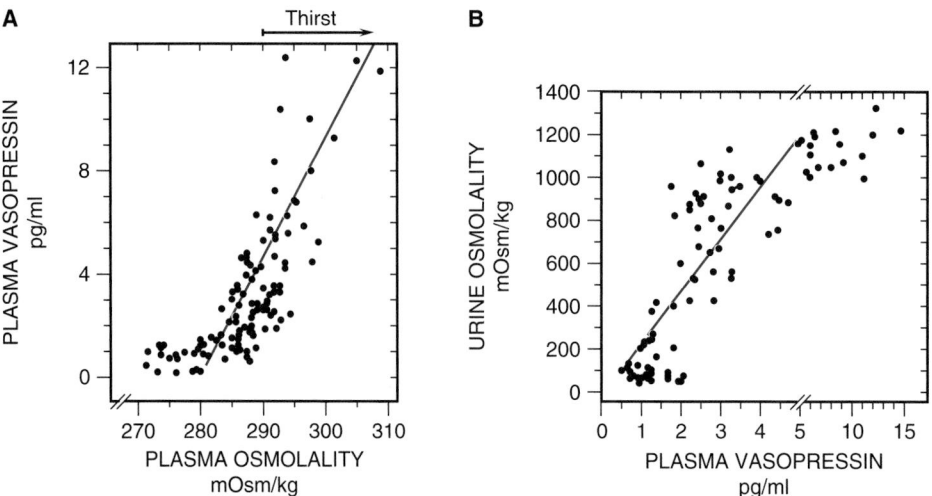

Figure 29–2. *A.* The relationship between plasma osmolality and plasma vasopressin levels. Plasma osmolality associated with thirst is indicated by arrow. *B.* The relationship between plasma vasopressin levels and urine osmolality. (From Robertson *et al.*, 1977, and Kovacs and Robertson, 1992, with permission.)

synthesis in the adrenal medulla stimulates catecholamine secretion from chromaffin cells and may promote adrenal cortical growth and stimulate aldosterone synthesis.

Regulation of Vasopressin Secretion. An increase in plasma osmolality is the principal physiological stimulus for vasopressin secretion by the posterior pituitary (Bankir, 2001). Severe hypovolemia/hypotension also is a powerful stimulus for vasopressin release. In addition, pain, nausea, and hypoxia can stimulate vasopressin secretion, and several endogenous hormones and pharmacological agents can modify vasopressin release.

Hyperosmolality. The relationship between plasma osmolality and plasma vasopressin concentration is shown in Figure 29–2A, and the relationship between plasma vasopressin levels and urine osmolality is illustrated in Figure 29–2B. The osmolality threshold for secretion is approximately 280 mOsm/kg. Below the threshold, vasopressin is barely detectable in plasma, and above the threshold, vasopressin levels are a steep and relatively linear function of plasma osmolality. A small increase in plasma osmolality leads to enhanced vasopressin secretion. Indeed, a 2% elevation in plasma osmolality causes a two- to threefold increase in plasma vasopressin levels, which, in turn, causes increased solute-free water reabsorption, with an increase in urine osmolality. Increases in plasma osmolality above 290 mOsm/kg lead to an intense desire for water (thirst). Thus the vasopressin system affords the organism longer thirst-free periods and, in the event that water is unavailable, allows the organism to survive longer periods of water deprivation. It is important to point out, however,

that above a plasma osmolality of approximately 290 mOsm/kg, plasma levels of vasopressin exceed 5 p*M*. Since urinary concentration is maximal (about 1200 mOsm/kg) when vasopressin levels exceed 5 p*M*, further defense against hypertonicity depends entirely on water intake rather than on decreases in water loss.

Several CNS structures are involved in osmotic stimulation of vasopressin release by the posterior pituitary; these structures are collectively referred to as the *osmoreceptive complex.* Although magnocellular neurons in the SON and PVN are osmosensitive, afferent inputs from other components of the osmoreceptive complex are required for a normal vasopressin response. The SON and PVN receive projections from the subfornical organ (SFO) and the organum vasculosum of the lamina terminalis (OVLT) either directly or indirectly *via* the median preoptic nucleus (MnPO). Subgroups of neurons in the SFO, OVLT, and MnPO are either osmoreceptors or osmoresponders (*i.e.,* are stimulated by osmoreceptive neurons located at other sites). Thus a web of interconnecting neurons contributes to osmotically induced vasopressin secretion.

Aquaporin 4, a water-selective channel, is associated with CNS structures involved in osmoregulation and may confer osmosensitivity. In the CNS, aquaporin 4 resides on glial and ependymal cells rather than on neurons, suggesting that osmotic status may be communicated to the neuronal cell by a glial–neuron interaction (Wells, 1998).

Hepatic Portal Osmoreceptors. An oral salt load activates hepatic portal osmoreceptors leading to increased vasopressin release. This mechanism augments plasma vasopressin levels even before the oral salt load increases plasma osmolality (Stricker *et al.*, 2002).

Hypovolemia and Hypotension. Vasopressin secretion also is regulated hemodynamically by changes in effective blood volume and/or arterial blood pressure (Robertson, 1992). Regardless of the cause (*e.g.*, hemorrhage, sodium depletion, diuretics, heart failure, hepatic cirrhosis with ascites, adrenal insufficiency, or hypotensive drugs), reductions in effective blood volume and/or arterial blood pressure may be associated with high circulating concentrations of vasopressin. However, unlike osmoregulation, hemodynamic regulation of vasopressin secretion is exponential; *i.e.*, small decreases (5% to 10%) in blood volume and/or pressure have little effect on vasopressin secretion, whereas larger decreases (20% to 30%) can increase vasopressin levels to 20 to 30 times normal levels (exceeding the concentration of vasopressin required to induce maximal antidiuresis). Vasopressin is one of the most potent vasoconstrictors known, and the vasopressin response to hypovolemia or hypotension serves as a mechanism to stave off cardiovascular collapse during periods of severe blood loss and/or hypotension. Hemodynamic regulation of vasopressin secretion does not disrupt osmotic regulation; rather, hypovolemia/hypotension alters the set point and slope of the plasma osmolality–plasma vasopressin relationship (Figure 29–3).

The neuronal pathways that mediate hemodynamic regulation of vasopressin release are different from those involved in osmoregulation. Baroreceptors in the left atrium, left ventricle, and pulmonary veins sense blood volume (filling pressures), and baroreceptors in the carotid sinus and aorta monitor arterial blood pressure. Nerve impulses reach brainstem nuclei predominantly through the vagal trunk and glossopharyngeal nerve; these signals are relayed to the solitary tract nucleus, then to the A_1-noradrenergic cell group in the caudal ventrolateral medulla, and finally to the SON and PVN.

Hormones and Neurotransmitters. Vasopressin-synthesizing magnocellular neurons have a large array of receptors on both perikarya and nerve terminals; therefore, vasopressin release can be accentuated or attenuated by chemical agents acting at both ends of the magnocellular neuron. Also, hormones and neurotransmitters can modulate vasopressin secretion by stimulating or inhibiting neurons in nuclei that project, either directly or indirectly, to the SON and PVN. Because of these complexities, the results of any given investigation may depend critically on the route of administration of the agent and on the experimental paradigm. In many cases, the precise mechanism by which a given agent modulates vasopressin secretion is either unknown or controversial, and the physiological relevance of modulation of vasopressin secretion by most hormones and neurotransmitters is unclear.

Nonetheless, several agents are known to stimulate vasopressin secretion, including acetylcholine (*via* nicotinic receptors), histamine (*via* H_1 receptors), dopamine (*via* both D_1 and D_2 receptors), glutamine, aspartate, cholecystokinin, neuropeptide Y, substance P, vasoactive intestinal polypeptide, prostaglandins, and angiotensin II. Inhibitors of vasopressin secretion include atrial natriuretic peptide, γ-aminobutyric acid, and opioids (particularly dynorphin *via* κ receptors). The affects of angiotensin II have received the most attention. Angiotensin II, applied directly to magnocellular neurons in the SON and PVN, increases neuronal excitability; when applied to the MnPO, angiotensin II indirectly stimulates magnocellular neurons in the SON and PVN. In addition, angiotensin II stimulates angiotensin-sensitive neurons in the OVLT and SFO (circumventricular nuclei lacking a blood–brain barrier) that project to the SON/PVN. Thus angiotensin II synthesized in the brain and circulating angiotensin may stimulate vasopressin release. Inhibition of the conversion of angiotensin II to angiotensin III blocks angiotensin II–induced vasopressin release, suggesting that angiotensin III is the main effector peptide of the brain renin–angiotensin system controlling vasopressin release (Reaux *et al.*, 2001).

Pharmacological Agents. A number of drugs alter urine osmolality by stimulating or inhibiting the secretion of vasopressin. In some cases the mechanism by which a drug alters vasopressin secretion involves direct effects on one or more CNS structures that regulate vasopressin secretion. In other cases vasopressin secretion is altered indirectly by the effects of a drug on blood volume, arterial blood pressure, pain, or nausea. In most cases the mechanism is not known. Stimulators of vasopressin secretion include vincristine, cyclophosphamide, tricyclic antidepressants, nicotine, epinephrine, and high doses of morphine. Lithium, which inhibits the renal effects of vasopressin, also enhances vasopressin secretion. Inhibitors of vasopressin secretion include ethanol, phenytoin, low doses of morphine, glucocorticoids, fluphenazine, haloperidol, promethazine, oxilorphan, and butorphanol. Carbamazepine has a renal action to produce antidiuresis in patients with central diabetes insipidus but actually inhibits vasopressin secretion *via* a central action.

BASIC PHARMACOLOGY OF VASOPRESSIN

Vasopressin Receptors. The cellular effects of vasopressin are mediated mainly by interactions of the hormone with the three types of receptors, V_{1a}, V_{1b}, and V_2. The V_{1a} receptor is the most widespread subtype of vasopressin receptor; it is found in vascular smooth muscle, the adrenal gland, myometrium, the bladder, adipocytes, hepatocytes, platelets, renal medullary interstitial cells, vasa recta in the renal microcirculation, epithelial cells in the

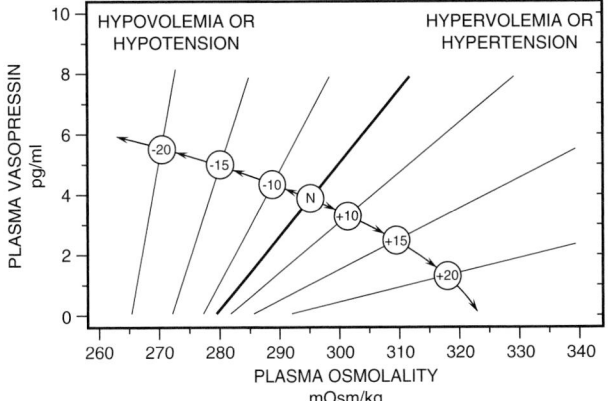

Figure 29–3. Interactions between osmolality and hypovolemia/hypotension. Numbers in circles refer to percentage increase (+) or decrease (−) in blood volume or arterial blood pressure. N indicates normal blood volume/blood pressure. (From Robertson, 1992, with permission.)

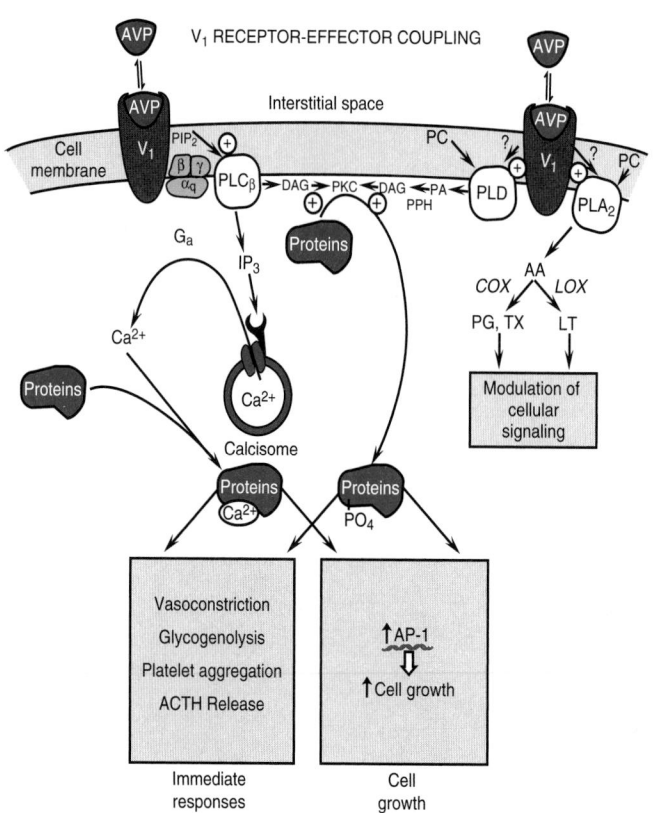

Figure 29–4. *Mechanism of V_1 receptor–effector coupling.* Binding of 8-arginine vasopressin (AVP) to V_1 vasopressin receptors (V_1) stimulates several membrane-bound phospholipases. Stimulation of the G_q–PLC–β pathway results in IP_3 formation, mobilization of intracellular Ca^{2+}, and activation of PKC. Activation of V_1 receptors also causes influx of extracellular Ca^{2+} by an unknown (?) mechanism. PKC and Ca^{2+}/calmodulin–activated protein kinases phosphorylate cell-type-specific proteins leading to cellular responses. A further component of the AVP response derives from the production of eicosanoids secondary to the activation of PLA_2; the resulting mobilization of arachidonic acid (AA) provides substrate for eicosanoid synthesis *via* the cyclooxygenase (COX) and lipoxygenase (LOX) pathways, leading to local production of prostaglandins (PG), thromboxanes (TX), and leukotrienes (LT), which may activate a variety of signaling pathways, including those linked to G_S and G_q. Biological effects mediated by the V_1 receptor include vasoconstriction, glycogenolysis, platelet aggregation, ACTH release, and growth of vascular smooth muscle cells. The effects of vasopressin on cell growth involve transcriptional regulation *via* the FOS/JUN AP-1 transcription complex.

renal cortical collecting-duct, spleen, testis, and many CNS structures. V_{1b} receptors have a more limited distribution and are found in the anterior pituitary, several brain regions, the pancreas, and the adrenal medulla. V_2 receptors are located predominantly in principal cells of the renal collecting-duct system but also are present on epithelial cells in the thick ascending limb and on vascular endothelial cells. Although originally defined by pharmacological criteria, vasopressin receptors now are defined by their primary amino acid sequences. The cloned vasopressin receptors are typical heptahelical G protein–coupled receptors. Manning and coworkers (1999) have synthesized novel hypotensive vasopressin peptide agonists that do not interact with V_{1a}, V_{1b}, or V_2 receptors and may stimulate a putative vasopressin vasodilatory receptor.

Finally, two additional putative receptors for vasopressin have been cloned. A vasopressin-activated Ca^{2+}-mobilizing receptor with one transmembrane domain binds vasopressin and increases intracellular Ca^{2+} (Serradeil-Le Gal *et al.*, 2002b). A dual angiotensin II–vasopressin heptahelical receptor activates adenylyl cyclase in response to both angiotensin II and vasopressin (Serradeil-Le Gal *et al.*, 2002b). The physiological roles of these putative vasopressin receptors are unclear.

V_1 Receptor–Effector Coupling. Figure 29–4 summarizes the current model of V_1 receptor–effector coupling. Vasopressin binding to V_1 receptors activates the G_q–PLC pathway, thereby increasing the generation of IP_3 and diacylglycerol (*see* Chapter 1 for further discussion of these signal-transduction pathways). These mediators, in turn, increase the intracellular Ca^{2+} concentration and activate protein kinase C, ultimately causing biological effects that include immediate responses (*e.g.,* vasoconstriction, glycogenolysis, platelet aggregation, and ACTH release) and growth of smooth muscle cells. This mitogenic effect involves activation of the AP-1 transcription factor and its c-fos and c-jun subunits. Other effects of V_1-receptor activation may be mediated by stimulation of small G proteins, activation of PLD and PLA_2, and activation of V_1-sensitive Ca^{2+} influx. Some effects of V_1-receptor activation are secondary to synthesis of prostaglandins and epoxyeicosatrienoic acids, which act through the eicosanoid receptors (*see* Chapter 25).

V_2 Receptor–Effector Coupling. Principal cells in the renal collecting duct have V_2 receptors on their basolateral membranes that couple to G_S to stimulate adenylyl cyclase activity (Figure 29–5) when vasopressin binds to V_2 receptors. The resulting increase in cellular cyclic AMP content and protein kinase A (PKA) activity triggers an increased rate of insertion of water channel–containing vesicles (WCVs) into the apical membrane and a decreased rate of endocytosis of WCVs from the apical membrane (Snyder *et al.,* 1992). The distribution of WCVs between the cytosolic compartment and the apical membrane compartment is thus shifted in favor of the apical membrane compartment (Nielsen *et al.,* 1999). Because WCVs contain preformed functional water channels (aquaporin 2), their net shift into apical membranes in response to V_2-receptor stimulation greatly increases the water permeability of the apical membrane.

Aquaporins are a family of water channel proteins that allow water molecules to cross biological membranes (Marples *et al.,* 1999; Nielsen *et al.,* 2001; Agre and Konzo, 2003). Aquaporins have six membrane domains connected by five loops (A to E; Figure 29–6). Loops B and E dip into the cell membrane, and the asparagine–proline–alanine sequences in each B and E loop interact to form a water pore. Aquaporins generally form tetramers in cell membranes. Of the 10 cloned mammalian aquaporins, at least 7 are found in the kidney. Aquaporin 1 is present in the apical and basolateral membrane of the proximal tubule and in the thin descending limb. Aquaporin 2 resides in the apical membrane and WCVs of the collecting-duct principal cells, whereas aquaporins 3 and 4 are present in the basolateral membrane of principal cells. Aquaporin 7 is in the apical brush border of the straight proximal tubule. Aquaporins 6 and 8 are located intracellulary in the collecting-duct principal cells. Aquaporin 2, the water channel in WCVs, is phosphorylated on serine 256 by PKA, ultimately leading to vasopressin-induced insertion of WCVs into apical membranes (Nishimoto *et al.,* 1999). PKA is targeted to WCVs by specific anchoring proteins (Klussmann and Rosenthal, 2001). In addition to increasing the insertion of aquaporin 2 into apical membranes in collecting-duct principal cells, vasopressin also increases the expression of aquaporin 2 mRNA and protein (Marples *et al.,* 1999), largely mediated by increased phosphorylation of the cyclic AMP–response element–binding protein (CREB) and increased transcription of the gene encoding aquaporin 2. Thus chronic dehydration leads to long-term up-regulation of aquaporin 2 and water transport in the collecting duct.

For maximum concentration of urine, large amounts of urea must be deposited in the interstitium of the inner medullary collecting duct. It is not surprising, therefore, that V_2-receptor activation also increases urea permeability by 400% in the terminal portions of the inner medullary collecting duct. The V_2 receptors increase urea permeability by activating a vasopressin-regulated urea transporter (termed *VRUT, UT1,* or *UT-A1*), most likely by PKA-induced phosphorylation (Sands, 2003). The kinetics of vasopressin-induced water and urea permeability differ, and vasopressin-induced regula-

V_2 RECEPTOR-EFFECTOR COUPLING

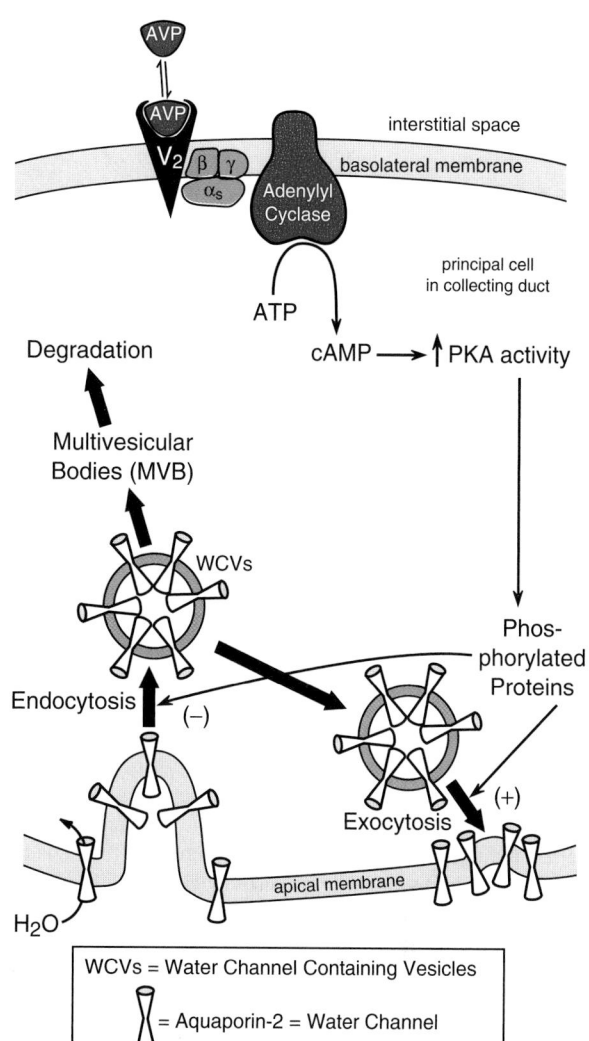

Figure 29–5. *Mechanism of V_2 receptor–effector coupling.* Binding of vasopressin (AVP) to the V_2 receptor activates the G_S–adenylyl cyclase–cAMP–PKA pathway and shifts the balance of aquaporin 2 trafficking toward the apical membrane of the principal cell of the collecting duct, thus enhancing water permeability. Although phosphorylation of serine 256 of aquaporin 2 is involved in V_2 receptor signaling, other proteins located both in the water channel–containing vesicles and the apical membrane of the cytoplasm also may be involved.

tion of VRUT does not entail vesicular trafficking to the plasma membrane (Inoue *et al.,* 1999).

In addition to increasing the water permeability of the collecting duct and the urea permeability of the inner medullary collecting duct, V_2-receptor activation also increases Na^+ transport in the thick ascending limb and collecting duct. Increased Na^+ transport in the thick ascending limb is mediated by three mechanisms that affect the Na^+–K^+–$2Cl^-$ symporter, *i.e.,* rapid phosphorylation of the sym-

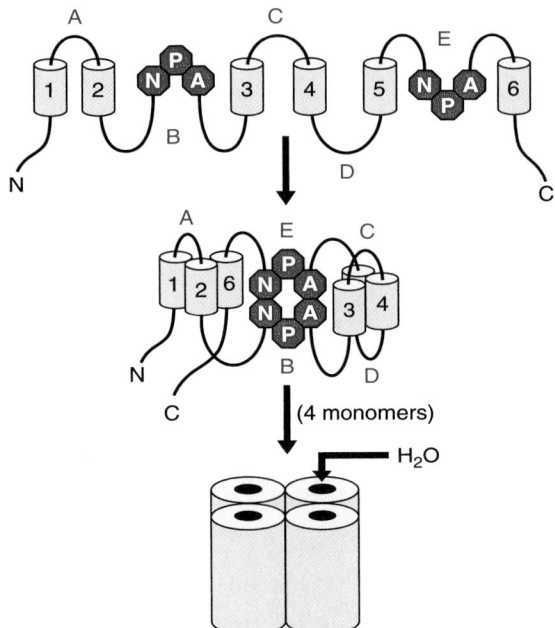

Figure 29–6. Structure of aquaporins. Aquaporins have six transmembrane domains, and the NH_2 and COOH termini are intracellular. Loops B and E each contain an asparagine–proline–alanine (NPA) sequence. Aquaporins fold with transmembrane domains 1, 2, and 6 in close proximity and transmembrane domains 3, 4 and 5 in juxtaposition. The long B and E loops dip into the membrane, and the NPA sequences align to create a pore through which water can diffuse. Most likely aquaporins form a tetrameric oligomer. At least seven aquaporins are expressed at distinct sites in the kidney. Aquaporin 1, abundant in the proximal tubule and descending thin limb, is essential for concentration of urine. Aquaporin 2, exclusively expressed in the principal cells of the connecting tubule and collecting duct, is the major vasopressin-regulated water channel. Aquaporin 3 and aquaporin 4 are expressed in the basolateral membranes of collecting-duct principal cells and provide exit pathways for water reabsorbed apically *via* aquaporin 2. Aquaporins 6 to 8 are also expressed in kidney; their functions remain to be clarified. Vasopressin regulates water permeability of the collecting duct by influencing the trafficking of aquaporin 2 from intracellular vesicles to the apical plasma membrane. Binding of AVP to V_2 receptors activates the G_s–adenylyl cyclase–cAMP–PKA pathway, leading to phosphorylation of ser256 on aquaporin 2. Phosphorylation (of three of the four monomers) promotes insertion of the tetramers into the apical membrane, increasing permeability to water. PKA also mediates longer-term regulation by enhancing transcription of the aquaporin 2 gene, thereby promoting aquaporin 2 synthesis. For details, *see* text and Nielsen *et al.*, 2001.

porter, translocation of the symporter into the luminal membrane, and increased expression of symporter protein (Ecelbarger *et al.*, 2001; Giménez and Forbush, 2003). Enhanced Na^+ transport in the collecting duct is mediated by increased expression of subunits of the epithelial sodium channel (Ecelbarger *et al.*, 2001). The multiple

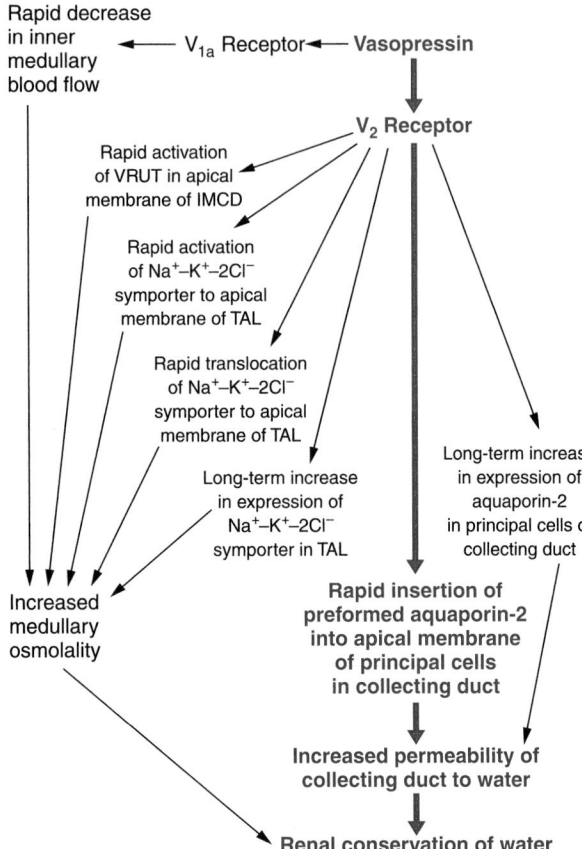

Figure 29–7. Mechanisms by which vasopressin increases the renal conservation of water. IMCD, inner medullary collecting duct; TAL, thick ascending limb; VRUT, vasopressin-regulated urea transporter. Thick and thin arrows denote major and minor pathways, respectively.

mechanisms by which vasopressin increases water reabsorption are summarized in Figure 29–7.

Renal Actions of Vasopressin. Several sites of vasopressin action in the kidney involve both V_1 and V_2 receptors (Bankir, 2001). V_1 receptors mediate contraction of mesangial cells in the glomerulus and contraction of vascular smooth muscle cells in the vasa recta and efferent arteriole. Indeed, V_1-receptor-mediated reduction of inner medullary blood flow contributes to the maximum concentrating capacity of the kidney (Franchini and Cowley, 1996) (Figure 29–7). V_1 receptors also stimulate prostaglandin synthesis by medullary interstitial cells. Since prostaglandin E_2 inhibits adenylyl cyclase in the collecting duct, stimulation of prostaglandin synthesis by V_1 receptors may counterbalance V_2-receptor-mediated antidiuresis. V_1 receptors on principal cells in the cortical collecting duct may inhibit V_2-receptor-mediated water flux *via* activation of protein kinase C (PKC). V_2 receptors mediate the most prominent response to vasopressin, *i.e.,* increased water permeability of the collecting duct. Indeed, vasopressin can increase water permeability in the collecting duct at concentrations as low as 50 f*M*. Thus V_2-receptor-mediated effects of vasopressin occur at concentrations far lower than are required to engage V_1-receptor-mediated actions. This differential sensitivity may not be due to differences in receptor affinities because cloned rat V_{1a} and V_2 receptors have similar affinities for vasopressin (K_d = 0.7 and 0.4 n*M*, respectively) but rather may be due to differential amplification of their signal-transduction pathways.

The collecting-duct system is critical for water conservation. By the time tubular fluid arrives at the cortical collecting duct, it has been rendered hypotonic by the upstream diluting segments of the nephron that reabsorb NaCl without reabsorbing water. In the well-hydrated subject, plasma osmolality is in the normal range, concentrations of vasopressin are low, the entire collecting duct is relatively impermeable to water, and the urine is dilute. Under conditions of dehydration, plasma osmolality is increased, concentrations of vasopressin are elevated, and the collecting duct becomes permeable to water. The osmotic gradient between the dilute tubular urine and the hypertonic renal interstitial fluid (which becomes progressively more hypertonic in deeper regions of the renal medulla) provides for the osmotic flux of water out of the collecting duct. The final osmolality of urine may be as high as 1200 mOsm/kg in human beings, and a significant saving of solute-free water thus is possible.

Other renal actions mediated by V_2 receptors include increased urea transport in the inner medullary collecting duct and increased Na^+ transport in the thick ascending limb; both effects contribute to the urine-concentrating ability of the kidney (Figure 29–7). V_2 receptors also increase Na^+ transport in the cortical collecting duct (Ecelbarger *et al.*, 2001), and this may synergize with aldosterone to enhance Na^+ reabsorption during hypovolemia.

Pharmacological Modification of the Antidiuretic Response to Vasopressin. *Nonsteroidal antiinflammatory drugs* (NSAIDs) (*see* Chapter 26), particularly *indomethacin*, enhance the antidiuretic response to vasopressin. Since prostaglandins attenuate antidiuretic responses to vasopressin and NSAIDs inhibit prostaglandin synthesis, reduced prostaglandin production probably accounts for the potentiation of vasopressin's antidiuretic response. *Carbamazepine* and *chlorpropamide* also enhance the antidiuretic effects of vasopressin by unknown mechanisms. In rare instances, chlorpropamide can induce water intoxication.

A number of drugs inhibit the antidiuretic actions of vasopressin. *Lithium* is of particular importance because of its use in the treatment of manic–depressive disorders. Lithium-induced polyuria is usually, but not always, reversible. Acutely, lithium appears to reduce V_2-receptor-mediated stimulation of adenylyl cyclase. Also, lithium increases plasma levels of parathyroid hormone, a partial antagonist to vasopressin. In most patients, the antibiotic *demeclocycline* attenuates the antidiuretic effects of vasopressin, probably owing to decreased accumulation and action of cyclic AMP.

Nonrenal Actions of Vasopressin. Vasopressin and related peptides are ancient hormones in evolutionary terms, and they are found in species that do not concentrate urine. Thus it is not surprising that vasopressin has nonrenal actions in mammals.

Cardiovascular System. The cardiovascular effects of vasopressin are complex, and vasopressin's role in physiological situations is ill-defined. Vasopressin is a potent vasoconstrictor (V_1-receptor-mediated), and resistance vessels throughout the circulation may be affected. Vascular smooth muscle in the skin, skeletal muscle, fat, pancreas, and thyroid gland appear most sensitive, with significant vasoconstriction also occurring in the gastrointestinal tract, coronary vessels, and brain. Despite the potency of vasopressin as a direct vasoconstrictor, vasopressin-induced pressor responses *in vivo* are minimal and occur only with vasopressin concentrations significantly higher than those required for maximal antidiuresis. To a large extent, this is due to circulating vasopressin actions on V_1 receptors to inhibit sympathetic efferents and potentiate baroreflexes. In addition, V_2 receptors cause vasodilation in some blood vessels.

A large body of data supports the conclusion that vasopressin helps to maintain arterial blood pressure during episodes of severe hypovolemia/hypotension. At present, there is no convincing evidence for a role of vasopressin in essential hypertension in human beings (Kawano *et al.*, 1997).

The effects of vasopressin on the heart (reduced cardiac output and heart rate) are largely indirect and result from coronary vasoconstriction, decreased coronary blood flow, and alterations in vagal and sympathetic tone. In humans, the effects of vasopressin on coronary blood flow can be demonstrated easily, especially if large doses are employed. The cardiac actions of the hormone are of more than academic interest. Some patients with coronary insufficiency experience angina even in response to the relatively small amounts of vasopressin required to control diabetes insipidus, and vasopressin-induced myocardial ischemia has led to severe reactions and even death.

Central Nervous System (CNS). It is likely that vasopressin plays a role as a neurotransmitter and/or neuromodulator. Vasopressin may participate in the acquisition of certain learned behaviors (Dantzer and Bluthé, 1993), in the development of some complex social processes (Young *et al.*, 1998), and in the pathogenesis of specific psychiatric diseases such as depression (Scott and Dinan, 2002). However, the physiological/pathophysiological relevance of these findings is controversial, and some of the actions of vasopressin on memory and learned behavior may be due to visceral autonomic effects. Many studies support a physiological role for vasopressin as a naturally occurring antipyretic factor (Cridland and Kasting, 1992). Although vasopressin can modulate CNS autonomic systems controlling heart rate, arterial blood pressure, respiration rate, and sleep patterns, the physiological significance of these actions is unclear. Finally, secretion of ACTH is enhanced by vasopressin released from parvicellular neurons in the PVN and secreted into the pituitary portal capillaries from axon terminals in the median eminence. Although vasopressin is not the principal corticotropin-releasing factor, vasopressin may provide for sustained activation of the hypothalamic–pituitary–adrenal axis during chronic stress (Aguilera and Rabadan-Diehl, 2000) (*see* Chapter 59). The CNS effects of vasopressin appear to be mediated predominantly by V_1 receptors.

Blood Coagulation. Activation of V_2 receptors by desmopressin or vasopressin increases circulating levels of procoagulant factor VIII and of von Willebrand factor. These effects are mediated by extrarenal V_2 receptors (Bernat *et al.*, 1997). Presumably, vasopressin stimulates the secretion of von Willebrand factor and of factor VIII from storage sites in vascular endothelium. However, since release of von Willebrand factor does not occur when desmopressin is applied directly to cultured endothelial cells or to isolated blood vessels, intermediate factors are likely to be involved.

Other Nonrenal Effects of Vasopressin. At high concentrations, vasopressin stimulates contraction of smooth muscle in the uterus (*via* oxytocin receptors) and gastrointestinal tract (*via* V_1 receptors). Vasopressin is stored in platelets, and activation of V_1 receptors stimulates platelet aggregation. Also, activation of V_1 receptors on hepatocytes stimulates glycogenolysis. The physiological significance of these effects of vasopressin in not known.

VASOPRESSIN RECEPTOR AGONISTS AND ANTAGONISTS

A number of vasopressinlike peptides occur naturally (Table 29–1). All are nonapeptides, contain cysteine residues in positions 1 and 6, have an intramolecular disulfide bridge between the two cysteine residues (essential for agonist activity), have additional conserved amino acids in positions 5, 7, and 9 (asparagine, proline, and glycine, respectively), contain a basic amino acid in position 8, and are amidated on the carboxyl terminus. In all mammals except swine, the neurohypophyseal peptide is 8-arginine vasopressin, and the terms *vasopressin, arginine vasopressin* (AVP), and *antidiuretic hormone* (ADH) are used interchangeably. The chemical structure of *oxytocin* is closely related to that of vasopressin: Oxytocin is [Ile³, Leu⁸]AVP. As discussed further in Chapter 55, oxytocin binds to specific oxytocin receptors on myoepithelial cells in the mammary gland and on smooth muscle cells in the uterus, causing milk ejection and uterine contraction, respectively. Inasmuch as vasopressin and oxytocin are structurally similar, it is not surprising that vasopressin and oxytocin agonists and antagonists can bind to each other's receptors. Therefore, most of the available peptide vasopressin agonists and antagonists have some affinity for oxytocin receptors; at high doses, they may block or mimic the effects of oxytocin.

Many vasopressin analogues were synthesized with the goal of increasing duration of action and selectivity for vasopressin receptor subtypes (V_1 *versus* V_2 vasopressin receptors, which mediate pressor responses and antidiuretic responses, respectively). Deamination at position 1 increases duration of action and increases antidiuretic activity without increasing vasopressor activity. Substitution of D-arginine for L-arginine greatly reduces vasopressor activity without reducing antidiuretic activity. Thus the antidiuretic-to-vasopressor ratio for 1-deamino-8-D-arginine vasopressin (Table 29–1), also called *desmopressin* (DDAVP), is approximately 3000 times greater than that for vasopressin, and desmopressin now is the preferred drug for the treatment of central diabetes insipidus. Substitution of valine for glutamine in position 4 further increases the antidiuretic selectivity, and the antidiuretic-to-vasopressor ratio for deamino[Val⁴, D-Arg⁸]AVP (Table 29–1) is approximately 11,000 times greater than that for vasopressin. Recently, Nakamura and colleagues (2000) synthesized a nonpeptide V_2-receptor agonist (Table 29–1).

Increasing V_1 selectivity has proved more difficult than increasing V_2 selectivity, but a limited number of agonists with modest selectivity for V_1 receptors have been developed (Table 29–1). Vasopressin receptors in the adenohypophysis that mediate vasopressin-induced ACTH release are neither classical V_1 nor V_2 receptors. Since the vasopressin receptors in the adenohypophysis appear to share a common signal-transduction mechanism with classical V_1 receptors, and since many vasopressin analogues with vasoconstrictor activity release ACTH, V_1 receptors have been subclassified into V_{1a} (vascular/hepatic) and V_{1b} (pituitary) receptors. V_{1b} receptors also are called V_3 *receptors*. Vasopressin analogues that are agonists selective for V_{1a} or V_{1b} receptors have been described (Table 29–1).

Chemistry of Vasopressin Receptor Antagonists. The impetus for the development of specific vasopressin receptor antagonists is the belief that such drugs may be useful in a number of clinical settings. Based on receptor physiology, selective V_{1a} antagonists may be beneficial when total peripheral resistance is increased (*e.g.*, congestive heart failure and hypertension), whereas selective V_2 antagonists could be useful whenever reabsorption of solute-free water is excessive (*e.g.*, the syndrome of inappropriate secretion of antidiuretic hormone and hyponatremia associated with a reduced effective blood volume). Combined V_{1a}/V_2 receptor antagonists might be beneficial in diseases associated with a combination of increased peripheral resistance and dilutional hyponatremia (*e.g.*, congestive heart failure).

Highly selective V_1 and V_2 peptide antagonists that are structural analogues of vasopressin have been synthesized (*see* Table 29–2 for examples), including both cyclic and

Table 29–2
Vasopressin Receptor Antagonists

I. PEPTIDE ANTAGONISTS

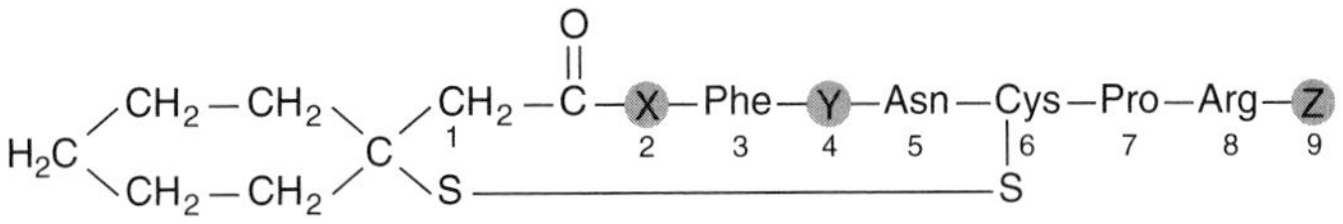

$$H_2C \begin{matrix} CH_2-CH_2 \\ \\ CH_2-CH_2 \end{matrix} C \begin{matrix} CH_2-C \\ | \\ S \end{matrix} \overset{O}{\underset{1}{\parallel}} \overset{}{X}-Phe-Y-Asn-Cys-Pro-Arg-Z$$

	X	Y	Z
A. *V_1-selective antagonists*			
V_{1a}-selective antagonist	Tyr—OMe	Gln	Gly (NH$_2$)
d(CH$_2$)$_5$[Tyr(Me)^2]AVP			
V_{1b}-selective antagonist	Tyr—OMe	Gln	Gly (NH$_2$)
dP [Tyr(Me)^2]AVP[*‡]			
B. *V_2-selective antagonists*[†]			
1. des Gly-NH$_2$^{9}-d(CH$_2$)$_5$[D-Ile^2, Ile^4]AVP	D-Ile	Ile	—
2. d(CH$_2$)$_5$[D-Ile^2, Ile^4, Ala-NH$_2$^{9}]AVP	D-Ile	Ile	Ala (NH$_2$)

II. NONPEPTIDE ANTAGONISTS

A. *V_{1a}-selective antagonists*

OPC-21268

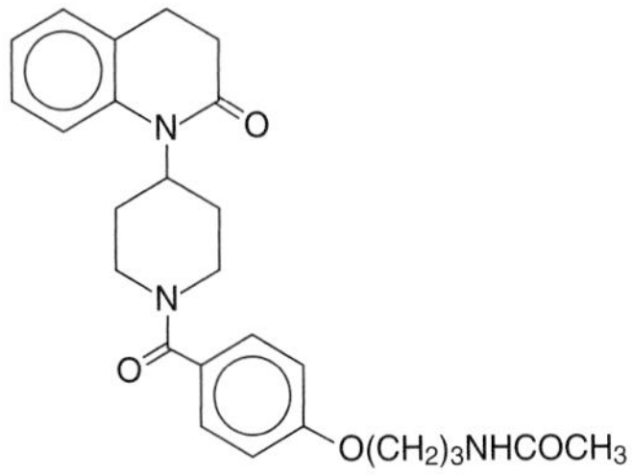

SR 49059 (relcovaptan)

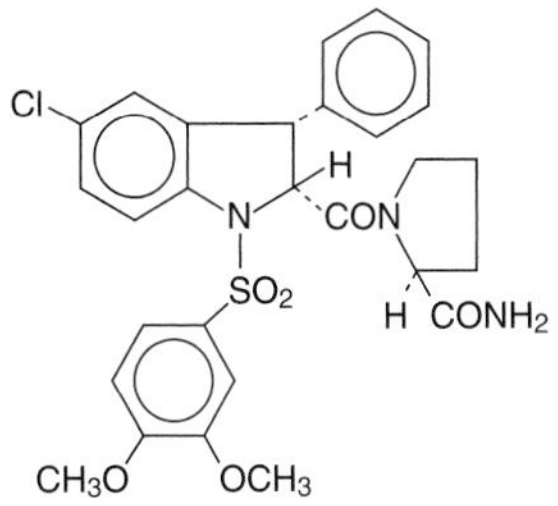

B. *V_{1b}-selective antagonists*

SSR 149415

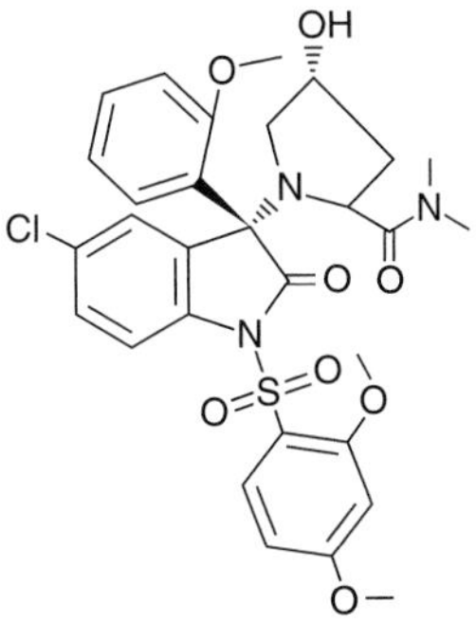

C. *V_2-selective antagonists*

SR 121463A

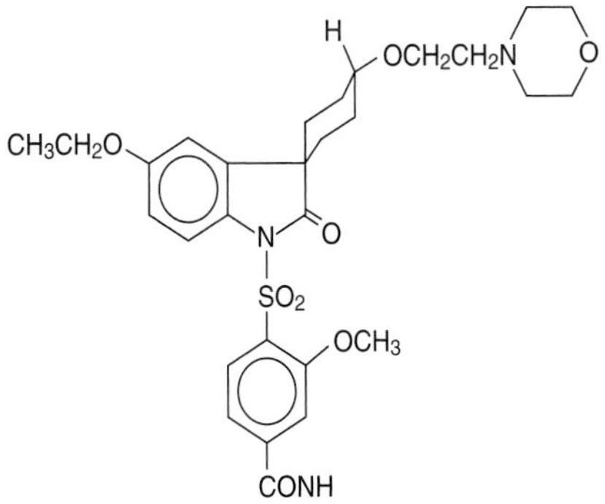

VPA-985 (lixivaptan)

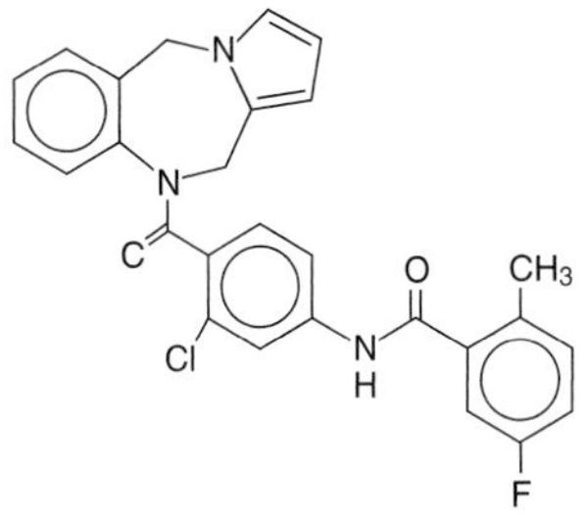

(Continued)

Table 29–2

Vasopressin Receptor Antagonists (Continued)

C. V_2-selective antagonists (cont.)
  OPC-31260 (mozavaptan)

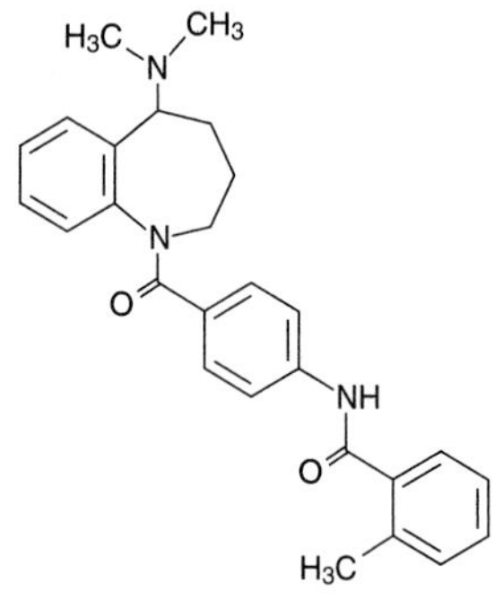

OPC-41061 (tolvaptan)

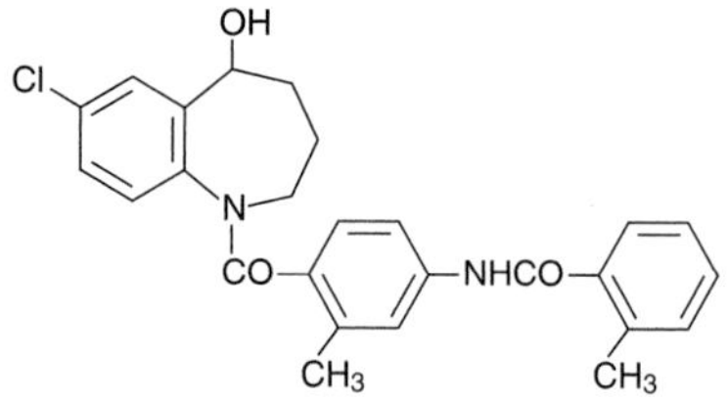

D. V_{1a}-/V_2-selective antagonists
  YM-471

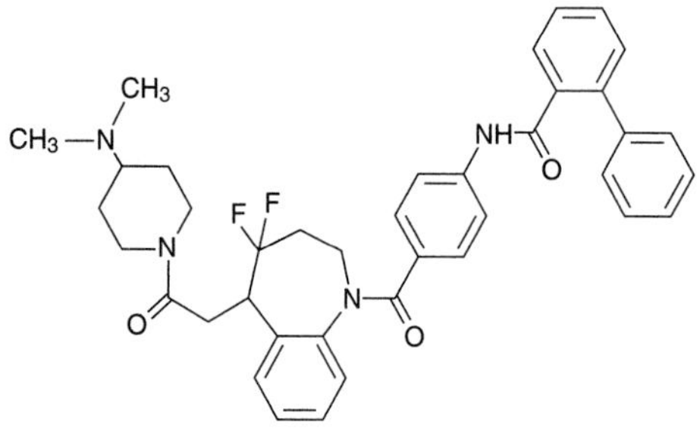

YM 087

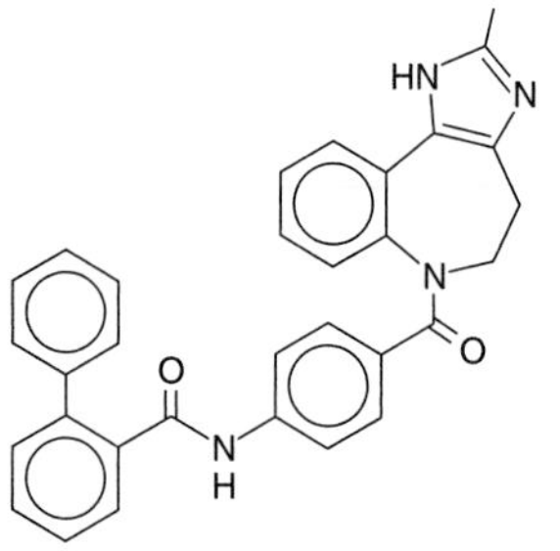

JTV-605

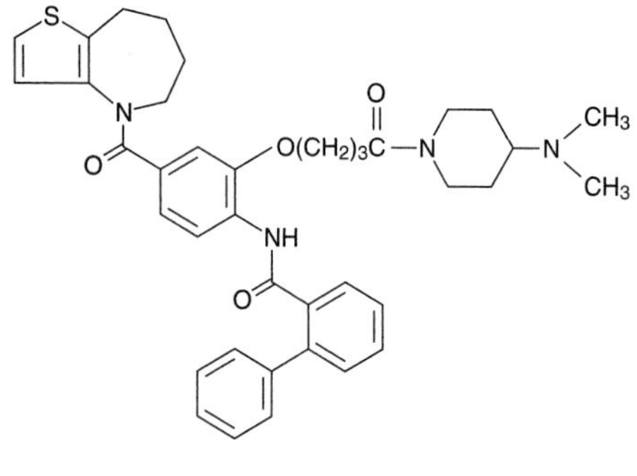

CL-385004

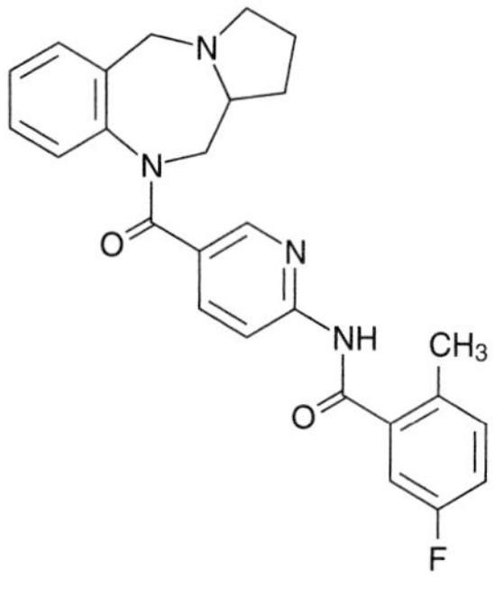

*Also blocks V_{1a} receptor, ‡

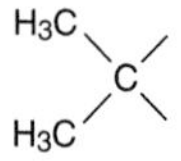

H_3C \ /
       C   rather than
H_3C / \

H_2C — CH_2 \ /
              C
H_2C — CH_2 /

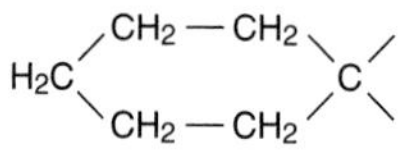

†V_2 antagonistic activity in rats; however, antagonistic activity may be less or nonexistent in other species. Also, with prolonged infusion may exhibit significant agonist activity.

linear peptides. [1-(β-Mercapto-β,β-cyclopentamethylene-proprionic acid),2-O-methyltyrosine]arginine vasopressin, also known as d(CH₂)₅[Tyr(Me)²]AVP, has a greater affinity for V_{1a} receptors than for either V_{1b} or V_2 receptors; this antagonist has been employed widely in physiological and pharmacological studies. Although [1-deaminopenicil-

lamine, 2-O-methyltyrosine]arginine vasopressin, also called dP[Tyr(Me)²]AVP, is a potent V_{1b} receptor antagonist with little affinity for the V_2 receptor, it also blocks V_{1a} receptors. No truly selective peptide V_{1b}-receptor antagonist is available. Peptide antagonists have limited oral activity, and the potency of peptide V_2 antagonists is species-dependent. Also, with prolonged infusion, peptide V_2 antagonists have significant agonist activity.

DISEASES AFFECTING THE VASOPRESSIN SYSTEM

Diabetes Insipidus (DI). DI is a disease of impaired renal conservation of water owing either to an inadequate secretion of vasopressin from the neurohypophysis (central DI) or to an insufficient renal response to vasopressin (nephrogenic DI). Very rarely, DI can be caused by an abnormally high rate of degradation of vasopressin by circulating vasopressinases. Pregnancy may accentuate or reveal central and/or nephrogenic DI by increasing plasma levels of vasopressinase and by reducing the renal sensitivity to vasopressin. Patients with DI excrete large volumes (more than 30 ml/kg per day) of dilute (less than 200 mOsm/kg) urine and, if their thirst mechanism is functioning normally, are polydipsic. In contrast to the sweet urine excreted by patients with diabetes mellitus, urine from patients with DI is tasteless, hence the name *insipidus*. The urinary taste test for DI has been supplanted by the approach of observing whether the patient is able to reduce urine volume and increase urine osmolality after a period of carefully observed fluid deprivation. Central DI can be distinguished from nephrogenic DI by administration of desmopressin, which will increase urine osmolality in patients with central DI but have little or no effect in patients with nephrogenic DI. DI can be differentiated from primary polydipsia by measuring plasma osmolality, which will be low to low-normal in patients with primary polydipsia and high to high-normal in patients with DI. For a more complete discussion of diagnostic procedures, *see* Robertson (2001).

Central DI. Head injury, either surgical or traumatic, in the region of the pituitary and/or hypothalamus may cause central DI. Postoperative central DI may be transient, permanent, or triphasic (recovery followed by permanent relapse). Other causes include hypothalamic or pituitary tumors, cerebral aneurysms, CNS ischemia, and brain infiltrations and infections (Robertson, 2001). Finally, central DI may be idiopathic or familial. Familial central DI usually is autosomal dominant (chromosome 20), and vasopressin deficiency occurs several months or years after birth and worsens gradually. Autosomal dominant central DI is linked to mutations in the vasopressin preprohormone gene that cause the prohormone to misfold and oligomerize improperly. The long-term result is accumulation of the mutant vasopressin precursor in the affected neuron because the precursor cannot move from the endoplasmic reticulum into the secretory pathway. Accumulation of mutant vasopressin precursor causes neuronal death, hence the dominant mode of inheritance (Robertson, 2001). Rarely, familial central DI is autosomal recessive owing to a mutation in the vasopressin peptide itself that gives rise to an inactive vasopressin mutant.

Antidiuretic peptides are the primary treatment for central DI, with desmopressin being the peptide of choice. For patients with central DI who cannot tolerate antidiuretic peptides because of side effects or allergic reactions, other treatment options are available. *Chlorpropamide*, an oral sulfonylurea, potentiates the action of small or residual amounts of circulating vasopressin and will reduce urine volume in more than half of all patients with central DI. A dose of 125 to 500 mg daily is particularly effective in patients with partial central DI. If polyuria is not controlled satisfactorily with chlorpropamide alone, addition of a thiazide diuretic (*see* Chapter 28) to the regimen usually results in an adequate reduction in the volume of urine. *Carbamazepine* (800 to 1000 mg daily in divided doses) and *clofibrate* (1 to 2 g daily in divided doses) also reduce urine volume in patients with central DI. Long-term use of these agents may induce serious adverse effects; therefore, carbamazepine and clofibrate are used rarely to treat central DI. The antidiuretic mechanisms of chlorpropamide, carbamazepine, and clofibrate are not clear. These agents are not effective in nephrogenic DI, which indicates that functional V_2 receptors are required for the antidiuretic effect. Since carbamazepine inhibits and chlorpropamide has little effect on vasopressin secretion, it is likely that carbamazepine and chlorpropamide act directly on the kidney to enhance V_2-receptor-mediated antidiuresis.

Nephrogenic DI. Nephrogenic DI may be congenital or acquired. Hypercalcemia, hypokalemia, postobstructive renal failure, lithium, foscarnet, clozapine, demeclocycline, and other drugs can induce nephrogenic DI. As many as one in three patients treated with lithium may develop nephrogenic DI. X-linked nephrogenic DI is caused by mutations in the gene encoding the V_2 receptor, which maps to Xq28. A number of missense, nonsense, and frame-shift mutations in the gene encoding the V_2 receptor have been identified in patients with this disorder (Knoers and Deen, 2001). Mutations in the V_2-receptor gene may cause impaired routing of the V_2 receptor to the cell surface, defective coupling of the receptor to G proteins, or decreased affinity of the receptor for vasopressin. The effects of these mutations range from a complete loss of responsiveness to vasopressin to a shift to the left of the concentration–response curve. Autosomal recessive and dominant nephrogenic DI result from inactivating mutations in aquaporin 2. These findings indicate that aquaporin 2 is essential for the antidiuretic effect of vasopressin in human beings.

Although the mainstay of treatment of nephrogenic DI is assurance of an adequate intake of water, drugs also can be used to reduce polyuria. *Amiloride* (*see* Chapter 28) blocks the uptake of lithium by the sodium channel in the collecting-duct system and is considered the drug of choice for lithium-induced nephrogenic DI despite the absence of Food and Drug Administration (FDA) approval. Paradoxically, *thiazide diuretics* reduce the polyuria of patients with DI and often are used to treat non-lithium-induced nephrogenic DI. The use of thiazide diuretics in infants with nephrogenic DI may be crucially important because uncontrolled polyuria may exceed the child's capacity to imbibe and absorb fluids. The antidiuretic mechanism of thiazides in DI is incompletely understood. It is possible that the natriuretic action of thiazides and resulting depletion of extracellular fluid volume play an important role in the thiazide-induced antidiuresis. In this regard, whenever extracellular fluid volume is reduced, compensatory mechanisms increase reabsorption of NaCl in the proximal tubule, reducing the volume delivered to the distal tubule. Consequently, less free water can be formed, which should diminish polyuria. However, studies in rats with vasopressin-deficient DI challenge this hypothesis (Grønbeck *et al.*, 1998). Nonetheless, the antidiuretic effects appear to parallel the ability of thiazides to cause natriuresis, and the drugs are given in doses similar to those used to mobilize edema fluid. In patients with DI, a 50% reduction of urine volume is a good response to thiazides. Moderate restriction of sodium intake can enhance the antidiuretic effectiveness of thiazides.

A number of case reports describe the effectiveness of indomethacin in the treatment of nephrogenic DI; however, other prostaglandin synthase inhibitors (*e.g., ibuprofen*) appear to be less effective. The mechanism of the effect may involve a decrease in glomerular filtration rate, an increase in medullary solute concentration, and/or enhanced proximal reabsorption of fluid. Also, since prostaglandins attenuate vasopressin-induced antidiuresis in patients with at least a partially intact V_2-receptor system, some of the antidiuretic response to indomethacin may be due to diminution of the prostaglandin effect and enhancement of the effects of vasopressin on the principal cells of the collecting duct.

Syndrome of Inappropriate Secretion of Antidiuretic Hormone (SIADH). SIADH is a disease of impaired water excretion with accompanying hyponatremia and hypo-osmolality caused by the *inappropriate* secretion of vasopressin. The clinical manifestations of plasma hypotonicity resulting from SIADH may include lethargy, anorexia, nausea and vomiting, muscle cramps, coma, convulsions, and death. A multitude of disorders can induce SIADH (Robertson, 2001), including malignancies, pulmonary diseases, CNS injuries/diseases (*e.g.*, head trauma, infections, and tumors), and general surgery. The three drug classes most commonly implicated in drug-induced SIADH include psychotropic medications (*e.g., fluoxetine,* haloperidol, and *tricyclic antidepressants*), sulfonylureas (*e.g.*, chloropropamide), and vinca alkaloids (*e.g., vincristine* and *vinblastine*). Other drugs strongly associated with SIADH include thiazide diuretics, clonidine, *enalapril, ifosphamide,* and *methyldopa.* In a normal individual, an elevation in plasma vasopressin *per se* does not induce plasma hypotonicity because the person simply stops drinking owing to an osmotically induced aversion to fluids. Therefore, plasma hypotonicity only occurs when excessive fluid intake (oral or intravenous) accompanies inappropriate secretion of vasopressin. Treatment of hypotonicity in the setting of SIADH includes water restriction, intravenous administration of hypertonic saline, loop diuretics (which interfere with the concentrating ability of the kidneys), and drugs that inhibit the effect of vasopressin to increase water permeability in the collecting ducts. To inhibit vasopressin's action in the collecting ducts, *demeclocycline*, a tetracycline, currently is the preferred drug.

Although lithium can inhibit the renal actions of vasopressin, it is effective in only a minority of patients, may induce irreversible renal damage when used chronically, and has a low therapeutic index. Therefore, lithium should be considered for use only in patients with symptomatic SIADH who cannot be controlled by other means or in whom tetracyclines are contraindicated, *e.g.*, patients with liver disease. It is important to stress that the majority of patients with SIADH do not require therapy because plasma Na$^+$ stabilizes in the range of 125 to 132 mM; such patients usually are asymptomatic. Only when symptomatic hypotonicity ensues, generally when plasma Na$^+$ levels drop below 120 mM, should therapy with demeclocycline be initiated. Since hypotonicity, which causes an influx of water into cells with resulting cerebral swelling, is the cause of symptoms, the goal of therapy is simply to increase plasma osmolality toward normal. For a more complete description of the diagnosis and treatment of SIADH, *see* Robertson (2001).

Other Water-Retaining States. In patients with congestive heart failure, cirrhosis, or nephrotic syndrome, *effective* blood volume often is reduced, and hypovolemia frequently is exacerbated by the liberal use of diuretics. Since hypovolemia stimulates vasopressin release, patients may become hyponatremic owing to vasopressin-mediated retention of water. The development of potent orally active V_2-receptor antagonists and specific inhibitors of water channels in the collecting duct would provide an effective therapeutic strategy not only in patients with SIADH but also in the much more common setting of hyponatremia in patients with heart failure, liver cirrhosis, and nephrotic syndrome.

CLINICAL SUMMARY; PHARMACOLOGY OF VASOPRESSIN PEPTIDES

Therapeutic Uses. Only two antidiuretic peptides are available for clinical use in the United States. (1) Vasopressin (synthetic 8-L-arginine vasopressin; PITRESSIN) is available as a sterile aqueous solution; it may be administered subcutaneously, intramuscularly, or intranasally. (2) *Desmopressin acetate* (synthetic 1-deamino-8-D-arginine vasopressin; DDAVP, others) is available as a sterile aqueous solution packaged for intravenous or subcutaneous injection, in a nasal solution for intranasal administration with either a nasal spray pump or rhinal tube delivery system, and in tablets for oral administration. The therapeutic uses of vasopressin and its congeners can be divided into two main categories according to the type of vasopressin receptor involved.

V_1-receptor-mediated therapeutic applications are based on the rationale that V_1 receptors cause contraction of gastrointestinal and vascular smooth muscle. V_1-receptor-mediated contraction of gastrointestinal smooth muscle has been used to treat postoperative ileus and abdominal distension and to dispel intestinal gas before abdominal roentgenography to avoid interfering gas shadows. V_1-receptor-mediated vasoconstriction of the splanchnic arterial vessels reduces blood flow to the portal system and thereby attenuates pressure and bleeding in esophageal varices (Burroughs, 1998). Although endoscopic variceal banding ligation is the treatment of choice for bleeding esophageal varices, V_1-receptor agonists have been used in an emergency setting until endoscopy can be performed (Vlavianos and Westaby, 2001). Simultaneous administration of nitroglycerin with V_1-receptor agonists may attenuate the cardiotoxic effects of V_1 agonists while enhancing their beneficial splanchnic effects . Also, V_1-receptor agonists have been used during abdominal surgery in patients with portal hypertension to diminish the risk of hemorrhage during the procedure. Finally, V_1-receptor-mediated vasoconstriction

has been used to reduce bleeding during acute hemorrhagic gastritis, burn wound excision, cyclophosphamide-induced hemorrhagic cystitis, liver transplant, cesarean section, and uterine myoma resection. The applications of V_1-receptor agonists can be accomplished with vasopressin; however, the use of vasopressin for all these indications is no longer recommended because of significant adverse reactions. Although not yet available in the United States, *terlipressin* (GLYPRESSIN) is preferred for bleeding esophageal varices because of increased safety compared with vasopressin (Vlavianos and Westaby, 2001). Moreover, terlipressin is effective in patients with hepatorenal syndrome, particularly when combined with albumin (Ortega *et al.*, 2002).

Vasopressin levels in patients with vasodilatory shock are inappropriately low, and such patients are extraordinarily sensitive to the pressor actions of vasopressin (Robin *et al.*, 2003). The combination of vasopressin and *norepinephrine* is superior to norepinephrine alone in the management of catecholamine-resistant vasodilatory shock (Dunser *et al.*, 2003). Although the efficacy of vasopressin in the resuscitation of patients with ventricular fibrillation or pulseless electrical activity is similar to that of epinephrine, vasopressin followed by epinephrine appears to be more effective than epinephrine alone in the treatment of patients with asystole (Wenzel *et al.*, 2004).

V_2-receptor-mediated therapeutic applications are based on the rationale that V_2 receptors cause water conservation and release of blood coagulation factors. Central but not nephrogenic DI can be treated with V_2-receptor agonists, and polyuria and polydipsia usually are well controlled. Some patients experience transient DI (*e.g.,* in head injury or surgery in the area of the pituitary); however, therapy for most patients with DI is lifelong. Desmopressin is the drug of choice for the vast majority of patients, and numerous clinical trials have demonstrated the efficacy and tolerability of desmopressin in both adults and children. The duration of effect from a single intranasal dose is from 6 to 20 hours; twice-daily administration is effective in most patients. There is considerable variability in the intranasal dose of desmopressin required to maintain normal urine volume, and the dosage must be tailored individually. The usual intranasal dosage in adults is 10 to 40 μg daily either as a single dose or divided into two or three doses. In view of the high cost of the drug and the importance of avoiding water intoxication, the schedule of administration should be adjusted to the minimal amount required. An initial dose of 2.5 μg can be used, with therapy first directed toward the control of nocturia. An equivalent or higher morning dose controls daytime polyuria in most patients, although a third dose occa-

sionally may be needed in the afternoon. In some patients, chronic allergic rhinitis or other nasal pathology may preclude reliable absorption of the peptide following nasal administration. Oral administration of desmopressin in doses 10 to 20 times the intranasal dose provides adequate blood levels of desmopressin to control polyuria. Subcutaneous administration of 1 to 2 μg daily of desmopressin also is effective in central DI.

Vasopressin has little, if any, place in the long-term therapy of DI because of its short duration of action and V_1-receptor-mediated side effects. Vasopressin can be used as an alternative to desmopressin in the initial diagnostic evaluation of patients with suspected DI and to control polyuria in patients with DI who recently have undergone surgery or experienced head trauma. Under these circumstances, polyuria may be transient, and long-acting agents may produce water intoxication.

An additional V_2-receptor-mediated therapeutic application is the use of desmopressin in bleeding disorders (Mannucci, 1997; Sutor, 1998). In most patients with type I von Willebrand's disease (vWD) and in some with type IIn vWD, desmopressin will elevate von Willebrand factor and shorten bleeding time. However, desmopressin generally is ineffective in patients with types IIa, IIb, and III vWD. Desmopressin may cause a marked transient thrombocytopenia in individuals with type IIb vWD and is contraindicated in such patients. Desmopressin also increases factor VIII levels in patients with mild to moderate hemophilia A. Desmopressin is not indicated in patients with severe hemophilia A, those with hemophilia B, or those with factor VIII antibodies. Using a test dose of nasal spray, the response of any given patient with type I vWD or hemophilia A to desmopressin should be determined at the time of diagnosis or 1 to 2 weeks before elective surgery to assess the extent of increase in factor VIII or von Willebrand factor. Desmopressin is employed widely to treat the hemostatic abnormalities induced by uremia. In patients with renal insufficiency, desmopressin shortens bleeding time and increases circulating levels of factor VIII coagulant activity, factor VIII–related antigen, and ristocetin cofactor. It also induces the appearance of larger von Willebrand factor multimers. Desmopressin is effective in some patients with liver cirrhosis–induced or drug-induced (*e.g., heparin, hirudin,* and *antiplatelet agents*) bleeding disorders. Desmopressin, given intravenously at a dose of 0.3 μg/kg, increases factor VIII and von Willebrand factor for more than 6 hours. Desmopressin can be given at intervals of 12 to 24 hours depending on the clinical response and the severity of bleeding. Tachyphylaxis to desmopressin usually occurs after several days (owing to depletion of factor VIII and von Wille-

brand factor storage sites) and limits its usefulness to preoperative preparation, postoperative bleeding, excessive menstrual bleeding, and emergency situations.

Another V_2-receptor-mediated therapeutic application is the use of desmopressin for primary nocturnal enuresis. Bedtime administration of desmopressin intranasal spray or tablets provides a high response rate that is sustained with long-term use, that is safe, and that accelerates the cure rate (van Kerrebroeck, 2002). Finally, desmopressin has been found to relieve post–lumbar puncture headache probably by causing water retention and thereby facilitating rapid fluid equilibration in the CNS.

Pharmacokinetics. When vasopressin and desmopressin are given orally, they are inactivated quickly by trypsin, which cleaves the peptide bond between amino acids 8 and 9. Inactivation by peptidases in various tissues (particularly the liver and kidneys) results in a plasma half-life of vasopressin of 17 to 35 minutes. Following intramuscular or subcutaneous injection, the antidiuretic effects of vasopressin last 2 to 8 hours. The plasma half-life of desmopressin has two components, a fast component of 6.5 to 9 minutes and a slow component of 30 to 117 minutes. Only 3% and 0.15%, respectively, of intranasally and orally administered desmopressin is absorbed.

Toxicity, Adverse Effects, Contraindications, Drug Interactions. Most adverse effects are mediated through the V_1 receptor acting on vascular and gastrointestinal smooth muscle; consequently, such adverse effects are much less common and less severe with desmopressin than with vasopressin. After the injection of large doses of vasopressin, marked facial pallor owing to cutaneous vasoconstriction is observed commonly. Increased intestinal activity is likely to cause nausea, belching, cramps, and an urge to defecate. Most serious, however, is the effect on the coronary circulation. Vasopressin should be administered only at low doses and with extreme caution in individuals suffering from vascular disease, especially coronary artery disease. Other cardiac complications include arrhythmia and decreased cardiac output. Peripheral vasoconstriction and gangrene have been encountered in patients receiving large doses of vasopressin.

The major V_2-receptor-mediated adverse effect is water intoxication, which can occur with desmopressin or vasopressin. In this regard, many drugs, including carbamazepine, chlorpropamide, morphine, tricyclic antidepressants, and NSAIDs, can potentiate the antidiuretic effects of these peptides. Several drugs such as lithium, demeclocycline, and ethanol can attenuate the antidiuretic response to desmopressin. Desmopressin and vasopressin should be used cautiously in disease states in which a rapid increase in extracellular water may impose risks (*e.g.,* in angina, hypertension, and heart failure) and should not be used in patients with acute renal failure. Patients receiving desmopressin to maintain hemostasis should be advised to reduce fluid intake. Also, it is imperative that these peptides not be administered to patients with primary or psychogenic polydipsia because severe hypotonic hyponatremia will ensue.

Mild facial flushing and headache are the most common adverse effects associated with desmopressin. Allergic reactions ranging from urticaria to anaphylaxis may occur with desmopressin or vasopressin. Intranasal administration may cause local adverse effects in the nasal passages, such as edema, rhinorrhea, congestion, irritation, pruritus, and ulceration.

Future Directions in Vasopressin Analogues

Nonpeptide vasopressin receptor antagonists and agonists are being developed for a wide range of clinical indications, including for V_{1a}-selective antagonists: dysmenorrhea, preterm labor, and Raynaud's syndrome; for V_{1b}-selective antagonists: stress-related disorders, anxiety, depression, ACTH-secreting tumors, and Cushing's syndrome; for V_2-selective and V_{1a}/V_2-selective antagonists: heart failure, SIADH, cirrhosis, hyponatremia, brain edema, nephrotic syndrome, diabetic nephropathy, and glaucoma; and for V_2-selective agonists: central DI, nocturnal enuresis, nocturnal polyuria, and urinary incontinence (Wong and Verbalis, 2001; Serradeil-Le Gal *et al.*, 2002b; Thibonnier *et al.*, 2001).

Preliminary data support several of the aforementioned indications for vasopressin receptor antagonists and agonists. SR 49059 is a V_{1a}-selective antagonist that has efficacy in primary dysmenorrhea (Brouard *et al.*, 2000), and SSR 149415 is a V_{1b}-selective antagonist that demonstrates anxiolytic activity in animal models of stress (Serradeil-Le Gal *et al.*, 2002a; Griebel *et al.*, 2002). Aquaretics are drugs that increase free-water clearance with minimal effects on electrolyte excretion. Recent randomized clinical trials demonstrate efficacy for *YM 087* (CONIVAPTAN) and *OPC-41067* (TOLVAPTAN), V_{1a}/V_2-selective antagonists, respectively, as aquaretics in heart failure patients (Udelson *et al.*, 2001; Gheorghiade *et al.*, 2003). The V_2-selective antagonist *VPA-985* (LIXIVAPTAN) is an effective aquaretic in patients with hyponatremia of various etiologies (Wong *et al.*, 2003). In contrast, the V_2-selective agonist *OPC-51803* has strong antidiuretic effects in animals and is being developed for central DI, nocturnal enuresis, and urinary incontinence (Naka-

mura *et al.*, 2003). It is likely that a number of nonpeptide vasopressin receptor antagonists and agonists will become available clinically in the near future.

BIBLIOGRAPHY

Bernat, A., Hoffmann, T., Dumas, A., *et al.* V_2 receptor antagonism of DDAVP-induced release of hemostatis factors in conscious dogs. *J. Pharmacol. Exp. Ther.,* **1997,** *282*:597–602.

Brouard, R., Bossmar, T., Fournie-Lloret, D., *et al.* Effect of SR49059, an orally active V_{1a} vasopressin receptor antagonist, in the prevention of dysmenorrhea. *Int. J. Obstet. Gynecol.,* **2000,** *107*:614–619.

Cridland, R.A., and Kasting, N.W. A critical role for central vasopressin in regulation of fever during bacterial infection. *Am. J. Physiol.,* **1992,** *263*:R1235–R1240.

Dunser, M.W., Mayr, A.J., Ulmer, H., *et al.* Arginine vasopressin in advanced vasodilatory shock: A prospective, randomized, controlled study. *Circulation,* **2003,** *107*:2313–2319.

Franchini, K.G., and Cowley, A.W., Jr. Renal cortical and medullary blood flow responses during water restriction: role of vasopressin. *Am. J. Physiol.,* **1996,** *270*:R1257–R1264.

Gheorghiade, M., Niazi, I., Ouyang, J., *et al.,* for the Tolvaptan Investigators. Vasopressin V_2-receptor blockade with TOLVAPTAN in patients with chronic heart failure: Results from a double-blind, randomized trial. *Circulation,* **2003,** *107*:2690–2696.

Giminz, I., and Forbush, B. Short-term stimulation of the renal Na–K–Cl cotransporter (NKCC2) by vasopressin involves phosphorylation and membrane translocation of the protein. *J. Biol. Chem.,* **2003,** *278*:26946–26951.

Griebel, G., Simiand, J., Serradeil-Le Gal, C., *et al.* Anxiolytic- and antidepressant-like effects of the nonpeptide vasopressin V_{1b} receptor agonist SSR149415 suggest an innovative approach for the treatment of stress-related disorders. *Proc. Natl. Acad. Sci., U.S.A.,* **2002,** *99*:6370–6375.

Grønbeck, L., Marples, D., Nielsen, S., and Christensen, S. Mechanism of antidiuresis caused by bendroflumethiazide in conscious rats with diabetes insipidus. *Br. J. Pharmacol.,* **1998,** *123*:737–745.

Hupf, H., Grimm, D., Riegger, G.A.J., and Schunkert, H. Evidence for a vasopressin system in the rat heart. *Circ. Res.,* **1999,** *84*:365–370.

Inoue, T., Terris, J., Ecelbarger, C.A., *et al.* Vasopressin regulates apical targeting of aquaporin-2 but not of UT1 urea transporter in renal collecting duct. *Am. J. Physiol.,* **1999,** *276*:F559–F566.

Kawano, Y., Matsuoka, H., Nishikimi, T., *et al.* The role of vasopressin in essential hypertension: Plasma levels and effects of the V_1 receptor antagonist OPC-21268 during different dietary sodium intakes. *Am. J. Hypertens.,* **1997,** *10*:1240–1244.

Nakamura, S., Hirano, T., Tsujimae, K., *et al.* Antidiuretic effects of a nonpeptide vasopressin V_2-receptor agonist OPC-51803 administered orally to rats. *J. Pharmacol. Exp. Ther.,* **2000,** *295*:1005–1011.

Nakamura, S., Hirano, T., Yamamura, Y., *et al.* Effects of OPC-51803, a novel, nonpeptide vasopressin V_2-receptor agonist, on micturition frequency in Brattleboro and aged rats. *J. Pharmacol. Sci.,* **2003,** *93*:484–488.

Nakamura, S., Yamamura, Y, Itoh, S., *et al.* Characterization of a novel nonpeptide vasopressin V_2-receptor agonist, OPC-51803, in cells transfected human vasopressin receptor subtypes. *Br. J. Pharmacol.,* **2000,** *129*:1700–1706.

Nishimoto, G., Zelenina, M., Li, D., *et al.* Arginine vasopressin stimulates phosphorylation of aquaporin-2 in rat renal tissue. *Am. J. Physiol.*, **1999**, *276*:F254–F259.

Ortega, R., Ginès, P., Uriz, J., *et al.* Terlipressin therapy with and without albumin for patients with hepatorenal syndrome: Results of a prospective, nonrandomized study. *Hepatology*, **2002**, *36*:941–948.

Serradeil-Le Gal, C., Wagnon, J., Simiand, J., *et al.* Characterization of (2S,4R)-1-[5-chloro-1-[2,4-dimethoxyphenyl)sulfonyl]-3-(2-methoxyphenyl)-2-oxo-2,3-dihydro-1H-indol-3-yl]-4-hydroxy-*N,N*-dimethyl-2-pyrrolidine carboxamide (SSR149415), a selective and orally active vasopressin V_{1b} receptor antagonist. *J. Pharmacol. Exp. Ther.*, **2002a**, *300*:1122–1130.

Snyder, H.M., Noland, T.D., and Breyer, M.D. cAMP-dependent protein kinase mediates hydro-osmotic effect of vasopressin in collecting duct. *Am. J. Physiol.*, **1992**, *263*:C147–C153.

Stricker, E.M., Callahan, J.B., Huang, W., and Sved, A.F. Early osmoregulatory stimulation of neurohypophyseal hormone secretion and thirst after gastric NaCl loads. *Am. J. Physiol. Regulatory Integrative Comp. Physiol.*, **2002**, *282*:R1710–R1717.

Udelson, J.E., Smith, W.B., Hendrix, G.H., *et al.* Acute hemodynamic effects of conivaptan, a dual V_{1A} and V_2 vasopressin receptor antagonist, in patients with advanced heart failure. *Circulation*, **2001**, *104*:2417–2423.

Wenzel, V., Krismer, A.C., Arntz, H.R., *et al.*, for the European Resuscitation Council Vasopressor during Cardiopulmonary Resuscitation Study Group. A comparison of vasopressin and epinephrine for out-of-hospital cardiopulmonary resuscitation. *New Engl. J. Med.*, **2004**, *350*:105–113.

Wong, F., Blei, A.T., Blendis, L.M., and Thuluvath, P.J. A vasopressin receptor antagonist (VPA-985) improves serum sodium concentration in patients with hyponatremia: A multicenter, randomized, placebo-controlled trial. *Hepatology*, **2003**, *37*:182–191.

MONOGRAPHS AND REVIEWS

Agre, P., and Konozo, D. Aquaporin water channels: molecular mechanisms for human disease. *FEBS Lett.*, **2003**, *555*:72–78.

Aguilera, G., and Rabadan-Diehl, C. Vasopressinergic regulation of the hypothalamic–pituitary–adrenal axis: Implications for stress adaptation. *Regul. Pept.*, **2000**, *96*:23–29.

Bankir, L. Antidiuretic action of vasopressin: Quantitative aspects and interaction between V_{1a} and V_2 receptor–mediated effects. *Cardiovasc. Res.*, **2001**, *51*(suppl.):372–390.

Burroughs, A.K. Pharmacological treatment of acute variceal bleeding. *Digestion*, **1998**, *59*:28–36.

Dantzer, R., and Bluthé, R.M. Vasopressin and behavior: from memory to olfaction. *Regul. Pept.*, **1993**, *45*:121–125.

David, J.L. Desmopressin and hemostasis. *Regul. Pept.*, **1993**, *45*:311–317.

Ecelbarger, C.A., Kim, G.H., Wade, J.B., and Knepper, M.A. Regulation of the abundance of renal sodium transporters and channels by vasopressin. *Exp. Neurol.*, **2001**, *171*:227–234.

Guillon, G., Grazzini, E., Andrez, M., *et al.* Vasopressin: a potent autocrine/paracrine regulator of mammal adrenal functions. *Endocr. Res.*, **1998**, *24*:703–710.

Klussman, E. and Rosenthal, W. Role and identification of protein kinase A anchoring proteins in vasopressin-mediated aquaporin-2 translocation. *Kidney Int.*, **2001**, *60*:446–449.

Knoers, N.V.A.M., and Deen, P.M.T. Molecular and cellular defects in nephrogenic diabetes insipidus. *Pediatr. Nephrol.*, **2001**, *16*:1146–1152.

Kovacs, L., and Robertson, G.L. Syndrome of inappropriate antidiuresis. *Endocrinol. Metab. Clin. North Am.*, **1992**, *21*:859–875.

Manning, M., Stoev, S., Cheng, L.L., *et al.* Discovery and design of novel vasopressin hypotensive peptide agonists. *J. Recept. Signal Transduct. Res.*, **1999**, *19*:631–644.

Mannucci, P.M. Desmopressin (DDAVP) in the treatment of bleeding disorders: The first 20 years. *Blood*, **1997**, *90*:2515–2521.

Marples, D., Frøkiaer, J., and Nielsen, S. Long-term regulation of aquaporins in the kidney. *Am. J. Physiol.*, **1999**, *276*:F331–F339.

Nielsen, S., Frøklaer, J., Marples, D, *et al.* Aquaporins in the kidney: from molecules to medicine. *Physiol. Rev.*, **2001**, *83*:205–244.

Nielsen, S., Kwon, T.H., Christensen, B.M., *et al.* Physiology and pathophysiology of renal aquaporins. *J. Am. Soc. Nephrol.*, **1999**, *10*:647–663.

Reaux, A., Fournie-Zaluski, M.C., and Llorens-Cortes, C. Angiotensin III: A central regulator of vasopressin release and blood pressure. *Trends Endocrinol. Metab.*, **2001**, *12*:157–162.

Robertson, G.L. Antidiuretic hormone, normal and disordered function. *Endocrinol. Metab. Clin. North Am.*, **2001**, *30*:671–694.

Robertson, G.L. Regulation of vasopressin secretion. In, *The Kidney: Physiology and Pathophysiology*, Vol. 2., 2d ed. (Seldin, D.W., and Giebisch, G., eds.) Raven Press, New York, **1992**, pp. 1595–1613.

Robertson, G.L., Athar, S., and Shelton, R.L. Osmotic control of vasopressin function. In, *Disturbances in Body Fluid Osmolality.* (Andreoli, T.E., Grantham, J.J., and Rector, F.C., eds.) American Physiological Society, Bethesda, MD, **1977**, pp. 125–148.

Robin, J.K., Oliver, J.A., and Landry, D.W. Vasopressin deficiency in the syndrome of irreversible shock. *J. Trauma*, **2003**, *54*(suppl.):149–154.

Sands, J.M. Molecular mechanisms of urea transport. *J. Membrane Biol.*, **2003**, *191*:149–163.

Scott, L.V., and Dinan, T.G. Vasopressin as a target for antidepressant development: An assessment of the available evidence. *J. Affect. Disorders*, **2002**, *72*:113–124.

Serradeil-Le Gal, C., Wagnon, J., Valette, G., *et al.* Nonpeptide vasopressin receptor antagonists: Development of selective and orally active V_{1a}, V_2, and V_{1b} receptor ligands. *Prog. Brain Res.*, **2002b**, *139*:197–210.

Sutor, A.H. Desmopressin (DDAVP) in bleeding disorders of childhood. *Semin. Thromb. Hemost.*, **1998**, *24*:555–566.

Thibonnier, M., Coles, P., Thibonnier, A., and Shoham, M. The basic and clinical pharmacology of nonpeptide vasopressin receptor antagonists. *Annu. Rev. Pharmacol. Toxicol.*, **2001**, *41*:175–202.

Van Kerrebroeck, P.E.V. Experience with the long-term use of desmopressin for nocturnal enuresis in children and adolescents. *Br. J. Urol. Int.*, **2002**, *89*:420–425.

Vlavianos, P., and Westaby, D. Management of acute variceal haemorrhage. *Eur. J. Gastroenterol. Hepatol.*, **2001**, *13*:335–342.

Wells, T. Vesicular osmometers, vasopressin secretion and aquaporin-4: A new mechanism for osmoreception? *Mol. Cell. Endocrinol.*, **1998**, *136*:103–107.

Wong, L.L. and Verbalis, J.G. Vasopressin V_2 receptor antagonists. *Cardiovasc. Res.*, **2001**, *51*:391–402.

Young, L.J., Wang, Z., and Insel, T.R. Neuroendocrine bases of monogamy. *Trends Neurosci.*, **1998**, *21*:71–75.

RENIN AND ANGIOTENSIN

Edwin K. Jackson

The renin–angiotensin system participates significantly in the pathophysiology of hypertension, congestive heart failure, myocardial infarction, and diabetic nephropathy. This realization has led to a thorough exploration of the renin–angiotensin system and the development of new approaches for inhibiting its actions. This chapter discusses the biochemistry, molecular and cellular biology, and physiology of the renin–angiotensin system; the pharmacology of drugs that interrupt the renin–angiotensin system; and the clinical utility of inhibitors of the renin–angiotensin system. Therapeutic applications of drugs covered in this chapter also are discussed in Chapters 31, 32, and 33.

THE RENIN–ANGIOTENSIN SYSTEM

History. In 1898, Tiegerstedt and Bergman found that crude saline extracts of the kidney contained a pressor substance that they named *renin.* Although their discovery had an obvious bearing on the problem of arterial hypertension and its relation to kidney disease, the finding generated little interest until 1934, when Goldblatt and his colleagues demonstrated that constriction of the renal arteries produced persistent hypertension in dogs. In 1940, Braun-Menéndez and his colleagues in Argentina and Page and Helmer in the United States reported that renin was an enzyme that acted on a plasma protein substrate to catalyze the formation of the actual pressor material, a peptide, that was named *hypertensin* by the former group and *angiotonin* by the latter. These two terms persisted for nearly 20 years until it was agreed to rename the pressor substance *angiotensin* and to call the plasma substrate *angiotensinogen.* In the mid-1950s, two forms of angiotensin were recognized, a decapeptide (angiotensin I) and an octapeptide (angiotensin II) formed by proteolytic cleavage of angiotensin I by an enzyme termed *angiotensin-converting enzyme* (ACE). The octapeptide was shown to be the more active form, and its synthesis in 1957 by Schwyzer and by Bumpus made the material available for intensive study.

In 1958, Gross suggested that the renin–angiotensin system was involved in the regulation of aldosterone secretion. It was soon shown that the kidneys are important for such regulation and that synthetic angiotensin potently stimulates the production of aldoster-

one in humans. Moreover, renin secretion increased with depletion of Na^+. Thus the renin–angiotensin system came to be recognized as a mechanism to stimulate aldosterone synthesis and secretion and an important homeostatic mechanism in the regulation of blood pressure and electrolyte composition.

In the early 1970s, polypeptides were discovered that either inhibited the formation of angiotensin II or blocked angiotensin II receptors; experimental studies with these inhibitors revealed important physiological and pathophysiological roles for the renin–angiotensin system. These findings inspired the development of a new and broadly efficacious class of antihypertensive drugs: the orally active ACE inhibitors. Subsequent studies with ACE inhibitors uncovered roles for the renin–angiotensin system in the pathophysiology of hypertension, heart 4failure, vascular disease, and renal failure, providing impetus for the development of additional classes of inhibitors of the renin–angiotensin system. In 1982 it was reported that derivatives of imidazole-5-acetic acid attenuated vasoconstriction induced by angiotensin II. Two of these compounds, S-8307 and S-8308, were shown subsequently to be selective and competitive antagonists of angiotensin II receptors. Refinements of these compounds yielded losartan, an orally active, highly selective, and potent nonpeptide angiotensin II receptor antagonist. Subsequently, many other angiotensin II receptor antagonists have been developed.

Components of the Renin–Angiotensin System

Overview. Angiotensin II, the most active angiotensin peptide, is derived from angiotensinogen in two proteolytic steps. First, renin, an enzyme released from the kidneys, cleaves the decapeptide angiotensin I from the amino terminus of angiotensinogen (renin substrate). Then angiotensin-converting enzyme (ACE) removes the carboxy-terminal dipeptide of angiotensin I to produce the octapeptide angiotensin II. Angiotensin II is degraded subsequently by further proteolysis. These enzymatic steps and amino acid sequences are summarized in Figure 30–1. Angiotensin II acts by binding to two heptahelical G protein–coupled receptors. All the components of the renin–angiotensin system are described below.

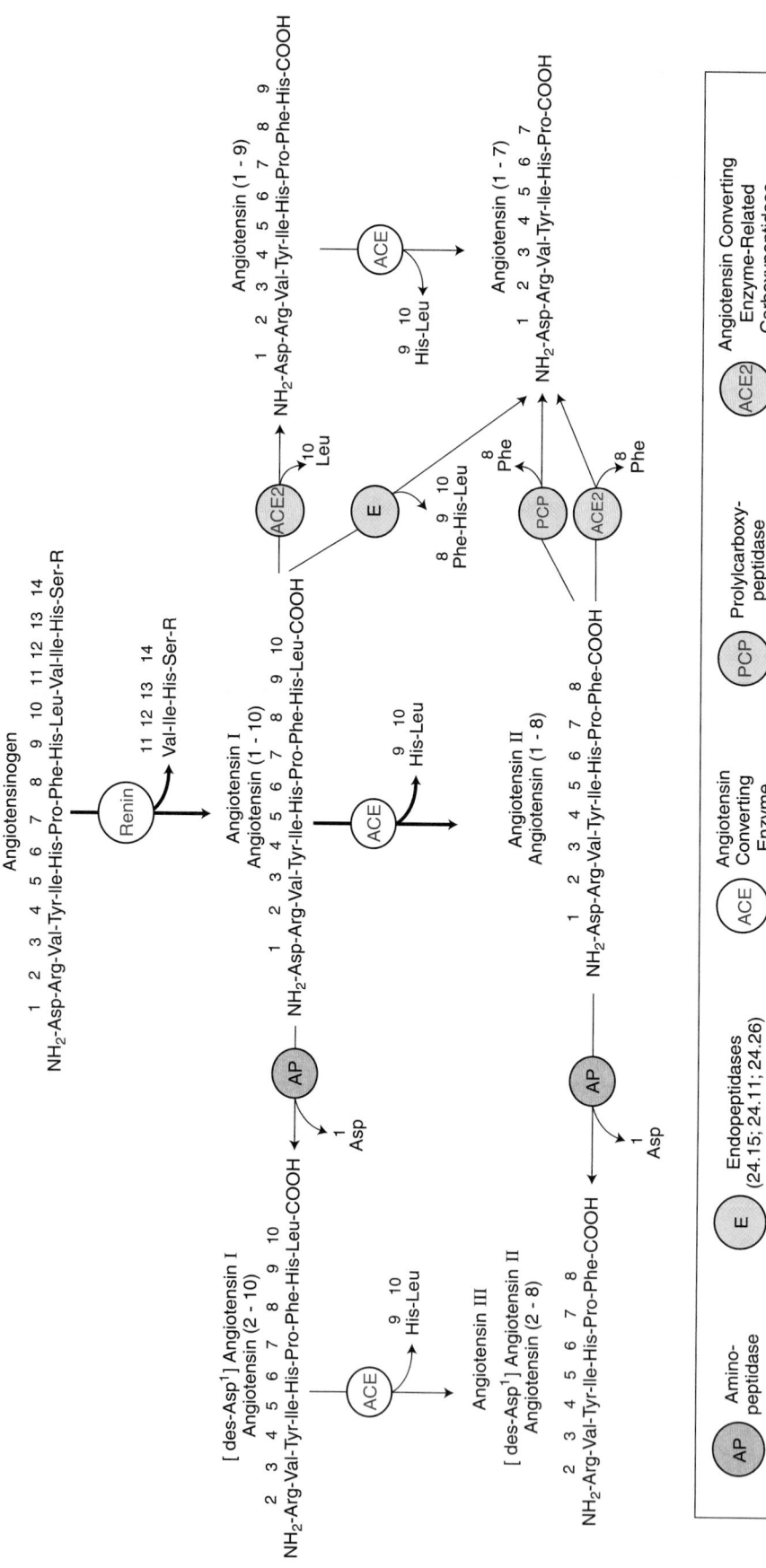

Figure 30–1. *Formation of angiotensin peptides.* The heavy arrows show the classical pathway, and the light arrows indicate alternative pathways. The structures of the angiotensins shown are those found in human beings, horses, rats, and pigs; the bovine form has valine in the 5 position. The N-terminal sequence of human angiotensinogen is depicted. AP, aminopeptidase; E, endopeptidases (24.15; 24.11; 24.26); ACE, angiotensin-converting enzyme; PCP, prolylcarboxylpeptidase.

Renin. The major determinant of the rate of angiotensin II production is the amount of renin released by the kidney. Renin is synthesized, stored, and secreted into the renal arterial circulation by the granular juxtaglomerular cells that lie in the walls of the afferent arterioles that enter the glomeruli. Renin is stored in granules within juxtaglomerular cells and is secreted by exocytosis (Friis *et al.*, 1999).

Renin is an aspartyl protease that attacks a restricted number of substrates. Its principal natural substrate is a circulating α_2-globulin, angiotensinogen, that is secreted by hepatocytes (*see* below). Renin cleaves the bond between residues 10 and 11 at the amino terminus of angiotensinogen to generate angiotensin I. The active form of renin is a glycoprotein that contains 340 amino acids. It is synthesized as a preproenzyme of 406 amino acid residues that is processed to prorenin, a mature but inactive form of the protein. Prorenin then is activated by an as yet uncharacterized enzyme that removes 43 amino acids from its amino terminus to yield active renin. Similar to other aspartyl proteases, renin has a bilobal structure with a cleft that forms the active site (Sielecki *et al.*, 1989). A truncated, nonsecreted form of renin is expressed in the brain from an alternative promoter within intron I of the renin gene (Lee-Kirsch *et al.*, 1999).

Both renin and prorenin are stored in the juxtaglomerular cells and, when released, circulate in the blood. The concentration of prorenin in the circulation is approximately tenfold greater than that of the active enzyme. The half-life of circulating renin is approximately 15 minutes. The physiological status of circulating prorenin is unclear.

Control of Renin Secretion (Figure 30–2). The secretion of renin from juxtaglomerular cells is controlled predominantly by three pathways: two acting locally within the kidney and the third acting through the central nervous system (CNS) and mediated by norepinephrine release from renal noradrenergic nerves. One intrarenal mechanism controlling renin release is the *macula densa pathway* (top of Figure 30–2A). The macula densa lies adjacent to the juxtaglomerular cells and is composed of specialized columnar epithelial cells in the wall of that portion of the cortical thick ascending limb that passes between the afferent and efferent arterioles of the glomerulus. A change in NaCl reabsorption by the macula densa results in the transmission to nearby juxtaglomerular cells of chemical signals that modify renin release. Increases in NaCl flux across the macula densa inhibit renin release, whereas decreases in NaCl flux stimulate renin release. Both adenosine and prostaglandins mediate the macula densa pathway; the former is released when NaCl transport increases, and the latter is released when NaCl transport decreases. Adenosine, acting *via* the A_1 adenosine receptor, inhibits renin release, and prostaglandins stimulate renin release.

Substantial evidence exists supporting a role for inducible cyclooxygenase (COX-2) and neuronal nitric oxide synthase (nNOS) in the mechanism of macula densa–stimulated renin release. Although constitutive cyclooxygenase (COX-1) is the most abundant cyclooxygenase isoform in the mammalian kidney, inducible COX-2 is the only cyclooxygenase form expressed in the macula densa, where it is up-regulated by chronic dietary sodium restriction (Harris *et al.*, 1994), a maneuver that increases renin release in part *via* the macula densa pathway. Renin release induced by a low-sodium diet is blunted by selective inhibition of COX-2 (Kammerl *et al.*, 2001) and is attenuated in COX-2 knockout mice (Yang *et al.*, 2000). Moreover, selective inhibition of COX-2 blocks macula densa–mediated renin release in the isolated perfused juxtaglomerular preparation (Traynor *et al.*, 1999). In a similar manner, the expression of nNOS in the macula densa is up-regulated by dietary sodium restriction (Singh *et al.*, 1996), and selective inhibition of nNOS reduces renin release in response to chronic dietary sodium restriction (Beierwaltes, 1997). The nNOS/NO pathway, in part, may mediate increases in COX-2 expression induced by a low-sodium diet (Cheng *et al.*, 2000). Together these findings suggest a biochemical interplay between COX-2 and nNOS in the regulation of macula densa–mediated renin release. Since NO reacts with superoxide anion to generate peroxynitrite, which markedly activates cyclooxygenase activity (Landino *et al.*, 1996), it is plausible that activation of macula densa–mediated renin release by sodium depletion involves the following events: up-regulation of nNOS and COX-2 in the macula densa, increased biosynthesis of NO and peroxynitrite in the macula densa, peroxynitrite-induced activation of COX-2 in the macula densa, increased prostaglandin production in the macula densa, and paracrine activation of prostaglandin receptors in neighboring juxtaglomerular cells. However, COX-2 expression in the macula densa is not attenuated in nNOS knockout mice (Theilig *et al.*, 2002), which suggests that other mechanisms can compensate for nNOS in the regulation of COX-2. Possible mechanisms by which the macula densa and autonomic nervous system regulate renin release are summarized in Figure 30–2B.

Although a change in NaCl transport by the macula densa is the key event that modulates the macula densa pathway, regulation of this pathway is more dependent on the luminal concentration of Cl^- than Na^+. NaCl transport into the macula densa is mediated by the Na^+–K^+–$2Cl^-$ symporter, and the half-maximal concentrations of Na^+ and Cl^- required for transport *via* this symporter are 2 to 3 and 40 mEq/L, respectively. Since the luminal concentration of Na^+ at the macula densa usually is much greater than the level required for half-maximal transport, physiological variations in luminal Na^+ concentrations at the macula densa have little effect on renin release (*i.e.*, the symporter remains saturated with respect to Na^+). On the other hand, physiological changes in Cl^- concentrations (20 to 60 mEq/L) at the macula densa profoundly affect macula densa–mediated renin release.

The second intrarenal mechanism controlling renin release is the *intrarenal baroreceptor pathway* (middle of Figure 30–2A). Increases and decreases in blood pressure in the preglomerular vessels inhibit and stimulate renin release, respectively. The immediate stimulus to secretion is believed to be reduced tension within the wall of the afferent arteriole. Increases and decreases in renal perfusion pressure may inhibit and stimulate, respectively, the release of renal prostaglandins, which may mediate in part the intrarenal baroreceptor pathway. In support of this conclusion, COX-2 inhibition decreases renin secretion and blood pressure in renin-dependent renovascular hypertension (Wang *et al.*, 1999). Biomechanical coupling *via* stretch-activated ion channels also may play a role in this pathway (Carey *et al.*, 1997).

The third mechanism, the *β-adrenergic receptor pathway* (bottom of Figure 30–2A), is mediated by the release of norepinephrine from postganglionic sympathetic nerves; activation of β_1-receptors on juxtaglomerular cells enhances renin secretion.

The three mechanisms regulating renin release are embedded in a physiological network. Increased renin secretion enhances the formation of angiotensin II, and angiotensin II stimulates angiotensin subtype 1 (AT_1) receptors on juxtaglomerular cells to inhibit renin release, an effect termed *short-loop negative feedback*. Angiotensin II also increases arterial blood pressure by stimulating AT_1 receptors. Increases in blood pressure inhibit renin release by (1) activating high-pressure baroreceptors, thereby reducing renal sympathetic

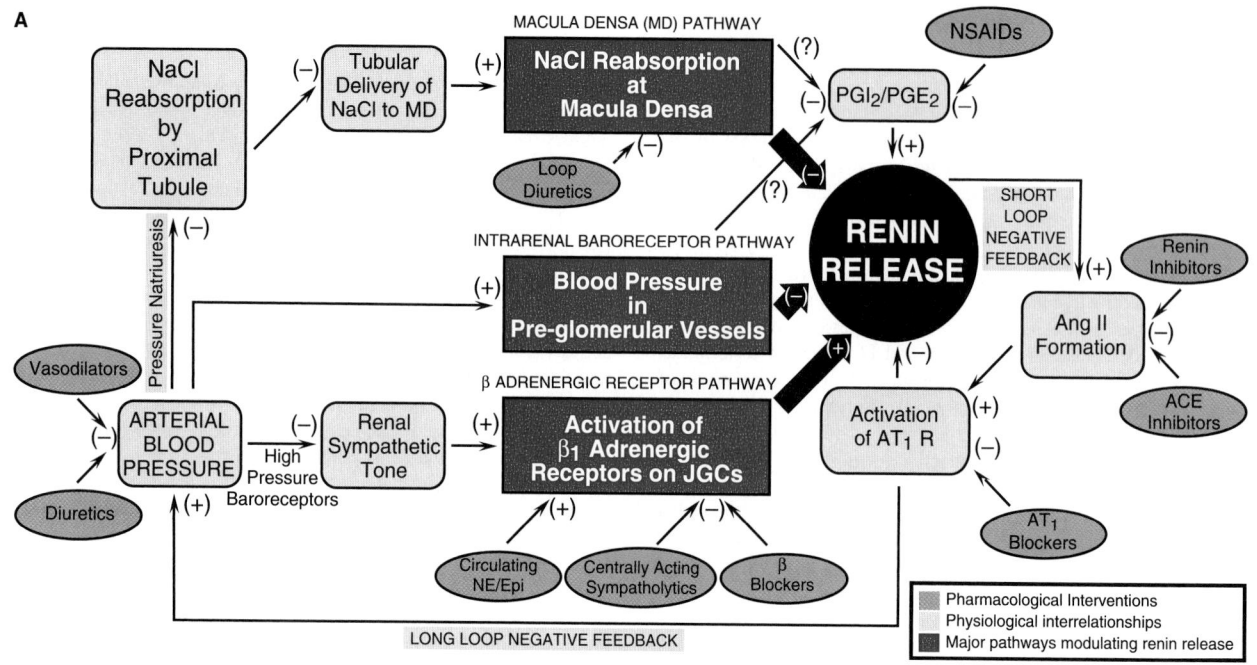

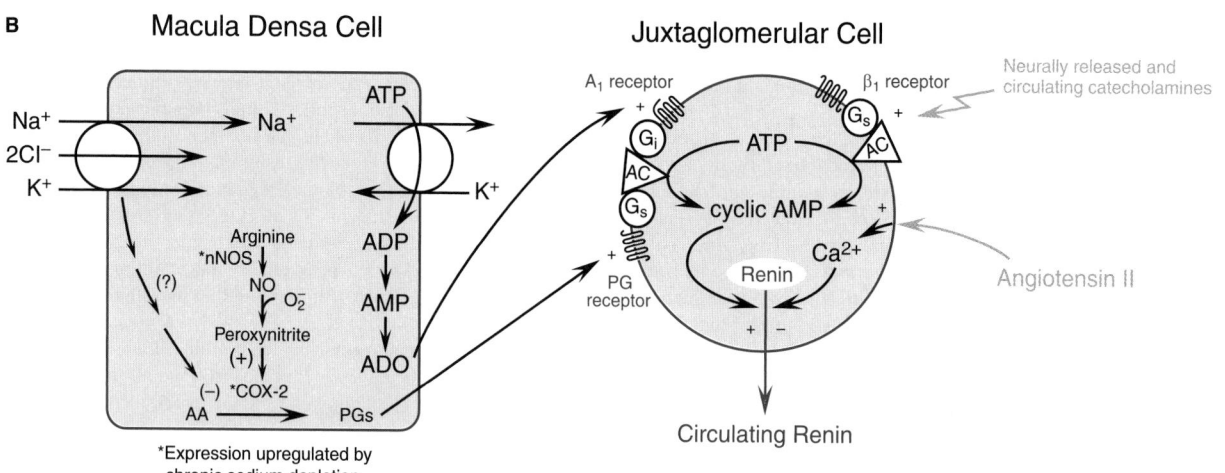

*Expression upregulated by
chronic sodium depletion

Figure 30–2. *A.* Schematic portrayal of the three major physiological pathways regulating renin release. *See* text for details. MD, macula densa; PGI_2/PGE_2 prostaglandins I_2 and E_2; NSAIDs, nonsteroidal antiinflammatory drugs; Ang II, angiotensin II; ACE, angiotensin-converting enzyme, AT_1 R, angiotensin subtype 1 receptor; NE/Epi, norepinephrine/epinephrine; JGCs, juxtaglomerular cells. *B.* Possible mechanisms by which the macula densa regulates renin release. Both acute changes in tubular delivery of NaCl to the macula densa and chronic changes in dietary sodium intake cause appropriate signals to be conveyed from macula densa to the juxtaglomerular cells. Chronic sodium depletion up-regulates neuronal nitric oxide synthase (nNOS) and inducible cyclooxygenase (COX-2) in the macula densa. nNOS increases nitric oxide (NO) production, and NO reacts with superoxide anion (O_2^-) to form peroxynitrite, an activator of COX-2. In addition, COX-2 may be rapidly, although indirectly, inhibited and stimulated by increases and decreases in NaCl transport, respectively, across the macula densa. Arachidonic acid (AA) is converted to prostaglandins (PGs), which diffuse to nearby juxtaglomerular cells to stimulate adenylyl cyclase (AC) *via* prostaglandin receptors, such as EP_4 and IP, that couple to G_s. Circulating and locally released catecholamines also stimulate adenylyl cyclase *via* β_1 receptors. Cyclic AMP (cAMP) augments renin release. Increased NaCl transport depletes ATP and increases adenosine (ADO) levels in the macula densa. ADO diffuses to the juxtaglomerular cells and activates the AT_1-G_i pathway, inhibiting AC and reducing cellular cAMP. Increased NaCl transport in the macula densa augments the efflux of ATP through basolateral maxianion channels, and ATP is converted to adenosine in the extracellular compartment and inhibits adenylyl cyclase *via* A_1 receptors. In addition, ATP released from the macula densa may inhibit renin release directly by binding to P2Y receptors coupled to G_q on juxtaglomerular cells. Activation of G_q increases intracellular Ca^{2+}, which inhibits renin release. Circulating angiotensin II (Ang II) binds to AT_1 receptors on juxtaglomerular cells and inhibits renin release *via* G_q-induced increases in intracellular Ca^{2+}.

tone, (2) increasing pressure in the preglomerular vessels, and (3) reducing NaCl reabsorption in the proximal tubule (pressure natriuresis), which increases tubular delivery of NaCl to the macula densa. The inhibition of renin release owing to angiotensin II–induced increases in blood pressure has been termed *long-loop negative feedback.*

The physiological pathways regulating renin release can be influenced by arterial blood pressure, dietary salt intake, and a number of pharmacological agents. In all these cases, renin release is affected by a complex interplay of the mechanisms summarized in Figure 30-2A. Loop diuretics (*see* Chapter 28) stimulate renin release in part by blocking the reabsorption of NaCl at the macula densa. *Nonsteroidal antiinflammatory drugs* (NSAIDs) (*see* Chapter 26) inhibit prostaglandin synthesis and thereby decrease renin release. ACE inhibitors, angiotensin-receptor blockers, and renin inhibitors interrupt both the short- and long-loop negative feedback mechanisms and therefore increase renin release. However, the effect of chronic inhibition of the renin–angiotensin system on renin release also involves COX-2 and nNOS. In this regard, chronic administration of ACE inhibitors up-regulates renocortical COX-2 and nNOS expression (Kammerl *et al.*, 2002), and the ability of chronic ACE inhibition to stimulate renin release is attenuated in COX-2 knockout mice (Cheng *et al.*, 2001). In general, diuretics and vasodilators increase renin release by decreasing arterial blood pressure. Centrally acting sympatholytic drugs, as well as β adrenergic receptor antagonists, decrease renin secretion by reducing activation of β adrenergic receptors on juxtaglomerular cells. Phosphodiesterase inhibitors stimulate renin release by increasing cyclic AMP in juxtaglomerular cells (Friis *et al.*, 2002).

Angiotensinogen. The substrate for renin is angiotensinogen, an abundant globular glycoprotein (MW = 55,000 to 60,000) containing 13% to 14% carbohydrate. High-molecular-weight (350,000 to 500,000) angiotensinogen also circulates in plasma and represents a complex of angiotensinogen with other proteins. Angiotensin I is cleaved from the amino terminus of angiotensinogen. The human angiotensinogen contains 452 amino acids and is synthesized as pre-angiotensinogen, which has a 24– or 33–amino acid signal peptide. Angiotensinogen is synthesized primarily in the liver, although angiotensinogen transcripts also are abundant in fat, certain regions of the CNS, and kidney. Angiotensinogen is synthesized and secreted continuously by the liver, and its synthesis is stimulated by inflammation, insulin, estrogens, glucocorticoids, thyroid hormone, and angiotensin II. During pregnancy, plasma levels of angiotensinogen increase severalfold owing to increased estrogen.

Circulating levels of angiotensinogen are approximately equal to the K_m of renin for its substrate (about 1 μM). Consequently, the rate of angiotensin II synthesis, and therefore blood pressure, can be influenced by changes in angiotensinogen levels. For instance, knockout mice lacking angiotensinogen are hypotensive (Tanimoto *et al.*, 1994), and there is a progressive relationship among the number of copies of the angiotensinogen gene, plasma levels of angiotensinogen, and arterial blood pressure (Kim *et al.*, 1995). Also, intravenous injection of angiotensinogen increases arterial blood pressure (Klett and Granger, 2001). Oral contraceptives containing estrogen increase circulating levels of angiotensinogen and can induce hypertension. Furthermore, a missense mutation in the angiotensinogen gene (a methionine to threonine at position 235 of angiotensinogen) that increases plasma levels of angiotensinogen is associated with essential (Jeunemaitre *et al.*, 1992; Caulfield *et al.*, 1994, 1995; Kunz *et al.*, 1997; Staessen *et al.*, 1999; Sethi *et al.*,

2001, 2003) and pregnancy-induced (Ward *et al.*, 1993) hypertension. Angiotensinogen has sequence homologies with the serpin protein family, and serpins have antiangiogenic properties. Both angiotensinogen and [des-angiotensin I]angiotensinogen also inhibit angiogenesis (Célérier *et al.*, 2002).

Angiotensin-Converting Enzyme (ACE, Kininase II, Dipeptidyl Carboxypeptidase). ACE is an ectoenzyme and glycoprotein with an apparent molecular weight of 170,000. Human ACE contains 1277 amino acid residues and has two homologous domains, each with a catalytic site and a Zn^{2+}-binding region. ACE has a large amino-terminal extracellular domain, a short carboxyl-terminal intracellular domain, and a 17–amino acid hydrophobic region that anchors the ectoenzyme to the cell membrane. Circulating ACE represents membrane ACE that has undergone proteolysis at the cell surface by a secretase (Beldent *et al.*, 1995). ACE is rather nonspecific and cleaves dipeptide units from substrates with diverse amino acid sequences. Preferred substrates have only one free carboxyl group in the carboxyl-terminal amino acid, and proline must not be the penultimate amino acid; thus the enzyme does not degrade angiotensin II. ACE is identical to kininase II, the enzyme that inactivates bradykinin and other potent vasodilator peptides. Although slow conversion of angiotensin I to angiotensin II occurs in plasma, the very rapid metabolism that occurs *in vivo* is due largely to the activity of membrane-bound ACE present on the luminal surface of endothelial cells throughout the vascular system.

The *ACE* gene encodes both somatic and testis-specific isozymes. The testis ACE is found exclusively in developing spermatids and mature sperm and is encoded by the second half of the ACE gene, driven by a testis-specific promoter. Testis ACE is involved in the transport of sperm in the oviduct and in binding of the sperm to the zonae pellucidae (Hagaman *et al.*, 1998). These effects of testis-specific ACE are not mediated by angiotensin II.

The *ACE* gene contains an insertion deletion polymorphism in intron 16 that explains 47% of the phenotypic variance in serum ACE levels (Rigat *et al.*, 1990). The deletion allele, associated with higher levels of serum ACE and increased metabolism of bradykinin (Murphey *et al.*, 2000), may confer an increased risk of ischemic heart disease (Cambien *et al.*, 1992; Gardemann *et al.*, 1995; Mattu *et al.*, 1995; Fatini *et al.*, 2000), coronary artery spasm (Oike *et al.*, 1995), restenosis after coronary stenting (Amant *et al.*, 1997; Ribichini *et al.*, 1998), vascular endothelial dysfunction (Butler *et al.*, 1999), left ventricular hypertrophy (Iwai *et al.*, 1994; Schunkert *et al.*, 1994), exercise-induced left ventricular growth (Montgomery *et al.*, 1997), carotid artery disease (Hosoi *et al.*, 1996; Losito *et al.*, 2000), ischemic stroke (Kario *et al.*, 1996), hypertension in males (O'Donnell *et al.*, 1998; Fornage *et al.*, 1998; Higaki *et al.*, 2000), diabetic nephropathy (Marre *et al.*, 1997; Hadjadj *et al.*, 2001), deterioration of renal function in immunoglobulin A (IgA) nephropathy (Yoshida *et al.*, 1995), renal artery stenosis (Olivieri *et al.*, 1999), and thrombosis in patients undergoing hip arthroplasty (Philipp *et al.*, 1998). Surprisingly, however, the deletion allele is more frequent in centenarians (Schachter *et al.*, 1994), a finding that may be explained by the strong association of the deletion allele with protection against Alzheimer's disease (Kehoe *et al.*, 1999).

Two groups independently discovered a novel angiotensin converting enzyme–related carboxypeptidase, now termed *ACE2* (Donoghue *et al.*, 2000; Tipnis *et al.*, 2000). Human ACE2 is 805 amino acids in length with a short putative signal sequence. ACE2 contains a single catalytic domain that is 42% identical to the two catalytic domains of ACE. ACE2 cleaves angiotensin I to angiotensin(1–9) and processes angiotensin II to angiotensin(1–7). ACE2 is not inhibited by the standard ACE inhibitors described in this chapter. In animals, reduced expression of ACE2 is associated with hypertension and defects in cardiac contractility (Crackower *et al.*, 2002). ACE2 also serves as a receptor for the SARS coronavirus (Li *et al.*, 2003). The physiological significance of ACE2 still is uncertain; it may serve as a counter-regulatory mechanism to oppose the effects of ACE (Yagil and Yagil, 2003).

Angiotensin Peptides. When given intravenously, angiotensin I is converted to angiotensin II so rapidly that the pharmacological responses to these two peptides are indistinguishable. However, angiotensin I *per se* is less than 1% as potent as angiotensin II on smooth muscle, heart, and the adrenal cortex. As shown in Figure 30–1, angiotensin III, also called [des-Asp¹]angiotensin II or angiotensin (2–8), can be formed either by the action of aminopeptidase on angiotensin II or by the action of ACE on [des-Asp¹]angiotensin I. Angiotensin III and angiotensin II cause qualitatively similar effects. Angiotensin II and angiotensin III stimulate aldosterone secretion with equal potency; however, angiotensin III is only 25% and 10% as potent as angiotensin II in elevating blood pressure and stimulating the adrenal medulla, respectively.

Angiotensin(1–7) is formed by multiple pathways (Figure 30–1). Angiotensin I can be metabolized to angiotensin(1–7) by metalloendopeptidase 24.15, endopeptidase 24.11, and prolylendopeptidase 24.26. Angiotensin II can be converted to angiotensin(1–7) by prolylcarboxypeptidase (Ferrario *et al.*, 1997). ACE2 converts angiotensin I to angiotensin(1–9) and angiotensin II to angiotensin(1–7); ACE metabolizes angiotensin(1–9) to angiotensin(1–7). ACE inhibitors increase tissue and plasma levels of angiotensin(1–7) both because angiotensin I levels are increased and diverted away from angiotensin II formation (Figure 30–1) and because ACE contributes importantly to the plasma clearance of angiotensin(1–7) (Yamada *et al.*, 1998). The pharmacological profile of angiotensin(1–7) is distinct from that of angiotensin II: Angiotensin(1–7) does not cause vasoconstriction, aldosterone release, or facilitation of noradrenergic neurotransmission. Angiotensin(1–7) releases vasopressin, stimulates prostaglandin biosynthesis, elicits depressor responses when microinjected into certain brainstem nuclei, dilates some blood vessels, and exerts a natriuretic action on the kidneys. Angiotensin(1–7) also inhibits proliferation of vascular smooth muscle cells (Tallant *et al.*, 1999). The effects of angiotensin(1–7) may be mediated by a specific angiotensin(1–7) receptor (Tallant *et al.*, 1997). The *Mas* protooncogene encodes an orphan G protein–coupled receptor that binds angiotensin(1–7) (Santos *et al.*, 2003). Ferrario and colleagues (1997) proposed that angiotensin(1–7) serves to counterbalance the actions of angiotensin II. Angiotensin(3–8), also called *angiotensin IV,* is yet another biologically active angiotensin peptide. Putative receptors for angiotensin(3–8) are detectable in a number of tissues (Swanson *et al.*, 1992), and the peptide stimulates the expression of plasminogen activator inhibitor-1 in endothelial (Kerins *et al.*, 1995) and proximal tubular (Gesualdo *et al.*, 1999) cells, although in vascular smooth muscle cells and cardiomyocytes, angiotensin II rather than angiotensin(3–8) mediates increased expression of plasminogen activator inhibitor-1 (Chen *et al.*, 2000). Angiotensin(3–8) also may be involved in memory acquisition and, like angiotensin(1–7), appears to counteract the effects of angiotensin II (de Gasparo *et al.*, 2000). The physiological significance of angiotensin(1–7) and angiotensin(3–8) remains uncertain.

There is considerable information on the structure–activity relationships of angiotensin-related peptides with regard to activity at

receptors for angiotensin II (Samanen and Regoli, 1994). In general, phenylalanine in position 8 is critical for most agonist activity, and the aromatic residues in positions 4 and 6, the guanido group in position 2, and the C-terminal carboxyl are thought to be involved in binding to the receptor site. Position 1 is not critical, but replacement of aspartic acid in position 1 with sarcosine enhances binding to angiotensin receptors and slows hydrolysis by rendering the peptide refractory to a subgroup of aminopeptidases (angiotensinase A). Such a substitution, combined with that of alanine or isoleucine in place of phenylalanine in position 8, yields potent angiotensin II receptor antagonists.

Angiotensinases. This term is applied to various peptidases that are involved in the degradation and inactivation of angiotensin peptides; none is specific. Among them are aminopeptidases, endopeptidases, and carboxypeptidases.

Local (Tissue) Renin–Angiotensin Systems. The traditional view of the renin–angiotensin system is that of a classical endocrine system. Circulating renin from the kidney acts on circulating angiotensinogen of hepatic origin to produce angiotensin I in the plasma, circulating angiotensin I is converted by plasma ACE and by pulmonary endothelial ACE to angiotensin II, and angiotensin II then is delivered to its target organs *via* the bloodstream, where it induces a physiological response. This traditional view is an oversimplification that must be expanded to include local (tissue) renin–angiotensin systems. In this regard it is important to distinguish between *extrinsic* and *intrinsic* local renin–angiotensin systems.

Extrinsic Local Renin–Angiotensin Systems. ACE is present on the luminal face of vascular endothelial cells throughout the circulation, and circulating renin of renal origin can be taken up (sequestered) by the arterial wall and by other tissues. Thus the conversion of hepatic angiotensinogen to angiotensin I and the conversion of angiotensin I (both circulating and locally produced) to angiotensin II may occur primarily within or at the surface of the blood vessel wall, not in the circulation *per se*. Indeed, many vascular beds produce angiotensins I and II locally, and a substantial fraction of local production does not occur in the plasma as it transverses the vascular bed (Danser *et al.*, 1991, 1994; Hilgers *et al.*, 2001). Local sequestration of renal renin in both vascular and cardiac tissues reportedly participates in the local production of angiotensins (Kato *et al.*, 1993; Taddei *et al.*, 1993; Danser *et al.*, 1994), a conclusion not universally accepted (Hu *et al.*, 1998).

Intrinsic Local Renin–Angiotensin Systems. Many tissues—including the brain, pituitary, blood vessels, heart, kidney, and adrenal gland—express mRNAs for renin, angiotensinogen, and/or ACE, and various cells cultured from these tissues produce renin, angiotensinogen, ACE, and angiotensins I, II, and III (Phillips *et al.*, 1993; Saavedra, 1992; Dzau, 1993; Baker *et al.*, 1992). Thus it appears that local renin–angiotensin systems exist independently of the renal/hepatic-based system. Although these local systems do not contribute significantly to circulating levels of active renin or angiotensins (Campbell *et al.*, 1991), local production of angiotensin II by intrinsic local renin–angiotensin systems may influence vascular, cardiac, and renal function and structure.

Alternative Pathways for Angiotensin Biosynthesis. Some tissues contain nonrenin angiotensinogen-processing enzymes that convert angiotensinogen to angiotensin I (nonrenin proteases) or directly to angiotensin II (*e.g.,* cathepsin G, tonin) and non-ACE angiotensin I–processing enzymes that convert angiotensin I to angiotensin II (*e.g.,* cathepsin G, chymostatin-sensitive angiotensin II–generating enzyme, heart chymase) (Dzau *et al.,* 1993). There is mounting evidence that chymase, possibly mast cell–derived, contributes to the local tissue conversion of angiotensin I to angiotensin II, particularly in the heart (Wolny *et al.,* 1997; Wei *et al.,* 1999) and kidneys (Hollenberg *et al.,* 1998); however, the role of chymase as a non-ACE angiotensin I–processing enzyme is species- and organ-dependent (Akasu *et al.,* 1998).

Angiotensin Receptors. The effects of angiotensins are exerted through specific heptahelical G protein–coupled receptors (de Gasparo *et al.,* 2000). The two subtypes of angiotensin receptors (Whitebread *et al.,* 1989; Chiu *et al.,* 1989) now are designated AT_1 and AT_2 (Bumpus *et al.,* 1991). The AT_1 receptor has a high affinity for losartan (and related biphenyl tetrazole derivatives), a low affinity for PD 123177 (and related 1-benzyl spinacine derivatives), and a low affinity for CGP 42112A (a peptide analog). In contrast, the AT_2 receptor has a high affinity for PD 123177 and CGP 42112A but a low affinity for losartan.

The AT_1 receptor is 359 amino acids long; the AT_2 receptor consists of 363 amino acids. The AT_1 and AT_2 receptors have little sequence homology. Most of the known biological effects of angiotensin II are mediated by the AT_1 receptor. Functional roles for the AT_2 receptors are poorly defined, but they may exert antiproliferative, proapoptotic, vasodilatory, and antihypertensive effects (Inagami *et al.,* 1999; Ardaillou, 1999; Horiuchi *et al.,* 1999; Siragy *et al.,* 2000; Moore *et al.,* 2001; Carey *et al.,* 2001). The complex effects of AT_2 receptor activation on vascular tone and biology may depend on such factors as species, organ, and vascular diameter (Henrion *et al.,* 2001). Although the AT_2 receptor generally is conceptualized as a cardiovascular protective receptor, its activation may contribute to cardiac fibrosis (Ichihara *et al.,* 2001).

The AT_2 receptor is distributed widely in fetal tissues, but its distribution is more restricted in adults. In adults, some tissues contain primarily either AT_1 receptors or AT_2 receptors, whereas other tissues contain the receptor subtypes in similar amounts. In this regard, tissue and species differences are the rule, not the exception (Timmermans *et al.,* 1993). The AT_1-receptor gene contains a polymorphism (A-to-C transversion in position 1166) that reportedly is associated with hypertension (Kainulainen *et al.,* 1999), hypertrophic cardiomyopathy (Osterop *et al.,* 1998), coronary artery vasoconstriction (Amant *et al.,* 1997), and aortic stiffness (Benetos *et al.,* 1996). Moreover, the C allele synergizes with the ACE deletion allele with regard to increased risk of coronary artery disease (Tiret *et al.,* 1994; Álvarez *et al.,* 1998). Preeclampsia is associated with the development of agonistic autoantibodies against the AT_1 receptor (Wallukat *et al.,* 1999). AT_1 receptors regulate their own expression by a mechanism involving phosphorylation of calreticulin. Phosphorylated calreticulin binds to and destabilizes AT_1-receptor mRNA (Nickenig *et al.,* 2002).

Angiotensin Receptor–Effector Coupling. AT_1 receptors activate a large array of signal-transduction systems to produce effects that vary with cell type and that are a combination of primary and secondary responses (Griendling *et al.,* 1997; Berk, 1999; Inagami, 1999; Blume *et al.,* 1999; Rocic *et al.,* 2001; Haendeler and Berk, 2000; Epperson *et al.,* 2004) (Figure 30–3). AT_1 receptors couple to several heterotrimeric G proteins, including G_q, $G_{12/13}$ and G_i. In most cell types, AT_1 receptors couple to G_q to activate the PLCβ–IP$_3$–Ca^{2+} pathway (*see* Chapter 1). Secondary to G_q activation, activation of PKC, PLA$_2$, and PLD and eicosanoid production may occur, as well as activation of

Ca^{2+}-dependent and MAP kinases and the Ca^{2+}–calmodulin–dependent activation of NOS. Activation of G_i may occur and will reduce the activity of adenylyl cyclase, lowering cellular cyclic AMP content; however, there also is evidence for $G_q \rightarrow G_s$ cross-talk such that activation of the AT_1–G_q–PLC pathway enhances cyclic AMP production (Meszaros *et al.,* 2000; Epperson *et al.,* 2004). The $\beta\gamma$ subunits of G_i and activation of $G_{12/13}$ lead to activation of tyrosine kinases and small G proteins such as Rho. Ultimately, through a combination of direct and secondary effects, the JAK/STAT pathway is activated, and a variety of transcriptional regulatory factors is induced, as summarized by Figure 30–3. By these mechanisms, angiotensin influences the expression of a host of gene products relating to cell growth and the production of components of the extracellular matrix. AT_1 receptors also stimulate the activity of a membrane-bound NADH/NADPH oxidase that generates superoxide anion. Catalase transforms the superoxide anion to hydrogen peroxide, which may contribute to biochemical effects (MAP kinase activation), expression of monocyte chemoattractant protein-1 and physiological effects [acute effects on renal function (López *et al.,* 2003), chronic effects on blood pressure (Landmesser *et al.,* 2002), and vascular hypertrophy (Wang *et al.,* 2001)]. Angiotensin II also induces the expression of a novel redox-sensitive gene product, Id3, that depresses the amount of cell-cycle inhibitors such as p21^{WAF1}, p27^{Kip1}, and p53 and increases cell growth (Mueller *et al.,* 2002). The relative importance of these myriad signal-transduction pathways in mediating biological responses to angiotensin II is tissue-specific. The presence of other receptors may alter the response to AT_1-receptor activation. For example, AT_1 receptors heterodimerize with bradykinin B$_2$ receptors, a process that enhances angiotensin II sensitivity in preeclampsia (AbdAlla *et al.,* 2001).

Less is known about AT_2 receptor–effector coupling. Signaling from AT_2 receptors is mediated largely by G_i (Hansen *et al.,* 2000). Consequences of AT_2-receptor activation include activation of phosphatases, potassium channels, and bradykinin and NO production and inhibition of calcium channel functions (Horiuchi *et al.,* 1999). The AT_2 receptor may bind directly to and antagonize the AT_1 receptor.

Functions and Effects of the Renin–Angiotensin System

The renin–angiotensin system plays a major role in both the short- and long-term regulation of arterial blood pressure. Modest increases in plasma concentrations of angiotensin II acutely raise blood pressure; on a molar basis, angiotensin II is approximately 40 times more potent than norepinephrine, and the EC$_{50}$ of angiotensin II for acutely raising arterial blood pressure is approximately 0.3 nmol/L. When a single moderate dose of angiotensin II is injected intravenously, systemic blood pressure begins to rise within seconds, peaks rapidly, and returns to normal within minutes (Figure 30–4). This *rapid pressor response* to angiotensin II is due to a swift increase in total peripheral resistance—a response that helps to maintain arterial blood pressure in the face of an acute hypotensive challenge (*e.g.,* blood loss or vasodilation). Although angiotensin II increases cardiac con-

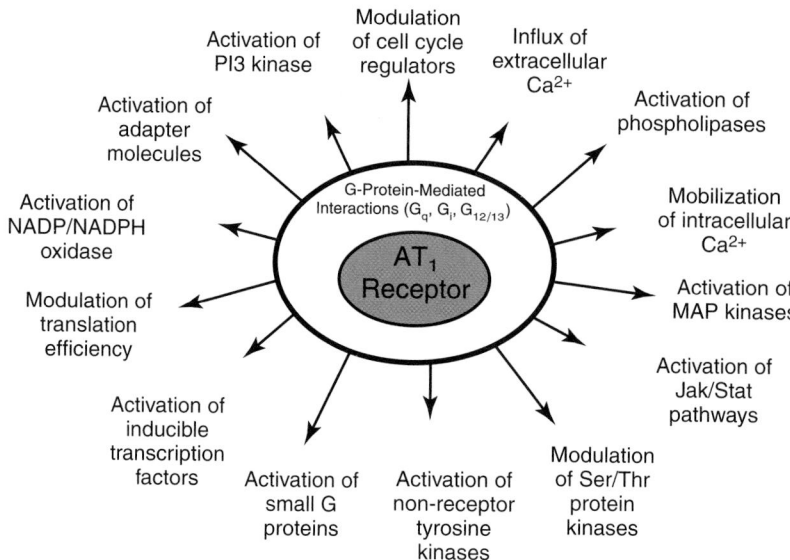

Figure 30–3. *Multiple mechanisms of AT₁ receptor–effector coupling.* AT₁ receptors couple to G_q, G_i, and $G_{12/13}$. Through effectors, second messengers, and signaling cascades, a large array of response pathways is subsequently engaged to produce immediate and long-term effects of angiotensin II.

tractility directly (*via* opening voltage-gated Ca^{2+} channels in cardiac myocytes) and increases heart rate indirectly (*via* facilitation of sympathetic tone, enhanced adrenergic neurotransmission, and adrenal catecholamine release), the rapid increase in arterial blood pressure activates a baroreceptor reflex that decreases sympathetic tone and increases vagal tone. Thus, depending on the physiological state, angiotensin II may increase, decrease, or not change cardiac contractility, heart rate, and cardiac output. Changes in cardiac output therefore contribute little, if at all, to the rapid pressor response induced by angiotensin II.

Angiotensin II also causes a *slow pressor response* that helps to stabilize arterial blood pressure over the long term. A continuous infusion of initially subpressor doses of angiotensin II gradually increases arterial blood pressure, with the maximum effect requiring days to achieve. This slow pressor response probably is mediated by a decrement in renal excretory function that shifts the renal pressure–natriuresis curve to the right (*see* below). Angiotensin II stimulates the synthesis of endothelin-1 and superoxide anion (Laursen *et al.*, 1997; Rajagopalan *et al.*, 1997; Ortiz *et al.*, 2001), which may contribute to the slow pressor response.

In addition to its effects on arterial blood pressure, angiotensin II significantly alters the morphology of the cardiovascular system, causing hypertrophy of vascular

and cardiac cells and increased synthesis and deposition of collagen by cardiac fibroblasts.

The effects of angiotensin II on total peripheral resistance, renal function, and cardiovascular structure are

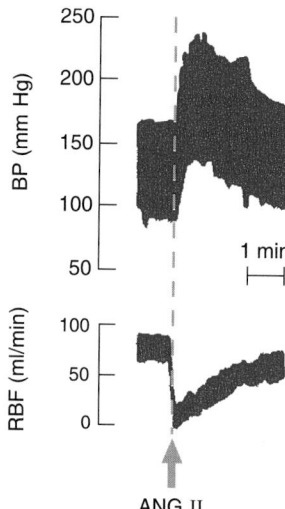

Figure 30–4. *Effect of a bolus intravenous injection of angiotensin II (0.05 μg/kg) on arterial blood pressure and renal blood flow in a conscious dog.* (From Zimmerman, 1979, with permission.)

mediated by a number of direct and indirect mechanisms, as summarized by Figure 30–5.

Mechanisms by Which Angiotensin II Increases Total Peripheral Resistance.
Angiotensin II increases total peripheral resistance (TPR) *via* direct and indirect effects on blood vessels.

Direct Vasoconstriction. Angiotensin II constricts precapillary arterioles and, to a lesser extent, postcapillary venules by activating AT_1 receptors located on vascular smooth muscle cells and stimulating the G_q–PLC–IP_3–Ca^{2+} pathway. Angiotensin II has differential effects on vascular beds. Direct vasoconstriction is strongest in the kidneys (Figure 30–4) and somewhat less in the splanchnic vascular bed; blood flow in these regions falls sharply when angiotensin II is infused. Angiotensin II–induced vasoconstriction is much less in vessels of the brain and still weaker in those of the lung and skeletal muscle. In these regions, blood flow actually may increase, especially following small changes in the concentration of the peptide, because the relatively weak vasoconstrictor response is opposed by the elevated systemic blood pressure. Nevertheless, high circulating concentrations of angiotensin II may decrease cerebral and coronary blood flow.

Enhancement of Peripheral Noradrenergic Neurotransmission. Angiotensin II facilitates peripheral noradrenergic neurotransmission by augmenting norepinephrine release from sympathetic nerve terminals, by inhibiting the reuptake of norepinephrine into nerve terminals, and by enhancing the vascular response to norepinephrine. High concentrations of the peptide stimulate ganglion cells directly. Facilitation of adrenergic transmission by endogenous angiotensin II occurs in animals with renin-dependent renovascular hypertension (Zimmerman *et al.*, 1987), and in humans, intracoronary angiotensin II potentiates sympathetic nervous system–induced coronary vasoconstriction (Saino *et al.*, 1997).

Effects on the Central Nervous System. Small amounts of angiotensin II infused into the vertebral arteries cause an increase in arterial blood pressure. This response—mediated by increased sympathetic outflow—reflects effects of the hormone on circumventricular nuclei that are not protected by a blood–brain barrier (*e.g.*, area postrema, subfornical organ, and organum vasculosum of the lamina terminalis). Circulating angiotensin II also attenuates baroreceptor-mediated reductions in sympathetic discharge, thereby increasing arterial pressure. The CNS is affected both by blood-borne angiotensin II and by angiotensin II formed within the brain (Saavedra,

1992; Bunnemann *et al.*, 1993). The brain contains all components of a renin–angiotensin system. Moreover, there is angiotensinlike immunoreactivity at many sites within the CNS, suggesting that angiotensin II serves as a neurotransmitter or modulator. In addition to increasing sympathetic tone, angiotensin II also causes a centrally mediated dipsogenic effect and enhances the release of vasopressin from the neurohypophysis. Increased drinking and vasopressin secretion result more consistently from intraventricular than from intravenous injections.

Release of Catecholamines from the Adrenal Medulla. Angiotensin II stimulates the release of catecholamines from the adrenal medulla by depolarizing chromaffin cells. Although this response usually is of minimal physiological importance, intense and dangerous reactions have followed the administration of angiotensin II to individuals with pheochromocytoma.

Mechanisms by Which Angiotensin II Alters Renal Function.
Angiotensin II has pronounced effects on renal function, reducing the urinary excretion of Na^+ and water while increasing the excretion of K^+. The overall effect of angiotensin II on the kidneys is to shift the renal pressure–natriuresis curve to the right (*see* below). Like the effects of angiotensin II on TPR, its effects on renal function are multifaceted.

Direct Effects of Angiotensin II on Sodium Reabsorption in the Renal Tubules. Very low concentrations of angiotensin II stimulate Na^+/H^+ exchange in the proximal tubule—an effect that increases Na^+, Cl^-, and bicarbonate reabsorption. Approximately 20% to 30% of the bicarbonate handled by the nephron may be affected by this mechanism (Liu and Cogan, 1987). Angiotensin II also increases the expression of the Na^+–glucose symporter in the proximal tubule (Bautista *et al.*, 2004). Paradoxically, at high concentrations, angiotensin II may inhibit Na^+ transport in the proximal tubule. Angiotensin II also directly stimulates the Na^+–K^+–$2Cl^-$ symporter in the thick ascending limb (Kovács *et al.*, 2002). The proximal tubule secretes angiotensinogen, and the connecting tubule releases renin, so a paracrine tubular renin–angiotensin system may contribute to Na^+ reabsorption (Rohrwasser *et al.*, 1999).

Release of Aldosterone from the Adrenal Cortex. Angiotensin II stimulates the zona glomerulosa of the adrenal cortex to increase the synthesis and secretion of aldosterone, and angiotensin II exerts trophic and permissive effects that augment responses to other stimuli (*e.g.*, ACTH and K^+). Increased output of aldosterone is elicited by concentrations of angiotensin II that have lit-

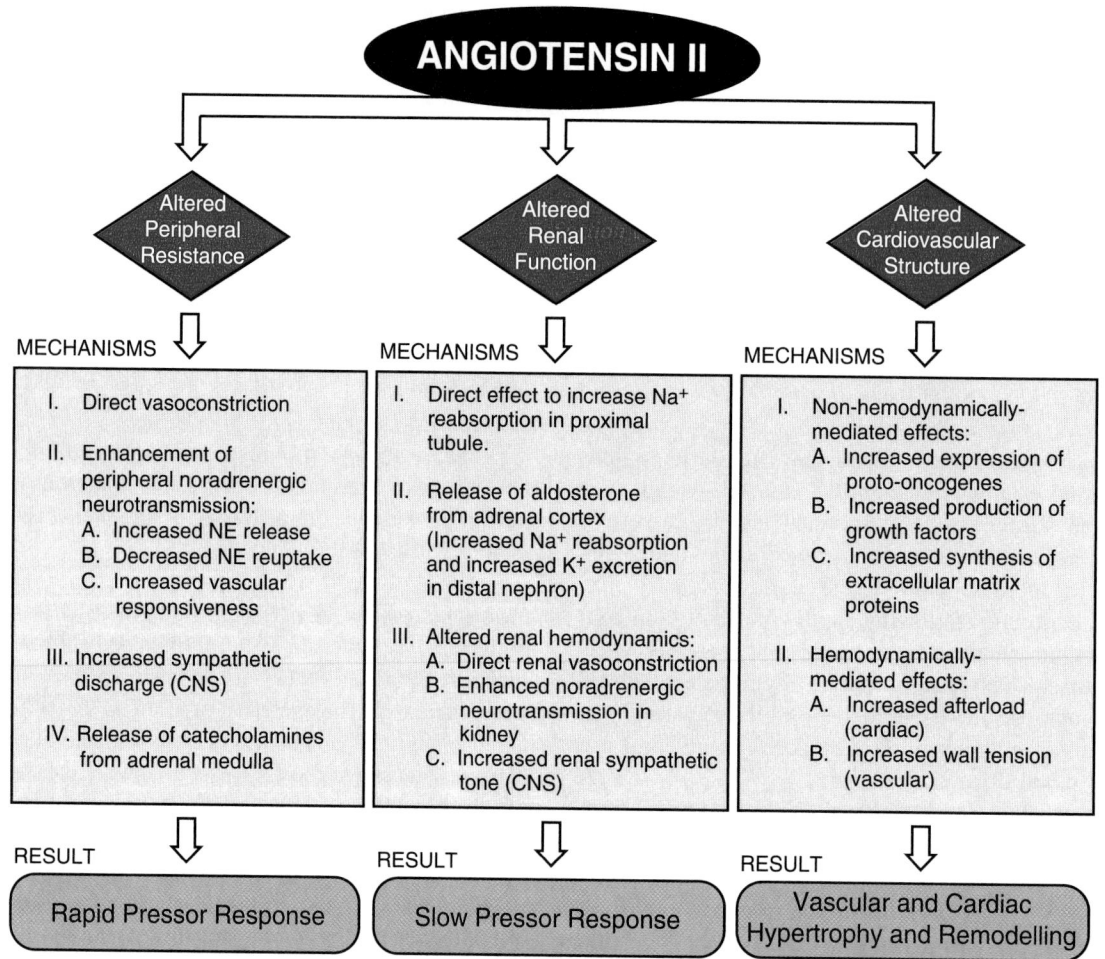

Figure 30–5. *Summary of the three major effects of angiotensin II and the mechanisms that mediate them.* NE, norepinephrine.

tle or no acute effect on blood pressure. As described in Chapters 28 and 59, aldosterone acts on the distal and collecting tubules to cause retention of Na^+ and excretion of K^+ and H^+. The stimulant effect of angiotensin II on aldosterone synthesis and release is enhanced under conditions of hyponatremia or hyperkalemia and is reduced when concentrations of Na^+ and K^+ in plasma are altered in the opposite directions. Such changes in sensitivity are due in part to alterations in the number of receptors for angiotensin II on zona glomerulosa cells, as well as to adrenocortical hyperplasia in the Na^+-depleted state.

Altered Renal Hemodynamics. Reductions in renal blood flow markedly attenuate renal excretory function, and angiotensin II reduces renal blood flow by directly constricting the renal vascular smooth muscle, by enhancing renal sympathetic tone (a CNS effect), and

by facilitating renal adrenergic transmission (an intrarenal effect). Angiotensin II–induced vasoconstriction of preglomerular microvessels is enhanced by endogenous adenosine owing to an interaction between the signal-transduction systems activated by AT_1 and the adenosine A_1 receptors (Hansen *et al.*, 2003). Autoradiographic and *in situ* hybridization studies indicate a high concentration of AT_1 receptors in the vasa recta of the renal medulla, and angiotensin II may reduce Na^+ excretion in part by diminishing medullary blood flow. Angiotensin II variably influences glomerular filtration rate (GFR) *via* several mechanisms: (1) constriction of the afferent arterioles, which reduces intraglomerular pressure and tends to reduce GFR, (2) contraction of mesangial cells, which decreases the capillary surface area within the glomerulus available for filtration and also tends to decrease GFR, and (3) constriction of efferent arterioles, which increases intraglomerular pressure and tends to increase GFR. The outcome of these opposing effects on GFR depends on the physiological state. Normally, GFR is slightly reduced by angiotensin II; however, during renal artery hypotension, the effects of angiotensin II on the efferent arteriole predominate so that angiotensin II increases GFR. Thus blockade of the renin–angiotensin system may cause acute renal failure in patients with bilateral renal artery stenosis or in patients with unilateral stenosis who have only a single kidney.

Mechanisms by Which Angiotensin II Alters Cardiovascular Structure.

Several cardiovascular diseases are accompanied by changes in the morphology of the heart and/or blood vessels that increase morbidity and mortality. Pathological alterations in cardiovascular structures may involve hypertrophy (an increase in tissue mass) and remodeling (redistribution of mass within a structure). Examples include (1) increased wall-to-lumen ratio in blood vessels (associated with hypertension), (2) concentric cardiac hypertrophy (also associated with hypertension), (3) eccentric cardiac hypertrophy and cardiac fibrosis (associated with congestive heart failure and myocardial infarction), and (4) thickening of the intimal surface of the blood vessel wall (associated with atherosclerosis and angioplasty). These morbid changes in cardiovascular structure are due to increased migration, proliferation (hyperplasia), and hypertrophy of cells, as well as to increased extracellular matrix. The cells involved include vascular smooth muscle cells, cardiac myocytes, and fibroblasts. The renin–angiotensin system may contribute importantly to the aforementioned morbid changes in cardiovascular structure. In this regard, angiotensin II (1) stimulates the migration (Bell and Madri, 1990; Dubey *et al.*, 1995), proliferation (Daemen *et al.*, 1991), and hypertrophy of vascular smooth muscle cells (Itoh *et al.*, 1993), (2) increases extracellular matrix production by vascular smooth muscle cells (Scott-Burden *et al.*, 1990), (3) causes hypertrophy of cardiac myocytes (Baker *et al.*, 1992), and (4) increases extracellular matrix production by cardiac fibroblasts (Villarreal *et al.*, 1993; Crawford *et al.*, 1994; Ostrom *et al.*, 2003).

Nonhemodynamically Mediated Effects of Angiotensin II on Cardiovascular Structure.

Angiotensin II stimulates migration, proliferation, hypertrophy, and/or synthetic capacity of vascular smooth muscle cells, cardiac myocytes, and fibroblasts in part by acting directly on cells to induce the expression of specific proto-oncogenes. In cell culture, angiotensin II rapidly (within minutes) increases steady-state levels of mRNA for c-*fos*, c-*jun*, c-*myc*, and egr-1. FOS and JUN, the proteins coded by c-*fos* and c-*jun*, combine to form AP-1, which alters the expression of several genes that stimulate cell growth (hypertrophy and hyperplasia), including basic fibroblast growth factor, platelet-derived growth factor, and transforming growth factor β. In addition, the expression of genes coding for extracellular matrix proteins, such as collagen, fibronectin, and tenascin, is increased.

Hemodynamically Mediated Effects of Angiotensin II on Cardiovascular Structure.

In addition to the direct cellular effects of angiotensin II on cardiovascular structure, changes in cardiac preload (volume expansion owing to Na^+ retention) and afterload (increased arterial blood pressure) probably contribute to cardiac hypertrophy and remodeling. Arterial hypertension also contributes to hypertrophy and remodeling of blood vessels.

Role of the Renin–Angiotensin System in Long-Term Maintenance of Arterial Blood Pressure Despite Extremes in Dietary Na+ Intake.

Arterial blood pressure is a major determinant of Na^+ excretion. This is illustrated graphically by plotting urinary Na^+ excretion *versus* mean arterial blood pressure (Figure 30–6), a plot known as the *renal pressure–natriuresis curve*. Over the long term, Na^+ excretion must equal Na^+ intake; therefore, the set point for long-term levels of arterial blood pressure can be obtained as the intersection of a horizontal line representing Na^+ intake with the renal pressure–natriuresis curve (Guyton, 1991). If the renal pressure–natriuresis

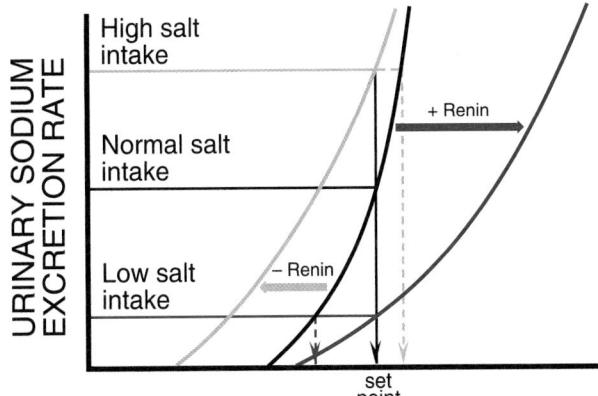

Figure 30–6. *Interactions among salt intake, the renal pressure–natriuresis mechanism, and the renin–angiotensin system to stabilize long-term levels of arterial blood pressure despite large variations in dietary sodium intake.* (Modified from Jackson *et al.*, 1985, with permission.)

curve were fixed, then long-term levels of arterial blood pressure would be greatly affected by dietary Na+ intake. However, as illustrated in Figure 30–6, the renin–angiotensin system plays a major role in maintaining a constant set point for long-term levels of arterial blood pressure despite extreme changes in dietary Na+ intake. When dietary Na+ intake is low, renin release is stimulated, and angiotensin II acts on the kidneys to shift the renal pressure–natriuresis curve to the right. Conversely, when dietary Na+ is high, renin release is inhibited, and the withdrawal of angiotensin II shifts the renal pressure–natriuresis curve to the left. Consequently, despite large swings in dietary Na+ intake, the intersection of salt intake with the renal pressure–natriuresis curve remains near the same set point. When modulation of the renin–angiotensin system is blocked by drugs, changes in salt intake markedly affect long-term levels of arterial blood pressure.

Other Effects of the Renin–Angiotensin System. Expression of the renin–angiotensin system is required for the development of normal kidney morphology, particularly the maturational growth of the renal papilla (Niimura *et al.*, 1995). Angiotensin II causes a marked anorexigenic effect and weight loss, and high circulating levels of angiotensin II may contribute to the anorexia, wasting, and cachexia of heart failure (Brink *et al.*, 1996).

Angiotensin and Vascular Disease

The renin–angiotensin system induces vascular disease by multiple mechanisms, including stimulating vascular smooth muscle cell migration, proliferation, and extracellular matrix production; increasing the release of plasminogen activator inhibitor-1 from vascular smooth muscle cells; enhancing the expression of monocyte chemoattractant protein-1 in vascular smooth muscle cells; augmenting the expression of adhesion proteins, such as intercellular adhesion molecule-1 (ICAM-1), integrins, and osteopontin, in vascular cells (Pastore *et al.*, 1999; Schnee and Hsueh, 2000); and stimulating the production of inflammatory chemokines and cytokines that enhance the migration of inflammatory cells (Ruiz-Ortego *et al.*, 2001). Angiotensin II markedly accelerates the development of atherosclerosis and aortic aneurysms in apolipoprotein E–deficient mice (Daugherty *et al.*, 2000: Weiss *et al.*, 2001), an animal model of atherosclerosis. Conversely, inhibition of the renin–angiotensin system attenuates the development of atherosclerosis in diabetic apolipoprotein E–deficient mice (Candido *et al.*, 2002).

INHIBITORS OF THE RENIN–ANGIOTENSIN SYSTEM

Angiotensin II itself has limited therapeutic utility and is not available for therapeutic use in the United States. Instead, clinical interest focuses on inhibitors of the renin–angiotensin system.

Angiotensin Converting Enzyme (ACE) Inhibitors

History. In the 1960s, Ferreira and colleagues found that the venoms of pit vipers contain factors that intensify responses to bradykinin. These bradykinin-potentiating factors proved to be a family of peptides that inhibit kininase II, an enzyme that inactivates bradykinin. Erdös and coworkers established that ACE and kininase II are the same enzyme, which catalyzes both the synthesis of angiotensin II, a potent pressor substance, and the destruction of bradykinin, a potent vasodilator.

Following the discovery of bradykinin-potentiating factors, the nonapeptide teprotide was synthesized and tested in human subjects. It lowered blood pressure in many patients with essential hypertension more consistently than did peptide angiotensin II-receptor antagonists, such as saralasin, which have partial agonist activity. Teprotide also exerted beneficial effects in patients with heart failure. These key observations encouraged the search for ACE inhibitors that would be active orally.

The orally effective ACE inhibitor *captopril* was developed by a rational approach that involved analysis of the inhibitory action of teprotide, inference about the action of ACE on its substrates, and analogy with carboxypeptidase A, which was known to be inhibited by D-benzylsuccinic acid. Ondetti, Cushman, and colleagues argued that inhibition of ACE might be produced by succinyl amino acids that corresponded in length to the dipeptide cleaved by ACE. This hypothesis proved to be true and led to the synthesis of a series of carboxy alkanoyl and mercapto alkanoyl derivatives that are potent competitive inhibitors of ACE. Most active was captopril (*see* Vane, 1999, for an insider's perspective on the discovery of ACE inhibitors).

Pharmacological Effects in Normal Laboratory Animals and Human Beings. The essential effect of these agents on the renin–angiotensin system is to inhibit the conversion of the relatively inactive angiotensin I to the active angiotensin II (or the conversion of [des-Asp¹]angiotensin I to angiotensin III). Thus ACE inhibitors attenuate or abolish responses to angiotensin I but not to angiotensin II (Figure 30–1). In this regard, ACE inhibitors are highly selective drugs. They do not interact directly with other components of the renin–angiotensin system, and their principal pharmacological and clinical effects apparently arise from suppression of synthesis of angiotensin II. Nevertheless, ACE is an enzyme with many substrates, and inhibition of ACE may induce effects unrelated to reducing the levels of angiotensin II. Since ACE inhibitors increase brady-kinin levels and bradykinin stimulates prostaglandin biosynthesis, bradykinin and/or prostaglandins may contribute to the pharmacological effects of ACE inhibitors. Indeed, some studies demonstrate that blockade of bradykinin receptors in humans attenuates the acute blood pressure reduction (Gainer *et al.*, 1998) and increase in forearm blood flow (Witherrow *et al.*, 2001) induced by ACE inhibition. However, other studies fail to demonstrate a role for bradykinin in the vascular or cardiac effects of ACE inhibitors (Davie *et al.*, 1999; Campbell *et al.*, 1999; Rhaleb *et al.*, 1999). ACE inhibitors increase by fivefold the circulating levels of the natural stem cell regulator *N*-acetyl-seryl-aspartyl-lysyl-proline (Ac-SDKP; Azizi *et al.*, 1997), which may contribute to the cardioprotective effects of ACE inhibitors (Rhaleb *et al.*, 2001). In addition, ACE inhibitors interfere with both short- and long-loop negative feedbacks on renin release (Figure 30–2A). Consequently, ACE inhibitors increase renin release and the rate of formation of angiotensin I. Since the metabolism of angiotensin I to angiotensin II is blocked by ACE inhibitors, angiotensin I is directed down alternative metabolic routes, resulting in the increased production of peptides such as angiotensin(1–7). Whether or not biologically active peptides such as angiotensin(1–7) contribute to the pharmacological effects of ACE inhibitors is unknown.

In healthy, Na^+-replete animals and human beings, a single oral dose of an ACE inhibitor has little effect on systemic blood pressure, but repeated doses over several days cause a small reduction in blood pressure. By contrast, even a single dose of these inhibitors lowers blood pressure substantially in normal subjects when they have been depleted of Na^+.

Clinical Pharmacology. Many ACE inhibitors have been synthesized. These drugs can be classified into three broad groups based on chemical structure: (1) sulfhydryl-containing ACE inhibitors structurally related to captopril (*e.g.*, fentiapril, pivalopril, zofenopril, and alacepril); (2) dicarboxyl-containing ACE inhibitors structurally related to enalapril (*e.g.*, lisinopril, benazepril, quinapril, moexipril, ramipril, trandolapril, spirapril, perindopril, pentopril, and cilazapril); and (3) phosphorus-containing ACE inhibitors structurally related to fosinopril. Many ACE inhibitors are ester-containing prodrugs that are 100 to 1000 times less potent but have a much better oral bioavailability than the active molecules.

Currently, 11 ACE inhibitors are available for clinical use in the United States (Figure 30-7). In general, ACE inhibitors differ with regard to three properties: (1) potency, (2) whether ACE inhibition is primarily a direct effect of the drug itself or the effect of an active metabolite, and (3) pharmacokinetics (*i.e.*, extent of absorption, effect of food on absorption, plasma half-life, tissue distribution, and mechanisms of elimination).

There is no compelling reason to favor one ACE inhibitor over another because all ACE inhibitors effectively block the conversion of angiotensin I to angiotensin II, and all have similar therapeutic indications, adverse-effect profiles, and contraindications. However, the Quality-of-Life Hypertension Study Group reported that although captopril and enalapril are indistinguishable with regard to antihypertensive efficacy and safety, captopril may have a more favorable effect on quality of life (Testa *et al.*, 1993). Since hypertension usually requires lifelong treatment, quality-of-life issues are an important consideration in comparing antihypertensive drugs. ACE inhibitors differ markedly in tissue distribution, and it is possible that this difference could be exploited to inhibit some local renin–angiotensin systems while leaving others relatively intact. Whether site-specific inhibition actually confers therapeutic advantages remains to be established.

With the notable exceptions of fosinopril and spirapril (which display balanced elimination by the liver and kidneys), ACE inhibitors are cleared predominantly by the kidneys. Therefore, impaired renal function significantly diminishes the plasma clearance of most ACE inhibitors, and dosages of these drugs should be reduced in patients with renal impairment. *Elevated plasma renin activity (PRA) renders patients hyperresponsive to ACE inhibitor–induced hypotension, and initial dosages of all ACE inhibitors should be reduced in patients with high plasma levels of renin (e.g., patients with heart failure and salt-depleted patients).*

Captopril (CAPOTEN). Captopril, the first ACE inhibitor to be marketed, is a potent ACE inhibitor with a K_i of 1.7 n*M*. It is the only ACE inhibitor approved for use in the United States that contains a sulfhydryl moiety. Given orally, captopril is absorbed rapidly and has a bioavailability of about 75%. Peak concentrations in plasma occur within an hour, and the drug is cleared rapidly with a half-life of approximately 2 hours. Most of the drug is eliminated in urine, 40% to 50% as captopril and the rest as captopril disulfide dimers and captopril–cysteine disulfide. The oral dose of captopril ranges from 6.25 to 150 mg two to three times daily, with 6.25 mg three times daily or 25 mg twice daily being appropriate for the initiation of therapy for heart failure or hypertension, respectively. Most patients should not receive daily doses in

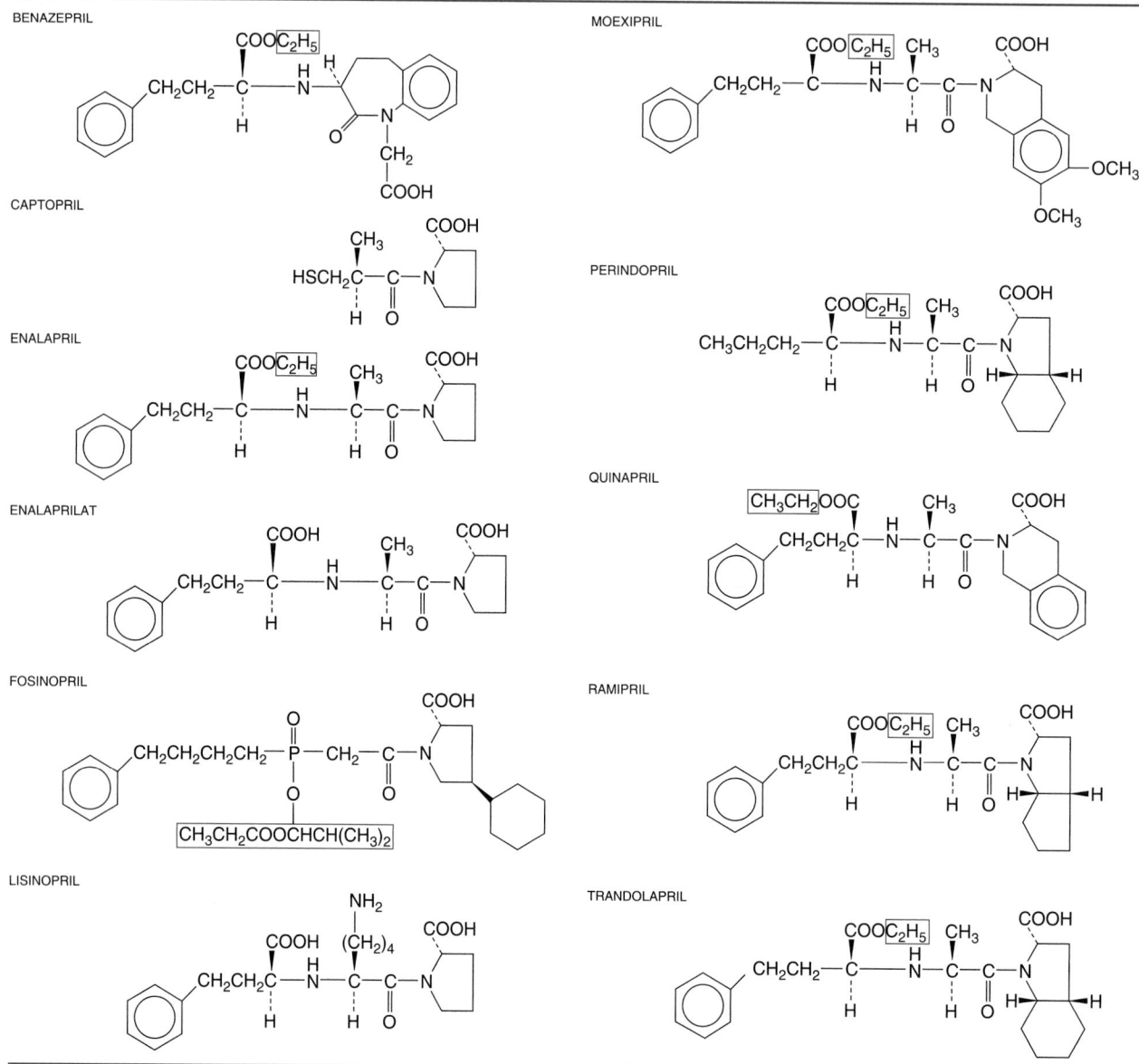

Figure 30–7. *Chemical structures of selected angiotensin-converting enzyme inhibitors.* Captopril, lisinopril, and enalaprilat are active molecules. Benazepril, enalapril, fosinopril, moexipril, perindopril, quinapril, ramipril, and trandolapril are relatively inactive until converted to their corresponding diacids. The structures enclosed within blue boxes are removed by esterases and replaced with a hydrogen atom to form the active molecule *in vivo* (*e.g.,* enalapril to enalaprilat or ramipril to ramiprilat).

excess of 150 mg. Since food reduces the oral bioavailability of captopril by 25% to 30%, the drug should be given 1 hour before meals.

Enalapril (VASOTEC). Enalapril maleate, the second ACE inhibitor approved in the United States, is a prodrug that is hydrolyzed by esterases in the liver to produce the active dicarboxylic acid, enalaprilat. *Enalapri-*

lat is a highly potent inhibitor of ACE with a K_i of 0.2 nM. Although it also contains a "proline surrogate," enalaprilat differs from captopril in that it is an analogue of a tripeptide rather than of a dipeptide. Enalapril is absorbed rapidly when given orally and has an oral bioavailability of about 60% (not reduced by food). Although peak concentrations of enalapril in plasma occur within an hour, enalaprilat concentrations peak only after 3 to 4 hours. Enalapril has a half-life of only 1.3 hours, but enalaprilat, because of tight binding to ACE, has a plasma half-life of about 11 hours. Nearly all the drug is eliminated by the kidneys as either intact enalapril or enalaprilat. The oral dosage of enalapril ranges from 2.5 to 40 mg daily (single or divided dosage), with 2.5 and 5 mg daily being appropriate for the initiation of therapy for heart failure and hypertension, respectively. The initial dose for hypertensive patients who are taking diuretics, are water- or Na^+-depleted, or have heart failure is 2.5 mg daily.

Enalaprilat (VASOTEC INJECTION). Enalaprilat is not absorbed orally but is available for intravenous administration when oral therapy is not appropriate. For hypertensive patients, the dosage is 0.625 to 1.25 mg given intravenously over 5 minutes. This dosage may be repeated every 6 hours.

Lisinopril (PRINIVIL, ZESTRIL). Lisinopril, the third ACE inhibitor approved for use in the United States, is the lysine analogue of enalaprilat; unlike enalapril, lisinopril itself is active. *In vitro,* lisinopril is a slightly more potent ACE inhibitor than is enalaprilat. Lisinopril is absorbed slowly, variably, and incompletely (about 30%) after oral administration (not reduced by food); peak concentrations in plasma are achieved in about 7 hours. It is cleared as the intact compound by the kidney, and its half-life in plasma is about 12 hours. Lisinopril does not accumulate in tissues. The oral dosage of lisinopril ranges from 5 to 40 mg daily (single or divided dosage), with 5 and 10 mg daily being appropriate for the initiation of therapy for heart failure and hypertension, respectively. A daily dose of 2.5 mg is recommended for patients with heart failure who are hyponatremic or have renal impairment.

Benazepril (LOTENSIN). Cleavage of the ester moiety by hepatic esterases transforms benazepril, a prodrug, into benazeprilat, an ACE inhibitor that *in vitro* is more potent than captopril, enalaprilat, or lisinopril. Benazepril is absorbed rapidly but incompletely (37%) after oral administration (only slightly reduced by food). Benazepril is nearly completely metabolized to benazeprilat and to the glucuronide conjugates of benazepril and benazeprilat, which are excreted into both the urine and bile; peak concentrations of benazepril and benazeprilat in plasma are achieved in about 0.5 to 1 hour and 1 to 2 hours, respectively. Benazeprilat has an effective half-life in plasma of about 10 to 11 hours. With the exception of the lungs, benazeprilat does not accumulate in tissues. The oral dosage of benazepril ranges from 5 to 80 mg daily (single or divided dosage).

Fosinopril (MONOPRIL). Fosinopril is the only ACE inhibitor approved for use in the United States that contains a phosphinate group that binds to the active site of ACE. Cleavage of the ester moiety by hepatic esterases transforms fosinopril, a prodrug, into fosinoprilat, an ACE inhibitor that *in vitro* is more potent than captopril yet less potent than enalaprilat. Fosinopril is absorbed slowly and incompletely (36%) after oral administration (rate but not extent reduced by food). Fosinopril is largely metabolized to fosinoprilat (75%) and to the glucuronide conjugate of fosinoprilat. These are excreted in both the urine and bile; peak concentrations of fosinoprilat in plasma are achieved in about 3 hours. Fosinoprilat has an effective half-life in plasma of about 11.5 hours, and its clearance is not significantly altered by renal impairment. The oral dosage of fosinopril ranges from 10 to 80 mg daily (single or divided dosage). The dose is reduced to 5 mg daily in patients with Na^+ or water depletion or renal failure.

Trandolapril (MAVIK). Approximately 10% and 70% of an oral dose of trandolapril is bioavailable (absorption rate but not extent is reduced by food) as trandolapril and trandolaprilat, respectively. Trandolaprilat is about eight times more potent than trandolapril as an ACE inhibitor. Trandolapril is metabolized to trandolaprilat and to inactive metabolites (mostly glucuronides of trandolapril and deesterification products), and these are recovered in the urine (33%, mostly trandolaprilat) and feces (66%). Peak concentrations of trandolaprilat in plasma are achieved in 4 to 10 hours. Trandolaprilat displays biphasic elimination kinetics with an initial half-life of about 10 hours (the major component of elimination), followed by a more prolonged half-life owing to slow dissociation of trandolaprilat from tissue ACE. Plasma clearance of trandolaprilat is reduced by both renal and hepatic insufficiency. The oral dosage ranges from 1 to 8 mg daily (single or divided dosage). The initial dose is 0.5 mg in patients who are taking a diuretic or who have renal impairment.

Quinapril (ACCUPRIL). Cleavage of the ester moiety by hepatic esterases transforms quinapril, a prodrug, into quinaprilat, an ACE inhibitor that *in vitro* is about as potent as benazeprilat. Quinapril is absorbed rapidly (peak concentrations are achieved in 1 hour, but the peak may be delayed after food), and the rate but not extent of oral absorption (60%) may be reduced by food. Quinapril is metabolized to quinaprilat and to other minor metabolites, and quinaprilat is excreted in the urine (61%) and feces (37%). Peak concentrations of quinaprilat in plasma are achieved in about 2 hours. Conversion of quinapril to quinaprilat is reduced in patients with diminished liver function. The initial half-life of quinaprilat is about 2 hours; a prolonged terminal half-life of about 25 hours may be due to high-affinity binding of the drug to tissue ACE. The oral dosage of quinapril ranges from 5 to 80 mg daily (single or divided dosage).

Ramipril (ALTACE). Cleavage of the ester moiety by hepatic esterases transforms ramipril into ramiprilat, an ACE inhibitor that *in vitro* is about as potent as benazeprilat and quinaprilat. Ramipril is absorbed rapidly (peak concentrations of ramipril achieved in 1 hour), and the rate but not extent of its oral absorption (50% to 60%) is reduced by food. Ramipril is metabolized to ramiprilat and to inactive metabolites (glucuronides of ramipril and ramiprilat and the diketopiperazine ester and acid) that are excreted predominantly by the kidneys. Peak concentrations of ramiprilat in plasma are achieved in about 3 hours. Ramiprilat displays triphasic elimination kinetics with half-lives of 2 to 4 hours, 9 to 18 hours, and greater than 50 hours. This triphasic elimination is due to extensive distribution to all tissues (initial half-life), clearance of free ramiprilat from plasma (intermediate half-life), and dissociation of ramiprilat from tissue ACE (terminal half-life). The oral dosage of ramipril ranges from 1.25 to 20 mg daily (single or divided dosage).

Moexipril (UNIVASC). Moexipril is another prodrug whose antihypertensive activity is almost entirely due to its deesterified metabolite, moexiprilat. Moexipril is absorbed incompletely, with bioavailability as moexiprilat of about 13%. Bioavailability is markedly decreased by food; therefore, the drug should be taken 1 hour before meals. The time to peak plasma concentration of moexiprilat is almost 1.5 hours, and the elimination half-life varies between 2 and 12 hours. The recommended dosage range is 7.5 to 30 mg daily in one or two divided doses. The dosage range is halved in patients who are taking diuretics or who have renal impairment.

Perindopril (ACEON). Perindopril erbumine is a prodrug, and 30% to 50% of systemically available perindopril is transformed to perindoprilat by hepatic esterases. Although the oral bioavailability of perindopril (75%) is not affected by food, the bioavailability of perindoprilat is reduced by approximately 35%. Perindopril is metabolized to perindoprilat and to inactive metabolites (glucuronides of perindopril and perindoprilat, dehydrated perindopril, and diastereomers of dehydrated perindoprilat) that are excreted predominantly by the kidneys. Peak concentrations of perindoprilat in plasma are achieved in 3 to 7 hours. Perindoprilat displays biphasic elimination kinetics with half-lives of 3 to 10 hours (the major component of elimination) and 30 to 120 hours (owing to slow dissociation of perindoprilat from tissue ACE). The oral dosage ranges from 2 to 16 mg daily (single or divided dosage).

Therapeutic Uses of ACE Inhibitors and Clinical Summary. Drugs that interfere with the renin–angiotensin system play a prominent role in the treatment of cardiovascular disease, the major cause of mortality in modern societies.

ACE Inhibitors in Hypertension (See Chapter 32). Inhibition of ACE lowers systemic vascular resistance and mean, diastolic, and systolic blood pressures in various hypertensive states. The effects are observed readily in animal models of renal and genetic hypertension. In human subjects with hypertension, ACE inhibitors commonly lower blood pressure, except when high blood pressure is due to primary aldosteronism. The initial change in blood pressure tends to be positively correlated with plasma renin activity (PRA) and angiotensin II plasma levels prior to treatment. However, several weeks into treatment, additional patients show a sizable reduction in blood pressure, and the antihypertensive effect then correlates poorly or not at all with pretreatment values of PRA. It is possible that increased local (tissue) production of angiotensin II and/or increased responsiveness of tissues to normal levels of angiotensin II in some hypertensive patients makes them sensitive to ACE inhibitors despite normal PRA. Regardless of the mechanisms, ACE inhibitors have broad clinical utility as antihypertensive agents.

The long-term fall in systemic blood pressure observed in hypertensive individuals treated with ACE inhibitors is accompanied by a leftward shift in the renal pressure–natriuresis curve (Figure 30–6) and a reduction in total peripheral resistance in which there is variable participation by different vascular beds. The kidney is a notable exception to this variability because increased renal blood flow owing to vasodilation is a relatively constant finding. This is not surprising because the renal vessels are exceptionally sensitive to the vasoconstrictor actions of angiotensin II. Increased renal blood flow occurs without an increase in GFR; thus the filtration fraction is reduced. Both the afferent and efferent arterioles are dilated. Blood flows in the cerebral and coronary beds, where autoregulatory mechanisms are powerful, generally are well maintained.

Besides causing systemic arteriolar dilatation, ACE inhibitors increase the compliance of large arteries, which contributes to a reduction of systolic pressure. Cardiac function in patients with uncomplicated hypertension generally is little changed, although stroke volume and cardiac output may increase slightly with sustained treatment. Baroreceptor function and cardiovascular reflexes are not compromised, and responses to postural changes and exercise are little impaired. Surprisingly, even when a substantial lowering of blood pressure is achieved, heart rate and concentrations of catecholamines in plasma generally increase only slightly, if at all. This perhaps reflects an alteration of baroreceptor function with increased arterial compliance and the loss of the normal tonic influence of angiotensin II on the sympathetic nervous system.

Aldosterone secretion in the general population of hypertensive individuals is reduced, but not seriously impaired, by ACE inhibitors. Aldosterone secretion is maintained at adequate levels by other steroidogenic stimuli, such as adrenocorticotropic hormone and K^+. The activity of these secretogogues on the zona glomerulosa of the adrenal cortex requires, at most, only very small trophic or permissive amounts of angiotensin II, which always are present because ACE inhibition never is complete. Excessive retention of K^+ is encountered only in patients taking supplemental K^+, in patients with renal impairment, or in patients taking other medications that reduce K^+ excretion.

ACE inhibitors alone normalize blood pressure in approximately 50% of patients with mild to moderate hypertension. Ninety percent of patients with mild to moderate hypertension will be controlled by the combination of an ACE inhibitor and either a Ca^{2+} channel blocker, a β adrenergic receptor blocker, or a diuretic (Zusman, 1993). Diuretics in particular augment the antihypertensive response to ACE inhibitors by rendering the patient's blood pressure renin-dependent.

There is increasing evidence that ACE inhibitors are superior to other antihypertensive drugs in hypertensive patients with diabetes, in whom they improve endothelial function (O'Driscoll *et al.*, 1997) and reduce cardiovascular events more so than do Ca^{2+} channel blockers (Estacio *et al.*, 1998; Tatti *et al.*, 1998) or diuretics and β adrenergic receptor antagonists (Hansson *et al.*, 1999).

ACE Inhibitors in Left Ventricular Systolic Dysfunction (See Chapter 33). Left ventricular systolic dysfunction ranges from a modest, asymptomatic reduction in systolic performance to a severe impairment of left ventricular systolic function with New York Heart Association grade IV congestive heart failure. It is now clear that unless contraindicated, ACE inhibitors should be given to all patients with impaired left ventricular systolic function whether or not they have symptoms of overt heart failure.

Several large prospective, randomized, placebo-controlled clinical studies support the usefulness of ACE inhibitors in patients with varying degrees of left ventricular systolic dysfunction. These studies are summarized in Table 30–1 and are described in more detail in Chapter 33. Collectively, these studies demonstrate that inhibition of ACE in patients with systolic dysfunction prevents or delays the progression of heart failure, decreases the incidence of sudden death and myocardial infarction, decreases hospitalization, and improves quality of life. The more severe the ventricular dysfunction, the greater is the benefit from ACE inhibition.

Although the mechanisms by which ACE inhibitors improve outcome in patients with systolic dysfunction are not completely understood, the induction of a more favorable hemodynamic state most likely plays an important role. Inhibition of ACE commonly reduces afterload and systolic wall stress, and both cardiac output and cardiac index increase, as do indices of stroke work and stroke volume. In systolic dysfunction, angiotensin II decreases arterial compliance, and this is reversed by ACE inhibition (Lage *et al.*, 2002). Heart rate generally is reduced. Systemic blood pressure falls, sometimes steeply at the outset, but tends to return toward initial levels. Renovascular resistance falls sharply, and renal blood flow increases. Natriuresis occurs as a result of the improved renal hemodynamics, the reduced stimulus to the secretion of aldosterone by angiotensin II, and the diminished direct effects of angiotensin II on the kidney. The excess volume of body fluids contracts, which reduces venous return to the right side of the heart. A further reduction results from venodilation and an increased capacity of the venous bed. Venodilation is a somewhat unexpected effect of ACE inhibition because angiotensin II has little acute venoconstrictor activity. Nevertheless, long-term infusion of angiotensin II increases venous tone, perhaps by central or peripheral interactions with the sympathetic nervous system. The response to ACE inhibitors also involves reductions of pulmonary arterial pressure, pulmonary capillary wedge pressure, and left atrial and left ventricular filling volumes and pressures. Consequently, preload and diastolic wall stress are diminished. The better hemodynamic performance results in increased exercise tolerance and suppression of the sympathetic nervous system (Grassi *et al.*, 1997). Cerebral and coronary blood flows usually are well maintained, even when systemic blood pressure is reduced.

The beneficial effects of ACE inhibitors in systolic dysfunction also involve improvements in ventricular geometry. In heart failure, ACE inhibitors reduce ventric-

Table 30–1
Summary of Clinical Trials with ACE Inhibitors in Heart Disease

STUDY	REFERENCE	ACE INHIBITOR	PATIENT GROUP	OUTCOME	COMMENT
CONSENSUS	CONSENSUS Trial Study Group, 1987	Enalapril vs. placebo ($n = 257$)	NYHA IV CHF	Decreased overall mortality	Reduced pump failure
SOLVD-Treatment	SOLVD Investigators, 1991	Enalapril vs. placebo ($n = 2569$)	NYHA II & III CHF	Decreased overall mortality	Reduced pump failure
V-HeFt II	Cohn et al., 1991	Enalapril vs. hydralazine-isosorbide ($n = 804$)	NYHA II & III CHF	Decreased overall mortality	Reduced sudden death
SAVE	Pfeffer et al., 1992	Captopril vs. placebo ($n = 2231$)	MI with asymptomatic LV dysfunction	Decreased overall mortality	Reduced pump failure and recurrent MI
Kleber et al.	Kleber et al., 1992	Captopril vs. placebo ($n = 170$)	NYHA II CHF	Decreased progression of CHF	Treatment for 2.7 years
SOLVD-Prevention	SOLVD Investigators, 1992	Enalapril vs. placebo ($n = 4228$)	Asymptomatic LV dysfunction	Decreased death + hospitalization due to CHF	Treatment for 14.6 to 62 months
CONSENSUS II	Swedberg et al., 1992	Enalaprilat, then enalapril vs. placebo ($n = 6090$)	MI	No change in survival	Hypotension following IV enalaprilat
AIRE	AIRE Study Investigators, 1993	Ramipril vs. placebo ($n = 2006$)	MI with overt CHF	Decreased overall mortality	Benefit in 30 days
ISIS-4	ISIS-4 Collaborative Group, 1995	Captopril vs. placebo ($n = 58,050$)	MI	Decreased overall mortality	Treatment for 1 month
GISSI-3	Gruppo Italiano, 1994	Lisinopril vs. open control ($n = 19,394$)	MI	Decreased overall mortality	Treatment for 6 weeks
TRACE	Køber et al., 1995	Trandolapril vs. placebo ($n = 1749$)	MI with LV dysfunction	Decreased overall mortality	Treatment for 24 to 50 months
SMILE	Ambrosioni et al., 1995	Zofenopril vs. placebo ($n = 1556$)	MI	Decreased overall mortality	Treatment for 6 weeks
FEST	Erhart et al., 1995	Fosinopril vs. placebo ($n = 308$)	NYHA II & III CHF	Increased exercise tolerance	Treatment for 12 months
TREND	Mancini et al., 1996	Quinapril vs. placebo ($n = 105$)	CAD	Improved coronary endothelial function	Treatment for 6 months

(Continued)

Table 30–1
Summary of Clinical Trials with ACE Inhibitors in Heart Disease (Continued)

STUDY	REFERENCE	ACE INHIBITOR	PATIENT GROUP	OUTCOME	COMMENT
FAMIS	Borghi *et al.*, 1997	Fosinopril vs. placebo ($n = 285$)	MI	Decreased overall mortality and incidence of CHF	Early (<9 hours) initiation of treatment Treatment for 3 months
QUIET	Cashin-Hemphill *et al.*, 1999	Quinapril vs. placebo ($n = 1750$)	Undergoing angioplasty	No change in progression of atherosclerosis	Treatment for 3 years
ATLAS	Parker *et al.*, 1999	Low vs. high dose lisinopril ($n = 3164$)	NYHA II–IV CHF	Reduced hospitalization with high dose	Treatment for 39–58 months
APRES	Kjøller-Hansen *et al.*, 2000	Ramipril vs. placebo ($n = 159$)	Revascularization with moderate LV dysfunction	Reduced cardiac death, MI, or clinical CHF	Treatment for 33 months
HOPE	Heart Outcomes Prevention Study Investigators, 2000	Ramipril vs. placebo ($n = 9297$)	CAD or high risk for CVD without CHF	Decreased CVD death, MI, stroke, overall mortality	Treatment for 5 years
PEACE	Pfeffer *et al.*, 2001	Trandolapril vs. placebo ($n = 8290$)	CAD without CHF	In progress as of 02/04	Treatment for 5.2 years
HOPE	Arnold *et al.*, 2003	Ramipril vs. placebo ($n = 9297$)	CAD or high risk for CVD without CHF	Decreased rate of development of CHF	Treatment for 4.5 years
EUROPA	European Trial, 2003	Perindopril vs. placebo ($n = 12,218$)	CAD without CHF	Decreased CVD death and MI	Treatment for 4.2 years

ABBREVIATIONS: MI, myocardial infarction; CAD, coronary artery disease; CHF, congestive heart failure; CVD, cardiovascular disease; LV, left ventricular; NYHA, New York Heart Association; IV, intravenous administration.

ular dilation and tend to restore the heart to its normal elliptical shape. ACE inhibitors may reverse ventricular remodeling *via* changes in preload/afterload, by preventing the growth effects of angiotensin II on myocytes, and by attenuating cardiac fibrosis induced by angiotensin II and aldosterone. Aldosterone levels are elevated in heart failure, and aldosterone markedly increases ACE expression in cultured neonatal rat cardiac myocytes (Harada *et al.*, 2001).

Although the role of ACE inhibitors in left ventricular systolic dysfunction is firmly established, whether these drugs improve diastolic dysfunction is an important open question. Infusions of enalaprilat into the left coronary arteries of patients with left ventricular hypertrophy significantly improve diastolic function (Friedrich *et al.*, 1994; Kyriakidis *et al.*, 1998).

ACE Inhibitors in Acute Myocardial Infarction. Several large prospective, randomized clinical studies involving thousands of patients (Table 30–1) provide convincing evidence that ACE inhibitors reduce overall mortality when treatment is begun during the peri-infarction period. The beneficial effects of ACE inhibitors in acute myocardial infarction are particularly large in hypertensive (Borghi *et al.*, 1999) and diabetic (Zuanetti *et al.*, 1997; Gustafsson *et al.*, 1999) patients. Unless contraindicated (*e.g.*, cardiogenic shock or severe hypotension), ACE inhibitors should be started immediately during the acute phase of myocardial infarction and can be administered along with thrombolytics, aspirin, and β adrenergic receptor antagonists (ACE Inhibitor Myocardial Infarction Collaborative Group, 1998). After several weeks, ACE-inhibitor therapy should be re-evaluated. In high-risk patients (*e.g.*, large infarct, systolic ventricular dysfunction), ACE inhibition should be continued long term.

ACE Inhibitors in Patients Who Are at High Risk of Cardiovascular Events. ACE inhibitors tilt the fibrinolytic balance toward a profibrinolytic state by reducing plasma levels of plasminogen activator inhibitor-1 (Vaughan *et al.*, 1997; Brown *et al.*, 1999) and improve endothelial vasomotor dysfunction in patients with coronary artery disease (Mancini *et al.*, 1996). The HOPE study demonstrated that patients at high risk of cardiovascular events benefited considerably from treatment with ACE inhibitors (Heart Outcomes Prevention Study Investigators, 2000). ACE inhibition significantly decreased the rate of myocardial infarction, stroke, and death in a broad range of patients who did not have left ventricular dysfunction but had evidence of vascular disease or diabetes and one other risk factor for cardiovascular disease. The EUROPA trial examined the effects of ACE inhibition in patients with coronary artery disease but without heart failure. Like the HOPE study, the EUROPA trial demonstrated that ACE inhibition reduced cardiovascular disease death and myocardial infarction (European Trial, 2003). The APRES study showed that the beneficial effects of ACE inhibition in patients at high risk of cardiovascular events were expressed even after coronary revascularization (Kjøller-Hansen *et al.*, 2000). Thus the HOPE, EUROPA, and APRES studies suggest that the use of ACE inhibitors should be expanded to the large population of patients at risk for ischemic cardiovascular events.

ACE Inhibitors in Chronic Renal Failure. Diabetes mellitus is the leading cause of renal disease. In patients with type 1 diabetes mellitus and diabetic nephropathy, captopril prevents or delays the progression of renal disease (Lewis *et al.*, 1993). Renoprotection in type 1 diabetes, as defined by changes in albumin excretion, also is observed with lisinopril (Euclid Study Group, 1997). The renoprotective effects of ACE inhibitors in type 1 diabetes is in part independent of blood pressure reduction. Specific renoprotection by ACE inhibitors is more difficult to demonstrate in type 2 diabetics, with some studies providing positive results (Ravid *et al.*, 1993, 1996, 1998), whereas others do not demonstrate blood pressure–independent renoprotection (Brenner and Zagrobelny, 2003). In addition to attenuating diabetic nephropathy, ACE

inhibitors also may decrease retinopathy progression in type 1 diabetics (Chaturvedi *et al.*, 1998). ACE inhibitors also attenuate the progression of renal insufficiency in patients with a variety of nondiabetic nephropathies (Maschio *et al.*, 1996; GISEN Group, 1997; Ruggenenti *et al.*, 1998, 1999b; Kshirsagar *et al.*, 2000; Praga *et al.*, 2003) and may arrest the decline in GFR even in patients with severe renal disease (Ruggenenti *et al.*, 1999a).

Several mechanisms participate in the renal protection afforded by ACE inhibitors. Increased glomerular capillary pressure induces glomerular injury, and ACE inhibitors reduce this parameter both by decreasing arterial blood pressure and by dilating renal efferent arterioles. ACE inhibitors increase the permeability selectivity of the filtering membrane, thereby diminishing exposure of the mesangium to proteinaceous factors that may stimulate mesangial cell proliferation and matrix production, two processes that contribute to expansion of the mesangium in diabetic nephropathy. Since angiotensin II is a growth factor, reductions in the intrarenal levels of angiotensin II may further attenuate mesangial cell growth and matrix production.

ACE Inhibitors in Scleroderma Renal Crisis. Before the use of ACE inhibitors, patients with scleroderma renal crisis generally died within several weeks. ACE inhibitors have improved considerably this otherwise grim prognosis (Steen and Medsger, 1990).

Adverse Effects of ACE Inhibitors. Serious untoward reactions to ACE inhibitors are rare, and in general, ACE inhibitors are well tolerated. Metabolic side effects are not encountered during long-term therapy with ACE inhibitors. The drugs do not alter plasma concentrations of uric acid or Ca^{2+} and actually may improve insulin sensitivity in patients with insulin resistance and decrease cholesterol and lipoprotein(a) levels in proteinuric renal disease.

Hypotension. A steep fall in blood pressure may occur following the first dose of an ACE inhibitor in patients with elevated PRA. In this regard, care should be exercised in patients who are salt-depleted, in patients being treated with multiple antihypertensive drugs, and in patients who have congestive heart failure. In such situations, treatment should be initiated with very small doses of ACE inhibitors, or salt intake should be increased and diuretics withdrawn before beginning therapy.

Cough. In 5% to 20% of patients, ACE inhibitors induce a bothersome, dry cough; it usually is not dose-related, occurs more frequently in women than in men, usually develops between 1 week and 6 months after initiation of therapy, and sometimes requires cessation of therapy. This adverse effect may be mediated by the accumulation in the lungs of bradykinin, substance P, and/or prostaglandins. Thromboxane antagonism (Malini *et al.*, 1997), aspirin (Tenenbaum *et al.*, 2000), and iron supplementation (Lee *et al.*, 2001) reduce cough induced by ACE inhibitors. Once ACE inhibitors are stopped, the cough disappears, usually within 4 days (Israili and Hall, 1992).

Hyperkalemia. Despite some reduction in the concentration of aldosterone, significant K^+ retention is rarely encountered in patients with normal renal function who are not taking other drugs that cause K^+ retention. However, ACE inhibitors may cause hyperkalemia in patients with renal insufficiency or in patients taking K^+-sparing diuretics, K^+ supplements, β adrenergic receptor blockers, or NSAIDs.

Acute Renal Failure. Angiotensin II, by constricting the efferent arteriole, helps to maintain adequate glomerular filtration when renal perfusion pressure is low. Consequently, inhibition of ACE can induce acute renal insufficiency in patients with bilateral renal artery stenosis, stenosis of the artery to a single remaining kidney, heart failure, or volume depletion owing to diarrhea or diuretics. Older patients with congestive heart failure are particularly susceptible to ACE inhibitor–induced acute renal failure. However, in nearly all patients who receive appropriate treatment, recovery of renal function occurs without sequelae (Wynckel *et al.*, 1998).

Fetopathic Potential. Although ACE inhibitors are not teratogenic during the early period of organogenesis (first trimester), continued administration of ACE inhibitors during the second and third trimesters can cause oligohydramnios, fetal calvarial hypoplasia, fetal pulmonary hypoplasia, fetal growth retardation, fetal death, neonatal anuria, and neonatal death. These fetopathic effects may be due in part to fetal hypotension. While ACE inhibitors are not contraindicated in women of reproductive age, *once pregnancy is diagnosed, it is imperative that ACE inhibitors be discontinued as soon as possible.* If necessary, an alternative antihypertensive regimen should be instituted. The fetus is not at risk of ACE inhibitor–induced pathology if ACE inhibitors are discontinued during the first trimester of pregnancy (Brent and Beckman, 1991).

Skin Rash. ACE inhibitors occasionally cause a maculopapular rash that may or may not itch. The rash may resolve spontaneously or may respond to a reduced dosage or a brief course of antihistamines. Although initially attributed to the presence of the sulfhydryl group in captopril, a rash also may occur with other ACE inhibitors, albeit less frequently.

Proteinuria. ACE inhibitors have been associated with proteinuria (more than 1 g/day); however, a causal relationship has been difficult to establish. In general, proteinuria is not a contraindication for ACE inhibitors because ACE inhibitors are renoprotective in certain renal diseases associated with proteinuria, *e.g.,* diabetic nephropathy.

Angioedema. In 0.1% to 0.5% of patients, ACE inhibitors induce a rapid swelling in the nose, throat, mouth, glottis, larynx, lips, and/or tongue. This untoward effect, called *angioedema,* apparently is not dose-related, and if it occurs, it does so within the first week of therapy, usually within the first few hours after the initial dose. Airway obstruction and respiratory distress may lead to death. Although the mechanism of angioedema is unknown, it may involve accumulation of bradykinin, induction of tissue-specific autoantibodies, or inhibition of complement 1–esterase inhibitor. Once ACE inhibitors are stopped, angioedema disappears within hours; meanwhile, the patient's airway should be protected, and if necessary, epinephrine, an antihistamine, and/or a glucocorticoid should be administered (Israili and Hall, 1992). African-Americans have a 4.5 times greater risk of ACE inhibitor–induced angioedema than do Caucasians (Brown *et al.,* 1996). Although it is rare, angioedema of the intestine (visceral angioedema) also has been reported in association with ACE inhibitors. Visceral angioedema is characterized by emesis, watery diarrhea, and abdominal pain. Most cases of visceral angioedema occur in the absence of oropharyngeal edema, and because the symptoms are nonspecific, diagnosis can be elusive.

Dysgeusia. An alteration in or loss of taste can occur in patients receiving ACE inhibitors. This adverse effect, which may occur more frequently with captopril, is reversible.

Neutropenia. Neutropenia is a rare but serious side effect of ACE inhibitors. Although the frequency of neutropenia is low, it occurs predominantly in hypertensive patients with collagen-vascular or renal parenchymal disease. If the serum creatinine concentration is 2 mg/dl or greater, the dose of ACE inhibitor should be kept low, and the patient should be counseled to seek medical evaluation if symptoms of neutropenia (*e.g.,* sore throat, fever) develop.

Glycosuria. An exceedingly rare and reversible side effect of ACE inhibitors is spillage of glucose into the urine in the absence of hyperglycemia (Cressman *et al.,* 1982). The mechanism is unknown.

Hepatotoxicity. Also exceedingly rare and reversible is hepatotoxicity, usually of the cholestatic variety (Hagley *et al.,* 1993). The mechanism is unknown.

Drug Interactions. Antacids may reduce the bioavailability of ACE inhibitors; capsaicin may worsen ACE inhibitor–induced cough; NSAIDs, including aspirin (Guazzi *et al.,* 1998), may reduce the antihypertensive response to ACE inhibitors; and K$^+$-sparing diuretics and K$^+$ supplements may exacerbate ACE inhibitor–induced hyperkalemia. ACE inhibitors may increase plasma levels of digoxin and lithium and may increase hypersensitivity reactions to allopurinol.

NONPEPTIDE ANGIOTENSIN II RECEPTOR ANTAGONISTS

History. Attempts to develop therapeutically useful angiotensin II receptor antagonists date to the early 1970s, and these initial endeavors concentrated on angiotensin peptide analogs. Saralasin, 1-sarcosine, 8-isoleucine angiotensin II, and other 8-substituted angiotensins were potent angiotensin II receptor antagonists but were of no clinical value because of lack of oral bioavailability and because all peptide angiotensin II receptor antagonists expressed unacceptable partial agonist activity.

Although initial efforts to develop nonpeptide angiotensin-receptor antagonists were unsuccessful, a breakthrough came in the early 1980s with the issuance of patents on a series of imidazole-5-acetic acid derivatives that attenuated pressor responses to angiotensin II in rats. Two compounds described in the patents, S-8307 and S-8308, later were found to be highly specific, albeit very weak, nonpeptide angiotensin II receptor antagonists that were devoid of partial agonist activity (Wong *et al.*, 1988; Chiu *et al.*, 1988). In an instructive example of drug design, molecular modeling of these lead compounds gave rise to the hypothesis that their structures would have to be extended to mimic more closely the pharmacophore of angiotensin II (Figure 30–8A). Through an insightful series of stepwise modifications (Figure 30–8B), the orally active, potent, and selective nonpeptide AT$_1$-receptor antagonist *losartan* was developed (Timmermans *et al.*, 1993). Losartan was approved for clinical use in the United States in 1995. Since then, six additional AT$_1$-receptor antagonists (Figure 30–9) have been approved. AT$_1$-receptor antagonists approved in the United States are either biphenylmethyl derivatives or thienylmethylacrylic acid derivatives (Figure 30–9). Although these AT$_1$-receptor antagonists are devoid of partial agonist activity, nonpeptide AT$_1$-receptor agonists have been synthesized, and structural modifications as minor as a methyl group can transform a potent antagonist into an agonist (Perlman *et al.*, 1997).

Pharmacological Effects. The angiotensin II receptor blockers (ARBs) available for clinical use bind to the AT$_1$ receptor with high affinity and generally are more than 10,000-fold selective for the AT$_1$ receptor *versus* the AT$_2$ receptor. The rank-order affinity of the AT$_1$ receptor for ARBs is candesartan = omesartan > irbesartan = eprosartan > telmisartan = valsartan = EXP 3174 (the active metabolite of losartan) > losartan. Although binding of ARBs to the AT$_1$ receptor is competitive, the inhibition by ARBs of biological responses to angiotensin II often is insurmountable; *i.e.,* the maximal response to angiotensin II cannot be restored in the presence of the ARB regard-

less of the concentration of angiotensin II added to the experimental preparation. Of the currently available ARBs, candesartan suppresses the maximal response to angiotensin II the most, whereas insurmountable blockade by irbesartan, eprosartan, telmisartan, and valsartan is less. Although losartan antagonism is surmountable, its active metabolite, EXP 3174, causes some degree of insurmountable blockade. The mechanism of insurmountable antagonism by ARBs may be due to slow dissociation kinetics of the compounds from the AT$_1$ receptor; however, a number of other factors may contribute, such as ARB-induced receptor internalization and alternative binding sites for ARBs on the AT$_1$ receptor (McConnaughey *et al.*, 1999). Regardless of the mechanism, insurmountable antagonism has the theoretical advantage of sustained receptor blockade even with increased levels of endogenous ligand and with missed doses of drug. Whether this theoretical advantage translates into an enhanced clinical performance remains to be determined.

The pharmacology of ARBs is well described (Timmermans *et al.*, 1993; Csajka *et al.*, 1997). ARBs potently and selectively inhibit, both *in vitro* and *in vivo,* most of the biological effects of angiotensin II, including angiotensin II–induced (1) contraction of vascular smooth muscle, (2) rapid pressor responses, (3) slow pressor responses, (4) thirst, (5) vasopressin release, (6) aldosterone secretion, (7) release of adrenal catecholamines, (8) enhancement of noradrenergic neurotransmission, (9) increases in sympathetic tone, (10) changes in renal function, and (11) cellular hypertrophy and hyperplasia. ARBs reduce arterial blood pressure in animals with renovascular and genetic hypertension, as well as in transgenic animals overexpressing the renin gene. ARBs, however, have little effect on arterial blood pressure in animals with low-renin hypertension (*e.g.,* rats with hypertension induced by NaCl and deoxycorticosterone).

A critical issue is whether or not ARBs are equivalent to ACE inhibitors with regard to therapeutic efficacy. Although both classes of drugs block the renin–angiotensin system, ARBs differ from ACE inhibitors in several important aspects: (1) *ARBs reduce activation of AT$_1$ receptors more effectively than do ACE inhibitors.* ACE inhibitors reduce the biosynthesis of angiotensin II produced by the action of ACE on angiotensin I but do not inhibit alternative non-ACE angiotensin II–generating pathways. Because ARBs block the AT$_1$ receptor, the actions of angiotensin II *via* the AT$_1$ receptor are inhibited regardless of the biochemical pathway leading to angiotensin II formation. (2) In contrast to ACE inhibitors, *ARBs permit activation of AT$_2$ receptors.* ACE inhibitors increase renin release; however, because ACE inhibitors

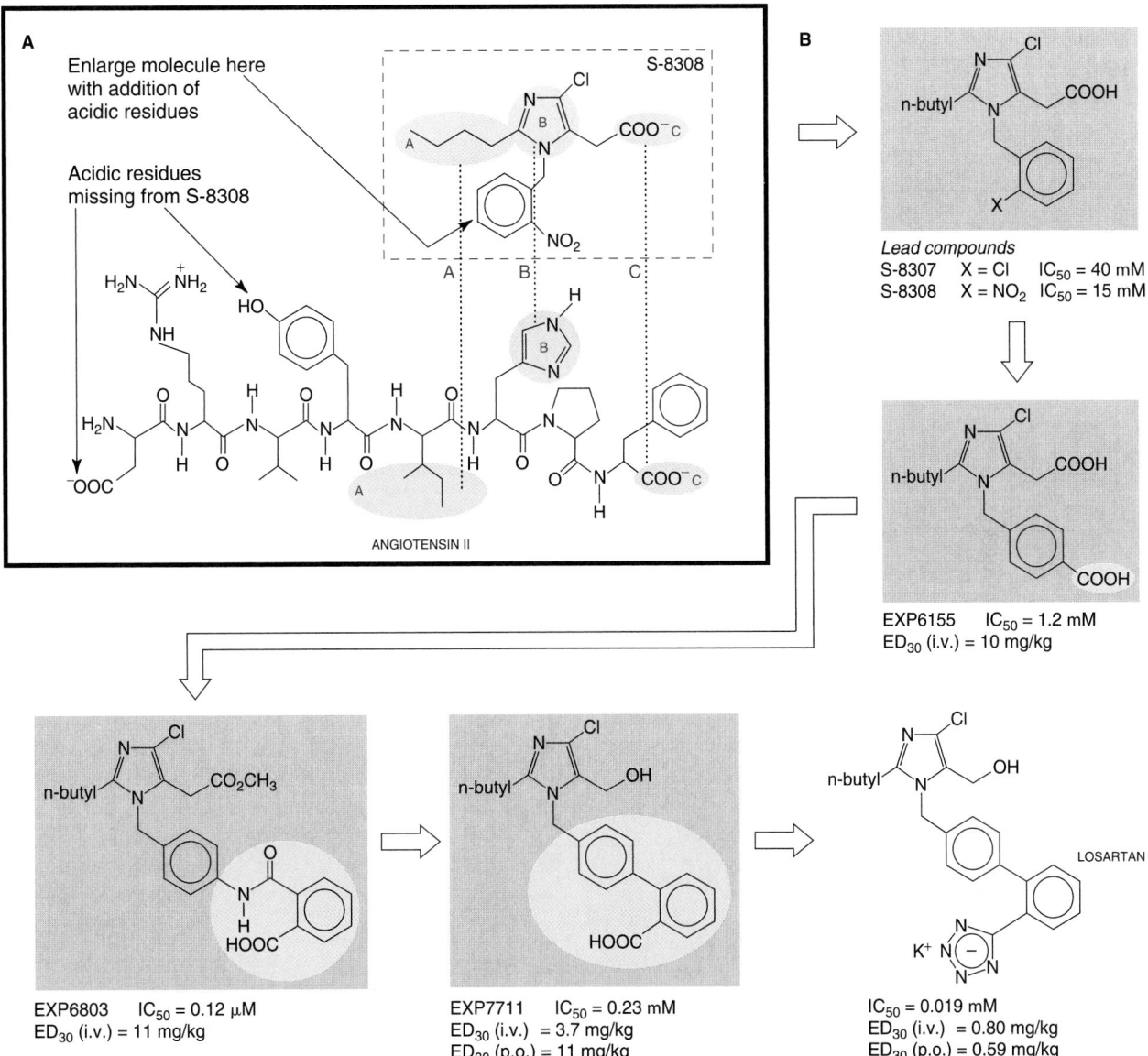

Figure 30–8. **A.** Hypothesized relationship between S-8308 (Takeda lead compound) and angiotensin II, and design strategies to enhance binding affinity of nonpeptide antagonists to the angiotensin II receptor. Letters indicate corresponding regions of S-8308 and angiotensin II. **B.** Pathway leading to the discovery of losartan. (Modified from Timmermans *et al.*, 1993, with permission.)

block the conversion of angiotensin I to angiotensin II, ACE inhibition is not associated with increased levels of angiotensin II. ARBs also stimulate renin release; however, with ARBs, this translates into a several-fold increase in circulating levels of angiotensin II. Because AT_2 receptors are not blocked by clinically available ARBs, this increased level of angiotensin II is available to activate AT_2 receptors. (3) *ACE inhibitors may increase angiotensin(1–7) levels more than do ARBs.* ACE is involved in the clearance of angiotensin(1–7), so inhibition of ACE

may increase angiotensin(1–7) levels more so than do ARBs. (4) *ACE inhibitors increase the levels of a number of ACE substrates, including bradykinin and Ac-SDKP.* ACE is a nondiscriminating enzyme that processes an array of substrates; inhibiting ACE therefore increases the levels of ACE substrates and decreases the levels of their corresponding products. Whether the pharmacological differences between ARBs and ACE inhibitors result in significant differences in therapeutic outcomes is an open question.

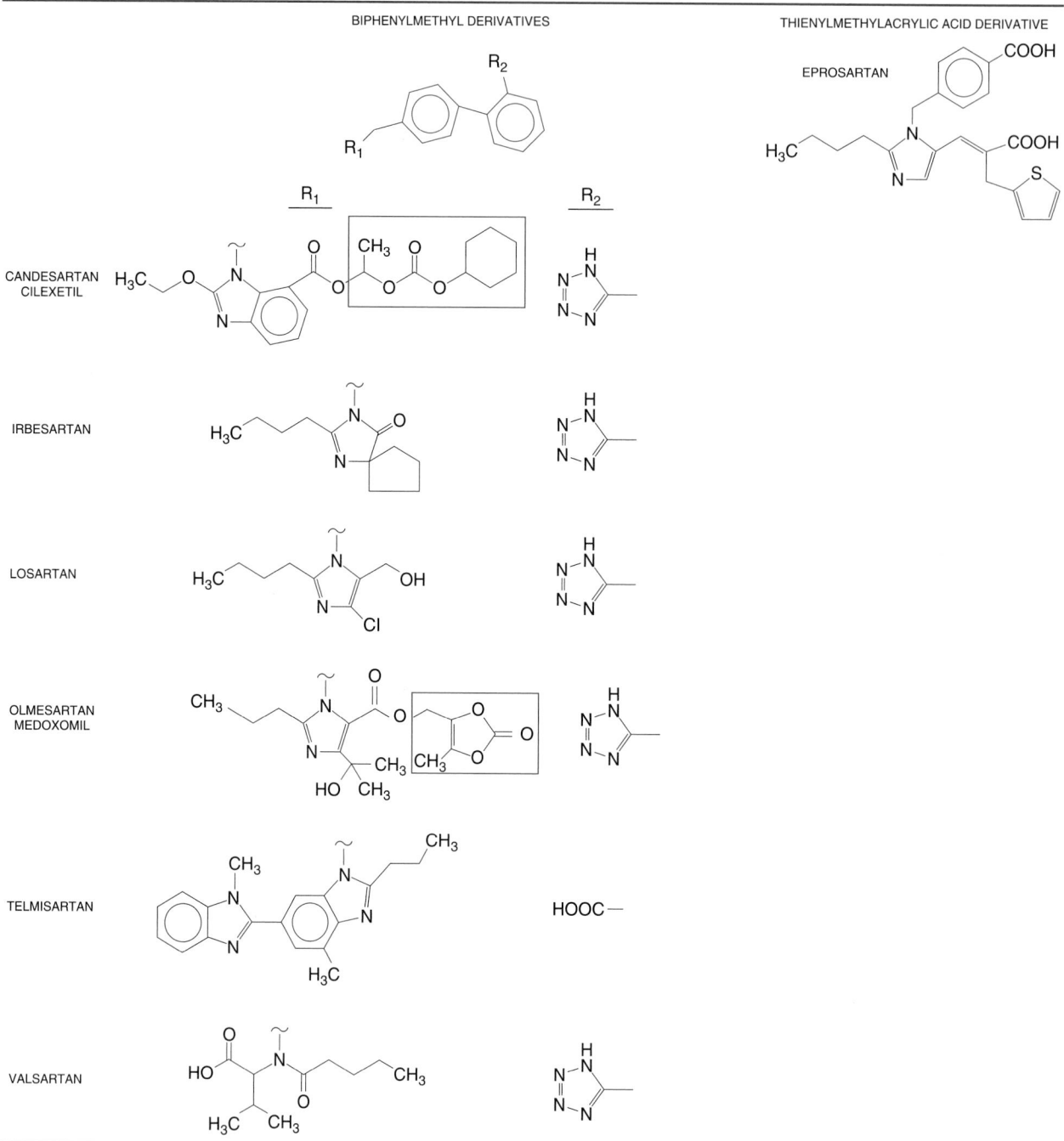

Figure 30–9. *FDA-approved angiotensin II-receptor antagonists.* Structures within blue boxes are removed by esterases and replaced with hydrogen atom to form the active molecule *in vivo.* ~ indicates point of attachment to biphenyl core.

Clinical Pharmacology. Oral bioavailability of ARBs generally is low (<50%, except for irbesartan, with 70% available), and protein binding is high (>90%).

Candesartan Cilexetil (ATACAND). Candesartan cilexetil is an inactive ester prodrug that is completely hydro-lyzed to the active form, candesartan, during absorption from the gastrointestinal tract. Peak plasma levels are obtained 3 to 4 hours after oral administration, and the plasma half-life is about 9 hours. Plasma clearance of candesartan is due to renal elimination (33%) and biliary excretion (67%). The plasma clearance of candesartan is affected by renal insufficiency but not by mild to moderate hepatic insufficiency. Candesartan cilexetil should be administered orally once or twice daily for a total daily dosage of 4 to 32 mg.

Eprosartan (*TEVETEN*). Peak plasma levels are obtained approximately 1 to 2 hours after oral administration, and the plasma half-life ranges from 5 to 9 hours. Eprosartan is metabolized in part to the glucuronide conjugate, and the parent compound and its glucuronide conjugate are cleared by renal elimination and biliary excretion. The plasma clearance of eprosartan is affected by both renal insufficiency and hepatic insufficiency. The recommended dosage of eprosartan is 400 to 800 mg/day in one or two doses.

Irbesartan (*AVAPRO*). Peak plasma levels are obtained approximately 1.5 to 2 hours after oral administration, and the plasma half-life ranges from 11 to 15 hours. Irbesartan is metabolized in part to the glucuronide conjugate, and the parent compound and its glucuronide conjugate are cleared by renal elimination (20%) and biliary excretion (80%). The plasma clearance of irbesartan is unaffected by either renal or mild to moderate hepatic insufficiency. The oral dosage of irbesartan is 150 to 300 mg once daily.

Losartan (*COZAAR*). Approximately 14% of an oral dose of losartan is converted to the 5-carboxylic acid metabolite EXP 3174, which is more potent than losartan as an AT_1-receptor antagonist. The metabolism of losartan to EXP 3174 and to inactive metabolites is mediated by CYP2C9 and CYP3A4. Peak plasma levels of losartan and EXP 3174 occur approximately 1 to 3 hours after oral administration, respectively, and the plasma half-lives are 2.5 and 6 to 9 hours, respectively. The plasma clearances of losartan and EXP 3174 (600 and 50 ml/min, respectively) are due to renal clearance (75 and 25 ml/min, respectively) and hepatic clearance (metabolism and biliary excretion). The plasma clearance of losartan and EXP 3174 is affected by hepatic but not renal insufficiency. Losartan should be administered orally once or twice daily for a total daily dose of 25 to 100 mg. In addition to being an ARB, losartan is a competitive antagonist of the thromboxane A_2 receptor and attenuates platelet aggregation (Levy *et al.*, 2000). Also, EXP3179, an active metabolite of losartan, reduces COX-2 mRNA up-regulation and COX-dependent prostaglandin generation (Krämer *et al.*, 2002).

Olmesartan Medoxomil (*BENICAR*). Olmesartan medoxomil is an inactive ester prodrug that is completely hydrolyzed to the active form, olmesartan, during absorption from the gastrointestinal tract. Peak plasma

levels are obtained 1.4 to 2.8 hours after oral administration, and the plasma half-life is between 10 and 15 hours. Plasma clearance of olmesartan is due to both renal elimination and biliary excretion. Although renal impairment and hepatic disease decrease the plasma clearance of olmesartan, no dose adjustment is required in patients with mild to moderate renal or hepatic impairment. The oral dosage of olmesartan medoxomil is 20 to 40 mg once daily.

Telmisartan (*MICARDIS*). Peak plasma levels are obtained approximately 0.5 to 1 hour after oral administration, and the plasma half-life is about 24 hours. Telmisartan is cleared from the circulation mainly by biliary secretion of intact drug. The plasma clearance of telmisartan is affected by hepatic but not renal insufficiency. The recommended oral dosage of telmisartan is 40 to 80 mg once daily.

Valsartan (*DIOVAN*). Peak plasma levels occur approximately 2 to 4 hours after oral administration, and the plasma half-life is about 9 hours. Food markedly decreases absorption. Valsartan is cleared from the circulation by the liver (about 70% of total clearance). The plasma clearance of valsartan is affected by hepatic but not renal insufficiency. The oral dosage of valsartan is 80 to 320 mg once daily.

Therapeutic Uses of Angiotensin II-Receptor Antagonists. All ARBs are approved for the treatment of hypertension. In addition, irbesartan and losartan are approved for diabetic nephropathy, losartan is approved for stroke prophylaxis, and valsartan is approved for heart failure patients who are intolerant of ACE inhibitors. The efficacy of ARBs in lowering blood pressure is comparable with that of other established antihypertensive drugs, with an adverse-effect profile similar to that of placebo (Mimran *et al.*, 1999). ARBs also are available as fixed-dose combinations with hydrochlorothiazide.

Losartan is well tolerated in patients with heart failure and is comparable to enalapril with regard to improving exercise tolerance (Lang *et al.*, 1997). The Evaluation of Losartan in the Elderly (ELITE) study reported that in elderly patients with heart failure, losartan was as effective as captopril in improving symptoms and reduced mortality more than did captopril (Pitt *et al.*, 1997). However, the greater reduction in mortality by losartan was not confirmed in the larger Losartan Heart Failure Survival Study (ELITE II) trial (Pitt *et al.*, 2000); in fact, captopril tended to have a more favorable effect on several outcome measures. The results of the OPTIMAAL trial support the conclusions of the ELITE II study favoring captopril over losartan (Dickstein *et al.*, 2002). However, the Valsartan in

Acute Myocardial Infarction (VALIANT) trial demonstrated that valsartan is as effective as captopril in patients with myocardial infarction complicated by left ventricular systolic dysfunction with regard to all-cause-mortality (Pfeffer *et al.*, 2003a). Both valsartan and candesartan reduce mortality and morbidity in heart failure patients (Cohn *et al.*, 2001; Maggioni *et al.*, 2002; Pfeffer *et al.*, 2003a, 2003b; Granger *et al.*, 2003). Current recommendations are to use ACE inhibitors as first-line agents for the treatment of heart failure and to reserve ARBs for treatment of heart failure in patients who cannot tolerate or have an unsatisfactory response to ACE inhibitors. At present, there is conflicting evidence regarding the advisability of combining an ARB and an ACE inhibitor in heart failure patients (Pfeffer *et al.*, 2003a; McMurray *et al.*, 2003).

In part *via* blood pressure–independent mechanisms, ARBs are renoprotective in type 2 diabetes mellitus (Brenner *et al.*, 2001; Lewis *et al.*, 2001; Parving *et al.*, 2001; Viberti *et al.*, 2002). Based on these results, many experts now consider them the drugs of choice for renoprotection in diabetic patients. The Losartan Intervention For Endpoint (LIFE) Reduction in Hypertension Study demonstrated the superiority of an ARB compared with a β_1 adrenergic receptor antagonist with regard to reducing stroke in hypertensive patients with left ventricular hypertrophy (Dahlöf *et al.*, 2002). Also, irebesartan appears to maintain sinus rhythm in patients with persistent, long-standing atrial fibrillation (Madrid *et al.*, 2002). Losartan is reported to be safe and highly effective in the treatment of portal hypertension in patients with cirrhosis and portal hypertension (Schneider *et al.*, 1999) without compromising renal function.

Adverse Effects. The incidence of discontinuation of ARBs owing to adverse reactions is comparable with that of placebo. Unlike ACE inhibitors, ARBs do not cause cough, and the incidence of angioedema with ARBs is much less than with ACE inhibitors. As with ACE inhibitors, ARBs have teratogenic potential and should be discontinued before the second trimester of pregnancy. ARBs should be used cautiously in patients whose arterial blood pressure or renal function is highly dependent on the renin–angiotensin system (*e.g.*, renal artery stenosis). In such patients, ARBs can cause hypotension, oliguria, progressive azotemia, or acute renal failure. ARBs may cause hyperkalemia in patients with renal disease or in patients taking K^+ supplements or K^+-sparing diuretics. ARBs enhance the blood pressure–lowering effect of other antihypertensive drugs, a desirable effect but one that may necessitate dosage adjustment.

BIBLIOGRAPHY

AbdAlla, S., Lother, H., Abdel-tawab, A.M., and Quitterer, U. The angiotensin II AT_2 receptor is an AT_1 receptor antagonist. *J. Biol. Chem.*, **2001**, *276*:39721–39726.

AbdAlla, S., Lother, H., El Massiery, A., and Quitterer, U. Increased AT_1 receptor heterodimers in preeclampsia mediate enhanced angiotensin II responsiveness. *Nature Med.*, **2002**, *7*:1003–1009.

ACE Inhibitor Myocardial Infarction Collaborative Group. Indications for ACE inhibitors in the early treatment of acute myocardial infarction: Systematic overview of individual data from 100,000 patients in randomized trials. *Circulation*, **1998**, *97*:2202–2212.

AIRE Study Investigators. Effect of ramipril on mortality and morbidity of survivors of acute myocardial infarction with clinical evidence of heart failure. *Lancet*, **1993**, *342*:821–828.

Akasu, M., Urata, H., Kinoshita, A., *et al.* Differences in tissue angiotensin II–forming pathways by species and organs in vitro. *Hypertension*, **1998**, *32*:514–520.

Álvarez, R., Reguero, J.R., Batalla, A., *et al.* Angiotensin-converting enzyme and angiotensin II receptor 1 polymorphisms: Association with early coronary disease. *Cardiovasc. Res.*, **1998**, *40*:375–379.

Amant, C., Bauters, C., Bodart, J.-C., *et al.* D allele of the angiotensin I–converting enzyme is a major risk factor for restenosis after coronary stenting. *Circulation*, **1997**, *96*:56–60.

Amant, C., Hamon, M., Bauters, C., *et al.* The angiotensin II type 1 receptor gene polymorphism is associated with coronary artery vasoconstriction. *J. Am. Coll. Cardiol.*, **1997**, *29*:486–490.

Ambrosioni, E., Borghi, C., and Magnani, B. The effect of the angiotensin-converting-enzyme inhibitor zofenopril on mortality and morbidity after anterior myocardial infarction. *New Engl. J. Med.*, **1995**, *332*:80–85.

Arnold, J.M.O., Yusuf, S., Young, J., *et al.*, on behalf of the HOPE Investigators. Prevention of heart failure in patients in the heart outcomes prevention evaluation (HOPE) study. *Circulation*, **2003**, *107*:1284–1290.

Azizi, M., Ezan, E., Nicolet, L., Grognet, J.-M., and Menard, J. High plasma level of *N*-acetyl-seryl-aspartyl-lysyl-proline: A new marker of chronic angiotensin-converting enzyme inhibition. *Hypertension*, **1997**, *30*:1015–1019.

Bautista, R., Manning, R., Martinez, F., *et al.* Antiotensin II–dependent increased expression of Na^+–glucose cotransporter in hypertension. *Am. J. Physiol. Renal Physiol.*, **2004**, *286*:F127–F133.

Beierwaltes, W.H. Macula densa stimulation of renin is reversed by selective inhibition of neuronal nitric oxide synthase. *Am. J. Physiol.*, **1997**, *272*:R1359–R1364.

Beldent, V., Michaud, A., Bonnefoy, C., Chauvet, M.-T., and Corvol, P. Cell surface localization of proteolysis of human endothelial angiotensin I–converting enzyme: Effect of the amino-terminal domain in the solubilization process. *J. Biol. Chem.*, **1995**, *270*:28962–28969.

Bell, L., and Madri, J.A. Influence of the angiotensin system on endothelial and smooth muscle cell migration. *Am. J. Pathol.*, **1990**, *137*:7–12.

Benetos, A., Gautier, S., Ricard, S., *et al.* Influence of angiotensin-converting enzyme and angiotensin II type 1 receptor gene polymorphisms on aortic stiffness in normotensive and hypertensive patients. *Circulation*, **1996**, *94*:698–703.

Borghi, C., Bacchelli, S., Esposti, D.D., *et al.* Effects of the administration of an angiotensin-converting enzyme inhibitor during the acute phase of myocardial infarction in patients with arterial hypertension. SMILE Study Investigators. Survival of Myocardial Infarction Long-term Evaluation. *Am. J. Hypertens.*, **1999**, *12*:665–672.

Borghi, C., Marino, P., Zardini, P., *et al.* Post acute myocardial infarction. The Fosinopril in Acute Myocardial Infarction Study (FAMIS). *Am. J. Hypertens.,* **1997,** *10*:247S–254S.

Brenner, B.M., Cooper, M.E., de Zeeuw, D., *et al.,* for the RENAAL Study Investigators. Effects of losartan on renal and cardiovascular outcomes in patients with type 2 diabetes and nephropathy. *New Engl. J. Med.,* **2001,** *345*:861–869.

Brink, M., Wellen, J., and Delafontaine, P. Angiotensin II causes weight loss and decreases circulating insulin-like growth factor I in rats through a pressor-independent mechanism. *J. Clin. Invest.,* **1996,** *97*:2509–2516.

Brown, N.J., Agirbasli, M., and Vaughan, D.E. Comparative effect of angiotensin-converting enzyme inhibition and angiotensin II type 1 receptor antagonism on plasma fibrinolytic balance in humans. *Hypertension,* **1999,** *34*:285–290.

Brown, N.J., Ray, W.A., Snowden, M., and Griffin, M.R. Black Americans have an increased rate of angiotensin converting enzyme inhibitor–associated angioedema. *Clin. Pharmacol. Ther.,* **1996,** *60*:8–13.

Butler, R., Morris, A.D., Burchell, B., and Struthers, A.D. *DD* angiotensin-converting enzyme gene polymorphism is associated with endothelial dysfunction in normal humans. *Hypertension,* **1999,** *33*:1164–1168.

Cambien, F., Poirier, O., Lecerf, L., *et al.* Deletion polymorphism in the gene for angiotensin-converting enzyme is a potent risk factor for myocardial infarction. *Nature,* **1992,** *359*:641–644.

Campbell, D.J., Duncan, A.-M., and Kladis, A. Angiotensin-converting enzyme inhibition modifies angiotensin but not kinin peptide levels in human atrial tissue. *Hypertension,* **1999,** *34*:171–175.

Campbell, D.J., Kladis, A., Skinner, S.L., and Whitworth, J.A. Characterization of angiotensin peptides in plasma of anephric man. *J. Hypertens.,* **1991,** *9*:265–274.

Candido, R., Jandeleit-Dahm, K.A., Cao, Z., *et al.* Prevention of accelerated atherosclerosis by angiotensin-converting enzyme inhibition in diabetic apolipoprotein E–deficient mice. *Circulation,* **2002,** *106*:246–253.

Carey, R.M., Howell, N.L., Jin, X.-H., and Siragy, H.M. Angiotensin type 2 receptor–mediated hypotension in angiotensin type 1 receptor–blocked rats. *Hypertension,* **2001,** *38*:1272–1277.

Carey, R.M., McGrath, H.E., Pentz, E.S., Gomez, R.A., and Barrett, P.Q. Biomechanical coupling in renin-releasing cells. *J. Clin. Invest.,* **1997,** *100*:1566–1574.

Cashin-Hemphill, L., Holmvang, G., Chan, R.C., *et al.* Angiotensin-converting enzyme inhibition as antiatherosclerotic therapy: No answer yet. QUIET Investigators. QUinapril Ischemic Event Trial. *Am. J. Cardiol.,* **1999,** *83*:43–47.

Caulfield, M., Lavender, P., Farrall, M., *et al.* Linkage of the angiotensinogen gene to essential hypertension. *New Engl. J. Med.,* **1994,** *330*:1629–1633.

Caulfield, M., Lavender, P., Newell-Price, J., *et al.* Linkage of the angiotensinogen gene locus to human essential hypertension in African Caribbeans. *J. Clin. Invest.,* **1995,** *96*:687–692.

Célérier, J., Cruz, A., Lamandé, N., Gasc, J.-M., and Corvol, P. Angiotensin and its cleaved derivatives inhibit angiogenesis. *Hypertension,* **2002,** 39:224–228.

Chaturvedi, N., Sjolie, A.K., Stephenson, J.M., *et al.* Effect of lisinopril on progression of retinopathy in normotensive people with type 1 diabetes. The EUCLID Study Group. EURODIAB Controlled Trial of Lisinopril in Insulin-Dependent Diabetes Mellitus. *Lancet,* **1998,** *351*:28–31.

Chen, H.-C., Bouchie, J.L., Perez, A.S., *et al.* Role of the angiotensin AT$_1$ receptor in rat aortic and cardiac *PAI*-1 gene expression. *Arterioscler. Thromb. Vasc. Biol.,* **2000,** *20*:2297–2302.

Cheng, H.-F., Wang, J.-L., Zhang, M.-Z., McKanna, J.A., and Harris, R.C. Nitric oxide regulates renal cortical cyclooxygenase-2 expression. *Am. J. Physiol. Renal Physiol.,* **2000,** *279*:F122–F129.

Cheng, H.-F., Wang, J.-L., Zhang, M.-Z., *et al.* Genetic deletion of COX-2 prevents increased renin expression in response to ACE inhibition. *Am. J. Physiol. Renal Physiol.,* **2001,** *280*:F449–F456.

Chiu, A.T., Carini, D.J., Johnson, A.L., *et al.* Non-peptide angiotensin II receptor antagonists: II. Pharmacology of S-8308. *Eur. J. Pharmacol.,* **1988,** *157*:13–21.

Chiu, A.T., Herblin, W.F., McCall, D.E., *et al.* Identification of angiotensin II receptor subtypes. *Biochem. Biophys. Res. Commun.,* **1989,** *165*:196–203.

Cohn, J.N., Johnson, G., Ziesche, S., *et al.* A comparison of enalapril with hydralazine–isosorbide dinitrate in the treatment of chronic congestive heart failure. *New Engl. J. Med.,* **1991,** *325*:303–310.

Cohn, J.N., and Tognoni, G., for the Valsartan Heart Failure Trial Investigators. A randomized trial of the angiotensin-receptor blocker valsartan in chronic heart failure. *New Engl. J. Med.,* **2001,** *345*:1667–1675.

CONSENSUS Trial Study Group. Effects of enalapril on mortality in severe congestive heart failure: Results of the Cooperative North Scandinavian Enalapril Survival Study (CONSENSUS). *New Engl. J. Med.,* **1987,** *316*:1429–1435.

Crackower, M.A., Sarao, R., Oudit, G.Y., *et al.* Angiotensin-converting enzyme 2 is an essential regulator of heart function. *Nature,* **2002,** *417*:822–828.

Crawford, D.C., Chobanian, A.V., and Brecher, P. Angiotensin II induces fibronectin expression associated with cardiac fibrosis in the rat. *Circ. Res.,* **1994,** *74*:727–739.

Cressman, M.D., Vidt, D.G., and Acker, C. Renal glycosuria and azotemia after enalapril maleate (MK-421). *Lancet,* **1982,** 2:440.

Daemen, M.J.M.P., Lombardi, D.M., Bosman, F.T., and Schwartz, S.M. Angiotensin II induces smooth muscle cell proliferation in the normal and injured rat arterial wall. *Circ. Res.,* **1991,** *68*:450–456.

Dahlöf, B., Devereux, R.B., Kjeldsen, S.E., *et al.,* for the LIFE Study Group. Cardiovascular morbidity and mortality in the losartan intervention for endpoint reduction in hypertension study (LIFE): A randomized trial against atenolol. *Lancet,* **2002,** *359*:995–1003.

Danser, A.H., Sassen, L.M., Admiraal, P.J., *et al.* Regional production of angiotensins I and II: Contribution of vascular kidney-derived renin. *J. Hypertens.,* **1991,** *9*(suppl):S234–S235.

Danser, A.H., van Kats, J.P., Admiraal, P.J., *et al.* Cardiac renin and angiotensins: Uptake from plasma versus in situ synthesis. *Hypertension,* **1994,** *24*:37–48.

Danser, A.H., Koning, M.M., Admiraal, P.J., *et al.* Production of angiotensins I and II at tissue sites in intact pigs. *Am. J. Physiol.,* **1992,** *263*:H429–H437.

Daugherty, A., Manning, M.W., and Cassis, L.A. Angiotensin II promotes atherosclerotic lesions and aneurysms in apolipoprotein E–deficient mice. *J. Clin. Invest.,* **2000,** *105*:1605–1612.

Davie, A.P., Dargie, H.J., and McMurray, J.J.V. Role of bradykinin in the vasodilator effects of losartan and enalapril in patients with heart failure. *Circulation,* **1999,** *100*:268–273.

Dickstein, K., and Kjekshus, J., and the *OPTIMAAL* Steering Committee, for the *OPTIMAAL* Study Group. Effects of losartan and captopril on mortality and morbidity in high-risk patients after acute myocardial infarction: The OPTIMAAL randomised trial. *Lancet,* **2002,** *360*:752–760.

Donoghue, M., Hsieh, F., Baronas, E., *et al.* A novel angiotensin-converting enzyme–related carboxypeptidase (ACE2) converts angiotensin I to angiotensin(1–9). *Circ. Res.,* **2000,** *87*:E1–E9.

Dubey, R.K., Jackson, E.K., and Luscher, T.F. Nitric oxide inhibits angiotensin II–induced migration of rat aortic smooth muscle cell: Role of cyclic nucleotides and angiotensin$_1$ receptors. *J. Clin. Invest.*, **1995**, *96*:141–149.

Erhardt, L., MacLean, A., Ilgenfritz, J., Gelperin, K., and Blumenthal, M. Fosinopril attenuates clinical deterioration and improves exercise tolerance in patients with heart failure. Fosinopril Efficacy/Safety Trial (FEST) Study Group. *Eur. Heart J.*, **1995**, *16*:1892–1899.

Estacio, R.O., Jeffers, B.W., Hiatt, W.R., *et al*. The effect of nisoldipine as compared with enalapril on cardiovascular outcomes in patients with non-insulin-dependent diabetes and hypertension. *New Engl. J. Med.*, **1998**, *338*:645–652.

EUCLID Study Group. Randomised, placebo-controlled trial of lisinopril in normotensive patients with insulin-dependent diabetes and normoalbuminuria or microalbuminuria. *Lancet*, **1997**, *349*:1787–1792.

EURopean trial On reduction of cardiac events with Perindopril in stable coronary Artery disease (EUROPA) Investigators. Efficacy of perindopril in reduction of cardiovascular events among patients with stable coronary artery disease: Randomised, double-blind, placebo-controlled, multicentre trial (the EUROPA study). *Lancet*, **2003**, *362*:782–788.

Fatini, C., Abbate, R., Pepe, G., *et al*. Searching for a better assessment of the individual coronary risk profile: The role of angiotensin-converting enzyme, angiotensin II type 1 receptor and angiotensinogen gene polymorphisms. *Eur. Heart J.*, **2000**, *21*:633–638.

Fornage, M., Amos, C.I., Kardia, S., *et al*. Variation in the region of the angiotensin-converting enzyme gene influences interindividual differences in blood pressure levels in young white males. *Circulation*, **1998**, *97*:1773–1779.

Friedrich, S.P., Lorell, B.H., Rousseau, M.F., *et al*. Intracardiac angiotensin-converting enzyme inhibition improves diastolic function in patients with left ventricular hypertrophy due to aortic stenosis. *Circulation*, **1994**, *90*:276l–2771.

Friis, U.G., Jensen, B.L., Aas, J.K., and Skøtt, O. Direct demonstration of exocytosis and endocytosis in single mouse juxtaglomerular cells. *Circ. Res.*, **1999**, *84*:929–936.

Friis, U.G., Jensen, B.L., Sethi, S., *et al*. Control of renin secretion from rat juxtaglomerular cells by cAMP-specific phosphodiesterases. *Circ. Res.*, **2002**, *90*:996–1003.

Gainer, J.V., Morrow, J.D., Loveland, A., King, D.J., and Brown, N.J. Effect of bradykinin-receptor blockade on the response to angiotensin-converting-enzyme inhibitor in normotensive and hypertensive subjects. *New Engl. J. Med.*, **1998**, *339*:1285–1292.

Gardemann, A., Weiss, T., Schwartz, O., *et al*. Gene polymorphism but not catalytic activity of angiotensin I–converting enzyme is associated with coronary artery disease and myocardial infarction in low-risk patients. *Circulation*, **1995**, *92*:2796–2799.

Gesualdo, L., Ranieri, E., Monno, R., *et al*. Angiotensin IV stimulates plasminogen activator inhibitor-I expression in proximal tubular epithelial cells. *Kidney Int.*, **1999**, *56*:461–470.

GISEN Group (Gruppo Italiano di Studi Epidemiologici in Nefrologia). Randomised, placebo-controlled trial of effect of ramipril on decline in glomerular filtration rate and risk of terminal renal failure in proteinuric, non-diabetic nephropathy. *Lancet*, **1997**, *349*:1857–1863.

Granger, C.B., McMurray, J.J.V., Yusuf, S., *et al*., for the CHARM Investigators and Committees. Effects of candesartan in patients with chronic heart failure and reduced left-ventricular systolic function intolerant to angiotensin-converting-enzyme inhibitors: The CHARM-alternative trial. *Lancet*, **2003**, *362*:772–776.

Grassi, G., Cattaneo, B.M., Seravalle, G., *et al*. Effects of chronic ACE inhibition on sympathetic nerve traffic and baroreflex control of circulation in heart failure. *Circulation*, **1997**, *96*:1173–1179.

Gruppo Italiano per lo Studio della Sopravvivenza nellíInfarto Miocardico. GISSI-3: Effects of lisinopril and transdermal glyceryl trinitrate singly and together on 6-week mortality and ventricular function after acute myocardial infarction. *Lancet*, **1994**, *343*:1115–1122.

Guazzi, M.D., Campodonico, J., Celeste, F., *et al*. Antihypertensive efficacy of angiotensin converting enzyme inhibition and aspirin counteraction. *Clin. Pharmacol. Ther.*, **1998**, *63*:79–86.

Gustafsson, I., Torp-Pedersen, C., Kober, L., Gustafsson, F., and Hildebrandt, P. Effect of the angiotensin-converting enzyme inhibitor trandolapril on mortality and morbidity in diabetic patients with left ventricular dysfunction after acute myocardial infarction. Trace Study Group. *J. Am. Coll. Cardiol.*, **1999**, *34*:83–89.

Hadjadj, S., Belloum, R., Bouhanick, B., *et al*. Prognostic value of angiotensin-I converting enzyme *I/D* polymorphism for nephropathy in type 1 diabetes mellitus: a prospective study. *J. Am. Soc. Nephrol.*, **2001**, *12*:541–549.

Hagaman, J.R., Moyer, J.S., Bachman, E.S., *et al*. Angiotensin-converting enzyme and male fertility. *Proc. Natl. Acad. Sci. USA*, **1998**, *95*:2552–2557.

Hansen, P.B., Hashimoto, S., Briggs, J., and Schnermann, J. Attenuated renovascular constrictor responses to angiotensin II in adenosine 1 receptor knockout mice. *Am. J. Physiol. Regul. Integr. Comp. Physiol.*, **2003**, *285*:R44–R49.

Hansen, J.L., Servant, G., Baranski, T.J., *et al*. Functional reconstitution of the angiotensin II type 2 receptor and G$_i$ activation. *Circ. Res.*, **2000**, *87*:753–759.

Hansson, L., Lindholm, L.H., Niskanen, L., *et al*. Effect of angiotensin-converting-enzyme inhibition compared with conventional therapy on cardiovascular morbidity and mortality in hypertension: The Captopril Prevention Project (CAPPP) randomised trial. *Lancet*, **1999**, *353*:611–616.

Harada, E., Yoshimura, M., Yasue, H., *et al*. Aldosterone induces angiotensin-converting-enzyme gene expression in cultural neonatal rat cardiocytes. *Circulation*, **2001**, *104*:137–139.

Harris, R.C., McKanna, J.A., Akai, Y., *et al*. Cyclooxygenase-2 is associated with the macula densa of rat kidney and increases with salt restriction. *J. Clin. Invest.*, **1994**, *94*:2504–2510.

Heart Outcomes Prevention Study Investigators. Effects of an angiotensin-converting-enzyme inhibitor ramipril on cardiovascular events in high-risk patients. The Heart Outcomes Prevention Evaluation Study Investigators. *New Engl. J. Med.*, **2000**, *342*:145–153 (published erratum appears in *New Engl. J. Med.*, **2000**, *342*:478).

Higaki, J., Baba, S., Katsuya, T., *et al*. Deletion allele of angiotensin-converting enzyme gene increases risk of essential hypertension in Japanese men. The Suita Study. *Circulation*, **2000**, *101*:2060–2065.

Hilgers, K.F., Veelken, R., Müller, D.N., *et al*. Renin uptake by the endothelium mediates vascular angiotensin formation. *Hypertension*, **2001**, *38*:243–248.

Hosoi, M., Nishizawa, Y., Kogawa, K., *et al*. Angiotensin-converting enzyme gene polymorphism is associated with carotid arterial wall thickness in non insulin-dependent diabetic patients. *Circulation*, **1996**, *94*:704–707.

Hu, L., Catanzaro, D.F., Pitarresi, T.-M., Laragh, J.H., and Sealey, J.E. Identical hemodynamic and hormonal responses to 14-day infusions of renin or angiotensin II in conscious rats. *J. Hypertens.*, **1998**, *16*:1285–1298.

Ichihara, S., Senbonmatsu, T., Price, E., Jr., *et al*. Angiotensin II type 2 receptor is essential for left ventricular hypertrophy and cardiac fibrosis in chronic angiotensin II–induced hypertension. *Circulation*, **2001**, *104*:346–351.

ISIS-4 (Fourth International Study of Infarct Survival) Collaborative Group. ISIS-4: A randomised factorial trial assessing early oral captopril, oral mononitrate, and intravenous magnesium sulphate in 58,050 patients with suspected acute myocardial infarction. *Lancet*, **1995**, *345*:669–685.

Itoh, H., Mukoyama, M., Pratt, R.E., Gibbons, G.H., and Dzau, V.J. Multiple autocrine growth factors modulate vascular smooth muscle cell growth response to angiotensin II. *J. Clin. Invest.*, **1993**, *91*:2268–2274.

Iwai, N., Ohmichi, N., Nakamura, Y., and Kinoshita, M. *DD* genotype of the angiotensin-converting enzyme gene is a risk factor for left ventricular hypertrophy. *Circulation*, **1994**, *90*:2622–2628.

Iyer, S.N., Lu, D., Katovich, M.J., and Raizada, M.K. Chronic control of high blood pressure in the spontaneously hypertensive rat by delivery of angiotensin type 1 receptor antisense. *Proc. Natl. Acad. Sci. U.S.A.*, **1996**, *93*:9960–9965.

Jeunemaitre, X., Soubrier, F., Kotelevtsev, Y.V., *et al*. Molecular basis of human hypertension: Role of angiotensinogen. *Cell*, **1992**, *71*:169–180.

Kainulainen, K., Perola, M., Terwilliger, J., *et al*. Evidence for involvement of the type 1 angiotensin II receptor locus in essential hypertension. *Hypertension*, **1999**, *33*:844–849.

Kammerl, M.C., Nüsing, R.M., Schweda, F., *et al*. Low sodium and furosemide-induced stimulation of the renin system in man is mediated by cyclooxygenase 2. *Clin. Pharmacol. Ther.*, **2001**, *70*:468–474.

Kammerl, M.C., Richthammer, W., Kurtz, A., and Kramer, B.K. Angiotensin II feedback is a regulator of renocortical renin, COX-2, and nNOS expression. *Am. J. Physiol. Regul. Integr. Comp. Physiol.*, **2002**, *282*:R1613–R1617.

Kario, K., Kanai, N., Saito, K., *et al*. Ischemic stroke and the gene for angiotensin-converting enzyme in Japanese hypertensives. *Circulation*, **1996**, *93*:1630–1633.

Kato, H., Iwai, N., Inui, H., *et al*. Regulation of vascular angiotensin release. *Hypertension*, **1993**, *21*:446–454.

Kehoe, P.G., Russ, C., McIlory, S., *et al*. Variation in *DCP1*, encoding ACE, is associated with susceptibility to Alzheimer disease. *Nature Genet.*, **1999**, *21*:71–72.

Kerins, D.M., Hao, Q., and Vaughan, D.E. Angiotensin induction of PAI-1 expression in endothelial cells is mediated by the hexapeptide angiotensin IV. *J. Clin. Invest.*, **1995**, *96*:2515–2520.

Kim, H.-S., Krege, J.H., Kluckman, K.D., *et al*. Genetic control of blood pressure and the angiotensinogen locus. *Proc. Natl. Acad. Sci. USA*, **1995**, *92*:2735–2739.

Kjøller-Hansen, L., Steffensen, R., and Grande, P. The Angiotensin-converting Enzyme inhibition Post Revascularization Study (APRES). *J. Am. Coll. Cardiol.*, **2000**, *35*:881–888.

Kleber, F.X., Niemoller, L., and Doering, W. Impact of converting enzyme inhibition on progression of chronic heart failure: Results of the Munich Mild Heart Failure Trial. *Br. Heart J.*, **1992**, *67*:289–296.

Klett, C.P.R., and Granger, J.P. Physiological elevation in plasma angiotensinogen increases blood pressure. *Am. J. Physiol. Regul. Integr. Comp. Physiol.*, **2001**, *281*:R1437–R1441.

Køber, L., Torp-Pedersen, C., Carlsen, J.E., *et al*. A clinical trial of the angiotensin-converting-enzyme inhibitor trandolapril in patients with left ventricular dysfunction after myocardial infarction. Trandolapril Cardiac Evaluation (TRACE) Study Group. *New Engl. J. Med.*, **1995**, *333*:1670–1676.

Kovács, G., Peti-Peterdi, J., Rosivall, L., and Bell, P.D. Angiotensin II directly stimulates macula densa Na–2Cl–K cotransport via apical AT_1 receptors. *Am. J. Pysiol. Renal Physiol.*, **2002**, *282*:F301–F306.

Krämer, C., Sunkomat, J., Witte, J., *et al*. Angiotensin II receptor-independent antiinflammatory and antiaggregatory properties of losartan: Role of the active metabolite EXP3179. *Circ. Res.*, **2002**, *90*:770–776.

Kshirsagar, A.V., Joy, M.S., Hogan, S.L., Falk, R.J., and Colindres, R.E. Effect of ACE inhibitors in diabetic and nondiabetic chronic renal disease: A systematic overview of randomized placebo-controlled trials. *Am. J. Kidney Dis.*, **2000**, *35*:695–707.

Kunz, R., Kreutz, R., Beige, J., Distler, A., and Sharma, A.M. Association between the angiotensinogen 235T-variant and essential hypertension in whites: A systematic review and methodological appraisal. *Hypertension*, **1997**, *30*:1331–1337.

Kyriakidis, M., Triposkiadis, F., Dernellis, J., *et al*. Effects of cardiac versus circulatory angiotensin-converting enzyme inhibition on left ventricular diastolic function and coronary blood flow in hypertrophic obstructive cardiomyopathy. *Circulation*, **1998**, *97*:1342–1347.

Lage, S.G., Kopel, L., Medeiros, C.C.J., Carvalho, R.T., and Creager, M.A. Angiotensin II contributes to arterial compliance in congestive heart failure. *Am. J. Physiol. Heart Circ. Physiol.*, **2002**, *283*:H1424–H1429.

Landino, L.M., Crews, B.C., Timmons, M.D., Morrow, J.D., and Marnett, L.J. Peroxynitrite, the coupling product of nitric oxide and superoxide, activates prostaglandin biosynthesis. *Proc. Natl. Acad. Sci. U.S.A.*, **1996**, *93*:15069–15074.

Landmesser, U., Cai, H., Dikalov, S., *et al*. Role of $p47^{phox}$ in vascular oxidative stress and hypertension caused by angiotensin II. *Hypertension*, **2002**, *40*:511–515.

Lang, R.M., Elkayam, U., Yellen, L.G., *et al*. Comparative effects of losartan and enalapril on exercise capacity and clinical status in patients with heart failure. The Losartan Pilot Exercise Study Investigators. *J. Am. Coll. Cardiol.*, **1997**, *30*:983–991.

Laursen, J.B., Rajagopalan, S., Galis, Z., *et al*. Role of superoxide in angiotensin II–induced but not catecholamine-induced hypertension. *Circulation*, **1997**, *95*:588–593.

Lee, S.-C., Park, S.W., Kim, D.-K., Lee, S.H., and Hong, K.P. Iron supplementation inhibits cough associated with ACE inhibitors. *Hypertension*, **2001**, *38*:166–170.

Lee-Kirsch, M.A., Gaudet, F., Cardoso, M.C., and Lindpaintner, K. Distinct renin isoforms generated by tissue-specific transcription initiation and alternative splicing. *Circ. Res.*, **1999**, *84*:240–246.

Levy, P.J., Yunis, C., Owen, J., *et al*. Inhibition of platelet aggregability by losartan in essential hypertension. *Am. J. Cardiol.*, **2000**, *86*:1188–1192.

Lewis, E.J., Hunsicker, L.G., Bain, R.P., and Rohde, R.D., The effect of angiotensin-converting-enzyme inhibition on diabetic nephropathy. *New Engl. J. Med.*, **1993**, *329*:1456–1462.

Lewis, E.J., Hunsicker, L.G., *et al*., for the Collaborative Study Group. Renoprotective effect of the angiotensin-receptor antagonist irbesartan in patients with nephropathy due to type 2 diabetes. *New Engl. J. Med.*, **2001**, *345*:851–860.

Li, W., Moore, M.J., Vasilieva, N., *et al*. Angiotensin-converting enzyme 2 is a functional receptor for the SARS coronavirus. *Nature*, **2003**, *426*:450–454.

Liu, F.-Y., and Cogan, M.G. Angiotensin II: A potent regulator of acidification in the rat early proximal convoluted tubule. *J. Clin. Invest.*, **1987**, *80*:272–275.

Lopez, B., Salom, M.G., Arregui, B., Valero, F., and Fenoy, F.J. Role of superoxide in modulating the renal effects of angiotensin II. *Hypertension*, **2003**, *42*:1150–1156.

Losito, A., Selvi, A., Jeffery, S., *et al*. Angiotensin-converting enzyme gene *I/D* polymorphism and carotid artery disease in renovascular hypertension. *Am. J. Hypertens.*, **2000**, *13*:128–133.

Madrid, A.H., Bueno, M.G., Rebollo, J.M.G., *et al.* Use of irbesartan to maintain sinus rhythm in patients with long-lasting persistent atrial fibrillation: A prospective and randomized study. *Circulation,* **2002,** *106*:331–336.

Maggioni, A.P., Anand, I., Gottlieb, S.O., *et al.,* on behalf of the Val-HeFT Investigators. Effects of valsartan on morbidity and mortality in patients with heart failure not receiving angiotensin-converting enzyme inhibitors. *J. Am. Coll. Cardiol.,* **2002,** *40*:1414–1421.

Malini, P.L., Strocchi, E., Zanardi, M., Milani, M., and Ambrosioni, E. Thromboxane antagonism and cough induced by angiotensin-converting-enzyme inhibitor. *Lancet,* **1997,** *350*:15–18.

Mancini, G.B.J., Henry, G.C., Macaya, C., *et al.* Angiotensin-converting enzyme inhibition with quinapril improves endothelial vasomotor dysfunction in patients with coronary artery disease. The TREND (Trial on Reversing ENdothelial Dysfunction) Study. *Circulation,* **1996,** *94*:258–265.

Marre, M., Jeunemaitre, X., Gallois, Y., *et al.* Contribution of genetic polymorphism in the renin–angiotensin system to the development of renal complications in insulin-dependent diabetes. Genetique de la Nephropathie Diabetique (GENEDIAB) study group. *J. Clin. Invest.,* **1997,** *99*:1585–1595.

Maschio, G., Alberti, D., Janin, G., *et al.* Effect of the angiotensin-converting-enzyme inhibitor benazepril on the progression of chronic renal insufficiency. The Angiotensin-Converting-Enzyme Inhibition in Progressive Renal Insufficiency Study Group. *New Engl. J. Med.,* **1996,** *334*:939–945.

Mattu, R.K., Needham, E.W., Galton, D.J., *et al.* A DNA variant at the angiotensin-converting enzyme gene locus associates with coronary artery disease in the Caerphilly Heart Study. *Circulation,* **1995,** *91*:270–274.

McMurray, J.J.V., Ostergren, J., Swedberg, K., *et al.,* for the CHARM Investigators and Committees. Effects of candesartan in patients with chronic heart failure and reduced left-ventricular systolic function taking angiotensin-converting-enzyme inhibitors: The CHARM-added trial. *Lancet,* **2003,** *362*:767–771.

Meszaros, J.G., Gonzalez, A.M., Endo-Mochizuki, Y., *et al.* Identification of G protein–coupled signaling pathways in cardiac fibroblasts: Cross-talk between G_q and G_s. *Am. J. Physiol.,* **2000,** *278*:154–162.

Montgomery, H.E., Clarkson, P., Dollery, C.M., *et al.* Association of angiotensin-converting enzyme gene *I/D* polymorphism with change in left ventricular mass in response to physical training. *Circulation,* **1997,** *96*:741–747.

Moore, A.F., Heiderstadt, N.T., Huang, E., *et al.* Selective inhibition of the renal angiotensin type 2 receptor increases blood pressure in conscious rats. *Hypertension,* **2001,** *37*:1285–1291.

Mueller, C., Baudler, S., Welzel, H., Bohm, M., and Nickenig, G. Identification of a novel redox-sensitive gene, *Id3,* which mediates angiotensin II–induced cell growth. *Circulation,* **2002,** *105*:2423–2428.

Mukoyama, M., Nakajima, M., Horiuchi, M., *et al.* Expression cloning of type 2 angiotensin II receptor reveals a unique class of seven-transmembrane receptors. *J. Biol. Chem.,* **1993,** *268*:24539–24542.

Murphey, L.J., Gainer, J.V., Vaughan, D.E., and Brown, N.J. Angiotensin-converting enzyme insertion/deletion polymorphism modulates the human in vivo metabolism of bradykinin. *Circulation,* **2000,** *102*:829–832.

Murphy, T.J., Alexander, R.W., Griendling, K.K., Runge, M.S., and Bernstein, K.E. Isolation of a cDNA encoding the vascular type-1 angiotensin II receptor. *Nature Med.,* **1991,** *351*:233–236.

Nickenig, G., Michaelsen, F., Muller, C., *et al.* Destabolization of AT_1 receptor mRNA by calreticulun. *Circ. Res.,* **2002,** *90*:53–58.

Niimura, F., Labosky, P.A., Kakuchi, J., *et al.* Gene targeting in mice reveals a requirement for angiotensin in the development and maintenance of kidney morphology and growth factor regulation. *J. Clin. Invest.,* **1995,** *96*:2947–2954.

O'Donnell, C.J., Lindpaintner, K., Larson, M.G., *et al.* Evidence for association and genetic linkage of the angiotensin-converting enzyme locus with hypertension and blood pressure in men but not women in the Framingham Heart Study. *Circulation,* **1998,** *97*:1766–1772.

O'Driscoll, G., Green, D., Rankin, J., Stanton, K., and Taylor, R. Improvement in endothelial function by angiotensin converting enzyme inhibition in insulin-dependent diabetes mellitus. *J. Clin. Invest.,* **1997,** *100*:678–684.

Oike, Y., Hata, A., Ogata, Y., *et al.* Angiotensin converting enzyme as a genetic risk factor for coronary artery spasm: Implication in the pathogenesis of myocardial infarction. *J. Clin. Invest.,* **1995,** *96*:2975–2979.

Olivieri, O., Trabetti, E., Grazioli, S., *et al.* Genetic polymorphisms of the renin–angiotensin system and atheromatous renal artery stenosis. *Hypertension,* **1999,** *34*:1097–1100.

Ortiz, M.C., Manriquez, M.C., Romero, J.C., and Juncos, J.A. Antioxidants block angiotensin II–induced increases in blood pressure and endothelin. *Hypertension,* **2001,** *38*:655–659.

Osterop, A.P.R.N., Kofflard, M.J.M., Sandkuijl, L.A., *et al.* AT_1 receptor A/C^{1166} polymorphism contributes to cardiac hypertrophy in subjects with hypertrophic cardiomyopathy. *Hypertension,* **1998,** *32*:825–830.

Ostrom, R.S., Naugle, J.E., Hase, M., *et al.* Angiotensin II enhances adenylyl cyclase signaling via Ca^{++}/calmodulin: G_q–G_s cross-talk regulates collagen production in cardiac fibroblasts. *J. Biol. Chem.,* **2003,** *278*:24461–24468.

Packer, M., Poole-Wilson, P.A., Armstrong, P.W., *et al.,* on behalf of the ATLAS Study Group. Comparative effects of low and high doses of the angiotensin-converting enzyme inhibitor, lisinopril, on morbidity and mortality in chronic heart failure. *Circulation,* **1999,** *100*:2312–2318.

Parving, H.-H., Lehnert, H., Brochner-Mortensen, J., *et al.,* for the Irbesartan in Patients with Type 2 Diabetes and Microalbuminuria Study Group. The effect of irbesartan on the development of diabetic nephropathy in patients with type 2 diabetes. *New Engl. J. Med.,* **2001,** *345*:870–878.

Pastore, L., Tessitore, A., Martinotti, S., *et al.* Angiotensin II stimulates intercellular adhesion molecule-1 (ICAM-1) expression by human vascular endothelial cells and increases soluble ICAM-1 release *in vivo. Circulation,* **1999,** *100*:1646–1652.

Perlman, S., Costa-Neto, C.M., Miyakawa, A.A., *et al.* Dual agonistic and antagonistic property of nonpeptide angiotensin AT_1 ligands: susceptibility to receptor mutations. *Mol. Pharmacol.,* **1997,** *51*:301–311.

Pfeffer, M.A., Braunwald, E., MoyÈ, L.A., *et al.* Effect of captopril on mortality and morbidity in patients with left ventricular dysfunction after myocardial infarction. *New Engl. J. Med.* **1992,** *327*:669–677.

Pfeffer, M.A., Domanski, M., Verter, J., *et al.,* for the PEACE Investigators. The continuation of the Prevention of Events with Angiotensin-Converting Enzyme inhibition (PEACE) trial. *Am. Heart J.,* **2001,** *142*:375–377.

Pfeffer, M.A., McMurray, J.J.V., Valazquez, E.J., *et al.,* for the Valsartan in Acute Myocardial Infarction Trial Investigators. Valsartan, captopril, or both in myocardial infarction complicated by heart failure, left ventricular dysfunction, or both. *New Engl. J. Med.,* **2003a,** *349:*1893–1906.

Pfeffer, M.A., Swedberg, K., Granger, C.B., *et al.,* for the CHARM Investigators and Committees. Effects of candesartan on mortality and morbidity in patients with chronic heart failure: The CHARM-overall programme. *Lancet,* **2003b,** *362:*759–766.

Philipp, C.S., Dilley, A., Saidi, P., *et al.* Deletion polymorphism in the angiotensin-converting enzyme gene as thrombophilic risk factor after hip arthroplasty. *Thromb. Haemost.,* **1998,** *80:*869–873.

Pitt, B., Segal, R., Martinez, F.A., *et al.* Randomised trial of losartan versus captopril in patients over 65 with heart failure (Evaluation of Losartan in the Elderly study, ELITE). *Lancet,* **1997,** *349:*747–752.

Pitt, B., Poole-Wilson, P.A., Segal, R., *et al.,* on behalf of the ELITE II investigators. Effect of losartan compared with captopril on mortality in patients with symptomatic heart failure: Randomized trial-the Losartan Heart Failure Survival Study ELITE II. *Lancet,* **2000,** *355:*1582–1587.

Praga, M., Gutierrez, E., Gonzalez, E., Morales, E., and Hernandez, E. Treatment of IgA nephropathy with ACE inhibitors: A randomized and controlled trial. *J. Am. Soc. Nephrol.,* **2003,** *14:*1578-1583.

Rajagopalan, S., Laursen, J.B., Borthayre, A., *et al.* Role for endothelin-1 in angiotensin II–mediated hypertension. *Hypertension,* **1997,** *30:*29–34.

Ravid, M., Brosh, D., Levi, Z., *et al.* Use of enalapril to attenuate decline in renal function in normotensive, normoalbuminuric patients with type 2 diabetes mellitus: A randomized, controlled trial. *Ann. Intern. Med.,* **1998,** *128:*982–988.

Ravid, M., Lang, R., Rachmani, R., and Lishner, M. Long-term renoprotective effect of angiotensin-converting enzyme inhibition in non-insulin-dependent diabetes mellitus: A 7-year follow-up study. *Arch. Intern. Med.,* **1996,** *156:*286–289.

Ravid, M., Savin, H., Jutrin, I., *et al.* Long-term stabilizing effect of angiotensin-converting enzyme inhibition on plasma creatinine and on proteinuria in normotensive type II diabetic patients. *Ann. Intern. Med.,* **1993,** *118:*577–581.

Rhaleb, N.E., Peng, H., Alfie, M.E., Shesely, E.G., and Carretero, O.A. Effect of ACE inhibitor on DOCA–salt– and aortic coarctation–induced hypertension in mice: Do kinin B2 receptors play a role? *Hypertension,* **1999,** *33:*329–334.

Rhaleb, N.-E., Peng, H., Yang, X.-P., *et al.* Long-term effect of *N*-acetyl-seryl-aspartyl-lysly-proline on left ventricular collagen deposition in rats with two-kidney, one-clip hypertension. *Circulation,* **2001,** *103:*3136–3141.

Ribichini, F., Steffenino, G., Dellavalle, A., *et al.* Plasma activity and insertion/deletion polymorphism of angiotensin I–converting enzyme: A major risk factor and a marker of risk for coronary stent restenosis. *Circulation,* **1998,** *97:*147–154.

Rigat, B., Hubert, C., Alhenc-Gelas, F., *et al.* An insertion/deletion polymorphism in the angiotensin I–converting enzyme gene accounting for half the variance of serum enzyme levels. *J. Clin. Invest.,* **1990,** *86:*1343–1346.

Rocic, P., Govindarajan, G., Sabri, A., and Lucchesi, P.A. A role for PKY2 in regulation of ERK1/2 MAP kinases and PI3–kinase by ANG II in vascular smooth muscle. *Am. J. Physiol. Cell Physiol.,* **2001,** *280:*C90–C99.

Rohrwasser, A., Morgan, T., Dillon, H.F., *et al.* Elements of a paracrine tubular renin–angiotensin system along the entire nephron. *Hypertension,* **1999,** *34:*1265–1274.

Ruggenenti, P., Perna, A., Benini, R., *et al.* In chronic nephropathies prolonged ACE inhibition can induce remission: Dynamics of time-dependent changes in GFR. Investigators of the GISEN Group. Gruppo Italiano Studi Epidemiologici in Nefrologia. *J. Am. Soc. Nephrol.,* **1999a,** *10:*997–1006.

Ruggenenti, P., Perna, A., Gherardi, G., *et al.* Renoprotective properties of ACE-inhibition in non-diabetic nephropathies with non-nephrotic proteinuria. *Lancet,* **1999b,** *354:*359–364.

Ruggenenti, P., Perna, A., Gherardi, G., *et al.* Renal function and requirement for dialysis in chronic nephropathy patients on long-term ramipril: REIN follow-up trial. Gruppo Italiano di Studi Epidemiologici in Nefrologia (GISEN). Ramipril Efficacy in Nephropathy. *Lancet,* **1998,** *352:*1252–1256.

Saino, A., Pomidossi, G., Perondi, R., *et al.* Intracoronary angiotensin II potentiates coronary sympathetic vasoconstriction in humans. *Circulation,* **1997,** *96:*148–153.

Santos, R.A., Simoes e Silva, A.C., Maric, C., *et al.* Angiotensin(1–7) is an endogenous ligand for the G protein–coupled receptor Mas. *Proc. Natl. Acad. Sci. U.S.A.,* **2003,** *100:*8258–8263.

Sasaki, K., Yamano, Y., Bardhan, S., *et al.* Cloning and expression of a complementary DNA encoding a bovine adrenal angiotensin II type-1 receptor. *Nature,* **1991,** *351:*230–233.

Schachter, F., Faure-Delanef, L., Guenot, F., *et al.* Genetic associations with human longevity at the APOE and ACE loci. *Nature Genet.,* **1994,** *6:*29–32.

Schneider, A.W., Kalk, J.F., and Klein, C.P. Effect of losartan, an angiotensin II receptor antagonist, on portal pressure in cirrhosis. *Hepatology,* **1999,** *29:*334–339.

Schunkert, H., Hense, H.-W., Holmer, S.R., *et al.* Association between a deletion polymorphism of the angiotensin-converting-enzyme gene and left ventricular hypertrophy. *New Engl. J. Med.,* **1994,** *330:*1634–1638.

Scott-Burden, T., Hahn, A.W.A., Resink, T.J., and Bühler, F.R. Modulation of extracellular matrix by angiotensin II: Stimulated glycoconjugate synthesis and growth in vascular smooth muscle cells. *J. Cardiovasc. Pharmacol.,* **1990,** *16*(suppl. 4):S36–S41.

Sethi, A.A., Nordestgaard, B.G., Agerholm-Larsen, B., *et al.* Angiotensinogen polymorphisms and elevated blood pressure in the general population. The Copenhagen City Heart Study. *Hypertension,* **2001,** *37:*875–881.

Sethi, A.A., Nordestgaard, B.G., Gronholdt, M.-L.M., *et al.* Angiotensinogen single nucleotide polymorphisms, elevated blood pressure, and risk of cardiovascular disease. *Hypertension,* **2003,** *41:*1202–1211.

Sielecki, A.R., Hayakawa, K., Fujinaga, M., *et al.* Structure of recombinant human renin, a target for cardiovascular-active drugs, at 2.5 Å resolution. *Science,* **1989,** *243:*1346–1351.

Singh, I., Grams, M., Wang, W.H., *et al.* Coordinate regulation of renal expression of nitric oxide synthase, renin, and angiotensinogen mRNA by dietary salt. *Am. J. Physiol.,* **1996,** *270:*F1027–F1037.

Siragy, H.M., de Gasparo, M., and Carey, R.M. Angiotensin type 2 receptor mediates valsartan-induced hypotension in conscious rats. *Hypertension,* **2000,** *35:*1074–1077.

SOLVD Investigators. Effect of enalapril on survival in patients with reduced left ventricular ejection fractions and congestive heart failure. *New Engl. J. Med.,* **1991,** *325:*293–302.

SOLVD Investigators. Effect of enalapril on mortality and the development of heart failure in asymptomatic patients with reduced left ventricular ejection fractions. *New Engl. J. Med.* **1992,** *327:*685–691 (published erratum in New Engl. J. Med., 1992, 329:1768).

Staessen, J.A., Kuznetsova, T., Wang, J.G., *et al.* M235T angiotensinogen gene polymorphism and cardiovascular renal risk. *J. Hypertens.,* **1999,** *17:*9–17.

Steen, V.D., and Medsger, T.A., Jr. Long-term outcomes of scleroderma renal crisis. *Ann. Intern. Med.*, **2000**, *17*:600-603.

Swanson, G.N., Hanesworth, J.M., Sardinia, M.F., *et al.* Discovery of a distinct binding site for angiotensin II(3–8), a putative angiotensin IV receptor. *Regul. Pept.*, **1992**, *40*:409–419.

Swedberg, K., Held, P., Kjekshus, J., *et al.* Effects of the early administration of enalapril on mortality in patients with acute myocardial infarction: Results of the Cooperative New Scandinavian Enalapril Survival Study II (CONSENSUS II). *New Engl. J. Med.*, **1992**, *327*:678–684.

Taddei, S., Virdis, A., Abdel-Haq, B., *et al.* Indirect evidence for vascular uptake of circulating renin in hypertensive patients. *Hypertension*, **1993**, *21*:852–860.

Tallant, E.A., Lu, X., Weiss, R.B., Chappell, M.C., and Ferrario, C.M. Bovine aortic endothelial cells contain an angiotensin-(1–7) receptor. *Hypertension*, **1997**, *29*:388–393.

Tanimoto, K., Sugiyama, F., Goto, Y., *et al.* Angiotensinogen-deficient mice with hypotension. *J. Biol. Chem.*, **1994**, *269*:31334–31337.

Tatti, P., Pahor, M., Byington, R.P., *et al.* Outcome results of the Fosinopril Versus Amlodipine Cardiovascular Events Randomized Trial (FACET) in patients with hypertension and NIDDM. *Diabetes Care*, **1998**, *21*:597–603.

Tenenbaum, A., Grossman, E., Shemesh, J., *et al.* Intermediate but not low doses of aspirin can suppress angiotensin-converting enzyme inhibitor–induced cough. *Am. J. Hypertens.*, **2000**, *13*:776–782.

Testa, M.A., Anderson, R.B., Nackley, J.F., Hollenberg, N.K., and the Quality-of-Life Hypertension Study Group. Quality of life and antihypertensive therapy in men: A comparison of captopril with enalapril. *New Engl. J. Med.*, **1993**, *328*:907–913.

Theilig, F., Campean, V., Paliege, A., *et al.* Epithelial COX-2 expression is not regulated by nitric oxide in rodent renal cortex. *Hypertension*, **2002**, *39*:848–853.

Tipnis, S.R., Hooper, N.M., Hyde, R., *et al.* A human homolog of angiotensin-converting enzyme: Cloning and functional expression as a captopril-insensitive carboxypeptidase. *J. Biol. Chem.*, **2000**, *275*:33238–33243.

Tiret, L., Bonnardeaux, A., Poirier, O., *et al.* Synergistic effects of angiotensin-converting enzyme and angiotensin-II type 1 receptor gene polymorphisms on risk of myocardial infarction. *Lancet*, **1994**, *344*:910–913.

Traynor, T.R., Smart, A., Briggs, J.P., and Schnermann, J. Inhibition of macula densa–stimulated renin secretion by pharmacological blockade of cyclooxygenase-2. *Am. J. Physiol.*, **1999**, *277*:F706–F710.

Vaughan, D.E., Rouleau, J.-L., Ridker, P.M., *et al.* Effects of ramipril on plasma fibrinolytic balance in patients with acute anterior myocardial infarction. HEART Study Investigators. *Circulation*, **1997**, *96*:442–447.

Viberti, G., and Wheeldon, N.M., for the MicroAlbuminuria Reduction with VALsartan (MARVAL) Study Investigators. Microalbuminuria reduction with valsartan in patients with type 2 diabetes mellitus: A blood pressure–independent effect. *Circulation*, **2002**, *106*:672–678.

Villarreal, F.J., Kim, N.N., Ungab, G.D., Printz, M.P., and Dillmann, W.H. Identification of functional angiotensin II receptors on rat cardiac fibroblasts. *Circulation*, **1993**, *88*:2849–286l.

Wallukat, G., Homuth, V., Fischer, T., *et al.* Patients with preeclampsia develop agonistic autoantibodies against the angiotensin AT_1 receptor. *J. Clin. Invest.*, **1999**, *103*:945–952.

Wang, H.D., Xu, S., Johns, D.G., *et al.* Role of NADPH oxidase in the vascular hypertrophic and oxidative stress response to angiotensin II in mice. *Circ. Res.*, **2001**, *88*:947–953.

Wang, J.-L., Cheng, H.-F., and Harris, R.C. Cyclooxygenase-2 inhibition decreases renin content and lowers blood pressure in a model of renovascular hypertension. *Hypertension*, **1999**, *34*:96–101.

Ward, K., Hata, A., Jeunemaitre, X., *et al.* A molecular variant of angiotensinogen associated with preeclampsia. *Nature Genet.*, **1993**, *4*:59–61.

Wei, C.-C., Meng, Q.C., Palmer, R., *et al.* Evidence for angiotensin-converting enzyme– and chymase-mediated angiotensin II formation in the interstitial fluid space of the dog heart in vivo. *Circulation*, **1999**, *99*:2583–2589.

Weiss, D., Kools, J.J., and Taylor, W.R. Angiotensin II–induced hypertension accelerates the development of atherosclerosis in ApoE-deficient mice. *Circulation*, **2001**, *103*:448–454.

Whitebread, S., Mele, M., Kamber, B., and de Gasparo, M. Preliminary biochemical characterization of two angiotensin II receptor subtypes. *Biochem. Biophys. Res. Commun.*, **1989**, *163*:284–291.

Witherow, F.N., Helmy A., Webb, D.J., Fox, K.A.A., and Newby, D.E. Bradykinin contributes to the vasodilator effects of chronic angiotensin-converting enzyme inhibition in patients with heart failure. *Circulation*, **2001**, *104*:2177–2181.

Wolny, A., Clozel, J.-P., Rein, J., *et al.* Functional and biochemical analysis of angiotensin II–forming pathways in the human heart. *Circ. Res.*, **1997**, *80*:219–227.

Wong, P.C., Chiu, A.T., Price, W.A., *et al.* Nonpeptide angiotensin II receptor antagonists: I. Pharmacological characterization of 2-*N*-butyl-4-chloro-1-(2-chlorobenzyl)imidazole-5-acetic acid, sodium salt (S-8307). *J. Pharmacol. Exp. Ther.*, **1988**, *247*:1–7.

Wynckel, A., Ebikili, B., Melin, J.-P., *et al.* Long-term follow-up of acute renal failure caused by angiotensin converting enzyme inhibitors. *Am. J. Hypertens.*, **1998**, *11*:1080–1086.

Yamada, K., Iyer, S.N., Chappell, M.C., Ganten, D., and Ferrario, C.M. Converting enzyme determines plasma clearance of angiotensin-(1–7). *Hypertension*, **1998**, *32*:496–502.

Yang, T., Endo, Y., Huang, Y.G., *et al.* Renin expression in COX-2-knockout mice on normal and low-salt diets. *Am. J. Physiol. Renal Physiol.*, **2000**, *279*:F819–F825.

Yoshida, H., Mitarai, T., Kawamura, T., *et al.* Role of the deletion of polymorphism of the angiotensin converting enzyme gene in the progression and therapeutic responsiveness of IgA nephropathy. *J. Clin. Invest.*, **1995**, *96*:2162–2169.

Zhang, G.-X., Kimura, S., Nishiyama, A., *et al.* ROS during the acute phase of Ang II hypertension participates in cardiovascular MAPK activation but not vasoconstriction. *Hypertension*, **2004**, *43*:117–124.

Zimmerman, B.G. Absence of adrenergic mediation of agonist response to [Sar^1,Ala^8]angiotensin II in conscious normotensive and hypertensive dogs. *Clin. Sci.*, **1979**, *57*:71–81.

Zimmerman, J.B., Robertson, D., and Jackson, E.K. Angiotensin II–noradrenergic interactions in renovascular hypertensive rats. *J. Clin. Invest.*, **1987**, *80*:443–457.

Zuanetti, G., Latini, R., Maggioni, A.P., *et al.* Effect of the ACE inhibitor lisinopril on mortality in diabetic patients with acute myocardial infarction: Data from the GISSI-3 study. *Circulation*, **1997**, *96*:4239–4245.

MONOGRAPHS AND REVIEWS

Ardaillou, R. Angiotensin II receptors. *J. Am. Soc. Nephrol.*, **1999**, *10*(suppl. 11):S30–S39.

Baker, K.M., Booz, G.W., and Dostal, D.E. Cardiac actions of angiotensin II: Role of an intracardiac renin–angiotensin system. *Annu. Rev. Physiol.*, **1992**, *54*:227–241.

Berk, B.C. Angiotensin II signal transduction in vascular smooth muscle: Pathways activated by specific tyrosine kinases. *J. Am. Soc. Nephrol.*, **1999**, *10*(suppl. 11):S62–S68.

Blume, A., Herdegen, T., and Unger, T. Angiotensin peptides and inducible transcription factors. *J. Mol. Med.*, **1999**, *77*:339–357.

Brenner, B.M., and Zagrobelny, J. Clinical renoprotection trials involving angiotensin II–receptor antagonists and angiotensin-converting-enzyme inhibitors. *Kidney Int.,* **2003,** *63*(suppl):S77–S85.

Brent, R.L., and Beckman, D.A. Angiotensin-converting enzyme inhibitors, an embryopathic class of drugs with unique properties: information for clinical teratology counselors. *Teratology,* **1991,** *43*:543–546.

Bumpus, F.M., Catt, K.J., Chiu, A.T., *et al.* Nomenclature for angiotensin receptors: A report of the nomenclature committee of the council for high blood pressure research. *Hypertension,* **1991,** *17*:720–721.

Bunnemann, B., Fuxe, K., and Ganten, D. The renin–angiotensin system in the brain: An update 1993. *Regul. Pept.,* **1993,** *46*:487–509.

Csajka, C., Buclin, T., Brunner, H.R., and Biollaz, J. Pharmacokinetic–pharmacodynamic profile of angiotensin II receptor antagonists. *Clin. Pharmacokinet.,* **1997,** *32*:1–29.

de Gasparo, M., Catt, K.J., Inagami, T., Wright, J.W., and Unger, T.H. International union of pharmacology: XXIII. The angiotensin II receptors. *Pharmacol. Rev.,* **2000,** *52*:415–472.

Dzau, V.J. Vascular renin–angiotensin system and vascular protection. *J. Cardiovasc. Pharmacol.,* **1993,** *22*(suppl.)5:S1–S9.

Dzau, V.J., Sasamura, H., and Hein, L. Heterogeneity of angiotensin synthetic pathways and receptor subtypes: Physiological and pharmacological implications. *J. Hypertens.,* **1993,** *11*:S13–S18.

Epperson, S., Gustafsson, A.B., Gonzalez, A.M., *et al.* Pharmacology of G-protein-linked signaling in cardiac fibroblasts. In, *Interstitial Fibrosis and Heart Failure.* (Villarreal, F.J., ed.) Springer, New York, **2004,** pp. 83–97.

Ferrario, C.M., Chappell, M.C., Tallant, E.A., Brosnihan, K.B., and Diz, D.I. Counterregulatory actions of angiotensin-(1–7). *Hypertension,* **1997,** *30*:535–541.

Griendling, K.K., Ushio-Fukai, M., Lassegue, B., and Alexander, R.W. Angiotensin II signaling in vascular smooth muscle: New concepts. *Hypertension,* **1997,** *29*:366–373.

Guyton, A.C. Blood pressure control: Special role of the kidneys and body fluids. *Science,* **1991,** *252*:1813–1816.

Haendeler, J., and Berk, B.C. Angiotensin II mediated signal transduction: Important role of tyrosine kinases. *Regul. Pept.,* **2000,** *95*:1–7.

Hagley, M.T., Hulisz, D.T., and Burns, C.M. Hepatotoxicity associated with angiotensin-converting enzyme inhibitors. *Ann. Pharmacother.,* **1993,** *27*:228–231.

Henrion, D., Kubis, N., and Levy, B.I. Physiological and pathophysiological functions of the AT_2 subtype receptor of angiotensin II: From large arteries to the microcirculation. *Hypertension,* **2001,** *38*:1150–1157.

Hollenberg, N.K., Fisher, N.D.L., and Price, D.A. Pathways for angiotensin II generation in intact human tissue: Evidence from comparative pharmacological interruption of the renin system. *Hypertension,* **1998,** *32*:387–392.

Horiuchi, M., Akishita, M., and Dzau, V.J. Recent progress in angiotensin II type 2 receptor research in the cardiovascular system. *Hypertension,* **1999,** *33*:613–621.

Inagami, T. Molecular biology and signaling of angiotensin receptors: An overview. *J. Am. Soc. Nephrol.,* **1999,** *10*(suppl. 11):S2–S7.

Inagami, T., Eguchi, S., Numaguchi, K., *et al.* Cross-talk between angiotensin II receptors and the tyrosine kinases and phosphatases. *J. Am. Soc. Nephrol.,* **1999,** *10*(suppl.11:S57–S61.

Israili, Z.H., and Hall, W.D. Cough and angioneurotic edema associated with angiotensin-converting enzyme inhibitor therapy: A review of the literature and pathophysiology. *Ann. Intern. Med.,* **1992,** *117*:234–242.

McConnaughey, M.M., McConnaughey, J.S., and Ingenito, A.J. Practical considerations of the pharmacology of angiotensin receptor blockers. *J. Clin. Pharmacol.,* **1999,** *39*:547–559.

Mimran, A., Ribstein, J., and DuCailar, G. Angiotensin II receptor antagonists and hypertension. *Clin. Exp. Hypertens.,* **1999,** *21*: 847–858.

Phillips, M.I., Speakman, E.A., and Kimura, B. Levels of angiotensin and molecular biology of the tissue renin angiotensin systems. *Regul. Pept.,* **1993,** *43*:1–20.

Ruiz-Ortego, M., Lorenzo, O., Ruperez, M., *et al.* Role of the renin–angiotensin system in vascular diseases: Expanding the field. *Hypertension,* **2001,** *38*:1382–1387.

Saavedra, J.M. Brain and pituitary angiotensin. *Endocr. Rev.,* **1992,** *13*:329–380.

Samanen, J., and Regoli, D. Structure–activity relationships of peptide angiotensin II receptor agonists and antagonists. In, *Angiotensin II Receptors:* Vol. 2. *Medicinal Chemistry.* (Ruffolo, R.R., Jr., ed.), CRC Press, Boca Raton, FL, **1994,** pp. 11–97.

Schnee, J.M., and Hsueh, W.A. Angiotensin II, adhesion, and cardiac fibrosis. *Cardiovasc. Res.,* **2000,** *46*:264–268.

Tallant, E.A., Diz, D.I., and Ferrario, C.M. State-of-the-art lecture: Antiproliferative actions of angiotensin-(1–7) in vascular smooth muscle. *Hypertension,* **1999,** *34*:950–957.

Timmermans, P.B.M.W.M., Wong, P.C., Chiu, A.T., *et al.* Angiotensin II receptors and angiotensin II receptor antagonists. *Pharmacol. Rev.,* **1993,** *45*:205–251.

Vane, J.R. The history of inhibitors of angiotensin converting enzyme. *J. Physiol. Pharmacol.,* **1999,** *50*:489–498.

von Lutterotti, N., Catanzaro, D.F., Sealey, J.E., and Laragh, J.H. Renin is not synthesized by cardiac and extrarenal vascular tissues: A review of experimental evidence. *Circulation,* **1994,** *89*:458–470.

Yagil, Y., and Yagil, C. Hypothesis: ACE2 modulates pressure in the mammalian organism. *Hypertension,* **2003,** *41*:871–873.

Zusman, R.M. Angiotensin-converting enzyme inhibitors: More different than alike? Focus on cardiac performance. *Am. J. Cardiol.,* **1993,** *72*:25H–36H.

TREATMENT OF MYOCARDIAL ISCHEMIA

Thomas Michel

PATHOPHYSIOLOGY OF ISCHEMIC HEART DISEASE

Angina pectoris, the primary symptom of ischemic heart disease, is caused by transient episodes of myocardial ischemia that are due to an imbalance in the myocardial oxygen supply–demand relationship. This imbalance may be caused by an increase in myocardial oxygen demand (which is determined by heart rate, ventricular contractility, and ventricular wall tension) or by a decrease in myocardial oxygen supply (primarily determined by coronary blood flow but occasionally modified by the oxygen-carrying capacity of the blood) or sometimes by both (Figure 31–1). Since blood flow is inversely proportional to the fourth power of the artery's luminal radius, the progressive decrease in vessel radius that characterizes coronary atherosclerosis can impair coronary blood flow and lead to symptoms of angina when myocardial oxygen demand increases, as with exertion (so-called typical angina pectoris). In some patients, anginal symptoms may occur without any increase in myocardial oxygen demand but rather as a consequence of abrupt reduction in blood flow, as might result from coronary thrombosis (unstable angina) or vasospasm (variant or Prinzmetal angina). Regardless of the precipitating factors, the sensation of angina is similar in most patients. Typical angina is experienced as a heavy, pressing substernal discomfort (rarely called "pain"), often radiating to the left shoulder, flexor aspect of the left arm, jaw, or epigastrium. However, a significant minority of patients notes discomfort in a different location or of a different character. Women, the elderly, and diabetics are more likely to have ischemia with atypical symptoms. In most patients with typical angina, whose symptoms are provoked by exertion, the symptoms are relieved by rest or by administration of sublingual *nitroglycerin*.

Angina pectoris is a common symptom, affecting more than 6 million Americans (Gibbons *et al.*, 2002). Angina pectoris may occur in a stable pattern over many years or may become unstable, increasing in frequency or severity and even occurring at rest. In typical stable angina, the pathological substrate is usually fixed atherosclerotic narrowing of an epicardial coronary artery, on which exertion or emotional stress superimposes an increase in myocardial oxygen consumption. In variant angina, focal or diffuse coronary vasospasm episodically reduces coronary flow. Patients also may display a mixed pattern of angina with the addition of altered vessel tone on a background of atherosclerotic narrowing. In most patients with unstable angina, rupture of an atherosclerotic plaque, with consequent platelet adhesion and aggregation, decreases coronary blood flow. Plaques with thinner fibrous caps are more "vulnerable" to rupture.

Myocardial ischemia also may be *silent*, with electrocardiographic, echocardiographic, or radionuclide evidence of ischemia appearing in the absence of symptoms. While some patients have only silent ischemia, most patients who have silent ischemia have symptomatic episodes as well. The precipitants of silent ischemia appear to be the same as those of symptomatic ischemia. We now know that the *ischemic burden, i.e.*, the total time a patient is ischemic each day, is greater in many patients than was recognized previously. In most trials, the agents that are efficacious in conventional angina are also efficacious in reducing silent ischemia. β Adrenergic receptor antagonists appear to be more effective than the Ca^{2+} channel blockers in the prevention of episodes. Therapy directed at abolishing all silent ischemia has not been shown to be of additional benefit over conventional therapy.

This chapter describes the pharmacological agents used in the treatment of angina. The major drugs are nitrovasodilators (*see* Chapter 33), β adrenergic receptor antagonists (*see* Chapter 10), Ca^{2+} channel antagonists (*see* Chapter 32), and in both stable and unstable angina, antiplatelet agents (*see* Chapters 26 and 54) as well as statins (HMG CoA-reductase inhibitors) (*see* Chapter 35), which may have a role in stabilizing the vulnerable plaque. All approved antianginal agents improve the balance of myocardial oxygen supply and demand, increasing supply by dilating the coronary vasculature or decreasing demand by

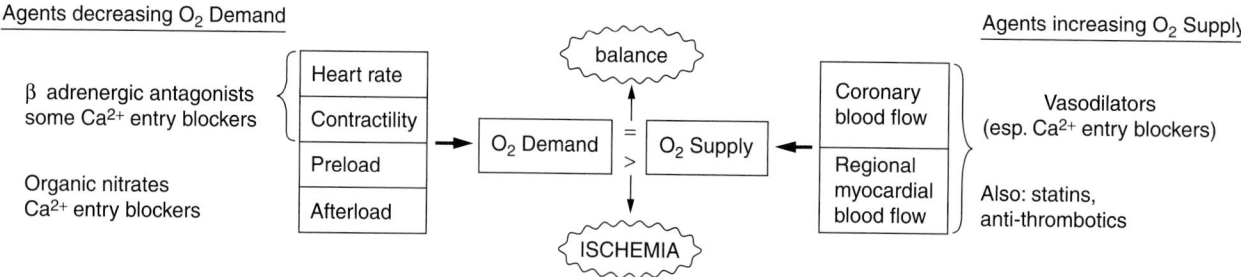

Figure 31–1. *Pharmacological modification of the major determinants of myocardial O₂ supply.* When myocardial O_2 requirements exceed O_2 supply, an ischemic episode results. This figure shows the primary hemodynamic sites of actions of pharmacological agents that can reduce O_2 demand (*left side*) or enhance O_2 supply (*right side*). Some classes of agents have multiple effects (*see* text). Stents, angioplasty, and coronary bypass surgery are mechanical interventions that increase O_2 supply. Both pharmacotherapy and mechanotherapy attempt to restore a dynamic balance between O_2 demand and O_2 supply.

reducing cardiac work (Figure 31–1). Increasing the cardiac extraction of oxygen from the blood is not a practical therapeutic goal. Drugs used in typical angina function principally by reducing myocardial oxygen demand by decreasing heart rate, myocardial contractility, and/or ventricular wall stress. By contrast, the principal therapeutic goal in unstable angina is to increase myocardial blood flow; strategies include the use of antiplatelet agents and *heparin* to reduce intracoronary thrombosis and coronary stents or coronary bypass surgery to restore flow by mechanical means. The therapeutic aim in variant or Prinzmetal angina is to prevent coronary vasoplasm.

Antianginal agents may provide prophylactic or symptomatic treatment, but β adrenergic receptor antagonists also reduce mortality apparently by decreasing the incidence of sudden cardiac death associated with myocardial ischemia and infarction. The treatment of cardiac risk factors can reduce the progression or even lead to the regression of atherosclerosis. *Aspirin* is used routinely in patients with myocardial ischemia, and daily aspirin use reduces the incidence of clinical events (Gibbons *et al.*, 2002; Libby *et al.*, 2002). Other antiplatelet agents such as oral *clopidogrel* and intravenous anti-integrin drugs such as *abciximab, tirofiban,* and *eptifibatide* have been shown to reduce morbidity in patients with angina who undergo coronary artery stenting (Yeghizarians *et al.*, 2000). Lipid-lowering drugs such as the statins reduce mortality in patients with hypercholesterolemia with or without known coronary artery disease (Libby *et al.*, 2002). Angiotensin-converting enzyme (ACE) inhibitors (*see* Chapter 29) also reduce mortality in patients with coronary disease (Yusuf *et al.*, 2000). Coronary artery bypass surgery and percutaneous coronary interventions such as angioplasty and coronary artery stent deployment can complement pharmacological treatment. In some subsets of patients, percutaneous or surgical revascularization may have a survival advantage over medical treatment alone. Intracoronary drug delivery using drug-eluting coronary stents represents an intersection of mechanical and pharmacological approaches in the treatment of coronary artery disease. Novel therapies that modify the expression of vascular or myocardial cell genes eventually may become an important part of the therapy of ischemic heart disease.

ORGANIC NITRATES

These agents are prodrugs that are sources of nitric oxide (NO). NO activates the soluble isoform of guanylyl cyclase, thereby increasing intracellular levels of cyclic GMP. In turn, this promotes the dephosphorylation of the myosin light chain and the reduction of cystolic (Ca^{2+}) and leads to the relaxation of smooth muscle cells in a broad range of tissues. The NO-dependent relaxation of vascular smooth muscle leads to vasodilation; NO-mediated guanylyl cyclase activation inhibits platelet aggregation and relaxes smooth muscle in the bronchi and gastrointestinal (GI) tract (Murad, 1996; Molina *et al.*, 1987; Thadani, 1992).

The broad biological response to nitrovasodilators suggests the existence of endogenous NO-modulated regulatory pathways; more than a century after the therapeutic use of nitrovasodilators, the enzymes responsible for endogenous NO synthesis were isolated and characterized. The endogenous synthesis of NO in humans is catalyzed by a family of NO synthases that oxidize the amino acid L-arginine to form NO (plus L-citrulline as a coproduct). There are three distinct mammalian NO synthase isoforms termed *nNOS, eNOS,* and *iNOS* (*see* Chapter 1), and they are involved in processes as diverse as neurotransmission, vasomotion, and immunomodulation (Lowenstein *et al.*, 1994). In several vascular disease states, pathways of endogenous NO-dependent regulation appear to be deranged (reviewed in Dudzinski *et al.*, 2005).

History. Nitroglycerin was first synthesized in 1846 by Sobrero, who observed that a small quantity placed on the tongue elicited a severe headache. In 1857, T. Lauder Brunton of Edinburgh administered *amyl nitrite,* a known vasodepressor, by inhalation and noted that anginal pain was relieved within 30 to 60 seconds. The action of amyl nitrite was transitory, however, and the dosage was difficult to adjust. Subsequently, William Murrell surmised that the action of nitroglycerin mimicked that of amyl nitrite and established the use of sublingual nitroglycerin for relief of the acute anginal attack and as a prophylactic agent to be taken prior to exertion. The empirical observation that organic nitrates could dramatically and safely alleviate the symptoms of angina pectoris led to their widespread acceptance by the medical profession. Basic investigations defined the role of NO in both the vasodilation produced by nitrates and endogenous vasodilation. The importance of NO as a signaling molecule in the cardiovascular system and elsewhere was recognized by the awarding of the 1998 Nobel Prize in medicine/physiology to Robert Furchgott, Louis Ignarro, and Ferid Murad.

Chemistry. Organic nitrates are polyol esters of nitric acid, whereas organic nitrites are esters of nitrous acid (Table 31–1). Nitrate esters ($—C—O—NO_2$) and nitrite esters ($—C—O—NO$) are characterized by a sequence of carbon–oxygen–nitrogen, whereas nitro compounds possess carbon–nitrogen bonds ($C—NO_2$). Thus *glyceryl trinitrate* is not a nitro compound, and it is erroneously called *nitroglycerin;* however, this nomenclature is both widespread and official. Amyl nitrite is a highly volatile liquid that must be administered by inhalation and is of limited therapeutic utility. Organic nitrates of low molecular mass (such as nitroglycerin) are moderately volatile, oily liquids, whereas the high-molecular-mass nitrate esters (*e.g., erythrityl tetranitrate, isosorbide dinitrate,* and *isosorbide mononitrate*) are solids. In the pure form (without an inert carrier such as lactose), nitroglycerin is explosive. The organic nitrates and nitrites, collectively termed *nitrovasodilators,* must be metabolized (reduced) to produce NO, the active principle of this class of compounds.

Pharmacological Properties

Mechanism of Action. Nitrites, organic nitrates, nitroso compounds, and a variety of other nitrogen oxide–containing substances (including *nitroprusside; see* Chapter 32) lead to the formation of the reactive free radical NO. The exact mechanism(s) of denitration of the organic nitrates to liberate NO remains an active area of investigation (Chen *et al.*, 2002). NO can activate guanylyl cyclase, increase the cellular level of cyclic GMP, activate PKG (the cyclic GMP–dependent protein kinase), and modulate the activities of cyclic nucleotide phosphodiesterases (PDEs 2, 3, and 5) in a variety of cell types. In smooth muscle, the net result is reduced phosphorylation of myosin light chain, reduced Ca^{2+} concentration in the cytosol, and relaxation. One important consequence of the NO-mediated increase in intracellular cyclic GMP is the activation of PKG, which catalyzes the phosphorylation

of various proteins in smooth muscle. Another important target of this kinase is the myosin light-chain phosphatase, which is activated on binding PKG (Surks et at., 1999) and leads to dephosphorylation of the myosin light chain and thereby promotes vasorelaxation (Waldman and Murad, 1987), Phosphorylation of the myosin light chain regulates the maintenance of the contractile state in smooth muscle. The pharmacological and biochemical effects of the nitrovasodilators appear to be identical to those of an endothelium-derived relaxing factor now known to be NO (Ignarro *et al.*, 1987; Murad, 1996; Furchgott, 1996). Although the soluble isoform of guanylyl cyclase remains the most extensively characterized molecular "receptor" for NO, it is increasingly clear that NO also forms specific adducts with thiol groups in proteins and with reduced glutathione to form nitrosothiol compounds with distinctive biological properties (Stamler *et al.*, 2001). The enzyme mitochondrial aldehyde dehydrogenase has been shown to catalyze the reduction of nitroglycerin to yield bioactive NO metabolites (Chen *et al.*, 2002), providing a potentially important clue to the biotransformation of organic nitrates in intact tissues. The regulation and pharmacology of eNOS have been reviewed recently (Dudzinski *et al.*, 2005).

Cardiovascular Effects. Hemodynamic Effects. The nitrovasodilators promote vascular smooth muscle relaxation. Low concentrations of nitroglycerin preferentially dilate the veins more than the arterioles. This venodilation decreases left and right ventricular chamber size and end-diastolic pressures but results in little change in systemic vascular resistance. Systemic arterial pressure may fall slightly, and heart rate is unchanged or may increase slightly in response to a decrease in blood pressure. Pulmonary vascular resistance and cardiac output are slightly reduced. Doses of nitroglycerin that do not alter systemic arterial pressure often produce arteriolar dilation in the face and neck, resulting in a flush, or dilation of meningeal arterial vessels, causing headache. The molecular basis for the differential response of arterial *versus* venous tissues to nitroglycerin remains incompletely understood; venous smooth muscle may be enriched in the enzyme that converts nitroglycerin to NO compared with arterial smooth muscle (Bauer and Fung, 1996).

Higher doses of organic nitrates cause further venous pooling and may decrease arteriolar resistance as well, thereby decreasing systolic and diastolic blood pressure and cardiac output and causing pallor, weakness, dizziness, and activation of compensatory sympathetic reflexes. The reflex tachycardia and peripheral arteriolar vasoconstriction tend to restore systemic vascular resistance;

Table 31–1
Organic Nitrates Available for Clinical Use

NONPROPRIETARY NAMES AND TRADE NAMES	CHEMICAL STRUCTURE	PREPARATIONS, USUAL DOSES, AND ROUTES OF ADMINISTRATION*
Nitroglycerin (glyceryl trinitrate; NITRO-BID, NITROSTAT, NITROL, NITRO-DUR, others)	H_2C—O—NO_2 HC—O—NO_2 H_2C—O—NO_2	T: 0.3 to 0.6 mg as needed S: 0.4 mg per spray as needed C: 2.5 to 9 mg two to four times daily B: 1 mg every 3 to 5 h O: 2.5 to 5 cm, topically to skin every 4 to 8 h D: 1 disc (2.5 to 15 mg) for 12 to 16 h per day IV: 10–20 μg/min; increments of 10 μg/min to a maximum of 400 μg/min
Isosorbide dinitrate (ISORDIL, SORBITRATE, DILATRATE-SR, others)		T: 2.5 to 10 mg every 2 to 3 h T(C): 5 to 10 mg every 2 to 3 h T(O): 5 to 40 mg every 8 h C: 40 to 80 mg every 12 h
Isosorbide-5-mononitrate (IMDUR, ISMO, others)		T: 10 to 40 mg twice daily C: 60 to 120 mg daily

*B, buccal (transmucosal) tablet; C, sustained-release capsule or tablet; D, transdermal disc or patch; Inh, inhalant; IV, intravenous injection; O, ointment; S, lingual spray; T, tablet for sublingual use; T(C), chewable tablet; T(O), oral tablet or capsule.

this is superimposed on sustained venous pooling. Coronary blood flow may increase transiently as a result of coronary vasodilation but may decrease subsequently if cardiac output and blood pressure decrease sufficiently.

In patients with autonomic dysfunction and an inability to increase sympathetic outflow (multiple-system atrophy and pure autonomic failure are the most common forms, much less commonly seen in the autonomic dysfunction associated with diabetes), the fall in blood pressure consequent to the venodilation produced by nitrates cannot be compensated. In these clinical contexts, nitrates may reduce arterial pressure and coronary perfusion pressure significantly, producing potentially life-threatening hypotension and even aggravating angina. The appropriate therapy in patients with orthostatic angina and normal coronary arteries is to correct the orthostatic hypotension by expanding volume (*fludrocortisone* and a high-sodium diet), to prevent venous pooling with fitted support garments, and to carefully titrate use of oral vasopressors. Since patients with autonomic dysfunction occasionally may have coexisting coronary artery disease, the coronary anatomy should be defined before therapy is undertaken.

Effects on Total and Regional Coronary Blood Flow. Ischemia is a powerful stimulus to coronary vasodilation, and regional blood flow is adjusted by autoregulatory mechanisms. In the presence of atherosclerotic coronary artery narrowing, ischemia distal to the lesion stimulates vasodilation; if the stenosis is severe, much of the capacity to dilate is used to maintain resting blood flow. When demand increases, further dilation may not be possible. After demonstration of direct coronary artery vasodilation in experimental animals, it became generally accepted that nitrates relieved anginal pain by dilating coronary arteries and thereby increasing coronary blood flow. In the presence of significant coronary stenoses, there is a disproportionate reduction in blood flow to the subendocardial regions of the heart, which are subjected to the greatest extravascular compression during systole; organic nitrates tend to restore blood flow in these regions toward normal.

The hemodynamic mechanisms responsible for these effects are not entirely clear. Most hypotheses have focused on the ability of organic nitrates to cause dilation and prevent vasoconstriction of large epicardial vessels without impairing autoregulation in the small vessels, which are responsible for about 90% of the overall coronary vascular resistance. The vessel diameter is an important determinant of the response to nitroglycerin; vessels larger than 200 μm in diameter are highly responsive, whereas those less than 100 μm respond minimally (Sellke *et al.*, 1990). Experimental evidence in patients undergoing coronary bypass surgery indicates that nitrates do have a relaxant effect on large coronary vessels. Collateral flow to ischemic regions also is increased. Moreover, analyses of coronary angiograms in humans have shown that sublingual nitroglycerin can dilate epicardial stenoses and reduce the resistance to flow through such areas (Brown *et al.*, 1981; Feldman *et al.*, 1981). The resulting increase in blood flow would be distributed preferentially to ischemic myocardial regions as a consequence of vasodilation induced by autoregulation. An important indirect mechanism for a preferential increase in subendocardial blood flow is the nitroglycerin-induced reduction in intracavitary systolic and diastolic pressures that oppose blood flow to the subendocardium (*see* below). To the extent that organic nitrates decrease myocardial requirements for oxygen (*see* below), the increased blood flow in ischemic regions could be balanced by decreased flow in non-ischemic areas, and an overall increase in coronary artery blood flow need not occur. Dilation of cardiac veins may improve the perfusion of the coronary microcirculation. Such redistribution of blood flow to subendocardial tissue is *not* typical of all vasodilators. *Dipyridamole,* for example, dilates resistance vessels nonselectively by distorting autoregulation and is ineffective in patients with typical angina.

In patients with angina owing to coronary artery spasm, the ability of organic nitrates to dilate epicardial coronary arteries, and particularly regions affected by spasm, may be the primary mechanism by which they are of benefit.

Effects on Myocardial Oxygen Requirements. By their effects on the systemic circulation, the organic nitrates also can reduce myocardial oxygen demand. The major determinants of myocardial oxygen consumption include left ventricular wall tension, heart rate, and myocardial contractility. Ventricular wall tension is affected by a number of factors that may be considered under the categories of preload and afterload. *Preload* is determined by the diastolic pressure that distends the ventricle (ventricular end-diastolic pressure). Increasing end-diastolic volume augments the ventricular wall tension (by the law of Laplace, tension is proportional to pressure times radius). Increasing venous capacitance with nitrates decreases

venous return to the heart, decreases ventricular end-diastolic volume, and thereby decreases oxygen consumption. An additional benefit of reducing preload is that it increases the pressure gradient for perfusion across the ventricular wall, which favors subendocardial perfusion. *Afterload* is the impedance against which the ventricle must eject. In the absence of aortic valvular disease, afterload is related to peripheral resistance. Decreasing peripheral arteriolar resistance reduces afterload and thus myocardial work and oxygen consumption.

Organic nitrates decrease both preload and afterload as a result of respective dilation of venous capacitance and arteriolar resistance vessels. They do not directly alter the inotropic or chronotropic state of the heart. Since nitrates reduce the primary determinants of oxygen demand, their net effect usually is to decrease myocardial oxygen consumption. In addition, an improvement in the lusitropic state of the heart may be seen with more rapid early diastolic filling (Breisblatt *et al.*, 1988). This may be secondary to the relief of ischemia rather than primary, or it may be due to a reflex increase in sympathetic activity. Nitrovasodilators also increase cyclic GMP in platelets, with consequent inhibition of platelet function (De Caterina *et al.*, 1988; Lacoste *et al.*, 1994) and decreased deposition of platelets in animal models of arterial wall injury (Lam *et al.*, 1988). While this may contribute to their antianginal efficacy, the effect appears to be modest and in some settings may be confounded by the potential of nitrates to alter the pharmacokinetics of heparin, reducing its antithrombotic effect.

When nitroglycerin is injected or infused directly into the coronary circulation of patients with coronary artery disease, anginal attacks (induced by electrical pacing) are not aborted even when coronary blood flow is increased. However, sublingual administration of nitroglycerin does relieve anginal pain in the same patients. Furthermore, venous phlebotomy that is sufficient to reduce left ventricular end-diastolic pressure can mimic the beneficial effect of nitroglycerin.

Patients are able to exercise for considerably longer periods after the administration of nitroglycerin. Nevertheless, with or without nitroglycerin, angina occurs at the same value of the *triple product* (aortic pressure × heart rate × ejection time, which is proportional to myocardial consumption of oxygen). The observation that angina occurs at the same level of myocardial oxygen consumption suggests that the beneficial effects of nitroglycerin result from reduced cardiac oxygen demand rather than an increase in the delivery of oxygen to ischemic regions of myocardium. However, these results do not preclude the possibility that a favorable redistribution of blood flow to ischemic subendocardial myocardium may contribute to relief of pain in a typical anginal attack, nor do they preclude the possibility that direct coronary vasodilation may be the major effect of nitroglycerin in situations where vasospasm compromises myocardial blood flow.

Mechanism of Relief of Symptoms of Angina Pectoris. The nitrate-induced relief of anginal pain has been ascribed to a decrease in cardiac work secondary to the fall in systemic arterial pressure. As described earlier, the ability of nitrates to dilate epicardial coronary arteries, even in areas of atherosclerotic stenosis, is modest, and the bulk of evidence continues to favor a reduction in myocardial work, and thus in myocardial oxygen demand, as their primary effect in chronic stable angina.

Paradoxically, high doses of organic nitrates may reduce blood pressure to such an extent that coronary flow is compromised; reflex tachycardia and adrenergic enhancement of contractility also occur. These effects may override the beneficial action of the drugs on myocardial oxygen demand and can aggravate ischemia. Additionally, sublingual nitroglycerin administration may produce bradycardia and hypotension probably owing to activation of the Bezold-Jarisch reflex.

Other Effects. The nitrovasodilators act on almost all smooth muscle. Bronchial smooth muscle is relaxed irrespective of the cause of the preexisting tone. The muscles of the biliary tract, including those of the gallbladder, biliary ducts, and sphincter of Oddi, are effectively relaxed. Smooth muscle of the GI tract, including that of the esophagus, can be relaxed and its spontaneous motility decreased by nitrates both *in vivo* and *in vitro*. The effect may be transient and incomplete *in vivo*, but abnormal "spasm" frequently is reduced. Indeed, many incidences of atypical chest pain and "angina" are due to biliary or esophageal spasm, and these too can be relieved by nitrates. Similarly, nitrates can relax ureteral and uterine smooth muscle, but these responses are of uncertain clinical significance.

Absorption, Fate, and Excretion. More than a century after the first use of organic nitrates to treat angina pectoris, their biotransformation remains the subject of active investigation. Studies in the 1970s suggested that nitroglycerin is reductively hydrolyzed by hepatic glutathione–organic nitrate reductase. More recent studies have implicated a mitochondrial aldehyde dehydrogenase enzyme in the biotransformation of nitroglycerin (Chen *et al.*, 2002). Other enzymatic and nonenzymatic pathways also may contribute to the biotransformation of nitrovasodilators. Despite uncertainties about the quantitative importance of the various pathways involved in nitrovasodilator metabolism, the pharmacokinetic properties of nitroglycerin and isosorbide dinitrate have been studied in some detail (Parker and Parker, 1998).

Nitroglycerin. In humans, peak concentrations of nitroglycerin are found in plasma within 4 minutes of sublingual administration; the drug has a half-life of 1 to 3 minutes. The onset of action of nitroglycerin may be even more rapid if it is delivered as a sublingual spray rather than as a sublingual tablet. Dinitrate metabolites, which have about one-tenth the vasodilator potency, appear to have half-lives of approximately 40 minutes.

   Isosorbide Dinitrate. The major route of metabolism of isosorbide dinitrate in humans appears to be by enzymatic denitration followed by glucuronide conjugation. Sublingual administration produces maximal plasma concentrations of the drug by 6 minutes, and the fall in concentration is rapid (half-life of approximately 45 minutes). The primary initial metabolites, isosorbide-2-mononitrate and isosorbide-5-mononitrate, have longer half-lives (3 to 6 hours) and are presumed to contribute to the therapeutic efficacy of the drug.

Isosorbide-5-Mononitrate. This agent is available in tablet form. It does not undergo significant first-pass metabolism and so has excellent bioavailability after oral administration. The mononitrate has a significantly longer half-life than does isosorbide dinitrate and has been formulated as a plain tablet and as a sustained-release preparation; both have longer durations of action than the corresponding dosage forms of isosorbide dinitrate.

Correlation of Plasma Concentrations of Drug and Biological Activity. Intravenous administration of nitroglycerin or long-acting organic nitrates in anesthetized animals produces the same transient (1 to 4 minutes) decrease in blood pressure. Since denitration markedly reduces the activity of the organic nitrates, their rapid clearance from blood indicates that the transient duration of action under these conditions correlates with the concentrations of the parent compounds. The rate of hepatic denitration is characteristic of each nitrate and is influenced by hepatic blood flow or the presence of hepatic disease. In experimental animals, injection of moderate amounts of organic nitrates into the portal vein results in little or no vasodepressor activity, indicating that a substantial fraction of drug can be inactivated by first-pass metabolism in the liver (isosorbide mononitrate is an exception).

Tolerance

Sublingual organic nitrates should be taken at the time of an anginal attack or in anticipation of exercise or stress. Such intermittent treatment provides reproducible cardiovascular effects. However, frequently repeated or continuous exposure to high doses of organic nitrates leads to a marked attenuation in the magnitude of most of their pharmacological effects (Thadani, 1994). The magnitude of tolerance is a function of dosage and frequency of use.

Tolerance may result from a reduced capacity of the vascular smooth muscle to convert nitroglycerin to NO, *true vascular tolerance,* or to the activation of mechanisms extraneous to the vessel wall, *pseudotolerance* (Münzel *et al.*, 1996). Multiple mechanisms have been proposed to account for nitrate tolerance, including volume expansion, neurohumoral activation, cellular depletion of sulfhydryl groups, and the generation of free radicals (Thadani, 1994; Rutherford, 1995; Parker and Parker, 1998). Inactivation of mitochondrial aldehyde dehydrogenase, an enzyme implicated in biotransformation of nitroglycerin, is seen in models of nitrate tolerance (Sydow *et al.*, 2004), potentially associated with oxidative stress (Parker, 2004). A reactive intermediate formed during the generation of NO from organic nitrates may itself damage and inactivate the enzymes of the activation pathway; tolerance could involve endothelium-derived superoxide (Münzel *et al.*, 1995). Clinical data relating to the ability of agents that modify the renin–angiotensin–aldosterone system to prevent nitrate tolerance are contradictory (Parker and Parker, 1998). Important to the interpretation of clinical trials, factors that may influence the ability of such modification to prevent nitrate tolerance include the dose, whether the ACE inhibitors or angiotensin-receptor antagonists were administered prior to the initiation of nitrates, and the tissue specificity of the agent. Despite experimental evidence that depletion of sulfhydryl groups may lead to impaired biotransformation of nitrates to NO and thereby result in nitrate tolerance, experimental results to date with sulfhydryl donors have been disappointing. Other changes that are observed in the setting of nitroglycerin tolerance include an enhanced response to vasoconstrictors such as angiotensin II, serotonin, and phenylephrine. Administration of nitroglycerin is associated with plasma volume expansion, which may be reflected by a decrease in hematocrit. Although diuretic therapy with *hydrochlorothiazide* can improve a patient's exercise duration, appropriately designed crossover trials have failed to demonstrate an effect of diuretics on nitrate tolerance (Parker *et al.*, 1996).

A more effective approach to restoring responsiveness is to interrupt therapy for 8 to 12 hours each day, which allows the return of efficacy. It is usually most convenient to omit dosing at night in patients with exertional angina either by adjusting dosing intervals of oral or buccal preparations or by removing cutaneous nitroglycerin. However, patients whose anginal pattern suggests its precipitation by increased left ventricular filling pressures (*i.e.,* occurring in association with orthopnea or paroxysmal nocturnal dyspnea) may benefit from continuing nitrates at night and omitting them during a quiet period of the day. Tolerance also has been seen with *isosorbide-5-mononitrate;* an eccentric twice-daily dosing schedule appears to maintain efficacy (Parker and Parker, 1998; Thadani *et al.*, 1992).

While these approaches appear to be effective, some patients develop an increased frequency of nocturnal angina when a nitrate-free interval is employed using nitroglycerin patches; such patients may require another class of antianginal agent during this period. Tolerance is not universal, and some patients develop only partial tolerance. The problem of anginal rebound during nitrate-free intervals is especially problematic in the treatment of unstable angina with intravenous nitroglycerin. As tolerance develops, increasing doses are required to achieve the same therapeutic effects; eventually, despite dose escalation, the drug loses efficacy.

A special form of nitroglycerin tolerance is observed in individuals exposed to nitroglycerin in the manufacture of explosives. If protection is inadequate, workers may experience severe headaches, dizziness, and postural weakness during the first several days of employment. Tolerance then develops, but headache and other symptoms may reappear after a few days away from the job—the

"Monday disease." The most serious effect of chronic exposure is a form of organic nitrate dependence. Workers without demonstrable organic vascular disease have been reported to have an increase in the incidence of acute coronary syndromes during the 24- to 72-hour periods away from the work environment (Parker *et al.*, 1995). Coronary and digital arteriospasm during withdrawal and its relaxation by nitroglycerin also have been demonstrated radiographically. Because of the potential problem of nitrate dependence, it seems prudent not to withdraw nitrates abruptly from a patient who has received such therapy chronically.

Toxicity and Untoward Responses

Untoward responses to the therapeutic use of organic nitrates are almost all secondary to actions on the cardiovascular system. Headache is common and can be severe. It usually decreases over a few days if treatment is continued and often can be controlled by decreasing the dose. Transient episodes of dizziness, weakness, and other manifestations associated with postural hypotension may develop, particularly if the patient is standing immobile, and may progress occasionally to loss of consciousness, a reaction that appears to be accentuated by *alcohol*. It also may be seen with very low doses of nitrates in patients with autonomic dysfunction. Even in severe nitrate syncope, positioning and other measures that facilitate venous return are the only therapeutic measures required. All the organic nitrates occasionally can produce drug rash.

Interaction of Nitrates with Phosphodiesterase 5 Inhibitors. Erectile dysfunction is a frequently encountered problem whose risk factors parallel those of coronary artery disease. Thus many men desiring therapy for erectile dysfunction already may be receiving (or may require, especially if they increase physical activity) antianginal therapy. The combination of *sildenafil* and other *phosphodiesterase 5* (PDE5) *inhibitors* with organic nitrate vasodilators can cause extreme hypotension.

Cells in the corpus cavernosum produce NO during sexual arousal in response to nonadrenergic, noncholinergic neurotransmission (Burnett *et al.*, 1992). NO stimulates the formation of cyclic GMP, which leads to relaxation of smooth muscle of the corpus cavernosum and penile arteries, engorgement of the corpus cavernosum, and erection. The accumulation of cyclic GMP can be enhanced by inhibition of the cyclic GMP–specific PDE5 family (Beavo *et al.*, 1994). Sildenafil (VIAGRA) and congeners inhibit PDE5 and have been demonstrated to improve erectile function in patients with erectile dysfunction (Goldstein *et al.*, 1998). Not surprisingly, PDE5 inhibitors have assumed the status of widely used recreational drugs. Since the introduction of sildenafil, two additional PDE5 inhibitors have been developed for use in therapy of erectile dysfunction. *Tadalafil* (CIALIS) and *vardenafil* (LEVITRA) share similar therapeutic efficacy and side-effect profiles with sildenafil; tadalafil has a longer time to onset of action and a longer therapeutic half-life than the other PDE5 inhibitors. Sildenafil has been the most thoroughly characterized of these compounds, but all three PDE5 inhibitors are contraindicated for patients taking organic nitrate vasodilators or α adrenergic receptor antagonists (*see* Chapter 10).

The side effects of sildenafil and other PDE5 inhibitors are largely predictable on the basis of their effects on PDE5. Headache, flushing, and rhinitis may be observed, as may dyspepsia owing to relaxation of the lower esophageal sphincter. Sildenafil and vardenafil also weakly inhibit PDE6, the enzyme involved in photoreceptor signal transduction (Beavo *et al.*, 1994), and can produce visual disturbances, most notably changes in the perception of color hue or brightness (Wallis *et al.*, 1999). Tadalafil inhibits PDE11, a widely distributed phosphodiesterase isoform, but the clinical importance of this effect is not clear. The most important toxicity of all these PDE5 inhibitors is hemodynamic. When given alone to men with severe coronary artery disease, these drugs have modest effects on blood pressure, producing less than a 10% fall in systolic, diastolic, and mean systemic pressures and in pulmonary artery systolic and mean pressures (Herrmann *et al.*, 2000). However, sildenafil, tadalafil, and vardenafil all have a significant and potentially dangerous interaction with organic nitrates, the therapeutic actions of which are mediated *via* their conversion to NO with resulting increases in cyclic GMP. In the presence of a PDE5 inhibitor, nitrates cause profound increases in cyclic GMP and can produce dramatic reductions in blood pressure. Compared with controls, healthy male subjects pretreated with sildenafil or the other PDE5 inhibitors exhibit a much greater decrease in systolic blood pressure when treated with sublingual *glyceryl trinitrate,* and in many subjects a fall of more than 25 mmHg was detected (Webb *et al.*, 1999). This drug class toxicity is the basis for the warning that PDE5 inhibitors should not be prescribed to patients receiving any form of nitrate (Cheitlin *et al.*, 1999) and dictates that patients should be questioned about the use of PDE5 inhibitors within 24 hours before nitrates are administered. A period of longer than 24 hours may be needed following administration of a PDE5 inhibitor for safe use of nitrates, especially with tadalafil because of its prolonged half-life. In the event that patients develop significant hypotension following combined administration of sildenafil and a nitrate, fluids and α adrenergic receptor agonists, if needed, should be used for support (Cheitlin *et al.*, 1999).

Sildenafil, tadalafil, and vardenafil are metabolized *via* cytochrome P450 (CYP3A4), and their toxicity may be enhanced in patients who receive other substrates of this enzyme, including macrolide and imidazole antibiotics, some statins, and antiretroviral agents (*see* individual chapters and Chapter 3). PDE5 inhibitors also may prolong cardiac repolarization by blocking the I_{Kr} (Geelen *et al.*, 2000). Although these interactions and effects are important clinically, the overall incidence and profile of adverse events observed with PDE5 inhibitors, when used without nitrates, are consistent with the expected background frequency of the same events in the treated population (Zusman *et al.*, 1999). In patients with coronary artery disease whose exercise capacity indicates that sexual activity is unlikely to precipitate angina and who are not currently taking nitrates, the use of PDE5 inhibitors can be considered. Such therapy needs to be individualized, and appropriate warnings must be given about the risk of toxicity if nitrates are taken subsequently for angina; this drug interaction may persist for approximately 24 hours for sildenafil and vardenafil and for considerably longer with tadalafil. Alternative nonnitrate antianginal therapy, such as β adrenergic receptor antagonists, should be used during these time periods (Cheitlin *et al.*, 1999).

Therapeutic Uses

Angina. Diseases that predispose to angina should be treated as part of a comprehensive therapeutic program with the primary goal being to prolong life. Conditions such as hypertension, anemia, thyrotoxicosis, obesity, heart failure, cardiac arrhythmias, and acute anxiety can precipitate anginal symptoms in many patients. The patient should be asked to stop smoking and overeating; hypertension and hyperlipidemia should be corrected (*see* Chapters 32 and 35); and daily aspirin (or clopidogrel or *ticlopidine* if aspirin is not tolerated) (*see* Chapter 54) should be prescribed. Exposure to sympathomimetic agents (*e.g.,* those in nasal decongestants) should be avoided. The use of drugs that modify the perception of pain is a poor approach to the treatment of angina because the underlying myocardial ischemia is not relieved.

Table 31–1 lists the preparations and dosages of the nitrites and organic nitrates. The rapidity of onset, the duration of action, and the likelihood of developing tolerance are related to the method of administration.

Sublingual Administration. Because of its rapid action, long-established efficacy, and low cost, nitroglycerin is the most useful drug of the organic nitrates given sublingually. The onset of action is within 1 to 2 minutes, but the effects are undetectable by 1 hour after administration. An initial dose of 0.3 mg nitroglycerin often relieves pain within 3 minutes. Absorption may be limited in patients with dentures or with dry mouths. Nitroglycerin tablets are stable but should be dispensed in glass containers and protected from moisture, light, and extremes of temperature. Active tablets usually produce a burning sensation under the tongue, but the absence of this sensation does not reliably predict loss of activity; elderly patients especially may be unable to detect the burning sensation. Anginal pain may be prevented when the drug is used prophylactically immediately prior to exercise or stress. The smallest effective dose should be prescribed. Patients should be instructed to seek medical attention immediately if three tablets taken over a 15-minute period do not relieve a sustained attack because this situation may be indicative of myocardial infarction or another cause of the pain. Patients also should be advised that there is no virtue in trying to avoid taking sublingual nitroglycerin for anginal pain. Other nitrates that can be taken sublingually do not appear to be longer acting than nitroglycerin because their half-lives depend only on the rate at which they are delivered to the liver. They are no more effective than nitroglycerin and often are more expensive.

Oral Administration. Oral nitrates often are used to provide prophylaxis against anginal episodes in patients who have more than occasional angina. They must be given in sufficient dosage to provide effective plasma levels after first-pass hepatic degradation. Low doses (*e.g.,* 5 to 10 mg isosorbide dinitrate) are no more effective than placebo in decreasing the frequency of anginal attacks or increasing exercise tolerance. In clinical studies, higher doses of either isosorbide dinitrate (*e.g.,* 20 mg or more orally every 4 hours) or sustained-release preparations of nitroglycerin decreased the frequency of anginal attacks and improved exercise tolerance. Effects peak at 60 to 90 minutes and last for 3 to 6 hours. Under these circumstances, the activities of less potent metabolites also may contribute to the therapeutic effect. Chronic oral administration of isosorbide dinitrate (120 to 720 mg daily) results in persistence of the parent compound and higher plasma concentrations of metabolites. However, these doses are more likely to cause troublesome side effects and tolerance. Prolonged (up to 4 hours) improvement of exercise tolerance can be demonstrated with a sustained-release oral form of nitroglycerin, but high doses (*e.g.,* 6.5 mg) of nitroglycerin are required.

Cutaneous Administration. Application of nitroglycerin ointment can relieve angina, prolong exercise capacity, and reduce ischemic ST-segment depression with exercise for 4 hours or more. Nitroglycerin ointment (2%) is applied to the skin (2.5 to 5 cm) as it is squeezed from the tube and then spread in a uniform layer; the dosage must be adjusted for each patient. Effects are apparent within 30 to 60 minutes (although absorption is variable) and last for 4 to 6 hours. The ointment is particularly useful for controlling nocturnal angina, which commonly develops within 3 hours after the patient goes to sleep. Transdermal nitroglycerin disks use a nitroglycerin-impregnated polymer (bonded to an adhesive bandage) that permits gradual absorption and a continuous plasma nitrate concentration over 24 hours. The onset of action is slow, with peak effects occurring at 1 to 2 hours. To avoid tolerance, therapy should be interrupted for at least 8 hours each day. With this regimen, long-term prophylaxis of ischemic episodes often can be attained.

Transmucosal or Buccal Nitroglycerin. This formulation is inserted under the upper lip above the incisors, where it adheres to the gingiva and dissolves gradually in a uniform manner. Hemodynamic effects are seen within 2 to 5 minutes, and it is therefore useful for short-term prophylaxis of angina. Nitroglycerin continues to be released into the circulation for a prolonged period, and exercise tolerance may be enhanced for up to 5 hours.

Congestive Heart Failure. The utility of nitrovasodilators to relieve pulmonary congestion and to increase cardiac output in congestive heart failure is addressed in Chapter 33.

Unstable Angina Pectoris and Non-ST-Segment-Elevation Myocardial Infarction. The term *unstable angina pectoris* has been used to describe a broad spectrum of clinical entities characterized by an acute or subacute worsening in a patient's anginal symptoms. The variable prognosis of unstable angina no doubt reflects the broad range of clinical entities subsumed by the term. More recently, efforts have been directed toward identifying patients with unstable angina on the basis of their risks for subsequent adverse outcomes such as myocardial infarction or death. The term *acute coronary syndrome* has been useful in this context: Common to most clinical presentations of acute coronary syndrome is disruption of a coronary plaque leading to local platelet aggregation and thrombosis at the arterial wall with subsequent partial or total occlusion of the vessel. There is some variability in the pathogenesis of unstable angina, with gradually progressive atherosclerosis accounting for some cases of new-onset exertional angina. Less commonly, vasospasm in minimally atherosclerotic coronary vessels may account for some cases where rest angina has not been preceded by symptoms of exertional angina. For the most part, the pathophysiological principles that underlie therapy for exertional angina—which are directed at decreasing myocardial oxygen *demand*—have limited efficacy in the treatment of acute coronary syndromes characterized by an insufficiency of myocardial oxygen (blood) *supply.*

Notably, the degree of coronary stenosis correlates poorly with the likelihood of plaque rupture. Drugs that reduce myocardial oxygen consumption by reducing ventricular preload (nitrates) or by reducing heart rate and ventricular contractility (using β adrenergic receptor antagonists) are efficacious, but additional therapies are directed at the atherosclerotic plaque itself and the consequences (or prevention) of its rupture. As discussed below, these therapies include combinations of (1) antiplatelet agents, including aspirin and clopidogrel; (2) anti-thrombin agents such as heparin and the thrombolytics; (3) anti-integrin therapies that directly inhibit platelet aggregation mediated by glycoprotein (GP)IIb/IIIa; (4) mechanopharmacological approaches with percutaneously deployed drug-delivering intracoronary stents; or (5) coronary bypass surgery for selected patients.

Along with nitrates and β adrenergic receptor antagonists, antiplatelet agents represent the cornerstone of therapy for acute coronary syndrome (Lange and Hills, 2004). Aspirin (*see* below) inhibits platelet aggregation and improves survival (Yeghiazarians *et al.*, 2000). Heparin (either unfractionated or low-molecular-weight) also appears to reduce angina and prevent infarction. These and related agents are discussed in detail in Chapters 26 and 54. Anti-integrin agents directed against the platelet integrin GPIIb/IIIa (including abciximab, tirofiban, and eptifibitide) are effective in combination with heparin, as discussed below. Nitrates are useful both in reducing vasospasm and in reducing myocardial oxygen consumption by decreasing ventricular wall stress. Intravenous administration of nitroglycerin allows high concentrations of drug to be attained rapidly. Because nitroglycerin is degraded rapidly, the dose can be titrated quickly and safely using intravenous administration. If coronary vasospasm is present, intravenous nitroglycerin is likely to be effective, although the addition of a Ca^{2+} channel blocker may be required to achieve complete control in some patients. Because of the potential risk of profound hypotension, nitrates should be withheld and alternate antianginal therapy administered if patients have consumed a PDE5 inhibitor within 24 hours (*see* above).

Acute Myocardial Infarction. Therapeutic maneuvers in myocardial infarction (MI) are directed at reducing the size of the infarct; preserving or retrieving viable tissue by reducing the oxygen demand of the myocardium; and preventing ventricular remodeling that could lead to heart failure.

Nitroglycerin is commonly administered to relieve ischemic pain in patients presenting with MI, but evidence that nitrates improve mortality in MI is sparse. Because they reduce ventricular preload through vasodilation, nitrates are effective in relief of pulmonary congestion. A decreased ventricular preload should be avoided in patients with right ventricular infarction because higher right-sided heart filling pressures are needed in this clinical context. Nitrates are relatively contraindicated in patients with systemic hypotension. According to the American Heart Association/American College of Cardiology (AHA/ACC) guidelines, "nitrates should not be used if hypotension limits the administration of β-blockers, which have more powerful salutary effects" (Antman *et al.*, 2004).

Since the proximate cause of MI is intracoronary thrombosis, reperfusion therapies are critically important, employing, when possible, direct percutaneous coronary interventions (PCIs) for acute MI, usually using drug-eluting intracoronary stents (Antman *et al.*, 2004). Thrombolytic agents are administered at hospitals where emergency PCI is not performed, but outcomes are better with direct PCI than with thrombolytic therapy (Antman *et al.*, 2004) (*see* discussion of thrombolytic and antiplatelet therapies in Chapter 54).

Variant (Prinzmetal) Angina. The large coronary arteries normally contribute little to coronary resistance. However, in variant angina, coronary constriction results in reduced blood flow and ischemic pain. Multiple mechanisms have been proposed to initiate vasospasm, including endothelial cell injury (Friesinger and Robertson, 1986). Whereas long-acting nitrates alone are occasionally efficacious in abolishing episodes of variant angina, additional therapy with Ca^{2+} channel blockers usually is required. Ca^{2+} channel blockers, but not nitrates, have been shown to influence mortality and the incidence of MI favorably in variant angina; they should be included in therapy.

Ca^{2+} CHANNEL ANTAGONISTS

Voltage-sensitive Ca^{2+} channels (L-type or slow channels) mediate the entry of extracellular Ca^{2+} into smooth muscle and cardiac myocytes and sinoatrial (SA) and atrioventricular (AV) nodal cells in response to electrical depolarization. In both smooth muscle and cardiac myocytes, Ca^{2+} is a trigger for contraction, albeit by different mechanisms. Ca^{2+} channel antagonists, also called *Ca^{2+} entry blockers,* inhibit Ca^{2+} channel function. In vascular smooth muscle, this leads to relaxation, especially in arterial beds. These drugs also may produce negative inotropic and chronotropic effects in the heart.

History. The work in the 1960s of Fleckenstein, Godfraind, and their colleagues led to the concept that drugs can alter cardiac and smooth muscle contraction by blocking the entry of Ca^{2+} into myocytes. Godfraind and associates showed that the effect of the diphenylpiperazine analogs *cinnarizine* and *lidoflazine* in preventing agonist-induced vascular smooth muscle contraction could be overcome by raising the concentration of Ca^{2+} in the extracellular medium; they used the term *calcium antagonist* to describe these agents (Godfraind *et al.*, 1986).

Hass and Hartfelder reported in 1962 that *verapamil,* a putative coronary vasodilator, possessed negative inotropic and chronotropic effects that were not seen with other vasodilatory agents, such as nitroglycerin. In 1967, Fleckenstein suggested that the negative inotropic effect resulted from inhibition of excitation–contraction coupling and that the mechanism involved reduced movement of Ca^{2+} into cardiac myocytes. A derivative of verapamil, *gallopamil,* and other compounds, such as

nifedipine, also were shown to block the movement of Ca^{2+} through the cardiac myocyte Ca^{2+} channel, or the slow channel (*see* Chapter 34), and thereby alter the plateau phase of the cardiac action potential. Subsequently, drugs in several chemical classes have been shown to alter cardiac and smooth muscle contraction by blocking or "antagonizing" the entry of Ca^{2+} through channels in the myocyte membrane.

Chemistry. The 10 Ca^{2+} channel antagonists that are approved for clinical use in the United States have diverse chemical structures. Five classes of compounds have been examined: phenylalkylamines, dihydropyridines, benzothiazepines, diphenylpiperazines, and a diarylaminopropylamine. At present, verapamil (a phenylalkylamine); *diltiazem* (a benzothiazepine); nifedipine, *amlodipine, felodipine, isradipine, nicardipine, nisoldipine,* and *nimodipine* (dihydropyridines); and *bepridil* (a diarylaminopropylamine ether used only for refractory angina) are approved for clinical use in the United States. Their structures and specificities are shown in Table 31–2. Although these agents are commonly grouped together as "calcium channel blockers," there are fundamental differences among verapamil, diltiazem, and the dihydropyridines, especially with respect to pharmacologic characteristics, drug interactions, and toxicities.

Mechanisms of Action. An increased concentration of cytosolic Ca^{2+} causes increased contraction in cardiac and vascular smooth muscle cells. The entry of extracellular Ca^{2+} is more important in initiating the contraction of cardiac myocytes (Ca^{2+}-induced Ca^{2+} release). The release of Ca^{2+} from intracellular storage sites also contributes to contraction of vascular smooth muscle, particularly in some vascular beds. Cytosolic Ca^{2+} concentrations may be increased by various contractile stimuli. Thus many hormones and neurohormones increase Ca^{2+} influx through so-called receptor-operated channels, whereas high external concentrations of K^+ and depolarizing electrical stimuli increase Ca^{2+} influx through voltage-sensitive, or "potential operated," channels. The Ca^{2+} channel antagonists produce their effects by binding to the α_1 subunit of the L-type Ca^{2+} channels and reducing Ca^{2+} flux through the channel.

Voltage-sensitive channels contain domains of homologous sequence that are arranged in tandem within a single large subunit. In addition to the major channel-forming subunit (termed α_1), Ca^{2+} channels contain several other associated subunits (termed α_2, β, γ, and δ) (Schwartz, 1992). Voltage-sensitive Ca^{2+} channels have been divided into at least three subtypes based on their conductances and sensitivities to voltage (Schwartz, 1992; Tsien *et al.*, 1988). The channels best characterized to date are the L, N, and T subtypes; P/Q and R channels also have been identified. Only the L-type channel is sensitive to the dihydropyridine Ca^{2+} channel blockers. Large divalent cations such as Cd^{2+} and Mn^{2+} block a wider range of Ca^{2+} channels. All approved Ca^{2+} channel blockers bind to the α_1 subunit of the L-type Ca^{2+} channel, which is the main pore-forming unit of the channel. This 200,000- to 250,000-dalton subunit is associated with a disulfide-linked $\alpha_2\delta$ subunit of approximately 140,000 daltons and an intracellular β subunit of 55,000 to 72,000 daltons. The α_1 subunits share a common topology of four homologous domains (I, II, III, and IV), each of which is composed of six putative transmembrane seg-

Table 31–2
Ca²⁺ Channel Blockers: Chemical Structures and Some Relative Cardiovascular Effects*

CHEMICAL STRUCTURE (NONPROPRIETARY AND TRADE NAMES)	VASODILATION (CORONARY FLOW)	SUPPRESSION OF CARDIAC CONTRACTILITY	SUPPRESSION OF AUTOMATICITY (SA NODE)	SUPPRESSION OF CONDUCTION (AV NODE)
Amlodipine (NORVASC)	5	1	1	0
Felodipine (PLENDIL)	5	1	1	0
Isradipine (DYNACIRC)	NR	NR	NR	NR
Nicardipine (CARDENE, others)	5	0	1	0
Nifedipine (ADALAT, PROCARDIA)	5	1	1	0
Diltiazem (CARDIZEM, DILACOR-XR, others)	3	2	5	4

(Continued)

Table 31–2
Ca²⁺ Channel Blockers: Chemical Structures and Some Relative Cardiovascular Effects* (Continued)

CHEMICAL STRUCTURE (NONPROPRIETARY AND TRADE NAMES)	VASODILATION (CORONARY FLOW)	SUPPRESSION OF CARDIAC CONTRACTILITY	SUPPRESSION OF AUTOMATICITY (SA NODE)	SUPPRESSION OF CONDUCTION (AV NODE)
Verapamil (CALAN, ISOPTIN, VERELAN, COVERA-HS)	4	4	5	5

*The relative cardiovascular effects are ranked from no effect (0) to most prominent (5). NR, not ranked. (Modified from Julian, 1987; Taira, 1987.)

ments (S1–S6). The $\alpha_2\delta$ and β subunits modulate the α_1 subunit. The phenylalkylamine Ca²⁺ channel blockers bind to transmembrane segment 6 of domain IV (IVS6), the benzothiazepine Ca²⁺ channel blockers bind to the cytoplasmic bridge between domain III (IIIS) and domain IV (IVS), and the dihydropyridine Ca²⁺ channel blockers bind to transmembrane segment of both domain III (IIIS6) and domain IV (IVS6). These three separate receptor sites are linked allosterically (Hockerman *et al.*, 1997; Abernethy and Schwartz, 1999). The vascular and cardiac effects of some of the Ca²⁺ channel blockers are summarized below and in Table 31–2.

Pharmacological Properties

Cardiovascular Effects. **Actions in Vascular Tissue.** Although there is some involvement of Na⁺ currents, depolarization of vascular smooth muscle cells depends primarily on the influx of Ca²⁺. At least three distinct mechanisms may be responsible for contraction of vascular smooth muscle cells. First, voltage-sensitive Ca²⁺ channels open in response to depolarization of the membrane, and extracellular Ca²⁺ moves down its electrochemical gradient (from approximately 1.5 to 120 mm) into the cell. After closure of Ca²⁺ channels, a finite period of time is required before the channels can open again in response to a stimulus. Second, agonist-induced contractions that occur without depolarization of the membrane result from stimulation of the PLC–IP₃ pathway, resulting in the release of intracellular Ca²⁺ from the sarcoplasmic reticulum (Berridge, 1993). This receptor-mediated release of intracellular Ca²⁺ may trigger further influx of extracellular Ca²⁺. Third, receptor-operated Ca²⁺ channels allow the entry of extracellular Ca²⁺ in response to receptor occupancy.

An increase in cytosolic Ca²⁺ results in enhanced binding of Ca²⁺ to calmodulin. The Ca²⁺–calmodulin

complex in turn activates myosin light-chain kinase, with resulting phosphorylation of the myosin light chain. Such phosphorylation promotes interaction between actin and myosin and contraction of smooth muscle. Ca²⁺ channel antagonists inhibit the voltage-dependent Ca²⁺ channels in vascular smooth muscle at significantly lower concentrations than are required to interfere with the release of intracellular Ca²⁺ or to block receptor-operated Ca²⁺ channels. All Ca²⁺ channel blockers relax arterial smooth muscle, but they have little effect on most venous beds and hence do not affect cardiac preload significantly.

Actions in Cardiac Cells. The mechanisms involved in excitation–contraction coupling in the cardiac muscle differ from those in vascular smooth muscle in that a portion of the two inward currents is carried by Na⁺ through the fast channel in addition to that carried by Ca²⁺ through the slow channel. Within the cardiac myocyte, Ca²⁺ binds to troponin, relieving the inhibitory effect of troponin on the contractile apparatus and permitting a productive interaction of actin and myosin leading to contraction. Thus Ca²⁺ channel blockers can produce a negative inotropic effect. Although this is true of all classes of Ca²⁺ channel blockers, the greater degree of peripheral vasodilation seen with the dihydropyridines is accompanied by a sufficient baroreflex-mediated increase in sympathetic tone to overcome the negative inotropic effect. Diltiazem also may inhibit mitochondrial Na⁺–Ca²⁺ exchange (Schwartz, 1992).

In the SA and AV nodes, depolarization largely depends on the movement of Ca²⁺ through the slow channel. The effect of a Ca²⁺ channel blocker on AV conduction and on the rate of the sinus node pacemaker depends on whether or not the agent delays the recovery of the slow channel (Schwarz, 1992). Although nifedipine reduces the slow inward current in a dose-dependent manner, it does not affect the rate of recovery of the slow Ca^{2+} channel. The channel blockade caused by nifedipine and related dihydropyridines also shows little dependence on the frequency of stimulation. At doses used clinically, nifedipine does not affect conduction through the node. In contrast, verapamil not only reduces the magnitude of the Ca^{2+} current through the slow channel but also decreases the rate of recovery of the channel. In addition, channel blockade caused by verapamil (and to a lesser extent by diltiazem) is enhanced as the frequency of stimulation increases, a phenomenon known as *frequency dependence* or *use dependence*. Verapamil and diltiazem depress the rate of the sinus node pacemaker and slow AV conduction; the latter effect is the basis for their use in the treatment of supraventricular tachyarrhythmias (*see* Chapter 34). Bepridil, like verapamil, inhibits both slow inward Ca^{2+} current and fast inward Na^+ current. It has a direct negative inotropic effect. Its electrophysiological properties lead to slowing of the heart rate, prolongation of the AV nodal effective refractory period, and importantly, prolongation of the QTc interval. Particularly in the setting of hypokalemia, the last effect can be associated with *torsades de pointes,* a potentially lethal ventricular arrhythmia (*see* Chapter 34).

Hemodynamic Effects. All the Ca^{2+} channel blockers approved for clinical use decrease coronary vascular resistance and increase coronary blood flow. The dihydropyridines are more potent vasodilators *in vivo* and *in vitro* than verapamil, which is more potent than diltiazem. The hemodynamic effects of these agents vary depending on the route of administration and the extent of left ventricular dysfunction.

Nifedipine given intravenously increases forearm blood flow with little effect on venous pooling; this indicates a selective dilation of arterial resistance vessels. The decrease in arterial blood pressure elicits sympathetic reflexes, with resulting tachycardia and positive inotropy. Nifedipine also has direct negative inotropic effects *in vitro*. However, nifedipine relaxes vascular smooth muscle at significantly lower concentrations than those required for prominent direct effects on the heart. Thus arteriolar resistance and blood pressure are lowered, contractility and segmental ventricular function are improved, and heart rate and cardiac output are increased modestly (Serruys *et al.*, 1983). After oral administration of nifedipine, arterial dilation increases peripheral blood flow; venous tone does not change.

The other dihydropyridines—amlodipine, felodipine, isradipine, nicardipine, nisoldipine, and nimodipine—share many of the cardiovascular effects of nifedipine. Amlodipine is a dihydropyridine that has a slow absorption and a prolonged effect. With a plasma half-

life of 35 to 50 hours, plasma levels and effect increase over 7 to 10 days of daily administration of a constant dose. Amlodipine produces both peripheral arterial vasodilation and coronary dilation, with a hemodynamic profile similar to that of nifedipine. However, there is less reflex tachycardia with amlodipine possibly because the long half-life produces minimal peaks and troughs in plasma concentrations (van Zwieten and Pfaffendorf, 1993; Taylor, 1994; Lehmann *et al.*, 1993). Felodipine may have even greater vascular specificity than does nifedipine or amlodipine. At concentrations producing vasodilation, there is no negative inotropic effect. Like nifedipine, felodipine indirectly activates the sympathetic nervous system, leading to an increase in heart rate (Todd and Faulds, 1992). Nicardipine has antianginal properties similar to those of nifedipine and may have selectivity for coronary vessels. Isradipine also produces the typical peripheral vasodilation seen with other dihydropyridines, but because of its inhibitory effect on the SA node, little or no rise in heart rate is seen. This inhibitory effect does not extend to the cardiac myocytes, however, because no cardiodepressant effect is seen. Despite the negative chronotropic effect, isradipine appears to have little effect on the AV node, so it may be used in patients with AV block or combined with a β adrenergic receptor antagonist. In general, because of their lack of myocardial depression and, to a greater or lesser extent, lack of negative chronotropic effect, dihydropyridines are less effective as monotherapy in stable angina than are verapamil, diltiazem, or a β adrenergic receptor antagonist. Nisoldipine is more than 1000 times more potent in preventing contraction of human vascular smooth muscle than in preventing contraction of human cardiac muscle *in vitro,* suggesting a high degree of vascular selectivity (Godfraind *et al.*, 1992). Although nisoldipine has a short elimination half-life, a sustained-release preparation has been developed that is efficacious as an antianginal agent. Nimodipine has high lipid solubility and was developed as an agent to relax the cerebral vasculature. It is effective in inhibiting cerebral vasospasm and has been used primarily to treat patients with neurological defects associated with cerebral vasospasm after subarachnoid hemorrhage.

Bepridil has been demonstrated to reduce blood pressure and heart rate in patients with stable exertional angina. It also produces an increase in left ventricular performance in patients with angina, but its side-effect profile (*see* below) limits its use to truly refractory patients.

Verapamil is a less potent vasodilator *in vivo* than are the dihydropyridines. Like the latter agents, verapamil causes little effect on venous resistance vessels at concentrations that produce arteriolar dilation. With doses of verapamil sufficient to produce peripheral arterial vasodilation, there are more direct negative chronotropic, dromotropic, and inotropic effects than with the dihydropyridines. Intravenous verapamil causes a decrease in arterial blood pressure owing to a decrease in vascular resistance, but the reflex tachycardia is blunted or abolished by the direct negative chronotropic effect of the drug. This intrinsic negative inotropic effect is partially offset by both a decrease in afterload and the reflex increase in adrenergic tone. Thus, in patients without congestive heart failure, ventricular performance is not impaired and actually may improve, especially if ischemia limits performance. In contrast, in patients with congestive heart failure, intravenous verapamil can cause a marked decrease in contractility and left ventricular function. Oral administration of verapamil reduces peripheral vascular resistance and blood pressure, often with minimal changes in heart rate. The relief of pacing-induced angina seen with verapamil is due primarily to a reduction in myocardial oxygen demand.

Intravenous administration of diltiazem can result initially in a marked decrease in peripheral vascular resistance and arterial blood pressure, which elicits a reflex increase in heart rate and cardiac output. Heart rate then falls below initial levels because of the direct negative chronotropic effect of the agent. Oral administration of diltiazem decreases both heart rate and mean arterial blood pressure. While diltiazem and verapamil produce similar effects on the SA and AV nodes, the negative inotropic effect of diltiazem is more modest.

The effects of Ca^{2+} channel blockers on diastolic ventricular relaxation (the lusitropic state of the ventricle) are complex. The direct effect of several of these agents, especially when given into the coronary arteries, is to impair relaxation (Amende *et al.*, 1983; Serruys *et al.*, 1983; Walsh and O'Rourke, 1985). Although several clinical studies have suggested an improvement in peak left ventricular filling rates when verapamil, nifedipine, nisoldipine, or nicardipine was given systemically (Bonow *et al.*, 1982; Paulus *et al.*, 1983), one must be cautious in extrapolating this change in filling rates to enhancement of relaxation. Because ventricular relaxation is so complex, the effect of even a single agent may be pleiotropic. If reflex stimulation of sympathetic tone increases cyclic AMP levels in myocytes, increased lusitropy will result that may outweigh a direct negative lusitropic effect. Likewise, a reduction in afterload will improve the lusitropic state. In addition, if ischemia is improved, the negative lusitropic effect of asymmetrical left ventricular contraction will be reduced. The sum total of these effects in any given patient cannot be determined *a priori*. Thus caution should be exercised in the use of Ca^{2+} channel blockers for this purpose; the ideal is to determine the end result objectively before committing the patient to therapy.

Absorption, Fate, and Excretion. Although the absorption of these agents is nearly complete after oral administration, their bioavailability is reduced, in some cases markedly, by first-pass hepatic metabolism. The effects of these drugs are evident within 30 to 60 minutes of an oral dose, with the exception of the more slowly absorbed and longer-acting agents amlodipine, isradipine, and felodipine. For comparison, peak effects of verapamil occur within 15 minutes of its intravenous administration. These agents all are bound extensively to plasma proteins (70% to 98%); their elimination half-lives vary widely and range from 1.3 to 64 hours. During repeated oral administration, bioavailability and half-life may increase because of saturation of hepatic metabolism. A major metabolite of diltiazem is desacetyldiltiazem, which has about one-half of diltiazem's potency as a vasodilator. *N*-Demethylation of verapamil results in production of norverapamil, which is biologically active but much less potent than the parent compound. The half-life of norverapamil is about 10 hours. The metabolites of the dihydropyridines are inactive or weakly active. In patients with hepatic cirrhosis, the bioavailabilities and half-lives of the Ca^{2+} channel blockers may be increased, and dosage should be decreased accordingly. The half-lives of these agents also may be longer in older patients. Except for diltiazem and nifedipine, all

the Ca^{2+} channel blockers are administered as racemic mixtures (Abernethy and Schwartz, 1999).

Toxicity and Untoward Responses. The most common side effects caused by the Ca^{2+} channel antagonists, particularly the dihydropyridines, are due to excessive vasodilation. Symptoms include dizziness, hypotension, headache, flushing, digital dysesthesia, and nausea. Patients also may experience constipation, peripheral edema, coughing, wheezing, and pulmonary edema. Nimodipine may produce muscle cramps when given in the large doses required for a beneficial effect in patients with subarachnoid hemorrhage. Less common side effects include rash, somnolence, and occasional minor elevations of liver function tests. These side effects usually are benign and may abate with time or with dose adjustment. Worsened myocardial ischemia has been observed in two studies with the dihydropyridine nifedipine (Schulz *et al.*, 1985; Egstrup and Anderson, 1993). In both these studies, worsening of angina was observed in patients with an angiographically demonstrable coronary collateral circulation. The worsening of angina may have resulted from excessive hypotension and decreased coronary perfusion, selective coronary vasodilation in nonischemic regions of the myocardium in a setting where vessels perfusing ischemic regions were already maximally dilated (*i.e.*, coronary steal), or an increase in oxygen demand owing to increased sympathetic tone and excessive tachycardia. In a study of monotherapy with an immediate-release formulation of nisoldipine, the dihydropyridine was not superior to placebo and was associated with a trend toward an increased incidence of serious adverse events, a process termed *proischemia* (Waters, 1991).

Although bradycardia, transient asystole, and exacerbation of heart failure have been reported with verapamil, these responses usually have occurred after intravenous administration of verapamil in patients with disease of the SA node or AV nodal conduction disturbances or in the presence of β adrenergic receptor blockade. The use of intravenous verapamil with a β adrenergic receptor antagonist is contraindicated because of the increased propensity for AV block and/or severe depression of ventricular function. Patients with ventricular dysfunction, SA or AV nodal conduction disturbances, and systolic blood pressures below 90 mmHg should not be treated with verapamil or diltiazem, particularly intravenously. Some Ca^{2+} channel antagonists can cause an increase in the concentration of digoxin in plasma, although toxicity from the cardiac glycoside rarely develops. The use of verapamil to treat digitalis toxicity thus is contraindicated; AV nodal conduction disturbances may be exacerbated. Bepridil, because of its anti-arrhythmic properties and its ability to prolong the QTc interval, can produce serious arrhythmic side effects. Especially in the setting of hypokalemia and/or bradycardia, polymorphic ventricular tachycardia (*torsades de pointes*), a potentially lethal arrhythmia, can be seen. Agranulocytosis also has been reported. Because of these serious side effects, bepridil should be reserved for patients refractory to all other appropriate medical and surgical therapy.

Several studies have raised concerns about the long-term safety of short-acting nifedipine (Opie *et al.*, 2000). The proposed mechanism for this adverse effect lies in abrupt vasodilation with reflex sympathetic activation. There does not appear to be either significant reflex tachycardia or long-term adverse outcomes from treatment with sustained-release forms of nifedipine or with dihydropyridine Ca^{2+} blockers such as amlodipine or felodipine, which have more favorable (slower) pharmacokinetics.

Therapeutic Uses

Variant Angina. Variant angina results from reduced flow rather than increased oxygen demand. Controlled clinical trials have demonstrated efficacy of the Ca^{2+} channel blocking agents for the treatment of variant angina (Gibbons *et al.*, 2002). These drugs can attenuate *ergonovine*-induced vasospasm in patients with variant angina, which suggests that protection in variant angina is due to coronary dilation rather than to alterations in peripheral hemodynamics.

Exertional Angina. Ca^{2+} channel antagonists also are effective in the treatment of exertional, or exercise-induced, angina. Their utility may result from an increase in blood flow owing to coronary arterial dilation, from a decrease in myocardial oxygen demand (secondary to a decrease in arterial blood pressure, heart rate, or contractility), or both. Numerous double-blind, placebo-controlled studies have shown that these drugs decrease the number of anginal attacks and attenuate exercise-induced ST-segment depression.

The *double product,* calculated as heart rate times systolic blood pressure, is an indirect measure of myocardial O_2 demand. Since these agents reduce the level of the double product at a given external workload, and because the value of the double product at peak exercise is not altered, the beneficial effect of Ca^{2+} channel blockers likely is due primarily to a decrease in O_2 demand rather than to an increase in coronary flow.

As described earlier, Ca^{2+} channel antagonists, particularly the dihydropyridines, may aggravate anginal symptoms in some patients when used without a β adrenergic receptor antagonist. This adverse effect is not prominent with verapamil or diltiazem because of their limited ability to induce marked peripheral vasodilation and reflex tachycardia. Concurrent therapy with nifedipine and the β adrenergic receptor antagonist *propranolol* or with amlodipine and any of several β adrenergic receptor antagonists has proven more effective than either agent given alone in exertional angina, presumably because the β adrenergic receptor antagonist suppresses reflex tachycardia (Gibbons *et al.*, 2002). This concurrent drug therapy is particularly attractive because the dihydropyridines, unlike verapamil and diltiazem, do not delay AV conduction and will not enhance the negative dromotropic effects associated with β adrenergic receptor blockade. Although concurrent administration of verapamil or diltiazem with a β adrenergic receptor antagonist also may reduce angina, the potential for AV block, severe bradycardia, and decreased left ventricular function requires that these combinations be used judiciously, especially if left ventricular function is compromised prior to therapy. Amlodipine produces less reflex tachycardia than does nifedipine probably because of a flatter plasma concentration profile. Isradipine, approximately equivalent to nifedipine in enhancing exercise tolerance, also produces less rise in heart rate, possibly because of its slow onset of action.

Unstable Angina. Medical therapy for unstable angina involves the administration of aspirin, which reduces mortality, nitrates, β adrenergic receptor blocking agents, and heparin, which are effective in controlling ischemic episodes and angina. Since vasospasm occurs in some patients with unstable angina (Yeghiazarians *et al.*, 2000), Ca^{2+} channel blockers offer an additional approach to the treatment of unstable angina. However, there is insufficient evidence to assess whether such treatment decreases mortality except when the underlying mechanism is vasospasm. In a randomized, double-blind clinical trial, the short-acting dihydropyridine nifedipine was found to be less effective than *metoprolol* (Muller *et al.*, 1984), and there are no studies supporting the administration of a dihydropyridine to patients with unstable angina. One small study of 121 patients reported a benefit of intravenous diltiazem compared with nitroglycerin on the end points of refractory angina and event-free survival (Göbel *et al.*, 1995). In contrast, therapy directed toward reduction of platelet function and thrombotic episodes clearly decreases morbidity and mortality in patients with unstable angina (*see* Chapters 26 and 54).

Myocardial Infarction. There is no evidence that Ca^{2+} channel antagonists are of benefit in the early treatment or secondary prevention of acute MI. In several trials, higher doses of the short-acting formulation of the dihydropyridine nifedipine had a detrimental effect on mortality

(Opie *et al.*, 2000; Yusuf, 1995; Furberg *et al.*, 1995). Diltiazem and verapamil may reduce the incidence of reinfarction in patients with a first non-Q-wave infarction who are not candidates for a β adrenergic receptor antagonist (Gibbons *et al.*, 2002), but β adrenergic receptor antagonists remain the drugs of first choice.

Other Uses. The use of Ca^{2+} channel antagonists as antiarrhythmic agents is discussed in Chapter 34; their use for the treatment of hypertension is discussed in Chapter 32; and use of amlodipine in the treatment of heart failure is reviewed in Chapter 33. Clinical trials are under way to evaluate the capacity of Ca^{2+} channel blockers to slow the progression of renal failure and to protect the transplanted kidney. Verapamil has been demonstrated to improve left ventricular outflow obstruction and symptoms in patients with hypertrophic cardiomyopathy. Verapamil also has been used in the prophylaxis of migraine headaches. While several studies suggest that dihydropyridines may suppress the progression of mild atherosclerosis, there is no evidence that this alters mortality or reduces the incidence of ischemic events. Nimodipine has been approved for use in patients with neurological deficits secondary to cerebral vasospasm after the rupture of a congenital intracranial aneurysm. Nifedipine, diltiazem, amlodipine, and felodipine appear to provide symptomatic relief in Raynaud's disease. The Ca^{2+} channel antagonists cause relaxation of the myometrium *in vitro* and may be effective in stopping preterm uterine contractions in preterm labor (*see* Chapter 55).

β ADRENERGIC RECEPTOR ANTAGONISTS

β Adrenergic receptor antagonists are effective in reducing the severity and frequency of attacks of exertional angina and in improving survival in patients who have had an MI. In contrast, these agents are not useful for vasospastic angina and, if used in isolation, may worsen the condition. Most β adrenergic receptor antagonists apparently are equally effective in the treatment of exertional angina (Gibbons *et al.*, 2002). *Timolol,* metoprolol, *atenolol,* and propranolol have been shown to exert cardioprotective effects. The effectiveness of β adrenergic receptor antagonists in the treatment of exertional angina is attributable primarily to a fall in myocardial oxygen consumption at rest and during exertion, although there also is some tendency for increased flow toward ischemic regions. The decrease in myocardial oxygen consumption is due to a negative chronotropic effect (particularly during exercise), a negative inotropic effect, and a reduction in arterial blood pressure (particularly systolic pressure) during exercise. Not all actions of β adrenergic receptor antagonists are beneficial in all patients. The decreases in heart rate and contractility

cause increases in the systolic ejection period and left ventricular end-diastolic volume; these alterations tend to increase O_2 consumption. However, the net effect of β adrenergic receptor blockade is usually to decrease myocardial O_2 consumption, particularly during exercise. Nevertheless, in patients with limited cardiac reserve who are critically dependent on adrenergic stimulation, β adrenergic receptor blockade can result in profound decreases in left ventricular function. Despite this, several β adrenergic receptor antagonists have been shown to reduce mortality in patients with congestive heart failure (*see* Chapter 33). Numerous β adrenergic receptor antagonists are approved for clinical use in the United States. Their pharmacology and the criteria for choosing a β_1-selective agent, an agent with intrinsic sympathomimetic activity, or a nonspecific agent are considered in detail in Chapter 10.

Therapeutic Uses

Unstable Angina. β Adrenergic receptor antagonists are effective in reducing recurrent episodes of ischemia and the risk of progression to acute MI (Braunwald *et al.*, 2002). Clinical trials have lacked sufficient statistical power to demonstrate beneficial effects of β adrenergic receptor antagonists on mortality. On the other hand, if the underlying pathophysiology is coronary vasospasm, nitrates and Ca^{2+} channel blockers may be effective, and β adrenergic receptor antagonists should be used with caution. In some patients, there is a combination of severe fixed disease and superimposed vasospasm; if adequate antiplatelet therapy and vasodilation have been provided by other agents and angina continues, the addition of a β adrenergic receptor antagonist may be helpful.

Myocardial Infarction. β Adrenergic receptor antagonists that do not have intrinsic sympathomimetic activity improve mortality in MI. They should be given early and continued indefinitely in patients who can tolerate them (Gibbons *et al.*, 2002).

COMPARISON OF ANTIANGINAL THERAPEUTIC STRATEGIES

In evaluating trials in which different forms of antianginal therapy are compared, careful attention must be paid to the patient population studied and to the pathophysiology and stage of the disease. An important placebo effect may be seen in these trials. The efficacy of antianginal treatment will depend on the severity of angina, the presence of coronary vasospasm, and myocardial O_2 demand. Optimally, the dose of each agent should be titrated to maximum benefit.

Task forces from the American College of Cardiology (ACC) and the American Heart Association (AHA) (Gibbons *et al.*, 2002) have published guidelines that are useful in the selection of appropriate initial therapy for patients with chronic stable angina pectoris. Patients with coronary artery disease should be treated with aspirin and a β adrenergic receptor blocking drug (particularly if there is a history of prior MI). The ACC/AHA guidelines also note that solid data support the use of ACE inhibitors in patients with coronary artery disease who also have left ventricular dysfunction and/or diabetes. Therapy of hypercholesterolemia is also indicated. Nitrates, for treatment of angina symptoms, and Ca^{2+} antagonists also may be used (Gibbons *et al.*, 2002). Table 31–3 summarizes the issues that the ACC/AHA task force considered to be relevant in choosing between β adrenergic receptor antagonists and Ca^{2+} channel blockers in patients with angina and other medical conditions. A meta-analysis of publications that compared two or more antianginal therapies has been conducted (Heidenreich *et al.*, 1999). Comparison of β adrenergic receptor antagonists with Ca^{2+} channel blockers showed that β adrenergic receptor antagonists are associated with fewer episodes of angina per week and a lower rate of withdrawal because of adverse events. However, there were no differences in time to ischemia during exercise or in the frequency of adverse events when Ca^{2+} channel blockers other than nifedipine were compared with β adrenergic receptor antagonists. There were no significant differences in outcome between the studies comparing long-acting nitrates and Ca^{2+} channel blockers and the studies comparing long-acting nitrates with β adrenergic receptor antagonists.

Combination Therapy. Since the different categories of antianginal agents have different mechanisms of action, it has been suggested that combinations of these agents would allow the use of lower doses, increasing effectiveness and reducing the incidence of side effects. However, despite the predicted advantages, combination therapy rarely achieves this potential and may be accompanied by serious side effects. Newer antianginal agents have distinct pharmacological mechanisms to reduce myocardial oxygen consumption (*e.g.*, ranolazine); some studies have suggested that these newer compounds may have additional efficacy in combination with other antianginal agents (Chaitman *et al.*, 2004).

Nitrates and β Adrenergic Receptor Antagonists. The concurrent use of organic nitrates and β adrenergic receptor antagonists can be very effective in the treatment of typical exertional angina. The additive efficacy is primarily a result of the blockade by one drug of a reflex effect elicited by the other. β Adrenergic receptor antagonists can block the baroreceptor-mediated reflex tachycardia and positive inotropic effects that are sometimes associated with nitrates, whereas nitrates, by increasing venous capacitance, can attenuate the increase in left ventricular end-diastolic volume associated with β adrenergic receptor blockade. Concurrent administration of nitrates also can alleviate the increase in coronary vascular resistance associated with blockade of β adrenergic receptors.

Ca^{2+} Channel Blockers and β Adrenergic Receptor Antagonists. Since there is a proven mortality benefit from the use of β adrenergic receptor antagonists in patients with heart disease, this class of drugs represents the first line of therapy. However, when angina is not controlled adequately by a β adrenergic receptor antagonist plus nitrates, additional improvement sometimes can be achieved by the addition of a Ca^{2+} channel blocker, especially if there is a component of coronary vasospasm. The differences among the chemical classes of Ca^{2+} channel blockers can lead to important adverse or salutary drug interactions with β adrenergic receptor antagonists. If the patient already is being treated with maximal doses of verapamil or diltiazem, it is difficult to demonstrate any additional benefit of β adrenergic receptor blockade, and excessive bradycardia, heart block, or heart failure may ensue. However, in patients treated with a dihydropyridine such as nifedipine or with nitrates, substantial reflex tachycardia often limits the effectiveness of these agents. A β adrenergic receptor antagonist may be a helpful addition in this situation, resulting in a lower heart rate and blood pressure with exercise. The efficacy of amlodipine is improved by combination with a β adrenergic receptor antagonist. However, in the Total Ischaemic Burden European Trial (TIBET), which compared the effects of atenolol, a sustained-release form of nifedipine, and their combination on exercise parameters and ambulatory ischemia in patients with mild angina, there were no differences between the agents, either singly or in combination, on any of the measured ischemic parameters (Fox *et al.*, 1996). On the other hand, in two studies of patients with more severe but still stable angina, atenolol and propranolol were shown to be superior to nifedipine, and the combination of propranolol and nifedipine was more effective than a β adrenergic receptor antagonist alone (Fox *et al.*, 1993).

Relative contraindications to the use of β adrenergic receptor antagonists for treatment of angina—bronchospasm, Raynaud's syndrome, or Prinzmetal angina—may lead to a choice to initiate therapy with a Ca^{2+} channel blocker. Fluctuations in coronary tone are important determinants of variant angina. It is likely that episodes of increased tone, such as those precipitated by cold and by emotion, superimposed on fixed disease have a role in the variable anginal threshold seen in some patients with otherwise chronic stable angina. Increased coronary tone also may be important in the anginal episodes occurring early after MI and after coronary angioplasty, and it probably accounts for those patients with unstable angina who respond to dihydropyridines. Atherosclerotic arteries have abnormal vasomotor responses to a number of stimuli (Dudzinski *et al.*, 2005), including exercise, other forms of sympathetic activation, and cholinergic agonists; in such vessels, stenotic segments actually may become more severely stenosed during exertion. This implies that the normal exercise-induced increase in coronary flow is lost in atherosclerosis. Similar exaggerated vascular contractile responses are seen in hyperlipidemia, even before anatomic evidence of atherosclerosis develops. Because of this, coronary vasodilators (nitrates and/or Ca^{2+} channel blockers) are an important part of the therapeutic program in the majority of patients with ischemic heart disease.

Ca^{2+} Channel Blockers and Nitrates. In severe exertional or vasospastic angina, the combination of a nitrate and a Ca^{2+} channel blocker may provide additional relief over that obtained with either type of agent alone. Since nitrates primarily reduce preload, whereas Ca^{2+} channel blockers reduce afterload, the net effect on reduction of oxygen demand should be additive. However, excessive vasodilation and hypotension can occur. The concurrent administration of a nitrate and nifedipine has been advocated in particular for patients

Table 31–3
Recommended Drug Therapy for Angina in Patients with Other Medical Conditions

CONDITION	RECOMMENDED TREATMENT (AND ALTERNATIVES) FOR ANGINA	DRUGS TO AVOID
Medical Conditions		
Systemic hypertension	β Adrenergic receptor antagonists (Ca^{2+} channel antagonists)	
Migraine or vascular headaches	β Adrenergic receptor antagonists (Ca^{2+} channel antagonists)	
Asthma or chronic obstructive pulmonary disease with bronchospasm	Verapamil or diltiazem	β Adrenergic receptor antagonists
Hyperthyroidism	β Adrenergic receptor antagonists	
Raynaud's syndrome	Long-acting, slow-release Ca^{2+} channel antagonists	β Adrenergic receptor antagonists
Insulin-dependent diabetes mellitus	β Adrenergic receptor antagonists (particularly if prior MI) or long-acting, slow-release Ca^{2+} channel antagonists	
Non-insulin-dependent diabetes mellitus	β Adrenergic receptor antagonists or long-acting, slow-release Ca^{2+} channel antagonists	
Depression	Long-acting, slow-release Ca^{2+} channel antagonists	β Adrenergic receptor antagonists
Mild peripheral vascular disease	β Adrenergic receptor antagonists or Ca^{2+} channel antagonists	
Severe peripheral vascular disease with rest ischemia	Ca^{2+} channel antagonists	β Adrenergic receptor antagonists
Cardiac Arrhythmias and Conduction Abnormalities		
Sinus bradycardia	Dihydropyridine Ca^{2+} channel antagonists	β Adrenergic receptor antagonists, diltiazem, verapamil
Sinus tachycardia (not due to heart failure)	β Adrenergic receptor antagonists	
Supraventricular tachycardia	Verapamil, diltiazem, or β adrenergic receptor antagonists	
Atrioventricular block	Dihydropyridine Ca^{2+} channel antagonists	β Adrenergic receptor antagonists, verapamil, diltiazem
Rapid atrial fibrillation (with digitalis)	Verapamil, diltiazem, or β adrenergic receptor antagonists	
Ventricular arrhythmias	β Adrenergic receptor antagonists	
Left Ventricular Dysfunction		
Congestive heart failure		
Mild (LVEF $\geq 40\%$)	β Adrenergic receptor antagonists	
Moderate to severe (LVEF $< 40\%$)	Amlodipine or felodipine (nitrates)	
Left-sided valvular heart disease		
Mild aortic stenosis	β Adrenergic receptor antagonists	
Aortic insufficiency	Long-acting, slow-release dihydropyridines	
Mitral regurgitation	Long-acting, slow-release dihydropyridines	
Mitral stenosis	β Adrenergic receptor antagonists	
Hypertrophic cardiomyopathy	β Adrenergic receptor antagonists, nondihydropyridine Ca^{2+} channel antagonists	Nitrates, dihydropyridine Ca^{2+} channel antagonists

SOURCE: Modified from Gibbons *et al.*, 1999. MI, myocardial infarction; LVEF, left ventricular ejection fraction.

with exertional angina with heart failure, the sick-sinus syndrome, or AV nodal conduction disturbances, but excessive tachycardia may be seen.

Ca²⁺ Channel Blockers, β Adrenergic Receptor Antagonists, and Nitrates. In patients with exertional angina that is not controlled by the administration of two types of antianginal agents, the use of all three may provide improvement, although the incidence of side effects increases significantly. The dihydropyridines and nitrates dilate epicardial coronary arteries; the dihydropyridines decrease afterload; the nitrates decrease preload; and the β adrenergic receptor antagonists decrease heart rate and myocardial contractility. Therefore, there is theoretical, and sometimes real, benefit with their combination, although adverse drug interactions may lead to clinically important events. For example, combining verapamil or diltiazem with a β adrenergic receptor antagonist greatly increases the risk of conduction system and left ventricular dysfunction–related side effects and should be undertaken only with extreme caution and only if no other alternatives exist.

ANTIPLATELET, ANTI-INTEGRIN, AND ANTITHROMBOTIC AGENTS

Aspirin reduces the incidence of MI and death in patients with unstable angina. In addition, low doses of aspirin appear to reduce the incidence of MI in patients with chronic stable angina. Aspirin, given in doses of 160 to 325 mg at the onset of treatment of MI, reduces mortality in patients presenting with unstable angina. The addition of clopidogrel to aspirin therapy reduces mortality in patients with acute coronary syndromes (Lange and Hillis, 2004). Heparin, in its unfractionated form and as low-molecular-weight heparin, also reduces symptoms and prevents infarction in unstable angina (Yeghiazarians *et al.*, 2000). Thrombin inhibitors, such as *hirudin* or *bivalirudin,* are being investigated; these agents directly inhibit even clot-bound thrombin, are not affected by circulating inhibitors, and function independently of antithrombin III. Thrombolytic agents, on the other hand, are of no benefit in unstable angina (Yeghiazarians *et al.*, 2000). Intravenous inhibitors of the platelet GPIIb/IIIa receptor (abciximab, tirofiban, and eptifibatide) are effective in preventing the complications of PCIs and in the treatment of patients presenting with acute coronary syndromes (Bhatt and Topol, 2000; Lange and Hillis, 2004).

TREATMENT OF CLAUDICATION AND PERIPHERAL VASCULAR DISEASE

Most patients with peripheral vascular disease also have coronary artery disease, and the therapeutic approaches for peripheral and coronary arterial diseases overlap. Mortality in patients with peripheral vascular disease is most commonly due to cardiovascular disease (Regensteiner and Hiatt, 2002), and treatment of coronary disease remains the central focus of therapy. Many patients with advanced peripheral arterial disease are more limited by the consequences of peripheral ischemia than by myocardial ischemia. In the cerebral circulation, arterial disease may be manifest as stroke or transient ischemic attacks. The painful symptoms of peripheral arterial disease in the lower extremities (claudication) typically are provoked by exertion, with increases in skeletal muscle O_2 demand exceeding blood flow impaired by proximal stenoses. When flow to the extremities becomes critically limiting, peripheral ulcers and rest pain from tissue ischemia can become debilitating.

Most of the therapies shown to be efficacious for treatment of coronary artery disease also have a salutary effect on progression of peripheral artery disease. Reductions in cardiovascular morbidity and mortality in patients with peripheral arterial disease have been documented with antiplatelet therapy using aspirin or with ADP antagonists such as clopidogrel or ticlopidine, administration of ACE inhibitors, and treatment of hyperlipidemia (Regensteiner and Hiatt, 2002). Interestingly, neither intensive treatment of diabetes mellitus nor antihypertensive therapy appears to alter the progression of symptoms of claudication. Other risk factor and lifestyle modifications remain cornerstones of therapy for patients with claudication: Physical exercise, rehabilitation, and smoking cessation have proven efficacy. Drugs used specifically in the treatment of lower extremity claudication include *pentoxyfylline* and *cilostazol* (Hiatt, 2001). Pentoxyfylline is a methylxanthine derivative that has been termed a *rheologic modifier* for its effects on increasing the deformability of red blood cells. However, the effects of pentoxifylline on lower extremity claudication appear to be modest. Cilostazol is an inhibitor of PDE3 and promotes accumulation of intracellular cyclic AMP in many cells, including blood platelets. Cilostazol-mediated increases in cyclic AMP inhibit platelet aggregation and promote vasodilation. The drug is metabolized by CYP3A4 and has important drug interactions with other drugs metabolized *via* this pathway (*see* Chapter 3). Cilostazol treatment improves symptoms of claudication but has no effect on cardiovascular mortality. As a PDE3 inhibitor, cilostazol is placed in the same drug class as *milrinone*, which had been used as an inotropic agent for patients with heart failure. Milrinone therapy was associated with an increase in sudden cardiac death, and the drug was withdrawn from the market. Cilostazol, therefore, is contraindicated in patients with heart failure, although it is not clear that cilastozol itself leads to increased mortality in such patients. Cilastozol has been reported to increase nonsustained ventricular tachycardia; headache is the most common side effect. Other treatments for claudication, including *naftidrofuryl, proprionyl levocarnitine,* and *prostaglandins,* have been explored in clinicals trials, and there is some evidence that some of these therapies may be efficacious.

MECHANOPHARMACOLOGICAL THERAPY: DRUG-ELUTING ENDOVASCULAR STENTS

Intracoronary stents can ameliorate angina and reduce adverse events in patients with acute coronary syndromes. However, the long-term efficacy of intracoronary stents is limited by subacute luminal restenosis within the stent, which occurs in a substantial minority of patients. The pathways that lead to "in-stent restenosis" are complex, but smooth muscle proliferation within the lumen of the stented artery is a common pathological finding (Schwartz and Henry, 2002). Local antiproliferative therapies at the time of stenting have been explored over many years, and the development of drug-eluting stents has had an important impact on clinical practice (Moses *et al.*, 2003; Stone *et al.*, 2004). Two drugs are currently being used in intravascular stents: *paclitaxel* (TAXOL) and *sirolimus* (RAPAMYCIN). Paclitaxel is a tricyclic diterpene that inhibits cellular proliferation by binding to and stabilizing polymerized microtubules. Sirolimus is a hydrophobic macrolide that binds to the cytosolic immunophilin FKBP12; the FKBP12–sirolimus complex inhibits the mammalian kinase target of RAPAMYCIN (mTOR), thereby inhibiting cell cycle progression (*see* Chapter 53). Paclitaxel and sirolimus differ markedly in their mechanisms of action but share common chemical properties as hydrophobic small molecules. Differences in the intracellular targets of these two drugs are associated with marked differences in their distribution in the vascular wall (Levin *et al.*, 2004). Stent-induced damage to the vascular endothelial cell layer can lead to thrombosis; patients typically are treated with antiplatelet agents, including clopidogrel (for up to 6 months) and aspirin (indefinitely), sometimes in conjunction with intravenously administered GPIIb/IIIa inhibitors. The inhibition of cellular proliferation by paclitaxel and sirolimus not only affects vascular smooth muscle cell proliferation but also attenuates the formation of an intact endothelial layer within the stented artery. Therefore, antiplatelet therapy (typically with clopidogrel)

is continued for several months after intracoronary stenting with drug-eluting stents. The rate of restenosis with drug-eluting stents is reduced markedly compared with "bare metal" stents, and the ongoing development of mechanopharmacological approaches likely will lead to novel approaches in intravascular therapeutics.

BIBLIOGRAPHY

Amende, I., Simon, R., Hood, W.P., Jr., Hetzer, R., and Lichtlen, P.R. Intracoronary nifedipine in human beings: Magnitude and time course of changes in left ventricular contraction/relaxation and coronary sinus blood flow. *J. Am. Coll. Cardiol.,* **1983,** 2:1141–1145.

Bauer, J.A., and Fung, H.L. Arterial versus venous metabolism of nitroglycerin to nitric oxide: A possible explanation of organic nitrate venoselectivity. *J. Cardiovasc. Pharmacol.,* **1996,** 28:371–374.

Bonow, R.O., Leon, M.B., Rosing, D.R., *et al.* Effects of verapamil and propranolol on left ventricular systolic function and diastolic filling in patients with coronary artery disease: Radionuclide angiographic studies at rest and during exercise. *Circulation,* **1982,** 65:1337–1350.

Breisblatt, W.M., Vita, N.A., Armuchastegui, M., Cohen, L.S., and Zaret, B.L. Usefulness of serial radionuclide monitoring during graded nitroglycerin infusion for unstable angina pectoris for determining left ventricular function and individualized therapeutic dose. *Am. J. Cardiol.,* **1988,** 61:685–690.

Brown, B.G., Bolson, E., Petersen, R.B., Pierce, C.D., and Dodge, H.T. The mechanisms of nitroglycerin action: Stenosis vasodilatation as a major component of the drug response. *Circulation,* **1981,** 64:1089–1097.

Burnett, A.L, Lowenstein, C.J., Bredt, D.S., Chang, T.S., and Snyder, S.H. Nitric oxide: A physiologic mediator of penile erection. *Science,* **1992,** 257:401–403.

Chaitman B.R., Pepine, C.J., Parker, J.O., *et al.* Effects of ranolazine with atenolol, amlodipine, or diltiazem on exercise tolerance and angina frequency in patients with severe chronic angina: A randomized, controlled trial. *JAMA* **2004,** 291:309–316.

Chen Z., Zhang, J., and Stamler, J.S. Identification of the enzymatic mechanism of nitroglycerin bioactivation. *Proc. Natl. Acad. Sci. U.S.A.,* **2002,** 99:8306–8311.

De Caterina, R., Giannessi, D., Mazzone, A., and Bernini, W. Mechanisms for the *in vivo* antiplatelet effects of isosorbide dinitrate. *Eur. Heart J.,* **1988,** 9(suppl A):45–49.

Deedwania, P.C., and Carbajal, E.V. Role of beta blockade in the treatment of myocardial ischemia. *Am. J. Cardiol.,* **1997,** 80:23J–28J.

Egstrup, K., and Andersen, P.E., Jr. Transient myocardial ischemia during nifedipine therapy in stable angina pectoris, and its relation to coronary collateral flow and comparison with metoprolol. *Am. J. Cardiol.,* **1993,** 71:177–183.

Feldman, R.L., Pepine, C.J., and Conti, C.R. Magnitude of dilatation of large and small coronary arteries of nitroglycerin. *Circulation,* **1981,** 64:324–333.

Fox, K.M., Mulcahy, D., Findlay, I., Ford, I., and Dargie, H.J. The Total Ischaemic Burden European Trial (TIBET): Effects of atenolol, nifedipine SR and their combination on the exercise test and the total ischaemic burden in 608 patients with stable angina. The TIBET Study Group. *Eur. Heart J.,* **1996,** 17:96–103.

Furberg, C.D., Psaty, B.M., and Meyer, J.V. Nifedipine: Dose-related increase in mortality in patients with coronary heart disease. *Circulation*, **1995**, *92*:1326–1331.

Furchgott, R.F. The discovery of endothelium-derived relaxing factor and its importance in the identification of nitric oxide. *JAMA*, **1996**, *276*:1186–1188.

Geelen, P., Drolet, B., Rail, J., *et al.* Sildenafil (VIAGRA) prolongs cardiac repolarization by blocking the rapid component of the delayed rectifier potassium current. *Circulation*, **2000**, *102*:275–277.

Göbel, E.J., Hautvast, R.W., van Gilst, W.H., *et al.* Randomised, double-blind trial of intravenous diltiazem versus glyceryl trinitrate for unstable angina pectoris. *Lancet*, **1995**, *346*:1653–1657.

Godfraind, T., Salomone, S., Dessy, C., *et al.* Selectivity scale of calcium antagonists in the human cardiovascular system based on *in vitro* studies. *J. Cardiovasc. Pharmacol.*, **1992**, *20*(suppl 5):S34–41.

Goldstein, I., Lue, T.F., Padma-Nathan, H., *et al.* Oral sildenafil in the treatment of erectile dysfunction. Sildenafil Study Group. *New Engl. J. Med.*, **1998**, *338*:1397–1404.

Heidenreich, P.A., McDonald, K.M., Hastie, T., *et al.* Meta-analysis of trials comparing beta-blockers, calcium antagonists, and nitrates for stable angina. *JAMA*, **1999**, *281*:1927–1936.

Herrmann, H.C., Chang, G., Klugherz, B.D., and Mahoney, P.D. Hemodynamic effects of sildenafil in men with severe coronary artery disease. *New Engl. J. Med.*, **2000**, *342*:1622–1626.

Lacoste, L.L., Theroux, P., Lidon, R.M., Colucci, R., and Lam, J.Y. Antithrombotic properties of transdermal nitroglycerin in stable angina pectoris. *Am. J. Cardiol.*, **1994**, *73*:1058–1062.

Lam, Y.T., Chesebro, J.H, and Fuster, V. Platelets, vasoconstriction, and nitroglycerin during arterial wall injury: A new antithrombotic role for an old drug. *Circulation*, **1988**, *78*:712–716.

Lehmann, G., Reiniger, G., Beyerle, A., and Rudolph, W. Pharmacokinetics and additional anti-ischaemic effectiveness of amlodipine, a once-daily calcium antagonist, during acute and long-term therapy of stable angina pectoris in patients pretreated with a beta-blocker. *Eur. Heart J.*, **1993**, *14*:1531–1535.

Levin, A.D., Vukmirovic, N., Hwang, C.W., and Edelman E.R. Specific binding to intracellular proteins determines arterial transport properties for rapamycin and paclitaxel. *Proc. Natl. Acad. Sci. U.S,A.*, **2004**, *101*:9463–9467.

Molina, C., Andresen, J.W., Rapoport, R.M., Waldman, S.A., and Murad, F. Effect of *in vivo* nitroglycerin therapy on endothelium-dependent and independent vascular relaxation and cyclic GMP accumulation in rat aorta. *J. Cardiovasc. Pharmacol.*, **1987**, *10*:371–378.

Moses J.W., Leon, M.B., Popma, J.J., *et al.* for the SIRIUS Investigators. Sirolimus-eluting stents versus standard stents in patients with stenosis in a native coronary artery. *New Engl. J. Med.*, **2003**, *349*:1315–1323.

Muller, J.E., Morrison, J., Stone, P.H., *et al.* Nifedipine therapy for patients with threatened and acute myocardial infarction: A randomized, double-blind, placebo-controlled comparison. *Circulation*, **1984**, *69*:740–747.

Münzel, T., Sayegh, H., Freeman, B.A., Tarpey, M.M., and Harrison, D.G. Evidence for enhanced vascular superoxide anion production in nitrate tolerance: A novel mechanism underlying tolerance and cross-tolerance. *J. Clin. Invest.*, **1995**, *95*:187–194.

Opie, L.H., Yusuf, S., and Kübler, W. Current status of safety and efficacy of calcium channel blockers in cardiovascular diseases: A critical analysis based on 100 studies. *Prog. Cardiovasc. Dis.*, **2000**, *43*:171–196.

Parker, J.D., Parker, A.B., Farrell, B., and Parker, J.O. Intermittent transdermal nitroglycerin therapy: Decreased anginal threshold during the nitrate-free interval. *Circulation*, **1995**, *91*:973–978.

Parker, J.D., Parker, A.B., Farrell, B., and Parker, J.O. Effects of diuretic therapy on the development of tolerance to nitroglycerin and exercise capacity in patients with chronic stable angina. *Circulation*, **1996**, *93*:691–696.

Paulus, W.J., Lorell, B.H., Craig, W.E., *et al.* Comparison of the effects of nitroprusside and nifedipine on diastolic properties in patients with hypertrophic cardiomyopathy: Altered left ventricular loading or improved muscle inactivation? *J. Am. Coll. Cardiol.*, **1983**, *2*:879–886.

Schwartz R.S., and Henry T.D. Pathophysiology of coronary artery restenosis. *Rev. Cardiovasc. Med.*, **2002**, *5*:S4–9.

Sellke, F.W., Myers, P.R., Bates, J.N., and Harrison, D.G. Influence of vessel size on the sensitivity of porcine coronary microvessels to nitroglycerin. *Am. J. Physiol.*, **1990**, *258*:H515–520.

Serruys, P.W., Hooghoudt, T.E., Reiger, J.H., *et al.* Influence of intracoronary nifedipine on left ventricular function, coronary vasomotility, and myocardial oxygen consumption. *Br. Heart. J.*, **1983**, *49*:427–441.

Stone, G W., Ellis, S.G., Cox, D.A., *et al.* The TAXUS-IV Investigators: A polymer-based, paclitaxel-eluting stent in patients with coronary artery disease. *New Engl. J. Med.*, **2004**, *350*:221–231.

Surks H.K., Mochizuki N., Kasai Y., *et al.* Regulation of myosin phosphatase by a specific interaction with cGMP-dependent protein kinase Iα. *Science*, **1999**, *286*:1583–1587.

Sydow, K., Daiber, A., Oelze, M., *et al.* Central role of mitochondrial aldehyde dehydrogenase and reactive oxygen species in nitroglycerin tolerance and cross-tolerance. *J. Clin. Invest.*, **2004**, *113*:482–489.

Thadani, U., Maranda, C.R., Amsterdam, E., *et al.* Lack of pharmacologic tolerance and rebound angina pectoris during twice-daily therapy with isosorbide-5-mononitrate. *Ann. Intern. Med.*, **1994**, *120*:353–359.

Tsien, R.W., Lipscombe, D., Madison, D.V., Bley, K.R., and Fox, A.P. Multiple types of neuronal calcium channels and their selective modulation. *Trends Neurosci.*, **1988**, *11*:431–438.

Wallis, R.M., Corbin, J.D., Francis, S.H., and Ellis, P. Tissue distribution of phosphodiestase families and the effects of sildenafil on tissue cyclic nucleotides, platelet function, and the contractile responses of trabeculae carneae and aortic rings *in vitro*. *Am. J. Cardiol.*, **1999**, *83*:3C–12C.

Walsh, R.A., and O'Rourke, R.A. Direct and indirect effects of calcium entry blocking agents on isovolumic left ventricular relaxation in conscious dogs. *J. Clin. Invest.*, **1985**, *75*:1426–1434.

Webb, D.J., Freestone, S., Allen, M.J., and Muirhead, G.J. Sildenafil citrate and blood-pressure-lowering drugs: Results of drug interaction studies with an organic nitrate and a calcium antagonist. *Am. J. Cardiol.*, **1999**, *83*:21C–28C.

Yusuf, S. Calcium antagonists in coronary artery disease and hypertension: Time for reevaluation? *Circulation*, **1995**, *92*:1079–1082.

Yusuf, S., Sleight, P., Pogue, J., *et al.* Effects of an angiotensin-converting enzyme inhibitor, ramipril, on cardiovascular events in high-risk patients. The Heart Outcomes Prevention Evaluation Study Investigators. *New Engl J. Med.*, **2000**, *342*:145–153.

MONOGRAPHS AND REVIEWS

Abernethy, D.R., and Schwartz, J.B. Calcium-antagonist drugs. *New Engl. J. Med.*, **1999**, *341*:1447–1457.

Antman, E.M., Anbe, D.R., Armstrong, P.W., *et al.* ACC/AHA guidelines for the management of patients with ST-elevation myocardial infarction—executive summary: A report of the American College of Cardiology/American Heart Association Task Force on Practice Guidelines (Writing Committee to Revise the 1999 Guidelines for the Management of Patients with Acute Myocardial Infarction). *Circulation*, **2004**, *110*:588–636.

Beavo, J.A., Conti, M., and Heaslip, R.J. Multiple cyclic nucleotide phosphodiesterases. *Mol. Pharmacol.*, **1994**, *46*:399–405.

Berridge, M.J. Inositol trisphosphate and calcium signalling. *Nature*, **1993**, *361*:315–325.

Bhatt, D.L., and Topol, E.J. Current role of platelet glycoprotein IIb/IIIa inhibitors in acute coronary syndromes. *JAMA*, **2000**, *284*:1549–1558.

Braunwald, E., Antman, E.M., Beasley, J.W., *et al.* and the American College of Cardiology and American Heart Association. ACC/AHA 2002 guideline update for the management of patients with unstable angina and non-ST-segment elevation myocardial infarction—summary article: A report of the American College of Cardiology/American Heart Association Task Force on Practice Guidelines (Committee on the Management of Patients with Unstable Angina). *J. Am. Coll. Cardiol.*, **2002**, *40*:1366–1374.

Cheitlin, M.D., Hutter, A.M., Jr., Brindis, R.G., *et al.* ACC/AHA expert consensus document: Use of sildenafil (VIAGRA) in patients with cardiovascular disease. American College of Cardiology/American Heart Association. *J. Am. Coll. Cardiol.*, **1999**, *33*:273–282.

Dudzinski D., Igarashi J., Greif, D. and Michel, T. The regulation and pharmacology of endothelial nitric oxide synthase. *Annu. Rev. Pharmacol. Toxicol.*, **2005**.

Friesinger, G.C., and Robertson, R.M. Vasospastic angina: A continuing search for mechanism(s). *J. Am. Coll. Cardiol.*, **1986**, *7*:30–31.

Gibbons, R.J., Abrams, J. Chatterjee, K., *et al.* ACC/AHA guideline update for the management of patients with chronic stable angina—summary article: A report of the American College of Cardiology/American Heart Association Task Force on practice guidelines. **2002;** available at *www.acc.org/clinical/guidelines/stable/stable*.

Gibbons, R.J., Chatterjee, K., Daley, J., *et al.* ACC/AHA/ACP-ASIM guidelines for the management of patients with chronic stable angina: A report of the American College of Cardiology/American Heart Association Task Force on Practice Guidelines. *J. Am. Coll. Cardiol.*, **1999**, *33*:2092–2197.

Godfraind, T., Miller, R., and Wibo, M. Calcium antagonism and calcium entry blockade. *Pharmacol. Rev.*, **1986**, *38*:321–416.

Hiatt, W.R. Medical treatment of peripheral arterial disease and claudication. *New Engl. J. Med.*, **2001**, *344*:1608–1621.

Hockerman, G.H., Peterson, B.Z., Johnson, B.D., and Catterall, W.A. Molecular determinants of drug binding and action on L-type calcium channels. *Annu. Rev. Pharmacol. Toxicol.*, **1997**, *37*:361–396.

Ignarro, L.J., Buga, G.M., Wood, K.S., Byrns, R.E., and Chaudhuri, G. Endothelium-derived relaxing factor produced and released from artery and vein is nitric oxide. *Proc. Natl. Acad. Sci. U.S.A.*, **1987**, *84*:9265–9269.

Julian, D.G. Symposium: Concluding remarks. *Am. J. Cardiol.*, **1987**, *59*:37J.

Lange, R.A, and Hillis, L.D. Antiplatelet therapy for ischemic heart disease. *New Engl. J. Med.*, **2004**, *350*:277–280.

Libby P., Ridker P.M., and Maseri A. Inflammation and atherosclerosis. *Circulation.*, **2002**, *105*:1135–1143.

Lowenstein, C.J., Dinerman, J.L., and Snyder, S.H. Nitric oxide: A physiologic messenger. *Ann. Intern. Med.*, **1994**, *120*:227–237.

Münzel, T., Kurz, S., Heitzer, T., and Harrison, D.G. New insights into mechanisms underlying nitrate tolerance. *Am. J. Cardiol.*, **1996**, *77*:24C–30C.

Murad, F. The 1996 Albert Lasker Medical Research Awards: Signal transduction using nitric oxide and cyclic guanosine monophosphate. *JAMA*, **1996**, *276*:1189–1192.

Parker, J.D. Nitrate tolerance, oxidative stress and mitochondrial function: Another worrisome chapter on the effects of organic nitrates. *J. Clin. Invest.*, **2004**, *113*:352–354.

Parker, J.D., and Parker, J.O. Nitrate therapy for stable angina pectoris. *New Engl. J. Med.*, **1998**, *338*:520–531.

Regensteiner, J.G., and Hiatt, W.R. Current medical therapies for patients with peripheral arterial disease: A critical review. *Am. J. Med.*, **2002**, *112*:49–57.

Rutherford, J.D. Nitrate tolerance in angina therapy: How to avoid it. *Drugs*, **1995**, *49*:196–199.

Schwartz, A. Molecular and cellular aspects of calcium channel antagonism. *Am. J. Cardiol.*, **1992**, *70*:6F–8F.

Stamler, J.S., Lamas, S., and Fang, F.C. Nitrosylation, the prototypic redox-based signaling mechanism. *Cell*, **2001**, *106*:675–683.

Taira, N. Differences in cardiovascular profile among calcium antagonists. *Am. J. Cardiol.*, **1987**, *59*:24B–29B.

Taylor, S.H. Usefulness of amlodipine for angina pectoris. *Am. J. Cardiol.*, **1994**, *73*:28A–33A.

Thadani, U. Role of nitrates in angina pectoris. *Am. J. Cardiol.*, **1992**, *70*:43B–53B.

Todd, P.A., and Faulds, D. Felodipine: A review of the pharmacology and therapeutic uses of the extended release formulation in cardiovascular disorders. *Drugs*, **1992**, *44*:251–277.

van Zwieten, P.A., and Pfaffendorf, M. Similarities and differences between calcium antagonists: Pharmacological aspects. *J. Hypertens. Suppl.*, **1993**, *11*:S3–11.

Waldman, S.A., and Murad, F. Cyclic GMP synthesis and function. *Pharmacol. Rev.*, **1987**, *39*:163–196.

Waters, D. Proischemic complications of dihydropyridine calcium channel blockers. *Circulation*, **1991**, *84*:2598–2600.

Yeghiazarians, Y., Braunstein, J.B., Askari, A., and Stone, P.H. Unstable angina pectoris. *New Engl. J. Med.*, **2000**, *342*:101–114.

Zusman, R.M., Morales, A., Glasser, D.B., and Osterloh, I.H. Overall cardiovascular profile of sildenafil citrate. *Am. J. Cardiol.*, **1999**, *83*:35C–44C.

THERAPY OF HYPERTENSION

Brian B. Hoffman

Hypertension is the most common cardiovascular disease. The prevalence of hypertension increases with advancing age; for example, about 50% of people between the ages of 60 and 69 years old have hypertension, and the prevalence is further increased beyond age 70 (Chobanian *et al.*, 2003).

Elevated arterial pressure causes pathological changes in the vasculature and hypertrophy of the left ventricle. As a consequence, hypertension is the principal cause of stroke, is a major risk factor for coronary artery disease and its attendant complications myocardial infarction and sudden cardiac death, and is a major contributor to cardiac failure, renal insufficiency, and dissecting aneurysm of the aorta.

Hypertension is defined conventionally as a sustained increase in blood pressure ≥140/90 mm Hg, a criterion that characterizes a group of patients whose risk of hypertension-related cardiovascular disease is high enough to merit medical attention. Actually, the risk of both fatal and nonfatal cardiovascular disease in adults is lowest with systolic blood pressures of less than 120 mm Hg and diastolic BP less than 80 mm Hg; these risks increase progressively with higher systolic and diastolic blood pressures. Recognition of this continuously increasing risk provides a simple definition of hypertension (Chobanian *et al.*, 2003) (Table 32–1). Although many of the clinical trials classify the severity of hypertension by diastolic pressure, progressive elevations of systolic pressure are similarly predictive of adverse cardiovascular events; at every level of diastolic pressure, risks are greater with higher levels of systolic blood pressure. Indeed, beyond age 50 years, systolic blood pressure predicts outcome better than diastolic blood pressure. Systolic blood pressure tends to rise disproportionately greater in the elderly due to decreased compliance in blood vessels associated with

aging and atherosclerosis. Isolated systolic hypertension (sometimes defined as systolic BP >140 to 160 mm Hg with diastolic BP <90 mm Hg) is largely confined to people >60 years of age.

At very high blood pressures (systolic ≥210 and/or diastolic ≥120 mm Hg), a subset of patients develops fulminant arteriopathy characterized by endothelial injury and a marked proliferation of cells in the intima, leading to intimal thickening and ultimately to arteriolar occlusion. This is the pathological basis of the syndrome of immediately life-threatening hypertension, which is associated with rapidly progressive microvascular occlusive disease in the kidney (with renal failure), brain (hypertensive encephalopathy), congestive heart failure, and pulmonary edema. These patients typically require in-hospital management on an emergency basis for prompt lowering of blood pressure. Interestingly, isolated retinal changes with papilledema in an otherwise asymptomatic patient with very high blood pressure (formerly called "malignant hypertension") may benefit from a more gradual lowering of blood pressure over days rather than hours.

The presence of pathologic changes in certain target organs heralds a worse prognosis than the same level of blood pressure in a patient lacking these findings. Thus, retinal hemorrhages, exudates, and papilledema indicate a far worse short-term prognosis for a given level of blood pressure. Left ventricular hypertrophy defined by electrocardiogram, or more sensitively by echocardiography, is associated with a substantially worse long-term outcome that includes a higher risk of sudden cardiac death. The risk of cardiovascular disease, disability, and death in hypertensive patients also is increased markedly by concomitant cigarette smoking, diabetes, or elevated low-density lipoprotein; the coexistence of hypertension with these risk factors increases cardiovascular morbidity and mortality to a degree that is compounded by each additional risk factor. Since the purpose of treating hypertension is to decrease cardiovascular risk, other dietary and pharmacological interventions may be required.

Pharmacological treatment of patients with hypertension associated with elevated diastolic pressures reduces morbidity and mortality from cardiovascular disease. Effective antihypertensive therapy markedly reduces the

Table 32–1
Criteria for Hypertension in Adults

	BLOOD PRESSURE (MM HG)	
CLASSIFICATION	*Systolic*	*Diastolic*
Normal	<120	and <80
Pre-hypertension	120–139	or 80–89
Hypertension, stage 1	140–159	or 90–99
Hypertension, stage 2	≥160	or ≤100

risk of strokes, cardiac failure, and renal insufficiency due to hypertension. However, reduction in risk of myocardial infarction may be less impressive.

Principles of Antihypertensive Therapy. Nonpharmacological therapy is an important component of treatment of all patients with hypertension. In some stage 1 hypertensives, blood pressure may be adequately controlled by a combination of weight loss (in overweight individuals), restricting sodium intake, increasing aerobic exercise, and moderating consumption of alcohol. These lifestyle changes, though difficult for many to implement, may facilitate pharmacological control of blood pressure in patients whose responses to lifestyle changes alone are insufficient.

Arterial pressure is the product of cardiac output and peripheral vascular resistance. Drugs lower blood pressure by actions on peripheral resistance, cardiac output, or both. Drugs may reduce the cardiac output by inhibiting myocardial contractility or by decreasing ventricular filling pressure. Reduction in ventricular filling pressure may be achieved by actions on the venous tone or on blood volume *via* renal effects. Drugs can reduce peripheral resistance by acting on smooth muscle to cause relaxation of resistance vessels or by interfering with the activity of systems that produce constriction of resistance vessels (*e.g.,* the sympathetic nervous system). In patients with isolated systolic hypertension, complex hemodynamics in a rigid arterial system contribute to increased blood pressure; drug effects may be mediated by changes in peripheral resistance but also *via* effects on large artery stiffness (Franklin, 2000). Antihypertensive drugs can be classified according to their sites or mechanisms of action (Table 32–2).

The hemodynamic consequences of long-term treatment with antihypertensive agents (Table 32–3) provide a rationale for potential complementary effects of concur-

Table 32–2
Classification of Antihypertensive Drugs by Their Primary Site or Mechanism of Action

Diuretics (Chapter 28)
  1. Thiazides and related agents (hydrochlorothiazide, chlorthalidone, *etc.*)
  2. Loop diuretics (furosemide, bumetanide, torsemide, ethacrynic acid)
  3. K^+-sparing diuretics (amiloride, triamterene, spironolactone)
Sympatholytic drugs (Chapters 9, 10, and 33)
  1. β Adrenergic antagonists (metoprolol, atenolol, *etc.*)
  2. α Adrenergic antagonists (prazosin, terazosin, doxazosin, phenoxybenzamine, phentolamine)
  3. Mixed adrenergic antagonists (labetalol, carvedilol)
  4. Centrally acting agents (methyldopa, clonidine, guanabenz, guanfacine)
  5. Adrenergic neuron blocking agents (guanadrel, reserpine)
Ca^{2+} channel blockers (Chapters 31 through 34) (verapamil, diltiazem, nimodipine, felodipine, nicardipine, isradipine, amlodipine)
Angiotensin converting enzyme inhibitors (Chapters 30 and 31), (captopril, enalapril, lisinopril, quinapril, ramipril, benazepril, fosinopril, moexipril, perindopril, trandolapril)
Angiotensin II–receptor antagonists (Chapters 30 and 33) (losartan, candesartan, irbesartan, valsartan, telmisartan, eprosartan)
Vasodilators (Chapter 33)
  1. Arterial (hydralazine, minoxidil, diazoxide, fenoldopam)
  2. Arterial and venous (nitroprusside)

rent therapy with two or more drugs. The simultaneous use of drugs with similar mechanisms of action and hemodynamic effects often produces little additional benefit. However, concurrent use of drugs from different classes is a strategy for achieving effective control of blood pressure while minimizing dose-related adverse effects.

It is generally not possible to predict the responses of individuals with hypertension to any specific drug. For example, for some antihypertensive drugs, on average about two-thirds of patients will have a meaningful clinical response, whereas about one-third of patients will not respond to the same drug. There is considerable interest in identifying genetic variation in order to improve selection of antihypertensive drugs in individual patients.

Table 32–3
Hemodynamic Effects of Long-Term Administration of Antihypertensive Agents

	HEART RATE	CARDIAC OUTPUT	TOTAL PERIPHERAL RESISTANCE	PLASMA VOLUME	PLASMA RENIN ACTIVITY
Diuretics	↔	↔	↓	–↓	↑
Sympatholytic agents					
Centrally acting	–↓	–↓	↓	–↑	–↓
Adrenergic neuron blockers	–↓	↓	↓	↑	–↑
α Adrenergic antagonists	–↑	–↑	↓	–↑	↔
β Adrenergic antagonists					
No ISA[*]	↓	↓	–↓	–↑	↓
ISA	↔	↔	↓	–↑	–↓
Arteriolar vasodilators	↑	↑	↓	↑	↑
Ca^{2+} channel blockers	↓ or ↑	↓ or ↑	↓	–↑	–↑
ACE inhibitors	↔	↔	↓	↔	↑
AT_1–receptor antagonists	↔	↔	↓	↔	↑

Changes are indicated as follows: ↑, increased; ↓, decreased; –↑, increased or no change; –↓, decreased or no change; ↔, unchanged. [*]ISA, intrinsic sympathomimetic activity. ACE, angiotensin converting enzyme; AT_1, the type 1 receptor for angiotensin II.

Polymorphisms in a number of genes involved in the metabolism of antihypertensive drugs have been identified, for example in the CYP family (phase I metabolism) and in phase II metabolism, such as catechol-O-methyltransferase. While these polymorphisms change the pharmacokinetics of specific drugs, it is not clear that there will be substantial differences in efficacy given the dose range available clinically for these drugs. Consequently, identification of polymorphisms that influence pharmacodynamic responses to antihypertensive drugs are of considerable interest. Polymorphisms influencing the actions of a number of classes of antihypertensive drugs, including angiotensin-converting enzyme inhibitors and diuretics, have been identified; so far, individual genes have not been found to have a major impact on pharmacodynamic responses. Genome-wide scanning may lead to identification of novel genes that are more clinically significant. Likewise, treatment may profit from an understanding of the molecular and genetic bases of hypertension (Garbers and Dubois, 1999).

DIURETICS

An early strategy for the management of hypertension was to alter Na^+ balance by restriction of salt in the diet. Pharmacological alteration of Na^+ balance became practical with the development of the orally active thiazide diuretics (*see* Chapter 28). These and related diuretic agents have antihypertensive effects when used alone, and they enhance the efficacy of virtually all other antihypertensive drugs. On account of these considerations, coupled with the very large favorable experience with

diuretics in randomized trials in patients with hypertension, this class of drugs remains very important in the treatment of hypertension.

The exact mechanism for reduction of arterial blood pressure by diuretics is not certain. Initially, the drugs decrease extracellular volume by interacting with a thiazide-sensitive Na-Cl cotransporter in the kidney, leading to a fall in cardiac output. However, the hypotensive effect is maintained during long-term therapy because of reduced vascular resistance; cardiac output returns to pretreatment values and extracellular volume returns almost to normal due to compensatory responses such as activation of the renin-angiotensin system. How this occurs is unknown; however, thiazides promote vasodilation in isolated vessels from laboratory animals and humans.

Hydrochlorothiazide may open Ca^{2+}-activated K^+ channels, leading to hyperpolarization of vascular smooth muscle cells, which leads in turn to closing of L-type Ca^{2+} channels and lower probability of opening, resulting in decreased Ca^{2+} entry and reduced vasoconstriction (Pickkers and Hughes, 1995). Hydrochlorothiazide also inhibits vascular carbonic anhydrase, which hypothetically may alter smooth-cell systolic pH and thereby cause opening of Ca^{2+}-activated K^+ channels with the consequences noted above (Pickkers *et al.*, 1999). The relevance of this intriguing finding to the observed antihypertensive effects of thiazides is speculative.

Benzothiadiazines and Related Compounds

Benzothiadiazines ("thiazides") and related diuretics are the most frequently used class of antihypertensive agents in the United States. Following the discovery of *chlorothiazide*, a number of oral diuretics were developed that have an aryl-sulfonamide structure and block the Na$^+$-Cl$^-$ cotransporter. Some of these are not benzothiadiazines but have structural features and molecular functions that are similar to the original benzothiadiazine compounds; thus, they are designated as members of the thiazide class of diuretics. For example, *chlorthalidone*, one of the nonbenzothiadiazines, is widely used in the treatment of hypertension. Because members of the thiazide class have the same pharmacological effects, they are generally interchangeable with appropriate adjustment of dosage (*see* Chapter 28). However, since the pharmacokinetics and pharmacodynamics of these drugs may differ, they may not necessarily have the same clinical efficacy in treating hypertension (Carter *et al.*, 2004).

Regimen for Administration of the Thiazide-Class Diuretics in Hypertension. When a thiazide-class diuretic is utilized as the sole antihypertensive drug (monotherapy), its dose-response curve for lowering blood pressure in patients with hypertension should be kept in mind. Antihypertensive effects can be achieved in many patients with as little as 12.5 mg of chlorthalidone (HYGROTON) or hydrochlorothiazide (HYDRODIURIL) daily. Furthermore, when used as monotherapy, the maximal daily dose of thiazide-class diuretics usually should not exceed 25 mg of hydrochlorothiazide or chlorthalidone (or equivalent). Even though more diuresis can be achieved with higher doses of these diuretics, evidence indicates that doses higher than this are not generally more efficacious in patients with normal renal function. These doses of hydrochlorothiazide are not at the top of the dose-response curve for adverse effects such as K$^+$ wasting and inhibition of uric acid excretion (*see* below), emphasizing the importance of knowledge about the dose-response relationships for both beneficial and adverse effects.

A large study comparing 25 and 50 mg of hydrochlorothiazide daily in an elderly population did not show a greater decrease in blood pressure with the larger dose (Medical Research Council Working Party, 1987). In the clinical trials of antihypertensive therapy in the elderly that demonstrated the best outcomes in cardiovascular morbidity and mortality, 25 mg of hydrochlorothiazide or chlorthalidone was the maximum dose given; if this dose did not achieve the target blood pressure reduction, treatment with a second drug was initiated (SHEP Cooperative Research Group, 1991; Dahlöf *et al.*, 1991; Medical Research Council Working Party, 1992). With respect to safety, a case-control study (Siscovick *et al.*, 1994) found a dose-dependent increase in the occurrence of sudden death at doses of hydrochlorothiazide greater than 25 mg daily. This finding supports the hypothesis proposed by the Multiple Risk Factor Intervention Trial Research Group (1982), suggesting that increased cardiovascular mortality is associated with higher diuretic doses. Taken together, clinical studies indicate that if adequate blood pressure reduction is not achieved with the 25-mg daily dose of hydro-

chlorothiazide or chlorthalidone, a second drug should be added rather than increasing the dose of diuretic. There is some concern that thiazide diuretics, especially at higher doses and in the absence of K$^+$-sparing diuretics or K$^+$ supplements, may increase the risk of sudden death. However, their overall therapeutic benefits are well established.

Urinary K$^+$ loss can be a problem with thiazides. Angiotensin converting enzyme (ACE) inhibitors and angiotensin receptor antagonists will attenuate diuretic-induced loss of potassium to some degree, and this is a consideration if a second drug is required to achieve further blood pressure reduction beyond that attained with the diuretic alone. Because the diuretic and hypotensive effects of these drugs are greatly enhanced when they are given in combination, care should be taken to initiate combination therapy with low doses of each of these drugs. Administration of ACE inhibitors or angiotensin receptor antagonists together with other K$^+$-sparing agents or with K$^+$ supplements requires great caution; combining K$^+$-sparing agents with each other or with K$^+$ supplementation can cause potentially dangerous hyperkalemia in some patients.

In contrast to the limitation on the dose of thiazide-class diuretics used as monotherapy, the treatment of severe hypertension that is unresponsive to three or more drugs may require larger doses of the thiazide-class diuretics. Indeed, hypertensive patients may become refractory to drugs that block the sympathetic nervous system or to vasodilator drugs, because these drugs engender a state in which the blood pressure is very volume-dependent. Therefore, it is appropriate to consider the use of thiazide-class diuretics in doses of 50 mg of daily hydrochlorothiazide equivalent when treatment with appropriate combinations and doses of three or more drugs fails to yield adequate control of the blood pressure. Alternatively, there may be a need to use higher-capacity diuretics such as *furosemide*, especially if renal function is not normal, in some of these patients. Dietary Na$^+$ restriction is a valuable adjunct to the management of such refractory patients and will minimize the dose of diuretic that is required. This can be achieved by a modest restriction of Na$^+$ intake to 2 g daily. More stringent Na$^+$ restriction is not feasible for most patients. Since the degree of K$^+$ loss relates to the amount of Na$^+$ delivered to the distal tubule, such restriction of Na$^+$ can minimize the development of hypokalemia and alkalosis. The effectiveness of thiazides as diuretics or antihypertensive agents is progressively diminished when the glomerular filtration rate falls below 30 ml/min. One exception is *metolazone*, which retains efficacy in patients with this degree of renal insufficiency.

Most patients will respond to thiazide diuretics with a reduction in blood pressure within about 4 weeks, although a minority will not achieve maximum reduction in arterial pressure for up to 12 weeks on a given dose. Therefore, doses should not be increased more often than every 4 to 6 weeks. There is no way to predict the antihypertensive response from the duration or severity of the hypertension in a given patient, although diuretics are unlikely to be effective as sole therapy in patients with stage 2 hypertension. Since the effect of thiazide diuretics is additive with that of other antihypertensive drugs, combination regimens that include these diuretics are common and rational. Diuretics also have the advantage of minimizing the retention of salt and water that is commonly caused by vasodilators and some sympatholytic drugs. Omitting or underutilizing a diuretic is a frequent cause of "resistant hypertension."

Adverse Effects and Precautions. The adverse effects of diuretics are discussed in Chapter 28. Some of these determine whether patients can tolerate and adhere to diuretic treatment. Erectile dysfunction is a troublesome adverse effect of the thiazide-class diuretics, and physicians should inquire specifically regarding its occurrence in conjunction with treatment with these drugs. Gout may be a consequence of the hyperuricemia induced by these diuretics. The occurrence of either of these adverse effects is a reason for considering alternative approaches to therapy. However, precipitation of acute gout is relatively uncommon with low doses of diuretics. Hydrochlorothiazide may cause rapidly developing, severe hyponatremia in some patients. Thiazides inhibit renal Ca^{2+} excretion, occasionally leading to hypercalcemia; although generally mild, this can be more severe in patients subject to hypercalcemia, such as those with primary hyperparathyroidism. The thiazide-induced decreased Ca^{2+} excretion may be used therapeutically in patients with osteoporosis or hypercalciuria.

Some other effects of thiazide diuretics are laboratory observations that are of concern primarily because they are putative *surrogate markers* for adverse drug effects on morbidity and mortality. *See* Chapter 5 for a discussion of the utility and problem of surrogate markers.

The effects of diuretic drugs on several surrogate markers for adverse outcomes merit consideration. The K^+ depletion produced by thiazide-class diuretics is dose-dependent and is variable among individuals, such that a subset of patients may become substantially K^+ depleted on diuretic drugs. Given chronically, even small doses lead to some K^+ depletion.

There are two types of ventricular arrhythmias that are thought to be enhanced by K^+ depletion. One of these is polymorphic ventricular tachycardia (*torsades de pointes*), which is induced by a number of drugs, including *quinidine*. Drug-induced polymorphic ventricular tachycardia is initiated by abnormal ventricular repolarization; because K^+

currents normally mediate repolarization, drugs that produce K^+ depletion potentiate polymorphic ventricular tachycardia. Accordingly, thiazide diuretics should not be given together with drugs that can cause polymorphic ventricular tachycardia (*see* Chapter 34).

The most important concern regarding K^+ depletion is its influence on ischemic ventricular fibrillation, the leading cause of sudden cardiac death and a major contributor to cardiovascular mortality in treated hypertensive patients. Studies in experimental animals have demonstrated that K^+ depletion lowers the threshold for electrically induced ventricular fibrillation in the ischemic myocardium and also increases spontaneous ischemic ventricular fibrillation (Curtis and Hearse, 1989). There is a positive correlation between diuretic dose and sudden cardiac death, and an inverse correlation between the use of adjunctive K^+-sparing agents and sudden cardiac death (Siscovick *et al.*, 1994). One controlled clinical trial demonstrated a significantly greater occurrence of sudden cardiac death in patients treated with 50 mg of hydrochlorothiazide daily in comparison with the β adrenergic receptor antagonist *metoprolol* (Medical Research Council Working Party, 1992).

Thiazide diuretics have been associated with changes in plasma lipids and glucose tolerance that have led to some concern. The clinical significance of the changes has been disputed. Nonetheless, recent clinical studies continue to demonstrate the efficacy of the thiazide diuretics in reducing cardiovascular risk (ALLHAT Officers, 2002).

All of the thiazide-like drugs cross the placenta, but they have not been shown to have direct adverse effects on the fetus. However, if administration of a thiazide is begun during pregnancy, there is a risk of transient volume depletion that may result in placental hypoperfusion. Since the thiazides appear in breast milk, they should be avoided by nursing mothers.

Other Diuretic Antihypertensive Agents

The thiazide diuretics are more effective antihypertensive agents than are the loop diuretics, such as furosemide and *bumetanide*, in patients who have normal renal function. This differential effect is most likely related to the short duration of action of loop diuretics, such that a single daily dose does not cause a significant net loss of Na^+ for an entire 24-hour period. Indeed, loop diuretics are frequently and inappropriately prescribed as a once-a-day medication in the treatment not only of hypertension, but also of congestive heart failure and ascites. The spectacular efficacy of the loop diuretics in producing a rapid and profound natriuresis can be detrimental for the treatment of hypertension. When a loop diuretic is given twice daily, the acute diuresis can be excessive and lead to more side effects than occur with a slower-acting, milder thiazide diuretic. Loop diuretics may be particularly useful in patients with azotemia or with severe edema associated with a vasodilator such as *minoxidil*.

Amiloride is a K⁺-sparing diuretic that has some efficacy in lowering blood pressure in patients with hypertension. *Spironolactone* also lowers blood pressure but has some significant adverse effects, especially in men (*e.g.*, impotence, gynecomastia, and benign prostatic hyperplasia). As a result of their capacity to inhibit loss of K⁺ in the urine, these drugs are used in the medical treatment of patients with hyperaldosteronism, a syndrome that can lead to hypokalemia. *Triamterene* is a K⁺-sparing diuretic that decreases the risk of hypokalemia in patients treated with a thiazide diuretic, but does not have efficacy in lowering blood pressure by itself. These agents should be used cautiously with frequent measurements of K⁺ concentrations in plasma in patients predisposed to hyperkalemia. Patients taking spironolactone, amiloride, or triamterene should be cautioned regarding the possibility that concurrent use of K⁺-containing salt substitutes could produce hyperkalemia. Renal insufficiency is a relative contraindication to the use of K⁺-sparing diuretics. *Concomitant use of an ACE inhibitor or an angiotensin-receptor antagonist magnifies the risk of hyperkalemia with these agents.*

Diuretic-Associated Drug Interactions

Since the antihypertensive effects of diuretics are frequently additive with those of other antihypertensive agents, a diuretic commonly is used in combination with other drugs. The K⁺- and Mg²⁺-depleting effects of the thiazides and loop diuretics also can potentiate arrhythmias that arise from *digitalis* toxicity. Corticosteroids can amplify the hypokalemia produced by the diuretics. All diuretics can decrease the clearance of Li⁺, resulting in increased plasma concentrations of Li⁺ and potential toxicity. Nonsteroidal antiinflammatory drugs (*see* Chapter 26) that inhibit the synthesis of prostaglandins reduce the antihypertensive effects of diuretics. The effects of selective cyclooxygenase-2 (COX-2) inhibitors on renal prostaglandin synthesis and function are similar to those of the traditional nonsteroidal antiinflammatory drugs. Nonsteroidal antiinflammatory drugs, β adrenergic receptor antagonists, and ACE inhibitors reduce plasma concentrations of aldosterone and can potentiate the hyperkalemic effects of a K⁺-sparing diuretic.

SYMPATHOLYTIC AGENTS

With the demonstration in 1940 that bilateral excision of the thoracic sympathetic chain could lower blood pressure, there was a search for effective chemical sympatholytic agents. Many of the early sympathetic drugs were poorly tolerated and had adverse side effects. A number of sympathetic agents are currently in use (Table 32–2). Antagonists of α and β adrenergic receptors are mainstays of antihypertensive therapy.

β Adrenergic Receptor Antagonists

β Adrenergic receptor antagonists were not expected to have antihypertensive effects when they were first investigated in patients with angina, their primary indication. However, *pronethalol*, a drug that was never marketed, was found to reduce arterial blood pressure in hypertensive patients with angina pectoris. This antihypertensive effect was subsequently demonstrated for *propranolol* and all other β adrenergic receptor antagonists. The pharmacology of these drugs is discussed in Chapter 10; characteristics relevant to their use in hypertension are described here.

Locus and Mechanism of Action. Antagonism of β adrenergic receptors affects the regulation of the circulation through a number of mechanisms, including a reduction in myocardial contractility, heart rate, and cardiac output. An important consequence of using β adrenergic receptors is blockade of the β receptors of the juxtaglomerular complex, reducing renin secretion and thereby diminishing production of circulating angiotensin II. This action likely contributes to the antihypertensive action of this class of drugs, in concert with the cardiac effects. β Adrenergic receptor antagonists may lower blood pressure by other mechanisms, including alteration of the control of the sympathetic nervous system at the level of the CNS, altered baroreceptor sensitivity, altered peripheral adrenergic neuron function, and increased *prostacyclin* biosynthesis. Because all β adrenergic receptor antagonists are effective antihypertensive agents and (+)-propranolol, the inactive isomer that has little β adrenergic receptor blocking activity, has no effect on blood pressure, the antihypertensive therapeutic effect of these agents is undoubtedly related to receptor blockade.

Pharmacological Effects. The β adrenergic blockers vary in their lipid solubility, selectivity for the β_1 adrenergic receptor subtype, presence of partial agonist or intrinsic sympathomimetic activity, and membrane-stabilizing properties. Despite these differences, all of the β adrenergic receptor antagonists are effective as antihypertensive agents. However, these differences do influence the clinical pharmacokinetics and spectrum of adverse effects of the various drugs. Drugs without intrinsic sympathomimetic activity produce an initial reduction in cardiac output and a reflex-induced rise in peripheral resistance, generally with no net change in arterial pressure. In patients who respond with a reduction in blood pressure, peripheral resistance gradually returns to pretreatment values or less. Generally, persistently reduced cardiac output and possibly decreased peripheral resistance accounts for the reduction in arterial pressure. Drugs with intrinsic sympathomimetic activity produce lesser decreases in resting heart rate and cardiac output; the fall in arterial pressure correlates with a fall in vascular resistance below pretreatment levels, possibly because of stimulation of vascular β_2 adrenergic receptors that mediate vasodilation. The clinical significance, if any, of these differences is unknown.

Adverse Effects and Precautions. The adverse effects of β adrenergic blocking agents are discussed in Chapter 10. These drugs should be avoided in patients with reactive airway disease (asthma) or with sinoatrial or atrioventricular (AV) nodal dysfunction or in combination with other drugs that inhibit AV conduction, such as *verapamil*. Patients with insulin-dependent diabetes also are better treated with other drugs.

β Receptor antagonists without intrinsic sympathomimetic activity increase concentrations of triglycerides in plasma and lower those of HDL cholesterol without changing total cholesterol concentrations. β Adrenergic blocking agents with intrinsic sympathomimetic activity have little or no effect on blood lipids or increase HDL cholesterol. The long-term consequences of these effects are unknown.

Sudden discontinuation of some β adrenergic blockers can produce a withdrawal syndrome that is likely due to up-regulation of β receptors during blockade, causing enhanced tissue sensitivity to endogenous catecholamines; this can exacerbate the symptoms of coronary artery disease. The result, especially in active patients, can be rebound hypertension. Thus, β adrenergic blockers should not be discontinued abruptly except under close observation; dosage should be tapered over 10 to 14 days prior to discontinuation.

Nonsteroidal antiinflammatory drugs such as *indomethacin* can blunt the antihypertensive effect of propranolol and probably other β receptor antagonists. This effect may be related to inhibition of vascular synthesis of prostacyclin, as well as to retention of Na^+ (Beckmann *et al.*, 1988).

Epinephrine can produce severe hypertension and bradycardia when a nonselective β receptor antagonist is present. The hypertension is due to the unopposed stimulation of α adrenergic receptors when vascular $β_2$ receptors are blocked; the bradycardia is the result of reflex vagal stimulation. Such paradoxical hypertensive responses to β adrenergic receptor antagonists have been observed in patients with hypoglycemia or pheochromocytoma, during withdrawal from *clonidine*, following administration of epinephrine as a therapeutic agent, or in association with the illicit use of cocaine.

Therapeutic Uses. The β receptor antagonists provide effective therapy for all grades of hypertension. Despite marked differences in their pharmacokinetic properties, the antihypertensive effect of all the β blockers is of sufficient duration to permit once or twice daily administration. Populations that tend to have a lesser antihypertensive response to β-blocking agents include the elderly and African-Americans. However, intraindividual differences in antihypertensive efficacy are generally much larger than statistical evidence of differences between racial or age-related groups. Consequently, these observations should not discourage the use of these drugs in individual patients in groups reported to be less responsive.

The β receptor antagonists do not usually cause retention of salt and water, and administration of a diuretic is not necessary to avoid edema or the development of tolerance. However, diuretics do have additive antihypertensive effects when combined with β blockers. The combination of a β receptor antagonist, a diuretic, and a vasodilator is effective for patients who require a third drug. β Adrenergic receptor antagonists are highly preferred drugs for hypertensive patients with conditions such as myocardial infarction, ischemic heart disease, or congestive heart failure.

$α_1$ Adrenergic Antagonists

The availability of drugs that selectively block $α_1$ adrenergic receptors without affecting $α_2$ adrenergic receptors adds another group of antihypertensive agents. The pharmacology of these drugs is discussed in detail in Chapter 10. *Prazosin* (MINIPRESS), *terazosin* (HYTRIN), and *doxazosin* (CARDURA) are the agents that are available for the treatment of hypertension.

Pharmacological Effects. Initially, $α_1$ adrenergic receptor antagonists reduce arteriolar resistance and increase venous capacitance; this causes a sympathetically mediated reflex increase in heart rate and plasma renin activity. During long-term therapy, vasodilation persists, but cardiac output, heart rate, and plasma renin activity return to normal. Renal blood flow is unchanged during therapy with an $α_1$ receptor antagonist. The $α_1$ adrenergic blockers cause a variable amount of postural hypotension, depending on the plasma volume. Retention of salt and water occurs in many patients during continued administration, and this attenuates the postural hypotension. $α_1$ Receptor antagonists reduce plasma concentrations of triglycerides and total LDL cholesterol and increase HDL cholesterol. These potentially favorable effects on lipids persist when a thiazide-type diuretic is given concurrently. The long-term consequences of these small, drug-induced changes in lipids are unknown.

Adverse Effects. The use of doxazosin as monotherapy for hypertension increased the risk for developing congestive heart failure (ALLHAT Officers, 2002). This may be a class effect that represents an adverse effect of all of the α_1 adrenergic receptor antagonists. However, this interpretation of the outcome of the ALLHAT study is controversial.

A major precaution regarding the use of the α_1 receptor antagonists for hypertension is the so-called first-dose phenomenon, in which symptomatic orthostatic hypotension occurs within 90 minutes of the initial dose of the drug or after a dosage increase. This effect may occur in up to 50% of patients, especially in patients who are already receiving a diuretic or an α receptor antagonist. After the first few doses, patients develop a tolerance to this marked hypotensive response.

Therapeutic Uses. α_1 Receptor antagonists are not recommended as monotherapy for hypertensive patients. Thus, they are used primarily in conjunction with diuretics, β blockers, and other antihypertensive agents. β Receptor antagonists enhance the efficacy of the α_1 blockers. α_1 Receptor antagonists are not the drugs of choice in patients with pheochromocytoma, because a vasoconstrictor response to epinephrine can still result from activation of unblocked vascular α_2 adrenergic receptors. α_1 Receptor antagonists are attractive drugs for hypertensive patients with benign prostatic hyperplasia, since they also improve urinary symptoms.

Combined α_1 and β Adrenergic Receptor Antagonists

Labetalol (NORMODYNE, TRANDATE) (*see* Chapter 10) is an equimolar mixture of four stereoisomers. One isomer is an α_1 antagonist (like prazosin), another is a nonselective β antagonist with partial agonist activity (like *pindolol*), and the other two isomers are inactive. Because of its capacity to block α_1 adrenergic receptors, labetalol given intravenously can reduce pressure sufficiently rapidly to be useful for the treatment of hypertensive emergencies. Labetalol has efficacy and side effects that would be expected with any combination of β and α_1 receptor antagonists; it also has the disadvantages that are inherent in fixed-dose combination products: the extent of α receptor antagonism compared to β receptor antagonism is somewhat unpredictable and varies from patient to patient.

Carvedilol (COREG) (*see* Chapters 10 and 33) is a β receptor antagonist with α_1 receptor antagonist activity. The drug has been approved for the treatment of hypertension and symptomatic heart failure. The ratio of α_1 to β receptor antagonist potency for carvedilol is approximately 1:10. Carvedilol undergoes oxidative metabolism and glucuronidation in the liver; the oxidative metabolism occurs *via* CYP2D6. Carvedilol reduces mortality in patients with systolic dysfunction and heart failure when used as an adjunct to therapy with diuretics and ACE inhibitors. It should not be given to those patients with decompensated heart failure who are dependent on sympathetic stimulation. As with labetalol, the long-term efficacy and side effects of carvedilol in hypertension are predictable based on its properties as a β and α_1 adrenergic receptor antagonist.

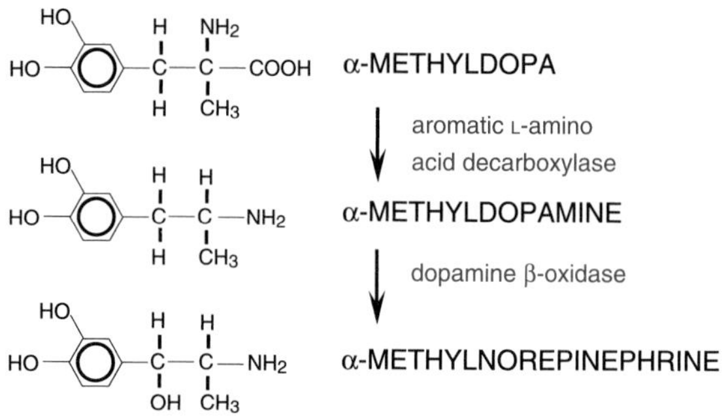

Figure 32–1. **The metabolism of methyldopa in adrenergic neurons. α-Methylnorepinephrine replaces norepinephrine in neurosecretory vesicles.**

Methyldopa

Methyldopa (ALDOMET) is a centrally acting antihypertensive agent. It is a prodrug that exerts its antihypertensive action *via* an active metabolite. Although used frequently as an antihypertensive agent in the past, methyldopa's significant adverse effects limit its current use in the United States to treatment of hypertension in pregnancy, where it has a record for safety.

Methyldopa (α-methyl-3,4-dihydroxy-L-phenylalanine), an analog of 3,4-dihydroxyphenylalanine (DOPA), is metabolized by the L-aromatic amino acid decarboxylase in adrenergic neurons to α-methyldopamine, which then is converted to α-methylnorepinephrine (Figure 32–1). α-Methylnorepinephrine is stored in the secretory vesicles of adrenergic neurons, substituting for norepinephrine (NE) itself. Thus, when the adrenergic neuron discharges its neurotransmitter, α-methylnorepinephrine is released instead of norepinephrine.

Because α-methylnorepinephrine is as potent as norepinephrine as a vasoconstrictor, its substitution for norepinephrine in peripheral adrenergic neurosecretory vesicles does not alter the vasoconstrictor response to peripheral adrenergic neurotransmission. Rather, α-methylnorepinephrine acts in the CNS to inhibit adrenergic neuronal outflow from the brainstem. Methylnorepinephrine probably acts as an agonist at presynaptic α_2 adrenergic receptors in the brainstem, attenuating NE release and thereby reducing the output of vasoconstrictor adrenergic signals to the peripheral sympathetic nervous system.

A body of evidence supports the conclusion that methyldopa acts in the brain *via* an active metabolite to lower blood pressure (Bobik *et al.*, 1988; Granata *et al.*, 1986; Reid, 1986). In experimental animals, the hypotensive effect of methyldopa is blocked by DOPA decarboxylase inhibitors that have access to the brain, but not by inhibitors that are excluded from the CNS. The hypotensive effect also is abolished by inhibitors of dopamine β-hydroxylase and by centrally acting α adrenergic receptor antagonists. Small doses of methyldopa that do not lower blood pressure when injected systemically elicit a hypotensive effect when injected into the vertebral artery. Selective microinjection of α-methylnorepinephrine into the C-1 area of the rostral ventrolateral medulla of the rat elicits a hypotensive response that is prevented by nonselective α receptor blockade and by α_2 receptor blockade. Presumably, methylnorepinephrine inhibits neurons in this area that are responsible for maintaining tonic discharge of peripheral sympathetic nerves and for transmission of baroreflex-initiated tone. The excess α adrenergic inhibition of sympathetic output may reflect the accumulation of methylnorepinephrine in quantities larger than the norepinephrine that it displaces. This model is feasible because methylnorepinephrine is not a substrate for monoamine oxidase, the enzyme principally responsible for norepinephrine degradation in the brain. In addition to inhibiting sympathetic output in the C-1 area of the rostral ventrolateral medulla, methylnorepinephrine may also exert inhibitory effects at other sites such as the solitary tract nucleus.

Pharmacological Effects.

Methyldopa reduces vascular resistance without causing much change in cardiac output or heart rate in younger patients with uncomplicated essential hypertension. In older patients, however, cardiac output may be decreased as a result of decreased heart rate and stroke volume; this is secondary to relaxation of veins and a reduction in preload. The fall in arterial pressure is maximal 6 to 8 hours after an oral or intravenous dose. Although the decrease in supine blood pressure is less than that in the upright position, symptomatic orthostatic hypotension is less common with methyldopa than with drugs that act exclusively on peripheral adrenergic neurons or autonomic ganglia; this is because methyldopa attenuates but does not completely block baroreceptor-mediated vasoconstriction. For this reason, it is well tolerated during surgical anesthesia. Any severe hypotension is reversible with volume expansion. Renal blood flow is maintained and renal function is unchanged during treatment with methyldopa.

Plasma concentrations of norepinephrine fall in association with the reduction in arterial pressure, and this reflects the decrease in sympathetic tone. Renin secretion also is reduced by methyldopa, but this is not a major effect of the drug and is not necessary for its hypotensive effects. Salt and water often are gradually retained with prolonged use of methyldopa, and this tends to blunt the antihypertensive effect. This has been termed "pseudotolerance," and can be overcome with concurrent use of a diuretic.

Absorption, Metabolism, and Excretion.

Since methyldopa is a prodrug that is metabolized in the brain to the active form, its concentration in plasma has less relevance for its effects than that for many other drugs. When administered orally, methyldopa is absorbed by an active amino acid transporter. Peak concentrations in plasma occur after 2 to 3 hours. The drug is distributed in a relatively small apparent volume (0.4 liter/kg) and is eliminated with a half-life of about 2 hours. The transport of methyldopa into the CNS is apparently also an active process. Methyldopa is excreted in the urine primarily as the sulfate conjugate (50% to 70%) and as the parent drug (25%). The remaining fraction is excreted as other metabolites, including methyldopamine, methylnorepinephrine, and O-methylated products of these catecholamines. The half-life of methyldopa is prolonged to 4 to 6 hours in patients with renal failure.

In spite of its rapid absorption and short half-life, the peak effect of methyldopa is delayed for 6 to 8 hours, even after intravenous administration, and the duration of action of a single dose is usually about 24 hours; this permits once- or twice-daily dosing. The discrepancy between the effects of methyldopa and the measured concentrations of the drug in plasma is most likely related to the time required for transport into the CNS, conversion to the active metabolite storage of α-methyl norepinephrine and its subsequent release in the vicinity of relevant α_2 receptors in the CNS. This is a good example of the potential for a complex relationship between a drug's pharmacokinetics and its pharmacodynamics. Patients with renal failure are more sensitive to the antihypertensive effect of methyldopa, but it is not known if this is due to alteration in excretion of the drug or to an increase in transport into the CNS.

Adverse Effects and Precautions.

In addition to lowering blood pressure, the active metabolite of methyldopa acts on α_2 adrenergic receptors in the brainstem to inhibit the centers that are responsible for wakefulness and alertness. Thus, methyldopa produces sedation that is largely transient. A diminution in psychic energy may persist in some patients, and depression occurs occasionally. Medullary centers that control salivation also are inhibited by α adrenergic receptors, and methyldopa may produce dryness of the mouth. Other side effects that are related to the pharmacological effects in the CNS include a reduction in libido, parkinsonian signs, and hyperprolactinemia that may become sufficiently pronounced to cause gynecomastia and galactorrhea. It seems possible that accumulation of α-methyldopamine in dopaminergic neurons could account for some central effects. In individuals who have sinoatrial node dysfunction, methyldopa may precipitate severe bradycardia and sinus arrest, including that which occurs with carotid sinus hypersensitivity.

Methyldopa also produces some adverse effects that are not related to its pharmacological action. Hepatotoxicity, sometimes associated with fever, is an uncommon but potentially serious toxic effect of methyldopa. Prompt diagnosis of hepatotoxicity requires a low threshold for considering the drug as a cause for hepatitis-like symptoms (*e.g.,* nausea, anorexia) and screening for hepatotoxicity (*e.g.,* with determination of hepatic transaminases) after 3 weeks and again 3 months after initiation of treatment. The incidence of methyldopa-induced hepatitis is unknown, but about 5% of patients will have transient increases in hepatic transaminases in plasma. Hepatic dysfunction usually is reversible with prompt discontinuation of the drug, but will recur if methyldopa is given again; a few cases of fatal hepatic necrosis have been reported. It is advisable to avoid the use of methyldopa in patients with hepatic disease.

Methyldopa can cause hemolytic anemia. At least 20% of patients who receive methyldopa for a year develop a positive Coombs test (antiglobulin test) that is due to autoantibodies directed against the Rh antigen on erythrocytes. The development of a positive Coombs test is not necessarily an indication to stop treatment with methyldopa; 1% to 5% of these patients will develop a hemolytic anemia that requires prompt discontinuation of the drug. The Coombs test may remain positive for as long as a year after discontinuation of methyldopa, but the hemolytic anemia usually resolves within a matter of weeks. Severe hemolysis may be attenuated by treatment with glucocorticoids. Adverse effects that are even more rare include leukopenia, thrombocytopenia, red cell aplasia, lupus erythematosus–like syndrome, lichenoid and granulomatous skin eruptions, myocarditis, retroperitoneal fibrosis, pancreatitis, diarrhea, and malabsorption.

Therapeutic Uses. Methyldopa is an effective antihypertensive agent that has been replaced by other drugs in many parts of the world. Methyldopa is a preferred drug for treatment of hypertension during pregnancy based on its effectiveness and safety for both mother and fetus.

The usual initial dose of methyldopa is 250 mg twice daily, and there is little additional effect with doses above 2 g per day. Administration of a single daily dose of methyldopa at bedtime minimizes sedative effects, but administration twice daily is required for some patients.

Clonidine, Guanabenz, and Guanfacine

The detailed pharmacology of the α_2 adrenergic agonists clonidine (CATAPRES), *guanabenz* (WYTENSIN), and *guanfacine* (TENEX) is discussed in Chapter 10. These drugs stimulate the α_{2A} subtype of α_2 adrenergic receptors in the brainstem, resulting in a reduction in sympathetic outflow from the CNS (Macmillan *et al.*, 1996). The decrease in plasma concentrations of norepinephrine

is correlated directly with the hypotensive effect (Goldstein *et al.*, 1985; Sorkin and Heel, 1986). Patients who have had a spinal cord transection above the level of the sympathetic outflow tracts do not display a hypotensive response to clonidine. At doses higher than those required to stimulate central α_{2A} receptors, these drugs can activate α_2 receptors of the α_{2B} subtype on vascular smooth muscle cells (Link *et al.*, 1996; MacMillan *et al.*, 1996). This effect accounts for the initial vasoconstriction that is seen when overdoses of these drugs are taken, and it has been postulated to be responsible for the loss of therapeutic effect that is observed with high doses (Frisk-Holmberg *et al.*, 1984; Frisk-Holmberg and Wibell, 1986). A major limitation in the use of these drugs is the paucity of information about their efficacy in reducing the risk of cardiovascular consequences of hypertension.

Pharmacological Effects. The α_2 adrenergic agonists lower arterial pressure by an effect on both cardiac output and peripheral resistance. In the supine position, when the sympathetic tone to the vasculature is low, the major effect is to reduce both heart rate and stroke volume; however, in the upright position, when sympathetic outflow to the vasculature is normally increased, these drugs reduce vascular resistance. This action may lead to postural hypotension. The decrease in cardiac sympathetic tone leads to a reduction in myocardial contractility and heart rate; this could promote congestive heart failure in susceptible patients.

Adverse Effects and Precautions. Many patients experience annoying and sometimes intolerable adverse effects with these drugs. Sedation and xerostomia are prominent adverse effects. The xerostomia may be accompanied by dry nasal mucosa, dry eyes, and parotid gland swelling and pain. Postural hypotension and erectile dysfunction may be prominent in some patients. Clonidine may produce a lower incidence of dry mouth and sedation when given transdermally, perhaps because high peak concentrations are avoided. Less common CNS side effects include sleep disturbances with vivid dreams or nightmares, restlessness, and depression. Cardiac effects related to the sympatholytic action of these drugs include symptomatic bradycardia and sinus arrest in patients with dysfunction of the sinoatrial node and AV block in patients with AV nodal disease or in patients taking other drugs that depress AV conduction. Some 15% to 20% of patients who receive transdermal clonidine may develop contact dermatitis.

Sudden discontinuation of clonidine and related α_2 adrenergic agonists may cause a withdrawal syndrome consisting of headache, apprehension, tremors, abdominal pain, sweating, and tachycardia. The arterial blood pressure may rise to levels above those that were present prior to treatment, but the syndrome may occur in the absence of an overshoot in pressure. Symptoms typically occur 18 to 36 hours after the drug is stopped and are associated with increased sympathetic discharge, as evidenced by elevated plasma and urine concentrations of catecholamines. The exact incidence of the withdrawal syndrome is not known, but it is likely dose related and more dangerous in patients with poorly controlled hypertension. Rebound hypertension also has been seen after discontinuation of transdermal administration of clonidine (Metz *et al.*, 1987).

Treatment of the withdrawal syndrome depends on the urgency of reducing the arterial blood pressure. In the absence of life-threatening target organ damage, patients can be treated by restoring the use of clonidine. If a more rapid effect is required, *sodium nitroprusside* or a combination of an α and β adrenergic blocker is appropriate. β Adrenergic blocking agents should not be used alone in this setting, since they may accentuate the hypertension by allowing unopposed α adrenergic vasoconstriction caused by activation of the sympathetic nervous system and elevated circulating catecholamines.

Because perioperative hypertension has been described in patients in whom clonidine was withdrawn the night before surgery, surgical patients who are being treated with an α_2 adrenergic agonist either should be switched to another drug prior to elective surgery or should receive their morning dose and/or transdermal clonidine prior to the procedure. All patients who receive one of these drugs should be warned of the potential danger of discontinuing the drug abruptly, and patients suspected of being nonadherent with medications should not be given α_2 adrenergic agonists for hypertension.

Adverse drug interactions with α_2 adrenergic agonists are rare. Diuretics predictably potentiate the hypotensive effect of these drugs. Tricyclic antidepressants may inhibit the antihypertensive effect of clonidine, but the mechanism of this interaction is not known.

Therapeutic Uses. The CNS effects are such that this class of drugs is not a leading option for monotherapy of hypertension. Indeed, there is no fixed place for these drugs in the treatment of hypertension. They effectively lower blood pressure in some patients who have not responded adequately to combinations of other agents. Enthusiasm for these drugs is diminished by the relative absence of evidence demonstrating reduction in risk of adverse cardiovascular events.

Clonidine has been used in hypertensive patients for the diagnosis of pheochromocytoma. The lack of suppression of the plasma concentration of norepinephrine to less than 500 pg/ml 3 hours after an oral dose of 0.3 mg of clonidine suggests the presence of such a tumor. A modification of this test, wherein overnight urinary excretion of norepinephrine and epinephrine is measured

after administration of a 0.3-mg dose of clonidine at bedtime, may be useful when results based on plasma norepinephrine concentrations are equivocal. Other uses for α_2 adrenergic agonists are discussed in Chapters 10, 13, and 23.

Guanadrel

Guanadrel (HYLOREL) specifically inhibits the function of peripheral postganglionic adrenergic neurons. The structure of guanadrel, which contains the strongly basic guanidine group, is:

GUANADREL

Locus and Mechanism of Action. Guanadrel is an exogenous false neurotransmitter that is accumulated, stored, and released like norepinephrine but is inactive at adrenergic receptors. The drug reaches its site of action by active transport into the neuron by the same transporter that is responsible for the reuptake of norepinephrine (*see* Chapter 6). In the neuron, guanadrel is concentrated within the adrenergic storage vesicle, where it replaces norepinephrine. During chronic administration, guanadrel acts as a "false neurotransmitter": it is present in storage vesicles, depletes the normal transmitter, can be released by stimuli that normally release norepinephrine but is inactive at adrenergic receptors. This replacement of norepinephrine with an inactive transmitter is probably the principal mechanism of action of guanadrel.

When given intravenously, guanadrel initially releases norepinephrine in an amount sufficient to increase arterial blood pressure. This is not noticeable with oral administration, since norepinephrine is released only slowly from the vesicles under this circumstance and is degraded within the neuron by monoamine oxidase. Nonetheless, because of the potential for norepinephrine release, guanadrel is contraindicated in patients with pheochromocytoma.

During adrenergic neuron blockade with guanadrel, effector cells become supersensitive to norepinephrine. The supersensitivity is similar to that produced by postganglionic sympathetic denervation.

Pharmacological Effects. Essentially all of the therapeutic and adverse effects of guanadrel result from functional sympathetic blockade. The antihypertensive effect is achieved by a reduction in peripheral vascular resistance that results from inhibition of α receptor–mediated vasoconstriction. Consequently, arterial pressure is reduced modestly in the supine position when sympathetic activity is usually low, but the pressure can fall to a greater extent during situations in which reflex sympathetic activation is a mechanism for maintaining arterial pressure, such as assumption of the upright posture, exercise, and depletion of plasma volume. Plasma volume often expands, which may diminish the antihypertensive efficacy of guanadrel and require administration of diuretic to restore the anti-hypertensive effect.

Absorption, Distribution, Metabolism, and Excretion. Guanadrel is rapidly absorbed, leading to maximal levels in plasma at 1 to 2 hours. Because guanadrel must be transported into and accumulate in adrenergic neurons, the maximum effect on blood pressure is not seen until 4 to 5 hours. Although the β phase of its elimination has an estimated half-life of 5 to 10 hours, this almost certainly does not reflect the longer half-life of drug stored at its site of action in the secretory vesicles of adrenergic neurons. The half-life of the pharmacological effect of guanadrel is determined by the drug's persistence in this neuronal pool and is probably at least 10 hours. Guanadrel is administered in a regimen of twice-daily doses.

Guanadrel is cleared from the body by both renal and nonrenal disposition. Its elimination is impaired in patients with renal insufficiency; total-body clearance was reduced by four- to fivefold in a group of patients with a creatinine clearance averaging 13 ml per minute.

Adverse Effects. Guanadrel produces undesirable effects that are related entirely to sympathetic blockade. Symptomatic hypotension during standing, exercise, ingestion of alcohol, or hot weather is the result of the lack of sympathetic compensation for these stresses. A general feeling of fatigue and lassitude is partially, but not entirely, related to postural hypotension. Sexual dysfunction usually presents as delayed or retrograde ejaculation. Diarrhea also may occur.

Because guanadrel is actively transported to its site of action, drugs that block or compete for the catecholamine transporter on the presynaptic membrane will inhibit the effect of guanadrel. Such drugs include the tricyclic antidepressants, *cocaine, chlorpromazine, ephedrine, phenylpropanolamine,* and *amphetamine* (*see* Chapter 6).

Therapeutic Uses. Because of the availability of a number of drugs that lower blood pressure without producing this degree of orthostatic hypotension, guanadrel is not employed in the monotherapy of hypertension and is used chiefly as an additional agent in patients who have not achieved a satisfactory antihypertensive effect on multiple other agents. The need to use this drug arises very rarely. The usual starting dose is 10 mg daily, and side effects can be minimized by not exceeding 20 mg daily.

Reserpine

Reserpine was the first drug that was found to interfere with the function of the sympathetic nervous system in human beings, and its use began the modern era of effective pharmacotherapy of hypertension.

Reserpine is an alkaloid extracted from the root of *Rauwolfia serpentina*, a climbing shrub indigenous to India. Ancient Hindu Ayurvedic writings describe medicinal uses of the plant; Sen and Bose described its use in the Indian biomedical literature. However, rauwolfia alkaloids were not used in western medicine until the mid-1950s. The structure of reserpine is:

RESERPINE

Locus and Mechanism of Action. Reserpine binds tightly to adrenergic storage vesicles in central and peripheral adrenergic neurons and remains bound for prolonged periods of time. The interaction inhibits the vesicular catecholamine transporter that facilitates vesicular storage. Thus, nerve endings lose their capacity to concentrate and store norepinephrine and dopamine. Catecholamines leak into the cytoplasm, where they are metabolized by intraneuronal monoamine oxidase, and little or no active transmitter is discharged from nerve endings when they are depolarized. The overall result is a pharmacological sympathectomy. A similar process occurs at storage sites for 5-hydroxytryptamine. Reserpine-induced depletion of biogenic amines correlates with evidence of sympathetic dysfunction and antihypertensive effects. Recovery of sympathetic function requires synthesis of new storage vesicles, which takes days to weeks after discontinuation of the drug. Since reserpine depletes amines in the CNS as well as in the peripheral adrenergic neuron, it is probable that its antihypertensive effects are related to both central and peripheral actions.

Pharmacological Effects. Both cardiac output and peripheral vascular resistance are reduced during long-term therapy with reserpine. Orthostatic hypotension may occur but does not usually cause symptoms. Heart rate and renin secretion fall. Salt and water are retained, which commonly results in "pseudotolerance."

Absorption, Metabolism, and Excretion. Few data are available on the pharmacokinetic properties of reserpine because of the lack of an assay capable of detecting low concentrations of the drug or its metabolites. Reserpine that is bound to isolated storage vesicles cannot be removed by dialysis, indicating that the binding is not in equilibrium with the surrounding medium. Because of the irreversible nature of reserpine binding, the amount of drug in plasma is unlikely to bear any consistent relationship to drug concentration at the site of action. Free reserpine is entirely metabolized; none of the parent drug is excreted unchanged.

Toxicity and Precautions. Most adverse effects of reserpine are due to its effect on the CNS. Sedation and inability to concentrate or perform complex tasks are the most common adverse effects. More serious is the occasional psychotic depression that can lead to suicide. Depression usually appears insidiously over many weeks or months and may not be attributed to the drug because of the delayed and gradual onset of symptoms. Reserpine must be discontinued at the first sign of depression; reserpine-induced depression may last several months after the drug is discontinued. The risk of depression is likely dose related. Depression appears to be uncommon, but not unknown, with doses of 0.25 mg per day or less. The drug should never be given to patients with a history of depression. Other adverse effects include nasal stuffiness and exacerbation of peptic ulcer disease, which is uncommon with small oral doses.

Therapeutic Uses. With the availability of newer drugs that are both effective and well tolerated, the use of reserpine has diminished because of its CNS side effects. Nonetheless, there has been some recent interest in using reserpine at low doses, in combination with diuretics, in the treatment of hypertension, especially in the elderly. Reserpine is used once daily with a diuretic, and several weeks are necessary to achieve a maximum effect. The daily dose should be limited to 0.25 mg or less, and as little as 0.05 mg per day may be efficacious when a diuretic is also used. One advantage of reserpine is that it is considerably less expensive than other antihypertensive drugs; thus, it is still used in developing nations.

Metyrosine

Metyrosine (DEMSER) is (–)-α-methyl-L-tyrosine. It has the structure shown below. Metyrosine inhibits tyrosine hydroxylase, the enzyme that catalyzes the conversion of tyrosine to DOPA and the rate-limiting step in catecholamine biosynthesis (*see* Chapter 6). At a dose of 1 to 4 g per day, metyrosine decreases catecholamine biosynthesis by 35% to 80% in patients with pheochromocytoma. The maximal decrease in synthesis occurs only after several days and may be assessed by measurements of urinary catecholamines and their metabolites.

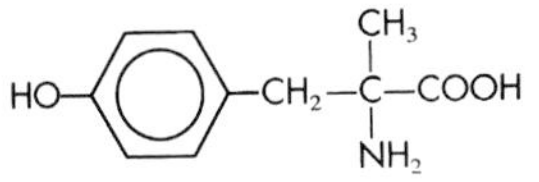

$$HO-\langle \rangle-CH_2-\overset{\overset{\displaystyle CH_3}{|}}{\underset{\underset{\displaystyle NH_2}{|}}{C}}-COOH$$

METYROSINE

Metyrosine is used as an adjuvant to *phenoxybenzamine* and other α adrenergic blocking agents for the management of malignant pheochromocytoma and in the preoperative preparation of patients for resection of pheochromocytoma. Metyrosine carries a risk of crystalluria, which can be minimized by maintaining a daily urine volume of more than 2 liters. Other adverse effects include orthostatic hypotension, sedation, extrapyramidal signs, diarrhea, anxiety, and psychic disturbances. Doses must be titrated carefully to achieve significant inhibition of catecholamine biosynthesis and yet minimize these substantive side effects.

CA²⁺ CHANNEL ANTAGONISTS

Ca^{2+} channel blocking agents are an important group of drugs for the treatment of hypertension. The general pharmacology of these drugs is presented in Chapter 31; their use in heart failure is discussed in Chapter 33; and their use in cardiac arrhythmias is covered in Chapter 34. Verapamil was the first clinically available calcium-channel blocker; it is a congener of *papaverine*. Many other calcium entry blockers with a wide range of structures are now available. The largest group, including *amlodipine, felodipine, isradipine*, and *nifedipine*, are termed dihydropyridines. *Diltiazem* is, with verapamil, the other

non-dihydropyridine available clinically. Interestingly, these different structures lead to differences in their sites and modes of action on calcium entry for reasons that are not well understood. Intracellular calcium flux is a final common path for a spectrum of cellular responses to a wide variety of stimuli. Given that the molecular basis of calcium channels is quite heterogeneous, coupled with the chemical heterogeneity of available calcium-channel blockers, the pharmacologic similarities of presently available dihydropyridines may mask differences in action that could be significant in terms of efficacy or adverse effects. The basis for their use in hypertension comes from the understanding that hypertension is generally the result of increased peripheral vascular resistance. Since contraction of vascular smooth muscle is dependent on the free intracellular concentration of Ca^{2+}, inhibition of transmembrane movement of Ca^{2+} through voltage-sensitive Ca^{2+} channels can decrease the total amount of Ca^{2+} that reaches intracellular sites. Ca^{2+}-calmodulin-dependent activation of myosin light chain kinase, resulting in phosphorylation of myosin light chains, causes an increase in actin-myosin ATPase activity and contraction (*see* Chapter 1). Indeed, all of the Ca^{2+} channel blockers lower blood pressure by relaxing arteriolar smooth muscle and decreasing peripheral vascular resistance (Weber, 2002). As a consequence of a decrease in peripheral vascular resistance, the Ca^{2+} channel blockers evoke a baroreceptor-mediated sympathetic discharge. In the case of the dihydropyridines, tachycardia may occur from the adrenergic stimulation of the sinoatrial node; this response is generally quite modest except when the drug is administered rapidly. Tachycardia is typically minimal to absent with verapamil and diltiazem because of the direct negative chronotropic effect of these two drugs. Indeed, the concurrent use of a β receptor antagonist drug may magnify negative chronotropic effects of these drugs or cause heart block in susceptible patients. Consequently, the concurrent use of β receptor antagonists with either verapamil or diltiazem may be problematic.

All Ca^{2+} channel blockers are effective when used alone for the treatment of mild to moderate hypertension; however, this class of drug is not currently viewed as appropriate for monotherapy of hypertension (Chobanian *et al.*, 2003). Patients with isolated systolic hypertension are an exception (*see* below).

The profile of adverse reactions to the Ca^{2+} channel blockers varies among the drugs in this class. Patients receiving immediate-release capsules of nifedipine develop headache, flushing, dizziness, and peripheral edema. However, short-acting formulations of nifedipine are not appropriate in the long-term treatment of hypertension.

Dizziness and flushing are much less of a problem with the sustained-release formulations and with the dihydropyridines having a long half-life and relatively constant concentrations of drug in plasma. The peripheral edema is not the result of generalized fluid retention; it most likely results from increased hydrostatic pressure in the lower extremities owing to precapillary dilation and reflex postcapillary constriction. Some other adverse effects of these drugs are due to actions in nonvascular smooth muscle. Contraction of the lower esophageal sphincter is inhibited by the Ca^{2+} channel blockers. For example, Ca^{2+} channel blockers can cause or aggravate gastroesophageal reflux. Constipation is a common side effect of verapamil, but it occurs less frequently with other Ca^{2+} channel blockers. Urinary retention is a rare adverse effect. Inhibition of sinoatrial node function by diltiazem and verapamil can lead to bradycardia and even sinoatrial node arrest, particularly in patients with sinoatrial node dysfunction; this effect is exaggerated by concurrent use of β adrenergic receptor antagonists.

Oral administration of nifedipine as an approach to urgent reduction of blood pressure has been abandoned. Sublingual administration does not achieve the maximum plasma concentration any more quickly than does oral administration. Moreover, in the absence of deleterious consequences of high arterial pressure, data do not support the rapid lowering of blood pressure. There is no place in the treatment of hypertension for the use of nifedipine or other dihydropyridine Ca^{2+} channel blockers with short half-lives when administered in a standard (immediate-release) formulation, because of the oscillation in blood pressure and concurrent surges in sympathetic reflex activity within each dosage interval.

Compared with other classes of antihypertensive agents, there is a greater frequency of achieving blood pressure control with Ca^{2+} channel blockers as monotherapy in elderly subjects and in African-Americans, population groups in which the low renin status is more prevalent. However, intrasubject variability is more important than relatively small differences between population groups. Ca^{2+} channel blockers are effective in lowering blood pressure and decreasing cardiovascular events in the elderly with isolated systolic hypertension (Staessen *et al.*, 1997). Indeed, these drugs may be a preferred treatment in these patients.

Significant drug-drug interactions may be encountered when Ca^{2+} channel blockers are used to treat hypertension. Verapamil blocks the P-glycoprotein drug transporter. Both the renal and hepatic disposition of *digoxin* occurs *via* this transporter. Accordingly, verapamil inhibits the elimination of digoxin and other drugs that are cleared from the body by the P-glycoprotein (*see* Chapter 2). When used with quinidine, Ca^{2+} channel blockers may cause excessive hypotension, particularly in patients with idiopathic hypertrophic subaortic stenosis.

ANGIOTENSIN-CONVERTING ENZYME INHIBITORS

Angiotensin II is an important regulator of cardiovascular function (*see* Chapter 30). The ability to reduce levels of angiotensin II with orally effective inhibitors of angiotensin-converting enzyme (ACE) represents an important advance in the treatment of hypertension. *Captopril* (CAPOTEN) was the first such agent to be developed for the treatment of hypertension. Since then, *enalapril* (VASOTEC), *lisinopril* (PRINIVIL), *quinapril* (ACCUPRIL), *ramipril* (ALTACE), *benazepril* (LOTENSIN), *moexipril* (UNIVASC), *fosinopril* (MONOPRIL), *trandolapril* (MAVIK), and *perindopril* (ACEON) also have become available. These drugs have proven to be very useful for the treatment of hypertension because of their efficacy and their very favorable profile of adverse effects, which enhances patient adherence. Chapter 30 presents the pharmacology of ACE inhibitors in detail.

The ACE inhibitors appear to confer a special advantage in the treatment of patients with diabetes, slowing the development and progression of diabetic glomerulopathy. They also are effective in slowing the progression of other forms of chronic renal disease, such as glomerulosclerosis, and many of these patients also have hypertension. An ACE inhibitor is the preferred initial agent in these patients. Patients with hypertension and ischemic heart disease are candidates for treatment with ACE inhibitors; administration of ACE inhibitors in the immediate post–myocardial infarction period has been shown to improve ventricular function and reduce morbidity and mortality (*see* Chapter 33).

The endocrine consequences of inhibiting the biosynthesis of angiotensin II are of importance in a number of facets of hypertension treatment. Because ACE inhibitors blunt the rise in aldosterone concentrations in response to Na^+ loss, the normal role of aldosterone to oppose diuretic-induced natriuresis is diminished. Consequently, ACE inhibitors tend to enhance the efficacy of diuretic drugs. This means that even very small doses of diuretics may substantially improve the antihypertensive efficacy of ACE inhibitors; conversely, the use of high doses of diuretics together with ACE inhibitors may lead to excessive reduction in blood pressure and to Na^+ loss in some patients.

The attenuation of aldosterone production by ACE inhibitors also influences K^+ homeostasis. There is only a very small and clinically unimportant rise in serum K^+ when these agents are used alone in patients with normal renal function. However, substantial retention of K^+ can occur in some patients with renal insufficiency. Furthermore, the potential for developing hyperkalemia should be considered when ACE inhibitors are used with other drugs that can cause K^+ retention, including the K^+-sparing diuretics (amiloride, triamterene, and spironolactone), nonsteroidal antiinflammatory drugs, K^+ supplements, and β receptor antagonists. Some patients with diabetic nephropathy may be at greater risk of hyperkalemia.

There are several cautions in the use of ACE inhibitors in patients with hypertension. Angioedema is a rare but serious and potentially fatal adverse effect of the ACE inhibitors. Patients starting treatment with these drugs should be explicitly warned to discontinue their use with the advent of any signs of angioedema. Due to the risk of severe fetal adverse effects, ACE inhibitors are contraindicated during pregnancy, a fact that should be communicated to women of childbearing age.

In most patients there is no appreciable change in glomerular filtration rate following the administration of ACE inhibitors. However, in renovascular hypertension, the glomerular filtration rate is generally maintained as the result of increased resistance in the postglomerular arteriole caused by angiotensin II. Accordingly, in patients with bilateral renal artery stenosis or stenosis in a sole kidney, the administration of an ACE inhibitor will reduce the filtration fraction and cause a substantial reduction in glomerular filtration rate. In some patients with preexisting renal disease, the glomerular filtration may decrease with an ACE inhibitor. More information is needed on how to balance the potential risk of reversible drug-induced impairment of glomerular filtration rate *versus* inhibition of the progression of kidney disease.

ACE inhibitors lower the blood pressure to some extent in most patients with hypertension. Following the initial dose of an ACE inhibitor, there may be a considerable fall in blood pressure in some patients; this response to the initial dose is a function of plasma renin activity prior to treatment. The potential for a large initial drop in blood pressure is the reason for using a low dose to initiate therapy, especially in patients who may have a very active renin-angiotensin system supporting blood pressure, such as patients with diuretic-induced volume contraction or congestive heart failure. With continuing treatment, there usually is a progressive fall in blood pressure that in most patients does not reach a maximum for several weeks. The blood pressure seen during chronic treatment is not strongly correlated with the pretreatment plasma renin activity. Young and middle-aged Caucasian patients have a higher probability of responding to ACE inhibitors; elderly African-American patients as a group are more resistant to the hypotensive effect of these drugs. While most ACE inhibitors are approved for once-daily dosing for hypertension, an significant fraction of patients have a response that lasts for less than 24 hours. These patients may require twice-daily dosing for adequate control of blood pressure. These drugs are discussed in detail in Chapter 30.

AT_1 ANGIOTENSIN II RECEPTOR ANTAGONISTS

The importance of angiotensin II in regulating cardiovascular function has led to the development of nonpeptide antagonists of the AT_1 angiotensin II receptor for clinical use. *Losartan* (COZAAR), *candesartan* (ATACAND), *irbesartan* (AVAPRO), *valsartan* (DIOVAN), *telmisartan* (MICARDIS), and *eprosartan* (TEVETEN) have been approved for the treatment of hypertension. The pharmacology of AT_1 receptor antagonists is presented in detail in Chapter 30. By antagonizing the effects of angiotensin II, these agents relax smooth muscle and thereby promote vasodilation, increase renal salt and water excretion, reduce plasma volume, and decrease cellular hypertrophy. Angiotensin II receptor antagonists also theoretically overcome some of the disadvantages of ACE inhibitors, which not only prevent conversion of angiotensin I to angiotensin II but also prevent ACE-mediated degradation of bradykinin and substance P.

There are two distinct subtypes of angiotensin II receptors, designated as type 1 (AT_1) and type 2 (AT_2). The AT_1 angiotensin II–receptor subtype is located predominantly in vascular and myocardial tissue and also in brain, kidney, and adrenal glomerulosa cells, which secrete aldosterone (*see* Chapter 30). The AT_2 subtype of angiotensin II receptor is found in the adrenal medulla, kidney, and in the CNS, and may play a role in vascular development (Horiuchi *et al.*, 1999). Because the AT_1 receptor mediates feedback inhibition of renin release, renin and angiotensin II concentrations are increased during AT_1-receptor antagonism. The clinical consequences of increased angiotensin II effects on an uninhibited AT_2 receptor are unknown; however, emerging data suggest that the AT_2 receptor may elicit antigrowth and antiproliferative responses.

Adverse Effects and Precautions. The adverse effects of AT_1 receptor antagonists may be considered in the context of those known to be associated with the ACE inhibitors. ACE inhibitors cause problems of two major types, those related to diminished concentrations of angiotensin II and those due to molecular actions independent of abrogating the function of angiotensin II.

Adverse effects of ACE inhibitors that result from inhibiting angiotensin II–related functions (*see* above) also occur with AT_1 receptor antagonists. These include hypotension, hyperkalemia, and reduced renal function, including that associated with bilateral renal artery stenosis and stenosis in the artery of a solitary kidney. Hypotension is most likely to occur in patients in whom the blood pressure is highly dependent on angiotensin II, including those with volume depletion (*e.g.,* with diuretics), renovascular hypertension, cardiac failure, and cirrhosis; in such patients initiation of treatment with low doses and attention to blood volume is essential. Hyperkalemia may occur in conjunction with other factors that alter K^+ homeostasis, such as renal insufficiency, ingestion of excess K^+, and the use of drugs that promote K^+ retention. Cough, an adverse effect of ACE inhibitors, is less frequent with angiotensin II receptor antagonists. Angioedema occurs very rarely.

AT_1 receptor antagonists should not be administered during pregnancy and should be discontinued as soon as pregnancy is detected.

Therapeutic Uses. When given in adequate doses, the AT_1 receptor antagonists appear to be as effective as ACE inhibitors in the treatment of hypertension. As with ACE inhibitors, these drugs may be less effective in African-American and low-renin patients.

The full effect of AT_1 receptor antagonists on blood pressure typically is not observed until about 4 weeks after the initiation of therapy. If blood pressure is not controlled by an AT_1 receptor antagonist alone, a low dose of a hydrochlorothiazide or other diuretic may be added. In several randomized, double-blind studies of patients with mild-to-severe hypertension, the addition of hydrochlorothiazide to an AT_1 receptor antagonist produced significant additional reductions in blood pressure in patients who demonstrated an insufficient response to hydrochlorothiazide alone. A smaller initial dosage is preferred for patients who have already received diuretics and therefore have an intravascular volume depletion, and for other patients whose blood pressure is highly dependent on angiotensin II. Given the different mechanisms by which they act, there is no assurance that the effects of ACE inhibitors and antagonists of the AT_1 receptor will be equivalent in preventing target organ damage in patients with hypertension.

VASODILATORS

Hydralazine

Hydralazine (APRESOLINE) was one of the first orally active antihypertensive drugs to be marketed in the United States; however, the drug initially was used infrequently because of tachycardia and tachyphylaxis. With a better understanding of the compensatory cardiovascular responses that accompany use of arteriolar vasodilators, hydralazine was combined with sympatholytic agents and diuretics with greater therapeutic success. Nonetheless, its role in the treatment of hypertension has markedly diminished on account of the subsequent introduction of new classes of antihypertensive drugs.

Numerous phthalazines have been synthesized in the hope of producing vasoactive agents, but only those with hydrazine moieties in the 1 or 4 position of the ring have vasodilatory activity. None of the analogs has any advantage over hydralazine. The structural formula of hydralazine (1-hydrazinophthalazine) is:

HYDRALAZINE

Locus and Mechanism of Action. Hydralazine causes direct relaxation of arteriolar smooth muscle. The molecular mechanisms mediating this action are not clear, but may ultimately involve a fall in intracellular calcium concentrations. While a variety of changes in cellular signaling pathways are influenced by hydralazine, precise molecular targets that explain its capacity to dilate arteries remain uncertain. The drug does not dilate epicardial coronary arteries or relax venous smooth muscle. Hydralazine-induced vasodilation is associated with powerful stimulation of the sympathetic nervous system, likely due to baroreceptor-mediated reflexes, which results in increased heart rate and contractility, increased plasma renin activity, and fluid retention; all of these effects counteract the antihypertensive effect of hydralazine. Although most of the sympathetic activity is due to a baroreceptor-mediated reflex, hydralazine may stimulate the release of norepinephrine from sympathetic nerve terminals and augment myocardial contractility directly.

Pharmacological Effects. Most of the effects of hydralazine are confined to the cardiovascular system. The decrease in blood pressure after administration of hydralazine is associated with a selective decrease in vascular resistance in the coronary, cerebral, and renal circulations, with a smaller effect in skin and muscle. Because of preferential dilation of arterioles over veins, postural hypotension is not a common problem; hydralazine lowers blood pressure equally in the supine and upright positions.

Absorption, Metabolism, and Excretion. Hydralazine is well absorbed through the gastrointestinal tract, but the systemic bioavailability is low (16% in fast acetylators and 35% in slow acetylators). Hydralazine is *N*-acetylated in the bowel and/or the liver. The half-life of hydralazine is 1 hour, and systemic clearance of the drug is about 50 ml/kg per minute.

The rate of acetylation is genetically determined; about half of the U.S. population acetylates rapidly and half do so slowly. The acetylated compound is inactive; thus, the dose necessary to produce a systemic effect is larger in fast acetylators. Since the systemic clearance exceeds hepatic blood flow, extrahepatic metabolism must occur. Indeed, hydralazine rapidly combines with circulating α-keto acids to form hydrazones, and the major metabolite recovered from the plasma is hydralazine pyruvic acid hydrazone. This metabolite has a longer half-life than hydralazine, but it does not appear to be very active. Although the rate of acetylation is an important determinant of the bioavailability of hydralazine, it does not play a role in the systemic elimination of the drug, probably because the hepatic clearance is so high that systemic elimination is principally a function of hepatic blood flow.

The peak concentration of hydralazine in plasma and the peak hypotensive effect of the drug occur within 30 to 120 minutes of ingestion. Although its half-life in plasma is about an hour, the duration of the hypotensive effect of hydralazine can last as long as 12 hours. There is no clear explanation for this discrepancy.

Toxicity and Precautions. Two types of adverse effects occur after the use of hydralazine. The first, which are extensions of the pharmacological effects of the drug, include headache, nausea, flushing, hypotension, palpitations, tachycardia, dizziness, and angina pectoris. Myocardial ischemia occurs because of the increased O_2 demand induced by the baroreceptor reflex-induced stimulation of the sympathetic nervous system and also because hydralazine does not dilate the epicardial coronary arteries; thus, the arteriolar dilation it produces may cause a "steal" of blood flow away from the ischemic region. Following parenteral administration to patients with coronary artery disease, the myocardial ischemia may be sufficiently severe and protracted to cause frank myocardial infarction. For this reason, parenteral administration of hydralazine is not advisable in hypertensive patients with coronary artery disease, hypertensive patients with multiple cardiovascular risk factors, or in older patients. In addition, if the drug is used alone, there may be salt retention with development of high-output congestive heart failure. When combined with a β adrenergic receptor blocker and a diuretic, hydralazine is better toler-

ated, although adverse effects such as headache are still commonly described and may necessitate discontinuation of the drug.

The second type of adverse effect is caused by immunological reactions, of which the drug-induced lupus syndrome is the most common. Administration of hydralazine also can result in an illness that resembles serum sickness, hemolytic anemia, vasculitis, and rapidly progressive glomerulonephritis. The mechanism of these autoimmune reactions is unknown.

The drug-induced lupus syndrome usually occurs after at least 6 months of continuous treatment with hydralazine, and its incidence is related to dose, sex, acetylator phenotype, and race. In one study, after 3 years of treatment with hydralazine, drug-induced lupus occurred in 10% of patients who received 200 mg daily, 5% who received 100 mg daily, and none who received 50 mg daily (Cameron and Ramsay, 1984). The incidence is four times higher in women than in men, and the syndrome is seen more commonly in Caucasians than in African-Americans. The rate of conversion to a positive antinuclear antibody test is faster in slow acetylators than in rapid acetylators, suggesting that the native drug or a nonacetylated metabolite is responsible. However, since the majority of patients with positive antinuclear antibody tests do not develop the drug-induced lupus syndrome, hydralazine need not be discontinued unless clinical features of the syndrome appear. These features are similar to those of other drug-induced lupus syndromes and consist mainly of arthralgia, arthritis, and fever. Pleuritis and pericarditis may be present, and pericardial effusion can occasionally cause cardiac tamponade. Discontinuation of the drug is all that is necessary for most patients with the hydralazine-induced lupus syndrome, but symptoms may persist in a few patients and administration of corticosteroids may be necessary.

Hydralazine also can produce a pyridoxine-responsive polyneuropathy. The mechanism appears to be related to the ability of hydralazine to combine with pyridoxine to form a hydrazone. This side effect is very unusual with doses ≤200 mg per day.

Therapeutic Uses. Hydralazine is no longer a first-line drug in the treatment of hypertension on account of its relatively unfavorable adverse-effect profile. It may have utility in the treatment of some patients with severe hypertension, can be part of evidence-based therapy in patients with congestive heart failure (in combination with nitrates for patients who cannot tolerate ACE inhibitors or AT_1 receptor antagonists), and in the treatment of hypertensive emergencies in pregnant women (especially preeclampsia) on account of extensive experience with the drug in that setting. Hydralazine should be used with the greatest of caution in elderly patients and in hypertensive patients with coronary artery disease because of the possibility of precipitation of myocardial ischemia due to reflex tachycardia. The usual oral dosage of hydralazine is 25 to 100 mg twice daily. Twice-daily administration is as effective as administration four times a day for control of blood pressure, regardless of acetylator phenotype. The maximum recommended dose of hydralazine is 200 mg per day to minimize the risk of drug-induced lupus syndrome.

K^+_{ATP} Channel Openers: Minoxidil

The discovery in 1965 of the hypotensive action of minoxidil (LONITEN) was a significant advance in the treatment of hypertension, since the drug has proven to be efficacious in patients with the most severe and drug-resistant forms of hypertension. The chemical structure of minoxidil is:

MINOXIDIL

Locus and Mechanism of Action. Minoxidil is not active *in vitro* but must be metabolized by hepatic sulfotransferase to the active molecule, minoxidil *N-O* sulfate; the formation of this active metabolite is a minor pathway in the metabolic disposition of minoxidil. Minoxidil sulfate relaxes vascular smooth muscle in isolated systems where the parent drug is inactive. Minoxidil sulfate activates the ATP-modulated K^+ channel. By opening K^+ channels in smooth muscle and thereby permitting K^+ efflux, it causes hyperpolarization and relaxation of smooth muscle (Leblanc *et al.*, 1989).

Pharmacological Effects. Minoxidil produces arteriolar vasodilation with essentially no effect on the capacitance vessels; the drug resembles hydralazine and *diazoxide* in this regard. Minoxidil increases blood flow to skin, skeletal muscle, the gastrointestinal tract, and the heart more than to the CNS. The disproportionate increase in blood flow to the heart may have a metabolic basis, in that administration of minoxidil is associated with a reflex increase in myocardial contractility and in cardiac output. The cardiac output can increase markedly, as much as three- to fourfold. The principal determinant of the elevation in cardiac output is the action of minoxidil on peripheral vascular resistance to enhance venous return to the heart; by inference from studies with other drugs, the increased venous return probably results from enhancement of flow in the regional vascular beds with a fast time constant for venous return to the heart (Ogilvie, 1985). The adrenergically mediated

increase in myocardial contractility contributes to the increased cardiac output, but is not the predominant causal factor.

The effects of minoxidil on the kidney are complex. Minoxidil is a renal artery vasodilator, but systemic hypotension produced by the drug occasionally can decrease renal blood flow. Renal function usually improves in patients who take minoxidil for the treatment of hypertension, especially if renal dysfunction is secondary to hypertension (Mitchell *et al.*, 1980). Minoxidil is a very potent stimulator of renin secretion; this effect is mediated by a combination of renal sympathetic stimulation and activation of the intrinsic renal mechanisms for regulation of renin release.

Discovery of K^+_{ATP} channels in a variety of cell types and in mitochondria is prompting consideration of K^+_{ATP} channel modulators as therapeutic agents in myriad cardiovascular diseases (Pollesello and Mebazaa, 2004) and may provide explanations for some of the effects of minoxidil noted in the previous section. Various K^+_{ATP} channels possess different regulatory sulfonylurea receptor subunits and thus exhibit tissue-specific responses. Recent studies suggest that certain actions of K^+_{ATP} channel openers can be influenced by hypercholesterolemia and by concurrent administration of sulfonylurea hypoglycemic agents (Miura and Miki, 2003).

Absorption, Metabolism, and Excretion. Minoxidil is well absorbed from the gastrointestinal tract. Although peak concentrations of minoxidil in blood occur 1 hour after oral administration, the maximal hypotensive effect of the drug occurs later, possibly because formation of the active metabolite is delayed.

Only about 20% of the absorbed drug is excreted unchanged in the urine, and the main route of elimination is by hepatic metabolism. The major metabolite of minoxidil is the glucuronide conjugate at the *N*-oxide position in the pyrimidine ring. This metabolite is less active than minoxidil, but it persists longer in the body. The extent of biotransformation of minoxidil to its active metabolite, minoxidil *N-O* sulfate, has not been evaluated in human beings. Minoxidil has a half-life in plasma of 3 to 4 hours, but its duration of action is 24 hours or occasionally even longer. It has been proposed that persistence of minoxidil in vascular smooth muscle is responsible for this discrepancy. However, without knowledge of the pharmacokinetic properties of the active metabolite, an explanation for the prolonged duration of action cannot be given.

Adverse Effects and Precautions. The adverse effects of minoxidil can be severe and are divided into three major categories: fluid and salt retention, cardiovascular effects, and hypertrichosis.

Retention of salt and water results from increased proximal renal tubular reabsorption, which is in turn secondary to reduced renal perfusion pressure and to reflex stimulation of renal tubular α adrenergic receptors. Similar antinatriuretic effects can be observed with the other arteriolar dilators (*e.g.*, diazoxide and hydralazine). Although administration of minoxidil causes increased secretion of renin and aldosterone, this is not an important mechanism for retention of salt and water in this case. Fluid retention usually can be controlled by the administration of a diuretic. However, thiazides may not be sufficiently efficacious, and it may be necessary to use a loop diuretic, especially if the patient has any degree of renal dysfunction. Retention of salt and water in patients taking minoxidil may be profound, requiring large doses of loop diuretics to prevent edema formation.

The cardiac consequences of the baroreceptor-mediated activation of the sympathetic nervous system during minoxidil therapy are similar to those seen with hydralazine; there is an increase in heart rate, myocardial contractility, and myocardial O_2 consumption. Thus, myocardial ischemia can be induced by minoxidil in patients with coronary artery disease. The cardiac sympathetic responses are attenuated by concurrent administration of a β adrenergic blocker. The adrenergically induced increase in renin secretion also can be ameliorated by a β receptor antagonist or an ACE inhibitor, with enhancement of blood pressure control.

The increased cardiac output evoked by minoxidil has particularly adverse consequences in those hypertensive patients who have left ventricular hypertrophy and diastolic dysfunction. Such poorly compliant ventricles respond suboptimally to increased volume loads, with a resulting increase in left ventricular filling pressure. This is probably a major contributor to the increased pulmonary artery pressure seen with minoxidil (and hydralazine) therapy in hypertensive patients, and is compounded by the retention of salt and water caused by minoxidil. Cardiac failure can result from minoxidil therapy in such patients; the potential for this complication can be reduced but not prevented by effective diuretic therapy. Pericardial effusion is an uncommon but serious complication of minoxidil. Although more commonly described in patients with cardiac failure and renal failure, pericardial effusion can occur in patients with normal cardiovascular and renal function. Mild and asymptomatic pericardial effusion is not an indication for discontinuing minoxidil, but the situation should be monitored closely to avoid progression to tamponade. Effusions usually clear when the drug is discontinued but can recur if treatment with minoxidil is resumed.

Flattened and inverted T waves frequently are observed in the electrocardiogram following the initiation of minoxidil treatment. These are not ischemic in origin and are seen with other drugs that activate K^+ channels. These drugs accelerate myocardial repolarization, shorten the refractory period, and one of them, *pinacidil*, lowers the ventricular fibrillation threshold and increases spontaneous ventricular fibrillation in the setting of myocardial ischemia (Chi *et al.*, 1990). The effect of minoxidil on the refractory period and ischemic ventricular fibrillation has not been investigated; whether or not such findings enhance the risk of ventricular fibrillation in human myocardial ischemia is unknown.

Hypertrichosis occurs in patients who receive minoxidil for an extended period and is probably a consequence of K^+ channel activation. Growth of hair occurs on the face, back, arms, and legs, and is particularly offensive to women. Frequent shaving or depilatory agents can be used to manage this problem. Topical minoxidil (ROGAINE) is marketed for the treatment of male pattern baldness. The topical use of minoxidil can cause measurable cardiovascular effects in some individuals (Leenen *et al.*, 1988).

Other side effects of the drug are rare and include rashes, Stevens-Johnson syndrome, glucose intolerance, serosanguineous bullae, formation of antinuclear antibodies, and thrombocytopenia.

Therapeutic Uses. Minoxidil is best reserved for the treatment of severe hypertension that responds poorly to other antihypertensive medications, especially in male patients with renal insufficiency (Campese, 1981). It has been used successfully in the treatment of hypertension in both adults and children. Minoxidil should never be used alone; it must be given concurrently with a diuretic to avoid fluid retention and with a sympatholytic drug (usually a β receptor antagonist) to control reflex cardiovascular effects. The drug usually is administered either once or twice a day, but some patients may require more frequent dosing for adequate control of blood pressure. The initial daily dose of minoxidil may be as little as 1.25 mg, which can be increased gradually to 40 mg in one or two daily doses.

Sodium Nitroprusside

Although sodium nitroprusside has been known since 1850 and its hypotensive effect in human beings was described in 1929, its safety and usefulness for the short-term control of severe hypertension were not demonstrated until the mid-1950s. Several investigators subsequently demonstrated that sodium nitroprusside also was effective in improving cardiac function in patients with left ventricular failure (*see* Chapter 34). The structural formula of sodium nitroprusside is:

$$2Na^+ \begin{bmatrix} & & CN & \\ & & | & CN \\ NC & \!\!-\!\!Fe\!\!-\!\! & CN \\ & ON & | \\ & & CN & \end{bmatrix}^{--}$$

SODIUM NITROPRUSSIDE

Locus and Mechanism of Action. Nitroprusside is a nitrovasodilator that acts by releasing nitric oxide (NO). NO activates the guanylyl cyclase–cyclic GMP–PKG pathway, leading to vasodilation (Murad, 1986; Linder *et al.*, 2005), mimicking the production of NO by vascular endothelial cells, which is impaired in many hypertensive patients (Ramchandra *et al.*, 2005). The mechanism of release of NO is not clear and likely involves both enzymatic and nonenzymatic pathways (Feelisch, 1998). Tolerance develops to *nitroglycerin* but not to nitroprusside (Fung, 2004). The pharmacology of the organic nitrates, including nitroglycerin, is presented in Chapter 31.

Pharmacological Effects. Nitroprusside dilates both arterioles and venules, and the hemodynamic response to its administration results from a combination of venous pooling and reduced arterial impedance. In subjects with normal left ventricular function, venous pooling affects cardiac output more than does the reduction of afterload; cardiac output tends to fall. In contrast, in patients with severely impaired left ventricular function and diastolic ventricular distention, the reduction of arterial impedance is the predominant effect, leading to a rise in cardiac output (*see* Chapter 33).

Sodium nitroprusside is a nonselective vasodilator, and regional distribution of blood flow is little affected by the drug. In general, renal blood flow and glomerular filtration are maintained, and plasma renin activity increases. Unlike minoxidil, hydralazine, diazoxide, and other arteriolar vasodilators, sodium nitroprusside usually causes only a modest increase in heart rate and an overall reduction in myocardial demand for oxygen.

Absorption, Metabolism, and Excretion. Sodium nitroprusside is an unstable molecule that decomposes under strongly alkaline conditions or when exposed to light. The drug must be given by continuous intravenous infusion to be effective. Its onset of action is within 30 seconds; the peak hypotensive effect occurs within 2 minutes, and when the infusion of the drug is stopped, the effect disappears within 3 minutes.

The metabolism of nitroprusside by smooth muscle is initiated by its reduction, which is followed by the release of cyanide and then nitric oxide (Bates *et al.*, 1991; Ivankovich *et al.*, 1978). Cyanide is further metabolized by liver rhodanase to thiocyanate, which is eliminated almost entirely in the urine. The mean elimination half-time for thiocyanate is 3 days in patients with normal renal function, and it can be much longer in patients with renal insufficiency.

Toxicity and Precautions. The short-term adverse effects of nitroprusside are due to excessive vasodilation, with hypotension and the consequences thereof. Close monitoring of blood pressure and the use of a continuous variable-rate infusion pump will prevent an excessive hemodynamic response to the drug in the majority of cases.

Less commonly, toxicity may result from conversion of nitroprusside to cyanide and thiocyanate. Toxic accumulation of cyanide leading to severe lactic acidosis usually occurs when sodium nitroprusside is infused at a rate greater than 5 μg/kg per minute, but also can occur in some patients receiving doses about 2 μg/kg per minute for a prolonged period. The limiting factor in the metabolism of cyanide appears to be the availability of sulfur-containing substrates in the body (mainly thiosulfate). The concomitant administration of *sodium thiosulfate* can prevent accumulation of cyanide in patients who are receiving higher-than-usual doses of sodium nitroprusside; the efficacy of the drug is unchanged (Schulz, 1984). The risk of thiocyanate toxicity increases when sodium nitroprusside is infused for more than 24 to 48 hours, especially if renal function is impaired. Signs and symptoms of thiocyanate toxicity include anorexia, nausea, fatigue, disorientation, and toxic psychosis. The plasma concentration of thiocyanate should be monitored during prolonged infusions of nitroprusside and should not be allowed to exceed 0.1 mg/ml. Rarely, excessive concentrations of thiocyanate may cause hypothyroidism by inhibiting iodine uptake by the thyroid gland. In patients with renal failure, thiocyanate can be removed readily by hemodialysis.

Nitroprusside can worsen arterial hypoxemia in patients with chronic obstructive pulmonary disease because the drug interferes with hypoxic pulmonary vasoconstriction and therefore promotes mismatching of ventilation with perfusion.

Therapeutic Uses. Sodium nitroprusside is used primarily to treat hypertensive emergencies, but can also be used in many situations when short-term reduction of cardiac preload and/or afterload is desired. Nitroprusside has been used to lower blood pressure during acute aortic dissection, to improve cardiac output in congestive heart failure, especially in hypertensive patients with pulmonary edema that does not respond to other treatment (*see* Chapter 33), and to decrease myocardial oxygen demand after acute myocardial infarction. In addition, nitroprusside is used to induce controlled hypotension during anesthesia in order to reduce bleeding in surgical procedures. In the treatment of acute aortic dissection, it is important to administer a β adrenergic receptor antagonist with nitroprusside, since reduction of blood pressure with nitroprusside alone can increase the rate of rise in pressure in the aorta as a result of increased myocardial contractility, thereby enhancing propagation of the dissection.

Sodium nitroprusside is available in vials that contain 50 mg. The contents of the vial should be dissolved in 2 to 3 ml of 5% dextrose in water. Addition of this solution to 250 to 1000 ml of 5% dextrose in water produces a concentration of 50 to 200 μg/ml. Because the compound decomposes in light, only fresh solutions should be used, and the bottle should be covered with an opaque wrapping. The drug must be administered as a controlled continuous infusion, and the patient must be closely observed. The majority of hypertensive patients respond to an infusion of 0.25 to 1.5 μg/kg per minute. Higher rates of infusion are necessary to produce controlled hypotension in normotensive patients under surgical anesthesia. Infusion of nitroprusside at rates exceeding 5 μg/kg per minute over a prolonged period can cause cyanide and/or thiocyanate poisoning. Patients who are receiving other antihypertensive medications usually require less nitroprusside to lower blood pressure. If infusion rates of 10 μg/kg per minute do not produce adequate reduction of blood pressure within 10 minutes, the rate of administration of nitroprusside should be reduced to minimize potential toxicity.

Diazoxide

Diazoxide (HYPERSTAT IV) is used in the treatment of hypertensive emergencies. Sodium nitroprusside is the drug of choice for this indication, but diazoxide may rarely be used if accurate infusion pumps are not available and/or close monitoring of blood pressure is not feasible. It also is administered orally (PROGLYCEM) to treat patients with various forms of hypoglycemia (*see* Chapter 60).

NONPHARMACOLOGICAL THERAPY OF HYPERTENSION

Nonpharmacological approaches to the reduction of blood pressure generally are advisable as the initial approach to treatment of patients with diastolic blood pressures in the range of 90 to 95 mm Hg. Furthermore, these approaches will augment the effectiveness of pharmacological therapy in patients with higher levels of blood pressure. Also, for patients with diastolic blood pressures in the range of 85 to 90 mm Hg, the epidemiological data on cardiovascular risks support the institution of nonpharmacological therapy. The indications and efficacy of various lifestyle modifications in hypertension are reviewed in a summary statement from the Joint National Committee (Chobanian *et al.*, 2003).

To maintain compliance with a therapeutic regimen, the intervention should not lessen the quality of life. All drugs have side effects. If minor alterations of normal activity or diet can reduce blood pressure to a satisfactory level, the complications of drug therapy can be avoided. In addition, nonpharmacological methods to lower blood pressure allow patients to participate actively in the management of their disease. Reduction of weight, restriction of salt, and moderation in the use of alcohol may reduce blood pressure and improve the efficacy of drug treatment. In addition, regular isotonic exercise also lowers blood pressure in hypertensive patients.

Reduction of Body Weight. Obesity and hypertension are closely associated, and the degree of obesity is positively correlated with the incidence of hypertension. Obese hypertensives may lower their blood pressure by losing weight regardless of a change in salt consumption (Maxwell *et al.*, 1984). The mechanism by which obesity causes hypertension is unclear, but increased secretion of insulin in obesity could result in insulin-mediated enhancement of renal tubular reabsorption of Na^+ and an expansion of extracellular volume. Obesity also is associated with increased activity of the sympathetic nervous system; this is reversed by weight loss. Maintenance of weight loss is difficult for many. A combination of aerobic physical exercise and dietary counseling may enhance compliance.

Sodium Restriction. Severe restriction of salt will lower the blood pressure in most hospitalized hypertensive patients. However, severe salt restriction is not practical from a standpoint of compliance. Several studies have shown that moderate restriction of salt intake to approximately 5 g per day (2 g Na^+) will, on average, lower blood pressure by 12 mm Hg systolic and 6 mm Hg diastolic. The higher the initial blood pressure, the greater the response. In addition, subjects over 40 years of age are more responsive to the hypotensive effect of moderate restriction of salt (Grobbee and Hofman, 1986). Even though not all hypertensive patients respond to restriction of salt, this intervention is likely benign and can easily be advised as an initial approach in all patients with mild hypertension. An additional benefit of salt restriction is improved responsiveness to some antihypertensive drugs.

Alcohol Restriction. Consumption of alcohol can raise blood pressure, but it is unclear how much alcohol must be consumed to observe this effect. Heavy consumption of alcohol increases the risk of cerebrovascular accidents but not coronary heart disease (Kagan *et al.*, 1985). In fact, small amounts of ethanol have been found to protect against the development of coronary artery disease. Hypertensive patients should be advised to restrict consumption of ethanol to no more than 30 ml per day (*see* Chapter 22).

Physical Exercise. Increased physical activity lowers rates of cardiovascular disease in men (Paffenbarger *et al.*, 1986). It is not known if this beneficial effect is secondary to an antihypertensive response to exercise. Lack of physical activity is associated with a higher incidence of hypertension (Blair *et al.*, 1984). Although consistent changes in blood pressure are not always observed, meticulously controlled studies have demonstrated that regular isotonic exercise reduces both systolic and diastolic blood pressures by approximately 10 mm Hg (Nelson *et al.*, 1986). The mechanism by which exercise can lower blood pressure is not clear. Regular isotonic exercise reduces blood volume and plasma catecholamines and elevates plasma concentrations of atrial natriuretic peptide. The beneficial effect of exercise can occur in subjects who demonstrate no change in body weight or salt intake during the training period.

Relaxation and Biofeedback Therapy. The fact that long-term stressful stimuli can cause sustained hypertension in animals has given credence to the possibility that relaxation therapy will lower blood pressure in some hypertensive patients. A few studies have generated positive results, but in general, relaxation therapy has inconsistent and modest effects on blood pressure (Jacob *et al.*, 1986). In addition, the long-term efficacy of such treatment has been difficult to demonstrate, presumably in part because patients must be highly motivated to respond to relaxation and biofeedback therapy. Only those few patients with mild hypertension who wish to use this method should be encouraged to try, and these patients should be closely followed and receive pharmacological treatment if necessary.

Potassium Therapy. There is a positive correlation between total body Na^+ and blood pressure and a negative correlation between total body K^+ and blood pressure in hypertensive patients (Lever *et al.*, 1981). In addition, dietary intake, plasma concentrations, and urinary excretion of K^+ are reduced in various populations of hypertensive subjects. Increased intake of K^+ might reduce blood pressure by increasing excretion of Na^+, suppressing renin secretion, causing arteriolar dilation (possibly by stimulating Na^+,K^+-ATPase activity, and decreasing intracellular concentrations of Ca^{2+}), and impairing responsiveness to endogenous vasoconstrictors. In hypertensive rats, supplementation with K^+ decreases blood pressure and reduces the incidence of stroke, regardless of blood pressure (Tobian, 1986). In mildly hypertensive patients, oral K^+ supplements of 48 mmol per day reduce both systolic and diastolic blood pressure (Siani *et al.*, 1987). Supplementation with K^+ also may protect against ventricular ectopy and stroke (Khaw and Barrett-Connor, 1987). Based on all of these data, it seems prudent to use a high-K^+ diet in conjunction with moderate restriction of Na^+ in the nonpharmacological treatment of hypertension. *However, a high-K^+ diet should not be recommended for patients on ACE inhibitors.*

Tobacco, Coffee, and Other Factors. Smoking *per se* does not cause hypertension, although cigarette smoking acutely raises blood pressure due to actions of nicotine. Smoking is a major risk factor for coronary heart disease. Hypertensive patients should have a great incentive to stop smoking. While clonidine has some efficacy in facilitating withdrawal from smoking, there is no evidence that preferential use of this drug in hypertensive smokers is desirable (*see* Chapter 23). Consumption of caffeine can raise blood pressure and elevate plasma concentrations of norepinephrine, but long-term consumption of caffeine causes tolerance to these effects and has not been associated with the development of hypertension. An increased intake of Ca^{2+} has been reported by some investigators to lower blood pressure. The mechanism of this effect is not understood, but suppression of the secretion of parathyroid hormone apparently is involved. However, supplemental Ca^{2+} does not lower blood pressure when populations of hypertensive subjects are studied. Although it is possible that there are some hypertensive patients who have a hypotensive response to Ca^{2+}, there is no easy way to identify such individuals. Supplemental use of Ca^{2+} for this purpose cannot be recommended at the present time (Kaplan, 1988).

SELECTION OF ANTIHYPERTENSIVE DRUGS IN INDIVIDUAL PATIENTS

Choice of antihypertensive drugs for individual patients may be complex; there are many sources of influence that modify therapeutic decisions. While results derived from randomized controlled clinical trials are the optimal foundation for rational therapeutics, it may be difficult to sort through the multiplicity of results and address how they apply to an individual patient. While therapeutic guidelines can be useful in reaching appropriate therapeutic decisions, it is often difficult for clinicians to apply guidelines at the point of care, and guidelines often do not provide enough information about recommended drugs. In addition, intense marketing of specific drugs to both clinicians and patients may confound optimal decision making. Moreover, persuading patients to continue taking sometimes expensive drugs for an asymptomatic disease is a challenge. Clinicians may be reluctant to prescribe and patients reluctant to consume the number of drugs that may be necessary to adequately control blood pressure. For these and other reasons, perhaps one-half of patients being treated for hypertension have not achieved therapeutic goals in blood pressure lowering.

Choice of an antihypertensive drug should be driven by likely benefit in an individual patient, taking into account concomitant diseases such as diabetes mellitus, problematic adverse effects of specific drugs, and cost.

Recent guidelines recommend diuretics as preferred initial therapy for most patients with uncomplicated stage 1 hypertension who are unresponsive to nonpharmacological measures. Patients are also commonly treated with other drugs: β receptor antagonists, ACE inhibitors/AT_1-receptor antagonists, and Ca^{2+} channel blockers. Patients with uncomplicated stage 2 hypertension will likely require the early introduction of a diuretic and another drug from a different class. Subsequently, doses can be titrated upward and additional drugs added in order to achieve goal blood pressures (blood pressure <140/90 mm Hg in uncomplicated patients). Some of these patients may require four different drugs to reach their goal.

A most important and high-risk group of patients with hypertension are those with compelling indications for specific drugs on account of other underlying serious cardiovascular disease (heart failure, post–myocardial infarction, or with high risk for coronary artery disease), chronic kidney disease, or diabetes (Chobanian *et al.*, 2003). For example, a hypertensive patient with congestive heart failure ideally should be treated with a diuretic, β receptor antagonist, ACE inhibitor/AT_1 receptor antagonist, and spironolactone because of the benefit of these drugs in congestive heart failure, even in the absence of hypertension. Similarly, ACE inhibitors/AT_1 receptor antagonists should be first-line drugs in the treatment of diabetics with hypertension in view of their well-established benefits in diabetic nephropathy.

Other patients may have less serious underlying diseases that could influence choice of antihypertensive drugs. For example, a hypertensive patient with symptomatic benign prostatic hyperplasia might benefit from having an α_1 receptor antagonist as part of his therapeutic program, since α_1 antagonists are efficacious in both diseases. Similarly, a patient with recurrent migraine attacks might particularly benefit from use of a β receptor antagonist since a number of drugs in this class are efficacious in preventing migraine attacks.

Patients with isolated systolic hypertension (systolic blood pressure >160 mm Hg and diastolic blood pressure <90 mm Hg) benefit particularly from diuretics and also from Ca^{2+} channel blockers. These should be first-line drugs in these patients in terms of efficacy, but compelling indications as above need to be taken into account.

These considerations have been addressed with regard to patients with hypertension that need treatment to reduce long-term risk, not patients in immediately life-threatening settings due to hypertension. While there are very limited clinical trial data, clinical judgment favors rapidly lowering blood pressure in patients with life-threatening complications of hypertension, such as patients with hypertensive encephalopathy or pulmonary edema due to severe hypertension. Rapid reduction in blood pressure has considerable risks for the patients; if blood pressure is decreased too quickly or extensively, cerebral blood flow may diminish due to adaptations in the cerebral circulation that protect the brain from the sequelae of very high blood pressures. The temptation to rapidly treat patients merely on the basis of increased blood pressure should be resisted. Appropriate therapeutic decisions need to encompass how well the patients' major organs are reacting to the very high blood pressures.

BIBLIOGRAPHY

ALLHAT Officers and Coordinators for the ALLHAT Collaborative Research Group. Major outcomes in high-risk hypertensive patients randomized to angiotensin-converting enzyme inhibitor or calcium channel blocker vs. diuretic: The Antihypertensive and Lipid-Lowering Treatment to Prevent Heart Attack Trial. *JAMA*, 2002, *288*:2981–2997.

Bates, J.N., Baker, M.T., Guerra, R. Jr., and Harrison, D.G. Nitric oxide generation from nitroprusside by vascular tissue. Evidence that reduction of the nitroprusside anion and cyanide loss are required. *Biochem. Pharmacol.*, 1991, *42*:S157–S165.

Beckmann, M.L., Gerber, J.G., Byyny, R.L., LoVerde, M., and Nies, A.S. Propranolol increases prostacyclin synthesis in patients with essential hypertension. *Hypertension*, 1988, *12*:582–588.

Blair, S.N., Goodyear, N.N., Gibbons, L.W., and Cooper, K.H. Physical fitness and incidence of hypertension in healthy normotensive men and women. *JAMA*, 1984, *252*:487–490.

Bobik, A., Oddie, C., Scott, P., Mill, G., and Korner, P. Relationships between the cardiovascular effects of α-methyldopa and its metabolism in pontomedullary noradrenergic neurons of the rabbit. *J. Cardiovasc. Pharmacol.*, 1988, *11*:529–537.

Cameron, H.A., and Ramsay, L.E. The lupus syndrome induced by hydralazine: a common complication with low dose treatment. *Br. Med. J. [Clin. Res. Ed.]*, 1984, *289*:410–412.

Chi, L., Uprichard, A.C., and Lucchesi B.R. Profibrillatory actions of pinacidil in a conscious canine model of sudden coronary death. *J. Cardiovasc. Pharmacol.*, 1990, *15*:452–464.

Curtis, M.J., and Hearse, D.J. Ischaemia-induced and reperfusion-induced arrhythmias differ in their sensitivity to potassium: implications for mechanisms of initiation and maintenance of ventricular fibrillation. *J. Mol. Cell. Cardiol.*, 1989, *21*:21–40.

Dahlöf, B., Lindholm, L.H., Hansson, L., *et al.* Morbidity and mortality in the Swedish Trial in Old Patients with Hypertension (STOP-Hypertension). *Lancet*, 1991, *338*:1281–1285.

Frisk-Holmberg, M., Paalzow, L., and Wibell, L. Relationship between the cardiovascular effects and steady-state kinetics of clonidine in hypertension. Demonstration of a therapeutic window in man. *Eur. J. Clin. Pharmacol.*, 1984, *26*:309–313.

Frisk-Holmberg, M., and Wibell, L. Concentration-dependent blood pressure effects of guanfacine. *Clin. Pharmacol. Ther.*, 1986, *39*:169–172.

Goldstein, D.S., Levinson, P.D., Zimlichman, R., *et al.* Clonidine suppression testing in essential hypertension. *Ann. Intern. Med.*, 1985, *102*:42–49.

Granata, A.R., Numao, Y., Kumada, M., and Reis, D.J. A1 noradrenergic neurons tonically inhibit sympathoexcitatory neurons of C1 area in rat brainstem. *Brain Res.*, 1986, *377*:127–146.

Horiuchi, M., Akishita, M., and Dzau, V.J. Recent progress in angiotensin II type 2 receptor research in the cardiovascular system. *Hypertension*, 1999, *33*:613–621.

Jacob, R.G., Shapiro, A.P., Reeves, R.A., *et al.* Relaxation therapy for hypertension. Comparison of effects with concomitant placebo, diuretic, and β-blocker. *Arch. Intern. Med.*, 1986, *146*:2335–2340.

Kagan, A., Popper, J.S., Rhoads, G.G., and Yano, K. Dietary and other risk factors for stroke in Hawaiian Japanese men. *Stroke*, 1985, *16*:390–396.

Khaw, K.T., and Barrett-Connor, E. Dietary potassium and stroke associated mortality. A 12-year prospective population study. *N. Engl. J. Med.*, 1987, *316*:235–240.

Kowaluk, E.A., Seth, P., and Fung, H.L. Metabolic activation of sodium nitroprusside to nitric oxide in vascular smooth muscle. *J. Pharmacol. Exp. Ther.*, 1992, *262*:916–922.

Leblanc, N., Wilde, D.W., Keef, K.D., and Hume, J.R. Electrophysiological mechanisms of minoxidil sulfate-induced vasodilation of rabbit portal vein. *Circ. Res.*, 1989, *65*:1102–1111.

Leenen, F.H., Smith, D.L., and Unger, W.P. Topical minoxidil: cardiac effects in bald man. *Br. J. Clin. Pharmacol.*, 1988, *26*:481–485.

Lever, A.F., Beretta-Piccoli, C., Brown, J.J., *et al.* Sodium and potassium in essential hypertension. *Br. Med. J. [Clin. Res. Ed.]*, 1981, *283*:463–468.

Linder, A., McCluskey, L., Cole, K., Lanning, K., and Webb R. Dynamic association of nitric oxide downstream signaling molecules with endothelial caveolin-1 in rat aorta. *J. Pharmacol. Exp. Therap.*, 2005, Epub ahead of print.

Link, R.E., Desai, K., Hein, L., *et al.* Cardiovascular regulation in mice lacking α_2-adrenergic receptor subtypes b and c. *Science*, 1996, *273*:803–805.

MacMillan, L.B., Hein, L., Smith, M.S., Piascik, M.T., and Limbird, L.E. Central hypotensive effects of the α_{2A}-adrenergic receptor subtype. *Science*, 1996, *273*:801–803.

Maxwell, M.H., Kushiro, T., Dornfield, L.P., Tuck, M.L., and Waks, A.U. BP changes in obese hypertensive subjects during rapid weight loss. Comparison of restricted v. unchanged salt intake. *Arch. Intern. Med.,* **1984,** *144:*1581–1584.

Medical Research Council Working Party. Comparison of the antihypertensive efficacy and adverse reactions to two doses of bendrofluazide and hydrochlorothiazide and the effect of potassium supplementation on the hypotensive action of bendrofluazide: substudies of the Medical Research Council's trials of treatment of mild hypertension: Medical Research Council Working Party. *J. Clin. Pharmacol.,* **1987,** *27:*271–277.

Medical Research Council Working Party. Medical Research Council trial of treatment of hypertension in older adults: principal results. MRC Working Party. *Br. Med. J.,* **1992,** *304:*405–412.

Metz, S., Klein, C., and Morton, N. Rebound hypertension after discontinuation of transdermal clonidine therapy. *Am. J. Med.,* **1987,** *82:*17–19.

Mitchell, H.C., Graham, R.M., and Pettinger, W.A. Renal function during long-term treatment of hypertension with minoxidil: comparison of benign and malignant hypertension. *Ann. Intern. Med.,* **1980,** *93:*676–681.

Multiple Risk Factor Intervention Trial Research Group. Multiple risk factor intervention trial. Risk factor changes and mortality results. *JAMA,* **1982,** *248:*1465–1477.

Murad, F. Cyclic guanosine monophosphate as a mediator of vasodilation. *J. Clin. Invest.,* **1986,** *78:*1–5.

Nelson, L., Jennings, G.L., Esler, M.D., and Korner, P.I. Effect of changing levels of physical activity on blood-pressure and haemodynamics in essential hypertension. *Lancet,* **1986,** *2:*473–476.

Ogilvie, R.I. Comparative effects of vasodilator drugs on flow distribution and venous return. *Can. J. Physiol. Pharmacol.,* **1985,** *63:*1345–1355.

Paffenbarger, R.S. Jr., Hyde, R.T., Wing, A.L., and Hsieh, C.C. Physical activity, all-cause mortality, and longevity of college alumni. *N. Engl. J. Med.,* **1986,** *314:*605–613.

Pickkers, P., and Hughes, A.D. Relaxation and decrease in $[Ca^{2+}]$ by hydrochlorothiazide in guinea pig isolated mesenteric arteries. *Br. J. Pharmacol.,* **1995,** *114:*703–707.

Pickkers, P., Garcha, R.S., Schachter, M., *et al.* Inhibition of carbonic anhydrase accounts for the direct vascular effects of hydrochlorothiazide. *Hypertension,* **1999,** *33:*1043–1048.

SHEP Cooperative Research Group. Prevention of stroke by antihypertensive drug treatment in older persons with isolated systolic hypertension. Final results of the Systolic Hypertension in the Elderly Program (SHEP). *JAMA,* **1991,** *265:*3255–3264.

Siani, A., Strazzullo, P., Russo, L., *et al.* Controlled trial of long-term oral potassium supplements in patients with mild hypertension. *Br. Med. J. [Clin. Res. Ed.],* **1987,** *294:*1453–1456.

Siscovick, D.S., Raghunathan, T.E., Psaty, B.M., *et al.* Diuretic therapy for hypertension and the risk of primary cardiac arrest. *N. Engl. J. Med.,* **1994,** *330:*1852–1857.

Staessen, J.A., Fagard, R., Thijs, L., *et al.* Randomised double-blind comparison of placebo and active treatment for older patients with isolated systolic hypertension. The Systolic Hypertension in Europe (Syst-Eur) Trial Investigators. *Lancet,* **1997,** *350:*757–764.

Tobian, L. High potassium diets markedly protect against stroke deaths and kidney disease in hypertensive rats, a possible legacy from prehistoric times. *Can. J. Physiol. Pharmacol.,* **1986,** *64:*840–848.

MONOGRAPHS AND REVIEWS

Ashcroft, F., and Gribble, F. New windows on the mechanism of K_{ATP} channel openers. *Trends Pharmacol. Sci.,* **2000,** *21:*439–445.

Campese, V.M. Minoxidil: a review of its pharmacological properties and therapeutic use. *Drugs,* **1981,** *22:*257–278.

Carter, B.L., Ernst, M.E., and Cohen, J.D. Hydrochlorothiazide versus chlorthalidone: evidence supporting their interchangeability. *Hypertension,* **2004,** *43:*4–9.

Chobanian, A.V., Bakris, G.L., Black, H.R., *et al.* Seventh Report of the Joint National Committee on Prevention, Detection, Evaluation, and Treatment of High Blood Pressure. *Hypertension,* **2003,** *42:*1206–1252.

Feelisch, M. The use of nitric oxide donors in pharmacological studies. *Naunyn Schmiedebergs Arch. Pharmacol.,* **1998,** *358:*113–122.

Franklin, S.S. Is there a preferred antihypertensive therapy for isolated systolic hypertension and reduced arterial compliance? *Curr. Hypertens. Rep.,* **2000,** *2:*253–259.

Fung, H-L. Biochemical mechanism of nitroglycerin action and tolerance: Is this old mystery solved? *Ann. Rev. Pharmacol. Toxicol.,* **2004,** *44:*67–85.

Garbers, D., and Dubois, S. The molecular basis of hypertension. *Ann. Rev. Biochem.,* **1999,** *68:*127–155.

Grobbee, D.E., and Hofman, A. Does sodium restriction lower blood pressure? *Br. Med. J. [Clin. Res. Ed.],* **1986,** *293:*27–29.

Ivankovich, A.D., Miletich, D.J., and Tinker, J.H. Sodium nitroprusside: metabolism and general considerations. *Int. Anesthesiol. Clin.,* **1978,** *16:*1–29.

Kaplan, N.M. Calcium and potassium in the treatment of essential hypertension. *Semin. Nephrol.,* **1988,** *8:*176–184.

Miura. T., and Miki, T. ATP-sensitive K^+ channel openers: old drugs with new clinical benefits for the heart. *Curr. Vasc. Pharmacol.,* **2003,** *1:*251–258.

Pollesello, P., and Mebazaa, A. ATP-dependent potassium channels as a key target for the treatment of myocardial and vascular dysfunction. *Curr. Opin. Crit. Care,* **2004,** *10:*436–441.

Ramachandra, R., Barrett, C., and Malpas, S. Nitric oxide and sympathetic nerve activity in the control of blood pressure. *Clin. Exp. Pharmacol. Physiol.,* **2005,** *32:*440–446.

Reid, J.L. α-Adrenergic receptors and blood pressure control. *Am. J. Cardiol.,* **1986,** *57:*6E–12E.

Schulz, V. Clinical pharmacokinetics of nitroprusside, cyanide, thiosulphate and thiocyanate. *Clin. Pharmacokinet.,* **1984,** *9:*239–251.

Sorkin, E.M., and Heel, R.C. Guanfacine. A review of its pharmacodynamic and pharmacokinetic properties, and therapeutic efficacy in the treatment of hypertension. *Drugs,* **1986,** *31:*301–336.

Weber, M.A. Calcium channel antagonists in the treatment of hypertension. *Am. J. Cardiovasc. Drugs,* **2002,** *2:*415–431.

PHARMACOTHERAPY OF CONGESTIVE HEART FAILURE

Thomas P. Rocco and James C. Fang

Congestive heart failure (CHF) is a major contributor to morbidity and mortality worldwide. There are approximately 5 million established cases of heart failure in the United States alone; a similar number of patients have asymptomatic left ventricular dysfunction and are therefore at risk to develop CHF. Heart failure accounts for more than half a million deaths annually in the United States; mortality in patients with advanced heart failure exceeds 50% at 1 year (American Heart Association, 2003). Fortunately, substantive advances in the understanding of CHF at the organ systems and cellular-molecular levels have driven important advances in the pharmacotherapy of heart failure that have revolutionized clinical practice. While palliation of symptoms and improvement in the quality of life remain important goals, it now is possible to approach therapy with the expectation that disease progression can be attenuated, and, in many instances, survival prolonged.

Historically, drug therapies have focused on the endpoint components of this syndrome, volume overload (congestion) and myocardial dysfunction (heart failure). Treatment strategies have typically emphasized the use of diuretics and cardiac glycosides, with investigative efforts directed at the development of new agents that improved contractile performance. While effective in providing relief of symptoms and in stabilizing patients with hemodynamic decompensation, such therapies have not been proven to improve survival. More recent work has provided greater insight into the induction and propagation of CHF, providing a conceptual framework in which heart failure is viewed as a consequence of disordered circulatory dynamics and pathologic cardiac remodeling. These developments have had a major positive impact on the treatment of CHF. Before discussing the clinical pharmacotherapy of heart failure, it is useful to establish a pathophysiologic framework through which its treatment can be approached.

Pathophysiology of Congestive Heart Failure

The principal function of the circulatory system is to deliver oxygenated blood to the periphery in response to aggregate local demand. Circulatory homeostasis therefore requires defense of both forward cardiac output and mean arterial pressure (MAP). The importance of the MAP derives from the fact that the systemic circulation consists of a number of parallel regional circulatory beds, each of which offers an intrinsic resistance to flow. Perfusion of these regional beds is determined by the inflow pressure (MAP) and is inversely proportional to the vascular resistance in the given subsegment of the circulation. This intrinsic resistance can be modulated to increase or decrease perfusion based on local and/or whole body demand for oxygen. The net effect is that the cardiac output delivered by the left ventricle is distributed, as required, to sites of demand *via* modulation of resistors in the peripheral circulatory beds. This local modulation of resistance is the mechanism by which blood flow is coupled to oxygen demand.

While local autoregulation determines the peripheral distribution of the cardiac output under physiologic circumstances, the circulation must also have the capacity to supersede local autoregulation when aggregate demand exceeds the delivery capacity of the cardiac output. The classic such example is hypovolemic shock, a situation in which forward cardiac output is reduced as a consequence of decreased intravascular volume. In this setting, both the sympathetic branch of the autonomic nervous system (*see*

Chapter 6) and the renin–angiotensin system (*see* Chapter 30) are activated; the vasoconstrictive effects of these systems substantially increase peripheral vascular resistance, leading to reduced flow to noncritical vascular beds. This redistribution of the cardiac output maintains perfusion to critical circulatory beds such as the CNS, the left ventricular myocardium, and the kidney. Concomitant with the redistribution of cardiac output, these neurohumoral systems also initiate a host of biological responses that increase the reabsorption of Na^+ and water. These compensatory mechanisms typically operate in the context of normal myocardial contractility and normal myocardial compliance, conditions that generally do not hold in the setting of heart failure and are best suited to the provision of short-term circulatory support to overcome transient, dynamic cardiovascular stress.

It is difficult to provide a comprehensive definition of CHF, since the term describes a final common pathway for the expression of myocardial dysfunction of diverse etiologies. While some emphasize the clinical distinction between systolic and diastolic heart failure, many patients exhibit abnormalities of both contractile performance and ventricular relaxation/filling. This is well illustrated by the fact that the rate and temporal partitioning of left ventricular diastolic filling are directly affected by impaired systolic contractile performance.

Despite the difficulties inherent in creating a unifying description to encompass these distinct clinical states, definitions of CHF have emerged that have been used in consensus guidelines developed to guide the evaluation and management of heart failure.

Congestive heart failure is the pathophysiologic state in which the heart is unable to pump blood at a rate commensurate with the requirements of metabolizing tissues, or can do so only from an elevated filling pressure (Braunwald and Bristow, 2000).

Heart failure is a complex of symptoms—fatigue, shortness of breath, and congestion—that are related to the inadequate perfusion of tissue during exertion and often to the retention of fluid. Its primary cause is an impairment of the heart's ability to fill or empty the left ventricle properly (Cohn, 1996).

Although inevitably incomplete, such definitions can provide a point of departure from which a pathophysiologic framework can be constructed. Integrating the above, one can define heart failure as a condition in which the heart fails to provide adequate forward output at normal filling pressures; this condition is typically associated with a clinical syndrome of reduced functional capacity and pulmonary and systemic venous congestion. It is important to reemphasize the fact that the failing heart

functions in the context of a systemic circulation that requires mechanisms by which both cardiac output and vascular resistance can be modulated.

The primary mechanism by which forward cardiac output is maintained is recruitment of preload reserve, a dynamic reduction of venous capacitance that results in "centralization" of peripheral blood volume and enhanced venous return, thereby increasing left ventricular end-diastolic volume (EDV). This increased left ventricular volume in turn leads to an increase in the length of left ventricular (LV) muscle fibers, thereby enhancing actin-myosin interaction and producing greater contractile force and increased LV stroke volume (SV); this fundamental relationship between left ventricular filling and stroke volume is the *Frank-Starling relationship* (the "normal" curve in Figure 33–1). This preload recruitment represents the primary mechanism intrinsic to the cardiovascular system by which cardiac output can be augmented. If preload recruitment does not provide sufficient forward cardiac output, the compensatory responses that

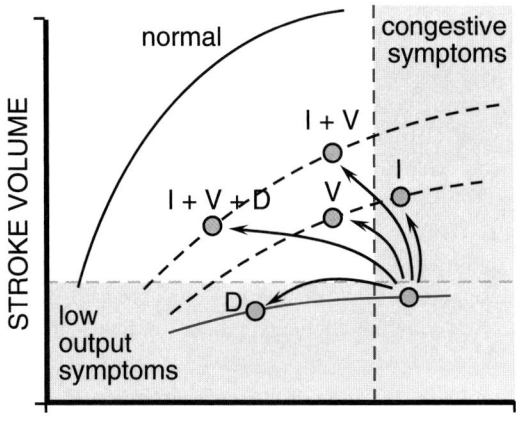

Figure 33–1. Hemodynamic responses to pharmacological interventions in heart failure. The relationships between diastolic filling pressure (or preload) and stroke volume (or ventricular performance) are illustrated for a normal heart (*black line*; the Frank-Starling relationship) and for a patient with heart failure due to predominant systolic dysfunction (*blue line*). Note that positive inotropic agents (I), such as cardiac glycosides or dobutamine, move patients to a higher ventricular function curve (*lower dashed line*), resulting in greater cardiac work for a given level of ventricular filling pressure. Vasodilators (V), such as ACE inhibitors or nitroprusside, also move patients to improved ventricular function curves while reducing cardiac filling pressures. Diuretics (D) improve symptoms of congestive heart failure by moving patients to lower cardiac filling pressures along the same ventricular function curve. Combinations of drugs often will yield additive effects on hemodynamics.

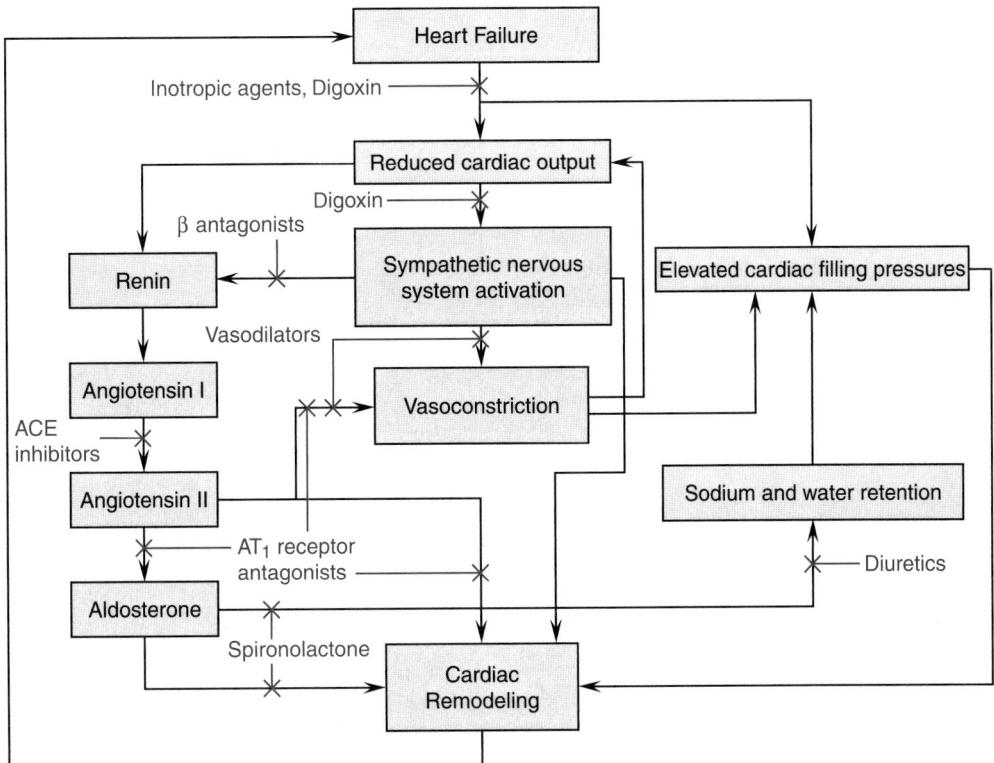

Figure 33–2. Pathophysiological mechanisms of heart failure and major sites of drug action. Heart failure is accompanied by compensatory neurohormonal responses including activation of the sympathetic nervous and renin–angiotensin systems. Although these responses initially help to maintain cardiovascular function by increasing ventricular preload and systemic vascular tone, with time they contribute to the progression of myocardial failure. Increased ventricular afterload, due to systemic vasoconstriction and chamber dilation, causes a depression in systolic function. In addition, increased afterload and the direct effects of angiotensin and norepinephrine on the ventricular myocardium cause pathological remodeling characterized by progressive chamber dilation and loss of contractile function. The figure illustrates several mechanisms that appear to play important roles in the pathophysiology of heart failure, and the sites of action of pharmacological therapies that have been shown to be of clinical value.

follow reflect the severity and duration of the hemodynamic stress.

In the case of acute circulatory stress (*e.g.*, myocardial infarction), neurohumoral systems are activated that support the circulation; principal among these are the sympathetic branch of the autonomic nervous system and the renin–angiotensin system. The net effect of activation of the sympathetic nervous system is increased myocardial contractility, enhanced myocardial relaxation, and increased heart rate (β adrenergic effects); activation of the sympathetic efferents also results in increases in systemic vascular resistance and MAP (α adrenergic effects). The renin–angiotensin system also supports cardiac output and mean arterial pressure. The system is activated by reduction of renal perfusion pressure, which increases renin secretion; renin cleaves circulating angiotensinogen to produce angiotensin I (Ang I); Ang I is converted to angiotensin II (Ang II) by the action of angiotensin-converting enzyme (ACE).

Ang II, a potent vasoconstrictor, thereby helps to maintain MAP; Ang II also leads to increased adrenal production of aldosterone, a mineralocorticoid that causes Na$^+$ and fluid retention, thereby expanding intravascular volume and increasing venous return. Thus, the sympathetic nervous system and renin–angiotensin system collaborate to maintain the MAP and cardiac output. Under physiologic conditions, these compensatory mechanisms operate in the context of normal myocardial contractility, normal myocardial compliance, and temporally constrained hemodynamic stress. In patients with CHF, these compensatory systems must operate under circumstances in which left ventricular performance is impaired and the hemodynamic stress is chronic. The intersections of compensatory mechanisms with pathophysiologic mechanisms, as well as sites of drug action, are shown in Figure 33–2.

In the setting of contractile dysfunction, the normal relationship between EDV and SV is shifted downward

(Figure 33–1), such that left ventricular SV may be reduced even if EDV is markedly increased. This increase in EDV results in higher diastolic and systolic wall stress and eventually leads to increases in left ventricular end-diastolic pressure and left atrial pressure; this in turn alters Starling forces in the pulmonary capillaries to favor transudation of fluid into the extravascular spaces of the pulmonary interstitium, producing interstitial and alveolar edema. In addition, the vasoconstrictive effectors of the sympathetic nervous system and the renin–angiotensin system lead to an increase in systemic vascular resistance, which contributes to an increased impedance to left ventricular ejection (increased afterload). The left ventricle becomes increasingly sensitive to the effects of afterload in the setting of contractile dysfunction; such increases in afterload ultimately produce substantial reductions in left ventricular stroke volume. The consequent reduction of cardiac output serves as an iterative stimulus to continued activation of the neurohumoral systems that stimulate the heart and constrict the vessels.

Hypertrophic Remodeling. It has long been presumed that the adult heart cannot respond to sustained hemodynamic stress by hyperplasia. In the face of such stress, however, signal transduction systems do exist that initiate the synthesis and spatial organization of new contractile proteins, a process known as *hypertrophic remodeling.*

In cases of chronic pressure overload, such as systemic arterial hypertension or valvular aortic stenosis, contractile proteins and new sarcomeres are added to existing cardiac myocytes in parallel to existing myofilaments. This leads to increased wall thickness and decreased chamber radius, resulting in reduction of systolic wall stress. Because LV ejection fraction is inversely proportional to systolic wall stress, this compensatory mechanism contributes to the maintenance of normal LV stroke volume. The disadvantage of concentric remodeling derives from the decrease in LV compliance that occurs as a consequence of this pattern of hypertrophy: LV diastolic pressure is increased at any given LV volume, predisposing to congestive symptoms.

In contrast, sustained increases of volume, such as left-sided valvular regurgitation, result in eccentric pattern hypertrophy. In this pattern of remodeling, new contractile proteins are added to existing myofilaments in series, leading to increased myocardial compliance and thereby attenuating diastolic wall stress. At the whole-organ level, this allows continued preload recruitment without significant elevation of LV diastolic pressure. As a result, total LV stroke volume is increased and forward cardiac output is maintained at normal filling pressures. This compensatory response does carry

some consequence: progressive LV dilation ultimately produces a secondary increase in systolic wall stress.

In circumstances of sustained pressure or volume loading, cardiomyocyte injury and whole-organ pump dysfunction supervene if the abnormal loading conditions are not corrected. This transition from compensated hypertrophy to contractile dysfunction has been referred to as the cardiomyopathy of chronic overload, the end result of maladaptive proliferative signaling (Katz, 1994; Villarreal, 2005).

Cellular Pathophysiology. At the cellular level, changes associated with the transition to contractile dysfunction include dysregulation of Ca^{2+} homeostasis, changes in the regulation and expression of the contractile proteins, and alterations in adrenergic signal transduction pathways.

Altered calcium homeostasis results in prolongation of the action potential and the Ca^{2+} transient. Mechanisms that increase the cytosolic concentration of Ca^{2+} include reduction of Ca^{2+} sequestration by the sarcoplasmic reticulum and increased Ca^{2+} uptake *via* the Na^+-Ca^{2+} exchanger. The derivative abnormalities of calcium handling can result in impairment of both myocardial contraction and relaxation.

Dysfunctional contractile proteins are produced by changes in the transcription of a number of genes in the cardiac myocyte. Available data indicate that myocytes enter a maladaptive proliferative phase in which fetal isoforms are expressed. Alterations of the contractile proteins associated with heart failure range from abnormalities of troponin and myosin that interfere with the rate of cross-bridge cycling to activation of collagenase/matrix metalloproteinases that disrupt the extracellular matrix that couples cellular elements.

Desensitization of the β receptor–G_s–adenylyl cyclase–cyclic AMP pathway is another major abnormality that has been described in the failing cardiac myocyte (Mann, 1999). The number of β receptors expressed at the cell surface is down-regulated, resulting in reduction of cyclic AMP production in response to β adrenergic stimulation. This reduction in β adrenergic signaling may reflect increased expression of both β adrenergic receptor kinase (which phosphorylates and thereby inhibits β receptors) and G_i, the inhibitory G protein. The expression of inducible nitric oxide (NO) synthase is increased in CHF; NO can have negative inotropic effects and can reduce cyclic AMP signaling. The net result of these alterations at the level of signaling *via* cyclic AMP–PKA is decreased phosphorylation of phospholamban, resulting in impaired Ca^{2+} uptake by the sarcoplasmic reticulum and consequent impairment of both contraction and relaxation.

Clinical Heart Failure

From the above discussion, one can delineate the following pathophysiologic sequence in response to myocardial failure. Initially, myocardial dysfunction and the attendant reduction of forward cardiac output lead to expansion of intravascular volume and activation of neurohumoral systems, particularly the sympathetic nervous system and the renin–angiotensin system. These compensatory responses maintain perfusion to vital organs by increasing left ventricular preload, stimulating myocardial contractility, and increasing arterial tone. While physiologic in the context of volume contraction, in the context of congestive failure, avid retention of Na^+ and water and vasoconstriction are pathologic (Weber, 2001). Acutely, these mechanisms help to sustain cardiac output by allowing the heart to operate at higher end-diastolic volumes, leading to increased stroke volume; concomitant peripheral vasoconstriction allows for regional redistribution of the cardiac output to critical perfusion beds. Unfortunately, each of these compensatory responses will also promote disease progression. Expansion of the intravascular volume and elevated ventricular chamber volumes will lead to increased diastolic and systolic wall stress; these changes in turn will lead to impaired myocardial energetics and will induce hypertrophic remodeling. Neurohumoral activation will lead to arterial and venous constriction; the former will increase left ventricular afterload (thereby compromising left ventricular stroke volume) and the latter will increase preload, thereby exacerbating both diastolic and systolic wall stress. In addition, the neurohumoral effectors (such as norepinephrine and Ang II) may act directly on the myocardium to promote unfavorable remodeling by causing myocyte apoptosis, abnormal gene expression, and alterations in the extracellular matrix (Colucci and Braunwald, 2000; Villarreal, 2005).

PHARMACOLOGICAL TREATMENT OF HEART FAILURE

The abnormalities of myocardial structure and function that underlie heart failure are often irreversible. As noted above, these abnormalities can serve as stimuli to the activation of biological responses that drive disease progression. It is perhaps not surprising that the syndrome of CHF is typically a chronic illness during which episodic, acute decompensation may occur. Drugs that reduce ventricular wall stress or inhibit the renin–angiotensin system (*e.g.,* selected vasodilators, ACE inhibitors, and aldosterone antagonists) or the sympathetic nervous system (*e.g.,* β adrenergic antagonists) can decrease pathological ventricular remodeling, attenuate disease progression, and decrease mortality in patients with heart failure due to systolic dysfunction. As a result, these drugs have become mainstays in the long-term treatment of heart failure. Some of the drugs that slow progression afford an immediate beneficial impact on hemodynamic function and symptoms (*e.g.,* vasodilators and ACE inhibitors). Other agents that attenuate disease progression can have an adverse effect on hemodynamic function and worsen symptoms in the short term and must therefore be used with caution (*e.g.,* β receptor antagonists). Figure 33–2 provides an overview of the pathophysiological mechanisms of heart failure and the sites of action of the major drug classes used in treatment.

The pharmacological treatment of heart failure for many years was limited to the use of digitalis glycosides and diuretics. Although *digitalis* has been supplanted by therapies that provide a mortality benefit (*e.g.,* ACE inhibitors), the clinical and investigative uses of the cardiac

glycosides have informed approaches to therapy and drug design and development. Similarly, while diuretics do not offer a mortality benefit, volume overload clearly remains a central component of the clinical syndrome and is often the factor that leads to initial diagnosis or to hospitalization for treatment of acute exacerbations.

The current approach to therapy for CHF involves preload reduction, afterload reduction, and enhancement of inotropic state (Figure 33–1). A variety of vasodilators will reduce preload and afterload (Table 33–1). Although a vasodilator's more prominent effect may be the reduction of either preload or afterload, most agents affect both, to differing extents.

Diuretics

Diuretics retain a central role in the pharmacological management of the "congestive" symptoms in patients with heart failure. The pharmacological properties of these agents are presented in detail in Chapter 28. Their importance in heart failure management reflects the central role of the kidney in the hemodynamic, hormonal, and autonomic responses to myocardial failure. The net effect of these responses is the retention of Na^+ and water and expansion of the extracellular fluid volume, allowing the heart to operate at higher end-diastolic volumes, and thereby to maintain LV stroke volume. However, this increase in end-diastolic volume results in higher end-diastolic filling pressures, increased ventricular chamber dimensions, and elevated wall stress. In turn, these changes result in pulmonary venous congestion and peripheral edema, ultimately limiting further augmentation of cardiac output. Elevated filling pressures are associated with enhanced activation of neurohumoral systems that can drive the progression of CHF (Hillege *et al.*, 2000).

Diuretics reduce extracellular fluid volume and ventricular filling pressure (or "preload"). Because patients with heart failure often operate on a "plateau" phase of the Starling curve (Figure 33–1), preload reduction can occur without concomitant reduction in cardiac output. Note that reduction in cardiac output can occur in patients who have had either sustained natriuresis and/or a rapid decline in intravascular volume. In this circumstance, diuretic therapy may augment neurohormonal activation due to volume depletion, with potentially deleterious effects on the progression of heart failure (McCurley *et al.*, 2004). For this reason, it is preferable to avoid the use of diuretics in the subset of patients with asymptomatic LV dysfunction and to use the minimal dose necessary to maintain euvolemia in patients with symptoms related to volume retention. Despite the efficacy

Table 33–1
Vasodilator Drugs Used to Treat Heart Failure

DRUG CLASS	EXAMPLES	MECHANISM OF VASODILATING ACTION	PRELOAD REDUCTION	AFTERLOAD REDUCTION
Organic nitrates	Nitroglycerin, isosorbide dinitrate	NO-mediated vasodilation	+++	+
Nitric oxide donors	Nitroprusside	NO-mediated vasodilation	+++	+++
Angiotensin-converting enzyme inhibitors	Captopril, enalapril, lisinopril	Inhibition of Ang II generation, decreased bradykinin degradation	++	++
Angiotensin receptor blockers	Losartan, candesartan	Blockade of AT_1 receptors	++	++
Phosphodiesterase inhibitors	Milrinone, inamrinone	Inhibition of cyclic AMP degradation	++	++
Direct-acting K^+-channel agonist	Hydralazine	Unknown	+	+++
	Minoxidil	Hyperpolarization of vascular smooth muscle cells	+	+++
α_1 Adrenergic antagonists	Doxazosin, prazosin	Selective α_1 adrenergic receptor blockade	+++	++
Nonselective α adrenergic antagonists	Phentolamine	Nonselective α adrenergic receptor blockade	+++	+++
Vasodilating β/α_1 adrenergic antagonists	Carvedilol, labetalol	Selective α_1 adrenergic receptor blockade	++	++
Ca^{2+} channel blockers	Amlodipine, nifedipine, felodipine	Inhibition of L-type Ca^{2+} channels	+	+++
β adrenergic agonists	Isoproterenol	Stimulation of vascular β_2 adrenergic receptors	+	++

ABBREVIATIONS: Ang II, angiotensin II; AT_1, type 1 Ang II receptor; NO, nitric oxide.

of diuretics in controlling congestive symptoms and improving exercise capacity, the use of diuretics, with the exception of aldosterone antagonists, does not reduce mortality in heart failure.

Dietary Sodium Restriction. All patients with clinically significant ventricular dysfunction, regardless of symptom status, should be advised to limit dietary intake of NaCl. Most patients will tolerate moderate reductions in salt intake (2 to 3 g/day total intake). More stringent salt restriction is seldom necessary and may be counterproductive, as it can lead to hyponatremia, hypokalemia, and hypochloremic metabolic alkalosis when combined with administration of loop diuretics.

Loop Diuretics. Of the loop diuretics currently available, *furosemide* (LASIX), *bumetanide* (BUMEX), and *torsemide* (DEMADEX) are widely used in the treatment of heart failure. Due to the increased risk of ototoxicity, *ethacrynic acid* (EDECRIN) should be reserved for patients who are allergic to sulfonamides or who have developed interstitial nephritis on alternative drugs.

Loop diuretics inhibit a specific ion transport protein, the Na^+-K^+-$2Cl^-$ symporter on the apical membrane of renal epithelial cells in the ascending limb of the loop of Henle (*see* Chapter 28). Their efficacy is dependent upon sufficient renal plasma flow and proximal tubular secretion to deliver the diuretics to their site of action. These drugs also reduce the tonicity of the medullary interstitium by preventing the resorption of solute in excess of water in the thick ascending limb of the loop of Henle. The increased delivery of Na^+ and fluid to distal nephron segments also markedly enhances K^+ secretion, particularly in the presence of elevated aldosterone levels, as is typically the case in heart failure.

The bioavailability of orally administered furosemide ranges from 40% to 70%. Higher doses of drug often are required to initiate diuresis in patients who present with worsening symptoms (Gottlieb, 2004); thus upward titration of dosage is required before furosemide is deemed ineffective. In contrast, the oral bioavailabilities of bumetanide and torsemide exceed 80%; as a result these agents provide more consistent absorption, albeit at a considerably greater cost. The pharmacologic actions of the loop diuretics are similar; thus, the use of the more expensive agents rarely is warranted (Brater, 1998).

Furosemide and bumetanide are short-acting drugs. The resultant postdose decline in renal tubular diuretic levels leads to avid renal Na^+ retention by all nephron segments. This can limit or prevent negative Na^+ balance and it is a common practice in CHF patients to administer two or more doses daily. This is an acceptable strategy for outpatient management of heart failure, provided there is adequate monitoring of daily weight and blood electrolyte levels.

Thiazide Diuretics. The thiazide diuretics (DIURIL, HYDRO-DIURIL, others) are most frequently used in the treatment of systemic hypertension; these drugs have a more restricted role in the treatment of CHF.

The principal site of action of the thiazide diuretics is the Na^+-Cl^- cotransporter of the epithelial cells in the distal convoluted tubule (*see* Chapter 28). This distal site of action permits rapid adjustment of water and solute absorption by more proximal nephron segments, limiting the utility of thiazide monotherapy in patients with more advanced disease. Thiazide diuretics are ineffective at glomerular filtration rates below 30 ml/min and are therefore not used in patients with significant impairment of renal function.

While thiazides have a limited role as single agents in the treatment of heart failure, they exhibit true synergism with loop diuretics: the natriuresis that follows coadministration exceeds the summed effects of the drugs administered individually. This synergism is the rationale for combination therapy in patients who appear refractory to loop diuretics. In general, thiazides are associated with a greater degree of potassium wasting for comparable volume reduction when compared to loop diuretics (Gottleib, 2004).

K^+-Sparing Diuretics. K^+-sparing diuretics (*see* Chapter 28) act principally in the collecting duct of the nephron and either inhibit apical membrane Na^+ conductance channels in epithelial cells (*e.g.*, *amiloride, triamterene*) or act as aldosterone antagonists (*e.g.*, *canrenone* [not commercially available in the United States], *spironolactone*, and *eplerenone*). These agents are relatively weak diuretics and therefore are not effective for volume reduction. Historically, these agents have been used to limit renal K^+ and Mg^{2+} wasting and/or to augment the diuretic response to other agents. There is now evidence that aldosterone antagonists improve survival in patients with advanced heart failure *via* a mechanism that is independent of diuresis (Pitt *et al.*, 1999; Pitt *et al.*, 2003).

Use of Diuretics in Clinical Practice. The majority of patients with heart failure will require chronic administration of a loop diuretic to maintain euvolemia. In patients with clinically evident fluid retention, furosemide typically is started at a dose of 40 mg once or twice per day, and the dosage is increased until an adequate diuresis is achieved. A larger initial dose may be required in patients with more

advanced heart failure or with concurrent azotemia. Serum electrolytes and renal function should be monitored frequently in patients with preexisting renal insufficiency or those in whom a rapid diuresis is desirable. Once fluid retention has resolved, the diuretic dose should be reduced to the minimal level necessary to maintain euvolemia. Electrolyte abnormalities and/or worsening azotemia may supervene before euvolemia is achieved. Hypokalemia may be corrected by potassium supplementation or addition of a potassium-sparing diuretic.

Aldosterone Antagonists

One of the principal features of CHF is marked activation of the renin–angiotensin–aldosterone system. In heart failure patients, plasma aldosterone concentrations may increase to as high as 20 times the normal level. Aldosterone has a range of biological effects beyond salt retention (Table 33–2), and antagonism of aldosterone's actions may be beneficial in patients with heart failure (Weber, 2001).

Clinical Use of Spironolactone in Heart Failure. The RALES Trial (Randomized Aldactone Evaluation Study) randomized patients with moderate-to-severe heart failure (New York Heart Association [NYHA] Class III to IV) to treatment with ≥25 mg daily of spirono-

Table 33–2
Potential Roles of Aldosterone in the Pathophysiology of Heart Failure

MECHANISM	PATHOPHYSIOLOGICAL EFFECT
Increased Na^+ and water retention	Edema, elevated cardiac filling pressures
K^+ and Mg^{2+} loss	Arrhythmogenesis and risk of sudden cardiac death
Reduced myocardial norepinephrine uptake	Potentiation of norepinephrine effects: myocardial remodeling and arrhythmogenesis
Reduced baroreceptor sensitivity	Reduced parasympathetic activity and risk of sudden cardiac death
Myocardial fibrosis, fibroblast proliferation	Remodeling and ventricular dysfunction
Alterations in Na^+ channel expression	Increased excitability and contractility of cardiac myocytes

lactone or placebo as an addition to conventional therapy; the large majority of patients were receiving concomitant ACE inhibitor therapy (Pitt *et al.*, 1999). Patients with serum creatinine concentrations >2.5 mg/dl (221 μM) were excluded from the study; a very small number of patients received 50 mg of spironolactone daily. Patients randomized to spironolactone had a significant (~30%) reduction in mortality and hospitalization for heart failure. The decrease in the risk of death was due to reductions in both progressive heart failure and sudden cardiac death. This risk reduction was achieved in the absence of a demonstrable diuretic effect, lending support to the hypothesis that aldosterone antagonists attenuate or reverse the pathologic remodeling that occurs in heart failure (Weber, 2001; Redfield *et al.*, 2003). Treatment generally was well tolerated; although 10% of men in the spironolactone group developed gynecomastia, withdrawal of treatment was necessary in less than 2%. Severe hyperkalemia occurred in only 2% of patients on spironolactone, and there were no clinically significant effects on renal function.

The RALES trial suggests that the beneficial effects of spironolactone are additive to those of ACE inhibitors; the use of spironolactone should be considered in patients with NYHA Class III and IV heart failure. Caution should be exercised when significant renal impairment is present. Treatment should be initiated at a dose of 12.5 or 25 mg daily. Higher doses should be avoided, as they may lead to hyperkalemia, particularly in patients receiving an ACE inhibitor (Juurlink *et al.*, 2004). Serum K$^+$ levels and electrolytes should be checked after initiation of treatment, and vigilance is warranted for potential drug interactions and medical disorders that may cause elevations in serum K$^+$ concentration (*e.g.*, potassium supplements, ACE inhibitors, and worsening renal function).

The findings of the RALES Trial were recently corroborated in the EPHESUS (Eplerenone Post-Acute Myocardial Infarction Heart Failure Efficacy and Survival) study (Pitt *et al.*, 2003). The EPHESUS data suggest that treatment with aldosterone antagonists is associated with mortality benefit in patients with heart failure due to left ventricular systolic dysfunction. The observations support the use of aldosterone antagonists in conjunction with inhibitors of the renin–angiotensin system and β receptor antagonists in patients with symptomatic heart failure. The role of aldosterone antagonists in patients with asymptomatic left ventricular dysfunction has not been established.

Diuretics in the Decompensated Patient. As discussed for the treatment of heart failure in the ambulatory patient, diuretics are important for the alleviation of intravascular and extravascular fluid overload. In patients with decompensated heart failure of a severity that warrants hospital admission, it is generally desirable to initiate diuresis by intravenous administration of a loop diuretic. This typically provides a more rapid and predictable diuresis than does enteral therapy. The loop diuretic may be administered as repetitive boluses titrated to achieve the desired response, or by constant infusion. An advantage of infusion is that the same total daily dose of diuretic, given as a continuous infusion, results in a more sustained natriuresis due to maintenance of high drug levels within the lumen of renal tubules (Dormans *et al.*, 1996). In addition, the risk of ototoxicity is reduced by continuous infusion when compared to repetitive, intermittent intravenous dosing (Lahav *et al.*, 1992). A typical continuous furosemide infusion is initiated with a 40-mg bolus injection followed by a constant infusion of 10 mg/hour, with upward titration of the infusion as necessary. When there is a poor response to monotherapy, coadministration of a thiazide agent is

warranted. If the poor response is due to reduced renal perfusion, short-term administration of sympathomimetic drugs or phosphodiesterase inhibitors to increase cardiac output may be required.

Diuretic Resistance in Heart Failure. The response to diuretics is often impaired in patients with CHF. This impaired response may itself be a manifestation of the Na$^+$ avidity and the volume retention that characterize advanced heart failure. While there may initially be a brisk response to once-daily dosing, a compensatory increase in Na$^+$ reabsorption during the remainder of the day may prevent effective diuresis; as a result, reduction of the dosing interval may be warranted. In advanced heart failure, edema, decreased motility of the bowel wall, and reduced splanchnic blood flow can result in delay or attenuation of peak diuretic effect. Patients who have impaired renal function typically require higher doses of diuretic to ensure adequate delivery of the drug to its site of action.

Following prolonged administration of a loop diuretic, a process of adaptation can occur in which there is a compensatory increase in Na$^+$ reabsorption in the distal nephron and blunting of net Na$^+$ and water loss. The more common causes of diuretic resistance are listed in Table 33–3. An increasing diuretic requirement may also be due to intravascular volume depletion following aggressive diuresis or to concurrent administration of vasoactive drugs; the possibility that diuretic resistance may be a manifestation of progressive heart failure must be considered. Invasive assessment of intracardiac filling pressures and cardiac output may be required to make these distinctions.

Vasodilators commonly employed as "unloading" agents in heart failure may reduce renal blood flow despite an increase in cardiac output; this occurs as a result of reduction in mean arterial pressure and redistribution of cardiac output to extrarenal circulatory beds. The net effect may be reduction of diuretic effectiveness. In addition, the presence of atherosclerotic renal artery stenosis in

Table 33–3
Causes of Diuretic Resistance in Heart Failure

Noncompliance with medical regimen; excess dietary Na$^+$ intake
Decreased renal perfusion and glomerular filtration rate due to:
Excessive intravascular volume depletion and hypotension due to aggressive diuretic or vasodilator therapy
Decline in cardiac output due to worsening heart failure, arrhythmias, or other primary cardiac causes
Selective reduction in glomerular perfusion pressure following initiation (or dose increase) of ACE inhibitor therapy
Nonsteroidal antiinflammatory drugs
Primary renal pathology (*e.g.*, cholesterol emboli, renal artery stenosis, drug-induced interstitial nephritis, obstructive uropathy)
Reduced or impaired diuretic absorption due to gut wall edema and reduced splanchnic blood flow

patients who receive vasodilator drugs may reduce renal perfusion pressure to levels below that necessary to maintain normal autoregulation and glomerular filtration.

The caveats about concomitant therapy merit particular emphasis when considering coadministration of diuretics and ACE inhibitors or AT_1 receptor antagonists. These inhibitors of the renin–angiotensin system can either augment or reduce the effectiveness of diuretics. A reduced response is observed most commonly in patients with decreased renal arterial perfusion pressure, due either to renal artery stenosis or to reduction of forward cardiac output. In such patients, a high level of Ang II–mediated glomerular efferent arteriolar tone is necessary to maintain glomerular filtration pressure. Pharmacologic antagonism of this intrarenal autoregulation may be accompanied by a decline in creatinine clearance and a derivative rise in the serum creatinine. In general, this is readily distinguished from the modest and limited rise in serum creatinine levels that commonly accompany administration of ACE inhibitors. Diuretic resistance that reflects poor forward cardiac output may require the use of positive inotropic agents (*e.g., dobutamine*) as vasodilator therapy is initiated.

Decreased responsiveness to loop diuretics in patients with known chronic heart failure should prompt an increase in the dose administered or the dosing frequency. If this is ineffective, a thiazide diuretic (*e.g., hydrochlorothiazide* or *metolazone*) administered with the loop diuretic is often effective (Ellison, 1991). However, this combination can result in an unpredictable and sometimes excessive diuresis, leading to intravascular volume depletion and renal K^+ wasting; the combination therefore should be used cautiously. Spironolactone also may be effective in these patients when combined with a loop diuretic. For a detailed discussion on the subject of diuretic resistance, see the review by Ellison (1999).

Metabolic Consequences of Diuretic Therapy. The side effects of diuretics are discussed in Chapter 28 (Gottlieb, 2004). With regard to diuretic use in heart failure, the most important adverse sequelae of diuretics are electrolyte abnormalities, including hyponatremia, hypokalemia, and hypochloremic metabolic alkalosis. The clinical importance, or even the existence, of significant Mg^{2+} deficiency with chronic diuretic use remains controversial (Bigger, 1994; Davies and Fraser, 1993). Both hypokalemia and renal Mg^{2+} wasting can be limited by administration of oral KCl supplements or a K^+-sparing diuretic.

Vasodilators

The rationale for the use of oral vasodilator drugs in the pharmacotherapy of CHF derived from the experience with the parenteral agents *phentolamine* and *nitroprusside* in patients with severe heart failure and elevated systemic vascular resistance (Cohn and Franciosa, 1977). Although a number of vasodilators may improve symptoms in heart failure, only the *hydralazine–isosorbide dinitrate* combination and antagonists of the renin–angiotensin system (ACE inhibitors and AT_1 receptor blockers) have been shown to improve survival in prospective randomized trials. The pharmacology of the vasodilators discussed in this chapter is considered in

more detail in Chapters 10, 30, and 32. Table 33–1 summarizes some properties of vasodilators used to treat heart failure.

A randomized, prospective trial verified the effectiveness of the isosorbide dinitrate–hydralazine combination in reducing mortality in patients with heart failure due to systolic dysfunction (Veterans Administration Cooperative Vasodilator-Heart Failure Trial I; V-HeFT I) (Cohn *et al.*, 1986). V-HeFT I also demonstrated that the mortality impact was agent-specific: the α receptor agonist *prazosin* was no better than placebo when compared to isosorbide plus hydralazine. In another trial, treatment with the ACE inhibitor *enalapril* was associated with reduction of mortality in patients with NYHA Class IV heart failure (CONSENSUS Trial Study Group, 1987). V-HeFT II, a trial that compared the isosorbide dinitrate–hydralazine combination to enalapril, indicated that vasodilators that antagonize the effects of angiotensin provide incremental survival benefit (Cohn *et al.*, 1991). Subsequent trials with ACE inhibitors and AT_1 receptor antagonists corroborated these early data and provided evidence supporting the use of ACE inhibitors and AT_1 receptor antagonists in patients with less advanced CHF and in those with asymptomatic left ventricular dysfunction.

Inhibitors of the Renin–Angiotensin System: ACE Inhibitors and AT_1 Receptor Antagonists

Renin–Angiotensin System Antagonists. The renin–angiotensin system (Figure 33–3) plays a central role in the pathophysiology of heart failure. Angiotensinogen is cleaved by kidney-derived renin to form the decapeptide angiotensin I (Ang I); ACE converts Ang I to the octapeptide Ang II. Ang II is a potent arterial vasoconstrictor and an important mediator of Na^+ and water retention through its effects on glomerular filtration pressure and aldosterone secretion. In addition, Ang II potentiates neural catecholamine release, is a secretagogue for catecholamine release from the adrenal medulla, is arrhythmogenic, promotes vascular hyperplasia and pathologic myocardial hypertrophy, and stimulates myocyte death. Consequently, the antagonism of Ang II forms one of the cornerstones of heart failure management (Weber, 2001).

ACE inhibitors suppress Ang II and aldosterone production, decrease sympathetic nervous system activity, and potentiate the effects of diuretics in heart failure. However, Ang II levels frequently return to baseline values following chronic treatment with ACE inhibitors (Juillerat *et al.*, 1990), due in part to production of Ang II through ACE-independent enzymes such as chymase, a tissue protease. The sustained clinical effectiveness of ACE inhibitors despite Ang II "escape" suggests that there are alternate mechanisms that contribute to the clinical effects of ACE inhibitors in heart failure. ACE is iden-

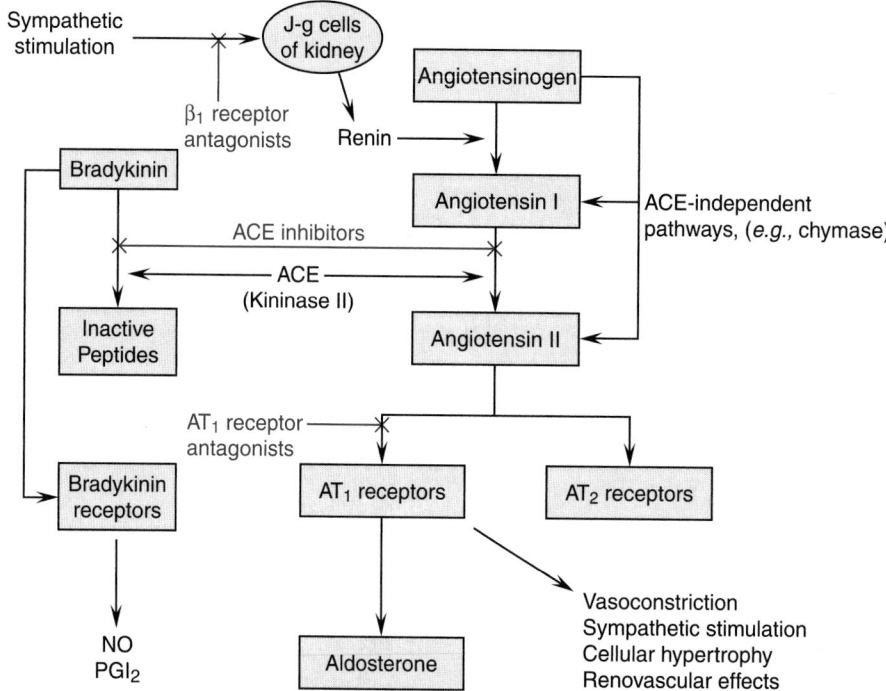

Figure 33–3. *The renin–angiotensin–aldosterone system.* Renin, excreted in response to β adrenergic stimulation of the juxta-glomerular (J-g) cells of the kidney, cleaves plasma angiotensinogen to produce angiotensin I (Ang I). Angiotensin II (Ang II) is formed through the cleavage of Ang I by angiotensin-converting enzyme (ACE). Most of the known biological effects of Ang II are mediated by the type 1 angiotensin receptor (AT_1). In general, the AT_2 receptor appears to counteract the effects of Ang II mediated by activation of the AT_1 pathway. Ang II also may be formed through ACE-independent pathways. These pathways, and possibly incomplete inhibition of tissue ACE, may account for persistence of angiotensin in patients treated with ACE inhibitors. AT_1 receptor antagonists have been postulated to provide more complete blockade of the renin-angiotensin-aldosterone system than ACE inhibition alone. ACE inhibition reduces bradykinin degradation, thus enhancing its levels and biological effects, including the production of nitric oxide (NO) and prostaglandin I_2 (PGI_2). Bradykinin may mediate some of the biological effects of ACE inhibitors.

tical to kininase II, which degrades bradykinin and other kinins that stimulate production of NO, cyclic GMP, and vasoactive eicosanoids; these vasodilator substances seem to oppose the effects of Ang II on the growth of vascular smooth muscle and cardiac fibroblasts and on production of extracellular matrix. Thus, the increased levels of bradykinin that result from ACE inhibition may play a role in the hemodynamic and anti-remodeling effects of ACE inhibitors.

ACE inhibitors are more potent arterial than venous dilators. In response to ACE inhibition, mean arterial pressure (MAP) may decrease or be unchanged; the change in MAP will be determined by the stroke volume response to afterload reduction. Heart rate typically is unchanged, even when there is a decrease in systemic arterial pressure, a response that likely reflects a decrease in sympathetic nervous system activity in response to ACE inhibition. The decrease in left ventricular afterload results in increased stroke volume and cardiac output.

Venodilation results in decreases in right and left heart filling pressures and end-diastolic volumes.

An alternative means of attenuating the hemodynamic and vascular impact of the renin–angiotensin system is through inhibition of angiotensin receptors. Most of the known clinical actions of angiotensin II, including its deleterious effects in heart failure, are mediated through the AT_1 angiotensin receptor. AT_2 angiotensin receptors, also present throughout the cardiovascular system, seem to mediate responses that counterbalance the biological effects of AT_1 receptor stimulation.

Due to their more distal site of action, AT_1 receptor antagonists may provide more potent reduction of the effects of angiotensin II than do ACE inhibitors. Furthermore, AT_1 receptor blockade may result in greater AT_2 receptor activation, as Ang II levels rise as a consequence of AT_1 receptor blockade. Note that blockade of AT_1 receptors does not alter bradykinin metabolism, which ACE inhibitors reduce.

Angiotensin-Converting Enzyme Inhibitors. The first orally active ACE inhibitor, *captopril* (CAPOTEN), was introduced in 1977, and five other ACE inhibitors—*enalapril* (VASOTEC), *ramipril* (ALTACE), *lisinopril* (PRINIVIL, ZESTRIL), *quinapril* (ACCUPRIL), and *fosinopril* (MONOPRIL)—are currently approved by the FDA for the treatment of heart failure. Data from numerous clinical trials involving well over 100,000 patients support the use of ACE inhibitors for the treatment of patients with heart failure of any severity, including the patient cohort with asymptomatic left ventricular dysfunction.

ACE-inhibitor therapy should be initiated at a low dose (*e.g.,* 6.25 mg of captopril or 5 mg of lisinopril), as some patients may experience an abrupt drop in blood pressure, particularly in the setting of volume contraction. Hypotension following drug administration can usually be reversed by intravascular volume expansion, although this may be counterproductive in patients with symptomatic heart failure. It is therefore reasonable to consider initiation of these drugs while congestive symptoms are present. ACE-inhibitor doses are customarily increased over several days in hospitalized patients or a few weeks in ambulatory patients, with careful observation of blood pressure, serum electrolytes, and serum creatinine levels.

There is no precisely defined relationship between dose and long-term clinical effectiveness of these drugs. However, it has been suggested that the target dose should in general be the doses used in clinical trials that have established drug efficacy in patients with heart failure. On this basis, target doses of these drugs would be 50 mg three times per day for captopril (Pfeffer *et al.*, 1992); 10 mg twice daily for enalapril (SOLVD Investigators, 1991; Cohn *et al.*, 1991); 10 mg once daily for lisinopril (GISSI-3, 1994); or 5 mg twice daily for ramipril (AIRE Study Investigators, 1993). In patients who have not achieved an adequate clinical response at these doses, further increases, as tolerated, may be of value. For instance, high-dose lisinopril (32.5 or 35 mg) reduced the combined endpoint of mortality and hospitalization when compared to lower doses of this agent in the ATLAS (Assessment of Treatment with Lisinopril and Survival) study (Packer *et al.*, 1999).

In patients with heart failure and reduced renal blood flow, ACE inhibitors, unlike other vasodilators, limit the kidney's ability to autoregulate glomerular perfusion pressure due to their selective effects on efferent arteriolar tone. If this occurs, the dose of ACE inhibitor should be reduced or another class of vasodilator added or substituted. Rarely, worsening of renal function following initiation of therapy with an ACE inhibitor will be due to the presence of bilateral renal artery stenosis. Preferably, the renal artery stenosis should be treated; if this is not technically or logistically feasible, another class of vasodilator should be substituted. Similarly, angioedema secondary to ACE inhibition should prompt immediate cessation of therapy. A small rise in serum K^+ levels occurs frequently with ACE inhibitors; this rise can be substantial in patients with renal impairment or in diabetic patients with type IV renal tubular acidosis (hyporeninemic hypoaldosteronism). Mild hyperkalemia is best managed by institution of a low-potassium diet, but may require adjustment of dosage. A troublesome cough may occur that is likely related to the effects of bradykinin. Substitution of an AT_1 receptor antagonist often alleviates this problem. The inability to use ACE inhibitors as a consequence of cardiorenal side effects (*e.g.,* excessive hypotension, progressive renal insufficiency, or

hyperkalemia) is itself a marker of poor prognosis in the CHF patient (Kittleson *et al.*, 2003).

Effect of ACE Inhibitors on Survival in Heart Failure. A number of placebo-controlled trials have demonstrated that ACE inhibitors improve survival in patients with overt heart failure due to systolic ventricular dysfunction, independent of the etiology. The CONSENSUS Study (Cooperative North Scandinavian Enalapril Survival Study, 1987) demonstrated a 40% reduction in mortality after 6 months in patients with severe heart failure randomized to enalapril rather than placebo. These results were extended to patients with mild-to-moderate heart failure in the treatment arm of the Studies On Left Ventricular Dysfunction (SOLVD Investigators, 1991) Trial, which reported a 16% reduction in mortality with enalapril treatment. ACE inhibitors are also more effective than other vasodilators. The second Veterans Administration Cooperative Vasodilator-Heart Failure Trial (V-HeFT II) (Cohn *et al.*, 1991) showed a small but clear incremental survival benefit in patients with mild-to-moderate heart failure with enalapril *vs.* the isosorbide dinitrate–hydralazine combination. A smaller randomized trial comparing captopril to hydralazine and isosorbide dinitrate in patients with moderate to severe heart failure also demonstrated a significant survival advantage in patients receiving the ACE inhibitor (Fonarow *et al.*, 1992).

These data have convinced many clinicians that ACE inhibitors improve survival of patients with symptomatic heart failure. Data from the prevention arm of the SOLVD Trial subsequently examined the impact of ACE inhibitors in asymptomatic patients with left ventricular systolic dysfunction (SOLVD Investigators, 1992). Although this study failed to demonstrate reduction in mortality among enalapril-treated patients, there was a statistically significant (29%) reduction in the combined endpoint of all-causes mortality/development of symptomatic heart failure.

Myocardial infarction is the leading cause of heart failure due to systolic dysfunction in industrialized countries. ACE inhibitors also prevent the development of clinically significant ventricular dysfunction and mortality following acute infarction. The Survival And Ventricular Enlargement trial (SAVE) (Pfeffer *et al.*, 1992) examined patients with recent, acute anterior myocardial infarction and ejection fractions of ≤40%; this study reported a 20% reduction in mortality and a 36% reduction in the rate of progression to severe heart failure at 12 months follow-up in the captopril-treated group. Two similar trials—AIRE Investigators (1993), and TRACE investigators (1995)—used two different ACE inhibitors in the post–myocardial infarct setting and found that both drugs improved mortality when compared to placebo. Both the SOLVD trials (Konstam *et al.*, 1992) and the SAVE trial (St. John Sutton *et al.*, 1994) demonstrated that enalapril and captopril, respectively, attenuated or prevented the increase in left ventricular end-diastolic/end-systolic volumes and the decline in LV ejection fraction that was observed in patients randomized to placebo. These benefits appear to accrue from all drugs in this class. ACE inhibitors appear to prevent the progression of heart failure after myocardial infarction by preventing adverse ventricular remodeling.

ACE inhibitors have been shown to be effective in specific patient subgroups, including women, African-Americans, and the elderly. Despite early reports to the contrary, analyses from the SOLVD database indicate that ACE inhibitors delay the progression of heart failure and improve mortality in African-Americans (Dries *et al.*, 2002).

AT_1 Receptor Antagonists. Activation of the AT_1 receptor mediates most of the deleterious effects of Ang II that have been described above. The receptor blockade provided by AT_1 antagonists provides a pharmacologic means by which to reduce the phenomenon of Ang II "escape" that occurs with ACE inhibitors. AT_1 receptor antagonism might also be expected to avoid the bradykinin-mediated side effects of ACE inhibition, principally cough and angioedema. These side effects, which occur in >10% of patients, represent an important limitation to the use of ACE inhibitors in clinical practice. It merits emphasis that angioedema has also been reported with AT_1 receptor antagonists and caution is therefore warranted when prescribing these agents to patients with a history of ACE inhibitor–associated angioedema.

The initial clinical application of AT_1 receptor antagonists was in the treatment of systemic hypertension, for which these agents are both effective and well-tolerated. Trial data also demonstrated that AT_1 antagonists provided additive antihypertensive effect when used in combination with ACE inhibitors. Several trials, including ELITE (Evaluation of Losartan in the Elderly) (Pitt *et al.*, 1997), SPICE (Study of Patients Intolerant of Converting Enzyme Inhibitors) (Bart, *et al.*, 1999) and CHARM (Candesartan in Heart Failure Assessment of Reduction in Morbidity and Mortality) (Doggrell, 2005), established that angiotensin-receptor blockers were well tolerated by patients with CHF. In ELITE, the effects of *losartan* (50 mg per day) and captopril (50 mg three times daily) were compared in elderly CHF patients (Pitt *et al.*, 1997). The drugs had similar effect on renal function; 10.5% of patients in both groups experienced ≥0.3-mg/dl increase in serum creatinine following initiation of therapy. Losartan was well tolerated; fewer patients in the losartan group discontinued therapy for side effects (12.5% *vs.* 20.8% in the captopril group) The principal side effect leading to discontinuation of ACE inhibitor therapy was cough. The SPICE Registry confirmed that AT_1 receptor antagonism is well tolerated in CHF patients; 83% of patients who were intolerant of an ACE inhibitor were able to tolerate treatment with *candesartan*.

The impact of AT_1 receptor antagonists with respect to mortality in heart failure patients was addressed in one arm of the CHARM study, a program of three separate studies of candesartan in heart failure. In the CHARM-Alternative trial, patients who were intolerant of ACE inhibitors were randomized to candesartan or placebo. Cardiovascular death and heart failure hospitalizations were significantly decreased in the active treatment arm (33% *vs.* 40%). These data support the use of AT_1 blockers as an alternative to ACE inhibitors in heart failure patients who do not tolerate ACE inhibition; furthermore, the data suggest that AT_1 antagonists provide a mortality benefit that is similar in magnitude to that achieved with ACE inhibitors.

Subsequent clinical trials have compared mortality in patients treated with ACE inhibitors or AT_1 receptor antagonists. The available data support the contention that AT_1 receptor antagonists provide an alternative to ACE inhibitors in the treatment of heart failure and provide comparable mortality benefits (Pitt *et al.*, 2000).

The combined use of ACE inhibitors and ARBs in the treatment of heart failure offers the intriguing possibility of additive therapeutic benefit by virtue of distinctive modes of angiotensin antagonism. Preliminary studies suggested that combined therapy with candesartan and enalapril had more favorable effects on hemodynamics, ventricular remodeling, and neurohormonal profile compared to therapy with either agent alone (McKelvie *et al.*, 1999). Two subsequent trials, Val-HeFT (Valsartan Heart Failure Trial) and

CHARM-Added, assessed combination therapy in chronic heart failure. Neither trial demonstrated an incremental mortality benefit with combination therapy, but each reported that combination therapy significantly reduced hospitalizations for heart failure.

The efficacy of AT_1 receptor antagonists (candesartan 32 mg once daily *vs.* placebo) has been studied in patients with diastolic heart failure in a clinical trial in patients with CHF who have preserved LV systolic function (the CHARM-Preserved Trial) (Yusuf, 2003). Although there was no significant difference in the primary endpoint of cardiovascular death or heart failure hospitalization, there were again fewer heart failure hospitalizations in the active treatment arm.

Thus, AT_1 receptor antagonists are well tolerated and effective in the treatment of hypertension and CHF. In patients with heart failure, AT_1 antagonists provide a mortality benefit that is similar to that provided by ACE inhibitors. AT_1 receptor antagonists should at present be viewed as the preferred alternative when ACE inhibitors cannot be tolerated. Current American Heart Association/American College of Cardiology guidelines suggest that the addition of an AT_1 blocker to a regimen that includes an ACE inhibitor can be considered in an effort to reduce hospitalizations, but conflicting evidence and divergence of opinion remain. Finally, AT_1 antagonists do appear to reduce hospitalization in patients with diastolic heart failure.

Nitrovasodilators. Nitrovasodilators have long been used in the treatment of heart failure and remain among the most widely used vasoactive medications in clinical practice. These drugs relax vascular smooth muscle by supplying NO and thereby activating soluble guanylyl cyclase. Thus, the drugs mimic the actions of endogenous NO, an intracellular and paracrine autocoid formed by the conversion of arginine to citrulline by a family of enzymes termed *NO synthases*. These enzymes are widely distributed and are found in endothelial and smooth muscle cells throughout the vasculature.

The basis for the differential sensitivity of selected regions of the vasculature to specific nitrovasodilators (*e.g.*, the sensitivity of the epicardial coronary arteries to *nitroglycerin*) remains controversial. Unlike nitroprusside, which is spontaneously converted to NO by reducing agents such as glutathione, nitroglycerin and other organic nitrates undergo a more complex enzymatic biotransformation to NO or bioactive *S*-nitrosothiols. The activities of specific enzyme(s) and cofactor(s) required for this biotransformation appear to differ among organs and at different levels of the vasculature within an organ (Napoli and Ignarro, 2003; Fung, 2004; Fukuto, *et al.*, 2005). The basic pharmacology of the organic nitrates is discussed in Chapter 31.

Organic Nitrates. Organic nitrates are available in a number of formulations that include rapid-acting nitroglycerin tablets or spray for sublingual administration, short-acting oral agents such as isosorbide dinitrate (ISOR-DIL, SORBITRATE, others), long-acting oral agents such as *isosorbide mononitrate* (IMDUR), topical preparations such as nitroglycerin ointment and transdermal patches, and intravenous nitroglycerin. The nitrate preparations are relatively safe and effective agents whose principal action in the treatment of congestive heart failure is reduction of left ventricular filling pressures. This preload reduction is due to an increase in peripheral venous capacitance. Nitrates will cause a decline in pulmonary and systemic vascular resistance, particularly at higher doses, although this response is less marked and less predictable than with nitroprusside. These drugs do have a selective vasodilator effect on the epicardial coronary vasculature and may enhance both systolic and diastolic ventricular function by increasing coronary flow; the clinical relevance of this coronary vasodilator effect in patients with epicardial coronary obstruction remains controversial.

Isosorbide dinitrate is more effective than placebo in improving exercise capacity and in reducing symptoms when administered to patients with chronic heart failure. However, the limited effects of these agents on the systemic vascular resistance and the problem of pharmacological tolerance limit the utility of organic nitrates as monotherapy in the treatment of CHF. In a number of small trials, isosorbide dinitrate has been shown to increase the clinical effectiveness of other vasodilators such as hydralazine, resulting in a sustained improvement in hemodynamics that exceeded that of either drug given alone. As noted previously, the combination of isosorbide dinitrate and hydralazine reduced overall mortality compared to placebo or the α_1 receptor antagonist prazosin in patients with mild-to-moderate heart failure concurrently treated with *digoxin* and diuretics (Cohn *et al.*, 1986). The mononitrate formulation has not been studied in chronic heart failure; the transdermal formulations are infrequently used in the treatment of CHF, reflecting concerns related to perfusion-dependent drug absorption in such patients.

Nitrate tolerance can limit the long-term effectiveness of these drugs in the treatment of CHF. Blood levels of these drugs should be permitted to fall to negligible levels for at least 6 to 8 hours each day. The timing of nitrate withdrawal can be adjusted to the patient's symptoms. Patients with recurrent orthopnea or paroxysmal nocturnal dyspnea, for example, would likely benefit most by using nitrates at night. *N-acetylcysteine* (MUCOMYST) may diminish tolerance to the hemodynamic effects of nitrates in heart failure (Mehra *et al.*, 1994). Likewise, hydralazine may decrease nitrate tolerance by an antioxidant effect that attenuates superoxide formation, thereby increasing the bioavailability of NO (Gogia *et al.*, 1995).

Hydralazine. The mechanism that underlies the vasodilator activity of hydralazine (APRESOLINE) remains poorly understood. The effects of this agent are not mediated through recognized neurohumoral systems and its mechanism of action at the cellular level in vascular smooth muscle is uncertain. Hydralazine is an effective antihypertensive drug (*see* Chapter 32), particularly when combined with agents that blunt compensatory increases in sympathetic tone and salt and water retention. In heart failure, hydralazine reduces right and left ventricular afterload by reducing pulmonary and systemic vascular resistance. This results in an augmentation of forward stroke volume and a reduction in ventricular systolic wall stress. Hydralazine

also appears to have moderate "direct" positive inotropic activity in cardiac muscle unrelated to afterload reduction. Hydralazine is effective in reducing renal vascular resistance and in increasing renal blood flow to a greater degree than are most other vasodilators, with the exception of ACE inhibitors. Reflecting these aggregate effects, hydralazine may be useful in heart-failure patients with renal dysfunction who cannot tolerate an ACE inhibitor. Hydralazine has minimal effects on venous capacitance and therefore is most effective when combined with agents with venodilating activity (*e.g.,* organic nitrates).

The combination of hydralazine (300 mg/day) and isosorbide dinitrate increased survival when compared to placebo or to the α_1 adrenergic antagonist prazosin in the landmark V-HeFT I Trial (Cohn *et al.*, 1986). Hydralazine, with or without nitrates, may provide additional hemodynamic improvement for patients with advanced heart failure who already are being treated with conventional doses of an ACE inhibitor, digoxin, and diuretics (Cohn, 1994). The combination preparation isosorbide dinitrate–hydralazine (BIDIL) was most recently investigated in the African-American Heart Failure Trial (A-HeFT). In this study of 1050 patients with NYHA Class III or IV heart failure, the isosorbide dinitrate–hydralazine combination (when added to standard therapy that included neurohumoral blockade) was associated with a significant (43%) reduction in all-cause mortality when compared to placebo.

There are several important limitations that constrain the use of hydralazine in the treatment of CHF. Although hydralazine therapy was associated with a greater increase in ejection fraction and exercise duration when compared to the ACE inhibitor enalapril, the latter drug was superior with respect to reduction of mortality (V-HeFT II, mortality 25% with hydralazine *vs.* 18% with enalapril). Side effects that may necessitate dose adjustment or withdrawal of hydralazine are common. In V-HeFT I, only 55% of patients were taking full doses of both hydralazine and isosorbide at 6 months. The lupus-like side effects associated with hydralazine are relatively uncommon (3.2% in V-HeFT I) and may be more likely to occur in patients with the "slow-acetylator" phenotype (*see* Chapter 3). Finally, compliance with the multidosing regimen may be difficult in CHF patients who are often taking multiple concurrent medications.

The oral bioavailability and pharmacokinetics of hydralazine are not altered significantly by heart failure unless there is severe hepatic congestion or hypoperfusion. Intravenous hydralazine is available but provides little practical advantage over oral formulations except for urgent use during pregnancy, a state in which relative or absolute contraindications exist for most other vasodilators. Hydralazine is typically started at a dose of 10 to 25 mg three or four times per day and the dosage up-titrated to 75 to 100 mg three or four times daily, as tolerated.

β Adrenergic Receptor Antagonists

Heart failure is characterized by sympathetic hyperactivation, a neurohumoral state that reflects biological responses that can be both compensatory and maladaptive. As detailed above, the sympathetic branch of the autonomic nervous system is activated as a physiological short-term compensatory response to hemodynamic stress. Sympathetic activation supports circulatory function by enhancing contractility (inotropy), augmenting ventricular relaxation and filling (lusitropy), and increasing heart rate (chronotropy). For many years, pharmacological approaches to the treatment of heart failure involved the use of drugs that would further stimulate sympathetic responses. These approaches reflected the viewpoint that the fundamental abnormality in CHF is the reduction of stroke volume/cardiac output that occurs as a consequence of myocardial dysfunction. Under this model, the use of β adrenergic receptor antagonists was judged to be contraindicated in patients with heart failure, and there was widespread use of drugs that further stimulate cardiac sympathetic pathways. Paradoxically, many of these sympathomimetics increased mortality in CHF patients, while an unexpected mortality benefit was seen with the administration of β adrenergic blocking drugs.

The use of sympathomimetic drugs such as dobutamine and *dopamine* was found to provide *short-term* relief of heart failure symptoms in patients with advanced ventricular dysfunction. It was presumed that the development of oral congeners of these sympathomimetic agents would represent a major advance in the pharmacotherapy of heart failure. This mechanistic hypothesis has been discredited by the results of a number of trials that have addressed the longer-term use of positive inotropic agents. These trials have been concordant in demonstrating increased mortality in CHF patients treated with drugs that amplify the β receptor/cyclic AMP–modulated Ca^{2+} signaling that underlies myocardial contraction and relaxation. These unexpected results underscore the critical observation that the salutary effects of a drug on hemodynamic function need not correlate with improved clinical outcomes. The recognition that sustained activation of sympathetic nerves in the context of myocardial injury contributes to the progression of contractile dysfunction is now well established and derives support from the demonstrable adverse consequences of long-term sympathetic stimulation (such as maladaptive proliferative signaling in the myocardium, direct cardiomyocyte toxicity, and myocyte apoptosis). The initial phase of the clinical investigation of β receptor antagonists in the treatment of heart failure encountered both skepticism regarding the underlying hypothesis and reluctance in clinical execution; the approach found support from empirical evidence in patients with heart failure and from the large database acquired in clinical trials of β blockers in patients with coronary artery disease and antecedent myocardial infarction (Gottlieb *et al.*, 1998).

Despite clinical and experimental evidence that β blockers can impair the inotropic performance of the ventricle, Waagstein and associates (1993) reported that β receptor antagonists (most commonly the β_1-selective agent *metoprolol*) improved symptoms, exercise tolerance, and measures of ventricular function over a period of several months in patients with heart failure due to idiopathic dilated cardiomyopathy (Swedberg, 1993). With few exceptions, clinical trials over the next decade reinforced these initial observations (Bristow, 2000). Although none of these studies was sufficiently powered to define the impact of β receptor antagonists on mortality in patients with heart failure, all demonstrated a consistent increase in left ventricular ejection fraction (Figure 33–4). Serial measurements indicate that a decrease in

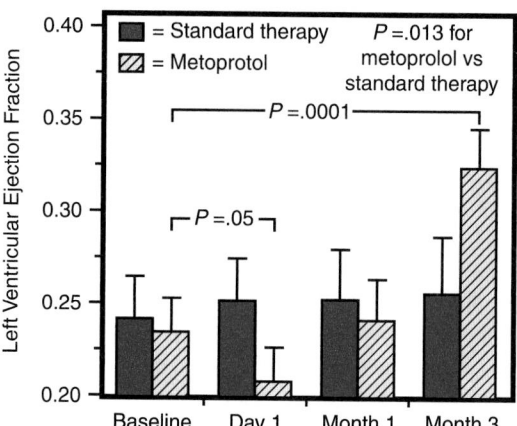

Figure 33–4. ***Time-dependent effects of metoprolol on left ventricular ejection fraction in patients with heart failure.*** In patients with severe left ventricular dysfunction, the initial administration of a low dose of metoprolol caused an immediate depression in ejection fraction (day 1). However, over time and despite uptitration of metoprolol to full therapeutic levels, ejection fraction returned to baseline (1 month), and by 3 months was significantly higher than at baseline. In the group given standard therapy, ejection fraction did not change significantly. An increase in left ventricular systolic function between 2 and 4 months after initiation of therapy is seen consistently with β receptor antagonists used in patients with heart failure. This observation confirms that the direct hemodynamic effect of a β adrenergic antagonist in patients with heart failure is to depress contractile function. Thus, the improvement in function with chronic therapy cannot be attributed to a direct hemodynamic effect, and likely reflects a beneficial effect of treatment on the biology of the myocardium. (Adapted with permission from Hall *et al.*, 1995.)

systolic function does occur immediately after initiation of a β antagonist in the CHF patient cohort, but systolic function recovers and improves beyond baseline levels over the ensuing 2 to 4 months (Hall *et al.*, 1995). It has been suggested that improved ventricular function with chronic β receptor antagonist therapy is due to attenuation or prevention of the β adrenergic receptor–mediated adverse effects of catecholamines on the myocardium (Eichhorn and Bristow, 1996).

Metoprolol. Metoprolol (LOPRESSOR, TOPROL XL, OTHERS) is a β_1-selective antagonist. The 25-mg extended-release tablet formulation is FDA approved for the management of mild-to-moderate heart failure.

A number of clinical trials have demonstrated the beneficial effects of β antagonist therapy in heart failure. In the Metoprolol in Dilated Cardiomyopathy Trial (Waagstein *et al.*, 1993), enrolled patients were receiving "optimal" medical management, including ACE inhibitors, and the mean dose of metoprolol was approximately 100 mg/day (achieved over a 6-week period of gradual upward titration that began at 10 mg/day). Although there was no difference in mortality between the treatment groups at 12 month follow-up, fewer patients in the β blocker arm required cardiac transplantation and there were significant improvements in ejection fraction, exercise tolerance, and quality of life (Waagstein *et al.*, 1993; Andersson *et al.*, 1994). In the MERIT-HF Trial (Metoprolol Randomized Intervention Trial in Congestive Heart Failure), patients (NYHA functional Class II to IV symptoms and an ejection fraction <40%) received metoprolol succinate (target dose, 200 mg per day) or placebo (MERIT-HF Study Group, 1999). β Blocker therapy decreased all-cause mortality by 34%, with this difference attributable to both reductions in sudden death and death from worsening heart failure. These beneficial effects on mortality were independent of age, sex, etiology of heart failure, or ejection fraction. Despite the relatively large target dose of metoprolol succinate (200 mg once daily), 64% of patients who received the β blocker achieved this goal (mean dose, ~160 mg per day).

Carvedilol. Carvedilol (COREG) is a nonselective β receptor antagonist and α_1-selective antagonist that is FDA approved for the management of mild-to-severe heart failure.

The U.S. Carvedilol Trial randomized patients with symptomatic heart failure (NHYA Classes II, III, and IV) and ejection fraction <35% to carvedilol or placebo (Packer *et al.*, 1996). All patients received concomitant ACE inhibitor therapy and were clinically and hemodynamically stable. Carvedilol (25 mg twice per day) was associated with significant (65%) reduction in all-cause mortality, an effect that was independent of age, sex, etiology of heart failure, or ejection fraction. The mortality benefit was due primarily to a decrease in deaths due to refractory pump failure, and to a lesser reduction in sudden cardiac death. There was a concomitant 27% reduction in hospitalization for heart failure exacerbations. The improvements in mortality and ejection fraction were dose related (Figure 33–5) (Bristow *et al.*, 1996). Exercise capacity (assessed by a 6-minute walk test) did not improve with carvedilol, but carvedilol did appear to slow the progression of heart failure in a subgroup of patients with good exercise capacity and mild symptoms at baseline (Colucci *et al.*, 1996). The Australia/New Zealand Carvedilol Trial, which studied patients with mild heart failure due to coronary artery disease, also reported a significant reduction (26%) in the combined endpoint of all-cause mortality and hospitalization (Australia/New Zealand Heart Failure Research Collaborative Group, 1997).

In the CAPRICORN Trial (Carvedilol Post Infarct Survival Control in LV Dysfunction Trial) (Dargie, 2001), patients with recent myocardial infarction (3 to 21 days prior to enrollment) and impaired systolic function (ejection fraction of <40%) were randomized to carvedilol (25 mg twice daily) or placebo. Patients with symptomatic heart failure and those with asymptomatic left ventricular dysfunction were included. Although there was no difference in the primary endpoint of all-cause mortality, carvedilol therapy was associated with a significant reduction in the combined endpoint of all-cause mortality and nonfatal myocardial infarction. At the opposite end of the spectrum, patients with symptomatic heart failure (at rest or with minimal exertion) and impaired systolic function (ejection fraction <25%) were randomized to carvedilol *vs.* placebo in the COPERNICUS Trial (Carvedilol Prospective Randomized Cumulative Survival Study) (Packer *et al.*, 2002a). Consistent with previous trials, there was a 35% decrease in all-cause mortality. Although the patients included in the trial had established heart failure, it merits emphasis that the placebo group mortality at 1 year

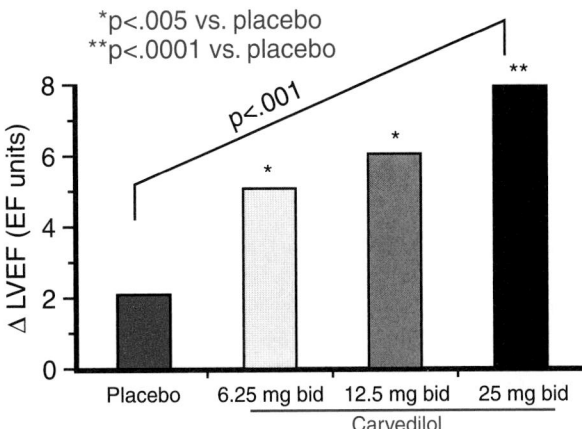

Figure 33–5. *Dose-dependent effect of carvedilol on left ventricular ejection fraction.* In the U.S. Carvedilol Trials Program, a subgroup of patients were randomized to placebo or carvedilol in the standard dose (25 mg twice per day bid), or in a reduced dose of 12.5 or 6.25 mg twice per day. After 6 months of treatment, left ventricular ejection fraction (ΔLVEF) increased with all three doses of carvedilol, but not with placebo. The increase in ejection fraction was strongly related to the dose of carvedilol. These data emphasize the importance of titrating doses of β receptor antagonists to the target or the highest tolerated dose. (Adapted with permission from Bristow *et al.*, 1996.)

was 18.5%, a finding that suggests that the cohort as a whole was not representative of patients with advanced heart failure.

Bisoprolol. Bisoprolol (ZEBETA) is also a β_1-selective antagonist. The CIBIS-II trial reported a 34% reduction in all-cause mortality in bisoprolol-treated patients that was due primarily to a decrease in sudden deaths (44% reduction) and to a lesser extent, a decrease in pump failure (26% reduction). The mortality benefit of bisoprolol was independent of the etiology of heart failure; β blocker therapy resulted in a significant (36%) decrease in hospitalizations for heart failure (CIBIS-II Investigators and Committee, 1999). In the United States, heart failure currently represents an off-label use for bisoprolol.

Mechanism of Action. The mechanisms by which β receptor antagonists affect clinical outcomes in patients with congestive heart failure have not been fully delineated. A consistent finding is a reduction in the incidence of sudden death, presumably reflecting a decrease in malignant ventricular arrhythmias. Thus, an antiarrhythmic benefit seems likely, possibly reflecting a reduced propensity to develop hypokalemia in the face of systemic β adrenergic blockade, or perhaps a direct consequence of the anti-ischemic effects of these drugs. Another consistent finding with β adrenergic blockade is an improvement in left ventricular structure and function with a decrease in chamber size and an increase in ejection fraction. This favorable remodeling is likely mediated by attenuating the molecular and cellular events that underlie pathological remodeling. Several lines of experimental evidence support this speculation. β adrenergic stimulation can cause apoptosis of cardiac myocytes (Communal *et al.*, 1998). In a mouse model of dilated cardiomyopathy, overexpression of the β_1 receptor in the myocardium is associated with myocyte apoptosis (Bisognano *et al.*, 2000). β Receptors may affect remodeling and turnover of extracellular matrix through their effects on myocardial gene expression. β Receptor antagonists could improve myocardial energetics (Eichhorn *et al.*, 1994) or reduce oxidative stress in the myocardium (Sawyer and Colucci, 2000). More recent data indicate that β antagonist therapy may attenuate the hyperphosphorylation of the ryanodine (RyR) receptor that has been linked to abnormal intracellular Ca^{2+} handling in experimental models of heart failure (Reiken *et al.*, 2001).

Clinical Use of β Adrenergic Receptor Antagonists in Heart Failure

The extensive body of data regarding the use of β receptor antagonists in chronic heart failure, reflecting more than 15,000 patients enrolled in controlled trials, provides compelling evidence that β antagonists improve symptoms, reduce hospitalization, and decrease mortality in patients with mild and moderate heart failure. Accordingly, β receptor antagonists are now recommended for routine use in patients with an ejection fraction <35% and NYHA Class II or III symptoms in conjunction with ACE inhibitor or angiotensin-receptor antagonist, and diuretics as required to palliate symptoms.

This general recommendation should be tempered by certain limitations in the experimental database. First, the large majority of the data that underlie this recommendation were obtained in relatively stable patients with mild-to-moderate symptoms. Therefore, the role of β receptor antagonists in patients with more severe symptoms, or with recent decompensation, is not yet clear. Likewise, the utility of β receptor blockade in patients with asymptomatic left ventricular dysfunction has not been studied. Finally, although it appears likely that the beneficial effects of these drugs are related to β receptor blockade, it cannot be assumed that all β receptor antagonists will exert similar effects. Thus, as discussed in Chapter 10, there is marked heterogeneity in pharmacological characteristics within this general class (*e.g.*, β adrenergic receptor selectivity, pharmacokinetics, direct or receptor-mediated vasodilation, and other non–receptor-mediated actions such antioxidant effects). These properties may play a role determining the overall efficacy of a given β receptor antagonist. Since β antagonists have the potential to worsen both ventricular function and symptoms in patients with heart failure, several caveats should be considered:

1. β Adrenergic receptor antagonists should be initiated at very low doses, generally less than one-tenth of the final target dose.
2. These drugs should be increased slowly, over the course of weeks, and under careful supervision. The rapid institution of the usual β adrenergic receptor–blocking doses used for hypertension or coronary artery disease may cause decompensation in many patients who otherwise would be able to tolerate a slower titration of dose. Even when therapy is initiated with low doses of a β antagonist,

there may be an increased tendency to retain fluid that will require adjustments in the diuretic regimen.
3. Although limited experience with NYHA Class IIIB and IV patients suggests that they may tolerate β blockers and benefit from their use, this group of patients should be approached with a high level of caution.
4. There is almost no experience in patients with new-onset, recently decompensated heart failure. There are theoretical reasons for caution in such patients, and at present they should not be treated with β blockers until after they have stabilized for several days to weeks.

Parenteral Vasodilators

The failing left ventricle is characterized by depression of myocardial contractility and increased sensitivity to alterations of left ventricular afterload. This latter attribute of the failing ventricle is manifest by a greater proportional reduction of stroke volume as the impedance to ejection is increased. Conversely, reduction in afterload in this setting can be associated with substantial increases in stroke volume. This increased afterload dependence underlies the beneficial effects of load reduction therapy in patients with heart failure due to systolic dysfunction (Figure 33–6).

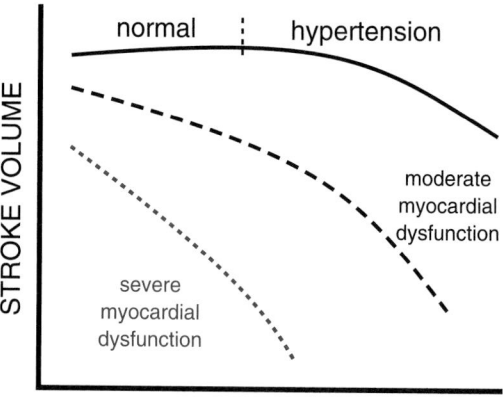

Figure 33–6. *Relationship between ventricular outflow resistance and stroke volume in patients with systolic ventricular dysfunction.* An increase in ventricular outflow resistance, a principal determinant of afterload, has little effect on stroke volume in normal hearts, as illustrated by the relatively flat curve. In contrast, in patients with systolic ventricular dysfunction, an increase in outflow resistance often is accompanied by a sharp decline in stroke volume. With more severe ventricular dysfunction, this curve becomes steeper. Because of this relationship, a reduction in systemic vascular resistance (one component of outflow resistance) in response to an arterial vasodilator may markedly increase stroke volume in patients with severe myocardial dysfunction. The resultant increase in stroke volume may be sufficient to offset the decrease in systemic vascular resistance, thereby preventing a fall in systemic arterial pressure. (Adapted with permission from Cohn and Franciosa, 1977.)

Sodium Nitroprusside. Sodium nitroprusside (NITRO-PRESS) is a prodrug and potent vasodilator that is effective in reducing both ventricular filling pressures and systemic vascular resistance. It has a rapid onset (2 to 5 minutes) and offset (quickly metabolized to cyanide and NO, the active vasodilator) of action and its dose can be titrated expeditiously to achieve the desired hemodynamic effect. For these reasons, nitroprusside is commonly used in intensive-care settings for rapid control of severe hypertension and for the management of decompensated heart failure. The basic pharmacologic properties of this drug are described in Chapter 32.

Several mechanisms contribute to the reduction of ventricular filling pressures after treatment with nitroprusside. This agent directly increases venous capacitance, resulting in a redistribution of blood volume from the central to the peripheral venous circulation. Nitroprusside also causes a fall in peripheral vascular resistance as well as an increase in aortic wall compliance and improves ventricular–vascular coupling; left ventricular afterload is decreased and cardiac output is thereby increased. This combination of preload and afterload reduction improves myocardial energetics by reducing wall stress. This improvement in myocardial energetics is contingent upon maintenance of a mean arterial pressure sufficient to drive coronary perfusion during diastole. Following the rapid withdrawal of nitroprusside, a transient deterioration in ventricular function associated with a rebound increase in systemic vascular resistance occurs.

Nitroprusside is particularly effective in patients with CHF due to elevations of systemic vascular resistance and/or mechanical complications that follow acute myocardial infarction (such as mitral regurgitation or left-to-right shunts through a ventricular septal defect). Thus, this drug is commonly used in cardiac care units.

As with most vasodilators, the most common adverse effect of nitroprusside is hypotension. In general, nitroprusside initiation in patients with severe heart failure results in increased cardiac output and a parallel increase in renal blood flow, improving both glomerular filtration and diuretic effectiveness. However, excessive reduction of systemic arterial pressure may limit or prevent an increase in renal blood flow in patients with more severe contractile dysfunction.

Cyanide produced during the biotransformation of nitroprusside is rapidly metabolized by the liver to thiocyanate, which is cleared by the kidney. Thiocyanate and/or cyanide toxicity is uncommon but may occur in the setting of hepatic or renal failure, or following prolonged high-dose infusion of the drug. Typical symptoms include unexplained abdominal pain, mental status changes, convulsions, or lactic acidosis. Methemoglobinemia is another unusual complication of prolonged, high-dose nitroprusside infusion and is due to the oxidation of hemoglobin by NO.

Intravenous Nitroglycerin. Intravenous nitroglycerin, like nitroprusside, is a vasoactive NO source that is commonly used in cardiac care units. Its structure and basic pharmacology are described in Chapter 31. Unlike nitroprusside, nitroglycerin is relatively selective for venous capacitance vessels, particularly at low infusion rates. Intravenous nitroglycerin is most often used in the treatment of acute coronary syndromes. In patients with CHF, intravenous nitroglycerin is most clearly indicated in the treatment of left heart failure due to acute myocardial ischemia. Parenteral nitroglycerin also is used in the treatment of nonischemic left heart failure when expeditious reduction of ventricular filling pressures is desired; nitroglycerin can be particularly useful in patients with symptomatic volume overload in whom effective diuresis has not been established. At higher infusion rates, this drug can also reduce systemic arterial resistance, although this effect is less predictable. Nitroglycerin therapy may be limited by headache and the development of nitrate tolerance, although the latter is generally overcome by uptitration of the infusion rate to maintain the desired response. Since nitroglycerin is administered in ethanol, high infusion rates can be associated with significant elevation of blood alcohol levels.

Nesiritide. Nesiritide (NATRECOR), a recombinant form of human brain natriuretic peptide (BNP), has been approved by the FDA for treatment of dyspnea due to congestive heart failure. The natriuretic peptides—atrial natriuretic peptide (ANP), BNP, and C-type natriuretic peptide—are a family of endogenous neurohormones that possess potent natriuretic, diuretic, and vasodilator properties. BNP is the agent that has found broad clinical application. It is secreted by ventricular cardiac myocytes in response to stretch; circulating levels of BNP correlate with the severity of heart failure. In the setting of heart failure, the effects of BNP counteract the effects of angiotensin and norepinephrine by producing vasodilation, natriuresis, and diuresis.

The BNP receptor is the extracellular domain of type A guanylyl cyclase, GC-A. GC-A is a monospanning membrane protein resembling the growth factor receptors, with guanylyl cyclase activity on the cytoplasmic tail. The active receptor–cyclase complex is a homodimer. Activation of GC-A by nesiritide (BNP) increases cyclic GMP content in target tissues, including vascular, endothelial, and smooth muscle cells. As with activation of the soluble guanylyl cyclase by NO derived from nitrovasodilators, elevated cyclic GMP leads to relaxation of vascular smooth muscle and vasodilation in both the venous and arterial systems. BNP is metabolized by specific clearance receptors, which facilitate its internalization and enzymatic degradation. It is also inactivated by neutral endopeptidases (NEP). The contribution of renal elimination of the drug is minor, and dose adjustment is not required in patients with renal dysfunction.

Nesiritide lowers right and left side cardiac filling pressures without a direct chronotropic or inotropic action. The hemodynamic response to nesiritide is characterized by decreased right atrial, pulmonary arterial, and pulmonary capillary wedge pressures; systemic vascular resistance is reduced and cardiac index is increased. Improvement in global clinical status, attenuation of dyspnea and fatigue, and enhanced diuretic responsiveness have been reported and corroborated. The 2002 VAMC Trial (Vasodilation in the Acute Management of CHF), compared nesiritide to intravenous nitroglycerin and placebo in the treatment of decompensated heart failure. Nesiritide was associated with greater reductions in pulmonary capillary wedge pressure at 3 and 24 hours. Improvements in dyspnea were comparable to nitroglycerin and better than placebo. In contrast to the effects of parenteral inotropic agents, nesiritide is not associated with increased ventricular or atrial arrhythmias. Thus, nesiritide may be preferable to inotropic drugs when treating refractory heart failure in patients at risk for arrhythmia.

Nesiritide therapy is initiated with a loading dose of 2 $\mu g/kg$ followed by an infusion rate of 0.01 $\mu g/kg$ per minute that can be increased in increments of 0.005 $\mu g/kg$ per minute to a maximum of 0.03 $\mu g/kg$ per minute. The primary side effect is hypotension that is reversible upon discontinuation of the drug. The half-life of the drug is 18 minutes; however, hypotensive effects may persist for a longer period than would be predicted on the basis of the elimination half-life. Although there is no specific systolic blood pressure below which nesiritide therapy is contraindicated, studies have typically excluded patients with systolic blood pressure ≤90 mm Hg; inotropic support may be preferred in such patients.

Vasopeptidase Inhibitors and BNP. Vasopeptidase inhibitors are a novel group of drugs that simultaneously inhibit ACE and neutral endopeptidases (NEP) and are effective antihypertensive agents. NEP is responsible for the enzymatic degradation of atrial and brain natriuretic peptides. Inhibitors of NEP therefore are expected to increase circulating levels of these natriuretic hormones and on this basis have been investigated as therapeutic agents in heart failure. Early studies suggest that vasopeptidase inhibitors are comparable to ACE inhibitors with respect to improving exercise capacity and decreasing symptoms. In the OVERTURE Trial (Omapatrilat Versus Enalapril Randomized Trial of Utility in Reducing Events), the vasopeptidase inhibitor omapatrilat did reduce the risk of death and hospitalization in chronic heart failure; the effect of omapatrilat was comparable to that of the ACE inhibitor, but was more frequently associated with symptomatic hypotension (Packer *et al.*, 2002b).

Cardiac Glycosides

The beneficial effects of cardiac glycosides in the treatment of heart failure have been attributed to a positive inotropic effect on failing myocardium and efficacy in controlling the ventricular rate response to atrial fibrillation. The cardiac glycosides also modulate autonomic nervous system activity, and it is likely that this mechanism contributes substantially to their efficacy in the management of heart failure. The cardiac glycosides possess a common molecular structure, a steroid nucleus containing an unsaturated lactone at the C17 position, and one or more glycosidic residues at C3 (Figure 33–7). However, the advent of alternative therapies that both palliate symptoms and improve survival has led to a more limited role for the cardiac glycosides in the pharmacotherapy of congestive heart failure. Only digoxin (LANOXIN, LANOXICAPS) is in widespread clinical use today.

Mechanisms of Action. *Inhibition of Na⁺,K⁺-ATPase.* All cardiac glycosides are potent and highly selective inhibitors of the active transport of Na^+ and K^+ across cell membranes. This biological effect is accomplished by binding to a specific site on the α subunit

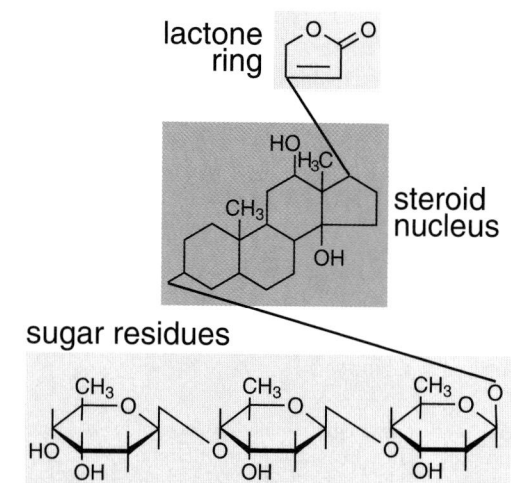

Figure 33–7. *Structure of digoxin.*

of Na^+,K^+-ATPase, the cellular Na^+ pump. The binding of cardiac glycosides to Na^+,K^+-ATPase and inhibition of the cellular ion pump is reversible and entropically driven. The regulation of Na^+,K^+-ATPase by cardiac glycosides has been reviewed in detail (Eichhorn and Gheorghiade, 2002).

Mechanism of the Positive Inotropic Effect. Both Na^+ and Ca^{2+} ions enter cardiac muscle cells during each depolarization (Figure 33–8). Ca^{2+} that enters the cell *via* the L-type Ca^{2+} channel during depolarization triggers the release of stored intracellular Ca^{2+} into the cytosol from the sarcoplasmic reticulum *via* the ryanodine receptor (RyR). This Ca^{2+}-induced Ca^{2+} release increases the level of cytosolic Ca^{2+} available to interact with the contractile proteins, thereby increasing the force of contraction. During myocyte repolarization and relaxation, cellular Ca^{2+} is re-sequestered by the sarcoplasmic reticular Ca^{2+}-ATPase (SERCA2), and also is removed from the cell by the Na^+-Ca^{2+} exchanger (NCX) and by a sarcolemmal Ca^{2+}-ATPase.

The capacity of the exchanger to extrude Ca^{2+} from the cell depends on the intracellular Na^+ concentration. Binding of cardiac glycosides to the sarcolemmal Na^+,K^+-ATPase and inhibition of cellular Na^+ pump activity results in a reduction in the rate of active Na^+ extrusion and a rise in cytosolic Na^+. This increase in intracellular Na^+ reduces the transmembrane Na^+ gradient that drives the extrusion of intracellular Ca^{2+} during myocyte repolarization. With reduced Ca^{2+} efflux and repeated entry of Ca^{2+} with each action potential, Ca^{2+} accumulates in the myocyte: Ca^{2+} uptake into the SR is increased; this increased Ca^{2+} becomes available for release from the SR onto troponin C and other Ca^{2+}-sensitive proteins of the contractile apparatus during the next cycle of excitation-contraction coupling, thereby augmenting myocyte contractility (Figure 33–8). This increase in releasable Ca^{2+} from the sarcoplasmic reticulum is the biological substrate through which cardiac glycosides enhance myocardial contractility. The cardiac glycoside binds preferentially to the phosphorylated form of the α subunit of the Na^+,K^+-ATPase. Extracellular K^+ promotes dephosphorylation of the enzyme as an initial step in this cation's active translocation into the cytosol, and also thereby decreases the affinity of the enzyme for cardiac glycosides. This explains in part the observation that increased extracellular K^+ reverses some of the toxic effects of the cardiac glycosides.

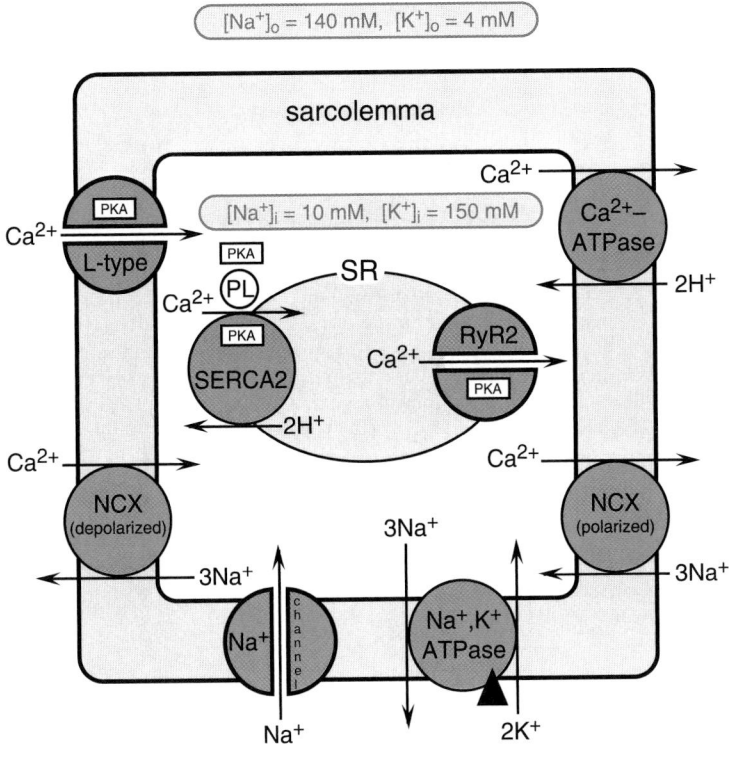

$[Na^+]_o = 140$ mM, $[K^+]_o = 4$ mM

sarcolemma

$[Na^+]_i = 10$ mM, $[K^+]_i = 150$ mM

Figure 33–8. *Sarcolemmal exchange of Na^+ and Ca^{2+} during cell depolarization and repolarization.* Na^+ and Ca^{2+} enter the cardiac myocyte *via* the Na^+ channel and the L-type Ca^{2+} channel during each cycle of membrane depolarization, triggering the release, through the ryanodine receptor (RyR), of larger amounts of Ca^{2+} from internal stores in the sarcoplasmic reticulum (SR). The resulting increase in intracellular Ca^{2+} interacts with troponin C and activates interactions between actin and myosin that result in sarcomere shortening. The electrochemical gradient for Na^+ across the sarcolemma is maintained by active transport of Na^+ out of the cell by the sarcolemmal Na^+,K^+-ATPase. The bulk of cytosolic Ca^{2+} is pumped back into the SR by a Ca^{2+}-ATPase, SERCA2. The remainder is removed from the cell by either a sarcolemmal Ca^{2+}-ATPase or a high capacity Na^+-Ca^{2+} exchange protein, NCX. NCX exchanges three Na^+ for every Ca^{2+}, using the electrochemical potential of Na^+ to drive Ca^{2+} extrusion. The direction of Na^+–Ca^{2+} exchange may reverse briefly during depolarization, when the electrical gradient across the sarcolemma is transiently reversed. β Receptor agonists and phosphodiesterase inhibitors, by increasing intracellular cyclic AMP levels, activate PKA, which phosphorylates target proteins, including phospholamban, the α subunit of the L-type Ca^{2+} channel and regulatory components of the RyR, as well as TnI, the inhibitory subunit of troponin (not shown). The effect of these phosphorylations is a positive inotropic effect: a faster rate of tension development to a higher level of tension, followed by a faster rate of relaxation. ▲ indicates site of cardiac glycoside binding. *See* text for mechanism of positive inotropic effect of cardiac glycosides.

Electrophysiological Actions. Atrial and ventricular myocytes, sinoatrial and atrioventricular (AV) nodal cells, and conduction fibers exhibit different responses to cardiac glycosides that are summations of direct responses and neurally-mediated reflex responses. At therapeutic serum or plasma concentrations (*i.e.,* 1 to 2 ng/ml), digoxin decreases automaticity and increases maximal diastolic resting membrane potential in atrial and AV nodal tissues, due to an increase in vagal tone and a decrease in sympathetic nervous system activity. In addition, there is prolongation of the effective refractory period and decreased conduction velocity in AV nodal tissue. These aggregate effects may cause sinus bradycardia or arrest and/or prolongation of AV conduction or higher-grade AV block. At higher concentrations, cardiac glycosides can increase sympathetic nervous system activity and directly affect automaticity in cardi-

ac tissue, actions that contribute to the genesis of atrial and ventricular arrhythmias. Increased intracellular Ca^{2+} loading and increased sympathetic tone increase the spontaneous (phase 4) rate of diastolic depolarization as well as delayed afterdepolarizations that may reach the threshold for generation of a propagated action potential. This simultaneous nonuniform increase in automaticity and depression of conduction in His-Purkinje and ventricular muscle fibers produces an electrophysiologic substrate that predisposes to serious ventricular arrhythmias, including ventricular tachycardia and ventricular fibrillation (*see* Chapter 34).

Regulation of Sympathetic Nervous System Activity. When cardiac output declines to a level that is inadequate to meet the demands of body tissues, increased sympathetic nervous system activity occurs as a compensatory response. This is due in part to a reduction in the sensitivity of the arterial baroreflex response to blood pressure, resulting in a decline in baroreflex-mediated tonic suppression of CNS-directed sympathetic activity (Ferguson *et al.*, 1989). This desensitization of the normal baroreflex arc also contributes to the sustained elevation in plasma norepinephrine, renin, vasopressin, and other indices of systemic neurohumoral activation that are present in heart failure.

A direct effect of cardiac glycosides on carotid baroreflex responsiveness to changes in carotid sinus pressure has been demonstrated in isolated preparations from animals with experimental heart failure (Wang *et al.*, 1990). In patients with moderate-to-advanced heart failure, infusion of a cardiac glycoside increased forearm blood flow and cardiac index and decreased heart rate; skeletal muscle sympathetic nerve activity, an indicator of the central sympathetic nervous system tone, was markedly reduced (Ferguson *et al.*, 1989). It is unlikely that these effects can be attributed to a direct inotropic effect of the drug, since dobutamine infusion did not suppress muscle sympathetic nerve activity in these patients despite comparable increases in cardiac output. Thus, the effects of digoxin in heart failure apparently include a reduction in neurohumoral activation that could represent an important contribution to the efficacy of cardiac glycosides in the treatment of heart failure.

Pharmacokinetics. The elimination half-life for digoxin is 36 to 48 hours in patients with normal or near-normal renal function. This permits once-a-day dosing; near steady-state blood levels are achieved one week after initiation of maintenance therapy. Digoxin is excreted by the kidney with a clearance rate that is proportional to the glomerular filtration rate. In patients with congestive heart failure and marginal cardiac reserve, an increase in cardiac output and renal blood flow with vasodilator therapy or sympathomimetic agents may increase renal digoxin clearance, necessitating adjustment of daily maintenance doses. Conversely, the half-life of the drug is increased substantially in patients with advanced renal insufficiency (to approximately 3.5 to 5 days); both the volume of distribution and the clearance rate of the drug are decreased in the elderly. As a result, the drug must be used with caution in patients with renal insufficiency and in the elderly.

Despite renal clearance, digoxin is not removed effectively by hemodialysis due to the drug's large (4 to 7 liters/kg) volume of distribution. The principal tissue reservoir is skeletal muscle and not adipose tissue, and thus dosing should be based on estimated lean body mass. Most digoxin tablets average 70% to 80% oral bioavailability; however, approximately 10% of the general population harbors the enteric bacterium *Eubacterium lentum*, which can convert digoxin into inactive metabolites, and this may account for some cases of apparent resistance to stan-

dard doses of oral digoxin. Liquid-filled capsules of digoxin (LANOXICAPS) have a higher bioavailability than do tablets (LANOXIN) and require dosage adjustment if a patient is switched from one dosage form to the other. Digoxin is available for intravenous administration, and maintenance doses can be given intravenously when oral dosing is impractical. Digoxin administered intramuscularly is erratically absorbed, causes local discomfort, and is not recommended. A number of drug interactions and clinical conditions can alter the pharmacokinetics of digoxin or alter patient susceptibility to the toxic manifestations of this drug. For example, chronic renal failure decreases the volume of distribution of digoxin, and therefore requires a decrease in maintenance dosage of the drug. Electrolyte disturbances, especially hypokalemia, acid–base imbalances, and the type of underlying heart disease also may alter a patient's susceptibility to toxic manifestations of digoxin.

Clinical Use of Digoxin in Heart Failure. The cardiac glycosides have long been used in the treatment of CHF. For a century, however, there has been controversy surrounding the efficacy of cardiac glycosides in the treatment of patients with heart failure who are in sinus rhythm. Despite widespread use of digoxin, objective data from randomized, controlled trials on the safety and efficacy of digoxin were lacking until the past decade.

The PROVED (Prospective Randomized study Of Ventricular failure and Efficacy of Digoxin) (Uretsky *et al.*, 1993) and RADIANCE (Randomized Assessment of Digoxin on Inhibition of Angiotensin Converting Enzyme) (Packer *et al.*, 1993) trials examined the effects of withdrawal of digoxin in stable patients with mild-to-moderate heart failure (*i.e.*, NYHA Class II and III) and systolic ventricular dysfunction (left ventricular ejection fraction <0.35%). All patients studied were in normal sinus rhythm. Withdrawal of digoxin resulted in a significant worsening of heart failure symptoms in patients who received placebo compared with patients who continued to receive active drug. Maximal treadmill exercise tolerance also declined significantly in patients withdrawn from digoxin in both trials, despite continuation of other medical therapies for heart failure.

The much larger Digoxin Investigation Group (DIG) trial studied the effect of digoxin therapy on survival in patients with heart failure (The Digitalis Investigation Group, 1997). Overall, there was no difference in mortality (from all causes) between the treatment groups. Over the 48 months of the study, fewer patients in the digoxin group died from or were hospitalized due to worsening heart failure; this benefit was seen at all levels of ejection fraction, but was greatest in patients with more severe degrees of heart failure. In a predefined substudy of patients with normal ejection fraction (*i.e.*, presumed to have diastolic heart failure), a similar pattern of benefit was seen with digoxin. Retrospective subgroup analyses suggest that the benefits of digoxin are optimized when serum concentrations are <1 ng/ml.

Use of Digoxin in Clinical Practice and Monitoring of Serum Levels. It is now recommended that digoxin be reserved for patients with heart failure who are in atrial fibrillation, or for patients in sinus rhythm who remain symptomatic despite maximal therapy with ACE inhibitors and β adrenergic receptor antagonists. The latter agents are viewed as first-line therapies on the basis of the proven mortality benefit. Most studies suggest that the maximal increase in contractility is apparent at serum levels of digoxin around 1.4 ng/ml or 1.8 nmol (Kelly and Smith, 1992a). The neurohormonal benefits of digoxin may occur at lower serum levels, between 0.5 and 1 ng/ml; higher serum concentrations are not associated with further decreases in neurohormonal activation or with increased clinical benefit. A retrospective subgroup analysis of the DIG trial suggested that the risk of death was greater with increasing serum concentrations, even at values that were within the traditional therapeutic range. Many authorities therefore advocate maintaining digoxin levels below 1 ng/ml (Gheorghiade *et al.*, 2004).

In summary, digoxin is no longer viewed as a first-line agent in the treatment of congestive heart failure. Despite this fact, it should be emphasized that digoxin, unlike virtually all other inotropic agents studied to date, does not have an adverse impact on mortality in CHF. Thus, digoxin is a therapeutic option in patients who remain symptomatic despite treatment with agents that improve survival. Digoxin may be unique among inotropic drugs by virtue of its neurohumoral effects, which include attenuation of sympathetic activation and reduction of renin release.

Digoxin Toxicity. The incidence and severity of digoxin toxicity have declined substantially in the past two decades, due in part to the development of alternative drugs for the treatment of supraventricular arrhythmias and heart failure, to the increased understanding of digoxin pharmacokinetics, to the monitoring of serum digoxin levels, and to the identification of important interactions between digoxin and other concomitantly administered drugs. Nevertheless, the recognition of digoxin toxicity remains an important consideration in the differential diagnosis of arrhythmias and neurological and gastrointestinal symptoms in patients receiving cardiac glycosides.

Vigilance for and early recognition of disturbances of impulse formation, conduction, or both are critically important. Among the more common electrophysiological manifestations are ectopic beats of AV junctional or ventricular origin, first-degree AV block, an excessively slow ventricular rate response to atrial fibrillation, or an accelerated AV junctional pacemaker. These often require only a dosage adjustment and appropriate monitoring. Sinus bradycardia, sinoatrial arrest or exit block, and second- or third-degree AV conduction delay usually respond to *atropine*, although temporary ventricular pacing may be necessary. Potassium administration should be considered for patients with evidence of increased AV junctional or ventricular automaticity, even when the serum K^+ is in the normal range, unless high-grade AV block also is present. *Lidocaine* or *phenytoin*, which have minimal effects on AV conduction, may be used for the treatment of worsening ventricular arrhythmias that threaten hemodynamic compromise (*see* Chapter 34). Electrical cardioversion carries an increased risk of inducing severe rhythm disturbances in patients with overt digitalis toxicity and should be used with particular caution. Note, too, that inhibition of the Na^+,K^+-ATPase activity of skeletal muscle can cause hyperkalemia.

Antidigoxin Immunotherapy. An effective antidote for life-threatening digoxin or *digitoxin* toxicity is available in the form of antidigoxin immunotherapy with purified Fab fragments from ovine antidigoxin antisera (DIGIBIND). A full neutralizing dose of Fab based on either the estimated total dose of drug ingested or the total body digoxin burden can be administered intravenously in saline solution over 30 to 60 minutes. For a more comprehensive review of the treatment of digitalis toxicity, see Kelly and Smith (1992b).

Parenteral Inotropic Agents

General Considerations. As noted earlier, patients with heart failure are most commonly hospitalized because of fluid retention that results in dyspnea and peripheral edema. Accordingly, relief of congestion through the use of diuretics and venodilators remains a therapeutic priority. A subset of these patients may present with clinical evidence of reduced forward cardiac output; the symptoms and signs associated with low output can range from fatigue, a common complaint, to azotemia and alterations in mental status. Patients who present with more severe decompensation typically require intensive therapy that may include parenteral inotropic agents; in extreme circumstances assisted ventilation and mechanical circulatory support may be required. Right heart catheterization and placement of a pulmonary artery catheter for continuous monitoring of intracardiac pressures can be helpful, particularly when volume status is unclear. In the setting of severe decompensation, the principal focus of initial therapy is to increase cardiac output by administration of agents that increase myocardial contractility.

β Adrenergic and Dopaminergic Agonists

Dopamine and dobutamine are the positive inotropic agents most often used for the short-term support of the circulation in advanced heart failure. These drugs act *via* stimulation of the cardiac myocyte dopamine D_1 receptor and β adrenergic receptor, leading to stimulation of the G_s–adenylyl cyclase–cyclic AMP–PKA pathway. The catalytic subunit of PKA phosphorylates a number of substrates that enhance Ca^{2+}-dependent contraction and speed relaxation (Figure 33–8). *Isoproterenol*, *epinephrine*, and *norepinephrine*, although useful in specific circumstances, have little role in the treatment of heart failure. The basic pharmacology of these and other adrenergic agonists is discussed in Chapter 10.

Dopamine. Dopamine, an endogenous catecholamine, has limited utility in the treatment of most patients with cardiogenic circulatory failure.

The pharmacological and hemodynamic effects of dopamine are dose dependent. At *low doses* (≤ 2 μg/kg per minute, based on estimated lean body mass), dopamine causes vasodilation by stimulating dopaminergic receptors on smooth muscle (causing cyclic AMP–dependent relaxation) and by stimulating presynaptic D_2 receptors on sympathetic nerves in the peripheral circulation (inhibiting norepinephrine release and reducing α adrenergic stimulation of vascular smooth muscle); these receptors are prominent in splanchnic and renal arterial beds. Dopamine infusion at this rate may increase renal blood flow and thereby help to maintain the glomerular filtration rate in patients who are refractory to diuretics; the clinical efficacy of this practice remains controversial. Dopamine also has direct effects on renal tubular epithelial cells that promote diuresis.

At *intermediate* infusion rates (2 to 5 μg/kg per minute), dopamine directly stimulates β receptors on the heart and vascular sympathetic neurons (enhancing cardiac contractility and neural norepinephrine release). At *higher* infusion rates (5 to 15 μg/kg per minute), peripheral arterial and venous constriction occur, mediated by α adrenergic receptor stimulation (*see* above). This effect may be desirable for support of a critically reduced arterial pressure in selected patients in whom circulatory failure is the result of vasodilation (*e.g.*, sepsis or anaphylaxis). However, high-dose dopamine infusion has little role in the treatment of patients with primary contractile dysfunction; in this setting, increased vasoconstriction will lead to increased afterload, further compromising left ventricular stroke volume, and forward cardiac output. Tachycardia, which is more pronounced with dopamine than with dobutamine, may provoke ischemia in patients with coronary artery disease.

Dobutamine. Dobutamine (DOBUTREX) is the β agonist of choice for the management of patients with systolic dysfunction and CHF. In the formulation available for clinical use, dobutamine is a racemic mixture that stimulates both β_1 and β_2 receptor subtypes. In addition, the (–) enantiomer is an agonist for α adrenergic receptors, whereas the (+) enantiomer is a very weak partial agonist. At infusion rates that result in a positive inotropic effect in humans, the β_1 adrenergic effect in the myocardium predominates. In the vasculature, the α adrenergic agonist effect of the (–) enantiomer appears to be negated by the partial agonism of the (+) enantiomer and the vasodilator effects of β_2 receptor stimulation. Thus, the principal hemodynamic effect of dobutamine is an increase in stroke volume due to its positive inotropic action. At doses that increase cardiac output, there is relatively little increase in heart rate. Dobutamine infusion generally causes a modest decrease in systemic resistance and intracardiac filling pressures (Figure 33–9). Dobutamine does not activate dopaminergic receptors. As such, the increase in renal blood flow that occurs in association with dobutamine is proportional to the increase in cardiac output.

Continuous infusion of dobutamine for up to several days in patients with severe clinical decompensation has been a common practice; pharmacological tolerance may limit efficacy during longer-term administration. Infusions are typically initiated at 2 to 3 μg/kg per minute, without a loading dose, and increased until the desired hemodynamic response is achieved. The blood pressure response to dobutamine is variable and is dependent on the relative effects of this agent on vascular tone and cardiac output. If cardiac output is significantly increased, heart rate may decline secondary to reflex withdrawal of sympathetic tone. The major side effects of dobutamine are excessive tachycardia and arrhythmias, which may require a reduction in dosage. Tolerance may occur after prolonged use, requiring substitution of an alternative drug such as a class III phosphodiesterase inhibitor. In patients who have been receiving a β receptor antagonist, the initial response to dobutamine may be attenuated.

Phosphodiesterase Inhibitors. The cyclic AMP–phosphodiesterase (PDE) inhibitors reduce the degradation of cellular cyclic AMP; the consequences are generally those of elevated cyclic AMP, much as would occur in response to a stimulator of adenylyl cyclase activity. In the heart, the result is positive inotropism. In the peripheral vasculature, the result is dilation of both resistance and capacitance vessels, leading to reduction of both afterload and preload. These combined effects on the myocardium and in the periphery underlie the classification of these drugs as "ino-dilators." The clinical use of older PDE inhibitors such as *theophylline* and *caffeine* is limited by their lack of isoform specificity and concomitant side effects. *Amrinone, milrinone,* and other PDE inhibitors with isoenzyme selectivity largely alleviate these side effects.

Inamrinone and Milrinone. Parenteral formulations of *inamrinone* (previous name amrinone) and milrinone have been approved for short-term support of the circulation in advanced heart failure. Both drugs are bipyridine derivatives and relatively selective inhibitors of PDE3, the cyclic GMP–inhibited cyclic AMP PDE. These drugs cause direct stimulation of myocardial contractility and acceleration of myocardial relaxation. In addition, they cause balanced arterial and venous dilation with a consequent fall in systemic and pulmonary vascular resistances, and left and right heart filling pressures. Cardiac output increases due to the stimulation of myocardial contractility and the decrease in left ventricular afterload. As a result of this dual mechanism of action, the increase in cardiac output with milrinone is greater than that seen with nitroprusside at doses that produce comparable reductions of systemic resistance. Conversely, the arterial and venous dilator effects of milrinone are greater than those of dobutamine at doses that produce comparable increases in cardiac output (Figure 33–10).

Both inamrinone and milrinone are effective for short-term treatment of patients with severe heart failure due to systolic dysfunction. Intravenous infusions of either drug should be initiated with a loading dose followed by a continuous infusion. For inamrinone, a 0.75-mg/kg bolus injection administered over 2 to 3 minutes is followed by a 2- to 20-μg/kg per minute infusion. The loading dose of milrinone is usually 50 μg/kg, and the continuous infusion rate ranges from 0.25 to 1 μg/kg per minute. The elimination half-lives of

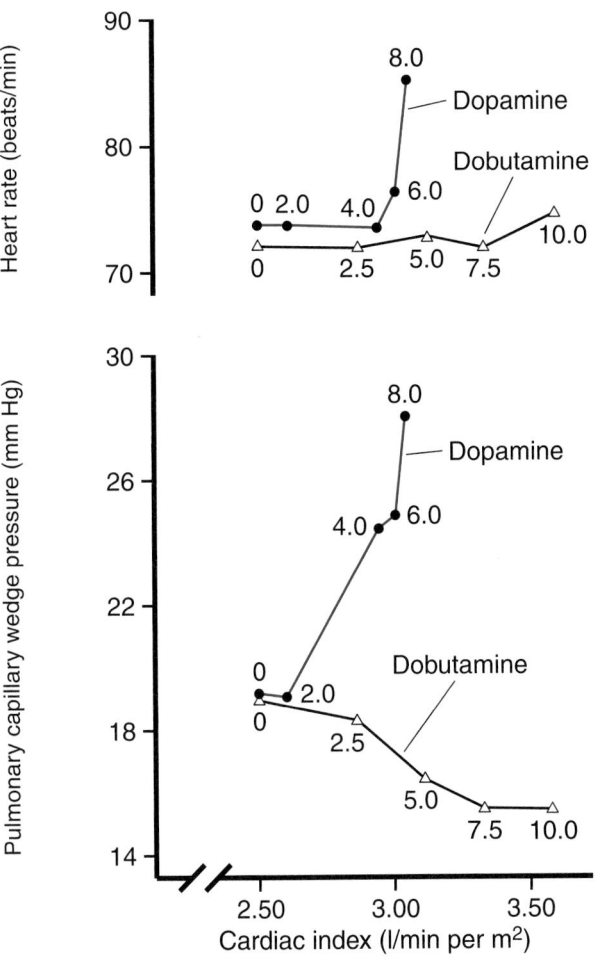

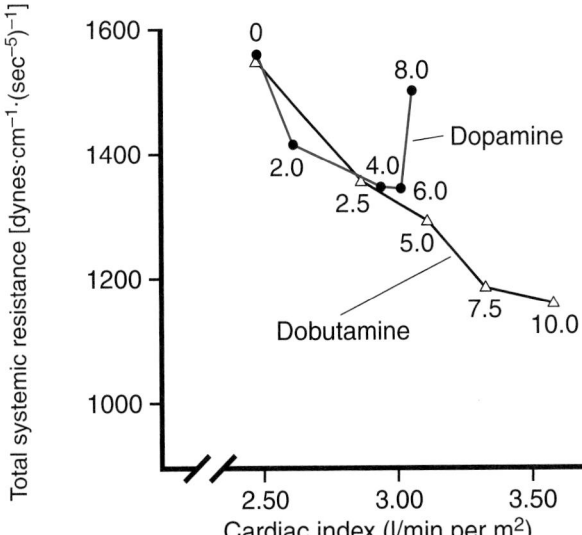

Figure 33–9. *Comparative hemodynamic effects of dopamine and dobutamine in patients with heart failure.* The numbers shown on the figures are infusion rates (μg/kg/min). Dobutamine increased cardiac output due to an increase in stroke volume (not shown); the drug also caused modest decreases in pulmonary capillary wedge pressure and systemic vascular resistance, reflecting both direct vasodilation (stimulation of β_2 receptors) and reflex withdrawal of sympathetic tone in response to improved cardiovascular function. At infusion rates >2 to 4 μg/kg/min, dopamine exerted a vasoconstrictor effect as evidenced by the increase in systemic vascular resistance. Dopamine also increased pulmonary capillary wedge pressure due to venoconstriction and a decrease in left ventricular function caused by the increase in afterload. (From Stevenson and Colucci [1996] with permission.)

inamrinone and milrinone in healthy subjects are 2 to 3 hours and 0.5 to 1 hour, respectively, and are approximately doubled in patients with severe heart failure. Clinically significant thrombocytopenia occurs in 10% of patients receiving inamrinone but is rare with milrinone. Because of its greater selectivity for PDE3 isoenzymes, shorter half-life, and more favorable side-effect profile, milrinone is the agent of choice among currently available PDE inhibitors for *short-term*, parenteral inotropic support. The vasodilating effects of the drug and its relatively protracted half-life limit use in patients with low systemic arterial pressure.

Chronic Positive Inotropic Therapy

Several oral inotropic agents have been developed and subsequently investigated in clinical trials. Some of these agents, particularly those of the PDE inhibitor class, have vasodilator actions in addition to their inotropic effects. While improvement in symptoms, functional status, and hemodynamic profile have been reported, the impact of these drugs on mortality during longer-term therapy has been disappointing. The dopaminergic agonist *ibopamine,* PDE inhibitors milrinone, inamrinone, and *vesnarinone,* and the benzimidazoline PDE inhibitor with calcium-sensitizing properties,

pimobendan, have been associated with increased mortality (Hampton *et al.*, 1997; Packer *et al.*, 1991; Cohn *et al.*, 1998). These observations underscore the conclusion stated earlier: *salutary effects on hemodynamic function do not translate into improved survival.* At present, digoxin is the only oral inotropic agent that is available for use in patients with CHF.

Continuous or intermittent outpatient therapy with dobutamine or milrinone, administered by a portable or home-based infusion pump through a central venous catheter, has been evaluated in patients with end-stage heart failure and symptoms refractory to other classes of drugs. There is as yet no convincing evidence that *chronic* parenteral inotropic therapy improves the quality or length of life. Furthermore, there are concerns that this form of therapy may actually hasten death (Gheorghiade *et al.*, 2000).

Diastolic Heart Failure

Epidemiologic studies of CHF indicate that approximately 30% to 40% of cases occur in patients with normal or preserved left ventricular systolic function.

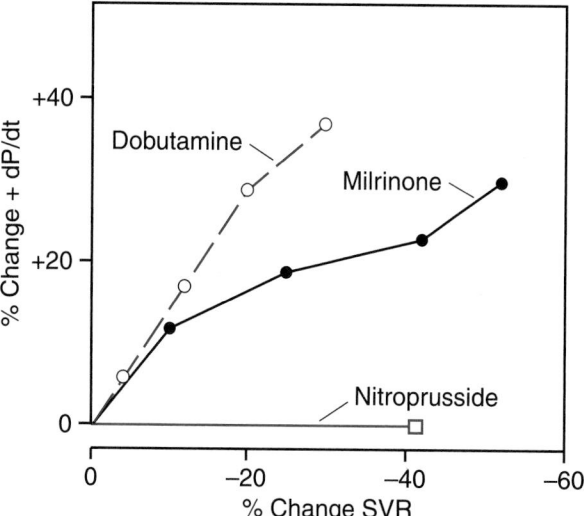

Figure 33–10. Comparative effects of dobutamine, milrinone, and nitroprusside on left ventricular contractility and systemic vascular resistance. Dobutamine, milrinone, and nitroprusside are parenteral agents used in the management of patients with severe heart failure. Shown are the effects of these drugs on left ventricular contractility, as reflected by left ventricular peak contractility (+dP/dt), and systemic vascular resistance (SVR) in patients with heart failure. Dobutamine and milrinone both increase left ventricular contractility due to their positive inotropic actions on the myocardium. Milrinone and dobutamine (to a lesser extent) also decrease SVR, indicating that they also exert a vasodilatory action. However, for a comparable increase in contractility, milrinone causes a greater decrease in SVR. Nitroprusside, a pure vasodilator, decreases SVR but had no effect on contractility. (Adapted with permission from Colucci *et al.*, 1986.)

Despite intact systolic function, such patients will present with typical signs and symptoms of heart failure, including dyspnea, impaired functional capacity, and pulmonary/systemic venous congestion. The pathogenesis of diastolic heart failure includes structural and functional abnormalities of the ventricle that are associated with impaired ventricular relaxation and impaired left ventricular distensibility (*i.e.,* abnormal LV compliance with increased chamber stiffness). These abnormalities in patients with diastolic heart failure are reflected in the LV pressure–volume relationship during diastole, which is shifted upward and to the left relative to normal subjects (Figure 33–11). Consonant with the definition of heart failure outlined above, the diagnosis of diastolic heart failure is made when the left ventricle is unable to fill to a volume that is sufficient to maintain normal cardiac output without exceeding the upper range of normal

diastolic pressure. In effect, the underlying problem in diastolic heart failure is the inability to fill (rather than to empty) the ventricle.

Over the last two decades, there has been a resurgence of interest in the diastolic phase of the cardiac cycle. In patients with primary diastolic dysfunction, the myocardial abnormality that accounts for abnormal filling is intrinsic; this is perhaps best illustrated by infiltrative disorders (restrictive cardiomyopathies) such as cardiac amyloidosis, hemochromatosis, sarcoidosis, and rare conditions such as endomyocardial fibrosis and Fabry's disease. It is also common to include familial hypertrophic cardiomyopathy among the disorders that are associated with clinical heart failure and intact systolic function.

Diastolic heart failure occurs more commonly as a secondary condition. This can occur as a consequence of excessive preload (*e.g.,* renal failure), excessive afterload (systemic hypertension), or changes in ventricular size, shape, and function that occur as a response to abnormal loading conditions. Diastolic heart failure can also occur in patients as a consequence of extramyocardial cardiac disease such as epicardial coronary artery disease or pericardial disease. With respect to secondary diastolic dysfunction, the disorder is more prevalent in women than men and increases in prevalence with advancing age. Systemic hypertension and diabetes are more common in such patients. The consensus view is that mortality in diastolic heart failure is less than that reported for age-matched patients with systolic dysfunction and CHF (5% to 8% *vs.* 10% to 15% annual mortality, respectively), although this remains controversial (Jones *et al.*, 2004).

Historically, hemodynamic findings obtained at cardiac catheterization were considered the gold standard for the diagnosis of diastolic heart failure: elevated intracardiac filling pressures; confirmation of preserved ejection fraction; and reduction of cardiac output at rest or subnormal increase in output during exercise. However, in the absence of invasive confirmation, the diagnosis should not be made until other conditions that can cause exertional dyspnea and exercise intolerance have been excluded. This caveat is particularly relevant in the era of widespread noninvasive evaluation of diastolic function. In one study, diastolic abnormalities (defined by echocardiographic criteria) were present in 28% of the study group, less than one-half of whom had clinical evidence of heart failure (American Heart Association, 2003).

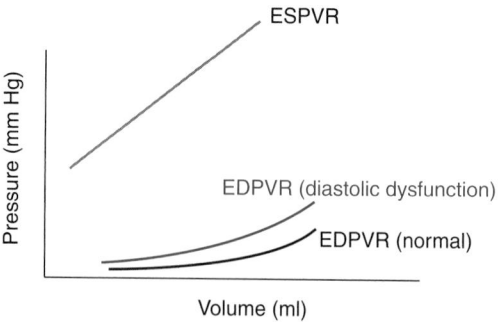

Figure 33–11. Diastolic dysfunction. EDPVR, end-diastolic pressure–volume relationship; ESPVR, end-systolic pressure–volume relationship. (Courtesy of Michael Parker, M.D.)

In contrast to the pharmacotherapy of patients with heart failure due to systolic dysfunction, there are few objective data upon which to base treatment decisions in patients with diastolic heart failure. There are no randomized, placebo-controlled trials to guide therapy in such patients, and one is therefore unable to initiate treatment in anticipation of attenuating disease progression or reducing mortality. It is, however, possible to make some general comments regarding mechanistic considerations in selecting treatment.

Patients with diastolic heart failure are typically dependent upon preload to maintain adequate cardiac output. While patients with symptomatic volume overload will benefit from careful modulation of intravascular volume, volume reduction should be accomplished gradually and treatment goals reassessed frequently. In addition to cautious volume management, it is important to maintain synchronous atrial contraction in such patients; this helps to maintain adequate left ventricular filling during the latter phase of diastole. As one might predict, cardiac function is often severely impaired if such patients develop atrial fibrillation; patients with diastolic heart failure will frequently experience clinical exacerbations coincident with conversion to atrial fibrillation, particularly in the context of suboptimal ventricular rate control. Meticulous control of the ventricular rate with drugs that slow AV conduction is mandatory (*see* Chapter 34) and restoration of sinus rhythm should be considered. It is also important to consider evaluation for and treatment of conditions that are associated with dynamic abnormalities of diastolic function, such as myocardial ischemia and poorly controlled systemic hypertension.

CLINICAL SUMMARY

Heart failure is a chronic illness that begins with a primary myocardial insult (that leads to loss of cardiomyocyte number or function) and that is progressive (through a course that is characterized by a variety of functional and structural compensations). In fact, this temporal progression of disease provides the basis for a revised classification system that is replacing the standard New York Heart Association categories that are based on patient functional status. Under this new construct (Figure 33–12), patients progress from a stage in which they are at risk to develop heart failure (Stage A) to a phase in which structural heart disease is established and demonstrable (Stage B). From this point of asymptomatic ventricular dysfunction, patients progress to a stage in which symptoms of the heart failure syndrome are present (Stage C); a subset of Stage C patients will progress to end-stage status (Stage D) in which symptoms refractory to medical therapy are present. Given that the syndrome of heart failure begins with a primary insult to the myocardium (such as infarction, excessive hemodynamic load, or inflammation), treatment should begin with prevention *via* the identification and remediation of risk factors that predispose to the development of

structural heart disease. For example, since coronary artery disease is the most common etiologic basis for systolic dysfunction and CHF, the prevention of myocardial infarction through risk factor modification (*e.g.,* lipid lowering, control of hypertension, and smoking cessation) is a critical therapeutic strategy with substantial public health implications.

Once structural heart disease is established (Stage B), compensatory mechanisms are activated that support cardiovascular function, but that also set the stage for disease progression. Symptoms are not present and this phase can therefore be referred to as the stage of asymptomatic ventricular dysfunction. Treatment in Stage B is directed at attenuation of sustained neurohormonal activation. With respect to therapy, it is advised that target doses of β blockers, ACE inhibitors, or AT_1 receptor antagonists be selected using the treatment guidelines applied in the clinical trials that established the morbidity and mortality benefits of these agents; it is axiomatic that the specific agent selected and the dosing regimen must be individualized.

After an asymptomatic period of variable duration, heart failure usually progresses to a symptomatic stage, with clinical manifestations reflecting specific hemodynamic profiles. Once symptoms ensue (Stage C), the goals of treatment include both relief of symptoms and prevention of disease progression. Drugs are selected that target the hemodynamic derangements that are thought to be responsible for symptoms. In addition to the use of diuretics and load-reducing therapies for relief of congestive symptoms, antagonism of the renin–angiotensin system and the sympathetic branch of the autonomic nervous system are indicated to prevent further myocardial injury, thereby attenuating disease progression. In the ambulatory patient in a compensated hemodynamic state, diuretics and organic nitrates are used to establish and maintain euvolemia; vasodilators are used to reduce the systemic vascular resistance in order to optimize forward cardiac output. While maintenance of forward cardiac output will help to attenuate neurohumoral activation, agents that antagonize the effects of Ang II and sympathetic stimulation are indicated; ACE inhibitors and AT_1 receptor antagonists are the agents of choice. If neither of these agents is tolerated, treatment with the hydralazine–isosorbide dinitrate combination should be initiated. Treatment with β blockers should be undertaken when hemodynamic stability is established and treatment with aldosterone antagonists considered in patients with preserved renal function. Digoxin is now primarily used for persistent symptoms in the ambulatory patient; this drug does have positive inotropic effects

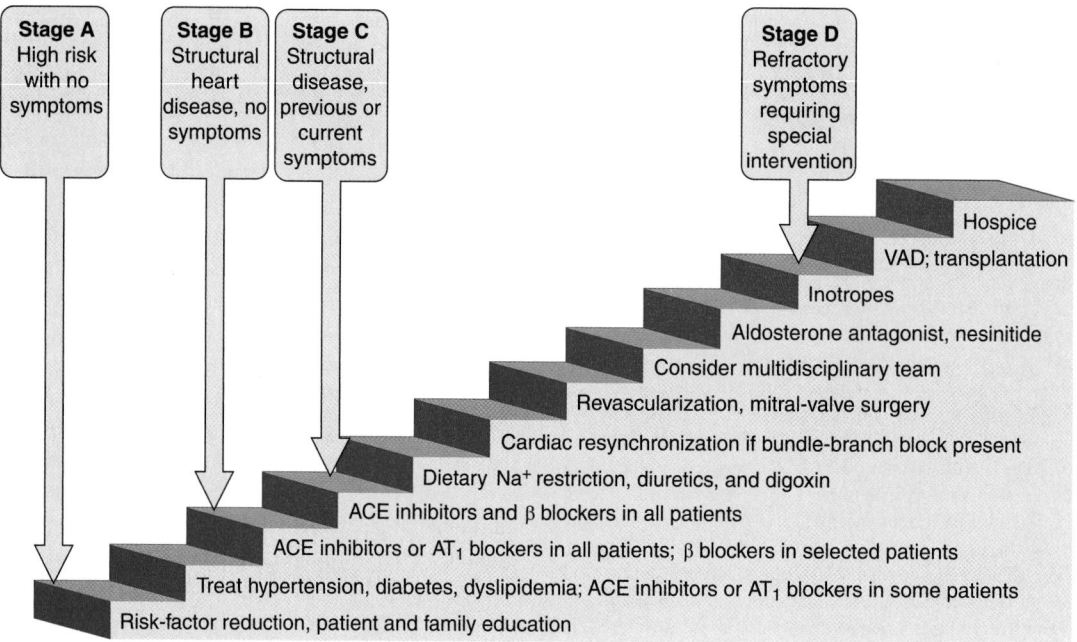

Figure 33–12. *Stages of heart failure.* (Reproduced with permission from Jessup and Brozena [2003].)

and independent effects that are mediated *via* neurohormonal antagonism. However, there are no data that cardiac glycosides decrease mortality.

In the symptomatic patient with hemodynamic decompensation, hospitalization may be required, since oral diuretic and vasodilator therapy alone may be inadequate to reestablish euvolemia and adequate peripheral perfusion. In such patients, parenteral vasodilators and inotropic agents may be required to restore forward cardiac output; such parenteral support may be required to reverse the avid retention of Na^+ and water that characterizes the decompensated state. Cardiac output can be increased by a number of distinctive therapeutic agents. In designing a treatment regimen, the clinician must consider the hemodynamic status of the individual patient. It is frequently possible to do so by qualitative assessment of the forward cardiac output (normal *versus* low), systemic vascular resistance (normal *versus* high), and intracardiac filling pressures (normal *versus* high); if assessment by physical examination is inconclusive, hemodynamic monitoring *via* bedside pulmonary artery catheterization can provide a more objective, quantitative assessment of these critical parameters of cardiac performance (Nohria *et al.*, 2003).

In patients with elevated systemic vascular resistance and normal-to-elevated systemic blood pressure, afterload reduction with nitroprusside is a logical treatment; it should be emphasized that nitroprusside will also increase venous capacitance, thereby decreasing preload as well. In the context of myocardial dysfunction, reduction of afterload will typically lead to improved forward cardiac output, based on the inverse relationship between impedance to ejection and stroke volume in the failing ventricle. Nitroprusside may also be effective when the systemic vascular resistance is elevated and systemic blood pressure is reduced; the caveat in this more complex hemodynamic setting is that the load reduction produced by nitroprusside must be counterbalanced by an increase in stroke volume. This derivative increase in stroke volume may not occur in the patient with advanced heart failure; rather, the result will be a further reduction in mean arterial pressure and the potential risk of peripheral organ hypoperfusion. An alternative approach would be the use of an inotropic-dilator drug such as milrinone; this drug will provide both preload and afterload reduction, and its concurrent positive inotropic effect may offset the reduction in mean arterial pressure that can occur from vasodilation alone.

In the decompensated patient who presents with heart failure and normal systemic vascular resistance, afterload reduction may be contraindicated in the short term. In such patients, treatment with a parenteral agent such as dobutamine may be preferable. The risk attendant to treatment with sympathomimetic drugs is related to the increase in myocardial O_2 consumption that may occur; this is of particular concern in patients with left heart failure that occurs as a direct consequence of myocardial ischemia. This clinical quandary has become less common in the era of aggressive myocardial revascularization; when it is encountered, coadministration of dobutamine with parenteral nitroglycerin should be considered.

In general, therapy in the patient with symptomatic pulmonary congestion should include diuresis to alleviate pulmonary and systemic vascular congestion. The administration of an oral or intravenous nitrate preparation may provide rapid symptomatic relief of pulmonary congestion by increasing venous capacitance. This treatment goal is desirable to reduce patient discomfort; an important ancillary impact of such treatment is the attenuation of the neurohumoral activation that accompanies elevation of intracardiac filling pressures and the attendant dyspnea. As previously noted, excessive preload reduction should be avoided given the dependence on preload that accompanies advanced myocardial dysfunction.

When advanced heart failure is unresponsive to these standard therapies, invasive hemodynamic monitoring may be required. Effective treatment of these patients is often complicated by concurrent renal insufficiency and hypotension, despite evidence of persistent elevation of intracardiac filling pressures. In this setting, selection of parenteral agents is guided by the data regarding systemic vascular resistance and filling pressures provided by the indwelling pulmonary artery catheter.

In patients who remain symptomatic and/or hemodynamically unstable (Stage D), referral to a specialized tertiary center with expertise in the evaluation and management of heart failure should be considered. At this advanced stage of disease, resource-intensive treatment (such as cardiac resynchronization therapy, mechanical assist devices, high-risk surgical interventions, or cardiac transplantation) or investigational therapies can be considered.

BIBLIOGRAPHY

AIRE (Acute Infarction Ramipril Efficacy) Study Investigators. Effect of ramipril on mortality and morbidity of survivors of acute myocardial infarction with clinical evidence of heart failure. *Lancet,* **1993,** *342:*821–828.

American Heart Association. *2004 Heart and Stroke Statistical Update,* American Heart Association, Dallas, **2003.**

Andersson, B., Hamm, C., Persson, S., *et al.* Improved exercise hemodynamic status in dilated cardiomyopathy after beta-adrenergic blockade treatment. *J. Am. Coll. Cardiol.,* **1994,** *23:*1397–1404.

Australia/New Zealand Heart Failure Research Collaborative Group. Randomised, placebo-controlled trial of carvedilol in patients with congestive heart failure due to ischaemic heart disease. *Lancet,* **1997,** *349:*375–380.

Bart, B.A., Ertl, G., Held, P., *et al.* Contemporary management of patients with left ventricular systolic dysfunction. Results from the Study of Patients Intolerant of Converting Enzyme Inhibitors (SPICE) Registry. *Eur Heart J.,* **1999,** *20:*1182–1190.

Bisognano, J.D., Weinberger, H.D., Bohlmeyer, T.J., *et al.* Myocardial-directed overexpression of the human β_1-adrenergic receptor in transgenic mice. *J. Mol. Cell. Cardiol.,* **2000,** *32:*817–830.

Bristow, M.R., Gilbert, E.M., Abraham, W.T., *et al.* Carvedilol produces dose-related improvements in left ventricular function and survival in subjects with chronic heart failure. MOCHA Investigators. *Circulation,* **1996,** *94:*2807–2816.

The Cardiac Insufficiency Bisoprolol Study II (CIBIS II): a randomized trial. CIBIS-II Investigators and Committee. *Lancet,* **1999,** *353:*9–13.

Cohn, J.N., Archibald, D.G., Ziesche, S., *et al.* Effect of vasodilator therapy on mortality in chronic congestive heart failure. Results of a Veterans Administration Cooperative Study. *N. Engl. J. Med.,* **1986,** *314:*1547–1552.

Cohn, J.N., Goldstein, S.O., Greenberg, B.H., *et al.* A dose-dependent increase in mortality with vesnarinone among patients with severe heart failure. Vesnarinone Trial Investigators. *N. Engl. J. Med.,* **1998,** *339:*1810–1816.

Cohn, J.N., Johnson, G., Ziesche, S., *et al.* A comparison of enalapril with hydralazine–isosorbide dinitrate in the treatment of chronic congestive heart failure. *N. Engl. J. Med.,* **1991,** *325:*303–310.

Colucci, W.S., Wright, R.F., and Braunwald, E. New positive inotropic agents in the treatment of congestive heart failure. Mechanisms of action and recent clinical developments. *N. Engl. J. Med.* **1986,** *314:*290–299.

Colucci, W.S., Packer, M., Bristow, M.R., *et al.* Carvedilol inhibits clinical progression in patients with mild symptoms of heart failure. U.S. Carvedilol Heart Failure Study Group. *Circulation,* **1996,** *94:*2800–2806.

Communal, C., Singh, K., Pimentel, D.R., and Colucci, W.S. Norepinephrine stimulates apoptosis in adult rat ventricular myocytes by activation of the β-adrenergic pathway. *Circulation,* **1998,** *98:*1329–1334.

CONSENSUS Trial Study Group. Effects of enalapril on mortality in severe congestive heart failure. Results of the Cooperative North Scandinavian Enalapril Survival Study (CONSENSUS). The CONSENSUS Trial Study Group. *N. Engl. J. Med.,* **1987,** *316:*1429–1435.

Dargie, H.J. Effect of carvedilol on outcome after myocardial infarction in patients with left ventricular dysfunction: the CAPRICORN randomized trial. *Lancet,* **2001,** *357:*1385–1390.

Davies, D.L., and Fraser, R. Do diuretics cause magnesium deficiency? *Br. J. Clin. Pharmacol.,* **1993,** *36:*1–10.

The Digitalis Investigation Group. The effect of digoxin on mortality and morbidity in patients with heart failure. *N. Engl. J. Med.,* **1997,** *336:*525–533.

Doggrell, S.A., CHARMed—the effects if candesartan in heart failure. *Expert Opin. Pharmacother.,* **2005,** *6:*513–516.

Dormans, T.P., van Meyel, J.J., Gerlag, P.G., *et al.* Diuretic efficacy of high dose furosemide in severe heart failure: bolus injection versus continuous infusion. *J. Am. Coll. Cardiol.,* **1996,** *28:*376–382.

Dries, D.L., Strong, M.H., Cooper, R.S., and Drazner, M.H. Efficacy of angiotensin-converting enzyme inhibition in reducing progression from asymptomatic left ventricular dysfunction to symptomatic heart failure in black and white patients. *J. Am. Coll. Cardiol.,* **2002,** *40:*311–317.

Eichhorn, E.J., Heesch, C.M., Barnett, J.H., *et al.* Effect of metoprolol on myocardial function and energetics in patients with nonischemic dilated cardiomyopathy: a randomized, double-blind, placebo-controlled study. *J. Am. Coll. Cardiol.,* **1994,** *24:*1310–1320.

Ellison, D.H. The physiologic basis of diuretic synergism: its role in treating diuretic resistance. *Ann. Intern. Med.,* **1991,** *114:*886–894.

Ferguson, D.W., Berg, W.J., Sanders, J.S., *et al.* Sympathoinhibitory responses to digitalis glycosides in heart failure patients. Direct evidence from sympathetic neural recordings. *Circulation,* **1989,** *80:*65–77.

Fonarow, G.C., Chelimsky-Fallick, C., Stevenson L.W., *et al.* Effect of direct vasodilation with hydralazine *versus* angiotensin-converting enzyme inhibition with captopril on mortality in advanced heart failure: the Hy-C trial. *J. Am. Coll. Cardiol.,* **1992,** *19:*842–850.

GISSI (Gruppo Italiano per lo Studio della Sopravvivenza nell'infarto Miocardico)-3. GISSI-3: effects of lisinopril and transdermal glyceryl trinitrate singly and together on 6-week mortality and ventricular function after acute myocardial infarction. *Lancet,* **1994,** *343:*1115–1122.

Gogia, H., Mehra, A., Parikh, S., *et al.* Prevention of tolerance to hemodynamic effects of nitrates with concomitant use of hydralazine in patients with chronic heart failure. *J. Am. Coll. Cardiol.,* **1995,** *26:*1575–1580.

Gottlieb, S.S., McCarter, R.J., and Vogel, R.A. Effect of β-blockade on mortality among high-risk and low-risk patients after myocardial infarction. *N. Engl. J. Med.,* **1998,** *339:*489–497.

Hall, S.A., Cigarroa, C.G., Marcoux, L., *et al.* Time course of improvement in left ventricular function, mass and geometry in patients with congestive heart failure treated with β-adrenergic blockade. *J. Am. Coll. Cardiol.,* **1995,** *25:*1154–1161.

Hampton, J.R., van Veldhuisen, D.J., Kleber, F.X., *et al.* Randomised study of effect of ibopamine on survival in patients with advanced severe heart failure. Second Prospective Randomised Study of Ibopamine on Mortality and Efficacy (PRIME II) Investigators. *Lancet,* **1997,** *349:*971–977.

Hillege, H.L., Girbes, A.R., deKam, P.J., *et al.* Renal function, neurohumoral activation, and survival in patients with chronic heart failure. *Circulation,* **2000,** *102:*203–210.

Jones, R., Francis, G.S., and Lauer, M.S. Predictors of mortality in patients with heart failure and preserved systolic function in The Digitalis Investigation Group trial. *J. Am. Coll. Cardiol.,* **2004,** *44:*1025–1029.

Juillerat, L., Nussberger, J., Menard, J., *et al.* Determinants of angiotensin II generation during converting enzyme inhibition. *Hypertension,* **1990,** *16:*564–572.

Juurlink, D.N., Mamdani, M.M., Lee, D.S., *et al.* Rates of hyperkalemia after publication of the Randomized Aldactone Evaluation Study. *N. Engl. J. Med.,* **2004,** *351:*543–551.

Kelly, R.A., and Smith, T.W. Use and misuse of digitalis blood levels. *Heart Dis. Stroke,* **1992a,** *1:*117–122.

Kelly, R.A., and Smith, T.W. Recognition and management of digitalis toxicity. *Am. J. Cardiol.,* **1992b,** *69:*108G–119G.

Kittleson, M., Hurwitz, S., Shah, M.R., *et al.* Development of circulatory-renal limitations to angiotensin-converting enzyme inhibitors identifies patients with severe heart failure and early mortality. *J. Am. Coll. Cardiol.,* **2003,** *41:*2029–2035.

Konstam, M.A., Rousseau, M.F., Kronenberg, M.W., *et al.* Effects of the angiotensin converting enzyme inhibitor enalapril on the long-term progression of left ventricular dysfunction in patients with heart failure. Studies of Left Ventricular Dysfunction (SOLVD) Investigators. *Circulation,* **1992,** *86:*431–438.

Korber, L., Torp-Pederson, C., Carlsen, J.E., *et al.* A clinical trial of the angiotensin-converting-enzyme inhibitor trandolapril in patients with left ventricular dysfunction after myocardial infarction. Trandolapril Cardiac Evaluation (TRACE) Study Group. *N. Engl. J. Med.,* **1995,** *333:*1670–1676.

Lahav, M., Regev, A., Ra'anani, P., and Theodor, E. Intermittent administration of furosemide *versus* continuous infusion preceded by a loading dose for congestive heart failure. *Chest,* **1992,** *102:*725–731.

McCurley, J.M., Hanlon, S.U., Wei, S.K., *et al.* Furosemide and the progression of left ventricular dysfunction in experimental heart failure. *J. Am. Coll. Cardiol.,* **2004,** *44:*1301–1307.

McKelvie, R.S., Yusuf, S., Pericak, D., *et al.* Comparison of candesartan, enalapril, and their combination in congestive heart failure: randomized evaluation of strategies for left ventricular dysfunction (RESOLVD) pilot study. The RESOLVD Pilot Study Investigators. *Circulation,* **1999,** *100:*1056–1064.

Mehra, A., Shotan, A., Ostrzega, E., *et al.* Potentiation of isosorbide dinitrate effects with *N*-acetylcysteine in patients with chronic heart failure. *Circulation,* **1994,** *89:*2595–2600.

MERIT-HF Study Group. Effect of metoprolol CR/XL in chronic heart failure: Metoprolol CR/XL Randomised Intervention Trial in Congestive Heart Failure (MERIT-HF). *Lancet,* **1999,** *353:*2001–2007.

Nohria, A., Tsang, S.W., Fang, C., *et al.* Clinical assessment identifies hemodynamic profiles that predict outcomes in patients admitted with heart failure. *J. Am. Coll. Cardiol.,* **2003,** *41:*1797–1804.

Packer, M., Bristow, M.R., Cohn, J.N., *et al.* The effect of carvedilol on morbidity and mortality in patients with chronic heart failure. U.S. Carvedilol Heart Failure Study Group. *N. Engl. J. Med.,* **1996,** *334:*1349–1355.

Packer, M., Califf, R.M., Konstam, M.A., *et al.,* for the OVERTURE study group. Comparison of omapatrilat and enalapril in patients with chronic heart failure. The Omapatrilat Versus Enalapril Trial of Utility in Reducing Events (OVERTURE). *Circulation,* **2002b,** *106:*920–926.

Packer, M., Carver, J.R., Rodeheffer, R.J., *et al.* Effect of oral milrinone on mortality in severe chronic heart failure. PROMISE Study Research Group. *N. Engl. J. Med.,* **1991,** *325:*1468–1475.

Packer, M., Fowler, M.B., Roecker, E.B., *et al.* Carvedilol Prospective Randomized Cumulative Survival (COPERNICUS) Study Group. Effects of carvedilol on morbidity of patients with severe chronic heart failure: results of the carvedilol prospective randomized cumulative survival (COPERNICUS) study. *Circulation,* **2002a,** *106:* 2194–2199.

Packer, M., Gheorghiade, M., Young, J.B., *et al.* Withdrawal of digoxin from patients with chronic heart failure treated with angiotensin-converting-enzyme inhibitors. RADIANCE Study. *N. Engl. J. Med.,* **1993,** *329:*1–7.

Packer, M., Poole-Wilson, P.A., Armstrong, P.W., *et al.* Comparative effects of low and high doses of the angiotensin converting enzyme inhibitor, lisinopril, on morbidity and mortality in chronic heart failure. Assessment of Treatment with Lisinopril and Survival (ATLAS) Study Group. *Circulation,* **1999,** *100:*2312–2318.

Pfeffer, M.A., Braunwald, E., Moye, L.A., *et al.* Effect of captopril on mortality and morbidity in patients with left ventricular dysfunction after myocardial infarction. Results of the Survival And Ventricular Enlargement trial. The SAVE Investigators. *N. Engl. J. Med.,* **1992,** *327:*669–677.

Pitt, B., Poole-Wilson, P.A., Segal, R., *et al.* Effect of losartan compared with captopril on mortality in patients with symptomatic heart failure: randomised trial—the Losartan Heart Failure Survival Study ELITE II. *Lancet,* **2000,** *355:*1582–1587.

Pitt, B., Remme, W., Zannad, F., *et al.,* and the Eplerenone Post-Acute Myocardial Infarction Heart Failure Efficacy and Survival Study Investigators. Eplerenone, a selective aldosterone blocker, in patients with left ventricular dysfunction after myocardial infarction. *N. Engl. J. Med.,* **2003,** *348:*1309–1321.

Pitt, B., Segal, R., Martinez, F.A., *et al.* Randomised trial of losartan versus captopril in patients over 65 with heart failure (Evaluation of Losartan in the Elderly Study, ELITE). *Lancet,* **1997,** *349:*747–752.

Pitt, B., Zannad, F., Remme, W.J., *et al.* The effect of spironolactone on morbidity and mortality in patients with severe heart failure. Randomized Aldactone Evaluation Study Investigators. *N. Engl. J. Med.,* **1999,** *341:*709–717.

Redfield, M.M., Jacobsen, S.J., Burnett, J.C., *et al.* Burden of systolic and diastolic ventricular dysfunction in the community: appreciating the scope of the heart failure epidemic. *JAMA,* **2003,** *289:*194–202.

Reiken, S., Gaburjanova, J., He, K., *et al.* β-Adrenergic receptor blockers restore cardiac calcium release channel (ryanodine receptor) structure and function in heart failure. *Circulation,* **2001,** *104:*2843–2848.

St. John Sutton, M., Pfeffer, M.A., Plappert, T., *et al.* Quantitative two-dimensional echocardiographic measurements are major predictors of adverse cardiovascular events after acute myocardial infarction. The protective effects of captopril. *Circulation,* **1994,** *89:*68–75.

Sawyer, D.B., and Colucci, W.S. Mitochondrial oxidative stress in heart failure: "oxygen wastage" revisited. *Circ. Res.,* **2000,** *86:*119–120.

Smith, T.W., Braunwald, E., and Kelly, R.A. The management of heart failure. In, *Heart Disease,* 4th ed. (Braunwald, E., ed.) Saunders, Philadelphia, **1992,** pp. 464–519.

Studies On Left Ventricular Dysfunction (SOLVD) Investigators. Effect of enalapril on mortality and the development of heart failure in asymptomatic patients with reduced left ventricular ejection fractions. *N. Engl. J. Med.,* **1992,** *327:*685–691. [Published erratum in *N. Engl. J. Med.,* **1992,** *327:*1768.]

Uretsky, B.F., Young, J.B., Shahidi, F.E., *et al.* Randomized study assessing the effect of digoxin withdrawal in patients with mild to moderate chronic congestive heart failure: results of the PROVED trial. PROVED Investigative Group. *J. Am. Coll. Cardiol.,* **1993,** *22:*955–962.

Waagstein, F., Bristow, M.R., Swedberg, K., *et al.* Beneficial effects of metoprolol in idiopathic dilated cardiomyopathy. Metoprolol in Dilated Cardiomyopathy (MDC) Trial Study Group. *Lancet,* **1993,** *342:*1441–1446.

Wang, W., Chen, J.S., and Zucker, I.H. Carotid sinus baroreceptor sensitivity in experimental heart failure. *Circulation,* **1990,** *81:*1959–1966.

Yusuf, S., Pfeffer, M., Swedberg, K., *et al.* CHARM Investigators and Committees. Effects of candesartan in patients with chronic heart failure and preserved left ventricular ejection fraction: the CHARM-Preserved Trial. *Lancet,* **2003,** *362:*777–781.

MONOGRAPHS AND REVIEWS

Bigger, J.T. Jr. Diuretic therapy, hypertension, and cardiac arrest. *N. Engl. J. Med.,* **1994,** *330:*1899–1900.

Brater, D.C. Diuretic therapy. *N. Engl. J. Med.,* **1998,** *339:*387–395.

Braunwald, E., and Bristow, M.R. Congestive heart failure: fifty years of progress. *Circulation,* **2000,** *102*(suppl. IV):14–23.

Bristow, M.R. β-Adrenergic receptor blockade in chronic heart failure. *Circulation,* **2000,** *101:*558–569.

Colucci, W.S., and Braunwald, E. Pathophysiology of heart failure. In, *Heart Disease,* 6th ed. (Braunwald, E., ed.) Saunders, Philadelphia, **2000.**

Cohn, J.N. The management of chronic heart failure. *N. Engl. J Med.,* **1996,** *335:*490–498.

Cohn, J.N. Treatment of infarct related heart failure: vasodilators other than ACE inhibitors. *Cardiovasc. Drugs Ther.,* **1994,** *8:*119–122.

Cohn, J.N., and Franciosa, J.A. Vasodilator therapy of cardiac failure. *N. Engl. J. Med.,* **1977,** *297:*254–258.

Eichhorn, E.J., and Bristow, M.R. Medical therapy can improve the biological properties of the chronically failing heart. A new era in the treatment of heart failure. *Circulation,* **1996,** *94:*2285–2296.

Eichhorn, E.J., and Gheorghiade, M. Digoxin. *Prog. Cardiovasc. Dis.,* **2002,** *44:*251–266.

Ellison, D.H. Diuretic resistance: physiology and therapeutics. *Semin. Nephrol.,* **1999,** *19:*581–597.

Fukuto, J., Switzer, C., Miranda, K., and Wink, D. Nitroxyl (HNO): Chemistry, biochemistry, and pharmacology. *Annu. Rev. Pharmacol. Toxicol.,* **2005,** *45:*335–355.

Fung, H-L. Biochemical mechanism of nitroglycerin action and tolerance: Is this old mystery solved? *Annu. Rev. Pharmacol. Toxicol.,* **2004,** *44:*67–85.

Gheorghiade, M., Adams, K.F., and Colucci, W.S. Digoxin in the management of cardiovascular disorders. *Circulation,* **2004,** *109:*2959–2964.

Gheorghiade, M., Cody, R.J., Francis, G.S., *et al.* Current medical therapy for advanced heart failure. *Heart Lung,* **2000,** *29:*16–32.

Gottleib, S.S. Management of volume overload in heart failure. In, *Heart Failure: A Companion to Braunwald's Heart Disease.* (Mann, D.L., ed.) Saunders, Philadelphia, **2004,** pp. 595–602.

Jessup, M., Brozena, S. Heart failure. *N. Engl. J. Med.,* **2003,** *348:*2007–2018.

Katz, A.M. The cardiomyopathy of overload: An unnatural growth response in the hypertrophied heart. *Ann. Intern. Med.,* **1994,** *121:*363–371.

Mann, D.L. Mechanisms and models in heart failure: a combinatorial approach. *Circulation,* **1999,** *100:*999–1008.

Napoli, C., and Ignarro, L. Nitric oxide-releasing drugs. *Annu. Rev. Pharmacol. Toxicol.,* **2003,** *43:*97–123.

Stevenson, L.W., and Colucci, W.S. Management of patients hospitalized with heart failure. In, *Cardiovascular Therapeutics: A Companion to Braunwald's Heart Disease.* (Smith, T.W., ed.) Saunders, Philadelphia, **1996,** pp. 199–209.

Swedberg, K. Initial experience with β blockers in dilated cardiomyopathy. *Am. J. Cardiol.,* **1993,** *71:*30C–38C.

Villarreal, F. *Interstitial Fibrosis in Heart Failure.* (Villarreal, F., ed.) Springer, New York, **2005.**

Weber, K.T. Aldosterone in congestive heart failure. *N. Engl. J. Med.,* **2001,** *345:*1689–1697.

ANTIARRHYTHMIC DRUGS

Dan M. Roden

Cardiac cells undergo depolarization and repolarization to form cardiac action potentials about sixty times per minute. The shape and duration of each action potential are determined by the activity of ion channel protein complexes in the membranes of individual cells, and the genes encoding most of these proteins now have been identified. Thus each heartbeat results from the highly integrated electrophysiological behavior of multiple proteins on multiple cardiac cells. Ion channel function can be perturbed by acute ischemia, sympathetic stimulation, or myocardial scarring to create abnormalities of cardiac rhythm, or arrhythmias. Available antiarrhythmic drugs suppress arrhythmias by blocking flow through specific ion channels or by altering autonomic function. An increasingly sophisticated understanding of the molecular basis of normal and abnormal cardiac rhythm may lead to identification of new targets for antiarrhythmic drugs and perhaps improved therapies.

Arrhythmias can range from incidental, asymptomatic clinical findings to life-threatening abnormalities. Mechanisms underlying cardiac arrhythmias have been identified in cellular and animal experiments. In some human arrhythmias, precise mechanisms are known, and treatment can be targeted specifically against those mechanisms. In other cases, mechanisms can be only inferred, and the choice of drugs is based largely on results of prior experience. Antiarrhythmic drug therapy can have two goals: termination of an ongoing arrhythmia or prevention of an arrhythmia. Unfortunately, antiarrhythmic drugs not only help to control arrhythmias but also can cause them, especially during long-term therapy. Thus, prescribing antiarrhythmic drugs requires that precipitating factors be excluded or minimized, that a precise diagnosis of the type of arrhythmia (and its possible mechanisms) be made, that the prescriber has reason to believe that drug therapy will be beneficial, and that the risks of drug therapy can be minimized.

PRINCIPLES OF CARDIAC ELECTROPHYSIOLOGY

The flow of ions across cell membranes generates the currents that make up cardiac action potentials. The factors that determine the magnitude of individual currents and their modulation by drugs can be explained at the cellular and molecular levels (Fozzard and Arnsdorf, 1991; Snyders *et al.*, 1991; Priori *et al.*, 1999). However, the action potential is a highly integrated entity: Changes in one current almost inevitably produce secondary changes in other currents. Most antiarrhythmic drugs affect more than one ion current, and many exert ancillary effects such as modification of cardiac contractility or autonomic nervous system function. Thus antiarrhythmic drugs usually exert multiple actions and can be beneficial or harmful in individual patients (Roden, 1994; Priori *et al.*, 1999).

The Cardiac Cell at Rest: A K+-Permeable Membrane

Ions move across cell membranes in response to electrical and concentration gradients, not through the lipid bilayer but through specific ion channels or transporters. The normal cardiac cell at rest maintains a transmembrane potential approximately 80 to 90 mV negative to the exterior; this gradient is established by pumps, especially the Na^+,K^+–ATPase, and fixed anionic charges within cells. There are both an electrical and a concentration gradient that would move Na^+ ions into resting cells (Figure 34–1). However, Na^+ channels, which allow Na^+ to move along this gradient, are closed at negative transmembrane potentials, so Na^+ does not enter normal resting cardiac cells. In contrast, a specific type of K^+ channel protein (the inward rectifier channel) is in an open conformation at negative potentials. Hence K^+ can move through these channels across the cell membrane at negative potentials in response to either electrical or concentration gradients (Figure 34–1). For each individual ion, there is an equilibrium potential E_x at which there is no net driving force for the ion to move across the membrane. E_x can be calculated using the Nernst equation:

$$E_x = -61 \log([x]_i / [x]_o) \qquad (34\text{--}1)$$

where $[x]_o$ is the extracellular concentration of the ion and $[x]_i$ is the intracellular concentration. For typical values for K^+, $[K]_o = 4$ mM and $[K]_i = 140$ mM, the calculated K^+ equilibrium potential E_K is –94 mV. There is thus no net force driving K^+ ions into or out of a cell when the transmembrane potential is –94 mV, which is close to the resting

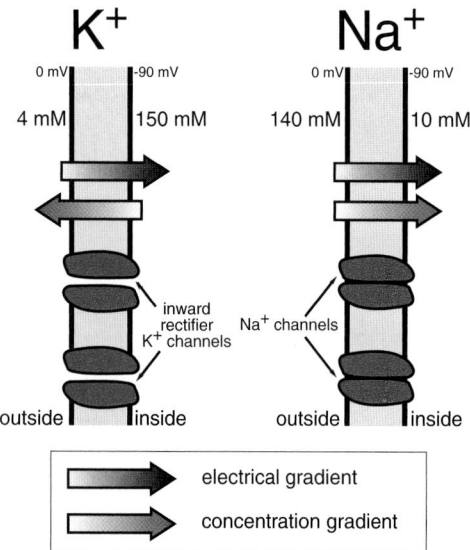

Figure 34–1. *Electrical and chemical gradients for K+ and for Na+ in a resting cardiac cell.* Inward rectifier K+ channels are open (*left*), allowing K+ ions to move across the membrane and the transmembrane potential to approach E_K. In contrast, Na+ does not enter the cell despite a large net driving force because Na+ channel proteins are in the closed conformation (*right*) in resting cells.

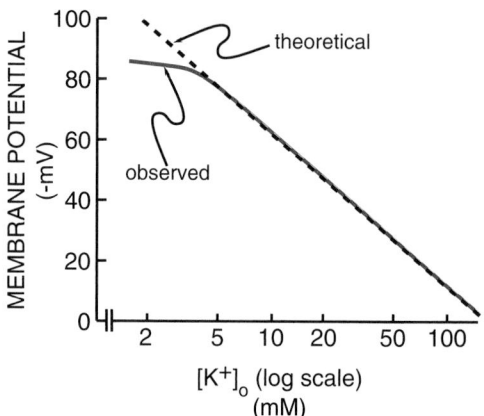

Figure 34–2. *The influence of extracellular K+ on theoretical E_K (dotted line) and on measured transmembrane potential (solid line).* At values of extracellular K+ of more than 4 mM, the two lines are identical, indicating that extracellular K+ is the major factor influencing resting potential.

potential. If $[K]_o$ is elevated to 10 mM, as might occur in diseases such as renal failure or myocardial ischemia, the calculated E_K rises to –70 mV. In this situation, there is excellent agreement between changes in theoretical E_K owing to changes in $[K]_o$ and the actual measured transmembrane potential (Figure 34–2), indicating that the normal cardiac cell at rest is permeable to K+ (because inward rectifier channels are open) and that $[K]_o$ is the major determinant of resting potential.

Na+ Channel Opening Initiates the Action Potential

If an atrial or ventricular cell at rest is depolarized above a threshold potential, Na+ channel proteins change conformation from the "closed" (resting) state to the "open" (conducting) state, allowing up to 10^7 Na+ ions per second to enter each cell and moving the transmembrane potential toward E_{Na} (+65 mV). This surge of Na+ ion movement lasts only about a millisecond, after which the Na+ channel protein rapidly changes conformation from the "open" state to an "inactivated," nonconducting state. Measuring Na+ current directly is technically demanding; the maximum upstroke slope of phase 0 (dV/dt_{max}, or V_{max}) of the action potential (Figure 34–3), which is proportional to Na+ current, is a convenient surrogate in some experimental settings. The traditional view is that Na+ channels, once inactivated, cannot reopen until they reassume the closed conformation. Electrophysiological techniques capable of measuring the behavior of individual ion channel proteins now are revealing some of the detailed mechanisms of these state transitions, and the findings obtained are changing some traditional views. For example, a small population of Na+ channels may continue to open during the action potential plateau in some cells (Figure 34–3). In fact, a defect in the structural region of the Na+ channel protein that has been implicated in control of channel inactivation causes one form of the congenital long QT syndrome, a disease associated with

abnormally long repolarization and serious arrhythmias (Roden and Spooner, 1999; Keating and Sanguinetti, 2001). In general, however, as the cell membrane repolarizes, the negative membrane potential moves Na+ channel proteins from inactivated to "closed" conformations. The relationship between Na+ channel availability and transmembrane potential is an important determinant of conduction and refractoriness in many cells, as discussed below.

The changes in transmembrane potential generated by the inward Na+ current produce, in turn, a series of openings (and in some cases subsequent inactivation) of other channels (Figure 34–3). For example, when a cell from the epicardium or the His–Purkinje conducting system is depolarized by the Na+ current, "transient outward" K+ channels change conformation to enter an open, or conducting, state; since the transmembrane potential at the end of phase 0 is positive to E_K, the opening of transient outward channels results in an outward, or repolarizing, K+ current (termed I_{TO}), which contributes to the phase 1 "notch" seen in action potentials from these tissues. Transient outward K+ channels, like Na+ channels, inactivate rapidly. During the phase 2 plateau of a normal cardiac action potential, inward, depolarizing currents, primarily through Ca^{2+} channels, are balanced by outward, repolarizing currents primarily through K+ ("delayed rectifier") channels. Delayed rectifier currents (collectively termed I_K) increase with time, whereas Ca^{2+} currents inactivate (and so decrease with time); as a result, cardiac cells repolarize (phase 3) several hundred milliseconds after the initial Na+ channel opening. Mutations in the genes encoding repolarizing K+ channels are responsible for the most common forms of the congenital long QT syndrome (Roden and Spooner, 1999; Keating and Sanguinetti, 2001). Identification of these specific channels has allowed more precise characterization of the pharmacological effects of antiarrhythmic drugs. A common mechanism whereby drugs prolong cardiac action potentials and provoke arrhythmias is inhibition of a specific delayed rectifier current, I_{Kr}, generated by expression of the *human ether-a-go-go related gene (HERG)*. The ion channel protein generated by *HERG* expression differs from other ion channels in important structural features that make it much more susceptible to drug block; understanding these structural constraints is an important first step to designing drugs lacking I_{Kr}-

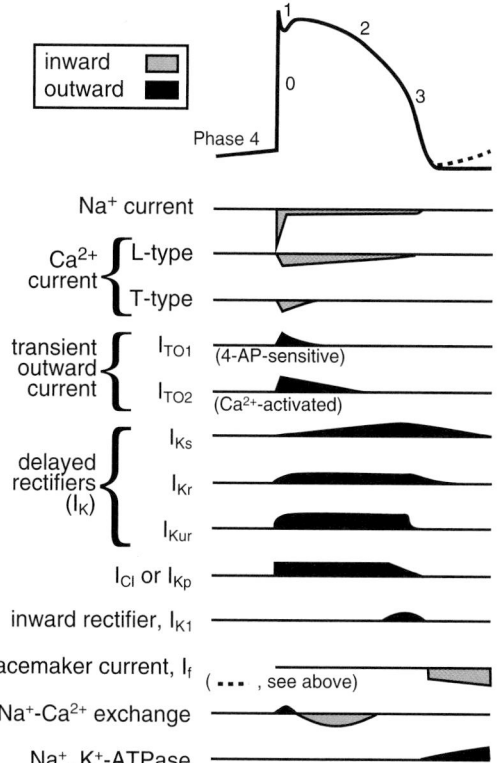

Figure 34–3. *The relationship between a hypothetical action potential from the conducting system and the time course of the currents that generate it.* The current magnitudes are not to scale; the Na$^+$ current is ordinarily 50 times larger than any other current, although the portion that persists into the plateau (phase 2) is small. Multiple types of Ca^{2+} current, transient outward current (I_{TO}), and delayed rectifier (I_K) have been identified. Each represents a different channel protein, usually associated with ancillary (function-modifying) subunits. 4-AP (4-aminopyridine) is a widely used *in vitro* blocker of K$^+$ channels. I_{TO2} may be a Cl$^-$ current in some species. Components of I_K have been separated on the basis of how rapidly they activate: slowly (I_{Ks}), rapidly (I_{Kr}), or ultrarapidly (I_{Kur}). The voltage-activated, time-independent current may be carried by Cl$^-$ (I_{Cl}) or K$^+$(I_{Kp}, *p* for plateau). For all currents shown here (with the possible exception of I_{TO2}), the genes encoding the major pore-forming proteins have been cloned. (Adapted from Task Force of the Working Group on Arrhythmias of the European Society of Cardiology, 1991, with permission.)

blocking properties (Mitcheson *et al.*, 2000). Avoiding I_{Kr}/*HERG* channel block has become a major issue in the development of new antiarrhythmic drugs (Roden, 2004).

Differing Action Potential Behaviors Among Cardiac Cells

This general description of the action potential and the currents that underlie it must be modified for certain cell types (Figure 34–4) pre-

sumably because of variability in the ion channel proteins expressed in individual cells. Endocardial ventricular cells lack a prominent transient outward current, whereas cells from the subendocardial His–Purkinje conducting system (and in some species from the midmyocardium) have very long action potentials (Antzelevitch *et al.*, 1991). Atrial cells have very short action potentials probably because I_{TO} is larger, and an additional repolarizing K$^+$ current, activated by the neurotransmitter acetylcholine, is present. As a result, vagal stimulation further shortens atrial action potentials. Cells of the sinus and atrioventricular (AV) nodes lack substantial Na$^+$ currents. In addition, these cells, as well as cells from the conducting system, normally display the phenomenon of spontaneous diastolic, or phase 4, depolarization and thus spontaneously reach threshold for regeneration of action potentials. The rate of spontaneous firing usually is fastest in sinus node cells, which therefore serve as the natural pacemaker of the heart. Specialized K$^+$ channels underlie the pacemaker current in the heart.

Modern molecular biological and electrophysiological techniques, by which the behavior of single ion channel proteins in an isolated patch of membrane can be studied, have refined the description of ion channels important for the normal functioning of cardiac cells and have identified channels that may be particularly important under pathological conditions. For example, we now know that transient outward and delayed rectifier currents actually result from multiple ion channel subtypes (Tseng and Hoffman, 1989; Sanguinetti and Jurkiewicz, 1990) (Figure 34–3) and that acetylcholine-evoked hyperpolarization results from activation of a K$^+$ channel formed by hetero-oligomerization of multiple, distinct channel proteins (Krapivinsky *et al.*, 1995).

The understanding that molecularly diverse entities subserve regulation of the cardiac action potential is important because drugs may target one channel subtype selectively. Furthermore, ancillary function-modifying proteins (the products of diverse genes) have been identified for most ion channels. In addition to the usual (L-type) Ca^{2+} channels, a second type of Ca^{2+} channel that is most prominent at relatively negative potentials, the T-type, has been identified in some cardiac cells (Bean, 1985). The T-type Ca^{2+} channel may be important in diseases such as hypertension and may play a role in pacemaker activity in some cells. A T-type-selective antihypertensive agent, *mibefradil,* was available briefly in the late 1990s but was withdrawn because it was involved in many serious, undesirable drug–drug interactions. Molecular cloning also has identified multiple isoforms, derived from separate genes, that underlie the L-type calcium channel. Specific channels that transport Cl$^-$ ions and result in repolarizing currents (I_{Cl}) have been identified in many species (Hume and Harvey, 1991); some of these are observed only under pathophysiological conditions. Some K$^+$ channels are quiescent when intracellular adenosine triphosphate (ATP) stores are normal and become active when these stores are depleted. Such ATP-inhibited K$^+$ channels may become particularly important in repolarizing cells during states of metabolic stress such as myocardial ischemia (Weiss *et al.*, 1991).

Maintenance of Intracellular Homeostasis

With each action potential, the cell interior gains Na$^+$ ions and loses K$^+$ ions. An ATP-requiring Na$^+$–K$^+$ exchange mechanism, or pump, is activated in most cells to maintain intracellular homeostasis. This Na$^+$,K$^+$–ATPase extrudes three Na$^+$ ions for every two K$^+$ ions shuttled from the exterior of the cell to the interior; as a result, the act of pumping itself generates a net outward (repolarizing) current.

Normally, intracellular Ca^{2+} is maintained at very low levels (<100 nM). In cardiac myocytes, the entry of Ca^{2+} during each

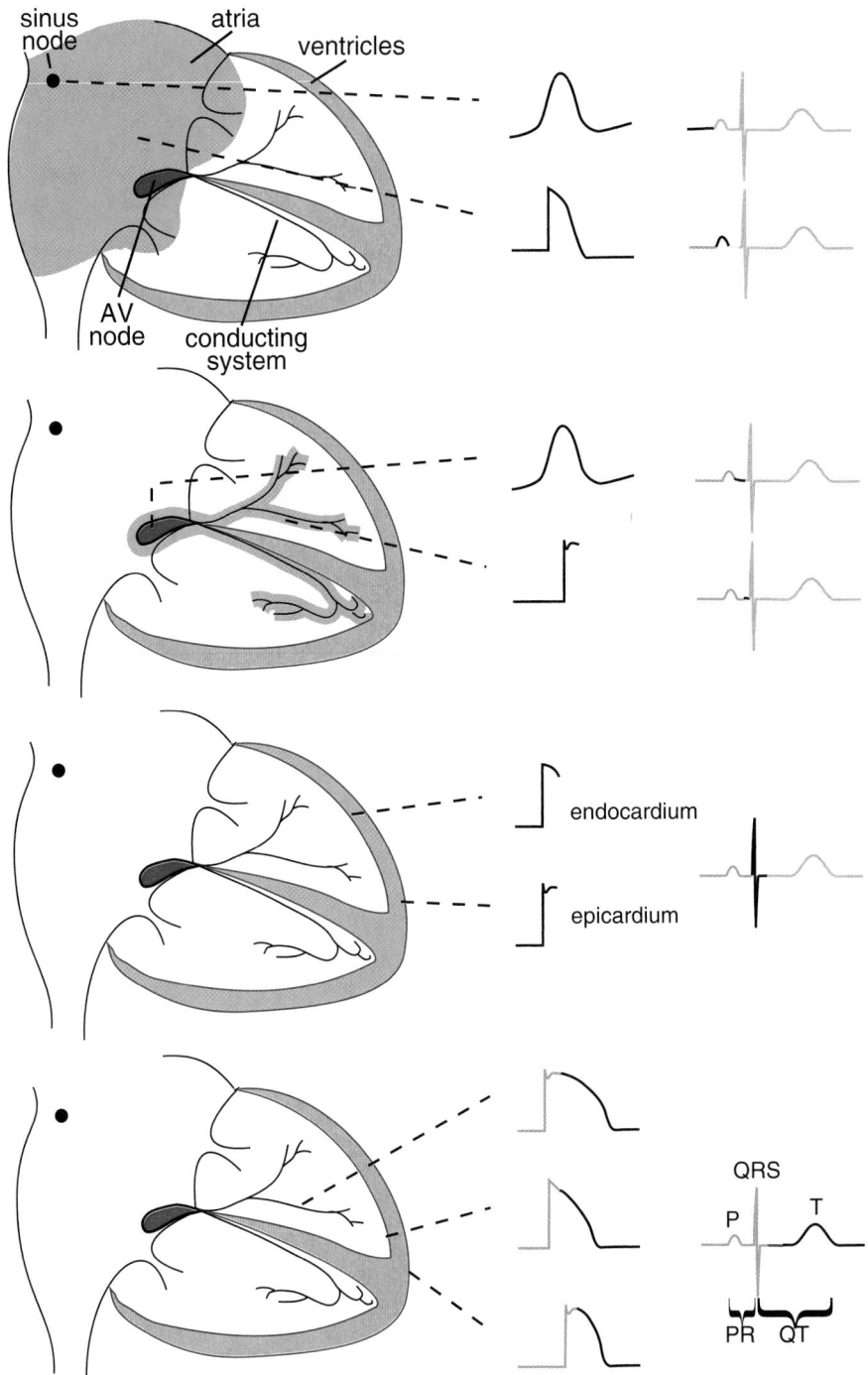

Figure 34–4. ***Normal impulse propagation.*** Action potentials from different regions of the heart are shown. In each panel, tissue that is depolarized is shown in light blue, and the portion of the electrocardiogram to which it contributes is shown in black.

action potential is a signal to the sarcoplasmic reticulum to release its Ca^{2+} stores. The resulting increase in intracellular Ca^{2+} then triggers Ca^{2+}-dependent contractile processes. Removal of intracellular Ca^{2+} occurs by both an ATP-dependent Ca^{2+} pump (which moves Ca^{2+} ions back to storage sites in the sarcoplasmic reticulum) and an electrogenic Na^+–Ca^{2+} exchange mechanism on the cell surface, which exchanges three Na^+ ions from the exterior for each Ca^{2+} ion extruded. Abnormal regulation of intracellular calcium, characterized by contractile dysfunction, is increasingly well described in heart failure and also may contribute to arrhythmias in this setting

(Pogwizd and Bers, 2004). The initial rise in Ca^{2+}, which serves as the trigger for Ca^{2+} release from intracellular stores, results from the opening of Ca^{2+} channels in the cell membrane or from Ca^{2+} entry through Na^+–Ca^{2+} exchange; *i.e.*, in response to phase 0 entry of Na^+, the Na^+–Ca^{2+} exchange protein may transiently extrude Na^+ ions in exchange for Ca^{2+} ions (Figure 34–3).

Impulse Propagation and the Electrocardiogram

Normal cardiac impulses originate in the sinus node. Impulse propagation in the heart depends on two factors: the magnitude of the depolarizing current (usually Na^+ current) and the geometry of cell–cell electrical connections. Cardiac cells are relatively long and thin and well coupled through specialized gap junction proteins at their ends, whereas lateral ("transverse") gap junctions are sparser. As a result, impulses spread along cells two to three times faster than across cells. This "anisotropic" (direction-dependent) conduction may be a factor in the genesis of certain arrhythmias described below (Priori *et al.*, 1999). Once impulses leave the sinus node, they propagate rapidly throughout the atria, resulting in atrial systole and the P wave of the surface electrocardiogram (ECG; Figure 34–4). Propagation slows markedly through the AV node, where the inward current (through Ca^{2+} channels) is much smaller than the Na^+ current in atria, ventricles, or the subendocardial conducting system. This conduction delay allows the atrial contraction to propel blood into the ventricle, thereby optimizing cardiac output. Once impulses exit the AV node, they enter the conducting system, where Na^+ currents are larger than in any other tissue. Hence propagation is correspondingly faster, up to 0.75 m/s longitudinally, and manifests as the QRS complex on the ECG as impulses spread from the endocardium to the epicardium, stimulating coordinated ventricular contraction. Ventricular repolarization results in the T wave of the ECG.

The ECG can be used as a rough guide to some cellular properties of cardiac tissue (Figure 34–4): (1) Heart rate reflects sinus node automaticity, (2) PR-interval duration reflects AV nodal conduction time, (3) QRS duration reflects conduction time in the ventricle, and (4) the QT interval is a measure of ventricular action potential duration.

Refractoriness: Fast-Response versus Slow-Response Tissue

If a single action potential, such as that shown in Figure 34–3, is restimulated very early during the plateau, no Na^+ channels are available to open, so no inward current results, and no action potential is generated: The cell is refractory. On the other hand, if a stimulus occurs after the cell has repolarized completely, Na^+ channels have recovered from inactivation, and a normal Na^+ channel–dependent upstroke results (Figure 34–5A). When a stimulus occurs during phase 3 of the action potential, the magnitude of the resultant Na^+ current depends on the number of Na^+ channels that have recovered from inactivation (Figure 34–5A), which, in turn, depends on the voltage at which the extra stimulus was applied. Thus, in atrial, ventricular, and His–Purkinje cells ("fast-response cells"), refractoriness is determined by the voltage-dependent recovery of Na^+ channels from inactivation. Refractoriness frequently is measured by assessing whether premature stimuli applied to tissue preparations (or the whole heart) result in propagated impulses. While the magnitude of the Na^+ current is one major determinant of such propagation, cellular geometry also is important in multicellular preparations. Ordinarily, each cell is connected to many neighbors so that impulses spread rapidly, and the heart acts like a single large cell, *i.e.*, a syncytium. However, if the

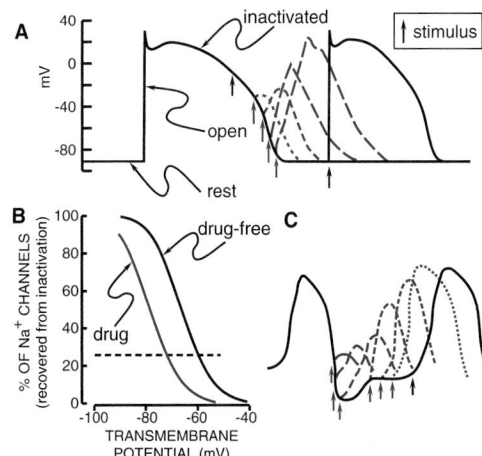

Figure 34–5. *Qualitative differences in responses of fast- and slow-response tissues to premature stimuli.* **A.** With a very early premature stimulus (*black arrow*) in fast-response tissue, all Na^+ channels still are in the inactivated state, and no upstroke results. As the action potential repolarizes, Na^+ channels recover from the inactivated to the resting state, from which opening can occur. The phase 0 upstroke slope of the premature action potentials (*blue*) are greater with later stimuli because recovery from inactivation is voltage-dependent. **B.** The relationship between transmembrane potential and degree of recovery of Na^+ channels from inactivation. The dotted line indicates 25% recovery. Most Na^+ channel–blocking drugs shift this relationship to the left. **C.** In slow-response tissues, premature stimuli delivered even after full repolarization of the action potential are depressed; recovery from inactivation is time-dependent.

geometric arrangement is such that a single cell must supply depolarizing current to many neighbors, conduction can fail. The *effective refractory period* (ERP) is the shortest interval at which a premature stimulus results in a propagated response and often is used to describe drug effects in intact tissue.

The situation is different in Ca^{2+} channel–dependent ("slow-response") tissue such as the AV node. The major factor controlling recovery from inactivation of Ca^{2+} channels is time (Figure 34–5C). Thus, even after a Ca^{2+} channel–dependent action potential has repolarized to its initial resting potential, not all Ca^{2+} channels are available for re-excitation. Therefore, an extra stimulus applied shortly after repolarization is complete generates a reduced Ca^{2+} current, which may propagate slowly to adjacent cells prior to extinction. An extra stimulus applied later will result in a larger Ca^{2+} current and faster propagation. Thus, in Ca^{2+} channel–dependent tissues, which include not only the AV node but also tissues whose underlying characteristics have been altered by factors such as myocardial ischemia, refractoriness is time-dependent, and propagation occurs slowly. Conduction that exhibits such dependence on the timing of premature stimuli is termed *decremental*. By contrast, conduction velocity in fast-response tissues is independent of prematurity until a stimulus shorter than the effective refractory period is applied, when it fails completely ("all-or-none response"). Slow conduction in the heart, a critical factor in the genesis of re-entrant arrhythmias (*see* below), also can occur when Na^+ currents are depressed by disease or membrane depolarization (*e.g.,* elevated [K]ₒ), resulting in decreased steady-state Na⁺ channel availability (Figure 34–5B).

MECHANISMS OF CARDIAC ARRHYTHMIAS

When the normal sequence of impulse initiation and propagation is perturbed, an arrhythmia occurs. Failure of impulse initiation may result in slow heart rates (bradyarrhythmias), whereas failure of impulses to propagate normally from atrium to ventricle results in dropped beats or "heart block" that usually reflects an abnormality in either the AV node or the His–Purkinje system. These abnormalities may be caused by drugs (Table 34–1) or by structural heart disease; in the latter case, permanent cardiac pacing may be required.

Abnormally rapid heart rhythms (tachyarrhythmias) are common clinical problems that may be treated with antiarrhythmic drugs. Three major underlying mechanisms have been identified: enhanced automaticity, triggered automaticity, and re-entry.

Enhanced Automaticity

Enhanced automaticity may occur in cells that normally display spontaneous diastolic depolarization—the sinus and AV nodes and the His–Purkinje system. β Adrenergic stimulation, hypokalemia, and mechanical stretch of cardiac muscle cells increase phase 4 slope and so accelerate pacemaker rate, whereas *acetylcholine* reduces pacemaker rate both by decreasing phase 4 slope and by hyperpolarization (making the maximum diastolic potential more negative). In addition, automatic behavior may occur in sites that ordinarily lack spontaneous pacemaker activity; *e.g.,* depolarization of ventricular cells (*e.g.,* by ischemia) may produce such "abnormal" automaticity. When impulses propagate from a region of enhanced normal or abnormal automaticity to excite the rest of the heart, arrhythmias result.

Afterdepolarizations and Triggered Automaticity

Under some pathophysiological conditions, a normal cardiac action potential may be interrupted or followed by an abnormal depolarization (Figure 34–6). If this abnormal depolarization reaches threshold, it may, in turn, give rise to secondary upstrokes that can propagate and create abnormal rhythms. These abnormal secondary upstrokes occur only after an initial normal, or "triggering," upstroke and so are termed *triggered rhythms.*

Two major forms of triggered rhythms are recognized. In the first case, under conditions of intracellular Ca²⁺ overload (*e.g.,* myocardial ischemia, adrenergic stress, digitalis intoxication, or heart failure), a normal action potential may be followed by a *delayed afterdepolarization* (DAD; Figure 34–6A). If this afterdepolarization reaches threshold, a secondary triggered beat or beats may occur. DAD amplitude is increased *in vitro* by rapid pacing, and clinical arrhythmias thought to correspond to DAD-mediated triggered beats are more frequent when the underlying cardiac rate is rapid (Priori *et al.*, 1999). In the second type of triggered activity, the key abnormality is marked prolongation of the cardiac action potential. When this occurs, phase 3 repolarization may be interrupted by an *early afterdepolarization* (EAD; Figure 34–6B). EAD-mediated triggering *in vitro* and clinical arrhythmias are most common when the underlying heart rate is slow, extracellular K⁺ is low, and certain drugs that prolong action potential duration (antiarrhythmics and others) are present. EAD-related triggered upstrokes probably reflect inward current through Na⁺ or Ca²⁺ channels. EADs are

induced much more readily in Purkinje cells and in midmyocardial (or M) cells than in epicardial or endocardial cells. When cardiac repolarization is markedly prolonged, polymorphic ventricular tachycardia with a long QT interval, known as the *torsades de pointes* syndrome, may occur. This arrhythmia is thought to be caused by EADs, which trigger functional re-entry (discussed below) owing to heterogeneity of action potential durations across the ventricular wall (Priori *et al.*, 1999). Congenital long QT syndrome, a disease in which *torsades de pointes* is common, can be caused by mutations in the genes encoding the Na⁺ channels or the channels underlying the repolarizing currents I_{Kr} and I_{Ks} (Roden and Spooner, 1999).

Re-entry

Anatomically Defined Re-entry. Re-entry can occur when impulses propagate by more than one pathway between two points in the heart, and those pathways have heterogeneous electrophysiological properties. Patients with Wolff–Parkinson–White (WPW) syndrome have accessory connections between the atrium and ventricle (Figure 34–7). With each sinus node depolarization, impulses can excite the ventricle *via* the normal structures (AV node) or the accessory pathway. However, the electrophysiological properties of the AV node and accessory pathways are different: Accessory pathways usually consist of fast-response tissue, whereas the AV node is composed of slow-response tissue. Thus, with a premature atrial beat, conduction may fail in the accessory pathway but continue, albeit slowly, in the AV node and then through the His–Purkinje system; there the propagating impulse may encounter the ventricular end of the accessory pathway when it is no longer refractory. The likelihood that the accessory pathway is no longer refractory increases as AV nodal conduction slows. When the impulse re-enters the atrium, it then can re-enter the ventricle *via* the AV node, re-enter the atrium *via* the accessory pathway, and so on (Figure 34–7). Re-entry of this type, referred to as *AV re-entrant tachycardia,* is determined by (1) the presence of an anatomically defined circuit, (2) heterogeneity in refractoriness among regions in the circuit, and (3) slow conduction in one part of the circuit. Similar "anatomically defined" re-entry commonly occurs in the region of the AV node (*AV nodal re-entrant tachycardia*) and in the atrium (*atrial flutter*). The term *paroxysmal supraventricular tachycardia* (PSVT) includes both AV re-entry and AV nodal re-entry, which share many clinical features. In some cases, it now is possible to identify and ablate critical portions of re-entrant pathways (or automatic foci), thus curing the patient and obviating the need for long-term drug therapy. Radiofrequency ablation is carried out through a catheter advanced to the interior of the heart and requires minimal convalescence.

Functionally Defined Re-entry. Re-entry also may occur in the absence of a distinct, anatomically defined pathway (Figure 34–8). For example, alterations in cell–cell coupling following acute myocardial infarction in dogs result in re-entrant ventricular tachycardia (VT) whose circuit depends not only on postinfarction scarring but also on the rapid longitudinal and slow transverse conduction properties of cardiac tissue (Wit *et al.*, 1990). If ischemia or other electrophysiological perturbations result in an area of sufficiently slow conduction in the ventricle, impulses exiting from that area may find the rest of the myocardium re-excitable, in which case fibrillation may ensue. Atrial or ventricular fibrillation is an extreme example of "functionally defined" (or "leading circle") re-entry: Cells are re-excited as soon as they are repolarized sufficiently to allow enough Na⁺ channels to recover from inactivation. In this

Table 34–1
Drug-Induced Cardiac Arrhythmias

ARRHYTHMIA	DRUG	LIKELY MECHANISM	TREATMENT*	CLINICAL FEATURES
Sinus bradycardia AV block	Digoxin	↑Vagal tone	Antidigoxin antibodies Temporary pacing	Atrial tachycardia may also be present
Sinus bradycardia AV block	Verapamil Diltiazem	Ca^{2+} channel block	Ca^{2+} Temporary pacing	
Sinus bradycardia AV block	β-Blockers Clonidine Methyldopa	Sympatholytic	Isoproterenol Temporary pacing	
Sinus tachycardia Any other tachycardia	β-Blocker withdrawal	Upregulation of β-receptors with chronic therapy; more receptors available for agonist after withdrawal of blocker	β-Blockade	Hypertension, angina also possible
↑ Ventricular rate in atrial flutter	Quinidine Flecainide Propafenone	Conduction slowing in atrium, with enhanced (quinidine) or unaltered AV conduction	AV nodal blockers	QRS complexes often widened at fast rates
↑ Ventricular rate in atrial fibrillation in patients with WPW syndrome	Digoxin Verapamil	↓ accessory pathway refractoriness	IV procainamide DC cardioversion	Ventricular rate can exceed 300/min
Multifocal atrial tachycardia	Theophylline	?↑ Intracellular Ca^{2+} and DADs	Withdraw theophylline ?Verapamil	Often in advanced lung disease
Polymorphic VT with ↑ QT interval (*torsades de pointes*)	Quinidine Sotalol Procainamide Disopyramide Dofetilide Ibutilide "Noncardioactive" drugs (*see* text) Amiodarone (rare)	EAD-related triggered activity	Cardiac pacing Isoproterenol Magnesium	Hypokalemia, bradycardia frequent Related to ↑ plasma concentrations, except for quinidine
Frequent or difficult to terminate VT ("incessant" VT)	Flecainide Propafenone Quinidine (rarer)	Conduction slowing in reentrant circuits	Na^+ bolus reported effective in some cases	Most often in patients with advanced myocardial scarring
Atrial tachycardia with AV block; ventricular bigeminy and others	Digoxin	DAD-related triggered activity (±↑ vagal tone)	Antidigoxin antibodies	Coexistence of abnormal impulses with abnormal sinus or AV nodal function
Ventricular fibrillation	Inappropriate use of IV verapamil	Severe hypotension and/or myocardial ischemia	Cardiac resuscitation (DC cardioversion)	Misdiagnosis of VT as PSVT → inappropriate use of verapamil

*In each of these cases, recognition and withdrawal of the offending drug(s) are mandatory.

ABBREVIATIONS: AV, atrioventricular; DAD, delayed afterdepolarization; DC, direct current; EAD, early afterdepolarization; WPW, Wolff–Parkinson–supraventricular tachycardia; IV, intravenous; ↑, increase; ↓, decrease; ?, unclear.

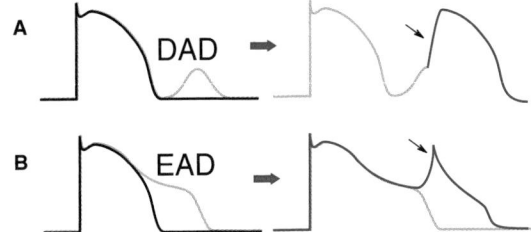

Figure 34–6. *Afterdepolarizations and triggered activity.* **A.** Delayed afterdepolarization (DAD) arising after full repolarization. A DAD that reaches threshold results in a triggered upstroke (*black arrow, right*). **B.** Early afterdepolarization (EAD) interrupting phase 3 repolarization. Under some conditions, triggered beat(s) can arise from an EAD (*black arrow, right*).

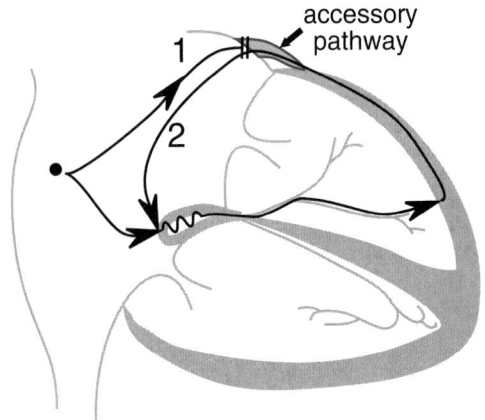

Figure 34–7. *Atrioventricular re-entrant tachycardia in the Wolff–Parkinson–White syndrome.* In these patients, an accessory atrioventricular connection is present (*light blue*). A premature atrial impulse blocks in the accessory pathway (1) and propagates slowly through the AV node and conducting system. On reaching the accessory pathway (by now no longer refractory), the impulse re-enters the atrium (2), where it then can re-enter the ventricle *via* the AV node and become self-sustaining (*see* Figure 34–9C). AV nodal blocking drugs readily terminate this tachycardia. Recurrences can be prevented by drugs that prevent atrial premature beats, by drugs that alter the electrophysiological characteristics of tissue in the circuit (*e.g.,* they prolong AV nodal refractoriness), and by nonpharmacological techniques that section the accessory pathway.

setting, neither organized activation patterns nor coordinated contractile activity is present.

Common Arrhythmias and Their Mechanisms

The primary tool for diagnosis of arrhythmias is the ECG, although more sophisticated approaches sometimes are used, such as recording from specific regions of the heart during artificial induction of arrhythmias by specialized pacing techniques. Table 34–2 lists common

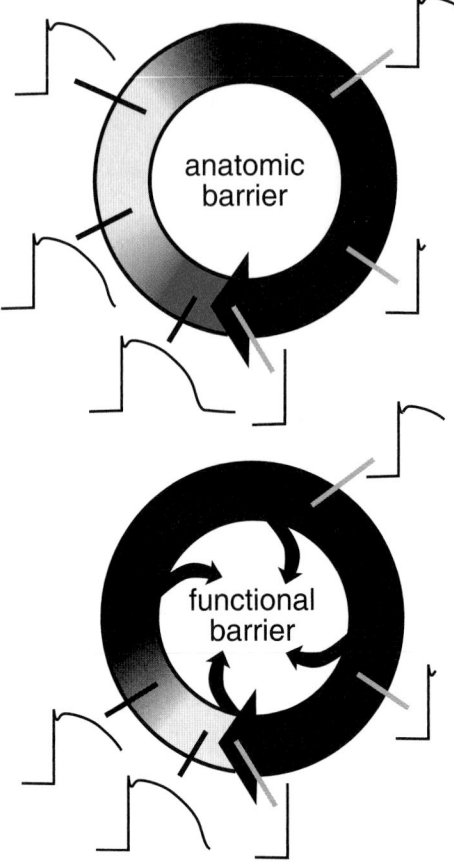

Figure 34–8. *Two types of re-entry.* The border of a propagating wavefront is denoted by a heavy black arrowhead. In anatomically defined re-entry (*top*), a fixed pathway is present (*e.g.,* Figure 34–7). The black area denotes tissue in the re-entrant circuit that is completely refractory because of the recent passage of the propagating wavefront; the gray area denotes tissue in which depressed upstrokes can be elicited (*see* Figure 34–5A), and the dark blue area represents tissue in which restimulation would result in action potentials with normal upstrokes. The dark blue area is termed an *excitable gap.* In functionally defined, or "leading circle," re-entry (*bottom*), there is no anatomic pathway and no excitable gap. Rather, the circulating wavefront creates an area of inexcitable tissue at its core. In this type of re-entry, the circuit does not necessarily remain in the same anatomic position during consecutive beats, and multiple such "rotors" may be present.

arrhythmias, their likely mechanisms, and approaches that should be considered for their acute termination and for long-term therapy to prevent recurrence. Examples of some arrhythmias discussed here are shown in Figure 34–9. Some arrhythmias, notably ventricular fibrillation (VF), are best treated not with drugs but with direct current (dc) cardioversion—the application of a large electric current across the chest. This technique also can be used to immediately restore normal rhythm in less serious cases; if the patient is conscious, a brief period of general anesthesia is required. Implantable cardioverter–defibrilla-

Table 34–2
A Mechanistic Approach to Antiarrhythmic Therapy

ARRHYTHMIA	COMMON MECHANISM	ACUTE THERAPY[a]	CHRONIC THERAPY[a]
Premature atrial, nodal, or ventricular depolarizations	Unknown	None indicated	None indicated
Atrial fibrillation	Disorganized "functional" reentry Continual AV node stimulation → irregular, often rapid, ventricular rate	1. Control ventricular response: AV nodal block[b] 2. Restore sinus rhythm: DC cardioversion	1. Control ventricular response: AV nodal block[b] 2. Maintain normal rhythm: K^+ channel block Na^+ channel block with $\tau_{recovery} > 1$ second
Atrial flutter	Stable reentrant circuit in the right atrium Ventricular rate often rapid and irregular	Same as atrial fibrillation	Same as atrial fibrillation AV nodal blocking drugs especially desirable to avoid ↑ ventricular rate Ablation in selected cases[c]
Atrial tachycardia	Enhanced automaticity, DAD-related automaticity, or reentry within the atrium	Same as atrial fibrillation	Same as atrial fibrillation Ablation of tachycardia "focus"[c]
AV nodal reentrant tachycardia (PSVT)	Reentrant circuit within or near AV node	*Adenosine AV nodal block Less commonly: ↑ vagal tone (digitalis, edrophonium, phenylephrine)	*AV nodal block Flecainide Propafenone *Ablation[c]
Arrhythmias associated with WPW syndrome:			
1. AV reentry (PSVT)	Reentry (Figure 34–7)	Same as AV nodal reentry	K^+ channel block Na^+ channel block with $\tau_{recovery} > 1$ second Ablation[c]
2. Atrial fibrillation with atrioventricular conduction *via* accessory pathway	Very rapid rate due to nondecremental properties of accessory pathway	*DC cardioversion *Procainamide	Ablation[c] K^+ channel block Na^+ channel block with $\tau_{recovery} > 1$ second (AV nodal blockers can be harmful)
VT in patients with remote myocardial infarction	Reentry near the rim of the healed myocardial infarction	Lidocaine Amiodarone Procainamide DC cardioversion	*ICD[d] *Amiodarone K^+ channel block Na^+ channel block
VT in patients without structural heart disease	DADs triggered by ↑ sympathetic tone	Adenosine[e] Verapamil[e] β-Blockers[e] DC cardioversion	Verapamil[e] β-Blockers[e]

(Continued)

Table 34–2
A Mechanistic Approach to Antiarrhythmic Therapy (Continued)

ARRHYTHMIA	COMMON MECHANISM	ACUTE THERAPY[a]	CHRONIC THERAPY[a]
VF	Disorganized reentry	*DC cardioversion Lidocaine Amiodarone Procainamide	*ICD[d] *Amiodarone K^+ channel block Na^+ channel block
Torsades de pointes, congenital or acquired; (often drug-related)	EAD-related triggered activity	Pacing Magnesium Isoproterenol	β-Blockade Pacing

*Indicates treatment of choice. [a]Acute drug therapy is administered intravenously; chronic therapy implies long-term oral use. [b]AV nodal block can be achieved clinically by adenosine, Ca^{2+} channel block, β adrenergic receptor blockade, or increased vagal tone (a major antiarrhythmic effect of digitalis glycosides). [c]Ablation is a procedure in which tissue responsible for the maintenance of a tachycardia is identified by specialized recording techniques and then selectively destroyed, usually by high-frequency radio waves delivered through a catheter placed in the heart. [d]ICD, implanted cardioverter/defibrillator. A device that can sense VT or VF and deliver pacing and/or cardioverting shocks to restore normal rhythm. [e]These may be harmful in reentrant VT and so should be used for acute therapy only if the diagnosis is secure.

ABBREVIATIONS: DAD, delayed afterdepolarization; EAD, early afterdepolarization; WPW, Wolff–Parkinson–White; PSVT, paroxysmal supraventricular tachycardia; VT, ventricular tachycardia; VF, ventricular fibrillation.

tors (ICDs), devices that are capable of detecting VF and automatically delivering a defibrillating shock, are used increasingly in patients judged to be at high risk for VF. Often drugs are used with these devices if defibrillating shocks, which are painful, occur frequently.

MECHANISMS OF ANTIARRHYTHMIC DRUG ACTION

Drug effects that may be antiarrhythmic can be demonstrated *in vitro* or in animal models, but the relationship between the multiple effects that drugs produce in patients and their effects on arrhythmias can be complex. A single arrhythmia may result from multiple mechanisms. Drugs may be antiarrhythmic by suppressing the initiating mechanism or by altering the re-entrant circuit. In some cases, drugs may suppress the initiator but nonetheless promote re-entry (*see* below).

Drugs may slow automatic rhythms by altering any of the four determinants of spontaneous pacemaker discharge (Figure 34–10): increase maximum diastolic potential, decrease phase 4 slope, threshold potential, or increase action potential duration. *Adenosine* and acetylcholine may increase maximum diastolic potential, and *β adrenergic receptor antagonists* (*β-blockers; see* Chapter 10) may decrease phase 4 slope. Block of Na^+ or Ca^{2+} channels usually results in altered threshold, and block of cardiac K^+ channels prolongs the action potential.

Antiarrhythmic drugs may block arrhythmias owing to DADs or EADs by two major mechanisms: (1) inhibition of the development of afterdepolarizations, and (2) interference with the inward current (usually through Na^+ or Ca^{2+} channels), which is responsible for the upstroke. Thus arrhythmias owing to *digitalis*-induced DADs may be inhibited by *verapamil* (which blocks the development of DAD) or by *quinidine* (which blocks Na^+ channels, thereby elevating the threshold required to produce the abnormal upstroke). Similarly, two approaches are used in arrhythmias related to EAD-induced triggered beats (Tables 34–1 and 34–2). EADs can be inhibited by shortening action potential duration; in practice, heart rate is accelerated by *isoproterenol* infusion or by pacing. Triggered beats arising from EADs can be inhibited by Mg^{2+}, without normalizing repolarization *in vitro* or QT interval, through mechanisms that are not well understood. In patients with a congenitally prolonged QT interval, *torsades de pointes* often occurs with adrenergic stress; therapy includes *β* adrenergic blockade (which does not shorten the QT interval) as well as pacing.

In anatomically determined re-entry, drugs may terminate the arrhythmia by blocking propagation of the action potential. Conduction usually fails in a "weak link" in the circuit. In the example of the WPW-related arrhythmia described earlier, the weak link is the AV node, and drugs that prolong AV nodal refractoriness and slow AV nodal conduction, such as Ca^{2+} channel blockers, *β* adrenergic

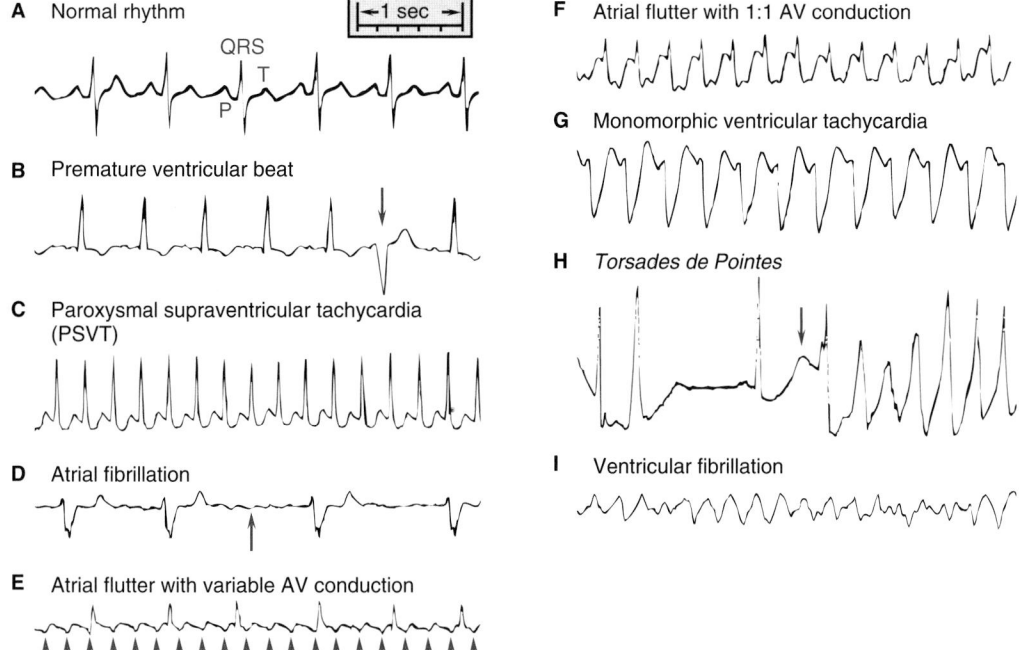

Figure 34–9. *ECGs showing normal and abnormal cardiac rhythms.* The P, QRS, and T waves in normal sinus rhythm are shown in panel *A*. Panel *B* shows a premature beat arising in the ventricle (*arrow*). Paroxysmal supraventricular tachycardia (PSVT) is shown in panel *C*; this is most likely re-entry using an accessory pathway (*see* Figure 34–7) or re-entry within or near the AV node. In atrial fibrillation (panel *D*), there are no P waves, and the QRS complexes occur irregularly (and at a slow rate in this example); electrical activity between QRS complexes shows small undulations (*arrow*) corresponding to fibrillatory activity in the atria. In atrial flutter (panel *E*), the atria beat rapidly, approximately 250 beats per minute (*arrows*) in this example, and the ventricular rate is variable. If a drug that slows the rate of atrial flutter is administered, 1:1 atrioventricular conduction (panel *F*) can occur. In monomorphic ventricular tachycardia (VT, panel *G*), identical wide QRS complexes occur at a regular rate, 180 beats per minute. The electrocardiographic features of the *torsades de pointes* syndrome (panel *H*) include a very long QT interval (>600 ms in this example, *arrow*), and ventricular tachycardia in which each successive beat has a different morphology (polymorphic VT). Panel *I* shows the disorganized electrical activity characteristic of ventricular fibrillation.

receptor antagonists, or digitalis glycosides, are likely to be effective. On the other hand, slowing conduction in functionally determined re-entrant circuits may change the pathway without extinguishing the circuit. In fact, slow conduction generally promotes the development of re-entrant arrhythmias, whereas the most likely approach for terminating functionally determined re-entry is prolongation of refractoriness (Task Force, 1991). In fast-response tissues, refractoriness is prolonged by delaying the recovery of Na⁺ channels from inactivation. Drugs that act by blocking Na⁺ channels generally shift the voltage dependence of recovery from block (Figure 34–5B) and so prolong refractoriness (Figure 34–11).

Drugs that increase action potential duration without direct action on Na⁺ channels (*e.g.*, by blocking delayed rectifier currents) also will prolong refractoriness (Singh,

1993) (Figure 34–11). In slow-response tissues, Ca²⁺ channel block prolongs refractoriness. Drugs that interfere with cell–cell coupling also theoretically should increase refractoriness in multicellular preparations; *amiodarone* may exert this effect in diseased tissue (Levine *et al.*, 1988). Acceleration of conduction in an area of slow conduction also could inhibit re-entry; *lidocaine* may exert such an effect, and peptides that suppress experimental arrhythmias by increasing gap junction conductance have been described.

State-Dependent Ion Channel Block

Mathematical models describing drug–channel interactions have been useful in understanding conditions under which drugs do or do not suppress arrhythmias. A

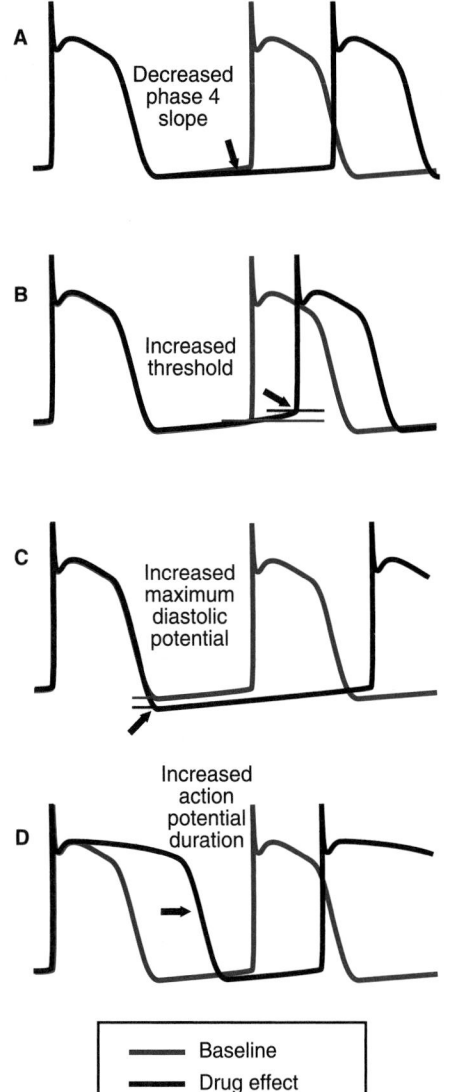

Figure 34–10. *Four ways to reduce the rate of spontaneous discharge in automatic tissues.* The thin horizontal line represents threshold potential.

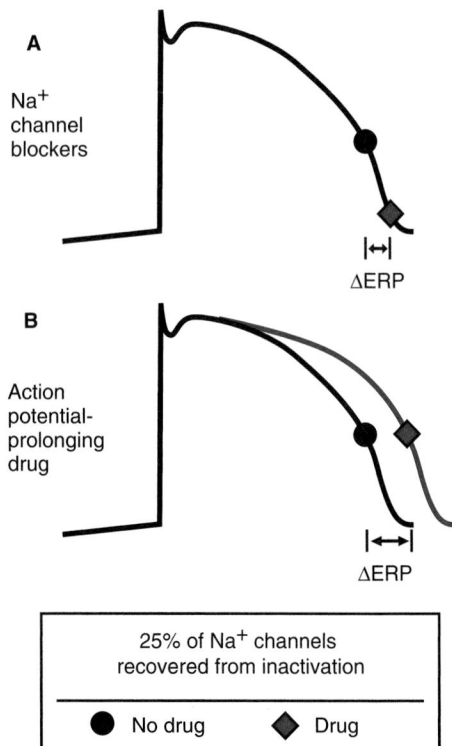

Figure 34–11. *Two ways to increase refractoriness in fast-response cells.* In this figure, the black dot indicates the point at which a sufficient number of Na$^+$ channels (an arbitrary 25%; *see* Figure 34–5B) have recovered from inactivation to allow a premature stimulus to produce a propagated response in the absence of a drug. Block of Na$^+$ channels (*A*) shifts voltage dependence of recovery (*see* Figure 34–5B) and so delays the point at which 25% of channels have recovered (*blue diamond*), prolonging refractoriness. Note that if the drug also dissociates slowly from the channel (*see* Figure 34–12), refractoriness in fast-response tissues actually can extend beyond full repolarization ("postrepolarization refractoriness"). Drugs that prolong the action potential (*B*) also will extend the point at which an arbitrary percentage of Na$^+$ channels have recovered from inactivation, even without directly interacting with Na$^+$ channels.

more recent advance has been the elucidation of molecular and structural determinants of ion channel permeation and drug block. This information likely will play an increasing role in analyzing the actions of available and new antiarrhythmic compounds (MacKinnon, 2003).

A key concept is that ion channel–blocking drugs bind to specific sites on the ion channel proteins to modify function (*e.g.*, decrease current) and that the affinity of the ion channel protein for the drug on its target site will vary as the ion channel protein shuttles among functional con-

formations (or ion channel "states") (Snyders *et al.*, 1991). Physicochemical characteristics, such as molecular weight and lipid solubility, are important determinants of state-dependent binding. State-dependent binding has been studied most extensively in the case of Na$^+$ channel–blocking drugs. Most useful agents of this type block open and/or inactivated Na$^+$ channels and have very little affinity for channels in the resting state. Thus, with each action potential, drugs bind to Na$^+$ channels and block them, and with each diastolic interval, drugs dissociate, and the block is released. Block may be due to a drug

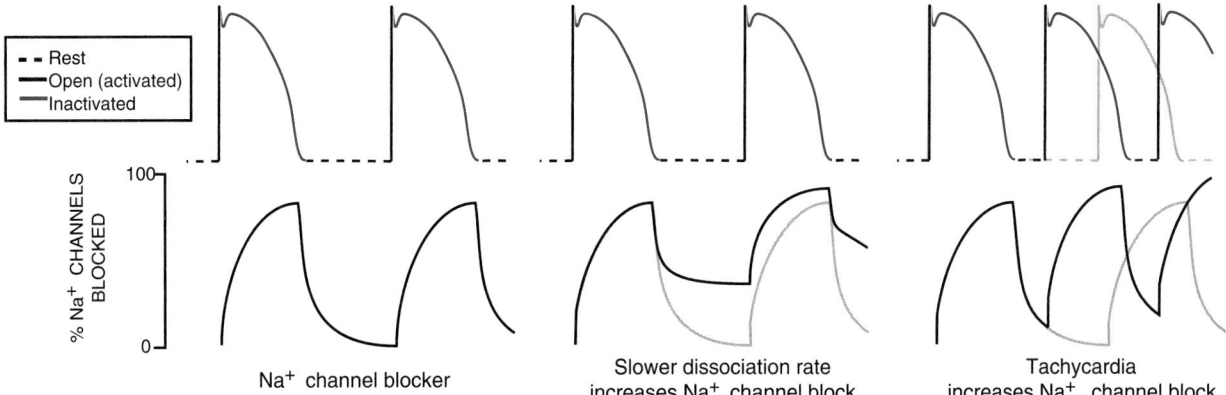

Figure 34–12. *Recovery from block of Na⁺ channels during diastole.* This recovery is the critical factor determining extent of steady-state Na⁺ channel block. Na⁺ channel blockers bind to (and block) Na⁺ channels in the open and/or inactivated states, resulting in phasic changes in the extent of block during the action potential. As shown in the middle panel, a decrease in the rate of recovery from block increases the extent of block. Different drugs have different rates of recovery, and depolarization reduces the rate of recovery. The right panel shows that increasing heart rate, which results in relatively less time spent in the rest state and also increases the extent of block. (Modified from Roden *et al.*, 1993, with permission.)

binding within the conduction pore or binding at a remote site that then induces allosteric changes in the ability of the channel protein to form a pore. As illustrated in Figure 34–12, the dissociation rate is a key determinant of steady-state block of Na⁺ channels. When heart rate increases, the time available for dissociation decreases, and steady-state Na⁺ channel block increases. The rate of recovery from block also slows as cells are depolarized, as in ischemia (Snyders *et al.*, 1991). This explains the finding that Na⁺ channel blockers depress Na⁺ current, and hence conduction, to a greater extent in ischemic tissues than in normal tissues. Open versus inactivated-state block also may be important in determining the effects of some drugs. Increased action potential duration, which results in a relative increase in time spent in the inactivated state, may increase block by drugs that bind to inactivated channels, such as lidocaine or amiodarone (Snyders *et al.*, 1991).

The rate of recovery from block often is expressed as a time constant ($\tau_{recovery}$, the time required to complete approximately 63% of an exponentially determined process to be complete; Courtney, 1987). In the case of drugs such as lidocaine, $\tau_{recovery}$ is so short (<<1 s) that recovery from block is very rapid, and substantial Na⁺ channel block occurs only in rapidly driven tissues, particularly in ischemia. Conversely, drugs such as *flecainide* have such long $\tau_{recovery}$ values (>10 s) that roughly the same number of Na⁺ channels is blocked during systole and diastole. As a result, marked slowing of conduction occurs even in normal tissues at normal rates.

Classifying Antiarrhythmic Drugs

Classifying drugs by common electrophysiological properties emphasizes the connection between basic electrophysiological actions and antiarrhythmic effects (Vaughan Williams, 1992). To the extent that the clinical actions of drugs can be predicted from their basic electrophysiological properties, such classification schemes have merit. However, as each compound is better characterized in a range of *in vitro* and *in vivo* test systems, it becomes apparent that differences in pharmacological effects occur even among drugs that share the same classification, some of which may be responsible for the observed clinical differences in responses to drugs of the same broad "class" (Table 34–3). An alternative way of approaching antiarrhythmic therapy is to attempt to classify arrhythmia mechanisms and then to target drug therapy to the electrophysiological mechanism most likely to terminate or prevent the arrhythmia (Task Force, 1991) (Table 34–2).

Na⁺ Channel Block. The extent of Na⁺ channel block depends critically on heart rate and membrane potential, as well as on drug-specific physicochemical characteristics that determine $\tau_{recovery}$ (Figure 34–12). The following description applies when Na⁺ channels are blocked, *i.e.,* at rapid heart rates in diseased tissue with a rapid-recovery drug such as lidocaine or even at normal rates in normal tissues with a slow-recovery drug such as flecainide. When Na⁺ channels are blocked, threshold for excitability is decreased; *i.e.,* greater membrane depolarization is required

Table 34–3
Major Electrophysiological Actions of Antiarrhythmic Drugs

DRUG	NA⁺ CHANNEL BLOCK		↑APD	Ca²⁺ CHANNEL BLOCK	AUTONOMIC EFFECTS	OTHER EFFECTS
	$\tau_{RECOVERY}$[1], SECONDS	STATE DEPENDENCE[1]				
Lidocaine	0.1	I > O				
Phenytoin	0.2	I				
Mexiletine*	0.3					
Tocainide*	0.4	O > I				
Procainamide	1.8	O	✓		Ganglionic blockade (especially intravenous)	✓: Metabolite prolongs APD
Quinidine	3	O	✓	(x)	α-Blockade, vagolytic	
Disopyramide†	9	O	✓		Anticholinergic	
Moricizine	~10	O ≈ I				
Propafenone†	11	O ≈ I	✓		β-Blockade (variable clinical effect)	
Flecainide*	11	O	(x)	(x)		
β-Blockers:						
Propanolol†					β-Blockade	Na⁺ channel block *in vitro*
Sotalol†			✓		β-Blockade	
Amiodarone	1.6	I	✓	(x)	Noncompetitive β-blockade	Antithyroid action
Dofetilide			✓			
Ibutilide			✓			
Verapamil*				✓		
Diltiazem*				✓		
Digoxin					✓:Vagal stimulation	✓: Inhibition of Na⁺,K⁺–ATPase
Adenosine				✓	✓:Adenosine receptor activation	✓: Activation of outward K⁺ current
Magnesium			?✓			Mechanism not well understood

✓indicates an effect that is important in mediating the clinical action of a drug. (x)indicates a demonstrable effect whose relationship to drug action in patients is less well established. *indicates drugs prescribed as racemates, and the enantiomers are thought to exert similar electrophysiological effects. †indicates racemates for which clinically relevant differences in the electrophysiological properties of individual enantiomers have been reported (*see* text). One approach to classifying drugs is:

Class	Major action
I	Na⁺ channel block
II	β-blockade
III	action potential prolongation (usually by K⁺ channel block)
IV	Ca²⁺ channel block

Drugs are listed here according to this scheme. It is important to bear in mind, however, that many drugs exert multiple effects that contribute to their clinical actions. It is occasionally clinically useful to subclassify Na⁺ channel blockers by their rates of recovery from drug-induced block ($\tau_{recovery}$) under physiological conditions. Since this is a continuous variable and can be modulated by factors such as depolarization of the resting potential, these distinctions can become blurred: class Ib, $\tau_{recovery}$ < 1 s; class Ia, $\tau_{recovery}$ 1–10 s; class Ic, $\tau_{recovery}$ > 10 s. These class and subclass effects are associated with distinctive ECG changes, characteristic "class" toxicities, and efficacy in specific arrhythmia syndromes (*see* text). [1]These data are dependent on experimental conditions, including species and temperature. The $\tau_{recovery}$ values cited here are from Courtney (1987), with the exception of moricizine, which was found by Lee and Rosen (1991) to have a value slightly less than that for flecainide. The state-dependence is from Snyders *et al.*, (1991).
ABBREVIATIONS: O, Open state blocker; I, inactivated state blocker; APD, action potential duration.

to bring Na^+ channels from the rest to open states. This change in threshold probably contributes to the clinical findings that Na^+ channel blockers tend to increase both pacing threshold and the energy required to defibrillate the fibrillating heart (Echt *et al.*, 1989). These deleterious effects may be important if antiarrhythmic drugs are used in patients with pacemakers or implanted defibrillators. Na^+ channel block decreases conduction velocity in fast-response tissue and increases QRS duration. Usual doses of flecainide prolong QRS intervals by 25% or more during normal rhythm, whereas lidocaine increases QRS intervals only at very fast heart rates. Drugs with $\tau_{recovery}$ values greater than 10 s (*e.g.*, flecainide) also tend to prolong the PR interval; it is not known whether this represents additional Ca^{2+} channel block (*see* below) or block of fast-response tissue in the region of the AV node. Drug effects on the PR interval also are highly modified by autonomic effects. For example, quinidine actually tends to shorten the PR interval largely as a result of its vagolytic properties. Action potential duration is either unaffected or shortened by Na^+ channel block; some Na^+ channel–blocking drugs do prolong cardiac action potentials but by other mechanisms, usually K^+ channel block (Table 34–3).

By increasing threshold, Na^+ channel block decreases automaticity (Figure 34–10B) and can inhibit triggered activity arising from DADs or EADs. Many Na^+ channel blockers also decrease phase 4 slope (Figure 34–10A). In anatomically defined re-entry, Na^+ channel blockers may decrease conduction sufficiently to extinguish the propagating re-entrant wavefront. However, as described earlier, conduction slowing owing to Na^+ channel block may exacerbate re-entry. Block of Na^+ channels also shifts the voltage dependence of recovery from inactivation (Figure 34–5B) to more negative potentials, thereby tending to increase refractoriness. Thus, whether a given drug exacerbates or suppresses re-entrant arrhythmias depends on the balance between its effects on refractoriness and on conduction in a particular re-entrant circuit. Lidocaine and *mexiletine* have short $\tau_{recovery}$ values and are not useful in atrial fibrillation or flutter, whereas quinidine, flecainide, *propafenone*, and similar agents are effective in some patients. Many of these agents owe part of their antiarrhythmic activity to blockade of K^+ channels.

Na$^+$ Channel–Blocker Toxicity. Conduction slowing in potential re-entrant circuits can account for toxicity to drugs that block the Na^+ channel (Table 34–1). For example, Na^+ channel block decreases conduction velocity and hence slows atrial flutter rate. Normal AV nodal function permits a greater number of impulses to penetrate the ventricle, and heart rate actually may increase (Figure 34–9). Thus atrial flutter rate may drop from 300 per minute, with

2:1 or 4:1 AV conduction (*i.e.*, a heart rate of 150 or 75 beats per minute), to 220 per minute, but with 1:1 transmission to the ventricle (*i.e.*, a heart rate of 220 beats per minute), with potentially disastrous consequences. This form of drug-induced arrhythmia is especially common during treatment with quinidine because the drug also increases AV nodal conduction through its vagolytic properties; flecainide and propafenone also have been implicated. Therapy with Na^+ channel blockers in patients with re-entrant ventricular tachycardia after a myocardial infarction can increase the frequency and severity of arrhythmic episodes. Although the mechanism is unclear, slowed conduction allows the re-entrant wavefront to persist within the tachycardia circuit. Such drug-exacerbated arrhythmia can be very difficult to manage, and deaths owing to intractable drug-induced ventricular tachycardia have been reported. In this setting, Na^+ infusion may be beneficial. Several Na^+ channel blockers (*e.g.*, *procainamide* and quinidine) have been reported to exacerbate neuromuscular paralysis by D-tubocurarine (*see* Chapter 9).

Action Potential Prolongation. Most drugs that prolong the action potential do so by blocking K^+ channels, although enhanced inward Na^+ current also can cause prolongation. Enhanced inward current may underlie QT prolongation (and arrhythmia suppression) by *ibutilide*. Block of cardiac K^+ channels increases action potential duration and reduces normal automaticity (Figure 34–10D). Increased action potential duration, seen as an increase in QT interval, increases refractoriness (Figure 34–11) and therefore should be an effective way of treating re-entry (Task Force, 1991; Singh, 1993). Experimentally, K^+ channel block produces a series of desirable effects: reduced defibrillation energy requirement, inhibition of ventricular fibrillation owing to acute ischemia, and increased contractility (Echt *et al.*, 1989; Roden, 1993). As shown in Table 34–3, most K^+ channel blocking drugs also interact with β adrenergic receptors (*sotalol*) or other channels (*e.g.*, amiodarone and quinidine). Amiodarone and sotalol appear to be at least as effective as drugs with predominant Na^+ channel–blocking properties in both atrial and ventricular arrhythmias. "Pure" action potential–prolonging drugs (*e.g.*, *dofetilide* and ibutilide) also are available (Murray, 1998; Torp-Pedersen *et al.*, 1999).

Toxicity of Drugs That Prolong QT Interval. Most of these agents disproportionately prolong cardiac action potentials when underlying heart rate is slow and can cause *torsades de pointes* (Table 34–1, Figure 34–9). While this effect usually is seen with QT-prolonging antiarrhythmic drugs, it can occur more rarely with drugs that are used for noncardiac indications. For such agents, the risk of *torsades de pointes* may become apparent only after widespread use postmarketing, and recognition of this risk has been a common cause for drug withdrawal (Roden, 2004). For unknown reasons, drug-induced *torsades de pointes* associated with antiarrhythmic drugs is significantly more common in women (Makkar *et al.*, 1993).

Ca^{2+} Channel Block. The major electrophysiological effects resulting from block of cardiac Ca^{2+} channels are in slow-response tissues, the sinus and AV nodes. Dihydropyridines, such as *nifedipine,* which are used commonly in angina and hypertension (*see* Chapters 31 and 32), preferentially block Ca^{2+} channels in vascular smooth muscle; their cardiac electrophysiological effects, such as heart rate acceleration, result principally from reflex sympathetic activation secondary to peripheral vasodilation. Only verapamil, *diltiazem,* and *bepridil* block Ca^{2+} channels in cardiac cells at clinically used doses. These drugs generally slow heart rate (Figure 34–10A), although hypotension, if marked, can cause reflex sympathetic activation and tachycardia. The velocity of AV nodal conduction decreases, so the PR interval increases. AV nodal block occurs as a result of decremental conduction, as well as increased AV nodal refractoriness. These latter effects form the basis of the antiarrhythmic actions of Ca^{2+} channel blockers in re-entrant arrhythmias whose circuit involves the AV node, such as AV re-entrant tachycardia (Figure 34–7).

Another important indication for antiarrhythmic therapy is to reduce ventricular rate in atrial flutter or fibrillation. Rare forms of ventricular tachycardia appear to be DAD-mediated and respond to verapamil (Sung *et al.*, 1983). Parenteral verapamil and diltiazem are approved for rapid conversion of PSVTs to sinus rhythm and for temporary control of rapid ventricular rate in atrial flutter or fibrillation. Oral verapamil may be used in conjunction with digoxin to control ventricular rate in chronic atrial flutter or fibrillation and for prophylaxis of repetitive PSVT. Unlike β adrenergic receptor antagonists, Ca^{2+} channel blockers have not been shown to reduce mortality after myocardial infarction (Singh, 1990). In contrast to other Ca^{2+} channel blockers, bepridil increases action potential duration in many tissues and can exert an antiarrhythmic effect in atria and ventricles. However, because bepridil can cause *torsades de pointes*, it is not prescribed widely and has been discontinued in the United States.

Verapamil and Diltiazem. The major adverse effect of intravenous verapamil or diltiazem is hypotension, particularly with bolus administration. This is a particular problem if the drugs are used mistakenly in patients with ventricular tachycardia (in which Ca^{2+} channel blockers usually are not effective) misdiagnosed as AV nodal re-entrant tachycardia (Stewart *et al.*, 1986). Hypotension also is frequent in patients receiving other vasodilators, including quinidine, and in patients with underlying left ventricular dysfunction, which the drugs can exacerbate. Severe sinus bradycardia or AV block also occurs, especially in susceptible patients, such as those also receiving β-blockers. With oral therapy, these adverse effects tend to be less severe. Constipation can occur with oral verapamil.

Verapamil (CALAN, ISOPTIN, VERELAN, COVERA-HS) is prescribed as a racemate. L-Verapamil is a more potent calcium channel blocker than is D-verapamil. However, with oral therapy, the L-enantiomer undergoes more extensive first-pass hepatic metabolism. For this reason, a given concentration of verapamil prolongs the PR interval to a greater extent when administered intravenously (where concentrations of the L- and D-enantiomers are equivalent) than when administered orally (Echizen *et al.*, 1985). *Diltiazem* (CARDIZEM, TIAZAC, DILACOR XR, and others) also undergoes extensive first-pass hepatic metabolism, and both drugs have metabolites that exert Ca^{2+} channel–blocking actions. In clinical practice, adverse effects during therapy with verapamil or diltiazem are determined largely by underlying heart disease and concomitant therapy; plasma concentrations of these agents are not measured routinely. Both drugs can increase serum digoxin concentration, although the magnitude of this effect is variable; excess slowing of ventricular response may occur in patients with atrial fibrillation.

Block of β Adrenergic Receptors. β Adrenergic stimulation increases the magnitude of the Ca^{2+} current and slows its inactivation, increases the magnitude of repolarizing K^+ and Cl^- currents (Sanguinetti *et al.*, 1991; Hume and Harvey, 1991), increases pacemaker current (thereby increasing sinus rate; DiFrancesco, 1993), and under pathophysiological conditions, can increase both DAD- and EAD-mediated arrhythmias. The increases in plasma epinephrine associated with severe stress (*e.g.*, acute myocardial infarction or resuscitation from cardiac arrest) lower serum K^+, especially in patients receiving chronic diuretic therapy (Brown *et al.*, 1983). β Adrenergic receptor antagonists inhibit these effects and can be antiarrhythmic by reducing heart rate, decreasing intracellular Ca^{2+} overload, and inhibiting afterdepolarization-mediated automaticity. Epinephrine-induced hypokalemia appears to be mediated by β_2 adrenergic receptors and is blocked by "noncardioselective" antagonists such as *propranolol* (*see* Chapter 10). In acutely ischemic tissue, β-blockers increase the energy required to fibrillate the heart, an antiarrhythmic action (Anderson *et al.*, 1983). Although the precise mechanisms have not been established, these effects may contribute to the reduced mortality observed in trials of chronic therapy with β-blockers—including propranolol, *timolol,* and *metoprolol*—after myocardial infarction (Singh, 1990). *Atenolol* and metoprolol have been shown to decrease mortality in the first week following myocardial infarction.

As with Ca^{2+} channel blockers and digitalis, β-blockers increase AV nodal conduction time (increased PR interval) and prolong AV nodal refractoriness; hence they are useful in terminating re-entrant arrhythmias that involve the AV node and in controlling ventricular response in atrial fibrillation or flutter. In many (but not all) patients with the congenital long QT syndrome, as well as in many other patients, arrhythmias are triggered by physical or emotional stress; β-blockers may be useful in these cases (Schwartz *et al.*, 2000; Roden and Spooner, 1999). β Adrenergic receptor antagonists also reportedly are effective in controlling arrhythmias owing to Na^+ channel blockers; this effect may be due in part to slowing of the heart rate, which then decreases the extent of rate-dependent conduction slowing by Na^+ channel block (Myerburg *et al.*, 1989). As described further in Chapter 10, adverse effects of β-blockade include fatigue, bronchospasm, hypotension, impotence, depression, aggravation of heart failure, worsening of symptoms owing to peripheral vascular disease, and masking of the symptoms of hypoglycemia in diabetic patients (*see* Chapters 10 and 32). In patients with arrhythmias owing to excess sympathetic stimulation (*e.g.*, pheochromocytoma or *clonidine* withdrawal), β-blockers can result in unopposed α adrenergic stimulation, with resulting severe hypertension and/or α adrenergic-mediated arrhythmias. In such patients, arrhythmias should be treated with both α and β adrenergic antagonists or with a drug such as labetalol that combines α- and β-blocking properties. Abrupt discontinuation of chronic β-blocker therapy can lead to "rebound" symptoms, including hypertension, increased angina, and arrhythmias; thus β-receptor antagonists are tapered over 2 weeks (*see* Chapters 10 and 31 to 33).

Selected β Adrenergic Receptor Blockers. It is likely that most β adrenergic antagonists share antiarrhythmic properties. Some, such as propranolol, also exert Na^+ channel–blocking ("membrane stabilizing") effects at high concentrations *in vitro*, but the clinical significance of this effect is uncertain. Similarly, drugs with intrinsic sympathomimetic activity may be less useful as antiarrhythmics, at least in theory (Singh, 1990). *Acebutolol* is as effective as quinidine in suppressing ventricular ectopic beats, an arrhythmia that many clinicians no longer treat. Sotalol (*see* below) is more effective for many

arrhythmias than are other β-blockers probably because of its K^+ channel–blocking actions. *Esmolol* (Frishman *et al.*, 1988) is a β_1-selective agent that is metabolized by erythrocyte esterases and so has a very short elimination half-life (9 minutes). Intravenous esmolol is useful in clinical situations in which immediate β adrenergic blockade is desired (*e.g.*, for rate control of rapidly conducted atrial fibrillation). Because of esmolol's very rapid elimination, adverse effects due to β adrenergic blockade—should they occur—dissipate rapidly when the drug is stopped. Although methanol is a metabolite of esmolol, methanol intoxication has not been a clinical problem.

PRINCIPLES IN THE CLINICAL USE OF ANTIARRHYTHMIC DRUGS

Drugs that modify cardiac electrophysiology often have a very narrow margin between the doses required to produce a desired effect and those associated with adverse effects. Moreover, antiarrhythmic drugs can induce new arrhythmias with possibly fatal consequences. Nonpharmacological treatments, such as cardiac pacing, electrical defibrillation, or ablation of targeted regions (Morady, 1999), are indicated for some arrhythmias; in other cases, no therapy is required, even though an arrhythmia is detected. Therefore, the fundamental principles of therapeutics described here must be applied to optimize antiarrhythmic therapy.

1. Identify and Remove Precipitating Factors

Factors that commonly precipitate cardiac arrhythmias include hypoxia, electrolyte disturbances (especially hypokalemia), myocardial ischemia, and certain drugs. Antiarrhythmics, including cardiac glycosides, are not the only drugs that can precipitate arrhythmias (Table 34–1). For example, *theophylline* can cause multifocal atrial tachycardia, which sometimes can be managed simply by reducing the dose of theophylline. *Torsades de pointes* can arise not only during therapy with action potential–prolonging antiarrhythmics but also with other drugs not ordinarily classified as having effects on ion channels. These include the antibiotic *erythromycin* (*see* Chapter 46); the antiprotozoal *pentamidine* (*see* Chapter 40); some antipsychotics, notably *thioridazine* (*see* Chapter 18); and certain tricyclic antidepressants (*see* Chapter 17).

2. Establish the Goals of Treatment

Some Arrhythmias Should Not Be Treated: The CAST Example. Abnormalities of cardiac rhythm are readily detectable by a variety of recording methods. However, the mere detection of an abnormality does not equate with the need for therapy. This was illustrated in the Cardiac Arrhythmias Suppression Trial (CAST). The presence of asymptomatic ventricular ectopic beats is a known marker for increased risk of sudden death owing to ventricular fibrillation in patients convalescing from myocardial infarction. In the CAST, patients whose ventricular ectopic beats were suppressed by the potent Na$^+$ channel blockers *encainide* (no longer marketed) or *flecainide* were randomly assigned to receive those drugs or placebo. Unexpectedly, the mortality rate was two- to threefold higher among patients treated with the drugs than those treated with placebo (CAST Investigators, 1989). While the explanation for this effect is not known, several lines of evidence suggest that in the presence of these drugs, transient episodes of myocardial ischemia and/or sinus tachycardia can cause marked conduction slowing (because these drugs have a very long $\tau_{recovery}$), resulting in fatal re-entrant ventricular tachyarrhythmias (Ruskin, 1989; Ranger *et al.*, 1989; Akiyama *et al.*, 1991). One consequence of this pivotal clinical trial was to re-emphasize the concept that therapy should be initiated only when a clear benefit to the patient can be identified. When symptoms are obviously attributable to an ongoing arrhythmia, there usually is little doubt that termination of the arrhythmia will be beneficial; when chronic therapy is used to prevent recurrence of an arrhythmia, the risks may be greater (Roden, 1994). *Among the antiarrhythmic drugs discussed here, only β adrenergic blockers and, to a lesser extent, amiodarone* (Connolly, 1999) *have been shown to reduce mortality during long-term therapy.*

Symptoms Due to Arrhythmias. Some patients with an arrhythmia may be asymptomatic; in this case, establishing any benefit for treatment will be very difficult. Some patients may present with presyncope, syncope, or even cardiac arrest, which may be due to brady- or tachyarrhythmias. Other patients may present with a sensation of irregular heartbeats (*i.e.*, palpitations) that can be minimally symptomatic in some individuals and incapacitating in others. The irregular heartbeats may be due to intermittent premature contractions or to sustained arrhythmias such as atrial fibrillation (which results in an irregular ventricular rate) (Figure 34–9). Finally, patients may present with symptoms owing to decreased cardiac output attributable to arrhythmias. The most common symptom is breathlessness either at rest or on exertion. Rarely, sustained tachycardias may produce no "arrhythmia" symptoms (such as palpitations) but will depress contractile function; these patients may present with congestive heart failure that can be controlled by treating the arrhythmia.

Choosing Among Therapeutic Approaches. In choosing among available therapeutic options, it is important to establish clear therapeutic goals. For example, three options are available in patients with atrial fibrillation: (1) Reduce the ventricular response using AV nodal blocking agents such as digitalis, verapamil, diltiazem, or β adrenergic antagonists (Table 34–1); (2) restore and maintain normal rhythm using drugs such as quinidine, flecainide, or amiodarone; or (3) decide not to implement antiarrhythmic therapy, especially if the patient truly is asymptomatic. Most patients with atrial fibrillation also benefit from anticoagulation to reduce stroke incidence regardless of symptoms (Singer, 1996) (*see* Chapter 54).

Factors that contribute to choice of therapy include not only symptoms but also the type and extent of structural heart disease, the QT interval prior to drug therapy, the coexistence of conduction system disease, and the presence of noncardiac diseases (Table 34–4). In the rare patient with the WPW syndrome and atrial fibrillation, the ventricular response can be extremely rapid and can be accelerated paradoxically by AV nodal blocking drugs such as digitalis or Ca^{2+} channel blockers; deaths owing to drug therapy have been reported under these circumstances.

Table 34–4
Patient-Specific Antiarrhythmic Drug Contraindications

CONDITION	EXCLUDE/USE WITH CAUTION
Cardiac	
Heart failure	Disopyramide, flecainide
Sinus or AV node dysfunction	Digoxin, verapamil, diltiazem, β adrenergic receptor antagonists, amiodarone
Wolff–Parkinson–White syndrome (risk of extremely rapid rate if atrial fibrillation develops)	Digoxin, verapamil, diltiazem
Infranodal conduction disease	Na$^+$ channel blockers, amiodarone
Aortic/subaortic stenosis	Bretylium
History of myocardial infarction	Flecainide
Prolonged QT interval	Quinidine, procainamide, disopyramide, sotalol, dofetilide, ibutilide, amiodarone
Cardiac transplant	Adenosine
Noncardiac	
Diarrhea	Quinidine
Prostatism, glaucoma	Disopyramide
Arthritis	Chronic procainamide
Lung disease	Amiodarone
Tremor	Mexiletine, tocainide (use discontinued in U.S.)
Constipation	Verapamil
Asthma, peripheral vascular disease, hypoglycemia	β Adrenergic blockers, propafenone

The frequency and reproducibility of arrhythmia should be established prior to initiating therapy because inherent variability in the occurrence of arrhythmias can be confused with a beneficial or adverse drug effect. Techniques for this assessment include recording cardiac rhythm for prolonged periods or evaluating the response of the heart to artificially induced premature beats. It is important to recognize that drug therapy may be only partially effective: A marked decrease in the duration of paroxysms of atrial fibrillation may be sufficient to render a patient asymptomatic even if an occasional episode still can be detected.

3. Minimize Risks

Antiarrhythmic Drugs Can Cause Arrhythmias. One well-recognized risk of antiarrhythmic therapy is the possibility of provoking new arrhythmias, with potentially life-threatening consequences. Antiarrhythmic drugs can provoke arrhythmias by different mechanisms (Table 34–1). These drug-provoked arrhythmias must be recognized because further treatment with antiarrhythmic drugs often exacerbates the problem, whereas withdrawal of the causative agent often is curative. Thus, establishing a precise diagnosis is critical, and targeting therapies at underlying mechanisms of the arrhythmias may be required. For example, treating a ventricular tachycardia with verapamil not only may be ineffective but also can cause catastrophic cardiovascular collapse (Stewart *et al.*, 1986).

Monitoring of Plasma Concentration. Some adverse effects of antiarrhythmic drugs result from excessive plasma drug concentrations. Measuring plasma concentration and adjusting the dose to maintain the concentration within a prescribed therapeutic range may minimize some adverse effects. In many patients, serious adverse reactions relate to interactions involving antiarrhythmic drugs (often at usual plasma concentrations), transient factors such as electrolyte disturbances or myocardial ischemia, and the type and extent of the underlying heart disease (Ruskin, 1989; Roden, 1994). Factors such as generation of unmeasured active metabolites, variability in elimination of enantiomers (which may exert differing pharmacological effects), and disease- or enantiomer-specific abnormalities in drug binding to plasma proteins can complicate the interpretation of plasma drug concentrations.

Patient-Specific Contraindications. Another way to minimize the adverse effects of antiarrhythmic drugs is to avoid certain drugs in certain patient subsets altogether. For example, patients with a history of congestive heart failure are particularly prone to develop heart failure during *disopyramide* therapy. In other cases, adverse effects of drugs may be difficult to distinguish from exacerbations of underlying disease. Amiodarone may cause interstitial lung disease; its use therefore is undesirable in a patient with advanced pulmonary disease in whom the development of this potentially fatal adverse effect would be difficult to detect. Specific diseases that constitute relative or absolute contraindications to specific drugs are listed in Table 34–4.

4. The Electrophysiology of the Heart as a "Moving Target"

Cardiac electrophysiology varies dynamically in response to external influences such as changing autonomic tone, myocardial ischemia, and myocardial stretch (Priori *et al.*, 1999). For example, myocardial ischemia results in changes in extracellular K^+ that make the resting potential less negative, inactivate Na^+ channels, decrease Na^+ current, and slow conduction (Weiss *et al.*, 1991). In addition, myocardial ischemia can result in the formation and release of metabolites such as lysophosphatidylcholine, which can alter ion channel function; ischemia also may activate channels that otherwise are quiescent, such as the ATP-inhibited K^+ channels. Thus, in response to myocardial ischemia, a normal heart may display changes in resting potential, conduction velocity, intracellular Ca^{2+} concentrations, and repolarization, any one of which then may create arrhythmias or alter response to antiarrhythmic therapy.

ANTIARRHYTHMIC DRUGS

Summaries of important electrophysiological and pharmacokinetic features of the drugs considered here are pre-

sented in Tables 34–3 and 34–5. Ca^{2+} channel blockers and β adrenergic antagonists were considered earlier and in Chapters 1 and 31 to 33. The drugs are presented in alphabetical order.

Adenosine. Adenosine (ADENOCARD) is a naturally occurring nucleoside that is administered as a rapid intravenous bolus for the acute termination of re-entrant supraventricular arrhythmias (Lerman and Belardinelli, 1991). Rare cases of ventricular tachycardia in patients with otherwise normal hearts are thought to be DAD-mediated and can be terminated by adenosine. Adenosine also has been used to produce controlled hypotension during some surgical procedures and in the diagnosis of coronary artery disease. Intravenous ATP appears to produce effects similar to those of adenosine.

ADENOSINE

Pharmacological Effects. The effects of adenosine are mediated by its interaction with specific G protein–coupled adenosine receptors (*see* Chapter 11). Adenosine activates acetylcholine-sensitive K^+ current in the atrium and sinus and AV nodes, resulting in shortening of action potential duration, hyperpolarization, and slowing of normal automaticity (Figure 34–10C). Adenosine also inhibits the electrophysiological effects of increased intracellular cyclic AMP that occur with sympathetic stimulation. Because adenosine thereby reduces Ca^{2+} currents, it can be antiarrhythmic by increasing AV nodal refractoriness and by inhibiting DADs elicited by sympathetic stimulation.

Administration of an intravenous bolus of adenosine to humans transiently slows sinus rate and AV nodal conduction velocity and increases AV nodal refractoriness. A bolus of adenosine can produce transient sympathetic activation by interacting with carotid baroreceptors (Biaggioni *et al.*, 1991); a continuous infusion can cause hypotension.

Adverse Effects. A major advantage of adenosine therapy is that adverse effects are short-lived because the drug is transported into cells and deaminated so rapidly. Transient asystole (lack of any cardiac rhythm whatsoever) is common but usually lasts less than 5 seconds and is

Table 34-5
Pharmacokinetic Characteristics and Doses of Antiarrhythmic Drugs

DRUG	BIOAVAILABILITY Reduced: 1st pass metabolism	PROTEIN BINDING >80%	ELIMINATION Renal	ELIMINATION Hepatic	ELIMINATION Other	ELIMINATION $t_{\frac{1}{2}}$*	ACTIVE METABOLITE(S)	THERAPEUTIC† PLASMA CONCENTRATION	USUAL DOSES‡ Loading Doses	USUAL DOSES‡ Maintenance Doses
Adenosine§					✓	<10 s	✓		6–12 mg (IV only)	
Amiodarone		✓		✓		Weeks		0.5–2 µg/ml	800–1600 mg/day × 2–4 weeks (IV: 100–300 mg)	100–400 mg/day
Digoxin	~80%		✓			36 h		0.5–2.0 ng/ml	1 mg over 12–24 h	0.125–0.375 mg q24h
Digitoxin	>80%	✓	✓	✓		7–9 days	(Digoxin)	10–30 ng/ml		0.05–0.3 mg q24h
Diltiazem	✓			✓		4 h	(x)		0.25–0.35 mg/kg over 10 min (IV)	5–15 mg/h (IV); 30–90 mg q6h; 120–300 mg q24h¶
Disopyramide	>80%		✓	✓		4–10 h	(x)	2–5 µg/ml		100–200 mg q6h; 200–400 mg q12h¶; 200–400 mg q12h¶
Dofetilide	>80%		✓	(x)		7–10 h				0.25–0.5 mg q12h¶¶
Esmolol					✓	5–10 min			0.5 mg/kg/min; may repeat × 2 (IV)	0.05–0.2 mg/kg/min (IV)
Flecainide	>80%		✓	✓		10–18 h		0.2–1 µg/ml		50–200 mg q12h
Ibutilide	✓					6 h			1 mg (IV) over 10 min; may repeat once 10 min later	
Lidocaine	✓	✓		✓		120 min	(x)	1.5–5 µg/ml	3–4 mg/kg over 20–30 min (IV)	1–4 mg/min (IV)
Mexiletine	>80%			✓		9–15 h		0.5–2 µg/ml		100–300 mg q8h
Moricizine	✓	✓		✓		2–3 h	(x)			200–300 mg q8h
Procainamide	>80%		✓	✓		3–4 h	✓	4–8 µg/ml	1 g (IV), given at 20 mg/min	1–4 mg/min (IV); 250–750 mg q3h; 500–1000 mg q6h¶
(N-Acetyl procainamide)	(>80%)		(✓)			(6–10 h)		(10–20 µg/ml)		

Table 34-5
Pharmacokinetic Characteristics and Doses of Antiarrhythmic Drugs (Continued)

DRUG	BIOAVAILABILITY Reduced: 1st pass metabolism	PROTEIN BINDING >80%	ELIMINATION Renal	ELIMINATION Hepatic	ELIMINATION Other	ELIMINATION $t_{\frac{1}{2}}$*	ACTIVE METABOLITE(S)	THERAPEUTIC† PLASMA CONCENTRATION	USUAL DOSES‡ Loading Doses	USUAL DOSES‡ Maintenance Doses
Propafenone	✓	✓		✓		2–32 h	✓	<1 µg/ml		150–300 mg q8h
Propranolol	✓	✓		✓		4 h	✓		1–3 mg (IV)	10–80 mg q6–8h; 80–240 mg q24h¶
Quinidine	>80%	~80%	(x)	✓		4–10 h	✓	2–5 µg/ml		324–648 mg (gluconate) q8h
Sotalol	>80%		✓			8 h		<5 µg/ml (?)		80–320 mg q12h
Tocainide	>80%		✓	✓		15 h		3–11 µg/ml		400–600 mg q8h
Verapamil	✓	✓		✓		3–7 h	✓		5–10 mg (IV)	80–120 mg q8h; 120–240 mg q24h¶

(x): metabolite or route of elimination probably of minor clinical importance. *The elimination half-life is one, but not the only, determinant of how frequently a drug must be administered to maintain a therapeutic effect and avoid toxicity (Chapter 5: Principles of Therapeutics). For some drugs with short elimination half-lives, infrequent dosing is nevertheless possible, *e.g.*, propranolol or verapamil. Formulations that allow slow release into the gastrointestinal tract of a rapidly eliminated compound (available for many drugs including procainamide, disopyramide, verapamil, diltiazem, and propranolol) also allow infrequent dosing. †The therapeutic range is bounded by a plasma concentration below which no therapeutic effect is likely, and an upper concentration above which the risk of adverse effects increases. As discussed in the text, many serious adverse reactions to antiarrhythmic drugs can occur at "therapeutic" concentrations in susceptible individuals. When only an upper limit is cited, a lower limit has not been well defined. Variable generation of active metabolites may further complicate the interpretation of plasma concentration data (Chapters 1: Pharmacokinetics: The Dynamics of Drug Absorption, Distribution, and Elimination and 5: Principles of Therapeutics). ‡Oral doses are presented unless otherwise indicated. Doses are presented as suggested ranges in adults of average build; lower doses are less likely to produce toxicity. Lower maintenance dosages may be required in patients with renal or hepatic disease. Loading doses are only indicated when a therapeutic effect is desired before maintenance therapy would bring drug concentrations into a therapeutic range, *i.e.*, for acute therapy (*e.g.*, lidocaine, verapamil, adenosine) or when the elimination half-life is extremely long (amiodarone). §Bioavailability reduced by incomplete absorption. ¶Indicates suggested dosage using slow-release formulation. ¶¶This drug is available only in a restricted distribution system (*see* text).

ABBREVIATIONS: IV, intravenous; q, every.

in fact the therapeutic goal. Most patients feel a sense of chest fullness and dyspnea when therapeutic doses (6 to 12 mg) of adenosine are administered. Rarely, an adenosine bolus can precipitate bronchospasm or atrial fibrillation presumably by heterogeneously shortening atrial action potentials.

Clinical Pharmacokinetics. Adenosine is eliminated with a half-life of seconds by carrier-mediated uptake, which occurs in most cell types, including the endothelium, and subsequent metabolism by adenosine deaminase. Adenosine probably is the only drug whose efficacy requires a rapid bolus dose, preferably through a large central intravenous line; slow administration results in elimination of the drug prior to its arrival at the heart.

The effects of adenosine are potentiated in patients receiving *dipyridamole,* an adenosine-uptake inhibitor, and in patients with cardiac transplants owing to denervation hypersensitivity. Methylxanthines (*see* Chapter 27) such as theophylline and caffeine block adenosine receptors; therefore, larger than usual doses are required to produce an antiarrhythmic effect in patients who have consumed these agents in beverages or as therapy.

Amiodarone. Amiodarone (CORDARONE, PACERONE) exerts a multiplicity of pharmacological effects, none of which is clearly linked to its arrhythmia-suppressing properties (Mason, 1987). Amiodarone is a structural analog of thyroid hormone, and some of its antiarrhythmic actions and its toxicity may be attributable to interaction with nuclear thyroid hormone receptors. Amiodarone is highly lipophilic, is concentrated in many tissues, and is eliminated extremely slowly; consequently, adverse effects may resolve very slowly. In the United States, the drug is indicated for oral therapy in patients with recurrent ventricular tachycardia or fibrillation resistant to other drugs. Oral amiodarone also is effective in maintaining sinus rhythm in patients with atrial fibrillation (Connolly, 1999). An intravenous form is indicated for acute termination of ventricular tachycardia or fibrillation (Kowey *et al.,* 1995) and is supplanting lidocaine as first-line therapy for out-of-hospital cardiac arrest (Dorian *et al.,* 2002). Trials of oral amiodarone have shown a modest beneficial effect on mortality after acute myocardial infarction (Amiodarone Trials Meta-Analysis Investigators, 1997). Despite uncertainties about its mechanisms of action and the potential for serious toxicity, amiodarone now is used very widely in the treatment of common arrhythmias such as atrial fibrillation (Roy *et al.,* 2000).

AMIODARONE

Pharmacological Effects. Studies of the acute effects of amiodarone in *in vitro* systems are complicated by its insolubility in water, necessitating the use of solvents such as dimethyl sulfoxide. Amiodarone's effects may be mediated by perturbation of the lipid environment of the ion channels (Herbette *et al.,* 1988). Amiodarone blocks inactivated Na^+ channels and has a relatively rapid rate of recovery (time constant $\approx$ 1.6 s) from block. It also decreases Ca^{2+} current and transient outward delayed rectifier and inward rectifier K^+ currents and exerts a noncompetitive adrenergic blocking effect. Amiodarone potently inhibits abnormal automaticity and, in most tissues, prolongs action potential duration. Amiodarone decreases conduction velocity by Na^+ channel block and by a poorly understood effect on cell–cell coupling that may be especially important in diseased tissue (Levine *et al.,* 1988). Prolongations of the PR, QRS, and QT intervals and sinus bradycardia are frequent during chronic therapy. Amiodarone prolongs refractoriness in all cardiac tissues; Na^+ channel block, delayed repolarization owing to K^+ channel block, and inhibition of cell–cell coupling all may contribute to this effect.

Adverse Effects. Hypotension owing to vasodilation and depressed myocardial performance are frequent with the intravenous form of amiodarone and may be due in part to the solvent. While depressed contractility can occur during long-term oral therapy, it is unusual. Despite administration of high doses that would cause serious toxicity if continued long-term, adverse effects are unusual during oral drug-loading regimens, which typically require several weeks. Occasional patients develop nausea during the loading phase, which responds to a decrease in daily dose.

Adverse effects during long-term therapy reflect both the size of daily maintenance doses and the cumulative dose (*i.e.,* to duration of therapy), suggesting that tissue accumulation may be responsible. The most serious adverse effect during chronic amiodarone therapy is pulmonary fibrosis, which can be rapidly progressive and fatal. Underlying lung disease, doses of 400 mg/day or more, and recent pulmonary insults such as pneumonia appear to be risk factors (Dusman *et al.,* 1990). Serial chest X-rays or pulmonary function studies may detect early amiodarone toxicity, but monitoring plasma concentrations has not been useful. With low doses, such as 200 mg/day or less used in atrial fibrillation, pulmonary toxicity is unusual. Other adverse effects during long-term therapy include corneal microdeposits (which often are asymptomatic), hepatic dysfunction, neuromuscular symptoms (most commonly peripheral neuropathy or proximal muscle weakness), photosensitivity, and hypo- or hyperthyroidism. The multiple effects of amiodarone on thyroid function are discussed further in Chapter 56. Treatment consists of withdrawal of the drug and supportive measures, including corticosteroids, for life-threatening pulmonary toxicity; reduction of dosage may be sufficient if the drug is deemed necessary and the adverse effect is not life-threatening. Despite the marked QT prolongation and bradycardia typical of chronic amiodarone therapy, *torsades de pointes* and other drug-induced tachyarrhythmias are unusual.

Clinical Pharmacokinetics. Amiodarone's oral bioavailability is approximately 30% presumably because of poor absorption. This incomplete bioavailability is important in calculating equivalent dosing regimens when converting from intravenous to oral therapy. The drug is distributed in lipid; *e.g.,* heart-tissue-to-plasma concentration ratios of greater than 20:1 and lipid-to-plasma ratios of greater than 300:1 have been reported. After the initiation of amiodarone therapy, increases in refractoriness, a marker of pharmacological effect, require several weeks to develop. Amiodarone undergoes hepatic metabolism by CYP3A4 to desethyl-amiodarone, a metabolite with pharmacological effects similar to those of the parent drug. When amiodarone therapy is withdrawn from a patient who has been receiving therapy for several years, plasma concentrations decline with a half-life of weeks to months. The mechanism whereby amiodarone and desethyl-amiodarone are eliminated is not well established.

A therapeutic plasma amiodarone concentration range of 0.5 to 2 μg/ml has been proposed. However, efficacy apparently depends as much on duration of therapy as on plasma concentration, and elevated plasma concentrations do not predict toxicity (Dusman *et al.,* 1990). Because of amiodarone's slow accumulation in tissue, a high-dose oral loading regimen (*e.g.,* 800 to 1600 mg/day) usually is administered for several weeks before maintenance therapy is started. Maintenance dose is adjusted based on adverse effects and the arrhythmias being treated. If the presenting arrhythmia is life-threatening, dosages of more than 300 mg/day normally are used unless unequivocal toxicity occurs. On the other hand, maintenance doses of 200 mg/day or less are used if recurrence of an arrhythmia would be tolerated, as in patients with atrial fibrillation. Because of its very slow elimination, amiodarone is administered once daily, and omission of one or two doses during chronic therapy rarely results in recurrence of arrhythmia.

Dosage adjustments are not required in hepatic, renal, or cardiac dysfunction. Amiodarone potently inhibits the hepatic metabolism or renal elimination of many compounds. Mechanisms identified to date include inhibition of CYP3A4 and CYP2C9 and P-glycoprotein (*see* Chapter 3). Dosages of warfarin, other antiarrhythmics (*e.g.,* flecainide, procainamide, and quinidine), or digoxin usually require reduction during amiodarone therapy.

Bretylium. *Bretylium* is a quaternary ammonium compound that prolongs cardiac action potentials and interferes with reuptake of norepinephrine by sympathetic neurons. In the past, bretylium was used to treat ventricular fibrillation and prevent its recurrence; the drug no longer is available.

Cardiac Glycosides. **Pharmacological Effects.** Digitalis glycosides exert positive inotropic effects and are used widely in heart failure (*see* Chapter 33). Their inotropic action results from increased intracellular Ca^{2+} (Smith, 1988), which also forms the basis for arrhythmias related to cardiac glycoside intoxication. Cardiac glycosides increase phase 4 slope (*i.e.,* increase the rate of automaticity), especially if $[K]_o$ is low. These drugs (*e.g.,* digoxin) also exert prominent vagotonic actions, resulting in inhibition of Ca^{2+} currents in the AV node and activation of acetylcholine-mediated K^+ currents in the atrium. Thus the major "indirect" electrophysiological effects of cardiac glycosides are hyperpolarization, shortening of atrial action potentials, and increases in AV nodal refractoriness. The latter action accounts for the utility of digitalis in terminating re-entrant arrhythmias involving the AV node and in controlling ventricular response in patients with atrial fibrillation. Cardiac glycosides may be especially useful in the latter situation because many such patients have heart failure, which can be exacerbated by other AV nodal blocking drugs such as Ca^{2+} channel blockers or β adrenergic receptor antagonists. However, sympathetic drive is increased markedly in many patients with advanced heart failure, so digitalis is not very effective in decreasing the rate; on the other hand, even a modest decrease in rate can ameliorate heart failure. Similarly, in other conditions in which high sympathetic tone drives rapid atrioventricular conduction (*e.g.,* chronic lung disease and thyrotoxicosis), digitalis therapy may be only marginally effective in slowing the rate. In heart transplant patients, in whom innervation has been ablated, cardiac glycosides are ineffective for rate control. Increased sympathetic activity and hypoxia can potentiate digitalis-induced changes in automaticity and DADs, thus increasing the risk of digitalis toxicity. A further complicating feature in thyrotoxicosis is increased digoxin clearance. The major ECG effects of cardiac glycosides are PR prolongation and a nonspecific alteration in ventricular repolarization (manifested by depression of the ST segment), whose underlying mechanism is not well understood.

Adverse Effects. Because of the low therapeutic index of cardiac glycosides, their toxicity is a common clinical problem (*see* Chapter 33). Arrhythmias, nausea, disturbances of cognitive function, and blurred or yellow vision are the usual manifestations. Elevated serum concentrations of digitalis, hypoxia (*e.g.,* owing to chronic lung disease), and electrolyte abnormalities (*e.g.,* hypokalemia, hypomagnesemia, and hypercalcemia) predispose patients to digitalis-induced arrhythmias. While digitalis intoxication can cause virtually any arrhythmia, certain types of arrhythmias are characteristic. Arrhythmias that should raise a strong suspicion of digitalis intoxication are those in which DAD-related tachycardias occur along with impairment of sinus node or AV nodal function. Atrial tachycardia with AV block is classic, but ventricular bigeminy (sinus beats alternating with beats of ventricular origin), "bidirectional" ventricular tachycardia (a very rare entity), AV junctional tachycardias, and various degrees of AV block also can occur. With severe intoxication (*e.g.,* with suicidal ingestion), severe hyperkalemia owing to poisoning of Na^+,K^+–ATPase and profound bradyarrhythmias, which may be unresponsive to pacing therapy, are seen. In patients with elevated serum digitalis levels, the risk of precipitating ventricular fibrillation by DC cardioversion probably is increased; in those with therapeutic blood levels, DC cardioversion can be used safely.

Minor forms of cardiac glycoside intoxication may require no specific therapy beyond monitoring cardiac rhythm until symptoms and signs of toxicity resolve. Sinus bradycardia and AV block often respond to intravenous atropine, but the effect is transient. Mg^{2+} has been used successfully in some cases of digitalis-induced tachycardia. Any serious arrhythmia should be treated with antidigoxin Fab fragments (DIGIBIND), which are highly effective in binding digoxin and digitoxin and greatly enhance their renal excretion (*see* Chapter 33). Serum glycoside concentrations rise markedly with antidigitalis antibodies, but these represent bound (pharmacologically inactive) drug. Temporary cardiac pacing may be required for advanced sinus node or AV node dysfunction. Digitalis exerts direct arterial vasoconstrictor effects, which can be especially deleterious in patients with advanced atherosclerosis who receive intravenous drug; mesenteric and coronary ischemia have been reported.

Clinical Pharmacokinetics. The most commonly used digitalis glycoside in the United States is *digoxin* (LANOXIN), although *digitoxin* (various generic preparations) also is used for chronic oral therapy. Digoxin tablets are incompletely (75%) bioavailable, but capsules are more than 90% bioavailable. In some patients, intestinal microflora may metabolize digoxin, markedly reducing bioavailability. In these patients, higher than usual doses are required for clinical efficacy; toxicity is a serious risk if antibiotics such as *tetracycline* or erythromycin are administered because these drugs can destroy intestinal microflora. Inhibition of P-glycoprotein (*see* below) also may play a role. Digoxin is 20% to 30% protein-bound. The antiarrhythmic effects of digoxin can be achieved with intravenous or oral therapy. However, digoxin undergoes relatively slow distribution to effector site(s); therefore, even with intravenous therapy, there is a lag of several hours between drug administration and the development of measurable antiarrhythmic effects such as PR-interval prolongation or slowing of the ventricular rate in atrial fibrillation. To avoid intoxication, a loading dose of approximately 1 to 1.5 mg digoxin is administered over 24 hours. Measurement of postdistribution serum digoxin concentration and adjustment of the daily dose (0.125 to 0.375 mg) to maintain concentrations of 0.5 to 2 ng/ml are useful during chronic digoxin therapy (Table 34–5). Some patients may require and tolerate higher concentrations, but with an increased risk of adverse effects.

DIGOXIN

DIGITOXIN

The elimination half-life of digoxin ordinarily is approximately 36 hours, so maintenance doses are administered once daily. Renal elimination of unchanged drug accounts for less than 80% of digoxin elimination. Digoxin doses should be reduced (or dosing interval increased) and serum concentrations monitored closely in patients with impaired excretion owing to renal failure or in patients who are hypothyroid. Digitoxin undergoes primarily hepatic metabolism and may be useful in patients with fluctuating or advanced renal dysfunction. Digitoxin metabolism is accelerated by drugs such as *phenytoin* and *rifampin* that induce hepatic metabolism (*see* Chapter 3). Digitoxin's elimination half-life is even longer than that of digoxin (about 7 days); it is highly protein-bound, and its therapeutic range is 10 to 30 ng/ml.

Amiodarone, quinidine, verapamil, diltiazem, *cyclosporine, itraconazole,* propafenone, and flecainide decrease digoxin clearance, likely by inhibiting P-glycoprotein, the major route of digoxin elimination (Fromm *et al.*, 1999). New steady-state digoxin concentrations are approached after 4 to 5 half-lives, *i.e.*, in about a week. Digitalis toxicity results so often with quinidine or amiodarone that it is routine to decrease the dose of digoxin if these drugs are started. In all cases, digoxin concentrations should be measured regularly and the dose adjusted if necessary. Hypokalemia, which can be caused by many drugs (*e.g.*, diuretics, *amphotericin B,* and corticosteroids), will potentiate digitalis-induced arrhythmias.

Disopyramide. Disopyramide (NORPACE, others) exerts electrophysiological effects very similar to those of quinidine, but the drugs have different adverse effect profiles (Morady *et al.*, 1982). Disopyramide is used to maintain sinus rhythm in patients with atrial flutter or atrial fibrillation and to prevent recurrence of ventricular tachycardia or ventricular fibrillation. Disopyramide is prescribed as a racemate. Its structure is given below.

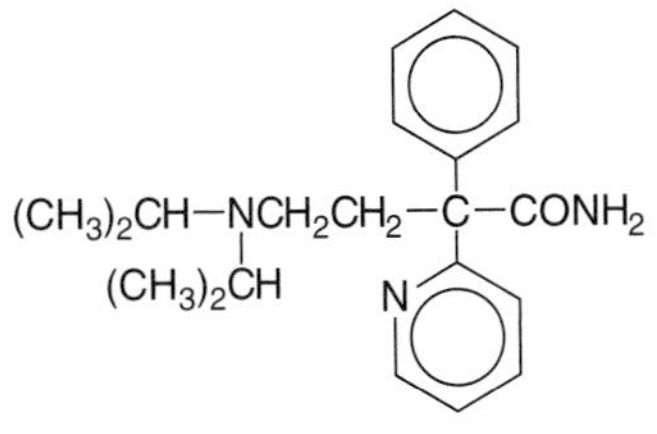

$$(CH_3)_2CH-NCH_2CH_2-\underset{N}{\overset{|}{C}}-CONH_2$$
$$(CH_3)_2CH$$

DISOPYRAMIDE

Pharmacological Actions and Adverse Effects. The *in vitro* electrophysiological actions of *S*-(+)-disopyramide are similar to those of quinidine. The *R*-(−)-enantiomer produces similar Na⁺ channel block but does not prolong cardiac action potentials. Unlike quinidine, racemic disopyramide is not an α adrenergic receptor antagonist, but it does exert prominent anticholinergic actions that account for many of its adverse effects. These include precipitation of glaucoma, constipation, dry mouth, and urinary retention; the latter is most common in males with prostatism but can occur in females. Disopyramide commonly depresses contractility, which can precipitate heart failure (Podrid *et al.*, 1980), and also can cause *torsades de pointes.*

Clinical Pharmacokinetics. Disopyramide is well absorbed. Binding to plasma proteins is concentration dependent, so a small increase in total concentration may represent a disproportionately larger increase in free drug concentration (Lima *et al.*, 1981). Disopyramide is eliminated by both hepatic metabolism (to a weakly active metabolite) and renal excretion of unchanged drug. The dose should be reduced in patients with renal dysfunction. Higher than usual dosages may be required in patients receiving drugs that induce hepatic metabolism, such as phenytoin.

Dofetilide. Dofetilide (TIKOSYN) is a potent and "pure" I_{Kr} blocker. As a result of this specificity, it has virtually no extracardiac pharmacological effects. Dofetilide is effective in maintaining sinus rhythm in patients with atrial fibrillation. In the DIAMOND studies (Torp-Pedersen *et al.*, 1999), dofetilide did not affect mortality in patients with advanced heart failure or in those convalescing from acute myocardial infarction. Dofetilide currently is available through a restricted distribution system that includes only physicians, hospitals, and other institutions that have received special educational programs covering proper dosing and treatment initiation.

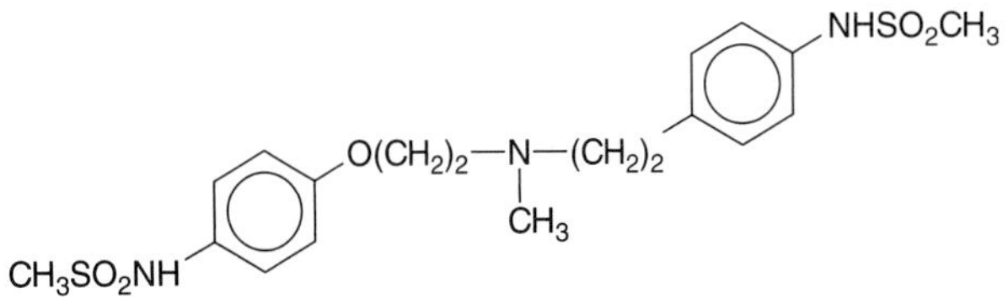

$$CH_3SO_2NH \quad O(CH_2)_2-N-(CH_2)_2 \quad NHSO_2CH_3$$
$$CH_3$$

DOFETILIDE

Adverse Effects. *Torsades de pointes* occurred in 1% to 3% of patients in clinical trials where strict exclusion criteria (*e.g.*, hypokalemia) were applied and continuous ECG monitoring was used to detect marked QT prolongation in the hospital. The incidence of this adverse effect during more widespread use of the drug, marketed since 2000, is unknown. Other adverse effects were no more common than with placebo during premarketing clinical trials.

Clinical Pharmacokinetics. Most of a dose of dofetilide is excreted unchanged by the kidneys. In patients with mild to moderate renal failure, decreases in dosage based on creatinine clearance are required to minimize the risk of *torsades de pointes*. The drug should not be used in patients with advanced renal failure or with inhibitors of renal cation transport. Dofetilide also undergoes minor hepatic metabolism.

Flecainide. The effects of flecainide (TAMBOCOR) therapy are thought to be attributable to the drug's very long $\tau_{recovery}$ from Na$^+$ channel block (Roden and Woosley, 1986a). In the CAST study, flecainide increased mortality in patients convalescing from myocardial infarction (CAST Investigators, 1989). However, it continues to be approved for the maintenance of sinus rhythm in patients with supraventricular arrhythmias, including atrial fibrillation, in whom structural heart disease is absent (Anderson *et al.*, 1989; Henthorn *et al.*, 1991).

CF$_3$CH$_2$O

—CONHCH$_2$—

OCH$_2$CF$_3$

FLECAINIDE

Pharmacological Effects. Flecainide blocks Na$^+$ current and delayed rectifier K$^+$ current (I_{Kr}) *in vitro* at similar concentrations, 1 to 2 μM (Ikeda *et al.*, 1985; Follmer and Colatsky, 1990). It also blocks Ca^{2+} currents *in vitro*. Action potential duration is shortened in Purkinje cells, probably owing to block of late-opening Na$^+$ channels, but prolonged in ventricular cells, probably owing to block of delayed rectifier current (Ikeda *et al.*, 1985). Flecainide does not cause EADs *in vitro* or *torsades de pointes*. In atrial tissue, flecainide disproportionately prolongs action potentials at fast rates, an especially desirable antiarrhythmic drug effect; this effect contrasts with that of quinidine, which prolongs atrial action potentials to a greater extent at slower rates (Wang *et al.*, 1990). Flecainide prolongs the duration of PR, QRS, and QT intervals even at normal heart rates.

Adverse Effects. Flecainide produces few subjective complaints in most patients; dose-related blurred vision is the most common noncardiac adverse effect. It can exacerbate congestive heart failure in patients with depressed left ventricular performance. The most serious adverse effects are provocation or exacerbation of potentially lethal arrhythmias. These include acceleration of ventricular rate in patients with atrial flutter, increased frequency of episodes of re-entrant ventricular tachycardia, and increased mortality in patients convalescing from myocardial infarction (Crijns *et al.*, 1988; CAST Investigators, 1989; Ranger *et al.*, 1989). As discussed earlier, it is like-

ly that all these effects can be attributed to Na$^+$ channel block. Flecainide also can cause heart block in patients with conduction system disease.

Clinical Pharmacokinetics. Flecainide is well absorbed. The elimination half-life is shorter with urinary acidification (10 hours) than with urinary alkalinization (17 hours), but it is nevertheless sufficiently long to allow dosing twice daily (Table 34–5). Elimination occurs by both renal excretion of unchanged drug and hepatic metabolism to inactive metabolites. The latter is mediated by the polymorphically distributed enzyme CYP2D6 (Gross *et al.*, 1989) (*see* Chapter 3). However, even in patients in whom this pathway is absent because of genetic polymorphism or inhibition by other drugs (*i.e.*, quinidine and fluoxetine), renal excretion ordinarily is sufficient to prevent drug accumulation. In the rare patient with renal dysfunction and lack of active CYP2D6, flecainide may accumulate to toxic plasma concentrations. Flecainide is a racemate, but there are no differences in the electrophysiological effects or disposition kinetics of its enantiomers (Kroemer *et al.*, 1989). Some reports have suggested that plasma flecainide concentrations greater than 1 μg/ml should be avoided to minimize the risk of flecainide toxicity; however, in susceptible patients, the adverse electrophysiological effects of flecainide therapy can occur at therapeutic plasma concentrations.

Ibutilide. Ibutilide (CORVERT) is an I_{Kr} blocker that in some systems also activates an inward Na$^+$ current (Murray, 1998). The action potential–prolonging effect of the drug may arise from either mechanism. Ibutilide is administered as a rapid infusion (1 mg over 10 minutes) for the immediate conversion of atrial fibrillation or flutter to sinus rhythm. The drug's efficacy rate is higher in patients with atrial flutter (50% to 70%) than in those with atrial fibrillation (30% to 50%). In atrial fibrillation, the conversion rate is lower in those in whom the arrhythmia has been present for weeks or months compared with those in whom it has been present for days. The major toxicity with ibutilide is *torsades de pointes,* which occurs in up to 6% of patients and requires immediate cardioversion in up to one-third of these. The drug undergoes extensive first-pass metabolism and so is not used orally. It is eliminated by hepatic metabolism and has a half-life of 2 to 12 hours (average of 6 hours).

OH   C$_2$H$_5$

CH$_3$SO$_2$NH — —C—(CH$_2$)$_3$—N—C$_7$H$_{15}$

H

IBUTILIDE

Lidocaine. Lidocaine (XYLOCAINE) is a local anesthetic that also is useful in the acute intravenous therapy of ventricular arrhythmias. When lidocaine was administered to all patients with suspected myocardial infarction, the incidence of ventricular fibrillation was reduced (Lie *et al.*, 1974). However, survival to hospital discharge tended to be decreased (Hine *et al.*, 1989) perhaps because of lidocaine-exacerbated heart block or congestive heart failure. Therefore, lidocaine no longer is administered routinely to all patients in coronary care units.

LIDOCAINE

Pharmacological Effects. Lidocaine blocks both open and inactivated cardiac Na^+ channels. *In vitro* studies suggest that lidocaine-induced block reflects an increased likelihood that the Na^+ channel protein assumes a nonconducting conformation in the presence of drug (Balser *et al.*, 1996). Recovery from block is very rapid, so lidocaine exerts greater effects in depolarized (*e.g.,* ischemic) and/or rapidly driven tissues. Lidocaine is not useful in atrial arrhythmias possibly because atrial action potentials are so short that the Na^+ channel is in the inactivated state only briefly compared with diastolic (recovery) times, which are relatively long (Snyders *et al.*, 1991). In some studies, lidocaine increased current through inward rectifier channels, but the clinical significance of this effect is not known. Lidocaine can hyperpolarize Purkinje fibers depolarized by low $[K]_o$ or stretch; the resulting increased conduction velocity may be antiarrhythmic in re-entry.

Lidocaine decreases automaticity by reducing the slope of phase 4 and altering the threshold for excitability. Action potential duration usually is unaffected or is shortened; such shortening may be due to block of the few Na^+ channels that inactivate late during the cardiac action potential. Lidocaine usually exerts no significant effect on PR or QRS duration; QT is unaltered or slightly shortened. The drug exerts little effect on hemodynamic function, although rare cases of lidocaine-associated exacerbations of heart failure have been reported, especially in patients with very poor left ventricular function.

Adverse Effects. When a large intravenous dose of lidocaine is administered rapidly, seizures can occur. When plasma concentrations of the drug rise slowly above the therapeutic range, as may occur during maintenance therapy, tremor, dysarthria, and altered levels of consciousness are more common. Nystagmus is an early sign of lidocaine toxicity.

Clinical Pharmacokinetics. Lidocaine is well absorbed but undergoes extensive though variable first-pass hepatic metabolism; thus oral use of the drug is inappropriate. In theory, therapeutic plasma concentrations of lidocaine may be maintained by intermittent intramuscular administration, but the intravenous route is preferred (Table 34–5). Lidocaine's metabolites, glycine xylidide (GX) and monoethyl GX, are less potent as Na^+ channel blockers than the parent drug. GX and lidocaine appear to compete for access to the Na^+ channel, suggesting that with infusions during which GX accumulates, lidocaine's efficacy may be diminished (Bennett *et al.*, 1988). With infusions lasting longer than 24 hours, the clearance of lidocaine falls—an effect that has been attributed to competition between parent drug and metabolites for access to hepatic drug-metabolizing enzymes.

Plasma concentrations of lidocaine decline biexponentially after a single intravenous dose, indicating that a multicompartment model is necessary to analyze lidocaine disposition. The initial drop in plasma lidocaine following intravenous administration occurs rapidly, with a half-life of approximately 8 minutes, and represents distribution from the central compartment to peripheral tissues. The terminal elimination half-life, usually approximately 100 to 120 minutes, represents drug elimination by hepatic metabolism. Lidocaine's efficacy depends on maintenance of therapeutic plasma concentrations in the central compartment. Therefore, the administration of a single bolus dose of lidocaine can result in transient arrhythmia suppression that dissipates rapidly as the drug is distributed and concentrations in the central compartment fall. To avoid this distribution-related loss of efficacy, a loading regimen of 3 to 4 mg/kg over 20 to 30 minutes is used—*e.g.,* an initial 100 mg followed by 50 mg every 8 minutes for three doses. Subsequently, stable concentrations can be maintained in plasma with an infusion of 1 to 4 mg/min, which replaces drug removed by hepatic metabolism. The time to steady-state lidocaine concentrations is approximately 8 to 10 hours. If the maintenance infusion rate is too low, arrhythmias may recur hours after the institution of apparently successful therapy. On the other hand, if the rate is too high, toxicity may result. In either case, routine measurement of plasma lidocaine concentration at the time of expected steady state is useful in adjusting maintenance infusion rate.

In heart failure, the central volume of distribution is decreased, so the total loading dose should be decreased. Since lidocaine clearance also is decreased, the rate of the maintenance infusion should be decreased. Lidocaine clearance also is reduced in hepatic disease, during treatment with *cimetidine* or β-blockers, and during prolonged infusions (Nies *et al.*, 1976). Frequent measurement of plasma lidocaine concentration and dose adjustment to ensure that plasma concentrations remain within the therapeutic range (1.5 to 5 μg/ml) are necessary to minimize toxicity in these settings. Lidocaine is bound to the acute-phase reactant α_1-acid glycoprotein. Diseases such as acute myocardial infarction are associated with increases in α_1-acid glycoprotein and protein binding and hence a decreased proportion of free drug. These findings may explain why some patients require and tolerate higher than usual total plasma lidocaine concentrations to maintain antiarrhythmic efficacy (Kessler *et al.*, 1984).

Mexiletine and Tocainide. *Mexiletine* (MEXITIL) and *tocainide* (TONOCARD; no longer marketed in the United States) are analogs of lidocaine that have been modified to reduce first-pass hepatic metabolism and permit chronic oral therapy (Roden and Woosley, 1986b; Campbell, 1987). Their electrophysiological actions are similar to those of lidocaine. Tremor and nausea, the major dose-related adverse effects, can be minimized by taking the drugs with food. Because tocainide can cause potentially fatal bone marrow aplasia and pulmonary fibrosis, it is used rarely; it is no longer available in the United States.

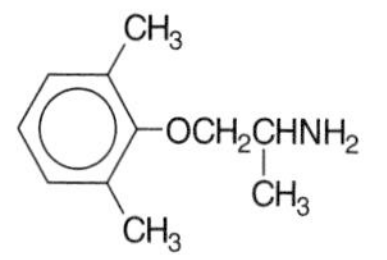

MEXILETINE

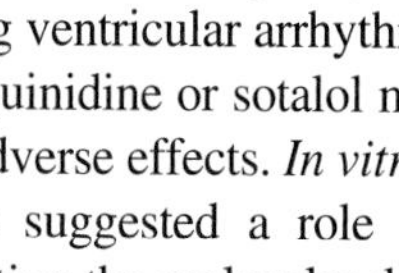

TOCAINIDE

Mexiletine undergoes hepatic metabolism, which is inducible by drugs such as phenytoin. Mexiletine is approved for treating ventricular arrhythmias; combinations of mexiletine with quinidine or sotalol may increase efficacy while reducing adverse effects. *In vitro* studies and clinical anecdotes have suggested a role for mexiletine (or flecainide) in correcting the molecular defect in the form of congenital long QT syndrome caused by abnormal Na$^+$ channel inactivation (Shimizu and Antzelevitch, 1997).

Moricizine. *Moricizine* (ETHMOZINE) is a phenothiazine analog with Na$^+$ channel–blocking properties used in the

chronic treatment of ventricular arrhythmias (Clyne *et al.*, 1992). In a randomized, double-blind trial (CAST II), moricizine increased mortality in patients shortly after a myocardial infarction and did not improve survival during long-term therapy (Cardiac Arrhythmia Suppression Trial II Investigators, 1992). Moricizine undergoes extensive first-pass hepatic metabolism; despite its short elimination half-life, its antiarrhythmic effect can persist for many hours after a single dose, suggesting that some of its metabolites may be active.

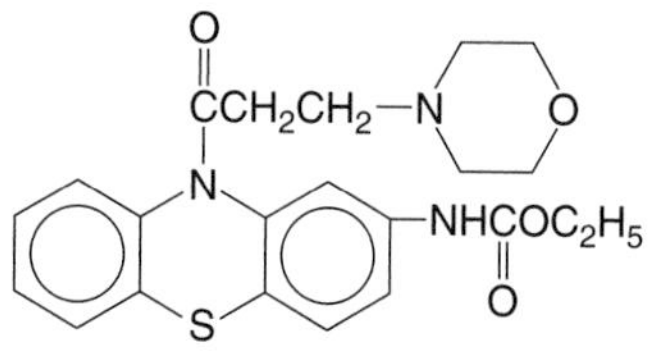

MORICIZINE

Procainamide. Procainamide (PROCAN SR, others) is an analog of the local anesthetic procaine. It exerts electrophysiological effects similar to those of quinidine but lacks quinidine's vagolytic and α adrenergic blocking activity. Procainamide is better tolerated than quinidine when given intravenously. Loading and maintenance intravenous infusions are used in the acute therapy of many supraventricular and ventricular arrhythmias. However, long-term oral treatment is poorly tolerated and often is stopped owing to adverse effects.

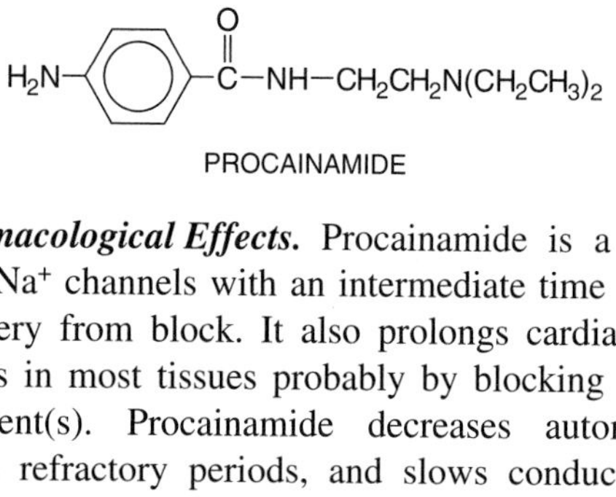

PROCAINAMIDE

Pharmacological Effects. Procainamide is a blocker of open Na$^+$ channels with an intermediate time constant of recovery from block. It also prolongs cardiac action potentials in most tissues probably by blocking outward K$^+$ current(s). Procainamide decreases automaticity, increases refractory periods, and slows conduction. Its major metabolite, *N*-acetyl procainamide, lacks the Na$^+$ channel–blocking activity of the parent drug but is equipotent in prolonging action potentials. Since the plasma concentrations of *N*-acetyl procainamide often exceed those of procainamide, increased refractoriness and QT prolongation during chronic procainamide therapy may be partly attributable to the metabolite. However, it is the parent drug that slows conduction and produces QRS-interval prolongation. Although hypotension may occur at high plasma concentrations, this effect usually is attributable to ganglionic blockade rather than to any negative inotropic effect, which is minimal.

Adverse Effects. Hypotension and marked slowing of conduction are major adverse effects of high concentrations (>10 $\mu g/ml$) of procainamide, especially during intravenous use. Dose-related nausea is frequent during oral therapy and may be attributable in part to high plasma concentrations of N-acetyl procainamide. *Torsades de pointes* can occur, particularly when plasma concentrations of N-acetyl procainamide rise to greater than 30 $\mu g/$ ml. Procainamide produces potentially fatal bone marrow aplasia in 0.2% of patients; the mechanism is not known, but high plasma drug concentrations are not suspected.

During long-term therapy, most patients will develop biochemical evidence of the drug-induced lupus syndrome, such as circulating antinuclear antibodies (Woosley *et al.*, 1978). Therapy need not be interrupted merely because of the presence of antinuclear antibodies. However, 25% to 50% of patients eventually develop symptoms of the lupus syndrome; common early symptoms are rash and small-joint arthralgias. Other symptoms of lupus, including pericarditis with tamponade, can occur, although renal involvement is unusual. The lupuslike symptoms resolve on cessation of therapy or during treatment with N-acetyl procainamide (*see* below).

Clinical Pharmacokinetics. Procainamide is eliminated rapidly ($t_{\frac{1}{2}}$ = 3 to 4 hours) by both renal excretion of unchanged drug and hepatic metabolism. The major pathway for hepatic metabolism is conjugation by N-acetyl transferase, whose activity is determined genetically, to form N-acetyl procainamide. N-Acetyl procainamide is eliminated by renal excretion ($t_{\frac{1}{2}}$ = 6 to 10 hours) and is not significantly converted back to procainamide. Because of the relatively rapid elimination rates of both the parent drug and its major metabolite, oral procainamide usually is administered as a slow-release formulation. In patients with renal failure, procainamide and/or N-acetyl procainamide can accumulate to potentially toxic plasma concentrations. Reduction of procainamide dose and dosing frequency and monitoring of plasma concentrations of both compounds are required in this situation. Because the parent drug and metabolite exert different pharmacological effects, the practice of using the sum of their concentrations to guide therapy is inappropriate.

In individuals who are "slow acetylators," the procainamide-induced lupus syndrome develops more often and earlier during treatment than among rapid acetylators (Woosley *et al.*, 1978). In addition, the symptoms of procainamide-induced lupus resolve during treatment with N-acetyl procainamide. Both these findings support results of *in vitro* studies suggesting that it is chronic

exposure to the parent drug (or an oxidative metabolite) that results in the lupus syndrome; these findings also provided one rationale for the further development of N-acetyl procainamide and its analogs as antiarrhythmic agents (Roden, 1993).

Propafenone. *Propafenone* (RYTHMOL) is an Na^+ channel blocker with a relatively slow time constant for recovery from block (Funck-Brentano *et al.*, 1990). Some data suggest that, like flecainide, propafenone also blocks K^+ channels. Its major electrophysiological effect is to slow conduction in fast-response tissues. The drug is prescribed as a racemate; while the enantiomers do not differ in their Na^+ channel–blocking properties, S-(+)-propafenone is a β adrenergic receptor antagonist *in vitro* and in some patients. Propafenone prolongs PR and QRS durations. Chronic therapy with oral propafenone is used to maintain sinus rhythm in patients with supraventricular tachycardias, including atrial fibrillation; like other Na^+ channel blockers, it also can be used in ventricular arrhythmias, but with only modest efficacy.

$$CH_2-CH_2-CO$$
$$O-CH_2-CHOH-CH_2$$
$$NH-C_3H_7$$

PROPAFENONE

Adverse effects during propafenone therapy include acceleration of ventricular response in patients with atrial flutter, increased frequency or severity of episodes of re-entrant ventricular tachycardia, exacerbation of heart failure, and the adverse effects of β adrenergic blockade, such as sinus bradycardia and bronchospasm (*see* above and Chapter 10).

Clinical Pharmacokinetics. Propafenone is well absorbed and is eliminated by both hepatic and renal routes. The activity of CYP2D6, an enzyme that functionally is absent in approximately 7% of Caucasians and African-Americans (*see* Chapter 3), is a major determinant of plasma propafenone concentration and thus the clinical action of the drug. In most subjects ("extensive metabolizers"), propafenone undergoes extensive first-pass hepatic metabolism to 5-hydroxy propafenone, a metabolite equipotent to propafenone as an Na^+ channel blocker but much less potent as a β adrenergic receptor antagonist. A second metabolite, N-desalkyl propafenone, is formed by non-CYP2D6-mediated metabolism and is a less potent blocker of Na^+ channels and β adrenergic receptors. CYP2D6-mediated metabolism of propafenone is saturable, so small increases in dose can increase plasma propafenone concentration disproportionately. In "poor metabolizer" subjects, in whom functional CYP2D6 is absent, first-pass hepatic metabolism is much less than in extensive metabolizers, and plasma propafenone concentrations will be much higher after an equal dose. The incidence of adverse effects during propafenone therapy is significantly higher in poor metabolizers.

CYP2D6 activity can be inhibited markedly by a number of drugs, including quinidine and fluoxetine. In extensive metabolizer subjects receiving such drugs or in poor metabolizer subjects, plasma propafenone concentrations of more than 1 μg/ml are associated with clinical effects of β adrenergic receptor blockade, such as reduction of exercise heart rate (Lee *et al.*, 1990). It is recommended that dosage in patients with moderate to severe liver disease should be reduced to approximately 20% to 30% of the usual dose, with careful monitoring. It is not known if propafenone doses must be decreased in patients with renal disease. A slow-release formulation allows twice-daily dosing.

Quinidine. As early as the 18th century, the bark of the cinchona plant was used to treat "rebellious palpitations" (Levy and Azoulay, 1994). Studies in the early 20th century identified quinidine, a diastereomer of the antimalarial quinine, as the most potent of the antiarrhythmic substances extracted from the cinchona plant, and by the 1920s, quinidine was used as an antiarrhythmic agent. Quinidine is used to maintain sinus rhythm in patients with atrial flutter or atrial fibrillation and to prevent recurrence of ventricular tachycardia or ventricular fibrillation (Grace and Camm, 1998).

CH$_2$=CH

HO

CH$_3$O

N

QUINIDINE

Pharmacological Effects. Quinidine (various generic preparations) blocks Na$^+$ current and multiple cardiac K$^+$ currents. It is an open-state blocker of Na$^+$ channels, with a time constant of recovery in the intermediate (~3 seconds) range; as a consequence, QRS duration increases modestly, usually by 10% to 20%, at therapeutic dosages. At therapeutic concentrations, quinidine commonly prolongs the QT interval up to 25%, but the effect is highly variable. At concentrations as low as 1 μM, quinidine blocks Na$^+$ current and the rapid component of delayed rectifier (I_{Kr}); higher concentrations block the slow component of delayed rectifier, inward rectifier, transient outward current, and L-type Ca^{2+} current.

Quinidine's Na$^+$ channel–blocking properties result in an increased threshold for excitability and decreased automaticity. As a consequence of its K$^+$ channel–blocking actions, quinidine prolongs action potentials in most cardiac cells, most prominently at slow heart rates. In some cells, such as midmyocardial cells and Purkinje cells, quinidine consistently elicits EADs at slow heart rates, particularly when [K]$_o$ is low (Priori *et al.*, 1999). Quinidine prolongs refractoriness in most tissues probably as a result of both prolongation of action potential duration and Na$^+$ channel blockade.

In intact animals and humans, quinidine also produces α adrenergic receptor blockade and vagal inhibition. Thus the intravenous use of quinidine is associated with marked hypotension and sinus tachycardia. Quinidine's vagolytic effects tend to inhibit its direct depressant effect on AV nodal conduction, so the effect of drug on the PR interval is variable. Moreover, quinidine's vagolytic effect can result in increased AV nodal transmission of atrial tachycardias such as atrial flutter (Table 34–1).

Adverse Effects. *Noncardiac.* Diarrhea is the most common adverse effect during quinidine therapy, occurring in 30% to 50% of patients; the mechanism is not known. Diarrhea usually occurs within the first several days of quinidine therapy but can occur later. Diarrhea-induced hypokalemia may potentiate *torsades de pointes* due to quinidine.

A number of immunological reactions can occur during quinidine therapy. The most common is thrombocytopenia, which can be severe but which resolves rapidly with discontinuation of the drug. Hepatitis, bone marrow depression, and lupus syndrome occur rarely. None of these effects is related to elevated plasma quinidine concentrations.

Quinidine also can produce cinchonism, a syndrome that includes headache and tinnitus. In contrast to other adverse responses to quinidine therapy, cinchonism usually is related to elevated plasma quinidine concentrations and can be managed by dose reduction.

Cardiac. Between 2% and 8% of patients who receive quinidine therapy will develop marked QT-interval prolongation and *torsades de pointes*. In contrast to effects of sotalol, *N*-acetyl procainamide, and many other drugs, quinidine-associated *torsades de pointes* generally occurs at therapeutic or even subtherapeutic plasma concentrations. The reasons for individual susceptibility to this adverse effect are not known.

At high plasma concentrations of quinidine, marked Na$^+$ channel block can occur, with resulting ventricular tachycardia. This adverse effect occurs when very high doses of quinidine are used to try to convert atrial fibrillation to normal rhythm; this aggressive approach to quinidine dosing has been abandoned, and quinidine-induced ventricular tachycardia is unusual.

Quinidine can exacerbate heart failure or conduction system disease. However, in most patients with congestive heart failure, quinidine is well tolerated, perhaps because of its vasodilating actions.

Clinical Pharmacokinetics. Quinidine is well absorbed and is 80% bound to plasma proteins, including albumin and, like lidocaine, the acute-phase reactant α_1-acid glycoprotein. As with lidocaine, greater than usual doses (and total plasma quinidine concentrations) may be required to maintain therapeutic concentrations of free quinidine in high-stress states such as acute myocardial infarction (Kessler *et al.*, 1984). Quinidine undergoes extensive hepatic oxidative metabolism, and approximately 20% is excreted unchanged by the kidneys. One metabolite, 3-hydroxyquinidine, is nearly as potent as quinidine in blocking cardiac Na$^+$ channels and prolonging cardiac action potentials. Concentrations of unbound 3-hydroxyquinidine equal to or exceeding those of quinidine are tolerated by some patients. Other metabolites are less potent than quinidine, and their plasma concentrations are lower; thus they are unlikely to contribute significantly to the clinical effects of quinidine.

There is substantial individual variability in the range of dosages required to achieve therapeutic plasma concentrations of 2 to 5 μg/ml. Some of this variability may be assay-dependent because not all assays exclude quinidine metabolites. In patients with advanced renal disease or congestive heart failure, quinidine clearance is decreased only modestly. Thus, dosage requirements in these patients are similar to those in other patients.

Drug Interactions. Quinidine is a potent inhibitor of CYP2D6. As a result, the administration of quinidine to patients receiving drugs that undergo extensive CYP2D6-mediated metabolism may result in altered drug effects owing to accumulation of parent drug and failure of metabolite formation. For example, inhibition of CYP2D6-mediated metabolism of *codeine* to its active metabolite *morphine* results in decreased analgesia. On the other hand, inhibition of CYP2D6-mediated metabolism of propafenone results in elevated plasma propafenone concentrations and increased β adrenergic receptor blockade. Quinidine reduces the clearance of digoxin and digitoxin; inhibition of P-glycoprotein–mediated digoxin transport has been implicated (Fromm *et al.*, 1999).

Quinidine metabolism is induced by drugs such as *phenobarbital* and phenytoin (Data *et al.*, 1976). In patients receiving these agents, very high doses of quinidine may be required to achieve therapeutic concentrations. If therapy with the inducing agent is then stopped, quinidine concentrations may rise to very high levels, and its dosage must be adjusted downward. Cimetidine and verapamil also elevate plasma quinidine concentrations, but these effects usually are modest.

Sotalol.　Sotalol (BETAPACE, BETAPACE AF) is a nonselective β adrenergic receptor antagonist that also prolongs cardiac action potentials by inhibiting delayed rectifier and possibly other K$^+$ currents (Hohnloser and Woosley, 1994). Sotalol is prescribed as a racemate; the L-enantiomer is a much more potent β adrenergic receptor antagonist than the D-enantiomer, but the two are equipotent as K$^+$ channel blockers. Its structure is shown below:

$$CH_3SO_2NH-\text{\textcircled{}}-\overset{\overset{\displaystyle OH}{|}}{CH}CH_2NHCH(CH_3)_2$$

SOTALOL

In the United States, racemic sotalol is approved for use in patients with both ventricular tachyarrhythmias and atrial fibrillation or flutter. Clinical trials suggest that it is at least as effective as most Na$^+$ channel blockers in ventricular arrhythmias (Mason, 1993).

Sotalol prolongs action potential duration throughout the heart and QT interval on the ECG. It decreases automaticity, slows AV nodal conduction, and prolongs AV refractoriness by blocking both K$^+$ channels and β adrenergic receptors, but it exerts no effect on conduction velocity in fast-response tissue. Sotalol causes EADs and triggered activity *in vitro* and can cause *torsades de pointes,* especially when the serum K$^+$ concentration is low. Unlike the situation with quinidine, the incidence of *torsades de pointes* seems to depend on the dose of sotalol; indeed, *torsades de pointes* is the major toxicity with sotalol overdose. Occasional cases occur at low dosages, often in patients with renal dysfunction, because sotalol is eliminated by renal excretion of unchanged drug. The other adverse effects of sotalol therapy are those associated with β adrenergic receptor blockade (*see* above and Chapter 10).

Magnesium.　The intravenous administration of 1 to 2 g MgSO$_4$ reportedly is effective in preventing recurrent episodes of *torsades de pointes,* even if the serum Mg^{2+} concentration is normal (Tzivoni *et al.*, 1988). However, controlled studies of this effect have not been performed. The mechanism of action is unknown because the QT interval is not shortened; an effect on the inward current, possibly a Ca^{2+} current, responsible for the triggered upstroke arising from EADs (*black arrow,* Figure 34–6B) is possible. Intravenous Mg^{2+} also has been used successfully in arrhythmias related to digitalis intoxication. Large placebo-controlled trials of intravenous magnesium to improve outcome in acute myocardial infarction have yielded conflicting results (Woods and Fletcher, 1994; ISIS-4 Collaborative Group, 1995). While oral Mg^{2+} supplements may be useful in preventing hypomagnesemia, there is no evidence that chronic Mg^{2+} ingestion exerts a direct antiarrhythmic action.

BIBLIOGRAPHY

Akiyama, T., Pawitan, Y., Greenberg, H., *et al.* Increased risk of death and cardiac arrest from encainide and flecainide in patients after non-Q-wave acute myocardial infarction in the Cardiac Arrhythmia Suppression Trial. The CAST Investigators. *Am. J. Cardiol.,* **1991,** *68*:1551–1555.

Amiodarone Trials Meta-Analysis Investigators. Effect of prophylactic amiodarone on mortality after acute myocardial infarction and in congestive heart failure—Meta-analysis of individual data from 6500 patients in randomised trials. *Lancet,* **1997,** *350*:1417–1424.

Anderson, J.L., Rodier, H.E., and Green, L.S. Comparative effects of β-adrenergic blocking drugs on experimental ventricular fibrillation threshold. *Am. J. Cardiol.,* **1983,** *51*:1196–1202.

Anderson, J.L., Gilbert, E.M., Alpert, B.L., *et al.* Prevention of symptomatic recurrences of paroxysmal atrial fibrillation in patients initially tolerating antiarrhythmic therapy: A multicenter, double-blind, crossover study of flecainide and placebo with transtelephonic monitoring. Flecainide Supraventricular Tachycardia Study Group. *Circulation,* **1989,** *80*:1557–1570.

Antzelevitch, C., Sicouri, S., Litovsky, S.H., *et al.* Heterogeneity within the ventricular wall: electrophysiology and pharmacology of epicardial, endocardial, and M cells. *Circ. Res.,* **1991,** *69*:1427–1449.

Balser, J.R., Nuss, H.B., Orias, D.W., *et al.* Local anesthetics as effectors of allosteric gating: Lidocaine effects on inactivation-deficient rat skeletal muscle Na channels. *J. Clin. Invest.,* **1996,** *98*:2874–2886.

Bean, B.P., Two kinds of calcium channels in canine atrial cells. Differences in kinetics, selectivity, and pharmacology. *J. Gen. Physiol.,* **1985,** *86*:1–30.

Bennett, P.B., Woosley, R.L., and Hondeghem, L.M. Competition between lidocaine and one of its metabolites, glycylxylidide, for cardiac sodium channels. *Circulation,* **1988,** *78*:692–700.

Biaggioni, I., Killian, T.J., Mosqueda-Garcia, R., *et al.* Adenosine increases sympathetic nerve traffic in humans. *Circulation,* **1991,** *83*:1668–1675.

Brown, M.J., Brown, D.C., and Murphy, M.B. Hypokalemia from β_2-receptor stimulation by circulating epinephrine. *New Engl. J. Med.,* **1983,** *309*:1414–1419.

Cardiac Arrhythmia Suppression Trial II Investigators. Effect of the antiarrhythmic agent moricizine on survival after myocardial infarction. *New Engl. J. Med.,* **1992,** *327*:227–233.

CAST Investigators. Preliminary report: Effect of encainide and flecainide on mortality in a randomized trial of arrhythmia suppression after myocardial infarction. *New Engl. J. Med.,* **1989,** *321*:406–412.

Crijns, H.J., van Gelder, I.C., and Lie, K.I. Supraventricular tachycardia mimicking ventricular tachycardia during flecainide treatment. *Am. J. Cardiol.,* **1988,** *62*:1303–1306.

Data, J.L., Wilkinson, G.R., and Nies, A.S. Interaction of quinidine with anticonvulsant drugs. *New Engl. J. Med.,* **1976,** *294*:699–702.

Dorian, P., Cass, D., Schwartz, B., *et al.* Amiodarone as compared with lidocaine for shock-resistant ventricular fibrillation. *New Engl. J. Med.,* **2002,** *346*:884–890.

Dusman, R.E., Stanton, M.S., Miles, W.M., *et al.* Clinical features of amiodarone-induced pulmonary toxicity. *Circulation,* **1990,** *82*:51–59.

Echizen, H., Vogelgesang, B., and Eichelbaum, M. Effects of D,L-verapamil on atrioventricular conduction in relation to its stereoselective first-pass metabolism. *Clin. Pharmacol. Ther.,* **1985,** *38*:71–76.

Echt, D.S., Black, J.N., Barbey, J.T., *et al.* Evaluation of antiarrhythmic drugs on defibrillation energy requirements in dogs: sodium channel block and action potential prolongation. *Circulation,* **1989,** *79*:1106–1117.

Follmer, C.H., and Colatsky, T.J. Block of delayed rectifier potassium current, I_K, by flecainide and E-4031 in cat ventricular myocytes. *Circulation,* **1990,** *82*:289–293.

Fromm, M.F., Kim, R.B., Stein, C.M., *et al.* Inhibition of P-glycoprotein-mediated drug transport: A unifying mechanism to explain the interaction between digoxin and quinidine. *Circulation,* **1999,** *99*:552–557.

Gross, A.S., Mikus, G., Fischer, C., *et al.* Stereoselective disposition of flecainide in relation to sparteine/debrisoquine metaboliser phenotype. *Br. J. Clin. Pharmacol.,* **1989,** *28*:555–566.

Henthorn, R.W., Waldo, A.L., Anderson, J.L., *et al.* Flecainide acetate prevents recurrence of symptomatic paroxysmal supraventricular tachycardia. The Flecainide Supraventricular Tachycardia Study Group. *Circulation,* **1991,** *83*:119–125.

Herbette, L.G., Trumbore, M., Chester, D.W., and Katz, A.M. Possible molecular basis for the pharmacokinetics and pharmacodynamics of three membrane-active drugs: Propranolol, nimodipine and amiodarone. *J. Mol. Cell Cardiol.,* **1988,** *20*:373–378.

Hine, L.K., Laird, N., Hewitt, P., and Chalmers, T.C. Meta-analytic evidence against prophylactic use of lidocaine in acute myocardial infarction. *Arch. Intern. Med.,* **1989,** *149*:2694–2698.

Hume, J.R., and Harvey, R.D. Chloride conductance pathways in heart. *Am. J. Physiol.,* **1991,** *261*:C399–C412.

Ikeda, N., Singh, B.N., Davis, L.D., and Hauswirth, O. Effects of flecainide on the electrophysiologic properties of isolated canine and rabbit myocardial fibers. *J. Am. Coll. Cardiol.,* **1985,** *5*:303–310.

ISIS-4 Collaborative Group. ISIS-4: a randomised factorial trial assessing early oral captopril, oral mononitrate, and intravenous magnesium sulphate in 58,050 patients with suspected acute myocardial infarction. ISIS-4 (Fourth International Study of Infarct Survival) Collaborative Group. *Lancet,* **1995,** *345*:669–685.

Keating, M.T., and Sanguinetti, M.C. Molecular and cellular mechanisms of cardiac arrhythmias. *Cell,* **2001,** *104*:569–580.

Kessler, K.M., Kissane, B., Cassidy, J., *et al.* Dynamic variability of binding of antiarrhythmic drugs during the evolution of acute myocardial infarction. *Circulation,* **1984,** *70*:472–478.

Kowey, P.R., Levine, J.H., Herre, J.M., *et al.* Randomized, double-blind comparison of intravenous amiodarone and bretylium in the treatment of patients with recurrent, hemodynamically destabilizing ventricular tachycardia or fibrillation. The Intravenous Amiodarone Multicenter Investigators Group. *Circulation.,* **1995,** *92*:3255–3263.

Krapivinsky, G., Gordon, E.A., Wickman, K., *et al.* The G protein–gated atrial K⁺ channel I_{KACh} is a heteromultimer of two inwardly rectifying K⁺-channel proteins. *Nature,* **1995,** *374*:135–141.

Kroemer, H.K., Turgeon, J., Parker, R.A., and Roden, D.M. Flecainide enantiomers: Disposition in human subjects and electrophysiologic actions in vitro. *Clin. Pharmacol. Ther.,* **1989,** *46*:584–590.

Lee, J.H., and Rosen, M.R. Use-dependent actions and effects on transmembrane action potentials of flecainide, encainide, and ethmozine in canine Purkinje fibers. *J. Cardiovasc. Pharmacol.,* **1991,** *18*:285–292.

Lee, J.T., Kroemer, H.K., Silberstein, D.J., *et al.* The role of genetically determined polymorphic drug metabolism in the beta-blockade produced by propafenone. *New Engl. J. Med.,* **1990,** *322*:1764–1768.

Lerman, B.B., and Belardinelli, L. Cardiac electrophysiology of adenosine: Basic and clinical concepts. *Circulation,* **1991,** *83*:1499–1509.

Levine, J.H., Moore, E.N., Kadish, A.H., *et al.* Mechanisms of depressed conduction from long-term amiodarone therapy in canine myocardium. *Circulation,* **1988,** *78*:684–691.

Lie, K.I., Wellens, H.J., van Capelle, F.J., and Durrer, D. Lidocaine in the prevention of primary ventricular fibrillation: A double-blind, randomized study of 212 consecutive patients. *New Engl. J. Med.,* **1974,** *291*:1324–1326.

Lima, J.J., Boudoulas, H., and Blanford, M. Concentration-dependence of disopyramide binding to plasma protein and its influence on kinetics and dynamics. *J. Pharmacol. Exp. Ther.,* **1981,** *219*:741–747.

MacKinnon, R. Potassium channels. *FEBS Lett.,* **2003,** *555*:62–65.

Makkar, R.R., Fromm, B.S., Steinman, R.T., *et al.* Female gender as a risk factor for torsades de pointes associated with cardiovascular drugs. *JAMA,* **1993,** *270*:2590–2597.

Mason, J.W. A comparison of seven antiarrhythmic drugs in patients with ventricular tachyarrhythmias. Electrophysiologic Study versus Electrocardiographic Monitoring Investigators. *New Engl. J. Med.,* **1993,** *329*:452–458.

Mitcheson, J.S., Chen, J., Lin, M., *et al.* A structural basis for drug-induced long QT syndrome. *Proc. Natl. Acad. Sci. U.S.A.,* **2000,** *97*:12329–12333.

Myerburg, R.J., Kessler, K.M., Cox, M.M., *et al.* Reversal of proarrhythmic effects of flecainide acetate and encainide hydrochloride by propranolol. *Circulation,* **1989,** *80*:1571–1579.

Nies, A.S., Shand, D.G., and Wilkinson, G.R. Altered hepatic blood flow and drug disposition. *Clin. Pharmacokinet.,* **1976,** *1*:135–155.

Podrid, P.J., Schoeneberger, A., and Lown, B. Congestive heart failure caused by oral disopyramide. *New Engl. J. Med.,* **1980,** *302*:614–617.

Pogwizd, S.M., and Bers, D.M. Cellular basis of triggered arrhythmias in heart failure. *Trends Cardiovasc. Med.,* **2004,** *14*:61–66.

Ranger, S., Talajic, M., Lemery, R., *et al.* Amplification of flecainide-induced ventricular conduction slowing by exercise: A potentially significant clinical consequence of use-dependent sodium channel blockade. *Circulation.,* **1989,** *79*:1000–1006.

Roden, D.M. Drug-induced prolongation of the QT Interval. *New Engl. J. Med.,* **2004,** *350*:1013–1022.

Roden, D.M. Antiarrhythmic drugs: Past, present and future. *J. Cardiovasc. Electrophysiol.,* **2003,** *14*:1389–1396.

Roy, D., Talajic, M., Dorian, P., *et al.* Amiodarone to prevent recurrence of atrial fibrillation. Canadian Trial of Atrial Fibrillation Investigators. *New Engl. J. Med.,* **2000,** *342*:913–920.

Ruskin, J.N. The cardiac arrhythmia suppression trial (CAST). *New Engl. J. Med.,* **1989,** *321*:386–388.

Sanguinetti, M.C., and Jurkiewicz, N.K. Two components of cardiac delayed rectifier K⁺ current: differential sensitivity to block by class III antiarrhythmic agents. *J. Gen. Physiol.,* **1990,** *96*:195–215.

Sanguinetti, M.C., Jurkiewicz, N.K., Scott, A., and Siegl, P.K. Isoproterenol antagonizes prolongation of refractory period by the class III antiarrhythmic agent E-4031 in guinea pig myocytes: Mechanism of action. *Circ. Res.,* **1991,** *68*:77–84.

Shimizu, W., and Antzelevitch, C. Sodium channel block with mexiletine is effective in reducing dispersion of repolarization and preventing *torsade des pointes* in LQT2 and LQT3 models of the long-QT syndrome. *Circulation,* **1997,** *96*:2038–2047.

Singer, D.E. Anticoagulation for atrial fibrillation: Epidemiology informing a difficult clinical decision. *Proc. Assoc. Am. Phys.,* **1996,** *108*:29–36.

Stewart, R.B., Bardy, G.H., and Greene, H.L. Wide complex tachycardia: Misdiagnosis and outcome after emergent therapy. *Ann. Intern. Med.,* **1986,** *104*:766–771.

Sung, R.J., Shapiro, W.A., Shen, E.N., *et al.* Effects of verapamil on ventricular tachycardias possibly caused by reentry, automaticity, and triggered activity. *J. Clin. Invest.,* **1983,** *72*:350–360.

Torp-Pedersen, C., Moller, M., Bloch-Thomsen, P.E., *et al.* Dofetilide in patients with congestive heart failure and left ventricular dysfunction. Danish Investigations of Arrhythmia and Mortality on Dofetilide Study Group. *New Engl. J. Med.,* **1999,** *341*:857–865.

Tseng, G.N., and Hoffman, B.F. Two components of transient outward current in canine ventricular myocytes. *Circ. Res.,* **1989,** *64*:633–647.

Tzivoni, D., Banai, S., Schuger, C., *et al.* Treatment of *torsade de pointes* with magnesium sulfate. *Circulation,* **1988,** *77*:392–397.

Wang, Z.G., Pelletier, L.C., Talajic, M., and Nattel, S. Effects of flecainide and quinidine on human atrial action potentials: Role of rate-dependence and comparison with guinea pig, rabbit, and dog tissues. *Circulation,* **1990,** *82*:274–283.

Weiss, J.N., Garfinkel, A., and Chen, P.S. Novel approaches to identifying antiarrhythmic drugs. *Trends Cardiovasc. Med.,* **2003,** *13*:326–330.

Weiss, J.N., Nademanee, K., Stevenson, W.G., and Singh, B. Ventricular arrhythmias in ischemic heart disease. *Ann. Intern. Med.,* **1991,** *114*:784–797.

Wenckebach, K.F. Cinchona derivates in the treatment of heart disorders. *JAMA,* **1923,** *81*:472–474.

Wit, A.L., Dillon, S.M., Coromilas, J., *et al.* Anisotropic reentry in the epicardial border zone of myocardial infarcts. *Ann. N.Y. Acad. Sci.,* **1990,** *591*:86–108.

Woods, K.L., and Fletcher, S. Long-term outcome after intravenous magnesium sulphate in suspected acute myocardial infarction: The second Leicester Intravenous Magnesium Intervention Trial (LIMIT-2). *Lancet,* **1994,** *343*:816–819.

Woosley, R.L., Drayer, D.E., Reidenberg, M.M., *et al.* Effect of acetylator phenotype on the rate at which procainamide induces antinuclear antibodies and the lupus syndrome. *New Engl. J. Med.,* **1978,** *298*:1157–1159.

MONOGRAPHS AND REVIEWS

Campbell, R.W. Mexiletine. *New Engl. J. Med.,* **1987,** *316*:29–34.

Clyne, C.A., Estes, N.A., III, and Wang, P.J. Moricizine. *New Engl. J. Med.,* **1992,** *327*:255–260.

Courtney, K.R. Progress and prospects for optimum antiarrhythmic drug design. *Cardiovasc. Drugs Ther.,* **1987,** *1*:117–123.

Connolly, S.J. Evidence-based analysis of amiodarone efficacy and safety. *Circulation,* **1999,** *100*:2025–2034.

DiFrancesco, D. Pacemaker mechanisms in cardiac tissue. *Annu. Rev. Physiol.,* **1993,** *55*:455–472.

Fozzard, H.A., and Arnsdorf, M.F. Cardiac electrophysiology. In, *The Heart and Cardiovascular System: Scientific Foundations.* (Fozzard,

H.A., Haber, E., Jennings, R.B., Katz, A.M., and Morgan, H.E., eds.) Raven Press, New York, **1991,** pp. 63–98.

Frishman, W.H., Murthy, S., and Strom, J.A. Ultra-short-acting β-adrenergic blockers. *Med. Clin. North Am.,* **1988,** *72:*359–372.

Funck-Brentano, C., Kroemer, H.K., Lee, J.T., and Roden, D.M. Propafenone. *New Engl. J. Med.,* **1990,** *322:*518–525.

Grace, A.A., and Camm, J. Quinidine. *New Engl. J. Med.,* **1998,** *338:* 35–45.

Hohnloser, S.H., and Woosley, R.L. Sotalol. *New Engl. J. Med.,* **1994,** *331:*31–38.

Levy, S., and Azoulay, S. Stories about the origin of quinquina and quinidine. *J. Cardiovasc. Electrophysiol.,* **1994,** *5:*635–636.

Mason, J.W. Amiodarone. *New Engl. J. Med.,* **1987,** *316:*455–466.

Morady, F. Radio-frequency ablation as treatment for cardiac arrhythmias. *New Engl. J. Med.,* **1999,** *340:*534–544.

Morady, F., Scheinman, M.M., and Desai, J. Disopyramide. *Ann. Intern. Med.,* **1982,** *96:*337–343.

Murray, K.T. Ibutilide. *Circulation,* **1998,** *97:*493–497.

Priori, S.G., Barhanin, J., Hauer, R.N., *et al.* Genetic and molecular basis of cardiac arrhythmias: Impact on clinical management. Study group on molecular basis of arrhythmias of the Working Group on Arrhythmias of the European Society of Cardiology. *Eur. Heart J.,* **1999,** *20:*174–195.

Roden, D.M. Current status of class III antiarrhythmic drug therapy. *Am. J. Cardiol.,* **1993,** *72:*44B–49B.

Roden, D.M. Risks and benefits of antiarrhythmic therapy. *New Engl. J. Med.,* **1994,** *331:*785–791.

Roden, D.M., Echt, D.S., Lee, J.T, and Murray, K.T. Clinical Pharmacology of antiarrhythmic agents. In, *Sudden Cardiac Death.* (Josephson, M.E., ed.) Blackwell Scientific, London, **1993,** pp. 182–185.

Roden, D.M., and Spooner, P.M. Inherited long QT syndromes: A paradigm for understanding arrhythmogenesis. *J. Cardiovasc. Electrophysiol.,* **1999,** *10:*1664–1683.

Roden, D.M., and Woosley, R.L. Drug therapy: Flecainide. *New Engl. J. Med.,* **1986a,** *315:*36–41.

Roden, D.M., and Woosley, R.L. Drug therapy: Tocainide. *New Engl. J. Med.,* **1986b,** *315:*41–45.

Schwartz, P.J., Priori, S.G., and Napolitano, C. Long QT syndrome. In, *Cardiac Electrophysiology: From Cell to Bedside,* 3d ed. (Zipes, D.P., and Jalife, J., eds.) Saunders, Philadelphia, **2000,** pp. 615–640.

Singh, B.N. Advantages of beta blockers versus antiarrhythmic agents and calcium antagonists in secondary prevention after myocardial infarction. *Am. J. Cardiol.,* **1990,** *66:*9C–20C.

Singh, B.N. Arrhythmia control by prolonging repolarization: the concept and its potential therapeutic impact. *Eur. Heart J.,* **1993,** *14*(suppl H):14–23.

Smith, T.W. Digitalis: Mechanisms of action and clinical use. *New Engl. J. Med.,* **1988,** *318:*358–365.

Snyders, D.J., Hondeghem, L.M., and Bennett, P.B. Mechanisms of drug-channel interaction. In, *The Heart and Cardiovascular System: Scientific Foundations.* (Fozzard, H.A., Haber, E., Jennings, R.B., Katz, A.M., and Morgan, H.E., eds.) Raven Press, New York, **1991,** pp. 2165–2193.

Task Force of the Working Group on Arrhythmias of the European Society of Cardiology. The Sicilian gambit: A new approach to the classification of antiarrhythmic drugs based on their actions on arrhythmogenic mechanisms. *Circulation,* **1991,** *84:*1831–1851.

Vaughan Williams, E.M. Classifying antiarrhythmic actions: by facts or speculation. *J. Clin. Pharmacol.,* **1992,** *32:*964–977.

DRUG THERAPY FOR HYPERCHOLESTEROLEMIA AND DYSLIPIDEMIA

Robert W. Mahley and Thomas P. Bersot

Hyperlipidemia is a major cause of atherosclerosis and atherosclerosis-associated conditions, such as coronary heart disease (CHD), ischemic cerebrovascular disease, and peripheral vascular disease. Although the incidence of these atherosclerosis-related events has declined in the United States, these conditions still account for the majority of morbidity and mortality among middle-aged and older adults. The incidence and absolute number of annual events will likely increase over the next decade because of the epidemic of obesity and the aging of the U.S. population. Dyslipidemias, including hyperlipidemia (hypercholesterolemia) and low levels of high-density-lipoprotein cholesterol (HDL-C), are major causes of increased atherogenic risk; both genetic disorders and lifestyle (sedentary behavior and diets high in calories, saturated fat, and cholesterol) contribute to the dyslipidemias seen in developed countries around the world. This chapter focuses on drug therapy: 3-hydroxy-3-methylglutaryl coenzyme A (HMG-CoA) reductase inhibitors—the statins—which are the most effective and best tolerated drugs currently in use for treating dyslipidemia, bile acid–binding resins, nicotinic acid (*niacin*), fibric acid derivatives, and the cholesterol absorption inhibitor *ezetimibe*. Despite the efficacy of drug therapy, alterations in lifestyle have a far greater potential for reducing vascular disease risk and at a lower cost.

Recognition that dyslipidemia is a risk factor has led to the development of drugs that reduce cholesterol levels. These drugs provide benefit in patients across the entire spectrum of cholesterol levels, primarily by reducing levels of low-density lipoprotein cholesterol (LDL-C). In well-controlled clinical trials, fatal and nonfatal CHD events and strokes were reduced by as much as 30% to 40% (Scandinavian Simvastatin Survival Study, 1994;

Shepherd *et al.*, 1995; The Long-Term Intervention with Pravastatin in Ischaemic Disease [LIPID] Study Group, 1998; Heart Protection Study Collaborative Group, 2002; Heart Protection Study Collaborative Group, 2003; Law *et al.*, 2003).

Clinical trial data support extending lipid-lowering therapy to high-risk patients whose major lipid risk factor is a reduced plasma level of HDL-C, even if their LDL-C level does not meet the existing threshold values for initiating hypolipidemic drug therapy (The Expert Panel, 2002). In patients with low HDL-C and average LDL-C levels, appropriate drug therapy reduced CHD endpoint events by 20% to 35% (Heart Protection Study Collaborative Group, 2002; Downs *et al.*, 1998; Rubins *et al.*, 1999). Since two-thirds of patients with CHD in the United States have low HDL-C levels (<40 mg/dl), it is important to include low-HDL patients in management guidelines for dyslipidemia, even if their LDL-C levels are in the normal range (Bersot *et al.*, 2003).

Severe hypertriglyceridemia (*i.e.,* triglyceride levels of >1000 mg/dl) requires therapy to prevent pancreatitis. Moderately elevated triglyceride levels (150 to 400 mg/dl) also are of concern because they often occur as part of the metabolic syndrome, which includes insulin resistance, obesity, hypertension, low HDL-C levels, and substantially increased CHD risk. The atherogenic dyslipidemia in patients with the metabolic syndrome is characterized by moderately elevated triglycerides, low HDL-C levels, and lipid-depleted LDL (sometimes referred to as "small, dense LDL") (Reaven, 2002; Reaven, 2003; Grundy *et al.*, 2004a; Grundy *et al.*, 2004c). The metabolic syndrome affects ~25% of adults and is common in CHD patients; hence, identification of moderate hypertriglyceridemia in a patient, even if the total cholesterol level is normal, should trigger an evaluation to identify this disorder (Ford *et al.*, 2002; The Expert Panel, 2002).

Hyperlipidemia (elevated levels of triglycerides or cholesterol) and reduced HDL-C levels occur as a consequence of several interrelated factors that affect the concentrations of the various plasma lipoproteins. These factors may be lifestyle or behavioral (*e.g.*, diet or exercise), genetic (*e.g.*, mutations in a gene regulating lipoprotein levels), or metabolic (*e.g.*, diabetes mellitus or other conditions that influence plasma lipoprotein metabolism). An understanding of these factors requires a brief description of lipoprotein metabolism. A more detailed description can be found elsewhere (Mahley *et al.*, 2003).

PLASMA LIPOPROTEIN METABOLISM

Lipoproteins are macromolecular assemblies that contain lipids and proteins. The lipid constituents include free and esterified cholesterol, triglycerides, and phospholipids. The protein components, known as apolipoproteins or apoproteins, provide structural stability to the lipoproteins, and also may function as ligands in lipoprotein–receptor interactions or as cofactors in enzymatic processes that regulate lipoprotein metabolism. In all spherical lipoproteins, the most water-insoluble lipids (cholesteryl esters and triglycerides) are core components, and the more polar, water-soluble components (apoproteins, phospholipids, and unesterified cholesterol) are located on the surface. The major classes of lipoproteins and a number of their properties are presented in Table 35–1.

Table 35–2 describes apoproteins that have well-defined roles in plasma lipoprotein metabolism. These apolipoproteins include apolipoprotein (apo) A-I, apoA-II, apoA-IV, apoA-V, apoB-100, apoB-48, apoC-I, apoC-II, apoC-III, apoE, and apo(a). Except for apo(a), the lipid-binding regions of all apoproteins contain structural features called amphipathic helices that interact with the polar, hydrophilic lipids (such as surface phospholipids) and with the aqueous plasma environment in which the lipoproteins circulate. Differences in the non–lipid-binding regions determine the functional specificities of the apolipoproteins.

Chylomicrons. Chylomicrons are synthesized from the fatty acids of dietary triglycerides and cholesterol absorbed from the small intestine by epithelial cells.

Intestinal cholesterol and plant sterol absorption is mediated by Niemann-Pick C1–like 1 protein (NPC1L1), which appears to be the target of ezetimibe, a cholesterol absorption inhibitor (Altmann *et al.*, 2004). Plant sterols, unlike cholesterol, are not normally esterified and incorporated into chylomicrons. Two ATP-binding cassette (ABC) half-transporters, ABCG5 and ABCG8, which reside on the apical plasma membrane of enterocytes, channel plant sterols back into the intestinal lumen, preventing their assimilation into the body (Graf *et al.*, 2002; Repa *et al.*, 2002). Patients with the autosomal recessive disorder sitosterolemia have mutations in either of the genes that encode ABCG5 and ABCG8. As a result, they absorb unusually large amounts of plant sterols, fail to excrete dietary sterols into the bile, and thus accumulate plant sterols in the blood and tissues; this accumulation is associated with tendon and subcutaneous xanthomas and a markedly increased risk of premature CHD (Berge *et al.*, 2000; Lee *et al.*, 2001). Triglyceride synthesis is regulated by diacylglycerol transferase, an enzyme that regulates triglyceride synthesis in many tissues (Buhman *et al.*, 2001). After their synthesis in the endoplasmic reticulum, triglycerides are transferred by microsomal triglyceride transfer protein (MTP) to the site where newly synthesized apoB-48 is available to form chylomicrons.

Dietary cholesterol is esterified by the type 2 isozyme of acyl coenzyme A:cholesterol acyltransferase (ACAT). ACAT-2 is found in the intestine and in the liver, where cellular free cholesterol is esterified before triglyceride-rich lipoproteins [chylomicrons and very-low-density lipoproteins (VLDL)] are assembled. In the intestine, ACAT-2 regulates the absorption of dietary cholesterol, and thus may be a potential pharmacological target for reducing blood cholesterol levels (Buhman *et al.*, 2001). Another ACAT enzyme, ACAT-1, is expressed in macrophages, including foam cells, adrenocortical cells, and skin sebaceous glands. Although ACAT-1 esterifies cholesterol and promotes foam-cell development, ACAT-1 knockout mice do not have reduced susceptibility to atherosclerosis (Buhman *et al.*, 2001).

Chylomicrons, the largest plasma lipoproteins, are the only lipoproteins that float to the top of a tube of plasma that has been allowed to stand undisturbed for 12 hours. The buoyancy of chylomicrons reflects their high fat content (98% to 99%), of which 85% is dietary triglyceride. In chylomicrons, the ratio of triglycerides to cholesterol is ~10 or greater. In normolipidemic individuals, chylomicrons are present in plasma for 3 to 6 hours after a fat-containing meal has been ingested. After a fast of 10 to 12 hours, no chylomicrons remain.

The apolipoproteins of chylomicrons include some that are synthesized by intestinal epithelial cells (apoB-48, apoA-I, and apoA-IV), and others acquired from HDL (apoE and apoC-I, C-II, and C-III) after chylomicrons have been secreted into the lymph and enter the plasma (Table 35–2). The apoB-48 of chylomicrons is one of two forms of apoB present in lipoproteins. ApoB-48, synthesized only by intestinal epithelial cells, is unique to chylomicrons. ApoB-100 is synthesized by the liver and incorporated into VLDL and intermediate-density lipoproteins (IDL) and LDL, which are products of VLDL catabolism. The apparent molecular weight of apoB-48 is 48% that of apoB-100, which accounts for the name "apoB-48." The amino acid sequence of apoB-48 is identical to the first 2152 of the 4536 residues of apoB-100. An RNA-editing mechanism unique to the intestine accounts for the premature termination of the translation of the apoB-100 mRNA (Anant and Davidson, 2001). ApoB-48 lacks the portion of the sequence of apoB-100 that allows apoB-100 to bind to the LDL receptor, so apoB-48 functions primarily as a structural component of chylomicrons.

Table 35–1
Characteristics of Plasma Lipoproteins

LIPOPROTEIN CLASS	DENSITY OF FLOTATION, G/ML	MAJOR LIPID CONSTITUENT	TG:CHOL RATIO	SIGNIFICANT APOPROTEINS	SITE OF SYNTHESIS	MECHANISM(S) OF CATABOLISM
Chylomicrons and remnants	<<1.006	Dietary triglycerides and cholesterol	10:1	B-48, E, A-I, A-IV, C-I, C-II, C-III	Intestine	Triglyceride hydrolysis by LPL ApoE-mediated remnant uptake by liver
VLDL	<1.006	"Endogenous" or hepatic triglycerides	5:1	B-100, E, C-I, C-II, C-III	Liver	Triglyceride hydrolysis by LPL
IDL	1.006–1.019	Cholesteryl esters and "endogenous" triglycerides	1:1	B-100, E, C-II, C-III	Product of VLDL catabolism	50% converted to LDL mediated by HL, 50% apoE-mediated uptake by liver 50% apoE-mediated uptake by liver
LDL	1.019–1.063	Cholesteryl esters	NS	B-100	Product of VLDL catabolism	ApoB-100–mediated uptake by LDL receptor (~75% in liver)
HDL	1.063–1.21	Phospholipids, cholesteryl esters	NS	A-I, A-II, E, C-I, C-II, C-III	Intestine, liver, plasma	Complex: Transfer of cholesteryl ester to VLDL and LDL Uptake of HDL cholesterol by hepatocytes
Lp(a)	1.05–1.09	Cholesteryl esters	NS	B-100, apo(a)	Liver	Unknown

Abbreviations: apo, apolipoprotein; CHOL, cholesterol; HDL, high-density lipoproteins; IDL, intermediate-density lipoproteins; Lp(a), lipoprotein(a); LDL, low-density lipoproteins; NS, not significant (triglyceride is less than 5% of LDL and HDL); TG, triglyceride; VLDL, very-low-density lipoproteins; HL, hepatic lipase; LPL, lipoprotein lipase.

935

Table 35–2
Apolipoproteins

APOLIPOPROTEIN	AVERAGE CONCENTRATION, MG/DL	CHROMOSOME	MOLECULAR MASS, KD	SITES OF SYNTHESIS	FUNCTIONS
ApoA-I	130	11	~29	Liver, intestine	Structural in HDL; LCAT cofactor; ligand of ABCA1 receptor; reverse cholesterol transport
ApoA-II	40	1	~17	Liver	Forms –S–S– complex with apoE-2 and E-3, which inhibits E-2 and E-3 binding to lipoprotein receptors
Apo A-V	<1	11	~40	Liver	Modulates triglyceride incorporation into hepatic VLDL; activates LPL
ApoB-100	85	2	~513	Liver	Structural protein of VLDL, IDL, LDL; LDL receptor ligand
ApoB-48	Fluctuates according to dietary fat intake	2	~241	Intestine	Structural protein of chylomicrons
ApoC-I	6	19	~6.6	Liver	LCAT activator. Modulates receptor binding of remnants
ApoC-II	3	19	8.9	Liver	Lipoprotein lipase cofactor
ApoC-III	12	11	8.8	Liver	Modulates receptor binding of remnants
ApoE	5	19	34	Liver, brain, skin, gonads, spleen	Ligand for LDL receptor and receptors binding remnants; reverse cholesterol transport (HDL with apoE)
Apo(a)	Variable (under genetic control)	6	Variable	Liver	Modulator of fibrinolysis

Abbreviations: apo, apolipoprotein; HDL, high-density lipoproteins; IDL, intermediate-density lipoproteins; LCAT, lecithin:cholesterol acyltransferase; LDL, low-density lipoproteins; LPL, lipoprotein lipase; VLDL, very-low-density lipoproteins.

After gaining entry to the circulation *via* the thoracic duct, chylomicrons are metabolized initially at the capillary luminal surface of tissues that synthesize lipoprotein lipase (LPL), a triglyceride hydrolase (Figure 35–1). These tissues include adipose tissue, skeletal and cardiac muscle, and breast tissue of lactating women. As the triglycerides are hydrolyzed by LPL, the resulting free fatty acids are taken up and utilized by the adjacent tissues. The interaction of chylomicrons and LPL requires apoC-II as an absolute cofactor. The absence of functional LPL or functional apoC-II prevents the hydrolysis of triglycerides in chylomicrons and results in severe hypertriglyceridemia and pancreatitis during childhood or even infancy (chylomicronemia syndrome). Potentially atherogenic roles for LPL have been identified that affect the metabolism and

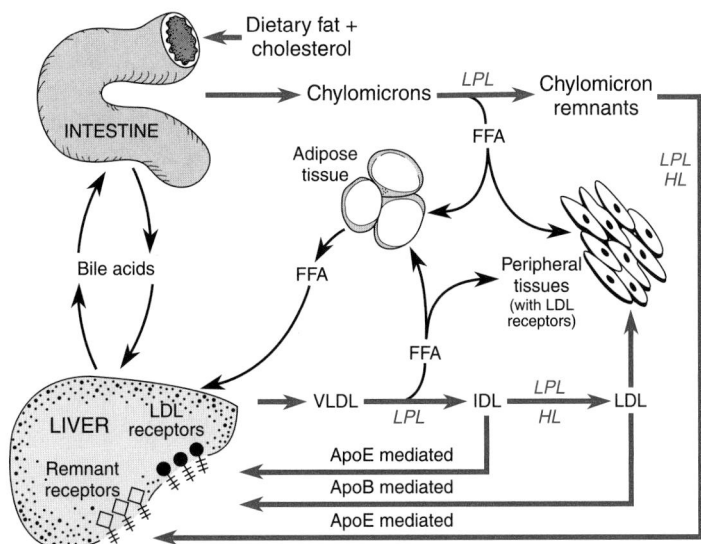

Figure 35–1. ***The major pathways involved in the metabolism of chylomicrons synthesized by the intestine and VLDL synthe-sized by the liver.*** Chylomicrons are converted to chylomicron remnants by the hydrolysis of their triglycerides by LPL. Chylomicron remnants are rapidly cleared from the plasma by the liver. "Remnant receptors" include the LDL receptor-related protein (LRP), LDL, and perhaps other receptors. FFA released by LPL is used by muscle tissue as an energy source or taken up and stored by adipose tissue. FFA, free fatty acid; HL, hepatic lipase; IDL, intermediate-density lipoproteins; LDL, low-density lipoproteins; LPL, lipopro-tein lipase; VLDL, very-low-density lipoproteins.

uptake of atherogenic lipoproteins by the liver and the arterial wall, and that impact the dyslipidemia of insulin resistance (Stein and Stein, 2003).

The concentration of chylomicrons can be controlled only by reducing dietary fat consumption. There is no cur-rent therapeutic approach that will enhance chylomicron catabolism except for insulin replacement in patients with type I diabetes mellitus. Insulin has a "permissive effect" on LPL-mediated triglyceride hydrolysis.

Chylomicron Remnants. After LPL-mediated removal of much of the dietary triglycerides, the chylomicron remnants, which still contain all of the dietary cholester-ol, detach from the capillary surface and within minutes are removed from the circulation by the liver in a multi-step process mediated by apoE (Figure 35–1) (Mahley and Huang, 1999; Mahley and Ji, 1999). First, the rem-nants are sequestered by the interaction of apoE with heparan sulfate proteoglycans on the surface of hepato-cytes and are processed by hepatic lipase (HL), further reducing the remnant triglyceride content. Next, apoE mediates remnant uptake by interacting with the hepatic LDL receptor or the LDL receptor–related protein (LRP) (Herz and Strickland, 2001). The multifunctional LRP recognizes a variety of ligands, including apoE, HL, and LPL, and several ligands unrelated to lipid metabolism.

In plasma lipid metabolism, the LRP is important because it is the back-up receptor responsible for the uptake of apoE-enriched remnants of chylomicrons and VLDL. Cell-surface heparan sulfate proteoglycans facil-itate the interaction of apoE-containing remnant lipopro-teins with the LRP, which mediates uptake by hepato-cytes (Mahley and Huang, 1999). Inherited absence of either functional HL (very rare) or functional apoE impedes remnant clearance by the LDL receptor and the LRP, increasing triglyceride- and cholesterol-rich rem-nant lipoproteins in the plasma (type III hyperlipopro-teinemia) (Mahley and Rall, 2001).

During the initial hydrolysis of chylomicron trigly-cerides by LPL, apoA-I and phospholipids are shed from the surface of chylomicrons and remain in the plasma. This is one mechanism by which nascent (precursor) HDL are generated. Chylomicron remnants are not pre-cursors of LDL, but the dietary cholesterol delivered to the liver by remnants increases plasma LDL levels by reducing LDL receptor–mediated catabolism of LDL by the liver.

Very-Low-Density Lipoproteins. VLDL are produced in the liver when triglyceride production is stimulated by an increased flux of free fatty acids or by increased *de novo* synthesis of fatty acids by the liver. VLDL particles are 40 to 100 nm in diameter and are large enough to cause plasma turbidity, but unlike chylomicrons, do not float spontaneously to the top of a tube of undisturbed plasma.

ApoB-100, apoE, and apoC-I, C-II, and C-III are synthesized constitutively by the liver and incorporated into VLDL (Table 35–2). If triglycerides are not available to form VLDL, the newly synthesized apoB-100 is degraded by hepatocytes. Triglycerides are synthesized in the endoplasmic reticulum, and along with other lipid constituents, are transferred by MTP to the site in the endoplasmic reticulum where newly synthesized apoB-100 is available to form nascent (precursor) VLDL. Small amounts of apoE and the C apoproteins are incorporated into nascent particles within the liver before secretion, but most of these apoproteins are acquired from plasma HDL after the VLDL are secreted by the liver.

ApoA-V modulates plasma triglyceride levels, possibly by affecting hepatic VLDL triglyceride secretion and by promoting LPL-mediated hydrolysis of chylomicrons and VLDL triglycerides (Oliva *et al.*, 2005). ApoA-V is produced solely by the liver, and despite its very low plasma concentration (~0.1% of the concentration of apoA-I), profoundly affects plasma triglyceride levels in mice and humans (van der Vliet *et al.*, 2001; Pennacchio *et al.*, 2002). Overexpression of apoA-V in transgenic mice reduces triglyceride levels by half, while inactivation of the apoA-V gene increases triglyceride levels fourfold (Pennacchio *et al.*, 2001). Polymorphisms in the human apoA-V gene are associated with significant variability in triglyceride levels, but the precise mechanism by which apoA-V modulates plasma triglyceride levels is unknown (Pennacchio *et al.*, 2002).

Without MTP, hepatic triglycerides cannot be transferred to apoB-100. As a consequence, patients with dysfunctional MTP fail to make any of the apoB-containing lipoproteins (VLDL, IDL, or LDL). MTP also plays a key role in the synthesis of chylomicrons in the intestine, and mutations of MTP that result in the inability of triglycerides to be transferred to either apoB-100 in the liver or apoB-48 in the intestine prevent VLDL and chylomicron production and cause the genetic disorder abetalipoproteinemia (Berriot-Varoqueaux *et al.*, 2000).

Plasma VLDL is then catabolized by LPL in the capillary beds in a process similar to the lipolytic processing of chylomicrons (Figure 35–1). When triglyceride hydrolysis is nearly complete, the VLDL remnants, usually termed IDL, are released from the capillary endothelium and reenter the circulation. ApoB-100 containing small VLDL and IDL (VLDL remnants), which have a half-life of less than 30 minutes, have two potential fates. About 40% to 60% are cleared from the plasma by the liver *via* interaction with LDL receptors and LRP, which recognize ligands (apoB-100 and apoE) on the remnants. LPL and HL convert the remainder of the IDL to LDL by removal of additional triglycerides. The C apoproteins and apoE redistribute to HDL. *Virtually all LDL particles in the plasma are derived from VLDL.*

ApoE plays a major role in the metabolism of triglyceride-rich lipoproteins (chylomicrons, chylomicron remnants, VLDL, and IDL) and has a number of major functions related to the binding and

uptake of plasma lipoproteins and to the redistribution of lipids locally among cells (Mahley and Huang, 1999; Mahley and Rall, 2000). About half of the apoE in the plasma of fasting subjects is associated with triglyceride-rich lipoproteins, and the other half is a constituent of HDL. ApoE controls the catabolism of the apoE-containing lipoproteins by mediating their binding to cell-surface heparan sulfate proteoglycans (especially in the liver) and to LDL receptors and the LRP (Mahley and Ji, 1999).

About three-fourths of the apoE in plasma is synthesized by the liver, and the remainder is synthesized by a variety of tissues. The brain is the second most abundant site of apoE mRNA synthesis, which occurs in both astrocytes and neurons (Mahley and Rall, 2000). ApoE also is synthesized by macrophages, where it appears to play a role in modulating cholesterol accumulation. In transgenic mice, overexpression of apoE by macrophages inhibits hypercholesterolemia-induced atherogenesis (Bellosta *et al.*, 1995; Hasty *et al.*, 1999).

Three alleles of the apoE gene (designated ε2, ε3, and ε4) occur with a frequency of ~8%, 77%, and 15%, respectively, and code for the three major forms of apoE: E2, E3, and E4. Consequently, there are three homozygous apoE phenotypes (E2/2, E3/3, and E4/4) and three heterozygous phenotypes (E2/3, E2/4, and E3/4). Approximately 60% of the population is homozygous for apoE3.

Single amino acid substitutions result from the genetic polymorphisms in the apoE gene (Mahley and Rall, 2000). ApoE2, with a cysteine at residue 158, differs from apoE3, which has arginine at this site. ApoE3, with a cysteine at residue 112, differs from apoE4, which has arginine at this site. These single amino acid differences affect both receptor binding and lipid binding of the three apoE isoforms. Both apoE3 and apoE4 can bind to the LDL receptor, but apoE2 binds much less effectively, and as a consequence causes the remnant lipoprotein dyslipidemia of type III hyperlipoproteinemia. ApoE2 and apoE3 bind preferentially to the phospholipids of HDL, whereas apoE4 binds preferentially to VLDL triglycerides.

Low-Density Lipoproteins. The LDL particles arising from the catabolism of IDL have a half-life of 1.5 to 2 days, which accounts for the higher plasma concentration of LDL than of VLDL and IDL. In subjects without hypertriglyceridemia, two-thirds of plasma cholesterol is found in the LDL. Plasma clearance of LDL particles is mediated primarily by LDL receptors; a small component is mediated by nonreceptor clearance mechanisms (Brown and Goldstein, 1986). More than 900 mutations of the LDL receptor gene have been identified in association with defective or absent LDL receptors that cause high levels of plasma LDL and familial hypercholesterolemia (Rader *et al.*, 2003). ApoB-100, the only apoprotein of LDL, is the ligand that binds LDL to its receptor. Residues 3000 to 3700 in the carboxyl-terminal sequence are critical for binding. Mutations in this region disrupt binding and are a cause of hypercholesterolemia (familial defective apoB-100) (Innerarity *et al.*, 1990). Autosomal recessive hypercholesterolemia closely resembles familial hypercholesterolemia, but is not caused by LDL receptor mutations; the autosomal recessive hypercholesterolemia protein is required for internalization of LDL receptor complexes to which LDL binds on the surface of hepatocytes (Rader *et al.*, 2003).

The liver expresses a large complement of LDL receptors and removes ~75% of all LDL from the plasma. Consequently, manipulation of hepatic LDL receptor expression is a most effective way to modulate plasma LDL-C levels. Thyroxine and estrogen enhance LDL receptor gene expression, which explains their LDL-C–lowering effects (Shin and Osborne, 2003).

The most effective dietary alteration (decreased consumption of saturated fat and cholesterol) and pharmacological treatment (statins) for hypercholesterolemia act by enhancing hepatic LDL receptor expression (Xie *et al.*, 2002). Regulation of LDL receptor expression is part of a complex process by which cells regulate their free cholesterol content. This regulatory process is mediated by transcription factors called *sterol regulatory element binding proteins* (SREBPs) and SREBP *cleavage activating protein* (Horton *et al.*, 2002). The SREBP cleavage activating protein is both a sensor of cellular cholesterol content and an escort of SREBPs. When cellular cholesterol content is reduced, SREBPs undergo proteolytic cleavage in the Golgi apparatus, and the amino-terminal domain, guided by the SREBP cleavage activating protein, translocates to the nucleus, where it activates expression of the LDL receptor and of other enzymes involved in cholesterol biosynthesis.

LDL become atherogenic when they are modified by oxidation (Witztum and Steinberg, 2001), a required step for LDL uptake by the scavenger receptors of macrophages. This process leads to foam-cell formation in arterial lesions. At least two scavenger receptors (SRs) are involved (SR-AI/II and CD36). Knocking out either receptor in transgenic mice retards the uptake of oxidized LDL by macrophages. Expression of the two receptors is regulated differently: SR-AI/II appears to be expressed more in early atherogenesis, and CD36 expression is greater as foam cells form during lesion progression (Dhaliwal and Steinbrecher, 1999; Nakata *et al.*, 1999). Despite the large body of evidence implicating oxidation of LDL as a requisite step during atherogenesis, controlled clinical trials have failed to show efficacy of antioxidant vitamins in preventing vascular disease (Yusuf, 2002; Brown *et al.*, 2002).

High-Density Lipoproteins. The metabolism of HDL is complex because of the multiple mechanisms by which HDL particles are modified in the plasma compartment and by which HDL particles are synthesized. ApoA-I is the major HDL apoprotein, and its plasma concentration is a more powerful inverse predictor of CHD risk than is the HDL-C level (Tall *et al.*, 2000; Mahley *et al.*, 2003).

ApoA-I synthesis is required for normal production of HDL. Mutations in the apoA-I gene that cause HDL deficiency are variable in their clinical expression and often are associated with accelerated atherogenesis (Assmann *et al.*, 2001). Conversely, overexpression of apoA-I in transgenic mice protects against experimentally induced atherogenesis.

Mature HDL can be separated by ultracentrifugation into HDL_2 (d = 1.063 to 1.125 g/ml), which are larger, more cholesterol-rich lipoproteins (70 to 100 Å in diameter), and HDL_3 (d = 1.125 to 1.21 g/ml), which are smaller particles (50 to 70 Å in diameter). In addition, two major subclasses of mature HDL particles in the plasma can be differentiated by their content of the major HDL apoproteins, apoA-I and apoA-II (Duriez and Fruchart, 1999). Mature HDL particles have α electrophoretic mobility. Some α-migrating HDL particles contain only apoA-I and no apoA-II and are called LpA-I HDL particles. Others contain both apoA-I and apoA-II and are called LpA-I/A-II HDL particles. LpA-I particles are larger than LpA-I/A-II and are primarily associated with HDL_2. LpA-I/A-II particles are smaller and are primarily associated with HDL_3. Patients with reduced HDL-C levels and CHD have lower levels of LpA-I, but not of LpA-I/A-II, than subjects with normal HDL-C levels (Duriez and Fruchart, 1999). This finding suggests that HDL particles containing apoA-I and apoA-II may not be atheroprotective. In fact, overexpression of apoA-II in transgenic mice enhances susceptibility to atherosclerosis (Schultz *et al.*, 1993). ApoA-II deficiency is not associated with any apparent deleterious effects in humans (Deeb *et al.*, 1990).

The precursor of most of the α-migrating plasma HDL is a discoidal particle containing apoA-I and phospholipid, called pre-β1 HDL because of its pre-β1 electrophoretic mobility. Pre-β1 HDL are synthesized by the liver and the intestine, and they also arise when surface phospholipids and apoA-I of chylomicrons and VLDL are lost as the triglycerides of these lipoproteins are hydrolyzed. Phospholipid transfer protein plays an important role in the transfer of phospholipids to HDL (Tall *et al.*, 2000).

Discoidal pre-β1 HDL can then acquire free (unesterified) cholesterol from the cell membranes of tissues, such as arterial wall macrophages, by an interaction with the class B, type I scavenger receptor (SR-BI), to which the apoA-I of HDL docks, so that free cholesterol can be transferred to or from the HDL particle (Williams *et al.*, 1999). SR-BI facilitates the movement of excess free cholesterol from cells with excess cholesterol (*e.g.,* foam cells in the arterial wall) (Williams *et al.*, 1999; Assmann and Nofer, 2003). Hepatic SR-BI facilitates the uptake of cholesteryl esters from the HDL without internalizing and degrading the lipoproteins. In mice, overexpression of SR-BI reduces susceptibility to atherosclerosis, and elimination of SR-BI significantly increases atherosclerosis (Krieger and Kozarsky, 1999). A homologue of SR-BI, CLA-1, has been identified in humans (Dhaliwal and Steinbrecher, 1999). Modulation of CLA-1 expression may offer new avenues for the management of atherogenesis (Krieger, 1999).

The membrane transporter ABCA1 facilitates the transfer of free cholesterol from cells to HDL (Attie *et al.*, 2001). When ABCA1 is defective, the acquisition of cholesterol by HDL is greatly diminished, and HDL levels are markedly reduced because poorly lipidated nascent HDL are metabolized rapidly. Loss-of-function mutations of ABCA1 cause the defect observed in Tangier disease, a genetic disorder characterized by extremely low levels of HDL and cholesterol accumulation in the liver, spleen, tonsils, and neurons of peripheral nerves. Transgenic animals overexpressing ABCA1 in the liver and macrophages have elevated plasma levels of HDL and apoA-I and reduced susceptibility to atherosclerosis (Vaisman *et al.*, 2001; Joyce *et al.*, 2002).

After free cholesterol is acquired by the pre-β1 HDL, it is esterified by lecithin:cholesterol acyltransferase. The newly esterified and nonpolar cholesterol moves into the core of the discoidal HDL. As the cholesteryl ester content increases, the HDL particle becomes spherical and less dense. These newly formed spherical HDL particles (HDL_3) further enlarge by accepting more free cholesterol, which is in turn esterified by lecithin:cholesterol acyltransferase. In this way, HDL_3 are converted to HDL_2, which are larger and less dense than HDL_3.

As the cholesteryl ester content of the HDL_2 increases, the cholesteryl esters of these particles begin to be exchanged for triglycerides derived from any of the triglyceride-containing lipoproteins (chylomicrons, VLDL, remnant lipoproteins, and LDL). This exchange is mediated by the cholesteryl ester transfer protein (CETP), and in humans accounts for the removal of about two-thirds of the cholesterol associated with HDL. The transferred cholesterol subsequently is metabolized as part of the lipoprotein into which it was transferred. The triglyceride that is transferred into HDL_2 is hydrolyzed in the liver by HL, a process that regenerates smaller, spherical HDL_3 particles that recirculate and acquire additional free cholesterol from tissues containing excess free cholesterol.

HL activity is regulated and modulates HDL-C levels. Both androgens and estrogens affect HL gene expression, but with opposite effects (Brinton, 1996). Androgens increase HL activity, which accounts for the lower HDL-C values observed in men than in women. Estrogens reduce HL activity, but their impact on HDL-C levels in women is substantially less than that of androgens on HDL-C levels in men. HL appears to have a pivotal role in regulating HDL-C levels, as HL activity is increased in many patients with low HDL-C levels.

HDL are protective lipoproteins that decrease the risk of CHD; thus, high levels of HDL are desirable. This protective effect may result from the participation of HDL in reverse cholesterol transport, the process by which excess cholesterol is acquired from cells and transferred to the liver for excretion (Assmann and Nofer, 2003). HDL also may protect against atherogenesis by mechanisms not directly related to reverse cholesterol transport. These functions include putative antiinflammatory, antioxidative, platelet antiaggregatory, anticoagulant, and profibrinolytic activities (Nofer *et al.*, 2002).

Lipoprotein(a). Lipoprotein(a) [Lp(a)] is composed of an LDL particle that has a second apoprotein in addition to apoB-100 (Ginsberg and Goldberg, 2001; Mahley *et al.*, 2003). The second apoprotein, apo(a), is attached to apoB-100 by at least one disulfide bond and does not function as a lipid-binding apoprotein. Apo(a) of Lp(a) is structurally related to plasminogen and appears to be atherogenic by interfering with fibrinolysis of thrombi on the surfaces of plaques.

HYPERLIPIDEMIA AND ATHEROSCLEROSIS

Despite a continuing decline in the incidence of atherosclerosis-related deaths in the past 39 years, deaths from CHD, cerebrovascular disease, and peripheral vascular disease accounted for 38.5% of the 2.4 million deaths in the United States during 2001. Two-thirds of atherosclerosis deaths were due to CHD. About 85% of CHD deaths occurred in individuals over 65 years of age. Among the 15% dying prematurely (below age 65), 80% died during their first CHD event. Among those dying of sudden cardiac death in 1997, 50% of the men and 64% of the women had previously been asymptomatic (American Heart Association, 2003). It is estimated that an average

of 11.5 years of life are lost as a consequence of having a myocardial infarction.

These statistics illustrate the importance of identifying and managing risk factors for CHD. *The major conventional risk factors are elevated LDL-C, reduced HDL-C, cigarette smoking, hypertension, type 2 diabetes mellitus, advancing age, and a family history of premature (men <55 years; women <65 years) CHD events in a first-degree relative.* Control of the modifiable risk factors is especially important in preventing premature CHD. Observational studies suggest that modifiable risk factors account for 85% of excess risk (risk over and above that of individuals with optimal risk-factor profiles) for premature CHD (Stamler *et al.*, 1986; Wilson *et al.*, 1998). The presence of one or more conventional risk factors in 90% of patients with CHD belies claims that a large percentage of CHD, perhaps as much as 50%, is not attributable to conventional risk factors (Canto and Iskandrian, 2003). Furthermore, these studies indicate that, when total cholesterol levels are below 160 mg/dl, CHD risk is markedly attenuated, even in the presence of additional risk factors (Grundy *et al.*, 1998). This pivotal role of hypercholesterolemia in atherogenesis gave rise to the almost universally accepted cholesterol-diet-CHD hypothesis: elevated plasma cholesterol levels cause CHD; diets rich in saturated (animal) fat and cholesterol raise cholesterol levels; and lowering cholesterol levels reduces CHD risk (Thompson and Barter, 1999). Although the relationship between cholesterol, diet, and CHD was recognized nearly 50 years ago, proof that cholesterol lowering was safe and prevented CHD death required extensive epidemiological studies and clinical trials.

Epidemiological Studies. Epidemiological studies have demonstrated the importance of the relationship between excess saturated fat consumption and elevated cholesterol levels. Reducing the consumption of dietary saturated fat and cholesterol is the cornerstone of population-based approaches to the management of hypercholesterolemia. In addition, it is clearly established that the higher the cholesterol level, the higher the CHD risk (Stamler *et al.*, 1986).

Clinical Trials. Studies of the efficacy of cholesterol lowering began in the 1960s, and the results of the earliest trials showed that modest reductions in total cholesterol and LDL-C were associated with reductions in fatal and nonfatal CHD events, but not total mortality (Illingworth and Durrington, 1999). It was not until the advent of a more efficacious class of cholesterol-lowering drugs, the statins, that cholesterol reduction therapy was finally proven to prevent CHD events and reduce total mortality (Scandinavian Simvastatin Survival Study, 1994). Subsequently, many trials of statins have documented the efficacy and safety of cholesterol-lowering therapy (Table 35–3) (Law *et al.*, 2003). Patients benefit regardless of gender, age, or baseline lipid values whether or not they have a prior history of vascular disease (Heart Protection Study Collaborative Group, 2002). Since publication of the 2001 National Cholesterol Education Program (NCEP) Adult Treatment Panel (ATP) III guidelines, clinical trials have been com-

Table 35–3
Results of Major Primary and Secondary Prevention Statin Trials

TRIAL	DURATION (years)	STATIN, DOSE	REDUCTION IN LDL-C (%)	Number of Subjects		CHD Death or Nonfatal MI		RELATIVE RISK REDUCTION (%)
				PLACEBO	DRUG	PLACEBO	DRUG	
Primary prevention trials								
WOSCOPS (Shepherd et al., 1995)	5	Pravastatin, 40 mg	26	3293	3302	248	174	30
AFCAPS (Downs et al., 1998)	5	Lovastatin, 20 or 40 mg	25	3301	3304	95	57	40
ASCOT-LLA (Sever et al., 2003)	3.3	Atorvastatin, 10 mg	35	5137	5168	137	86	38
Secondary prevention trials								
4S (Scandinavian Simvastatin Survival Study, 1994)	5.4	Simvastatin, 20 or 40 mg	34	2223	2221	627	431	31
HPS (Heart Protection Study Collaborative Group, 2002)	5	Simvastatin, 40 mg	30	10267	10269	1212	898	26
CARE (Sacks et al., 1996)	5	Pravastatin, 40 mg	32	2078	2081	274	212	23
LIPID (The Long-Term Intervention with Pravastatin in Ischaemic Disease (LIPID) Study Group, 1998)	5	Pravastatin, 40 mg	28	4502	4512	715	557	22
PROSPER (Shepherd et al., 2002)	3.2	Pravastatin, 40 mg	34	1259	1306	211	166	24

Table 35–4

Treatment Based on LDL-C Levels (2004 Revision of NCEP Adult Treatment Panel III Guidelines)

RISK CATEGORY	LDL-C GOAL	Adults	
		THERAPEUTIC LIFESTYLE CHANGE	DRUG THERAPY
Very high risk Atherosclerosis-induced CHD plus one of: (a) multiple risk factors, (b) diabetes mellitus, (c) a poorly controlled single factor, (d) acute coronary syndrome, (e) metabolic syndrome	<70 mg/dl*	No threshold	No threshold
High risk CHD or CHD equivalent	<100 mg/dl*	No threshold	No threshold
Moderately high risk 2+ risk factors 10-year risk: 10%–20%	<130 mg/dl (Optional <100 mg/dl)	≥100 mg/dl	≥130 mg/dl (100–129 mg/dl)[†]
Moderate risk 2+ risk factors 10-year risk <10%	<130 mg/dl	≥130 mg/dl	>160 mg/dl
0–1 risk factor	<160 mg/dl	≥160 mg/dl	≥190 mg/dl (Optional: 160–189 mg/dl)[‡]

*If pretreatment LDL-C is near or below LDL-C goal value, then a statin dose sufficient to lower LDL-C by 30%–40% should be prescribed. [†]Patients in this category include those with a 10-year risk of 10%–20% and one of the following: (a) age >60 years; (b) three or more risk factors; (c) a severe risk factor; (d) triglycerides >200 mg/dl and HDL-C <40 mg/dl; (e) metabolic syndrome; (f) highly sensitive C-reactive protein (CRP) >3 mg/l; (g) coronary calcium score (age/gender adjusted) >75th percentile. [‡]Patients include those with (a) any severe single risk factor; (b) multiple major risk factors; (c) 10-year risk >8%. *Abbreviations:* CHD, coronary heart disease; CHD equivalent, peripheral vascular disease, abdominal aortic aneurysm, symptomatic carotid artery disease, >20% 10-year CHD risk, or diabetes mellitus; LDL-C, low-density-lipoprotein cholesterol; NCEP, National Cholesterol Education Program.

pleted that have prompted a revision in the ATP III guidelines (Illingworth and Durrington, 1999; The Expert Panel, 2002).

The key features of the revision include abandoning the concept of a threshold LDL-C level that must be exceeded before initiating cholesterol-lowering drug therapy in CHD or CHD equivalent patients; adopting a new target LDL-C level (<70 mg/dl) for very high-risk patients; and employing a "standard statin dose" (a dosage sufficient to lower LDL-C by 30% to 40%) as a minimum therapy when initiating cholesterol-lowering therapy with statins (Grundy et al., 2004b) (Table 35–4).

The clinical trials that provide information about threshold LDL-C levels, which must be exceeded before initiating cholesterol-lowering drug therapy for CHD patients, include the Cholesterol and Recurrent Events (CARE) and Long-Term Intervention with Pravastatin in Ischaemic Disease (LIPID) trial that employed *pravastatin* (40 mg daily) or placebo, and the Heart Protection Study (HPS) in which *simvastatin* (40 mg daily) was the treatment (Sacks *et al.*, 2000). The LIPID and CARE trials were secondary prevention studies lasting 5 years. There was no reduction in CHD events associated with taking pravastatin (40 mg daily) among the 20% of patients with baseline LDL-C <125 mg/dl. The results of these two clinical trials provided the only data per-

taining to CHD patients with low baseline LDL-C levels (<125 mg/dl) when the ATP III guidelines were published in 2001. The lack of treatment effect in this group accounts for the recommendation that cholesterol-lowering drug therapy be optional, not mandatory, for CHD patients with baseline LDL-C levels below 130 mg/dl (The Expert Panel, 2002). The HPS was a large secondary prevention trial comparing simvastatin (40 mg daily) to placebo. All subjects, including the 17.5% with baseline LDL-C <100 mg/dl (mean baseline LDL-C, 97 mg/dl; mean on-treatment LDL-C, 65 mg/dl) experienced a 24% reduction in the relative risk of sustaining a vascular event (Heart Protection Study Collaborative Group, 2002). Due to this outcome of the HPS, ATP III guidelines abandoned the concept of a threshold value for LDL-C that must be exceeded before prescribing cholesterol-lowering drug therapy for CHD patients (Grundy *et al.*, 2004b). Comparing the proven benefit of simvastatin (40 mg daily; ~41% reduction of LDL-C) in HPS to the lack of benefit of pravastatin (40 mg daily; ~34% reduction of LDL-C) in CARE and LIPID among patients with LDL-C <125 mg/dl, it is apparent that CHD patients with low baseline LDL-C levels require dosages of statins sufficient to lower LDL-C by at least 40%.

The new target of LDL-C <70 mg/dl for very high-risk patients was based on the outcome of the HPS, which showed that CHD patients with baseline LDL-C levels below 100 mg/dl benefited from statin therapy, and the outcome of the Pravastatin or Atorvastatin Evaluation and Infection Therapy—Thrombolysis in Myocardial Infarction (PROVE IT–TIMI) 22 trial (Cannon *et al.*, 2004). This study compared the benefit of "intensive" LDL-C lowering with *atorvastatin*, 80 mg daily, versus "standard" LDL-C lowering with pravastatin, 40 mg daily, in hospitalized patients with acute coronary syndrome. Intensive treatment with atorvastatin, 80 mg daily, lowered the median LDL-C level to 62 mg/dl, and standard treatment with pravastatin, 40 mg daily, lowered median LDL-C to 95 mg/dl. High-intensity treatment with atorvastatin was associated with a 16% reduction in the relative risk of sustaining a primary endpoint event (a composite of death, nonfatal myocardial infarction, rehospitalization for unstable angina, revascularization, and stroke) after only 2 years of treatment. Taken together the results of HPS and PROVE IT suggest that LDL-C <70 mg/dl is indicated for patients with low baseline LDL-C levels (~100 mg/dl) and for high-risk acute coronary syndrome patients similar to those in the PROVE IT trial (Grundy *et al.*, 2004b). Other trials involving patients treated intensively or with standard therapy are nearly complete and will provide additional information about the value of lowering LDL-C to values substantially lower than 100 mg/dl.

The results of the clinical trials suggest that CHD risk is reduced by 1% for every 1% reduction in LDL-C. Consequently, use of minimal doses of statins to produce small LDL-C reductions that barely attain LDL-C goals would minimize the treatment benefit associated with standard doses of statins that lower LDL-C by up to 40% (Grundy *et al.*, 2004b). Thus, current recommendations for statin therapy are that LDL-C levels should be lowered by 30% to 40% from baseline as well as achieving a specific LDL-C goal (Grundy *et al.*, 2004b).

National Cholesterol Education Program (NCEP) Guidelines for Treatment: Managing Patients with Dyslipidemia

The current NCEP guidelines for management of patients are of two types. One is a population-based approach to reduce CHD risk, which includes recommendations to increase exercise (to expend ~2000 calories/week) and to lower blood cholesterol by dietary recommendations: reduce total calories from fat to less than 30% and from saturated and trans fats to less than 10%; consume less than 300 mg of cholesterol per day; eat a variety of oily fish twice a week (Kris-Etherton *et al.*, 2002) and oils/foods rich in α-linolenic acid (canola, flaxseed, and soybean oils, flaxseed, and walnuts); and maintain desirable body weight. The second is the patient-based approach that focuses on lowering LDL-C levels as the primary goal of therapy (The Expert Panel, 2002; Grundy *et al.*, 2004b).

The guidelines for the management of adults 20 years and older recommend a complete fasting lipoprotein profile (total cholesterol, LDL-C, HDL-C, and triglycerides). The classification of lipid levels is shown in Table 35–5. If the values for total cholesterol, LDL-C, and triglycerides are in the lowest category and the HDL-C level is

Table 35–5
*Classification of Plasma Lipid Levels**

Total cholesterol	
<200 mg/dl	Desirable
200–239 mg/dl	Borderline high
≥240 mg/dl	High
HDL-C	
<40 mg/dl	Low (consider <50 mg/dl as low for women)
>60 mg/dl	High
LDL-C	
<70 mg/dl	Optimal for very high risk (minimal goal for CHD equivalent patients)
<100 mg/dl	Optimal
100–129 mg/dl	Near optimal
130–159 mg/dl	Borderline high
160–189 mg/dl	High
≥190 mg/dl	Very high
Triglycerides	
<150 mg/dl	Normal
150–199 mg/dl	Borderline high
200–499 mg/dl	High
≥500 mg/dl	Very high

Abbreviations: HDL-C, high-density-lipoprotein cholesterol; LDL-C, low-density-lipoprotein cholesterol. *2001 National Cholesterol Education Program guidelines.

not low, lifestyle recommendations (diet and exercise) should be made to ensure maintenance of a normal lipid profile. Other vascular disease risk factors (Table 35–6), if present, should be assessed and treated individually. For patients with elevated levels of total cholesterol, LDL-C, or triglycerides, or reduced HDL-C values, further treatment is based on the patient's risk-factor status (Table 35–6), LDL-C levels (Table 35–4), and calculation of the Framingham risk score (Table 35–7) of primary prevention patients with two or more risk factors.

All patients who meet the criteria for lipid-lowering therapy should receive instruction about therapeutic lifestyle change. Dietary restrictions include less than 7% of calories from saturated and trans fatty acids, less than 200 mg of cholesterol daily, up to 20% of calories from monounsaturated fatty acids, up to 10% of calories from polyunsaturated fat, and total fat calories ranging between 25% and 35% of all calories. Two oily fish meals per week are especially important for post–myocardial infarction patients due to a substantial reduction in the risk of sudden cardiac death (Kris-Etherton *et al.*, 2002). Patients with CHD or a CHD equivalent (symptomatic peripheral or

Table 35–6
Risk Factors for Coronary Heart Disease**

Age
  Male >45 years or female >55 years
Family history of premature CHD
  A first-degree relative (male below 55 years or
    female below 65 years when the first CHD
    clinical event occurs)
Current cigarette smoking
  Defined as smoking within the preceding 30 days
Hypertension
  Blood pressure ≥140/90 or use of antihypertensive
    medication, irrespective of blood pressure
Low HDL-C
  <40 mg/dl (consider <50 mg/dl as "low" for women)
Obesity†
  Body mass index >25 kg/m² and waist circumference
    above 40 inches (men) or 35 inches (women)

Abbreviations: CHD, coronary heart disease; HDL-C, high-density-lipoprotein cholesterol. *Diabetes mellitus is considered to be a CHD-
equivalent disorder; therefore, the lipid management of diabetes patients
is the same as that for patients with established vascular disease (American Diabetes Association, 1999). †Obesity was returned to the list of
CHD risk factors in 1998, although it was not included as a risk factor in
the 2001 NCEP guidelines (Pi-Sunyer et al., 1998).

carotid vascular disease, abdominal aortic aneurysm, >20%
10-year CHD risk, or diabetes mellitus) should immediately start appropriate lipid-lowering drug therapy irrespective
of their baseline LDL-C level (Heart Protection Study Collaborative Group, 2002; Grundy *et al.*, 2004b). Patients
without CHD or CHD equivalent should be managed with
lifestyle advice (diet, exercise, weight management) for 3
to 6 months before drug therapy is implemented.

Before drug therapy is initiated, secondary causes of
hyperlipidemia should be excluded. Most secondary causes (Table 35–8) can be excluded by ascertaining the
patient's medication history and by measuring serum creatinine, liver function tests, fasting glucose, and thyroid-
stimulating hormone levels. Treatment of the disorder
causing secondary dyslipidemia may preclude the necessity of treatment with hypolipidemic drugs.

Risk Assessment Using Framingham Risk Scores

The 2001 NCEP guidelines (The Expert Panel, 2002;
Grundy *et al.*, 2004b) and those of the European Atherosclerosis Society (Wood *et al.*, 1998) employ risk assessment tables devised from the Framingham Heart Study in
an attempt to match the intensity of treatment to the severity of CHD risk in patients without a prior history of
symptomatic atherosclerotic vascular disease. High risk or
"CHD equivalent" status is defined as >20% chance of
sustaining a CHD event in the next 10 years. The tables
used to determine a patient's absolute risk do not take into
account risk associated with a family history of premature
CHD or obesity. As a consequence, the risk may be seriously underestimated, resulting in insufficiently aggressive management (Lloyd-Jones *et al.*, 2004). After calculation of the risk score, more aggressive therapy should be
considered for obese patients or for patients with a family
history of premature CHD. It is also unlikely that the
Framingham risk model is appropriate for assessing risk
in all ethnic groups (Bersot *et al.*, 2003; Liu *et al.*, 2004).

Arterial Wall Biology and Plaque Stability

More effective lipid-lowering agents and a better understanding of atherogenesis have helped to prove that aggressive lipid-lowering therapy has many beneficial effects

Table 35–7
Guidelines Based on LDL-C and Total Cholesterol:HDL-C Ratio for Treatment of Low HDL-C Patients

RISK CATEGORY	Goals				Lifestyle Change Initiated for				Drug Therapy Initiated for			
	LDL-C		TC:HDL-C		LDL-C		TC:HDL-C		LDL-C		TC:HDL-C	
CHD or equivalent	<100	and	<3.5		≥100	or	≥3.5		≥100	or	≥3.5	
2+ risk factors	<130	and	<4.5		≥130	or	≥4.5		≥130	or	≥6.0	
0–1 risk factor	<160	and	<5.5		≥160	or	≥5.5		≥160	or	≥7.0	

Abbreviations: CHD, coronary heart disease; HDL-C, high-density lipoprotein cholesterol; LDL-C, low-density-lipoprotein cholesterol; TC, total cholesterol.

Table 35–8
Secondary Causes of Dyslipidemia

DISORDER	MAJOR LIPID EFFECT
Diabetes mellitus	Triglycerides > cholesterol; low HDL-C
Nephrotic syndrome	Triglycerides usually > cholesterol
Alcohol use	Triglycerides > cholesterol
Contraceptive use	Triglycerides > cholesterol
Estrogen use	Triglycerides > cholesterol
Glucocorticoid excess	Triglycerides > cholesterol
Hypothyroidism	Cholesterol > triglycerides
Obstructive liver disease	Cholesterol > triglycerides

Abbreviation: HDL-C, high-density-lipoprotein cholesterol.

over and above those obtained by simply decreasing lipid deposition in the arterial wall. Arteriographic trials have shown that, although aggressive lipid lowering results only in very small increases in lumen diameter, it promptly decreases acute coronary events (Cannon *et al.*, 2004; Brown *et al.*, 1993). Lesions causing less than 60% occlusion are responsible for more than two-thirds of the acute events. Aggressive lipid-lowering therapy may prevent acute events through its positive effects on the arterial wall; it corrects endothelial dysfunction, corrects abnormal vascular reactivity (spasm), and increases plaque stability.

Atherosclerotic lesions containing a large lipid core, large numbers of macrophages, and a poorly formed fibrous cap (Brown *et al.*, 1993; Libby, 2002; Corti *et al.*, 2003) are prone to plaque rupture and acute thrombosis. Aggressive lipid lowering appears to alter plaque architecture, resulting in less lipid, fewer macrophages, and a larger collagen and smooth muscle cell–rich fibrous cap. Stabilization of plaque susceptibility to thrombosis appears to be a direct result of LDL-C lowering or an indirect result of changes in cholesterol and lipoprotein metabolism or arterial wall biology (*see* "Potential Cardioprotective Effects Other Than LDL Lowering," below).

Whom and When to Treat? Large-scale trials with statins have provided new insights into which patients with dyslipidemia should be treated and when treatment should be initiated.

Gender. Both men and women benefit from lipid-lowering therapy (Heart Protection Study Collaborative Group, 2002). Statins, rather than hormone-replacement therapy, are now the recommended first-line drug thera-

py for lowering lipids in postmenopausal women. This recommendation reflects the increased CHD morbidity in older women with established CHD who were treated with hormone-replacement therapy (Mosca *et al.*, 1999) (*see* Chapter 57).

Age. Age >45 years in men and >55 years in women is considered to be a CHD risk factor. The statin trials have shown that patients >65 years of age benefit from therapy as much as do younger patients (Law *et al.*, 2003). Old age *per se* is not a reason to refrain from initiating drug therapy in an otherwise healthy person.

Cerebrovascular Disease Patients. In most observational studies, plasma cholesterol levels correlate positively with the risk of ischemic stroke. In clinical trials, statins reduced stroke and transient ischemic attacks in patients with and without CHD (Heart Protection Study Collaborative Group, 2004).

Peripheral Vascular Disease Patients. Statins are beneficial in patients with peripheral vascular disease (Heart Protection Study Collaborative Group, 2002).

Hypertensive Patients and Smokers. The risk reduction for coronary events in hypertensive patients and in smokers is similar to that in subjects without these risk factors (Heart Protection Study Collaborative Group, 2002; Sever *et al.*, 2003).

Type 2 Diabetes Mellitus. Patients with type 2 diabetes benefit very significantly from aggressive lipid lowering (*see* "Treatment of Type 2 Diabetes," below) (Heart Protection Study Collaborative Group, 2003).

Post–Myocardial Infarction or Revascularization Patients. As soon as CHD is diagnosed, it is essential to begin lipid-lowering therapy (NCEP guidelines: LDL-C goal <70 mg/dl for very high-risk patients) (Grundy *et al.*, 2004b). Compliance with drug therapy is greatly enhanced if treatment is initiated in the hospital (Fonarow and Gawlinski, 2000). It remains to be determined if statin therapy alters restenosis after angioplasty; however, the NHLBI Post Coronary Artery Bypass Graft trial showed that statin therapy improved the long-term outcome after bypass surgery and that the lower the LDL-C, the better (The Post Coronary Artery Bypass Graft Trial Investigators, 1997).

Can Cholesterol Levels Be Lowered Too Much? Are there total and LDL cholesterol levels below which adverse health consequences begin to increase? Observational studies initially were confusing. In the United States and western Europe, low cholesterol levels were associated with an increase in noncardiac mortality from chronic pulmonary disease, chronic liver disease, cancer (many primary sites), and hemorrhagic stroke. However, more recent data indicate that it is the noncardiac diseases that cause the low plasma cholesterol levels and not the low cholesterol levels that cause the noncardiac diseases (Law *et al.*, 1994). One exception may be hemorrhagic stroke. In the Multiple Risk Factor Intervention Trial (MRFIT), hemorrhagic stroke occurred more frequently in hypertensive patients with total cholesterol levels below 160 mg/dl; however, the increased incidence of hemorrhagic stroke was more than offset by reduced CHD risk due to the low cholesterol levels (Neaton *et al.*, 1992). In addition, in a study of the Chinese population, in which cholesterol levels rarely exceeded 160 mg/dl, lower levels of total cholesterol were not associated with increases in hemorrhagic stroke or any other cause of noncardiac mortality (Chen *et al.*, 1991).

Abetalipoproteinemia and hypobetalipoproteinemia, two rare disorders associated with extremely low total cholesterol levels, are instructive because affected individuals have reduced CHD risk and no increase in noncardiac mortality (Welty *et al.*, 1998). Patients who are homozygous for the mutations that cause these disorders have total cholesterol levels below 50 mg/dl and triglyceride levels below 25 mg/dl.

Individuals consuming very low levels of total fat (less than 5% of total calories) and vegetarians, who consume no animal fat, usually have total cholesterol levels below 150 mg/dl and have no increase in noncardiac mortality (Appleby *et al.*, 1999).

Based on the lack of harm associated with low total cholesterol levels in these various groups, reducing cholesterol levels to similarly low levels with drugs does not appear to be contraindicated (Grundy *et al.*, 2004b). With the advent of more efficacious cholesterol-lowering agents, it soon may be possible to test the benefits and risks of lowering total cholesterol levels below 150 mg/dl. Whether even lower cholesterol levels will translate into a further reduction in clinical events (Figure 35–2) is not known, but many researchers are optimistic.

Treatment of Type 2 Diabetes

Diabetes mellitus is an independent predictor of high risk for CHD. CHD morbidity is two to four times higher in patients

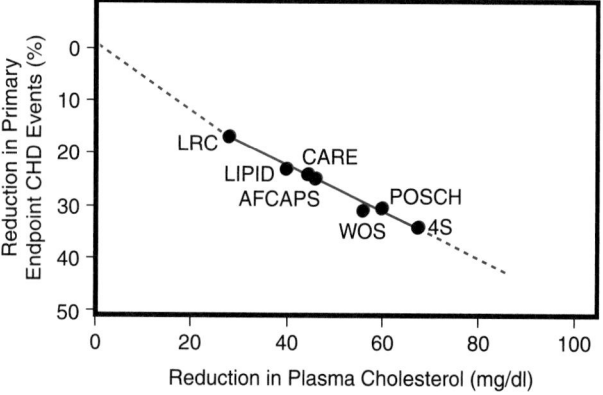

Figure 35–2. ***Reduction in coronary heart disease events in clinical trials is associated with the extent of cholesterol lowering. As more potent cholesterol-reducing agents become available, will it be possible to reduce events by 50% or more in a typical 5-year trial?*** AFCAPS, Air Force/Texas Coronary Atherosclerosis Prevention Study; CARE, Cholesterol and Recurrent Events trial; LIPID, Long-Term Intervention with Pravastatin in Ischaemic Disease (LIPID) study; LRC, Lipid Research Clinics Coronary Primary Prevention Trial; POSCH, Program on the Surgical Control of the Hyperlipidemias; 4S, Scandinavian Simvastatin Survival Study; WOS, West of Scotland Coronary Prevention Study. (Adapted from Thompson and Barter, 1999, and used by permission of Lippincott Williams & Wilkins.)

with diabetes than in nondiabetics, and the mortality from CHD is up to 100% higher in diabetic patients over a 6-year period (Grundy *et al.*, 1999). Glucose control is essential but provides only minimal benefit with respect to CHD prevention. Aggressive treatment of diabetic dyslipidemia through diet, weight control, and drugs is critical in reducing risk.

Diabetic dyslipidemia is usually characterized by high triglycerides, low HDL-C, and moderate elevations of total cholesterol and LDL-C. In fact, diabetics without diagnosed CHD have the same level of risk as nondiabetics with established CHD (Haffner, 1998). Thus, the dyslipidemia treatment guidelines for diabetic patients are the same as for patients with CHD, irrespective of whether the diabetic patient has had a CHD event (The Expert Panel, 2002). The first line of treatment for diabetic dyslipidemia usually should be a statin (Grundy *et al.*, 1999; American Diabetes Association, 2004).

Clinical trials with simvastatin, pravastatin, and *lovastatin* have clearly established that diabetics profit from cholesterol lowering as much as other subgroups (Heart Protection Study Collaborative Group, 2003; American Diabetes Association, 2004). A 3-year arteriographic study demonstrated a 40% decrease of focal coronary stenoses in type 2 diabetics treated with *fenofibrate* ($p = 0.029$) (Diabetes Atherosclerosis Intervention Study Investigators, 2001).

Metabolic Syndrome

There is an increased CHD risk associated with the insulin-resistant, prediabetic state described under the rubric of "metabolic syndrome." This syndrome consists of a constellation of five CHD risk factors (Table 35–9). The prevalence of metabolic syndrome among patients with premature vascular disease may be as high as 50% (Solymoss *et al.*, 2003). Treatment should focus on weight loss and increased physical activity, since being overweight or obese usually precludes optimal risk factor reduction. Specific treatment of increased LDL-C and triglyceride levels and low HDL-C levels should also be undertaken.

Treatment of Hypertriglyceridemia

There is increased CHD risk associated with the presence of triglyceride levels above 150 mg/dl. Three categories of hypertriglyceridemia are recognized (Table 35–5), and treatment is recommended based on the degree of elevation. Weight loss, increased exercise, and alcohol restriction are important for all hypertriglyceridemic patients. The LDL-C goal should be ascertained based on each patient's risk factors or CHD status (Table 35–4). If triglycerides remain above 200 mg/dl after the LDL-C goal is reached, further reduction in triglycerides may be

Table 35–9
Clinical Identification of the Metabolic Syndrome

RISK FACTOR	DEFINING LEVEL
Abdominal obesity*	Waist circumference[†]
Men	>102 cm (>40 in)
Women	>88 cm (>35 in)
Triglycerides	≥150 mg/dl
HDL-C	
Men	<40 mg/dl
Women	<50 mg/dl
Blood pressure	≥130/≥85 mm Hg
Fasting glucose	>110 mg/dl[†]

The 2001 NCEP guidelines define the metabolic syndrome as the presence of three or more of these risk factors. *Abbreviation:* HDL-C, high-density-lipoprotein cholesterol. *Overweight and obesity are associated with insulin resistance and the metabolic syndrome. However, the presence of abdominal obesity is more highly correlated with the metabolic risk factors than is an elevated body mass index. Therefore, the simple measurement of waist circumference is recommended to identify the body weight component of the metabolic syndrome. [†]Some male patients can develop multiple metabolic risk factors when the waist circumference is only marginally increased [e.g., 94–102 cm (37–39 in.)]. Such patients may have a strong genetic contribution to insulin resistance, and like men with categorical increases in waist circumference, they should benefit from changes in life habits.

achieved by increasing the dose of a statin or of niacin. Combination therapy (statin plus niacin or statin plus fibrate) may be required, but caution is necessary with these combinations to avoid myopathy (*see* "Statins in Combination with Other Lipid-Lowering Drugs," below).

Treatment of Low HDL-C. The most frequent risk factor for premature CHD is low HDL-C. In one study of men with angiographically documented CHD, ~60% had HDL-C levels of <35 mg/dl and only 25% had LDL-C >160 mg/dl (Genest *et al.*, 1991). In a separate study of older men with CHD, 38% had HDL-C levels <35 mg/dl and two-thirds had HDL-C <40 mg/dl (Rubins *et al.*, 1995). Subjects with "normal" cholesterol levels of <200 mg/dl but with low HDL-C (<40 mg/dl) have as much CHD risk as subjects with higher total cholesterol levels (230 to 260 mg/dl) and more normal HDL-C (40 to 49 mg/dl) (Castelli *et al.*, 1986).

In patients with low HDL-C, the total cholesterol:HDL-C ratio is a particularly useful predictor of CHD risk. A favorable ratio is ≤3.5 and a ratio of >4.5 is associated with increased risk (Castelli, 1994). American men, who are a high-risk group, have a typical ratio of ~4.5. Patients with low HDL-C may have what are considered to be "normal" total and LDL cholesterol levels; however, because of their low HDL-C levels, such patients may be at high risk based on the total cholesterol:HDL-C ratio (*e.g.,* a total cholesterol, 180 mg/dl; HDL-C, 30 mg/dl; ratio, 6). A desirable total cholesterol level in low-HDL-C patients may be considerably lower than 200 mg/dl, especially since low-HDL-C patients may also have moderately elevated triglycerides, which may reflect increased levels of atherogenic remnant lipoproteins (Grundy, 1998). Patients with average or low LDL-C, low HDL-C, and high total cholesterol:HDL-C ratios have benefitted from treatment. See Table 35–10 for a summary of trial results (Downs *et al.*, 1998; Rubins *et al.*, 1999).

The treatment of low HDL-C patients focuses on lowering LDL-C to the target level based on the patient's risk

Table 35–10
Benefit of Lipid-Lowering Therapy in Patients with Low HDL-C and "Normal" LDL-C Levels

	AFCAPS/TexCAPS (Lovastatin, 30 mg Once Daily)		VA HIT (Gemfibrozil, 0.6 g Twice Daily)	
	BASELINE	ON TREATMENT	BASELINE	ON TREATMENT
Total cholesterol (mg/dl)	228	184	175	170
LDL-C (mg/dl)	156	115	111	115
HDL-C (mg/dl)	37	39	32	35
Triglycerides (mg/dl)	163	143	161	122
Total cholesterol:HDL-C ratio	6.2	4.7	5.5	4.9
Primary event reduction	37%		22%	

Abbreviations: AFCAPS/TexCAPS, Air Force/Texas Coronary Atherosclerosis Prevention Study; HDL-C, high-density-lipoprotein cholesterol; LDL-C, low-density-lipoprotein cholesterol; VA HIT, Veterans Affairs High Density Lipoprotein Intervention Trial.

factor or CHD status (Table 35–4) *and* a reduction of VLDL cholesterol (estimated by dividing the plasma triglyceride level by 5) below 30 mg/dl. Satisfactory treatment results are a ratio of total cholesterol:HDL-C that is 3.5 or less. Patients with total cholesterol:HDL-C ratios >4.5 are at risk even if their "non-HDL-C" levels (LDL-C and VLDL cholesterol) are at the goal values recommended by the 2001 NCEP guidelines. Consequently, it is useful to base treatment of patients with low HDL-C levels on both LDL-C levels and the total cholesterol:HDL-C ratio (Tables 35–7 and 35–10) (Bersot *et al.*, 2003).

DRUG THERAPY OF DYSLIPIDEMIA

Statins

The statins are the most effective and best-tolerated agents for treating dyslipidemia. These drugs are competitive inhibitors of 3-hydroxy-3-methylglutaryl coenzyme A (HMG-CoA) reductase, which catalyzes an early, rate-limiting step in cholesterol biosynthesis. Higher doses of the more potent statins (*e.g.*, atorvastatin and simvastatin) also can reduce triglyceride levels caused by elevated VLDL levels. Some statins also are indicated for raising HDL-C levels, although the clinical significance of these effects on HDL-C remains to be proven.

Multiple well-controlled clinical trials have documented the efficacy and safety of simvastatin, pravastatin, lovastatin, and atorvastatin in reducing fatal and nonfatal CHD events, strokes, and total mortality (Table 35–3) (Law *et al.*, 2003). Rates of adverse events in statin trials were the same in the placebo groups and in the groups receiving the drug. This was true with regard to noncardiac illness and the two laboratory tests, hepatic transaminases and creatine kinase (CK), that are commonly monitored in patients taking statins (Law *et al.*, 2003).

History. Statins were isolated from a mold, *Penicillium citrinum,* and identified as inhibitors of cholesterol biosynthesis in 1976 by Endo and colleagues. Subsequent studies by Brown and Goldstein established that statins act by inhibiting HMG-CoA reductase. The first statin studied in humans was *compactin,* renamed *mevastatin,* which demonstrated the therapeutic potential of this class of drugs. However, Alberts and colleagues at Merck developed the first statin approved for use in humans, lovastatin (formerly known as mevinolin), which was isolated from *Aspergillus terreus.* Five other statins are also available. Pravastatin and simvastatin are chemically modified derivatives of lovastatin (Figure 35–3). Atorvastatin, *fluvastatin,* and *rosuvastatin* are structurally distinct synthetic compounds.

Chemistry. The structural formulas of the original statin (mevastatin) and the six statins currently available in the United States are shown in

Figure 35–3 along with the reaction (conversion of HMG-CoA to mevalonate) catalyzed by HMG-CoA reductase, the enzyme they competitively inhibit. The statins possess a side group that is structurally similar to HMG-CoA. Mevastatin, lovastatin, simvastatin, and pravastatin are fungal metabolites, and each contains a hexahydronaphthalene ring. Lovastatin differs from mevastatin in having a methyl group at carbon 3. There are two major side chains. One is a methylbutyrate ester (lovastatin and pravastatin) or a dimethylbutyrate ester (simvastatin). The other contains a hydroxy acid that forms a six-membered analog of the intermediate compound in the HMG-CoA reductase reaction (Figure 35–3). Fluvastatin, atorvastatin, and rosuvastatin are entirely synthetic compounds containing a heptanoic acid side chain that forms a structural analog of the HMG-CoA intermediate. As a result of their structural similarity to HMG-CoA, statins are reversible competitive inhibitors of the enzyme's natural substrate, HMG-CoA. The inhibition constant (K_i) of the statins is in the 1 nmol range; the dissociation constant of HMG-CoA is three orders of magnitude higher.

Lovastatin and simvastatin are lactone prodrugs that are modified in the liver to active hydroxy acid forms. Since they are lactones, they are less soluble in water than are the other statins, a difference that appears to have little if any clinical significance. Pravastatin (an acid in the active form), fluvastatin (sodium salt), and atorvastatin and rosuvastatin (calcium salts), are all administered in the active, open-ring form.

Mechanism of Action. Statins exert their major effect—reduction of LDL levels—through a mevalonic acid–like moiety that competitively inhibits HMG-CoA reductase. By reducing the conversion of HMG-CoA to mevalonate, statins inhibit an early and rate-limiting step in cholesterol biosynthesis.

Statins affect blood cholesterol levels by inhibiting hepatic cholesterol synthesis, which results in increased expression of the LDL receptor gene. In response to the reduced free cholesterol content within hepatocytes, membrane-bound SREBPs are cleaved by a protease and translocated to the nucleus. The transcription factors then bind the sterol-responsive element of the LDL receptor gene, enhancing transcription and increasing the synthesis of LDL receptors (Horton *et al.*, 2002). Degradation of LDL receptors also is reduced. The greater number of LDL receptors on the surface of hepatocytes results in increased removal of LDL from the blood, thereby lowering LDL-C levels.

Some studies suggest that statins also can reduce LDL levels by enhancing the removal of LDL precursors (VLDL and IDL) and by decreasing hepatic VLDL production (Aguila-Salinas *et al.*, 1998). Since VLDL remnants and IDL are enriched in apoE, a statin-induced increase in the number of LDL receptors, which recognize both apoB-100 and apoE, enhances the clearance of these LDL precursors. The reduction in hepatic VLDL production induced by statins is thought to be mediated by reduced synthesis of cholesterol, a required component of VLDL (Thompson, 1996). This mechanism also likely accounts for the triglyceride-lowering effect of statins (Ginsberg, 1998) and may account for the reduction (~25%) of LDL-C levels in patients with homozygous familial hypercholesterolemia treated with 80 mg of atorvastatin or simvastatin.

Triglyceride Reduction by Statins. Triglyceride levels >250 mg/dl are reduced substantially by statins, and the percent reduction

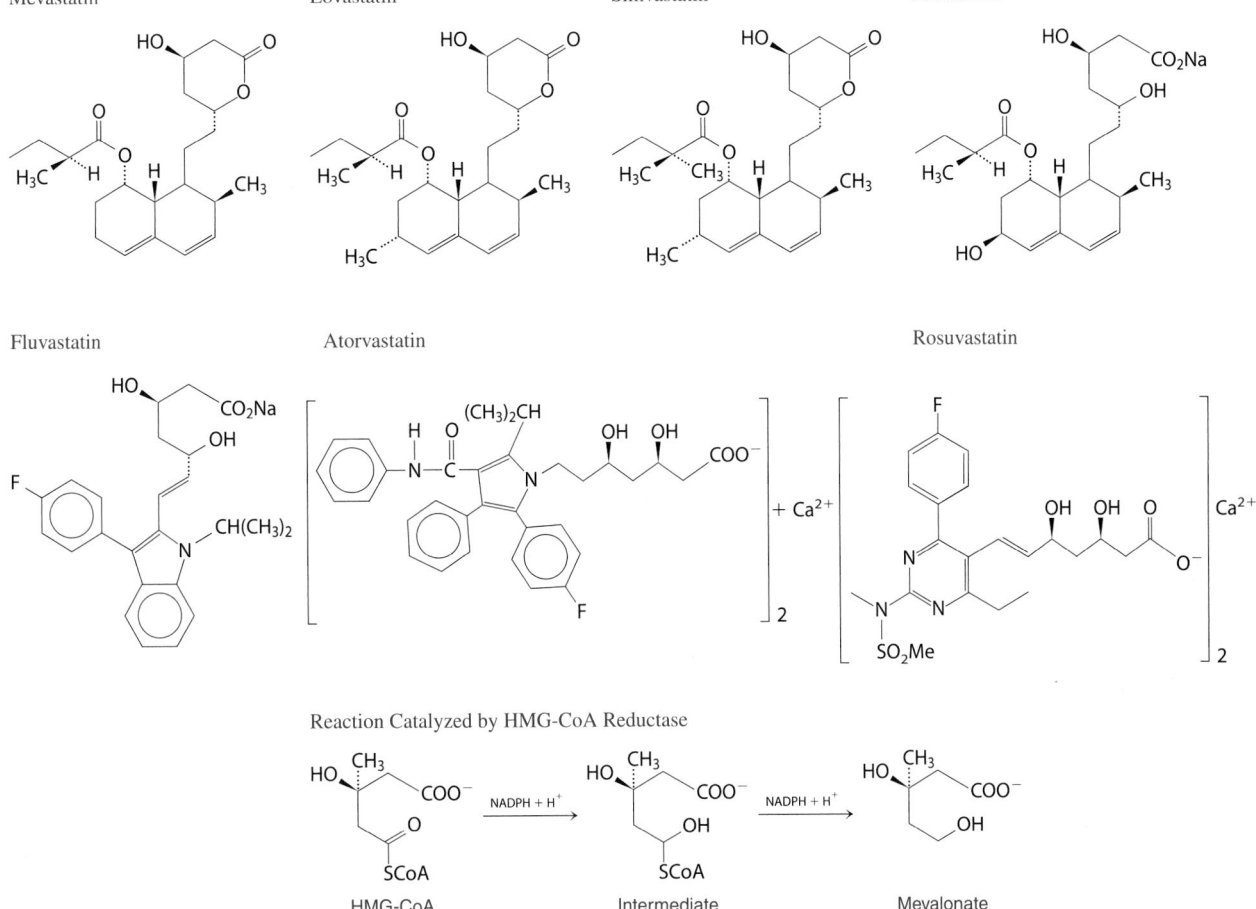

Figure 35–3. *Chemical structures of the statins and the reaction catalyzed by 3-hydroxy-3-methylglutaryl coenzyme A (HMG-CoA) reductase.*

achieved is similar to the percent reduction in LDL-C (Stein *et al.*, 1998). Accordingly, hypertriglyceridemic patients taking the highest doses of the most potent statins (simvastatin and atorvastatin, 80 mg/day; rosuvastatin, 40 mg/day) experience a 35% to 45% reduction in LDL-C and a similar reduction in fasting triglyceride levels (Bakker-Arkema *et al.*, 1996; Ose *et al.*, 2000; Hunninghake *et al.*, 2004). If baseline triglyceride levels are below 250 mg/dl, reductions in triglycerides do not exceed 25% irrespective of the dose or statin used (Stein *et al.*, 1998). Similar reductions (35% to 45%) in triglycerides can be accomplished with doses of fibrates or niacin (*see* below), although these drugs do not reduce LDL-C to the same extent as atorvastatin or simvastatin at the 80-mg dose.

Effect of Statins on HDL-C Levels. Most studies of patients treated with statins have systematically excluded patients with low HDL-C levels. In studies of patients with elevated LDL-C levels and gender-appropriate HDL-C levels (40 to 50 mg/dl for men; 50 to 60 mg/dl for women), an increase in HDL-C of 5% to 10% was observed, irrespective of the dose or statin employed. However, in patients with reduced HDL-C levels (<35 mg/dl), statins may differ in their effects on HDL-C levels. Simvastatin, at its highest dose of 80 mg, increases HDL-C and apoA-I levels more than a comparable

dose of atorvastatin (Crouse *et al.*, 2000). In preliminary studies of patients with hypertriglyceridemia and low HDL-C, rosuvastatin appears to raise HDL-C levels by as much as 15% to 20% (Hunninghake *et al.*, 2004). More studies are needed to ascertain whether the effects of statins on HDL-C in patients with low HDL-C levels are clinically significant.

Effects of Statins on LDL-C Levels. Statins lower LDL-C by 20% to 55%, depending on the dose and statin used. In large trials comparing the effects of the various statins, equivalent doses appear to be 5 mg of simvastatin = ~15 mg of lovastatin = ~15 mg of pravastatin = ~40 mg of fluvastatin (Pedersen and Tobert, 1996); 20 mg of simvastatin = ~10 mg of atorvastatin (Jones *et al.*, 1998; Crouse *et al.*, 1999), and 20 mg of atorvastatin = 10 mg of rosuvastatin (Jones *et al.*, 2003). Analysis of dose-response relationships for all statins demonstrates that the efficacy of LDL-C lowering is log-linear; LDL-C is reduced by ~6% (from baseline) with each doubling of the dose (Pedersen and Tobert, 1996; Jones *et al.*, 1998). Maximal effects on plasma cholesterol levels are achieved within 7 to 10 days.

Table 35–11 provides information on the statin doses required to reduce LDL-C by 20% to 55%. The fractional reductions achieved with the various doses are the same regardless of the absolute value of the

Table 35–11
Doses (mg) of Statins Required to Achieve Various Reductions in Low-Density-Lipoprotein Cholesterol from Baseline

	20%–25%	26%–30%	31%–35%	36%–40%	41%–50%	51%–55%
Atorvastatin	—	—	10	20	40	80
Fluvastatin	20	40	80			
Lovastatin	10	20	40	80		
Pravastatin	10	20	40			
Rosuvastatin	—	—	—	5	10	20, 40
Simvastatin	—	10	20	40	80	

baseline LDL-C level. The statins are effective in almost all patients with high LDL-C levels. The exception is patients with homozygous familial hypercholesterolemia, who have very attenuated responses to the usual doses of statins because both alleles of the LDL receptor gene code for dysfunctional LDL receptors; the partial response in these patients is due to a reduction in hepatic VLDL synthesis associated with the inhibition of HMG-CoA reductase–mediated cholesterol synthesis. Statin therapy does not reduce Lp(a) levels (Kostner et al., 1989).

Potential Cardioprotective Effects Other Than LDL Lowering. Although the statins clearly exert their major effects on CHD by lowering LDL-C and improving the lipid profile as reflected in plasma cholesterol levels (Figure 35–2) (Thompson and Barter, 1999), a multitude of potentially cardioprotective effects are being ascribed to these drugs (Liao and Laufs, 2005). However, the mechanisms of action for non–lipid-lowering roles of statins have not been established, and it is not known whether these potential pleiotropic effects represent a class-action effect, differ among statins, or are biologically or clinically relevant. Until these questions are resolved, selection of a specific statin should not be based on any one of these effects. Nevertheless, the potential importance of the nonlipid roles of statins merits discussion.

Statins and Endothelial Function. A variety of studies have established that the vascular endothelium plays a dynamic role in vasoconstriction/relaxation. Hypercholesterolemia adversely affects the processes by which the endothelium modulates arterial tone. Statin therapy enhances endothelial production of the vasodilator nitric oxide, leading to improved endothelial function after a month of therapy (O'Driscoll et al., 1997; Laufs et al., 1998). However, similar results have been observed after a single acute reduction of LDL levels by apheresis (Tamai et al., 1997). In nonhuman primates fed a high-cholesterol diet, statin therapy improved endothelial function independent of significant changes in plasma cholesterol levels (Williams et al., 1998).

Statins and Plaque Stability. The vulnerability of plaques to rupture and thrombosis is of greater clinical relevance than the degree of stenosis they cause (Corti et al., 2003). Statins may affect plaque stability in a variety of ways. They reportedly inhibit monocyte infiltration into the artery wall in a rabbit model (Bustos et al., 1998) and inhibit macrophage secretion of matrix metalloproteinases in vitro (Bellosta et al., 1998). The metalloproteinases degrade extracellular matrix components and thus weaken the fibrous cap of atherosclerotic plaques.

Statins also appear to modulate the cellularity of the artery wall by inhibiting proliferation of smooth muscle cells and enhancing apoptotic cell death (Corsini et al., 1998). It is debatable whether these effects would be beneficial or harmful if they occurred in vivo. Reduced proliferation of smooth muscle cells and enhanced apoptosis could retard initial hyperplasia and restenosis, but also could weaken the fibrous cap and destabilize the lesion. Interestingly, statin-induced suppression of cell proliferation and the induction of apoptosis have been extended to tumor biology. The effects of statins on isoprenoid biosynthesis and protein phenylation associated with reduced synthesis of the cholesterol precursor mevalonate may alter the development of malignancies (Davignon and Laaksonen, 1999; Wong et al., 2002; Li et al., 2003).

Statins and Inflammation. Appreciation of the importance of inflammatory processes in atherogenesis is growing (Libby, 2002), and statins may have an antiinflammatory role (Libby and Aikawa, 2003). Statins decreased the risk of CHD and levels of C-reactive protein (CRP, an independent marker for inflammation and high CHD risk) independently of cholesterol lowering (Libby and Aikawa, 2003; Libby and Ridker, 2004). Body weight and the metabolic syndrome are associated with elevated levels of highly sensitive CRP, leading some to suggest that the CRP may simply be a marker of obesity and insulin resistance (Pearson et al., 2003). It remains to be determined whether the C-reactive protein is simply a marker of inflammation or if it contributes to the pathogenesis of atherosclerosis. The clinical utility of measuring CRP with "highly sensitive" assays appears to be limited to those primary prevention subjects with a moderate (10% to 20%) 10-year risk of sustaining a CHD event. Values of highly sensitive CRP above 3 mg/L suggests that such patients should be managed as secondary prevention patients (Pearson et al., 2003).

Statins and Lipoprotein Oxidation. Oxidative modification of LDL appears to play a key role in mediating the uptake of lipoprotein cholesterol by macrophages and in other processes, including cytotoxicity within lesions (Steinberg, 1997). Statins reduce the susceptibility of lipoproteins to oxidation both in vitro and ex vivo (Hussein et al., 1997).

Statins and Coagulation. Statins reduce platelet aggregation (Hussein et al., 1997) and reduce the deposition of platelet thrombi in the porcine aorta model (Lacoste et al., 1995). In addition, the different statins have variable effects on fibrinogen levels, the significance of which remains to be determined (Rosenson and Tangney, 1998). Elevated plasma fibrinogen levels are associated with an increase in the incidence of CHD (Ernst and Resch, 1993); however, it remains to be determined whether fibrinogen is a contributor to or a marker of disease.

Absorption, Metabolism, and Excretion. *Absorption from the Small Intestine.* After oral administration, intestinal absorption of the statins varies between 30% and 85%. All the statins, except simvastatin and lovastatin, are administered in the β-hydroxy acid form, which is the form that inhibits HMG-CoA reductase. Simvastatin and lovastatin are administered as inactive lactones, which must be transformed in the liver to their respective β-hydroxy acids, simvastatin acid (SVA) and lovastatin acid (LVA). There is extensive first-pass hepatic uptake of all statins, but the mechanisms by which they enter the liver differ. Atorvastatin, pravastatin, and rosuvastatin uptake is mediated by the organic anion transporter 2 (OATP2) (Hsiang *et al.*, 1999; Schneck *et al.*, 2004). The highly lipophilic lactone forms of simvastatin and lovastatin are thought to enter the liver by simple diffusion (Ohtawa *et al.*, 1999). Due to extensive first-pass hepatic uptake, systemic bioavailability of the statins and their hepatic metabolites varies between 5% and 30% of administered doses. The metabolites of all statins, except fluvastatin and pravastatin, have some HMG-CoA reductase inhibitory activity (Bellosta *et al.*, 2004). Under steady-state conditions, small amounts of the parent drug and its metabolites produced in the liver can be found in the systemic circulation. After the lactones of simvastatin and lovastatin are transformed in the liver to SVA and LVA, small amounts of these active inhibitors of HMG-CoA reductase can be found in the systemic circulation as well as small amounts of the lactone forms. In the plasma, greater than 95% of statins and their metabolites are protein bound with the exception of pravastatin and its metabolites, which are only 50% bound.

After an oral dose, plasma concentrations of statins peak in 1 to 4 hours. The half-lives of the parent compounds are 1 to 4 hours, except in the case of atorvastatin and rosuvastatin, which have half-lives of about 20 hours. The longer half-lives of atorvastatin and rosuvastatin may contribute to their greater cholesterol-lowering efficacy (Corsini *et al.*, 1999). The liver biotransforms all statins, and more than 70% of statin metabolites are excreted by the liver with subsequent elimination in the feces (Bellosta *et al.*, 2004). As noted below, inhibition by other drugs of OATP2 activity (which transports several statins into hepatocytes) and inhibition or induction of CYP3A4 by a variety of pharmacologic agents provide rationales for drug-drug interactions involving statins.

Adverse Effects and Drug Interactions. *Hepatotoxicity.* Initial postmarketing surveillance studies of the statins revealed an elevation in hepatic transaminase to values greater than three times the upper limit of normal, with an incidence as great as 1%. The incidence appeared to be dose related. However, as of 2003, in the placebo-controlled outcome trials in which 10- to 40-mg doses of simvastatin, lovastatin, fluvastatin, atorvastatin, or pravastatin were used, the incidence of threefold elevations in hepatic transaminases was 1% to 3% in the active drug treatment groups and 1.1% in placebo patients (Law *et al.*, 2003). No cases of liver failure occurred in these trials. Although serious hepatotoxicity is rare, 30 cases of liver failure associated with statin use were reported to the FDA between 1987 and 2000, a rate of about one case per million person-years of use (Law *et al.*, 2003). It is therefore reasonable to measure alanine aminotransferase (ALT) at baseline and thereafter when clinically indicated. Patients taking 80-mg doses (or 40 mg of rosuvastatin) should have their ALT checked after 3 months. If the ALT values are normal, it is not necessary to repeat the ALT test unless clinically indicated.

Myopathy. The major adverse effect of clinical significance associated with statin use is myopathy. Between 1987 and 2001, the FDA recorded 42 deaths from rhabdomyolysis induced by statins (except *cerivastatin*, which has been withdrawn from the market worldwide). This is a rate of one death per million prescriptions (30-day supply). In the statin trials described above (under hepatotoxicity), rhabdomyolysis occurred in eight active drug recipients *versus* five placebo subjects. Among active drug recipients, 0.17% had CK values exceeding 10 times the upper limit of normal, the value commonly used to define statin-induced rhabdomyolysis; among placebo-treated subjects, the incidence was 0.13%. Only 13 out of 55 drug-treated subjects and 4 out of 43 placebo subjects with greater than tenfold elevations of CK reported any muscle symptoms (Law *et al.*, 2003).

The incidence of myopathy is quite low (~0.01%), but the risk of myopathy and rhabdomyolysis increases in proportion to plasma statin concentrations (Omar *et al.*, 2001). Consequently, factors inhibiting statin catabolism are associated with increased myopathy risk, including advanced age (especially >80 years of age), hepatic or renal dysfunction, perioperative periods, multisystem disease (especially in association with diabetes mellitus), small body size, and untreated hypothyroidism (Pasternak *et al.*, 2002; Thompson *et al.*, 2003). Concomitant use of drugs that diminish statin catabolism is associated with myopathy and rhabdomyolysis in 50% to 60% of cases (Thompson *et al.*, 2003). The most common statin interactions occurred with fibrates, especially *gemfibrozil*, 38%; *cyclosporine*, 4%; *digoxin*, 5%; *warfarin*, 4%; macrolide antibiotics, 3%, *mibefradil*, 2%; and azole antifungals, 1% (Thompson *et al.*, 2003). Other drugs that increase the risk of statin-induced myopathy include niacin (rare), HIV protease inhibitors, *amiodarone*, and *nefazodone* (Pasternak *et al.*, 2002).

There are a variety of pharmacokinetic mechanisms by which these drugs increase myopathy risk when administered concomitantly with statins. Gemfibrozil, the drug most commonly associated with statin-induced myopathy, inhibits both uptake of the active hydroxy acid forms of statins into hepatocytes by OATP2 and interferes with the transformation of most statins by CYPs and glucuronidases. Primarily due to inhibition of OATP2-mediated hepatic uptake, coadministration of gemfibrozil nearly doubles the plasma concentration of rosuvastatin (Schneck *et al.*, 2004). This occurs despite the fact that gemfibrozil has little effect on rosuvastatin glucuronidation or oxidation, which are important pathways in the catabolism of the other statins (Prueksaritanont *et al.*, 2002a; Prueksaritanont *et al.*, 2002b; Prueksaritanont *et al.*, 2002c). Other fibrates, especially fenofibrate, do not interfere with the glucuronidation of statins and pose less risk of myopathy when used in combination with statin therapy (for reviews of statin interactions with other drugs, *see* Corsini, 2003; Bellosta *et al.*, 2004). Concomitant therapy with simvastatin, 80 mg daily, and fenofibrate, 160 mg daily, results in no clinically significant pharmacokinetic interaction (Bergman *et al.*, 2004). Similar results were obtained in a study of low-dose rosuvastatin, 10 mg daily, plus fenofibrate, 67 mg three times a day (Martin *et al.*, 2003). When statins are administered with niacin, the myopathy is probably caused by an enhanced inhibition of skeletal muscle cholesterol synthesis (a pharmacodynamic interaction) (Christians *et al.*, 1998).

Other drugs that interfere with statin oxidation are those metabolized primarily by CYP3A4 and include certain macrolide antibiotics (*e.g., erythromycin*); azole antifungals (*e.g., itraconazole*); cyclosporine; a phenylpiperazine antidepressant, nefazodone; and HIV protease inhibitors (Christians *et al.*, 1998; Corsini, 2003; Bellosta *et al.*, 2004). These pharmacokinetic interactions are associated with increased plasma concentrations of statins and their active metabolites. Atorvastatin, lovastatin, and simvastatin are primarily metabolized by CYP3A4. Fluvastatin is mostly (50% to 80%) metabolized by CYP2C9 to inactive metabolites, but CYP3A4 and CYP2C8 also contribute to its metabolism. Pravastatin, however, is not metabolized to any appreciable extent by the CYP system (Corsini *et al.*, 1999) and is excreted unchanged in the urine. Pravastatin, fluvastatin, and rosuvastatin are not extensively metabolized by CYP3A4. Pravastatin and fluvastatin may be less likely to cause myopathy when used with one of the predisposing drugs. However, because cases of myopathy have been reported with both drugs, the benefits of combined therapy with any statin should be carefully weighed against the risk of myopathy. Although rosuvastatin is not transformed to any appreciable extent by oxidation, cases of myopathy have been reported, particularly in association with concomitant use of gemfibrozil (Schneck *et al.*, 2004).

The myopathy syndrome is characterized by intense myalgia similar to flu-related myalgia, first in the arms and thighs and then in the entire body, along with weakness and fatigue. Symptoms progress as long as the patient continues to take the statin. Myoglobinuria, renal failure, and death have been reported (Staffa *et al.*, 2002). Serum CK levels in affected patients typically are tenfold higher than the upper limit of normal. As soon as myopathy is suspected, a blood sample should be drawn to document the presence of a significantly elevated (approaching tenfold elevation) CK level, since many patients complain of muscle pain unrelated to true statin-induced myopathy. The statin, and any other drug suspected of contributing to myopathy, should be discontinued if true myopathy is suspected, even if it is not possible to measure CK activity to document the presence of myopathy. Rhabdomyolysis should be excluded and renal function monitored.

Since myopathy rarely occurs in the absence of combination therapy, routine CK monitoring is not recommended unless the statins are used with one of the predisposing drugs. Such monitoring is not sufficient to protect patients, as myopathy can occur months to years after combined therapy is initiated. As a rule, statins may be used in combination with one of these predisposing drugs with reduced risk of myopathy if the statin is administered at no more than 25% of its maximal dose (Christians *et al.*, 1998; Corsini, 2003; Bellosta *et al.*, 2004). This dose would be 10 mg for rosuvastatin and 20 mg for all other statins.

Early concerns about statin-induced eye pathology have not been substantiated (Bradford *et al.*, 1991). Likewise, speculation that the more lipid-soluble statins might penetrate to the CNS and cause effects there has proven unfounded; except as they affect statin uptake by hepatic OATP2 (*see* above), differences in lipid solubility among statins do not appear to be clinically relevant.

Pregnancy. *The safety of statins during pregnancy has not been established.* Women wishing to conceive should not take statins. During their childbearing years, women taking statins should use highly effective contraception (*see* Chapter 57). Nursing mothers also are advised to avoid taking statins.

Therapeutic Uses. Each statin has a low recommended starting dose that reduces LDL-C by 20% to 30%. Dyslipidemic patients frequently remain on their initial dose, are not titrated to achieve their target LDL-C level, and thus remain undertreated. For this reason, it is advisable to start each patient on a dose that will achieve the patient's target goal for LDL-C lowering. For example, a patient with a baseline LDL-C of 150 mg/dl and a goal of 100 mg/dl requires a 33% reduction

in LDL-C and should be started on a dose expected to provide it (Table 35–11).

Hepatic cholesterol synthesis is maximal between midnight and 2:00 A.M. Thus, statins with half-lives of 4 hours or less (all but atorvastatin and rosuvastatin) should be taken in the evening.

The manufacturer's initial recommended dose of lovastatin (MEVACOR) is 20 mg and is slightly more effective if taken with the evening meal than if it is taken at bedtime, although bedtime dosing is preferable to missing doses. The dose of lovastatin may be increased every 3 to 6 weeks up to a maximum of 80 mg per day. The 80-mg dose is slightly (2% to 3%) more effective if given as 40 mg twice daily. Lovastatin, at 20 mg, is marketed in combination with 500, 750, or 1000 mg of extended-release niacin (ADVICOR). Few patients are appropriate candidates for this fixed-dose combination (*see* section on nicotinic acid, below). Alternate-day statin therapy has been associated with nearly equivalent efficacy, as judged by serum lipid profiles and reduced cost, and has been proposed as a means to enhance compliance; clinical trials are needed to evaluate the efficacy of alternate-day dosing with regard to reducing clinical events.

The approved starting dose of simvastatin (ZOCOR) for most patients is 20 mg at bedtime unless the required LDL-C reduction exceeds 45% or the patient is a high-risk secondary prevention patient, in which case a 40-mg starting dose is indicated. The maximal dose is 80 mg, and the drug should be taken at bedtime. In patients taking cyclosporine, fibrates, or niacin, the daily dose should not exceed 20 mg.

Pravastatin (PRAVACHOL) therapy is initiated with a 20- or 40-mg dose that may be increased to 80 mg. This drug should be taken at bedtime. Since pravastatin is a hydroxy acid, it is bound by bile-acid sequestrants, which reduces its absorption. Practically, this is rarely a problem since the resins should be taken before meals and pravastatin should be taken at bedtime. Pravastatin is also marketed in combination with buffered aspirin (PRAVIGARD). The small advantage of combining these two drugs should be weighed against the disadvantages inherent in fixed-dose combinations.

The starting dose of fluvastatin (LESCOL) is 20 or 40 mg, and the maximum is 80 mg per day. Like pravastatin, it is administered as a hydroxy acid and should be taken at bedtime, several hours after ingesting a bile-acid sequestrant (if the combination is used).

Atorvastatin (LIPITOR) has a long half-life, which allows administration of this statin at any time of the day. The starting dose is 10 mg, and the maximum is 80 mg per day.

Atorvastatin is marketed in combination with the Ca^{2+}-channel blocker amlodipine (CADUET), for patients with hypertension or angina as well as hypercholesterolemia. The physician should weigh any advantage of combination against the associated risks and disadvantages.

Rosuvastatin (CRESTOR) is available in doses ranging between 5 and 40 mg. It has a half-life of 20 to 30 hours and may be taken at any time of day. Since experience with rosuvastatin is limited, treatment should be initiated with 5 to 10 mg daily, increasing stepwise, if needed, until the incidence of myopathy is better defined. If the combination of gemfibrozil with rosuvastatin is used, the dose of rosuvastatin should not exceed 10 mg. Rosuvastatin at a dose of 80 mg (dose not approved by the FDA) was noted to cause proteinuria and hematuria and isolated cases of renal failure. Other statins have also been observed to cause proteinuria, apparently by inhibiting tubular protein reabsorption. Whether statin-induced proteinuria is harmful or beneficial, especially in patients with chronic kidney disease, remains to be determined (Agarwal, 2004). The significance and etiology of the hematuria caused by the 80-mg dose of rosuvastatin remains to be determined.

The choice of statins should be based on efficacy (reduction of LDL-C) and cost. Three drugs (lovastatin, simvastatin, and pravastatin) have been used safely in clinical trials involving thousands of subjects for 5 or more years. The documented safety records of these statins should be considered, especially when initiating therapy in younger patients. Once drug treatment is initiated, it is almost always lifelong. Baseline determinations of alanine aminotransferase (ALT) and repeat testing at 3 to 6 months are recommended. If ALT is normal after the initial 3 to 6 months, then it need not be repeated more than once every 6 to 12 months. Creatine kinase (CK) measurements are not routinely necessary unless the patient also is taking a drug that enhances the risk of myopathy. Because myopathy may develop months to years after the start of combined therapy, it is unlikely that routine monitoring for the accompanying rise in CK will consistently herald the onset, even if monitoring is performed every 3 to 4 months.

Statin Use by Children. Some statins have been approved for use in children with heterozygous familial hypercholesterolemia. Atorvastatin, lovastatin, and simvastatin are indicated for children age 11 or older. Pravastatin is approved for children age 8 or older.

Statins in Combination with Other Lipid-Lowering Drugs. Statins, in combination with the bile acid–binding resins *cholestyramine* and *colestipol*, produce 20% to 30% greater reductions in LDL-C than can be achieved with statins alone (Tikkanen, 1996). Preliminary data indicate that *colesevelam hydrochloride* plus a statin lowers LDL-C by 8% to 16% more than statins alone. Niacin also can enhance the effect of statins, but the occurrence of myopathy increases when statin doses greater than 25% of maximum (*e.g.,* 20 mg of simvastatin or atorvastatin) are used with niacin (Guyton and Capuzzi, 1998). The combination of a fibrate (*clofibrate*, gemfibrozil, or fenofibrate) with a statin is particularly useful in patients with hypertriglyceridemia and high LDL-C levels. This combination increases the risk of myopathy but usually is safe with a fibrate at its usual maximal dose and a statin at no more than 25% of its maximal dose (Tikkanen, 1996; Athyros *et al.*, 1997). Fenofibrate, which is least likely to interfere with statin metabolism, appears to be the safest fibrate to use with statins (Prueksaritanont *et al.*, 2002b).

Triple therapy with resins, niacin, and statins can reduce LDL-C by up to 70% (Malloy *et al.*, 1987). VYTORIN, a fixed combination of simvastatin (10, 20, 40, or 80 mg) and ezetimibe (10 mg), decreased LDL-C levels by up to 60% at 24 weeks.

Bile-Acid Sequestrants

The two established bile-acid sequestrants or resins (cholestyramine and colestipol) are among the oldest of the hypolipidemic drugs, and they are probably the safest, since they are not absorbed from the intestine. These resins are also recommended for patients 11 to 20 years of age. Because statins are so effective as monotherapy, the resins are most often used as second agents if statin therapy does not lower LDL-C levels sufficiently. When used with a statin, cholestyramine and colestipol usually are prescribed at submaximal doses. Maximal doses can reduce LDL-C by up to 25% but are associated with unacceptable gastrointestinal side effects (bloating and constipation) that limit compliance. Colesevelam is a newer bile-acid sequestrant that is prepared as an anhydrous gel and taken as a tablet. It lowers LDL-C by 18% at its maximum dose. The safety and efficacy of colesevelam have not been studied in pediatric patients or pregnant women.

Cholestyramine was used in the Coronary Primary Prevention Trial, one of the first studies to document that lowering LDL-C prevents heart disease events (Lipid Research Clinics Program, 1984). Cholestyramine therapy reduced total cholesterol by 13% and LDL-C by 20%, compared with diet-induced reductions of 5% in total cholesterol and 8% in LDL-C. CHD events (fatal and nonfatal) were reduced by 19%, suggesting that a 1% reduction in total cholesterol is associated with at least a 2% reduction in CHD events.

Chemistry. Figure 35–4 shows the structure of these agents. Cholestyramine and colestipol are anion-exchange resins. Cholestyramine, a polymer of styrene and divinylbenzene with active sites formed from trimethylbenzylammonium groups, is a quaternary amine. Colestipol, a copolymer of diethylenetriamine and 1-chloro-2,3-epoxypropane, is a mixture of tertiary and quaternary diamines. Cholestyramine and colestipol are hygroscopic powders administered as chloride salts and are insoluble in water. Colesevelam is a polymer, poly(allylamine hydrochloride), cross-linked with epichlorohydrin and alkylated with 1-bromodecane and (6-bromohexyl)-trimethylammonium bromide. It is a hydrophilic gel and insoluble in water.

Mechanism of Action. The bile-acid sequestrants are highly positively charged and bind negatively charged bile acids. Because of their large size, the resins are not absorbed, and the bound bile acids are excreted in the

Cholestyramine

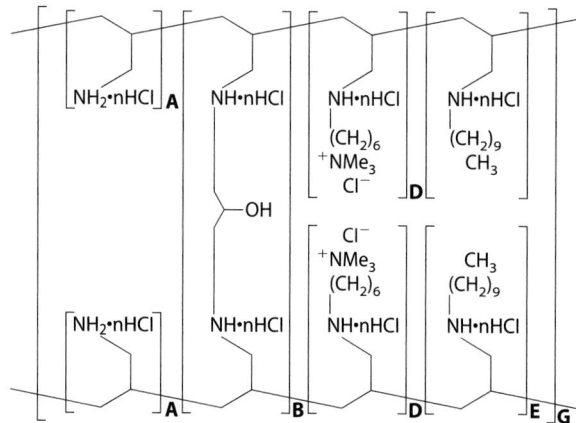

Colestipol

Colesevelam

A = Primary Amines
B = Cross-linked Amines
D = Quaternary Ammonium Alkylated Amines
E = Decalkylated Amines
n = Fraction of Protonated Amines
G = Extended Polymeric Network

Figure 35–4. *Structures of cholestyramine, colestipol, and colesevelam.*

stool. Since over 95% of bile acids are normally reabsorbed, interruption of this process depletes the pool of bile acids, and hepatic bile-acid synthesis increases. As a result, hepatic cholesterol content declines, stimulating the production of LDL receptors, an effect similar to that of statins. The increase in hepatic LDL receptors increases LDL clearance and lowers LDL-C levels, but this effect is partially offset by the enhanced cholesterol

synthesis caused by upregulation of HMG-CoA reductase (Shepherd *et al.*, 1980). Inhibition of reductase activity by a statin substantially increases the effectiveness of the resins.

The resin-induced increase in bile-acid production is accompanied by an increase in hepatic triglyceride synthesis, which is of consequence in patients with significant hypertriglyceridemia (baseline triglyceride level >250 mg/dl). In such patients, bile-acid sequestrant therapy may cause striking increases in triglyceride levels. An initial report suggests that colesevelam may not raise triglyceride levels significantly (Davidson *et al.*, 1999); until this issue is resolved, use of colesevelam to lower LDL-C levels in hypertriglyceridemic patients should be accompanied by frequent (every 1 to 2 weeks) monitoring of fasting triglyceride levels until the triglyceride level is stable, or the use of colesevelam in these patients should be avoided.

Effects on Lipoprotein Levels. The reduction in LDL-C by resins is dose-dependent. Doses of 8 to 12 g of cholestyramine or 10 to 15 g of colestipol are associated with 12% to 18% reductions in LDL-C. Maximal doses (24 g of cholestyramine, 30 g of colestipol) may reduce LDL-C by as much as 25%, but will cause GI side effects that are poorly tolerated by most patients. One to two weeks is sufficient to attain maximal LDL-C reduction by a given resin dose. In patients with normal triglyceride levels, triglycerides may increase transiently and then return to baseline. HDL-C levels increase 4% to 5%. Statins plus resins or niacin plus resins can reduce LDL-C by as much as 40% to 60%. Colesevelam, in doses of 3 to 3.75 g, reduces LDL-C levels by 9% to 19%.

Adverse Effects and Drug Interactions. The resins are generally safe, as they are not systemically absorbed. Since they are administered as chloride salts, rare instances of hyperchloremic acidosis have been reported. Severe hypertriglyceridemia is a contraindication to the use of cholestyramine and colestipol since these resins increase triglyceride levels (Crouse, 1987). At present, there are insufficient data on the effect of colesevelam on triglyceride levels.

Cholestyramine and colestipol both are available as a powder that must be mixed with water and drunk as a slurry. The gritty sensation is unpleasant to patients initially but can be tolerated. Colestipol is available in a tablet form that reduces the complaint of grittiness but not the gastrointestinal symptoms. Colesevelam is available as a hard capsule that absorbs water and creates a soft, gelatinous material that allegedly minimizes the potential for gastrointestinal irritation.

Patients taking cholestyramine and colestipol complain of bloating and dyspepsia. These symptoms can be substantially reduced if the drug is completely suspended in liquid several hours before ingestion (*e.g.*, evening doses can be mixed in the morning and refrigerated; morning doses can be mixed the previous evening and refrigerated). Constipation may occur but sometimes can be prevented by adequate daily water intake and psyllium, if necessary. Colesevelam may be less likely to cause the dyspepsia, bloating, and constipation observed in patients treated with cholestyramine or colestipol (Davidson *et al.*, 1999).

Cholestyramine and colestipol bind and interfere with the absorption of many drugs, including some thiazides, *furosemide*, *propranolol*, *l-thyroxine*, digoxin, warfarin, and some of the statins

(Farmer and Gotto, 1994). The effect of cholestyramine and colestipol on the absorption of most drugs has not been studied. For this reason, it is wise to administer all drugs either 1 hour before or 3 to 4 hours after a dose of cholestyramine or colestipol. Colesevelam does not appear to interfere with the absorption of fat-soluble vitamins or of drugs such as digoxin, lovastatin, warfarin, *metoprolol, quinidine,* and *valproic acid.* The maximum concentration and the AUC of sustained-release *verapamil* are reduced by 31% and 11%, respectively, when the drug is coadministered with colesevelam. Since the effect of colesevelam on the absorption of other drugs has not been tested, it seems prudent to recommend that patients take other medications 1 hour before or 3 or 4 hours after a dose of colesevelam.

Therapeutic Uses. Cholestyramine resin (QUESTRAN, others) is available in bulk (with scoops that measure a 4-g dose) or in individual packets of 4 g. Additional flavorings are added to increase palatability. The "light" preparations contain artificial sweeteners rather than sucrose. Colestipol hydrochloride (COLESTID, others) is available in bulk, in individual packets containing 5 g of colestipol, or as 1-g tablets.

Resins should never be taken in the dry form. The powdered forms of cholestyramine (4 g per dose) and colestipol (5 g per dose) are either mixed with a fluid (water or juice) and drunk as a slurry or mixed with crushed ice in a blender. Ideally, patients should take the resins before breakfast and before supper, starting with one scoop or packet twice daily, and increasing the dosage after several weeks or longer as needed and as tolerated. Patients generally will not take more than two doses (scoops or packets) twice a day.

Colesevelam hydrochloride (WELCHOL) is available as a solid tablet containing 0.625 g of colesevelam. The starting dose is either three tablets taken twice daily with meals or all six tablets taken with a meal. The tablets should be taken with a liquid. The maximum daily dose is 7 tablets (4.375 g).

Niacin (Nicotinic Acid)

Niacin, *nicotinic acid* (pyridine-3-carboxylic acid), one of the oldest drugs used to treat dyslipidemia, favorably affects virtually all lipid parameters (Knopp, 1998).

NICOTINIC ACID   NICOTINAMIDE

Niacin is a water-soluble B-complex vitamin that functions as a vitamin only after its conversion to NAD or NADP, in which it occurs as an amide. Both niacin and its amide may be given orally as a source of niacin for its functions as a vitamin but only niacin affects lipid levels. The hypolipidemic effects of niacin require larger doses than are required for its vitamin effects. Niacin is the best agent available for increasing HDL-C (increments of 30% to 40%); it also lowers triglycerides by 35% to 45% (as effectively as fibrates and the more potent statins) and reduces LDL-C levels by 20% to 30% (Knopp *et al.,* 1985; Vega and Grundy, 1994; Martin-Jadraque *et al.,* 1996). Niacin also is the only lipid-lowering drug that reduces Lp(a) levels significantly, by about 40% (Carlson *et al.,* 1989); however, adequate control of other lipid abnormalities renders an elevation of Lp(a) harmless (Maher *et al.,* 1995). Estrogen and neomycin also significantly lower Lp(a) levels (Espeland *et al.,* 1998; Shlipak *et al.,* 2000). Despite its salutary effect on lipids, niacin has side effects that limit its use (*see* "Adverse Effects," below).

Mechanism of Action. In adipose tissue, niacin inhibits the lipolysis of triglycerides by hormone-sensitive lipase, which reduces transport of free fatty acids to the liver and decreases hepatic triglyceride synthesis. Niacin and related compounds (*e.g.,* 5-methylpyrazine-2-carboxylic-4-oxide, *acipimox*) may exert their effects on lipolysis by inhibiting adipocyte adenylyl cyclase. A GPCR for niacin has been identified and designated as HM74A (Wise *et al.,* 2003); its mRNA is highly expressed in the adipose tissue and spleen, sites of high-affinity nicotinic acid binding (Lorenzen *et al.,* 2001). Niacin stimulates the HM74A (HM74b)-G_i–adenylyl cyclase pathway in adipocytes, inhibiting cAMP production and decreasing hormone-sensitive lipase activity, triglyceride lipolysis, and release of free fatty acids. Niacin may also inhibit a rate-limiting enzyme of triglyceride synthesis, diacylglycerol acetyltransferase 2 (Ganji, *et al.,* 2004). Identification of the nicotinic acid receptor may permit the development of new compounds that may affect fatty acid metabolism, dyslipidemia, and ultimately, atherogenesis (Karpe and Frayn, 2004).

In the liver, niacin reduces triglyceride synthesis by inhibiting both the synthesis and esterification of fatty acids, effects that increase apoB degradation (Jin *et al.,* 1999). Reduction of triglyceride synthesis reduces hepatic VLDL production, which accounts for the reduced LDL levels. Niacin also enhances LPL activity, which promotes the clearance of chylomicrons and VLDL triglycerides. Niacin raises HDL-C levels by decreasing the fractional clearance of apoA-I in HDL rather than by enhancing HDL synthesis. This effect is due to a reduction in the hepatic clearance of HDL-apoA-I, but not of cholesteryl esters, thereby increasing the apoA-I content of plasma and augmenting reverse cholesterol transport (Jin *et al.,* 1997). In macrophages, niacin stimulates expression of the scavenger receptor CD36 and the cholesterol exporter ABCA1. The net effect of niacin on monocytic cells ("foam cells") is HDL-mediated reduction of cellular cholesterol content (Rubic *et al.,* 2004).

Effects on Plasma Lipoprotein Levels. Regular or crystalline niacin in doses of 2 to 6 g per day reduces triglycerides by 35% to 50%, and the maximal effect occurs within 4 to 7 days (Figge *et al.*, 1988). Reductions of 25% in LDL-C levels are possible with doses of 4.5 to 6 g per day, but 3 to 6 weeks are required for maximal effect. HDL-C increases less in patients with low HDL-C levels (<35 mg/dl) than in those with higher levels. Average increases of 15% to 30% occur in patients with low HDL-C levels; greater increases may occur in patients with normal HDL-C levels at baseline (Vega and Grundy, 1994; Sprecher, 2000). Combination therapy with resins can reduce LDL-C levels by as much as 40% to 60% (Malloy *et al.*, 1987).

Absorption, Fate, and Excretion. The pharmacological doses of regular (crystalline) niacin used to treat dyslipidemia are almost completely absorbed, and peak plasma concentrations (up to 0.24 mmol) are achieved within 30 to 60 minutes. The half-life is about 60 minutes, which accounts for the necessity of twice- or thrice-daily dosing. At lower doses, most niacin is taken up by the liver; only the major metabolite, nicotinuric acid, is found in the urine. At higher doses, a greater proportion of the drug is excreted in the urine as unchanged nicotinic acid (Iwaki *et al.*, 1996).

Adverse Effects. Two of niacin's side effects, flushing and dyspepsia, limit patient compliance. The cutaneous effects include flushing and pruritus of the face and upper trunk, skin rashes, and acanthosis nigricans. Flushing and associated pruritus are prostaglandin-mediated (Stern *et al.*, 1991). Flushing is worse when therapy is initiated or the dosage is increased, but ceases in most patients after 1 to 2 weeks of a stable dose. Taking an aspirin each day alleviates the flushing in many patients. Flushing recurs if only one or two doses are missed, and the flushing is more likely to occur when niacin is consumed with hot beverages (coffee, tea) or with ethanol-containing beverages. Flushing is minimized if therapy is initiated with low doses (100 to 250 mg twice daily) and if the drug is taken after breakfast or supper. Dry skin, a frequent complaint, can be dealt with by using skin moisturizers, and acanthosis nigricans can be dealt with by using lotions or creams containing *salicylic acid*. Dyspepsia and rarer episodes of nausea, vomiting, and diarrhea are less likely to occur if the drug is taken after a meal. Patients with any history of peptic ulcer disease should not take niacin because it can reactivate ulcer disease.

The most common, medically serious side effects are hepatotoxicity, manifested as elevated serum transaminases and hyperglycemia. Both regular (crystalline) niacin and sustained-release niacin, which was developed to reduce flushing and itching, have been reported to cause severe liver toxicity, and sustained-release niacin can cause fulminant hepatic failure (Tatò *et al.*, 1998). An extended-release niacin (NIASPAN), appears to be less likely to cause severe hepatotoxicity (Capuzzi *et al.*, 1998), perhaps simply because it is administered once daily instead of more frequently (Guyton *et al.*, 1998). The incidence of flushing and pruritus with this preparation is not substantially different from that with regular niacin. Severe hepatotoxicity is more likely to occur when patients take more than 2 g of sustained-release, over-the-counter preparations. Affected patients experience flu-like fatigue and weakness. Usually, aspartate transaminase and ALT are elevated, serum albu-

min levels decline, and total cholesterol and LDL-C levels decline substantially. In fact, reductions in LDL-C of 50% or more in a patient taking niacin should be viewed as a sign of niacin toxicity (Tatò *et al.*, 1998).

In patients with diabetes mellitus, niacin should be used cautiously, since niacin-induced insulin resistance can cause severe hyperglycemia (Knopp *et al.*, 1985; Henkin *et al.*, 1991; Schwartz, 1993). Niacin use in patients with diabetes mellitus often mandates a change to insulin therapy. In a study of patients with type 2 diabetes taking NIASPAN, 4% stopped taking the drug because of inadequate glycemic control (Grundy *et al.*, 2002). If niacin is prescribed for patients with known or suspected diabetes, blood glucose levels should be monitored at least weekly until proven to be stable. Niacin also elevates uric acid levels and may reactivate gout. A history of gout is a relative contraindication for niacin use. Rarer reversible side effects include toxic amblyopia and toxic maculopathy. Atrial tachyarrhythmias and atrial fibrillation have been reported, more commonly in elderly patients. *Niacin, at doses used in humans, has been associated with birth defects in experimental animals and should not be taken by pregnant women.*

Therapeutic Uses. Niacin is indicated for hypertriglyceridemia and elevated LDL-C; it is especially useful in patients with both hypertriglyceridemia and low HDL-C levels. There are two commonly available forms of niacin. Crystalline niacin (immediate-release or regular) refers to niacin tablets that dissolve quickly after ingestion. Sustained-release niacin refers to preparations that continuously release niacin for 6 to 8 hours after ingestion. NIASPAN is the only preparation of niacin that has been approved by the FDA for treating dyslipidemia and that requires a prescription.

Crystalline niacin tablets are available over the counter in a variety of strengths from 50- to 500-mg tablets. To minimize the flushing and pruritus, it is best to start with a low dose (*e.g.,* 100 mg twice daily taken after breakfast and supper). The dose may be increased stepwise every 7 days by 100 to 200 mg to a total daily dose of 1.5 to 2 g. After 2 to 4 weeks at this dose, transaminases, serum albumin, fasting glucose, and uric acid levels should be measured. Lipid levels should be checked and the dose increased further until the desired effect on plasma lipids is achieved. After a stable dose is attained, blood should be drawn every 3 to 6 months to monitor for the various toxicities.

Since concurrent use of niacin and a statin can cause myopathy, the statin should be administered at no more than 25% of its maximal dose. Patients also should be instructed to discontinue therapy if flulike muscle aches occur. Routine measurement of CK in patients taking niacin and statins does not assure that severe myopathy will be detected before onset of symptoms, as patients have developed myopathy after several years of concomitant use of niacin with a statin.

Over-the-counter, sustained-release niacin preparations and NIASPAN are effective up to a total daily dose of 2 g per day. All doses of sustained-release niacin, but particularly doses above 2 g per day, have been reported to cause hepatotoxicity, which may occur soon after beginning therapy or after several years of use (Knopp *et al.*, 1985). The potential for severe liver damage should preclude its use in most patients, including those who have taken an equivalent dose of crystalline niacin safely for many years and are considering switching to a sustained-release preparation (Tatò *et al.*, 1998). NIASPAN may be less likely to cause hepatotoxicity.

Fibric Acid Derivatives: PPAR Activators

History. In 1962, Thorp and Waring reported that ethyl chlorophenoxyisobutyrate lowered lipid levels in rats. In 1967, the ester form (clofibrate) was approved for use in the United States and became the most widely prescribed hypolipidemic drug. Its use declined dramatically, however, after the World Health Organization reported that, despite a 9% reduction in cholesterol levels, clofibrate treatment did not reduce fatal cardiovascular events, although nonfatal infarcts were reduced (Committee of Principal Investigators, 1978). Total mortality was significantly greater in the clofibrate group. The increased mortality was due to multiple causes, including cholelithiasis. Interpretation of these negative results was clouded by failure to analyze the data according to the intention-to-treat principle. A later analysis demonstrated that the apparent increase in noncardiac mortality did not persist in the clofibrate-treated patients after discontinuation of the drug (Heady *et al.*, 1992). Clofibrate use was virtually abandoned after publication of the results of the 1978 WHO trial. Clofibrate as well as two other fibrates, gemfibrozil and fenofibrate, remain available in the United States.

Two subsequent trials involving only men have reported favorable effects of gemfibrozil therapy on fatal and nonfatal cardiac events without an increase in morbidity or mortality (Frick *et al.*, 1987; Rubins *et al.*, 1999). A third trial of men and women reported fewer events in a subgroup characterized by high triglyceride and low HDL-C levels (Haim *et al.*, 1999).

Chemistry. Clofibrate, the prototype of the fibric acid derivatives, is the ethyl ester of *p*-chlorophenoxyisobutyrate. Gemfibrozil is a nonhalogenated phenoxypentanoic acid and thus is distinct from the halogenated fibrates. A number of fibric acid analogs (*e.g.,* fenofibrate, *bezafibrate,* and *ciprofibrate*) have been developed and are used in Europe and elsewhere (*see* Figure 35–5 for structural formulas).

Mechanism of Action. Despite extensive studies in humans, the mechanisms by which fibrates lower lipoprotein levels, or raise HDL levels, remain unclear (Illingworth, 1991). Recent studies suggest that many of the effects of these compounds on blood lipids are mediated by their interaction with peroxisome proliferator activated receptors (PPARs) (Kersten *et al.*, 2000), which regulate gene transcription. Three PPAR isotypes (α, β, and γ) have been identified. Fibrates bind to PPARα, which is expressed primarily in the liver and brown adipose tissue and to a lesser extent in kidney, heart, and skeletal muscle. Fibrates reduce triglycerides through PPARα-mediated stimulation of fatty acid oxidation, increased LPL synthesis, and reduced expression of apoC-III. An increase in LPL would enhance the clearance of triglyceride-rich lipoproteins. A reduction in hepatic production of apoC-III, which serves as an inhibitor of lipolytic processing and receptor-mediated clearance, would enhance the clearance of VLDL. Fibrate-mediated increases in HDL-C are due to PPARα stimulation of apoA-I and apoA-II expression (Staels and Auwerx, 1998), which increases HDL levels. Fenofibrate is more effective than gemfibrozil at increasing HDL levels (Rader, 2003).

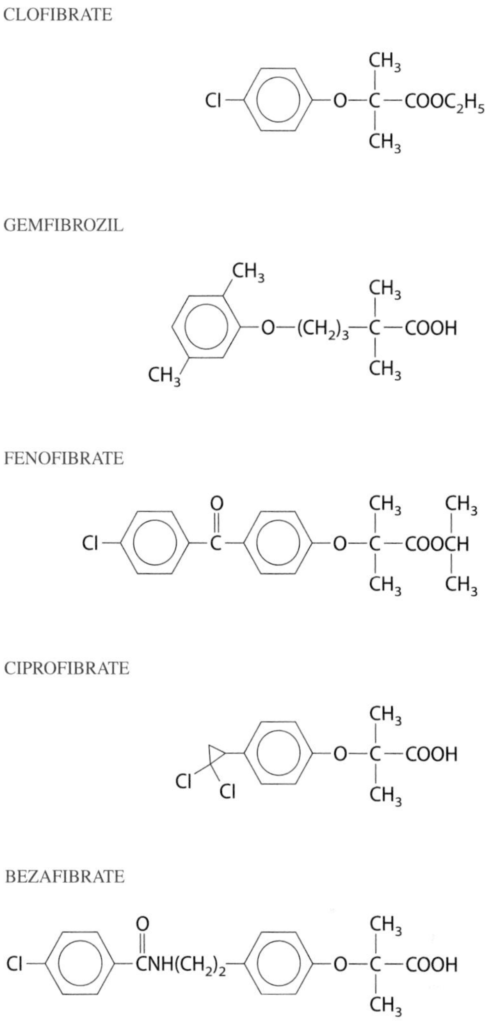

Figure 35–5. Structures of the fibric acids.

LDL levels rise in many patients treated with gemfibrozil, especially those with hypertriglyceridemia. However, LDL levels are unchanged or fall in others, especially those whose triglyceride levels are not elevated or who are taking a second-generation agent, such as fenofibrate, bezafibrate, or ciprofibrate. The decrease in LDL levels may be due in part to changes in the cholesterol and triglyceride contents of LDL that are mediated by CETP; such changes can alter the affinity of LDL for the LDL receptor. There also is evidence that a PPARα-mediated increase in hepatic SREBP-1 production enhances hepatic expression of LDL receptors (Kersten *et al.*, 2000). Lastly, fibrates reduce the plasma concentration of small, dense, more easily oxidized LDL particles (Yuan *et al.*, 1994; Vakkilainen *et al.*, 2003).

Most of the fibric acid agents have potential antithrombotic effects, including inhibition of coagulation and enhancement of fibrinolysis. These salutary effects also could alter cardiovascular outcomes by mechanisms unrelated to any hypolipidemic activity (Watts and Dimmitt, 1999).

Effects on Lipoprotein Levels. The effects of the fibric acid agents on lipoprotein levels differ widely, depending on the starting lipoprotein profile, the presence or absence of a genetic hyperlipoproteinemia, the associated environmental influences, and the specific fibrate used.

Patients with type III hyperlipoproteinemia (dysbetalipoproteinemia) are among the most sensitive responders to fibrates (Mahley and Rall, 2001). Elevated triglyceride and cholesterol levels are dramatically lowered, and tuberoeruptive and palmar xanthomas may regress completely. Angina and intermittent claudication also improve (Kuo *et al.*, 1988).

In patients with mild hypertriglyceridemia (*e.g.,* triglycerides <400 mg/dl), fibrate treatment decreases triglyceride levels by up to 50% and increases HDL-C concentrations about 15%; LDL-C levels may be unchanged or increase. The second-generation agents, such as fenofibrate, bezafibrate, and ciprofibrate, lower VLDL levels to a degree similar to that produced by gemfibrozil, but they also are more likely to decrease LDL levels by 15% to 20%. In patients with more marked hypertriglyceridemia (*e.g.,* 400 to 1000 mg/dl), a similar fall in triglycerides occurs, but LDL increases of 10% to 30% are seen frequently. Normotriglyceridemic patients with heterozygous familial hypercholesterolemia usually experience little change in LDL levels with gemfibrozil; with the other fibric acid agents, reductions as great as 20% may occur in some patients.

Fibrates usually are the drugs of choice for treating severe hypertriglyceridemia and the chylomicronemia syndrome. While the primary therapy is to remove alcohol and as much fat from the diet as possible, fibrates help both by increasing triglyceride clearance and by decreasing hepatic triglyceride synthesis. In patients with chylomicronemia syndrome, fibrate maintenance therapy and a low-fat diet keep triglyceride levels well below 1000 mg/dl and thus prevent episodes of pancreatitis.

In a 5-year study of hyperlipidemic men, gemfibrozil reduced total cholesterol by 10% and LDL-C by 11%, raised HDL-C levels by 11%, and decreased triglycerides by 35% (Frick *et al.*, 1987). Overall, there was a 34% decrease in the sum of fatal plus nonfatal cardiovascular events without any effect on total mortality. No increased incidence of gallstones or cancers was observed. Subgroup analysis suggested that the greatest benefit occurred in the subjects with the highest levels of VLDL or combined VLDL and LDL and in those with the lowest HDL-C levels (<35 mg/dl). Gemfibrozil may have affected the outcome by influencing platelet function, coagulation factor synthesis, or LDL size. In a recent secondary prevention trial, gemfibrozil reduced fatal and nonfatal CHD events by 22% despite a lack of effect on LDL-C levels. HDL-C levels increased by 6%, which may have contributed to the favorable outcome (Rubins *et al.*, 1999).

Absorption, Fate, and Excretion. All of the fibrate drugs are absorbed rapidly and efficiently (>90%) when given with a meal but less efficiently when taken on an empty stomach. The ester bond is hydrolyzed rapidly, and peak plasma concentrations are attained within 1 to 4 hours. More than 95% of these drugs in plasma are bound to protein, nearly exclusively to albumin. The half-lives of fibrates differ significantly (Miller and Spence, 1998), ranging from 1.1 hours (gemfibrozil) to 20 hours (fenofibrate). The drugs are widely distributed throughout the body, and concentrations in liver, kidney, and intestine exceed the plasma level. Gemfibrozil is transferred across the placenta. The fibrate drugs are excreted predominantly as glucuronide conjugates; 60% to 90% of an oral dose is excreted in the urine, with smaller amounts appearing in the feces. Excretion of these drugs is impaired in renal failure, though excretion of gemfibrozil is less severely compromised in renal insufficiency than is excretion of other fibrates

(Evans *et al.*, 1987). Nevertheless, the use of fibrates is contraindicated in patients with renal failure.

Adverse Effects and Drug Interactions. Fibric acid compounds usually are well tolerated (Miller and Spence, 1998). Side effects may occur in 5% to 10% of patients but most often are not sufficient to cause discontinuation of the drug. Gastrointestinal side effects occur in up to 5% of patients. Other side effects are reported infrequently and include rash, urticaria, hair loss, myalgias, fatigue, headache, impotence, and anemia. Minor increases in liver transaminases and alkaline phosphatase have been reported. Clofibrate, bezafibrate, and fenofibrate have been reported to potentiate the action of oral anticoagulants, in part by displacing them from their binding sites on albumin. Careful monitoring of the prothrombin time and reduction in dosage of the anticoagulant may be appropriate when treatment with a fibrate is begun.

A myopathy syndrome occasionally occurs in subjects taking clofibrate, gemfibrozil, or fenofibrate, and may occur in up to 5% of patients treated with a combination of gemfibrozil and higher doses of statins. To diminish the risk of myopathy, statin doses should be reduced when combination therapy of a statin plus a fibrate is employed. Several drug interactions may contribute to this adverse response. Gemfibrozil inhibits hepatic uptake of statins by OATP2. Gemfibrozil also competes for the same glucuronosyl transferases that metabolize most statins. As a consequence, levels of both drugs may be increased when they are coadministered. (Prueksaritanont *et al.*, 2002b; Prueksaritanont *et al.*, 2002c). Patients taking this combination should be instructed to be aware of the potential symptoms and should be followed at 3-month intervals with careful history and determination of CK values until a stable pattern is established. Patients taking fibrates with rosuvastatin should be followed especially closely even if low doses (5 to 10 mg) of rosuvastatin are employed until there is more experience with and knowledge of the safety of this specific combination. Fenofibrate is glucuronidated by enzymes that are not involved in statin glucuronidation. Thus, fenofibrate-statin combinations are less likely to cause myopathy than combination therapy with gemfibrozil and statins.

All of the fibrates increase the lithogenicity of bile. Clofibrate use has been associated with increased risk of gallstone formation; gemfibrozil and fenofibrate reportedly do not increase biliary tract disease.

Renal failure is a relative contraindication to the use of fibric acid agents, as is hepatic dysfunction. Combined statin-fibrate therapy should be avoided in patients with compromised renal function. Gemfibrozil should be used with caution and at a reduced dosage to treat the hyperlipidemia of renal failure. *Fibrates should not be used by children or pregnant women.*

Therapeutic Uses. Clofibrate is available for oral administration. The usual dose is 2 g per day in divided doses. This compound is little used but may be useful in patients who do not tolerate gemfibrozil or fenofibrate. Gemfibrozil (LOPID) is usually administered as a 600-mg dose taken twice a day, 30 minutes before the morning and evening meals. The TRICOR brand of fenofibrate is available in tablets or 48 and 145 mg. The usual daily dose is 145 mg. Generic fenofibrate (LOFIBRA) is available in capsules containing 67, 134, and 200 mg. TRICOR, 145 mg, and LOFIBRA, 200 mg, are equivalent doses.

Fibrates are the drugs of choice for treating hyperlipidemic subjects with type III hyperlipoproteinemia as well as subjects with severe hypertriglyceridemia (triglycerides >1000 mg/dl) who are at risk for pancreatitis. Fibrates appear to have an important role in subjects with high triglycerides and low HDL-C levels associated with the metabolic syndrome or type 2 diabetes mellitus (Robins, 2001). When fibrates are used in such patients, the LDL levels need to be monitored; if LDL levels rise, the addition of a low dose of a statin may be needed. Many experts now treat such patients first with a statin (Heart Protection Study Collaborative Group, 2003), and then add a fibrate, based on the reported benefit of gemfibrozil therapy (Rubins *et al.*, 1999). However, statin-fibrate combination therapy has not been evaluated in outcome studies (American Diabetes Association, 2004). If this combination is used, there should be careful monitoring for myopathy.

Ezetimibe and the Inhibition of Dietary Cholesterol Uptake

Ezetimibe is the first compound approved for lowering total and LDL-C levels that inhibits cholesterol absorption by enterocytes in the small intestine (van Heek *et al.*, 2000). It lowers LDL-C levels by about 18% and is used primarily as adjunctive therapy with statins. Outcome studies employing ezetimibe with statins are beginning, but no results are anticipated for several years (Baigent and Landry, 2003).

History. Ezetimibe (SCH58235) was developed by pharmaceutical chemists studying inhibition of intestinal acyl coenzyme A:cholesterol acyltransferase (ACAT) (Burnett *et al.*, 1994). Several compounds were found to inhibit cholesterol absorption, but by inhibiting intestinal cholesterol absorption rather than ACAT (van Heek *et al.*, 1997).

EZETIMIBE

Mechanism of Action. Recent data indicate that ezetimibe inhibits a specific transport process in jejunal enterocytes, which take up cholesterol from the lumen. The putative transport protein is NPC1L1 (Altmann *et al.*, 2004; Davis *et al.*, 2004). In wild-type mice, ezetimibe inhibits cholesterol absorption by about 70%; in NPC1L1 knockout mice, cholesterol absorption is 86% lower than in wild-type mice, and ezetimibe has no effect on cholesterol absorption (Altmann *et al.*, 2004). Ezetimibe does not affect intestinal triglyceride absorption. In human subjects, ezetimibe reduced cholesterol absorption by 54%, precipitating a compensatory increase in cholesterol synthesis, which can be inhibited with a cholesterol synthesis inhibitor such as a statin (Sudhop *et al.*, 2002). There is also a substantial reduction of plasma levels of plant sterols (campesterol and sitosterol concentrations are reduced by 48% and 41%, respective-

ly), indicating that ezetimibe also inhibits intestinal absorption of plant sterols.

The consequence of inhibiting intestinal cholesterol absorption is a reduction in the incorporation of cholesterol into chylomicrons. The reduced cholesterol content of chylomicrons diminishes the delivery of cholesterol to the liver by chylomicron remnants. The diminished remnant cholesterol content may decrease atherogenesis directly, as chylomicron remnants are very atherogenic lipoproteins. In experimental animal models of remnant dyslipidemia, ezetimibe profoundly diminished diet-induced atherosclerosis (Davis *et al.*, 2001a).

Reduced delivery of intestinal cholesterol to the liver by chylomicron remnants stimulates expression of the hepatic genes regulating LDL receptor expression and cholesterol biosynthesis. The greater expression of hepatic LDL receptors enhances LDL-C clearance from the plasma. Indeed, ezetimibe reduces LDL-C levels by 15% to 20% (Gagné *et al.*, 2002; Knopp *et al.*, 2003). Fasting triglyceride levels decrease about 5%, and HDL-C levels increase about 1% to 2% (Dujovne *et al.*, 2002).

Combination Therapy (Ezetimibe Plus Statins). The maximal efficacy of ezetimibe for lowering LDL-C is between 15% and 20% when used as monotherapy (Gagné *et al.*, 2002; Knopp *et al.*, 2003). This reduction is equivalent to, or less than, that attained with 10- to 20-mg doses of most statins. Consequently, the role of ezetimibe as monotherapy of patients with elevated LDL-C levels appears to be limited to the small group of statin-intolerant patients.

The actions of ezetimibe are complementary to those of statins. Statins, which inhibit cholesterol biosynthesis, increase intestinal cholesterol absorption (Miettinen and Gylling, 2003). Ezetimibe, which inhibits intestinal cholesterol absorption, enhances cholesterol biosynthesis by as much as 3.5 times in experimental animals (Davis *et al.*, 2001b). Dual therapy with these two classes of drugs prevents the enhanced cholesterol synthesis induced by ezetimibe and the increase in cholesterol absorption induced by statins. This combination provides additive reductions in LDL-C levels irrespective of the statin employed (Ballantyne *et al.*, 2003; Melani *et al.*, 2003; Ballantyne *et al.*, 2004). There is a further reduction of 15% to 20% in LDL-C when ezetimibe is combined with any statin at any dose. Increasing statin dosages from the usual starting dose of 20 mg to 80 mg normally yields only an additional 12% reduction in LDL-C, whereas adding ezetimibe, 10 mg daily, to 20 mg of a statin will reduce LDL-C by an additional 18% to 20%.

A combination tablet containing ezetimibe, 10 mg, and various doses of simvastatin (10, 20, 40, and 80 mg) has been approved (VYTORIN). At the highest simvastatin dose (80 mg), plus ezetimibe (10 mg), average LDL-C reduction was 60%, which is greater than can be attained with any statin as monotherapy (Feldman *et al.*, 2004).

Absorption, Fate, and Excretion. Ezetimibe is highly water insoluble, precluding studies of its bioavailability. After ingestion, it is glucuronidated in the intestinal epithelium, absorbed, and enters an enterohepatic recirculation (Patrick *et al.*, 2002). Pharmacokinetic studies indicate that about 70% is excreted in the feces and about 10% in the urine (as a glucuronide conjugate) (Patrick *et al.*, 2002). Bile acid sequestrants inhibit absorption of ezetimibe, and the two agents should not be administered together. Otherwise, no significant drug interactions have been reported.

Adverse Effects and Drug Interactions. Other than rare allergic reactions, specific adverse effects have not been observed in patients taking ezetimibe. The safety of ezetimibe during pregnancy has not been established. With doses of ezetimibe sufficient to increase exposure 10 to 150 times compared with a 10-mg dose in humans, fetal skeletal abnormalities were noted in rats and rabbits. *Since all statins are contraindicated in pregnant and nursing women, combination products containing ezetimibe and a statin should not be used by women in childbearing years in the absence of contraception.*

Therapeutic Uses. Ezetimibe (ZETIA) is available as a 10-mg tablet that may be taken at any time during the day, with or without food. Ezetimibe may be taken with any medication other than bile acid sequestrants, which inhibit its absorption.

Inhibitors of Cholesteryl Ester Transfer Protein

The cholesteryl ester transfer protein (CETP) is a plasma glycoprotein synthesized by the liver that mediates the transfer of cholesteryl esters from the larger subfractions of HDL (HDL_2) to triglyceride-rich lipoproteins and LDL in exchange for a molecule of triglyceride. Enrichment of HDL_2 with triglycerides enhances its catabolism by the liver. In animal models, inhibition of CETP results in higher HDL levels, decreased LDL levels, and resistance to developing atherosclerosis. Observational studies of humans with CETP gene mutations associated with reduced CETP activity indicate that HDL levels are increased and LDL levels are lower in affected patients. However, there are reports of both increased and decreased prevalence of CHD, or no effect on CHD prevalence in patients with naturally occurring CETP mutations.

Clinical trials of CETP inhibitors in human subjects are under way (*see* review by Forrester *et al.*, 2005). Two CETP inhibitors, JTT-705 and *torcetrapib*, are being tested (de Grooth *et al.*, 2002; Brousseau *et al.*, 2004; Clark *et al.*, 2004). JTT-705 forms a disulfide bond with CETP, and torcetrapib is thought to stabilize the association of CETP with its lipoprotein substrate, creating a nonfunctional complex. The levels of HDL-C are increased by 45% to 106% in normal subjects and in patients with low HDL-C levels. Further studies of the safety of these compounds and proof that this approach prevents clinical vascular disease are required before CETP inhibitors can be routinely used in managing dyslipidemic patients.

CLINICAL SUMMARY

Patients with any type of dyslipidemia (*e.g.*, elevated levels of cholesterol, low levels of HDL-C with or without hypercholesterolemia, or moderately elevated triglyceride levels with low HDL-C levels) are at risk of developing atherosclerosis-induced vascular disease. Maintaining ideal body weight, eating a diet low in saturated fat and cholesterol, and regular exercise are the cornerstones of managing dyslipidemia. In the absence of vascular disease, type 2 diabetes mellitus, or metabolic syndrome, adoption of these behaviors will alleviate the need for cholesterol-lowering medications in many subjects. Patients should be treated to achieve target lipid values after assessing their future risk for a vascular disease event. In virtually every type of dyslipidemic patient, statins have been proven to reduce the risk of subsequent CHD events and nonhemorrhagic stroke. For this reason, statin therapy should be the first-line choice when choosing between classes of lipid-lowering agents.

A second principle is to treat with statin doses adequate to reduce the patient's lipid values to goal levels. Most patients are not adequately treated and do not reach goal values. Safety is greatly enhanced if doctors discuss with their patients the rare but serious side effects of hepatotoxicity and rhabdomyolysis with associated renal failure. In patients requiring combination therapy, long-term compliance may be improved in a subset of patients by using a fixed-dose preparation: lovastatin plus extended-release niacin (ADVICOR) or simvastatin plus ezetimibe (VYTORIN).

Finally, patients with low HDL-C levels may not receive the maximum benefit of lipid-lowering therapy as prescribed by the ATP III guidelines based on levels of LDL-C or non-HDL-C. For this reason, treatment of patients with low HDL-C levels should be based on both LDL-C levels and the ratio of total cholesterol:HDL-C (Table 35–7).

BIBLIOGRAPHY

Agarwal, R. Statin induced proteinuria: Renal injury or renoprotection. *J. Am. Soc. Nephrol.*, **2004**, *15:*2502–2503.

Aguila-Salinas, C.A., Barrett, H., and Schonfeld, G. Metabolic modes of action of the statins in the hyperlipoproteinemias. *Atherosclerosis*, **1998**, *141:*203–207.

Altmann, S.W., Davis, H.R., Jr., Zhu, L.J., *et al.* Niemann-Pick C1 like 1 protein is critical for intestinal cholesterol absorption. *Science*, **2004**, *303:*1201–1204.

American Diabetes Association. Management of dyslipidemia in adults with diabetes. *Diabetes Care*, **1999**, *22*(suppl 1):S56–S59.

American Diabetes Association. Dyslipidemia management in adults with diabetes. *Diabetes Care*, **2004**, *27*(suppl 1):S68–S71.

American Heart Association. *Heart Disease and Stroke Statistics—2004 Update.* American Heart Association, Dallas, TX, **2003.**

Anant, S., and Davidson, N.O. Molecular mechanisms of apolipoprotein B mRNA editing. *Curr. Opin. Lipidol.*, **2001**, *12:*159–165.

Appleby, P.N., Thorogood, M., Mann, J.I., and Key, T.J. The Oxford Vegetarian Study: an overview. *Am. J. Clin. Nutr.*, **1999**, *70*(suppl):525S–531S.

Assmann, G., and Nofer, J.R. Atheroprotective effects of high-density lipoproteins. *Annu. Rev. Med.,* 2003, *54:*321–341.

Assmann, G., von Eckardstein, A., and Brewer, H.B., Jr. Familial analphalipoproteinemia: Tangier disease. In, *The Metabolic and Molecular Bases of Inherited Disease,* 8th ed., Vol. 2. (Scriver, C.R., Beaudet, A.L., Sly, W.S., *et al.,* eds.) McGraw-Hill, New York, 2001, pp. 2937–2960.

Athyros, V.G., Papageorgiou, A.A., Hatzikonstandinou, H.A., *et al.* Safety and efficacy of long-term statin-fibrate combinations in patients with refractory familial combined hyperlipidemia. *Am. J. Cardiol.,* 1997, *80:*608–613.

Attie, A.D., Kastelein, J.P., and Hayden, M.R. Pivotal role of ABCA1 in reverse cholesterol transport influencing HDL levels and susceptibility to atherosclerosis. *J. Lipid Res.,* 2001, *42:*1717–1726.

Baigent, C., and Landry, M. Study of Heart and Renal Protection (SHARP). *Kidney Int. Suppl.,* 2003, *63:*S207–S210.

Bakker-Arkema, R.G., Davidson, M.H., Goldstein, R.J., *et al.* Efficacy and safety of a new HMG-CoA reductase inhibitor, atorvastatin, in patients with hypertriglyceridemia. *JAMA,* 1996, *275:*128–133.

Ballantyne, C.M., Blazing, M.A., King, T.R., Brady, W.E., and Palmisano, J. Efficacy and safety of ezetimibe co-administered with simvastatin compared with atorvastatin in adults with hypercholesterolemia. *Am. J. Cardiol.,* 2004, *93:*1487–1494.

Ballantyne, C.M., Houri, J., Notarbartolo, A., *et al.* Effect of ezetimibe coadministered with atorvastatin in 628 patients with primary hypercholesterolemia: A prospective, randomized, double-blind trial. *Circulation,* 2003, *107:*2409–2415.

Bellosta, S., Mahley, R.W., Sanan, D.A., *et al.* Macrophage-specific expression of human apolipoprotein E reduces atherosclerosis in hypercholesterolemic apolipoprotein E–null mice. *J. Clin. Invest.,* 1995, *96:*2170–2179.

Bellosta, S., Paoletti, R., and Corsini, A. Safety of statins: focus on clinical pharmacokinetics and drug interactions. *Circulation,* 2004, *109:*III50–III57.

Bellosta, S., Via, D., Canavesi, M., *et al.* HMG-CoA reductase inhibitors reduce MMP-9 secretion by macrophages. *Arterioscler. Thromb. Vasc. Biol.,* 1998, *18:*1671–1678.

Berge, K.E., Tian, H., Graf, G.A., Yu, L., *et al.* Accumulation of dietary cholesterol in sitosterolemia caused by mutations in adjacent ABC transporters. *Science,* 2000, *290:*1771–1775.

Bergman, A.J., Murphy, G., Burke, J., *et al.* Simvastatin does not have a clinically significant pharmacokinetic interaction with fenofibrate in humans. *J. Clin. Pharmacol.,* 2004, *44:*1054–1062.

Berriot-Varoqueaux, N., Aggerbeck, L.P., Samson-Bouma, M.E., and Wetterau, J.R. The role of the microsomal triglyceride transfer protein in abetalipoproteinemia. *Annu. Rev. Nutr.,* 2000, *20:*663–697.

Bersot, T.P., Pépin, G.M., and Mahley, R.W. Risk determination of dyslipidemia in populations characterized by low levels of high-density lipoprotein cholesterol. *Am. Heart J.,* 2003, *146:*1052–1059.

Bradford, R.H., Shear, C.L., Chremos, A.N., *et al.* Expanded Clinical Evaluation of Lovastatin (EXCEL) study results. I. Efficacy in modifying plasma lipoproteins and adverse event profile in 8245 patients with moderate hypercholesterolemia. *Arch. Intern. Med.,* 1991, *151:*43–49.

Brinton, E.A. Oral estrogen replacement therapy in postmenopausal women selectively raises levels and production rates of lipoprotein A-I and lowers hepatic lipase activity without lowering the fractional catabolic rate. *Arterioscler. Thromb. Vasc. Biol.,* 1996, *16:*431–440.

Brousseau, M.E., Schaefer, E.J., Wolfe, M.L., *et al.* Effects of an inhibitor of cholesteryl ester transfer protein on HDL cholesterol. *N. Engl. J. Med.,* 2004, *350:*1505–1515.

Brown, B.G., Cheung, M.C., Lee, A.C., Zhao, X.Q., and Chait, A. Antioxidant vitamins and lipid therapy: end of a long romance? *Arterioscler. Thromb. Vasc. Biol.,* 2002, *22:*1535–1546.

Brown, M.S., and Goldstein, J.L. A receptor-mediated pathway for cholesterol homeostasis. *Science,* 1986, *232:*34–47.

Brown, B.G., Zhao, X.Q., Sacco, D.E., and Albers, J.J. Lipid lowering and plaque regression. New insights into prevention of plaque disruption and clinical events in coronary disease. *Circulation,* 1993, *87:*1781–1791.

Buhman, K.K., Chen, H.C., and Farese, R.V., Jr. The enzymes of neutral lipid synthesis. *J. Biol. Chem.,* 2001, *276:*40369–40372.

Burnett, D.A., Caplan, M.A., Davis, H.R., Jr., Burrier, R.E., and Clader, J.W. 2-Azetidinones as inhibitors of cholesterol absorption. *J. Med. Chem.,* 1994, *37:*1733–1736.

Bustos, C., Hernández-Presa, M.A., Ortego, M., *et al.* HMG-CoA reductase inhibition by atorvastatin reduces neointimal inflammation in a rabbit model of atherosclerosis. *J. Am. Coll. Cardiol.,* 1998, *32:*2057–2064.

Cannon, C.P., Braunwald, E., McCabe, C.H., *et al.* Intensive versus moderate lipid lowering with statins after acute coronary syndromes. *N. Engl. J. Med.,* 2004, *350:*1495–1504.

Canto, J.G., and Iskandrian, A.E. Major risk factors for cardiovascular disease: debunking the "only 50%" myth. *JAMA,* 2003, *290:*947–949.

Capuzzi, D.M., Guyton, J.R., Morgan, J.M., *et al.* Efficacy and safety of an extended-release niacin (Niaspan): a long-term study. *Am. J. Cardiol.,* 1998, *82:*74U–81U.

Carlson, L.A., Hamsten, A., and Asplund, A. Pronounced lowering of serum levels of lipoprotein Lp(a) in hyperlipidaemic subjects treated with nicotinic acid. *J. Intern. Med.,* 1989, *226:*271–276.

Castelli, W.P. The folly of questioning the benefits of cholesterol reduction. *Am. Fam. Physician,* 1994, *49:*567–572.

Castelli, W.P., Garrison, R.J., Wilson, P.W., *et al.* Incidence of coronary heart disease and lipoprotein cholesterol levels. The Framingham Study. *JAMA,* 1986, *256:*2835–2838.

Chen, Z., Peto, R., Collins, R., *et al.* Serum cholesterol concentration and coronary heart disease in population with low cholesterol concentrations. *BMJ,* 1991, *303:*276–282.

Christians, U., Jacobsen, W., and Floren, L.C. Metabolism and drug interactions of 3-hydroxy-3-methylglutaryl coenzyme A reductase inhibitors in transplant patients: are the statins mechanistically similar? *Pharmacol. Ther.,* 1998, *80:*1–34.

Clark, R.W., Sutfin, T.A., Ruggeri, R.B., *et al.* Raising high-density lipoprotein in humans through inhibition of cholesteryl ester transfer protein: an initial multidose study of torcetrapib. *Arterioscler. Thromb. Vasc. Biol.,* 2004, *24:*490–497.

Committee of Principal Investigators. A co-operative trial in the primary prevention of ischaemic heart disease using clofibrate. Report from the Committee of Principal Investigators. *Br. Heart J.,* 1978, *40:*1069–1118.

Corsini, A., Bellosta, S., Baetta, R., *et al.* New insights into the pharmacodynamic and pharmacokinetic properties of statins. *Pharmacol. Ther.,* 1999, *84:*413–428.

Corsini, A., Pazzucconi, F., Arnaboldi, L., *et al.* Direct effects of statins on the vascular wall. *J. Cardiovasc. Pharmacol.,* 1998, *31:*773–778.

Corsini, A. The safety of HMG-CoA reductase inhibitors in special populations at high cardiovascular risk. *Cardiovasc. Drugs Ther.,* 2003, *17:*265–285.

Corti, R., Fuster, V., and Badimon, J.J. Pathogenetic concepts of acute coronary syndromes. *J. Am. Coll. Cardiol.,* 2003, *41*(suppl):7S–14S.

Crouse, J.R. III, Frohlich, J., Ose, L., Mercuri, M., and Tobert, J.A. Effects of high doses of simvastatin and atorvastatin on high-density lipoprotein cholesterol and apolipoprotein A-I. *Am. J. Cardiol.,* **1999,** *83:*1476–1477.

Crouse, J.R., III. Hypertriglyceridemia: A contraindication to the use of bile acid binding resins. *Am. J. Med.,* **1987,** *83:*243–248.

Crouse, J.R., Kastelein, J., Isaacsohn, J., *et al.* A large, 36 week study of the HDL-C raising effects and safety of simvastatin versus atorvastatin. *Atherosclerosis,* **2000,** *151:*8–9.

Davidson, M.H., Dillon, M.A., Gordon, B., *et al.* Colesevelam hydrochloride cholestagel: a new, potent bile acid sequestrant associated with a low incidence of gastrointestinal side effects. *Arch. Intern. Med.,* **1999,** *159:*1893–1900.

Davignon, J., and Laaksonen, R. Low-density lipoprotein-independent effects of statins. *Curr. Opin. Lipidol.,* **1999,** *10:*543–559.

Davis, H.R., Jr., Compton, D.S., Hoos, L., and Tetzloff, G. Ezetimibe, a potent cholesterol absorption inhibitor, inhibits the development of atherosclerosis in ApoE knockout mice. *Arterioscler. Thromb. Vasc. Biol.,* **2001a,** *21:*2032–2038.

Davis, H.R., Jr., Pula, K.K., Alton, K.B., Burrier, R.E., and Watkins, R.W. The synergistic hypercholesterolemic activity of the potent cholesterol absorption inhibitor, ezetimibe, in combination with 3-hydroxy-3-methylglutaryl coenzyme A reductase inhibitors in dogs. *Metabolism,* **2001b,** *50:*1234–1241.

Davis, H.R., Jr., Zhu, L.J., Hoos, L.M., *et al.* Niemann-Pick C1 Like 1 (NPC1L1) is the intestinal phytosterol and cholesterol transporter and a key modulator of whole-body cholesterol homeostasis. *J. Biol. Chem.,* **2004,** *279:*33586–33592.

Deeb, S.S., Takata, K., Peng, R.L., Kajiyama, G., and Albers, J.J. A splice-junction mutation responsible for familial apolipoprotein A-II deficiency. *Am. J. Hum. Genet.,* **1990,** *46:*822–827.

Dhaliwal, B.S., and Steinbrecher, U.P. Scavenger receptors and oxidized low density lipoproteins. *Clin. Chim. Acta,* **1999,** *286:*191–205.

Diabetes Atherosclerosis Intervention Study Investigators. Effect of fenofibrate on progression of coronary-artery disease in type 2 diabetes: the Diabetes Atherosclerosis Intervention Study, a randomised study. *Lancet,* **2001,** *357:*905–910.

Downs, J.R., Clearfield, M., Weis, S., *et al.* Primary prevention of acute coronary events with lovastatin in men and women with average cholesterol levels: results of AFCAPS/TexCAPS. *JAMA,* **1998,** *279:*1615–1622.

Dujovne, C.A., Ettinger, M.P., McNeer, J.F., *et al.* Efficacy and safety of a potent new selective cholesterol absorption inhibitor, ezetimibe, in patients with primary hypercholesterolemia. *Am. J. Cardiol.,* **2002,** *90:*1092–1097.

Duriez, P., and Fruchart, J.C. High-density lipoprotein subclasses and apolipoprotein A-I. *Clin. Chim. Acta,* **1999,** *286:*97–114.

Ernst, E., and Resch, K.L. Fibrinogen as a cardiovascular risk factor: a meta-analysis and review of the literature. *Ann. Intern. Med.,* **1993,** *118:*956–963.

Espeland, M.A., Marcovina, S.M., Miller, V., *et al.* Effect of postmenopausal hormone therapy on lipoprotein(a) concentration. PEPI Investigators. Postmenopausal Estrogen/Progestin Interventions. *Circulation,* **1998,** *97:*979–986.

Evans, J.R., Forland, S.C., and Cutler, R.E. The effect of renal function on the pharmacokinetics of gemfibrozil. *J. Clin. Pharmacol.,* **1987,** *27:*994–1000.

Farmer, J.A., and Gotto, A.M., Jr. Antihyperlipidaemic agents. Drug interactions of clinical significance. *Drug Saf.,* **1994,** *11:*301–309.

Feldman, T., Koren, M., Insull, W., Jr., *et al.* Treatment of high-risk patients with ezetimibe plus simvastatin co-administration versus simvastatin alone to attain National Cholesterol Education Program Adult Treatment Panel III low-density lipoprotein cholesterol goals. *Am. J. Cardiol.,* **2004,** *93:*1481–1486.

Figge, H.L., Figge, J., Souney, P.F., Mutnick, A.H., and Sacks, F. Nicotinic acid: a review of its clinical use in the treatment of lipid disorders. *Pharmacotherapy,* **1988,** *8:*287–294.

Fonarow, G.C., and Gawlinski, A. Rationale and design of the Cardiac Hospitalization Atherosclerosis Management Program at the University of California Los Angeles. *Am. J. Cardiol.,* **2000,** *35:*10A–17A.

Ford, E.S., Giles, W.H., and Dietz, W.H. Prevalence of the metabolic syndrome among US adults: findings from the third National Health and Nutrition Examination Survey. *JAMA,* **2002,** *287:*356–359.

Forrester, J., Makkar, R., and Shah, P. Increasing high-density lipoprotein cholesterol in dyslipidemia by cholesterol ester transfer protein inhibition. *Circulation* **2005,** *111:*1847–1854.

Frick, M.H., Elo, O., Haapa, K., *et al.* Helsinki Heart Study: primary-prevention trial with gemfibrozil in middle-aged men with dyslipidemia. Safety of treatment, changes in risk factors, and incidence of coronary heart disease. *N. Engl. J. Med.,* **1987,** *317:*1237–1245.

Gagné, C., Bays, H.E., Weiss, S.R., *et al.* Efficacy and safety of ezetimibe added to ongoing statin therapy for treatment of patients with primary hypercholesterolemia. *Am. J. Cardiol.,* **2002,** *90:*1084–1091.

Ganji, H., Tavintharan, S., Zhu, D., *et al.* Niacin noncompetitively inhibits DGAT2 but not DGAT1 activity in HepG2 cells. *J. Lipid Res.,* **2004,** *45:*1835–1845.

Genest, J.J., McNamara, J.R., Salem, D.N., and Schaefer, E.J. Prevalence of risk factors in men with premature coronary artery disease. *Am. J. Cardiol.,* **1991,** *67:*1185–1189.

Ginsberg, H.N. Effects of statins on triglyceride metabolism. *Am. J. Cardiol.,* **1998,** *81:*32B–35B.

Graf, G.A., Li, W.P., Gerard, R.D., *et al.* Coexpression of ATP-binding cassette proteins ABCG5 and ABCG8 permits their transport to the apical surface. *J. Clin. Invest.,* **2002,** *110:*659–669.

de Grooth, G.J., Kuivenhoven, J.A., Stalenhoef, A.F., *et al.* Efficacy and safety of a novel cholesteryl ester transfer protein inhibitor, JTT-705, in humans: a randomized phase II dose-response study. *Circulation,* **2002,** *105:*2159–2165.

Grundy, S.M., Balady, G.J., Criqui, M.H., *et al.* Primary prevention of coronary heart disease: guidance from Framingham: a statement for healthcare professionals from the AHA Task Force on Risk Reduction. American Heart Association. *Circulation,* **1998,** *97:*1876–1887.

Grundy, S.M., Benjamin, I.J., Burke, G.L., *et al.* Diabetes and cardiovascular disease: a statement for healthcare professionals from the American Heart Association. *Circulation,* **1999,** *100:*1134–1146.

Grundy, S.M., Brewer, H.B., Jr., Cleeman, J.I., Smith, S.C., Jr., and Lenfant, C. Definition of metabolic syndrome: Report of the National Heart, Lung, and Blood Institute/American Heart Association conference on scientific issues related to definition. *Circulation,* **2004a,** *109:*433–438.

Grundy, S.M., Cleeman, J.I., Merz, C.N., *et al.* Implications of recent clinical trials for the National Cholesterol Education Program Adult Treatment Panel III guidelines. *Circulation,* **2004b,** *110:*227–239.

Grundy, S.M., Hansen, B., Smith, S.C., Jr., Cleeman, J.I., and Kahn, R.A. Clinical management of metabolic syndrome: report of the American Heart Association/National Heart, Lung, and Blood Institute/American Diabetes Association conference on scientific issues related to management. *Circulation,* **2004c,** *109:*551–556.

Grundy, S.M. Hypertriglyceridemia, atherogenic dyslipidemia, and the metabolic syndrome. *Am. J. Cardiol.,* **1998,** *81:*18B–25B.

Grundy, S.M., Vega, G.L., McGovern, M.E., *et al.* Efficacy, safety, and tolerability of once-daily niacin for the treatment of dyslipidemia associated with type 2 diabetes: results of the assessment of diabetes control and evaluation of the efficacy of niaspan trial. *Arch. Intern. Med.,* **2002,** *162:*1568–1576.

Guyton, J.R., and Capuzzi, D.M. Treatment of hyperlipidemia with combined niacin-statin regimens. *Am. J. Cardiol.,* **1998,** *82:*82U–84U.

Guyton, J.R., Goldberg, A.C., Kreisberg, R.A., Sprecher, D.L., Superko, H.R., and O'Connor, C.M. Effectiveness of once-nightly dosing of extended-release niacin alone and in combination for hypercholesterolemia. *Am. J. Cardiol.,* **1998,** *82:*737–743.

Haffner, S.M. Management of dyslipidemia in adults with diabetes. *Diabetes Care,* **1998,** *21:*160–178.

Haim, M., Benderly, M., Brunner, D., *et al.* Elevated serum triglyceride levels and long-term mortality in patients with coronary heart disease: the Bezafibrate Infarction Prevention (BIP) registry. *Circulation,* **1999,** *100:*475–482.

Hasty, A.H., Linton, M.F., Brandt, S.J., *et al.* Retroviral gene therapy in ApoE-deficient mice: ApoE expression in the artery wall reduces early foam cell lesion formation. *Circulation,* **1999,** *99:*2571–2576.

Heady, J.A., Morris, J.N., and Oliver, M.F. WHO clofibrate/cholesterol trial: clarifications. *Lancet,* **1992,** *340:*1405–1406.

Heart Protection Study Collaborative Group. Effects of cholesterol-lowering with simvastatin on stroke and other major vascular events in 20,536 people with cerebrovascular disease or other high-risk conditions. *Lancet,* **2004,** *363:*757–767.

Heart Protection Study Collaborative Group. MRC/BHF Heart Protection Study of cholesterol lowering with simvastatin in 20,536 high-risk individuals: a randomised placebo-controlled trial. *Lancet,* **2002,** *360:*7–22.

Heart Protection Study Collaborative Group. MRC/BHF Heart Protection Study of cholesterol-lowering with simvastatin in 5963 people with diabetes: A randomised placebo-controlled trial. *Lancet,* **2003,** *361:*2005–2016.

van Heek, M., Farley, C., Compton, D.S., *et al.* Comparison of the activity and disposition of the novel cholesterol absorption inhibitor, SCH58235, and its glucuronide, SCH60663. *Br. J. Pharmacol.,* **2000,** *129:*1748–1754.

van Heek, M., France, C.F., Compton, D.S., *et al.* In vivo metabolism-based discovery of a potent cholesterol absorption inhibitor, SCH58235, in the rat and rhesus monkey through the identification of the active metabolites of SCH48461. *J. Pharmacol. Exp. Ther.,* **1997,** *283:*157–163.

Henkin, Y., Oberman, A., Hurst, D.C., and Segrest, J.P. Niacin revisited: clinical observations on an important but underutilized drug. *Am. J. Med.,* **1991,** *91:*239–246.

Herz, J., and Strickland, D.K. LRP: a multifunctional scavenger and signaling receptor. *J. Clin. Invest.,* **2001,** *108:*779–784.

Horton, J.D., Goldstein, J.L., and Brown, M.S. SREBPs: Activators of the complete program of cholesterol and fatty acid synthesis in the liver. *J. Clin. Invest.,* **2002,** *109:*1125–1131.

Hsiang, B., Zhu, Y., Wang, Z., *et al.* A novel human hepatic organic anion transporting polypeptide (OATP2). Identification of a liver-specific human organic anion transporting polypeptide and identification of rat and human hydroxymethylglutaryl-CoA reductase inhibitor transporters. *J. Biol. Chem.,* **1999,** *274:*37161–37168.

Hunninghake, D.B., Stein, E.A., Bays, H.E., *et al.* Rosuvastatin improves the atherogenic and atheroprotective lipid profiles in patients with hypertriglyceridemia. *Coron. Artery Dis.,* **2004,** *15:*115–123.

Hussein, O., Rosenblat, M., Schlezinger, S., Keidar, S., and Aviram, M. Reduced platelet aggregation after fluvastatin therapy is associated with altered platelet lipid composition and drug binding to the platelets. *Br. J. Clin. Pharmacol.,* **1997,** *44:*77–84.

Illingworth, D.R., and Durrington, P.N. Dyslipidemia and atherosclerosis: how much more evidence do we need? *Curr. Opin. Lipidol.,* **1999,** *10:*383–386.

Illingworth, D.R. Fibric acid derivatives. In, *Drug Treatment of Hyperlipidemia.* (Rifkind, B.M., ed.) Marcel Dekker, New York, **1991,** pp. 103–138.

Innerarity, T.L., Mahley, R.W., Weisgraber, K.H., *et al.* Familial defective apolipoprotein B100: a mutation of apolipoprotein B that causes hypercholesterolemia. *J. Lipid Res.,* **1990,** *31:*1337–1349.

Iwaki, M., Ogiso, T., Hayashi, H., Tanino, T., and Benet, L.Z. Acute dose-dependent disposition studies of nicotinic acid in rats. *Drug Metab. Dispos.,* **1996,** *24:*773–779.

Jin, F.Y., Kamanna, V.S., and Kashyap, M.L. Niacin accelerates intracellular ApoB degradation by inhibiting triacylglycerol synthesis in human hepatoblastoma (HepG2) cells. *Arterioscler. Thromb. Vasc. Biol.,* **1999,** *19:*1051–1059.

Jin, F.Y., Kamanna, V.S., and Kashyap, M.L. Niacin decreases removal of high-density lipoprotein apolipoprotein A-I but not cholesterol ester by Hep G2 cells. Implication for reverse cholesterol transport. *Arterioscler. Thromb. Vasc. Biol.,* **1997,** *17:*2020–2028.

Jones, P.H., Davidson, M.H., Stein, E.A., *et al.* Comparison of the efficacy and safety of rosuvastatin versus atorvastatin, simvastatin, and pravastatin across doses (STELLAR trial). *Am. J. Cardiol.,* **2003,** *92:*152–160.

Jones, P., Kafonek, S., Laurora, I., and Hunninghake, D. Comparative dose efficacy study of atorvastatin versus simvastatin, pravastatin, lovastatin, and fluvastatin in patients with hypercholesterolemia (the CURVES study). *Am. J. Cardiol.,* **1998,** *81:*582–587.

Joyce, C.W., Amar, M.J., Lambert, G., *et al.* The ATP binding cassette transporter A1 (ABCA1) modulates the development of aortic atherosclerosis in C57BL/6 and apoE-knockout mice. *Proc. Natl. Acad. Sci. USA,* **2002,** *99:*407–412.

Karpe, F., and Frayn, K.N. The nicotinic acid receptor—a new mechanism for an old drug. *Lancet,* **2004,** *363:*1892–1894.

Kersten, S., Desvergne, B., and Wahli, W. Roles of PPARs in health and disease. *Nature,* **2000,** *405:*421–424.

Knopp, R.H. Clinical profiles of plain versus sustained-release niacin (Niaspan) and the physiologic rationale for nighttime dosing. *Am. J. Cardiol.,* **1998,** *82:*24U–28U.

Knopp, R.H., Dujovne, C.A., Le Beaut, A., *et al.* Evaluation of the efficacy, safety, and tolerability of ezetimibe in primary hypercholesterolaemia: a pooled analysis from two controlled phase III clinical studies. *Int. J. Clin. Pract.,* **2003,** *57:*363–368.

Knopp, R.H., Ginsberg, J., Albers, J.J., *et al.* Contrasting effects of unmodified and time-release forms of niacin on lipoproteins in hyperlipidemic subjects: Clues to mechanism of action of niacin. *Metabolism,* **1985,** *34:*642–650.

Kostner, G.M., Gavish, D., Leopold, B., *et al.* HMG CoA reductase inhibitors lower LDL cholesterol without reducing Lp(a) levels. *Circulation,* **1989,** *80:*1313–1319.

Krieger, M. Charting the fate of the "good cholesterol": Identification and characterization of the high-density lipoprotein receptor SR-BI. *Annu. Rev. Biochem.,* **1999,** *68:*523–558.

Krieger, M., and Kozarsky, K. Influence of the HDL receptor SR-BI on atherosclerosis. *Curr. Opin. Lipidol.,* **1999,** *10:*491–497.

Kris-Etherton, P.M., Harris, W.S., and Appel, L.J. American Heart Association, Nutrition Committee. Fish consumption, fish oil, omega-3 fatty acids, and cardiovascular disease. *Circulation,* **2002,** *106:*2747–2757.

Kuo, P.T., Wilson, A.C., Kostis, J.B., Moreyra, A.B., and Dodge, H.T. Treatment of type III hyperlipoproteinemia with gemfibrozil to retard progression of coronary artery disease. *Am. Heart J.,* **1988,** *116:*85–90.

Lacoste, L., Lam, J.Y., Hung, J., *et al.* Hyperlipidemia and coronary disease. Correction of the increased thrombogenic potential with cholesterol reduction. *Circulation,* **1995,** *92:*3172–3177.

Laufs, U., La Fata, V., Plutzky, J., and Liao, J.K. Upregulation of endothelial nitric oxide synthase by HMG CoA reductase inhibitors. *Circulation,* **1998,** *97:*1129–1135.

Law, M.R., Thompson, S.G., and Wald, N.J. Assessing possible hazards of reducing serum cholesterol. *BMJ,* **1994,** *308:*373–379.

Law, M.R., Wald, N.J., and Rudnicka, A.R. Quantifying effect of statins on low density lipoprotein cholesterol, ischaemic heart disease, and stroke: Systematic review and meta-analysis. *BMJ,* **2003,** *326:*1423.

Lee, M.H., Lu, K., Hazard, S., *et al.* Identification of a gene, *ABCG5,* important in the regulation of dietary cholesterol absorption. *Nat. Genet.,* **2001,** *27:*79–83.

Li, H.Y., Appelbaum, F.R., Willman, C.L., Zager, R.A., and Banker, D.E. Cholesterol-modulating agents kill acute myeloid leukemia cells and sensitize them to therapeutics by blocking adaptive cholesterol responses. *Blood,* **2003,** *101:*3628–3634.

Liao, J., and Laufs, U. Pleiotropic effects of statins. *Annu. Rev. Pharmacol.,* **2005,** *45:*89–118.

Libby, P. Inflammation in atherosclerosis. *Nature,* **2002,** *420:*868–874.

Libby, P., and Ridker, P.M. Inflammation and atherosclerosis: Role of C-reactive protein in risk assessment. *Am. J. Med.,* **2004,** *116*(suppl):9S–16S.

Lipid Research Clinics Program. The Lipid Research Clinics Coronary Primary Prevention Trial results. II. The relationship of reduction in incidence of coronary heart disease to cholesterol lowering. *JAMA,* **1984,** *252:*2545–2548.

Liu, J., Hong, Y., D'Agostino, R.B., Sr., *et al.* Predictive value for the Chinese population of the Framingham CHD risk assessment tool compared with the Chinese Multi-provincial Cohort Study. *JAMA,* **2004,** *291:*2591–2599.

Lloyd-Jones, D.M., Nam, B.H., D'Agostino, R.B., Sr., *et al.* Parental cardiovascular disease as a risk factor for cardiovascular disease in middle-aged adults: a prospective study of parents and offspring. *JAMA,* **2004,** *291:*2204–2211.

Lorenzen, A., Stannek, C., Lang, H., *et al.* Characterization of a G protein-coupled receptor for nicotinic acid. *Mol. Pharmacol.,* **2001,** *59:*349–357.

Maher, V.M., Brown, B.G., Marcovina, S.M., *et al.* Effects of lowering elevated LDL cholesterol on the cardiovascular risk of lipoprotein(a). *JAMA,* **1995,** *274:*1771–1774.

Mahley, R.W., and Huang, Y. Apolipoprotein E: from atherosclerosis to Alzheimer's disease and beyond. *Curr. Opin. Lipidol.,* **1999,** *10:*207–217.

Mahley, R.W., and Ji, Z.S. Remnant lipoprotein metabolism: key pathways involving cell-surface heparan sulfate proteoglycans and apolipoprotein E. *J. Lipid Res.,* **1999,** *40:*1–16.

Mahley, R.W., and Rall, S.C., Jr. Apolipoprotein E: far more than a lipid transport protein. *Annu. Rev. Genomics Hum. Genet.,* **2000,** *1:*507–537.

Mahley, R.W., and Rall, S.C., Jr. Type III hyperlipoproteinemia (dysbetalipoproteinemia): The role of apolipoprotein E in normal and abnormal lipoprotein metabolism. In, *The Metabolic and Molecular Bases of Inherited Disease,* 8th Ed., Vol. 2. (Scriver, C.R., Beaudet, A.L., Sly, W.S., *et al.* eds.) McGraw-Hill, New York, **2001,** pp. 2835–2862.

Mahley, R.W., Weisgraber, K.H., and Farese, R.V., Jr. Disorders of lipid metabolism. In, *Williams Textbook of Endocrinology,* 10th ed. (Larsen, P.R., Kronenberg, H.M., Melmed, S., and Polonsky, K.S., eds.) Saunders, Philadelphia, **2003,** pp. 1642–1705.

Malloy, M.J., Kane, J.P., Kunitake, S.T., and Tun, P. Complementarity of colestipol, niacin, and lovastatin in treatment of severe familial hypercholesterolemia. *Ann. Intern. Med.,* **1987,** *107:*616–623.

Martin, P.D., Dane, A.L., Schneck, D.W., and Warwick, M.J. An open-label, randomized, three-way crossover trial of the effects of coadministration of rosuvastatin and fenofibrate on the pharmacokinetic properties of rosuvastatin and fenofibric acid in healthy male volunteers. *Clin. Ther.,* **2003,** *25:*459–471.

Martin, P.D., Warwick, M.J., Dane, A.L., *et al.* Metabolism, excretion, and pharmacokinetics of rosuvastatin in healthy adult male volunteers. *Clin. Ther.,* **2003,** *25:*2822–2835.

Martin-Jadraque, R., Tato, F., Mostaza, J.M., Vega, G.L., and Grundy, S.M. Effectiveness of low-dose crystalline nicotinic acid in men with low high-density lipoprotein cholesterol levels. *Arch. Intern. Med.,* **1996,** *156:*1081–1088.

Melani, L., Mills, R., Hassman, D., *et al.* Efficacy and safety of ezetimibe coadministered with pravastatin in patients with primary hypercholesterolemia: a prospective, randomized, double-blind trial. *Eur. Heart J.,* **2003,** *24:*717–728.

Miettinen, T.A., and Gylling, H. Synthesis and absorption markers of cholesterol in serum and lipoproteins during a large dose of statin treatment. *Eur. J. Clin. Invest.,* **2003,** *33:*976–982.

Miller, D.B., and Spence, J.D. Clinical pharmacokinetics of fibric acid derivatives (fibrates). *Clin. Pharmacokinet.,* **1998,** *34:*155–162.

Mosca, L., Grundy, S.M., Judelson, D., *et al.* Guide to Preventive Cardiology for Women. AHA/ACC Scientific Statement Consensus panel statement. *Circulation,* **1999,** *99:*2480–2484.

Nakata, A., Nakagawa, Y., Nishida, M., *et al.* CD36, a novel receptor for oxidized low-density lipoproteins, is highly expressed on lipid-laden macrophages in human atherosclerotic aorta. *Arterioscler. Thromb. Vasc. Biol.,* **1999,** *19:*1333–1339.

Neaton, J.D., Blackburn, H., Jacobs, D., *et al.* and Multiple Risk Factor Intervention Trial Research Group. Serum cholesterol level and mortality findings for men screened in the Multiple Risk Factor Intervention Trial. *Arch. Intern. Med.,* **1992,** *152:*1490–1500.

Nofer, J.R., Kehrel, B., Fobker, M., *et al.* HDL and arteriosclerosis: Beyond reverse cholesterol transport. *Atherosclerosis,* **2002,** *161:*1–16.

O'Driscoll, G., Green, D., and Taylor, R.R. Simvastatin, an HMG–coenzyme A reductase inhibitor, improves endothelial function within one month. *Circulation,* **1997,** *95:*1126–1131.

Ohtawa, M., Masuda, N., Akasaka, I., *et al.* Cellular uptake of fluvastatin, an inhibitor of HMG-CoA reductase, by rat cultured hepatocytes and human aortic endothelial cells. *Br. J. Clin. Pharm.,* **1999,** *47:*383–389.

Oliva, C.P., Pisciotta, L., Volti, G.I., *et al.* Inherited apoprotein A-V deficiency in severe hypertriglyceridemia. *Arterioscler. Thromb. Vasc. Biol.,* **2005,** in press.

Omar, M.A., Wilson, J.P., and Cox, T.S. Rhabdomyolysis and HMG-CoA reductase inhibitors. *Ann. Pharmacother.,* **2001,** *35:*1096–1107.

Ose, L., Davidson, M.H., Stein, E.A., *et al.* Lipid-altering efficacy and safety of simvastatin 80 mg/day: Long-term experience in a large group of patients with hypercholesterolemia. World Wide Expanded Dose Simvastatin Study Group. *Clin. Cardiol.,* **2000,** *23:*39–46.

Pasternak, R.C., Smith, S.C., Jr., Bairey-Merz, C.N., *et al.* ACC/AHA/NHLBI Clinical Advisory on the Use and Safety of Statins. *Circulation,* **2002,** *106:*1024–1028.

Patrick, J.E., Kosoglou, T., Stauber, K.L., *et al.* Disposition of the selective cholesterol absorption inhibitor ezetimibe in healthy male subjects. *Drug Metab. Dispos.,* **2002,** *30:*430–437.

Pearson, T.A., Mensah, G.A., Alexander, R.W., *et al.* Markers of inflammation and cardiovascular disease: application to clinical and public health practice: a statement for healthcare professionals from the Centers for Disease Control and Prevention and the American Heart Association. *Circulation,* 2003, *107:*499–511.

Pedersen, T.R., and Tobert, J.A. Benefits and risks of HMG-CoA reductase inhibitors in the prevention of coronary heart disease. A reappraisal. *Drug Saf.,* **1996,** *14:*11–24.

Pennacchio, L.A., Olivier, M., Hubacek, J.A., *et al.* An apolipoprotein influencing triglycerides in humans and mice revealed by comparative sequencing. *Science,* 2001, *294:*169–173.

Pennacchio, L.A., Olivier, M., Hubacek, J.A., *et al.* Two independent apolipoprotein A5 haplotypes influence human plasma triglyceride levels. *Hum. Mol. Genet.,* 2002, *11:*3031–3038.

Pi-Sunyer, F.X., Becker, D.M., Bouchard, C., *et al. Clinical Guidelines on the Identification, Evaluation, and Treatment of Overweight and Obesity in Adults. The Evidence Report.* U.S. Department of Health and Human Services, Public Health Service, National Institutes of Health (NIH Publ. No. 98-4083), Bethesda, MD, **1998,** pp. 58–59.

Prueksaritanont, T., Subramanian, R., Fang, X., *et al.* Glucuronidation of statins in animals and humans: A novel mechanism of statin lactonization. *Drug Metab. Dispos.,* **2002a,** *30:*505–512.

Prueksaritanont, T., Tang, C., Qiu, Y., *et al.* Effects of fibrates on metabolism of statins in human hepatocytes. *Drug Metab. Disp.,* **2002b,** *30:*1280–1287.

Prueksaritanont, T., Zhao, J.J., Ma, B., *et al.* Mechanistic studies on metabolic interactions between gemfibrozil and statins. *J. Pharmacol. Exp. Ther.,* **2002c,** *301:*1042–1051.

Rader, D.J., Cohen, J., and Hobbs, H.H. Monogenic hypercholesterolemia: new insights in pathogenesis and treatment. *J. Clin. Invest.,* **2003,** *111:*1795–1803.

Rader, D.J. Effects of nonstatin lipid drug therapy on high-density lipoprotein metabolism. *Am. J. Cardiol.,* **2003,** *91*(suppl):18E–23E.

Reaven, G.M. Importance of identifying the overweight patient who will benefit the most by losing weight. *Ann. Intern. Med.,* **2003,** *138:*420–423.

Reaven, G. Metabolic syndrome. Pathophysiology and implications for management of cardiovascular disease. *Circulation,* **2002,** *106:*286–288.

Repa, J.J., Berge, K.E., Pomajzl, C., *et al.* Regulation of ATP-binding cassette sterol transporters ABCG5 and ABCG8 by the liver X receptors α and β. *J. Biol. Chem.,* **2002,** *277:*18793–18800.

Robins, S.J. Targeting low high-density lipoprotein cholesterol for therapy: lessons from the Veterans Affairs High-Density Lipoprotein Intervention Trial. *Am. J. Cardiol.,* **2001,** *88:*19N–23N.

Rosenson, R.S., and Tangney, C.C. Antiatherothrombotic properties of statins: implications for cardiovascular event reduction. *JAMA,* **1998,** *279:*1643–1650.

Rubic, T., Trottmann, M., and Lorenz, R.L. Stimulation of CD36 and the key effector of reverse cholesterol transport ATP-binding cassette A1 in monocytoid cells by niacin. *Biochem. Pharmacol.,* **2004,** *67:*411–419.

Rubins, H.B., Robins, S.J., Collins, D., *et al.* Distribution of lipids in 8,500 men with coronary artery disease. Department of Veterans Affairs HDL Intervention Trial Study Group. *Am. J. Cardiol.,* **1995,** *75:*1196–1201.

Rubins, H.B., Robins, S.J., Collins, D., *et al.* Gemfibrozil for the secondary prevention of coronary heart disease in men with low levels of high-density lipoprotein cholesterol. Veterans Affairs High-Density Lipoprotein Cholesterol Intervention Trial Study Group. *N. Engl. J. Med.,* **1999,** *341:*410–418.

Sacks, F.M., Pfeffer, M.A., Moye, L.A., *et al.* The effect of pravastatin on coronary events after myocardial infarction in patients with average cholesterol levels. Cholesterol and Recurrent Events Trial Investigators. *N. Engl. J. Med.,* **1996,** *335:*1001–1009.

Sacks, F.M., Tonkin, A.M., Shepherd, J., *et al.* Effect of pravastatin on coronary disease events in subgroups defined by coronary risk factors: the Prospective Pravastatin Pooling Project. *Circulation,* **2000,** *102:*1893–1900.

Scandinavian Simvastatin Survival Study. Randomised trial of cholesterol lowering in 4444 patients with coronary heart disease: the Scandinavian Simvastatin Survival Study (4S). *Lancet,* **1994,** *344:*1383–1389.

Schneck, D.W., Birmingham, B.K., Zalikowski, J.A., *et al.* The effect of gemfibrozil on the pharmacokinetics of rosuvastatin. *Clin. Pharmacol. Ther.,* **2004,** *75:*455–463.

Schultz, J.R., Verstuyft, J.G., Gong, E.L., Nichols, A.V., and Rubin, E.M. Protein composition determines the anti-atherogenic properties of HDL in transgenic mice. *Nature,* **1993,** *365:*762–764.

Schwartz, M.L. Severe reversible hyperglycemia as a consequence of niacin therapy. *Arch. Intern. Med.,* **1993,** *153:*2050–2052.

Sever, P.S., Dahlöf, B., Poulter, N.R., *et al.* Prevention of coronary and stroke events with atorvastatin in hypertensive patients who have average or lower-than-average cholesterol concentrations, in the Anglo-Scandinavian Cardiac Outcomes Trial–Lipid Lowering Arm (ASCOT-LLA): a multicentre randomised controlled trial. *Lancet,* **2003,** *361:*1149–1158.

Shepherd, J., Blauw, G.J., Murphy, M.B., *et al.* Pravastatin in elderly individuals at risk of vascular disease (PROSPER): a randomised controlled trial. *Lancet,* **2002,** *360:*1623–1630.

Shepherd, J., Cobbe, S.M., Ford, I., *et al.* Prevention of coronary heart disease with pravastatin in men with hypercholesterolemia. West of Scotland Coronary Prevention Study Group. *N. Engl. J. Med.,* **1995,** *333:*1301–1307.

Shepherd, J., Packard, C.J., Bicker, S., Lawrie, T.D.V., and Morgan, H.G. Cholestyramine promotes receptor-mediated low-density-lipoprotein catabolism. *N. Engl. J. Med.,* **1980,** *302:*1219–1222.

Shin, D.J., and Osborne, T.F. Thyroid hormone regulation and cholesterol metabolism are connected through Sterol Regulatory Element-Binding Protein-2 (SREBP-2). *J. Biol. Chem.,* **2003,** *278:*34114–34118.

Shlipak, M.G., Simon, J.A., Vittinghoff, E., *et al.* Estrogen and progestin, lipoprotein(a), and the risk of recurrent coronary heart disease events after menopause. *JAMA,* **2000,** *283:*1845–1852.

Solymoss, B.C., Bourassa, M.G., Lespérance, J., *et al.* Incidence and clinical characteristics of the metabolic syndrome in patients with coronary artery disease. *Coron. Artery Dis.,* **2003,** *14:*207–212.

Sprecher, D.L. Raising high-density lipoprotein cholesterol with niacin and fibrates: a comparative review. *Am. J. Cardiol.,* **2000,** *86*(suppl):46L–50L.

Staels, B., and Auwerx, J. Regulation of apo A-I gene expression by fibrates. *Atherosclerosis,* **1998,** *137*(suppl):S19–S23.

Staffa, J.A., Chang, J., and Green, L. Cerivastatin and reports of fatal rhabdomyolysis. *N. Engl. J. Med.,* **2002,** *346:*539–540.

Stamler, J., Wentworth, D., and Neaton, J.D. Is relationship between serum cholesterol and risk of premature death from coronary heart disease continuous and graded? Findings in 356,222 primary screenees of the Multiple Risk Factor Intervention Trial (MRFIT). *JAMA,* **1986,** *256:*2823–2828.

Stein, E.A., Lane, M., and Laskarzewski, P. Comparison of statins in hypertriglyceridemia. *Am. J. Cardiol.,* **1998,** *81:*66B–69B.

Stein, Y., and Stein, O. Lipoprotein lipase and atherosclerosis. *Atherosclerosis,* **2003,** *170:*1–9.

Steinberg, D. Low density lipoprotein oxidation and its pathobiological significance. *J. Biol. Chem.,* **1997,** *272:*20963–20966.

Stern, R.H., Spence, J.D., Freeman, D.J., and Parbtani, A. Tolerance to nicotinic acid flushing. *Clin. Pharmacol. Ther.,* **1991,** *50:*66–70.

Sudhop, T., Lütjohann, D., Kodal, A., *et al.* Inhibition of intestinal cholesterol absorption by ezetimibe in humans. *Circulation,* **2002,** *106:*1943–1948.

Tall, A.R., Jiang, X.C., Luo, Y., and Silver, D. 1999 George Lyman Duff memorial lecture: lipid transfer proteins, HDL metabolism, and atherogenesis. *Arterioscler. Thromb. Vasc. Biol.,* **2000,** *20:*1185–1188.

Tamai, O., Matsuoka, H., Itabe, H., *et al.* Single LDL apheresis improves endothelium-dependent vasodilatation in hypercholesterolemic humans. *Circulation,* **1997,** *95:*76–82.

Tatò, F., Vega, G.L., and Grundy, S.M. Effects of crystalline nicotinic acid-induced hepatic dysfunction on serum low-density lipoprotein cholesterol and lecithin cholesteryl acyl transferase. *Am. J. Cardiol.,* **1998,** *81:*805–807.

The Expert Panel. Third Report of the National Cholesterol Education Program (NCEP) Expert Panel on Detection, Evaluation, and Treatment of High Blood Cholesterol in Adults (Adult Treatment Panel III). Final report. *Circulation,* **2002,** *106:*3143–3421.

The Long-Term Intervention with Pravastatin in Ischaemic Disease (LIPID) Study Group. Prevention of cardiovascular events and death with pravastatin in patients with coronary heart disease and a broad range of initial cholesterol levels. *N. Engl. J. Med.,* **1998,** *339:*1349–1357.

The Post Coronary Artery Bypass Graft Trial Investigators. The effect of aggressive lowering of low-density lipoprotein cholesterol levels and low-dose anticoagulation on obstructive changes in saphenous-vein coronary-artery bypass grafts. *N. Engl. J. Med.,* **1997,** *336:*153–162.

Thompson, G.R., and Barter, P.J. Clinical lipidology at the end of the millennium. *Curr. Opin. Lipidol.,* **1999,** *10:*521–526.

Thompson, P.D., Clarkson, P., and Karas, R.H. Statin-associated myopathy. *JAMA,* **2003,** *289:*1681–1690.

Thompson, G.R., Nauumova, R.P., and Watts, G.F. Role of cholesterol in regulating apolipoprotein D secretion by the liver. *J. Lipid Res.,* **1996,** *37:*439–447.

Tikkanen, M.J. Statins: Within-group comparisons, statin escape and combination therapy. *Curr. Opin. Lipidol.,* **1996,** *7:*385–388.

Vaisman, B.L., Lambert, G., Amar, M., *et al.* ABCA1 overexpression leads to hyperalphalipoproteinemia and increased biliary cholesterol excretion in transgenic mice. *J. Clin. Invest.,* **2001,** *108:*303–309.

Vakkilainen, J., Steiner, G., Ansquer, J.C., *et al.* Relationships between low-density lipoprotein particle size, plasma lipoproteins, and progression of coronary artery disease: the Diabetes Atherosclerosis Intervention Study (DAIS). *Circulation,* **2003,** *107:*1733–1737.

Vega, G.L., and Grundy, S.M. Lipoprotein responses to treatment with lovastatin, gemfibrozil, and nicotinic acid in normolipidemic

patients with hypoalphalipoproteinemia. *Arch. Intern. Med.,* **1994,** *154:*73–82.

van der Vliet, H.N., Sammels, M.G., Leegwater, A.C., *et al.* Apolipoprotein A-V: a novel apolipoprotein associated with an early phase of liver regeneration. *J. Biol. Chem.,* **2001,** *276:*44512–44520.

Watts, G.F., and Dimmitt, S.B. Fibrates, dyslipoproteinaemia and cardiovascular disease. *Curr. Opin. Lipidol.,* **1999,** *10:*561–574.

Welty, F.K., Lahoz, C., Tucker, K.L., *et al.* Frequency of ApoB and ApoE gene mutations as causes of hypobetalipoproteinemia in the Framingham offspring population. *Arterioscler. Thromb. Vasc. Biol.,* **1998,** *18:*1745–1751.

Williams, D.L., Connelly, M.A., Temel, R.E., *et al.* Scavenger receptor BI and cholesterol trafficking. *Curr. Opin. Lipidol.,* **1999,** *10:*329–339.

Williams, J.K., Sukhova, G.K., Herrington, D.M., and Libby, P. Pravastatin has cholesterol-lowering independent effects on the artery wall of atherosclerotic monkeys. *J. Am. Coll. Cardiol.,* **1998,** *31:*684–691.

Wilson, P.W., D'Agostino, R.B., Levy, D., *et al.* Prediction of coronary heart disease using risk factor categories. *Circulation,* **1998,** *97:*1837–1847.

Wise, A., Foord, S.M., Fraser, N.J., *et al.* Molecular identification of high and low affinity receptors for nicotinic acid. *J. Biol. Chem.,* **2003,** *278:*9869–9874.

Witztum, J.L., and Steinberg, D. The oxidative modification hypothesis of atherosclerosis: Does it hold for humans? *Trends Cardiovasc. Med.,* **2001,** *11:*93–102.

Wong, W.W., Dimitroulakos, J., Minden, M.D., and Penn, L.Z. HMG-CoA reductase inhibitors and the malignant cell: the statin family of drugs as triggers of tumor-specific apoptosis. *Leukemia,* **2002,** *16:*508–519.

Wood, D., De Backer, G., Faergeman, O., *et al.* Prevention of coronary heart disease in clinical practice. Recommendations of the Second Joint Task Force of European and Other Societies on Coronary Prevention. *Eur. Heart J.,* **1998,** *19:*1434–1503.

Xie, C., Woollett, L.A., Turley, S.D., and Dietschy, J.M. Fatty acids differentially regulate hepatic cholesteryl ester formation and incorporation into lipoproteins in the liver of the mouse. *J. Lipid Res.,* **2002,** *43:*1508–1519.

Yuan, J., Tsai, M.Y., and Hunninghake, D.B. Changes in composition and distribution of LDL subspecies in hypertriglyceridemic and hypercholesterolemic patients during gemfibrozil therapy. *Atherosclerosis,* **1994,** *110:*1–11.

Yusuf, S. Two decades of progress in preventing vascular disease. *Lancet,* **2002,** *360:*2–3.

PHARMACOTHERAPY OF GASTRIC ACIDITY, PEPTIC ULCERS, AND GASTROESOPHAGEAL REFLUX DISEASE

Willemijntje A. Hoogerwerf and Pankaj Jay Pasricha

The acid-peptic diseases are those disorders in which gastric acid and pepsin are necessary, but usually not sufficient, pathogenic factors. While inherently caustic, acid and pepsin in the stomach normally do not produce damage or symptoms because of intrinsic defense mechanisms. Barriers to the reflux of gastric contents into the esophagus comprise the primary esophageal defense. If these protective barriers fail and reflux occurs, dyspepsia and/or erosive esophagitis may result. Therapies are directed at decreasing gastric acidity, enhancing the lower esophageal sphincter, or stimulating esophageal motility (*see* Chapter 37). In the stomach, mucus and bicarbonate, stimulated by the local generation of prostaglandins, protect the gastric mucosa. If these defenses are disrupted, a gastric or duodenal ulcer may form. The treatment and prevention of these acid-related disorders are accomplished either by decreasing the level of gastric acidity or by enhancing mucosal protection. The appreciation that an infectious agent, *Helicobacter pylori*, plays a key role in the pathogenesis of acid-peptic diseases has stimulated new approaches to prevention and therapy.

PHYSIOLOGY OF GASTRIC SECRETION

Gastric acid secretion is a complex, continuous process in which multiple central and peripheral factors contribute to a common endpoint: the secretion of H^+ by parietal cells. Neuronal (acetylcholine, ACh), paracrine (histamine), and endocrine (gastrin) factors all regulate acid secretion (Figure 36–1). Their specific receptors (M_3, H_2, and CCK_2 receptors, respectively) are on the basolateral membrane of parietal cells in the body and fundus of the stomach. The H_2 receptor is a GPCR that activates the G_s–adenylylcyclase–cyclic AMP–PKA pathway. ACh and gastrin signal through GPCRs that couple to the G_q–PLC-IP_3–Ca^{2+} pathway in parietal cells. In parietal cells, the cyclic AMP and the Ca^{2+}-dependent pathways activate H^+,K^+-ATPase (the proton pump), which exchanges hydrogen and potassium ions across the parietal cell membrane. This pump generates the largest known ion gradient in vertebrates, with an intracellular pH of about 7.3 and an intracanalicular pH of about 0.8.

The most important structures for CNS stimulation of gastric acid secretion are the dorsal motor nucleus of the vagal nerve, the hypothalamus, and the solitary tract nucleus. Efferent fibers originating in the dorsal motor nuclei descend to the stomach *via* the vagus nerve and synapse with ganglion cells of the enteric nervous system. ACh release from postganglionic vagal fibers directly stimulates gastric acid secretion through muscarinic M_3 receptors on the

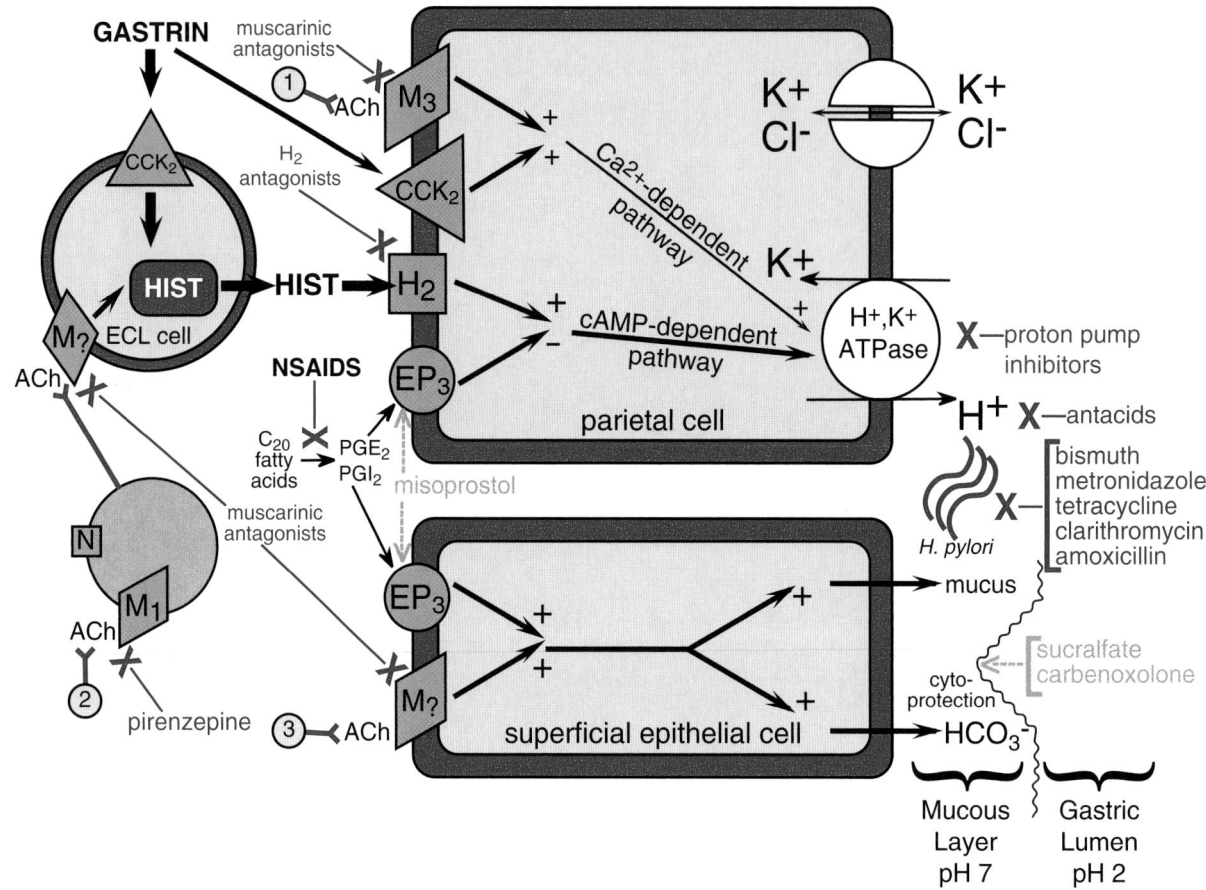

Figure 36–1. *Physiological and pharmacological regulation of gastric secretion: the basis for therapy of acid-peptic disorders.*
Shown are the interactions among an enterochromaffin-like (ECL) cell that secretes histamine, a parietal cell that secretes acid, and a superficial epithelial cell that secretes cytoprotective mucus and bicarbonate. Physiological pathways, shown in solid black, may be stimulatory (+) or inhibitory (–). *1* and *3* indicate possible inputs from postganglionic cholinergic fibers, while *2* shows neural input from the vagus nerve. Physiological agonists and their respective membrane receptors include: acetylcholine (ACh), muscarinic (M), and nicotinic (N) receptors; gastrin, cholecystokinin receptor 2 (CCK_2); histamine (HIST), H_2 receptor; and prostaglandin E_2 (PGE_2), EP_3 receptor. Drug actions are indicated by dashed lines. A blue X indicates targets of pharmacological antagonism. A light blue dashed arrow indicates a drug action that mimics or enhances a physiological pathway. Shown in blue are drugs used to treat acid-peptic disorders. NSAIDs are nonsteroidal antiinflammatory drugs and are ulcerogenic.

basolateral membrane of parietal cells. The CNS predominantly modulates the activity of the enteric nervous system *via* ACh, stimulating gastric acid secretion in response to the sight, smell, taste, or anticipation of food (the "cephalic" phase of acid secretion). ACh also indirectly affects parietal cells by increasing the release of histamine from the enterochromaffin-like (ECL) cells in the fundus of the stomach and of gastrin from G cells in the gastric antrum.

ECL cells, the source of gastric histamine secretion, usually are in close proximity to parietal cells. Histamine acts as a paracrine mediator, diffusing from its site of release to nearby parietal cells, where it activates H_2 receptors. The critical role of histamine in gastric acid secretion is dramatically demonstrated by the efficacy of H_2-receptor antagonists in decreasing gastric acid secretion (*see* below).

Gastrin, which is produced by antral G cells, is the most potent inducer of acid secretion. Multiple pathways stimulate gastrin

release, including CNS activation, local distention, and chemical components of the gastric contents. Gastrin stimulates acid secretion indirectly by inducing the release of histamine by ECL cells; a direct effect on parietal cells also plays a lesser role.

Somatostatin (SST), which is produced by antral D cells, inhibits gastric acid secretion. Acidification of the gastric luminal pH to <3 stimulates SST release, which in turn suppresses gastrin release in a negative feedback loop. SST-producing cells are decreased in patients with *H. pylori* infection, and the consequent reduction of SST's inhibitory effect may contribute to excess gastrin production.

Gastric Defenses Against Acid. The extremely high concentration of H^+ in the gastric lumen requires robust defense mechanisms to protect the esophagus and the stomach. The primary esophageal defense is the lower esophageal sphincter, which prevents reflux of acidic gastric contents into the esophagus. The stomach protects itself from acid damage by a number of mechanisms that require adequate mucosal blood flow, perhaps because of the high metabolic activity and oxygen requirements of the gastric mucosa. One key defense is the secretion of a mucus layer that protects gastric epithelial cells. Gastric mucus is soluble when secreted but quickly forms an insoluble gel that coats the mucosal surface of the stomach, slows ion diffusion, and prevents mucosal damage by macromolecules such as pepsin. Mucus production is stimulated by prostaglandins E_2 and I_2, which also directly inhibit gastric acid secretion by parietal cells. Thus, alcohol, aspirin, and other drugs that inhibit prostaglandin formation decrease mucus secretion and predispose to the development of acid-peptic disease. A second important part of the normal mucosal defense is the secretion of bicarbonate ions by superficial gastric epithelial cells. Bicarbonate neutralizes the acid in the region of the mucosal cells, thereby raising pH and preventing acid-mediated damage.

Figure 36–1 outlines the rationale and pharmacological basis for the therapy of acid-peptic diseases. The proton pump inhibitors are used most commonly, followed by the histamine H_2-receptor antagonists.

PROTON PUMP INHIBITORS

Chemistry; Mechanism of Action; Pharmacology. The most potent suppressors of gastric acid secretion are inhibitors of the gastric H^+,K^+-ATPase (proton pump) (Figure 36–2A). In typical doses, these drugs diminish the daily production of acid (basal and stimulated) by 80% to 95%. Five proton pump inhibitors are available for clinical use: *omeprazole* (PRILOSEC, RAPINEX, ZEGERID) and its S-isomer, *esomeprazole* (NEXIUM), *lansoprazole* (PREVACID), *rabeprazole* (ACIPHEX), and *pantoprazole* (PROTONIX). These drugs have different substitutions on their pyridine and/or benzimidazole groups but are remarkably similar in their pharmacological properties (*see* Appendix II). Omeprazole is a racemic mixture of R- and S-isomers; the S-isomer, esomeprazole (S-omeprazole), is eliminated less rapidly than R-omeprazole, which theoretically provides a therapeutic advantage because of the increased half-life. Despite claims to the contrary, all proton pump inhibitors have equivalent efficacy at comparable doses.

Proton pump inhibitors are prodrugs that require activation in an acid environment. After absorption into the systemic circulation, the prodrug diffuses into the parietal cells of the stomach and accumulates in the acidic secretory canaliculi. Here, it is activated by proton-catalyzed formation of a tetracyclic sulfenamide (Figure 36–2), trapping the drug so that it cannot diffuse back across the canalicular membrane. The activated form then binds covalently with sulfhydryl groups of cysteines in the H^+,K^+-ATPase, irreversibly inactivating the pump molecule. Acid secretion resumes only after new pump mole-

cules are synthesized and inserted into the luminal membrane, providing a prolonged (up to 24- to 48-hour) suppression of acid secretion, despite the much shorter plasma half-lives (0.5 to 2 hours) of the parent compounds. Because they block the final step in acid production, the proton pump inhibitors are effective in acid suppression regardless of other stimulating factors.

To prevent degradation of proton pump inhibitors by acid in the gastric lumen, oral dosage forms are supplied in different formulations: (1) enteric-coated drugs contained inside gelatin capsules (omeprazole, esomeprazole, and lansoprazole); (2) enteric-coated granules supplied as a powder for suspension (lansoprazole); (3) enteric-coated tablets (pantoprazole, rabeprazole, and omeprazole); and (4) powdered drug combined with sodium bicarbonate (omeprazole). The delayed-release and enteric-coated tablets dissolve only at alkaline pH, while admixture of omeprazole with sodium bicarbonate simply neutralizes stomach acid; both strategies substantially improve the oral bioavailability of these acid-labile drugs. Until recently, the requirement for enteric coating posed a challenge to the administration of proton pump inhibitors in patients for whom the oral route of administration is not available (Freston *et al.*, 2003). These patients and those requiring immediate acid suppression now can be treated parenterally with pantoprazole or lansoprazole, both of which are approved for intravenous administration in the United States. A single intravenous bolus of 80 mg of pantoprazole inhibits acid production by 80% to 90% within an hour, and this inhibition persists for up to 21 hours, permitting once-daily dosing to achieve the desired degree of hypochlorhydria. The FDA-approved dose of intravenous pantoprazole for gastroesophageal reflux disease is 40 mg daily for up to 10 days. Higher doses (*e.g.*, 160 to 240 mg in divided doses) are used to manage hypersecretory conditions such as the Zollinger-Ellison syndrome. An intravenous formulation of esomeprazole is available in Europe but not in the United States.

Pharmacokinetics. Since an acidic pH in the parietal cell acid canaliculi is required for drug activation, and since food stimulates acid production, these drugs ideally should be given about 30 minutes before meals. Concurrent administration of food may reduce somewhat the rate of absorption of proton pump inhibitors, but this effect is not thought to be clinically significant. Concomitant use of other drugs that inhibit acid secretion, such as H_2-receptor antagonists, might be predicted to lessen the effectiveness of the proton pump inhibitors, but the clinical relevance of this potential interaction is unknown.

Once in the small bowel, proton pump inhibitors are rapidly absorbed, highly protein bound, and extensively metabolized by hepatic CYPs, particularly CYP2C19 and CYP3A4. Several variants of CYP2C19 have been identified. Asians are more likely than Cau-

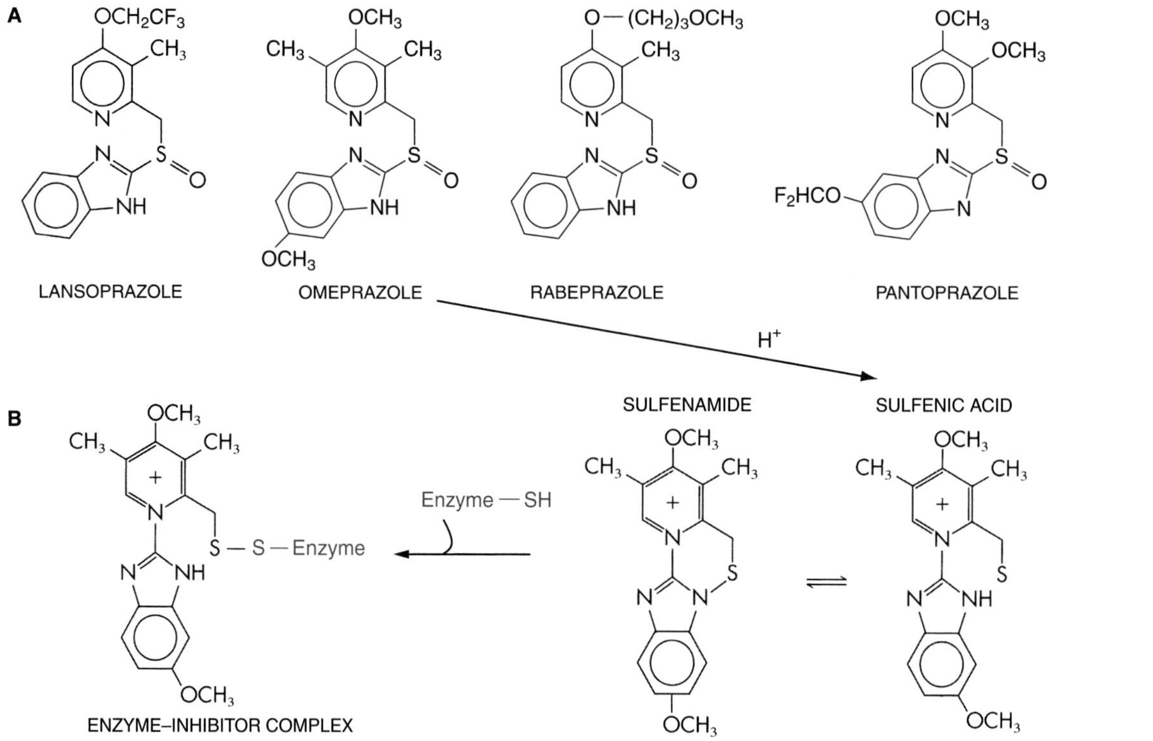

Figure 36–2. *Proton pump inhibitors.* **A.** Inhibitors of gastric H⁺,K⁺-ATPase (proton pump). **B.** Conversion of omeprazole to a sulfenamide in the acidic secretory canaliculi of the parietal cell. The sulfenamide interacts covalently with sulfhydryl groups in the proton pump, thereby irreversibly inhibiting its activity. The other three proton pump inhibitors undergo analogous conversions.

casians or African-Americans to have the CYP2C19 genotype that correlates with slow metabolism of proton pump inhibitors (23% *vs.* 3%, respectively), which has been suggested to contribute to heightened efficacy and/or toxicity in this ethnic group (Dickson and Stuart, 2003). Although the CYP2C19 genotype is correlated with the magnitude of gastric acid suppression by proton pump inhibitors in patients with gastroesophageal reflux disease, there is no evidence that the CYP2C19 genotype predicts clinical efficacy of these drugs (Chong and Ensom, 2003).

Because not all pumps or all parietal cells are active simultaneously, maximal suppression of acid secretion requires several doses of the proton pump inhibitors. For example, it may take 2 to 5 days of therapy with once-daily dosing to achieve the 70% inhibition of proton pumps that is seen at steady state (Wolfe and Sachs, 2000). More frequent initial dosing (*e.g.,* twice daily) will reduce the time to achieve full inhibition but is not proven to improve patient outcome. Since the proton pump inhibition is irreversible, acid secretion will be suppressed for 24 to 48 hours, or more, until new proton pumps are synthesized and incorporated into the luminal membrane of parietal cells.

Chronic renal failure does not lead to drug accumulation with once-a-day dosing of the proton pump inhibitors. Hepatic disease substantially reduces the clearance of esomeprazole and lansoprazole. Thus, in patients with severe hepatic disease, dose reduction is recommended for esomeprazole and should be considered for lansoprazole.

Adverse Effects and Drug Interactions. Proton pump inhibitors generally cause remarkably few adverse effects. The most common side effects are nausea, abdominal pain, constipation, flatulence, and diarrhea. Subacute myopathy, arthralgias, headaches, and skin rashes also have been reported. As noted above, proton pump inhibitors are metabolized by hepatic CYPs and therefore may interfere with the elimination of other drugs cleared by this route. Proton pump inhibitors have been observed to interact with *warfarin* (esomeprazole, lansoprazole, omeprazole, and rabeprazole), *diazepam* (esomeprazole and omeprazole), and *cyclosporine* (omeprazole and rabeprazole). Among the proton pump inhibitors, only omeprazole inhibits CYP2C19 (thereby decreasing the clearance of *disulfiram, phenytoin,* and other drugs) and induces the expression of CYP1A2 (thereby increasing the clearance of *imipramine,* several antipsychotic drugs, *tacrine,* and *theophylline*).

Chronic treatment with omeprazole decreases the absorption of vitamin B₁₂, but the clinical relevance of this effect is not clear. Loss of gastric acidity also may affect the bioavailability of such drugs as *ketoconazole, ampicillin* esters, and iron salts.

Hypergastrinemia is more frequent and more severe with proton pump inhibitors than with H₂-receptor antagonists, and gastrin levels of >500 ng/L occur in approximately 5% to 10% of users with chronic omeprazole administration. This hypergastrinemia may predispose to rebound hypersecretion of gastric acid upon discontinuation of therapy (*see* below) and also may promote the growth of gastrointestinal tumors. In rats, long-term administration of proton pump inhibitors causes hyperplasia of enterochromaffin-like cells and the development of gastric carcinoid tumors. Although the gastrin levels observed in rats are about tenfold higher than those seen in human beings, this finding has raised concerns about the possibility of similar complications of proton pump inhibitors in humans, for which there is no unequivocal evidence. The proton pump inhibitors have a track record of approximately 25 years of use worldwide without the emergence of major safety concerns (Klinkenberg-Knol *et al.*, 1994; Kuipers and Meuwissen, 2000).

Therapeutic Uses. Proton pump inhibitors are used principally to promote healing of gastric and duodenal ulcers and to treat gastro*e*sophageal *r*eflux *d*isease (GERD), including erosive esophagitis, which is either complicated or unresponsive to treatment with H_2-receptor antagonists. Proton pump inhibitors also are the mainstay in the treatment of pathological hypersecretory conditions, including the Zollinger-Ellison syndrome. Lansoprazole is FDA approved for treatment and prevention of recurrence of nonsteroidal antiinflammatory drug (NSAID)-associated gastric ulcers in patients who continue NSAID use. In addition, all proton pump inhibitors are FDA approved for reducing the risk of duodenal ulcer recurrence associated with *H. pylori* infections. Therapeutic applications of proton pump inhibitors are further discussed below under "Specific Acid-Peptic Disorders and Therapeutic Strategies."

Use in Children. In children, omeprazole is safe and effective for treatment of erosive esophagitis and GERD. Younger patients generally have increased metabolic capacity, which may explain the need for higher dosages of omeprazole per kilogram in children compared to adults.

H_2-RECEPTOR ANTAGONISTS

The description of selective histamine H_2-receptor blockade was a landmark in the treatment of acid-peptic disease (Black, 1993). Before the availability of the H_2-receptor antagonists, the standard of care was simply acid neutralization in the stomach lumen, generally with inadequate results. The long history of safety and efficacy with the H_2-receptor antagonists eventually led to their availability without a prescription. Increasingly, however, proton pump inhibitors are replacing the H_2-receptor antagonists in clinical practice.

Chemistry; Mechanism of Action; Pharmacology. The H_2-receptor antagonists inhibit acid production by reversibly competing with histamine for binding to H_2

receptors on the basolateral membrane of parietal cells. Four different H_2-receptor antagonists, which differ mainly in their pharmacokinetics (*see* Appendix II) and propensity to cause drug interactions, are available in the United States (Figure 36–3): *cimetidine* (TAGAMET), *ranitidine* (ZANTAC), *famotidine* (PEPCID), and *nizatidine* (AXID). These drugs are less potent than proton pump inhibitors but still suppress 24-hour gastric acid secretion by about 70%. The H_2-receptor antagonists predominantly inhibit basal acid secretion, which accounts for their efficacy in suppressing nocturnal acid secretion. Because the most important determinant of duodenal ulcer healing is the level of nocturnal acidity, evening dosing of H_2-receptor antagonists is adequate therapy in most instances. Ranitidine and nizatidine also may stimulate GI motility, but the clinical importance of this effect is unknown.

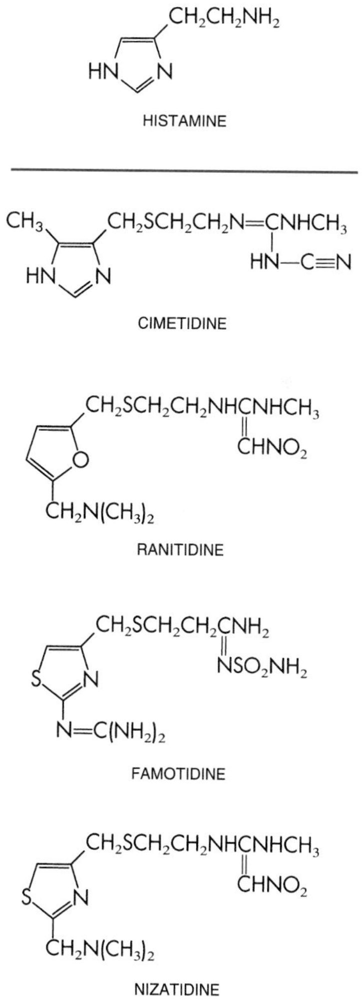

Figure 36–3. Histamine and H_2-receptor antagonists.

All four H_2-receptor antagonists are available as prescription and over-the-counter formulations for oral administration. Intravenous and intramuscular preparations of cimetidine, ranitidine, and famotidine also are available. When the oral or nasogastric routes are not an option, these drugs can be given in intermittent intravenous boluses or by continuous intravenous infusion (Table 36–1). The latter provides better control of gastric pH, but is not proven to be more effective in preventing clinically significant bleeding in critically ill patients.

Pharmacokinetics. The H_2-receptor antagonists are rapidly absorbed after oral administration, with peak serum concentrations within 1 to 3 hours. Absorption may be enhanced by food or decreased by antacids, but these effects probably are unimportant clinically. Therapeutic levels are achieved rapidly after intravenous dosing and are maintained for 4 to 5 hours (cimetidine), 6 to 8 hours (ranitidine), or 10 to 12 hours (famotidine). Unlike proton pump inhibitors, only a small percentage of H_2-receptor antagonists are protein-bound. Small amounts (from <10% to ~35%) of these drugs undergo metabolism in the liver, but liver disease *per se* is not an indication for dose adjustment. The kidneys excrete these drugs and their metabolites by filtration and renal tubular secretion, and it is important to reduce doses of H_2-receptor antagonists in patients with decreased creatinine clearance. Neither hemodialysis nor peritoneal dialysis clears significant amounts of the drugs.

Adverse Reactions and Drug Interactions. Like the proton pump inhibitors, the H_2-receptor antagonists generally are well tolerated, with a low (<3%) incidence of adverse effects. Side effects usually are minor and include diarrhea, headache, drowsiness, fatigue, muscular pain, and constipation. Less common side effects include those affecting the CNS (confusion, delirium, hallucinations, slurred speech, and headaches), which occur primarily with intravenous administration of the drugs or in elderly subjects. Long-term use of cimetidine at high doses—seldom used clinically today—decreases testosterone binding to the androgen receptor and inhibits a CYP that hydroxylates estradiol. Clinically, these effects can cause galactorrhea in women and gynecomastia, reduced sperm count, and impotence in men. Several reports have associated H_2-receptor antagonists with various blood dyscrasias, including thrombocytopenia. H_2-receptor antagonists cross the placenta and are excreted in breast milk. Although no major teratogenic risk has been associated with these agents, caution nevertheless is warranted when they are used in pregnancy (*see* below).

All agents that inhibit gastric acid secretion may alter the rate of absorption and subsequent bioavailability of the H_2-receptor antagonists (*see* "Antacids," below). Drug interactions with H_2-receptor antagonists occur mainly with cimetidine, and its use has decreased markedly. Cimetidine inhibits CYPs (*e.g.*, CYP1A2, CYP2C9, and CYP2D6), and thereby can increase the levels of a variety of drugs that are substrates for these enzymes. Ranitidine also interacts with hepatic CYPs, but with an affinity of only 10% of that of cimetidine; thus, ranitidine interferes only minimally with hepatic metabolism of other drugs. Famotidine and nizatidine are even safer in this regard, with no significant drug interactions mediated by inhibiting hepatic CYPs. Slight increases in blood-alcohol concentration may result from concomitant use of H_2-receptor antagonists, but this is unlikely to be clinically significant.

Therapeutic Uses. The major therapeutic indications for H_2-receptor antagonists are to promote healing of gastric and duodenal ulcers, to treat uncomplicated GERD, and to prevent the occurrence of stress ulcers. More information about the therapeutic applications of H_2-receptor antagonists is provided below under "Specific Acid-Peptic Disorders and Therapeutic Strategies."

TOLERANCE AND REBOUND WITH ACID-SUPPRESSING MEDICATIONS

Tolerance to the acid-suppressing effects of H_2-receptor antagonists is well described and may account for a diminished therapeutic effect with continued drug administration (Sandevik *et al.*, 1997). Tolerance can develop within 3 days of starting treatment and may be resistant to increased doses of the medications. Diminished sensitivity to these drugs may result from the effect of the secondary hypergastrinemia to stimulate histamine release from ECL cells. Proton pump inhibitors, despite even greater elevations of endogenous gastrin, do not cause this phenomenon, probably because their site of action is distal to the action of histamine on acid release. On the other hand, rebound increases in gastric acidity can occur

Table 36–1
Intravenous Doses of H_2-Receptor Antagonists

	CIMETIDINE	RANITIDINE	FAMOTIDINE
Intermittent bolus	300 mg every 6–8 hours	50 mg every 6–8 hours	20 mg every 12 hours
Continuous infusion	37.5–100 mg/hour	6.25–12.5 mg/hour	1.7–2.1 mg/hour

when either of these drug classes is discontinued, possibly reflecting changes in function and justifying a gradual drug taper or the substitution of alternatives (*e.g.*, antacids) in at-risk patients.

AGENTS THAT ENHANCE MUCOSAL DEFENSE

Prostaglandin Analogs: Misoprostol

Chemistry; Mechanism of Action; Pharmacology. Prostaglandin E_2 (PGE_2) and prostacyclin (PGI_2) are the major prostaglandins synthesized by the gastric mucosa. They bind to the EP_3 receptor on parietal cells (*see* Chapter 26) and stimulate the G_i pathway, thereby decreasing intracellular cyclic AMP and gastric acid secretion. PGE_2 also can prevent gastric injury by cytoprotective effects that include stimulation of mucin and bicarbonate secretion and increased mucosal blood flow. Although smaller doses than those required for acid suppression can protect the gastric mucosa in laboratory animals, this has not been convincingly demonstrated in humans; acid suppression appears to be the most important effect clinically (Wolfe and Sachs, 2000). Since NSAIDs diminish prostaglandin formation by inhibiting cyclooxygenase, synthetic prostaglandin analogs offer a logical approach to reducing NSAID-induced mucosal damage (*see* below). *Misoprostol* (15-deoxy-16-hydroxy-16-methyl-PGE_1; CYTOTEC) is a synthetic analog of prostaglandin E_1. Structural modifications include an additional methyl ester group at C1 that increases potency and duration of antisecretory effect, and transfer of a hydroxyl group from C15 to C16 and addition of a methyl group that increases oral bioactivity, duration of antisecretory action, and safety. The degree of inhibition of gastric acid secretion by misoprostol is directly related to dose; oral doses of 100 to 200 μg significantly inhibit basal acid secretion (up to 85% to 95% inhibition) or food-stimulated acid secretion (up to 75% to 85% inhibition). The usual recommended dose for ulcer prophylaxis is 200 μg four times a day.

Pharmacokinetics. Misoprostol is rapidly absorbed after oral administration and then is rapidly and extensively de-esterified to form misoprostol acid, the principal and active metabolite of the drug. Some of this conversion may occur in the parietal cells. A single dose inhibits acid production within 30 minutes; the therapeutic effect peaks at 60 to 90 minutes and lasts for up to 3 hours. Food and antacids decrease the rate of misoprostol absorption, resulting in delayed and decreased peak plasma concentrations of the active metabolite. The free acid is excreted mainly in the urine, with an elimination half-life of about 20 to 40 minutes.

Adverse Effects. Diarrhea, with or without abdominal pain and cramps, occurs in up to 30% of patients who take misoprostol. Apparently dose-related, it typically begins within the first 2 weeks after therapy is initiated and often resolves spontaneously within a week; more severe or protracted cases may necessitate drug discontinuation. *Misoprostol can cause clinical exacerbations of inflammatory bowel disease* (*see* Chapter 38) *and should be avoided in patients with this disorder. Misoprostol is contraindicated during pregnancy* because it can increase uterine contractility.

Therapeutic Use. Misoprostol is FDA approved to prevent NSAID-induced mucosal injury. However, it rarely is used because of its adverse effects and the inconvenience of four-times-daily dosing. The proton pump inhibitors and H_2-receptor antagonists also are used to diminish the gastrointestinal side effects of NSAIDs, but only lansoprazole holds an FDA approved indication for this purpose.

SUCRALFATE

Chemistry; Mechanism of Action; Pharmacology. In the presence of acid-induced damage, pepsin-mediated hydrolysis of mucosal proteins contributes to mucosal erosion and ulcerations. This process can be inhibited by sulfated polysaccharides. *Sucralfate* (CARAFATE) consists of the octasulfate of sucrose to which $Al(OH)_3$ has been added. In an acid environment (pH <4), sucralfate undergoes extensive cross-linking to produce a viscous, sticky polymer that adheres to epithelial cells and ulcer craters for up to 6 hours after a single dose. In addition to inhibiting hydrolysis of mucosal proteins by pepsin, sucralfate may have additional cytoprotective effects, including stimulation of local production of prostaglandins and epidermal growth factor. Sucralfate also binds bile salts; thus, some clinicians use sucralfate to treat individuals with the syndromes of biliary esophagitis or gastritis (the existence of which is controversial).

Therapeutic Uses. The use of sucralfate to treat peptic acid disease has diminished in recent years. Nevertheless, because increased gastric pH may be a factor in the development of nosocomial pneumonia in critically ill patients, sucralfate may offer an advantage over proton pump inhibitors and H_2-receptor antagonists for the prophylaxis

Table 36–2
Composition and Neutralizing Capacities of Popular Antacid Preparations

PRODUCT	Al(OH)$_3$*	Mg(OH)$_2$*	CaCO$_3$*	SIMETHICONE*	ACID NEUTRALIZING CAPACITY[†]
Tablets					
Gelusil	200	200	0	25	10.5
Maalox Quick Dissolve	0	0	600	0	12
Mylanta Double Strength	400	400	0	40	23
Riopan Plus Double Strength	Magaldrate, 1080			20	30
Calcium Rich Rolaids		80	412	0	11
Tums EX	0	0	750	0	15
Liquids					
Maalox TC	600	300	0	0	28
Milk of Magnesia	0	400	0	0	14
Mylanta Maximum Strength	400	400	0	40	25
Riopan	Magaldrate, 540			0	15

*Contents, milligrams per tablet or per 5 ml. [†]Acid-neutralizing capacity, milliequivalents per tablet or per 5 ml. The United States marketplace for antacids is fluid. The current trend of "reusing" well-known brand names to introduce new products that contain an active ingredient different from expected is a source of confusion that can present a danger to patients. Medication safety experts encourage clinical practitioners to refer to the active ingredient(s) in conjunction with the proprietary (brand) name when selecting OTC products.

of stress ulcers (*see* below). Due to its unique mechanism of action, sucralfate also has been used in several other conditions associated with mucosal inflammation/ulceration that may not respond to acid suppression, including oral mucositis (radiation and aphthous ulcers) and bile reflux gastropathy. Administered by rectal enema, sucralfate also has been used for radiation proctitis and solitary rectal ulcers.

Since it is activated by acid, sucralfate should be taken on an empty stomach 1 hour before meals. The use of antacids within 30 minutes of a dose of sucralfate should be avoided. The usual dose of sucralfate is 1 g four times daily (for active duodenal ulcer) or 1 g twice daily (for maintenance therapy).

Adverse Effects. The most common side effect of sucralfate is constipation (about 2%). As some aluminum can be absorbed, sucralfate should be avoided in patients with renal failure who are at risk for aluminum overload. Likewise, aluminum-containing antacids should not be combined with sucralfate in these patients. Sucralfate forms a viscous layer in the stomach that may inhibit absorption of other drugs, including phenytoin, digoxin, cimetidine, ketoconazole, and fluoroquinolone antibiotics. Sucralfate therefore should be taken at least 2 hours after the administration of other drugs. The "sticky" nature of the viscous gel produced by sucralfate in the stomach also may be responsible for the development of bezoars in some patients, particularly in those with underlying gastroparesis.

ANTACIDS

Although hallowed by tradition, the antacids largely have been replaced by more effective and convenient drugs. Nevertheless, they continue to be used by patients for a variety of indications, and some knowledge of their pharmacology is important for the medical professional (*see* Table 36–2 for a comparison of some commonly used antacid preparations).

Many factors, including palatability, determine the effectiveness and choice of antacid. Although sodium bicarbonate effectively neutralizes acid, it is very water-soluble and rapidly absorbed from the stomach, and the alkali and sodium loads may pose a risk for patients with cardiac or renal failure. Depending on particle size and crystal structure, $CaCO_3$ rapidly and effectively neutralizes gastric H^+, but the release of CO_2 from bicarbonate- and carbonate-containing antacids can cause belching, nausea, abdominal distention, and flatulence. Calcium also may induce rebound acid secretion, necessitating more frequent administration.

Combinations of Mg^{2+} (rapidly reacting) and Al^{3+} (slowly reacting) hydroxides provide a relatively balanced and sustained neutralizing capacity and are preferred by most experts. *Magaldrate* is a hydroxymagnesium aluminate complex that is converted rapidly in gastric acid to $Mg(OH)_2$ and $Al(OH)_3$, which are absorbed poorly and thus provide a sustained antacid effect. Although fixed combinations of magnesium and aluminum theoretically counteract the adverse effects of each other on the bowel (Al^{3+} can relax gastric smooth muscle, producing delayed gastric emptying and constipation, while Mg^{2+} exerts the opposite effects), such balance is not always achieved in practice.

Simethicone, a surfactant that may decrease foaming and hence esophageal reflux, is included in many antacid preparations. However, other fixed combinations, particularly those with aspirin, that are marketed for "acid indigestion" are irrational choices, are potentially unsafe in patients predisposed to gastroduodenal ulcers, and should not be used.

The relative effectiveness of antacid preparations is expressed as milliequivalents of acid-neutralizing capacity (defined as the quantity of 1N HCl, expressed in milliequivalents, that can be brought to pH 3.5 within 15 minutes); according to FDA requirements, antacids must have a neutralizing capacity of at least 5 mEq per dose. Due to discrepancies between *in vitro* and *in vivo* neutralizing capacities, antacid doses in practice are titrated simply to relieve symptoms. For uncomplicated ulcers, antacids are given orally 1 and 3 hours after meals and at bedtime. This regimen, providing about 120 mEq of a Mg-Al combination per dose, may be almost as effective as conventional dosing with an H_2-receptor antagonist. For severe symptoms or uncontrolled reflux, antacids can be given as often as every 30 to 60 minutes. In general, antacids should be administered in suspension form, as this probably has a greater neutralizing capacity than do powder or tablet dosage forms. If tablets are used, they should be thoroughly chewed for maximum effect.

Antacids are cleared from the empty stomach in about 30 minutes. However, the presence of food is sufficient to elevate gastric pH to about 5 for approximately 1 hour and to prolong the neutralizing effects of antacids for about 2 to 3 hours.

Antacids vary in the extent to which they are absorbed, and hence in their systemic effects. In general, most antacids can elevate urinary pH by about one pH unit. Antacids that contain Al^{3+}, Ca^{2+}, or Mg^{2+} are absorbed less completely than are those that contain $NaHCO_3$. With normal renal function, the modest accumulations of Al^{3+} and Mg^{2+} do not pose a problem; with renal insufficiency, however, absorbed Al^{3+} can contribute to osteoporosis, encephalopathy, and proximal myopathy. About 15% of orally administered Ca^{2+} is absorbed, causing a transient hypercalcemia. Although

this is not a problem in normal patients, the hypercalcemia from as little as 3 to 4 g of $CaCO_3$ per day can be problematic in patients with uremia. In the past, when large doses of $NaHCO_3$ and $CaCO_3$ were administered commonly with milk or cream for the management of peptic ulcer, the *milk-alkali syndrome* (alkalosis, hypercalcemia, and renal insufficiency) occurred frequently. Today, this syndrome is rare and generally results from the chronic ingestion of large quantities of Ca^{2+} (five to forty 500-mg tablets per day of calcium carbonate) taken with milk. Patients may be asymptomatic or may present with the insidious onset of hypercalcemia, reduced secretion of parathyroid hormone, retention of phosphate, precipitation of Ca^{2+} salts in the kidney, and renal insufficiency.

By altering gastric and urinary pH, antacids may affect a number of drugs (*e.g.*, thyroid hormones, allopurinol, and imidazole antifungals, by altering rates of dissolution and absorption, bioavailability, and renal elimination). Al^{3+} and Mg^{2+} antacids also are notable for their propensity to chelate other drugs present in the GI tract, forming insoluble complexes that pass through the GI tract without absorption. Thus, it generally is prudent to avoid concurrent administration of antacids and drugs intended for systemic absorption. Most interactions can be avoided by taking antacids 2 hours before or after ingestion of other drugs.

OTHER ACID SUPPRESSANTS AND CYTOPROTECTANTS

The M_1 muscarinic receptor antagonists *pirenzepine* and *telenzepine* (*see* Chapter 7) can reduce basal acid production by 40% to 50% and long have been used to treat patients with peptic ulcer disease in countries other than the United States. The ACh receptor on the parietal cell itself is of the M_3 subtype, and these drugs are believed to suppress neural stimulation of acid production *via* actions on M_1 receptors of intramural ganglia (Figure 36–1). Because of their relatively poor efficacy, significant and undesirable anticholinergic side effects, and risk of blood disorders (pirenzepine), they rarely are used today.

In the hope of providing more rapid onset of action and sustained acid suppression, reversible inhibitors of the gastric H^+,K^+-ATPase (*e.g.*, the pyrrolopyridazine derivative AKU517) are being developed for clinical use. Antagonists of the CCK2 gastrin receptor on parietal cells also are under study. The precise role that these agents will play in the therapy of acid-peptic disorders in the future is yet to be determined.

Rebamipide (2-(4-chlorobenzoylamino)-3-[2(1*H*)-quinolinon-4-yl]-propionic acid) is used for ulcer therapy in parts of Asia. It appears to exert a cytoprotective effect both by increasing prostaglandin generation in gastric mucosa and by scavenging reactive oxygen species. *Ecabet* (GASTROM; 12-sulfodehydroabietic acid monosodium), which appears to increase the formation of PGE_2 and PGI_2, also is used for ulcer therapy, mostly in Japan. *Carbenoxolone*, a derivative of glycyrrhizic acid found in licorice root, has been used with modest success for ulcer therapy in Europe. Its exact mechanism of action is not clear, but it may alter the composition and quantity of mucin. Unfortunately, carbenoxolone inhibits the type I isozyme of 11β-hydroxysteroid dehydrogenase, which protects the mineralocorticoid receptor from activation by cortisol in the distal nephron; it therefore causes hypokalemia and hypertension due to excessive mineralocorticoid receptor activation (*see* Chapter 59). *Bismuth compounds* (*see* Chapter 37) may be as effective as cimetidine in patients with peptic ulcers and are frequently prescribed in combination with antibiotics to eradicate *H. pylori* and prevent ulcer recurrence. Bismuth compounds bind to the base of the ulcer, promote mucin and bicarbonate production, and have significant antibacterial effects. Bismuth compounds are an important component of many anti-*Helicobacter* regimens (*see* below); however, given the availability of more effective drugs, bismuth compounds seldom are used alone as cytoprotective agents.

SPECIFIC ACID-PEPTIC DISORDERS AND THERAPEUTIC STRATEGIES

The success of acid-suppressing agents in a variety of conditions is critically dependent upon their ability to keep intragastric pH above a certain target, generally pH 3 to 5; this target varies to some extent with the disease being treated (Figure 36–4).

Gastroesophageal Reflux Disease

In the United States, gastroesophageal reflux disease (GERD) is common, and it is estimated that one in five adults has symptoms of heartburn or gastroesophageal regurgitation at least once a week. Although most cases follow a relatively benign course, GERD in some individuals can cause severe erosive esophagitis; serious

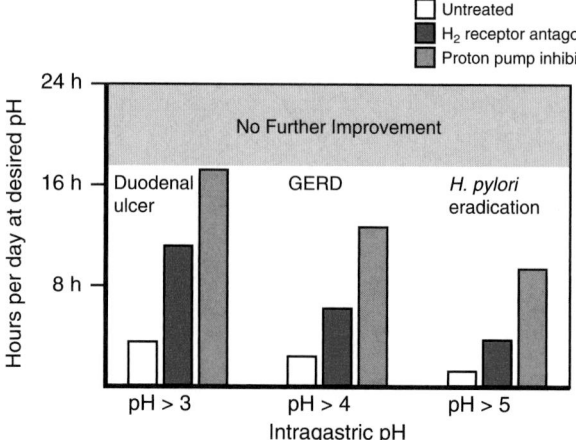

Figure 36–4. *Comparative success of therapy with proton pump inhibitors and H$_2$-receptor antagonists.* Data show the effects of a proton pump inhibitor (given once daily) and an H$_2$-receptor antagonist (given twice daily) in elevating gastric pH to the target ranges (*i.e.*, pH 3 for duodenal ulcer, pH 4 for GERD, and pH 5 for antibiotic eradication of *H. pylori*). (Adapted from Wolfe and Sachs, 2000, with permission.)

sequelae include stricture formation and Barrett's metaplasia (replacement of squamous by intestinal columnar epithelium), which, in turn, is associated with a small but significant risk of adenocarcinoma. Most of the symptoms of GERD reflect injurious effects of the refluxed acid-peptic content on the esophageal epithelium, providing the rationale for suppression of gastric acid. The goals of GERD therapy are complete resolution of symptoms and healing of esophagitis. Proton pump inhibitors clearly are more effective than H$_2$-receptor antagonists in achieving these goals. Healing rates after 4 weeks and 8 weeks of therapy with protein pump inhibitors are approximately 80% and 90%, respectively, while the corresponding healing rates with H$_2$-receptor antagonists are 50% and 75%, respectively. Indeed, proton pump inhibitors are so effective that their empirical use is advocated as a therapeutic trial in patients in whom GERD is suspected to play a role in the pathogenesis of symptoms. Because of the wide clinical spectrum associated with GERD, the therapeutic approach is best tailored to the level of severity in the individual patient (Figure 36–5). In general, the optimal dose for each patient is determined based upon symptom control, and routine measurement of esophageal pH to guide dosing is not recommended. Strictures associated with GERD also respond better to proton pump inhibitors than to H$_2$-receptor antagonists; indeed, the use of

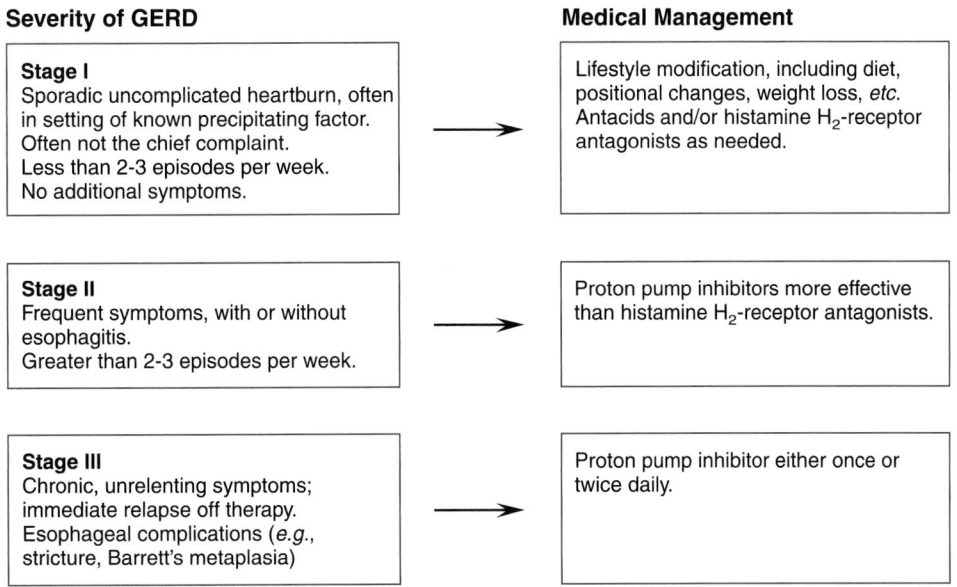

Figure 36–5. *General guidelines for the medical management of gastroesophageal reflux disease (GERD).* Only medications that suppress acid production or that neutralize acid are shown. (Adapted from Wolfe and Sachs, 2000, with permission.)

proton pump inhibitors reduces the requirement for esophageal dilation. Unfortunately, one of the other complications of GERD, Barrett's esophagus, appears to be more refractory to therapy, as neither acid suppression nor antireflux surgery has been shown convincingly to produce regression of metaplasia or to decrease the incidence of tumors.

Regimens for the treatment of GERD with proton pump inhibitors and histamine H_2-receptor antagonists are listed in Table 36–3. Although some patients with mild GERD symptoms may be managed by nocturnal doses of H_2-receptor antagonists, twice-daily dosing usually is required. Antacids are recommended only for the patient with mild, infrequent episodes of heartburn. In general, prokinetic agents (*see* Chapter 37) are not particularly useful for GERD, either alone or in combination with acid-suppressant medications.

GERD is a chronic disorder that requires long-term therapy. Some experts advocate "step-down" approaches that attempt to maintain symptomatic remission by either decreasing the dose of the proton pump inhibitor or switching to an H_2-receptor antagonist. Other experts have advocated intermittent, "on-demand" therapy with proton pump inhibitors for symptomatic relief in patients who have responded initially but continue to have symptoms. However, many patients will maintain their requirement for proton pump inhibitors, and several studies suggest that these

drugs are better than H_2-receptor antagonists for maintaining remission in GERD.

Severe Symptoms and Nocturnal Acid Breakthrough. In patients with severe symptoms or extraintestinal manifestations of GERD,

Table 36–3
Antisecretory Drug Regimens for Treatment and Maintenance of GERD

DRUG	DOSAGE
H_2-Receptor Antagonists	
Cimetidine	400*/800* mg *bid*
Famotidine	20/40 mg *bid*
Nizatidine	150*/300* mg *bid*
Ranitidine	150/300 mg *bid*
Proton Pump Inhibitors	
Esomeprazole	20/40 mg daily/40* mg *bid*
Lansoprazole	30*/60* mg daily/30* mg *bid*
Omeprazole	20/40* mg daily/20* mg *bid*
Pantoprazole	40/80* mg daily/40* mg *bid*
Rabeprazole	20/40* mg daily/20* mg *bid*

bid, twice daily. *Indicates unlabeled use.

twice-daily dosing with a proton pump inhibitor may be needed. However, it is difficult if not impossible to render patients achlorhydric—even on twice-daily doses of proton pump inhibitors—and two-thirds or more of subjects will continue to make acid, particularly at night. This phenomenon, called *nocturnal acid breakthrough,* has been invoked as a cause of refractory symptoms in some patients with GERD. However, decreases in gastric pH at night while on therapy generally are not associated with acid reflux into the esophagus, and the rationale for suppressing nocturnal acid secretion (even if feasible) remains to be established. Nevertheless, patients with continuing symptoms on twice-daily proton pump inhibitors are often treated by adding an H_2-receptor antagonist at night. While this can further suppress acid production, the effect is short-lived, probably due to the development of tolerance, as described above (Fackler *et al.*, 2002).

Therapy for Extraintestinal Manifestations of GERD. With varying levels of evidence, acid reflux has been implicated in a variety of atypical symptoms, including noncardiac chest pain, asthma, laryngitis, chronic cough, and other ear, nose, and throat conditions. Proton pump inhibitors have been used with some success in certain patients with these disorders, generally in higher doses and for longer periods of time than those used for patients with more classic symptoms of GERD.

GERD and Pregnancy. Heartburn is estimated to occur in 30% to 50% of pregnancies, with an incidence approaching 80% in some populations (Richter, 2003). In the vast majority of cases, GERD ends soon after delivery and thus does not represent an exacerbation of a preexisting condition. Nevertheless, because of its high prevalence and the fact that it can contribute to the nausea of pregnancy, treatment often is required. Treatment choice in this setting is complicated by the paucity of data for the most commonly used drugs. In general, most drugs used to treat GERD fall in FDA Category B, with the exception of omeprazole (FDA Category C).

Mild cases of GERD during pregnancy should be treated conservatively; antacids or sucralfate are considered the first-line drugs. If symptoms persist, H_2-receptor antagonists can be used, with ranitidine having the most established track record in this setting. Proton pump inhibitors are reserved for women with intractable symptoms or complicated reflux disease. In these situations, lansoprazole is considered the preferred choice among the proton pump inhibitors, based on animal data and available experience in pregnant women.

Peptic Ulcer Disease

The pathophysiology of peptic ulcer disease is best viewed as an imbalance between mucosal defense factors (bicarbonate, mucin, prostaglandin, nitric oxide, and other peptides and growth factors) and injurious factors (acid and pepsin). On average, patients with duodenal ulcers produce more acid than do control subjects, particularly at night (basal secretion). Although patients with gastric ulcers have normal or even diminished acid production, ulcers rarely if ever occur in the complete absence of acid. Presumably, a weakened mucosal defense and reduced bicarbonate production

contribute to the injury from the relatively lower levels of acid in these patients. *H. pylori* and exogenous agents such as nonsteroidal antiinflammatory drugs (NSAIDs) interact in complex ways to cause an ulcer. Up to 60% of peptic ulcers are associated with *H. pylori* infection of the stomach. This infection may lead to impaired production of somatostatin by D cells, and in time, decreased inhibition of gastrin production, resulting in increased acid production and reduced duodenal bicarbonate production.

NSAIDs also are very frequently associated with peptic ulcers (in up to 60% of patients, particularly those with complications such as bleeding). Topical injury by the luminal presence of the drug appears to play a minor role in the pathogenesis of these ulcers, as evidenced by the fact that ulcers can occur with very low doses of aspirin (10 mg) or with parenteral administration of NSAIDs. The effects of these drugs are instead mediated systemically; the critical element is suppression of the constitutive form of cyclooxygenase-1 (COX-1) in the mucosa and decreased production of the cytoprotective prostaglandins PGE_2 and PGI_2.

Table 36–4 summarizes current recommendations for drug therapy of gastroduodenal ulcers. Proton pump inhibitors relieve symptoms of duodenal ulcers and promote healing more rapidly than do H_2-receptor antagonists, although both classes of drugs are very effective in this setting. Peptic ulcer represents a chronic disease, and recurrence within 1 year is expected in the majority of patients who do not receive prophylactic acid suppression. With the appreciation that *H. pylori* plays a major etiopathogenic role in the majority of peptic ulcers (*see* below), prevention of relapse is focused on eliminating this organism from the stomach. Chronic acid suppression, once the mainstay of ulcer prevention, now is used mainly in patients who are *H. pylori*–negative or, in some cases, for maximum prevention of recurrence in patients who have had life-threatening complications.

Intravenous pantoprazole or lansoprazole clearly is the preferred therapy in patients with acute bleeding ulcers. The theoretical benefit of maximal acid suppression in this setting is to accelerate healing of the underlying ulcer. In addition, a higher gastric pH enhances clot formation and retards clot dissolution.

Treatment of Helicobacter pylori *Infection.* *H. pylori,* a gram-negative rod, has been associated with gastritis and the subsequent development of gastric and duodenal ulcers, gastric adenocarcinoma, and gastric B-cell lymphoma (Suerbaum and Michetti, 2002). Because of the

Table 36–4
Recommendations for Treatment of Gastroduodenal Ulcers

DRUG	ACTIVE ULCER	MAINTENANCE THERAPY
H₂-Receptor Antagonists		
Cimetidine	800 mg at bedtime/400 mg twice daily	400 mg at bedtime
Famotidine	40 mg at bedtime	20 mg at bedtime
Nizatidine/ranitidine	300 mg after evening meal or at bedtime/150 mg twice daily	150 mg at bedtime
Proton Pump Inhibitors		
Lansoprazole	15 mg (DU; NSAID risk reduction) daily	
	30 mg (GU including NSAID-associated) daily	
Omeprazole	20 mg daily	
Rabeprazole	20 mg daily	
Prostaglandin Analogs		
Misoprostol	200 μg four times daily (NSAID-associated ulcer prevention)[*]	

DU, duodenal ulcer; GU, gastric ulcer. [*]Only misoprostol 800 μg/day has been directly shown to reduce the risk of ulcer complications such as perforation, hemorrhage, or obstruction (Rostom *et al.*, 2004).

critical role of *H. pylori* in the pathogenesis of peptic ulcers, to eradicate this infection is standard care in patients with gastric or duodenal ulcers. Provided that patients are not taking NSAIDs, this strategy almost completely eliminates the risk of ulcer recurrence. Eradication of *H. pylori* also is indicated in the treatment of mucosa-associated lymphoid tissue lymphomas of the stomach, which can regress significantly after such treatment.

Many regimens for *H. pylori* eradication have been proposed. Evidence-based literature review suggests that the ideal regimen in this setting should achieve a cure rate of at least 80%. Five important considerations influence the selection of an eradication regimen (Graham, 2000) (Table 36–5). First, single-antibiotic regimens are ineffective in eradicating *H. pylori* infection and lead to microbial resistance. Combination therapy with two or three antibiotics (plus acid-suppressive therapy) is associated with the highest rate of *H. pylori* eradication. Second, a proton pump inhibitor or H₂-receptor antagonist significantly enhances the effectiveness of *H. pylori* antibiotic regimens containing *amoxicillin* or *clarithromycin*. Third, a regimen of 10 to 14 days of treatment appears to be better than shorter treatment regimens; in the United States, a 14-day course of therapy generally is preferred. Fourth, poor patient compliance is linked to the medication-related side effects experienced by as many as half of patients taking triple-agent regimens, and to the inconvenience of three- or four-drug regimens administered several times per day. Packaging that combines the daily doses into one convenient unit is avail-

able and may improve patient compliance (Table 36–5). Finally, the emergence of resistance to clarithromycin and *metronidazole* increasingly is recognized as an important factor in the failure to eradicate *H. pylori*. Clarithromycin resistance is related to mutations that prevent binding of the antibiotic to the ribosomes of the pathogen and is an all-or-none phenomenon. In contrast, metronidazole resistance is relative rather than absolute and may involve several adaptations by the bacteria. In the presence of *in vitro* evidence of resistance to metronidazole, amoxicillin should be used instead. In areas with a high frequency of resistance to clarithromycin and metronidazole, a 14-day, quadruple-drug regimen (three antibiotics combined with a proton pump inhibitor) generally is effective therapy.

NSAID-Related Ulcers. Chronic NSAID users have a 2% to 4% risk of developing a symptomatic ulcer, gastrointestinal bleeding, or perforation. Ideally, NSAIDs should be discontinued in patients with an ulcer if at all possible. If continued therapy is needed, selective COX-2 inhibitors may be considered, although this does not eliminate the risk of subsequent ulcer formation and the possible association of these drugs with adverse cardiovascular events mandates caution (*see* Chapter 25). Healing of ulcers despite continued NSAID use is possible with the use of acid-suppressant agents, usually at higher doses and for a considerably longer duration than standard regimens (*e.g.,* 8 weeks or longer). Again, proton pump inhibitors are superior to H₂-receptor antagonists and misoprostol in promoting the healing of active ulcers (healing rates of 80% to 90% for proton pump inhibitors *versus* 60% to 75% for the H₂-receptor antagonists), and in preventing recurrence of gastric and duodenal ulcers in the setting of continued NSAID administration (Lanza, 1998).

Table 36–5
Therapy of Helicobacter pylori *Infection*

Triple therapy × 14 days: [Proton pump inhibitor + clarithromycin 500 mg + (metronidazole 500 mg or amoxicillin 1 g)] twice a day. (Tetracycline 500 mg can be substituted for amoxicillin or metronidazole.)

Quadruple therapy × 14 days: Proton pump inhibitor twice a day + metronidazole 500 mg three times daily + (bismuth subsalicylate 525 mg + tetracycline 500 mg four times daily)

or

H_2-receptor antagonist twice a day + (bismuth subsalicylate 525 mg + metronidazole 250 mg + tetracycline 500 mg) four times daily

Dosages:

Proton pump inhibitors:	H_2-receptor antagonists:
Omeprazole: 20 mg	Cimetidine: 400 mg
Lansoprazole: 30 mg	Famotidine: 20 mg
Rabeprazole: 20 mg	Nizatidine: 150 mg
Pantoprazole: 40 mg	Ranitidine: 150 mg
Esomeprazole: 40 mg	

See Howden and Hunt, 1998.

Stress-Related Ulcers. Stress ulcers are ulcers of the stomach or duodenum that occur in the context of a profound illness or trauma requiring intensive care. The etiology of stress-related ulcers differs somewhat from that of other peptic ulcers, involving acid and mucosal ischemia. Because of limitations on the oral administration of drugs in many patients with stress-related ulcers, intravenous H_2-receptor antagonists have been used extensively to reduce the incidence of GI hemorrhage due to stress ulcers. Now that intravenous preparations of proton pump inhibitors are available, it is likely that they will prove to be equally beneficial. *However, there is some concern over the risk of pneumonia secondary to gastric colonization by bacteria in an alkaline milieu.* In this setting, sucralfate appears to provide reasonable prophylaxis against bleeding without increasing the risk of aspiration pneumonia. This approach also appears to provide reasonable prophylaxis against bleeding, but is less convenient (Cook *et al.*, 1998).

Zollinger-Ellison Syndrome. Patients with this syndrome develop pancreatic or duodenal gastrinomas that stimulate the secretion of very large amounts of acid, sometimes in the setting of multiple endocrine neoplasia, type I. This can lead to severe gastroduodenal ulceration and other consequences of uncontrolled hyperchlorhydria. Proton pump inhibitors clearly are the drugs of choice, usually given at twice the routine dosage for peptic ulcers with the therapeutic goal of reducing acid secretion to 1 to 10 mmol/h.

Nonulcer Dyspepsia. This term refers to ulcer-like symptoms in patients who lack overt gastroduodenal ulceration. It may be associated with gastritis (with or without *H. pylori*) or with NSAID use, but the pathogenesis of this syndrome remains controversial.

Although empirical treatment with acid-suppressive agents is used routinely in patients with nonulcer dyspepsia, there is no convincing evidence of their benefit in controlled trials.

CLINICAL SUMMARY

The control of acid-peptic disease represents a major triumph for modern pharmacology. Proton pump inhibitors are considered superior for acid suppression in most clinically significant acid-peptic diseases, including gastroesophageal reflux disease, peptic ulcers, and NSAID-induced ulcers. Proton pump inhibitors also are employed in combination with antibiotics to eradicate infection with *H. pylori* and thereby play a role in preventing recurrent peptic ulcers. These agents largely have replaced the use of misoprostol and sucralfate, although the latter still is a low-cost alternative for prophylaxis against stress ulcers. The delay in maximal inhibition of acid secretion with the proton pump inhibitors (3 to 5 days) makes them less suited for use on an as-needed basis for symptom relief. In this setting, H_2-receptor antagonists, while less effective than proton pump inhibitors in suppressing acid secretion, have a more rapid onset of action that makes them useful for patient-directed management of mild or infrequent symptoms.

BIBLIOGRAPHY

Black, J. Reflections on the analytical pharmacology of histamine H_2-receptor antagonists. *Gastroenterology,* **1993,** *105:*963–968.

Chong, E., and Ensom, M.H. Pharmacogenetics of the proton pump inhibitors: a systematic review. *Pharmacotherapy,* **2003,** *23:*460–471.

Cook, D., Guyatt, G., Marshall, J., *et al.* Comparison of sucralfate and ranitidine for the prevention of upper gastrointestinal bleeding in patients requiring mechanical ventilation. Canadian Critical Care Trials Group. *N. Engl. J. Med.,* **1998,** *338:*791–797.

Dickson, E.J., and Stuart, R.C. Genetics of response to proton pump inhibitor therapy: clinical implications. *Am. J. Pharmacogenomics,* **2003,** *3:*303–315.

Fackler, W.K., Ours, T.M., Vaezi, M.F., and Richter, J.E. Long-term effect of H2RA therapy on nocturnal gastric acid breakthrough. *Gastroenterology,* **2002,** *122:*625–632.

Freston, J., Chiu, Y.L., Pan, W.J., Lukasik, N., and Taubel, J. Oral bioavailability of pantoprazole suspended in sodium bicarbonate solution. *Am. J. Health Syst. Pharm.,* **2003,** *60:*1324–1329.

Graham, D.Y. Therapy of *Helicobacter pylori*: current status and issues. *Gastroenterology,* **2000,** *118:*S2–S8.

Howden, C.W., and Hunt, R.H. Guidelines for the management of *Helicobacter pylori* infection. Ad Hoc Committee on the Practice Parameters of the American College of Gastroenterology. *Am. J. Gastroenterol.,* **1998,** *93:*2330–2338.

Klinkenberg-Knol, E.C., Festen, H.P., Jansen, J.B., *et al.* Long-term treatment with omeprazole for refractory esophagitis: efficacy and safety. *Ann. Intern. Med.,* **1994,** *121:*161–167.

Kuipers, E.J., and Meuwissen, S.G. The efficacy and safety of long-term omeprazole treatment for gastroesophageal reflux disease. *Gastroenterology,* **2000,** *118:*795–798.

Lanza, F.L. A guideline for the treatment and prevention of NSAID-induced ulcers. Members of the Ad Hoc Committee on Practice Parameters of the American College of Gastroenterology. *Am. J. Gastroenterol.,* **1998,** *93:*2037–2046.

Richter, J.E. Gastroesophageal reflux disease during pregnancy. *Gastroenterol. Clin. North Am.,* **2003,** *32:*235–261.

Rostom, A., Dube, C., Wells, G., *et al.* Prevention of NSAID-induced gastroduodenal ulcers. In, *The Cochrane Library, Issue 2.* John Wiley & Sons, Ltd., Chichester, UK, **2004.**

Sandevik, A.K., Brenna, E., and Waldum, H.L. Review article: the pharmacological inhibition of gastric acid secretion-tolerance and rebound. *Aliment. Pharmacol. Ther.,* **1997,** *11:*1013–1018.

Suerbaum, S., and Michetti, P. *Helicobacter pylori* infection. *N. Engl. J. Med.,* **2002,** *347:*1175–1186.

Wolfe, M.M., and Sachs, G. Acid suppression: optimizing therapy for gastroduodenal ulcer healing, gastroesophageal reflux disease, and stress-related erosive syndrome. *Gastroenterology,* **2000,** *118:*S9–S31.

TREATMENT OF DISORDERS OF BOWEL MOTILITY AND WATER FLUX; ANTIEMETICS; AGENTS USED IN BILIARY AND PANCREATIC DISEASE

Pankaj Jay Pasricha

The longer I live, the more I am convinced that half the unhappiness in the world proceeds from little stoppages, from a duct choked up, from food pressing in the wrong place, from a vexed duodenum or an agitated pylorus.

—Sydney Smith (1771–1845)

INTRODUCTION TO GASTROINTESTINAL MOTILITY

The gastrointestinal tract is in a continuous contractile, absorptive, and secretory state. The control of this state is complex, with contributions by the muscle itself, local nerves (*i.e.,* the enteric nervous system, ENS), the central nervous system (CNS), and humoral pathways (Furness and Sanger, 2002; Galligan, 2002; Hansen, 2003). Of these, perhaps the most important regulator of physiological gut function is the ENS (Figure 37–1), which is an autonomous collection of nerves within the wall of the GI tract, organized into two connected networks of neurons: the *myenteric (Auerbach's) plexus,* found between the circular and longitudinal muscle layers, and the *submucosal (Meissner's) plexus,* found below the epithelium. The former is responsible for motor control, while the latter regulates secretion, fluid transport, and vascular flow.

The ENS is responsible for the largely autonomous nature of most gastrointestinal activity. This activity is organized into relatively distinct programs that respond to input from the local environment of the gut and the CNS. Each program consists of a series of complex, but coordinated, patterns of secretion and movement that show regional and temporal variation. The fasting program of the gut is called the MMC (*migrating myoelectric complex* when referring to electrical activity and *migrating motor complex* when referring to the accompanying contractions) and consists of a series of four phasic activities. The most characteristic, phase III, consists of clusters of rhythmic contractions that occupy short segments of the intestine for a period of 6 to 10 minutes before proceeding caudally. One whole MMC cycle (*i.e.,* all four phases) takes about 80 to 110 minutes. The migrating motor complex occurs in the fasting state, during which it helps sweep debris caudad in the gut. The migrating motor complex cycles continually in animals that feed constantly, but is interrupted by another pattern of contractions—the fed program—in intermittently feeding animals such as humans. The fed program consists of high-frequency (12 to 15 per minute) contractions that are either propagated for short segments (*propulsive*) or are irregular and not propagated (*mixing*).

The basic motor tool used by the ENS to integrate its programs is the peristaltic reflex. Physiologically, peristalsis is a series of reflex responses to a bolus in the lumen of a given segment of the intestine; the ascending excitatory reflex results in contraction of the circular muscle on the oral side of the bolus, while the descending inhibitory reflex results in relaxation on the anal side. The net pressure gradient moves the bolus caudad. Three neural elements, responsible for sensory, relay, and effector functions, are required to produce these reflexes. Luminal factors stimulate sensory elements in the mucosa, leading to a coordinated pattern of muscle activity that is directly controlled by the motor neurons of the myenteric plexus to provide the effector component of the peristaltic reflex. Motor neurons receive input from ascending and descending interneurons (which constitute the relay and programming systems) that are of two broad types, excitatory and inhibitory. The primary neurotransmitter of the excitatory motor neurons is acetylcholine (ACh), although tachy-

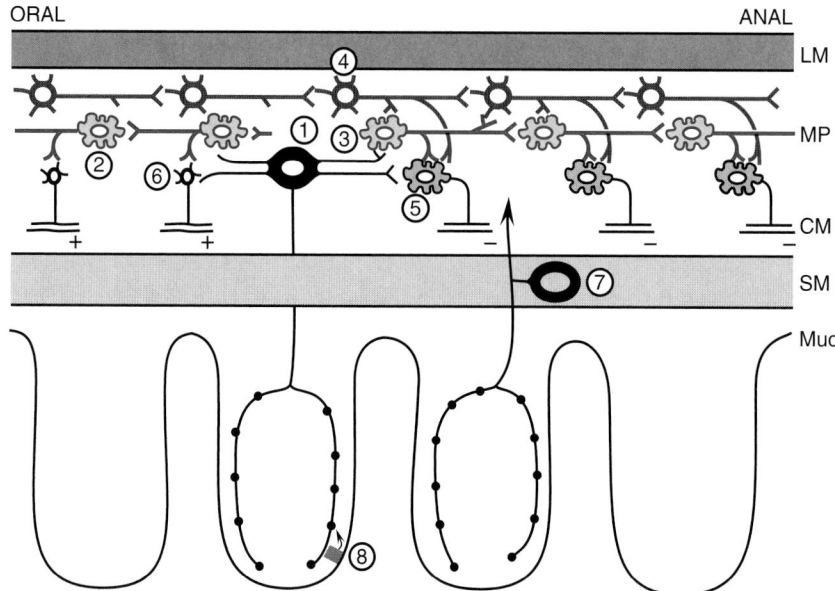

Figure 37–1. *The neuronal network that initiates and generates the peristaltic response.* Mucosal stimulation leads to release of serotonin by enterochromaffin cells (8), which excites the intrinsic primary afferent neuron (1), which then communicates with ascending (2) and descending (3) interneurons in the local reflex pathways. The reflex results in contraction at the oral end *via* the excitatory motor neuron (6) and aboral relaxation *via* the inhibitory motor neuron (5). The migratory myoelectric complex (*see* text) is shown here as being conducted by a different chain of interneurons (4). Another intrinsic primary afferent neuron with its cell body in the submucosa also is shown (7). MP, myenteric plexus; CM, circular muscle; LM, longitudinal muscle; SM, submucosa; Muc, mucosa. (Adapted from Kunze and Furness, 1999, with permission.)

kinins, co-released by these neurons, also play a role. The principal neurotransmitter in the inhibitory motor neurons appears to be nitric oxide (NO), although important contributions may also be made by ATP, vasoactive intestinal peptide, and pituitary adenylyl cyclase–activating peptide (PACAP), all of which are variably coexpressed with NO synthase.

This view of nerve–muscle interaction within the GI tract may be oversimplified, and other cell types may be important. One of these is the interstitial cell of Cajal, distributed within the gut wall and responsible for setting the electrical rhythm, and hence the pace of contractions, in various regions of the gut. These cells also may translate or modulate neuronal communication to the muscle, by mechanisms yet to be worked out.

Excitation-Contraction Coupling in GI Smooth Muscle

Control of tension in gastrointestinal smooth muscle is in large part dependent on the intracellular Ca^{2+} concentration. In general, there are two types of excitation-contraction coupling. Ionotropic receptors can mediate changes in membrane potential, which in turn activate voltage-dependent Ca^{2+} channels to trigger an influx of Ca^{2+} (electromechanical coupling); metabotropic receptors activate various signal transduction pathways to release Ca^{2+} from intracellular stores (pharmacomechanical coupling). Inhibitory receptors also exist on smooth muscle and generally act *via* PKA and PKG, whose kinase activities can lead to hyperpolarization, decreased cytosolic $[Ca^{2+}]$, and reduced interaction of actin and myosin. As an example, NO may induce relaxation *via* activation

of guanylyl cyclase, GMP–pathway, and the opening of several types of K^+ channels.

OVERVIEW OF FUNCTIONAL AND MOTILITY DISORDERS OF THE BOWEL

Gastrointestinal motility disorders are a complex and heterogeneous group of syndromes whose pathophysiology is not completely understood. Typical motility disorders include achalasia of the esophagus (impaired relaxation of the lower esophageal sphincter associated with defective esophageal peristalsis that results in dysphagia and regurgitation), gastroparesis (delayed gastric emptying), myopathic and neuropathic forms of intestinal dysmotility, and others. These disorders can be congenital, idiopathic, or secondary to systemic diseases (*e.g.,* diabetes mellitus or scleroderma). This term also has traditionally (and perhaps inaccurately) included disorders—such as irritable bowel syndrome (*see* below) and noncardiac chest pain—in which disturbances in pain processing or sensory function may be more important than any associated motor patterns. For most of these disorders, treatment remains empirical and symptom-based, reflecting our ignorance of the specific derangements in pathophysiology involved.

PROKINETIC AGENTS AND OTHER STIMULANTS OF GI CONTRACTILITY

Direct activation of muscarinic receptors, such as with the older cholinomimetic agents (see Chapter 7), is not a very effective strategy for treating GI motility disorders because these agents enhance contractions in a relatively uncoordinated fashion that produces little or no net propulsive activity. By contrast, *prokinetic* agents are medications that enhance coordinated GI motility and transit of material in the GI tract. Although ACh, when released from primary motor neurons in the myenteric plexus, is the principal immediate mediator of muscle contractility, most of the clinically useful prokinetic agents act "upstream" of ACh, at receptor sites on the motor neuron itself, or even more indirectly, on neurons one or two orders removed from it. Although pharmacologically and chemically diverse, these agents appear to enhance the release of excitatory neurotransmitter at the nerve-muscle junction without interfering with the normal physiological pattern and rhythm of motility. Coordination of activity among the segments of the gut, necessary for propulsion of luminal contents, therefore is maintained.

Agents useful clinically in altering GI motility are considered below.

Cholinergic Agents

Choline Derivatives. The effects of ACh on smooth muscle are mediated in large part by two types of G protein–coupled muscarinic receptors (mAChRs), M_2 and M_3 (see Chapter 7), that are present in the GI tract in a 4:1 ratio, respectively. Although less abundant, the M_3 receptor is more important; its activation increases intracellular Ca^{2+}, an effect mediated by the G_q-PLC-IP_3 pathway. ACh itself is not used pharmacologically because it affects all classes of cholinergic receptors (nicotinic and muscarinic) and is degraded rapidly by acetylcholinesterase. Modification of the structure of ACh has yielded drugs such as *bethanechol* that have increased receptor selectivity and that resist enzymatic hydrolysis. In addition to its lack of real prokinetic efficacy, bethanechol has significant side effects resulting from its broad muscarinic effects on contractility and secretion in the GI tract and other organs. These side effects include bradycardia, flushing, diarrhea and cramps, salivation, and blurred vision.

Acetylcholinesterase Inhibitors. These drugs inhibit the degradation of ACh by its esterase (see Chapter 8), thereby allowing ACh to accumulate at sites of release. Unlike muscarinic receptor agonists, these parasympathomimetic drugs do not stimulate muscle directly, but rather accelerate GI transit times by enhancing the contractile effects of ACh released at synaptic and neuromuscular junctions. Among these cholinergic muscle stimulants, *neostigmine methylsulfate* has been used off-label for some gastroenterological disorders, particularly those associated with acute colonic pseudo-obstruction (Ogilvie's syndrome) and paralytic ileus. The usual dose in the acute setting is 2 to 2.5 mg of neostigmine methylsulfate administered by IV push over 3 minutes with continuous monitoring of ECG, blood pressure, and O_2 saturation. Atropine should be available in case of severe bradycardia (heart rate of less than 50 bpm).

Dopamine-Receptor Antagonists

Dopamine is present in significant amounts in the GI tract and has several inhibitory effects on motility, including reduction of lower esophageal sphincter and intragastric pressures. These effects, which apparently result from suppression of ACh release from myenteric motor neurons, are mediated by D_2 dopaminergic receptors. By antagonizing the inhibitory effect of dopamine on myenteric motor neurons, dopamine receptor antagonists are effective as prokinetic agents; they have the additional advantage of relieving nausea and vomiting by antagonism of dopamine receptors in the chemoreceptor trigger zone (see below). Examples of such agents are *metoclopramide* and *domperidone*.

Metoclopramide. **Chemistry, Mechanism of Action, and Pharmacological Properties.** Metoclopramide (REGLAN) and other substituted benzamides are derivatives of *para*-aminobenzoic acid and are structurally related to *procainamide*. The chemical structure of metoclopramide is:

METOCLOPRAMIDE

The mechanisms of action of metoclopramide are complex and involve 5-HT_4-receptor agonism, vagal and central 5-HT_3-antagonism, and possible sensitization of muscarinic receptors on smooth muscle, in addition to dopamine receptor antagonism. Metoclopramide is one of the oldest true prokinetic agents; its administration results in coordinated contractions that enhance transit. Its effects are confined largely to the upper digestive tract, where it increases lower esophageal sphincter tone and stimulates antral and small intestinal contractions. Despite having *in vitro* effects on the contractility of colonic smooth muscle, metoclopramide has no clinically significant effects on large-bowel motility.

Pharmacokinetics. Metoclopramide is absorbed rapidly after oral ingestion, undergoes sulfation and glucuronide conjugation by the liver, and is excreted principally in the urine, with a half-life of 4 to 6 hours. Peak concentrations occur within 1 hour after a single oral dose; the duration of action is 1 to 2 hours.

Therapeutic Use. Metoclopramide has been used in patients with gastroesophageal reflux disease to produce symptomatic relief of, but not healing of, associated esophagitis. It clearly is less effective than modern acid-suppressive medications, such as proton pump inhibitors or histamine H_2-receptor antagonists, and now rarely is used in this setting. Metoclopramide is indicated more often in symptomatic patients with gastroparesis, in whom it may cause mild to modest improvements of gastric emptying (Tonini *et al.*, 2004). Metoclopramide injection is used as an adjunctive measure in medical or diagnostic procedures such as intestinal intubation or contrast radiography of the GI tract. Although it has been used in patients with postoperative ileus, its ability to improve transit in disorders of small-bowel motility appears to be limited. *In general, its greatest utility lies in its ability to ameliorate the nausea and vomiting that often accompany GI dysmotility syndromes.* Metoclopramide has also been used in the treatment of persistent hiccups, but its efficacy in this condition is equivocal at best.

Metoclopramide is available in oral dosage forms (tablets and solution) and as a parenteral preparation for intravenous or intramuscular use. The usual initial oral dose range is 10 mg, 30 minutes before each meal and at bedtime. The onset of action is within 30 to 60 minutes after an oral dose. In patients with severe nausea, an initial dose of 10 mg can be given intramuscularly (onset of action 10 to 15 minutes) or intravenously (onset of action 1 to 3 minutes). For prevention of chemotherapy-induced emesis, metoclopramide can be given as an infusion of 1 to 2 mg per kg of body weight, administered over at least 15 minutes, beginning 30 minutes before the chemotherapy is begun and repeated as needed every 2 or 3 hours. Alternatively, a continuous intravenous infusion may be given (3 mg/kg of body weight before chemotherapy, followed by 0.5 mg/kg of body weight per hour for 8 hours). The usual pediatric dose for gastroparesis is 0.1 to 0.2 mg/kg of body weight per dose, given 30 minutes before meals and at bedtime.

Adverse Effects. The major side effects of metoclopramide include extrapyramidal effects, such as those seen with the phenothiazines (*see* Chapter 18). Dystonias, usually occurring acutely after intravenous administration, and parkinsonian-like symptoms that may occur several weeks after initiation of therapy generally respond to treatment with anticholinergic or antihistaminic drugs and are reversible upon discontinuation of metoclopramide. Tardive dyskinesia also can occur with chronic treatment (months to years) and may be irreversible. Extrapyramidal effects appear to occur more commonly in children and young adults and at higher doses. Like other dopamine antagonists, metoclopramide also can cause galactorrhea by blocking the inhibitory effect of dopamine on prolactin

release, but this adverse effect is relatively infrequent in clinical practice. Methemoglobinemia has been reported occasionally in premature and full-term neonates receiving metoclopramide.

Domperidone; D_2 Receptor Antagonists

In contrast to metoclopramide, domperidone predominantly antagonizes the dopamine D_2 receptor without major involvement of other receptors. It is not available for use in the United States but has been used elsewhere (MOTILIUM, others) and has modest prokinetic activity in doses of 10 to 20 mg three times a day. Although it does not readily cross the blood–brain barrier to cause extrapyramidal side effects, domperidone exerts effects in the parts of the CNS that lack this barrier, such as those regulating emesis, temperature, and prolactin release. As is the case with metoclopramide, domperidone does not appear to have any significant effects on lower gastrointestinal motility. Other D_2-receptor antagonists being explored as prokinetic agents include *levosulpiride,* the levoenantiomer of *sulpiride.*

Serotonin Receptor Modulators

Serotonin (5-HT) plays an important role in the normal motor and secretory function of the gut (Talley, 2001) (*see* Chapter 11). Indeed, more than 90% of the total 5-HT in the body exists in the GI tract. The enterochromaffin cell, a specialized cell lining the mucosa of the gut, produces most of this 5-HT and rapidly releases 5-HT in response to chemical and mechanical stimulation (*e.g.,* food boluses; noxious agents such as cis-platinum; certain microbial toxins; adrenergic, cholinergic, and purinergic receptor agonists). 5-HT triggers the peristaltic reflex (Figure 37–1) by stimulating intrinsic sensory neurons in the myenteric plexus (*via* variant 5-HT receptors, 5-HT_{1p}, and *via* 5-HT_4 receptors), as well as extrinsic vagal and spinal sensory neurons (*via* 5-HT_3 receptors). Additionally, stimulation of submucosal intrinsic afferent neurons activates secretomotor reflexes resulting in epithelial secretion. 5-HT receptors also are found on other neurons in the enteric nervous system, where they can be either stimulatory (5-HT_3 and 5-HT_4) or inhibitory (5-HT_{1a}). In addition, serotonin also stimulates the release of other neurotransmitters, depending upon the receptor subtype. Thus, 5-HT_1 stimulation of the gastric fundus results in release of nitric oxide and reduces smooth muscle tone. 5-HT_4 stimulation of excitatory motor neurons enhances ACh release at the neuromuscular junction, and both 5-HT_3 and 5-HT_4 receptors facilitate interneuronal sig-

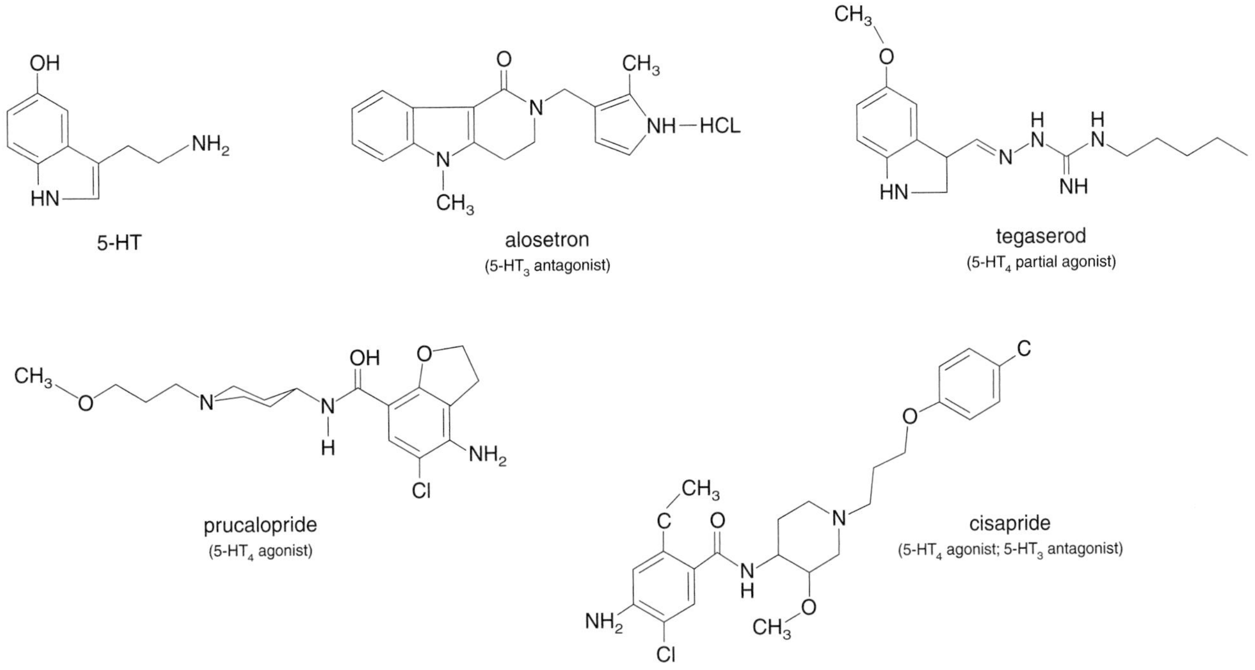

Figure 37–2. *Ligands of 5-HT$_3$ and 5-HT$_4$ receptors modulating gastrointestinal motility.*

naling. Developmentally, 5-HT acts as a neurotrophic factor for enteric neurons *via* the 5-HT$_{2B}$ and 5-HT$_3$ receptors.

Reuptake of serotonin by enteric neurons and epithelium is mediated by the same mechanism as 5-HT reuptake by serotonergic neurons in the CNS. This reuptake therefore also is blocked by selective serotonin reuptake inhibitors (*see* Chapter 17), which explains the common side effect of diarrhea that accompanies the use of these agents. In recent years, modulation of the multiple, complex, and sometimes opposing effects of 5-HT on gut motor function has become a major target for drug development.

Tegaserod Maleate. ***Chemistry, Mechanism of Action, and Pharmacological Properties.*** *Tegaserod* (ZELNORM), an aminoguanidine indole, is structurally related to serotonin and is a partial 5-HT$_4$ agonist with negligible affinity for other receptor subtypes (Figure 37–2). Tegaserod has multiple effects on the GI tract. It stimulates motility and accelerates transit in the esophagus, stomach, small bowel, and ascending colon. It also stimulates chloride secretion. Thus far, the clinical efficacy of tegaserod has been proven only in female patients with constipation-predominant irritable bowel syndrome (*see* below); however, the drug is being tested in a variety of other conditions,

including gastroparesis. In patients with constipation, tegaserod results in a statistically significant but mild-to-modest improvement in stool frequency, with less consistent effects on other parameters such as stool form, bloating, and pain. The absolute improvement is modest at best, with a difference of only about one to two bowel movements per week between the drug and placebo groups. It is not clear that the drug has any greater efficacy in this regard than other agents used for constipation. Males with constipation also may respond to tegaserod, but existing studies did not include enough men to demonstrate a statistically significant effect.

In clinical trials, tegaserod also reduced bloating (a prominent symptom in patients with irritable bowel syndrome) and pain, but it is not clear whether this represents an independent effect on sensory nerves or simply a consequence of decreased fecal or air distention of the colon. As yet, there is no evidence for significant modulation of nociceptive signaling by 5-HT$_4$ receptors.

Tegaserod is available for oral administration in 2-mg and 6-mg tablets and is approved for use in women with constipation-dominant irritable bowel syndrome at a dose of 6 mg twice daily. Tegaserod also has been approved for the treatment of chronic constipation. Higher doses have been suggested for other prokinetic effects (*e.g.,* stimulation of gastric emptying) but such uses have not been validated clinically.

After oral administration, tegaserod is partially absorbed from the gut, reaching peak plasma levels after 1 to 1.3 hours. Absorption is slowed by the presence of food in the stomach, so tegaserod is best taken on an empty stomach. Once in circulation, tegaserod is approximately 98% bound to plasma proteins. Tegaserod is degraded by acid hydrolysis before absorption from the stomach, and by oxidation and glucuronidation in the liver to three inactive N-glucuronide metabolites. Approximately two-thirds of the orally administered dose of tegaserod is excreted unchanged in feces, with the remainder excreted in urine; the drug has an estimated half-life of about 11 hours.

Diarrhea and headache are the most common side effects of tegaserod, occurring in about 10% of patients. Tegaserod does not appear to have any significant cardiac toxicity, and no clinically relevant drug-drug interactions have been identified. No dosage adjustment is required in elderly patients or those with mild-to-moderate hepatic or renal impairment; however, tegaserod should not be used in patients with severe hepatic or renal impairment.

Cisapride. *Cisapride* (PROPULSID) is a substituted piperidinyl benzamide (Figure 37–2) that appears to stimulate 5-HT$_4$ receptors and increase adenylyl cyclase activity within neurons. It also has weak 5-HT$_3$ antagonistic properties and may directly stimulate smooth muscle. Until recently, it was a commonly used prokinetic agent, particularly for gastroesophageal reflux disease and gastroparesis. However, it no longer is generally available in the United States because of its potential to induce serious and occasionally fatal cardiac arrhythmias, including ventricular tachycardia, ventricular fibrillation, and *torsades de pointes*. These arrhythmias result from a prolonged QT interval through an interaction with pore-forming subunits of the HERG K$^+$ channel. HERG K$^+$ channels conduct the rapid delayed rectifier K$^+$ current that is important for normal repolarization of the ventricle (*see* Chapter 34). Cisapride-induced ventricular arrhythmias occur most often when the drug is combined with other drugs that inhibit CYP3A4 (*see* Chapter 3); such combinations inhibit the metabolism of cisapride and lead to high plasma concentrations of the drug. Due to its association with ventricular arrhythmias, cisapride is contraindicated in patients with a history of prolonged QT interval, renal failure, ventricular arrhythmias, ischemic heart disease, congestive heart failure, respiratory failure, uncorrected electrolyte abnormalities (*e.g.,* hypokalemia and hypomagnesemia), or concomitant medications known to prolong the QT interval. At this time, cisapride is available only through an investigational, limited-access program for patients who have failed all standard therapeutic modalities and undergone a thorough diagnostic evaluation, including an electrocardiogram.

Other 5-HT$_4$-Receptor Modulators. *Prucalopride* (Figure 37–2) is a benzofuran derivative and a specific 5-HT$_4$-receptor agonist that facilitates cholinergic neurotransmission. It enhances colonic contractility in experimental animals, and preliminary studies suggest that it accelerates colonic transit in human beings. Another investigational agent in this class, *mosapride,* is under development.

Motilin Agonists: Macrolides and Erythromycin.
Chemistry, Pharmacological Effects, and Mechanism of Action. Motilin is a 22–amino acid peptide hormone found in the gastrointestinal M cells, as well as in some enterochromaffin cells of the upper small bowel. Motilin is a potent contractile agent of the upper GI tract. Motilin levels fluctuate in association with the migrating motor complex and appear to be responsible for the amplification, if not the actual induction, of phase III activity. In addition, motilin receptors are found on smooth muscle cells and enteric neurons. The effects of motilin can be mimicked by *erythromycin,* a discovery that arose from the frequent occurrence of GI side effects with the use of this antibiotic. This property is shared to varying extents by other macrolide antibiotics (*see* Chapter 46), including *oleandomycin, azithromycin,* and *clarithromycin.* In addition to its motilin-like effects, which are most pronounced at higher doses (250 to 500 mg), erythromycin at lower doses (*e.g.,* 40 to 80 mg) also may act by other poorly defined mechanisms that may involve cholinergic facilitation.

Erythromycin induces phase III migrating motor complex activity in dogs and increases smooth muscle contractility. It has multiple effects on upper GI motility, increasing lower esophageal pressure and stimulating gastric and small-bowel contractility. By contrast, it has little or no effect on colonic motility. At doses higher than 3 mg/kg, it can produce a spastic type of contraction in the small bowel, resulting in cramps, impairment of transit, and vomiting.

Therapeutic Use. The best-established use of erythromycin as a prokinetic agent is in patients with diabetic gastroparesis, where it can improve gastric emptying in the short term. Erythromycin-stimulated gastric contractions can be intense and result in "dumping" of relatively undigested food into the small bowel. This potential disadvantage can be exploited clinically to clear the stomach of undigestible residue such as plastic tubes or bezoars. Anecdotally, erythromycin also has been of benefit in patients with small-bowel dysmotility such as that seen in scleroderma, ileus, or pseudo-obstruction. Rapid development of tolerance to erythromycin, possibly by down-regulation of the motilin receptor, and undesirable (in this context) antibiotic effects have limited the use of this drug as a prokinetic agent. Several nonantibiotic synthetic analogs of erythromycin and peptide analogs of motilin have been developed; to date, the clinical results have been disappointing.

A standard dose of erythromycin for gastric stimulation is 3 mg/kg intravenously or 200 to 250 mg orally every 8 hours. For small-bowel stimulation, a smaller dose (*e.g.,* 40 mg intravenously) may be more useful, as higher doses may actually retard motility of this organ.

Miscellaneous Agents for Stimulating Motility.
The gastrointestinal hormone cholecystokinin (CCK) is released from the intestine in response to meals and delays gastric emptying. *Dexloxiglumide* is a CCK$_1$ (or CCK-A)–receptor antagonist that can improve gastric emptying and is being investigated in Europe as a treatment for gastroparesis and for constipation-dominant irritable bowel syndrome. Clonidine also has been reported to be of benefit in patients with gastroparesis. *Octreotide acetate* (SANDOSTATIN), a somatostatin analogue, also is used in some patients with intestinal dysmotility (*see* below).

In some disorders of motility, effective treatment does not necessarily require a "neuroenteric" approach. One such example is gastroesophageal reflux disease. Acid reflux is associated with transient lower esophageal sphincter relaxations that occur in the absence of a swallow. Since the damage to the esophagus ultimately is inflicted by acid, the most effective therapy for gastroesophageal reflux disease still is the suppression of acid production by the stomach (*see* Chapter 36). Neither metoclopramide nor cisapride by itself is particularly effective in gastroesophageal reflux disease. However, a

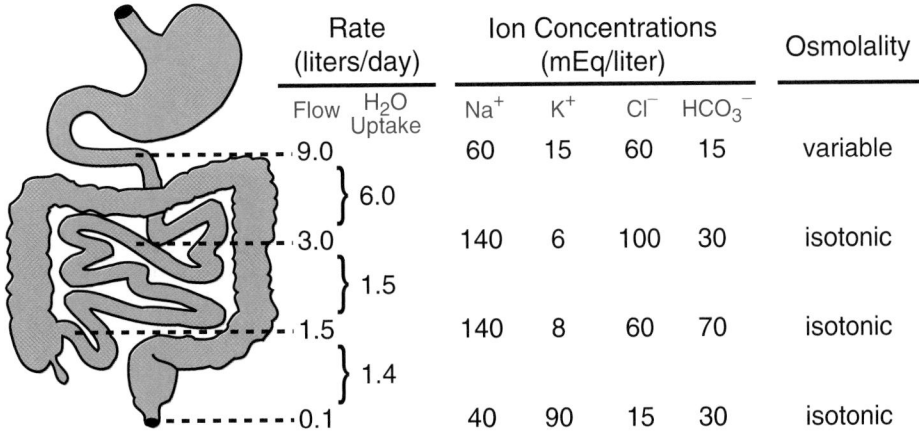

	Rate (liters/day)		Ion Concentrations (mEq/liter)				Osmolality
	Flow	H_2O Uptake	Na^+	K^+	Cl^-	HCO_3^-	
	9.0		60	15	60	15	variable
		6.0					
	3.0		140	6	100	30	isotonic
		1.5					
	1.5		140	8	60	70	isotonic
		1.4					
	0.1		40	90	15	30	isotonic

Figure 37–3. *The approximate volume and composition of fluid that traverses the small and large intestines daily.* Of the 9 liters of fluid presented to the small intestine each day, 2 liters are from the diet and 7 liters are from secretions (salivary, gastric, pancreatic, and biliary). The absorptive capacity of the colon is 4 to 5 liters per day.

new approach under investigation relies on suppression of the transient lower esophageal sphincter relaxations, as achieved by CCK_1-receptor antagonists (such as *loxiglumide*), GABA agonists (such as *baclofen*), and inhibitors of NO synthesis.

Other Agents That Suppress Motility.
Smooth muscle relaxants such as organic nitrates and Ca^{2+} channel antagonists (*see* Chapter 31) often produce temporary, if partial, relief of symptoms in motility disorders such as achalasia, in which the lower esophageal sphincter fails to relax, resulting in a functional obstruction to the passage of food and severe difficulty in swallowing. A more recent approach relies on the use of *botulinum toxin,* injected directly into the lower esophageal sphincter *via* an endoscope, in doses of 80 to 200 units (Zhao and Pasricha, 2003). This potent agent inhibits ACh release from nerve endings (*see* Chapter 9) and can produce partial paralysis of the sphincter muscle, with significant improvements in symptoms and esophageal clearance. However, its effects dissipate over a period of several months, requiring repeated injections. Botulinum toxin also is being used increasingly in other gastrointestinal conditions such as chronic anal fissures.

LAXATIVES, CATHARTICS, AND THERAPY FOR CONSTIPATION

Overview of GI Water and Electrolyte Flux. Fluid content is the principal determinant of stool volume and consistency; water normally accounts for 70% to 85% of total stool weight. Net stool fluid content reflects a balance between luminal input (ingestion and secretion of water and electrolytes) and output (absorption) along the length of the GI tract. The daily challenge for the gut is to extract water, minerals, and nutrients from the luminal contents, leaving behind a manageable pool of fluid for proper

expulsion of waste material *via* the process of defecation. Normally about 8 to 9 liters of fluid enter the small intestine daily from exogenous and endogenous sources (Figure 37–3). Net absorption of the water occurs in the small intestine in response to osmotic gradients that result from the uptake and secretion of ions and the absorption of nutrients (mainly sugars and amino acids), with only about 1 to 1.5 liters crossing the ileocecal valve. The colon then extracts most of the remaining fluid, leaving about 100 ml of fecal water daily.

Under normal circumstances, these quantities are well within the range of the total absorptive capacity of the small bowel (about 16 liters) and colon (4 to 5 liters). Neurohumoral mechanisms, pathogens, and drugs can alter these processes, resulting in changes in either secretion or absorption of fluid by the intestinal epithelium. Altered motility also contributes in a general way to this process, as the extent of absorption parallels transit time. With decreased motility and excess fluid removal, feces can become inspissated and impacted, leading to constipation. When the capacity of the colon to absorb fluid is exceeded, diarrhea will occur.

Constipation: General Principles of Pathophysiology and Treatment. Scientific definitions rely mostly on stool number; most surveys have found the normal stool frequency on a Western diet to be at least 3 times a week. However, patients use the term *constipation* not only for decreased frequency, but also for difficulty in initiation or passage, passage of firm or small-volume feces, or a feeling of incomplete evacuation. By questionnaire, 25% of the population of the United States, more commonly women and elderly people, complain of constipation. A survey of bowel habits of adults in the United States showed that 18% of respondents used laxatives at least once a month, but nearly one-third of users did not have constipation. Approximately 2.5 million physician visits per year are attributed to constipation.

Constipation has many reversible or secondary causes, including lack of dietary fiber, drugs, hormonal disturbances, neurogenic disorders, and systemic illnesses. In most cases of chronic constipation, no specific cause is found. Up to 60% of patients presenting with constipation will have normal colonic transit. These patients either have irritable bowel syndrome or define constipation in terms other than stool frequency (*e.g.,* changes in consistency, excessive straining, or a feeling of incomplete evacuation). In the rest, attempts usually are made to categorize the underlying pathophysiology either as a disorder of delayed colonic transit because of an underlying defect in colonic motility, or less commonly, as an isolated disorder of defecation or evacuation (outlet disorder) due to dysfunction of the neuromuscular apparatus of the recto-anal region. Colonic motility is responsible for mixing luminal contents to promote absorption of water and moving them from proximal to distal segments by means of propulsive contractions. Mixing in the colon is accomplished in a way similar to that in the small bowel: by short- or long-duration, stationary (nonpropulsive) contractions. Propulsive contractions in the colon include giant migrating contractions, also known as colonic mass actions or mass movements, which propagate caudally over extended lengths in the colon and evoke mass transfer of feces from the right to the left colon once or twice a day. Disturbances in motility therefore may have complex effects on bowel movements. "Decreased motility" of the mass action type and "increased motility" of the nonpropulsive type may lead to constipation. In any given patient, the predominant factor often is not obvious. Consequently, the pharmacological approach to constipation remains empirical and is based, in most cases, on nonspecific principles.

In many cases, constipation can be corrected by adherence to a fiber-rich (20 to 30 g daily) diet, adequate fluid intake, appropriate bowel habits and training, and avoidance of constipating drugs. However, the association between constipation and either fluid intake or exercise has not withstood scientific scrutiny. Constipation related to medications can be corrected by use of alternative drugs where possible, or adjustment of dosage. If nonpharmacological measures alone are inadequate or unrealistic (*e.g.,* because of elderly age or infirmity), they may be supplemented with bulk-forming agents or osmotic laxatives. When stimulant laxatives are used, they should be administered at the lowest effective dosage and for the shortest period of time to avoid abuse. In addition to perpetuating dependence on drugs, the laxative habit may lead to excessive loss of water and electrolytes; secondary aldosteronism may occur if volume depletion is prominent. Steatorrhea, protein-losing enteropathy with hypoalbuminemia, and osteomalacia due to excessive loss of calcium in the stool have been reported.

In addition to treating constipation, laxatives frequently are employed before surgical, radiological, and endoscopic procedures where an empty colon is desirable.

The terms *laxatives, cathartics, purgatives, aperients,* and *evacuants* often are used interchangeably. There is a

distinction, however, between *laxation* (the evacuation of formed fecal material from the rectum) and *catharsis* (the evacuation of unformed, usually watery fecal material from the entire colon). Most of the commonly used agents promote laxation, but some are actually cathartics that act as laxatives at low doses.

Laxatives generally act in one of the following ways: (1) enhancing retention of intraluminal fluid by hydrophilic or osmotic mechanisms; (2) decreasing net absorption of fluid by effects on small- and large-bowel fluid and electrolyte transport; or (3) altering motility by either inhibiting segmenting (nonpropulsive) contractions or stimulating propulsive contractions. Based on their actions, laxatives can be classified as shown in Table 37–1; their known effects on motility and secretion are listed in Table 37–2. However, recent studies indicate considerable overlap among these traditional categories. A variety of laxatives, both osmotic agents and stimulants, increase the activity of NO synthase and the biosynthesis of platelet-activating factor in the gut. Platelet-activating factor is a phospholipid proinflammatory mediator that stimulates colonic secretion and GI motility (Izzo *et al.*, 1998). Nitric oxide also may stimulate intestinal secretion and inhibit segmenting contractions in the colon, thereby promoting laxation. Agents that reduce the expression of NO synthase or its activity can prevent the laxative effects of castor oil, cascara, and bisacodyl (but not senna), as well as magnesium sulfate.

An alternate way to classify laxatives is by the pattern of effects produced by the usual clinical dosage (Table 37–3).

Table 37–1
Classification of Laxatives

1. **Luminally active agents**
   a. Hydrophilic colloids; bulk-forming agents (bran, psyllium, *etc.*)
   b. Osmotic agents (nonabsorbable inorganic salts or sugars)
   c. Stool-wetting agents (surfactants) and emollients (docusate, mineral oil)
2. **Nonspecific stimulants or irritants (with effects on fluid secretion and motility)**
   Diphenylmethanes (bisacodyl)
   Anthraquinones (senna and cascara)
   Castor oil
3. **Prokinetic agents (acting primarily on motility)**
   5-HT$_4$ receptor agonists
   Opioid receptor antagonists

Table 37–2
Summary of Effects of Some Laxatives on Bowel Function

AGENT	SMALL BOWEL		COLON		
	Transit Time	Mixing Contractions	Propulsive Contractions	Mass Actions	Stool Water
Dietary fiber	↓	?	↑	?	↑
Magnesium	↓	—	↑	↑	↑↑
Lactulose	↓	?	?	?	↑↑
Metoclopramide	↓	?	↑	?	—
Cisapride	↓	?	↑	?	↑
Erythromycin	↓	?	?	?	?
Naloxone	↓	↓	—	—	↑
Anthraquinones	↓	↓	↑	↑	↑↑
Diphenylmethanes	↓	↓	↑	↑	↑↑
Docusates	—	?	?	?	—

KEY: ↑, increased; ↓, decreased; ?, no data available; —, no effect on this parameter. Modified from Kreek, 1994, with permission.

Dietary Fiber and Supplements

Under normal circumstances, the bulk, softness, and hydration of feces depend on the fiber content of the diet. Fiber is defined as that part of food that resists enzymatic digestion and reaches the colon largely unchanged. Colonic bacteria ferment fiber to varying degrees, depending on its chemical nature and water solubility. Fermentation of fiber has two important effects: (1) it produces short-chain fatty acids that are trophic for colonic epithelium, and (2) it increases bacterial mass. Although fermentation of fiber generally decreases stool water, short-chain fatty acids also may have a prokinetic effect, and increased bacterial mass may contribute to increased stool volume. On the other hand, fiber that is not fermented can attract water and increase stool bulk. The net effect on bowel movement therefore varies with different compositions of dietary fiber (Table 37–4). In general, insoluble, poorly fermentable fibers, such as lignin, are most effective in increasing stool bulk and transit.

Table 37–3
Classification and Comparison of Representative Laxatives

LAXATIVE EFFECT AND LATENCY IN USUAL CLINICAL DOSAGE		
Softening of Feces, 1 To 3 Days	Soft or Semifluid Stool, 6 To 8 Hours	Watery Evacuation, 1 To 3 Hours
Bulk-forming laxatives Bran Psyllium preparations Methylcellulose Calcium polycarbophil	*Stimulant laxatives* Diphenylmethane derivatives Bisacodyl	*Osmotic laxatives** Sodium phosphates Magnesium sulfate Milk of magnesia Magnesium citrate
Surfactant laxatives Docusates Poloxamers Lactulose	Anthraquinone derivatives Senna Cascara sagrada	*Castor oil*

*Employed in high dosage for rapid cathartic effect and in lower dosage for laxative effect.

Table 37–4
Properties of Different Dietary Fibers

TYPE OF FIBER	WATER SOLUBILITY	% FERMENTED
Nonpolysaccharides		
Lignin	Poor	0
Cellulose	Poor	15
Noncellulose polysaccharides		
Hemicellulose	Good	56–87
Mucilages and gums	Good	85–95
Pectins	Good	90–95

Bran, the residue left when flour is made from cereals, contains more than 40% dietary fiber. Wheat bran, with its high lignin content, is most effective at increasing stool weight. Fruits and vegetables contain more *pectins* and *hemicelluloses,* which are more readily fermentable and produce less effect on stool transit. *Psyllium husk,* derived from the seed of the plantago herb (*Plantago ovata;* known as ispaghula or isabgol in many parts of the world), is a component of many commercial products for constipation (META-MUCIL, others). Psyllium husk contains a hydrophilic mucilloid that undergoes significant fermentation in the colon, leading to an increase in colonic bacterial mass. The usual dose is 2.5 to 4 g (1 to 3 teaspoonfuls in 250 ml of fruit juice), titrated upwards until the desired goal is reached. A variety of semisynthetic celluloses—*e.g., methylcellulose* (CITRUCEL, others) and the hydrophilic resin *calcium polycarbophil* (FIBERCON, FIBERALL, others), a polymer of acrylic acid resin—also are available. These poorly fermentable compounds absorb water and increase fecal bulk.

Fiber is contraindicated in patients with obstructive symptoms and in those with megacolon or megarectum. Fecal impaction should be treated before initiating fiber supplementation. Bloating is the most common side effect of soluble fiber products (perhaps due to colonic fermentation), but it usually decreases with time. Calcium polycarbophil preparations release Ca^{2+} in the GI tract and thus should be avoided by patients who must restrict their intake of calcium or who are taking tetracycline. Sugar-free bulk laxatives may contain aspartame and are contraindicated in patients with phenylketonuria. Allergic reactions to psyllium have been reported.

Osmotically Active Agents

Saline Laxatives. Laxatives containing magnesium cations or phosphate anions commonly are called *saline laxatives*: magnesium sulfate, magnesium hydroxide, magnesium citrate, sodium phosphate. Their cathartic action is believed to result from osmotically mediated water retention, which then stimulates peristalsis. Other mechanisms may contribute to their effects, including the production of inflammatory mediators. Magnesium-containing laxatives may stimulate the release of cholecystokinin, which leads to intraluminal fluid and electrolyte accumulation and to increased intestinal motility. It is estimated that for every additional mEq of Mg^{2+} in the intestinal lumen, fecal weight increases by about 7 g. The usual dose of magnesium salts contains 40 to 120 mEq of Mg^{2+} and produces 300 to 600 ml of stool within 6 hours. The intensely bitter taste of some preparations may induce nausea and can be masked with citrus juices.

Phosphate salts are better absorbed than magnesium-based agents and therefore need to be given in larger doses to induce catharsis. The most frequently employed preparation of sodium phosphate is an oral solution (FLEET PHOSPHO-SODA), which contains 1.8 g of dibasic sodium phosphate and 4.8 g of monobasic sodium phosphate in 10 ml. The usual adult dose is 20 to 30 ml taken with ample water. For colonic preparation before a procedure, larger doses are used, typically in the form of two doses of 45 ml each, a few hours apart, the evening before the procedure. A newer preparation of phosphate salts (VISICOL) is available in tablet form, containing 1.5 g total sodium phosphate per tablet. For colon preparation, two doses of 20 tablets each (30 g sodium phosphate) are recommended before the procedure. Adequate fluid intake (1 to 3 L) is essential for any oral sodium phosphate regimen used for colonic preparation. Sodium phosphate also can be given as an enema for laxative purposes (*see* below).

Magnesium- and phosphate-containing preparations are tolerated reasonably well by most patients. However, they must be used with caution or avoided in patients with renal insufficiency, cardiac disease, or preexisting electrolyte abnormalities, and in patients on diuretic therapy. Patients taking more than 45 ml of oral sodium phosphate as a prescribed bowel preparation may experience electrolyte shifts that pose a risk for the development of symptomatic dehydration, renal failure, metabolic acidosis, tetany from hypocalcemia, and even death in medically vulnerable populations.

Nondigestible Sugars and Alcohols. Lactulose (CEPHULAC, CHRONULAC, others) is a synthetic disaccharide of galactose and fructose that resists intestinal disaccharidase activity.

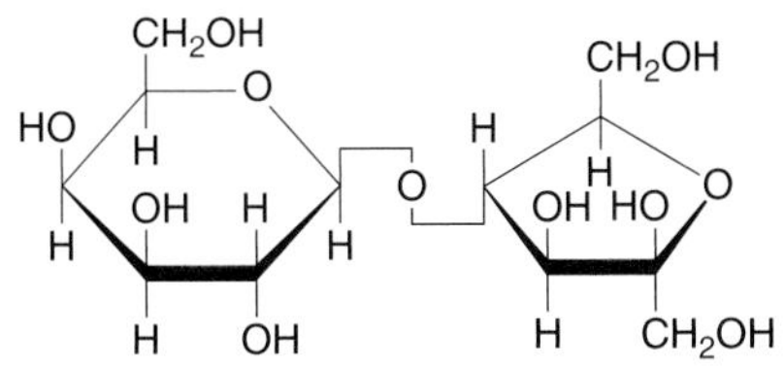

LACTULOSE

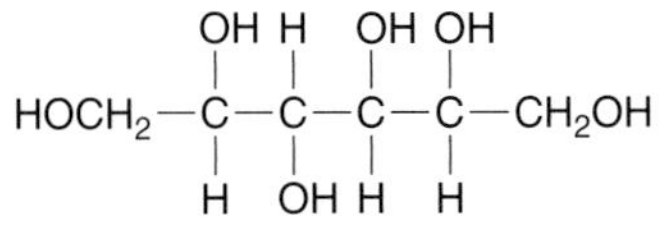

SORBITOL

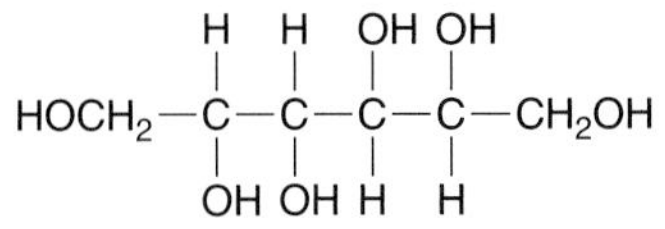

MANNITOL

This and other nonabsorbable sugars such as *sorbitol* and *mannitol,* whose structures are shown above, are hydrolyzed in the colon to short-chain fatty acids, which stimulate colonic propulsive motility by osmotically drawing water into the lumen. Sorbitol and lactulose are equally efficacious in the treatment of constipation caused by opioids and *vincristine,* of constipation in the elderly, and of idiopathic chronic constipation. They are available as 70% solutions, which are given in doses of 15 to 30 ml at night, with increases as needed up to 60 ml per day in divided doses. Effects may not be seen for 24 to 48 hours after dosing is begun. Abdominal discomfort or distention and flatulence are relatively common in the first few days of treatment but usually subside with continued administration. A few patients dislike the sweet taste of the preparations; dilution with water or administering the preparation with fruit juice can mask the taste.

Lactulose also is used to treat hepatic encephalopathy. Patients with severe liver disease have an impaired capacity to detoxify ammonia coming from the colon, where it is produced by bacterial metabolism of fecal urea. The drop in luminal pH that accompanies hydrolysis to short-chain fatty acids in the colon results in "trapping" of the ammonia by its conversion to the polar ammonium ion. Combined with the increases in colonic transit, this therapy significantly lowers circulating ammonia levels. The therapeutic goal in this condition is to give sufficient amounts of lactulose (usually 20 to 30 g, 3 to 4 times per day) to produce two to three soft stools a day with a pH of 5 to 5.5.

Polyethylene Glycol–Electrolyte Solutions. Long-chain *polyethylene glycols* (PEGs; molecular weight ~3350 daltons) are poorly absorbed, and PEG solutions are retained in the lumen by virtue of their high osmotic nature. When used in high volume, aqueous solutions of PEGs (COLYTE, GOLYTELY, others) produce an effective catharsis and are used widely for colonic cleansing for radiological, surgical, and endoscopic procedures (4 liters of this solution taken over 3 hours, beginning at least 4 hours before the procedure). To avoid net transfer of ions across the intestinal wall, these preparations contain an isotonic mixture of sodium sulfate, sodium bicarbonate, sodium chloride, and potassium chloride. The osmotic activity of the PEG molecules retains the added water and the electrolyte concentration assures little or no net ionic shifts.

PEGs are also increasingly being used in smaller doses (250 to 500 ml daily) for the treatment of constipation in difficult cases. A powder form of polyethylene glycol 3350 (MIRALAX) is now available for the short-term treatment (2 weeks or less) of occasional constipation, although the agent has been prescribed safely for longer periods in clinical practice. The usual dose is 17 g of powder per day in 8 ounces of water. This preparation does not contain electrolytes, so larger volumes may represent a risk for ionic shifts. As with other laxatives, prolonged, frequent, or excessive use may result in dependence or electrolyte imbalance.

Stool-Wetting Agents and Emollients

Docusate salts are anionic surfactants that lower the surface tension of the stool to allow mixing of aqueous and fatty substances, softening the stool and permitting easier defecation. However, these agents also stimulate intestinal fluid and electrolyte secretion (possibly by increasing mucosal cyclic AMP) and alter intestinal mucosal permeability. *Docusate sodium* (diocytl sodium sulfosuccinate; COLACE, DOXINATE, others) and *docusate calcium* (dioctyl calcium sulfosuccinate; SURFAK, others), are available in several dosage forms. Despite their widespread use, these agents have marginal, if any, efficacy in most cases of constipation.

Mineral oil is a mixture of aliphatic hydrocarbons obtained from petrolatum. The oil is indigestible and absorbed only to a limited extent. When mineral oil is taken orally for 2 to 3 days, it penetrates and softens the stool and may interfere with resorption of water. The side effects of mineral oil preclude its regular use and include: interference with absorption of fat-soluble substances (such as vitamins), elicitation of foreign-body reactions in the intestinal mucosa and other tissues, and leakage of oil past the anal sphincter. Rare complications such as lipid pneumonitis due to aspiration also can occur, so "heavy" mineral oil should not be taken at bedtime and "light" (topical) mineral oil should never be administered orally.

Stimulant (Irritant) Laxatives

Stimulant laxatives have direct effects on enterocytes, enteric neurons, and GI smooth muscle that only now are beginning to be understood. These agents probably induce a limited low-grade inflammation in the small and large bowel to promote accumulation of water and electrolytes and stimulate intestinal motility. Mechanisms include activation of prostaglandin–cyclic AMP and NO–cyclic GMP pathways, platelet-activating factor production (*see* above), and perhaps inhibition of Na$^+$,K$^+$-ATPase. Included in this group are *diphenylmethane derivatives, anthraquinones, and ricinoleic acid.*

Diphenylmethane Derivatives. Phenolphthalein, once among the most popular components of laxatives, has been withdrawn from the market in the United States because of potential carcinogenicity. *Oxyphenisatin,* another older drug, was withdrawn due to hepatotoxicity. *Sodium picosulfate* (LUBRILAX, SUR-LAX) is a diphenylmethane derivative widely available outside of the United States. It is hydrolyzed by colonic bacteria to its active form, and hence acts locally only in the colon. Effective doses of the diphenylmethane derivatives vary as much as four- to eightfold in individual patients. Consequently, recommended doses may be ineffective in some patients but may produce cramps and excessive fluid secretion in others.

Bisacodyl is the only diphenylmethane derivative available in the United States. It is marketed as an enteric-coated preparation (DULCOLAX, CORRECTOL, others) and as a suppository for rectal administration. The usual oral daily dose of bisacodyl is 10 to 15 mg for adults and 5 to 10 mg for children ages 6 to 12 years old. The drug requires hydrolysis by endogenous esterases in the bowel for activation, and so the laxative effects after an oral dose usually are not produced in less than 6 hours; taken at bedtime, it will produce its effect the next morning. Suppositories work much more rapidly, within 30 to 60 minutes. Due to the possibility of developing an atonic nonfunctioning colon, bisacodyl should not be used for more than 10 consecutive days.

Bisacodyl is mainly excreted in the stool; about 5% is absorbed and excreted in the urine as a glucuronide. Overdosage can lead to catharsis and fluid and electrolyte deficits. The diphenylmethanes can damage the mucosa and initiate an inflammatory response in the small bowel and colon. To avoid drug activation in the stomach with consequent gastric irritation and cramping, patients should

swallow tablets without chewing or crushing and avoid milk or antacid medications within 1 hour of the ingestion of bisacodyl.

Anthraquinone Laxatives. These derivatives of plants such as *aloe, cascara,* and *senna* share a tricyclic anthracene nucleus modified with hydroxyl, methyl, or carboxyl groups to form monoanthrones, such as rhein and frangula. Monoanthrones are irritating to the oral mucosa; however, the process of aging or drying converts them to more innocuous dimeric (dianthrones) or glycoside forms. This process is reversed by bacterial action in the colon to generate the active forms. Senna (SENOKOT, EX-LAX) is obtained from the dried leaflets on pods of *Cassia acutifolia* or *Cassia angustifolia* and contains the rhein dianthrone glycosides *sennoside A* and *B. Cascara sagrada* ("sacred bark"; COLAMIN, SAGRADA-LAX) is obtained from the bark of the buckthorn tree and contains the glycosides *barbaloin* and *chrysaloin.* Barbaloin is also found in aloe. The rhubarb plant also produces anthraquinone compounds that have been used as laxatives. Anthraquinones can also be synthesized; however, the synthetic monoanthrone *danthron* was withdrawn from the United States market because of concerns over possible carcinogenicity. In addition, all aloe and cascara sagrada products sold as laxatives have been withdrawn from the United States market because of failure to demonstrate scientific evidence of efficacy and safety.

Anthraquinone laxatives can produce giant migrating colonic contractions and induce water and electrolyte secretion. They are poorly absorbed in the small bowel, but because they require activation in the colon, the laxative effect is not noted until 6 to 12 hours after ingestion. Active compounds are absorbed to a variable degree from the colon and excreted in the bile, saliva, milk, and urine.

The adverse consequences of long-term use of these agents have limited their use. A melanotic pigmentation of the colonic mucosa (*melanosis coli*) has been observed in patients using anthraquinone laxatives for long periods (at least 4 to 9 months). Histologically, this is caused by the presence of pigment-laden macrophages within the lamina propria. The condition is benign and reversible on discontinuation of the laxative. These agents also have been associated with the development of "cathartic colon," which can be seen in patients (typically women) who have a long-standing history (typically years) of laxative abuse. Regardless of whether a definitive causal relationship can be demonstrated between the use of these agents and colonic pathology, it is clear that they should not be recommended for chronic or long-term use.

Castor Oil. An age-old home remedy, *castor oil* (PURGE, NEOLOID, others) is derived from the bean of the castor plant, *Ricinus communis,* and contains two well-known noxious ingredients: an extremely toxic protein, *ricin,* and an oil composed chiefly of the triglyceride of ricinoleic acid. The triglyceride is hydrolyzed in the small bowel by the action of lipases into glycerol and the active agent, ricinoleic acid, which acts primarily in the small intestine to stimulate secretion of fluid and electrolytes and speed intestinal transit. When taken on an empty stomach, as little as 4 ml of castor oil may produce a laxative effect within 1 to 3 hours; however, the usual dose for a cathartic effect is 15 to 60 ml for adults. Because of its unpleasant taste and its potential toxic effects on intestinal epithelium and enteric neurons, castor oil is seldom recommended now.

Prokinetic and Other Agents for Constipation

Although several of the agents described above stimulate motility, they do so in nonspecific or indirect ways. By contrast, the term *prokinetic* generally is reserved for agents that enhance GI transit *via* interaction with specific receptors involved in the regulation of motility. Currently available prokinetic agents are not very useful in the treatment of constipation. However, newer agents, particularly the more potent 5-HT$_4$-receptor agonists such as tegaserod, may be useful for the treatment of chronic constipation. Another potentially useful agent is *misoprostol,* a synthetic prostaglandin analog primarily used for protection against gastric ulcers resulting from the use of nonsteroidal antiinflammatory agents (*see* Chapter 36). Prostaglandins can stimulate colonic contractions, particularly in the descending colon, and this may account for the diarrhea that limits the usefulness of misoprostol as a gastroprotectant. On the other hand, this property may be utilized for therapeutic gain in patients with intractable constipation. Another prostaglandin analog, RU-0211, is under development. *Colchicine,* a microtubule formation inhibitor used for gout (*see* Chapter 26), also has been shown to be effective in constipation (mechanism unknown), but its toxicity has limited widespread use. A novel biological agent, *neurotrophin-3* (NT-3), recently was shown to be effective in improving frequency and stool consistency and decreasing straining, again by an unknown mechanism of action.

Enemas and Suppositories

Enemas commonly are employed, either by themselves or as adjuncts to bowel preparation regimens, to empty the distal colon or rectum of retained solid material. Bowel distention by any means will produce an evacuation reflex in most people, and almost any form of enema, including normal saline solution, can achieve this. Specialized enemas contain additional substances that either are osmotically active or irritant; however, their safety and efficacy have not been studied in a rigorous manner. Repeated enemas with tap water or other hypotonic solutions can cause hyponatremia; repeated enemas with sodium phosphate–containing solution can cause hypocalcemia. Phosphate-containing enemas also are known to alter the appearance of rectal mucosa.

Glycerin is a trihydroxy alcohol that is absorbed orally, but acts as a hygroscopic agent and lubricant when given rectally. The resultant water retention stimulates peristalsis and usually produces a bowel movement in less than an hour. Glycerin is for rectal use only and is given in a single daily dose as a 2- or 3-g rectal suppository or as 5 to 15 ml of an 80% solution in enema form. Rectal glycerin may cause local discomfort, burning, or hyperemia and (minimal) bleeding. Some glycerin suppositories contain sodium stearate, which can cause local irritation.

ANTIDIARRHEAL AGENTS

Diarrhea: General Principles and Approach to Treatment. Diarrhea (Greek and Latin: *dia,* through, and *rheein,* to flow or run) does not require any definition to people who suffer from "the too rapid evacuation of too fluid stools." Scientists usually define diarrhea as excessive fluid weight, with 200 g per day representing the upper limit of normal stool water weight for healthy adults in the western world. Since stool weight is largely determined by stool water, most cases of diarrhea result from disorders of intestinal water and electrolyte transport.

An appreciation and knowledge of the underlying causative processes in diarrhea facilitates effective treatment. From a mechanistic perspective, diarrhea can be caused by an increased osmotic load within the intestine (resulting in retention of water within the lumen); excessive secretion of electrolytes and water into the intestinal lumen; exudation of protein and fluid from the mucosa; and altered intestinal motility resulting in rapid transit (and decreased fluid absorption). In most instances, multiple processes are affected simultaneously, leading to a net increase in stool volume and weight accompanied by increases in fractional water content.

Many patients with sudden onset of diarrhea have a benign, self-limited illness requiring no treatment or evaluation. In severe cases, dehydration and electrolyte imbalances are the principal risk, particularly in infants, children, and frail elderly patients. *Oral rehydration therapy* therefore is a cornerstone for patients with acute illnesses resulting in significant diarrhea. This is of particular importance in developing countries, where the use of such therapy saves many thousands of lives every year. This therapy exploits the fact that nutrient-linked cotransport of water and electrolytes remains intact in the small bowel in most cases of acute diarrhea. Sodium and chloride absorption is linked to glucose uptake by the enterocyte; this is followed by movement of water in the same direction. A balanced mixture of glucose and electrolytes in volumes matched to losses therefore can prevent dehydration. This can be provided by many commercial premixed formulas using glucose-electrolyte or rice-based physiological solutions.

Pharmacotherapy of diarrhea should be reserved for patients with significant or persistent symptoms. Nonspecific antidiarrheal agents typically do not address the underlying pathophysiology responsible for the diarrhea; their principal utility is to provide symptomatic relief in mild cases of acute diarrhea. Many of these agents act by decreasing intestinal motility and should be avoided as much as possible in acute diarrheal illnesses caused by invasive organisms. In such cases, these agents may mask the clinical picture, delay clearance of organisms, and increase the risk of systemic invasion by the infectious organisms; they also may induce local complications such as toxic megacolon.

Bulk-Forming and Hydroscopic Agents.

Hydrophilic and poorly fermentable colloids or polymers such as *carboxymethylcellulose* and calcium polycarbophil absorb water and increase stool bulk (calcium polycarbophil absorbs 60 times its weight in water). They usually are used for constipation (*see* above), but are sometimes useful in mild chronic diarrheas in patients suffering with irritable bowel syndrome. The mechanism of this effect is not clear, but they may work as gels to modify stool texture and viscosity and to produce a perception of decreased stool fluidity. Some of these agents also may bind bacterial toxins and bile salts. Clays such as *kaolin* (a hydrated aluminum silicate) and other silicates such as *attapulgite* (magnesium aluminum disilicate; DIASORB) bind water avidly (attapulgite absorbs eight times its weight in water) and also may bind enterotoxins. However, this effect is not selective and may involve other drugs and nutrients; hence these agents are best avoided within 2 to 3 hours of taking other medications. A mixture of kaolin and pectin (a plant polysaccharide) is a popular over-the-counter remedy (KAOPECTOLIN) and may provide useful symptomatic relief of mild diarrhea.

Bile Acid Sequestrants.

Cholestyramine, colestipol, and *colesevalam* effectively bind bile acids and some bacterial toxins. Cholestyramine is useful in the treatment of bile salt–induced diarrhea, as in patients with resection of the distal ileum. In these patients, there is partial interruption of the normal enterohepatic circulation of bile salts, resulting in excessive concentrations reaching the colon and stimulating water and electrolyte secretion (*see* below). Patients with extensive ileal resection (usually more than 100 cm) eventually develop net bile salt depletion, which can produce steatorrhea because of inadequate micellar formation required for fat absorption. In such patients, the use of cholestyramine will aggravate the diarrhea. The drug also has had an historic role in treating mild antibiotic-associated diarrhea and mild colitis due to *Clostridium difficile.* However, its use in infectious diarrheas generally is discouraged, as it may decrease clearance of the pathogen from the bowel.

In patients suspected of having bile salt–induced diarrhea, a trial of cholestyramine can be given at a dose of 4 g of the dried resin (contained in either 9 g [QUESTRAN, others] or 5 g [QUESTRAN LIGHT, others] of powder) four times a day. If successful, the dose may be titrated down to achieve the desired stool frequency.

Cholestyramine resin also is helpful for the relief of pruritus associated with partial biliary obstruction and in conditions such as primary biliary cirrhosis. In such conditions, excessive bile acids are thought to be deposited in the skin and cause irritation. Cholestyramine increases fecal excretion of bile acids and reduces circulating and eventually systemic levels with relief of pruritus in about 1 to 3 weeks.

Bismuth.

Bismuth compounds have been used to treat a variety of gastrointestinal diseases and symptoms for centuries, although their mechanism of action remains poorly understood. PEPTO-BISMOL (*bismuth subsalicylate*) is an over-the-counter preparation estimated to be used by 60% of American households. It is a crystal complex consisting of trivalent bismuth and salicylate suspended in a mixture of magnesium aluminum silicate clay. In the low pH of the stomach, the bismuth subsalicylate reacts with hydrochloric acid to form bismuth oxychloride and salicylic acid. While 99% of the bismuth passes unaltered and unabsorbed into the feces, the salicylate is absorbed in the stomach and small intestine. Thus, caution should be used in patients taking salicylates for other indications.

Bismuth is thought to have antisecretory, antiinflammatory, and antimicrobial effects. Nausea and abdominal cramps also are relieved by bismuth. The clay in PEPTO-BISMOL also may have some additional benefits in diarrhea, but this is not clear. Bismuth subsalicylate has been used extensively for the prevention and treatment of traveler's diarrhea, but it also is effective in other forms of episodic diarrhea and in acute gastroenteritis. Today, the most common antibacterial use of this agent is in the treatment of *Helicobacter pylori* (*see* Chapter 36). A recommended dose of the bismuth subsalicylate (30 ml of regular strength PEPTO-BISMOL liquid or 2 tablets) contains approximately equal amounts of bismuth and salicylate (262 mg each). For control of indigestion, nausea, or diarrhea, the dose is repeated every 30 to 60 minutes, as needed, up to eight times a day. Bismuth products have a long track record of safety at recommended doses, although impaction may occur in infants and debilitated patients. Dark stools (sometimes mistaken for melena) and black staining of the tongue in association with bismuth compounds are caused by bismuth sulfide formed in a reaction between the drug and bacterial sulfides in the gastrointestinal tract.

Antimotility and Antisecretory Agents

Opioids.

Opioids continue to be widely used in the treatment of diarrhea. They act by several different mechanisms, mediated principally through either μ- or δ-opioid receptors on enteric nerves, epithelial cells, and muscle (*see* Chapter 21). These mechanisms include effects on intestinal motility (μ receptors), intestinal secretion (δ receptors), or absorption (μ and δ receptors). Commonly used antidiarrheals such as *diphenoxylate, difenoxin,* and *loperamide* act principally *via* peripheral μ-opioid receptors and are preferred over opioids that penetrate the CNS.

Loperamide. Loperamide (IMODIUM, IMODIUM A-D, others), a piperidine butyramide derivative with μ-receptor activity, is an orally active antidiarrheal agent. The drug is 40 to 50 times more potent than morphine as an antidiarrheal agent and penetrates the CNS poorly. It increases small intestinal and mouth-to-cecum transit times. Loperamide also increases anal sphincter tone, an effect that may be of therapeutic value in some patients who suffer from anal incontinence. In addition, loperamide has antisecretory activity against cholera toxin and some forms of *E. coli* toxin, presumably by acting on G_i-linked receptors and countering the increase in cellular cyclic AMP generated in response to the toxins.

Because of its effectiveness and safety, loperamide is marketed for over-the-counter distribution and is available in capsule, solution, and chewable forms. It acts quickly after an oral dose, with peak plasma levels achieved within 3 to 5 hours. It has a half-life of about 11 hours and undergoes extensive hepatic metabolism. The usual adult dose is 4 mg initially followed by 2 mg after each subsequent loose stool, up to 16 mg per day. If clinical improvement in acute diarrhea does not occur within 48 hours, loperamide should be discontinued. Recommended maximum daily doses for children are 3 mg for ages 2 to 5 years, 4 mg for ages 6 to 8 years, and 6 mg for ages 8 to 12 years. Loperamide is not recommended for use in children younger than 2 years of age.

Loperamide has been shown to be effective against traveler's diarrhea, used either alone or in combination with antimicrobial agents (*trimethoprim, trimethoprim-sulfamethoxazole,* or a *fluoroquinolone*). Loperamide also has been used as adjunct treatment in almost all forms of chronic diarrheal disease, with few adverse effects. Loperamide lacks significant abuse potential and is more effective in treating diarrhea than diphenoxylate (*see* below). Overdosage, however, can result in CNS depression (especially in children) and paralytic ileus. In patients with active inflammatory bowel disease involving the colon (*see* Chapter 38), loperamide should be used with great caution, if at all, to prevent development of toxic megacolon.

Loperamide N-*oxide,* an investigational agent, is a site-specific prodrug; it is chemically designed for controlled release of loperamide in the intestinal lumen, thereby reducing systemic absorption.

Diphenoxylate and Difenoxin. Diphenoxylate and its active metabolite difenoxin (diphenoxylic acid) are piperidine derivatives that are related structurally to meperidine. As antidiarrheal agents, diphenoxylate and difenoxin are somewhat more potent than morphine. Both compounds are extensively absorbed after oral administration, with peak levels achieved within 1 to 2 hours. Diphenoxylate is rapidly deesterified to difenoxin, which is eliminated with a half-life of about 12 hours. Both drugs can produce CNS effects when used in higher doses (40 to 60 mg per day) and thus have a potential for abuse and/or addiction. They are available in preparations containing small doses of atropine (considered subtherapeutic) to discourage abuse and deliberate overdosage: 25 μg of *atropine sulfate* per tablet with either 2.5 mg diphenoxylate hydrochloride (LOMOTIL) or 1 mg of difenoxin hydrochloride (MOTOFEN). The usual dosage is two tablets initially, then one tablet every 3 to 4 hours. With excessive use or overdose, constipation and (in inflammatory conditions of the colon) toxic megacolon may develop. In high doses, these drugs cause CNS effects as well as anticholinergic effects from the atropine (dry mouth, blurred vision, *etc.*) (*see* Chapter 7).

Other opioids used for diarrhea include codeine (in doses of 30 mg given three or four times daily) and opium-containing compounds. *Paregoric* (camphorated opium tincture) contains the equivalent of 2 mg of morphine per 5 ml (0.4 mg/ml); *deodorized tincture of opium,* which is 25 times stronger, contains the equivalent of 50 mg of morphine per 5 ml (10 mg/ml). The two tinctures sometimes are confused in prescribing and dispensing, resulting in dangerous overdoses. The antidiarrheal dose of opium tincture for adults is 0.6 ml (equivalent to 6 mg morphine) four times daily; the adult dose of paregoric is 5 to 10 ml (equivalent to 2 or 4 mg morphine) one to four times daily. Paregoric is used in children at a dose of 0.25 to 0.5 ml/kg (equivalent to 0.1 to 0.2 mg morphine/kg) one to four times daily.

Enkephalins are endogenous opioids that are important enteric neurotransmitters. Enkephalins inhibit intestinal secretion without affecting motility. *Racecadotril* (acetorphan), a dipeptide inhibitor of enkephalinase, reinforces the effects of endogenous enkephalins on the δ-opioid receptor to produce an antidiarrheal effect.

a_2 Adrenergic Receptor Agonists. a_2 Adrenergic receptor agonists such as *clonidine* can interact with specific receptors on enteric neurons and enterocytes, thereby stimulating absorption and inhibiting secretion of fluid and electrolytes and increasing intestinal transit time. These agents may have a special role in diabetics with chronic diarrhea, in whom autonomic neuropathy can lead to loss of noradrenergic innervation. Oral clonidine (beginning at 0.1 mg twice a day) has been used in these patients; the use of a topical preparation (*e.g.,* CATAPRES TTS, two patches a week) may result in more steady plasma levels of the drug. Clonidine also may be useful in patients with diarrhea caused by opiate withdrawal. Side effects such as hypotension, depression, and perceived fatigue may be dose limiting in susceptible patients.

Octreotide and Somatostatin. Octreotide (SANDOSTATIN) (*see* Chapter 55) is an octapeptide analog of somatostatin that is effective in inhibiting the severe secretory diarrhea brought about by hormone-secreting tumors of the pancreas and the gastrointestinal tract. Its mechanism of action appears to involve inhibition of hormone secretion, including serotonin and various other GI peptides (*e.g.,* gastrin, vasoactive intestinal polypeptide, insulin, secretin, *etc.*). Octreotide has been used, with varying success, in other forms of secretory diarrhea such as chemotherapy-induced diarrhea, diarrhea associated with human immunodeficiency virus (HIV), and diabetes-associated diarrhea. Its greatest utility, however, may be in the "dumping syndrome" seen in some patients after gastric surgery and pyloroplasty. In this condition, octreotide inhibits the release of hormones (triggered by rapid passage of food into the small intestine) that are responsible for distressing local and systemic effects.

Octreotide has a half-life of 1 to 2 hours and is administered either subcutaneously or intravenously as a bolus dose. Standard initial therapy with octreotide is 50 to 100 μg, given subcutaneously two or three times a day, with titration to a maximum dose of 500 μg three times a day based on clinical and biochemical responses. A long-acting preparation of octreotide acetate enclosed in biodegradable microspheres (SANDOSTATIN LAR DEPOT) is available for use in the treatment of diarrheas associated with carcinoid tumors and vasoactive intestinal peptide–secreting tumors, as well as in the treatment of acromegaly (*see* Chapter 55). This preparation is injected intramuscularly once per month in a dose of 20 or 30 mg. Side effects of octreotide depend on the duration of therapy. Short-term therapy leads to transient nausea, bloating, or pain at sites of injection. Long-term therapy can lead to gallstone formation and hypo- or hyperglycemia. Another long-acting somatostatin analog, *lanreotide* (SOMATULIN, others), is available in Europe but not in the United States; another, *vapreotide,* is under development. *Somatostatin* (STILAMIN) also is available in Europe but not in the United States.

Use in Variceal Bleeding. Vasoactive agents have been used to control variceal bleeding. Traditionally, *vasopressin* has been used (*see* Chapter 29), but its significant side effects—such as myocardial ischemia, peripheral vascular disease, and the release of plasminogen activator and factor VIII—have led to its decline. Somatostatin and octreotide are effective in reducing hepatic blood flow, hepatic venous wedge pressure, and azygos blood flow. These agents constrict the splanchnic arterioles by a direct action on vascular smooth muscle and by inhibiting the release of peptides contributing to the hyperdynamic circulatory syndrome of portal hypertension. Octreotide also may act through the autonomic nervous system. These agents can control bleeding acutely and decrease bleeding-related mortality, with an efficacy comparable to endoscopic therapy or balloon tamponade. The major advantage of somatostatin and octreotide over vasopressin is their safety. Because of the short half-life of somatostatin (1 to 2 minutes), it can be given only by intravenous infusion (a 250-μg bolus dose followed by 250 μg hourly). For patients with variceal bleeding, therapy with octreotide usually is initiated while the patient is awaiting endoscopy. It

is given intravenously as an infusion of 25 to 50 μg/hour for 48 hours after a bolus of 100 μg. Some clinicians give 100 μg subcutaneously every 6 to 8 hours for an additional 72 hours until the patient has had the second endoscopic treatment.

Use in Intestinal Dysmotility. Octreotide has complex and apparently conflicting effects on GI motility, including inhibition of antral motor activity and colonic tone. However, octreotide also can rapidly induce phase III activity of the migrating motor complex in the small bowel to produce longer and faster contractions than those occurring spontaneously. Its use has been shown to result in improvement in selected patients with scleroderma and small-bowel dysfunction.

Use in Pancreatitis. Both somatostatin and octreotide inhibit pancreatic secretion and have been used for the prophylaxis and treatment of acute pancreatitis. The rationale for their use is to "put the pancreas to rest" so as not to aggravate inflammation by the continuing production of proteolytic enzymes, to reduce intraductal pressures, and to ameliorate pain. Octreotide probably is less effective than somatostatin in this regard because it may cause an increase in sphincter of Oddi pressure and perhaps also have a deleterious effect on pancreatic blood flow. Although some studies have suggested that these agents improve mortality in patients with acute pancreatitis, definitive data are lacking.

OTHER AGENTS

Calcium channel blockers such as *verapamil* and *nifedipine* (*see* Chapter 31) reduce motility and may promote intestinal electrolyte and water absorption. Constipation, in fact, is a significant side effect of these drugs. However, because of their systemic effects and the availability of other agents, they seldom if ever are used for diarrheal illnesses.

Berberine is a plant alkaloid that has been used for millennia in traditional Indian and Chinese medicine. It is produced by several genera of the families Ranuculaceae and Berberidaceae (*e.g., Berberis, Mahonia,* and *Coptis*) and has complex pharmacological actions that include antimicrobial actions, stimulation of bile flow, inhibition of ventricular tachyarrhythmias, and possible antineoplastic activity. It is used most commonly in bacterial diarrhea and cholera, but is also apparently effective against intestinal parasites. The antidiarrheal effects in part may be related to its antimicrobial activity, as well as its ability to inhibit smooth muscle contraction and delay intestinal transit by antagonizing the effects of acetylcholine (by competitive and noncompetitive mechanisms) and blocking the entry of Ca^{2+} into cells. In addition, it inhibits intestinal secretion.

Chloride channel blockers are effective antisecretory agents *in vitro* but are too toxic for human use and have not proven to be effective antidiarrheal agents *in vivo*. Calmodulin inhibitors, which include *chlorpromazine*, also are antisecretory. *Zaldaride maleate,* a new drug in this class, may be effective in traveler's diarrhea by reducing secretion without affecting intestinal motility.

IRRITABLE BOWEL SYNDROME

Irritable bowel syndrome, a condition that affects up to 15% of the population in the United States, is perhaps one of the more challenging nonfatal illnesses seen by gastroenterologists (Mertz, 2003). Patients may complain of a variety of symptoms, the most characteristic of which is recurrent abdominal pain associated with altered bowel movements. The pathophysiology of this condition is not clear; it appears to result from a varying combination of disturbances in visceral motor and sensory function, often associated with significant affective disorders. The disturbances in bowel function, which can be either constipation or diarrhea or both at different times, have led to the classical interpretation of irritable bowel syndrome as being a "motility disorder," but motor disturbances cannot explain the entire clinical picture. Recently, more emphasis has been devoted to the pathogenesis of pain in these patients, and there now is considerable evidence to suggest a specific enhancement of visceral (as opposed to somatic) sensitivity to noxious, as well as physiological stimuli in this syndrome. The etiopathogenesis of this visceral hypersensitivity probably is multifactorial; a popular hypothesis is that transient visceral injury in genetically predisposed individuals leads to long-lasting sensitization of the neural pain circuit despite complete resolution of the initiating event. Increasingly, this concept is being extended to other so-called functional disorders of the gut characterized by unexplained pain, including noncardiac chest pain and nonulcer dyspepsia. These disorders, also considered for many years to arise from motor disturbances, may in fact represent part of a spectrum of a new syndrome of "visceral hyperalgesia."

Many patients can be managed satisfactorily with a strong patient-physician relationship, simple counseling, and adjunctive measures, including dietary restrictions and fiber supplementation; overt psychological abnormalities should be treated appropriately. Despite these measures, a significant proportion of patients remain plagued by severe symptoms, and drug therapy is attempted almost invariably. However, there are very few effective pharmacological options for these patients, a situation that in part reflects our limited understanding of the pathogenesis of this syndrome.

The pharmacological approach to irritable bowel syndrome reflects its multifaceted nature. Treatment of bowel symptoms (either diarrhea or constipation) is predominantly symptomatic and nonspecific. Patients with mild symptoms often are started on fiber supplements; this approach may work for constipation and diarrhea (by binding water). Patients with episodic, discrete pain episodes often are treated with agents that may reduce smooth muscle contractility in the gut. These so-called antispasmodics include anticholinergic agents, Ca^{2+} channel antagonists, and peripheral opioid receptor antagonists. The use of most such drugs is hallowed by years of tradition, but seldom has been subjected to critical assessment; however, these drugs may be modestly effective in a subset of patients and are useful adjuncts.

In recent years, an increasing emphasis is being placed on the pharmacological treatment of visceral sensitivity. Although the biological basis of visceral hyperalgesia in irritable bowel syndrome patients is not known, a possible role for serotonin has been suggested

based on its known involvement in sensitization of nociceptor neurons in inflammatory conditions. This has led to the development of specific receptor modulators, such as tegaserod and *alosetron* (Figure 37–2). *Buspirone* and *sumatriptan* are serotonin 5-HT$_1$ receptor agonists (*see* Chapter 11) that can reduce gastric and colonic sensitivity to distention and are being evaluated in clinical trials.

The most effective class of agents in this regard has been the tricyclic antidepressants (*see* Chapter 17), which can have neuromodulatory and analgesic properties independent of their antidepressant effect. Tricyclic antidepressants have a proven track record in the management of chronic "functional" visceral pain. Effective analgesic doses of these drugs (*e.g.*, 25 to 75 mg per day of *nortryptiline*) are significantly lower than those required to treat depression. Although changes in mood usually do not occur at these doses, there may be some diminution of anxiety and restoration of sleep patterns, which can be considered desirable effects in this group of patients. Selective serotonin reuptake inhibitors have fewer side effects and have been advocated particularly for patients with functional constipation as they can increase bowel movements and even cause diarrhea. However, they probably are not as effective as tricyclic antidepressants in the management of visceral pain.

a_2 Adrenergic receptor agonists, such as clonidine (*see* Chapter 10), also can increase visceral compliance and reduce distention-induced pain. The somatostatin analog octreotide (*see* above) has selective inhibitory effects on peripheral afferent nerves projecting from the gut to the spinal cord in healthy human beings and has been shown to blunt the perception of rectal distention in patients with irritable bowel syndrome. *Fedotozine,* an investigational opioid that appears to be a peripherally active, selective κ-receptor antagonist, produces marginal improvement in symptoms in patients with irritable bowel syndrome and functional dyspepsia. The lack of CNS effects is an advantage in such patients in whom chronic medication use is anticipated. Other agents of unproven value include leuprolide, a gonadotropin-releasing hormone analog (*see* Chapter 55).

Alosetron and Other 5-HT$_3$ Antagonists

The 5-HT$_3$ receptor participates in several important processes in the gut, including sensitization of spinal sensory neurons, vagal signaling of nausea, and peristaltic reflexes. Some of these effects in experimental models are potentially conflicting, with release of excitatory and inhibitory neurotransmitters. However, the clinical effect of 5-HT$_3$ antagonism is a general reduction in GI contractility with decreased colonic transit, along with an increase in fluid absorption. In general, therefore, these antagonists produce the opposite effects seen with 5-HT$_4$ agonists such as tegaserod. Although they also may blunt visceral sensation, a direct effect on spinal afferents has not been fully established. Alosetron (LOTRONEX) was the first agent in this class specifically approved for the treatment of diarrhea-predominant irritable bowel syndrome in women. Alosetron is a much more potent antagonist of the 5-HT$_3$ receptor than *ondansetron* (*see* below) and causes significant (though modest) improvements in abdominal pain as well as stool frequency, consistency, and urgency in these patients. Shortly after its initial release, alosetron was withdrawn from the U.S. market because of an unusually high incidence of ischemic colitis (up to 3 per 1000 patients), leading to surgery and even death in a small number of cases. The mechanism of this effect is not fully established, but may result from the drug's ability to suppress intestinal relaxation, thereby causing severe spasm in segments of the colon in susceptible individuals. It is not clear whether this is a nonspecific effect or involves serotoninergic mechanisms. Nevertheless, the FDA has recently reapproved this drug for diarrhea-predominant irritable bowel syndrome under a limited distribution system. However, concerns about the consequences of prescribing this drug are important, and the manufacturer requires a prescription program that includes physician certification and an elaborate patient education and consent protocol before dispensing.

Alosetron is rapidly absorbed from the GI tract; its duration of action (about 10 hours) is longer than expected from its half-life of 1.5 hours. It is metabolized by hepatic CYPs. The drug should be started at 1 mg per day for the first 4 weeks, and advanced to a maximum of 1 mg twice daily if an adequate response is not achieved.

Other 5-HT₃ antagonists currently available in the United States are approved for nausea and vomiting (*see* below). Newer agents in this category, such as *cilansetron,* have considerable promise for functional bowel disorders and are being tested.

ANTISPASMODICS AND OTHER AGENTS

Anticholinergic agents ("spasmolytics" or "antispasmodics") often are used in patients with irritable bowel syndrome. The most common agents of this class available in the United States are nonspecific antagonists of the muscarinic receptor (*see* Chapter 7) and include the tertiary amines *dicyclomine* (BENTYL) and *hyoscyamine* (LEVSIN, others) and the quaternary ammonium compounds *glycopyrrolate* (ROBINUL) and *methscopolamine* (PAMINE). The advantage of the latter two compounds is that they have a limited propensity to cross the blood–brain barrier and hence a lower risk for neurological side effects such as light-headedness, drowsiness, or nervousness. These agents typically are given either on an as-needed basis (with the onset of pain) or before meals to prevent the pain and fecal urgency that predictably occur in some patients with irritable bowel syndrome (with presumed exaggerated gastrocolic reflex).

Dicyclomine is given in doses of 10 to 20 mg orally every 4 to 6 hours as necessary. Hyoscyamine is available in many forms, including oral capsules, tablets, elixir, drops, a nonaerosol spray (0.125 to 0.25 mg every 4 hours as needed), and an extended-release form for oral use (0.375 mg every 12 hours as needed). Glycopyrrolate also comes in extended-release tablets (2 mg once or twice a day), in addition to a standard-release form (1 mg up to three times a day). Methscopolamine is provided as 2.5-mg tablets and the dose is 1 or 2 tablets, three to four times a day.

Other Drugs. *Clidinium bromide,* another quaternary ammonium compound with antimuscarinic activity, is used in a fixed combination with *chlordiazepoxide hydrochloride* (2.5 mg of clidinium and 5 mg of chlordiazepoxide; LIBRAX); however, such combinations are of limited value in patients with irritable bowel syndrome because of the risk of habituation and rebound withdrawal. *Cimetropium,* another antimuscarinic compound that reportedly is

effective in patients with irritable bowel syndrome, is not available in the United States. *Otilonium bromide,* also not available in the United States, has been used extensively for patients with irritable bowel syndrome in other parts of the world. It is a quaternary ammonium salt with antimuscarinic effects that also appears to block Ca²⁺ channels and neurokinin NK-2 receptors. *Mebeverine hydrochloride* is a derivative of hydroxybenzamide that appears to have a direct effect on the smooth muscle cell, blocking K⁺, Na⁺, and Ca²⁺ channels. It is widely used outside of the United States as an antispasmodic agent for patients with irritable bowel syndrome.

ANTINAUSEANTS AND ANTIEMETIC AGENTS

Nausea and Vomiting

The act of emesis and the sensation of nausea that accompanies it generally are viewed as protective reflexes that serve to rid the stomach and intestine of toxic substances and prevent their further ingestion. Vomiting is a complex process that consists of a pre-ejection phase (gastric relaxation and retroperistalsis), retching (rhythmic action of respiratory muscles preceding vomiting and consisting of contraction of abdominal and intercostal muscles and diaphragm against a closed glottis), and ejection (intense contraction of the abdominal muscles and relaxation of the upper esophageal sphincter). This is accompanied by multiple autonomic phenomena including salivation, shivering, and vasomotor changes. During prolonged episodes, marked behavioral changes including lethargy, depression, and withdrawal may occur. The process appears to be coordinated by a central emesis center in the lateral reticular formation of the mid-brainstem adjacent to both the chemoreceptor trigger zone (CTZ) in the area postrema (AP) at the bottom of the fourth ventricle and the solitary tract nucleus (STN) of the vagus nerve. The lack of a blood–brain barrier allows the CTZ to monitor blood and cerebrospinal fluid constantly for toxic substances and to relay information to the emesis center to trigger nausea and vomiting. The emesis center also receives information from the gut, principally by the vagus nerve (*via* the STN) but also by splanchnic afferents *via* the spinal cord. Two other important inputs to the emesis center come from the cerebral cortex (particularly in anticipatory nausea or vomiting) and the vestibular apparatus (in motion sickness). In turn, the center sends out efferents to the nuclei responsible for respiratory, salivary, and vasomotor activity, as well as to striated and smooth muscle involved in the act. The CTZ has high concentrations of receptors for serotonin (5-HT₃), dopamine (D₂), and opioids, while the STN is rich in receptors for enkephalin, histamine, and ACh, and also contains

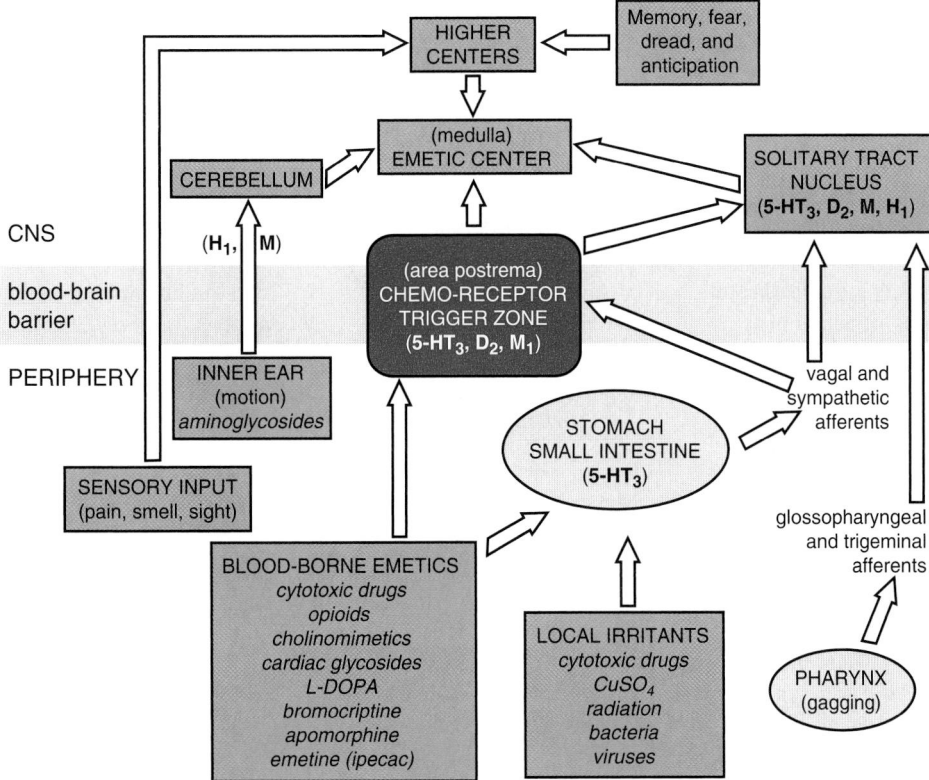

Figure 37–4. ***Pharmacologist's view of emetic stimuli.*** Myriad signaling pathways lead from the periphery to the emetic center. Stimulants of these pathways are noted in *italics.* These pathways involve specific neurotransmitters and their receptors (**bold** type). Receptors are shown for dopamine (D_2), acetylcholine (muscarinic, M), histamine (H_1), and 5-hydroxytryptamine (5-HT_3). Some of these receptors also may mediate signaling in the emetic center.

5-HT_3 receptors. A variety of these neurotransmitters are involved in nausea and vomiting (Figure 37–4), and an understanding of their nature has allowed a rational approach to the pharmacological treatment of nausea and vomiting (Scuderi, 2003).

Antiemetics generally are classified according to the predominant receptor on which they are proposed to act (Table 37–5). However, considerable overlap among these mechanisms exists, particularly for the older agents (Table 37–6). For treatment and prevention of the nausea and emesis associated with cancer chemotherapy, several antiemetic agents from different pharmacological classes may be used in combination (Table 37–7). The individual classes of agents are presented below.

5-HT₃-Receptor Antagonists

Chemistry, Pharmacological Effects, and Mechanism of Action. Ondansetron (ZOFRAN) is the prototypical drug in this class. Since their introduction in the early 1990s, the 5-HT_3-receptor antagonists have become the most widely used drugs for chemotherapy-induced emesis. Other agents in this class include *granisetron* (KYTRIL), *dolasetron* (ANZEMET), *palonosetron* (ALOXI; intravenous use only) and *tropisetron*

(available in some countries but not in the United States). The differences among these agents are related mainly to their chemical structures, 5-HT_3 receptor affinities, and pharmacokinetic profiles (Table 37–8).

There is evidence that effects at peripheral and central sites contribute to the efficacy of these agents. 5-HT_3 receptors are present in several critical sites involved in emesis, including vagal afferents, the STN (which receives signals from vagal afferents), and the area postrema itself (Figure 37–4). Serotonin is released by the enterochromaffin cells of the small intestine in response to chemotherapeutic agents and may stimulate vagal afferents (*via* 5-HT_3 receptors) to initiate the vomiting reflex. Experimentally, vagotomy has been shown to prevent cisplatin-induced emesis. However, the highest concentrations of 5-HT_3 receptors in the CNS are found in the STN and CTZ, and antagonists of 5-HT_3 receptors also may suppress nausea and vomiting by acting at these sites.

Pharmacokinetics. The antiemetic effects of these drugs persist long after they disappear from the circulation, suggesting their continuing interaction at the receptor level. In fact, all of these drugs can be administered effectively just once a day.

These agents are absorbed well from the GI tract. Ondansetron is extensively metabolized in the liver by CYP1A2, CYP2D6, and CYP3A4, followed by glucuronide or sulfate conjugation. Patients with hepatic dysfunction have reduced plasma clearance, and some adjustment in the dosage is advisable. Although ondansetron clearance

Table 37–5
General Classification of Antiemetic Agents

ANTIEMETIC CLASS	EXAMPLES	TYPE OF VOMITING MOST EFFECTIVE AGAINST
5-HT$_3$ receptor antagonists*	Ondansetron	Cytotoxic drug induced emesis
Centrally acting dopamine receptor antagonists	Metoclopramide*† Promethazine‡	Cytotoxic drug induced emesis
Histamine H$_1$ receptor antagonists	Cyclizine	Vestibular (motion sickness)
Muscarinic receptor antagonists	Hyoscine (scopolamine)	Motion sickness
Neurokinin receptor antagonists	Investigational	Cytotoxic drug induced emesis (delayed vomiting)
Cannabinoid receptor agonists	Dronabinol	Cytotoxic drug induced emesis

*The most effective agents for chemotherapy-induced nausea and vomiting are the 5-HT$_3$ antagonists and metoclopramide. In addition to their use as single agents, they are often combined with other drugs to improve efficacy as well as reduce the incidence of side effects. †Also has some peripheral activity at 5-HT$_3$ receptors. ‡Also has some antihistaminic and anticholinergic activity.

Table 37–6
Receptor Specificity of Antiemetic Agents

PHARMACOLOGIC CLASS Drugs in Class	DOPAMINE (D$_2$)	ACETYLCHOLINE (Muscarinic)	HISTAMINE	SEROTONIN
Anticholinergics				
Scopolamine	+	++++	+	–
Antihistamines				
Cyclizine	+	+++	++++	–
Dimenhydrinate, diphenhydramine, hydroxyzine	+	++	++++	–
Medizine	+	+++	++++	–
Promethazine	++	++	++++	–
Antiserotonins				
Dolasetron, granisetron, ondansetron, palonosetron, ramosetron	–	–	–	++++
Benzamides				
Domperidone	++++	–	–	+
Metoclopramide	+++	–	–	++
Butyrophenones				
Droperidol	++++	–	+	+
Haloperidol	++++	–	+	–
Phenothiazines				
Chlorpromazine	++++	++	++++	+
Fluphenazine	++++	+	++	–
Perphenazine	++++	+	++	+
Prochlorperazine	++++	++	++	+
Steroids				
Betamethasone, dexamethasone	–	–	–	–

For details, see Scuderi, 2003. Plus signs indicate some (+) to considerable (++++) interaction. (–) indicates no effect.

Table 37–7

A. Some Antiemetic Regimens Used in Cancer Chemotherapy

ANTIEMETIC AGENT	INITIAL DOSE
For Severe Chemotherapy-Induced Emesis *(Several Antiemetic Agents Used in Combination)*	
Dexamethasone	20 mg IV
Metoclopramide	3 mg/kg body weight IV every 2 h × 2
Diphenhydramine	25–50 mg IV every 2 h × 2
Lorazepam	1–2 mg IV
Dexamethasone	20 mg IV
Ondansetron	32 mg IV daily, in divided doses
For Moderate Chemotherapy-Induced Emesis *(Antiemetic Agents Used Singly)*	
Prochlorperazine	5–10 mg orally or IV, or 25 mg by rectal suppository
Thiethylperazine	10 mg orally, IM, or by rectal suppository
Dexamethasone	10–20 mg IV
Ondansetron	8 mg orally or 10 mg IV
Dronabinol	10 mg orally

B. Useful Combinations of Antiemetic Agents for Improved Antiemetic Effect

PRIMARY AGENT	SUPPLEMENTAL AGENT
5-HT$_3$ receptor antagonist	Corticosteroid, phenothiazine, butyrophenone
Substituted benzamide	Corticosteroid ± muscarinic receptor antagonist
Phenothiazine/ butyrophenone	Corticosteroid
Corticosteroid	Benzodiazepine
Cannabinoid	Corticosteroid

C. Useful Combinations of Antiemetic Agents Providing Decreased Toxicity of the Primary Agent

PRIMARY AGENT	SUPPLEMENTAL AGENT
Substituted benzamide	H$_1$ receptor antagonist, corticosteroid, benzodiazepine
Phenothiazine/ butyrophenone	H$_1$ receptor antagonist
Cannabinoid	Phenothiazine

ABBREVIATIONS: H, histamine, 5-HT, serotonin; IV, intravenous; IM, intramuscular. SOURCE: All combination regimens are from Grunberg and Hesketh, 1993, with permission.

also is reduced in elderly patients, no adjustment in dosage for age is recommended. Granisetron also is metabolized predominantly by the liver, a process that appears to involve the CYP3A family, as it is inhibited by *ketoconazole*. Dolasetron is converted rapidly by plasma carbonyl reductase to its active metabolite, hydrodolasetron. A portion of this compound then undergoes subsequent biotransformation by CYP2D6 and CYP3A4 in the liver, while about one-third of it is excreted unchanged in the urine. Palonosetron is metabolized principally by CYP2D6 and excreted in the urine as the metabolized and the unchanged form in about equal proportions.

Therapeutic Use. These agents are most effective in treating chemotherapy-induced nausea and in treating nausea secondary to upper abdominal irradiation, where all three agents appear to be equally efficacious. They also are effective against hyperemesis of pregnancy, and to a lesser degree, postoperative nausea, but not against motion sickness. Unlike other agents in this class, palonosetron also may be helpful in delayed emesis (*see* below), perhaps a reflection of its long half-life.

These agents are available as tablets, oral solution, and intravenous preparations for injection. For patients on cancer chemotherapy, these drugs can be given in a single intravenous dose (Table 37–8) infused over 15 minutes, beginning 30 minutes before chemotherapy, or in two to three divided doses, with the first usually given 30 minutes before and subsequent doses at various intervals after chemotherapy. The drugs also can be used intramuscularly or orally.

Adverse Effects. In general, these drugs are very well tolerated, with the most common adverse effects being constipation or diarrhea, headache, and light-headedness. As a class, these agents have been shown experimentally to induce minor electrocardiographic changes, but these are not expected to be clinically significant in most cases.

Dopamine-Receptor Antagonists

Phenothiazines such as *prochlorperazine, thiethylperazine,* and chlorpromazine (*see* Chapter 18) are among the most commonly used "general purpose" antinauseants and antiemetics. Their effects in this regard are complex, but their principal mechanism of action is dopamine D$_2$ receptor antagonism at the CTZ. Compared to metoclopramide or ondansetron (*see* above), these drugs do not appear to be as uniformly effective in cancer chemotherapy–induced emesis. On the other hand, they also possess antihistaminic and anticholinergic activities, which are of value in other forms of nausea, such as motion sickness.

Antihistamines

Histamine H$_1$-receptor antagonists are primarily useful for motion sickness and postoperative emesis. They act

Table 37–8
5-HT₃ Antagonists in Chemotherapy-Induced Nausea/Emesis

DRUG	CHEMICAL NATURE	RECEPTOR INTERACTIONS	$T_{\frac{1}{2}}$	DOSE (IV)
Ondansetron	Carbazole derivative	5-HT₃ antagonist and weak 5-HT₄ antagonist	3.9 hours	0.15 mg/kg
Granisetron	Indazole	5-HT₃ antagonist	9–11.6 hours	10 μg/kg
Dolasetron	Indole moiety	5-HT₃ antagonist	7–9 hours	0.6–3 mg/kg
Palonosetron	Isoquinoline	5-HT₃ antagonist; highest affinity for 5-HT₃ receptor in this class	40 hours	0.25 mg
Ramosetron	Benzidazolyl derivative	5-HT₃ antagonist	5.8 hours	300 μg/kg

on vestibular afferents and within the brainstem. *Cyclizine, hydroxyzine, promethazine,* and *diphenhydramine* are examples of this class of agents. Cyclizine has additional anticholinergic effects that may be useful for patients with abdominal cancer. For a detailed discussion of these drugs, *see* Chapter 24.

Anticholinergic Agents

The most commonly used muscarinic receptor antagonist is *scopolamine* (hyoscine), which can be injected as the hydrobromide, but usually is administered as the free base in the form of a transdermal patch (TRANSDERM-SCOP). Its principal utility is in the prevention and treatment of motion sickness, although it has been shown to have some activity in postoperative nausea and vomiting, as well. In general, anticholinergic agents have no role in chemotherapy-induced nausea. For a detailed discussion of these drugs, *see* Chapter 7.

DRONABINOL

Dronabinol (delta-9-tetrahydrocannabinol; MARINOL) is a naturally occurring cannabinoid that can be synthesized chemically or extracted from the marijuana plant, *Cannabis sativa.* The exact mechanism of the antiemetic action of dronabinol is unknown but probably relates to stimulation of the CB₁ subtype of cannabinoid receptors on neurons in and around the vomiting center.

Pharmacokinetics. Dronabinol is a highly lipid-soluble compound that is absorbed readily after oral administration; its onset of action occurs within an hour, and peak levels are achieved within 2 to 4 hours. It undergoes extensive first-pass metabolism with limited systemic bioavailability after single doses (only 10% to 20%). Active and inactive metabolites are formed in the liver; the principal active metabolite is 11-OH-delta-9-tetrahydrocannabinol.

These metabolites are excreted primarily *via* the biliary-fecal route, with only 10% to 15% excreted in the urine. Both dronabinol and its metabolites are highly bound (>95%) to plasma proteins. Because of its large volume of distribution, a single dose of dronabinol can result in detectable levels of metabolites for several weeks.

Therapeutic Use. Dronabinol is a useful prophylactic agent in patients receiving cancer chemotherapy when other antiemetic medications are not effective. It also can stimulate appetite and has been used in patients with acquired immunodeficiency syndrome (AIDS) and anorexia. As an antiemetic agent, it is administered at an initial dose of 5 mg/m² given 1 to 3 hours before chemotherapy and then every 2 to 4 hours afterward for a total of four to six doses. If this is not adequate, incremental increases in dose can be made up to a maximum of 15 mg/m². For other indications, the usual starting dose is 2.5 mg twice a day; this can be titrated up to 20 mg a day.

Adverse Effects. Dronabinol has complex effects on the CNS, including a prominent central sympathomimetic activity. This can lead to palpitations, tachycardia, vasodilation, hypotension, and conjunctival injection (bloodshot eyes). Patient supervision is necessary because marijuana-like "highs" (*e.g.,* euphoria, somnolence, detachment, dizziness, anxiety, nervousness, panic, etc.) can occur, as can more disturbing effects such as paranoid reactions and thinking abnormalities. After abrupt withdrawal of dronabinol, an abstinence syndrome manifest by irritability, insomnia, and restlessness can occur. Because of its high affinity for plasma proteins, dronabinol can displace other plasma protein-bound drugs, whose doses may have to be adjusted as a consequence. Dronabinol should be prescribed with great caution to persons with a history of substance abuse (alcohol, drugs) because it also may be abused by these patients.

Glucocorticoids and Antiinflammatory Agents

Glucocorticoids such as *dexamethasone* can be useful adjuncts (Table 37–7) in the treatment of nausea in patients with widespread cancer, possibly by suppressing peritumoral inflammation and prostaglandin production. A similar mechanism has been invoked to explain beneficial effects of nonsteroidal antiinflammatory drugs in the nausea and vomiting induced by systemic irradiation. For a detailed discussion of these drugs, *see* Chapters 26 and 59.

Benzodiazepines

Benzodiazepines, such as *lorazepam* and *alprazolam,* by themselves are not very effective antiemetics, but their sedative, amnesic, and anti-anxiety effects can be helpful in reducing the anticipatory component of nausea and vomiting in patients. For a detailed discussion of these drugs, *see* Chapter 16.

Substance P Receptor Antagonists

APREPITANT

The nausea and vomiting associated with cisplatin (*see* Chapter 51) has two components: an acute phase that universally is experienced (within 24 hours after chemotherapy) and a delayed phase that affects only some patients (on days 2 to 5). 5-HT receptor antagonists are not very effective against delayed emesis. Antagonists of the NK_1 receptors for substance P, such as *aprepitant* (EMEND), have antiemetic effects in delayed nausea and improve the efficacy of standard antiemetic regimens in patients receiving multiple cycles of chemotherapy. Substance P belongs to the tachykinin family of neurotransmitters and is in vagal afferent fibers innervating the STN and area postrema. The tachykinins represent a novel, promising target for new antinauseant drugs.

After absorption, aprepitant is bound extensively to plasma proteins (>95%); it is metabolized avidly, primarily by hepatic CYP3A4, and is excreted in the stools; its half-life is 9 to 13 hours. Aprepitant has the potential to interact with other substrates of CYP3A4, requiring adjustment of other drugs, including dexamethasone, *methylprednisolone* (whose dose may need to be reduced by 50%), and *warfarin.* Aprepitant is contraindicated in

patients on cisapride (*see* above) or *pimozide,* in whom life-threatening QT prolongation has been reported.

Aprepitant is supplied in 80- and 125-mg capsules and is administered for 3 days in conjunction with highly emetogenic chemotherapy along with a 5-HT$_3$-receptor antagonist and a corticosteroid. The recommended adult dosage of aprepitant is 125 mg administered 1 hour before chemotherapy on day one, followed by 80 mg once daily in the morning on days 2 and 3 of the treatment regimen.

AGENTS USED FOR MISCELLANEOUS GASTROINTESTINAL DISORDERS

Chronic Pancreatitis and Steatorrhea

Pancreatic Enzymes. Chronic pancreatitis is a debilitating syndrome that results in symptoms from loss of glandular function (exocrine and endocrine) and inflammation (pain). Because there is no cure for chronic pancreatitis, the goals of pharmacological therapy are prevention of malabsorption and palliation of pain. The cornerstone of therapy for malabsorption still is the use of pancreatic enzymes. Although also used for pain, these agents are much less effective for this symptom.

Enzyme Formulations. The two common preparations of pancreatic enzymes for replacement therapy are obtained from the pancreas of the hog (S*us scrofa* Linne var. *domesticus* Gray). *Pancreatin* (DONNAZYME, others) contains amylase, lipase, and protease and has one-twelfth of the lipolytic activity of *pancrelipase,* on a weight-by-weight basis. Pancrelipase is more commonly used and is available in uncoated forms, as well as capsules containing enteric-coated microspheres and enteric-coated microtablets, which withstand gastric acid (lipase is inactivated by acid) and disintegrate at pH > 6. Familiarity with these two classes of preparations is important clinically (Table 37–9).

Replacement Therapy for Malabsorption. Fat malabsorption (steatorrhea) and protein maldigestion occur when the pancreas loses more than 90% of its ability to produce digestive enzymes. The resultant diarrhea and malabsorption can be managed reasonably well if 30,000 USP units of pancreatic lipase are delivered to the duodenum during a 4-hour period with and after meals; this represents about 10% of the normal pancreatic output. Alternatively, one can titrate the dosage to the fat content of the diet, with approximately 8000 USP units of lipase activity required for each 17 g of dietary fat. Available preparations of pancreatic enzymes (Table 37–10) contain up to 20,000 units of lipase and 75,000 units of protease, and the typical dose of pancrelipase is 1 to 3 capsules or tablets with or just before meals and snacks, adjusted until a satisfactory symptomatic response is obtained. The loss of pancreatic amylase does not present a problem because of other sources of this enzyme (*e.g.,* salivary glands). Patients using uncoated preparations require concomitant pharmacological control of gastric acid production with a proton pump inhibitor (*see* Chapter 36).

Enzymes for Pain. Pain is the other cardinal symptom of chronic pancreatitis. The rationale for its treatment with pancreatic enzymes is based on the principle of negative feedback inhibition of the pan-

Table 37–9
Comparison of Uncoated and Enteric-Coated Pancreatic Enzyme Preparations[*]

	UNCOATED PREPARATIONS	ENTERIC-COATED PREPARATIONS
Number of tablets or capsules required per dose	2–8	2–3
Acid suppression required	Yes	No
Site of delivery	Duodenum	More distal small bowel and beyond
Symptoms relieved	Pain; malabsorption	Malabsorption

[*]The major components of these preparations are a lipase and a protease (*see* Table 37–10).

creas by the presence of duodenal proteases. The release of cholecys-tokinin (CCK), the principal secretagogue for pancreatic enzymes, is triggered by CCK-releasing monitor peptide in the duodenum, which normally is denatured by pancreatic trypsin. In chronic pancreatitis, trypsin insufficiency leads to persistent activation of this peptide and an increased release of CCK, which is thought to cause pancreatic pain because of continuous stimulation of pancreatic enzyme output and increased intraductal pressure. Delivery of active proteases to the duodenum (which can be done reliably only with uncoated preparations) therefore is important for the interruption of this loop. Although enzymatic therapy has become firmly entrenched for the treatment of painful pancreatitis, the evidence supporting this practice is equivocal at best.

Table 37–10
Pancreatic Enzyme Formulations

BRAND NAME	LIPASE[*]	PROTEASE[*]	AMYLASE
Conventional (uncoated)			
VIOKASE 8	8,000	30,000	30,000
VIOKASE 16	16,000	60,000	60,000
KUZYME HP	8,000	30,000	30,000
Enteric coated			
PANCREASE			
MT 4	4,000	12,000	12,000
MT 10	10,000	30,000	30,000
MT 16	16,000	48,000	48,000
CREON			
5	5,000	18,750	16,600
10	10,000	37,500	33,200
20	20,000	75,000	66,400
ULTRASE			
MT 12	12,000	39,000	39,000
MT 18	18,000	58,500	58,500
MT 20	20,000	65,000	65,000

[*]U.S. Pharmacopeia units per tablet or capsule. *See* Forsmark and Toskes, 2000.

In general, pancreatic enzyme preparations are tolerated extremely well by patients. For patients with hypersensitivity to pork protein, bovine enzymes are available. Hyperuricosuria in patients with cystic fibrosis can occur, and malabsorption of folate and iron has been reported. In the past, products with higher lipase content were available, but these were withdrawn after reports associating their use with the development of colonic strictures in patients with cystic fibrosis.

Octreotide (*see* above, and Chapter 55) also has been used, with questionable efficacy, to decrease refractory abdominal pain in patients with chronic pancreatitis. In the future, CCK antagonists may assume a therapeutic role.

BILE ACIDS

Bile acids and their conjugates are essential components of bile that are synthesized from cholesterol in the liver. The major bile acids in human adults are depicted in Figure 37–5. Bile acids induce bile flow, feedback-inhibit cholesterol synthesis, promote intestinal excretion of cholesterol, and facilitate the dispersion and absorption of lipids and fat-soluble vitamins. After secretion into the biliary tract, bile acids are largely (95%) reabsorbed in the intestine (mainly in the terminal ileum), returned to the liver, and then again secreted in bile (enterohepatic circulation). *Cholic acid, chenodeoxycholic acid,* and *deoxycholic acid* constitute 95% of bile acids, while *lithocholic acid* and *ursodeoxycholic acid* are minor constituents. The bile acids exist largely as glycine and taurine conjugates, the salts of which are called *bile salts.* Colonic bacteria convert primary bile acids (cholic and chenodeoxycholic acid) to secondary acids (mainly deoxycholic and lithocholic acid) by sequential deconjugation and dehydroxylation. These secondary bile acids also are absorbed in the colon and join the primary acids in the enterohepatic pool.

Dried bile from the Himalayan bear (Yutan) has been used for centuries in China to treat liver disease. Ursodeoxycholic acid (UDCA; ursodiol, ACTIGALL) (Figure 37–5) is a hydrophilic, dehydroxylated bile acid that is formed by epimerization of the bile acid chenodeoxycholic acid (CDCA; chenodiol) in the gut by intestinal bacteria; it com-

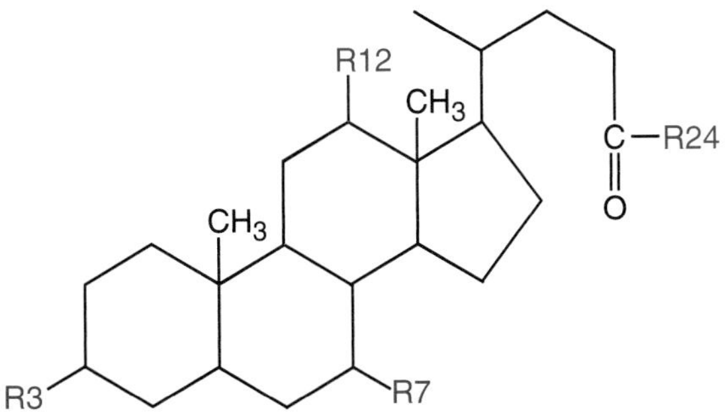

Bile Acid	R3	R7	R12	R24
Cholic acid	–OH	–OH	–OH	
Chenodeoxycholic acid	–OH	–OH	–H	glycine (75%)
Deoxycholic acid	–OH	–H	–OH	taurine (24%)
Lithocholic acid	–SO₃⁻ /–OH	–H	–H	–OH (<1%)
Ursodeoxycholic acid	–OH	◄OH	–H	

Figure 37–5. *Major bile acids in adults.*

prises approximately 1% to 3% of the total bile acid pool in human beings, but is present at much higher concentrations in bears. When administered orally, litholytic bile acids such as chenodiol and ursodiol can alter relative concentrations of bile acids, decrease biliary lipid secretion, and reduce the cholesterol content of the bile so that it is less lithogenic. Ursodiol also may have cytoprotective effects on hepatocytes and effects on the immune system that account for some of its beneficial effects in cholestatic liver diseases.

Bile acids were first used therapeutically for gallstone dissolution; use for this indication requires a functional gallbladder because the modified bile must enter the gallbladder to interact with gallstones. To be amenable to dissolution, the gallstones must be composed of cholesterol monohydrate crystals and generally must be smaller than 15 mm in diameter to provide a favorable ratio of surface to size. For these reasons, the overall efficacy of litholytic bile acids in the treatment of gallstones has been disappointing (partial dissolution occurs in 40% to 60% of patients completing therapy and is complete in only 33% to 50% of these). While a combination of chenodiol and ursodiol probably is better than either agent alone, ursodiol is preferred as a single agent because of its greater efficacy and less-frequent side effects (*e.g.,* hepatotoxicity).

Primary biliary cirrhosis is a chronic, progressive, cholestatic liver disease of unknown etiology that typically affects middle-aged to elderly women. Ursodiol (administered at 13 to 15 mg/kg per day in two divided doses) reduces the concentration of primary bile acids and improves biochemical and histological features of primary biliary cirrhosis. Ursodiol also has been used in a variety of other cholestatic liver diseases, including primary sclerosing cholangitis, and in cystic fibrosis; in general, it is less effective in these conditions than in primary biliary cirrhosis.

ANTIFLATULENCE AGENTS

"Gas" is a common but relatively vague gastrointestinal complaint, used in reference not only to flatulence and eructation, but also bloating or fullness. Although few if any symptoms can be directly attributable to excessive intestinal gas, over-the-counter and herbal preparations that are touted as antiflatulent are very popular. One of these is *simethicone,* a mixture of siloxane polymers stabilized with silicon dioxide:

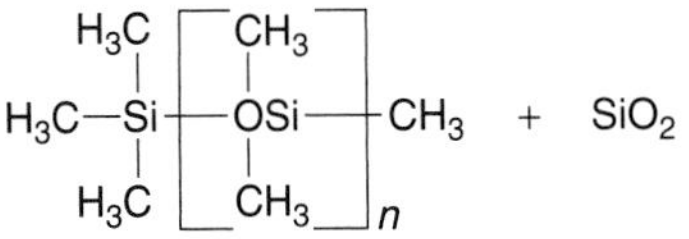

Simethicone is an inert, nontoxic insoluble liquid. Because of its ability to collapse bubbles by forming a thin layer on their surface, it is an effective antifoaming agent. Although it may be effective in diminishing gas volumes in the GI tract, it is not clear whether this accomplishes a therapeutic effect.

Simethicone is available in chewable tablets, liquid-filled capsules, or suspensions, either by itself or in combination with other over-the-counter medications including antacids and other digestants. The usual dosage in adults is 40 to 125 mg four times daily.

CLINICAL SUMMARY

GI Motility Disorders. As a group these are difficult disorders to treat because of a lack of effective therapeutic options. For patients with gastroparesis, first-line therapy consists of metoclopramide, which accelerates gastric emptying and also has antiemetic effects. Erythromycin, a motilin agonist, also has been used for these patients, but is most effective in the short-term. The role of newer agents such as tegaserod in this condition is under investigation. For patients with small-bowel dysmotility, the choices are even more limited: Metoclopramide and erythromycin generally do not work; therapy with octreotide may benefit a subset of patients.

Constipation. Although many choices exist for this condition, most therapies are empirical and nonspecific. Constipation often can be addressed by simple measures such as increasing fiber intake, avoiding constipating medications, and the judicious use of osmotic laxatives on an as-needed basis. For more persistent symptoms, a specific prokinetic 5-HT₄-receptor agonist, tegaserod, may be used with modest efficacy in women who also have irritable bowel syndrome. Stimulant laxatives, although effective, should be avoided for long-term use. Patients with chronic constipation who do not respond to simple measures should undergo further testing to discover uncommon but specific disorders of colonic or anorectal motility.

Diarrhea. In most cases, an attempt should be made to find the underlying cause and target it specifically. If no such cause is found, chronic diarrhea can be treated empirically, with the simplest approach being bulk-forming and hygroscopic agents, followed by opioids such as loperamide or diphenoxylate/difenoxin.

Irritable Bowel Syndrome. This common syndrome requires a combination of pharmacological and behavioral approaches. Antispasmodics are useful by themselves in mild cases and as adjuncts in a regimen that includes tricyclic antidepressants for more persistent pain.

Nausea and Vomiting. The discovery of the 5-HT$_3$ receptor antagonists has led to a major advance in the treatment of nausea and vomiting, especially in the postchemotherapy and postoperative settings. Anticholinergics are most effective in motion sickness. Antihistamines and related drugs still are useful for empiric treatment of nausea from a variety of causes. Dronabinol may be an effective agent for more refractory cases. The clinical utility of newer agents such as aprepitant in situations other than postchemotherapy nausea will be tested in coming years.

BIBLIOGRAPHY

Forsmark, C.E., and Toskes, P.P. Treatment of chronic pancreatitis. In, *Therapy of Digestive Disorders: A Companion to Sleisenger and Fordtran's Gastrointestinal and Liver Disease.* (Wolfe, M.M., and Cohen, S., eds.) Saunders, Philadelphia, **2000,** pp. 235–245.

Furness, J.B., and Sanger, G.J. Intrinsic nerve circuits of the gastrointestinal tract: identification of drug targets. *Curr. Opinion Pharmacol.,* **2002,** *2:*612–622.

Galligan, J. Pharmacology of synaptic transmission in the enteric nervous system. *Curr. Opin. Pharmacol.,* **2002,** *2:*623–629.

Grunberg, S.M., and Hesketh, P.J. Control of chemotherapy-induced emesis. *N. Engl. J. Med.,* **1993,** *329:*1790–1796.

Hansen, M.B. The enteric nervous system I: organization and classification. *Pharmacol. Toxicol.,* **2003,** *92:*105–113.

Izzo, A.A., Gaginella, T.S., Mascolo, N., and Capasso, F. Recent findings on the mode of action of laxatives: the role of platelet activating factor and nitric oxide. *Trends Pharmacol. Sci.,* **1998,** *19:*403–405.

Kreek, M.J. Constipation syndromes. In, *A Pharmacological Approach to Gastrointestinal Disorders.* (Lewis, J.H., ed.) Williams & Wilkins, Baltimore, **1994,** pp. 179–208.

Kunze, W.A., and Furness, J.B. The enteric nervous system and regulation of intestinal motility. *Annu. Rev. Physiol.,* **1999,** *61:*117–142.

Mertz, H.R. Drug therapy: irritable bowel syndrome. *N. Engl. J. Med.,* **2003,** *349:*2136–2146.

Scuderi, P.E. Pharmacology of anti-emetics. *Int. Anesthesiol. Clin.,* **2003,** *41:*41–66.

Talley, N.J. Serotoninergic neuroenteric modulators. *Lancet,* **2001,** *358:*2061–2068.

Tonini, M., Cipollina, L., Poluzzi, E., *et al.* Review article: clinical implications of enteric and central D$_2$ receptor blockade by antidopaminergic gastrointestinal prokinetics. *Aliment. Pharmacol. Ther.,* **2004,** *19:*379–390.

Zhao, X., and Pasricha, P.J. Botulinum toxin for spastic GI disorders: a systematic review. *Gastrointest. Endosc.,* **2003,** *57:*219–235.

PHARMACOTHERAPY OF INFLAMMATORY BOWEL DISEASE

Joseph H. Sellin and Pankaj Jay Pasricha

Inflammatory bowel disease (IBD) is a spectrum of chronic idiopathic inflammatory intestinal conditions. IBD causes significant gastrointestinal symptoms that include diarrhea, abdominal pain, bleeding, anemia, and weight loss. IBD also is associated with a spectrum of extraintestinal manifestations, including arthritis, ankylosing spondylitis, sclerosing cholangitis, uveitis, iritis, pyoderma gangrenosum, and erythema nodosum.

IBD conventionally is divided into two major subtypes: ulcerative colitis and Crohn's disease. Ulcerative colitis is characterized by confluent mucosal inflammation of the colon starting at the anal verge and extending proximally for a variable extent (*e.g.,* proctitis, left-sided colitis, or pancolitis). Crohn's disease, by contrast, is characterized by transmural inflammation of any part of the gastrointestinal tract but most commonly the area adjacent to the ileocecal valve. The inflammation in Crohn's disease is not necessarily confluent, frequently leaving "skip areas" of relatively normal mucosa. The transmural nature of the inflammation may lead to fibrosis and strictures or, alternatively, fistula formation.

Medical therapy for IBD is problematic. Because no unique abnormality has been identified, current therapy for IBD seeks to dampen the generalized inflammatory response; however, no agent can reliably accomplish this, and the response of an individual patient to a given medicine may be limited and unpredictable. Based on this variable response, clinical trials generally employ standardized quantitative assessments of efficacy that take into account both clinical and laboratory parameters (*e.g.,* the Crohn's Disease Activity Index). The disease also exhibits marked fluctuations in activity—even in the absence of therapy—leading to a significant "placebo effect" in therapeutic trials.

Specific goals of pharmacotherapy in IBD include controlling acute exacerbations of the disease, maintaining remission, and treating specific complications such as fistulas. Specific drugs may be better suited for one or the other of these aims (Table 38–1). For example, steroids remain the treatment of choice for moderate to severe flares but are inappropriate for long-term use because of side effects and their inability to maintain remission. Other immunosuppressives, such as *azathioprine,* that require several weeks to achieve their therapeutic effect have a limited role in the acute setting but are preferred for long-term management.

For many years *glucocorticoids* and *sulfasalazine* were the mainstays of medical therapy for IBD. More recently, medicines used in other immune/inflammatory conditions, such as azathioprine and *cyclosporine,* have been adapted for IBD therapy. A more thorough appreciation of the intricacies of the inflammatory response and improved biotechnology have led to the development of biological agents that can target single steps in the immune cascade. Drug delivery to the appropriate site(s) along the gastrointestinal tract also has been a major challenge, and second-generation agents have been created with improved drug delivery, increased efficacy, and decreased side effects.

PATHOGENESIS OF INFLAMMATORY BOWEL DISEASE

Crohn's disease and ulcerative colitis are chronic idiopathic inflammatory disorders of the GI tract; a summary of proposed pathogenic events and potential sites of therapeutic intervention is shown in Figure 38–1. While

Table 38–1
Medications Commonly Used to Treat Inflammatory Bowel Disease

CLASS/Drug	CROHN'S DISEASE					ULCERATIVE COLITIS			
	ACTIVE DISEASE			MAINTENANCE		ACTIVE DISEASE			MAINTENANCE
	Mild–Moderate	Moderate–Severe	Fistula	Medical Remission	Surgical Remission	Distal Colitis	Mild–Moderate	Moderate–Severe	
Mesalamine									
Enema	+[a]	–	–	–	–	+	+[b]	–	+
Oral	+	+	–	+/–	+[c]	+	+	–	+
Antibiotics (metronidazole, ciprofloxacin, others)	+	+	+	?	+[c]	–	–	–	+[c]
Corticosteroids, classic and novel									
Enema, foam, suppository	+[a]	–	–	–	–	+	+[b]	–	–
Oral	+	+	–	–	–	+	+	+	–
Intravenous	–	+	–	–	–	+[d]	–	+	–
Immunomodulators									
6-MP/AZA	–	+	+	+	+[c]	+[d]	–	+[d]	+[d]
Methotrexate	–	+	?	?	?	–	–	–	–
Cyclosporine	–	+[d]	+[d]	–	–	+[d]	–	+[d]	–
Biological response modifiers									
Infliximab	+[d]	+	+	+[c]	?	?	?	?	?

[a]Distal colonic disease only. [b]For adjunctive therapy. [c]Some data to support use; remains controversial. [d]Selected patients. ABBREVIATIONS: 6-MP, 6-mercaptopurine; AZA, azathioprine. From Sands, 1999, with permission.

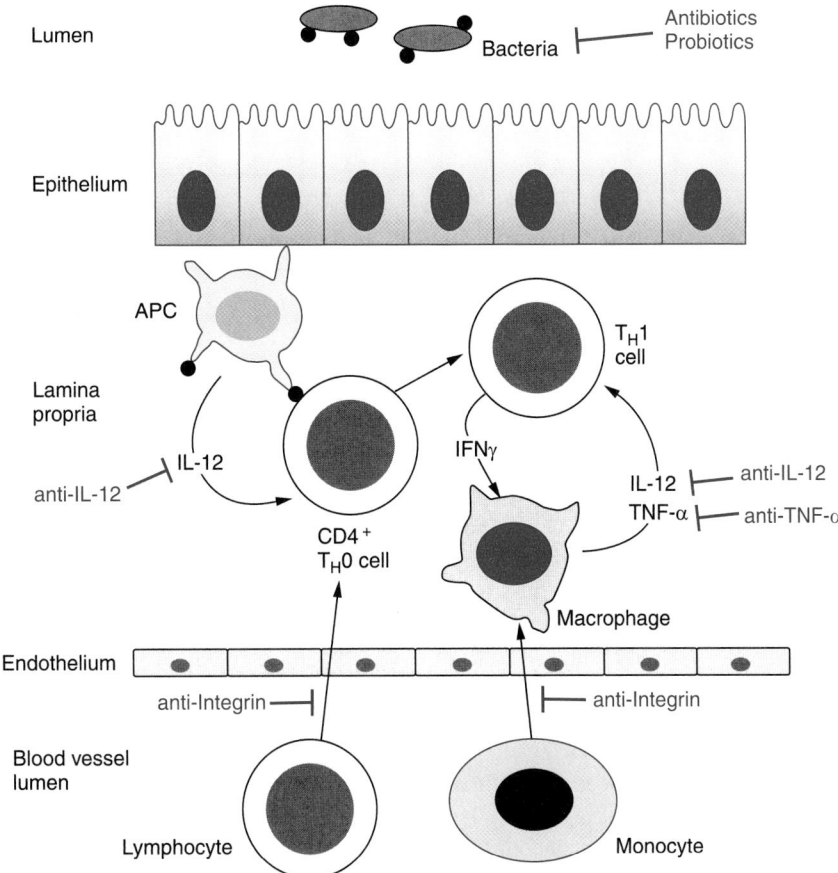

Figure 38–1. ***Proposed pathogenesis of inflammatory bowel disease and target sites for pharmacological intervention.*** Shown are the interactions among bacterial antigens in the intestinal lumen and immune cells in the intestinal wall. If the endothelial barrier is impaired, bacterial antigens (dark circles) can gain access to antigen-presenting cells (APCs) in the lamina propria. These cells then present the antigen(s) to CD4+ lymphocytes and also secrete IL-12, thereby inducing the differentiation of T_H1 cells in Crohn's disease (or type 2 helper T cells in ulcerative colitis). The T_H1 cells produce a characteristic array of lymphokines, including IFN-γ, which in turn activates macrophages. Macrophages positively regulate T_H1 cells by secreting additional IL-12 and TNF-α. In addition to general immunosuppressants that affect multiple sites of inflammation (*e.g.,* glucocorticoids, thioguanine derivatives, methotrexate, and cyclosporine), more specific sites for therapeutic intervention involve the intestinal bacteria (antibiotics and probiotics) and therapy directed at TNF-α (*see* text for further details).

Crohn's disease and ulcerative colitis share a number of gastrointestinal and extraintestinal manifestations and can respond to a similar array of drugs, emerging evidence suggests that they result from fundamentally distinct pathogenetic mechanisms (Bouma and Strober, 2003). Histologically, the transmural lesions in Crohn's disease exhibit marked infiltration of lymphocytes and macrophages, granuloma formation, and submucosal fibrosis, whereas the superficial lesions in ulcerative colitis have lymphocytic and neutrophilic infiltrates. Within the diseased bowel in Crohn's disease, the cytokine profile includes increased levels of interleukin-12 (IL-12), interferon-γ, and tumor necrosis factor-α (TNF-α), findings characteristic of T-helper 1 (T_H1)–mediated inflammatory processes. In contrast, the inflammatory response in ulcerative colitis resembles more closely that mediated by the T_H2 pathway.

Important insights into pathogenesis also have emerged from genetic analyses of Crohn's disease. Mutations in a gene called *nucleotide-binding oligomerization domain-2* (*NOD2,* also called *CARD15*) are associated with both familial and sporadic Crohn's disease in Caucasians (Hugot *et al.*, 2001; Ogura *et al.*, 2001). *NOD2* is expressed in monocytes, granulocytes, dendritic cells, and epithelial cells. It is proposed to function as an intracellular sensor for bacterial infection by recognizing peptidoglycans, thereby playing an important role in the natural immunity to bacterial pathogens. Consistent with this model, other studies have identified bacterial antigens, including pseudomonal protein I2 (Dalwadi *et al.*, 2001) and a flagellin protein (Lodes *et al.*, 2004), as dominant superantigens that induce the T_H1 response in Crohn's disease (shown as bacterial products in Figure 38–1). Thus these converging experimental approaches are generating novel insights into the pathogenesis of Crohn's disease that soon may translate into novel therapeutic approaches to IBD. The major therapeutic agents available for IBD are described below.

MESALAMINE (5-ASA)-BASED THERAPY

Chemistry, Mechanism of Action, and Pharmacological Properties. First-line therapy for mild to moderate ulcerative colitis generally involves *mesalamine* (5-aminosalicylic acid, or 5-ASA). As shown in Figure 38–2, the archetype for this class of medications is sulfasalazine (AZULFIDINE), which consists of 5-ASA linked to *sulfapyridine* by an azo bond. Although this drug was developed originally as therapy for rheumatoid arthritis, clinical trials serendipitously demonstrated a beneficial effect on the gastrointestinal symptoms of subjects with concomitant ulcerative colitis. Sulfasalazine represents one of the first examples of an oral drug that is delivered effectively to the distal gastrointestinal tract. Given individually, either 5-ASA or sulfapyridine is absorbed in the upper gastrointestinal tract; the azo linkage in sulfasalazine prevents absorption in the stomach and small intestine, and the individual components are not liberated for absorption until colonic bacteria cleave the bond. 5-ASA is now regarded as the therapeutic moiety, with little, if any, contribution by sulfapyridine.

Although mesalamine is a salicylate, its therapeutic effect does not appear to be related to cyclooxygenase inhibition; indeed, traditional nonsteroidal antiinflammatory drugs actually may exacerbate IBD. Many potential sites of action have been demonstrated *in vitro* for either sulfasalazine or mesalamine: inhibition of the production of IL-1 and TNF-α, inhibition of the lipoxygenase pathway, scavenging of free radicals and oxidants, and inhibition of NF-κB, a transcription factor pivotal to production of inflammatory mediators. Specific mechanisms of action of these drugs have not been identified.

Although not active therapeutically, sulfapyridine causes many of the side effects observed in patients taking sul-

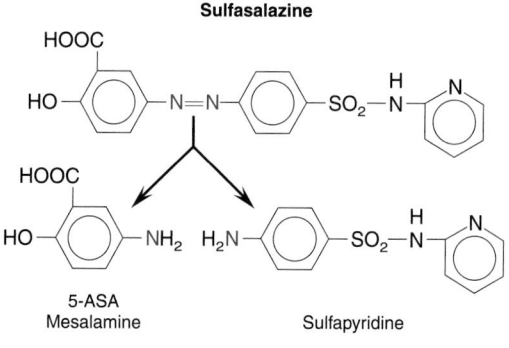

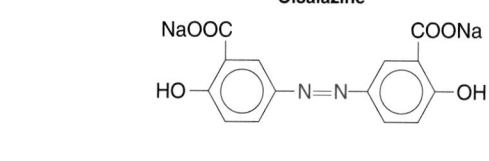

Figure 38–2. *Structures of sulfasalazine and related agents.* The blue N atoms indicate the diazo linkage that is cleaved to generate the active moiety.

fasalazine. To preserve the therapeutic effect of 5-ASA without the side effects of sulfapyridine, several second-generation 5-ASA compounds have been developed (Figures 38–2, 38–3, and 38–4). They are divided into two groups: prodrugs and coated drugs. Prodrugs contain the same azo bond as sulfasalazine but replace the linked sulfapyridine with either another 5-ASA (*olsalazine,* DIPENTUM) or an inert compound (*balsalazide,* COLAZIDE). Thus, these compounds act at similar sites along the gastrointestinal tract as does sulfasalazine. The alternative approaches employ either a delayed-release formulation (PENTASA) or a

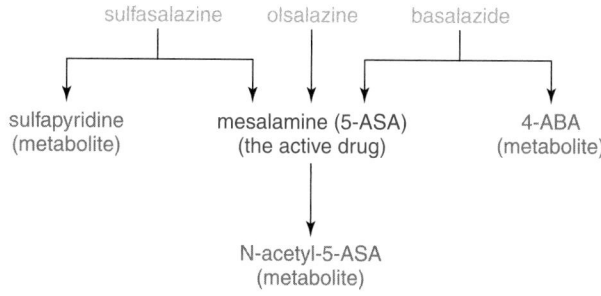

Figure 38–3. *Metabolic fates of the different oral formulations of mesalamine (5-ASA).* Chemical structures are in Figure 38–2.

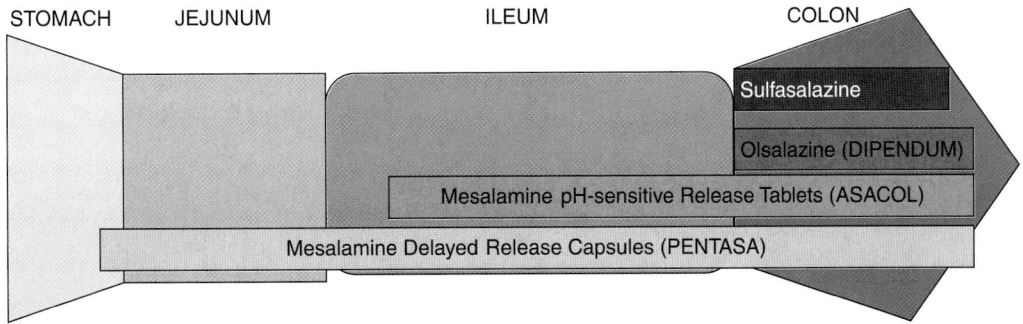

Figure 38–4. *Sites of release of mesalamine (5-ASA) in the GI tract from different oral formulations.*

pH-sensitive coating (ASACOL). Delayed-release mesalamine is released throughout the small intestine and colon, whereas pH-sensitive mesalamine is released in the terminal ileum and colon. These different distributions of drug delivery have potential therapeutic implications.

Oral sulfasalazine is of proven value in patients with mild or moderately active ulcerative colitis, with response rates in the range of 60% to 80% (Prantera *et al.*, 1999). The usual dose is 4 g/day in four divided doses with food; to avoid adverse effects, the dose is increased gradually from an initial dose of 500 mg twice a day. Doses as high as 6 g/day can be used but cause an increased incidence of side effects. For patients with severe colitis, sulfasalazine is of less certain value, even though it is often added as an adjunct to systemic glucocorticoids. Regardless of disease severity, the drug plays a useful role in preventing relapses once remission has been achieved. In general, newer 5-ASA preparations have similar therapeutic efficacy in ulcerative colitis with fewer side effects. Because they lack the dose-related side effects of sulfapyridine, the newer formulations can be used to provide higher doses of mesalamine with some improvement in disease control. The usual doses to treat active disease are 800 mg three times a day for ASACOL and 1 g four times a day for PENTASA. Lower doses are used for maintenance (*e.g.*, ASACOL, 800 mg twice a day). Although some studies have suggested that a given preparation may be superior in treating colonic disease, there is no consensus on this issue.

The efficacy of 5-ASA preparations (*e.g.*, sulfasalazine) in Crohn's disease is less striking, with modest benefit at best in controlled trials. Sulfasalazine has not been shown to be effective in maintaining remission and has been replaced by newer 5-ASA preparations. Some studies have reported that both ASACOL and PENTASA are more effective than placebo in inducing remission in patients with Crohn's disease (particularly colitis), although higher doses than those typically used in ulcerative colitis are required. The role of mesalamine in maintenance therapy for Crohn's disease is controversial, and there is no clear benefit of continued 5-ASA therapy in patients who achieve medical remission (Camma *et al.*, 1997). Because they largely bypass the small intestine, the second-generation 5-ASA prodrugs such as olsalazine and balsalazide do not have a significant effect in small bowel Crohn's disease.

Topical preparations of mesalamine suspended in a wax matrix suppository (ROWASA) or in a suspension enema (CANASA) are effective in active proctitis and distal ulcerative colitis, respectively. They appear to be superior to topical *hydrocortisone* in this setting, with response rates of 75% to 90%. Mesalamine enemas (4 g/60 ml)

should be used at bedtime and retained for at least 8 hours; the suppository (500 mg) should be used two to three times a day with the objective of retaining it for at least 3 hours. Response to local therapy with mesalamine may occur within 3 to 21 days; however, the usual course of therapy is from 3 to 6 weeks. Once remission has occurred, lower doses are used for maintenance.

Pharmacokinetics. Approximately 20% to 30% of orally administered sulfasalazine is absorbed in the small intestine. Much of this is taken up by the liver and excreted unmetabolized in the bile; the rest (about 10%) is excreted unchanged in the urine. The remaining 70% reaches the colon, where, if cleaved completely by bacterial enzymes, it generates 400 mg mesalamine for every gram of the parent compound. Thereafter, the individual components of sulfasalazine follow different metabolic pathways. Sulfapyridine, which is highly lipid-soluble, is absorbed rapidly from the colon. It undergoes extensive hepatic metabolism, including acetylation and hydroxylation, conjugation with glucuronic acid, and excretion in the urine. The acetylation phenotype of the patient determines plasma levels of sulfapyridine and the probability of side effects; rapid acetylators have lower systemic levels of the drug and fewer adverse effects. By contrast, only 25% of mesalamine is absorbed from the colon, and most of the drug is excreted in the stool. The small amount that is absorbed is acetylated in the intestinal mucosal wall and the liver and then excreted in the urine. Intraluminal concentrations of mesalamine therefore are very high (around 1500 μg/ml or 10 mM in patients taking a typical dose of 3 g/day).

The pH-sensitive coating of ASACOL (EUDAGRIT-S) limits gastric and small intestinal absorption of 5-ASA, as assessed by urinary, ileostomal, and fecal measurements of the various metabolites. The pharmacokinetics of PENTASA differ somewhat. The ethylcellulose-coated microgranules are released in the upper gastrointestinal tract as discrete, prolonged-release units of mesalamine. Acetylated mesalamine can be detected in the circulation within an hour after ingestion, indicating some rapid absorption, but some intact microgranules also can be detected in the colon. Because it is released in the small bowel, a greater fraction of PENTASA is absorbed systemically compared with the other 5-ASA preparations.

Adverse Effects. Side effects of sulfasalazine occur in 10% to 45% of patients with ulcerative colitis and are related primarily to the sulfa moiety. Some are dose-related, including headache, nausea, and fatigue. These reactions can be minimized by giving the medication with meals or by decreasing the dose. Allergic reactions include rash, fever, Stevens-Johnson syndrome, hepatitis, pneumonitis, hemolytic anemia, and bone marrow suppression. Sulfasalazine reversibly decreases the number and motility of sperm but does not impair female fertility. It also inhibits intestinal folate absorption; therefore, folate usually is given with sulfasalazine.

The newer mesalamine formulations generally are well tolerated, and side effects are relatively infrequent and minor. Headache, dyspepsia, and skin rash are the most common. Diarrhea appears to be particularly common with olsalazine (occurring in 10% to 20% of patients); this may be related to its ability to stimulate chloride and fluid secretion in the small bowel. Nephrotoxicity, although rare, is a more serious concern. Mesalamine has been associated with interstitial nephritis; while its pathogenic role is controversial, renal function should be monitored in all patients receiving these drugs. Both sulfasalazine and its metabolites cross the placenta but have not been shown to harm the fetus. Although they have not been studied as thoroughly, the newer formulations also appear to be safe in pregnancy. The risks to the fetus from the consequences of uncontrolled IBD in pregnant women are believed to outweigh the risks associated with the therapeutic use of these agents (*see* below).

GLUCOCORTICOIDS

The effects of glucocorticoids on the inflammatory response are numerous and well documented (*see* Chapters 52 and 59). Although glucocorticoids are universally recognized as effective in acute exacerbations, their use in either ulcerative colitis or Crohn's disease involves considerable challenges and pitfalls, and they are indicated only for moderate to severe IBD. Because the same issues have an impact on steroid use in both ulcerative colitis and Crohn's disease, they are addressed together.

The response to steroids in individual patients with IBD divides them into three general classes: steroid-responsive, steroid-dependent, and steroid-unresponsive. Steroid-responsive patients improve clinically, generally within 1 to 2 weeks, and remain in remission as the steroids are tapered and then discontinued. Steroid-dependent patients also respond to glucocorticoids but then experience a relapse of symptoms as the steroid dose is tapered. Steroid-unresponsive patients do not improve even with prolonged high-dose steroids. Approximately 40% of patients are steroid-responsive, 30% to 40% have only a partial response or become steroid-dependent, and 15% to 20% of patients do not respond to steroid therapy.

Steroids sometimes are used for prolonged periods to control symptoms in steroid-dependent patients. However, the failure to respond to steroids with prolonged remission (*i.e.,* a disease relapse) should prompt consideration of alternative therapies, including immunosuppressives and *infliximab* (*see* below). Steroids are not effective in maintaining remission in either ulcerative colitis or Crohn's disease (Steinhart *et al.,* 2003); thus their significant side effects (*see* Chapter 59) have led to increased

emphasis on limiting the duration and cumulative dose of steroids in IBD.

The approach to steroid therapy in IBD differs somewhat from that in diseases such as asthma or rheumatoid arthritis. Initial doses are between 40 to 60 mg *prednisone* or equivalent per day; higher doses generally are no more effective. The glucocorticoid dose in IBD is tapered over weeks to months. Even with these slow tapers, however, efforts should be made to minimize the duration of steroid therapy.

Glucocorticoids induce remission in the majority of patients with either ulcerative colitis or Crohn's disease (Faubion *et al.,* 2001). Oral prednisone is the preferred agent for moderate to severe disease, and the typical dose is 40 to 60 mg once a day. Most patients improve substantially within 5 days of initiating treatment; others require treatment for several weeks before remission occurs. For more severe cases, glucocorticoids are given intravenously. Generally, *methylprednisolone* or *hydrocortisone* is used for intravenous therapy, although some experts believe that *corticotropin* (ACTH) is more effective in patients who have not previously received any steroids.

Glucocorticoid enemas are useful in patients whose disease is limited to the rectum (proctitis) and left colon. Hydrocortisone is available as a retention enema (100 mg/60 ml), and the usual dose is one 60-ml enema per night for 2 or 3 weeks. When administered optimally, the drug can reach up to or beyond the descending colon. Patients with distal disease usually respond within 3 to 7 days. Absorption, while less than with oral preparations, is still substantial (up to 50% to 75%). Hydrocortisone also can be given once or twice daily as a 10% foam suspension (CORTIFOAM) that delivers 80 mg hydrocortisone per application; this formulation can be useful in patients with very short areas of distal proctitis and difficulty retaining fluid.

Budesonide (ENTOCORT ER) is an enteric-release form of a synthetic steroid that is used for ileocecal Crohn's disease (Greenberg *et al.,* 1994; McKeage and Goa, 2002). It is proposed to deliver adequate steroid therapy to a specific portion of inflamed gut while minimizing systemic side effects owing to extensive first-pass hepatic metabolism to inactive derivatives. Topical therapy (*e.g.,* enemas and suppositories) also is effective in treating colitis limited to the left side of the colon. While the topical potency of budesonide is 200 times higher than that of hydrocortisone, its oral systemic bioavailability is only 10%. In some studies, budesonide was associated with a lower incidence of systemic side effects than prednisone, although data also indicate that systemic steroids are more effective in patients with higher Crohn's Disease Activity Index scores. Budesonide (9 mg/day for 10 to 12 weeks) is effective in the acute management of mild-to-moderate exacerbations of Crohn's disease, but its role in maintaining remission has not been fully delineated (Hofer, 2003).

A significant number of patients with IBD fail to respond adequately to glucocorticoids and are either steroid-resistant or steroid-dependent. The reasons for this failure are poorly understood but may involve complications such as fibrosis or strictures in Crohn's disease, which will not respond to antiinflammatory measures alone; local complications such as abscesses, in which case the use of steroids may lead to uncontrolled sepsis; and intercurrent infections with organisms such as cytomegalovirus and *Clostridium difficile*. Steroid failures also may be related to specific pharmacogenomic factors such as up-regulation of the multidrug resistance (*mdr*) gene (Farrell *et al.*, 2000) or altered levels of corticosteroid-binding globulin.

IMMUNOSUPPRESSIVE AGENTS

Several drugs developed initially for cancer chemotherapy or as immunosuppressive agents in organ transplants have been adapted for treatment of IBD. While their initial use in IBD was based on their immunosuppressive effects, their specific mechanisms of action are unknown. Increasing clinical experience has defined specific roles for each of these medicines as mainstays in the pharmacotherapy of IBD. However, both real and potential side effects mandate a careful assessment of potential risks and benefits in each patient.

Thiopurine Derivatives

The cytotoxic thiopurine derivatives *mercaptopurine* (6-MP, PURINETHOL) and azathioprine (IMMURAN) (*see* Chapters 51 and 52) are used to treat patients with severe IBD or those who are steroid-resistant or steroid-dependent (Pearson *et al.*, 1995). These thiopurine antimetabolites impair purine biosynthesis and inhibit cell proliferation. Both are prodrugs: Azathioprine is converted to mercaptopurine, which is subsequently metabolized to 6-thioguanine nucleotides that are the presumed active moiety (Figure 38–5). These drugs generally are used interchangeably with appropriate dose adjustments, typically azathioprine (2 to 2.5 mg/kg) or mercaptopurine (1.5 mg/kg). As discussed below, the pathways by which they are metabolized are clinically relevant, and specific assays can be used to assess clinical response and to avoid side effects. Because of concerns about side effects, these drugs were used initially only in Crohn's disease, which lacks a surgical curative option. They now are considered equally effective in Crohn's disease and ulcerative colitis. These drugs effectively maintain remission in both diseases; they also may prevent (or, more typically, delay) recurrence of Crohn's disease after surgical resection. Finally, they are used successfully to treat fistulas in Crohn's disease. The clinical response to azathioprine or mercaptopurine may take weeks to months, such that other drugs with a more rapid onset of action (*e.g.,* mesalamine, glucocorticoids, or infliximab) are preferred in the acute setting.

The decision to initiate immunosuppressive therapy depends on an accurate assessment of the risk/benefit ratio. In general, physicians who treat IBD believe that the long-term risks of azathioprine–mercaptopurine are lower than those of steroids. Thus, these purines are

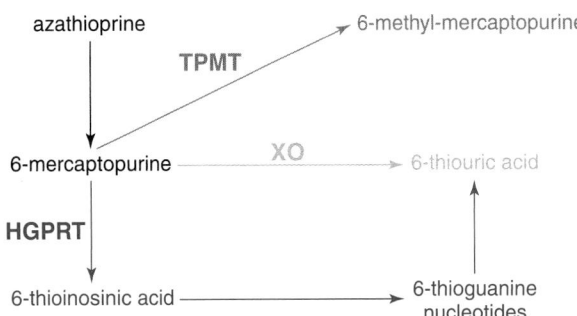

Figure 38–5. *Metabolism of azathioprine and 6-mercaptopurine.* TPMT = thiopurine methyltransferase; XO = xanthine oxidase; HGPRT = hypoxanthine–guanine phosphoribosyl transferase. The activities of these enzymes vary among humans because genetic polymorphisms are expressed differentially, explaining responses and side effects when azathioprine–mercaptopurine therapy is employed. *See* text for details.

used in steroid-unresponsive or steroid-dependent disease and in patients who have had recurrent flares of disease requiring repeated courses of steroids. Additionally, patients who have not responded adequately to mesalamine but are not acutely ill may benefit by conversion from glucocorticoids to immunosuppressive drugs. Immunosuppressives therefore may be viewed as steroid-sparing agents.

Adverse effects of azathioprine–mercaptopurine can be divided into three general categories: idiosyncratic, dose-related, and possible. Although the therapeutic effects of azathioprine–mercaptopurine often are delayed, their side effects occur at any time after initiation of treatment and can affect up to 10% of patients. The most serious idiosyncratic reaction is pancreatitis, which affects approximately 5% of patients treated with these drugs. Fever, rash, and arthralgias are seen occasionally, whereas nausea and vomiting are somewhat more frequent. The major dose-related side effect is bone marrow suppression, and circulating blood counts should be monitored closely when therapy is initiated and at less frequent intervals during maintenance therapy (*e.g.,* every 3 months). Elevations in liver function tests also may be dose-related. Although keeping drug levels in the appropriate range diminishes these adverse effects, they can occur even with therapeutic serum levels of 6-thioguanine nucleotides. The serious side effect of cholestatic hepatitis is relatively rare. Although the increased risk of infection is a significant concern with immunosuppressives, especially if pancytopenia occurs, infections are linked more closely to concomitant glucocorticoid therapy than to the immunosuppressives (Aberra *et al.*, 2003).

There is some concern that the immunosuppressive agents may increase the risk of hematological malignancies. Immunosuppressive regimens given in the setting of cancer chemotherapy or organ transplants have been associated with an increased incidence of malignancy, particularly non-Hodgkin's lymphoma. Definitive conclusions about the causative roles of azathioprine–mercaptopurine in lymphomas are complicated by the possible increased incidence of lymphomas in IBD *per se* and by the relative rarity of these cancers. The increased risk, if any, must be relatively small.

Pharmacogenetics. Favorable responses to azathioprine–mercaptopurine are seen in up to two-thirds of patients.

Recent insights into the metabolism of the thiopurine agents and appreciation of genetic polymorphisms in these pathways have provided new insights into variability in response rates and side effects. As shown in Figure 38–4, mercaptopurine has three metabolic fates: (1) conversion by xanthine oxidase to 6-thiouric acid; (2) metabolism by thiopurine methyltransferase (TPMT) to 6-methyl-mercaptopurine (6-MMP); and (3) conversion by hypoxanthine–guanine phosphoribosyl transferase (HGPRT) to 6-thioguanine nucleotides and other metabolites. The relative activities of these different pathways may explain, in part, individual variations in efficacy and side effects of these immunosuppressives.

The plasma half-life of mercaptopurine is limited by its relatively rapid (*i.e.,* within 1 to 2 hours) uptake into erythrocytes and other tissues. Following this uptake, differences in TPMT activity determine the drug's fate. Approximately 80% of the United States population has what is considered "normal" metabolism, whereas one in 300 individuals has minimal TPMT activity. In the latter setting, mercaptopurine metabolism is shifted away from 6-methyl-mercaptopurine and driven toward 6-thioguanine nucleotides, which can severely suppress the bone marrow. About 10% of people have intermediate TPMT activity; given a similar dose, these individuals will tend to have higher 6-thioguanine levels than the normal metabolizers. Finally, approximately 10% of the population is considered rapid metabolizers. In these individuals, mercaptopurine is shunted away from 6-thioguanine nucleotides toward 6-MMP, which has been associated with abnormal liver function tests. In addition, relative to normal metabolizers, the 6-thioguanine levels of these rapid metabolizers are lower for an equivalent oral dose, possibly reducing therapeutic response. Given this variability, some experts evaluate an individual's TPMT activity status prior to initiating treatment with thiopurines and also measure 6-thioguanine/6-MMP levels in individuals not responding to therapy. To avoid these complexities, treatment with 6-thioguanine was explored; unfortunately, 6-thioguanine is associated with a high incidence of an uncommon liver abnormality, hepatic nodular regeneration, and associated portal hypertension; 6-thioguanine therapy of IBD therefore has been abandoned.

Xanthine oxidase in the small intestine and liver converts mercaptopurine to thiouric acid, which is inactive as an immunosuppressive. Inhibition of xanthine oxidase by *allopurinol* diverts mercaptopurine to more active metabolites such as 6-thioguanine and increases both immunosuppressive and potential toxic effects. Thus patients on mercaptopurine should be warned about potentially serious interactions with medications used to treat gout or hyperuricemia, and the dose should be decreased to 25% of the standard dose in subjects who are already taking allopurinol.

Methotrexate

Methotrexate was engineered to inhibit dihydrofolate reductase, thereby blocking DNA synthesis and causing cell death. First used in cancer treatment, methotrexate subsequently was recognized to have beneficial effects in autoimmune diseases such as rheumatoid arthritis and psoriasis (*see* Chapter 62 for a discussion of the use of methotrexate in dermatologic disorders). The antiinflammatory effects of methotrexate may involve mechanisms in addition to inhibition of dihydrofolate reductase.

As with azathioprine–mercaptopurine, methotrexate generally is reserved for patients whose IBD is either steroid-resistant or steroid-dependent. In Crohn's disease, it both induces and maintains remission, generally with a more rapid response than that seen with mercaptopurine or azathioprine (Feagin *et al.,* 1995). Only limited studies have examined the role of methotrexate in ulcerative colitis.

Therapy of IBD with methotrexate differs somewhat from its use in other autoimmune diseases. Most important, higher doses (*e.g.,* 15 to 25 mg/week) are given parenterally. The increased efficacy with parenteral administration may reflect the unpredictable intestinal absorption at higher doses of methotrexate. For unknown reasons, the incidence of methotrexate-induced hepatic fibrosis in patients with IBD is lower than that seen in patients with psoriasis.

Cyclosporine

The calcineurin inhibitor cyclosporine is a potent immunomodulator used most frequently after organ transplantation (*see* Chapter 52). It is effective in specific clinical settings in IBD, but the high frequency of significant adverse effects limits its use as a first-line medication.

Cyclosporine is effective in severe ulcerative colitis that has failed to respond adequately to glucocorticoid therapy. Between 50% and 80% of these severely ill patients improve significantly (generally within 7 days) in response to intravenous cyclosporine (2 to 4 mg/kg per day), sometimes avoiding emergent colectomy. Careful monitoring of cyclosporine levels is necessary to maintain a therapeutic level in whole blood between 300 and 400 ng/ml.

Oral cyclosporine is less effective as maintenance therapy in IBD, perhaps because of its limited intestinal absorption. In this setting, long-term therapy with NEORAL (a microemulsion formulation of cyclosporine with increased oral bioavailability) may be more effective, but this has not been studied fully. The calcineurin inhibitors can be used to treat fistulous complications of Crohn's disease. A significant, rapid response to intravenous cyclosporine has been observed; however, frequent relapses accompany oral cyclosporine therapy, and other medical strategies are required to maintain fistula closure. Thus the calcineurin inhibitors generally are used to treat specific problems over a short term while providing a bridge to longer-term therapy (Sandborn, 1995).

Other immunomodulators are also being evaluated in IBD include *tacrolimus* (FK 506, PROGRAF) and *mycophenolate mofetil* (CELLCEPT) (*see* Chapter 52).

ANTI-TNF THERAPY

Infliximab (REMICADE, cA2), a chimeric immunoglobulin (25% mouse, 75% human) that binds to and neutralizes TNF-α, represents a new class of therapeutic agents for treating IBD (Targan *et al.,* 1997). Although a great many of both pro- and antiinflammatory cytokines are generated in the inflamed gut in IBD (Figure 38–1), there is some rationale for targeting TNF-α because it is one of the principal cytokines mediating the T_H1 immune response characteristic of Crohn's disease.

Infliximab (5 mg/kg infused intravenously at intervals of several weeks to months) decreases the frequency of acute flares in approximately two-thirds of patients with moderate to severe Crohn's disease and also facilitates the closing of enterocutaneous fistulas associated with Crohn's disease (Present *et al.*, 1999). Its longer-term role in Crohn's disease is evolving, but emerging evidence supports its efficacy in maintaining remission (Rutgeerts *et al.*, 2004) and in preventing recurrence of fistulas (Sands *et al.*, 2004).

Although infliximab was designed specifically to target TNF-α, it also may have more complex actions. *Etaneracept,* another anti-TNF-α therapy that uses a circulating receptor to clear soluble TNF-α, blocks its biologic effects but is ineffective in Crohn's disease. Infliximab binds membrane-bound TNF-α and may cause lysis of these cells by antibody-dependent or cell-mediated cytotoxicity. Thus, infliximab may deplete specific populations of subepithelial inflammatory cells. These effects, together with its mean terminal plasma half-life of 8 to 10 days, may explain the prolonged clinical effects of infliximab.

The use of infliximab as a biologic response modifier raises several important considerations. Both acute (fever, chills, urticaria, or even anaphylaxis) and subacute (serum sickness–like) reactions may develop after infliximab infusion. Anti–double-stranded DNA antibodies develop in 9% of patients, but a frank lupus-like syndrome occurs only rarely. Antibodies to infliximab can decrease its clinical efficacy; strategies to minimize the development of these antibodies (*e.g.,* treatment with glucocorticoids or other immunosuppressives) may be critical to preserving infliximab efficacy for either recurrent or chronic therapy (Farrell *et al.*, 2003). Other proposed strategies to overcome the problem of "antibody resistance" include increasing the dose of infliximab or decreasing the interval between infusions.

Infliximab therapy is associated with increased incidence of respiratory infections; of particular concern is potential reactivation of tuberculosis or other granulomatous infections with subsequent dissemination. The FDA recommends that candidates for infliximab therapy should be tested for latent tuberculosis with purified protein derivative, and patients who test positive should be treated prophylactically with *isoniazid.* However, anergy with a false-negative skin test has been noted in some patients with Crohn's disease, and some experts routinely perform chest radiographs to look for active or latent pulmonary disease. Infliximab also is contraindicated in patients with severe congestive heart failure (New York Heart Association classes III and IV) and should be used cautiously in class I or II patients. As with the immunosuppressives, there is concern about the possible increased incidence of non-Hodgkin's lymphoma, but a causal role has not been established. Finally, the significant cost of infliximab is an important consideration in some patients.

Additional anti-TNF therapies are being evaluated in treating Crohn's disease, including a more humanized monoclonal antibody (CDP571) that should be less antigenic, and *thalidomide* (THALOMID), a drug with significant anti-TNF-α effects (*see* Chapter 52). Despite the fact that ulcerative colitis does not appear to have a T_H1-type immune response mediated through TNF-α, some studies have shown a beneficial effect of TNF-α modulation in this disorder as well. Clearly, this area of IBD therapy is evolving rapidly as new drugs emerge and clinical experience increases.

ANTIBIOTICS AND PROBIOTICS

An emerging concept is that a balance in the gastrointestinal tract normally exists among the mucosal epithelium, the normal gut flora, and the immune response (McCracken and Lorenz, 2001). Moreover, there are experimental and clinical data that colonic bacteria may either initiate or perpetuate the inflammation of IBD (Sartor, 1999), and—as discussed earlier under "Pathogenesis of Inflammatory Bowel Disease"—recent studies have implicated specific bacterial antigens in the pathogenesis of Crohn's disease. Thus, certain bacterial strains may be either pro- (*e.g., Bacteroides*) or antiinflammatory (*e.g., Lactobacillus*), prompting attempts to manipulate the colonic flora in patients with IBD. Traditionally, antibiotics have been used to this end, most prominently in Crohn's disease. More recently, probiotics have been used to treat specific clinical situations in inflammatory bowel disease (*see* below).

Antibiotics can be used as either (1) adjunctive treatment along with other medications for active inflammatory bowel disease; (2) treatment for a specific complication of Crohn's disease; or (3) prophylaxis for recurrence in postoperative Crohn's disease. *Metronidazole* (Sutherland *et al.*, 1991), *ciprofloxacin* (Arnold *et al.*, 2002), and *clarithromycin* are the antibiotics used most frequently. They are more beneficial in Crohn's disease involving the colon than in disease restricted to the ileum. Specific Crohn's disease–related complications that may benefit from antibiotic therapy include intra-abdominal abscess and inflammatory masses, perianal disease (including fistulas and perirectal abscesses), small bowel bacterial overgrowth secondary to partial small bowel obstruction, secondary infections with organisms such as *C. difficile,* and postoperative complications. Metronidazole may be particularly effective for the treatment of perianal disease. Postoperatively, metronidazole and related compounds have been shown to delay the recurrence of Crohn's disease. In one study, a 3-month course of metronidazole (20 mg/kg per day) prolonged the time to both endoscopic and clinical recurrence (Rutgeerts *et al.*, 1995). The significant side effects of prolonged systemic antibiotic use must be balanced against their potential benefits, and definitive data to support their routine use are lacking.

Probiotics are a mixture of putatively beneficial lyophilized bacteria given orally. Although probiotics are a promising alternative to more conventional therapies for inflammatory bowel disease, their role in treating ulcerative colitis and Crohn's disease requires further evaluation. In one study, probiotics diminished the occurrence of pouchitis, a common inflammatory condition that occurs in surgically created ileal reservoirs after total proctocolectomy for ulcerative colitis (Gionchetti *et al.*, 2003).

SUPPORTIVE THERAPY IN INFLAMMATORY BOWEL DISEASE

Analgesic, anticholinergic, and antidiarrheal agents play supportive roles in reducing symptoms and improving quality of life. These drugs should be individualized based on a patient's symptoms and are supplementary to antiinflammatory medications. Oral *iron, folate,* and *vitamin B*$_{12}$ should be administered as indicated. *Loperamide* or *diphenoxylate* (*see* Chapter 37) can be used to reduce the frequency of bowel movements and relieve rectal urgency in patients with mild disease; these agents are contraindicated in patients with severe disease because they may predispose to the development of toxic megacolon. *Cholestyramine* can be used to prevent bile salt–induced colonic secretion in patients who have undergone limited ileocolic resections. Anticholinergic agents (*dicyclomine hydrochloride,* etc.; *see* Chapter 7) are used to reduce abdominal cramps, pain, and rectal urgency. As with the antidiarrheal agents, they are contraindicated in severe disease or when obstruction is suspected. Care should be taken to differentiate exacerbation of IBD from symptoms that may be related to coexistent functional bowel disease (*see* Chapter 37).

THERAPY OF INFLAMMATORY BOWEL DISEASE DURING PREGNANCY

IBD is a chronic disease that affects women in their reproductive years; thus the issue of pregnancy often has a significant impact on medical management. The effects of IBD on pregnancy and the effects of pregnancy on IBD are beyond the scope of this chapter. In general, decreased disease activity increases fertility and improves pregnancy outcomes. At the same time, limiting medication during pregnancy is always desired but sometimes conflicts with the goal of controlling the disease.

Mesalamine and glucocorticoids are FDA category B drugs that are used frequently in pregnancy and generally are considered safe, whereas methotrexate is clearly contraindicated in pregnant patients. The use of thiopurine immunosuppressives is more controversial. Because these medications are given long term, both their initiation and discontinuation are major management decisions. Although there are no controlled trials of these medications in pregnancy, considerable experience has emerged over the last several years. There does not appear to be an increase in adverse outcomes in pregnant patients maintained on thiopurine-based immunosuppressives (Francella *et al.*, 2003). Nonetheless, decisions regarding the use of these

medications in patients contemplating pregnancy are complex and necessarily must involve consideration of the risks and benefits involved.

CLINICAL SUMMARY

The treatment of IBD in any given patient may have several different goals, such as relief of symptoms, induction of remission in patients with active disease, prevention of relapse (*i.e.,* maintenance therapy), healing of fistulas, and avoidance of emergent surgery. Further, therapy may be tailored to some extent to the severity and location of disease. Acute exacerbations of ulcerative colitis are treated with colonic-release preparations of 5-ASA and, in most patients with significant inflammation, with glucocorticoids. For milder cases involving only the rectum, these drugs may be given topically (by enema). Maintenance therapy for patients with ulcerative colitis is principally in the form of 5-ASA compounds, which generally are effective and safe. In patients who relapse on these preparations, purine metabolites (*e.g.,* azathioprine–mercaptopurine) may be used. Other approaches being tested in this setting include the use of probiotic bacteria.

Drugs used in mild-to-moderately active Crohn's disease include sulfasalazine, budesonide, and oral corticosteroids. In contrast to their use in ulcerative colitis, the role of 5-ASA preparations in maintenance therapy of Crohn's disease is limited. Patients who relapse frequently may be treated with immunosuppressive agents (azathioprine–mercaptopurine or methotrexate). Steroid-dependent patients may be treated with long-term budesonide. Infliximab is particularly useful in closing fistulas associated with Crohn's disease but increasingly is used in acute flares of this condition. Its role in maintaining patients in remission is being evaluated but must be balanced against the risk of side effects. Antibiotics, particularly metronidazole, may be useful adjuncts for the acute treatment of complications associated with Crohn's disease (including perianal disease) but are not established as a routine therapy in this disorder.

BIBLIOGRAPHY

Aberra, F.N., Lewis, J.D., Hass, D., *et al.* Corticosteroids and immunomodulators: postoperative infectious complication risk in inflammatory bowel disease. *Gastroenterology* **2003**, *125*:320–327.

Arnold G.L., Beaves, M.R., Pryjdun, V.O., and Mook, W.J. Preliminary study of ciprofloxacin in active Crohn's disease. *Inflamm. Bowel Dis.* **2002**, 8:10–15.

Bouma G., and Strober W. The immunological and genetic basis of inflammatory bowel disease. *Nature Rev. Immunol.* **2003**, *3*:521–533.

Camma, C., Giunta, M., Rosselli, M., and Cottone, M. Mesalamine in the maintenance treatment of Crohn's disease: A meta-analysis adjusted for confounding variables. *Gastroenterology* **1997**, *113*:1465–1473.

Dalwadi, H., Wei, B., Kronenberg, M., Sutton, C.L., and Braun, J. The Crohn's disease–associated bacterial protein I2 is a novel enteric T-cell superantigen. *Immunity* **2001**, *15*:149–158.

Farrell, R.J., Murphy, A., Long, A., *et al.* High multidrug resistance (P-glycoprotein 170) expression in inflammatory bowel disease patients who fail medical therapy. *Gastroenterology* **2000**, *118*:279–288.

Farrell, R.J., Alsahli, M., Jeen, Y.T., *et al.* Intravenous hydrocortisone premedication reduces antibodies to infliximab in Crohn's disease: A randomized, controlled trial. *Gastroenterology* **2003**, *124*:917–924.

Faubion, W.A., Jr., Loftus, E.V., Harmsen, W.S., Zinmeister, A.R., and Sandborn, W.J. The natural history of corticosteroid therapy for inflammatory bowel disease: A population-based study. *Gastroenterology* **2001**, *121*:255–260.

Feagan, B.G., Rochon, J., Fedorak, R.N., *et al.* Methotrexate for the treatment of Crohn's disease. *New. Eng. J. Med.* **1995**, 332:292-297.

Francella, A., Dyan, A., Bodian C., *et al.* The safety of 6-mercaptopurine for childbearing patients with inflammatory bowel disease: A retrospective cohort study. *Gastroenterology* **2003**, *124*:9–17.

Gionchetti, P., Rizzello, F., Helwig, U., *et. al.* Prophylaxis of pouchitis onset with probiotic therapy, a double-blind, placebo-controlled trial. *Gastroenterology* **2003**, *124*:1202–1209.

Greenberg, G.R., Feagan, B.R., Martin, F., *et al.* Oral budesonide for active Crohn's disease. *New Eng. J. Med.* **1994**, *331*:836–841.

Hofer, K.N. Oral budesonide in management of Crohn's disease. *Ann. Pharmacother.* **2003**, *37*:1457–1464.

Hugot, J.P., Chamaillard, M., Zouali, H. *et al.* Association of NOD2 leucine-rich repeat variants with susceptibility to Crohn's disease. *Nature* **2001**, *411*:599–603.

Lodes, M.J., Cong, Y., Elson, C.O. *et al.* Bacterial flagellin is a dominant antigen in Crohn's disease. *J. Clin. Invest.* **2004**, *113*:1296–1306.

McCracken, V.J., and Lorenz, R.G. The gastrointestinal ecosystem: A precarious alliance among epithelium, immunity, and microbiota. *Cell Microbiol.* **2001**, *3*:1–11.

McKeage, K., and Goa, K.L. Budesonide (ENTOCORT EC capsules). *Drugs* **2002**, *62*:2263–2282.

Ogura, Y., Bonen, D.K., Inohara N. *et al.* A frameshift mutation in *NOD2* associated with susceptibility to Crohn's disease. *Nature* **2001**, *411*:603–606.

Pearson, D.C., May, G.R., Fick, G.H., and Sutherland, L.R. Azathioprine and mercaptopurine in Crohn's disease: A meta-analysis. *Ann. Intern. Med.* **1995**, *123*:132–142.

Prantera, C., Cottone, M., Pallone, F., *et al.* Mesalamine in the treatment of mild to moderate active Crohn's ileitis: Results of a randomized, multicenter trial. *Gastroenterology* **1999**, *116*:521–526.

Present, D.H., Rutgeerts, P., Targan, S., *et al.* Infliximab for the treatment of fistulas in patients with Crohn's disease. *New Eng. J. Med.* **1999**, *340*:1398–1405.

Rutgeerts, P., Hiele, M., Geboes, K., *et al.* Controlled trial of metronidazole treatment for prevention of Crohn's recurrence after ileal resection. *Gastroenterology* **1995**, *108*:1617–1621.

Rutgeerts, P., Feagan, B.F., Lichtenstein, G.R., *et al.* Comparison of scheduled and episodic treatment strategies of infliximab in Crohn's disease. *Gastroenterology* **2004**, *126*:402–413.

Sandborn. W.J. A critical review of cyclosporine therapy in inflammatory bowel disease. *Inflamm. Bowel Dis.* **1995**, *1*:48–63.

Sands, B.E., Anderson, F.H., Bernstein, C.N. *et al.* Infliximab maintenance therapy for fistulizing Crohn's disease. *New Engl. J. Med.* **2004**, *350*:876–885.

Sartor, R.B. Microbial factors in the pathogenesis of Crohn's disease, ulcerative colitis and experimental intestinal inflammation. In: *Inflammatory Bowel Disease,* 5th ed. (Kirsner, J.B., Hanauer, S., eds.) Saunders, Philadelphia, **1999**, pp. 153–178.

Steinhart, A.H., Ewe, K., Griffiths, A.M., Modigliani, R., and Thomsen, O.O. Corticosteroids for maintenance of remission in Crohn's disease. *Cochrane Database Syst. Rev.* **2003**, CD000301.

Sutherland, L., Singleton, J., Sessions, J. *et al.* Double blind, placebo-controlled trial of metronidazole in Crohn's disease. *Gut* **1991**, *32*:1071–1075.

Targan, S.R., Hanauer, S.B., van Deventer, S.J., *et al.* A short-term study of chimeric monoclonal antibody cA2 to tumor necrosis factor alpha for Crohn's disease. *New Eng. J. Med.* **1997**, *337*:1029–1035.

CHEMOTHERAPY OF PROTOZOAL INFECTIONS
Malaria

Theresa A. Shapiro and Daniel E. Goldberg

Malaria, especially that caused by *Plasmodium falciparum*, is the world's most devastating human parasitic infection. Malaria afflicts nearly 500 million people and causes some 2 million deaths each year (Breman, 2001). Infection with *P. falciparum*, which preferentially affects children younger than 5 years of age, pregnant women, and nonimmune individuals, is responsible for nearly all this mortality. Although mosquito-transmitted malaria now is rare in North America, Europe, and Russia, its increasing prevalence in many other parts of the world poses a major international health and economic burden and a serious risk to travelers from nonendemic areas.

Inexpensive and safe drugs, insecticides, and ultimately, vaccines still are needed to combat malaria. In the 1950s, attempts to eradicate this scourge failed primarily because of the development of resistance to insecticides. Since 1960, transmission of malaria has risen in most regions where the infection is endemic, drug-resistant strains of *P. falciparum* have spread, and the degree of drug resistance has increased. More recently, chloroquine-resistant strains of *P. vivax* also have been documented.

The discovery by Trager and Jensen of techniques for continuous maintenance of *P. falciparum in vitro* led to practical assays to screen for antimalarial drug candidates.

This important advance, together with the availability of the sequence of the entire *P. falciparum* genome (Gardner *et al.*, 2002), is revealing new molecular targets for antimalarial drug action and for vaccine development. To understand the actions and therapeutic uses of antimalarial drugs, it is essential to know the biology of the malaria parasite in humans.

BIOLOGY OF MALARIAL INFECTION

Nearly all human malaria is caused by four species of obligate intracellular protozoa of the genus *Plasmodium*. Although malaria can be transmitted by transfusion of infected blood, congenitally, and by sharing needles, infection usually is transmitted by the bite of infected female *Anopheline* mosquitoes. Sporozoites from the mosquito salivary glands rapidly enter the circulation after a bite and localize *via* specific recognition events in hepatocytes, where they transform, multiply, and develop into tissue schizonts (Figure 39–1). This primary asymptomatic tissue (preerythrocytic or exoerythrocytic) stage of infection lasts for 5 to 15 days, depending on the *Plasmodium* species. Tissue schizonts then rupture, each

releasing thousands of merozoites that enter the circulation, invade erythrocytes, and initiate the erythrocytic
cycle. Once the tissue schizonts burst in *P. falciparum* and
P. malariae infections, no forms of the parasite remain in
the liver. However, in *P. vivax* and *P. ovale* infections,
tissue parasites (hypnozoites) persist that can produce
relapses of erythrocytic infection months to years after the
primary attack. Once plasmodia enter the erythrocytic
cycle, they cannot reinvade the liver; thus, there is no tissue stage of infection for malaria contracted by transfusion. In erythrocytes, most parasites undergo asexual
development from young ring forms to trophozoites and
finally to mature schizonts. Schizont-containing erythrocytes rupture, each releasing 6 to 32 merozoites depending on the *Plasmodium* species. It is this process that produces febrile clinical attacks. The merozoites invade more
erythrocytes to continue the cycle, which proceeds until
death of the host or modulation by drugs or acquired partial immunity. The periodicity of parasitemia and febrile
clinical manifestations depends on the timing of schizogo-
ny of a generation of erythrocytic parasites. For *P. falciparum, P. vivax,* and *P. ovale,* it takes about 48 hours to
complete this process; for *P. malariae,* about 72 hours is
required.

For erythrocyte invasion, merozoites bind to specific ligands
on the red cell surface (*see* Miller *et al.*, 2002; Sibley, 2004). *P.
falciparum* has a family of binding proteins that can recognize a
number of host cell molecules, including glycophorins A, B, and
C, as well as band 3. It is able to invade all stages of erythrocytes
and therefore can achieve high parasitemias. *P. vivax* is more
selective in its binding; it needs to recognize the Duffy chemokine
receptor protein as well as reticulocyte-specific proteins; thus, it
will not establish infection in Duffy-negative individuals and will
only invade reticulocytes. Because of this restricted subpopulation
of suitable erythrocytes, *P. vivax* rarely exceeds 1% parasitemia in
the bloodstream. *P. ovale* is similar to *P. vivax* in its predilection
for young red blood cells, but the mechanism of its erythrocyte
recognition is unknown. *P. malariae* recognizes only senescent red
cells, maintains a very low parasitemia, and typically causes an
indolent infection.

P. falciparum assembles cytoadherence proteins (the PfEMPs
encoded by a highly variable family of *var* genes) into structures
called *knobs* on the erythrocyte surface. This allows the parasitized
erythrocyte to bind to the vascular endothelium, to avoid the spleen,
and to grow in a lower oxygen environment. For the patient, the
consequences are microvascular blockage in the brain and organ
beds and local release of cytokines and direct vascular mediators
such as nitric oxide, leading to cerebral malaria (*see* Craig and
Scherf, 2001, and Miller *et al.*, 2002, for reviews).

Some erythrocytic parasites differentiate into sexual forms
known as *gametocytes*. After infected blood is ingested by a
female mosquito, exflagellation of the male gametocyte is followed by fertilization of the female gametocyte in the insect gut.
The resulting zygote, which develops as an oocyst in the gut wall,
eventually gives rise to sporozoites, which invade the salivary

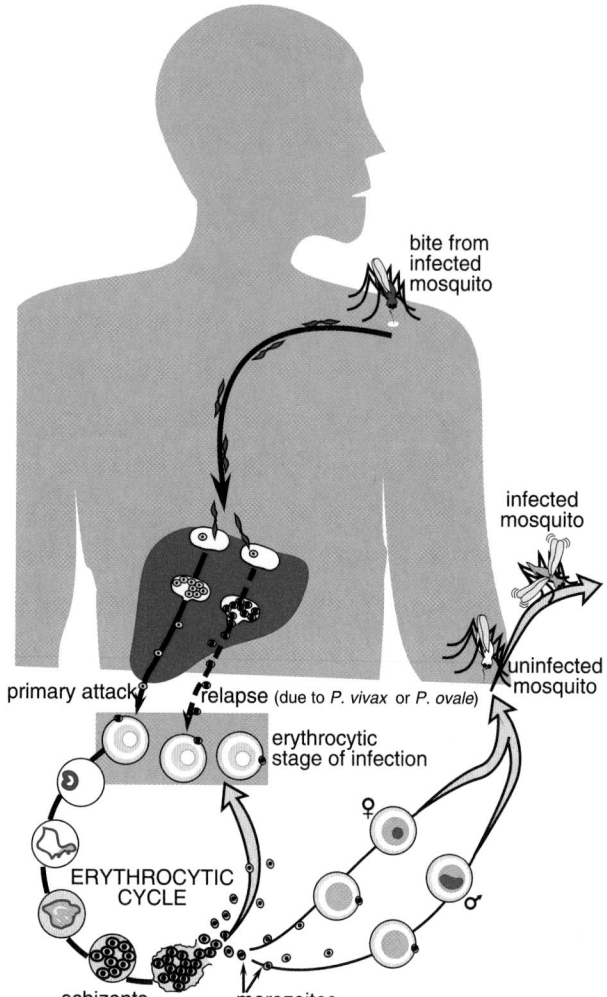

Figure 39–1. *Life cycle of malaria parasites.*

gland of the mosquito. The insect then can infect a human host by
taking a blood meal.

Symptomatic malaria is typified by high spiking fevers that may
have a periodic pattern (*see* above), chills, headache, myalgias, malaise, and gastrointestinal symptoms. In addition, each *Plasmodium*
species causes a distinct illness: (1) *P. falciparum* is the most dangerous. By invading erythrocytes of any age, sequestering in the
vasculature, and producing endotoxin-like products, this species can
cause an overwhelming parasitemia, hypoglycemia, and shock with
multiorgan failure. Delay in treatment may lead to death. If treated
early, the infection usually responds within 48 hours. If treatment is
inadequate, *recrudescence* of infection may result. (2) *P. vivax*
infection has a low mortality rate in untreated adults and is characterized by relapses caused by the reactivation of latent tissue forms.
(3) *P. ovale* causes a malarial infection with a periodicity and
relapses similar to those of *P. vivax,* but it is milder. (4) *P. malariae*
causes a generally indolent infection that is common in localized
areas of the tropics. Clinical attacks may occur years or decades
after infection.

CLASSIFICATION OF ANTIMALARIAL AGENTS

Antimalarials can be categorized by the stage of the parasite that they affect and by their intended use for either prophylaxis or treatment. The various stages of the malaria life cycle that occur in humans differ from one another not only in their morphology and metabolism but also in their drug sensitivity. For this reason, the classification of antimalarial drugs is best done in the context of the life cycle (Figure 39–2).

The tabulated spectrum of activity leads to several generalizations. The first relates to prophylaxis: *Since none of the drugs kills sporozoites, it is not truly possible to prevent infection but only to prevent the development of symptomatic malaria caused by the asexual erythrocytic forms.* The second relates to treatment of an established infection: *None of the antimalarials is effective against all liver and red cell stages of the life cycle that may coexist in the same patient. Complete cure therefore may require more than one drug.*

The patterns of clinically useful activity fall into three general classes. Class I agents are not reliable against primary or latent liver stages or against *P. falciparum* gametocytes. Their action is directed against the asexual erythrocytic forms. These drugs will treat, or prevent, clinically symptomatic malaria. When used prophylactically, the class I drugs must be taken for several weeks after exposure until parasites complete the liver phase and become susceptible to therapy. The spectrum is somewhat expanded for the class II agents, which target not only the asexual erythrocytic forms but also the primary liver stages of *P. falciparum.* This additional activity shortens to several days the required period for postexposure prophylaxis. Finally, primaquine is unique in its spectrum of activity, which includes reliable efficacy against primary and latent liver stages as well as gametocytes. Primaquine has no place in the treatment of symptomatic malaria but rather is used most commonly to eradicate the hypnozoites of *P. vivax* and *P. ovale,* which are responsible for relapsing infections.

Aside from their antiparasitic activity, the utility of antimalarials for prophylaxis or therapy is dictated by their

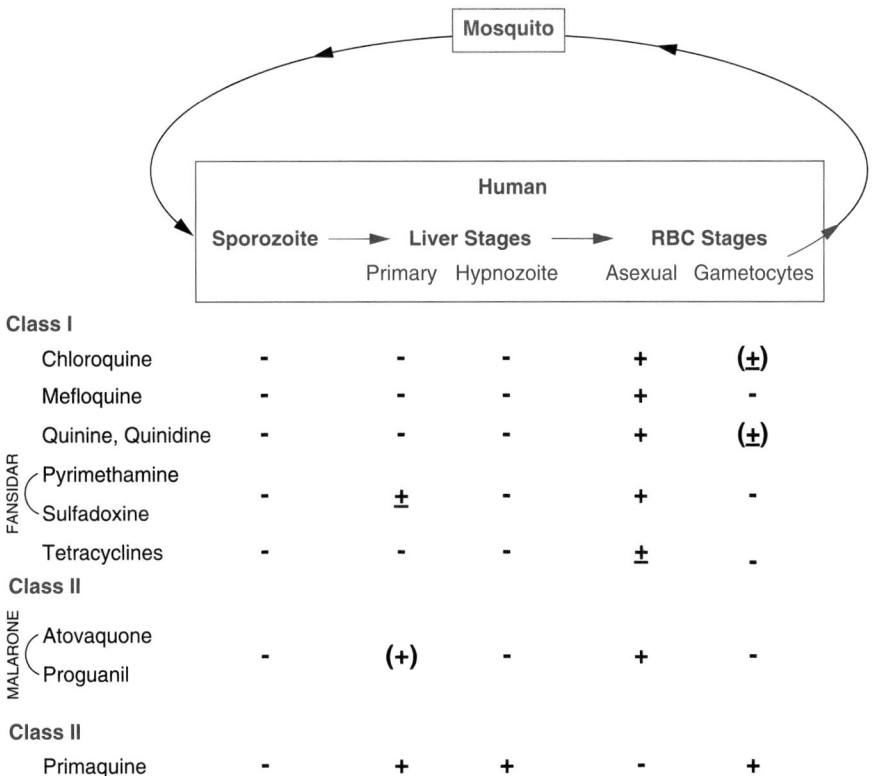

Figure 39–2. Spectrum of clinically useful activity for antimalarial drugs. For atovaquone and proguanil, reliable activity against the primary liver stage has been shown for *P. falciparum* only; for the class I agents, activity against gametocytes does not include *P. falciparum.*

pharmacokinetics and safety. Thus, quinine and primaquine, which have short half-lives and common toxicities, generally are reserved for treatment of established infection and not used for prophylaxis in a healthy traveler. In contrast, chloroquine is relatively safe and has a one-week half-life that is convenient for prophylactic dosing (in those few areas still reporting chloroquine-sensitive malaria).

Older classifications of the antimalarials are defined extensively in the 10th edition of this book. Briefly, causal prophylactics act on the initial hepatic stages, drugs for terminal prophylaxis and radical cure target hypnozoites, and agents for suppressive prophylaxis or cure target the asexual red cell forms.

Regimens currently recommended for *chemoprophylaxis* in nonimmune individuals are given in Table 39–1, whereas regimens for the *treatment* of malaria in nonimmune individuals are given in Table 39–2. Individual agents are discussed in more detail below.

ARTEMISININ AND DERIVATIVES

History. Artemisinin is a sesquiterpene lactone endoperoxide derived from the weed *qing hao* (*Artemisia annua*), also called *sweet wormwood* or *annual wormwood*. The Chinese have ascribed medicinal value to this plant for more than 2000 years (Klayman, 1985). As early as 340 A.D., Ge Hong prescribed tea made from *qing hao* as a remedy for fevers, and in 1596, Li Shizhen recommended it to relieve the symptoms of malaria. By 1972, Chinese scientists had extracted and crystallized the major antimalarial ingredient, *qinghaosu,* now known as *artemisinin.* Three semisynthetic derivatives with improved potency and bioavailability have since largely replaced the use of artemisinin. These include *dihydroartemisinin,* a reduced product; *artemether,* an oil-soluble methyl ether; and *artesunate,* the water-soluble hemisuccinate ester of dihydroartemisinin; their structures are:

ARTEMISININ

DIHYDROARTEMISININ

ARTEMETHER

ARTESUNATE

As a class, the artemisinins are potent and fast-acting antimalarials with no clinical evidence of resistance. They are particularly well suited for the treatment of severe *P. falciparum* malaria and now play a key role in the combination therapy of drug-resistant infections. Millions of patients, especially in China and Southeast Asia, have been treated with endoperoxides, which generally are regarded to be safe. However, these agents have not been approved by the FDA for marketing in the United States, and inactive counterfeits that closely mimic genuine drugs are common (Newton *et al.*, 2003b).

Antiparasitic Activity. Extensive structure–activity studies have confirmed the requirement for an endoperoxide moiety for antimalarial activity (O'Neill and Posner, 2004). These compounds act rapidly against the asexual erythrocytic stages of *P. vivax* and *P. falciparum.* Their potency *in vivo* is ten- to one hundredfold greater than that of other antimalarials (White, 1997). They are not cross-resistant with other drugs; indeed, sensitivity to the artemisinins may be increased paradoxically in chloroquine-resistant parasites. When used alone, the artemisinins are associated with a high level of parasite recrudescence; the reason for this is not clear but may be related to their rapid metabolism or perhaps to a post-antibiotic-like effect on the parasite. They have gametocytocidal activity but do not affect either primary or latent liver stages.

The current model of artemisinin action involves two steps (Meshnick, 2001). First, heme iron within the parasite catalyzes cleavage of the endoperoxide bridge. This is followed by rearrangement to produce a carbon-centered radical that alkylates and damages macromolecules in the parasite, likely including the ortholog of sarco/endoplasmic reticulum Ca^{2+}–ATPase (Eckstein-Ludwig *et al.*, 2003). Artemisinin and its derivatives exhibit antiparasitic activity *in vitro* against other protozoa, including *Leishmania major* and *Toxoplasma gondii,* and have been used alone or in combination in patients with schistosomiasis (Utzinger *et al.*, 2003).

Absorption, Fate, and Excretion. The semisynthetic artemisinins have been formulated for several dosing routes, including oral (dihydroartemisinin, artesunate, and artemether), intramuscular (artesunate and artemether), intravenous (artesunate), and rectal (artesunate). In general, disposition of the artemisinins is incompletely understood (Giao and de Vries, 2001). Absorption after oral dosing typically is 30% or less. Peak plasma levels occur within minutes of artesunate administration and at 2 to 6 hours after artemether administration. The endoperoxides are not highly bound to plasma proteins, although the linkage may be covalent. Both artesunate and artemether are converted extensively to dihydroartemisinin, which provides much of their antimalarial activity and has a plasma half-life of just 1 to 2 hours; its major urinary metabolite is a glucuronide.

With repeated dosing, artemisinin and artesunate induce their own cytochrome P450 (CYP)–mediated metabolism, which may enhance clearance by up to fivefold. The complex and important

These regimens, based on Centers for Disease Control and Prevention (CDC) recommendations current at the time of writing, may change over time. Up-to-date information should be obtained from the CDC at *www.cdc.gov/travel/*. Recommendations and available treatments vary in other countries.

***Prophylaxis for infections with chloroquine-sensitive* P. falciparum,[†] P. vivax, P. malariae, *and* P. ovale**

Chloroquine phosphate (ARALEN) is available for oral administration. Adults take 500 mg chloroquine phosphate (300 mg base) weekly starting 1–2 weeks before entering an endemic area and continuing for 4 weeks after leaving. The pediatric dosage is 8.3 mg/kg chloroquine phosphate (5 mg base per kg, up to the maximum adult dose) taken orally by the same schedule. *Note: Primaquine phosphate* is used to eradicate latent tissue forms of *P. vivax* and *P. ovale* and effect a radical cure after individuals leave areas endemic for these infections (*see* Table 39–2 and text).

***Prophylaxis for infections with drug-resistant strains of* P. falciparum[‡] *or* P. vivax.[§]** *Note:* The choice of regimen depends on the local geographic profile of drug resistance and other factors (*see* text).

Preferred regimens:

Atovaquone–proguanil (MALARONE) is available for oral dosing only as a fixed-combination tablet containing 250 mg atovaquone and 100 mg proguanil hydrochloride (adult tablet) or 62.5 mg atovaquone and 25 g proguanil hydrochloride (pediatric tablet). Adults and children over 40 kg should take one adult tablet per day beginning 1–2 days prior to exposure and continuing for 7 days after exposure. Smaller children should be dosed on the same schedule: 11–20 kg, 1 pediatric tablet daily; 21–30 kg, 2 pediatric tablets; 31–40 kg, 3 pediatric tablets. *Note:* For *P. vivax* malaria, atovaquone–proguanil may not be as effective as mefloquine. Atovaquone–proguanil is not recommended for children under 11 kg, pregnant women, or those breast-feeding infants. Contraindicated in persons with severe renal impairment.

Mefloquine hydrochloride (LARIAM) is available for oral administration only. Tablets marketed in the United States contain 250 mg mefloquine hydrochloride, equivalent to 228 mg mefloquine base (this may vary in Canada and elsewhere). The dosing below is expressed in mg salt. Adults and children over 45 kg body weight take 250 mg weekly starting 1–2 weeks before entering an endemic area and ending 4 weeks after leaving. Pediatric doses, taken by the same schedule, are 5 mg/kg for children up to 15 kg (may have to be prepared by a pharmacist); 62.5 mg ($^1/_4$ tablet) for 15–19 kg; 125 mg ($^1/_2$ tablet) for 20–30 kg; 187.5 mg ($^3/_4$ tablet) for 31–45 kg. *Note:* Mefloquine is *not* recommended for children weighing less than 5 kg or individuals with a history of seizures, severe neuropsychiatric disturbances, sensitivity to quinoline antimalarials, or cardiac conduction abnormalities.

Doxycycline hyclate (VIBRAMYCIN, others). Formulations of doxycycline are available in capsules, coated tablets, and liquid preparations for oral administration. The adult dose of doxycycline is 100 mg daily. For children over 8 years of age, the dosage is 2 mg/kg given once daily, up to the adult dose. Prophylaxis with doxycycline should begin 1 day before travel to an endemic area and end 4 weeks after leaving. This regimen is used in geographical areas where highly multidrug-resistant strains of *P. falciparum* are prevalent. *Note:* Doxycycline should not be given to children younger than 8 years of age or to pregnant women. Doxycycline is contraindicated in individuals who are hypersensitive to any tetracycline. Prophylaxis with doxycycline can be combined with the chloroquine phosphate regimen shown above for chloroquine-sensitive malaria. This strategy often is used in geographic areas where infection with more than one *Plasmodium* species is likely.

Primaquine phosphate USP. Tablets marketed in the United States contain 15 mg primaquine base per tablet (this may vary elsewhere); doses below are expressed as primaquine base. Primaquine may be used in special circumstances, such as when preferred agents cannot be tolerated or for multidrug-resistant *P. falciparum*. This should be done with caution and in consultation with malaria experts, such as those available through the CDC at 770-488-7788. The adult dose is 30 mg base (two tablets) daily starting several days before exposure and continued for 7 days after exposure. The same regimen at a dose of 0.6 mg/kg base is used for children. Primaquine is contraindicated in G6PD deficiency or pregnancy (*see* text).

Other regimens:

The mefloquine, doxycycline, or chloroquine prophylactic regimens listed above may be used together with a self-treatment regimen. The latter should be used for prompt treatment of presumed malaria if, for example, the traveler is in a very remote area. *Medical attention should be sought immediately.* The preferred regimen is *atovaquone–proguanil* (MALARONE). Adults and children greater than 41 kg should take 4 adult tablets as a single daily dose for three consecutive days; smaller children also should take adult tablets once daily for three consecutive days: 11–20 kg, 1 tablet; 21–30 kg, 2 tablets; 31–40 kg, 3 tablets.

*No chemoprophylactic regimen is always effective in preventing malaria. Recommended drug regimens always should be used in conjunction with other protective measures to avoid mosquito bites (*see* text). [†]These strains now exist only in Mexico, Central America west of the Panama Canal Zone, the Caribbean, and parts of South America and the Middle East; *see* Figure 39–4. [‡]These strains exist in other geographical areas endemic for *P. falciparum* malaria; *see* Figure 39–4. [§]Papua New Guinea and Indonesia are the two areas where chloroquine-resistant *P. vivax* are highly prevalent, resulting in a high failure rate with prophylaxis. Resistant *P. vivax* also has been found sporadically in India, Burma, and Central and South America.

Table 39–2
Regimens for Treatment of Malaria in the United States

These regimens, modified from CDC recommendations current at the time of writing, may change over time. Up-to-date information should be obtained from the CDC at *www.cdc.gov/travel/*. Recommendations and available treatments vary in other countries.

Treatment of severe malarial infections

Note: Infections with *P. falciparum* in nonimmune or pregnant patients constitute medical emergencies because they can progress rapidly to a fatal outcome.[*] Chemotherapy should be initiated promptly and not await parasitological confirmation. Parenteral therapy with *quinidine gluconate* is advised for severely ill patients who cannot take oral medication; the regimen is identical for all species of *Plasmodium*. Exchange transfusion may benefit some patients.

Preferred regimen:

Quinidine gluconate is given intravenously to both adults and children starting with a loading dose of 10 mg of the salt per kg dissolved in 300 ml of normal saline and infused over 1 to 2 hours (maximum dose 600 mg of the salt). This is followed by continuous infusion at the rate of 0.02 mg of the salt per kg per minute for at least 24 hours and until oral therapy with quinine sulfate is feasible. During administration of quinidine gluconate, blood pressure (for hypotension) and ECG (for widening of the QRS complex and lengthening of the QT interval) should be monitored continuously and total blood glucose (for hypoglycemia) periodically. These complications, if severe, may warrant temporary discontinuation of the drug.

Quinine sulfate can be substituted for quinidine gluconate once patients can take oral medication. The dose for adults is 650 mg of the salt given every 8 hours. The pediatric dose is 10 mg of the salt per kg given every 8 hours. Therapy with quinidine/quinine usually is given for 3 to 7 days depending on the species of *Plasmodium* and geographical profile of drug resistance (7 days for *P. falciparum* in Southeast Asia). Previous use of mefloquine may mandate dosage reduction (*see* text).

Adjunctive therapy:

For optimal clinical response, any one of the following regimens should be used together with oral quinine sulfate therapy. The particular choice depends on the geographical profile of antimalarial drug resistance.

Doxycycline hyclate (VIBRAMYCIN, others). The adult dose is 100 mg taken orally twice a day for 7 days. For children over 8 years of age, the dosage is 2 mg/kg, increasing up to the adult dose and given by the same schedule. *Tetracycline* may be substituted if doxycycline hyclate is unavailable. Adults receive 250 mg every 6 hours for 7 days, whereas the pediatric dosage is 6.25 mg/kg every 6 hours for 7 days. *Note:* Because of adverse effects on bones and teeth, tetracyclines should not be given to children younger than 8 years of age or to pregnant women. These drugs are contraindicated in individuals who are hypersensitive to any tetracycline.

Clindamycin. The adult or pediatric dosage is 20 mg (base) per kg orally per day divided into three or four doses for 7 days.

Pyrimethamine–sulfadoxine (FANSIDAR). This combination is available for oral use only in tablets containing 25 mg pyrimethamine and 500 mg sulfadoxine. One dose is taken by mouth on the last day of quinine sulfate therapy: Adults take 3 tablets; children 5–10 kg, 0.5 tablet; 11–14 kg, 0.75 tablet; 15–20 kg, 1 tablet; 21–30 kg, 1.5 tablets; 31–40 kg, 2 tablets; 41–50 kg, 2.5 tablets; over 50 kg, 3 tablets. Owing to extensive drug resistance, pyrimethamine–sulfadoxine should be used as an adjunct treatment primarily in young children or women who are not able to tolerate clindamycin.

Other oral treatment regimens for infections with chloroquine-resistant P. vivax[†] and drug-resistant strains of P. falciparum[‡]

If quinine-based therapy cannot be used, mefloquine currently is the preferred alternative (except for Southeast Asia) but could be supplanted in this role by atovaquone–proguanil once more experience is obtained.

Mefloquine hydrochloride (LARIAM, MEPHAQUINE). The adult dose is 750 mg of the salt taken by mouth followed 6–12 hours later by 500 mg. The corresponding pediatric dose for children weighing less than 45 kg is 15 mg of the salt per kg followed 6–12 hours later by 10 mg of the salt per kg. (*Note:* The pediatric dosage is not approved by the FDA.) The initial dose should be repeated *only* if vomiting occurs within the first hour. Therapeutic doses of mefloquine may induce gastrointestinal and neuropsychiatric symptoms. Because of its long half-life and potential for serious drug interactions, extreme caution is advised in using certain antimalarial agents (*e.g.*, quinine or halofantrine) with or shortly after mefloquine. (*See* text for further details.)

(Continued)

Table 39–2
Regimens for Treatment of Malaria in the United States (Continued)

> *Atovaquone–proguanil hydrochloride* (MALARONE). A fixed-dose combination of these drugs is available in tablets containing 250 mg atovaquone and 100 mg proguanil hydrochloride. The dose for adults is 1000 mg atovaquone plus 400 mg proguanil hydrochloride taken by mouth once each day for 3 days. The pediatric dose for children weighing 11 to 20 kg is 250 mg atovaquone plus 100 mg proguanil hydrochloride; 21 to 30 kg, 500 mg atovaquone plus 200 mg proguanil hydrochloride; 31 to 40 kg, 750 mg atovaquone plus 300 mg proguanil hydrochloride. These doses are given once daily for 3 days with food to increase drug bioavailability. If vomiting occurs within 30 minutes, the dose should be repeated. If nausea is severe, the dose may be split in half and given twice daily. Experience with children weighing under 11 kg is limited, but if necessary, pediatric tablets are available. Consult CDC recommendations for dosages.
>
> **Oral treatment of infections with P. vivax, P. malariae, P. ovale,** *and chloroquine-sensitive* **P. falciparum**[‡]
>
> *Chloroquine phosphate* (ARALEN) is available in 250- and 500-mg tablets (equivalent to 150 and 300 mg base, respectively) for oral administration. The adult dosage is two 500-mg tablets immediately, followed by one 500-mg tablet at 6, 24, and 48 hours. The dosage for children is 16.7 mg/kg (10 mg base per kg) immediately, followed by 8.3 mg/kg (5 mg base per kg) at 6, 24, and 48 hours, not to exceed the adult dosage.
>
> *Prevention of relapse:*
>
> To eradicate latent tissue forms of *P. vivax* and *P. ovale* that persist to cause relapses of infection, primaquine phosphate is supplied in tablets containing either 13.2 or 26.3 mg of the salt (7.5 or 15 mg base, respectively) for oral administration only. Therapy with primaquine is started after the acute attack (about day 4) at doses of 52.6 mg (30 mg base) daily for 14 days. Pediatric doses are 1.06 mg/kg (0.6 mg base per kg) daily, also for 14 days. The same primaquine regimen also can be used during the last 2 weeks of chloroquine phosphate prophylaxis for individuals who have left areas endemic for *P. vivax* or *P. ovale* infection. Alternatively, adults using chloroquine for prophylaxis against *P. vivax* or *P. ovale* may take 500 mg chloroquine phosphate (300 mg base) together with 78.9 mg primaquine phosphate (45 mg base) weekly for 8 weeks starting after leaving an endemic area to achieve a "radical" cure. Primaquine is contraindicated in pregnancy and in severe G6PD deficiency (*see* text).

[*]Emergency advice is available from the Division of Parasitic Diseases, Centers for Disease Control and Prevention (CDC) (telephone: 770-488-7788).
[†]Papua New Guinea and Indonesia are the two areas where chloroquine-resistant *P. vivax* are highly prevalent, resulting in a high failure rate. Resistant *P. vivax* also has been found sporadically in India, Burma, and Central and South America. Currently, patients acquiring *P. vivax* infections from regions other than Papua New Guinea and Indonesia should be treated with chloroquine. [‡]*See* Figure 39–4.

questions of metabolic interaction between artemisinins and the other antimalarials with which they almost always are coadministered remain largely to be studied (Giao and de Vries, 2001); however, there appear to be no clinically significant pharmacokinetic or toxic interactions between the artemisinin compounds and mefloquine.

Therapeutic Uses. Given their rapid and potent activity against even multidrug-resistant parasites, the artemisinins are valuable for the initial treatment of severe *P. falciparum* infections. In this setting, intravenous artesunate compared favorably with a standard quinine regimen in terms of efficacy and safety (Newton *et al.*, 2003a). The artemisinins generally are not used alone because of their incomplete efficacy and to prevent the selection of resistant parasites. However, in a series of trials in Africa, South America, and Asia, artesunate has proven exceedingly useful when combined with other

antimalarials for the first-line treatment of malaria (Adjuik *et al.*, 2004). Artemisinin combination treatment (ACT) now is espoused because the addition of endoperoxides effects a rapid and substantial reduction of parasite burden, reduces the likelihood of resistance, and may decrease disease transmission by reducing gametocyte carriage. Artemisinins should not be used for prophylaxis because of their short half-life, incompletely characterized safety in healthy subjects, and unreliability when used alone.

Toxicity and Contraindications. Despite a relative lack of formal safety studies in humans, after three decades and use in millions of people, the artemisinins enjoy a reputation of safety (Taylor and White, 2004). There nevertheless remains a pressing need for systematic human safety data, especially in children (Johann-Liang and Albrecht, 2003). In preclinical toxicity studies, the principal target organs are brain, liver, bone marrow, and fetus.

Neurotoxicity in rats and dogs is most evident in brainstem nuclei and is more pronounced for the lipophilic derivatives. In patients, the many neurological changes that occur in severe malaria confound the evaluation of neurotoxicity; however, no systematic changes were attributable to treatment in patients older than 5 years of age. As in animals, dose-related and reversible changes have been seen in reticulocyte and neutrophil counts and in transaminase levels in patients. About 1 in 3000 patients develops an allergic reaction. The artemisinins are potent embryotoxins in animals. Only a few small studies have monitored the outcome of pregnancies in women treated with endoperoxides, but to date there are no reported increases in congenital or developmental abnormalities (McGready *et al.*, 1998). The question of early fetal loss in humans has not been studied. Given the current state of safety information, the artemisinins should be used with caution in very young children and pregnant women.

ATOVAQUONE

History. Based on the antiprotozoal activity of hydroxynaphthoquinones, atovaquone (MEPRON) was developed as a promising synthetic derivative with potent activity against *Plasmodium* species and the opportunistic pathogens *Pneumocystis carinii* and *Toxoplasma gondii* (Hudson *et al.*, 1991). After limited clinical trials, the FDA approved this compound in 1992 for treatment of mild-to-moderate *P. carinii* pneumonia in patients intolerant to *trimethoprim–sulfamethoxazole* (*see* Chapter 43). Subsequent clinical studies in patients with uncomplicated *P. falciparum* malaria revealed that atovaquone produced good initial responses but also high rates of relapse with parasites that were extremely atovaquone-resistant (Looareesuwan *et al.*, 1996). In contrast, use of proguanil with atovaquone evoked high cure rates with few relapses (of atovaquone-sensitive parasites) and minimal toxicity (Looareesuwan *et al.*, 1996, 1999b). A fixed combination of atovaquone with proguanil (MALARONE) now is available in the United States for malaria prophylaxis and treatment. Atovaquone has some efficacy against brain and eye infections with *T. gondii*, and its use in combination with other antiparasitic agents is still being explored. Atovaquone has the chemical structure shown below:

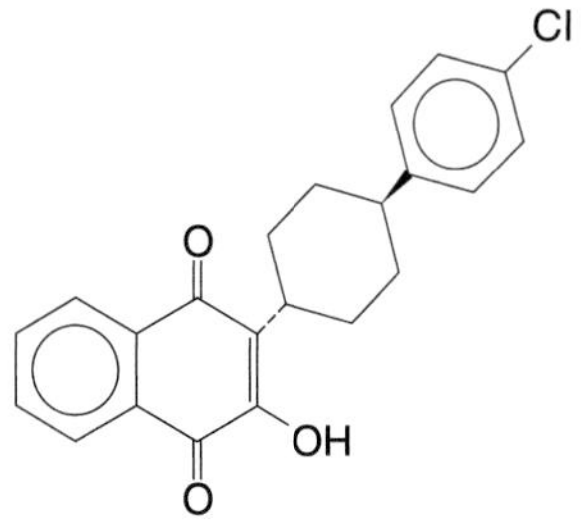

ATOVAQUONE

Antiparasitic Effects, Mechanism, and Resistance. Atovaquone is a highly lipophilic analog of *ubiquinone.* In animal models and *in vitro* systems, it has potent activity against blood stages of plasmodia, tachyzoite and cyst

forms of *T. gondii,* the fungus *P. carinii,* and *Babesia* species (Hughes *et al.*, 1990; Hudson *et al.*, 1991; Hughes and Oz, 1995). It is active against liver stages of *P. falciparum* (Shaprio *et al.*, 1999) but not against *P. vivax* hypnozoites (Berman *et al.*, 2001). Atovaquone is highly potent against *P. falciparum* both in culture (IC_{50} 0.7 to 4.3 nM) and in *Aotus* monkeys (Hudson *et al.*, 1991). This compound interferes with mitochondrial functions, such as ATP and pyrimidine biosynthesis, in susceptible malaria parasites. Thus, atovaquone acts selectively at the cytochrome bc_1 complex of malaria mitochondria to inhibit electron transport and collapse the mitochondrial membrane potential (*see* Vaidya and Mather, 2000). Synergism between proguanil and atovaquone appears to be due to the capacity of proguanil as a biguanide to enhance the membrane-collapsing activity of atovaquone (Srivastava and Vaidya, 1999). Atovaquone likewise affects mitochondrial function in permeabilized *T. gondii* tachyzoites (Vercesi *et al.*, 1998).

Resistance to atovaquone in *P. falciparum* develops readily *in vitro* and *in vivo* (Vaidya and Mather, 2000). Mutations in resistant organisms have been mapped to the mitochondrially encoded cytochrome b gene, particularly the region encoding the ubiquinol oxidation catalytic domain. Similar mutations have been reported in resistant isolates of rodent malaria species, as well as in *T. gondii* and perhaps *P. carinii*. The ease of selection of resistant mutants is at odds with the remarkable stability of the *P. falciparum* mitochondrial genome sequence across disparate isolates. It has been proposed that atovaquone action in the mitochondria generates mutagenic reactive oxygen species *via* electron transport blockade. This raises the interesting possibility that drug action promotes drug resistance. Resistance can be prevented by using proguanil in combination with atovaquone. It remains to be seen how long this will be effective. Atovaquone–proguanil treatment failure with drug-resistant organisms already has been documented (Fivelman *et al.*, 2002; Wichmann *et al.*, 2004).

Absorption, Fate, and Excretion. Absorption after a single oral dose is slow, erratic, and variable; increased two- to threefold by fatty food; and dose-limited above 750 mg. More than 99% of the drug is bound to plasma protein, and cerebrospinal fluid (CSF) levels are less than 1% of those in plasma. Plasma level–time profiles often show a double peak, albeit with considerable variability; the first peak appears in 1 to 8 hours, whereas the second occurs 1 to 4 days after a single dose. This pattern suggests an enterohepatic circulation, as does the long half-life, averaging 1.5 to 3 days. Humans do not metabolize atovaquone significantly. It is excreted in bile, and more than 94% of the drug is recovered unchanged in feces; only traces appear in the urine (Rolan *et al.*, 1997). Clearance of atovaquone may vary among different ethnic populations treated for *P. falciparum* malaria (Hussein *et al.*, 1997).

Therapeutic Uses. Atovaquone is used with a biguanide for prophylaxis and treatment of malaria to obtain optimal clinical results and avoid emergence of drug-resistant plasmodial strains. A tablet containing a fixed dose of 250 mg atovaquone and 100 mg proguanil hydrochloride, taken orally, has been highly effective and safe in a 3-day regimen for treating mild-to-moderate attacks of drug-resistant *P. falciparum* malaria (Looareesuwan *et al.*, 1999a). The same regimen followed by primaquine appears to be fairly effective in treatment of *P. vivax* malaria (Looareesuwan *et al.*, 1999b; Lacy *et al.*, 2002), but experience in treatment of non–*P. falciparum* malaria is limited and should be reserved for chloroquine-resistant *P. vivax* cases in which quinine and mefloquine cannot be used. Atovaquone–proguanil also is useful for malaria prophylaxis, which can be discontinued 1 week after leaving the endemic area because both components have hepatic-phase activity. Here, as for treatment, experience in non–*P. falciparum* malaria is somewhat limited (Ling *et al.*, 2002).

Opportunistic infections owing to the fungus *P. carinii* or the protozoan *T. gondii* are especially serious threats to immunocompromised patients such as those with human immunodeficiency virus (HIV) infection and acquired immune deficiency syndrome (AIDS). Atovaquone remains an alternative for prophylaxis and treatment of pulmonary *P. carinii* infection in patients who can take oral medication but cannot tolerate trimethoprim–sulfamethoxazole or parenteral *pentamidine* (*see* Chapters 43 and 48 and the ninth edition of this book). *T. gondii* infections in these patients, especially cerebral lesions, have shown only limited dose-related positive responses to prolonged regimens of atovaquone (Torres *et al.*, 1997). *Toxoplasma* chorioretinitis in immunocompetent patients probably responds better to this drug (Pearson *et al.*, 1999). Atovaquone also is used in combination with *azithromycin* for infections owing to *Babesia* species (Krause, 2003).

Toxicity. Atovaquone causes few side effects that require cessation of therapy. The most common reactions are abdominal pain, nausea, vomiting, diarrhea, headache, and rash. Vomiting and diarrhea may result in therapeutic failure owing to decreased drug absorption. However, readministration of this drug within an hour of vomiting still may evoke a positive therapeutic response in patients with *P. falciparum* malaria (Looareesuwan *et al.*, 1999a). Patients treated with atovaquone exhibit occasional and usually transient abnormalities of serum transaminase or amylase levels.

Precautions and Contraindications. While atovaquone seems remarkably safe, the drug needs further evaluation in pediatric patients weighing less than 11 kg, pregnant women, and lactating mothers. Accordingly, the drug is not recommended in these individuals. Routine tests for carcinogenicity, mutagenicity, and teratogenicity have been negative. Further experience is necessary, especially regarding rare or long-term toxicity. Atovaquone may compete with certain drugs for binding to plasma proteins, and therapy with *rifampin*, a potent inducer of CYP–mediated drug metabolism, can reduce plasma levels of atovaquone substantially,

whereas plasma levels of rifampin are raised. Coadministration with *tetracycline* is associated with a 40% reduction in plasma concentration of atovaquone.

DIAMINOPYRIMIDINES

History. Based on their structural analogy with the antimalarial proguanil (*see* Proguanil below), in the late 1940s a large series of 2,4-diaminopyrimidines was tested for inhibitory activity against malaria parasites. Pyrimethamine (DARAPRIM) exhibited potent activity and was chosen by Hitchings for further development. Earlier studies, designed to overcome the ready selection of drug-resistant parasites, first described the profound antimalarial synergism that occurs when a sulfonamide is coadministered with proguanil. Accordingly, pyrimethamine was formulated and marketed as a fixed combination with *sulfadoxine,* a sulfonamide whose pharmacokinetics match those of pyrimethamine. For several decades this combination (FANSIDAR) has been used extensively for malaria therapy, especially against chloroquine-resistant strains of *P. falciparum.* Unfortunately, widespread resistance now seriously compromises its utility, and pyrimethamine–sulfadoxine is no longer recommended for prophylaxis because of the unacceptable risk of toxicity (*see* below). Because of its low cost, pyrimethamine–sulfadoxine still has some utility in the treatment of *P. falciparum* malaria in parts of Africa (Winstanley, 2001). Pyrimethamine has the following chemical structure:

PYRIMETHAMINE

Antiprotozoal Effects. **Antimalarial Actions.** Pyrimethamine is a slow-acting blood schizontocide with antimalarial effects *in vivo* similar to those of proguanil (*see* below). However, pyrimethamine has greater antimalarial potency, and its half-life is much longer than that of *cycloguanil,* the active metabolite of proguanil. Pyrimethamine's efficacy against hepatic forms of *P. falciparum* is less than that of proguanil, and at therapeutic doses, pyrimethamine fails to eradicate the latent tissue forms of *P. vivax* or gametocytes of any plasmodial species.

Action against Other Protozoa. High doses of pyrimethamine given concurrently with *sulfadiazine* is the preferred therapy for infection with *T. gondii* in infants and immunosuppressed individuals (*see* Chapter 40).

Mechanisms of Antimalarial Action and Resistance. The 2,4-diaminopyrimidines inhibit dihydrofolate reductase of plasmodia at concentrations far lower than those required to produce comparable inhibition of the mammalian enzymes (Ferone *et al.*, 1969). Unlike its counterpart in human cells, the dihydrofolate reductase in malaria parasites resides on the same polypeptide chain as thymidylate synthase and, importantly, is not upregulated in the face of inhibition. The latter property contributes to the selective toxicity of the antifolates (Zhang and Rathod, 2002).

Synergism between pyrimethamine and the sulfonamides or sulfones has been attributed to inhibition of two steps in an essential metabolic pathway, although other mechanisms may contribute. The two steps involved are the utilization of *p*-aminobenzoic acid for the synthesis of dihydropteroic acid, which is catalyzed by dihydropteroate synthase and inhibited by sulfonamides, and the reduction of dihydrofolate to tetrahydrofolate, which is catalyzed by dihydrofolate reductase and inhibited by pyrimethamine. Inhibition by antifolates is manifested late in the life cycle of malarial parasites by failure of nuclear division at the time of schizont formation in erythrocytes and liver.

Several factors may affect the therapeutic response to antifolates, including host immunity to the parasite (which augments efficacy) and dietary *p*-aminobenzoic acid or folate, both of which can be imported by the malaria parasite and which can reduce drug efficacy substantially (Wang *et al.*, 1997). Resistance to pyrimethamine has developed in regions of prolonged or extensive drug use and can be attributed entirely to mutations in dihydrofolate reductase–thymidylate synthetase (Gregson and Plowe, 2005). This gene has been cloned and sequenced in strains of *P. falciparum* that are either sensitive or resistant to pyrimethamine. Several different mutations have been identified that introduce single-amino-acid changes linked to pyrimethamine resistance; these changes decrease the binding affinity of pyrimethamine for its active site in the dihydrofolate reductase moiety. The key mutation associated with pyrimethamine resistance is the substitution of asparagine for serine at position 108 (S108N). In clinical isolates from the field or with recombinant protein, it can be shown that a stepwise accumulating series of additional mutations at Arg[50], Ile[51], Arg[59], and Leu[164] is associated with progressively increasing resistance. Interestingly, the pattern of amino acid substitutions is different in parasites resistant to cycloguanil, even though cross-resistance can occur between these structurally related inhibitors of plasmodial dihydrofolate reductase.

Absorption, Fate, and Distribution. After oral administration, pyrimethamine is slowly but completely absorbed; it reaches peak plasma levels in about 2 to 6 hours. The compound binds to plasma proteins and accumulates mainly in kidneys, lungs, liver, and spleen. It is eliminated slowly with a half-life in plasma of about 80 to 95 hours. Concentrations that are suppressive for responsive plasmodial strains remain in the blood for about 2 weeks, but these are lower in patients with malaria (Winstanley *et al.*, 1992). Several metabolites of pyrimethamine appear in the urine, but their identities and antimalarial properties have not been fully characterized. Pyrimethamine also is excreted in the milk of nursing mothers.

Therapeutic Uses. Pyrimethamine is virtually always given with either a sulfonamide or sulfone to enhance its antifolate activity, but it still acts slowly relative to the quinoline blood schizontocides, and its prolonged elimination encourages the selection of resistant parasites. The use of pyrimethamine should be restricted to the treatment of chloroquine-resistant *P. falciparum* malaria in areas where resistance to antifolates has not yet fully developed. Pyrimethamine together with a short-acting sulfonamide such as sulfadiazine also may be used as an adjunct to quinine to treat an acute malarial attack. Dosage regimens for this indication are given in Table 39–2. Pyrimethamine–sulfadoxine is no longer recommended for prophylaxis because of toxicity owing to the accompanying sulfonamide (*see* below).

High doses of pyrimethamine plus sulfadiazine are the treatment of choice for infections with *T. gondii* in immunocompromised adults; if such patients are left untreated, these infections progress rapidly to a fatal outcome (Kasper, 2001) (*see* Chapter 40). Initial therapy consists of an oral loading dose of 200 mg followed by 50 to 75 mg pyrimethamine daily for 4 to 6 weeks along with 4 to 6 g sulfadiazine daily in four divided doses. *Leucovorin* (folinic acid), 10 to 15 mg daily, should be taken for the same period to prevent bone marrow toxicity (*see* below). For subsequent long-term suppressive therapy, lower doses of pyrimethamine (25 to 50 mg daily) and sulfadiazine (2 to 4 g daily) may suffice. To deal with toxicity, pyrimethamine often has been used with agents such as *clindamycin, spiramycin,* or other *macrolides* (*see* Kasper, 2001). Infants with congenital, placentally transmitted toxoplasmosis usually respond positively to oral pyrimethamine (0.5 to 1.0 mg/kg daily) and oral sulfadiazine (100 mg/kg daily) given over a one year period.

Toxicity, Precautions, and Contraindications. Antimalarial doses of pyrimethamine alone cause little toxicity except occasional skin rashes and depression of hematopoiesis. Excessive doses produce a megaloblastic anemia resembling that of folate deficiency that responds readily to drug withdrawal or treatment with folinic acid. At high doses, pyrimethamine is teratogenic in animals, and in humans, trimethoprim–sulfamethoxazole therapy is associated with birth defects (Hernandez-Diaz *et al.*, 2000), but such toxicity has not been studied systematically for pyrimethamine in humans.

Sulfonamides or sulfones rather than pyrimethamine usually account for the toxicity associated with coadministration of these antifolate drugs (*see* Chapter 43). The combination of pyrimethamine (25 mg) and sulfadoxine (500 mg) (FANSIDAR) is no longer recommended for antimalarial prophylaxis because in about 1 in 5000 to 1 in 8000 individuals it causes severe and even fatal cutaneous reactions such as erythema multiforme, Stevens-Johnson syndrome, and toxic epidermal necrolysis. This combination also has been associated with serum sickness–type reactions, urticaria, exfoliative dermatitis, and hepatitis. Pyrimethamine–sulfadoxine is contraindicated for individuals with previous reactions to sulfonamides, for lactating mothers, and for infants younger than 2 months of age. Administration of pyrimethamine with *dapsone* (MALOPRIM), a drug combination unavailable in the United States, occasionally has been associated with agranulocytosis. Higher doses of pyrimethamine

(75 mg daily) used along with sulfadiazine (4 to 6 g daily) to treat toxoplasmosis produce skin rashes, bone marrow suppression, and renal toxicity in about 40% of immunocompromised patients. However, much of this toxicity probably is due to sulfadiazine (*see* Kasper, 2001).

PROGUANIL

History. Proguanil (PALUDRINE) is the common name for *chloroguanide,* a biguanide derivative that emerged in 1945 as a product of British antimalarial drug research. The antimalarial activity of proguanil eventually was ascribed to cycloguanil, a cyclic triazine metabolite and selective inhibitor of the bifunctional plasmodial dihydrofolate reductase–thymidylate synthetase. Indeed, investigation of compounds bearing a structural resemblance to cycloguanil resulted in the development of antimalarial dihydrofolate reductase inhibitors such as pyrimethamine. Accrued evidence also indicates that proguanil itself has intrinsic antimalarial activity independent of its effect on parasite dihydrofolate reductase–thymidylate synthetase (*see* Fidock and Wellems, 1997).

Chemistry. Proguanil and its triazine metabolite cycloguanil have the following chemical structures:

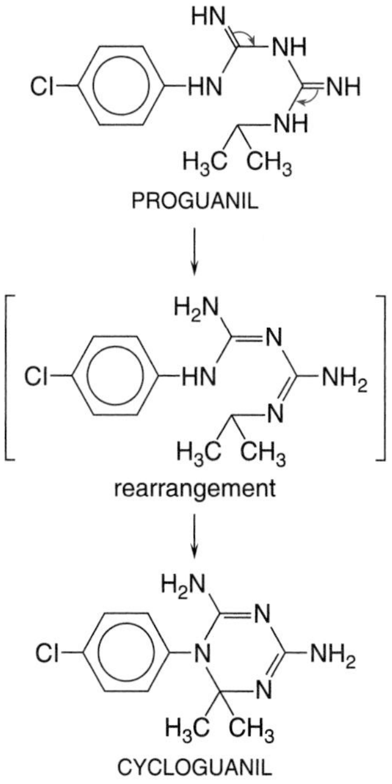

PROGUANIL

rearrangement

CYCLOGUANIL

Proguanil has the widest margin of safety of a large series of antimalarial biguanide analogs examined. Dihalogen substitution in positions 3 and 4 of the benzene ring yields *chlorproguanil* (LAPUDRINE), a more potent prodrug than proguanil that also is used clinically. Cycloguanil is structurally related to pyrimethamine.

Antimalarial Actions. In sensitive *P. falciparum* malaria, proguanil exerts activity against both the prima-

ry liver stages and the asexual red cell stages, thus adequately controlling the acute attack and usually eradicating the infection. Proguanil also is active against acute *P. vivax* malaria, but because the latent tissue stages of *P. vivax* are unaffected, relapses may occur after the drug is withdrawn. Proguanil treatment does not destroy gametocytes, but fertilized gametes encysted in the gut of the mosquito fail to develop normally.

Mechanisms of Antimalarial Action and Resistance. The active triazine metabolite of proguanil selectively inhibits the bifunctional dihydrofolate reductase–thymidylate synthetase of sensitive plasmodia, causing inhibition of DNA synthesis and depletion of folate cofactors. By cloning and sequencing dihydrofolate reductase–thymidylate synthetase genes from sensitive and resistant *P. falciparum,* investigators found that certain amino acid changes near the dihydrofolate reductase–binding site are linked to resistance to either cycloguanil, pyrimethamine, or both.

Specifically, resistance to cycloguanil (and chlorcycloguanil) can be linked to mutations leading to paired Val[16]/Thr[108] substitutions in plasmodial dihydrofolate reductase, such resistance being especially enhanced by an additional substitution at Leu[164]. This pattern differs from that typically observed for pyrimethamine resistance described earlier. However, overlapping resistance to cycloguanil and pyrimethamine indicates that mutation patterns leading to the final resistance phenotype may be quite complex. Thus, genetic analyses of resistant *P. falciparum* strains, together with novel expression and assay systems, represent a powerful approach for identifying and monitoring new generations of antimalarials directed at vulnerable plasmodia biochemical targets (Sibley *et al.,* 2001).

The presence of plasmodial dihydrofolate reductase is not required for the intrinsic antimalarial activity of proguanil or chlorproguanil (Fidock and Wellems, 1997), but the molecular basis for this direct activity still is unknown. Proguanil as the biguanide accentuates the mitochondrial membrane-potential-collapsing action of atovaquone against *P. falciparum* but displays no such activity by itself (Srivastava and Vaidya, 1999) (*see* Atovaquone, above). In contrast to cycloguanil, resistance to the intrinsic antimalarial activity of proguanil itself, either alone or in combination with atovaquone, has yet to be well documented.

Absorption, Fate, and Excretion. Proguanil is slowly but adequately absorbed from the GI tract. After a single oral dose, peak concentrations of the drug in plasma usually are attained within 5 hours. The mean plasma elimination half-life is about 12 to 20 hours or longer depending on the rate of metabolism. Metabolism of proguanil in mammals cosegregates with mephenytoin oxidation polymorphism (Ward *et al.,* 1991) controlled by isoforms in the CYP2C subfamily. Only about 3% of Caucasians are deficient in this oxidation phenotype, as contrasted with about 20% of

Asians and Kenyans. Proguanil is oxidized to two major metabolites, cycloguanil and an inactive 4-chlorophenylbiguanide. On a 200-mg daily dosage regimen, extensive metabolizers develop plasma levels of cycloguanil that are above the therapeutic range, whereas poor metabolizers may not (Helsby *et al.*, 1993). Proguanil itself does not accumulate appreciably in tissues during long-term administration, except in erythrocytes, where its concentration is about three times that in plasma. Accumulation in infected erythrocytes could be critical for the intrinsic antimalarial effects of proguanil either by itself or with atovaquone. The inactive 4-chlorophenyl-biguanide metabolite is not readily detected in plasma but appears in increased quantities in the urine of poor proguanil metabolizers. In humans, from 40% to 60% of the absorbed proguanil is excreted in urine either as the parent drug or as the active metabolite.

Therapeutic Uses. Proguanil as a single agent is not available in the United States but is prescribed as such in England and Europe for Caucasians traveling to malarious areas. Strains of *P. falciparum* resistant to proguanil emerge rapidly in areas where the drug is used exclusively, but breakthrough infections also may result from deficient conversion of this compound to its active antimalarial metabolite. Proguanil is ineffective against multidrug-resistant strains of *P. falciparum* in Thailand and New Guinea. The drug can protect against certain strains of *P. falciparum* in sub-Saharan Africa that are resistant to chloroquine and pyrimethamine–sulfadoxine.

Proguanil is effective and well tolerated when given orally once daily for 3 days in combination with atovaquone for the treatment of malarial attacks owing to chloroquine- and multidrug-resistant strains of *P. falciparum* and *P. vivax* (*see* Atovaquone, above). Indeed, this drug combination (MALARONE) has been successful in Southeast Asia, where highly drug-resistant strains of *P. falciparum* prevail. *P. falciparum* readily develops clinical resistance to monotherapy with either proguanil or atovaquone, but resistance to the combination is uncommon unless the strain is initially resistant to atovaquone. In contrast, some strains resistant to proguanil do respond to proguanil plus atovaquone.

Toxicity and Side Effects. In prophylactic doses of 200 to 300 mg daily, proguanil causes few untoward effects except occasional nausea and diarrhea. Large doses (1 g or more daily) may cause vomiting, abdominal pain, diarrhea, hematuria, and the transient appearance of epithelial cells and casts in the urine. Gross accidental or deliberate overdose (as much as 15 g) has been followed by complete recovery. Doses as high as 700 mg twice daily have been taken for more than 2 weeks without serious toxicity. Proguanil is considered safe for use during pregnancy. It is remarkably safe when used in conjunction with other antimalarial drugs such as chloroquine, atovaquone, tetracyclines, and other antifolates.

QUINOLINES AND RELATED COMPOUNDS

Quinolines have been the mainstay of antimalarial chemotherapy starting with quinine nearly 400 years ago. In the last century, legions of related compounds were synthesized and tested for antimalarial activity. From these programs have come a number of drugs that are useful for the prophylaxis and treatment of malaria. The most important of these are shown in Figure 39–3.

Chloroquine and Hydroxychloroquine

History. Chloroquine (ARALEN) is one of a large series of 4-aminoquinolines investigated as part of the extensive cooperative program of antimalarial research in the United States during World War II. Beginning in 1943, thousands of compounds were synthesized and tested for activity. Chloroquine eventually proved most promising and was released for field trial. When hostilities ceased, it was discovered that the compound had been synthesized and studied as early as 1934 under the name of RESOCHIN by the Germans but rejected because of toxicity in avian models.

Chemistry. The structure of chloroquine is shown in Figure 39–3. The D, L, and DL forms of chloroquine have equal potency in duck malaria, but the D-isomer is somewhat less toxic than the L-isomer in mammals. A chlorine atom attached to position 7 of the quinoline ring confers the greatest antimalarial activity in both avian and human malarias. Research on the structure–activity relationships of chloroquine and related alkaloid compounds continues in an effort to find new, effective antimalarials with improved safety profiles that can be used successfully against chloroquine- and multidrug-resistant strains of *P. falciparum* (examples include the bisquinolines and short-chain chloroquines).

Hydroxychloroquine (PLAQUENIL), in which one of the *N*-ethyl substituents of chloroquine is β-hydroxylated, is essentially equivalent to chloroquine against *P. falciparum* malaria. This analog is preferred over chloroquine for treatment of mild rheumatoid arthritis and lupus erythematosus because, given in the high doses required, it may cause less ocular toxicity than chloroquine (Easterbrook, 1999).

*Pharmacological Effects. **Antimalarial Actions**.* Chloroquine is highly effective against erythrocytic forms of *P. vivax, P. ovale, P. malariae,* and chloroquine-sensitive strains of *P. falciparum*. It is the prophylaxis and treatment of choice when these organisms are involved. It exerts activity against gametocytes of the first three plasmodial species but not against those of *P. falciparum*. The drug has no activity against latent tissue forms of *P. vivax* or *P. ovale*.

Other Effects. Chloroquine or its analogs are used for therapy of conditions other than malaria. Their use to treat hepatic amebiasis is

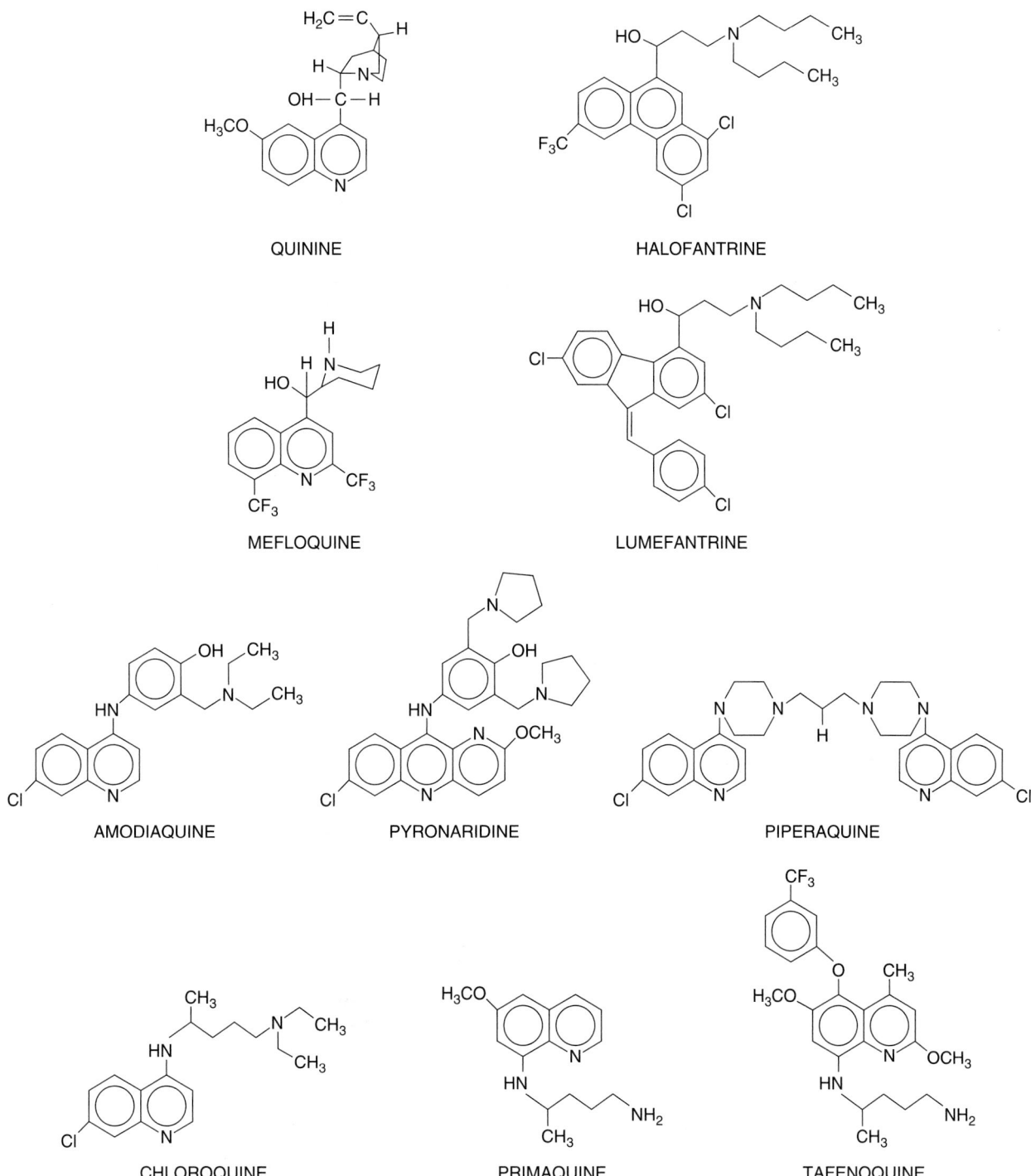

Figure 39–3. *Chemical structure of antimalarial quinolines and related compounds.*

described in Chapter 40. Chloroquine and hydroxychloroquine have been used as secondary drugs to treat a variety of chronic diseases because both alkaloids concentrate in lysosomes and have antiinflammatory properties. Thus, these compounds, often together with other agents, have clinical efficacy in rheumatoid arthritis, systemic lupus erythematosus, discoid lupus, sarcoidosis, and photosensitivity diseases such as porphyria cutanea tarda and severe polymorphous light eruption (Danning and Boumpas, 1998; Fazzi, 2003; Sarkany, 2001).

Mechanisms of Antimalarial Action and Resistance to Chloroquine and Other Antimalarial Quinolines. Asexual malaria parasites flourish in host erythrocytes by digesting hemoglobin in their acidic food vacuoles, a process that generates free radicals and heme (ferriprotoporphyrin IX) as highly reactive by-products. Perhaps aided by histidine-rich proteins and lipids, heme is sequestered as an insoluble unreactive malarial pigment termed *hemozoin*. Many theories for the mechanism of action of chloroquine have been advanced (Tilley *et al.*, 2001). The weight of the current evidence suggests that quinolines interfere with heme handling. Chloroquine concentrates in the food vacuoles of susceptible plasmodia, where it binds to heme as it is released during hemoglobin degradation and disrupts heme sequestration. Failure to inactivate heme or even enhanced toxicity of drug–heme complexes is thought to kill the parasites *via* oxidative damage to membranes, digestive proteases, and possibly other critical biomolecules. Other quinolines such as quinine, *amodiaquine*, and mefloquine, as well as other aminoalcohol analogs (*lumefantrine, halofantrine*) and Mannich base analogs (*pyronaridine*), may act by a similar mechanism, although differences in their actions have been proposed (Sullivan *et al.*, 1998; Tilley *et al.*, 2001).

Resistance of erythrocytic asexual forms of *P. falciparum* to antimalarial quinolines, especially chloroquine, now is common in most parts of the world (Figure 39–4). More than 5 years ago, Fitch and coworkers noted that chloroquine-sensitive *P. falciparum* parasites concentrated the drug to higher levels than did chloroquine-resistant organisms (Fitch *et al.*, 1979). Reasons for the relatively reduced levels of chloroquine in food vacuoles of chloroquine-resistant parasites have yet to be completely clarified. These could include differences in plasmodial uptake and transport of chloroquine to food vacuoles as well as differences in vacuolar influx, efflux, and trapping of drug (Tilley *et al.*, 2001).

The studies of Wellems and colleagues (Carlton *et al.*, 2001) have identified a gene (*crt*, for chloroquine resistance transporter) with alleles that confer chloroquine resistance on *P. falciparum* in culture. These alleles correlate with resistance in clinical field strains. Multiple mutations appear to be needed to confer resistance. Interestingly, different alleles confer resistance in African, Asian, and South American strains (Sidhu *et al.*, 2002). Papua New Guinea isolates have the South American pattern (Mehlotra *et al.*, 2001). The *crt* gene appears to encode a transporter that resides in the food vacuole membrane. Its physiological function is unknown, and its mechanism of action in conferring resistance to chloroquine is poorly understood. Chloroquine-resistant *P. vivax* isolates do not appear to have significant alterations in their *crt* ortholog and may have a different resistance mechanism. Isogenic strains of *P. falciparum* expressing sensitive or resistant *crt* alleles have similar sensitivity to amodiaquine, suggesting that this agent is not acted on by the chloroquine resistance mechanism (Sidhu *et al.*, 2002). The P-

glycoprotein transporter encoded by *Pfmdr1* and perhaps other transporters may play a modulatory role in chloroquine resistance (Mu *et al.*, 2003), and the glutathione system also could play a role (Ginsburg and Golenser, 2003).

Absorption, Fate, and Excretion. Chloroquine is well absorbed from the GI tract and rapidly from intramuscular and subcutaneous sites. The drug distributes relatively slowly into a very large apparent volume (over 100 L/kg) (*see* Krishna and White, 1996). This is due to extensive sequestration of chloroquine in tissues, particularly liver, spleen, kidney, lung, melanin-containing tissues, and to a lesser extent, brain and spinal cord. Chloroquine binds moderately (60%) to plasma proteins and undergoes appreciable biotransformation *via* hepatic CYPs to two active metabolites, desethylchloroquine and bisdesethylchloroquine (*see* Ducharme and Farinotti, 1996). These metabolites may reach concentrations in plasma 40% and 10% of that of chloroquine, respectively. The renal clearance of chloroquine is about half of its total systemic clearance. Unchanged chloroquine and its major metabolite account for more than 50% and 25% of the urinary drug products, respectively, and the renal excretion of both compounds is increased by acidification of the urine.

Both in adults and in children, chloroquine exhibits complex pharmacokinetics such that plasma levels of the drug shortly after dosing are determined primarily by the rate of distribution rather than the rate of elimination (*see* Krishna and White, 1996). Because of extensive tissue binding, a loading dose is required to achieve effective concentrations in plasma. After parenteral administration, rapid entry together with slow exit of chloroquine from a small central compartment can result in transiently high and potentially lethal concentrations of the drug in plasma. Hence, parenteral chloroquine is given either slowly by constant intravenous infusion or in small divided doses by the subcutaneous or intramuscular route. Chloroquine is safer when given orally because the rates of absorption and distribution are more closely matched; peak plasma levels are achieved in about 3 to 5 hours after dosing by this route. The half-life of chloroquine increases from a few days to weeks as plasma levels decline, reflecting the transition from slow distribution to even slower elimination from extensive tissue stores. The terminal half-life ranges from 30 to 60 days, and traces of the drug can be found in the urine for years after a therapeutic regimen.

Therapeutic Uses. Chloroquine is inexpensive and safe, but its usefulness has declined in those parts of the world where strains of *P. falciparum* have emerged that are relatively or absolutely resistant to its action. Except in areas where resistant strains of *P. vivax* are reported (Table 39–2), chloroquine is very effective in prophylaxis or treatment of acute attacks of malaria caused by *P. vivax*, *P. ovale*, and *P. malariae*. Chloroquine has no activity against primary or latent liver stages of the parasite. To prevent relapses in *P. vivax* and *P. ovale* infections, primaquine can be given either with chloroquine or reserved for use until after a patient leaves an endemic area. Chloroquine rapidly controls the clinical symptoms and parasitemia of acute malarial attacks. Most patients become completely afebrile within 24 to 48 hours after receiving therapeutic doses, and thick smears of periph-eral blood generally are negative by 48 to 72 hours. If patients fail to respond during the second day of chloro-quine therapy, resistant strains of *P. falciparum* should be suspected and therapy instituted with quinine or another rapidly acting blood schizontocide. Although chloroquine can be given safely by parenteral routes to comatose or vomiting patients until the drug can be taken orally, quinidine gluconate usually is given in the United States. In comatose children, chloroquine is well absorbed and effective when given through a nasogastric tube. Tables 39–1 and 39–2 provide information about recommended prophylactic and therapeutic dosage regi-mens involving the use of chloroquine. These regimens are subject to modification according to clinical judg-ment, geographic patterns of chloroquine resistance, and regional usage.

Toxicity and Side Effects. Taken in proper doses, chloroquine is an extraordinarily safe drug; however, its safety margin is narrow, and a single dose of 30 mg/kg may be fatal (Taylor and White, 2004). Acute chloroquine toxicity is encountered most frequently when therapeutic or high doses are administered too rapidly by parenteral routes (*see* above). Toxic manifestations relate primar-ily to the cardiovascular system and the CNS. Cardiovascular effects include hypotension, vasodilation, suppressed myocardial function, cardiac arrhythmias, and eventual cardiac arrest. Confu-sion, convulsions, and coma indicate CNS dysfunction. Chloro-quine doses of more than 5 g given parenterally usually are fatal. Prompt treatment with mechanical ventilation, epinephrine, and diazepam may be lifesaving.

Doses of chloroquine used for oral therapy of the acute malarial attack may cause GI upset, headache, visual disturbances, and urticar-ia. Pruritus also occurs, most commonly among dark-skinned persons. Prolonged medication with suppressive doses occasionally causes side effects such as headache, blurring of vision, diplopia, confusion, convulsions, lichenoid skin eruptions, bleaching of hair, widening of the QRS interval, and T-wave abnormalities. These complications usually disappear soon after the drug is withheld. Rare instances of hemolysis and blood dyscrasias have been reported. Chloroquine may cause discoloration of nail beds and mucous membranes. Chloroquine can interfere with the immunogenicity of certain vaccines (Horowitz and Carbonaro, 1992; Pappaioanou *et al.*, 1986).

High daily doses (>250 mg) leading to cumulative total doses of more than 1 g of base per kilogram of chloroquine or hydroxychlo-roquine, such as those used for treatment of diseases other than malaria, can result in irreversible retinopathy and ototoxicity. Retin-opathy presumably is related to drug accumulation in melanin-rich tissues and can be avoided if the daily dose is 250 mg or less (*see* Rennie, 1993). Prolonged therapy with high doses of 4-aminoquino-line also can cause toxic myopathy, cardiopathy, and peripheral neu-ropathy; these reactions improve if the drug is withdrawn promptly (Estes *et al.*, 1987). Rarely, neuropsychiatric disturbances, including suicide, may be related to overdose.

Precautions and Contraindications. This topic has been reviewed by Taylor and White (2004). Chloroquine is not recommended for treating individuals with epilepsy or myasthenia gravis. The drug

should be used cautiously if at all in the presence of hepatic disease or severe gastrointestinal, neurological, or blood disorders. The dose must be adjusted in renal failure. In rare cases, chloroquine can cause hemolysis in patients with glucose-6-phosphate dehydrogen-ase (G6PD) deficiency (*see* Primaquine below). Concomitant use of *gold* or *phenylbutazone* (no longer available in the United States) with chloroquine should be avoided because of the tendency of all three agents to produce dermatitis. Chloroquine should not be pre-scribed for patients with psoriasis or other exfoliative skin condi-tions because it causes severe reactions. It should not be used for malaria in patients with porphyria cutanea tarda but is used in small-er doses for treatment of the underlying disease (*see* Chapter 63). Chloroquine is an inhibitor of CYP2D6 and interacts with a variety of different agents. It should not be given with mefloquine because of increased risk of seizures. Most important, this antimalarial opposes the action of anticonvulsants and increases the risk of ven-tricular arrhythmias from coadministration with *amiodarone* or halofantrine. By increasing plasma levels of *digoxin* and *cyclospor-ine,* chloroquine also can increase the risk of toxicity from these agents. For patients receiving long-term, high-dose therapy, oph-thalmological and neurological evaluations are recommended every 3 to 6 months.

Quinine and Quinidine.

History. The medicinal use of qui-nine dates back more than 350 years (Rocco, 2003). Quinine is the chief alkaloid of cinchona, the powdered bark of the South American cinchona tree, otherwise known as Peruvian, Jesuit's, or Cardinal's bark. It had been used by indigenous Peruvians to treat shivering. In 1633, an Augustinian monk named Calancha, of Lima, Peru, first wrote that a powder of cinchona "given as a beverage, cures the fevers and tertians." By 1640, cinchona was used to treat fevers in Europe. The Jesuit fathers were the main importers and distributors of cinchona in Europe.

For almost two centuries the bark was employed for medicine as a powder, extract, or infusion. In 1820, Pelletier and Caventou iso-lated quinine from cinchona. Quinine still is a mainstay for treating attacks of chloroquine- and multidrug-resistant *P. falciparum* malar-ia (Table 39–2). However, multitherapy with other antimalarials is beginning to supplant quinine regimens because of increasing resis-tance of *P. falciparum* to quinine together with its toxicity.

Chemistry. Cinchona contains a mixture of more than 20 struc-turally related alkaloids, the most important of which are quinine and quinidine. Both compounds contain a quinoline group attached through a secondary alcohol linkage to a quinuclidine ring (Figure 39–3). A methoxy side chain is attached to the quinoline ring and a vinyl to the quinuclidine. They differ only in the steric configuration at two of the three asymmetrical centers: the carbon bearing the sec-ondary alcohol group and at the quinuclidine junction. Although quinine and quinidine have been synthesized, the procedures are complex; hence they still are obtained from natural sources. Quini-dine is both somewhat more potent as an antimalarial and more toxic than quinine (Karle *et al.*, 1992; Krishna and White, 1996) (cardiovascular effects are considered in Chapter 34). Structure–activity relationships of the cinchona alkaloids are detailed in earlier editions of this book. Such studies provided the basis for the discov-ery of more recent antimalarials such as mefloquine.

Pharmacological Effects. *Antimalarial Actions.* Quinine acts primarily against asexual erythrocytic forms; it has lit-tle effect on hepatic forms of malarial parasites. The alka-

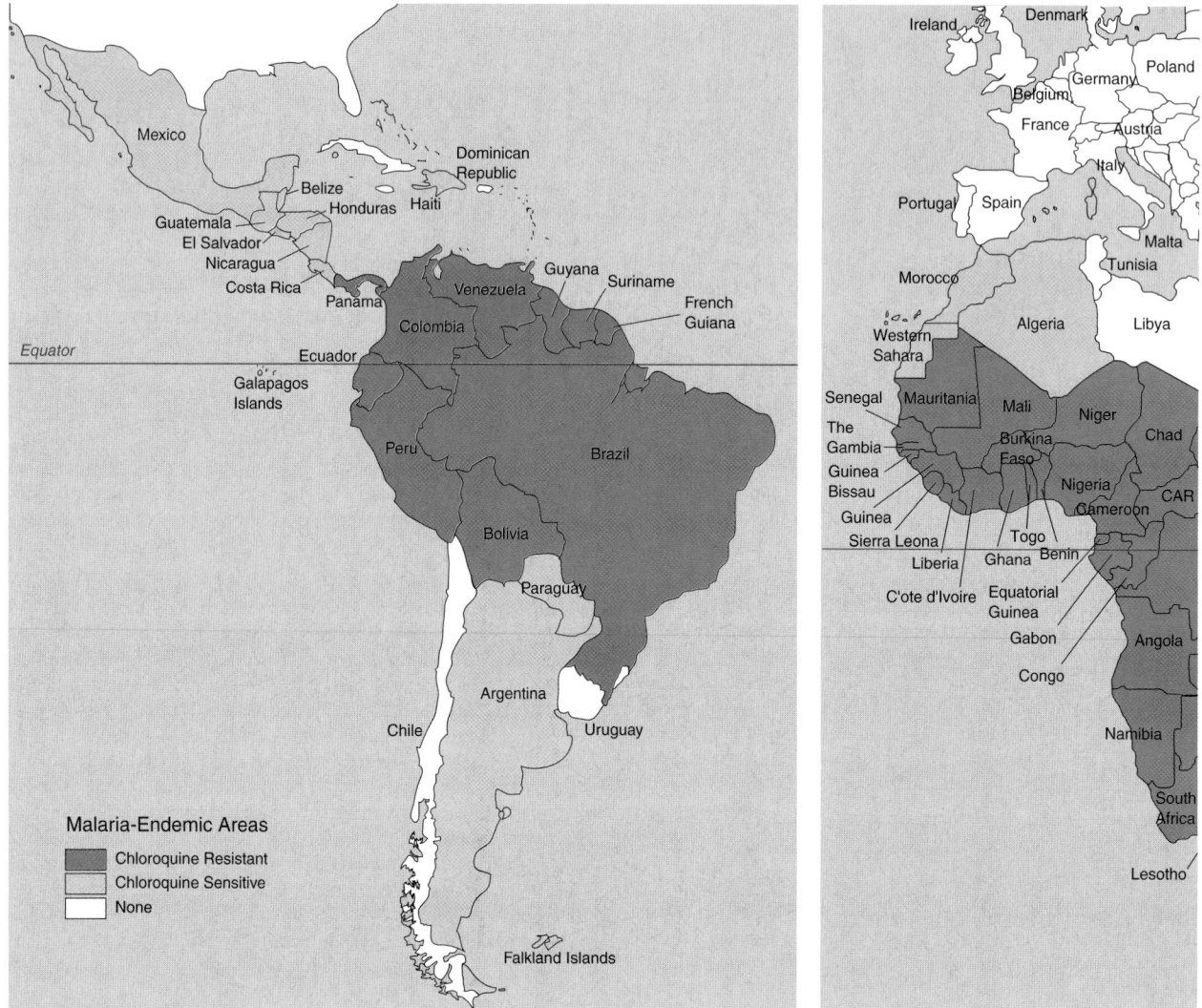

Figure 39–4. *Distribution of malaria and chloroquine-resistant* **Plasmodium falciparum,** *2002.* From Centers for Disease Control and Prevention.

loid also is gametocidal for *P. vivax* and *P. malariae* but not for *P. falciparum*. Quinine is more toxic and less effective than chloroquine against malarial parasites susceptible to both drugs. However, quinine, along with its stereoisomer quinidine, is especially valuable for the parenteral treatment of severe illness owing to drug-resistant strains of *P. falciparum*, even though these strains have become more resistant to both agents in certain parts of Southeast Asia and South America. Because of its toxicity and short half-life, quinine generally is not used for prophylaxis.

The mechanism of the antimalarial action of quinine and related quinoline antimalarials is reviewed under Chloroquine above. The basis of *P. falciparum* resistance to quinine is complex. Patterns of

P. falciparum resistance to quinine more closely resemble those of resistance to mefloquine and halofantrine rather than to chloroquine. Amplification of *pfmdr1* in *P. falciparum,* implicated in resistance to mefloquine and halofantrine, also can confer resistance to quinine *in vitro*. However, the correlation is inconsistent (Dorsey *et al.*, 2001; Sidhu *et al.*, 2002). Quinine and quinidine sensitivity also can diverge in different strains (Sidhu *et al.*, 2002). Recent evidence suggests the participation of a number of different transporter genes in conferring resistance to quinine (Mu *et al.*, 2003).

Action on Skeletal Muscle. Quinine and related cinchona alkaloids exert effects on skeletal muscle that have clinical implications. Quinine increases the tension response to a single maximal stimulus delivered to muscle directly or through nerves, but it also increases the refrac-

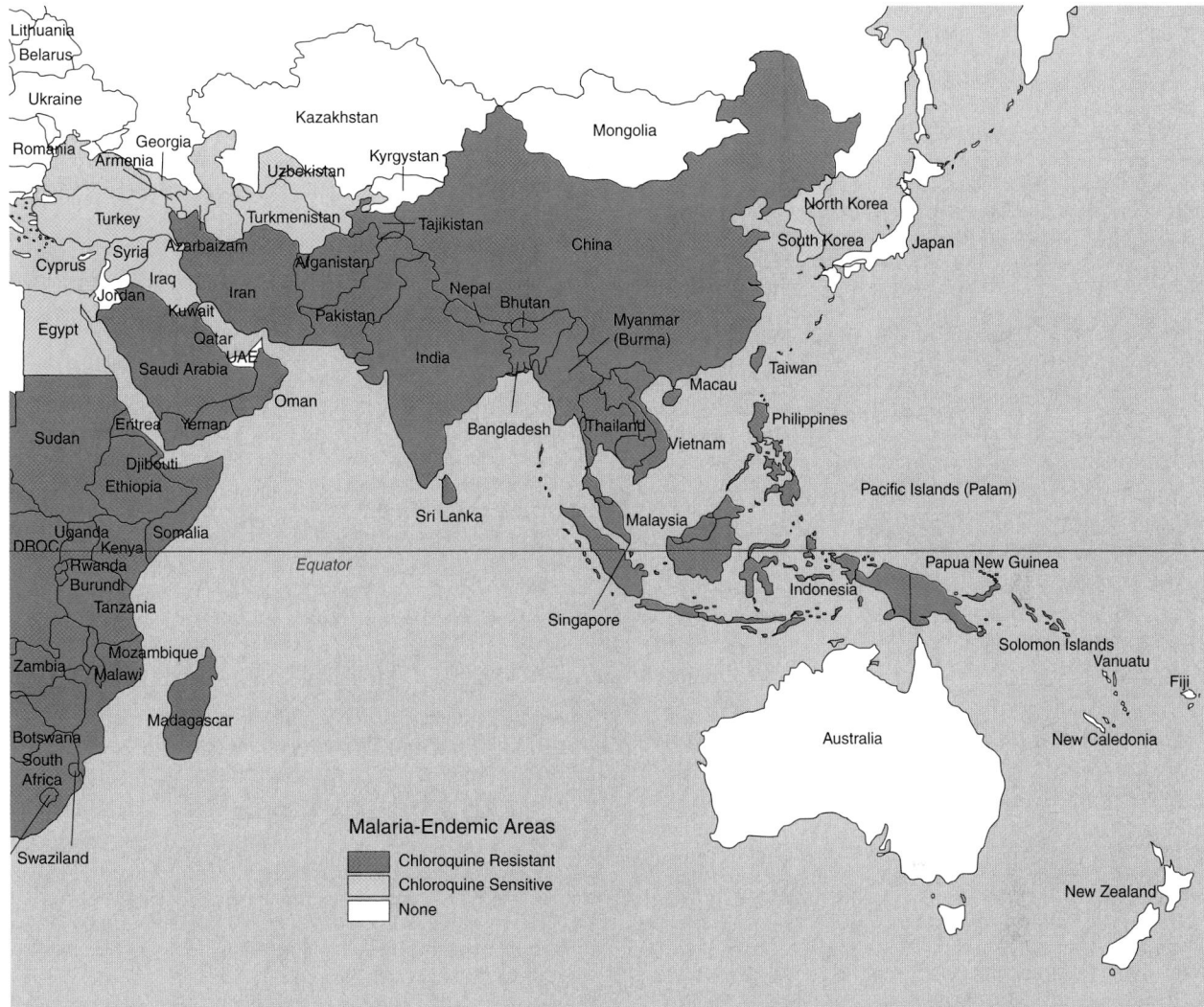

Figure 39–4. *(continued) Distribution of malaria and chloroquine-resistant* **Plasmodium falciparum, *2002.*** From Centers for Disease Control and Prevention.

tory period of muscle so that the response to tetanic stimulation is diminished. The excitability of the motor endplate region decreases so that responses to repetitive nerve stimulation and to acetylcholine are reduced. Thus, quinine can antagonize the actions of *physostigmine* on skeletal muscle as effectively as *curare*. Quinine also may produce alarming respiratory distress and dysphagia in patients with myasthenia gravis. Quinine may cause symptomatic relief of myotonia congenita. This disease is the pharmacological antithesis of myasthenia gravis such that drugs effective in one syndrome aggravate the other.

Absorption, Fate, and Excretion. Quinine is readily absorbed when given orally or intramuscularly. In the former case, absorption occurs mainly from the upper small intestine and is more than 80% complete, even in patients with marked diarrhea. After an oral dose, plasma levels of quinine reach a maximum in 3 to 8 hours and, after distributing into an apparent volume of about 1.5 L/kg in healthy individuals, decline with a half-life of about 11 hours after termination of therapy. As reviewed by Krishna and White (1996), the pharmacokinetics of quinine may change according to the severity of malarial infection. Values for both the apparent volume of distribution and the systemic clearance of quinine decrease, the latter more than the former, so that the average elimination half-life increases from 11 to 18 hours. After standard therapeutic doses, peak plasma levels of quinine may reach 15 to 20 mg/L in severely ill Thai patients without causing major toxicity (*see* below); in contrast, levels greater than 10 mg/L produce severe drug reactions in self-poisoning. The high levels of plasma α_1-acid glycoprotein produced in severe malaria may prevent toxicity by binding the drug and thereby reducing the free fraction of quinine. Concentrations of quinine are lower in erythrocytes (33% to 40%) and CSF (2% to 5%) than in plasma, and the drug readily reaches fetal tissues.

The cinchona alkaloids are metabolized extensively, especially by hepatic CYP3A4 (Zhao et al., 1996), so only about 20% of an administered dose is excreted unaltered in the urine. There is no accumulation of the drugs in the body on continued administration. However, the major metabolite of quinine, 3-hydroxyquinine, retains some antimalarial activity and can accumulate and possibly cause toxicity in patients with renal failure (Newton et al., 1999). Renal excretion of quinine itself is more rapid when the urine is acidic.

Therapeutic Uses. Treatment of Malaria.
It is a telling commentary of the current state of antimalarial therapy that quinine is the treatment of choice for drug-resistant P. falciparum malaria despite its antiquity and considerable toxicity. In severe illness, the prompt use of loading doses of intravenous quinine (or quinidine, where IV quinine is not available, as in the United States) is imperative and can be lifesaving. Oral medication to maintain therapeutic concentrations then is given as soon as it can be tolerated and is continued for 5 to 7 days. Especially for treatment of infections with multidrug-resistant strains of P. falciparum, slower-acting blood schizontocides such as a sulfonamide or a tetracycline are given concurrently to enhance the efficacy of quinine. Formulations of quinine and quinidine and specific regimens for their use in the treatment of P. falciparum malaria are shown in Table 39–2.

Recommendations shown in Table 39–2 are derived from practice and should be modified as appropriate. In a series of studies over the past two decades, White and associates derived rational regimens, including the institution of loading doses, for the use of quinine and quinidine in the treatment of P. falciparum malaria in Southeast Asia (see Krishna and White, 1996). Between 0.2 and 2.0 mg/L has been estimated as the therapeutic range for "free" quinine. Regimens needed to achieve this target may vary based on patient age, severity of illness, and the responsiveness of P. falciparum to the drug. For example, lower doses are more effective in treating children in Africa than adults in Southeast Asia because the pharmacokinetics of quinine differ in the two populations, as does the susceptibility of P. falciparum to the drug (Krishna and White, 1996). Dosage regimens for quinidine are similar to those for quinine, although quinidine binds less to plasma proteins and has a larger apparent volume of distribution, greater systemic clearance, and shorter terminal elimination half-life than quinine (see Krishna and White, 1996; Miller

et al., 1989). It has been suggested (Thompson et al., 2003) that the dose of quinidine currently recommended by the Centers for Disease Control and Prevention (10 mg salt per kilogram initially, followed by 0.02 mg salt per kilogram per minute) may be too low and really should be 10 and 0.02 mg of base (60% of the salt is base). Clinical data on which to base a firm recommendation are lacking.

Treatment of Nocturnal Leg Cramps. Recumbency leg muscle cramps (night cramps) reportedly have been relieved by quinine in a dose of 200 to 300 mg (available until 1995 in products that did not require a prescription) before retiring. In some individuals, only a brief period of quinine therapy has been said to be required to provide relief, but in others, even large doses of the drug were ineffective. In 1995, the FDA issued a ruling that required drug manufacturers to stop marketing over-the-counter quinine products for nocturnal leg cramps. The FDA stated, as the basis for the ruling, that there were inadequate data to support the safety and effectiveness of quinine for use in treating nocturnal leg cramps.

Toxicity and Side Effects. The fatal oral dose of quinine for adults is about 2 to 8 g. Quinine is associated with a triad of dose-related toxicities when it is given at full therapeutic or excessive doses. These are cinchonism, hypoglycemia, and hypotension. Mild forms of cinchonism—consisting of tinnitus, high-tone deafness, visual disturbances, headache, dysphoria, nausea, vomiting, and postural hypotension—occur very frequently and disappear soon after the drug is withdrawn. Hypoglycemia also is common, mostly in the treatment of severe malaria, but can be life-threatening if not treated promptly with intravenous glucose. Hypotension is more rare but also serious and most often is associated with excessively rapid intravenous infusions of quinine or quinidine. Prolonged medication or high single doses also may produce GI, cardiovascular, and dermal manifestations. These and other drug-associated toxicities are discussed below.

Hearing and vision are particularly affected. Functional impairment of the eighth nerve results in tinnitus, decreased auditory acuity, and vertigo. Visual signs consist of blurred vision, disturbed color perception, photophobia, diplopia, night blindness, constricted visual fields, scotomata, mydriasis, and even blindness (Bateman and Dyson, 1986). The visual and auditory effects probably are the result of direct neurotoxicity, although secondary vascular changes may have a role. Marked spastic constriction of the retinal vessels occurs; the retina is ischemic, the discs are pale, and retinal edema may ensue. In severe cases, optic atrophy results.

Gastrointestinal symptoms also are prominent in cinchonism. Nausea, vomiting, abdominal pain, and diarrhea result from the local irritant action of quinine, but the nausea and emesis also have a central basis. The skin often is hot and flushed, and sweating is prominent. Rashes appear frequently. Angioedema, especially of the face, is observed occasionally.

Quinine and quinidine, even at therapeutic doses, may cause hyperinsulinemia and severe hypoglycemia through their powerful stimulatory effect on pancreatic beta cells. Despite treatment with glucose infusions, this complication can be serious and possibly life threatening, especially in pregnancy and prolonged severe infection.

Hypoglycemia is seen occasionally in uninfected patients who take quinine (Limburg *et al.*, 1993).

Quinine rarely causes cardiovascular complications unless therapeutic plasma concentrations are exceeded (Krishna and White, 1996). QTc prolongation is mild and does not appear to be affected by concurrent mefloquine treatment. However, severe hypotension is predictable when quinine is administered too rapidly by the intravenous route. Acute overdosage also may cause serious and even fatal cardiac dysrhythmias such as sinus arrest, junctional rhythms, AV block, and ventricular tachycardia and fibrillation (Bateman and Dyson, 1986). Quinidine is even more cardiotoxic than quinine; its effects on the heart are discussed in detail in Chapter 34. Cardiac monitoring of patients on intravenous quinidine is advisable where possible.

When small doses of cinchona alkaloids cause toxic manifestations, the individual usually is hypersensitive to the drug. Cutaneous flushing and pruritus, often accompanied by skin rashes, fever, gastric distress, dyspnea, ringing in the ears, and visual impairment, are the usual expressions of hypersensitivity. Hemoglobinuria and asthma from quinine may occur more rarely. "Blackwater fever"—the triad of massive hemolysis, hemoglobinemia, and hemoglobinuria leading to anuria, renal failure, and even death—is a rare type of hypersensitivity reaction to quinine therapy that occurs in pregnancy and in the treatment of malaria. Quinine may cause milder hemolysis upon occasion, especially in people with G6PD deficiency. Symptomatic thrombocytopenic purpura by an antibody- and complement-dependent mechanism also is rare, but this reaction can occur even in response to ingestion of tonic water, which has about one-twenty-fifth the therapeutic oral dose per 12 oz ("cocktail purpura"). Other rare reactions to the drug include hypoprothrombinemia, leukopenia, and agranulocytosis. High doses of quinine used to terminate pregnancy may cause fetal abnormalities.

Precautions, Contraindications, and Interactions. Quinine must be used with considerable caution, if at all, in patients who manifest hypersensitivity to the drug, especially when this takes the form of cutaneous, angioedematous, visual, or auditory symptoms. Quinine should be discontinued immediately if evidence of hemolysis appears. The drug should not be used in patients with tinnitus or optic neuritis. In patients with cardiac dysrhythmias, the administration of quinine requires the same precautions as for quinidine (*see* Chapter 34). Quinine appears to be fairly safe in pregnancy and is used commonly for treatment of malaria in this circumstance, but caution must be used to monitor the elevated risk of hypoglycemia.

Because parenteral solutions of quinine are highly irritating, the drug should not be given subcutaneously; concentrated solutions may cause abscesses when injected intramuscularly or thrombophlebitis when infused intravenously. Absorption of quinine from the gastrointestinal tract can be delayed by antacids containing aluminum. Quinine and quinidine can delay the absorption and elevate plasma levels of digoxin and related cardiac glycosides (*see* Chapters 33 and 34). Likewise, the alkaloid may raise plasma levels of *warfarin* and related anticoagulants. The action of quinine at neuromuscular junctions will enhance the effect of neuromuscular blocking agents and oppose the action of acetylcholinesterase inhibitors (*see* above). Prochlorperazine can amplify quinine's cardiotoxicity, as can halofantrine. The renal clearance of quinine can be decreased by *cimetidine* and increased by acidification of the urine and by rifampin.

Mefloquine

History and Chemistry. Mefloquine (LARIAM) is a product of the Malaria Research Program established in 1963 by the Walter Reed Institute for Medical Research to develop promising new compounds to combat emerging strains of drug-resistant *P. falciparum*. Of many 4-quinoline methanols tested based on their structural similarity to quinine, mefloquine (Figure 39–3) displayed high antimalarial activity in animal models and emerged from clinical trials as safe and highly effective against drug-resistant strains of *P. falciparum* (Schmidt *et al.*, 1978). Mefloquine was first used to treat chloroquine-resistant *P. falciparum* malaria in Thailand, where it was formulated with pyrimethamine–sulfadoxine (FANSIMEF) to delay development of drug-resistant parasites. This strategy failed largely because slow elimination of mefloquine fostered the selection of resistant parasites at subtherapeutic drug concentrations (*see* White, 1999). Mefloquine is used for the prophylaxis and chemotherapy of drug-resistant *P. falciparum* and *P. vivax* malaria.

Antimalarial Actions.
Mefloquine exists as a racemic mixture of four optical isomers with about the same antimalarial potency. It is a highly effective blood schizontocide. Mefloquine has no activity against early hepatic stages and mature gametocytes of *P. falciparum* or latent tissue forms of *P. vivax*. The drug may have some sporontocidal activity but is not used clinically for this purpose.

Mechanisms of Antimalarial Action and Resistance. The exact mechanism of action of mefloquine is unknown but may be similar to that of chloroquine (*see* Chloroquine, above). Certain isolates of *P. falciparum* exhibit resistance to mefloquine. The molecular basis of this resistance is not fully understood and is clearly multifactorial. The chloroquine-resistant alleles of the *pfcrt* gene actually confer increased sensitivity to mefloquine and some other quinolines (Sidhu *et al.*, 2002). Amplification of the *pfmdr1* gene is associated with resistance to mefloquine and quinine (Dorsey *et al.*, 2001). Correlation of mefloquine resistance with these changes is not absolute, suggesting that other factors yet to be determined are involved. The stereoselectivity of mefloquine resistance (and action) has yet to be characterized.

Absorption, Fate, and Excretion. Mefloquine is taken orally because parenteral preparations cause severe local reactions. The drug is well absorbed, a process enhanced by the presence of food. Probably owing to extensive enterogastric and enterohepatic circulation, plasma levels of mefloquine rise in a biphasic manner to their peak in about 17 hours. The drug is widely distributed, highly bound (~98%) to plasma proteins, and slowly eliminated with a terminal half-life of about 20 days. The biotransformation of mefloquine has not been well characterized in humans, although several metabolites are formed. Plasma levels of the inactive mefloquine 4-carboxylic acid exceed those of mefloquine itself and decline at about the same rate. Excretion is mainly by the fecal route; only about 10% of mefloquine appears unchanged in the urine. The stereoisomers of mefloquine exhibit quite different pharmacokinetic characteristics that relate to their biodisposition (Hellgren *et al.*, 1997). However, changes in the pharmacokinetics of racemic mefloquine that can occur as a result of age, ethnicity, pregnancy, and malarial illness do not substantially affect dosing regimens (*see* Palmer *et al.*, 1993; Schlagenhauf, 1999).

Therapeutic Uses

Mefloquine should be reserved for the prevention and treatment of malaria caused by drug-resistant *P. falciparum* and P. vivax. The drug is especially useful as a prophylactic agent for nonimmune travelers who stay for only brief periods in areas where these infections are endemic (Table 39–1). In areas where malaria is due to drug-resistant strains of *P. falciparum*, recent evidence indicates that mefloquine is more effective when used in combination with an artemisinin compound (*see* Artemisinin, above).

Toxicity and Side Effects. The adverse effects of mefloquine have been reviewed in detail (Schlagenhauf, 1999; Taylor and White, 2004). Mefloquine given orally generally is well tolerated, particularly at prophylaxis dosages. Different trials vary widely with regard to frequency and severity of side effects. In part, this may be due to the varied populations studied. Early vomiting occurs more frequently at treatment dosages. Dividing the dose improves tolerance. The full dose should be repeated if vomiting occurs within the first hour. Nausea, late vomiting, dizziness, and neuropsychiatric side effects are increased at treatment dosages. Estimates for frequency of severe CNS toxicity after mefloquine treatment range up to 0.5% and include seizures, confusion or decreased sensorium, acute psychosis, and disabling vertigo. Such symptoms generally are reversible on drug discontinuation. At prophylactic dosages, the risk of serious neuropsychiatric effects is estimated to be about 0.01% (about the same as for chloroquine). Mild-to-moderate toxicities (*e.g.,* disturbed sleep, dysphoria, headache, GI disturbances, and dizziness) occur even at prophylactic dosages. Whether these symptoms are more common than with other antimalarial regimens is debated. Adverse effects usually are manifest after the first to third doses and often abate even with continued treatment. Reports of cardiac abnormalities, hemolysis, and agranulocytosis are rare.

Contraindications and Interactions. At very high doses, mefloquine causes teratogenesis and developmental abnormalities in rodents. Mefloquine is approved for use during pregnancy by the CDC and after the first trimester by the WHO. However, there have been studies suggesting an increased rate of still births with mefloquine use, especially during the first trimester (Taylor and White, 2004). The significance of these data has been debated, but it is fair to say that the evidence for mefloquine's safety in pregnancy is not fully convincing, and alternatives should be sought. Pregnancy also should be avoided for 3 months after mefloquine use because of the prolonged half-life of this agent. The drug is contraindicated for patients with a history of seizures, severe neuropsychiatric disturbances, or adverse reactions to quinoline antimalarials such as quinine, quinidine, halofantrine, mefloquine, and chloroquine. Although mefloquine can be taken safely 12 hours after a last dose of quinine, taking quinine shortly after mefloquine can be very hazardous because the latter is eliminated so slowly. Treatment with or after

halofantrine or within 2 months of prior mefloquine administration is contraindicated. Mefloquine is reported to increase the risk of seizures in epileptic patients controlled by *valproate,* and it may compromise adequate immunization by live typhoid vaccine. Until more data become available, caution is advised for use of mefloquine along with drugs that can perturb cardiac conduction. Recent studies do not indicate that mefloquine compromises the performance of tasks that require good motor coordination, for example, driving or operating machinery (Schlagenhauf, 1999). Even so, the WHO advises against use of mefloquine for patients in occupations that require great dexterity, such as pilots.

Primaquine

History. The weak plasmodicidal activity of methylene blue, first discovered by Ehrlich in 1891, later was exploited to develop the 8-aminoquinoline antimalarials. From a large series of quinoline derivatives synthesized with methoxy and substituted 8-amino groups, pamaquine was the first introduced into medicine. During World War II the search for more potent and less toxic 8-aminoquinoline antimalarials led to the selection of primaquine. This compound, in contrast with other antimalarials, acts on tissue stages (exoerythrocytic) of plasmodia in the liver to prevent and cure relapsing malaria. The striking hemolysis that may follow primaquine therapy led directly to the landmark discovery of G6PD deficiency, the first genetic disorder associated with an enzyme (Carson *et al.*, 1956) (*see* Chapter 4). Hemolysis remains notoriously identified with primaquine therapy, and there is a pressing need for alternatives to this important drug. 8-Aminoquinoline shows promise but needs more evaluation (Kain and Jong, 2003; Wiesner *et al.*, 2003b). The chemical structure of primaquine is shown in Figure 39–3.

Antimalarial Actions. Primaquine destroys primary and latent hepatic stages of *P. vivax* and *P. ovale* and thus has great clinical value for preventing relapses of *P. vivax* or *P. ovale* malaria. The drug will not treat ongoing attacks of malaria, even though it displays some activity against the erythrocytic stages. The 8-aminoquinolines exert a marked gametocidal effect against all four species of plasmodia that infect humans, especially *P. falciparum.* Some strains of *P. vivax* exhibit partial resistance to the action of primaquine (Smoak *et al.*, 1997), which makes it imperative that strict adherence to drug regimen be maintained and that other liver-stage antimalarials be developed.

Mechanism of Antimalarial Action. Little is known about the antimalarial action of the 8-aminoquinolines. Primaquine may be converted to electrophiles that act as oxidation–reduction mediators (*see* below). Such activity could contribute to antimalarial effects by generating reactive oxygen species or by interfering with electron transport in the parasite (Bates *et al.*, 1990).

Absorption, Fate, and Excretion. Primaquine causes marked hypotension after parenteral administration and therefore is given only by the oral route. Absorption from the gastrointestinal tract is nearly complete. After a single dose, the plasma concentration reaches a maximum within 3 hours and then falls with an apparent elimination half-life of 6 hours. The apparent volume of distribution is several times that of total-body water. Primaquine is metabolized rapidly (Brueckner *et al.*, 2001); only a small fraction of an administered dose is excreted as the parent drug. Many oxidative metabolites of primaquine have been observed, but 8-(3-carboxyl-1-methylpropylamino)-6-methoxyquinoline is the major metabolite in human plasma. After a single dose, this metabolite reaches concentrations more than ten times those of primaquine; it is eliminated more slowly and accumulates with multiple doses.

Therapeutic Uses. Primaquine is used primarily for the terminal prophylaxis and radical cure of *P. vivax* and *P. ovale* (relapsing) malarias because of its high activity against the latent tissue forms of these plasmodial species. The compound is given together with a blood schizontocide, usually chloroquine, to eradicate erythrocytic stages of these plasmodia and reduce the possibility of emerging drug resistance. For terminal prophylaxis, primaquine regimens are initiated shortly before or immediately after the patient leaves an endemic area (Table 39–1). Radical cure of *P. vivax* or *P. ovale* malaria can be achieved if the drug is given either during the long-term latent period of infection or during an acute attack. Limited studies also have shown efficacy in prevention of *P. falciparum* and *P. vivax* malaria when primaquine is taken prophylactically (Taylor and White, 2004). The drug generally is well tolerated when taken for up to 1 year.

Toxicity and Side Effects. Primaquine is fairly innocuous when given to most Caucasians in the usual therapeutic doses. Primaquine can cause mild-to-moderate abdominal distress in some individuals; these symptoms often are alleviated by taking the drug at mealtime. Mild anemia, cyanosis (methemoglobinemia), and leukocytosis are less common. High doses (60 to 240 mg daily) accentuate the abdominal symptoms and cause methemoglobinemia in most subjects. Methemoglobinemia can occur even with usual doses of primaquine and can be severe in individuals with congenital deficiency of nicotinamide adenine dinucleotide (NADH) methemoglobin reductase (Coleman and Coleman, 1996). Chloroquine and dapsone may be synergistic with primaquine in producing methemoglobinemia in these patients. Granulocytopenia and agranulocytosis are rare complications of therapy and usually are associated with overdosage. Also rare are hypertension, arrhythmias, and symptoms referable to the CNS.

Therapeutic or higher doses of primaquine may cause acute hemolysis and hemolytic anemia in humans with G6PD deficiency (Taylor and White, 2004). This X-linked condition, primarily owing to amino acid substitutions in the G6PD enzyme, affects more than 200 million people worldwide. More than 400 genetic variants have been identified that are associated with variable responses to oxidative stress. About 11% of African-Americans have the A– variant of G6PD, which makes them vulnerable to hemolysis caused by pro-oxidant drugs such as primaquine. Sensitivity of erythrocytes to pri-

maquine can be even more severe in some Caucasian ethnic groups, including Sardinians, Sephardic Jews, Greeks, and Iranians. These populations have a G6PD variant in which two amino acid substitutions impair both enzyme stability and activity. Because primaquine sensitivity is inherited by a gene on the X chromosome, hemolysis often is of intermediate severity in heterozygous females who have two populations of red cells, one normal and the other deficient in G6PD. Owing to "variable penetrance," such females may be affected less frequently than predicted. Primaquine is the prototype of more than 50 drugs, including antimalarial sulfonamides and other substances known to cause hemolysis in susceptible individuals with G6PD deficiency (*see* Chapter 4).

Precautions and Contraindications. Patients should be tested for G6PD deficiency before they receive primaquine. Primaquine has been used cautiously in subjects with the A– form of G6PD deficiency, although benefits of treatment may not necessarily outweigh the risks. The drug should not be used in patients with more severe deficiency. The CDC recommend use only when a normal G6PD level has been documented. If a daily dose of more than 30 mg primaquine base (more than 15 mg in possibly sensitive patients) is given, repeated blood counts and at least gross examination of the urine for hemoglobin should be undertaken. Primaquine should not be used in pregnant women and can be used only in lactating mothers whose infants have a normal G6PD level.

Primaquine is contraindicated for acutely ill patients suffering from systemic disease characterized by a tendency to granulocytopenia; very active forms of rheumatoid arthritis and lupus erythematosus are examples of such conditions. Primaquine should not be given to patients receiving other potentially hemolytic drugs or agents capable of depressing the myeloid elements of the bone marrow.

Other Quinolines and Related Antimalarials

A number of quinolines and structurally related antimalarials are available outside the United States or are in development. Amodiaquine is a congener of chloroquine (Figure 39–3) that is no longer recommended in the United States for chemoprophylaxis of *P. falciparum* malaria because its use is associated with hepatic toxicity and agranulocytosis. It is inexpensive and has substantial activity in chloroquine-resistant strains; its use in endemic areas with few alternatives is being debated and reevaluated (Olliaro and Mussano, 2003). *Isoquine* is an isomer of amodiaquine that may yield fewer toxic metabolites and is being assessed (Olliaro and Taylor, 2003). Pyronaridine is a Mannich-base antimalarial that is structurally related to amodiaquine (Figure 39–3). This compound, developed by the Chinese in the 1970s, was shown to be well tolerated and effective against *P. falciparum* and *P. vivax* malarias. However, it cannot be recommended for routine use at this time because of a lack of standardized dosage regimens and because its possible long-term toxicity has yet to be evaluated adequately (Winstanley, 2001). This drug currently is being developed in combination with artesunate (Olliaro and Taylor, 2003). *Piperaquine* is a bisquinoline (shown in Figure 39–3) that has been used extensively in Asia. It has activity against chloroquine-resistant parasites and currently is being assessed as a combination with dihydroartemisinin (Ridley, 2002; Tran *et al.*, 2004). Halofantrine (HALFAN) is a phenanthrene methanol antimalarial drug (Figure 39–3) with blood schizontocidal properties similar to those of the quinoline antimalarials. This compound was developed originally to treat acute malarial attacks caused by drug-resistant strains of *P. falciparum*. Because halofantrine displays erratic bioavailability, potentially lethal cardiotoxicity, and extensive cross-resistance with mefloquine, its use generally is not recommended. Details of the history, pharmacology, and toxicology of halofantrine are presented in the ninth edition of this book. Lumefantrine is a drug with structural similarities to mefloquine and halofantrine (Figure 39–3). It is marketed in combination with artemether (CO-ARTEM) for treatment of malaria (Ridley, 2002). It appears to be effective and well tolerated, but experience is limited.

SULFONAMIDES AND SULFONES

Shortly after their introduction into therapeutics, the sulfonamides were found to have antimalarial activity, a property investigated extensively during World War II. The sulfones also were shown to be effective; the first trial of dapsone was against *P. falciparum* in 1943. The sulfonamides are used together with pyrimethamine and often in addition to quinine to treat chloroquine-resistant *P. falciparum* malaria, especially in parts of Africa. The sulfonamides and sulfones are slow-acting blood schizontocides that are more active against *P. falciparum* than *P. vivax*. As *p*-aminobenzoate analogs that competitively inhibit the dihydropteroate synthase of *P. falciparum,* the sulfonamides are used together with an inhibitor of parasite dihydrofolate reductase to enhance their antiplasmodial action. The synergistic "antifolate" combination of sulfadoxine, a long-acting sulfonamide, with pyrimethamine (FANSIDAR) is used to treat malarial attacks in parts of Africa. The sulfone dapsone given with the biguanide chlorproguanil also has been effective for therapy of chloroquine-resistant *P. falciparum* malaria.

The future of the antimalarial antifolates appears bleak unless they are used together with more effective, rapidly acting drugs, *e.g.*, an artemisinin derivative. Long-term use of pyrimethamine–sulfadoxine, for example, is no longer recommended for prophylaxis of *P. falciparum* malaria because of potentially serious toxicity from the sulfonamide (Bjorkman and Phillips-Howard, 1991) (*see* Diaminopyrimidines, above, and Chapter 43). Moreover, resistance of *P. falciparum* to the antifolates is prevalent and develops rapidly on exposure to these agents, rendering them ineffective in many parts of the world. Mutations that cause amino acid substitutions at several different loci in the dihydropteroate synthase of *P. falciparum* confer resistance to sulfadoxine and raise the K_i values for other sulfonamides and dapsone as well. These and other mutations that accumulate during exposure to sulfonamides, together with dihydrofolate reductase mutations associated with pyrimethamine and cycloguanil resistance, can severely compromise therapy of *P. falciparum* malaria with antifolate combinations (Sibley *et al.*, 2001).

TETRACYCLINES

The tetracyclines are slow-acting blood schizontocides that are used alone for short-term prophylaxis in areas with chloroquine and mefloquine resistance. Tetracyclines are particularly useful for the treatment of the acute malarial attack owing to multidrug-resistant strains of *P. falciparum* that also show partial resistance to quinine. Their relative slowness of action makes them ineffective as single agents for malaria treatment. As an adjunct to quinine or quinidine, they are quite useful therapy (*see* Quinine, above). Several tetracyclines appear equivalent, but *tetracycline* or *doxycycline* usually is recommended. Clindamycin is an alternative. Tetracyclines have shown marked activity against primary tissue schizonts of chloroquine-resistant *P. falciparum*. Doxycycline is used alone by travelers for short-term prophylaxis of multidrug-resistant strains. Dosage regimens for tetracyclines and doxycycline are listed in Tables 39–1 and 39–2. Because of their adverse effects on bones and teeth, tetracyclines should not be given to pregnant women or children younger than 8 years of age. Photosensitivity reactions or drug-induced superinfections may mandate discontinuation of therapy or prophylaxis with these agents (*see* Chapter 46).

PRINCIPLES AND GUIDELINES FOR PROPHYLAXIS AND CHEMOTHERAPY OF MALARIA

Pharmacological control of malaria poses a difficult challenge because *P. falciparum,* which causes nearly all the deaths from human malaria, has become progressively more resistant to available antimalarial drugs. Fortunately, chloroquine still is effective against malarias caused by *P. ovale, P. malariae,* most strains of *P. vivax,* and chloroquine-sensitive strains of *P. falciparum* found in some geographic areas. However, chloroquine-resistant strains of *P. falciparum* now prevail in all endemic areas except Mexico, Central America west of the Panama Canal Zone, the Caribbean, and parts of South America and the Middle East (Figure 39–4). Except for parts of Africa, extensive geographic overlap also exists between chloroquine resistance and resistance to pyrimethamine–sulfadoxine, an inexpensive combination of antifolate drugs used widely for the treatment of *P. falciparum* malaria. Multidrug-resistant *P. falciparum* malaria, especially prevalent and severe in Southeast Asia and Oceania, now is well established in South America and threatens Africa. These infections may not respond adequately even to mefloquine or quinine.

Genetic studies indicate that isolates of *P. falciparum* from patients in highly endemic areas contain many parasite clones with different drug-resistance phenotypes (Druilhe *et al.*, 1998). A patient with severe malaria may have 10^{12} parasites, so it is easy to understand how single point mutations conferring resistance can arise in virtually every patient and double mutations can arise occasionally. Compounding the situation, parasites that already have developed drug-resistant traits might be even more prone to acquiring resistance to new unrelated antimalarial agents by a hypermutation mechanism (Rathod *et al.*, 1997). Therefore, drugs or drug combinations that are to be successful must not be susceptible to single-point-mutation resistance. Intense chloroquine use for decades preceded development of resistance to this agent likely because multiple mutations were necessary to confer resistance. Resistance also can be promoted by free radicals generated by atovaquone treatment in the mitochondria of the parasite; this is thought to promote development of resistance to this drug (*see* Atovaquone, above). Pharmacokinetics also can be a determinant in the generation of resistance. Drugs with a long half-life are more likely to select out resistant parasites (White, 2004). On a population level, the fitness of resistant parasites is an important parameter—if mutation causes a reduced ability to survive or grow, the parasites are less likely to spread. On the other side, in the case of antifolates, treatment actually induces gametocytogenesis, which promotes propagation and may explain the sweep of particular resistance alleles across Africa. These considerations strongly suggest using regimens consisting of two or more agents to treat drug-resistant *P. falciparum* malaria (White, 1999, 2004). Promising examples of such regimens include artemisinin combination treatments (ACT) (*see* Artemisinin, above) and proguanil together with atovaquone. Current recommendations for drugs and dosing regimens for the prophylaxis and therapy of malaria in nonimmune individuals are shown in Tables 39–1 and 39–2. These will change and should serve only as general guidelines to be modified appropriately according to the status and habitat of the patient; the geographic origin, species, and drug-resistance profile of infecting parasites; and the agents used locally for malaria control.

The following section presents an overview of the chemoprophylaxis and chemotherapy of malaria. For more details about individual drugs and their clinical applications, the reader should consult the text and references, especially Thompson and colleagues (2003), Kain and Jong (2003), and Suh and colleagues (2004) for prophylaxis and treatment; Taylor and White (2004) for toxicity; and Stauffer and Fischer (2003) for treatment of children. The latest information about malaria risk areas and prophylaxis is available from the CDC (*www.cdc.gov/travel/travel*). Consultation and emergency advice about treatment are available 24 hours a day from the duty officer, Division of Parasitic Diseases, CDC.

Importantly, *drugs should not replace simple, inexpensive measures for malaria prevention.* Individuals visiting malarious areas should take appropriate steps to prevent mosquito bites. Avoiding exposure to mosquitoes at dusk and dawn, usually times of maximal feeding, is one such measure. Others include wearing long-sleeved dark clothes, using insect repellents containing at least 30% *N,N'*-diethylmetatoluamide (DEET) (Fradin and Day, 2002), and sleeping in well-screened rooms or under bed nets impregnated with a pyrethrin insecticide such as permethrin (Kain and Jong, 2003).

A number of regimens are available for malaria chemoprophylaxis. In general, dosing should be started before exposure, ideally before the traveler leaves home, to establish therapeutic blood levels and to detect early signs or symptoms of intolerance so that the regimen can be modified before departure. As described earlier, the duration of postexposure dosing is dictated by the spectrum of drug action (Figure 39–2). In those few areas where chloroquine-sensitive strains of *P. falciparum* are found, chloroquine still is suitable for prophylaxis. It also remains the drug of choice for prophylaxis and control of infections due to *P. vivax, P. ovale,* and *P. malariae.* In areas where chloroquine-resistant malaria is endemic, mefloquine and atovaquone–proguanil are the regimens of choice for prophylaxis. There is more experience with mefloquine and more evidence for its efficacy against *P. vivax,* which is a consideration in areas where this species coexists with *P. falciparum.* However, there are more contraindications to the use of mefloquine and perhaps more toxicity (*see* Mefloquine, above). Doxycycline is an alternative chemoprophylactic agent. In cases where mefloquine, atovaquone–proguanil, and doxycycline all are contraindicated, primaquine is a possibility for prophylaxis. Primaquine, like atovaquone–proguanil, is active against liver stages and can be discontinued shortly after leaving the endemic area. Attempts at radical cure of *P. vivax* malaria with primaquine should be delayed until the patient leaves an endemic area.

A malarial attack should be viewed as a medical emergency, especially for vulnerable populations such as nonimmune travelers, pregnant women, and young children. Treatment with a rapidly acting blood schizontocide must be instituted promptly if *P. falciparum* malaria is suspected from a travel history and clinical findings. One should not wait for a definitive parasitological diagnosis in such patients because their clinical status may deteriorate rapidly. Moreover, the clinical presentation may be atypical, and thick blood smears may fail to reveal plasmodia in early stages of this infection. Chloroquine is the drug of choice for *P. vivax, P. ovale, P. malariae,* and chloroquine-sensitive strains of *P. falciparum*. The oral route of administration is used whenever possible, but chloroquine can be given intramuscularly or even intravenously if suitable precautions are taken, although quinine and quinidine usually are the parenteral drugs of choice (*see* above). Within 48 to 72 hours of initiating therapy, patients should show marked clinical improvement and a substantial decrease in parasitemia as monitored by daily thick blood smears. Lack of such a response or failure to clear parasites from the blood by 7 days is indicative of drug resistance. If chloroquine-resistant *P. falciparum* malaria is suspected, either from the travel history or from lack of response to chloroquine, the preferred treatment is quinine. For multidrug-resistant *P. falciparum* malaria, quinine is given together with other effective but slower-acting blood schizontocides such as antifolates or tetracyclines (Table 39–2) (*see* above). Again, the oral route of drug administration is preferred, but intravenous preparations should be given until oral medication can be taken. For parenteral therapy in the U.S., quinidine gluconate must be substituted for quinine dihydrochloride, which is no longer available. Exchange transfusion may be of additional value in severe *P. falciparum* malaria with high parasitemia (Miller *et al.*, 1989).

Attacks of malaria may recur during or after a course of antimalarial chemotherapy, even in the absence of reinfection. Recurrent attacks caused by *P. vivax*, *P. ovale*, or *P. malariae* usually are well controlled by another course of chloroquine combined with or followed by a course of primaquine in the case of *P. vivax* or *P. ovale*. Some patients with *P. vivax* infection may require more than one course of primaquine to effect a radical cure. Recrudescence of *P. falciparum* malarial attacks or parasitemia after appropriate treatment with chloroquine usually denotes infection with chloroquine-resistant plasmodia (for clinical classification of drug resistance, *see* Bruce-Chwatt *et al.*, 1986). Quinine together with a slower-acting drug such as doxycycline in Southeast Asia or with antifolate antimalarials (*e.g.*, pyrimethamine–sulfadoxine) in Africa has combated this problem successfully (Table 39–2). However, the 7-day course of treatment that often is required, the toxic doses of quinine needed to overcome increasingly drug-resistant parasites, and poor patient compliance compromise the utility of these regimens. Mefloquine is a good alternative to quinine for geographical areas where resistance is lacking, but mefloquine cannot be given parenterally. Moreover, toxic doses of mefloquine may be needed to eradicate parasites that exhibit *in vitro* cross-resistance to quinine. Especially promising compounds for treatment of multidrug-resistant *P. falciparum* malaria are the artemisinin compounds. As the most rapidly acting and potent blood schizontocides known, these endoperoxides markedly reduce parasite burden in a single life cycle and, when used to initiate therapy, make ideal partners for other drugs such as quinolines or antifolates. Parasite resistance has not been seen to date probably because of their rapid action and very short half-lives (*see* above). Success against multidrug-resistant *P. falciparum* malaria also has been achieved with atovaquone–proguanil.

However, this combination is relatively expensive, and treatment failure owing to resistance already is being reported (*see* Atovaquone, above).

Malarial infection, especially with *P. falciparum*, is a severe threat to children and pregnant women. With appropriate adjustments and safety precautions, the treatment of children generally is the same as for adults. However, tetracyclines should not be given except in an emergency to children younger than 8 years of age, and atovaquone–proguanil has been approved only for children weighing more than 11 kg. Pregnant women should be urged not to travel to endemic areas if possible. While chloroquine and proguanil may be used during pregnancy, safety documentation is not as complete as would be desired. Antifolates, tetracyclines, the artemisinins, atovaquone, and primaquine should be avoided. Quinine and quinidine can be used with appropriate caution given to the frequently accompanying hypoglycemia. Mefloquine can be used if necessary, but safety data are not quite reassuring.

In lactating mothers, treatment with most compounds is acceptable, but use of atovaquone–proguanil is not recommended. Also, the infant must be tested and found to have a normal G6PD level before using primaquine. For prophylaxis in long-term travelers (Hughes *et al.*, 2003), chloroquine is safe at the doses used, but some recommend yearly retinal examinations. Mefloquine and doxycycline are well tolerated. Atovaquone–proguanil has been studied for up to 20 weeks but probably is acceptable for years based on experience with the individual components.

NEW TARGETS

Genome analysis has suggested a number of new targets, many of which are shared with bacteria and/or plants but not mammals. The apicoplast, a specialized organelle of algal origin, appears to be important for lipid and heme biosynthesis (Ralph *et al.*, 2004). It is a major focus of current drug-development efforts. Furthest along is an inhibitor of apicoplast DoxP isoprenoid biosynthesis, fosmidomycin (Wiesner *et al.*, 2003a). This agent, developed as an antibacterial drug, has shown efficacy in combination with clindamycin against *P. falciparum* malaria in limited trials. Inhibition of phospholipid metabolism, proteases involved in hemoglobin degradation, and protein prenylation also are being studied actively, among other pathways (*see* Rosenthal *et al.*, 2002; Ridley, 2002).

CLINICAL SUMMARY

Agents available in the United States as antimalarials include quinolines, atovaquone, diaminopyrimidines, sulfa drugs, and tetracyclines. Long-acting quinolines such as chloroquine and mefloquine are used for prophylaxis and treatment, although resistance to chloroquine now is widespread, whereas toxicity and increasing resistance limit mefloquine's utility. Short-acting quinolines such as quinine and quinidine are important for the treatment of severe and drug-resistant malaria. Primaquine is a quinoline with activity against the latent hepatic phase of some malaria parasites and is used for radical cure of these infections. Atovaquone is a hydroxynaphthoquinone that is useful for prophylaxis and treatment when combined with proguanil (MALARONE). Diaminopyrimidines are used in combination with sulfa drugs (pyrimethamine–sulfadoxine, FANSIDAR) in therapy of chloroquine-resistant malaria or with atovaquone (as above). Tetracyclines can be used for treatment as an adjunct to other agents such as quinine or as a prophylaxis in regions where multidrug resistance occurs. The artemisinins, currently not approved for use in the United States, are a group of potent antimalarials that are used in combination treatments for drug-resistant malaria infections. Many promising combinations are being explored.

BIBLIOGRAPHY

Adjuik, M., Babiker, A., Garner, P., *et al.* Artesunate combinations for treatment of malaria: Meta-analysis. *Lancet, 2004, 363*:9–17.

Bates, M.D., Meshnick, S.R., Sigler, C.I., *et al. In vitro* effects of primaquine and primaquine metabolites on exoerythrocytic stages of *Plasmodium berghei. Am. J. Trop. Med. Hyg.,* **1990,** *42*:532–537.

Berman, J.D., Nielsen, R., Chulay, J.D., *et al.* Causal prophylactic efficacy of atovaquone–proguanil (MALARONE) in a human challenge model. *Trans. R. Soc. Trop. Med. Hyg.,* **2001,** *95*:429–432.

Bjorkman, A., and Phillips-Howard, P.A. Adverse reactions to sulfa drugs: Implications for malaria chemotherapy. *Bull. WHO,* **1991,** *69*:297–304.

Carson, P.E., Flanagan, C.L., Ickes, C.E., and Alving, A.S. Enzymatic deficiency in primaquine-sensitive erythrocytes. *Science,* **1956,** *124*:484–485.

Craig, A., and Scherf, A. Molecules on the surface of the *Plasmodium falciparum* infected erythrocyte and their role in malaria pathogenesis and immune evasion. *Mol. Biochem. Parasitol.,* **2001,** *115*:129–143.

Dorsey, G., Kamya, M.R., Singh, A., and Rosenthal, P.J. Polymorphisms in the *Plasmodium falciparum pfcrt* and *pfmdr-1* genes and clinical response to chloroquine in Kampala, Uganda. *J. Infect. Dis.,* **2001,** *183*:1417–1420.

Druilhe, P., Daubersies, P., Patarapotikul, J., *et al.* A primary malarial infection is composed of a very wide range of genetically diverse but related parasites. *J. Clin. Invest.,* **1998,** *101*:2008–2016.

Eckstein-Ludwig, U., Webb, R.J., Van Goethem, I.D., *et al.* Artemisinins target the SERCA of *Plasmodium falciparum. Nature,* **2003,** *424*:957–961.

Estes, M.L., Ewing-Wilson, D., Chou, S.M., *et al.* Chloroquine neuromyotoxicity: Clinical and pathologic perspective. *Am. J. Med.,* **1987,** *82*:447–455.

Ferone, R., Burchall, J.J., and Hitchings, G.H. *Plasmodium berghei* dihydrofolate reductase: Isolation, properties, and inhibition by antifolates. *Mol. Pharmacol.,* **1969,** *5*:49–59.

Fidock, D.A., and Wellems, T.E. Transformation with human dihydrofolate reductase renders malaria parasites insensitive to WR99210 but does not affect the intrinsic activity of proguanil. *Proc. Natl. Acad. Sci. U.S.A.,* **1997,** *94*:10931–10936.

Fitch, C.D., Chan, R.L., and Chevli, R. Chloroquine resistance in malaria: Accessibility of drug receptors to mefloquine. *Antimicrob. Agents Chemother.,* **1979,** *15*:258–262.

Fivelman, Q.L., Butcher, G.A., Adagu, I.S., Warhurst, D.C., and Pasvol, G. Malarone treatment failure in *in vivo* confirmation of resistance of *Plasmodium falciparum* isolate from Lagos, Nigeria. *Malar. J.,* **2002,** *1*:1.

Fradin, M.S., and Day, J.F. Comparative efficacy of insect repellents against mosquito bites. *New Engl. J. Med.,* **2002,** *347*:13–18.

Gardner, M.J., Hall, N., Fung, E., *et al.* Genome sequence of the human malaria parasite *Plasmodium falciparum. Nature,* **2002,** *419*:498–511.

Hellgren, U., Berggren-Palme, I., Bergqvist, Y., and Jerling, M. Enantioselective pharmacokinetics of mefloquine during long-term intake of the prophylactic dose. *Br. J. Clin. Pharmacol.,* **1997,** *44*:119–124.

Helsby, N.A., Edwards, G., Breckenridge, A.M., and Ward, S.A. The multiple-dose pharmacokinetics of proguanil. *Br. J. Clin. Pharmacol.,* **1993,** *35*:653–656.

Hernandez-Diaz, S., Werler, M.M., Walker, A.M., and Mitchell, A.A. Folic acid antagonists during pregnancy and the risk of birth defects. *New Engl. J. Med.,* **2000,** *343*:1608–1614.

Horowitz, H., and Carbonaro, C.A. Inhibition of the *Salmonella typhi* oral vaccine strain, Ty21a, by mefloquine and chloroquine. *J. Infect. Dis.,* **1992,** *166*:1462–1464.

Hudson, A.T., Dickins, M., Ginger, C.D., *et al.* 566C80: A potent broad-spectrum antiinfective agent with activity against malaria and opportunistic infections in AIDS patients. *Drugs Exp. Clin. Res.,* **1991,** *17*:427–435.

Hughes, W.T., Gray, V.L., Gutteridge, W.E., *et al.* Efficacy of a hydroxynaphthoquinone, 566C80, in experimental *Pneumocystis carinii* pneumonitis. *Antimicrob. Agents Chemother.,* **1990,** *34*:225–228.

Hughes, W.T., and Oz, H.S. Successful prevention and treatment of babesiosis with atovaquone. *J. Infect. Dis.,* **1995,** *172*:1042–1046.

Hussein, Z., Eaves, J., Hutchinson, D.B., and Canfield, C.J. Population pharmacokinetics of atovaquone in patients with acute malaria caused by *Plasmodium falciparum. Clin. Pharmacol. Ther.,* **1997,** *61*:518–530.

Johann-Liang, R., and Albrecht, R. Safety evaluations of drugs containing artemisinin derivatives for the treatment of malaria. *Clin. Infect. Dis.,* **2003,** *36*:1626–1627.

Karle, J.M., Karle, I.L., Gerena, L., and Milhous, W.K. Stereochemical evaluation of the relative activities of the cinchona alkaloids against *Plasmodium falciparum. Antimicrob. Agents Chemother.,* **1992,** *36*:1538–1544.

Lacy, M.D., Maguire, J.D., Barcus, M.J., *et al.* Atovaquone/proguanil therapy for *Plasmodium falciparum* and *Plasmodium vivax* malaria in

Indonesians who lack clinical immunity. *Clin. Infect. Dis.,* **2002,** *35*:92–95.

Limburg, P.J., Katz, H., Grant, C.S., and Service, F.J. Quinine-induced hypoglycemia. *Ann. Intern Med.,* **1993,** *119*:218–219.

Ling, J., Baird, J.K., Fryauff, D.J., *et al.* and Naval Medical Research Unit 2 Clinical Trials Team. Randomized, placebo-controlled trial of atovaquone/proguanil for the prevention of *Plasmodium falciparum* or *Plasmodium vivax* malaria among migrants to Papua, Indonesia. *Clin. Infect Dis.,* **2002,** *35*:825–833.

Looareesuwan, S., Viravan, C., Webster, H.K., *et al.* Clinical studies of atovaquone, alone or in combination with other antimalarial drugs, for treatment of acute uncomplicated malaria in Thailand. *Am. J. Trop. Med. Hyg.,* **1996,** *54*:62–66.

Looareesuwan, S., Wilairatana, P., Glanarongran, R., *et al.* Atovaquone and proguanil hydrochloride followed by primaquine for treatment of *Plasmodium vivax* malaria in Thailand. *Trans. R. Soc. Trop. Med. Hyg.,* **1999b,** *93*:637–640.

McGready, R., Cho, T., Cho, J.J., *et al.* Artemisinin derivatives in the treatment of falciparum malaria in pregnancy. *Trans. R. Soc. Trop. Med. Hyg.,* **1998,** *92*:430–433.

Mehlotra, R.K., Fujioka, H., Roepe, P.D., *et al.* Evolution of a unique *Plasmodium falciparum* chloroquine-resistance phenotype in association with *pfcrt* polymorphism in Papua New Guinea and South America. *Proc. Natl. Acad. Sci. U.S.A.,* **2001,** *98*:12689–12694.

Miller, K.D., Greenberg, A.E., and Campbell, C.C. Treatment of severe malaria in the United States with a continuous infusion of quinidine gluconate and exchange transfusion. *New Engl. J. Med.,* **1989,** *321*:65–70.

Mu, J., Ferdig, M.T., Feng, X., *et al.* Multiple transporters associated with malaria parasite responses to chloroquine and quinine. *Mol. Microbiol.,* **2003,** *49*:977–989.

Newton, P., Keeratithakul, D., Teja-Isavadharm, P., *et al.* Pharmacokinetics of quinine and 3-hydroxyquinine in severe falciparum malaria with acute renal failure. *Trans. R. Soc. Trop. Med. Hyg.,* **1999,** *93*:69–72.

Newton, P.N., Angus, B.J., Chierakul, W., *et al.* Randomized comparison of artesunate and quinine in the treatment of severe falciparum malaria. *Clin. Infect. Dis.,* **2003a,** *37*:7–16.

Newton, P.N., Dondorp, A., Green, M., *et al.* Counterfeit artesunate antimalarials in Southeast Asia. *Lancet,* **2003b,** *362*:169.

Pappaioanou, M., Fishbein, D.B., Dreesen, D.W., *et al.* Antibody response to preexposure human diploid-cell rabies vaccine given concurrently with chloroquine. *New Engl. J. Med.,* **1986,** *314*:280–284.

Pearson, P.A., Piracha, A.R., Sen, H.A., and Jaffe, G.J. Atovaquone for the treatment of toxoplasma retinochoroiditis in immunocompetent patients. *Ophthalmology,* **1999,** *106*:148–153.

Rathod, P.K., McErlean, T., and Lee, P.C. Variations in frequencies of drug resistance in *Plasmodium falciparum. Proc. Natl. Acad. Sci. U.S.A.,* **1997,** *94*:9389–9393.

Rolan, P.E., Mercer, A.J., Tate, E., *et al.* Disposition of atovaquone in humans. *Antimicrob. Agents Chemother.,* **1997,** *41*:1319–1321.

Schmidt, L.H., Crosby, R., Rasco, J., and Vaughan, D. Antimalarial activities of various 4-quinolonemethanols with special attention to WR-142,490 (mefloquine). *Antimicrob. Agents Chemother.,* **1978,** *13*:1011–1030.

Shapiro, T.A., Ranasinha, C.D., Kumar, N., and Barditch-Crovo, P. Prophylactic activity of atovaquone against *Plasmodium falciparum* in humans. *Am. J. Trop. Med. Hyg.,* **1999,** *60*:831–836.

Sidhu, A.B., Verdier-Pinard, D., and Fidock, D.A. Chloroquine resistance in *Plasmodium falciparum* malaria parasites conferred by *pfcrt* mutations. *Science,* **2002,** *298*:210–213.

Smoak, B.L., DeFraites, R.F., Magill, A.J., *et al. Plasmodium vivax* infections in U.S. Army troops: Failure of primaquine to prevent relapse in studies from Somalia. *Am. J. Trop. Med. Hyg.,* **1997,** *56*:231–234.

Srivastava, I.K., and Vaidya, A.B. A mechanism for the synergistic antimalarial action of atovaquone and proguanil. *Antimicrob. Agents Chemother.,* **1999,** *43*:1334–1339.

Stauffer, W., and Fischer, P.R. Diagnosis and treatment of malaria in children. *Clin. Infect. Dis.,* **2003,** *37*:1340–1348.

Sullivan, D.J. Jr., Matile, H., Ridley, R.G., and Goldberg, D.E. A common mechanism for blockade of heme polymerization by antimalarial quinolines. *J. Biol. Chem.,* **1998,** *273*:31103–31107.

Torres, R.A., Weinberg, W., Stansell, J., *et al.* Atovaquone for salvage treatment and suppression of toxoplasmic encephalitis in patients with AIDS. Atovaquone/Toxoplasmic Encephalitis Study Group. *Clin. Infect. Dis.,* **1997,** *24*:422–429.

Tran, T.H., Dolecek, C., Pfam, P.M., *et al.* Dihydroartemisinin–piperaquine against multidrug-resistant *Plasmodium falciparum* malaria in Vietnam: Randomised clinical trial. *Lancet,* **2004,** *363*:18–22.

Vaidya, A.B. and Mather, M.W. Atovaquone resistance in malaria parasites. *Drug Resist. Updat.,* **2000,** *3*:283–287.

Vercesi, A.E., Rodrigues, C.O., Uyemura, S.A., *et al.* Respiration and oxidative phosphorylation in the apicomplexan parasite *Toxoplasma gondii. J. Biol. Chem.,* **1998,** *273*:31040–31047.

Wang, P., Sims, P.F., and Hyde, J.E. A modified *in vitro* sulfadoxine susceptibility assay for *Plasmodium falciparum* suitable for investigating Fansidar resistance. *Parasitology,* **1997,** *115*:223–230.

Ward, S.A., Helsby, N.A., Skjelbo, E., *et al.* The activation of the biguanide antimalarial proguanil co-segregates with the mephenytoin oxidation polymorphism: A panel study. *Br. J. Clin. Pharmacol.,* **1991,** *31*:689–692.

White, N. Antimalarial drug resistance and combination chemotherapy. *Philos. Trans. R. Soc. Lond. B. Biol. Sci.,* **1999,** *354*:739–749.

Wichmann, O., Muehlen, M., Gruss, H., *et al.* Malarone treatment failure not associated with previously described mutations in the cytochrome b gene. *Malar. J.,* **2004,** *3*:14.

Winstanley, P.A., Watkins, W.M., Newton, C.R., *et al.* The disposition of oral and intramuscular pyrimethamine/sulphadoxine in Kenyan children with high parasitaemia but clinically non-severe falciparum malaria. *Br. J. Clin. Pharmacol.,* **1992,** *33*:143–148.

Zhang, K., and Rathod, P.K. Divergent regulation of dihydrofolate reductase between malaria parasite and human host. *Science,* **2002,** *296*:545–547.

Zhao, X.J., Yokoyama, H., Chiba, K., *et al.* Identification of human cytochrome P450 isoforms involved in the 3-hydroxylation of quinine by human liver microsomes and nine recombinant human cytochromes P450. *J. Pharmacol. Exp. Ther.,* **1996,** *279*:1327–1334.

MONOGRAPHS AND REVIEWS

Bateman, D.N., and Dyson, E.H. Quinine toxicity. *Adverse Drug React. Acute Poison. Rev.,* **1986,** *5*:215–233.

Breman, J.G. The ears of the hippopotamus: Manifestations, determinants, and estimates of the malaria burden. *Am. J. Trop. Med. Hyg.,* **2001,** *64*:1–11.

Bruce-Chwatt, L.J., Black, R.H., Canfield, C.J., *et al. Chemotherapy of Malaria.* World Health Organization, Geneva, **1986.**

Brueckner, R.P., Ohrt, C., Baird, J.K., and Milhous, W.K. 8-Aminoquinolines. In, *Antimalarial Chemotherapy: Mechanisms of Action, Resistance, and New Directions in Drug Discovery.* (Rosenthal, P.J., ed.) Humana Press, Totowa, NJ, **2001,** pp. 123–151.

Carlton, J.M., Fidock, D.A., Djimde, A., *et al.* Conservation of a novel vacuolar transporter in *Plasmodium* species and its central role in chloroquine resistance of *P. falciparum*. *Curr. Opin. Microbiol.,* **2001,** *4*:415–420.

Coleman, M.D., and Coleman, N.A. Drug-induced methaemoglobinaemia. Treatment issues. *Drug Saf.,* **1996,** *14*:394–405.

Danning, C.L., and Boumpas, D.T. Commonly used disease-modifying antirheumatic drugs in the treatment of inflammatory arthritis: An update on mechanisms of action. *Clin. Exp. Rheumatol.,* **1998,** *16*:595–604.

Ducharme, J., and Farinotti, R. Clinical pharmacokinetics and metabolism of chloroquine: Focus on recent advancements. *Clin. Pharmacokinet.,* **1996,** *31*:257–274.

Easterbrook, M. Detection and prevention of maculopathy associated with antimalarial agents. *Int. Ophthalmol. Clin.,* **1999,** *39*:49–57.

Fazzi, P. Pharmacotherapeutic management of pulmonary sarcoidosis. *Am. J. Respir. Med.,* **2003,** *2*:311–320.

Giao, P.T., and de Vries, P.J. Pharmacokinetic interactions of antimalarial agents. *Clin. Pharmacokinet.,* **2001,** *40*:343–373.

Ginsburg, H., and Golenser, J. Glutathione is involved in the antimalarial action of chloroquine and its modulation affects drug sensitivity of human and murine species of *Plasmodium*. *Redox Rep.,* **2003,** *8*:276–279.

Gregson, A., and Plowe, C. Mechanisms of resistance of malaria parasites to antifolates. *Pharmacol. Rev.* **2005,** *57*:117–145.

Hughes, C., Tucker, R., Bannister, B., and Bradley, D.J., and Health Protection Agency Advisory Committee on Malaria Prevention for UK Travellers. Malaria prophylaxis for long-term travellers. *Commun. Dis. Public Health,* **2003,** *6*:200–208.

Kain, K.C., and Jong, E.C. Malaria prevention. In, *The Travel and Tropical Medicine Manual.* (Jong, E.C. and McMullen, R., eds.) Saunders, Philadelphia, **2003,** pp.52–74.

Kasper, L.H. *Toxoplasma* infection. In, *Harrison's Principles of Internal Medicine,* 15th ed. (Braunwald, E., Hauser, S.L., Fauci, A.S., *et al.,* eds.) McGraw-Hill, New York, **2001,** pp. 1222–1227.

Klayman, D.L. Qinghaosu (artemisinin): An antimalarial drug from China. *Science,* **1985,** *228*:1049–1055.

Krause, P.J. Babesiosis diagnosis and treatment. *Vector Borne Zoonotic Dis.,* **2003,** *3*:45–51.

Krishna, S., and White, N.J. Pharmacokinetics of quinine, chloroquine and amodiaquine: Clinical implications. *Clin. Pharmacokinet.,* **1996,** *30*:263–299.

Looareesuwan, S., Chulay, J.D., Canfield, C.J., and Hutchinson, D.B. Malarone (atovaquone and proguanil hydrochloride): A review of its clinical development for treatment of malaria. Malarone Clinical Trials Study Group. *Am. J. Trop. Med. Hyg.,* **1999a,** *60*:533–541.

Meshnick, S.R. Artemisinin and its derivatives. In, *Antimalarial Chemotherapy: Mechanisms of Action, Resistance, and New Directions in Drug Discovery.* (Rosenthal, P.J., ed.) Humana Press, Totowa, NJ, **2001,** pp. 191–201.

Miller, L.H., Baruch, D.I., Marsh, K., and Doumbo, O.K. The pathogenic basis of malaria. *Nature,* **2002,** *415*:673–679.

O'Neill, P.M., and Posner, G.H. A medicinal chemistry perspective on artemisinin and related endoperoxides. *J. Med. Chem.,* **2004,** *47*:2945–2964.

Olliaro, P., and Mussano, P. Amodiaquine for treating malaria. *Cochrane Database Syst. Rev.,* **2003,** CD000016.

Olliaro, P.L., and Taylor, W.R. Antimalarial compounds: From bench to bedside. *J. Exp. Biol.,* **2003,** *206*:3753–3759.

Palmer, K.J., Holliday, S.M., and Brogden, R.N. Mefloquine: A review of its antimalarial activity, pharmacokinetic properties and therapeutic efficacy. *Drugs,* **1993,** *45*:430–475.

Ralph, S.A., Van Dooren, G.G., Waller, R.F., *et al.* Tropical infectious diseases: Metabolic maps and functions of the *Plasmodium falciparum* apicoplast. *Nature Rev. Microbiol.,* **2004,** *2*:203–216.

Rennie, I.G. Clinically important ocular reactions to systemic drug therapy. *Drug Saf.,* **1993,** *9*:196–211.

Ridley, R.G. Medical need, scientific opportunity and the drive for antimalarial drugs. *Nature,* **2002,** *415*:686–693.

Rocco, F. *The Miraculous Fever-Tree: Malaria and the Quest for a Cure that Changed the World.* HarperCollins, New York, **2003.**

Rosenthal, P.J., Sijwali, P.S., Singh, A., and Shenai, B.R. Cysteine proteases of malaria parasites: Targets for chemotherapy. *Curr. Pharm. Des.,* **2002,** *8*:1659–1672.

Sarkany, R.P. The management of porphyria cutanea tarda. *Clin. Exp. Dermatol.,* **2001,** *26*:225–232.

Schlagenhauf, P. Mefloquine for malaria chemoprophylaxis 1992–1998: A review. *J. Travel Med.,* **1999,** *6*:122–133.

Sibley, C.H., Hyde, J.E., Simms, P.F., *et al.* Pyrimethamine–sulfadoxine resistance in *Plasmodium falciparum*: What next? *Trends Parasitol.,* **2001,** *17*:582–588.

Sibley, L.D. Intracellular parasite invasion strategies. *Science,* **2004,** *304*:248–253.

Suh, K.N., Kain, K.C., and Keystone, J.S. Malaria. *Can. Med. Assoc. J.,* **2004,** *170*:1693–1702.

Taylor, W.R., and White, N.J. Antimalarial drug toxicity: A review. *Drug Saf.,* **2004,** *27*:25–61.

Thompson, M.J., White, N.J., and Jong, E.C. Malaria diagnosis and treatment. In, *The Travel and Tropical Medicine Manual.* (Jong, E.C. and McMullen, R., eds.) Saunders, Philadelphia, **2003,** pp. 269–288.

Tilley, L., Loria, P., and Foley, M. Chloroquine and other quinoline antimalarials. In, *Antimalarial Chemotherapy: Mechanisms of Action, Resistance, and New Directions in Drug Discovery.* (Rosenthal, P.J., ed.) Humana Press, Totowa, NJ, **2001,** pp. 87–121.

Utzinger, J., Keiser, J., Shuhua, X., *et al.* Combination chemotherapy of schistosomiasis in laboratory studies and clinical trials. *Antimicrob. Agents Chemother.,* **2003,** *47*:1487–1495.

White, N.J. Assessment of the pharmacodynamic properties of antimalarial drugs *in vivo*. *Antimicrob. Agents Chemother.,* **1997,** *41*:1413–1422.

White, N.J. Antimalarial drug resistance. *J. Clin. Invest.,* **2004,** *113*:1084–1092.

Wiesner, J., Borrmann, S., and Jomaa, H. Fosmidomycin for the treatment of malaria. *Parasitol. Res.,* **2003a,** *90*(suppl.):71–76.

Wiesner, J., Ortmann, R., Jomaa, H., and Schlitzer, M. New antimalarial drugs. *Angew. Chem. Int. Ed. Engl.,* **2003b,** *42*:5274–5293.

Winstanley, P. Modern chemotherapeutic options for malaria. *Lancet Infect. Dis.,* **2001,** *1*:242–250.

CHEMOTHERAPY OF PROTOZOAL INFECTIONS
Amebiasis, Giardiasis, Trichomoniasis, Trypanosomiasis, Leishmaniasis, and Other Protozoal Infections

Margaret A. Phillips and Samuel L. Stanley, Jr.

Humans host a wide variety of protozoal parasites that can be transmitted by insect vectors, directly from other mammalian reservoirs or from one person to another. Because protozoa multiply rapidly in their hosts and effective vaccines are unavailable, chemotherapy has been the only practical way to both treat infected individuals and reduce transmission. The immune system plays a crucial role in protecting against the pathological consequences of protozoal infections. Thus, opportunistic infections with protozoa are prominent in infants, individuals with cancer, transplant recipients, those receiving immunosuppressive drugs or extensive antibiotic therapy, and persons with advanced human immunodeficiency virus (HIV) infection. Treatment of protozoal infections in immunocompromised individuals is especially difficult, and the outcome is often unsatisfactory.

Most antiprotozoal drugs have been in use for years despite major advances in bioscience relevant to parasite biology, host defenses, and mechanisms of disease. Satisfactory agents for treating important protozoal infections such as African trypanosomiasis (sleeping sickness) and chronic Chagas' disease still are lacking. Many effective antiprotozoal drugs are toxic at therapeutic doses, a problem exacerbated by increasing drug resistance. Development of drug resistance also poses a serious threat to better-tolerated antiprotozoal agents in current use. Unfortunately, many of these diseases afflict the poor in developing countries, and there is little economic incentive for pharmaceutical companies to develop new antiparasitic drugs. In fact, there are only a few new agents available, and one, *nitazoxanide*,

represents the first drug developed and approved specifically for protozoal infections (other than malaria) in a decade. Scientists and physicians working in this field must be creative and have turned to drugs developed originally for other indications (*e.g., amphotericin* and *miltefosine* for leishmaniasis), to investigational drugs made available directly from the Centers for Disease Control and Prevention (CDC), or to agents developed for veterinary use to discover new antiparasitic therapies.

This chapter briefly describes important human protozoal infections other than malaria and the drugs used to treat them.

INTRODUCTION TO PROTOZOAL INFECTIONS OF HUMAN BEINGS

Amebiasis. Amebiasis affects about 10% of the world's population, causing invasive disease in about 50 million people and death in about 100,000 of these annually. In the United States, amebiasis is seen most commonly in the states that border Mexico and among individuals living in poverty, crowded conditions, and areas with poor sanitation. Two morphologically identical but genetically distinct species of *Entamoeba* (*i.e., E. histolytica* and *E. dispar*) have been isolated from infected persons. While the proportions vary worldwide, *E. dispar* accounts for approximately 90% of human infections, with *E. histolytica* responsible for only 10%. However, only *E. histolytica* is capable of causing disease and thus requires treatment. The two organisms can be differentiated by antigen-detection enzyme-linked immunosorbent assays (ELISAs) or by polymerase chain reaction (PCR)–based diagnostics. Humans are the only known hosts for these protozoa, which are transmitted almost exclusively by the fecal–oral route. Ingested *E. histolytica* cysts from contaminated food or water survive acid gastric contents and transform into *trophozoites* that reside in the large intestine. The outcome of *E. histolytica* infection is variable. Many individuals remain asymptomatic but excrete the infectious cyst form, making them a source for further infections. In other individuals, *E. histolytica* trophozoites invade into the colonic mucosa with resulting colitis and bloody diarrhea (amebic dysentery). In a smaller proportion of patients, *E. histolytica* trophozoites invade through the colonic mucosa, reach the portal circulation, and travel to the liver, where they establish an amebic liver abscess.

The cornerstone of therapy for amebiasis is the nitroimidazole compound *metronidazole* or its analogs *tinidazole* and *ornidazole*. Metronidazole and tinidazole are the only nitroimidazoles available in the United States and are the drugs of choice for the treatment of amebic colitis, amebic liver abscess, and any other extraintestinal form of amebiasis. Other agents, such as dehydroemetine and chloroquine, are now used rarely in the treatment of amebic colitis or amebic liver abscess and are reserved for only very unusual cases where metronidazole is contraindicated. Because metronidazole is so well absorbed in the gut, levels may not be therapeutic in the colonic lumen, and it is less effective against cysts. Hence patients with amebiasis (amebic colitis or amebic liver abscess) also should receive a luminal agent to eradicate any *E. histolytica* trophozoites residing within the gut lumen. Luminal agents are also used to treat asymptomatic individuals found to be infected with *E. histolytica*. The nonabsorbed aminoglycoside *paromomycin* and the 8-hydroxyquinoline compound iodoquinol are two effective luminal agents. *Diloxanide furoate*, previously considered the luminal agent of choice for amebiasis, is no longer available in the United States. Nitazoxanide (ALINIA), a drug approved in the United States for the treatment of cryptosporidiosis and giardiasis, is also active against *E. histolytica*.

Giardiasis. Giardiasis, caused by the flagellated protozoan *Giardia intestinalis*, is prevalent worldwide and is the most commonly reported intestinal protozoal infection in the United States (Farthing, 1996). Infection results from ingestion of the cyst form of the parasite, which is found in fecally contaminated water or food. *Giardia* is a zoonosis, and cysts shed from animals or from infected humans can contaminate recreational and drinking water supplies. *Giardia* was the most common cause of waterborne outbreaks of diarrhea in the United States between 1978 and 1991 (Lengerich *et al.*, 1994). Human-to-human transmission *via* the fecal–oral route is especially common among children in day-care centers and nurseries, as well as among institutionalized individuals and male homosexuals.

Infection with *Giardia* results in one of three syndromes: an asymptomatic carrier state, acute self-limited diarrhea, or chronic diarrhea. Asymptomatic infection is most common; these individuals excrete *Giardia* cysts and serve as a source for new infections. Most adults with symptomatic infection will develop an acute self-limited illness with watery, foul-smelling stools, abdominal distension, and flatus. However, a significant proportion of these individuals go on to develop a chronic diarrhea syndrome (>2 weeks of illness) with signs of malabsorption (steatorrhea) and weight loss.

The diagnosis of giardiasis is made by identification of cysts or trophozoites in fecal specimens or of trophozoites in duodenal contents. Chemotherapy with a 5-day course of metronidazole usually is successful, although therapy may have to be repeated or

prolonged in some instances. A single dose of tinidazole (TINDAMAX) probably is superior to metronidazole for the treatment of giardiasis. The nonabsorbed aminoglycoside paromomycin has been used to treat pregnant women to avoid any possible mutagenic effects of the other drugs. Nitazoxanide, *N-(nitrothiazolyl) salicylamide,* and tinidazole were approved recently for the treatment of giardiasis in immune-competent children younger than 12 years of age. They join *furazolidone* as the only drugs currently approved by the Food and Drug Administration (FDA) for the treatment of giardiasis.

Trichomoniasis. Trichomoniasis is caused by the flagellated protozoan *Trichomonas vaginalis*. This organism inhabits the genitourinary tract of the human host, where it causes vaginitis in women and, uncommonly, urethritis in men. Trichomoniasis is a sexually transmitted disease, with more than 200 million people infected worldwide and at least 3 million women infected in the United States annually. Infection with *Trichomonas* has been associated with an increased risk of acquiring HIV infection.

Only *trophozoite* forms of *T. vaginalis* have been identified in infected secretions. Metronidazole remains the drug of choice for the treatment of trichomoniasis. However, treatment failures owing to metronidazole-resistant organisms are becoming more frequent (Dunne *et al.*, 2003). Tinidazole, another nitroimidazole that was approved recently by the FDA, appears to be better tolerated than metronidazole and has been used successfully at higher doses to treat metronidazole-resistant *T. vaginalis* (Sobel *et al.*, 2001). Nitazoxanide shows activity against *T. vaginalis in vitro* but has not undergone clinical trials and is not licensed for the treatment of trichomoniasis.

Toxoplasmosis. Toxoplasmosis is a cosmopolitan zoonotic infection caused by the obligate intracellular protozoan *Toxoplasma gondii* (Montoya and Liesenfeld, 2004). Although cats and other feline species are the natural hosts, tissue cysts (*bradyzoites*) have been recovered from all mammalian species examined. The four most common routes of infection in humans are (1) ingestion of undercooked meat containing tissue cysts; (2) ingestion of vegetable matter contaminated with soil containing infective *oocysts;* (3) direct oral contact with feces of cats shedding oocysts; and (4) transplacental fetal infection with *tachyzoites* from acutely infected mothers.

Primary infection with *T. gondii* produces clinical symptoms in about 10% of immunocompetent individuals. The acute illness is usually self-limiting, and treatment rarely is required. Individuals who are immunocompromised, however, are at risk of developing toxoplasmic encephalitis from reactivation of tissue cysts deposited in the brain. The vast majority of cases of toxoplasmic encephalitis are seen in patients with AIDS, in whom the disease is fatal if it is not recognized and treated appropriately. Clinical manifestations of congenital toxoplasmosis vary widely, but chorioretinitis, which may present decades after perinatal exposure, is the most commonly recognized finding. The primary treatment for toxoplasmic encephalitis consists of the antifolates *pyrimethamine* and *sulfadiazine* along with *folinic acid* (LEUCOVORIN). However, therapy must be discontinued in about 40% of cases because of toxicity owing primarily to the sulfa compound. In this instance, *clindamycin* can be substituted for sulfadiazine without loss of efficacy. Alternative regimens combining *azithromycin, clarithromycin, atovaquone,* or *dapsone* with either *trimethoprim–sulfamethoxazole* or pyrimethamine and folinic acid are less toxic but also less effective than the combination of pyrimethamine and sulfadiazine.

Spiramycin, which concentrates in placental tissue, is used for the treatment of acute acquired toxoplasmosis in pregnancy to prevent transmission to the fetus. If fetal infection is detected, the combination of pyrimethamine, sulfadiazine, and folinic acid is administered to the mother (only after the first 12 to 14 weeks of pregnancy) and to the newborn in the postnatal period.

Cryptosporidiosis. Cryptosporidia are coccidian protozoan parasites that can cause diarrhea in a number of animal species, including humans (Ramirez *et al.,* 2004). Their taxonomy is evolving, but *Cryptosporidium parvum* and the newly named *C. hominis* appear to account for almost all infections in humans. Infectious *oocysts* in feces may be spread either by direct human-to-human contact or by contaminated water supplies, the latter being recognized as an established route of epidemic infection. Groups at risk include travelers, children in day-care facilities, male homosexuals, animal handlers, veterinarians, and other healthcare personnel. Immunocompromised individuals are especially vulnerable. After ingestion, the mature oocyte is digested, releasing *sporozoites* that invade host epithelial cells, penetrating the cell membrane but not actually entering the cytoplasm. In most individuals, infection is self-limited. However, in AIDS patients and other immunocompromised individuals, the severity of voluminous, secretory diarrhea may require hospitalization and supportive therapy to prevent severe electrolyte imbalance and dehydration.

The most effective therapy for cryptosporidiosis in AIDS patients is restoration of their immune function through highly active antiretroviral therapy (HAART) (*see* Chapter 50). *Nitazoxanide* has shown activity in treating cryptosporidiosis in immunocompetent children and is possibly effective in immunocompetent adults as well (Rossignol *et al.,* 2001). Its efficacy in children and adults with HIV infection and AIDS is not clearly established, and it appears that the lower their CD4 count, the less likely a patient is to respond to nitazoxanide (Rossignol *et al.,* 1998; Bailey and Erramouspe, 2004). Nevertheless, it is currently the only drug approved for the treatment of cryptosporidiosis in the United States. *Paromomycin* or the combination of paromomycin and *azithromycin* has been used to treat cryptosporidiosis in AIDS patients, but in a randomized, controlled trial, paromomycin alone was no more effective than placebo for this indication (Hewitt *et al.,* 2000).

Trypanosomiasis. African trypanosomiasis, or "sleeping sickness," is caused by subspecies of the hemoflagellate *Trypanosoma brucei* that are transmitted by bloodsucking tsetse flies of the genus *Glossinia.* Largely restricted to Central Africa, it causes serious human illness and also threatens livestock (*nagana*), leading to protein malnutrition. In humans, the infection is fatal unless treated. Owing to strict surveillance, vector control, and early therapy, the prevalence of African sleeping sickness declined to its nadir in the early 1960s. However, relaxation of these measures, together with massive population displacement and breakdowns in societal infrastructure owing to armed conflict, led to a resurgence of this disease in the 1990s (Welburn and Odiit, 2002; Abel *et al.,* 2004; Kennedy, 2004). An estimated 300,000 to 500,000 Africans carry the infection, and over 60 million people are at risk for the disease. It is extremely rare in travelers returning to the United States and can be difficult to diagnose in its more chronic form (Lejon *et al.,* 2003). The parasite is entirely extracellular, and early human infection is characterized by the finding of replicating parasites in the bloodstream without

central nervous system (CNS) involvement (stage 1). Symptoms of early-stage disease include febrile illness, lymphadenopathy, splenomegaly, and occasional myocarditis that result from systemic dissemination of the parasites. Stage 2 disease is characterized by CNS involvement. There are two types of African trypanosomiasis, the East African (Rhodesian) and West African (Gambian), caused by *T. brucei rhodesiense* and *T. brucei gambiense,* respectively. *T. brucei rhodesiense* produces a progressive and rapidly fatal form of disease marked by early involvement of the CNS and terminal cardiac failure; *T. brucei gambiense* causes illness that is characterized by later involvement of the CNS and a more long-term course that progresses to the classical symptoms of sleeping sickness over months to years. Neurological symptoms include confusion, poor coordination, sensory deficits, disruption of the sleep cycle, and eventual progression into coma and death.

There are four drugs used for the treatment of sleeping sickness, and only one, *eflornithine,* has been developed since the 1950s (Fries and Fairlamb, 2003; Fairlamb, 2003; Legros *et al.,* 2002; Bouteille *et al.,* 2003). Standard therapy for early-stage disease is *pentamidine* for *T. brucei gambiense* and suramin for *T. brucei rhodesiense.* These agents are not effective against late-stage disease, and the standard treatment of the CNS phase is *melarsoprol,* which is a highly toxic agent that causes a fatal reactive encephalopathy in about 2% to 10% of treated patients. Moreover, resistance to this agent is leading to increasing numbers of treatment failures (Maser *et al.,* 2003). All three compounds must be given parenterally over long periods (Pépin and Milord, 1994). Eflornithine, which was developed originally as an anticancer agent, offers the only alternative for the treatment of late-stage disease. This compound is an irreversible inhibitor of ornithine decarboxylase, a key enzyme in polyamine metabolism. It has shown marked efficacy against both early and late stages of human *T. brucei gambiense* infection (Pépin and Milord, 1994; Fries and Fairlamb, 2003; Burri and Brun, 2003). It notably has significantly fewer side effects than melarsoprol, and it has been shown to be effective in patients who have failed melarsoprol therapy. However, this agent is expensive and difficult to administer, leading to availability problems that have restricted its use. Further, it is ineffective as monotherapy for infections of *T. brucei rhodesiense* (*see* below). Although *T. brucei* offers a variety of attractive molecular targets for selective pharmacological intervention, few have been turned to practical advantage despite their promise in experimental systems and animal models (Wang, 1995; Fries and Fairlamb, 2003; Fairlamb, 2003).

American trypanosomiasis, or *Chagas' disease,* a zoonotic infection caused by *Trypanosoma cruzi,* affects about 18 to 20 million people from Mexico to Argentina and Chile (Urbina and Docambo, 2003; Rodriques-Coura and deCastro; Fairlamb, 2003), where the chronic form of the disease in adults is a major cause of cardiomyopathy, megaesophagus, megacolon, and death. Bloodsucking triatomid bugs infesting poor rural dwellings most commonly transmit this infection to young children; transplacental transmission also may occur in endemic areas.

Reactivation of disease also may occur in patients who are immunosuppressed after organ transplantation or because of infection (*e.g.,* AIDS, leukemia, and other neoplasias). Occurrences of *T. cruzi* infection in transplant patients or through blood transfusions have been reported in the United States, where up to 300,000 immigrants are estimated to carry the disease. Acute infection is evidenced by a raised tender skin nodule (*chagoma*) at the site of inoculation; other signs may be absent or range from fever, adenitis, skin rash, and hepatosplenomegaly to, albeit rarely, acute myocarditis and death. Invading metacyclic *trypomastigotes* penetrate host cells, especially macrophages, where they proliferate as *amastigotes*. The latter then differentiate into trypomastigotes that enter the bloodstream. Circulating trypomastigotes do not multiply until they invade other cells or are ingested by an insect vector during a blood meal. After recovery from the acute infection that lasts a few weeks to months, individuals usually remain asymptomatic for years despite sporadic parasitemia. During this period, their blood can transmit the parasites to transfusion recipients and accidentally to laboratory workers. An increasing fraction of adults develops overt chronic disease of the heart and gastrointestinal tract as they age. Progressive destruction of myocardial cells and neurons of the myenteric plexus results from the special tropism of *T. cruzi* for muscle cells. Whether an undefined autoimmune response also contributes to the pathogenesis of Chagas' disease is controversial, especially because recent studies with improved techniques indicate the presence of *T. cruzi* at sites of cardiac lesions. However, immunological defenses, especially cell-mediated immunity, do play a role in modulating the course of disease. Two nitroheterocyclic drugs, *nifurtimox* (available under an investigational new drug protocol from the CDC drug service) and *benznidazole* are used to treat this infection. Both agents suppress parasitemia and can cure the acute phase of Chagas' disease in 60% to 80% of cases. Their value in treating the chronic infection, however, is controversial. Several studies demonstrate that treatment can result in parasitological cure even in advanced cases, and importantly, even when patients remain positive for parasites by PCR and serological testing, treatment with these two drugs can reduce clinical symptoms. The recommendations of the Pan American Health Organization and the World Health Organization (WHO) are that patients with either acute- or recent chronic-phase disease should be treated. For patients with late chronic-phase disease (>10 years), parasitological cure is less likely, and there is no consensus on how to manage these patients. Both drugs are toxic and must be taken for long periods. Field isolates vary with respect to their susceptibility to nifurtimox and benznidazole. Moreover, resistance to both compounds can be induced in the laboratory. While both drugs can generate intracellular free radicals, their mechanisms of action and resistance are not well understood. Clearly, new drugs with better potency against parasites in the chronic phase and with reduced toxicities are needed. A number of triazole antifungal agents that inhibit sterol biosynthesis have been shown to have good activity against *T. cruzi* in animal models, and inhibitors of a cysteine protease (cruzipain) are currently being evaluated for the treatment of Chagas' disease by the Institute for One World Health. In the absence of new drugs, however, alternative measures such as improved vector control and housing accommodations have been used to reduce the transmission of Chagas' disease substantially in Brazil, Chile, and Venezuela (World Health Organization, 1999).

Leishmaniasis. Leishmaniasis is a complex vector-borne zoonosis caused by about 20 different species of obligate intramacrophage protozoa of the genus *Leishmania* (Croft and Coombs, 2003; Fairlamb, 2003; Meyerhoff, 1999). Small mammals and canines generally serve as reservoirs for these pathogens, which can be transmitted to humans by the bites of some 30 different species of female phlebotomine sandflies. Various forms of leishmaniasis

affect people in southern Europe and many tropical and subtropical regions throughout the world. Flagellated extracellular free *promastigotes,* regurgitated by feeding flies, enter the host, where they attach to and become phagocytized by tissue macrophages. There they transform into *amastigotes,* which reside and multiply within phagolysosomes until the cell bursts. Released amastigotes then propagate the infection by invading more macrophages. Amastigotes taken up by feeding sandflies transform back into promastigotes, thereby completing the transformation cycle. The particular localized or systemic disease syndrome caused by *Leishmania* depends on the species or subspecies of infecting parasite, the distribution of infected macrophages, and especially the host's immune response. In increasing order of systemic involvement and potential clinical severity, major syndromes of human leishmaniasis have been classified into *cutaneous, mucocutaneous, diffuse cutaneous,* and *visceral (kala azar)* forms. Leishmaniasis increasingly is becoming recognized as an AIDS-associated opportunistic infection (Berman, 1997).

The classification, clinical features, course, and chemotherapy of the various human leishmaniasis syndromes have been reviewed recently, in addition to the biochemistry and immunology of the parasite and host germane to chemotherapy (Herwaldt, 1999; Croft and Coombs, 2003). Cutaneous forms of leishmaniasis generally are self-limiting, with cures occurring within 3 to 18 months after infection. However, this form of the disease can leave disfiguring scars. The mucocutaneous, diffuse cutaneous, and visceral forms of the disease do not resolve without therapy. Visceral leishmaniasis caused by *L. donovani* is fatal unless treated. The list of current drugs useful for the treatment of all forms of leishmaniasis has been described recently in several reviews (Berman, 2003; Croft and Coombs, 2003; Fries and Fairlamb, 2003). The classic therapy for all species of *Leishmania* is *pentavalent antimony;* however, increasing resistance to this compound has been encountered. Liposomal *amphotericin B* is a highly effective agent for visceral leishmaniasis, and it is currently the drug of choice for antimony-resistant disease, although the high cost has been a barrier to its clinical use (*see* Chapter 48). Importantly, treatment of leishmania is currently undergoing major changes owing to the success of the first orally active agent, *miltefosine*, in clinical trials (Sundar *et al.,* 2002; Jha *et al.,* 1999). Miltefosine was approved in India for the treatment of visceral leishmaniasis in 1992. The drug also appears to have promise for the treatment of the cutaneous disease and for the treatment of dogs, which serve as an important animal reservoir of the disease. Paromomycin and pentamidine both have been used with success as parenteral agents for visceral disease, although the usefulness of pentamidine has been limited by toxicity. Topical formulations of paromomycin, recently combined with *gentamicin,* have also shown effectiveness against cutaneous disease in studies conducted by the Walter Reed Institute of Research.

Other Protozoal Infections. Just a few of the many less common protozoal infections of humans are highlighted here.

Babesiosis, caused by either *Babesia microti* or *B. divergens,* is a tick-borne zoonosis that superficially resembles malaria in that the parasites invade erythrocytes, producing a febrile illness, hemolysis, and hemoglobinuria. This infection usually is mild and self-limiting but can be severe or even fatal in asplenic or severely immunocompromised individuals. Currently recommended therapy is with a combination of *clindamycin* and *quinine,* but a combination of azithromycin and atovaquone was found to be as effective in treating adults with babesiosis and was associated with fewer adverse effects (Krause *et al.*, 2000).

Balantidiasis, caused by the ciliated protozoan *Balantidium coli,* is an infection of the large intestine that may be confused with amebiasis. Unlike amebiasis, however, this infection usually responds to *tetracycline* therapy.

Isospora belli, a coccidian parasite, causes diarrhea in AIDS patients, and responds to treatment with *trimethroprim–sulfamethoxazole. Cyclospora cayetanensis,* another coccidian parasite, causes self-limited diarrhea in normal hosts and can cause prolonged diarrhea in individuals with AIDS. It too is susceptible to trimethroprim–sulfamethoxazole. Microsporidia are spore-forming unicellular eukaryotic fungal parasites that can cause a number of disease syndromes, including diarrhea in immunocompromised individuals. Infections with microsporidia of the *Encephalitozoon* genus, including *E. hellum, E. intestinalis,* and *E. cuniculi,* have been treated successfully with *albendazole,* a derivative of *benzamidole* and inhibitor of β-tubulin polymerization (Gross, 2003) (*see* Chapter 41). Immunocompromised individuals with intestinal microsporidiosis owing to *E. bieneusi* (which does not respond as well to albendazole) have been treated successfully with the antibiotic *fumagillin* (Molina *et al.*, 2002).

AMPHOTERICIN

The pharmacology, formulation, and toxicology of amphotericin are presented in Chapter 48. Only those features of the drug pertinent to its use in leishmaniasis are described here.

Antiprotozoal Effects. In 1997, the FDA approved liposomal amphotericin B (AMBISOME) for the treatment of visceral leishmaniasis. Amphotericin is a highly effective antileishmanial agent that cures nearly 100% of the cases of visceral leishmaniasis in clinical studies, and it has become the drug of choice for antimonial-resistant cases (Berman, 2003; Fries and Fairlamb, 2003). The drug has not been useful against cutaneous or mucosal leishmaniasis, which likely has its basis in pharmacokinetic considerations. The lipid preparations of the drug have reduced toxicity, but the cost of the drug and the difficulty of administration remain a problem in endemic regions.

The mechanism of action of amphotericin against leishmania is similar to the basis for the drug's antifungal activities (*see* Chapter 48). Amphotericin complexes with ergosterol precursors in the cell membrane, forming pores that allow ions to enter the cell. Leishmania has similar sterol composition to fungal pathogens, and the drug binds to these sterols preferentially over the host cholesterol. No significant resistance to the drug has been encountered after nearly 30 years of use as an antifungal agent.

Therapeutic Uses. The recommended dose for the treatment of visceral leishmaniasis is 3 mg/kg per day intravenously for days 1 to 5, 14, and 21, with the dose being increased to 4 mg/kg and extended to days 1 to 5, 10, 17, 24, 31, and 38 for immunosuppressed patients (Fairlamb, 2003). Shorter courses of the drug have been tested with good efficacy and provide a potential alternative with lower cost. Cure rates of 93% and 89% were found for 5-day dosing of 7.5 and 3.75 mg/kg, respectively, and a single injection of 5 mg/kg cured 91% of patients in a 46-person trial (Berman, 2003).

CHLOROQUINE

The pharmacology and toxicology of chloroquine are presented in Chapter 39. Only those features of the drug pertinent to its use in amebiasis are described here.

Chloroquine is directly toxic to *E. histolytica* trophozoites and is highly concentrated within the liver, making it an effective therapy for amebic liver abscess. However, it is not as effective as metronidazole and should be used to treat amebic liver abscess only when metronidazole or another nitroimidazole compound is either contraindicated or not available. Chloroquine is not effective against intestinal amebiasis because it is absorbed in the small bowel and attains low concentrations in the colonic lumen and wall. Anyone receiving chloroquine for the treatment of amebic liver abscess also should receive a luminal agent (paromomycin or iodoquinol) to eliminate *E. histolytica* intestinal colonization.

The conventional course of treatment with chloroquine phosphate for extraintestinal amebiasis in adults is 1 g/day for 2 days, followed by 500 mg/day for at least 2 to 3 weeks. Because of the low toxicity of this drug, this dose can be increased or the schedule can be repeated if necessary.

DILOXANIDE FUROATE

Diloxanide furoate (FURAMIDE) is the furoate ester of diloxanide, a derivative of dichloroacetamide. Diloxanide furoate is a very effective luminal agent for the treatment of *E. histolytica* infection but is no longer available in the United States. The reader is referred to the 10th edition of this book for further details on this agent.

EFLORNITHINE

History. Eflornithine (α-difluoromethylornithine, DFMO, ORNIDYL) is an irreversible catalytic (suicide) inhibitor of ornithine decarboxylase, the enzyme that catalyzes the first and rate-limiting step in the biosynthesis of polyamines (Marton and Pegg, 1995; Igarashi and Kashiwagi, 2000; Seiler, 2003). The polyamines—putrescine, spermidine, and in mammals, spermine—are required for cell division and for normal cell differentiation. In trypanosomes, spermidine additionally is required for the synthesis of trypanothione, which is a conjugate of spermidine and glutathione that replaces many of the functions of glutathione in the parasite cell (Fries and Fairlamb, 2003; Fairlamb, 2003). Both in animal models and *in vitro,* eflornithine arrests the growth of several types of tumor cells, providing the basis for its clinical evaluation as an antitumor agent (Seiler, 2003). The discovery that eflornithine cured rodent infections with *T. brucei* first focused attention on protozoal polyamine biosynthesis as a potential target for chemotherapeutic attack (Bacchi *et al.*, 1980). Eflornithine currently is used to treat West African (Gambian) trypanosomiasis caused by *T. brucei gambiense* (Fries and Fairlamb, 2003; Fairlamb, 2003; Pépin and Milord,

1994; Mpia and Pépin, 2002; Burri and Brun, 2003). The drug usually is curative even for late CNS stages of infection resistant to arsenical trypanocides. In contrast, this compound is largely ineffective for East African trypanosomiasis, and its high cost, coupled with production shortages and the difficult treatment regimen, had limited its application in the field (Burri and Brun, 2003). However, recent studies have sparked renewed interest in the potential of eflornithine as both a chemopreventive agent for people at high risk for various types of epithelial cancers (Meyskens and Gerner, 1999) and for its use to reduce facial hair in woman (Wickware, 2002). The marketing of the compound for this latter use has enabled a stable supply of the drug to be provided to the WHO through 2006. Eflornithine is no longer available for systemic use in the United States but may be available for treatment of Gambian trypanosomiasis by special request from the WHO. The chemical structure of eflornithine is:

$$
\begin{array}{c}
NH_2 \\
| \\
CH_2 \\
| \\
CH_2 \\
| \\
F \quad CH_2 \\
| \quad\quad | \\
H-C-C-NH_2 \\
| \quad\quad | \\
F \quad COOH
\end{array}
$$

EFLORNITHINE

Antitrypanosomal Effects. The effects of eflornithine have been evaluated both on drug-susceptible and drug-resistant *T. brucei in vitro* and in infections with these parasites in rodent models (Fries and Fairlamb, 2003; Fairlamb, 2003). Eflornithine is a cytostatic agent that has multiple biochemical effects on trypanosomes, all of which are a consequence of polyamine depletion. The polyamine putrescine is depleted to undetectable levels, whereas both spermidine and trypanothine levels are reduced by 25% to 50%, and methionine metabolism is altered. Depletion of the polyamines, or of trypanothione, would be expected to be lethal to the cells based on genetic studies that have disrupted the biosynthetic genes in the pathway. As a consequence, macromolecular biosynthesis is depressed, and the parasites transform from the long, slender dividing forms into the short, stumpy nonreplicating forms. These latter parasites are unable to synthesize variable cell surface glycoprotein and eventually are cleared by the immune system.

The molecular mechanism of eflornithine action clearly has been established to be inhibition of ornithine decarboxylase, whereas the mechanisms of selective toxicity are still debated (Fries and Fairlamb, 2003; Fairlamb, 2003, Wang, 1997). Eflornithine irreversibly inhibits both mammalian and trypanosomal ornithine decarboxylases, thereby preventing the synthesis of putrescine, a precursor of polyamines needed for cell division. Eflornithine inactivates the enzyme through covalent labeling of an active-site cysteine residue, and an X-ray structure of the *T. brucei* enzyme bound to the drug has been reported (Grishin *et al.*, 1999). A number of studies demonstrate conclusively that ornithine decarboxylase is the target of eflornithine action that leads to cell death. Mutant bloodstream trypanosomes lacking ornithine decarboxylase or wild-type trypanosomes treated with eflornithine cannot replicate, and mice inoculated with these null parasites become resistant to infection by wild-type parasites (Li *et al.*, 1998; Mutomba *et al.*, 1999). The

product of the ornithine decarboxylase reaction, putrescine, rescues the growth deficit in both the mutant parasites and eflornithine-treated cells. The null mutant parasites grown with putrescine are not affected by eflornithine, demonstrating the selectivity of the drug for the target enzyme.

The mechanisms of selective toxicity between the host and parasite, or between the different species of *T. brucei,* are less clear (Wang, 1995; Fries and Fairlamb, 2003). The parasite and human enzymes are equally susceptible to inhibition by eflornithine; however, the mammalian enzyme is turned over rapidly, whereas the parasite enzyme is stable, and this difference likely plays a role in the selective toxicity. In addition, mammalian cells may be able to replenish polyamine pools through uptake of extracellular polyamines, whereas the slender bloodstream forms of human trypanosomes divide within human blood, which contains only very low levels of these essential compounds. Further, the parasites lack efficient transport mechanisms.

T. brucei rhodesiense cells are less sensitive to eflornithine inhibition than *T. brucei gambiense* cells, and studies *in vitro* suggest that the effective doses are increased by 10 to 20 times in the refractory cells (Matovu *et al.*, 2001). The molecular basis for the higher dose requirement in *T. brucei rhodesiense* is still poorly understood; however, it has been postulated to involve differences both in enzyme stability and in the metabolism of *S*-adenosylmethionine compared with the sensitive *T. brucei gambiense* cell lines (Fries and Fairlamb, 2003).

Absorption, Fate, and Excretion. Eflornithine is given by either the intravenous or the oral route; its bioavailability after oral administration is about 54%. Peak plasma levels are achieved about 4 hours after an oral dose, and the elimination half-life averages about 200 minutes. The drug does not bind to plasma proteins but is well distributed and penetrates into the cerebrospinal fluid (CSF). The last property is especially important in late-stage African trypanosomiasis, where CSF:plasma ratios exceeding 0.9 have been reported. Over 80% of eflornithine is cleared by the kidney largely in unchanged form. There is some evidence that eflornithine displays dose-dependent pharmacokinetics at the highest doses used clinically (Burri and Brun, 2003).

Therapeutic Uses. Experience with the use of eflornithine for the treatment of West African trypanosomiasis owing to *T. brucei gambiense* has been well summarized (Van Nieuwenhove, 1992; Pépin *et al.*, 2000; Mpia and Pépin, 2002). Most patients reported had advanced disease with CNS complications, and many had received arsenicals prior to treatment with eflornithine. The preferred regimen for adult patients was found to be 100 mg/kg given intravenously every 6 hours for 14 days. Virtually all patients improved on this regimen unless they were extremely ill, and the WHO reported improval rates exceeding 90% in late-stage patients. Clinical trials have been conducted on a 7-day course, which was found to be effective for relapsing cases. A higher risk of treatment failure overall was found in patients who were stuporous on admission or were older (Pépin *et al.*, 2000). Children younger than 12 years of age required higher doses of eflornithine, probably because they clear the drug more rapidly than do adults and because the drug does not reach the CNS as well. To avoid early convulsions, which could be more frequent in children receiving higher doses, a regimen using the current intravenous dosage (400 mg/kg per day) in the first few days, followed by an increase for the second part of therapy, has been proposed (Milord *et al.*, 1993). A recent study combining eflornithine with melarsoprol suggests that the drugs may act synergistically (Mpia and Pépin, 2002); however, the potential for improving treatment by combining eflornithine with other antitrypanosomal agents remains unexplored.

Equal doses of eflornithine were less effective when given by the oral route probably because of limited bio-availability. The problem cannot be overcome simply by increasing the oral dose because of ensuing osmotic diarrhea.

The WHO is currently revisiting this question and plans to initiate clinical trials to assess efficacy of oral treatment regimens (Legros *et al.*, 2002). Eflornithine has proven to be less successful for treating AIDS patients with West African trypanosomiasis, presumably because host defenses play a critical role in clearing drug-treated *T. brucei gambiense* from the bloodstream. Even high doses of eflornithine failed to improve East African trypanosomiasis owing to *T. brucei rhodesiense,* consistent with the relatively short half-life and high activity of ornithine decarboxylase in these parasites.

Toxicity and Side Effects. Eflornithine causes severe adverse effects in treated patients (Burri and Brun, 2003; Van Nieuwenhove, 1992); however, they are generally reversible on withdrawal of the drug. Anemia (48%), diarrhea (39%), and leukopenia (27%) are the most common complications in patients receiving intravenous medication. Diarrhea is both dose-related and dose-limiting, especially after oral administration of the drug. Convulsions occur early in about 7% of treated patients, but they do not appear to recur despite continuation of therapy. Other complications—such as thrombocytopenia, alopecia, vomiting, abdominal pain, dizziness, fever, anorexia, and headache—occur in less than 10% of treated patients. Reversible hearing loss can occur after prolonged therapy with oral doses. While this has been a problem in the use of eflornithine for cancer chemotherapy, hearing loss has not been observed during the treatment of sleeping sickness.

Therapeutic doses of eflornithine are large and require coadministration of substantial volumes of intravenous fluid. This can pose practical limitations in remote settings and cause fluid overload in susceptible patients.

EMETINE AND DEHYDROEMETINE

The use of emetine, an alkaloid derived from *ipecac* ("Brazil root"), as a direct-acting systemic amebicide dates from the early part of the twentieth century. Dehydroemetine (MEBADIN) has similar pharmacological properties but is considered to be less toxic. Although both drugs were once used widely to treat severe invasive intestinal amebiasis and extraintestinal amebiasis, they have been replaced by metronidazole, which is as effective and far safer. Thus, emetine and dehydroemetine should not be used unless metronidazole is contraindicated. In the United States, dehydroemetine is available under an investigational new drug protocol from the CDC drug service. Details of the pharmacology and toxicology of emetine and dehydroemetine are presented in the fifth and earlier editions of this book.

FUMAGILLIN

Fumagillin (FUMIDIL B, others) is an acyclic polyene macrolide produced by the fungus *Aspergillus fumigatus*. Its structure is shown below:

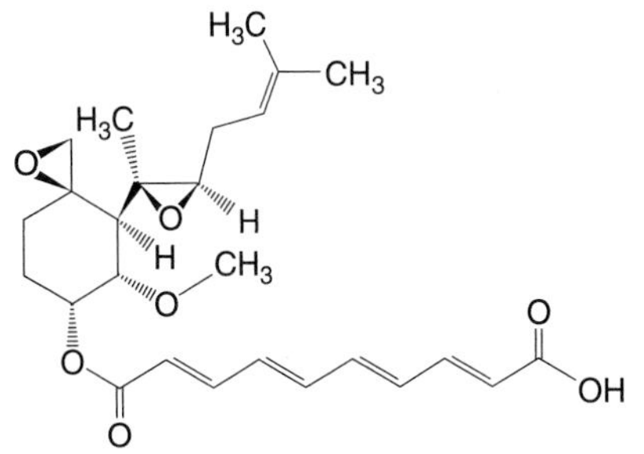

FUMAGILLIN

Both fumagillin and its synthetic analog *TNP-470* are toxic to microsporidia, and fumagillin is used widely to treat the microsporidian *Nosema apis*, a pathogen of honey bees. Fumagillin has some activity against *E. histolytica* and was tested as a drug for amebiasis more than five decades ago. Both fumagillin and TNP-470 also inhibit angiogenesis and suppress tumor growth, and TNP-470 is undergoing clinical trials as an anticancer agent (*see* Chapter 51). Human methionine–aminopeptidase-2 has been identified as the target for fumagillin's antitumor activity, and a gene encoding methionine–aminopeptidase-2 has been found in the genome of the microsporidian parasite *E. cuniculi*. Fumagillin is used topically to treat keratoconjunctivitis caused by *E. hellem* at a dose of 3 to 10 mg/ml in a balanced salt suspension. For the treatment of intestinal microsporidiosis caused by *E. bieneusi*, fumagillin was used at a dose of 20 mg orally three times daily for 2 weeks (Molina *et al.*, 2002). Adverse effects of fumagillin may include abdominal cramps, nausea, vomiting, and diarrhea. Reversible thrombocytopenia and neutropenia also have been reported (Molina *et al.*, 2002). Fumagillin has not been approved for the systemic treatment of microsporidia infection in the United States.

8-HYDROXYQUINOLINES

The halogenated 8-hydroxyquinolines *iodoquinol* (diiodohydroxyquin) and *clioquinol* (iodochlorhydroxyquin) have been used as luminal agents to eliminate intestinal colonization with *E. histolytica*. Iodoquinol (YODOXIN) is the safer of the two agents and is the only one available for use as an oral agent in the United States. When used at appropriate doses (never to exceed 2 g/day and duration of therapy not greater than 20 days in adults), adverse effects are unusual. However, the use of these drugs, especially at doses exceeding 2 g/day, for long periods is associated with significant risk. The most important toxic reaction, which has been ascribed primarily to clioquinol, is subacute myelo-optic neuropathy. This disease is a myelitis-like illness that was first described in epidemic form (thousands of afflicted patients) in Japan; only sporadic cases have been reported elsewhere, but the actual prevalence is undoubtedly higher. Peripheral neuropathy is a less severe manifestation of neurotoxicity owing to these drugs. Administration of iodoquinol in high doses to children with chronic diarrhea has been associated with optic atrophy and permanent loss of vision. Because of its superior adverse-event profile, paromomycin is preferred by many authorities as the luminal agent used to treat amebiasis; however, iodoquinol is a reasonable alternative. Iodoquinol is used in combination with metronidazole to treat individuals with amebic colitis or amebic liver abscess but may be used as a single agent for asymptomatic individuals found to be infected with *E. histolytica*. For adults, the recommended dose of iodoquinol is 650 mg orally three times daily for 20 days, whereas children receive 10 mg/kg of body weight orally three times a day (not to exceed 2 g/day) for 20 days.

The pharmacology and toxicology of the 8-hydroxyquinolines are described in greater detail in the fifth and earlier editions of this book.

MELARSOPROL

History. In 1949, Friedheim demonstrated that melarsoprol, the dimercaptopropanol derivative of melarsen oxide, was effective in the treatment of late-stage trypanosomiasis. It was considerably safer than other trypanocides available at the time. Despite the fact that it causes an often fatal encephalopathy in 2% to 10% of the patients, it has remained a first-line drug in the treatment of late (CNS) stages of both West and East African trypanosomiasis. The continued use of melarsoprol in the field is indicative of the paucity of alternative therapies for the disease.

Chemistry and Preparation. Melarsoprol has the following chemical structure:

MELARSOPROL

Melarsoprol (Mel B; ARSOBAL), consisting of two stereoisomers in a 3:1 ratio (Ericsson *et al.*, 1997), is insoluble in water and is supplied as a 3.6% (w/v) solution in propylene glycol for intravenous administration. It is available in the United States only from the CDC.

Antiprotozoal Effects. Melarsoprol has many wide-ranging nonspecific effects on both the trypanosome and host cells (Fries and Fairlamb, 2003). Melarsoprol is a prodrug and is metabolized rapidly (half-life of 30 minutes) to melarsen oxide, the active form of the drug. Arsenoxides react avidly and reversibly with vicinal sulfhydryl groups, including those of proteins, and thereby inactivate a great number and variety of enzymes. The same nonspecific mechanisms by which melarsoprol is lethal to parasites are probably responsible for its toxicity to host tissues. However, susceptible African trypanosomes actively concentrate melarsoprol *via* an unusual purine transporter, which may account for the small level of selective toxicity that is achieved (de Koning, 2001; Fairlamb, 2003).

The basis for the trypanocidal action of melarsoprol is not understood, probably owing to its high reactivity with many biomolecules. Disruption of energy metabolism by inhibition of glycolytic enzyme was long thought to explain its trypanocidal activity. Other evidence suggests, however, that this is not a primary effect. Melarsoprol reacts with trypanothione, the spermidine–glutathione adduct that substitutes for glutathione in these parasites. Binding of melarsoprol to trypanothione results in formation of melarsen oxide–trypanothione adduct (Mel T), a compound that is a potent competitive inhibitor of trypanothione reductase, the enzyme responsible for maintaining trypanothione in its reduced form.

Both the sequestering of trypanothione and the inhibition of trypanothione reductase would be expected to have lethal consequences to the cell. However, critical evidence directly linking melarsoprol's action on the trypanothione system to parasite death is still lacking (Fries and Fairlamb, 2003; Fairlamb, 2003).

The number of treatment failures owing to increasing resistance of trypanosomes to melarsoprol has risen sharply in recent years. Failure rates as high as 27% in Uganda and Angola have been reported (Burri and Keiser, 2001; Welburn and Odiit, 2002). *In vitro* analysis of field isolates indicates that resistant strains are tenfold less sensitive to the drug than sensitive strains (Brun *et al.*, 2001; Matovu *et al.*, 2001).

Resistance to melarsoprol is likely to involve transport defects, although the situation is complicated by evidence for multiple transport mechanisms of the drug (de Koning, 1991; Maser *et al.*, 2003; Bray *et al.*, 2003). The best-characterized transporter is an unusual adenine–adenosine transporter termed the *P2 transporter* that has activity on melarsoprol as well as pentamidine and *berenil*. Cross-resistance between these compounds is observed frequently. Point mutations in this transporter are found in melarsoprol-resistant field isolates. However, null mutant cell lines that lack this transporter were resistant to berenil but had only twofold resistance to melarsoprol and pentamidine. The evidence for at least one additional common transporter for these drugs is strong; however, it remains to be identified and characterized.

Absorption, Fate, and Excretion. Melarsoprol is always administered intravenously. A small but therapeutically significant amount of the drug enters the CSF and has a lethal effect on trypanosomes infecting the CNS. The compound is excreted rapidly, with 70% to 80% of the arsenic appearing in the feces (Pépin and Milord, 1994).

et al., 1997). Resistance of anaerobic bacteria to metronidazole is being recognized increasingly and has important clinical consequences. In the case of *Bacteroides* spp., metronidazole resistance has been linked to a family of nitroimidazole (*nim*) resistance genes, *nimA, -B, -C, -D, -E*, and *-F*, that can be encoded chromosomally or episomally (Gal and Brazier, 2004). The exact mechanisms underlying resistance are not known, but *nim* genes appear to encode a nitroimidazole reductase capable of converting a 5-nitroimidazole to a 5-aminoimidazole, thus stopping the formation of the reactive nitroso group responsible for microbial killing. Metronidazole has been used widely for the treatment of the microaerophilic organism *Helicobacter pylori*, the major cause of ulcer disease and gastritis worldwide. However, *Helicobacter* can develop resistance to metronidazole rapidly. Multiple mechanisms probably are operating, but there are data associating loss-of-function mutations in an oxygen-independent NADPH nitroreductase (*rdxA* gene) with resistance to metronidazole (Mendz and Mègraud, 2002).

Absorption, Fate, and Excretion. The pharmacokinetic properties of metronidazole and its two major metabolites have been investigated intensively (Lamp *et al.*, 1999). Preparations of metronidazole are available for oral, intravenous, intravaginal, and topical administration. The drug usually is absorbed completely and promptly after oral intake, reaching concentrations in plasma of 8 to 13 μg/ml within 0.25 to 4 hours after a single 500-mg dose. (Mean effective concentrations of the compound are 8 μg/ml or less for most susceptible protozoa and bacteria.) A linear relationship between dose and plasma concentration pertains for doses of 200 to 2000 mg. Repeated doses every 6 to 8 hours result in some accumulation of the drug; systemic clearance exhibits dose dependence. The half-life of metronidazole in plasma is about 8 hours, and its volume of distribution is approximately that of total-body water. Less than 20% of the drug is bound to plasma proteins. With the exception of the placenta, metronidazole penetrates well into body tissues and fluids, including vaginal secretions, seminal fluid, saliva, and breast milk. Therapeutic concentrations also are achieved in CSF.

After an oral dose, over 75% of labeled metronidazole is eliminated in the urine largely as metabolites; only about 10% is recovered as unchanged drug. The liver is the main site of metabolism, and this accounts for over 50% of the systemic clearance of metronidazole. The two principal metabolites result from oxidation of side chains, a hydroxy derivative and an acid. The hydroxy metabolite has a longer half-life (about 12 hours) and contains nearly 50% of the antitrichomonal activity of metronidazole. Formation of glucuronides also is observed. Small quantities of reduced metabolites, including ring-cleavage products, are formed by the gut flora. The urine of some patients may be reddish brown owing to the presence of unidentified pigments derived from the drug. Oxidative metabolism of metronidazole is induced by *phenobarbital, prednisone, rifampin,* and possibly *ethanol. Cimetidine* appears to inhibit hepatic metabolism of the drug.

Therapeutic Uses. The uses of metronidazole for antiprotozoal therapy have been reviewed extensively (Freeman *et al.*, 1997; Johnson, 1993; Stanley, 2003; Nash, 2001). Metronidazole cures genital infections with *T. vaginalis* in both females and males in more than 90% of cases. The preferred treatment regimen is 2 g metronidazole as a single oral dose for both males and females. For patients who cannot tolerate a single 2-g dose, an alternative regimen is a 250-mg dose given three times daily or a 375-mg dose given twice daily for 7 days. When repeated courses or higher doses of the drug are required for uncured or recurrent infections, it is recommended that intervals of 4 to 6 weeks elapse between courses. In such cases, leukocyte counts should be carried out before, during, and after each course of treatment.

Treatment failures owing to the presence of metronidazole-resistant strains of *T. vaginalis* are becoming increasingly common. Most of these cases can be treated successfully by giving a second 2-g dose to both patient and sexual partner. In addition to oral therapy, the use of a topical gel containing 0.75% metronidazole or a 500- to 1000-mg vaginal suppository will increase the local concentration of drug and may be beneficial in refractory cases (Heine and McGregor, 1993).

Metronidazole is an effective amebicide and is the agent of choice for the treatment of all symptomatic forms of amebiasis, including amebic colitis and amebic liver abscess. The recommended dose is 500 to 750 mg metronidazole taken orally three times daily for 7 to 10 days. The daily dose for children is 35 to 50 mg/kg given in three divided doses for 7 to 10 days.

While standard recommendations are for 7 to 10 days' duration of therapy, amebic liver abscess has been treated successfully by short courses (2.4 g daily as a single oral dose for 2 days) of metronidazole or tinidazole (Stanley, 2003). *E. histolytica* persist in most patients who recover from acute amebiasis after metronidazole therapy, so it is recommended that all such individuals also be treated with a luminal amebicide.

Although effective for the therapy of giardiasis, metronidazole has yet to be approved for treatment of this infection in the United States. Favorable responses have been noted with doses similar to or lower than those used for trichomoniasis; the usual regimen is 250 mg given three times daily for 5 days for adults and 15 mg/kg given three times a day for 5 days for children. A daily dose of 2 g for 3 days also has been used successfully.

Metronidazole is a relatively inexpensive, highly versatile drug with clinical efficacy against a broad spectrum of anaerobic and microaerophilic bacteria. It is used for the treatment of serious infections owing to susceptible anaerobic bacteria, including *Bacteroides, Clostridium, Fusobacterium, Peptococcus, Peptostreptococcus, Eubacterium,* and *Helicobacter.* The drug is also given in combination with other antimicrobial agents to treat polymicrobial infections with aerobic and anaerobic bacteria. Metronidazole achieves clinically effective levels in bones, joints, and the CNS. Metronidazole can be given intravenously when oral administration is not possible. A loading dose of 15 mg/kg is followed 6 hours later by a maintenance dose of 7.5 mg/kg every 6 hours, usually for 7 to 10 days. Metronidazole is used as a component of prophylaxis of postoperative mixed bacterial infections (Song and Glenny, 1998) and is used as a single agent to treat bacterial vaginosis. It is used in combination with other antibiotics and a proton pump inhibitor in regimens to treat infection with *H. pylori* (Suerbaum and Michetti, 2002) (*see* Chapter 36).

Metronidazole is being used increasingly as primary therapy for *Clostridium difficile* infection, the major cause of pseudomembranous colitis. Given at doses of 250 to 500 mg orally three times daily for 7 to 14 days (or even longer), metronidazole is an effective and cost-saving alternative to oral *vancomycin* therapy. Finally, metronidazole is used in the treatment of patients with Crohn's disease who have perianal fistulas, and it can help control colonic (but not small bowel) Crohn's disease. However, high doses (750 mg three times daily) for prolonged periods may be necessary, and neurotoxicity may be limiting (Podolsky, 2002). Metronidazole and other nitroimidazoles can sensitize hypoxic tumor cells to the effects of ionizing radiation, but these drugs are not used clinically for this purpose.

Toxicity, Contraindications, and Drug Interactions. The toxicity of metronidazole has been reviewed (Raether and Hanel, 2003). Side effects only rarely are severe enough to discontinue therapy. The most common are headache, nausea, dry mouth, and a metallic taste. Vomiting, diarrhea, and abdominal distress are experienced occasionally. Furry tongue, glossitis, and stomatitis occurring during therapy may be associated with an exacerbation of candidiasis. Dizziness, vertigo, and very rarely, encephalopathy, convulsions, incoordination, and ataxia are neurotoxic effects that warrant discontinuation of metronidazole. The drug also should be withdrawn if numbness or paresthesias of the extremities occur. Reversal of serious sensory neuropathies may be slow or incomplete. Urticaria, flushing, and pruritus are indicative of drug sensitivity that can require withdrawal of metronidazole. Metronidazole is a rare cause of Stevens-Johnson syndrome (toxic epidermal necrolysis), but a recent report described a high rate of this syndrome among individuals receiving high doses of metronidazole and concurrent therapy with the antihelminthic *mebendazole* (Chen *et al.*, 2003).

Dysuria, cystitis, and a sense of pelvic pressure also have been reported. Metronidazole has a well-documented disulfiram-like effect, and some patients will experience abdominal distress, vomiting, flushing, or headache if they drink alcoholic beverages during or within 3 days of therapy with this drug. Patients should be cautioned to avoid consuming alcohol during metronidazole treatment even though the risk of a severe reaction is low. By the same token, metronidazole and *disulfiram* or any disulfiram-like drug should not be taken together because confusional and psychotic states may occur. Although related chemicals have caused blood dyscrasias, only a temporary neutropenia, reversible after discontinuation of therapy, occurs with metronidazole.

Metronidazole should be used with caution in patients with active disease of the CNS because of its potential neurotoxicity. The drug also may precipitate CNS signs of *lithium* toxicity in patients receiving high doses of lithium. Plasma levels of metronidazole can be elevated by drugs such as cimetidine that inhibit hepatic microsomal metabolism. Moreover, metronidazole can prolong the prothrombin time of patients receiving therapy with *coumadin* anticoagulants. The dosage of metronidazole should be reduced in patients with severe hepatic disease.

Given in high doses for prolonged periods, metronidazole is carcinogenic in rodents; it also is mutagenic in bacteria (Raether and Hanel, 2003). Mutagenic activity is associated with metronidazole and several of its metabolites found in the urine of patients treated with therapeutic doses of the drug. However, there is no evidence that therapeutic doses of metronidazole pose any significant increased risk of cancer to human patients. There is conflicting evidence about the teratogenicity of metronidazole in animals. While metronidazole has been taken during all stages of pregnancy with no apparent adverse effects, its use during the first trimester generally is not advised.

MILTEFOSINE

History. Miltefosine (IMPAVIDO) is an alkylphosphocholine (APC) analog that was developed originally as an anticancer agent. Its antiprotozoal activity was discovered in the 1980s during the time that it was being evaluated for cancer chemotherapy. In 1992 it was approved in India as the first orally active treatment available for visceral leishmaniasis. It has been highly curative against the parasite in the studies conducted to date, and it is hoped that this compound will revolutionize the treatment of this fatal disease (Croft and Combs, 2003; Berman, 2003). Studies also suggest that it is effective against the cutaneous forms of the disease (Soto *et al.*, 2004). Miltefosine has the following chemical structure:

MILTEFOSINE

Antiprotozoal Effects. *In vitro* analysis of a large number of alkylglycerophosphoethanolamines (AGPEs), alkylglycerophosphocholines (AGPCs), and APCs, originally developed as anticancer agents, demonstrated that a number of these compounds had potent antileishmanial activity against cultured promastigote or amastigote parasites (Croft *et al.*, 2003). Of the APCs, miltefosine demonstrated the best activity against both stages of parasites. The potency of miltefosine varies for different

Leishmania spp., with *L. donovani* being the most sensitive (ED_{50} values of 1.2 to 5 μM against amastigotes) and *L. major* being the least sensitive (ED_{50} values of 8 to 40 μM against amastigotes). Several phospholipid analogs also had good potency against cultured *T. cruzi* parasites, whereas they were relatively inactive against *T. brucei*. *In vivo*, miltefosine had the best activities of the tested APCs, and by 5 days of treatment with 20 mg/kg orally, it gave greater than 95% suppression of *L. donovani* and *L. infantum* amastigotes in the affected organs of mice. It also had good activity when administered as a 6% ointment to skin lesions of *L. mexicana* or *L. major* on *BALB/c* mice.

In phase II human studies against visceral leishmaniasis, 95% to 98% cure rates were observed with a 100 mg/day oral dose for 28 to 42 days (Croft *et al.*, 2003). Phase III studies of drug efficacy in India on larger numbers of patients continued to demonstrate a greater than 95% rate of parasitological cure, and the drug is effective against antimonial-resistant cases and in immunocompromised patients (Sundar *et al.*, 2002; Jha *et al.*, 1999). These studies have led to the conclusion that oral miltefosine is a safe and effective treatment for visceral leishmaniasis. Further analyses of efficacy in regions of the world other than India, however, are needed. Recent studies of oral miltefosine also have shown greater than 95% efficacy against cutaneous leishmaniasis (Soto *et al.*, 2004). Miltefosine is the first orally available therapy for leishmaniasis and may revolutionize the treatment of this disease.

The mechanism of action of miltefosine is not yet understood. Potential targets in mammalian cells include protein kinase C; phosphatidylcholine biosynthesis, where miltefosine inhibits CTP:phosphocholine-cytidylyltransferase; and sphingomyelin biosynthesis, where increased levels of cellular ceramide may trigger apoptosis (Croft *et al.*, 2003). *Leishmania* studies suggest the drug may alter ether–lipid metabolism, cell signaling, or glycosylphosphatidylinosital anchor biosynthesis. A transporter for miltefosine has been cloned recently by functional rescue of a laboratory-generated resistant strain of *L. donovani* (Perez-Victoria *et al.*, 2003). The transporter is a P-type ATPase that belongs to the aminophospholipid translocase subfamily, and the basis for the drug resistance appears to be point mutation in the transporter leading to decreased drug uptake.

Absorption, Fate, and Excretion. Miltefosine is well absorbed orally and distributed throughout the human body. Plasma concentrations are proportional to the dose, and maximum serum concentrations for dosing of 50 to 150 mg/kg per day were 20 to 80 μg/ml with a half-life of 6 to 8 days. No differences between sexes or between adults and children were observed in the pharmacokinetic parameters.

Therapeutic Uses. Oral miltefosine is registered for use in India for the treatment of visceral leishmaniasis in adults at a dose of 100 mg/kg daily (for patients weighing more than 25 kg) for 28 days. A similar dosing schedule has shown efficacy against cutaneous disease. Efficacy and tolerance in children also have been

assessed on a limited number of patients; children should be administered 2.5 mg/kg per day. The compound cannot be given intravenously because it has hemolytic activity.

Toxicity and Side Effects. Vomiting and diarrhea have been reported as frequent side effects in up to 60% of the patients. Elevations in hepatic transaminases and serum creatinine also have been reported. These effects are typically mild and resolve quickly. They are generally reversible once the drug is withdrawn. The drug is contraindicated in pregnant women. Women should receive a negative pregnancy test prior to treatment, and birth control is required during and for at least 2 months after treatment. In rats, a possible effect on male fertility was noted; clinical trials to assess this risk in humans are ongoing. However, early studies have not indicated that male fertility problems detected in animal models will be observed in humans.

NIFURTIMOX

History. Nitrofurans and nitroimidazole analogs were shown to be effective in experimental infections with American trypanosomiasis caused by *T. cruzi*. Of these, nifurtimox and benznidazole were introduced in the late 1970s and are currently used clinically to treat the disease. Nifurtimox (Bayer 2502, LAMPIT), which is a nitrofuran analog, is no longer available commercially but can be obtained in the United States from the CDC. Benznidazole (Roche 7-1051, ROCHAGAN), which is a nitroimidazole analog, can only be obtained from the manufacturer.

Antiprotozoal Effects. Nifurtimox and benznidazole are trypanocidal against both the trypomastigote and amastigote forms of *T. cruzi*. Nifurtimox also has activity against *T. brucei* and can be curative against both early- and late-stage disease (Pépin *et al.*, 1995). Further evaluation of its potential for use alone or in combination with suramin or melarsoprol for this disease is ongoing at the WHO.

The trypanocidal action of nifurtimox derives from its ability to undergo activation by partial reduction to nitro radical anions. Transfer of electrons from the activated drug then regenerates the native nitrofuran and forms superoxide radical anions and other reactive oxygen species such as hydrogen peroxide and hydroxyl radical (Fairlamb, 2003). Reaction of free radicals with cellular macromolecules results in cellular damage that includes lipid peroxidation and membrane injury, enzyme inactivation, and damage to DNA. Nifurtimox also may produce damage to mammalian tissues by formation of radicals and redox cycling. The mechanism of action of benznidazole also requires a one-electron transfer that occurs in the cell. The generated nitro anion radicals then form covalent attachments to macromolecules leading to cellular damage that kills the parasites (Fries and Fairlamb, 2003; Urbina and Docampo, 2003).

Absorption, Fate, and Excretion. Nifurtimox is well absorbed after oral administration, with peak plasma levels observed after about 3.5 hours (Paulos *et al.*, 1989). Despite this, only low concentrations of the drug (10 to 20 μM) are present in plasma, and less than 0.5% of the dose is excreted in urine. The elimination half-life is only about 3 hours. High concentrations of several unidentified metabolites are found, however, and nifurtimox clearly undergoes rapid biotransformation, probably *via* a presystemic first-pass effect. Whether the metabolites have any trypanocidal activity is unknown.

Therapeutic Uses. Nifurtimox and benznidazole are employed in the treatment of American trypanosomiasis (Chagas' disease) caused by *T. cruzi* (Urbina and Docampo, 2003; Rodreques-Coura and de Castro, 2002; Fries and Fairlamb, 2003). However, because of toxicity issues, benznidazole is the preferred treatment. Both drugs markedly reduce the parasitemia, morbidity, and mortality of acute Chagas' disease, with parasitological cures being obtained in 80% of these cases. Parasitological cure is defined by a negative result in polymerase chain reaction (PCR) and serological tests for the parasite. In the chronic form of the disease, parasitological cures are still possible in up to 50% of the patients, although the drug is less effective than in the acute stage. However, even in the absence of a complete parasitological cure, treatment of chronic infections also reduces the clinical symptoms of the disease. Treatment with nifurtimox or benznidazole has no effect on irreversible organ lesions. While a component of tissue destruction may be autoimmune in nature, the continued presence of parasites in the infected organs of patients with chronic disease argues that Chagas' disease should be treated as a parasitic disease. The clinical response of the acute illness to drug therapy varies with geographical region; parasite strains present in Argentina, southern Brazil, Chile, and Venezuela appear to be more susceptible than those in central Brazil. Despite these uncertainties, treatment of all seropositive individuals is recommended and should be initiated as soon as possible, although many physicians still are uncomfortable treating the chronic stage of the disease because of the toxicity. Therapy with nifurtimox or benznidazole should start promptly after exposure for persons at risk of *T. cruzi* infection from laboratory accidents or from blood transfusions.

Both drugs are given orally. For nifurtimox, adults with acute infection should receive 8 to 10 mg/kg per day in four divided doses for 90 to 120 days. Children 1 to 10 years of age with acute Chagas' disease should receive 15 to 20 mg/kg per day in four divided doses for 90 days; for individuals 11 to 16 years old, the daily dose is 12.5 to 15 mg/kg given according to the same schedule. For benznidazole, the recommended treatment is 5 to 7 mg/kg per day in two divided doses for 30 to 90 days, with children up to 12 years receiving 10 mg/kg per day. Gastric upset and weight loss can occur during treatment. If the latter occurs, dosage should be reduced. The ingestion of alcohol should be avoided during treatment because the incidence of side effects may increase.

Toxicity and Side Effects. Children tolerate nifurtimox and benznidazole better than do adults. Nonetheless, drug-related side effects are common. They range from hypersensitivity reactions—such as dermatitis, fever, icterus, pulmonary infiltrates, and anaphylaxis—to dose- and age-dependent complications primarily referable to the gastrointestinal tract and both the peripheral and central nervous systems (Brener, 1979). Nausea and vomiting are common, as are myalgia and weakness. Peripheral neuropathy and gastrointestinal symptoms are especially common after prolonged treatment; the latter complication may lead to weight loss and preclude further therapy. Headache, psychic disturbances, paresthesias, polyneuritis, and CNS excitability are less frequent. Leukopenia and decreased sperm counts also have been reported. Because of the seriousness of Chagas' disease and the lack of superior drugs, there are few absolute contraindications to the use of these drugs.

NITAZOXANIDE

History. *Nitatzoxanide* (*N*-[nitrothiazolyl] salicylamide, ALINA) is an oral synthetic broad-spectrum antiparasitic agent that was synthesized originally in the 1980s based on the structure of the antihelminthic *niclosamide* (*see* Chapter 41). It was found initially to have activity against tapeworms (Rossignol and Maisonneuve, 1984); subsequent *in vitro* studies suggested that it was effective against a number of intestinal helminths and protozoans. Following several controlled clinical trials in children with diarrhea, nitazoxanide received FDA approval in 2002 for the treatment of cryptosporidiosis and giardiasis in children.

Chemistry. Nitazoxanide has the following chemical structure:

NITAZOXANIDE

Antimicrobial Effects. Nitazoxanide and its active metabolite, tizoxanide (desacetyl-nitazoxanide), inhibit the growth of sporozoites and oocytes of *C. parvum* and inhibit the growth of the trophozoites of *G. intestinalis*, *E. histolytica*, and *T. vaginalis in vitro* (Adagu *et al.*, 2002). Activity against other protozoans, including *Blastocystis hominis*, *Isospora belli*, and *Cyclospora cayetanensis* also has been reported. Nitazoxanide also demonstrated activity against the intestinal helminths: *Hymenolepsis nana*, *Trichuris trichura*, *Ascaris lumbricoides*, *Enterobius vermicularis*, *Ancylostoma duodenale*, *Strongyloides stercoralis*, and the liver fluke *Fasciola hepatica*. Effects against some anaerobic or microaerophilic bacteria, including *Clostridium* spp. and *H. pylori,* also have been reported.

Mechanism of Action and Resistance. While the exact mechanisms remain unclear, nitazoxanide appears to interfere with the PFOR enzyme-dependent electron-transfer reaction. This reaction is essential in anaerobic metabolism. Nitazoxanide does not appear to produce DNA mutations, suggesting that its mode of action is different from that of the nitroimidazoles (*e.g.,* metronidazole). No resistance to nitazoxanide in infectious agents previously known to be susceptible to the drug has yet been reported.

Absorption, Fate, and Excretion. Following oral administration, nitazoxanide is hydrolyzed rapidly to its active metabolite tizoxanide, which undergoes conjugation primarily to tizoxanide glucuronide. Bioavailability after an oral dose is excellent, and maximum plasma concentrations of the metabolites are detected within 1 to 4 hours of administration of the parent compound. Tizoxanide is greater than 99.9% bound to plasma proteins. Tizoxanide is excreted in the urine, bile, and feces, whereas tizoxanide glucuronide is excreted in the urine and bile. The pharmacokinetics of nitazoxanide in individuals with impaired hepatic or renal function have not been studied.

Therapeutic Uses. In the United States, nitazoxanide is currently available only as an oral suspension. It is approved for the treatment of *G. intestinalis* infection in children under the age of 12 (therapeutic efficacy of 85% to 90% for clinical response) and for the treatment of diarrhea in children under 12 caused by cryptosporidia (therapeutic efficacy ranging from 56% to 88% for clinical response) (Amadi *et al.*, 2002; Rossignol *et al.*, 2001). The efficacy of nitazoxanide in children (or adults) with cryptosporidia infection and AIDS has not been clearly established. For children between the ages of 12 and 47 months, the recommended dose is 100 mg nitazoxanide every 12 hours for 3 days; for children between 4 and 11 years of age, the dose is 200 mg nitazoxanide every 12 hours for 3 days. A 500-mg tablet, suitable for adult dosing (every 12 hours), is not yet available in the United States.

Nitazoxanide has been used as a single agent to treat mixed infections with intestinal parasites (protozoa and helminths) in several trials. Effective parasite clearance (based on negative follow-up fecal samples) after nitazoxanide treatment was shown for *G. intestinalis*, *E. histolytica/E. dispar*, *B. hominis*, *C. parvum*, *C. cayetanensis*, *I. belli*, *H. nana*, *T. trichura*, *A. lumbricoides*, and *E. vermicularis* (Diaz *et al.*, 2003; Romero-Cabello *et al.*, 1997), although

more than one course of therapy was required in some cases. Nitazoxanide may have some efficacy against *Fasciola hepatica* infections (Favennec *et al.*, 2003), and has been used to treat infections with *G. intestinalis* that is resistant to metronidazole and albendazole (Abboud *et al.*, 2001).

Toxicity and Side Effects. To date, adverse effects appear to be rare with nitazoxanide. Abdominal pain, diarrhea, vomiting, and headache have been reported, but rates were no different from those in patients receiving placebo. A greenish tint to the urine is seen in most individuals taking nitazoxanide. Nitazoxanide is considered a category B agent for use in pregnancy based on animal teratogenicity and fertility studies, but there is no clinical experience with its use in pregnant women or nursing mothers.

PAROMOMYCIN

Paromomycin (aminosidine, HUMATIN) is an aminoglycoside of the neomycin/kanamycin family (*see* Chapter 45) that is used as an oral agent to treat *E. histolytica* infection. Paromomycin also has been used orally to treat cryptosporidiosis and giardiasis. A topical formulation has been used to treat trichomoniasis, and parenteral administration has been used for visceral leishmaniasis. The structure of paromomycin is:

PAROMOMYCIN

Paromomycin shares the same mechanism of action as neomycin and kanamycin (binding to the 30S ribosomal subunit) and has the same spectrum of antibacterial activity. Paromomycin is available only for oral use in the United States. Following oral administration, 100% of the drug is recovered in the feces, and even in cases of compromised gut integrity, there is little evidence for clinically significant absorption of paromomycin. *Parenteral administration carries the same risks of nephrotoxicity and ototoxicity seen with other aminoglycosides.*

Paromomycin has become the drug of choice for treating intestinal colonization with *E. histolytica*. It is used in combination with metronidazole to treat amebic colitis and amebic liver abscess and can be used as a single agent for asymptomatic individuals found to have *E. histolytica* intestinal colonization. Recommended dosing for adults and children is 25 to 35 mg/kg per day orally in three divided doses. Adverse effects are rare with oral usage but include abdominal pain and cramping, epigastric pain, nausea and vomiting, steatorrhea, and diarrhea. Rarely, rash and headache have been reported. Paromomycin has been used to treat cryptosporidiosis in AIDS patients both as a single agent (oral doses of 500 mg three times daily or 1 g orally twice daily for 14 to 28 days followed by 500 mg orally twice daily) and in combination with azithromycin (paromomycin 1 g orally twice daily plus azithromycin 600 mg orally once daily for 4 weeks, followed by paromomycin alone for 8 weeks). While still recommended by some authorities, in a randomized, controlled trial, paromomycin was no more effective than placebo in treating individuals with cryptosporidiosis and AIDS (Hewitt *et al.*, 2000). Paromomycin has been advocated as a treatment for giardiasis in pregnant women, especially during the first trimester, when metronidazole is contraindicated and as an alternative agent for metronidazole-resistant isolates of *G. intestinalis*. While there is limited clinical experience, response rates of 55% to 90% have been reported (Gardner and Hill, 2001). Dosing in adults is 500 mg orally three times daily for 10 days, whereas children have been treated with 25 to 30 mg/kg per day in three divided oral doses. Paromomycin formulated as a 6.25% cream has been used to treat vaginal trichomoniasis in patients who had failed metronidazole therapy or could not receive metronidazole. Some cures have been reported, but vulvovaginal ulcerations and pain have complicated treatment (Nyirjesy *et al.*, 1998).

Paromomycin as a topical formulation containing 15% paromomycin in combination with either a patented base from Walter Reed Army Institute of Research or 12% *methylbenzonium chloride* has shown variable efficacy in clinical trials for the treatment of cutaneous leishmaniasis (Berman, 2003). Paromomycin has been administered parenterally (doses of 16 to 18 mg/kg per day) alone or in combination with antimony to treat visceral leishmaniasis. In one study, cure rates of 89% with paromomycin alone were reported, and cure rates of 94% were seen with combination therapy. These results compared favorably with the cure rate for antimony alone (69% in this study) in an endemic area where antimony resistance is common (Thakur *et al.*, 2000).

PENTAMIDINE

History. Pentamidine is a positively charged aromatic diamine that was discovered in 1937 as a fortuitous consequence of the search for hypoglycemic compounds that might compromise parasite energy metabolism. Of the compounds tested, three were found to possess outstanding activity: *stilbamidine, pentamidine,* and *promamidine.* Pentamidine was the most useful clinically because of its relative stability, lower toxicity, and ease of administration. Pentamidine is a broad-spectrum agent with activity against several species of pathogenic protozoa and some fungi. Alone or in combination with suramin, pentamidine is used for the treatment of early-stage *T. brucei gambiense* infection (Docampo and Moreno, 2003; Nok, 2003). Pentamidine is an alternative agent for the treatment of antimony-resistant visceral leishmaniasis, although the availability of newer, less toxic agents, (*e.g.,* liposomal preparations of amphotericin and miltefosine) may decrease its use (Berman, 2003). Pentamidine is also used as an alternative agent for the treatment and prophylaxis of pneumocystis pneumonia caused by the ascomycetous fungus *Pneumocystis jiroveci* (formerly known as *Pneumocystis carinii*) (Thomas and Limper, 2004). *T. brucei rhodesiense* is refractory to treatment by pentamidine for unexplained reasons. *Diminazene* (BERENIL) is a related diamidine that is used as an inexpensive alternative to pentamidine for the treatment of early African trypanoso-

miasis in some endemic areas despite the fact that it is *approved for veterinary use only.*

Chemistry. Pentamidine has the following chemical structure:

$$HN=C(NH_2)-C_6H_4-OCH_2(CH_2)_3CH_2O-C_6H_4-C(=NH)NH_2$$

PENTAMIDINE

Pentamidine as the di-isethionate salt is marketed for injection (PENTAM 300) or for use as an aerosol (NEBUPENT). One milligram of pentamidine base is equivalent to 1.74 mg of the pentamidine isethionate. The di-isethionate salt is highly water soluble; however, solutions should be used promptly after preparation because pentamidine is unstable in solution.

Antiprotozoal and Antifungal Effects. The positively charged aromatic diamidines are toxic to a number of different protozoa yet show rather marked selectivity of action. They are effective for the treatment of *T. brucei gambiense* sleeping sickness but not *T. brucei rhodesiense* or *T. cruzi* infections. Additionally, they are useful for the treatment of antimony-resistant leishmania infections.

The diamidines also are fungicidal. Activity *in vitro* against *Blastomyces dermatitidis* led to the successful therapeutic trial of these drugs in systemic blastomycoses. The use of amphotericin B, however, has reduced the value of the diamidines in the treatment of this disease. At near-therapeutic levels, pentamidine kills nonreplicating forms of *P. jiroveci* in culture (Pifer *et al.*, 1983), but other evidence suggests that pentamidine exerts a biostatic rather than biocidal effect (Vöhringer and Arastéh, 1993).

Mechanism of Action and Resistance. The mechanism of action of the diamidines is unknown. The dicationic compounds appear to display multiple effects on any given parasite and act by disparate mechanisms in different parasites (Wang, 1995; Fairlamb, 2003). In *T. brucei,* for example, the diamidines are concentrated *via* an energy-dependent high-affinity uptake system to millimolar concentrations in cells; this selective uptake is essential to their efficacy. The best-characterized diamidine transporter is the same purine (P2) adenine and adenosine transporter used by the melamine-based arsenicals, which explains the cross-resistance to diamidines exhibited by certain arsenical-resistant strains of *T. brucei* generated in the laboratory (Fairlamb, 2003; de Koning, 2001; Maser *et al.,* 2003; Bray *et al.,* 2003). However, it is becoming increasingly clear that multiple transporters are responsible for pentamidine uptake, and this may account for the fact that little resistance to this drug is observed in field isolates despite years of use as a prophylactic agent. Although failure to concentrate diamidines is the usual cause of pentamidine resistance *in vitro,* other mechanisms also may be involved (Fairlamb, 2003).

The positively charged hydrophobic diamidines may exert their trypanocidal effects by reacting with a variety of negatively charged intracellular targets such as membrane phospholipids, enzymes, RNA, and DNA. Indeed, ribosomal aggregation, inhibition of DNA and protein synthesis, and inhibition of several enzymes—along with seeming loss of trypanosomal kinetoplast DNA—all have been reported (Fairlamb, 2003). The loss of kinetoplast DNA may be mediated through inhibition of topoisomerase II, a hypothesis that is supported by recent studies using interference RNA to knock down levels of the protein. This latter effect cannot account for the broad antimicrobial activity of the drug and thus cannot fully explain its mechanism of action. Inhibition of *S*-adenosyl-L-methionine decarboxylase *in vitro* suggested that pentamidine might interfere with polyamine biosynthesis; however, polyamine levels are not affected in intact cells, suggesting that inhibition of this enzyme plays no role in the toxicity of the drug (Fairlamb, 2003). Inhibition of a plasma Ca^{2+},Mg^{2+}-ATPase also has been reported (Fairlamb, 2003).

In *Leishmania,* pentamidine accumulates within the mitochondria, and disintegration of the kinetoplast and collapse of the mitochondrial membrane potential are early effects of the drug. An important role for mitochondria as the target for pentamidine's antileishmanial activities is also suggested by studies of pentamidine-resistant parasites, where resistance was not associated with decreased drug uptake into the parasite but linked to decreased concentrations of the drug within mitochondria (Bray et al., 2003).

Absorption, Fate, and Excretion. The pharmacokinetics and biodisposition of pentamidine isethionate have been studied most extensively in AIDS patients with *P. jiroveci* infections (Vöhringer and Arastéh, 1993); information from patients with Gambian trypanosomiasis is more limited (Pépin and Milord, 1994; Bronner et al., 1995; Bouteille et al., 2003). Pentamidine isethionate is fairly well absorbed from parenteral sites of administration. Following a single intravenous dose, the drug disappears from plasma with an apparent half-life of several minutes to a few hours and maximum plasma concentrations after intramuscular injection occurring at 1 hour. The half-life of elimination is very slow, lasting from weeks to months, and the drug is 70% bound to plasma proteins. This highly charged compound is poorly absorbed orally and does not cross the blood–brain barrier, explaining why it is ineffective against late-stage trypanosomiasis.

After multiple parenteral doses, the liver, kidney, adrenal, and spleen contain the highest concentrations of drug, whereas only traces are found in the brain (Donnelly et al., 1988). The lungs contain intermediate but therapeutic concentrations after five daily doses of 4 mg/kg. Inhalation of pentamidine aerosols is used for prophylaxis of *Pneumocystis* pneumonia; delivery of drug by this route results in little systemic absorption and decreased toxicity compared with intravenous administration in both adults and children (Leoung et al., 1990; Hand et al., 1994). The actual dose delivered to the lungs depends on both the size of particles generated by the nebulizer and the patient's ventilatory patterns.

Therapeutic Uses. Pentamidine isethionate usually is given by intramuscular injection or by slow intravenous infusion over 60 minutes in single doses of 1.7 to 4.5 mg/kg per day for a series of 10 days. However, alternative dosing schedules are common, and the coadministration

of suramin on alternate days provides an alternative means of treating *T. brucei gambiense* infections (Pépin and Milord, 1994). Because of failure to penetrate the CNS, pentamidine is not used to treat *T. brucei rhodesiense,* which affects the brain early in the course of infection. The drug is also ineffective in *T. brucei gambiense* infections once the CNS is involved.

Pentamidine has been used successfully in courses of 12 to 15 intramuscular doses of 2 to 4 mg/kg either daily or every other day to treat visceral leishmaniasis (kala azar caused by *L. donovani*). This compound provides an alternative to antimonials or lipid formulations of amphotericin B for patients who cannot tolerate the latter agents. Pentamidine isethionate given as four intramuscular doses of 3 mg/kg every other day has enjoyed some success in the treatment of cutaneous leishmaniasis (Oriental sore caused by *L. tropica*) but is not used routinely to treat this infection (Berman, 1997).

Pentamidine is one of several drugs or drug combinations used to treat or prevent *Pneumocystis* infection. *Pneumocystis* pneumonia (PCP) is a major cause of mortality in individuals with HIV infection and AIDS and can occur in patients who are immunosuppressed by other mechanisms (*e.g.,* high-dose corticosteroids or underlying malignancy). The availability of highly active antiretroviral therapy (HAART) has reduced the number of cases of PCP significantly within the United States and Europe and greatly reduced the number of individuals requiring prophylaxis for PCP. Trimethoprim–sulfamethoxazole is the drug of choice for the treatment and prevention of PCP (*see* Chapter 43). Pentamidine is reserved for two indications. Pentamidine given intravenously as a 4 mg/kg single daily dose for 21 days is used to treat severe PCP in individuals who cannot tolerate trimethorprim–sulfamethoxazole and are not candidates for alternative agents such as atovaquone or the combination of clindamycin and *primaquine*. Pentamidine has been recommended as a "salvage" agent for individuals with PCP who failed to respond to initial therapy (usually trimethoprim–sulfamethoxazole), but a meta-analysis suggested that pentamidine is less effective than other therapies (specifically the combination of clindamycin and primaquine or atovaquone) for this indication (Smego et al., 2001). Pentamidine administered as an aerosol preparation is used for the prevention of PCP in at-risk individuals who cannot tolerate trimethoprim–sulfamethoxazole and are not deemed candidates for either dapsone (alone or in combination with pyrimethamine) or atovaquone. Candidates for PCP prophylaxis are individuals with HIV infection and a CD4 count of less than 200/mm^3 and individuals with HIV infection and persistent unexplained fever or oropharyngeal candidiasis. Secondary prophylaxis is recommended for everyone with a documented PCP episode. For prophylaxis, pentamidine isethionate is given monthly as a 300-mg dose in a 5% to 10% nebulized solution over 30 to 45 minutes. While the monthly dosage regimen is convenient, aerosolized pentamidine has several disadvantages, including its failure to treat any extrapulmonary sites of *Pneumocystis,* the lack of efficacy against any other potential opportunistic pathogens (compared with trimethoprim–sulfamethoxazole), and a slightly increased risk for pneumothorax. Long-term aerosolized pentamidine prophylaxis (5 years or more) has not been associated with the development of any pulmonary disease (Obaji *et al.*, 2003). For individuals who receive HAART and develop CD4 counts persistently above 200/mm^3 for 3 months, primary or secondary PCP prophylaxis can be stopped.

Toxicity and Side Effects. Pentamidine is a toxic agent, and approximately 50% of individuals receiving the drug at recommended doses (4 mg/kg per day) will show some adverse effect. Intravenous administration of pentamidine may be associated with hypotension, tachycardia, and headache. These effects are probably secondary to the ability of pentamidine to bind imidazoline receptors (*see* Chapter 10) and can be ameliorated by slowing the rate of the intravenous infusion (Wood *et al.*, 1998). As noted earlier, the diamidines were designed originally for use as hypoglycemics, and pentamidine retains that property. Hypoglycemia, which can be life threatening, may occur at any time during pentamidine treatment, even weeks into therapy. Careful monitoring of blood sugar is key. Paradoxically, pancreatitis, hyperglycemia, and the development of insulin-dependent diabetes have been seen in some patients. Pentamidine is nephrotoxic (almost 25% of treated patients will show signs of renal dysfunction), and if the serum creatinine concentration rises more than 1.0 to 2.0 mg/dl, it may be necessary to withhold the drug temporarily or change to an alternative agent. Individuals developing pentamidine-induced renal dysfunction are at higher risk for hypoglycemia. Other adverse effects include skin rashes, thrombophlebitis, anemia, neutropenia, and elevation of hepatic enzymes. Intramuscular administration of pentamidine, while effective, is associated with the development of sterile abscesses at the injection site, which can become infected secondarily. For this reason, most authorities recommend intravenous administration. Aerosolized pentamidine is associated with few adverse events.

QUINACRINE

Quinacrine is an acridine derivative used widely during World War II as an antimalarial agent. Although it has been replaced by newer and safer antimalarial drugs (*see* Chapter 39), *quinacrine hydrochloride* is very effective against *G. lamblia,* producing cure rates of at least 90%. However, quinacrine is no longer available in the United States. For a description of the pharmacology and toxicology of quinacrine, consult the fifth and earlier editions of this book.

SODIUM STIBOGLUCONATE

History. Antimonial compounds were introduced in 1945 and have been used for therapy of leishmaniasis and other protozoal

infections (Berman, 2003; Fairlamb, 2003; Croft and Coombs, 2003). The first trivalent antimonial compound used to treat cutaneous leishmaniasis and kala azar was *antimony potassium tartrate* (tartar emetic), which was both toxic and difficult to administer. Tartar emetic and other trivalent arsenicals eventually were replaced by pentavalent antimonial derivatives of phenylstibonic acid. An early member of this family of compounds was *sodium stibogluconate* (sodium antimony gluconate, PENTOSTAM). This drug is used widely today and, together with *meglumine antimonate* (GLUCANTIME), a pentavalent antimonial compound preferred in French-speaking countries, has been the mainstay of the treatment of leishmaniasis. However, increasing resistance to antimonials has reduced their efficacy, and both lipid-based amphotericin and miltefosine are being used increasingly in their place (Fries and Fairlamb, 2003; Croft and Coombs, 2003; Berman, 2003).

Chemistry. Sodium stibogluconate has the following chemical structure:

SODIUM STIBOGLUCONATE

Clinical formulations of sodium stibogluconate actually consist of multiple uncharacterized molecular forms, some of which have higher molecular masses than the compound shown (Fairlamb, 2003). Typical preparations contain 30% to 34% pentavalent antimony by weight as well as *m*-chlorocresol added as a preservative. In the United States, sodium stibogluconate is no longer available.

Antiprotozoal Effects and Drug Resistance. The mechanism of the antileishmanial action of sodium stibogluconate remains an active area of research, and recent studies have provided interesting new insights. These studies support the old hypothesis that relatively nontoxic pentavalent antimonials act as prodrugs. These compounds are reduced to the more toxic Sb^{3+} species that kill amastigotes within the phagolysosomes of macrophages. This reduction preferentially occurs in the intracellular amastigote stage, and recently an enzyme, As^{5+} reductase, was characterized that is able to reduce Sb^{5+} to the active Sb^{3+} form. Furthermore, the overexpression of this enzyme in promastigotes increased their sensitivity to the drugs (Zhou *et al.*, 2004). Classically, it was thought that the antiparasitic effects of antimonials occurred through inhibition of glucose catabolism and fatty acid oxidation; however, recent studies strongly suggest that the drugs operate by interfering with the trypanothione redox system. In drug-sensitive cell lines, Sb^{3+} induces a rapid efflux of trypanothione and glutathione from the cells, and it also inhibits trypanothione reductase, thereby causing a significant loss of thiol reduction potential in the cells (Wyllie *et al.*, 2004). This hypothesis is further supported by the observation that laboratory-generated resistance to antimonials leads to overexpression of glutathione and polyamine biosynthetic enzymes, resulting in increased trypanothione levels, which conjugate to the drug. Elevated levels of ABC transporters, which are involved in the efflux of these conjugates, also were observed (Croft, 2001).

Absorption, Fate, and Excretion. The pentavalent antimonials attain much higher concentrations in plasma than do the trivalent compounds. Consequently, most of a single dose of sodium stibogluconate is excreted in the urine within 24 hours. Its pharmacokinetic behavior is similar whether the drug is given intravenously or intramuscularly; it is not active orally (Pamplin *et al.*, 1981; Chulay *et al.*, 1988). The agent is absorbed rapidly, distributed in an apparent volume of about 0.22 L/kg, and eliminated in two phases. The first has a short half-life of about 2 hours, and the second is much slower ($t_{\frac{1}{2}}$ = 33 to 76 hours). The prolonged terminal elimination phase may reflect conversion of the pentavalent antimonial (Sb^{5+}) to the more toxic trivalent (Sb^{3+}) form that is concentrated and slowly released from tissues. Indeed, about 20% of the plasma antimony is present in the trivalent form after pentavalent antimonial administration. Sequestration of antimony in macrophages also may contribute to the prolonged antileishmanial effect after plasma antimony levels have dropped below the minimal inhibitory concentration observed *in vitro*.

Therapeutic Uses. The changing use of sodium stibogluconate, meglumine antimonate, and other agents for the chemotherapy of leishmaniasis has been reviewed extensively (Berman, 2003; Croft and Coombs, 2003; Fries and Fairlamb, 2003). Sodium stibogluconate is given parenterally, with the dosage regimen individualized depending on the local responsiveness of a particular form of leishmaniasis to this compound. The standard course is 20 mg/kg per day for 20 days for cutaneous disease and for 28 days for visceral disease. Prolonged dosage schedules with maximally tolerated doses are now needed for successful therapy of visceral, mucosal, and some cutaneous forms of leishmaniasis, in part to overcome increasing clinical resistance to antimonial drugs. Even high-dose regimens may no longer produce satisfactory results. Increased resistance has greatly compromised the effectiveness of these drugs, and treatment failure rates of as high as 60% have been observed in parts of India. This is in contrast to previous cure rates of 85% to 90% for both visceral and cutaneous disease. Amphotericin B is the recommended alternative for treatment of either visceral leishmaniasis (kala azar) in India or mucosal leishmaniasis in general,

although the newly approved orally active compound miltefosine is likely to see much wider use in the coming years.

Children usually tolerate the drug well, and the dose per kilogram is the same as that given to adults. Patients who respond favorably show clinical improvement within 1 to 2 weeks of initiation of therapy. The drug may be given on alternate days or for longer intervals if unfavorable reactions occur in especially debilitated individuals. Patients infected with HIV present a challenge because they usually relapse after successful initial therapy with either pentavalent antimonials or amphotericin B.

Toxicity and Side Effects. The toxicity of the pentavalent antimonials is best evaluated in patients without systemic disease, *i.e.*, visceral leishmaniasis. In general, high-dose regimens of sodium stibogluconate are fairly well tolerated; toxic reactions usually are reversible, and most subside despite continued therapy. Effects noted most commonly include pain at the injection site after intramuscular administration; chemical pancreatitis in nearly all patients; elevation of serum hepatic transaminase levels; bone marrow suppression manifested by decreased red cell, white cell, and platelet counts in the blood; muscle and joint pain; weakness and malaise; headache; nausea and abdominal pain; and skin rashes. Changes in the electrocardiogram that include T-wave flattening and inversion and prolongation of the QT interval found in patients with systemic disease are uncommon in other forms of leishmaniasis (Navin *et al.*, 1992; Berman, 1997; Sundar *et al.*, 1998). Reversible polyneuropathy has been reported. Hemolytic anemia and renal damage are rare manifestations of antimonial toxicity, as are shock and sudden death.

SURAMIN

History. Based on the trypanocidal activity of the dyes *trypan red, trypan blue,* and *afridol violet,* research in Germany resulted in the introduction of suramin into therapy in 1920. Today, the drug is used primarily for treatment of African trypanosomiasis; it has no clinical utility against American trypanosomiasis. Although suramin is effective in clearing adult filariae in *onchocerciasis,* it has been replaced by *ivermectin* for the treatment of this condition (*see* Chapter 41). Suramin is a potent inhibitor of retroviral reverse transcriptase *in vitro,* but it is ineffective in HIV infection. Drug-associated adrenal insufficiency, along with the antiproliferative activity of suramin, stimulated the experimental use of high doses, alone or with other compounds, for the therapy of adrenocortical hyperfunction, adrenocortical carcinoma, and a variety of other metastatic tumors (Voogd *et al.*, 1993; Frommel, 1997). The antiparasitic and antineoplastic properties of suramin, along with its clinical uses and limitations, have been the topic of numerous reviews (Voogd *et al.*, 1993; Pépin and Milord, 1994; Barrett and Barrett, 2000).

Chemistry and Preparation. *Suramin sodium* (BAYER 205, formerly GERMANIN, others) has the following chemical structure:

SURAMIN SODIUM

The drug is soluble in water, but solutions deteriorate quickly in air; only freshly prepared solutions should be used. In the United States, suramin is available only from the CDC.

Antiparasitic Effects. Suramin is a relatively slowly acting trypanocide (>6 hours *in vitro*) with high clinical activity against both *T. brucei gambiense* and *T. brucie rhodesiense* and an unknown mechanism of action (Fairlamb, 2003; Bouteille, 2003). Selective toxicity is likely to result from the ability of the parasite to take up the drug by receptor-mediated endocytosis of the protein-bound drug, with low-density lipoproteins being the most important interacting proteins for this event (Fries and Fairlamb, 2003). Suramin reacts reversibly with a variety of biomolecules *in vitro,* inhibiting many trypanosomal and mammalian enzymes and receptors unrelated to its antiparasitic effects, including purinergic and AMPA receptors (Fairlamb, 2003; Suzuki *et al.*, 2004). Compartmentation protects many vital molecules, such as the glycolytic enzymes inside trypanosomal glycosomes, from suramin because this compound does not cross membrane barriers by passive diffusion. However, the chemical structure of suramin may confer transport specificity because removal of its two methyl groups results in the loss of trypanocidal activity *in vivo* but not *in vitro* (Morty *et al.*, 1998). Suramin-treated trypanosomes exhibit damage to intracellular membrane structures other than lysosomes, but whether or not this relates to the drug's primary action is unknown. Inhibition of a trypanosomal cytosolic serine oligopeptidase may account for at least part of the activity of suramin, but it is also a potent inhibitor of dihydrofolate reductase, thymidine kinase, and several of the glycolytic enzymes. The synergism that has been observed between eflornithine and suramin also has led to speculation that it may inhibit polyamine biosynthesis (Fries and Fair-

lamb, 2003). No clear consensus for the mechanism of action has emerged, and the lack of any significant field resistance points to multiple potential targets.

Suramin is the only microfilaricide used clinically, albeit rarely now, for the treatment of human onchocerciasis. This compound displays delayed but prolonged filaricidal activity against both adult male and female worms and lesser but significant activity against microfilariae. Its mechanism of action against *Onchocerca volvulus* is unknown (Voogd *et al.*, 1993).

Absorption, Fate, and Excretion. Because it is not absorbed after oral intake, suramin is given intravenously to avoid local inflammation and necrosis associated with subcutaneous or intramuscular injections. After its administration, the drug displays complex pharmacokinetics with marked interindividual variability. The concentration in plasma falls fairly rapidly after a few hours, but the drug is 99.7% serum bound and has a terminal elimination half-life of about 90 days. Suramin is not appreciably metabolized, and renal clearance accounts for elimination of about 80% of the compound from the body. This large polar anion does not enter cells readily, and tissue concentrations are uniformly lower than those in plasma. In experimental animals, however, the kidneys contain considerably more suramin than do other organs. Such retention may account for the fairly frequent occurrence of albuminuria following injection of the drug in human beings. Very little suramin penetrates the CSF, consistent with its lack of efficacy once the CNS has been invaded by trypanosomes. The dose-dependent prolonged persistence of suramin in the circulation explains why the drug has been used for prophylaxis of African trypanosomiasis.

Therapeutic Uses. Suramin is used to treat African trypanosomiasis but is of no value in South American trypanosomiasis caused by *T. cruzi*. It is used as the first-line therapy for early-stage *T. brucei rhodesiense* infection and as an alternative to pentamidine for early-stage *T. brucei gambiense*. Because no drug resistance has been observed after over 80 years of use, it is also an ideal drug for prophylaxis.

Because only small amounts of the drug enter the brain, suramin is used primarily to treat early stages (before CNS involvement) of African trypanosomiasis (Pépin and Milord, 1994). For therapy of early West African infections, this drug is more effective when given by intravenous regimens that also include intramuscular injections of pentamidine. In contrast, suramin alone appears superior for therapy of early East African disease. Suramin will clear the hemolymphatic system of trypanosomes even in late-stage disease, so it is often administered before initiating melarsoprol to reduce the risk of reactive encephalopathy associated with the administration of that arsenical (*see* above). In animal models, suramin has been found to display synergism with other trypanocides, including eflornithine. However, suramin–

eflornithine therapy has been disappointing against late-stage human *T. brucei rhodesiense* infection (Clerinx *et al.*, 1998).

Suramin is given by slow intravenous injection as a 10% aqueous solution. Treatment of active African trypanosomiasis should not be started until 24 hours after diagnostic lumbar puncture to ensure no CNS involvement, and caution is required if the patient has onchocerciasis (river blindness) because of the potential for eliciting a Mazzotti reaction (*i.e.,* pruritic rash, fever, malaise, lymph node swelling, eosinophilia, arthralgias, tachycardia, hypotension, and possibly permanent blindness). The normal single dose for adults with *T. brucei rhodesiense* infection is 1 g. It is advisable to employ a test dose of 200 mg initially to detect sensitivity, after which the normal dose is given on days 1, 3, 7, 14, and 21. The pediatric dose is 20 mg/kg, given according to the same schedule. Patients in poor condition should be treated with lower doses during the first week. When suramin and pentamidine are used to treat early-stage *T. brucei gambiense* infection, Pépin and Milord (1994) recommend suramin (20 mg/kg, up to a maximum of 1 g) given intravenously on days 1 and 13 and pentamidine isethionate (4 mg/kg) given intramuscularly on days 1, 3, 5, 13, 15, and 17. However, suramin and pentamidine may lose their advantage over pentamidine alone for the treatment of Gambian trypanosomiasis if there is even minimal evidence of CNS involvement (Pépin and Khonde, 1996). Patients who relapse after suramin therapy should be treated with melarsoprol (Pépin and Milord, 1994).

Suramin is effective for the prophylaxis of African trypanosomiasis. Chemoprophylaxis is not recommended for travelers on occasional brief visits to endemic areas because the risk of serious drug toxicity outweighs the risk of acquiring the disease (*see* below). For chemoprophylaxis, the single dose of 1 g is repeated weekly for 5 or 6 weeks.

Toxicity and Side Effects. Suramin can cause a variety of untoward reactions that vary in intensity and frequency and tend to be more severe in debilitated patients. Fortunately, the most serious immediate reaction consisting of nausea, vomiting, shock, and loss of consciousness is rare (about 1 in 2000 patients). Malaise, nausea, and fatigue are also common immediate reactions. Parasite destruction may cause febrile episodes and skin hypersensitivity rashes that are reduced by pretreatment with glucocorticoids; concomitant onchocerciasis optimally should be treated first with ivermectin to minimize these reactions (*see* Chapter 41). The most common problem encountered after several doses of suramin is renal toxicity, manifested by albuminuria, and delayed neurological complications, including headache, metallic taste, paresthesias, and peripheral neuropathy. These complications usually disappear spontaneously despite continued therapy. At higher doses over long periods of treatment used for cancer chemotherapy, suramin-induced coagulopathy is the most common toxicity observed, whereas development of a severe polyradiculoneuropathy is the most serious complication (Voogd *et al.*, 1993). Other, less prevalent reac-

tions include vomiting, diarrhea, stomatitis, chills, abdominal pain, and edema. Laboratory abnormalities noted in 12% to 26% of patients with AIDS include leukopenia and occasional agranulocytosis, thrombocytopenia, proteinuria, and elevations of plasma creatinine, transaminases, and bilirubin, which are reversible. Unexpected findings in patients with AIDS include adrenal insufficiency and vortex keratopathy.

Precautions and Contraindications. Patients receiving suramin should be followed closely. Therapy should not be continued in patients who show intolerance to initial doses, and the drug should be employed with great caution in individuals with renal insufficiency. Moderate albuminuria is common during control of the acute phase, but persisting, heavy albuminuria calls for caution as well as modification of the treatment schedule. If casts appear, treatment with suramin should be discontinued. The occurrence of palmar-plantar hyperesthesia may presage peripheral neuritis.

BIBLIOGRAPHY

Abboud, P., Lemee, V., Gargala, G., *et al.* Successful treatment of metronidazole- and albendazole-resistant giardiasis with nitazoxanide in a patient with acquired immunodeficiency syndrome. *Clin. Infect. Dis.,* **2001,** *32*:1792–1794.

Abel, P.M., Kiala, G., Loa, V., *et al.* Retaking sleeping sickness control in Angola. *Trop. Med. Int. Health.,* **2004,** *9*:141–148 (erratum in *Trop. Med. Int. Health.,* **2004,** *9*:314).

Adagu, I.S., Nolder, D., Warhurst, D.C., and Rossignol, J.F. *In vitro* activity of nitazoxanide and related compounds against isolates of *Giardia intestinalis, Entamoeba histolytica,* and *Trichomonas vaginalis. J. Antimicrob. Chemother.,* **2002,** *49*:103–111.

Amadi, B., Mwiya, M., Musuku, J., *et al.* Effect of nitazoxanide on morbidity and mortality in Zambian children with cryptosporidiosis: A randomized, controlled trial. *Lancet,* **2002,** *360*:1375–1380.

Bacchi, C.J., Nathan, H.C., Hunter, S.H., McCann, P.P., and Sjoerdsma, A. Polyamine metabolism: A potential therapeutic target in trypanosomes. *Science,* **1980,** *210*:332–334.

Bailey, J.M., and Erramouspe, J. Nitazoxanide treatment for giardiasis and cryptosporidiosis in children. *Ann. Pharmocother.,* **2004,** *38*:634–640.

Bronner, U., Gustafsson, L.L., Doua, F., *et al.* Pharmacokinetics and adverse reactions after a single dose of pentamidine in patients with *Trypanosoma gambiense* sleeping sickness. *Br. J. Clin. Pharmacol.,* **1995,** *39*:289–295.

Brun, R., Schumacher, R., Schmid, C., Kunz, C., and Burri, C. The phenomenon of treatment failures in human African trypanosomiasis. *Trop. Med. Int. Health,* **2001,** *6*:906–914.

Burri, C., and Keiser, J. Pharmacokinetic investigations in patients from northern Angola refractory to melarsoprol treatment. *Trop. Med. Int. Health,* **2001,** *6*:412–420.

Chen, K.T., Twu, S.J., Chang, H.J., and Lin, R.S. Outbreak of Stevens-Johnson syndrome/toxic epidermal necrolysis associated with mebendazole and metronidazole use among Filipino laborers in Taiwan. *Am. J. Public Health.* **2003,** 93:489–492.

Chulay, J.D., Fleckenstein, L., and Smith, D.H. Pharmacokinetics of antimony during treatment of visceral leishmaniasis with sodium stibogluconate or meglumine antimoniate. *Trans. R. Soc. Trop. Med. Hyg.,* **1988,** 82:69–72.

Clerinx, J., Taelman, H., Bogaerts, J., and Vervoort, T. Treatment of late-stage rhodesiense trypanosomiasis using suramin and eflornithine: report of six cases. *Trans. R. Soc. Trop. Med. Hyg.,* **1998,** 92:449–450.

Diaz, E., Mondragon, J., Ramirez E., and Bernal, R. Epidemiology and control of intestinal parasites with nitazoxanide in children in Mexico. *Am. J. Trop. Med. Hyg.,* **2003,** 68:384–385.

Donnelly, H., Bernard, E.M., Rothkotter, H., Gold, J.W., and Armstrong, D. Distribution of pentamidine in patients with AIDS. *J. Infect. Dis.,* **1988,** *157*:985–989.

Dunne, R.L., Dunn, L.A., Upcroft, P., O'Donoghue, P.J., and Upcroft, J.A. Drug resistance in the sexually transmitted protozoan *Trichomonas vaginalis. Cell Res.,* **2003,** 13:239–249.

Ericsson, O., Schweda, E.K., Bronner, U., *et al.* Determination of melarsoprol in biological fluids by high-performance liquid chromatography and characterisation of two stereoisomers by nuclear magnetic resonance spectroscopy. *J. Chromatogr. B. Biomed. Sci. Appl.,* **1997,** 690:243–251.

Favennec, L., Jave-Ortiz, J., Gargala, G., *et al.* Double-blind, randomized, placebo-controlled study of nitazoxanide in the treatment of fascioliasis in adults and children from northern Peru. *Aliment. Pharmacol. Therm.,* **2003,** 17:265–270.

Frommel, T.O. Suramin is synergistic with vinblastine in human colonic tumor cell lines: Effect of cell density and timing of drug delivery. *Anticancer Res.,* **1997,** 17:2065–2071.

Gal, M., and Brazier, J.S. Metronidazole resistance in *Bacteroides* spp. carrying *nim* genes and the selection of slow-growing metronidazole-resistant mutants. *J. Antimicrob. Chemother.,* **2004,** 54:109–116.

Grishin, N.V., Osterman, A.L., Brooks, H.B., Phillips, M.A., and Goldsmith, E.J. The X-ray structure of ornithine decarboxylase from *Trypanosoma brucei:* The native structure and the structure in complex with α-difluoromethylornithine. *Biochemistry,* **1999,** 38:15174–15184.

Gross, U. Treatment of microsporidiosis including albendazole. *Parasitol. Res.,* **2003,** 90(suppl):14–18.

Hand, I.L., Wiznia, A.A., Porricolo, M., Lambert, G., and Caspe, W.B. Aerosolized pentamidine for prophylaxis of *Pneumocystis carinii* pneumonia in infants with human immunodeficiency virus infection. *Pediatr. Infect. Dis. J.,* **1994,** 13:100–104.

Hewitt R.G., Yiannoutsos, C.T., Higgs, E.S., *et al.* Paromomycin: no more effective than placebo for treatment of cryptosporidiosis in patients with advanced human immunodeficiency virus infection. AIDS Clinical Trial Group. *Clin. Infect. Dis.,* **2000,** 31:1084–1092.

Jha, T.K., Sundar, S., Thakur, C.P., *et al.* Miltefosine, an oral agent, for the treatment of Indian visceral leishmaniasis. *New Engl. J. Med.,* **1999,** *341*:1795–800.

Krause, P.J., Lepore, T., Sikand, V.K., *et al.* Atovaquone and azithromycin for the treatment of babesiosis. *New Engl. J. Med.,* **2000,** *343*:1454–1458.

Lejon, V., Boelaert, M., Jannin, J., Moore, A., and Buscher, P. The challenge of *Trypanosoma brucei gambiense* sleeping sickness diagnosis outside of Africa. *Lancet Infect. Dis.,* **2003,** 3:804–808.

Leoung, S.G., Feigal, D.W., Jr., Montgomery, A.B., *et al.* Aerosolized pentamidine for prophylaxis against *Pneumocystis carinii* pneumonia: The San Francisco community prophylaxis trial. *New Engl. J. Med.,* **1990,** *323*:769–775.

Li, F., Hua, S.B., Wang, C.C., and Gottesdiener, K.M. *Trypanosoma brucei brucei:* Characterization of an ODC null bloodstream form mutant and the action of α-difluoromethylornithine. *Exp. Parasitol.,* **1998,** 88:255–257.

Matovu, E., Enyaru, J.C., Legros, D., *et al.* Melarsoprol refractory *T. b. gambiense* from Omugo, northwestern Uganda. *Trop. Med. Int. Health,* **2001,** 6:407–411.

Meyerhoff, A. U.S. Food and Drug Administration approval of AmBicome (liposomal amphotericin B) for the treatment of visceral leishmaniasis. *Clin. Infect. Dis.,* **1999,** 28:42–48.

Meyskens, F.L., Jr., and Gerner, E.W. Development of difluoromethylornithine (DFMO) as a chemopreventative agent. *Clin. Cancer Res.,* **1999,** 5:945–951.

Milord, F., Loko, L., Éthier, L., Mpia, B., and Pépin, J. Eflornithine concentrations in serum and cerebrospinal fluid of 63 patients treated for *Trypanosoma brucei gambiense* sleeping sickness. *Trans. R. Soc. Trop. Med. Hyg.,* **1993,** 87:473–477.

Molina, J.M., Tourneur, M., Sarfati, C., *et al.* Fumagillin treatment of intestinal microsporidiosis. *New Engl. J. Med.,* **2002,** *346*:1963–1969.

Morty, R.E., Troeberg, L., Pike, R.N., *et al.* A trypanosome oligopeptidase as a target for the trypanocidal agents pentamidine, diminazene, and suramin. *FEBS Lett.,* **1998,** *433*:251–256.

Mpia B., Pepin, J. Combination of eflornithine and melarsoprol for melarsoprol-resistant Gambian trypanosomiasis. *Trop. Med. Int. Health.* **2002,** 7:775–779.

Mutomba, M.C., Li F., Gottesdiener K.M., and Wang C.C. A *Trypanosoma brucei* bloodstream form mutant deficient in ornithine decarboxylase can protect against wild-type infection in mice. *Exp. Parasitol.,* **1999,** *91*:176–84.

Navin, T.R., Arana, B.A., Arana, F.E., Berman, J.D., and Chajón, J.F. Placebo-controlled clinical trial of sodium stibogluconate (PENTOSTAM) versus ketoconazole for treating cutaneous leishmaniasis in Guatemala. *J. Infect. Dis.,* **1992,** *165*:528–534.

Nyirjesy, P., Sobel, J.D., Weitz, M.V., Leaman, D.J., and Gelone, S.P. Difficult-to-treat trichomoniasis: Results with paromomycin cream. *Clin. Infect. Dis.* **1998,** 26:986–988.

Obaji, J., Lee-Pack, L.R., Gutierrez, C., and Chan, C.K. The pulmonary effects of long-term exposure to aerosol pentamidine: A 5-year surveillance study in HIV-infected patients. *Chest,* **2003,** *123*:1983–1987.

Pamplin, C.L., Desjardins, R., Chulay, J., *et al.* Pharmacokinetics of antimony during sodium stibogluconate therapy for cutaneous leishmaniasis. *Clin. Pharmacol. Ther.,* **1981,** 29:270–271.

Paulos, C., Paredes, J., Vasquez, I., *et al.* Pharmacokinetics of a nitrofuran compound, nifurtimox, in healthy volunteers. *Int. J. Clin. Pharmacol. Ther. Toxicol.,* **1989,** 27:454–457.

Pépin, J., and Khonde, N. Relapses following treatment of early-stage *Trypanosoma brucei gambiense* sleeping sickness with a combination of pentamidine and suramin. *Trans. R. Soc. Trop. Med. Hyg.,* **1996,** 90:183–186.

Pépin, J., Mpia, B., and Iloasebe, M. *Trypanosoma brucei gambiense* African trypanosomiasis: Differences between men and women in severity of disease and response to treatment. *Trans. R. Soc. Trop. Med. Hyg.,* **2002,** 96:421–426.

Pépin, J., Khonde, N., Maiso, F., *et al.* Short-course eflornithine in Gambian trypanosomiasis: A multicentre randomized, controlled trial. *Bull. WHO,* **2000,** 78:1284–1295.

Pépin, J., Milord, F., Khonde, A.N., *et al.* Risk factors for encephalopathy and mortality during melarsoprol treatment of *Trypanosoma brucei gambiense* sleeping sickness. *Trans. R. Soc. Trop. Med. Hyg.,* **1995,** 89:92–97.

Perez-Victoria, F.J., Gamarro, F., Ouellette, M., and Castanys, S. Functional cloning of the miltefosine transporter: A novel P-type phospholipid translocase from leishmania involved in drug resistance. *J. Biol. Chem.*, **2003**, *278*:49965–49971.

Pifer, L.L., Pifer, D.D., and Woods, D.R. Biological profile and response to antipneumocystis agents of *Pneumocystis carinii* in cell culture. *Antimicrob. Agents Chemother.*, **1983**, *24*:674–678.

Quon, D.V., d'Oliveira, C.E., and Johnson, P.J. Reduced transcription of the ferredoxin gene in metronidazole-resistant *Trichomonas vaginalis*. *Proc. Natl. Acad. Sci. U.S.A.*, **1992**, *89*:4402–4406.

Romero-Cabello, R., Guerrero, L.R., Munoz-Garcia, M.R., and Geyne-Cruz, A. Nitazoxanide for the treatment of intestinal protozoan and helminthic infections in Mexico. *Trans. R. Soc. Trop. Med. Hyg.*, **1997**, *91*:701–703.

Rossignol, J.F., and Maisonneuve, H. Nitazoxanide in the treatment of *Taenia saginata* and *Hymenolepis nana* infections. *Am. J. Trop. Med. Hyg.*, **1984**, *33*:511–512.

Rossignol, J.F., Ayoub A., and Ayers, M.S. Treatment of diarrhea caused by *Cryptosporidium parvum:* A prospective, randomized, double-blind, placebo-controlled study of nitazoxanide. *J. Infect. Dis.*, **2001**, *184*:103–106.

Rossignol, J.F., Hidalgo, H., Feregrino, M., *et al.* A double-"blind," placebo-controlled study of nitazoxanide in the treatment of cryptosporidial diarrhoea in AIDS patients in Mexico. *Trans. R. Soc. Trop. Med. Hyg.*, **1998**, *92*:663–666.

Samarawickrema, N.A., Brown, D.M. Upcroft, J.A., Thammapalerd, N., and Upcroft, P. Involvement of superoxide dismutase and pyruvate: ferredoxin oxidoreductase in mechanisms of metronidazole resistance in *Entamoeba histolytica*. *J. Antimicrob. Agents Chemother.*, **1997**, *40*:833–840.

Smego, R.A., Jr., Nagar, S., Maloba, B., and Popara, M. A meta-analysis of salvage therapy for *Pneumocystis carinii* pneumonia. *Arch. Intern. Med.*, **2001**, *161*:1529–1533.

Sobel, J.D., Nyirjesy, P., and Brown, W. Tinidazole therapy for metronidazole-resistant vaginal trichomoniasis. *Clin. Infect. Dis.*, **2001**, *33*:1341–1346.

Soto, J., Arana, B.A., Toledo, J., *et al.* Miltefosine for New World cutaneous leishmaniasis. *Clin. Infect. Dis.*, **2004**, *38*:1266–1272.

Sundar, S., Jha, T.K., Thakur, C.P., *et al.* Oral miltefosine for Indian visceral leishmaniasis. *New Engl. J. Med.*, **2002**, *347*:1739–1746.

Sundar, S., Sinha, P.R., Agrawal, N.K., *et al.* A cluster of cases of severe cardiotoxicity among kala-azar patients treated with a high-osmolarity lot of sodium antimony gluconate. *Am. J. Trop. Med. Hyg.*, **1998**, *59*:139–143.

Suzuki, E., Kessler, M., Montgomery, K., and Arai, A. Divergent effects of the purinoceptor antagonists suramin and pyridoxal-5'-phosphate-6-(2-naphthylazo-6'-nitro-4',8' disulfonate) (PPNDS) on α-amino-3-hydroxy-5-methyl-4-isoxazole proprionic acid (AMPA) receptors. *Mol. Pharmacol.*, **2004**, *66*:1738–1747.

Thakur, C.P., Kanyok, T.P., Pandey, A.K., *et al.* A prospective, randomized, comparative open-label trial of the safety and efficacy of paromomycin (aminosidine) plus sodium stibogluconate versus sodium stibogluconate alone for the treatment of visceral leishmaniasis. *Trans. R. Soc. Trop. Med. Hyg.* **2000**, *94*:429–431.

Upcroft, J.A., Campbell, R.W., Benakli, K., Upcroft, P., and Vanelle, P. Efficacy of new 5-nitroimidazoles against metronidazole-susceptible and -resistant *Giardia, Trichomonas,* and *Entamoeba* spp. *Antimicrob. Agents Chemother.*, **1999**, *43*:73–76.

Wassmann, C., Hellberg, A., Tannich, E., and Bruchhaus, I. Metronidazole resistance in the protozoan parasite *Entamoeba histolytica* is associated with increased expression of iron-containing superoxide dismutase and peroxiredoxin and decreased expression of ferredoxin 1 and flavin reductase. *J. Biol. Chem.*, **1999**, *274*:26051–26056.

Wickware, P. Resurrecting the resurrection drug. *Nature Med.*, **2002**, *8*:908–909.

Wood, D.H., Hall, J.E., Rose, B.G., and Tidwell, R.R. 1,5-Bis(4-amidinophenoxy)pentane (pentamidine) is a potent inhibitor of [³H]idazoxan binding to imidazoline I₂ binding sites. *Eur. J. Pharmacol.*, **1998**, *353*:97–103.

World Health Organization. Chile and Brazil to be certified free of transmission of Chagas' disease. *TDR News*, **1999**, *59*:10.

Wyllie, S., Cunningham, M.L., and Fairlamb, A.H. Dual action of antimonial drugs on thiol redox metabolism in the human pathogen *Leishmania donovani*. *J. Biol. Chem.*, **2004**, *279*:39925–39932.

Yarlett, N., Yarlett, N.C., and Lloyd, D. Metronidazole-resistant clinical isolates of *Trichomonas vaginalis* have lowered oxygen affinities. *Mol. Biochem. Parasitol.*, **1986**, *19*:111–116.

Zhou, Y., Messier, N., Ouellette, M., Rosen, B.P., and Mukhopadhyay, R. *Leishmania* major LmACR2 is a pentavalent antimony reductase that confers sensitivity to the drug pentostam. *J. Biol. Chem.*, **2004**, *279*:37445–37551.

MONOGRAPHS AND REVIEWS

Barrett, S.V., and Barrett, M.P. Anti–sleeping sickness drugs and cancer chemotherapy. *Parasitol. Today,* **2000**, *16*:7–9.

Berman, J. Current treatment approaches to leishmaniasis. *Curr. Opin. Infect. Dis.*, **2003**, *16*:396–401.

Berman, J.D. Human leishmaniasis: Clinical, diagnostic, and chemotherapeutic developments in the last 10 years. *Clin. Infect. Dis.*, **1997**, *24*:684–703.

Bouteille, B., Oukem, O., Bisser, S., and Dumas, M. Treatment perspectives for human African trypanosomiasis. *Fundam. Clin. Phamacol.*, **2003**, *17*:171–181.

Bray, P.G., Barrett, M.P., Ward, S.A., and deKoning, H.P. Pentamidine uptake and resistance in pathogenic protozoa: Past, present and future. *Trends. Parasitol.*, **2003**, *19*:232–239.

Brener, Z. Present status of chemotherapy and chemoprophylaxis of human trypanosomiasis in the western hemisphere. *Pharmacol. Ther.*, **1979**, *7*:71–90.

Burri, C., and Brun, R. Eflornithine for the treatment of human African trypanosomiasis. *Parasitol. Res.*, **2003**, *90*(suppl):49–52.

Croft, S.L., and Coombs, G.H. Leishmaniasis: Current chemotherapy and recent advances in the search for novel drugs. *Trends. Parasitol.*, **2003**, *19*:502–508.

Croft, S.L. Monitoring drug resistance in leishmaniasis. *Trop. Med. Int. Health,* **2001**, *6*:899–905.

deKoning, H.P. Transporters in African trypanosomes: Role in drug action and resistance. *Int. J. Parasitol.*, **2001**, *31*:512–522.

Docampo, R., and Moreno, S.N. Current chemotherapy of human African trypanosomiasis. *Parasitol Res.*, **2003**, *90*(suppl):10–13.

Fairlamb, A.H. Chemotherapy of human African trypanosomiasis: Current and future prospects. *Trends Parasitol.*, **2003**, *19*:488–494.

Farthing, M.J. Giardiasis. *Gastroenterol. Clin. North Am.*, **1996**, *25*:493–515.

Freeman, C.D., Klutman, N.E., and Lamp, K.C. Metronidazole: A therapeutic review and update. *Drugs*, **1997**, *54*:679–708.

Fries, D.S., and Fairlamb, A.H. Antiprotozoal agents. In, *Burger's Medicinal Chemistry and Drug Discovery*, 6th ed. (D.J. Abraham, ed.) Wiley, Hoboken, NJ, **2003**.

Gardner, T.B., and Hill, D.R. Treatment of giardiasis. *Clin. Microbiol. Rev.*, **2001**, *14*:114–128.

Heine, P., and McGregor, J.A. *Trichomonas vaginalis*: A reemerging pathogen. *Clin. Obstet. Gynecol.*, **1993**, *36*:137–144.

Herwaldt, B.L. Leishmaniasis. *Lancet*, **1999**, *354*:1191–1199.

Igarashi, K., and Kashiwagi, K. Polyamines: Mysterious modulators of cellular functions. *Biochem. Biophys. Res. Commun.,* **2000,** *271*:559–564.

Johnson, P.J. Metronidazole and drug resistance. *Parasitol. Today,* **1993,** *9*:183–186.

Kennedy, P.G. Human African trypanosomiasis of the CNS: Current issues and challenges. *J. Clin. Invest.,* **2004,** *113*:496–504.

Lamp, K.C., Freeman, C.D., Klutman, N.E., and Lacy, M.K. Pharmaco-kinetics and pharmacodynamics of the nitroimidazole antimicrobials. *Clin. Pharmacokinet.,* **1999,** *36*:353–373.

Land, K.M., and Johnson, P.J. Molecular mechanisms underlying metronidazole resistance in trichomonads. *Exp. Parasitol.,* **1997,** *87*:305–308.

Legros, D., Ollivier, G., Gastellu-Etchegorry, M., *et al.* Treatment of human African trypanosomiasis: Present situation and needs for research and development. *Lancet Infect. Dis.,* **2002,** *2*:437–440.

Lengerich, E.J., Addiss, D.G., and Juranek, D.D. Severe giardiasis in the United States. *Clin. Infect. Dis.,* **1994,** *18*:760–763.

Marton, L.J., and Pegg, A.E. Polyamines as targets for therapeutic intervention. *Annu. Rev. Phamacol. Toxicol.,* **1995,** *35*:55–91.

Maser, P., Luscher, A., and Kaminsky, R. Drug transport and drug resistance in African trypanosomes. *Drug Resist. Update,* **2003,** *6*:281–290.

Mendz, G.L., and Mègraud, F. Is the molecular basis of metronidazole resistance in microaerophilic organisms understood? *Trends. Microbiol.,* **2002,** *10*:370–375.

Montoya, J.G., and Liesenfeld, O. Toxoplasmosis. *Lancet,* **2004,** *363*:1965–1976.

Nash, T.E. Treatment of *Giardia lamblia* infections. *Pediatr. Infect. Dis. J.,* **2001,** *20*:193–195.

Nok, A.J. Arsenicals (melarsoprol), pentamidine and suramin in the treatment of human African trypanosomiasis. *Paristol. Res.,* **2003,** *90*:71–79.

Pépin, J., and Milord, F. The treatment of human African trypanosomiasis. *Adv. Parasitol.,* **1994,** *33*:1–47.

Podolsky, D.K. Inflammatory bowel disease. *New Engl. J. Med.,* **2002,** *347*:417–429.

Raether, W., and Hänel, H. Nitroheterocyclic drugs with broad-spectrum activity. *Parasitol. Res.,* **2003,** *90*(suppl):19–39.

Ramirez, N.E., Ward, L.A., and Sreevatsan, S. A review of the biology and epidemiology of cryptosporidiosis in humans and animals. *Microbes Infect.,* **2004,** *6*:773–785.

Rodriques-Coura, J., and de Castro, S.L. A critical review on Chagas' disease chemotherapy. *Mem. Inst. Oswaldo Cruz,* **2002,** *97*:3–24.

Samuelson, J. Why metronidazole is active against both bacteria and parasites. *Antimicrob. Agents Chemother.,* **1999,** *43*:1533–1541.

Seiler, N. Thirty years of polyamine-related approaches to cancer therapy: Retrospect and prospect. 1. Selective enzyme inhibitors. *Curr. Drug Targets,* **2003,** *4*:537–564.

Song, F., and Glenny, A.M. Antimicrobial prophylaxis in colorectal surgery: A systematic review of randomized, controlled trials. *Health Technol. Assess.,* **1998,** *2*:1–110.

Stanley, S.L., Jr. Amoebiasis. *Lancet,* **2003,** *361*:1025–1034.

Suerbaum, S., and Michetti, P. *Helicobacter pylori* infection. *New Engl. J. Med.,* **2002,** *347*:1175–1186.

Thomas, C.F., Jr., and Limper, A.H. *Pneumocystis* pneumonia. *New Engl. J. Med.,* **2004,** *350*:2487–2498.

Upcroft, J.A., and Upcroft, P. Keto-acid oxidoreductases in the anaerobic protozoa. *J. Eukaryot. Microbiol.,* **1999,** *46*:447–449.

Upcroft, P., and Upcroft, J.A. Drug targets and mechanisms of resistance in the anaerobic protozoa. *Clin. Microbiol. Rev.,* **2001,** *14*:150–164.

Urbina, J.A., and Docampo, R. Specific chemotherapy of Chagas' disease: Controversies and advances. *Trends Parasitol.,* **2003,** *19*:495–501.

Van Nieuwenhove, S. Advances in sleeping sickness therapy. *Ann. Soc. Belg. Med. Trop.,* **1992,** *72*(suppl 1):39–51.

Vöhringer, H.F., and Arastéh, K. Pharmacokinetic optimisation in the treatment of *Pneumocystis carinii* pneumonia. *Clin. Pharmacokinet.,* **1993,** *24*:388–412.

Voogd, T.E., Vansterkenburg, E.L., Wilting, J., and Janssen, L.H. Recent research on the biological activity of suramin. *Pharmacol. Rev.,* **1993,** *45*:177–203.

Wang, C.C. Molecular mechanisms and therapeutic approaches to the treatment of African trypanosomiasis. *Annu. Rev. Pharmacol. Toxicol.,* **1995,** *35*:93–127.

Wang, C.C. Validating targets for antiparasitic chemotherapy. *Parasitology,* **1997,** *114*(suppl):31–44.

Welburn S.C., and Odiit, M. Recent developments in human African trypanosomiasis. *Curr. Opin. Infect. Dis.,* **2002,** *15*:477–84.

CHEMOTHERAPY OF HELMINTH INFECTIONS

Alex Loukas and Peter J. Hotez

Infections with helminths, or parasitic worms, affect more than two billion people worldwide. In regions of rural poverty in the tropics, where prevalence is greatest, simultaneous infection with more than one type of helminth is common. The relative incidence of common helminthic infections in humans worldwide is illustrated in Figure 41–1.

Primarily as a result of stepped-up advocacy by the World Health Organization (WHO), the World Bank, and smaller nongovernmental organizations such as the London-based Partnership for Child Development (PCD), there is increasing appreciation for the impact of helminth infections on the health and education of school-aged children (Savioli *et al.*, 2002). These organizations have promoted the periodic and frequent use of anthelmintic drugs in schools as a means to control morbidity caused by soil-transmitted helminths and schistosomes in developing countries. In addition, there is interest in eliminating arthropod-borne helminth infections by interrupting their transmission through the widespread use of anthelmintics. Control programs using anthelmintics could become the world's largest health programs (Horton, 2003).

Worms pathogenic for humans are Metazoa, classified into roundworms (nematodes) and two types of flatworms, flukes (trematodes) and tapeworms (cestodes). These biologically diverse eukaryotes vary with respect to life cycle, bodily structure, development, physiology, localization within the host, and susceptibility to chemotherapy. Immature forms invade humans *via* the skin or gastrointestinal tract and evolve into well-differentiated adult worms with characteristic tissue distributions. With few exceptions, such as *Strongyloides* and *Echinococcus*, these organisms cannot complete their life cycle and replicate themselves within the human host. Therefore, the extent of exposure to these parasites dictates the severity of infection, and reduction in the number of adult organisms by chemotherapy is sustained unless reinfection occurs. The prevalence of parasitic helminths typically displays a negative binomial distribution within an infected population such that relatively few persons carry heavy parasite burdens. Without treatment, those individuals are most likely to become ill and to perpetuate infection within their community.

Anthelmintics are drugs that act either locally to expel worms from the gastrointestinal tract or systemically to eradicate adult helminths or developmental forms that invade organs and tissues. Due to discovery and development of anthelmintics, particularly for veterinary applications, physicians now have effective, and in some cases broad-spectrum, agents that will cure or control most human infections caused by either flukes or intestinal helminths. But cysticercosis, echinococcosis, filariasis, and trichinosis are examples of systemic infections caused by tissue-dwelling helminths that at best respond only partially to currently available drugs. Because metazoan parasites generally are long-lived and have relatively complex life cycles, acquired resistance to anthelmintics in humans has yet to become a major factor limiting clinical efficacy. However, based on extensive use of anthelmintics, such as the benzimidazoles in veterinary medicine, the potential for drug resistance among helminths in humans cannot be discounted.

This chapter first describes the recommended chemotherapy for common human infections caused by helminths and then discusses the properties of specific anthelmintics.

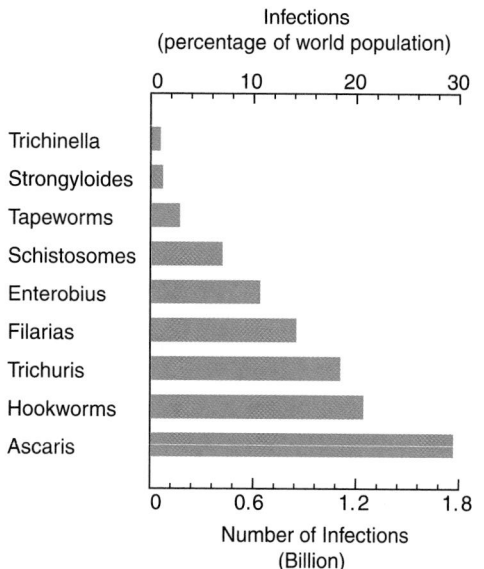

Figure 41–1. *Relative incidence of helminth infections worldwide.*

TREATMENT OF HELMINTH INFECTIONS

Nematodes (Roundworms)

The major nematode parasites of humans include the soil-transmitted helminths (STHs; sometimes referred to as "geohelminths") and the filarial nematodes.

The major STH infections, which include ascariasis, trichuriasis, and hookworm infection, are among the most prevalent infections in developing countries. Because STH worm burdens are higher in school-aged children than in any other single group, the WHO and the PCD advocate using schools and schoolteachers to administer broad-spectrum anthelmintics on a periodic and frequent basis. The most widely used agents employed for reducing morbidity are the benzimidazole anthelmintics (BZAs), either *albendazole* (ALBENZA and ZENTEL) or *mebendazole* (VERMOX) (*see* Table 41–1). A single dose of a BZA reduces worm burdens and subsequently improves host iron and hemoglobin status, physical growth, cognition, educational achievement, and school absenteeism, as well as having a positive influence on the entire community, namely through a reduction in the spread of ascariasis and trichuriasis (Bundy *et al.*, 1990; Savioli *et al.*, 2002; Hotez *et al.*, 2004a; Hotez *et al.*, 2005). In 2001, the World Health Assembly adopted a resolution urging that by 2010 member states should regularly administer anthelmintics to

75% of all school-age children at risk for morbidity (World Health Organization, 2002). Concerns with this recommendation include: (1) the sheer scope of the undertaking (Horton, 2003); (2) the high rates of posttreatment STH reinfection that occur in areas of high transmission (Albonico *et al.*, 1995); (3) the possibility that widespread treatment will lead to the emergence of BZA drug resistance (Albonico, 2003; Albonico *et al.*, 2003); and (4) the observation that focusing exclusively on school-aged children would miss populations that are vulnerable to hookworm infection, such as preschool children and women of reproductive age (Brooker *et al.*, 2004; Hotez *et al.*, 2004a).

In addition to targeting STH infections among school-aged children, there is an ongoing attempt to employ anthelmintics that eliminate lymphatic filariasis (LF) and onchocerciasis (river blindness) over the next 10 to 20 years (Molyneux and Zagaria, 2002; Molyneux *et al.*, 2003). The term *elimination* refers to the reduction of disease incidence to zero or close to zero, with a requirement for ongoing control efforts (Hotez *et al.*, 2004b). The major goal for LF and onchocerciasis elimination is to interrupt arthropod-borne transmission by administering combination therapy with either *diethylcarbamazine* and albendazole (in LF-endemic regions such as India and Egypt), or *ivermectin* and albendazole (in LF regions where onchocerciasis and/or loiasis are co-endemic). These drugs target the microfilarial stages of the parasite, which circulate in blood and are taken up by arthropod vectors where further parasite development takes place. Both control programs rely heavily on the generosity of major drug companies that donate ivermectin and albendazole (Molyneux *et al.*, 2003; Burnham and Mebrahtu, 2004).

Ascaris lumbricoides* and *Toxocara canis. *Ascaris lumbricoides*, known as the "roundworm," parasitizes an estimated 1.2 billion people worldwide (de Silva *et al.*, 2003). Ascariasis may affect from 70% to 90% of persons in some tropical regions, but it also is seen in temperate climates. People become infected by ingesting food or soil contaminated with embryonated *A. lumbricoides* eggs. The highest ascaris worm burdens occur in school-aged children in whom the parasite can cause intestinal obstruction or hepatobiliary ascariasis (Crompton, 2001).

More effective, less toxic compounds largely have replaced the older ascaricides. Mebendazole, *pyrantel pamoate* (ANTIMINTH, others), and albendazole are preferred agents. *Piperazine* also is effective but is used less often because of occasional neurotoxicity and hypersensitivity reactions. Cure with any of these drugs can be achieved in nearly 100% of cases, and all infected persons should be treated. Mebendazole and albendazole are preferred for therapy of asymptomatic to moderate ascariasis. Both of these benzimidazoles are ascaricidal and have a broad spectrum of activity against mixed

Table 41–1
Structure of the Benzimidazoles

R₁	R₂	DERIVATIVE
N=\\—S (thiazole ring)	H—	Thiabendazole
—NHCO₂CH₃	(phenyl)—C=O	Mebendazole
—NHCO₂CH₃	CH₃CH₂CH₂S—	Albendazole

infections with other gastrointestinal nematodes. Albendazole is useful against infections with some systemic nematodes and some cestodes as well. Both compounds should be used with caution to treat heavy *Ascaris* infections, alone or with hookworms. In rare instances, hyperactive ascarids may migrate to unusual loci and cause serious complications such as appendicitis, occlusion of the common bile duct, intestinal obstruction, and intestinal perforation with peritonitis. Therapy with nonascaricidal agents such as pyrantel is preferred by some clinicians for heavy *Ascaris* infections because this agent paralyzes the worms prior to their expulsion. Surgery still may be required despite the use of these agents. Pyrantel is considered safe for use during pregnancy, whereas the BZAs should be avoided during the first trimester (*see* below). Pyrantel and albendazole are considered "investigational" drugs for treatment of ascariasis in the United States, even though they are approved for other indications.

Toxocariasis, a zoonotic infection caused by the canine ascarid *Toxocara canis*, is a common helminthiasis in North America and Europe. Possibly, it has displaced pinworm as the most common helminthic infection in the United States (Sharghi *et al.*, 2000). The three major syndromes caused by *T. canis* infection are visceral larva migrans (VLM), ocular larva migrans (OLM), and covert toxocariasis (CT). CT has been postulated to represent an underappreciated cause of asthma and seizures (Sharghi *et al.*, 2000; Sharghi *et al.*, 2001). The specific treatment of VLM is reserved for patients with severe, persistent, or progressive symptoms (Hotez *et al.*, 2005). Albendazole is the drug of choice. In contrast, the role of anthelmintic drugs for the treatment of OLM and CT is controversial. In the case of the former, surgical management often is indicated, sometimes accompanied by systemic or topical steroids (Sabrosa and de Souza, 2001).

Hookworm. *Necator americanus, Ancylostoma duodenale.* These closely related hookworm species infect 740 million people in developing countries (de Silva *et al.*, 2003). *N. americanus* is the predominant hookworm worldwide, especially in the Americas, sub-Saharan

Africa, South China, and Southeast Asia, whereas *A. duodenale* is focally endemic in Egypt, and parts of northern India and China. Infection also occurs farther north in unusual but relatively warm settings such as mines and large mountain tunnels, hence the term *miner's disease* and *tunnel disease*. Hookworm larvae live in the soils and penetrate exposed skin. After reaching the lungs, the larvae migrate to the oral cavity and are swallowed. After attaching to the jejunal mucosa, the derived adult worms feed on host blood. There is a direct correlation between the number of hookworms (hookworm burden) as determined by quantitative fecal egg counts and fecal blood loss. In individuals with low iron reserves, the correlation extends to hookworm burden and degree of iron-deficiency anemia (Hotez *et al.*, 2004a). Unlike heavy *Ascaris* and *Trichuris* infections, which occur predominantly in children, heavy hookworm infections also occur in adults, including women of reproductive age. In some endemic areas, the heaviest hookworm burdens occur exclusively in adult populations.

Although iron supplementation (and transfusion in severe cases) often is helpful in individuals with severe iron-deficiency anemia, the major treatment goal is to remove blood-feeding adult hookworms from the intestines. Albendazole and mebendazole now are agents of first choice against both *A. duodenale* and *N. americanus*, and both benzimidazoles have the advantage of effectiveness against other roundworms when there is multiple infection. When used in a single dose, albendazole is superior to mebendazole at removing adult hookworms from the GI tract. Oral albendazole is the drug of choice for treating *cutaneous larva migrans* or "creeping eruption," which is due most commonly to skin migration by larvae of the dog hookworm, *A. braziliense*. Oral ivermectin or topical *thiabendazole* also can be used.

Trichuris trichiura. *Trichuris* (whipworm) infection occurs in an estimated 795 million people in developing countries (de Silva *et al.*, 2003). The infection is acquired by ingestion of embryonated eggs. In children, heavy *Trichuris* worm burdens can lead to colitis, *Trichuris* dysentery syndrome, and rectal prolapse (Bundy and Cooper, 1989). Mebendazole and albendazole are considered the safest and most effective agents for treatment of whipworm, alone or together with *Ascaris* and hookworm infections. Pyrantel pamoate is ineffective against *Trichuris*.

Strongyloides stercoralis. *S. stercoralis*, sometimes called the threadworm or dwarf threadworm, is exceptional among helminths because it can replicate and cause cycles of larval reinfection within the human host. The organism infects more than 200 million people worldwide, most frequently in the tropics and other hot, humid locales. In the United States, strongyloidiasis is endemic in the Appalachian region. It also is found in institutionalized individuals living in unsanitary conditions and in immigrants, travelers, and military personnel who lived in endemic areas. Infective larvae in fecally contaminated soil penetrate the skin or mucous membranes, travel to the lungs, and ultimately mature into adult worms in the small intestine, where they reside. Most infected individuals are asymptomatic, while some experience skin rashes and gastrointestinal symptoms. Life-threatening, systemic disease due to massive larval hyperinfection can occur in immunosuppressed persons, even decades after the initial infection. Most deaths caused by parasites in the United States probably are due to *Strongyloides* hyperinfection. Ivermectin is the best drug for treating intestinal strongyloidiasis. Hyperinfection may require prolonged or repeated therapy. Effective benzimidazole compounds, listed in order of decreasing efficacy, are thiabendazole and albendazole. Thiabendazole shows efficacy comparable to that of ivermectin but is far more toxic.

Enterobius vermicularis. *Enterobius*, the pinworm, is one of the most common helminth infections in temperate climates, including the United States. This parasite rarely causes serious complications; pruritus in the perianal and perineal regions, however, can be severe, and scratching may cause secondary infection. In female patients, worms may wander into the genital tract and penetrate into the peritoneal cavity. Salpingitis or even peritonitis may ensue. Because the infection is easily distributed throughout members of a family, a school, or an institution, the physician must decide whether to treat all individuals in close contact with an infected person, and more than one course of therapy may be required.

Pyrantel pamoate, mebendazole, and albendazole are highly effective. Single oral doses of each should be repeated after 2 weeks. When their use is combined with rigid standards of personal hygiene, a very high proportion of cures can be obtained. Treatment is simple and almost devoid of side effects.

Trichinella spiralis. *T. spiralis* is ubiquitous, regardless of climate, and can live outside its hosts. It is found in Canada, Eastern Europe, and now less frequently the United States. The infection results from eating raw or insufficiently cooked flesh of infected animals, especially pigs. When released by acid stomach contents, encysted larvae mature into adult worms in the intestine. Adults then produce infectious larvae that invade tissues, especially skeletal muscle and heart. Severe infection can be fatal, but more typically causes marked muscle pain and cardiac complications. Fortunately, infection is readily preventable. All pork, including pork sausages, should be thoroughly cooked before being eaten. The encysted larvae are killed by exposure to heat of 60°C for 5 minutes.

Albendazole and mebendazole appear to be effective against the intestinal forms of *T. spiralis* that are present early in infection. The efficacy of these agents or any anthelmintic agent on larvae that have migrated to muscle is questionable. Glucocorticoids may be of considerable value in controlling the acute and dangerous manifestations of established infection, although steroids can alter the metabolism of albendazole (*see* below).

***Wuchereria bancrofti* and *Brugia* Species (Lymphatic Filariasis).** Adult worms that cause human filariasis dwell either in the lymphatic system (*Wuchereria bancrofti, Brugia malayi, Brugia timori*) or other tissues (*Mansonella* species). Spread by the bites of infected mosquitoes, lymphatic filariasis (LF) affects nearly 120 million people, about 90% of them infected with *W. bancrofti* and most of the rest with *B. malayi*. Of the 120 million infections worldwide, approximately 40 million people in 80 countries have clinical disease (Molyneux and Zagaria, 2002). The major endemic regions are sub-Saharan Africa, the Indian subcontinent, Southeast Asia and the Pacific region, and the tropical regions of the Americas. In LF, host reactions to the adult worms initially cause lymphatic inflammation manifested by fevers, lymphangitis, and lymphadenitis; this can progress to lymphatic obstruction typified by lymphedema, hydrocele, and elephantiasis. A reaction to microfilariae, *tropical pulmonary eosinophilia*, also occurs in some persons. In 1997, the World Health Assembly passed a resolution calling on WHO member states to support the global elimination of LF. This led to the establishment of the Global Program for the Elimination of LF, which recommended that all at-risk individuals be treated once yearly with an oral two-drug combination (Molyneux and Zagaria, 2002). For most countries, the WHO recommends albendazole and diethylcarbamazine. The exceptions are in many parts of sub-Saharan Africa, where loiasis and onchocerciasis are co-endemic, and in Yemen, where albendazole and ivermectin are the drugs of choice (Molyneux *et al.*, 2003). These drugs clear circulating microfilariae from infected subjects (Molyneux and Zagaria, 2002), thereby reducing the likelihood that mosquitoes will transmit LF to other individuals. To date the number of serious adverse events from LF-control mass chemotherapy programs has been remarkably low and recently was estimated at 1 out of 4.5 million (Molyneux *et al.*, 2003).

Diethylcarbamazine also is the drug of choice for the direct treatment of LF adult worms. However, the effect on the adult worms is variable; best results are achieved in *W. bancrofti* and *B. malayi* infections if chemotherapy is started early, before lymphatic obstruction has occurred. Diethylcarbamazine decreases the incidence of filarial lymphangitis, but it is unclear whether it reverses lymphatic damage or other chronic manifestations of LF. In longstanding elephantiasis, surgical measures are required to improve lymph drainage and remove redundant tissue. Filariasis caused by *Mansonella* species, transmitted largely by midges, is variably responsive to chemotherapy, but does not usually result in serious pathology.

***Loa loa* (loiasis).** Transmitted by deerflies, *L. loa* is a tissue-migrating filarial parasite found in large river regions of Central and West Africa. Adult worms in subcutaneous tissues typically cause episodic "Calabar" swellings and allergic reactions, but also can penetrate the conjunctivae and skin. Rarely, encephalopathy, cardiopathy, or nephropathy occur in association with heavy infection. Diethylcarbamazine currently is the best single drug for the treatment of loiasis, but it is advisable to start with a small initial dose to diminish host reactions that result from destruction of microfilariae. Glucocorticoids often are required to control acute reactions. In rare instances, serious cerebral reactions occur in the treatment of loiasis, probably due to destruction of microfilariae in the brain or cerebral vasculature. If headache is severe and there is other evidence of an adult *L. loa* near the orbit, extra caution for initial dosing is advised. The potential complications of unmonitored diethylcarbamazine treatment of loiasis are the major reason that this agent is not recommended for mass chemoprophylaxis of LF in regions of sub-Saharan Africa where *L. loa* is co-endemic.

***Onchocerca volvulus* (Onchocerciasis or River Blindness).** Transmitted by blackflies near fast-flowing streams and rivers, *O. volvulus* infects about 17 million people in 22 countries in sub-Saharan Africa (Molyneux *et al.*, 2003), and less than 100,000 people in parts of Mexico, Guatemala, and South America. Some cases also occur in Yemen. Inflammatory reactions, primarily to microfilariae rather than adult worms, affect the subcutaneous tissues, lymph nodes, and eyes. Onchocerciasis is a leading cause of infectious blindness worldwide, and results from the cumulative destruction of microfilariae in the eyes, a process that evolves over decades.

Ivermectin is the best single drug for control and treatment of onchocerciasis. Diethylcarbamazine is no longer recommended. Both agents kill only microfilariae of *O. volvulus*, but ivermectin produces far milder systemic reactions and few if any ocular complications. With diethylcarbamazine, such reactions are likely to be severe, particularly in cases in which there are lesions of the eye. Ivermectin treatments clear microfilariae in the tissues, prevent the development of blindness, and interrupt onchocerciasis transmission, a cornerstone of control. Widespread use of ivermectin from 1974 through 2002 through the Mectizan donation plan resulted in the prevention of 600,000 cases of blindness. Since then, the Nongovernmental Development Organizations Group for Onchocerciasis Control (which includes UNICEF, The Carter Center, Lion Clubs, and Helen Keller International, among others) has proposed ivermectin treatment for at least 40 million additional people (www.who.int/pbd/blindness/onchocerciasis). Although *suramin* (*see* Chapter 40) is lethal to adult *O. volvulus*, treatment with this relatively toxic agent probably is unwarranted. Less toxic macrofilaricides are needed.

Dracunculus medinensis. Known as the guinea, dragon, or Medina worm, this parasite causes dracunculiasis, an infection in decline that is most commonly found in rural Sudan and West Africa. People become infected by drinking water containing copepods that carry infective larvae. After about 1 year, the adult female worms migrate and emerge through the skin, usually of the lower legs or feet.

There is no suitable anthelmintic that acts directly against *D. medinensis*. Traditional treatment for this disabling condition is to draw the live adult female worm out day by day by rolling it onto a small piece of wood. This procedure risks severe infection if rupture occurs. *Metronidazole*, 250 mg given three times a day for 10 days, can provide symptomatic and functional relief by facilitating removal of the worm through indirect suppression of host inflammatory responses. Through the advocacy and work of the Carter Center, strategies such as filtering drinking water and reducing contact of infected individuals with water have markedly reduced the transmission and prevalence of dracunculiasis in most endemic regions.

Cestodes (Flatworms)

Taenia saginata. Humans are the definitive hosts for *Taenia saginata*, known as the beef tapeworm. This most common form of tapeworm usually is detected after passage of proglottids from the intestine. It is cosmopolitan, occurring most commonly in sub-Saharan Africa and the Middle East, where undercooked or raw beef is consumed. Preventable by cooking beef to 60°C for over 5 minutes, this infection rarely produces serious clinical disease, but it must be distinguished from that produced by *Taenia solium*.

Praziquantel is the drug of choice for treatment of infection by *T. saginata*, although *niclosamide* also is used because it is cheap and available. Both are very effective, simple to administer, and comparatively free from side effects. Assessment of cure can be difficult because the worm (segments as well as scolex) usually is passed in a partially digested state. If the parasitological diagnosis is uncertain, praziquantel is the preferred drug because of the danger of cysticercosis (*see* below).

Taenia solium. *Taenia solium*, or pork tapeworm, also has a cosmopolitan distribution; immigrant populations are a common source of infection in the United States. This cestode causes two types of infection. The intestinal form with adult tapeworms is caused by eating undercooked meat containing cysticerci; this can be prevented by proper cooking of infected meat. *Cysticercosis*, the far more dangerous systemic form that usually coexists with the intestinal form, is caused by invasive larval forms of the parasite (Garcia and Del Brutto, 2000). This infection by parasite eggs usually results either from ingestion of fecally contaminated infectious material, or from eggs liberated from a gravid segment passing upward into the duodenum, where the outer layers are digested. In either case, larvae

gain access to the circulation and tissues exactly as in their cycle in the intermediate host, usually the pig. The seriousness of the resulting disease depends on the particular tissue involved. Invasion of the brain (neurocysticercosis) is common and dangerous. Epilepsy, meningitis, and increased intracranial pressure can develop, depending on the inflammatory reactions to the cysticerci and/or their size and location. Praziquantel is preferred for treatment of intestinal infections with *T. solium*. Albendazole and praziquantel are the drugs of choice for treating cysticercosis, although most studies suggest that albendazole is more effective. Chemotherapy is appropriate only when it is directed at live cysticerci causing pathology; pretreatment with glucocorticoids is advised strongly in this situation to minimize inflammatory reactions to dying parasites (Evans *et al.*, 1997). Anthelmintic treatment can shrink brain cysts but also can have adverse consequences leading to seizures and hydrocephalus. One trial found that there was insufficient evidence to determine whether cysticidal therapy in neurocysticercosis is associated with beneficial effects (Salinas and Prasad, 2000). Some investigators and physicians advocate use of cysticidal therapy for patients with multiple cysts or viable cysts (as determined by absence of ring enhancement on contrast neuroimaging studies).

Diphyllobothrium latum. *Diphyllobothrium latum*, the fish tapeworm, is found most commonly in rivers and lakes of the northern hemisphere. In North America, the pike is the most common second intermediate host. The eating of inadequately cooked, infested fish introduces the larvae into the human intestine; the larvae can develop into adult worms up to 25 meters long. Most infected individuals are asymptomatic. The most frequent manifestations include abdominal symptoms and weight loss, while megaloblastic anemia develops due to a deficiency of vitamin B_{12}, which is taken up by the parasite. Therapy with praziquantel readily eliminates the worm and ensures hematological remission.

Hymenolepis nana. *Hymenolepis nana*, the dwarf tapeworm, is the smallest and most common tapeworm parasitizing humans. Infection with this cestode is cosmopolitan, more prevalent in tropical than temperate climates, and most common among institutionalized children, including those in the southern United States. *H. nana* is the only cestode that can develop from ovum to mature adult in humans without an intermediate host. Cysticerci develop in the villi of the intestine and then regain access to the intestinal lumen where larvae mature into adults. Treatment therefore must be adapted to this cycle of autoinfection. Praziquantel is effective against *H. nana* infections, but higher doses than those used for other tapeworm infections usually are required. In addition, therapy may have to be repeated. Treatment failure or reinfection is indicated by the appearance of eggs in the stool about 4 weeks after the last dose. Albendazole is partially efficacious against *H. nana*; in 277 cases from 11 studies, 69.5% of patients were cured by albendazole (400 mg daily for 3 days) (Horton, 2000).

Echinococcus Species. Humans serve as one of several intermediate hosts for larval forms of *Echinococcus* species that cause "cystic" (*E. granulosus*) and "alveolar" (*E. multilocularis* and *E. vogeli*) hydatid disease. Dogs are definitive hosts for these tapeworms. Parasite eggs from canine stools are a major worldwide cause of disease in associated livestock (*e.g.*, sheep and goats). *E. granulosus* produces unilocular, slowly growing cysts, most often in liver and lung, whereas *E. multilocularis* creates multilocular invasive cysts, predominantly in the same organs. Removal of the cysts by surgery is the preferred treatment, but leakage from ruptured cysts may spread disease to other organs. Prolonged regimens of albendazole, either alone or as an adjunct to surgery, are reportedly of some benefit. However, some patients are not cured despite multiple courses of therapy. Treatment of infected dogs with praziquantel eradicates adult worms and interrupts transmission of these infections. New treatment methods, such as percutaneous puncture, aspiration, injection of scolicidal agents, and re-aspiration–based techniques, have received much attention, and yield rates of cure and relapse equivalent to those following surgery. Adjunct treatment with BZAs now is considered the cornerstone of the interdisciplinary approach to controlling cystic echinococcosis (Kern, 2003).

Trematodes (Flukes)

Schistosoma haematobium, Schistosoma mansoni, Schistosoma japonicum. These are the main species of blood flukes that cause human schistosomiasis; less common species are *Schistosoma intercalatum* and *Schistosoma mekongi*. The infection affects about 200 million people, and more than 600 million are considered at risk. Schistosomiasis is widely distributed over the South American continent and certain Caribbean islands (*S. mansoni*), much of Africa and the Arabian Peninsula (*S. mansoni* and *S. haematobium*), and China, the Philippines, and Indonesia (*S. japonicum*). Infected snails act as intermediate hosts for freshwater transmission of the infection, which continues to spread as the development of agricultural and water resources increases. Schistosomiasis, or schistosomal disease, which generally correlates with the intensity of infection, primarily involves the liver, spleen, and gastrointestinal tract (*S. mansoni* and *S. japonicum*) or the lower genitourinary tract (*S. haematobium*). Heavy infections with *S. haematobium* are associated with squamous cell carcinoma of the bladder in some endemic regions. Chronic infections can result in portosystemic shunting due to granuloma formation and periportal fibrosis in the liver.

Praziquantel is the drug of choice for treating all species of schistosomes that infect humans. The drug is safe and effective when given in single or divided oral doses on the same day. These properties make praziquantel especially suitable for population-based chemotherapy. Moreover, repeated chemotherapy with praziquantel is thought to accelerate protective immune responses by increasing exposure to antigens released from dying worms that induce a T-helper type-2 response (Mutapi *et al.*, 1998). Although not effective clinically against *S. haematobium* and *S. japonicum, oxamniquine* is effective for treatment of *S. mansoni* infections, particularly in South America, where the sensitivity of most strains may permit single-dose therapy. However, resistance has been reported, in both the field and the laboratory, and higher doses of the drug are required to treat African strains than to treat Brazilian strains of *S. mansoni*. *Metrifonate* has been used with considerable success in the treatment of *S. haematobium* infections, but the drug is not effective against *S. mansoni* and *S. japonicum*. Metrifonate is relatively inexpensive and can be used in conjunction with oxamniquine for treatment of mixed infections with *S. haematobium* and *S. mansoni*.

The artemisinin derivative *artemether* (*see* Chapter 39) shows promise as an anti-schistosomal agent. Artemether targets the larval schistosomula stages of the parasite. Clinical trials confirmed that artemether (oral dose of 6 mg/kg once every 2 to 3 weeks) significantly reduced the incidence and intensity of schistosome infections without adverse reactions. Combined treatment of animals harboring juvenile and adult schistosome worms with artemether and praziquantel resulted in significantly higher worm burden reductions than each drug administered singly (Xiao *et al.*, 2002). There is concern, however, that widespread use of artemether as an anthelmintic may induce drug-resistant malaria in areas where multidrug resistant plasmodia still respond to artemether therapy.

Paragonimus westermani and Other Paragonimus Species. Called lung flukes, a number of *Paragonimus* species, of which *P. westermani* is the most common, are pathogenic for humans and carnivores. Found in the Far East and on the African and South American continents, these parasites have two intermediate hosts: snails and crustaceans. Humans become infected by eating raw or undercooked crabs or crayfish. Disease is caused by reactions to adult worms in the lungs and ectopic sites. Although these flukes are rather refractory to praziquantel *in vitro*, the drug is effective when used clinically. *Bithionol* is considered a second-line agent. *Triclabendazole* recently was shown to be efficacious in animals, and when a small number of human patients were treated with 10 mg/kg daily for 3 days, all were cured (Gao *et al.*, 2003).

Clonorchis sinensis, Opisthorchis viverrini, Opisthorchis felineus. These closely related trematodes exist in the Far East (*C. sinensis*, "the Chinese liver fluke," and *O. viverrini*) and parts of Eastern Europe (*O. felineus*). Metacercariae released from poorly cooked infected cyprinoid fish mature into adult flukes that inhabit the human biliary system. Heavy infections can cause obstructive liver disease, inflammatory gallbladder pathology associated with cholangiocarcinoma, and obstructive pancreatitis. One-day therapy with praziquantel is highly effective against these parasites.

Fasciola hepatica. Humans are only accidentally infected with *F. hepatica*, the large liver fluke that exists worldwide and primarily affects herbivorous ruminants such as cattle and sheep. Eating contaminated freshwater plants such as watercress initiates the infection. Migratory larvae penetrate the intestine, invade the liver from the peritoneum, and eventually reside in the biliary tract. The acute illness is characterized by fever, urticaria, and abdominal symptoms, whereas chronic infection resembles that caused by other hepatic flukes. However, unlike *O. viverrini*, *F. hepatica* infection is not associated with cholangiocarcinoma. Unlike infections with other flukes, fascioliasis does not usually respond to praziquantel. Previously the recommended drug was bithionol, which may be obtained from the Centers for Disease Control and Prevention Drug Service. However, triclabendazole, given as a single oral dose of 10 mg/kg, or in cases of severe infection 20 mg/kg divided into two doses, now is the drug of choice for human fascioliasis. In the United States, this agent is available only from the manufacturer (Novartis). The cure rate among a cohort of Turkish patients was 78%, and the addition of another course(s) increased this to 90%. No significant side effects were reported (Saba *et al.*, 2004).

Fasciolopsis buski, Heterophyes heterophyes, Metagonimus yokogawai, Nanophyetus salmincola. Obtained by eating contaminated water chestnuts and other caltrops in Southeast Asia, *F. buski* is one of the largest parasites causing human infection. Undercooked fish transmit infection with the other, much smaller gastrointestinal trematodes that are widely distributed geographically. Abdominal symptoms produced by reactions to these flukes usually are mild, but heavy infections with *F. buski* can cause intestinal obstruction and peritonitis. Infections with all the intestinal trematodes respond well to single-day therapy with praziquantel.

ANTHELMINTIC DRUGS

Benzimidazoles (BZAs)

History. The discovery by Brown and coworkers that thiabendazole possessed potent activity against gastrointestinal nematodes sparked development of the BZAs as broad-spectrum anthelmintic agents against parasites of both veterinary and human medical importance. Of the hundreds of derivatives tested, those most therapeutically useful have modifications at the 2 and/or 5 positions of the benzimidazole ring system (Townsend and Wise, 1990). Three compounds, thiabendazole, mebendazole, and albendazole, have been used extensively for the treatment of human helminth infections. The chemical structures of these drugs are shown in Table 41–1.

Thiabendazole, which contains a thiazole at position 2, is active against a wide range of nematodes that infect the GI tract. However, its clinical use against these organisms has declined markedly because of thiabendazole's toxicity relative to that of other equally effective drugs. Mebendazole, the prototype benzimidazole carbamate, was introduced for the treatment of intestinal roundworm infections as a result of research carried out more than 30 years ago. Albendazole is a newer benzimidazole carbamate that is used worldwide, primarily against a variety of intestinal and tissue nematodes, but also against larval forms of certain cestodes (de Silva *et al.*, 1997; Venkatesan, 1998). Albendazole has become the drug of choice for treating cysticercosis (Sotelo and Jung, 1998; Garcia and Del Brutto, 2000) and cystic hydatid disease (Horton, 1997). When used yearly in conjunction with either ivermectin or diethylcarbamazine, single doses of albendazole have shown considerable promise for global control of lymphatic filariasis and related tissue filarial infections (Molyneux and Zagaria, 2002; Molyneux *et al.*, 2003). Albendazole is not effective against *F. hepatica*.

Anthelmintic Action. BZAs produce many biochemical changes in susceptible nematodes including inhibition of mitochondrial fumarate reductase, reduced glucose transport, and uncoupling of oxidative phosphorylation, but their primary action likely is to inhibit microtubule polymerization by binding to β-tubulin (Lacey, 1988; Lacey, 1990; Prichard, 1994). The selective toxicity of these agents results because the BZAs bind parasite β-tubulin with much higher affinity than they do the mammalian protein. Studies on BZA-resistant worms, such as the free-living nematode *Caenorhabditis elegans* (Driscoll *et al.*, 1989) and the sheep nematode *Haemonchus contortus,* have provided insights into the mechanisms of BZA action (Lacey, 1990; Prichard, 1994). In particular, both laboratory-derived and field-isolated strains of benzimidazole-resistant *H. contortus* display reduced high-affinity drug binding to β-tubulin (Lubega and Prichard, 1991) and alterations in β-tubulin isotype gene expression (Kwa *et al.*, 1993; Kwa *et al.*, 1995; Roos, 1997) that correlate with drug resistance. Thus, the two identified mechanisms of drug resistance in nematodes involve both a progressive loss of "susceptible" β-tubulin gene isotypes together with emergence of a "resistant" isotype with a conserved point mutation that encodes a tyrosine instead of a phenylalanine at position 200 of β-tubulin (Roos, 1997; Sangster and Gill, 1999). While this mutation may not be required for BZA resistance in all parasites, *e.g.*, *G. lamblia* (Upcroft *et al.*, 1996), development of novel BZA analogs that target this form of resistance in parasitic nematodes will be challenging because tyrosine also is present at position 200 of human β-tubulin. Although BZA resistance currently is widespread among livestock nematodes, to date there has been no evidence for its emergence among human nematodes. However, the recent observa-

tion that the efficacy of mebendazole can diminish in some settings with frequent and periodic use (Albonico *et al.*, 2003), and the plans for the widespread use of BZAs to control LF caused by STH (Horton, 2003), suggest that global monitoring for downstream BZA resistance could become critically important.

The BZAs, exemplified by mebendazole and albendazole, are versatile anthelmintic agents, particularly against gastrointestinal nematodes, where their action is not dictated by systemic drug concentration. Appropriate doses of mebendazole and albendazole are highly effective in treating the major STH infections (ascariasis, enterobiasis, trichuriasis, and hookworm) as well as less common human nematode infections. These drugs are active against both larval and adult stages of nematodes that cause these infections, and they are ovicidal for *Ascaris* and *Trichuris*. Immobilization and death of susceptible gastrointestinal parasites occur slowly, and their clearance from the GI tract may not be complete until several days after treatment. Accumulating evidence indicates that removal of STHs in children by a single-dose treatment with either albendazole or mebendazole improves their health, as evidenced by posttreatment catch-up growth and improved iron status (Stephenson *et al.*, 1989; Hotez, 2000; Hotez *et al.*, 2005). In addition, BZA treatment of STH infections also produces improvements in childhood intellectual and cognitive development (Drake *et al.*, 2000). These observations have led to advocacy for the implementation of large-scale STH control programs that target school-aged children (Savioli *et al.*, 2002; World Health Organization, 2002). Albendazole is superior to mebendazole in curing hookworm and trichuriasis infections in children (de Silva *et al.*, 1997; de Silva *et al.*, 2003; Bennett and Guyatt, 2000), especially when used as a single dose (Albonico *et al.*, 2003). Moreover, albendazole is more effective than mebendazole against strongyloidiasis (Liu and Weller, 1993), cystic hydatid disease caused by *Echinococcus granulosus* (Horton, 1997; Davis *et al.*, 1989), and neurocysticercosis caused by larval forms of *Taenia solium* (Evans *et al.*, 1997; Garcia and Del Brutto, 2000). The BZAs probably are active against the intestinal stages of *Trichinella spiralis* in humans, but probably do not affect the larval stages in tissues. Albendazole is highly effective against the migrating forms of dog and cat hookworms that cause cutaneous larval migrans, although thiabendazole can be used topically for this purpose. Regimens in which albendazole with either ivermectin or diethylcarbamazine are given as single annual doses show great promise for the elimination of LF (Molyneux and Zagaria, 2002). Such combined therapy has the additional benefit of reducing STH worm burdens in school-aged children (Albonico *et al.*, 1999). Certain microsporidial species that cause intestinal infections in HIV-infected individuals respond partially (*Enterocytozoon bieneusi*) or completely (*Encephalitozoon intestinalis* and related *Encephalitozoon* species) to albendazole; albendazole's sulfoxide metabolite appears to be especially effective against these parasites *in vitro* (Katiyar and Edlind, 1997). Albendazole also has some efficacy against anaerobic protozoa such as *Trichomonas vaginalis* and *Giardia lamblia* (Ottesen *et al.*, 1999). While BZAs have antifungal activity, their clinical use against human mycoses is limited.

Absorption, Fate, and Excretion.
BZAs have only limited solubility in water; minor differences in solubility consequently have a major effect on absorption.

Thiabendazole is absorbed rapidly after oral ingestion and reaches peak concentrations in plasma after about 1 hour. Most of the drug is excreted in the urine within 24 hours as 5-hydroxythiabendazole, conjugated either as the glucuronide or the sulfate. In contrast, tablet formulations of mebendazole are poorly and erratically absorbed, and concentrations of the drug in plasma are low and do not reflect the dosage taken. The low systemic bioavailability (22%) of mebendazole results from a combination of poor absorption and rapid first-pass hepatic metabolism. Coadministration of *cimetidine* will increase plasma levels of mebendazole, possibly due to inhibition of first-pass CYP-mediated metabolism (Dayan, 2003). Mebendazole is about 95% bound to plasma proteins and is extensively metabolized. The major metabolites, methyl-5-(α-hydroxybenzyl)-2-benzimidazole carbamate and 2-amino-5-benzoylbenzimidazole, have lower rates of clearance than does mebendazole. Mebendazole, rather than its metabolites, appears to be the active drug form (Gottschall *et al.*, 1990). Conjugates of mebendazole and its metabolites have been found in bile, but little unchanged mebendazole appears in the urine.

Albendazole is variably and erratically absorbed after oral administration; absorption is enhanced by the presence of fatty foods and possibly by bile salts. A fatty meal or eating enhances absorption by up to fivefold in humans (Dayan, 2003). After a 400-mg oral dose, albendazole cannot be detected in plasma, because the drug is rapidly metabolized in the liver and possibly in the intestine, to albendazole sulfoxide, which has potent anthelmintic activity (Marriner *et al.*, 1986; Moroni *et al.*, 1995; Redondo *et al.*, 1999). Both the (+) and (–) enantiomers of albendazole sulfoxide are formed, but the (+) enantiomer reaches much higher peak plasma concentrations in humans and is cleared much more slowly than the (–) form (Delatour *et al.*, 1991; Marques *et al.*, 1999). Total sulfoxide attains peak plasma concentrations of about 300 ng/ml, but with wide interindividual variation. Albendazole sulfoxide is about 70% bound to plasma proteins and has a highly variable plasma half-life ranging from about 4 to 15 hours (Delatour *et al.*, 1991; Jung *et al.*, 1992; Marques *et al.*, 1999). It is well distributed into various tissues including hydatid cysts, where it reaches a concentration of about one-fifth that in plasma (Marriner *et al.*, 1986; Morris *et al.*, 1987). This probably explains why albendazole is more effective than mebendazole for treating hydatid cyst disease, and possibly other tissue-dwelling helminths. Formation of albendazole sulfoxide is catalyzed by both microsomal flavin monooxygenase and CYP isoforms in the liver and possibly also in the intestine (Redondo *et al.*, 1999). Hepatic flavin monooxygenase activity appears associated with (+) albendazole sulfoxide formation, whereas CYPs preferentially produce the (–) sulfoxide metabolite (Delatour *et al.*, 1991). Both sulfoxide derivatives are oxidized further to the nonchiral sulfone metabolite of albendazole, which is pharmacologically inactive; this reaction favors the (–) sulfoxide and probably becomes rate limiting in determining the clearance and plasma half-life of the bioactive (+) sulfoxide metabolite (Delatour *et al.*, 1991). Induction of enzymes involved in sulfone formation from the (+) sulfoxide could account for some of the wide variation noted in plasma half-lives of albendazole sulfoxide. Indeed, in animal models, BZAs can induce their own metabolism (Gleizes *et al.*, 1991). Albendazole metabolites are excreted mainly in the urine.

Therapeutic Uses. The introduction of thiabendazole (MINTEZOL) was a major advance in the therapy of cuta-

neous larva migrans (creeping eruption) and *Strongyloides stercoralis* infection. The majority of patients experience marked relief of symptoms of creeping eruption, and a high percentage of cures are achieved after topical treatment with 15% thiabendazole in a water-soluble cream base applied to the affected area two or three times per day for 5 days (Davies *et al.*, 1993). A common regimen for therapy of strongyloidiasis is 25 mg/kg of thiabendazole given twice daily after meals for 2 days; the total daily dose should not exceed 3 g. This schedule should be extended for 5 to 7 days for treatment of disseminated strongyloidiasis or until the parasites have been eliminated. As a first-line drug for the treatment of strongyloidiasis, thiabendazole has been largely replaced by ivermectin (*see* "Ivermectin," below). Thiabendazole given at a dosage of 25 mg/kg twice daily for 7 days may produce some benefit for early trichinosis, but has no effect on migrating or muscle-stage larvae. Thiabendazole also is effective in gastrointestinal nematode infections, but because of its toxicity, it should no longer be used for those infections.

Mebendazole is highly effective against gastrointestinal nematode infections and is particularly valuable for the treatment of mixed infections. Mebendazole always is taken orally, and the same dosage schedule applies to adults and children more than 2 years of age. For treatment of enterobiasis, a single 100-mg tablet is taken; a second should be given after 2 weeks. For control of ascariasis, trichuriasis, or hookworm infections, the recommended regimen is 100 mg of mebendazole taken in the morning and evening for 3 consecutive days (or a single 500-mg tablet administered once). If the patient is not cured 3 weeks after treatment, a second course should be given. The 3-day mebendazole regimen is more effective than single doses of either mebendazole (500 mg) or albendazole (400 mg), which also have been used successfully to control these mixed infections. A single dose of albendazole appears superior to a single dose of mebendazole against hookworms (de Silva *et al.*, 1997; Bennett and Guyatt, 2000). A single dose of mebendazole achieves a cure rate against hookworm of only 21% (Bennett and Guyatt, 2000). Moreover, the efficacy of mebendazole against hookworm may diminish with frequent and repeated use (Albonico *et al.*, 2003), which may reflect emerging BZA drug resistance.

Infections with *Capillaria philippinensis* are also resistant to treatment with mebendazole, and a 10-day treatment regimen with albendazole (400 mg/day) is considered the drug of choice, although 400 mg/day of mebendazole given in two divided doses for at least 20 days produced few relapses in patients with relapses after thiabendazole (Cross, 1992). Mebendazole has been used to treat cystic hydatid disease, although surgery should be performed first, and chemotherapy with albendazole now is considered to be superior (Horton, 1997).

Like mebendazole, albendazole provides safe and highly effective therapy against infections with gastrointestinal nematodes, including mixed infections of *Ascaris*, *Trichuris*, and hookworms. For treatment of STH infections (enterobiasis, ascariasis, trichuriasis, and hookworm), albendazole is taken as a single oral 400-mg dose by adults and children more than 2 years of age. In children between the ages of 12 and 24 months, the WHO recommends a reduced dose of 200 mg. Cure rates for light to moderate *Ascaris* infections typically are more than 97%, although heavy infections may require therapy for 2 to 3 days. A 400-mg dose of albendazole appears to be superior to a 500-mg dose of mebendazole for curing hookworm infections and reducing egg counts (Sacko *et al.*, 1999; Bennett and Guyatt, 2000). At a dose of 400 mg daily for 3 days, albendazole exhibits highly variable efficacy against strongyloidiasis; both thiabendazole and ivermectin are more effective in treating this infection.

Albendazole is the drug of choice for treating cystic hydatid disease due to *Echinococcus granulosus*. While the drug provides only a modest cure rate when used alone, it produces superior results when used before and after either surgery to remove cysts or aspiration/injection of cysts with protoscolicidal agents (Horton, 1997; Schantz, 1999). A typical dosage regimen for adults is 400 mg given twice a day (for children 15 mg/kg per day with a maximum of 800 mg) for 1 to 6 months. This regimen often is used as adjunctive therapy for either surgical resection or percutaneous drainage. While still the best drug available, albendazole appears to be just marginally effective against alveolar echinococcosis caused by *E. multilocularis* (Venkatesan, 1998); therefore surgical intervention is usually required.

Albendazole also is the preferred treatment of neurocysticercosis caused by larval forms of *Taenia solium* (Evans *et al.*, 1997; Sotelo and Jung, 1998; Garcia and Del Brutto, 2000). The recommended dosage is 400 mg given twice a day for adults for 8 to 30 days, depending on the number, type, and location of the cysts. For children, the dose is 15 mg/kg per day (maximum 800 mg) in two doses for 8 to 30 days. For both adults and children, the course can be repeated as necessary, as long as liver and bone marrow toxicities are monitored. Glucocorticoids are usually given for several days before initiating albendazole therapy to reduce the incidence of side effects

resulting from inflammatory reactions to dead and dying cysticerci. Such pretreatment also increases plasma levels of albendazole sulfoxide. Therapy with either albendazole or praziquantel should include consultation with a neurologist and/or neurosurgeon regarding anticonvulsant therapy, the possible development of complications of arachnoiditis, vasculitis, or cerebral edema, and the need for surgical intervention should obstructive hydrocephalus occur. Albendazole, 400 mg per day, also has shown efficacy for therapy of microsporidial intestinal infections in patients with AIDS.

Albendazole has been combined with either diethylcarbamazine or ivermectin in programs directed toward controlling LF (Ottesen *et al.*, 1999; Molyneux and Zagaria, 2002). By annual dosing with combination therapy for 4 to 6 years, the strategy is to maintain the microfilaremia at such low levels that transmission cannot occur. The period of therapy is estimated to correspond to the duration of fecundity of adult worms. Albendazole is given with diethylcarbamazine to control LF in most parts of the world. However, to avoid serious reactions to dying microfilariae, the albendazole/ivermectin combination is recommended in locations where filariasis coexists with either onchocerciasis or loiasis. Recently, the benefits of adding albendazole to either diethylcarbamazine or ivermectin for LF control were evaluated (Addiss *et al.*, 2004). It was concluded that there currently is insufficient reliable research to confirm or refute whether adding albendazole has an effect on LF.

Toxicity, Side Effects, Precautions, and Contraindications. Overall, the BZAs have excellent safety profiles. To date millions of children have been treated in mass deworming chemotherapy programs. Overall, the incidence of side effects, primarily mild GI symptoms, occurs in only 1% of treated children (Urbani and Albonico, 2003).

The clinical utility of thiabendazole in adults is compromised by its toxicity. Side effects frequently encountered with therapeutic doses include anorexia, nausea, vomiting, and dizziness. Less frequently, diarrhea, fatigue, drowsiness, giddiness, or headache occur. Occasional fever, rashes, erythema multiforme, hallucinations, sensory disturbances, and Stevens-Johnson syndrome have been reported. Angioedema, shock, tinnitus, convulsions, and intrahepatic cholestasis are rare complications of therapy. Some patients excrete a metabolite that imparts an odor to the urine much like that occurring after ingestion of asparagus. Crystalluria without hematuria has been reported on occasion; it promptly subsides with discontinuation of therapy. Transient leukopenia has been noted in a few patients on thiabendazole therapy. There are no absolute contraindications to the use of thiabendazole. Because CNS side effects occur frequently, activities requiring mental alertness should be avoided during therapy. Thiabendazole has hepatotoxic potential and should be used with caution in patients with hepatic disease or decreased hepatic function. The effects of thiabendazole in pregnant women have not been studied adequately, so it should be used in pregnancy only when the potential benefit justifies the risk.

Unlike thiabendazole, mebendazole does not cause significant systemic toxicity in routine clinical use, even in the presence of anemia and malnutrition. This probably reflects its low systemic bioavailability. Transient symptoms of abdominal pain, distention, and diarrhea have occurred in cases of massive infestation and expulsion of gastrointestinal worms. Rare side effects in patients treated with high doses of mebendazole include allergic reactions, alopecia, reversible neutropenia, agranulocytosis, and hypospermia. Reversible elevation of serum transaminases is not uncommon in this population. Mebendazole treatment may be associated with occipital seizures (Wilmshurst and Robb, 1998). Mebendazole is a potent embryotoxin and teratogen in laboratory animals; effects may occur in pregnant rats at single oral doses as low as 10 mg/kg. Thus, despite a lack of evidence for teratogenicity in humans, it generally is advised that mebendazole not be given to pregnant women or to children less than 2 years of age (*see* below for exceptions and further explanation). It also should not be used in patients who have experienced allergic reactions to the agent.

Like mebendazole, albendazole produces few side effects when used for short-term therapy of gastrointestinal helminthiasis, even in patients with heavy worm burdens. Transient mild GI symptoms (epigastric pain, diarrhea, nausea, and vomiting) occur in approximately 1% of treated individuals. Dizziness, and headache occur on occasion. In school-age mass treatments, the incidence of side effects with albendazole is very low (Horton, 2000). Allergic phenomena rarely occur (edema 7/10,000; rashes 2/10,000; and urticaria 1/10,000) but these usually resolve after 48 hours. In children with asymptomatic trichuriasis, albendazole reportedly impaired growth in children with low levels of infection (Forrester *et al.*, 1998); to date, this observation has not been confirmed.

Even in long-term therapy of cystic hydatid disease and neurocysticercosis, albendazole is well tolerated by most patients. The most common side effect is an increase in serum aminotransferase activity; rarely jaundice or chemical cholestasis may be noted, but enzyme activities return to normal after therapy is completed. A recent pharmacoepidemiologic analysis concluded that long-term treatment of echinococcosis or cysticercosis with high-dose albendazole accounted for most of the adverse drug reactions attributed to anthelmintic therapy (Bagheri *et al.*, 2004). Therefore, liver function tests should be monitored during protracted albendazole therapy, and the drug is not recommended for patients with cirrhosis (Davis *et al.*, 1989). Especially if not pretreated with glucocorticoids, some patients with neurocysticercosis may experience serious neurological sequelae that depend on the location of inflamed cysts with dying cysticerci. Other side effects during extended therapy include gastrointestinal pain, severe headaches, fever, fatigue, loss of hair, leukopenia, and thrombocytopenia. Albendazole is teratogenic and embryotoxic in animals and it should not be given to pregnant women. The safety of albendazole in children less than 2 years of age has not been established.

The BZAs as a group display remarkably few clinically significant interactions with other drugs. The most versatile member of this family, albendazole, probably induces its own metabolism, and plasma levels of its sulfoxide metabolites can be increased by coadministration of glucocorticoids and possibly praziquantel. Caution is advised when using high doses of albendazole together with general inhibitors of hepatic CYPs. As indicated above, coadministration of cimetidine can increase the bioavailability of mebendazole.

Use in Pregnancy. Because of the ongoing and anticipated widespread use of BZAs in global control programs for both STH and filarial infections, there is a high level of interest about their use in young children and in the second and third trimesters of pregnancy.

As indicated above, both albendazole and mebendazole are embryotoxic and teratogenic in pregnant rats, and are not generally recommended for use in pregnancy (Hotez *et al.*, 2005). However, in postmarketing surveys on women who inadvertently consumed mebendazole during the first trimester, the incidence of spontaneous abortion and malformations did not exceed that of the general population; comparable studies with albendazole are not available. A review of the risk of congenital abnormalities from BZAs concluded that their use during pregnancy was not associated with an increased risk of major congenital defects; nonetheless, it is recommended that treatment should be avoided during the first trimester of pregnancy (Urbani and Albonico, 2003). Because hookworm occurs in an estimated 44 million pregnant women in developing countries (Bundy *et al.*, 1995), some of whom develop iron-deficiency anemia leading to adverse pregnancy outcomes, BZA treatment would be beneficial during the second and third trimesters of pregnancy (World Health Organization, 2002). There is no evidence that maternal BZA therapy presents a risk to breast-fed infants (Urbani and Albonico, 2003).

Use in Young Children. The BZAs have not been extensively studied in children under 2 years of age. The WHO convened an informal consultation on the use of BZAs in young children in 2002 and concluded that they may be used to treat children past the first year of life if the risks from adverse consequences caused by STHs are justified (Montresor *et al.*, 2003). The WHO recommends a reduced dose of 200 mg of albendazole in children between the ages of 12 and 24 months.

Diethylcarbamazine. Diethylcarbamazine is a first-line agent for control and treatment of lymphatic filariasis and for therapy of tropical pulmonary eosinophilia caused by *Wuchereria bancrofti* and *Brugia malayi* (Ottesen and Ramachandran, 1995). Although this agent is partially effective against onchocerciasis and loiasis, it can cause serious reactions to affected microfilariae in both infections. For this reason, ivermectin has replaced diethylcarbamazine for therapy of onchocerciasis. Despite its toxicity, diethylcarbamazine remains the best drug available to treat loiasis. Annual single doses of both diethylcarbamazine and albendazole show considerable promise for the control of lymphatic filariasis in geographic regions where onchocerciasis and loiasis are not endemic (Molyneux and Zagaria, 2002; Molyneux *et al.*, 2003).

Chemistry. Diethylcarbamazine (HETRAZAN) is formulated as the water-soluble citrate salt containing 51% by weight of the active base. Because the compound is tasteless, odorless, and stable to heat, it also can be taken in the form of fortified table salt containing 0.2% to 0.4% by weight of the base. The drug is available outside the United States. In the United States it can be obtained from the CDC. Diethylcarbamazine has the following chemical structure:

$$H_3C-N \underset{\text{DIETHYLCARBAMAZINE}}{\overset{O}{\underset{}{\boxed{}}}N-C-N \overset{C_2H_5}{\underset{C_2H_5}{}}}$$

DIETHYLCARBAMAZINE

Anthelmintic Action. Microfilarial forms of susceptible filarial species are most affected by diethylcarbamazine, which elicits rapid disappearance of these developmental forms of *W. bancrofti, B. malayi,* and *L. loa* from human blood. The drug causes microfilariae of *O. volvulus* to disappear from skin but does not kill microfilariae in nodules that contain the adult (female) worms. It does not affect the microfilariae of *W. bancrofti* in a hydrocele, despite penetration into the fluid. The mechanism of action of diethylcarbamazine on susceptible microfilariae is not well understood, but the drug appears to exert a direct effect on *W. bancrofti* microfilariae by causing organelle damage and apoptosis (Peixoto *et al.*, 2004). There is evidence that diethylcarbamazine kills worms of adult *L. loa* and probably adult *W. bancrofti* and *B. malayi* as well. However, it has little action against adult *O. volvulus.* The mechanism of filaricidal action of diethylcarbamazine against adult worms is unknown. Some studies suggest that diethylcarbamazine compromises intracellular processing and transport of certain macromolecules at the plasma membrane (Spiro *et al.*, 1986). The drug also may affect specific immune and inflammatory responses of the host by undefined mechanisms (Mackenzie and Kron, 1985; Martin *et al.*, 1997).

Absorption, Fate, and Excretion. Diethylcarbamazine is absorbed rapidly from the gastrointestinal tract. Peak plasma levels occur within 1 to 2 hours after a single oral dose, and the plasma half-life varies from 2 to 10 hours, depending on the urinary pH. Metabolism is both rapid and extensive. A major metabolite, diethylcarbamazine-*N*-oxide, is bioactive. Diethylcarbamazine is excreted by both urinary and extraurinary routes; more than 50% of

an oral dose appears in acidic urine as the unchanged drug, but this value is decreased when the urine is alkaline. Indeed, alkalinizing the urine can elevate plasma levels, prolong the plasma half-life, and increase both the therapeutic effect and toxicity of diethylcarbamazine (Awadzi *et al.*, 1986). Therefore, dosage reduction may be required for people with renal dysfunction or sustained alkaline urine.

Therapeutic Uses. Dosages of diethylcarbamazine citrate used to prevent or treat filarial infections have evolved empirically and vary according to local experience. Recommended regimens differ according to whether the drug is used for population-based chemotherapy, control of filarial disease, or prophylaxis against infection.

W. bancrofti, B. malayi, and *B. timori.* The standard regimen for the treatment of LF traditionally has been a 12-day, 72-mg/kg (6 mg/kg per day) course of diethylcarbamazine. In the United States, it is common practice to administer small test doses of 50 to 100 mg (1 to 2 mg/kg for children) over a 3-day period prior to beginning the 12-day regimen. However, a single dose of 6 mg/kg had comparable macrofilaricidal and microfilaricidal efficacy to the standard regimen (Addiss and Dreyer, 2000). Single-dose therapy may be repeated every 6 to 12 months, as necessary.

Although diethylcarbamazine does not usually reverse existing lymphatic damage, the early treatment of asymptomatic individuals may prevent new lymphatic damage. In men, the effect of the drug can be monitored by scrotal ultrasound approximately 2 to 4 weeks following treatment. Repeat treatment sometimes is recommended if microfilariae remain in the circulation or if adult worms remain on the ultrasound (Addiss and Dreyer, 2000). Expanded use of ultrasound also has facilitated the identification of infected individuals who are microfilaria-negative on blood examination. These individuals also benefit from diethylcarbamazine treatment. During acute episodes of lymphangitis, treatment with diethylcarbamazine is not recommended until acute symptoms subside (Addiss and Dreyer, 2000).

Supportive treatment is critical for the successful management of LF. This includes prevention of secondary bacterial infections through attention to hygiene, wearing shoes to prevent foot injury, and avoidance of lymphostasis through exercise and limb elevation (Addiss and Dreyer, 2000). Attention to hygiene, prevention of secondary bacterial infections, and physiotherapy sometimes can reverse elephantiasis and lymphedema of the leg.

For mass treatment with the objective of reducing microfilaremia to subinfective levels for mosquitoes, the introduction of diethylcarbamazine into table salt (0.2% to 0.4% by weight of the base) has markedly reduced the prevalence, severity, and transmission of lymphatic filariasis in many endemic areas (Gelband, 1994). A major advance was the discovery that diethylcarbamazine given annually as a single oral dose of 6 mg/kg was most effective in reducing microfilaremia when coadministered with either albendazole (400 mg) or ivermectin (0.2 to 0.4 mg/kg) (Ottesen *et al.*, 1999). Adverse reactions to microfilarial destruction, greater after the oral diethylcarbamazine tablet than the table salt preparation, usually are well tolerated. However, mass chemotherapy with diethylcarbamazine should *not* be used in regions where onchocerciasis or loiasis coexist because, even in the table salt formulation, the drug may induce severe reactions related to parasite burden in these infections.

Ovolvulus and Lloa. Diethylcarbamazine is contraindicated for the treatment of onchocerciasis because it causes severe reactions related to microfilarial destruction, including worsening ocular lesions (*see* below). For purposes of LF control, use of diethylcarbamazine is considered contraindicated in areas where onchocerciasis is endemic (Molyneux *et al.*, 2003). Such reactions are far less severe in response to ivermectin, the preferred drug for this infection. Despite its drawbacks, diethylcarbamazine remains the best available drug for therapy of loiasis. Treatment is initiated with test doses of 50 mg (1 mg/kg in children) daily for 2 to 3 days, escalating to maximally tolerated daily doses of 9 mg/kg in three doses for a total of 2 to 3 weeks.

Low test doses are used, often accompanied by pretreatment with glucocorticoids or antihistamines, to minimize reactions to dying microfilariae and adult worms; these reactions consist of severe allergic reactions, and occasionally meningoencephalitis and coma from invasion of the CNS by microfilariae. Repeated courses of diethylcarbamazine treatment, separated by 3 to 4 weeks, may be required to cure loiasis. Ivermectin is not a good alternative to diethylcarbamazine for treatment of loiasis, but albendazole may prove to be useful in patients who either fail therapy with diethylcarbamazine or who cannot tolerate the drug (Klion *et al.*, 1999).

Diethylcarbamazine is clinically effective against microfilariae and adult worms of *Dipetalonema streptocerca*, but filariasis due to *Mansonella perstans, M. ozzardi*, or *Dirofilaria immitis* responds minimally to this agent. Diethylcarbamazine is no longer recommended as a first-line drug for the treatment of toxocariasis.

Toxicity and Side Effects. Below a daily dose of 8 to 10 mg/kg, direct toxic reactions to diethylcarbamazine are rarely severe and usually disappear within a few days despite continuation of therapy. These reactions include anorexia, nausea, headache, and at high doses, vomiting. Major adverse

effects result directly or indirectly from the host response to destruction of parasites, primarily microfilariae.

Reactions typically are most severe in patients heavily infected with *O. volvulus*, less serious in *B. malayi* or *L. loa* infections, and mild in bancroftian filariasis, but the drug occasionally induces retinal hemorrhages and severe encephalopathy in patients heavily infected with *L. loa*. In patients with onchocerciasis, the *Mazzotti reaction* typically occurs within a few hours after the first dose and includes intense itching, enlargement and tenderness of the lymph nodes, and sometimes a papular rash, fever, tachycardia, arthralgias, and headache. This reaction persists for 3 to 7 days and then subsides, after which high doses sometimes can be tolerated. Ocular complications include limbitis, punctate keratitis, uveitis, and atrophy of the retinal pigment epithelium (Rivas-Alcala *et al.*, 1981; Dominguez-Vazquez *et al.*, 1983). In patients with bancroftian or brugian filariasis, nodular swellings may occur along the course of the lymphatics, and there often is an accompanying lymphadenitis. This reaction also subsides within a few days. Almost all patients receiving therapy exhibit a leukocytosis, first evident on the second day, reaching its peak on the fourth or fifth day, and gradually subsiding over a period of a few weeks. Reversible proteinuria may occur, and the eosinophilia so frequently observed in patients with filariasis can be intensified by therapy with diethylcarbamazine. Delayed reactions to more mature dying filarial forms include lymphangitis, swelling and lymphoid abscesses in bancroftian and brugian filariasis, and small skin wheals in loiasis. Diethylcarbamazine appears to be safe for use during pregnancy.

Precautions and Contraindications. Population-based chemotherapy with diethylcarbamazine should be avoided in areas where onchocerciasis or loiasis is endemic, although the drug can be used to protect foreign travelers from these infections. Pretreatment with glucocorticoids and antihistamines often is undertaken to minimize indirect reactions to diethylcarbamazine that result from dying microfilariae. Dosage reduction must be considered for patients with impaired renal function or persistent alkaline urine.

Doxycycline

The discovery that filarial parasites, including *W. bancrofti* and *O. volvulus,* harbor bacterial symbionts of the genus *Wolbachia* has led to efforts to examine the effect of antibiotics for treating filarial infections (Taylor and Hoerauf, 2001). For instance, a 6-week regimen of doxycycline (100 mg daily) was found to result in sterility of adult female *Onchocerca* worms (Hoerauf *et al.*, 2000). Studies using shorter treatment courses and alternative antibiotics including rifampicin are in progress. It will be of interest to determine whether anti-*Wolbachia* therapy exerts an antimacrofilaricidal effect, or whether this approach could be applied to mass-treatment strategies (Molyneux *et al.*, 2003).

Ivermectin

History. In the mid-1970s, surveys of natural products revealed that a fermentation broth of the soil actinomycete *Streptomyces avermitilis* ameliorated infection with *Nem-*

atospiroides dubius in mice. Isolation of the anthelmintic components from cultures of this organism led to discovery of the *avermectins*, a novel class of 16-membered lactones (Campbell, 1989). Ivermectin (MECTIZAN; STROMECTOL; 22,23-dihydroavermectin B_{1a}) is a semisynthetic analog of avermectin B_{1a} (abamectin), an insecticide developed for crop management. Ivermectin now is used extensively to control and treat a broad spectrum of infections caused by parasitic nematodes (roundworms) and arthropods (insects, ticks, and mites) that plague livestock and domestic animals (Campbell and Benz, 1984; Campbell, 1993). In 1996, the FDA approved the use of ivermectin in humans for treatment of onchocerciasis, the filarial infection responsible for river blindness, and for therapy of intestinal strongyloidiasis. Ivermectin taken as a single oral dose every 6 to 12 months continues to serve as the mainstay of major programs to control onchocerciasis. In addition, annual oral doses of ivermectin, either taken alone or specifically when taken together with annual oral doses of albendazole, markedly reduce microfilaremia in lymphatic filariasis due to *W. bancrofti* or *B. malayi* (Ottesen *et al.*, 1999; Plaisier *et al.*, 2000; Molyneux and Zagaria, 2002; Molyneux *et al.*, 2003) (*see* "Benzimidazoles," above). Currently The Global Alliance to Eliminate Lymphatic Filariasis advocates diethylcarbamazine (6 mg/kg) plus albendazole (400 mg) (www.filariasis.org). The two-drug regimen now is featured in programs to control LF and is preferred in regions where LF coexists with either onchocerciasis or loiasis. Ivermectin is the drug of choice against intestinal strongyloidiasis and is effective against several other human infections caused by intestinal nematodes (Naquira *et al.*, 1989; Gann *et al.*, 1994; de Silva *et al.*, 1997). The agent also has been used successfully against human scabies and head lice.

Chemistry. The milbemycins are macrocyclic lactone analogs of the avermectins. Some of these compounds have antiparasitic activity similar to that of the avermectins and probably act by similar mechanisms (Fisher and Mrozik, 1992; Arena *et al.*, 1995).

The chemical structure of ivermectin is shown below.

IVERMECTIN

Antiparasitic Activity and Resistance. Several reviews have focused on the antiparasitic action of and resistance to the avermectins and related milbemycins (Cully *et al.*, 1996; Sangster, 1996; Martin *et al.*, 1997; Sangster and Gill, 1999). Ivermectin is effective and highly potent against at least some developmental stages of many parasitic nematodes and insects that affect animals and humans. The drug immobilizes affected organisms by inducing a tonic paralysis of the musculature. Studies of *Caenorhabditis elegans* indicate that avermectins induce paralysis *via* a group of glutamate-gated Cl^- channels found only in invertebrates. There is close correlation among activation and potentiation by avermectins and milbemycin D of glutamate-sensitive Cl^- current, nematicidal activity, and membrane binding affinity (Arena *et al.*, 1995; Cully *et al.*, 1996). Moreover, glutamate-gated Cl^- channels are expressed in the pharyngeal muscle cells of these worms, consistent with the marked and potent inhibitory effect of avermectins on the feeding behavior of the organisms (Sangster and Gill, 1999). Therefore, ivermectin probably binds to glutamate-activated Cl^- channels found in nematode nerve or muscle cells, which causes hyperpolarization by increasing permeability of chloride ions through the cell membrane; this results in paralysis of the parasite (Ikeda, 2003). The basis for resistance or relative unresponsiveness to avermectin action shown by different nematodes, especially those species parasitizing livestock, is complex. Several different avermectin-"resistant" developmental and physiological phenotypes have been described, but definitive relationships among these phenotypes and native avermectin receptor subtypes, locations, numbers, and binding affinities require clarification (Sangster and Gill, 1999; Hejmadi *et al.*, 2000). Alterations in genes encoding ATP-dependent P-glycoprotein transporters that bind avermectins and in those encoding putative components of the glutamate-gated Cl^- channel have been associated with the development of resistance in *Haemonchus contortus* (Xu *et al.*, 1998; Blackhall *et al.*, 1998). A large increase in low-affinity glutamate binding has been detected in ivermectin-resistant nematodes, but how this relates to drug resistance is unclear (Hejmadi *et al.*, 2000). Glutamate-gated Cl^- channels probably are one site of ivermectin action in insects and crustaceans, too (Duce and Scott, 1985; Scott and Duce, 1985; Zufall *et al.*, 1989). Avermectins also bind with high affinity to γ-aminobutyric acid (GABA)-gated and other ligand-gated Cl^- channels in nematodes such as *Ascaris* and in insects, but the physiological consequences are less well defined. Lack of high-affinity avermectin receptors in cestodes and trematodes may explain why these helminths are not sensitive to ivermectin (Shoop *et al.*, 1995). Avermectins also interact with GABA receptors in mammalian brain, but their affinity for invertebrate receptors is about one hundredfold higher (Schaeffer and Haines, 1989).

In humans infected with *O. volvulus*, ivermectin causes a rapid, marked decrease in microfilarial counts in the skin and ocular tissues that lasts for 6 to 12 months (Greene *et al.*, 1987; Newland *et al.*, 1988). The drug has little discernible effect on adult parasites, even at doses as high as 800 μg/kg (Molyneux *et al.*, 2003), but affects developing larvae and blocks egress of microfilariae from the uterus of adult female worms (Awadzi *et al.*, 1985; Court *et al.*, 1985). By reducing microfilariae in the skin, ivermectin decreases transmission to the *Simulium* black fly vector (Cupp *et al.*, 1986; Cupp *et al.*, 1989). Regular treatment with ivermectin also has been conjectured to act prophylactically against the development of *Onchocerca* infection (Molyneux *et al.*, 2003).

Ivermectin also is effective against microfilaria but not against adult worms of *W. bancrofti*, *B. malayi*, *L. loa*, and *M. ozzardi* (de Silva *et al.*, 1997). The drug exhibits excellent efficacy in humans against *Ascaris lumbricoides*, *Strongyloides stercoralis*, and cutaneous larva migrans. Other gastrointestinal nematodes are either partially affected (*Trichuris trichura* and *Enterobius vermicularis*) or unresponsive (*Necator americanus* and *Ancylostoma duodenale*) (Naquira *et al.*, 1989; de Silva *et al.*, 1997).

Absorption, Fate, and Excretion. In humans, peak levels of ivermectin in plasma are achieved within 4 to 5 hours after oral administration. The long terminal half-life of about 57 hours in adults primarily reflects a low systemic clearance (about 1 to 2 liters/hour) and a large apparent volume of distribution (*see* Appendix II). Ivermectin is about 93% bound to plasma proteins (Klotz *et al.*, 1990). The drug is extensively converted by hepatic CYP3A4 to at least 10 metabolites, mostly hydroxylated and demethylated derivatives (Zeng *et al.*, 1998). Virtually no ivermectin appears in human urine in either unchanged or conjugated form (Krishna and Klotz, 1993). In animals, ivermectin is recovered in feces, nearly all as unchanged drug, and the highest tissue concentrations occur in liver and fat. Extremely low levels are found in brain, even though ivermectin would be expected to penetrate the blood–brain barrier on the basis of its lipid solubility. Studies in transgenic mice suggest that a P-glycoprotein efflux pump in the blood–brain barrier prevents ivermectin from entering the CNS (Schinkel *et al.*, 1994). This and the limited affinity of ivermectin for CNS receptors may explain the paucity of CNS side effects and the relative safety of this drug in humans.

Therapeutic Uses. Onchocerciasis. Single oral doses of ivermectin (150 μg/kg) given every 6 to 12 months are considered effective, safe, and practical for reducing the number of circulating microfilariae in adults and children 5 years of age or older (Goa *et al.*, 1991). Widespread use of ivermectin therefore has become a mainstay of onchocerciasis control programs in the Americas and in sub-Saharan Africa. Equally important, such therapy results in reversal of lymphadenopathy and acute inflammatory changes in ocular tissues and arrests the development of further ocular pathology due to microfilariae. Marked reduction of microfilariae in the skin and ocular tissues is noted within a few days and lasts for 6 to 12 months; the dose then should be repeated. Cure is not attained, because ivermectin has little effect on adult *O. volvulus*. Ivermectin has been used since 1987 as the mainstay for onchocerciasis control programs in all 34 countries in Africa and in the Middle

East and Latin America, where the disease is endemic. Nearly 20 million people have received at least one dose of the drug, and many have received 6 to 9 doses (Dull and Meredith, 1998). Since 1991, the Onchocerciasis Elimination Programme in the Americas (OEPA) has been highly effective in reducing transmission in the endemic nations of the Americas, Brazil, Colombia, Ecuador, Guatemala, Mexico, and Venezuela through biannual treatment with ivermectin (Molyneux *et al.*, 2003). Through the African Programme for Onchocerciasis Control, there is an interest in extending biannual ivermectin coverage to the endemic regions of sub-Saharan Africa. Annual doses of the drug are quite safe and substantially reduce transmission of this infection (Brown, 1998; Boatin *et al.*, 1998). How long such therapy should continue still is unknown.

The possibility that high-dose ivermectin could be used as an agent against the adult stage worms (macrofilaricide) has been investigated (Molyneux *et al.*, 2003). However, the high-dose regimens appear to offer no benefit over standard doses, and they are accompanied by unexpected side effects of mild visual changes (Molyneux *et al.*, 2003).

Lymphatic Filariasis. Initial studies indicated that single annual doses of ivermectin (400 μg/kg) are both effective and safe for mass chemotherapy of infections with *W. bancrofti* and *B. malayi* (Ottesen and Ramachandran, 1995). Ivermectin is as effective as diethylcarbamazine for controlling lymphatic filariasis, and unlike the latter agent, can be used in regions where onchocerciasis, loiasis, or both infections are endemic. Although ivermectin as a single agent can reduce *W. bancrofti* microfilaremia, the duration of treatment required to eliminate LF at 65% coverage presumably would be longer than 6 years (Molyneux *et al.*, 2003). More recent evidence indicates that a single annual dose of ivermectin (200 μg/kg) and a single annual dose of albendazole (400 mg) are even more effective in controlling lymphatic filariasis than either drug alone (www.filariasis.org). The duration of treatment is for at least 5 years based on the estimated fecundity of the adult worms. This dual-drug regimen also reduces infections with intestinal nematodes. Facilitated by corporate donation of ivermectin and albendazole, the drug combination now serves as the treatment standard for mass chemotherapy and control of lymphatic filariasis (Ottesen *et al.*, 1999) (*see* "Benzimidazoles," above).

Infections with Intestinal Nematodes. The finding that a single dose of 150 to 200 μg/kg of ivermectin can cure human strongyloidiasis is encouraging, especially because this drug also is effective against coexisting ascariasis, trichuriasis, and enterobiasis (Naquira *et al.*, 1989). A single dose of 100 µg/kg of ivermectin is as effective as traditional treatment of intestinal strongyloidiasis with thiabendazole, and less toxic (Gann *et al.*, 1994; Keiser and Nutman, 2004). In a Phase III trial in Japan, 49 of 50 *S. stercoralis*–infected patients were cured after they received 200 µg/kg of ivermectin orally twice at an interval of 2 weeks (Ikeda, 2003). In *Strongyloides* hyperinfection syndrome, ivermectin has been used successfully, including cases that were unresponsive to thiabendazole (Keiser and Nutman, 2004).

Other Indications. Although ivermectin has activity against microfilaria but not against adult worms of *L. loa* and *M. ozzardi*, it is not used clinically to treat infections with these parasites. Taken as a single 200-µg/kg oral dose, ivermectin is a first-line drug for treatment of cutaneous larva migrans caused by dog or cat hookworms. Similar doses also are safe and highly effective against human head lice and scabies, the latter even in HIV-infected individuals (de Silva *et al.*, 1997).

Toxicity, Side Effects, and Precautions.

Ivermectin is well tolerated by uninfected humans and other mammals. In animals, signs of CNS toxicity, including lethargy, ataxia, mydriasis, tremors, and eventually death, occur only at very high doses; dogs, particularly collie breeds, are especially vulnerable (Campbell and Benz, 1984). In infected humans, ivermectin toxicity nearly always results from Mazzotti-like reactions to dying microfilariae; the intensity and nature of these reactions relate to the microfilarial burden and the duration and type of filarial infection.

After treatment of *O. volvulus* infections with ivermectin, these side effects usually are limited to mild itching and swollen, tender lymph nodes, which arise in 5% to 35% of people, last just a few days, and are relieved by aspirin and antihistamines (Goa *et al.*, 1991). Rarely, more severe reactions occur that include high fever, tachycardia, hypotension, prostration, dizziness, headache, myalgia, arthralgia, diarrhea, and facial and peripheral edema; these may respond to glucocorticoid therapy. Ivermectin induces milder side effects than does diethylcarbamazine, and unlike the latter, seldom exacerbates ocular lesions in onchocerciasis. The drug can cause rare but serious side effects including marked disability and encephalopathies in patients coinfected with heavy burdens of *L. loa* microfilaria (Gardon *et al.*, 1997). *Loa* encephalopathy is associated with ivermectin treatment of individuals with *Loa* microfilaremia levels ≥30,000 microfilariae per milliliter of blood (Molyneux *et al.*, 2003). Most of the cases of *Loa* encephalopathy in association with ivermectin chemotherapy have been recorded in the central province of Cameroon (Molyneux *et al.*, 2003). There is little evidence that ivermectin is teratogenic or carcinogenic.

Because of its effects on GABA receptors in the CNS, ivermectin is contraindicated in conditions associated with an impaired blood–brain barrier (*e.g.*, African trypanosomiasis and meningitis). Caution also is advised about coadministration of ivermectin with other agents that depress CNS activity. A recent analysis of the experience of epileptics who received ivermectin indicated that such individuals should not be excluded from onchocerciasis treatment programs (Twum-Danso, 2004). Possible adverse interactions of ivermectin with other drugs that are extensively metabolized by hepatic CYP3A4 have yet to be evaluated. Ivermectin is not approved for use in children less than 5 years old or in pregnant women, but both populations undoubtedly have been exposed to the drug in mass treatment programs. Lactating women taking the drug secrete low levels in their milk; the consequences for nursing infants are unknown.

Metrifonate

Metrifonate (trichlorfon; BILARCIL) is an organophosphorus compound used first as an insecticide and later as an anthelmintic, especially for treatment of schistosomiasis haematobium. Metrifonate has the following chemical structure:

METRIFONATE

Metrifonate is a prodrug; at physiological pH, it is converted nonenzymatically to *dichlorvos* (2,2-dichlorovinyl dimethyl phosphate, DDVP), a potent cholinesterase inhibitor (Hinz *et al.*, 1996). However, inhibition of cholinesterase alone is unlikely to explain the antischistosomal properties of metrifonate (Bloom, 1981). *In vitro*, dichlorvos is about equally potent as an inhibitor of both *S. mansoni* and *S. haematobium* acetylcholinesterases, yet metrifonate is effective clinically only against infections with *S. haematobium*. The molecular basis for this species-selective effect is not understood. More complete information on the pharmacology and therapeutic uses of metrifonate can be found in the 10th edition of this book.

Niclosamide

Niclosamide (NICLOCIDE), a halogenated salicylanilide derivative, was introduced in the 1960s for human use as a taeniacide. This compound was considered as a second-choice drug to praziquantel for treating human intestinal infections with *Taenia saginata*, *Diphyllobothrium latum*, *Hymenolepis nana*, and most other cestodes because it was cheap, effective, and readily available in many parts of the world. However, therapy with niclosamide poses a risk to people infected with *T. solium*, because ova released from drug-damaged gravid worms develop into larvae that can cause cysticercosis, a dangerous infection that responds poorly to chemotherapy. Niclosamide is no longer approved for use in the United States. More complete information on the pharmacology and therapeutic uses of niclosamide can be found in the ninth edition of this book.

Oxamniquine

Oxamniquine (VANSIL) is a 2-aminomethyltetrahydroquinoline derivative that is used as a second-choice drug to praziquantel for the treatment of schistosomiasis. Most strains of *S. mansoni* are highly susceptible to oxamniquine, but *S. haematobium* and *S. japonicum* are virtually unaffected by therapeutic doses. Because of a low incidence of mild side effects together with normally high efficacy after a single oral dose, oxamniquine continues to be used in *S. mansoni* control programs, especially in South America. More details on the pharmacology and therapeutic uses of oxamniquine can be found in the ninth edition of this book.

Piperazine

The discovery of the anthelmintic properties of piperazine usually is credited to Fayard (1949), but these first were observed by Boismare, a Rouen pharmacist whose recipe is quoted in Fayard's thesis. A large number of substituted piperazine derivatives exhibit anthelmintic activity, but apart from diethylcarbamazine, none has found a place in human therapeutics. Piperazine, a cyclic secondary amine, has the following chemical structure:

PIPERAZINE

Piperazine is highly effective against *Ascaris lumbricoides* and *Enterobius vermicularis*. The predominant effect of piperazine on *Ascaris* is a flaccid paralysis that results in expulsion of the worm by peristalsis. Affected worms recover if incubated in drug-free medium. Piperazine acts as a GABA-receptor agonist. By increasing chloride ion conductance of *Ascaris* muscle membrane, the drug produces hyperpolarization and reduced excitability that leads to muscle relaxation and flaccid paralysis (Martin, 1985). The basis for its selectivity of action is not clear, but studies like those done on ivermectin (Arena *et al.*, 1995) could help resolve this issue. More complete information on the pharmacology and therapeutic uses of piperazine may be found in the 10th edition of this book.

Praziquantel

History. Praziquantel (BILTRICIDE, DISTOCIDE) is a pyrazinoisoquinoline derivative developed after this class of compounds was discovered to have anthelmintic activity in 1972. In animals and humans, infections with many different cestodes and trematodes respond favorably to this agent, whereas nematodes generally are unaffected (Symposium, 1981; Andrews, 1985). Treatment with praziquantel of patients coinfected with schistosomes and hookworms reduced hookworm prevalence and infection intensities (egg counts) significantly (Utzinger *et al.*, 2002). Praziquantel has the following chemical structure:

PRAZIQUANTEL

The (−) isomer is responsible for most of the drug's anthelmintic activity.

Anthelmintic Action. After rapid and reversible uptake, praziquantel has two major effects on adult schistosomes. At the lowest effective concentrations, it causes increased muscular activity, followed by contraction and spastic paralysis. Affected worms detach from blood vessel walls, resulting in a rapid shift from the mesenteric veins to the liver. At slightly higher therapeutic concentrations, praziquantel causes tegumental damage, which exposes a number of tegumental antigens (Redman *et al.*, 1996). Comparisons of stage-specific susceptibility of *S. mansoni* to praziquantel *in vitro* and *in vivo* indicate that the clinical efficacy of this drug correlates better with tegumental action (Xiao *et al.*, 1985). Studies in laboratory animals have shown that praziquantel is less effective against *S. mansoni* and *S. japonicum* in immunosuppressed mice (Fallon *et al.*, 1996). Whether or not host immune status is important for clinical efficacy of praziquantel in humans is not known.

The tegument of schistosomes seems to be the primary site of action of praziquantel. The drug causes an influx of Ca^{2+} across the tegument, and the effect is blocked in Ca^{2+}-free medium. A number of praziquantel-sensitive sites have been suggested as possible targets, but the precise molecular mechanism of action remains elusive (Redman *et al.*, 1996). Praziquantel also produces a variety of biochemical changes, but most appear to be secondary to its primary tegumental action (Andrews, 1985). Nearly all available information about the action of praziquantel has come from studies on schistosomes. Although it generally is assumed that the anthelmintic action of praziquantel against other trematodes and cestodes is the same as for schistosomes, direct evidence is lacking.

Absorption, Fate, and Excretion. Praziquantel is readily absorbed after oral administration, so that maximal levels in human plasma occur in 1 to 2 hours. The pharmacokinetics of praziquantel are dose-related. Extensive first-pass metabolism to many inactive hydroxylated and conjugated products limits the bioavailability of this drug and results in plasma concentrations of metabolites at least one hundredfold higher than that of praziquantel. The drug is about 80% bound to plasma proteins. Its plasma half-life is 0.8 to 3 hours, depending on the dose, compared with 4 to 6 hours for its metabolites, but this may be prolonged in patients with severe liver disease, including those with hepatosplenic schistosomiasis. About 70% of an oral dose of praziquantel is recovered as metabolites in the urine within 24 hours; most of the remainder is metabolized in the liver and eliminated in the bile.

Therapeutic Uses. Praziquantel is approved in the United States only for therapy of schistosomiasis and liver fluke infections, but elsewhere, this remarkably versatile and safe drug also is used to treat infections with many other trematodes and cestodes. Praziquantel should be stored at temperatures below 30°C and swallowed with water without chewing because of its bitter taste.

Praziquantel is the drug of choice for treating schistosomiasis caused by all *Schistosoma* species that infect humans. Although dosage regimens vary, a single oral dose of 40 mg/kg or three doses of 20 mg/kg each, given 4 to 6 hours apart, generally produce cure rates of 70% to 95% and consistently high reductions (over 85%) in egg counts. Tablets of 600 mg currently are available from generic manufacturers; on average, treatment of a school-aged child in Africa requires 2.5 tablets (World Health Organization, 2002).

The absence of weighing scales in Africa and elsewhere in developing countries led to the innovative development of "tablet poles" to determine dosing. Tablet poles operate by measuring height to the nearest centimeter and then determining five height intervals that correspond to 1.5, 2, 2.5, 3, and 4 tablets of praziquantel (World Health Organization, 2002 and www.who.int/wormcontrol). In China, 200-mg tablets typically are used and the number of tablets is modified accordingly. A 600-mg/5-ml praziquantel syrup is available in Egypt (World Health Organization, 2002).

Strains of *S. mansoni* and *S. japonicum* resistant to praziquantel have been selected in laboratory studies (Fallon *et al.*, 1996). Moreover, decreased clinical efficacy of praziquantel against infections with *S. mansoni* has been reported in two human populations, one in a focal area of high transmission in northern Senegal (van Lieshout *et al.*, 1999) and the other in Egypt, where 1% to 2% of patients were not cured after two or three treatments with praziquantel (Ismail *et al.*, 1999). However, praziquantel-tolerant or -resistant schistosome strains currently do not limit its clinical usefulness (Fallon *et al.*, 1996).

Three doses of 25 mg/kg taken 4 to 8 hours apart on the same day result in high rates of cure for infections with either the liver flukes *Clonorchis sinensis* and *Opisthorchis viverrini*, or the intestinal flukes *Fasciolopsis buski*, *Heterophyes heterophyes*, and *Metagonimus yokogawai*. The same three-dose regimen used for 2 days is highly effective against infections with the lung fluke, *Paragonimus westermani*. Infections with *Fasciola hepatica* are unresponsive to high doses, even though praziquantel penetrates this trematode. The reason for the insensitivity of *F. hepatica* to praziquantel is unknown.

Low doses of praziquantel can be used successfully to treat intestinal infections with adult cestodes, for example, a single oral dose of 25 mg/kg for *Hymenolepis nana* and 10 to 20 mg/kg for *Diphyllobothrium latum*, *Taenia saginata*, or *T. solium*. Retreatment after 7 to 10 days is advisable for individuals heavily infected with *H. nana*. While albendazole is preferred for therapy of human cysticercosis, the tissue infection with intermediate cyst larvae of *T. solium*, prolonged high-dose therapy with praziquantel remains an alternative treatment (Evans *et al.*, 1997). Neither the "cystic" nor "alveolar" hydatid diseases caused by larval stages of *Echinococcus*

tapeworms respond to praziquantel; here, too, albendazole is effective (Horton, 1997; Schantz, 1999).

Toxicity, Precautions, and Interactions. Abdominal discomfort, particularly pain and nausea, diarrhea, headache, dizziness, and drowsiness may occur shortly after taking praziquantel; these direct effects are transient and dose-related. Indirect effects such as fever, pruritus, urticaria, rashes, arthralgia, and myalgia are noted occasionally. Such side effects and increases in eosinophilia often relate to parasite burden. In neurocysticercosis, inflammatory reactions to praziquantel may produce meningismus, seizures, mental changes, and cerebrospinal fluid pleocytosis. These effects usually are delayed in onset, last 2 to 3 days, and respond to appropriate symptomatic therapy such as analgesics and anticonvulsants.

Praziquantel is considered safe in children over 4 years of age, who probably tolerate the drug better than do adults. Low levels of the drug appear in the maternal milk, but there is no evidence that this compound is mutagenic or carcinogenic. High doses of praziquantel increase abortion rates in rats, but a retrospective study showed that treatment of pregnant women in Sudan resulted in no significant differences between treated and untreated women in the rates of abortion or preterm deliveries. Moreover, no congenital abnormalities were noted by clinical examination in any of the babies born to either group (Adam *et al.*, 2004).

The bioavailability of praziquantel is reduced by inducers of hepatic CYPs such as carbamazepine and phenobarbital; predictably, coadministration of the CYP inhibitor cimetidine has the opposite effect (Bittencourt *et al.*, 1992; Dachman *et al.*, 1994). Dexamethasone reduces the bioavailability of praziquantel, but the mechanism is not understood. Under certain conditions, praziquantel may increase the bioavailability of albendazole (Homeida *et al.*, 1994).

Praziquantel is contraindicated in ocular cysticercosis because the host response can irreversibly damage the eye. Shortly after taking the drug, driving, operating machinery, and other tasks requiring mental alertness should be avoided. The half-life of praziquantel can be prolonged in patients with severe hepatic disease; dosage adjustment in such patients may be required (Mandour *et al.*, 1990).

Pyrantel Pamoate

Pyrantel pamoate first was introduced into veterinary practice as a broad-spectrum anthelmintic directed against pinworm, roundworm, and hookworm infections. Its effectiveness and lack of toxicity led to its trial against related intestinal helminths in humans. *Oxantel pamoate,* an *m*-oxyphenol analog of pyrantel, is effective for single-dose treatment of trichuriasis. Pyrantel is employed as the pamoate salt and has the following chemical structure:

PYRANTEL

Antihelmintic Action. Pyrantel and its analogs are depolarizing neuromuscular blocking agents. They open nonselective cation channels and induce marked, persistent activation of nicotinic acetylcholine receptors, which results in spastic paralysis of the worm (Robertson *et al.*, 1994). Pyrantel also inhibits cholinesterases. It causes a slowly developing contracture of isolated preparations of *Ascaris* at 1% of the concentration of acetylcholine required to produce the same effect. In single muscle cells of this helminth, pyrantel causes depolarization and increased spike-discharge frequency, accompanied by increases in tension. Pyrantel is effective against hookworm, pinworm, and roundworm; unlike its analog oxantel, it is ineffective against *Trichuris trichiura.*

Absorption, Fate, and Excretion. Pyrantel pamoate is poorly absorbed from the gastrointestinal tract, a property that contributes to its selective action on gastrointestinal nematodes. Less than 15% is excreted in the urine as parent drug and metabolites. The major proportion of an administered dose is recovered in the feces.

Therapeutic Uses. Pyrantel pamoate is an alternative to mebendazole in the treatment of ascariasis and enterobiasis. High cure rates have been achieved after a single oral dose of 11 mg/kg, to a maximum of 1 g. Pyrantel also is effective against hookworm infections caused by *Ancylostoma duodenale* and *Necator americanus,* although repeated doses are needed to cure heavy infections by *N. americanus.* The drug should be used in combination with oxantel for mixed infections with *T. trichiura.* In the case of pinworm, it is wise to repeat the treatment after an interval of 2 weeks. In the United States, pyrantel is sold as an over-the-counter pinworm treatment (PIN-X).

Precautions. When given parenterally, pyrantel can produce complete neuromuscular blockade in animals; only very large oral doses produce toxic effects. Transient and mild GI symptoms occasionally are observed in humans, as are headache, dizziness, rash, and fever. Pyrantel pamoate has not been studied in pregnant women. Thus, its use in pregnant patients and children less than 2 years of age is not recommended. Because pyrantel pamoate and piperazine are mutually antagonistic with respect to their neuromuscular effects on parasites, they should not be used together.

BIBLIOGRAPHY

Adam, I., el Elwasila, T., and Homeida, M. Is praziquantel therapy safe during pregnancy? *Trans. R. Soc. Trop. Med. Hyg.,* **2004,** *98:*540–543.

Albonico, M., Bickle, Q., Ramsan, M., *et al.* Efficacy of mebendazole and levamisole alone or in combination against intestinal nematode infections after repeated targeted mebendazole treatment in Zanzibar. *Bull. WHO.,* **2003,** *81:*343–352.

Albonico, M., Smith, P.G., Ercole, E., *et al.* Rate of reinfection with intestinal nematodes after treatment of children with mebendazole or albendazole in a highly endemic area. *Trans. R. Soc. Trop. Med. Hyg.,* **1995,** *89:*538–541.

Arena, J.P., Liu, K.K., Paress, P.S., *et al.* The mechanism of action of avermectins in *Caenorhabditis elegans:* correlation between activation of glutamate-sensitive chloride current, membrane binding, and biological activity. *J. Parasitol.,* **1995,** *81:*286–294.

Awadzi, K., Adjepon-Yamoah, K.K., Edwards, G., *et al.* The effect of moderate urine alkalinisation on low dose diethylcarbamazine therapy in patients with onchocerciasis. *Br. J. Clin. Pharmacol.,* **1986,** *21:*669–676.

Awadzi, K., Dadzie, K.Y., Shulz-Key, H., *et al.* The chemotherapy of onchocerciasis X. An assessment of four single dose treatment regimes of MK-933 (ivermectin) in human onchocerciasis. *Ann. Trop. Med. Parasitol.,* **1985,** *79:*63–78.

Bittencourt, P.R., Gracia, C.M., Martins, R., *et al.* Phenytoin and carbamazepine decreased oral bioavailability of praziquantel. *Neurology,* **1992,** *42:*492–496.

Blackhall, W.J., Liu, H.Y., Xu, M., Prichard, R.K., and Beech, R.N. Selection at a P-glycoprotein gene in ivermectin- and moxidectin-selected strains of *Haemonchus contortus. Mol. Biochem. Parasitol.,* **1998,** *95:*193–201.

Bloom, A. Studies of the mode of action of metrifonate and DDVP in schistosomes—cholinesterase activity and the hepatic shift. *Acta Pharmacol. Toxicol. (Copenh.),* **1981,** *49(suppl 5):*109–113.

Boatin, B.A., Hougard, J.M., Alley, E.S., *et al.* The impact of Mectizan on the transmission of onchocerciasis. *Ann. Trop. Med. Parasitol.,* **1998,** *92(suppl 1):*S46–S60.

Court, J.P., Bianco, A.E., Townson, S., Ham, P.J., and Friedheim, E. Study on the activity of antiparasitic agents against *Onchocerca lienalis* third stage larvae *in vitro. Trop. Med. Parasitol.,* **1985,** *36:*117–119.

Cupp, E.W., Bernardo, M.J., Kiszewski, A.E., *et al.* The effects of ivermectin on transmission of *Onchocerca volvulus. Science,* **1986,** *231:*740–742.

Cupp, E.W., Onchoa, A.O., Collins, R.C., *et al.* The effect of multiple ivermectin treatments on infection of *Simulium ochraceum* with *Onchocerca volvulus. Am. J. Trop. Med. Hyg.,* **1989,** *40:*501–506.

Dachman, W.D., Adubofour, K.O., Bikin, D.S., *et al.* Cimetidine-induced rise in praziquantel levels in a patient with neurocysticercosis being treated with anticonvulsants. *J. Infect. Dis.,* **1994,** *169:*689–691.

Davies, H.D., Sakuls, P., and Keystone, J.S. Creeping eruption. A review of clinical presentation and management of 60 cases presenting to a tropical disease unit. *Arch. Dermatol.,* **1993,** *129:*588–591.

Davis, A., Dixon, H., and Pawlowski, Z.S. Multicentre clinical trials of benzimidazole-carbamates in human cystic echinococcosis (phase 2). *Bull. World Health Organ.,* **1989,** *67:*503–508.

Delatour, P., Benoit, E., Besse, S., and Boukraa, A. Comparative enantioselectivity in the sulfoxidation of albendazole in man, dogs and rats. *Xenobiotica,* **1991,** *21:*217–221.

Dominguez-Vazquez, A., Taylor, H.R., Greene, B.M., *et al.* Comparison of flubendazole and diethylcarbamazine in treatment of onchocerciasis. *Lancet,* **1983,** *1:*139–143.

Driscoll, M., Dean, E., Reilly, E., Bergholz, E., and Chalfie, M. Genetic and molecular analysis of *Caenorhabditis elegans* β-tubulin that conveys benzimidazole sensitivity. *J. Cell Biol.,* **1989,** *109:*2993–3003.

Duce, I.R., and Scott, R.H. Actions of dihydroavermectin B_{1a} on insect muscle. *Br. J. Pharmacol.,* **1985,** *85:*395–401.

Fayard, C. Ascaridiose et piperazine. Thesis, Paris, **1949.** (Quoted from *Semin. Hop. Paris, 1949, 35:*1778.)

Forrester, J.E., Bailar III, J.C., Esrey, S.A., *et al.* Randomised trial of albendazole and pyrantel in symptomless trichuriasis in children. *Lancet,* **1998,** *352:*1103–1108.

Gann, P.H., Neva, F.A., and Gam, A.A. A randomized trial of single- and two-dose ivermectin *versus* thiabendazole for treatment of strongyloidiasis. *J. Infect. Dis.,* **1994,** *169:*1076–1079.

Gao, J., Liu, Y., Wang, X., and Hu, P. Triclabendazole in the treatment of *Paragonimiasis skrjabini. Chin. Med. J.,* **2003,** *116:*1683–1686.

Gardon, J., Gardon-Wendel, N., Demanga-Ngangue, *et al.* Serious reactions after mass treatment of onchocerciasis with ivermectin in an area endemic for *Loa loa* infection. *Lancet,* **1997,** *350:*18–22.

Gelband, H. Diethylcarbamazine salt in the control of lymphatic filariasis. *Am. J. Trop. Med. Hyg.,* **1994,** *50:*655–662.

Gleizes, C., Eeckhoutte, C., Pineau, T., Alvinerie, M., and Galtier, P. Inducing effect of oxfendazole on cytochrome P450IA2 in rabbit liver. Consequences on cytochrome P450-dependent monooxygenases. *Biochem. Pharmacol.,* **1991,** *41:*1813–1820.

Goa, K.L., McTavish, D., and Clissold, S.P. Ivermectin. A review of its antifilarial activity, pharmacokinetic properties and clinical efficacy in onchocerciasis. *Drugs,* **1991,** *42:*640–658.

Greene, B.M., White, A.T., Newland, H.S., *et al.* Single dose therapy with ivermectin for onchocerciasis. *Trans. Assoc. Am. Physicians,* **1987,** *100:*131–138.

Hejmadi, M.V., Jagannathan, S., Delany, N.S., Coles, G.C., and Wolstenholme, A.J. L-glutamate binding sites of parasitic nematodes: association with ivermectin resistance? *Parasitology,* **2000,** *120:*535–545.

Hinz, V.C., Grewig, S., and Schmidt, B.H. Metrifonate induces cholinesterase inhibition exclusively via slow release of dichlorvos. *Neurochem. Res.,* **1996,** *21:*331–337.

Homeida, M., Leahy, W., Copeland, S., Ali, M.M., and Harron, D.W. Pharmacokinetic interaction between praziquantel and albendazole in Sudanese men. *Ann. Trop. Med. Parasitol.,* **1994,** *88:*551–559.

Ismail, M., Botros, S., Metwally, A., *et al.* Resistance to praziquantel: direct evidence from *Schistosoma mansoni* isolated from Egyptian villagers. *Am. J. Trop. Med. Hyg.,* **1999,** *60:*932–935.

Jung, H., Hurtado, M., Sanchez, M., Medina, M.T., and Sotelo, J. Clinical pharmacokinetics of albendazole in patients with brain cysticercosis. *J. Clin. Pharmacol.,* **1992,** *32:*28–31.

Katiyar, S.K., and Edlind, T.D. *In vitro* susceptibilities of the AIDS-associated microsporidian *Encephalitozoon intestinalis* to albendazole, its sulfoxide metabolite, and 12 additional benzimidazole derivatives. *Antimicrob. Agents Chemother.,* **1997,** *41:*2729–2732.

Kern, P. *Echinococcus granulosus* infection: clinical presentation, medical treatment and outcome. *Langenbecks Arch. Surg.,* **2003,** *388:*413–420.

Klion, A.D., Horton, J., and Nutman, T.B. Albendazole therapy for loiasis refractory to diethylcarbamazine treatment. *Clin. Infect. Dis.,* **1999,** *29:*680–682.

Klotz, U., Ogbuokiri, J.E., and Okonkwo, P.O. Ivermectin binds avidly to plasma proteins. *Eur. J. Clin. Pharmacol.,* **1990,** *39:*607–608.

Krishna, D.R., and Klotz, U. Determination of ivermectin in human plasma by high-performance liquid chromatography. *Arzneimittelforshung,* **1993,** *43:*609–611.

Kwa, M.S., Kooyman, F.N., Boersema, J.H., and Roos, M.H. Effect of selection for benzimidazole resistance in *Haemonchus contortus* on β-tubulin isotype 1 and isotype 2 genes. *Biochem. Biophys. Res. Commun.,* **1993,** *191:*413–419.

Kwa, M.S., Veenstra, J.G., Van Dijk, M., and Roos, M.H. Beta-tubulin genes from the parasitic nematode *Haemonchus contortus* modulate drug resistance in *Caenorhabditis elegans. J. Mol. Biol.,* **1995,** *246:*500–510.

Lacey, E. The role of the cytoskeletal protein, tubulin, in the mode of action and mechanism of drug resistance to benzimidazoles. *Int. J. Parasitol.,* **1988,** *18:*885–936.

van Lieshout, L., Stelma, F.F., Guisse, F., *et al.* The contribution of host-related factors to low cure rates of praziquantel for the treatment of *Schistosoma mansoni* in Senegal. *Am. J. Trop. Med. Hyg.,* **1999,** *61:*760–765.

Lubega, G.W., and Prichard, R.K. Beta-tubulin and benzimidazole resistance in the sheep nematode *Haemonchus contortus. Mol. Biochem. Parasitol.,* **1991,** *47:*129–137.

Mandour, M.E., el Turabi, H., Homeida, M.M., *et al.* Pharmacokinetics of praziquantel in healthy volunteers and patients with schistosomiasis. *Trans. R. Soc. Trop. Med. Hyg.,* **1990,** *84:*389–393.

Marques, M.P., Takayanagui, O.M., Bonato, P.S., Santos, S.R., and Lanchote, V.L. Enantioselective kinetic disposition of albendazole sulfoxide in patients with neurocysticercosis. *Chirality,* **1999,** *11:*218–223.

Marriner, S.E., Morris, D.L., Dickson, B., and Bogan, J.A. Pharmacokinetics of albendazole in man. *Eur. J. Clin. Pharmacol.,* **1986,** *30:*705–708.

Martin, R.J. γ-Aminobutyric acid- and piperazine-activated single-channel currents from *Ascaris suum* body muscle. *Br. J. Pharmacol.,* **1985,** *84:*445–461.

Moroni, P., Buronfosse, T., Longin-Sauvageon, C., Delatour, P., and Benoit, E. Chiral sulfoxidation of albendazole by the flavin adenine dinucleotide-containing and cytochrome P450–dependent monooxygenases from rat liver microsomes. *Drug Metab. Dispos.,* **1995,** *23:*160–165.

Morris, D.L., Chinnery, J.B., Georgiou, G., Stamatakis, G., and Golematis, B. Penetration of albendazole sulfoxide into hydatid cysts. *Gut,* **1987,** *28:*75–80.

Mutapi, F., Ndhlovu, P.D., Hagan, P., *et al.* Chemotherapy accelerates the development of acquired immune responses to *Schistosoma haematobium* infection. *J. Infect. Dis.,* **1998,** *178:*289–293.

Naquira, C., Jimenez, G., Guerra, J.G., *et al.* Ivermectin for human strongyloidiasis and other intestinal helminths. *Am. J. Trop. Med. Hyg.,* **1989,** *40:*304–309.

Newland, H.S., White, A.T., Greene, B.M., *et al.* Effect of single-dose ivermectin therapy on human *Onchocerca volvulus* infection with onchocercal ocular involvement. *Br. J. Ophthalmol.,* **1988,** *72:*561–569.

Peixoto, C.A., Rocha, A., Aguiar-Santos, A., and Florencio, M.S. The effects of diethylcarbamazine on the ultrastructure of *Wuchereria bancrofti in vivo* and *in vitro. Parasitol. Res.,* **2004,** *92:*513–517.

Plaisier, A.P., Stolk, W.A., van Oortmarssen, G.J., and Habbema, J.D. Effectiveness of annual ivermectin treatment for *Wuchereria bancrofti* infection. *Parasitol. Today,* **2000,** *16:*298–302.

Redondo, P.A., Alvarez, A.I., Garcia, J.L., *et al.* Presystemic metabolism of albendazole: experimental evidence of an efflux process of albendazole sulfoxide to intestinal lumen. *Drug Metab. Dispos.,* **1999,** *27:*736–740.

Rivas-Alcala, A.R., Greene, B.M., Taylor, H.R., *et al.* Chemotherapy of onchocerciasis: a controlled comparison of mebendazole, levamisole, and diethylcarbamazine. *Lancet,* **1981,** *2:*485–490.

Robertson, S.J., Pennington, A.J., Evans, A.M., and Martin, R.J. The action of pyrantel as an agonist and an open-channel blocker at acetylcholine receptors in isolated *Ascaris suum* muscle vesicles. *Eur. J. Pharmacol.,* **1994,** *271:*273–282.

Sacko, M., De Clercq, D., Behnke, J.M., *et al.* Comparison of the efficacy of mebendazole, albendazole and pyrantel in treatment of hookworm infections in the southern region of Mali, West Africa. *Trans. R. Soc. Trop. Med. Hyg.,* **1999,** *93:*195–203.

Schaeffer, J.M., and Haines, H.W. Avermectin binding in *Caenorhabditis elegans.* A two-state model for the avermectin binding site. *Biochem. Pharmacol.,* **1989,** *38:*2329–2338.

Schantz, P.M. Editorial response: Treatment of cystic echinococcosis—improving but still limited. *Clin. Infect. Dis.,* **1999,** *29:*310–311.

Schinkel, A.H., Smit, J.J., van Tellingen, O., *et al.* Disruption of the mouse *mdr1a* P-glycoprotein gene leads to a deficiency in the blood–brain barrier and to increased sensitivity to drugs. *Cell,* **1994,** *77:*491–502.

Scott, R.H., and Duce, I.R. Effects of 22,23-dihydroavermectin on locust (*Schistocerca gregaria*) muscles may involve several sites of action. *Pest. Science,* **1985,** *16:*599–604.

Sharghi, N., Schantz, P.M., Caramico, L., *et al.* Environmental exposure to *Toxocara* as a possible risk factor for asthma: a clinic-based case-control study. *Clin. Infect. Dis.,* **2001,** *32:*E111–E116.

Shoop, W.L., Ostlind, D.A., Roher, S.P., *et al.* Avermectins and milbemycins against *Fasciola hepatica: in vivo* drug efficacy and *in vitro* receptor binding. *Int. J. Parasitol.,* **1995,** *25:*923–927.

Sotelo, J., and Jung, H. Pharmacokinetic optimisation of the treatment of neurocysticercosis. *Clin. Pharmacokinet.,* **1998,** *34:*503–515.

Spiro, R.C., Parsons, W.G., Perry, S.K., *et al.* Inhibition of post-translational modification and surface expression of a melanoma-associated chondroitin sulfate proteoglycan by diethylcarbamazine or ammonium chloride. *J. Biol. Chem.,* **1986,** *261:*5121–5129.

Stephenson, L.S., Latham, M.C., Kurz, K.M., Kinoti, S.N., and Brigham, H. Treatment with a single dose of albendazole improves growth of Kenyan schoolchildren with hookworm, *Trichuris trichiura,* and *Ascaris lumbricoides. Am. J. Trop. Med. Hyg.,* **1989,** *41:*78–87.

Upcroft, J., Mitchell, R., Chen, N., and Upcroft, P. Albendazole resistance in *Giardia* is correlated with cytoskeletal changes but not with a mutation at amino acid 200 in β-tubulin. *Microb. Drug Resist.,* **1996,** *2:*303–308.

Wilmshurst, J.M., and Robb, S.A. Can mebendazole cause lateralized occipital seizures? *Eur. J. Paediatr. Neurol.,* **1998,** *2:*323–324.

Xiao, S.H., Catto, B.A., and Webster, L.T., Jr. Effects of praziquantel on different developmental stages of *Schistosoma mansoni in vitro* and *in vivo. J. Infect. Dis.,* **1985,** *151:*1130–1137.

Xu, M., Molento, M., Blackhall, W., *et al.* Ivermectin resistance in nematodes may be caused by alteration of P-glycoprotein homolog. *Mol. Biochem. Parasitol.,* **1998,** *91:*327–335.

Zeng, Z., Andrew, N.W., Arison, B.H., Luffer-Atlas, D., and Wang, R.W. Identification of cytochrome P4503A4 as the major enzyme responsible for the metabolism of ivermectin by human liver microsomes. *Xenobiotica,* **1998,** *28:*313–321.

Zufall, F., Franke, C., and Hatt, H. The insecticide avermectin B$_{1a}$ activates a chloride channel in crayfish muscle membrane. *J. Exp. Biol.,* **1989,** *142:*191–205.

MONOGRAPHS AND REVIEWS

Addiss, D., Critchley, J., Ejere, H., *et al.* International Filariasis Review Group. *Cochrane Database Syst. Rev.,* **2004,** CD003753.

Addiss, D.G., and Dreyer, G. Treatment of lymphatic filariasis. In, *Lymphatic Filariasis.* (Nutman, T.B., ed.) Imperial College Press, London, **2000,** pp. 151–1919.

Albonico, M., Crompton, D.W., and Savioli, L. Control strategies for human intestinal nematode infections. *Adv. Parasitol.,* **1999,** *42:*277–341.

Albonico, M. Methods to sustain drug efficacy in helminth control programmes. *Acta Trop.,* **2003,** *86:*233–242.

Andrews, P. Praziquantel: mechanisms of anti-schistosomal activity. *Pharmacol. Ther.,* **1985,** *29:*129–156.

Bagheri, H., Simiand, E., Montastruc, J.L., and Magnaval, J.F. Adverse drug reactions to anthelmintics. *Ann. Pharmacother.,* **2004,** *38:*383–388.

Bennett, A., and Guyatt, H. Reducing intestinal nematode infection: efficacy of albendazole and mebendazole. *Parasitol. Today,* **2000,** *16:*71–74.

Brown, K.R. Changes in the use profile of Mectizan: 1987–1997. *Ann. Trop. Med. Parasitol.,* **1998,** *92(suppl 1):*S61–S64.

Brooker, S., Bethony, J., and Hotez, P.J. Hookworm infection in the 21st Century. *Adv. Parasitol.,* **2004,** *58:*197–228.

Bundy, D.A., Chan, M.S., and Savioli, L. Hookworm infection in pregnancy. *Trans. R. Soc. Trop. Med. Hyg.,* **1995,** *89:*521–522.

Bundy, D.A., and Cooper, E.S. *Trichuris* and trichuriasis in humans. *Adv. Parasitol.,* **1989,** *28:*107–173.

Bundy, D.A., Wong, M.S., Lewis, L.L., and Horton, J. Control of geohelminths by delivery of targeted chemotherapy through schools. *Trans. R. Soc. Trop. Med. Hyg.,* **1990,** *84:*115–120.

Burnham, G., and Mebrahtu, T. The delivery of ivermectin (Mectizan). *Trop. Med. Int. Health,* **2004,** *9:*A26–A44.

Campbell, W.C., ed. *Ivermectin and Abamectin.* Springer-Verlag, New York, **1989.**

Campbell, W.C. Ivermectin, an antiparasitic agent. *Med. Res. Rev.,* **1993,** *13:*61–79.

Campbell, W.C., and Benz, G.W. Ivermectin: a review of efficacy and safety. *J. Vet. Pharmacol. Ther.,* **1984,** *7:*1–16.

Crompton, D.W. *Ascaris* and ascariasis. *Adv. Parasitol.,* **2001,** *48:*285–375.

Cross, J.H. Intestinal capillariasis. *Clin. Microbiol. Rev.,* **1992,** *5:*120–129.

Cully, D.F., Wilkinson, H., Vassilatis, D.K., Etter, A., and Arena, J.P. Molecular biology and electrophysiology of glutamate-gated chloride channels of invertebrates. *Parasitology,* **1996,** *113(suppl):*S191–S200.

Dayan, A.D. Albendazole, mebendazole and praziquantel. Review of non-clinical toxicity and pharmacokinetics. *Acta Trop.,* **2003,** *86:*141–159.

Drake, L.J., Jukes, M.C.H., Sternberg, R.J., and Bundy, D.A.P. Geohelminth infections (ascariasis, trichuriasis, and hookworm): cognitive and developmental impacts. *Semin. Pediatr. Infect. Dis.,* **2000,** *11:*245–251.

Dull, H.B., and Meredith, S.E. The Mectizan Donation Programme—a 10-year report. *Ann. Trop. Med. Parasitol.,* **1998,** *92(suppl 1):*S69–S71.

Evans, C., Garcia, H.H., Gilman, R.H., and Friedland, J.S. Controversies in the management of cysticercosis. *Emerg. Infect. Dis.,* **1997,** *3:*403–405.

Fallon, P.G., Tao, L.F., Ismail, M.M., and Bennett, J.L. Schistosome resistance to praziquantel: fact or artifact? *Parasitol. Today,* **1996,** *12:*316–320.

Fisher, M.H., and Mrozik, H. The chemistry and pharmacology of avermectins. *Annu. Rev. Pharmacol. Toxicol.,* **1992,** *32:*537–553.

Garcia, H.H., and Del Brutto, O.H. *Taenia solium* cysticercosis. *Infect. Dis. Clin. North Am.,* **2000,** *14:*97–119.

Gottschall, D.W., Theodorides, V.J., and Wang, R. The metabolism of benzimidazole anthelmintics. *Parasitol. Today,* **1990,** *6:*115–124.

Hoerauf, A., Volkmann, L., Hamelmann, C., *et al.* Endosymbiotic bacteria in worms as targets for a novel chemotherapy in filariasis. *Lancet,* **2000,** *355:*1242–1243.

Horton, J. Albendazole: a review of anthelmintic efficacy and safety in humans. *Parasitology,* **2000,** *121:*S113–S132.

Horton, J. Global anthelmintic chemotherapy programs: learning from history. *Trends Parasitol.,* **2003,** *19:*405–409.

Horton, R.J. Albendazole in treatment of human cystic echinococcosis: 12 years of experience. *Acta Trop.,* **1997,** *64:*79–93.

Hotez, P.J., Bethony, J., and Brooker, S. Soil-transmitted helminth infections. In, *Current Pediatric Therapy,* 18th ed. (Burg, F.D., Ingelfinger, J.R., Polin, Gershon, A.A. eds.), Elsevier, **2005,** in press.

Hotez, P.J., Brooker, S., Bethony, J., *et al.* Current concepts: hookworm infection. *N. Engl. J. Med.,* **2004a,** *351:*799–807.

Hotez, P.J. Pediatric geohelminth infections. *Semin. Pediatr. Infect. Dis.,* **2000,** *11:*236–244.

Hotez, P.J., Remme, J.H.F., Buss, P., *et al.* Combating tropical infectious diseases: report of the disease control priorities in developing countries project. *Clin. Infect. Dis.,* **2004b,** *38:*871–878.

Ikeda, T. Pharmacological effects of ivermectin, an antiparasitic agent for intestinal strongyloidiasis: its mode of action and clinical efficacy. *Nippon Yakurigauku Zasshi,* **2003,** *122:*527–538.

Keiser, P.B., and Nutman, T. Strongyloides stercoralis in the immunocompromised population. *Clin. Microbiol. Rev.,* **2004,** *17:*208–217.

Lacey, E. The mode of action of benzimidazoles. *Parasitol. Today,* **1990,** *6:*112–115.

Liu, L.X., and Weller, P.F. Strongyloidiasis and other intestinal nematode infections. *Infect. Dis. Clin. North. Am.,* **1993,** *7:*655–682.

Mackenzie, C.D., and Kron, M.A. Diethylcarbamazine: a review of its action in onchocerciasis, lymphatic filariasis and inflammation. *Trop. Dis. Bull.,* **1985,** *82:*R1–R37.

Martin, R.J., Robertson, A., and Bjorn, H. Target sites of anthelmintics. *Parasitology,* **1997,** *114(suppl):*S111–S124.

Molyneux, D.H., Bradley, M., Hoerauf, A., Kyelem, D., and Taylor, M.J. Mass drug treatment for lymphatic filariasis and onchocerciasis. *Trends. Parasitol.,* **2003,** *19:*516–522.

Molyneux, D.H., and Zagaria, N. Lymphatic filariasis elimination: progress in global programme development. *Ann. Trop. Med. Parasitol.,* **2002,** *96(Suppl. 2):*S15–S40.

Montresor, A., Awasthi, S., and Crompton, D.W. Use of benzimidazoles in children younger than 24 months for the treatment of soil-transmitted helminthiasis. *Acta Trop.,* **2003,** *86:*223–232.

Ottesen, E.A., Ismail, M.M., and Horton, J. The role of albendazole in programmes to eliminate lymphatic filariasis. *Parasitol. Today,* **1999,** *15:*382–386.

Ottesen, E.A., and Ramachandran, C.P. Lymphatic filariasis infection and disease: control strategies. *Parasitol. Today,* **1995,** *11:*129–131.

Prichard, R. Anthelmintic resistance. *Vet. Parasitol.,* **1994,** *54:*259–268.

Redman, C.A., Robertson, A., Fallon, P.G., *et al.* Praziquantel: an urgent and exciting challenge. *Parasitol. Today,* **1996,** *12:*14–20.

Roos, M.H. The role of drugs in the control of parasitic nematode infections: must we do without? *Parasitology,* **1997,** *114(suppl):*S137–S144.

Saba, R., Korkmaz, M., Inan, D., *et al.* Human fascioliasis. *Clin. Microbiol. Infect.,* **2004,** *10:*385–387.

Sabrosa, N.A., and de Souza, E.C. Nematode infections of the eye: toxocariasis and diffuse unilateral subacute neuroretinitis. *Curr. Opin. Ophthalmol.,* **2001,** *12:*450–454.

Salinas, R., and Prasad, K. Drugs for treating neurocysticercosis (tapeworm infection of the brain). *Cochrane Database Syst. Rev.,* **2000,** *2:*CD000215.

Sangster, N.C. Pharmacology of anthelmintic resistance. *Parasitology,* **1996,** *113(suppl):*S201–S216.

Sangster, N.C., and Gill, J. Pharmacology of anthelmintic resistance. *Parasitol. Today,* **1999,** *15:*141–146.

Savioli, L., Stansfield, S., Bundy, D.A., *et al.* Schistosomiasis and soil-transmitted helminth infections: forging control efforts. *Trans. R. Soc. Trop. Med. Hyg.,* **2002,** *96:*577–579.

Sharghi, N., Schantz, P., and Hotez, P.J. Toxocariasis: an occult cause of childhood asthma, seizures, and neuropsychological deficit? *Semin. Pediatr. Infect. Dis.,* **2000,** *11:*257–260.

de Silva, N.R., Brooker, S., Hotez, P.J., *et al.* Soil-transmitted helminth infections: updating the global picture. *Trends Parasitol.,* **2003,** *19:*547–551.

de Silva, N., Guyatt, H., and Bundy, D. Anthelminitics. A comparative review of their clinical pharmacology. *Drugs,* **1997,** *53:*769–788.

Symposium. (Various authors.) Biltricide symposium on African schistosomiasis. (Classen, H.G., and Schramm, V., eds.) *Arzneimittelforschung,* **1981,** *31:*535–618.

Taylor, M.J., and Hoerauf, A. A new approach to the treatment of filariasis. *Curr. Opin. Infect. Dis.,* **2001,** *14:*727–731.

Townsend, L.B., and Wise, D.S. The synthesis and chemistry of certain anthelmintic benzimidazoles. *Parasitol. Today,* **1990,** *6:*107–112.

Twum-Danso, N.A. Mass treatment of onchocerciasis with ivermectin: should people with epilepsy and/or growth-retardation syndromes be excluded? *Ann. Trop. Med. Parasitol.,* **2004,** *98:*99–114.

Urbani, C., and Albonico, M. Anthelminthic drug safety and drug administration in the control of soil-transmitted helminthiasis in community campaigns. *Acta Trop.,* **2003,** *86:*215–223.

Utzinger, J., Vounatsou, P., N'Goran, E.K., Tanner, M., and Booth, M. Reduction in the prevalence and intensity of hookworm infections after praziquantel treatment for schistosomiasis infection. *Int. J. Parasitol.,* **2002,** *32:*759–765.

Venkatesan, P. Albendazole. *J. Antimicrob. Chemother.,* **1998,** *41:*145–147.

World Health Organization. *Prevention and Control of Schistosomiasis and Soil-Transmitted Helminthiasis,* Report of a WHO Expert Committee. WHO Technical Report Series 912, **2002,** Geneva.

Xiao, S., Tanner, M., N'Goran, E.K., *et al.* Recent investigations of artemether, a novel agent for the prevention of schistosomiasis japonica, mansoni and haematobia. *Acta Trop.,* **2002,** *82:*175–181.

SECTION VIII
Chemotherapy of Microbial Diseases

CHAPTER

42

GENERAL PRINCIPLES OF ANTIMICROBIAL THERAPY

Henry F. Chambers

Antimicrobial agents are among the most commonly used and misused of all drugs. The inevitable consequence of the widespread use of antimicrobial agents has been the emergence of antibiotic-resistant pathogens, fueling an ever-increasing need for new drugs. However, the pace of antimicrobial drug development has slowed dramatically, with only a handful of new agents, few of which are novel, being introduced into clinical practice each year. Reducing inappropriate antibiotic use is thought to be the best way to control resistance. Although awareness of the consequences of antibiotic misuse is increasing, overprescribing remains widespread, driven largely by patient demand, time pressure on clinicians, and diagnostic uncertainty. If the gains in the treatment of infectious diseases are to be preserved, clinicians must be wiser and more selective in the use of antimicrobial agents.

This chapter reviews the general classes of antimicrobial drugs, their mechanisms of action, and mechanisms of bacterial resistance. It also discusses principles for the selection of an appropriate antibiotic, the use of antibiotic combinations, and the role of chemoprophylaxis. This chapter offers a philosophical and a practical approach to the appropriate use of antimicrobial agents and discusses the factors that influence the outcome of such treatment. Also emphasized is the frequent misuse of antimicrobial agents owing to lack of identification of the responsible microor-

ganism, which can lead to superinfection or drug resistance. The pharmacological properties and uses of individual classes of antimicrobials are discussed in Chapters 43 through 50.

Definition and Characteristics. In the strictest sense, antibiotics are antibacterial substances produced by various species of microorganisms (bacteria, fungi, and actinomycetes) that suppress the growth of other microorganisms. Common usage often extends the term *antibiotics* to include synthetic antimicrobial agents, such as *sulfonamides* and *quinolones*. Antibiotics differ markedly in physical, chemical, and pharmacological properties, in antimicrobial spectra, and in mechanisms of action. Knowledge of molecular mechanisms of bacterial replication has greatly facilitated rational development of compounds that can interfere with their replication.

Classification and Mechanism of Action. Antimicrobial agents are classified based on chemical structure and proposed mechanism of action, as follows: (1) agents that inhibit synthesis of bacterial cell walls, including the β-lactam class (*e.g.*, penicillins, cephalosporins, and carbapenems) and dissimilar agents such as *cycloserine, vancomycin,* and *bacitracin;* (2) agents that act directly on the cell membrane of the microorganism, increasing permeability and leading to leakage of intracellular compounds, including detergents such as *polymyxin;* polyene antifungal agents (*e.g., nystatin* and *amphotericin B*) which bind to cell-wall sterols; and the lipopeptide daptomycin (Carpenter and Chambers, 2004); (3) agents that disrupt function of 30S or 50S ribosomal subunits to reversibly inhibit protein synthesis, which generally are bacteriostatic (*e.g.*, *chloramphenicol,* the *tetracyclines, erythromycin, clindamycin, streptogramins,* and *linezolid*); (4) agents that bind to the 30S ribosomal subunit and alter protein synthesis, which generally are bactericidal (*e.g.*, the *aminoglycosides*); (5) agents that affect bacterial nucleic acid metabolism, such as the rifamycins (*e.g., rifampin* and *rifabutin*), which inhibit RNA polymerase, and the quinolones, which inhibit topoisomerases; and (6) the antimetabolites, including *trimethoprim* and the *sulfonamides*, which block essential enzymes of folate metabolism. There are several classes of antiviral agents, including: (1) nucleic acid analogs, such as *acyclovir* or *ganciclovir*, which selectively inhibit viral DNA polymerase, and *zidovudine* or *lamivudine*, which inhibit HIV reverse transcriptase; (2) nonnucleoside HIV reverse transcriptase inhibitors, such as *nevirapine* or *efavirenz;* (3) inhibitors of other essential viral enzymes, *e.g.*, inhibitors of HIV protease or influenza neuraminidase; and (4) fusion inhibitors such as enfuvirtide. Additional categories likely will emerge as more complex mechanisms are elucidated. The precise mechanism of action of some antimicrobial agents still is unknown.

Factors That Determine the Susceptibility and Resistance of Microorganisms to Antimicrobial Agents.
Successful antimicrobial therapy of an infection ultimately depends on the concentration of antibiotic at the site of infection. This concentration must be sufficient to inhibit growth of the offending microorganism. If host defenses are intact and active, a minimum inhibitory effect, such as that provided by *bacteriostatic* agents (*i.e.*, agents that interfere with growth or replication of the microorganism but do not kill it) may be sufficient. On the other hand, if host defenses are impaired, antibiotic-mediated killing (*i.e.*, a *bactericidal* effect) may be required to eradicate the infection. The concentration of drug at the site of infection not only must inhibit the organism but also must remain below the level that is toxic to human cells. If this can be achieved, the microorganism is considered susceptible to the antibiotic. If an inhibitory or bactericidal concentration exceeds that which can be achieved safely *in vivo*, then the microorganism is considered resistant to that drug.

The achievable serum concentration for an antibiotic guides selection of the breakpoint for designating a microorganism as either susceptible or resistant by *in vitro* susceptibility testing. However, the concentration at the site of infection may be considerably lower than achievable serum concentrations (*e.g.*, vitreous fluid of the eye or cerebrospinal fluid). Local factors (*e.g.*, low pH, high protein concentration, and anaerobic conditions) also may impair drug activity. Thus, the drug may be only marginally effective or ineffective in such cases even though standardized *in vitro* tests would likely report the microorganism as "sensitive." Conversely, concentrations of drug in urine may be much higher than those in plasma. Microorganisms that might otherwise be considered "resistant" may be eradicated when infection is limited to the urinary tract.

Bacterial Resistance to Antimicrobial Agents. The recent emergence of antibiotic resistance in bacterial pathogens, both nosocomially and in the community, is a very serious development that threatens the end of the antibiotic era. Today, more than 70% of the bacteria associated with hospital-acquired infections in the United States are resistant to one or more of the drugs previously used to treat them. Penicillin-resistant strains of pneumococci account for 50% or more of isolates in some European countries, and the proportion of such strains is rising in the United States. The worldwide emergence of *Haemophilus* and gonococci that produce β-lactamase is a major therapeutic problem. *Methicillin*-resistant strains of *Staphylococcus aureus* are endemic in hospitals and are isolated increasingly from community-acquired infections (Naimi *et al.*, 2003; Vandenesch *et al.*, 2003). Multiple-drug-resistant strains of *S. aureus* with intermediate susceptibility to antibiotics and high-level resistance to vancomycin have been reported (Hiramatsu *et al.*, 1997; Smith *et al.*, 1999; Weigel *et al.*, 2003). There now are strains of enterococci, *Pseudomonas,* and *Enterobacter* that are resistant to all available antibiotics. Epidemics of multiple-drug-resistant strains of *Mycobacterium tuberculosis* have been reported in the United States.

The rampant spread of antibiotic resistance mandates a more responsible approach to antibiotic use. The Centers for Disease Control and Prevention has outlined a series of steps to prevent or diminish antimicrobial resistance. Important components include appropriate use of vaccination, judicious use and proper attention to indwelling catheters, early involvement of infectious disease experts, choosing antibiotic therapy based on local patterns of susceptibilities of organisms, proper antiseptic technique to ensure infection rather than contamination, appropriate use of prophylactic antibiotics in surgical procedures, infection control procedures to isolate the pathogen, and strict compliance to hand hygiene (Anonymous, 2002a, 2002b).

For an antibiotic to be effective, it must reach its target in an active form, bind to the target, and interfere with its function. Accordingly, bacterial resistance to an antimicrobial agent is attributable to three general mechanisms: (1) The drug does not reach its target, (2) the drug is not active, or (3) the target is altered (Davies, 1994; Spratt, 1994; Li and Nikaido, 2004).

The outer membrane of gram-negative bacteria is a permeable barrier that excludes large polar molecules from entering the cell. Small polar molecules, including many antibiotics, enter the cell through protein channels called *porins*. Absence of, mutation in, or loss of a favored porin channel can slow the rate of drug entry into a cell or prevent entry altogether, effectively reducing drug concentration at the target site. If the target is intracellular and the drug requires active transport across the cell membrane, a mutation or phenotypic change that shuts down this transport mechanism can confer resistance. For example, *gentamicin,* which targets the ribosome, is actively transported across the cell membrane using energy provided by the membrane electrochemical gradient. This gradient is generated by respiratory enzymes that couple electron transport and oxidative phosphorylation. A mutation in an enzyme in this pathway or anaerobic conditions (oxygen is the terminal electron acceptor of this pathway, and its absence reduces the membrane potential energy) slows entry of gentamicin into the cell, resulting in resistance. Bacteria also have efflux pumps that can transport drugs out of the cell. Resistance to numerous drugs, including tetracycline, chloramphenicol, fluoroquinolones, macrolides, and *β*-lactam antibiotics, is mediated by an efflux pump mechanism (Li and Nikaido, 2004). Figure 42–1 depicts the multiple membrane and periplasm components that reduce the intracellular concentrations of *β*-lactam antibiotics and cause resistance.

Drug inactivation is the second general mechanism of drug resistance. Bacterial resistance to aminoglycosides and to *β*-lactam antibiotics usually is due to production of an aminoglycoside-modifying enzyme or *β*-lactamase, respectively. A variation of this mechanism is failure of the bacterial cell to activate a prodrug. This is the basis of the most common type of resistance to *isoniazid* in *M. tuberculosis* (Bertrand *et al.*, 2004).

The third general mechanism of drug resistance is target alteration. This may be due to mutation of the natural target (*e.g.*, fluoroquinolone resistance), target modification (*e.g.*, ribosomal protection type of resistance to macrolides and tetracyclines), or acquisition of a resistant form of the native, susceptible target (*e.g.*, staphylococcal

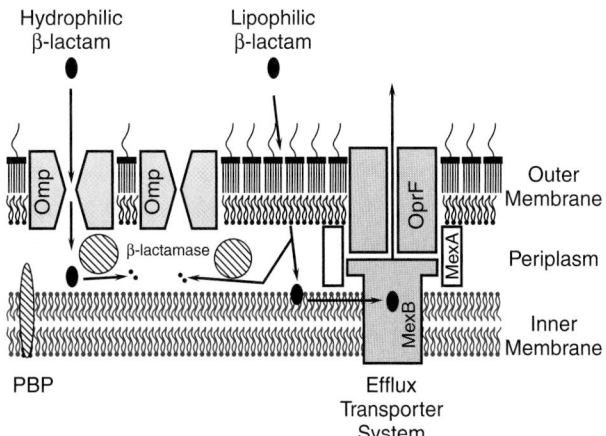

Figure 42–1. *Model depicting the interaction among components mediating resistance to β-lactam antibiotics in Pseudomonas aeruginosa. (Courtesy of Hiroshi Nikaido.)* Most β-lactam antibiotics are hydrophilic and must cross the outer membrane barrier of the cell *via* outer membrane protein (Omp) channels, or porins. The channel has size and charge selectivity such that some Omps slow or block transit of the drug. If an Omp permitting drug entry is altered by mutation, is missing, or is deleted, then drug entry is slowed or prevented. β-Lactamase concentrated between the inner and outer membranes in the periplasmic space constitutes an enzymatic barrier that works in concert with the porin permeability barrier. If the antibiotic is a good substrate for β-lactamase, it will be destroyed rapidly even if the outer membrane is relatively permeable to the drug. If the rate of drug entry is slow, then a relatively inefficient β-lactamase with a slow turnover rate can hydrolyze just enough drug that an effective concentration cannot be achieved. If the target (PBP, penicillin-binding protein) has low binding affinity for the drug or is altered, then the minimum concentration for inhibition is elevated, further contributing to resistance. Finally, β-lactam antibiotics (and other polar antibiotics) that enter the cell and avoid β-lactamase destruction can be taken up by an efflux transporter system (*e.g.,* MexA, MexB, and OprF) and pumped across the outer membrane, further reducing the intracellular concentration of active drug.

methicillin resistance caused by production of a low-affinity penicillin-binding protein) (Nakajima, 1999; Hooper, 2002; Lim and Strynadka, 2002).

Drug resistance may be acquired by mutation and selection, with passage of the trait *vertically* to daughter cells. For mutation and selection to be successful in generating resistance, the mutation cannot be lethal and should not appreciably alter virulence. For the trait to be passed on, the original mutant or its progeny also must disseminate and replicate; otherwise, the mutation will be lost until it is "rediscovered" by some other mutant arising from within a wild-type population.

Drug resistance more commonly is acquired by *horizontal transfer* of resistance determinants from a donor cell, often of another bacterial species, by transduction, transformation, or conjugation. Resistance acquired by horizontal transfer can disseminate rapidly and widely either by clonal spread of the resistant strain or by subsequent transfers to other susceptible recipient strains. For example, the plasmid-encoded staphylococcal β-lactamase gene is distributed widely among many unrelated strains, including enterococci (Murray, 1992). Plasmid-encoded class A β-lactamases of gram-negative bacteria also have spread widely to *Escherichia coli, Neisseria gonorrhoeae,* and *Haemophilus* spp. Horizontal transfer of resistance offers several advantages over mutation-selection. Lethal mutation of an essential gene is avoided; the level of resistance often is higher than that produced by mutation, which tends to yield incremental changes; the gene, which still can be transmitted vertically, can be mobilized and rapidly amplified within a population by transfer to susceptible cells; and the resistance gene can be eliminated when it no longer offers a selective advantage.

Mutation-Selection. Mutation and antibiotic selection of the resistant mutant are the molecular basis for resistance to *streptomycin* (ribosomal mutation), quinolones (gyrase or topoisomerase IV gene mutation), rifampin (RNA polymerase gene mutation), and linezolid (ribosomal RNA mutation). This mechanism underlies all drug resistance in *M. tuberculosis* (Riska *et al.*, 2000). Mutations may occur in the gene encoding (1) the target protein, altering its structure so that it no longer binds the drug; (2) a protein involved in drug transport; (3) a protein important for drug activation or inactivation, in the case of extended-spectrum β-lactamases (Bush, 2001); or (4) in a regulatory gene or promoter affecting expression of the target, a transport protein, or an inactivating enzyme. Mutations are not caused by drug exposure *per se*. They are random events that confer a survival advantage when drug is present. However, certain drugs that induce the bacterial SOS system of DNA repair proteins that accommodate potentially lethal stress (*e.g.*, fluoroquinolones) may facilitate resistance gene transfer or increase the mutation frequency by induction of error-prone polymerases (Goodman, 2002; Chopra *et al.*, 2003; Beaber *et al.*, 2004). Any large population of antibiotic-susceptible bacteria is likely to contain rare mutants that are only slightly less susceptible than the parent. Through sequential acquisition of more mutations, clinically significant resistance may emerge. High-level resistance of *E. coli* to fluoroquinolones is due to such an accumulation of multiple stepwise mutations. In some instances, a single-step mutation results in a high degree of resistance. For example, a point mutation within the drug-binding domain in the β subunit of bacterial RNA polymerase confers high-level resistance to rifampin.

Horizontal Gene Transfer. Horizontal transfer of resistance genes is greatly facilitated by and is largely dependent on mobile genetic elements. The role of plasmids and transducing phages as carriers of resistance genes and transfer elements is discussed in more detail

below. Other mobile elements, transposable elements, integrons, and gene cassettes also participate in the process. Transposable elements are of three general types: insertion sequences, transposons, and transposable phages; two of these, insertion sequences and transposons, are important for resistance. *Insertion sequences* (Mahillon and Chandler, 1998) are short segments of DNA encoding enzymatic functions (*e.g.*, transposase and resolvase) for site-specific recombination with inverted repeat sequences at either end. They can copy themselves and insert themselves into the chromosome or a plasmid. Insertion sequences do not encode resistance, but they function as sites for integration of other resistance-encoding elements, *e.g.*, plasmids or transposons.

Transposons are basically insertion sequences that also code for other functions, one of which can be drug resistance. Since transposons move between chromosome and plasmid, the resistance gene can hitchhike its way onto a transferable element out of the host and into a recipient. Transposons are mobile elements that excise and integrate in the bacterial genomic or plasmid DNA (*i.e.*, from plasmid to plasmid, from plasmid to chromosome, or from chromosome to plasmid).

Integrons (Fluit and Schmitz, 2004) are not formally mobile and do not copy themselves, but they encode an integrase and provide a specific site into which mobile gene cassettes integrate. *Gene cassettes* encode resistance determinants, usually lacking a promoter, with a downstream repeat sequence. The integrase recognizes this repeat sequence and directs insertion of the cassette into position behind a strong promoter that is present on the integron. Integrons may be located within transposons or in plasmids, and therefore may be mobilizable, or located on the chromosome.

Another type of gene cassette, *SCCmec* (*S*taphylococcal *C*hromosomal *C*assette), has been described in methicillin-resistant strains of staphylococci (Katayama, *et al.*, 2000). The methicillin resistance gene *mecA* is located within this cassette along with recombinase genes. The recombinases both excise and integrate the cassette element, which exists as a circular intermediate that is not self-replicating, into a very specific site in the staphylococcal chromosome. How this element is transferred and the role of excision–mobilization in this process are not known.

Transduction. Transduction is acquisition of bacterial DNA from a phage (a virus that propagates in bacteria) that has incorporated DNA from a previous host bacterium within its outer protein coat. If the DNA includes a gene for drug resistance, the newly infected bacterial cell may acquire resistance. Transduction is particularly important in the transfer of antibiotic resistance among strains of *S. aureus.*

Transformation. Transformation is the uptake and incorporation into the host genome by homologous recombination of free DNA released into the environment by other bacterial cells. Transformation is the molecular basis of penicillin resistance in pneumococci and *Neisseria* (Spratt, 1994). Penicillin-resistant pneumococci produce altered penicillin-binding proteins (PBPs) that have low-affinity binding of penicillin. Nucleotide sequence analysis of the genes encoding these altered PBPs indicates that they are mosaics in which blocks of foreign DNA from a closely related species of streptococcus have been imported and incorporated into the resident PBP gene.

Conjugation. Conjugation is gene transfer by direct cell-to-cell contact through a sex pilus or bridge. This complex and fascinating mechanism for the spread of antibiotic resistance is extremely important because multiple resistance genes can be transferred in a single event. The transferable genetic material consists of two different sets of plasmid-encoded genes that may be on the same or different plasmids. One set encodes the actual resistance; the second encodes genes necessary for the bacterial conjugation process.

Conjugative plasmids tend to be rather large (50 kilobases or more). They combine elements of plasmid DNA rolling-circle replication (only a single strand is transferred, and it replicates in the host) with a type IV bacterial secretion system. Plasmid transfer requires an origin of transfer demarcating the site within the plasmid where transfer will occur, DNA replicating enzymes, and coupling proteins that direct the DNA across two cell membranes on its way from the host into the recipient. Genes encoding the resistance determinants may be located on transposons.

Conjugation with genetic exchange between nonpathogenic and pathogenic microorganisms probably occurs in the GI tracts of human beings and animals. The efficiency of transfer is low; however, antibiotics can exert a powerful selective pressure to allow emergence of the resistant strain. Genetic transfer by conjugation is common among gram-negative bacilli, and resistance is conferred on a susceptible cell as a single event. Enterococci also contain a broad range of host-range conjugative plasmids that are involved in the transfer and spread of resistance genes among gram-positive organisms. Vancomycin resistance in enterococci is mediated by a conjugative plasmid (Arthur and Courvalin, 1993; Murray, 2000). Vancomycin resistance in *S. aureus* is due to conjugative transfer of vanA-type vancomycin resistance genes encoded on a transposon from *Enterococcus faecalis* donor into a methicillin-resistant strain of *S. aureus* with subsequent integration of the transposon into a resident staphylococcal conjugative plasmid (Weigel *et al.*, 2003).

Selection of an Antimicrobial Agent

Optimal and judicious selection of antimicrobial agents for the therapy of infectious diseases requires clinical judgment and detailed knowledge of pharmacological and microbiological factors. Antibiotics have three general uses: empirical therapy, definitive therapy, and prophylactic or preventive therapy. When used as empirical, or initial, therapy, the antibiotic should cover all the likely pathogens because the infecting organism(s) has not yet been defined. Either combination therapy or, preferably, treatment with a single broad-spectrum agent may be employed. However, once the infecting microorganism is identified, definitive antimicrobial therapy should be instituted with a narrow-spectrum, low-toxicity agent to complete the course of treatment. Failure to document the bacterial etiology so that a narrow-spectrum agent can be used and failure to narrow the spectrum when an organism has been identified are two common ways in which antibiotics are misused.

The first consideration in selecting an antimicrobial agent is whether it is even indicated. *The reflex action to associate fever with treatable infections and prescribe antimicrobial therapy without further evaluation is irrational and potentially dangerous.* The diagnosis may be masked if therapy is started and appropriate cultures are not obtained. Antibiotics are potentially toxic, and antimi-crobial agents promote selection of resistant microorganisms. Of course, definitive identification of a bacterial infection before treatment is initiated often is not possible. In the absence of a clear indication, antibiotics often may be used if disease is severe and if it seems likely that withholding therapy will result in failure to manage a potentially serious or life-threatening infection.

Initiation of optimal empirical antibiotic therapy requires knowledge of the most likely infecting microorganisms and their susceptibilities to antimicrobial drugs. Selection of an antibiotic regimen should rely on the clinical presentation, which may suggest the specific microorganism, and knowledge of the microorganisms most likely to cause specific infections in a given host. In addition, simple and rapid laboratory techniques are available for the examination of infected tissues. The most valuable and time-tested method for immediate identification of bacteria is examination of the infected secretion or body fluid with Gram's stain. Such tests help to narrow the list of potential pathogens and permit more rational selection of initial antibiotic therapy. However, in many situations, identification of the morphology of the infecting organism is not adequate to arrive at a specific bacteriological diagnosis, and the selection of a single narrow-spectrum antibiotic may be inappropriate, particularly if the infection is life threatening. Broad antimicrobial coverage is then indicated, pending isolation and identification of the microorganism. *Whenever the clinician is faced with initiating therapy on a presumptive bacteriological diagnosis, cultures of the presumed site of infection and blood, if bacteremia is a possibility, should be taken prior to the institution of drug therapy.* For definitive therapy, the regimen should be changed to a more specific and narrow-spectrum antimicrobial agent once an organism has been isolated and results of susceptibility tests are known.

Testing for Microbial Sensitivity to Antimicrobial Agents. Bacterial strains, even from the same species, may vary widely in sensitivity to antibiotics. Information about the antimicrobial susceptibility of the infecting microorganism is important for appropriate drug selection. Several tests are available for determination of bacterial sensitivity to antimicrobial agents. The most commonly used are disk-diffusion tests, agar- or broth-dilution tests, and automated test systems.

The disk-diffusion technique provides only qualitative or semi-quantitative information on antimicrobial susceptibility. The test is performed by applying commercially available filter-paper disks impregnated with a specific amount of the drug onto an agar surface, over which a culture of the microorganism has been streaked. After 18 to 24 hours of incubation, the size of the clear zone of inhibition around the disk is measured. The diameter of the zone depends on the activity of the drug against the test strain. Standardized values for zone sizes for each bacterial species and each antibiotic permit classification of the clinical isolate as resistant, intermediate, or susceptible.

Dilution tests employ antibiotics in serially diluted concentrations in solid agar or broth medium containing a culture of the test microorganism. The lowest concentration of the agent that prevents visible growth after 18 to 24 hours of incubation is known as the *minimal inhibitory concentration* (MIC).

Automated systems also use a broth-dilution method. The optical density of a broth culture of the clinical isolate incubated in the presence of drug is determined. If the density of the culture exceeds a threshold optical density, then growth has occurred at that concentration of drug. The MIC is the concentration at which the optical density remains below the threshold.

Pharmacokinetic Factors. In vitro activity, although critical, is only a guide as to whether an antibiotic is likely to be effective for an infection. Successful therapy also depends on achieving a drug concentration that is sufficient to inhibit or kill bacteria at the site of the infection without harming the patient. To accomplish this therapeutic goal, several pharmacokinetic and host factors must be evaluated.

The location of the infection to a large extent may dictate the choice of drug and the route of administration. The minimal drug concentration achieved at the infected site should be approximately equal to the MIC for the infecting organism, although in most instances it is advisable to achieve multiples of this concentration if possible. However, there is evidence to suggest that even subinhibitory concentrations of antibiotics may enhance phagocytosis (Nosanchuk *et al.*, 1999) and may be effective. Although this may explain why some infections are cured even when inhibitory concentrations are not achieved, it should be the aim of antimicrobial therapy to produce antibacterial concentrations of drug at the site of infection during the dosing interval. This can be achieved only if the pharmacokinetic and pharmacodynamic principles presented in Chapter 1 are understood and employed.

Access of antibiotics to sites of infection depends on multiple factors. If the infection is in the cerebrospinal fluid (CSF), the drug must pass the blood–brain barrier. Antimicrobial agents that are polar at physiological pH generally penetrate poorly; some, such as *penicillin G,* are actively transported out of the CSF by an anion transport mechanism in the choroid plexus. The concentrations of penicillins and cephalosporins in the CSF usually are only 0.5% to 5% of steady-state concentrations determined simultaneously in plasma. However, the integrity of the blood–brain barrier is diminished during active bacterial infection; tight junctions in cerebral capillaries open, leading to a marked increase in the penetration of even polar

drugs (Quagliarello and Scheld, 1997). As the infection is eradicated and the inflammatory reaction subsides, penetration returns to normal. Since this may occur while viable microorganisms persist in the CSF, drug dosage should not be reduced as the patient improves.

Penetration of drugs into sites of infection almost always depends on passive diffusion. The rate of penetration is thus proportional to the concentration of free drug in the plasma or extracellular fluid. Drugs that are extensively bound to protein thus may not penetrate to the same extent as those bound to a lesser extent. Drugs that are highly protein bound also may have reduced activity because only the unbound fraction of drug is free to interact with its target.

Traditionally, the dose and dosing frequency of antibiotics have been selected to achieve antibacterial activity at the site of infection for most of the dosing interval. However, controversy exists as to whether the therapeutic effect achieved from relatively constant antibacterial activity is superior to that from high peak concentrations followed by periods of subinhibitory activity. To a certain extent, this depends on whether a drug exhibits concentration- or time-dependent growth inhibition (Craig, 1998). The activity of β-lactam antibiotics, for example, is primarily time-dependent, whereas that of aminoglycosides is concentration-dependent. Activity also may depend on the specific organism and the site of infection. Studies in animals with meningitis suggest that pulse dosing (intermittent administration) of β-lactam antibiotics may be more efficacious than continuous exposure (Täuber *et al.*, 1989), but constant activity apparently is superior in other experimental infections. Experimental data suggest that aminoglycosides are at least as efficacious and less toxic when given in a single, large daily dose than when given more frequently (Barclay *et al.*, 1999). Studies in patients also suggest that continuous administration of aminoglycosides may cause unnecessary toxicity.

Knowledge of the status of the individual patient's renal and hepatic function also is essential, especially when excessive plasma or tissue concentrations of the drugs may cause serious toxicity. Most antimicrobial agents and their metabolites are eliminated primarily by the kidneys. Nomograms are available to facilitate adjustment of dosage of many such agents in patients with renal insufficiency. These are discussed in the chapters dealing with the individual drugs and in Appendix II. One must be particularly careful when using aminoglycosides, vancomycin, or *flucytosine* in patients with impaired renal function because these drugs are eliminated exclusively by renal mechanisms, and their toxicity correlates with their concentration in plasma and tissue. If renal toxicity of a drug that is cleared by the kidney occurs and care is not exercised, a vicious cycle may ensue. For drugs that are metabolized or excreted by the liver (*e.g.,* erythromycin, chloramphenicol, metronidazole, and clindamycin), dosages may have to be reduced in patients with hepatic disease.

Route of Administration. The discussion of choice of routes of administration that appears in Chapter 1 obviously applies to antimicrobial agents. While oral administration is preferred whenever possible, parenteral administration of antibiotics usually is recommended in seriously ill patients in whom predictable concentrations of drug must be achieved. Specific factors that govern the choice of route of administration for individual agents are discussed in the chapters that follow.

Host Factors. Innate host factors can be the prime determinants not only of the type of drug selected but also of its dosage, route of administration, risk and nature of untoward effects, and therapeutic effectiveness.

Host Defense Mechanisms. A critical determinant of the therapeutic effectiveness of antimicrobial agents is the functional state of host defense mechanisms. Both humoral and cellular immunity are important. Inadequacy of type, quality, and quantity of the immunoglobulins; alteration of the cellular immune system; or a qualitative or quantitative defect in phagocytic cells may result in therapeutic failure despite the use of otherwise appropriate and effective drugs. In the immunocompetent host, merely halting multiplication of the microorganisms with a bacteriostatic agent frequently is sufficient to cure the infection. If host defenses are impaired, bacteriostatic activity may be inadequate, and a bactericidal agent may be required for cure. Examples include bacterial endocarditis, where phagocytic cells are absent from the infected site; bacterial meningitis, where phagocytic cells are ineffective because of lack of opsonins in CSF; and disseminated bacterial infections in neutropenic patients, where the total mass of phagocytic cells is reduced. Patients with acquired immune deficiency syndrome (AIDS) have impaired cellular immune responses, and therapy for various opportunistic infections in these patients often is suppressive but not curative. For example, most AIDS patients with bacteremia owing to *Salmonella* will respond to conventional therapy, but this infection may relapse even after prolonged treatment (Gordon *et al.,* 2002). Similarly, treatment of disseminated atypical mycobacterial infection is recommended as long as CD4 counts are below 100 cells/μl (Kaplan *et al.,* 2002).

Local Factors. Cure of an infection with antibiotics depends on an understanding of how local factors at the site of infection affect the antimicrobial activity of the drug. Antimicrobial activity may be reduced significantly in pus, which contains phagocytes, cellular debris, and proteins that can bind drugs or create conditions unfavorable to drug action (Konig *et al.,* 1998). Low pH, characteristic of the fluid in abscesses and in other confined infected sites (pleural space, CSF, and urine), and anaerobic conditions can reduce the antimicrobial activity of some agents markedly, particularly the aminoglycosides. In addition, penetration of antimicrobial agents into infected areas such as abscess cavities can be impaired because the vascular supply is reduced. Successful therapy of abscesses usually requires drainage.

The presence of a foreign body in an infected site markedly reduces the likelihood of successful antimicrobial therapy. Prosthetic material (*e.g.,* prosthetic cardiac valves, prosthetic joints, pacemakers, vascular grafts, and various vascular and CNS shunts) promotes formation of a bacterial biofilm that impairs phagocytosis (Leid *et al.,* 2002). Conditions within the biofilm, where bacterial densities often are high, slow bacterial growth. Because rapidly growing cells are more susceptible to antibiotics than slowly growing or stationary cells, antimicrobial activity is reduced, favoring bacterial persistence (Lewis, 2001). Infections associated with foreign bodies thus are characterized by frequent relapses and failure, even with long-term, high-dose antibiotic therapy. Successful therapy usually requires removal of the foreign material.

Intracellular pathogens, *e.g., Salmonella, Brucella, Toxoplasma, Listeria,* and *M. tuberculosis,* are protected from the action of antimicrobial agents that penetrate into cells poorly. Certain antibiotics—*e.g.,* fluoroquinolones, isoniazid, trimethoprim–sulfamethoxazole, and rifampin—penetrate cells well and can achieve intracellular concentrations that inhibit or kill pathogens residing within cells.

Age. The age of the patient is an important determinant of antimicrobial drug pharmacokinetics. Mechanisms of elimination, especially renal excretion and hepatic biotransformation, are poorly developed in the newborn, especially the premature infant. Failure to make adjustments for such differences can have disastrous consequences (*e.g., see* discussion of the gray-baby syndrome, caused by chloramphenicol, in Chapter 46). Elderly patients clear drugs eliminated by the kidneys less well because of reduced creatinine clearance. They also may metabolize drugs less rapidly, predisposing them to elevated and potentially toxic concentrations of drugs when compared with younger patients. Elderly patients therefore are more likely to suffer toxicity at otherwise safe concentrations of drugs, as is the case for aminoglycoside ototoxicity.

Developmental factors also may determine the type of untoward response to a drug. Tetracyclines bind avidly to developing teeth and bones, and their use in young children can result in retardation of bone growth and discoloration or hypoplasia of tooth enamel.

Fluoroquinolones accumulate in the cartilage of developing bone, affecting its growth. Kernicterus may follow the use of sulfonamides in newborn infants because this class of drugs competes effectively with bilirubin for binding sites on plasma albumin. Achlorhydria in young children and in the elderly or antacid therapy may alter absorption of orally administered antimicrobial agents (*e.g.*, increased absorption of penicillin G and decreased absorption of *ketoconazole* and *itraconazole*).

Genetic Factors. Certain genetic or metabolic abnormalities must be considered when prescribing antibiotics. A number of drugs (*e.g.*, sulfonamides, *nitrofurantoin,* chloramphenicol, and *nalidixic acid*) may produce acute hemolysis in patients with glucose-6-phosphate dehydrogenase deficiency. Patients who acetylate isoniazid rapidly may have subtherapeutic concentrations of the drug in plasma.

Pregnancy. Pregnancy may impose an increased risk of reaction to antimicrobial agents for both mother and fetus. Hearing loss in the child has been associated with administration of streptomycin to the mother during pregnancy. Tetracyclines can affect the bones and teeth of the fetus. Pregnant women receiving tetracycline may develop fatal acute fatty necrosis of the liver, pancreatitis, and associated renal damage. Pregnancy also may affect the pharmacokinetics of various antibiotics.

The lactating female can pass antimicrobial agents to her nursing child. Both nalidixic acid and the sulfonamides in breast milk have been associated with hemolysis in children with glucose-6-phosphate dehydrogenase deficiency. In addition, sulfonamides, even in the small amounts received from breast milk, may predispose the nursing child to kernicterus.

Drug Allergy. Antibiotics, especially β-lactams, are notorious for provoking allergic reactions. Patients with a history of atopy seem particularly susceptible to the development of these reactions. Sulfonamides, trimethoprim, nitrofurantoin, and erythromycin also have been associated with hypersensitivity reactions, especially rash. A history of anaphylaxis (immediate hypersensitivity reaction) or hives and laryngeal edema (accelerated reaction) precludes use of the drug in all but extreme, life-threatening situations. Skin testing, particularly of the penicillins, may be of value in predicting life-threatening reactions. Antimicrobial agents, like other drugs, can cause drug fever, which can be mistaken for a sign of continued infection.

Comorbid Conditions. Patients predisposed to seizures are at risk for localized or major motor seizures while taking high doses of penicillin G. This neurotoxicity of penicillin and other β-lactam antibiotics correlates with high concentrations of drug in the CSF and typically occurs in patients with impaired renal function who are given large doses of the drugs. Isoniazid causes a peripheral neuropathy that is preventable and reversible by administration of *pyridoxine*. Diabetics and HIV-infected patients, who are prone to neuropathy because of their underlying diseases, and alcoholics, who often are malnourished, are particularly predisposed. Oncology and HIV-infected patients often have bone marrow suppression, which makes them particularly susceptible to hematologic side effects of antibiotics. Patients with myasthenia gravis or other neuromuscular problems are susceptible to the neuromuscular blocking effect of the aminoglycosides.

Therapy with Combined Antimicrobial Agents

The simultaneous use of two or more antimicrobial agents is recommended in specifically defined situations based on pharmacological rationale. However, selection of an appropriate combination requires an understanding of the potential for interaction between the antimicrobial agents. Interactions may affect either the microorganism or the patient. Antimicrobial agents acting at different targets may enhance or impair overall antimicrobial activity. A combination of drugs also may have additive or superadditive toxicities. For example, vancomycin given alone usually has minimal nephrotoxicity. However, when vancomycin is given with an aminoglycoside, the toxicity of the aminoglycoside is increased (Rybak *et al.*, 1999).

Methods of Testing Antimicrobial Activity of Drug Combinations. Two methods are used to measure antimicrobial activity of drug combinations. The first employs serial twofold dilutions of antibiotics in broth inoculated with a standard number of the test microorganism in a checkerboard array so that a large number of antibiotic concentrations in different proportions can be tested simultaneously (Figure 42–2). The concentrations of each drug, singly and in combination, that prevent visible growth are determined after an 18- to 24-hour incubation. *Synergism* is defined as inhibition of growth by a combination of drugs at concentrations less than or equal to 25% of the MIC of each drug acting alone. This implies that one drug is affecting the microorganism in such a way that it becomes more sensitive to the inhibitory effect of the other. If one-half the inhibitory concentration of each drug is required to produce inhibition, the result is called *additive* [fractional inhibitory concentration (FIC) index = 1] (Figure 42–2), suggesting that the two drugs are working independently of each other. If more than one-half the MIC of each drug is necessary to produce the inhibitory effect, the drugs are said to be *antagonistic* (FIC index >1). When the drugs are tested for a variety of proportionate drug concentrations, as with the checkerboard technique, an isobologram may be constructed (Figure 42–2). Synergism is shown by a concave curve, the additive effect by a straight line, and antagonism by a convex curve. Since the endpoint is growth inhibition, not killing, synergism by this method may not indicate enhanced bactericidal effect.

The second method for evaluating drug combinations is the time–kill curve, which assays bactericidal activity. Identical cultures are incubated simultaneously with antibiotics added singly or in combination. Quantitative subcultures are taken over time to determine the number of bacteria remaining. If a combination of antibiotics is more bactericidal than either drug alone, typically defined as at least a hundredfold reduction in the inoculum for the combination compared with the most active single agent, the result is termed *synergism*. If the combination kills

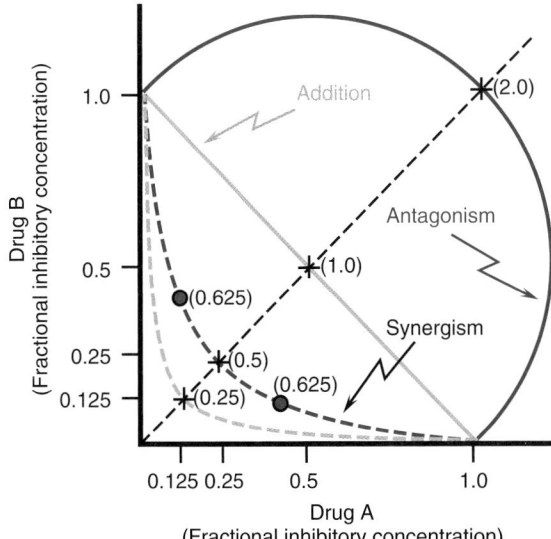

Figure 42–2. *Effect of combinations of two antimicrobial agents to inhibit bacterial growth.* The effects are expressed as isobols and fractional inhibitory concentration (FIC) indices. Based on the minimum inhibitory concentration (MIC), the FIC index is equal to the sum of the values of FIC for the individual drugs:

$$FIC\ index\ =\ \frac{(MIC\ of\ A\ with\ B)}{(MIC\ of\ A\ alone)}+\frac{(MIC\ of\ B\ with\ A)}{(MIC\ of\ B\ alone)}$$

Points on concave isobols (FIC index < 1) are indicative of synergistic interaction between the two agents, and points on convex isobols (FIC index > 1) represent antagonism. The nature of the interaction is adequately revealed by testing combinations lying along the black dashed line (marked +). *See* text for further explanation.

fewer bacteria than the most active drug alone, *antagonism* is said to occur. If the combination kills the same number of bacteria or results in less than a hundredfold reduction in the inoculum compared with the most active single drug, the result is called *indifference*.

Bacteriostatic antibiotics (*e.g.*, tetracyclines, erythromycin, and chloramphenicol) frequently antagonize the action of bactericidal drugs (*e.g.*, β-lactam antibiotics, vancomycin, and aminoglycosides) because bacteriostatic antibiotics inhibit cell division and protein synthesis, which are required for the bactericidal effect of most bactericidal agents. Bactericidal drugs in combination tend to be additive or synergistic. For example, an inhibitor of cell wall synthesis and an aminoglycoside are synergistic against many bacterial species. Rifampin combinations appear to be an exception to this general rule. Although it is bactericidal, rifampin inhibits protein synthesis, which may account for its indifferent or antagonistic effect *in vitro* when combined with other bactericidal antibiotics.

The clinical relevance of this phenomenon is not clear because rifampin combinations are effective clinically.

Indications for the Clinical Use of Combinations of Antimicrobial Agents. Use of a combination of antimicrobial agents may be justified (1) for empirical therapy of an infection in which the cause is unknown, (2) for treatment of polymicrobial infections, (3) to enhance antimicrobial activity (*i.e.*, synergism) for a specific infection, or (4) to prevent emergence of resistance.

Empirical Therapy of Severe Infections in Which a Cause Is Unknown. Empirical therapy of infection probably is the most common reason for using a combination of antibiotics. Knowledge of the type(s) of infection(s), the microbiology, and the spectrum of activity of the several potentially useful antimicrobial agents is essential for selection of a rational and effective regimen (Anonymous, 2001). Severe illness and less certainty as to the particular infection or the causative agent may mandate broad coverage initially. More than one agent may be required to ensure that the regimen includes an agent that is active against the potential pathogens. For example, in the treatment of community-acquired pneumonia, a macrolide is used for atypical organisms such as *Mycoplasma,* and *cefuroxime* is used for pneumococci and gram-negative pathogens. Prolonged administration of empirical broad-spectrum coverage or multiple antibiotics, however, should be avoided; it often is unnecessary (*e.g.*, when the infection is caused by a single pathogen or no infection is documented) and unnecessarily expensive. Moreover, toxicity, superinfection, and selection of multiple-drug-resistant microorganisms may result. Inappropriately broad coverage often is continued because adequate cultures were not obtained prior to the initiation of therapy or because of the misconception that a broad-spectrum regimen is superior to a narrow-spectrum regimen. Although reluctance to change antimicrobial agents is understandable when a favorable clinical response has occurred, *the goal should be to use the most selectively active drug that produces the fewest adverse effects, which includes adverse affects on host normal flora.*

Treatment of Polymicrobial Infections. Treatment of intra-abdominal, hepatic, and brain abscesses and some genital tract infections may require the use of a drug combination to eradicate these typically mixed aerobic–anaerobic infections. These and other mixed infections may be caused by two or more microorganisms that are sufficiently different in antimicrobial susceptibility such that no single agent can provide the required coverage.

Enhancement of Antibacterial Activity in the Treatment of Specific Infections. Antimicrobial agents administered together may produce a synergistic effect. Synergistic combinations of antimicrobial agents have been shown to be better than single-agent therapy in relatively few infections.

Perhaps the best-documented example of the utility of a synergistic combination of antimicrobial agents is in the treatment of enterococcal endocarditis (Wilson *et al.*, 1995). *In vitro*, penicillin alone is bacteriostatic against enterococci, whereas a combination of penicillin and streptomycin or gentamicin is bactericidal. Treatment of enterococcal endocarditis with penicillin alone frequently results in relapses, whereas combination therapy is curative.

The combination of penicillin and streptomycin or gentamicin also is synergistic *in vitro* against strains of *viridans* streptococci. This combination eradicates bacteria from infected valvular vegetations more rapidly than does penicillin alone in animal models. A 2-week course of treatment with the combination is just as effective as a 4-week penicillin-only regimen for patients with streptococcal endocarditis. β-Lactam antibiotic–aminoglycoside combinations have been recommended in the therapy of infections with *Pseudomonas aeruginosa*. *In vitro*, an antipseudomonal β-lactam plus an aminoglycoside is synergistic against most strains of *P. aeruginosa*. This combination is more active than either drug alone in animal models. Some but not all clinical studies suggest that outcome is improved when a β-lactam plus an aminoglycoside combination is used for serious pseudomonal infections (Paul *et al.*, 2004; Hilf *et al.*, 1989; Leibovici *et al.*, 1997). Combination therapy has been advocated for the treatment of infections caused by other gram-negative rods. However, the benefits of using a drug combination over a single, effective agent remain largely unproven (Barriere, 1992; Rybak and McGrath, 1996).

The combination of a sulfonamide and an inhibitor of dihydrofolate reductase, such as trimethoprim, is synergistic owing to the blocking of sequential steps in microbial folate synthesis. A fixed combination of sulfamethoxazole and trimethoprim, which is active against organisms that may be resistant to sulfonamides alone, is effective for the treatment of urinary tract infections, *Pneumocystis* pneumonia, typhoid fever, shigellosis, and certain infections owing to ampicillin-resistant *Haemophilus influenzae*.

The combination of flucytosine and amphotericin B is synergistic against *Cryptococcus neoformans in vitro* and in animal models of infection. This combination also has been shown to sterilize the CSF more rapidly than amphotericin B alone in AIDS patients with cryptococcal meningitis (van der Horst *et al.*, 1997).

Prevention of the Emergence of Resistant Microorganisms. The theoretical basis for combination therapy of tuberculosis is to prevent the emergence of resistant mutants that might result from monotherapy. For example, if the frequency of mutation for the acquisition of resistance to one drug is 10^{-7} and that for a second drug is 10^{-6}, the probability of two simultaneous, independent mutations in a single cell is the product of the two frequencies, 10^{-13}. The number of organisms that would have to be present for such a mutant to occur is several orders of magnitude greater than that likely to be encountered clinically. The concomitant use of two or more active agents vastly improves cure rates by preventing the development of resistance. Other examples supporting the concept of combination therapy include infections that are treated with rifampin, such as staphylococcal osteomyelitis or prosthetic valve endocarditis (Zimmerli *et al.*, 1998), in which a second agent is added to prevent emergence of rifampin-resistant mutants, and combination therapy of *Helicobacter pylori* infection (Taylor *et al.*, 1997). Other than for these specific examples, few data document that drug combinations improve outcome by preventing the emergence of resistance.

Disadvantages of Combinations of Antimicrobial Agents. Disadvantages of antimicrobial combinations include increased risk of toxicity from two or more agents, selection of multiple-drug-resistant microorganisms, eradication of normal host flora with subsequent superinfection, and increased cost to the patient. Although antagonism of one antibiotic by another has been a frequent observation *in vitro*, well-documented clinical examples of this phenomenon are relatively rare. The most notable of these involves the therapy of pneumococcal meningitis. Lepper and Dowling reported in 1951 that the fatality rate among patients with pneumococcal meningitis who were treated with penicillin alone was 21%, whereas patients treated with a combination of penicillin and *chlortetracycline* had a fatality rate of 79%. Nonetheless, because the addition of a bacteriostatic drug to a bactericidal drug frequently results in a bacteriostatic effect, antagonism between antibiotics probably is relatively unimportant when host defenses are adequate. On the other hand, if achieving a bactericidal effect is critical for cure of the infection (*e.g.*, meningitis, endocarditis, and gram-negative infections in neutropenic patients), such antibiotic antagonism could adversely affect outcome.

The Prophylaxis of Infection with Antimicrobial Agents

Chemoprophylaxis is highly effective in some clinical settings. In others, it accounts for some of the most flagrant misuses of antimicrobials, is totally without value, and may be deleterious. Use of antimicrobial compounds to prevent infections remains controversial in numerous situations. *In general, if a single, effective, nontoxic drug is used to prevent infection by a specific microorganism or to eradicate an early infection, then chemoprophylaxis frequently is successful. On the other hand, if the aim of prophylaxis is to prevent colonization or infection by any or all microorganisms present in the environment of a patient, then prophylaxis often fails.*

Prophylaxis may be used to protect healthy persons from acquisition of or invasion by specific microorganisms to which they are exposed. Successful examples of this practice include rifampin administration to prevent meningococcal meningitis in people who are in close contact with a case, prevention of gonorrhea or syphilis after contact with an infected person, and the intermittent use of trimethoprim–sulfamethoxazole to prevent recurrent urinary tract infections usually caused by *E. coli*.

Antimicrobial prophylaxis, often with an oral fluoroquinolone, is used to prevent a variety of infections in patients undergoing organ transplantation or receiving cancer chemotherapy. Although specific infections often can be prevented, superinfections with opportunistic fungal pathogens or multiple-drug-resistant bacteria can be a problem. Moreover, the infection rate may be lowered without changing overall outcomes. Prophylaxis is recommended for primary and secondary prevention of opportunistic infections in AIDS patients whose CD4 counts are below certain thresholds, *e.g.*, less than 200 cells/μl for the prevention of *Pneumocystis* pneumonia and less than 50 cells/μl for prevention of atypical mycobacterial infection (Kaplan *et al.*, 2002).

Chemoprophylaxis is recommended for patients with valvular or other structural lesions of the heart predisposing to endocarditis who are undergoing dental, surgical, or other procedures that produce a high incidence of bacteremia (Dajani *et al.*, 1997). Clinical data suggesting that dental procedures have a minimal, if indeed any, role in causing endocarditis (Strom *et al.*, 1998) have challenged some of the recommendations for chemoprophylaxis, but the recommendations nevertheless remain the standard of care. A procedure that injures a mucous membrane where there are large numbers of bacteria (such as in the oropharyngeal or gastrointestinal tract) will produce transient bacteremia. Streptococci from the mouth, enterococci from the gastrointestinal or genitourinary tract, and staphylococci from the skin commonly enter the bloodstream and may adhere to an abnormal or damaged valve surface, producing endocarditis. Chemoprophylaxis is directed against these microorganisms. Therapy, generally as a single dose, should begin 1 hour before the procedure for oral drugs and 30 minutes for parental drugs. Criteria have been established for the selection of specific drugs and patients who should receive chemoprophylaxis for various procedures (Table 42–1).

The most extensive and probably best-studied use of chemoprophylaxis is to prevent wound infections after various surgical procedures (Bratzler and Houck, 2004) (Table 42–1). Wound infection results when a critical number of bacteria are present in the wound at the time of closure. Several factors determine the size of this critical inoculum, including virulence of the bacteria, the presence of devitalized or poorly vascularized tissue, the presence of a foreign body, and the status of the host. Antimicrobial agents directed against the invading microorganisms may reduce the number of viable bacteria below the critical level and thus prevent infection.

Several factors are important for the effective and judicious use of antibiotics for surgical prophylaxis. First, antimicrobial activity must be present at the wound site at the time of its closure. Thus the drug should be given preoperatively (1 hour before incision) and perhaps intraoperatively for prolonged procedures to ensure that therapeutic levels are maintained during the entire procedure. Second, the antibiotic must be active against the most likely contaminating microorganisms. Thus cephalosporins are used commonly in this form of chemoprophylaxis. Third, prolonged administration of drugs after the surgical procedure is unwarranted and potentially harmful. No data suggest that the incidence of wound infections is lower if antimicrobial treatment is continued after the day of surgery (Bratzler and Houck, 2004). Use beyond 24 hours not only is unnecessary but also leads to the development of more resistant flora and superinfections caused by antibiotic-resistant strains. Chemoprophylaxis should be limited to operative procedures for which there are data supporting its use. A number of studies indicate that it can be justified in dirty or contaminated surgical procedures (*e.g.*, resection of the colon), where the incidence of wound infections is high. These include less than 10% of all surgical procedures. In clean surgical procedures, which account for approximately 75% of the total, the expected incidence of wound infection is less than 5%, and antibiotics should not be used routinely. When the surgery involves insertion of a prosthetic implant (*e.g.*, prosthetic valve, vascular graft, prosthetic joint), cardiac surgery, or neurosurgical procedures, the complications of infection are so drastic that most authorities currently agree to chemoprophylaxis with these indications. Of course, the use of systemic antibiotics for chemoprophylaxis during surgical procedures does not reduce the need for sterile and skilled surgical technique.

Superinfections

All individuals who receive therapeutic doses of antibiotics undergo alterations in the normal microbial population of the intestinal, upper respiratory, and genitourinary tracts; as a result, some develop *superinfection,* defined as the appearance of bacteriological and clinical evidence of a new infection during the chemotherapy of a primary one. This phenomenon is relatively common and potentially very dangerous because the microorganisms respon-

Table 42–1
Guidelines for Prophylactic Antibiotics in Surgical Procedures

Antibiotics should be administered 30 to 60 minutes prior to incision and may need to be readministered to maintain effective serum drug concentrations during prolonged procedures. A single preoperative antibiotic dose is usually sufficient prophylaxis. Continuation of antibiotics for up to 24 hours may be considered in some cases (for example, contaminated cases, surgery of long duration, implantation of prosthetic material).

NATURE OF SURGERY	PROBABLE PATHOGEN(S)	RECOMMENDED DRUG(S) (ADULT DOSAGE)	TIME OF ADMINISTRATION
I. Clean			
A. Thoracic, cardiac, vascular, and orthopedic; neurosurgery	*S. aureus**, congulase-negative staphylococci, gram-negative bacilli, *Pseudomonas*	Cefazolin (1 g IV) Vancomycin* (1 g IV)	At induction of anesthesia
B. Ophthalmic		Gentamicin or neomycin-gramacidin-polymixin B ophthalmic drops; multiple drugs at intervals for first 24 hours	
II. Clean-Contaminated			
A. Head and neck (potentially entering esophageal lumen)	*S. aureus* and oral anaerobes	Cefazolin (1 to 2 g IV) or clindamycin (600 mg IV) ± gentamicin (1.5 mg/kg IV)	At induction of anesthesia
B. Abdominal—cholecystectomy and high-risk gastroduodenal or biliary		Cefazolin (1 g IV)	At induction of anesthesia
C. Abdominal—appendectomy		Cefoxitin or cefotetan (1 g IV)	At induction of anesthesia
D. Colorectal Preoperative lavage recommended, plus antimicrobial treatment		Go-LYTELY electrolyte solution (4 liters)	Preoperative day
1. Oral antimicrobial prophylaxis		Erythromycin stearate (1 g PO) *or* metronidazole (500 mg PO) **plus** neomycin (1 g PO)	At 1 P.M., 2 P.M., and 11 P.M. on the preoperative day
2. Parenteral antimicrobial prophylaxis	Patients who have not received lavage and oral prophylaxis should receive parenteral antibiotics for ≤24 hours to cover enteric aerobes (including *E. coli*, *Klebsiella* spp.) and enteric anaerobes (including *B. fragilis*, *Clostridium* spp., anaerobic cocci, and *Fusobacterium* spp.)	Cefotetan (1 g every 12 hours for 2 doses) Ceftizoxime (1 g every 12 hours for 2 doses) Cefoxitin (1 g every 4 to 8 hours for 3 doses)	

(Continued)

Table 42–1
Guidelines for Prophylactic Antibiotics in Surgical Procedures (Continued)

NATURE OF SURGERY	PROBABLE PATHOGEN(S)	RECOMMENDED DRUG(S) (ADULT DOSAGE)	TIME OF ADMINISTRATION
II. Clean-Contaminated (Continued)			
E. Gynecological			
1. Vaginal or abdominal hysterectomy and high-risk cesarean section (following labor or ruptured membrane only)		Cefazolin (1 g IV)	At induction of anesthesia or postcord clamp
2. High-risk abortion, first trimester		Penicillin G (2 million units IV) *or* doxycycline (300 mg PO)	
3. High-risk abortion, second trimester		Cefazolin (1 g IV)	
F. Urology		Prophylactic antibiotics have not been shown to reduce the incidence of wound infection after urological procedures. Bacteriuria is the most common postoperative complication; only patients with evidence of infected urine should be treated with antibiotics directed against the specific pathogens isolated.	
III. Trauma-Contaminated Wounds			
A. Extremity	Antimicrobial coverage for Group A streptococci, staphylococci, and *Clostridium* spp.	Cefazolin (1 g every 8 hours IV) Vancomycin (1 g every 12 hours IV)†	
B. Ruptured viscus—abdomen/bowel injury		Cefotetan (1 g every 12 hours) *or* ceftizoxime (1 g every 12 hours) *or* cefoxitin (1 g every 6 hours) *or* clindamycin (600 mg IV every 8 hours) + gentamicin (1.5 mg/kg IV every 8 hours)† for ≤5 days	
C. Bites (cats and human)	Aerobic and anaerobic streptococci from skin and oral flora. Infection of animal bites additionally may be caused by *Pasteurella multocida*, which is penicillin-sensitive	Amoxicillin/clavulanate (750/125 mg twice a day for 5 days *or* doxycycline 100 mg PO twice a day for 5 days)	

*Recommended for hospitals with a high prevalence of infections caused by methicillin-resistant staphylococci or for serious allergy to β-lactams.
†For serious β-lactam allergy. *Abbreviations:* IV, intravenous administration; PO, oral administration

sible for the new infection can be drug-resistant strains of Enterobacteriaceae, *Pseudomonas*, and *Candida* or other fungi. Superinfection is due to removal of the inhibitory influence of the normal flora, which produce antibacterial substances and also presumably compete for essential nutrients. The broader the antibacterial spectrum and the longer the period of antibiotic treatment, the greater is the alteration in the normal microflora, and the greater is the possibility that a single, typically drug-resistant microorganism will become predominant, invade the host, and produce infection. *The most specific and narrowest spectrum antimicrobial agent should be chosen to treat infections whenever feasible.*

The fact that harmful effects may follow the therapeutic or prophylactic use of anti-infective agents should not discourage the physician from their administration in any situation in which they are definitely indicated. However, the clinician should use restraint in prescribing antimicrobial drugs in instances where evidence of infection is entirely lacking or, at most, only suggestive.

Misuses of Antibiotics

The purpose of this introductory chapter has been to lay the groundwork for the maximally effective use of antimicrobial drugs. Therefore, a brief discussion of the misuse and overuse of antimicrobial agents is in order. Organizations such as the Centers for Disease Control and Prevention have outlined a number of steps to optimize the use of antimicrobial agents and to prevent drug resistance and the transmission of infections (Anonymous, 2002a, 2002b).

Treatment of Nonresponsive Infections. A common misuse of these agents is in infections that have been proved by experimental and clinical observation to be nonresponsive to treatment with antimicrobial agents (Nyquist *et al.*, 1998). Most of the diseases caused by viruses are self-limited and do not respond to any of the currently available anti-infective compounds. Thus, antimicrobial therapy of measles, mumps, and at least 90% of infections of the upper respiratory tract and many GI infections is ineffective and, therefore, useless.

Therapy of Fever of Unknown Origin. Fever of undetermined cause may persist for only a few days to a week or for a longer period. Both of these are treated frequently and inappropriately with empirical antimicrobial agents. Fever of short duration, in the absence of localizing signs, probably is associated with undefined viral infections. Antimicrobial therapy is unnecessary, and resolution of

fever occurs spontaneously within a week or less. Fever persisting for 2 or more weeks, commonly referred to as *fever of unknown origin,* has a variety of causes, of which only about one-quarter are infections (de Kleijn *et al.,* 1997). Some of these infections (*e.g.,* tuberculosis or disseminated fungal infections) may require treatment with antimicrobial agents that are not used commonly for bacterial infections. Others, such as occult abscesses, may require surgical drainage or prolonged courses of pathogen-specific therapy, as in the case of bacterial endocarditis. Inappropriately administered antimicrobial therapy may mask an underlying infection, delay the diagnosis, and by rendering cultures negative, prevent identification of the infectious pathogen. Noninfectious causes, including regional enteritis, lymphoma, renal cell carcinoma, hepatitis, collagen–vascular disorders, and drug fever, do not respond to antimicrobial agents at all. Rather than embarking on a course of empirical antimicrobial therapy for fever of unknown origin, the physician should search for its cause.

Improper Dosage. Dosing errors, which can be the wrong frequency of administration or the use of either an excessive or a subtherapeutic dose, are common. Although antimicrobial drugs are among the safest and least toxic of drugs used in medical practice, excessive amounts can result in significant toxicities, including seizures (*e.g.,* penicillin), vestibular damage (*e.g.,* aminoglycosides), and renal failure (*e.g.,* aminoglycosides), especially in patients with impaired drug excretion or metabolism. The use of too low a dose may result in treatment failure and is most likely to select for microbial resistance.

Inappropriate Reliance on Chemotherapy Alone. Infections complicated by abscess formation, the presence of necrotic tissue, or the presence of a foreign body often cannot be cured by antimicrobial therapy alone. Drainage, débridement, and removal of the foreign body are at least as important as the choice of antimicrobial agent. For example, the patient with pneumonia and empyema often fails to be cured even with administration of large doses of an effective drug unless the infected pleural fluid is drained. The patient with *S. aureus* bacteremia owing to an intravascular device will continue to have fevers and positive blood cultures and is at risk of dying unless the device is removed. As a general rule, when an appreciable quantity of pus, necrotic tissue, or a foreign body is present, the most effective treatment is an antimicrobial agent given in adequate dose plus a properly performed surgical procedure.

Lack of Adequate Bacteriological Information. Antimicrobial therapy administered to hospitalized patients too often is given in the absence of supporting microbiological data. Bacterial cultures and Gram stains of infected material are obtained too infrequently, and the results, when available, often are disregarded in the selection and application of drug therapy. *Frequent use of drug combinations or drugs with the broadest spectra is a cover for diagnostic imprecision.* The agents are selected more likely by habit than for specific indications, and the dosages employed are routine rather than individualized on the basis of the clinical situation, microbiological information, and the pharmacological considerations presented in this and subsequent chapters of this section.

BIBLIOGRAPHY

Anonymous. The choice of antibacterial drugs. *Med. Lett. Drugs. Ther.*, **2001**, *43*:69–78.

Anonymous. Guideline for hand hygiene in health-care settings: Recommendations of the Healthcare Infection Control Practices Advisory Committee. *M.M.W.R.*, **2002a**, *51*:RR-16.

Anonymous. Guideline for the prevention of intravascular catheter-related infections. *M.M.W.R.*, **2002b**, *51*:RR-10.

Arthur, M., and Courvalin, P. Genetics and mechanisms of glycopeptide resistance in enterococci. *Antimicrob. Agents Chemother.*, **1993**, *37*:1563–1571.

Barclay, M.L., Kirkpatrick, C.M., and Begg, E.J. Once daily aminoglycoside therapy: Is it less toxic than multiple daily doses and how should it be monitored? *Clin. Pharmacokinet.*, **1999**, *36*:89–98.

Barriere, S.L. Bacterial resistance to β-lactams, and its prevention with combination antimicrobial therapy. *Pharmacotherapy*, **1992**, *12*:397–402.

Beaber, J.W., Hochhut, B., *et al.* SOS response promotes horizontal dissemination of antibiotic resistance genes. *Nature*, **2004**, *427*:72–74.

Bertrand, T., Eady, N.A., *et al.* Crystal structure of *Mycobacterium tuberculosis* catalase-peroxidase. *J. Biol. Chem.*, **2004**, *1*:1.

Bratzler, D.W., and Houck, P.M. Antimicrobial prophylaxis for surgery: An advisory statement from the National Surgical Infection Prevention Project. *Clin. Infect. Dis.*, **2004**, *38*:1706–1715.

Bush, K. New β-lactamases in gram-negative bacteria: Diversity and impact on the selection of antimicrobial therapy. *Clin. Infect. Dis.*, **2001**, *32*:1085–1089.

Carpenter, C.F., and Chambers, H.F. Daptomycin: Another novel agent for treating infections due to drug-resistant gram-positive pathogens. *Clin. Infect. Dis.*, **2004**, *38*:994–1000.

Chopra, I., O'Neill, A.J., *et al.* The role of mutators in the emergence of antibiotic-resistant bacteria. *Drug Resist. Update*, **2003**, *6*:137–145.

Craig, W.A. Pharmacokinetic/pharmacodynamic parameters: Rationale for antibacterial dosing of mice and men. *Clin. Infect. Dis.*, **1998**, *26*:1–10.

Dajani, A.S., Taubert, K.A., Wilson, W., *et al.* Prevention of bacterial endocarditis: Recommendations by the American Heart Association. *JAMA*, **1997**, *277*:1794–1801.

Davies, J. Inactivation of antibiotics and the dissemination of resistance genes. *Science*, **1994**, *264*:375–382.

de Kleijn, E.M., Vandenbroucke, J.P., and van der Meer, J.W. Fever of unknown origin (FUO): I. A prospective multicenter study of 167 patients with epidemiologic entry criteria. The Netherlands FUO Study Group. *Medicine*, **1997**, *76*:392–400.

Fluit, A.C., and Schmitz, F.J. Resistance integrins and super-integrons. *Clin. Microbiol. Infect.*, **2004**, *10*:272–288.

Goodman, M.F. Error-prone repair DNA polymerases in prokaryotes and eukaryotes. *Ann. Rev. Biochem.*, **2002**, *71*:17–50.

Gordon, M.A. Banda, H.T., *et al.* Non-typhoidal *Salmonella* bacteraemia among HIV-infected Malawian adults: High mortality and frequent recrudescence. *AIDS*, **2002**, *16*:1633–1641.

Hilf, M., Yu, V.L., Sharp, J., *et al.* Antibiotic therapy for *Pseudomonas aeruginosa* bacteremia: Outcome correlations in a prospective study of 200 patients. *Am. J. Med.*, **1989**, *87*:540–546.

Hiramatsu, K., Hanaki, H., Ino, T., *et al.* Methicillin-resistant *Staphylococcus aureus* clinical strain with reduced vancomycin susceptibility. *J. Antimicrob. Chemother.*, **1997**, *40*:135–136.

Hooper, D.C. Fluoroquinolone resistance among gram-positive cocci. *Lancet Infect. Dis.*, **2002**, *2*:530–538.

Kaplan, J.E., Masur, H., *et al.* Guidelines for preventing opportunistic infections among HIV-infected persons: Recommendations of the U.S. Public Health Service and the Infectious Diseases Society of America. *M.M.W.R. Recomm. Rep.*, **2002**, *51*(RR-8):1–52.

Katayama, Y., Ito, T., *et al.* A new class of genetic element, staphylococcus cassette chromosome mec, encodes methicillin resistance in *Staphylococcus aureus*. *Antimicrob. Agents Chemother.*, **2000**, *44*:1549–1555.

Konig, C., Simmen, H.P., and Blaser, J. Bacterial concentrations in pus and infected peritoneal fluid—implications for bactericidal activity of antibiotics. *J. Antimicrob. Chemother.*, **1998**, *42*:227–232.

Leibovici, L., Paul, M., Poznanski, O., *et al.* Monotherapy versus β-lactam–aminoglycoside combination treatment for gram-negative bacteremia: A prospective, observational study. *Antimicrob. Agents Chemother.*, **1997**, *41*:1127–1133.

Leid, J.G., Shirtliff, M.E., *et al.* Human leukocytes adhere to, penetrate, and respond to *Staphylococcus aureus* biofilms. *Infect. Immun.*, **2002**, *70*:6339–6345.

Lewis, K. Riddle of biofilm resistance. *Antimicrob. Agents Chemother.*, **2001**, *45*:999–1007.

Li, X.Z., and Nikaido, H. Efflux-mediated drug resistance in bacteria. *Drugs*, **2004**, *64*:159–204.

Lim, D., and Strynadka, N.C. Structural basis for the β-lactam resistance of PBP2a from methicillin-resistant *Staphylococcus aureus*. *Nature Struct. Biol.*, **2002**, *9*:870–876.

Mahillon, J., and Chandler, M. Insertion sequences. *Microbiol. Mol. Biol. Rev.*, **1998**, *62*:725–774.

Murray, B.E. β-Lactamase-producing enterococci. *Antimicrob. Agents Chemother.*, **1992**, *36*:2355–2359.

Murray, B.E. Vancomycin-resistant enterococcal infections. *New Engl. J. Med.*, **2000**, *342*:710–721.

Naimi, T.S., LeDell, K.H., *et al.* Comparison of community- and health care-associated methicillin-resistant *Staphylococcus aureus* infection. *JAMA*, **2003**, *290*:2976–2984.

Nakajima, Y. Mechanisms of bacterial resistance to macrolide antibiotics. *J. Infect. Chemother.*, **1999**, *5*:61–74.

Nosanchuk, J.D., Cleare, W., Franzot, S.P., and Casadevall, A. Amphotericin B and fluconazole affect cellular charge, macrophage phagocytosis, and cellular morphology of *Cryptococcus neoformans* at subinhibitory concentrations. *Antimicrob. Agents Chemother.*, **1999**, *43*:233–239.

Nyquist, A.C., Gonzales, R., Steiner, J.F., and Sande, M.A. Antibiotic prescribing for children with colds, upper respiratory tract infections, and bronchitis. *JAMA,* **1998,** *279*:875–877.

Paul, M., Benuri-Silbiger, I., *et al.* β-Lactam monotherapy versus β-lactam–aminoglycoside combination therapy for sepsis in immunocompetent patients: Systematic review and meta-analysis of randomised trials. *Br. Med. J.,* **2004,** *328*:668.

Quagliarello, V.J., and Scheld, W.M. Treatment of bacterial meningitis. *New Engl. J. Med.,* **1997,** *336*:708–716.

Riska, P.F., Jacobs, W.R., Jr., *et al.* Molecular determinants of drug resistance in tuberculosis. *Int. J. Tuberc. Lung Dis.,* **2000,** *4*(2 suppl 1):S4–S10.

Rybak, M.J., Abate, B.J., *et al.* Prospective evaluation of the effect of an aminoglycoside dosing regimen on rates of observed nephrotoxicity and ototoxicity. *Antimicrob. Agents Chemother.,* **1999,** *43*:1549–1555.

Rybak, M.J., and McGrath, B.J. Combination antimicrobial therapy for bacterial infections: Guidelines for the clinician. *Drugs,* **1996,** *52*:390–405.

Smith, T.L., Pearson, M.L., Wilcox, K.R., *et al.* Emergence of vancomycin resistance in *Staphylococcus aureus*. Glycopeptide–Intermediate *Staphylococcus aureus* Working Group. *New Engl. J. Med.,* **1999,** *340*:493–501.

Spratt, B.G. Resistance to antibiotics mediated by target alterations. *Science,* **1994,** *264*:388–393.

Strom, B.L., Abrutyn, E., Berlin, J.A., *et al.* Dental and cardiac risk factors for infective endocarditis: A population-based, case-control study. *Ann. Intern. Med.,* **1998,** *129*:761–769.

Täuber, M.G., Kunz, S., Zak, O., and Sande, M.A. Influence of antibiotic dose, dosing interval and duration of therapy on outcome in experimental pneumococcal meningitis in rabbits. *Antimicrob. Agents Chemother.,* **1989,** *33*:418–423.

Taylor, J.L., Zagari, M., Murphy, K., and Freston, J.W. Pharmacoeconomic comparison of treatments for the eradication of *Helicobacter pylori. Arch. Intern. Med.,* **1997,** *157*:87–97.

van der Horst, C.M., Saag, M.S., Cloud, G.A., *et al.* Treatment of cryptococcal meningitis associated with the acquired immunodeficiency syndrome. National Institute of Allergy and Infectious Diseases Mycoses Study Group and AIDS Clinical Trials Group. *New Engl. J. Med.,* **1997,** *337*:15–21.

Vandenesch, F., Naimi, T., *et al.* Community-acquired methicillin-resistant *Staphylococcus aureus* carrying Panton-Valentine leukocidin genes: Worldwide emergence. *Emerg. Infect. Dis.,* **2003,** *9*:978–984.

Weigel, L.M., Clewell, D.B., *et al.* Genetic analysis of a high-level vancomycin-resistant isolate of *Staphylococcus aureus. Science,* **2003,** *302*:1569–1571.

Wilson, W.R., Karchmer, A.W., Dajani, A.S., *et al.* Antimicrobial treatment of adults with infective endocarditis due to streptococci, enterococci, staphylococci, and HACEK microorganisms. American Heart Association. *JAMA,* **1995,** *274*:1706–1713.

Zimmerli, W., Widmer, A.F., Blatter, M., Frei, R., and Ochsner, P.E. Role of rifampin for treatment of orthopedic implant-related staphylococcal infections: A randomized, controlled trial. Foreign-Body Infection (FBI) Study Group. *JAMA,* **1998,** *279*:1537–1541.

SULFONAMIDES, TRIMETHOPRIM– SULFAMETHOXAZOLE, QUINOLONES, AND AGENTS FOR URINARY TRACT INFECTIONS

William A. Petri, Jr.

SULFONAMIDES

The sulfonamide drugs were the first effective chemotherapeutic agents to be employed systemically for the prevention and cure of bacterial infections in humans. The considerable medical and public health importance of their discovery and their subsequent widespread use were quickly reflected in the sharp decline in morbidity and mortality figures for treatable infectious diseases. The advent of *penicillin* and subsequently of other antibiotics has diminished the usefulness of the sulfonamides, and they presently occupy a relatively small place in the therapeutic armamentarium of the physician. However, the introduction in the mid-1970s of the combination of *trimethoprim* and *sulfamethoxazole* has increased the use of sulfonamides for the prophylaxis and treatment of specific microbial infections.

History. Investigations at the I. G. Farbenindustrie resulted, in 1932, in the patenting of PRONTOSIL and several other azo dyes containing a sulfonamide group. Prompted by the knowledge that synthetic azo dyes had been studied for their action against streptococci, Domagk tested the new compounds and observed that mice with streptococcal and other infections could be protected by PRONTOSIL. In 1933, the first clinical case study was reported by Foerster, who gave PRONTOSIL to a 10-month-old infant with staphylococcal septicemia and obtained a dramatic cure. Little attention was paid elsewhere to these epoch-making advances in chemotherapy until Colebrook and Kenny, as well as Buttle and coworkers, reported their favorable clinical results with PRONTOSIL and its active metabolite, sulfanilamide, in puerperal sepsis and meningococcal infections. These two reports awakened the medical profession to the new field of antibacterial chemotherapy, and experimental and clinical articles soon appeared in profusion. The

development of the carbonic anhydrase inhibitor–type diuretics and the sulfonylurea hypoglycemic agents followed from observations made with the sulfonamide antibiotics. For discovering the chemotherapeutic value of PRONTOSIL Domagk was awarded the Nobel Prize in Medicine for 1938.

Chemistry. The term *sulfonamide* is employed herein as a generic name for derivatives of *para*-aminobenzenesulfonamide (sulfanilamide); the structural formulas of selected members of this class are shown in Figure 43–1. Most of them are relatively insoluble in water, but their sodium salts are readily soluble. The minimal structural prerequisites for antibacterial action are all embodied in sulfanilamide itself. The —SO_2NH_2 group is not essential as such, but the important feature is that the sulfur is linked directly to the benzene ring. The *para*-NH_2 group (the N of which has been designated as N4) is essential and can be replaced only by moieties that can be converted *in vivo* to a free amino group. Substitutions made in the amide NH_2 group (the N of which has been designated as N1) have variable effects on antibacterial activity of the molecule. However, substitution of heterocyclic aromatic nuclei at N1 yields highly potent compounds.

Effects on Microbes

Sulfonamides have a wide range of antimicrobial activity against both gram-positive and gram-negative bacteria. However, resistant strains have become common, and the usefulness of these agents has diminished correspondingly. In general, the sulfonamides exert only a bacteriostatic effect, and cellular and humoral defense mechanisms of the host are essential for final eradication of the infection.

Antibacterial Spectrum. Resistance to sulfonamides is increasingly a problem. Microorganisms that may be susceptible *in vitro* to sulfonamides include *Streptococcus pyo-*

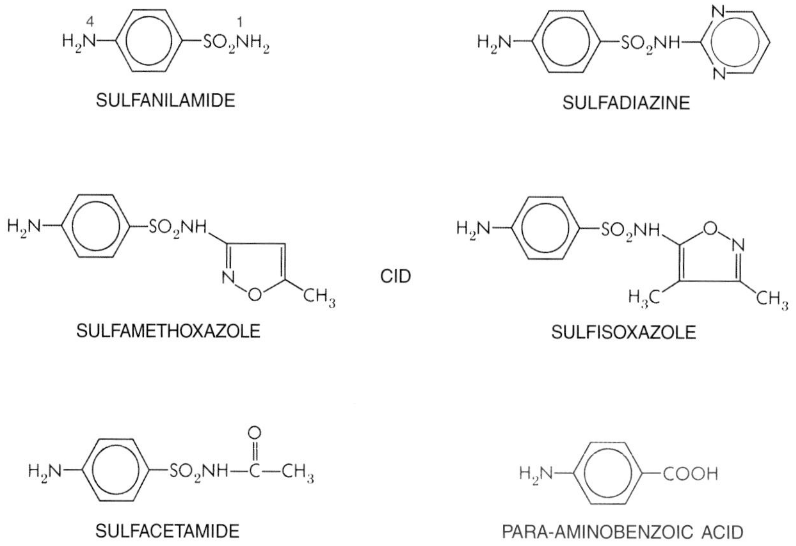

SULFANILAMIDE

SULFADIAZINE

SULFAMETHOXAZOLE   CID

SULFISOXAZOLE

SULFACETAMIDE

PARA-AMINOBENZOIC ACID

Figure 43–1. *Structural formulas of selected sulfonamides and para-aminobenzoic acid.* The N of the *para*-NH$_2$ group is designated as N4; that of the amide NH$_2$, as N1.

genes, *Streptococcus pneumoniae, Haemophilus influenzae, Haemophilus ducreyi, Nocardia, Actinomyces, Calymmatobacterium granulomatis,* and *Chlamydia trachomatis.* Minimal inhibitory concentrations (MICs) range from 0.1 μg/ml for *C. trachomatis* to 4 to 64 μg/ml for *Escherichia coli.* Peak plasma drug concentrations achievable *in vivo* are approximately 100 to 200 μg/ml.

Although sulfonamides were used successfully for the management of meningococcal infections for many years, the majority of isolates of *Neisseria meningitidis* of serogroups B and C in the United States and group A isolates from other countries are now resistant. A similar situation prevails with respect to *Shigella.* Strains of *E. coli* isolated from patients with urinary tract infections (community-acquired) often are resistant to sulfonamides, which are no longer the therapy of choice for such infections.

Mechanism of Action. Sulfonamides, structural analogs and competitive antagonists of *para*-aminobenzoic acid (PABA), prevent normal bacterial utilization of PABA for the synthesis of folic acid (pteroylglutamic acid). More specifically, sulfonamides are competitive inhibitors of dihydropteroate synthase, the bacterial enzyme responsible for the incorporation of PABA into dihydropteroic acid, the immediate precursor of folic acid (Figure 43–2). Sensitive microorganisms are those that must synthesize their own folic acid; bacteria that can use preformed folate are not affected. Bacteriostasis induced by sulfonamides is counteracted by PABA competitively. Sulfonamides do not affect mammalian cells by this mechanism because they require preformed folic acid and cannot synthesize it. Thus, mammalian cells are comparable to sulfonamide-insensitive bacteria that use preformed folate.

Synergists of Sulfonamides. One of the most active agents that exerts a synergistic effect when used with a sulfonamide is trimethoprim (*see* Bushby and Hitchings, 1968). This compound is a potent and selective competitive inhibitor of microbial dihydrofolate reductase, the enzyme that reduces dihydrofolate to tetrahydrofolate. It is this reduced form of folic acid that is required for one-carbon transfer reactions. The simultaneous administration of a sulfonamide and trimethoprim thus introduces sequential blocks in the pathway by which microorganisms synthesize tetrahydrofolate from precursor molecules (Figure 43–2). The expectation that such a combination would yield synergistic antimicrobial effects has been realized both *in vitro* and *in vivo* (*see* below).

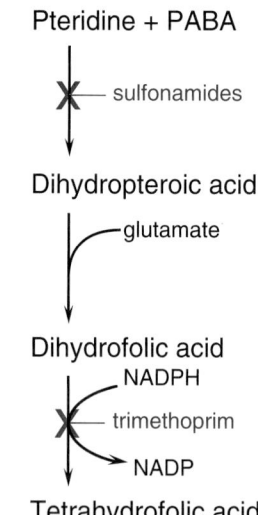

Figure 43–2. *Steps in folate metabolism blocked by sulfonamides and trimethoprim.*

Acquired Bacterial Resistance to Sulfonamides. Bacteria resistant to sulfonamides is presumed to originate by random mutation and selection or by transfer of resistance by plasmids (*see* Chapter 42). Such resistance, once it is maximally developed, usually is persistent and irreversible, particularly when produced *in vivo*. Acquired resistance to sulfonamide usually does not involve cross-resistance to antimicrobial agents of other classes. The *in vivo* acquisition of resistance has little or no effect on either virulence or antigenic characteristics of microorganisms.

Resistance to sulfonamide probably is the consequence of an altered enzymatic constitution of the bacterial cell; the alteration may be characterized by (1) a lower affinity for sulfonamides by dihydropteroate synthase, (2) decreased bacterial permeability or active efflux of the drug, (3) an alternative metabolic pathway for synthesis of an essential metabolite, or (4) an increased production of an essential metabolite or drug antagonist. For example, some resistant staphylococci may synthesize 70 times as much PABA as do the susceptible parent strains. Nevertheless, an increased production of PABA is not a constant finding in sulfonamide-resistant bacteria, and resistant mutants may possess enzymes for folate biosynthesis that are less readily inhibited by sulfonamides. Plasmid-mediated resistance is due to plasmid-encoded drug-resistant dihydropteroate synthetase.

Absorption, Fate, and Excretion

Except for sulfonamides especially designed for their local effects in the bowel (*see* Chapter 38), this class of drugs is absorbed rapidly from the gastrointestinal tract. Approximately 70% to 100% of an oral dose is absorbed, and sulfonamide can be found in the urine within 30 minutes of ingestion. Peak plasma levels are achieved in 2 to 6 hours, depending on the drug. The small intestine is the major site of absorption, but some of the drug is absorbed from the stomach. Absorption from other sites, such as the vagina, respiratory tract, or abraded skin, is variable and unreliable, but a sufficient amount may enter the body to cause toxic reactions in susceptible persons or to produce sensitization.

All sulfonamides are bound in varying degree to plasma proteins, particularly to albumin. The extent to which this occurs is determined by the hydrophobicity of a particular drug and its pK_a; at physiological pH, drugs with a high pK_a exhibit a low degree of protein binding, and *vice versa*.

Sulfonamides are distributed throughout all tissues of the body. The diffusible fraction of sulfadiazine is distributed uniformly throughout the total-body water, whereas *sulfisoxazole* is confined largely to the extracellular space. The sulfonamides readily enter pleural, peritoneal, synovial, ocular, and similar body fluids and may reach concentrations therein that are 50% to 80% of the simultaneously determined concentration in blood. Since the protein content of such fluids usually is low, the drug is present in the unbound active form.

After systemic administration of adequate doses, *sulfadiazine* and sulfisoxazole attain concentrations in cerebrospinal fluid that may be effective in meningeal infections. At steady state, the concentration ranges between 10% and 80% of that in the blood. However, because of the emergence of sulfonamide-resistant microorganisms, these drugs are used rarely for the treatment of meningitis.

Sulfonamides pass readily through the placenta and reach the fetal circulation. The concentrations attained in the fetal tissues are sufficient to cause both antibacterial and toxic effects.

The sulfonamides undergo metabolic alterations *in vivo*, especially in the liver. The major metabolic derivative is the N4-acetylated sulfonamide. Acetylation, which occurs to a different extent with each agent, is disadvantageous because the resulting products have no antibacterial activity and yet retain the toxic potential of the parent substance.

Sulfonamides are eliminated from the body partly as the unchanged drug and partly as metabolic products. The largest fraction is excreted in the urine, and the half-life of sulfonamides in the body thus depends on renal function. In acid urine, the older sulfonamides are insoluble and may precipitate, forming crystalline deposits that can cause urinary obstruction (*see* below). Small amounts are eliminated in the feces, bile, milk, and other secretions.

Pharmacological Properties of Individual Sulfonamides

The sulfonamides may be classified into three groups on the basis of the rapidity with which they are absorbed and excreted: (1) agents that are absorbed and excreted rapidly, such as sulfisoxazole and sulfadiazine; (2) agents that are absorbed very poorly when administered orally and hence are active in the bowel lumen, such as *sulfasalazine*; (3) agents that are used mainly topically, such as *sulfacetamide, mafenide*, and *silver sulfadiazine*; and (4) long-acting sulfonamides, such as *sulfadoxine*, that are absorbed rapidly but excreted slowly (Table 43–1).

Rapidly Absorbed and Eliminated Sulfonamides. *Sulfisoxazole.* Sulfisoxazole (GANTRISIN, others) is a rapidly absorbed and excreted sulfonamide with excellent antibacterial activity. Since its high solubility eliminates much of the renal toxicity inherent in the use of older sulfonamides, it has essentially replaced the less-soluble agents.

Sulfisoxazole is bound extensively to plasma proteins. Following an oral dose of 2 to 4 g, peak concentrations in plasma of 110 to 250 μg/ml are found in 2 to 4 hours. From 28% to 35% of sulfisoxazole in the blood and about 30% in the urine is in the acetylated

Table 43–1
Classes of Sulfonamides

CLASS	SULFONAMIDE	SERUM HALF-LIFE HOURS
Absorbed and excreted rapidly	Sulfisoxazole	5–6
	Sulfamethoxazole	11
	Sulfadiazine	10
Poorly absorbed– active in bowel lumen	Sulfasalazine	—
Topically used	Sulfacetamide	—
	Silver sulfadiazine	—
Long-acting	Sulfadoxine	100–230

form. Approximately 95% of a single dose is excreted by the kidney in 24 hours. Concentrations of the drug in urine thus greatly exceed those in blood and may be bactericidal. The concentration in cerebrospinal fluid averages about a third of that in the blood.

Sulfisoxazole acetyl is tasteless and hence preferred for oral use in children. Sulfisoxazole acetyl is marketed in combination with *erythromycin ethylsuccinate* (PEDIAZOLE, others) for use in children with otitis media. The urine becomes orange-red soon after ingestion of this mixture because of the presence of phenazopyridine, an orange-red dye.

Fewer than 0.1% of patients receiving sulfisoxazole suffer serious toxic reactions. The untoward effects produced by this agent are similar to those which follow the administration of other sulfonamides, as discussed below. Because of its relatively high solubility in the urine as compared with sulfadiazine, sulfisoxazole only infrequently produces hematuria or crystalluria (0.2% to 0.3%). Despite this, patients taking this drug should ingest an adequate quantity of water. Sulfisoxazole and all sulfonamides that are absorbed must be used with caution in patients with impaired renal function. Like all sulfonamides, sulfisoxazole may produce hypersensitivity reactions, some of which are potentially lethal. Sulfisoxazole currently is preferred over other sulfonamides by most clinicians when a rapidly absorbed and rapidly excreted sulfonamide is indicated.

Sulfamethoxazole. Sulfamethoxazole is a close congener of sulfisoxazole, but its rates of enteric absorption and urinary excretion are slower. It is administered orally and employed for both systemic and urinary tract infections. Precautions must be observed to avoid sulfamethoxazole crystalluria because of the high percentage of the acetylated, relatively insoluble form of the drug in the urine. The clinical uses of sulfamethoxazole are the same as those for sulfisoxazole. It also is marketed in fixed-dose combinations with trimethoprim (*see* below).

Sulfadiazine. Sulfadiazine given orally is absorbed rapidly from the GI tract, and peak blood concentrations are reached within 3 to 6 hours after a single dose. Following an oral dose of 3 g, peak concentrations in plasma are 50 μg/ml. About 55% of the drug is bound to plasma protein at a concentration of 100 μg/ml when plasma protein levels are normal. Therapeutic concentrations

are attained in cerebrospinal fluid within 4 hours of a single oral dose of 60 mg/kg.

Sulfadiazine is excreted quite readily by the kidney in both the free and acetylated forms, rapidly at first and then more slowly over a period of 2 to 3 days. It can be detected in the urine within 30 minutes of oral ingestion. About 15% to 40% of the excreted sulfadiazine is in acetylated form. This form of the drug is excreted more readily than the free fraction, and the administration of alkali accelerates the renal clearance of both forms by further diminishing their tubular reabsorption.

In adults and children who are being treated with sulfadiazine, every precaution must be taken to ensure fluid intake adequate to produce a urine output of at least 1200 ml in adults and a corresponding quantity in children. If this cannot be accomplished, sodium bicarbonate may be given to reduce the risk of crystalluria.

Poorly Absorbed Sulfonamides. Sulfasalazine (AZULFIDINE) is very poorly absorbed from the GI tract. It is used in the therapy of ulcerative colitis and regional enteritis, but relapses tend to occur in about one-third of patients who experience a satisfactory initial response. *Corticosteroids* are more effective in treating acute attacks, but sulfasalazine is preferred to corticosteroids for the treatment of patients who are mildly or moderately ill with ulcerative colitis (*see* Chapter 38). The drug also is being employed as the first approach to treatment of relatively mild cases of regional enteritis and granulomatous colitis. Sulfasalazine is broken down by intestinal bacteria to *sulfapyridine,* an active sulfonamide that is absorbed and eventually excreted in the urine, and *5-aminosalicylate,* which reaches high levels in the feces. 5-Aminosalicylate is the effective agent in inflammatory bowel disease, whereas sulfapyridine is responsible for most of the toxicity. Toxic reactions include Heinz-body anemia, acute hemolysis in patients with glucose-6-phosphate dehydrogenase deficiency, and agranulocytosis. Nausea, fever, arthralgias, and rashes occur in up to 20% of patients treated with the drug; desensitization has been an effective treatment. Sulfasalazine can cause a reversible infertility in males owing to changes in sperm number and morphology. There is no evidence that the compound alters the intestinal microflora of patients with ulcerative colitis.

Sulfonamides for Topical Use. *Sulfacetamide.* Sulfacetamide is the N1-acetyl-substituted derivative of *sulfanilamide.* Its aqueous solubility (1:140) is approximately 90 times that of sulfadiazine. Solutions of the sodium salt of the drug (ISOPTO-CETAMIDE, others) are employed extensively in the management of ophthalmic infections. Although topical sulfonamide for most purposes is discouraged because of lack of efficacy and a high risk of sensitization, sulfacetamide has certain advantages. Very high aqueous concentrations are not irritating to the eye and are effective against susceptible microorganisms. A 30% solution of the sodium salt has a pH of 7.4, whereas the solutions of sodium salts of other sulfonamides are highly alkaline. The drug penetrates into ocular fluids and tissues in high concentration. Sensitivity reactions to sulfacetamide are rare, but the drug should not be used in patients with known hypersensitivity to sulfonamides.

Silver Sulfadiazine. Silver sulfadiazine (SILVADENE, others) inhibits the growth *in vitro* of nearly all pathogenic bacteria and fungi, including some species resistant to sulfonamides. The compound is used topically to reduce microbial colonization and the incidence of infections of wounds from burns. It should not be used to treat an established deep infection. Silver is released slowly from the preparation in concentrations that are selectively toxic to the microorganisms. However, bacteria may develop resistance to silver sulfadiazine. Although little silver is absorbed, the plasma concentration of sulfadiazine may approach therapeutic levels if a large surface area is involved. Adverse reactions—burning, rash, and itching—are infrequent. Silver sulfadiazine is considered by most authorities to be one of the agents of choice for the prevention of burn infection.

Mafenide. This sulfonamide (α-amino-*p*-toluene-sulfonamide) is marketed as *mafenide acetate* (SULFAMYLON). When applied topically, it is effective for the prevention of colonization of burns by a large variety of gram-negative and gram-positive bacteria. It should not be used in treatment of an established deep infection. Superinfection with *Candida* occasionally may be a problem. The cream is applied once or twice daily to a thickness of 1 to 2 mm over the burned skin. Cleansing of the wound and removal of debris should be carried out before each application of the drug. Therapy is continued until skin grafting is possible. Mafenide is rapidly absorbed systemically and converted to *para*-carboxyben-zenesulfonamide. Studies of absorption from the burn surface indicate that peak plasma concentrations are reached in 2 to 4 hours. Adverse effects include intense pain at sites of application, allergic reactions, and loss of fluid by evaporation from the burn surface because occlusive dressings are not used. The drug and its primary metabolite inhibit carbonic anhydrase, and the urine becomes alkaline. Metabolic acidosis with compensatory tachypnea and hyperventilation may ensue; these effects limit the usefulness of mafenide.

Long-Acting Sulfonamides. *Sulfadoxine* (N1-[5,6-dimethoxy-4-pyrimidiny] sulfanilamide) has a particularly long half-life (7 to 9 days). It is used in combination with *pyrimethamine* (500 mg sulfadoxine plus 25 mg pyrimethamine as FANSIDAR) for the prophylaxis and treatment of malaria caused by *mefloquine*-resistant strains of *Plasmodium falciparum* (*see* Chapter 39). Because of severe and sometimes fatal reactions, including the Stevens-Johnson syndrome, the drug should be used for prophylaxis only where the risk of resistant malaria is high.

Sulfonamide Therapy

The number of conditions for which the sulfonamides are therapeutically useful and constitute drugs of first choice has been reduced sharply by the development of more effective antimicrobial agents and by the gradual increase in the resistance of a number of bacterial species to this class of drugs. However, introduction of the combination of trimethoprim and sulfamethoxazole has revived the use of sulfonamides.

Urinary Tract Infections. Since a significant percentage of urinary tract infections in many parts of the world are caused by sulfonamide-resistant microorganisms, sulfonamides are no longer a therapy of first choice. Trimethoprim–sulfamethoxazole, a quinolone, trimethoprim, *fosfomycin,* or *ampicillin* are the preferred agents. However, sulfisoxazole may be used effectively in areas where the prevalence of resistance is not high or when the organism is known to be sensitive. The usual dosage is 2 to 4 g initially followed by 1 to 2 g, orally four times a day for 5 to 10 days. Patients with acute pyelonephritis with high fever and other severe constitutional manifestations are at risk of bacteremia and shock and should not be treated with a sulfonamide.

Nocardiosis. Sulfonamides are of value in the treatment of infections due to *Nocardia* spp. A number of instances of complete recovery from the disease after adequate treatment with a sulfonamide have been recorded. Sulfisoxazole or sulfadiazine may be given in dosages of 6 to 8 g daily. Concentrations of sulfonamide in plasma should be 80 to 160 μg/ml. This schedule is continued for several months after all manifestations have been controlled. The administration of sulfonamide together with a second antibiotic has been recommended, especially for advanced cases, and ampicillin, erythromycin, and *streptomycin* have been suggested for this purpose. The clinical response and the results of sensitivity testing may be helpful in choosing a companion drug. Notably, there are no clinical data to show that combination therapy is better than therapy with a sulfonamide alone. Trimethoprim–sulfamethoxazole also has been effective, and some authorities consider it to be the drug of choice.

Toxoplasmosis. The combination of *pyrimethamine* and sulfadiazine is the treatment of choice for toxoplasmosis (Montoya and Remington, 2000) (*see* Chapter 40). Pyrimethamine is given as a loading dose of 75 mg followed by 25 mg orally per day, with sulfadiazine 1 g orally every 6 hours, plus folinic acid 10 mg orally each day for at least 3 to 6 weeks. Patients should receive at least 2 L of fluid intake daily to prevent crystalluria during therapy.

Use of Sulfonamides for Prophylaxis. The sulfonamides are as efficacious as oral penicillin in preventing streptococcal infections and recurrences of rheumatic fever among susceptible subjects. Despite the efficacy of sulfonamides for long-term prophylaxis of rheumatic fever, their toxicity and the possibility of infection by drug-resistant streptococci make sulfonamides less desirable than penicillin for this purpose. They should be used, however, without hesitation in patients who are hypersensitive to penicillin. If untoward responses occur, they usually do so during the first 8 weeks of therapy; serious reactions after this time are rare. White blood cell counts should be carried out once weekly during the first 8 weeks.

Untoward Reactions to Sulfonamides

The untoward effects that follow the administration of sulfonamides are numerous and varied; the overall incidence of reactions is about 5%. Certain forms of toxicity may be related to individual differences in sulfonamide metabolism (Shear *et al.*, 1986).

Disturbances of the Urinary Tract. Although the risk of crystalluria was relatively high with the older, less soluble sulfonamides, the incidence of this problem is very low with more soluble agents such as sulfisoxazole. Crystalluria has occurred in dehydrated patients with the acquired immune deficiency syndrome (AIDS) who were receiving sulfadiazine for *Toxoplasma* encephalitis. Fluid intake should be sufficient to ensure a daily urine volume of at least 1200 ml (in adults). Alkalinization of the urine may be desirable if urine volume or pH is unusually low because the solubility of sulfisoxazole increases greatly with slight elevations of pH.

Disorders of the Hematopoietic System. *Acute Hemolytic Anemia.* The mechanism of the acute hemolytic anemia produced by sulfonamides is not always readily apparent. In some cases it has been thought to be a sensitization phenomenon. In other instances the hemolysis is related to an erythrocytic deficiency of glucose-6-phosphate dehydrogenase activity. Hemolytic anemia is rare after treatment with sulfadiazine (0.05%); its exact incidence following therapy with sulfisoxazole is unknown.

Agranulocytosis. Agranulocytosis occurs in about 0.1% of patients who receive sulfadiazine; it also can follow the use of other sulfonamides. Although return of granulocytes to normal levels may be delayed for weeks or months after sulfonamide is withdrawn, most patients recover spontaneously with supportive care.

Aplastic Anemia. Complete suppression of bone-marrow activity with profound anemia, granulocytopenia, and thrombocytopenia is an extremely rare occurrence with sulfonamide therapy. It probably results from a direct myelotoxic effect and may be fatal. However, reversible suppression of the bone marrow is quite common in patients with limited bone marrow reserve (*e.g.,* patients with AIDS or those receiving myelosuppressive chemotherapy).

Hypersensitivity Reactions. The incidence of other hypersensitivity reactions to sulfonamides is quite variable. Among the skin and mucous membrane manifestations attributed to sensitization to sulfonamide are morbilliform, scarlatinal, urticarial, erysipeloid, pemphigoid, purpuric, and petechial rashes, as well as erythema nodosum, erythema multiforme of the Stevens-Johnson type, Behçet's syndrome, exfoliative dermatitis, and photosensitivity. These hypersensitivity reactions occur most often after the first week of therapy but may appear earlier in previously sensitized individuals. Fever, malaise, and pruritus frequently are present simultaneously. The incidence of untoward dermal effects is about 2% with sulfisoxazole, although patients with AIDS manifest a higher frequency of rashes with sulfonamide treatment than do other individuals. A syndrome similar to serum sickness may appear after several days of sulfonamide therapy. Drug fever is a common untoward manifestation of sulfonamide treatment; the incidence approximates 3% with sulfisoxazole.

Focal or diffuse necrosis of the liver owing to direct drug toxicity or sensitization occurs in fewer than 0.1% of patients. Headache, nausea, vomiting, fever, hepatomegaly, jaundice, and laboratory evidence of hepatocellular dysfunction usually appear 3 to 5 days after sulfonamide administration is started, and the syndrome may progress to acute yellow atrophy and death.

Miscellaneous Reactions. Anorexia, nausea, and vomiting occur in 1% to 2% of persons receiving sulfonamides, and these manifestations probably are central in origin. The administration of sulfonamides to newborn infants, especially if premature, may lead to the displacement of bilirubin from plasma albumin. In newborn infants, free bilirubin can become deposited in the basal ganglia and subthalamic nuclei of the brain, causing an encephalopathy called *kernicterus.* Sulfonamides should not be given to pregnant women near term because these drugs pass through the placenta and are secreted in milk.

Drug Interactions. The most important interactions of the sulfonamides involve those with the oral anticoagulants, the sulfonylurea hypoglycemic agents, and the hydantoin anticonvulsants. In each case, sulfonamides can potentiate the effects of the other drug by mechanisms that appear to involve primarily inhibition of metabolism and, possibly, displacement from albumin. Dosage adjustment may be necessary when a sulfonamide is given concurrently.

TRIMETHOPRIM–SULFAMETHOXAZOLE

The introduction of trimethoprim in combination with sulfamethoxazole constitutes an important advance in the development of clinically effective antimicrobial agents and represents the practical application of a theoretical consideration; *i.e.,* if two drugs act on sequential steps in the pathway of an obligate enzymatic reaction in bacteria (Figure 43–2), the result of their combination will be synergistic (*see* Hitchings, 1961). In much of the world the combination is known as *cotrimoxazole.* In addition to its combination with sulfamethoxazole (BACTRIM, SEPTRA, others), trimethoprim also is available as a single-entity preparation (PROLOPRIM, others).

Chemistry. Sulfamethoxazole was discussed earlier in this chapter, and its structural formula is shown in Figure 43–1. The history of trimethoprim, a diaminopyrimidine, is discussed in Chapter 39. Its structural formula is:

TRIMETHOPRIM

Antibacterial Spectrum. The antibacterial spectrum of trimethoprim is similar to that of sulfamethoxazole, although the former drug usually is 20 to 100 times more potent than the latter. Most gram-negative and gram-positive microorganisms are sensitive to trimethoprim, but resistance can develop when the drug is used alone. *Pseudomonas aeruginosa, Bacteroides fragilis,* and enterococci usually are resistant. There is significant variation in the susceptibility of Enterobacteriaceae to trimethoprim in different geographical locations because of the spread of resistance mediated by plasmids and transposons.

Efficacy of Trimethoprim–Sulfamethoxazole in Combination. *Chlamydia diphtheriae* and *N. meningitidis* are susceptible to trimethoprim–sulfamethoxazole. Although most *S. pneumoniae* are susceptible, there has been a disturbing increase in resistance (*see* below). From 50% to 95% of strains of *Staphylococcus aureus, Staphylococcus epidermidis, S. pyogenes,* the *viridans* group of streptococci, *E. coli, Proteus mirabilis, Proteus morganii, Proteus rettgeri, Enterobacter* spp., *Salmonella, Shigella, Pseudomonas pseudomallei, Serratia,* and *Alcaligenes* spp. are inhibited. Also sensitive are *Klebsiella* spp., *Brucella abortus, Pasteurella haemolytica, Yersinia pseudotuberculosis, Yersinia enterocolitica,* and *Nocardia asteroides.* Methicillin-resistant strains of *S. aureus,* although also resistant to trimethoprim or sulfamethoxazole alone, may be susceptible to the combination. A synergistic interaction between the components of the preparation is apparent even when microorganisms are resistant to sulfonamide with or without moderate resistance to trimethoprim. However, a maximal degree of synergism occurs when microorganisms are sensitive to both components. The activity of trimethoprim–sulfamethoxazole *in vitro* depends on the medium in which it is determined; *e.g.,* low concentrations of thymidine almost completely abolish the antibacterial activity.

Mechanism of Action. The antimicrobial activity of the combination of trimethoprim and sulfamethoxazole results from its actions on two steps of the enzymatic pathway for the synthesis of tetrahydrofolic acid. Sulfonamide inhibits the incorporation of *para*-aminobenzoic acid (PABA) into folic acid, and trimethoprim prevents the reduction of dihydrofolate to tetrahydrofolate (Figure 43–2). Tetrahydrofolate is essential for one-carbon transfer reactions, *e.g.,* the synthesis of thymidylate from deoxyuridylate. Selective toxicity for microorganisms is achieved in two ways. Mammalian cells use preformed folates from the diet and do not synthesize the compound. Furthermore, trimethoprim is a highly selective inhibitor of dihydrofolate reductase of lower organisms: About 100,000 times more drug is required to inhibit human reductase than the bacterial enzyme. This relative selectivity is vital because this enzymatic function is essential to all species.

The synergistic interaction between sulfonamide and trimethoprim is predictable from their respective mechanisms. There is an optimal ratio of the concentrations of the two agents for synergism that equals the ratio of the minimal inhibitory concentrations of the drugs acting independently. While this ratio varies for different bacteria, the most effective ratio for the greatest number of microorganisms is 20 parts sulfamethoxazole to 1 part trimethoprim. The combination thus is formulated to achieve a sulfamethoxazole concentration *in vivo* that is 20 times greater than that of trimethoprim. The pharmacokinetic properties of the sulfonamide chosen to be in combination with trimethoprim are critical because relative constancy of the concentrations of the two compounds in the body is desired.

Bacterial Resistance. Bacterial resistance to trimethoprim–sulfamethoxazole is a rapidly increasing problem, although resistance is lower than it is to either of the agents alone. Resistance often is due to the acquisition of a plasmid that codes for an altered dihydrofolate reductase. The development of resistance is a problem for the treatment of many different bacterial infections. In a survey of children with otitis media in Memphis, Tennessee, 29% of isolates were penicillin-resistant, and 25% of these also were resistant to trimethoprim–sulfamethoxazole (Centers for Disease Control and Prevention, 1994a). In another survey, approximately 50% of *Shigella sonnei* isolates from The Netherlands were resistant (Voogd *et al.,* 1992). Emergence of trimethoprim–sulfamethoxazole–resistant *S. aureus* and Enterobacteriaceae is a special problem in AIDS patients receiving the drug for prophylaxis of *Pneumocystis jiroveci* (formerly called *Pneumocystis carinii*) pneumonia (Martin *et al.,* 1999).

Absorption, Distribution, and Excretion. The pharmacokinetic profiles of sulfamethoxazole and trimethoprim

are closely but not perfectly matched to achieve a constant ratio of 20:1 in their concentrations in blood and tissues. The ratio in blood is often greater than 20:1, and that in tissues is frequently less. After a single oral dose of the combined preparation, trimethoprim is absorbed more rapidly than sulfamethoxazole. The concurrent administration of the drugs appears to slow the absorption of sulfamethoxazole. Peak blood concentrations of trimethoprim usually occur by 2 hours in most patients, whereas peak concentrations of sulfamethoxazole occur by 4 hours after a single oral dose. The half-lives of trimethoprim and sulfamethoxazole are approximately 11 and 10 hours, respectively.

When 800 mg sulfamethoxazole is given with 160 mg trimethoprim (the conventional 5:1 ratio) twice daily, the peak concentrations of the drugs in plasma are approximately 40 and 2 $\mu g/ml$, the optimal ratio. Peak concentrations are similar (46 and 3.4 $\mu g/ml$) after intravenous infusion of 800 mg sulfamethoxazole and 160 mg trimethoprim over a period of 1 hour.

Trimethoprim is distributed and concentrated rapidly in tissues, and about 40% is bound to plasma protein in the presence of sulfamethoxazole. The volume of distribution of trimethoprim is almost nine times that of sulfamethoxazole. The drug readily enters cerebrospinal fluid and sputum. High concentrations of each component of the mixture also are found in bile. About 65% of sulfamethoxazole is bound to plasma protein.

About 60% of administered trimethoprim and from 25% to 50% of administered sulfamethoxazole are excreted in the urine in 24 hours. Two-thirds of the sulfonamide is unconjugated. Metabolites of trimethoprim also are excreted. The rates of excretion and the concentrations of both compounds in the urine are reduced significantly in patients with uremia.

Therapeutic Uses. *Urinary Tract Infections.* Treatment of uncomplicated lower urinary tract infections with trimethoprim–sulfamethoxazole often is highly effective for sensitive bacteria. The preparation has been shown to produce a better therapeutic effect than does either of its components given separately when the infecting microorganisms are of the family Enterobacteriaceae. Single-dose therapy (320 mg trimethoprim plus 1600 mg sulfamethoxazole in adults) has been effective in some cases for the treatment of acute uncomplicated urinary tract infections, but a minimum of 3 days of therapy is more likely to be effective (Zinner and Mayer, 2000; Stamm and Hooton, 1993).

The combination appears to have special efficacy in chronic and recurrent infections of the urinary tract. Small doses (200 mg sulfamethoxazole plus 40 mg trimethoprim per day or two to four times these amounts once or twice per week) appear to be effective in reducing the number of recurrent urinary tract infections in adult females. This effect may be related to the presence of therapeutic concentrations of trimethoprim in vaginal secretions. Enterobacteriaceae surrounding the urethral orifice may be eliminated or markedly reduced in number, thus diminishing the chance of an ascending reinfection. Trimethoprim also is found in therapeutic concentrations in prostatic secretions, and trimethoprim–sulfamethoxazole is often effective for the treatment of bacterial prostatitis.

Bacterial Respiratory Tract Infections. Trimethoprim–sulfamethoxazole is effective for acute exacerbations of chronic bronchitis. Administration of 800 to 1200 mg sulfamethoxazole plus 160 to 240 mg trimethoprim twice a day appears to be effective in decreasing fever, purulence and volume of sputum, and sputum bacterial count. Trimethoprim–sulfamethoxazole should *not* be used to treat streptococcal pharyngitis because it does not eradicate the microorganism. It is effective for acute otitis media in children and acute maxillary sinusitis in adults caused by susceptible strains of *H. influenzae* and *S. pneumoniae.*

Gastrointestinal Infections. The combination is an alternative to *fluoroquinolone* for treatment of shigellosis because many strains of the causative agent now are resistant to *ampicillin;* however, resistance to trimethoprim–sulfamethoxazole is increasingly common. It also is a second-line drug (*ceftriaxone* or a fluoroquinolone is the preferred treatment) for typhoid fever, but resistance is an increasing problem. In adults, trimethoprim-sulfamethoxazole appears to be effective when the dose is 800 mg sulfamethoxazole plus 160 mg trimethoprim every 12 hours for 15 days.

Trimethoprim–sulfamethoxazole appears to be effective in the management of carriers of sensitive strains of *Salmonella typhi* and other *Salmonella* spp. One proposed schedule is the administration of 800 mg sulfamethoxazole plus 160 mg trimethoprim twice a day for 3 months; however, failures have occurred. The presence of chronic disease of the gallbladder may be associated with a high incidence of failure to clear the carrier state. Acute diarrhea owing to sensitive strains of enteropathogenic *E. coli* can be treated or prevented with either trimethoprim or trimethoprim plus sulfamethoxazole (Hill and Pearson, 1988). However, antibiotic treatment (either trimethoprim–sulfamethoxazole or *cephalosporin*) of diarrheal illness owing to enterohemorrhagic *E. coli* O157:H7 may increase the risk of hemolytic-uremic syndrome, perhaps by increasing the release of Shiga toxin by the bacteria (Wong *et al.*, 2000).

Infection by **Pneumocystis jiroveci.** High-dose therapy (trimethoprim 15 mg/kg per day plus sulfamethoxazole 100 mg/kg per day in three or four divided doses) is effective for this severe infection in patients with AIDS (Thomas and Limper, 2004). This combination compares favorably with *pentamidine* for treatment of this disease. Adjunctive corticosteroids should be given at the onset of anti-*Pneumocystis* therapy in patients with a P_{O_2} of less than 70 mm Hg or an alveolar–arterial gradient of greater than 35 mm Hg (Lane *et al.*, 1994). However, the incidence of side effects is high for both regimens (Sattler and Remington, 1981; Lane *et al.*, 1994). Lower-dose oral therapy with 800 mg sulfamethoxazole plus 160 mg trimethoprim (given twice daily) has been used successfully in AIDS patients with less severe pneumonia (P_{O_2} > 60 mm Hg) (Medina *et al.*, 1990). Prophylaxis with 800 mg sulfamethoxazole and 160 mg trimethoprim once daily or three times a week is effective in preventing pneumonia caused by this organism in patients with AIDS (Schneider *et al.*, 1992; Gallant *et al.*, 1994). Adverse reactions are less frequent with the lower prophylactic doses of trimethoprim–sulfamethoxazole. The most common problems are rash, fever, leukopenia, and hepatitis.

Prophylaxis in Neutropenic Patients. Several studies have demonstrated the effectiveness of low-dose therapy (150 mg/m^2 of body surface area of trimethoprim and 750 mg/m^2 of body surface area of sulfamethoxazole) for the prophylaxis of infection by *P. carinii* (*see* Hughes *et al.*, 1977). In addition, significant protection against sepsis caused by gram-negative bacteria was noted when 800 mg sulfamethoxazole and 160 mg trimethoprim were given twice daily to severely neutropenic patients. The emergence of resistant bacteria may limit the usefulness of trimethoprim–sulfamethoxazole for prophylaxis (Gualtieri *et al.*, 1983).

Miscellaneous Infections. *Nocardia* infections have been treated successfully with the combination, but failures also have been reported. Although a combination of *doxycycline* and streptomycin or *gentamicin* now is considered to be the treatment of choice for brucellosis, trimethoprim–sulfamethoxazole may be an effective substitute for the doxycycline combination. Trimethoprim–sulfamethoxazole also has been used successfully in the treatment of Whipple's disease, infection by *Stenotrophomonas maltophilia,* and infection by the intestinal parasites *Cyclospora* and *Isospora.* Wegener's granulomatosis may respond, depending on the stage of the disease. Trimethoprim–sulfamethoxazole also has been used to treat methicillin-resistant strains of *S. aureus.*

Untoward Effects. There is no evidence that trimethoprim–sulfamethoxazole, when given in the recommended doses, induces folate deficiency in normal persons. However, the margin between toxicity for bacteria and that for human beings may be relatively narrow when the cells of the patient are deficient in folate. In such cases, trimethoprim–sulfamethoxazole may cause or precipitate megaloblastosis, leukopenia, or thrombocytopenia. In routine use, the combination appears to exert little toxicity. About 75% of the untoward effects involve the skin. However, trimethoprim–sulfamethoxazole has been reported to cause up to three times as many dermatological reactions as does sulfisoxazole when given alone (5.9% *versus* 1.7%) (Arndt and Jick, 1976). Exfoliative dermatitis, Stevens-Johnson syndrome, and toxic epidermal necrolysis (Lyell's syndrome) are rare, occurring primarily in older individuals. Nausea and vomiting constitute the bulk of GI reactions; diarrhea is rare. Glossitis and stomatitis are relatively common. Mild and transient jaundice has been noted and appears to have the histological features of allergic cholestatic hepatitis. CNS reactions consist of headache, depression, and hallucinations, manifestations known to be produced by sulfonamides. Hematological reactions, in addition to those just mentioned, are various anemias (including aplastic, hemolytic, and macrocytic), coagulation disorders, granulocytopenia, agranulocytosis, purpura, Henoch-Schönlein purpura, and sulfhemoglobinemia. Permanent impairment of renal function may follow the use of trimethoprim–sulfamethoxazole in patients with renal disease, and a reversible decrease in creatinine clearance has been noted in patients with normal renal function.

Patients with AIDS frequently have hypersensitivity reactions when trimethoprim–sulfamethoxazole is administered (Gordin *et al.*, 1984). These adverse reactions include rash, neutropenia, Stevens-Johnson syndrome, Sweet's syndrome, and pulmonary infiltrates. It may be possible to continue therapy in such patients following rapid oral desensitization (Gluckstein and Ruskin, 1995).

THE QUINOLONES

The first quinolone, *nalidixic acid,* was isolated as a by-product of the synthesis of *chloroquine*. It has been available for the treatment of urinary tract infections for many years. The introduction of fluorinated 4-quinolones, such as *ciprofloxacin* (CIPRO), *moxifloxacin* (AVELOX), and *gatifloxacin* (TEQUIN) represents a particularly important therapeutic advance because these agents have broad antimicrobial activity and are effective after oral administration for the treatment of a wide variety of infectious diseases (Table 43–2). Relatively few side effects appear to accompany the use of these fluoroquinolones, and microbial resistance to their action does not develop rapidly (*see* Andriole, 1993; Hooper, 2000a). Rare and potentially fatal side effects, however, have resulted in the withdrawal from the market of *temafloxacin* (immune hemolytic anemia), *trovafloxacin* (hepatotoxicity), *grepafloxacin* (cardiotoxicity), and *clinafloxacin* (phototoxicity). In all these cases, the side effects were so infrequent as to be missed by prerelease clinical trials and detected only by postmarketing surveillance (Sheehan and Chew, 2003).

Chemistry. The compounds that currently are available for clinical use in the United States are quinolones containing a carboxylic acid moiety at position 3 of the primary ring structure. Many of the newer fluoroquinolones also contain a fluorine substituent at position 6 and a piperazine moiety at position 7 (Table 43–2).

Mechanism of Action. The quinolone antibiotics target bacterial DNA gyrase and topoisomerase IV (Drlica and Zhao, 1997). For many gram-positive bacteria (such as *S. aureus*), topoisomerase IV is the primary activity inhibited by the quinolones. In contrast, for many gram-negative bacteria (such as *E. coli*), DNA gyrase is the primary quinolone target (Hooper, 2000a; Alovero *et al.*, 2000). The individual strands of double-helical DNA must be separated to permit DNA replication or transcription. However, anything that separates the strands results in "overwinding" or excessive positive supercoiling of the DNA in front of the point of separation. To combat this mechanical obstacle, the bacterial enzyme DNA gyrase is responsible for the continuous introduction of negative supercoils into DNA. This is an ATP-dependent reaction requiring that both strands of the DNA be cut to permit passage of a segment of DNA through the break; the break then is resealed.

The DNA gyrase of *E. coli* is composed of two 105,000-dalton A subunits and two 95,000-dalton B subunits encoded by the *gyrA* and *gyrB* genes, respectively. The A subunits, which carry out the strand-cutting function of the gyrase, are the site of action of the quinolones (Figure 43–3). The drugs inhibit gyrase-mediated DNA supercoiling at concentrations that correlate well with those required to inhibit bacterial growth (0.1 to 10 μg/ml). Mutations of the gene that encodes the A subunit polypeptide can confer resistance to these drugs (Hooper, 2000a).

Topoisomerase IV also is composed of four subunits encoded by the *parC* and *parE* genes in *E. coli* (Drlica and Zhao, 1997; Hooper, 2000a). Topoisomerase IV separates interlinked (catenated) daughter DNA molecules that are the product of DNA replication. Eukaryotic cells do not contain DNA gyrase. However, they do contain a conceptually and mechanistically similar type II DNA topoisomerase that removes positive supercoils from eukaryotic DNA to prevent its tangling during replication. This enzyme is the target for some antineoplastic agents (*see* Chapter 51). Quinolones inhibit eukaryotic type II topoisomerase only at much higher concentrations (100 to 1000 μg/ml) (Mitscher and Ma, 2003).

Antibacterial Spectrum. The fluoroquinolones are potent bactericidal agents against *E. coli* and various species of *Salmonella, Shigella, Enterobacter, Campylobacter,* and *Neisseria* (*see* Eliopoulos and Eliopoulos, 1993). Minimal inhibitory concentrations of the fluoroquinolones for 90% of these strains (MIC_{90}) usually are less than 0.2 μg/ml. Ciprofloxacin is more active than *norfloxacin* (NOROXIN) against *P. aeruginosa;* values of MIC_{90} range from 0.5 to 6 μg/ml. Fluoroquinolones also have good activity against staphylococci, but not against methicillin-resistant strains (MIC_{90} = 0.1 to 2 μg/ml).

Activity against streptococci is limited to a subset of the quinolones, including *levofloxacin* (LEVAQUIN), *gatifloxacin* (TEQUIN), and *moxifloxacin* (AVELOX) (Hooper, 2000a; Eliopoulos and Eliopoulos, 1993). Several intracellular bacteria are inhibited by fluoroquinolones at concentrations that can be achieved in plasma; these include species of *Chlamydia, Mycoplasma, Legionella, Brucella,* and *Mycobacterium* (including *Mycobacterium tuberculosis*) (Leysen *et al.*, 1989; Alangaden and Lerner, 1997). Ciprofloxacin, *ofloxacin* (FLOXIN), and *pefloxacin* have MIC_{90} values from 0.5 to 3 μg/ml for *M. fortuitum, M. kansasii,* and *M. tuberculosis;* ofloxacin and pefloxacin are active in animal models of leprosy (Hooper, 2000a). However, clinical experience with these pathogens remains limited.

Several of the new fluoroquinolones have activity against anaerobic bacteria, including *garenoxacin* and *gemifloxacin* (Medical Letter, 2000).

Resistance to quinolones may develop during therapy *via* mutations in the bacterial chromosomal genes encoding DNA gyrase or topoisomerase IV or by active transport of the drug out of the bacteria (Oethinger *et al.*, 2000). No quinolone-modifying or -inactivating activities have been identified in bacteria (Gold and Moellering, 1996). Resistance has increased after the introduction of fluoroquinolones, especially in *Pseudomonas* and staphylococci (Pegues *et al.*, 1998; Peterson *et al.*, 1998). Increasing fluoroquinolone resistance also is being observed in *C. jejuni, Salmonella, N. gonorrhoeae,* and *S. pneumoniae* (Smith *et al.*, 1999; Centers for Disease Control and Prevention, 1994b; Thornsberry *et al.*, 1997; Mølbak *et al.*, 1999).

As mentioned in Chapter 42, the pharmacokinetic and pharmacodynamic parameters of antimicrobial agents are important in preventing the selection and spread of resistant strains and have led to description of the mutation-prevention concentration, which is the lowest concentration of antimicrobial that prevents selection of resistant bac-

Table 43–2
Structural Formulas of Selected Quinolones and Fluoroquinolones

CONGENER	R_1	R_6	R_7	X
Nalidixic acid	—C_2H_5	—H	—CH_3	—N—
Cinoxacin (*N replaces C2*)	—C_2H_5	(Fused dioxolo ring)*		—CH—
Norfloxacin	—C_2H_5	—F		—CH—
Ciprofloxacin		—F		—CH—
Ofloxacin		—F		—CH—
Sparfloxacin (*—NH₂ on C5*)		—F		
Fleroxacin	—CH_2—CH_2—F	—F		
Pefloxacin	—C_2H_5	—F		—CH—
Levofloxacin		—F		
Garenoxacin		—H		
Gemifloxacin		—F		—N—

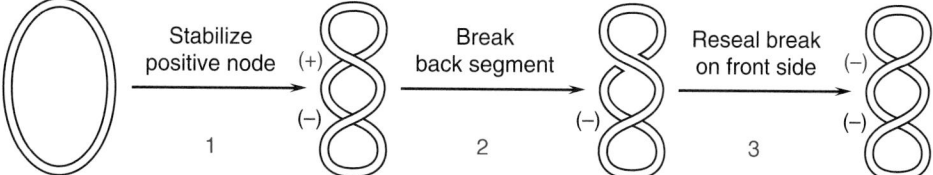

Figure 43–3. *Model of the formation of negative DNA supercoils by DNA gyrase.* The enzyme binds to two segments of DNA (1), creating a node of positive (+) superhelix. The enzyme then introduces a double-strand break in the DNA and passes the front segment through the break (2). The break is then resealed (3), creating a negative (−) supercoil. Quinolones inhibit the nicking and closing activity of the gyrase and also block the decatenating activity of topoisomerase IV. (Reprinted from Cozzarelli, 1980, with permission.)

teria from high bacterial inocula. β-Lactams are time-dependent agents without significant postantibiotic effects, resulting in bacterial eradication when unbound serum concentrations exceed MICs of these agents against infecting pathogens for more than 40% to 50% of the dosing interval. By contrast, fluoroquinolones are concentration-dependent agents, resulting in bacterial eradication when unbound serum area-under-the-curve-to-MIC ratios exceed 25 to 30. These observations are now being used to assess the roles of current agents, develop new formulations, and assess potency of new antimicrobials.

Absorption, Fate, and Excretion. The quinolones are well absorbed after oral administration and are distributed widely in body tissues. Peak serum levels of the fluoroquinolones are obtained within 1 to 3 hours of an oral dose of 400 mg, with peak levels ranging from 1.1 *μg/ml* for *sparfloxacin* to 6.4 *μg/ml* for *levofloxacin.* Relatively low serum levels are reached with norfloxacin and limit its usefulness to the treatment of urinary tract infections. Food does not impair oral absorption but may delay the time to peak serum concentrations. Oral doses in adults are 200 to 400 mg every 12 hours for ofloxacin, 400 mg every 12 hours for norfloxacin and pefloxacin, and 250 to 750 mg every 12 hours for ciprofloxacin. Bioavailability of the fluoroquinolones is greater than 50% for all agents and greater than 95% for several. The serum half-life ranges from 3 to 5 hours for norfloxacin and ciprofloxacin to 20 hours for sparfloxacin. The volume of distribution of quinolones is high, with concentrations of quinolones in urine, kidney, lung and prostate tissue, stool, bile, and macrophages and neutrophils higher than serum levels. Quinolone concentrations in cerebrospinal fluid, bone, and prostatic fluid are lower than in serum. Pefloxacin and ofloxacin levels in ascites fluid are close to serum levels, and ciprofloxacin, ofloxacin, and pefloxacin have been detected in human breast milk.

Most quinolones are cleared predominantly by the kidney, and dosages must be adjusted for renal failure. Exceptions are pefloxacin and moxifloxacin, which are metabolized predominantly by the liver and should not be used in patients with hepatic failure. None of the agents is removed efficiently by peritoneal dialysis or hemodialysis.

Therapeutic Uses. Urinary Tract Infections. Nalidixic acid is useful only for urinary tract infections caused by susceptible microorganisms. The fluoroquinolones are significantly more potent and have a much broader spectrum of antimicrobial activity. Norfloxacin is approved for use in the United States only for urinary tract infections. Comparative clinical trials indicate that the fluoroquinolones are more efficacious than trimethoprim–sulfamethoxazole for the treatment of urinary tract infections (Hooper and Wolfson, 1991; Warren *et al.*, 1999).

Prostatitis. Norfloxacin, ciprofloxacin, and ofloxacin all have been effective in uncontrolled trials for the treatment of prostatitis caused by sensitive bacteria. Fluoroquinolones administered for 4 to 6 weeks appear to be effective in patients not responding to trimethoprim–sulfamethoxazole (Hooper and Wolfson, 1991).

Sexually Transmitted Diseases. The quinolones are contraindicated in pregnancy. Fluoroquinolones lack activity for *Treponema pallidum* but have activity *in vitro* against *N. gonorrhoeae, C. trachomatis,* and *H. ducreyi.* For chlamydial urethritis/cervicitis, a 7-day course of ofloxacin or sparfloxacin is an alternative to a 7-day treatment with doxycycline or a single dose of azithromycin; other available quinolones have not been reliably effective. A single oral dose of a fluoroquinolone such as ofloxacin or ciprofloxacin is effective treatment for sensitive strains of *N. gonorrhoeae,* but increasing resistance to fluoroquinolones has led to ceftriaxone being the first-line agent for this infection (Newman *et al.*, 2004). Pelvic inflammatory disease has been treated effectively with a 14-day course of ofloxacin combined with an antibiotic with activity against anaerobes (clindamycin or metronidazole) (Centers for Disease Control and Prevention, 1998). Chancroid (infection by *H. ducreyi*) can be treated with 3 days of ciprofloxacin.

Gastrointestinal and Abdominal Infections. For traveler's diarrhea (frequently caused by enterotoxigenic *E. coli*), the quinolones are equal to trimethoprim–sulfamethoxazole in effectiveness, reducing the duration of loose stools by 1 to 3 days (DuPont and Ericsson, 1993). Norfloxacin, ciprofloxacin, and ofloxacin given for 5 days all have been effective in the treatment of patients with shigellosis, with even shorter courses effective in many cases (Bennish *et al.*, 1992). Norfloxacin is superior to tetracyclines in decreasing the duration of diarrhea in cholera (Bhattacharya *et al.*, 1990). Ciprofloxacin and ofloxacin treatment cures most patients with enteric fever caused by *S. typhi,* as well as bacteremic nontyphoidal infections in AIDS patients, and it clears chronic fecal carriage. Shigellosis is treated effectively with either ciprofloxacin or *azithromycin* (Khan *et al.*, 1997). The *in vitro* ability of the quinolones to induce the Shiga toxin *stx2* gene (the cause of the hemolytic-uremic syndrome) in *E. coli* suggests that the quinolones should not be used for Shiga toxin–producing *E. coli* (Miedouge *et al.*, 2000). Ciprofloxacin and ofloxacin have been less effective in treating episodes of peritonitis occurring in patients on chronic ambulatory peritoneal dialysis likely owing to the higher MICs for these drugs for the coagulase-negative staphylococci that are a common cause of peritonitis in this setting.

Respiratory Tract Infections. The major limitation to the use of quinolones for the treatment of community-acquired pneumonia and bronchitis had been the poor *in vitro* activity of ciprofloxacin, ofloxacin, and norfloxacin against *S. pneumoniae* and anaerobic bacteria. However, many of the newer fluoroquinolones, including gatifloxacin and moxifloxacin, have excellent activity against *S. pneumoniae*. Initial clinical experience with some of these newer quinolones shows comparable efficacy to β-lactam antibiotics (Aubier *et al.*, 1998; File *et al.*, 1997). The fluoroquinolones have *in vitro* activity against the rest of the commonly recognized respiratory pathogens, including *H. influenzae, Moraxella catarrhalis, S. aureus, M. pneumoniae, Chlamydia pneumoniae,* and *Legionella pneumophila.* Either a fluoroquinolone (ciprofloxacin or levofloxacin) or azithromycin is the antibiotic of choice for *L. pneumophila* (Yu, 2000). Fluoroquinolones have been very effective at eradicating both *H. influenzae* and *M. catarrhalis* from sputum. Mild to moderate respiratory exacerbations owing to *P. aeruginosa* in patients with cystic fibrosis have responded to oral fluoroquinolone therapy. Emerging clinical data are demonstrating a clear role for the newer fluoroquinolones as single agents for treatment of community-acquired pneumonia (Hooper, 2000a). However, on the horizon is a decreasing susceptibility of *S. pneumoniae* to fluoroquinolones (Chen *et al.*, 1999; Wortmann and Bennett, 1999).

Bone, Joint, and Soft Tissue Infections. The treatment of chronic osteomyelitis requires prolonged (weeks to months) antimicrobial therapy with agents active against *S. aureus* and gram-negative rods. The fluoroquinolones, by virtue of their oral administration and appropriate antibacterial spectrum for these infections, may be used appropriately in some cases (Gentry and Rodriguez-Gomez, 1991); recommended doses are 500 mg every 12 hours or, if severe, 750 mg twice daily. Bone and joint infections may require treatment for 4 to 6 weeks or more. Dosage should be reduced for patients with severely impaired renal function. Ciprofloxacin should not be given to children or pregnant women. Clinical cures have been as high as 75% in chronic osteomyelitis in which gram-negative rods predominated (Hooper, 2000a). Failures have been associated with the development of resistance in *S. aureus, P. aeruginosa,* and *Serratia marcescens.* In diabetic foot infections, which are commonly caused by a mixture of bacteria including gram-negative rods, anaerobes, streptococci, and staphylococci, the fluoroquinolones in combination with an agent with antianaerobic activity are a reasonable choice. Ciprofloxacin as sole therapy is effective in 50% of diabetic foot infections (Peterson *et al.*, 1989).

Other Infections. Ciprofloxacin received wide usage for the prophylaxis of anthrax and has been shown to be effective for the treatment of tularemia (Chocarro *et al.*, 2000; Swartz, 2001). The quinolones may be used as part of multiple-drug regimens for the treatment of multidrug-resistant tuberculosis and for the treatment of atypical mycobacterial infections as well as *M. avium* complex infections in AIDS (*see* Chapter 47). In neutropenic cancer patients with fever, the combination of a quinolone with an *aminoglycoside* is comparable to β-lactam–aminoglycoside combinations; quinolones are less effective when used alone (Meunier *et al.*, 1991). Quinolones, when used as prophylaxis in neutropenic patients, have decreased the incidence of gram-negative rod bacteremias (GIMEMA Infection Program, 1991). Ciprofloxacin plus *amoxicillin–clavulanate* has been shown recently to be effective as an oral empirical therapy for fever in low-risk patients with granulocytopenia secondary to cancer chemotherapy (Kern *et al.*, 1999; Freifeld *et al.*, 1999).

Adverse Effects. Quinolones and fluoroquinolones generally are well tolerated (Mandell, 2003). The most common adverse reactions involve the GI tract, with 3% to 17% of patients reporting mostly mild nausea, vomiting, and/or abdominal discomfort. Diarrhea and antibiotic-associated colitis have been unusual. CNS side effects, predominately mild headache and dizziness, have been seen in 0.9% to 11% of patients. Rarely, hallucinations, delirium, and seizures have occurred, predominantly in patients who also were receiving *theophylline* or a nonsteroidal antiinflammatory drug. Ciprofloxacin and pefloxacin inhibit the metabolism of theophylline, and toxicity from elevated concentrations of the methylxanthine may occur (Schwartz *et al.*, 1988). Nonsteroidal antiinflammatory drugs may augment displacement of γ-aminobutyric acid (GABA) from its receptors by the quinolones (Halliwell *et al.*, 1993). Rashes, including photosensitivity reactions, also can occur. Achilles tendon rupture or tendinitis has occurred rarely. Renal disease, hemodialysis, and steroid use may be predisposing factors (Mandell, 2003). All these agents can produce arthropathy in several species of immature animals. Traditionally, the use of quinolones in children has been contraindicated for this reason. However, children with cystic fibrosis given ciprofloxacin, norfloxacin, and nalidixic acid have had few, and reversible, joint symptoms (Burkhardt *et al.*, 1997). Therefore, in some cases the benefits may outweigh the risks of quinolone therapy in children.

Leukopenia, eosinophilia, and mild elevations in serum transaminases occur rarely. QT_c interval (QT interval corrected for heart rate) prolongation has been observed with sparfloxacin and to a lesser extent with gatifloxacin and moxifloxacin. Quinolones probably should be used only with caution in patients on class III (*amiodarone*) and class IA (*quinidine, procainamide*) antiarrhythmics (*see* Chapter 34).

ANTISEPTIC AND ANALGESIC AGENTS FOR URINARY TRACT INFECTIONS

The urinary tract antiseptics inhibit the growth of many species of bacteria. They cannot be used to treat systemic infections because effective concentrations are not achieved in plasma with safe doses. However, because they are concentrated in the renal tubules, they can be administered orally to treat infections of the urinary tract. Furthermore, effective antibacterial concentrations reach the renal pelves and the bladder. Treatment with such drugs can be thought of as local therapy: Only in the kidney and bladder, with the rare exceptions mentioned below, are adequate therapeutic levels achieved (*see* Hooper, 2000b).

Methenamine. *Methenamine* is a urinary tract antiseptic and prodrug that owes its activity to its capacity to generate formaldehyde.

Chemistry. Methenamine is hexamethylenetetramine (hexamethylenamine). It has the following structure:

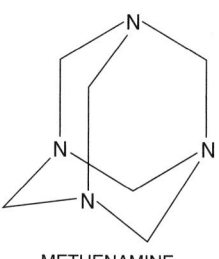

METHENAMINE

The compound decomposes in water to generate formaldehyde, according to the following reaction:

$$NH_4(CH_2)_6 + 6H_2O + 4H^+ \rightarrow 4NH_4^+ + 6HCHO$$

At pH 7.4, almost no decomposition occurs; however, the yield of formaldehyde is 6% of the theoretical amount at pH 6 and 20% at pH 5. Thus, acidification of the urine promotes the formaldehyde-dependent antibacterial action. The reaction is fairly slow, and 3 hours are required to reach 90% completion (Strom and Jun, 1993).

Antimicrobial Activity. Nearly all bacteria are sensitive to free formaldehyde at concentrations of about 20 $\mu g/ml$. Urea-splitting microorganisms (*e.g., Proteus* spp.) tend to raise the pH of the urine and thus inhibit the release of formaldehyde. Microorganisms do not develop resistance to formaldehyde.

Pharmacology and Toxicology. Methenamine is absorbed orally, but 10% to 30% decomposes in the gastric juice unless the drug is protected by an enteric coating. Because of the ammonia produced, methenamine is contraindicated in hepatic insufficiency. Excretion in the urine is nearly quantitative. When the urine pH is 6 and the daily urine volume is 1000 to 1500 ml, a daily dose of 2 g will yield a concentration of 18 to 60 $\mu g/ml$ of formaldehyde; this is more than the MIC for most urinary tract pathogens. Various poorly metabolized acids can be used to acidify the urine. Low pH alone is bacteriostatic, so acidification serves a double function. The acids commonly used are *mandelic acid* and *hippuric acid* (UREX, HIPREX).

Gastrointestinal distress frequently is caused by doses greater than 500 mg four times a day, even with enteric-coated tablets. Painful and frequent micturition, albuminuria, hematuria, and rashes may result from doses of 4 to 8 g/day given for longer than 3 to 4 weeks. Once the urine is sterile, a high dose should be reduced. Because systemic methenamine has low toxicity at the typically used doses, renal insufficiency does not constitute a contraindication to the use of methenamine alone, but the acids given concurrently may be detrimental. Methenamine mandelate is contraindicated in renal insufficiency. Crystalluria from the mandelate moiety can occur. Methenamine combines with sulfamethizole and perhaps other sulfonamides in the urine, which results in mutual antagonism.

Therapeutic Uses and Status. Methenamine is not a primary drug for the treatment of acute urinary tract infections, but it is of value for chronic suppressive treatment (Stamm and Hooton, 1993). The agent is most useful when the causative organism is *E. coli,* but it usually can suppress the common gram-negative offenders and often *S. aureus* and *S. epidermidis* as well. *Enterobacter aerogenes* and *Proteus vulgaris* are usually resistant. Urea-splitting bacteria (mostly *Proteus*) make it difficult to control the urine pH. The physician should strive to keep the pH below 5.5.

Nitrofurantoin. *Nitrofurantoin* (FURADANTIN, MACROBID, others) is a synthetic nitrofuran that is used for the prevention and treatment of infections of the urinary tract. Its structural formula is:

NITROFURANTOIN

Antimicrobial Activity. Enzymes capable of reducing nitrofurantoin appear to be crucial for its activation. Highly reactive interme-

diates are formed, and these seem to be responsible for the observed capacity of the drug to damage DNA. Bacteria reduce nitrofurantoin more rapidly than do mammalian cells, and this is thought to account for the selective antimicrobial activity of the compound. Bacteria that are susceptible to the drug rarely become resistant during therapy. Nitrofurantoin is active against many strains of *E. coli* and enterococci. However, most species of *Proteus* and *Pseudomonas* and many species of *Enterobacter* and *Klebsiella* are resistant. Nitrofurantoin is bacteriostatic for most susceptible microorganisms at concentrations of 32 $\mu g/ml$ or less and is bactericidal at concentrations of 100 $\mu g/ml$ and more. The antibacterial activity is higher in an acidic urine.

Pharmacology and Toxicity. Nitrofurantoin is absorbed rapidly and completely from the GI tract. The macrocrystalline form of the drug is absorbed and excreted more slowly. Antibacterial concentrations are not achieved in plasma following ingestion of recommended doses because the drug is eliminated rapidly. The plasma half-life is 0.3 to 1 hour; about 40% is excreted unchanged into the urine. The average dose of nitrofurantoin yields a concentration in urine of approximately 200 $\mu g/ml$. This concentration is soluble at pH >5, but the urine should not be alkalinized because this reduces antimicrobial activity. The rate of excretion is linearly related to the creatinine clearance, so in patients with impaired glomerular function, the efficacy of the drug may be decreased and the systemic toxicity increased. Nitrofurantoin colors the urine brown.

The most common untoward effects are nausea, vomiting, and diarrhea; the macrocrystalline preparation is better tolerated. Various hypersensitivity reactions occur occasionally. These include chills, fever, leukopenia, granulocytopenia, hemolytic anemia [associated with glucose-6-phosphate dehydrogenase deficiency (Gait, 1990)], cholestatic jaundice, and hepatocellular damage. Chronic active hepatitis is an uncommon but serious side effect (Black *et al.*, 1980; Tolman, 1980). Acute pneumonitis with fever, chills, cough, dyspnea, chest pain, pulmonary infiltration, and eosinophilia may occur within hours to days of the initiation of therapy; these symptoms usually resolve quickly after discontinuation of the drug. More insidious subacute reactions also may be noted, and interstitial pulmonary fibrosis can occur in patients taking the drug chronically. This appears to be due to generation of oxygen radicals as a result of redox cycling of the drug in the lung. Elderly patients are especially susceptible to the pulmonary toxicity of nitrofurantoin (*see* Holmberg *et al.*, 1980). Megaloblastic anemia is rare. Various neurological disorders are observed occasionally. Headache, vertigo, drowsiness, muscular aches, and nystagmus are readily reversible, but severe polyneuropathies with demyelination and degeneration of both sensory and motor nerves have been reported; signs of denervation and muscle atrophy result. Neuropathies are most likely to occur in patients with impaired renal function and in persons on long-continued treatment. Toxic reactive metabolites may contribute to some adverse reactions (Spielberg and Gordon, 1981).

The oral dosage of nitrofurantoin for adults is 50 to 100 mg four times a day with meals and at bedtime. Alternatively, the daily dosage is better expressed as 5 to 7 mg/kg in four divided doses (not to exceed 400 mg). A single 50- to 100-mg dose at bedtime may be sufficient to prevent recurrences. The daily dose for children is 5 to 7 mg/kg but may be as low as 1 mg/kg for long-term therapy (Lohr *et al.*, 1977). A course of therapy should not exceed 14 days, and repeated courses should be separated by rest periods. Pregnant women, individuals with impaired renal function (creatinine clearance < 40 ml/min), and children younger than 1 month of age should not receive nitrofurantoin.

Nitrofurantoin is approved only for the treatment of urinary tract infections caused by microorganisms known to be susceptible to the drug. Currently, bacterial resistance to nitrofurantoin is more frequent than resistance to fluoroquinolones or trimethoprim–sulfamethoxazole, making nitrofurantoin a second-line agent for treatment of urinary tract infections (Stamm and Hooton, 1993). Nitrofurantoin also is not recommended for treatment of pyelonephritis or prostatitis. However, nitrofurantoin is effective for prophylaxis of recurrent urinary tract infections (Brumfitt and Hamilton-Miller, 1995).

Phenazopyridine. *Phenazopyridine hydrochloride* (PYRIDIUM, others) is *not* a urinary antiseptic. However, it does have an analgesic action on the urinary tract and alleviates symptoms of dysuria, frequency, burning, and urgency. The usual dose is 200 mg three times daily. The compound is an azo dye, which colors urine orange or red; the patient should be so informed. Gastrointestinal upset is seen in up to 10% of patients and can be reduced by administering the drug with food; overdosage may result in methemoglobinemia. Phenazopyridine has been marketed since 1925 and has had dual prescription/over-the-counter (OTC) marketing status since 1951. As part of their ongoing review of OTC drug products, the FDA is currently in the process of evaluating products containing less than 200 mg phenazopyridine to determine whether these products generally are recognized as safe and effective as urinary analgesics. The outcome of this evaluation will determine the continued availability of OTC phenazopyridine products in the United States. Products containing 200 mg phenazopyridine are sold by prescription, but their long-term availability in the marketplace also may be affected by the FDA's final OTC ruling.

BIBLIOGRAPHY

Alovero, F.L., Pan, X. S., Morris, J.E., Manzo, R.H., and Fisher, L.M. Engineering the specificity of antibacterial fluoroquinolones: benzenesulfonamide modifications at C-7 of ciprofloxacin change its primary target in *Streptococcus pneumoniae* from topoisomerase IV to gyrase. *Antimicrob. Agents Chemother.*, **2000**, *44*:320–325.

Arndt, K.A., and Jick, H. Rates of cutaneous reactions to drugs: A report from the Boston Collaborative Drug Surveillance Program. *JAMA*, **1976**, *235*:918–923.

Aubier, M., Verster, R., Reganney, C., Geslin, P., and Vercken, J.B. Once-daily sparfloxacin versus high-dosage amoxicillin in the treatment of community-acquired, suspected pneumococcal pneumonia in adults. Sparfloxacin European Study Group. *Clin. Infect. Dis.*, **1998**, *26*:1312–1320.

Bennish, M.L., Salam, M.A., Khan, W.A., and Khan, A.M. Treatment of shigellosis: III. Comparison of one- or two-dose ciprofloxacin with standard 5-day therapy. A randomized, blinded trial. *Ann. Intern. Med.*, **1992**, *117*:727–734.

Bhattacharya, S.K., Bhattacharya, M.K., Dutta, P., *et al.* Double-blind, randomized, controlled clinical trial of norfloxacin for cholera. *Antimicrob. Agents Chemother.*, **1990**, *34*:939–940.

Black, M., Rabin, L., and Schatz, N. Nitrofurantoin-induced chronic active hepatitis. *Ann. Intern. Med.*, **1980**, *92*:62–64.

Brumfitt, W., and Hamilton-Miller, J.M. A comparative trial of low dose cefaclor and macrocrystalline nitrofurantoin in the prevention of recurrent urinary tract infection. *Infection*, **1995**, *23*:98–102.

Burkhardt, J.E., Walterspeil, J.N., and Schaad, U.B. Quinolone arthropathy in animals versus children. *Clin. Infect. Dis.*, **1997**, *25*:1196–1204.

Bushby, S.R., and Hitchings, G.H. Trimethoprim, a sulphonamide potentiator. *Br. J. Pharmacol.*, **1968**, *33*:72–90.

Centers for Disease Control and Prevention. Drug-resistant *Streptococcus pneumoniae*—Kentucky and Tennessee, 1993. *M.M.W.R.*, **1994a**, *43*:23–26 and 31.

Centers for Disease Control and Prevention. Decreased susceptibility of *Neisseria gonorrhoeae* to fluoroquinolones—Ohio and Hawaii, 1992–1994. *M.M.W.R.*, **1994b**, *43*:325–327.

Centers for Disease Control and Prevention. 1998 guidelines for treatment of sexually transmitted diseases. *M.M.W.R.*, **1998**, *47*:1–111.

Chen, D.K., McGeer, A., de Azavedo, J.C., and Low, D.E. Decreased susceptibility of *Streptococcus pneumoniae* to fluoroquinolones in Canada. Canadian Bacterial Surveillance Network. *New Engl. J. Med.*, **1999**, *341*:233–239.

Chocarro, A., Gonzalez, A, and Garcia, I. Treatment of tularemia with ciprofloxacin. *Clin. Infect. Dis.*, **2000**, *31*:623.

Eliopoulos, G.M., and Eliopoulos, C.T. Activity *in vitro* of the quinolones. In, *Quinolone Antimicrobial Agents,* 2d ed. (Hooper, D.C., and Wolfson, J.S., eds.) American Society for Microbiology, Washington, **1993**, pp. 161–193.

File, T.M., Jr., Segreti, J., Dunbar, L., *et al.* A multicenter, randomized study comparing the efficacy and safety of intravenous and/or oral levofloxacin versus ceftriaxone and/or cefuroxime axetil in treatment of adults with community-acquired pneumonia. *Antimicrob. Agents Chemother.*, **1997**, *41*:1965–1972.

Freifeld, A., Marchigiani, D., Walsh, T., *et al.* A double-blind comparison of empirical oral and intravenous antibiotic therapy for low-risk febrile patients with neutropenia during cancer chemotherapy. *New Engl. J. Med.*, **1999**, *341*:305–311.

Gait, J.E. Hemolytic reactions to nitrofurantoin in patients with glucose-6-phosphate dehydrogenase deficiency: theory and practice. *D.I.C.P.*, **1990**, *24*:1210–1213.

Gentry, L.O., and Rodriguez-Gomez, G. Ofloxacin versus parenteral therapy for chronic osteomyelitis. *Antimicrob. Agents Chemother.*, **1991**, *35*:538–541.

GIMEMA Infection Program. Prevention of bacterial infection in neutropenic patients with hematologic malignancies: A randomized, multicenter trial comparing norfloxacin with ciprofloxacin. Gruppo Italiano Malattie Ematologiche Maligne dell'Adulto. *Ann. Intern. Med.*, **1991**, *115*:7–12.

Gluckstein, D., and Ruskin, J. Rapid oral desensitization to trimethoprim–sulfamethoxazole (TMP-SMZ): Use in prophylaxis for *Pneumocystis carinii* pneumonia in patients with AIDS who were previously tolerant to TMP-SMZ. *Clin. Infect. Dis.*, **1995**, *20*:849–853.

Gordin, F.M., Simon, G.L., Wofsy, C.B., and Mills, J. Adverse reactions to trimethoprim–sulfamethoxazole in patients with acquired immunodeficiency syndrome. *Ann. Intern. Med.*, **1984**, *100*:495–499.

Gualtieri, R.J., Donowitz, G.R., Kaiser, D.L., Hess, C.E., and Sande, M.A. Double-blind randomized study of prophylactic trimethoprim–sulfamethoxazole in granulocytopenic patients with hematologic malignancies. *Am. J. Med.*, **1983**, *74*:934–940.

Halliwell, R.F., Davey, P.G., and Lambert, J.J. Antagonism of GABA$_A$ receptors by 4-quinolones. *J. Antimicrob. Chemother.*, **1993**, *31*:457–462.

Hitchings, G.H. A biochemical approach to chemotherapy. *Ann. N.Y. Acad. Sci.*, **1961**, *23*:700–708.

Holmberg, L., Boman, G., Bottiger, L.E., *et al.* Adverse reactions to nitrofurantoin: Analysis of 921 reports. *Am. J. Med.*, **1980**, *69*:733–738.

Hughes, W.T., Kuhn, S., Chaudhary, S., *et al.* Successful chemoprophylaxis for *Pneumocystis carinii* pneumonitis. *New Engl. J. Med.,* **1977,** *297*:1419–1426.

Kern, W.V., Cometta, A., De Bock, R., *et al.* Oral versus intravenous empirical antimicrobial therapy for fever in patients with granulocytopenia who are receiving cancer chemotherapy. International Antimicrobial Therapy Cooperative Group of the European Organization for Research and Treatment of Cancer. *New Engl. J. Med.,* **1999,** *341*:312–318.

Khan, W.A., Seas, C., Dhar, U., Salam, M.A., and Bennish, M.L. Treatment of shigellosis: V. Comparison of azithromycin and ciprofloxacin. A double-blind, randomized, controlled trial. *Ann. Intern. Med.,* **1997,** *126*:697–703.

Leysen, D.C., Haemers, A., and Pattyn, S.R. Mycobacteria and the new quinolones. *Antimicrob. Agents Chemother.,* **1989,** *33*:1–5.

Lohr, J.A., Nunley, D.H., Howards, S.S., and Ford, R.F. Prevention of recurrent urinary tract infections in girls. *Pediatrics,* **1977,** *59*:562–565.

Martin, J.N., Rose, D.A., Hadley, W.K., *et al.* Emergence of trimethoprim–sulfamethoxazole resistance in the AIDS era. *J. Infect. Dis.,* **1999,** *180*:1809–1818.

Medina, I., Mills, J., Leoung, G., *et al.* Oral therapy for *Pneumocystis carinii* pneumonia (PCP) in the acquired immune deficiency syndrome: A controlled trial of trimethoprim–sulfamethoxazole versus trimethoprim–dapsone. *New Engl. J. Med.,* **1990,** *323*:776–782.

Meunier, F., Zinner, S.H., Gaya, H., *et al.* Prospective, randomized evaluation of ciprofloxacin versus piperacillin plus amikacin for empiric antibiotic therapy of febrile granulocytopenic cancer patients with lymphomas and solid tumors. The European Organization for Research on Treatment of Cancer International Antimicrobial Therapy Cooperative Group. *Antimicrob. Agents Chemother.,* **1991,** *35*:873–878.

Miedouge, M., Hacini, J., Grimont, F., and Watine, J. Shiga toxin–producing *Escherichia coli* urinary tract infection associated with hemolytic-uremic syndrome in an adult and possible adverse effect of ofloxacin therapy. *Clin. Infect. Dis.,* **2000,** *30*:395–396.

Mølbak, K., Baggesen, D.L., Aarestrup, F.M., *et al.* An outbreak of multidrug-resistant, quinolone-resistant *Salmonella enterica* serotype typhimurium DT104. *New Engl. J. Med.,* **1999,** *341*:1420–1425.

Newman, L.M., Wang, S.A., Ohye, R.G., *et al.* The epidemiology of fluoroquinolone-resistant *Neisseria gonorrhoeae* in Hawaii, 2001. *Clin. Infect. Dis.,* **2004,** *38*:649–654.

Oethinger, M., Kern, W.V., Jellen-Ritter, A.S., McMurry, L.M., and Levy, S.B. Ineffectiveness of topoisomerase mutations in mediating clinically significant fluoroquinolone resistance in *Escherichia coli* in the absence of the AcrAB efflux pump. *Antimicrob. Agents Chemother.,* **2000,** *44*:10–13.

Peterson, L.R., Lissack, L.M., Canter, K., *et al.* Therapy of lower extremity infections with ciprofloxacin in patients with diabetes mellitus, peripheral vascular disease, or both. *Am. J. Med.,* **1989,** *86*:801–808.

Peterson, L.R., Postelnick, M., Pozdol, T.L., Reisberg, B., and Noskin, G.A. Management of fluoroquinolone resistance in *Pseudomonas aeruginosa:* Outcome of monitored use in a referral hospital. *Int. J. Antimicrob. Agents,* **1998,** *10*:207–214.

Pegues, D.A., Colby, C., Hibberd, P.L., *et al.* The epidemiology of resistance to ofloxacin and oxacillin among clinical coagulase-negative staphylococcal isolates: Analysis of risk factors and strain types. *Clin. Infect. Dis.,* **1998,** *26*:72–79.

Sattler, F.R., and Remington, J.S. Intravenous trimethoprim–sulfamethoxazole therapy for *Pneumocystis carinii* pneumonia. *Am. J. Med.,* **1981,** *70*:1215–1221.

Schneider, M.M., Hoepelman, A.I., Eeftinck Schattenkerk, J.K., *et al.* A controlled trial of aerosolized pentamidine or trimethoprim–sulfamethoxazole as primary prophylaxis against *Pneumocystis carinii* pneumonia in patients with human immunodeficiency virus infection. The Dutch AIDS Treatment Group. *New Engl. J. Med.,* **1992,** *327*:1836–1841.

Schwartz, J., Jauregui, L., Lettieri, J., and Bachmann, K. Impact of ciprofloxacin on theophylline clearance and steady-state concentrations in serum. *Antimicrob. Agents Chemother.,* **1988,** *32*:75–77.

Shear, N.H., Spielberg, S.P., Grant, D.M., Tang, B.K., and Kalow, W. Differences in metabolism of sulfonamides predisposing to idiosyncratic toxicity. *Ann. Intern. Med.,* **1986,** *105*:179–184.

Smith, K.E., Besser, J.M., Hedberg, C.W., *et al.* Quinolone-resistant *Campylobacter jejuni* infections in Minnesota, 1992–1998. Investigation team. *New Engl. J. Med.,* **1999,** *340*:1525–1532.

Spielberg, S.P., and Gordon, G.B. Nitrofurantoin cytotoxicity. *In vitro* assessment of risk based on glutathione metabolism. *J. Clin. Invest.,* **1981,** *67*:37–41.

Strom, J.G., Jr., and Jun, H.W. Effect of urine pH and ascorbic acid on the rate of conversion of methenamine to formaldehyde. *Biopharm. Drug Dispos.,* **1993,** *14*:61–69.

Swartz, M.N. Recognition and management of anthrax: An update. *New Engl. J. Med.,* **2001,** *345*:1621–1626.

Thomas, C.F., and Limpor, A.H. *Pneumocystis* pneumonia. *New Engl. J. Med.,* **2004,** *350*:2487–2498.

Thornsberry, C., Ogilvie, P., Kahn, J., and Mauriz, Y. Surveillance of antimicrobial resistance in *Streptococcus pneumoniae, Haemophilus influenzae,* and *Moraxella catarrhalis* in the United States in 1996–1997 respiratory season. The Laboratory Investigator Group. *Diagn. Microbiol. Infect. Dis.,* **1997,** *29*:249–257.

Tolman, K.G. Nitrofurantoin and chronic active hepatitis. *Ann. Intern. Med.,* **1980,** *92*:119–120.

Voogd, C.E., Schot, C.S., van Leeuwen, W.J., and van Klingeren, B. Monitoring of antibiotic resistance in shigellae isolated in The Netherlands 1984–1989. *Eur. J. Clin. Microbiol. Infect. Dis.,* **1992,** *11*:164–167.

Weidner, W., Schiefer, H.G., and Dalhoff, A. Treatment of chronic bacterial prostatitis with ciprofloxacin: Results of a one-year follow-up study. *Am. J. Med.,* **1987,** *82*:280–283.

Wong, C.S., Jelacic, S., Habeeb, R.L., Watkins, S.L., and Tarr, P.L. The risk of the hemolytic-uremic syndrome after antibiotic treatment of *Escherichia coli* O157:H7. *New Engl. J. Med.,* **2000,** *342*:1930–1936.

Wortmann, G.W., and Bennett, S.P. Fatal meningitis due to levofloxacin-resistant *Streptococcus pneumoniae. Clin. Infect. Dis.,* **1999,** *29*:1599–1600.

Yu, V.L. *Legionella pneumophila* (Legionnaires' disease). In, *Mandell, Douglas, and Bennett's Principles and Practice of Infectious Diseases,* 5th ed. (Mandell, G.L., Bennett, J.E., and Dolin, R., eds.) Churchill Livingstone, New York, **2000,** pp. 2424–2435.

MONOGRAPHS AND REVIEWS

Alangaden, G.J., and Lerner, S.A. The clinical use of fluoroquinolones for the treatment of mycobacterial diseases. *Clin. Infect. Dis.,* **1997,** *25*:1213–1221.

Andriole, V.T. The future of the quinolones. *Drugs,* **1993,** *45*(suppl 3):1–7.

Cozzarelli, N.R. DNA gyrase and the supercoiling of DNA. *Science,* **1980,** *207*:953–960.

Drlica, K., and Zhao, X. DNA gyrase, topoisomerase IV, and the 4-quinolones. *Microbiol. Mol. Biol. Rev.,* **1997,** *61*:377–392.

DuPont, H.L., and Ericsson, C.D. Prevention and treatment of traveler's diarrhea. *New Engl. J. Med.,* **1993,** *328*:1821–1827.

Gallant, J.E., Moore, R.D., and Chaisson, R.E. Prophylaxis for opportunistic infections in patients with HIV infection. *Ann. Intern. Med.,* **1994,** *120*:932–944.

Gold, H.S., and Moellering, R.C., Jr. Antimicrobial-drug resistance. *New Engl. J. Med.,* **1996,** *335*:1445–1453.

Hill, D.R., and Pearson, R.D. Health advice for international travel. *Ann. Intern. Med.,* **1988,** *108*:839–852.

Hooper, D.C. Quinolones. In, *Mandell, Douglas, and Bennett's Principles and Practice of Infectious Diseases,* 5th ed. (Mandell, G.L., Bennett, J.E., and Dolin, R., eds.) Churchill Livingstone, New York, **2000a,** pp. 404–423.

Hooper, D.C. Urinary tract agents: Nitrofurantoin and methenamine. In, *Mandell, Douglas, and Bennett's Principles and Practice of Infectious Diseases,* 5th ed. (Mandell, G.L., Bennett, J.E., and Dolin, R., eds.) Churchill Livingstone, New York, **2000b,** pp. 423–428.

Hooper, D.C., and Wolfson, J.S. Fluoroquinolone antimicrobial agents. *New Engl. J. Med.,* **1991,** *324*:384–394.

Lane, H.C., Laughon, B.E., Falloon, J., *et al.* N.I.H. conference: Recent advances in the management of AIDS-related opportunistic infections. *Ann. Intern. Med.,* **1994,** *120*:945–955.

Mandell, L.A. Improved safety profile of newer fluoroquinolone. In, *Fluoroquinolone Antibiotics.* (Ronald, A.R., and Low, D.E., eds.) Birkhauser, Basel, **2003,** pp. 73–86.

Medical Letter. Gatifloxacin and moxifloxacin: Two new fluoroquinolones. *Med. Lett. Drugs Ther.,* **2000,** *42*:15–17.

Mitscher, L.A., and Ma, Z. Structure-activity relationships of quinolones. In, *Fluoroquinolone Antibiotics.* (Ronald, A.R., and Low, D.E., eds.) Birkhauser, Basel, **2003,** pp. 11–48.

Montoya, J.G., and Remington, J.S. *Toxoplasma gondii.* In, *Mandell, Douglas, and Bennett's Principles and Practice of Infectious Diseases,* 5th ed. (Mandell, G.L., Bennett, J.E., and Dolin, R., eds.) Churchill Livingstone, New York, **2000,** pp. 2858–2888.

Sheehan, G., and Chew, N.S.Y. The history of quinolones. In, *Fluoroquinolone Antibiotics.* (Ronald, A.R., and Low, D.E., eds.) Birkhauser, Basel, **2003,** pp. 1–10.

Stamm, W.E., and Hooton, T.M. Management of urinary tract infection in adults. *New Engl. J. Med.,* **1993,** *329*:1328–1334.

Warren, J.W., Abruytyn, E., Hebel, J.R., *et al.* Guidelines for antimicrobial treatment of uncomplicated acute bacterial cystitis and acute pyelonephritis in women. Infectious Diseases Society of America. *Clin. Infect. Dis.,* **1999,** *29*:745–758.

Zinner, S.H., and Mayer, K.H. Sulfonamides and trimethoprim. In, *Mandell, Douglas, and Bennett's Principles and Practice of Infectious Diseases,* 5th ed. (Mandell, G.L., Bennett, J.E., and Dolin, R., eds.) Churchill Livingstone, New York, **2000,** pp. 394–404.

PENICILLINS, CEPHALOSPORINS, AND OTHER β-LACTAM ANTIBIOTICS

William A. Petri, Jr.

The β-lactam antibiotics are useful and frequently prescribed antimicrobial agents that share a common structure and mechanism of action—inhibition of synthesis of the bacterial peptidoglycan cell wall. This class includes penicillins G and V, which are highly active against susceptible gram-positive cocci; penicillinase-resistant penicillins such as nafcillin, which are active against penicillinase-producing *Staphylococcus aureus; ampicillin* and other agents with an improved gram-negative spectrum, especially when combined with a β-lactamase inhibitor; and extended-spectrum penicillins with activity against *Pseudomonas aeruginosa,* such as piperacillin.

The β-lactams also include the cephalosporin antibiotics, which are classified by generation: First-generation agents have excellent gram-positive and modest gram-negative activity; second-generation agents have somewhat better activity against gram-negative organisms and include some agents with antianaerobe activity; third-generation agents have activity against gram-positive organisms and much more activity against the Enterobacteriaceae, with a subset active against *P. aeruginosa*; and fourth-generation agents encompass the antimicrobial spectrum of all the third-generation agents and have increased stability to hydrolysis by inducible chromosomal β-lactamases.

β-Lactamase inhibitors such as *clavulanate* are used to extend the spectrum of penicillins against β-lactamase-producing organisms. Carbapenems, including *imipenem* and *meropenem,* have the broadest antimicrobial spectrum of any antibiotic, whereas the *monobactam aztreonam* has a gram-negative spectrum resembling that of the *aminoglycosides.*

Bacterial resistance against the β-lactam antibiotics continues to increase at a dramatic rate. Mechanisms of resistance include not only production of β-lactamases that destroy the antibiotics but also alterations in or acquisition of novel penicillin-binding proteins and decreased entry and/or active efflux of the antibiotic.

THE PENICILLINS

The penicillins constitute one of the most important groups of antibiotics. Although numerous other antimicrobial agents have been produced since the first penicillin became available, these still are used widely, and major antibiotics and new derivatives of the basic penicillin nucleus still are being produced. Many of these have unique advantages such that members of this group of antibiotics are currently the drugs of choice for a large number of infectious diseases.

History. The history of the brilliant research that led to the discovery and development of penicillin is well chronicled. In 1928, while studying *Staphylococcus* variants in the laboratory at St. Mary's Hospital in London, Alexander Fleming observed that a mold contaminating one of his cultures caused the bacteria in its vicinity to undergo lysis. Broth in which the fungus was grown was markedly inhibitory for many microorganisms. Because the mold belonged to the genus *Penicillium,* Fleming named the antibacterial substance *penicillin.*

A decade later, penicillin was developed as a systemic therapeutic agent by the concerted research of a group of investigators at Oxford University headed by Florey, Chain, and Abraham. By May 1940, the crude material then available was found to produce dramatic therapeutic effects when administered parenterally to mice with experimentally produced streptococcal infections. Despite great obstacles to its laboratory production, enough penicillin was accumulated by 1941 to conduct therapeutic trials in several patients desperately ill with staphylococcal and streptococcal infections refractory to all other therapy. At this stage, the crude, amorphous penicillin was only about 10% pure, and it required nearly 100 L of the broth in which the mold had been grown to obtain enough of the antibiotic to treat one patient for 24 hours. Bedpans actually were

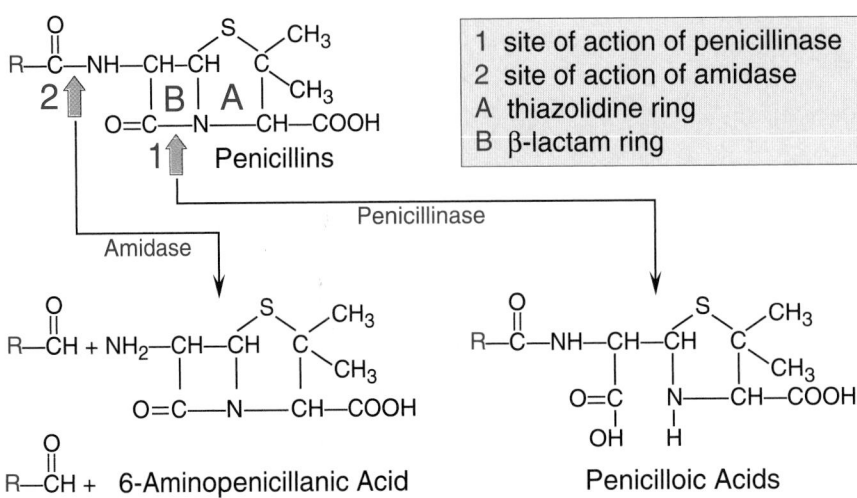

Figure 44–1. Structure of penicillins and products of their enzymatic hydrolysis.

used by the Oxford group for growing cultures of *Penicillium notatum*. Case 1 in the 1941 report from Oxford was that of a policeman who was suffering from a severe mixed staphylococcal and streptococcal infection. He was treated with penicillin, some of which had been recovered from the urine of other patients who had been given the drug. It is said that an Oxford professor referred to penicillin as a remarkable substance grown in bedpans and purified by passage through the Oxford Police Force.

A vast research program soon was initiated in the United States. During 1942, 122 million units of penicillin were made available, and the first clinical trials were conducted at Yale University and the Mayo Clinic, with dramatic results. By the spring of 1943, 200 patients had been treated with the drug. The results were so impressive that the surgeon general of the U.S. Army authorized trial of the antibiotic in a military hospital. Soon thereafter, penicillin was adopted throughout the medical services of the U.S. Armed Forces.

The deep-fermentation procedure for the biosynthesis of penicillin marked a crucial advance in the large-scale production of the antibiotic. From a total production of a few hundred million units a month in the early days, the quantity manufactured rose to over 200 trillion units (nearly 150 tons) by 1950. The first marketable penicillin cost several dollars per 100,000 units; today, the same dose costs only a few cents.

Chemistry. The basic structure of the penicillins, as shown in Figure 44–1, consists of a thiazolidine ring (A) connected to a β-lactam ring (B) to which is attached a side chain (R). The penicillin nucleus itself is the chief structural requirement for biological activity; metabolic transformation or chemical alteration of this portion of the molecule causes loss of all significant antibacterial activity. The side chain (Table 44–1) determines many of the antibacterial and pharmacological characteristics of a particular type of penicillin. Several natural penicillins can be produced depending on the chemical composition of the fermentation medium used to culture *Penicillium*. Penicillin G (benzylpenicillin) has the greatest antimicrobial activity of these and is the only natural penicillin used clinically. For penicillin G, the side chain (R in Figure 44–1) is a phenyl-methyl substituent (Table 44–1).

Semisynthetic Penicillins. The discovery that 6-aminopenicillanic acid could be obtained from cultures of *P. chrysogenum* that were depleted of side-chain precursors led to the development of the semisynthetic penicillins. Side chains can be added that alter the susceptibility of

the resulting compounds to inactivating enzymes (β-lactamases) and that change the antibacterial activity and the pharmacological properties of the drug. 6-Aminopenicillanic acid is now produced in large quantities with the aid of an amidase from *P. chrysogenum* (Figure 44–1). This enzyme splits the peptide linkage by which the side chain of penicillin is joined to 6-aminopenicillanic acid. Table 44–1 shows the variety of side chains that have been added to 6-aminopenicillanic acid to produce the medicinal penicillins in current use; the table also summarizes their major therapeutic properties (*e.g.,* absorption following oral administration, resistance to penicillinase, and antimicrobial spectrum).

Unitage of Penicillin. The international unit of penicillin is the specific penicillin activity contained in 0.6 μg of the crystalline sodium salt of penicillin G. One milligram of pure penicillin G sodium thus equals 1667 units; 1.0 mg of pure penicillin G potassium represents 1595 units. The dosage and the antibacterial potency of the semisynthetic penicillins are expressed in terms of weight.

Mechanism of Action of the Penicillins and Cephalosporins. The β-lactam antibiotics can kill susceptible bacteria. Although knowledge of the mechanism of this action is incomplete, numerous researchers have supplied information that allows understanding of the basic phenomenon (*see* Ghuysen, 1991; Bayles, 2000).

The cell walls of bacteria are essential for their normal growth and development. Peptidoglycan is a heteropolymeric component of the cell wall that provides rigid mechanical stability by virtue of its highly cross-linked latticework structure (Figure 44–2). In gram-positive microorganisms, the cell wall is 50 to 100 molecules thick, but it is only 1 or 2 molecules thick in gram-negative bacteria (Figure 44–3). The peptidoglycan is composed of glycan chains, which are linear strands of two alternating amino sugars (*N*-acetylglucosamine and *N*-acetylmuramic acid) that are cross-linked by peptide chains.

The biosynthesis of the peptidoglycan involves about 30 bacterial enzymes and may be considered in three stages. The first stage, precursor formation, takes place in the cytoplasm. The product, uridine diphosphate (UDP)–acetylmuramyl-pentapeptide, accumulates in cells when subsequent synthetic stages are inhibited. The last reaction in the synthesis of this compound is the addition of a dipeptide, D-alanyl-D-alanine. Synthesis of the dipeptide involves prior racemization of L-alanine and condensation catalyzed by D-alanyl-D-alanine synthetase.

Table 44–1
Chemical Structures and Major Properties of Various Penicillins

$$R-\overset{\overset{\textstyle O}{\textstyle \|}}{C}-NH_2-CH-CH \quad \overset{\textstyle S}{\diagup} \quad \overset{\textstyle CH_3}{\underset{\textstyle CH_3}{C}}$$

$$O=C-N-\ -CH-COOH$$

Penicillins are substituted 6-aminopenicillanic acids

R	NONPROPRIETARY NAME	MAJOR PROPERTIES		
		Absorption after Oral Administration	Resistance to Penicillinase	Useful Antimicrobial Spectrum
—CH₂— (phenyl)	Penicillin G	Variable (poor)	No	
		Streptococcus species, [**] Enterococci, [**] *Listeria, Neisseria meningitidis*, many anaerobes (not *Bacteroides fragilis*),[***] spirochetes, *Actinomyces, Erysipelothrix* spp., *Pasteurella multocida*[***]		
—OCH₂— (phenyl)	Penicillin V	Good	No	
(dimethoxyphenyl)	Methicillin	Poor (not given orally)	Yes	
(isoxazolyl ring)	Oxacillin ($R_1 = R_2 = H$)			
	Cloxacillin ($R_1 = Cl; R_2 = H$)	Good	Yes	
	Dicloxacillin ($R_1 = R_2 = Cl$)	Indicated only for non-methicillin-resistant strains of *Staphylococcus aureus* and *Staphylococcus epidermidis*. Compared to other penicillins, these penicillinase-resistant penicillins lack activity against *Listeria monocytogenes* and *Enterococcus* spp.		
(dimethoxynaphthyl)	Nafcillin	Variable	Yes	
R_1—(phenyl)—CH—NH₂	Ampicillin[†] ($R_1 = H$)	Good	No	
	Amoxicillin ($R_1 = OH$)	Excellent		
		Extends spectrum of penicillin to include sensitive strains of Enterobacteriaceae[***] *Escherichia coli, Proteus mirabilis, Salmonella, Shigella, Haemophilus influenzae*,[***] and *Helicobacter pylori*.		
		Superior to penicillin for treatment of *Listeria monocytogenes* and sensitive enterococci. Amoxicillin most active of all oral β-lactams against penicillin-resistant *Streptococcus pneumoniae*		

(Continued)

Table 44–1
Chemical Structures and Major Properties of Various Penicillins (Continued)

R	NONPROPRIETARY NAME	Absorption after Oral Administration	Resistance to Penicillinase	Useful Antimicrobial Spectrum
		MAJOR PROPERTIES		
(structure: phenyl–CH(COOR₁))	Carbenicillin (R₁ = H)	Poor (not given orally)		
	Carbenicillin indanyl (R₁ = 5-indanol)	Good	No	
		Less active than ampicillin against *Streptococcus* species, *Enterococcus faecalis*, *Klebsiella*, and *Listeria monocytogenes*. Activity against *Pseudomonas aeruginosa* is inferior to that of mezlocillin and piperacillin		
(structure: thienyl–CH(COOH))	Ticarcillin	Poor (not given orally)	No	
(structure: phenyl–CH(NHCO–imidazolidinone–SO₂CH₃))	Mezlocillin	Poor (not given orally)	No	
(structure: phenyl–CH(NHCO–piperazinedione–C₂H₅))	Piperacillin	Poor (not given orally)	No	
		Extends spectrum of ampicillin to include *Psuedomonas aeruginosa*,[‡] Enterobacteriaceae,[***] Bacteroides species[***]		

[*]Equivalent to R in Figure 45–1. [**]Many strains are resistant due to altered penicillin-binding proteins. [***]Many strains are resistant due to production of β-lactamases. [†]There are other congeners of ampicillin; *see* the text. [‡]Some strains are resistant due to decreased entry or active efflux.

D-Cycloserine is a structural analog of D-alanine and acts as a competitive inhibitor of both the racemase and the synthetase (*see* Chapter 47).

During reactions of the second stage, UDP-acetylmuramyl-pentapeptide and UDP-acetylglucosamine are linked (with the release of the uridine nucleotides) to form a long polymer.

The third and final stage involves completion of the cross-link. This is accomplished by a transpeptidation reaction that occurs outside the cell membrane. The transpeptidase itself is membrane-bound. The terminal glycine residue of the pentaglycine bridge is linked to the fourth residue of the pentapeptide (D-alanine), releasing the fifth residue (also D-alanine) (Figure 44–2). It is this last step in peptidoglycan synthesis that is inhibited by the β-lactam antibiotics and glycopeptide antibiotics such as *vancomycin* (by a different mechanism than the β-lactams; *see* Chapter 45). Stereomodels reveal that the conformation of penicillin is very similar to that of D-alanyl-D-alanine. The transpeptidase probably is acylated by penicillin; that is, penicilloyl enzyme apparently is formed, with cleavage of the —CO—N— bond of the β-lactam ring.

Although inhibition of the transpeptidase just described is demonstrably important, there are additional, related targets for the actions of penicillins and cephalosporins; these are collectively termed *penicillin-binding proteins* (PBPs). All bacteria have several such entities; for example, *S. aureus* has four PBPs, whereas *Escherichia coli* has at least seven. The PBPs vary in their affinities for different β-lactam antibiotics, although the interactions eventually become covalent. The higher-molecular-weight PBPs of *E. coli* (PBPs 1a and 1b) include the transpeptidases responsible for synthesis of the peptidoglycan. Other PBPs in *E. coli* include those that are necessary for maintenance of the rodlike shape of the bacterium and for septum formation at division. Inhibition of the transpeptidases causes spheroplast formation and rapid lysis. However, inhibition of the activities of other PBPs may cause delayed lysis (PBP 2) or the production of long, filamentous forms of the bacterium (PBP 3). The lethality of penicillin for bacteria appears to involve both lytic and nonlytic mechanisms. Penicillin's disruption of the balance between PBP-mediated peptidoglycan assem-

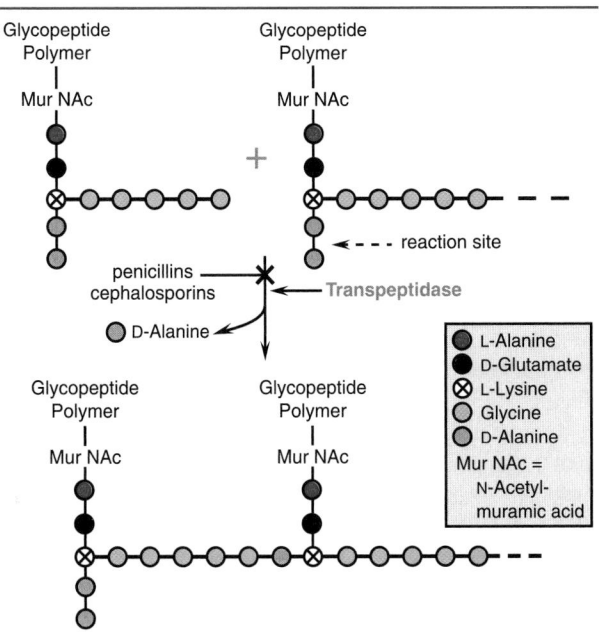

Figure 44–2. *Action of β-lactam antibiotics in* **Staphylococcus aureus.** The bacterial cell wall consists of glycopeptide polymers linked via bridges between amino acid side chains. In *S. aureus*, the bridge is (Gly)$_5$-D-Ala between lysines. The cross-linking is catalyzed by a transpeptidase, the enzyme that penicillins and cephalosporins inhibit.

bly and murein hydrolase activity results in autolysis. Nonlytic killing by penicillin may involve holin-like proteins in the bacterial membrane that collapse the membrane potential (Bayles, 2000).

Mechanisms of Bacterial Resistance to Penicillins and Cephalosporins. Although all bacteria with cell walls contain PBPs, β-lactam antibiotics cannot kill or even inhibit all bacteria because by various mechanisms bacteria can be resistant to these agents. The microorganism may be intrinsically resistant because of structural differences in the PBPs that are the targets of these drugs. Furthermore, a sensitive strain may acquire resistance of this type by the development of high-molecular-weight PBPs that have decreased affinity for the antibiotic. Because the β-lactam antibiotics inhibit many different PBPs in a single bacterium, the affinity for β-lactam antibiotics of several PBPs must decrease for the organism to be resistant. Altered PBPs with decreased affinity for β-lactam antibiotics are acquired by homologous recombination between PBP genes of different bacterial species. Four of the five high-molecular-weight PBPs of the most highly penicillin-resistant *Streptococcus pneumoniae* isolates have decreased affinity for β-lactam antibiotics as a result of interspecies homologous recombination events (Figure 44–4). In contrast, isolates with high-level resistance to third-generation cephalosporins contain alterations of only two of the five high-molecular-weight PBPs because the other PBPs have inherently low affinity for the third-generation cephalosporins. Penicillin resistance in *Streptococcus sanguis* and other *viridans* streptococci apparently emerged as a result of replacement of its PBPs with resistant PBPs from *S. pneumoniae* (Carratalá *et al.*, 1995). Methicillin-resistant *S. aureus* are resistant *via* acquisition of an additional high-molecular-weight

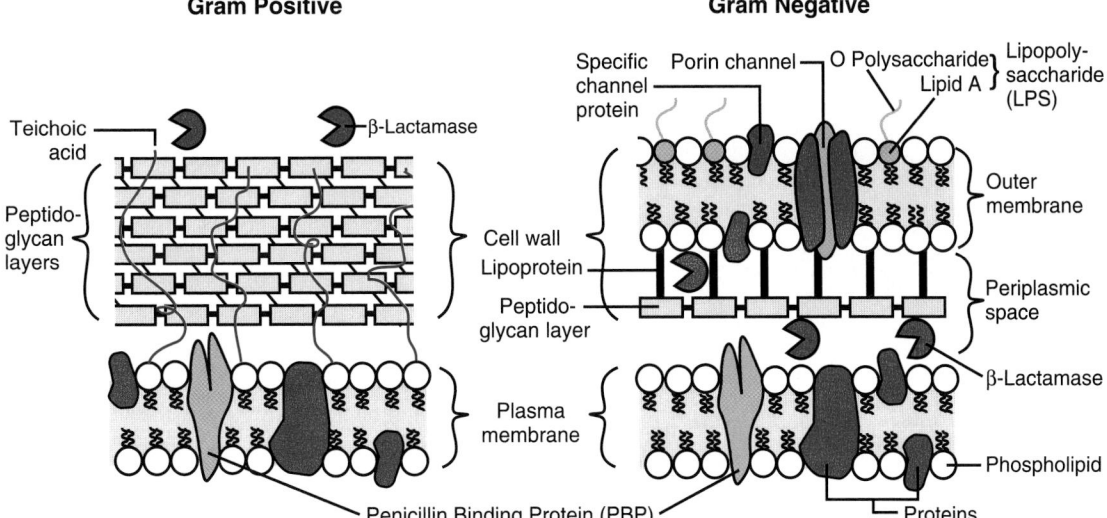

Figure 44–3. *Comparison of the structure and composition of gram-positive and gram-negative cell walls. (Adapted from Tortora et al., 1989, with permission.)*

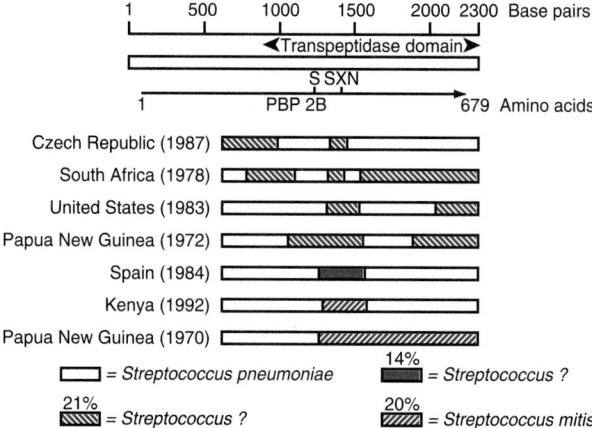

Figure 44–4. *Mosaic PBP 2B genes in penicillin-resistant pneumococci.* The divergent regions in the PBP 2B genes of seven resistant pneumococci from different countries are shown. These regions have been introduced from at least three sources, one of which appears to be *Streptococcus mitis.* The approximate percent sequence divergence of the divergent regions from the PBP 2B genes of susceptible pneumococci is shown. (Reprinted from Spratt, 1994, with permission.)

PBP (*via* a transposon from an unknown organism) with a very low affinity for all β-lactam antibiotics. The gene (*MecA*) encoding this new PBP also is present in and responsible for methicillin resistance in the coagulase-negative staphylococci (Spratt, 1994).

Other instances of bacterial resistance to the β-lactam antibiotics are caused by the inability of the agent to penetrate to its site of action (Jacoby, 1994) (Figure 44–5). In

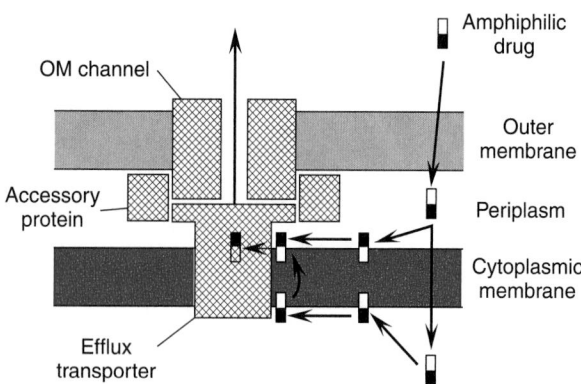

Figure 44–5. *Antibiotic efflux pumps of gram-negative bacteria.* Multidrug efflux pumps traverse both the inner and outer membranes of gram-negative bacteria. The pumps are composed of a minimum of three proteins and are energized by the proton motive force. Increased expression of these pumps is an important cause of antibiotic resistance. (Reprinted from Nikaido, 1998, with permission.)

gram-positive bacteria, the peptidoglycan polymer is very near the cell surface (Figure 44–3). Some gram-positive bacteria have polysaccharide capsules that are external to the cell wall, but these structures are not a barrier to the diffusion of the β-lactams; the small β-lactam antibiotic molecules can penetrate easily to the outer layer of the cytoplasmic membrane and the PBPs, where the final stages of the synthesis of the peptidoglycan take place. The situation is different with gram-negative bacteria. Their surface structure is more complex, and their inner membrane, which is analogous to the cytoplasmic membrane of gram-positive bacteria, is covered by the outer membrane, lipopolysaccharide, and capsule (Figure 44–3). The outer membrane functions as an impenetrable barrier for some antibiotics (*see* Nakae, 1986). Some small hydrophilic antibiotics, however, diffuse through aqueous channels in the outer membrane that are formed by proteins called *porins.* Broader-spectrum penicillins, such as ampicillin and amoxicillin, and most of the cephalosporins diffuse through the pores in the *E. coli* outer membrane significantly more rapidly than can penicillin G. The number and size of pores in the outer membrane vary among different gram-negative bacteria. An extreme example is *P. aeruginosa,* which is intrinsically resistant to a wide variety of antibiotics because it lacks the classical high-permeability porins (Nikaido, 1994). Active efflux pumps serve as another mechanism of resistance, removing the antibiotic from its site of action before it can act (Nikaido, 1998) (Figure 44–5). This is an important mechanism of β-lactam resistance in *P. aeruginosa, E. coli,* and *Neisseria gonorrhoeae.*

Bacteria also can destroy β-lactam antibiotics enzymatically. β-Lactamases are capable of inactivating certain of these antibiotics and may be present in large quantities (Figures 44–1 and 44–3). Different microorganisms elaborate a number of distinct β-lactamases, although most bacteria produce only one form of the enzyme. The substrate specificities of some of these enzymes are relatively narrow, and these often are described as either penicillinases or cephalosporinases. Other "extended spectrum" enzymes are less discriminant and can hydrolyze a variety of β-lactam antibiotics. β-Lactamases are grouped into four classes: A through D. Class A β-lactamases include the extended-spectrum β-lactamases (ESBLs) and degrade penicillins, some cephalosporins, and, in some instances, carbapenems. Class A and D enzymes are inhibited by the commercially available β-lactamase inhibitors, such as clavulanate and *tazobactam.* Class B β-lactamases are Zn^{2+}-dependent enzymes that destroy all β-lactams except aztreonam, whereas class C β-lactamases are active against cephalosporins. Class D includes cloxacillin-degrading enzymes (Bush, 2001).

In general, gram-positive bacteria produce and secrete a large amount of β-lactamase (Figure 44–3). Most of these enzymes are penicillinases. The information for staphylococcal penicillinase is encoded in a plasmid, and this may be transferred by bacteriophage to other bacteria. The enzyme is inducible by substrates, and 1% of the dry weight of the bacterium can be penicillinase. In gram-negative bacteria, β-lactamases are found in relatively small amounts but are located in the periplasmic space between the inner and outer cell membranes (Figure 44–3). Since the enzymes of cell wall synthesis are on the outer surface of the inner membrane, these β-lactamases are strategically located for maximal protection of the microbe. β-Lactamases of gram-negative bacteria are encoded either in chromosomes or in plasmids, and they may be constitutive or inducible. The plasmids can be transferred between bacteria by conjugation. These enzymes can hydrolyze penicillins, cephalosporins, or both (*see* Davies, 1994). However, there is an inconsistent correlation between the susceptibility of an antibiotic to inactivation by β-lactamase and the ability of that antibiotic to kill the microorganism.

Other Factors That Influence the Activity of β-Lactam Antibiotics. Microorganisms adhering to implanted prosthetic devices (*e.g.,* catheters, artificial joints, prosthetic heart valves, etc.) produce biofilms. Bacteria in biofilms produce extracellular polysaccharides and, in part owing to decreased growth rates, are much less sensitive to antibiotic therapy (Donlan, 2001). The density of the bacterial population and the age of an infection influence the activity of β-lactam antibiotics. The drugs may be several thousand times more potent when tested against small bacterial inocula than when tested against a dense culture. Many factors are involved. Among these are the greater number of relatively resistant microorganisms in a large population, the amount of β-lactamase produced, and the phase of growth of the culture. The clinical significance of this effect of inoculum size is uncertain. The intensity and duration of penicillin therapy needed to abort or cure experimental infections in animals increase with the duration of the infection. The primary reason is that the bacteria are no longer multiplying as rapidly as they do in a fresh infection. These antibiotics are most active against bacteria in the logarithmic phase of growth and have little effect on microorganisms in the stationary phase, when there is no need to synthesize components of the cell wall.

The presence of proteins and other constituents of pus, low pH, or low oxygen tension does not appreciably decrease the ability of β-lactam antibiotics to kill bacteria. However, bacteria that survive inside viable cells of the host generally are protected from the action of the β-lactam antibiotics.

Classification of the Penicillins and Summary of Their Pharmacological Properties

It is useful to classify the penicillins according to their spectra of antimicrobial activity (Table 44–1) (*see* Chambers, 2000).

1. *Penicillin G* and its close congener *penicillin V* are highly active against sensitive strains of gram-positive cocci, but they are readily hydrolyzed by penicillinase. Thus they are ineffective against most strains of *S. aureus.*

2. The penicillinase-resistant penicillins [*methicillin* (discontinued in the United States), *nafcillin, oxacillin, cloxacillin* (not currently marketed in the United States), and *dicloxacillin*] have less potent antimicrobial activity against microorganisms that are sensitive to penicillin G, but they are the agents of first choice for treatment of penicillinase-producing *S. aureus* and *S. epidermidis* that are not methicillin-resistant.

3. *Ampicillin, amoxicillin,* and others make up a group of penicillins whose antimicrobial activity is extended to include such gram-negative microorganisms as *Haemophilus influenzae, E. coli,* and *Proteus mirabilis.* Frequently these drugs are administered with a β-lactamase inhibitor such as *clavalanate* or *salbactam* to prevent hydrolysis by broad-spectrum β-lactamases that are found with increasing frequency in clinical isolates of these gram-negative bacteria.

4. The antimicrobial activity of *carbenicillin* (discontinued in the United States), its indanyl ester (*carbenicillin indanyl*), and *ticarcillin* is extended to include *Pseudomonas, Enterobacter,* and *Proteus* spp. These agents are inferior to ampicillin against gram-positive cocci and *Listeria monocytogenes* and are less active than piperacillin against *Pseudomonas.*

5. *Mezlocillin, azlocillin* (both discontinued in the United States), and *piperacillin* have excellent antimicrobial activity against *Pseudomonas, Klebsiella,* and certain other gram-negative microorganisms. Piperacillin retains the activity of ampicillin against gram-positive cocci and *L. monocytogenes.*

Although the pharmacological properties of the individual drugs are discussed in detail below, certain generalizations are useful. Following absorption of orally administered penicillins, these agents are distributed widely throughout the body. Therapeutic concentrations of penicillins are achieved readily in tissues and in secretions such as joint fluid, pleural fluid, pericardial fluid, and bile. Penicillins do not penetrate living phagocytic cells to a significant extent, and only low concentrations of these drugs are found in prostatic secretions, brain tissue, and intraocular fluid. Concentrations of penicillins in cerebrospinal fluid (CSF) are variable but are less than 1% of those in plasma when the meninges are normal. When there is inflammation, concentrations in CSF may increase to as much as 5% of the plasma value. Penicillins are eliminated rapidly, particularly by glomerular filtration and renal tubular secretion, such that their half-lives in the body are short; values of 30 to 90 minutes are typical. Concentrations of these drugs in urine thus are high.

Penicillin G and Penicillin V

Antimicrobial Activity. The antimicrobial spectra of penicillin G *(benzylpenicillin)* and penicillin V (the phenoxymethyl derivative) are very similar for aerobic gram-positive microorganisms. However, penicillin G is 5 to 10 times more active against *Neisseria* spp. that are sensitive to penicillins and against certain anaerobes.

Penicillin G has activity against a variety of species of gram-positive and gram-negative cocci, although many bacteria previously sensitive to the agent are now resistant. Most streptococci (but not enterococci) are very susceptible to the drug; concentrations of less than 0.01 $\mu g/ml$ usually are effective. However, penicillin-resistant *viridans* streptococci (Carratalá *et al.*, 1995) and *S. pneumoniae* are becoming more common. During 1997, 13.6% of *S. pneumoniae* sterile-site isolates had high-level [minimal inhibitory concentration (MIC) ≥ 2 $\mu g/ml$)] and 11.4% of isolates had low-level (MIC ≥ 0.12 $\mu g/ml$) penicillin resistance, for a total of 25% of isolates (Centers for Disease Control and Prevention, 1999, 2002). Penicillin-resistant pneumococci are especially common in pediatric populations, such as children attending day-care centers. Many penicillin-resistant pneumococci also are resistant to third-generation cephalosporins.

Whereas most strains of *S. aureus* were highly sensitive to penicillin G when this agent was first employed therapeutically, more than 90% of strains of staphylococci isolated from individuals inside or outside of hospitals are now resistant to penicillin G. Most strains of *S. epidermidis* also are resistant to penicillin. Unfortunately, penicillinase-producing strains of gonococci that are highly resistant to penicillin G have become widespread. With rare exceptions, meningococci are quite sensitive to penicillin G.

Although the vast majority of strains of *Corynebacterium diphtheriae* are sensitive to penicillin G, some are highly resistant. The presence of chromosomally encoded β-lactamase in *Bacillus anthracis* is the reason that penicillin was not used for prophylaxis of anthrax exposure, although most isolates are susceptible. Most anaerobic microorganisms, including *Clostridium* spp., are highly sensitive. *Bacteroides fragilis* is an exception, displaying resistance to penicillins and cephalosporins by virtue of expressing a broad-spectrum cephalosporinase. Some strains of *Prevotella melaninogenicus* also have acquired this trait. *Actinomyces israelii, Streptobacillus moniliformis, Pasteurella multocida,* and *L. monocytogenes* are inhibited by penicillin G. Most species of *Leptospira* are moderately susceptible to the drug. One of the most exquisitely sensitive microorganisms is *Treponema pallidum. Borrelia burgdorferi,* the organism responsible for Lyme disease, also is susceptible. None of the penicillins is effective against amebae, plasmodia, rickettsiae, fungi, or viruses.

Absorption. Oral Administration of Penicillin G. About one-third of an orally administered dose of penicillin G is absorbed from the intestinal tract under favorable conditions. Gastric juice at pH 2 rapidly destroys the antibiotic. The decrease in gastric acid production with aging accounts for better absorption of penicillin G from the gastrointestinal tract of older individuals. Absorption is rapid, and maximal concentrations in blood are attained in 30 to 60 minutes. The peak value is approximately 0.5

unit/ml (0.3 $\mu g/ml$) after an oral dose of 400,000 units (about 250 mg) in an adult. Ingestion of food may interfere with enteric absorption of all penicillins, perhaps by adsorption of the antibiotic onto food particles. Thus oral penicillin G should be administered at least 30 minutes before a meal or 2 hours after. Despite the convenience of oral administration of penicillin G, this route should be used only in infections in which clinical experience has proven its efficacy.

Oral Administration of Penicillin V. The virtue of penicillin V in comparison with penicillin G is that it is more stable in an acidic medium and therefore is better absorbed from the gastrointestinal tract. On an equivalent oral-dose basis, penicillin V (K^+ salt; VEETIDS) yields plasma concentrations two to five times greater than those provided by penicillin G. The peak concentration in the blood of an adult after an oral dose of 500 mg is nearly 3 $\mu g/ml$. Once absorbed, penicillin V is distributed in the body and excreted by the kidney in a manner similar to that of penicillin G.

Parenteral Administration of Penicillin G. After intramuscular injection, peak concentrations in plasma are reached within 15 to 30 minutes. This value declines rapidly because the half-life of penicillin G is 30 minutes.

Many means for prolonging the sojourn of the antibiotic in the body and thereby reducing the frequency of injections have been explored. *Probenecid* blocks renal tubular secretion of penicillin, but it is used rarely for this purpose (*see* below). More commonly, repository preparations of penicillin G are employed. The two such compounds currently favored are *penicillin G procaine* (WYCILLIN, others) and *penicillin G benzathine* (BICILLIN L-A, PERMAPEN). Such agents release penicillin G slowly from the area in which they are injected and produce relatively low but persistent concentrations of antibiotic in the blood.

Penicillin G procaine suspension is an aqueous preparation of the crystalline salt that is only 0.4% soluble in water. Procaine combines with penicillin mole for mole; a dose of 300,000 units thus contains approximately 120 mg procaine. When large doses of penicillin G procaine are given (*e.g.,* 4.8 million units), procaine may reach toxic concentrations in the plasma. If the patient is believed to be hypersensitive to procaine, 0.1 ml of 1% solution of procaine should be injected intradermally as a test. The anesthetic effect of the procaine accounts in part for the fact that injections of penicillin G procaine are virtually painless.

The injection of 300,000 units of penicillin G procaine produces a peak concentration in plasma of about 0.9 $\mu g/ml$ within 1 to 3 hours; after 24 hours, the concentration is reduced to 0.1 $\mu g/ml$, and by 48 hours it has fallen to 0.03 $\mu g/ml$. A larger dose (600,000 units) yields somewhat higher values that are maintained for as long as 4 to 5 days.

Penicillin G benzathine suspension is the aqueous suspension of the salt obtained by the combination of 1 mol of an ammonium base and 2 mol of penicillin G to yield *N,N'*-dibenzylethylenediamine dipenicillin G. The salt itself is only 0.02% soluble in water. The long persistence of penicillin in the blood after a suitable intramuscular dose reduces cost, need for repeated injections, and local trauma. The local anesthetic effect of penicillin G benzathine is comparable with that of penicillin G procaine.

Penicillin G benzathine is absorbed very slowly from intramuscular depots and produces the longest duration of detectable antibiotic of all the available repository penicillins. For example, in adults, a dose of 1.2 million units given intramuscularly produces a concentration in plasma of 0.09 *μg*/ml on the first, 0.02 *μg*/ml on the fourteenth, and 0.002 *μg*/ml on the thirty-second day after injection. The average duration of demonstrable antimicrobial activity in the plasma is about 26 days.

Distribution. Penicillin G is distributed widely throughout the body, but the concentrations in various fluids and tissues differ widely. Its apparent volume of distribution is about 0.35 L/kg. Approximately 60% of the penicillin G in plasma is reversibly bound to albumin. Significant amounts appear in liver, bile, kidney, semen, joint fluid, lymph, and intestine.

While probenecid markedly decreases the tubular secretion of the penicillins, this is not the only factor responsible for the elevated plasma concentrations of the antibiotic that follow its administration. Probenecid also produces a significant decrease in the apparent volume of distribution of the penicillins.

Cerebrospinal Fluid. Penicillin does not readily enter the CSF when the meninges are normal. However, when the meninges are acutely inflamed, penicillin penetrates into the CSF more easily. Although the concentrations attained vary and are unpredictable, they are usually in the range of 5% of the value in plasma and are therapeutically effective against susceptible microorganisms.

Penicillin and other organic acids are secreted rapidly from the CSF into the bloodstream by an active transport process. Probenecid competitively inhibits this transport and thus elevates the concentration of penicillin in CSF. In uremia, other organic acids accumulate in the CSF and compete with penicillin for secretion; the drug occasionally reaches toxic concentrations in the brain and can produce convulsions.

Excretion. Under normal conditions, penicillin G is eliminated rapidly from the body mainly by the kidney but in small part in the bile and by other routes. Approximately 60% to 90% of an intramuscular dose of penicillin G in aqueous solution is eliminated in the urine, largely within the first hour after injection. The remainder is metabolized to penicilloic acid. The half-life for elimination of penicillin G is about 30 minutes in normal adults. Approximately 10% of the drug is eliminated by glomeru-

lar filtration and 90% by tubular secretion. Renal clearance approximates the total renal plasma flow. The maximal tubular secretory capacity for penicillin in the normal adult male is about 3 million units (1.8 g) per hour.

Clearance values are considerably lower in neonates and infants because of incomplete development of renal function; as a result, after doses proportionate to surface area, the persistence of penicillin in the blood is several times as long in premature infants as in children and adults. The half-life of the antibiotic in children younger than 1 week of age is 3 hours; by 14 days of age it is 1.4 hours. After renal function is fully established in young children, the rate of renal excretion of penicillin G is considerably more rapid than in adults.

Anuria increases the half-life of penicillin G from a normal value of 0.5 hour to about 10 hours. When renal function is impaired, 7% to 10% of the antibiotic may be inactivated each hour by the liver. Patients with renal shutdown who require high-dose therapy with penicillin can be treated adequately with 3 million units of aqueous penicillin G followed by 1.5 million units every 8 to 12 hours. The dose of the drug must be readjusted during dialysis and the period of progressive recovery of renal function. If, in addition to renal failure, hepatic insufficiency also is present, the half-life will be prolonged even further.

Therapeutic Uses. ***Pneumococcal Infections.*** Penicillin G remains the agent of choice for the management of infections caused by sensitive strains of *S. pneumoniae*. However, strains of pneumococci resistant to usual doses of penicillin G are being isolated more frequently in several countries, including the United States (*see* Centers for Disease Control and Prevention, 1999; Fiore *et al.*, 2000).

Pneumococcal Pneumonia. Until it is highly likely or established that the infecting isolate of pneumococcus is penicillin-sensitive, pneumococcal pneumonia should be treated with a third-generation cephalosporin or with 20 million to 24 million units of penicillin G daily by constant intravenous infusion. If the organism is sensitive to penicillin, then the dose can be reduced (Medical Letter, 2004). For parenteral therapy of sensitive isolates of pneumococci, penicillin G or penicillin G procaine is favored. Although oral treatment with 500 mg penicillin V given every 6 hours for treatment of pneumonia owing to penicillin-sensitive isolates has been used with success in this disease, it cannot be recommended for routine initial use because of the existence of resistance. Therapy should be continued for 7 to 10 days, including 3 to 5 days after the patient's temperature has returned to normal.

Pneumococcal Meningitis. Until it is established that the infecting pneumococcus is penicillin-sensitive, pneumococcal meningitis should be treated with a combination of vancomycin and a third-generation cephalosporin (John, 1994; Catalan *et al.*, 1994). *Dexamethasone* given at the same time as antibiotics was associated with an improved outcome (de Gans and van de Beek, 2002). Prior to the appearance of penicillin resistance, penicillin treatment reduced the death rate in this disease from nearly 100% to about 25%. The recommended therapy is 20 million to 24 million units of penicillin G daily by constant intravenous infusion or divided into boluses given every 2 to 3 hours. The usual duration of therapy is 14 days.

Streptococcal Infections. *Streptococcal Pharyngitis (Including Scarlet Fever).* This is the most common disease produced by *S. pyogenes* (group A β-hemolytic streptococcus). Penicillin-resistant isolates have yet to be observed for *S. pyogenes* (Tomasz, 1986). The preferred oral therapy is with penicillin V, 500 mg every 6 hours for 10 days. Equally good results are produced by the administration of 600,000 units of penicillin G procaine intramuscularly once daily for 10 days or by a single injection of 1.2 million units of penicillin G benzathine. Parenteral therapy is preferred if there are questions of patient compliance. Penicillin therapy of streptococcal pharyngitis reduces the risk of subsequent acute rheumatic fever; however, current evidence suggests that the incidence of glomerulonephritis that follows streptococcal infections is not reduced to a significant degree by treatment with penicillin.

Streptococcal Toxic Shock and Necrotizing Fascitis. These are life-threatening infections associated with toxin production and are treated optimally with penicillin plus *clindamycin* (to decrease toxin synthesis) (Bisno and Stephens, 1996).

Streptococcal Pneumonia, Arthritis, Meningitis, and Endocarditis. While uncommon, these conditions should be treated with penicillin G when they are caused by *S. pyogenes;* daily doses of 12 million to 20 million units are administered intravenously for 2 to 4 weeks. Such treatment of endocarditis should be continued for a full 4 weeks.

Infections Caused by Other Streptococci. The *viridans* streptococci are the most common cause of infectious endocarditis. These are nongroupable β-hemolytic microorganisms that are increasingly resistant to penicillin G (MIC >0.1 μg/ml). Since enterococci also may be β-hemolytic, and certain other β-hemolytic strains may be relatively resistant to penicillin, it is important to determine quantitative microbial sensitivities to penicillin G in patients with endocarditis. Patients with penicillin-sensitive *viridans* group streptococcal endocarditis can be treated successfully with 1.2 million units of procaine penicillin G given four times daily for 2 weeks or with daily doses of 12 million to 20 million units of intravenous penicillin G for 2 weeks, both regimens in combination with *streptomycin* 500 mg intramuscularly every 12 hours or *gentamicin* 1 mg/kg every 8 hours. Some physicians prefer a 4-week course of treatment with penicillin G alone.

Enterococcal endocarditis is one of the few diseases treated optimally with two antibiotics. The recommended therapy for penicillin- and aminoglycoside-sensitive enterococcal endocarditis is 20 million units of penicillin G or 12 g ampicillin daily administered intravenously in combination with a low dose of gentamicin. Therapy usually should be continued for 6 weeks, but selected patients with a short duration of illness (<3 months) have been treated successfully in 4 weeks (Wilson *et al.*, 1984).

Infections with Anaerobes. Many anaerobic infections are caused by mixtures of microorganisms. Most are sensitive to penicillin G. An exception is the *B. fragilis* group, in which up to 75% of strains may be resistant to high concentrations of this antibiotic. Pulmonary and periodontal infections (with the exception of β-lactamase-producing *Prevotella melaninogenica*) usually respond well to penicillin G, although a multicenter study indicated that clindamycin is more effective than penicillin for therapy of lung abscess (Levison *et al.*, 1983). Mild-to-moderate infections at these sites may be treated with oral medication (either penicillin G or penicillin V 400,000 units four times daily). More severe infections should be treated with 12 million to 20 million units of penicillin G intravenously. Brain abscesses also frequently contain several species of anaerobes, and most authorities prefer to treat such disease with high

doses of penicillin G (20 million units per day) plus *metronidazole* or *chloramphenicol*. Some physicians add a third-generation cephalosporin for activity against aerobic gram-negative bacilli.

Staphylococcal Infections. The vast majority of staphylococcal infections are caused by microorganisms that produce penicillinase. A patient with a staphylococcal infection who requires treatment with an antibiotic should receive one of the penicillinase-resistant penicillins—*e.g.*, nafcillin or oxacillin (Swartz, 2004).

So-called methicillin-resistant staphylococci are resistant to penicillin G, all the penicillinase-resistant penicillins, and the cephalosporins. Isolates occasionally may appear to be sensitive to various cephalosporins *in vitro,* but resistant populations arise during therapy and lead to failure (Chambers *et al.*, 1984). Vancomycin, *linezolid, quinupristin–dalfopristin,* and *daptomycin* are active for infections caused by these bacteria, although reduced susceptibility to vancomycin has been observed (Centers for Disease Control and Prevention, 2004).

Meningococcal Infections. Penicillin G remains the drug of choice for meningococcal disease. Patients should be treated with high doses of penicillin given intravenously, as described for pneumococcal meningitis. Penicillin-resistant strains of *N. meningitides* have been reported in Britain and Spain but are infrequent at present. In 1997, 97% of *N. meningitides* isolates analyzed from the United States were penicillin-sensitive (Rosenstein *et al.*, 2000). The occurrence of penicillin-resistant strains should be considered in patients who are slow to respond to treatment (Sprott *et al.*, 1988, Mendelman *et al.*, 1988). It should be remembered that penicillin G does not eliminate the meningococcal carrier state, and its administration thus is ineffective as a prophylactic measure.

Gonococcal Infections. Gonococci gradually have become more resistant to penicillin G, and penicillins are no longer the therapy of choice, unless it is known that gonococcal strains in a particular geographical area are susceptible. Uncomplicated gonococcal urethritis is the most common infection, and a single intramuscular injection of 250 mg *ceftriaxone* is the recommended treatment (Sparling and Handsfield, 2000).

Gonococcal arthritis, disseminated gonococcal infections with skin lesions, and gonococcemia should be treated with ceftriaxone 1 g daily given either intramuscularly or intravenously for 7 to 10 days. Ophthalmia neonatorum also should be treated with ceftriaxone for 7 to 10 days (25 to 50 mg/kg per day intramuscularly or intravenously).

Syphilis. Therapy of syphilis with penicillin G is highly effective. Primary, secondary, and latent syphilis of less than 1 year's duration may be treated with penicillin G procaine (2.4 million units per day intramuscularly) plus probenecid (1.0 g/day orally) for 10 days or with 1 to 3 weekly intramuscular doses of 2.4 million units of penicillin G benzathine (three doses in patients with HIV infection). Patients with late latent syphilis, neurosyphilis, or cardiovascular syphilis may be treated with a variety of regimens. Since the latter two conditions are potentially lethal and their progression can be halted (but not reversed), intensive therapy with 20 million units of penicillin G daily for 10 days is recommended. Since there are no proven alternatives for treating syphilis in pregnant women, penicillin-allergic individuals must be acutely desensitized to prevent anaphylaxis (Centers for Disease Control and Prevention, 2002).

Infants with congenital syphilis discovered at birth or during the postnatal period should be treated for at least 10 days with 50,000 units/kg daily of aqueous penicillin G in two divided doses or 50,000 units/kg of procaine penicillin G in a single daily dose (Tramont, 2000).

Most patients (70% to 90%) with secondary syphilis develop the Jarisch-Herxheimer reaction. This also may be seen in patients with other forms of syphilis. Several hours after the first injection of penicillin, chills, fever, headache, myalgias, and arthralgias may develop. The syphilitic cutaneous lesions may become more prominent, edematous, and brilliant in color. Manifestations usually persist for a few hours, and the rash begins to fade within 48 hours. It does not recur with the second or subsequent injections of penicillin. This reaction is thought to be due to release of spirochetal antigens with subsequent host reactions to the products. *Aspirin* gives symptomatic relief, and therapy with penicillin should not be discontinued.

Actinomycosis. Penicillin G is the agent of choice for the treatment of all forms of actinomycosis. The dose should be 12 million to 20 million units of penicillin G intravenously per day for 6 weeks. Some physicians continue therapy for 2 to 3 months with oral penicillin V (500 mg four times daily). Surgical drainage or excision of the lesion may be necessary before cure is accomplished.

Diphtheria. There is no evidence that penicillin or any other antibiotic alters the incidence of complications or the outcome of diphtheria; specific antitoxin is the only effective treatment. However, penicillin G eliminates the carrier state. The parenteral administration of 2 to 3 million units per day in divided doses for 10 to 12 days eliminates the diphtheria bacilli from the pharynx and other sites in practically 100% of patients. A single daily injection of penicillin G procaine for the same period produces comparable results.

Anthrax. Strains of *Bacillus anthracis* resistant to penicillin have been recovered from human infections. When penicillin G is used, the dose should be 12 million to 20 million units per day.

Clostridial Infections. Penicillin G is the agent of choice for gas gangrene; the dose is in the range of 12 million to 20 million units per day given parenterally. Adequate débridement of the infected areas is essential. Antimicrobial drugs probably have no effect on the ultimate outcome of tetanus. Débridement and administration of human tetanus immune globulin may be indicated. Penicillin is administered, however, to eradicate the vegetative forms of the bacteria that may persist.

Fusospirochetal Infections. Gingivostomatitis, produced by the synergistic action of *Leptotrichia buccalis* and spirochetes that are present in the mouth, is readily treatable with penicillin. For simple "trench mouth," 500 mg penicillin V given every 6 hours for several days is usually sufficient to clear the disease.

Rat-Bite Fever. The two microorganisms responsible for this infection, *Spirillum minor* in the Orient and *Streptobacillus moniliformis* in America and Europe, are sensitive to penicillin G, the therapeutic agent of choice. Since most cases due to *Streptobacillus* are complicated by bacteremia and, in many instances, by metastatic infections, especially of the synovia and endocardium, the dose should be large; a daily dose of 12 million to 15 million units given parenterally for 3 to 4 weeks has been recommended.

Listeria Infections. Ampicillin (with gentamicin for immunosuppressed patients with meningitis) and penicillin G are the drugs of choice in the management of infections owing to *L. monocytogenes*. The recommended dose of ampicillin is 1 to 2 g intravenously every 4 hours. The recommended dose of penicillin G is 15 million to 20 million units parenterally per day for at least 2 weeks. When endocarditis is the problem, the dose is the same, but the duration of treatment should be no less than 4 weeks.

Lyme Disease. Although a *tetracycline* is the usual drug of choice for early disease, *amoxicillin* is effective; the dose is 500 mg three times daily for 21 days. Severe disease is treated with a third-generation cephalosporin or 20 million units of intravenous penicillin G daily for 14 days.

Erysipeloid. The causative agent of this disease, *Erysipelothrix rhusiopathiae,* is sensitive to penicillin. The uncomplicated infection responds well to a single injection of 1.2 million units of penicillin G benzathine. When endocarditis is present, penicillin G, 12 million to 20 million units per day, has been found to be effective; therapy should be continued for 4 to 6 weeks.

Pasteurella multocoda. Pasteurella multocoda is the cause of wound infections after a cat or dog bite. It is uniformly susceptible to penicillin G and ampicillin and resistant to penicillinase-resistant penicillins and first-generation cephalosporins (Goldstein *et al.,* 1988). When the infection causes meningitis, a third-generation cephalosporin is preferred because the MICs are slightly lower than for penicillin.

Prophylactic Uses of the Penicillins. The demonstrated effectiveness of penicillin in eradicating microorganisms was followed quickly and quite naturally by attempts to prove that it also was effective in preventing infection in susceptible hosts. As a result, the antibiotic has been administered in almost every situation in which a risk of bacterial invasion has been present. As prophylaxis has been investigated under controlled conditions, it has become clear that penicillin is highly effective in some situations, useless and potentially dangerous in others, and of questionable value in still others (*see* Chapter 42).

Streptococcal Infections. The administration of penicillin to individuals exposed to *S. pyogenes* affords protection from infection. The oral ingestion of 200,000 units of penicillin G or penicillin V twice a day or a single injection of 1.2 million units of penicillin G benzathine is effective. Indications for this type of prophylaxis include outbreaks of streptococcal disease in closed populations, such as boarding schools or military bases. Patients with extensive deep burns are at high risk of severe wound infections with *S. pyogenes;* "low dose" prophylaxis for several days appears to be effective in reducing the incidence of this complication.

Recurrences of Rheumatic Fever. The oral administration of 200,000 units of penicillin G or penicillin V every 12 hours produces a striking decrease in the incidence of recurrences of rheumatic fever in susceptible individuals. Because of the difficulties of compliance, parenteral administration is preferable, especially in children. The intramuscular injection of 1.2 million units of penicillin G benzathine once a month yields excellent results. In cases of hypersensitivity to penicillin, *sulfisoxazole* or *sulfadiazine,* 1 g twice a day for adults, also is effective; for children weighing under 27 kg, the dose is halved. Prophylaxis must be continued throughout the year. The duration of such treatment is an unsettled question. It has been suggested that prophylaxis should be continued for life because instances of acute rheumatic fever have been observed in the fifth and sixth decades. However, the necessity for such prolonged prophylaxis has not been established and may be unnecessary for certain young adults judged to be at low risk for recurrence (Berrios *et al.,* 1993).

Syphilis. Prophylaxis for a contact with syphilis consists of a course of therapy as described for primary syphilis. A serological test for syphilis should be performed at monthly intervals for at least 4 months thereafter.

Surgical Procedures in Patients with Valvular Heart Disease.
About 25% of cases of subacute bacterial endocarditis follow dental
extractions. This observation, together with the fact that up to 80%
of persons who have teeth removed experience a transient bacteremia, emphasizes the potential importance of chemoprophylaxis for
those who have congenital or acquired valvular heart disease of any
type and need to undergo dental procedures. Since transient bacterial invasion of the bloodstream occurs occasionally after surgical
procedures (*e.g.*, tonsillectomy and genitourinary and gastrointestinal procedures) and during childbirth, these, too, are indications for
prophylaxis in patients with valvular heart disease. Whether the
incidence of bacterial endocarditis actually is altered by this type of
chemoprophylaxis remains to be determined.

Detailed recommendations for adults and children with valvular heart disease have been formulated (*see* Dajani *et al.*, 1997;
Durack, 2000).

The Penicillinase-Resistant Penicillins

The penicillins described in this section are resistant to
hydrolysis by staphylococcal penicillinase. Their appropriate use should be restricted to the treatment of infections
that are known or suspected to be caused by staphylococci
that elaborate the enzyme—which now includes the vast
majority of strains of this bacterium that are encountered
clinically. These drugs are much less active than is penicillin G against other penicillin-sensitive microorganisms,
including non-penicillinase-producing staphylococci.

The role of the penicillinase-resistant penicillins as
the agents of choice for most staphylococcal disease is
changing with the increasing incidence of isolates of so-called methicillin-resistant microorganisms. As commonly used, this term denotes resistance of these bacteria
to all the penicillinase-resistant penicillins and cephalosporins. Hospital-acquired strains usually are resistant
to the aminoglycosides, tetracyclines, *erythromycin,* and
clindamycin as well. Vancomycin is considered the drug
of choice for such infections. Some physicians use a
combination of vancomycin and *rifampin,* especially for
life-threatening infections and those involving foreign
bodies. Community-acquired methicillin-resistant strains
are less likely to be resistant to other classes of antibiotics with the exception of macrolides (Okuma *et al.*,
2002). Methicillin-resistant *S. aureus* contains an additional high-molecular-weight PBP with a very low affinity for β-lactam antibiotics (Spratt, 1994). From 40% to
60% of strains of *S. epidermidis* also are resistant to the
penicillinase-resistant penicillins by the same mechanism. As with methicillin-resistant *S. aureus,* these strains
may appear to be susceptible to cephalosporins on disk-sensitivity testing, but there usually is a significant population of microbes that is resistant to cephalosporins and
that emerges during such therapy. Vancomycin also is the
drug of choice for serious infection caused by methicillin-

resistant *S. epidermidis;* rifampin is given concurrently
when a foreign body is involved.

The Isoxazolyl Penicillins: Oxacillin, Cloxacillin, and Dicloxacillin.

These three congeneric semisynthetic penicillins are similar pharmacologically and thus conveniently are considered together. Their structural formulas
are shown in Table 44–1. All are relatively stable in an
acidic medium and are absorbed adequately after oral
administration. All are markedly resistant to cleavage by
penicillinase. These drugs are not substitutes for penicillin
G in the treatment of diseases amenable to it, and they are
not active against enterococci or *Listeria.* Furthermore,
because of variability in intestinal absorption, oral administration is not a substitute for the parenteral route in the
treatment of serious staphylococcal infections that require
a penicillin unaffected by penicillinase.

Pharmacological Properties. The isoxazolyl penicillins are
potent inhibitors of the growth of most penicillinase-producing staphylococci. This is their valid clinical use. Dicloxacillin is the most
active, and many strains of *S. aureus* are inhibited by concentrations
of 0.05 to 0.8 μg/ml. Comparable values for cloxacillin and oxacillin
are 0.1 to 3 and 0.4 to 6 μg/ml, respectively. These differences may
have little practical significance, however, because dosages (*see*
below) are adjusted accordingly. These agents are, in general, less
effective against microorganisms susceptible to penicillin G, and
they are not useful against gram-negative bacteria.

These agents are absorbed rapidly but incompletely (30% to 80%)
from the gastrointestinal tract. Absorption of the drugs is more efficient
when they are taken on an empty stomach; preferably they are administered 1 hour before or 2 hours after meals to ensure better absorption.
Peak concentrations in plasma are attained by 1 hour and approximately 5 to 10 μg/ml after the ingestion of 1 g oxacillin. Slightly higher concentrations are achieved after the administration of 1 g cloxacillin,
whereas the same oral dose of dicloxacillin yields peak plasma concentrations of 15 μg/ml. There is little evidence that these differences are
of clinical significance. All these congeners are bound to plasma albumin to a great extent (approximately 90% to 95%); none is removed
from the circulation to a significant degree by hemodialysis.

The isoxazolyl penicillins are excreted rapidly by the kidney.
Normally, about one-half of any of these drugs is excreted in the
urine in the first 6 hours after a conventional oral dose. There also is
significant hepatic elimination of these agents in the bile. The half-lives for all are between 30 and 60 minutes. Intervals between doses
of oxacillin, cloxacillin, and dicloxacillin do not have to be altered
for patients with renal failure. The above-noted differences in plasma concentrations produced by the isoxazolyl penicillins are related
mainly to differences in rate of urinary excretion and degree of
resistance to degradation in the liver.

Nafcillin. This semisynthetic penicillin is highly resistant to penicillinase and has proven effective against infections caused by penicillinase-producing strains of *S. aureus.* Its structural formula is shown
in Table 44–1.

Pharmacological Properties. Nafcillin is slightly more active
than oxacillin against penicillin G–resistant *S. aureus* (most strains
are inhibited by 0.06 to 2 μg/ml). While it is the most active of the

penicillinase-resistant penicillins against other microorganisms, it is not as potent as penicillin G.

Nafcillin is variably inactivated in the acidic medium of the gastric contents. Its oral absorption is irregular regardless of whether the drug is taken with meals or on an empty stomach; injectable preparations therefore should be used. The peak plasma concentration is about 8 μg/ml 60 minutes after a 1-g intramuscular dose. Nafcillin is about 90% bound to plasma protein. Peak concentrations of nafcillin in bile are well above those found in plasma. Concentrations of the drug in CSF appear to be adequate for therapy of staphylococcal meningitis.

The Aminopenicillins: Ampicillin, Amoxicillin, and Their Congeners

These agents have similar antibacterial activity and a spectrum that is broader than the antibiotics heretofore discussed. They all are destroyed by β-lactamase (from both gram-positive and gram-negative bacteria).

Antimicrobial Activity. Ampicillin and the related aminopenicillins are bactericidal for both gram-positive and gram-negative bacteria. The meningococci and *L. monocytogenes* are sensitive to this class of drugs. Many pneumococcal isolates have varying levels of resistance to ampicillin. Penicillin-resistant strains should be considered ampicillin/amoxicillin-resistant. *H. influenzae* and the *viridans* group of streptococci exhibit varying degrees of resistance. Enterococci are about twice as sensitive to ampicillin on a weight basis as they are to penicillin G (MIC for ampicillin averages 1.5 μg/ml). Although most strains of *N. gonorrhoeae, E. coli, P. mirabilis, Salmonella,* and *Shigella* were highly susceptible when ampicillin was first used in the early 1960s, an increasing percentage of these species now is resistant. From 30% to 50% of *E. coli,* a significant number of *P. mirabilis,* and practically all species of *Enterobacter* presently are insensitive. Resistant strains of *Salmonella* (plasmid mediated) have been recovered with increasing frequency in various parts of the world. Most strains of *Shigella* now are resistant. Most strains of *Pseudomonas, Klebsiella, Serratia, Acinetobacter,* and indole-positive *Proteus* also are resistant to this group of penicillins; these antibiotics are less active against *B. fragilis* than is penicillin G. However, concurrent administration of a β-lactamase inhibitor such as clavulanate or *sulbactam* markedly expands the spectrum of activity of these drugs (*see* below).

Ampicillin. This drug is the prototype of the group. Its structural formula is shown in Table 44–1.

Pharmacological Properties. Ampicillin (PRINCIPEN, others) is stable in acid and is well absorbed after oral administration. An oral dose of 0.5 g produces peak concentrations in plasma of about 3 μg/ml at 2 hours. Intake of food prior to ingestion of ampicillin diminishes absorption. Intramuscular injection of 0.5 or 1 g sodium ampicillin yields peak plasma concentrations of about 7 or 10 μg/ml, respectively, at 1 hour; these decline exponentially, with a half-life of approximately 80 minutes. Severe renal impairment markedly prolongs the persistence of ampicillin in the plasma. Peritoneal dialysis is ineffective in

removing the drug from the blood, but hemodialysis removes about 40% of the body store in about 7 hours. Adjustment of the dose of ampicillin is required in the presence of renal dysfunction. Ampicillin appears in the bile, undergoes enterohepatic circulation, and is excreted in appreciable quantities in the feces.

Amoxicillin. This drug, a penicillinase-susceptible semisynthetic penicillin, is a close chemical and pharmacological relative of ampicillin (Table 44–1). The drug is stable in acid and is designed for oral use. It is absorbed more rapidly and completely from the gastrointestinal tract than is ampicillin, which is the major difference between the two. The antimicrobial spectrum of amoxicillin is essentially identical to that of ampicillin, with the important exception that amoxicillin appears to be less effective than ampicillin for shigellosis.

Peak plasma concentrations of amoxicillin (AMOXIL, others) are 2 to 2½ times greater for amoxicillin than for ampicillin after oral administration of the same dose; they are reached at 2 hours and average about 4 μg/ml when 250 mg is administered. Food does not interfere with absorption. Perhaps because of more complete absorption of this congener, the incidence of diarrhea with amoxicillin is less than that following administration of ampicillin. The incidence of other adverse effects appears to be similar. While the half-life of amoxicillin is similar to that for ampicillin, effective concentrations of orally administered amoxicillin are detectable in the plasma for twice as long as with ampicillin, again because of the more complete absorption. About 20% of amoxicillin is protein-bound in plasma, a value similar to that for ampicillin. Most of a dose of the antibiotic is excreted in an active form in the urine. Probenecid delays excretion of the drug.

Therapeutic Indications for the Aminopenicillins.

Upper Respiratory Infections. Ampicillin and amoxicillin are active against *S. pyogenes* and many strains of *S. pneumoniae* and *H. influenzae,* which are major upper respiratory bacterial pathogens. The drugs constitute effective therapy for sinusitis, otitis media, acute exacerbations of chronic bronchitis, and epiglottitis caused by sensitive strains of these organisms. Amoxicillin is the most active of all the oral β-lactam antibiotics against both penicillin-sensitive and penicillin-resistant *S. pneumoniae* (Friedland and McCracken, 1994). Based on the increasing prevalence of pneumococcal resistance to penicillin, an increase in dose of oral amoxicillin (from 40 to 45 up to 80 to 90 mg/kg per day) for empirical treatment of acute otitis media in children is recommended (Dowell *et al.,* 1999). Ampicillin-resistant *H. influenzae* may be a problem in many areas.

The addition of a β-lactamase inhibitor (amoxicillin–clavulanate or ampicillin–sulbactam) extends the spectrum to β-lactamase-producing *H. influenzae* and Enterobacteriaceae. Bacterial pharyngitis should be treated with penicillin G or penicillin V because *S. pyogenes* is the major pathogen.

Urinary Tract Infections. Most uncomplicated urinary tract infections are caused by Enterobacteriaceae, and *E. coli* is the most common species; ampicillin often is an effective agent, although resistance is increasingly common. Enterococcal urinary tract infections are treated effectively with ampicillin alone.

Meningitis. Acute bacterial meningitis in children is most frequently due to *S. pneumoniae* or *N. meningitidis.* Since 20% to 30% of strains of *S. pneumoniae* now may be resistant to this antibiotic, ampicillin is not indicated for single-agent treatment of meningitis. Ampicillin has excellent activity against *L. monocytogenes,* a cause of meningitis in immunocompromised persons. Thus the combination of ampicillin and vancomycin plus a third-generation cephalosporin is a rational regimen for empirical treatment of suspected bacterial meningitis.

Salmonella Infections. Disease associated with bacteremia, disease with metastatic foci, and the enteric fever syndrome (including typhoid fever) respond favorably to antibiotics. A *fluoroquinolone* or ceftriaxone is considered by some to be the drug of choice, but the administration of *trimethoprim–sulfamethoxazole* or high doses of ampicillin (12 g/day for adults) also is effective. In some geographical areas, resistance to ampicillin is common. The typhoid carrier state has been eliminated successfully in patients without gallbladder disease with ampicillin, trimethoprim–sulfamethoxazole, or *ciprofloxacin.*

Antipseudomonal Penicillins: The Carboxypenicillins and the Ureidopenicillins

The carboxypenicillins, *carbenicillin* and *ticarcillin* and their close relatives, are active against some isolates of *P. aeruginosa* and certain indole-positive *Proteus* spp. that are resistant to ampicillin and its congeners. They are ineffective against most strains of *S. aureus, Enterococcus faecalis, Klebsiella,* and *L. monocytogenes. B. fragilis* is susceptible to high concentrations of these drugs, but penicillin G is actually more active on the basis of weight. The ureidopenicillins, *mezlocillin* and *piperacillin,* have superior activity against *P. aeruginosa* compared with carbenicillin and ticarcillin. In addition, mezlocillin and piperacillin are useful for treatment of infections with *Klebsiella.* The carboxypenicillins and the ureidopenicillins are sensitive to destruction by β-lactamases.

Carbenicillin and Carbenicillin Indanyl. *Carbenicillin.* This drug is a penicillinase-susceptible derivative of 6-aminopenicillanic acid. Its structural formula is shown in Table 44–1. Carbenicillin was the first penicillin with activity against *P. aeruginosa* and some *Proteus* strains that are resistant to ampicillin. Because carbenicillin is supplied as a disodium salt, it contains about 5 mEq Na$^+$ per gram of drug, and this will result in the administration of more than 100 mEq Na$^+$ when patients are treated for *P. aeruginosa* infections. Carbenicillin has been superseded by ticarcillin or piperacillin (*see* below).

Preparations of carbenicillin may cause adverse effects in addition to those which follow the use of other penicillins (*see* below). Congestive heart failure may result from the administration of excessive Na$^+$. Hypokalemia may occur because of obligatory excretion of cation with the large amount of nonreabsorbable anion (carbenicillin) presented to the distal renal tubule. The drug interferes with platelet function, and bleeding may occur because of abnormal aggregation of platelets.

Carbenicillin Indanyl Sodium (GEOCILLIN). This congener is the indanyl ester of carbenicillin; it is acid stable and is suitable for oral administration. After absorption, the ester is converted rapidly to carbenicillin by hydrolysis of the ester linkage. The antimicrobial spectrum of the drug is therefore that of carbenicillin. Although the concentration of carbenicillin reached in the serum is not high enough to treat a systemic *Pseudomonas* infection, the active moiety is excreted rapidly in the urine, where it achieves effective concentrations. Thus the only use of this drug is for the management of urinary tract infections caused by *Proteus* spp. other than *P. mirabilis* and by *P. aeruginosa.*

Ticarcillin (TICAR). This semisynthetic penicillin (Table 44–1) is very similar to carbenicillin, but it is two to four times more active against *P. aeruginosa.* Ticarcillin is inferior to piperacillin for the treatment of serious infections caused by *Pseudomonas.*

Mezlocillin. This ureidopenicillin is more active against *Klebsiella* than is carbenicillin; its activity against *Pseudomonas in vitro* is similar to that of ticarcillin. It is more active than ticarcillin against *E. faecalis. Mezlocillin sodium* (MEZLIN) has been discontinued in the United States.

Piperacillin. Piperacillin (PIPRACIL) extends the spectrum of ampicillin to include most strains of *P. aeruginosa,* Enterobacteriaceae (non-β-lactamase-producing), many *Bacteroides* spp., and *E. faecalis.* In combination with a β-lactamase inhibitor (*piperacillin–tazobactam,* ZOSYN) it has the broadest antibacterial spectrum of the penicillins. Pharmacokinetic properties are reminiscent of the other ureidopenicillins. High biliary concentrations are achieved.

Therapeutic Indications. Piperacillin and related agents are important agents for the treatment of patients with serious infections caused by gram-negative bacteria. Such patients frequently have impaired immunological defenses, and their infections often are acquired in the hospital. Therefore, these penicillins find their greatest use in treating bacteremias, pneumonias, infections following burns, and urinary tract infections owing to microorganisms resistant to penicillin G and ampicillin; the bacteria especially responsible include *P. aeruginosa,* indole-positive strains of *Proteus,* and *Enterobacter* spp. Since *Pseudomonas* infections are common in neutropenic patients, therapy for severe bacterial infections in such individuals should include a β-lactam antibiotic such as piperacillin with good activity against these microorganisms.

Untoward Reactions to Penicillins

Hypersensitivity Reactions. Hypersensitivity reactions are by far the most common adverse effects noted with the penicillins, and these agents probably are the most common cause of drug allergy. Allergic reactions complicate between 0.7% and 4% of all treatment courses. There is no convincing evidence that any single penicillin differs from the group in its potential for causing true allergic reactions. In approximate order of decreasing frequency, manifestations of allergy to penicillins include maculopapular rash, urticarial rash, fever, bronchospasm, vasculitis, serum sickness, exfoliative dermatitis, Stevens–Johnson syndrome, and anaphylaxis (Weiss and Adkinson, 2000). The overall incidence of such reactions to the penicillins varies from 0.7% to 10% in different studies.

Hypersensitivity reactions may occur with any dosage form of penicillin; allergy to one penicillin exposes the patient to a greater risk of reaction if another is given. On the other hand, the occurrence of an untoward effect does not necessarily imply repetition on subsequent exposures. Hypersensitivity reactions may appear in the absence of a previous known exposure to the drug. This may be caused by unrecognized prior exposure to penicillin in the environment (*e.g.,* in foods of animal origin or from the fungus-producing penicillin). Although elimination of the antibiotic usually results in rapid clearing of the allergic manifestations, they may persist for 1 or 2 weeks or longer after therapy has been stopped. In some cases, the reaction is mild and disappears even when the penicillin is continued; in others, immediate cessation of penicillin treatment is required. In a few instances, it is necessary to interdict the future use of penicillin because of the risk of death, and the patient should be so warned. It must be stressed that fatal episodes of anaphylaxis have followed the ingestion of very small doses of this antibiotic or skin testing with minute quantities of the drug.

Penicillins and their breakdown products act as haptens after covalent reaction with proteins. The most abundant breakdown product is the penicilloyl moiety [major determinant moiety (MDM)], which is formed when the β-lac-

tam ring is opened. A large percentage of IgE-mediated reactions are to the MDM, but at least 25% of reactions are to other breakdown products, and the severities of the reactions to the various components are comparable. These products are formed *in vivo* and can be found in solutions of penicillin prepared for administration. The terms *major* and *minor determinants* refer to the frequency with which antibodies to these haptens appear to be formed. They do not describe the severity of the reaction that may result. In fact, anaphylactic reactions to penicillin usually are mediated by IgE antibodies against the minor determinants.

Antipenicillin antibodies are detectable in virtually all patients who have received the drug and in many who have never knowingly been exposed to it. Recent treatment with the antibiotic induces an increase in major-determinant-specific antibodies that are skin sensitizing. The incidence of positive skin reactors is three to four times higher in atopic than in nonatopic individuals. Clinical and immunological studies suggest that immediate allergic reactions are mediated by skin-sensitizing or IgE antibodies, usually of minor-determinant specificities. Accelerated and late urticarial reactions usually are mediated by major-determinant–specific skin-sensitizing antibodies. The recurrent-arthralgia syndrome appears to be related to the presence of skin-sensitizing antibodies of minor-determinant specificities. Some maculopapular and erythematous reactions may be due to toxic antigen–antibody complexes of major-determinant-specific IgM antibodies. Accelerated and late urticarial reactions to penicillin may terminate spontaneously because of the development of blocking antibodies.

Skin rashes of all types may be caused by allergy to penicillin. Scarlatiniform, morbilliform, urticarial, vesicular, and bullous eruptions may develop. Purpuric lesions are uncommon and usually are the result of a vasculitis; thrombocytopenic purpura may occur very rarely. Henoch–Schönlein purpura with renal involvement has been a rare complication. Contact dermatitis is observed occasionally in pharmacists, nurses, and physicians who prepare penicillin solutions. Fixed-drug reactions also have occurred. More severe reactions involving the skin are exfoliative dermatitis and exudative erythema multiforme of either the erythematopapular or vesiculobullous type; these lesions may be very severe and atypical in distribution and constitute the characteristic Stevens–Johnson syndrome. The incidence of skin rashes appears to be highest following the use of ampicillin, being about 9%; rashes follow the administration of ampicillin in nearly all patients with infectious mononucleosis. When *allopurinol* and ampicillin are administered concurrently, the incidence of rash also increases. Ampicillin-induced skin eruptions in such patients may represent a "toxic" rather than a truly allergic reaction. Positive skin reactions to the major and minor determinants of penicillin sensitization may be absent. The rash may clear even while administration of the drug is continued.

The most serious hypersensitivity reactions produced by the penicillins are angioedema and anaphylaxis. Angioedema, with marked swelling of the lips, tongue, face, and periorbital tissues, frequently accompanied by asthmatic breathing and "giant hives," has been observed after topical, oral, or systemic administration of penicillins of various types.

Acute anaphylactic or anaphylactoid reactions induced by various preparations of penicillin constitute the most important immediate danger connected with their use. Among all drugs, the penicillins are most often responsible for this type of untoward effect. Anaphylactoid reactions may occur at any age. Their incidence is thought to be 0.004% to 0.04% in persons treated with penicillins (Kucers and Bennett, 1987). About 0.001% of patients treated with these agents die from anaphylaxis. It has been estimated that there are at least 300 deaths per year due to this complication of therapy. About 70% have had penicillin previously, and one-third of these reacted to it on a prior occasion. Anaphylaxis most often has followed the injection of penicillin, although it also has been observed after oral ingestion of the drug and even has resulted from the intradermal instillation of a very small quantity for the purpose of testing for the presence of hypersensitivity. The clinical pictures that develop vary in severity. The most dramatic is sudden, severe hypotension and rapid death. In other instances, bronchoconstriction with severe asthma; abdominal pain, nausea, and vomiting; extreme weakness and a fall in blood pressure; or diarrhea and purpuric skin eruptions have characterized the anaphylactic episodes.

Serum sickness varies from mild fever, rash, and leukopenia to severe arthralgia or arthritis, purpura, lymphadenopathy, splenomegaly, mental changes, electrocardiographic abnormalities suggestive of myocarditis, generalized edema, albuminuria, and hematuria. It is mediated by IgG antibodies. This reaction is rare, but when it occurs, it appears after penicillin treatment has been continued for 1 week or more; it may be delayed, however, until 1 or 2 weeks after the drug has been stopped. Serum sickness caused by penicillin may persist for a week or longer.

Vasculitis of the skin or other organs may be related to penicillin hypersensitivity. The Coombs reaction frequently becomes positive during prolonged therapy with a penicillin or cephalosporin, but hemolytic anemia is rare. Reversible neutropenia may occur. It is not known if this is truly a hypersensitivity reaction; it has been noted with all the penicillins and has been seen in up to 30% of patients treated with 8 to 12 g nafcillin for longer than 21 days. The bone marrow shows an arrest of maturation.

Fever may be the only evidence of a hypersensitivity reaction to the penicillins. It may reach high levels and be maintained, remittent, or intermittent; chills occur occasionally. The febrile reaction usually disappears within 24 to 36 hours after administration of the drug is stopped but may persist for days.

Eosinophilia is an occasional accompaniment of other allergic reactions to penicillin. At times, it may be the sole abnormality, and eosinophils may reach levels of 10% to 20% or more of the total number of circulating white blood cells.

Penicillins rarely cause interstitial nephritis; methicillin has been implicated most frequently. Hematuria, albuminuria, pyuria, renal cell and other casts in the urine, elevation of serum creatinine, and even oliguria have been noted. Biopsy shows a mononuclear infiltrate with eosinophilia and tubular damage. IgG is present in the interstitium. This reaction usually is reversible.

Management of the Patient Potentially Allergic to Penicillin. Evaluation of the patient's history is the most practical way to avoid the use of penicillin in patients who are at the greatest risk of adverse reaction. Most patients who give a history of allergy to penicillin should be treated with a different type of antibiotic. Unfortunately, there is no totally reliable means to confirm a history of penicillin allergy (Romano *et al.*, 2003). Skin testing for IgE-mediated immediate-type responses is compromised by the lack of a commercially available minor-determinant mixture. Skin testing using major and minor penicillin determinants to predict allergic reactions to synthetic penicillins is useful if the reagents are generally available. An NIAID multicenter study used major and minor determinants for skin testing. Of 726 patients with a history of penicillin allergy, 566 had negative skin tests. Of those, only 7 of 566 (1.2%) had possibly IgE-mediated immediate or accelerated penicillin allergy when given penicillin (Sogn *et al.*, 1992). Radioallergosorbent tests (RASTs) for IgE antipenicilloyl determinants suffer from the same limitations as skin tests (Weiss and Adkinson, 2000).

Occasionally, *desensitization* is recommended for penicillin-allergic patients who must receive the drug. This procedure consists of administering gradually increasing doses of penicillin in the hope of avoiding a severe reaction and should be performed only in an intensive care setting. This may result in a subclinical anaphylactic discharge and the binding of all IgE before full doses are administered. Penicillin may be given in doses of 1, 5, 10, 100, and 1000 units intradermally in the lower arm, with 60-minute intervals between doses. If this is well tolerated, then 10,000 and 50,000 units may be given subcutaneously. Desensitization also may be accomplished by the oral administration of penicillin. When full doses are reached, penicillin should not be discontinued and then restarted because immediate reactions may recur (*see* Weiss and Adkinson, 2000, for details). The patient should be observed constantly during the desensitizing procedure, an intravenous line must be in place, and epinephrine and equipment and expertise for artificial ventilation must be on hand. It must be emphasized that this procedure may be dangerous, and its efficacy is unproven.

Patients with life-threatening infections (*e.g.*, endocarditis or meningitis) may be continued on penicillin despite the development of a maculopapular rash, although alternative antimicrobial agents should be used whenever possible. The rash often resolves as therapy is continued, perhaps owing to the development of blocking antibodies of the IgG class. The rash may be treated with *antihistamines* or *glucocorticoids*, although there is no evidence that this therapy is efficacious. Rarely, exfoliative dermatitis with or without vasculitis develops in these patients if therapy with penicillin is continued.

Other Adverse Reactions. The penicillins have minimal direct toxicity. Apparent toxic effects that have been reported include bone marrow depression, granulocytopenia, and hepatitis. The last-named effect is rare but is seen most commonly following the administration of oxacillin and nafcillin. The administration of penicillin G, carbenicillin, piperacillin, or ticarcillin has been associated with a potentially significant defect of hemostasis that appears to be due to an impairment of platelet aggregation; this may be caused by interference with the binding of aggregating agents to platelet receptors (Fass *et al.*, 1987).

Most common among the irritative responses to penicillin are pain and sterile inflammatory reactions at the sites of intramuscular injections—reactions that are related to concentration. Serum transaminases and lactic dehydrogenase may be elevated as a result of local damage to muscle. In some individuals who receive penicillin intravenously, phlebitis or thrombophlebitis develops. Many persons who take various penicillin preparations by mouth experience nausea, with or without vomiting, and some have mild to severe diarrhea. These manifestations often are related to the dose of the drug.

When penicillin is injected accidentally into the sciatic nerve, severe pain occurs and dysfunction in the area of distribution of this nerve develops and persists for weeks. Intrathecal injection of penicillin G may produce arachnoiditis or severe and fatal encephalopathy. Because of this, intrathecal or intraventricular administration of penicillins should be avoided. The parenteral administration of large doses of penicillin G (>20 million units per day, or less with renal insufficiency) may produce lethargy, confusion, twitching, multifocal myoclonus, or localized or generalized epileptiform seizures. These are most apt to occur in the presence of renal insufficiency, localized lesions of the central nervous system (CNS), or hyponatremia. When the concentration of penicillin G in CSF exceeds 10 μg/ml, significant dysfunction of the CNS is frequent. The injection of 20 million units of penicillin G potassium, which contains 34 mEq of K[+], may lead to severe or even fatal hyperkalemia in persons with renal dysfunction.

Injection of penicillin G procaine may result in an immediate reaction, characterized by dizziness, tinnitus, headache, hallucinations, and sometimes seizures. This is due to the rapid liberation of toxic concentrations of procaine. It has been reported to occur in 1 of 200 patients receiving 4.8 million units of penicillin G procaine to treat venereal disease.

Reactions Unrelated to Hypersensitivity or Toxicity. Regardless of the route by which the drug is administered, but most strikingly when it is given by mouth, penicillin changes the composition of the microflora by eliminating sensitive microorganisms. This phenomenon is usually of no clinical significance, and the normal microflora are reestablished shortly after therapy is stopped. In some persons, however, superinfection results from the changes in flora. Pseudomembranous colitis, related to overgrowth and production of a toxin by *Clostridium difficile*, has followed oral and, less commonly, parenteral administration of penicillins.

THE CEPHALOSPORINS

History and Source. *Cephalosporium acremonium*, the first source of the cephalosporins, was isolated in 1948 by Brotzu from the sea near a sewer outlet off the Sardinian coast. Crude filtrates from cultures of this fungus were found to inhibit the *in vitro* growth of *S. aureus* and to cure staphylococcal infections and typhoid fever in human beings. Culture fluids in which the Sardinian fungus was cultivated were found to contain three distinct antibiotics, which were named *cephalosporin P, N*, and *C*. With isolation of the active nucleus of cephalosporin C, 7-aminocephalosporanic acid, and with the addition of side chains, it became possible to produce semisynthetic compounds with antibacterial activity very much greater than that of the parent substance.

Chemistry. Cephalosporin C contains a side chain derived from D-α-aminoadipic acid, which is condensed with a dihydrothiazine β-lactam ring system (7-aminocephalosporanic acid). Compounds containing 7-aminocephalosporanic acid are relatively stable in dilute acid and highly resistant to penicillinase regardless of the nature of their side chains and their affinity for the enzyme.

Cephalosporin C can be hydrolyzed by acid to 7-aminocephalosporanic acid. This compound subsequently has been modified by the addition of different side chains to create a whole family of cephalosporin antibiotics. It appears that modifications at position 7 of the β-lactam ring are associated with alteration in antibacterial activity and that substitutions at position 3 of the dihydrothiazine ring are associated with changes in the metabolism and pharmacokinetic properties of the drugs.

The *cephamycins* are similar to the cephalosporins but have a methoxy group at position 7 of the β-lactam ring of the 7-aminocephalosporanic acid nucleus. The structural formulas of representative cephalosporins and cephamycins are shown in Table 44–2.

Table 44–2
Names, Structural Formulas, Dosage, and Dosage Forms of Selected Cephalosporins and Related Compounds

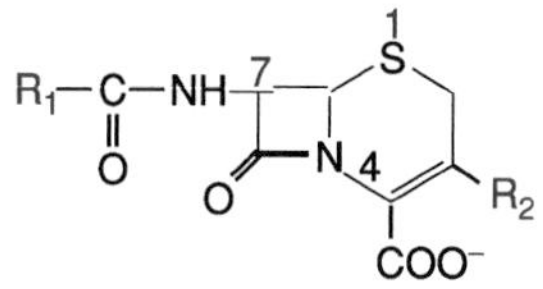

Cephim nucleus

COMPOUND (TRADE NAMES)	R_1	R_2	DOSAGE FORMS,* ADULT DOSAGE FOR SEVERE INFECTION, AND $t_{\frac{1}{2}}$
First-generation			
Cefazolin (ANCEF, KEFZOL, others)	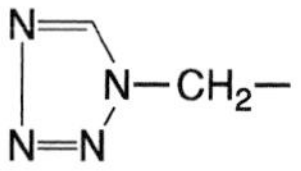	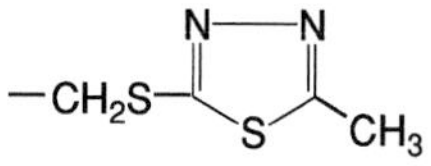	I: 1 to 1.5 g every 6 hours $t_{\frac{1}{2}}$ = about 2 hours
Cephalexin (KEFLEX, others)	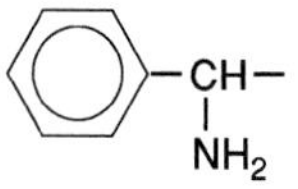	$-CH_3$	O: 1 g every 6 hours $t_{\frac{1}{2}}$ = 0.9 hour
Cefadroxil (DURICEF)	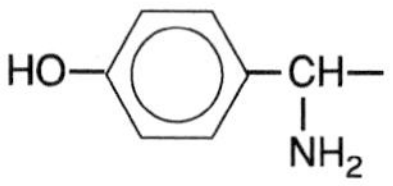	$-CH_3$	O: 1 g every 12 hours $t_{\frac{1}{2}}$ = 1.1 hours
Second-generation			
Cefoxitin[†] (MEFOXIN)	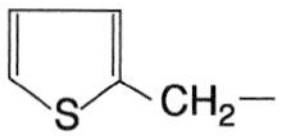	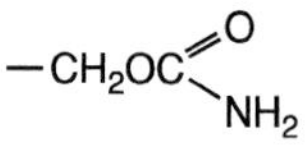	I: 2 g every 4 hours or 3 g every 6 hours $t_{\frac{1}{2}}$ = 0.7 hours
Cefaclor (CECLOR)	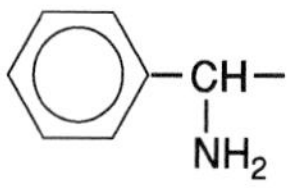	$-Cl$	O: 1 g every 8 hours $t_{\frac{1}{2}}$ = 0.7 hours
Cefprozil (CEFZIL)	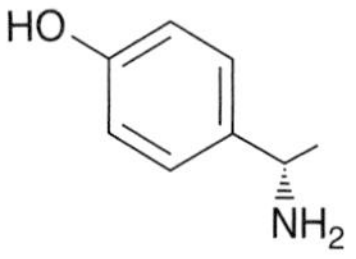	$CH=CH-CH_2$	O: 500 mg every 12 hours $t_{\frac{1}{2}}$ = 1.3 hours
Cefuroxime (ZINACEF) Cefuroxime acetil[‡] (CEFTIN)	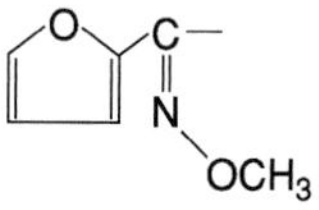	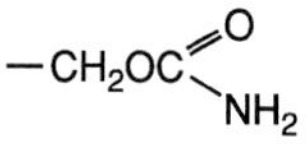	I: up to 3 g every 8 hours $t_{\frac{1}{2}}$ = 1.7 hours T: 500 mg every 12 hours
Loracarbef[¶] (LORABID)	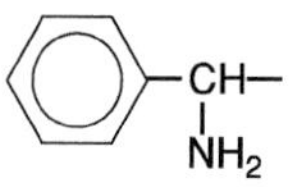	$-Cl$	O: 200 to 400 mg every 12 hours $t_{\frac{1}{2}}$ = 1.1 hours
Cefotetan (CEFOTAN)	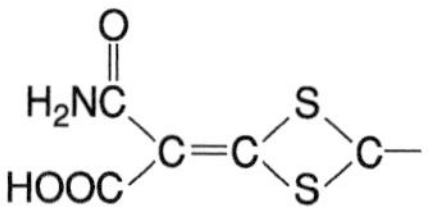	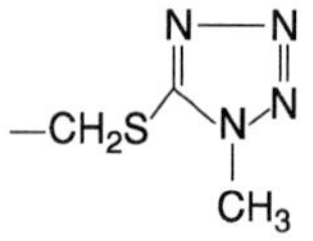	I: 2 to 3 g every 12 hours $t_{\frac{1}{2}}$ = 3.3 hours
Ceforanide (PRECEF)	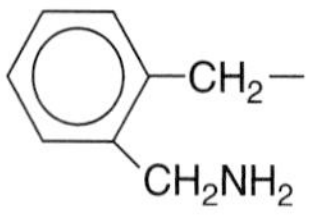		I: 1 g every 12 hours $t_{\frac{1}{2}}$ = 2.6 hours

(Continued)

Table 44–2

Names, Structural Formulas, Dosage, and Dosage Forms of Selected Cephalosporins and Related Compounds (Continued)

COMPOUND (TRADE NAMES)	R_1	R_2	DOSAGE FORMS,* ADULT DOSAGE FOR SEVERE INFECTION, AND $t_{\frac{1}{2}}$
Third-generation			
Cefotaxime (CLAFORAN)	(aminothiazole–OCH₃ oxime structure)	$-CH_2OC(=O)CH_3$	I: 2 g every 4 to 8 hours; $t_{\frac{1}{2}} = 1.1$ hours
Cefpodoxime proxetil§ (VANTIN)	(aminothiazole–OCH₃ oxime structure)	$-CH_2OCH_3$	O: 200 to 400 mg every 12 hours; $t_{\frac{1}{2}} = 2.2$ hours
Cefibuten (CEDAX)	(aminothiazole–COOH structure)	$-H$	O: 400 mg every 24 hours; $t_{\frac{1}{2}} = 2.4$ hours
Cefdinir (OMNICEF)	(aminothiazole–OH oxime structure)	$CH=CH_2$	O: 300 mg every 12 hours or 600 mg every 24 hours; $t_{\frac{1}{2}} = 1.7$ hours
Cefditoren pivoxil (SPECTRACEF)	(aminothiazole–OCH₃ oxime structure)	(methylthiazole structure)	O: 400 mg every 12 hours; $t_{\frac{1}{2}} = 1.6$ hours
Ceftizoxime (CEFIZOX)	(aminothiazole–OCH₃ oxime structure)	$-H$	I: 3 to 4 g every 8 hours; $t_{\frac{1}{2}} = 1.8$ hours
Ceftriaxone (ROCHEPHIN)	(aminothiazole–OCH₃ oxime structure)	$-CH_2S-$ (triazinone structure)	I: 2 g every 12 to 24 hours; $t_{\frac{1}{2}} = 8$ hours
Cefoperazone (CEFOBID)	(HO-phenyl–CH–NHCO–piperazinedione–C_2H_5 structure)	$-CH_2S-$ (methyltetrazole structure)	I: 1.5 to 4 g every 6 to 8 hours; $t_{\frac{1}{2}} = 2.1$ hours
Ceftazidime (HORTAZ, others)	(aminothiazole–OC(CH₃)₂ oxime structure)	$-CH_2$ (pyridinium structure)	I: 2 g every 8 hours; $t_{\frac{1}{2}} = 1.8$ hours
Fourth-generation			
Cefepime (MAXIPIME)	(aminothiazole–OCH₃ oxime structure)	$-CH_2N^+$ (methylpyrrolidinium structure)	I: 2 g every 8 hours; $t_{\frac{1}{2}} = 2$ hours

*T, tablet; C, capsule; O, oral suspension; I, injection †Cefoxitin, a cophamycin, has a –OCH₃ group at position 7 of cephem nucleus. ‡Cefuroxime axctil is the acetyloxyethyl ester of cefuroxime. ¶Loracarbef, a carbacephem, has a carbon instead of sulfur at position 1 of cephem nucleus. §Cefpodoxime proxetil has a –COOCH(CH₃)OCOOCH(CH₃)₂ group at position 4 of cephem nucleus.

Table 44–3
Cephalosporin Generations

EXAMPLES	USEFUL SPECTRUM[a]
First Generation	
Cefazolin (ANCEF, ZOLICEF, others)	Streptococci[b]; *Staphylococcus aureus.*[c]
Cephalexin monohydrate (KEFTAB)	
Cefadroxil (DURACEF)	
Cephradine (VELOSEF)	
Second Generation	
Cefuroxime (ZINACEF)	*Escherichia coli, Klebsiella, Proteus, Haemophilus influenzae, Moraxella catarrhalis.* Not as active against gram-positive organisms as first-generation agents.
Cefuroxime axetil (CEFTIN)	
Cefprozil (CEFZIL)	Inferior activity against *S. aureus* compared to cefuroxime but with added activity against *Bacteroides fragilis* and other *Bacteroides* spp.
Cefmetazole (ZEFAZONE)	
Loracarbef (LORABID)	
Third Generation	
Cefotaxime (CLAFORAN)	Enterobacteriaceae[d]; *Pseudomonas aeruginosa*[e]; *Serratia; Neisseria gonorrhoeae;* activity for *S. aureus, Streptococcus pneumoniae,* and *Streptococcus pyogenes*[f] comparable to first-generation agents. Activity against *Bacteroides* spp. inferior to that of cefoxitin and cefotetan.
Ceftriaxone (ROCEPHIN)	
Cefdinir (OMNICEF)	
Cefditoren pivoxil (SPECTRACEF)	
Ceftibuten (CEDAX)	
Cefpodoxime proxetil (VANTIN)	
Ceftizoxime (CEFIZOX)	
Cefoperazone (CEFOBID)	} Active against *Pseudomonas*
Ceftazidime (FORTAZ, others)	
Fourth Generation	
Cefepine (MAXIPINE)	Comparable to third-generation but more resistant to some β-lactamases.

[a]All cephalosporins lack activity against enterococci, *Listeria monocytogenes, Legionella* spp., methicillin-resistant *S. aureus, Xanthomonas maltophilia,* and *Acinetobacter* species. [b]Except for penicillin-resistant strains. [c]Except for methicillin-resistant strains. [d]Resistance to cephalosporins may be induced rapidly during therapy by de-repression of bacterial chromosomal β-lactamases, which destroy the cephalosporins. [e]Ceftazidime only. [f]Ceftazidime lacks significant gram-positive activity. Cefotaxime is most active in class against *S. aureus* and *S. pyogenes.*

Mechanism of Action. Cephalosporins and cephamycins inhibit bacterial cell wall synthesis in a manner similar to that of penicillin. This was discussed in detail earlier.

Classification. The large number of cephalosporins makes a system of classification most desirable. Although cephalosporins may be classified by their chemical structure, clinical pharmacology, resistance to β-lactamase, or antimicrobial spectrum, the well-accepted system of classification by "generations" is very useful, although admittedly somewhat arbitrary (Table 44–3).

Classification by generations is based on general features of antimicrobial activity (*see* Karchmer, 2000). The *first-generation* cephalosporins, epitomized by *cephalothin* and *cefazolin,* have good activity against gram-positive bacteria and relatively modest activity against gram-negative microorganisms. Most gram-positive cocci (with

the exception of enterococci, methicillin-resistant *S. aureus,* and *S. epidermidis*) are susceptible. Most oral cavity anaerobes are sensitive, but the *B. fragilis* group is resistant. Activity against *Moraxella catarrhalis, E. coli, K. pneumoniae,* and *P. mirabilis* is good. The *second-generation* cephalosporins have somewhat increased activity against gram-negative microorganisms but are much less active than the third-generation agents. A subset of second-generation agents (*cefoxitin, cefotetan,* and *cefmetazole*) also is active against the *B. fragilis* group. *Third-generation* cephalosporins generally are less active than first-generation agents against gram-positive cocci, but they are much more active against the Enterobacteriaceae, including β-lactamase-producing strains. A subset of third-generation agents (*ceftazidime* and *cefoperazone*) also is active against *P. aeruginosa* but less active than other third-generation agents against gram-positive cocci.

Therapeutic Uses. Imipenem–cilastatin is effective for a wide variety of infections, including urinary tract and lower respiratory infections; intra-abdominal and gynecological infections; and skin, soft tissue, bone, and joint infections. The drug combination appears to be especially useful for the treatment of infections caused by cephalosporin-resistant nosocomial bacteria, such as *Citrobacter freundii* and *Enterobacter* spp. It would be prudent to use imipenem for empirical treatment of serious infections in hospitalized patients who have recently received other β-lactam antibiotics because of the increased risk of infection with cephalosporin- and/or penicillin-resistant bacteria. Imipenem should not be used as monotherapy for infections owing to *P. aeruginosa* because of the risk of resistance developing during therapy.

Meropenem. Meropenem (MERREM IV) is a dimethyl-carbamoyl pyrolidinyl derivative of *thienamycin*. It does not require coadministration with cilastatin because it is not sensitive to renal dipeptidase. Its toxicity is similar to that of imipenem except that it may be less likely to cause seizures (0.5% of meropenem- and 1.5% of imipenem-treated patients seized). Its *in vitro* activity is similar to that of imipenem, with activity against some imipenem-resistant *P. aeruginosa* but less activity against gram-positive cocci. Clinical experience with meropenem demonstrates therapeutic equivalence with imipenem.

Ertapenem. Ertapenem (INVANZ) differs from imipenem and meropenem by having a larger serum half-life that allows once-daily dosing and by having inferior activity against *P. aeruginosa* and *Acinetobacter* spp. Its spectrum of activity against gram-positive organisms, Enterobacteriaceae, and anaerobes makes it attractive for use in intra-abdominal and pelvic infections (Solomkin *et al.*, 2003).

Aztreonam. Aztreonam (AZACTAM) is a monocyclic β-lactam compound (a monobactam) isolated from *Chromobacterium violaceum* (Sykes *et al.*, 1981). Its structural formula is as follows:

AZTREONAM

Aztreonam interacts with penicillin-binding proteins of susceptible microorganisms and induces the formation of long filamentous bacterial structures. The compound is resistant to many of the β-lactamases that are elaborated by most gram-negative bacteria.

The antimicrobial activity of aztreonam differs from those of other β-lactam antibiotics and more closely resembles that of an aminoglycoside. Aztreonam has activity only against gram-negative bacteria; it has no activity against gram-positive bacteria and anaerobic organisms. However, activity against Enterobacteriaceae is excellent, as is that against *P. aeruginosa*. It is also highly active *in vitro* against *H. influenzae* and gonococci.

Aztreonam is administered either intramuscularly or intravenously. Peak concentrations of aztreonam in plasma average nearly 50 μg/ml after a 1-g intramuscular dose. The half-life for elimination is 1.7 hours, and most of the drug is recovered unaltered in the urine. The half-life is prolonged to about 6 hours in anephric patients.

Aztreonam generally is well tolerated. Interestingly, patients who are allergic to penicillins or cephalosporins appear not to react to aztreonam, with the exception of ceftazidime.

The usual dose of aztreonam for severe infections is 2 g every 6 to 8 hours. This should be reduced in patients with renal insufficiency. Aztreonam has been used successfully for the therapy of a variety of infections. One of its notable features is little allergic cross-reactivity with β-lactam antibiotics, with the possible exception of ceftazidine (Perez Pimiento *et al.*, 1998), with which it has considerable structural similarity. Aztreonam is therefore quite useful for treating gram-negative infections that normally would be treated with a β-lactam antibiotic were it not for the history of a prior allergic reaction.

β-LACTAMASE INHIBITORS

Certain molecules can inactivate β-lactamases, thus preventing the destruction of β-lactam antibiotics that are substrates for these enzymes. β-Lactamase inhibitors are most active against plasmid-encoded β-lactamases (including the enzymes that hydrolyze ceftazidime and cefotaxime), but they are inactive at clinically achievable concentrations against the type I chromosomal β-lactamases induced in gram-negative bacilli (such as *Enterobacter, Acinetobacter,* and *Citrobacter*) by treatment with second- and third-generation cephalosporins.

Clavulanic acid is produced by *Streptomyces clavuligerus;* its structural formula is as follows:

CLAVULANIC ACID

It has poor intrinsic antimicrobial activity, but it is a "suicide" inhibitor that irreversibly binds β-lactamases produced by a wide range of gram-positive and gram-negative microorganisms. Clavulanic acid is well absorbed by mouth and also can be given parenterally. It has been combined with amoxicillin as an oral preparation (AUGMENTIN) and with ticarcillin as a parenteral preparation (TIMENTIN).

Amoxicillin plus clavulanate is effective *in vitro* and *in vivo* for β-lactamase-producing strains of staphylococci, *H. influenzae*, gonococci, and *E. coli*. Amoxicillin–clavulanate plus ciprofloxacin has been shown to be an effective oral treatment for low-risk, febrile patients with neutropenia from cancer chemotherapy (Freifeld *et al.*, 1999; Kern *et al.*, 1999). It also is effective in the treatment of acute otitis media in children, sinusitis, animal or human bite wounds, cellulitis, and diabetic foot infections. The addition of clavulanate to ticarcillin (TIMENTIN) extends its spectrum such that it resembles imipenem to include aerobic gram-negative bacilli, *S. aureus*, and *Bacteroides* spp. There is no increased activity against *Pseudomonas* spp. (Bansal *et al.*, 1985). The dosage should be adjusted for patients with renal insufficiency. The combination is especially useful for mixed nosocomial infections and is used often with an aminoglycoside.

Sulbactam is another β-lactamase inhibitor similar in structure to clavulanic acid. It may be given orally or parenterally along with a β-lactam antibiotic. It is available for intravenous or intramuscular use combined with ampicillin (UNASYN). Dosage must be adjusted for patients with impaired renal function. The combination has good activity against gram-positive cocci, including β-lactamase-producing strains of *S. aureus*, gram-negative aerobes (but not *Pseudomonas*), and anaerobes; it also has been used effectively for the treatment of mixed intra-abdominal and pelvic infections.

Tazobactam is a penicillanic acid sulfone β-lactamase inhibitor. In common with the other available inhibitors, it has poor activity against the inducible chromosomal β-lactamases of Enterobacteriaceae but has good activity against many of the plasmid β-lactamases, including some of the extended-spectrum class. It has been combined with piperacillin as a parenteral preparation (ZOSYN) (*see* Bryson and Brogden, 1994).

The combination of piperacillin and tazobactam does not increase the activity of piperacillin against *P. aeruginosa* because resistance is due to either chromosomal β-lactamases or decreased permeability of piperacillin into the periplasmic space. Because the currently recommended dose (3 g piperacillin per 375 mg tazobactam every 4 to 8 hours) is less than the recommended dose of piperacillin when used alone for serious infections (3 to 4 g every 4 to 6 hours), concern has been raised that piperacillin–tazobactam may prove ineffective in the treatment of some *P. aeruginosa* infections that would have responded to piperacillin. The combination of piperacillin plus tazobactam should be equivalent in antimicrobial spectrum to ticarcillin plus clavulanate.

BIBLIOGRAPHY

Bansal, M.B., Chuah, S.K., and Thadepalli, H. *In vitro* activity and *in vivo* evaluation of ticarcillin plus clavulanic acid against aerobic and anaerobic bacteria. *Am. J. Med.*, 1985, *79*:33–38.

Barriere, S.L., and Mills, J. Ceforanide: Antibacterial activity, pharmacology, and clinical efficacy. *Pharmacotherapy*, 1982, *2*:322–327.

Barriere, S.L. Pharmacology and pharmacokinetics of cefprozil. *Clin. Infect. Dis.*, 1992, *14*(suppl. 2):S184–S188.

Baumgartner, J.D., and Glauser, M.P. Single daily dose treatment of severe refractory infections with ceftriaxone: Cost savings and possible parenteral outpatient treatment. *Arch. Intern. Med.*, 1983, *143*:1868–1873.

Bennett, S., Wise, R., Weston, D., and Dent, J. Pharmacokinetics and tissue penetration of ticarcillin combined with clavulanic acid. *Antimicrob. Agents Chemother.*, 1983, *23*:831–834.

Berrios, X., del Campo, E., Guzman, B., and Bisno, A.L. Discontinuing rheumatic fever prophylaxis in selected adolescents and young adults: A prospective study. *Ann. Intern. Med.*, 1993, *118*:401–406.

Brogden, R.N., and Ward, A. Ceftriaxone: A reappraisal of its antibacterial activity and pharmacokinetic properties, and an update on its therapeutic use with particular reference to once-daily administration. *Drugs*, 1988, *35*:604–645.

Carratalá, J., Alcaide, F., Fernandez-Sevilla, A., *et al.* Bacteremia due to *viridans* streptococci that are highly resistant to penicillin: Increase among neutropenic patients with cancer. *Clin. Infect. Dis.*, 1995, *20*:1169–1173.

Catalan, M.J., Fernandez, J.M., Vazquez, A., *et al.* Failure of cefotaxime in the treatment of meningitis due to relatively resistant *Streptococcus pneumoniae*. *Clin. Infect. Dis.*, 1994, *18*:766–769.

Centers for Disease Control and Prevention. Geographic variation in penicillin resistance in *Streptococcus pneumoniae*—Selected sites, United States, 1997. *M.M.W.R.*, 1999, *48*:656–661.

Centers for Disease Control and Prevention. Multidrug-resistant *Streptococcus pneumoniae* in a child care center—Southwest Georgia, December 2000. *M.M.W.R.*, 2002, *50*:1156–1158.

Centers for Disease Control and Prevention. Sexually transmitted diseases guidelines. *M.M.W.R.*, 2002, *51*:1–80.

Centers for Disease Control and Prevention. Vancomycin-intermediate/resistant *Staphyloccocus aureus*. *M.M.W.R.*, 2004, *53*:322–323 and http://www.cdc.gov/ncidod/hip/vanco/VANCO.HTM.

Chambers, H.F., Hackbarth, C.J., Drake, T.A., Rusnak, M.G., and Sande, M.A. Endocarditis due to methicillin-resistant *Staphylococcus aureus* in rabbits: Expression of resistance to beta-lactam antibiotics *in vivo* and *in vitro*. *J. Infect. Dis.*, 1984, *149*:894–903.

Dajani, A.S., Taubert, K.A., Wilson, W., *et al.* Prevention of bacterial endocarditis. *JAMA*, 1997, *277*:1794–1801.

deGans, J., and van de Beek, D. Dexamethasone in adults with bacterial meningitis. *New Engl. J. Med.*, 2002, *347*:1549–1556.

del Rio, M.A., Chrane, D., Shelton, S., McCracken, G.H., Jr., and Nelson, J.D. Ceftriaxone versus ampicillin and chloramphenicol for treatment of bacterial meningitis in children. *Lancet*, 1983, *1*:1241–1244.

Dowell, S.F., Butler, J.C., Giebink, G.S., *et al.* Acute otitis media: Management and surveillance in an era of pneumococcal resistance—a report from the Drug-resistant *Streptococcus pneumoniae* Therapeutic Working Group. *Pediatr. Infect. Dis. J.*, 1999, *18*:1–9.

Edmond, M.B., Wallace, S.E., McClish, D.K., *et al.* Nosocomial bloodstream infections in United States hospitals: A three-year analysis. *Clin. Infect. Dis.*, 1999, *29*:239–244.

Fass, R.J., Copelan, E.A., Brandt, J.T., Moeschberger, M.L., and Ashton, J.J. Platelet-mediated bleeding caused by broad-spectrum penicillins. *J. Infect. Dis.*, 1987, *155*:1242–1248.

Fiore, A.E., Moroney, J.F., Farley, M.M., *et al.* Clinical outcomes of meningitis caused by *Streptococcus pneumoniae* in the era of antibiotic resistance. *Clin. Infect. Dis.*, 2000, *30*:71–77.

Freifeld, A., Marchigiani, D., Walsh, T., *et al.* A double-blind comparison of empirical oral and intravenous antibiotic therapy for low-risk febrile patients with neutropenia during cancer chemotherapy. *New Engl. J. Med.,* **1999,** *341*:305–311.

Friedland, I.R., and McCracken, G.H., Jr. Management of infections caused by antibiotic-resistant *Streptococcus pneumoniae. New Engl. J. Med.,* **1994,** *331*:377–382.

Goldstein, E.J., Citron, D.M., and Richwald, G.A. Lack of *in vitro* efficacy of oral forms of certain cephalosporins, erythromycin, and oxacillin against *Pasteurella multocida. Antimicrob. Agents Chemother.,* **1988,** *32*:213–215.

Haas, D.W., Stratton, C.W., Griffin, J.P., Weeks, L., and Alls, S.C. Diminished activity of ceftizoxime in comparison to cefotaxime and ceftriaxone against *Streptococcus pneumoniae. Clin. Infect. Dis.,* **1995,** *20*:671–676.

Hamilton-Miller, J.M., and Brumfitt, W. Activity of ceftazidime (GR 20263) against nosocomially important pathogens. *Antimicrob. Agents Chemother.,* **1981,** *19*:1067–1069.

John, C.C. Treatment failure with use of a third-generation cephalosporin for penicillin-resistant pneumococcal meningitis: Case report and review. *Clin. Infect. Dis.,* **1994,** *18*:188–193.

Jones, R.N., Pfaller, M.A., Doern, G.V., Erwin, M.E., and Hollis, R.J. Antimicrobial activity and spectrum investigation of eight broadspectrum β-lactam drugs: A 1997 surveillance trial in 102 medical centers in the United States. Cefepime Study Group. *Diagn. Microbiol. Infect. Dis.,* **1998,** *30*:215–228.

Jorgensen, J.H., Doern, G.V., Maher, L.A., Howell, A.W., and Redding, J.S. Antimicrobial resistance among respiratory isolates of *Haemophilus influenzae, Moraxella catarrhalis,* and *Streptococcus pneumoniae* in the United States. *Antimicrob. Agents Chemother.,* **1990,** *34*:2075–2080.

Kern, W.V., Cometta, A., De Bock, R., *et al.* Oral versus intravenous empirical antimicrobial therapy for fever in patients with granulocytopenia who are receiving cancer chemotherapy. International Antimicrobial Therapy Cooperative Group of the European Organization for Research and Treatment of Cancer. *New Engl. J. Med.,* **1999,** *341*:312–318.

Levison, M.E., Mangura, C.T., Lorber, B., *et al.* Clindamycin compared with penicillin for the treatment of anaerobic lung abscess. *Ann. Intern. Med.,* **1983,** *98*:466–471.

Mendelman, P.M., Campos, J., Chaffin, D.O., *et al.* Relative penicillin G resistance in *Neisseria meningitidis* and reduced affinity of penicillinbinding protein 3. *Antimicrob. Agents Chemother.,* **1988,** *32*:706–709.

Neu, H.C., Aswapokee, N., Aswapokee, P., and Fu, K.P. HR 756, a new cephalosporin active against gram-positive and gram-negative aerobic and anaerobic bacteria. *Antimicrob. Agents Chemother.,* **1979,** *15*:273–281.

Neu, H.C., Turck, M., and Phillips, I. Ceftizoxime, a broad-spectrum β-lactamase stable cephalosporin. *J. Antimicrob. Chemother.,* **1982,** *10*(suppl. C): 1–355.

Nikaido, H. Antibiotic resistance caused by gram-negative multidrug efflux pumps. *Clin. Infect. Dis.,* **1998,** *27*(suppl. I):S32–S41.

Okuma, K., Iwakawa, K., and Turnidge, J. D. Dissemination of new methicillin-resistant *Staphylococcus aureus* clones in the community. *J. Clin. Microbiol.,* **2002,** *40*:4289–4294.

Perez Pimiento, A., Gomez Martinez, M., Minguez Mena, A., *et al.* Aztreonam and ceftazidime: Evidence of *in vivo* cross allergenicity. *Allergy,* **1998,** *53*:624–625.

Phillips, I., Wise, R., and Leigh, D.A. Cefotetan: A new cephamycin. *J. Antimicrob. Chemother.,* **1983,** *11*(suppl.):1–239.

Rosenstein, N.E., Stocker, S.A., Popovic, T., Tenover, F.C., and Perkins, B.A. Antimicrobial resistance of *Neisseria meningitidis* in the United

States, 1997. The Active Bacterial Core Surveillance (ABCs) Team. *Clin. Infect. Dis.,* **2000,** *30*:212–213.

Sahm, D.F., Marsilio, M.K., and Piazza, G. Antimicrobial resistance in key bloodstream bacterial isolates: Electronic surveillance with the Surveillance Network Database—USA. *Clin. Infect. Dis.,* **1999,** *29*:259–263.

Sanders, C.S. Cefepime: The next generation? *Clin. Infect. Dis.,* **1993,** *17*:369–379.

Sattler, F.R., Weitekamp, M.R., and Ballard, J.O. Potential for bleeding with the new β-lactam antibiotics. *Ann. Intern. Med.,* **1986,** *105*:924–931.

Schaad, U.B., Suter, S., Gianella-Borradori, A., *et al.* A comparison of ceftriaxone and cefuroxime for the treatment of bacterial meningitis in children. *New Engl. J. Med.,* **1990,** *322*:141–147.

Sogn, D.D., Evans, R., Shepherd, G.M., *et al.* Results of the NIAID collaborative clinical trial to test the predictive value of skin testing with major and minor penicillin derivatives in hospitalized adults. *Arch. Intern. Med.,* **1992,** *152*:1025–1032.

Solomkin, J.S., Yellin, A.E., Rutstein, O.D., *et al.* Ertapenem vs. piperacillin/tazobactam in the treatment of complicated intra-abdominal infections: Results of a double-blind, randomized comparative phase III trial. *Ann. Surg.,* **2003,** *237*:235–242.

Sprott, M.S., Kearns, A.M., and Field, J.M. Penicillin-insensitive *Neisseria meningitidis. Lancet,* **1988,** *1*:1167.

Sykes, R.B., Cimarusti, C.M., Bonner, D.P., *et al.* Monocyclic β-lactam antibiotics produced by bacteria. *Nature,* **1981,** *291*:489–491.

Tomasz, A. Penicillin-binding proteins and the antibacterial effectiveness of β-lactam antibiotics. *Rev. Infect. Dis.,* **1986,** *8*(suppl. 3):S260–S278.

Wade, J.C., Smith, C.R., Petty, B.G., *et al.* Cephalothin plus an aminoglycoside is more nephrotoxic than methicillin plus an aminoglycoside. *Lancet,* **1978,** *2*:604–606.

Wexler, H.M., and Finegold, S.M. *In vitro* activity of cefotetan compared with that of other antimicrobial agents against anaerobic bacteria. *Antimicrob. Agents Chemother.,* **1988,** *32*:601–604.

Wilson, W.R., Wilkowske, C.J., Wright, A.J., Sande, M.A., and Geraci, J.E. Treatment of streptomycin-susceptible and streptomycinresistant enterococcal endocarditis. *Ann. Intern. Med.,* **1984,** *100*:816–823.

MONOGRAPHS AND REVIEWS

Bank, N.U., and Kammer, R.B. Hematologic complications associated with β-lactam antibiotics. *Rev. Infect. Dis.,* **1983,** *5*:S380–S398.

Barradell, L.B., and Bryson, H.M. Cefepime: A review of its antibacterial activity, pharmacokinetic properties and therapeutic use. *Drugs,* **1994,** *47*:471–505.

Bayles, K.W. The bactericidal action of penicillin: New clues to an unsolved mystery. *Trends Microbiol.,* **2000,** *8*:81274–81278.

Bisno, A.L., Stevens, D.L. Streptococcal infections of skin and soft tissues. *New Engl. J. Med.,* **1996,** *334*:240–245.

Bryson, H.M., and Brogden, R.N. Piperacillin/tazobactam: A review of its antibacterial activity, pharmacokinetic properties and therapeutic potential. *Drugs,* **1994,** *47*:506–535.

Bush, K. New β-lactamases in gram-negative bacteria: Diversity and impact on the selection of antimicrobial therapy. *Clin. Infect. Dis.,* **2001,** *32*:1085–1089.

Chambers, H.F. Penicillins. In, *Mandell, Douglas, and Bennett's Principles and Practice of Infectious Diseases,* 5th ed. (Mandell, G.L., Bennett, J.E., and Dolin, R., eds.) Churchill Livingstone, Philadelphia, **2000,** pp. 261–274.

Davies, J. Inactivation of antibiotics and the dissemination of resistance genes. *Science,* **1994,** *264*:375–382.

Donlan, R.M. Biofilm formation: A clinically relevant microbiologic process. *Clin. Infect. Dis.,* **2001,** *33*:1387–1392.

Durack, D.T. Prophylaxis of infective endocarditis. In, *Mandell, Douglas, and Bennett's Principles and Practice of Infectious Diseases,* 5th ed. (Mandell, G.L., Bennett, J.E., and Dolin, R., eds.) Churchill Livingstone, Philadelphia, **2000,** pp. 917–925.

Ghuysen, J.M. Serine *β*-lactamases and penicillin-binding proteins. *Annu. Rev. Microbiol.,* **1991,** *45*:37–67.

Jacoby, G.A. Prevalence and resistance mechanisms of common bacterial respiratory pathogens. *Clin. Infect. Dis.,* **1994,** *18*:951–957.

Kammer, R.B. Host effects of *β*-lactam antibiotics. In, *Contemporary Issues in Infectious Diseases,* Vol. 1: *New Dimensions in Antimicrobial Therapy.* (Root, R.K., and Sande, M.A., eds.) Churchill Livingstone, New York, **1984,** pp. 101–119.

Karchmer, A.W. Cephalosporins. In, *Mandell, Douglas, and Bennett's Principles and Practice of Infectious Diseases,* 5th ed. (Mandell, G.L., Bennett, J.E., and Dolin, R., eds.) Churchill Livingstone, Philadelphia, **2000,** pp. 274–291.

Kucers, A., and Bennett, N.M. *The Use of Antibiotics*: *A Comprehensive Review with Clinical Emphasis.* Lippincott, Philadelphia, **1987.**

Medical Letter. Antimicrobial prophylaxis for surgery: Treatment guidelines. *Med. Lett.,* **2004,** *2*:27–32.

Medical Letter. Choice of antibacterial drugs: Treatment guidelines. *Med. Lett.,* **2004,** *2*:13–26.

Nakae, T. Outer-membrane permeability of bacteria. *Crit. Rev. Microbiol.,* **1986,** *13*:1–62.

Nikaido, H. Prevention of drug access to bacterial targets: Permeability barriers and active efflux. *Science,* **1994,** *264*:382–388.

Quagliarello, V., Scheld, W.M. Drug therapy: Treatment of bacterial meningitis. *New Engl. J. Med.,* **1997,** *336*:708–716.

Romano, A., Mondino, C., Viola, M., and Montuschi, P. Immediate allergic reactions to *β*-lactams: Diagnosis and therapy. *Int. J. Immunopathol. Pharmacol.,* **2003,** *16*:19–23.

Sparling, P.F. and Handsfield, H.H. *Neisseria gonorrhoeae.* In, *Mandell, Douglas, and Bennett's Principles and Practice of Infectious Diseases,* 5th ed. (Mandell, G.L., Bennett, J.E., and Dolin, R., eds.) Churchill Livingstone, Philadelphia, **2000,** pp. 2242–2258.

Spratt, B.G. Resistance to antibiotics mediated by target alterations. *Science,* **1994,** *264*:388–393.

Swartz, M.N. Cellulitis. *New Engl. J. Med.,* **2004,** *350*:904–912.

Tortora, G.J., Funke, B.R., and Case, C.L. *Microbiology: An Introduction,* 3d ed. Benjamin/Cummings, New York, **1989,** p. 83.

Tramont, E.C. *Treponema pallidum* (syphilis). In, *Mandell, Douglas, and Bennett's Principles and Practice of Infectious Diseases,* 5th ed. (Mandell, G.L., Bennett, J.E., and Dolin, R., eds.) Churchill Livingstone, Philadelphia, **2000,** pp. 2474–2490.

Weiss, M.E., and Adkinson, N.F., Jr. *β*-Lactam allergy. In, *Mandell, Douglas, and Bennett's Principles and Practice of Infectious Diseases,* 5th ed. (Mandell, G.L., Bennett, J.E., and Dolin, R., eds.) Churchill Livingstone, Philadelphia, **2000,** pp. 299–305.

AMINOGLYCOSIDES

Henry F. Chambers

The aminoglycoside group includes *gentamicin, tobramycin, amikacin, netilmicin, kanamycin, streptomycin,* and *neomycin.* These drugs are used primarily to treat infections caused by aerobic gram-negative bacteria; streptomycin is an important agent for the treatment of tuberculosis. In contrast to most inhibitors of microbial protein synthesis, which are bacteriostatic, the aminoglycosides are bactericidal inhibitors of protein synthesis. Mutations affecting proteins in the bacterial ribosome, the target for these drugs, can confer marked resistance to their action. However, most commonly resistance is due to acquisition of plasmids or transposon-encoding genes for aminoglycoside-metabolizing enzymes or from impaired transport of drug into the cell. Thus there can be cross-resistance between members of the class.

These agents contain amino sugars linked to an aminocyclitol ring by glycosidic bonds (Figure 45–1). They are polycations, and their polarity is responsible in part for pharmacokinetic properties shared by all members of the group. For example, none is absorbed adequately after oral administration, inadequate concentrations are found in cerebrospinal fluid (CSF), and all are excreted relatively rapidly by the normal kidney. Although aminoglycosides are widely used and important agents, serious toxicity limits their usefulness. All members of the group share the same spectrum of toxicity, most notably nephrotoxicity and ototoxicity, which can involve the auditory and vestibular functions of the eighth cranial nerve.

History and Source. Aminoglycosides are natural products or semisynthetic derivatives of compounds produced by a variety of soil actinomycetes. Streptomycin was first isolated from a strain of *Streptomyces griseus.* Gentamicin and netilmicin are broad-spectrum antibiotics derived from species of the actinomycete *Micromonospora.* The difference in spelling (-*micin*) compared with the other aminoglycoside antibiotics (-*mycin*) reflects this difference in origin. Tobramycin is one of several components of an aminoglycoside complex (*nebramycin*) that is produced by *S. tenebrarius* (Higgins and Kastner, 1967). It is most similar in antimicrobial activity and toxicity to gentamicin. In contrast to the other aminoglycosides, amikacin, a derivative of kanamycin, and netilmicin, a derivative of *sisomicin,* are semisynthetic products. Other aminoglycoside antibiotics have been developed (*e.g., arbekacin, isepamicin,* and *sisomicin*), but they have not been introduced into clinical practice in the United States because numerous potent, less toxic alternatives (*e.g.,* broad-spectrum β-lactam antibiotics and quinolones) are available.

Chemistry. The aminoglycosides consist of two or more amino sugars joined in glycosidic linkage to a hexose nucleus, which usually is in a central position (Figure 45–1). This hexose, or aminocyclitol, is either streptidine (found in streptomycin) or 2-deoxystreptamine (found in all other available aminoglycosides). These compounds thus are aminoglycosidic aminocyclitols, although the simpler term *aminoglycoside* is used commonly to describe them. A related compound, *spectinomycin,* is an aminocyclitol that does not contain amino sugars; it is discussed in Chapter 46.

The aminoglycoside families are distinguished by the amino sugars attached to the aminocyclitol. In the neomycin family, which includes *neomycin B* and *paromomycin,* an aminoglycoside used orally for the treatment of intestinal parasitic infections, there are three amino sugars attached to the central 2-deoxystreptamine. The kanamycin and gentamicin families have only two such amino sugars. Neomycin B has the following structural formula:

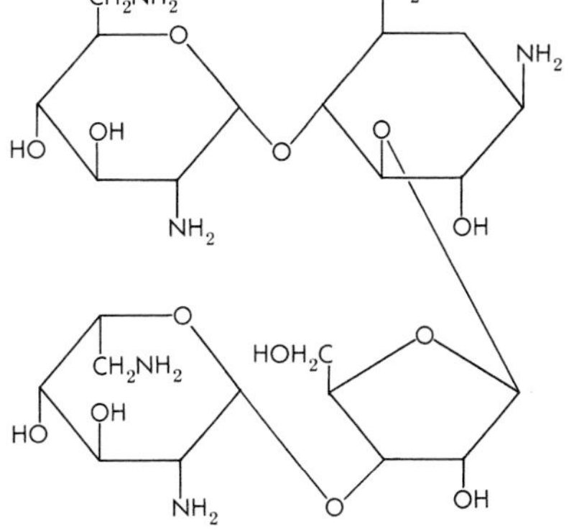

NEOMYCIN B

In the kanamycin family, which includes *kanamycins A* and *B*, amikacin, and tobramycin, two amino sugars are linked to a centrally located 2-deoxystreptamine moiety; one of these is a 3-aminohexose (Figure 45–1). The structural formula of kanamycin A, which is the major component of the commercial product, is as follows:

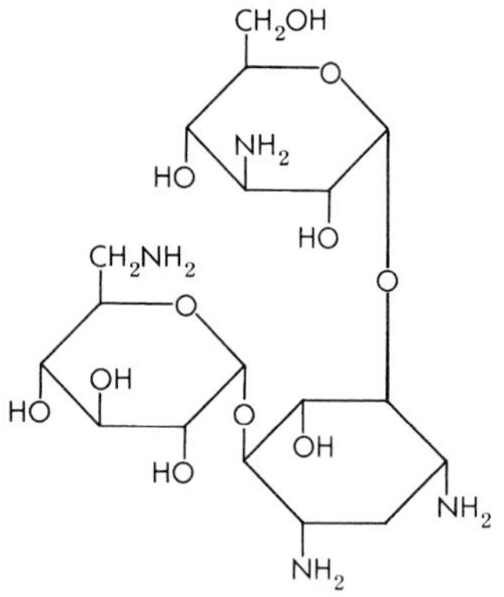

KANAMYCIN A

Amikacin is a semisynthetic derivative prepared from kanamycin A by acylation of the 1-amino group of the 2-deoxystreptamine moiety with 2-hydroxy-4-aminobutyric acid.

The gentamicin family, which includes *gentamicins C_1, C_{1a}*, and *C_2*, sisomicin, and netilmicin (the 1-*N*-ethyl derivative of sisomicin), contains a different 3-amino sugar (garosamine). Variations in methylation of the other amino sugar result in the different components of gentamicin (Figure 45–1). These modifications appear to have little effect on biological activity.

Streptomycin differs from the other aminoglycoside antibiotics in that it contains streptidine rather than 2-deoxystreptamine, and the aminocyclitol is not in a central position. The structural formula of streptomycin is as follows:

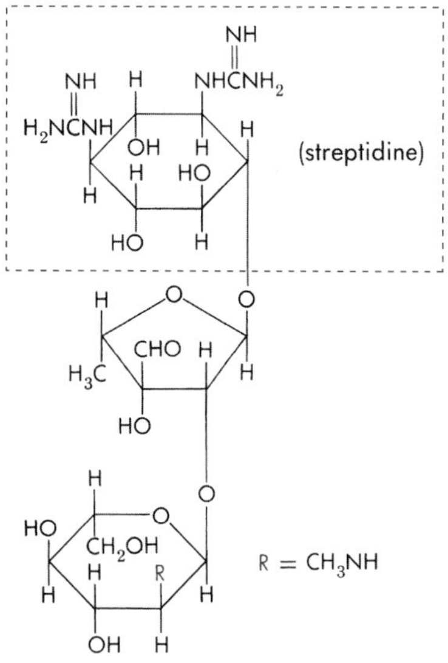

STREPTOMYCIN

Mechanism of Action. The aminoglycoside antibiotics are rapidly bactericidal. Bacterial killing is concentration-dependent: The higher the concentration, the greater is the rate at which bacteria are killed. A post-antibiotic effect, *i.e.*, residual bactericidal activity persisting after the serum concentration has fallen below the minimum inhibitory concentration (MIC), also is characteristic of aminoglycoside antibiotics; the duration of this effect also is concentration dependent. These properties probably account for the efficacy of once-daily dosing regimens of aminoglycosides. Although much is known about their capacity to inhibit protein synthesis and decrease the fidelity of translation of mRNA at the ribosome (Shannon and Phillips, 1982), the precise mechanism responsible for the rapidly lethal effect of aminoglycosides on bacteria is unknown.

Aminoglycosides diffuse through aqueous channels formed by porin proteins in the outer membrane of gram-negative bacteria to enter the periplasmic space. Transport of aminoglycosides across the cytoplasmic (inner) membrane depends on electron transport in part because of a requirement for a membrane electrical potential (interior negative) to drive permeation of these antibiotics. This phase of transport has been termed *energy-dependent phase I* (EDP_1). It is rate-limiting and can be blocked or inhibited by divalent cations (*e.g.*, Ca^{2+} and Mg^{2+}), hyperosmolarity, a reduction in pH, and anaerobic conditions. The last two conditions impair the ability of the bacteria to maintain the membrane potential, which is the driving force necessary for transport. Thus the antimicrobial activity of aminoglycosides is reduced markedly in the anaerobic environment of an abscess, in hyperosmolar acidic urine, and in other conditions that limit EDP_1. Once inside the cell, aminoglycosides bind to polysomes and interfere with protein synthesis by causing misreading and premature termination of mRNA translation (Figure 45–2). The resulting aberrant proteins may be inserted into the cell membrane, leading to altered permeability and further stimulation of aminoglycoside transport (Busse *et al.*, 1992). This phase of aminoglycoside transport, termed *energy-dependent phase II* (EDP_2), is poorly understood; however, EDP_2 may link to disruption of the structure of the cytoplasmic membrane, perhaps by the aberrant proteins. This concept is consistent with the observed progression of the leakage of small ions, followed by larger molecules and, eventually, by proteins from the bacterial cell prior to aminoglycoside-induced death. This progressive disruption of the cell envelope, as well as other vital cell processes, may help to explain the lethal action of aminoglycosides (Bryan, 1989).

The primary intracellular site of action of the aminoglycosides is the 30S ribosomal subunit, which consists of 21 proteins and a single 16S molecule of RNA. At least three of these ribosomal pro-

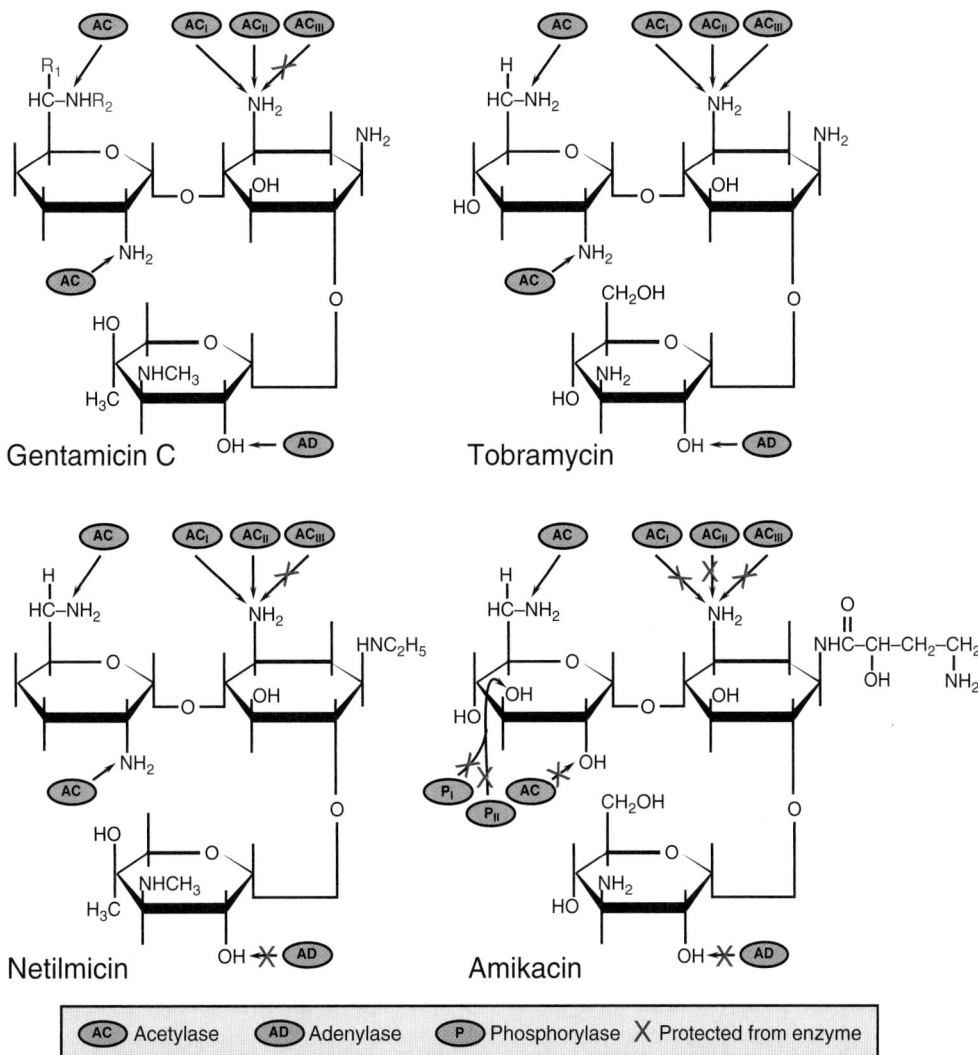

Gentamicin C

Tobramycin

Netilmicin

Amikacin

| AC Acetylase | AD Adenylase | P Phosphorylase | X Protected from enzyme |

Figure 45–1. *Sites of activity of various plasmid-mediated enzymes capable of inactivating aminoglycosides.* The symbol X indicates regions of the molecules that are protected from the designated enzyme. In gentamicin C_1, $R_1=R_2=CH_3$; in gentamicin C_2, $R_1=CH_3$, $R_2=H$; in gentamicin C_{1a}, $R_1=R_2=H$. (Modified with permission from Moellering, 1977.)

teins, and perhaps the 16S ribosomal RNA as well, contribute to the streptomycin-binding site, and alterations of these molecules markedly affect the binding and subsequent action of streptomycin. For example, a single amino acid substitution of asparagine for lysine at position 42 of one ribosomal protein (S_{12}) prevents binding of the drug; the resulting mutant is totally resistant to streptomycin. Substitution of glutamine for lysine creates a mutant that actually requires streptomycin for survival. The other aminoglycosides also bind to the 30S ribosomal subunit; however, they also appear to bind to several sites on the 50S ribosomal subunit (Davis, 1988).

Aminoglycosides disrupt the normal cycle of ribosomal function by interfering, at least in part, with the initiation of protein synthesis, leading to the accumulation of abnormal initiation complexes, or *streptomycin monosomes,* shown schematically in Figure 45–2B (Luzzatto *et al.,* 1969). Aminoglycosides also cause misreading of the mRNA template and incorporation of incorrect amino acids into the growing polypeptide chains. Aminoglycosides vary in their

capacity to cause misreading presumably owing to differences in their affinities for specific ribosomal proteins. Although there appears to be a strong correlation between bactericidal activity and the ability to induce misreading (Hummel and Böck, 1989), it remains to be established that this is the primary mechanism of aminoglycoside-induced cell death.

Microbial Resistance to the Aminoglycosides. Bacteria may be resistant to aminoglycosides because of failure of the antibiotic to penetrate intracellularly, low affinity of the drug for the bacterial ribosome, or inactivation of the drug by microbial enzymes. Clinically, drug inactivation is the most common mechanism for acquired microbial resistance to aminoglycosides. The genes encoding aminoglycoside-modifying enzymes are acquired primarily by conju-

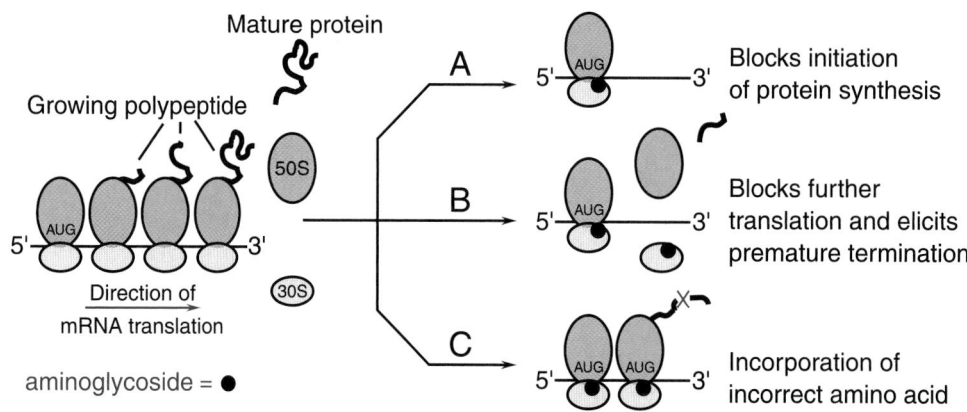

Figure 45–2. *Effects of aminoglycosides on protein synthesis.* **A.** Aminoglycoside (represented by closed circles) binds to the 30S ribosomal subunit and interferes with initiation of protein synthesis by fixing the 30S–50S ribosomal complex at the start codon (AUG) of mRNA. As 30S–50S complexes downstream complete translation of mRNA and detach, the abnormal initiation complexes, so-called streptomycin monosomes, accumulate, blocking further translation of the message. Aminoglycoside binding to the 30S subunit also causes misreading of mRNA, leading to **B.** premature termination of translation with detachment of the ribosomal complex and incompletely synthesized protein or **C.** incorporation of incorrect amino acids (indicated by the X), resulting in the production of abnormal or nonfunctional proteins.

gation and transfer of resistance plasmids (Davies, 1994) (*see* Chapter 42). These enzymes phosphorylate, adenylate, or acetylate specific hydroxyl or amino groups (Figure 45–1). Amikacin is a suitable substrate for only a few of these inactivating enzymes (Figure 45–1); thus strains that are resistant to multiple other drugs tend to be susceptible to amikacin. The metabolites of the aminoglycosides may compete with the unaltered drug for transport across the inner membrane, but they are incapable of binding effectively to ribosomes and interfering with protein synthesis.

A significant percentage of clinical isolates of *Enterococcus faecalis* and *E. faecium* are highly resistant to all aminoglycosides. Infections caused by aminoglycoside-resistant strains of enterococci can be especially difficult to treat because of the loss of the synergistic bactericidal activity between a *penicillin* or *vancomycin* and an aminoglycoside (Spera and Farber, 1992; Vemuri and Zervos, 1993) and because these strains often also are cross-resistant to vancomycin and penicillin. Resistance to gentamicin indicates cross-resistance to tobramycin, amikacin, kanamycin, and netilmicin because the inactivating enzyme is bifunctional and can modify all these aminoglycosides (Murray, 1999). Owing to differences in the chemical structures of streptomycin and other aminoglycosides, this enzyme does not modify streptomycin, which is inactivated by another enzyme; consequently, gentamicin-resistant strains of enterococci may be susceptible to streptomycin. Natural resistance to aminoglycosides may be caused by failure of the drug to penetrate the cytoplasmic (inner) membrane. Penetration of drug across the outer membrane of gram-negative microorganisms into the periplasmic space can be slow, but resistance on this

basis is unimportant clinically. Transport of aminoglycosides across the cytoplasmic membrane is an oxygen-dependent active process. Strictly anaerobic bacteria thus are resistant to these drugs because they lack the necessary transport system. Similarly, facultative bacteria are resistant when they are grown under anaerobic conditions (Mates *et al.*, 1983). Resistance owing to mutations that alter ribosomal structure is relatively uncommon. Missense mutations in *Escherichia coli* that substitute a single amino acid in a crucial ribosomal protein may prevent binding of streptomycin. Although highly resistant to streptomycin, these strains are not widespread in nature. Similarly, only 5% of strains of *Pseudomonas aeruginosa* exhibit such ribosomal resistance to streptomycin. It has been estimated that approximately half the streptomycin-resistant strains of enterococci are ribosomally resistant (Eliopoulos *et al.*, 1984). Because ribosomal resistance usually is specific for streptomycin, these strains of enterococci remain sensitive to a combination of penicillin and gentamicin *in vitro*.

Antibacterial Spectrum of the Aminoglycosides. The antibacterial activity of gentamicin, tobramycin, kanamycin, netilmicin, and amikacin is directed primarily against aerobic gram-negative bacilli. Kanamycin, like streptomycin, has a more limited spectrum compared with other aminoglycosides; in particular, it should not be used to treat infections caused by *Serratia* or *P. aeruginosa*. Aminoglycosides have little activity against anaerobic microorganisms or facultative bacteria under anaerobic conditions. Their action against most gram-positive bacteria is limited, and they should not be used as single agents to

Table 45–1

Typical Minimal Inhibitory Concentrations of Aminoglycosides That Will Inhibit 90% (MIC_{90}) of Clinical Isolates for Several Species

SPECIES	MIC_{90} $\mu g/ml$				
	KANAMYCIN	GENTAMICIN	NETILMICIN	TOBRAMYCIN	AMIKACIN
Citrobacter freundii	8	0.5	0.25	0.5	1
Enterobacter spp.	4	0.5	0.25	0.5	1
Escherichia coli	16	0.5	0.25	0.5	1
Klebsiella pneumoniae	32	0.5	0.25	1	1
Proteus mirabilis	8	4	4	0.5	2
Providencia stuartii	128	8	16	4	2
Pseudomonas aeruginosa	>128	8	32	4	2
Serratia spp.	>64	4	16	16	8
Enterococcus faecalis	—	32	2	32	≥64
Staphylococcus aureus	2	0.5	0.25	0.25	16

SOURCE: Adapted with permission from Wiedemann and Atkinson, 1991.

treat infections caused by gram-positive bacteria. In combination with a cell wall–active agent, such as a penicillin or vancomycin, an aminoglycoside (streptomycin and gentamicin have been tested most extensively) produces a synergistic bactericidal effect *in vitro* against enterococci, streptococci, and staphylococci. Clinically, the superiority of aminoglycoside combination regimens over β-lactams alone is not proven except in relatively few infections (discussed below).

The aerobic gram-negative bacilli vary in their susceptibility to the aminoglycosides (Table 45–1). Tobramycin and gentamicin exhibit similar activity against most gram-negative bacilli, although tobramycin usually is more active against *P. aeruginosa* and some *Proteus* spp. Many gram-negative bacilli that are resistant to gentamicin because of plasmid-mediated inactivating enzymes also will be resistant to tobramycin. Amikacin and, in some instances, netilmicin retain their activity against gentamicin-resistant strains because they are a poor substrate for many of the aminoglycoside-inactivating enzymes.

ABSORPTION, DISTRIBUTION, DOSING, AND ELIMINATION OF THE AMINOGLYCOSIDES

Absorption. The aminoglycosides are highly polar cations and therefore are very poorly absorbed from the gastrointestinal tract. Less than 1% of a dose is absorbed after either oral or rectal administration. The drugs are not inactivated in the intestine and are eliminated quantitatively in the feces. Long-term oral or rectal administration of aminoglycosides may result in accumulation to toxic concentrations in patients with renal impairment. Absorption of gentamicin from the gastrointestinal tract may be increased by gastrointestinal disease (*e.g.*, ulcers or inflammatory bowel disease). Instillation of these drugs into body cavities with serosal surfaces also may result in rapid absorption and unexpected toxicity, *i.e.*, neuromuscular blockade. Similarly, intoxication may occur when aminoglycosides are applied topically for long periods to large wounds, burns, or cutaneous ulcers, particularly if there is renal insufficiency.

All the aminoglycosides are absorbed rapidly from intramuscular sites of injection. Peak concentrations in plasma occur after 30 to 90 minutes and are similar to those observed 30 minutes after completion of an intravenous infusion of an equal dose over a 30-minute period. These concentrations typically range from 4 to 12 $\mu g/ml$ following a 1.5 to 2 mg/kg dose of gentamicin, tobramycin, or netilmicin and from 20 to 35 $\mu g/ml$ following a 7.5 mg/kg dose of amikacin or kanamycin. In critically ill patients, especially those in shock, absorption of drug may be reduced from intramuscular sites because of poor perfusion.

Distribution. Because of their polar nature, the aminoglycosides do not penetrate into most cells, the central nervous system (CNS), and the eye. Except for streptomycin, there is negligible binding of aminoglycosides to plasma albumin. The apparent volume of distribution of these drugs is 25% of lean body weight and approximates the volume of extracellular fluid.

Concentrations of aminoglycosides in secretions and tissues are low. High concentrations are found only in the renal cortex and the endolymph and perilymph of the inner ear; the high concentration in these sites likely contribute to the nephrotoxicity and ototoxicity caused by these drugs. As a result of active hepatic secretion, concentrations in bile approach 30% of those found in plasma, but this represents a very minor excretory route for the aminoglycosides. Penetration into respiratory secretions is poor (Levy, 1986). Diffusion into pleural and synovial fluid is relatively slow, but concentrations that approximate those in the plasma may be achieved after repeated administration. Inflammation increases the penetration of aminoglycosides into peritoneal and pericardial cavities.

Concentrations of aminoglycosides achieved in CSF with parenteral administration usually are subtherapeutic. In experimental animals and human beings, concentrations in CSF in the absence of inflammation are less than 10% of those in plasma; this value may approach 25% when there is meningitis (Strausbaugh *et al.*, 1977). Intrathecal or intraventricular administration of aminoglycosides has been used to achieve therapeutic levels, but the availability of third- and fourth-generation cephalosporins has made this unnecessary in most cases. Penetration of aminoglycosides into ocular fluids is so poor that effective therapy of bacterial endophthalmitis requires periocular and intraocular injections of the drugs.

Administration of aminoglycosides to women late in pregnancy may result in accumulation of drug in fetal plasma and amniotic fluid. Streptomycin and tobramycin can cause hearing loss in children born to women who receive the drug during pregnancy. Insufficient data are available regarding the other aminoglycosides; it is therefore recommended that they be used with caution during pregnancy and only for strong clinical indications in the absence of suitable alternatives.

Dosing. Recommended doses of individual aminoglycosides in the treatment of specific infections are given in later sections of this chapter. Current practice is to give the total daily dose as a single injection, although historically it was administered as two or three equally divided doses. Numerous studies have shown that administration of the total dose once daily is associated with less toxicity and is just as effective as multiple-dose regimens (Buijk *et al.*, 2002; Charnas *et al.*, 1997; Gilbert *et al.*, 1998; Rybak *et al.*, 1999). This diminished toxicity is probably due to a threshold effect from accumulation of drug in the inner ear or in the kidney. More drug accumulates with higher plasma concentrations, particularly at trough, and with prolonged periods of exposure. Elimination of aminoglycoside from these organs occurs more slowly when plasma concentrations are relatively high (Figure 45–3). A once-daily dosing regimen, despite the higher peak concentration, provides a longer period when concentrations fall below the threshold for toxicity than does a multiple-dose regimen (12 hours *versus* less than 3 hours total in the example shown), accounting for its lower toxicity. Aminoglycoside bactericidal activity, on the other hand, is related directly to the peak concentration achieved because aminoglycosides cause concentration-dependent killing and a concentration-dependent postantibiotic effect. This enhanced activity at higher concentrations probably accounts for the equivalent efficacy of a once-daily regimen compared with a multiple-dose regimen despite the relatively prolonged periods of time that plasma concentrations are "subtherapeutic," *i.e.*, below the MIC.

Numerous studies in a variety of clinical settings employing virtually every commonly used aminoglycoside have demonstrated that once-daily regimens are as safe or safer than multiple-dose regimens with equal efficacy (Ferriols-Lisart and Alos-Alminana, 1996; Bailey *et al.*, 1997; Charnas *et al.*, 1997; Freeman *et al.*, 1997; Deamer, 1998). Once-daily dosing also costs less and is administered more easily. For these reasons, administration of aminoglycosides as a single daily dose generally is preferred; exceptions include use in pregnancy, neonatal and pediatric infections (Rastogi *et al.*, 2002; Knoderer, *et al.*, 2003), and low-dose combination therapy of bacterial endocarditis because data documenting equivalent

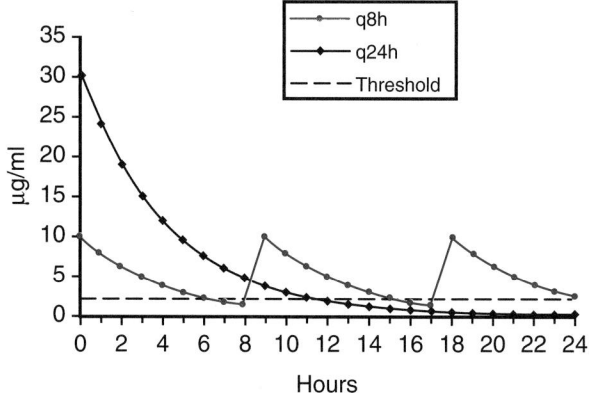

Figure 45–3. *Plasma concentrations (μg/ml) after administration of 5.1 mg/kg of gentamicin intravenously to a hypothetical patient either as a single dose (q24h) or as three divided doses (q8h).* The threshold for toxicity has been chosen to correspond to a plasma concentration of 2 μg/ml, the maximum recommended. The once-daily regimen produces a threefold higher plasma concentration, which enhances efficacy that otherwise might be compromised due to prolonged sub-MIC concentrations later in the dosing interval compared with the every-8-hours regimen. The once-daily regimen provides a 12-hour period during which plasma concentrations are below the threshold for toxicity, thereby minimizing the toxicity that otherwise might result from the high plasma concentrations early on. The every-8-hours regimen, in contrast, provides only a brief period during which plasma concentrations are below the threshold for toxicity.

safety and efficacy are inadequate. Once-daily dosing also should be avoided in patients with creatinine clearances of less than 20 to 25 ml/min because accumulation is likely to occur. Less frequent dosing (*e.g.*, every 48 hours) is more appropriate for these patients.

Whether once-daily or multiple-daily dosing is chosen, the dose must be adjusted for patients with creatinine clearances of below 80 to 100 ml/min (Table 45–2), and plasma concentrations must be monitored. Use of nomograms may be helpful in selecting initial doses, but variability in aminoglycoside clearance among patients is too large for these to be relied on for more than a few days (Bartal, *et al.*, 2003). If it is anticipated that the patient will be treated with an aminoglycoside for more than 3 to 4 days, then plasma concentrations should be monitored to avoid drug accumulation. In addition, aminoglycosides generally should not be used as single agents except for urinary tract infections because of relatively poor tissue penetration and poorer outcomes associated with aminoglycoside monotherapy (Leibovici *et al.*, 1997).

For twice- or thrice-daily dosing regimens, both peak and trough plasma concentrations are determined. The trough sample is obtained just before a dose, and the peak sample is obtained 60 minutes after intramuscular injection or 30 minutes after an intravenous infusion given over 30 minutes. The peak concentration documents that the dose produces therapeutic concentrations, generally accepted to be 4 to 10 μg/ml for gentamicin, netilmicin, and tobramycin and 15 to 30 μg/ml for amikacin and streptomycin (Gilbert *et al.*, 1999). The trough concentration is used to avoid toxicity by monitoring for accumulation of drug. Trough concentrations should be less than 1 to

Table 45–2

Algorithm for Dose Reduction of Aminoglycosides Based on Calculated Creatinine Clearance

CREATININE CLEARANCE, ML/MIN	% OF MAXIMUM DAILY DOSE*	FREQUENCY OF DOSING
100	100	
75	75	
50	50	Every 24 hours
25	25	
20	80	
10	60	Every 48 hours
<10	40	

*The maximum adult daily dose for amikacin, kanamycin, and streptomycin is 15 mg/kg; for gentamicin and tobramycin, 5.5 mg/kg; and for netilmicin, 6.5 mg/kg.

2 μg/ml for gentamicin, netilmicin, and tobramycin and 5 to 10 μg/ml for amikacin and streptomycin.

Monitoring of aminoglycoside plasma concentrations also is important when using a once-daily dosing regimen, although peak concentrations are not determined routinely (these will be three to four times higher than the peak achieved with a multiple-daily-dosing regimen). Several approaches may be used to determine that drug is being cleared and not accumulating. The simplest method is to obtain a trough sample 24 hours after dosing and adjust the dose to achieve the recommended plasma concentration, e.g., below 1 to 2 μg/ml in the case of gentamicin or tobramycin. This approach probably is the least desirable. An undetectable trough concentration could reflect grossly inadequate dosing in patients who clear the drug rapidly with prolonged periods (perhaps well over half the dosing interval) during which concentrations are subtherapeutic. In contrast, a 24-hour trough concentration target of 1 to 2 μg/ml actually would increase aminoglycoside exposure compared with a multiple-daily-dosing regimen (Barclay et al., 1999), which defeats the goal of providing a washout with concentrations of 0 to 1 μg/ml between 18 to 24 hours after a dose. A second approach relies on nomograms to target a range of concentrations in a sample obtained earlier in the dosing interval. For example, if the plasma concentration from a sample obtained 8 hours after a dose of gentamicin is between 1.5 and 6 μg/ml, then the concentration at 18 hours will be less than 1 μg/ml (Chambers et al., 1998). Target ranges of 1 to 1.5 μg/ml for gentamicin at 18 hours for patients with creatinine clearances above 50 ml/min and 1 to 2.5 μg/ml for those with clearances below 50 ml/min also have been used (Gilbert et al., 1998). This method also tends to be inaccurate, particularly when conditions that alter aminoglycoside clearance are present (Bartal et al., 2003; Toschlog et al., 2003). The most accurate method for monitoring plasma levels for dose adjustment is to measure the concentration in two plasma samples drawn several hours apart (e.g., at 2 and 12 hours after a dose). The clearance then can be calculated and the dose adjusted to achieve the desired target range.

Elimination. The aminoglycosides are excreted almost entirely by glomerular filtration, and urine concentrations of 50 to 200 μg/ml are achieved. A large fraction of a parenterally administered dose is excreted unchanged during the first 24 hours, with most of this appearing in the first 12 hours. The half-lives of the aminoglycosides in plasma are similar and vary between 2 and 3 hours in patients with normal renal function. Renal clearance of aminoglycosides is approximately two-thirds of the simultaneous creatinine clearance; this observation suggests some tubular reabsorption of these drugs.

After a single dose of an aminoglycoside, disappearance from the plasma exceeds renal excretion by 10% to 20%; however, after 1 to 2 days of therapy, nearly 100% of subsequent doses eventually is recovered in the urine. This lag period probably represents saturation of binding sites in tissues. The rate of elimination of drug from these sites is considerably longer than from plasma; the half-life for tissue-bound aminoglycoside has been estimated to range from 30 to 700 hours (Schentag and Jusko, 1977). For this reason, small amounts of aminoglycosides can be detected in the urine for 10 to 20 days after drug administration is discontinued. Aminoglycoside bound to renal tissue exhibits antibacterial activity and protects experimental animals against bacterial infections of the kidney even when the drug no longer can be detected in serum (Bergeron et al., 1982).

The concentration of aminoglycoside in plasma produced by the initial dose depends only on the volume of distribution of the drug. Since the elimination of aminoglycosides depends almost entirely on the kidney, a linear relationship exists between the concentration of creatinine in plasma and the half-life of all aminoglycosides in patients with moderately compromised renal function. In anephric patients, the half-life varies from 20 to 40 times that determined in normal individuals. *Because the incidence of nephrotoxicity and ototoxicity is related to the concentration to which an aminoglycoside accumulates, it is critical to reduce the maintenance dosage of these drugs in patients with impaired renal function.* The size of the individual dose, the interval between doses, or both can be altered. There is no conclusive information on the best approach, and even the currently accepted therapeutic range has been questioned (McCormack and Jewesson, 1992). The most consistent plasma concentrations are achieved when the loading dose is given in milligrams per kilogram of body weight; and since aminoglycosides are distributed minimally in fatty tissue, the lean or expected body weight should be used. Methods for calculation of dosage are described in Appendix II.

There are obvious difficulties in using any of these approaches for ill patients with rapidly changing renal function (Lesar et al., 1982). In addition, even when known factors are taken into consideration, concentrations of aminoglycosides achieved in plasma after a given dose vary widely among patients. If the extracellular volume is expanded, the volume of distribution is increased, and concentrations will be reduced. For unknown reasons, aminoglycoside clearances are increased and half-lives are reduced in patients with cystic fibrosis; the volume of distribution is increased in patients with leukemia (Rosenthal et al., 1977; Spyker et al., 1978). Patients with anemia (hematocrit <25%) have a concentration in plasma that is higher than expected probably because of reduction in the number of binding sites on red blood cells.

Determination of the concentration of drug in plasma is an essential guide to the proper administration of aminoglycosides. In patients with life-threatening systemic infections, aminoglycoside concentrations should be determined several times per week (more frequently if renal function is changing) and should be determined within 24 to 48 hours of a change in dosage.

Aminoglycosides can be removed from the body by either hemodialysis or peritoneal dialysis. Approximately 50% of the administered dose is removed in 12 hours by hemodialysis, which has been used for the treatment of overdosage. As a general rule, a dose equal to half the loading dose administered after each hemodialysis should maintain the plasma concentration in the desired range; however, a number of variables make this a rough approximation at best. Continuous arteriovenous hemofiltration (CAVH) and continuous venovenous hemofiltration (CVVH) will result in aminoglycoside clearances approximately equivalent to 15 and 15 to 30 ml/min of creatinine clearance, respectively, depending on the flow rate. The amount of aminoglycoside removed can be replaced by administering approximately 15% to 30% of the maximum daily dose (Table 45–2) each day. Frequent monitoring of plasma drug concentrations is again crucial.

Peritoneal dialysis is less effective than hemodialysis in removing aminoglycosides. Clearance rates are approximately 5 to 10 ml/min for the various drugs but are highly variable. If a patient who requires dialysis has bacterial peritonitis, a therapeutic concentration of the aminoglycoside probably will not be achieved in the peritoneal fluid because the ratio of the concentration in plasma to that in peritoneal fluid may be 10:1 (Smithivas *et al.*, 1971). Thus it is recommended that antibiotic be added to the dialysate to achieve concentrations equal to those desired in plasma. For intermittent dosing *via* peritoneal dialysate, 2 mg/kg of amikacin is added to the bag once a day. The corresponding dose for gentamicin, netilmicin, or tobramycin is 0.6 mg/kg. For continuous dosing, the dose for amikacin is 12 mg/L (25 mg/L loading dose in the first bag), and the dose for gentamicin, netilmicin, or tobramycin is 4 mg/L in each bag (8 mg/L loading dose). This should be preceded by administration of a loading dose, either parenterally or in dialysis fluid.

Although excretion of aminoglycosides is similar in adults and children older than 6 months of age, half-lives of the drugs may be prolonged significantly in the newborn: 8 to 11 hours in the first week of life in newborns weighing less than 2 kg and approximately 5 hours in those weighing more than 2 kg (Yow, 1977). Thus it is critically important to monitor concentrations of aminoglycosides during treatment of neonates (Philips *et al.*, 1982).

Aminoglycosides can be inactivated by various penicillins *in vitro* (Konishi *et al.*, 1983) and in patients with end-stage renal failure (Blair *et al.*, 1982), thus making dosage recommendations even more difficult. Amikacin appears to be the least affected by this interaction.

UNTOWARD EFFECTS OF THE AMINOGLYCOSIDES

All aminoglycosides have the potential to produce reversible and irreversible vestibular, cochlear, and renal toxicity. These side effects complicate the use of these compounds and make their proper administration difficult.

Ototoxicity. Vestibular and auditory dysfunction can follow the administration of any of the aminoglycosides. Studies of animals and human beings have documented progressive accumulation of these drugs in the perilymph and endolymph of the inner ear. Accumulation occurs predominantly when concentrations in plasma are high. Diffusion back into the bloodstream is slow; the half-lives of the aminoglycosides are five to six times longer in the otic fluids than in plasma. Back-diffusion is concentration dependent and is facilitated at the trough concentration of drug in plasma. Ototoxicity is more likely to occur in patients with persistently elevated concentrations of drug in plasma. However, even a single dose of tobramycin has been reported to produce slight temporary cochlear dysfunction during periods when the concentration in plasma is at its peak (Wilson and Ramsden, 1977). Ototoxicity has been linked to mutations in a mitochondrial ribosomal RNA gene, indicating that a genetic predisposition exists for this side effect (Bates, 2003). Oxidant stress probably plays a role, and *ras* activation has been implicated (Battaglia *et al.*, 2003). Ototoxicity is largely irreversible and results from progressive destruction of vestibular or cochlear sensory cells, which are highly sensitive to damage by aminoglycosides (Brummett, 1983). Studies in guinea pigs exposed to large doses of gentamicin reveal degeneration of the type I sensory hair cells in the central part of the crista ampullaris (vestibular organ) and fusion of individual sensory hairs into giant hairs (Wersäll *et al.*, 1973). Similar studies with gentamicin and tobramycin also demonstrate loss of hair cells in the cochlea of the organ of Corti (Theopold, 1977). With increasing dosage and prolonged exposure, damage progresses from the base of the cochlea, where high-frequency sounds are processed, to the apex, which is necessary for the perception of low frequencies. While these histological changes correlate with the ability of the cochlea to generate an action potential in response to sound, the biochemical mechanism for ototoxicity is poorly understood. Early changes induced by aminoglycosides have been shown in experimental ototoxicity to be reversible by Ca^{2+}. Once sensory cells are lost, however, regeneration does not occur; retrograde degeneration of the auditory nerve follows, resulting in irreversible hearing loss. It has been suggested that aminoglycosides interfere with the active transport system essential for the maintenance of the ionic balance of the endolymph (Neu and Bendush, 1976). This would lead to alteration in the normal concentrations of ions in the labyrinthine fluids, with impairment of electrical activity and nerve conduction. Eventually, the electrolyte changes, or perhaps the drugs themselves, damage the hair cells irreversibly. The degree of permanent dysfunction correlates with the number of destroyed or altered sensory hair cells and is thought to be related to sustained exposure to the drug. Interestingly, total dose and duration of aminoglycoside exposure and other risk factors, such as advanced age, bacteremia, liver disease, and renal disease, that reasonably might predispose one to ototoxicity have not been proven to do so (de Jager and van Altena, 2002). Repeated courses of aminoglycosides, each probably resulting in the loss of more cells, seem to lead to deafness. Drugs such as *ethacrynic acid* and *furosemide* potentiate the ototoxic effects of the aminoglycosides in animals (Brummett, 1983); data implicating furosemide are less convincing in humans (Moore *et al.*, 1984a). Hearing loss following exposure to these agents also is more likely to develop in patients with preexisting auditory impairment. Although all aminoglycosides are capable of affecting cochlear and vestibular function, some preferential toxicity is evident. Streptomycin and gentamicin produce predominantly vestibular effects, whereas amikacin, kanamycin, and neomycin primarily affect auditory function; tobramycin affects both equally. The incidence of ototoxicity is extremely difficult to determine. Data from audiometry suggest that the incidence may be as high as 25% (Moore *et al.*, 1984a; de Jager and van Altena, 2002). The relative incidence appears to be equal for tobramycin, gentamicin, and amikacin. Initial studies in laboratory animals and human beings suggested that netilmicin is less ototoxic than other aminoglycosides (Lerner *et al.*, 1983); however, the incidence of ototoxicity from netilmicin is not negligible—such complications developed in 10% of patients in one clinical trial of netilmicin.

The incidence of vestibular toxicity is particularly high in patients receiving streptomycin; nearly 20% of individuals who received 500 mg twice daily for 4 weeks for enterococcal endocarditis developed clinically detectable irreversible vestibular damage (Wilson *et al.*, 1984). In addition, up to 75% of patients who received 2 g streptomycin for more than 60 days showed evidence of nystagmus or postural imbalance.

Since the initial symptoms may be reversible, it is recommended that patients receiving high doses and/or prolonged courses of aminoglycosides be monitored carefully for ototoxicity; however, deafness may occur several weeks after therapy is discontinued.

Clinical Symptoms of Cochlear Toxicity. A high-pitched tinnitus often is the first symptom of toxicity. If the drug is not discontinued, auditory impairment may develop after a few days. The tinnitus may persist for several days to 2 weeks after therapy is stopped. Since perception of sound in the high-frequency range (outside the conversational range) is lost first, the affected individual is not always aware of the difficulty, and it will not be detected unless careful audiometric examination is carried out. If the hearing loss progresses, the lower sound ranges are affected, and conversation becomes difficult.

Clinical Symptoms of Vestibular Toxicity. Moderately intense headache lasting 1 or 2 days may precede the onset of labyrinthine dysfunction. This is followed immediately by an acute stage in which nausea, vomiting, and difficulty with equilibrium develop and persist for 1 to 2 weeks. Prominent symptoms include vertigo in the upright position, inability to perceive termination of movement ("mental pastpointing"), and difficulty in sitting or standing without visual cues. Drifting of the eyes at the end of a movement so that both focusing and reading are difficult, a positive Romberg test, and rarely, pendular trunk movement and spontaneous nystagmus are outstanding signs. The acute stage ends suddenly and is followed by the appearance of manifestations consistent with chronic labyrinthitis, in which, although symptomless while in bed, the patient has difficulty when attempting to walk or make sudden movements; ataxia is the most prominent feature. The chronic phase persists for approximately 2 months; it is gradually superseded by a compensatory stage in which symptoms are latent and appear only when the eyes are closed. Adaptation to the impairment of labyrinthine function is accomplished by the use of visual cues and deep proprioceptive sensation for determining movement and position. It is more adequate in the young than in the old but may not be sufficient to permit the high degree of coordination required in many special trades. Recovery from this phase may require 12 to 18 months, and most patients have some permanent residual damage. Although there is no specific treatment for the vestibular deficiency, early discontinuation of the drug may permit recovery before irreversible damage of the hair cells.

Nephrotoxicity. Approximately 8% to 26% of patients who receive an aminoglycoside for more than several days will develop mild renal impairment that is almost always reversible (Smith *et al.*, 1980). The toxicity results from accumulation and retention of aminoglycoside in the proximal tubular cells (Aronoff *et al.*, 1983; Lietman and Smith, 1983). The initial manifestation of damage at this site is excretion of enzymes of the renal tubular brush border (Patel *et al.*, 1975). After several days, there is a defect in renal concentrating ability, mild proteinuria, and the appearance of hyaline and granular casts. The glomerular filtration rate is reduced after several additional days (Schentag *et al.*, 1979). The nonoliguric phase of renal insufficiency is thought to be due to the effects of aminoglycosides on the distal portion of the nephron with a reduced sensitivity of the collecting-duct epithelium to endogenous antidiuretic hormone (Appel, 1982). While severe acute tubular necrosis may occur rarely, the most common significant finding is a mild rise in plasma creatinine (5 to 20 μg/ml; 40 to 175 μM). Hypokalemia, hypocalcemia, and hypophosphatemia are seen very infrequently. The impairment in renal function is almost always reversible because the proximal tubular cells have the capacity to regenerate.

Several variables appear to influence nephrotoxicity from aminoglycosides. Toxicity correlates with the total amount of drug administered. Consequently, toxicity is more likely to be encountered with longer courses of therapy. Continuous infusion is more nephrotoxic in animals than is intermittent dosing (Powell *et al.*, 1983); constantly elevated concentrations of drug in plasma above a critical level, which is manifest by elevated trough serum concentrations, correlate with toxicity in human beings (Keating *et al.*, 1979).

The nephrotoxic potential varies among individual aminoglycosides. The relative toxicity correlates with the concentration of drug found in the renal cortex in experimental animals. Neomycin, which concentrates to the greatest degree, is highly nephrotoxic in human beings and should not be administered systemically. Streptomycin does not concentrate in the renal cortex and is the least nephrotoxic. Most of the controversy has concerned the relative toxicities of gentamicin and tobramycin. Gentamicin is concentrated in the kidney to a greater degree than is tobramycin, but several controlled clinical trials have given different estimates of their relative nephrotoxicities (Smith *et al.*, 1980; Fong *et al.*, 1981; Keys *et al.*, 1981). If differences between the renal toxicity of these two aminoglycosides do exist in human beings, they appear to be slight. Comparative studies with amikacin, sisomicin, and netilmicin are not conclusive. Other drugs, such as *amphotericin B, vancomycin, angiotensin-converting enzyme inhibitors, cisplatin,* and *cyclosporine,* may potentiate aminoglycoside-induced nephrotoxicity (Wood *et al.*, 1986). Furosemide enhances the nephrotoxicity of aminoglycosides in rats if there is concurrent fluid depletion (Mitchell *et al.*, 1977). Clinical studies have not proven conclusively that furosemide itself potentiates nephrotoxicity (Smith and Lietman, 1983), but volume depletion and wasting of K^+ that accompany its use have been incriminated.

Advanced age, liver disease, diabetes mellitus, and septic shock have been suggested as risk factors for the development of nephrotoxicity from aminoglycosides, but data are not convincing (Moore *et al.*, 1984b). Note, however, that renal function in the elderly patient is overestimated by measurement of creatinine concentration in plasma, and overdosing will occur if this value is used as the only guide in this patient population (Baciewicz *et al.*, 2003).

Even though aminoglycosides consistently alter the structure and function of renal proximal tubular cells, these effects usually are reversible. The most important result of this toxicity may be reduced excretion of the drug, which, in turn, predisposes to ototoxicity. Monitoring drug concentrations in plasma is useful, particularly during prolonged and/or high-dose therapy. However, it never has been proven that toxicity can be prevented by avoiding excessive peak or trough concentrations of aminoglycosides. In fact, experience with once-daily dosing regimens strongly suggests that high peaks (*e.g.*, 25 μg/ml or higher) do not increase toxicity.

The biochemical events leading to tubular cell damage and glomerular dysfunction are poorly understood but may involve perturbations of the structure of cellular membranes. Aminoglycosides inhibit various phospholipases, sphingomyelinases, and ATPases, and they alter the function of mitochondria and ribosomes (Queener *et al.*, 1983; Humes *et al.*, 1984). Because of the ability of cationic aminoglycosides to interact with anionic phospholipids, these drugs may impair the synthesis of membrane-derived autacoids and intracellular second messengers such as prostaglandins, inositol phosphates, and diacylglycerol. Derangements of prostaglandin metabolism may explain the relationship between tubular damage and reduction in glomerular filtration rate. Others have observed morphological changes in glomerular endothelial cells (decreased number of endothelial fenestrations) (Luft and Evan, 1980) and reduction in the glomerular capillary ultrafiltration coefficient in animals receiving aminoglycosides (Baylis *et al.*, 1977).

Ca^{2+} has been shown to inhibit the uptake and binding of aminoglycosides to the renal brush-border luminal membrane *in vitro,* and supplementary dietary Ca^{2+} attenuates experimental nephrotoxicity (Bennett *et al.*, 1982). Aminoglycosides eventually are internalized by pinocytosis. Morphologically, there is clear evidence of accumulation of drug in liposomes, a means by which aminoglycosides are trapped, concentrated (up to 50 times the plasma concentration) (Aronoff *et al.*, 1983), and prepared for extrusion into the urine as multilamellar phospholipid structures called *myeloid bodies* (Swan, 1997).

Neuromuscular Blockade. An unusual toxic reaction of acute neuromuscular blockade and apnea has been attributed to the aminoglycosides. The order of decreasing potency for blockade is neomycin, kanamycin, amikacin, gentamicin, and tobramycin. In humans, neuromuscular blockade generally has occurred after intrapleural or intraperitoneal instillation of large doses of an aminoglycoside; however, the reaction can follow intravenous, intramuscular, and even oral administration of these agents. Most episodes have occurred in association with anesthesia or the administration of other neuromuscular blocking agents. Patients with myasthenia gravis are particularly susceptible to neuromuscular blockade by aminoglycosides (*see* Chapter 8).

Aminoglycosides may inhibit prejunctional release of acetylcholine while also reducing postsynaptic sensitivity to the transmitter

(Sokoll and Gergis, 1981), but Ca^{2+} can overcome this effect, and the intravenous administration of a calcium salt is the preferred treatment for this toxicity (Singh *et al.*, 1978). Inhibitors of acetylcholinesterase (*e.g., edrophonium* and *neostigmine*) also have been used with varying degrees of success.

Other Effects on the Nervous System. The administration of streptomycin may produce dysfunction of the optic nerve, including scotomas, presenting as enlargement of the blind spot. Among the less common toxic reactions to streptomycin is peripheral neuritis. This may be due either to accidental injection of a nerve during the course of parenteral therapy or to toxicity involving nerves remote from the site of antibiotic administration. Paresthesia, most commonly perioral but also present in other areas of the face or in the hands, occasionally follows the use of the antibiotic and usually appears within 30 to 60 minutes after injection of the drug. It can persist for several hours.

Other Untoward Effects. In general, the aminoglycosides have little allergenic potential; anaphylaxis and rash are unusual. Rare hypersensitivity reactions—including skin rashes, eosinophilia, fever, blood dyscrasias, angioedema, exfoliative dermatitis, stomatitis, and anaphylactic shock—have been reported. Parenterally administered aminoglycosides are not associated with pseudomembranous colitis, probably because they do not disrupt the normal anaerobic flora. Other reactions that have been attributed to individual drugs are discussed below.

STREPTOMYCIN

Streptomycin is used for the treatment of certain unusual infections generally in combination with other antimicrobial agents. Because it generally is less active than other members of the class against aerobic gram-negative rods, it has fallen into disuse. Streptomycin may be administered by deep intramuscular injection or intravenously. Intramuscular injection may be painful, with a hot, tender mass developing at the site of injection. The dose of streptomycin is 15 mg/kg per day for patients with creatinine clearances above 80 ml/min. It typically is administered as a 1000-mg single daily dose or 500 mg twice daily, resulting in peak serum concentrations of approximately 50 to 60 and 15 to 30 μg/ml and trough concentrations of less than 1 and 5 to 10 μg/ml, respectively. The total daily dose should be reduced in direct proportion to the reduction in creatinine clearance for creatinine clearances above 30 ml/min (Table 45–2).

Therapeutic Uses. **Bacterial Endocarditis.** Streptomycin and penicillin in combination are synergistically bactericidal *in vitro* and in animal models of infection against strains of enterococci, group D streptococci, and the various oral streptococci of the *viridans* group. A combination of penicillin G and streptomycin may be indicated for treatment of streptococcal endocarditis (Wilson *et al.*, 1995). The combination of penicillin G, which by itself is only bacteriostatic against enterococci, and streptomycin is effective for enterococcal endocarditis. Streptomycin rarely is used for this indication, however, having been replaced almost entirely by gentamicin, because its toxicity is primarily renal and reversible, whereas that of streptomycin is vestibular and irreversible. Gentamicin also should be used when the strain of enterococcus is resistant to streptomycin (MIC >2 mg/ml). Similarly, streptomycin should be used instead of gentamicin when the strain is resistant to the latter and susceptibility has been demonstrated to streptomycin, which may occur because the enzymes that inactivate these two aminoglycosides are different.

Tularemia. Streptomycin (or gentamicin) is the drug of choice for the treatment of tularemia (Ellis *et al.*, 2002). Most cases respond to the administration of 1 g (15 to 25 mg/kg) streptomycin per day (in divided doses) for 7 to 10 days. Fluoroquinolones and tetracyclines also are effective, although the failure rate may be higher with tetracyclines.

Plague. Streptomycin is effective agent for the treatment of all forms of plague. The recommended dose is 2 g/day in two divided doses for 7 to 10 days. Gentamicin is probably as efficacious (Boulanger *et al.*, 2004).

Tuberculosis. In the treatment of tuberculosis, streptomycin always should be used in combination with at least one or two other drugs to which the causative strain is susceptible. The dose for patients with normal renal function is 15 mg/kg per day as a single intramuscular injection for 2 to 3 months and then 2 or 3 times a week thereafter.

GENTAMICIN

Gentamicin is an important agent for the treatment of many serious gram-negative bacillary infections. It is the aminoglycoside of first choice because of its low cost and reliable activity against all but the most resistant gram-negative aerobes. Gentamicin preparations are available for parenteral, ophthalmic, and topical administration.

Therapeutic Uses of Gentamicin and Other Aminoglycosides. Gentamicin, tobramycin, amikacin, and netilmicin can be used interchangeably for the treatment of most of the following infections and therefore are discussed together. For most indications, gentamicin is the preferred agent because of long experience with its use and its relatively low cost. Many different types of infections can be treated successfully with these aminoglycosides; however, owing to their toxicities, prolonged use should be restricted to the therapy of life-threatening infections and those for which a less toxic agent is contraindicated or less effective.

The typical recommended intramuscular or intravenous dose of *gentamicin sulfate* (GARAMYCIN) for adults is a loading dose of 2 mg/kg and then 3 to 5 mg/kg per day, one-third being given every 8 hours when administered as a multiple-daily-dosing regimen. The once-daily dose is 5 to 7 mg/kg given over 30 to 60 minutes for patients with normal renal function (and below this range if renal function is impaired). The upper limit of this dose range may be required to achieve therapeutic levels for trauma or burn patients, those with septic shock, and others in whom drug clearance is more rapid or volume of distribution is larger than normal. Several dosage schedules have been suggested for newborns and infants: 3 mg/kg once daily for preterm newborns younger than 35 weeks' gestation (Rastogi *et al.*, 2002; Hansen *et al.*, 2003); 4 mg/kg once daily for newborns older than 35 weeks' gestation; 5 mg/kg daily in two divided doses for neonates with severe infections; and 2 to 2.5 mg/kg every 8 hours for children up to 2 years of age. Peak plasma concentrations range from 4 to 10 μg/ml (dosing: 1.7 mg/kg every 8 hours) and 16 to 24 μg/ml (dosing: 5.1 mg/kg once daily). It should be emphasized that the recommended doses of gentamicin do not always yield desired concentrations. Periodic determinations of the plasma concentration of aminoglycosides are recommended strongly, especially in seriously ill patients, to confirm that drug concentrations are in the desired range (*see* sections on dosing above for more details). Although it has not been established exactly what plasma concentration is toxic, trough concentrations continually above 2 μg/ml have been associated with toxicity (Raveh *et al.*, 2002).

Aminoglycosides frequently are used in combination with a penicillin or a cephalosporin for the therapy of proven or suspected serious gram-negative microbial infections, especially those due to *P. aeruginosa, Enterobacter, Klebsiella, Serratia,* and other species resistant to less toxic antibiotics, including urinary tract infections, bacteremia, infected burns, osteomyelitis, pneumonia, peritonitis, and otitis. With few exceptions (*e.g.,* enterococcal endocarditis) (Le and Bayer, 2003), the superiority of aminoglycoside combination therapy over an effective single-drug regimen has not been demonstrated. Because of their toxicity with prolonged administration, aminoglycosides should not be used for more than a few days unless deemed essential for a successful or improved outcome. Aminoglycosides never must be mixed in the same solution with penicillins because the penicillin inactivates the aminoglycoside to a significant degree (Konishi *et al.*, 1983). Similar incompatibilities exist *in vitro* to different degrees between gentamicin and *heparin, amphotericin B,* and the various cephalosporins.

Urinary Tract Infections. Aminoglycosides usually are not indicated for the treatment of uncomplicated urinary tract infections, although a single intramuscular dose of gentamicin (5 mg/kg) has been effective in curing more than 90% of uncomplicated infections of the lower urinary tract (Varese *et al.*, 1980). However, as strains of *E. coli* have acquired resistance to β-lactams, *trimethoprim–sulfamethoxazole,* and *fluoroquinolones,* use of aminoglycosides may increase. In the seriously ill patient with pyelonephritis, an aminoglycoside alone or in combination with a β-lactam antibiotic offers broad and effective initial coverage. Once the microorganism is isolated and its sensitivities to antibiotics are determined, the aminoglycoside should be discontinued if the infecting microorganism is sensitive to less toxic antibiotics.

Pneumonia. The organisms that cause community-acquired pneumonia will be susceptible to broad-spectrum β-lactam antibiotics, macrolides, or a fluoroquinolone, and usually it is not necessary to add an aminoglycoside. Therapy with an aminoglycoside alone is likely to be ineffective; therapeutic concentrations are difficult to achieve owing to relatively poor penetration of drug into inflamed tissues and the associated conditions of low oxygen tension and low pH—both of which interfere with aminoglycoside antibacterial activity. Aminoglycosides are ineffective for the treatment of pneumonia due to anaerobes or *S. pneumoniae,* which are common causes of community-acquired pneumonia. They should not be considered as effective single-drug therapy for any aerobic gram-positive cocci (including *S. aureus* or streptococci), the microorganisms commonly responsible for suppurative pneumonia or lung abscess. Thus gentamicin (or other aminoglycosides) never should be used as the sole agent to treat pneumonia acquired in the community or as the initial treatment for pneumonia acquired in the hospital (Kunin, 1977).

An aminoglycoside in combination with a β-lactam antibiotic may be used for empirical therapy of hospital-acquired pneumonia in which multiple-drug-resistant gram-negative aerobes are a likely causative agent. However, provided the companion drug is active against the causative agent, there is generally no benefit from adding an aminoglycoside. One exception may be the treatment of pneumonia caused by *P. aeruginosa,* for which combination therapy generally is recommended, with the goal of preventing the emergence of resistance.

Meningitis. Availability of third-generation cephalosporins, especially *cefotaxime* and *ceftriaxone,* has reduced the need for treatment with aminoglycosides in most cases of meningitis, except for infections caused by gram-negative organisms that are resistant to β-lactam antibiotics (*e.g.,* species of *Pseudomonas* and *Acinetobacter*). If therapy with an aminoglycoside is necessary, in adults, 5 mg of a preservative-free formulation of gentamicin (or equivalent dose of another aminoglycoside) is administered directly intrathecally once daily (Barnes *et al.,* 2003).

Peritoneal Dialysis–Associated Peritonitis. Patients who develop peritonitis as a result of peritoneal dialysis may be treated with aminoglycoside diluted into the dialysis fluid to a concentration of 4 to 8 mg/L for gentamicin, netilmicin, or tobramycin or 6 to 12 mg/L for amikacin. Intravenous or intramuscular administration of drug is unnecessary because serum and peritoneal fluid will equilibrate rapidly.

Bacterial Endocarditis. "Synergistic" or low-dose gentamicin (3 mg/kg per day in three divided doses) in combination with a penicillin or vancomycin has been recommended in certain circumstances for treatment of bacterial endocarditis. There is good evidence that penicillin and gentamicin in combination are effective as a short-course (*i.e.,* 2-week) regimen for uncomplicated native-valve streptococcal endocarditis. In cases of enterococcal endocarditis, concomitant administration of penicillin and gentamicin for 4 to 6 weeks has been recommended because of an unacceptably high relapse rate with penicillin alone. A large case series from Sweden, however, found that cure rates were not substantially affected by shortening the duration of aminoglycoside therapy to a median duration of 15 days (Olaison and Schadewitz, 2002). A 2-week regimen of gentamicin or tobramycin in combination with *nafcillin* is effective for the treatment of selected cases of staphylococcal tricuspid valve endocarditis in injection drug users (Chambers *et al.,* 1988), although the need to including the aminoglycoside is not established (Le and Bayer, 2003).

Aminoglycosides have no clinically proven benefit in treatment of staphylococcal mitral or aortic valve endocarditis. Because of toxicity and limited, if any, clinical benefit, aminoglycoside combination therapy has fallen from favor as a first-line regimen for treatment of endocarditis.

Sepsis. Inclusion of an aminoglycoside in an empirical regimen used to be recommended commonly for the febrile patient with granulocytopenia and for infections suspected to be caused by *P. aeruginosa.* Numerous studies using potent broad-spectrum β-lactams (*e.g.,* carbapenems and antipseudomonal cephalosporins) have demonstrated no benefit from adding an aminoglycoside to the regimen. Most

authorities continue to recommend combination therapy of documented non–urinary tract *P. aeruginosa* infections, particularly pneumonia with bacteremia. If there is concern that an infection may be caused by a multiple-drug-resistant organism that may be susceptible only to an aminoglycoside, then adding this antibiotic to the regimen is reasonable. Evidence that aminoglycosides are beneficial for other gram-negative infections is weak if the isolate is susceptible to other antibiotics. To avoid toxicity, aminoglycosides should be used briefly and sparingly as long as other alternatives are available.

Topical Applications. Gentamicin is absorbed slowly when it is applied topically in an ointment and somewhat more rapidly when it is applied as a cream. When the antibiotic is applied to large areas of denuded body surface, as may be the case in burned patients, plasma concentrations can reach 4 μg/ml, and 2% to 5% of the drug used may appear in the urine.

Untoward Effects. Like other aminoglycosides, the most important and serious side effects of the use of gentamicin are nephrotoxicity and irreversible ototoxicity. Intrathecal or intraventricular administration is used rarely because it may cause local inflammation and can result in radiculitis and other complications.

TOBRAMYCIN

The antimicrobial activity, pharmacokinetic properties, and toxicity profile of tobramycin (NEBCIN) are very similar to those of gentamicin. Tobramycin may be given either intramuscularly or intravenously. Dosages and serum concentrations are identical with those for gentamicin. Tobramycin (TOBREX) also is available in ophthalmic ointments and solutions.

Therapeutic Uses. Indications for the use of tobramycin are the same as those for gentamicin. The superior activity of tobramycin against *P. aeruginosa* makes it the preferred aminoglycoside for treatment of serious infections caused by this organism. It usually should be used concurrently with an antipseudomonal β-lactam antibiotic. In contrast to gentamicin, tobramycin shows poor activity in combination with penicillin against many strains of enterococci. Most strains of *E. faecium* are highly resistant. Tobramycin is ineffective against mycobacteria.

Untoward Effects. Tobramycin, like other aminoglycosides, causes nephrotoxicity and ototoxicity. Studies in experimental animals suggest that tobramycin may be less toxic to hair cells in the cochlear and vestibular end organs and cause less renal tubular damage than does gentamicin. However, clinical data are less convincing.

AMIKACIN

The spectrum of antimicrobial activity of amikacin (AMIKIN) is the broadest of the group. Because of its resistance to many of the aminoglycoside-inactivating enzymes, it has a special role in hospitals where gentamicin- and tobramycin-resistant microorganisms are prevalent. Amikacin is similar to kanamycin in dosage and pharmacokinetic properties.

The recommended dose of amikacin is 15 mg/kg per day as a single daily dose or divided into two or three equal portions, which must be reduced for patients with renal failure. The drug is absorbed rapidly after intramuscular injection, and peak concentrations in plasma approximate 20 μg/ml after injection of 7.5 mg/kg. An intravenous infusion of the same dose over a 30-minute period produces a peak concentration in plasma of nearly 40 μg/ml at the end of the infusion, which falls to about 20 μg/ml 30 minutes later. The concentration 12 hours after a 7.5 mg/kg dose typically is between 5 and 10 μg/ml. A 15 mg/kg once-daily dose produces peak concentrations that are between 50 and 60 μg/ml and a trough of less than 1 μg/ml.

Therapeutic Uses. Amikacin has become the preferred agent for the initial treatment of serious nosocomial gram-negative bacillary infections in hospitals where resistance to gentamicin and tobramycin has become a significant problem. Amikacin is active against the vast majority of aerobic gram-negative bacilli in the community and the hospital. This includes most strains of *Serratia, Proteus,* and *P. aeruginosa.* It is active against nearly all strains of *Klebsiella, Enterobacter,* and *E. coli* that are resistant to gentamicin and tobramycin. Most resistance to amikacin is found among strains of *Acinetobacter, Providencia,* and *Flavobacter* and strains of *Pseudomonas* other than *P. aeruginosa*; these all are unusual pathogens. Like tobramycin, amikacin is less active than gentamicin against enterococci and should not be used. Amikacin is not active against the majority of gram-positive anaerobic bacteria. It is active against *M. tuberculosis* (99% of strains inhibited by 4 μg/ml), including streptomycin-resistant strains and atypical mycobacteria. It has been used in the treatment of disseminated atypical mycobacterial infection in acquired immunodeficiency syndrome (AIDS) patients.

Untoward Effects. As with the other aminoglycosides, amikacin causes ototoxicity and nephrotoxicity. Auditory deficits are produced most commonly.

NETILMICIN

Netilmicin (NETROMYCIN) is the latest of the aminoglycosides to be marketed. It is similar to gentamicin and tobramycin in its pharmacokinetic properties and dosage. Its antibacterial activity is broad against aerobic gram-negative bacilli. Like amikacin, it is not metabolized by the majority of the aminoglycoside-inactivating enzymes, and it therefore may be active against certain bacteria that are resistant to gentamicin.

The recommended dose of netilmicin for complicated urinary tract infections in adults is 1.5 to 2 mg/kg every 12 hours. For other serious systemic infections, a total daily dose of 4 to 7 mg/kg is administered as a single dose or two to three divided doses. Children should receive 3 to 7 mg/kg per day in two to three divided doses; neonates receive 3.5 to 5 mg/kg per day as a single daily dose

(Gosden *et al.,* 2001). The distribution and elimination of netilmicin, gentamicin, and tobramycin are very similar. An intravenous infusion of 2 mg/kg netilmicin given over a 60-minute period results in a peak plasma concentration of approximately 11 μg/ml (Luft *et al.,* 1978). The half-time for elimination is usually 2 to 2.5 hours in adults and increases with renal insufficiency.

Therapeutic Uses. Netilmicin is useful for the treatment of serious infections owing to susceptible Enterobacteriaceae and other aerobic gram-negative bacilli. It is effective against certain gentamicin-resistant pathogens, with the exception of enterococci (Panwalker *et al.,* 1978).

Untoward Effects. As with other aminoglycosides, netilmicin also may produce ototoxicity and nephrotoxicity. Animal models have suggested that netilmicin may be less toxic than other aminoglycosides (Luft *et al.,* 1976), but this remains to be proven in humans (Tange *et al.,* 1995).

KANAMYCIN

The use of kanamycin has declined markedly because its spectrum of activity is limited compared with other aminoglycosides, and it is among the most toxic.

Kanamycin sulfate (KANTREX) is available for injection and oral use. The parenteral dose for adults is 15 mg/kg per day (two to four equally divided and spaced doses), with a maximum of 1.5 g/day. Children may be given up to 15 mg/kg per day.

Therapeutic Uses. Kanamycin is all but obsolete, and there are few indications for its use. Kanamycin has been employed to treat tuberculosis in combination with other effective drugs. It has no therapeutic advantage over streptomycin or amikacin and probably is more toxic; either should be used instead, depending on susceptibility of the isolate.

Prophylactic Uses. Kanamycin can be administered orally as adjunctive therapy in cases of hepatic encephalopathy. The dose is 4 to 6 g/day for 36 to 72 hours; quantities as large as 12 g/day (in divided doses) have been given.

Untoward Effects. Kanamycin is ototoxic and nephrotoxic. Like neomycin (*see* below), its oral administration can cause malabsorption and superinfection. The untoward effects of the oral administration of aminoglycosides are considered under "Neomycin" below.

NEOMYCIN

Neomycin is a broad-spectrum antibiotic. Susceptible microorganisms usually are inhibited by concentrations of 5 to 10 μg/ml or less. Gram-negative species that are highly sensitive are *E. coli, Enterobacter aerogenes, Klebsiella pneumoniae,* and *Proteus vulgaris.* Gram-positive microorganisms that are inhibited include *S. aureus* and *E. faecalis*. *M. tuberculosis* also is sensitive to neomycin. Strains of *P. aeruginosa* are resistant to neomycin.

Neomycin sulfate is available for topical and oral administration. Neomycin and *polymyxin B* have been used for irrigation of the bladder. For this purpose, 1 ml of a preparation (NEOSPORIN G.U. IRRIGANT) containing 40 mg neomycin and 200,000 units polymyxin B per milliliter is diluted in 1 L of 0.9% sodium chloride solution and is used for continuous irrigation of the urinary bladder through appropriate catheter systems. The goal is to prevent bacteriuria and bacteremia associated with the use of indwelling catheters. The bladder usually is irrigated at the rate of 1 L every 24 hours.

Neomycin currently is available in many brands of creams, ointments, and other products alone and in combination with polymyxin, *bacitracin,* other antibiotics and a variety of corticosteroids. There is no evidence that these topical preparations shorten the time required for healing of wounds or that those containing a steroid are more effective.

Therapeutic Uses. Neomycin has been used widely for topical application in a variety of infections of the skin and mucous membranes caused by microorganisms susceptible to the drug. These include infections associated with burns, wounds, ulcers, and infected dermatoses. However, such treatment does not eradicate bacteria from the lesions.

The oral administration of neomycin (usually in combination with erythromycin base) has been employed primarily for "preparation" of the bowel for surgery. For therapy of hepatic encephalopathy, a daily dose of 4 to 12 g (in divided doses) by mouth is given, provided that renal function is normal. Because renal insufficiency is a complication of hepatic failure and neomycin is nephrotoxic, it is used rarely for this indication. *Lactulose* is a much less toxic agent and is preferred (*see* Chapter 37).

Absorption and Excretion. Neomycin is poorly absorbed from the gastrointestinal tract and is excreted by the kidney, as are the other aminoglycosides. An oral dose of 3 g produces a peak plasma concentration of 1 to 4 μg/ml; a total daily intake of 10 g for 3 days yields a blood concentration below that associated with systemic toxicity if renal function is normal. Patients with renal insufficiency may accumulate the drug. About 97% of an oral dose of neomycin is not absorbed and is eliminated unchanged in the feces.

Untoward Effects. Hypersensitivity reactions, primarily skin rashes, occur in 6% to 8% of patients when neomycin is applied topically. Individuals sensitive to this agent may develop cross-reactions when exposed to other aminoglycosides. The most important toxic effects of neomycin are renal damage and nerve deafness; this is why the drug is no longer available for parenteral administration. Toxicity has been reported in patients with normal renal function after topical application or irrigation of wounds with 0.5% neomycin solution. Neuromuscular blockade with respiratory paralysis also has occurred after irrigation of wounds or serosal cavities.

The most important adverse effects resulting from the oral administration of neomycin are intestinal malabsorption and superinfection. Individuals treated with 4 to 6 g/day of the drug by mouth sometimes develop a spruelike syndrome with diarrhea, steatorrhea, and azotorrhea. Overgrowth of yeasts in the intestine also may

occur; this is not associated with diarrhea or other symptoms in most cases.

CLINICAL SUMMARY

The role of aminoglycosides in the treatment of bacterial infections has diminished steadily as alternative drugs have become available. The aminoglycosides are narrow-spectrum agents, with their activity limited mainly to gram-negative aerobes. Compared with other antibacterials, aminoglycosides are among the most toxic, particularly if used for prolonged periods of time; serum concentrations must be monitored to avoid drug accumulation. These agents are first-line therapy for only a limited number of very specific, often historically prominent infections, such as plague, tularemia, and tuberculosis. Gentamicin or amikacin may have a role as a backup agent in the treatment of nosocomial infections caused by multidrug-resistant gram-negative pathogens such as *Pseudomonas* or *Acinetobacter*. Gentamicin also may be useful for the treatment of serious urinary tract infections caused by enteric organisms that have acquired resistance to sulfa drugs, penicillins, cephalosporins, and fluoroquinolones. Although gentamicin has been recommended for use in combination with vancomycin or a β-lactam to enhance bactericidal effect (*i.e.,* synergism), the clinical benefit of such combinations is unproven for most infections. Because more effective and less toxic alternatives usually are available, aminoglycosides should be used sparingly and reserved for specific indications, as noted earlier. If an aminoglycoside must be used, the duration of therapy should be kept to a minimum to avoid toxicity, and serum concentrations should be monitored.

BIBLIOGRAPHY

Appel, G.B. Aminoglycoside nephrotoxicity: Physiologic studies of the sites of nephron damage. In, *The Aminoglycosides: Microbiology, Clinical Use, and Toxicity.* (Whelton, A., and Neu, H.C., eds.) Marcel Dekker, New York, **1982,** pp. 269–282.

Aronoff, G.R., Pottratz, S.T., Brier, M.E., *et al.* Aminoglycoside accumulation kinetics in rat renal parenchyma. *Antimicrob. Agents Chemother.,* **1983,** *23:*74–78.

Baciewicz, A.M., Sokos, D.R., and Cowan, R.I. Aminoglycoside-associated nephrotoxicity in the elderly. *Ann. Pharmacother.,* **2003,** *37:*182–186.

Bailey, T.C., Little, J.R., Littenberg, B., Reichley, R.M., and Dunagan, W.C. A meta-analysis of extended-interval dosing versus multiple daily dosing of aminoglycosides. *Clin. Infect. Dis.,* **1997,** *24:*786–795.

Barclay, M.L., Kirkpatrick, C.M., and Begg, E.J. Once-daily aminoglycoside therapy: Is it less toxic than multiple daily doses and how should it be monitored? *Clin. Pharmacokinet.,* **1999,** *36:*89–98.

Barnes, B.J., Wiederhold, N.P., Micek, S.T., Polish, L.B., and Ritchie, D.J. *Enterobacter cloacae* ventriculitis successfully treated with cefepime and gentamin: Case report and review of the literature. *Pharmacotherapy*, **2003**, *23*:537–542.

Bartal, C., Danon, A., Schlaeffer, F., *et al.* Pharmacokinetic dosing of aminoglycosides: A controlled trial. *Am. J. Med.*, **2003**, *114*:194–198.

Bates, D.E. Aminoglycoside ototoxicity. *Drugs Today (Barc.)*, **2003**, *39*:277–285.

Battaglia, A., Pak, K., and Brors, D., *et al.* Involvement of *ras* activation in toxic hair cell damage of the mammalian cochlea. *Neuroscience*, **2003**, *122*:1025–1035.

Baylis, C., Rennke, H.R., and Brenner, B.M. Mechanisms of the defect in glomerular ultrafiltration associated with gentamicin administration. *Kidney Int.*, **1977**, *12*:344–353.

Bennett, W.M., Elliott, W.C., Houghton, D.C., *et al.* Reduction of experimental gentamicin nephrotoxicity in rats by dietary calcium loading. *Antimicrob. Agents Chemother.*, **1982**, *22*:508–512.

Bergeron, M.G., Bastille, A., Lessard, C., and Gagnon, P.M. Significance of intrarenal concentrations of gentamicin for the outcome of experimental pyelonephritis in rats. *J. Infect. Dis.*, **1982**, *146*:91–96.

Blair, D.C., Duggan, D.O., and Schroeder, E.T. Inactivation of amikacin and gentamicin by carbenicillin in patients with end-stage renal failure. *Antimicrob. Agents Chemother.*, **1982**, *22*:376–379.

Boulanger, L.L., Ettestad, P., Fogarty, J.D., *et al.* Gentamicin and tetracyclines for the treatment of human plague: Review of 75 cases in new Mexico, 1985–1999. *Clin. Infect. Dis.*, **2004**, *38*:663–669.

Brummett, R.E. Animal models of aminoglycoside antibiotic ototoxicity. *Rev. Infect. Dis.*, **1983**, *5*(suppl. 2):S294–S303.

Buijk, S.E., Mouton, J.W., Gyssens, I.C., Verbrugh, H.A., and Bruining, H.A. Experience with a once-daily dosing program of aminoglycosides in critically ill patients. *Intensive Care Med.*, **2002**, *28*:936–942.

Busse, H.J., Wöstmann, C., and Bakker, E.P. The bactericidal action of streptomycin: membrane permeabilization caused by the insertion of mistranslated proteins into the cytoplasmic membrane of *Escherichia coli* and subsequent caging of the antibiotic inside the cells due to degradation of these proteins. *J. Gen. Microbiol.*, **1992**, *138*:551–561.

Chambers, H.F., Miller, R.T., and Newman, M.D. Right-sided *Staphylococcus aureus* endocarditis in intravenous drug abusers: Two-week combination study. *Ann. Intern. Med.*, **1988**, *109*:619–624.

Charnas, R., Luthi, A.R., and Ruch, W. Once-daily ceftriaxone plus amikacin vs. three-times-daily ceftazidime plus amikacin for treatment of febrile neutropenic children with cancer. Writing Committee for the International Collaboration on Antimicrobial Treatment of Febrile Neutropenia in Children. *Pediatr. Infect. Dis. J.*, **1997**, *16*:346–353.

de Jager, P., and van Altena, R. Hearing loss and nephrotoxicity in long-term aminoglycoside treatment in patients with tuberculosis. *Int. J. Tuberc. Lung Dis.*, **2002**, *6*:622–627.

Deamer, R.L. Single daily dosing of aminoglycosides. *Am. Fam. Phys.*, **1998**, *58*:1747–1750.

Eliopoulos, G.M., Farber, B.F., Murray, B.E., Wennersten, C., and Moellering, R.C., Jr. Ribosomal resistance of clinical enterococcal to streptomycin isolates. *Antimicrob. Agents Chemother.*, **1984**, *25*:398–399.

Ellis, J., Oyston, P.C., Green, M., and Titball, R.W. Tularemia. *Clin. Microbiol. Rev.*, **2002**, *15*:631–646.

Ferriols-Lisart, R., and Alos-Alminana, M. Effectiveness and safety of once-daily aminoglycosides: A meta-analysis. *Am. J. Health Syst. Pharm.*, **1996**, *53*:1141–1150.

Fong, I.W., Fenton, R.S., and Bird, R. Comparative toxicity of gentamicin versus tobramycin: A randomized, prospective study. *J. Antimicrob. Chemother.*, **1981**, *7*:81–88.

Freeman, C.D., Nicolau, D.P., Belliveau, P.P., and Nightingale, C.H. Once-daily dosing of aminoglycosides: Review and recommendations for clinical practice. *J. Antimicrob. Chemother.*, **1997**, *39*:677–686.

Gilbert, D.N., Lee, B.L., Dworkin, R.J., *et al.* A randomized comparison of the safety and efficacy of once-daily gentamicin or thrice-daily gentamicin in combination with ticarcillin–clavulanate. *Am. J. Med.*, **1998**, *105*:182–191.

Gosden, P.E., Bedford, K.A., Dixon, J.J., *et al.* Pharmacokinetics of once-a-day netilmicin (4.5 mg/kg) in neonates. *J. Chemother.*, **2001**, *13*:270–276.

Hansen, A., Forbes, P., Arnold, A., and O'Rourke, E. Once-daily gentamicin dosing for the preterm and term newborn: Proposal for a simple regimen that achieves target levels. *J. Perinatol.*, **2003**, *23*:635–639.

Higgins, C.E., and Kastner, R.E. Nebramycin, a new broad-spectrum antibiotic complex: II. Description of *Streptomyces tenebrarius*. *Antimicrob. Agents Chemother.*, **1967**, *7*:324–331.

Humes, H.D., Sastrasinh, M., and Weinberg, J.M. Calcium is a competitive inhibitor of gentamicin–renal membrane binding interactions, and dietary calcium supplementation protects against gentamicin nephrotoxicity. *J. Clin. Invest.*, **1984**, *73*:134–147.

Hummel, H., and Böck, A. Ribosomal changes resulting in antimicrobial resistance. In, *Microbial Resistance to Drugs. Handbook of Experimental Pharmacology.* Vol. 91. (Bryan, L.E., ed.) Springer-Verlag Berlin, **1989**, pp. 193–226.

Keating, M.J., Bodey, G.P., Valdivieso, M., and Rodriguez, V. A randomized comparative trial of three aminoglycosides—comparison of continuous infusions of gentamicin, amikacin, and sisomicin combined with carbenicillin in the treatment of infections in neutropenic patients with malignancies. *Medicine*, **1979**, *58*:159–170.

Keys, T.F., Kurtz, S.B., Jones, J.D., and Muller, S.M. Renal toxicity during therapy with gentamicin or tobramycin. *Mayo Clin. Proc.*, **1981**, *56*:556–559.

Knoderer, C.A., Everett, J.A., and Buss, W.F. Clinical issues surrounding once-daily aminoglycoside dosing in children. *Pharmacotherapy*, **2003**, *23*:44–56.

Konishi, H., Goto, M., Nakamoto, Y., *et al.* Tobramycin inactivation by carbenicillin, ticarcillin, and piperacillin. *Antimicrob. Agents Chemother.*, **1983**, *23*:653–657.

Kunin, C.M. Blunder drug for pneumonia (letter). *New Engl. J. Med.*, **1977**, *297*:113–114.

Le, T., and Bayer, A.S. Combination antibiotic therapy for infective endocarditis. *Clin. Infect. Dis.*, **2003**, *36*:615–621.

Leibovici, L., Paul, M., Poznanski, O., *et al.* Monotherapy *versus* β-lactam–aminoglycoside combination treatment for gram-negative bacteremia: A prospective, observational study. *Antimicrob. Agents Chemother.*, **1997**, *41*:1127–1133.

Lerner, A.M., Reyes, M.P., Cone, L.A., *et al.* Randomised, controlled trial of the comparative efficacy, auditory toxicity, and nephrotoxicity of tobramycin and netilmicin. *Lancet*, **1983**, *1*:1123–1126.

Lesar, T.S., Rotschafer, J.C., Strand, L.M., *et al.* Gentamicin dosing errors with four commonly used nomograms. *JAMA*, **1982**, *248*:1190–1193.

Levy, J. Antibiotic activity in sputum. *J. Pediatr.*, **1986**, *108*:841–846.

Lietman, P.S., and Smith, C.R. Aminoglycoside nephrotoxicity in humans. *J. Infect. Dis.*, **1983**, *5*(suppl. 2):S284–S292.

Luft, F.C., Brannon, D.R., Stropes, L.L., *et al.* Pharmacokinetics of netilmicin in patients with renal impairment and in patients on dialysis. *Antimicrob. Agents Chemother.*, **1978**, *14*:403–407.

Luft, F.C., and Evan, A.P. Comparative effects of tobramycin and gentamicin on glomerular ultrastructure. *J. Infect. Dis.*, **1980**, *142*:910–914.

Luft, F.C., Yum, M.N., and Kleit, S.A. Comparative nephrotoxicities of netilmicin and gentamicin in rats. *Antimicrob. Agents Chemother.,* **1976,** *10*:845–849.

Luzzatto, L., Apirion, D., and Schlessinger, D. Polyribosome depletion and blockage of the ribosome cycle by streptomycin in *Escherichia coli. J. Mol. Biol.,* **1969,** *42*:315–335.

Mates, S.M., Patel, L., Kaback, H.R., and Miller, M.H. Membrane potential in anaerobically growing *Staphylococcus aureus* and its relationship to gentamicin uptake. *Antimicrob. Agents Chemother.,* **1983,** *23*:526–530.

McCormack, J.P., and Jewesson, P.J. A critical reevaluation of the "therapeutic range" of aminoglycosides. *Clin. Infect. Dis.,* **1992,** *14*:320–339.

Mitchell, C.J., Bullock, S., and Ross, B.D. Renal handling of gentamicin and other antibiotics by the isolated perfused rat kidney: Mechanism of nephrotoxicity. *J. Antimicrob. Chemother.,* **1977,** *3*:593–600.

Moore, R.D., Smith, C.R., and Lietman, P.S. Risk factors for the development of auditory toxicity in patients receiving aminoglycosides. *J. Infect. Dis.,* **1984a,** *149*:23–30.

Moore, R.D., Smith, C.R., Lipsky, J.J., *et al.* Risk factors for nephrotoxicity in patients with aminoglycosides. *Ann. Intern. Med.,* **1984b,** *100*:352–357.

Murry, K.R., McKinnon, P.S., Mitrzyk, B., and Rybak, M.J. Pharmacodynamic characterization of nephrotoxicity associated with once-daily aminoglycoside. *Pharmacotherapy,* **1999,** *19*:1252–1260.

Olaison, L., Schadewitz, K., and Swedish Society of Infectious Diseases Quality Assurance Study Group for Endocarditis. Enterococcal endocarditis in Sweden, 1995–1999: Can shorter therapy with aminoglycosides be used? *Clin. Infect. Dis.,* **2002,** *34*:159–166.

Panwalker, A.P., Malow, J.B., Zimelis, V.M., and Jackson, G.G. Netilmicin: Clinical efficacy, tolerance, and toxicity. *Antimicrob. Agents Chemother.,* **1978,** *13*:170–176.

Patel, V., Luft, F.C., Yum, M.N., *et al.* Enzymuria in gentamicin-induced kidney damage. *Antimicrob. Agents Chemother.,* **1975,** *7*:364–369.

Philips, J.B., III, Satterwhite, C., Dworsky, M.E., and Cassady, G. Recommended amikacin doses in newborns often produce excessive serum levels. *Pediatr. Pharmacol. (New York),* **1982,** *2*:121–125.

Powell, S.H., Thompson, W.L., Luthe, M.A., *et al.* Once-daily vs. continuous aminoglycoside dosing: efficacy and toxicity in animal and clinical studies of gentamicin, netilmicin, and tobramycin. *J. Infect. Dis.,* **1983,** *147*:918–932.

Queener, S.F., Luft, F.C., and Hamel, F.G. Effect of gentamicin treatment on adenylate cyclase and Na+,K+-ATPase activities in renal tissues of rats. *Antimicrob. Agents Chemother.,* **1983,** *24*:815–818.

Rastogi, A., Agarwal, G., Pyati, S., and Pildes, R.S. Comparison of two gentamicin dosing schedules in very low birth weight infants. *Pediatr. Infect. Dis. J.,* **2002,** *21*:234–240.

Raveh, D., Kopyt, M., Hite, Y., *et al.* Risk factors for nephrotoxicity in elderly patients receiving once-daily aminoglycosides. *Q. J. Med.,* **2002,** *95*:291–297.

Rosenthal, A., Button, L.N., and Khaw, K.T. Blood volume changes in patients with cystic fibrosis. *Pediatrics,* **1977,** *59*:588–594.

Rybak, M.J., Abate, B.J., Kang, S.L., *et al.* Prospective evaluation of the effect of an aminoglycoside dosing regimen on rates of observed nephrotoxicity and ototoxicity. *Antimicrob. Agents Chemother.,* **1999,** *43*:1549–1555.

Schentag, J.J., Gengo, F.M., Plaut, M.E., *et al.* Urinary casts as an indicator of renal tubular damage in patients receiving aminoglycosides. *Antimicrob. Agents Chemother.,* **1979,** *16*:468–474.

Schentag, J.J., and Jusko, W.J. Renal clearance and tissue accumulation of gentamicin. *Clin. Pharmacol. Ther.,* **1977,** *22*:364–370.

Singh, Y.N., Harvey, A.L., and Marshall, I.G. Antibiotic-induced paralysis of the mouse phrenic nerve—hemidiaphragm preparation and reversibility by calcium and by neostigmine. *Anesthesiology,* **1978,** *48*:418–424.

Smith, C.R., and Lietman, P.S. Effect of furosemide on aminoglycoside-induced nephrotoxicity and auditory toxicity in humans. *Antimicrob. Agents Chemother.,* **1983,** *23*:133–137.

Smith, C.R., Lipsky, J.J., Laskin, O.L., *et al.* Double-blind comparison of the nephrotoxicity and auditory toxicity of gentamicin and tobramycin. *New Engl. J. Med.,* **1980,** *302*:1106–1109.

Smithivas, T., Hyams, P.J., Matalon, R., *et al.* The use of gentamicin in peritoneal dialysis: I. Pharmacologic results. *J. Infect. Dis.,* **1971,** *124*(suppl.):77–83.

Spera, R.V., Jr., and Farber, B.F. Multiply-resistant *Enterococcus faecium:* The nosocomial pathogen of the 1990s. *JAMA,* **1992,** *268*:2563–2564.

Spyker, D.A., Sande, M.A., and Mandell, G.L. Tobramycin pharmacokinetics in patients with cystic fibrosis and leukemia. In, *Eighteenth Interscience Conference on Antimicrobial Agents and Chemotherapy.* American Society for Microbiology, Washington, **1978,** p. 345.

Strausbaugh, L.J., Mandaleris, C.D., and Sande, M.A. Comparison of four aminoglycoside antibiotics in the therapy of experimental *E. coli* meningitis. *J. Lab. Clin. Med.,* **1977,** *89*:692–701.

Tange, R.A., Dreschler, W.A., Prins, J.M., *et al.* Ototoxicity and nephrotoxicity of gentamicin vs. netilmicin in patients with serious infections: A randomized clinical trial. *Clin. Otolaryngol.,* **1995,** *20*:118–1123.

Theopold, H.M. Comparative surface studies of ototoxic effects of various aminoglycoside antibiotics on the organ of Corti in the guinea pig: A scanning electron microscopic study. *Acta Otolaryngol. (Stockh.),* **1977,** *84*:57–64.

Varese, L.A., Graziolo, F., Viretto, A., and Antoniola, P. Single-dose (bolus) therapy with gentamicin in management of urinary tract infection. *Int. J. Pediatr. Nephrol.,* **1980,** *1*:104–105.

Vemuri, R.K., and Zervos, M.J. Enterococcal infections: The increasing threat of nosocomial spread and drug resistance. *Postgrad. Med J.,* **1993,** *93*:121–124, 127–128.

Wersäll, J., Bjorkroth, B., Flock, A., and Lundquist, P.G. Experiments on the ototoxic effects of antibiotics. *Adv. Otorhinolaryngol.,* **1973,** *20*:14–41.

Wiedemann, B., and Atkinson, B.A. Susceptibility to antibiotics: Species incidence and trends. In, *Antibiotics in Laboratory Medicine,* 3d ed. (Lorian, V., ed.) Williams & Wilkins, Baltimore, **1991,** pp. 962–1208.

Wilson, P., and Ramsden, R.T. Immediate effects of tobramycin on human cochlea and correlation with serum tobramycin levels. *Br. Med. J.,* **1977,** *1*:259–261.

Wilson, W.R., Karchmer, A.W., Dajani, A.S., *et al.* Antibiotic treatment of adults with infective endocarditis due to streptococci, enterococci, staphylococci, and HACEK microorganisms. American Heart Association. *JAMA,* **1995,** *274*:1706–1713.

Wilson, W.R., Wilkowske, C.J., Wright, A.J., Sande, M.A., and Geraci, J.E. Treatment of streptomycin-susceptible and streptomycin-resistant enterococcal endocarditis. *Ann. Intern. Med.,* **1984,** *100*:816–823.

Wood, C.A., Kohlhepp, S.J., Kohnen, P.W., *et al.* Vancomycin enhancement of experimental tobramycin nephrotoxicity. *Antimicrob. Agents Chemother.,* **1986,** *30*:20–24.

Yow, M.D. An overview of pediatric experience with amikacin. *Am. J. Med.,* **1977,** *62*:954–958.

MONOGRAPHS AND REVIEWS

Bryan, L.E. Cytoplasmic membrane transport and antimicrobial resistance. In, *Microbial Resistance to Drugs: Handbook of Experimental Pharmacology,* Vol. 91. (Bryan, L.E., ed.) Springer-Verlag, Berlin, **1989,** pp. 35–57.

Chambers, H.F., Hadley, W.K., and Jawetz, E. Aminoglycosides and spectinomycin. In, *Basic and Clinical Pharmacology,* 7th ed. (Katzung, B.G., ed.) Appleton & Lange, Stamford, CT, **1998,** pp. 752–760.

Davies, J. Inactivation of antibiotics and the dissemination of resistance genes. *Science,* **1994,** *264*:375–382.

Davis, B.B. The lethal action of aminoglycosides. *J. Antimicrob. Chemother.,* **1988,** *22*:1–3.

Gilbert, D.N., Moellering, R.C., Jr., and Sande, M.A. *The Sanford Guide to Antimicrobial Therapy 1999,* 29th ed. Antimicrobial Therapy, Inc., Hyde Park, VT, **1999.**

Moellering, R.C., Jr. Microbiological considerations in the use of tobramycin and related aminoglycosidic aminocyclitol antibiotics. *Med. J. Aust.,* **1977,** *2*(suppl):4–8.

Murray, B.E. New aspects of antimicrobial resistance and the resulting therapeutic dilemmas. *J. Infect. Dis.,* **1991,** *163*:1184–1194.

Neu, H.C., and Bendush, C.L. Ototoxicity of tobramycin: A clinical overview. *J. Infect. Dis.,* **1976,** *134*:S206–S218.

Shannon, K., and Phillips, I. Mechanisms of resistance to aminoglycosides in clinical isolates. *J. Antimicrob. Chemother.,* **1982,** *9*:91–102.

Sokoll, M.D., and Gergis, S.D. Antibiotics and neuromuscular function. *Anesthesiology,* **1981,** *55*:148–159.

Swan, S.K. Aminoglycoside nephrotoxicity. *Semin. Nephrol.,* **1997,** *17*:27–33.

Toschlog, E.A., Blount, K.P., Rotondo, M.F., *et al.* Clinical predictors of subtherapeutic aminoglycoside levels in trauma patients undergoing once-daily dosing. *J. Trauma,* **2003,** *55*:255–260; discussion 260–262.

PROTEIN SYNTHESIS INHIBITORS AND MISCELLANEOUS ANTIBACTERIAL AGENTS

Henry F. Chambers

The antimicrobial agents discussed in this chapter are: (1) bacteriostatic, protein-synthesis inhibitors that target the ribosome, such as *tetracyclines, chloramphenicol, macrolides, ketolides, clindamycin, quinupristin/dalfopristin, linezolid,* and *spectinomycin*; (2) glycopeptides (*vancomycin* and *teicoplanin*) and lipopeptides (*daptomycin*); and (3) miscellaneous compounds acting by diverse mechanisms with limited indications: *bacitracin, polymyxin,* and *mupirocin*.

TETRACYCLINES

History. *Chlortetracycline,* the prototype of this class, was introduced in 1948, but is no longer marketed in the United States. Because of their activity against *Rickettsia,* gram-positive and gram-negative bacteria, aerobes, anaerobes, and *Chlamydia,* tetracyclines became known as "broad-spectrum" antibiotics. They are sufficiently similar to permit discussion as a group.

Source and Chemistry. *Oxytetracycline* is a natural product elaborated by *Streptomyces rimosus.* Tetracycline is a semisynthetic derivative of chlortetracycline. *Demeclocycline* is the product of a mutant strain of *Strep. aureofaciens,* and *methacycline* (not available in the United States), *doxycycline,* and *minocycline* all are semisynthetic derivatives. The tetracyclines are close congeners of polycyclic naphthacenecarboxamide. Their structural formulas are shown in Table 46–1.

Effects on Pathogenic Microorganisms. Tetracyclines are bacteriostatic antibiotics with activity against a wide range of aerobic and anaerobic gram-positive and gram-negative bacteria. They also are effective against some microorganisms, such as *Rickettsia, Coxiella burnetii, Mycoplasma pneumoniae, Chlamydia* spp., *Legionella*

spp., *Ureaplasma,* some atypical mycobacteria, and *Plasmodium* spp., that are resistant to cell-wall-active antimicrobial agents. They are not active against fungi. Demeclocycline, tetracycline, oxytetracycline, minocycline, and doxycycline are available in the United States for systemic use. Chlortetracycline and oxytetracycline are used in ophthalmic preparations. Methacycline is not available. Other derivatives are available in other countries. The more lipophilic drugs, minocycline and doxycycline, usually are the most active by weight, followed by tetracycline. Resistance of a bacterial strain to any one member of the class may result in cross-resistance to other tetracyclines. Bacterial strains with tetracycline minimum inhibitory concentrations (MICs) ≤4 μg/ml are considered susceptible except for *Haemophilus influenzae* and *Streptococcus pneumoniae,* whose susceptibility breakpoints (defined as the upper limit of the concentration at which bacteria are still considered susceptible to a given drug) are ≤2 μg/ml, and *Neisseria gonorrhoeae,* with a breakpoint of ≤0.25 μg/ml.

Bacterial Susceptibilities. Tetracyclines intrinsically are more active against gram-positive than gram-negative microorganisms, but acquired resistance is common. The prevalence of resistant strains varies in different regions. For example, approximately 10% of *Streptococcus pneumoniae* isolates in the United States are resistant to tetracycline *versus* 40% in the Asia-Pacific region (Hoban *et al.,* 2001). Susceptibilities of staphylococci, enterococci, and hemolytic streptococci are variable: *Bacillus anthracis* and *Listeria monocytogenes* are susceptible, *H. influenzae* is generally susceptible, but many Enterobacteriaceae have acquired resistance. Although all strains of *Pseudomonas aeruginosa* are resistant, 90% of strains of *Burkholderia pseudomallei* (the cause of melioidosis) are sensitive. Most strains of *Brucella* also are susceptible. Tetracyclines remain useful for infections caused by *Haemophilus ducreyi* (chancroid), *Brucella, Vibrio cholerae* and

Table 46–1

Structural Formulas of the Tetracyclines

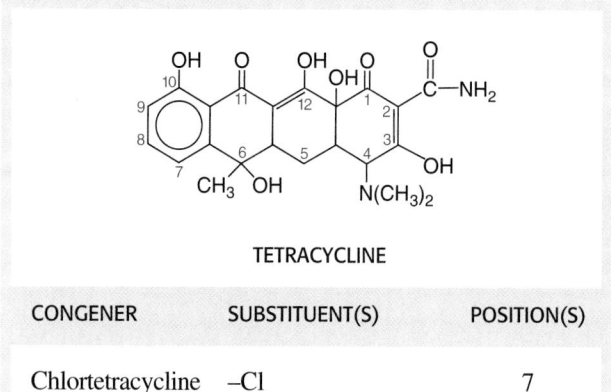

TETRACYCLINE

CONGENER	SUBSTITUENT(S)	POSITION(S)
Chlortetracycline	–Cl	7
Oxytetracycline	–OH,–H	5
Demeclocycline	–OH,–H; –Cl	6; 7
Methacycline	–OH,–H; CH₂	5; 6
Doxycycline	–OH,–H; –CH₃, –H	5; 6
Minocycline	–H,–H; –N(CH₃)₂	6; 7

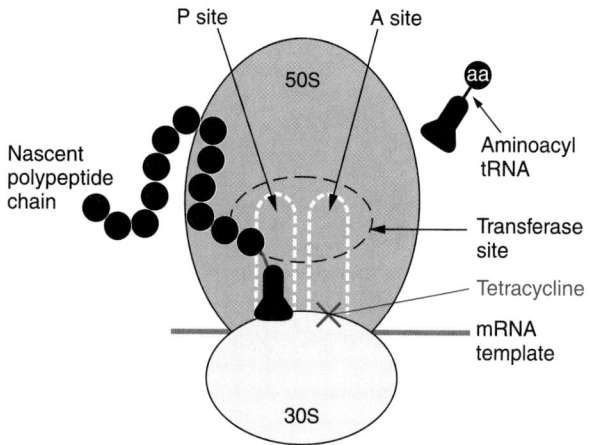

Figure 46–1. *Inhibition of bacterial protein synthesis by tetracyclines.* Messenger RNA (mRNA) attaches to the 30S subunit of bacterial ribosomal RNA. The P (peptidyl) site of the 50S ribosomal RNA subunit contains the nascent polypeptide chain; normally, the aminoacyl tRNA charged with the next amino acid (aa) to be added to the chain moves into the A (acceptor) site, with complementary base pairing between the anticodon sequence of tRNA and the codon sequence of mRNA. *Tetracyclines* inhibit bacterial protein synthesis by binding to the 30S subunit and blocking tRNA binding to the A site.

V. vulnificus, and inhibit the growth of *Legionella pneumophila, Campylobacter jejuni, Helicobacter pylori, Yersinia pestis, Yersinia enterocolitica, Francisella tularensis,* and *Pasteurella multocida.* Strains of *Neisseria gonorrhoeae* no longer are predictably susceptible to tetracycline, which is not recommended for treatment of gonococcal infections. The tetracyclines are active against many anaerobic and facultative microorganisms. The MIC breakpoint for susceptible anaerobic bacteria is 8 μg/ml. A variable number of anaerobes (*e.g., Bacteroides* spp., *Propionibacterium, Peptococcus*) are sensitive to doxycycline, but other antibiotics (*e.g.,* chloramphenicol, clindamycin, *metronidazole,* and certain β-lactam antibiotics) have better activity. Tetracycline is active against *Actinomyces* and is a drug of choice for treating actinomycosis.

Rickettsiae. All tetracyclines are highly effective against the rickettsiae responsible for Rocky Mountain spotted fever, murine typhus, epidemic typhus, scrub typhus, rickettsialpox, and Q fever (*C. burnetii*).

Miscellaneous Microorganisms. The tetracyclines are active against many spirochetes, including *Borrelia recurrentis, Borrelia burgdorferi* (Lyme disease), *Treponema pallidum* (syphilis), and *Treponema pertenue.* Tetracyclines are active against *Chlamydia* and *Mycoplasma.* Some nontuberculosis strains of mycobacteria (*e.g., M. marinum*) also are susceptible.

Effects on Intestinal Flora. Many of the tetracyclines are incompletely absorbed from the gastrointestinal tract, and high concentrations in the bowel can markedly alter enteric flora. Sensitive aerobic and anaerobic coliform microorganisms and gram-positive spore-forming bacteria are suppressed markedly during long-term tetracycline regimens. As the fecal coliform count declines, overgrowth of tetracycline-resistant microorganisms occurs, particularly of yeasts (*Candida* spp.), enterococci, *Proteus,* and *Pseudomonas.* Tetracycline occasionally produces pseudomembranous colitis caused by *Clostridium difficile.*

Mechanism of Action.

Tetracyclines inhibit bacterial protein synthesis by binding to the 30S bacterial ribosome and preventing access of aminoacyl tRNA to the acceptor (A) site on the mRNA-ribosome complex (Figure 46–1). These drugs enter gram-negative bacteria by passive diffusion through the hydrophilic channels formed by the porin proteins of the outer cell membrane and by active transport *via* an energy-dependent system that pumps all tetracyclines across the cytoplasmic membrane. Entry of these drugs into gram-positive bacteria requires metabolic energy, but is not as well understood.

Resistance to the Tetracyclines.

Resistance is primarily plasmid-mediated and often is inducible. The three main resistance mechanisms are: (1) decreased accumulation of tetracycline as a result of either decreased antibiotic influx or acquisition of an energy-dependent efflux pathway; (2) production of a ribosomal protection protein that displaces tetracycline from its target, a "protection" that also may occur by mutation; and (3) enzymatic inactivation of tetracyclines. Cross resistance, or lack thereof, among tetracyclines depends on which mechanism is operative. For example, *S. aureus* strains that are tetracycline-resistant on the basis of efflux mediated by *tetK* still may be susceptible to minocycline. Tetracycline resistance due to a ribosomal protection mechanism (*tetM*) produces cross-resistance to doxycycline and minocycline because the target site protected is the same for all tetracyclines.

The glycylcyclines are synthetic analogues of the tetracyclines, with the most promising compound being the *9-tert*-butyl-glyclyamido derivative of minocycline, *tigecycline*. The glycylcyclines exhibit antibacterial activities typical of earlier tetracyclines, and also display activity against tetracycline-resistant organisms containing genes responsible for efflux mechanisms or ribosomal protection. The glycyclcyclines also appear to be active against other resistant pathogens including methicillin-resistant *S. aureus* and *S. epidermidis*, penicillin-resistant *S. pneumoniae*, and vancomycin-resistant enterococci.

Absorption, Distribution, and Excretion. **Absorption.** Oral absorption of most tetracyclines is incomplete. The percentage of an oral dose that is absorbed with an empty stomach is low for chlortetracycline (30%); intermediate for oxytetracycline, demeclocycline, and tetracycline (60% to 80%); and high for doxycycline (95%) and minocycline (100%). The percentage of unabsorbed drug rises as the dose increases. Absorption mostly takes place in the stomach and upper small intestine and is greater in the fasting state. Absorption of tetracyclines is impaired by the concurrent ingestion of dairy products; aluminum hydroxide gels; calcium, magnesium, and iron or zinc salts; and bismuth subsalicylate. Thus, milk, milk products, antacids, Pepto-Bismol, and dietary Fe and Zn supplements will interfere with tetracycline absorption. The decreased absorption apparently results from chelation of divalent and trivalent cations.

Variable absorption of orally administered tetracyclines leads to a wide range of plasma concentrations in different individuals. Oxytetracycline and tetracycline are incompletely absorbed. After a single oral dose, the peak plasma concentration is attained in 2 to 4 hours. These drugs have half-lives in the range of 6 to 12 hours and frequently are administered two to four times daily. The administration of 250 mg every 6 hours produces peak plasma concentrations of 2 to 2.5 μg/ml. Increasing the dosage above 1 g every 6 hours does not further increase plasma concentrations. Demeclocycline, which also is incompletely absorbed, can be administered in lower daily dosages than the above-mentioned congeners because its half-life of 16 hours provides effective plasma concentrations for 24 to 48 hours.

Oral doses of oxycycline and minocycline are well absorbed (90% to 100%) and have half-lives of 16 to 18 hours; they therefore can be administered less frequently and at lower doses than tetracycline, oxytetracycline, or demeclocycline. After an oral dose of 200 mg of doxycycline, a maximum plasma concentration of 3 μg/ml is achieved at 2 hours, and the plasma concentration remains above 1 μg/ml for 8 to 12 hours. Plasma concentrations are equivalent whether doxycycline is given orally or parenterally. Food, including dairy products, does not interfere with the absorption of doxycycline or minocycline.

Distribution. Tetracyclines distribute widely throughout the body and into tissues and secretions, including urine and prostate. They accumulate in reticuloendothelial cells of the liver, spleen, and bone marrow, and in bone, dentine, and enamel of unerupted teeth (*see* below).

Inflammation of the meninges is not required for the passage of tetracyclines into the cerebrospinal fluid (CSF). Penetration of these drugs into most other fluids and tissues is excellent. Concentrations in synovial fluid and the mucosa of the maxillary sinus approach that in plasma. Tetracyclines cross the placenta and enter the fetal circulation and amniotic fluid. Relative to the maternal circulation, tetracycline concentrations in umbilical cord plasma and amniotic fluid are 60% and 20%, respectively. Relatively high concentrations of these drugs also are found in breast milk.

Excretion. With the exception of doxycycline, the primary route of elimination for most tetracyclines is the kidney, although they also are concentrated in the liver and excreted in bile. After biliary excretion, they are partially reabsorbed *via* enterohepatic recirculation. Elimination *via* the intestinal tract occurs even when the drugs are given parenterally. Minocycline is an exception and is significantly metabolized by the liver. Comparable amounts of tetracycline (*i.e.*, 20% to 60%) are excreted in the urine within 24 hours following oral or intravenous administration. Approximately 10% to 35% of a dose of oxytetracycline is excreted in active form in the urine, where it can be detected within 30 minutes and reaches a peak concentration about 5 hours after administration. The rate of renal clearance of demeclocycline is less than half that of tetracycline. Decreased hepatic function or obstruction of the common bile duct reduces the biliary excretion of these agents, resulting in longer half-lives and higher plasma concentrations. Because of their enterohepatic circulation, these drugs may remain in the body for a long time after cessation of therapy.

Minocycline is recovered from urine and feces in significantly lower amounts than are the other tetracyclines, and it appears to be metabolized to a considerable extent. Renal clearance of minocycline is low. The drug persists in the body long after its administration is stopped, possibly due to retention in fatty tissues. Nonetheless, the half-life of minocycline is not prolonged in patients with hepatic failure.

Doxycycline at recommended doses does not accumulate significantly in patients with renal failure and thus is one of the safest of the tetracyclines for use in patients with renal impairment. The drug is excreted in the feces. Its half-life may be significantly shortened by concurrent therapy with barbiturates, phenytoin, rifampin, or other inducers of hepatic microsomal enzymes.

Routes of Administration and Dosage. A wide variety of tetracyclines are available for oral, parenteral, and topical administration. As indicated earlier, only tetracycline, oxytetracycline (TERRAMYCIN, others), demeclocycline (DECLOMYCIN), minocycline (MINOCIN, others), and doxycycline (VIBRAMYCIN, others) are available in the United States.

Oral Administration. The oral dose of tetracycline ranges from 1 to 2 g per day in adults. Children older than 8 years of age should receive 25 to 50 mg/kg daily in two to four divided doses. The recommended dose of demeclocycline is 150 mg every 6 hours or 300 mg every 12 hours for adults and 6 to 12 mg/kg in two to four divided doses for children older than 8 years of age. Demeclocycline is used rarely as an antimicrobial agent because of its higher risks of photosensitivity reactions and nephrogenic diabetes insipidus (*see* Untoward Effects, below). The dose of doxycycline for adults is 100 mg 12 hours apart on the first day and then 100 mg once a day, or twice daily when severe infection is present; for children older than 8 years of age the dose is 4 to 5 mg/kg per day in two divided doses the first day, then 2 to 2.5 mg/kg given once or twice daily. The dose of minocycline for adults is 200 mg initially, followed by 100 mg every 12 hours; for children, it is 4 mg/kg initially followed by 2 mg/kg every 12 hours.

Gastrointestinal distress, nausea, and vomiting can be minimized by administration of tetracyclines with food. As mentioned previously, dairy products; antacids containing calcium, aluminum, zinc, magnesium, or silicate; vitamins with iron; sulcralfate (which contains aluminum); and bismuth subsalicylate will interfere with tetracycline absorption and should be avoided (*see* Chapter 36). Cholestyramine and colestipol also bind orally administered tetracyclines and interfere with their absorption. Generally, tetracyclines should be administered 2 hours before or 2 hours after meals and other drugs that interfere with their absorption.

Parenteral Administration. Doxycycline, the preferred parenteral tetracycline in the United States, is indicated in severe illness, in patients unable to ingest medication, or when the oral drug causes significant nausea and vomiting. Tetracyclines should not be administered intramuscularly because of local irritation and poor absorption.

The usual intravenous dose of doxycycline is 200 mg in one or two infusions on the first day and 100 mg once or twice daily on subsequent days. For children who weigh less than 45 kg, the dose is 4.4 mg/kg on the first day, after which it is reduced by half. The total daily dose of intravenous tetracycline (no longer available in the United States) for most acute infections is 1 g (or 2 g for severe infection), divided into equal doses and administered at 6- or 12-hour intervals. This dose, which should not be exceeded, may cause adverse effects in some patients (*see* Toxic Effects). The low pH of tetracycline, but not doxycycline or minocycline, invariably causes phlebitis if infused into a peripheral vein. The intravenous dose of minocycline for adults is 200 mg, followed by 100 mg every 12 hours. Children older than 8 years of age should receive an initial dose of 4 mg/kg, followed by 2 mg/kg every 12 hours. Each 100 mg of minocycline must be diluted with 500 to 1000 ml of compatible fluid and slowly infused over 6 hours to minimize toxicity.

Local Application. Except for local use in the eye, topical use of the tetracyclines is not recommended. Their use in ophthalmic therapy is discussed in Chapter 63. Minocycline sustained-release microspheres for subgingival administration are used in dentistry as an adjunct to scaling and root planing procedures to reduce pocket depth in patients with adult periodontitis.

Therapeutic Uses. The tetracyclines have been used extensively to treat infectious diseases and as an additive to animal feeds to facilitate growth. These uses have increased bacterial resistance to tetracyclines, but the drugs remain useful for infections caused by rickettsiae, mycoplasmas, and chlamydiae. Doxycycline is useful for treatment of respiratory tract infections because it covers atypical organisms and because respiratory pathogens increasingly are resistant to other drug classes.

Rickettsial Infections. Tetracyclines are effective and may be life-saving in rickettsial infections, including Rocky Mountain spotted fever, recrudescent epidemic typhus (Brill's disease), murine typhus, scrub typhus, rickettsialpox, and Q fever. Clinical improvement often is evident within 24 hours after initiation of therapy. Doxycycline is the drug of choice for treatment of suspected or proven Rocky Mountain spotted fever in adults and in children, including those younger than 9 years of age, in whom the risk of staining of permanent teeth is outweighed by the seriousness of this potentially fatal infection (Masters *et al.*, 2003).

Mycoplasma Infections. *Mycoplasma pneumoniae* is sensitive to the tetracyclines. Treatment of pneumonia with tetracycline shortens the duration of fever, cough, malaise, fatigue, pulmonary rales, and radiological abnormalities in the lungs. Mycoplasma may persist in the sputum after cessation of therapy, despite rapid resolution of the active infection.

Chlamydia. *Lymphogranuloma Venereum.* Doxycycline (100 mg twice daily for 21 days) is first-line therapy for treatment of this infection. The size of buboes decreases within 4 days, and inclusion and elementary bodies entirely disappear from the lymph nodes within one week. Rectal pain, discharge, and bleeding of lymphogranulomatous proctitis are decreased markedly. When relapses occur, treatment is resumed with full doses and is continued for longer periods.

Pneumonia, bronchitis, or sinusitis caused by *Chlamydia pneumoniae* responds to tetracycline therapy. The tetracyclines also are of value in cases of psittacosis. Drug therapy for 10 to 14 days usually is adequate.

Trachoma. Doxycycline (100 mg twice daily for 14 days) or tetracycline (250 mg four times daily for 14 days) is effective for this infection. However, this disease is important in early childhood before the complete calcification of the permanent teeth, and tetracyclines therefore often are contraindicated (*see* "Untoward Effects," below). *Azithromycin* (*see* section on macrolides), which is effective as a single dose, is preferred.

Nonspecific Urethritis. Nonspecific urethritis is often due to *Chlamydia trachomatis.* Doxycycline, 100 mg every 12 hours for 7 days, is effective; however, azithromycin is usually preferred because it can be given as a single 1-g dose.

Sexually Transmitted Diseases. Because of resistance, doxycycline no longer is recommended for gonococcal infections. If coinfection with *C. trachomatis* has not been excluded, then either doxycycline or azithromycin should be administered in addition to an agent effective for gonococcal urethritis (Centers for Disease Control and Prevention, 2002).

C. trachomatis often is a coexistent pathogen in acute pelvic inflammatory disease, including endometritis, salpingitis, parametritis, and/or peritonitis. Doxycycline, 100 mg intravenously twice daily, is recommended for at least 48 hours after substantial clinical improvement, followed by oral therapy at the same dosage to complete a 14-day course. Doxycycline usually is combined with *cefoxitin* or *cefotetan* (*see* Chapter 44) to cover anaerobes and facultative aerobes.

Acute epididymitis is caused by infection with *C. trachomatis* or *N. gonorrhoeae* in men less than 35 years of age. Effective regimens include a single injection of ceftriaxone (250 mg) plus doxycycline, 100 mg orally twice daily for 10 days. Sexual partners of patients with any of the above conditions also should be treated.

Nonpregnant, penicillin-allergic patients who have primary, secondary, or latent syphilis can be treated with a tetracycline regimen such as doxycycline 100 mg orally twice daily for 2 weeks. Tetracyclines should not be used for treatment of neurosyphilis.

Anthrax. Doxycycline 100 mg every 12 hours (2.2 mg/kg every 12 hours for children weighing less than 45 kg) is indicated for prevention or treatment of anthrax. It should be used in combination with another agent when treating inhalational or gastrointestinal infection. The recommended duration of therapy is 60 days for exposures occurring as an act of bioterrorism.

Bacillary Infections. *Brucellosis.* Tetracyclines in combination with rifampin or streptomycin are effective for acute and chronic infections caused by *Brucella melitensis, Brucella suis,* and *Brucella abortus.* Effective regimens are doxycycline, 200 mg per day, plus rifampin, 600 to 900 mg daily for 6 weeks, or the usual dose of doxycycline plus streptomycin 1 g daily, intramuscularly. Relapses usually respond to a second course of therapy.

Tularemia. Although streptomycin is preferable, tetracyclines also are effective in tularemia (Ellis *et al.,* 2002). Both the ulceroglandular and typhoidal types of the disease respond well.

Cholera. Doxycycline (300 mg as a single dose) is effective in reducing stool volume and eradicating *Vibrio cholerae* from the stool within 48 hours. Antimicrobial agents, however, are not substitutes for fluid and electrolyte replacement in this disease. In addition, some strains of *V. cholerae* are resistant to tetracyclines.

Other Bacillary Infections. Therapy with the tetracyclines is often ineffective in infections caused by *Shigella, Salmonella,* or other Enterobacteriaceae because of a high prevalence of drug-resistant strains in many areas. Resistance limits the usefulness of tetracyclines for travelers' diarrhea.

Coccal Infections. Because of resistance, tetracyclines fell into disuse for infections caused by staphylococci, streptococci, or meningococci. However, community strains of methicillin-resistant *S. aureus* often are susceptible to tetracycline, doxycycline, or minocycline, which appear to be effective for uncomplicated skin and soft-tissue infections. Approximately 85% of strains of *S. pneumoniae* are susceptible to tetracyclines, and doxycycline remains an effective agent for empirical therapy of community-acquired pneumonia (Bartlett *et al.,* 1998).

Urinary Tract Infections. Tetracyclines are no longer recommended for routine treatment of urinary tract infections because many enteric organisms that cause these infections, including *E. coli,* are resistant.

Other Infections. Actinomycosis, although most responsive to *penicillin G,* may be successfully treated with a tetracycline. Minocycline is an alternative for the treatment of nocardiosis, but a sulfonamide should be used concurrently. Yaws and relapsing fever respond favorably to the tetracyclines. Tetracyclines are useful in the acute treatment and for prophylaxis of leptospirosis (*Leptospira* spp.). *Borrelia* spp., including *B. recurrentis* (relapsing fever) and *B. burgdorferi* (Lyme disease), respond to therapy with a tetracycline. The tetracyclines have been used to treat susceptible atypical mycobacterial pathogens, including *M. marinum*.

Acne. Tetracyclines have been used to treat acne. They may act by inhibiting propionibacteria, which reside in sebaceous follicles and metabolize lipids into irritating free fatty acids. The relatively low doses of tetracycline used for acne (*e.g.*, 250 mg orally twice a day) apparently are associated with few side effects.

Untoward Effects. **Toxic Effects.** *Gastrointestinal.* All tetracyclines can produce gastrointestinal irritation, most commonly after oral administration. Epigastric burning and distress, abdominal discomfort, nausea, vomiting, and diarrhea may occur. Tolerability can be improved by administering the drug with food, but tetracyclines should not be taken with dairy products or antacids. Tetracycline has been associated with esophagitis, esophageal ulcers, and pancreatitis. *Pseudomembranous colitis caused by overgrowth of* Clostridium difficile *is a potentially life-threatening complication* (*see* below).

Photosensitivity. Demeclocycline, doxycycline, and other tetracyclines to a lesser extent may produce mild-to-severe photosensitivity reactions in the skin of treated individuals exposed to sunlight. Onycholysis and pigmentation of the nails may develop with or without accompanying photosensitivity.

Hepatic Toxicity. Oxytetracycline and tetracycline are the least hepatotoxic of these agents. Hepatic toxicity typically develops in patients receiving 2 g or more of drug per day parenterally, but this effect also may occur when large quantities are administered orally. Pregnant women are particularly susceptible to tetracycline-induced hepatic damage.

Renal Toxicity. Tetracyclines may aggravate azotemia in patients with renal disease because of their catabolic effects. Doxycycline has fewer renal side effects than do other tetracyclines. Nephrogenic diabetes insipidus has been observed in some patients receiving demeclocycline, and this phenomenon has been exploited for the treatment of the syndrome of inappropriate secretion of antidiuretic hormone (*see* Chapter 29).

Fanconi syndrome, characterized by nausea, vomiting, polyuria, polydipsia, proteinuria, acidosis, glycosuria, and aminoaciduria, has been observed in patients ingesting outdated and degraded tetracycline. These symptoms presumably result from a toxic effect on proximal renal tubules.

Effects on Teeth. Children receiving long- or short-term therapy with a tetracycline may develop permanent brown discoloration of the teeth. The larger the drug dose relative to body weight, the more intense the enamel discoloration. The duration of therapy appears to be less important than the total quantity of antibiotic administered. The risk of this untoward effect is highest when a tetracycline is given to neonates and babies before the first dentition. However, pigmentation of the permanent teeth may develop if the drug is given between the ages of 2 months and 5 years, when these teeth are being calcified. The deposition of the drug in the teeth and bones probably is due to its chelating property and the formation of a tetracycline–calcium orthophosphate complex.

Treatment of pregnant patients with tetracyclines may produce discoloration of the teeth in their children. The period of greatest danger to the teeth is from midpregnancy to about 4 to 6 months of the postnatal period for the deciduous anterior teeth, and from a few months to 5 years of age for the permanent anterior teeth, when the crowns are being formed. However, children up to 8 years old may be susceptible to this complication of tetracycline therapy.

Miscellaneous Effects. Tetracyclines are deposited in the skeleton during gestation and throughout childhood and may depress bone growth in premature infants. This is readily reversible if the period of exposure to the drug is short.

Thrombophlebitis frequently follows intravenous administration. This irritative effect of tetracyclines has been used therapeutically in patients with malignant pleural effusions, where drug is instilled into the pleural space in a procedure called pleurodesis.

Long-term tetracycline therapy may produce leukocytosis, atypical lymphocytes, toxic granulation of granulocytes, and thrombocytopenic purpura.

The tetracyclines may cause increased intracranial pressure (pseudotumor cerebri) in young infants, even when given in the usual therapeutic doses. Except for the elevated pressure, the spinal fluid is normal. The pressure promptly returns to normal when therapy is discontinued, and this complication rarely occurs in older individuals.

Patients receiving minocycline may experience vestibular toxicity, manifested by dizziness, ataxia, nausea, and vomiting. The symptoms occur soon after the initial dose and generally disappear within 24 to 48 hours after drug administration is stopped. Long-term use of minocycline can pigment the skin, producing a brownish discoloration. Doxycycline currently is being studied as an inhibitor of matrix metalloproteinases (Villareal *et al.*, 2003), an action unrelated to its effects on bacterial protein synthesis.

Hypersensitivity Reactions. Various skin reactions, including morbilliform rashes, urticaria, fixed drug eruptions, and generalized exfoliative dermatitis, rarely may follow the use of any of the tetracyclines. Among the more severe allergic responses are angioedema and anaphylaxis; anaphylactoid reactions can occur even after the oral use of these agents. Other hypersensitivity reactions are burning of the eyes, cheilosis, atrophic or hypertrophic glossitis, pruritus ani or vulvae, and vaginitis. Although the exact cause of these reactions is unknown, they can persist for weeks or months after cessation of tetracycline therapy. Fever of varying degrees and eosinophilia may occur when these agents are administered. Asthma also has been observed. Cross-sensitization among the various tetracyclines is common.

Biological Effects Other Than Allergic or Toxic. Like all antimicrobial agents, the tetracyclines administered orally or parenterally may lead to the development of superinfections caused by strains of bacteria or fungi resistant to these agents. Vaginal, oral, and even systemic infections are observed. The incidence of these infections appears to be much higher with the tetracyclines than with the penicillins.

Pseudomembranous colitis, caused by an overgrowth of toxin-producing *C. difficile,* is characterized by severe diarrhea, fever, and stools containing shreds of mucous membrane and a large number of neutrophils. The toxin is cytotoxic to mucosal cells and causes shallow ulcerations that can be seen by sigmoidoscopy. Discontinuation of the drug, combined with the oral administration of metronidazole, usually is curative.

To decrease the incidence of toxic effects, observe the following precautions in the use of the tetracyclines: Do not administer them to pregnant patients; do not use them for treatment of common infections in children younger than 8 years of age; and discard unused supplies of these antibiotics. Inform patients of these precautions.

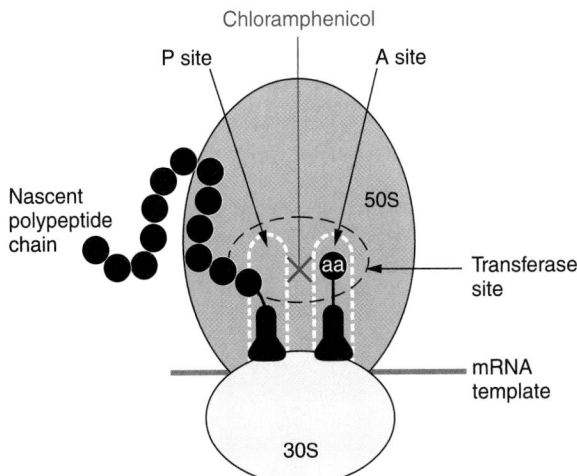

Figure 46–2. Inhibition of bacterial protein synthesis by chloramphenicol. Chloramphenicol binds to the 50S ribosomal subunit at the peptidyltransferase site and inhibits the transpeptidation reaction. Chloramphenicol binds to the 50S ribosomal subunit near the site of action of clindamycin and the macrolide antibiotics. These agents interfere with the binding of chloramphenicol and thus may interfere with each other's actions if given concurrently. *See* Figure 46–1 and its legend for additional information.

CHLORAMPHENICOL

History and Source. Chloramphenicol, an antibiotic produced by *Streptomyces venezuelae,* was introduced into clinical practice in 1948. With the drug's wide use, it became evident that chloramphenicol could cause serious and fatal blood dyscrasias. For this reason, chloramphenicol is now reserved for treatment of life-threatening infections (*e.g.*, meningitis, rickettsial infections) in patients who cannot take safer alternatives because of resistance or allergies (Wareham and Wilson, 2002).

Chemistry. Chloramphenicol has the following structural formula:

$$O_2N-\text{\textbigcirc}-\underset{\underset{\text{CHLORAMPHENICOL}}{}}{\overset{\overset{OH}{|}}{C}H}\overset{\overset{CH_2OH}{|}}{C}H-NH-\overset{\overset{O}{\|}}{C}-CHCl_2$$

The antibiotic is unique among natural compounds in that it contains a nitrobenzene moiety and is a derivative of dichloroacetic acid. The biologically active form is levorotatory.

Mechanism of Action. Chloramphenicol inhibits protein synthesis in bacteria, and to a lesser extent, in eukaryotic cells. The drug readily penetrates bacterial cells, probably by facilitated diffusion. Chloramphenicol acts primarily by binding reversibly to the 50S ribosomal sub-

unit (near the binding site for the macrolide antibiotics and clindamycin, which chloramphenicol inhibits competitively). Although binding of tRNA at the codon recognition site on the 30S ribosomal subunit is undisturbed, the drug apparently prevents the binding of the amino acid–containing end of the aminoacyl tRNA to the acceptor site on the 50S ribosomal subunit. The interaction between peptidyltransferase and its amino acid substrate cannot occur, and peptide bond formation is inhibited (Figure 46–2).

Chloramphenicol also can inhibit mitochondrial protein synthesis in mammalian cells, perhaps because mitochondrial ribosomes resemble bacterial ribosomes (both are 70S) more than they do the 80S cytoplasmic ribosomes of mammalian cells. The peptidyltransferase of mitochondrial ribosomes, but not of cytoplasmic ribosomes, is inhibited by chloramphenicol. Mammalian erythropoietic cells are particularly sensitive to the drug.

Antimicrobial Actions. Chloramphenicol possesses a broad spectrum of antimicrobial activity. Strains are considered sensitive if they are inhibited by concentrations of 8 μg/ml or less, except *N. gonorrhoeae, S. pneumoniae,* and *H. influenzae,* which have lower MIC breakpoints. Chloramphenicol is bacteriostatic against most species, although it may be bactericidal against *H. influenzae, Neisseria meningitidis,* and *S. pneumoniae.* More than 95% of strains of the following gram-negative bacteria are inhibited *in vitro* by 8 μg/ml or less of chloramphenicol: *H. influenzae, N. meningitidis, N. gonorrhoeae, Brucella* spp., and *Bordetella pertussis*. Likewise, most anaerobic bacteria, including gram-positive cocci and *Clostridium* spp., and gram-negative rods including *B. fragilis*, are inhibited by this concentration of the drug. Some aerobic gram-positive cocci, including *Streptococcus pyogenes, Streptococcus agalactiae* (group B streptococci), and *S. pneumoniae*, are sensitive to 8 μg/ml. Strains of *S. aureus* tend to be less susceptible, with MICs greater than 8 μg/ml. Chloramphenicol is active against *Mycoplasma, Chlamydia*, and *Rickettsia*.

The Enterobacteriaceae are variably sensitive to chloramphenicol. Most strains of *Escherichia coli* (75% or more) and *Klebsiella pneumoniae* are susceptible. *Proteus mirabilis* and indole-positive *Proteus* spp. are susceptible. *P. aeruginosa* is resistant to even very high concentrations of chloramphenicol. Strains of *V. cholerae* have remained largely susceptible to chloramphenicol. Strains of *Shigella* and *Salmonella* resistant to multiple drugs, including chloramphenicol, are prevalent. Of special concern is the increasing prevalence of multiple-drug-resistant strains of *Salmonella* serotype typhi, particularly for strains acquired outside the United States.

Resistance to Chloramphenicol. Resistance to chloramphenicol usually is caused by a plasmid-encoded acetyltransferase that inactivates the drug. Resistance also can result from decreased permeability and from ribosomal mutation. Acetylated derivatives of chloramphenicol fail to bind to bacterial ribosomes.

Absorption, Distribution, Fate, and Excretion.   Chloramphenicol (CHLOROMYCETIN) is absorbed rapidly from the gastrointestinal tract, and peak concentrations of 10 to 13 μg/ml occur within 2 to 3 hours after the administration of a 1-g dose. The preparation of chloramphenicol for parenteral use is the water-soluble, inactive prodrug sodium succinate. Similar concentrations of chloramphenicol succinate in plasma are achieved after intravenous and intramuscular administration. Hydrolysis of chloramphenicol succinate by esterases occurs *in vivo*. Chloramphenicol succinate is rapidly cleared from plasma by the kidneys; this may reduce overall bioavailability of the drug, since as much as 30% of the dose may be excreted before hydrolysis. Poor renal function in the neonate and other states of renal insufficiency result in increased plasma concentrations of chloramphenicol succinate. Decreased esterase activity has been observed in the plasma of neonates and infants, prolonging time to peak concentrations of active chloramphenicol (up to 4 hours) and extending the period over which renal clearance of chloramphenicol succinate can occur.

Chloramphenicol is widely distributed in body fluids and readily reaches therapeutic concentrations in CSF, where values are approximately 60% of those in plasma (range, 45% to 99%) in the presence or absence of meningitis. The drug actually may accumulate in the brain. Chloramphenicol is present in bile, milk, and placental fluid. It also is found in the aqueous humor after subconjunctival injection.

Hepatic metabolism to the inactive glucuronide is the major route of elimination. This metabolite and chloramphenicol itself are excreted in the urine following filtration and secretion. Patients with cirrhosis or otherwise impaired hepatic function have decreased metabolic clearance, and dosage should be adjusted in these individuals. The half-life of chloramphenicol correlates with plasma bilirubin concentrations. About 50% of chloramphenicol is bound to plasma proteins; such binding is reduced in cirrhotic patients and in neonates. Half-life is not altered significantly by renal insufficiency or hemodialysis, and dosage adjustment usually is not required. However, if the dose of chloramphenicol has been reduced because of cirrhosis, clearance by hemodialysis may be significant. This effect can be minimized by administering the drug at the end of hemodialysis. Significant variability in the metabolism and pharmacokinetics of chloramphenicol in neonates, infants, and children necessitates monitoring of drug concentrations in plasma.

Therapeutic Uses. *Therapy with chloramphenicol must be limited to infections for which the benefits of the drug outweigh the risks of the potential toxicities. When other antimicrobial drugs that are equally effective and potentially less toxic are available, they should be used instead of chloramphenicol (Wareham and Wilson, 2002).*

Typhoid Fever. Third-generation cephalosporins and quinolones are drugs of choice for the treatment of typhoid fever because they are less toxic and because many strains of *Salmonella typhi* often are resistant to chloramphenicol (Parry, 2003).

The adult dose of chloramphenicol for typhoid fever is 1 g every 6 hours for 4 weeks. Although intravenous and oral routes have been used, the response is more rapid with oral administration. Provided that the primary isolate is sensitive, relapses respond satisfactorily to retreatment.

Bacterial Meningitis. Third-generation cephalosporins have replaced chloramphenicol in the therapy of bacterial meningitis (Quagliarello and Scheld, 1997). Chloramphenicol remains an alternative drug for the treatment of meningitis caused by *H. influenzae, N. meningitidis,* and *S. pneumoniae* in patients who have severe allergy to β-lactams and in developing countries (Fuller *et al.*, 2003). The total daily dose for children should be 50 to 75 mg/kg of body weight, divided into four equal doses given intravenously every 6 hours for 2 weeks. Results with chloramphenicol used for pneumococcal meningitis may be unsatisfactory, because some strains are inhibited but not killed. Moreover, penicillin-resistant strains frequently also are resistant to chloramphenicol (Hoban *et al.*, 2001). In the rare situation in which chloramphenicol must be used to treat pneumococcal meningitis, lumbar puncture should be repeated 2 to 3 days after treatment is initiated to ensure that an adequate response has occurred. Higher doses of chloramphenicol (100 mg/kg per day) sometimes may be required.

Anaerobic Infections. Chloramphenicol is quite effective against most anaerobic bacteria, including *Bacteroides* spp., and it is effective for treatment of serious intra-abdominal infections or brain abscesses. However, equally effective and less toxic alternatives are available, and chloramphenicol is rarely indicated.

Rickettsial Diseases. The tetracyclines usually are the preferred agents for the treatment of rickettsial diseases. However, in patients allergic to these drugs, in those with reduced renal function, in pregnant women, and in children younger than 8 years of age who require prolonged or repeated courses of therapy, chloramphenicol may be the drug of choice. Rocky Mountain spotted fever, epidemic, murine, scrub, and recrudescent typhus, and Q fever respond well to chloramphenicol. For adults, a dose of 50 mg/kg per day is recommended for all the rickettsial diseases. The daily dose of chloramphenicol for children with these diseases is 75 mg/kg, divided into equal portions and given every 6 to 8 hours; if chloramphenicol palmitate is used (not available in the United States), the daily maintenance dose may be as high as 100 mg/kg, given at the same intervals. Therapy should be continued until the general condition has improved and the patient is afebrile for 24 to 48 hours.

Brucellosis. Chloramphenicol is not as effective as the tetracyclines in the treatment of brucellosis. When a tetracycline is contraindicated, 750 to 1000 mg of chloramphenicol orally every 6 hours is recommended. Relapses usually respond to retreatment.

Untoward Effects.
Chloramphenicol inhibits the synthesis of proteins of the inner mitochondrial membrane, probably by inhibiting the ribosomal peptidyltransferase. These include subunits of cytochrome *c* oxidase, ubiquinone-cytochrome *c* reductase, and the proton-translocating ATPase critical for aerobic metabolism. Much of the toxicity observed with this drug can be attributed to these effects.

Hypersensitivity Reactions. Although relatively uncommon, macular or vesicular skin rashes result from hypersensitivity to chloramphenicol. Fever may appear simultaneously or be the sole manifestation. Angioedema is a rare complication. Jarisch-Herxheimer reactions may occur after institution of chloramphenicol therapy for syphilis, brucellosis, and typhoid fever.

Hematological Toxicity. The most important adverse effect of chloramphenicol is on the bone marrow. Chloramphenicol affects the hematopoietic system in two ways: a dose-related toxicity that presents as anemia, leukopenia, or thrombocytopenia; and an idiosyncratic response manifested by aplastic anemia, leading in many cases to fatal pancytopenia. Pancytopenia seems to occur more commonly in individuals who undergo prolonged therapy and especially in those who are exposed to the drug on more than one occasion. A genetic predisposition is suggested by the occurrence of pancytopenia in identical twins. Although the incidence of the reaction is low— 1 in approximately 30,000 or more courses of therapy— the fatality rate is high when bone-marrow aplasia is complete, and there is an increased incidence of acute leukemia in those who recover. Aplastic anemia accounts for approximately 70% of cases of blood dyscrasias due to chloramphenicol, while hypoplastic anemia, agranulocy-

tosis, and thrombocytopenia make up the remainder. The exact biochemical mechanism has not yet been elucidated but is hypothesized to involve conversion of the nitro group to a toxic intermediate by intestinal bacteria.

The risk of aplastic anemia does not contraindicate the use of chloramphenicol in situations in which it may be life-saving. The drug should never be used, however, in undefined situations or in diseases readily, safely, and effectively treatable with other antimicrobial agents.

Dose-related, reversible erythroid suppression probably reflects an inhibitory action of chloramphenicol on mitochondrial protein synthesis in erythroid precursors, which in turn impairs iron incorporation into heme. Leukopenia and thrombocytopenia also may occur. Bone marrow suppression occurs regularly when plasma concentrations are 25 μg/ml or higher and is observed with the use of large doses of chloramphenicol, prolonged treatment, or both. Dose-related suppression of the bone marrow may progress to fatal aplasia if treatment is continued, but most cases of bone marrow aplasia develop suddenly, without prior dose-related marrow suppression. Some patients who developed chronic bone marrow hypoplasia after chloramphenicol treatment subsequently developed acute myeloblastic leukemia.

The administration of chloramphenicol in the presence of hepatic disease frequently depresses erythropoiesis. About one-third of patients with severe renal insufficiency exhibit the same reaction.

Toxic and Irritative Effects. Nausea and vomiting, unpleasant taste, diarrhea, and perineal irritation may follow the oral administration of chloramphenicol. Among the rare toxic effects produced by this antibiotic are blurring of vision and digital paresthesias. Tissues that have a high rate of oxygen consumption may be particularly susceptible to chloramphenicol effects on mitochondrial enzyme systems; encephalopathy and cardiomyopathy have been reported.

Neonates, especially if premature, may develop a serious illness termed *gray baby syndrome* if exposed to excessive doses of chloramphenicol. This syndrome usually begins 2 to 9 days (average of 4 days) after treatment is started. Within the first 24 hours, vomiting, refusal to suck, irregular and rapid respiration, abdominal distention, periods of cyanosis, and passage of loose, green stools occur. The children all are severely ill by the end of the first day, and in the next 24 hours turn an ashen-gray color and become flaccid and hypothermic. A similar "gray syndrome" has been reported in adults who were accidentally overdosed with the drug. Death occurs in about 40% of patients within 2 days of initial symptoms. Those who recover usually exhibit no sequelae.

Two mechanisms apparently are responsible for chloramphenicol toxicity in neonates: (1) a developmental deficiency of glucuronyl transferase, the hepatic enzyme that metabolizes chloramphenicol, in the first 3 to 4 weeks of life; and (2) inadequate renal excretion of unconjugated drug. At the onset of the clinical syndrome, chloramphenicol concentrations in plasma usually exceed 100 $\mu g/$ml, although they may be as low as 75 $\mu g/ml$. Children 2 weeks of age or younger should receive chloramphenicol in a daily dose no larger than 25 mg/kg of body weight; after this age, full-term infants may be given daily quantities up to 50 mg/kg. Toxic effects have not been observed in the newborns when as much as 1 g of the antibiotic has been given every 2 hours to the mothers during labor.

Chloramphenicol is removed only minimally from the blood by either peritoneal dialysis or traditional hemodialysis. Thus, exchange transfusion and charcoal hemoperfusion have been used to treat overdose with chloramphenicol in infants.

Drug Interactions. Chloramphenicol inhibits hepatic cytochrome P450 isozymes (CYPs) and thereby prolongs the half-lives of drugs that are metabolized by this system, including *warfarin, dicumarol, phenytoin, chlorpropamide,* antiretroviral protease inhibitors, *rifabutin,* and *tolbutamide.* Severe toxicity and death have occurred because of failure to recognize such effects.

Conversely, other drugs may alter the elimination of chloramphenicol. Concurrent administration of *phenobarbital* or *rifampin,* which potently induce CYPs, shortens the half-life of the antibiotic and may result in subtherapeutic drug concentrations.

MACROLIDES (ERYTHROMYCIN, CLARITHROMYCIN, AND AZITHROMYCIN)

History and Source. *Erythromycin* was discovered in 1952 by McGuire and coworkers in the metabolic products of a strain of *Streptomyces erythreus. Clarithromycin* and azithromycin are semisynthetic derivatives of erythromycin.

Chemistry. Macrolide antibiotics contain a many-membered lactone ring (14-membered rings for erythromycin and clarithromycin and a 15-membered ring for azithromycin) to which are attached one or more deoxy sugars. Clarithromycin differs from erythromycin only by methylation of the hydroxyl group at the 6 position, and azithromycin differs by the addition of a methyl-substituted nitrogen atom into the lactone ring. These structural modifications improve acid stability and tissue penetration and broaden the spectrum of activity. The structural formulas of the macrolides are as follows:

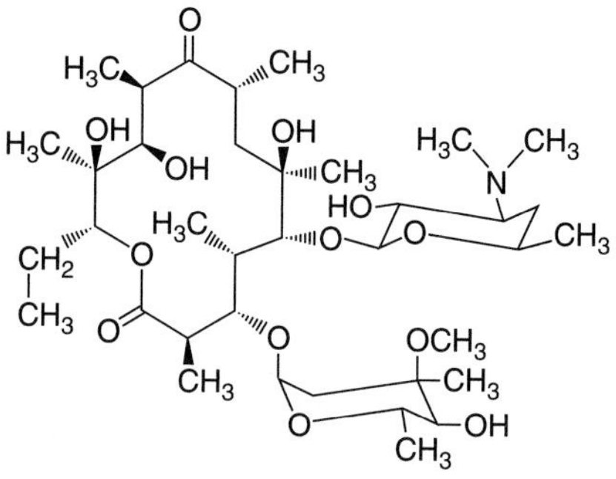

ERYTHROMYCIN

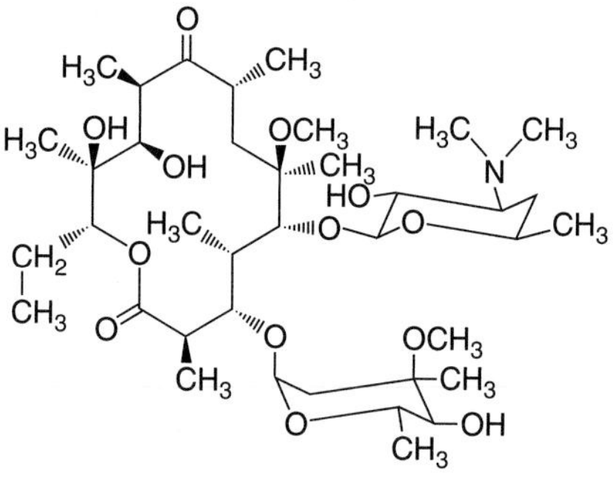

CLARITHROMYCIN

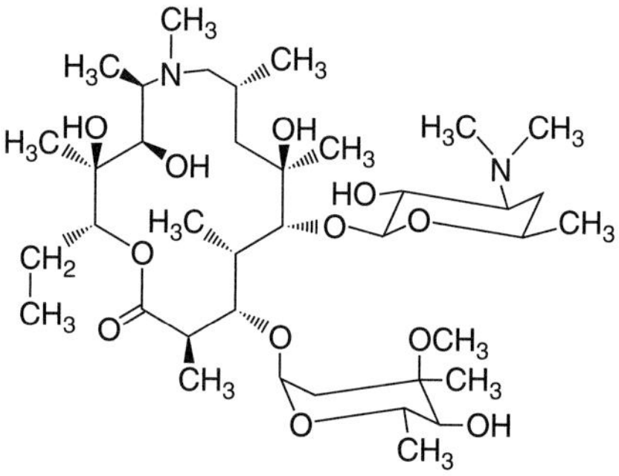

AZITHROMYCIN

Antibacterial Activity. Erythromycin usually is bacteriostatic, but may be bactericidal in high concentrations against very susceptible organisms. The antibiotic is most active *in vitro* against aerobic gram-positive cocci and bacilli. Susceptible strains of *S. pyogenes, S. pneumoniae,* and viridans streptococci have MICs that range from 0.015 to 1 $\mu g/ml$. Macrolide resistance is common among streptococci. Because the mechanisms producing resistance to erythromycin affect all macrolides, cross-resistance among them is complete. The prevalence of macrolide resistance among group A streptococcal isolates, which can be as high as 40%, is related to consumption of macrolide antibiotics within the population. Macrolide resistance among *S. pneumoniae* often coexists with penicillin resistance. Only 5% of penicillin-susceptible strains are macrolide-resistant, whereas 50% or more of penicillin-resistant strains may be macrolide-resistant. Staphylococci are not reliably sensitive to erythromycin. Macrolide-resistant strains of *S. aureus* are potentially cross-resistant to clindamycin and streptogramin B (quinupristin). Gram-positive bacilli also are sensitive to erythromycin; typical MICs are 1 µg/ml for *Clostridium perfringens,* from 0.2 to 3 µg/ml for *Corynebacterium diphtheriae,* and from 0.25 to 4 µg/ml for *Listeria monocytogenes.*

Erythromycin is inactive against most aerobic enteric gram-negative bacilli. It has modest activity *in vitro* against other gram-negative organisms, including *H. influenzae* (MIC, 1 to 32 µg/ml) and *N. meningitidis* (MIC, 0.4 to 1.6 µg/ml), and good activity against most strains of *N. gonorrhoeae* (MIC, 0.12 to 2 µg/ml). Useful antibacterial activity also is observed against *Pasteurella multocida, Borrelia* spp., and *Bordetella pertussis.* Resistance is common for *B. fragilis* (the MIC ranging from 2 to 32 µg/ml). Macrolides are usually active against *Campylobacter jejuni* (MIC, 0.5 to 4 µg/ml). Erythromycin is active against *M. pneumoniae* (MIC, 0.004 to 0.02 µg/ml) and *Legionella pneumophila* (MIC, 0.01 to 2 µg/ml). Most strains of *C. trachomatis* are inhibited by 0.06 to 2 µg/ml of erythromycin. Some of the atypical mycobacteria, including *M. scrofulaceum,* are sensitive to erythromycin *in vitro; M. kansasii* and *M. avium-intracellulare* vary in sensitivity. *M. fortuitum* is resistant. Macrolides have no effect on viruses, yeasts, or fungi.

Clarithromycin is slightly more potent than erythromycin against sensitive strains of streptococci and staphylococci, and has modest activity against *H. influenzae* and *N. gonorrhoeae.* Clarithromycin has good activity against *M. catarrhalis, Chlamydia* spp., *L. pneumophila, B. burgdorferi, Mycoplasma pneumoniae,* and *H. pylori.*

Azithromycin generally is less active than erythromycin against gram-positive organisms and slightly more active than either erythromycin or clarithromycin against *H. influenzae* and *Campylobacter* spp. Azithromycin is very active against *M. catarrhalis, P. multocida, Chlamydia* spp., *M. pneumoniae, L. pneumophila, B. burgdorferi, Fusobacterium* spp., and *N. gonorrhoeae.*

In general, organisms are considered susceptible to clarithromycin and azithromycin at MICs ≤2 µg/ml. An exception is *H. influenzae,* with MIC breakpoints of ≤8 µg/ml and ≤4 µg/ml for clarithromycin and azithromycin, respectively.

Azithromycin and clarithromycin have enhanced activity against *M. avium-intracellulare,* as well as against some protozoa (e.g., *Toxoplasma gondii, Cryptosporidium,* and *Plasmodium* spp.). Clarithromycin has good activity against *Mycobacterium leprae.*

Mechanism of Action.
Macrolide antibiotics are bacteriostatic agents that inhibit protein synthesis by binding reversibly to 50S ribosomal subunits of sensitive microorganisms (Figure 46–3), at or very near the site that binds chloramphenicol (Figure 46–2). Erythromycin does not inhibit peptide bond formation *per se,* but rather inhibits the translocation step wherein a newly synthesized peptidyl tRNA molecule moves from the acceptor site on the ribosome to the peptidyl donor site. Gram-positive bacteria accumulate about 100 times more erythromycin than do gram-negative bacteria. Cells are considerably more permeable to the un-ionized form of the drug, which probably explains the increased antimicrobial activity at alkaline pH.

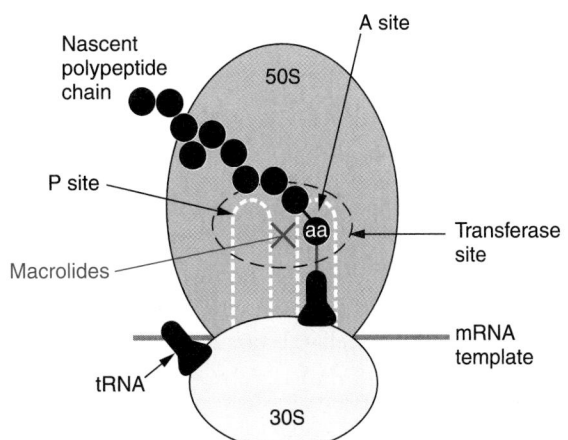

Figure 46–3. *Inhibition of bacterial protein synthesis by the macrolide antibiotics erythromycin, clarithromycin, and azithromycin.* Macrolide antibiotics are bacteriostatic agents that inhibit protein synthesis by binding reversibly to the 50S ribosomal subunits of sensitive organisms. Erythromycin appears to inhibit the translocation step wherein the nascent peptide chain temporarily residing at the A site of the transferase reaction fails to move to the P, or donor, site. Alternatively, macrolides may bind and cause a conformational change that terminates protein synthesis by indirectly interfering with transpeptidation and translocation. *See* Figure 46–1 and its legend for additional information.

Resistance to macrolides usually results from one of four mechanisms: (1) drug efflux by an active pump mechanism (encoded by *mrsA, mefA,* or *mefE* in staphylococci, group A streptococci, or *S. pneumoniae,* respectively); (2) ribosomal protection by inducible or constitutive production of methylase enzymes, mediated by expression of *ermA, ermB,* and *ermC,* which modify the ribosomal target and decrease drug binding; (3) macrolide hydrolysis by esterases produced by Enterobacteriaceae (Lina *et al.,* 1999; Nakajima, 1999); and (4) chromosomal mutations that alter a 50S ribosomal protein (found in *B. subtilis, Campylobacter* spp., mycobacteria, and gram-positive cocci).

The MLS$_B$ (macrolide-lincosamide-streptogramin B) phenotype is conferred by *erm* genes, which encode methylases that modify the macrolide binding of the ribosome. Because macrolides, lincosamides, and type B streptogramins share the same ribosomal binding site, constitutive expression of *erm* confers cross-resistance to all three drug classes. If resistance is due to inducible expression of *erm,* there is resistance to the macrolides, which are inducers of *erm,* but not to lincosamides and streptogramin B, which are not inducers. Cross-resistance can still occur if constitutive mutants are selected by exposure to lincosamides or streptogramin B. Efflux-mediated resistance to macrolides may not result in cross-resistance to lincosamides or streptogramin B because they are structurally dissimilar to macrolides and are not substrates of the macrolide pump.

Absorption, Distribution, and Excretion. *Absorption.*

Erythromycin base is incompletely but adequately absorbed from the upper small intestine. Because it is inactivated by gastric acid, the drug is administered as enteric-coated tablets, as capsules containing enteric-coated pellets that dissolve in the duodenum, or as an ester. Food, which increases gastric acidity, may delay absorption.

Peak serum concentrations are 0.3 to 0.5 $\mu g/ml$, 4 hours after oral administration of 250 mg of the base, and 0.3 to 1.9 $\mu g/ml$ after a single dose of 500 mg. Esters of erythromycin base (*e.g.,* stearate, estolate, and ethylsuccinate) have improved acid stability, and their absorption is less altered by food. A single, oral 250-mg dose of erythromycin estolate produces peak serum concentrations of approximately 1.5 $\mu g/ml$ after 2 hours, and a 500-mg dose produces peak concentrations of 4 $\mu g/ml$. Peak serum concentrations of erythromycin ethylsuccinate are 1.5 $\mu g/ml$ (0.5 $\mu g/ml$ of base) 1 to 2 hours after administration of a 500-mg dose. These peak values include the inactive ester and the free base, the latter of which comprises 20% to 35% of the total. The concentration of microbiologically active erythromycin base in serum therefore is similar for the various preparations.

Higher concentrations of erythromycin can be achieved by intravenous administration. Values are approximately 10 $\mu g/ml$ 1 hour after intravenous administration of 500 to 1000 mg of erythromycin lactobionate.

Clarithromycin is absorbed rapidly from the gastrointestinal tract after oral administration, but first-pass metabolism reduces its bioavailability to 50% to 55%. Peak concentrations occur approximately 2 hours after drug administration. Clarithromycin may be given with or without food, but the extended-release form, typically given once-daily as a 1-g dose, should be administered with food to improve bioavailability. Steady-state peak concentrations in plasma of 2 to 3 $\mu g/ml$ are achieved after 2 hours with a regimen of 500 mg every 12 hours, or after 2 to 4 hours with two 500-mg extended-release tablets given once daily.

Azithromycin administered orally is absorbed rapidly and distributes widely throughout the body, except to the brain and CSF. Concomitant administration of aluminum and magnesium hydroxide antacids decreases the peak serum drug concentrations but not overall bioavailability. Azithromycin should not be administered with food. A 500-mg loading dose will produce a peak plasma drug concentration of approximately 0.4 $\mu g/ml$. When this loading dose is followed by 250-mg once-daily for 4 days, the steady-state peak drug concentration is 0.24 $\mu g/ml$. Azithromycin also can be administered intravenously, producing plasma concentrations of 3 to 4 $\mu g/ml$ after a 1-hour infusion of 500 mg.

Distribution. Erythromycin diffuses readily into intracellular fluids, achieving antibacterial activity in essentially all sites except the brain and CSF. Erythromycin penetrates into prostatic fluid, achieving concentrations approximately 40% of those in plasma. Concentrations in middle ear exudate reach only 50% of serum

concentrations and thus may be inadequate for the treatment of otitis media caused by *H. influenzae.* Protein binding is approximately 70% to 80% for erythromycin base and even higher, 96%, for the estolate. Erythromycin traverses the placenta, and drug concentrations in fetal plasma are about 5% to 20% of those in the maternal circulation. Concentrations in breast milk are 50% of those in serum.

Clarithromycin and its active metabolite, 14-hydroxyclarithromycin, distribute widely and achieve high intracellular concentrations throughout the body. Tissue concentrations generally exceed serum concentrations. Concentrations in middle-ear fluid are 50% higher than simultaneous serum concentrations for clarithromycin and the active metabolite. Protein binding of clarithromycin ranges from 40% to 70% and is concentration dependent.

Azithromycin's unique pharmacokinetic properties include extensive tissue distribution and high drug concentrations within cells (including phagocytes), resulting in much greater concentrations of drugs in tissue or secretions compared to simultaneous serum concentrations. Tissue fibroblasts act as the natural reservoir for the drug *in vivo.* Protein binding is 50% at very low plasma concentrations and less at higher concentrations.

Elimination. Only 2% to 5% of orally administered erythromycin is excreted in active form in the urine; this value is from 12% to 15% after intravenous infusion. The antibiotic is concentrated in the liver and is excreted in the bile, which may contain as much as 250 $\mu g/ml$ when serum concentrations are very high. The serum elimination half-life of erythromycin is approximately 1.6 hours. Although the half-life may be prolonged in patients with anuria, dosage reduction is not routinely recommended in renal-failure patients. The drug is not removed significantly by either peritoneal dialysis or hemodialysis.

Clarithromycin is eliminated by renal and nonrenal mechanisms. It is metabolized in the liver to several metabolites, the active 14-hydroxy metabolite being the most significant. Primary metabolic pathways are oxidative *N*-demethylation and hydroxylation at the 14 position. The elimination half-lives are 3 to 7 hours for clarithromycin and 5 to 9 hours for 14-hydroxyclarithromycin. Metabolism is saturable, resulting in nonlinear pharmacokinetics with higher dosages; longer half-lives are observed after larger doses. The amount of clarithromycin excreted unchanged in the urine ranges from 20% to 40%, depending on the dose administered and the formulation (tablet *versus* oral suspension). An additional 10% to 15% of a dose is excreted in the urine as 14-hydroxyclarithromycin. Although the pharmacokinetics of clarithromycin are altered in patients with either hepatic or renal dysfunction, dose adjustment is not necessary unless the creatinine clearance is less than 30 ml per minute.

Azithromycin undergoes some hepatic metabolism to inactive metabolites, but biliary excretion is the major route of elimination. Only 12% of drug is excreted unchanged in the urine. The elimination half-life, 40 to 68 hours, is prolonged because of extensive tissue sequestration and binding.

Therapeutic Uses. Depending on the nature and severity of the infection, the usual oral dose of erythromycin (*erythromycin base;* E-MYCIN, others) for adults ranges from 1 to 2 g per day, in equally divided and spaced amounts, usually given every 6 hours. Daily doses of erythromycin as large as 8 g orally, given for 3 months, have been well tolerated. Food should not be taken concurrently, if possible, with erythromycin base or the stearate formulations, but this is not necessary with *erythromycin estolate* or *erythromycin ethylsuccinate* (E.E.S., others). The oral dose of erythromycin for children is 30 to 50 mg/kg per day, divided into four portions; this dose may be doubled for severe infections. Intramuscular administration of erythromycin is not recommended because of pain upon injection. Intravenous administration is generally reserved for the therapy of severe infections, such as legionellosis. The usual dose is 0.5 to 1 g every 6 hours; 1 g of erythromycin gluceptate has been given intravenously every 6 hours for as long as 4 weeks with no adverse effects except for thrombophlebitis at the site of injection. *Erythromycin lactobionate* (ERYTHROCIN LACTOBIONATE-I.V.) is available for intravenous injection.

Clarithromycin (BIAXIN FILMTABS, BIAXIN XL FILMTABS, and BIAXIN granules for suspension) usually is given twice daily at a dose of 250 mg for children older than 12 years and adults with mild to moderate infection. Larger doses (*e.g.,* 500 mg twice daily) are indicated for more severe infection such as pneumonia or when infection is caused by more resistant organisms such as *H. influenzae.* Children younger than 12 years old have received 7.5 mg/kg twice daily in clinical studies. The 500-mg, extended-release formulation is given as two tablets once daily. Clarithromycin (500 mg) is also packaged with *lansoprazole* (30 mg) and *amoxicillin* (1 g) as a combination regimen (PREVPAC) that is administered twice daily for 14 days to eradicate *H. pylori* and to reduce the associated risk of duodenal ulcer recurrence (*see* Chapter 36).

Azithromycin (ZITHROMAX tablet, oral suspension, and powder for intravenous injection) should be given 1 hour before or 2 hours after meals when administered orally.

For outpatient therapy of community-acquired pneumonia, pharyngitis, or skin and skin-structure infections, a loading dose of 500 mg is given on the first day, then 250 mg per day is given for days 2 through 5. Treatment or prophylaxis of *M. avium-intracellulare* infection in AIDS patients requires higher doses: 500 mg daily in combination with one or more other agents for treatment, or 1200 mg once weekly for primary prevention (Kovacs and Masur, 2000). Azithromycin is useful in treatment of sexually transmitted diseases, especially during pregnancy when tetracyclines are contraindicated. The treatment of uncomplicated nongonococcal urethritis presumed to be caused by *C. trachomatis* consists of a single 1-g dose of azithromycin. This dose also is effective for chancroid. Azithromycin (1 g a week for 3 weeks) is an alternative regimen for treatment of granuloma inguinale or lymphogranuloma venereum.

In children, the recommended dose of azithromycin oral suspension for acute otitis media and pneumonia is 10 mg/kg on the first day (maximum 500 mg) and 5 mg/kg (maximum 250 mg per day) on days 2 through 5. The dose for tonsillitis or pharyngitis is 12 mg/kg per day, up to 500 mg total, for 5 days.

Mycoplasma pneumoniae Infections. A macrolide or tetracycline is the drug of choice for mycoplasma infections. Erythromycin reduces the duration of fever caused by *M. pneumoniae* and accelerates the rate of clearing of the chest radiographs.

Legionnaires' Disease. Erythromycin has been considered as the drug of choice for treatment of pneumonia caused by *L. pneumophila, L. micdadei,* or other *Legionella* spp. Because of excellent *in vitro* activity, superior tissue concentration, the ease of administration as a single daily dose, and better tolerability compared to erythromycin, azithromycin (or a fluoroquinolone) has supplanted erythromycin as the first-line agent for treatment of legionellosis (Garey and Amsden, 1999). The recommended dose is 500 mg daily, intravenously or orally, for a total of 10 to 14 days.

Chlamydial Infections. Chlamydial infections can be treated effectively with any of the macrolides. A single 1-g dose of azithromycin is recommended for patients with uncomplicated urethral, endocervical, rectal, or epididymal infections because of the ease of compliance. During pregnancy, erythromycin base, 500 mg four times daily for 7 days, is recommended as first-line therapy for chlamydial urogenital infections. Azithromycin, 1 g orally as a single dose, is a suitable alternative. Erythromycin base is preferred for chlamydial pneumonia of infancy and ophthalmia neonatorum (50 mg/kg per day in four divided doses for 10 to 14 days). Azithromycin, 1 g a week for 3 weeks, may be effective for lymphogranuloma venereum.

Pneumonia caused by *Chlamydia pneumoniae* responds to macrolides, fluoroquinolones, and tetracyclines in standard doses for community-acquired pneumonia. No comparative trials have been conducted to determine which agent, if any, is most efficacious. Duration of therapy also is ill defined. In practice, a specific etiological diagnosis rarely is made and length of treatment, typically 7 to 10 days, often is determined empirically based on clinical response.

Diphtheria. Erythromycin 250 mg four times daily for 7 days is very effective for acute infections or for eradicating the carrier state. The other macrolides also are likely to be effective; because clinical experience with them is lacking, they are not FDA approved for this indication. The presence of an antibiotic does not alter the course of an acute infection with the diphtheria bacillus or the risk of complications. Antitoxin is indicated in the treatment of acute infection.

Pertussis. Erythromycin is the drug of choice for treating persons with *B. pertussis* disease and for postexposure prophylaxis of household members and close contacts. A 7-day regimen of erythromycin estolate (40 mg/kg per day, maximum 1 g/day) is as effective as the 14-day regimens traditionally recommended (Halperin *et al.*, 1997). Clarithromycin and azithromycin also are effective (Bace *et al.*, 1999). If administered early in the course of whooping cough, erythromycin may shorten the duration of illness; it has little influence on the disease once the paroxysmal stage is reached, although it may eliminate the microorganisms from the nasopharynx. Nasopharyngeal cultures should be obtained from people with pertussis who do not improve with erythromycin therapy, since resistance has been reported.

Streptococcal Infections. Pharyngitis, scarlet fever, erysipelas, and cellulitis caused by *S. pyogenes* and pneumonia caused by *S. pneumoniae* respond to macrolides. They are valuable alternatives for treatment of patients who have a serious allergy to penicillin. Unfortunately, macrolide-resistant strains are increasingly encountered. Penicillin-resistant strains of *S. pneumoniae* also are very likely to be resistant to macrolides.

Staphylococcal Infections. Erythromycin has been an alternative agent for the treatment of relatively minor infections caused by either penicillin-sensitive or penicillin-resistant *S. aureus*. However, many strains of *S. aureus* are resistant to macrolides, and they no longer can be relied upon unless *in vitro* susceptibility has been documented.

Campylobacter Infections. The treatment of gastroenteritis caused by *C. jejuni* with erythromycin (250 to 500 mg orally four times a day for 7 days) hastens eradication of the microorganism from the stools and reduces the duration of symptoms. Availability of fluoroquinolones, which are highly active against *Campylobacter* species and other enteric pathogens, largely has replaced the use of erythromycin for this disease in adults. Erythromycin remains useful for treatment of *Campylobacter* gastroenteritis in children.

Helicobacter pylori Infection. Clarithromycin 500 mg, in combination with omeprazole, 20 mg, and amoxicillin, 1 g, each administered twice daily for 10 to 14 days, is effective for treatment of peptic ulcer disease caused by *H. pylori* (Peterson *et al.*, 2000). Numerous other regimens, some effective as 7-day treatments, have been studied and also are effective. The more effective regimens generally include three agents, one of which usually is clarithromycin (*see* Chapter 36).

Tetanus. Erythromycin (500 mg orally every 6 hours for 10 days) may be given to eradicate *Clostridium tetani* in patients with tetanus who are allergic to penicillin. However, the mainstays of therapy are débridement, physiological support, tetanus antitoxin, and drug control of convulsions.

Syphilis. Erythromycin has been used in the treatment of early syphilis in patients who are allergic to penicillin, but it no longer is recommended. Tetracyclines are the recommended alternative in penicillin-allergic patients. During pregnancy it is recommended that patients be desensitized to penicillin.

Mycobacterial Infections. Clarithromycin or azithromycin is recommended as first-line therapy for prophylaxis and treatment of dis-

seminated infection caused by *M. avium-intracellulare* in AIDS patients and for treatment of pulmonary disease in non–HIV-infected patients (Kovacs and Masur, 2000). Azithromycin (1.2 g once weekly) or clarithromycin (500 mg twice daily) is recommended for primary prevention for AIDS patients with fewer than 50 CD4 cells per mm³. Single-agent therapy should not be used for treatment of active disease or for secondary prevention in AIDS patients. Clarithromycin (500 mg twice daily) plus ethambutol (15 mg/kg once daily) with or without rifabutin is an effective combination regimen. Azithromycin (500 mg once daily) may be used instead of clarithromycin, but clarithromycin appears to be slightly more efficacious (Ward *et al.*, 1998). Clarithromycin also has been used with minocycline for the treatment of *Mycobacterium leprae* in lepromatous leprosy.

Other Infections. Clarithromycin and azithromycin have been used in the treatment of toxoplasmosis encephalitis and diarrhea due to *Cryptosporidium* in AIDS patients. Rigorous clinical trials demonstrating efficacy of macrolides for these infections are lacking.

Prophylactic Uses. Penicillin is the drug of choice for the prophylaxis of recurrences of rheumatic fever. Erythromycin is an effective alternative for individuals who are allergic to penicillin.

Erythromycin has been recommended as an alternative to penicillin in allergic patients for prevention of bacterial endocarditis after dental or respiratory-tract procedures. Clindamycin has replaced erythromycin for use in penicillin-allergic patients. Clarithromycin or azithromycin as a single 500-mg dose also may be used (Dajani *et al.*, 1997).

Untoward Effects. Serious untoward effects are rarely caused by erythromycin. Among the allergic reactions observed are fever, eosinophilia, and skin eruptions, which may occur alone or in combination; each disappears shortly after therapy is stopped. Cholestatic hepatitis is the most striking side effect. It is caused primarily by erythromycin estolate and rarely by the ethylsuccinate or the stearate. The illness starts after about 10 to 20 days of treatment and is characterized initially by nausea, vomiting, and abdominal cramps. The pain often mimics that of acute cholecystitis. These symptoms are followed shortly thereafter by jaundice, which may be accompanied by fever, leukocytosis, eosinophilia, and elevated transaminases in plasma. Biopsy of the liver reveals cholestasis, periportal infiltration by neutrophils, lymphocytes, and eosinophils, and occasionally, necrosis of neighboring parenchymal cells. Findings usually resolve within a few days after cessation of drug therapy and rarely are prolonged. The syndrome may represent a hypersensitivity reaction to the estolate ester.

Oral administration of erythromycin, especially of large doses, frequently is accompanied by epigastric distress, which may be quite severe. Intravenous administration of erythromycin may cause similar symptoms, with abdominal cramps, nausea, vomiting, and diarrhea. Erythromycin stimulates gastrointestinal motility by acting on motilin receptors. Because of this property, erythromycin is used postoperatively to promote peristalsis; it has been exploited to speed gastric emptying in patients with gastroparesis (*see* Chapter 37). The gastrointestinal symptoms are dose-related and occur more commonly in children and young adults; they may be reduced by prolonging the infusion time to 1 hour or by pretreatment with glycopyrrolate (Bowler *et al.*, 1992). Intravenous infusion of 1-g doses, even when dissolved in a large volume, often is followed by thrombophlebitis. This can be minimized by slow rates of infusion.

Erythromycin has been reported to cause cardiac arrhythmias, including QT prolongation with ventricular tachycardia. Most patients have had underlying cardiac disease, or the arrhythmias were associated with combination drug therapies that included erythromycin (*e.g.,* cisapride or *terfenadine* plus erythromycin; *see* Chapter 34).

Transient auditory impairment is a potential complication of treatment with erythromycin; it has been observed to follow intravenous administration of large doses of the gluceptate or lactobionate (4 g per day) or oral ingestion of large doses of the estolate.

Drug Interactions. Erythromycin and clarithromycin inhibit CYP3A4 and are associated with clinically significant drug interactions (Periti *et al.*, 1992). Erythromycin potentiates the effects of *carbamazepine*, corticosteroids, *cyclosporine*, *digoxin*, ergot alkaloids, *theophylline*, *triazolam*, *valproate*, and warfarin, probably by interfering with CYP-mediated metabolism of these drugs (*see* Chapter 3). Clarithromycin, which is structurally related to erythromycin, has a similar drug interaction profile. Azithromycin, which differs from erythromycin and clarithromycin because of its 15-membered lactone ring structure, and *dirithromycin*, which is a longer-acting 14-membered lactone ring analog of erythromycin analog, appear to be free of these drug interactions. Caution is advised, nevertheless, when using azithromycin in conjunction with drugs known to interact with erythromycin.

KETOLIDES (TELITHROMYCIN)

Source and Chemistry. Ketolides, of which *telithromycin* (KETEK) is the only one currently approved, are semisynthetic derivatives of erythromycin (Ackermann and Rodloff, 2003). Telithromycin differs from erythromycin in that a 3-keto group replaces the α-L-cladinose of the 14-member macrolide ring, and there is a substituted carbamate at C11-C12. These modifications render ketolides less susceptible to methylase-mediated (*erm*) and efflux-mediated (*mef* or *msr*) mechanisms of resistance. Ketolides therefore are active against many macrolide-resistant gram-positive strains. The structural formula of telithromycin is:

TELITHROMYCIN

Antibacterial Activity. Ketolides and macrolides have very similar antibacterial properties. Telithromycin is active against staphylococci, streptococci, *S. pneumoniae*, *Haemophilus* spp., *Moraxella catarrhalis*, mycoplasma, chlamydia, and *Legionella*. It is slightly more active by weight than erythromycin. MIC breakpoints for telithromycin are ≤ 0.25 μg/ml for *S. aureus*, ≤ 1 μg/ml for *S. pneumoniae*, and ≤ 4 μg/ml for *H. influenzae*.

Mechanism of Action and Resistance. Ketolides and macrolides have the same ribosomal target site. The principal difference between the two is that structural modifications within ketolides neutralize the common resistance mechanisms that make macrolides ineffective (Nilius and Ma, 2002). Introduction of the 3-keto function converts a methylase-inducing macrolide into a noninducing ketolide. This moiety also prevents drug efflux, probably because it generates a less-desirable substrate. The carbamate substitution at C11-C12 enhances binding to the ribosomal target site, even when the site is methylated, by introducing an extra interaction of the ketolide with the ribosome. Inducible and constitutive methylase-producing strains of *S. pneumoniae* are therefore telithromycin-susceptible. However, constitutive methylase-producing strains of *S. aureus* and *S. pyogenes* are telithromycin-resistant because the strength of the ketolide interaction with the fully methylated ribosomal binding site is insufficient to overcome resistance. Constitutive methylase producers can be selected from strains with the inducible *erm* phenotype.

Absorption, Distribution, and Excretion. Telithromycin is formulated as a 400-mg tablet for oral administration. There is no parenteral form. It is well absorbed with approximately 60% bioavailability. Peak serum concentrations, averaging 2 μg/ml following a single, 800-mg oral dose, are achieved within 30 minutes to 4 hours. With a half-life of 9.8 hours, the drug can be given once daily. It is 60% to 70% bound by serum protein, principally albumin. It penetrates well into most tissues, exceeding plasma concentrations by approximately two- to tenfold or more. Telithromycin is concentrated into macrophages and white blood cells, where concentrations of 40 μg/ml (500 times the simultaneous plasma concentration) are maintained 24 hours after dosing. The drug is cleared primarily by hepatic metabolism, 50% by CYP3A4 and 50% by CYP-independent metabolism. No adjustment of the dose is required for hepatic failure or mild-to-moderate renal failure. No dose has been established for patients in whom creatinine clearance is less than 30 ml/minute, although a reduction in dosage probably is advisable (Shi *et al.*, 2004).

Therapeutic Uses. Given its spectrum of activity and based on its noninferiority against a number of comparators, telithromycin is approved for treatment of respiratory tract infections, including acute exacerbation of chronic bronchitis (5-day regimen), acute bacterial sinusitis (5-day regimen), and community-acquired pneumonia (7- to 10-day regimen). Although telithromycin is not indicated for treatment of severe pneumonia or bacteremia, almost 90% of patients who proved to have pneumococcal bacteremia were clinically cured after taking it. In premarketing trials of telithromycin on patients with community-acquired pneumonia caused by multiple-drug-resistant strains of *S. pneumoniae* (resistant to penicillins, cephalosporins, macrolides, tetracyclines, or trimethoprim-sulfamethoxazole) over 90% of patients were cured.

Untoward Effects. Telithromycin generally is well tolerated. Nausea, vomiting, and diarrhea are the most common side effects, occurring in 3% to 10% of treatment courses. Visual disturbances due to slowed accommodation occur in about 1% of treatment courses, and include blurred vision, difficulty focusing, and diplopia. Reversible hepatic dysfunction with elevated transaminases or hepatitis has been reported. Pseudomembranous colitis has been reported. Telithromycin is not recommended for routine use in patients with myasthenia gravis due to reports of disease exacerbation in telithromycin-treated patients.

Telithromycin may cause clinically significant QTc prolongation and increased risk of ventricular arrhythmia in predisposed patients (*see* Chapter 34). It should not be used in patients with prolonged QT syndrome, uncorrected hypokalemia or hypomagnesemia, profound bradycardia, or in patients receiving certain antiarrhythmics (*e.g.*, *quinidine*, *procainamide*, *amiodarone*) or other agents that prolong QTc (*e.g.*, cisapride, *pimozide*).

Telithromycin has several clinically significant drug interactions similar to those for erythromycin. It is both a substrate and a strong inhibitor of CYP3A4. Coadministration of rifampin, a potent inducer of CYP, decreases the serum concentrations of telithromycin by 80%. CYP3A4 inhibitors (*e.g.*, *itraconazole*) increase peak serum concentrations of telithromycin. Serum concentrations of CYP3A4 substrates (*e.g.*, pimozide, cisapride, *midazolam*, statins, cyclosporine, phenytoin) are increased by telithromycin. Telithromycin also increases peak serum concentrations of *metoprolol* and digoxin.

CLINDAMYCIN

Chemistry. Clindamycin is a derivative of the amino acid *trans*-L-4-*n*-propylhygrinic acid, attached to a sulfur-containing derivative of an octose. It is a congener of *lincomycin*, and its structural formula is:

CLINDAMYCIN

Mechanism of Action. Clindamycin binds exclusively to the 50S subunit of bacterial ribosomes and suppresses protein synthesis. Although clindamycin, erythromycin, and chloramphenicol are not structurally related, they act at sites in close proximity (Figures 46–2 and 46–3), and binding by one of these antibiotics to the ribosome may inhibit the interaction of the others. There are no clinical indications for the concurrent use of these antibiotics. Macrolide resistance due to ribosomal methylation by *erm*-encoded enzymes also may produce resistance to clindamycin. However, because clindamycin does not induce the methylase, there is cross-resistance only if the enzyme is produced constitutively. Clindamycin is not a substrate for macrolide efflux pumps; thus strains that are resistant to macrolides by this mechanism are susceptible to clindamycin. Altered metabolism occasionally causes clindamycin resistance (Bozdogan *et al.*, 1999).

Antibacterial Activity. Bacterial strains are susceptible to clindamycin at MICs of ≤0.5 μg/ml. Clindamycin generally is similar to erythromycin in its *in vitro* activity against susceptible strains of pneumococci, *S. pyogenes,* and viridans streptococci. Ninety percent or more of strains of streptococci, including some that are macrolide-resistant, remain susceptible to clindamycin, with MICs less than 0.5 *μg/ml* (Doern *et al.*, 1998). Methicillin-susceptible strains of *S. aureus* usually are susceptible to clindamycin, but methicillin-resistant strains of *S. aureus* and coagulase-negative staphylococci frequently are resistant.

Clindamycin is more active than erythromycin or clarithromycin against anaerobic bacteria, especially *B. fragilis*; some strains are inhibited by <0.1 *μg/ml*, and most are inhibited by 2 *μg/ml*. The MICs for other anaerobes are as follows: *Bacteroides melaninogenicus,* 0.1 to 1 *μg/ml; Fusobacterium,* <0.5 *μg/ml* (although most strains of *Fusobacterium varium* are resistant); *Peptostreptococcus,* <0.1 to 0.5 *μg/ml; Peptococcus,* 1 to 100 *μg/ml* (with 10% of strains resistant); and *C. perfringens,* <0.1 to 8 *μg/ml.* From 10% to 20% of clostridial species other than *C. perfringens* are resistant. Resistance to clindamycin in *Bacteroides* spp. increasingly is encountered (Hedberg and Nord, 2003). Strains of *Actinomyces israelii* and *Nocardia asteroides* are sensitive. Essentially all aerobic gram-negative bacilli are resistant.

With regard to atypical organisms and parasites, *M. pneumoniae* is resistant. *Chlamydia* spp. are variably sensitive, although the clinical relevance is not established. Clindamycin plus *primaquine* and clindamycin plus *pyrimethamine* are second-line regimens for *Pneumocystis jiroveci* pneumonia and *T. gondii* encephalitis, respectively. Clindamycin has been used for treatment of babesiosis.

Absorption, Distribution, and Excretion. Absorption.

Clindamycin is nearly completely absorbed following oral administration. Peak plasma concentrations of 2 to 3 *μg/ml* are attained within 1 hour after the ingestion of 150 mg. The presence of food in the stomach does not reduce absorption significantly. The half-life of the antibiotic is about 2.9 hours, and modest accumulation of drug is thus expected if it is given every 6 hours.

Clindamycin palmitate, an oral preparation for pediatric use, is an inactive prodrug that is hydrolyzed rapidly *in vivo.* Its rate and extent of absorption are similar to those of clindamycin. After several oral doses at 6-hour intervals, children attain plasma concentrations of 2 to 4 *μg/ml* with the administration of 8 to 16 *μg/kg.*

The phosphate ester of clindamycin, which is given parenterally, also is rapidly hydrolyzed *in vivo* to the active parent compound. After intramuscular injection, peak concentrations in plasma are not attained until 3 hours in adults and 1 hour in children; these values approximate 6 *μg/ml* after a 300-mg dose and 9 μg/ml after a 600-mg dose in adults.

Distribution. Clindamycin is widely distributed in many fluids and tissues, including bone. Significant concentrations are not attained in CSF, even when the meninges are inflamed. Concentrations sufficient to treat cerebral toxoplasmosis are achievable (Gatti *et al.*, 1998). The drug readily crosses the placental barrier. Ninety percent or more of clindamycin is bound to plasma proteins. Clindamycin accumulates in polymorphonuclear leukocytes, alveolar macrophages, and in abscesses.

Excretion. Only about 10% of the clindamycin administered is excreted unaltered in the urine, and small quantities are found in the feces. However, antimicrobial activity persists in feces for 5 or more days after parenteral therapy with clindamycin is stopped; growth of clindamycin-sensitive microorganisms in colonic contents may be suppressed for up to 2 weeks.

Clindamycin is inactivated by metabolism to *N*-demethylclindamycin and clindamycin sulfoxide, which are excreted in the urine and bile. Accumulation of clindamycin can occur in patients with severe hepatic failure, and dosage adjustments thus may be required.

Therapeutic Uses. The oral dose of clindamycin (*clindamycin hydrochloride;* CLEOCIN) for adults is 150 to 300 mg every 6 hours; for severe infections, it is 300 to 600 mg every 6 hours. Children should receive 8 to 12 mg/kg per day of *clindamycin palmitate hydrochloride* (CLEOCIN PEDIATRIC) in three or four divided doses (some physicians recommend 10 to 30 mg/kg per day in six divided doses) or for severe infections, 13 to 25 mg/kg per day. However, children weighing 10 kg or less should receive 1/2 teaspoonful of clindamycin palmitate hydrochloride (37.5 mg) every 8 hours as a minimal dose.

For serious infections due to aerobic gram-positive cocci and the more sensitive anaerobes (not generally including *B. fragilis, Peptococcus,* and *Clostridium* spp. other than *C. perfringens*), intravenous or intramuscular administration is recommended in dosages of 600 to 1200 mg per day, divided into three or four equal doses for adults. *Clindamycin phosphate* (CLEOCIN PHOSPHATE) is available for intramuscular or intravenous use. For more severe infections, particularly those proven or suspected to be caused by *B. fragilis, Peptococcus,* or *Clostridium* species other than *C. perfringens,* parenteral administration of 1.2 to 2.4 g per day of clindamycin is suggested. Daily doses as high as 4.8 g have been given intravenously to adults. Children should receive 10 to 40 mg/kg per day in three or four divided doses; in severe infections, a minimal daily dose of 300 mg is recommended, regardless of body weight.

Although a number of infections with gram-positive cocci will respond favorably to clindamycin, *the high incidence of diarrhea and the occurrence of pseudomembranous colitis limit its use to infections in which it is clearly superior to other agents.* Clindamycin is particularly valuable for the treatment of infections with anaerobes, especially those due to *B. fragilis.* Clindamycin is not predictably useful for the treatment of bacterial brain abscesses, since penetration into the CSF is poor; metronidazole, in combination with penicillin or a third-generation cephalosporin, is preferred.

On the basis of one clinical trial which found that clindamycin (600 mg intravenously every 8 hours) was superior to penicillin (1 million units intravenously every 4 hours; Levison *et al.*, 1983), clindamycin has replaced penicillin as the drug of choice for treatment of lung abscess and anaerobic lung and pleural space infections.

Clindamycin (600 to 1200 mg given intravenously every 6 hours) in combination with pyrimethamine (a 200-mg loading dose followed by 75 mg orally each day) and *leucovorin* (folinic acid, 10 mg/day) is effective for acute treatment of encephalitis caused by *T. gondii* in patients with AIDS. Clindamycin (600 mg intravenously every 8 hours, or 300 to 450 mg orally every 6 hours for less severe disease) in combination with primaquine (15 mg of base once daily) is useful for the treatment of mild to moderate cases of *P. jiroveci* pneumonia in AIDS patients.

Clindamycin also is available as a topical solution, gel, or lotion (CLEOCIN T, others) and as a vaginal cream (CLEOCIN). It is effective topically (or orally) for acne vulgaris and bacterial vaginosis.

Untoward Effects. The reported incidence of diarrhea associated with the administration of clindamycin ranges from 2% to 20%. A number of patients (variously reported as 0.01% to 10%) have developed pseudomembranous colitis caused by the toxin from the organism *C. difficile.* This colitis is characterized by abdominal pain, diarrhea, fever, and mucus and blood in the stools. Proctoscopic examination reveals white to yellow plaques on the mucosa of the colon. *This syndrome may be lethal.* Discontinuation of the drug, combined with administration of metronidazole orally or intravenously usually is curative, but relapses can occur. Agents that inhibit peristalsis, such as opioids, may prolong and worsen the condition.

Skin rashes occur in approximately 10% of patients treated with clindamycin and may be more common in patients with HIV infection. Other reactions, which are uncommon, include exudative erythema multiforme (Stevens-Johnson syndrome), reversible elevation of aspartate aminotransferase and alanine aminotransferase, granulocytopenia, thrombocytopenia, and anaphylactic reactions. Local thrombophlebitis may follow intravenous administration of the drug. Clindamycin can inhibit neuromuscular transmission and may potentiate the effect of a neuromuscular blocking agent administered concurrently.

QUINUPRISTIN/DALFOPRISTIN

Quinupristin/dalfopristin (SYNERCID) is a combination of quinupristin, a streptogramin B, with dalfopristin, a streptogramin A, in a 30:70 ratio. These compounds are semisynthetic derivatives of naturally occurring pristinamycins, produced by *Streptomyces pristinaespiralis.* *Pristinamycin* has been available in France for more than 30 years for oral treatment of staphylococcal infections. Quinupristin and dalfopristin are more soluble derivatives of pristinamycin IA and pristinamycin IIA, respectively, and therefore are suitable for intravenous administration. Their chemical structures are:

QUINUPRISTIN

DALFOPRISTIN

Antibacterial Activity. Quinupristin/dalfopristin is active against gram-positive cocci, including *S. pneumoniae,* beta- and alpha-hemolytic strains of streptococci, *E. faecium* (but not *E. faecalis*), and coagulase-positive and coagulase-negative strains of staphylococci. The combination is largely inactive against gram-negative organisms, although *Moraxella catarrhalis* and *Neisseria* spp. are susceptible. It also is active against organisms responsible for atypical pneumonia, *M. pneumoniae, Legionella* spp., and *Chlamydia pneumoniae.* The combination is bactericidal against streptococci and many strains of staphylococci, but bacteriostatic against *E. faecium.* MICs for strains of streptococci, including penicillin-susceptible and penicillin-resistant strains of *S. pneumoniae,* are 0.25 to 1 μg/ml. MICs typically are <1 μg/ml for both methicillin-susceptible and methicillin-resistant strains of staphylococci and for vancomycin-intermediate *S. aureus* strains. MICs for *E. faecium* are 1 μg/ml or less for both vancomycin-susceptible and vancomycin-resistant strains, but for *E. faecalis* are 8 μg/ml or higher.

Mechanism of Action. Quinupristin and dalfopristin are protein synthesis inhibitors that bind the 50S ribosomal subunit. Quinupristin binds at the same site as macrolides and has a similar effect, with inhibition of polypeptide elongation and early termination of protein synthesis. Dalfopristin binds at a site nearby, resulting in a conformational change in the 50S ribosome, synergistically enhancing the binding of quinupristin at its target site. Dalfopristin directly interferes with polypeptide-chain formation. In many bacterial species, the net result of the cooperative and synergistic binding of these two molecules to the ribosome is bactericidal activity.

Resistance to quinupristin is mediated by MLS type B resistance determinants (*e.g., ermA* and *ermC* in staphylococci and *ermB* in enterococci), encoding a ribosomal methylase that prevents binding of drug to its target; or *vgb* or *vgbB,* which encode lactonases that inactivate type B streptogramins (Allignet *et al.,* 1998; Bozdogan and Leclercq, 1999). Resistance to dalfopristin is mediated by *vat, vatB, vatC, vatD,* and *satA,* which encode acetyltransferases that inactivate type A streptogramins (Allignet *et al.,* 1998; Allignet and El Solh, 1999; Soltani *et al.,* 2000); or staphylococcal genes *vga* and *vgaB,* which encode ATP-binding efflux proteins that pump type A streptogramins out of the cell (Allignet *et al.,* 1998; Bozdogan and Leclercq, 1999). These resistance determinants are located on plasmids that may be transferable by conjugative mobilization (Allignet *et al.,* 1998). Resistance to quinupristin/dalfopristin always is associated with a resistance gene for type A streptogramins. Genes encoding resistance to type B streptogramins also may be present, but are not sufficient by themselves to produce resistance. Methylase-encoding *erm* genes, however, can render the combination bacteriostatic instead of bactericidal, making it ineffective in certain infections in which bactericidal activity is necessary for cure, such as endocarditis.

Absorption, Distribution, and Excretion. The combination of quinupristin/dalfopristin is administered only by intravenous infusion over at least 1 hour. It is incompatible with saline and heparin and should be dissolved in 5% dextrose in water. Steady-state peak serum concentrations in healthy male volunteers are approximately 3 μg/ml of quinupristin and 7 μg/ml of dalfopristin with a 7.5-mg/kg dose administered every 8 hours. The half-life is 0.85 hour for quinupristin and 0.7 hour for dalfopristin. The volume of distribution is 0.87 L/kg for quinupristin and 0.71 L/kg for dalfopristin. Hepatic metabolism by conjugation is the prin-

cipal means of clearance for both compounds, with 80% of an administered dose eliminated by biliary excretion. Renal elimination of active compound accounts for most of the remainder. No dosage adjustment is necessary for renal insufficiency. Pharmacokinetics are not significantly altered by peritoneal dialysis or hemodialysis. The area under the plasma concentration curve of active component and its metabolites is increased by 180% for quinupristin and 50% for dalfopristin by hepatic insufficiency. No adjustment is recommended unless the patient is unable to tolerate the drug, in which case the dosing frequency should be reduced from 8 hours to 12 hours.

Therapeutic Uses. Quinupristin/dalfopristin is approved in the United States for treatment of infections caused by vancomycin-resistant strains of *E. faecium* and complicated skin and skin-structure infections caused by methicillin-susceptible strains of *S. aureus* or *S. pyogenes* (Nichols *et al.,* 1999). In Europe it also is approved for treatment of nosocomial pneumonia and infections caused by methicillin-resistant strains of *S. aureus* (Fagon *et al.,* 2000). In open-label, nonrandomized studies, clinical and microbiological cure rates for a variety of infections caused by vancomycin-resistant *E. faecium* were approximately 70% with quinupristin/dalfopristin at a dose of 7.5 mg/kg every 8 to 12 hours (Moellering *et al.,* 1999). Quinupristin/dalfopristin should be reserved for treatment of serious infections caused by multiple-drug-resistant gram-positive organisms such as vancomycin-resistant *E. faecium.*

Untoward Effects. The most common side effects are infusion-related events, such as pain and phlebitis at the infusion site and arthralgias and myalgias. Phlebitis and pain can be minimized by infusion of drug through a central venous catheter. Arthralgias and myalgias, which are more likely to be a problem in patients with hepatic insufficiency and may be due to accumulation of metabolites, are managed by reducing the infusion frequency to every 12 hours. Quinupristin/dalfopristin inhibits CYP3A4. The concomitant administration of other CYP3A4 substrates (*see* Chapter 3) with quinupristin/dalfopristin may raise blood pressure and/or result in significant toxicity. Examples include antihistamines (*e.g., azelastine* and *clemastine*); some anticonvulsants (*e.g., fosphenytoin* and *felbamate*), macrolide antibiotics; some fluoroquinolones (*e.g., moxifloxacin* and *ketoconazole*); some antimalarials (*e.g., chloroquine, mefloquine,* and *quinine*); some antidepressants (*e.g., fluoxetine, imipramine, venlafaxine*); some antipsychotics (*e.g., haloperidol, risperidone,* and *quetiapine*); *tacrolimus*; and *doxepin.* Appropriate caution and monitoring are recommended for drugs in which the toxic therapeutic window is narrow or for drugs that prolong the QTc interval.

LINEZOLID

Linezolid (ZYVOX) is a synthetic antimicrobial agent of the oxazolidinone class (Clemett and Markham, 2000; Diekema and Jones, 2000; Hamel *et al.*, 2000). Its chemical structure is:

LINEZOLID

Antibacterial Activity. Linezolid is active against gram-positive organisms including staphylococci, streptococci, enterococci, gram-positive anaerobic cocci, and gram-positive rods such as *Corynebacterium* spp. and *Listeria monocytogenes*. It has poor activity against most gram-negative aerobic or anaerobic bacteria. It is bacteriostatic against enterococci and staphylococci and bactericidal against streptococci. MICs are ≤2 µg/ml against strains of *E. faecium*, *E. faecalis*, *S. pyogenes*, *S. pneumoniae*, and viridans strains of streptococci. MICs are ≤4 µg/ml for strains of *S. aureus* and coagulase-negative staphylococci. *Mycobacterium tuberculosis* is moderately susceptible, with MICs of 2 µg/ml. Because of its unique mechanism of action, linezolid is active against strains that are resistant to multiple other agents, including penicillin-resistant strains of *S. pneumoniae;* methicillin-resistant, vancomycin-intermediate, and vancomycin-resistant strains of staphylococci; and vancomycin-resistant strains of enterococci.

Mechanism of Action. Linezolid inhibits protein synthesis by binding to the P site of the 50S ribosomal subunit and preventing formation of the larger ribosomal-fMet-tRNA complex that initiates protein synthesis. As mentioned above, there is no cross-resistance with other drug classes. Resistance in enterococci and staphylococci is due to point mutations of the 23S rRNA (Wilson *et al.*, 2003). Since multiple copies of 23S rRNA genes are present in bacteria, resistance generally requires mutations in two or more copies.

Absorption, Distribution, and Excretion. Linezolid is well absorbed after oral administration and may be administered without regard to food. With oral bioavailability approaching 100%, dosing for oral and intravenous preparations is the same. Peak serum concentrations average 12 to 14 µg/ml 1 to 2 hours after a single 600-mg dose in adults and approximately 20 µg/ml at steady state with dosing every 12 hours. The half-life is approximately 4 to 6 hours. Linezolid is 30% protein-bound and distributes widely to well-perfused tissues, with a 0.6 to 0.7 L/kg volume of distribution.

Linezolid is broken down by nonenzymatic oxidation to aminoethoxyacetic acid and hydroxyethyl glycine derivatives. Approximately 80% of the dose of linezolid appears in the urine, 30% as active compound, and 50% as the two primary oxidation products. Ten percent of the administered dose appears as oxidation products in feces. Although serum concentrations and half-life of the parent compound are not appreciably altered by renal insufficiency, oxidation products accumulate in renal insufficiency, with half-lives increasing by approximately 50% to 100%. The clinical significance of this is unknown, and no dose adjustment in renal insufficiency is currently recommended. Linezolid and its breakdown products are eliminated by dialysis; therefore the drug should be administered after hemodialysis. One case report noted sustained therapeutic concentrations of linezolid in peritoneal dialysis fluid with oral administration of 600 mg of linezolid twice daily (DePestel *et al.*, 2003).

Therapeutic Uses. Linezolid is FDA approved for treatment of infections caused by vancomycin-resistant *E. faecium;* nosocomial pneumonia caused by methicillin-susceptible and-resistant strains of *S. aureus;* community-acquired pneumonia caused by penicillin-susceptible strains of *S. pneumoniae;* complicated skin and skin-structure infections caused by streptococci and methicillin-susceptible and -resistant strains of *S. aureus;* and uncomplicated skin and skin-structure infections (Clemett and Markham, 2000). In noncomparative studies, linezolid (600 mg twice daily) has had clinical and microbiological cure rates in the range of 85% to 90% in treatment of a variety of infections (soft tissue, urinary tract, and bacteremia) caused by vancomycin-resistant *E. faecium*. A 200-mg, twice-daily dose was less effective, with a clinical and microbiological cure rates of approximately 75% and 59%, respectively. The 600-mg, twice-daily dose therefore should be used for treatment of infections caused by enterococci. A 400-mg, twice-daily dosage regimen is recommended only for treatment of uncomplicated skin and skin-structure infections.

In randomized, comparative studies, cure rates with linezolid (~60%) were similar to those with vancomycin for nosocomial pneumonia caused by methicillin-resistant or -susceptible *S. aureus* (Rubinstein *et al.*, 2001; Wunderink *et al.*, 2003a). A post-hoc analysis suggested that linezolid may be superior to vancomycin for nosocomial pneumonia caused by methicillin-resistant *S. aureus*, but this needs to be confirmed in a prospective randomized trial (Wunderink *et al.*, 2003b). Efficacy of linezolid also was similar to that of either oxacillin or vancomycin for skin and skin-structure infections, the majority of microbiologically documented cases being caused by *S. aureus*. Although relatively few patients with *S.*

aureus bacteremia have been treated, linezolid appears to be comparable in efficacy to vancomycin for methicillin-resistant strains. Linezolid also may be an effective alternative for patients with methicillin-resistant *S. aureus* infections who are failing vancomycin therapy or whose isolates have reduced susceptibility to vancomycin (Howden *et al.*, 2004). Linezolid is bacteriostatic for staphylococci and enterococci; it probably should not be used for treatment of suspected endocarditis.

Linezolid should be reserved as an alternative agent for treatment of infections caused by multiple-drug-resistant strains. It should not be used when other agents are likely to be effective (e.g., community-acquired pneumonia, even though it has the indication). Indiscriminant use and overuse will hasten selection of resistant strains and the eventual loss of this valuable new agent.

Untoward Effects. The drug seems to be well tolerated, with generally minor side effects (*e.g.*, gastrointestinal complaints, headache, rash). Myelosuppression, including anemia, leukopenia, pancytopenia, and thrombocytopenia, has been reported in patients receiving linezolid. Thrombocytopenia or a significant reduction in platelet count has been associated with linezolid in 2.4% of treated patients, and its occurrence is related to duration of therapy. Platelet counts should be monitored in patients with risk of bleeding, preexisting thrombocytopenia, or intrinsic or acquired disorders of platelet function (including those potentially caused by concomitant medication) and in patients receiving courses of therapy lasting beyond 2 weeks. Linezolid is a weak, nonspecific inhibitor of monoamine oxidase. Patients receiving concomitant therapy with an adrenergic or serotonergic agent or consuming more than 100 mg of tyramine a day may experience palpitations, headache, or hypertensive crisis. Peripheral and optic neuropathy, which seem to be reversible upon drug discontinuation, have been reported with prolonged use. Linezolid is neither a substrate nor an inhibitor of CYPs.

SPECTINOMYCIN

Source and Chemistry. Spectinomycin is an antibiotic produced by *Streptomyces spectabilis*. The drug is an aminocyclitol; its structural formula is as follows:

SPECTINOMYCIN

Antibacterial Activity and Mechanism. Spectinomycin is active against a number of gram-negative bacterial species, but it is inferior to other drugs to which such microorganisms are suscep-

tible. *Its only therapeutic use is in the treatment of gonorrhea caused by strains resistant to first-line drugs, or if there are contraindications to the use of these drugs.*

Spectinomycin selectively inhibits protein synthesis in gram-negative bacteria. The antibiotic binds to and acts on the 30S ribosomal subunit. Its action is similar to that of the aminoglycosides, but spectinomycin is not bactericidal and does not cause misreading of messenger RNA. Bacterial resistance may be mediated by mutations in the 16S ribosomal RNA or by modification of the drug by adenylyltransferase (Clark *et al.*, 1999).

Absorption, Distribution, and Excretion. Spectinomycin is rapidly absorbed after intramuscular injection. A single dose of 2 g produces peak serum concentrations of 100 μg/ml at 1 hour. Eight hours after injection, the concentration is approximately 15 μg/ml. The drug is not significantly bound to plasma protein, and all of an administered dose is recovered in the urine within 48 hours.

Therapeutic Uses. The Centers for Disease Control and Prevention recommends *ceftriaxone, cefixime, ciprofloxacin, ofloxacin*, or *levofloxacin* for the treatment of uncomplicated gonococcal infection (Centers for Disease Control, 2002). However, spectinomycin is recommended as an alternative regimen in patients who are intolerant or allergic to β-lactam antibiotics and quinolones. Spectinomycin also is useful in pregnancy when patients are intolerant to β-lactams and when quinolones are contraindicated. The recommended dose for men and women is a single, deep intramuscular injection of 2 g. One of the disadvantages of this regimen is that spectinomycin has no effect on incubating or established syphilis, and it is not active against *Chlamydia* spp. It also is less effective for pharyngeal infections, and followup cultures to document cure should be obtained.

Untoward Effects. Spectinomycin, when given as a single intramuscular injection, produces few significant untoward effects. Urticaria, chills, and fever have been noted after single doses, as have dizziness, nausea, and insomnia. The injection may be painful.

POLYMYXIN B AND COLISTIN

Because of the extreme nephrotoxicity associated with parenteral administration of these drugs, they are rarely if ever used except topically.

Source and Chemistry. The polymyxins, discovered in 1947, are a group of closely related antibiotics elaborated by various strains of *Bacillus polymyxa. Colistin* is produced by *Bacillus (Aerobacillus) colistinus*. These drugs, which are cationic detergents, are relatively simple, basic peptides with molecular masses of about 1000 daltons. The structural formula for polymyxin B, which is a mixture of polymyxins B$_1$ and B$_2$, is:

Polymyxin B$_1$: R = (+)-methyloctanoyl
Polymyxin B$_2$: R = 6-methylheptanoyl
DAB = α,γ-diaminobutyric acid

Colistin (polymyxin E) has a similar structure; it is available as colistin sulfate for oral use and as colistimethate sodium for parenteral administration (not recommended).

Antibacterial Activity and Mechanism of Action. The antimicrobial activities of polymyxin B and colistin are similar and are restricted to gram-negative bacteria, including *Enterobacter, E. coli, Klebsiella, Salmonella, Pasteurella, Bordetella,* and *Shigella,* which usually are sensitive to concentrations of 0.05 to 2 μg/ml. Most strains of *P. aeruginosa* are inhibited by less than 8 μg/ml *in vitro. Proteus* spp. are intrinsically resistant.

Polymyxins are surface-active, amphipathic agents. They interact strongly with phospholipids and disrupt the structure of cell membranes. The permeability of the bacterial membrane changes immediately on contact with the drug. Sensitivity to polymyxin B apparently is related to the phospholipid content of the cell wall–membrane complex. The cell walls of certain resistant bacteria may prevent access of the drug to the cell membrane.

Polymyxin B binds to the lipid A portion of endotoxin (the lipopolysaccharide of the outer membrane of gram-negative bacteria) and inactivates this molecule. Polymyxin B attenuates pathophysiologic consequences of the release of endotoxin in several experimental systems, but the clinical utility of polymyxin B for this indication has not yet been established.

Absorption, Distribution, and Excretion. Polymyxin B and colistin are not absorbed when given orally and are poorly absorbed from mucous membranes and the surfaces of large burns. They are cleared renally, and modification of the dose is required in patients with impaired renal function.

Therapeutic Uses. Polymyxin B sulfate is available for ophthalmic, otic, and topical use in combination with a variety of other compounds. Colistin is available as otic drops. Parenteral preparations are still marketed, but they generally are not recommended and are rarely used. However, colistin may be useful as a salvage regimen for treatment of infections caused by multiple-drug-resistant organisms such as *Stenotrophomonas maltophilia, Acinetobacter* spp., or *P. aeruginosa,* when other alternatives have been exhausted (Linden *et al.,* 2003; San Gabriel *et al.,* 2004).

Infections of the skin, mucous membranes, eye, and ear due to polymyxin B–sensitive microorganisms respond to local application of the antibiotic in solution or ointment. External otitis, frequently due to *Pseudomonas,* may be cured by the topical use of the drug. *P. aeruginosa* is a common cause of infection of corneal ulcers; local application or subconjunctival injection of polymyxin B often is curative.

Untoward Effects. Polymyxin B applied to intact or denuded skin or mucous membranes produces no systemic reactions because of its almost complete lack of absorption from these sites. Hypersensitization is uncommon with topical application. Polymyxins interfere with neurotransmission at the neuromuscular junction, resulting in muscle weakness and apnea. Other neurological reactions include paresthesias, vertigo, and slurred speech. Polymyxins are nephrotoxic, and administration with aminoglycosides should be avoided if possible.

VANCOMYCIN

History and Source. Vancomycin is a glycopeptide antibiotic produced by *Streptococcus orientalis. Teicoplanin,* also a glycopeptide, is available in Europe (Biavasco *et al.,* 1997).

Chemistry. Vancomycin is a complex and unusual tricyclic glycopeptide with a molecular mass of about 1500 daltons. Its structural formula is:

VANCOMYCIN

Antibacterial Activity. Vancomycin is primarily active against gram-positive bacteria. Strains are considered susceptible at MICs of ≤4 μg/ml. *S. aureus* and *S. epidermidis,* including strains resistant to methicillin, usually are inhibited by concentrations of 1 to 4 μg/ml. *S. pyogenes, S. pneumoniae,* and viridans streptococci are highly susceptible to vancomycin. *Bacillus* spp., including *B. anthracis,* are inhibited by 2 μg/ml or less. *Corynebacterium* spp. (diphtheroids) are inhibited by less than 0.04 to 3.1 μg/ml of vancomycin; most species of *Actinomyces,* by 5 to 10 μg/ml; and *Clostridium* spp., by 0.39 to 6 μg/ml. Essentially all species of gram-negative bacilli and mycobacteria are resistant to vancomycin.

Mechanisms of Action and Resistance. Vancomycin inhibits the synthesis of the cell wall in sensitive bacteria by binding with high affinity to the D-alanyl-D-alanine terminus of cell wall precursor units (Figure 46–4). The drug is bactericidal for dividing microorganisms.

Strains of enterococci once were uniformly susceptible to vancomycin. Vancomycin-resistant strains of enterococci, primarily *Enterococcus faecium,* have emerged as major nosocomial pathogens in hospitals in the United States. Vancomycin resistance determinants in *E. faecium* and *E. faecalis* are located on a transposon that is part of a conjugative plasmid, rendering it readily transferable among enterococci, and potentially, other gram-positive bacteria. These strains typically are resistant to multiple antibiotics, including *streptomycin, gentamicin,* and *ampicillin,* effectively eliminating these as alternative therapeutic agents. Resistance to streptomycin and gentamicin

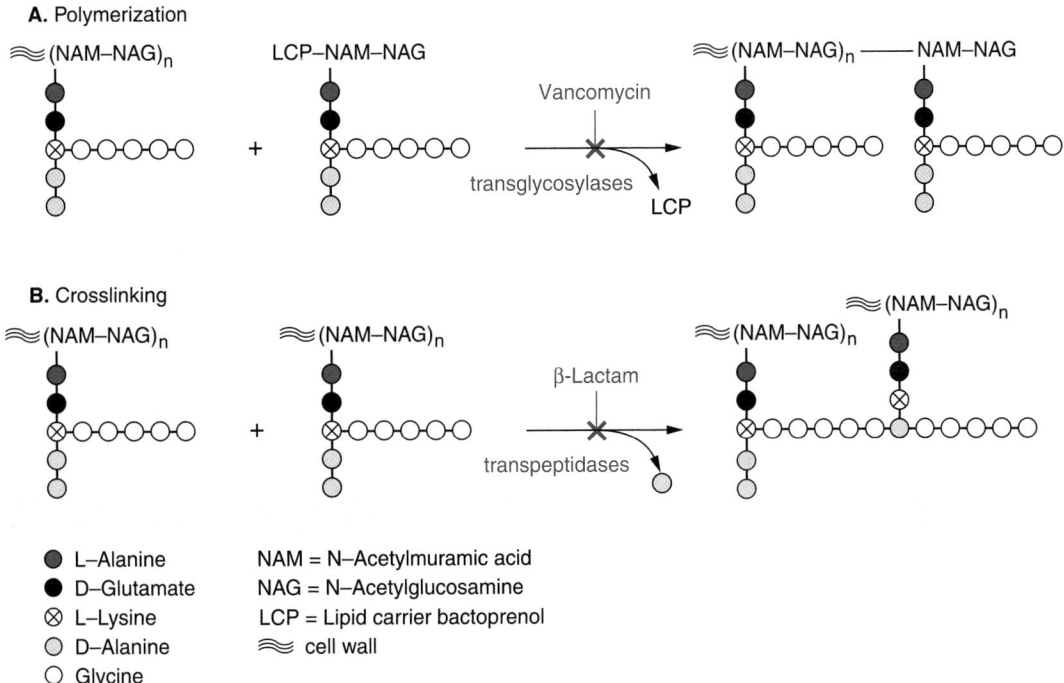

Figure 46–4. Inhibition of bacterial cell wall synthesis. Vancomycin inhibits the polymerization or transglycosylase reaction (*A*) by binding to the D-alanyl-D-alanine terminus of the cell wall precursor unit attached to its lipid carrier and blocks linkage to the glycopeptide polymer (indicated by the subscript n). These (NAM–NAG)$_n$ peptidoglycan polymers are located within the cell wall. *Van A*-type resistance is due to expression of enzymes that modify cell wall precursor by substituting a terminal D-lactate for D-alanine, reducing vancomycin binding affinity by 1000 times. β-Lactam antibiotics inhibit the cross-linking or transpeptidase reaction (*B*) that links glycopeptide polymer chains by formation of a cross-bridge with the stem peptide (the five glycines in this example) of one chain, displacing the terminal D-alanine of an adjacent chain.

is of special concern, because the combination of an aminoglycoside with a cell-wall-synthesis inhibitor is the only reliably bactericidal regimen for treatment of enterococcal endocarditis.

Enterococcal resistance to vancomycin is the result of alteration of the D-alanyl-D-alanine target to D-alanyl-D-lactate or D-alanyl-D-serine (Arias *et al.*, 2000), which bind vancomycin poorly, due to the lack of a critical site for hydrogen bonding. Several enzymes within the *van* gene cluster are required for this target alteration to occur.

Several phenotypes of resistance to vancomycin have been described. The *Van A* phenotype confers inducible resistance to teicoplanin and vancomycin in *E. faecium* and *E. faecalis*. The *Van B* phenotype, which tends to be a lower level of resistance, also has been identified in *E. faecium* and *E. faecalis*. The trait is inducible by vancomycin but not teicoplanin, and consequently, many strains remain susceptible to teicoplanin. The *Van C* phenotype, the least important clinically and least well characterized, confers resistance only to vancomycin, is constitutive, and is present in no species of enterococci other than *E. faecalis* and *E. faecium*. *Van D* and *Van E* gene clusters also have been identified, and presumably others will follow.

S. aureus and coagulase-negative staphylococci may express reduced or "intermediate" susceptibility to vancomycin (MIC, 8 to 16

μg/ml) (Hiramatsu *et al.*, 1997; Smith *et al.*, 1999; Garrett *et al.*, 1999) or high-level resistance (MIC ≥32 μg/ml; Centers for Disease Control, 2004). Intermediate resistance is associated with (and may be preceded by) a heterogeneous phenotype in which a small proportion of cells within the population (1 in 10⁵ to 1 in 10⁶) will grow in the presence of vancomycin concentrations above 4 μg/ml. The genetic and biochemical basis of the intermediate phenotype is not well understood. Intermediate strains produce an abnormally thick cell wall, and resistance may be due to false targets for vancomycin. Several genetic elements and multiple mutations are involved, and many of the genes that have been implicated encode enzymes of the cell-wall biosynthetic pathway (Sieradzki and Tomasz, 1999; Sieradzki *et al.*, 1999).

The first high-level vancomycin-resistant *S. aureus* strain (MIC ≥32 μg/ml) was isolated in June 2002 (Weigel *et al.*, 2003). This strain, like others that have subsequently been isolated, harbored a conjugative plasmid into which the *Van A* transposon, Tn1546, was integrated as a consequence of an interspecies horizontal gene transfer from *E. faecalis* to a methicillin-resistant strain of *S. aureus*.

Infections caused by intermediate strains have failed to respond to vancomycin clinically and in animal models (Climo *et al.*, 1999; Moore *et al.*, 2003). Prior treatment courses and low vancomycin levels may predispose patients to infection and treatment failure with vancomycin-intermediate strains. These strains typically are resistant to methicillin and multiple other antibiotics; their emergence is a major concern because until recently vancomycin has been the only antibiotic to which staphylococci were reliably susceptible.

Absorption, Distribution, and Excretion. Vancomycin is poorly absorbed after oral administration. For parenteral therapy, the drug should be administered intravenously, never intramuscularly. A single intravenous dose of 1 g in adults produces plasma concentrations of 15 to 30 μg/ml 1 hour after a 1- to 2-hour infusion. The drug has a serum elimination half-life of about 6 hours. Approximately 30% of vancomycin is bound to plasma protein. Vancomycin appears in various body fluids, including the CSF when the meninges are inflamed (7% to 30%); bile; and pleural, pericardial, synovial, and ascitic fluids. About 90% of an injected dose is excreted by glomerular filtration. The drug accumulates if renal function is impaired, and dosage adjustments must be made under these circumstances. The drug can be cleared rapidly from plasma with high-flux methods of hemodialysis.

Therapeutic Uses. Vancomycin hydrochloride (VANCOCIN, others) is marketed for *intravenous* use as a sterile powder for solution. It should be diluted and infused over at least a 60-minute period to avoid infusion-related adverse reactions (*see* below). The usual dose of vancomycin for adults is 30 mg/kg per day in 2 to 3 divided doses. This dose will yield average steady-state serum concentrations of 15 μg/ml. The "therapeutic range" for this agent is somewhat controversial. A target trough serum concentration of 5 to 15 μg/ml, 10 to 20 μg/ml for more serious infections such as endocarditis or meningitis, is recommended. Doses above 30 mg/kg per day may be required to achieve these trough concentrations, and up to 60 mg/kg per day has been suggested for use in meninigitis (Quagliarello and Scheld, 1997). *The "peak" concentration, which need not be monitored routinely, as the distribution phase of the drug is long, should generally remain below 60 μg/ml to avoid ototoxicity.*

Pediatric doses are as follows: for newborns during the first week of life, 15 mg/kg initially, followed by 10 mg/kg every 12 hours; for infants 8 to 30 days old, 15 mg/kg followed by 10 mg/kg every 8 hours; for older infants and children, 10 mg/kg every 6 hours.

Alteration of dosage is required for patients with impaired renal function. The drug has been used effectively in functionally anephric patients and dialysis patients by the administration of 1 g (approximately 15 mg/kg) every 5 to 7 days. Because there is so much variation in how well vancomycin is dialyzed with different membranes, it is recommended that blood levels be monitored to decide how frequently the drug needs to be administered to maintain therapeutic concentrations.

Vancomycin can be administered orally to patients with pseudomembranous colitis, although metronidazole is preferred.

The dose for adults is 125 to 250 mg every 6 hours; the total daily dose for children is 40 mg/kg, given in three to four divided doses. *Vancomycin hydrochloride for oral solution* is available for this purpose, as are capsules.

Vancomycin should be employed only to treat serious infections and is particularly useful in the management of infections due to methicillin-resistant staphylococci, including pneumonia, empyema, endocarditis, osteomyelitis, and soft-tissue abscesses and in severe staphylococcal infections in patients who are allergic to penicillins and cephalosporins. However, vancomycin is less rapidly bactericidal than any of the antistaphylococcal β-lactams (*e.g.*, *nafcillin* or *cefazolin*) and therefore may be less efficacious clinically (Levine *et al.*, 1991). Treatment with vancomycin is effective and convenient when there is disseminated staphylococcal infection or localized infection of a shunt in a patient with irreversible renal disease who is being maintained by hemodialysis or peritoneal dialysis, because the drug can be administered once weekly or in the dialysis fluid. Intraventricular administration of vancomycin (*via* a shunt or reservoir) has been necessary in a few cases of CNS infections due to susceptible microorganisms that did not respond to intravenous therapy alone.

Administration of vancomycin is an effective alternative for the treatment of endocarditis caused by viridans streptococci in patients who are allergic to penicillin. In combination with an aminoglycoside, it may be used for enterococcal endocarditis in patients with serious penicillin allergy. Vancomycin also is effective for the treatment of infections caused by *Corynebacterium* spp. Vancomycin has become an important antibiotic in the management of known or suspected penicillin-resistant pneumococcal infections (Friedland and McCracken, 1994).

Untoward Effects. Among the hypersensitivity reactions produced by vancomycin are macular skin rashes and anaphylaxis. Phlebitis and pain at the site of intravenous injection are relatively uncommon. Chills, rash, and fever may occur. Rapid intravenous infusion may cause erythematous or urticarial reactions, flushing, tachycardia, and hypotension. The extreme flushing that can occur is sometimes called "red-neck" or "red-man" syndrome. This is not an allergic reaction but a direct toxic effect of vancomycin on mast cells, causing them to release histamine.

Auditory impairment, sometimes permanent, may follow the use of this drug. Ototoxicity is associated with excessively high concentrations of the drug in plasma (60 to 100 μg/ml). Nephrotoxicity, formerly quite common probably because of less pure formulations of the drug, has become an unusual side effect when appropriate doses are used, as judged by renal function and determinations of blood levels of the drug. Caution must be exercised, however, when ototoxic or nephrotoxic drugs, such as aminoglycosides, are administered concurrently or in patients with impaired renal function.

TEICOPLANIN

Source and Chemistry. Teicoplanin is a glycopeptide antibiotic produced by *Actinoplanes teichomyetius*. The drug actually is a mixture of six closely related compounds: one compound has a terminal hydrogen at the oxygen indicated by an asterisk; five compounds have an R substituent of either a decanoic acid [*n*-, 8-methyl-, 9-methyl, (*Z*)-4-] or of a nonanoic acid [8-methyl]. Although not FDA approved for use in the United States, it is available in Europe. It is similar to vancomycin in chemical structure, mechanism of action, spectrum of activity, and route of elimination (*i.e.*, primarily renal). Its structure is:

TEICOPLANIN

Mechanisms of Action and Resistance. Teicoplanin, like vancomycin, inhibits cell-wall synthesis by binding with high affinity to the D-alanyl-D-alanine terminus of cell wall precursor units (Figure 46–4), and it is active only against gram-positive bacteria. It is reliably bactericidal against susceptible strains, except for enterococci. It is active against methicillin-susceptible and methicillin-resistant staphylococci, which typically have MICs of <4 μg/ml. The MICs for *Listeria monocytogenes, Corynebacterium* spp., *Clostridium* spp., and anaerobic gram-positive cocci range from 0.25 to 2 μg/ml. Nonviridans and viridans streptococci, *S. pneumoniae,* and enterococci are inhibited by concentrations ranging from 0.01 to 1 μg/ml. Some strains of staphylococci, coagulase-positive and coagulase-negative, as well as enterococci and other organisms that are intrinsically resistant to vancomycin (*i.e., Lactobacillus* spp. and *Leuconostoc* spp.), are resistant to teicoplanin.

The mechanisms of resistance to teicoplanin in strains of staphylococci have not been elucidated, but resistance can emerge in a previously susceptible strain during a course of therapy. The *Van A* phenotype of vancomycin-resistant enterococci also determines resistance to teicoplanin. The mechanism is the same as for vancomycin: alteration of the cell-wall target so that the glycopeptide does not bind. Strains of enterococci with *Van B* resistance often are susceptible to teicoplanin, which is a poor inducer of the enzymes responsible for the cell-wall alteration. *Van C* strains of enterococci, which in general are not human pathogens, are susceptible to teicoplanin.

Absorption, Distribution, and Excretion. The primary differences between vancomycin and teicoplanin are: teicoplanin can be administered safely by intramuscular injection; it is highly bound by plasma proteins (90% to 95%); and it has an extremely long serum elimination half-life (up to 100 hours in patients with normal renal function). The dose of teicoplanin in adults is 6 to 30 mg/kg per day, with the higher dosages reserved for treatment of serious staphylococcal infec-

tions. Once-daily dosing is possible for the treatment of most infections because of the prolonged serum elimination half-life. As with vancomycin, teicoplanin doses must be adjusted in patients with renal insufficiency. For functionally anephric patients, administration once weekly has been appropriate, but serum drug concentrations should be monitored to determine that the therapeutic range has been maintained (*e.g.*, trough concentration of 15 to 20 μg/ml).

Therapeutic Uses. Teicoplanin has been used to treat a wide variety of infections, including osteomyelitis and endocarditis, caused by methicillin-resistant and methicillin-susceptible staphylococci, streptococci, and enterococci. Teicoplanin has been found to be comparable to vancomycin in efficacy, except for treatment failures from low doses used for such serious infections as endocarditis. Teicoplanin is not as efficacious as antistaphylococcal penicillins for treating bacteremia and endocarditis caused by methicillin-susceptible *S. aureus*, with teicoplanin cure rates of 60% to 70% *versus* 85% to 90% for the penicillins. The efficacy of teicoplanin against *S. aureus* may be improved by the addition of an aminoglycoside (*e.g.*, gentamicin 1 mg/kg every 8 hours in patients with normal renal function) to provide a synergistic effect. Strains of streptococci are uniformly susceptible to teicoplanin. This drug has been very effective in a once-daily regimen for patients with streptococcal osteomyelitis or endocarditis. Teicoplanin is among the most active drugs against enterococci. Limited experience indicates that it is effective, although only bacteriostatic, for serious enterococcal infections. It should be combined with gentamicin to achieve a bactericidal effect in the treatment of enterococcal endocarditis.

Untoward Effects. The main side effect reported for teicoplanin is skin rash, which is more common in higher dosages. Hypersensitivity reactions, drug fever, and neutropenia also have been reported. Ototoxicity has occurred rarely.

DAPTOMYCIN

Source and Chemistry. Daptomycin (CUBICIN) is a cyclic lipopeptide antibiotic derived from *Streptomyces roseosporus*. Discovered more than 20 years ago, its clinical development has been resumed in response to increasing need for bactericidal antibiotics effective against vancomycin-resistant gram-positive bacteria (Carpenter and Chambers, 2004). Its structural formula is:

DAPTOMYCIN

Antibacterial Activity. Daptomycin is a bactericidal antibiotic selectively active against aerobic, facultative, and anaerobic gram-positive bacteria (Jevitt *et al.*, 2003; Streit *et al.*, 2004). The MIC susceptibility breakpoint for staphylococci and streptococci is ≤1 μg/ml; for enterococci it is ≤4 μg/ml. Approximately 90% of strains of staphylococci and streptococci are inhibited at concentrations of 0.25 to 0.5 μg/ml; the corresponding values for *E. faecalis* and *E. faecium* are 0.5 to 1 and 2 to 4 μg/ml, respectively. Daptomycin may be active against vancomycin-resistant strains, although MICs tend to be higher for these organisms than for their vancomycin-susceptible counterparts. MICs of *Corynebacterium* spp., *Peptostreptococcus*, propionibacteria, and *Clostridium perfringens* are ≤0.5 to 1 μg/ml (Goldstein *et al.*, 2004). *Actinomyces* spp. are inhibited over the concentration range of 4 to 32 μg/ml. *In vitro* activity of daptomycin is Ca^{2+}-dependent, and MIC tests should be performed in medium containing 50 mg/L calcium.

Mechanisms of Action and Resistance. Daptomycin binds to bacterial membranes resulting in depolarization, loss of membrane potential, and cell death. It has concentration-dependent bactericidal activity. Due to its unique mechanism of action, cross-resistance with other antibiotic classes seems not occur, and there are no known resistance mechanisms. There were two cases (one *S. aureus* and one *E. faecalis*) among more than 1000 cases treated in which resistance emerged during therapy. Staphylococci with decreased susceptibility to vancomycin have higher daptomycin MICs than fully susceptible strains (Jevitt *et al.*, 2003).

Absorption, Fate, and Excretion. Daptomycin is poorly absorbed orally and should only be administered intravenously. Direct toxicity to muscle precludes intramuscular injection. The steady-state peak serum concentration following intravenous administration of 4 mg/kg in healthy volunteers is approximately 58 μg/ml. Daptomycin displays linear pharmacokinetics at doses up to 8 mg/kg. It is reversibly bound to albumin; protein binding is 92%. The serum half-life is 8 to 9 hours in normal subjects, permitting once-daily dosing. Approximately 80% of the administered dose is recovered in urine; a small amount is excreted in feces. Dosage adjustment is required for creatinine clearance below 30 ml/minute; this is accomplished by administering the recommended dose every 48 hours. For hemodialysis patients the dose should be administered immediately after dialysis.

Daptomycin neither inhibits nor induces CYPs, and there are no important drug-drug interactions. However, caution is recommended when administering daptomycin in conjunction with aminoglycosides or statins because of potential risks of nephrotoxicity and myopathy, respectively.

Therapeutic Uses. Daptomycin is indicated for treatment of complicated skin and skin-structure infections caused by methicillin-susceptible and methicillin-resistant strains of *S. aureus*, hemolytic streptococci, and vancomycin-susceptible *E. faecalis* (Carpenter and Chambers, 2004). Its efficacy is comparable to that of vancomycin. Efficacy in more serious infections, such as endocarditis or complicated bacteremia, has not been demonstrated, although clinical trials are under way. Daptomycin was inferior to comparators for treatment of community-acquired pneumonia and is not indicated for this infection.

Untoward Effects. Skeletal muscle damage occurs in dogs given daptomycin at doses above 10 mg/kg. Peripheral neuropathic effects with axonal degeneration occurred at higher doses. In humans, ele-

vations of creatine kinase may occur; this does not require discontinuation of the drug unless there are findings of an otherwise unexplained myopathy. In Phase 1 and 2 clinical trials, a few patients had evidence of possible neuropathy, although this was not observed in Phase 3 studies.

BACITRACIN

Source and Chemistry. Bacitracin is an antibiotic produced by the Tracy-I strain of *Bacillus subtilis*. The bacitracins are a group of polypeptide antibiotics; multiple components have been demonstrated in the commercial products. The major constituent is bacitracin A. Its probable structural formula is:

BACITRACIN

A unit of the antibiotic is equivalent to 26 μg of the USP standard.

Mechanism of Action; Antibacterial Activity. Bacitracin inhibits the synthesis of the bacterial cell wall. A variety of gram-positive cocci and bacilli, *Neisseria*, *H. influenzae*, and *Treponema pallidum* are sensitive to 0.1 unit or less of bacitracin per milliliter. *Actinomyces* and *Fusobacterium* are inhibited by concentrations of 0.5 to 5 units/ml. Enterobacteriaceae, *Pseudomonas, Candida* spp., and *Nocardia* are resistant to the drug.

Therapeutic Uses. While bacitracin previously has been employed parenterally, current use is restricted to topical application.

Bacitracin is available in ophthalmic and dermatologic ointments; the antibiotic also is available as a powder for the preparation of topical solutions. The ointments are applied directly to the involved surface one or more times daily. A number of topical preparations of bacitracin, to which *neomycin* or polymyxin or both have been added, are available, and some contain the three antibiotics plus hydrocortisone.

Topical bacitracin alone or in combination with other antimicrobial agents has no established value in the treatment of furunculosis, pyoderma, carbuncle, impetigo, and superficial and deep abscesses. For open infections such as infected eczema and infected dermal ulcers, the local application of the antibiotic may be of some help in eradicating sensitive bacteria. Unlike several other antibiotics used topically, bacitracin rarely produces hypersensitivity. Suppurative conjunctivitis and infected corneal ulcer respond well to the topical use of bacitracin when caused by susceptible bacteria. Bacitracin has been used with limited success for eradication of nasal carriage of staphylococci. Oral bacitracin has been used with some success for the treatment of antibiotic-associated diarrhea caused by *C. difficile*. Bacitracin is used by neurosurgeons to irrigate the meninges intraoperatively as an alternative to vancomycin. It has no direct toxicity on neurons.

Untoward Effects. Serious nephrotoxicity results from the parenteral use of this antibiotic. Hypersensitivity reactions rarely result from topical application.

MUPIROCIN

Source and Chemistry. Mupirocin (BACTROBAN) is derived from a fermentation product of *Pseudomonas fluorescens*. It is for topical use only. Its structural formula is:

MUPIROCIN

Antibacterial Activity. Mupirocin is active against many gram-positive and selected gram-negative bacteria. It has good activity with MICs ≤1 μg/ml against *Streptococcus pyogenes* and methicillin-susceptible and methicillin-resistant strains of *S. aureus*. It is bactericidal at concentrations achieved with topical application.

Mechanism of Action and Resistance. Mupirocin inhibits bacterial protein synthesis by reversible binding and inhibition of isoleucyl transfer-RNA synthetase. There is no cross-resistance with other classes of antibiotics. Low-level resistance, which is not clinically significant, is due to mutations of the host gene encoding isoleucyl transfer-RNA synthetase or an extra chromosomal copy of a gene encoding a modified isoleucyl transfer-RNA synthetase (Ramsey *et al.*, 1996; Udo *et al.*, 2001). High-level resistance (MIC >1 mg/ml) is mediated by a plasmid or chromosomal copy of *mupA*, which encodes a "bypass" synthetase that binds mupirocin poorly (Udo *et al.*, 2001).

Absorption, Fate, and Excretion. Systemic absorption through intact skin or skin lesions is minimal. Any mupirocin that is absorbed is rapidly metabolized to inactive monic acid.

Therapeutic Uses. Mupirocin is available as a 2% cream and a 2% ointment for dermatologic use and as a 2% ointment for intranasal use. The dermatologic preparations are indicated for treatment of traumatic skin lesions and impetigo secondarily infected with *S. aureus* or *S. pyogenes*.

The nasal ointment is approved for eradication of *S. aureus* nasal carriage. Mupirocin is highly effective in eradicating *S. aureus* carriage (Laupland and Conly, 2003). Because *S. aureus* colonization often precedes infection, eradication of carriage by intranasal application of mupirocin might reduce the risk of later infection. However, two clinical trials failed to demonstrate that mupirocin prophylaxis reduces nosocomial *S. aureus* infections (Kalmeijer *et al.*, 2002; Wertheim *et al.*, 2004).

A third large study found that *S. aureus* nasal carriers had fewer *S. aureus* nosocomial infections of any site, but failed to show a reduction in *S. aureus* surgical site infections, the primary endpoint of the study (Perl *et al.*, 2002). The accumulated evidence indicates that patients who stand to benefit from mupirocin prophylaxis are those with proven *S. aureus* nasal colonization plus risk factors for

distant infection or a history of skin or soft tissue infections. General inpatient populations and individuals lacking specific risk factors for *S. aureus* infection are not likely to benefit from mupirocin prophylaxis.

Untoward Effects. Mupirocin may cause irritation and sensitization at the site of application. Contact with the eyes should be avoided because mupirocin causes tearing, burning, and irritation that may take several days to resolve. Systemic reactions to mupirocin occur rarely, if at all. Polyethylene glycol present in the ointment can be absorbed from damaged skin. Application of the ointment to large surface areas should be avoided in patients with moderate to severe renal failure to avoid accumulation of polyethylene glycol.

CLINICAL SUMMARY

Doxycycline, the most important member of the tetracyclines, is useful as a broad-spectrum agent that treats sexually transmitted diseases, rickettsial infections, plague, brucellosis, tularemia, and spirochetal infections. The emergence of resistance to other antibiotic classes among common bacterial pathogens has enhanced the utility of doxycycline for respiratory tract infections, given its activity against *S. pneumoniae*, *Haemophilus* spp., and atypical pneumonia pathogens; and for skin and soft-tissue infections caused by community strains of methicillin-resistant *S. aureus*, for which minocycline also is particularly active.

Macrolides and ketolides are useful for treatment of respiratory tract infections because they are active against the common pathogens of community-acquired pneumonia, including *S. pneumoniae*, *Haemophilus* spp., *Chlamydia*, mycoplasma, and *Legionella*. They generally are well-tolerated, orally bioavailable, and except for erythromycin, effective in once- or twice-daily dosing. All except azithromycin have important drug interactions because they inhibit hepatic CYPs.

Chloramphenicol is rarely used in the United States and Europe because it can cause irreversible bone marrow toxicity and because less-toxic drugs are readily available. However, it continues to be an important antibiotic in developing nations because it is inexpensive and highly effective for a broad range of infections.

Spectinomycin is indicated only for the treatment of gonococcal infection when a β-lactam or fluoroquinolone cannot be used. Clindamycin has excellent activity against gram-positive cocci, but principally is used to treat anaerobic infections. Vancomycin, daptomycin, quinupristin/dalfopristin, and linezolid are indicated for the treatment of gram-positive infections caused by drug-resistant organisms such as penicillin-resistant pneumococci and methicillin-resistant staphylococci. Quinupristin/dalfopristin and linezolid are indicated for the treatment of vancomycin-resistant *E. faecium* infections. These drugs, along with daptomycin, also are active against vancomycin-insensitive strains of *S. aureus*, although sufficient data demonstrating clinical efficacy are lacking.

Polymyxins, bacitracin, and mupirocin are useful for the topical treatment of minor skin infections. Colistin (poly-myxin E) can be administered systemically and is active against drug-resistant gram-negative bacteria, including *Pseudomonas*, *Stenotrophomonas*, and *Acinetobacter*; its significant toxicity makes it an agent of last resort. Mupirocin is effective for eradication of *S. aureus* nasal colonization.

BIBLIOGRAPHY

Ackermann, G., and Rodloff, A.C. Drugs of the 21st century: telithro-mycin (HMR 3647)—the first ketolide. *J. Antimicrob. Chemother.*, **2003**, *51*:497–511.

Allignet, J., and El Solh, N. Comparative analysis of staphylococcal plasmids carrying three streptogramin-resistance genes: vat-vgb-vga. *Plasmid*, **1999**, *42*:134–138.

Allignet, J., Liassine, N., and el Solh, N. Characterization of a staphy-lococcal plasmid related to pUB110 and carrying two novel genes, vatC and vgbB, encoding resistance to streptogramins A and B and similar antibiotics. *Antimicrob. Agents Chemother.*, **1998**, *42*:1794–1798.

Arias, C.A., Courvalin, P., and Reynolds, P.E. van C cluster of vanco-mycin-resistant *Enterococcus gallinarum* BM4174. *Antimicrob. Agents Chemother.*, **2000**, *44*:1660–1666.

Bace, A., Zrnic, T., Begovac, J., et al. Short-term treatment of pertussis with azithromycin in infants and young children. *Eur. J. Clin. Micro-biol. Infect. Dis.*, **1999**, *18*:296–298.

Bartlett, J.G., Breiman, R.F., Mandell, L.A., and File, T.M. Jr. Commu-nity-acquired pneumonia in adults: guidelines for management. *Clin. Infect. Dis.*, **1998**, *26*:811–838.

Biavasco, F., Vignaroli, C., Lupidi, R., et al. In vitro antibacterial activi-ty of LY333328, a new semisynthetic glycopeptide. *Antimicrob. Agents Chemother.*, **1997**, *41*:2165–2172.

Bowler, W.A., Hostettler, C., Samuelson, D., et al. Gastrointestinal side effects of intravenous erythromycin: incidence and reduction with prolonged infusion time and glycopyrrolate pretreatment. *Am. J. Med.*, **1992**, *92*:249–253.

Bozdogan, B., and Leclercq, R. Effects of genes encoding resistance to streptogramins A and B on the activity of quinupristin-dalfopristin against *Enterococcus faecium*. *Antimicrob. Agents Chemother.*, **1999**, *43*:2720–2725.

Bozdogan, B., Berrezouga, L., et al. A new resistance gene, linB, con-ferring resistance to lincosamides by nucleotidylation in *Enterococ-cus faecium* HM1025. *Antimicrob. Agents Chemother.*, **1999**, *43*:925–929.

Centers for Disease Control and Prevention. Sexually transmitted diseas-es treatment guidelines. *MMWR Recomm. Rpt.*, **2002**, *51*(RR6):1–78.

Centers for Disease Control and Prevention. Vancomycin-resistant *Sta-phylococcus aureus*—New York. *MMWR Morb. Mortal. Wkly. Rep.* **2004**, *53*:322–323.

Clark, N.C., Olsvik, O., Swenson, J.M., et al. Detection of a streptomy-cin/spectinomycin adenylyltransferase gene (aadA) in *Enterococcus faecalis*. *Antimicrob. Agents Chemother.*, **1999**, *43*:157–160.

Climo, M.W., Patron, R.L., and Archer, G.L. Combinations of vancomy-cin and β-lactams are synergistic against staphylococci with reduced susceptibilities to vancomycin. *Antimicrob. Agents Chemother.*, **1999**, *43*:1747–1753.

Dajani, A.S., Taubert, K.A., Wilson, W., et al. Prevention of bacterial endocarditis: recommendations by the American Heart Association. *Clin. Infect. Dis.*, **1997**, *25*:1448–1458.

DePestel, D.D., Peloquin, C.A., and Carver, P.L. Peritoneal dialysis fluid concentrations of linezolid in the treatment of vancomycin-resis-tant *Enterococcus faecium* peritonitis. *Pharmacotherapy*, **2003**, *23*:1322–1326.

Doern, G.V., Pfaller, M.A., Kugler, K., et al. Prevalence of antimicrobi-al resistance among respiratory tract isolates of *Streptococcus pneu-moniae* in North America: 1997 results from the SENTRY antimicro-bial surveillance program. *Clin. Infect. Dis.*, **1998**, *27*:764–770.

Fagon, J., Patrick, H., Haas, D.W., et al. Treatment of gram-positive nosocomial pneumonia. Prospective randomized comparison of quin-upristin/dalfopristin versus vancomycin. Nosocomial Pneumonia Group. *Am. J. Respir. Crit. Care Med.*, **2000**, *161*:753–762.

Friedland, I.R., and McCracken, G.H. Jr. Management of infections caused by antibiotic-resistant *Streptococcus pneumoniae*. *N. Engl. J. Med.*, **1994**, *331*:377–382.

Fuller, D.G., Duke, T. et al. Antibiotic treatment for bacterial meningitis in children in developing countries. *Ann. Trop. Paediatr.*, **2003**, *23*:233–253.

Garey, K.W., and Amsden, G.W. Intravenous azithromycin. *Ann. Phar-macother.*, **1999**, *33*:218–228.

Garrett, D.O., Jochimsen, E., Murfitt, K., et al. The emergence of decreased susceptibility to vancomycin in *Staphylococcus epidermi-dis*. *Infect. Control Hosp. Epidemiol.*, **1999**, *20*:167–170.

Gatti, G., Malena, M., Casazza, R., et al. Penetration of clindamycin and its metabolite N-demethylclindamycin into cerebrospinal fluid fol-lowing intravenous infusion of clindamycin phosphate in patients with AIDS. *Antimicrob. Agents Chemother.*, **1998**, *42*:3014–3017.

Goldstein, E.J., Citron, D.M., et al. In vitro activities of the new semi-synthetic glycopeptide telavancin (TD-6424), vancomycin, daptomy-cin, linezolid, and four comparator agents against anaerobic gram-positive species and *Corynebacterium* spp. *Antimicrob. Agents Chemother.*, **2004**, *48*:2149–2152.

Halperin, S.A., Bortolussi, R., Langley, J.M., et al. Seven days of eryth-romycin estolate is as effective as fourteen days for the treatment of *Bordetella pertussis* infections. *Pediatrics*, **1997**, *100*:65–71.

Hedberg, M., and Nord, C.E. Antimicrobial susceptibility of *Bacteroides fragilis* group isolates in Europe. *Clin. Microbiol. Infect.*, **2003**, *9*:475–488.

Hiramatsu, K., Aritaka, N., Hanaki, H., et al. Dissemination in Japanese hospitals of strains of *Staphylococcus aureus* heterogeneously resis-tant to vancomycin. *Lancet*, **1997**, *350*:1670–1673.

Hoban, D.J., Doern, G.V., et al. Worldwide prevalence of antimicrobial resistance in *Streptococcus pneumoniae*, *Haemophilus influenzae*, and *Moraxella catarrhalis* in the SENTRY Antimicrobial Surveil-lance Program, 1997–1999. *Clin. Infect. Dis.*, **2001**, *32*:S81–S93.

Howden, B.P., Ward, P.B., et al. Treatment outcomes for serious infections caused by methicillin-resistant *Staphylococcus aureus* with reduced van-comycin susceptibility. *Clin. Infect. Dis.*, **2004**, *38*:521–528.

Jevitt, L.A., Smith, A.J., *et al. In vitro* activities of Daptomycin, Linezolid, and Quinupristin-Dalfopristin against a challenge panel of Staphylococci and Enterococci, including vancomycin-intermediate *Staphylococcus aureus* and vancomycin-resistant *Enterococcus faecium*. *Microb. Drug Resist.*, **2003,** *9:*389–393.

Kalmeijer, M.D., Coertjens, H., *et al.* Surgical site infections in orthopedic surgery: the effect of mupirocin nasal ointment in a double-blind, randomized, placebo-controlled study. *Clin. Infect. Dis.*, **2002,** *35:*353–358.

Kovacs, J.A., and Masur, H. Prophylaxis against opportunistic infections in patients with human immunodeficiency virus infection. *N. Engl. J. Med.*, **2000,** *342:*1416–1429.

Laupland, K.B., and Conly, J.M. Treatment of *Staphylococcus aureus* colonization and prophylaxis for infection with topical intranasal mupirocin: an evidence-based review. *Clin. Infect. Dis.*, **2003,** *37:*933–938.

Levine, D.P., Fromm, B.S., and Reddy, B.R. Slow response to vancomycin or vancomycin plus rifampin in methicillin-resistant *Staphylococcus aureus* endocarditis. *Ann. Intern. Med.*, **1991,** *115:*674–680.

Levison, M.E., Mangura, C.T., Lorber, B., *et al.* Clindamycin compared with penicillin for the treatment of anaerobic lung abscess. *Ann. Intern. Med.*, **1983,** *98:*466–471.

Lina, G., Quaglia, A., *et al.* Distribution of genes encoding resistance to macrolides, lincosamides, and streptogramins among staphylococci. *Antimicrob. Agents Chemother.*, **1999,** *43:*1062–1066.

Linden, P.K., Kusne, S., *et al.* Use of parenteral colistin for the treatment of serious infection due to antimicrobial-resistant *Pseudomonas aeruginosa. Clin. Infect. Dis.*, **2003,** *37:*154–160.

Masters, E.J., Olson, G.S., *et al.* Rocky Mountain spotted fever: a clinician's dilemma. *Arch. Intern. Med.*, **2003,** *163:*769–774.

Moellering, R.C., Linden, P.K., Reinhardt, J., *et al.* The efficacy and safety of quinupristin/dalfopristin for the treatment of infections caused by vancomycin-resistant *Enterococcus faecium. J. Antimicrob. Chemother.*, **1999,** *44:*251–261.

Moore, M.R., Perdreau-Remington, F., *et al.* Vancomycin treatment failure associated with heterogeneous vancomycin-intermediate *Staphylococcus aureus* in a patient with endocarditis and in the rabbit model of endocarditis. *Antimicrob. Agents Chemother.*, **2003,** *47:*1262–1266.

Nakajima, Y. Mechanisms of bacterial resistance to macrolide antibiotics. *J. Infect. Chemother.*, **1999,** *5:*61–74.

Nichols, R.L., Graham, D.R., Barriere, S.L., *et al.* Treatment of hospitalized patients with complicated gram-positive skin and skin structure infections: two randomized, multicentre studies of quinupristin/dalfopristin versus cefazolin, oxacillin or vancomycin. Synercid Skin and Skin Structure Infection Group. *J. Antimicrob. Chemother.*, **1999,** *44:*263–273.

Nilius, A.M., and Ma, Z. Ketolides: the future of the macrolides? *Curr. Opin. Pharmacol.*, **2002,** *2:*493–500.

Parry, C.M. Antimicrobial drug resistance in *Salmonella enterica. Curr. Opin. Infect. Dis.*, **2003,** *16:*467–472.

Periti, P., Mazzei, T., Mini, E., and Novelli, A. Pharmacokinetic drug interactions of macrolides. *Clin. Pharmacokinet.*, **1992,** *23:*106–131.

Perl, T.M., Cullen, J.J., *et al.* Intranasal mupirocin to prevent postoperative *Staphylococcus aureus* infections. *N. Engl. J. Med.*, **2002,** *346:*1871–1877.

Peterson, W.L., Fendrick, A.M., Cave, D.R., *et al. Helicobacter pylori–*related disease: guidelines for testing and treatment. *Arch. Intern. Med.*, **2000,** *160:*1285–1291.

Quagliarello, V.J., and Scheld, W.M. Treatment of bacterial meningitis. *N. Engl. J. Med.*, **1997,** *336:*708–716.

Ramsey, M.A., Bradley, S.F. *et al.* Identification of chromosomal location of mupA gene, encoding low-level mupirocin resistance in staphylococcal isolates. *Antimicrob. Agents Chemother.*, **1996,** *40:*2820–2823.

Rubinstein, E., Cammarata, S., *et al.* Linezolid (PNU-100766) versus vancomycin in the treatment of hospitalized patients with nosocomial pneumonia: a randomized, double-blind, multicenter study. *Clin. Infect. Dis.*, **2001,** *32:*402–412.

San Gabriel, P., Zhou, J., *et al.* Antimicrobial susceptibility and synergy studies of *Stenotrophomonas maltophilia* isolates from patients with cystic fibrosis. *Antimicrob. Agents Chemother.*, **2004,** *48:*168–171.

Shi, J., Montay, G., *et al.* Pharmacokinetics and safety of the ketolide telithromycin in patients with renal impairment. *J. Clin. Pharmacol.*, **2004,** *44:*234–244.

Sieradzki, K., and Tomasz, A. Gradual alterations in cell wall structure and metabolism in vancomycin-resistant mutants of *Staphylococcus aureus. J. Bacteriol.*, **1999,** *181:*7566–7570.

Sieradzki, K., Wu, S.W., and Tomasz, A. Inactivation of the methicillin resistance gene mecA in vancomycin-resistant *Staphylococcus aureus. Microb. Drug Resist.*, **1999,** *5:*253–237.

Smith, T.L., Pearson, M.L., Wilcox, K.R., *et al.* Emergence of vancomycin resistance in *Staphylococcus aureus.* Glycopeptide-Intermediate *Staphylococcus aureus* Working Group. *N. Engl. J. Med.*, **1999,** *340:*493–501.

Soltani, M., Beighton, D., Philpott-Howard, J., and Woodford, N. Mechanisms of resistance to quinupristin-dalfopristin among isolates of *Enterococcus faecium* from animals, raw meat, and hospital patients in Western Europe. *Antimicrob. Agents Chemother.*, **2000,** *44:*433–436.

Streit, J.M., Jones, R.N., *et al.* Daptomycin activity and spectrum: a worldwide sample of 6737 clinical Gram-positive organisms. *J. Antimicrob. Chemother.* **2004,** *53:*669–674.

Udo, E.E., Jacob, L.E., *et al.* Genetic analysis of methicillin-resistant *Staphylococcus aureus* expressing high- and low-level mupirocin resistance. *J. Med. Microbiol.*, **2001,** *50:*909–915.

Villareal, F.J., Griffin, M., Owens, J., *et al.* Early short-term treatment with doxycycline modulates post-infarction left ventricular remodeling. *Circulation*, **2003,** *108:*1487–1492.

Ward, T.T., Rimland, D., Kauffman, C., *et al.* Randomized, open-label trial of azithromycin plus ethambutol vs. clarithromycin plus ethambutol as therapy for *Mycobacterium avium* complex bacteremia in patients with human immunodeficiency virus infection. Veterans Affairs HIV Research Consortium. *Clin. Infect. Dis.*, **1998,** *27:*1278–1285.

Weigel, L.M., Clewell, D.B., *et al.* Genetic analysis of a high-level vancomycin-resistant isolate of *Staphylococcus aureus. Science*, **2003,** *302:*1569–1571.

Wertheim, H.F., Vos, M.C., *et al.* Mupirocin prophylaxis against nosocomial *Staphylococcus aureus* infections in nonsurgical patients: a randomized study. *Ann. Intern. Med.*, **2004,** *140:*419–425.

Wilson, P., Andrews J.A., *et al.* Linezolid resistance in clinical isolates of *Staphylococcus aureus. J. Antimicrob. Chemother.*, **2003,** *51:*186–188.

Wunderink, R.G., Cammarata, S.K., *et al.* Continuation of a randomized, double-blind, multicenter study of linezolid versus vancomycin in the treatment of patients with nosocomial pneumonia. *Clin. Ther.*, **2003a,** *25:*980–992.

Wunderink, R.G., Rello, J., *et al.*, Linezolid *vs.* vancomycin: analysis of two double-blind studies of patients with methicillin-resistant *Staphylococcus aureus* nosocomial pneumonia. *Chest*, **2003b,** *124:*1789–1797.

MONOGRAPHS AND REVIEWS

Carpenter, C.F., and Chambers, H.F. Daptomycin: another novel agent for treating infections due to drug-resistant gram-positive pathogens. *Clin. Infect. Dis.*, **2004,** *38:*994–1000.

Clemett, D., and Markham, A. Linezolid. *Drugs,* **2000,** *59:*815–827; discussion, 828.

Diekema, D.I., and Jones, R.N. Oxazolidinones: a review. *Drugs,* **2000,** *59:*7–16.

Ellis, J., Oyston, P.C., *et al.* Tularemia. *Clin. Microbiol. Rev.* **2002,** *15:*631–646.

Hamel, J.C., Stapert, D., Moerman, J.K., and Ford, C.W. Linezolid, critical characteristics. *Infection,* **2000,** *28:*60–64.

Wareham, D.W., and Wilson, P. Chloramphenicol in the 21st century. *Hosp. Med.*, **2002,** *63:*157–161.

CHEMOTHERAPY OF TUBERCULOSIS, *MYCOBACTERIUM AVIUM* COMPLEX DISEASE, AND LEPROSY

William A. Petri, Jr.

Mycobacterial organisms cause tuberculosis, *Mycobacterium avium* complex (MAC) disease, and leprosy. Tuberculosis remains the primary worldwide cause of death due to infectious disease. A number of characteristics of mycobacteria make these diseases chronic and necessitate prolonged treatment. Mycobacteria grow slowly and may be dormant in the host for long periods; thus, they are relatively resistant to the effects of antibiotics. Many antibacterial agents do not penetrate the cell walls of mycobacteria, and a portion of mycobacteria can reside inside macrophages, adding another permeability barrier that effective agents must cross. Mycobacteria are agile in developing resistance to single chemotherapeutic agents. As a consequence, effective therapy of mycobacterial infections requires a prolonged course (months to years) of multiple drugs. Issues of patient compliance and drug toxicity are important, as are drug interactions, especially in patients being treated concurrently for HIV and tuberculosis or MAC infection. This chapter provides an overview of drugs used for first- and second-line treatment of tuberculosis and discusses therapeutic strategies evolving as resistance to available agents increases. Prophylaxis and treatment of *M. avium* infection in the setting of HIV coinfection are also discussed. In addition, this chapter covers the five clinically recognized forms of leprosy and the drug combinations used for their treatment.

The essential elements of the treatment of mycobacterial disease are to always treat with at least 2 different drugs to which the organism is susceptible and to treat for sufficient duration to prevent relapse (Leibert and Rom, 2004).

Drugs used in the treatment of tuberculosis can be divided into two major categories (Table 47–1). "First-line"

agents combine the greatest level of efficacy with an acceptable degree of toxicity; these include *isoniazid, rifampin, ethambutol, streptomycin*, and *pyrazinamide*. The large majority of patients with tuberculosis can be treated successfully with these drugs. Excellent results for patients with non–drug-resistant tuberculosis can be obtained with a 6-month course of treatment; for the first 2 months, isoniazid, rifampin, ethambutol, and pyrazinamide are given, followed by isoniazid and rifampin for the remaining 4 months. Administration of rifampin in combination with isoniazid for 9 months also is effective therapy for all forms of disease caused by strains of *Mycobacterium tuberculosis* susceptible to both agents (Bass *et al.*, 1994). Occasionally, because of microbial resistance, it may be necessary to resort to "second-line" drugs in addition; thus, treatment may be initiated with 5 to 6 drugs. This category of agents includes *moxifloxacin* or *gatifloxacin, ethionamide, aminosalicylic acid, cycloserine, amikacin, kanamycin, capreomycin*, and *linezolid* (Iseman, 1993). In HIV-infected patients receiving protease inhibitors and/or nonnucleoside reverse transcriptase inhibitors, drug interactions with the rifamycins (rifampin, *rifapentine, rifabutin*) are an important concern. Directly observed therapy, in which a health care worker actually witnesses the ingestion of medications, improves the outcome of tuberculosis treatment regimens (Havlir and Barnes, 1999).

Isoniazid is ineffective in the treatment of leprosy or *M. avium* complex infection. Lepromatous (multibacillary) leprosy is treated with *dapsone, clofazimine*, and rifampin for a minimum of 2 years, while tuberculoid (paucibacillary) leprosy is treated with dapsone and rifampin for 6 months.

Table 47–1

Drugs Used in the Treatment of Tuberculosis, Mycobacterium avium *Complex, and Leprosy*

MYCOBACTERIAL SPECIES	FIRST-LINE THERAPY	ALTERNATIVE AGENTS
M. tuberculosis	Isoniazid + rifampin*+ pyrazinamide + ethambutol or streptomycin	Moxifloxacin or gatifloxacin; cycloserine; capreomycin; kanamycin; amikacin; ethionamide; clofazimine; aminosalicylic acid
M. avium complex	Clarithromycin or azithromycin + ethambutol with or without rifabutin	Rifabutin; rifampin; ethionamide; cycloserine; moxifloxacin or gatifloxacin
M. kansasii	Isoniazid + rifampin*+ ethambutol	Trimethoprim-sulfamethoxazole; ethionamide; cycloserine; clarithromycin; amikacin; streptomycin; moxifloxacin or gatifloxacin
M. fortuitum complex	Amikacin + doxycycline	Cefoxitin; rifampin; a sulfonamide; moxifloxacin or gatifloxacin; clarithromycin; trimethoprim-sulfamethoxazole; imipenem
M. marinum	Rifampin + ethambutol	Trimethoprim-sulfamethoxazole; clarithromycin; minocycline; doxycycline
M. leprae	Dapsone + rifampin ± clofazimine	Minocycline; moxifloxacin or gatifloxacin; clarithromycin; ethionamide

*In HIV-infected patients, the substitution of rifabutin for rifampin minimizes drug interactions with the HIV protease inhibitors and nonnucleoside reverse transcriptase inhibitors.

Antimicrobial agents with activity against MAC include rifabutin, *clarithromycin, azithromycin,* streptomycin, and fluoroquinolones. Clarithromycin and azithromycin are more effective than rifabutin for prophylaxis of *M. avium* complex infection in patients with AIDS. Clarithromycin or azithromycin, in combination with ethambutol (to prevent development of resistance), is effective treatment for *M. avium* complex infection in HIV-infected individuals.

I. DRUGS FOR TUBERCULOSIS

ISONIAZID

Isoniazid (isonicotinic acid hydrazide; NYDRAZID, others) is still considered the primary drug for the chemotherapy of tuberculosis. All patients with disease caused by isoniazid-sensitive strains of the tubercle bacillus should receive the drug if they can tolerate it.

History. The discovery of isoniazid was fortuitous; in 1945 Chorine reported that nicotinamide possesses tuberculostatic action. Examination of the compounds related to nicotinamide revealed that many pyridine derivatives possess tuberculostatic activity; among these were congeners of isonicotinic acid. Because the thiosemicarbazones were known to inhibit *M. tuberculosis,* the thiosemicarbazone of isonicotinaldehyde was synthesized and studied. The starting material for this synthesis was the methyl ester of isonicotinic acid, and the first intermediate was isonicotinylhydrazide (isoniazid).

Chemistry. Isoniazid is the hydrazide of isonicotinic acid; the structural formula is:

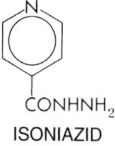

ISONIAZID

The isopropyl derivative of isoniazid, iproniazid (1-isonicotinyl-2-isopropylhydrazide), also inhibits the multiplication of the tubercle bacillus. This compound, which potently inhibits monoamine oxidase, is too toxic for use in human beings. However, its study led to the use of monoamine oxidase inhibitors for the treatment of depression (*see* Chapter 17).

Antibacterial Activity. Isoniazid is bacteriostatic for "resting" bacilli, but is bactericidal for rapidly dividing microorganisms. The minimal tuberculostatic concentration is 0.025 to 0.05 $\mu g/ml$. The bacteria undergo one or two divisions before multiplication is arrested. The drug is remarkably selective for mycobacteria, and concentrations in excess of 500 $\mu g/ml$ are required to inhibit the growth of other microorganisms.

Isoniazid is highly effective for the treatment of experimentally induced tuberculosis in animals and is strikingly superior to streptomycin. Unlike streptomycin, isoniazid penetrates cells with ease and is just as effective against bacilli growing within cells as it is against those growing in culture media.

Among the various nontuberculous (atypical) mycobacteria, only *M. kansasii* is sometimes susceptible to isoniazid. However, sensitivity always must be tested *in vitro*, since the inhibitory concentration required may be rather high.

Bacterial Resistance. When tubercle bacilli are grown *in vitro* in increasing concentrations of isoniazid, mutants are readily selected that are resistant to the drug, even when the drug is present in enormous concentrations. However, cross-resistance between isoniazid and other agents used to treat tuberculosis (except ethionamide, which is structurally related to isoniazid) does not occur. The most common mechanism of isoniazid resistance is mutations in catalase-peroxidase (*katg*) that decrease its activity, preventing conversion of the prodrug isoniazid to its active metabolite (Blanchard, 1996). Another mechanism of resistance is related to a mutation in the mycobacterial *inhA* and *KasA* genes involved in mycolic acid biosynthesis (Banerjee *et al.*, 1994). Mutations in NADH dehydrogenase (*ndh*) also confer isoniazid resistance (Miesel *et al.*, 1998). Interestingly, isoniazid-resistant strains of *M. tuberculosis* appear to be less virulent in animal models (Zhang, 2004).

As with the other agents described, treatment with isoniazid alone selects for isoniazid-resistant bacteria and leads to the emergence *in vivo* of resistant strains. The shift from primarily sensitive to mainly insensitive microorganisms occasionally occurs within a few weeks after therapy is started; however, the time of appearance of isoniazid resistance varies considerably from one case to another. Approximately 1 in 10^6 tubercle bacilli will be genetically resistant to isoniazid; since tuberculous cavities may contain as many as 10^7 to 10^9 microorganisms, it is not surprising that treatment with isoniazid alone selects for these resistant bacteria. The incidence of primary resistance to isoniazid in the United States until recently had been fairly stable at 2% to 5% of isolates of *M. tuberculosis*. Resistance currently is estimated at 8% of isolates, but may be much higher in certain populations, including Asian and Hispanic immigrants and in large urban areas and coastal or border communities (Centers for Disease Control, 1999; Iseman, 1993).

Mechanism of Action. Isoniazid is a prodrug; mycobacterial catalase-peroxidase converts isoniazid into an active metabolite. A primary action of isoniazid is to inhibit the biosynthesis of mycolic acids—long, branched lipids that are attached to a unique polysaccharide, arabino galactan, to form part of the mycobacterial cell wall. The mechanism of action of isoniazid is complex, with resistance mapping to mutations in at least five different genes (*katG* [coding for the catalase-peroxidase that activates the prodrug isoniazid], *inhA, ahpC, kasA,* and *ndh*) (*see* above). The preponderance of evidence points to *inhA* as the primary drug target. Indeed, the catalase-peroxidase–activated isoniazid, but not the prodrug, binds to the *inhA* gene product enoyl-ACP reductase of

fatty acid synthase II, which converts Δ^2-unsaturated fatty acids to saturated fatty acids in the mycolic acid biosynthetic pathway (Vilcheze *et al.*, 2000). Mycolic acids are unique to mycobacteria, explaining the high degree of selectivity of the antimicrobial activity of isoniazid. Mutations of the *katG* gene that result in an inactive catalase-peroxidase cause high-level isoniazid resistance, since the prodrug cannot be activated by the catalase-peroxidase (Blanchard, 1996). Isoniazid also inhibits mycobacterial catalase-peroxidase (the isoniazid-activating enzyme), which may increase the likelihood of damage to the mycobacteria from reactive oxygen species and H_2O_2. Exposure to isoniazid leads to a loss of acid-fastness and a decrease in the quantity of methanol-extractable lipids in the microorganisms.

Absorption, Distribution, and Excretion. Isoniazid is readily absorbed when administered either orally or parenterally. Aluminum-containing antacids may interfere with absorption. Peak plasma concentrations of 3 to 5 $\mu g/ml$ develop 1 to 2 hours after oral ingestion of usual doses.

Isoniazid diffuses readily into all body fluids and cells. The drug is detectable in significant quantities in pleural and ascitic fluids; concentrations in the cerebrospinal fluid (CSF) with inflamed meninges are similar to those in the plasma (Holdiness, 1985). Isoniazid penetrates well into caseous material. The concentration of the agent is initially higher in the plasma and muscle than in the infected tissue, but the latter retains the drug for a long time in quantities well above those required for bacteriostasis.

From 75% to 95% of a dose of isoniazid is excreted in the urine within 24 hours, mostly as metabolites. The main excretory products in humans result from enzymatic acetylation (acetylisoniazid) and enzymatic hydrolysis (isonicotinic acid). Small quantities of an isonicotinic acid conjugate (probably isonicotinyl glycine), one or more isonicotinyl hydrazones, and traces of *N*-methylisoniazid also are detectable in the urine.

The distribution of slow and rapid inactivators of the drug is bimodal owing to differences in the levels and activity of the genetically polymorphic arylamine *N*-acetyltransferase type 2 (NAT2) (Figure 47–1). The activity of NAT2 enzyme translated from variant alleles is decreased mostly by the impaired stability or a decrease in Vmax. At least 36 NAT2 alleles have been identified, although many may not be clinically important (Kinzig-Schippers *et al.*, 2005). As an autosomal recessive trait, only individuals bearing two variant alleles are expected to be prone to impaired acetylation capacity (Meisel, 2002). The rate of acetylation significantly alters the concentrations of the drug that are achieved in plasma and its half-life in the circulation. The half-life of the drug may be prolonged by hepatic insufficiency.

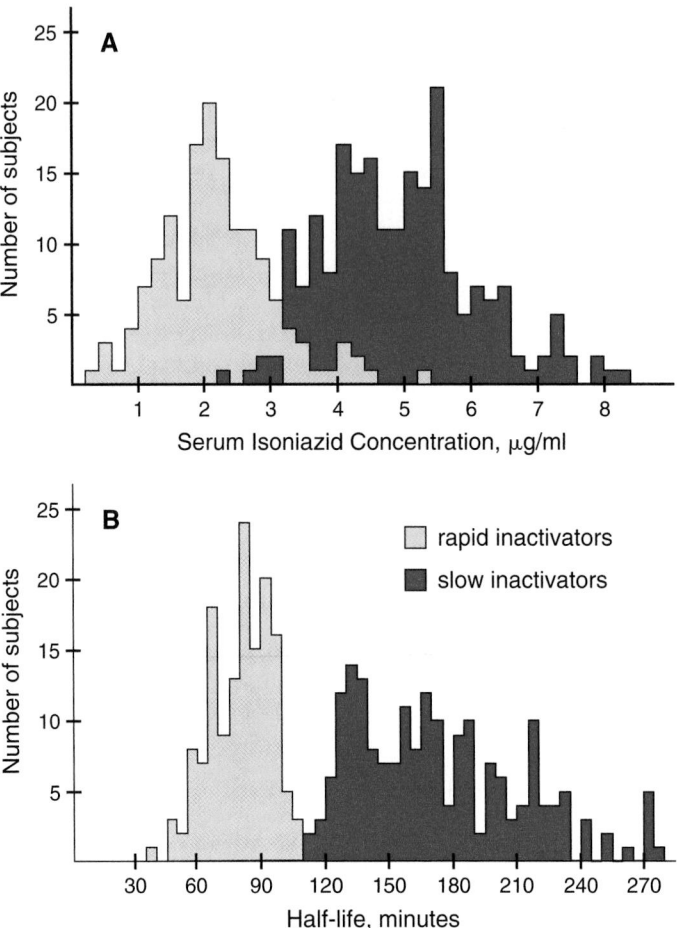

Figure 47–1. *Bimodal distribution of serum isoniazid concentrations and half-lives in a large group of Finnish patients.* More than 300 patients were given intravenous injections of 5 mg/kg of isoniazid. Serum drug concentrations were assayed at multiple times after injection. *A.* The distribution of the serum concentrations of isoniazid 180 minutes after injection; the light blue histograms represent rapid inactivators, and the dark blue histograms, slow inactivators. *B.* The distribution of serum half-lives of isoniazid for patients of each group. (Reproduced with permission from Tiitinen, 1969.)

The frequency of each acetylation phenotype is dependent upon race but is not influenced by sex or age. Fast acetylation is found in Inuit and Japanese. Slow acetylation is the predominant phenotype in most Scandinavians, Jews, and North African Caucasians. The incidence of "slow acetylators" among various racial types in the United States is about 50%. Since high acetyltransferase activity (fast acetylation) is inherited as an autosomal dominant trait, "fast acetylators" of isoniazid are either heterozygous or homozygous. The average concentration of active isoniazid in the circulation of fast acetylators is about 30% to 50% of that in slow acetylators. In the whole population, the half-life of isoniazid varies from less than 1 to more than 4 hours (Figure 47–1). The mean half-life in fast acetylators is approximately 70 minutes, whereas 2 to 5 hours is characteristic of slow acetylators. Because isoniazid is relatively nontoxic, a sufficient amount of drug can be administered to fast acetylators to achieve a therapeutic effect equal to that seen in slow acetylators. A dosage reduction is recommended for slow acetylators with hepatic failure. The clearance of isoniazid is dependent only to a small degree on the status of renal function, but patients who are slow inactivators of the drug may accumulate toxic concentrations if their renal function is impaired.

Therapeutic Uses. Isoniazid is still the most important drug worldwide for the treatment of all types of tuberculosis. Toxic effects can be minimized by prophylactic therapy with *pyridoxine* and careful surveillance of the patient. For treatment of active infections, the drug must be used concurrently with another agent, although it is used alone for prophylaxis.

Isoniazid is available for oral and parenteral administration. The commonly used total daily dose of isoniazid is 5 mg/kg, with a maximum of 300 mg; oral and intramuscular doses are identical. Isoniazid usually is given orally in a single daily dose but may be given in two divided doses. Although doses of 10 to 20 mg/kg, with a maximum of 600 mg, occasionally are used in severely ill patients, there is no evidence that this regimen is more effective. Children should receive 10 to 20 mg/kg per day (300 mg maximum). Isoniazid may be used as intermittent therapy for tuberculosis; after a minimum of 2 months of daily therapy with isoniazid, rifampin, and pyrazinamide, for sensitive strains of *M. tuberculosis,* patients may be treated with twice-weekly doses of isoniazid (15 mg/kg orally) plus rifampin (10 mg/kg, up to 600 mg per dose) for 4 months.

Pyridoxine, vitamin B$_6$, (10 to 50 mg per day) should be administered with isoniazid to minimize the risks of peripheral neuropathy and central nervous system toxicity (*see* below) in malnourished patients and those predisposed to neuropathy (*e.g.,* the elderly, pregnant women, HIV-infected individuals, diabetics, alcoholics, and uremics) (Snider, 1980).

Untoward Effects. The incidence of adverse reactions to isoniazid was estimated to be 5.4% among more than 2000 patients treated with the drug; the most prominent of these reactions were rash (2%), fever (1.2%), jaundice (0.6%), and peripheral neuritis (0.2%). Hypersensitivity to isoniazid may result in fever, various skin eruptions, hepatitis, and morbilliform, maculopapular, purpuric, and urticarial rashes. Hematological reactions also may occur (agranulocytosis, eosinophilia, thrombocytopenia, anemia). Vasculitis associated with antinuclear antibodies may appear during treatment but disappears when the drug is stopped. Arthritic symptoms (back pain; bilateral proximal interphalangeal joint involvement; arthralgia of the knees, elbows, and wrists; and the "shoulder-hand" syndrome) have been attributed to this agent.

If pyridoxine is not given concurrently, peripheral neuritis (most commonly paresthesias of feet and hands) is the most common reaction to isoniazid and occurs in about 2% of patients receiving 5 mg/kg of the drug daily. Higher doses may result in peripheral neuritis in 10% to 20% of patients. Neuropathy is more frequent in slow acetylators and in individuals with diabetes mellitus, poor nutrition, or anemia. The prophylactic administration of pyridoxine prevents the development not only of peripheral neuritis, but also of most other nervous system disorders in practically all instances, even when therapy lasts as long as 2 years.

Isoniazid may precipitate convulsions in patients with seizure disorders, and rarely, in patients with no history of seizures. Optic neuritis and atrophy also have occurred during therapy with the drug. Muscle twitching, dizziness, ataxia, paresthesias, stupor, and toxic encephalopathy that may be fatal are other manifestations of the neurotoxicity of isoniazid. A number of mental abnormalities may appear during the use of this drug, including euphoria, transient impairment of memory, separation of ideas and reality, loss of self-control, and florid psychoses.

Isoniazid is known to inhibit the parahydroxylation of *phenytoin,* and signs and symptoms of toxicity occur in approximately 27% of patients given both drugs, particularly in those who are slow acetylators (Miller *et al.,* 1979). Concentrations of phenytoin in plasma should be monitored and adjusted if necessary. The dosage of isoniazid should not be changed.

Although jaundice has been known for some time to be an untoward effect of exposure to isoniazid, not until the early 1970s did it become apparent that severe hepatic injury leading to death may occur in some individuals receiving this drug (Garibaldi *et al.,*

1972). Additional studies in adults and children have confirmed this observation; the characteristic pathological process is bridging and multilobular necrosis. Continuation of the drug after symptoms of hepatic dysfunction have appeared tends to increase the severity of damage. The mechanisms responsible for this toxicity are unknown, although acetylhydrazine, which is a metabolite of isoniazid, causes hepatic damage in adults. Hence, patients who are rapid acetylators of isoniazid might be expected to be more likely to develop hepatotoxicity than slow acetylators; whether this is true, however, is unresolved. A contributory role of alcoholic hepatitis has been noted, but chronic carriers of the hepatitis B virus tolerate isoniazid (McGlynn *et al.,* 1986). Age appears to be the most important factor in determining the risk of isoniazid-induced hepatotoxicity. Hepatic damage is rare in patients less than 20 years old; the complication is observed in 0.3% of those 20 to 34 years old, and the incidence increases to 1.2% and 2.3% in individuals 35 to 49 and older than 50 years of age, respectively (Bass *et al.,* 1994; Comstock, 1983). Up to 12% of patients receiving isoniazid may have elevated plasma aspartate and alanine transaminase activities (Bailey *et al.,* 1974). Patients receiving isoniazid should be carefully evaluated at monthly intervals for symptoms of hepatitis (anorexia, malaise, fatigue, nausea, and jaundice) and warned to discontinue the drug if such symptoms occur. Some clinicians also prefer to determine serum aspartate aminotransferase activities at monthly intervals in high-risk individuals (ages 7 to 35, excessive alcohol intake, history of liver disease, etc.) (Byrd *et al.,* 1979), and recommend that an elevation greater than five times normal is cause for drug discontinuation. Most hepatitis occurs 4 to 8 weeks after the start of therapy. Isoniazid should be administered with great care to those with preexisting hepatic disease.

Among miscellaneous reactions associated with isoniazid therapy are dryness of the mouth, epigastric distress, methemoglobinemia, tinnitus, and urinary retention. In persons predisposed to pyridoxine-deficiency anemia, the administration of isoniazid may result in dramatic anemia, but treatment with large doses of vitamin B$_6$ gradually returns the blood to normal in such cases. A drug-induced syndrome resembling systemic lupus erythematosus has also been reported. Overdose of isoniazid, as in attempted suicide, may result in nausea, vomiting, dizziness, slurred speech, and visual hallucinations followed by coma, seizures, metabolic acidosis, and hyperglycemia. Pyridoxine is an antidote in this setting; it should be given in a dose that approximates the amount of isoniazid ingested.

RIFAMPIN AND OTHER RIFAMYCINS

The rifamycins (rifampin, rifabutin, rifapentine) are a group of structurally similar, complex macrocyclic antibiotics produced by *Amycolatopsis mediterranei* (Farr, 2000); rifampin (RIFADIN; RIMACTANE) is a semisynthetic derivative of one of these—rifamycin B. Rifamycins were first isolated by Lepetit Research Laboratories from cultures obtained from a pine forest near Nice, France (Vernon, 2004).

Chemistry. Rifampin is soluble in organic solvents and in water at acidic pH. It has the following structure:

RIFAMPIN

Antibacterial Activity. Rifampin inhibits the growth of most gram-positive bacteria as well as many gram-negative microorganisms such as *Escherichia coli, Pseudomonas,* indole-positive and indole-negative *Proteus,* and *Klebsiella.* Rifampin is very active against *Staphylococcus aureus* and coagulase-negative staphylococci. The drug also is highly active against *Neisseria meningitidis* and *Haemophilus influenzae;* minimal inhibitory concentrations range from 0.1 to 0.8 μg/ml. Rifampin inhibits the growth of *Legionella* species in cell culture and in animal models.

Rifampin in concentrations of 0.005 to 0.2 μg/ml inhibits the growth of *M. tuberculosis in vitro.* Among nontuberculous mycobacteria, *M. kansasii* is inhibited by 0.25 to 1 μg/ml. The majority of strains of *Mycobacterium scrofulaceum, Mycobacterium intracellulare,* and *M. avium* are suppressed by concentrations of 4 μg/ml, but certain strains may be resistant to 16 μg/ml. *Mycobacterium fortuitum* is highly resistant to the drug. Rifampin increases the *in vitro* activity of streptomycin and isoniazid, but not that of ethambutol, against *M. tuberculosis.*

Bacterial Resistance. Microorganisms, including mycobacteria, may develop resistance to rifampin rapidly *in vitro* as a one-step process, and one of every 10^7 to 10^8 tubercle bacilli is resistant to the drug. Microbial resistance to rifampin is due to an alteration of the target of this drug, DNA-dependent RNA polymerase, with resistance in most cases being due to mutations between codons 507 and 533 of the polymerase *rpoB* gene (Blanchard, 1996); the mutations reduce binding of the drug to the polymerase. As a consequence, the antibiotic must not be used alone in the chemotherapy of tuberculosis. When rifampin has been used to eradicate the meningococcal carrier state, failures have been due to the appearance of drug-resistant bacteria after treatment for as few as 2 days. Certain rifampin-resistant bacterial mutants have decreased virulence. Tuberculosis caused by rifampin-resistant mycobacteria has been described in patients who had not received prior chemotherapy, but this is very rare (usually less than 1%; Cauthen *et al.,* 1988).

Mechanism of Action.
Rifampin inhibits DNA-dependent RNA polymerase of mycobacteria and other microorganisms by forming a stable drug–enzyme complex, leading to suppression of initiation of chain formation (but not chain elongation) in RNA synthesis. More specifically, the β subunit of this complex enzyme is the site of action of the drug, although rifampin binds only to the holoenzyme. Nuclear RNA polymerases from a variety of eukaryotic cells do not bind rifampin, and RNA synthesis is correspondingly unaffected in eukaryotic cells.

High concentrations of rifamycin antibiotics can inhibit RNA synthesis in mammalian mitochondria, viral DNA–dependent RNA polymerases, and reverse transcriptases. Rifampin is bactericidal for both intracellular and extracellular microorganisms.

Absorption, Distribution, and Excretion. The oral administration of rifampin produces peak concentrations in plasma in 2 to 4 hours; after ingestion of 600 mg, this value is about 7 μg/ml, but there is considerable variability. Aminosalicylic acid may delay the absorption of rifampin and cause a failure to reach adequate plasma concentrations. If aminosalicylate and rifampin are used concurrently, they should be given separately at an interval of 8 to 12 hours.

Following absorption from the gastrointestinal tract, rifampin is eliminated rapidly in the bile, and an enterohepatic circulation ensues. During this time, the drug is progressively deacetylated, such that after 6 hours, nearly all of the antibiotic in the bile is in the deacetylated form, which retains essentially full antibacterial activity. Intestinal reabsorption is reduced by deacetylation (as well as by food), and thus metabolism facilitates elimination of the drug. The half-life of rifampin varies from 1.5 to 5 hours and is increased by hepatic dysfunction; the half-life may be decreased in patients receiving isoniazid concurrently who are slow inactivators of isoniazid. The half-life of rifampin is progressively shortened by about 40% during the first 14 days of treatment, owing to induction of hepatic microsomal enzymes that accelerate rifampin deacetylation. Up to 30% of a dose of the drug is excreted in the urine and 60% to 65% in the feces; less than half of this may be unaltered antibiotic. Adjustment of dosage is not necessary in patients with impaired renal function.

Rifampin is distributed throughout the body and is present in effective concentrations in many organs and body fluids, including the CSF. This is perhaps best exemplified by the fact that the drug may impart an orange-red color to the urine, feces, saliva, sputum, tears, and sweat; patients should be so warned. (For various aspects of rifampin metabolism, *see* Furesz, 1970; Farr, 2000.)

Therapeutic Uses. Rifampin for oral administration is available alone and as a fixed-dose combination with isoniazid (150 mg of isoniazid, 300 mg of rifampin; RIFAMATE) or with isoniazid and pyrazinamide (50 mg of isoniazid, 120 mg of rifampin, and 300 mg pyrazinamide; RIFATER). A parenteral form of rifampin is available for use when the drug cannot be taken by mouth. *Rifampin and isoniazid are the most effective drugs available for the treatment of tuberculosis.*

The dose of rifampin for treatment of tuberculosis in adults is 600 mg, given once daily, either 1 hour before or 2 hours after a meal. Children should receive 10 mg/kg given in the same way. Doses of 15 mg/kg or higher are associated with increased hepatotoxicity in children (Centers for Disease Control, 1980). Rifampin, like isoniazid, should never be used alone for the treatment of tuberculosis because of the rapidity with which resistance may develop. Despite the long list of untoward effects from rifampin, their incidence is low, and treatment seldom has to be interrupted.

The use of rifampin in the chemotherapy of tuberculosis is detailed below. Rifampin also is indicated for the prophylaxis of meningococcal disease and *H. influenzae* meningitis. To prevent meningococcal disease, adults may be treated with 600 mg twice daily for 2 days or 600 mg once daily for 4 days; children should receive 10 to 15 mg/kg, to a maximum of 600 mg.

Untoward Effects. Rifampin generally is well tolerated. When given in usual doses, fewer than 4% of patients with tuberculosis have significant adverse reactions; the most common are rash (0.8%), fever (0.5%), and nausea and vomiting (1.5%) (Grosset and Leventis, 1983). Rarely, hepatitis and deaths due to liver failure have been observed in patients who received other hepatotoxic agents in addition to rifampin, or who had preexisting liver disease. Hepatitis from rifampin rarely occurs in patients with normal hepatic function; likewise, the combination of isoniazid and rifampin appears generally safe in such patients (Gangadharam, 1986). However, chronic liver disease, alcoholism, and old age appear to increase the incidence of severe hepatic problems when rifampin is given alone or concurrently with isoniazid.

Rifampin should not be administered on an intermittent schedule (less than twice weekly) and/or in daily doses of 1.2 g or greater because this is associated with frequent side effects. A flulike syndrome with fever, chills, and myalgias develops in 20% of patients so treated. The syndrome also may include eosinophilia, interstitial nephritis, acute tubular necrosis, thrombocytopenia, hemolytic anemia, and shock.

Because rifampin potently induces CYP1A2, 2C9, 2C19, and 3A4, its administration results in a decreased half-life for a number of compounds, including HIV protease and non-nucleoside reverse transcriptase inhibitors, *digitoxin*, *digoxin*, *quinidine*, *disopyramide*, *mexiletine*, *tocainide*, *ketoconazole*, *propranolol*, *metoprolol*, *clofibrate*, *verapamil*, *methadone*, *cyclosporine*, corticosteroids, oral anticoagulants, *theophylline*, barbiturates, oral contraceptives, *halothane*, *fluconazole*, and the sulfonylureas (Farr, 2000).

Rifabutin (*see* below) has less effect on the metabolism of many of the HIV protease inhibitors. The significant interaction between rifampin and oral anticoagulants of the *coumarin* type leads to a decrease in efficacy of these agents. This effect appears about 5 to 8 days after rifampin administration is started and persists for 5 to 7 days after it is stopped (*see* Chapter 54). The ability of rifampin to enhance the catabolism of a variety of steroids leads to the decreased effectiveness of oral contraceptives, and can induce adrenal insufficiency in patients with marginal adrenocortical reserve (*see* Chapter 59). The increased metabolism of methadone and other narcotics has led to reports of precipitation of withdrawal syndromes and inadequate pain control unless the dose is increased. Rifampin may reduce biliary excretion of contrast media used for visualization of the gallbladder (Baciewicz *et al.*, 1987).

Gastrointestinal disturbances produced by rifampin (epigastric distress, nausea, vomiting, abdominal cramps, diarrhea) have occasionally required discontinuation of the drug. Various symptoms related to the nervous system also have been noted, including fatigue, drowsiness, headache, dizziness, ataxia, confusion, inability to concentrate, generalized numbness, pain in the extremities, and muscular weakness. Hypersensitivity reactions include fever, pruritus, urticaria, various types of skin eruptions, eosinophilia, and soreness of the mouth and tongue. Hemolysis, hemoglobinuria, hematuria, renal insufficiency, and acute renal failure have been observed rarely; these also are thought to be hypersensitivity reactions. Thrombocytopenia, transient leukopenia, and anemia have occurred during therapy. Since the potential teratogenicity of rifampin is unknown and the drug is known to cross the placenta, it is best to avoid the use of this agent during pregnancy.

Graber and associates (1973) noted immunoglobulin light-chain proteinuria (either kappa, lambda, or both) in about 85% of patients with tuberculosis treated with rifampin. None of the patients had symptoms or electrophoretic patterns compatible with myeloma. However, renal failure has been associated with light-chain proteinuria (Warrington *et al.*, 1977).

Rifampin is effective for chemoprophylaxis of meningococcal disease and meningitis due to *H. influenzae* in household contacts of patients with such infections. Combined with a β-lactam antibiotic or vancomycin, rifampin may be useful for therapy in selected cases of staphylococcal endocarditis (on both natural and prosthetic valves) or osteomyelitis, especially those caused by staphylococci "tolerant" to penicillin. Rifampin may be indicated for treatment of infections in patients with inadequate leukocytic bactericidal activity and for eradication of the staphylococcal nasal carrier state in patients with chronic furunculosis.

Rifabutin (MYCOBUTIN) is a rifampin derivative used in tuberculosis-infected HIV patients treated concurrently with protease inhibitors because rifabutin is a less potent inducer of CYPs. It has the same mechanism of action as rifampin and is discussed further in the section on drugs for *Mycobacterium avium* complex. Unique side effects of rifabutin include polymyalgia, pseudojaundice, and anterior uveitis (Vernon, 2004). About one-fourth of rifampin-resistant *M. tuberculosis* isolates are rifabutin-sensitive, so it may have a role in the treatment of multidrug-resistant tuberculosis.

Rifapentine (PRIFTIN) has a longer half-life than rifampin and rifabutin, which allows once-weekly dosing.

Compared to rifabutin and rifampin, it is intermediate in its induction of CYPs (Vernon, 2004). Its use in the treatment of tuberculosis in HIV-infected patients was associated with the selection of rifamycin resistance; rifabutin is therefore preferred in this situation (Vernon, 2004).

ETHAMBUTOL

Chemistry. Ethambutol is a water-soluble and heat-stable compound; its structural formula is:

$$H-\underset{\underset{C_2H_5}{|}}{\overset{\overset{CH_2OH}{|}}{C}}-NH-CH_2-CH_2-HN-\underset{\underset{CH_2OH}{|}}{\overset{\overset{C_2H_5}{|}}{C}}-H$$

ETHAMBUTOL

Antibacterial Activity, Mechanism of Action, Resistance. Nearly all strains of *M. tuberculosis* and *M. kansasii* as well as a number of strains of MAC are sensitive to ethambutol (Pablos-Méndez *et al.*, 1998). The sensitivities of other nontuberculous organisms are variable. Ethambutol has no effect on other bacteria. It suppresses the growth of most isoniazid- and streptomycin-resistant tubercle bacilli. Resistance to ethambutol develops very slowly *in vitro*.

Mycobacteria take up ethambutol rapidly when the drug is added to cultures that are in the exponential growth phase. However, growth is not significantly inhibited before about 24 hours. Ethambutol inhibits arabinosyl transferases involved in cell wall biosynthesis. Bacterial resistance to the drug develops *in vivo via* single amino acid mutations in the *embA* gene when ethambutol is given in the absence of other effective agents (Belanger *et al.*, 1996).

Absorption, Distribution, and Excretion. About 75% to 80% of an orally administered dose of ethambutol is absorbed from the gastrointestinal tract. Concentrations in plasma are maximal in humans 2 to 4 hours after the drug is taken and are proportional to the dose. A single dose of 25 mg/kg produces a plasma concentration of 2 to 5 μg/ml at 2 to 4 hours. The drug has a half-life of 3 to 4 hours. Within 24 hours, 75% of an ingested dose of ethambutol is excreted unchanged in the urine; up to 15% is excreted in the form of two metabolites, an aldehyde and a dicarboxylic acid derivative. Renal clearance of ethambutol is approximately 7 ml·min^{-1}·kg^{-1}; thus it is evident that the drug is excreted by tubular secretion in addition to glomerular filtration.

Therapeutic Uses. Ethambutol (*ethambutol hydrochloride*; MYAMBUTOL) has been used with notable success in the therapy of tuberculosis of various forms when given concurrently with isoniazid. Because of a lower incidence of toxic effects and better acceptance by patients, ethambutol has essentially replaced aminosalicylic acid.

Ethambutol is available for oral administration in tablets containing the D isomer. The usual adult dose of ethambutol is 15 mg/kg given once a day. Some physicians prefer to treat with 25 mg/kg per day for the first 60 days and then to reduce the dose to 15 mg/kg per day, particularly for those who have received previous therapy. Ethambutol accumulates in patients with impaired renal function, and adjustment of dosage is necessary.

Ethambutol is not recommended for children under 5 years of age, in part because of concern about the ability to test their visual acuity (*see* below). Children from ages 6 to 12 years should receive 10 to 15 mg/kg per day.

The use of ethambutol in the chemotherapy of tuberculosis is described below.

Untoward Effects. The most important side effect is optic neuritis, resulting in decreased visual acuity and loss of ability to differentiate red from green. The incidence of this reaction is proportional to the dose of ethambutol and is observed in 15% of patients receiving 50 mg/kg per day, in 5% of patients receiving 25 mg/kg per day, and in fewer than 1% of patients receiving daily doses of 15 mg/kg (the recommended dose for treatment of tuberculosis). The intensity of the visual difficulty is related to the duration of therapy after the decreased visual acuity first becomes apparent and may be unilateral or bilateral. Tests of visual acuity and red-green discrimination prior to the start of therapy and periodically thereafter are thus recommended. Recovery usually occurs when ethambutol is withdrawn; the time required is a function of the degree of visual impairment.

Ethambutol produces very few untoward reactions. Fewer than 2% of nearly 2000 patients who received daily doses of 15 mg/kg of ethambutol had adverse reactions: 0.8% experienced diminished visual acuity, 0.5% had a rash, and 0.3% developed drug fever. Other side effects that have been observed are pruritus, joint pain, gastrointestinal upset, abdominal pain, malaise, headache, dizziness, mental confusion, disorientation, and possible hallucinations. Numbness and tingling of the fingers owing to peripheral neuritis are infrequent. Anaphylaxis and leukopenia are rare.

Therapy with ethambutol results in an increased concentration of urate in the blood in about 50% of patients, owing to decreased renal excretion of uric acid. The effect may be detectable as early as 24 hours after a single dose or as late as 90 days after treatment is started. This untoward effect is possibly enhanced by isoniazid and pyridoxine (Postlethwaite *et al.*, 1972).

STREPTOMYCIN

The pharmacology of streptomycin, including its adverse effects and its uses in infections other than tuberculosis, are discussed in Chapter 45. Only features of the drug related to its antibacterial activity and therapeutic effects in the management of mycobacterial diseases are considered here.

History. Streptomycin was the first clinically available effective drug for the treatment of tuberculosis. At first it was given in large doses, but problems related to toxicity and the development of resistant microorganisms seriously limited its usefulness. The antibiotic was then administered in smaller quantities, but streptomycin administered alone still proved to be far from ideal for the management of all forms of the disease. However, the discovery of other compounds that, when administered concurrently with streptomycin, reduced the rate at which microorganisms became drug-resistant enabled physicians to treat tuberculosis effectively with streptomycin. It is now the least used of the first-line agents in the therapy of tuberculosis.

Antibacterial Activity. Streptomycin is bactericidal for the tubercle bacillus *in vitro*. Concentrations as low as 0.4 μg/ml may inhibit growth. The vast majority of strains of *M. tuberculosis* are sensitive to 10 μg/ml. *M. kansasii* is frequently sensitive, but other nontuberculous mycobacteria are only occasionally susceptible.

The activity of streptomycin *in vivo* is essentially suppressive. When the antibiotic is administered to experimental animals prior to inoculation with the tubercle bacillus, the development of disease is not prevented. Infection progresses until the animals' immunological mechanisms respond. The presence of viable microorganisms in abscesses and in the regional lymph nodes adds support to the concept that the activity of streptomycin *in vivo* is to suppress, not to eradicate, the tubercle bacillus. This property of streptomycin may be related to the observation that the drug does not readily enter living cells and thus cannot kill intracellular microbes.

Bacterial Resistance. Large populations of all strains of tubercle bacilli include a number of cells that are markedly resistant to streptomycin because of mutation. However, primary resistance to the antibiotic is found in only 2% to 3% of isolates of *M. tuberculosis*. Selection for resistant tubercle bacilli occurs *in vivo* as it does *in vitro*. In general, the longer therapy is continued, the greater the incidence of resistance to streptomycin. When streptomycin was used alone, as many as 80% of patients harbored insensitive tubercle bacilli after 4 months of treatment; many of these microorganisms were not inhibited by concentrations of drug as high as 1 mg/ml.

Therapeutic Uses. Since other effective agents have become available, the use of streptomycin for the treatment of pulmonary tuberculosis has been sharply reduced. Many clinicians prefer to give 4 drugs, of which streptomycin may be one, for the most serious forms of tuberculosis, such as disseminated disease or meningitis.

For tuberculosis, adults should be given 15 mg/kg per day in divided doses given by intramuscular injection every 12 hours, not to exceed 1 g per day. Children should receive 20 to 40 mg/kg per day in divided doses every 12 to 24 hours, not to exceed 1 g per day. Therapy usually is discontinued after 2 to 3 months, or sooner if cultures become negative.

Untoward Effects. Untoward effects of streptomycin are considered in detail in Chapter 45. In one series of 515 patients with tuberculosis who were treated with this aminoglycoside, 8.2% had adverse reactions; half of these involved the auditory and vestibular functions of the eighth cranial nerve. Other relatively frequent problems included rash (in 2%) and fever (in 1.4%).

PYRAZINAMIDE

Chemistry. Pyrazinamide is the synthetic pyrazine analog of nicotinamide. It has the following structural formula:

PYRAZINAMIDE

Antibacterial Activity. Pyrazinamide exhibits bactericidal activity *in vitro* only at a slightly acidic pH. Activity at acid pH is ideal, since *M. tuberculosis* resides in an acidic phagosome within the macrophage (Jacobs, 2000). Tubercle bacilli within monocytes *in vitro* are inhibited or killed by the drug at a concentration of 12.5 μg/ml. Resistance develops rapidly if pyrazinamide is used alone. The target of pyrazinamide appears to be the mycobacterial fatty acid synthase I gene involved in mycolic acid biosynthesis (Zimhony *et al.*, 2000).

Absorption, Distribution, and Excretion. Pyrazinamide is well absorbed from the gastrointestinal tract and widely distributed throughout the body. The oral administration of 500 mg produces plasma concentrations of about 9 to 12 μg/ml at 2 hours and 7 μg/ml at 8 hours. The plasma half-life is 9 to 10 hours in patients with normal renal function. The drug is excreted primarily by renal glomerular filtration. Pyrazinamide is distributed widely—including to the CNS, lungs, and liver—after oral administration. Penetration of the drug into the CSF is excellent. Pyrazinamide is hydrolyzed to pyrazinoic acid and subsequently hydroxylated to 5-hydroxypyrazinoic acid, the major excretory product.

Therapeutic Uses. Pyrazinamide has become an important component of short-term (6-month) multiple-drug therapy of tuberculosis (British Thoracic Association, 1982; Bass *et al.*, 1994). Pyrazinamide is available in tablets for oral administration. The daily dose for adults is 15 to 30 mg/kg orally, given as a single dose. The maximum quantity to be given is 2 g per day, regardless of weight. Children should receive 15 to 30 mg/kg per day; daily doses also should not exceed 2 g. Pyrazinamide has been safe and effective when administered twice or thrice weekly (at increased dosages).

Untoward Effects. Injury to the liver is the most serious side effect of pyrazinamide. When a dose of 40 to 50 mg/kg is administered orally, signs and symptoms of hepatic disease appear in about 15% of patients, with jaundice in 2% to 3% and death due to hepatic necrosis in rare instances. Elevations of plasma alanine and aspartate aminotransferases are the earliest abnormalities produced by the drug. Regimens employed currently (15 to 30 mg/kg per day) are much safer. Prior to pyrazinamide administration all patients should undergo studies of hepatic function and these studies should be repeated at frequent intervals during the entire period of treatment. If evidence of significant hepatic damage becomes apparent, therapy must be stopped. Pyrazinamide should not be given to individuals with any degree of hepatic dysfunction unless this is absolutely unavoidable.

The drug inhibits excretion of urate, resulting in hyperuricemia in nearly all patients; acute episodes of gout have occurred. Other untoward effects that have been observed with pyrazinamide are arthralgias, anorexia, nausea and vomiting, dysuria, malaise, and fever. While some international organizations recommend the use of pyrazinamide in pregnancy, this is not the case in the United States because of inadequate data on teratogenicity (Bass *et al.*, 1994).

QUINOLONES

The fluoroquinolones, which are discussed in Chapter 43, are highly active against *M. tuberculosis* as well as nontuberculous mycobacteria and are important components of treatment regimens of multidrug-resistant tuberculosis (Drlica *et al.*, 2004) (Table 47–1). The C-8-methoxy-fluoroquinolones, such as gatifloxacin (TEQUIN) and moxifloxacin (AVELOX), are the most active and therefore least likely to result in the development of quinolone resistance. Unfortunately, when resistance develops to one fluoroquinolone in mycobacteria, cross-resistance develops within this entire class of antibiotics. Thus the most active fluoroquinolones should be used, and only in combination with other antimycobacterial agents, to prevent resistance from developing (Ginsberg *et al.*, 2003).

LINEZOLID

Linezolid (ZYVOX), which is discussed in Chapter 46, is highly active *in vitro* against *M. tuberculosis* and some nontuberculous mycobacteria (Wallace *et al.*, 2001; Alcala *et al.*, 2003). Clinical experience with its use to treat these infections is limited at present.

INTERFERON-γ

Interferon-γ (IFN-γ) (ACTIMMUNE) activates macrophages to kill *M. tuberculosis*. Aerosol delivery of IFN-γ to the lungs of patients with multidrug-resistant tuberculosis results in wide pulmonary distribution and enhanced local immune stimulation (Condos *et al.*, 2004). IFN-γ is discussed further in Chapter 52.

ETHIONAMIDE

Chemistry. Synthesis and study of a variety of congeners of thioisonicotinamide revealed that an α-ethyl derivative—ethionamide

(TRECATOR-SC)—is considerably more effective than the parent compound. It has the following structural formula:

ETHIONAMIDE

Antibacterial Activity, Resistance. The multiplication of *M. tuberculosis* is suppressed by concentrations of ethionamide ranging from 0.6 to 2.5 $\mu g/ml$. Resistance can develop rapidly *in vitro* and *in vivo* when ethionamide is used as a single-agent treatment, and can include low-level cross-resistance to isoniazid. A concentration of 10 $\mu g/ml$ or less will inhibit approximately 75% of photochromogenic mycobacteria; the scotochromogens are more resistant. Ethionamide is very effective in the treatment of experimental tuberculosis in animals, although its activity varies greatly with the animal model studied.

Mechanism of Action. In the manner of isoniazid, ethionamide is also an inactive prodrug that is activated by a mycobacterial redux system. EtaA, an NADPH-specific, FAD-containing monooxygenase, converts ethionamide to a sulfoxide, and thence to 2-ethyl-4-aminopyridine (Vannelli *et al.*, 2002). Although these products are not toxic to mycobacteria, it is believed that a closely related and transient intermediate is the active antibiotic. Ethionamide inhibits mycobacterial growth by inhibiting the activity of the *inhA* gene product, the enoyl-ACP reductase of fatty acid synthase II (Larsen *et al.*, 2002). This is the same enzyme that activated isoniazid inhibits. Although the exact mechanisms of inhibition may differ, the results are the same: inhibition of mycolic acid biosynthesis and consequent impairment of cell-wall synthesis. Recent advances in understanding the mechanisms of activation and action of thioamides (Fraaije, *et al.*, 2004) may suggest new agents for treating mycobacterial infections.

Absorption, Distribution, and Excretion. The oral administration of 1 g of ethionamide yields peak concentrations in plasma of about 20 $\mu g/ml$ in 3 hours; the concentration at 9 hours is 3 $\mu g/ml$. The half-life of the drug is about 2 hours. Approximately 50% of patients are unable to tolerate a single dose larger than 500 mg because of gastrointestinal disturbance. Ethionamide is rapidly and widely distributed; the concentrations in the blood and various organs are approximately equal. Significant concentrations are present in CSF. Ethionamide is cleared by hepatic metabolism; like aminosalicylic acid, ethionamide inhibits the acetylation of isoniazid *in vitro*. Less than 1% of ethionamide is excreted in an active form in the urine.

Therapeutic Uses. *Ethionamide is a secondary agent, to be used concurrently with other drugs only when therapy with primary agents is ineffective or contraindicated.*

Ethionamide is administered only orally. The initial dosage of ethionamide for adults is 250 mg twice daily; it is increased by 125 mg per day every 5 days until a dose of 15 to 20 mg/kg per day is achieved. The maximal dose is 1 g daily. The drug is best taken with meals in divided doses in order to minimize gastric irritation. Children should receive 15 to 20 mg/kg per day in two divided doses, not to exceed 1 g per day.

Untoward Effects. The most common reactions to ethionamide are anorexia, nausea and vomiting, gastric irritation, and a variety of neurologic symptoms. Severe postural hypotension, mental depression, drowsiness, and asthenia are common. Convulsions and peripheral neuropathy are rare. Other reactions referable to the nervous system include olfactory disturbances, blurred vision, diplopia, dizziness, paresthesias, headache, restlessness, and tremors. Pyridoxine (vitamin B_6) relieves the neurologic symptoms and its concomitant administration is recommended. Severe allergic skin rashes, purpura, stomatitis, gynecomastia, impotence, menorrhagia, acne, and alopecia also have been observed. A metallic taste also may be noted. Hepatitis has been associated with the use of the drug in about 5% of cases. The signs and symptoms of hepatotoxicity clear when treatment is stopped. Hepatic function should be assessed at regular intervals in patients receiving ethionamide.

AMINOSALICYLIC ACID

Chemistry. The structural formula of aminosalicylic acid (*p*-aminosalicylic acid, PAS) is:

AMINOSALICYLIC ACID

Antibacterial Activity. Aminosalicylic acid is bacteriostatic. *In vitro*, most strains of *M. tuberculosis* are sensitive to a concentration of 1 μg/ml. The antimicrobial activity of aminosalicylic acid is highly specific, and microorganisms other than *M. tuberculosis* are unaffected. Most nontuberculous mycobacteria are not inhibited by the drug. Aminosalicylic acid alone is of little value in the treatment of tuberculosis in humans.

Bacterial Resistance. Strains of tubercle bacilli insensitive to several hundred times the usual bacteriostatic concentration of aminosalicylic acid can be produced *in vitro*. Resistant strains of tubercle bacilli also emerge in patients treated with aminosalicylic acid, but much more slowly than with streptomycin.

Mechanism of Action. Aminosalicylic acid is a structural analog of *para*-aminobenzoic acid, and its mechanism of action appears to be very similar to that of the sulfonamides (*see* Chapter 43). Nonetheless, the sulfonamides are ineffective against *M. tuberculosis,* and aminosalicylic acid is inactive against sulfonamide-susceptible bacteria. This differential sensitivity presumably reflects differences in the enzymes responsible for folate biosynthesis in the various microorganisms.

Absorption, Distribution, and Excretion. Aminosalicylic acid is readily absorbed from the gastrointestinal tract. A single oral dose of 4 g of the free acid produces maximal concentrations in plasma of about 75 μg/ml within 1.5 to 2 hours. The sodium salt is absorbed even more rapidly. The drug appears to be distributed throughout the total body water and reaches high concentrations in pleural fluid and caseous tissue but CSF levels are low. The drug has a half-life of about 1 hour, and concentrations in plasma are negligible within 4 to 5 hours after a single conventional dose. Over 80% of the drug is excreted in the urine; more than 50% is in the form of the acetylated compound; the largest portion of the remainder is made up of the free acid. Excretion of aminosalicylic acid is greatly retarded by renal dysfunction, and the use of the drug is not recommended in such patients. Probenecid decreases the renal excretion of this agent.

Therapeutic Uses. Aminosalicylic acid (PASER) is a second-line agent. Its importance in the management of pulmonary and other forms of tuberculosis has markedly decreased since more active and better-tolerated drugs, such as rifampin and ethambutol, have been developed (*see* Chemotherapy of Tuberculosis, below).

It is administered orally in a daily dose of 10 to 12 g. Because it is a gastric irritant, the drug is best administered after meals, with the daily dose being divided into 2 to 4 equal portions. Children should receive 150 to 300 mg/kg per day in 3 to 4 divided doses.

Untoward Effects. The incidence of untoward effects associated with the use of aminosalicylic acid is approximately 10% to 30%. Gastrointestinal problems—including anorexia, nausea, epigastric pain, abdominal distress, and diarrhea—are predominant and often limit patient adherence. Patients with peptic ulcers tolerate the drug especially poorly. Hypersensitivity reactions to aminosalicylic acid are seen in 5% to 10% of patients. High fever may develop abruptly, with intermittent spiking, or it may appear gradually and be low-grade. Generalized malaise, joint pains, and sore throat may be present at the same time. Skin eruptions of various types appear as isolated reactions or accompany the fever. Among the hematological abnormalities that have been observed are leukopenia, agranulocytosis, eosinophilia, lymphocytosis, an atypical mononucleosis syndrome, and thrombocytopenia. Acute hemolytic anemia may appear in some instances.

CYCLOSERINE

Cycloserine (SEROMYCIN) is a broad-spectrum antibiotic produced by *Streptococcus orchidaceus*. It was first isolated from a fermentation brew in 1955 and was later synthesized. Currently, cycloserine is used in conjunction with other tuberculostatic drugs in the treatment of pulmonary or extrapulmonary tuberculosis when primary agents (isoniazid, rifampin, ethambutol, pyrazinamide, streptomycin) have failed.

Chemistry. Cycloserine is D-4-amino-3-isoxazolidone; the structural formula is:

CYCLOSERINE

The drug is stable in alkaline solution but is rapidly destroyed when exposed to neutral or acidic pH.

Antibacterial Activity. Cycloserine is inhibitory for *M. tuberculosis* in concentrations of 5 to 20 μg/ml *in vitro*. There is no cross-resistance between cycloserine and other tuberculostatic agents. While the antibiotic is effective in experimental infections caused by other microorganisms, studies *in vitro* reveal no suppression of growth in cultures made in conventional media, which contain D-alanine; this amino acid blocks the antibacterial activity of cycloserine.

Mechanism of Action. Cycloserine and D-alanine are structural analogs; thus, cycloserine inhibits reactions in which D-alanine is involved in bacterial cell-wall synthesis (*see* Chapter 44). The use of medium free of D-alanine reveals that the antibiotic inhibits the growth *in vitro* of enterococci, *E. coli, S. aureus, Nocardia* species, and *Chlamydia.*

Absorption, Distribution, and Excretion. When given orally, 70% to 90% of cycloserine is rapidly absorbed. Peak concentrations in plasma are reached 3 to 4 hours after a single dose and are in the range of 20 to 35 μg/ml in children who receive 20 mg/kg; only small quantities are present after 12 hours. Cycloserine is distributed throughout body fluids and tissues. There is no appreciable blood–brain barrier to the drug, and CSF concentrations are approximately the same as those in plasma. About 50% of a parenteral dose of cycloserine is excreted unchanged in the urine in the first 12 hours; a total of 65% is recoverable in the active form over a period of 72 hours. Very little of the antibiotic is metabolized. The drug may accumulate to toxic concentrations in patients with renal insufficiency; it may be removed from the circulation by dialysis.

Therapeutic Uses. Cycloserine should be used only when retreatment is necessary or when microorganisms are resistant to other drugs. When cycloserine is employed to treat tuberculosis, it must be given together with other effective agents. Cycloserine is available for oral administration. The usual dose for adults is 250 to 500 mg twice daily.

Untoward Effects. Reactions to cycloserine most commonly involve the central nervous system. Symptoms tend to appear within the first 2 weeks of therapy and usually disappear when the drug is withdrawn. Among the central manifestations are somnolence, headache, tremor, dysarthria, vertigo, confusion, nervousness, irritability, psychotic states with suicidal tendencies, paranoid reactions, catatonic and depressed reactions, twitching, ankle clonus, hyperreflexia, visual disturbances, paresis, and tonic-clonic or absence seizures. Large doses of cycloserine or the concomitant ingestion of alcohol increases the risk of seizures. Cycloserine is contraindicated in individuals with a history of epilepsy and should be used with caution in individuals with a history of depression, as suicide is a risk.

OTHER DRUGS

The agents in this section are similar in several aspects. They are all second-line drugs that are used only for treatment of disease caused by resistant *M. tuberculosis* or by nontuberculous mycobacteria. They all must be given parenterally, and they have similar pharmacokinetics and toxicity. *Since these agents are potentially ototoxic and nephrotoxic, no two drugs from this group should be employed simultaneously, and these drugs should not be*

used in combination with streptomycin. Streptomycin, an aminoglycoside that is discussed in Chapter 45, inhibits the growth of *M. tuberculosis in vitro* at a concentration of 10 μg/ml or less.

Amikacin also is an aminoglycoside (*see* Chapter 45). It is extremely active against several mycobacterial species and has a role in the treatment of disease caused by nontuberculous mycobacteria (Brown and Wallace, 2000).

Capreomycin (CAPASTAT) is an antimycobacterial cyclic peptide elaborated by *Streptococcus capreolus*. It consists of 4 active components—capreomycins IA, IB, IIA, and IIB. The agent used clinically contains primarily IA and IB. Bacterial resistance to capreomycin develops when it is given alone; such microorganisms show cross-resistance with kanamycin and *neomycin*. Capreomycin is used only in conjunction with other appropriate antitubercular drugs in treatment of pulmonary tuberculosis when bactericidal agents cannot be tolerated or when causative organisms have become resistant.

Capreomycin must be given intramuscularly. The recommended daily dose is 15 to 30 mg/kg per day or up to 1 g for 60 to 120 days, followed by 1 g two to three times a week. The adverse reactions associated with the use of capreomycin are hearing loss, tinnitus, transient proteinuria, cylindruria, and nitrogen retention. Severe renal failure is rare. Eosinophilia is common. Leukocytosis, leukopenia, rashes, and fever have also been observed. Injections of the drug may be painful.

CHEMOTHERAPY OF TUBERCULOSIS

The availability of effective agents has so altered the treatment of tuberculosis that most patients are now treated in the ambulatory setting, often after diagnosis and initial therapy in a general hospital. Prolonged bed rest is not necessary or even helpful in speeding recovery. Patients must, however, be seen at frequent intervals to follow the course of their disease and treatment. The local health department must be notified of all cases. Contacts should be investigated for the possibility of disease and for the appropriateness of prophylactic therapy with isoniazid.

The majority of cases of previously untreated tuberculosis in the United States is caused by microorganisms that are sensitive to isoniazid, rifampin, ethambutol, and pyrazinamide. *To prevent the development of resistance to these agents that frequently occurs, treatment must include at least 2 drugs to which the bacteria are sensitive.* The preferred standard 6-month treatment program for drug-sensitive tuberculosis in adults and children consists of isoniazid, rifampin, pyrazinamide, and ethambutol for 2 months, followed by isoniazid and rifampin (for sensitive organisms) for 4 additional months. The combination of isoniazid and rifampin for 9 months is equally effective for drug-sensitive tuberculosis. Because of the increasing frequency of drug resistance, the Centers for Disease Control and Prevention (CDC) has recommended that initial therapy should be with a 4-drug regimen (isoniazid, rifampin, pyrazinamide, and ethambutol or streptomycin) pending sensitivity results. Directly observed therapy is the most effective approach to ensure treatment completion rates of about 90% (Chaulk and Kazandjian, 1998).

Drug interactions are a special concern in patients receiving highly active antiretroviral therapy. The rifamycins accelerate the metabolism of protease inhibitors and non-nucleoside reverse transcriptase inhibitors. Of the rifamycins, rifabutin has the least effect on *indinavir* and *nelfinavir* serum levels, and is therefore the current agent of choice in this setting.

Patients infected with the human immunodeficiency virus (HIV) may benefit from longer (9- to 12-month) treatment regimens (Havlir and Barnes, 1999). Treatment should be initiated with at least a 4-drug regimen consisting of isoniazid, rifabutin, pyrazinamide, and ethambutol or streptomycin. In patients with a high likelihood of infection with multidrug-resistant strains, an initial 5- or 6-drug regimen may be appropriate (Lane *et al.*, 1994; Gallant *et al.*, 1994). Treatment should be continued for at least 6 months after three negative cultures have been obtained. If isoniazid or rifampin cannot be used, therapy should be continued for at least 18 months (12 months after cultures become negative). Chemoprophylaxis (*see* below) should be undertaken if a patient with HIV infection has a positive tuberculin test (induration ≥5 mm), a history of a positive tuberculin skin test that was not treated with chemoprophylaxis, or recent close contact with a potentially infectious patient with tuberculosis. Isoniazid does not reduce the incidence of tuberculosis in anergic patients with HIV, so the earlier recommendation to treat such patients with chemoprophylaxis has been abandoned (Gordin *et al.*, 1997).

Therapy of Specific Types of Tuberculosis. Therapy for uncomplicated drug-sensitive pulmonary tuberculosis consists of isoniazid (5 mg/kg, up to 300 mg per day), rifampin (10 mg/kg per day, up to 600 mg daily), pyrazinamide (15 to 30 mg/kg per day or a maximum of 2 g per day), and a fourth agent. The fourth agent may be either ethambutol (usual adult dose of 15 mg/kg once per day) or streptomycin (1 g daily). The dosage of streptomycin is reduced to 1 g twice weekly after 2 months. Some physicians prefer to institute ethambutol therapy with a dose of 25 mg/kg per day for the first 60 days, and then to reduce the dose to 15 mg/kg per day, particularly for those who have received previous therapy. Pyridoxine, 15 to 50 mg per day, also should be included for most adults to minimize adverse reactions to isoniazid (Snider, 1980). Isoniazid, rifampin, pyrazinamide, and ethambutol or streptomycin are given for 2 months; isoniazid and rifampin are then continued for 4 additional months. Children are treated similarly; doses are isoniazid, 10 mg/kg per day (300 mg maximum); rifampin, 10 to 20 mg/kg per day (600 mg maximum); pyrazinamide, 15 to 30 mg/kg per day (2 g

maximum; Bass *et al.*, 1994). The multidrug regimen of isoniazid, rifampin, and ethambutol is considered safe during pregnancy.

Clinical improvement is readily discernible in the vast majority of patients with pulmonary tuberculosis if the treatment is appropriate. Efficacy usually becomes obvious within the first 2 weeks of therapy and is evidenced by a reduction of fever, decrease in cough, weight gain, and increase in the sense of well-being. Progressive radiological improvement also is evident. Over 90% of patients who receive optimal treatment will have negative cultures within 3 to 6 months, depending on the severity of the disease. Cultures that remain positive after 6 months frequently yield resistant microorganisms; the value of using an alternative therapeutic program should then be considered.

Failure of chemotherapy may be due to (1) irregular or inadequate therapy (resulting in persistent or resistant mycobacteria) caused by poor patient adherence to the protracted therapeutic regimen; (2) the use of a single drug, with interruption necessitated by toxicity or hypersensitivity; (3) an inadequate initial regimen; or (4) the primary resistance of the microorganism.

Problems in Chemotherapy. *Bacterial Resistance to Drugs.* One of the more important problems in the chemotherapy of tuberculosis is bacterial resistance. The primary reason for development of drug resistance is poor patient adherence. To prevent noncompliance and the attendant development of drug-resistant tuberculosis, directly observed therapy is advisable for most patients, in which a health care provider observes the patient ingest the medications 2 to 5 times weekly (Barnes and Barrows, 1993; Chaulk and Kazandjian, 1998).

Where drug resistance is suspected but sensitivities are not yet known (as in patients who have undergone several courses of treatment), therapy should be instituted with 5 or 6 drugs, including 2 or 3 that the patient has not received in the past. Such a regimen might include isoniazid, rifampin, pyrazinamide, ethambutol, streptomycin, and ethionamide. Some physicians include isoniazid in the therapeutic regimen, even if microorganisms are resistant, because of some evidence that disease with isoniazid-resistant mycobacteria does not "progress" during such therapy. Others prefer to discontinue isoniazid to lessen the possibility of toxicity. Therapy should be continued for at least 24 months.

Nontuberculous (Atypical) Mycobacteria. These microorganisms (not including *M. avium* complex, which is discussed later) have been recovered from a variety of lesions in humans (Brown and Wallace, 2000). Because they frequently are resistant to many of the commonly used agents, they must be examined for sensitivity *in vitro* and drug therapy selected on this basis (Table 47–1). In some instances, surgical removal of the infected tissue followed by long-term treatment with effective agents is necessary.

M. kansasii causes disease similar to that caused by *M. tuberculosis,* but it may be milder. The microorganisms may be resistant to isoniazid. Therapy with isoniazid, rifampin, and ethambutol has been successful (Lane *et al.*, 1994). *M. marinum* causes skin lesions. A combination of rifampin and ethambutol is probably effective; *minocycline* (Loria, 1976) or tetracycline is active *in vitro* and is used by some physicians (Izumi *et al.*, 1977). *M. scrofulaceum* is an uncommon cause of cervical lymphadenitis. Surgical excision still seems to be the therapy of choice (Lincoln and Gilberg, 1972). Microbes of the *M. fortuitum* complex (including *Mycobacterium chelonae*) are usually saprophytes, but they may cause chronic lung disease and infections of skin and soft tissues. The microorganisms are highly resistant to most drugs, but amikacin, *cefoxitin*, and tetracyclines are active *in vitro* (Sanders *et al.*, 1977; Sanders, 1982).

Chemoprophylaxis of Tuberculosis. The chemoprophylaxis of tuberculosis is the practice of treating latent infection to prevent progression to active disease. Latent infection may be diagnosed by a positive delayed-type hypersensitivity reaction to a purified protein derivative (PPD) of tuberculosis injected intradermally (the "tuberculin test"). There are several approaches to the chemoprophylaxis of tuberculosis. The classical prophylaxis with 12 months of isoniazid resulted in a 75% reduction in the risk of active tuberculosis (from an incidence of 14.3% to 3.6% over 5 years). A 6-month course of isoniazid therapy was nearly as effective, with a 65% risk reduction and a lower incidence of isoniazid-induced hepatitis (International Union Against Tuberculosis, 1982). Currently the CDC recommends isoniazid for 6 to 9 months or rifampin for 4 months if isoniazid cannot be used (Centers for Disease Control, 2001). A 2-month regimen of daily rifampin and pyrazinamide was shown to be as effective as 12 months of isoniazid in one study of HIV-infected individuals (Halsey *et al.*, 1998). However, severe hepatotoxicity resulting in the deaths of 5 of the estimated 10,000 non–HIV-infected individuals has resulted in the rifampin-plus-pyrazinamide regimen being used only in exceptional circumstances (*e.g.*, PPD conversion after exposure to isoniazid-resistant *M. tuberculosis*) and only with intensive monitoring for liver injury during treatment (Centers for Disease Control, 2001; Leibert and Rom, 2004).

Prophylactic therapy can effectively prevent the development of active tuberculosis in certain instances (Haas, 2000). There are 4 categories of patients for whom prophylactic therapy should be considered: those exposed to tuberculosis but who have no evidence of infection; those with infection (positive tuberculin test: induration >5 mm [HIV infected or other immunosuppressed patients and recent contacts of TB patients]); those with infection positive tuberculin test (induration >10 mm reaction to 5 units of PPD [not immunocompromised but with risk factors for TB]) and no apparent disease; and those with a history of tuberculosis but in whom the disease is currently "inactive" (Centers for Disease Control, 2001; Bass *et al.*, 1994; Wilkinson *et al.*, 1998; Gordin *et al.*, 1997; Gallant *et al.*, 1994). The main risk of chemoprophylaxis is isoniazid-induced hepatitis, which is much less common (as low as 1/100,000 for severe isoniazid hepatitis) (Nolan *et al.*, 1999) with current approaches to monitoring patients for liver injury due to isoniazid. Monitored isoniazid prophylaxis minimizes the risk of toxicity even in patients over the age of 35 (Salpeter *et al.*, 1997; Centers for Disease Control, 2001).

Household contacts and other close associates of patients with tuberculosis who have negative tuberculin tests should receive isoniazid for at least 6 months after the contact has been broken, regardless of age. This is especially important for children. If the tuberculin skin test becomes positive, therapy should be continued for 12 months.

Patients with old "inactive" tuberculosis who have not received adequate chemotherapy in the past should be considered for 1 year of treatment with isoniazid (Comstock, 1983). HIV-infected intravenous drug abusers with a positive skin test have an approximately 8% chance per year of developing active tuberculosis (Selwyn *et al.*, 1989). Isoniazid prophylaxis in HIV-infected persons appears to be as effective as in nonimmunocompromised persons (Wilkinson *et al.*, 1998). The CDC recommends that isoniazid prophylaxis be continued for 12 months. Persons infected with HIV who are exposed to multidrug-resistant tuberculosis should receive prophylaxis with rifampin and pyrazinamide (with close monitoring for hepatic toxicity; Centers for Disease Control, 2001) or high-dose ethambutol and pyrazinamide, with or without a fluoroquinolone (Gallant *et al.*, 1994).

Prophylaxis with isoniazid is contraindicated for patients who have active hepatic disease or who have had reactions to the drug. In these individuals rifampin for 4 months can be given (Centers for Disease Control, 2001). In pregnant women, prophylaxis usually should be delayed until after delivery. For prophylaxis, isoniazid generally is given to adults in a daily dose of 300 mg. Children should receive 10 mg/kg to a maximal daily dose of 300 mg. Pyridoxine should be coadministered in individuals susceptible to isoniazid-induced neuropathy (*see* above).

II. DRUGS FOR *MYCOBACTERIUM AVIUM* COMPLEX

Before the advent of highly active antiretroviral therapy (HAART, *see* Chapter 50) and the use of prophylactic regimens, disseminated infection with MAC bacteria occurred in 15% to 40% of patients with HIV infection. Infections with MAC now are greatly reduced (Benson, 1997–98). Patients with *M. avium* complex infection usually are in advanced stages of HIV disease, with CD4 T-lymphocyte counts below 100/mm^3 and symptoms of fever, night sweats, weight loss, and anemia at the time of diagnosis. In non–HIV-infected persons, MAC infection usually is limited to the lungs and presents with a chronic productive cough and chest roentgenograms showing evidence of limited, diffuse, and/or cavitary disease (Havlir and Ellner, 2000). Although standard antimycobacterial agents have little activity against MAC, new antimicrobial agents with activity against MAC recently have become available. These agents currently are in use for both the prevention and treatment of MAC in patients with AIDS.

RIFABUTIN

Rifabutin is a derivative of rifamycin, which shares a common mechanism of action (inhibition of mycobacterial RNA polymerase), but is more active than rifampin *in vitro* and in experimental murine tuberculosis.

Chemistry. Rifabutin is soluble in organic solvents and at low concentrations (0.19 mg/ml) in water. It has the following structure:

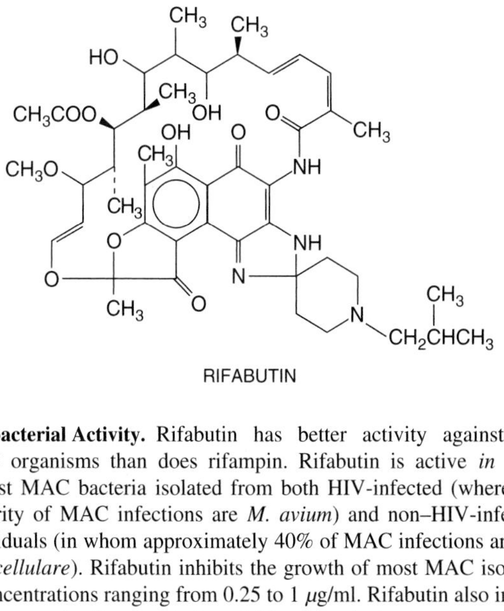

RIFABUTIN

Antibacterial Activity. Rifabutin has better activity against the MAC organisms than does rifampin. Rifabutin is active *in vitro* against MAC bacteria isolated from both HIV-infected (where the majority of MAC infections are *M. avium*) and non–HIV-infected individuals (in whom approximately 40% of MAC infections are *M. intracellulare*). Rifabutin inhibits the growth of most MAC isolates at concentrations ranging from 0.25 to 1 μg/ml. Rifabutin also inhibits the growth of many strains of *M. tuberculosis* at concentrations of $\leq$0.125 μg/ml.

Bacterial Resistance. Cross-resistance between rifampin and rifabutin is common in *M. tuberculosis,* although some strains have been identified that are resistant to rifampin yet sensitive to rifabutin. Of 225 *M. avium* strains that were resistant to 10 μg/ml of rifampin, 80% were sensitive to 1 μg/ml rifabutin (Heifets *et al.*, 1985).

Absorption, Distribution, Metabolism, and Excretion. The oral administration of 300 mg of rifabutin produces a peak plasma concentration of approximately 0.4 μg/ml at 2 to 3 hours. The drug is metabolized by hepatic CYPs and eliminated in a biphasic manner with a mean

terminal half-life of 45 hours (range of 16 to 96 hours). Because rifabutin is a lipophilic drug, concentrations are substantially higher (five- to tenfold) in tissue than in plasma. Following absorption from the GI tract, rifabutin is eliminated in the urine and bile. Adjustment of dosage is not necessary in patients with impaired renal function. Rifabutin is a weaker inducer of hepatic CYPs than is rifampin.

Therapeutic Uses. Rifabutin is effective for the prevention of MAC infection in HIV-infected individuals. At a dose of 300 mg per day, rifabutin decreased the frequency of MAC bacteremia (2%) (Nightingale *et al.*, 1993). However, azithromycin or clarithromycin are more effective and less likely to interact with HAART drugs. Rifabutin also is commonly substituted for rifampin in the treatment of tuberculosis in HIV-infected patients, as it has a less profound CYP-dependent interaction with indinavir and nelfinavir (Haas, 2000). Rifabutin also is used in combination with clarithromycin and ethambutol for the therapy of MAC disease (Shafran *et al.*, 1996).

Untoward Effects. Rifabutin generally is well tolerated in persons with HIV infection; primary reasons for discontinuation of therapy include rash (4%), gastrointestinal intolerance (3%), and neutropenia (2%) (Nightingale *et al.*, 1993). Overall, neutropenia occurred in 25% of patients with severe HIV infection who received rifabutin. Uveitis and arthralgias have occurred in patients receiving rifabutin doses greater than 450 mg daily in combination with clarithromycin or fluconazole. Patients should be cautioned to discontinue the drug if visual symptoms (pain or blurred vision) occur. Like rifampin, the drug causes an orange-tan discoloration of skin, urine, feces, saliva, tears, and contact lenses. Rarely, thrombocytopenia, a flulike syndrome, hemolysis, myositis, chest pain, and hepatitis have occurred in patients treated with rifabutin.

Although a less potent inducer of CYPs than rifampin, rifabutin does induce hepatic microsomal enzymes, with its administration decreasing the half-life of a number of different compounds, including *zidovudine, prednisone*, digitoxin, quinidine, ketoconazole, propranolol, phenytoin, sulfonylureas, and *warfarin*. It has less effect than does rifampin on serum levels of indinavir and nelfinavir.

MACROLIDES

The macrolides clarithromycin and azithromycin are extremely valuable agents for the treatment of MAC and other nontuberculous mycobacteria. Clarithromycin alters the metabolism of many other drugs that are metabolized at the cytochrome P450 system, leading to many potential drug interactions. A discussion of the pharmacology of the macrolides is presented in Chapter 46. Only features of the macrolides related to their use in the treatment of MAC infections are considered here.

Antibacterial Activity. Clarithromycin is approximately fourfold more active than azithromycin against MAC bacteria *in vitro* and is active against most nontuberculous mycobacteria with the exception of *Mycobacterium simiae* at ≤4 μg/ml. Azithromycin's lower potency may be compensated for *in vivo* by its greater intracellular penetration: Tissue levels generally exceed plasma levels by one hundredfold.

Bacterial Resistance. Use of clarithromycin or azithromycin alone in the therapy of MAC infection is associated with the development of resistance after prolonged treatment. For this reason, these drugs should not be used as monotherapy of MAC infection.

Therapeutic Uses. Clarithromycin (500 mg twice daily) or azithromycin (500 mg daily) is used in combination with ethambutol, with or without rifabutin, for treatment of MAC infection (Shafran *et al.*, 1996). Treatment should be continued throughout the lifetime of an HIV-infected individual (U.S. Public Health Service, 1999). Azithromycin has minimal potential for affecting drugs metabolized by CYP3A4.

Untoward Effects. The high doses used to treat MAC infections can occasionally cause tinnitus, dizziness, and reversible hearing loss.

QUINOLONES

The quinolones (*e.g., ciprofloxacin, levofloxacin*, moxifloxacin, and gatifloxacin) are discussed in detail in Chapter 43. These drugs have inhibitory activity against MAC bacteria *in vitro* (at concentrations of ≤100 μg/ml). Minimal inhibitory concentrations for *M. fortuitum* and *M. kansasii* are ≤3 μg/ml for these quinolones but *M. chelonae* usually are resistant. Single-agent therapy of *M. fortuitum* infection with ciprofloxacin has been associated with the development of resistance. Ciprofloxacin, 750 mg twice daily or 500 mg three times daily, has been used as part of a 4-drug regimen (with clarithromycin, rifabutin, and amikacin) as salvage therapy for MAC infections in HIV-infected patients, with improvement in symptoms (Havlir and Ellner, 2000). Multidrug-resistant tuberculosis has been treated with ofloxacin, 300 or 800 mg each day, in combination with second-line agents. Moxifloxacin and gatifloxacin are more active *in vitro* than the older fluoroquinolones and would be expected to be useful agents clinically.

AMIKACIN

The antibacterial activity and pharmacology of amikacin are discussed fully in Chapter 45. Amikacin may have a role as a third or fourth agent in a multiple-drug regimen for MAC treatment. Most isolates of MAC are inhibited *in vitro* by 8 to 32 μg/ml of amikacin.

CHEMOTHERAPY OF *MYCOBACTERIUM AVIUM* COMPLEX

Initial pessimism about the treatment of MAC infection has lifted with the availability of clarithromycin and azithromycin. Both of these agents have excellent activity against many strains of MAC, with clinical responses (decrease or elimination of bacteremia, resolution of fever and night sweats) demonstrated even with single-drug therapy. Single-agent therapy, however, has been associated with the emergence of resistant strains. Most clinicians treat disseminated MAC infections with clarithromycin or azithromycin plus ethambutol (Haas, 2000; Shafran *et al.*, 1996). In some situations, and with unclear benefits, rifabutin, clofazimine, and/or a quinolone are added to the above regimen. Drug interactions and adverse drug reactions are common with multiple-drug regimens and necessitated drug discontinuation in 46% of patients in one study (Kemper *et al.*, 1992). Clinical improvement should be expected in the first 1 to 2 months of treatment, with sterilization of blood cultures seen as late as 3 months into therapy. Therapy of MAC infection in HIV-infected individuals should continue for life if the therapy is associated with clinical and microbiological improvement (U.S. Public Health Service, 1999). Isoniazid and pyrazinamide have no role in the treatment of MAC infection.

Prophylaxis of MAC infection with clarithromycin or azithromycin should be strongly considered for HIV-infected persons whose CD4 cell count is less than 50/mm^3. Clarithromycin and azithromycin are well-tolerated medications that have proven effective at reducing the incidence of MAC infection in this population. With the advent of HAART, it would be a reasonable decision to stop prophylaxis in a patient who responds to anti-HIV therapy with a sustained CD4$^+$ T-lymphocyte count greater than 100/mm^3 and a sustained suppression of HIV plasma RNA (U.S. Public Health Service, 1999).

III. DRUGS FOR LEPROSY

Largely due to a World Health Organization global initiative to eliminate leprosy (Hansen's disease) as a public health problem by 2005, between 1985 and 2003 the number of leprosy patients worldwide plummeted by nearly 90% to around 534,000. The cornerstone of the WHO's global elimination strategy is the provision of effective multidrug chemotherapy, namely dapsone, rifampin, and clofazimine (Table 47–1), free of charge, to all leprosy patients in the world. The ongoing success of the strategy is evident; by the end of 2003, all but 10 of the 22 countries considered endemic for leprosy in 1985 had achieved elimination (defined as a prevalence rate of <1 case per 10,000 inhabitants) of the disease (World Health Organization, 2004). The history of the development of multidrug therapy against leprosy has been published by the WHO (Sansarricq, 2004).

SULFONES

The sulfones are derivatives of 4,4′-diaminodiphenylsulfone (dapsone), all of which have certain pharmacological properties in common. They are discussed here as a class; only dapsone and *sulfoxone* are considered individually.

History. The sulfones first attracted interest because of their chemical relationship to the sulfonamides. In the 1940s, sulfones were found to be effective in suppressing experimental infections with the tubercle bacillus and for rat leprosy; this finding was soon followed by successful clinical trials in human leprosy. The sulfones are currently the most important drugs for the treatment of this disorder.

Chemistry. All clinically useful sulfones are derivatives of dapsone. Despite the study and development of a large variety of sulfones, dapsone remains the agent most useful clinically.

Antibacterial Activity, Mechanism of Action, and Resistance. Because *Mycobacterium leprae* does not grow on artificial media, conventional methods cannot be applied to determine its susceptibility to potential therapeutic agents *in vitro*. Therefore, *in vivo* assays with rat footpads have been used to test agents. Dapsone is bacteriostatic, but not bactericidal, for *M. leprae,* and the estimated sensitivity to the drug is between 1 and 10 μg/ml for microorganisms recovered from untreated patients (Levy and Peters, 1976). *M. leprae* may become resistant to the drug during therapy.

The mechanism of action of the sulfones is the same as that of the sulfonamides: they are competitive inhibitors of dihydropteroate synthase and prevent the normal bacterial utilization of *para*-amino-benzoic acid. Both possess approximately the same range of antibacterial activity and both are antagonized by *para*-aminobenzoic acid.

Dapsone-resistant strains of *M. leprae* are termed *secondary* if they emerge during therapy. Secondary resistance usually is seen in lepromatous (multibacillary) patients treated with a single drug. The incidence is as high as 19% (WHO Expert Committee on Leprosy, 1998). Partial-to-complete primary resistance (seen in previously untreated patients) has been described in 2.5% to 40% of patients, depending on geographical location (Centers for Disease Control, 1982); some authorities question the clinical significance of primary resistance (Gelber *et al.*, 1990; Gelber and Rea, 2000).

Therapeutic Uses. Dapsone is available for oral administration. Several dosage schedules have been recommended (Gelber and Rea, 2000). Daily therapy with 100 mg has been successful in adults. Therapy usually is begun with smaller amounts, and doses are increased to those recommended over 1 to 2 months. Therapy

should be continued for at least 3 years and may be necessary for the lifetime of the patient.

Untoward Effects. The untoward reactions induced by various sulfones are very similar, with the most common being hemolysis of varying degree. This develops in almost every individual treated with 200 to 300 mg of dapsone per day. Doses of 100 mg or less in normal healthy persons and 50 mg or less in healthy individuals with a glucose-6-phosphate dehydrogenase deficiency do not cause hemolysis. Methemoglobinemia also is common, and Heinz-body formation may occur. A genetic deficiency in the NADH-dependent methemoglobin reductase can result in severe methemoglobinemia after administration of dapsone. While diminished red-cell survival usually occurs during the use of sulfones and is presumed to be a dose-related effect of their oxidizing activity, hemolytic anemia is unusual unless the patient also has a disorder of either the erythrocytes or the bone marrow. The hemolysis may be so severe that manifestations of hypoxia become striking.

Anorexia, nausea, and vomiting may follow the oral administration of sulfones. Isolated instances of headache, nervousness, insomnia, blurred vision, paresthesias, reversible peripheral neuropathy (thought to be due to axonal degeneration), drug fever, hematuria, pruritus, psychosis, and a variety of skin rashes have been reported (Rapoport and Guss, 1972). An infectious mononucleosis-like syndrome, which may be fatal, occurs occasionally. The sulfones may induce an exacerbation of lepromatous leprosy by a process thought to be analogous to the Jarisch-Herxheimer reaction. This "sulfone syndrome" may develop 5 to 6 weeks after initiation of treatment in malnourished people. Its manifestations include fever, malaise, exfoliative dermatitis, jaundice with hepatic necrosis, lymphadenopathy, methemoglobinemia, and anemia.

If proper precautions are observed, the sulfones may be given safely for many years in doses adequate for the successful therapy of leprosy. Treatment should be initiated with a small dose and the quantity then increased gradually. Patients must be under consistent and prolonged laboratory and clinical supervision. The reactions induced by the sulfones, especially those related to exacerbation of the leprosy, may be very severe and may require the cessation of treatment as well as the institution of specific measures to reduce the threat to life.

Absorption, Distribution, and Excretion. Dapsone is absorbed rapidly and nearly completely from the gastrointestinal tract. The disubstituted sulfones, such as sulfoxone, are absorbed incompletely when administered orally, and large amounts are excreted in the feces. Peak concentrations of dapsone in plasma are reached within 2 to 8 hours after administration; the mean half-life of elimination is about 20 to 30 hours. Twenty-four hours after oral ingestion of 100 mg, plasma concentrations range from 0.4 to 1.2 μg/ml, and a dose of 100 mg of dapsone per day produces an average of 2 μg of "free" dapsone per gram of blood or nonhepatic tissue. About 70% of the drug is bound to plasma protein. Concentrations in plasma following conventional doses of sulfoxone sodium are 10 to 15 μg/ml. These values fall relatively rapidly; however, appreciable quantities are still present at 8 hours.

The sulfones are distributed throughout total body water and are present in all tissues. They tend to be retained in skin and muscle and especially in liver and kidney; traces of the drug are present in these organs up to 3 weeks after therapy is stopped. The sulfones are retained in the circulation for a long time because of intestinal reabsorption from the bile; periodic interruption of treatment is advisable for this reason. Dapsone is acetylated in the liver, and the rate of acetylation is genetically determined; the same enzyme carries out the acetylation of isoniazid. Daily administration of 50 to 100 mg results in serum levels exceeding the usual minimal inhibitory concentrations, even in rapid acetylators, in whom the serum half-life of dapsone is shorter than usual.

Approximately 70% to 80% of a dose of dapsone is excreted in the urine. The drug is present in urine as an acid-labile mono-*N*-glucuronide and mono-*N*-sulfamate in addition to an unknown number of unidentified metabolites. *Probenecid* decreases the urinary excretion of the acid-labile dapsone metabolites significantly and that of free dapsone to a lesser extent (Goodwin and Sparell, 1969).

RIFAMPIN

Rifampin has been discussed above with regard to its use in tuberculosis. This antibiotic is rapidly bactericidal for *M. leprae*, and the minimal inhibitory concentration is <1 μg/ml. Infectivity of patients is reversed rapidly by therapy that includes rifampin. Because of the prevalence of resistance to dapsone, the WHO Expert Committee on Leprosy (1998) now recommends a regimen of multiple drugs, including rifampin.

CLOFAZIMINE

Clofazimine (LAMPRENE) is a phenazine dye with the following structural formula:

CLOFAZIMINE

The biochemical basis for the antimicrobial actions of clofazimine remains to be established. Clofazimine appears to preferentially bind to GC-rich mycobacterial DNA (Morrison and Marley, 1976) and also increase mycobacterial phospholipase A_2 activity and inhibit microbial K^+ transport (Steel *et al.*, 1999). It is weakly bactericidal against *M. intracellulare*. The drug also exerts an anti-inflammatory effect and prevents the development of erythema nodosum leprosum. Clofazimine is now recommended as a component of multiple-drug therapy for leprosy (*see* below). The compound also is useful for treatment of chronic skin ulcers (Buruli ulcer) produced by *Mycobacterium ulcerans*.

Clofazimine is absorbed by the oral route and appears to accumulate in tissues. Human leprosy from which dapsone-resistant bacilli have been recovered has been treated with clofazimine with good results. However, unlike dapsone-sensitive microorganisms, in which killing occurs immediately after dapsone is administered, dapsone-resistant strains do not exhibit an appreciable effect until 50 days after initiation of therapy with clofazimine. The daily dose of clofazimine is usually 100 mg. Patients treated with clofazimine may develop red discoloration of the skin, which may be very distressing to light-skinned individuals. Eosinophilic enteritis has also been described as an adverse reaction to the drug.

MISCELLANEOUS AGENTS

Thalidomide has been shown effective for the treatment of erythema nodosum leprosum (Okafor, 2003). It has immunomodulatory actions and inhibits tumor necrosis factor-α (*see* Chapter 52), but the mechanism of action against leprosy is not established. Doses of 100 to 300 mg per day have been effective. *Because of the marked teratogenicity of thalidomide, its prescribing and dispensing is restricted to physicians and patients enrolled in the System for Thalidomide Education and Prescribing Safety (STEPS) oversight program.* This oversight program is designed to help ensure a zero-tolerance policy for thalidomide exposure during pregnancy.

Ethionamide has been discussed above as an agent for treatment of tuberculosis. It can be used as a substitute for clofazimine in oral doses of 250 to 375 mg per day. Newer agents that appear promising based on animal trials and limited experience in patients include minocycline, clarithromycin, *pefloxacin* (an investigational fluoroquinolone in the United States), and *ofloxacin* (Gelber and Rea, 2000).

CHEMOTHERAPY OF LEPROSY

Five clinical types of leprosy are recognized. At one end of the spectrum is *tuberculoid leprosy*. This form of the disease is characterized by skin macules with clear centers and well-defined margins; these are almost always anesthetic. *M. leprae* is rarely found in smears made from quiescent lesions but may appear during activity. Virchow cells are not demonstrable. Noncaseating foci with giant cells of the Langhans variety are present. The patient's cell-mediated immune responses are normal, and the lepromin test (intradermal injection of a suspension of heat-killed, bacillus-laden tissue) is invariably positive. The disease is characterized by prolonged remissions with periodic reactivation.

At the other end of the spectrum is the widely disseminated *lepromatous* form of the disease. Patients with this disease have markedly impaired cell-mediated immunity and are frequently anergic; the lepromin test causes no reaction. Lepromatous disease is characterized by diffuse or ill-defined, localized infiltration of the skin, which becomes thickened, glossy, and corrugated; areas of decreased sensation may appear. *M. leprae* is demonstrable in smears, and granulomas containing bacteria-laden histiocytes (Virchow cells) are present. As the disease progresses, large nerve trunks are involved and anesthesia, atrophy of skin and muscle, absorption of small bones, ulceration, and spontaneous amputations may occur. Three intermediate forms of the disease are recognized: borderline tuberculoid disease, borderline lepromatous disease, and borderline disease (Gelber and Rea, 2000).

Patients with tuberculoid leprosy may develop "reversal reactions," which are manifestations of delayed hypersensitivity to antigens of *M. leprae*. Cutaneous ulcerations and deficits of peripheral nerve function may occur. Early therapy with corticosteroids or clofazimine is effective.

Reactions in the lepromatous form of the disease (erythema nodosum leprosum) are characterized by the appearance of raised, tender, intracutaneous nodules, severe constitutional symptoms, and high fever. This reaction may be triggered by several conditions, but is often associated with therapy. It is thought to be an Arthus-type reaction related to release of microbial antigens in patients harboring large numbers of bacilli. Treatment with clofazimine or thalidomide is effective.

The outlook for persons with leprosy has been remarkably altered by successful chemotherapy, surgical procedures that help to restore function and repair disfigurement, and a striking change in the attitude of the public toward patients who have this infection. The social stigma of individuals with this affliction gradually is being replaced by the attitude that considers leprosy a disease caused by a bacterium. Patients with leprosy can be classified as "infectious" or "noninfectious" on the basis of the type and duration of disease and effects of therapy. Thus, even "infectious" patients need not be hospitalized provided that adequate medical supervision and therapy are maintained, the home environment meets specific conditions, and the local health officer concurs in the disposition of the case.

Therapy, when effective, heals ulcers and mucosal lesions in months. Cutaneous nodules respond more slowly, and it may take years to eradicate bacteria from mucous membranes, skin, and nerves. The degree of residual pigmentation or depigmentation, atrophy, and scarring depends upon the extent of the initial involvement. Severe ocular lesions show little response to the sulfones. If treatment is initiated before ocular disease is evident, the latter may be prevented. Keratoconjunctivitis and corneal ulceration may be secondary to nerve involvement.

The World Health Organization now recommends therapy with multiple drugs for all patients with leprosy (WHO Expert Committee on Leprosy, 1998). The reasons for using combinations of agents include reduction in the development of resistance, the need for adequate therapy when primary resistance already exists, and reduction in the duration of therapy. Dosage recommendations for control programs take a number of practical constraints into account. For patients with large populations of bacteria (multibacillary forms)— including lepromatous disease, borderline lepromatous disease, and borderline disease—the following regimen is suggested: dapsone, 100 mg daily; plus clofazimine, 50 mg daily (unsupervised); plus rifampin, 600 mg, and clofazimine, 300 mg, once a month under supervision for 1 to 5 years. Some prefer to treat lepromatous leprosy with daily dapsone (100 mg) and daily rifampin (450 to 600 mg) (Gelber and Rea, 2000). All drugs are given orally. The minimal duration of therapy is 2 years, and treatment should continue until acid-fast bacilli are not detected in lesions.

Patients with a small population of bacteria (paucibacillary disease), including those with tuberculoid, borderline tuberculoid, and indeterminate disease, should be treated with dapsone, 100 mg daily, plus rifampin, 600 mg once monthly (under supervision), for a minimum of 6 months. Relapses are treated by repeating the regimen. A recent clinical trial suggests that single-dose multidrug therapy with rifampin (600 mg), ofloxacin (400 mg), and minocycline (100 mg) may be as effective (Single Lesion Multicentre Trial Group, 1997). More prolonged treatment programs are recommended for patients in the United States (Gelber and Rea, 2000).

CLINICAL SUMMARY

Combination therapy is almost always the desirable approach for myobacterial disease to ensure effective eradication and to prevent the emergence of resistance. Isoniazid, rifampin, ethambutol, streptomycin, and pyrazinamide are first-line agents for the treatment of tuberculosis. The use of immunomodulators such as interferon-γ to increase macrophage killing of the intracellular bacterium is a potentially interesting new avenue for treatment. Antimi-

crobial agents with excellent activity against *Mycobacterium avium* complex include rifabutin, clarithromycin, azithromycin, and fluoroquinolones. Drug interactions and adverse drug reactions, however, are common with multiple-drug regimens, and clinical monitoring is important. Considerable progress has been achieved in eliminating leprosy through the use of multiple-drug chemotherapy including dapsone, rifampin, and clofazimine. Thalidomide also has been found to have activity in patients with leprosy.

BIBLIOGRAPHY

Alcala, L., Ruiz-Serrano, M.J., Perez-Fernandez Turegano, C., *et al.* In vitro activities of linezolid against clinical isolates of *Mycobacterium tuberculosis* that are susceptible or resistant to first-line antituberculous drugs. *Antimicrob. Agents Chemother.,* **2003**, *47:*416–417.

Baciewicz, A.M., Self, T.H., and Bekemeyer, W.B. Update on rifampin drug interactions. *Arch. Intern. Med.,* **1987**, *147:*565–568.

Bailey, W.C., Weill, H., DeRouen, T.A., *et al.* The effect of isoniazid on transaminase levels. *Ann. Intern. Med.,* **1974**, *81:*200–202.

Banerjee, A., Dubnau, E., Quemard, A., *et al.* inhA, a gene encoding a target for isoniazid and ethionamide in *Mycobacterium tuberculosis.* *Science,* **1994**, *263:*227–230.

Belanger, A.E., Besra, G.S., Ford, M.E., *et al.* The *embAB* genes of *Mycobacterium avium* encode an arabinosyl transferase involved in cell wall arabinan biosynthesis that is a target for the antimycobacterial drug ethambutol. *Proc. Natl. Acad. Sci. U.S.A.,* **1996**, *93:*11919–11924.

Benson, C.A. Disseminated *Mycobacterium avium* complex infection: implications of recent chemical trials on prophylaxis and treatment. *AIDS Clin. Rev.,* **1997–98**, 271–287.

British Thoracic Association. A controlled trial of six months chemotherapy in pulmonary tuberculosis. Second report: results during the twenty-four months after the end of chemotherapy. *Am. Rev. Respir. Dis.,* **1982**, *126:*460–462.

Byrd, R.B., Horn, B.R., Solomon, D.A., and Griggs, G.W. Toxic effects of isoniazid in tuberculosis chemoprophylaxis. Role of biochemical monitoring in 1,000 patients. *JAMA,* **1979**, *241:*1239–1241.

Cauthen, G.M., Kilburn, J.O., Kelly, G.D., and Good, R.C. Resistance to anti-tuberculosis drugs in patients with and without prior treatment: survey of 31 state and large city laboratories, 1982–1986. *Am. Rev. Respir. Dis.,* **1988**, *137*(suppl):260.

Centers for Disease Control and Prevention. Adverse drug reactions among children treated for tuberculosis. *M.M.W.R. Morb. Mortal. Wkly. Rep.,* **1980**, *29:*589–591.

Centers for Disease Control and Prevention. Increase in prevalence of leprosy caused by dapsone-resistant *Mycobacterium leprae. M.M.W.R. Morb. Mortal. Wkly. Rep.,* **1982**, *30:*637–638.

Centers for Disease Control and Prevention. Tuberculosis elimination revisited: obstacles, opportunities, and a renewed commitment. Advisory Council for the Elimination of Tuberculosis (ACET). *M.M.W.R. Morb. Mortal. Wkly. Rep.,* **1999**, *48:*1–13.

Centers for Disease Control and Prevention. Update: fatal and severe liver injuries associated with rifampin and pyrazinamide for latent tuberculosis infection, and revisions in American Thoracic/CDC recommendations-United States, 2001. *M.M.W.R. Morb. Mortal. Wkly. Rep.,* **2001**, *50:*733-735.

Chaulk, C.P., and Kazandjian, V.A. Directly observed therapy for treatment completion of pulmonary tuberculosis: Consensus Statement of the Public Health Tuberculosis Guidelines Panel. *JAMA*, **1998**, *279*:943–948.

Comstock, G.W. New data on preventive treatment with isoniazid. *Ann. Intern. Med.*, **1983**, *98*:663–665.

Condos, R., Hull, F.P., Schluger, N.W., *et al*. Regional deposition of aerosolized interferon-gamma in pulmonary tuberculosis. *Chest*, **2004**, *125*:2416–2155.

Fraaije, M.W., *et al*. The Prodrug Activator EtaA from *M. tuberculosis* is a Baeyer-Villiger monooxygenase. *J. Biol. Chem.*, **2004**, *279*:3354–3360.

Furesz, S. Chemical and biological properties of rifampicin. *Antibiot. Chemother.*, **1970**, *16*:316–351.

Gangadharam, P.R. Isoniazid, rifampin, and hepatotoxicity. *Am. Rev. Respir. Dis.*, **1986**, *133*:963–965.

Garibaldi, R.A., Drusin, R.E., Ferebee, S.H., and Gregg, M.B. Isoniazid-associated hepatitis. Report of an outbreak. *Am. Rev. Respir. Dis.*, **1972**, *106*:357–365.

Gelber, R.H., Rea, T.H., Murray, L.P., *et al*. Primary dapsone-resistant Hansen's disease in California. Experience with over 100 *Mycobacterium leprae* isolates. *Arch. Dermatol.*, **1990**, *126*:1584–1586.

Goodwin, C.S., and Sparell, G. Inhibition of dapsone excretion by probenecid. *Lancet*, **1969**, *2*:884–885.

Gordin, F.M., Matts, J.P., Miller, C., *et al*. A controlled trial of isoniazid in persons with anergy and human immunodeficiency virus infection who are at risk for tuberculosis. Terry Beirn Community Programs for Clinical Research on AIDS. *N. Engl. J. Med.*, **1997**, *337*:315–320.

Graber, C.D., Jebaily, J., Galphin, R.L., and Doering, E. Light chain proteinuria and humoral immunocompetence in tuberculous patients treated with rifampin. *Am. Rev. Respir. Dis.*, **1973**, *107*:713–717.

Grosset, J., and Leventis, S. Adverse effects of rifampin. *Rev. Infect. Dis.*, **1983**, *5*:S440–S446.

Halsey, N.A., Coberly, J.S., Desormeaux, J., *et al*. Randomised controlled trial of isoniazid *versus* rifampin and pyrazinamide for prevention of tuberculosis in HIV-1 infection. *Lancet*, **1998**, *351*:786–792.

Heifets, L.B., Iseman, M.D., Lindholm-Levy, P.J., and Kanes, W. Determination of ansamycin MICs for *Mycobacterium avium* complex in liquid medium by radiometric and conventional methods. *Antimicrob. Agents Chemother.*, **1985**, *28*:570–575.

Holdiness, M.R. Cerebrospinal fluid pharmacokinetics of antituberculosis antibiotics. *Clin. Pharmacokinet.*, **1985**, *10*:532–534.

International Union Against Tuberculosis (IUAT). Efficacy of various durations of isoniazid preventive therapy for tuberculosis: five years follow-up in the IUAT trial. *Bull. World Health Organ.*, **1982**, *60*:555–564.

Izumi, A.K., Hanke, C.W., and Higaki, M. *Mycobacterium marinum* infections treated with tetracycline. *Arch. Dermatol.*, **1977**, *113*:1067–1068.

Kemper, C.A., Meng, T.C., Nussbaum, J., *et al*. Treatment of *Mycobacterium avium* complex bacteremia in AIDS with a four-drug oral regimen: rifampin, ethambutol, clofazimine and ciprofloxacin. The California Collaborative Treatment Group. *Ann. Intern. Med.*, **1992**, *116*:466–472.

Kinzig-Schippers, M., Tomalik-Scharte, D., Jetter, A., et al. Should we use *N*-acetyltransferase type 2 genotyping to personalize isoniazid doses? *Antimicrob. Agents Chemother.* **2005**, *49*:1733–1738.

Larsen, M.H., *et al*. Overexpression of inhA, but not kasA, confers resistance to isoniazid and ethionamide in *Mycobacterium smegmatis, M. bovis* BCG and *M. tuberculosis. Mol Microbiol.*, **2002**, *46*:453–466.

Levy, L., and Peters, J.H. Susceptibility of *Mycobacterium leprae* to dapsone as a determinant of patient response to acedapsone. *Antimicrob. Agents Chemother.*, **1976**, *9*:102–112.

Lincoln, E.M., and Gilberg, L.A. Disease in children due to mycobacteria other than *Mycobacterium tuberculosis. Am. Rev. Respir. Dis.*, **1972**, *105*:683–714.

Loria, P.R. Minocycline hydrochloride treatment for atypical acid-fast infection. *Arch. Dermatol.*, **1976**, *112*:517–519.

McGlynn, K.A., Lustbader, E.D., Sharrar, R.G., Murphy, E.C., and London, W.T. Isoniazid prophylaxis in hepatitis B carriers. *Am. Rev. Respir. Dis.*, **1986**, *134*:666–668.

Meisel, P. Arylamine *N*-acetyltransferases and drug response. *Pharmacogenomics*, **2002**, *3*:349–366.

Miesel, L., Weisbrod, T., Marcinkeviciene, J.A., *et al*. NADH dehydrogenase defects confer resistance to isoniazid and conditional lethality in *Mycobacterium smegmatis. J. Bacteriol.*, **1998**, *180*:2459–2467.

Miller, R.R., Porter, J., and Greenblatt, D.J. Clinical importance of the interaction of phenytoin and isoniazid: a report from the Boston Collaborative Drug Surveillance Program. *Chest*, **1979**, *75*:356–358.

Morrison, N.E., and Marley, G.M. Clofazimine binding studies with deoxyribonucleic acid. *Int. J. Lepr. Other Mycobact. Dis.*, **1976**, *44*:475–481.

Nightingale, S.D., Cameron, D.W., Gordin, F.M., *et al*. Two controlled trials of rifabutin prophylaxis against *Mycobacterium avium* complex infection in AIDS. *N. Engl. J. Med.*, **1993**, *329*:828–833.

Nolan, C.M., Goldberg, S.V., Buskin, S.E. Hepatotoxicity associated with isoniazid preventive therapy. *JAMA*, **1999**, *281*:1014–1018.

Okafor, M.C. Thalidomide for erythema nodosum leprosum and other applications. *Pharmacotherapy*, **2003**, *23*:481–493.

Pablos-Méndez, A., Raviglione, M.C., Laszlo, A., *et al*. Global surveillance for antituberculosis-drug resistance, 1994–1997. World Health Organization-International Union against Tuberculosis and Lung Disease Working Group on Anti-Tuberculosis Drug Resistance Surveillance. *N. Engl. J. Med.*, **1998**, *338*:1641–1649.

Postlethwaite, A.E., Bartel, A.G., and Kelley, W.N. Hyperuricemia due to ethambutol. *N. Engl. J. Med.*, **1972**, *286*:761–762.

Rapoport, A.M., and Guss, S.B. Dapsone-induced peripheral neuropathy. *Arch. Neurol.*, **1972**, *27*:184–186.

Salpeter, S.R., Sanders, G.D., Salpeter, E.E., and Owens, D.K. Monitored isoniazid prophylaxis for low risk tuberculin reactors older than 35 years of age: a risk-benefit and cost-effectiveness analysis. *Ann. Intern. Med.*, **1997**, *127*:1051–1061.

Sanders, W.E., Jr., Hartwig, E.C., Schneider, N.J., Cacciatore, R., and Valdez, H. Susceptibility of organisms in the *Mycobacterium fortuitum* complex to antituberculous and other antimicrobial agents. *Antimicrob. Agents Chemother.*, **1977**, *12*:295–297.

Sanders, W.E., Jr. Lung infection caused by rapidly growing mycobacteria. *J. Respir. Dis.*, **1982**, *3*:30–38.

Sansarricq, H. Multidrug against leprosy: development and implementation over the past 25 years. World Health Organization, Geneva, **2004**. Available at www.who.int/lep/

Selwyn, P.A., Hortel, D., Lewis, V.A., *et al*. A prospective study of the risk of tuberculosis among intravenous drug users with human immunodeficiency virus infection. *N. Engl. J. Med.*, **1989**, *320*:545–555.

Shafran, S.D., Singer, J., Zarowny, D.P., *et al*. A comparison of two regimens for the treatment of *Mycobacterium avium* complex bacteremia in AIDS: rifabutin, ethambutol, and clarithromycin *versus* rifampin, ethambutol, clofazimine, and ciprofloxacin. Canadian HIV Trials Network Protocol 010 Study Group. *N. Engl. J. Med.*, **1996**, *335*:377–383.

Single Lesion Multicentre Trial Group. Efficacy of single-dose multi-drug therapy for the treatment of single-lesion paucibacillary leprosy. *Lepr. Rev.,* **1997,** *68:*341–349.

Snider, D.E., Jr. Pyridoxine supplementation during isoniazid therapy. *Tubercle,* **1980,** *61:*191–196.

Steel, H.C., Matlola, N.M., and Anderson, R. Inhibition of potassium transport and growth of mycobacteria exposed to clofazimine and B669 is associated with a calcium-independent increase in microbial phospholipase A$_2$ activity. *J. Antimicrob. Chemother.,* **1999,** *44:*209-216.

Tiitinen, H. Isoniazid and ethionamide serum levels and inactivation in Finnish subjects. *Scand. J. Resp. Dis.,* **1969,** *50:*110–124.

U.S. Public Health Service. 1999 USPHS/IDSA guidelines for the prevention of opportunistic infections in persons infected with human immunodeficiency virus. U.S. Public Health Service (USPHS) and Infectious Diseases Society of America (IDSA). *M.M.W.R. Morb. Mortal. Wkly. Rep.,* **1999,** *48:*1–59, 61–66.

Vannelli, T.A., Dykman, A., and Ortiz de Montellano, P.R. The antituberculosis drug ethionamide is activated by a flavoprotein monooxygenase. *J Biol Chem.,* **2002,** *277:*12824–12829.

Vilcheze, C., Morbidoni, H.R., Weisbrod, T.R., *et al.* Inactivation of the *inhA*-encoded fatty acid synthase II (FASII) enoyl-acyl carrier protein reductase induces accumulation of the FASI end products and cell lysis of *Mycobacterium smegmatis. J. Bacteriol.,* **2000,** *182:*4059–4067.

Wallace, R.J., Brown-Elliott, B.A., Ward, S.C., *et al.* Activities of linezolid against rapidly growing mycobacteria. *Antimicrob. Agents Chemother.,* **2001,** *43:*764–767.

Warrington, R.J., Hogg, G.R., Paraskevas, F., and Tse, K.S. Insidious rifampin-associated renal failure with light-chain proteinuria. *Arch. Intern. Med.,* **1977,** *137:*927–930.

Wilkinson, D., Squire, S.B., and Garner, P. Effect of preventive treatment for tuberculosis in adults infected with HIV: systematic review of randomised placebo controlled trials. *Br. Med. J.,* **1998,** *317:*625–629.

World Health Organization Expert Committee on Leprosy. *World Health Organ. Tech. Rep. Ser.,* **1998,** *874:*1–43.

World Health Organization. Leprosy Elimination Project Status Report 2003 (Draft). World Health Organization, Geneva, **2004.** Available at: www.who.int/lep/.

Zimhony, O., Cox, J.S., Welch, J.T., Vilcheze, C., and Jacobs, W.R., Jr. Pyrazinamide inhibits the eukaryotic-like fatty acid synthetase I (FASI) of *Mycobacterium tuberculosis. Nat. Med.,* **2000,** *6:*1043–1047.

MONOGRAPHS AND REVIEWS

American Thoracic Society and Centers for Disease Control. Targeted tuberculin testing and treatment of latent tuberculosis infection. *Am. J. Respir. Crit. Care Med.,* **2000,** *161:*S221–S247.

Barnes, P.F., and Barrows, S.A. Tuberculosis in the 1990s. *Ann. Intern. Med.,* **1993,** *119:*400–410.

Bass, J.B., Jr., Farer, L.S., Hopewell, P.C., *et al.* Treatment of tuberculosis and tuberculosis infections in adults and children. American Thoracic Society and The Centers for Disease Control and Prevention. *Am. J. Respir. Crit. Care Med.,* **1994,** *149:*1359–1374.

Blanchard, J.S. Molecular mechanisms of drug resistance in *Mycobacterium tuberculosis. Annu. Rev. Biochem.,* **1996,** *65:*215–239.

Brown, B.A., and Wallace, R.J., Jr. Infections due to nontuberculous mycobacteria. In, *Mandell, Douglas and Bennett's Principles and Practice of Infectious Diseases,* 5th ed. (Mandell, G.L., Bennett, J.E., and Dolin, R., eds.) Churchill Livingstone, Philadelphia, **2000,** pp. 2630–2636.

Drlicka, K., Lu, T., Malik, M., and Zhoa, X. Fluoroquinolones as antituberculosis agents. In, *Tuberculosis,* 2nd ed. (Rom, W.N., and Gray, S.M., eds.) Lippincott Williams & Wilkins, Philadelphia, **2004,** pp. 791–807.

Farr, B.F. Rifamycins. In, *Mandell, Douglas and Bennett's Principles and Practice of Infectious Diseases,* 5th ed. (Mandell, G.L., Bennett, J.E., and Dolin, R., eds.) Churchill Livingstone, Philadelphia, **2000,** pp. 348–361.

Gallant, J.E., Moore, R.D., and Chaisson, R.E. Prophylaxis for opportunistic infections in patients with HIV infection. *Ann. Intern. Med.,* **1994,** *120:*932–944.

Gelber, R.H., and Rea, T.E. *Mycobacterium leprae* (leprosy, Hansen's disease). In, *Mandell, Douglas and Bennett's Principles and Practice of Infectious Diseases,* 5th ed. (Mandell, G.L., Dolin, R., and Bennett, J.E., eds.) Churchill Livingstone, Philadelphia, **2000,** pp. 2608–2616.

Ginsberg, A.S., Grosset, J.H., and Bishai, W.R. Fluoroquinolones, tuberculosis and resistance. *Lancet Infect. Dis.,* **2003,** *3:*432–442.

Haas, D.W. *Mycobacterium tuberculosis.* In, *Mandell, Douglas and Bennett's Principles and Practice of Infectious Diseases,* 5th ed. (Mandell, G.L., Dolin, R., and Bennett, J.E., eds.) Churchill Livingstone, Philadelphia, **2000,** pp. 2576–2607.

Havlir, D.V., and Barnes, P.F. Tuberculosis in patients with human immunodeficiency virus infection. *N. Engl. J. Med.,* **1999,** *340:*367–373.

Havlir, D.V., and Ellner, J.J. *Mycobacterium avium* complex. In, *Mandell, Douglas and Bennett's Principles and Practice of Infectious Diseases,* 5th ed. (Mandell, C.L., Dolin, R., and Bennett, J.E., eds.) Churchill Livingstone, Philadelphia, **2000,** pp. 2616–2630.

Iseman, M.D. Treatment of multidrug-resistant tuberculosis. *N. Engl. J. Med.,* **1993,** *329:*784–791. [Published erratum in *N. Engl. J. Med.,* **1993,** *329:*1435 (error in Table 4).]

Jacobs, W.R., Jr. *Mycobacterium tuberculosis:* a once genetically intractable organism. In, *Molecular Genetics of Mycobacteria.* (Hatfall, G.F., and Jacobs, W.R., Jr., eds.) ASM Press, Washington, D.C., **2000.**

Lane, H.C., Laughon, B.E., Falloon, J., *et al.* Recent advances in the management of AIDS-related opportunistic infections. *Ann. Intern. Med.,* **1994,** *120:*945–955.

Leibert, W., and Rom, W.N. Principles of tuberculosis management. In, *Tuberculosis,* 2nd ed. (Rom, W.N., and Gray, S.M., eds.) Lippincott, Williams & Wilkins, Philadelphia, **2004,** pp. 713–728.

Vernon, A.A. Rifamycin antibiotics, with a focus on newer agents. In, *Tuberculosis,* 2nd ed. (Rom, W.N., and Gray, S.M., eds.) Lippincott, Williams & Wilkins, Philadelphia, **2004,** pp. 759–771.

Zhang, Y. Isoniazid. In, *Tuberculosis,* 2nd ed. (Rom, W.N., and Gray, S.M., eds.) Lippincott, Williams & Wilkins, Philadelphia, **2004,** pp. 739–758.

ANTIMICROBIAL AGENTS
Antifungal Agents

John E. Bennett

Antifungal agents described in this chapter are discussed under two major headings, systemic and topical, although this distinction is somewhat arbitrary. The imidazole, triazole, and polyene antifungal agents may be used either systemically or topically, while many superficial mycoses can be treated either systemically or topically. Although *Pneumocystis jiroveci*, responsible for life-threatening pneumonia in immunocompromised patients, is a fungus and not a protozoan, its treatment is discussed elsewhere because the drugs used are primarily antibacterial or antiprotozoal rather than antifungal.

The last several decades have produced a remarkable growth in the number of antifungal agents (Table 48–1). Azole antifungal agents have dominated antifungal drug development and clinical use. Although the era of developing new azoles is drawing to a close, use of this class of compounds remains huge because of their broad spectrum, oral bioavailability, and low toxicity.

Another area of antifungal drug development has been lipid formulations of *amphotericin B*. Compared with the original deoxycholate formulation (conventional amphotericin B; C-AMB), the lipid formulations have markedly reduced renal toxicity, with more variable reduction in infusion-related chills and fever. It remains unclear whether any lipid preparation is more effective in any mycosis than the C-AMB preparation given at full dosages.

The most recent class of antifungal drugs to be developed has been the echinocandins, which were reported to have anti-*Candida* activity two decades ago. Limitations of spectrum, lack of oral bioavailability, and difficulty in synthesis of soluble congeners have inhibited development of this class.

Promising preclinical studies have been published with nikkomycins, which inhibit chitin synthesis, and sordarins, natural products that inhibit fungal growth by blocking elongation factor 2 (Herreros *et al.*, 1998). No clinical studies with these agents are in progress. Currently the major pharmaceutical companies have very limited or no programs for development of antifungal drugs, a situation that does not bode well for the future.

SYSTEMIC ANTIFUNGAL AGENTS

Amphotericin B

Chemistry. Amphotericin B is one of a family of some 200 polyene macrolide antibiotics. Those studied to date share the characteristics of four to seven conjugated double bonds, an internal cyclic ester, poor aqueous solubility, substantial toxicity on parenteral administration, and a common mechanism of antifungal action. Amphotericin B (*see* structure below) is a heptaene macrolide containing seven conjugated double bonds in the *trans* position and 3-amino-3,6-dideoxymannose (mycosamine) connected to the main ring by a glycosidic bond. The amphoteric behavior for which the drug is named derives from the presence of a carboxyl group on the main ring and a primary amino group on mycosamine; these groups confer aqueous solubility at extremes of pH. X-ray crystallography has shown the molecule to be rigid and rod-shaped, with the hydrophilic hydroxyl groups of the macrolide ring forming an opposing face to the lipophilic polyenic portion.

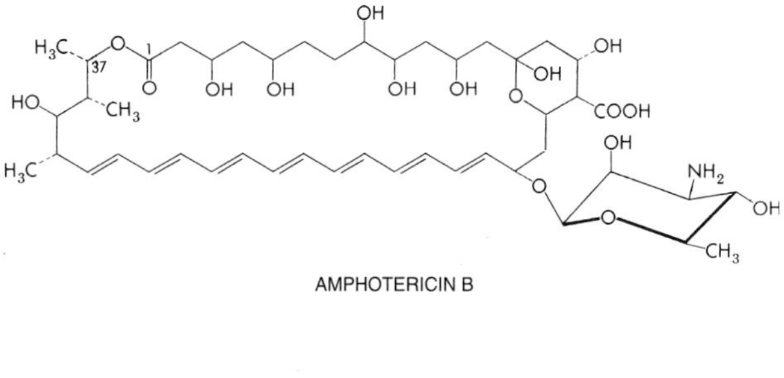

AMPHOTERICIN B

Table 48–1
Treatment of Mycoses

DEEP MYCOSES	DRUGS	SUPERFICIAL MYCOSES	DRUGS
Invasive aspergillosis		***Candidiasis***	
Immunosuppressed	Voriconazole, amphotericin B	*Vulvovaginal*	*Topical* Butoconazole, clotrimazole, miconazole, nystatin, terconazole, tioconazole
Nonimmunosuppressed	Voriconazole, amphotericin B, itraconazole		*Oral* Fluconazole
Blastomycosis		*Oropharyngeal*	*Topical* Clotrimazole, nystatin
Rapidly progressive or CNS	Amphotericin B		
Indolent and non-CNS	Itraconazole		*Oral (systemic)* Fluconazole, itraconazole
Candidiasis		*Cutaneous*	*Topical* Amphotericin B, clotrimazole, ciclopirox, econazole, ketoconazole, miconazole, nystatin
Deeply invasive or esophageal	Amphotericin B, fluconazole, caspofungin		
Coccidioidomycosis			
Rapidly progressing	Amphotericin B		
Indolent	Itraconazole, fluconazole	***Ringworm***	*Topical* Butenafine, ciclopirox, clotrimazole, econazole, haloprogin, ketoconazole, miconazole, naftifine, oxiconazole, sertaconazole, sulconazole, terbinafine, tolnaftate, undecylenate
Meningeal	Fluconazole, intrathecal amphotericin B		
Cryptococcosis			
Non-AIDS and initial AIDS	Amphotericin B, flucytosine		
Maintenance AIDS	Fluconazole		*Systemic* Griseofulvin, itraconazole, terbinafine
Histoplasmosis			
Chronic pulmonary	Itraconazole		
Disseminated			
Rapidly progressing or CNS	Amphotericin B		
Indolent non-CNS	Itraconazole		
Maintenance AIDS	Itraconazole		
Mucormycosis	Amphotericin B		
Pseudallescheriasis	Voriconazole, itraconazole		
Sporotrichosis			
Cutaneous	Itraconazole		
Extracutaneous	Amphotericin B, itraconazole		

Drug Formulations. Amphotericin B is insoluble in water but was formulated for intravenous infusion by complexing it with the bile salt deoxycholate. The complex is marketed as a lyophilized powder (FUNGIZONE) containing 50 mg of amphotericin B, 41 mg of deoxycholate, and a small amount of sodium phosphate buffer. The amphotericin B–deoxycholate complex (C-AMB) forms a colloid in water, with particles largely below 0.4 μm in diameter. Filters in intravenous infusion lines that trap particles above 0.22 μm in diameter will remove significant amounts of drug. Addition of electrolytes to infusion solutions causes the colloid to aggregate.

The amphipathic nature of amphotericin B has made it possible to create lipid formulations for intravenous infusion. Three such formulations of amphotericin B are marketed in the United States. Amphotericin B colloidal dispersion (ABCD, AMPHOTEC, AMPHOCIL) contains roughly equimolar amounts of amphotericin B and cholesteryl sulfate. Like C-AMB, ABCD forms a colloidal solution when dispersed in aqueous solution. In aqueous solution, ABCD particles are disk-shaped; they are 115 nm wide by 4 nm thick. ABCD provides much lower blood levels than C-AMB in mice and human beings. In mice, 41% to 80% of 14 daily doses can be recovered in the liver. In a randomized, double-blind study in patients with neutropenic fever comparing daily ABCD (4 mg/kg) with C-AMB (0.8 mg/kg), chills and hypoxia were significantly more common with ABCD (79.8% and 12%, respectively) than with C-AMB (65.4% and 2.9%), requiring withdrawal of 4.6% of the study patients receiving ABCD, compared with only 0.9% of those receiving C-AMB (White *et al.*, 1998). Hypoxia was associated with severe febrile reactions. In a randomized, double-blind comparison of ABCD (6 mg/kg) and C-AMB (1 to 1.5 mg/kg) in invasive aspergillosis patients, the 95% confidence limits on the difference in efficacy between the two drugs was within 20% (Bowden *et al.*, 2002). ABCD was less nephrotoxic than C-AMB (49% *vs.* 15%) but caused more fever (27% *vs.* 16%) and chills (53% *vs.* 30%). Administration of the recommended ABCD dose over 3 to 4 hours and use of premedication to reduce febrile reactions are advised, particularly with initial infusions. ABCD is approved only for patients with invasive aspergillosis who are not responding to or are unable to tolerate C-AMB.

A small, unilamellar vesicle formulation of amphotericin B (AMBISOME) also is available. Amphotericin B (50 mg) is combined with 350 mg of lipid in an approximately 10% molar ratio. The lipid contains hydrogenated soy lecithin (phosphatidylcholine), cholesterol, and distearoylphosphatidylglycerol in a 10:5:4 molar ratio. The drug is supplied as a lyophilized powder, which is reconstituted with sterile water for injection. With complete dispersion, particle size is about 80 nm. Blood levels following intravenous infusion are almost equivalent to those obtained with C-AMB, and because AMBISOME can be given at higher doses, blood levels have been achieved that exceed those obtained with C-AMB. Amphotericin B accumulation in the liver and spleen is higher with AMBISOME than with C-AMB. In a series of 23 patients receiving 3 mg/kg daily for an average of 27 days, the average serum creatinine rise was 34%, with nephrotoxicity requiring dose reduction in only one patient (Coker *et al.*, 1993). Adverse effects include nephrotoxicity, hypokalemia, and infusion-related reactions, such as fever, chills, hypoxia, hypotension, and hypertension, but these uncommonly lead to drug discontinuation. Infusion-related pain in the back, abdomen, or chest occurs in occasional patients, usually with the first few doses. Anaphylaxis also has been reported. Most of the information about the efficacy of AMBISOME comes from open studies that make comparisons difficult. Blinded, randomized trials of C-AMB and AMBISOME as empirical therapy or prophylaxis in febrile neutropenic patients have found equivalent results, but these studies cast no light on efficacy in established infections. Studies comparing AMBISOME with C-AMB for disseminated histoplasmosis or cryptococcal meningitis in AIDS patients, using either drug as a short course followed by prolonged azole therapy, have not yet established efficacy against those mycoses. AMBISOME is approved for empiric therapy of fever in the neutropenic host not responding to appropriate antibacterial agents, as well as for salvage therapy of aspergillosis, cryptococcosis, and candidiasis. The recommended daily intravenous dose for empiric therapy is 3 mg/kg; for treatment of mycoses, the dosage is 3 to 5 mg/kg. AMBISOME also is effective in visceral leishmaniasis at doses of 3 to 4 mg/kg daily. The drug is administered in 5% dextrose in water, with initial doses being infused over 2 hours. If well tolerated, infusion duration can be shortened to 1 hour. Doses of 7.5 to 10 mg/kg have been used in small numbers of patients but are associated with a higher rate of azotemia and hypokalemia.

The third lipid formulation is amphotericin B lipid complex (ABLC, ABELCET). This preparation of dimyristoylphosphatidylcholine and dimyristoylphosphatidylglycerol in a 7:3 mixture with

approximately 35 mol% amphotericin B forms ribbonlike sheets that range in size from 1.6 to 11 μm. Blood levels of amphotericin B are much lower with ABLC than with the same dose of C-AMB. In open, noncomparative trials, ABLC has seemed to be effective in a variety of mycoses, with the possible exception of cryptococcal meningitis (Sharkey *et al.*, 1996). ABLC is given in a dose of 5 mg/kg in 5% dextrose in water, infused once daily over 2 hours. The drug is approved for salvage therapy of deep mycoses.

The cost of the lipid formulations of amphotericin B is 20 to 50 times that of C-AMB, raising formidable cost-benefit issues. A systematic review of the literature concluded that the three lipid formulations collectively reduced the risk of the patient's serum creatinine doubling during therapy by 58% (Barrett *et al.*, 2003). In patients at high risk for nephrotoxicity, ABLC is more nephrotoxic than AMBISOME (Wingard *et al.*, 2000). In some patients, the additive burden of amphotericin B nephrotoxicity can help precipitate advanced renal failure, with attendant morbidity and financial burden. Infusion-related reactions are not consistently reduced with the use of lipid preparations. ABCD causes more infusion-related reactions than C-AMB. Although AMBISOME reportedly causes fewer infusion-related reactions than ABLC during the first dose (Wingard *et al.*, 2000), the difference depends on whether premedication is given and varies considerably between patients. Infusion-related reactions typically decrease with subsequent infusions.

Antifungal Activity. Amphotericin B has useful clinical activity against *Candida* spp., *Cryptococcus neoformans, Blastomyces dermatitidis, Histoplasma capsulatum, Sporothrix schenckii, Coccidioides immitis, Paracoccidioides braziliensis, Aspergillus* spp., *Penicillium marneffei,* and the agents of mucormycosis.

Amphotericin B has limited activity against the protozoa *Leishmania braziliensis* and *Naegleria fowleri.* The drug has no antibacterial activity.

Mechanism of Action. The antifungal activity of amphotericin B depends principally on its binding to a sterol moiety, primarily ergosterol that is present in the membrane of sensitive fungi. By virtue of their interaction with these sterols, polyenes appear to form pores or channels that increase the permeability of the membrane, allowing leakage of a variety of small molecules (Figure 48–1).

Fungal Resistance. Some isolates of *Candida lusitaniae* have appeared to be relatively resistant to amphotericin B. *Aspergillus terreus* may be more resistant to amphotericin B than other *Aspergillus* species, although the host's immune response is the most significant factor in determining outcome in invasive aspergillosis (Steinbach *et al.*, 2004). Mutants selected *in vitro* for nystatin or amphotericin B resistance replace ergosterol with certain precursor sterols. The rarity of significant amphotericin B resistance arising during therapy has left it unclear whether ergosterol-deficient mutants retain sufficient pathogenicity to survive in deep tissue.

Absorption, Distribution, and Excretion. Gastrointestinal absorption of all amphotericin B formulations is negligible. Repeated daily intravenous infusions to adults of 0.5 mg/kg of C-AMB result in concentrations in plasma of about 1 to 1.5 μg/ml at the end of the infusion; these concentrations fall to about 0.5 to 1 μg/ml within 24 hours. The drug is released from its complex with deoxycholate

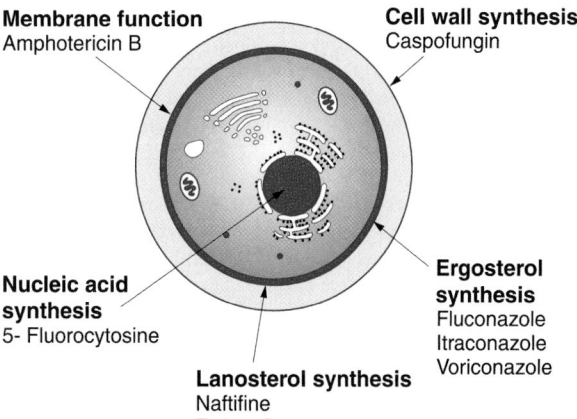

Figure 48–1. *Mechanism of action of amphotericin, imidazoles, triazoles, and allylamines in fungi.* Amphotericin B and other polyenes, such as nystatin, bind to ergosterol in fungal cell membranes and increase membrane permeability. The imidazoles and triazoles, such as itraconazole and fluconazole, inhibit 14-α-sterol demethylase, prevent ergosterol synthesis, and lead to the accumulation of 14-α-methylsterols. The allylamines, such as naftifine and terbinafine, inhibit squalene epoxidase and prevent ergosterol synthesis. The echinocandins, such as caspofungin, inhibit the formation of glucans in the fungal cell wall.

in the bloodstream, and the amphotericin B that remains in plasma is more than 90% bound to proteins, largely β-lipoprotein. Approximately 2% to 5% of each dose appears in the urine when patients are on daily therapy. Drug elimination apparently is unchanged in anephric patients and in patients receiving hemodialysis. Hepatic or biliary disease has no known effect on metabolism of the drug in humans. At least one-third of an injected dose can be recovered unchanged by methanolic extraction of tissue at autopsy; the highest concentrations are found in liver and spleen, with lesser amounts in kidney and lung. Concentrations of amphotericin B (C-AMB) in fluids from inflamed pleura, peritoneum, synovium, and aqueous humor are approximately two-thirds of trough concentrations in plasma. Little amphotericin B penetrates into cerebrospinal fluid (CSF), vitreous humor, or normal amniotic fluid. Because of extensive binding to tissues, there is a terminal phase of elimination with a half-life of about 15 days.

Therapeutic Uses. The usual therapeutic dose of C-AMB is 0.5 to 0.6 mg/kg, administered in 5% glucose over 4 hours. *Candida* esophagitis in adults responds to 0.15 to 0.2 mg/kg daily. Rapidly progressive mucormycosis or invasive aspergillosis is treated with doses of 1 to 1.2 mg/kg daily until progression is arrested. Double-dose alternate-day therapy may be more convenient but is not less toxic and therefore is rarely indicated.

Intrathecal infusion of amphotericin B C-AMB is useful in patients with meningitis caused by *Coccidioides*. The drug can be injected into the CSF of the lumbar spine, cisterna magna, or lateral cerebral ventricle. Regardless of the injection site, treatment is initiated with 0.05 to 0.1 mg and increased on a three-times-weekly schedule to 0.5 mg, as tolerated. Therapy is then continued on a twice-weekly schedule. Fever and headache are common reactions that may be decreased by intrathecal administration of 10 to 15 mg of hydrocortisone. Other less common but more serious problems that attend the use of intrathecal injections depend at least partially on the injection site. Local injections of amphotericin B into a joint or peritoneal dialysate fluid commonly produce irritation and pain. Intraocular injection following pars plana vitrectomy has been used successfully for fungal endophthalmitis.

Intravenous administration of amphotericin B is the treatment of choice for mucormycosis and is used for initial treatment of cryptococcal meningitis, severe or rapidly progressing histoplasmosis, blastomycosis, coccidioidomycosis, and penicilliosis marneffei, as well as in patients not responding to azole therapy of invasive aspergillosis, extracutaneous sporotrichosis, fusariosis, alternariosis, and trichosporonosis. Amphotericin B (C-AMB or AMBISOME) is often given to selected patients with profound neutropenia who have fever that does not respond to broad-spectrum antibacterial agents over 5 to 7 days. Amphotericin B given once weekly has been used to prevent relapse in patients with AIDS who have been treated successfully for cryptococcosis or histoplasmosis.

Bladder irrigation with 50 μg/ml of amphotericin B in sterile water is effective for *Candida* cystitis. Relapse is common if the catheter remains in the bladder or there is significant postvoiding residual urine. Inhalational administration of amphotericin B has not been successful in treatment of pulmonary mycoses. Topical amphotericin B is useful only in cutaneous candidiasis (*see* below).

Untoward Effects. The major acute reaction to intravenous amphotericin B formulations is fever and chills. Tachypnea and respiratory stridor or modest hypotension also may occur, but true bronchospasm or anaphylaxis is rare. Patients with preexisting cardiac or pulmonary disease may tolerate the metabolic demands of the reaction poorly and develop hypoxia or hypotension. Although the reaction ends spontaneously in 30 to 45 minutes, meperidine may shorten it. Pretreatment with oral acetaminophen or use of intravenous hydrocortisone hemisuccinate, 0.7 mg/kg, at the start of the infusion decreases reactions. Febrile reactions abate with subsequent infusions. Infants, children, and patients receiving therapeutic doses of glucocorticoids are less prone to reactions.

Azotemia occurs in 80% of patients who receive C-AMB for deep mycoses (Carlson and Condon, 1994). Toxicity is dose-dependent and transient and is increased by concurrent therapy with other nephrotoxic agents, such as aminoglycosides or cyclosporine. Although permanent histological changes in renal tubules occur even during short courses of C-AMB, permanent functional impairment is uncommon in adults with normal renal function prior to treatment unless the cumulative dose exceeds 3 to 4 g. Renal tubular acidosis and renal wasting of K^+ and Mg^{2+} also may be seen during and for several weeks after therapy. Supplemental K^+ is required in one-third of patients on prolonged therapy. An increase in intrarenal vascular resistance is the major cause of nephrotoxicity in amphotericin B–treated rats. In patients and experimental animals, saline loading has decreased nephrotoxicity, even in the absence of water or salt deprivation. Administration of 1 L of normal saline intravenously on the day that C-AMB is to be given has been recommended for adults who are able to tolerate the Na⁺ load and who are not already receiving that amount in intravenous fluids. Azotemia occurs much less frequently with lipid preparations of amphotericin, and saline loading is not recommended.

Hypochromic, normocytic anemia is usual with C-AMB; the average hematocrit declined to 27% in one study. Decreased production of erythropoietin is the probable mechanism. Patients with low plasma erythropoietin may respond to administration of recombinant erythropoietin. Anemia reverses slowly following cessation of therapy. Headache, nausea, vomiting, malaise, weight loss, and phlebitis at peripheral infusion sites are common side effects. Thrombocytopenia or mild leukopenia is observed rarely. Hepatotoxicity is not firmly established with any amphotericin B formulation. Arachnoiditis has been observed as a complication of injection C-AMB into the CSF.

Flucytosine

Chemistry. *Flucytosine* is a fluorinated pyrimidine related to *fluorouracil* and *floxuridine*. It is 5-fluorocytosine, the formula of which is as follows:

FLUCYTOSINE

Antifungal Activity. Flucytosine has clinically useful activity against *Cryptococcus neoformans*, *Candida* spp., and the agents of chromoblastomycosis. Within these species, determination of susceptibility *in vitro* has been extremely dependent on the method employed, and susceptibility testing performed on isolates obtained prior to treatment has not correlated with clinical outcome.

Mechanism of Action. All susceptible fungi are capable of deaminating flucytosine to 5-fluorouracil, a potent antimetabolite that is used in cancer chemotherapy (Figure 48–2) (*see* Chapter 51). Fluorouracil is metabolized first to 5-fluorouracil-ribose monophosphate (5-FUMP) by the enzyme uracil phosphoribosyl transferase (UPRTase, also called uridine monophosphate pyrophosphorylase). As in mammalian cells, 5-FUMP then is either incorporated into RNA (*via* synthesis of 5-fluorouridine triphosphate) or metabolized to 5-fluoro-2'-deoxyuridine-5'-monophosphate (5-FdUMP), a potent inhibitor of thymidylate synthetase. DNA synthesis is impaired as the ultimate result of this latter reaction. The selective action of flucytosine is due to the lack or low levels of cytosine deaminase in mammalian cells, which prevents metabolism to fluorouracil.

Fungal Resistance. Drug resistance arising during therapy (secondary resistance) is an important cause of therapeutic failure when flucytosine is used alone for cryptococcosis and candidiasis. In chromoblastomycosis, resurgence of lesions after an initial response has led to the presumption of secondary drug resistance. In isolates of *Cryptococcus* and *Candida* species, secondary drug resistance has been accompanied by a change in the minimal inhibitory concentration from less than 2.5 μg/ml to more than 360 μg/ml. The

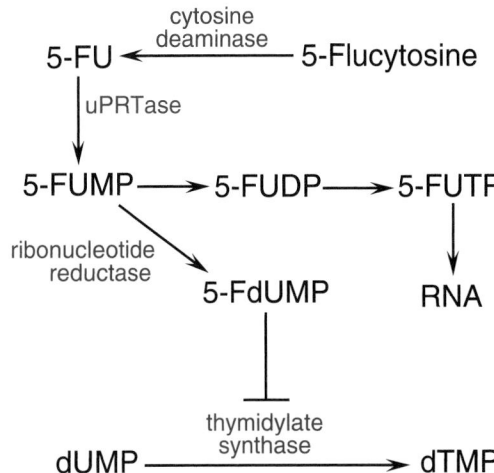

Figure 48–2. *Action of flucytosine in fungi.* 5-Flucytosine is transported by cytosine permease into the fungal cell, where it is deaminated to 5-fluorouracil (5-FU). The 5-FU is then converted to 5-fluorouracil-ribose monophosphate (5-FUMP) and then is either converted to 5-fluorouridine triphosphate (5-FUTP) and incorporated into RNA or converted by ribonucleotide reductase to 5-fluoro-2'-deoxyuridine-5'-monophosphate (5-FdUMP), which is a potent inhibitor of thymidylate synthase. 5-FUDP, 5-fluorouridine-5'-diphosphate; dUMP, deoxyuridine-5'-monophosphate; dTMP, deoxyuridine-5'-monophosphate.

mechanism for this resistance can be loss of the permease necessary for cytosine transport or decreased activity of either UPRTase or cytosine deaminase (Figure 48–2). In *Candida albicans*, substitution of thymine for cytosine at nucleotide 301 in the gene encoding UPRTase (*FUR1*) causes a cysteine to become an arginine, modestly increasing flucytosine resistance (Dodgson *et al.*, 2004). Flucytosine resistance is further increased if both *FUR1* alleles in the diploid fungus are mutated. This specific mutation has been found only in a group of genetically related isolates called "Clade 1," and its clinical significance is unknown.

Absorption, Distribution, and Excretion. Flucytosine is absorbed rapidly and well from the gastrointestinal tract. It is widely distributed in the body, with a volume of distribution that approximates total body water, and is minimally bound to plasma proteins. The peak plasma concentration in patients with normal renal function is approximately 70 to 80 μg/ml, achieved 1 to 2 hours after a dose of 37.5 mg/kg. Approximately 80% of a given dose is excreted unchanged in the urine; concentrations in the urine range from 200 to 500 μg/ml. The half-life of the drug is 3 to 6 hours in normal individuals. In renal failure, the half-life may be as long as 200 hours. The clearance of flucytosine is approximately equivalent to that of creatinine. Because of its obligate renal excretion, modification of dosage is necessary in patients with decreased renal function, and concentrations of drug in plasma should be measured periodically. Peak concentrations should range between 50 and 100 μg/ml. Flucytosine is cleared by hemodialysis, and patients undergoing such treatment should receive a single dose of 37.5 mg/kg after dialysis; the drug also is removed by peritoneal dialysis.

Flucytosine concentration in CSF is about 65% to 90% of that found simultaneously in the plasma. The drug also appears to penetrate into the aqueous humor.

Therapeutic Uses. Flucytosine (ANCOBON) is given orally at 100 mg/kg per day, in four divided doses at 6-hour intervals. Dosage must be adjusted for decreased renal function. Flucytosine is used predominantly in combination with amphotericin B. Flucytosine caused no added toxicity when added to 0.7 mg/kg of amphotericin B for the initial 2 weeks of therapy of cryptococcal meningitis in AIDS patients. Although the CSF colony count diminished more rapidly with combination therapy, there was no apparent impact on mortality or morbidity (van der Horst *et al.*, 1997; Brouwer *et al.*, 2004). An all-oral regimen of flucytosine plus *fluconazole* also has been advocated for therapy of AIDS patients with cryptococcosis, but the combination has substantial gastrointestinal toxicity with no evidence that flucytosine adds benefit to the regimen (Larsen *et al.*, 1994). In cryptococcal meningitis of non-AIDS patients, the role of flucytosine is more conjectural. The addition of flucytosine to 6 weeks or more of therapy with C-AMB runs the risk of substantial bone marrow suppression or colitis if the flucytosine dose is not promptly adjusted downward as amphotericin B–induced azotemia occurs. It is now common practice in HIV-negative patients with cryptococcal meningitis is to begin with C-AMB or AMBISOME plus flucytosine and change to fluconazole after the patient has improved (Pappas *et al.*, 2001). Prospective study of this regimen is needed in HIV-negative patients, where the goal is cure and not just suppression of symptoms.

Untoward Effects. Flucytosine may depress the bone marrow and lead to leukopenia and thrombocytopenia; patients are more prone to this complication if they have an underlying hematological disorder, are being treated with radiation or drugs that injure the bone marrow, or have a history of treatment with such agents. Other untoward effects—including rash, nausea, vomiting, diarrhea, and severe enterocolitis—have been noted. In approximately 5% of patients, plasma levels of hepatic enzymes are elevated, but this effect reverses when therapy is stopped. Toxicity is more frequent in patients with AIDS or azotemia (including those who are receiving amphotericin B concurrently) and when plasma drug concentrations exceed 100 μg/ml. Toxicity may result from conversion of flucytosine to 5-fluorouracil by the microbial flora in the intestinal tract of the host.

Imidazoles and Triazoles

The azole antifungals include two broad classes, imidazoles and triazoles, which share the same antifungal spectrum and mechanism of action. The systemic triazoles are metabolized more slowly and have less effect on human sterol synthesis than do the imidazoles. Because of these advantages, new congeners under development are mostly triazoles. Of the drugs now on the market in the United States, *clotrimazole, miconazole, ketoconazole, econazole, buto-*

conazole, oxiconazole, sertaconazole, and *sulconazole* are imidazoles; *terconazole, itraconazole,* fluconazole, *voriconazole,* and *posaconazole* (an experimental drug) are triazoles. The topical use of azole antifungals is described in the second section of this chapter. The structure of a triazole is as follows:

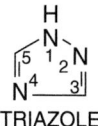

TRIAZOLE

Antifungal Activity. Azoles as a group have clinically useful activity against *Candida albicans, Candida tropicalis, Candida parapsilosis, Candida glabrata, Cryptococcus neoformans, Blastomyces dermatitidis, Histoplasma capsulatum, Coccidioides* species, *Paracoccidioides brasiliensis,* and ringworm fungi (dermatophytes). *Aspergillus* spp., *Scedosporium apiospermum* (*Pseudallescheria boydii*), *Fusarium,* and *Sporothrix schenckii* are intermediate in susceptibility. *Candida krusei* and the agents of mucormycosis are resistant. Thus, these drugs do not have any useful antibacterial or antiparasitic activity, with the possible exception of antiprotozoal effects against *Leishmania major* and the investigational azole, posaconazole, which has some *in vitro* activity against mucormycosis.

Mechanism of Action. At concentrations achieved following systemic administration, the major effect of imidazoles and triazoles on fungi is inhibition of 14-α-sterol demethylase, a microsomal cytochrome P450 (CYP) enzyme (Figure 48–1). Imidazoles and triazoles thus impair the biosynthesis of ergosterol for the cytoplasmic membrane and lead to the accumulation of 14-α-methylsterols. These methylsterols may disrupt the close packing of acyl chains of phospholipids, impairing the functions of certain membrane-bound enzyme systems such as ATPase and enzymes of the electron transport system and thus inhibiting growth of the fungi.

Some azoles (*e.g.,* clotrimazole) directly increase permeability of the fungal cytoplasmic membrane, but the concentrations required are likely only obtained with topical use.

Azole resistance has emerged gradually during prolonged azole therapy, causing clinical failure in patients with far-advanced HIV infection and oropharyngeal or esophageal candidiasis. The primary mechanism of resistance in *C. albicans* is accumulation of mutations in *ERG11*, the gene coding for the 14-α-sterol demethylase. These mutations protect heme in the enzyme pocket from binding to the azole, but allow access of the natural substrate for the enzyme, lanosterol. Cross resistance is conferred to all azoles. Increased azole efflux by both ATP-binding cassette (ABC) and major facilitator superfamily transporters can add to fluconazole resistance in

C. albicans and *C. glabrata.* Increased production of 14-α-sterol demethylase is another potential cause of resistance. Mutation of the C5,6 sterol reductase gene *ERG3* also can increase azole resistance in some species.

Ketoconazole

Ketoconazole, administered orally, has been replaced by itraconazole for the treatment of all mycoses except when the lower cost of ketoconazole outweighs the advantage of itraconazole. Itraconazole lacks ketoconazole's corticosteroid suppression, while retaining most of ketoconazole's pharmacological properties and expanding the antifungal spectrum. Ketoconazole sometimes is used to inhibit excessive production of glucocorticoids in patients with Cushing's syndrome (*see* Chapter 59).

Itraconazole

This synthetic triazole is an equimolar racemic mixture of four diastereoisomers (two enantiomeric pairs), each possessing three chiral centers. The structural formula, which is shown below, is closely related to the imidazole ketoconazole:

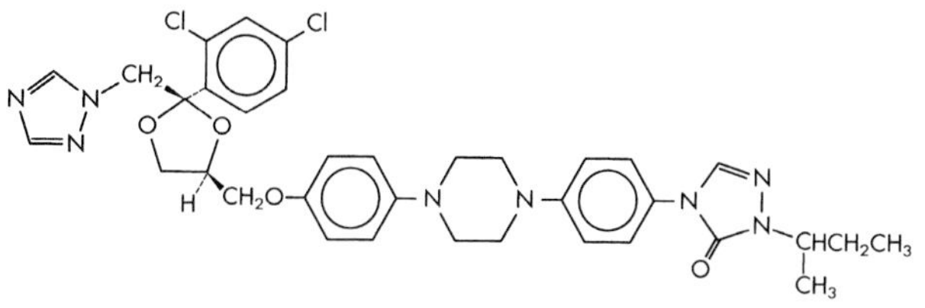

ITRACONAZOLE

Absorption, Distribution, and Excretion. Itraconazole (SPORONOX) is available as a capsule and two solution formulations, one for oral and one for intravenous administration. The capsule form of the drug is best absorbed in the fed state, but the oral solution is better absorbed in the fasting state, providing peak plasma concentrations that are more than 150% of those obtained with the capsule. Both the oral solution and intravenous formulation are solubilized in a 40:1 weight ratio of itraconazole hydroxypropyl-β-cyclodextrin, so that administration of 200 mg of itraconazole provides 8 g of this excipient. Itraconazole is metabolized in the liver. It is both a substrate for and a potent inhibitor of CYP3A4. Itraconazole is present in plasma with an approximately equal concentration of a biologically active metabolite, hydroxy-itraconazole. Bioassays may report up to 3.3 times as much itraconazole in plasma as do physical methods such as high-performance liquid chromatography, depending on the susceptibility of

the bioassay organism to hydroxy-itraconazole. The native drug and metabolite are >99% bound to plasma proteins. Neither appears in urine or CSF. The half-life of itraconazole at steady state is approximately 30 to 40 hours. Steady-state levels of itraconazole are not reached for 4 days and those of hydroxy-itraconazole for 7 days; thus, loading doses are recommended when treating deep mycoses. Severe liver disease will increase itraconazole plasma concentrations, but azotemia and hemodialysis have no effect. Some 80% to 90% of intravenously administered hydroxypropyl-β-cyclodextrin is excreted in the urine, and the compound accumulates in the presence of azotemia. Intravenous administration of itraconazole is contraindicated in patients with a creatinine clearance below 30 ml/min because of concern about potential hydroxypropyl-β-cyclodextrin toxicity. Itraconazole is not carcinogenic but is teratogenic in rats, and is contraindicated for the treatment of onychomycosis during pregnancy or for women contemplating pregnancy (category C).

Drug Interactions. Table 48–2 lists known interactions of itraconazole with other drugs, a list that is still expanding. Many of the interactions can result in serious toxicity from the companion drug, inducing potentially fatal cardiac arrhythmias when used with *quinidine* or *cisapride* (only available under a restricted program in the United States). Other interactions may decrease itraconazole concentrations below therapeutic levels.

Therapeutic Uses. Itraconazole given as a capsule is the drug of choice for patients with indolent, nonmeningeal infections due to *B. dermatitidis, H. capsulatum, P. brasiliensis,* and *C. immitis.* This dosage form also is useful in therapy of indolent invasive aspergillosis outside the CNS, particularly after the infection has been stabilized with amphotericin B. The intravenous formulation is approved for the initial 2 weeks of therapy with blastomycosis, histoplasmosis, and indolent aspergillosis, and for empirical therapy of febrile neutropenic patients not responding to antibacterial antibiotics and at high risk of fungal infections. The intravenous route would be most appropriate for patients unable to tolerate the oral formulation or unable to absorb itraconazole because of decreased gastric acid production. Approximately half the patients with distal subungual onychomycosis respond to itraconazole (Evans and Sigurgeirsson, 1999). Although not an approved use, itraconazole is a reasonable choice for treatment of pseudallescheriasis, an infection not responding to amphotericin B therapy, as well as cutaneous and extracutaneous sporotrichosis, tinea corporis, and extensive tinea versicolor. HIV-infected patients with disseminated histoplasmosis or *Penicillium marneffei* infections have a decreased incidence of relapse if given prolonged itraconazole "maintenance" therapy. It is as yet unclear whether patients responding to highly active antiretroviral therapy (HAART) will require less than lifelong therapy for *P. marneffei* and disseminated histoplasmosis (*see* Chapter 50). Itraconazole is not recommended for maintenance therapy of cryptococcal meningitis in HIV-infected patients because of a high incidence of relapse. Long-term therapy has been used in non-HIV–infected patients with allergic bronchopulmonary aspergillosis to decrease the dose of glucocorticoids and reduce attacks of acute bronchospasm (Salez *et al.,* 1999).

Table 48–2
Interactions of Itraconazole with Other Drugs

OTHER DRUG CONCENTRATION INCREASED	ITRACONAZOLE CONCENTRATION DECREASED
Alfentanil	Drugs that decrease gastric
Alprazolam	acidity
Amprenavir	H_2-receptor blockers
Atorvastatin	Proton pump blockers
Buspirone	Simultaneous antacids
Busulfan	(includes didanosine
Cerivastatin	buffer)
Cisapride	Carbamazepine
Cyclophosphamide	Isoniazid
Cyclosporine	Nevirapine
Delavirdine	Phenobarbital
Diazepam	Phenytoin
Digoxin	Rifampin, rifabutin
Dihydropyridine Ca^{2+}	St. John's wort
channel blockers	
Docetaxel	**ITRACONAZOLE**
Felodipine	**CONCENTRATION INCREASED**
Haloperidol	
Indinavir	Amprenavir
Loratidine	Clarithromycin
Lovastatin	Grapefruit juice
Methylprednisolone	Indinavir
Midazolam	Lopinavir
Nisoldipine	Ritonavir
Phenytoin	
Pimozide	
Quinidine	
Ritonavir	
Saquinavir	
Sildenafil	
Simvastatin	
Sirolimus	
Sulfonylureas (gly-	
buride, others)	
Tacrolimus	
Terfenadine	
Trimetrexate	
Triazolam	
Verapamil	
Vinca alkaloids (vin-	
cristine, vinblastine)	
Warfarin	

Itraconazole solution is effective and approved for use in oropharyngeal and esophageal candidiasis. Because the oral solution preparation has more gastrointestinal side effects than do fluconazole tablets, itraconazole solution usually is reserved for patients not responding to fluconazole who are not receiving protease inhibitors or other drugs that make itraconazole contraindicated. Itraconazole capsules and oral solution are not bioequivalent and should not be used interchangeably.

Untoward Effects. Adverse effects of itraconazole therapy can occur as a result of interactions with many other drugs (Table 48–2). Serious hepatotoxicity has rarely led to hepatic failure and death. If symptoms of hepatotoxicity occur, the drug should be discontinued and liver function assessed. Itraconazole causes a dose-dependent inotropic effect that can lead to congestive heart failure in patients with impaired ventricular function. In the absence of interacting drugs, itraconazole capsules are well tolerated at 200 mg daily. Gastrointestinal distress occasionally prevents use of 400 mg per day. In one series of patients receiving 50 to 400 mg per day, nausea and vomiting were recorded in 10%, hypertriglyceridemia in 9%, hypokalemia in 6%, increased serum aminotransferase in 5%, rash in 2%, and at least one side effect in 39%. Occasionally, rash necessitates drug discontinuation, but most adverse effects can be handled with dose reduction. Profound hypokalemia has been seen in patients receiving 600 mg or more daily and in those who recently have received prolonged amphotericin B therapy. Doses of 300 mg twice daily have led to other side effects, including adrenal insufficiency, lower limb edema, hypertension, and in at least one case, rhabdomyolysis. Doses above 400 mg per day are not recommended for long-term use.

Intravenous itraconazole has all the adverse effects of capsules but generally is well tolerated, except for chemical phlebitis. A dedicated catheter port is required, and infusion durations less than 1 hour are not recommended. Toxicity from high plasma levels of hydroxypropyl-β-cyclodextrin in azotemic patients has not been reported, but pending further studies, the intravenous formulation is contraindicated in patients with a creatinine clearance below 30 ml/min.

The oral solution of itraconazole is well tolerated but has all the adverse effects of itraconazole capsules. Anaphylaxis has been observed rarely, as well as severe rash, including Stevens-Johnson syndrome. Some patients complain of the taste, and gastrointestinal side effects are common, although adherence is generally unimpaired. Diarrhea, abdominal cramps, anorexia, and nausea are more common than with the capsules.

Dosage. In treating deep mycoses, a loading dose of 200 mg of itraconazole is administered three times daily for the first 3 days. For maintenance therapy, two 100-mg capsules are given twice daily with food. The divided doses are alleged to increase the area under the plasma concentration *versus* time curve (AUC), even though the half-life is about 30 hours. For maintenance therapy of HIV-infected patients with disseminated histoplasmosis, 200 mg once daily is used. Onychomycosis can be treated with either 200 mg once daily for 12 weeks or 200 mg twice daily for 1 week out of each month—so-called pulse therapy (Evans and Sigurgeirsson, 1999). Retention of active drug in the nail keratin permits intermittent treatment. Daily therapy is preferred by some authorities for infections likely to be more refractory, but costs twice as much as pulse therapy. Once-daily *terbinafine* (250 mg), however, is slightly superior to pulse therapy with itraconazole (*see* below). A loading dose of itraconazole is given as a 200-mg intravenous infusion over 1 hour twice daily for 2 days, followed by 200 mg once daily for 12 days. Itraconazole oral solution should be taken fasting in a dose of 100 mg (10 ml) once daily and swished vigorously in the mouth before swallowing to optimize any topical effect. Patients with oropharyngeal or esophageal thrush are given 100 mg of the solution twice a day for 2 to 4 weeks.

Fluconazole

Fluconazole is a fluorinated bistriazole. Its structure is as follows:

FLUCONAZOLE

Absorption, Distribution, and Excretion. Fluconazole is almost completely absorbed from the gastrointestinal tract. Plasma concentrations are essentially the same whether the drug is given orally or intravenously, and its bioavailability is unaltered by food or gastric acidity. Peak plasma concentrations are 4 to 8 μg/ml after repetitive doses of 100 mg. Renal excretion accounts for over 90% of elimination, and the elimination half-time is 25 to 30 hours. Fluconazole diffuses readily into body fluids, including breast milk, sputum, and saliva; concentrations in CSF can reach 50% to 90% of the simultaneous values in plasma. The dosage interval should be increased from 24 to 48 hours with a creatinine clearance of 21 to 40 ml/min and to 72 hours at 10 to 20 ml/min. A dose of 100 to 200 mg should be given after each hemodialysis. About 11% to 12% of drug in the plasma is protein bound.

Drug Interactions. Fluconazole is an inhibitor of CYP3A4 and CYP2C9. Fluconazole significantly increases plasma concentrations of *amprenavir*, cisapride, *cyclosporine, phenytoin,* sulfonylureas (*glipizide, tolbutamide,* others), *tacrolimus, theophylline, telithromycin,* and *warfarin.* Patients who receive more than 400 mg daily or azotemic patients who have elevated fluconazole blood levels may experience drug interactions not otherwise seen. Rifampin decreases the fluconazole AUC by about 25%, which ordinarily would not be significant. Drugs that decrease gastric acidity do not significantly lower fluconazole blood levels.

Therapeutic Uses. *Candidiasis.* Fluconazole, 200 mg on the first day and then 100 mg daily for at least 2 weeks, is effective in oropharyngeal candidiasis. Esophageal candidiasis responds to 100 to 200 mg daily, and this dose also has been used to decrease candiduria in high-risk patients. A single dose of 150 mg is effective in uncomplicated vaginal candidiasis. A dose of 400 mg daily decreases the incidence of deep candidiasis in allogeneic bone marrow transplant recipients and is useful in treating candidemia of nonimmunosuppressed patients. Fluconazole is not proven to be effective treatment for deep candidiasis in profoundly neutropenic patients. In patients who have not been receiving fluconazole prophylaxis, the drug has been used successfully as empirical treatment of febrile neutropenia in patients not responding to antibacterial agents and who are not judged to be at high risk of fungal infections. Based on resistance *in vitro, Candida krusei* would not be expected to respond to fluconazole or other azoles.

Cryptococcosis. Fluconazole, 400 mg daily, is used for the initial 8 weeks in the treatment of cryptococcal meningitis in patients with AIDS after the patient's clinical condition has been stabilized with intravenous amphotericin B. After 8 weeks, the dose is decreased to 200 mg daily and continued indefinitely. If the patient responds to HAART, has a CD4 count maintained above 100 to 200/mm^3 for at least 6 months, and is asymptomatic from cryptococcal meningitis, it is reasonable to discontinue maintenance fluconazole as long as the CD4 response is maintained. A lumbar CSF with negative culture and no cryptococcal antigen provides additional assurance that the infection is inactive. For AIDS patients with cryptococcal meningitis who are alert and oriented and have other favorable prognostic signs, initial therapy with 400 mg daily may be considered. Fluconazole 400 mg daily has been recommended as continuation therapy in non-AIDS patients with cryptococcal meningitis who have responded to an initial course of C-AMB or AMBISOME and for patients with pulmonary cryptococcosis (Saag *et al.,* 2000).

Other Mycoses. Fluconazole is the drug of choice for treatment of coccidioidal meningitis because of much less morbidity than with intrathecal amphotericin B. In other forms of coccidioidomycosis, fluconazole is comparable to itraconazole. Fluconazole has activity against histoplasmosis, blastomycosis, sporotrichosis, and ringworm, but response is less than with equivalent doses of itraconazole. Fluconazole is not effective in the prevention or treatment of aspergillosis. As with other azoles, with the possible exception of posaconazole, there is no activity in mucormycosis.

Untoward Effects. Nausea and vomiting may occur at doses above 200 mg daily. Patients receiving 800 mg daily may require parenteral antiemetics. Side effects in patients receiving more than 7 days of drug, regardless of dose, include the following: nausea 3.7%, headache 1.9%, skin rash 1.8%, vomiting 1.7%, abdominal pain 1.7%, and diarrhea 1.5%. Reversible alopecia may occur with prolonged therapy at 400 mg daily. Rare cases of deaths due to hepatic failure or Stevens-Johnson syndrome have been reported. Fluconazole is teratogenic in rodents and has been associated with skeletal and cardiac deformities in three infants born to two women taking high doses during pregnancy. Thus the drug should be avoided during pregnancy (category C).

Dosage. Fluconazole (DIFLUCAN, others) is marketed in the United States as tablets of 50, 100, 150, and 200 mg for oral administration, powder for oral suspension providing 10 and 40 mg/ml, and intravenous solutions containing 2 mg/ml in saline and in dextrose solution. Dosage is 50 to 800 mg once daily and is identical for oral and intravenous administration. Children are treated with 3 to 6 mg/kg once daily.

Voriconazole

Voriconazole (VFEND; UK-109,495) is a triazole with a structure similar to fluconazole but has increased activity *in vitro*, an expanded spectrum, and poor aqueous solubility (pregnancy risk category C). The structure is shown below:

VORICONAZOLE

Absorption, Distribution, and Excretion. Oral bioavailability is 96% and protein binding 56% (Jeu *et al.*, 2003). Gastric acid is not necessary for absorption. Volume of distribution is high (4.6 L/kg), with extensive drug distribution in tissues. Metabolism occurs through the hepatic CYPs, particularly CYP2C19 and to a lesser extent CYP2C9. CYP3A4 plays a limited role. Less than 2% of native drug is recovered from urine, though 80% of the inactive metabolites are secreted in the urine. The oral dose does not have to be adjusted for azotemia or hemodialysis. Peak plasma concentrations after oral doses of 200 mg orally twice daily are about 3 μg/ml. CSF concentrations of 1 to 3 μg/ml have been reported in a patient with fungal meningitis.

Plasma elimination half-life is 6 hours. Voriconazole exhibits nonlinear metabolism so that higher doses cause greater-than-linear increases in drug exposure. Genetic polymorphisms in CYP2C19 can cause up to fourfold differences in drug exposure; 15% to 20% of Asians are homozygous poor metabolizers, compared to 2% of Caucasians and African-Americans. Patients older than 65 years had 86% higher plasma AUC than patients aged 18 to 45. Patients with mild or moderate hepatic insufficiency had an average AUC that was 223% of age- and weight-matched controls. Patients with cirrhosis should receive the same loading dose of voriconazole but half the maintenance dose. There are no data to guide dosing in patients with severe hepatic insufficiency.

The intravenous formulation of voriconazole contains sulfobutyl ether β-cyclodextrin (SBECD). When voriconazole is given intravenously, SBECD is excreted completely by the kidney. Significant accumulation of SBECD occurs with a creatinine clearance below 50 ml/min. Because toxicity of SBECD at high plasma concentrations is unclear, oral voriconazole is preferred in azotemic patients.

Drug Interactions. Voriconazole is metabolized by, and inhibits, CYP2C19, CYP2C9, and CYP3A4. The affinity of voriconazole is highest for CYP2C19, followed in rank order by CYP2C9 and CYP3A4. The major metabolite of voriconazole, the voriconazole N-oxide, also inhibits the metabolic activity of CYP2C9, CYP3A4, and to a lesser extent, CYP2C19. Inhibitors or inducers of these three enzymes may increase or decrease voriconazole plasma concentrations, respectively. In addition, there is potential for voricona-

zole and its major metabolite to increase the plasma concentrations of other drugs metabolized by these enzymes.

Coadministration with *rifampin, rifabutin,* or *ritonavir* is contraindicated because of accelerated voriconazole metabolism. *Efavirenz* and perhaps other nonnucleoside reverse transcriptase inhibitors (NNRTIs) significantly increase voriconazole metabolism and slow the metabolism of the NNRTI. When given with phenytoin, the voriconazole dose should be doubled. Drugs that significantly accumulate in patients receiving voriconazole include cyclosporine, tacrolimus, phenytoin, rifabutin, warfarin, and *sirolimus*. Because the sirolimus AUC increases elevenfold when voriconazole is given, coadministration is contraindicated. *Omeprazole* dose should be reduced by half if 40 mg or more per day is given. Until more experience with voriconazole is gained, it is prudent to be observant for the drug interactions known to occur with other azoles (Table 48–2).

Therapeutic Uses. In an open, randomized trial, voriconazole provided superior efficiency to C-AMB in the primary therapy of invasive aspergillosis (Herbrecht *et al.*, 2002). In a secondary analysis, survival also was superior in the voriconazole arm. Voriconazole was compared to AMBISOME in an open randomized trial in the empirical therapy of neutropenic patients whose fever did not respond to more than 96 hours of antibacterial therapy. Because the 95% confidence interval in this noninferiority trial permitted the possibility that voriconazole might be more than 10% worse than AMBISOME, the FDA did not approve voriconazole for this use (Walsh *et al.*, 2002). However, in a secondary analysis, there were fewer breakthrough infections with voriconazole (1.9%) than with AMBISOME (5%). Voriconazole is approved for use in esophageal candidiasis on the basis of a double-blind, randomized comparison with fluconazole (Ally *et al.*, 2001). Voriconazole is also approved for use as salvage therapy in patients with *Pseudallescheria boydii* (*Scedosporium apiospermum*) and *Fusarium* infections.

Untoward Effects. Voriconazole is teratogenic in animals and contraindicated in pregnancy (class D). Although voriconazole is generally well tolerated, occasional cases of hepatotoxicity have been reported and liver function should be monitored. Voriconazole, like some other azoles, causes a prolongation of the QTc interval, which can become significant in patients with other risk factors for *torsades de pointes*. Patients must be warned about possible visual effects. Approximately 30% of patients note transient visual changes beginning about half an hour after administration and lasting for another half hour. Blurred vision, altered color perception, and photophobia have been reported. Activities that require keen vision should be avoided when vision is altered. No sequelae occur. Uncommonly, transient visual hallucinations or confusion occur. Patients receiving their first intravenous infusion have had anaphylactoid reactions, with faintness, nausea, flushing, feverishness, and rash. In such patients, the infusion should be stopped. Rash has been reported in 5.8% of patients.

Dosage. Voriconazole for intravenous infusion is packaged as 200 mg with 3.2 g SBECD. Treatment is usually initiated with an intravenous infusion of 6 mg/kg every 12 hours for two doses, followed by 4 mg/kg every 12 hours. It should be administered at 3 mg/kg per hour, not as a bolus. As the patient improves, oral administration is continued as 200 mg every 12 hours. Patients failing to respond may be given 300 mg every 12 hours. Voriconazole is available as 50- or 200-mg tablets or a suspension of 40 mg/ml when hydrated. The tablets, but not the suspension, contain lactose. Because high-fat meals reduce voriconazole bioavailability, oral drug should be given either 1 hour before or 1 hour after meals.

Echinocandins

Screening natural products of fungal fermentation in the 1970s led to the discovery that *echinocandins* had activity against *Candida* and that the biologic activity was directed against formation of $\beta(1,3)$ D-glucans in the cell wall (Wiederhold and Lewis, 2003). Selection of different echinocandins and their chemical modifications led first to the discovery of *cilofungin*. Clinical trials were stopped because of toxicity from the solubilizing agent. Further research has led to one drug approved for clinical use, *caspofungin*, and two compounds that are in development: *anidulafungin* and *micafungin*. All have the same mechanism of action but differing pharmacologic properties. Susceptible fungi include *Candida* species and *Aspergillus* species. *In vitro* resistance can be conferred in *C. albicans* by mutation in one of the genes that encodes $\beta(1,3)$ D-glucan synthase. Azole-resistant isolates of *C. albicans* remain susceptible to echinocandins.

Caspofungin Acetate. Caspofungin acetate (cancidas, MK-0991) is a water-soluble, semisynthetic lipopeptide synthesized from the fermentation product of *Glarea lozoyensis* (Keating and Figgit, 2003; Johnson and Perfect, 2003). The chemical structure for caspofungin is shown below. The fermentation product is called pneumocandin B_0 because of its activity against cysts of *Pneumocystis jiroveci*. In susceptible yeasts, caspofungin causes lysis. In *Aspergillus*, hyphal tips become bulbous and may rupture, but hyphal growth continues sufficiently to negate use of the usual growth-inhibition endpoints for MIC estimation. It is not known if other endpoints correlate with *in vivo* activity, making it unwise to refer to caspofungin's *in vitro* activity against molds. Animal models have shown promising activity against *Aspergillus* species as well as many species of *Candida*. These models do not suggest activity against *Cryptococcus neoformans* or *Histoplasma capsulatum*.

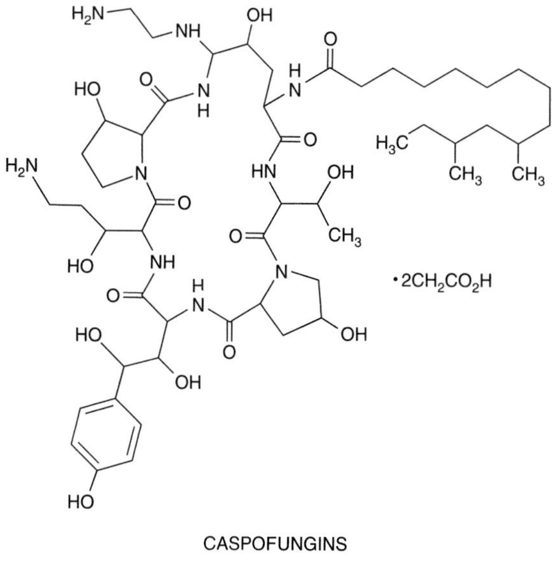

CASPOFUNGINS

Absorption, Distribution, and Excretion. Caspofungin is not absorbed through the gastrointestinal tract. After intravenous injection, caspofungin is eliminated from the bloodstream with a half-life of 9 to 11

hours. Catabolism is largely by hydrolysis and *N*-acetylation, with excretion of the metabolites in the urine and feces. Mild and moderate hepatic insufficiency increases the AUC by 55% and 76%, respectively. About 97% of serum drug is bound to albumin. Only clinically insignificant amounts of bioactive drug are present in urine, and no dose adjustment is necessary for renal insufficiency or hemodialysis.

Drug Interactions. The only potentially significant interaction yet found was a 35% increase in the caspofungin AUC by cyclosporine. Some subjects also developed increased serum aminotransferases, but it is unclear whether the modest increase in caspofungin AUC was responsible. Repeated administration of caspofungin (100 mg per day) has been well tolerated.

Therapeutic Use. Caspofungin is approved for patients with invasive aspergillosis who are failing or intolerant of approved drugs, such as amphotericin B formulations or voriconazole. Approval was based on a study of 63 patients in a noncomparative salvage trial. Caspofungin is also approved for esophageal candidiasis, based on randomized trials that found noninferiority to fluconazole and C-AMB (Villanueva *et al.*, 2001). Efficacy in fluconazole failures has not been reported but would be anticipated because there is no cross resistance. A blinded, randomized clinical trial of caspofungin in deeply invasive candidiasis found noninferiority to C-AMB, leading to approval for that indication (Mora-Duarte *et al.*, 2002). Most patients in that multicenter study were not neutropenic and had catheter-acquired candidemia. Too few patients were infected with *C. glabrata* to judge activity against that species. Efficacy was comparable to that of fluconazole in the same patient population. Caspofungin is also approved for the treatment of persistently febrile neutropenic patients with suspected fungal infections.

Untoward Effects. Caspofungin has been remarkably well tolerated, with the exception of phlebitis at the infusion site. Histamine-like effects have been reported with rapid infusions. Other symptoms have been equivalent to those observed in patients receiving fluconazole in the comparator arm.

Dosage. Caspofungin is administered intravenously once daily over 1 hour. In candidemia and salvage therapy of aspergillosis, the initial dose is 70 mg, followed by 50 mg daily. The dose may be increased to 70 mg daily in patients failing to respond. Esophageal candidiasis is treated with 50 mg daily.

Griseofulvin

Chemistry. The structural formula of *griseofulvin* is as follows:

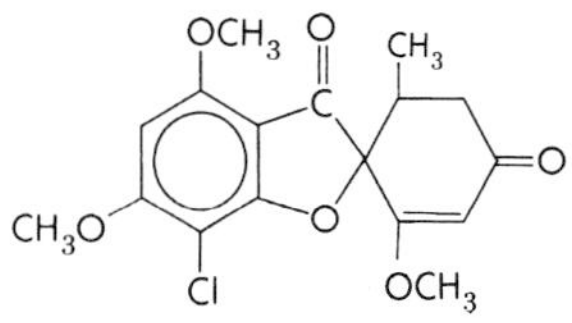

GRISEOFULVIN

The drug is practically insoluble in water.

Antifungal Activity. Griseofulvin is fungistatic *in vitro* for various species of the dermatophytes *Microsporum*, *Epidermophyton*, and *Trichophyton*. The drug has no effect on bacteria or on other fungi.

Resistance. Although failure of ringworm lesions to improve is not rare, isolates from these patients usually are still susceptible to griseofulvin *in vitro.*

Mechanism of Action. A prominent morphological manifestation of the action of griseofulvin is the production of multinucleate cells as the drug inhibits fungal mitosis. In mammalian cells treated with high concentrations, griseofulvin causes disruption of the mitotic spindle by interacting with polymerized microtubules. Although the effects of the drug are thus similar to those of *colchicine* and the vinca alkaloids, its binding sites on the microtubular protein are distinct. In addition to its binding to tubulin, griseofulvin also may bind to a microtubule-associated protein.

Absorption, Distribution, and Excretion. The oral administration of a 0.5-g dose of griseofulvin produces peak plasma concentrations of approximately 1 μg/ml in about 4 hours. Blood levels are quite variable, however. Some studies have shown improved absorption when the drug is taken with a fatty meal. Since the rates of dissolution and disaggregation limit the bioavailability of griseofulvin, microsized and ultramicrosized powders are now used in preparations (FULVI-CIN U/F and GRIS-PEG, respectively). Although the bioavailability of the ultramicrocrystalline preparation is said to be 50% greater than that of the conventional microsized powder, this may not always be true. Griseofulvin has a half-life in plasma of about 1 day, and approximately 50% of the oral dose can be detected in the urine within 5 days, mostly in the form of metabolites. The primary metabolite is 6-methylgriseofulvin. Barbiturates decrease griseofulvin absorption from the gastrointestinal tract.

Griseofulvin is deposited in keratin precursor cells; when these cells differentiate, the drug is tightly bound to, and persists in, keratin, providing prolonged resistance to fungal invasion. For this reason, the new growth of hair or nails is the first to become free of disease. As the fungus-containing keratin is shed, it is replaced by normal tissue. Griseofulvin is detectable in the stratum corneum of the skin within 4 to 8 hours of oral administration. Sweat and transepidermal fluid loss play an important role in the transfer of the drug in the stratum corneum. Only a very small fraction of a dose of the drug is present in body fluids and tissues.

Therapeutic Uses. Mycotic disease of the skin, hair, and nails due to *Microsporum, Trichophyton,* or *Epidermophyton* responds to griseofulvin therapy. Infections that are readily treatable with this agent include infections of the hair (tinea capitis) caused by *Microsporum canis, Microsporum audouinii, Trichophyton schoenleinii,* and *Trichophyton verrucosum;* "ringworm" of the glabrous skin; tinea cruris and tinea corporis caused by *M. canis, Trichophyton rubrum, T. verrucosum,* and *Epidermophyton floccosum;* and tinea of the hands (*T. rubrum* and *T. mentagrophytes*) and beard (*Trichophyton* species). Griseofulvin also is highly effective in "athlete's foot" or epidermophytosis involving the skin and nails, the vesicular form of which is most commonly due to *T. mentagrophytes* and the hyperkeratotic type to *T. rubrum.* However, topical therapy is preferred (*see* below). *T. rubrum* and *T. mentagrophytes* infections may require higher-than-conventional doses. Since very high doses of griseofulvin are carcinogenic and teratogenic in laboratory animals, the drug should not be used systemically to treat trivial infections that respond to topical therapy.

Dosage. The recommended daily dose of griseofulvin is 5 to 15 mg/kg for children and 500 mg to 1 g for adults. Doses of 1.5 to 2 g daily may be used for short periods in severe or extensive infec-

tions. Best results are obtained when the daily dose is divided and given at 6-hour intervals, although the drug often is given twice per day. Treatment must be continued until infected tissue is replaced by normal hair, skin, or nails, which requires 1 month for scalp and hair ringworm, 6 to 9 months for fingernails, and at least a year for toenails. Itraconazole or terbinafine is preferred for onychomycosis. Griseofulvin is not effective in treatment of subcutaneous or deep mycoses.

Untoward Effects. The incidence of serious reactions associated with the use of griseofulvin is very low. One of the minor effects is headache, which is sometimes severe and usually disappears as therapy is continued. The incidence of headache may be as high as 15%. Other nervous system manifestations include peripheral neuritis, lethargy, mental confusion, impairment of performance of routine tasks, fatigue, syncope, vertigo, blurred vision, transient macular edema, and augmentation of the effects of alcohol. Among the side effects involving the alimentary tract are nausea, vomiting, diarrhea, heartburn, flatulence, dry mouth, and angular stomatitis. Hepatotoxicity also has been observed. Hematologic effects include leukopenia, neutropenia, punctate basophilia, and monocytosis; these often disappear despite continued therapy. Blood studies should be carried out at least once a week during the first month of treatment or longer. Common renal effects include albuminuria and cylindruria without evidence of renal insufficiency. Reactions involving the skin are cold and warm urticaria, photosensitivity, lichen planus, erythema, erythema multiforme–like rashes, and vesicular and morbilliform eruptions. Serum sickness syndromes and severe angioedema develop rarely during treatment with griseofulvin. Estrogenlike effects have been observed in children. A moderate but inconsistent increase of fecal protoporphyrins has been noted with chronic use.

Griseofulvin induces hepatic CYPs, thus increasing the rate of metabolism of warfarin; adjustment of the dosage of the latter agent may be necessary in some patients. The drug may reduce the efficacy of low-estrogen oral contraceptive agents, probably by a similar mechanism.

Terbinafine

Terbinafine is a synthetic allylamine, structurally similar to the topical agent *naftifine*. Its structural formula is shown below:

TERBINAFINE

Terbinafine is well absorbed, but bioavailability is decreased to about 40% because of first-pass metabolism in the liver. Proteins bind more than 99% of the drug in plasma. Drug accumulates in skin, nails, and fat. The initial half-life is about 12 hours but extends to 200 to 400 hours at steady state. Drug can be found in plasma for 4 to 8 weeks after prolonged therapy. Terbinafine is not recommended in patients with marked azotemia or hepatic failure, because in the latter condition, terbinafine plasma levels are increased by unpredictable amounts. Rifampin decreases and cimetidine increases plasma terbinafine concentrations. The drug is well tolerated, with a low incidence of gastrointestinal distress, headache, or rash. Rarely, hepatotoxicity, severe neutropenia, Stevens-Johnson syndrome, or toxic epidermal necrolysis may occur. The drug is contraindicated in pregnancy (category B). It is recommended that systemic terbinafine therapy for onychomycosis be postponed until after pregnancy is complete. Its mechanism of action is probably inhibition of fungal squalene epoxidase, blocking ergosterol biosynthesis.

Terbinafine (LAMISIL), given as one 250-mg tablet daily, is at least as effective for nail onychomycosis as 200 mg daily of itraconazole, and slightly more effective than pulse itraconazole therapy (*see* above) (Evans, 1999). Duration of treatment varies with the site being treated but typically is 3 months. Although not approved for this use, terbinafine (250 mg daily) also is effective in ringworm elsewhere on the body. No pediatric formulation is available, so there is little experience with the drug in tinea capitis, usually a disease of children. The topical use of terbinafine is discussed in the following section.

Topical Antifungal Agents

Topical treatment is useful in many superficial fungal infections—*i.e.*, those confined to the stratum corneum, squamous mucosa, or cornea. Such diseases include dermatophytosis (ringworm), candidiasis, tinea versicolor, piedra, tinea nigra, and fungal keratitis. Topical administration of antifungal agents usually is not successful for mycoses of the nails (onychomycosis) and hair (tinea capitis) and has no place in the treatment of subcutaneous mycoses, such as sporotrichosis and chromoblastomycosis. The efficacy of topical agents in the treatment of superficial mycoses depends not only on the type of lesion and the mechanism of action of the drug, but also on the viscosity, hydrophobicity, and acidity of the formulation. Regardless of formulation, penetration of topical drugs into hyperkeratotic lesions often is poor. Removal of thick, infected keratin is sometimes a useful adjunct to therapy and is the principal mode of action of Whitfield's ointment (*see* below).

A plethora of topical agents is available for the treatment of superficial mycoses. Many of the older drugs—including *gentian violet, carbol-fuchsin, acrisorcin, triacetin, sulfur, iodine,* and *aminacrine*—are now rarely indicated and are not discussed here. Among the topical agents, the preferred formulation for cutaneous application usually is a cream or solution. Ointments are messy and are too occlusive for macerated or fissured intertriginous lesions. The use of powders, whether applied by shake containers or aerosols, is largely confined to the feet and moist lesions of the groin and other intertriginous areas.

The systemic agents used for the treatment of superficial mycoses are discussed above. Some of these agents also are administered topically; their uses are described here and also in Chapter 62.

Imidazoles and Triazoles for Topical Use

As discussed above, these closely related classes of drugs are synthetic antifungal agents that are used both topically and systemically. Indications for their topical use include ringworm, tinea versicolor, and mucocutaneous candidiasis. Resistance to imidazoles or triazoles is very rare among the fungi that cause ringworm. Selection of one of these agents for topical use should be based on cost and availability, since testing *in vitro* for fungal susceptibility to these drugs does not predict clinical responses.

Cutaneous Application. The preparations for cutaneous use described below are effective for tinea corporis, tinea pedis, tinea cruris, tinea versicolor, and cutaneous candidiasis. They should be applied twice a day for 3 to 6 weeks. Despite some activity *in vitro* against bacteria, this effect is not clinically useful. The cutaneous formulations are not suitable for oral, vaginal, or ocular use.

Vaginal Application. Vaginal creams, suppositories, and tablets for vaginal candidiasis are all used once a day for 1 to 7 days, preferably at bedtime to facilitate retention. None is useful in trichomoniasis, despite some activity *in vitro*. Most vaginal creams are administered in 5-g amounts. Three vaginal formulations—clotrimazole tablets, miconazole suppositories, and terconazole cream—come in both low- and high-dose preparations. A shorter duration of therapy is recommended for the higher dose of each. These preparations are administered for 3 to 7 days. Approximately 3% to 10% of the vaginal dose is absorbed. Although some imidazoles are teratogenic in rodents, no adverse effects on the human fetus have been attributed to the vaginal use of imidazoles or triazoles. The most common side effect is vaginal burning or itching. A male sexual partner may experience mild penile irritation. Cross-allergenicity among these compounds is assumed to exist, based on their structural similarities.

Oral Use. Use of the oral troche of clotrimazole is properly considered as topical therapy. The only indication for this 10-mg troche is oropharyngeal candidiasis. Antifungal activity is due entirely to the local concentration of the drug; there is no systemic effect.

Clotrimazole

Clotrimazole has the following structure:

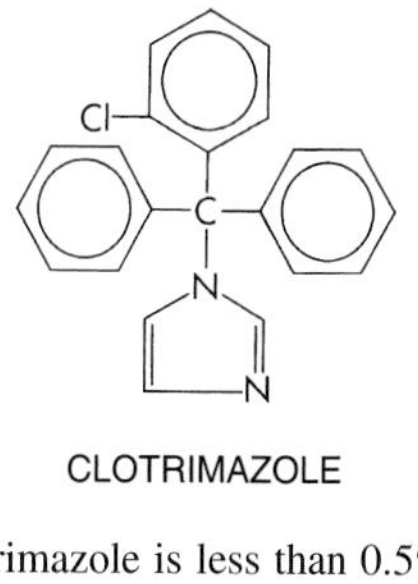

CLOTRIMAZOLE

Absorption of clotrimazole is less than 0.5% after application to the intact skin; from the vagina, it is 3% to 10%. Fungicidal concentrations remain in the vagina for as long as 3 days after application of the drug. The small amount absorbed is metabolized in the liver and excreted in bile. In adults, an oral dose of 200 mg per day will give rise initially to plasma concentrations of 0.2 to 0.35 μg/ml, followed by a progressive decline.

In a small fraction of recipients, clotrimazole on the skin may cause stinging, erythema, edema, vesication, desquamation, pruritus, and urticaria. When it is applied to the vagina, about 1.6% of recipients complain of a mild burning sensation, and rarely of lower abdominal cramps, a slight increase in urinary frequency, or skin rash. Occasionally, the sexual partner may experience penile or urethral irritation. By the oral route, clotrimazole can cause gastrointestinal irritation. In patients using troches, the incidence of this side effect is about 5%.

Therapeutic Uses. Clotrimazole is available as a 1% cream, lotion, and solution (LOTRIMIN, MYCELEX, others), 1% or 2% vaginal cream or vaginal tablets of 100, 200, or 500 mg (GYNE-LOTRIMIN, MYCELEX-G, others), and 10-mg troches (MYCELEX, others). On the skin, applications are made twice a day. For the vagina, the standard regimens are one 100-mg tablet once a day at bedtime for 7 days, one 200-mg tablet daily for 3 days, one 500-mg tablet inserted only once, or 5 g of cream once a day for 3 days (2% cream) or 7 days (1% cream). For nonpregnant females, one 200-mg tablet may be used once a day for 3 days. Troches are to be dissolved slowly in the mouth five times a day for 14 days.

Clotrimazole has been reported to cure dermatophyte infections in 60% to 100% of cases. The cure rates in cutaneous candidiasis are 80% to 100%. In vulvovaginal candidiasis, the cure rate is usually above 80% when the 7-day regimen is used. A 3-day regimen of 200 mg once a day appears to be similarly effective, as does single-dose treatment (500 mg). Recurrences are common after all regimens. The cure rate with oral troches for oral and pharyngeal candidiasis may be as high as 100% in the immunocompetent host.

Econazole

Econazole, the deschloro derivative of miconazole, has the following structure:

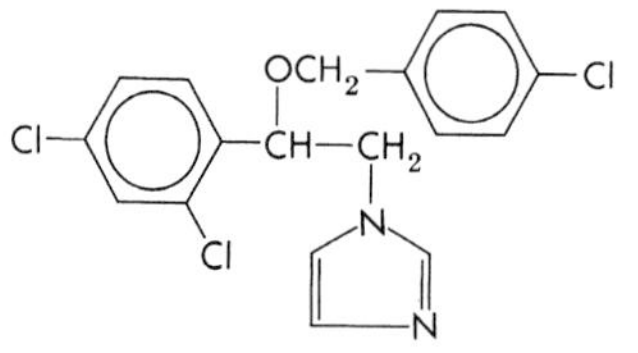

ECONAZOLE

Econazole readily penetrates the stratum corneum and is found in effective concentrations down to the mid-dermis. However, less than 1% of an applied dose appears to be absorbed into the blood. Approximately 3% of recipients have local erythema, burning, stinging, or itching.

Econazole nitrate (SPECTAZOLE, others) is available as a water-miscible cream (1%) to be applied twice a day.

Miconazole

Miconazole is a very close chemical congener of econazole, with the following structure:

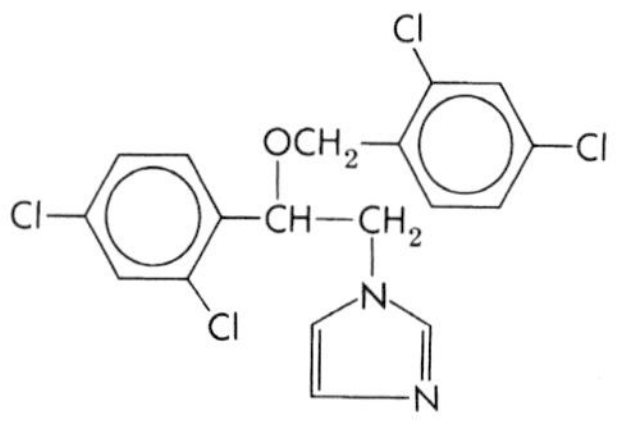

MICONAZOLE

Miconazole readily penetrates the stratum corneum of the skin and persists there for more than 4 days after application. Less than 1% is absorbed into the blood. Absorption is no more than 1.3% from the vagina.

Adverse effects from topical application to the vagina include burning, itching, or irritation in about 7% of recipients, and infrequently, pelvic cramps (0.2%), headache, hives, or skin rash. Irritation, burning, and maceration are rare after cutaneous application. Miconazole is considered safe for use during pregnancy, although some authors avoid its vaginal use during the first trimester.

Therapeutic Uses. Miconazole nitrate is available as a dermatologic ointment, cream, solution, spray, or powder (MICATIN, MONISTAT-DERM, others). To avoid maceration, only the lotion should be applied to intertriginous areas. It is available as a 2% and 4% vaginal cream, and as 100-mg, 200-mg, or 1200-mg vaginal suppositories (MONISTAT 7, MONISTAT 3, others), to be applied high in the vagina at bedtime for 7, 3, or 1 day(s), respectively.

In the treatment of tinea pedis, tinea cruris, and tinea versicolor, the cure rate may be over 90%. In the treatment of vulvovaginal candidiasis, the mycologic cure rate at the end of 1 month is about 80% to 95%. Pruritus sometimes is relieved after a single application. Some vaginal infections caused by *Candida glabrata* also respond.

Terconazole and Butoconazole

Terconazole (TERAZOL, others) is a ketal triazole with structural similarities to ketoconazole. Its structure is as follows:

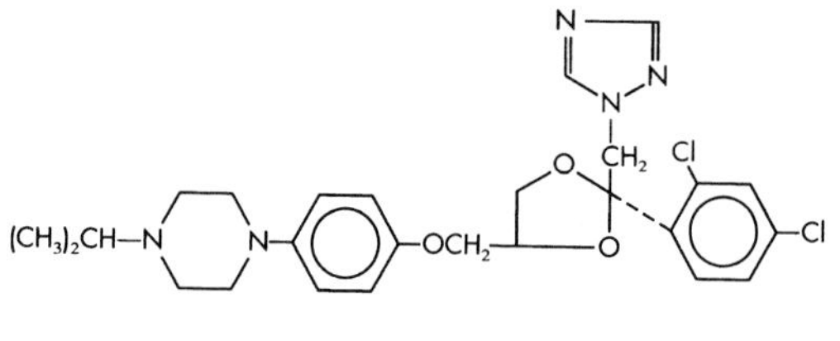

TERCONAZOLE

The mechanism of action of terconazole is similar to that of the imidazoles. The 80-mg vaginal suppository is inserted at bedtime for 3 days, while the 0.4% vaginal cream is used for 7 days and the 0.8% cream for 3 days. Clinical efficacy and patient acceptance of both preparations are at least as good as for clotrimazole in patients with vaginal candidiasis.

Butoconazole is an imidazole that is pharmacologically quite comparable to clotrimazole. Its structural formula is as follows:

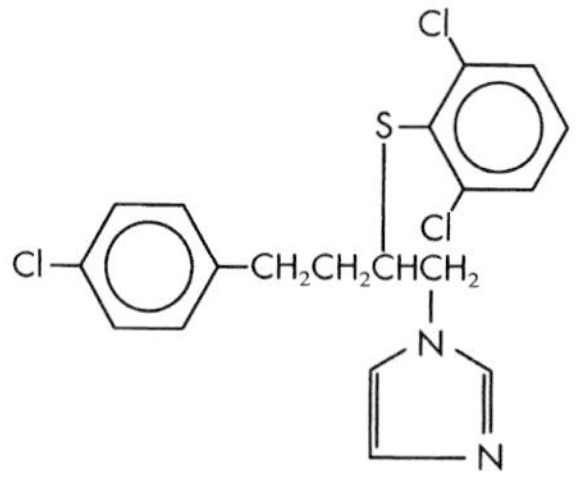

BUTOCONAZOLE

Butoconazole nitrate (MYCELEX 3, others) is available as a 2% vaginal cream; it is used at bedtime in nonpregnant females. Because of the slower response during pregnancy, a 6-day course is recommended (during the second and third trimester).

Tioconazole

Tioconazole (VAGISTAT 1, others) is an imidazole that is marketed for treatment of *Candida* vulvovaginitis. A single 4.6-g dose of ointment (300 mg) is given at bedtime.

Oxiconazole, Sulconazole, and Sertaconazole

These imidazole derivatives are used for the topical treatment of infections caused by the common pathogenic dermatophytes. Oxiconazole nitrate (OXISTAT) is available as a cream and lotion; sulconazole nitrate (EXELDERM) is supplied as a solution and cream. Sertaconazole (ERTACZO) is a 2% cream marketed for tinea pedis.

Ciclopirox Olamine

Ciclopirox olamine (LOPROX) has broad-spectrum antifungal activity. The chemical structure is as follows:

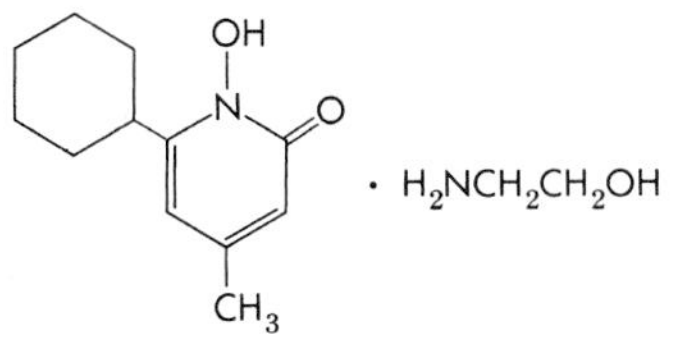

CICLOPIROX OLAMINE

It is fungicidal to *C. albicans, E. floccosum, M. canis, T. mentagrophytes,* and *T. rubrum.* It also inhibits the growth of *Malassezia furfur.* After application to the skin, it penetrates through the epidermis into the dermis, but even under occlusion, less than 1.5% is absorbed into the systemic circulation. Because the half-life is 1.7 hours, no systemic accumulation occurs. The drug penetrates into hair follicles and sebaceous glands. It can sometimes cause hypersensitivity. It is available as a 0.77% cream and lotion for the treatment of cutaneous candidiasis and for tinea corporis, cruris, pedis, and versicolor. Cure rates in the dermatomycoses and candidal infections have been variously reported to be 81% to 94%. No topical toxicity has been noted.

Ciclopirox is also sold as a 0.77% gel and a 1% shampoo for the treatment of seborrheic dermatitis of the scalp, and an 8% topical solution (PENLAC NAIL LACQUER) is sold for the treatment of onychomycosis.

Haloprogin

Haloprogin is a halogenated phenolic ether with the following structure:

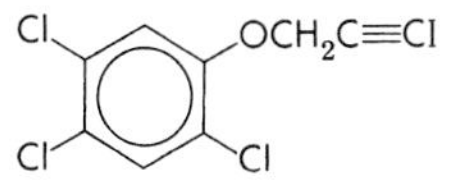

HALOPROGIN

It is fungicidal to various species of *Epidermophyton, Pityrosporum, Microsporum, Trichophyton,* and *Candida.* During treatment with this drug, irritation, pruritus, burning sensations, vesiculation, increased maceration, and "sensitization" (or exacerbation of the lesion) occasionally occur, especially on the foot if occlusive

footgear is worn. Haloprogin is poorly absorbed through the skin; it is converted to trichlorophenol in the body. The systemic toxicity from topical application appears to be low.

Haloprogin (HALOTEX) cream or solution is applied twice a day for 2 to 4 weeks. Its principal use is against tinea pedis, for which the cure rate is about 80%; it is thus approximately equal in efficacy to *tolnaftate* (*see* below). It also is used against tinea cruris, tinea corporis, tinea manuum, and tinea versicolor. Haloprogin is no longer available in the United States.

Tolnaftate

Tolnaftate is a thiocarbamate with the following structure:

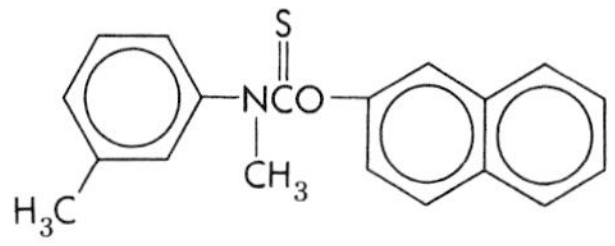

TOLNAFTATE

Tolnaftate is effective in the treatment of most cutaneous mycoses caused by *T. rubrum, T. mentagrophytes, T. tonsurans, E. floccosum, M. canis, M. audouinii, Microsporum gypseum,* and *M. furfur,* but it is ineffective against *Candida.* In tinea pedis, the cure rate is around 80%, compared with about 95% for miconazole. Toxic or allergic reactions to tolnaftate have not been reported.

Tolnaftate (AFTATE, TINACTIN, others) is available in a 1% concentration as a cream, gel, powder, aerosol powder, and topical solution, or as a topical aerosol liquid. The preparations are applied locally twice a day. Pruritus is usually relieved in 24 to 72 hours. Involution of interdigital lesions caused by susceptible fungi is very often complete in 7 to 21 days.

Naftifine

Naftifine is an allylamine with the following structure:

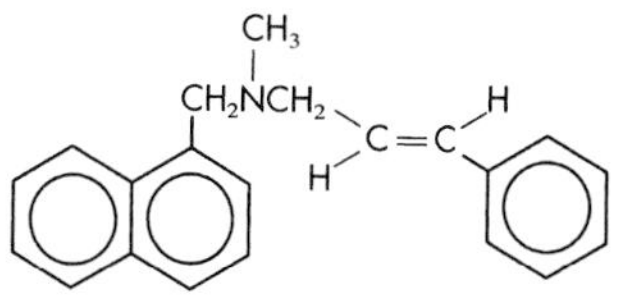

NAFTIFINE

Naftifine is representative of the allylamine class of synthetic agents that inhibit squalene-2,3-epoxidase and thus inhibit fungal biosynthesis of ergosterol. The drug has broad-spectrum fungicidal activity *in vitro.* Naftifine hydrochloride (NAFTIN) is available as a 1% cream or gel. It is effective for the topical treatment of tinea cruris and tinea corporis; twice-daily application is recommended. The drug is well tolerated, although local irritation has been observed in 3% of treated patients. Allergic contact dermatitis also has been reported. Naftifine also may be efficacious for cutaneous candidiasis and tinea versicolor, although the drug is not approved for these uses.

Terbinafine

Terbinafine 1% cream or spray is applied twice daily and is effective in tinea corporis, tinea cruris, and tinea pedis. Terbinafine is less active against *Candida* species and *Malassezia furfur,* but the cream also can be used in cutaneous candidiasis and tinea versicolor. In European studies, oral terbinafine has appeared to be effective in treatment of ringworm, and in some cases of onychomycosis. The systemic use of terbinafine is discussed above.

Butenafine

Butenafine hydrochloride (MENTAX) is a benzylamine derivative with a mechanism of action similar to that of terbinafine and naftifine. Its spectrum of antifungal activity and use also are similar to those of the allylamines.

Polyene Antifungal Antibiotics

Nystatin. *Nystatin* was discovered in the New York State Health Laboratory and was named accordingly; it is a tetraene macrolide produced by *Streptomyces noursei*. Nystatin is structurally similar to amphotericin B and has the same mechanism of action. Nystatin is not absorbed from the gastrointestinal tract, skin, or vagina. A liposomal formulation (NYOTRAN) is in clinical trials for candidemia.

Nystatin (MYCOSTATIN, NILSTAT, others) is useful only for candidiasis and is supplied in preparations intended for cutaneous, vaginal, or oral administration for this purpose. Infections of the nails and hyperkeratinized or crusted skin lesions do not respond. Topical preparations include ointments, creams, and powders, all of which contain 100,000 units/g. Powders are preferred for moist lesions and are applied two or three times a day. Creams or ointments are used twice daily. Combinations of nystatin with antibacterial agents or corticosteroids also are available. Allergic reactions to nystatin are very uncommon.

Vaginal tablets containing 100,000 units of the drug are inserted once daily for 2 weeks. Although the tablets are well tolerated, imidazoles or triazoles are more effective agents than nystatin for vaginal candidiasis.

An oral suspension that contains 100,000 units/ml of nystatin is given four times a day. Premature and low-birth-weight neonates should receive 1 ml of this preparation, infants 2 ml, and children or adults 4 to 6 ml per dose. Older children and adults should be instructed to swish the drug around the mouth and then swallow. If not otherwise instructed, the patient may expectorate the bitter liquid and fail to treat the infected mucosa in the posterior pharynx or esophagus. Nystatin suspension is usually effective for oral candidiasis of the immunocompetent host. Other than the bitter taste and occasional complaints of nausea, adverse effects are uncommon. A 200,000-unit troche (mycostatin pastilles) is available for the treatment of oral candidiasis, and a 500,000-unit oral tablet is sold for the treatment of nonesophageal membrane gastrointestinal candidiasis.

Amphotericin B. Topical amphotericin B (FUNGIZONE) also is used for cutaneous candidiasis. A lotion, cream, and ointment are marketed; these preparations all contain 3% amphotericin B and are applied to the lesion two to four times daily. The systemic use of amphotericin B is discussed above.

Miscellaneous Antifungal Agents

Undecylenic Acid. *Undecylenic acid* is 10-undecenoic acid, an 11-carbon unsaturated compound. It is a yellow liquid with a characteristic rancid odor. It is primarily fungistatic, although fungicidal activity may be observed with long exposure to high concentrations of the agent. The drug is active against a variety of fungi, including

those that cause ringworm. Undecylenic acid (DESENEX, others) is available in a foam, ointment, cream, powder, spray powder, soap, and liquid. *Zinc undecylenate* is marketed in combination with other ingredients. The zinc provides an astringent action that aids in the suppression of inflammation. Compound undecylenic acid ointment contains both undecylenic acid (about 5%) and zinc undecylenate (about 20%). *Calcium undecylenate* (CALDESENE, CRUEX) is available as a powder.

Undecylenic acid preparations are used in the treatment of various dermatomycoses, especially tinea pedis. Concentrations of the acid as high as 10%, as well as those of the acid and salt in the compound ointment, may be applied to the skin. The preparations as formulated are usually not irritating to tissue, and sensitization to them is uncommon. It is of undoubted benefit in retarding fungal growth in tinea pedis, but the infection frequently persists despite intensive treatment with preparations of the acid and the zinc salt. At best, the clinical "cure" rate is about 50%, which is much lower than that obtained with the imidazoles, haloprogin, or tolnaftate. Efficacy in the treatment of tinea capitis is marginal, and the drug is no longer used for that purpose. Undecylenic acid preparations also are approved for use in the treatment of diaper rash, tinea cruris, and other minor dermatologic conditions.

Benzoic Acid and Salicylic Acid. An ointment containing benzoic and salicylic acids is known as *Whitfield's ointment*. It combines the fungistatic action of benzoate with the keratolytic action of salicylate. It contains benzoic acid and salicylic acid in a ratio of 2:1 (usually 6% to 3%) and is used mainly in the treatment of tinea pedis. Since benzoic acid is only fungistatic, eradication of the infection occurs only after the infected stratum corneum is shed, and continuous medication is required for several weeks to months. The salicylic acid accelerates the desquamation. The ointment also is sometimes used to treat tinea capitis. Mild irritation may occur at the site of application.

BIBLIOGRAPHY

Ally, R., Schürmann, D., Kreisel, W., *et al.*, for the Esophageal Candidiasis Study Group. A randomized, double-blind, double-dummy, multicenter trial of voriconazole and fluconazole in the treatment of esophageal candidiasis in immunocompromised patients. *Clin. Infect. Dis.*, **2001**, *33*:1447–1454.

Barrett, J.P., Vardulaki, K.A., Conlon, C., *et al.*, for the Amphotericin B Systematic Review Study Group. A systematic review of the antifungal effectiveness and tolerability of amphotericin B formulations. *Clin. Ther.*, **2003**, *25*:1295–1320.

Bowden, R., Chandrasekar, P., White, M.H., *et al.* A double-blind, randomized, controlled trial of amphotericin B colloidal dispersion versus amphotericin B for treatment of invasive aspergillosis in immunocompromised patients. *Clin. Infect. Dis.*, **2002**, *35*:359–366.

Brouwer, A.E., Rajanuwong, A., Chierakul, W., *et al.* Combination antifungal therapies for HIV-associated cryptococcal meningitis: a randomised trial. *Lancet*, **2004**, *363*:1764–1767.

Carlson, M.A., and Condon, R.E. Nephrotoxicity of amphotericin B. *J. Am. Coll. Surg.*, **1994**, *179*:361–381.

Coker, R.J., Viviani, M., Gazzard, B.G., *et al.* Treatment of cryptococcosis with liposomal amphotericin B (AmBisome) in 23 patients with AIDS. *AIDS*, **1993**, *7*:829–835.

Dodgson, A.R., Dodgson, K.J., Pujol, C., Pfaller, M.A., and Soll, D.R. Clade-specific flucytosine resistance is due to a single nucleotide change in the *FUR1* gene of *Candida albicans*. *Antimicrob. Agents Chemother.*, **2004,** *48:*2223–2227.

Evans, E.G., and Sigurgeirsson, B. Double blind, randomised study of continuous terbinafine compared with intermittent itraconazole in treatment of toenail onychomycosis. The LION Study Group. *B.M.J.*, **1999,** *318:*1031–1035.

Herbrecht, R., Denning, D.W., Patterson, T.F., *et al.* Voriconazole versus amphotericin B for primary therapy of invasive aspergillosis. *N. Engl. J. Med.*, **2002,** *347:*408–415.

Herreros, E., Martinez, C.M., Almela, M.J., *et al.* Sordarins: *in vitro* activities of new antifungal derivatives against pathogenic yeasts, *Pneumocystis carinii*, and filamentous fungi. *Antimicrob. Agents Chemother.*, **1998,** *42:*2863–2869.

van der Horst, C.M., Saag, M.S., Cloud, G.A., *et al.* Treatment of cryptococcal meningitis associated with the acquired immunodeficiency syndrome. National Institute of Allergy and Infectious Diseases Mycoses Study Group and AIDS Clinical Trials Group. *N. Engl. J. Med.*, **1997,** *337:*15–21.

Jeu, L., Piacenti, F.J., Lyakhovetskiy, A.G., and Fung, H.B. Voriconazole. *Clin. Ther.*, **2003,** *25:*1321–1381.

Johnson, M.D., and Perfect, J.R. Caspofungin: first approved agent in a new class of antifungals. *Expert Opin. Pharmacother.*, **2003,** *4:*807–823.

Keating, G., and Figgitt, D. Caspofungin: a review of its use in oesophageal candidiasis, invasive candidiasis and invasive aspergillosis. *Drugs.*, **2003,** *63:*2235–2263.

Larsen, R.A., Bozzette, S.A., Jones, B.E., *et al.* Fluconazole combined with flucytosine for treatment of cryptococcal meningitis in patients with AIDS. *Clin. Infect. Dis.*, **1994,** *19:*741–745.

Mora-Duarte, J., Betts, R., Rotstein, C., *et al.* Comparison of caspofungin and amphotericin B for invasive candidiasis. *N. Engl. J. Med.*, **2002,** *347:*2020–2029.

Pappas, P.G., Perfect, J.R., Cloud, G.A., *et al.* Cryptococcosis in human immunodeficiency virus-negative patients in the era of effective azole therapy. *Clin. Infect. Dis.*, **2001,** *33:*690–699.

Saag, M.S., Graybill, R.J., Larsen, R.A., *et al.* Practice guidelines for the management of cryptococcal disease. Infectious Diseases Society of America. *Clin. Infect. Dis.*, **2000,** *30:*710–718.

Salez, F., Brichet, A., Desurmont, S., *et al.* Effects of itraconazole therapy in allergic bronchopulmonary aspergillosis. *Chest*, **1999,** *116:*1665–1668.

Sharkey, P.K., Graybill, J.R., Johnson, E.S., *et al.* Amphotericin B lipid complex compared with amphotericin B in the treatment of cryptococcal meningitis in patients with AIDS. *Clin. Infect. Dis.*, **1996,** *22:*315–321.

Steinbach, W.J., Perfect, J.R., Schell, W.A., Walsh, T.J., and Benjamin, D.K., Jr. *In vitro* analyses, animal models, and 60 clinical cases of invasive *Aspergillus terreus* infection. *Antimicrob. Agents Chemother.*, **2004,** *48:*3217–3225.

Villanueva, A., Arathoon, E.G., Gotuzzo, E., *et al.* A randomized double-blind study of caspofungin versus amphotericin for the treatment of candidal esophagitis. *Clin. Infect. Dis.*, **2001,** *33:*1529–1535.

Walsh, T.J., Pappas, P., Winston, D.J., *et al.,* for the National Institute of Allergy and Infectious Diseases Mycoses Study Group. Voriconazole compared with liposomal amphotericin B for empirical antifungal therapy in patients with neutropenia and persistent fever. *N. Engl. J. Med.*, **2002,** *346:*225–234.

White, M.H., Bowden, R.A., Sandler, E.S., *et al.* Randomized, double-blind clinical trial of amphotericin B colloidal dispersion *vs.* amphotericin B in the empirical treatment of fever and neutropenia. *Clin. Infect. Dis.*, **1998,** *27:*296–302.

Wiederhold, N.P., and Lewis, R.E. The echinocandin antifungals: an overview of the pharmacology, spectrum and clinical efficacy. *Expert Opin. Invest. Drugs*, **2003,** *12:*1313–1333.

Wingard, J.R, White, M.H., Anaissie, E., *et al.* A randomized, double-blind comparative trial evaluating the safety of liposomal amphotericin B versus amphotericin B lipid complex in the empirical treatment of febrile neutropenia. *Clin. Infect. Dis.*, **2000,** *31:*1155–1163.

ANTIVIRAL AGENTS (NONRETROVIRAL)

Frederick G. Hayden

Viruses are obligate intracellular parasites that consist of either double- or single-stranded DNA or RNA enclosed in a protein coat called a *capsid.* Some viruses also possess a lipid envelope that, like the capsid, may contain antigenic glycoproteins. Most viruses contain or encode enzymes essential for viral replication inside a host cell, and they usurp the metabolic machinery of their host cell. The discovery of novel antiviral inhibitors often is linked to a better understanding of the molecular events in viral replication. Table 49–1 outlines the stages of viral replication and the classes of antiviral agents that could act at each stage of replication. Effective antiviral agents inhibit virus-specific replicative events or preferentially inhibit virus-directed rather than host cell–directed nucleic acid or protein synthesis. However, host cell molecules that are essential to viral replication also may offer targets for developing new short-term therapies. This chapter provides information about the antiviral activity, pharmacology, and clinical uses of specific antiviral agents for non–human immunodeficiency virus (non-HIV) infections.

Figure 49–1 provides a schematic diagram of the replicative cycle of a DNA virus (*A*) and an RNA virus (*B*). DNA viruses (and the diseases they cause) include poxviruses (smallpox), herpesviruses (chickenpox, shingles, oral and genital herpes), adenoviruses (conjunctivitis, sore throat), hepadnaviruses [hepatitis B (HBV)], and papillomaviruses (warts). Typically, DNA viruses enter into the host cell nucleus, where the viral DNA is transcribed into mRNA by host cell polymerase; mRNA is translated in the usual host cell fashion into virus-specific proteins. One exception to this strategy is poxvirus, which has its own RNA polymerase and consequently replicates in the host cell cytoplasm.

For RNA viruses, the replication strategy in the host cell relies either on enzymes in the virion (the whole infective viral particle) to synthesize its mRNA or on the viral RNA serving as its own mRNA. The mRNA is translated into various viral proteins, including RNA polymerase, which directs the synthesis of more viral mRNA and genomic RNA (Figure 49–1B). Most RNA viruses complete their replication in the cytoplasm, but some, such as influenza, are transcribed in the host cell nucleus. Examples of RNA viruses (and the diseases they cause) include rubella virus (German measles), rhabdoviruses (rabies), picornaviruses (poliomyelitis, meningitis, colds, hepatitis A), arenaviruses (meningitis, Lassa fever), flaviviruses (West Nile meningoencephalitis, yellow fever, hepatitis C), orthomyxoviruses (influenza), paramyxoviruses (measles, mumps), and coronaviruses [colds, severe acute respiratory syndrome (SARS)].

One group of RNA viruses that deserves special mention is retroviruses, responsible for diseases such as acquired immunodeficiency syndrome (AIDS) (*see* Chapter 50) and T-cell leukemias [human T-cell lymphotropic virus I (HTLV-I)]. In retroviruses, the virus contains a reverse-transcriptase enzyme activity that makes a DNA copy of the viral RNA template. The DNA copy is then integrated into the host genome, at which point it is referred to as a *provirus* and is transcribed into both genomic RNA and mRNA for translation into viral proteins. The polymerase of hepadnaviruses possesses reverse-transcriptase activity, and nucleoside antiretroviral agents often are inhibitory for HBV.

Experiences from the development of antiviral agents have provided useful general insights with practical implications:

1. Although many compounds show antiviral activity *in vitro,* most affect some host cell function and are associated with unacceptable toxicity in human beings.

Table 49–1
Stages of Virus Replication and Possible Targets of Action of Antiviral Agents

STAGE OF REPLICATION	CLASSES OF SELECTIVE INHIBITORS
Cell entry	
Attachment	Soluble receptor decoys, antireceptor antibodies, fusion protein
Penetration	inhibitors
Uncoating	Ion channel blockers, capsid stabilizers
Release of viral genome	
Transcription of viral genome*	Inhibitors of viral DNA polymerase, RNA polymerase, reverse
Transcription of viral messenger RNA	transcriptase, helicase, primase, or integrase
Replication of viral genome	
Translation of viral proteins	Interferons, antisense oligonucleotides, ribozymes
Regulatory proteins (early)	Inhibitors of regulatory proteins
Structural proteins (late)	
Posttranslational modifications	
Proteolytic cleavage	Protease inhibitors
Myristoylation, glycosylation	
Assembly of virion components	Interferons, assembly protein inhibitors
Release	Neuraminidase inhibitors, antiviral antibodies, cytotoxic
Budding, cell lysis	lymphocytes

*Depends on specific replication strategy of virus, but virus-specified enzyme required for part of process.

2. Effective agents typically have a restricted spectrum of antiviral activity and target a specific viral protein, most often an enzyme involved in viral nucleic acid synthesis (polymerase or transcriptase) or viral protein processing (protease).

3. Single-nucleotide changes leading to critical amino acid substitutions in a target protein often are sufficient to cause antiviral drug resistance. Indeed, the selection of a drug-resistant variant indicates that a drug has a specific mechanism of antiviral action.

4. Current agents inhibit active replication, so viral replication may resume following drug removal. Effective host immune responses remain essential for recovery from infection. Clinical failures of antiviral therapy may occur with drug-sensitive virus in highly immunocompromised patients or following emergence of drug-resistant variants.

5. Most drug-resistant viruses are recovered from immunocompromised patients with high viral replicative loads and repeated or prolonged courses of antiviral treatment. (Influenza A virus is an exception.)

6. Current antiviral agents do not eliminate nonreplicating or latent virus, although some drugs have been used effectively for chronic suppression of disease reactivation.

7. Clinical efficacy depends on achieving inhibitory concentrations at the site of infection, usually within infected cells. For example, nucleoside analogs must be taken up and phosphorylated intracellularly for activity; consequently, concentrations of critical enzymes or competing substrates influence antiviral effects in cells of different types and in different metabolic states.

8. *In vitro* sensitivity tests for antiviral agents are not standardized, except for selected viruses (*e.g.,* herpes simplex virus), and results depend on the assay system, cell type, viral inoculum, and laboratory. Therefore, clear relationships among drug concentrations active *in vitro,* those achieved in blood or other body fluids, and clinical response have not been established for most antiviral agents.

Despite the clinical caveats implicit in these general principles, there are a number of useful antiviral agents and treatment strategies. Table 49–2 summarizes currently approved antiviral drugs. Their pharmacological properties are presented below, class by class, as listed in the table.

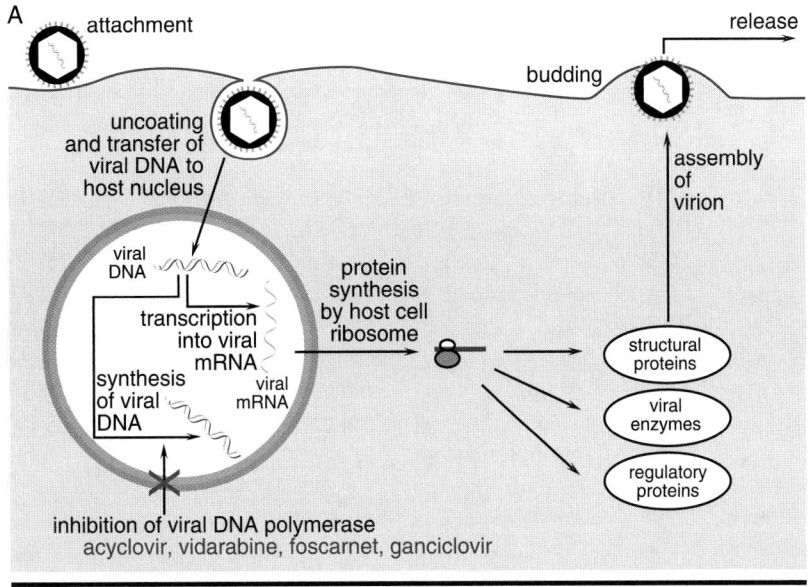

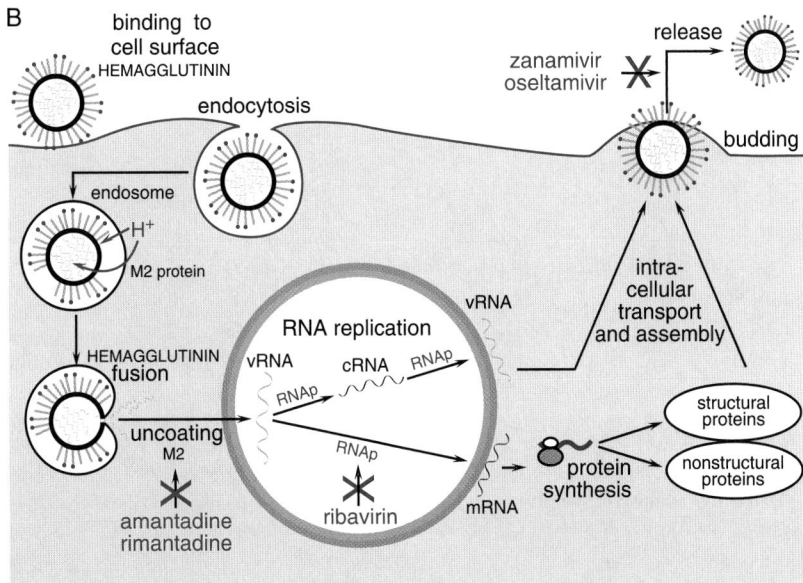

Figure 49–1. *Replicative cycles of DNA (A) and RNA (B) viruses.* The replicative cycles of herpesvirus (*A*) and influenza (*B*) are examples of DNA-encoded and RNA-encoded viruses, respectively. Sites of action of antiviral agents also are shown. Key: mRNA = messenger RNA; cDNA = complementary DNA; vRNA = viral RNA; DNAp = DNA polymerase; RNAp = RNA polymerase; cRNA = complementary RNA. An X on top of an arrow indicates a block to virus growth. *A.* Replicative cycles of herpes simplex virus, a DNA virus, and the probable sites of action of antiviral agents. Herpesvirus replication is a regulated multistep process. After infection, a small number of immediate-early genes are transcribed; these genes encode proteins that regulate their own synthesis and are responsible for synthesis of early genes involved in genome replication, such as thymidine kinases, DNA polymerases, etc. After DNA replication, the bulk of the herpesvirus genes (called *late genes*) are expressed and encode proteins that either are incorporated into or aid in the assembly of progeny virions. *B.* Replicative cycles of influenza, an RNA virus, and the loci for effects of antiviral agents. The mammalian cell shown is an airway epithelial cell. The M2 protein of influenza virus allows an influx of hydrogen ions into the virion interior, which in turn promotes dissociation of the RNP segments and release into the cytoplasm (uncoating). Influenza virus mRNA synthesis requires a primer cleared from cellular mRNA and used by the viral RNAp complex. The neuraminidase inhibitors zanamivir and oseltamivir specifically inhibit release of progeny virus. Small capitals indicate virus proteins.

Table 49–2
Nomenclature of Antiviral Agents

GENERIC NAME	OTHER NAMES	TRADE NAMES (USA)	DOSAGE FORMS AVAILABLE
Antiherpesvirus agents			
Acyclovir	ACV, acycloguanosine	ZOVIRAX	IV, O, T, ophth*
Cidofovir	HPMPC, CDV	VISTIDE	IV
Famciclovir	FCV	FAMVIR	O
Foscarnet	PFA, phosphonoformate	FOSCAVIR	IV, O*
Fomivirsen	ISIS 2922	VITRAVENE	Intravitreal
Ganciclovir	GCV, DHPG	CYTOVENE	IV, O, intravitreal
Idoxuridine	IDUR	HERPES, STOXIL, DENDRID	Ophth
Penciclovir	PCV	DENAVIR	T, IV*
Trifluridine	TFT, trifluorothymidine	VIROPTIC	Ophth
Valacyclovir		VALTREX	O
Valganciclovir		VALCYTE	O
Anti-influenza agents			
Amantadine		SYMMETREL	O
Oseltamivir	GS4104	TAMIFLU	O
Rimantadine		FLUMADINE	O
Zanamivir	GC167	RELENZA	Inhaled
Antihepatitis agents			
Adefovir dipivoxil	Bis-pom-PMEA	HEPSERA	O
Interferon-alfa		INTRON A, ROFERON A, INFERGEN, ALFERON N, WELLFERON*	Injected
Lamivudine	3TC	EPIVIR	O
Pegylated interferon alfa		PEGASYS, PEG-INTRON	SC
Other antiviral agents			
Ribavirin		VIRAZOLE, REBETOL, COPEGUS	O, inhaled, IV
Imiquimod		ALDARA	Topical

*Not currently approved for use in USA. ABBREVIATIONS: IV, intravenous; O, oral; T, topical; ophth, ophthalmic.

ANTIHERPESVIRUS AGENTS

Infection with herpes simplex virus type 1 (HSV-1) typically causes diseases of the mouth, face, skin, esophagus, or brain. Herpes simplex virus type 2 (HSV-2) usually causes infections of the genitals, rectum, skin, hands, or meninges. Both cause serious infections in neonates. HSV infection may be a primary one in a naive host, a nonprimary initial one in a host previously infected by other viruses, or the consequence of activation of a latent infection.

The first systemically administered antiherpesvirus agent, *vidarabine,* was approved by the Food and Drug Administration (FDA) in 1977. However, its toxicities restricted its use to life-threatening infections of HSV and varicella-zoster virus (VZV). The discovery and development of *acyclovir,* approved in 1982, provided the first effective treatment for less severe HSV and VZV infections in ambulatory patients. Intravenous acyclovir is superior to vidarabine in terms of efficacy and toxicity in HSV encephalitis and in VZV infections of immunocompromised patients. Acyclovir is the prototype of a group of antiviral agents that are phosphorylated intracellularly by a viral kinase and subsequently by host cell enzymes to become inhibitors of viral DNA synthesis. Other agents employing this strategy include *penciclovir* and *ganciclovir.*

Acyclovir and Valacyclovir

Chemistry and Antiviral Activity. Acyclovir (9-[(2-hydroxy-ethoxy)methyl]-9H-guanine) is an acyclic guanine nucleoside analog that lacks a 3′-hydroxyl on the side chain. *Valacyclovir* is the L-valyl ester prodrug of acyclovir.

ACYCLOVIR

Acyclovir's clinically useful antiviral spectrum is limited to herpesviruses. *In vitro,* acyclovir is most active against HSV-1 (0.02 to 0.9 μg/ml), approximately half as active against HSV-2 (0.03 to 2.2 μg/ml), a tenth as potent against VZV (0.8 to 4.0 μg/ml) and Epstein-Barr virus (EBV), and least active against cytomegalovirus (CMV) (generally greater than 20 μg/ml) and human herpesvirus (HHV-6) (Wagstaff *et al.,* 1994). Uninfected mammalian cell growth generally is unaffected by high acyclovir concentrations (>50 μg/ml).

Mechanisms of Action and Resistance. Acyclovir inhibits viral DNA synthesis *via* a mechanism outlined in Figure 49–2 (Elion, 1986). Its selectivity of action depends on interaction with two distinct viral proteins: HSV thymidine kinase and DNA polymerase. Cellular uptake and initial phosphorylation are facilitated by HSV thymidine kinase. The affinity of acyclovir for HSV thymidine kinase is about 200 times greater than for the mammalian enzyme. Cellular enzymes convert the monophosphate to acyclovir triphosphate, which is present in forty- to one hundredfold higher concentrations in HSV-infected than in uninfected cells and competes for endogenous deoxyguanosine triphosphate (dGTP). The immunosuppressive agent *mycophenolate mofetil* (*see* Chapter 52) potentiates the antiherpes activity of acyclovir and related agents by depleting intracellular dGTP pools. Acyclovir triphosphate competitively inhibits viral DNA polymerases and, to a much smaller extent, cellular DNA polymerases. Acyclovir triphosphate also is incorporated into viral DNA, where it acts as a chain terminator because of the lack of a 3′-hydroxyl group. By a mechanism termed *suicide inactivation,* the terminated DNA template containing acyclovir binds the viral DNA polymerase and leads to its irreversible inactivation.

Acyclovir resistance in HSV has been linked to one of three mechanisms: absence or partial production of viral thymidine kinase, altered thymidine kinase substrate specificity (*e.g.,* phosphorylation of thymidine but not acyclo-vir), or altered viral DNA polymerase. Alterations in viral enzymes are caused by point mutations and base insertions or deletions in the corresponding genes. Resistant variants are present in native virus populations, and heterogeneous mixtures of viruses occur in isolates from treated patients. The most common resistance mechanism in clinical HSV isolates is absent or deficient viral thymidine kinase activity; viral DNA polymerase mutants are rare. Phenotypic resistance typically is defined by *in vitro* inhibitory concentrations of greater than 2 to 3 μg/ml, which predict failure of therapy in immunocompromised patients.

Acyclovir resistance in VZV isolates is caused by mutations in VZV thymidine kinase and less often by mutations in viral DNA polymerase.

Absorption, Distribution, and Elimination. The oral bioavailability of acyclovir ranges from 10% to 30% and decreases with increasing dose (Wagstaff *et al.,* 1994). Peak plasma concentrations average 0.4 to 0.8 μg/ml after 200-mg doses and 1.6 μg/ml after 800-mg doses. Following intravenous dosing, peak and trough plasma concentrations average 9.8 and 0.7 μg/ml after 5 mg/kg every 8 hours and 20.7 and 2.3 μg/ml after 10 mg/kg every 8 hours, respectively.

Valacyclovir is converted rapidly and virtually completely to acyclovir after oral administration in healthy adults. This conversion is thought to result from first-pass intestinal and hepatic metabolism through enzymatic hydrolysis. Unlike acyclovir, valacyclovir is a substrate for intestinal and renal peptide transporters. The relative oral bioavailability of acyclovir increases three- to fivefold to approximately 70% following valacyclovir administration (Stein-grimsdottir *et al.,* 2000). Peak acyclovir concentrations average 5 to 6 μg/ml following single 1000-mg doses of oral valacyclovir and occur approximately 2 hours after dosing. Peak plasma concentrations of valacyclovir are only 4% of acyclovir levels. Less than 1% of an administered dose of valacyclovir is recovered in the urine, and most is eliminated as acyclovir.

Acyclovir distributes widely in body fluids, including vesicular fluid, aqueous humor, and cerebrospinal fluid. Compared with plasma, salivary concentrations are low, and vaginal secretion concentrations vary widely. Acyclovir is concentrated in breast milk, amniotic fluid, and placenta. Newborn plasma levels are similar to maternal ones. Percutaneous absorption of acyclovir after topical administration is low.

The mean plasma $t_{\frac{1}{2}}$ of elimination of acyclovir is about 2.5 hours, with a range of 1.5 to 6 hours in adults with normal renal function. The elimination $t_{\frac{1}{2}}$ of acyclovir is about 4 hours in neonates and increases to 20 hours in anuric patients (Wagstaff *et al.,* 1994). Renal excretion of unmetabolized acyclovir by glomerular filtration and tubular secretion is the principal route of elimination. Less than 15% is excreted as 9-carboxymethoxymethylguanine or minor metabolites. The pharmacokinetics of oral acyclovir and valacyclovir appear to be similar in pregnant and nonpregnant women (Kimberlin *et al.,* 1998).

Untoward Effects. Acyclovir generally is well tolerated. Topical acyclovir in a polyethylene glycol base may cause mucosal irritation and transient burning when applied to genital lesions.

Oral acyclovir has been associated infrequently with nausea, diarrhea, rash, or headache and very rarely with renal insufficiency

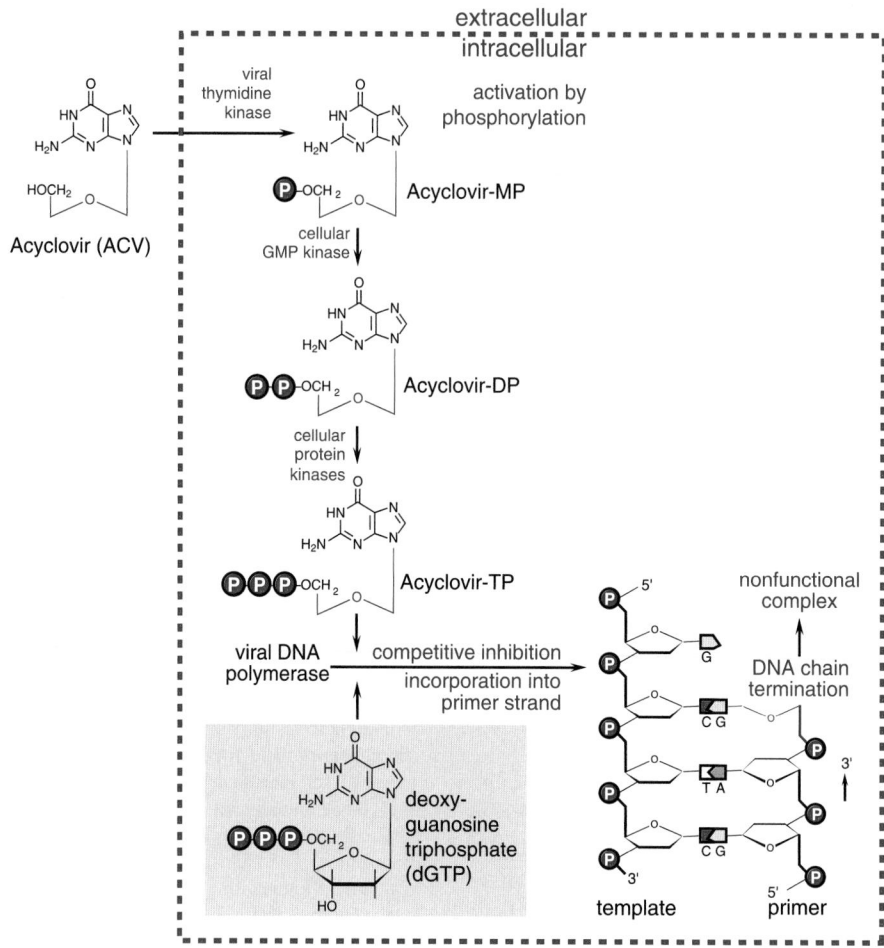

Figure 49–2. *Conversion of acyclovir to acyclovir triphosphate leading to DNA chain termination.* Acyclovir is converted to the monophosphate (MP) derivative by a herpesvirus thymidine kinase. Acyclovir-MP is then phosphorylated to acyclovir-DP and acyclovir-TP by cellular enzymes. Uninfected cells convert very little or no drug to the phosphorylated derivatives. Thus, acyclovir is selectively activated in cells infected with herpesviruses that code for appropriate thymidine kinases. Incorporation of acyclovir-MP from acyclovir-TP into the primer strand during viral DNA replication leads to chain termination and formation of an inactive complex with the viral DNA polymerase. (Adapted from Elion, 1986, with permission.)

or neurotoxicity. Valacyclovir also may be associated with headache, nausea, diarrhea, nephrotoxicity, and central nervous system (CNS) symptoms. High doses of valacyclovir have been associated with confusion and hallucinations, nephrotoxicity, and uncommonly, severe thrombocytopenic syndromes, sometimes fatal, in immunocompromised patients (Feinberg *et al.*, 1998). Acyclovir has been associated with neutropenia in neonates. Chronic acyclovir suppression of genital herpes has been used safely for up to 10 years. No excess frequency of congenital abnormalities has been recognized in infants born to women exposed to acyclovir during pregnancy (Ratanajamit *et al.*, 2003).

The principal dose-limiting toxicities of intravenous acyclovir are renal insufficiency and CNS side effects. Preexisting renal insufficiency, high doses, and high acyclovir plasma levels (>25 μg/ml) are risk factors for both. Reversible renal dysfunction occurs in approximately 5% of patients, probably related to high

urine levels causing crystalline nephropathy. Manifestations include nausea, emesis, flank pain, and increasing azotemia. Rapid infusion, dehydration, and inadequate urine flow increase the risk. Infusions should be given at a constant rate over at least an hour. Nephrotoxicity usually resolves with drug cessation and volume expansion. Neurotoxicity occurs in 1% to 4% of patients and may be manifested by altered sensorium, tremor, myoclonus, delirium, seizures, or extrapyramidal signs. Phlebitis following extravasation, rash, diaphoresis, nausea, hypotension, and interstitial nephritis also have been described. Hemodialysis may be useful in severe cases.

Severe somnolence and lethargy may occur with combinations of *zidovudine* and acyclovir. Concomitant *cyclosporine* and probably other nephrotoxic agents enhance the risk of nephrotoxicity. *Probenecid* decreases the acyclovir renal clearance and prolongs the plasma $t_{\frac{1}{2}}$ of elimination. Acyclovir may decrease the renal clearance of other drugs eliminated by active renal secretion, such as *methotrexate*.

Therapeutic Uses. In immunocompetent persons, the clinical benefits of acyclovir and valacyclovir are greater in initial HSV infections than in recurrent ones, which typically are milder in severity (Whitley and Gnann, 1992). These drugs are particularly useful in immunocompromised patients because these individuals experience both more frequent and more severe HSV and VZV infections. Since VZV is less susceptible than HSV to acyclovir, higher doses must be used for treating varicella or zoster infections than for HSV infections. Oral valacyclovir is as effective as oral acyclovir in HSV infections and more effective for treating herpes zoster.

Herpes Simplex Virus Infections. In initial genital HSV infections, oral acyclovir (200 mg five times daily or 400 mg three times daily for 7 to 10 days) and valacyclovir (1000 mg twice daily for 7 to 10 days) are associated with significant reductions in virus shedding, symptoms, and time to healing (Kimberlin and Rouse, 2004). Intravenous acyclovir (5 mg/kg every 8 hours) has similar effects in patients hospitalized with severe primary genital HSV infections. Topical acyclovir is much less effective than systemic administration. None of these regimens reproducibly reduces the risk of recurrent genital lesions. Patient-initiated acyclovir (200 mg five times daily or 400 mg three times daily for 5 days or 800 mg three times daily for 2 days) or valacyclovir (500 mg twice daily for 3 or 5 days) shortens the manifestations of recurrent genital HSV episodes by 1 to 2 days. Frequently recurring genital herpes can be suppressed effectively with chronic oral acyclovir (400 mg twice daily or 200 mg three times daily) or with valacyclovir (500 mg or, for very frequent recurrences, 1000 mg once daily). During use, the rate of clinical recurrences decreases by about 90%, and subclinical shedding is markedly reduced, although not eliminated. Valacyclovir suppression of genital herpes reduces the risk of transmitting infection to a susceptible partner by about 50% over an 8-month period (Corey *et al.*, 2004). Chronic suppression may be useful in those with disabling recurrences of herpetic whitlow or HSV-related erythema multiforme.

Oral acyclovir is effective in primary herpetic gingivostomatitis (600 mg/m^2 four times daily for 10 days in children) but provides only modest clinical benefit in recurrent orolabial herpes. Short-term, high-dose valacyclovir (2 g twice over one day) shortens the duration of recurrent orolabial herpes by about one day (Anonymous, 2002). Topical acyclovir cream is modestly effective in recurrent labial (Spruance *et al.*, 2002) and genital herpes simplex virus infections. Preexposure acyclovir prophylaxis (400 mg twice daily for one week) reduces the overall risk of recurrence by 73% in those with sun-induced recurrences of HSV infections. Acyclovir during the last month of pregnancy reduces the likelihood of viral shedding and frequency of cesarean section in women with primary or recurrent genital herpes (Sheffield *et al.*, 2003).

In immunocompromised patients with mucocutaneous HSV infection, intravenous acyclovir (250 mg/m^2 every 8 hours for 7 days) shortens healing time, duration of pain, and the period of virus shedding. Oral acyclovir (800 mg five times per day) and valacyclovir (1000 mg twice daily) for 5 to 10 days are also effective. Recurrences

are common after cessation of therapy and may require long-term suppression. In those with very localized labial or facial HSV infections, topical acyclovir may provide some benefit. Intravenous acyclovir may be beneficial in viscerally disseminating HSV in immunocompromised patients and in patients with HSV-infected burn wounds.

Systemic acyclovir prophylaxis is highly effective in preventing mucocutaneous HSV infections in seropositive patients undergoing immunosuppression. Intravenous acyclovir (250 mg/m^2 every 8 to 12 hours) begun prior to transplantation and continuing for several weeks prevents HSV disease in bone marrow transplant recipients. For patients who can tolerate oral medications, oral acyclovir (400 mg five times daily) is effective, and long-term oral acyclovir (200 to 400 mg three times daily for 6 months) also reduces the risk of VZV infection (Steer *et al.*, 2000). In HSV encephalitis, acyclovir (10 mg/kg every 8 hours for a minimum of 10 days) reduces mortality by over 50% and improves overall neurologic outcome compared with vidarabine. Higher doses (15 to 20 mg/kg every 8 hours) and prolonged treatment (up to 21 days) are recommended by many experts. Intravenous acyclovir (20 mg/kg every 8 hours for 21 days) is more effective than lower doses in viscerally invasive neonatal HSV infections (Kimberlin *et al.*, 2001). In neonates and immunosuppressed patients and, rarely, in previously healthy persons, relapses of encephalitis following acyclovir may occur. The value of continuing long-term suppression with valacyclovir after completing intravenous acyclovir is under study.

An ophthalmic formulation of acyclovir (not available in the United States) is at least as effective as topical vidarabine or *trifluridine* in herpetic keratoconjunctivitis.

Infection owing to resistant HSV is rare in immunocompetent persons; however, in immunocompromised hosts, acyclovir-resistant HSV isolates can cause extensive mucocutaneous disease and, rarely, meningoencephalitis, pneumonitis, or visceral disease. Resistant HSV can be recovered from 6% to 17% of immunocompromised patients receiving acyclovir treatment (Bacon *et al.*, 2003). Recurrences after cessation of acyclovir usually are due to sensitive virus but may be due to acyclovir-resistant virus in AIDS patients. In patients with progressive disease, intravenous *foscarnet* therapy is effective, but vidarabine is not (Chilukuri and Rosen, 2003).

Varicella-Zoster Virus Infections. If begun within 24 hours of rash onset, oral acyclovir has therapeutic effects in varicella of children and adults. In children weighing up to 40 kg, acyclovir (20 mg/kg, up to 800 mg per dose, four times daily for 5 days) reduces fever and new lesion formation by about one day. Routine use in uncomplicated pediatric varicella is not recommended but should be considered in those at risk of moderate-to-severe illness (persons over 12 years old, secondary household cases, those with chronic cutaneous or pulmonary disorders, or those receiving *corticosteroids* or long-term *salicylates*) (Committee on Infectious Diseases American Academy of Pediatrics, 2003). In adults treated within 24 hours, oral acyclovir (800 mg five times daily for 7 days) reduces the time to crusting of lesions by approximately 2 days, the maximum number of lesions by one-half, and the duration of fever (Wallace *et al.*, 1992). Intravenous acyclovir appears to be effective in varicella pneumonia or encephalitis of previously healthy adults. Oral acyclovir (10 mg/kg four times daily) given between 7 and 14 days after exposure may reduce the risk of varicella.

In older adults with localized herpes zoster, oral acyclovir (800 mg five times daily for 7 days) reduces pain and healing times if treatment can be initiated within 72 hours of rash onset. A reduction in ocular complications, particularly keratitis and anterior uveitis, occurs with treatment of zoster ophthalmicus. Prolonged acyclovir and concurrent *prednisone* for 21 days speed zoster healing and improve quality-of-life measures compared with each therapy alone. Valacyclovir (1000 mg three times daily for 7 days) provides more prompt relief of zoster-associated pain than acyclovir in older adults (≥50 years) with zoster (Beutner *et al.*, 1995).

In immunocompromised patients with herpes zoster, intravenous acyclovir (500 mg/m² every 8 hours for 7 days) reduces viral shedding, healing time, and the risks of cutaneous dissemination and visceral complications, as well as the length of hospitalization, in disseminating zoster. In immunosuppressed children with varicella, intravenous acyclovir decreases healing time and the risk of visceral complications.

Acyclovir-resistant VZV isolates uncommonly have been recovered from HIV-infected children and adults who may manifest chronic hyperkeratotic or verrucous lesions and sometimes meningoradiculitis. Intravenous foscarnet also appears to be effective for acyclovir-resistant VZV infections.

Other Viruses. Acyclovir is ineffective therapeutically in established cytomegalovirus (CMV) infections but has been used for CMV prophylaxis in immunocompromised patients. High-dose intravenous acyclovir (500 mg/m² every 8 hours for one month) in CMV-seropositive bone marrow transplant recipients is associated with about 50% lower risk of CMV disease and, when combined with prolonged oral acyclovir (800 mg four times daily through 6 months), improves survival (Prentice *et al.*, 1994). Following engraftment, valacyclovir (2000 mg four times daily to day 100) appears as effective as intravenous ganciclovir prophylaxis in such patients (Winston *et al.*, 2003). High-dose oral acyclovir or valacyclovir (2000 mg four times daily) suppression for 3 months may reduce the risk of CMV disease and its sequelae in certain solid-organ transplant recipients (Lowance *et al.*, 1999), but oral *valganciclovir* is the preferred agent for mismatched graft recipients (Pereyra and Rubin, 2004). Compared with acyclovir, high-dose valacyclovir reduces CMV disease in advanced HIV infection but is associated with greater toxicity and possibly shorter survival (Feinberg *et al.*, 1998).

In infectious mononucleosis, acyclovir is associated with transient antiviral effects but no clinical benefits. EBV-related oral hairy leukoplakia may improve with acyclovir. Oral acyclovir in conjunction with systemic corticosteroids appears beneficial in treating Bell's palsy, but valacyclovir is ineffective in acute vestibular neuritis.

Cidofovir

Chemistry and Antiviral Activity. Cidofovir (1-[(S)-3-hydroxy-2-(phosphonomethoxy)-propyl]cytosine dihydrate) is a cytidine nucleotide analog with inhibitory activity against human herpes, papilloma, polyoma, pox, and adenoviruses (Hitchcock *et al.*, 1996).

CIDOFOVIR

In vitro inhibitory concentrations range from greater than 0.2 to 0.7 µg/ml for CMV, 0.4 to 33 µg/ml for HSV, and 0.02 to 17 µg/ml for adenoviruses. Because cidofovir is a phosphonate that is phosphorylated by cellular but not virus enzymes, it inhibits acyclovir-resistant thymidine kinase (TK)–deficient or TK-altered HSV or VZV strains, ganciclovir-resistant CMV strains with UL97 mutations but not those with DNA polymerase mutations, and some foscarnet-resistant CMV strains. Cidofovir synergistically inhibits CMV replication in combination with ganciclovir or foscarnet. Ether lipid esters of cidofovir are orally active in animal models of poxvirus and CMV infections (Kern *et al.*, 2004).

Mechanisms of Action and Resistance. Cidofovir inhibits viral DNA synthesis by slowing and eventually terminating chain elongation. Cidofovir is metabolized to its active diphosphate form by cellular enzymes; the levels of phosphorylated metabolites are similar in infected and uninfected cells. The diphosphate acts as both a competitive inhibitor with respect to dCTP and as an alternative substrate for viral DNA polymerase. The diphosphate has a prolonged intracellular half-life and competitively inhibits its CMV and HSV DNA polymerases at concentrations one-eighth to one six-hundredth of those required to inhibit human DNA polymerases (Hitchcock *et al.*, 1996). A phosphocholine metabolite has a prolonged intracellular half-life (~87 hours) and may serve as an intracellular reservoir of drug. The prolonged intracellular half-life of cidofovir diphosphate allows infrequent dosing regimens, and single doses are effective in experimental HSV, varicella, and poxvirus infections.

Cidofovir resistance in CMV is due to mutations in viral DNA polymerase. Low-level resistance to cidofovir develops in up to about 30% of retinitis patients by 3 months of therapy. Highly ganciclovir-resistant CMV isolates that possess DNA polymerase and UL97 kinase mutations are resistant to cidofovir, and prior ganciclovir therapy may select for cidofovir resistance. Some foscarnet-resistant CMV isolates show cross-resistance to cidofovir, and triple-drug-resistant variants with DNA polymerase mutations occur.

Absorption, Distribution, and Elimination. Cidofovir is dianionic at physiological pH and has very low oral bioavailability (Cundy, 1999). The plasma levels after intravenous dosing decline in a biphasic pattern with a terminal half-life that averages about 2.6 hours. The volume of distribution approximates total-body water. Penetration into the CNS or eye has not been well characterized, but cerebrospinal fluid (CSF) levels are low. Extemporaneously compounded topical cidofovir gel may result in low plasma concentrations (<0.5 µg/ml) in patients with large mucocutaneous lesions.

Cidofovir is cleared by the kidney *via* glomerular filtration and tubular secretion. Over 90% of the dose is recovered unchanged in the urine without significant metabolism in human beings. The probenecid-sensitive organic anion transporter 1 mediates uptake of cidofovir into proximal renal tubular epithelial cells (Ho *et al.*, 2000). High-dose probenecid (2 g 3 hours before and 1 g 2 and 8 hours after each infusion) blocks tubular transport of cidofovir and reduces renal clearance and associated nephrotoxicity. At cidofovir doses of 5 mg/kg, peak plasma concentrations increase from 11.5 to 19.6 μg/ml with probenecid, and renal clearance is reduced to the level of glomerular filtration. Elimination relates linearly to creatinine clearance, and the half-life increases to 32.5 hours in patients on chronic ambulatory peritoneal dialysis (CAPD). Both CAPD and hemodialysis remove over 50% of the administered dose (Cundy, 1999).

Untoward Effects. Nephrotoxicity is the principal dose-limiting side effect of intravenous cidofovir. Proximal tubular dysfunction includes proteinuria, azotemia, glycosuria, metabolic acidosis, and uncommonly, Fanconi's syndrome. Concomitant oral probenecid (*see* above) and saline prehydration reduce the risk of renal toxicity. On maintenance doses of 5 mg/kg every 2 weeks, up to 50% of patients develop proteinuria, 10% to 15% show an elevated serum creatinine concentration, and 15% to 20% develop neutropenia. Anterior uveitis that is responsive to topical corticosteroids and cycloplegia occurs commonly and ocular hypotony occurs infrequently with intravenous cidofovir. Concurrent probenecid administration is associated with gastrointestinal upset, constitutional symptoms, and hypersensitivity reactions, including fever, rash, and uncommonly, anaphylactoid manifestations. Administration with food and pretreatment with *antiemetics, antihistamines,* and/or *acetaminophen* may improve tolerance.

Probenecid but not cidofovir alters zidovudine pharmacokinetics such that zidovudine doses should be reduced when probenecid is present, as should the doses of drugs similarly affected by probenecid [*e.g., β-lactam antibiotics, nonsteroidal antiinflammatory drugs* (NSAIDs), *acyclovir, lorazepam, furosemide,* methotrexate, *theophylline,* and *rifampin*]. Concurrent nephrotoxic agents are contraindicated, and an interval of at least 7 days before beginning cidofovir treatment is recommended after prior exposure to an *aminoglycoside,* intravenous *pentamidine, amphotericin B,* foscarnet, NSAID, or contrast dye. Cidofovir and oral ganciclovir are poorly tolerated in combination at full doses.

Topical application of cidofovir is associated with dose-related application-site reactions (*e.g.,* burning, pain, and pruritus) in up to one-third of patients and occasionally ulceration. Intravitreal cidofovir may cause vitreitis, hypotony, and visual loss and is contraindicated.

Preclinical studies indicate that cidofovir has mutagenic, gonadotoxic, embryotoxic, and teratogenic effects. Because cidofovir is carcinogenic in rats, it is considered a potential human carcinogen. It may cause infertility and is classified as pregnancy category C.

Therapeutic Uses. Intravenous cidofovir is approved for the treatment of CMV retinitis in HIV-infected patients. Intravenous cidofovir (5 mg/kg once a week for 2 weeks followed by dosing every 2 weeks) increases the time to progression of CMV retinitis in previously untreated patients and in those failing or intolerant of ganciclovir and foscarnet therapy. CMV viremia may persist during cido-

fovir administration. Maintenance doses of 5 mg/kg are more effective but less well tolerated than 3 mg/kg doses. Intravenous cidofovir has been used for treating acyclovir-resistant mucocutaneous HSV infection, adenovirus disease in transplant recipients (Ljungman *et al.*, 2003), and progressive multifocal leukoencephalopathy or extensive molluscum contagiosum in HIV patients. Reduced doses (0.25 to 1 mg/kg every 2 to 3 weeks) without probenecid may be beneficial in BK virus nephropathy in renal transplant patients (Vats *et al.*, 2003).

Extemporaneously compounded topical cidofovir gel eliminates virus shedding and lesions in some HIV-infected patients with acyclovir-resistant mucocutaneous HSV infections and has been used in treating anogenital warts and molluscum contagiosum in immunocompromised patients and cervical intraepithelial neoplasia in women. Intralesional cidofovir induces remissions in adults and children with respiratory papillomatosis.

Docosanol

Docosanol is a long-chain saturated alcohol that has been approved by the FDA as a 10% over-the-counter cream for the treatment of recurrent orolabial herpes. Docosanol inhibits the *in vitro* replication of many lipid-enveloped viruses, including HSV, at millimolar concentrations. It does not inactivate HSV directly but appears to block fusion between the cellular and viral envelope membranes and inhibit viral entry into the cell. Topical treatment beginning within 12 hours of prodromal symptoms or lesion onset reduces healing time by about one day and appears to be well tolerated (Anonymous, 2000). Treatment initiation at papular or later stages provides no benefit.

Famciclovir and Penciclovir

Chemistry and Antiviral Activity. Famciclovir is the diacetyl ester prodrug of 6-deoxy penciclovir and lacks intrinsic antiviral activity. *Penciclovir* (9-[4-hydroxy-3-hydroxymethylbut-1-yl] guanine) is an acyclic guanine nucleoside analog. The side chain differs structurally in that the oxygen has been replaced by a carbon, and an additional hydroxymethyl group is present. The structure of penciclovir is

PENCICLOVIR

Penciclovir is similar to acyclovir in its spectrum of activity and potency against HSV and VZV (Safrin *et al.*, 1997). The inhibitory concentrations of penciclovir depend on cell type but are usually within twofold of those of acyclovir for HSV and VZV. It also is inhibitory for HBV.

Mechanisms of Action and Resistance. Penciclovir is an inhibitor of viral DNA synthesis. In HSV- or VZV-infected cells, penciclovir is phosphorylated initially by viral thymidine kinase. Penciclovir triphosphate serves as a competitive inhibitor of viral DNA polymerase (Safrin *et al.*, 1997) (Figure 49–2). Although penciclovir triphosphate is approximately one one-hundredth times as potent as acyclovir triphosphate in inhibiting viral DNA polymerase, it is present in much higher concentrations and for more prolonged periods in infected cells than acyclovir triphosphate. The prolonged intracellular $t_{\frac{1}{2}}$ of penciclovir triphosphate, 7 to 20 hours, is associated with prolonged antiviral effects. Because penciclovir has a 3′-hydroxyl group, it is not an obligate chain terminator but does inhibit DNA elongation.

Resistant variants owing to thymidine kinase or DNA polymerase mutations can be selected by passage *in vitro*, but the occurrence of resistance during clinical use is currently low (Bacon *et al.*, 2003). Thymidine kinase–deficient, acyclovir-resistant herpes viruses are cross-resistant to penciclovir.

Absorption, Distribution, and Elimination. Oral penciclovir has low (5%) bioavailability. In contrast, famciclovir is well absorbed orally and converted rapidly to penciclovir by deacetylation of the side chain and oxidation of the purine ring during and following absorption from the intestine (Gill and Wood, 1996). The bioavailability of penciclovir is 65% to 77% following oral administration of famciclovir. Food slows absorption but does not reduce overall bioavailability. After single 250- or 500-mg doses of famciclovir, the peak plasma concentration of penciclovir averages 1.6 and 3.3 μg/ml, respectively. A small quantity of the 6-deoxy precursor but no famciclovir is detectable in plasma. After intravenous infusion of penciclovir at 10 mg/kg, peak plasma levels average 12 μg/ml. The volume of distribution is about twice the volume of total-body water. The plasma $t_{\frac{1}{2}}$ of elimination of penciclovir averages about 2 hours, and over 90% is excreted unchanged in the urine, probably by both filtration and active tubular secretion. Following oral famciclovir administration, nonrenal clearance accounts for about 10% of each dose, primarily through fecal excretion, but penciclovir (60% of dose) and its 6-deoxy precursor (<10% of dose) are eliminated primarily in the urine. The plasma half-life averages 9.9 hours in renal insufficiency (Cl_{cr} < 30 ml/min); hemodialysis efficiently removes penciclovir. Lower peak plasma concentrations of penciclovir but no reduction in overall bioavailability occur in compensated chronic hepatic insufficiency (Boike *et al.*, 1994).

Untoward Effects. Oral famciclovir is well tolerated but may be associated with headache, diarrhea, and nausea. Urticaria, rash, and hallucinations or confusional states (predominantly in the elderly) have been reported. Topical penciclovir, which is formulated in 40% propylene glycol and a cetomacrogol base, is associated infrequently with application-site reactions (~1%). The short-term tolerance of famciclovir is comparable with that of acyclovir.

Penciclovir is mutagenic at high concentrations *in vitro*. Although studies in laboratory animals indicate that chronic famciclovir administration is tumorigenic and decreases spermatogenesis and fertility in rodents and dogs, long-term administration (1 year) does not affect spermatogenesis in men. No teratogenic effects have been observed in animals, but safety during pregnancy has not been established.

No clinically important drug interactions have been identified to date with famciclovir or penciclovir (Gill and Wood, 1996).

Therapeutic Uses. Oral famciclovir, topical penciclovir, and intravenous penciclovir are approved for managing HSV and VZV infections in various countries (Sacks and Wilson, 1999). Oral famciclovir (250 mg three times a day for 7 to 10 days) is as effective as acyclovir in treating first-episode genital herpes (Kimberlin and Rouse, 2004). In patients with recurrent genital HSV, patient-initiated famciclovir treatment (125 or 250 mg twice a day for 5 days) reduces healing time and symptoms by about one day. Famciclovir (250 mg twice a day for up to 1 year) is effective for suppression of recurrent genital HSV, but single daily doses are less effective. Higher doses (500 mg twice a day) reduce HSV recurrences in HIV-infected persons. Intravenous penciclovir (5 mg/kg every 8 or 12 hours for 7 days) is comparable with intravenous acyclovir for treating mucocutaneous HSV infections in immunocompromised hosts (Lazarus *et al.*, 1999). In immunocompetent persons with recurrent orolabial HSV, topical 1% penciclovir cream (applied every 2 hours while awake for 4 days) shortens healing time and symptoms by about one day (Raborn *et al.*, 2002).

In immunocompetent adults with herpes zoster of 3 days' duration or less, famciclovir (500 mg three times a day for 10 days) is at least as effective as acyclovir (800 mg five times daily) in reducing healing time and zoster-associated pain, particularly in those 50 years of age and older. Famciclovir is comparable with valacyclovir in treating zoster and reducing associated pain in older adults (Tyring *et al.*, 2000). Famciclovir (500 mg three times a day for 7 to 10 days) also is comparable with high-dose oral acyclovir in treating zoster in immunocompromised patients and in those with ophthalmic zoster (Tyring *et al.*, 2001).

Famciclovir is associated with dose-related reductions in HBV DNA and transaminase levels in patients with chronic HBV hepatitis but is less effective than *lamivudine* (Lai *et al.*, 2002). Famciclovir is also ineffective in treating lamivudine-resistant HBV infections owing to emergence of multiply resistant variants.

Fomivirsen

Fomivirsen, a 21-base phosphorothioate oligionucleotide, is the first FDA-approved antisense therapy for viral infections. It is complementary to the messenger RNA sequence for the major immediate-early transcriptional region of CMV and inhibits CMV replication through sequence-specific and nonspecific mechanisms, including inhibition of virus binding to cells. Fomivirsen is active against CMV strains resistant to ganciclovir, foscarnet, and cidofovir. CMV variants with tenfold reduced susceptibility to fomivirsen have been selected by *in vitro* passage.

Fomivirsen is given by intravitreal injection in the treatment of CMV retinitis for patients intolerant of or unresponsive to other therapies. Following injection, it is cleared slowly from the vitreous ($t_{\frac{1}{2}}$ of approximately 55 hours) through distribution to the retina and probable exonuclease digestion (Geary *et al.*, 2002). Local metabolism by exonucleases accounts for elimination. In HIV-infected patients with refractory, sight-threatening CMV retinitis, fomivirsen injections (330 μg weekly for 3 weeks and then every 2 weeks or on days 1 and 15 followed by monthly) significantly delay time to retinitis progression (Vitravene Study Group, 2002). Ocular side effects include iritis in up to one-quarter of patients, which can be managed with topical corticosteroids; vitritis; cataracts; and increases in intraocular pressure in 15% to 20% of patients. Recent cidofovir use may increase the risk of inflammatory reactions.

Foscarnet

Chemistry and Antiviral Activity. Foscarnet (trisodium phosphonoformate) is an inorganic pyrophosphate analog that is inhibitory for all herpesviruses and HIV (Wagstaff and Bryson, 1994).

$$\overset{\overset{\displaystyle O}{\|}}{(NaO)_2PCOONa}$$

FOSCARNET SODIUM

In vitro inhibitory concentrations are generally 100 to 300 μM for CMV and 80 to 200 μM for other herpesviruses, including most ganciclovir-resistant CMV and acyclovir-resistant HSV and VZV strains. Combinations of foscarnet and ganciclovir synergistically inhibit CMV replication *in vitro*. Concentrations of 500 to 1000 μM reversibly inhibit the proliferation and DNA synthesis of uninfected cells.

Mechanisms of Action and Resistance. Foscarnet inhibits viral nucleic acid synthesis by interacting directly with herpesvirus DNA polymerase or HIV reverse transcriptase (Chrisp and Clissold, 1991) (Figure 49–1B). It is taken up slowly by cells and does not undergo significant intracellular metabolism. Foscarnet reversibly blocks the pyrophosphate binding site of the viral polymerase in a noncompetitive manner and inhibits cleavage of pyrophosphate from deoxynucleotide triphosphates. Foscarnet has approximately one hundredfold greater inhibitory effects against herpesvirus DNA polymerases than against cellular DNA polymerase α.

Herpesviruses resistant to foscarnet have point mutations in the viral DNA polymerase and are associated with three- to sevenfold reductions in foscarnet activity *in vitro*.

Absorption, Distribution, and Elimination. Oral bioavailability of foscarnet is low. Following an intravenous infusion of 60 mg/kg every 8 hours, peak and trough plasma concentrations are approximately 450 to 575 and 80 to 150 μM, respectively. Vitreous levels approximate those in plasma, and CSF levels average 66% of those in plasma at steady state.

Over 80% of foscarnet is excreted unchanged in the urine by glomerular filtration and probably tubular secretion. Plasma clearance decreases proportionally with creatinine clearance, and dose adjustments are indicated for small decreases in renal function. Plasma elimination is complex, with initial bimodal half-lives totaling 4 to 8 hours and a prolonged terminal $t_{\frac{1}{2}}$ for elimination averaging 3 to 4 days. Sequestration in bone with gradual release accounts for the fate of an estimated 10% to 20% of a given dose. Foscarnet is cleared efficiently by hemodialysis (~50% of a dose).

Untoward Effects. Foscarnet's major dose-limiting toxicities are nephrotoxicity and symptomatic hypocalcemia. Increases in serum creatinine occur in up to one-half of patients but are reversible after cessation in most patients. High doses, rapid infusion, dehydration, prior renal insufficiency, and concurrent nephrotoxic drugs are risk factors. Acute tubular necrosis, crystalline glomerulopathy, nephrogenic diabetes insipidus, and interstitial nephritis have been described. Saline loading may reduce the risk of nephrotoxicity.

Foscarnet is highly ionized at physiological pH, and metabolic abnormalities are very common. These include increases or decreases in Ca^{2+} and phosphate, hypomagnesemia, and hypokalemia. Decreased serum ionized Ca^{2+} may cause paresthesia, arrhythmias, tetany, seizures, and other CNS disturbances. Concomitant intravenous *pentamidine* administration increases the risk of symptomatic hypocalcemia. Parenteral *magnesium sulfate* does not alter foscarnet-induced hypocalcemia or symptoms (Huycke *et al.*, 2000).

CNS side effects include headache in approximately 25% of patients, tremor, irritability, seizures, and hallucinosis. Other reported side effects are generalized rash, fever, nausea or emesis, anemia, leukopenia, abnormal liver function tests, electrocardiographic changes, infusion-related thrombophlebitis, and painful genital ulcerations. Topical foscarnet may cause local irritation and ulceration, and oral foscarnet may cause gastrointestinal disturbance. Preclinical studies indicate that high foscarnet concentrations are mutagenic and may cause tooth and skeletal abnormalities in developing laboratory animals. Safety in pregnancy or childhood is uncertain.

Therapeutic Uses. Intravenous foscarnet is effective for treatment of CMV retinitis, including ganciclovir-resistant infections, other types of CMV infection, and acyclovir-resistant HSV and VZV infections (Wagstaff and Bryson, 1994). Foscarnet is poorly soluble in aqueous solutions and requires large volumes for administration.

In CMV retinitis in AIDS patients, foscarnet (60 mg/kg every 8 hours or 90 mg/kg every 12 hours for 14 to 21 days followed by chronic maintenance at 90 to 120 mg/kg every day in one dose) is associated with clinical stabilization in about 90% of patients (Wagstaff and Bryson, 1994). A comparative trial of foscarnet with ganciclovir found comparable control of CMV retinitis in AIDS patients but improved overall survival in the foscarnet-treated group (Anonymous, 1992). This improved survival with foscarnet may be related to the drug's intrinsic anti-HIV activity, but patients stop taking foscarnet over three times as often as ganciclovir because of side effects. A combination of foscarnet and ganciclovir is more effective than either drug alone in refractory retinitis; combinations may be useful in treating ganciclovir-resistant CMV infections in solid-organ transplant patients. Foscarnet benefits other CMV syndromes in AIDS or transplant patients but is ineffective as monotherapy in treating CMV pneumonia in bone marrow transplant patients. When used for preemptive therapy of CMV viremia in bone marrow transplant recipients, foscarnet (60 mg/kg every 12 hours for 2 weeks followed by 90 mg/kg daily for 2 weeks) is as effective as intravenous ganciclovir and causes less neutropenia (Reusser *et al.*, 2002). When used for CMV infections, foscarnet may reduce the risk of Kaposi's sarcoma in HIV-infected patients. Intravitreal injections of foscarnet also have been used.

In acyclovir-resistant mucocutaneous HSV infections, lower doses of foscarnet (40 mg/kg every 8 hours for 7 days or longer) are associated with cessation of viral shedding and with complete healing of lesions in about three-quarters of patients. Foscarnet also appears to be effective in acyclovir-resistant VZV infections. Topical foscarnet cream is ineffective in treating recurrent genital HSV in immunocompetent persons but appears to be useful in chronic acyclovir-resistant infections in immunocompromised patients.

Resistant clinical isolates of herpesviruses have emerged during therapeutic use and may be associated with poor clinical response to foscarnet treatment.

Ganciclovir and Valganciclovir

Chemistry and Antiviral Activity. Ganciclovir (9-[1,3-dihydroxy-2-propoxymethyl] guanine) is an acyclic guanine nucleoside analog that is similar in structure to acyclovir except in having an additional hydroxymethyl group on the acyclic side chain. Valganciclovir is the L-valyl ester prodrug of ganciclovir. The structure of ganciclovir is

GANCICLOVIR

This agent has inhibitory activity against all herpesviruses but is especially active against CMV (Noble and Faulds, 1998). Inhibitory concentrations are similar to those of acyclovir for HSV and VZV but 10 to 100 times lower for human CMV strains (0.2 to 2.8 μg/ml).

Inhibitory concentrations for human bone marrow progenitor cells are similar to those inhibitory for CMV replication, a finding predictive of ganciclovir's myelotoxicity during clinical use. Inhibition of human lymphocyte blastogenic responses also occurs at clinically achievable concentrations of 1 to 10 μg/ml.

Mechanisms of Action and Resistance. Ganciclovir inhibits viral DNA synthesis. It is monophosphorylated intracellularly by viral thymidine kinase during HSV infection and by a viral phosphotransferase encoded by the UL97 gene during CMV infection. Ganciclovir diphosphate and ganciclovir triphosphate are formed by cellular enzymes. At least tenfold higher concentrations of ganciclovir triphosphate are present in CMV-infected than in uninfected cells. The triphosphate is a competitive inhibitor of deoxyguanosine triphosphate incorporation into DNA and preferentially inhibits viral rather than host cellular DNA polymerases. Ganciclovir is incorporated into both viral and cellular DNA. Incorporation into viral DNA causes eventual cessation of DNA chain elongation (Figures 49–1B and 49–2).

Intracellular ganciclovir triphosphate concentrations are tenfold higher than those of acyclovir triphosphate and decline much more slowly with an intracellular $t_{\frac{1}{2}}$ of elimination exceeding 24 hours. These differences may account in part for ganciclovir's greater anti-CMV activity and provide the rationale for single daily doses in suppressing human CMV infections.

CMV can become resistant to ganciclovir by one of two mechanisms: reduced intracellular ganciclovir phosphorylation owing to mutations in the viral phosphotransferase encoded by the UL97 gene and mutations in viral DNA polymerase (Gilbert *et al.*, 2002). Resistant CMV clinical isolates have 4 to more than 20 times increases in inhibitory concentrations. Resistance has been associated primarily with impaired phosphorylation but sometimes only with DNA polymerase mutations. Highly resistant variants with dual UL97 and polymerase mutations are cross-resistant to cidofovir and variably to foscarnet. Ganciclovir also is much less active against acyclovir-resistant thymidine kinase–deficient HSV strains.

Absorption, Distribution, and Elimination. The oral bioavailability of ganciclovir averages 6% to 9% following ingestion with food. Peak and trough plasma levels are about 0.5 to 1.2 and 0.2 to 0.5 μg/ml, respectively, after 1000-mg doses every 8 hours. Oral valganciclovir is well absorbed and hydrolyzed rapidly to ganciclovir; the bioavailability of ganciclovir averages 61% following valganciclovir (Curran and Noble, 2001). Food increases the bioavailability of valganciclovir by about 25%, and peak ganciclovir concentrations average 6.1 $\mu g/ml$ after 875-mg doses. High oral valganciclovir doses in the fed state provide ganciclovir exposures comparable with intravenous dosing (Brown *et al.*, 1999). Following intravenous administration of 5 mg/kg doses of ganciclovir, peak and trough plasma concentrations average 8 to 11 and 0.6 to 1.2 $\mu g/ml$, respectively. Following intravenous dosing, vitreous fluid levels are similar to or higher than those in plasma and average about 1 $\mu g/ml$. Vitreous levels decline with a half-life of 23 to 26 hours. Intraocular sustained-release ganciclovir implants provide vitreous levels of about 4.1 $\mu g/ml$.

The plasma half-life is about 2 to 4 hours in patients with normal renal function. Over 90% of ganciclovir is eliminated unchanged by renal excretion through glomerular filtration and tubular secretion. Consequently, the plasma $t_{\frac{1}{2}}$ increases almost linearly as creatinine clearance declines and may reach 28 to 40 hours in those with severe renal insufficiency.

Untoward Effects. Myelosuppression is the principal dose-limiting toxicity of ganciclovir. Neutropenia occurs in about 15% to 40% of patients and thrombocytopenia in 5% to 20% (Faulds and Heel, 1990). Neutropenia is observed most commonly during the second week of treatment and usually is reversible within 1 week of drug cessation. Persistent fatal neutropenia has occurred. Oral valganciclovir is associated with headache and gastrointestinal disturbance (*i.e.,* nausea, pain, and diarrhea) in addition to the toxicities associated with intravenous ganciclovir, including neutropenia. Recombinant *granulocyte colony-stimulating factor* (G-CSF, *filgrastim, lenograstim*) may be useful in treating ganciclovir-induced neutropenia (*see* Chapter 53).

CNS side effects occur in 5% to 15% of patients and range in severity from headache to behavioral changes to convulsions and coma. About one-third of patients have had to interrupt or prematurely stop intravenous ganciclovir therapy because of bone marrow or CNS toxicity. Infusion-related phlebitis, azotemia, anemia, rash, fever, liver function test abnormalities, nausea or vomiting, and eosinophilia also have been described.

Teratogenicity, embryotoxicity, irreversible reproductive toxicity, and myelotoxicity have been observed in animals at ganciclovir dosages comparable with those used in human beings. Ganciclovir is classified in pregnancy category C.

Zidovudine and probably other cytotoxic agents increase the risk of myelosuppression, as do nephrotoxic agents that impair ganciclovir excretion. Probenecid and possibly acyclovir reduce renal clearance of ganciclovir. *Zalcitabine* increases oral ganciclovir exposure by an average of 22%. Oral ganciclovir increases the absorption and peak plasma concentrations of *didanosine* by approximately twofold and that of zidovudine by about 20%.

Therapeutic Uses. Ganciclovir is effective for treatment and chronic suppression of CMV retinitis in immunocompromised patients and for prevention of CMV disease in transplant patients. In CMV retinitis, initial induction treatment (5 mg/kg intravenously every 12 hours for 10 to 21 days) is associated with improvement or stabilization in about 85% of patients (Faulds and Heel, 1990). Reduced viral excretion is usually evident by 1 week, and funduscopic improvement is seen by 2 weeks. Because of the high risk of relapse, AIDS patients with retinitis require suppressive therapy with high doses of ganciclovir (30 to 35 mg/ kg per week). Oral ganciclovir (1000 mg three times daily) is effective for suppression of retinitis after initial intravenous treat-

ment. Oral valganciclovir (900 mg twice daily for 21 days initial treatment) is comparable with intravenous dosing for initial control and sustained suppression (900 mg daily) of CMV retinitis (Martin *et al.*, 2002).

Intravitreal ganciclovir injections have been used in some patients, and an intraocular sustained-release ganciclovir implant (VITRASERT) is more effective than systemic dosing in suppressing retinitis progression.

Ganciclovir therapy (5 mg/kg every 12 hours for 14 to 21 days) may benefit other CMV syndromes in AIDS patients or solid-organ transplant recipients (Infectious Disease Community of Practice *et al.*, 2004). Response rates of 67% or higher have been found in combination with a decrease in immunosuppressive therapy. The duration of therapy depends on demonstrating clearance of viremia; early switch from intravenous ganciclovir to oral valganciclovir is feasible. Recurrent CMV disease occurs commonly after initial treatment. In bone marrow transplant recipients with CMV pneumonia, ganciclovir alone appears ineffective. However, ganciclovir combined with intravenous immunoglobulin or CMV immunoglobulin reduces the mortality of CMV pneumonia by about one-half. Ganciclovir treatment may benefit infants with congenital CMV disease (Michaels *et al.*, 2003), and further studies are in progress.

Ganciclovir has been used for both prophylaxis and preemptive therapy of CMV infections in transplant recipients (Pillay, 2000; Pereyra and Rubin, 2004). In bone marrow transplant recipients, preemptive ganciclovir treatment (5 mg/kg every 12 hours for 7 to 14 days followed by 5 mg/kg every day to days 100 to 120 after transplant) starting when CMV is isolated from bronchoalveolar lavage or from other sites is highly effective in preventing CMV pneumonia and appears to reduce mortality in these patients. Initiation of ganciclovir at the time of engraftment also reduces CMV disease rates but does not improve survival in part because of infections owing to ganciclovir-related neutropenia.

Intravenous ganciclovir, oral ganciclovir, and oral valganciclovir reduce the risk of CMV disease in solid-organ transplant recipients (Pereyra and Rubin, 2004; Infectious Disease Community of Practice *et al.*, 2004). Oral ganciclovir (1000 mg three times daily for 3 months) reduces CMV disease risk in liver transplant recipients, including high-risk patients with primary infection or those receiving antilymphocyte antibodies. Oral valganciclovir prophylaxis generally is more effective than high-dose oral acyclovir. Oral valganciclovir (900 mg once daily) provides somewhat greater antiviral effects and similar reductions in CMV disease as oral ganciclovir in mismatched solid-organ transplant recipients (Paya *et al.*, 2004).

In advanced HIV disease, oral ganciclovir (1000 mg three times daily) may reduce the risk of CMV disease and possibly mortality in those not receiving didanosine (Brosgart *et al.*, 1998). The addition of oral high-dose ganciclovir (1500 mg three times daily) to the intraocular ganciclovir implant further delays the time to retinitis progression and reduces the risk of new CMV disease and possibly the risk of Kaposi's sarcoma.

Ganciclovir resistance emerges in a minority of transplant patients, especially mismatched solid-organ recipients (Limaye *et al.*, 2000), and is associated with poorer prognosis. The use of antithymocyte globulin and prolonged ganciclovir exposure are risk factors. Recovery of ganciclovir-resistant CMV isolates has been associated with progressive CMV disease in AIDS and other immunocompromised patients. Over one-quarter of retinitis patients have resistant isolates by 9 months of therapy, and resistant CMV has been recovered from CSF, vitreous fluid, and visceral sites.

A ganciclovir ophthalmic gel formulation appears to be effective in treating HSV keratitis (Colin *et al.*, 1997). Oral ganciclovir reduces HBV DNA levels and aminotransferase levels in chronic hepatitis B (Hadziyannis *et al.*, 1999).

Systemic ganciclovir has been studied in conjunction with suicide gene therapy expressing HSV thymidine kinase for treatment of brain tumors and a variety of other malignancies.

Idoxuridine

Idoxuridine (5-iodo-2′-deoxyuridine) is an iodinated thymidine analog that inhibits the *in vitro* replication of various DNA viruses, including herpesviruses and poxviruses (Prusoff, 1988). Its structure is

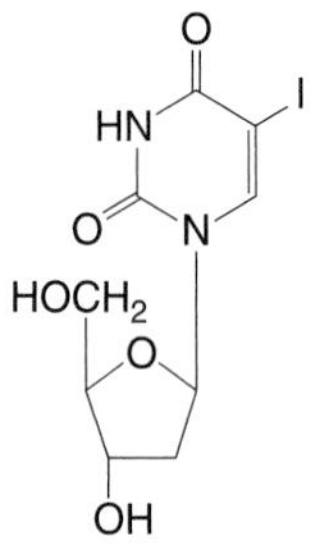

IDOXURIDINE

Inhibitory concentrations of idoxuridine for HSV-1 are 2 to 10 μg/ml, at least tenfold higher than those of acyclovir. Idoxuridine lacks selectivity, in that low concentrations inhibit the growth of uninfected cells. The triphosphate inhibits viral DNA synthesis and is incorporated into both viral and cellular DNA. Such altered DNA is more susceptible to breakage and also leads to faulty transcription. Resistance to idoxuridine develops readily *in vitro* and occurs in viral isolates recovered from idoxuridine-treated patients with HSV keratitis.

In the United States, idoxuridine is approved only for topical treatment of HSV keratitis, although idoxuridine formulated in *dimethylsulfoxide* is available outside the United States for topical treatment of herpes labialis, genitalis, and zoster. In ocular HSV infections, topical idoxuridine is more effective in epithelial infections, especially initial episodes, than in stromal infections. Adverse reactions include pain, pruritus, inflammation, and edema involving the eye or lids; rarely do allergic reactions occur.

Trifluridine

Trifluridine (5-trifluoromethyl-2′-deoxyuridine) is a fluorinated pyrimidine nucleoside that has *in vitro* inhibitory activity against HSV types 1 and 2, CMV, vaccinia, and to a lesser extent, certain adenoviruses. Its structure is

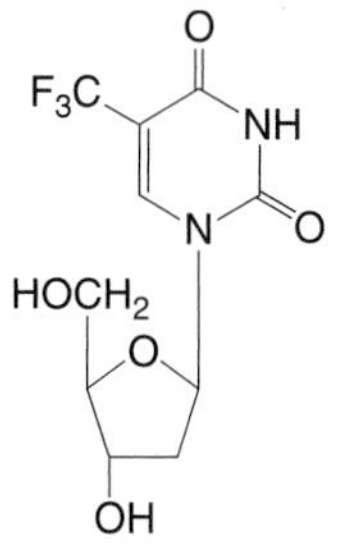

TRIFLURIDINE

Concentrations of trifluridine of 0.2 to 10 μg/ml inhibit replication of herpesviruses, including acyclovir-resistant strains. Trifluridine also inhibits cellular DNA synthesis at relatively low concentrations.

Trifluridine Inhibition of Viral DNA Synthesis. Trifluridine monophosphate irreversibly inhibits thymidylate synthase, and trifluridine triphosphate is a competitive inhibitor of thymidine triphosphate incorporation into DNA; trifluridine is incorporated into viral and cellular DNA. Trifluridine-resistant HSV with altered thymidine kinase substrate specificity can be selected *in vitro,* and resistance in clinical isolates has been described.

Trifluridine currently is approved in the United States for treatment of primary keratoconjunctivitis and recurrent epithelial keratitis owing to HSV types 1 and 2. Topical trifluridine is more active than idoxuridine and comparable with vidarabine in HSV ocular infections. Adverse reactions include discomfort on instillation and palpebral edema. Hypersensitivity reactions, irritation, and superficial punctate or epithelial keratopathy are uncommon. Topical trifluridine also appears to be effective in some patients with acyclovir-resistant HSV cutaneous infections.

ANTI-INFLUENZA AGENTS

Amantadine and Rimantadine

Chemistry and Antiviral Activity. Amantadine (1-adamantanamine hydrochloride) and its α-methyl derivative *rimantadine* (α-methyl-1-adamantane methylamine hydrochloride) are uniquely configured tricyclic amines.

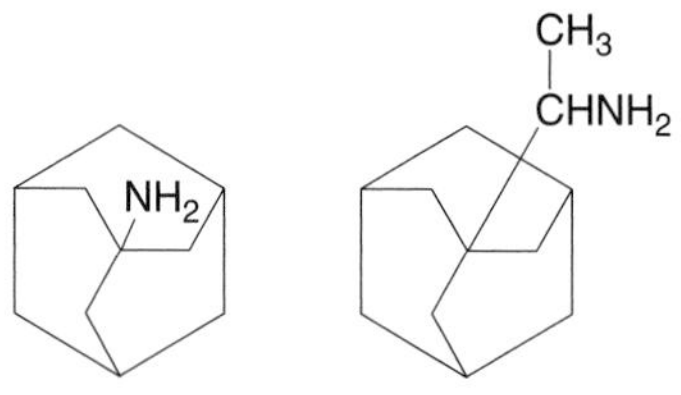

AMANTADINE   RIMANTADINE

Low concentrations of either agent specifically inhibit the replication of influenza A viruses (Hayden and Aoki, 1999). Depending on the assay method and strain, inhibitory concentrations of the drugs range from about 0.03 to 1.0 μg/ml for influenza A viruses. Rimantadine generally is 4 to 10 times more active than amantadine. Concentrations of 10 μg/ml or greater inhibit other enveloped viruses but are not achievable in human beings and may be cytotoxic. Rimantadine is inhibitory *in vitro* for *Trypanosoma brucei*, a cause of African sleeping sickness, at concentrations of 1 to 2.5 μg/ml. These agents do not inhibit hepatitis C virus (HCV) enzymes or internal ribosomal entry site–mediated translation but block the ion channel activity of the HCV p7 protein *in vitro* (Griffin *et al.*, 2003).

Mechanisms of Action and Resistance.

Amantadine and rimantadine share two mechanisms of antiviral action. They inhibit an early step in viral replication, probably viral uncoating; for some strains, they also have an effect on a late step in viral assembly probably mediated through altering hemagglutinin processing. The primary locus of action is the influenza A virus M2 protein, an integral membrane protein that functions as an ion channel. By interfering with this function of the M2 protein, the drugs inhibit the acid-mediated dissociation of the ribonucleoprotein complex early in replication and potentiate acidic pH–induced conformational changes in the hemagglutinin during its intracellular transport later in replication.

Primary drug resistance is uncommon (<1% to 2.5%) in field isolates but occurs in some avian and swine influenza viruses, including recent H5N1 human isolates.

Resistance is selected readily by virus passage in the presence of drug and is seen commonly (30% or more) in isolates recovered during treatment (Hayden, 1996). Resistance with over one hundredfold increases in inhibitory concentrations has been associated with single-nucleotide changes leading to amino acid substitutions in the transmembrane region of M2 (Hayden, 1996). Amantadine and rimantadine share cross-susceptibility and resistance.

Absorption, Distribution, and Elimination. Amantadine and rimantadine are well absorbed after oral administration (Hayden and Aoki, 1999) (Table 49–3). Peak plasma concentrations of amantadine average 0.5 to 0.8 μg/ml on a 100-mg twice-daily regimen in healthy young adults. Comparable doses of rimantadine give peak and trough plasma concentrations of approximately 0.4 to 0.5 and 0.2 to 0.4 μg/ml, respectively. The elderly require only one-half the weight-adjusted dose of amantadine needed for young adults to achieve equivalent trough plasma levels of 0.3 μg/ml. Both drugs have very large volumes of distribution. Nasal secretion and salivary levels of amantadine approximate those found in the serum. Amantadine is excreted in breast milk. Rimantadine concentrations in nasal mucus average 50% higher than those in plasma.

Amantadine is excreted largely unmetabolized in the urine through glomerular filtration and probably tubular secretion. The plasma $t_{\frac{1}{2}}$ of elimination is about 12 to 18 hours in young adults. Because amantadine's elimination is highly dependent on renal function, the elimination $t_{\frac{1}{2}}$ increases up to twofold in the elderly and even more in those with renal impairment. Dose adjustments are advisable in those with mild decrements in renal function. In contrast, rimantadine is metabolized extensively by hydroxylation, conjugation, and glucuronidation prior to renal excretion. Following oral administration, the elimination $t_{\frac{1}{2}}$ of rimantadine averages 24 to 36 hours, and 60% to 90% is excreted in the urine as metabolites. Renal clearance of unchanged rimantadine is similar to creatinine clearance.

Table 49–3
Pharmacological Characteristics of Antivirals for Influenza

	AMANTADINE	RIMANTADINE	ZANAMIVIR	OSELTAMIVIR
Spectrum (types of influenza)	A	A	A, B	A, B
Route/formulations	Oral (tablet/capsule/syrup)	Oral (tablet/syrup)	Inhaled (powder) Intravenous*	Oral (capsule/syrup)
Oral bioavailability	> 90%	> 90%	< 5%[†]	~ 80%[‡]
Effect of meals on AUC	Negligible	Negligible	Not applicable	Negligible
Plasma $t_{\frac{1}{2},elim}$, h	12–18	24–36	2.5–5	6–10[‡]
Protein binding, %	67%	40%	< 10%	3%[‡]
Metabolism, %	< 10%	~ 75%	Negligible	Negligible[‡]
Renal excretion, % (parent drug)	>90%	~ 25%	100%	95%[‡]
Dose adjustments	$Cl_{cr} \leq 50$ Age $\geq$ 65 yrs	$Cl_{cr} \leq 10$ Age $\geq$ 65 years	None	$Cl_{cr} \leq 30$

*Investigational at present. [†]Systemic absorption 4% to 17% after inhalation. [‡]For antivirally active oseltamivir carboxylate (GS4071).

Untoward Effects. The most common side effects related to amantadine and rimantadine are minor dose-related gastrointestinal and CNS complaints (Hayden and Aoki, 1999). These include nervousness, light-headedness, difficulty concentrating, insomnia, and loss of appetite or nausea. CNS side effects occur in approximately 5% to 33% of patients treated with amantadine at doses of 200 mg/day but are significantly less frequent with rimantadine. The neurotoxic effects of amantadine appear to be increased by concomitant ingestion of antihistamines and psychotropic or anticholinergic drugs, especially in the elderly. Amantadine dose reductions are required in older adults (100 mg/day) because of decreased renal function, but 20% to 40% of infirm elderly will experience side effects even at this lower dose. At comparable doses of 100 mg/day, rimantadine is significantly better tolerated in nursing home residents than is amantadine (Keyser *et al.*, 2000).

High amantadine plasma concentrations (1.0 to 5.0 μg/ml) have been associated with serious neurotoxic reactions, including delirium, hallucinosis, seizures, and coma, and cardiac arrhythmias. Exacerbations of preexisting seizure disorders and psychiatric symptoms may occur with amantadine and possibly with rimantadine. Amantadine is teratogenic in animals. The safety of these drugs has not been established in pregnancy (pregnancy category C).

Therapeutic Uses. Amantadine and rimantadine are effective for the prevention and treatment of influenza A virus infections. Seasonal prophylaxis with either drug (a total of 200 mg/day in one or two divided doses in young adults) is about 70% to 90% protective against influenza A illness (Hayden and Aoki, 1999). Efficacy has been shown during pandemic influenza (Hayden, 2001), in preventing nosocomial influenza, and in curtailing nosocomial outbreaks. Doses of 100 mg/day are better tolerated and still appear to be protective against influenzal illness. Postexposure prophylaxis with either drug provides protection of exposed family contacts if ill young children are not concurrently treated (Hayden, 1996).

Seasonal prophylaxis is an alternative in high-risk patients if the influenza vaccine cannot be administered or may be ineffective (*i.e.,* in immunocompromised patients). Prophylaxis should be started as soon as influenza is identified in a community or region and should be continued throughout the period of risk (usually 4 to 8 weeks) because any protective effects are lost several days after cessation of therapy. Alternatively, the drugs can be started in conjunction with immunization and continued for 2 weeks until protective immune responses develop.

In uncomplicated influenza A illness of adults, early amantadine or rimantadine treatment (200 mg/day for 5 days) reduces the duration of fever and systemic complaints by 1 to 2 days, speeds functional recovery, and sometimes decreases the duration of virus shedding (Hayden and Aoki, 1999). In children, rimantadine treatment may be associated with less illness and lower viral titers during the first 2 days of treatment, but rimantadine-treated children have more prolonged shedding of virus. The optimal dose and duration of therapy have not been established in children for either agent. It also is uncertain whether treatment reduces risk of complications in high-risk patients or is useful in patients with established pulmonary complications.

Resistant variants have been recovered from approximately 30% of treated children or outpatient adults by the fifth day of therapy (Hayden, 1996). Resistant variants also arise commonly in immunocompromised patients (Englund *et al.*, 1998). Illnesses owing to apparent transmission of resistant virus associated with failure of drug prophylaxis have been documented in contacts of drug-treated

ill persons in households and in nursing homes (Hayden, 1996). Resistant variants appear to be pathogenic and can cause typical disabling influenzal illness.

The discovery that amantadine also is useful in treating parkinsonism was due to serendipity. This application is discussed in Chapter 20. Amantadine and rimantadine have been used alone or in combination with *interferon* and other agents in treating chronic hepatitis C with inconsistent results (Smith *et al.*, 2004).

Oseltamivir

Chemistry and Antiviral Activity. Oseltamivir carboxylate [(3*R*, 4*R*, 5*S*)-4-acetylamino-5-amino-3(1-ethylpropoxyl)-1-cyclohexene-1-carboxylic acid] is a transition-state analog of sialic acid that is a potent selective inhibitor of influenza A and B virus neuraminidases. The structure is

OSELTAMIVIR CARBOXYLATE

Oseltamivir phosphate is an ethyl ester prodrug that lacks antiviral activity. Oseltamivir carboxylate has an antiviral spectrum and potency similar to that of *zanamivir* (*see* below). It inhibits amantadine- and rimantadine-resistant influenza A viruses and some zanamivir-resistant variants.

Mechanisms of Action and Resistance. Influenza neuraminidase cleaves terminal sialic acid residues and destroys the receptors recognized by viral hemagglutinin, which are present on the cell surface, in progeny virions, and in respiratory secretions (Gubareva *et al.*, 2000). This enzymatic action is essential for release of virus from infected cells. Interaction of oseltamivir carboxylate with the neuraminidase causes a conformational change within the enzyme's active site and inhibits its activity. Inhibition of neuraminidase activity leads to viral aggregation at the cell surface and reduced virus spread within the respiratory tract.

Influenza variants selected *in vitro* for resistance to oseltamivir carboxylate contain hemagglutinin and/or neuraminidase mutations. The most commonly recognized variants (mutations at positions 292 in N2 and 274 in N1 neuraminidases) have reduced infectivity and virulence in animal models. Outpatient oseltamivir therapy has been associated with recovery of resistant variants in about 0.5% of adults and 5.5% of children (Roberts, 2001); a higher frequency (~18%) occurs in hospitalized children.

Absorption, Distribution, and Elimination. Oral oseltamivir phosphate is absorbed rapidly (Table 49–3) and cleaved by esterases in the gastrointestinal tract and liver to the active carboxylate. Low blood levels of the phosphate are detectable, but exposure is only 3% to 5% of that of the metabolite. The bioavailability of the carboxylate is estimated to be approximately 80% (He *et al.*, 1999). The time to maximum plasma concentrations of the carboxylate is about 2.5 to 5 hours. Food does not decrease bioavailability but reduces the risk of gastrointestinal intolerance. After 75-mg doses, peak plasma concentrations average 0.07 μg/ml for oseltamivir phosphate and 0.35 μg/ml for the carboxylate. The carboxylate has a volume of distribution similar to extracellular water. Bronchoalveolar lavage levels in animals and middle ear fluid and sinus concentrations in humans are comparable with plasma levels. Following oral administration, the plasma half-life of oseltamivir phosphate is 1 to 3 hours and that of the carboxylate ranges from 6 to 10 hours. Both the prodrug and active metabolite are eliminated primarily unchanged through the kidney. Probenecid doubles the plasma half-life of the carboxylate, which indicates tubular secretion by the anionic pathway.

Untoward Effects. Oral oseltamivir is associated with nausea, abdominal discomfort, and, less often, emesis, probably owing to local irritation. Gastrointestinal complaints usually are mild-to-moderate in intensity, typically resolve in 1 to 2 days despite continued dosing, and are preventable by administration with food. The frequency of such complaints is about 10% to 15% when oseltamivir is used for the treatment of influenza illness and less than 5% when used for prophylaxis. An increased frequency of headache was reported in one prophylaxis study in elderly adults.

Oseltamivir phosphate and the carboxylate do not interact with the cytochrome P450 enzymes (CYPs) *in vitro*. Their protein binding is low. No clinically significant drug interactions have been recognized to date. Oseltamivir does not appear to impair fertility or to be teratogenic in animal studies, but safety in pregnancy is uncertain (pregnancy category C). Very high doses have been associated with increased mortality, perhaps related to increased brain concentrations, in unweaned rats, and oseltamivir is not approved for use in children younger than 1 year of age.

Therapeutic Uses. Oral oseltamivir is effective in the treatment and prevention of influenza A and B virus infections. Treatment of previously healthy adults (75 mg twice daily for 5 days) or children aged 1 to 12 years (weight-adjusted dosing) with acute influenza reduces illness duration by about 1 to 2 days, speeds functional recovery, and reduces the risk of complications leading to antibiotic use by 40% to 50% (Cooper *et al.*, 2003; Whitley *et al.*, 2001). Treatment is associated with approximate halving of the risk of subsequent hospitalization in adults (Kaiser *et al.*, 2003). When used for prophylaxis during the influenza season, oseltamivir (75 mg once daily) is effective (approximately 70% to 90%) in reducing the likelihood of influenza illness in both unimmunized working adults and in immunized nursing home residents (Cooper *et al.*, 2003); short-term use (7 to 10 days) protects against influenza in household contacts (Hayden *et al.*, 2004).

Zanamivir

Chemistry and Antiviral Activity. Zanamivir (4-guanidino-2,4-dideoxy-2,3-dehydro-*N*-acetyl neuraminic acid) is a sialic acid analog that potently and specifically inhibits the neuraminidases of influenza A and B viruses. Depending on the strain, zanamivir competitively inhibits influenza neuraminidase activity at concentrations of approximately 0.2 to 3 ng/ml but affects neuraminidases from other pathogens and mammalian sources only at 10^6-fold higher concentrations. Zanamivir inhibits *in vitro* replication of influenza A and B viruses, including amantadine- and rimantadine-resistant strains and several oseltamivir-resistant variants. It is active after topical administration in animal models of influenza. Its structure is:

ZANAMIVIR

Mechanisms of Action and Resistance. Like oseltamivir, zanamivir inhibits viral neuraminidase and thus causes viral aggregation at the cell surface and reduced spread of virus within the respiratory tract (Gubareva *et al.*, 2000).

In vitro selection of viruses resistant to zanamivir is associated with mutations in the viral hemagglutinin and/or neuraminidase. Hemagglutinin variants generally have mutations in or near the receptor binding site that make them less dependent on neuraminidase action for release from cells *in vitro*, although they typically retain susceptibility *in vivo*. Hemagglutinin variants are cross-resistant to other neuraminidase inhibitors. Neuraminidase variants contain mutations in the enzyme active site that diminish binding of zanamivir, but the altered enzymes show reduced activity or stability. Zanamivir-resistant variants usually have decreased infectivity in animals. Resistance emergence has not been documented with zanamivir in immunocompetent hosts to date but has been seen rarely in highly immunocompromised patients (Gubareva *et al.*, 2000).

Absorption, Distribution, and Elimination. The oral bioavailability of zanamivir is low (<5%) (Table 49–3), and the commercial form is delivered by oral inhalation of dry powder in a lactose carrier. The proprietary inhaler device is breath-actuated and requires a cooperative patient. Following inhalation of the dry powder, approximately 15% is deposited in the lower respiratory tract and about 80% in the oropharynx (Cass *et al.*, 1999). Overall bioavailability is less than 20%, and plasma levels after 10-mg inhaled doses average about 35 to 100 ng/ml in adults and children (Peng *et al.*, 2000). Median zanamivir concentrations in induced sputum samples are 1336 ng/ml at 6 hours and 47 ng/ml at 24 hours after a single 10-mg dose in healthy volunteers (Peng *et al.*, 2000). The plasma half-life of zanamivir averages 2.5 to 5 hours after oral inhalation but only 1.7 hours following intravenous dosing. Over 90% is eliminated in the urine without recognized metabolism.

Untoward Effects. Topically applied zanamivir generally is well tolerated in ambulatory adults and children with influenza. Wheezing and bronchospasm have been reported in some influenza-infected patients without known airway disease, and acute deteriorations in lung function, including fatal outcomes, have occurred in those with underlying asthma or chronic obstructive airway disease. Tolerability in more serious bronchopulmonary disorders or in intubated patients is uncertain. Zanamivir is not generally recommended for treatment of patients with underlying airway disease (*e.g.*, asthma or chronic obstructive pulmonary disease) because of the risk of serious adverse events.

Preclinical studies of zanamivir revealed no evidence of mutagenic, teratogenic, or oncogenic effects (pregnancy category C). No clinically significant drug interactions have been recognized to date. Zanamivir does not diminish the immune response to injected influenza vaccine.

Therapeutic Uses. Inhaled zanamivir is effective for the prevention and treatment of influenza A and B virus infections. Early zanamivir treatment (10 mg twice daily for 5 days) of febrile influenza in ambulatory adults and children aged 5 years and older shortens the time to illness resolution by 1 to 3 days (Cooper *et al.*, 2003; Hedrick *et al.*, 2000) and in adults reduces by 40% the risk of lower respiratory tract complications leading to antibiotic use (Kaiser *et al.*, 2000). Once-daily inhaled, but not intranasal, zanamivir is highly protective against community-acquired influenza illness (Cooper *et al.*, 2003), and when given for 10 days, it protects against household transmission (Hayden *et al.*, 2004). Intravenous zanamivir is protective against experimental human influenza but has not been studied in treating natural influenza.

ANTIHEPATITIS AGENTS

A number of agents are available for treatment of hepatitis B virus (HBV) and hepatitis C virus (HCV) infections. Several agents (*e.g.*, interferons and *ribavirin*) have other uses as well.

Adefovir

Chemistry and Antiviral Activity. Adefovir dipivoxil (9-[2-[bis[(pivaloyloxy)methoxy]phosphinyl]methoxyl]ethyl]adenine, bis-POM PMEA) is a diester prodrug of adefovir, an acyclic phosphonate nucleotide analog of adenosine monophosphate. Its structure is:

ADEFOVIR DIPIVOXIL

It is inhibitory *in vitro* against a range of DNA and RNA viruses, but its clinical use is limited to HBV infections (De Clercq, 2003). Inhibitory concentrations for HBV range from 0.2 to 1.2 μM in cell culture, and it is active against lamivudine-resistant HBV strains. Oral adefovir dipivoxil shows dose-dependent inhibition of hepadnavirus replication in animal models. *In vitro* combinations of adefovir and lamivudine or other anti-HBV nucleosides show enhanced antihepadnavirus activity *in vitro* (Delaney *et al.*, 2004), and trials of dual therapy are in progress.

Mechanisms of Action and Resistance. Adefovir dipivoxil enters cells and is deesterified to adefovir. Adefovir is converted by cellular enzymes to the diphosphate, which acts as a competitive inhibitor of viral DNA polymerases and reverse transcriptases with respect to deoxyadenosine triphosphate and also serves as a chain terminator of viral DNA synthesis (Cundy, 1999). Its selectivity relates to a higher affinity for HBV DNA polymerase compared with cellular polymerases. The intracellular $t_{\frac{1}{2}}$ of the diphosphate is prolonged, ranging from 5 to 18 hours, so once-daily dosing is feasible. Adefovir resistance has been detected in a small proportion (~4%) of chronically infected HBV patients during 3 years of treatment. Such variants have unique point mutations in the HBV polymerase but retain susceptibility to lamivudine. The consequences of the emergence of resistance remain to be determined.

Absorption, Distribution, and Elimination. The parent compound has low oral bioavailability (<12%), whereas the dipivoxil prodrug is absorbed rapidly and hydrolyzed by esterases in the intestine and blood to adefovir with liberation of pivalic acid (Cundy *et al.*, 1995). Adefovir bioavailability is approximately 30% to 60%. After 10-mg doses of the prodrug, peak serum concentrations of adefovir average 0.02 μg/ml, and the prodrug is not detectable. Food does not affect bioavailability. Adefovir has low protein binding (<5%) and has a volume of distribution similar to body water (~0.4 L/kg).

Adefovir is eliminated unchanged by renal excretion through a combination of glomerular filtration and tubular secretion. After oral administration of adefovir dipivoxil, about 30% to 45% of the dose is recovered within 24 hours, and the serum $t_{\frac{1}{2}}$ of elimination ranges from 5 to 7.5 hours. Clearance dose reductions are indicated for Cl_{Cr} values of less than 50 ml/min. Adefovir is removed by hemodialysis, but the effects of peritoneal dialysis or severe hepatic insufficiency on pharmacokinetics are unreported.

Pivalic acid is a product of adefovir dipivoxil metabolism that can cause reduced free carnitine levels. Although L-carnitine has been given in some HIV studies, supplementation generally is not recommended at the doses of adefovir dipivoxil used in chronic HBV infection.

Untoward Effects. Adefovir dipivoxil causes dose-related nephrotoxicity and tubular dysfunction, manifested by azotemia and hypophosphatemia, acidosis, glycosuria, and proteinuria that usually are reversible months after discontinuation. The lower dose (10 mg/day) used in chronic HBV infection patients has been associated with few adverse events (*e.g.,* headache, abdominal discomfort, diarrhea, and asthenia) and negligible renal toxicity compared with a threefold higher dose (Hadziyannis *et al.,* 2003; Marcellin *et al.,* 2003). Adverse events lead to premature discontinuation in about 2% of patients. After 2 years of dosing, the risk of serum creatinine levels rising above 0.5 mg/dl is about 2% but is higher in those with preexisting renal insufficiency. Adefovir is transported efficiently into tubular epithelium by a probenecid-sensitive human organic anion transporter (hOAT1), and the diphosphate's inhibitory effects on renal adenyl cyclase may contribute to nephrotoxicity. Acute, sometimes severe exacerbations of hepatitis can occur in patients stopping adefovir or other anti-HBV therapies. Close monitoring is necessary, and resumption of antiviral therapy may be required in some patients.

No clinically important drug interactions have been recognized to date, although drugs that reduce renal function or compete for active tubular secretion could decrease adefovir clearance. *Ibuprofen* increases adefovir exposure modestly. An increased risk of lactic acidosis and steatosis may exist when adefovir is used in conjunction with nucleoside analogs or other antiretroviral agents.

Adefovir is genotoxic, and high doses cause renal tubular nephropathy, hepatotoxicity, and toxicity to lymphoid tissues in animals. Adefovir dipivoxil is not associated with reproductive toxicity, although high intravenous doses of adefovir cause maternal and embryotoxicity with fetal malformations in rats (pregnancy category C).

Therapeutic Uses. Adefovir dipivoxil is approved for treatment of chronic HBV infections. In patients with HBV e-antigen (HbeAg)–positive chronic hepatitis B, adefovir dipivoxil (10 mg/day) results in over one hundredfold reduced serum HBV DNA levels and, in about one-half of patients, improved hepatic histology and normalization of aminotransferase levels by 48 weeks (Marcellin *et al.,* 2003). Continued therapy is associated with increasing frequencies of aminotransferase normalization and HbeAg seroconversion (De Clercq, 2003). In patients with HbeAg-negative chronic HBV, adefovir is associated with similar biochemical and histologic benefits (Hadziyannis *et al.,* 2003). Regression of cirrhosis may occur in some patients.

In patients with lamivudine-resistant HBV infections, adefovir dipivoxil monotherapy results in sustained reductions in serum HBV DNA levels, but lamivudine alone or added to adefovir is not beneficial (Peters *et al.,* 2004). In patients with dual HIV and lamivudine-resistant HBV infections, adefovir dipivoxil (10 mg/day) causes significant HBV DNA level reductions (Benhamou *et al.,* 2001), and it also has been used successfully in patients with lamivudine-resistant HBV infections both before and following liver transplantation. The optimal duration of treatment in different popu-

lations, possible long-term effects on HBV complications, and combined use with other anti-HBV agents are under study.

Interferons

Classification and Antiviral Activity. Interferons (IFNs) are potent cytokines that possess antiviral, immunomodulating, and antiproliferative activities (Samuel, 2001; Biron, 2001) (*see* Chapter 52). These proteins are synthesized by host cells in response to various inducers and, in turn, cause biochemical changes leading to an antiviral state in cells. Three major classes of human interferons with significant antiviral activity currently are recognized: α (>18 individual species), β, and γ. Clinically used recombinant α IFNs (Table 49–2) are nonglycosylated proteins of approximately 19,500 daltons.

IFN-α and IFN-β may be produced by nearly all cells in response to viral infection and a variety of other stimuli, including double-stranded RNA and certain cytokines (*e.g.,* interleukin 1, interleukin 2, and tumor necrosis factor). IFN-γ production is restricted to T-lymphocytes and natural killer cells responding to antigenic stimuli, mitogens, and specific cytokines. IFN-α and IFN-β exhibit antiviral and antiproliferative actions; stimulate the cytotoxic activity of lymphocytes, natural killer cells, and macrophages; and up-regulate class I major histocompatibility (MHC) antigens and other surface markers. IFN-γ has less antiviral activity but more potent immunoregulatory effects, particularly macrophage activation, expression of class II MHC antigens, and mediation of local inflammatory responses.

Most animal viruses are inhibited by IFNs, although many DNA viruses are relatively insensitive. Considerable differences in sensitivity to the effects of IFNs exist among different viruses and assay systems. The biological activity of IFN usually is measured in terms of antiviral effects in cell culture and generally is expressed as international units (IU) relative to reference standards.

Mechanisms of Action. Following binding to specific cellular receptors, IFNs activate the JAK-STAT signal-transduction pathway and lead to the nuclear translocation of a cellular protein complex that binds to genes containing an IFN-specific response element. This, in turn, leads to synthesis of over two dozen proteins that contribute to viral resistance mediated at different stages of viral penetration (Samuel, 2001; Der *et al.,* 1998) (Figure 49–3). Inhibition of protein synthesis is the major inhibitory effect for many viruses. IFN-induced proteins include 2´-5´-oligoadenylate [2-5(A)] synthetase and a protein kinase, either of which can inhibit protein synthesis in the presence of double-stranded RNA. The 2-5(A) synthetase produces adenylate

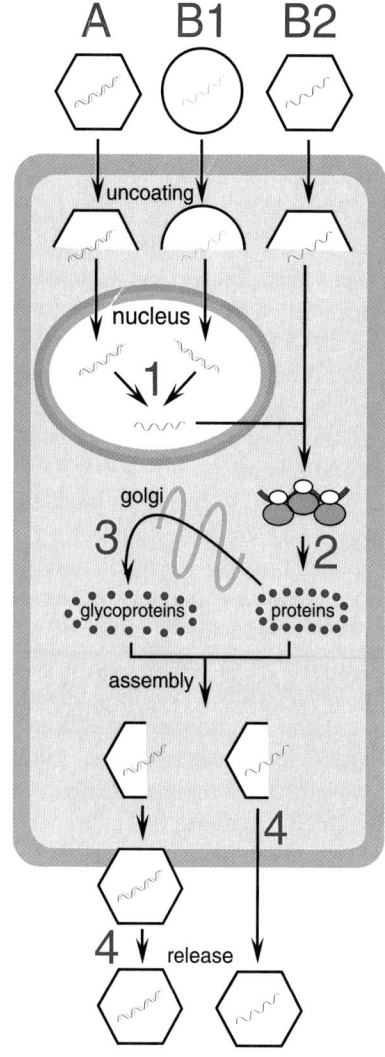

Viruses
A. DNA
B. RNA
  1. orthomyxoviruses and retroviruses
  2. picornaviruses and most RNA viruses

IFN Effects
1. transcription inhibition
   activates Mx protein
   blocks mRNA synthesis

2. translation inhibition
   activates methylase, thereby reducing
   mRNA cap methylation

   activates 2'5' oligoadenylate synthetase
   —> 2'5'A —> inhibits mRNA splicing
   and activates RNaseL —> cleaves
   viral RNA

   activates protein kinase P1 —> blocks
   eIF-2α function —> inhibits initiation
   of mRNA translation

   activates phosphodiesterase —> blocks
   tRNA function

3. protein processing inhibition
   inhibits glycosyltransferase, thereby reducing
   protein glycosylation

4. virus maturation inhibition
   inhibits glycosyltransferase, thereby reducing
   glycoprotein maturation

   causes membrane changes —> blocks
   budding

Figure 49–3. *Interferon-mediated antiviral activity occurs via multiple mechanisms.* The binding of IFN to specific cell surface receptor molecules signals the cell to produce a series of antiviral proteins. The stages of viral replication that are inhibited by various IFN-induced antiviral proteins are shown. Most of these act to inhibit the translation of viral proteins (mechanism 2), but other steps in viral replication also are affected (mechanisms 1, 3, and 4). The roles of these mechanisms in the other actions of IFNs are under study. *Key:* IFN = interferon; mRNA = messenger RNA; Mx = specific cellular protein; tRNA = transfer RNA; RNase L = latent cellular endoribonuclease; $2'5'A$ = $2'-5'$-oligoadenylates; eIF-2α = protein synthesis initiation factor. (Modified from Baron *et al.*, 1992, with permission.)

oligomers that activate a latent cellular endoribonuclease (RNase L) to cleave both cellular and viral single-stranded RNAs. The protein kinase selectively phosphorylates and inactivates a protein involved in protein synthesis, eukaryotic initiation factor 2 (eIF-2). IFN-induced protein kinase also may be an important effector of apoptosis. In addition, IFN induces a phosphodiesterase that cleaves a portion of transfer RNA and thus prevents peptide elongation. A given virus may be inhibited at several steps, and the principal inhibitory effect differs among virus families. Certain

viruses are able to counter IFN effects by blocking production or activity of selected IFN-inducible proteins. For example, IFN resistance in hepatitis C virus is attributable to inhibition of the IFN-induced protein kinase, among other mechanisms.

Complex interactions exist between IFNs and other parts of the immune system, so IFNs may ameliorate viral infections by exerting direct antiviral effects and/or by modifying the immune response to infection (Biron, 2001). For example, IFN-induced expression of MHC antigens may contribute to the antiviral actions of IFN by enhancing the lytic effects of cytotoxic T-lymphocytes. Conversely, IFNs may mediate some of the systemic symptoms associated with viral infections and contribute to immunologically mediated tissue damage in certain viral diseases.

Absorption, Distribution, and Elimination. Oral administration does not result in detectable IFN levels in serum or increases in 2-5(A) synthetase activity in peripheral blood mononuclear cells (used as a marker of IFN's biologic activity) (Wills, 1990). After intramuscular or subcutaneous injection of IFN-α, absorption exceeds 80%. Plasma levels are dose-related, peaking at 4 to 8 hours and returning to baseline by 18 to 36 hours. Levels of 2-5(A) synthetase in peripheral blood mononuclear cells show increases beginning at 6 hours and lasting through 4 days after a single injection. An antiviral state in peripheral blood mononuclear cells peaks at 24 hours and decreases slowly to baseline by 6 days after injection. Intramuscular or subcutaneous injections of IFN-β result in negligible plasma levels, although increases in 2-5(A) synthetase levels may occur. After systemic administration, low levels of IFN are detected in respiratory secretions, CSF, eye, and brain.

Because IFNs induce long-lasting cellular effects, their activities are not easily predictable from usual pharmacokinetic measures. After intravenous dosing, clearance of IFN from plasma occurs in a complex manner (Bocci, 1992). With subcutaneous or intramuscular dosing, the plasma $t_{\frac{1}{2}}$ of elimination of IFN-α ranges from approximately 3 to 8 hours. Elimination from the blood relates to distribution to the tissues, cellular uptake, and catabolism primarily in the kidney and liver. Negligible amounts are excreted in the urine. Clearance of IFN-α2 is reduced by 64% to 79% in hemodialysis patients.

Attachment of IFN proteins to large, inert polyethylene glycol (PEG) molecules (pegylation) slows absorption, decreases clearance, and provides higher and more prolonged serum concentrations that enable once-weekly dosing (Bruno *et al.*, 2004). Two pegylated IFNs are available commercially: *peginterferon alfa-2a* and *peginterferon alfa-2b*. PegIFN alfa-2b has a straight-chain 12,000-dalton type of PEG that increases the plasma $t_{\frac{1}{2}}$ from approximately 2 to 3 hours to approximately 30 to 54 hours (Glue *et al.*, 2000). PegIFN alfa-2a consists of an ester derivative of a branched-chain 40,000-dalton PEG bonded to IFN-α2a and has a plasma $t_{\frac{1}{2}}$ averaging about 80 to 90 hours. PegIFN alfa-2a is more stable and dispensed in solution, whereas pegIFN alfa-2b requires reconstitution prior to use. For pegIFN alfa-2a, peak serum concentrations occur up to 120 hours after dosing and remain detectable throughout the weekly dosing interval (Bruno *et al.*, 2004); steady-state levels occur 5 to 8 weeks after initiation of weekly dosing (Keating and Curran, 2003). For pegIFN alfa-2a, dose-related maximum plasma concentrations occur at 15 to 44 hours after dosing and decline by 96 to 168 hours. These differences in pharmacokinetics may be associated with differences in antiviral effects (Bruno *et al.*, 2004). Increasing PEG size is associated with longer $t_{\frac{1}{2}}$ and less renal clearance. About 30% of pegIFN alfa-2b is cleared renally; pegIFN alfa-2a also is cleared primarily by the liver. Dose reductions in both pegylated IFNs are indicated in end-stage renal disease.

Untoward Effects. Injection of IFN doses of 1 to 2 million units (MU) or greater usually is associated with an acute influenzalike syndrome beginning several hours after injection. Symptoms include fever, chills, headache, myalgia, arthralgia, nausea, vomiting, and diarrhea (Dusheiko, 1997). Fever usually resolves within

12 hours. Tolerance develops gradually in most patients. Febrile responses can be moderated by pretreatment with various antipyretics. Up to one-half of patients receiving intralesional therapy for genital warts experience the influenzal illness initially, as well as discomfort at the injection site, and leukopenia.

The principal dose-limiting toxicities of systemic IFN are myelosuppression with granulocytopenia and thrombocytopenia; neurotoxicity manifested by somnolence, confusion, behavioral disturbance, and rarely, seizures; debilitating neurasthenia and depression; autoimmune disorders including thyroiditis; and uncommonly, cardiovascular effects with hypotension and tachycardia. The risk of depression appears to be higher in chronically infected HCV than in HBV patients (Marcellin *et al.*, 2004). Elevations in hepatic enzymes and triglycerides, alopecia, proteinuria and azotemia, interstitial nephritis, autoantibody formation, pneumonia, and hepatotoxicity may occur. Alopecia and personality change are common in IFN-treated children (Sokal *et al.*, 1998). The development of serum neutralizing antibodies to exogenous IFNs may be associated infrequently with loss of clinical responsiveness. IFN may impair fertility, and safety during pregnancy is not established.

IFN reduces the metabolism of various drugs by the hepatic CYPs and significantly increases levels of drugs such as theophylline. IFNs can increase the hematologic toxicity of drugs such as zidovudine and ribavirin and may increase the neurotoxicity and cardiotoxic effects of other drugs.

Pegylated IFNs are tolerated about as well as standard IFNs, with discontinuation rates ranging from 2% to 11%, although the frequencies of fever, nausea, injection-site inflammation, and neutropenia may be somewhat higher. Laboratory abnormalities, including severe neutropenia and the need for dose modifications, are higher in HIV-coinfected persons (Torriani, 2004).

Therapeutic Uses. Recombinant, natural, and pegylated IFNs currently are approved in the United States, depending on the specific IFN type, for treatment of condyloma acuminatum, chronic HCV infection, chronic HBV infection, Kaposi's sarcoma in HIV-infected patients, other malignancies, and multiple sclerosis.

Hepatitis B Virus. In patients with chronic HBV infection, parenteral administration of various IFNs is associated with loss of HBV DNA, loss of HBeAg and development of anti-HBe antibody, and biochemical and histological improvement in about 25% to 50% of the patients. Lasting responses require moderately high IFN doses and prolonged administration (typically 5 MU/day or 10 MU in adults and 6 MU/m^2 in children three times per week for 4 to 6 months) (Sokal *et al.*, 1998). Plasma HBV DNA and polymerase activity decline promptly in most patients, but complete disappearance is sustained in only about one-third of patients or less. Low pretherapy serum HBV DNA levels and high aminotransferase levels are predictors of response. Sustained responses are infrequent in those with vertically acquired infection, anti-HBe positivity, or concurrent immunosuppression owing to HIV. PegIFN alfa-2a appears superior to conventional IFN alfa-2a in HbeAg-positive patients (Cooksley *et al.*, 2003), and treatment (180 mg once weekly for 24 weeks) is associated with normalization of aminotransferases in about 60% and sustained viral suppression in about 20% of HBeAg-negative patients (Marcellin *et al.*, 2004). Responses with seroconversion to anti-HBe usually are associated with aminotransferase elevations and often a hepatitis-like illness during the second or third month of therapy, likely related to immune clearance of infected hepatocytes. High-dose IFN can cause myelosuppression and clinical deterioration in those with decompensated liver disease.

Remissions in chronic hepatitis B induced by IFN are sustained in over 80% of patients treated and frequently are followed by loss of HBV surface antigen (HbsAg), histological improvement or stabilization, and reduced risk of liver-related complications and mortality (Lau *et al.*, 1997). IFN may benefit some patients with nephrotic syndrome and glomerulonephritis owing to chronic HBV infection. Antiviral effects and improvements occur in about one-half of chronic hepatitis D virus (HDV) infections, but relapse is common unless HbsAg disappears. IFN does not appear to be beneficial in acute HBV or HDV infections.

Hepatitis C Virus. In chronic HCV infection, IFN alfa-2b monotherapy (3 MU three times a week) is associated with an approximate 50% to 70% rate of aminotransferase normalization and loss of plasma viral RNA, but relapse rates are high, and sustained virologic remission (absence of detectable HCV RNA) is observed in only about 10% to 25% of patients. Sustained viral responses are associated with long-term histologic improvement and probably reduced risk of hepatocellular carcinoma and hepatic failure (Coverdale *et al.*, 2004). Viral genotype and pretreatment RNA level influence response to treatment, but early viral clearance is the best predictor of sustained response. Failure to achieve an early viral response (nondetectable HCV RNA or reduction $\geq 2 \log_{10}$ compared with baseline at 12 weeks) predicts lack of sustained viral response with continued treatment (Seeff and Hoofnagle, 2002). Nonresponders generally do not benefit from IFN monotherapy retreatment, but they and patients relapsing after monotherapy often respond to combined pegylated IFN and ribavirin treatment (*see* below). IFN treatment may benefit HCV-associated cryoglobulinemia and glomerulonephritis. IFN administration during acute HCV infection appears to reduce the risk of chronicity (Alberti *et al.*, 2002).

Pegylated IFNs are superior to conventional thrice-weekly IFN monotherapy in inducing sustained remissions in treatment-naive patients. Monotherapy with pegIFN alfa-2a (180 μg subcutaneously weekly for 48 weeks) or pegIFN alfa-2b (weight-adjusted doses of 1.5 μg/kg per week) is associated with sustained response in 30% to 39%, including stable cirrhotic patients (Heathcote *et al.*, 2000), and is a treatment option in patients unable to take ribavirin. Studies of prolonged (4 years) maintenance monotherapy with pegylated IFNs are in progress for those not responding to IFN–ribavirin combinations.

The efficacy of conventional and pegylated IFNs is enhanced by the addition of ribavirin to the treatment regimens, particularly for genotype 1 infections. Combined therapy with pegIFN alfa-2a (180 μg once weekly for 48 weeks) and ribavirin (1000 to 1200 mg/day in divided doses) gives higher sustained viral response rates than IFN–ribavirin combinations in previously untreated patients (Fried *et al.*, 2002). A shorter duration of therapy (24 weeks) and lower ribavirin dose (800 mg/day) are effective in genotype 2 and 3 infections, but prolonged therapy and higher ribavirin doses are needed for genotype 1 and 4 infections (Hadziyannis *et al.*, 2004). Approximately 15% to 20% of those failing to respond to combined IFN–ribavirin will have sustained responses to combined pegIFN–ribavirin. Histologic improvement may occur in patients who do not achieve sustained viral responses. In patients with compensated cirrhosis, treatment may reverse cirrhotic changes and possibly reduce the risk of hepatocellular carcinoma (Poynard *et al.*, 2002).

Papillomavirus. In refractory condylomata acuminata (genital warts), intralesional injection of various natural and recombinant IFNs is associated with complete clearance of injected warts in 36% to 62% of patients, but other treatments are preferred (Wiley *et al.*, 2002). Relapse occurs in 20% to 30% of patients. Verruca vulgaris may respond to intralesional IFN-α. Intramuscular or subcutaneous administration is associated with some regression in wart size but greater toxicity. Systemic IFN may provide adjunctive benefit in recurrent juvenile laryngeal papillomatosis and in treating laryngeal disease in older patients.

Other Viruses. IFNs have been shown to have virologic and clinical effects in various herpesvirus infections including genital HSV infections, localized herpes-zoster infection of cancer patients or of older adults, and CMV infections of renal transplant patients. However, IFN generally is associated with more side effects and inferior clinical benefits compared with conventional antiviral therapies. Topically applied IFN and trifluridine combinations appear active in acyclovir-resistant mucocutaneous HSV infections.

In HIV-infected persons, IFNs have been associated with antiretroviral effects. In advanced infection, however, the combination of zidovudine and IFN is associated with only transient benefit and excessive hematological toxicity. IFN-α (3 MU three times weekly) is effective for treatment of HIV-related thrombocytopenia resistant to zidovudine therapy.

Except for adenovirus, IFN has broad-spectrum antiviral activity against respiratory viruses *in vitro*. However, prophylactic intranasal IFN-α is protective only against rhinovirus colds, and chronic use is limited by the occurrence of nasal side effects. Intranasal IFN is therapeutically ineffective in established rhinovirus colds. Systemically administered IFN-α may be beneficial in early treatment of SARS (Loutfy *et al.*, 2003).

Lamivudine

Chemistry and Antiviral Activity. Lamivudine, the (–)-enantiomer of 2′,3′-dideoxy-3′-thiacytidine, is a nucleoside analog that inhibits HIV reverse transcriptase and HBV DNA polymerase. Its use as an antiretroviral agent is discussed in Chapter 50. It inhibits HBV replication *in vitro* by 50% at concentrations of 4 to 7 ng/ml with negligible cellular cytotoxicity. Cellular enzymes convert lamivudine to the triphosphate, which competitively inhibits HBV DNA polymerase and causes chain termination. The intracellular $t_{\frac{1}{2}}$ of the triphosphate averages 17 to 19 hours in HBV-infected cells, so infrequent dosing is possible.

LAMIVUDINE

Mechanisms of Action and Resistance. Lamivudine triphosphate is a potent inhibitor of the DNA polymerase/reverse transcriptase of HBV, and oral lamivudine is active in animal models of hepadnavirus infection. Lamivudine shows enhanced antiviral activity in combination with adefovir or penciclovir against hepadnaviruses. Point mutations in the *YMDD* motif of HBV DNA polymerase result in a 40 to 10^4 times reduction in *in vitro* susceptibility (Ono *et al.*, 2001). Lamivudine resistance confers cross-resistance to related agents such as *emtricitabine* and *clevudine* and is often associated with an additional non-*YMDD* mutation that confers cross-resistance to famciclovir. Lamivudine-resistant HBV retains susceptibility to adefovir and partially to entecavir (Ono *et al.*, 2001). Viruses bearing *YMDD* mutations are less replication competent *in vitro* than wild-type HBV. However, lamivudine resistance is associated with elevated HBV DNA levels, decreased likelihood of HbeAg loss or seroconversion, hepatitis exacerbations, and progressive fibrosis and graft loss in transplant recipients (Dienstag *et al.*, 2003; Lai *et al.*, 2002).

Absorption, Distribution, and Elimination. Following oral administration, lamivudine is absorbed rapidly with a bioavailability of about 80% in adults (Johnson *et al.*, 1999). Peak plasma levels average approximately 1000 ng/ml after 100-mg doses. Lamivudine is distributed widely in a volume comparable with total-body water. The plasma $t_{\frac{1}{2}}$ of elimination averages about 9 hours, and approximately 70% of the dose is excreted unchanged in the urine. About 5% is metabolized to an inactive *trans*-sulfoxide metabolite. In HBV-infected children, doses of 3 mg/kg per day provide plasma exposure and trough plasma levels comparable with those in adults receiving 100 mg daily (Sokal *et al.*, 2000). Dose reductions are indicated for moderate renal insufficiency (creatinine clearance < 50 ml/min). *Trimethoprim* decreases the renal clearance of lamivudine.

Untoward Effects. At the doses used for chronic HBV infection, lamivudine generally has been well tolerated. Aminotransferase rises after therapy occur more often in lamivudine recipients, and flares in post-treatment aminotransferase elevations (>500 IU/ml) occur in about 15% of patients after cessation.

Therapeutic Uses. Lamivudine is approved for the treatment of chronic HBV hepatitis in adults and children. In adults, doses of 100 mg/day for 1 year cause suppression of HBV DNA levels, normalization of aminotransferase levels in 41% or more of patients, and reductions in hepatic inflammation in over 50% of patients (Dienstag *et al.*, 1999; Lai *et al.*, 2002). Seroconversion with antibody to HbeAg occurs in fewer than 20% of recipients at 1 year. In children aged 2 to 17 years, lamivudine (3 mg/kg per day to a maximum of 100 mg for 1 year) is associated with normalization of aminotransferase levels in about one-half and seroconversion to anti-Hbe in about one-fifth of cases (Jonas *et al.*, 2002). In those without emergence of resistant variants, prolonged therapy is associated with sustained suppression of HBV DNA, continued histological improvement, and an increased proportion of patients experiencing a virological response (loss of HbeAg and undetectable HBV DNA). Prolonged therapy is associated with an approximate halving of the risk of clinical progression and development of hepatocellular carcinoma in those with advanced fibrosis or cirrhosis (Liaw *et al.*, 2004). However, the frequency of lamivudine-resistant variants increases progressively with continued drug administration, and frequencies of 38%, 53%, and 67% have been found after 2, 3, and 4 years of treatment, respectively (Liaw *et al.*, 2004). The risk of

resistance development is higher after transplantation and in HIV/HBV-coinfected patients.

Combined use of IFN or pegIFN alfa-2a with lamivudine has not improved responses in HBeAg-positive patients consistently. The addition of lamivudine to pegINF alfa-2a for 1 year of therapy does not improve post-treatment response rates in HBeAg-negative patients (Marcellin *et al.*, 2004). In HIV and HBV coinfections, higher lamivudine doses are associated with antiviral effects and uncommonly anti-HBe seroconversion. Administration of lamivudine before and after liver transplantation may suppress recurrent HBV infection.

Ribavirin

Chemistry and Antiviral Activity. Ribavirin (1-β-D-ribo-fur-anosyl-$1H$-1,2,4-triazole-3-carboxamide) is a purine nucleoside analog with a modified base and D-ribose sugar.

RIBAVIRIN

Ribavirin inhibits the replication of a wide range of RNA and DNA viruses, including orthomyxo-, paramyxo-, arena-, bunya-, and flaviviruses *in vitro*. *In vitro* inhibitory concentrations range from 3 to 10 μg/ml for influenza, parainfluenza, and respiratory syncytial (RSV) viruses. Similar concentrations may reversibly inhibit macromolecular synthesis and proliferation of uninfected cells, suppress lymphocyte responses, and alter cytokine profiles *in vitro*.

Mechanisms of Action and Resistance. The antiviral mechanism of ribavirin is incompletely understood but relates to alteration of cellular nucleotide pools and inhibition of viral messenger RNA synthesis (Tam *et al.*, 2002). Intracellular phosphorylation to the mono-, di-, and triphosphate derivatives is mediated by host cell enzymes. In both uninfected and RSV-infected cells, the predominant derivative (>80%) is the triphosphate, which has an intracellular $t_{\frac{1}{2}}$ of less than 2 hours.

Ribavirin monophosphate competitively inhibits cellular inosine-5′-phosphate dehydrogenase and interferes with the synthesis of GTP and thus nucleic acid synthesis in general. Ribavirin triphosphate also competitively inhibits the GTP-dependent 5′ capping of viral messenger RNA and specifically influenza virus transcriptase activity. Ribavirin appears to have multiple sites of action, and some of these (*e.g.,* inhibition of GTP synthesis) may potentiate others (*e.g.,* inhibition of GTP-dependent enzymes). Ribavirin also may enhance viral mutagenesis to an extent that some viruses may be inhibited in effective replication, so-called lethal mutagenesis (Hong and Cameron, 2002).

Emergence of viral resistance to ribavirin has not been documented in most viruses but has been reported in Sindbis and HCV (Young *et al.*, 2003); it has been possible to select cells that do not phosphorylate it to its active forms.

Absorption, Distribution, and Elimination. Ribavirin is actively taken up by nucleoside transporters in the proximal small bowel; oral bioavailability averages approximately 50% (Glue, 1999). Extensive accumulation occurs in plasma, and steady state is reached by about 4 weeks. Food increases plasma levels substantially (Glue, 1999). Following single or multiple oral doses of 600 mg, peak plasma concentrations average approximately 0.8 and 3.7 μg/ml, respectively. After intravenous doses of 1000 and 500 mg, plasma concentrations average approximately 24 and 17 μg/ml, respectively. With aerosol administration, plasma levels increase with the duration of exposure and range from 0.2 to 1.0 μg/ml after 5 days (Englund *et al.*, 1990). Levels in respiratory secretions are much higher but vary up to one thousandfold.

The apparent volume of distribution for ribavirin is large (~10 L/kg) owing to its cellular uptake. Plasma protein binding is negligible. The elimination of ribavirin is complex. The plasma $t_{\frac{1}{2}}$ increases to approximately 200 to 300 hours at steady state. Erythrocytes concentrate ribavirin triphosphate; the drug exits red cells gradually, with a $t_{\frac{1}{2}}$ of approximately 40 days. Hepatic metabolism and renal excretion of ribavirin and its metabolites are the principal routes of elimination. Hepatic metabolism involves deribosylation and hydrolysis to yield a triazole carboxamide. Ribavirin clearance decreases threefold in those with advanced renal insufficiency (Cl_{cr} = 10 to 30 ml/min); the drug should be used cautiously in patients with creatinine clearances of less than 50 ml/min.

Untoward Effects. Aerosolized ribavirin may cause conjunctival irritation, rash, transient wheezing, and occasional reversible deterioration in pulmonary function. When used in conjunction with mechanical ventilation, equipment modifications and frequent monitoring are required to prevent plugging of ventilator valves and tubing with ribavirin. Techniques to reduce environmental exposure of health care workers are recommended (Shults *et al.*, 1996).

Systemic ribavirin causes dose-related reversible anemia owing to extravascular hemolysis and suppression of bone marrow. Associated increases occur in reticulocyte counts and in serum bilirubin, iron, and uric acid concentrations. High ribavirin triphosphate levels may cause oxidative damage to membranes, leading to erythrophagocytosis by the reticuloendothelial system. Bolus intravenous infusion may cause rigors. About 20% of chronic HCV infection patients receiving combination IFN–ribavirin therapy discontinue treatment early because of side effects. In addition to IFN toxicities, oral ribavirin increases the risk of fatigue, cough, rash, pruritus, nausea, insomnia, dyspnea, depression, and particularly, anemia.

Preclinical studies indicate that ribavirin is teratogenic, embryotoxic, oncogenic, and possibly gonadotoxic. To prevent possible teratogenic effects, up to 6 months is required for washout following cessation of long-term treatment (Glue, 1999).

Pregnant women should not directly care for patients receiving ribavirin aerosol (FDA pregnancy category X).

Ribavirin inhibits the phosphorylation and antiviral activity of pyrimidine nucleoside HIV reverse-transcriptase inhibitors such as zidovudine and stavudine but increases the activity of purine nucleoside reverse-transcriptase inhibitors (*e.g.,* didanosine) *in vitro*. It appears to increase the risk of mitochondrial toxicity from didanosine.

Therapeutic Uses. Oral ribavirin in combination with injected pegIFN alfa-2a or -2b has become standard treatment for chronic HCV infection (Seeff and Hoofnagle, 2002). Ribavirin monotherapy for 6 or 12 months reversibly decreases aminotransferase elevations to normal in about 30% of patients but does not affect HCV RNA levels. Combination therapy with pegIFN alfa-2a and oral ribavirin (500 mg, or 600 mg if weight is greater than 75 kg, twice daily for 24 to 48 weeks) increases the likelihood of sustained biochemical and virologic responses to about 56% depending on genotype (Fried *et al.*, 2002). The combination is superior to IFN or pegIFN monotherapy and combinations of pegIFN alfa-2 and ribavirin in both treatment-naive patients and those not responding to, or relapsing after, IFN monotherapy. A longer duration of therapy (48 weeks) appears necessary in those with genotype 1 infections, whereas 24 weeks' therapy is adequate in genotype 2 and 3 infections (Hadziyannis *et al.*, 2004). Combined ribavirin and pegIFN alfa-2a or -2b is effective in achieving sustained viral responses in a minority of HCV/HIV-coinfected patients (Torriani, 2004). Combined therapy has been used in the management of recurrent HCV infection after liver transplantation.

Ribavirin aerosol is approved in the United States for treatment of RSV bronchiolitis and pneumonia in hospitalized children. Aerosolized ribavirin (usual dose of 20 mg/ml as the starting solution in the drug reservoir of the small particle aerosol generator unit for 18 hours' exposure per day for 3 to 7 days) may reduce some illness measures, but its use generally is not recommended (Committee on Infectious Diseases American Academy of Pediatrics, 2003). No consistent beneficial effects on duration of hospitalization, ventilatory support, mortality, or long-term pulmonary function have been found. High-dose, reduced-duration therapy (60 mg/ml in the drug reservoir of the small particle aerosol generator unit for 2 hours three times daily) has been used (Englund *et al.*, 1990). Aerosol ribavirin combined with intravenous immunoglobulin appears to reduce mortality of RSV infection in bone marrow transplant and other highly immunocompromised patients (Ghosh *et al.*, 2000).

Intravenous and/or aerosol ribavirin has been used occasionally in treating severe influenza virus infection and in the treatment of immunosuppressed patients with adenovirus, vaccinia, parainfluenza, or measles virus infections. Aerosolized ribavirin is associated with reduced duration of fever but no other clinical or antiviral effects in influenza infections in hospitalized children. Intravenous ribavirin decreases mortality in Lassa fever and has been used in treating other arenavirus-related hemorrhagic fevers. Intravenous ribavirin is beneficial in hemorrhagic fever with renal syndrome owing to hantavirus infection but appears ineffective in hantavirus-associated cardiopulmonary syndrome or SARS. Oral ribavirin has been used for the treatment and prevention of Crimean–Congo hemorrhagic fever and treatment of Nipah virus infections (Mar-

Table 49–4
Examples of Antiviral Agents in Clinical Development

VIRUS	AGENT	CLASSIFICATION/SITE OF ACTION	ROUTE	COMMENT
Hepatitis B virus	Entecavir	Nucleoside RT/DNAp inhibitor	O	Less inhibitory for lamivudine-resistant HBV
	Clevudine	Nucleoside RT/DNAp inhibitor	O	Not inhibitory for lamivudine-resistant HBV
	Emtricitabine	Nucleoside RT/DNAp inhibitor	O	Approved for HIV; not inhibitory for lamivudine-resistant HBV
	Telbivudine	Nucleoside RT/DNAp inhibitor	O	Not inhibitory for lamivudine-resistant HBV
	Tenofovir	Nucleotide RT/DNAp inhibitor	O	Approved for HIV; inhibitory for lamivudine-resistant HBV and active in HBV/HIV coinfections
Hepatitis C virus	Viramidine	Nucleoside analog	O	Ribavirin analog with antiviral and immunomodulatory activities
	BILN 2061	NS4A protease inhibitor	O	
	NM283	RNA polymerase inhibitor	O	Valine ester prodrug of ribonucleoside analog
Herpes simplex	Resiquimod	Immune modulator	Topical	
Cytomegalovirus	Maribavir	DNA synthesis inhibitor	O	Novel antiviral action, inhibits UL97 and nuclear egress of virions
Rhinovirus	sICAM-1	Soluble receptor decoy	Intranasal	
	Pleconaril	Capsid binder	Intranasal	
Influenza virus	Peramivir	Neuraminidase inhibitor	O	
	R-118958	Neuraminidase inhibitor	Inhaled	Long acting in murine model

ABBREVIATIONS: RT, reverse transcriptase; DNAp, DNA polymerase; O, oral.

dani *et al.*, 2003). Intravenous ribavirin is investigational in the United States.

OTHER AGENTS

Imiquimod

Imiquimod [1-(2-methylpropyl)-1*H*-imidazo[4,5-*c*]quino-lin-4 amine] is a novel immunomodulatory agent that is effective for topical treatment of condylomata acuminata and certain other dermatologic conditions (Skinner, 2003). It lacks direct antiviral or antiproliferative effects *in vitro* but rather induces cytokines and chemokines with antiviral and immunomodulating effects. Imiquimod shows antiviral activity in animal models after systemic or topical administration. When applied topically as a 5% cream to genital warts in humans, it induces local IFN-α, -β, and -γ and TNF-α responses and causes reductions in viral load and wart size. When applied topically

(three times weekly for up to 16 weeks), imiquimod cream is associated with complete clearance of treated genital and perianal warts in about 50% of patients, with response rates being higher in women than in men (Wiley *et al.*, 2002; Skinner, 2003). The median time to clearance is 8 to 10 weeks; relapses are not uncommon. Application is associated with local erythema in about 20% of patients, excoriation/flaking in 18% to 26%, itching in 10% to 20%, burning in 5% to 12%, and less often, erosions or ulcerations.

STRATEGIES UNDER DEVELOPMENT

Table 49–4 summarizes some of the antiviral agents that are in clinical development, excluding those for HIV infection.

More satisfactory antiviral therapies likely will come in part from the identification of agents with improved pharmacokinetic properties, greater potency, and/or improved toxicity profiles compared with existing ones. New drug-delivery techniques that improve pharmacokinetic properties (*e.g.,* prodrugs to enhance oral bioavailability, carrier molecules to alter absorption and/or degradation) or target particular tissues or cell types are receiving particular attention in drug development. For example, ether lipid esters of cidofovir provide increased cellular uptake and *in vitro* antiviral activity, enhanced oral bioavailability, reduced nephrotoxicity, and activity in animal models of CMV and poxvirus infections (Kern *et al.*, 2004).

As in other areas of antimicrobial chemotherapy, the combined use of antiviral agents has been studied as a means of increasing antiviral activity, reducing drug dosage and the associated risk of toxicity, and preventing or modifying the development of drug resistance. Because viral isolates may be mixtures of sensitive and resistant viruses or viruses with different resistance mutations, treatment with combinations of drugs may provide broader activity than treatment with single agents. Drug combinations may constrain the mutability of the virus, enhance susceptibility to a second agent, or diminish viral replicative capacity.

Future therapeutic breakthroughs probably also will depend on the identification of new molecular targets in viral replication and novel therapeutic modalities. The first antisense oligonucleotide has been approved for a human viral infection (*fomivirsen* for CMV retinitis), but important problems regarding potency, selectivity, and delivery to target cells remain to be solved. An antiviral strategy increasingly used in laboratory studies is RNA interference, a process of gene silencing in which introduced double-stranded RNA (dsRNA) leads to sequence-specific degradation of messenger RNA. Antiviral effects using small interfering RNAs (siRNAs) have been shown in cell culture for a range of viruses, including HCV, influenza, RSV, picornaviruses, and SARS coronavirus in humans and for several in animals, including influenza (Ge *et al.*, 2003). *In vivo* application of this approach is limited by the technical challenges of achieving intracellular delivery of sufficient siRNA, so the clinical potential of RNA interference remains to be determined.

Other approaches that may prove to be useful involve agents to moderate host immunopathological responses, agents to boost host immune responses, and virus-specific immunotherapies (*e.g.,* monoclonal antibodies, therapeutic vaccines) to supplement host responses.

BIBLIOGRAPHY

Alberti, A., Boccato, S., Vario, A., and Benvegnu, L. Therapy of acute hepatitis C. *Hepatology,* **2002,** *36:*S195–200.

Anonymous. Valacyclovir (Valtrex) for herpes labialis. *Med. Lett. Drugs Ther.,* **2002,** *44:*95–96.

Anonymous. Mortality in patients with the acquired immunodeficiency syndrome treated with either foscarnet or ganciclovir for cytomegalovirus retinitis. Studies of Ocular Complications of AIDS Research Group, in Collaboration With the AIDS Clinical Trials Group (published erratum appears in New Engl. J. Med., 1992, Apr. 23;326:1172). *New Engl. J. Med.,* **1996,** *326:*213–220.

Anonymous. Docosanol cream (Abreva) for recurrent herpes labialis. *Med. Lett. Drugs Ther.,* **2000,** *42:*108.

Bacon, T.H, Levin, M.J., Leary, J.J., *et al.* Herpes simplex virus resistance to acyclovir and penciclovir after two decades of antiviral therapy. *Clin. Microbiol. Rev.,* **2003,** *16:*114–128.

Baron, S., Coppenhaver, D.H., and Dianzani, F., *et al.* Introduction to the interferon system. In, *Interferons: Principles and Medical Applications.* (Baron, S., Dianzani, F., Stanton, G.J., *et al.,* eds.) University of Texas Medical Branch Dept. of Microbiology, Galveston, TX, **1992,** pp. 1–15.

Benhamou, Y., Bochet, M., Thibault, V., *et al.* Safety and efficacy of adefovir dipivoxil in patients co-infected with HIV-1 and lamivudine-resistant hepatitis B virus: An open-label pilot study. *Lancet,* **2001,** *358:*718–723.

Beutner, K., Friedman, D., Forszpaniak, C., *et al.* Valaciclovir compared with acyclovir for improved therapy for herpes zoster in immunocompetent adults. *Antimicrob. Agents Chemother.,* **1995,** *39:*1546–1553.

Biron, C., Interferons alpha and beta as immune regulators: A new look. *Immunity,* **2001,** *14:*661–664.

Bocci, V. Physiochemical and biologic properties of interferons and their potential uses in drug delivery systems. *Crit. Rev. Ther. Drug Carrier Syst.,* **1992,** *9:*91–133.

Boike, S., Pue, M., Audet, P., *et al.* Pharmacokinetics of famciclovir in subjects with chronic hepatic disease. *J. Clin. Pharmacol.,* **1994,** *34:*1199–1207.

Brosgart, C., Louis, T., Hillman D., *et al.* A randomized, placebo-controlled trial of the safety and efficacy of oral ganciclovir for prophylaxis of cytomegalovirus disease in HIV-infected individuals. Terry Beirn Community Programs for Clinical Research on AIDS. *AIDS,* **1998,** *12:*269–277.

Brown, F., Banken, L., Saywell, K., and Arum, I. Pharmacokinetics of valganciclovir and ganciclovir following multiple oral dosages of valganciclovir in HIV- and CMV-seropositive volunteers. *Clin. Pharmacokinet.,* **1999,** *37:*167–176.

Bruno, R., Sacchi, P., Ciappina, V., *et al.* Viral dynamics and pharmacokinetics of peginterferon alpha-2a and peginterferon alpha-2b in naive patients with chronic hepatitis C: A randomized, controlled study. *Antiviral Ther.,* **2004,** *9:*491–497.

Cass, L., Efthymiopoulos, C., and Bye, A. Pharmacokinetics of zanamivir after intravenous, oral, inhaled or intranasal administration to healthy volunteers. *Clin. Pharmacokinet.,* **1999,** *36:*1–11.

Chilukuri, S., and Rosen, T. Management of acyclovir-resistant herpes simplex virus. *Dermatol. Clin.,* **2003,** *21:*311–320.

Chrisp, P., and Clissold, S.P. Foscarnet: A review of its antiviral activity, pharmacokinetic properties and therapeutic use in immunocompromised patients with cytomegalovirus retinitis. *Drugs,* **1991,** *41:*104–129.

Colin, J., Hoh, H., Easty, D., *et al.* Ganciclovir ophthalmic gel (Virgan: 0.15%) in the treatment of herpes simplex keratitis. *Cornea,* **1997,** *16:*393–399.

Committee on Infectious Diseases, American Academy of Pediatrics, *Red Book: 2003 Report of the Committee on Infectious Diseases.* American Academy of Pediatrics, Elk Grove Village, IL, **2003.**

Cooksley, W., Piratvisuth, T., Lee, S., *et al.* Peginterferon alpha-2a (40 kDa): An advance in the treatment of hepatitis B e antigen–positive chronic hepatitis B. *J. Viral Hepat.,* **2003,** *10*:298-305.

Cooper, N., Sutton, A., Abrams, K., *et al.* Effectiveness of neuraminidase inhibitors in treatment and prevention of influenza A and B: Systematic review and meta-analyses of randomised, controlled trials. *Br. Med. J.,* **2003,** *326*:1235–1239.

Corey, L., Wald, A., Patel, R., *et al.* Once-daily valacyclovir to reduce the risk of transmission of genital herpes. *New Engl. J. Med.,* **2004,** *350*:11–20.

Coverdale, S., Khan, M., Byth, K., *et al.* Effects of interferon treatment response on liver complications of chronic hepatitis C: 9-year follow-up study. *Am. J. Gastroenterol.,* **2004,** *99*:636–644.

Cundy, K. Clinical pharmacokinetics of the antiviral nucleotide analogues cidofovir and adefovir. *Clin. Pharmacokinet.,* **1999,** *36*:127–143.

Curran, M., and Noble, S. Valganciclovir. *Drugs,* **2001,** *61*:1145–1150.

De Clercq, E. Clinical potential of the acyclic nucleoside phosphonates cidofovir, adefovir, and tenofovir in treatment of DNA virus and retrovirus infections. *Clin. Microbiol. Rev.,* **2003,** *16*:569–596.

Delaney, W., Yang, H., Miller, M., *et al.* Combinations of adefovir with nucleoside analogs produce additive antiviral effects against hepatitis B virus *in vitro. Antimicrob. Agents Chemother.,* **2004,** *48*:3702–3710.

Der, S., Zhou, A., Williams, B., and Silverman, R. Identification of genes differentially regulated by interferon alpha, beta, or gamma using oligonucleotide arrays. *Proc. Natl. Acad. Sci. U.S.A.,* **1998,** *95*:15623–15628.

Dienstag, J., Goldin, R., Heathcote, E., *et al.* Histological outcome during long-term lamivudine therapy. *Gastroenterology,* **2003,** *124*:105–117.

Dienstag, J., Schiff, E., Wright, T., *et al.* Lamivudine as initial treatment for chronic hepatitis B in the United States. *New Engl. J. Med.,* **1999,** *341*:1256–1263.

Dusheiko, G. Side effects of Alpha interferon in chronic hepatitis C. *Hepatology,* **1997,** *26*:112S–121S.

Elion, G.B. History, mechanism of action, spectrum and selectivity of nucleoside analogs. In, *Antiviral Chemotherapy: New Directions for Clinical Application and Research.* (Mills, J., and Corey, L., eds.) Elsevier, New York, **1986,** pp. 118–137.

Englund, J., Piedra, P., Jefferson, L., *et al.* High-dose, short-duration ribavirin aerosol therapy in children with suspected respiratory syncytial virus infection. *J. Pediatr.,* **1990,** *117*:313–320.

Faulds, D., and Heel, R. Ganciclovir: A review of its antiviral activity, pharmacokinetic properties and therapeutic efficacy in cytomegalovirus infections. *Drugs,* **1990,** *39*:597–638.

Feinberg, J., Hurwitz, S., Cooper, D., *et al.* A randomized, double-blind trial of valaciclovir prophylaxis for cytomegalovirus disease in patients with advanced human immunodeficiency virus infection. AIDS Clinical Trials Group Protocol 204/Glaxo Wellcome 123-014 International CMV Prophylaxis Study Group. *J. Infect. Dis.,* **1998,** *177*:48–56.

Fried, M., Shiffman, M., Reddy, K., *et al.* Peginterferon alfa-2a plus ribavirin for chronic hepatitis C virus infection. *New Engl. J. Med.,* **2002,** *347*:975–982.

Ge, Q., McManus, M., Nguyen, T., *et al.* RNA interference of influenza virus production by directly targeting mRNA for degradation and indirectly inhibiting all viral RNA transcription. *Proc. Natl. Acad. Sci. U.S.A.,* **2003,** *100*:2718–2723.

Geary, R., Henry, S., and Grillone, L. Fomivirsen: clinical pharmacology and potential drug interactions. *Clin. Pharmacokinet.,* **2002,** *41*:255–260.

Ghosh, S., Champlin, R.I., Englund, J., *et al.* Respiratory syncytial virus upper respiratory tract illnesses in adult blood and marrow transplant recipients: Combination therapy with aerosolized ribavirin and intravenous immunoglobulin. *Bone Marrow Transplant.,* **2000,** *25*:751–755.

Gilbert. C., Bestman-Smith, J., and Boivin, G. Resistance of herpesviruses to antiviral drugs: Clinical impacts and molecular mechanisms. *Drug Resist. Update,* **2002,** *5*:88–114.

Gill, K.S., and Wood, M.J. The clinical pharmacokinetics of famciclovir. *Clin. Pharmacokinet.,* **1996,** *31*:1–8.

Glue, P. The clinical pharmacology of ribavirin. *Semin. Liver Dis.,* **1999,** *19*(suppl 1):17–24.

Glue, P., Fang, J., Rouzier-Panis, R., *et al.* Pegylated interferon-alpha2b: Pharmacokinetics, pharmacodynamics, safety, and preliminary efficacy data. Hepatitis C Intervention Therapy Group. *Clin. Pharmacol. Ther.,* **2000,** *68*:556–567.

Griffin, S., Beales, L., Clarke, D., *et al.* The P7 protein of hepatitis C virus forms an ion channel that is blocked by the antiviral drug, amantadine. *FEBS Lett.,* **2003,** *535*:34–38.

Gubareva, L., Hayden, F., and Kaiser, L. Influenza virus neuraminidase inhibitors. *Lancet,* **2000,** *355*:827–835.

Hadziyannis S.J., Manesis E.K., and Papakonstantinou, A. Oral ganciclovir treatment in chronic hepatitis B virus infection: a pilot study. *J. Hepatol.,* **1999,** *31*:210–214.

Hadziyannis, S., Sette, H., Morgan, T., *et al.* Peginterferon-alpha2a and ribavirin combination therapy in chronic hepatitis C: A randomized study of treatment duration and ribavirin dose. *Ann. Intern. Med.,* **2004,** *140*:346–355.

Hadziyannis, S., Tassopoulos, N., Heathcote, E., *et al.* Adefovir dipivoxil for the treatment of hepatitis B e antigen–negative chronic hepatitis B. *New Engl. J. Med.,* **2003,** *348*:800–807.

Hayden, F. Perspectives on antiviral use during pandemic influenza. *Phil. Trans. Soc. Lond.,* **2001,** *356*:1877–1884.

Hayden, F. Antiviral drugs (other than antiretrovirals), in *Mandell, Douglas, and Bennett's Principles and Practice of Infectious Diseases.* (Mandell G., Bennett, J. and Dolin, R. eds) Churchill-Livingstone, Philadelphia, **2004,** pp. 310–347.

Hayden, F. Amantadine and rimantadine: Clinical aspects, in *Antiviral Drug Resistance.* (Richman, D. ed.) Wiley, New York, **1996,** pp. 59–77.

Hayden, F., and Aoki, F. Amantadine, rimantadine, and related agents, in *Antimicrobial Therapy and Vaccines.* (Yu, V., Merigan, T., White, N., and Barriere, S. eds.) Williams & Wilkins, Baltimore, **1999,** pp. 1344–1365.

Hayden, F., Belshe, R., Villanueva, C., *et al.* Management of influenza in households: A prospective, randomized comparison of oseltamivir treatment with or without post-exposure prophylaxis. *J. Infect. Dis.,* **2004,** *189*:440–449.

He, G., Massarella, J., and Ward, P. Clinical pharmacokinetics of the prodrug oseltamivir and its active metabolite Ro 64-0802. *Clin. Pharmacokinet.,* **1999,** *37*:471–484.

Heathcote, J., Shiffman, M., Cooksley, G., *et al.* Peginterferon alfa-2a in patients with chronic hepatitis C and cirrhosis. *New Engl. J. Med.,* **2000,** *343*:1673–1680.

Hedrick, J., Barzilai, A., Behre, U., *et al.* Zanamivir for treatment of symptomatic influenza A and B infection in children five to twelve years of age: A randomized, controlled trial. *Pediatr. Infect. Dis. J.,* **2000,** *19*:410–417.

Hitchcock, M., Jaffe, H., Martin, J., and Stagg, R. Cidofovir, a new agent with potent anti-herpesvirus activity. *Antiviral Chem. Chemother.,* **1996,** *7*:115–127.

Ho, E., Lin, D., Mendel, D., and Cihlar, T. Cytotoxicity of antiviral nucleotides adefovir and cidofovir is induced by the expression of human renal organic anion transporter 1. *J. Am. Soc. Nephrol.*, **2000**, *11*:383–393.

Hong, Z., and Cameron, C. Pleiotropic mechanisms of ribavirin antiviral activities. *Prog. Drug Res.*, **2002**, *59*:41–69.

Infectious Disease Community of Practice, American Society of Transplantation, Guidelines for the prevention and management of infectious complications of solid organ transplantation: Cytomegalovirus. *Am. J. Transplant.*, **2004**, *4*(suppl 10):51–58.

Johnson, M., Moore, K., Yuen, G., et al. Clinical pharmacokinetics of lamivudine. *Clin. Pharmacokinet.*, **1999**, *36*:41–66.

Jonas, M., Kelly, D., Mizerski, J., et al. Clinical trial of lamivudine in children with chronic hepatitis B. *N.ewEngl. J. Med.*, **2002**, *346*:1706–1713.

Kaiser, L., Keene, O., Hammond, J., et al. Impact of zanamivir on antibiotics use for respiratory events following acute influenza in adolescents and adults. *Arch. Intern. Med.*, **2000**, *160*:3234–3240.

Kaiser, L., Wat, C., Mills, T., et al. Impact of oseltamivir treatment on influenza-related lower respiratory tract complications and hospitalizations. *Arch. Intern. Med.*, **2003**, *163*:1667–1672.

Keating, G., and Curran, M. Peginterferon-alpha-2a (40 kDa) plus ribavirin: A review of its use in the management of chronic hepatitis C. *Drugs*, **2003**, *63*:701–730.

Kern, E., Collins, D., Wan, W., et al. Oral treatment of murine cytomegalovirus infections with ether lipid esters of cidofovir. *Antimicrob. Agents Chemother.*, **2004**, *48*:3516–3522.

Keyser, L., Karl, M., Nafziger, A., and Bertino, J., Jr. Comparison of central nervous system adverse effects of amantadine and rimantadine used as sequential prophylaxis of influenza A in elderly nursing home patients. *Arch. Intern. Med.*, **2000**, *160*:1485–1488.

Kimberlin, D., Weller, S., Whitley, R., et al. Pharmacokinetics of oral valacyclovir and acyclovir in late pregnancy. *Am. J. Obstet. Gynecol.*, **1998**, *179*:846–851.

Kimberlin, D.W., Lin, C.Y., Jacobs, R.F., et al. Safety and efficacy of high-dose intravenous acyclovir in the management of neonatal herpes simplex virus infections. *Pediatrics*, **2001**, *108*:230–238.

Kimberlin, D., and Rouse, D. Clinical practice: Genital herpes. *New Engl. J. Med.*, **2004**, *350*:1970–1977.

Lai, C., Yuen, M., Hui, C., et al. Comparison of the efficacy of lamivudine and famciclovir in Asian patients with chronic hepatitis B: Results of 24 weeks of therapy. *J. Med. Virol.*, **2002**, *67*:334–338.

Lau, D., Everhart, J., Kleiner, D., et al. Long-term follow-up of patients with chronic hepatitis B treated with interferon alfa. *Gastroenterology*, **1997**, *113*:1660–1667.

Lazarus, H., Belanger, R., Candoni, A., et al. Intravenous penciclovir for treatment of herpes simplex infections in immunocompromised patients: Results of a multicenter, acyclovir-controlled trial. The Penciclovir Immunocompromised Study Group. *Antimicrob. Agents Chemother.*, **1999**, *43*:1192–1197.

Liaw, Y., Sung, J., Chow, W., et al. Lamivudine for patients with chronic hepatitis B and advanced liver disease. *New Engl. J. Med.*, **2004**, *351*:1521–1531.

Limaye, A., Corey, L., Koelle, D., et al. Emergence of ganciclovir-resistant cytomegalovirus disease among recipients of solid-organ transplants. *Lancet*, **2000**, *356*:645–649.

Ljungman, P., Ribaud, P., Eyrich, M., et al. Cidofovir for adenovirus infections after allogeneic hematopoietic stem cell transplantation: A survey by the Infectious Diseases Working Party of the European Group for Blood and Marrow Transplantation. *Bone Marrow Transplant.*, **2003**, *31*:481–486.

Loutfy, M.R., Blatt, L M., Siminovitch, K.A., et al. Interferon alfacon-1 plus corticosteroids in severe acute respiratory syndrome: A preliminary study. *JAMA*, **2003**, *290*:3222–3228.

Lowance, D., Neumayer, H., Legendre C.M., et al. Valacyclovir for the prevention of cytomegalovirus disease after renal transplantation. *New Engl. J. Med.*, **1999**, *340*:1462–1470.

Marcellin P., Chang T.T., Lim, S.G., et al. Adefovir dipivoxil for the treatment of hepatitis B e antigen–positive chronic hepatitis B. *New Engl. J. Med.*, **2003**, *348*:808–816.

Marcellin, P., Lau, G.K., and Bonino, F. Peginterferon alfa-2a alone, lamivudine alone, and the two in combination in patients with HBeAg-negative chronic hepatitis B. *New Engl. J. Med.*, **2004**, *351*:1206–1217.

Mardani, M., Jahromi, M.K., Naieni, K.H., and Zeinali, M. The efficacy of oral ribavirin in the treatment of Crimean-Congo hemorrhagic fever in Iran. *Clin. Infect. Dis.*, **2003**, *36*:1613–1618.

Martin, D.F., Sierra-Madero, J., Walmsley, S., et al. A controlled trial of valganciclovir as induction therapy for cytomegalovirus retinitis. *New Engl. J. Med.*, **2002**, *346*:1119–1126.

Michaels, M.G., Greenberg, D.P., Sabo, D.L., and Wald, E.R. Treatment of children with congenital cytomegalovirus infection with ganciclovir. *Pediatr. Infect. Dis.*, **2003**, *22*:504–509.

Noble, S., and Faulds, D. Ganciclovir: An update of its use in the prevention of cytomegalovirus infection and disease in transplant recipients. *Drugs*, **1998**, *56*:115–146.

Ono, S.K., Kato, N., Shiratori, Y., et al. The polymerase L528M mutation cooperates with nucleotide binding-site mutations, increasing hepatitis B virus replication and drug resistance. *J. Clin. Invest.*, **2001**, *107*:449–455.

Paya, C., Humar, A., Dominguez, E., et al. Efficacy and safety of valganciclovir vs. oral ganciclovir for prevention of cytomegalovirus disease in solid organ transplant recipients. *Am. J. Transplant.*, **2004**, *4*:611–620.

Peng, A.W., Milleri, S., and Stein, D.S. Direct measurement of the anti-influenza agent zanamivir in the respiratory tract following inhalation. *Antimicrob. Agents Chemother.*, **2000**, *44*:1974–1976.

Pereyra, F., and Rubin, R.H. Prevention and treatment of cytomegalovirus infection in solid organ transplant recipients. *Curr. Opin. Infect. Dis.*, **2004**, *17*:357–361.

Peters, M.G., Hann, H., Martin, P., et al. Adefovir dipivoxil alone or in combination with lamivudine in patients with lamivudine-resistant chronic hepatitis B. *Gastroenterology*, **2004**, *126*:91–101.

Pillay, D. Management of herpes virus infections following transplantation. *J. Antimicrob. Chemother.*, **2000**, *45*:729–748.

Poynard, T., McHutchison, J., Manns, M., et al. Impact of pegylated interferon alfa-2b and ribavirin on liver fibrosis in patients with chronic hepatitis C. *Gastroenterology*, **2002**, *122*:1303–1313.

Prentice, H.G., Gluckman, E., Powles, R.L., et al. Impact of long-term acyclovir on cytomegalovirus infection and survival after allogeneic bone marrow transplantation. European Acyclovir for CMV Prophylaxis Study Group. *Lancet*, **1994**, *343*:749–753.

Prusoff, W.H. Idoxuridine or how it all began. In, *Clinical Use of Antiviral Drugs.* (DeClercq, E., ed.) Martinus Nijhoff Publishing, Boston, **1988**, pp. 15–24.

Raborn, G.W., Martel, A.Y., Lassonde, M., et al. Effective treatment of herpes simplex labialis with penciclovir cream: combined results of two trials. *J. Am. Dent. Assoc.*, **2002**, *133*:303–309.

Ratanajamit, C., Vinther, S., Jepsen, P., et al. Adverse pregnancy outcome in women exposed to acyclovir during pregnancy: a population-based observational study. *Scand. J. Infect. Dis.*, **2003**, *35*:255–259.

Reusser, P., Einsele, H., Lee, J., *et al*. Randomized multicenter trial of foscarnet versus ganciclovir for preemptive therapy of cytomegalovirus infection after allogeneic stem cell transplantation. *Blood,* **2002,** *99*:1159–1164.

Roberts, N.A. Treatment of influenza with neuraminidase inhibitors: Virological implications. *Philos. Trans. R. Soc. Lond. B. Biol. Sci.,* **2001,** *356*:1895–1897.

Sacks, S.L., and Wilson, B. Famciclovir/penciclovir. *Adv. Exp. Med. Biol.,* **1999,** *458*:135–147.

Safrin, S., Cherrington, J. M., and Jaffe, H. S. Clinical uses of cidofovir. *Rev. Med. Virol.,* **1997,** *7*:145–156.

Samuel, C.E. Antiviral actions of interferons. *Clin. Microbiol. Rev.,* **2001,** *14*:778–809.

Seeff, L.B. and Hoofnagle, J. H. National Institutes of Health Consensus Development Conference statement: Management of hepatitis C. *Hepatology,* **2002,** *36*(5 suppl 1):S1–2.

Sheffield, J.S., Hollier, L.M., Hill, J.B., Stuart, G.S., and Wendel, G.D. Acyclovir prophylaxis to prevent herpes simplex virus recurrence at delivery: A systematic review. *Obstet. Gynecol.,* **2003,** *102*:1396–1403.

Shults, R.A., Baron, S., Decker, J., Deitchman, S.D., and Connor, J.D. Health care worker exposure to aerosolized ribavirin: Biological and air monitoring. *J. Occup. Environ. Med.,* **1996,** *38*:257–263.

Skinner, R.B., Jr. Imiquimod. *Dermatol. Clin.,* **2003,** *21*:291–300.

Smith, J.P., Riley, T.R., Devenyi, A.M., Bingaman, S.I., and Kunselman, A.M. Amantadine therapy for chronic hepatitis C: A randomized, double-blind, placebo-controlled trial. *J. Gen. Intern. Med.,* **2004,** 19:662–668.

Sokal, E.M., Conjeevaram, H.S., Roberts, E.A., *et al*. Interferon alfa therapy for chronic hepatitis B in children: A multinational randomized, controlled trial. *Gastroenterology,* **1998,** *114*:988–995.

Sokal, E.M., Roberts, E.A., Mieli-Vergani, G., *et al*. Dose ranging study of the pharmacokinetics, safety, and preliminary efficacy of lamivudine in children and adolescents with chronic hepatitis B. *Antimicrob. Agents Chemother.,* **2000,** *44*:590–597.

Spruance, S.L., Nett, R., Marbury, T., *et al*. Acyclovir cream for treatment of herpes simplex labialis: Results of two randomized, double-blind, vehicle-controlled, multicenter clinical trials. *Antimicrob. Agents Chemother.,* **2002,** *46*:2238–2243.

Steer, C.B., Szer, J., Sasadeusz, J., *et al*. Varicella-zoster infection after allogeneic bone marrow transplantation: Incidence, risk factors and prevention with low-dose aciclovir and ganciclovir. *Bone Marrow Transplant.,* **2000,** *25*:657–664.

Steingrimsdottir, H., Gruber, A., Palm, C., *et al*. Bioavailability of aciclovir after oral administration of acyclovir and its prodrug valaciclovir to patients with leukopenia after chemotherapy. *Antimicrob. Agents Chemother.,* **2000,** *44*:207–209.

Tam, R.C., Lau, J.Y., and Hong, Z. Mechanisms of action of ribavirin in antiviral therapies. *Antiviral Chem. Chemother.,* **2002,** *12*:261–272.

Torriani, F.J., Rodriguez-Torres, M., Rockstroh, J.K., *et al*. Peginterferon alfa-2a plus ribavirin for chronic hepatitis C virus infection in HIV-infected patients. *New Engl. J. Med.,* **2004,** 351:438–450.

Tyring, S., Engst, R., and Corriveau, C. Famciclovir for ophthalmic zoster: A randomised aciclovir controlled study. *Br. J. Ophthalmol.,* **2001,** *85*:576–581.

Tyring, S.K., Beutner, K, Tucker, B.A., Anderson, W.C., and Crooks, J. Antiviral therapy for herpes zoster. *Arch. Fam. Med.,* **2000,** *9*:863–869.

Vats, A., Shapiro, R., Singh, R., *et al*. Quantitative viral load monitoring and cidofovir therapy for the management of BK virus–associated nephropathy in children and adults. *Transplantation,* **2003,** *75*:105–112.

Vitravene Study Group. Randomized dose-comparison studies of intravitreous fomivirsen for treatment of cytomegalovirus retinitis that has reactivated or is persistently active despite other therapies in patients with aids. *Am. J. Ophthalmol.,* **2002,** *133*:475–483.

Wagstaff, A.J., and Bryson, H.M. Foscarnet: A reappraisal of its antiviral activity, pharmacokinetic properties and therapeutic use in immunocompromised patients with viral infections. *Drugs,* **1994,** *48*:199–226.

Wagstaff, A.J., Faulds, D., and Goa, K.L. Aciclovir: A reappraisal of its antiviral activity, pharmacokinetic properties and therapeutic efficacy. *Drugs,* **1994,** *47*:153–205.

Wallace, M.R., Bowler, W.A., Murray, N.B., Brodine, S.K., and Oldfield, E.C. Treatment of adult varicella with oral acyclovir. A randomized, placebo-controlled trial. *Ann. Intern. Med.,* **1992,** *117*:358–363.

Whitley, R.J., and Gnann, J.J. Acyclovir: A decade later. *New Engl. J. Med.,* **1992,** *327*:782–789.

Whitley, R.J., Hayden, F.G., Reisinger, K., *et al*. Oral oseltamivir treatment of influenza in children. *Pediatr. Infect. Dis. J.,* **2001,** *20*:127–133.

Wiley, D.J., Douglas, J., Beutner, K., *et al*. External genital warts: Diagnosis, treatment, and prevention. *Clin. Infect. Dis.,* **2002,** *35*:S210–S224.

Wills, R.J. Clinical pharmacokinetics of interferons. *Clin. Pharmacokinet.,* **1990,** *19*:390–399.

Winston, D.J., Yeager, A. M., Chandrasekar, P.H., *et al*. Randomized comparison of oral valacyclovir and intravenous ganciclovir for prevention of cytomegalovirus disease after allogeneic bone marrow transplantation. *Clin. Infect. Dis.,* **2003,** *36*:749–758.

Young, K.C., Lindsay, K.L, and Lee, K.J. Identification of a ribavirin-resistant NS5B mutation of hepatitis C virus during ribavirin monotherapy. *Hepatology,* **2003,** *38*:869–878.

ANTIRETROVIRAL AGENTS AND TREATMENT OF HIV INFECTION

Charles Flexner

I. OVERVIEW OF HIV INFECTION

Combination antiretroviral therapy prolongs life and prevents progression of disease caused by human immunodeficiency virus (HIV). The pharmacotherapy of HIV infection is a rapidly moving field. In 2004, there were 20 antiretroviral drugs available in the United States. Since three-drug combinations are the minimum standard of care for this infection, current agents constitute at least 1140 possible regimens. The long-term management of a patient on antiretroviral therapy can be daunting, even for an experienced healthcare provider. Knowing the essential features of the pathophysiology of this disease and how chemotherapeutic agents affect the virus and the host is critical in developing a rational approach to therapy. *Unique features of this drug class include the need for lifelong administration to control virus replication and the possibility of rapid emergence of permanent drug resistance if these agents are not used properly.*

In 2004, an estimated 42 million people were living with HIV infection worldwide, with the majority in resource-poor countries. Increasingly, the public health impact of this epidemic has shifted to those regions least able to afford treatment. Fewer than 5% of those who would benefit from combination antiretroviral therapy were receiving it, even though such treatment is known to reduce the complications of infection and prolong life (Lee *et al.*, 2001). The causes of maldistribution of effective antiretroviral therapy are complex, including social and economic inequities, patient and provider choice, and shortcomings in the convenience and tolerability of available regimens. Regardless, these drugs have the capacity

to improve the quality of human health substantially and to produce near-normal life expectancies for some patients with a previously lethal disease (Lee *et al.*, 2001).

PATHOGENESIS OF HIV-RELATED DISEASE

Human immunodeficiency viruses (HIV) are lentiviruses, a family of mammalian retroviruses evolved to establish chronic persistent infection with gradual onset of clinical symptoms. Unlike herpesviruses, replication is constant following infection, and although some infected cells may harbor nonreplicating but infectious virus for years, there generally is no true period of viral latency following infection (Greene and Peterlin, 2002). Humans and chimpanzees are the only known hosts for these viruses.

There are two major families of HIV. Most of the epidemic involves HIV-1; HIV-2 is a close relative whose distribution is concentrated in western Africa. HIV-1 is genetically diverse, with at least five distinct subfamilies or clades. HIV-1 and HIV-2 have similar *in vitro* sensitivity to most antiretroviral drugs, although the nonnucleoside reverse transcriptase inhibitors (NNRTIs) are HIV-1-specific and have no activity against HIV-2. Within HIV-1 isolates, clade *per se* does not seem to have a major effect on drug sensitivity.

Virus Structure. HIV is a typical retrovirus with a small RNA genome of 9300 base pairs. Two copies of the genome are contained in a nucleocapsid core surrounded by a lipid bilayer, or envelope, that is derived from the host cell plasma membrane (Figure 50–1). The

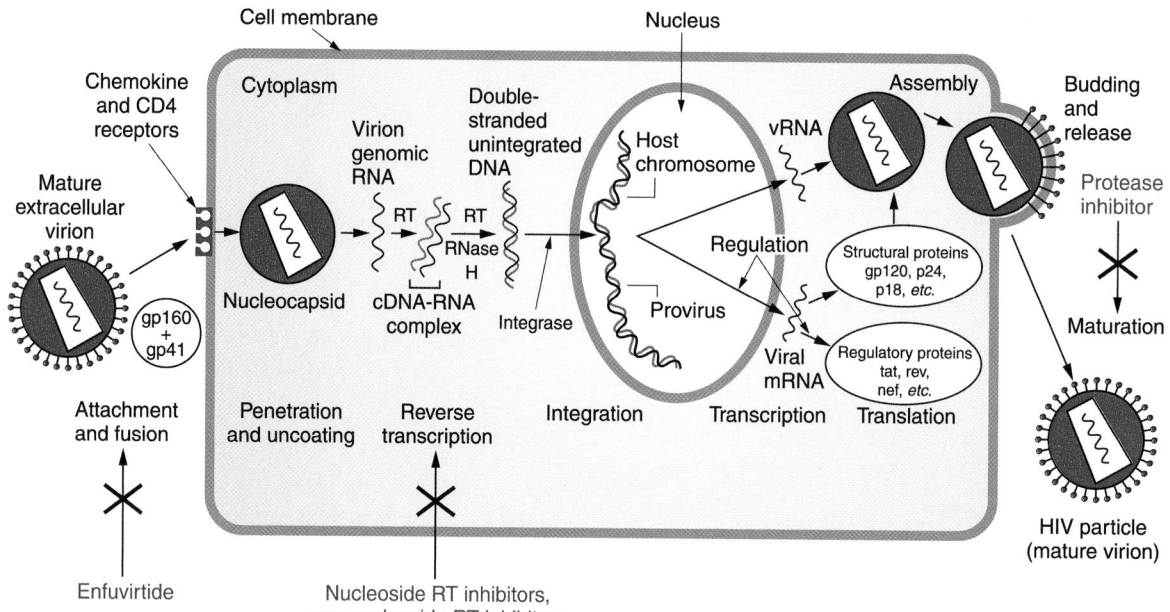

Figure 50–1. *Replicative cycle of HIV-1 showing the sites of action of available antiretroviral agents.* Available antiretroviral agents are shown in blue. Key: RT, reverse transcriptase; cDNA, complementary DNA; mRNA, messenger RNA; RNase H, ribonuclease H; gp120 + gp41, extracellular and intracellular domains, respectively, of envelope glycoprotein. (Adapted from Hirsch and D'Aquila, 1993.)

viral genome encodes three major open reading frames: *gag* encodes a polyprotein that is processed to release the major structural proteins of the virus; *pol* overlaps *gag* and encodes three important enzyme activities—an RNA-dependent DNA polymerase or reverse transcriptase with RNAase activity, protease, and the viral integrase; and *env* encodes the large transmembrane envelope protein responsible for cell binding and entry. Several small genes encode regulatory proteins that enhance virion production or combat host defenses. These include *tat*, *rev*, *nef*, and *vpr* (Greene and Peterlin, 2002).

Virus Life Cycle. HIV tropism is controlled by the envelope protein gp160 (env) (Figure 50–1). The major target for env binding is the CD4 receptor present on lymphocytes and macrophages, although cell entry also requires binding to a coreceptor, generally the chemokine receptor CCR5 or CXCR4 (Greene and Peterlin, 2002). CCR5 is present on macrophage lineage cells. Most infected individuals harbor predominately the CCR5-tropic virus; it is believed that this virus is responsible for sexual transmission of HIV and that the initial cells infected in sexual transmission express this coreceptor. A shift from CCR5 to CXCR4 utilization is associated with advancing disease, and the affinity of

HIV-1 for CXCR4 allows infection of T-lymphocytes (Berger *et al.*, 1999). A phenotypic switch from CCR5 to CXCR4 heralds accelerated loss of CD4+ helper T cells and increased risk of immunosuppression. Whether coreceptor switch is a cause or a consequence of advancing disease is still unknown.

The gp41 domain of env controls the fusion of the virus lipid bilayer with that of the host cell. Following fusion, full-length viral RNA enters the cytoplasm, where it undergoes replication to a short-lived RNA–DNA duplex; the original RNA is degraded by RNase H to allow creation of a full-length double-stranded DNA copy of the virus (Figure 50–1). Because the HIV reverse transcriptase is error-prone and lacks a proofreading function, mutation is quite frequent and estimated to occur at approximately three bases out of every full-length (9300-base-pair) replication (Coffin, 1995). Virus DNA is transported into the nucleus, where it is integrated into a host chromosome by the viral integrase in a random or quasi-random location (Greene and Peterlin, 2002).

Following integration, the virus may remain in a quiescent state, not producing RNA or protein but replicating as the cell divides. When a cell that harbors the virus is activated, viral RNA and proteins are produced. Structural proteins assemble around full-length genomic RNA to form a nucleocapsid (Figure 50–1). The transmembrane envelope and other structural proteins assemble at the cell surface, concentrated in cholesterol-rich lipid rafts. The nucleocapsid cores are directed to these sites and bud through the cell membrane, creating a new enveloped HIV particle containing two complete single-stranded RNA genomes. Reverse transcriptase is incorporated into this particle so that replication can begin immediately after the virus enters a new cell (Greene and Peterlin, 2002).

How the Virus Causes Disease. Sexual acquisition of HIV infection is thought to be mediated by one or, at most, a handful of infectious virus particles. Soon after infection, there is a rapid burst of replication peaking at 2 to 4 weeks, with 10^9 or more cells becoming infected. This peak is associated with a transient dip in the number of peripheral CD4+ (helper) T-lymphocytes. As a result of new host immune responses and target cell depletion, the number of infectious virions as reflected by the plasma HIV RNA concentration (also know as *viral load*) declines to a quasi-steady state. This level of virus activity has been termed the *set point* and reflects the interplay between host immunity and the pathogenicity of the infecting virus (Coffin, 1995). Most viruses are derived from CD4+ cells that turn over with a half-life of 2.2 days (Perelson *et al.*, 1996). Thus, in the average infected individual, several billion infectious virus particles are produced every few days.

Eventually, the host CD4+ T-lymphocyte count begins a steady decline, accompanied by a rise in the plasma HIV RNA concentration. Once the peripheral CD4 cell count falls below 200 cells/mm³, there is an increasing risk of opportunistic diseases and ultimately death. Sexual acquisition of CCR5-tropic HIV-1 is associated with a median time to clinical disease (usually an opportunistic infection such as *Pneumocystis carinii* pneumonia) of 8 to 10 years. Some patients, termed *long-term nonprogressors,* can harbor HIV for more than two decades without significant decline in peripheral CD4 cell count or clinical immunosuppression; this may reflect a combination of favorable host immunogenetics and immune responses (Fauci, 1996).

An important question relevant to treatment is whether HIV disease is a consequence purely of CD4+ lymphocyte depletion or other factors. Most natural history data suggest the former, although both the amount of virus measurable in the patient's circulation and the CD4 cell count are independent predictors of disease progression (Mellors *et al.*, 1996, 1997). Regardless, successful therapy is based on inhibition of HIV replication; treatments designed specifically to boost the host immune system without exerting a direct antiviral effect have had no reliable clinical benefit.

HISTORY OF ANTIRETROVIRAL THERAPY

The rapid discovery and development of combinations of antiretroviral agents capable of long-term control of HIV replication were remarkable achievements. Cooperation between government and academic researchers, the pharmaceutical industry, and regulatory agencies in the United States and Europe quickly converted bench observations into new treatment modalities. The identification of HIV as the causative agent of acquired immune deficiency syndrome (AIDS) in 1985 and the immediate availability of its complete genome (Fisher *et al.*, 1985) paved the way for the development of selective inhibitors.

The first effective antiretroviral agent, *zidovudine,* was synthesized by Horwitz in 1964 as a false nucleoside with disappointing anticancer activity. The drug was shown by Osterag in 1972 to inhibit the *in vitro* replication of a murine type D retrovirus (McLeod and Hammer, 1992). Mitsuya and Broder, working in Bethesda in 1985, reported that this drug had potent *in vitro* anti-HIV activity (Mitsuya *et al.*, 1985). Clinical studies of zidovudine began that same year, and by 1987 this drug was approved and marketed for the control of HIV infection based on the results of a small but definitive randomized clinical trial (Fischl *et al.*, 1987). Large numbers of nucleoside analogs already had been synthesized as potential anticancer and immunomodulatory drugs, and this made it possible for similar compounds to be tested efficiently and approved.

Selective nonnucleoside reverse transcriptase inhibitors (NNRTIs) were identified by iterative screening using purified viral enzyme (Pauwels *et al.*, 1990). The clinical development of these drugs was hindered by the rapid emergence of drug resistance (Wei *et al.*, 1995). However, three drugs in this category were approved by 1998 (Table 50–1). HIV protease inhibitors were the products of rational drug design, relying on technology developed to identify transition-state peptidomimetic antagonists of proteases in the renin–angiotensin cascade (Flexner, 1998). Highly selective antagonists of the HIV protease were reported as early as 1987. Phase I trials of the first of these drugs, *saquinavir,* began in 1989, and this drug was approved for prescription use in 1995. Two additional protease inhibitors, *ritonavir* and *indinavir,* were approved within the next 4 months.

Table 50–1
Antiretroviral Agents Approved for Use in the United States

GENERIC NAME [U.S. TRADE NAME]	ABBREVIATION; CHEMICAL NAMES
Nucleoside reverse transcriptase inhibitors	
Zidovudine [RETROVIR]*	ZDV; azidothymidine (AZT)
Didanosine [VIDEX; VIDEX EC]	ddI; dideoxyinosine
Stavudine [ZERIT; ZERIT XR]	d4T; didehydrodeoxythymidine
Zalcitabine [HIVID]	DDC; dideoxycytidine
Lamivudine [EPIVIR]*	3TC; dideoxythiacytidine
Abacavir [ZIAGEN]*	ABC; cyclopropylaminopurinylcyclopentene
Tenofovir disoproxil [VIREAD]*	TDF; phosphinylmethoxypropyladenine (PMPA)
Emtricitabine [EMTRIVA]*	FTC; fluorooxathiolanyl cytosine
Nonnucleoside reverse transcriptase inhibitors	
Nevirapine [VIRAMUNE]	NVP
Efavirenz [SUSTIVA]	EFV
Delavirdine [RESCRIPTOR]	DLV
Protease inhibitors	
Saquinavir [INVIRASE; FORTOVASE]	SQV
Indinavir [CRIXIVAN]	IDV
Ritonavir [NORVIR]	RTV
Nelfinavir [VIRACEPT]	NFV
Amprenavir [AGENERASE]	APV
Lopinavir [KALETRA][†]	LPV/r
Atazanavir [REYATAZ]	ATV
Fosamprenavir [LEXIVA]	FPV
Fusion inhibitor	
Enfuvirtide [FUZEON]	T-20

*A fixed-dose coformulation of zidovudine + lamivudine is available as COMBIVIR; a fixed-dose coformulation of zidovidine + lamivudine + abacavir is available as TRIZIVIR; a fixed-dose coformulation of abacavir with lamivudine is available as EPZICOM; a fixed-dose coformulation of tenofovir with emtricitabine is available as TRUVADA. [†]Lopinavir is only available as part of a fixed-dose coformulation with ritonavir (KALETRA).

Innovation in drug approval and regulation facilitated the availability of multiple agents capable of fighting this infection. In 1989, the U.S. Food and Drug Administration (FDA) agreed to make promising agents available to patients with advanced disease through an expanded access program. The capacity to assess plasma HIV RNA concentration and CD4 cell count and proof of the relevance of those measures in place of mortality and morbidity (Mellors *et al.*, 1996), made it possible to collapse the time frame for clinical drug development. The most promising drug combinations were identified by their effect on these surrogate endpoints in clinical trials as short as 6 months in duration.

Today, a detailed understanding of the molecular basis of drug resistance guides the search for new agents and informs the selection of combination strategies for existing drugs. The large number of possible drug combinations has given patients more chances at virus control but also complicates the practice of HIV medicine. Current challenges include access to effective long-term treatment in resource-poor countries and identification of new drugs for treatment-experienced patients with resistance to approved drugs. Although many steps in the virus life cycle are potential points for antiviral intervention, only three are targeted by available agents: virus–cell fusion, reverse transcription, and proteolytic processing (Figure 50–1).

PRINCIPLES OF HIV CHEMOTHERAPY

Current treatment assumes that all aspects of disease derive from the direct toxic effects of HIV on host cells, mainly CD4+ T-lymphocytes. This viewpoint is based on studies demonstrating the importance of high plasma HIV RNA concentration (Mellors *et al.*, 1996) and low CD4+ lymphocyte count (Mellors *et al.*, 1997) as predictors of disease progression and mortality. Validation has come from evidence that treatment regimens associated with long-term suppression of HIV replication (as measured by decreased plasma HIV RNA) and repletion of peripheral CD4 cells are clinically beneficial (Lee *et al.*, 2001). The goal of therapy is to suppress virus replication as much as possible for as long as possible.

Deciding when to start antiretroviral therapy has been a shifting target during the epidemic. Zidovudine, the first antiretroviral drug, was approved initially only for patients with advanced, symptomatic disease. In this population, zidovudine monotherapy dramatically reduced HIV-associated mortality after only 6 months of treatment compared with placebo (Fischl *et al.*, 1987). The clinical benefit of this drug in patients with less advanced disease or no symptoms was more difficult to demonstrate, and two large comparative trials showed no benefit of early *versus* delayed initiation of therapy (Hamilton *et al.*, 1992; Concorde Coordinating Committee, 1994).

The more substantial antiretroviral effects of the HIV protease inhibitors and NNRTIs (Ho *et al.*, 1995; Wei *et al.*, 1995) prompted a new look at early and widespread treatment of infected persons. Because these agents caused a rapid 99% to 99.9% decline in plasma HIV RNA concentration (as opposed to the 70% drop caused by zidovudine), it was thought erroneously that combining these drugs with nucleoside analogs might eradicate the virus from infected individuals after only a few years of treatment (Perelson *et al.*, 1996). Because newer agents increased CD4 cell counts to normal or near-normal levels, some felt that earlier institution of therapy might preserve the immune system before it could be further ravaged by the virus. The concept of "hit early, hit hard" led many patients to seek combination therapy regardless of disease stage or symptoms.

Several findings reversed this enthusiasm for universal treatment (Harrington and Carpenter, 2000). First, a number of studies indicated the low likelihood that HIV could be eradicated with drug therapy. A reservoir of long-lived quiescent T cells harboring infectious HIV DNA integrated into the host chromosome was identified independently by several groups of investigators (Chun *et al.*, 1998; Finzi *et al.*, 1997). Infectious HIV could be produced by these quiescent cells after chemical activation *ex vivo* (and presumably if the cells were activated by immune stimuli *in vivo*), but the nonreplicating form of the viral genome was not susceptible to drugs. Recent estimates suggest that at least some of these cells will survive for decades and probably for the life of the patient (Siliciano *et al.*, 2003) regardless of treatment.

More recent natural history studies point to the low risk of short-term disease progression when the CD4 cell count is greater than 350 cells/mm^3 or plasma HIV RNA concentrations are less than 50,000 copies/ml (Phair *et al.*, 2002). The toxic risks of long-term combination chemotherapy, the need for nearly perfect adherence to prescribed regimens, the inconvenience of some regimens, and the high cost of lifelong treatment point to a risk–benefit ratio that favors treating only patients with low CD4 counts and/or very high viral load (Table 50–2). As simpler, less toxic, and better-tolerated drug regimens become available, there may be renewed interest in earlier initiation of treatment.

Drug resistance is also a more extensive and serious problem than imagined originally. There is a high likelihood that any infected individual will harbor viruses with single-amino-acid mutations conferring some degree of resistance to any known antiretroviral drug because of the high mutation rate of HIV and the tremendous number of infectious virions (Coffin, 1995). As a consequence, treatment with only a single antiretroviral drug inevitably provokes the emergence of drug-resistant virus, in some cases within a few weeks (Wei *et al.*, 1995). Drug therapy does not cause mutation but provides the necessary selective pressure to promote growth of drug-resistant viruses that arise naturally (Coffin, 1995). A combination of active agents therefore is required to prevent drug resistance, analogous to strategies employed in the treatment of tuberculosis (*see* Chapter 47). Intentional drug holidays, also known as *structured treatment interruptions,* allow the virus to replicate anew and increase the risk of drug resistance and disease progression (Lawrence *et al.*, 2003) and therefore are not recommended. This reflects the ability of the virus to persist indefinitely in the face of effective therapy (Kieffer *et al.*, 2004). As more clinical safety data accumulate, there may be further exploration of treatment interruptions as a strategy for lowering drug costs and toxicity in selected patients. At present, all antiretroviral therapy outside the research setting is combination therapy. The current standard of care is to use at least three drugs simultaneously for the entire duration of treatment (Table 50–2). The expected outcome of initial therapy in a previously untreated patient is an undetectable viral load (plasma HIV RNA of less than 50 copies/ml) within 24 weeks of starting treatment (Department of Health and Human Services, 2004). In prospective comparative trials, two-drug regimens were more effective than single-drug regimens (Fischl *et al.*, 1995; Hammer *et al.*, 1996; Saag *et al.*, 1998), and three-drug regimens are more effective still (Collier *et al.*, 1996; Gulick *et al.*, 1997; Hammer *et al.*, 1997). Mathematical models of HIV replication suggest that three is the minimum number of agents required to guarantee effective long-term suppression of HIV replication without resistance (Muller and Bonhoeffer, 2003). In treatment-naive patients, a regimen containing a nonnucleoside plus two nucleoside reverse transcriptase inhibitors was as effective as a regimen containing an additional nucleoside (Shafer *et al.*, 2003), indicating the equivalence of these three-drug and four-drug regimens. Four or more drugs often are used simultaneously in pretreated patients harboring drug-resistant virus (Piketty *et al.*, 1999), but the number of agents a patient can take is limited by toxicity and inconvenience.

Pharmacodynamic synergy is probably not an important consideration in regimen selection, although most prescribers prefer to use drugs that attack at least two different molecular sites. This could include nucleoside reverse transcriptase inhibitors that target the active site of the enzyme combined with a nonnucleoside inhibitor that binds to a different site on the same enzyme or an inhibitor of a

Table 50–2
U.S. Department of Health and Human Services Guidelines for Initiating Therapy in Treatment-Naive HIV-Infected Patients, 2004

A. Patient Characteristics

CLINICAL CATEGORY	CD4 COUNT	PLASMA HIV RNA	RECOMMENDATION
AIDS-defining illness* or severe symptoms	Any value	Any value	Treat.
Asymptomatic	<200 cells/mm^3	Any value	Treat.
Asymptomatic	>200 cells/mm^3, but <350 cells/mm^3	Any value	Offer treatment, following full discussion of pros and cons with each patient.
Asymptomatic	>350 cells/mm^3	>100,000 copies/ml	Most physicians recommend deferring therapy, but some will treat.
Asymptomatic	>350 cells/mm^3	<100,000 copies/ml	Defer therapy.

B. Preferred and Alternative Regimens

PREFERRED REGIMENS		NUMBER OF PILLS PER DAY
NNRTI-based	EFV + (3TC or FTC) + (AZT or TDF) (not for use in first trimester of pregnancy or in women with high pregnancy potential)	2–3
PI-based	LPV/r + (3TC or FTC) + AZT	8–9

ALTERNATIVE REGIMENS		NUMBER OF PILLS PER DAY
NNRTI-based	EFV + (3TC or FTC) + (ABC or ddI or d4T)	2–4
	NVP + (3TC or FTC) + (AZT or d4T or ddI or ABC or TDF)	3–6
PI-based	ATV + (3TC or FTC) + (AZT or d4T or ABC or ddI) or (TDF + RTV 100 mg/d)	3–6
	FosAPV + (3TC or FTC) + (AZT or d4T or ABC or TDF or ddI)	5–8
	FosAPV/RTV† + (3TC or FTC) + (AZT or d4T or ABC or TDF or ddI)	5–8
	IDV/RTV† + (3TC or FTC) + (AZT or d4T or ABC or TDF or ddI)	7–12
	LPV/r + (3TC or FTC) + (d4T or ABC or TDF or ddI)	7–10
	NFV + (3TC or FTC) + (AZT or d4T or ABC or TDF or ddI)	5–8
	SQV/RTV† + (3TC or FTC) + (AZT or d4T or ABC or TDF or ddI)	13–16
3 NRTI-based‡	ABC + AZT + 3TC, only when a preferred or an alternative NNRTI- or a PI-based regimen cannot or should not be used	2

(Continued)

Table 50–2

U.S. Department of Health and Human Services Guidelines for Initiating Therapy in Treatment-Naive HIV-Infected Patients, 2004 (Continued)

REGIMENS THAT SHOULD NOT BE USED	RATIONALE
AZT + d4T	Pharmacologic antagonism between AZT and d4T
ABC + TDF + 3TC once daily as a triple-NRTI regimen	High rate of early virological nonresponse seen in treatment-naive patients
TDF + ddI + 3TC combination once daily as a triple-NRTI regimen	High rate of early virological nonresponse seen in treatment-naive patients
ATV + IDV	Potential additive hyperbilirubinemia
ddI + DDC	Additive peripheral neuropathy
FTC + 3TC	Similar resistance profile with no potential benefit
3TC + DDC	*In vitro* antagonism
SQV hard-gel capsule as single protease inhibitor	Poor oral bioavailability and inferior antiretroviral activity when compared with other protease inhibitors
d4T + DDC	Additive peripheral neuropathy

ABBREVIATIONS: EFV, efavirenz; 3TC, lamivudine; AZT, zidovudine; TDF, tenofovir disoproxil fumarate; d4T, stavudine; LPV/r, lopinavir/ritonavir coformulation; FTC, emtricitabine; NVP, nevirapine; ddI, didanosine; ATV, atazanavir; fosAPV, fosamprenavir; RTV, ritonavir; IDV, indinavir; NFV, nelfinavir; SQV, saquinavir *Higher incidence of lipoatrophy, hyperlipidemia, and mitochondrial toxicities reported with d4T than with other NRTIs. *AIDS-defining illness per Centers for Disease Control, 1993. Severe symptoms include unexplained fever or diarrhea > 2–4 weeks, oral candidiasis, or >10% unexplained weight loss. †Low-dose (100–400 mg) ritonavir per day. ‡The triple-NRTI regimen had reduced efficacy compared with NNRTI-based regimens in one large controlled clinical trial and should be used only when an NNRTI- or PI-based regimen cannot or should not be used as first-line therapy. SOURCE: Adapted from Panel on Clinical Practices for Treatment of HIV Infection, 2004.

different enzyme, the HIV protease (Table 50–2). The preceeding regimens have similar long-term efficacy. However, a three-drug regimen containing a single drug class is not as effective as a two-class regimen in treatment-naive patients. In one large randomized, controlled trial, 89% of patients taking two nucleoside analogs plus an NNRTI had undetectable plasma HIV RNA at 32 weeks as compared with 79% of those taking three nucleosides (Gulick *et al.*, 2004). Whether this reflects the inferiority of attacking only a single viral target or the inferiority of the specific drugs involved has yet to be determined. Nonetheless, enthusiasm for single-class therapy is limited at present. Regimens containing three or four different drug classes are reserved for treatment-experienced patients who have failed multiple previous regimens. This acknowledges the benefit of reserving at least one drug class for future treatment in case of failure (Department of Health and Human Services, 2004).

Failure of an antiretroviral regimen involves a persistent increase in plasma HIV RNA concentrations in a previously undetectable patient despite continued treatment or failure to reduce plasma HIV RNA significantly in a patient who has taken a prescribed regimen for more than 12 weeks (Department of Health and Human Services, 2004). This indicates resistance to one or more drugs in the regimen and necessitates a change in treatment. Once resistance occurs, resistant strains remain in tissues indefinitely, even though the resistant virus may not be detectable in the plasma. The selection of new agents is informed by the patient's treatment history, as well as viral resistance testing, preferably obtained while the patient is still taking a failing regimen to facilitate proper recovery and characterization of the patient's virus (Kuritzkes, 2004). Treatment failure generally requires the implementation of a completely new combination

of drugs. Adding a single agent to a three-drug regimen sometimes is employed as a form of treatment intensification for patients whose viral load has fallen but is not undetectable. However, adding a single effective agent to a failing regimen is functional monotherapy if the patient is resistant to all drugs in the regimen.

The risk of failing a regimen depends on the percent of prescribed doses taken in any given period of treatment. After a median of 6 months of treatment, virologic failure occurred in 22% of those taking 95% or more of their antiretroviral doses but in more than half of those taking less than 95% of prescribed doses (Paterson *et al.*, 2000). This places an important educational burden on the health care provider and requires exceptional patient responsibility. Resistance owing to poor adherence probably is inescapable for a virus that is persistent, prolific, and error-prone in its replication because these three qualities nearly guarantee drug resistance if drugs are not taken as recommended. Despite the availability of highly effective and well-tolerated drugs, long-term success, as defined by the percent of patients with an undetectable plasma HIV RNA after 1 year, is only 30% to 50% in patients treated outside clinical trials in the United States (Lucas *et al.*, 1999). This relatively low effectiveness reflects in part the type of patient seen in urban clinical care settings but also indicates the extreme degree of adherence to prescribed medications needed to maintain suppression of HIV.

One recent concern of long-term therapy is the development of a metabolic syndrome characterized by insulin resistance, fat redistribution, and hyperlipidemia and known as the *HIV lipodystrophy syndrome*. Lipodystrophy occurs in 10% to 40% of treated patients and has been seen with most drug combinations used in clinical trials. The pathogenesis is somewhat mysterious but involves pheno-typic and metabolic changes similar to those seen with other human lipodystrophy syndromes (Garg, 2004). Clinical features include peripheral fat wasting (lipoatrophy), central fat accumulation including enlarged breasts and buffalo hump, insulin resistance and hyperglycemia, and elevations in serum cholesterol and triglyc-erides. Switching from one drug regimen to another may not reverse the symptoms, emphasizing its ubiquitous nature and possible role of HIV infection *per se.* Treatment is symptom-directed and should include management of hyperlipidemias as recommended by the American Heart Association (*see* Chapter 35). Lipodystrophy has been associated with an increased risk of in myocardial infarction in virologically controlled patients, emphasizing the importance of car-diovascular risk factor reduction (Sekhar *et al.*, 2004).

II. DRUGS USED TO TREAT HIV INFECTION

NUCLEOSIDE AND NUCLEOTIDE REVERSE TRANSCRIPTASE INHIBITORS

The HIV-encoded, RNA-dependent DNA polymerase, also called *reverse transcriptase,* converts viral RNA into proviral DNA that is then incorporated into a host cell chromosome. Available inhibitors of this enzyme are either nucleoside/nucleotide analogs or nonnucleoside inhibitors (Figure 50–2 and Table 50–3).

Like all available antiretroviral drugs, nucleoside and nucleotide reverse transcriptase inhibitors prevent infection of susceptible cells but have no impact on cells that already harbor HIV. Nucleoside and nucleotide analogs must enter cells and undergo phosphorylation to generate synthetic substrates for the enzyme (Table 50–3). The fully phosphor-ylated analogs block replication of the viral genome both by competitively inhibiting incorporation of native nucle-otides and by terminating elongation of nascent proviral DNA because they lack a 3-hydroxyl group.

All but one of the drugs in this class are nucleosides that must be triphosphorylated at the 5′-hydroxyl to exert activity. The sole exception, *tenofovir,* is a nucleotide monophosphate analog that requires two additional phosphates to acquire full activity. These compounds inhibit both HIV-1 and HIV-2, and several have broad-spectrum activity against other human and animal retroviruses; *emtricitabine, lamivudine, zalcitabine,* and tenofovir are active against hepatitis B virus (HBV) *in vitro,* and tenofovir also has activity against herpesviruses (De Clercq, 2003).

The selective toxicity of these drugs depends on their ability to inhibit the HIV reverse transcriptase without inhibiting host cell DNA polymerases. Although the intracellular triphosphates for all these drugs have low affinity for human DNA polymerase-α and -β, some are capable of inhibiting human DNA polymerase-γ, which is

the mitochondrial enzyme. As a result, the important toxicities com-mon to this class of drugs result in part from the inhibition of mito-chondrial DNA synthesis (Chen *et al.*, 1991; Lee *et al.*, 2003). These toxicities include anemia, granulocytopenia, myopathy, peripheral neuropathy, and pancreatitis. Lactic acidosis with or without hepatomegaly and hepatic steatosis is a rare but potentially fatal complication seen with *stavudine,* zidovudine, *didanosine,* and zalcitabine; it is probably not associated independently with the other drugs (Tripuraneni *et al.*, 2004). Phosphorylated emtricitabine, lamivudine, and tenofovir have low affinity for DNA polymerase-γ and are largely devoid of mitochondrial toxicity.

The chemical structures of the eight currently approved nucleo-side and nucleotide reverse transcriptase inhibitors are shown in Figure 50–2; their pharmacokinetic properties are summarized in Table 50–3. Phosphorylation pathways for these eight drugs are summarized in Figure 50–3. Most nucleoside and nucleotide reverse transcriptase inhibitors are eliminated from the body primarily by renal excretion. Zidovudine and *abacavir,* however, are cleared mainly by hepatic glucuronidation. Most of the parent compounds are eliminated rapidly from the plasma, with elimination half-lives of 1 to 10 hours (Table 50–3). Tenofovir, however, has a plasma half-life of 14 to 17 hours. Despite rapid clearance from the plasma, the critical pharmacological pathway for these agents is production and elimination of the intracellular nucleoside triphosphate or nucle-otide diphosphate, which is the active anabolite. In general, the phosphorylated anabolites are eliminated from cells much more gradually than the parent drug is eliminated from the plasma. Esti-mated elimination half-lives for intracellular triphosphates range from 2 to 50 hours (Table 50–3). This allows for less frequent dos-ing than would be predicted from plasma half-lives of the parent compounds. All approved nucleoside and nucleotide reverse tran-scriptase inhibitors are dosed once or twice daily, with the exception of zalcitabine, which is dosed every 8 hours.

These drugs generally are not involved in clinically significant pharmacokinetic drug interactions because they are not substrates for hepatic cytochrome P450 enzymes (CYPs). However, tenofovir increases concentrations of concurrent didanosine by 25% to 40% perhaps through inhibition of purine nucleoside phosphorylase, and a reduction of the didanosine dose is recommended when these agents are given together (Chapman *et al.*, 2003). Tenofovir also may reduce the concentrations of some concurrently administered HIV protease inhibitors by 25% or more, although the pharmacological mechanisms responsible for these drug interactions are unknown.

High-level resistance to nucleoside reverse transcriptase inhibi-tors, especially thymidine analogs, occurs slowly as compared with NNRTIs and protease inhibitors. Zidovudine resistance was noted in only one-third of treated subjects after 1 year of monotherapy (Fischl *et al.*, 1995). High-level resistance can occur rapidly with lamivudine and emtricitabine. In most cases, high-level resistance requires accumulation of a minimum of three to four codon substi-tutions, although a recently described two-amino-acid insertion is associated with resistance to all drugs in this class (Gallant *et al.*, 2003). Cross-resistance is common but often confined to drugs hav-ing similar chemical structures; for example, zidovudine is a thymi-dine analog, and a zidovudine-resistant isolate is much more likely to be cross-resistant to the thymidine analog stavudine than to the cytosine analog lamivudine.

When used investigationally as monotherapy, most of these drugs induce only a 30% to 90% mean peak decrease in plasma con-centrations of HIV RNA; abacavir, however, can cause up to a 99% decrease (Hervey and Perry, 2000). CD4 lymphocyte count increas-

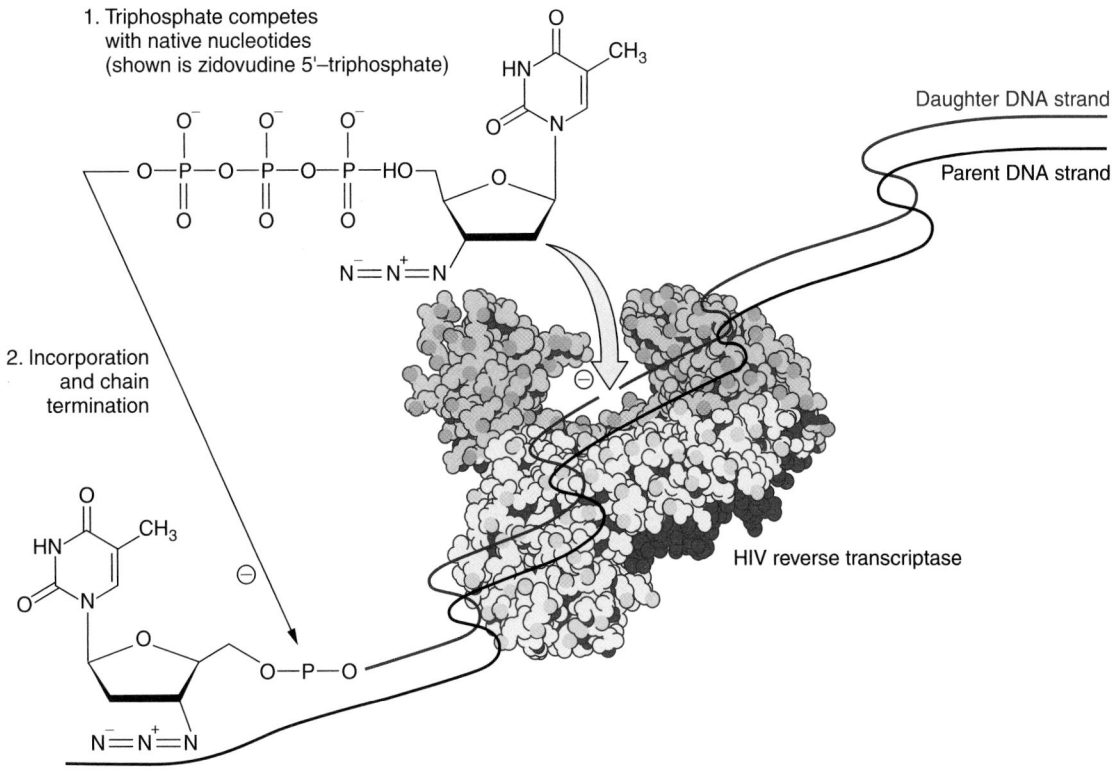

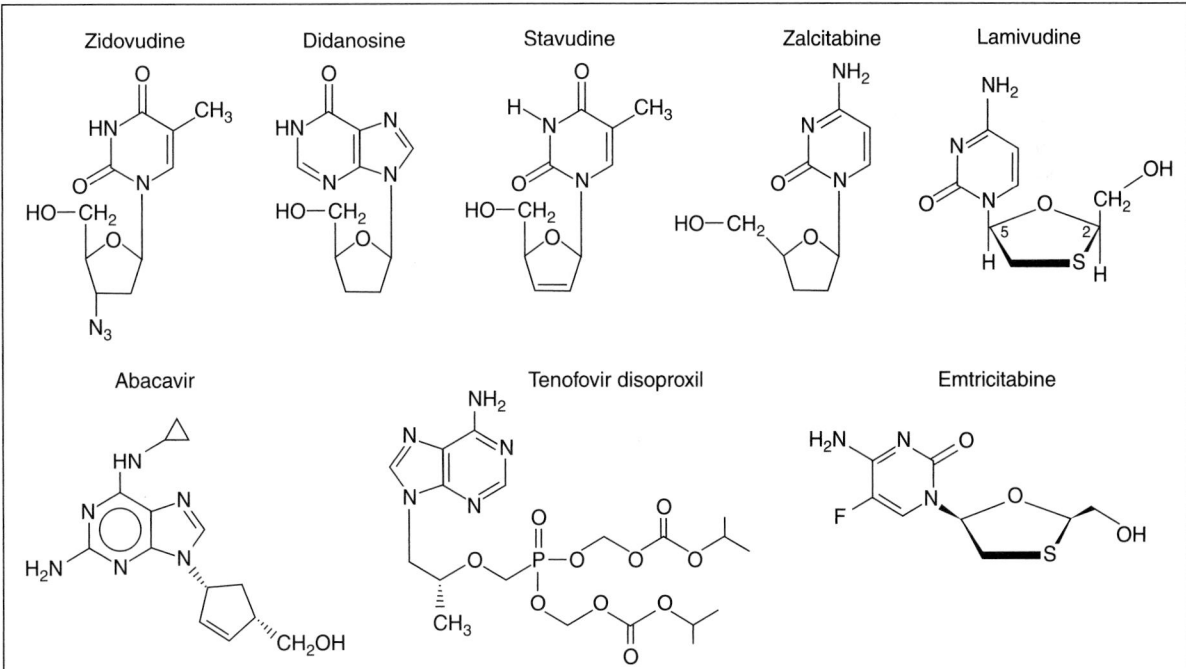

Figure 50–2. *Structures and mechanism of nucleoside and nucleotide reverse transcriptase inhibitors.*

Table 50–3

Pharmacokinetic Properties of Nucleoside and Nucleotide Reverse Transcriptase Inhibitors*

PARAMETER	ZIDOVUDINE	LAMIVUDINE	STAVUDINE†	DIDANOSINE‡	ABACAVIR	ZALCITABINE	TENOFOVIR	EMTRICITABINE
Oral bioavailability, %	64	86–87	86	42	83	88	25	93
Effect of meals on AUC	↓24% (high fat)	↔	↔	↓55% (acidity)	↔	↓14%	↑40% (high fat)	↔
Plasma $t_{\frac{1}{2}}$elim, h	1.0	5–7	1.1–1.4	1.5	0.8–1.5	1–2	14–17	10
Intracellular $t_{\frac{1}{2}}$elim of triphosphate, h	3–4	12–18	3.5	25–40	21	2–3	10–50	39
Plasma protein binding, %	20–38	<35	<5	<5	50	<5	<8	<4
Metabolism, %	60–80 (glucuronidation)	<36	ND	50 (purine metabolism)	>80 (dehydrogenation and glucuronidation)	20	ND	13
Renal excretion of parent drug, %	14	71	39	18–36	<5	60–80	70–80	86

ABBREVIATIONS: AUC, area under plasma concentration–time curve; $t_{\frac{1}{2}}$elim, half-life of elimination; ↑, increase; ↓, decrease; ↔, no effect; ND, not determined. *Reported mean values in adults with normal renal and hepatic function. †Parameters reported for the stavudine capsule formulation. ‡Parameters reported for the didanosine chewable tablet formulation.

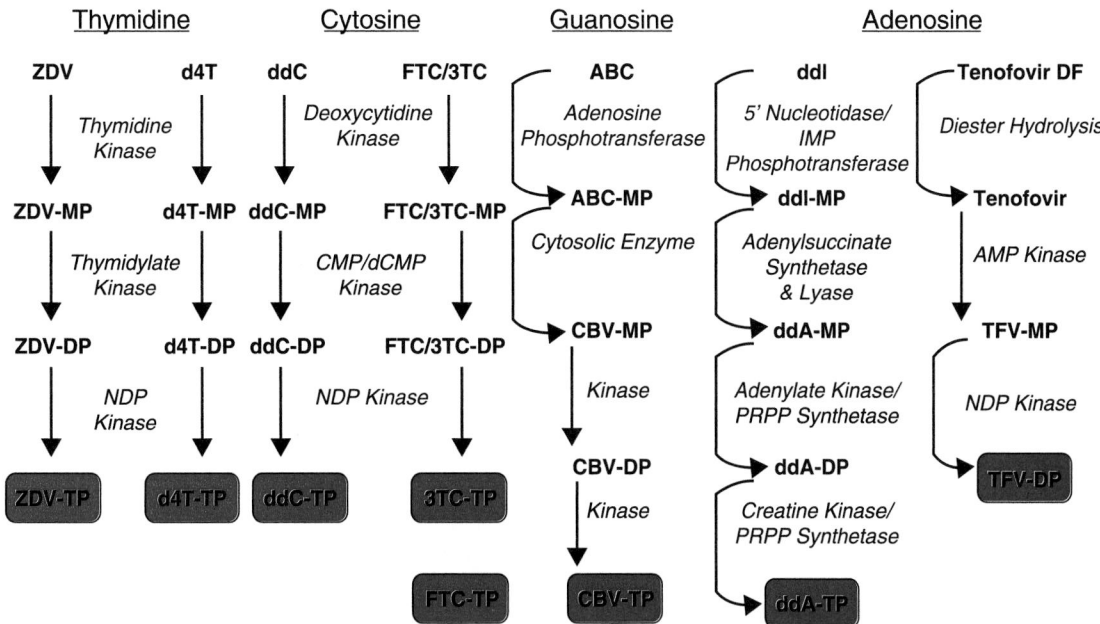

Figure 50–3. *Intracellular activation of nucleoside analog reverse transcriptase inhibitors.* Drugs and phosphorylated anabolites are abbreviated; the enzymes responsible for each conversion are spelled out. The active antiretroviral anabolite for each drug is shown in the blue box. Key: ZDV, zidovudine; d4T, stavudine; ddC, dideoxycytidine; FTC, emtricitabine; 3TC, lamivudine; ABC, abacavir; ddI, didanosine; DF, disoproxil fumarate; MP, monophosphate; DP, diphosphate; TP, triphosphate; AMP, adenosine monophosphate; CMP, cytosine monophosphate; dCMP, deoxycytosine monophosphate; IMP, inosine 5′-monophosphate; PRPP, phosphoribosyl pyrophosphate; NDP, nucleoside diphosphate. (Adapted from Khoo *et al.*, 2002.)

es are also modest with nucleoside monotherapy (mean increases of 50 to 100 cells/mm³, depending on disease stage). Nonetheless, these drugs remain a critical component of therapy, and nearly all patients taking antiretroviral therapy are currently taking at least one agent from this class. Although modest in their own antiviral potency, several nucleoside analogs have favorable safety and tolerability profiles and are useful in suppressing the emergence of HIV isolates resistant to the more potent drugs in combination regimens.

Zidovudine

Chemistry and Antiviral Activity. Zidovudine (3′-azido-3′-deoxythymidine) is a synthetic thymidine analog with potent *in vitro* activity against a broad spectrum of retroviruses including HIV-1, HIV-2, and human T-cell lymphotrophic viruses (HTLV) I and II (McLeod and Hammer, 1992). Its IC_{50} against laboratory and clinical isolates of HIV-1 ranges from 10 to 48 nM. Zidovudine is active in lymphoblastic and monocytic cell lines but is substantially less active in chronically infected cells (Geleziunas *et al.*, 1993) probably because it has no impact on cells already infected with HIV. Zidovudine appears to be more active in lymphocytes than in monocyte–macrophage cells because of enhanced phosphorylation in the former. For the same reason, the drug is more potent in activated than in resting lymphocytes because the phos-

phorylating enzyme, thymidine kinase, is S-phase-specific (Gao *et al.*, 1994).

Mechanism of Action and Resistance. Intracellular zidovudine is phosphorylated by thymidine kinase to zidovudine 5′-monophosphate, which is then phosphorylated by thymidylate kinase to the diphosphate and by nucleoside diphosphate kinase to zidovudine 5′-triphosphate (Furman *et al.*, 1986) (Figure 50–3). Because the conversion of zidovudine 5′-monophosphate to diphosphate is very inefficient, high concentrations of the monophosphate accumulate inside the cell (Slusher *et al.*, 1992) and may serve as a precursor depot for formation of triphosphate. As a consequence, there is little correlation between extracellular concentrations of parent drug and intracellular concentrations of triphosphate (Dudley, 1995), and higher plasma concentrations of zidovudine do not increase intracellular triphosphate concentrations proportionately. Zidovudine 5′-triphosphate terminates the elongation of proviral DNA because it is incorporated by reverse transcriptase into nascent DNA but lacks a 3′-hydroxyl group. The monophosphate competitively inhibits cellular thymidylate kinase, and this may reduce the amount of intracellular thymidine triphosphate (Furman *et al.*, 1986). Although this latter effect could increase antiviral activity, it also may contribute to toxicity. Zidovudine 5′-triphosphate only weakly inhibits cellular DNA polymerase-α but is a more potent inhibitor of mitochondrial polymerase-γ.

Resistance to zidovudine is associated with mutations at reverse transcriptase codons 41, 44, 67, 70, 118, 210, 215, and 219 (Gallant *et al.*, 2003). These mutations are referred to as *thymidine analog mutations* (TAMs) because of their ability to confer cross-resistance to other thymidine analogs such as stavudine. Two clusters of resistance mutations occur commonly. Using the single-letter amino-acid symbols: the pattern of 41L, 210W, and 215Y is associated with high-level resistance to zidovudine, as well as cross-resistance to other drugs in this class, including tenofovir and abacavir. The pattern 67N, 70R, 215F, and 219Q pattern is less common and is also associated with lower levels of resistance and cross-resistance. TAMs associated with resistance to zidovudine and stavudine promote excision of the incorporated triphosphate anabolites through pyrophosphorolysis (Naeger *et al.*, 2002). Mutations accumulated gradually when zidovudine was used as the sole antiretroviral agent, and clinical resistance developed in only 31% of patients after 1 year of zidovudine monotherapy (Fischl *et al.*, 1995). Cross-resistance to multiple nucleoside analogs has been reported following prolonged therapy and has been associated with a mutation cluster involving codons 62, 75, 77, 116, and 151. In addition, a recently described mutation at codon 69 (typically T69S) followed by a two-amino-acid insertion produces cross-resistance to all current nucleoside and nucleotide analogs (Gallant *et al.*, 2003).

Absorption, Distribution, and Elimination. Zidovudine is absorbed rapidly and reaches peak plasma concentrations within 1 hour (Dudley, 1995). Like other nucleoside analogs, the elimination half-life of the parent compound (about 1 hour) is considerably shorter than that of the intracellular triphosphate, which is 3 to 4 hours (Table 50–3). Failure to recognize this led to serious overdosing of the drug when it was first approved; the recommended dose was 250 mg every 4 hours in 1987, compared with 300 mg twice a day presently.

Zidovudine undergoes rapid first-pass hepatic metabolism by conversion to 5-glucuronyl zidovudine. This limits systemic bioavailability to about 64%. Food may slow absorption but does not alter the *AUC* (area under the plasma concentration–time curve) (Table 50–3), and the drug can be administered regardless of food intake (Dudley, 1995). Total urinary recoveries of zidovudine and its glucuronide metabolite are 14% and 74%, respectively. The pharmacokinetic profile of zidovudine is not altered significantly during pregnancy, and drug concentrations in the newborn approach those of the mother (Watts *et al.*, 1991). Zidovudine is not bound to plasma proteins to a significant degree. Parent drug crosses the blood–brain barrier relatively well and achieves a cerebrospinal fluid (CSF)–plasma ratio of approximately 0.6. Zidovudine also is detectable in breast milk, semen, and fetal tissue (Gillet *et al.*, 1989; Watts *et al.*, 1991). Zidovudine concentrations are higher in the male genital tract than in the peripheral circulation, suggesting active transport or trapping.

Untoward Effects. Patients initiating zidovudine treatment often complain of fatigue, malaise, myalgia, nausea, anorexia, headache, and insomnia. These symptoms usually resolve within the first few weeks of treatment. Bone marrow suppression, mainly anemia and granulocytopenia, occurs most often in individuals with advanced HIV disease and very low CD4 counts and also was more common with the higher doses used when the drug was first approved. In such patients, anemia may develop within 4 weeks of starting therapy and probably reflects toxic effects on erythroid stem cells. Anemia can be managed by administering recombinant human erythropoietin. Erythrocytic macrocytosis is seen in approximately 90% of all patients but usually is not associated with anemia. Neutropenia is uncommon but can be managed with recombinant granulocyte or granulocyte–macrophage colony-stimulating factors (*see* Chapter 53).

Chronic zidovudine administration has been associated with nail hyperpigmentation. Skeletal muscle myopathy can occur and is associated with depletion of mitochondrial DNA, most likely as a consequence of inhibition of DNA polymerase-γ (Arnaudo *et al.*, 1991). Serious hepatic toxicity, with or without steatosis and lactic acidosis, is rare but can be fatal. Risk factors for the lactic acidosis–steatosis syndrome include female sex, obesity, and prolonged exposure to the drug (Tripuraneni *et al.*, 2004).

Drug Interactions and Precautions. Zidovudine is not a substrate or inhibitor of CYPs. However, *probenecid, fluconazole, atovaquone,* and *valproic acid* may increase plasma concentrations of zidovudine probably through inhibition of glucuronosyl transferase (Dudley, 1995). The clinical significance of these interactions is unknown because intracellular triphosphate levels may be unchanged despite higher plasma concentrations. Zidovudine can cause bone marrow suppression and should be used cautiously in patients with preexisting anemia or granulocytopenia and in those taking other marrow-suppressive drugs. Stavudine and zidovudine compete for intracellular phosphorylation and should not be used concomitantly. Three clinical trials found a significantly worse virologic outcome in patients taking these two drugs together as compared with either agent used alone (Havlir *et al.*, 2000).

Therapeutic Uses. Zidovudine is FDA approved for the treatment of adults and children with HIV infection and for preventing mother-to-child transmission of HIV infection; it is also recommended for postexposure prophylaxis in HIV-exposed healthcare workers, also in combination with other antiretroviral agents.

Zidovudine is more effective when combined with other antiretroviral drugs. Zidovudine combined with lamivudine, didanosine, or zalcitabine is more effective than zidovudine alone (Hammer *et al.*, 1996). Greater benefit is achieved when zidovudine is combined with two nucleoside analogs (Saag *et al.*, 1998). The current standard of care for treatment-naive patients (Table 50–2B) is to combine zidovudine with a potent protease inhibitor and another nucleoside analog (Hammer *et al.*, 1997) or with an NNRTI and another nucleoside analog (Staszewski *et al.*, 1999).

The M184V substitution in the reverse transcriptase gene associated with the use of lamivudine or emtricitabine greatly restores sensitivity to zidovudine (Gallant *et al.*, 2003). The combination of zidovudine and lamivudine produces greater long-term suppression of plasma HIV RNA than does zidovudine alone (Eron *et al.*, 1995). As a result, this agent is often combined with lamivudine in clinical practice.

Zidovudine monotherapy reduced the risk of perinatal transmission of HIV by 67% (Connor *et al.*, 1994), and combining zidovudine with other antiretroviral drugs is even more efficacious in this setting. Zidovudine is also recommended as a component of combination therapy administered to healthcare workers soon after exposure to contaminated blood or body fluids to prevent HIV transmission (Cardo *et al.*, 1997). Despite being the oldest antiretroviral drug, zidovudine remains a popular component of combination regimens. This is a consequence of broad experience with the drug and its well-known tolerability, toxicity, and efficacy profiles. Zidovudine is available in coformulated tablets with lamivudine or with lamivudine and abacavir.

Didanosine

Chemistry and Antiviral Activity. Didanosine (2′,3′-dideoxyinosine) is a purine nucleoside analog active against HIV-1, HIV-2, and other retroviruses including HTLV-1 (Perry and Noble, 1999). Its IC_{50} against HIV-1 ranges from 10 nM in monocytes–macrophage cells, to 10 μM in lymphoblast cell lines.

Mechanism of Action and Resistance. Didanosine is transported into cells by a nucleobase carrier and undergoes initial phosphorylation by 5′-nucleotidase and inosine 5′-monophosphate phosphotransferase (Dudley, 1995; Khoo *et al.*, 2002). Didanosine 5′-monophosphate is then converted to dideoxyadenosine 5′-monophosphate by adenylosuccinate synthetase and adenylosuccinate lyase (Figure 50–3). Adenylate kinase and phosphoribosyl pyrophosphate synthetase produce dideoxyadenosine 5′-diphosphate, which is converted to the triphosphate by creatine kinase and phosphoribosyl pyrophosphate synthetase. Dideoxyadenosine 5′-triphosphate is the active anabolite of didanosine, which therefore functions as an antiviral adenosine analog. Dideoxyadenosine 5′-triphosphate terminates the elongation of proviral DNA because it is incorporated by reverse transcriptase into nascent HIV DNA but lacks a 3′-hydroxyl group.

Resistance to didanosine is associated with mutations at reverse transcriptase codons 65 and 74. The L74V substitution, which reduces susceptibility 5 to 26 times *in vitro*, is seen most commonly in patients failing to respond to didanosine. Other nucleoside analog mutations, including thymidine analog mutations, can contribute to didanosine resistance even though the drug does not appear to select for these mutations *de novo*. The reverse transcriptase insertion mutations at codon 69 produce cross-resistance to all current nucleoside analogs, including didanosine (Gallant *et al.*, 2003). The M184V mutation seen in response to emtricitabine and lamivudine reduces didanosine susceptibility *in vitro* but probably plays no role in clinical resistance to this drug.

Absorption, Distribution, and Elimination. Didanosine is acid labile and is degraded at low gastric pH (Dudley, 1995). An antacid buffer is used in most formulations to improve bioavailability. Chewable tablets contain calcium carbonate and magnesium hydroxide, whereas the powder form contains citrate–phosphate buffer. The pediatric powder formulation lacks buffer and is reconstituted with purified water and mixed with a liquid antacid preparation. Food decreases didanosine bioavailability (*AUC*) by approximately 55%, so all formulations of didanosine must be administered at least 30 minutes before or 2 hours after eating (Perry and Noble, 1999). This complicates dosing of didanosine in combination with antiretroviral drugs that must be given with food, as is the case for most HIV protease inhibitors. The enzyme purine nucleoside phosphorylase

(PNP) probably contributes to the presystemic clearance of didanosine because tenofovir, which inhibits PNP, greatly increases concentrations of orally administered didanosine (Robbins *et al.*, 2003). PNP converts didanosine to hypoxanthine, which is ultimately converted to uric acid.

Peak plasma concentrations of didanosine are seen approximately 1 hour after oral administration of the chewable tablets or powder formulations and 2 hours after delayed-release capsules. The plasma elimination half-life of parent drug is approximately 1.5 hours, but the estimated intracellular half-life of dideoxyadenosine 5′-triphosphate is substantially longer, 25 to 40 hours (Perry and Noble, 1999). As a result, didanosine can be administered once daily. Didanosine is excreted both by glomerular filtration and by tubular secretion and does not undergo metabolism to a significant degree. Drug doses therefore must be adjusted in patients with renal insufficiency or renal failure (Jayasekara *et al.*, 1999).

Didanosine is not protein bound to a significant degree. The cerebrospinal penetration of didanosine is less than that of zidovudine, with a CSF–plasma ratio of 0.2, but the clinical significance of this is unclear. Didanosine has been detected in placental and fetal circulation at a small fraction of concentrations in maternal circulation (Dancis *et al.*, 1993).

Untoward Effects. The most serious toxicities associated with didanosine include peripheral neuropathy and pancreatitis, both of which are thought to be a consequence of mitochondrial toxicity. Up to 20% of patients reported peripheral neuropathy in early clinical trials (Perry and Noble, 1999). As with other dideoxynucleosides, peripheral neuropathy is more common with higher doses or concentrations of didanosine and is more prevalent in patients with underlying HIV-related neuropathy or in those receiving other neurotoxic drugs. Typically, this is a symmetrical distal sensory neuropathy that begins in the feet and lower extremities but may involve the hands as it progresses (stocking/glove distribution). Patients complain of pain, numbness, and tingling in the affected extremities. If the drug is stopped as soon as symptoms appear, the neuropathy will stabilize and should improve or resolve. Retinal changes and optic neuritis also have been reported with didanosine, and patients should undergo periodic retinal examinations.

Acute pancreatitis is a rare but potentially fatal complication of didanosine. Acute pancreatitis is associated with higher doses and concentrations of didanosine but has occurred in up to 7% of patients using the recommended dose of 200 mg twice daily (Perry and Noble, 1996). Pancreatitis is more common with advanced HIV disease, and other risk factors include a previous history of pancreatitis, alcohol or illicit drug use, and hypertriglyceridemia. Combining didanosine with stavudine, which is also associated with peripheral neuropathy and pancreatitis, increases the risk and severity of both toxicities (Havlir *et al.*, 2001; Moore *et al.*, 2000).

As with other dideoxynucleosides and zidovudine, serious hepatic toxicity—with or without steatosis, hepatomegaly, and lactic acidosis—occurs very rarely but can be fatal. Risk factors for the lactic acidosis–steatosis syndrome include female sex, obesity, and prolonged exposure to the drug (Tripuraneni *et al.*, 2004).

Other reported adverse effects include elevated hepatic transaminases, headache, and asymptomatic hyperuricemia. Diarrhea is reported more frequently with didanosine than with other nucleoside analogs and has been attributed to the antacid in the buffered oral preparations (Perry and Noble, 1999). Didanosine chewable tablets contain 36.5 mg phenylalanine and should be avoided in those with phenylketonuria. Buffered powder for oral solution contains 1.4 g sodium per packet and should be used cautiously in those on sodium-restricted diets.

Drug Interactions and Precautions. Buffering agents included in didanosine formulations can interfere with the bioavailability of some coadministered drugs because of altered pH or chelation with cations in the buffer. For example, the *ciprofloxacin AUC* is decreased by up to 98% when given with didanosine, and concentrations of *ketoconazole* and *itraconazole,* whose absorption is pH-dependent, also are diminished (Piscitelli and Gallicano, 2001). A 200-mg dose of buffered didanosine reduced the indinavir *AUC* by 84%. These interactions generally can be avoided by separating administration of didanosine from that of other agents by at least 2 hours. The enteric-coated formulation of didanosine does not alter ciprofloxacin or indinavir absorption.

Didanosine is excreted renally, and shared renal excretory mechanisms provide a basis for drug interactions with didanosine. Oral *ganciclovir* can increase plasma didanosine concentrations approximately twofold and may be associated with an increase in didanosine toxicity. *Allopurinol* can increase the didanosine *AUC* more than fourfold and should be avoided. Tenofovir increases the didanosine *AUC* by 44% to 60% and also may increase the risk of didanosine toxicity. If these two drugs must be given together, it is recommended to decrease the didanosine dose from 400 to 250 mg once daily (Chapman *et al.,* 2003). *Methadone* decreases the didanosine *AUC* by 57% to 63% (Rainey *et al.,* 2000) possibly as a consequence of altered gastrointestinal motility and delayed absorption, although this has not been associated with a higher risk of failing didanosine treatment.

Didanosine should be avoided in patients with a history of pancreatitis or neuropathy because the risk and severity of both complications increase. Coadministration of other drugs that cause pancreatitis or neuropathy also will increase the risk and severity of these symptoms. For this reason, stavudine and zalcitabine should be avoided or used only with great caution. *Ethambutol, isoniazid, vincristine, cisplatin,* and *pentamidine* also should be avoided.

The combination of didanosine and *hydroxyurea* was used to exploit a beneficial interaction that creates a favorable intracellular ratio of concentrations of dideoxyadenosine 5′-triphosphate to deoxythymidine 5′-triphosphate (Frank *et al.,* 2004). Although this combination may boost didanosine antiviral activity modestly, it increases toxicity substantially, producing peripheral neuropathy and fatal pancreatitis, and should be avoided (Havlir *et al.,* 2001; Moore *et al.,* 2000).

Therapeutic Use. Didanosine is FDA approved for adults and children with HIV infection in combination with other antiretroviral agents. Didanosine reduced disease progression and death in early monotherapy studies, although HIV plasma RNA concentrations generally fell at most by 90% when the drug was used as a sole agent (Dolin *et al.,* 1995). Didanosine combined with another nucleoside analog reduced clinical disease progression and afforded greater viral suppression compared with zidovudine monotherapy (Hammer *et al.,* 1996; Saravolatz *et al.,* 1996). Didanosine has long-term efficacy when combined with other nucleoside analogs and HIV protease inhibitors or NNRTIs (Table 50–2). Didanosine as a component of combination therapy

also has beneficial effects in infants and children (Luzuriaga *et al.,* 1997).

Stavudine

Chemistry and Antiviral Activity. Stavudine (2′,3′-didehydro-2′,3′-dideoxythymidine, d4T) is a synthetic thymidine analog reverse transcriptase inhibitor that is active *in vitro* against HIV-1 and HIV-2. Its IC_{50} in lymphoblastoid and monocytic cell lines and in primary mononuclear cells ranges from 0.009 to 4 μM (Hurst and Noble, 1999).

Mechanism of Action and Resistance. Intracellular stavudine is phosphorylated by thymidine kinase to stavudine 5′-monophosphate, which is then phosphorylated by thymidylate kinase to the diphosphate and by nucleoside diphosphate kinase to stavudine 5′-triphosphate (Hurst and Noble, 1999) (Figure 50–3). Unlike zidovudine monophosphate, stavudine monophosphate does not accumulate in the cell, and the rate-limiting step in activation appears to be generation of the monophosphate. Stavudine 5′-triphosphate terminates the elongation of proviral DNA because it is incorporated by reverse transcriptase into nascent DNA but lacks a 3′-hydroxyl group. Like zidovudine, stavudine is most potent in activated cells probably because thymidine kinase is an S-phase-specific enzyme (Gao *et al.,* 1994). Stavudine and zidovudine are antagonistic *in vitro,* and thymidine kinase has a higher affinity for zidovudine than for stavudine (Merrill *et al.,* 1996).

Stavudine resistance is seen most frequently with mutations at reverse transcriptase codons 41, 44, 67, 70, 118, 210, 215, and 219 (Gallant *et al.,* 2003), which are the same mutations associated with zidovudine resistance. Clusters of resistance mutations that include M41L, K70R, and T215Y are associated with a lower level of *in vitro* resistance than seen with zidovudine but are found in up to 38% of patients who fail to respond to stavudine. TAMs associated with resistance to zidovudine and stavudine promote excision of the incorporated triphosphate anabolites through pyrophosphorolysis (Naeger *et al.,* 2002). As with zidovudine, resistance mutations for stavudine appear to accumulate slowly. Cross-resistance to multiple nucleoside analogs has been reported following prolonged therapy and has been associated with a mutation cluster involving codons 62, 75, 77, 116, and 151. In addition, a recently described mutation at codon 69 (typically T69S) followed by a 2-amino-acid insertion produces cross-resistance to all current nucleoside and nucleotide analogs (Gallant *et al.,* 2003).

Absorption, Distribution, and Elimination. Stavudine is well absorbed and reaches peak plasma concentrations within 1 hour (Hurst and Noble, 1999). Bioavailability is not affected by food. The drug undergoes active tubular secretion, and renal elimination accounts for about 40% of parent drug. Stavudine concentrations are higher in patients with low body weight, and the dose should be decreased from 40 to 30 mg twice daily in patients weighing less than 60 kg. Dose also should be adjusted in patients with renal insufficiency (Jayasekara *et al.,* 1999). A sustained-release formulation that can be given once daily was approved recently by the FDA.

Plasma protein binding is less than 5%. The drug penetrates well into the CSF, achieving concentrations that are about 40% of those in plasma. Stavudine also readily crosses the human placenta and reaches concentrations in the circulation of fetal macaques that are about 80% of those in the mother (Odinecs *et al.*, 1996). Placental concentrations of stavudine are about half those of zidovudine, possibly reflecting stavudine's lower lipid solubility.

Untoward Effects. The most common serious toxicity of stavudine is peripheral neuropathy. Neuropathy occurred in up to 71% of patients in initial monotherapy trials with a dose of 4 mg/kg per day. With the current recommended dose of 40 mg twice daily, the neuropathy incidence is about 12% (Hurst and Noble, 1999). Although this is thought to reflect mitochondrial toxicity, stavudine is a less potent inhibitor of DNA polymerase-γ than either didanosine or zalcitabine, suggesting that other mechanisms may be involved (Cui *et al.*, 1997). As with other dideoxynucleosides, peripheral neuropathy is more common with higher doses or concentrations of stavudine and is more prevalent in patients with underlying HIV-related neuropathy or in those receiving other neurotoxic drugs. Stavudine is also associated with a progressive motor neuropathy characterized by weakness and in some cases respiratory failure, similar to Guillain-Barré syndrome (HIV Neuromuscular Syndrome Study Group, 2004).

Lactic acidosis and hepatic steatosis have been associated with stavudine use. This may be more common when stavudine and didanosine are combined. Elevated serum lactate is more common with stavudine than with zidovudine or abacavir (Tripuraneni *et al.*, 2004), although the relationship to relative risk of hepatic steatosis is unknown. Acute pancreatitis is not highly associated with stavudine but is more common when stavudine is combined with didanosine than when didanosine is given alone (Havlir *et al.*, 2001; Moore *et al.*, 2000).

Stavudine recently has been implicated in the etiology of HIV lipodystrophy syndrome, especially lipoatrophy. Of all nucleoside analogs, stavudine use is associated most strongly with fat wasting (Mallal *et al.*, 2000; Heath *et al.*, 2001). Whether this is a consequence of the extensive use of this agent combined with its mitochondrial toxicity or reflects a pathogenetic mechanism that has yet to be discovered remains to be determined. Other reported adverse effects include elevated hepatic transaminases, headache, nausea, and rash, although these side effects are almost never severe enough to cause discontinuation of the drug.

Drug Interactions and Precautions. Stavudine is largely renally cleared and is not subject to metabolic drug interactions. The incidence and severity of peripheral neuropathy may be increased when stavudine is combined with other neuropathic medications, and therefore drugs such as ethambutol, isoniazid, *phenytoin,* and vincristine should be avoided. Combining stavudine with didanosine leads to increased risk and severity of peripheral neuropathy and potentially fatal pancreatitis; therefore, *these two drugs should not be used together under most circumstances* (Havlir *et al.*, 2001; Moore *et al.*, 2000). Stavudine and zidovudine compete for intracellular phosphorylation and should not be used concomitantly. Three clinical trials found a significantly worse virologic outcome in patients taking these two drugs together as compared with either agent used alone (Havlir *et al.*, 2000).

Therapeutic Use. In early monotherapy trials, stavudine reduced plasma HIV RNA by 70% to 90% and delayed disease progression compared with continued zidovudine therapy (Spruance *et al.*, 1997). Lamivudine improves the long-term virologic response to stavudine, possibly reflecting the benefits of the M184V mutation (Kuritzkes *et al.*, 1999).

Many large prospective clinical trials have demonstrated potent and durable suppression of viremia and sustained increases in CD4+ cell counts when stavudine is combined with other nucleoside analogs plus NNRTIs or protease inhibitors (Hurst and Noble, 1999). The drug therefore remains a common component of antiretroviral regimens.

Zalcitabine

Chemistry and Antiviral Activity. Zalcitabine (2',3'-dideoxycytidine. ddC) is a synthetic cytosine analog reverse transcriptase inhibitor. It is active against HIV-1, HIV-2, and hepatitis B virus (HBV). The *in vitro* IC_{50} of zalcitabine against HIV-1 ranges from 2 nM in monocytes–macrophage cell lines to 0.5 μM in human peripheral blood mononuclear cells. Zalcitabine has considerably more antiretroviral activity in monocytes–macrophage cell lines than other nucleoside analogs, but the potential clinical utility of this observation is uncertain.

Mechanisms of Action and Resistance. Zalcitabine enters cells by both carrier-mediated transport and passive diffusion (Adkins *et al.*, 1997). It is converted to the monophosphate by deoxycytidine kinase and undergoes further phosphorylation by deoxycytidine monophosphate kinase and nucleoside diphosphate kinase to yield dideoxycytidine 5'-triphosphate, which is the active anabolite (Adkins *et al.*, 1997) (Figure 50–3). Zalcitabine is more efficiently phosphorylated in resting cells and therefore is more potent in resting cells than other nucleoside analogs (Gao *et al.*, 1993), although the clinical relevance of this is unknown. As with other dideoxynucleoside analogs, dideoxycytidine 5'-triphosphate terminates the elongation of proviral DNA because it is incorporated by reverse transcriptase into nascent HIV DNA but lacks a 3'-hydroxyl group. Zalcitabine inhibits human DNA polymerases-β and -γ and also decreases intracellular deoxycytidine triphosphate pools, factors that may contribute to its cellular and host toxicity (Chen *et al.*, 1991).

High-level resistance has not been reported in patients receiving zalcitabine as a sole nucleoside analog or in combination with zidovudine (Adkins *et al.*, 1997). However, low-to-moderate *in vitro* resistance is seen with four mutations associated with zalcitabine use that occur at reverse transcriptase codons 65, 69, 74, and 184 (Gallant *et al.*, 2003). The K65R substitution is associated with cross-resistance to didanosine, abacavir, and tenofovir, as well as the cytosine analogs lamivudine and emtricitabine. The M184V substitution is also associated with the use of lamivudine or emtricitabine and enhances HIV-1 sensitivity to zidovudine *in vitro*; the presence of this mutation is associated with improved long-term suppression of viremia when zidovudine is combined with lamivudine or emtricitabine, although a similar effect has not been demonstrated for the combination of zalcitabine and zidovudine. The T69D substitution is unique to zalcitabine but overlaps a recently described mutation at codon 69 (typically T69S) followed by a 2-amino-acid insertion that produces cross-resistance to all current nucleoside and nucleotide analogs (Gallant *et al.*, 2003).

Absorption, Distribution, and Elimination. The oral bioavailability of zalcitabine is greater than 80%, and 60% to 80% of the parent compound is recovered unchanged in the urine (Adkins *et al.*, 1997). Food has a negligible effect on oral bioavailability. Clearance is greatly diminished in patients with compromised renal function, and daily doses should be reduced in this population (Jayasekara *et al.*, 1999). The half-life of intracellular dideoxycytidine 5′-triphosphate is estimated to be 2 to 3 hours. It is therefore recommended that zalcitabine be administered every 8 hours in patients with normal renal function. The CSF–plasma concentration ratio ranges from 0.09 to 0.37, although the clinical significance of CSF penetration is not known.

Untoward Effects. Zalcitabine toxicities are similar to those of the other dideoxynucleoside analogs didanosine and stavudine. Severe peripheral neuropathy has been reported in up to 15% of patients. Peripheral neuropathy is dose-related and more common with preexisting HIV-associated neuropathy and advanced HIV disease. This is a symmetrical distal sensory neuropathy that begins in the feet but may progress to a stocking/glove distribution. Other specific risk factors for neuropathy include alcohol consumption, diabetes, and low vitamin B_{12} concentrations (Fichtenbaum *et al.*, 1995). If the drug is stopped as soon as symptoms appear, the neuropathy usually stabilizes and should improve or resolve. Pancreatitis occurs rarely with zalcitabine therapy and appears to be less frequent than with didanosine (Saravolatz *et al.*, 1996).

One toxicity unique to zalcitabine is oral ulceration and stomatitis, suggesting that this drug may have toxicity in rapidly dividing mucosal cells. Ulcerations of the buccal mucosa, soft palate, tongue, or pharynx occur in up to 4% of patients (Adkins *et al.*, 1997) but may resolve with continued therapy. An erythematous maculopapular rash is reported commonly during the first 14 days of therapy but generally is self-limited and mild. Other reported toxicities include cardiomyopathy, arthralgias, myalgias, and elevated hepatic transaminases.

Drug Interactions and Precautions. Lamivudine inhibits the intracellular phosphorylation of zalcitabine (Veal *et al.*, 1996) and antagonizes zalcitabine's antiretroviral activity *in vitro* (Merrill *et al.*, 1996), although the clinical significance of this interaction is unknown. Probenecid increases the zalcitabine *AUC* by about 50% probably through inhibition of tubular secretion; *cimetidine* increases the *AUC* by 36% *via* an unknown mechanism (Adkins *et al.*, 1997). Zalcitabine should be avoided in patients with a history of pancreatitis or neuropathy because the risk and severity of both complications increase. Coadministration of other drugs that cause pancreatitis or neuropathy also will increase the risk and severity of these symptoms. Ethambutol, isoniazid, vincristine, cisplatin, and pentamidine, as well as the antiretroviral drugs didanosine and stavudine, therefore should be avoided.

Therapeutic Use. Zalcitabine has long-term efficacy in three-drug combination regimens. For example, the combination of zalcitabine, zidovudine, and saquinavir was superior to two-drug regimens in a prospective, randomized clinical trial (Collier *et al.*, 1996). Zalcitabine is used infrequently in the United States because it is the only nucleoside analog that still must be administered every 8 hours, carries significant toxicity risks, and has inferior antiviral activity compared with more convenient agents.

Lamivudine

Chemistry and Antiviral Activity. Lamivudine [(−)2′, 3′-dideoxy, 3′-thiacytidine, 3TC] is a cytosine analog reverse transcriptase inhibitor that is active against HIV-1, HIV-2, and HBV. The molecule has two chiral centers and is manufactured as the pure 2R, *cis*(−)-enantiomer (Figure 50–2). The racemic mixture from which lamivudine originates has antiretroviral activity but is less potent and substantially more toxic than the pure (−)-enantiomer. Compared with the (+)-enantiomer, the phosphorylated (−)-enantiomer is more resistant to cleavage from nascent RNA/DNA duplexes by cellular 3′-5′ exonucleases, which may contribute to its greater potency (Skalski *et al.*, 1993). The IC_{50} of lamivudine against laboratory strains of HIV-1 ranges from 2 to 670 nM, although the IC_{50} in primary human peripheral blood mononuclear cells is as high as 15 μM (Perry and Faulds, 1997).

Mechanism of Action and Resistance. Lamivudine enters cells by passive diffusion, where it is converted to the monophosphate by deoxycytidine kinase, and undergoes further phosphorylation by deoxycytidine monophosphate kinase and nucleoside diphosphate kinase to yield lamivudine 5′-triphosphate, which is the active anabolite (Perry and Faulds, 1997) (Figure 50–3). The intracellular triphosphate acts as a competitive inhibitor of reverse transcriptase and is incorporated into HIV DNA to cause chain termination. Lamivudine is phosphorylated more efficiently in resting cells, which may explain its reduced potency in primary peripheral blood mononuclear cells as compared with cell lines (Gao *et al.*, 1994). Lamivudine has low affinity for human DNA polymerases, explaining its low toxicity to the host.

High-level resistance to lamivudine occurs with single-amino-acid substitutions, M184V or M184I. These mutations can reduce *in vitro* sensitivity to lamivudine by up to one thousandfold (Perry and Faulds, 1997). The same mutations confer high-level cross-resistance to emtricitabine and a lesser degree of resistance to zalcitabine and abacavir (Gallant *et al.*, 2003). The M184V mutation restores zidovudine susceptibility in zidovudine-resistant HIV (Larder *et al.*, 1995) and also partially restores tenofovir susceptibility in tenofovir-resistant HIV harboring the K65R mutation (Wainberg *et al.*, 1999). The same K65R mutation confers resistance to lamivudine and the other cytosine analogs emtricitabine and zalcitabine, as well as didanosine, stavudine, and abacavir.

HIV-1 isolates harboring the M184V mutation have increased transcriptional fidelity *in vitro* (Wainberg *et al.*, 1996) and decreased replication capacity (Miller *et al.*, 1999). Variants with the M184I mutation are even more impaired with regard to *in vitro* replication (Larder *et al.*, 1995) and usually are replaced in lamivudine-treated patients by the M184V mutation. The reduced fitness of lamivudine-resistant viruses harboring these mutations and their ability to prevent or partially reverse the effect of thymidine analog mutations may contribute to the sustained virologic benefits of zidovudine and lamivudine combination therapy (Eron *et al.*, 1995).

Although the use of lamivudine to treat HBV infection is discussed in Chapter 49, some parallels in drug resistance are worth noting. High-level resistance to lamivudine occurs with a single mutation in the HBV DNA polymerase gene; as with HIV, this consists of a methionine-to-valine substitution (M2041V) in the enzyme active site. Resistance to lamivudine occurs in up to 90% of HIV/HBV coinfected patients after 4 years of treatment. However, virologic benefits persist in some treated patients harboring lamivudine-resistant HBV possibly because the mutated virus has substantially reduced replicative capacity (Leung *et al.*, 2001).

Absorption, Distribution, and Elimination. The oral bioavailability of lamivudine is greater than 80% and is not affected by food. Although lamivudine was marketed originally with a recommended dose of 150 mg twice daily based on the short plasma half-life of the parent compound, the intracellular half-life of lamivudine 5′-triphosphate is 12 to 18 hours, and the drug is now approved for use once daily at 300 mg (Moore *et al.*, 1999). Lamivudine is excreted primarily unchanged in the urine, and dose adjustment is recommended for patients with a creatinine clearance of less than 50 ml/min (Jayasekara *et al.*, 1999). Lamivudine does not bind significantly to plasma proteins and freely crosses the placenta into the fetal circulation. Like zidovudine, lamivudine concentrations are higher in the male genital tract than in the peripheral circulation, suggesting active transport or trapping. Central nervous system (CNS) penetration appears to be poor, with a CSF–plasma concentration ratio of 0.15 or less (Perry and Faulds, 1997). The clinical significance of the low CSF penetration is unknown.

Untoward Effects. Lamivudine is one of the least toxic antiretroviral drugs and has few significant adverse effects. Neutropenia, headache, and nausea have been reported at higher than recommended doses. Pancreatitis has been reported in pediatric patients, but this has not been confirmed in controlled trials of adults or children. Because lamivudine also has activity against HBV and substantially lowers plasma HBV DNA concentrations, caution is warranted in using this drug in patients coinfected with HBV; discontinuation of lamivudine may be associated with a rebound of HBV replication and exacerbation of hepatitis.

Drug Interactions and Precautions. Lamivudine inhibits the intracellular phosphorylation of the cytosine analog zalcitabine (Veal *et al.*, 1996) and antagonizes zalcitabine's antiretroviral activity *in vitro* (Merrill *et al.*, 1996), although the clinical significance of this interaction is unknown. Since lamivudine and emtricitabine have nearly identical resistance and activity patterns, there is no rationale for their combined use. Lamivudine is synergistic with most other nucleoside analogs *in vitro* (Merrill *et al.*, 1996; Veal *et al.*, 1996). Trimethoprim–sulfamethoxazole increases the lamivudine plasma *AUC* by 43% presumably through inhibition of renal tubular secretion (Moore *et al.*, 1996). However, the effect on intracellular triphosphate concentrations is unknown, and dose adjustment is not recommended.

Therapeutic Use. In early monotherapy studies, initial declines in plasma HIV-1 RNA concentrations of up to 90% occurred within 14 days but rebounded rapidly with emergence of lamivudine-resistant HIV (Perry and Faulds, 1997). Patients randomized to the combination of lamivudine plus zidovudine had substantially better mean decreases in plasma HIV-1 RNA at 52 weeks (97% *versus* 70% decrease in copies/ml) and increases in CD4+ lymphocyte counts (+61 *versus* −53 cells/mm^3) compared with those receiving zidovudine alone (Eron *et al.*, 1995). In a large randomized, double-blind trial, combining lamivudine with zidovudine or stavudine caused about a twelvefold further decline in viral load at 24 weeks compared with zidovudine or stavudine monotherapy (Kuritzkes *et al.*, 1999); in the same trial, combining lamivudine with didanosine conferred no additional benefits. Many trials have confirmed the value of using lamivudine in three-drug regimens with other nucleoside analogs, protease inhibitors, and/or NNRTIs. Lamivudine has been effective in combination with other antiretroviral drugs in both treatment-naive and experienced patients (Perry and Faulds, 1997) and is a common component of therapy (Table 50–2B), given its safety, convenience, and efficacy.

Abacavir

Chemistry and Antiviral Activity. Abacavir is a synthetic carbocyclic purine analog [(1S, cis)-4-[2-amino-6-(cyclopropylamino)-9H-purin-9-yl)]-2-cyclopentene-1-methanol] (Figure 50–2). Abacavir is converted inside cells to an active metabolite, carbovir 5′-triphosphate (Figure 50–3), which is a potent inhibitor of the HIV-1 reverse transcriptase. [*Carbovir,* a related guanine analog, was withdrawn from clinical development owing to poor oral bioavailability (Hervey and Perry, 2000)]. The IC$_{50}$ of abacavir for primary clinical HIV-1 isolates is 0.26 μM, and its IC$_{50}$ for laboratory strains ranges from 0.07 to 5.8 μM.

Mechanisms of Action and Resistance. Abacavir is the only approved antiretroviral that is active as a guanosine analog. It is initially monophosphorylated by adenosine phosphotransferase. The monophosphate is then converted to (−)-carbovir 3′-monophosphate, which is then phosphorylated to the di- and triphosphates by cellular kinases (Figure 50–3). Carbovir 5′-triphosphate terminates the elongation of proviral DNA because it is incorporated by reverse transcriptase into nascent DNA but lacks a 3′-hydroxyl group.

Clinical resistance to abacavir is associated with four specific codon substitutions: K65R, L74V, Y115F, and M184V (Gallant *et al.*, 2003). Individually, these substitutions produce only modest (two- to fourfold) resistance to abacavir compared to virus *in vitro* but in combination can reduce susceptibility by up to tenfold. The Y115F mutation is seen uniquely with abacavir. The L74V mutation is associated with cross-resistance to the purine analog didanosine and the cytosine analog zalcitabine. K65R confers cross-resistance to all nucleosides except zidovudine. An alternate pathway for abacavir resistance involves mutations at codons 41, 210, and 215, which have been associated with a reduced likelihood of virologic response. Abacavir sensitivity is greatly reduced by the multinucleoside resistance clusters, including that associated with the Q151M substitution, as well as the two-amino-acid insertion following codon 69 (Gallant *et al.*, 2003).

Absorption, Distribution, and Elimination. Abacavir's oral bioavailability is greater than 80% regardless of food intake (Table 50–3). Abacavir is eliminated by metabolism to the 5′-carboxylic acid derivative catalyzed by alcohol dehydrogenase and by glucuronidation to the 5′-glucuronide. These metabolites account for 30% and 36% of elimination, respectively (Hervey and Perry, 2000). Abacavir is not a substrate or inhibitor of CYPs. Abacavir is 50% bound to plasma proteins, and the CSF–plasma AUC is approximately 0.3. Although the introduced dose of abacavir was 300 mg twice daily, carbovir triphosphate accumulates inside the cell and has a reported elimination half-life of up to 21 hours (Hervey and Perry, 2000) (Table 50–2); thus a regimen of 600 mg once daily is approved.

Untoward Effects. The most important adverse effect of abacavir is a unique and potentially fatal hypersensitivity syndrome. This syndrome is characterized by fever, abdominal pain, and other gastrointestinal complaints; a mild maculopapular rash; and malaise or fatigue. Respiratory complaints (cough, pharyngitis, dyspnea), musculoskeletal complaints, headache, and paresthesias are reported less commonly. Median time to onset of symptoms is 11 days, and 93% of cases occur within 6 weeks of initiating therapy (Hetherington *et al.*, 2002). The presence of concurrent fever, abdominal pain, and rash within 6 weeks of starting abacavir is diagnostic and necessitates immediate discontinuation of the drug. Patients having only one of these symptoms may be observed to see if additional symptoms appear. Unlike many hypersensitivity syndromes, this condition worsens with continued treatment. *Abacavir can never be restarted once discontinued for hypersensitivity because reintroduction of the drug leads to rapid recurrence of severe symptoms, accompanied by hypotension, a shocklike state, and possibly death.* The reported mortality rate of restarting abacavir in sensitive individuals is 4% (Hervey and Perry, 2000).

Abacavir hypersensitivity occurs in 2% to 9% of patients depending on the population studied. The cause is a genetically mediated immune response linked to both the *HLA-B*5701* locus and the M493T allele in the heat-shock locus *Hsp70-Hom* (Martin *et al.*, 2004). One of the strongest pharmacogenetic associations ever described, the latter gene is implicated in antigen presentation, and this haplotype is associated with aberrant tumor necrosis factor-α release after exposure of human lymphocytes to abacavir *ex vivo*. In one Caucasian population, the combination of these two markers occurred in 94.4% of cases and less than 0.5% of controls for a positive predictive value of 93.8% and a negative predictive value of 99.5% (Martin *et al.*, 2004). Other genes may be involved because the syndrome is much less common in populations with a low prevalence of *HLA-B*5701* (*e.g.*, African-Americans), but it can occur in patients lacking this HLA type (Hetherington *et al.*, 2002).

In those without true hypersensitivity, abacavir is a well-tolerated drug. Carbovir 5′-triphosphate is a weak inhibitor of human DNA polymerases, including DNA polymerase-γ (Hervey and Perry, 2000). Abacavir therefore has not been associated with adverse events thought to be due to mitochondrial toxicity, such as myelosuppression, peripheral neuropathy, and pancreatitis.

Drug Interactions and Precautions. Abacavir is not associated with any clinically significant pharmacokinetic drug interactions. However, a large dose of *ethanol* (0.7 g/kg) increased the abacavir plasma AUC by 41% and prolonged the elimination half-life by 26% (McDowell *et al.*, 2000) possibly owing to competition for alcohol dehydrogenase. Patients starting abacavir must be warned about the symptoms of abacavir hypersensitivity and instructed to seek medical help immediately if symptoms occur.

Therapeutic Use. In initial monotherapy studies, abacavir reduced HIV plasma RNA concentrations up to 300 times more than that seen with other antiretroviral nucleosides, and increased CD4+ lymphocyte counts by 80 to 200 cells/mm^3 (Hervey and Perry, 2000). Abacavir is not a more potent inhibitor of HIV replication than other nucleosides *in vitro*, and the mechanism for its more potent *in vivo* activity is unexplained.

Abacavir is effective in combination with other nucleoside analogs, NNRTIs, and protease inhibitors. Adding abacavir to zidovudine and lamivudine results in a substantially greater decrease in plasma HIV-l RNA than seen with the two-drug regimen of zidovudine plus lamivudine in adults (Hervey and Perry, 2000) and children (Saez-Llorens *et al.*, 2001). Adding abacavir to stable antiretroviral therapy can result in additional antiviral effect, but treatment-experienced patients are much less likely to benefit from this drug if there are multiple preexisting nucleoside resistance mutations.

Abacavir is available in a coformulation with zidovudine and lamivudine for twice-daily dosing. However, the combination of abacavir, zidovudine, and lamivudine was somewhat less effective in a randomized, double-blind, placebo-controlled trial in 1147 treatment-naive patients than was the combination of zidovudine, lamivudine, and *efavirenz* or the four-drug regimen of zidovudine, lamivudine, abacavir, and efavirenz; 79% of patients in the abacavir, zidovudine, lamivudine group had undetectable plasma HIV RNA at 32 weeks as compared with 89% with the other regimens (Gulick *et al.*, 2004). Abacavir is also available in a coformulation with lamivudine for once-daily dosing.

Tenofovir

Chemistry and Antiviral Activity. Tenofovir is a derivative of adenosine 5′-monophosphate lacking a complete ribose ring and is the only nucleotide analog currently marketed for the treatment of HIV infection. Because the parent compound had very poor oral bioavailability, tenofovir is available only as the disoproxil fumarate prodrug, which has improved oral absorption and cellular penetration substantially. Like lamivudine and emtricitabine, tenofovir is active against HIV-1, HIV-2, and HBV. The IC_{50} of tenofovir disoproxil fumarate against laboratory strains of HIV-1 ranges from 2 to 7 nM, making the prodrug about one hundredfold more active *in vitro* than the parent compound (Chapman *et al.*, 2003).

Mechanism of Action and Resistance. Tenofovir disoproxil fumarate is hydrolyzed rapidly to tenofovir and then is phosphorylated by cellular kinases to its active metabolite, tenofovir diphosphate (Figure 50–3); the active moiety is, in fact, a triphosphate compound because the parent drug starts out as the monophosphate. The intracellular diphosphate is a competitive inhibitor of viral reverse transcriptases and is incorporated into HIV DNA to cause chain termination because it has an incomplete ribose ring. Although tenofovir diphosphate has broad-spectrum activity against viral DNA polymerases, it has low affinity for human DNA polymerases-α, -β, and -γ, which is the basis for its selective toxicity.

Virus replication in the presence of suboptimal concentrations of drug can select for mutations conferring resistance to tenofovir. Specific resistance occurs with a single substitution at codon 65 of reverse transcriptase (K65R). This mutation reduces *in vitro* sensitivity by only three- to fourfold but has been associated with clinical failure of tenofovir-containing regimens (Chapman *et al.*, 2003). Tenofovir sensitivity and virologic efficacy also are reduced in patients harboring HIV isolates with high-level resistance to zidovudine or stavudine, specifically those having three or more TAMs, including M41L or L120W. However, HIV variants that are resistant to zidovudine show only partial resistance to tenofovir, possibly a reflection of the much less efficient excision of tenofovir diphosphate by pyrophosphorolysis (Naeger *et al.*, 2002). The M184V mutation associated with lamivudine or emtricitabine resistance partially restores susceptibility in tenofovir-resistant HIV harboring the K65R mutation (Wainberg *et al.*, 1999).

The K65R mutation was reported in only 2% to 3% of tenofovir-treated patients in initial clinical studies, and this mutation usually was not associated with treatment failure. Patients failing most tenofovir-containing regimens are more likely to harbor genotypic resistance to the other drugs in the regimen. Notable exceptions are once-daily combination regimens of three nucleosides, specifically tenofovir plus didanosine and lamivudine and tenofovir plus abacavir and lamivudine. Both these regimens were associated with very high early rates of virologic failure or nonresponse, and at the time of failure, the K65R mutation was present in 36% to 64% of virus isolated from patients participating in these trials (Department of Health and Human Services, 2004).

Absorption, Distribution, and Elimination. Tenofovir disoproxil fumarate has an oral bioavailability of 25%. A high-fat meal increases the oral bioavailability to 39%, but the drug can be taken without regard to food (Chapman *et al.*, 2003). Tenofovir is not bound significantly to plasma proteins. The plasma elimination half-life ranges from 14 to 17 hours (Bang and Scott, 2003). The reported half-life of intracellular tenofovir diphosphate is 11 hours in activated peripheral blood mononuclear cells and 49 hours or longer in resting cells (Chapman *et al.*, 2003). The drug therefore can be dosed once daily. Tenofovir undergoes both glomerular filtration and active tubular secretion. Between 70% and 80% of an intravenous dose of tenofovir is recovered unchanged in the urine. Doses should be decreased in those with renal insufficiency (Chapman *et al.*, 2003).

Untoward Effects. Tenofovir generally is well tolerated, with few significant adverse effects reported except for flatulence. In placebo-controlled, double-blinded trials, the drug had no other adverse effects reported more frequently than with placebo after treatment for up to 24 weeks; tenofovir was significantly less toxic than stavudine. Unlike the antiviral nucleotides *adefovir* and *cidofovir* (*see* Chapter 49), tenofovir is not toxic to human renal tubular cells *in vitro* (Chapman *et al.*, 2003). However, rare episodes of acute renal failure and Fanconi syndrome have been reported with tenofovir, and this drug should be used

with caution in patients with preexisting renal disease. Because tenofovir also has activity against HBV and may lower plasma HBV DNA concentrations, caution is warranted in using this drug in patients coinfected with HBV; discontinuation of tenofovir may be associated with a rebound of HBV replication and exacerbation of hepatitis.

Drug Interactions and Precautions. Tenofovir is not metabolized to a significant extent by CYPs and is not known to inhibit or induce these enzymes. However, tenofovir has been associated with a few potentially important pharmacokinetic drug interactions. A 300-mg dose of tenofovir increased the didanosine *AUC* by 44% to 60% probably as a consequence of inhibition of the enzyme purine nucleoside phosphorylase by both tenofovir and tenofovir monophosphate (Robbins *et al.*, 2003). These two drugs probably should not be used together, or if this is essential, the dose of didanosine should be reduced from 400 to 250 mg/day (Chapman *et al.*, 2003). Although tenofovir is not known to induce CYPs, it has been reported to reduce the *atazanavir AUC* by approximately 26%. In addition, low-dose ritonavir (100 mg twice daily) increases the tenofovir *AUC* by 34%, and atazanavir increases the tenofovir *AUC* by 25%. The mechanism of these interactions is unknown.

Therapeutic Use. Tenofovir is FDA approved for treating HIV infection in adults in combination with other antiretroviral agents. The use of tenofovir in antiretroviral-experienced patients resulted in a further sustained decrease in HIV plasma RNA concentrations of 4.5 to 7.4 times relative to placebo after 48 weeks of treatment (Chapman *et al.*, 2003). Several large trials have confirmed the antiretroviral activity of tenofovir in three-drug regimens with other agents, including other nucleoside analogs, protease inhibitors, and/or NNRTIs. In a randomized, double-blind comparison trial in which treatment-naive patients also received lamivudine and efavirenz, tenofovir 300 mg once daily was as effective and less toxic than stavudine 40 mg twice daily (Gallant *et al.*, 2004).

Emtricitabine

Chemistry and Antiviral Activity. Emtricitabine is a cytosine analog that is chemically related to lamivudine and shares many of that drug's pharmacodynamic properties. Like lamivudine, it has two chiral centers and is manufactured as the enantiomerically pure (2R,5S)-5-fluoro-1-[2-(hydroxymethyl)-1,3-oxathiolan-5-yl]cytosine (FTC) (Figure 50–2). Emtricitabine is active against HIV-1, HIV-2, and HBV. The IC$_{50}$ of emtricitabine against laboratory strains of HIV-1 ranges from 2 to 530 nM, although, on average, the drug is about 10 times more active *in vitro* than lamivudine (Bang and Scott, 2003).

Mechanism of Action and Resistance. Emtricitabine enters cells by passive diffusion and is phosphorylated by deoxycytidine kinase and cellular kinases to its active metabolite, emtricitabine 5′-triphosphate (Figure 50–3). The intracellular triphosphate acts as a competitive inhibitor of reverse transcriptase and is incorporated into HIV DNA to cause chain termination. Like lamivudine, emtricitabine has low affinity for human DNA polymerases, explaining its low toxicity to the host.

High-level resistance to emtricitabine occurs with the same mutation (methionine-to-valine substitution at codon 184) affecting lamivudine, although this appears to occur less frequently with emtricitabine. In three studies, M184V occurred about half as frequently with emtricitabine-containing regimens as with lamivudine, and patients presenting with virologic failure were two to three times as likely to have wild-type virus at the time of failure as compared with lamivudine (Bang and Scott, 2003). The M184V mutation restores zidovudine susceptibility to zidovudine-resistant HIV and also partially restores tenofovir susceptibility to tenofovir-resistant HIV harboring the K65R mutation (Wainberg *et al.*, 1999). The same K65R mutation confers resistance to emtricitabine and the other cytosine analogs lamivudine and zalcitabine, as well as didanosine, stavudine, and abacavir.

Absorption, Distribution, and Elimination. Emtricitabine is absorbed rapidly and has an oral bioavailability of 93%. Food reduces the C_{max} but does not affect the *AUC,* and the drug can be taken without regard to meals. Emtricitabine is not bound significantly to plasma proteins. Compared with other nucleoside analogs, the drug has a slow systemic clearance and long elimination half-life of 8 to 10 hours (Bang and Scott, 2003). In addition, the estimated half-life of the intracellular triphosphate is very long, up to 39 hours in one report. This provides the pharmacokinetic rationale for once-daily dosing of this drug. Emtricitabine is excreted primarily unchanged in the urine, undergoing glomerular filtration and active tubular secretion.

Untoward Effects. Emtricitabine is one of the least toxic antiretroviral drugs and, like its chemical relative lamivudine, has few significant adverse effects and no effect on mitochondrial DNA *in vitro* (Bang and Scott, 2003). Prolonged exposure has been associated with hyperpigmentation of the skin, especially in sun-exposed areas. Elevated hepatic transaminases, hepatitis, and pancreatitis have been reported, but these have occurred in association with other drugs known to cause these toxicities. Since emtricitabine also has *in vitro* activity against HBV, caution is warranted in using this drug in patients coinfected with HBV; discontinuation of lamivudine, which is closely related to emtricitabine, has been associated with a rebound of HBV replication and exacerbation of hepatitis.

Drug Interactions and Precautions. Emtricitabine is not metabolized to a significant extent by CYPs, and it is not susceptible to any known metabolic drug interactions. The possibility of a pharmacokinetic interaction involving renal tubular secretion, such as that between trimethoprim and lamivudine, has not been investigated for emtricitabine, although the drug does not alter the pharmacokinetics of tenofovir.

Therapeutic Use. Emtricitabine is FDA approved for treating HIV infection in adults in combination with other antiretroviral agents. Two small monotherapy trials showed that the maximal antiviral effect of emtricitabine (mean 1.9 log unit decrease in plasma HIV RNA concentration) was achieved with a dose of 200 mg/day. Several

large trials have confirmed the antiretroviral activity of emtricitabine in three-drug regimens with other agents, including nucleoside or nucleotide analogs, protease inhibitors, and/or NNRTIs. In two randomized comparison studies, emtricitabine- and lamivudine-based triple-combination regimens had similar efficacy (Bang and Scott, 2003).

NONNUCLEOSIDE REVERSE TRANSCRIPTASE INHIBITORS

Nonnucleoside reverse transcriptase inhibitors (NNRTIs) include a variety of chemical substrates that bind to a hydrophobic pocket in the p66 subunit of the HIV-1 reverse transcriptase. The NNRTI-binding pocket is not essential for the function of the enzyme and is distant from the active site. These compounds induce a conformational change in the three-dimensional structure of the enzyme that greatly reduces its activity, and thus they act as noncompetitive inhibitors (Spence *et al.*, 1995). Unlike nucleoside and nucleotide reverse transcriptase inhibitors, these compounds do not require intracellular phosphorylation to attain activity. Because the binding site for NNRTIs is virus-strain-specific, the approved agents are active against HIV-1 but not HIV-2 or other retroviruses and should not be used to treat HIV-2 infection (Harris and Montaner, 2000). These compounds also have no activity against host cell DNA polymerases. The two most commonly used agents in this category, efavirenz and *nevirapine,* are quite potent and transiently decrease plasma HIV RNA concentrations by two orders of magnitude or more when used as sole agents (Havlir *et al.*, 1995; Wei *et al.*, 1995). The chemical structures of the three approved NNRTIs are shown in Figure 50–4, and their pharmacokinetic properties are summarized in Table 50–4.

All three approved NNRTIs are eliminated from the body by hepatic metabolism. Nevirapine and *delavirdine* are primarily substrates for the CYP3A4 isoform, whereas efavirenz is a substrate for CYP2B6 (Smith *et al.*, 2001) and CYP3A4. The steady-state elimination half-lives of efavirenz and nevirapine range from 24 to 72 hours, allowing daily dosing. Efavirenz and nevirapine are moderately potent inducers of hepatic drug-metabolizing enzymes including CYP3A4, whereas delavirdine is a CYP3A4 inhibitor. Pharmacokinetic drug interactions are thus an important consideration with this class of compounds and represent a potential toxicity.

The NNRTIs are more susceptible to high-level drug resistance than other classes of antiretroviral drugs because a single-amino-acid change in the NNRTI-binding pocket (usually in codons 103 or 181) renders the virus resistant to all available drugs in the class. Unlike nucleoside analogs or protease inhibitors, NNRTIs can induce resistance and virologic relapse within a few days or weeks

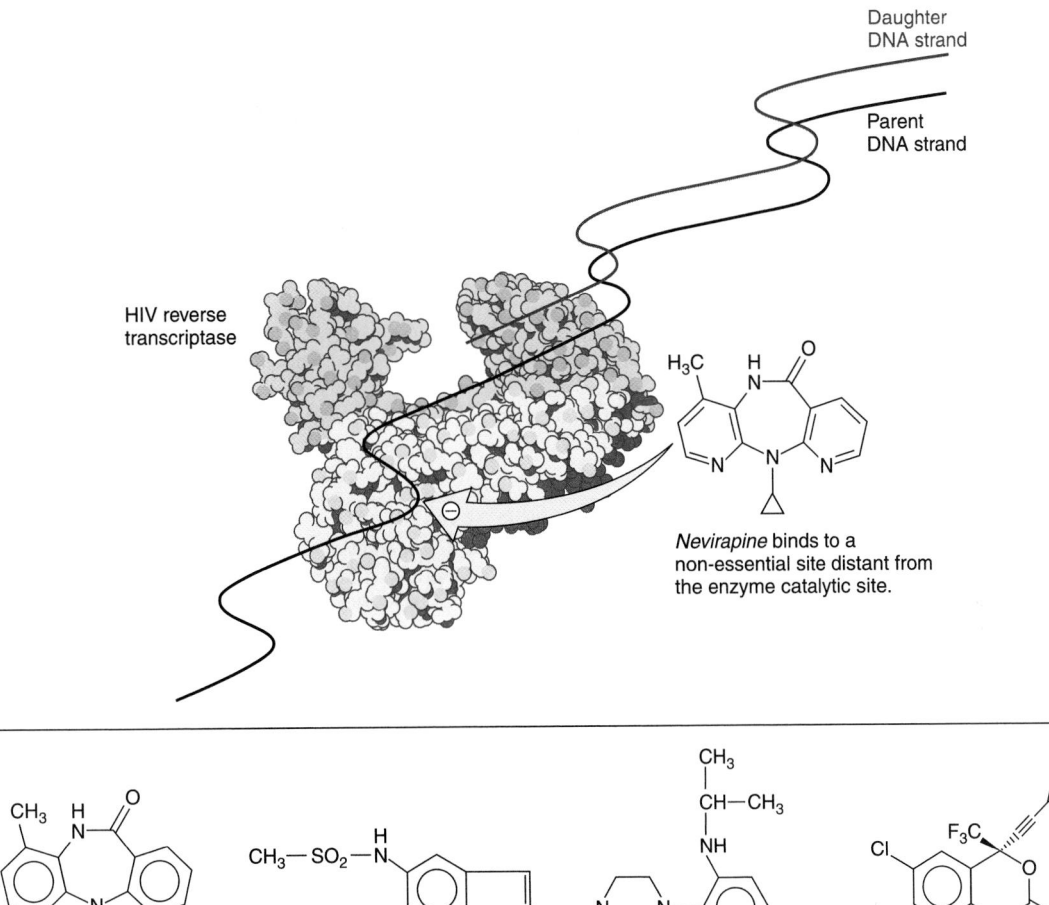

Figure 50–4. *Structures and mechanism of nonnucleoside reverse transcriptase inhibitors.*

Table 50–4
Pharmacokinetic Properties of Nonnucleoside Reverse Transcriptase Inhibitors

PARAMETER	NEVIRAPINE†	EFAVIRENZ†	DELAVIRDINE
Oral bioavailability, %	90–93	50	85
Effect of meals on *AUC*	↔	↑17–28%	↔
Plasma $t_{\frac{1}{2}}$,elim, h	25–30	40–55	2–11
Plasma protein binding, %	60	99	98
Metabolism	CYP3A4 > CYP2B6	CYP2B6 > CYP3A4	CYP3A4
Renal excretion of parent drug, %	<3	<3	<5
Autoinduction of metabolism	Yes	Yes	No
Inhibition of CYP3A	No	Yes	Yes

ABBREVIATIONS: *AUC*, area under plasma concentration–time curve; $t_{\frac{1}{2}}$,elim, half-life of elimination; ↑, increase; ↓, decrease; ↔, no effect. *Reported mean values in adults with normal renal and hepatic function. †Values at steady state after multiple oral doses.

if given as monotherapy (Wei *et al.*, 1995). Exposure to even a single dose of nevirapine in the absence of other antiretroviral drugs is associated with resistance mutations in up to one-third of patients (Eshleman *et al.*, 2004). *These agents are potent and highly effective but must be combined with at least two other active agents to avoid resistance* (Table 50–2B).

The use of efavirenz or nevirapine in combination with other antiretroviral drugs is associated with favorable long-term suppression of viremia and elevation of CD4+ lymphocyte counts (Harris and Montaner, 2000). Efavirenz in particular is a common component of first regimens for treatment-naive patients in recognition of its convenience, tolerability, and potency. Rashes occur frequently with all NNRTIs, usually during the first 4 weeks of therapy. These generally are mild and self-limited, although rare cases of potentially fatal Stevens-Johnson syndrome have been reported with nevirapine and efavirenz. Fat accumulation can be seen after long-term use of NNRTIs (Mallal *et al.*, 2000; Heath *et al.*, 2001), and fatal hepatitis has been associated with nevirapine use.

Nevirapine

Chemistry and Antiviral Activity. Nevirapine is a dipyridodiazepinone NNRTI with potent activity against HIV-1. The *in vitro* IC_{50} of this drug ranges from 10 to 100 nM. Like other compounds in this class, nevirapine does not have significant activity against HIV-2 or other retroviruses (Harris and Montaner, 2000).

Mechanism of Action and Resistance. Nevirapine is a noncompetitive inhibitor that binds to a site on the HIV-1 reverse transcriptase that is distant from the active site, inducing a conformational change that disrupts catalytic activity. Since the target site is HIV-1-specific and is not essential for the enzyme, resistance can develop rapidly. A single mutation at either codon 103 or codon 181 of reverse transcriptase decreases susceptibility more than one hundredfold (Kuritzkes, 2004). Nevirapine resistance is also associated with mutations at codons 100, 106, 108, 188, and 190, but either the K103N or the Y181C mutation is sufficient to produce clinical treatment failure (Eshleman *et al.*, 2004). *Cross-resistance extends to all FDA-approved NNRTIs with the most common mutations. Therefore, any patient who fails treatment with one NNRTI because of a specific resistance mutation should be considered to have failed the entire class.*

Absorption, Distribution, and Elimination. Nevirapine is well absorbed, and its bioavailability is not altered by food or antacids (Smith *et al.*, 2001). The drug readily crosses the placenta and has been found in breast milk, a feature that has encouraged use of nevirapine for prevention of mother-to-child transmission of HIV (Mirochnick *et al.*, 1998).

Nevirapine is eliminated mainly by oxidative metabolism involving CYP3A4 and CYP2B6. Less than 3% of the parent drug is eliminated unchanged in the urine (Smith *et al.*, 2001). Nevirapine has a long elimination half-life of 25 to 30 hours at steady state. The drug is a moderate inducer of CYPs, including CYP3A4; thus the drug induces its own metabolism, which decreases the half-life from 45 hours following the first dose to 25 to 30 hours after 2 weeks. To compensate for this, it is recommended that the drug be initiated at a dose of 200 mg once daily for 14 days, with the dose then increased to 200 mg twice daily if no adverse reactions have

occurred. Because of its long half-life, current clinical studies are investigating once-daily dosing of nevirapine.

Untoward Effects. The most frequent adverse event associated with nevirapine is rash, which occurs in approximately 16% of patients. Mild macular or papular eruptions commonly involve the trunk, face, and extremities and generally occur within the first 6 weeks of therapy. Pruritus is also common. In the majority of patients, the rash resolves with continued administration of drug. Up to 7% of patients discontinue therapy owing to rash, and administration of glucocorticoids may cause a more severe rash. Life-threatening Stevens-Johnson syndrome is rare but occurs in up to 0.3% of recipients (Harris and Montaner, 2000).

Elevated hepatic transaminases occur in up to 14% of patients. Clinical hepatitis occurs in up to 1% of patients. Severe and fatal hepatitis has been associated with nevirapine use, and this may be more common in women, especially during pregnancy (Dieterich *et al.*, 2004). Other reported side effects include fever, fatigue, headache, somnolence, and nausea.

Drug Interactions and Precautions. Because nevirapine induces CYP3A4, this drug may lower plasma concentrations of coadministered CYP3A4 substrates. Methadone withdrawal has been reported in patients receiving nevirapine (Altice *et al.*, 1999), presumably as a consequence of enhanced methadone clearance. Plasma *ethinyl estradiol* and *norethindrone* concentrations decrease by 20% with nevirapine, and alternative methods of birth control are advised (Smith *et al.*, 2001). Nevirapine also can reduce concentrations of some coadministered HIV protease inhibitors (Table 50–5).

Therapeutic Use. Nevirapine is FDA approved for the treatment of HIV-1 infection in adults and children in combination with other antiretroviral agents. In original monotherapy studies, a rapid fall in plasma HIV RNA concentrations of 99% or greater was followed by a return toward baseline within 8 weeks because of rapid emergence of resistance (Havlir *et al.*, 1995; Wei *et al.*, 1995). Nevirapine therefore never should be used as a single agent or as the sole addition to a failing regimen. The three-drug regimen of nevirapine, zidovudine, and didanosine reduced the plasma HIV RNA concentration to undetectable levels (<400 copies/ml) in 52% of antiretroviral-naive adults (Montaner *et al.*, 1998).

Single-dose nevirapine has been used commonly in pregnant HIV-infected women to prevent mother-to-child transmission. A single oral intrapartum dose of 200 mg nevirapine followed by a single dose given to the newborn reduced neonatal HIV infection to 13% compared with 21.5% infection with a more complicated zidovudine regimen (Guay *et al.*, 1999). Although this regimen is very inexpensive and generally well tolerated, the high prevalence of nevirapine resistance following the single oral dose (Eshleman *et al.*, 2004), coupled with the recent recognition of fatal nevirapine hepatitis, has prompted a reexamination of the role this regimen should play in the prevention of vertical transmission.

Table 50–5
Drug Interactions Between Nonnucleoside Reverse Transcriptase Inhibitors and HIV Protease Inhibitors*

	EFFECT OF NNRTI ON PLASMA AUC OF PI (% CHANGE)			EFFECT OF PI ON PLASMA AUC OF NNRTI (% CHANGE)		
	Delavirdine	Nevirapine	Efavirenz	Delavirdine	Nevirapine	Efavirenz
Saquinavir[†]	↑120–400%	↓24–38%	↓62%	↔	↔	↓12%
Indinavir	↑53%	↓31%	↓30–31%	↔	↔	↔
Ritonavir	↑70%	↔	↑18%	↔	↔	↑21%
Nelfinavir	↑107%	↔	↑20%	↓31%	↔	↓12%
Amprenavir	↑130%	NR	↓35%	↓61%	NR	↔
Fosamprenavir	NR	NR	↓13%	NR	NR	NR
Lopinavir[‡]	NR	↓27%	↓19–25%	NR	↑8–9%	↓16
Atazanavir	NR	NR	↓74%	NR	NR	NR

ABBREVIATIONS: NNRTI, nonnucleoside reverse transcriptase inhibitor; PI, HIV protease inhibitor; AUC, area under the plasma concentration–time curve; ↑, increase, ↓, decrease; ↔, no change; NR, not reported. *Reported mean change in the AUC of the standard dose of the affected drug by the standard dose of the affecting drug; studies using modified dosing regimens were dose-normalized. [†]Parameters reported for the saquinavir soft-gel capsule formulation. [‡]Lopinavir is only available in a coformulation with ritonavir.

Delavirdine

Chemistry and Antiviral Activity. Delavirdine is a bis-heteroarylpiperazine NNRTI that selectively inhibits HIV-1. The *in vitro* IC_{50} ranges from 6 to 30 nM for laboratory HIV-1 isolates to 1 to 700 nM for clinical isolates (Scott and Perry, 2000). Delavirdine does not have significant activity against HIV-2 or other retroviruses.

Mechanism of Action and Resistance. Delavirdine is a noncompetitive inhibitor that binds to a peripheral site on the HIV-1 reverse transcriptase and induces a conformational change that disrupts catalytic activity. The delavirdine–reverse transcriptase complex is stabilized by hydrogen bonding to the lysine at codon 103 and strong hydrophobic interactions with the proline at position 236 (Spence *et al.*, 1995). Since the target site is HIV-1-specific and is not essential for the enzyme, resistance can develop rapidly. A single mutation at either codon 103 or codon 181 of reverse transcriptase decreases susceptibility more than one hundredfold (Kuritzkes, 2004). Delavirdine resistance also is associated with mutations at codons 106, 188, and 236, but either the K103N or the Y181C mutation is sufficient to produce clinical treatment failure. Cross-resistance extends to all FDA-approved NNRTIs with the most common mutations. Therefore, any patient who fails treatment with one NNRTI because of a specific resistance mutation should be considered to have failed the entire class.

Absorption, Distribution, and Elimination. Delavirdine is well absorbed, especially at pH less than 2. Antacids, histamine H_2-receptor antagonists, proton pump inhibitors, and achlorhydria may decrease its absorption. Standard meals do not alter the delavirdine AUC, and the drug can be administered irrespective of food (Smith *et al.*, 2001). The drug may have nonlinear pharmacokinetics because the plasma half-life increases with increasing doses (Scott and Perry, 2000).

Delavirdine clearance is primarily through oxidative metabolism by CYP3A4, with less than 5% of a dose recovered unchanged in the urine. At the recommended dose of 400 mg three times daily, the mean elimination half-life is 5.8 hours, but it ranges from 2 to 11 hours because of the considerable interpatient variability in clearance (Smith *et al.*, 2001). Delavirdine is 98% bound to plasma proteins, mainly albumin. The penetration of delavirdine into CSF and semen is poor, possibly reflecting extensive plasma protein binding.

Untoward Effects. As with all drugs in this class, the most common side effect of delavirdine is rash, which occurs in 18% to 36% of subjects. Rash usually is seen in the first few weeks of treatment and often resolves despite continued therapy. The rash may be macular, papular, erythematous, or pruritic and usually involves the trunk and extremities. Fewer than 5% of patients discontinue delavirdine because of rash. Severe dermatitis, including *erythema multiforme* and Stevens-Johnson syndrome, has been reported but is rare. Elevated hepatic transaminases also have been reported, but delavirdine use is not associated with fatal hepatitis. Neutropenia also may occur rarely (Para *et al.*, 1999).

Drug Interactions and Precautions. Delavirdine is both a substrate for and an inhibitor of CYP3A4 and can alter the metabolism of other CYP3A4 substrates. Delavirdine therefore should be avoided with certain CYP3A4 substrates with a low therapeutic index, including *amiodarone, propafenone, ergot derivatives, pimozide, triazolam,* and *midazolam.* Delavirdine is a weak inhibitor of CYP2C9, CYP2D6, and CYP2C19 *in vitro.* Potent inducers of CYP3A4, such as *carbamazepine, phenobarbital,* phenytoin, *rifabutin,* and *rifampin,* may decrease delavirdine concentrations and should be avoided. Delavirdine increases the plasma concentrations of most HIV protease inhibitors (Table 50–5) and could be used to modestly enhance the pharmacokinetic profile or reduce the dose of these agents (Scott and Perry, 2000).

Therapeutic Use. Initial monotherapy studies with delavirdine produced only transient decreases in plasma HIV RNA concentrations owing to rapid emergence of resistance. Later studies of delavirdine in combination with nucleoside analogs showed sustained decreases in HIV-1 RNA (Friedland *et al.*, 1999; Para *et al.*, 1999). Delavirdine is not used as widely as other NNRTIs in large measure because of its short half-life and requirement for thrice-daily dosing.

Efavirenz

Chemistry and Antiviral Activity. Efavirenz is a 1,4-dihydro-2H-3,1-benzoxazin-2-one NNRTI (Figure 50–4) with potent activity against HIV-1. The *in vitro* IC_{50} of this drug ranges from 3 to 9 nM (Young *et al.*, 1995). Like other compounds in this class, efavirenz does not have significant activity against HIV-2 or other retroviruses.

Mechanism of Action and Resistance. Efavirenz is a noncompetitive inhibitor that binds to a site on the HIV-1 reverse transcriptase that is distant from the active site, thus inducing a conformational change that disrupts catalytic activity. Because the target site is HIV-1-specific and is not essential for the enzyme, resistance can develop rapidly. The most common resistance mutation seen clinically is at codon 103 of reverse transcriptase (K103N), and this decreases susceptibility up to one hundredfold or greater (Kuritzkes, 2004). Additional resistance mutations have been seen at codons 100, 106, 108, 181, 188, 190, and 225, but either the K103N or Y181C mutation is sufficient to produce clinical treatment failure. Cross-resistance extends to all FDA-approved NNRTIs.

Absorption, Distribution, and Elimination. Efavirenz is well absorbed from the gastrointestinal tract and reaches peak plasma concentrations within 5 hours. There is diminished absorption of the drug with increasing doses. Bioavailability (*AUC*) is increased by 22% with a high-fat meal. Efavirenz is more than 99% bound to plasma proteins and, as a consequence, has a low CSF–plasma ratio of 0.01 (Smith *et al.*, 2001). The clinical significance of this low CNS penetration is unclear, especially since the major toxicities of efavirenz involve the CNS. It is recommended that the drug be taken initially on an empty stomach at bedtime to reduce side effects.

Efavirenz is cleared *via* oxidative metabolism, mainly by CYP2B6 and to a lesser extent by CYP3A4. The parent drug is not excreted renally to a significant degree (Smith *et al.*, 2001). Efavirenz is cleared slowly, with an elimination half-life of 40 to 55 hours at steady state. This safely allows once-daily dosing.

Untoward Effects. Rash occurs frequently with efavirenz, in up to 27% of adult patients (Adkins and Noble, 1998). Rash usually occurs within the first few weeks of treatment and rarely requires drug discontinuation. Life-threatening skin eruptions such as Stevens-Johnson syndrome have been reported during postmarketing experience with efavirenz but are rare.

The most important adverse effects of efavirenz involve the CNS. Up to 53% of patients report some CNS or psychiatric side effects, but fewer than 5% discontinue the drug for this reason. CNS symptoms may occur with the first dose and may last for hours. More severe symptoms may require weeks to resolve. Patients commonly report dizziness, impaired concentration, dysphoria, vivid or disturbing dreams, and insomnia. Episodes of frank psychosis

(depression, hallucinations, and/or mania) have been associated with initiating efavirenz. Fortunately, CNS side effects generally become more tolerable and resolve within the first 4 weeks of therapy.

Other side effects reported with efavirenz include headache, increased hepatic transaminases, and elevated serum cholesterol. False-positive urine screening tests for marijuana metabolites also can occur depending on the assay used (Adkins and Noble, 1998).

Efavirenz is the only antiretroviral drug that is unequivocally teratogenic in primates. When efavirenz was administered to pregnant cynomolgus monkeys, 25% of fetuses developed malformations. In six cases where women were exposed to efavirenz during the first trimester of pregnancy, fetuses or infants had significant malformations, mainly of the brain and spinal cord. *Women of childbearing potential therefore should use two methods of birth control and avoid pregnancy while taking efavirenz.*

Drug Interactions and Precautions. Efavirenz is a moderate inducer of hepatic enzymes, especially CYP3A4. It undergoes limited auto-induction, but because of its long half-life, there is no need to alter drug dose during the first few weeks of treatment. Efavirenz decreases concentrations of phenobarbital, phenytoin, and carbamazepine; the methadone *AUC* is reduced by 33% to 66% at steady state (Adkins and Noble, 1998). Rifampin concentrations are unchanged by concurrent efavirenz, but rifampin may reduce efavirenz concentrations. Efavirenz reduces the rifabutin *AUC* by 38% on average. Efavirenz has a variable effect on HIV protease inhibitors (Table 50–5). Indinavir, saquinavir, and *amprenavir* concentrations are reduced, but ritonavir and *nelfinavir* concentrations are increased (Adkins and Noble, 1998). Drugs that induce CYP2B6 or CYP3A4 (*e.g.,* phenobarbital, phenytoin, and carbamazepine) would be expected to increase the clearance of efavirenz and should be avoided.

Therapeutic Use. Efavirenz was the first antiretroviral agent approved by the FDA for once-daily administration. Initial short-term monotherapy studies showed substantial decreases in plasma HIV RNA, but the drug should only be used in combination with other effective agents and should not be added as the sole new agent to a failing regimen. In antiretroviral-naive patients receiving efavirenz, zidovudine, and lamivudine, 70% achieved undetectable plasma HIV-1 RNA compared with 48% of those receiving indinavir plus zidovudine and lamivudine (Staszewski *et al.*, 1999). Much of this difference appeared to be the consequence of improved patient adherence to the efavirenz regimen. Efavirenz also has been used effectively in patients who have failed previous antiretroviral therapy in combination with other active drugs (Falloon *et al.*, 2000; Piketty *et al.*, 1999). In pediatric HIV infection, 60% of children failing prior therapy with a nucleoside reverse transcriptase inhibitor had sustained virologic benefit after 48 weeks of treatment with efavirenz, nelfinavir, and a nucleoside analog (Starr *et al.*, 1999).

Efavirenz is used widely in the developed world because of its convenience, effectiveness, and long-term tolerability. To date, no antiretroviral regimen has produced better long-term treatment responses than any efavirenz-containing regimen in randomized, prospective clinical trials. As a result, efavirenz plus two nucleoside reverse transcriptase inhibitors was one of two regimens preferred in 2004 for treatment-naive patients (Table 50–2).

HIV PROTEASE INHIBITORS

HIV protease inhibitors are peptidelike chemicals that competitively inhibit the action of the virus aspartyl protease (Figure 50–5). This protease is a homodimer consisting of two 99-amino-acid monomers; each monomer contributes an aspartic acid residue that is essential for catalysis (Pearl and Taylor, 1987). The preferred cleavage site for this enzyme is the N-terminal side of proline residues, especially between phenylalanine and proline. Human aspartyl proteases (*i.e.,* renin, pepsin, gastricsin, and cathepsins D and E) contain only one polypeptide chain and are not significantly inhibited by HIV protease inhibitors. These drugs prevent proteolytic cleavage of HIV gag and pol polyproteins that include essential structural (p17, p24, p9, and p7) and enzymatic (reverse transcriptase, protease, and integrase) components of the virus. This prevents the metamorphosis of HIV virus particles into their mature infectious form (Flexner, 1998). Infected patients treated with HIV protease inhibitors as sole agents experienced a one hundred- to one thousand-fold mean decrease in plasma HIV RNA concentrations within 12 weeks, an effect similar in magnitude to that produced by NNRTIs (Ho *et al.*, 1995).

The clearance of all approved HIV protease inhibitors is mainly through hepatic oxidative metabolism. All but one of these drugs are substrates predominately for CYP3A4. Nelfinavir's major metabolite, M8, is formed by CYP2C19, and M8 is then cleared by CYP3A4. Elimination half-lives of the HIV protease inhibitors range from 1.8 to 10 hours (Table 50–6), and most of these drugs can be dosed once or twice daily. Pharmacokinetic properties are characterized by high interindividual variability, which may reflect differential activity of intestinal and hepatic CYP450 isoforms (Back *et al.*, 2002; Rendic and Di Carlo, 1997).

Most HIV protease inhibitors are substrates for the P-glycoprotein drug transporter (P-gp), which is an efflux pump encoded by the *mdr1* gene. P-gp in capillary endothelial cells of the blood–brain barrier limits the penetration of HIV protease inhibitors into the brain (Kim *et al.*, 1998), although the low CSF–plasma drug concentration ratio characteristic of these drugs also may reflect extensive binding to plasma proteins. Most HIV protease inhibitors penetrate less well into semen than do nucleoside reverse transcriptase inhibitors and NNRTIs. Virologic responses in plasma, CSF, and semen usually are concordant (Taylor *et al.*, 1999), and the clinical significance of P-gp and protein-binding effects is unclear.

An important toxicity common to all approved HIV protease inhibitors is the potential for metabolic drug interactions (Tables 50–5 and 50–7). Most of these drugs inhibit CYP3A4 at clinically achieved concentrations, although the magnitude of inhibition varies greatly, with ritonavir being by far the most potent (Piscitelli and Gallicano, 2001). Ritonavir, nelfinavir, and amprenavir are also moderate inducers of hepatic enzymes including CYP3A4 and glucuronosyl *S*-transferase. Concentrations of all approved HIV protease inhibitors may be reduced in the presence of other CYP inducers. Patients and care providers must be vigilant about the possibility of clinically significant pharmacokinetic drug interactions in patients receiving these drugs. Nausea, vomiting, and diarrhea are also common, although symptoms generally resolve within 4 weeks of starting treatment.

It is a common practice to combine HIV protease inhibitors with a low dose of ritonavir to take advantage of that drug's remarkable capacity to inhibit CYP3A4 metabolism (Flexner, 2000). Although the approved dose of ritonavir for antiretroviral treatment is 600 mg twice daily, doses of 100 or 200 mg twice daily are sufficient to inhibit CYP3A4 and increase the concentrations of concurrently administered CYP3A4 substrates. Furthermore, lower doses of ritonavir are much better tolerated. The enhanced pharmacokinetic profile of HIV protease inhibitors administered with ritonavir reflects inhibition of both first-pass and systemic clearance, resulting in improved oral bioavailability and a longer elimination half-life of the coadministered drug. This allows a reduction in both drug dose and dosing frequency while increasing systemic concentrations (Flexner, 2000). Combinations of amprenavir, *fosamprenavir,* or atazanavir with ritonavir are approved for once-daily administration, and other once-daily dual protease inhibitor combinations are under investigation. *Lopinavir* is available only in a coformulation with ritonavir that is designed to take advantage of this beneficial pharmacokinetic drug interaction.

The speed with which HIV develops resistance to protease inhibitors is intermediate between that of nucleoside analogs and NNRTIs. In initial monotherapy studies, the median time to rebound in HIV plasma RNA concentrations of one log or greater was 3 to 4 months (Flexner, 1998). In contrast to NNRTIs, high-level resistance to these drugs generally requires accumulation of a minimum of four to five codon substitutions, which may take

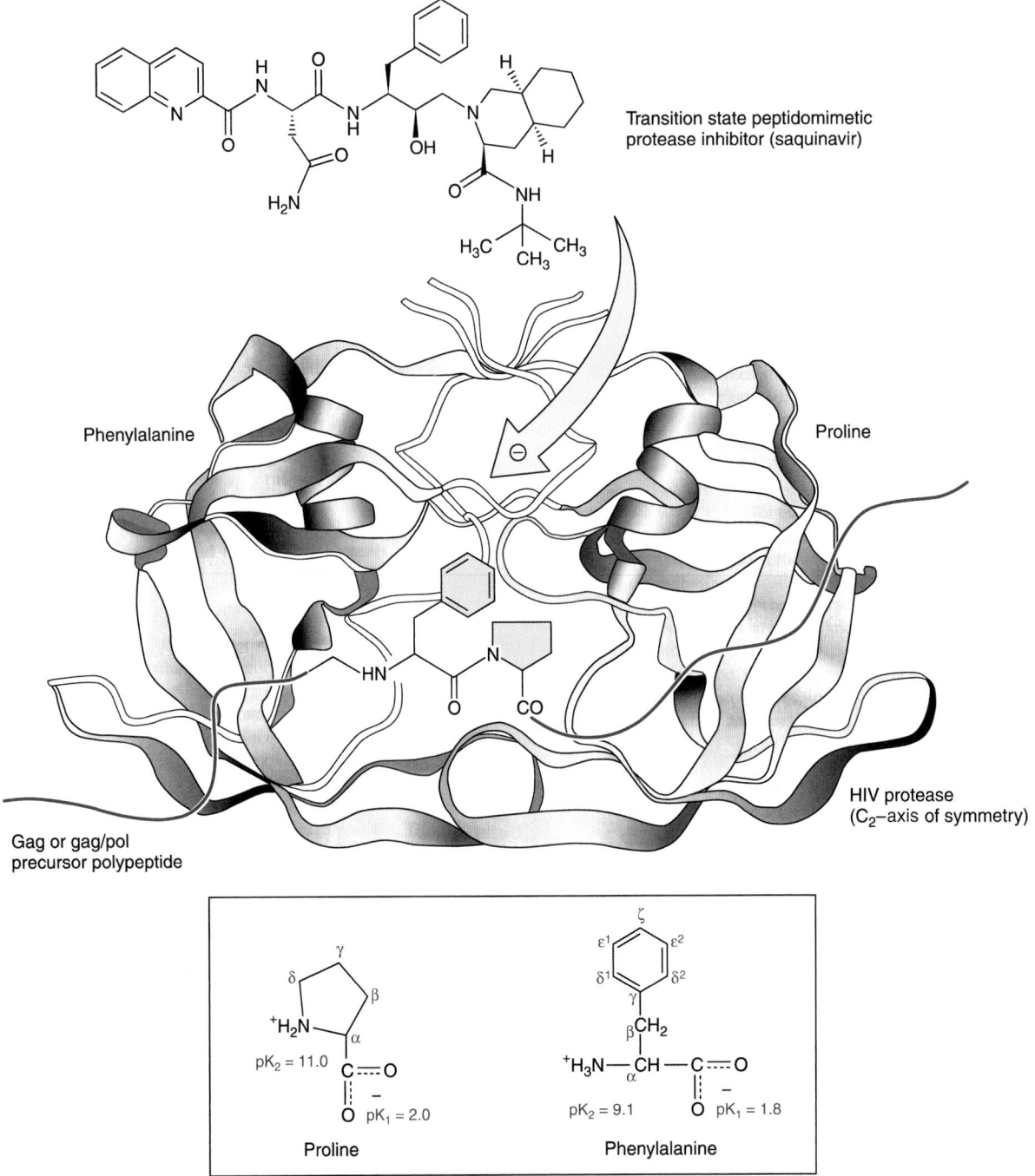

Transition state peptidomimetic protease inhibitor (saquinavir)

Phenylalanine

Proline

HIV protease (C₂–axis of symmetry)

Gag or gag/pol precursor polypeptide

Proline

Phenylalanine

Figure 50–5. *Mechanism of action of an HIV protease inhibitor.*

many months. Initial (primary) resistance mutations in the enzymatic active site confer only a three- to fivefold drop in sensitivity to most drugs, although primary mutations have a more pronounced effect on atazanavir and nelfinavir. However, these are followed by secondary mutations often distant from the active site that compensate for the reduction in proteolytic efficiency. Resistance to one HIV protease inhibitor occurs often, with the patient retaining sensitivity to other drugs in the class, although accumulation of secondary resistance mutations decreases the likelihood of long-term response to the next agent used (Flexner, 1998; Kuritzkes, 2004).

Table 50–6
Pharmacokinetic Properties of HIV-1 Protease Inhibitors*

PARAMETER	SAQUINAVIR†	INDINAVIR	RITONAVIR	NELFINAVIR	AMPRENAVIR	FOSAMPRENAVIR	LOPINAVIR‡	ATAZANAVIR
Oral bioavailability, %	13	60–65	>60	20–80 (formulation- and food-dependent)	35–90 (dose-dependent)	ND	ND	ND
Effect of meals on AUC	↑570% (high fat)	↓77% (high fat)	↑13% (capsule)	↑100–200%	↓21% (high fat)	↔	↑48% (moderate fat)	↑70% (light meal)
Plasma $t_{\frac{1}{2}}$,elim, h	1–2	1.8	3–5	3.5–5	7.1–10.6	7.7	5–6	6.5–7.9
Plasma protein binding, %	98	60	98–99	>98	90	90	98–99	86
Metabolism, %	CYP3A4	CYP3A4	CYP3A4 > CYP2D6	CYP2C19 > CYP3A4	CYP3A4	CYP3A4	CYP3A4	CYP3A4
Autoinduction of metabolism	No	No	Yes	Yes	No	No	Yes	No
Renal excretion of parent drug, %	<3	9–12	3.5	1–2	<3	1	<3	7
Inhibition of CYP3A4	+	++	+++	++	++	++	+++	++

ABBREVIATIONS: *AUC*, area under plasma concentration–time curve; $t_{\frac{1}{2}}$,elim, half-life of elimination; ↑, increase; ↓, decrease; ↔, no effect; CYP, cytochrome P450 isoform; ND, not determined; +, weak; ++, moderate; +++, substantial. *Reported mean values in adults with normal renal and hepatic function. †Parameters reported for the saquinavir soft-gel capsule formulation. ‡Lopinavir is only available in a coformulation with ritonavir.

Table 50-7
Drug Interactions Between HIV Protease Inhibitors*

DRUG EXERTING EFFECT	Drug Affected (Change in Plasma AUC)							
	SAQUINAVIR†	INDINAVIR	RITONAVIR	NELFINAVIR	AMPRENAVIR	FOSAMPRENAVIR	LOPINAVIR‡	ATAZANAVIR
Saquinavir†	—	↔	↔	↑18%	↓32%	NR	↔	NR
Indinavir	↑360–620%	—	↔	↑83%	↑33%	NR	↔	NR
Ritonavir	↑1590–1700%	↑320–500%	—	↑150%	↑220–230%	↑110%	↑46%§	↑240%
Nelfinavir	↑330–390%	↑51%	↔	—	↔	NR	NR	NR
Amprenavir	↓19%	↓38%	↔	↑15%	—	NR	↓15–37%	NR
Fosamprenavir	NR	NR	NR	NR	NR	—	↔	NR
Lopinavir‡	↑1290–1890%	↑84%	↔	NR	↑180%	↓26%	—	NR
Atazanavir	↑450%	NR	NR	NR	NR	NR	NR	—

ABBREVIATIONS: *AUC*, area under the plasma concentration–time curve; ↑, increase, ↓, decrease; ↔, no change; NR, not reported. *Reported mean change in the *AUC* of the standard dose of the affected drug by the standard dose of the affecting drug; studies using modified dosing regimens were dose-normalized. †Parameters reported for the saquinavir soft-gel capsule formulation. ‡Lopinavir is only available in a coformulation with ritonavir. §This represents the impact of additional ritonavir (100 mg bid) on the *AUC* of lopinavir in the coformulation of 400 mg lopinavir with 100 mg ritonavir bid.

HIV protease inhibitors produce favorable long-term suppression of viremia, elevation of CD4+ lymphocyte counts, reduced disease progression, and improved survival when combined with other active antiretroviral drugs (Flexner, 1998). With potent activity and favorable resistance profiles, these drugs are a common component of regimens for treatment-experienced patients. However, the virologic benefits of these drugs must be balanced against short- and long-term toxicities, including the risk of insulin resistance and lipodystrophy (Garg, 2004). In addition, dosing of some agents in this class may require as many as 18 capsules per day (Table 50–2), which makes adherence problematic.

Saquinavir

Chemistry and Antiviral Activity. Saquinavir is a peptidomimetic hydroxyethylamine HIV protease inhibitor. It is a transition-state analog of a phenylalanine–proline cleavage site in one of the native substrate sequences for the HIV aspartyl protease and was the product of a rational drug-design program (Roberts *et al.*, 1990). Saquinavir inhibits both HIV-1 and HIV-2 replication and has an *in vitro* IC_{50} in peripheral blood lymphocytes that ranges from 3.5 to 10 nM (Noble and Faulds, 1996).

Mechanisms of Action and Resistance. Saquinavir is selectively toxic by potently inhibiting the HIV-encoded protease but not host-encoded aspartyl proteases. Saquinavir reversibly binds to the active site of HIV protease, preventing polypeptide processing and subsequent virus maturation. Virus particles are produced in the presence of saquinavir but are noninfectious.

Virus replication in the presence of saquinavir selects for drug-resistant virus. The primary saquinavir resistance mutation occurs at HIV protease codon 90 (a leucine-to-methionine substitution), although primary resistance also has been reported with a glycine-to-valine substitution at codon 48. Secondary resistance mutations occur at codons 36, 46, 82, 84, and others, and these are associated with clinical saquinavir resistance as well as cross-resistance to other HIV protease inhibitors (Ives *et al.*, 1997). As is typical of HIV protease inhibitors, high-level resistance requires accumulation of multiple resistance mutations.

Absorption, Distribution, and Elimination. Saquinavir is marketed in two formulations, a hard-gelatin (INVIRASE) and a soft-gelatin (FORTOVASE) capsule. Fractional oral bioavailability of the original hard-gelatin capsule was only about 4% owing mainly to extensive first-pass metabolism (Flexner, 1998). The soft-gelatin capsule formulation has threefold greater oral bioavailability, although the hard-gel capsule is used when this drug is combined with ritonavir (Perry and Noble, 1998) (*see* below). The bioavailability of saquinavir is increased up to sixfold with a high-calorie, high-fat meal. Saquinavir has nonlinear pharmacokinetics with increasing dose; for example, tripling the oral dose of saquinavir is associated with an eightfold increase in *AUC*. Substances that inhibit intestinal but not hepatic CYP3A4, such as grapefruit juice, increase the saquinavir *AUC* by threefold at most (Flexner, 2000).

Saquinavir is metabolized primarily by intestinal and hepatic CYP3A4 (Fitzsimmons and Collins, 1997). Its metabolites are not known to be active against HIV-1. Saquinavir and its metabolites are eliminated through the biliary system and feces (>95% of drug), with minimal urinary excretion (<3%). Saquinavir's short half-life requires administration every 8 hours. However, saquinavir metabolism is exquisitely sensitive to inhibition by ritonavir (Table 50–7); thus saquinavir is usefully combined with low doses of ritonavir to allow once- or twice-daily administration. Low doses of ritonavir increase the saquinavir steady-state *AUC* by twenty- to thirtyfold (Flexner, 2000).

Untoward Effects. The most frequent side effects of saquinavir are gastrointestinal and include nausea, vomiting, diarrhea, and abdominal discomfort. Diarrhea and other gastrointestinal side effects may be more prevalent with the soft-gelatin formulation. Most side effects of saquinavir are mild and short-lived, although long-term use is associated with lipodystrophy.

Precautions and Interactions. Of all the HIV protease inhibitors, saquinavir is the least potent inhibitor of CYP3A4. Nonetheless, it is recommended that the drug not be coadministered with ergot derivatives, triazolam, midazolam, or other CYP3A4 substrates with a low therapeutic index. Saquinavir clearance is increased with CYP3A4 induction; thus coadministration of rifampin, nevirapine, or efavirenz lowers saquinavir concentrations and should be avoided (Flexner, 1998). The effect of nevirapine or efavirenz on saquinavir may be partially or completely reversed with ritonavir.

Therapeutic Use. In initial clinical trials, hard-gelatin capsules of saquinavir mesylate at the approved dose (600 mg three times daily) produced only modest virologic effect most likely because of poor oral bioavailability. Greater activity was achieved by increasing the dose fourfold, to 1200 mg six times daily (Schapiro *et al.*, 1996). When combined with ritonavir and nucleoside analogs, saquinavir produces viral load reductions comparable with those of other HIV protease inhibitor regimens (Flexner, 2000).

Ritonavir

Chemistry and Antiviral Activity. Ritonavir is a peptidomimetic HIV protease inhibitor designed to complement the C_2-symmetry of the enzyme active site (Flexner, 1998) (Figure 50–5). Ritonavir is active against both HIV-1 and HIV-2, although it may be slightly less active against the latter. Its IC_{50} for wild-type HIV-1 variants in the absence of human serum ranges from 4 to 150 nM.

Mechanisms of Action and Resistance. Ritonavir reversibly binds to the active site of the HIV protease, preventing polypeptide processing and subsequent virus maturation. Virus particles are produced in the presence of ritonavir but are noninfectious.

In patients treated with ritonavir as the sole protease inhibitor, virus replication in the presence of drug selects for drug-resistance mutations (Molla *et al.*, 1996). The primary ritonavir resistance mutation is usually at protease codon 82 (several possible substitutions for valine) or codon 84 (isoleucine-to-valine substitution). Additional mutations associated with increasing resistance occur at codons 20, 32, 46, 54, 63, 71, 84, and 90. High-level resistance requires accumulation of multiple mutations.

Absorption, Distribution, and Elimination. Absorption of ritonavir is rapid and is only slightly affected by food, depending on the formulation. The overall absorption of ritonavir from the capsule formulation increases by 13% when the capsule is taken with meals, but the bioavailability of the oral solution decreases by 7% (Flexner, 1998). Interindividual variability in pharmacokinetics is high, with a greater than sixfold variability in trough concentrations among patients given 600 mg ritonavir every 12 hours (Hsu *et al.*, 1998).

Ritonavir is metabolized primarily by CYP3A4 and to a lesser extent by CYP2D6. Ritonavir and its metabolites are mainly eliminated in feces (86% of parent drug and metabolites), with only 3% of drug eliminated unchanged in the urine. Ritonavir is 98% to 99% bound to plasma proteins, mainly to α_1-acid glycoprotein. Physiological concentrations of α_1-acid glycoprotein increase the *in vitro* IC_{50} by a factor of 10, whereas albumin increases the IC_{50} by a factor of four (Molla *et al.*, 1998).

Untoward Effects. The major side effects of ritonavir are gastrointestinal and include nausea, vomiting, diarrhea, anorexia, abdominal pain, and taste perversion. These side effects are dose-dependent and are less common with lower doses. Gastrointestinal toxicity may be reduced if the drug is taken with meals. Peripheral and perioral paresthesias also are common. These side effects generally abate within a few weeks of starting therapy.

Ritonavir induces its own metabolism, and gradual dose escalation over the first 2 weeks may minimize early intolerance. When ritonavir is used as the sole protease inhibitor, it should be initiated at 300 mg every 12 hours and escalated gradually to 600 mg every 12 hours by day 14 of therapy. Ritonavir causes dose-dependent elevations in serum total cholesterol and triglycerides, as well as other signs of lipodystrophy, and could increase the long-term risk of atherosclerosis in some patients.

Precautions and Interactions. Ritonavir is one of the most potent known inhibitors of CYP3A4, markedly increasing the plasma concentration and prolonging the elimination of many drugs including amiodarone, propafenone, ergot derivatives, pimozide, triazolam, and midazolam. This drug should be avoided or used with caution in combination with any CYP3A4 substrate, especially those with a narrow therapeutic index (Flexner, 1998). Ritonavir is also a weak inhibitor of CYP2D6. Potent inducers of CYP3A4 activity such as rifampin may lower ritonavir concentrations and should be avoided or dosage adjustments considered. The capsule and solution formulations of ritonavir contain alcohol and should not be administered with *disulfiram* or *metronidazole* (*see* Chapter 22).

Ritonavir is a moderate inducer of CYP3A4, glucuronosyl *S*-transferase, and possibly other hepatic enzymes. The concentrations of some drugs therefore will be decreased in the presence of ritonavir. Ritonavir reduces the ethinyl estradiol *AUC* by 40%, and alternative forms of contraception should be used (Piscitelli and Gallicano, 2001).

Therapeutic Use. Among patients with susceptible strains of HIV-1, ritonavir as a sole agent lowers plasma HIV-1

RNA concentrations by one hundred- to one thousandfold (Ho *et al.*, 1995). In a double-blind, randomized, placebo-controlled trial in 1090 patients with advanced HIV disease, the addition of ritonavir to current therapy reduced HIV-related mortality and disease progression by about 50% over a median of 6 months of follow-up (Cameron *et al.*, 1998). Ritonavir is used infrequently as the sole protease inhibitor in combination regimens because of gastrointestinal toxicity. However, numerous clinical trials have shown efficacy for ritonavir in various dual protease inhibitor combinations (Flexner, 2000).

Use of Ritonavir as a CYP3A4 Inhibitor. Ritonavir inhibits the metabolism of all current HIV protease inhibitors (Table 50–7) and is frequently combined with most of these drugs, with the exception of nelfinavir, to enhance their pharmacokinetic profile and allow a reduction in dose and dosing frequency of the coadministered drug (Flexner, 2000). Ritonavir also overcomes the deleterious effect of food on indinavir bioavailability. Under most circumstances, low doses of ritonavir (100 or 200 mg twice daily) are just as effective at inhibiting CYP3A4 and are much better tolerated than the 600-mg twice-daily treatment dose. The positive impact of low-dose ritonavir on the pharmacokinetics of lopinavir made possible the development and eventual approval of that drug, which is a component of one of two preferred starting regimens recommended by the U.S. Department of Health and Human Services in 2004 (Table 50–2).

Indinavir

Chemistry and Antiviral Activity. Indinavir is a peptidomimetic hydroxyethylene HIV protease inhibitor (Plosker and Noble, 1999). It is formulated as the sulfate salt to yield better solubility and more consistent plasma concentrations as compared with the free base. The molecule was based on a renin inhibitor with some similarity to a phenylalanine–proline cleavage site in the HIV gag polyprotein (Vacca *et al.*, 1994), although indinavir is not itself a renin inhibitor. Indinavir is tenfold more potent against the HIV-1 protease than that of HIV-2, and its 95% inhibitory concentration (IC_{95}) for wild-type HIV-1 ranges from 25 to 100 nM.

Mechanisms of Action and Resistance. Indinavir is selectively toxic by potently inhibiting the HIV-encoded protease but not host-encoded aspartyl proteases. Indinavir reversibly binds to the active site of HIV protease, preventing polypeptide processing and subsequent virus maturation. Virus particles are produced in the presence of indinavir but are noninfectious.

Viral replication in the presence of indinavir selects for drug-resistant virus. The primary indinavir resistance mutations occur at HIV protease codons 46 (a methionine-to-isoleucine or leucine), 82, and 84. However, secondary resistance mutations can accumulate at codons 10, 20, 24, 46, 54, 63, 71, 82, 84, and 90, and these are associated with clinical indinavir resistance as well as cross-resistance to other HIV protease inhibitors (Condra *et al.*, 1995).

Absorption, Distribution, and Elimination. Indinavir is absorbed rapidly after oral administration, with peak concentrations achieved in approximately 1 hour. Unlike other drugs in this class, food can adversely affect indinavir bioavailability; a high-calorie, high-fat meal reduces plasma concentrations by 75% (Plosker and Noble, 1999). Absorption is unaffected by light low-fat meals. Therefore, indinavir must be taken while fasting or with a low-fat meal. Indinavir has the lowest protein binding of the HIV protease inhibitors, with only 60% of drug bound to plasma proteins (Plosker and Noble, 1999). As a consequence, indinavir has higher fractional CSF penetration than other drugs in this class, although the clinical significance of this is unknown.

Indinavir undergoes extensive hepatic metabolism by CYP3A4. Indinavir and its metabolites are eliminated primarily in feces (81% of parent drug and metabolites). Plasma indinavir concentrations may increase with moderate liver disease, and dose reduction may be required. The short half-life of indinavir makes thrice-daily (every 8 hours) dosing necessary. However, indinavir clearance is greatly reduced by low doses of ritonavir, which also overcomes the deleterious effect of food on bioavailability (Flexner, 2000). This allows indinavir to be dosed twice daily regardless of meals.

Untoward Effects. A unique and common adverse effect of indinavir is crystalluria and nephrolithiasis. This stems from the poor solubility of the drug, which is lower at pH 7.4 than at pH 3.5 (Plosker and Noble, 1999). Precipitation of indinavir and its metabolites in urine can cause renal colic, and nephrolithiasis occurs in approximately 3% of patients. Patients must drink sufficient fluids to maintain dilute urine and prevent renal complications. Risk of nephrolithiasis is related to higher plasma drug concentrations, which presumably produce higher urine concentrations, regardless of whether or not the drug is combined with ritonavir (Dieleman *et al.*, 1999).

Indinavir frequently causes unconjugated hyperbilirubinemia, and 10% of patients develop an indirect serum bilirubin concentration of greater than 2.5 mg/dl (Plosker and Noble, 1999). This is generally asymptomatic and is not associated with serious long-term sequelae. As with other HIV protease inhibitors, prolonged administration of indinavir is associated with the HIV lipodystrophy syndrome, especially fat accumulation. Indinavir has been associated with hyperglycemia and can induce a relative state of insulin resistance in healthy HIV-seronegative volunteers following a single 800-mg dose (Noor *et al.*, 2002). Dermatologic complications have been reported, including hair loss, dry skin, dry and cracked lips, and ingrown toenails (Plosker and Noble, 1999). Gastrointestinal side effects are less common with indinavir than with other HIV protease inhibitors.

Precautions and Interactions. Patients taking indinavir should drink at least 2 L of water daily to prevent renal complications. Since indinavir solubility decreases at higher pH, antacids or other buffering agents *should not* be taken at the same time. Didanosine formulations containing an antacid buffer should not be taken within 2 hours before or 1 hour after indinavir. Like most other HIV protease inhibitors, indinavir is metabolized by CYP3A4 and is a moderately potent CYP3A4 inhibitor. Indinavir should not be coadministered with other CYP3A4 substrates that have a narrow therapeutic index.

Indinavir raises rifabutin concentrations and increases rifabutin toxicity; the rifabutin daily dose, therefore, should be reduced by 50% (Hamzeh *et al.*, 2003). Drugs that induce CYP3A4 may lower indinavir concentrations and should be avoided. Rifampin lowers the indinavir *AUC* by 90% and is contraindicated (Flexner, 1998); efavirenz, nevirapine, and rifabutin lower indinavir levels less substantially (by 25% to 35%) and may necessitate an increased indinavir dose (Hamzeh *et al.*, 2003).

Therapeutic Use. Large clinical trials have demonstrated both virologic and survival benefit of indinavir three times daily in combination with zidovudine and lamivudine (Gulick *et al.*, 1997; Hammer *et al.*, 1997). Twice-daily administration of the same total daily dose of indinavir (without ritonavir) was less efficacious (Haas *et al.*, 2000), possibly reflecting inadequate trough concentrations with less frequent dosing. However, when combined with ritonavir and nucleoside analogs, twice-daily indinavir produces viral load reductions comparable with those of other HIV protease inhibitor regimens (Flexner, 2000).

Nelfinavir

Chemistry and Antiviral Activity. Nelfinavir is a nonpeptidic protease inhibitor that is active against both HIV-1 and HIV-2 and is formulated as the mesylate salt of a basic amine (Bardsley-Elliot and Plosker, 2000) (Figure 50–6). The mean IC_{95} for HIV-1 in various *in vitro* assays is 59 nM. Like most drugs in this class, nelfinavir was a product of rational drug design (Roberts *et al.*, 1990).

Mechanisms of Action and Resistance. Nelfinavir reversibly binds to the active site of the HIV protease, preventing polypeptide processing and subsequent virus maturation.

Viral replication in the presence of nelfinavir selects for drug resistance. The primary nelfinavir resistance mutation is unique to this drug and occurs at HIV protease codon 30 (aspartic acid–to–asparagine substitution); this mutation results in a sevenfold decrease in susceptibility. Isolates with only this mutation retain full sensitivity to other HIV protease inhibitors (Bardsley-Elliot and Plosker, 2000). Less commonly, a primary resistance mutation occurs at position 90, which can confer cross-resistance. In addition, secondary resistance mutations can accumulate at codons 35, 36, 46, 71, 77, 88, and 90, and these are associated with further resistance to nelfinavir, as well as cross-resistance to other HIV protease inhibitors.

Absorption, Distribution, and Elimination. Nelfinavir is absorbed more slowly than other HIV-1 protease inhibitors, with peak concentrations achieved in 2 to 4 hours. As a result, drug concentrations continue to fall for 2 to 3 hours after taking the next dose of drug. Nelfinavir absorption is very sensitive to food effects; a moderate-fat meal increases the *AUC* two- to threefold, and higher concentrations are achieved with high-fat meals (Bardsley-Elliot and Plosker, 2000). Intraindividual and interindividual variabilities in plasma nelfinavir concentrations are considerable largely as a consequence of variable absorption. Originally approved at a dose of 750 mg

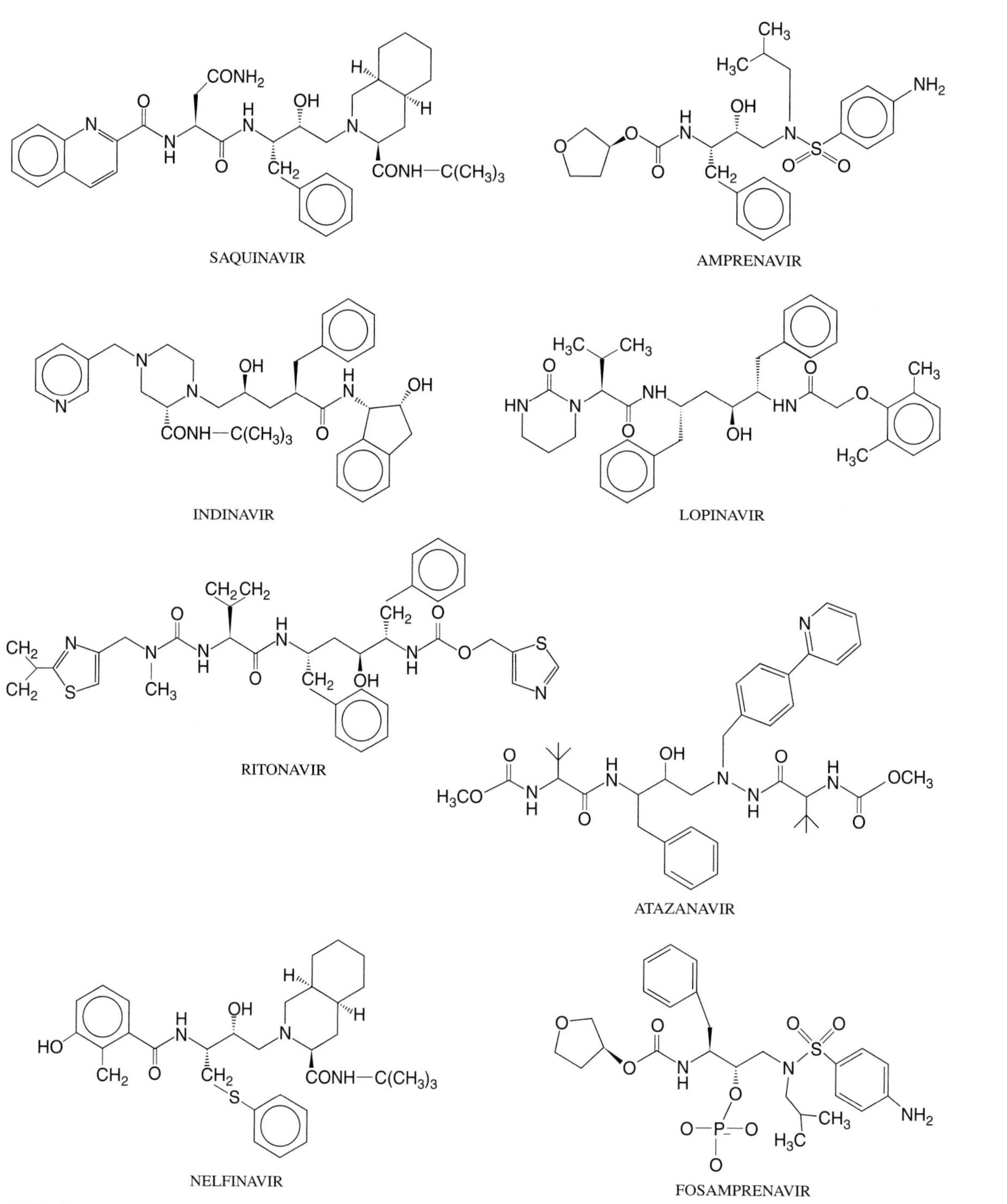

Figure 50-6. *Structure of HIV protease inhibitors.*

three times daily, nelfinavir is now administered at a dose of 1250 mg twice daily using a reduced-volume 625-mg tablet.

Nelfinavir undergoes oxidative metabolism in the liver primarily by CYP2C19 but also by CYP3A4 and CYP2D6. Its major hydroxy-*t*-butylamide metabolite, M8, is formed by CYP2C19 and has *in vitro*

antiretroviral activity similar to that of the parent drug. This is the only known active metabolite of an HIV protease inhibitor. M8 concentrations are 30% to 40% those of parent drug. Nelfinavir and its metabolites are eliminated primarily in feces, with less than 2% of drug excreted unchanged in the urine. Moderate or severe liver disease may prolong the half-life and increase plasma concentrations of the parent drug while lowering plasma concentrations of M8. Nelfinavir induces its own metabolism, and average trough concentrations after 1 week of therapy are approximately one-half those at day 2 of therapy (Bardsley-Elliot and Plosker, 2000).

Nelfinavir is greater than 98% bound to plasma proteins, mostly to albumin and α_1-acid glycoprotein. It is present in CSF at less than 1% of plasma concentrations at least in part owing to its extensive binding to plasma proteins and possibly to export by P-gp at the blood–brain barrier (Aweeka *et al.*, 1999).

Untoward Effects. The most important side effect of nelfinavir is diarrhea or loose stools, which resolve in most patients within the first 4 weeks of therapy. Up to 20% of patients report chronic occasional diarrhea lasting more than 3 months, although fewer than 2% of patients discontinue the drug because of diarrhea. Nelfinavir augments intestinal calcium-dependent chloride channel secretory responses *in vitro*, and electrolyte analysis of stool is most consistent with a secretory diarrhea (Rufo *et al.*, 2004). Otherwise, nelfinavir is generally well tolerated but has been associated with glucose intolerance, elevated cholesterol levels, and elevated triglycerides.

Precautions and Interactions. Because nelfinavir is metabolized by CYP2C19 and CYP3A4, concomitant administration of agents that induce these enzymes may be contraindicated (as with rifampin) or may necessitate an increased nelfinavir dose (as with rifabutin). Nelfinavir is a moderate inhibitor of CYP3A4 and may alter plasma concentrations of other CYP3A4 substrates. Nelfinavir inhibits CYP3A4 less than does ritonavir and does not appear to inhibit other CYP isoforms. Nelfinavir is also an inducer of hepatic drug-metabolizing enzymes, reducing the *AUC* of ethinyl estradiol by 47% and norethindrone by 18% (Flexner, 1998). Combination oral contraceptives therefore should not be used as the sole form of contraception in patients taking nelfinavir. Nelfinavir reduces the zidovudine *AUC* by 35%, suggesting induction of glucuronosyl *S*-transferase.

Therapeutic Use. Nelfinavir is indicated for the treatment of HIV infection in adults and children in combination with other antiretroviral drugs. Large clinical trials have demonstrated both virologic and clinical benefit when patients naive to HIV protease inhibitors and lamivudine received nelfinavir in combination with zidovudine and lamivudine (Bardsley-Elliot and Plosker, 2000). Recent large randomized, comparative trials have found that long-term virologic suppression with nelfinavir-based combination regimens is statistically significantly inferior to those using lopinavir–ritonavir (Cvetkovic and Goa, 2003), atazanavir, or efavirenz. This could reflect the unpredictable nature of nelfinavir absorption. Nelfinavir is well tolerated in pregnant HIV-infected women and shows no evidence of teratogenesis. The drug also has been used in HIV-infected patients with significant hepatic dysfunction without evidence of untoward toxicity despite higher drug concentrations (Khaliq *et al.*, 2000).

Amprenavir and Fosamprenavir

Chemistry and Antiviral Activity. Amprenavir is an *N,N*-disubstituted (hydroxyethyl) amino sulfonamide nonpeptide HIV protease inhibitor (Adkins and Faulds, 1998). Although developed using a sophisticated structure-based drug-design program, the same compound was identified previously using a more traditional high-throughput screen of an available chemical library (Werth, 1994). Amprenavir is the only available HIV protease inhibitor that contains a sulfonamide moiety, which may play a role in its dermatological side effects. The drug is active against both HIV-1 and HIV-2, with an IC_{90} for wild-type HIV-1 of approximately 80 nM.

Fosamprenavir is a phosphonooxy prodrug of amprenavir that has the advantage of greatly increased water solubility and improved oral bioavailability (Ellis *et al.*, 2004). This allows reduction in the pill burden from 16 capsules to 4 tablets per day. The original amprenavir formulation contained D-α-tocopheryl polyethylene glycol, which delivered a high daily dose of vitamin E; this excipient is not required with fosamprenavir. Fosamprenavir is as effective, more convenient, and generally better tolerated than amprenavir, and as a result, amprenavir 150-mg capsules were removed from the market at the end of 2004.

Mechanisms of Action and Resistance. Amprenavir is an active-site inhibitor of HIV protease. Virus replication in the presence of amprenavir selects for drug-resistant virus. Amprenavir's primary resistance mutation occurs at HIV protease codon 50; this isoleucine-to-valine substitution confers only twofold decreased susceptibility *in vitro*. Primary resistance occurs less frequently at codon 84. Secondary resistance mutations occur at codons 10, 32, 46, 47, 54, 73, and 90, which greatly increase resistance and cross-resistance. The same resistance patterns occur with fosamprenavir treatment (Ellis *et al.*, 2004).

Absorption, Distribution, and Elimination. Amprenavir is absorbed rapidly after oral administration. Taking amprenavir with a standard meal reduces the plasma *AUC* by only 13%, and the drug therefore can be administered without regard to food. Fosamprenavir is dephosphorylated rapidly to amprenavir in the intestinal mucosa. The phosphorylated prodrug is approximately 2000 times more water-soluble than amprenavir, allowing a more compact formulation. Meals have no significant effect on fosamprenavir pharmacokinetics (Ellis *et al.*, 2004). Amprenavir is 90% bound to plasma proteins, mostly α_1-acid glycoprotein. This binding is relatively weak, and physiological concentrations of α_1-acid glycoprotein increase the *in vitro* IC_{50} only three- to fivefold.

Amprenavir clearance is mainly by hepatic CYP3A4, and excretion is *via* the biliary route. Amprenavir is a moderate inhibitor and inducer of CYP3A4. Ritonavir increases amprenavir concentrations by inhibiting CYP3A4, allowing lower amprenavir doses. The daily amprenavir dose may be reduced from 1200 to 600 mg twice daily when 100-mg twice-daily ritonavir also is given or to 1200 mg once daily when 200 mg ritonavir also is given once daily (Flexner, 2000). Similar dose reductions are achieved by combining fosamprenavir with ritonavir.

Untoward Effects. The most common adverse effects associated with amprenavir are gastrointestinal and include nausea, vomiting, diarrhea, or loose stools. Hyperglycemia, fatigue, paresthesias, and headache also have been reported. Amprenavir is the HIV protease inhibitor that is most likely to produce skin eruptions; in one study of amprenavir monotherapy, rash occurred in 5 of 35 patients over 24 weeks and began within 7 to 12 days of starting therapy (Adkins and Faulds, 1998). Amprenavir is reported to have fewer effects on plasma lipid profiles compared with ritonavir-based protease inhibitor regimens. Fosamprenavir has a similar toxicity profile, but gastrointestinal side effects are much less frequent than with amprenavir, and rash also may be less frequent (19% *versus* 27%) (Ellis *et al.*, 2004).

Precautions and Interactions. Inducers of hepatic CYP3A4 activity (*e.g.,* rifampin and efavirenz) may lower plasma amprenavir concentrations. Because amprenavir is both a CYP3A4 inhibitor and inducer, metabolic drug interactions can occur and may be unpredictable. For example, atorvastatin, ketoconazole, and rifabutin concentrations increase significantly with amprenavir, whereas delavirdine and methadone concentrations decrease. Fosamprenavir is expected to have a drug-interaction potential similar to that of amprenavir.

Therapeutic Use. Clinical trials have demonstrated long-term virologic benefit in treatment-naive patients receiving amprenavir (1200 mg every 12 hours) in combination with zidovudine and lamivudine (Adkins and Faulds, 1998). Similar results are seen when amprenavir is combined with ritonavir.

One comparative trial found that an amprenavir-based regimen was less effective than an indinavir-based regimen, with HIV RNA values of less than 400 copies/ml in only 30% of the amprenavir-treated patients compared with 49% of the indinavir-treated patients after 48 weeks (Ellis *et al.*, 2004). This may reflect poor adherence to amprenavir owing to high pill burden and side effects. Several large randomized trials have established a better track record for fosamprenavir, showing equivalent or superior long-term viral RNA effects as nelfinavir in treatment-naive patients. However, in one comparative trial in treatment-experienced patients, fosamprenavir combined with ritonavir was marginally inferior to the lopinavir–ritonavir coformulation (Ellis *et al.*, 2004).

Lopinavir

Chemistry and Antiviral Activity. Lopinavir is a peptidomimetic HIV protease inhibitor that is structurally similar to ritonavir (Figure 50–6) but is three- to tenfold more potent against HIV-1 *in vitro*. Lopinavir is active against both HIV-1 and HIV-2; its IC_{50} for wild-type HIV variants

in the presence of 50% human serum ranges from 65 to 290 nM. Lopinavir is available only in coformulation with low doses of ritonavir, which is used to inhibit CYP3A4 metabolism and increase concentrations of lopinavir.

Mechanisms of Action and Resistance. Lopinavir is selectively toxic by potently inhibiting the HIV-encoded protease but not host-encoded aspartyl proteases. Protease-specific resistance mutations are identified with less frequency in patients taking lopinavir than with other HIV protease inhibitors. Treatment-naive patients who fail a first regimen containing lopinavir generally do not have HIV protease mutations but may have genetic resistance to the other drugs in the regimen (Cvetkovic *et al.*, 2003). For treatment-experienced patients, accumulation of four or more HIV protease inhibitor resistance mutations is associated with a reduced likelihood of virus suppression after starting lopinavir (Kuritzkes, 2004). Mutations associated with lopinavir failure in treatment-experienced patients include those at HIV protease codons 10, 20, 24, 32, 33, 36, 46, 47, 50, 53, 54, 63, 71, 73, 82, 84, and 90 (Cvetkovic *et al.*, 2003). There is no evidence that exposure to the low doses of ritonavir in the lopinavir–ritonavir coformulation selects for ritonavir-specific resistance mutations.

Absorption, Distribution, and Elimination. Lopinavir is only available as a coformulation with low doses of ritonavir. When administered orally without ritonavir, lopinavir plasma concentrations were exceedingly low mainly owing to first-pass metabolism. Both the first-pass metabolism and systemic clearance of lopinavir are very sensitive to inhibition by ritonavir. A single 50-mg dose of ritonavir increased the lopinavir *AUC* by 77 times compared with that produced with 400 mg lopinavir alone; 100 mg ritonavir increased the lopinavir *AUC* by 155-fold. Lopinavir trough concentrations were increased fifty to one hundredfold by coadministration of low doses of ritonavir (Cvetkovic *et al.*, 2003). Multiple-dose pharmacokinetic studies have not been conducted with lopinavir in the absence of ritonavir. Adding 100 mg ritonavir twice daily to the lopinavir–ritonavir coformulation (a total of 200 mg twice daily of ritonavir) has only a modest further effect on lopinavir concentrations, increasing the mean steady-state *AUC* by 46%.

Lopinavir is absorbed rapidly after oral administration. A moderate- to high-fat meal increases oral bioavailability by up to 50%, and it is therefore recommended that the drug be taken with food. Although the capsules contain lopinavir–ritonavir in a fixed 4:1 ratio, the observed plasma concentration ratio for these two drugs following oral administration is nearly 20:1, reflecting the sensitivity of lopinavir to the inhibitory effect of ritonavir on CYP3A4. Lopinavir undergoes extensive hepatic oxidative metabolism by CYP3A4. Approximately 90% of total drug in plasma is the parent compound, and less than 3% of a dose is eliminated unchanged in the urine. Both lopinavir and ritonavir are highly bound to plasma proteins, mainly to α_1-acid glycoprotein, and therefore have a low fractional penetration into CSF and semen. Unlike ritonavir, the *in vitro* IC_{50} of lopinavir is not affected by physiological concentrations of albumin (Molla *et al.*, 1998).

Untoward Effects. The most common adverse events reported with the lopinavir–ritonavir coformulation have been gastrointestinal, including loose stools, diarrhea, nausea, and vomiting. These are less frequent and less severe than those reported with the 600-mg twice-daily standard dose of ritonavir. The most common laboratory abnormalities include elevated total cholesterol and triglycerides. Because the same adverse effects occur with ritonavir, it is unclear whether the side effects are due to ritonavir, lopinavir, or both.

Precautions and Interactions. Because lopinavir metabolism is highly dependent on CYP3A4, concomitant administration of agents that induce CYP3A4, such as rifampin, may lower plasma lopinavir concentrations considerably. St. John's wort is a known inducer of CYP3A4, leading to lower concentrations of lopinavir and possible loss of antiviral effectiveness. Coadministration of other antiretrovirals that can induce CYP3A4, including amprenavir, nevirapine or efavirenz, may require increasing the dose of lopinavir (Cvetkovic *et al.*, 2003).

Although lopinavir is a weak inhibitor of CYP3A4 *in vitro*, the ritonavir in the coformulated capsule strongly inhibits CYP3A4 activity and probably dwarfs any lopinavir effect. Ritonavir increases concentrations of a number of drugs with narrow therapeutic indices (*e.g.*, midazolam, triazolam, propafenone, and ergot derivatives), and coadministration of these agents should be avoided. The liquid (but not capsule) formulation of lopinavir contains 42% ethanol and should not be administered with disulfiram or metronidazole (*see* Chapter 22). Ritonavir is also a moderate CYP inducer at the dose employed in the coformulation and can adversely decrease concentrations of some coadministered drugs, *e.g.*, oral contraceptives. There is no direct proof that lopinavir is a CYP inducer *in vivo*; however, concentrations of some coadministered drugs, *e.g.*, amprenavir and phenytoin, are lower with the lopinavir–ritonavir coformulation than would have been expected with low-dose ritonavir alone (Cvetkovic *et al.*, 2003).

Therapeutic Use. In comparative clinical trials, lopinavir has antiretroviral activity at least comparable with that of other potent HIV protease inhibitors and better than that of nelfinavir. A lopinavir-based regimen was one of the two preferred regimens for treatment-naive HIV-infected adults in 2004 (Table 50–2). Lopinavir also has considerable and sustained antiretroviral activity in patients who failed previous HIV protease inhibitor–containing regimens. In one study, 70 subjects who had failed therapy with one previous HIV protease inhibitor were treated for 2 weeks with lopinavir, followed by the addition of nevirapine. At 48 weeks, 60% of subjects had plasma HIV-1 RNA levels of less than 50 copies/ml despite substantial phenotypic resistance to other HIV protease inhibitors (Cvetkovic *et al.*, 2003). Because plasma concentrations of lopinavir generally are much higher than those required to suppress HIV replication *in vitro*, the drug may be capable of suppressing HIV isolates with low-level protease inhibitor resistance.

Atazanavir

Chemistry and Antiviral Activity. Atazanavir is an aza-peptide protease inhibitor with a C_2-symmetric chemical structure that is active against both HIV-1 and HIV-2 (Goldsmith and Perry, 2003) (Figure 50–6). The IC_{50} for

HIV-1 in various *in vitro* assays ranges from 2 to 15 nM. In the presence of 40% human serum, the *in vitro* IC_{50} is increased three- to fourfold (Goldsmith and Perry, 2003). Like most drugs in this class, atazanavir was a product of rational drug design based on the X-ray crystal structure of a peptide–enzyme complex (Roberts *et al.*, 1990).

Mechanisms of Action and Resistance. Atazanavir reversibly binds to the active site of HIV protease, preventing polypeptide processing and subsequent virus maturation. Viral replication in the presence of atazanavir selects for drug resistance. The primary atazanavir resistance mutation occurs at HIV protease codon 50 and confers approximately ninefold decreased susceptibility. This is an isoleucine-to-leucine substitution (I50L) that is distinct from the isoleucine-to-valine substitution selected by amprenavir. This mutation was present in 100% of viruses isolated from patients failing therapy in one clinical trial (Goldsmith and Perry, 2003). Isolates with only this mutation are still susceptible to inhibition by other protease inhibitors. Sensitivity to atazanavir is affected by various primary and secondary mutations that accumulate in patients who have failed other HIV protease inhibitors, with high-level resistance more likely if five or more additional mutations are present (Colonno *et al.*, 2003).

Absorption, Distribution, and Elimination. Atazanavir is absorbed rapidly after oral administration, with peak concentrations occurring about 2 hours after dosing. Atazanavir absorption is sensitive to food: A light meal increases the *AUC* by 70%, whereas a high-fat meal increases the *AUC* by 35% (Goldsmith and Perry, 2003). It is therefore recommended that the drug be administered with food, which also decreases the interindividual variability in pharmacokinetics. Absorption may be pH-dependent because proton pump inhibitors substantially reduce atazanavir concentrations after oral dosing.

Atazanavir undergoes oxidative metabolism in the liver primarily by CYP3A4, which accounts for most of the elimination of this drug. Only 7% of the parent drug is excreted unchanged in the urine. The mean elimination half-life of atazanavir at the standard 400-mg once-daily dose is approximately 7 hours; however, the drug has nonlinear pharmacokinetics, and the half-life increases to nearly 10 hours at a dose of 600 mg (Goldsmith and Perry, 2003). Atazanavir is 86% bound to plasma proteins, both to albumin and α_1-acid glycoprotein. It is present in CSF at less than 3% of plasma concentrations but has excellent penetration into seminal fluid (Goldsmith and Perry, 2003).

Untoward Effects. Like indinavir, atazanavir frequently causes unconjugated hyperbilirubinemia, although this is mainly a cosmetic side effect and is not associated with other hepatotoxicity. Approximately 40% of subjects receiving 400 mg atazanavir once daily in initial clinical trials developed a significant increase in total bilirubin (Goldsmith and Perry, 2003), although only 5% developed jaundice. Other side effects reported with atazanavir include diarrhea and nausea, mainly during the first few weeks of therapy. Overall, 6% of patients discontinued atazanavir because of side effects during 48 weeks of treatment. Patients treated with atazanavir in randomized clinical trials had significantly lower fasting triglyceride and cholesterol concentrations than patients treated with nelfinavir or efavirenz (Goldsmith and Perry, 2003), suggesting a reduced propensity to cause these side effects. In addition, atazanavir is not known to cause glucose intolerance or changes in insulin sensitivity.

Precautions and Interactions. Because atazanavir is metabolized by CYP3A4, concomitant administration of agents that induce this enzyme (*e.g.,* rifampin) is contraindicated. Efavirenz 600 mg once daily reduced the atazanavir *AUC* by 74%. Atazanavir is a moderate inhibitor of CYP3A4 and may alter plasma concentrations of other CYP3A4 substrates. Atazanavir inhibits CYP3A4 less than does ritonavir and does not appear to inhibit other CYP isoforms. Atazanavir is not known to induce hepatic drug-metabolizing enzymes.

Ritonavir significantly increases the atazanavir *AUC* and reduces atazanavir systemic clearance. Ritonavir 100 mg once daily increases the atazanavir 300-mg once-daily steady-state *AUC* by 2.5 times and increases the C_{min} 6.5 times (Goldsmith and Perry, 2003). Low-dose ritonavir also counters the effect of efavirenz on the atazanavir *AUC;* the *AUC* of atazanavir 300 mg with ritonavir 100 mg and efavirenz 600 mg is 30% higher than the *AUC* of atazanavir 400 mg alone.

Proton pump inhibitors reduce atazanavir concentrations substantially with concomitant administration. These drugs and H_2 blockers should be avoided in patients receiving atazanavir.

Therapeutic Use. In randomized clinical trials in treatment-naive patients, virologic and CD4 effects of atazanavir were similar to those of nelfinavir (Goldsmith and Perry, 2003) and, in one study, similar to those of efavirenz plus nucleoside analogs (Squires *et al.,* 2004). However, in treatment-experienced patients, atazanavir 400 mg once daily without ritonavir was inferior to the lopinavir–ritonavir coformulation given twice daily; 81% of lopinavir–ritonavir–treated patients had plasma HIV RNA concentrations less than 400 copies/ml at week 24 compared with 61% of atazanavir-treated patients. The combination of atazanavir and low-dose ritonavir had a similar viral-load effect as the lopinavir–ritonavir coformulation in one study (Goldsmith and Perry, 2003), suggesting that this drug should be combined with ritonavir in treatment-experienced patients—and perhaps in treatment-naive patients with high baseline viral load—in order to take advantage of the enhanced pharmacokinetic profile.

ENTRY INHIBITORS

Enfuvirtide is the only available HIV entry inhibitor, although there are a number of investigational drugs in this class. Enfuvirtide is a large, synthetic HIV-derived peptide that was investigated originally as a possible vaccine component in part because of a high degree of sequence conservation among HIV-1 strains. This peptide turned out to have potent anti-HIV activity *in vitro,* a property eventually attributed to selective inhibition of HIV-mediated membrane fusion (Jiang *et al.,* 1993; Wild *et al.,* 1994). Enfuvirtide is expensive to manufacture and must be administered by subcutaneous injection twice daily. Thus cost and route of administration may limit its

use. In contrast, most investigational entry inhibitors are orally available small molecules.

Enfuvirtide

Chemistry and Antiviral Activity. Enfuvirtide is a 36-amino-acid synthetic peptide whose sequence is derived from a part of the transmembrane gp41 region of HIV-1 that is involved in fusion of the virus membrane lipid bilayer with that of the host cell. Enfuvirtide is not active against HIV-2 but has a broad range of potencies against HIV-1 laboratory and clinical isolates. The reported *in vitro* IC_{50} ranges from 0.1 nM to 1.7 μM depending on the HIV-1 strain and testing method employed (Dando and Perry, 2003).

Mechanisms of Action and Resistance. Enfuvirtide has a unique mechanism of antiretroviral action. The peptide blocks the interaction between the N36 and C34 sequences of the gp41 glycoprotein by binding to a hydrophobic groove in the N36 coil (Sodroski, 1999). This prevents formation of a six-helix bundle critical for membrane fusion and viral entry into the host cell. Enfuvirtide inhibits infection of CD4+ cells by free virus particles, as well as cell-to-cell transmission of HIV *in vitro.* Enfuvirtide retains activity against viruses that have become resistant to antiretroviral agents of other classes because of its unique mechanism of action.

HIV can develop resistance to this drug through specific mutations in the enfuvirtide-binding domain of gp41 (Rimsky *et al.,* 1998). Of the patients experiencing virologic failure during enfuvirtide treatment, 94% had mutations in the gp41 region associated with enfuvirtide resistance *in vitro.* The most common mutations involve a V38A or N43D substitution. Single-amino-acid substitutions can confer up to 450 times resistance *in vitro,* although high-level clinical resistance is usually associated with two or more amino acid changes (Dando and Perry, 2003).

Absorption, Distribution, and Elimination. Enfuvirtide is the only approved antiretroviral drug that must be administered parenterally. The bioavailability of subcutaneous enfuvirtide is 84% compared with an intravenous dose (Dando and Perry, 2003). Peak concentrations after subcutaneous administration occur on average 4 hours after dosing, with an average apparent volume of distribution of 5.5 L. Pharmacokinetics of the subcutaneous drug are not affected by site of injection.

A deamidated metabolite at the C-terminal phenylalanine is present in humans with an *AUC* that is 2% to 15% that of the parent drug (Dando and Perry, 2003), and no other significant metabolites are detected. The major route of elimination for enfuvirtide has not been determined. The mean elimination half-life of parenteral drug is 3.8 hours, necessitating twice-daily administration. Enfuvirtide is 98% bound to plasma proteins, mainly albumin.

Untoward Effects. The most prominent adverse effects of enfuvirtide are injection-site reactions. In 98% of patients, one or more local side effects including pain, erythema, and induration at the site of injection are seen; 80% of patients develop nodules or cysts (Dando and Perry, 2003). Between 4% and 5% of patients discontinue treatment because of local reactions. Use of enfuvirtide has been associated with a higher incidence of lymphadenopathy and pneumonia in at least one study. Whether these are direct drug effects, a secondary consequence of drug-related immune dysfunction, or effects from another mechanism is currently the subject of investigation. Enfuvirtide suppresses interleukin 12 production *in vitro* by more than 90% at concentrations equal to or less than those required to inhibit HIV replication (Braun *et al.*, 2001), although the role this might play in clinical immunosuppression is unclear.

Precautions and Interactions. Enfuvirtide is not metabolized to a significant extent (*see* above) and is not known to alter the concentrations of any coadministered drugs. Ritonavir, rifampin, or ritonavir plus saquinavir did not alter enfuvirtide concentrations (Dando and Perry, 2003).

Therapeutic Use. Enfuvirtide is approved by the FDA for use only in treatment-experienced adults who have evidence of HIV replication despite ongoing antiretroviral therapy. In phase III clinical trials involving heavily pre-treated patients with documented multidrug-resistant HIV-1, the administration of enfuvirtide (90 mg subcutaneously twice daily) in combination with an optimized background regimen was associated with undetectable (<50 copies/ml) plasma HIV-1 RNA concentrations after 24 weeks of treatment in twice as many patients as those who used the optimized background regimen alone (12.2% to 19.6% *versus* 5.3% to 7.3%) (Lalezari *et al.*, 2003; Lazzarin *et al.*, 2003). Treatment response appears to be much more likely in patients with at least two other active drugs in the regimen, based on history and HIV genotype. Given the cost, inconvenience, and cutaneous toxicity of this drug, enfuvirtide generally is reserved for patients who have failed all other feasible antiretroviral regimens.

CURRENT TREATMENT GUIDELINES; CLINICAL SUMMARY

Several expert panels issue periodic recommendations for best combinations of antiretroviral drugs for treatment-naive and treatment-experienced patients. In the United States, the Panel on Clinical Practices for Treatment of HIV Infection convened by the Department of Health and Human Services (DHHS) issues updated guidelines approximately every 6 months. The October 2004 DHHS guidelines for initiating therapy in treatment-naive HIV-infected patients are summarized in Table 50–2. These recommendations are based on a consensus assessment of the results of published clinical trials regarding when to initiate treatment, when to change treatment regimens, and which regimens perform best in terms of antiviral efficacy, safety, and tolerability.

Practitioners need to be aware that guidelines are intended to provide general guidance rather than absolute recommendations for an average uncomplicated patient and may

Table 50–8
New Classes of Antiretroviral Agents in Clinical Development

DRUG CLASS	EXAMPLES
Entry inhibitors	
Attachment inhibitors	BMS-488043, PRO-542, TNX-355
Chemokine receptor antagonists	
CCR5 antagonists	AK-602, AMD-887, GSK-873140, PRO-140, SCH-417690, TAK-220, UK-427,857
CXCR4 antagonists	AMD-3100, AMD-070, KRH-2731
Integrase inhibitors	L-870810
Inhibitors of gag processing	PA-457
Regulatory protein antagonists	
Vif inhibitors	Mifepristone
Immune modifiers	
Therapeutic HIV vaccines	MRK Ad5 gag (replication-deficient adenovirus vector)

need to be modified based on intercurrent disease, concurrent medications, and other circumstances. U.S. guidelines sometimes are contradicted by guidelines designed for use in other countries or specific patient populations; these differences may reflect the different priorities given to drug costs and the importance of long-term toxicities.

Current treatment guidelines center around two important questions: when to start therapy in treatment-naive individuals and when to change therapy in individuals who are failing their current regimen. In each of these settings, there is a complex algorithm of possible drug choices depending on patient and virus demographics. The specific drugs recommended may change from year to year as new choices become available (Table 50–8) and clinical research data accumulate. However, *it is likely that future treatment guidelines will continue to be driven by the important principles mentioned earlier: (1) combination therapy in order to prevent the emergence of resistant virus; (2) emphasis on regimen convenience, tolerability, and adherence in order to chronically suppress HIV replication; and (3) the need for life-long treatment under most circumstances.*

Treatment guidelines are not sufficient to dictate all aspects of patient management. It is therefore imperative that prescribers of antiretroviral therapy maintain a comprehensive and current fund of knowledge regarding this disease and its pharmacotherapy. Because the treatment of HIV infection is a long-lived and complex affair, and because mistakes can have dire and irreversible consequences for the patient, the use of these drugs should be limited to those with specialized training.

BIBLIOGRAPHY

Altice, F.L., Friedland, G.H., and Cooney, E.L. Nevirapine induced opiate withdrawal among injection drug users with HIV infection receiving methadone. *AIDS,* **1999,** *13*:957–962.

Arnaudo, E., Dalakas, M., Shanske, S., *et al.* Depletion of muscle mitochondrial DNA in AIDS patients with zidovudine-induced myopathy. *Lancet,* **1991,** *337*:508–510.

Aweeka, F., Jayewardene, A., Staprans, S., *et al.* Failure to detect nelfinavir in the cerebrospinal fluid of HIV-1-infected patients with and without AIDS dementia complex. *J. Acquir. Immune Defic. Syndr. Hum. Retrovirol.,* **1999,** *20*:39–43.

Braun, M.C., Wang, J.M., Lahey, E., *et al.* Activation of the formyl peptide receptor by the HIV-derived peptide T-20 suppresses interleukin-12 p70 production by human monocytes. *Blood,* **2001,** *97*:3531–3536.

Cameron, D.W., Heath-Chiozzi, M., Danner, S., *et al.* Randomised, placebo-controlled trial of ritonavir in advanced HIV-1 disease. The Advanced HIV Disease Ritonavir Study Group. *Lancet,* **1998,** *351*:543–549.

Cardo, D.M., Culver, D.H., Ciesielski, C.A., *et al.* A case-control study of HIV seroconversion in health care workers after percutaneous exposure. Centers for Disease Control and Prevention Needlestick Surveillance Group. *New Engl. J. Med.,* **1997,** *337*:1485–1490.

Chen, C.H., Vazquez-Padua, M., and Cheng, Y.C. Effect of anti–human immunodeficiency virus nucleoside analogs on mitochondrial DNA and its implication for delayed toxicity. *Mol. Pharmacol.,* **1991,** *39*:625–628.

Chun, T.W., Engel, D., Berrey, M.M., *et al.* Early establishment of a pool of latently infected, resting CD4(+) T cells during primary HIV-1 infection. *Proc. Natl. Acad. Sci. U.S.A.,* **1998,** *95*:8869–8873.

Coffin, J.M. HIV population dynamics *in vivo*: Implications for genetic variation, pathogenesis, and therapy. *Science,* **1995,** *267*:483–489.

Collier, A.C., Coombs, R.W., Schoenfeld, D.A., *et al.* Treatment of human immunodeficiency virus infection with saquinavir, zidovudine, and zalcitabine. AIDS Clinical Trials Group. *New Engl. J. Med.,* **1996,** *334*:1011–1017.

Colonno, R.J., Thiry, A., Limoli, K., and Parkin, N. Activities of atazanavir (BMS-232632) against a large panel of human immunodeficiency virus type 1 clinical isolates resistant to one or more approved protease inhibitors. *Antimicrob. Agents Chemother.,* **2003,** *47*:1324–1333.

Concorde Coordinating Committee. Concorde: MRC/ANRS randomized, double-blind, controlled trial of immediate and deferred zidovudine in symptom-free HIV infection. *Lancet,* **1994,** *343*:871–881.

Condra, J.H., Schleif, W.A., Blahy, O.M., *et al. In vivo* emergence of HIV-1 variants resistant to multiple protease inhibitors. *Nature,* **1995,** *374*:569–571.

Connor, E.M., Sperling, R.S., Gelber, R., *et al.* Reduction of maternal–infant transmission of human immunodeficiency virus type 1 with zidovudine treatment. Pediatric AIDS Clinical Trials Group Protocol 076 Study Group. *New Engl. J. Med.,* **1994,** *331*:1173–1180.

Cui, L., Locatelli, L., Xie, M.Y., and Sommadossi, J.P. Effect of nucleoside analogs on neurite regeneration and mitochondrial DNA synthesis in PC-12 cells. *J. Pharmacol. Exp. Ther.,* **1997,** *280*:1228–1234.

Dancis, J., Lee, J.D., Mendoza, S., and Liebes, L. Transfer and metabolism of dideoxyinosine by the perfused human placenta. *J. Acquir. Immune Defic. Syndr.,* **1993,** *6*:2–6.

De Clercq, E. Clinical potential of the acyclic nucleoside phosphonates cidofovir, adefovir, and tenofovir in treatment of DNA virus and retrovirus infections. *Clin. Microbiol. Rev.,* **2003,** *16*:569–596.

Dieleman, J.P., Gyssens, I.C., van der Ende, M.E., *et al.* Urological complaints in relation to indinavir plasma concentrations in HIV-infected patients. *AIDS,* **1999,** *13*:473–478.

Dieterich, D.T., Robinson, P.A., Love, J., and Stern, J.O. Drug-induced liver injury associated with the use of nonnucleoside reverse-transcriptase inhibitors. *Clin. Infect. Dis.,* **2004,** *38*:S80–89.

Dolin, R., Amato, D.A., Fischl, M.A., *et al.* Zidovudine compared with didanosine in patients with advanced HIV type 1 infection and little or no previous experience with zidovudine. AIDS Clinical Trials Group. *Arch. Intern. Med.,* **1995,** *155*:961–974.

Eron, J.J., Benoit, S.L., Jemsek, J., *et al.* Treatment with lamivudine, zidovudine, or both in HIV-positive patients with 200 to 500 CD4+ cells per cubic millimeter. North American HIV Working Party. *New Engl. J. Med.,* **1995,** *333*:1662–1669.

Eshleman, S.H., Guay, L.A., Mwatha, A., *et al.* Comparison of nevirapine (NVP) resistance in Ugandan women 7 days vs. 6–8 weeks after single-dose NVP prophylaxis: HIVNET 012. *AIDS Res. Hum. Retroviruses,* **2004,** *20*:595–599.

Falloon, J., Piscitelli, S., Vogel, S., *et al.* Combination therapy with amprenavir, abacavir, and efavirenz in human immunodeficiency virus (HIV)–infected patients failing a protease-inhibitor regimen: Pharmacokinetic drug interactions and antiviral activity. *Clin. Infect. Dis.,* **2000,** *30*:313–318.

Fichtenbaum, C.J., Clifford, D.B., and Powderly, W.G. Risk factors for dideoxynucleoside-induced toxic neuropathy in patients with the human immunodeficiency virus infection. *J. Acquir. Immune Defic. Syndr. Hum. Retrovirol.,* **1995,** *10*:169–174.

Finzi, D., Hermankova, M., Pierson, T., *et al.* Identification of a reservoir for HIV-1 in patients on highly active antiretroviral therapy. *Science,* **1997,** *278*:1295–1300.

Fischl, M.A., Richman, D.D., Grieco, M.H., *et al.* The efficacy of azidothymidine (AZT) in the treatment of patients with AIDS and AIDS-related complex: A double-blind, placebo-controlled trial. *New Engl. J. Med.,* **1987,** *317*:185–191.

Fischl, M.A., Stanley, K., Collier, A.C., *et al.* Combination and monotherapy with zidovudine and zalcitabine in patients with advanced HIV disease. The NIAID AIDS Clinical Trials Group. *Ann. Intern. Med.,* **1995,** *122*:24–32.

Fisher, A.G., Collalti, E., Ratner, L., *et al.* A molecular clone of HTLV-III with biological activity. *Nature,* **1985,** *316*:262–265.

Fitzsimmons, M.E., and Collins, J.M. Selective biotransformation of the human immunodeficiency virus protease inhibitor saquinavir by human small-intestinal cytochrome P4503A4: Potential contribution to high first-pass metabolism. *Drug Metab. Dispos.,* **1997,** *25*:256–266.

Frank, I., Bosch, R.J., Fiscus, S., *et al.,* for the ACTG 307 Protocol Team. Activity, safety, and immunologic effects of hydroxyurea added to didanosine in antiretroviral naïve and experienced HIV-1 infected subjects: A randomized, placebo-controlled trial, ACTG 307. *AIDS Res. Hum. Retroviruses,* **2004,** *20*:916–926.

Friedland, G.H., Pollard, R., Griffith, B., *et al.* Efficacy and safety of delavirdine mesylate with zidovudine and didanosine compared with two-drug combinations of these agents in persons with HIV disease with CD4 counts of 100 to 500 cells/mm^3 (ACTG 261). ACTG 261 Team. *J. Acquir. Immune Defic. Syndr.,* **1999,** *21*:281–292.

Furman, P.A., Fyfe, J.A., St. Clair, M.H., *et al.* Phosphorylation of 3'-azido-3'-deoxythymidine and selective interaction of the 5'-triphosphate with human immunodeficiency virus reverse transcriptase. *Proc. Natl. Acad. Sci. U.S.A.,* **1986,** *83*:8333–8337.

Gallant, J.E., Staszewski, S., Pozniak, A.L., *et al.,* for the 903 Study Group. Efficacy and safety of tenofovir DF vs stavudine in combination therapy in antiretroviral-naive patients: A 3-year randomized trial. *JAMA,* **2004,** *292*:191–201.

Gao, W.Y., Shirasaka, T., Johns, D.G., *et al.* Differential phosphorylation of azidothymidine, dideoxycytidine, and dideoxyinosine in resting and activated peripheral blood mononuclear cells. *J. Clin. Invest.,* **1993,** *91*:2326–2333.

Gao, W.Y., Agbaria, R., Driscoll, J.S., and Mitsuya, H. Divergent anti-human immunodeficiency virus activity and anabolic phosphorylation of 2',3'-dideoxynucleoside analogs in resting and activated human cells. *J. Biol. Chem.,* **1994,** *269*:12633–12638.

Geleziunas, R., Arts, E.J., Boulerice, F., *et al.* Effect of 3'-azido-3'-deoxythymidine on human immunodeficiency virus type 1 replication in human fetal brain macrophages. *Antimicrob. Agents Chemother.,* **1993,** *37*:1305–1312.

Gillet, J.Y., Garraffo, R., Abrar, D., *et al.* Fetoplacental passage of zidovudine. *Lancet,* 1989, *2*:269–270.

Guay, L.A., Musoke, P., Fleming, T., *et al.* Intrapartum and neonatal single-dose nevirapine compared with zidovudine for prevention of mother-to-child transmission of HIV-1 in Kampala, Uganda: HIVNET 012 randomised trial. *Lancet,* **1999,** *354*:795–802.

Gulick, R.M., Mellors, J.W., Havlir, D., *et al.* Treatment with indinavir, zidovudine, and lamivudine in adults with human immunodeficiency virus infection and prior antiretroviral therapy. *New Engl. J. Med.,* **1997,** *337*:734–739.

Gulick, R.M., Ribaudo, H.J., Shikuma, C.M., *et al.,* for the AIDS Clinical Trials Group Study A5095 Team. Triple-nucleoside regimens versus efavirenz-containing regimens for the initial treatment of HIV-1 infection. *New Engl. J. Med.,* **2004,** *350*:1850–1861.

Haas, D.W., Arathoon, E., Thompson, M.A., *et al.,* for the Protocol 054/069 Study Teams. Comparative studies of two-times-daily versus three-times-daily indinavir in combination with zidovudine and lamivudine. *AIDS,* **2000,** *14*:1973–1978.

Hamilton, J.D., Hartigan, P.M., Simberkoff, M.S., *et al.* A controlled trial of early versus late treatment with zidovudine in symptomatic human immunodeficiency virus infection: Results of the Veterans Affairs Cooperative Study. *New Engl. J. Med.,* **1992,** *326*:437–443.

Hammer, S.M., Katzenstein, D.A., Hughes, M.D., *et al.* A trial comparing nucleoside monotherapy with combination therapy in HIV-infected adults with CD4 cell counts from 200 to 500 per cubic millimeter. AIDS Clinical Trials Group Study 175 Study Team. *New Engl. J. Med.,* **1996,** *335*:1081–1090.

Hammer, S.M., Squires, K.E., Hughes, M.D., *et al.* A controlled trial of two nucleoside analogues plus indinavir in persons with human immunodeficiency virus infection and CD4 cell counts of 200 per cubic millimeter or less. AIDS Clinical Trials Group 320 Study Team. *New Engl. J. Med.,* **1997,** *337*:725–733.

Hamzeh, F.M., Benson, C., Gerber, J., *et al.,* for the AIDS Clinical Trials Group 365 Study Team. Steady-state pharmacokinetic interaction of modified-dose indinavir and rifabutin. *Clin. Pharmacol. Ther.,* **2003,** *73*:159–169.2

Havlir, D., McLaughlin, M.M., and Richman, D.D. A pilot study to evaluate the development of resistance to nevirapine in asymptomatic human immunodeficiency virus-infected patients with CD4 cell counts of >500/mm^3: AIDS Clinical Trials Group Protocol 208. *J. Infect. Dis.,* **1995,** *172*:1379–1383.

Havlir, D.V., Tierney, C., Friedland, G.H., *et al. In vivo* antagonism with zidovudine plus stavudine combination therapy. *J. Infect. Dis.,* **2000,** *182*:321–325.

Havlir, D.V., Gilbert, P.B., Bennett, K., *et al.,* for the ACTG 5025 Study Group. Effects of treatment intensification with hydroxyurea in HIV-infected patients with virologic suppression. *AIDS,* **2001,** *15*:1379–1388.

Heath, K.V., Hogg, R.S., Chan, K.J., *et al.* Lipodystrophy-associated morphological, cholesterol and triglyceride abnormalities in a population-based HIV/AIDS treatment database. *AIDS,* **2001,** *15*:231–239.

Hetherington, S., Hughes, A.R., Mosteller, M., *et al.* Genetic variations in HLA-B region and hypersensitivity reactions to abacavir. *Lancet,* **2002,** *359*:1121–1122.

HIV Neuromuscular Syndrome Study Group. HIV-associated neuromuscular weakness syndrome. *AIDS,* **2004,** *18*:1403–1412.

Ho, D.D., Neumann, A.U., Perelson, A.S., *et al.* Rapid turnover of plasma virions and CD4 lymphocytes in HIV-1 infection. *Nature,* **1995,** *373*:123–126.

Ives, K.J., Jacobsen, H., Galpin, S.A., *et al.* Emergence of resistant variants of HIV in *vivo* during monotherapy with the proteinase inhibitor saquinavir. *J. Antimicrob. Chemother.,* **1997,** *39*:771–779.

Jiang, S., Lin, K., Strick, N., and Neurath, A.R. HIV-1 inhibition by a peptide. *Nature,* **1993,** *365*:113.

Khaliq, Y., Gallicano, K., Seguin, I., *et al.* Single- and multiple-dose pharmacokinetics of nelfinavir and CYP2C19 activity in human immunodeficiency virus–infected patients with chronic liver disease. *Br. J. Clin. Pharmacol.,* **2000,** *50*:108–115.

Kieffer, T.L., Finucane, M.M., Nettles, R.E., *et al.* Genotypic analysis of HIV-1 drug resistance at the limit of detection: Virus production without evolution in treated adults with undetectable HIV loads. *J. Infect. Dis.,* **2004,** *189*:1452–1465.

Kim, R.B., Fromm, M.F., Wandel, C., *et al.* The drug transporter P-glycoprotein limits oral absorption and brain entry of HIV-1 protease inhibitors. *J. Clin. Invest.,* **1998,** *101*:289–294.

Kuritzkes, D.R., Marschner, I., Johnson, V.A., *et al.* Lamivudine in combination with zidovudine, stavudine, or didanosine in patients with HIV-1 infection: A randomized, double-blind, placebo-controlled trial. National Institute of Allergy and Infectious Disease AIDS Clinical Trials Group Protocol 306 Investigators. *AIDS,* **1999,** *13*:685–694.

Lalezari, J.P., Henry, K., O'Hearn, M., *et al.* Enfuvirtide, an HIV-1 fusion inhibitor, for drug-resistant HIV infection in North and South America. *New Engl. J. Med.,* **2003,** *348*:2175–2185.

Larder, B.A., Kemp, S.D., and Harrigan, P.R. Potential mechanism for sustained antiretroviral efficacy of AZT-3TC combination therapy. *Science,* **1995,** *269*:696–699.

Lawrence, J., Mayers, D.L., Hullsiek, K.H., *et al.,* for the 064 Study Team of the Terry Beirn Community Programs for Clinical Research on AIDS. Structured treatment interruption in patients with multi-drug-resistant human immunodeficiency virus. *New Engl. J. Med.,* **2003,** *349*:837–846.

Lazzarin, A., Clotet, B., Cooper, D., *et al.* Efficacy of enfuvirtide in patients infected with drug-resistant HIV-1 in Europe and Australia. *New Engl. J. Med.,* **2003,** *348*:2186–2195.

Lee, L.M., Karon, J.M., Selik, R., *et al.* Survival after AIDS diagnosis in adolescents and adults during the treatment era, United States, 1984–1997. *JAMA,* **2001,** *285:*1308–1315.

Lee, H., Hanes, J., and Johnson, K.A. Toxicity of nucleoside analogues used to treat AIDS and the selectivity of the mitochondrial DNA polymerase. *Biochemistry,* **2003,** *42:*14711–14719.

Leung, N.W., Lai, C.L., Chang, T.T., *et al.,* on behalf of the Asia Hepatitis Lamivudine Study Group. Extended lamivudine treatment in patients with chronic hepatitis B enhances hepatitis B e antigen seroconversion rates: Results after 3 years of therapy. *Hepatology,* **2001,** *33:*1527–1532.

Lucas, G.M., Chaisson, R.E., and Moore, R.D. Highly active antiretroviral therapy in a large urban clinic: Risk factors for virologic failure and adverse drug reactions. *Ann. Intern. Med.,* **1999,** *131:*81–87.

Luzuriaga, K., Bryson, Y., Krogstad, P., *et al.* Combination treatment with zidovudine, didanosine, and nevirapine in infants with human immunodeficiency virus type 1 infection. *New Engl. J. Med.,* **1997,** *336:*1343–1349.

Mallal, S.A., John, M., Moore, C.B., *et al.* Contribution of nucleoside analogue reverse transcriptase inhibitors to subcutaneous fat wasting in patients with HIV infection. *AIDS,* **2000,** *14:*1309–1316.

Martin, A.M., Nolan, D., Gaudieri, S., *et al.* Predisposition to abacavir hypersensitivity conferred by HLA-B*5701 and a haplotypic Hsp70-Hom variant. *Proc. Natl. Acad. Sci. U.S.A.,* **2004,** *101:*4180–4185.

McDowell, J.A., Chittick, G.E., Stevens, C.P., *et al.* Pharmacokinetic interaction of abacavir (1592U89) and ethanol in human immunodeficiency virus–infected adults. *Antimicrob. Agents Chemother.,* **2000,** *44:*1686–1690.

Mellors, J.W., Munoz, A., Giorgi, J.V., *et al.* Plasma viral load and CD4+ lymphocytes as prognostic markers of HIV-1 infection. *Ann. Intern. Med.,* **1997,** *126:*946–954.

Mellors, J.W., Rinaldo, C.R., Jr., Gupta, P., *et al.* Prognosis in HIV-1 infection predicted by the quantity of virus in plasma. *Science,* **1996,** *272:*1167–1170.

Merrill, D.P., Moonis, M., Chou, T.C., and Hirsch, M.S. Lamivudine or stavudine in two- and three-drug combinations against human immunodeficiency virus type 1 replication *in vitro. J. Infect. Dis.,* **1996,** *173:*355–364.

Miller, M.D., Anton, K.E., Mulato, A.S., *et al.* Human immunodeficiency virus type 1 expressing the lamivudine-associated M184V mutation in reverse transcriptase shows increased susceptibility to adefovir and decreased replication capability *in vitro. J. Infect. Dis.,* **1999,** *179:*92–100.

Mirochnick, M., Fenton, T., Gagnier, P., *et al.* Pharmacokinetics of nevirapine in human immunodeficiency virus type 1–infected pregnant women and their neonates. Pediatric AIDS Clinical Trials Group Protocol 250 Team. *J. Infect. Dis.,* **1998,** *178:*368–374.

Mitsuya, H., Weinhold, K.J., Furman, P.A., *et al.* 3'-Azido-3'-deoxythymidine (BW A509U): An antiviral agent that inhibits the infectivity and cytopathic effect of human T-lymphotropic virus type III/lymphadenopathy-associated virus *in vitro. Proc. Natl. Acad. Sci. U.S.A.,* **1985,** *82:*7096–7100.

Molla, A., Korneyeva, M., Gao, Q., *et al.* Ordered accumulation of mutations in HIV protease confers resistance to ritonavir. *Nature Med.,* **1996,** *2:*760–766.

Molla, A., Vasavanonda, S., Kumar, G., *et al.* Human serum attenuates the activity of protease inhibitors toward wild-type and mutant human immunodeficiency virus. *Virology,* **1998,** 250:255–262.

Montaner, J.S., Reiss, P., Cooper, D., *et al.* A randomized, double-blind trial comparing combinations of nevirapine, didanosine, and zidovu-dine for HIV-infected patients: The INCAS Trial. Italy, the Netherlands, Canada and Australia Study. *JAMA,* **1998,** *279:*930–937.

Moore, K.H., Yuen, G.J., Raasch, R.H., *et al.* Pharmacokinetics of lamivudine administered alone and with trimethoprim–sulfamethoxazole. *Clin. Pharmacol. Ther.,* **1996,** *59:*550–558.

Moore, K.H., Barrett, J.E., Shaw, S., *et al.* The pharmacokinetics of lamivudine phosphorylation in peripheral blood mononuclear cells from patients infected with HIV-1. *AIDS,* **1999,** *13:*2239–2250.

Moore, R.D., Wong, W.M., Keruly, J.C., and McArthur, J.C. Incidence of neuropathy in HIV-infected patients on monotherapy versus those on combination therapy with didanosine, stavudine and hydroxyurea. *AIDS,* **2000,** *14:*273–278.

Naeger, L.K., Margot, N.A., and Miller, M.D. ATP-dependent removal of nucleoside reverse transcriptase inhibitors by human immunodeficiency virus type 1 reverse transcriptase. *Antimicrob. Agents Chemother.,* **2002,** *46:*2179–2184.

Noor, M.A., Seneviratne, T., Aweeka, F.T., *et al.* Indinavir acutely inhibits insulin-stimulated glucose disposal in humans: A randomized, placebo-controlled study. *AIDS,* **2002,** *16:*F1–8.

Odinecs, A., Nosbisch, C., Keller, R.D., *et al. In vivo* maternal-fetal pharmacokinetics of stavudine (2',3'-didehydro-3'-deoxythymidine) in pigtailed macaques (*Macaca nemestrina*). *Antimicrob. Agents Chemother.,* **1996,** *40:*196–202.

Para, M.F., Meehan, P., Holden-Wiltse, J., *et al.* ACTG 260: A randomized, phase I–II, dose-ranging trial of the anti–human immunodeficiency virus activity of delavirdine monotherapy. The AIDS Clinical Trials Group Protocol 260 Team. *Antimicrob. Agents Chemother.,* **1999,** *43:*1373–1378.

Paterson, D.L., Swindells, S., Mohr, J., *et al.* Adherence to protease inhibitor therapy and outcomes in patients with HIV infection. *Ann. Intern. Med.,* **2000,** *133:*21–30.

Pauwels, R., Andries, K., Desmyter, J., *et al.* Potent and selective inhibition of HIV-1 replication *in vitro* by a novel series of TIBO derivatives. *Nature,* **1990,** *343:*470–474.

Pearl, L.H., and Taylor, W.R. A structural model for the retroviral proteases. *Nature,* **1987,** *329:*351–354.

Perelson, A.S., Neumann, A.U., Markowitz, M., *et al.* HIV-1 dynamics *in vivo*: Virion clearance rate, infected cell life-span, and viral generation time. *Science,* **1996,** *271:*1582–1586.

Phair, J.P., Mellors, J.W., Detels, R., *et al.* Virologic and immunologic values allowing safe deferral of antiretroviral therapy. *AIDS,* **2002,** *16:*2455–2459.

Piketty, C., Race, E., Castiel, P., *et al.* Efficacy of a five-drug combination including ritonavir, saquinavir and efavirenz in patients who failed on a conventional triple-drug regimen: Phenotypic resistance to protease inhibitors predicts outcome of therapy. *AIDS,* **1999,** *13:*F71–77.

Rainey, P.M., Friedland, G., McCance-Katz, E.F., *et al.* Interaction of methadone with didanosine and stavudine. *J. Acquir. Immune Defic. Syndr.,* **2000,** *24:*241–248.

Rimsky, L.T., Shugars, D.C., and Matthews, T.J. Determinants of human immunodeficiency virus type 1 resistance to gp41-derived inhibitory peptides. *J. Virol.,* **1998,** *72:*986–993.

Robbins, B.L., Wilcox, C.K., Fridland, A., and Rodman, J.H. Metabolism of tenofovir and didanosine in quiescent or stimulated human peripheral blood mononuclear cells. *Pharmacotherapy,* **2003,** *23:*695–701.

Rufo, P., Lin, P.W., Andrade, A., *et al.* Diarrhea-associated HIV-1 aspartyl protease-inhibitors potentiate muscarinic activation of Cl⁻ secretion by T84 cells *via* prolongation of cytosolic Ca^{2+} signaling. *Am. J. Physiol. Cell Physiol.,* **2004,** *286:*998–1008.

Saag, M.S., Sonnerborg, A., Torres, R.A., *et al.* Antiretroviral effect and safety of abacavir alone and in combination with zidovudine in HIV-infected adults. Abacavir Phase 2 Clinical Team. *AIDS,* **1998,** *12:*F203–209.

Saez-Llorens, X., Nelson, R.P., Jr., Emmanuel, P., *et al.* A randomized, double-blind study of triple nucleoside therapy of abacavir, lamivudine, and zidovudine versus lamivudine and zidovudine in previously treated human immunodeficiency virus type 1–infected children. The CNAA3006 Study Team. *Pediatrics,* **2001,** *107:*E4.

Saravolatz, L.D., Winslow, D.L., Collins, G., *et al.* Zidovudine alone or in combination with didanosine or zalcitabine in HIV-infected patients with the acquired immunodeficiency syndrome or fewer than 200 CD4 cells per cubic millimeter. Investigators for the Terry Beirn Community Programs for Clinical Research on AIDS. *New Engl. J. Med.,* **1996,** *335:*1099–1106.

Schapiro, J.M., Winters, M.A., Stewart, F., *et al.* The effect of high-dose saquinavir on viral load and CD4+ T-cell counts in HIV-infected patients. *Ann. Intern. Med.,* **1996,** *124:*1039–1050.

Shafer, R.W., Smeaton, L.M., Robbins, G.K., *et al.,* for the AIDS Clinical Trials Group 384 Team. Comparison of four-drug regimens and pairs of sequential three-drug regimens as initial therapy for HIV-1 infection. *New Engl. J. Med.,* **2003,** *349:*2304–2315.

Siliciano, J.D., Kajdas, J., Finzi, D., *et al.* Long-term follow-up studies confirm the stability of the latent reservoir for HIV-1 in resting CD4+ T cells. *Nature Med.,* **2003,** *9:*727–728.

Skalski, V., Chang, C.N., Dutschman, G., and Cheng, Y.C. The biochemical basis for the differential anti–human immunodeficiency virus activity of two cis enantiomers of 2′,3′-dideoxy-3′-thiacytidine. *J. Biol. Chem.,* **1993,** *268:*23234–23238.

Slusher, J.T., Kuwahara, S.K., Hamzeh, F.M., *et al.* Intracellular zidovudine (ZDV) and ZDV phosphates as measured by a validated combined high-pressure liquid chromatography–radioimmunoassay procedure. *Antimicrob. Agents Chemother.,* **1992,** *36:*2473–2477.

Spence, R.A., Kati, W.M., Anderson, K.S., and Johnson, K.A. Mechanism of inhibition of HIV-1 reverse transcriptase by nonnucleoside inhibitors. *Science,* **1995,** *267:*988–993.

Spruance, S.L., Pavia, A.T., Mellors, J.W., *et al.* Clinical efficacy of monotherapy with stavudine compared with zidovudine in HIV-infected, zidovudine-experienced patients: A randomized, double-blind, controlled trial. Bristol-Myers Squibb Stavudine/019 Study Group. *Ann. Intern. Med.,* **1997,** *126:*355–363.

Squires, K., Lazzarin, A., Gatell, J.M., *et al.* Comparison of once-daily atazanavir with efavirenz, each in combination with fixed-dose zidovudine and lamivudine, as initial therapy for patients infected with HIV. *J. Acquir. Immune Defic. Syndr.,* **2004,** *36:*1011–1019.

Starr, S.E., Fletcher, C.V., Spector, S.A., *et al.* Combination therapy with efavirenz, nelfinavir, and nucleoside reverse-transcriptase inhibitors in children infected with human immunodeficiency virus type 1. Pediatric AIDS Clinical Trials Group 382 Team. *New Engl. J. Med.,* **1999,** *341:*1874–1881.

Staszewski, S., Morales-Ramirez, J., Tashima, K.T., *et al.* Efavirenz plus zidovudine and lamivudine, efavirenz plus indinavir, and indinavir plus zidovudine and lamivudine in the treatment of HIV-1 infection in adults. Study 006 Team. *New Engl. J. Med.,* **1999,** *341:*1865–1873.

Taylor, S., Back, D.J., Workman, J., *et al.* Poor penetration of the male genital tract by HIV-1 protease inhibitors. *AIDS,* **1999,** *13:*859–860.

Tripuraneni, N.S., Smith, P.R., Weedon, J., *et al.* Prognostic factors in lactic acidosis syndrome caused by nucleoside reverse transcriptase inhibitors: Report of eight cases and review of the literature. *AIDS Patient Care STDs,* **2004,** *18:*379–384.

Vacca, J.P., Dorsey, B.D., Schleif, W.A., *et al.* L-735,524: An orally bioavailable human immunodeficiency virus type 1 protease inhibitor. *Proc. Natl. Acad. Sci. U.S.A.,* **1994,** *91:*4096–4100.

Veal, G.J., Hoggard, P.G., Barry, M.G., *et al.* Interaction between lamivudine (3TC) and other nucleoside analogues for intracellular phosphorylation. *AIDS,* **1996,** *10:*546–548.

Volberding, P.A., Lagakos, S.W., Koch, M.A., *et al.* Zidovudine in asymptomatic human immunodeficiency virus infection: A controlled trial in persons with fewer than 500 CD4-positive cells per cubic millimeter. The AIDS Clinical Trials Group of the National Institute of Allergy and Infectious Diseases. *New Engl. J. Med.,* **1990,** *322:*941–949.

Wainberg, M.A., Drosopoulos, W.C., Salomon, H., *et al.* Enhanced fidelity of 3TC-selected mutant HIV-1 reverse transcriptase. *Science,* **1996,** *271:*1282–1285.

Wainberg, M.A., Miller, M.D., Quan, Y., *et al. In vitro* selection and characterization of HIV-1 with reduced susceptibility to PMPA. *Antivir. Ther.,* **1999,** *4:*87–94.

Watts, D.H., Brown, Z.A., Tartaglione, T., *et al.* Pharmacokinetic disposition of zidovudine during pregnancy. *J. Infect. Dis.,* **1991,** *163:*226–232.

Wei, X., Ghosh, S.K., Taylor, M.E., *et al.* Viral dynamics in human immunodeficiency virus type 1 infection. *Nature,* **1995,** *373:*117–122.

Wild, C.T., Shugars, D.C., Greenwell, T.K., *et al.* Peptides corresponding to a predictive alpha-helical domain of human immunodeficiency virus type 1 gp41 are potent inhibitors of virus infection. *Proc. Natl. Acad. Sci. U.S.A.,* **1994,** *91:*9770–9774.

Young, S.D., Britcher, S.F., Tran, L.O., *et al.* L-743,726 (DMP-266): A novel, highly potent nonnucleoside inhibitor of the human immunodeficiency virus type 1 reverse transcriptase. *Antimicrob. Agents Chemother.,* **1995,** *39:*2602–2605.

MONOGRAPHS AND REVIEWS

Adkins, J.C., and Faulds, D. Amprenavir. *Drugs,* **1998,** *55:*837–842.

Adkins, J.C., and Noble, S. Efavirenz. *Drugs,* **1998,** *56:*1055–1064.

Adkins, J.C., Peters, D.H., and Faulds, D. Zalcitabine: An update of its pharmacodynamic and pharmacokinetic properties and clinical efficacy in the management of HIV infection. *Drugs,* **1997,** *53:*1054–1080.

Back, D., Gatti, G., Fletcher, C., *et al.* Therapeutic drug monitoring in HIV infection: Current status and future directions. *AIDS,* **2002,** *16:*S5–35.

Bang, L.M. and Scott, L.J. Emtricitabine: An antiretroviral agent for HIV infection. *Drugs,* **2003,** *63:*2413–2424.

Bardsley-Elliot, A. and Plosker, G.L. Nelfinavir: an update on its use in HIV infection. *Drugs,* **2000,** *59:*581–620.

Berger, E.A., Murphy, P.M., and Farber, J.M. Chemokine receptors as HIV-1 coreceptors: Roles in viral entry, tropism, and disease. *Annu. Rev. Immunol.,* **1999,** *17:*657–700.

Chapman, T., McGavin, J., and Noble, S. Tenofovir disoproxil fumarate. *Drugs,* **2003,** *63:*1597–1608.

Cvetkovic, R.S., and Goa, K.L. Lopinavir–ritonavir: A review of its use in the management of HIV infection. *Drugs,* **2003,** *63:*769–802.

Dando, T.M., and Perry, C.M. Enfuvirtide. *Drugs,* **2003,** *63:*2755–2766.

Department of Health and Human Services (DHHS). Guidelines for the use of antiretroviral agents in HIV-1 infected adults and adolescents. Available at *http://www.aidsinfo.nih.gov/guidelines/adult/AA_032304.pdf;* last updated March 23, **2004.**

Dudley, M.N. Clinical pharmacokinetics of nucleoside antiretroviral agents. *J. Infect. Dis.,* **1995,** *171:*S99–112.

Ellis, J.M, Ross, J.W., and Coleman, C.I. Fosamprenavir: A novel protease inhibitor and prodrug of amprenavir. *Formulary,* **2004,** *19:*151–160.

Fauci, A.S. Host factors and the pathogenesis of HIV-induced disease. *Nature,* **1996,** *384*:529–534.

Flexner, C. HIV-protease inhibitors. *New Engl. J. Med.,* **1998,** *338*:1281–1292.

Flexner, C. Dual protease inhibitor therapy in HIV-infected patients: Pharmacologic rationale and clinical benefits. *Annu. Rev. Pharmacol. Toxicol.,* **2000,** *40*:649–674.

Gallant, J.E., Gerondelis, P.Z., Wainberg, M.A., *et al.* Nucleoside and nucleotide analogue reverse transcriptase inhibitors: A clinical review of antiretroviral resistance. *Antivir. Ther.,* **2003,** *8*:489–506.

Garg, A. Acquired and inherited lipodystrophies. *N. Engl. J. Med.,* **2004,** *350*:1220–1234.

Goldsmith, D.R., and Perry, C.M. Atazanavir. *Drugs,* **2003,** *63*:1679–1693.

Greene, W.C., and Peterlin, B.M. Charting HIV's remarkable voyage through the cell: Basic science as a passport to future therapy. *Nature Med.,* **2002,** *8*:673–680.

Harrington, M., and Carpenter, C.C. Hit HIV-1 hard, but only when necessary. *Lancet,* **2000,** *355*:2147–2152.

Harris, M., and Montaner, J.S. Clinical uses of non-nucleoside reverse transcriptase inhibitors. *Rev. Med. Virol.,* **2000,** *10*:217–229.

Hervey, P.S., and Perry, C.M. Abacavir: A review of its clinical potential in patients with HIV infection. *Drugs,* **2000,** *60*:447–479.

Hirsch, M.S., and D'Aquila, R.T. Therapy for human immunodeficiency virus infection. *New Engl. J. Med.,* **1993,** *328*:1686–1695.

Hsu, A., Granneman, G.R., and Bertz, R.J. Ritonavir: Clinical pharmacokinetics and interactions with other anti-HIV agents. *Clin. Pharmacokinet.,* **1998,** *35*:275–291.

Hurst, M., and Noble, S. Stavudine: An update of its use in the treatment of HIV infection. *Drugs,* **1999,** *58*:919–949.

Jayasekara, D., Aweeka, F.T., Rodriguez, R., *et al.* Antiviral therapy for HIV patients with renal insufficiency. *J. Acquir. Immune Defic. Syndr.,* **1999,** *21*:384–395.

Khoo, S.H., Back, D.J., and Merry, C. Pharmacology. In, *Practical Guidelines in Antiviral Therapy.* (Boucher, C.A.B. and Galasso, G.A.J., eds.) Elsevier, Amsterdam, **2002,** pp. 13–35.

Kuritzkes, D.R. Preventing and managing antiretroviral drug resistance. *AIDS Patient Care STDs,* **2004,** *18*:259–273.

McLeod, G.X., and Hammer, S.M. Zidovudine: Five years later. *Ann. Intern. Med.,* **1992,** *117*:487–501.

Muller, V., and Bonhoeffer, S. Mathematical approaches in the study of viral kinetics and drug resistance in HIV-1 infection. *Curr. Drug Targets Infect. Disord.,* **2003,** *3*:329–344.

Noble, S., and Faulds, D. Saquinavir: A review of its pharmacology and clinical potential in the management of HIV infection. *Drugs,* **1996,** *52*:93–112.

Panel on Clinical Practices for Treatment of HIV Infection, convened by the Department of Health and Human Services (DHHS). Guidelines for the use of antiretroviral agents in HIV-1-infected adults and adolescents, March 23, **2004.** Available at *http://www.aidsinfo.nih.gov/ guidelines/adult/AA_032304.pdf.*

Perry, C.M., and Faulds, D. Lamivudine: A review of its antiviral activity, pharmacokinetic properties and therapeutic efficacy in the management of HIV infection. *Drugs,* **1997,** *53*:657–680.

Perry, C.M., and Noble, S. Saquinavir soft-gel capsule formulation: A review of its use in patients with HIV infection. *Drugs,* **1998,** *55*:461–486.

Perry, C.M. and Noble, S. Didanosine: An updated review of its use in HIV infection. *Drugs,* **1999,** *58*:1099–1135.

Piscitelli, S.C., and Gallicano, K.D. Interactions among drugs for HIV and opportunistic infections. *New Engl. J. Med.,* **2001,** *344*:984–996.

Plosker, G.L., and Noble, S. Indinavir: A review of its use in the management of HIV infection. *Drugs,* **1999,** *58*:1165–1203.

Rendic, S., and Di Carlo, F.J. Human cytochrome P450 enzymes: A status report summarizing their reactions, substrates, inducers, and inhibitors. *Drug Metab. Rev.,* **1997,** *29*:413–580.

Roberts, N.A., Martin, J.A., Kinchington, D., *et al.* Rational design of peptide-based HIV proteinase inhibitors. *Science,* **1990,** *248*:358–361.

Scott, L.J., and Perry, C.M. Delavirdine: A review of its use in HIV infection. *Drugs,* **2000,** *60*:1411–1444.

Sekhar, R.V., Jahoor, F., Pownall, H.J., *et al.* Cardiovascular implications of HIV-associated dyslipidemic lipodystrophy. *Curr. Atheroscler. Rep.,* **2004,** *6*:173–179.

Smith, P.F., DiCenzo, R., and Morse, G.D. Clinical pharmacokinetics of non-nucleoside reverse transcriptase inhibitors. *Clin. Pharmacokinet.,* **2001,** *40*:893–905.

Sodroski, J.G. HIV-1 entry inhibitors in the side pocket. *Cell,* **1999,** *99*:243–246.

Werth, B. *The Billion Dollar Molecule: One Company's Quest for the Perfect Drug.* Simon & Schuster, New York, **1994.**

CHAPTER

51

ANTINEOPLASTIC AGENTS

Bruce A. Chabner, Philip C. Amrein, Brian J. Druker, M. Dror Michaelson,
Constantine S. Mitsiades, Paul E. Goss, David P. Ryan, Sumant Ramachandra,
Paul G. Richardson, Jeffrey G. Supko, Wyndham H. Wilson

The practice of cancer medicine has changed dramatically in the past four decades, as curative treatments have been identified for a number of previously fatal malignancies such as testicular cancer, lymphomas, and leukemia. New drugs have entered clinical use for disease presentations that were previously either untreatable or amenable only to local therapies such as surgery and irradiation. At present, adjuvant chemotherapy routinely follows local treatment of breast, colorectal, and lung cancer, and chemotherapy is employed as part of a multimodal approach to the initial treatment of many other tumors, including locally advanced stages of head and neck, lung, and esophageal cancer, soft tissue sarcomas, and pediatric solid tumors. Genetic therapies, vaccines, and other manipulations of the immune system are under active investigation, and drugs now are in common use for restoring bone marrow function after chemotherapy, induction of differentiation in tumor tissues, and inhibition of angiogenesis. At the same time, chemotherapic drugs have found expanded utility in noncancerous diseases. The same drugs used for cytotoxic antitumor therapy have become important components of immunosuppressive regimens for rheumatoid arthritis (*methotrexate* and *cyclophosphamide*), organ transplantation (methotrexate and *azathioprine*), sickle cell anemia (*5-azacytadine* and *hydroxyurea*), anti-infective chemotherapy (*trimetrexate* and *leucovorin*), and psoriasis (methotrexate).

While their range of uses has grown, few categories of medication have a narrower therapeutic index and a greater potential for causing harmful side effects than do the antineoplastic drugs. A thorough understanding of their pharmacology, drug interactions, and clinical pharmacokinetics is essential for safe and effective use in humans. The diversity of agents useful in treatment of neoplastic disease is summarized in Table 51–1.

Traditionally, cancer drugs were discovered through large-scale testing of synthetic chemicals and natural products against rapidly proliferating animal tumor systems, primarily murine leukemias (Chabner and Roberts, 2005). Most of the agents discovered in the first two decades of cancer chemotherapy (1950 to 1970) interacted with DNA or its precursors, inhibiting the synthesis of new genetic material or causing irreparable damage to DNA itself. In recent years, the discovery of new agents has extended from the more conventional natural products such as *paclitaxel* and semisynthetic agents such as *etoposide*, both of which target the proliferative process, to entirely new fields of investigation. These new fields represent the harvest of new knowledge about cancer biology, leading to the discovery of drugs that inhibit novel molecular targets. One such agent, *all*-trans-*retinoic acid*, elicits differentiation and can be used to promote remission in acute promyelocytic leukemia (APL) through its interaction with the unique fusion protein produced by the (15:17) RAR-PML translation, even after failure of standard chemotherapy. Initial success in characterizing unique tumor antigens and oncogenes has introduced new therapeutic opportunities. Thus, the *bcr-abl* translocation in chronic myelocytic leukemia

Table 51–1
Chemotherapeutic Agents Useful in Neoplastic Disease

CLASS	TYPE OF AGENT	NONPROPRIETARY NAMES (OTHER NAMES)	DISEASE*
Alkylating agents	Nitrogen mustards	Mechlorethamine	Hodgkin's disease; non-Hodgkin's lymphoma
		Cyclophosphamide Ifosfamide	Acute and chronic lymphocytic leukemia; Hodgkin's disease; non-Hodgkin's lymphoma; multiple myeloma; neuroblastoma; breast, ovary, lung cancer; Wilms' tumor; cervix, testis cancer; soft-tissue sarcoma
		Melphalan (L-sarcolysin)	Multiple myeloma; breast, ovarian cancer
		Chlorambucil	Chronic lymphocytic leukemia; primary macroglobulinemia; Hodgkin's disease; non-Hodgkin's lymphoma
	Ethyleneimines and methylmelamines	Altretamine	Ovarian cancer
		Thiotepa	Bladder, breast, ovarian cancer
	Methylhydrazine derivative	Procarbazine (*N*-methylhydrazine, MIH)	Hodgkin's disease
	Alkyl sulfonate	Busulfan	Chronic myelogenous leukemia
	Nitrosoureas	Carmustine (BCNU)	Hodgkin's disease; non-Hodgkin's lymphoma; primary brain tumor; melanoma
		Streptozocin (streptozotocin)	Malignant pancreatic insulinoma; malignant carcinoid
	Triazenes	Dacarbazine (DTIC; dimethyltriazenoimidazole carboxamide), temozolomide	Malignant melanoma; Hodgkin's disease; soft-tissue sarcomas; glioma; melanoma
	Platinum coordination complexes	Cisplatin, carboplatin, oxaliplatin	Testicular, ovarian, bladder, esophageal, lung, colon cancer
Antimetabolites	Folic acid analogs	Methotrexate (amethopterin)	Acute lymphocytic leukemia; choriocarcinoma; breast, head, neck, and lung cancer; osteogenic sarcoma; bladder cancer
		Pemetrexed	Mesothelioma, lung cancer
	Pyrimidine analogs	Fluorouracil (5-fluorouracil; 5-FU), capecitabine	Breast, colon, esophageal, stomach, pancreas, head and neck; premalignant skin lesion (topical)
		Cytarabine (cytosine arabinoside)	Acute myelogenous and acute lymphocytic leukemia; non-Hodgkin's lymphoma
		Gemcitabine	Pancreatic, ovarian, lung cancer
	Purine analogs and related inhibitors	Mercaptopurine (6-mercaptopurine; 6-MP)	Acute lymphocytic and myelogenous leukemia
		Pentostatin (2'-deoxycoformycin), cladribine, fludarabine	Hairy cell leukemia; chronic lymphocytic leukemia; small cell non-Hodgkin's lymphoma

(Continued)

Table 51–1
Chemotherapeutic Agents Useful in Neoplastic Disease (Continued)

CLASS	TYPE OF AGENT	NONPROPRIETARY NAMES (OTHER NAMES)	DISEASE*
Natural products	Vinca alkaloids	Vinblastine, vinorelbine	Hodgkin's disease; non-Hodgkin's lymphoma: breast, lung, and testis cancer
		Vincristine	Acute lymphocytic leukemia; neuroblastoma; Wilms' tumor; rhabdomyosarcoma; Hodgkin's disease; non-Hodgkin's lymphoma
	Taxanes	Paclitaxel, docetaxel	Ovarian, breast, lung, bladder, head and neck cancer
	Epipodophyllotoxins	Etoposide	Testis, small-cell lung, and other lung cancer; breast cancer; Hodgkin's disease; non-Hodgkin's lymphomas; acute myelogenous leukemia; Kaposi's sarcoma
		Teniposide	Same as etoposide; also acute lymphoblastic leukemia in children
	Camptothecins	Topotecan, irinotecan	Ovarian cancer; small-cell lung cancer; colon and lung cancer
	Antibiotics	Dactinomycin (actinomycin D)	Choriocarcinoma; Wilms' tumor; rhabdomyosarcoma; testis; Kaposi's sarcoma
		Daunorubicin (daunomycin, rubidomycin)	Acute myelogenous and acute lymphocytic leukemia
		Doxorubicin	Soft-tissue, osteogenic, and other sarcoma; Hodgkin's disease; non-Hodgkin's lymphoma; acute leukemia; breast, genitourinary, thyroid, lung, stomach cancer; neuroblastoma and other childhood sarcoma
	Anthracenedione	Mitoxantrone	Acute myelogenous leukemia; breast and prostate cancer
		Bleomycin	Testis, and cervical cancer; Hodgkin's disease; non-Hodgkin's lymphoma
		Mitomycin (mitomycin C)	Stomach, anal, and lung cancer
	Enzymes	L-Asparaginase	Acute lymphocytic leukemia
Miscellaneous agents	Substituted urea	Hydroxyurea	Chronic myelogenous leukemia; polycythemia vera; essential thrombocytosis
	Differentiating agents	Tretinoin, arsenic trioxide	Acute promyelocytic leukemia
	Protein tyrosine kinase inhibitor	Imatinib	Chronic myelocytic leukemia; gastrointestinal stromal tumors; hypereosinophilia syndrome
		Gefitinib	Non-small-cell lung cancer
	Proteasome inhibitor	Bortezomib	Multiple myeloma

(Continued)

Table 51–1
Chemotherapeutic Agents Useful in Neoplastic Disease (Continued)

CLASS	TYPE OF AGENT	NONPROPRIETARY NAMES (OTHER NAMES)	DISEASE*
	Biological response modifiers	Interferon-alfa, interleukin 2	Hairy cell leukemia; Kaposi's sarcoma; melanoma; carcinoid; renal cell; ovary; bladder; non-Hodgkin's lymphoma; mycosis fungoides; multiple myeloma; chronic myelogenous leukemia; malignant melanoma
	Antibodies (*see* Tables 51–3 and 51–4)		
Hormones and antagonists	Adrenocortical suppressants	Mitotane (*o,p'*-DDD) Aminoglutethimide	Adrenal cortex cancer Breast cancer
	Adrenocorticosteroids	Prednisone (several other equivalent preparations available; *see* Chapter 59)	Acute and chronic lymphocytic leukemia; non-Hodgkin's lymphoma; Hodgkin's disease; breast cancer
	Progestins	Hydroxyprogesterone caproate, medroxyprogesterone acetate, megestrol acetate	Endometrial, breast cancer
	Estrogens	Diethylstilbestrol, ethinyl estradiol (other preparations available; *see* Chapter 57)	Breast, prostate cancer
	Anti-estrogens	Tamoxifen, toremifene	Breast cancer
	Aromatase inhibitors	Anastrozole, letrozole, exemestane	Breast cancer
	Androgens	Testosterone propionate, fluoxymesterone (other preparations available; *see* Chapter 58)	Breast cancer
	Anti-androgen	Flutamide	Prostate cancer
	Gonadotropin-releasing hormone analog	Leuprolide	Prostate cancer

*Neoplasms are carcinomas unless otherwise indicated.

(CML) encodes a tyrosine kinase essential to cell proliferation and survival. Inhibition of the kinase by *imatinib* (STI-571), a new molecularly targeted drug, has become the standard treatment for CML, producing hematologic and cytogenic remission in the majority of patients. Similarly targeted immunological approaches use monoclonal antibodies against tumor-associated antigens such as the her-2/neu receptor in breast cancer cells, often in conjunction with cytotoxic drugs (Slamon *et al.*, 2001). These examples emphasize that both the strategy for drug evaluation and the routine care of cancer patients are likely to undergo revolutionary changes as entirely new treatment approaches arise from new knowledge of cancer biology. Figure 51–1 outlines some of the common targets for chemotherapeutic agents currently used for neoplastic disease. New clinical trial designs, aimed at determining effects of new drugs at the molecular level, increasingly will employ urinary and blood markers of tumor proliferation, angiogenesis, and other bio-

logical endpoints. Imaging of molecular, metabolic, or physiologic effects of drugs will become increasingly important in establishing that drugs effectively engage their targets (Fox *et al.*, 2002).

While molecularly targeted drugs have had outstanding success in CML and APL, it is unlikely that new therapies will replace cytotoxics in the near future. When used in combination and in early stages of disease, the cytotoxics have become increasingly effective. At the same time, their toxicities have become more manageable with the development of better antinausea drugs and with granulocyte colony-stimulating factor (G-CSF) and erythropoietin to restore marrow function (*see* Chapter 53). Finally, a greater insight into the mechanisms of tumor cell resistance to chemotherapy has led to the more rational construction of drug regimens and the earlier use of intensive therapies. Drug-resistant cells may be selected from the larger tumor population by exposure to low-dose, single-agent chemotherapy. The resistance that arises

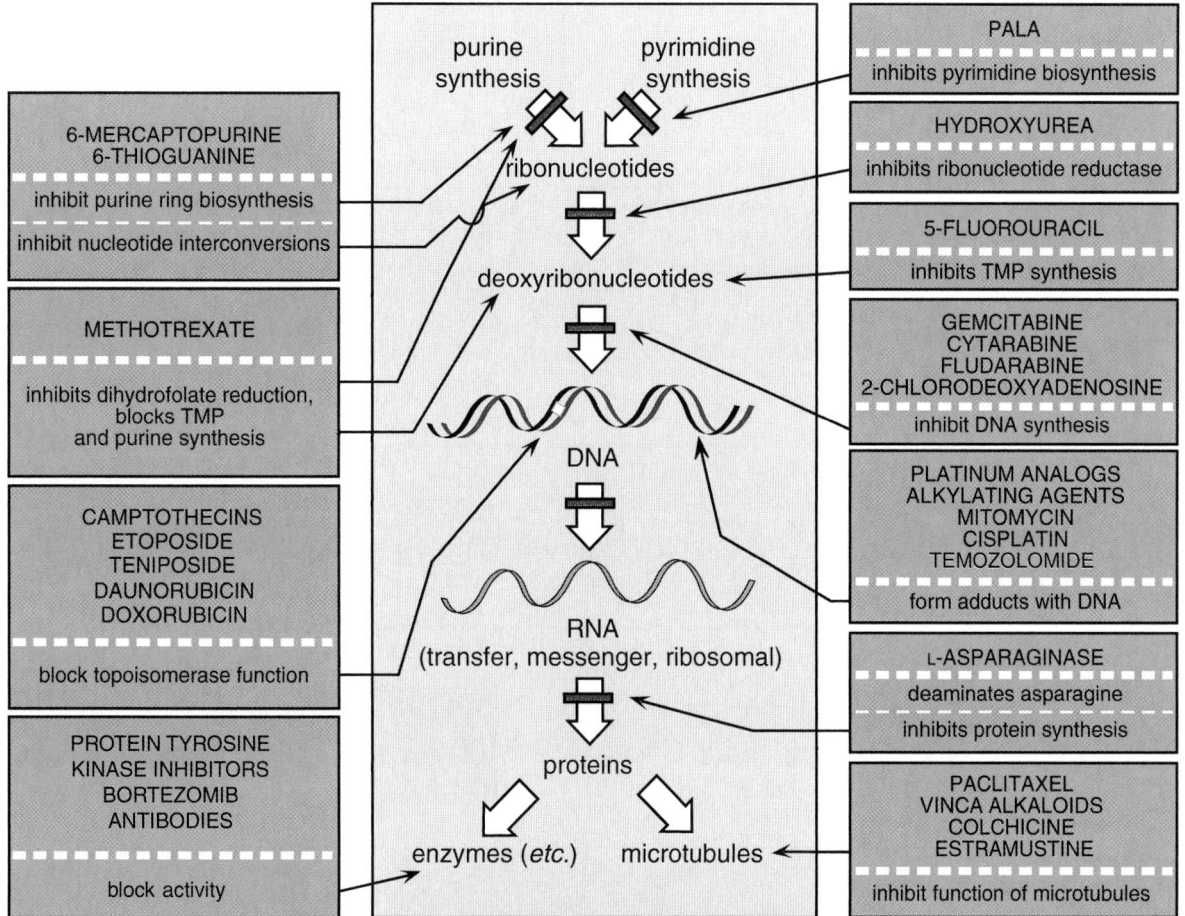

Figure 51–1. *Summary of the mechanisms and sites of action of some chemotherapeutic agents useful in neoplastic disease.* PALA = *N*-phosphonoacetyl-L-aspartate; TMP = thymidine monophosphate.

may be specific for the selecting agent, such as the loss of a necessary activating enzyme (deoxycytidine kinase for cytosine arabinoside), or may affect broader categories of disease, such as the overexpression of a general drug-efflux pump, the P-glycoprotein, a product of the *MDR* gene. This membrane protein is one of several ATP-dependent transporters that confer resistance to a broad range of natural products used in cancer treatment (Borst and Oude Elfrink, 2002; *see* also Chapter 2). More recently, it has become appreciated that mutations that raise the threshold for programmed cell death (apoptosis), such as the loss of the p53 tumor suppressor oncogene, enhanced activity of a mutated EGF receptor, or increased expression of the anti-apoptotic bcl-2, may lead to drug resistance (Ibrado *et al.*, 1996). Drug discovery efforts now are directed toward lowering the threshold for apoptosis in tumor cells, and restoring tumor cell sensitivity to drugs.

In designing specific regimens for clinical use, a number of factors must be taken into account. Drugs are most effective in combination, and may be synergistic because of their biochemical interactions. It is more effective to combine drugs that do not share common mechanisms of resistance and that do not overlap in their major toxicities. Cytotoxic drugs should be used as close as possible to their maximum individual doses and should be given as frequently as possible to discourage tumor regrowth and to maximize dose intensity, the dose given per unit time, a key parameter in the success of chemotherapy (Citron *et al.*, 2003). Since the tumor cell population in patients with clinically detectable disease exceeds 1 g, or 10^9 cells, and since each cycle of therapy kills less than 99% of the cells, it is necessary to repeat treatments in multiple cycles to eradicate the tumor cells.

The Cell Cycle. An understanding of cell-cycle kinetics is essential for the proper use of antineoplastic agents (Figure 51–2). Many of the most effective cytotoxic agents act by damaging DNA. Their toxicity is greater during the S, or DNA synthetic, phase of the cell cycle, while others, such as the vinca alkaloids and taxanes, block the formation of a

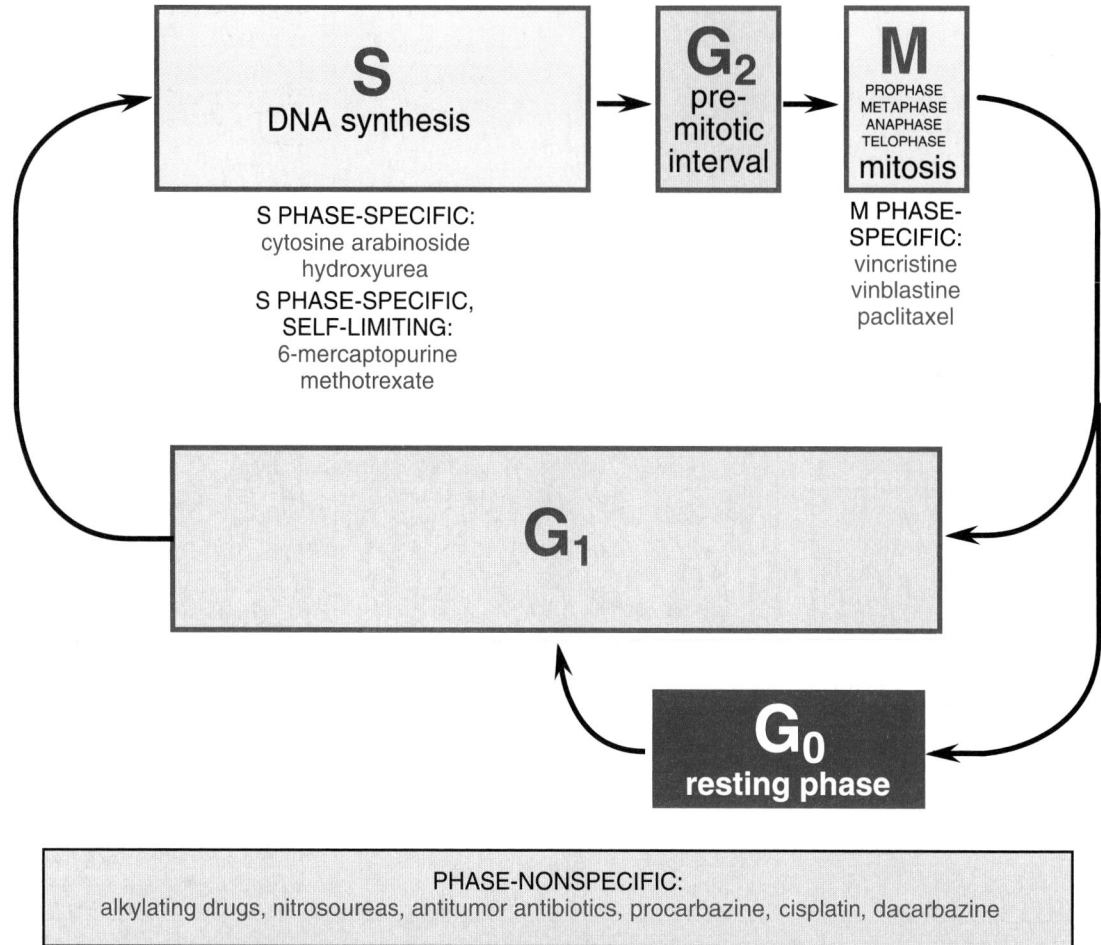

***Figure 51–2.** The cell cycle and the relationship of antitumor drug action to the cycle.* G_1 is the gap period between mitosis and the beginning of DNA synthesis. Resting cells (cells that are not preparing for cell division) are said to be in a subphase of G_1, G_0. S is the period of DNA synthesis, G_2 the premitotic interval, and M the period of mitosis. Examples of cell cycle–dependent anticancer drugs are listed in blue below the phase in which they act. Drugs that are cytotoxic for cells at any point in the cycle are called cycle-phase–nonspecific drugs. (Modified from Pratt *et al.*, 1994 with permission.)

functional mitotic spindle in M phase. These agents have activity against cells that pass through the most vulnerable phase of the cell cycle. Accordingly, human neoplasms that currently are most susceptible to chemotherapeutic measures are those with a high percentage of cells undergoing division. Similarly, normal tissues that proliferate rapidly (bone marrow, hair follicles, and intestinal epithelium) are subject to damage by most cytotoxic drugs, which often limits their usefulness. Conversely, slowly growing tumors with a small growth fraction (for example, carcinomas of the colon or non–small cell lung cancer) often are less responsive to cycle-specific drugs.

Although differences in the duration of the cell cycle occur between cells of various types, all cells display a similar pattern during the division process: (1) a phase that precedes DNA synthesis (G_1); (2) a DNA synthesis phase (S); (3) an interval following the termination of DNA synthesis (G_2); and (4) the mitotic phase (M) in which the cell, containing a double complement of DNA, divides into two daughter G_1 cells. Each of these daughter cells may immediately re-enter the cell cycle or pass into a nonproliferative stage, referred to as G_0. The G_0 cells of certain specialized tissues may differentiate into functional cells that no longer are capable of division. On the other hand, many cells, especially those in slow-growing tumors, may remain in the G_0 state for prolonged periods, only to re-enter the division cycle at a later time. Each transition in the cell cycle is controlled by the activity of specific cyclin-dependent kinases (CDKs), which are activated by their corresponding small regulatory proteins called cyclins, and inhibited by proteins such as p16. Mutations or loss of p16 or other components of the so-called retinoblastoma pathway such as retinoblastoma protein itself, or enhanced cyclin or CDK activity, will lead to relentless proliferation in tumor cells. Consequently, CDKs and their effector proteins have become attractive molecular targets for new antineoplastic agents.

Because of the central importance of DNA to the identity and functionality of a cell, elaborate mechanisms have evolved to monitor DNA integrity. If a cell expresses normal p53 protein, DNA damage activates a normal checkpoint function and damaged cells undergo apoptosis, or programmed cell death, when they reach the G_1/S boundary. If the p53 gene product is mutated or absent and the checkpoint function fails, damaged cells will not be diverted to the apoptotic pathway but will proceed through S phase. At the G_2-M interface, other checkpoint proteins monitor DNA integrity and may delay progression into M phase. Absence or mutation of these checkpoints allows cells to pass through mitosis and survive DNA damage (Lane and Fischer, 2004). These cells can proceed through S phase and some will emerge as a mutated and potentially drug-resistant population. *Thus, an understanding of cell-cycle kinetics and the controls of normal and malignant cell growth is crucial to the design of current therapeutic regimens and the search for new drugs.*

Achieving Therapeutic Balance and Efficacy. The treatment of most cancer patients requires a skillful interdigitation of multiple modalities of treatment, including surgery and irradiation, with drugs. Each of these forms of treatment carries its own risks and benefits. It is obvious that not all drug regimens are appropriate for all patients. Numerous factors must be considered, such as renal and hepatic function, bone marrow reserve, general performance status, and concurrent medical problems. Beyond those considerations, however, are less quantifiable factors such as the likely natural history of the tumor being treated, the patient's willingness to undergo difficult and potentially dangerous treatments, the patient's physical and emotional tolerance for side effects, and the likely long-term gains and risks involved.

One of the greatest challenges of therapeutics is to adjust dose to achieve a therapeutic, but nontoxic, outcome. While it is customary to base dose on body surface area for individual patients, this practice is not based on solid data (Sawyer and Ratain, 2001). Dose adjustment based on renal function or on pharmacokinetic monitoring does help meet specific targets such as desired drug concentration in plasma or area under the

concentration–time curve (AUC), a measure of tissue exposure to the agent in question.

Two important examples of improved therapy based on pharmacokinetic targeting are the following:

1. Calvert and Egorin showed that the thrombocytopenia caused by *carboplatin* was a direct function of AUC, which in turn was determined by renal clearance of the parent drug. They devised a formula for targeting a desired AUC based on creatinine clearance (Calvert *et al.*, 1995; Calvert and Egorin, 2002).
2. Relling and colleagues determined that therapeutic success was related to achieving targeted methotrexate concentrations in plasma during high-dose therapy for pediatric acute lymphoblastic leukemia (ALL). Monitoring of steady-state levels of methotrexate allowed dose adjustment and improvement in outcome (Relling *et al.*, 1999).

Molecular tests increasingly are being employed to identify patients likely to benefit from treatment and those at highest risk of toxicity (Chabner and Roberts, 2005). Pretreatment testing to select patients for response to treatment has become standard practice for hormonal therapy of breast cancer and for treatment with antibodies such as *trastuzumab* (her-2/neu receptor) and *rituximab* (CD20). However, in the use of traditional cytotoxic therapy, molecular testing has not been routinely employed. Inherited differences in protein sequence or expression levels (polymorphisms) occur commonly in the population, and affect either toxicity or response. In *fluorouracil* therapy, polymorphisms of drug target genes affect both response rates and toxicity. Tandem repeats in the promoter region of the gene encoding thymidylate synthase, the target of 5-fluorouracil, determine the level of expression of the enzyme. Increased numbers of repeats are associated with increased gene expression, a lower incidence of toxicity, and a decreased rate of response in patients with colorectal cancer (Pullarkat *et al.*, 2001). Polymorphisms of the dihydropyrimidine dehydrogenase gene, which is responsible for degradation of 5-fluorouracil, are associated with decreased enzyme activity and a significant risk of overwhelming drug toxicity, particularly in the rare individual homozygous for the polymorphic genes (Van Kuilenburg *et al.*, 2002). Other polymorphisms appear to affect the clearance and therapeutic activity of cancer drugs, including methotrexate, *irinotecan*, and *6-mercaptopurine* (*see* below) (Watters and McLeod, 2002).

Other aspects of molecular biology are entering into clinical decision-making in oncology. Gene expression profiling, in which the level of messenger RNA from thousands of genes are randomly surveyed for associations with tumor progression, response, or treatment outcome, have revealed tumor profiles that are highly associated with metastasis (Ramaswamy *et al.*, 2003) or with drug response. Perhaps the best example is the high correlation of HOX B13, a transcription factor, with disease recurrence in patients receiving adjuvant hormonal therapy in breast cancer (Ma *et al.*, 2004). An alternative approach, detailed sequencing of the drug target, has revealed that activating mutations in the epidermal growth factor receptor (EGFR) gene are associated with a high rate of response to *gefitinib* (IRESSA), an EGFR inhibitor, in patients with adenocarcinoma of the lung (Lynch *et al.*, 2004). Molecular tests to select patients for specific treatments undoubtedly will shorten the required time for drug testing and approval, improve the outcome of cancer therapy, and realize savings in the cost and toxicity of ineffective drugs (Chabner and Roberts, 2005; Park *et al.*, 2004).

Despite efforts to anticipate the development of complications, anticancer agents have variable pharmacokinetics and toxicity in individual patients. The causes of this variability are not always clear and often may be related to interindividual differences in drug metabolism, drug interactions, or bone marrow reserves. In dealing with toxicity, the physician must provide vigorous supportive care, including, where indicated, platelet transfusions, antibiotics, and hematopoietic growth factors (*see* Chapter 53). Other delayed toxicities affecting the heart, lungs, or kidneys may be irreversible, leading to permanent organ damage or death. Fortunately, such toxicities can be minimized by adherence to standardized protocols and the guidelines for drug use.

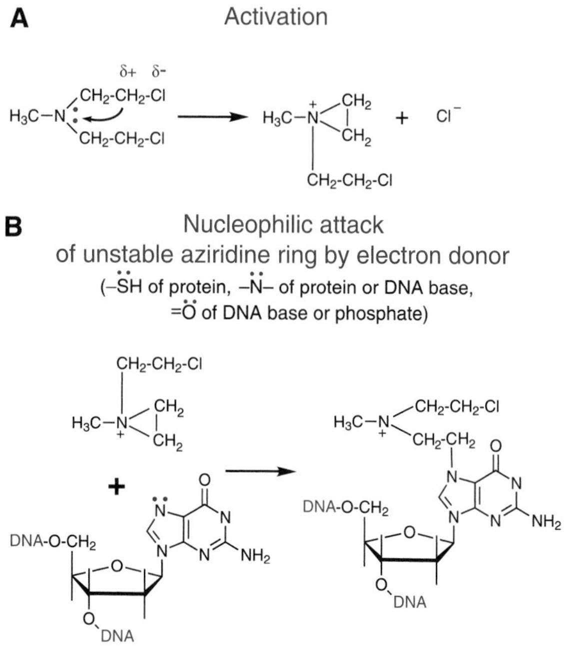

I. ALKYLATING AGENTS

The pervasive toxic effects of sulfur mustard gas were noted as the result of its use in World War I. A potent vesicant, the gas caused a topical burn to skin, eyes, lungs, and mucosa, and after massive exposure, aplasia of the bone marrow, lymphoid tissue, and ulceration of the gastrointestinal tract. Early clinical experiments with topically applied sulfur mustard led to regression of penile tumors. Thereafter, Goodman, Gilman and colleagues at Yale, working in a consortium organized by the U.S. Department of Defense, confirmed the antineoplastic action of the nitrogen mustards against a murine lymphosarcoma. In 1942, they began clinical studies of several mustards in patients with lymphoma, launching the modern era of cancer chemotherapy (Gilman and Philips, 1946).

At present five major types of alkylating agents are used in the chemotherapy of neoplastic diseases: (1) the nitrogen mustards; (2) the ethyleneimines; (3) the alkyl sulfonates; (4) the nitrosoureas; and (5) the triazenes. In addition, for pedagogical reasons, the methylhydrazine and platinum complexes are included under alkylating agents, even though the latter do not formally alkylate DNA and exhibit a different means to form covalent adducts with DNA.

Chemistry. The chemotherapeutic alkylating agents have in common the property of becoming strong electrophiles through the formation of carbonium ion intermediates or related transition complexes. These reactive intermediates form covalent linkages by alkylation of various nucleophilic moieties such as phosphate, ami-

Figure 51–3. Mechanism of action of alkylating agents.

no, sulfhydryl, hydroxyl, carboxyl, and imidazole groups. Their chemotherapeutic and cytotoxic effects are directly related to the alkylation of DNA. The 7 nitrogen atom of guanine is particularly susceptible to the formation of a covalent bond with bifunctional alkylating agents and may well represent the key target that determines their biological effects. Other atoms in the purine and pyrimidine bases of DNA, including N1 and N3 of adenine, N3 of cytosine, and O6 of guanine, react to form bonds with these agents, as do the amino and sulfhydryl groups of proteins.

The possible actions of alkylating agents on DNA are illustrated in Figure 51–3 with *mechlorethamine* (nitrogen mustard). First, one 2-chloroethyl side chain undergoes a first-order (S_N1) intramolecular cyclization, with release of Cl$^-$ and formation of a highly reactive ethyleniminium intermediate (Figure 51–3). The tertiary amine then is converted to an unstable quaternary ammonium compound, which can react avidly, through formation of a carbonium ion, with a variety of high electron density sites. This reaction proceeds as a second-order (S_N2) nucleophilic substitution. Alkylation of the N7 of guanine residues in DNA (Figure 51–3), a highly favored reaction, may exert several effects of considerable biological importance. Normally, guanine residues in DNA exist predominantly as the keto tautomer and readily make Watson-Crick base pairs by hydrogen bonding with cytosine residues. However, when the N7 of guanine is alkylated (to become a quaternary ammonium nitrogen), the guanine residue is more acidic and the enol tautomer is favored. The modified guanine can mispair with thymine residues during DNA synthesis, leading to the substitution of an adenine–thymine base pair for a guanine–cytosine base pair. Second, alkylation of the N7 labilizes the imidazole ring, making possible the opening of the imidazole ring or depurination by excision of guanine residues. Either of these changes must be repaired. Third, with bifunctional alkylating agents such as nitrogen mustard, the second 2-chloroethyl side chain can undergo a similar cyclization reaction and alkylate a second guanine residue or another nucleophilic moiety, resulting in

MECHLORETHAMINE

CYCLOPHOSPHAMIDE

IFOSFAMIDE

MELPHALAN

CHLORAMBUCIL

Figure 51–4. *Nitrogen mustards employed in therapy.*

the cross-linking of two nucleic acid chains or the linking of a nucleic acid to a protein, alterations that would cause a major disruption in nucleic acid function. Any of these effects could adequately explain both the mutagenic and the cytotoxic effects of alkylating agents. However, cytotoxicity of bifunctional alkylators correlates very closely with interstrand cross-linkage of DNA (Garcia *et al.*, 1988).

The ultimate cause of cell death related to DNA damage is not known. Specific cellular responses include cell-cycle arrest and attempts to repair DNA. Alternatively, recognition of extensively damaged DNA by p53 can trigger apoptosis. Mutations of p53 lead to alkylating-agent resistance (Kastan, 1999).

Structure–Activity Relationship. The alkylating agents used in chemotherapy share the capacity to contribute alkyl groups to biologically vital macromolecules such as DNA. Modification of the basic chloroethylamine structure changes reactivity, lipophilicity, active transport across biological membranes, sites of macromolecular attack, and mechanisms of DNA repair, all of which properties determine drug activity *in vivo*. With several of the most valuable agents (*e.g.*, cyclophosphamide and *ifosfamide*), the active alkylating moieties are generated *in vivo* after metabolism.

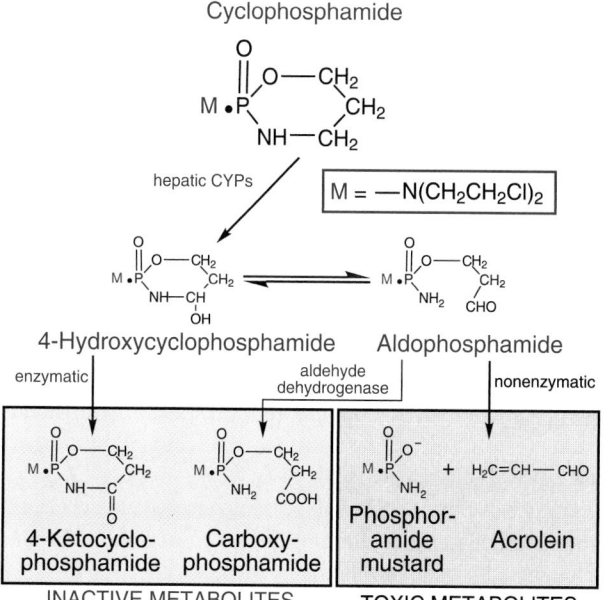

Figure 51–5. *Metabolism of cyclophosphamide.*

The biological activity of nitrogen mustards is based upon the presence of the *bis*-(2-chloroethyl) grouping. While mechlorethamine has been widely used in the past, linkage of the *bis*-(2-chloroethyl) group to election-rich substitutions such as unsaturated ring systems has yielded more stable drugs with greater selective killing of tumor cells. *Bis*-(2-chloroethyl) groups have been linked to amino acids (phenylalanine) and substituted phenyl groups (aminophenol butyric acid, as in *chlorambucil*) in an effort to make a more stable and orally available form. The rationale for the synthesis of cyclophosphamide can be found in previous editions of this textbook. The structures of important nitrogen mustards are shown in Figure 51–4.

A classical example of the role of host metabolism in the activation of an alkylating agent is seen with cyclophosphamide, now the most widely used agent of this class. The drug undergoes metabolic activation (hydroxylation) by cytochrome P450 isoenzyme 2B (CYP2B) (Figure 51–5), with subsequent transport of the activated intermediate to sites of action, as discussed below. The selectivity of cyclophosphamide against certain malignant tissues may result in part from the capacity of normal tissues, such as liver, to protect themselves against cytotoxicity by enzymatic degradation of the activated intermediates *via* aldehyde dehydrogenase, glutathione transferase, and other pathways.

Ifosfamide is an oxazaphosphorine, similar to cyclophosphamide. Cyclophosphamide has two chloroethyl groups on the exocyclic nitrogen atom, whereas one of the two-chloroethyl groups of ifosfamide is on the cyclic phosphoamide nitrogen of the oxazaphosphorine ring. Ifosfamide is activated in the liver by CYP3A4. The activation of ifosfamide proceeds more slowly, with greater production of dechlorinated metabolites and chloroacetaldehyde. These differences in metabolism likely account for the higher doses of ifosfamide required for equitoxic effects, the greater neurotoxicity of ifosfamide, and the possible differences in antitumor spectrum of the two agents (Furlanut and Franceschi, 2003).

Although initially considered an antimetabolite, the triazene derivative 5-(3,3-dimethyl-1-triazeno)-imidazole-4-carboxamide, usually referred to as *dacarbazine* or DTIC, functions through alkylation. Its structural formula is:

DACARBAZINE

Dacarbazine requires initial activation by the CYP system of the liver through an *N*-demethylation reaction. In the target cell, spontaneous cleavage of the metabolite, methyltriazenoimidazolecarboxamide (MTIC) yields an alkylating moiety, a methyl diazonium ion. A related triazene, *temozolomide,* undergoes spontaneous, nonenzymatic activation to MTIC, and has significant activity against gliomas. Its structure is:

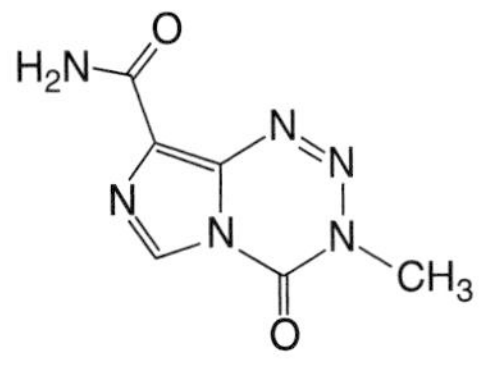

TEMOZOLOMIDE

The nitrosoureas, which include compounds such as 1,3-*bis*-(2-chloroethyl)-1-nitrosourea (*carmustine*; BCNU), 1-(2-chloroethyl)-3-cyclohexyl-1-nitrosourea (*lomustine*; CCNU), and its methyl derivative (*semustine*; methyl-CCNU), as well as the antibiotic *streptozocin* (streptozotocin), exert their cytotoxicity through the spontaneous breakdown to an alkylating intermediate, the 2-chloroethyl diazonium ion. The structural formula of carmustine is:

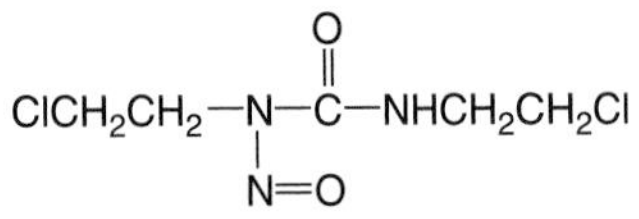

CARMUSTINE (BCNU)

The 2-chloroethyl diazonium ion, a strong electrophile, can alkylate a variety of substances; guanine, cytidine, and adenine adducts have been identified (Ludlum, 1990). Displacement of the halogen atom can then lead to interstrand or intrastrand cross-linking of the DNA. The formation of the cross-links after the initial alkylation reaction is relatively slow and can be interrupted by the DNA repair enzyme O^6-alkyl, alkyl guanine transferase (AGT) (Dolan *et al.,* 1990), which displaces the chloroethyl adduct from its binding to guanine in a suicide reaction. The same enzyme, when expressed in human gliomas, produces resistance to nitrosoureas (Middleton and Margison, 2003) and various methylating agents, including DTIC, temozolomide, and *procarbazine.* As with the nitrogen mustards, interstrand cross-linking appears to be the primary lesion responsible for the cytotoxicity of nitrosoureas (Ludlum, 1990). The reactions of the nitrosoureas with macromolecules are shown in Figure 51–6.

Since the formation of the ethyleniminium ion constitutes the initial reaction of the nitrogen mustards, it is not surprising that stable ethyleneimine derivatives have antitumor activity. Several compounds of this type, including *triethylenemelamine* (TEM) and *triethylene thiophosphoramide* (thiotepa), have been used clinically. In standard doses, thiotepa produces little toxicity other than myelosuppression; it also is used for high-dose chemotherapy regimens, in which it causes both mucosal and central nervous system toxicity. *Altretamine* (hexamethylmelamine; HMM) is mentioned here because of its chemical similarity to TEM. The methylmelamines are *N*-demethylated by hepatic microsomes (Friedman, 2001) with the release of formaldehyde, and there is a direct relationship between the degree of the demethylation and their activity against murine tumors.

Esters of alkanesulfonic acids alkylate DNA through the release of methyl radicals. *Busulfan* is of value in the treatment of CML and in high-dose chemotherapy; its structural formula is:

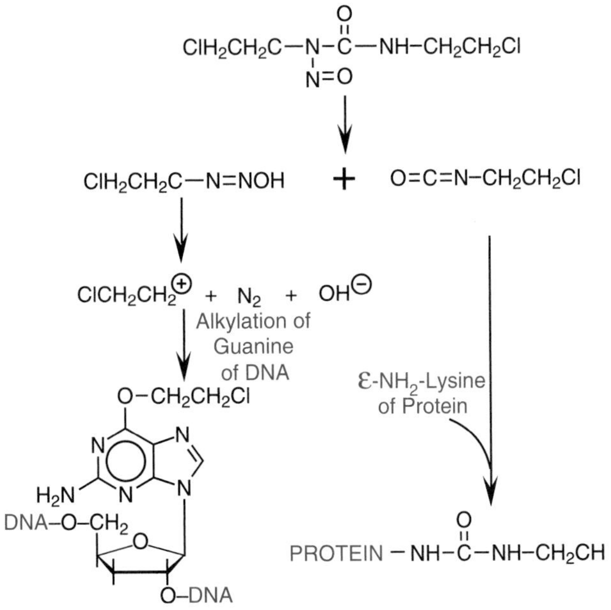

Figure 51–6. *Degradation of carmustine (BCNU) with generation of alkylating and carbamoylating intermediates.*

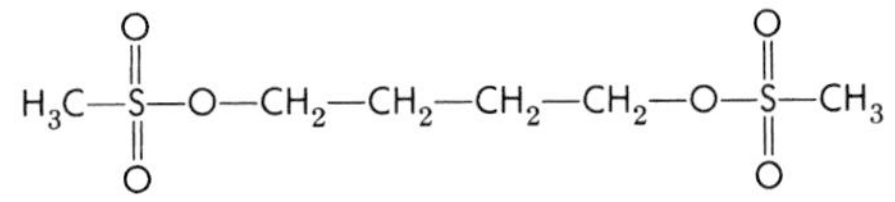

BUSULFAN

Pharmacological Actions

Cytotoxic Actions. The most important pharmacological actions of the alkylating agents are those that disturb DNA synthesis and cell division. The capacity of these drugs to interfere with DNA integrity and function and to induce cell death in rapidly proliferating tissues provides the basis for their therapeutic and toxic properties. Whereas certain alkylating agents may have damaging effects on tissues with normally low mitotic indices—for example, liver, kidney, and mature lymphocytes—these tissues usually are affected in a delayed time frame. Acute effects are manifest primarily against rapidly proliferating tissues. Lethality of DNA alkylation depends on the recognition of the adduct, the creation of DNA strand breaks by repair enzymes, and an intact apoptotic response. The actual mechanism(s) of cell death related to DNA alkylation are not yet well characterized.

In nondividing cells, DNA damage activates a checkpoint that depends on the presence of a normal p53 gene. Cells thus blocked in the G_1/S interface either repair DNA alkylation or undergo apoptosis. Malignant cells with mutant or absent p53 fail to suspend cell-cycle progression, do not undergo apoptosis (Fisher, 1994), and exhibit resistance to these drugs.

While DNA is the ultimate target of all alkylating agents, a crucial distinction must be made between the bifunctional agents, in which cytotoxic effects predominate, and the monofunctional methylating agents (procarbazine, temozolomide), which have greater capacity for mutagenesis and carcinogenesis. This suggests that the cross-linking of DNA strands represents a much greater threat to cellular survival than do other effects, such as single-base alkylation and the resulting depurination and chain scission. On the other hand, the more frequent methylation may be bypassed by DNA polymerases, leading to mispairing reactions that permanently modify DNA sequence. These new sequences are transmitted to subsequent generations, and may result in mutagenesis or carcinogenesis. Some methylating agents, such as procarbazine, are highly carcinogenic.

The DNA repair systems play an important role in removing adducts, and thereby determine the selectivity of action against particular cell types, and acquired resistance to alkylating agents. Alkylation of a single strand of DNA (mono adducts) is repaired by the nucleotide excision repair pathway, while the less frequent cross-links require participation of nonhomologous end joining, an error-prone pathway, or the error-free homologenous recombination pathway. After drug infusion in humans, mono adducts appear rapidly and peak within 2 hours of drug exposure, while cross-links peak at 8 hours. The half-lives for repair of adducts varies among normal tissues and tumors; in peripheral blood mononuclear cells, both mono adducts and cross-links disappear with a half-life of 12 to 16 hours (Souliotis *et al.*, 2003).

The homologous end-joining pathway has multiple components: sensors of DNA integrity (such as p53); activation signals such as the ataxia-telangiectasia-mutated (ATM) and ataxia-telangiectasia and rad-related (ATR) proteins; the activated repair complex composed of Fanconi anemia proteins and BRCA2, which localize at the site of DNA damage and initiate removal of the cross-linked segment of DNA; and homologous recombination, which allows resynthesis of the damaged DNA sequence followed by religation of the repaired sequences (Wang *et al.*, 2001). The process depends on the presence and accurate functioning of multiple proteins. Their absence or mutation, as in Fanconi anemia or ataxia telangiectasia, leads to extreme sensitivity to DNA cross-linking agents such as *mitomycin, cisplatin*, or classical alkylators (Venkitaraman, 2004).

Other repair enzymes specific for removing methyl and ethyl adducts from the O6 of guanine (AGT) and from the N3 of adenine and N7 of guanine (3-methyladenine-DNA glycosylase) have been identified (Matijasevic *et al.*, 1993). High expression of AGT protects cells from cytotoxic effects of nitrosoureas and methylating agents and confers drug resistance, while methylation and silencing of the gene in brain tumors is associated with high response rates to BCNU and improved survival (Esteller and Herman, 2004).

Detailed information is lacking on mechanisms of cellular uptake of alkylating agents. Mechlorethamine enters murine tumor cells by an active transport system, the natural substrate of which is choline. *Melphalan*, an analog of phenylalanine, is taken up by at least two active transport systems that carry leucine and other neutral amino acids. The highly lipophilic drugs, including nitrosoureas, carmustine, and lomustine, diffuse into cells passively.

Mechanisms of Resistance to Alkylating Agents. Resistance to an alkylating agent develops rapidly when it is used as a single agent. Specific biochemical changes implicated in the development of resistance include:

1. Decreased permeation of actively transported drugs (mechlorethamine and melphalan);
2. Increased intracellular concentrations of nucleophilic substances, principally thiols such as glutathione, which can conjugate with and detoxify electrophilic intermediates;
3. Increased activity of DNA repair pathways, which may differ for the various alkylating agents. Thus, increased activity of the complex nucleotide excision repair (NER) pathway seems to correlate with resistance to most chloroethyl and platinum adducts (Taniguchi *et al.*, 2003). AGT activity determines response to BCNU and to methylating drugs such as the triazenes, procarbazine and busulfan (Middleton and Margison, 2003); and
4. Increased rates of metabolism of the activated forms of cyclophosphamide and ifosfamide to their inactive keto and carboxy metabolites by aldehyde dehydrogenase (Figure 51–5).

To reverse cellular changes that lead to resistance, strategies have been devised that are effective in selected experimental tumors. These include the use of compounds that deplete glutathione, such as L-*buthionine-sulfoximine;* sulfhydryl compounds such as amifostine (WR-2721) that selectively detoxify alkylating species in normal cells and thereby prevent toxicity; O^6-*benzylguanine*, which inactivates the guanine O^6-alkyl transferase DNA repair enzyme; and compounds such as *ethacrynic acid* that inhibit the enzymes (glutathione transferases) that conjugate thiols with alkylating agents. While each of these modalities has experimental evidence to support its use, they all have the potential of increasing toxicity, and their clinical efficacy has not yet been proven. O^6-benzylguanine has advanced to phase II trials used in conjunction with carmustine or procarbazine against malignant gliomas (Middleton and Margison, 2003).

TOXICITIES OF ALKYLATING AGENTS

Bone Marrow Toxicity

The alkylating agents differ in their patterns of antitumor activity and in the sites and severity of their side effects. Most cause dose-limiting toxicity to bone marrow elements, and to a lesser extent, intestinal mucosa. Most alkylating agents, including nitrogen mustard, melphalan, chlorambucil, cyclophosphamide, and ifosfamide, cause acute myelosuppression, with a nadir of the peripheral blood granulocyte count at 6 to 10 days and recovery in 14 to 21 days. Cyclophosphamide has lesser effects on peripheral blood platelet counts than do the other agents. Busulfan suppresses all blood elements, particularly stem cells, and

Table 51–2
Dose-Limiting Extramedullary Toxicities of Single Alkylating Agents

DRUG	MTD,* mg/m²	FOLD INCREASE OVER STANDARD DOSE	MAJOR ORGAN TOXICITIES
Cyclophosphamide	7000	7	Cardiac, hepatic VOD
Ifosfamide	16,000	2.7	Renal, CNS, hepatic VOD
Thiotepa	1000	18	GI, CNS, hepatic VOD
Melphalan	180	5.6	GI, hepatic VOD
Busulfan	640	9	GI, hepatic VOD
Carmustine (BCNU)	1050	5.3	Lung, hepatic VOD
Cisplatin	200	2	PN, renal
Carboplatin	2000	5	Renal, PN, hepatic VOD

*Maximum tolerated dose (MTD; cumulative) in treatment protocols. Abbreviations: GI, gastrointestinal; CNS, central nervous system; PN, peripheral neuropathy; VOD, veno-occlusive disease.

may produce a prolonged and cumulative myelosuppression lasting months or even years. For this reason, it is used as a preparative regimen in allogenic bone marrow transplantation. Carmustine and other chloroethylnitrosoureas cause delayed and prolonged suppression of both platelets and granulocytes, reaching a nadir 4 to 6 weeks after drug administration and reversing slowly thereafter.

Both cellular and humoral immunity are suppressed by alkylating agents, which have been used to treat various autoimmune diseases. Immunosuppression is reversible at doses used in most anticancer protocols.

Mucosal Toxicity

In addition to effects on the hematopoietic system, alkylating agents are highly toxic to dividing mucosal cells, leading to oral mucosal ulceration and intestinal denudation. The mucosal effects are particularly significant in high-dose chemotherapy protocols associated with bone marrow reconstitution, as they predispose to bacterial sepsis arising from the gastrointestinal tract. In these protocols, cyclophosphamide, melphalan, and thiotepa have the advantage of causing less mucosal damage than the other agents. In high-dose protocols, however, a number of additional toxicities become limiting. They are listed in Table 51–2.

Neurotoxicity

CNS toxicity is manifest in the form of nausea and vomiting, particularly after intravenous administration of nitrogen mustard or BCNU. Ifosfamide is the most neurotoxic of this class of agents, producing altered mental status, coma, generalized seizures, and cerebellar ataxia. These

side effects have been linked to the release of chloroacetaldehyde from the phosphate-linked chloroethyl side chain of ifosfamide. High-dose busulfan may cause seizures; in addition, it accelerates the clearance of *phenytoin*, an antiseizure medication (*see* Chapter 19).

Other Organ Toxicities

While mucosal and bone marrow toxicities occur predictably and acutely with conventional doses of these drugs, other organ toxicities may occur after prolonged or high-dose use; these effects can appear after months or years, and may be irreversible and even lethal. All alkylating agents have caused pulmonary fibrosis, usually several months after treatment. In high-dose regimens, particularly those employing busulfan or BCNU, vascular endothelial damage may precipitate veno-occlusive disease (VOD) of the liver, an often fatal side effect that is successfully reversed by the investigational drug *defibrotide* (Richardson, 2003). The nitrosoureas and ifosfamide, after multiple cycles of therapy, may lead to renal failure. Cyclophosphamide and ifosfamide release a nephrotoxic and urotoxic metabolite, acrolein, which causes a severe hemorrhagic cystitis, a side effect that in high-dose regimens can be prevented by coadministration of *2-mercaptoethanesulfonate* (mesna or MESNEX), which conjugates acrolein in urine. Ifosfamide in high doses for transplant causes a chronic, and often irreversible, renal toxicity. Proximal, and less commonly distal, tubules may be affected, with difficulties in Ca^{2+} and Mg^{2+} reabsorption, glycosuria, and renal tubular acidosis. Nephrotoxicity is correlated with the total dose of drug received and increases in frequency in children less than 5 years of age. The syndrome has been attributed to chloroacetaldehyde and/or acrolein excreted in the urine (Skinner, 2003).

The more unstable alkylating agents (particularly mechlorethamine and the nitrosoureas) have strong vesicant properties, damage veins with repeated use, and if extravasated, produce ulceration. Most alkylating agents cause alopecia.

Finally, all alkylating agents have toxic effects on the male and female reproductive systems, causing an often permanent amenorrhea, particularly in perimenopausal women, and an irreversible azoospermia in men.

Leukemogenesis

As a class of drugs, the alkylating agents are highly leukemogenic. Acute nonlymphocytic leukemia, often associated with partial or total deletions of chromosome 5 or 7, peaks in incidence about 4 years after therapy and may affect up to 5% of patients treated on regimens containing alkylating drugs (Levine and Bloomfield, 1992). It often is preceded by a period of neutropenia or anemia, and bone marrow morphology consistent with myelodysplasia. Melphalan, the nitrosoureas, and the methylating agent procarbazine have the greatest propensity to cause leukemia, while it is less common with cyclophosphamide.

CLINICAL PHARMACOLOGY

Nitrogen Mustards

The chemistry and the pharmacological actions of the alkylating agents as a group, and of the nitrogen mustards, have been presented above. Only the unique pharmacological characteristics of the individual agents are considered below.

Mechlorethamine. Mechlorethamine was the first clinically used nitrogen mustard and is the most reactive of the drugs in this class.

Absorption and Fate. Severe local reactions of exposed tissues necessitate rapid intravenous injection of mechlorethamine for most clinical uses. In either water or body fluids, at rates affected markedly by pH, mechlorethamine rapidly undergoes chemical degradation as it combines with either water or cellular nucleophiles, and the parent compound disappears within minutes from the bloodstream.

Therapeutic Uses. Mechlorethamine HCl (MUSTARGEN) was formerly used primarily in the combination chemotherapy regimen MOPP (mechlorethamine, *vincristine* [ONCOVIN], procarbazine, and *prednisone*) in patients with Hodgkin's disease. It is given by intravenous bolus administration in doses of 6 mg/m^2 on days 1 and 8 of the 28-day cycles of each course of treatment. It has been largely replaced by cyclophosphamide, melphalan, and other more stable alkylating agents.

It also is used topically for treatment of cutaneous T-cell lymphoma as a solution that is rapidly mixed and applied to affected areas of skin.

Clinical Toxicity. The major acute toxic manifestations of mechlorethamine are nausea and vomiting, lacrimation, and myelosuppression. Leukopenia and thrombocytopenia limit the amount of drug that can be given in a single course.

Like other alkylating agents, nitrogen mustard blocks reproductive function and may produce menstrual irregularities or premature ovarian failure in women and oligospermia in men. Since fetal abnormalities can be induced, this drug as well as other alkylating agents should not be used in the first trimester of pregnancy and should only be used with caution in later stages of pregnancy. Breast-feeding must be terminated before therapy with mechlorethamine is initiated.

Local reactions to extravasation of mechlorethamine into the subcutaneous tissue result in a severe, brawny, tender induration that may persist for a long time. If the local reaction is unusually severe, a slough may result. If it is obvious that extravasation has occurred, the involved area should be promptly infiltrated with a sterile isotonic solution of sodium thiosulfate (167 mM); an ice compress then should be applied intermittently for 6 to 12 hours. Thiosulfate reacts avidly with nitrogen mustard and thereby protects tissue constituents.

Cyclophosphamide. ***Pharmacological and Cytotoxic Actions.*** The general cytotoxic action of this drug is similar to that of other alkylating agents. The drug is not a vesicant, and produces no local irritation.

Absorption, Fate, and Excretion. Cyclophosphamide is well absorbed orally. The drug is activated by CYP2B (Xie *et al.*, 2003) to 4-hydroxycyclophosphamide (Figure 51–5), which is in a steady state with the acyclic tautomer aldophosphamide. A closely related oxazaphosphorine, ifosfamide, is hydroxylated by CYP3A4. This difference may account for the somewhat slower activation of ifosfamide *in vivo*, and the interpatient variability in toxicity of both molecules. The rate of metabolic activation of cyclophosphamide exhibits significant interpatient variability and increases with successive doses in high-dose regimens, but appears to be saturable above infusion rates of 4 g/90 minutes and concentrations of parent compound above 150 μM (Chen *et al.*, 1995). 4-Hydroxycyclophosphamide may be oxidized further by aldehyde oxidase, either in liver or in tumor tissue, and perhaps by other enzymes, yielding the inactive metabolites carboxyphosphamide and 4-ketocyclophosphamide, and ifosfamide is inactivated in an analogous reaction. The active cyclophosphamide metabolites such as 4-hydroxycyclophosphamide and its tautomer, aldophosphamide, are carried in the circulation to tumor cells where aldophosphamide cleaves spontaneously, generating stoichiometric amounts of phosphoramide mustard and acrolein. Phosphoramide mustard is responsible for antitumor effects, while acrolein causes hemorrhagic cystitis often seen during therapy with cyclophosphamide. As mentioned above, cystitis can be reduced in intensity or prevented by the parenteral coadministration of mesna. Mesna does not negate the systemic antitumor activity of the drug.

For routine clinical use, ample fluid intake is recommended and vigorous intravenous hydration is required during high-dose treatment. Brisk hematuria in a patient receiving daily oral therapy should lead to immediate drug discontinuation. Refractory bladder hemorrhage may require cystectomy for control of bleeding.

The syndrome of inappropriate secretion of antidiuretic hormone has been observed in patients receiving cyclophosphamide, usually at doses higher than 50 mg/kg (DeFronzo *et al.*, 1973) (*see* Chapter 29). It is important to be aware of the possibility of water intoxication, since these patients usually are vigorously hydrated to prevent bladder toxicity.

Pretreatment with CYP inducers such as phenobarbital enhances the rate of activation of the azoxyphosphorenes but does not alter total exposure to active metabolites over time and does not affect toxicity or therapeutic activity in humans (Jao *et al.*, 1972). Cyclophosphamide can be used in full doses in patients with renal dysfunction, as it is eliminated by hepatic metabolism.

Urinary and fecal recovery of unchanged cyclophosphamide is minimal after intravenous administration. Maximal concentrations in plasma are achieved 1 hour after oral administration, and the half-life of parent drug in plasma is about 7 hours.

Therapeutic Uses. Cyclophosphamide (CYTOXAN, NEO-SAR, others) is administered orally or intravenously. Recommended doses vary widely, and published protocols for the dosage of cyclophosphamide and other chemotherapeutic agents and for the method and sequence of administration should be consulted.

As a single agent, a daily oral dose of 100 mg/m^2 for 14 days has been recommended as adjuvant therapy for breast cancer, and for patients with lymphomas and chronic lymphocytic leukemia. A higher dosage of 500 mg/m^2 intravenously every 2 to 4 weeks in combination with other drugs often is employed in the treatment of breast cancer and lymphomas. The neutrophil nadir of 500 to 1000 cells per mm^3 generally serves as a guide to dosage adjustments in prolonged therapy. In regimens associated with bone marrow or peripheral stem cell rescue, cyclophosphamide may be given in total doses of 5 to 7 g/m^2 over a 3- to 5-day period. Gastrointestinal ulceration, cystitis (counteracted by mesna and diuresis), and less commonly pulmonary, renal, hepatic, and cardiac toxicities (a hemorrhagic myocardial necrosis) may occur after high-dose therapy with total doses above 200 mg/kg.

The clinical spectrum of activity for cyclophosphamide is very broad. It is an essential component of many effective drug combinations for non-Hodgkin's lymphomas, ovarian cancers, and solid tumors in children. Complete remissions and presumed cures have been reported when cyclophosphamide was given as a single agent for Burkitt's lymphoma. It frequently is used in combination with methotrexate (or *doxorubicin*) and fluorouracil as adjuvant therapy after surgery for carcinoma of the breast.

Because of its potent immunosuppressive properties, cyclophosphamide has been used to prevent organ rejection after transplantation. It has activity in nonneoplastic disorders associated with altered immune reactivity, including Wegener's granulomatosis, rheumatoid arthritis, and the nephrotic syndrome. Caution is advised when the drug is considered for use in these conditions, not only because of its acute toxic effects but also because of its potential for inducing sterility, teratogenic effects, and leukemia.

Ifosfamide. Ifosfamide (IFEX), an analog of cyclophosphamide, also is activated by ring hydroxylation in the liver. Severe urinary tract and CNS toxicity limited the use of ifosfamide when it first was introduced in the early 1970s. However, adequate hydration and coadministration of mesna have reduced its bladder toxicity.

Therapeutic Uses. Ifosfamide is approved for use in combination for germ cell testicular cancer and is widely used to treat pediatric and adult sarcomas. It is a common component of high-dose chemotherapy regimens with bone marrow or stem cell rescue; in these regimens, in total doses of 12 to 14 g/m^2, it may cause severe neurological toxicity, including hallucinations, coma, and death, with symptoms appearing 12 hours to 7 days after beginning the ifosfamide infusion. This toxicity is thought to result from a metabolite, chloroacetaldehyde.

Although the clinical experience is limited, administration of methylene blue, 50 mg, the day before ifosfamide and three times per day during drug infusion, lowers the incidence of neurotoxicity from a high of 30% to near zero (Nicolao and Giometto, 2003). In addition, ifosfamide causes nausea, vomiting, anorexia, leukopenia, nephrotoxicity, and veno-occlusive disease of the liver.

In nonmyeloablative regimens, ifosfamide is infused intravenously over at least 30 minutes at a dose of up to 1.2 g/m^2 per day for 5 days. Intravenous mesna is given as bolus injections in a dosage equal to 20% of the ifosfamide dosage concomitantly and again 4 and 8 hours later, for a total mesna dose of 60% of the ifosfamide dose. Alternatively, mesna may be given concomitantly in a single dose equal to the ifosfamide dose. Patients also should receive at least 2 L of oral or intravenous fluid daily. Treatment cycles usually are repeated every 3 to 4 weeks.

Pharmacokinetics. The parent compound, ifosfamide, has an elimination half-life in plasma of approximately 15 hours after doses of 3.8 to 5 g/m^2 and a somewhat shorter half-life at lower doses, although its pharmacokinetics are highly variable from patient to patient due to variable rates of hepatic metabolism.

Toxicity. Ifosfamide has virtually the same toxicity profile as cyclophosphamide, although it causes greater platelet suppression, neurotoxicity, nephrotoxicity, and in the absence of mesna, urothelial damage.

Melphalan. *Pharmacological and Cytotoxic Actions.*
The general pharmacological and cytotoxic actions of melphalan, the phenylalanine derivative of nitrogen mustard, are similar to those of other mechlorethamine. The drug is not a vesicant.

Absorption, Fate, and Excretion. When given orally, melphalan is absorbed in an incomplete and variable manner, and 20% to 50% of the drug is recovered in the stool. The drug has a half-life in plasma of approximately 45 to 90 minutes, and 10% to 15% of an administered dose is excreted unchanged in the urine (Alberts *et al.*, 1979). Patients with decreased renal failure may develop unexpectedly severe myelosuppression (Cornwell *et al.*, 1982).

Therapeutic Uses. Oral *melphalan* (ALKERAN) for multiple myeloma is used in doses of 6 to 8 mg daily for a period of 4 days, in combination with other agents. A rest period of up to 4 weeks should then intervene. The usual intravenous dose is 15 mg/m^2 infused over 15 to 20 minutes. Doses are repeated at 2-week intervals for four doses and then at 4-week intervals based on response and tolerance. Dosage adjustments should be considered based on blood cell counts and in patients with renal impairment.

Melphalan also may be used in myeloablative regimens followed by bone marrow or peripheral blood stem cell reconstitution. For this use, the dose is 180 to 200 mg/m^2.

Clinical Toxicity. The clinical toxicity of melphalan is mostly hematological and is similar to that of other alkylating agents. Nausea and vomiting are less frequent. Alopecia does not occur at standard doses, and changes in renal or hepatic function have not been observed.

Chlorambucil. *Pharmacological and Cytotoxic Actions.*
The cytotoxic effects of chlorambucil on the bone marrow, lymphoid organs, and epithelial tissues are similar to those observed with the nitrogen mustards. As an orally

administered agent, chlorambucil is well tolerated in small daily doses, and provides flexible titration of blood counts. Nausea and vomiting may result from single oral doses of 20 mg or more.

Absorption, Fate, and Excretion. Oral absorption of chlorambucil is adequate and reliable. The drug has a half-life in plasma of approximately 1.5 hours, and it is almost completely metabolized (Alberts *et al.*, 1979) to phenyl acetic acid mustard and to decomposition products.

Therapeutic Uses. In treating chronic lymphocytic leukemia (CLL), the standard initial daily dosage of chlorambucil (LEUKE-RAN) is 0.1 to 0.2 mg/kg, given once daily and continued for 3 to 6 weeks. With a fall in the peripheral total leukocyte count or clinical improvement, the dosage is titrated to maintain neutrophils and platelets at acceptable levels. Maintenance therapy (usually 2 mg daily) often is required to maintain clinical remission.

It is a standard agent for patients with chronic lymphocytic leukemia and primary (Waldenström's) macroglobulinemia, and may be used for follicular lymphoma.

Clinical Toxicity. In CLL, chlorambucil may be given orally for months or years, achieving its effects gradually and often without significant toxicity to a compromised bone marrow.

Although it is possible to induce marked hypoplasia of the bone marrow with excessive doses of chlorambucil administered over long periods, its myelosuppressive action usually is moderate, gradual, and rapidly reversible. GI discomfort, azoospermia, amenorrhea, pulmonary fibrosis, seizures, dermatitis, and hepatotoxicity may rarely be encountered. A marked increase in the incidence of acute myelocytic leukemia (AML) and other tumors was noted in a large controlled study of its use for the treatment of polycythemia vera by the National Polycythemia Vera Study Group and in patients with breast cancer receiving chlorambucil as adjuvant chemotherapy (Lerner, 1978).

MISCELLANEOUS ALKYLATING DRUGS

While nitrogen mustards containing chlorethyl groups constitute the most widely used class of alkylating agents, alternative structures with greater chemical stability and defined activity in specific types of cancer continue to have value in clinical practice.

Ethylenimines and Methylmelamines

Altretamine. **Pharmacology and Cytotoxic Effects.** Altretamine (HEXALEN), formerly known as hexamethylmelamine, is structurally similar to the alkylating agent triethylenemelamine (*tretamine*). However, *in vitro* tests for alkylating activity of altretamine and its metabolites have been negative, and the precise mechanism of the cytotoxic action of altretamine is unknown. It is used as a palliative treatment for persistent or recurrent ovarian cancer following treatment failure with a cisplatin- or alkylating agent–

based combination. A review of the pharmacodynamic and pharmacokinetic properties and clinical use has been published by Lee and Faulds (1995). The usual dose of altretamine as a single agent in ovarian cancer is 260 mg/m^2 daily in four divided doses, for 14 or 21 consecutive days out of a 28-day cycle, for up to 12 cycles.

Absorption, Fate and Excretion. Following oral administration, altretamine is well absorbed from the GI tract and undergoes rapid demethylation in the liver. Peak plasma levels, which vary widely, are reached between 0.5 and 3 hours. The principal metabolites are pentamethylmelamine and tetramethylmelamine, which are highly bound to plasma proteins (75% and 50%, respectively) and excreted *via* the urine. The elimination half-life is reported to be 4 to 10 hours (Damia and D'Incalci, 1995).

Clinical Toxicities. The main toxicities of altretamine are myelosuppression and neurotoxicity. Altretamine causes both peripheral and central neurotoxicity. CNS symptoms include ataxia, depression, confusion, drowsiness, hallucinations, dizziness, and vertigo. Neurologic toxicity appears to be reversible upon discontinuation of therapy and may be prevented or decreased by concomitant administration of *pyridoxine*, although this remains unproven. Peripheral blood counts and a neurologic examination should be performed prior to the initiation of each course of therapy. Therapy should be interrupted for at least 14 days, and subsequently restarted at a lower dose of 200 mg/m^2 daily, if the white cell count falls below 2000 cells/mm^3 or the platelet count below 75,000 cells/mm^3 or if neurotoxic or intolerable gastrointestinal symptoms occur. If neurologic symptoms fail to stabilize on the reduced dose schedule, altretamine should be discontinued. Nausea and vomiting also are common side effects and may be dose-limiting. Renal toxicity also may be dose-limiting. Other rare adverse effects include rashes, alopecia, and hepatic toxicity. Severe, life-threatening orthostatic hypotension developed in patients who received amitriptyline, imipramine, or phenelzine concurrently with altretamine (Bruckner and Schleifer, 1983).

Thiotepa. **Pharmacological and Cytotoxic Effects.** Thiotepa (THIOPLEX) is composed of three ethyleneimine groups stabilized by attachment to the nucleophilic thiophosphoryl base. Its current use is primarily for high-dose chemotherapy regimens.

Both thiotepa and its desulfurated primary metabolite, triethylenephosphoramide (TEPA), to which it is rapidly converted by hepatic CYPs (Ng and Waxman, 1991), form DNA cross-links. The aziridine rings open after protonation of the ring-nitrogen, leading to a reactive molecule.

Absorption, Fate, and Excretion. TEPA becomes the predominant form of the drug present in plasma within hours of thiotepa administration. The parent compound has a plasma half-life of 1.2 to 2 hours, as compared to a longer half-life of 3 to 24 hours for TEPA. Thiotepa pharmacokinetics are essentially the same in children as in adults at conventional doses (up to 80 mg/m^2), and drug and metabolite half-lives are unchanged in children receiving high-dose therapy of 300 mg/m^2 per day for 3 days. Less than 10% of the administered drug appears in urine as the parent drug or the primary metabolite. Multiple secondary metabolites and chemical degradation products account for the remainder of parent.

Clinical Toxicities. The toxicities of thiotepa are essentially the same as those of the other alkylating agents, namely myelosuppression, and to a lesser extent mucositis. Myelosuppression tends to develop somewhat later than with cyclophosphamide, with leukopenic nadirs at 2 weeks and platelet nadirs at 3 weeks. In high-dose regimens thiotepa produces neurotoxic symptoms, including coma and seizures.

Alkyl Sulfonates

Busulfan. ***Pharmacological and Cytotoxic Actions.*** Busulfan exerts few pharmacological actions other than myelosuppression at conventional doses, and prior to the advent of imatinib mesylate (GLEEVEC), often was used in the chronic phase of CML to suppress granulocyte counts. In some patients a severe and prolonged pancytopenia resulted. In high-dose regimens, pulmonary fibrosis, gastrointestinal mucosal damage, and veno-occlusive disease of the liver become important.

Absorption, Fate, and Excretion. Busulfan is well absorbed after oral administration in doses of 2 to 6 mg/day, and has a plasma half-life of 2 to 3 hours. The drug is conjugated to glutathione by glutathione S-transferase A1A and further degraded by CYP-dependent pathways, and its major urinary metabolite is methane sulfonic acid. In high doses, children under 18 years of age clear the drug two to four times faster than adults, and tolerate higher doses (Vassal *et al.*, 1993). A dose of 40 mg/m^2 given every 6 hours for 4 days has been suggested for children weighing less than 20 kg.

An intravenous preparation is available for high-dose regimens. With doses of 1 mg/kg every 6 hours for 4 days, peak drug concentrations reach up to 10 μM in adults, but are 1 to 5 μM in children 1 to 3 years of age, because of faster clearance. There is significant variability in busulfan clearance among patients. Veno-occlusive disease is associated with high AUC and peak drug levels (AUC >1500 μM x min) and slow clearance, leading to recommendations for dose adjustment based on drug level monitoring (Grochow, 1993). A target of C_{ss} = 600 to 900 ng/ml in adults or AUC <1000 μM x min in children appears to achieve an appropriate balance between toxicity and therapeutic benefit (Witherspoon *et al.*, 2001; Tran *et al.*, 2000).

Therapeutic Uses. In treating CML, the initial oral dose of busulfan (MYLERAN, BUSULFEX) varies with the total leukocyte count and the severity of the disease; daily doses from 2 to 8 mg for adults (~60 μg/kg or 1.8 mg/m^2 for children) are used to initiate therapy and are adjusted appropriately to subsequent hematological and clinical responses, with the aim of reduction of the total leukocyte count to ≤10,000 cells/mm^3. A decrease in the leukocyte count is not usually seen during the first 10 to 15 days of treatment and the leukocyte count may actually increase; during this period an increase in leukocyte count should not be interpreted as drug resistance nor should the dose be increased. Because the leukocyte count may fall for more than a month after discontinuing the drug, it is recommended that busulfan be withdrawn when the total leukocyte count has declined to ~15,000 cells/mm^3. A normal leukocyte count usually is achieved within 12 to 20 weeks. During remission, daily treatment resumes when the total leukocyte count reaches ~50,000

cells/mm^3. Daily maintenance doses are 1 to 3 mg. In high-dose therapy, doses of 1 mg/kg are given every 6 hours for 4 days, with adjustment based on pharmacokinetics.

High doses of busulfan also have been used effectively in combination with high doses of cyclophosphamide to prepare leukemia patients for bone marrow transplantation. In high-dose regimens, as a component of conditioning before bone marrow or peripheral blood progenitor cell replacement support, busulfan is given at 0.8 mg/kg every 6 hours for 4 days. Anticonvulsants must be used concomitantly to protect against acute CNS toxicities, including tonic-clonic seizures, which may occur several hours after each dose. Busulfan induces the metabolism of phenytoin. In patients requiring antiseizure medication, non-enzyme inducing drugs such as *lorazepam* are recommended as an alternative to phenytoin. When phenytoin is used concurrently, plasma busulfan levels should be monitored and the busulfan dose adjusted accordingly.

Clinical Toxicity. The major toxic effects of busulfan are related to its myelosuppressive properties, and prolonged thrombocytopenia may be a hazard. Occasional patients experience nausea, vomiting, and diarrhea. Long-term use leads to impotence, sterility, amenorrhea, and fetal malformation. Rarely, patients develop asthenia and hypotension, a syndrome resembling Addison's disease, but without abnormalities of corticosteroid production.

High-dose busulfan causes veno-occlusive disease of the liver in up to 10% of patients, as well as seizures, hemorrhagic cystitis, permanent alopecia, and cataracts. The coincidence of veno-occlusive disease and hepatotoxicity is increased by its coadministration with drugs that inhibit CYPs, including imidazoles and *metronidazole*, possibly through inhibition of the clearance of busulfan and/or its toxic metabolites (Nilsson *et al.*, 2003).

Nitrosoureas

The nitrosoureas have an important role in the treatment of brain tumors and find occasional use in treating lymphomas and in high-dose regimens with bone marrow reconstitution. They function as bifunctional alkylating agents but differ in both pharmacological and toxicological properties from conventional nitrogen mustards. Carmustine (BCNU) and lomustine (CCNU) are highly lipophilic, and thus readily cross the blood–brain barrier, an important property in the treatment of brain tumors. Unfortunately, with the exception of streptozocin, nitrosoureas cause profound and delayed myelosuppression with recovery 4 to 6 weeks after a single dose. Long-term treatment with the nitrosoureas, especially semustine (methyl-CCNU), has resulted in renal failure. As with other alkylating agents, the nitrosoureas are highly carcinogenic and mutagenic. They generate both alkylating and carbamoylating moieties as illustrated in Figure 51–6.

Carmustine (BCNU). ***Pharmacological and Cytotoxic Actions.*** Carmustine's major action is its alkylation of DNA at the O^6-guanine position, an adduct repaired by AGT. Methylation of the AGT promoter region inhibits its expression in about 30% of primary gliomas, and is associated with sensitivity to nitrosoureas. In high doses with bone marrow rescue, it produces hepatic veno-occlusive disease, pulmonary fibrosis, renal failure, and secondary leukemia (Tew *et al.*, 2001).

Absorption, Fate, and Excretion. Carmustine is unstable in aqueous solution and in body fluids. After intravenous infusion, it disappears from the plasma with a highly variable half-life of 15 to 90 minutes or longer (Levin *et al.*, 1978). Approximately 30% to 80% of the drug appears in the urine within 24 hours as degradation products. The entry of alkylating metabolites into the cerebrospinal fluid (CSF) is rapid, and their concentrations in the CSF are 15% to 30% of the concurrent plasma values.

Therapeutic Uses. When used alone, carmustine (BICNU) usually is administered intravenously at doses of 150 to 200 mg/m^2, given by infusion over 1 to 2 hours and repeated at 6 weeks.

Because of its ability to cross the blood–brain barrier, carmustine is used with procarbazine in the treatment of malignant gliomas. An implantable carmustine wafer (GLIADEL) is available for use as an adjunct to surgery and radiation in newly diagnosed high-grade malignant glioma patients and as an adjunct to surgery for recurrent glioblastoma multiforme.

Streptozocin. This antibiotic has a methylnitrosourea (MNU) moiety attached to the 2 carbon of glucose. It has a high affinity for cells of the islets of Langerhans and causes diabetes in experimental animals.

Absorption, Fate, and Excretion. After intravenous infusions of 200 to 1600 mg/m^2, peak concentrations of streptozocin in the plasma are 30 to 40 μg/ml; the half-life of the drug is approximately 15 minutes. Only 10% to 20% of a dose is recovered intact in the urine.

Therapeutic Uses. Streptozocin (ZANOSAR) is useful in the treatment of human pancreatic islet cell carcinoma and malignant carcinoid tumors. It is administered intravenously, 500 mg/m^2 once daily for 5 days; this course is repeated every 6 weeks. Alternatively, 1000 mg/m^2 can be given weekly for 2 weeks, and the weekly dose then can be increased to a maximum of 1500 mg/m^2, depending on tolerance.

Clinical Toxicity. Nausea is frequent. Mild, reversible renal or hepatic toxicity occurs in approximately two-thirds of cases; in less than 10% of patients, renal toxicity may be cumulative with each dose and may be fatal. A serial determination of urinary protein excretion is an early sign of tubular damage and impending renal failure. Streptozocin should not be given with other nephrotoxic drugs. Hematological toxicity—anemia, leukopenia, or thrombocytopenia—occurs in 20% of patients.

Triazenes

Dacarbazine (DTIC). Dacarbazine functions as a methylating agent after metabolic activation in the liver. Its active metabolite is a monomethyl triazeno metabolite, MTIC, and it kills cells in all phases of the cell cycle. Resistance has been ascribed to the removal of methyl groups from the O^6-guanine bases in DNA by AGT.

Absorption, Fate, and Excretion. Dacarbazine is administered intravenously. After an initial rapid phase of disappearance (half-life of about 20 minutes), dacarbazine is removed from plasma with a terminal half-life of about 5 hours (Loo *et al.*, 1976). The half-life is prolonged in the presence of hepatic or renal disease. Almost 50% of the compound is excreted intact in the urine by tubular secretion. Elevated urinary concentrations of 5-aminoimidazole-4-carboxamide are derived from the catabolism of dacarbazine, rather than by inhibition of *de novo* purine biosynthesis.

Therapeutic Uses. Dacarbazine (DTIC-DOME, others) for malignant melanoma is given in doses of 3.5 mg/kg per day, intravenously, for a 10-day period, repeated every 28 days. Alternatively, 250 mg/m^2 can be given daily for 5 days and repeated every 3 weeks. Extravasation of the drug may cause tissue damage and severe pain.

At present, dacarbazine is employed in combination regimens for the treatment of Hodgkin's disease. It is less effective against malignant melanoma and adult sarcomas.

Clinical Toxicity. The toxicity of DTIC includes nausea and vomiting in more than 90% of patients; vomiting usually develops 1 to 3 hours after treatment and may last up to 12 hours. Myelosuppression, with both leukopenia and thrombocytopenia, usually is mild to moderate. A flulike syndrome consisting of chills, fever, malaise, and myalgias, may occur during treatment with DTIC. Hepatotoxicity, alopecia, facial flushing, neurotoxicity, and dermatologic reactions also have been reported.

Temozolomide. Temozolomide (TEMODAR) is a recently introduced triazene that has significant activity in patients with malignant gliomas, where it is the standard agent in combination with radiation therapy. Temozolomide, like dacarbazine, forms the methylating metabolite MTIC and kills cells in all phases of the cell cycle.

Absorption, Fate, and Excretion. Temozolomide is administered orally and its bioavailability approaches 100%. Maximum drug concentration reaches 5 μg/ml, or about 10 μM in plasma, approximately 1 hour after administration of a dose of 200 mg, and declines with an elimination half-life of 1.2 hours. The primary active metabolite MTIC reaches a maximum plasma concentration of 150 ng/ml 90 minutes after a dose, and declines with a half-life of 2 hours. Little intact drug is recovered in the urine, the primary urinary metabolite being the inactive imidazole carboxamide (Baker *et al.*, 1999). The pharmacokinetics of temozolomide are linear over the dose range of 100 to 260 mg/m^2.

Clinical Toxicity. The toxicities of temozolomide mirror those of DTIC.

Methylhydrazines

Procarbazine. The methylhydrazine derivatives were synthesized in a search for inhibitors of monoamine neurotransmitters (Bollag, 1963). Several compounds in this series were discovered to have anticancer activity, but only procarbazine (*N*-isopropyl-α-(2-methylhydrazino)-*p*-toluamide), an agent useful in Hodgkin's disease and malignant brain tumors, has won a place in clinical chemotherapy. The structural formula for procarbazine is:

PROCARBAZINE

Cytotoxic Action. The antineoplastic activity of procarbazine results from its conversion to highly reactive alkylating species, which methylate DNA by CYP-mediated hepatic oxidative metabolism (Erikson *et al.*, 1989; Swaffar *et al.*, 1989). The activation pathways are complex and not fully understood. The first step involves oxidation of the hydrazine function, yielding the azo metabolite, which exists in equilibrium with its hydrazone tautomer. *N*-oxidation of azoprocarbazine generates the isomeric benzylazoxy and methylazoxy metabolites, the latter of which liberates an entity resembling diazomethane, a potent methylating reagent (Swaffar *et al.*, 1989). Free-radical intermediates also may be involved in cytotoxicity. Activated procarbazine can produce chromosomal damage, including chromatid breaks and translocations, consistent with its mutagenic and carcinogenic actions. Exposure to procarbazine leads to inhibition of DNA, RNA, and protein synthesis *in vivo*. Resistance to procarbazine develops rapidly when it is used as a single agent. One mechanism results from the increased ability to repair methylation of guanine *via* guanine-O^6-alkyl transferase (Souliotis *et al.*, 1990).

Absorption, Fate, and Excretion. The pharmacokinetic behavior of procarbazine has not yet been thoroughly defined. Early studies using radiotracer techniques and other indirect methods demonstrated that procarbazine is efficiently absorbed from the gastrointestinal tract and that it rapidly distributes into the CNS (Oliverio *et al.*, 1964). The drug and its metabolites are predominantly eliminated in the urine, with *N*-isopropyl-terephthalamic acid being the major metabolite, accounting for about 25% of doses given either orally or intravenously to humans (Oliverio *et al.*, 1964). Mass spectrometric methods have identified the azo, methylazoxy, and benzylazoxy metabolites of the drug in the plasma of a cancer patient treated with oral procarbazine (Shiba and Weinkam, 1982). A marked decrease in the apparent clearance of the drug upon repeated daily oral administration has been observed (Shiba and Weinkam, 1982). In brain cancer patients, the concurrent use of antiseizure drugs that induce hepatic CYPs did not significantly alter the pharmacokinetics of the parent drug (He *et al.*, 2004). This is somewhat surprising, because of the established role of CYPs in the bioactivation of procarbazine and the observation that its activity against tumors growing in mice is significantly enhanced by pretreatment with enzyme-inducing drugs, including *phenobarbital* and phenytoin (Shiba and Weinkam, 1983).

Therapeutic Uses. The recommended dose of procarbazine (MATULANE) for adults is 100 mg/m^2 daily for 10 to 14 days in combination regimens. The drug rarely is used alone. Procarbazine is used in combination with mechlorethamine, vincristine, and prednisone (the MOPP regimen) for the treatment of Hodgkin's disease (DeVita, 1981). Alternative regimens with less leukemogenic potential have largely replaced MOPP. Of primary importance, procarbazine lacks cross-resistance with other mustard-type alkylating agents. Procarbazine has been used in combination with lomustine and vincristine (the PCV regimen) since the 1970s for treating patients with newly diagnosed or recurrent primary brain tumors (Grossman, 1997).

Clinical Toxicity. The most common toxic effects include leukopenia and thrombocytopenia, which begin during the second week of therapy and reverse within 2 weeks off treatment. GI symptoms such as mild nausea and vomiting occur in most patients; gastrointestinal symptoms and neurological and dermatological manifestations have been noted in 5% to 10% of cases.

Behavioral disturbances also have been reported. Because of augmentation of sedative effects, the concomitant use of CNS depressants should be avoided. Since procarbazine is a weak monoamine oxidase inhibitor, hypertensive reactions may result from its use concurrently with sympathomimetic agents, tricyclic antidepressants, or ingestion of foods with high tyramine content. Procarbazine has disulfiram-like actions (*see* Chapter 22), and therefore the ingestion of alcohol should be avoided. Procarbazine is highly carcinogenic, mutagenic, and teratogenic, and its use in MOPP therapy is associated with a 5% to 10% risk of acute leukemia; the greatest risk is for patients who also receive radiation therapy (Tucker *et al.*, 1988). Procarbazine also is a potent immunosuppressive agent and it causes infertility, particularly in males.

PLATINUM COORDINATION COMPLEXES

The platinum coordination complexes were first identified as potential antiproliferative agents in 1965 by Rosenberg and coworkers. They observed that a current delivered between platinum electrodes produced inhibition of *E. coli* proliferation. The inhibitory effects on bacterial replication later were ascribed to the formation of inorganic platinum-containing compounds in the presence of ammonium and chloride ions. *Cis*-diamminedichloro-platinum (II) (cisplatin) was the most active of these substances in experimental tumor systems and has proven to be of great clinical value. Since that discovery, many platinum-containing compounds have been synthesized and tested. Carboplatin was approved for treatment of ovarian cancers in 1989, and *oxaliplatin* was approved by the FDA for colon cancer in 2003 (Ibrahim *et al.*, 2004). As a group, these agents have broad antineoplastic activity, and have become the foundation for treatment of testicular cancer, ovarian cancer, and cancers of the head and neck, bladder, esophagus, lung, and colon. Although cisplatin and other platinum complexes do not form carbonium ion intermediates like other alkylating agents and/or formally alkylate DNA, they covalently bind to nucleophilic sites on DNA and share many pharmacological attributes, justifying their inclusion in the alkylating agent class.

Chemistry. Cisplatin and carboplatin are divalent inorganic, water-soluble, platinum-containing complexes, while oxaliplatin, which does not display cross-resistance in some experimental tumors, is tetravalent. In each case, the coordination of di- or tetravalent platinum with various organic adducts reduces its renal toxicity and stabilizes the metal ion, as compared to the inorganic divalent platinum ion. The structural formulas of cisplatin, carboplatin, and oxaliplatin are:

CISPLATIN

CARBOPLATIN

OXALIPLATIN

Mechanism of Action. Cisplatin, carboplatin, and oxaliplatin enter cells by diffusion, and by an active Cu^{2+} transporter (Kruh, 2003). Inside the cell, the chloride atoms of cisplatin may be displaced and the compound may be inactivated directly by reaction with nucleophiles such as thiols. Chloride is replaced by water, yielding a positively charged molecule. In the primary cytotoxic reaction, the aquated species of the drug then reacts with nucleophilic sites on DNA and proteins. Aquation is favored at the low concentrations of chloride inside the cell and in the urine. High concentrations of chloride stabilize the drug, explaining the effectiveness of chloride diuresis in preventing nephrotoxicity (*see* below). Hydrolysis of carboplatin removes the bidentate cyclobutanedicarboxylato group; this activation reaction occurs slowly.

The platinum complexes can react with DNA, forming both intrastrand and interstrand cross-links. The N7 of guanine is a particularly reactive site, leading to platinum cross-links between adjacent guanines on the same DNA strand; guanine–adenine cross-links also readily form and may be critical to cytotoxicity (Parker *et al.*, 1991). The formation of interstrand cross-links is less favored. DNA adducts formed by cisplatin inhibit DNA replication and transcription and lead to breaks and miscoding, and if recognized by p53 and other checkpoint proteins, induction of apoptosis. Although no conclusive association between platinum-DNA adduct formation and efficacy has been documented, the ability of patients to form and sustain platinum adducts appears to be an important predictor of clinical response (Reed *et al.*, 1986). Preclinical data suggest that the formation of the platinum-adenosine-to-guanosine adduct may be the most critical adduct in terms of cytotoxicity.

The specificity of cisplatin with regard to phase of the cell cycle appears to differ among cell types, although the effects of cross-linking are most pronounced during the S phase. Cisplatin is mutagenic, teratogenic, and carcinogenic. The use of cisplatin- or carboplatin-based chemotherapy for women with ovarian cancer is associated with a fourfold increased risk of developing secondary leukemia (Travis *et al.*, 1999).

Resistance to Platinum Analogs

The causes of tumor cell resistance to cisplatin and its analogs are incompletely understood. The various analogs differ in their degree of cross-resistance with cisplatin in experimental tumor systems. Carboplatin shares cross-resistance with cisplatin in most experimental tumors, while oxaliplatin and other tetravalent analogs do not. A number of factors influence cisplatin sensitivity in experimental cells, including intracellular drug accumulation and intracellular levels of glutathione and other sulfhydryls such as metallothionein that bind to and inactivate the drug (Meijer *et al.*, 1990), and

rates of repair of DNA adducts (Parker *et al.*, 1991). Repair of cisplatin-DNA adducts occurs through the nucleotide excision repair (NER) pathway (Reed, 1998). Inhibition or loss of NER increases sensitivity to cisplatin in ovarian cancer patients (Taniguchi *et al.*, 2003), while overexpression of NER components is associated with poor response to cisplatin-based therapy in lung cancer (Rosell *et al.*, 2003).

Resistance to cisplatin, but not oxaliplatin, appears to be partly mediated through loss of function in the mismatch repair (MMR) proteins (Vaisman *et al.*, 1998). MMR proteins, particularly hMLH1, hMLH2, or hMSH6, recognize platinum-DNA adducts and initiate apoptosis. Loss of MMR has been associated in some studies with resistance to cisplatin *in vitro* (Mello, 1996). Through an hMLH1-dependent event, cisplatin induces overexpression of p73, a member of the p53 family, as well as c-ABL tyrosine kinase, and consequently activates apoptosis (Gong *et al.*, 1999). In response to cisplatin exposure, apoptosis is not induced in cells deficient in MMR or in cells unable to upregulate c-ABL tyrosine kinase. By contrast, MMR repair proficiency is not required for oxaliplatin cytotoxicity (Fink *et al.*, 1996).

In the absence of effective repair of DNA-platinum adducts, sensitive cells cannot replicate or transcribe affected portions of the DNA strand. However, it is clear that some DNA polymerases are able to bypass adducts. It remains unproven whether these polymerases contribute to resistance. Cisplatin resistance related to loss of active uptake has been demonstrated in yeast; overexpression of copper efflux transporters, ATP7A and ATP7B, has been described in human tumors, and correlates with poor survival after cisplatin-based therapy for ovarian cancer (Kruh, 2003).

Cisplatin

Absorption, Fate, and Excretion. After intravenous administration, cisplatin has an initial plasma elimination half-life of 25 to 50 minutes; concentrations of total (bound and unbound) drug fall thereafter, with a half-life of 24 hours or longer. More than 90% of the platinum in the blood is covalently bound to plasma proteins. The unbound fraction, composed predominantly of parent drug, is cleared within minutes. High concentrations of cisplatin are found in the tissues of the kidney, liver, intestine, and testes, but there is poor penetration into the CNS. Only a small portion of the drug is excreted by the kidney during the first 6 hours; by 24 hours up to 25% is excreted, and by 5 days up to 43% of the administered dose is recovered in the urine, mostly covalently bound to protein and peptides. Biliary or intestinal excretion of cisplatin is minimal.

Therapeutic Uses. Cisplatin (PLATINOL-AQ, others) is given only by the intravenous route. The usual dose is 20 mg/m² per day for 5 days, 20 to 30 mg weekly for 3 to 4 weeks, or 100 mg/m², given once every 4 weeks. *To prevent renal toxicity, it is important to establish a chloride diuresis by the infusion of 1 to 2 liters of normal saline prior to treatment.* The appropriate amount of cisplatin then is diluted in a solution of dextrose and saline and administered intravenously over a period of 4 to 6 hours. Since aluminum reacts with and inactivates cisplatin, it is important not to use needles or other infusion equipment that contain aluminum when preparing or administering the drug.

Cisplatin, in combination with *bleomycin*, etoposide, ifosfamide, or *vinblastine* cures 90% of patients with testicular cancer. Used with paclitaxel, cisplatin induces complete response in the majority of patients with carcinoma of the ovary. Cisplatin produces responses in cancers of the bladder, head and neck, cervix, and endometrium; all forms of carcinoma of the lung; anal and rectal carcinomas; and neoplasms of childhood. Interestingly, the drug also sensitizes cells to radiation therapy and enhances control of locally advanced lung, esophageal, and head and neck tumors when given with irradiation.

Clinical Toxicities. Cisplatin-induced nephrotoxicity has been largely abrogated by adequate pretreatment hydration and diuresis. *Amifostine* (ETHYOL) is a thiophosphate cytoprotective agent that is labeled for the reduction of renal toxicity associated with repeated administration of cisplatin. Amifostine is dephosphorylated by alkaline phosphatase to a pharmacologically active free thiol metabolite. Faster dephosphorylation and preferential uptake by normal tissues results in a higher concentration of the thiol metabolite available to scavenge reactive cisplatin metabolites in normal tissues. Amifostine also is used to reduce xerostomia in patients undergoing irradiation for head and neck cancer, where the radiation port includes a substantial portion of the parotid glands. A review of the clinical status of amifostine as a cytoprotectant has been published.

Ototoxicity caused by cisplatin is unaffected by diuresis and is manifested by tinnitus and high-frequency hearing loss. The ototoxicity can be unilateral or bilateral, tends to be more frequent and severe with repeated doses, and may be more pronounced in children. Marked nausea and vomiting occur in almost all patients and usually can be controlled with 5-hydroxytryptamine (5-HT$_3$) antagonists, neurokinin-1 (NK1) receptor antagonists, and high-dose corticosteroids (*see* Chapter 37). At higher doses or after multiple cycles of treatment, cisplatin causes a progressive peripheral motor and sensory neuropathy, which may worsen after discontinuation of the drug and may be aggravated by subsequent or simultaneous treatment with taxanes or other neurotoxic drugs. Cisplatin causes mild-to-moderate myelosuppression, with transient leukopenia and thrombocytopenia. Anemia may become prominent after multiple cycles of treatment. Electrolyte disturbances, including hypomagnesemia, hypocalcemia, hypokalemia, and hypophosphatemia, are common. Hypocalcemia and hypomagnesemia secondary to renal electrolyte wasting may produce tetany if untreated. Routine measurement of Mg^{2+} concentrations in plasma is recommended. Hyperuricemia, hemolytic anemia, and cardiac abnormalities are rare side effects. Anaphylactic-like reactions, characterized by facial edema, bronchoconstriction, tachycardia, and hypotension, may occur within minutes after administration and should be treated by intravenous injection of epinephrine and with corticosteroids or antihistamines. Cisplatin has been associated with the development of AML, usually 4 years or more after treatment.

Carboplatin

The mechanisms of action and resistance and the spectrum of clinical activity of carboplatin (CBDCA, JM-8) are similar to those of cisplatin (*see* above). However, the two drugs differ significantly in their chemical, pharmacokinetic, and toxicological properties.

Because carboplatin is much less reactive than cisplatin, the majority of drug in plasma remains in its parent form, unbound to proteins. Most drug is eliminated *via* renal excretion, with a half-life in plasma of about 2 hours. A small fraction of platinum does become irreversibly bound to plasma proteins, and disappears slowly, with a half-life of 5 days or more.

Carboplatin is relatively well tolerated clinically, with less nausea, neurotoxicity, ototoxicity, and nephrotoxicity than that associated with cisplatin. Instead, the dose-limiting toxicity is myelosuppression, primarily evident as thrombocytopenia.

Carboplatin and cisplatin appear to be equally effective in the treatment of suboptimally debulked ovarian cancer, non–small cell lung cancer, and extensive stage small cell lung cancer; however, carboplatin may be less effective than cisplatin in germ cell, head and neck, and esophageal cancers (Go and Adjei, 1999). Carboplatin is an effective alternative for responsive tumors in patients unable to tolerate cisplatin because of impaired renal function, refractory nausea, significant hearing impairment, or neuropathy, but doses must be adjusted for renal function. In addition, it may be used in high-dose therapy with bone marrow or peripheral stem cell rescue. The dose of carboplatin should be adjusted in proportion to the reduction in creatinine clearance for patients with a creatinine clearance below 60 ml/min (Van Echo *et al.*, 1989; Calvert *et al.*, 1989; Calvert and Egarin, 2002). The following formula has been proposed for calculation of dose:

$$\text{Dose (mg)} = \text{AUC} \times (\text{GFR} + 25) \qquad (51–1)$$

where the target AUC (area under the plasma concentration–time curve) is in the range of 5 to 7 mg/ml per minute for acceptable toxicity in patients receiving single-agent carboplatin (GFR = glomerular filtration rate).

Carboplatin (PARAPLATIN) is administered as an intravenous infusion over at least 15 minutes, using the above-mentioned formula, and is given once every 28 days. Carboplatin currently has FDA approval for use in combination with paclitaxel or cyclophosphamide in patients with advanced ovarian cancer and lung cancer.

Oxaliplatin

Absorption, Fate and Excretion. Oxaliplatin, like cisplatin, has a very brief half-life in plasma, probably as a result of its rapid uptake by tissues and its reactivity. Maximum concentrations in plasma range from 1 to 1.5 μg platinum/ml for patients receiving 80 to 130 mg/m^2 intravenously, and decline thereafter with an initial half-life of 0.28 hours. While the ultrafiltrable component has a slow terminal clearance from plasma (half-life of 273 hours), most of the low-molecular-weight platinum species represent inactive degradation products. These metabolites undergo renal excretion at a rate dependent on the creatinine clearance. However, no dose adjustment is required for patients with creatinine clearances of greater than 20 ml/min, as decreased renal function does not affect the rapid chemical inactivation of the drug and its toxicity at doses of 65 to 130 mg/m^2 (Takimoto *et al.*, 2003).

Therapeutic Uses. Oxaliplatin exhibits a wide range of antitumor activity that differs from other platinum agents, and includes gastric and colorectal cancer. Oxaliplatin's effectiveness in colorectal cancer is perhaps due to its MMR-independent effects. It also suppresses expression of thymidylate synthase (TS), the target enzyme of 5-fluorouracil (5-FU) action, which may promote synergy of these two drugs. In combination with 5-fluorouracil, it is approved for treatment of patients with advanced colorectal cancer.

Clinical Toxicity. The dose-limiting toxicity of oxaliplatin is a peripheral neuropathy. An acute form often is triggered by exposure to cold, and manifests as paresthesias and/or dysesthesias in the upper and lower extremities, mouth, and throat. A second type of peripheral neuropathy is more closely related to cumulative dose and similar to that seen with cisplatin; 75% of patients receiving a cumulative dose of 1560 mg/m^2 experience some neurotoxicity. Hematologic toxicity is mild to moderate, and nausea is well controlled with $5-HT_3$ receptor antagonists (*see* Chapter 37). Oxaliplatin is unstable in the presence of chloride or alkaline solutions.

II. ANTIMETABOLITES

FOLIC ACID ANALOGS

Antifolate chemotherapy occupies a special place in the history of cancer treatment, as this class of drugs produced the first striking, although temporary, remissions in leukemia (Farber *et al.*, 1948), and the first cure of a solid tumor, choriocarcinoma (Berlin *et al.*, 1963). These advances provided great impetus to the development of chemotherapy for cancer. Interest in folate antagonists further increased with the development of curative combination therapy for childhood acute lymphocytic leukemia; in this therapy, methotrexate played a critical role in both systemic treatment and intrathecal therapy. Introduction of high-dose regimens with "rescue" of host toxicity by the reduced folate, leucovorin (folinic acid, citrovorum factor, 5-formyl tetrahydrofolate, N^5-formyl FH_4), further extended the effectiveness of this drug to both systemic and CNS lymphomas, osteogenic sarcoma, and leukemias. Most recently, *pemetrexed*, an analogue that differs from methotrexate in its transport properties and sites of action, has proven useful in treating mesothelioma and lung cancer.

Recognition that methotrexate, an inhibitor of dihydrofolate reductase, also directly inhibits the folate-dependent enzymes of *de novo* purine and thymidylate synthesis focused attention on the development of antifolate analogs that specifically target these other folate-dependent enzymes (Figure 51–7). Replacement of the N5 and/or N8 nitrogens of the pteridine ring and the N10 nitrogen of the bridge between the pteridine and benzoate rings of folate, as well as various side-chain substitutions, have generated a series of new inhibitors.

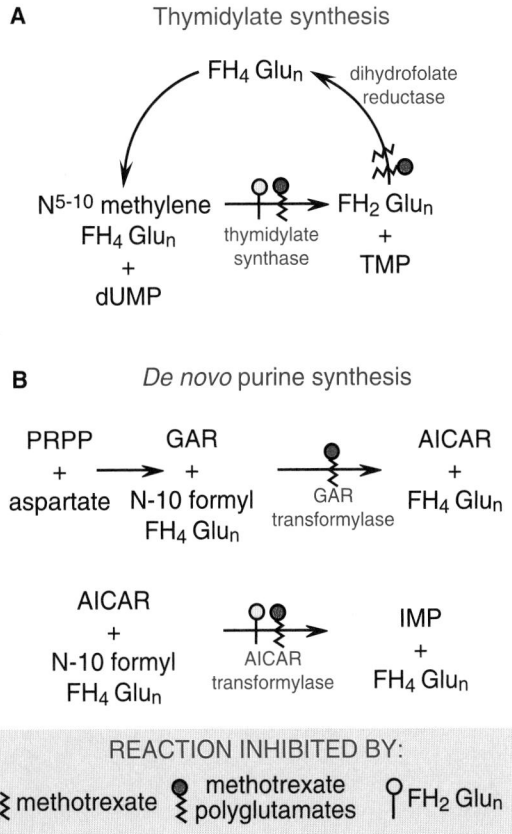

Figure 51–7. Sites of action of methotrexate and its polyglutamates. AICAR, aminoimidazole carboxamide; TMP, thymidine monophosphate; dUMP, deoxyuridine monophosphate; FH_2Glu_n, dihydrofolate polyglutamate; FH_4Glu_n, tetrahydrofolate polyglutamate; GAR, glycinamide ribonucleotide; IMP, inosine monophosphate; PRPP, 5-phosphoribosyl-1-pyrophosphate.

These new agents have greater capacity for transport into tumor cells, and exert their primary inhibitory effect on thymidylate synthase (*raltitrexed,* TOMUDEX), early steps in purine biosynthesis (*lometrexol*) or both (the multitargeted antifolate, pemetrexed) (Vogelzang *et al.*, 2003).

Aside from its antineoplastic activity, methotrexate also has been used with benefit in the therapy of psoriasis (*see* Chapter 62). Additionally, methotrexate inhibits cell-mediated immune reactions and is employed as an immunosuppressive agent to suppress graft-*versus*-host disease in allogenic bone marrow and organ transplantation and for the treatment of dermatomyositis, rheumatoid arthritis, Wegener's granulomatosis, and Crohn's disease (*see* Chapters 38 and 52).

Structure–Activity Relationship. Folic acid is an essential dietary factor. It is converted by enzymatic reduction to a series of tetrahydrofolate cofactors that provide carbon groups for the synthesis of precursors of DNA (thymidylate and purines) and RNA (purines). The biological functions and therapeutic applications of folic acid are further described in Chapter 53.

The primary target of methotrexate is the enzyme dihydrofolate reductase (DHFR) (Figure 51–7). Inhibition of DHFR leads to partial depletion of the tetrahydrofolate cofactors (5-10 methylene tetrahydrofolic acid and N-10 formyl tetrahydrofolic acid) required for the respective synthesis of thymidylate and purines. In addition, methotrexate, like its physiologic counterparts (the folates), undergoes conversion to a series of polyglutamates (MTX-PGs) in both normal and tumor cells. These MTX-PGs constitute an intracellular storage form of folates and folate analogs, and dramatically increase inhibitory potency of the analog for additional sites, including thymidylate synthase (TS) and two early enzymes in the purine biosynthetic pathway (Figure 51–7). Finally, the dihydrofolic acid polyglutamates that accumulate in cells behind the blocked DHFR reaction also act as inhibitors of TS and other enzymes (Figure 51–7) (Allegra et al., 1987b). Inhibitors of DHFR differ in their relative potency for blocking enzymes from different species. Agents have been identified that have little effect on the human enzyme, but have strong activity against bacterial and parasitic infections (see discussions of trimethoprim, Chapter 43; pyrimethamine, Chapter 39). By contrast, methotrexate is an effective inhibitor of DHFR in all species investigated. Crystallographic studies have revealed the structural basis for the high affinity of methotrexate for DHFR (Blakley and Sorrentino, 1998) and the species specificity of the various DHFR inhibitors (Matthews et al., 1985).

Because folic acid and many of its analogs are polar, they cross the blood–brain barrier poorly and require specific transport mechanisms to enter mammalian cells (Elwood, 1989). Three inward folate transport systems are found on mammalian cells: (1) a folate receptor, which has high affinity for folic acid but much reduced ability to transport methotrexate and other analogs (Elwood, 1989); (2) the reduced folate transporter, the major transit protein for methotrexate, raltitrexed, pemetrexed, and most analogs (Westerhof et al., 1995); and (3) a poorly characterized transporter that is active at low pH. The importance of transport in determining drug sensitivity is illustrated by the finding that the reduced folate transporter is highly expressed in the hyperdiploid subtype of acute lymphoblastic leukemia, due to the presence of multiple copies of chromosome 21, on which its gene resides; these cells have extreme sensitivity to methotrexate (Pui et al., 2004). Once in the cell, additional glutamyl residues are added to the molecule by the enzyme folylpolyglutamate synthetase. Intracellular methotrexate polyglutamates have been identified with up to six glutamyl residues. Since these higher polyglutamates are strongly charged and cross cellular membranes poorly, if at all, polyglutamation serves as a mechanism of entrapment and may account for the prolonged retention of methotrexate in chorionic epithelium (where it is a potent abortifacient), in tumors derived from this tissue, such as choriocarcinoma cells, and in normal tissues subject to cumulative drug toxicity, such as liver. Polyglutamylated folates and analogs have substantially greater affinity than the monoglutamate form for folate-dependent enzymes that are required for purine and thymidylate synthesis, and have at least equal affinity for DHFR.

New folate antagonists have been identified that are better substrates for the reduced folate carrier. Pemetrexed appears to have significant advantages in clinical chemotherapy (see below). In efforts to bypass the obligatory membrane transport system and to facilitate penetration of the blood–brain barrier, lipid-soluble folate antagonists also have been synthesized. Trimetrexate (NEUTREXIN) (Figure 51–8) was one of the first to be tested for clinical activity. The analog has modest antitumor activity, primarily in combination with leucovorin rescue. However, it is beneficial in the treatment of Pneumocystis jiroveci (Pneumocystis carinii) pneumonia (Allegra et al., 1987a), where leucovorin provides differential rescue of the host but not the parasite.

The most important new folate analog, MTA or pemetrexed (ALIMTA) (Figure 51–8), is a pyrrole-pyrimidine folate analog (Tay-

lor et al., 1992). It is avidly transported into cells via the reduced folate carrier, but also may gain entry by a unique folate transport activity found in mesothelioma cell lines (Wang et al., 2002). It readily is converted to polyglutamates that inhibit TS and glycine amide ribonucleotide transformylase, as well as dihydrofolate reductase. It has shown activity against colon cancer, mesothelioma, and non–small cell lung cancer, and has been approved for treatment of mesothelioma (Vogelzang et al., 2003).

Mechanism of Action. To function as a cofactor in one-carbon transfer reactions, folate must first be reduced by DHFR to tetrahydrofolate (FH_4). Single-carbon fragments are added enzymatically to FH_4 in various configurations and then may be transferred in specific synthetic reactions. In a key metabolic event catalyzed by TS (Figure 51–7), deoxyuridine monophosphate (dUMP) is converted to thymidine monophosphate (TMP), an essential component of DNA. In this reaction, a one-carbon group is transferred to dUMP from 5,10-methylene FH_4, and the reduced folate cofactor is oxidized to dihydrofolate (FH_2). To function again as a cofactor, FH_2 must be reduced to FH_4 by DHFR. Inhibitors such as methotrexate, with a high affinity for DHFR (K_i ~0.01 to 0.2 nM), prevent the formation of FH_4 and allow a vast accumulation of the toxic inhibitory substrate, FH_2 polyglutamate, behind the blocked reaction. The one-carbon transfer reactions crucial for the de novo synthesis of purine nucleotides and thymidylate cease, with the subsequent interruption of the synthesis of DNA and RNA. The toxic effects of methotrexate may be terminated by administering leucovorin, a fully reduced folate coenzyme, which repletes the intracellular pool of tetrahydrofolate cofactors.

As with most antimetabolites, methotrexate is only partially selective for tumor cells and is toxic to all rapidly dividing normal cells, such as those of the intestinal epithelium and bone marrow. Folate antagonists kill cells during the S phase of the cell cycle and are most effective when cells are proliferating rapidly.

Pemetrexed and its polyglutamates have a somewhat different spectrum of biochemical actions. Like methotrexate, it inhibits DHFR, but as a polyglutamate, even more potently glycinamide ribonucleotide formyltransferase (GART) and TS. Unlike methotrexate, it produces little change in the pool of reduced folates, indicating that the distal sites of inhibition (TS and GART) predominate. Its pattern of deoxynucleotide depletion, as studied in cell lines, also differs, with little effect on deoxyadenosine triphosphate (dATP), a profile more characteristic of primary TS inhibition (Chen et al., 1998). Like methotrexate, it induces p53 and cell-cycle arrest, but this effect does not seem to depend on downstream induction of p21.

Mechanisms of Resistance to Antifolates. In experimental systems, different biochemical mechanisms of acquired resistance to methotrexate affect each known step in methotrexate action, including: (1) impaired transport of methotrexate into cells (Assaraf et al., 2003; Trippett et al., 1992); (2) production of altered forms of DHFR that have decreased affinity for the inhibitor (Srimatkandada et al., 1989); (3) increased concentrations of intracellular DHFR through gene amplification or altered gene regulation (Matherly et al., 1997); (4) decreased ability to synthesize methotrexate polyglutamates (Li et al., 1992); and (5) increased expression of a drug efflux transporter, of the MRP (multidrug resistance protein) class (Stashenko et al., 1980).

DHFR levels in leukemic cells increase within 24 hours after treatment of patients with methotrexate; this likely reflects induction of new enzyme synthesis. The unbound DHFR protein may bind to its own message and inhibit translational efficiency of its own synthesis,

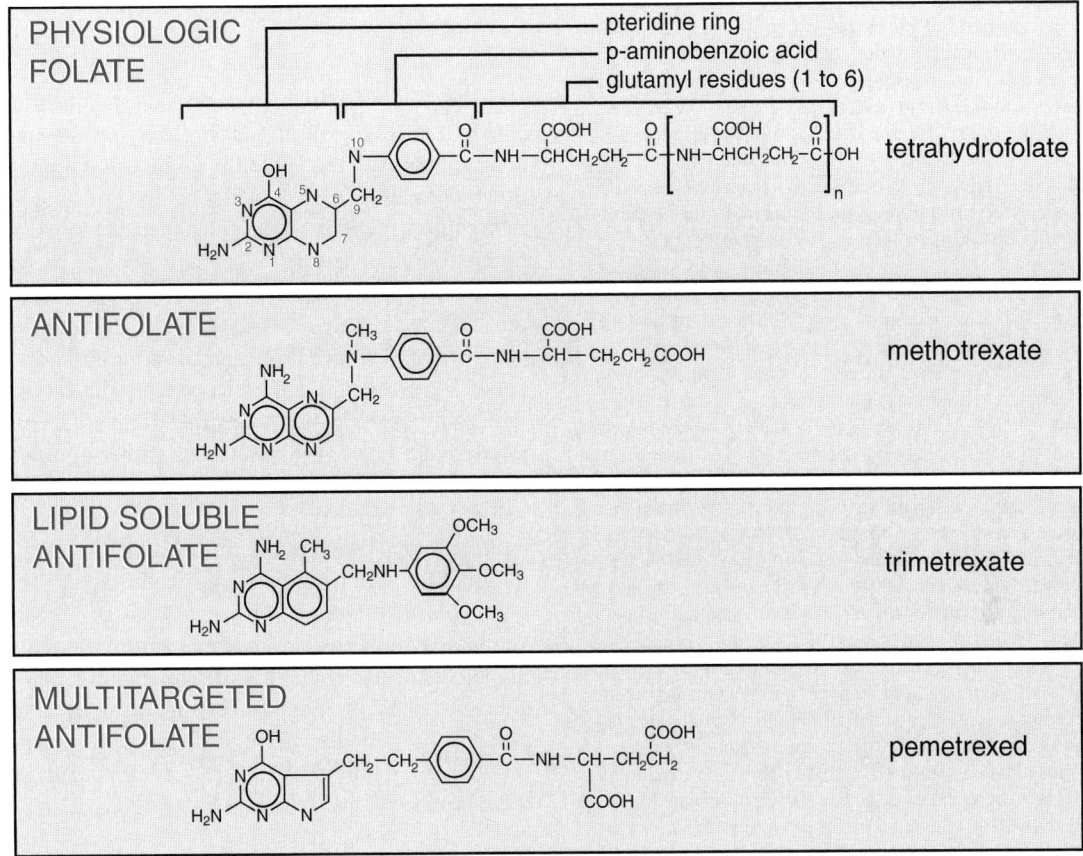

Figure 51–8. *The structure–activity bases for antifolate action.*

while the DHFR-MTX complex is ineffective in blocking the DHFR translation. With longer periods of drug exposure, tumor cell populations emerge that contain markedly increased levels of DHFR. These cells contain multiple gene copies of DHFR either in mitotically unstable double-minute chromosomes (extrachromosomal elements formed by amplification of DHFR genes in response to methotrexate treatment) or in stably integrated, homogeneously staining chromosomal regions or amplicons. First identified as an explanation for resistance to methotrexate (Schimke *et al.*, 1978), gene amplification of a target protein has since been implicated in the resistance to many antitumor agents, including 5-fluorouracil and *pentostatin* (2′-deoxycoformycin) (Stark and Wahl, 1984), and has been observed in patients with lung cancer (Curt *et al.*, 1985) and leukemia (Goker *et al.*, 1995).

To overcome resistance, high doses of methotrexate may permit entry of drug into transport-defective cells and may permit the intracellular accumulation of methotrexate in concentrations that inactivate high levels of DHFR.

The understanding of resistance to pemetrexed is incomplete. In various cell lines, resistance to this agent seems to arise either from TS amplification, changes in purine biosynthetic pathways, or both (Schultz *et al.*, 1999).

General Toxicity and Cytotoxic Action. The primary toxic effects of methotrexate and other folate antagonists used in cancer chemotherapy are exerted against rapidly dividing cells of the bone marrow and GI epithelium. Mucositis, myelosuppression, and thrombocytopenia reach their maximum in 5 to 10 days after drug administration, and except in instances of altered drug excretion, reverse rapidly thereafter.

In addition to its acute toxicities, methotrexate can cause pneumonitis, characterized by patchy inflammatory infiltrates that regress upon discontinuation of the drug. In some cases, patients can be rechallenged with drug without toxicity. The etiology is not clearly allergic.

A second toxicity of particular significance in chronic administration to patients with psoriasis or rheumatoid arthritis is hepatic fibrosis and cirrhosis. Increased hepatic portal fibrosis is detected with higher frequency than in control patients after 6 months or longer of continuous oral methotrexate treatment of psoriasis. Its presence mandates discontinuation of methotrexate. Acute, reversible elevation of hepatic enzymes is detected in serum after high-dose administration but rarely is associated with permanent changes.

Folic acid antagonists are toxic to developing embryos. Methotrexate is highly effective when used with the prostaglandin analog *misoprostol* in inducing abortion in first-trimester pregnancy (Hausknecht, 1995).

Absorption, Fate, and Excretion. Methotrexate is readily absorbed from the gastrointestinal tract at doses of less than 25 mg/m^2, but larger doses are absorbed incompletely and are routinely administered intravenously. Peak concentrations in the plasma of 1 to 10

μM are obtained after doses of 25 to 100 mg/m^2, and concentrations of 0.1 to 1 mM are achieved after high-dose infusions of 1.5 to 20 g/m^2. After intravenous administration, the drug disappears from plasma in a triphasic fashion (Sonneveld *et al.*, 1986). The rapid distribution phase is followed by a second phase, which reflects renal clearance (half-life of about 2 to 3 hours). A third phase has a half-life of approximately 8 to 10 hours. This terminal phase of disappearance, if unduly prolonged by renal failure, may be responsible for major toxic effects of the drug on the marrow, GI epithelium, and skin. Distribution of methotrexate into body spaces, such as the pleural or peritoneal cavity, occurs slowly. However, if such spaces are expanded (*e.g.*, by ascites or pleural effusion), they may act as a site of storage and slow release of drug, with resultant prolonged elevation of plasma concentrations and more severe toxicity.

Approximately 50% of methotrexate is bound to plasma proteins and may be displaced from plasma albumin by a number of drugs, including sulfonamides, salicylates, *tetracycline*, *chloramphenicol*, and phenytoin; caution should be used if these are given concomitantly. Up to 90% of a given dose is excreted unchanged in the urine within 48 hours, mostly within the first 8 to 12 hours. A small amount of methotrexate also is excreted in the stool. Metabolism of methotrexate in humans is usually minimal. After high doses, however, metabolites are readily detectable; these include 7-hydroxy-methotrexate, which is potentially nephrotoxic. Renal excretion of methotrexate occurs through a combination of glomerular filtration and active tubular secretion. Therefore, the concurrent use of drugs that reduce renal blood flow (*e.g.*, nonsteroidal antiinflammatory agents), that are nephrotoxic (*e.g.*, cisplatin), or that are weak organic acids (*e.g.*, *aspirin* or *piperacillin*) can delay drug excretion and lead to severe myelosuppression (Thyss *et al.*, 1986). Particular caution must be exercised in treating patients with renal insufficiency. In such patients, the dose should be adjusted in proportion to decreases in renal function, and high-dose regimens should be avoided if possible.

Methotrexate is retained in the form of polyglutamates for long periods—for example, for weeks in the kidneys and for several months in the liver.

It is important to emphasize that concentrations of methotrexate in CSF are only 3% of those in the systemic circulation at steady state; hence, neoplastic cells in the CNS probably are not killed by standard dosage regimens. When high doses of methotrexate are given (>1.5 g/m^2; *see* below), cytotoxic concentrations of methotrexate may be attained in the CNS.

Pharmacogenetics may influence the response to antifolates and their toxicity. The C677T substitution in methylenetetrahydrofolate reductase reduces the activity of the enzyme that generates methylenetetrahydrofolate, the cofactor for TS, and thereby increases methotrexate toxicity (Pullarkat *et al.*, 2001). The presence of this polymorphism in leukemic cells confers increased sensitivity to methotrexate, and might also modulate the toxicity and therapeutic effect of pemetrexed, a predominant TS inhibitor. Likewise, polymorphisms in the promoter region of TS govern the translation efficiency of this message, and by governing the intracellular levels of TS, modulate the response and toxicity of both antifolates (Pui *et al.*, 2004) and fluoropyrimidines (Pullarkat *et al.*, 2001).

Therapeutic Uses. Methotrexate (*amethopterin;* RHEUMATREX, TREXALL, others) has been used in the treatment of severe, disabling psoriasis in doses of 2.5 mg orally for 5 days, followed by a rest period of at least 2 days, or 10 to 25 mg intravenously weekly. It also is used intermittently at low dosage to induce remission in refractory rheumatoid arthritis (Hoffmeister, 1983). Complete awareness of the pharmacology and toxic potential of methotrexate is a prerequisite for its use in these non-neoplastic disorders.

Methotrexate is a critical drug in the management of acute lymphoblastic leukemia (ALL) in children. It is of great value in remission induction and consolidation, used in high doses, and in the maintenance of remissions in this highly curable disease. For maintenance therapy, it is administered intermittently at doses of 30 mg/m^2 intramuscularly weekly in two divided doses or in 2-day "pulses" of 175 to 525 mg/m^2 at monthly intervals. Outcome of treatment in children correlates inversely with the rate of drug clearance. During methotrexate infusion, high steady-state levels are associated with a lower leukemia relapse rate (Pui *et al.*, 2004). Methotrexate is of limited value in the types of leukemia seen in adults, except for treatment and prevention of leukemic meningitis. The intrathecal administration of methotrexate has been employed for treatment or prophylaxis of meningeal leukemia or lymphoma and for treatment of meningeal carcinomatosis. This route of administration achieves high concentrations of methotrexate in the CSF and is also effective in patients whose systemic disease has become resistant to methotrexate. The recommended intrathecal dose in all patients over 3 years of age is 12 mg (Bleyer, 1978). The dose is repeated every 4 days until malignant cells no longer are evident in the CSF. Leucovorin may be administered to counteract the toxicity of methotrexate that escapes into the systemic circulation, although this generally is not necessary. Since methotrexate administered into the lumbar space distributes poorly over the cerebral convexities, the drug may be more effective when given *via* an intraventricular Ommaya reservoir. Methotrexate is of established value in choriocarcinoma and related trophoblastic tumors of women; cure is achieved in approximately 75% of advanced cases treated sequentially with methotrexate and *dactinomycin*, and in more than 90% when early diagnosis is made. In the treatment of choriocarcinoma, 1 mg/kg of methotrexate is administered intramuscularly every other day for four doses, alternating with leucovorin (0.1 mg/kg every other day). Courses are repeated at 3-week intervals, toxicity permitting, and urinary β-human chorionic gonadotropin titers are used as a guide for persistence of disease.

Beneficial effects also are observed in the combination therapy of Burkitt's and other non-Hodgkin's lymphomas, and methotrexate is a component of regimens for carcinomas of the breast, head and neck, ovary, and bladder. High-dose methotrexate with leucovorin rescue (HDM-L) is a component of the standard regimen for adjuvant therapy of osteosarcoma, produces a high complete response rate in CNS lymphomas, and is a part of standard curative therapy for childhood ALL. A 6- to 72-hour infusion of relatively large doses of methotrexate may be employed every 2 to 4 weeks (from 1 to 7.5 g/m^2 or more), but only when leucovorin rescue is used. Such regimens produce cytotoxic concentrations of drug in the CSF and protect against leukemic meningitis. A typical regimen includes the infusion of 7.5 g/m^2 methotrexate for 6 hours followed by leucovorin at a dose of 15 mg/m^2 every 6 hours for seven doses, with the goal of rescuing normal cells to prevent toxicity. Other dosage regimens also are used.

The administration of HDM-L has the potential for renal toxicity, probably related to the precipitation of the drug, a weak acid, in the acidic tubular fluid. Thus, vigorous hydration and alkalinization of urine pH are required prior to drug administration. HDM-L should be performed only by experienced clinicians who are familiar with hydration regimens and who have access to laboratories that monitor concentrations of methotrexate in plasma. If methotrexate values measured 48 hours after drug administration are 1 μM or higher, higher doses (100 mg/m^2) of leucovorin must be given until the plasma concentration of methotrexate falls below a level of 50 nM (Stoller *et al.*, 1977). With appropriate hydration and urine alkalinization, and in patients with normal renal function, the incidence of nephrotoxicity following HDM-L approaches 2% (Widemann *et al.*, 2004). In patients who become oliguric, intermittent hemodialysis is ineffective in reducing methotrexate levels. Continuous-flow hemodialysis can eliminate methotrexate at a rate approximating 50% of the clearance rate in patients with intact renal function (Wall *et al.*, 1996). Alternatively, a methotrexate-cleaving enzyme, carboxypeptidase G2, can be obtained from the Cancer Therapy Evaluation Program at the National Cancer Institute. When administered intravenously, it rapidly clears the drug (DeAngelis *et al.*, 1996). Methotrexate concentrations in plasma fall by 99% or greater within 5 to 15 minutes following enzyme administration, with insignificant rebound. Carboxypeptidase G2 also has received limited evaluation as the sole rescue for high-dose methotrexate, without leucovorin, and was effective. Systemically administered carboxypeptidase G2 has little effect on methotrexate levels in the CSF.

At present, the only FDA-approved indication for pemetrexed is for second-line therapy in mesothelioma; it also is used, however, for refractory non–small cell lung cancer. Promising results have been published in its first-line use with cisplatin in both tumors (Scagliotti *et al.*, 2003; Manegold, 2004).

Clinical Toxicities. As previously stated, the primary toxicities of antifolates affect the bone marrow and the intestinal epithelium. Such patients may be at risk for spontaneous hemorrhage or life-threatening infection, and they may require prophylactic transfusion of platelets and broad-spectrum antibiotics if febrile. Side effects usually reverse completely within 2 weeks, but prolonged myelosuppression may occur in patients with compromised renal function who have delayed excretion of the drug. The dosage of methotrexate (and likely pemetrexed) must be reduced in proportion to any reduction in creatinine clearance.

Additional toxicities of methotrexate include alopecia, dermatitis, interstitial pneumonitis, nephrotoxicity, defective oogenesis or spermatogenesis, abortion, and teratogenesis. Elevation of hepatic enzymes is a consistent finding with high-dose methotrexate, but usually is reversible. On the other hand, low-dose methotrexate may lead to cirrhosis after long-term continuous treatment, as in patients with psoriasis. Intrathecal administration of methotrexate often causes meningismus and an inflammatory response in the CSF. Seizures, coma, and death may occur rarely. Leucovorin does not reverse neurotoxicity.

Pemetrexed toxicity mirrors that of methotrexate, with the additional feature of a prominent erythematous and pruritic rash in 40% of patients. *Dexamethasone*, 4 mg twice-daily on days –1, 0, and +1, markedly diminishes this toxicity. Unpredictably severe myelosuppression with pemetrexed, seen especially in patients with preexisting homocystinemia and possibly reflecting folate deficiency, is largely eliminated by concurrent administration of low doses of *folic acid*, 350 to 1000 mg per day, beginning 1 to 2 weeks prior to pemetrexed and continuing while the drug is administered. Intramuscular vitamin B$_{12}$ (1 mg) is given with the first dose of pemetrexed to correct possible B$_{12}$ deficiency. There is no evidence that these small doses of folate and B$_{12}$ compromise the therapeutic effect (Scagliotti *et al.*, 2003).

PYRIMIDINE ANALOGS

The antimetabolites as a class encompass a diverse group of drugs that inhibit RNA and DNA function in a variety of ways. Some, such as the fluoropyrimidines and the purine base analogs (6-mercaptopurine and *6-thioguanine*) inhibit the synthesis of essential precursors of DNA. Others, particularly the cytidine and adenosine nucleoside analogs, become incorporated into DNA and block its further elongation and its function. Other metabolic effects of these analogs may contribute to their cytotoxicity and even their ability to induce differentiation.

To understand the role of these drugs, it is useful to review the nomenclature of the DNA bases and their metabolic intermediates. Four bases, shown in Figure 51–9, form DNA; these include two pyrimidines, thymine and cytosine; and two purines, guanine and adenine. The base composition of RNA differs in that it incorporates uracil instead of thymine. Uracil may serve as a precursor of deoxythymidine monophosphate; in the final step of this conversion, TS adds a methyl group to the 5 position of deoxyuridine monophosphate. Cells can make these bases *de novo* and convert them to their active deoxynucleoside triphosphates (dNTPs). The dNTPs then act as substrates for DNA polymerase and become linked in 3′-5′ phosphate ester bonds to form DNA strands; their base sequence provides the code for subsequent RNA and protein sequences.

As an alternative to synthesis of new precursor molecules, cells can salvage either free bases or their deoxynucleosides (Figure 51–9), which are found in the systemic circulation, presumably the products of degradation of DNA. Certain bases, such as uracil, guanine, and their analogs, can be taken up by cells and converted intracellularly to (deoxy) nucleotides by the addition of deoxyribose and phosphate groups. Other bases, including cytosine, thymine, and adenine, cannot be activated by mammalian cells, which lack the ability to add the necessary ribose or deoxy ribose groups to these particular bases; however, preformed deoxy-

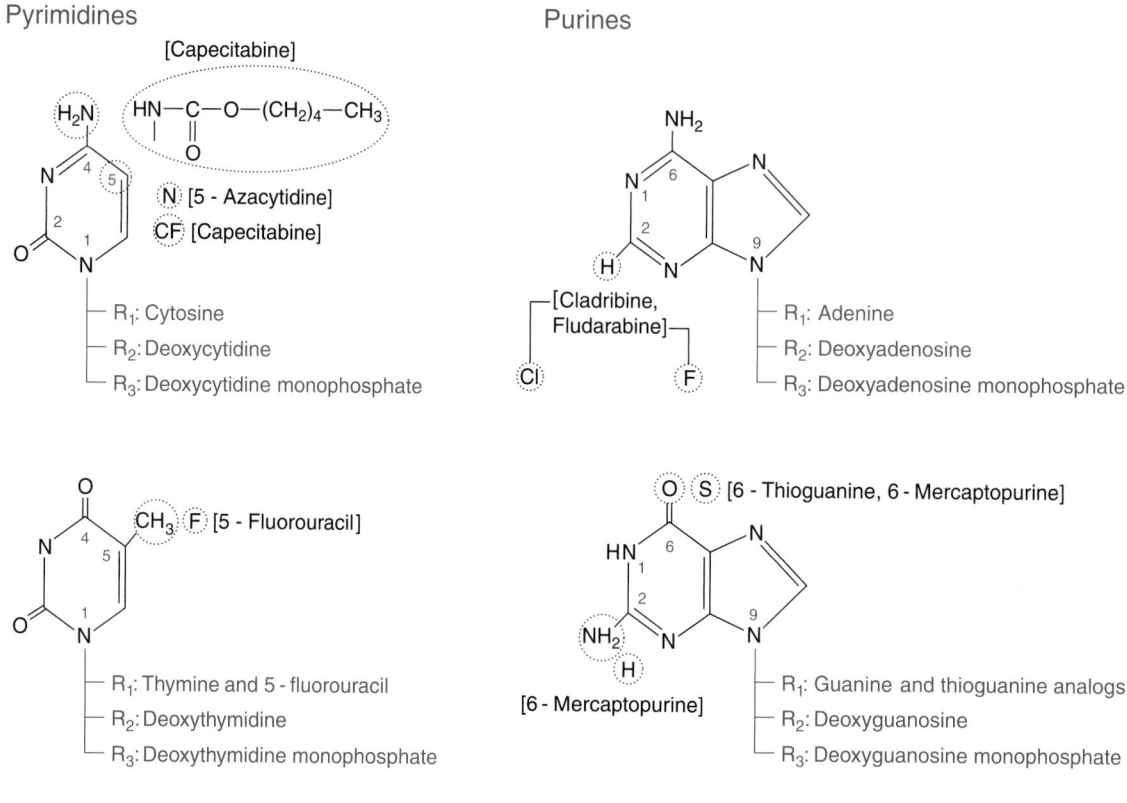

Figure 51–9. Chemical structures of the four bases incorporated into DNA and their analogs. Shown here are the chemical structures of the four bases that become incorporated into DNA, as well as the various modifications found in analogs that function as cytotoxic chemotherapeutic drugs. These modifications involve not only substitutions on the bases but changes in the deoxyribose ring to which the bases are attached (indicated by the asterisk). Some compounds, such as capecitabine and fludarabine, contain multiple substitutions. Others, such as 5-azacytidine, have ribose, rather than deoxyribose, at R_2. The rationale for these substitutions and their effect on DNA synthesis and function are discussed in the text.

nucleosides containing a deoxyribose linked to cytosine or adenine are readily transported into cells and activated by conversion to deoxynucleotides by intracellular kinases.

The limitations of cell uptake and conversion to active triphosphates determine the form in which specific analogs have been synthesized, varying from base analogs such as 5-FU to nucleosides such as cytosine arabinoside, and even to nucleotides such as fludarabine phosphate. Uracil and guanine analogs, containing substitutions on the base itself, are efficiently taken up into cells and converted to dNTPs. Some are useful drugs, such as 5-FU or 6-thioguanine. Because of the inability to activate cytosine or adenine

FLUOROPYRIMIDINE ANALOGS

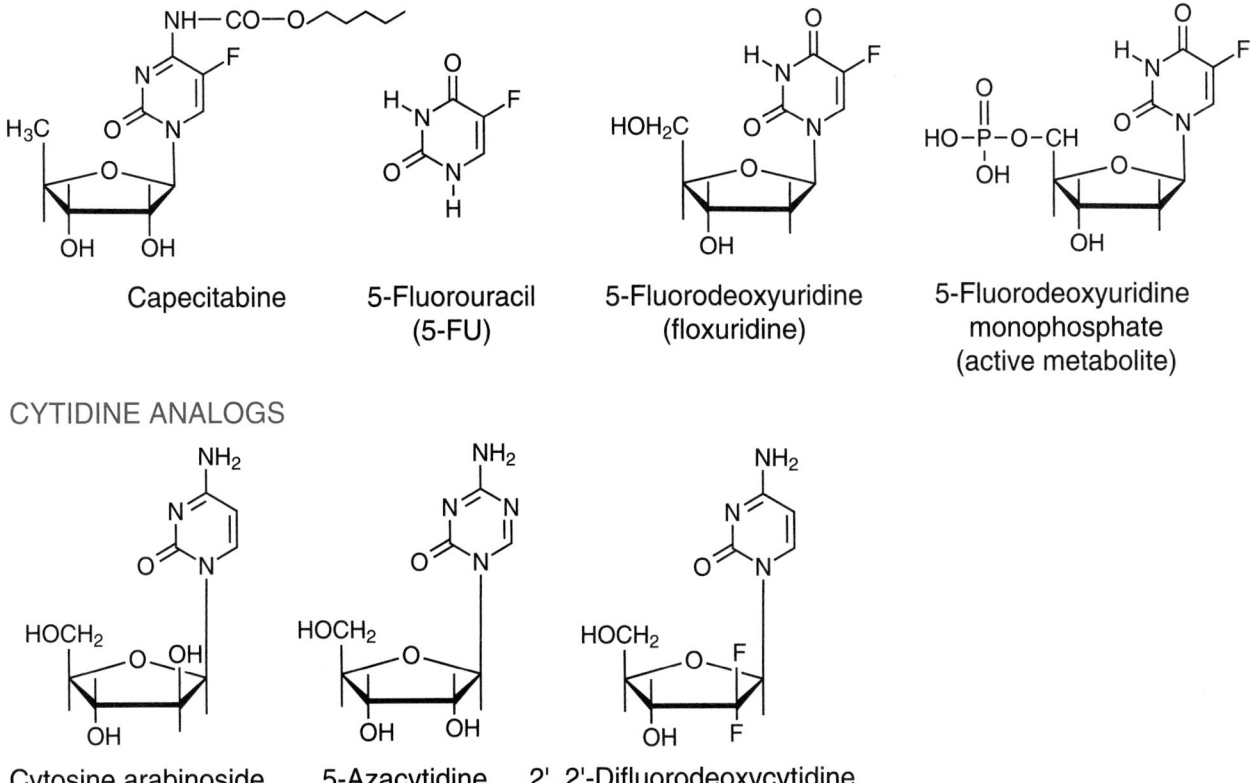

Capecitabine   5-Fluorouracil   5-Fluorodeoxyuridine   5-Fluorodeoxyuridine
                     (5-FU)   (floxuridine)   monophosphate
                                                           (active metabolite)

CYTIDINE ANALOGS

Cytosine arabinoside   5-Azacytidine   2′, 2′-Difluorodeoxycytidine
(cytarabine; AraC)   (gemcitabine)

Figure 51–10. *Structures of available pyrimidine analogs.*

bases, analogs of cytosine and adenine are synthesized as nucleosides, in which form (*cytosine arabinoside* [*cytarabine*; Ara-C] and *gemcitabine*, for example) they are readily transported into cells and converted by kinases to the active dNTPs (Figure 51–10). *Fludarabine phosphate*, a nucleotide, is dephosphorylated rapidly in plasma, releasing the nucleoside that is readily taken up by cells. Analogs may differ from the physiologic bases by alterations in purine or pyrimidine ring or by altering the sugar attached to the base, as in the arabinoside Ara-C, or by altering both the base and sugar, as in fludarabine phosphate.

General Mechanism of Action of Pyrimidine Antimetabolites. The best-characterized agents in this class are the halogenated pyrimidines, a group that includes fluorouracil (5-fluorouracil, or 5-FU), *floxuridine* (5-fluoro-2′-deoxyuridine, or 5-FUdR), and *idoxuridine* (5-iodode-oxyuridine) (*see* Chapter 49). If one compares the van der Waals radii of the various 5-position substituents, the dimension of the fluorine atom resembles that of hydrogen, whereas the bromine and iodine atoms are larger and close in size to the methyl group. Thus, iododeoxyuridine behaves as an analog of thymidine, and its primary biological action results from its phosphorylation and ultimate incorporation into DNA in place of thymidylate. In 5-FU, the

smaller fluorine at position 5 allows the molecule to mimic uracil biochemically. However, the fluorine–carbon bond is much tighter than that of C—H and prevents the methylation of the 5 position of 5-FU by thymidylate synthase. Instead, in the presence of the physiological cofactor 5,10-methylene tetrahydrofolate, the fluoropyrimidine locks the enzyme in an inhibited state and prevents the synthesis of thymidylate, a required DNA precursor.

A number of 5-FU analogs have reached the clinic. The most important of these is *capecitabine* (N4-pentoxycarbonyl-5′-deoxy-5-fluorocytidine) (Figure 51–10), a drug active against colon and breast cancers. This orally administered agent is converted to 5′-deoxy-5-fluorocytidine by carboxylesterase activity in liver and other normal and malignant tissues. From that point, it is converted to 5′-deoxy-fluorodeoxyuridine by the ubiquitous cytidine deaminase. The final step in its activation occurs when thymidine phosphorylase cleaves off the 5′-deoxy sugar, leaving intracellular 5-FU. Tumors with elevated thymidine phosphorylase activity seem particularly susceptible to this drug (Ishikawa *et al.*, 1998).

Analogs of cytidine also are potent antitumor agents. Nucleotides in RNA and DNA contain ribose and 2′-deoxyribose, respectively. The replacement of the ribose of cytidine with arabinose has yielded a useful chemotherapeutic agent, cytarabine (Ara-C). As may be seen in Figure 51–10, the hydroxyl group in Ara-C is attached to the 2′-carbon in the β, or upward, configuration, as compared with the α, or downward, position of the 2′-hydroxyl in

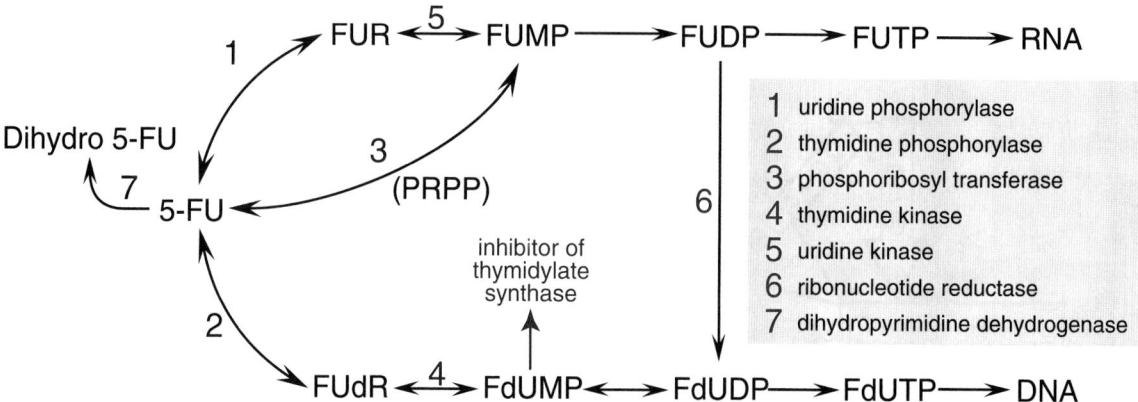

Figure 51–11. *Activation pathways for 5-fluorouracil (5-FU) and 5-floxuridine (FUR).* FUDP, floxuridine diphosphate; FUMP, floxuridine monophosphate; FUTP, floxuridine triphosphate; FUdR, fluorodeoxyuridine; FdUDP, fluorodeoxyuridine diphosphate; FdUMP, fluorodeoxyuridine monophosphate; FdUTP, fluorodeoxyuridine triphosphate; PRPP, 5-phosphoribosyl-1-pyrophosphate.

ribose. The arabinose analog is recognized enzymatically as a 2′-deoxyriboside; it is phosphorylated to a nucleoside triphosphate that competes with deoxycytidine triphosphate (dCTP) for incorporation into DNA (Chabner, 2001). When incorporated into DNA, it blocks elongation of the DNA strand and its template function.

Other cytidine analogs have received extensive clinical evaluation. *Azacitidine* (5-azacytidine) and its deoxyanalog, *decitabine*, inhibit DNA methyltransferase. They have antileukemic as well as differentiating actions. A newer analog, 2′,2′-difluorodeoxycytidine (gemcitabine) (Figure 51–10), becomes incorporated into DNA and inhibits the elongation of nascent DNA strands. It has useful activity in various human solid tumors, including pancreatic, lung, and ovarian cancer.

Fluorouracil and Floxuridine (Fluorodeoxyuridine)

Mechanism of Action. Fluorouracil (5-FU) requires enzymatic conversion to the nucleotide (ribosylation and phosphorylation) in order to exert its cytotoxic activity (Figure 51–11). Several routes are available for the formation of floxuridine monophosphate (FUMP). 5-FU may be converted to fluorouridine by uridine phosphorylase and then to FUMP by uridine kinase, or it may react directly with 5-phosphoribosyl-1-pyrophosphate (PRPP), in a reaction catalyzed by orotate phosphoribosyl transferase, to form FUMP. Many metabolic pathways are available to FUMP. As the triphosphate FUTP it may be incorporated into RNA. An alternative reaction sequence crucial for antineoplastic activity involves reduction of FUDP by ribonucleotide reductase to the deoxynucleotide level and formation of fluorodeoxyuridine monophosphate (FdUMP). 5-FU also may be converted by thymidine phosphorylase to the deoxyriboside fluorodeoxyuridine (FUdR), and then by thymidine kinase to fluorodeoxyuridine monophosphate (FdUMP), a potent inhibitor of thymidylate synthesis. This complex metabolic pathway for the generation of FdUMP may be bypassed through administration of floxuridine (fluorodeoxyuridine; FUdR), which is converted directly to FdUMP by thymidine kinase. FUdR is rarely used in clinical practice.

The interaction between FdUMP and TS blocks the synthesis of thymidine triphosphate (TTP), a necessary constituent of DNA (Figure 51–12). The folate cofactor, 5,10-methylenetetrahydrofolate, and FdUMP form a covalently bound ternary complex with TS. This inhibited complex resembles the transition state formed during the normal enzymatic reaction when dUMP is converted to thymidylate.

While the physiological complex of TS-folate-dUMP progresses to the synthesis of thymidylate by transfer of the methylene group and two hydrogen atoms from folate to dUMP, this reaction is blocked in the inhibited complex of TS-FdUMP-folate by the stability of the fluorine carbon bond on FdUMP; sustained inhibition of the enzyme results (Santi *et al.*, 1974).

5-FU also is incorporated into both RNA and DNA. In 5-FU–treated cells, both fluorodeoxyuridine triphosphate (FdUTP) and deoxyuridine triphosphate (dUTP) (the substrate that accumulates behind the blocked thymidylate synthase reaction) incorporate into DNA in place of the depleted physiological TTP. The significance of the incorporation of FdUTP and dUTP into DNA is unclear (Canman *et al.*, 1993). Presumably, the incorporation of deoxyuridylate and/or fluorodeoxyuridylate into DNA would call into action the excision–repair process. This process may result in DNA strand breakage because DNA repair requires TTP, but this substrate is

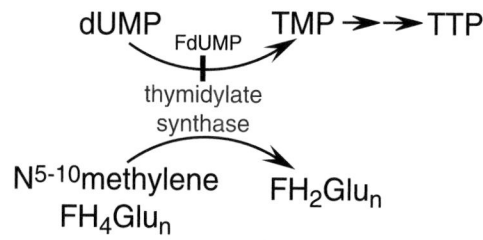

Other actions of 5-FU nucleotides:
· Inhibition of RNA processing
· Incorporation into DNA

Figure 51–12. *Site of action of 5-fluoro-2′-deoxyuridine-5′-phosphate (5-FdUMP).* 5-FU, 5-fluorouracil; dUMP, deoxyuridine monophosphate; TMP, thymidine monophosphate; TTP, thymidine triphosphate; FdUMP, fluorodeoxyuridine monophosphate; FH$_2$Glu$_n$, dihydrofolate polyglutamate; FH$_4$Glu$_n$, tetrahydrofolate polyglutamate.

lacking as a result of thymidylate synthase inhibition. 5-FU incorporation into RNA also causes toxicity as the result of major effects on both the processing and functions of RNA (Danenberg *et al.*, 1990).

A number of biochemical mechanisms have been identified that are associated with resistance to the cytotoxic effects of 5-FU or FUdR. These mechanisms include loss or decreased activity of the enzymes necessary for activation of 5-FU, amplification of TS (Washtein, 1982), and mutation of TS to a form that is not inhibited by FdUMP (Barbour *et al.*, 1990).

Both experimental studies and clinical trials support the position that the response to 5-FU correlates significantly with low levels of the degradative enzymes dihydrouracil dehydrogenase and thymidine phosphorylase, and a low level of expression of TS (Van Triest *et al.*, 2000). TS levels are finely controlled by an autoregulatory feedback mechanism wherein the unbound enzyme interacts with and inhibits the translational efficiency of its own mRNA, which provides for the rapid TS modulation needed for cellular division. When TS is bound to FdUMP, inhibition of translation is relieved, and levels of free TS rise, restoring thymidylate synthesis. Thus, TS autoregulation may be an important mechanism by which malignant cells become insensitive to the effects of 5-FU (Chu *et al.*, 1991).

Some malignant cells appear to have insufficient concentrations of 5,10-methylene tetrahydrofolate, and thus cannot form maximal levels of the inhibited ternary complex with TS. Addition of exogenous folate in the form of 5-formyl-tetrahydrofolate (leucovorin) increases formation of the complex and has enhanced responses to 5-FU in clinical trials (Grogan *et al.*, 1993). It is unclear the degree to which these mechanisms contribute to clinical resistance to 5-FU and its derivatives.

In addition to leucovorin, a number of other agents have been combined with 5-FU in attempts to enhance the cytotoxic activity through biochemical modulation. Methotrexate, by inhibiting purine synthesis and increasing cellular pools of PRPP, enhances the activation of 5-FU and increases antitumor activity of 5-FU when given prior to but not following 5-FU. In clinical trials, the combination of cisplatin and 5-FU has yielded impressive responses in tumors of the upper aerodigestive tract, but the molecular basis of their interaction is not well understood (Grem, 2001). Oxaliplatin is commonly used with 5-FU and leucovorin for treating metastatic colorectal cancer. The mechanism responsible for the synergistic clinical effect of adding oxaliplatin to 5-FU has not been fully elucidated. Experimental studies indicate that oxaliplatin may inhibit catabolism of 5-FU, perhaps by inhibiting dihydropyrimidine dehydrogenase (Fischel *et al.*, 2002). In addition, oxaliplatin also may inhibit expression of TS. Perhaps the most important interaction is the enhancement of irradiation by fluoropyrimidines, the basis for which is unclear. 5-FU with simultaneous irradiation is curative therapy for anal cancer and enhances local tumor control in head and neck, cervical, rectal, gastroesophageal, and pancreatic cancer.

Absorption, Fate, and Excretion. 5-FU is administered parenterally, since absorption after ingestion of the drug is unpredictable and incomplete. Metabolic degradation occurs in many tissues, particularly the liver. 5-FU is inactivated by reduction of the pyrimidine ring; this reaction is carried out by dihydropyrimidine dehydrogenase (DPD), which is found in liver, intestinal mucosa, tumor cells, and other tissues. Inherited deficiency of this enzyme leads to greatly increased sensitivity to the drug (Milano *et al.*, 1999). The rare individual who totally lacks this enzyme may experience profound drug toxicity following conventional doses of the drug. DPD deficiency can be detected either by enzymatic or molecular assays

using peripheral white blood cells, or by determining the plasma ratio of 5-FU to its metabolite, 5-fluoro-5,6-dihydrouracil, which is ultimately degraded to β-fluoro-alanine.

Rapid intravenous administration of 5-FU produces plasma concentrations of 0.1 to 1 mM; plasma clearance is rapid (half-life of 10 to 20 minutes). Urinary excretion of a single dose of 5-FU given intravenously amounts to only 5% to 10% in 24 hours. Although the liver contains high concentrations of DPD, dosage does not have to be modified in patients with hepatic dysfunction, presumably because of degradation of the drug at extrahepatic sites or by vast excess of this enzyme in the liver. Given by continuous intravenous infusion for 24 to 120 hours, 5-FU achieves plasma concentrations in the range of 0.5 to 8 μM. 5-FU enters the CSF in minimal amounts. Concentrations greater than 0.01 μM are sustained for up to 12 hours following conventional doses (Grem, 2001).

Capecitabine is well absorbed orally. It is rapidly de-esterified and deaminated, yielding high plasma concentrations of 5′-deoxy-fluorodeoxyuridine (5′-dFdU), which disappears with a half-life of about 1 hour. 5-FU levels are less than 10% of those of 5′-dFdU, reaching a maximum of 0.3 mg/L or 1μM at 2 hours. The conversion of 5′-dFdU to 5-FU by thymidine phosphorylase occurs in liver, peripheral tissues, and tumors. Liver dysfunction delays the conversion of the parent compound to 5′-dFdU and 5-FU, but there is no consistent effect on toxicity (Twelves *et al.*, 1999).

Therapeutic Uses. **5-Fluorouracil.** 5-Fluorouracil produces partial responses in 10% to 20% of patients with metastatic colon carcinomas, upper gastrointestinal tract carcinomas, and breast carcinomas. The administration of 5-FU in combination with leucovorin in the adjuvant setting is associated with a survival advantage for patients with colorectal cancers and gastric cancers.

For average-risk patients in good nutritional status with adequate hematopoietic function, the weekly dosage regimen employs 500 to 600 mg/m^2 with leucovorin once each week for 6 of 8 weeks. Other regimens use daily doses of 500 mg/m^2 for 5 days, repeated in monthly cycles. When used with leucovorin, doses of daily 5-FU for 5 days must be reduced to 375 to 425 mg/m^2 because of mucositis and diarrhea. 5-FU is increasingly used as a biweekly loading dose followed by a 48-hour continuous infusion, a schedule that has less overall toxicity as well as superior response rates and progression-free survival for patients with metastatic colon cancer (De Gramont *et al.*, 1998).

Floxuridine (FUdR). FUdR (fluorodeoxyuridine; FUDR) is used primarily by continuous infusion into the hepatic artery for treatment of metastatic carcinoma of the colon or following resection of hepatic metastases (Kemeny *et al.*, 1999); the response rate to such infusion is 40% to 50%, or double that observed with intravenous administration. Intrahepatic arterial infusion for 14 to 21 days may be used with minimal systemic toxicity. However, there is a significant risk of biliary sclerosis if this route is used for multiple cycles of therapy. Treatment should be discontinued at the earliest manifestation of toxicity (usually stomatitis or diarrhea) because the maximal effects of bone marrow suppression and gut toxicity will not be evident until days 7 to 14.

Capecitabine (XELODA). Capecitabine is approved by the FDA for the treatment of (1) metastatic breast cancer in patients who have not responded to a regimen of paclitaxel and an anthracycline antibiotic; (2) metastatic breast cancer when used in combination with *docetaxel* in patients who have had a prior anthracycline-containing regimen; and (3) metastatic colorectal cancer for patients in whom fluoropyrimidine monotherapy is preferred. The recommended dose is 2500 mg/m^2 daily, given orally in two divided doses with food, for 2 weeks followed by a rest period of 1 week. This cycle is then repeated two more times.

Combination Therapy. Higher response rates are seen when 5-FU is used in combination with other agents, such as cyclophosphamide and methotrexate (breast cancer), cisplatin (head and neck cancer), and with oxaliplatin or irinotecan in colon cancer. The combination of 5-FU and oxaliplatin or irinotecan has become the standard first-line treatment for patients with metastatic colorectal cancer (Goldberg, 2004). The use of 5-FU in combination regimens has improved survival in the adjuvant treatment for breast cancer (Early Breast Cancer Trialists' Collaborative Group, 1988), and with oxaliplatin and leucovorin, for colorectal cancer (Andre, 2004). 5-FU also is a potent radiation sensitizer. Beneficial effects also have been reported when combined with irradiation for cancers of the esophagus, stomach, pancreas, cervix, anus, and head and neck. 5-FU is used widely with very favorable results for the topical treatment of premalignant keratoses of the skin and multiple superficial basal cell carcinomas.

Clinical Toxicities. The clinical manifestations of toxicity caused by 5-FU and floxuridine are similar and may be difficult to anticipate because of their delayed appearance. The earliest untoward symptoms during a course of therapy are anorexia and nausea; these are followed by stomatitis and diarrhea, which constitute reliable warning signs that a sufficient dose has been administered. Mucosal ulcerations occur throughout the gastrointestinal tract and may lead to fulminant diarrhea, shock, and death, particularly in patients who are DPD deficient. The major toxic effects of bolus-dose regimens result from the myelosuppressive action of 5-FU. The nadir of leukopenia usually is between days 9 and 14 after the first injection of drug. Thrombocytopenia and anemia also may occur. Loss of hair, occasionally progressing to total alopecia, nail changes, dermatitis, and increased pigmentation and atrophy of the skin may be encountered. Hand-foot syndrome consisting of erythema, desquamation, pain, and sensitivity to touch of the palms and soles also can occur. Neurological manifestations, including an acute cerebellar syndrome, have been reported, and myelopathy has been observed after the intrathecal administration of 5-FU. Cardiac toxicity, particularly acute chest pain with evidence of ischemia in the electrocardiogram, also may occur. In general, myelosuppression, mucositis, and diarrhea occur less often with infusional regimens than bolus regimens, while hand-foot syndrome occurs more often with infusional regimens than bolus regimens. The low therapeutic indices of these agents emphasize the need for very skillful supervision by physicians familiar with the action of the fluorinated pyrimidines and the possible hazards of chemotherapy.

Capecitabine causes much the same spectrum of toxicities as 5-FU (diarrhea, myelosuppression), but the hand-foot syndrome

occurs more frequently and may require dose reduction or cessation of therapy.

CYTIDINE ANALOGS

Cytarabine (Cytosine Arabinoside; Ara-C)

Cytarabine (1-β-D-arabinofuranosylcytosine; Ara-C) is the most important antimetabolite used in the therapy of acute myelocytic leukemia (AML). It is the single most effective agent for induction of remission in this disease.

Mechanism of Action. This compound is an analog of 2'-deoxycytidine with the 2'-hydroxyl in a position *trans* to the 3'-hydroxyl of the sugar, as shown in Figure 51–9. The 2'-hydroxyl hinders rotation of the pyrimidine base around the nucleosidic bond and interferes with base stacking.

Ara-C penetrates cells by a carrier-mediated process shared by physiological nucleosides. Several candidate carriers bring nucleosides into cells. In infants and adults with ALL and the t(4;11) MLL translocation, high-dose Ara-C is particularly effective; in these patients, the nucleoside transporter, hENT1, is highly expressed (Pui *et al.*, 2004), and its expression correlates with sensitivity to Ara-C. hENT1 inhibition by nitrobenzylmercaptopurine riboside (NBMPR) prevents Ara-C toxicity to both ALL and AML cells. At extracellular drug concentrations above 10 μM (levels achievable with high-dose Ara-C), the nucleoside transporter no longer limits drug accumulation, and intracellular metabolism to a triphosphate becomes rate limiting.

As with most purine and pyrimidine antimetabolites, Ara-C must be "activated" by conversion to the 5'-monophosphate nucleotide (Ara-CMP), a reaction catalyzed by deoxycytidine kinase. Ara-CMP can then react with appropriate deoxynucleotide kinases to form the diphosphate and triphosphates (Ara-CDP and Ara-CTP). Ara-CTP competes with the physiological substrate deoxycytidine 5'-triphosphate (dCTP) for incorporation into DNA by DNA polymerases. The incorporated Ara-CMP residue is a potent inhibitor of DNA polymerase, both in replication and repair. Inhibition of DNA synthesis correlates with the total Ara-C incorporated into DNA. Thus, incorporation of about five molecules of Ara-C per 10^4 bases of DNA decreases cellular clonogenicity by about 50% (Kufe *et al.*, 1984).

Ara-C induces terminal differentiation of leukemic cells in tissue culture, an effect that is accompanied by decreased c-*myc* oncogene expression (Bianchi Scarra *et al.*, 1986). These changes in morphology, differentiation, and oncogene expression occur at concentrations above the threshold for cytotoxicity and may simply represent terminal injury of cells. However, molecular analysis of bone marrow specimens from some leukemic patients in remission after Ara-C therapy has revealed persistence of leukemic markers, suggesting that differentiation may have occurred.

The contribution of each of the above actions to cellular death caused by Ara-C is not fully understood. Fragmentation of DNA is observed in Ara-C–treated cells, and there is cytological and biochemical evidence for apoptosis in both tumor and normal tissues (Smets, 1994).

Ara-C exposure activates a complex system of secondary intracellular signals that determine whether a cell survives or undergoes apoptosis. It activates the transcription factor AP-1 and stimulates the formation of ceramide, a potent inducer of apoptosis. On the other hand, it promotes an increase in PKC and the cell damage response factor NF-κB in leukemic cells. Finally, the level of expression of BCL-2 and BCL-X$_L$ proteins correlates with relative sensitivity to Ara-C (Ibrado et al., 1996). Thus, the lethal actions may depend on its relative effects on pro-apoptotic and damage response pathways.

In addition to transport and biochemical factors that determine response, cell kinetic properties exert an important influence on the results of Ara-C treatment. It is likely that continued inhibition of DNA synthesis for a duration equivalent to at least one cell cycle is necessary to expose cells during the S, or DNA-synthetic, phase of the cycle. The mean cycle time of acute myelocytic leukemia cells is 1 to 2 days. The optimal interval between bolus doses of Ara-C is about 8 to 12 hours, a schedule that maintains intracellular concentrations of Ara-CTP at inhibitory levels for at least one cell cycle. Typical schedules for administration of Ara-C employ bolus doses every 12 hours for 5 to 7 days or a continuous infusion for 7 days.

Particular subtypes of AML derive benefit from high-dose Ara-C treatment; these include t(8;21), inv(16), t(9;16), and del(16), all of which involve core-binding factors that regulate hematopoiesis (Widemann, 1997).

Mechanisms of Resistance to Cytarabine. Response to Ara-C is strongly influenced by the relative activities of anabolic and catabolic enzymes that determine the proportion of drug converted to Ara-CTP. The rate-limiting enzyme is deoxycytidine kinase, which produces Ara-CMP. An important degradative enzyme is cytidine deaminase, which deaminates Ara-C to a nontoxic metabolite, arauridine. Cytidine deaminase is found in high activity in many tissues, including some human tumors. A second degradative enzyme, dCMP deaminase, converts Ara-CMP to the inactive metabolite, Ara-UMP. Increased synthesis and retention of Ara-CTP in leukemic cells is associated with a longer duration of complete remission in patients with AML (Preisler et al., 1985). As discussed above, the ability of cells to transport Ara-C also affects the clinical response.

Because drug concentration in plasma rapidly falls below the level needed to saturate transport and activation processes, clinicians have employed high-dose regimens (2 to 3 g/m^2 every 12 hours for 6 doses) to achieve 20- to 50 times higher serum levels with improved results in remission induction and consolidation (Mayer et al., 1994) for AML.

Absorption, Fate, and Excretion. Due to the presence of high concentrations of cytidine deaminase in the gastrointestinal mucosa and liver, only about 20% of the drug reaches the circulation after oral Ara-C administration; thus, the drug must be given intravenously. Peak concentrations of 2 to 50 μM are measurable in plasma after intravenous injection of 30 to 300 mg/m^2 but disappear rapidly (half-life of 10 minutes) from plasma. Less than 10% of the injected dose is excreted unchanged in the urine within 12 to 24 hours, while most appears as the inactive deaminated product, arabinosyl uracil. Higher concentrations of Ara-C are found in CSF after continuous infusion than after rapid intravenous injection. After intrathecal administration of the drug at a dose of 50 mg/m^2, relatively little deamination occurs, even after 7 hours, and peak concentrations of 1 to 2 μM are achieved that decline slowly with a half-life of approximately 3.4 hours. Concentrations above the threshold for cytotoxicity (0.4 μM) are maintained in the CSF for 24 hours or longer. More recently, a formulation of Ara-C (DEPOCYT) has been developed for sustained release into the cerebrospinal fluid. After a standard 50-mg dose, cytarabine concentration is maintained at cytotoxic levels for an average of 12 days, thus avoiding the need for repeated lumbar punctures. A possible benefit in terms of time to neurologic progression was suggested in a preliminary study comparing the administration of the sustained-release formulation, 50 mg every 2 weeks, with the standard intrathecal formulation in patients with lymphomatous meningitis (Glantz et al., 1999). It also appears to give equivalent results to standard intrathecal methotrexate in patients with carcinomatous meningitis (Cole et al., 2003).

Therapeutic Uses. Two standard dosage schedules are recommended for administration of cytarabine (CYTOSAR-U, TARABINE PFS, others): (1) rapid intravenous infusion of 100 mg/m^2 every 12 hours for 5 to 7 days; or (2) continuous intravenous infusion of 100 to 200 mg/m^2 daily for 5 to 7 days. In general, children tolerate higher doses than do adults. Intrathecal doses of 30 mg/m^2 every 4 days have been used to treat meningeal leukemia. The intrathecal administration of 50 to 70 mg of the liposomal formulation of cytarabine (DEPOCYT) every 2 weeks seems to be equally effective as the every-four-day regimen.

Conventional cytarabine is indicated for induction and maintenance of remission in acute nonlymphocytic leukemia and is useful in the treatment of other leukemias, such as ALL, AML, and CML in the blast phase. Intrathecal cytarabine is indicated for meningeal leukemia. A depot formulation of cytarabine is indicated for the intrathecal treatment of lymphomatous meningitis and may be useful for carcinomatous meningitis.

Clinical Toxicities. Cytarabine is a potent myelosuppressive agent capable of producing acute, severe leukopenia, thrombocytopenia, and anemia with striking megaloblastic changes. Other toxic manifestations include gastrointestinal disturbances, stomatitis, conjunctivitis, reversible hepatic enzyme elevations, noncardiogenic pulmonary edema, and dermatitis. Cerebellar toxicity, manifest as ataxia and slurred speech, and cerebral toxicity, including seizures, dementia, and coma, may follow intrathecal administration or high-dose systemic administration to patients older than 50 years of age and/or patients with poor renal function.

Azacitidine (5-Azacytidine)

5-Azacytidine and the closely related investigational drug decitabine (2′-dexoy-5-azacytidine), have antileukemic activity and induce differentiation. 5-Azacytidine is approved for treatment of myelodysplasia, for which it induces normalization of bone marrow in 15% to 20% of patients and a reduction in transfusion requirement in one-third of patients. It becomes incorporated into RNA and DNA and inhibits methylation of DNA, inducing the expression of silenced genes. Thus, it also is used for inducing fetal hemoglobin synthesis in sickle cell anemia, although it has been largely replaced for this indication by hydroxyurea. It undergoes very rapid deamination by cytidine deaminase, the product hydrolyzing to inactive metabolites. Its major toxicities include myelosuppression, and rather severe nausea and vomiting when given intravenously in large doses (150 to 200 mg/m^2 per day for 5 days). In low-dose daily subcutaneous regimens for myelodysplasia, 30 mg/m^2 per day, it is well tolerated.

Gemcitabine

Gemcitabine (2′,2′ difluorodeoxycytidine; dFdC), a difluoro analog of deoxycytidine, has become an important drug for patients with metastatic pancreatic cancer, non–small cell lung cancer, ovarian, bladder, esophageal, and head and neck cancer (Hertel *et al.*, 1990).

Mechanism of Action. Gemcitabine enters cells *via* active nucleoside transporters (Mackey *et al.*, 1998). Intracellularly, deoxycytidine kinase phosphorylates gemcitabine to produce difluorodeoxycytidine monophosphate (dFdCMP), from which point it is converted to difluorodeoxycytidine di- and triphosphate (dFdCDP and dFdCTP). While its anabolism and effects on DNA in general mimic those of cytarabine, there are differences in kinetics of inhibition, additional sites of action, effects of incorporation into DNA, and spectrum of clinical activity (Iwasaki *et al.*, 1997). Unlike cytarabine, the cytotoxicity of gemcitabine is not confined to the S phase of the cell cycle, and the drug is equally effective against confluent cells and cells in logarithmic growth phase. The cytotoxic activity may be a result of several actions on DNA synthesis: dFdCTP competes with dCTP as a weak inhibitor of DNA polymerase; dFdCDP is a potent inhibitor of ribonucleotide reductase, resulting in depletion of deoxyribonucleotide pools necessary for DNA synthesis; and dFdCTP is incorporated into DNA and after the incorporation of one more additional nucleotide leads to DNA strand termination (Heinemann *et al.*, 1988). This "extra" nucleotide may be important in hiding the dFdCTP from DNA repair enzymes, as the incorporated dFdCMP appears to be resistant to repair. The ability of cells to incorporate dFdCTP into DNA is critical for gemcitabine-induced apoptosis (Huang and Plunkett, 1995).

Absorption, Fate, and Elimination. Gemcitabine is administered as an intravenous infusion. The pharmacokinetics of the parent compound are largely determined by deamination, and the predominant urinary elimination product is the inactive metabolite difluorodeoxyuridine (dFdU). Gemcitabine has a short plasma half-life of approximately 15 minutes, with women and elderly subjects having slower clearance (Abbruzzese *et al.*, 1991). Clearance is dose-independent but can vary widely among individuals.

Similar to that of cytarabine, conversion of gemcitabine to dFdCMP by deoxycytidine kinase is saturated at infusion rates of approximately 10 mg/m^2 per minute, which produce plasma drug concentrations in the range of 15 to 20 μM (Grunewald *et al.*, 1991; Grunewald *et al.*, 1992). In an attempt to increase dFdCTP formation, the duration of infusion at this maximum concentration has been extended to 150 minutes. In contrast to a fixed infusion duration of 30 minutes, the 150-minute infusion produces a higher level of dFdCTP within peripheral blood mononuclear cells, increases the degree of myelosuppression, but has uncertain effects on antitumor activity (Tempero *et al.*, 2003).

The activity of dFdCTP on DNA repair mechanisms may allow for increased cytotoxicity of other chemotherapeutic agents, particularly platinum compounds. Preclinical studies of tumor cell lines

show that cisplatin-DNA adducts are enhanced in the presence of gemcitabine, presumably through suppression of nuclear excision repair (Van Moorsel *et al.*, 1999).

Therapeutic Uses. The standard dosing schedule for gemcitabine (GEMZAR) is a 30-minute intravenous infusion of 1 to 1.2 g/m^2 on days 1, 8, and 15 of each 28-day cycle.

Clinical Toxicities. The principal toxicity of gemcitabine is myelosuppression. In general, the longer-duration infusions lead to greater myelosuppression. Nonhematologic toxicities including a flu-like syndrome, asthenia, and mild elevation in liver transaminases may occur in 40% or more of patients. Although severe nonhematologic toxicities are rare, interstitial pneumonitis may occur and is responsive to steroids. Rarely, patients on gemcitabine treatment for many months may develop a slowly progressive hemolytic uremic syndrome, necessitating drug discontinuation. (Humphreys *et al.*, 2004). Gemcitabine is a very potent radiosensitizer and should not be used with radiotherapy except in closely monitored clinical trials (Lawrence *et al.*, 1999).

PURINE ANALOGS

The pioneering studies of Hitchings and Elion begun in 1942 identified analogues of naturally occurring purine bases with antileukemic and immunosuppressant properties. Their work led to the development of drugs used not only in the treatment of malignant diseases (mercaptopurine, thioguanine), but also for immunosuppression (azathioprine) and antiviral chemotherapy (*acyclovir, ganciclovir, vidarabine,* and *zidovudine*) (Figure 51–13). The hypoxanthine analog *allopurinol,* a potent inhibitor of xanthine oxidase, is an important by-product of this effort (*see* Chapter 26). Other purine analogs have found important use in cancer therapy. These include pentostatin (2′-deoxycoformycin), the first effective agent against hairy cell leukemia. Pentostatin has largely been replaced by another adenosine analog, *cladribine*, while the closely related fludarabine phosphate has become a standard treatment for chronic lymphocytic leukemia (CLL) and follicular lymphomas (Beutler, 1992).

6-Thiopurine Analogs

Structure–Activity Relationship. 6-Mercaptopurine (6-MP) and 6-thioguanine (6-TG) are approved agents for human leukemias, and function as analogs of the natural purines, hypoxanthine and guanine. The substitution of sulfur for oxygen on C6 of the purine ring creates compounds that are readily converted to nucleotides in normal and malignant cells. Nucleotides formed from 6-MP and 6-TG inhibit *de novo* purine synthesis and also become incorporated into nucleic acids. The structural formula of 6-MP and other purine analogs is shown in Figure 51–13.

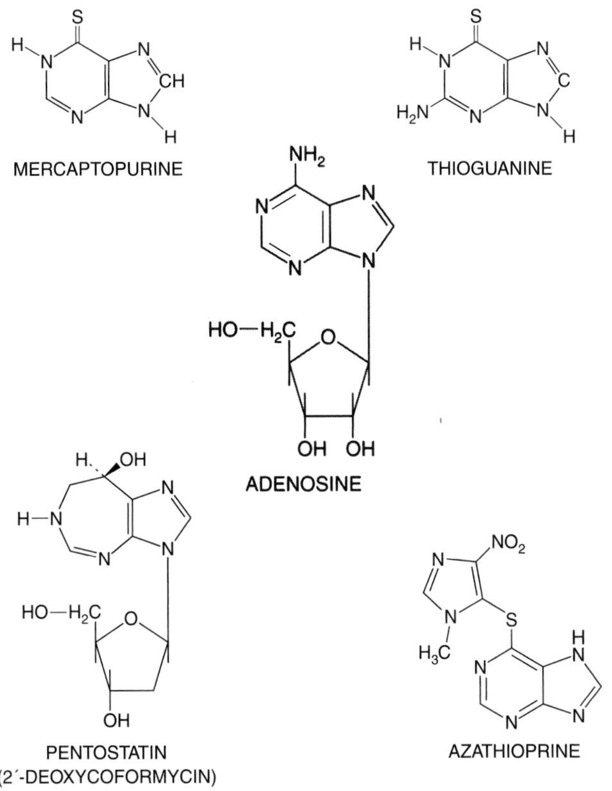

Figure 51–13. *Structural formulas of adenosine and various purine analogs.*

Mechanism of Action. Both 6-TG and 6-MP are excellent substrates for hypoxanthine guanine phosphoribosyl transferase (HGPRT) and are converted in a single step to the ribonucleotides 6-thioguanosine-5′-monophosphate (6-thioGMP) and 6-thioinosine-5′-monophosphate (T-IMP), respectively. Because T-IMP is a poor substrate for guanylyl kinase, the enzyme that converts guanosine monophosphate (GMP) to guanosine diphosphate (GDP), T-IMP accumulates intracellularly. Small amounts of 6-MP, however, also can be incorporated into cellular DNA in the form of thioguanine deoxyribonucleotide. T-IMP inhibits the first step in the *de novo* synthesis of the purine base. The formation of ribosyl-5-phosphate, as well as conversion of inosine-5′-monophosphate (IMP) to adenine and guanine nucleotides, also are inhibited. Of these, the most important point of attack seems to be the reaction of glutamine and 5-phosphoribosyl-1-pyrophosphate (PRPP) to form ribosyl-5-phosphate, the first committed step in the *de novo* pathway.

Despite extensive investigations, the role of incorporation of thiopurines into cellular DNA in the production of either the therapeutic or toxic effects remains unknown (Bo *et al.*, 1999). The incidence of pregnancy-related complications, however, was significantly increased when fathers used mercaptopurine within 3 months of conception (Rajapakse *et al.*, 2000). These compounds can cause marked inhibition of the coordinated induction of various enzymes required for DNA synthesis, as well as potentially critical alterations in the synthesis of polyadenylate-containing RNA (Giverhaug *et al.*, 1999).

Mechanisms of Resistance to the Thiopurine Antimetabolites. As with other tumor-inhibiting antimetabolites, acquired resistance is a major obstacle with the purine analogs. The most commonly encountered mechanism of 6-MP resistance observed *in vitro* is deficiency or complete lack of the activating enzyme, HGPRT.

Another mechanism of 6-MP resistance identified in cells from leukemic patients is an increase in particulate alkaline phosphatase activity. Other potential mechanisms for resistance to 6-MP include (1) decreased drug transport; (2) alteration in allosteric inhibition of ribosylamine 5-phosphate synthase; (3) altered recognition of DNA breaks and mismatches induced by 6-MP; and (4) increased activity of multidrug resistance protein 5, which exports nucleoside analogs (Wijnholds *et al.*, 2000).

Mercaptopurine Pharmacokinetics and Toxicity.
Absorption of mercaptopurine is incomplete after oral ingestion and bioavailability is reduced by first-pass metabolism by xanthine oxidase in the liver. Oral bioavailability is only 10% to 50%, with great interpatient variability and decreased absorption in the presence of food or oral antibiotics. Thus, when used in combination with other drugs, doses should be titrated according to the white blood cell and platelet counts. Bioavailability is increased when mercaptopurine is combined with high-dose methotrexate (Innocenti *et al.*, 1996).

After an intravenous dose, the half-life of the drug in plasma is relatively short (about 50 minutes in adults), due to rapid metabolic degradation by xanthine oxidase and by thiopurine methyltransferase. Restricted brain distribution of mercaptopurine results from an efficient efflux transport system in the blood–brain barrier (Deguchi *et al.*, 2000). In addition to the HGPRT-catalyzed anabolism of mercaptopurine, there are two other pathways for its metabolism. The first involves methylation of the sulfhydryl group and subsequent oxidation of the methylated derivatives. Expression of the enzyme thiopurine methyltransferase reflects the inheritance of polymorphic alleles (Relling *et al.*, 1999); up to 15% of the Caucasian population have decreased enzyme activity. Low levels of erythrocyte thiopurine methyltransferase activity are associated with increased drug toxicity in individual patients and a lower risk of relapse (Pui *et al.*, 2004). High concentrations of 6-methylmercaptopurine nucleotides are formed following 6-MP administration. Substantial amounts of the mono-, di-, and triphosphate nucleotides of 6-methylmercaptopurine ribonucleoside (6-MMPR) have been identified in cells in the blood and bone marrow of patients treated with mercaptopurine or azathioprine. They are less potent than 6-MP nucleotides as metabolic inhibitors, and their significance in contributing to the activity of 6-MP is not known. A relatively large percentage of the administered sulfur is excreted as inorganic sulfate, the result of enzymatic desulfuration.

The second major pathway for 6-MP metabolism involves its oxidation by xanthine oxidase to 6-thiouric acid, an inactive metabolite. Oral doses of 6-MP should be reduced by 75% in patients receiving the xanthine oxidase inhibitor allopurinol.

Therapeutic Uses. The initial average daily oral dose of mercaptopurine (6-mercaptopurine; PURINETHOL) is 50 to 100 mg/m², and is adjusted according to white blood cell count and platelet count. The total dose required to produce depression of the bone marrow in patients with nonhematological malignancies is about 45 mg/kg and may range from 18 to 100 mg/kg.

Hyperuricemia with hyperuricosuria may occur during treatment; the accumulation of uric acid presumably reflects the destruction of cells with release of purines that are oxidized by xanthine oxidase and an inhibition of the conversion of inosinic acid to nucleic acid precursors. This circumstance may be an indication for the use of allopurinol. Special caution must be employed if mercaptopurine or its imidazolyl derivative, azathioprine, is used with allopurinol, because the associated delay in catabolism of the purine analog (*see* above) increases the likelihood of severe toxicity. Patients treated simultaneously with both drugs should receive approximately 25% of the usual dose of mercaptopurine.

The combination of methotrexate and 6-MP appears to be synergistic, based on the effects of methotrexate inhibition of purine biosynthesis. By inhibiting the earliest steps in purine synthesis, methotrexate elevates the intracellular concentration of PRPP, which is required for 6-MP activation.

Clinical Toxicities. The principal toxicity of 6-MP is bone marrow depression, although in general this side effect develops more gradually than with folic acid antagonists; accordingly, thrombocytopenia, granulocytopenia, or anemia may not be encountered for several weeks. When depression of normal bone marrow elements occurs, dose reduction usually results in prompt recovery. Anorexia, nausea, or vomiting is seen in approximately 25% of adults, but stomatitis and diarrhea are rare; manifestations of gastrointestinal effects are less frequent in children than in adults. Jaundice and hepatic enzyme elevations occur in up to one-third of adult patients treated with 6-MP, and usually resolve upon discontinuation of therapy. Their appearance has been associated with bile stasis and hepatic necrosis on biopsy. The long-term complications associated with the use of 6-MP and its derivative, azathioprine, are opportunistic infection and an increased incidence of squamous cell malignancies of skin (Korelitz *et al.*, 1999). Teratogenic effects during the first trimester are associated with chronic 6-MP, and AML has been reported after prolonged use of 6-MP for Crohn's disease (Heizer and Peterson, 1998).

Fludarabine Phosphate

A fluorinated deamination-resistant nucleotide analog of the antiviral agent vidarabine (9-β-D-arabinofuranosyl-adenine), this compound is active in CLL and low-grade lymphomas (Zinzani *et al.*, 2000). After rapid extracellular dephosphorylation to the nucleoside fludarabine, it is rephosphorylated intracellularly by deoxycytidine kinase to the active triphosphate derivative. This antimetabolite inhibits DNA polymerase, DNA primase, DNA ligase, and ribonucleotide reductase, and is incorporated into DNA and RNA. The triphosphate nucleotide is an effective chain terminator when incorporated into DNA (Kamiya *et al.*, 1996), and the incorporation of fludarabine into RNA inhibits RNA function, RNA processing, and mRNA translation (Plunkett

and Gandhi, 1993). A major effect of this drug may be its activation of apoptosis, which may explain its activity against indolent lymphoproliferative disease, where only a small fraction of cells are in S phase (Dighiero, 1996). In experimental tumors, resistance to fludarabine is associated with decreased activity of deoxycytidine kinase, the enzyme that phosphorylates the drug (Mansson *et al.*, 2003).

The structural formulas of fludarabine phosphate and a related adenosine analog, cladribine, are:

	R_1	R_2	R_3
FLUDARABINE–5'–PHOSPHATE	F	O‖HO–P–OH	—OH
CLADRIBINE	Cl	H	H

Absorption, Fate, and Excretion. Fludarabine phosphate is administered intravenously and is rapidly converted to fludarabine in the plasma. The terminal half-life of fludarabine is approximately 10 hours. The compound is primarily eliminated by renal excretion, and approximately 23% appears in the urine as fludarabine because of its relative resistance to deamination by adenosine deaminase.

Therapeutic Uses. Fludarabine phosphate (FLUDARA) is available for intravenous use. The recommended dose of fludarabine phosphate is 20 to 30 mg/m^2 daily for 5 days. The drug is administered intravenously by infusion during a period of 30 minutes to 2 hours. Dosage may need to be reduced in renal impairment. Treatment may be repeated every 4 weeks, and at these doses gradual improvement usually occurs during a period of two to three cycles.

Fludarabine phosphate is used primarily for the treatment of patients with CLL, although experience is accumulating that suggests effectiveness in B-cell lymphomas refractory to standard therapy. In CLL patients previously refractory to a regimen containing a standard alkylating agent, response rates of 32% to 48% have been reported. Activity also has been seen with indolent non-Hodgkin's lymphoma, promyelocytic leukemia, cutaneous T-cell lymphoma, and Waldenström's macroglobulinemia. In patients with previously untreated low-grade lymphomas, fludarabine phosphate in combination with either cyclophosphamide or with dexamethasone and *mitoxantrone*, has resulted in a high rate of response. (Emmanouilides *et al.*, 1998). There is growing interest in its use as a potent immunosuppressive agent, with high-dose alkylators, in nonmyeloablative stem cell transplantation (Taussig *et al.*, 2003).

Clinical Toxicities. Toxic manifestations include myelosuppression, nausea and vomiting, chills and fever, malaise, anorexia, and weakness. Lymphopenia and thrombocytopenia are dose limiting and possibly cumulative (Malspeis *et al.*, 1990). CD4-positive T cells are depleted with therapy. Opportunistic infections and tumor lysis syndrome have been reported (Cheson *et al.*, 1999). Peripheral neuropathy may occur at standard doses. Altered mental status, seizures, optic neuritis, and coma have been observed at higher doses and in older patients. Rarely, CLL patients may develop an acute hemolytic anemia or pure red cell aplasia during fludarabine treatment. Severe pneumonitis that is responsive to corticosteroids has been encountered (Stoica *et al.*, 2002). Because a significant fraction of drug (about one-quarter) is eliminated in the urine, patients with compromised renal function should be treated with caution, and initial doses should be reduced in proportion to serum creatinine levels.

Cladribine

An adenosine deaminase-resistant purine analog, cladribine (2-chlorodeoxyadenosine; 2-CdA) has demonstrated potent activity in hairy cell leukemia, CLL, and low-grade lymphomas. After intracellular phosphorylation by deoxycytidine kinase and conversion to cladribine triphosphate, it is incorporated into DNA. It produces DNA strand breaks and depletion of NAD and ATP, as well as apoptosis, and is a potent inhibitor of ribonucleotide reductase (Beutler, 1992). The drug does not require cell division to be cytotoxic. Resistance is associated with loss of the activating enzyme, deoxycytidine kinase, or escape of ribonucleotide reductase from inhibition (Cardoen *et al.*, 2001).

The structural formula of cladribine is shown above with that of fludarabine-5′-phosphate.

Absorption, Fate, and Excretion. Cladribine is moderately well absorbed orally (55%), but is routinely administered intravenously. The drug is excreted by the kidneys, with a terminal half-life in plasma of 6.7 hours (Liliemark and Juliusson, 1991). Cladribine crosses the blood–brain barrier and reaches CSF concentrations of about 25% of those seen in plasma. In patients with meningeal involvement, however, CSF concentrations can approach those in plasma.

Therapeutic Uses. Cladribine (LEUSTATIN) is administered as a single course of 0.09 mg/kg per day for 7 days by continuous intravenous infusion.

Cladribine is considered the drug of choice in hairy cell leukemia. Eighty percent of patients achieve a complete response after a single course of therapy (Dearden *et al.*, 1999). The drug also is active in CLL, and is a secondary agent in other leukemias and low-grade lymphomas, Langerhans cell histiocytosis, cutaneous T-cell lymphomas including mycosis fungoides and the Sézary syndrome, and Waldenström's macroglobulinemia (Tondini *et al.*, 2000; Saven and Burian, 1999).

Clinical Toxicities. The major dose-limiting toxicity of cladribine is myelosuppression. Cumulative thrombocytopenia may occur with repeated courses. Opportunistic infections are common and are correlated with decreased CD4+ cell counts. Other toxic effects include nausea, infections, high fever, headache, fatigue, skin rashes, and tumor lysis syndrome. Neurological and immunosuppressive adverse effects are less evident than with pentostatin at clinically active doses.

Pentostatin (2′-Deoxycoformycin)

Pentostatin, a transition-state analog of the intermediate in the adenosine deaminase (ADA) reaction, is a potent inhibitor of ADA. Its effects mimic the phenotype of genetic ADA deficiency, which is associated with severe immunodeficiency affecting both T- and B-cell functions. It was isolated from fermentation cultures of *Streptomyces antibioticus*. Inhibition of ADA by pentostatin leads to accumulation of intracellular adenosine and deoxyadenosine nucleotides, which can block DNA synthesis by inhibiting ribonucleotide reductase. Deoxyadenosine also inactivates *S*-adenosyl homocysteine hydrolase. The resulting accumulation of *S*-adenosyl homocysteine is particularly toxic to lymphocytes. Pentostatin also can inhibit RNA synthesis, and its triphosphate derivative is incorporated into DNA, resulting in strand breakage (Stoica *et al.*, 2002). In combination with 2′-deoxyadenosine, it is capable of inducing apoptosis in human monocytoid leukemia cells (Niitsu *et al.*, 1998). Although the precise mechanism of cytotoxicity is not known, it is probable that the imbalance in purine nucleotide pools accounts for its antineoplastic effect in hairy cell leukemia and T-cell lymphomas.

The structural formula of pentostatin (2′-deoxycoformycin) is shown in Figure 51–13.

Absorption, Fate, and Excretion. Pentostatin is administered intravenously, and a single dose of 4 mg/m² has been reported to have a mean terminal half-life of 5.7 hours. The drug is eliminated almost entirely by renal excretion. Proportional reduction of dosage is recommended in patients with renal impairment as measured by reduced creatinine clearance.

Therapeutic Uses. Pentostatin (NIPENT) is available for intravenous use. The recommended dosage is 4 mg/m² administered every other week. After hydration with 500 to 1000 ml of 5% dextrose in half-normal (0.45%) saline, the drug is administered by rapid intravenous injection or by infusion during a period of up to 30 minutes, followed by an additional 500 ml of fluids. Extravasation does not produce tissue necrosis.

Pentostatin is extremely effective in producing complete remissions in hairy cell leukemia (Grever *et al.*, 2003). Complete responses of 58% and partial responses of 28% have been reported, even in patients who were refractory to interferon-alfa. Activity also is seen against CLL, CML, promyelocytic leukemia, cutaneous T-cell lymphoma, non-Hodgkin's lymphoma, and Langerhans cell histiocytosis (Dillman, 1994; Cortes *et al.*, 1997). Pentostatin has no significant activity against solid tumors or multiple myeloma.

Clinical Toxicities. Toxic manifestations include myelosuppression, gastrointestinal symptoms, skin rashes, and abnormal liver function studies at standard (4 mg/m^2) doses. Depletion of normal T cells occurs at these doses, and neutropenic fever and opportunistic infections have been reported (Steis *et al.*, 1991). Immunosuppression may persist for several years after discontinuation of pentostatin therapy. At higher doses (10 mg/m^2), major renal and neurological complications are encountered. The use of pentostatin in combination with fludarabine phosphate may result in severe or even fatal pulmonary toxicity.

III. NATURAL PRODUCTS

ANTIMITOTIC DRUGS

Vinca Alkaloids

History. The beneficial properties of the Madagascar periwinkle plant, *Catharanthus roseus* (formerly called *Vinca rosea*), a species of myrtle, have been described in medicinal folklore. While exploring claims that extracts of the periwinkle might have beneficial effects in diabetes mellitus, Noble and coworkers observed granulocytopenia and bone marrow suppression in rats. Purified alkaloids caused regression of an acute lymphocytic leukemia in mice. These extracts yielded four active dimeric alkaloids: vinblastine, vincristine, *vinleurosine,* and *vinrosidine.* Vinblastine and vincristine are important clinical agents for treatment of leukemias, lymphomas, and testicular cancer. A closely related derivative, *vinorelbine,* has important activity against lung cancer and breast cancer (Budman, 1997).

Chemistry. The vinca alkaloid antimitotic agents are asymmetrical dimeric compounds; the structures of vinblastine, vincristine, vindesine, and vinorelbine are:

	R$_1$	R$_2$	R$_3$
Structure **A**			
VINBLASTINE	—CH$_3$	—C(=O)—OCH$_3$	—O—C(=O)—CH$_3$
VINCRISTINE	—CH(=O)	—C(=O)—OCH$_3$	—O—C(=O)—CH$_3$
VINDESINE	—CH$_3$	—C(=O)—NH$_2$	—OH
Structure **B**			
VINORELBINE	—CH$_3$	—C(=O)—OCH$_3$	—O—C(=O)—CH$_3$

Mechanism of Action. The vinca alkaloids are cell-cycle–specific agents, and in common with other drugs such as *colchicine, podophyllotoxin,* and *taxanes,* block cells in mitosis. The biological activities of the vincas can be explained by their ability to bind specifically to β-tubulin and to block its ability to polymerize with α-tubulin into microtubules. When cells are incubated with vinblastine, the microtubules dissolve and highly regular crystals form, containing 1 mole of bound vinblastine per mole of tubulin. Cell division is arrested in metaphase. In the absence of an intact mitotic spindle, duplicated chromosomes cannot align along the division plate. They disperse throughout the cytoplasm (exploded mitosis) or may clump in unusual groupings, such as balls or stars. Cells blocked in mitosis undergo changes characteristic of apoptosis (Smets, 1994).

In addition to their key role in the formation of mitotic spindles, microtubules are found in high concentration in the brain and are essential to other cellular functions such as movement, phagocytosis, and axonal transport. Side effects of the vinca alkaloids, such as their neurotoxicity, may be due to disruption of these functions.

Drug Resistance. Despite their structural similarity, the vinca alkaloids have unique individual patterns of clinical effectiveness (*see* below). However, in most experimental systems, they share cross-resistance. Their antitumor effects are blocked by multidrug resistance, in which tumor cells become cross-resistant to a wide range of chemically dissimilar agents after exposure to a single (natural product) drug. Such multidrug-resistant tumor cells display cross-resistance to vinca alkaloids, the epipodophyllotoxins, anthracyclines, and taxanes. Chromosomal abnormalities consistent with gene amplification have been observed in resistant cells in culture, and the cells contain markedly increased levels of the P-glycoprotein, a membrane efflux pump that transports drugs from the cells (Endicott and Ling, 1989). Calcium channel blockers such as *verapamil* can reverse resistance of this type. Other membrane transporters such as the multidrug resistance–associated protein (MRP) (Kuss *et al.*, 1994), and the closely related breast cancer resistance protein, may mediate multidrug resistance. Still other forms of resistance to vinca alkaloids stem from mutations in β-tubulin or in the relative expression of isoforms of β-tubulin; both changes prevent the effective binding of the inhibitors to their target.

Cytotoxic Actions. Vincristine is a standard component of regimens for treating pediatric leukemias, lymphomas, and solid tumors. In large-cell non-Hodgkin's lymphomas, vincristine remains an important agent, particularly when used in the CHOP regimen with cyclophosphamide, doxorubicin, and prednisone. As mentioned previously, vincristine is more useful for remission induction in lymphocytic leukemia. Vincristine also is a standard component of a number of regimens used to treat pediatric solid tumors such as Wilms' tumor, neuroblastoma, and rhabdomyosarcoma.

Vinblastine is employed in treating bladder cancer, testicular carcinomas, and Hodgkin's disease. Vinorelbine has activity against non–small cell lung cancer and breast cancer. The very limited myelosuppressive action of vincristine makes it a valuable component of a number of combination therapy regimens for leukemia and lymphoma, while the lack of neurotoxicity of vinblastine is a decided advantage in lymphomas and in combination with cisplatin against testicular cancer. Vinorelbine, which causes a mild neurotoxicity as well as myelosuppression, has an intermediate toxicity profile.

Myelosuppression. The nadir of leukopenia following vinblastine or vinorelbine occurs 7 to 10 days following drug administration. Vincristine in standard doses, 1.4 to 2 mg/m², causes little reduction of formed elements in the blood. All three agents cause hair loss and local cellulitis if extravasated. A syndrome of hyponatremia due to inappropriate secretion of antidiuretic hormone occurs rarely after vincristine administration (*see* Chapter 29).

Neurological Toxicity. While all three derivatives may cause neurotoxic symptoms, vincristine has predictable cumulative effects. Numbness and tingling of the extremities and loss of deep tendon reflexes constitute the most common and earliest signs and are followed by motor weakness. The sensory changes do not usually warrant an immediate reduction in drug dose, but loss of motor function should lead to a reevaluation of the therapeutic plan, and under most circumstances, discontinuation of the drug. Rarely, patients may experience vocal cord paralysis or loss of extraocular muscle function. High-dose vincristine causes severe constipation or obstipation. Inadvertent intrathecal vincristine administration produces devastating and invariably fatal central neurotoxicity, with seizures and irreversible coma (Williams *et al.*, 1983).

Absorption, Fate, and Excretion. The liver extensively metabolizes all three agents, and the conjugates and metabolites are excreted in the bile (Zhou and Rahmani, 1992; Robieux *et al.*, 1996). Only a small fraction of a dose (less than 15%) is found in the urine unchanged. In patients with hepatic dysfunction (bilirubin >3 mg/dl), a 75% reduction in dose of any of the vinca alkaloids is advisable, although firm guidelines for dose adjustment have not been established. The pharmacokinetics of each of the three drugs are similar, with elimination half-lives of 1 and 20 hours for vincristine,

3 and 23 hours for vinblastine, and 1 and 45 hours for vinorelbine (Marquet *et al.*, 1992).

Vinblastine

Therapeutic Uses. Vinblastine sulfate (VELBAN, others) is given intravenously; special precautions must be taken against subcutaneous extravasation, since this may cause painful irritation and ulceration. The drug should not be injected into an extremity with impaired circulation. After a single dose of 0.3 mg/kg of body weight, myelosuppression reaches its maximum in 7 to 10 days. If a moderate level of leukopenia (approximately 3000 cells per mm³) is not attained, the weekly dose may be increased gradually by increments of 0.05 mg/kg of body weight. In regimens designed to cure testicular cancer, vinblastine is used in doses of 0.3 mg/kg every 3 weeks.

The most important clinical use of vinblastine is with bleomycin and cisplatin (*see* below) in the curative therapy of metastatic testicular tumors (Williams and Einhorn, 1985), although it has been supplanted by etoposide or ifosfamide in this disease. It is a component of the standard curative regimen for Hodgkin's disease, (ABVD; dacarbazine, vinblastine, doxorubicin, and bleomycin). It also is active in Kaposi's sarcoma, neuroblastoma, and Letterer-Siwe disease (histiocytosis X), as well as in carcinoma of the breast and choriocarcinoma.

Clinical Toxicities. The nadir of the leukopenia that follows the administration of vinblastine usually occurs within 7 to 10 days, after which recovery ensues within 7 days. Other toxic effects of vinblastine include neurological manifestations as described above. Gastrointestinal disturbances including nausea, vomiting, anorexia, and diarrhea may be encountered. The syndrome of inappropriate secretion of antidiuretic hormone has been reported. Loss of hair, stomatitis, and dermatitis occur infrequently. Extravasation during injection may lead to cellulitis and phlebitis. Local injection of hyaluronidase and application of moderate heat to the area may be of help by dispersing the drug.

Vincristine

Therapeutic Uses. Vincristine sulfate (ONCOVIN, VINCASAR PFS, others) used together with glucocorticoids is the treatment of choice to induce remissions in childhood leukemia; common dosages for these drugs are vincristine, intravenously, 2 mg/m² of body surface area weekly, and prednisone, orally, 40 mg/m² daily. Adult patients with Hodgkin's disease or non-Hodgkin's lymphomas usually receive vincristine as part of a complex protocol. When used in the MOPP regimen (*see* below), the recommended dose of vincristine is 1.4 mg/m². Vincristine seems to be tolerated better by children than by adults, who may experience severe, progressive neurological toxicity. Administration of the drug more frequently than every 7 days or at higher doses seems to increase the toxic manifestations without proportional improvement in the response rate. Maintenance therapy with vincristine is not recommended in children with leukemia. Precautions also should be used to avoid extravasation during intravenous administration of vincristine.

In large-cell lymphoma, a liposomal formulation of vincristine (ONCO-TCS), given in doses of 2 mg/m², appears to have less neurotoxicity and retains activity in patients who relapse after vincristine therapy. It has the expected pharmacokinetic advantage of slower elimination and greater tissue distribution as compared to the unmodified drug (Krishna *et al.*, 2001).

Clinical Toxicities. The clinical toxicity of vincristine is mostly neurological, as described above. The more severe neurological manifestations may be avoided or reversed by either suspending therapy or reducing the dosage upon occurrence of motor dysfunction. Severe constipation, sometimes resulting in colicky abdominal pain and obstruction, may be prevented by a prophylactic program of laxatives and hydrophilic (bulk-forming) agents and usually is a problem only with doses above 2 mg/m².

Alopecia occurs in about 20% of patients given vincristine; however, it is always reversible, frequently without cessation of therapy. Although less common than with vinblastine, leukopenia may occur with vincristine, and thrombocytopenia, anemia, polyuria, dysuria, fever, and gastrointestinal symptoms have been reported occasionally. The syndrome of inappropriate secretion of antidiuretic hormone occasionally has been observed during vincristine therapy. In view of the rapid action of the vinca alkaloids, it is advisable to prevent hyperuricemia by the administration of allopurinol.

Vinorelbine

Vinorelbine (NAVELBINE, others) is administered in normal saline as an intravenous infusion of 30 mg/m² given over 6 to 10 minutes. A lower dose (20 to 25 mg/m²) may be required for patients who have received prior chemotherapy. When used alone, it is initially given every week until progression of disease or dose-limiting toxicity. When used with cisplatin for the treatment of non–small cell lung carcinoma, it is given every 3 weeks. Like the other vincas, it is eliminated by hepatic metabolism, and has an elimination half-life of 24 hours. Its primary toxicity is granulocytopenia, with only modest thrombocytopenia and less neurotoxicity than other vinca alkaloids. It may cause allergic reactions and mild, reversible changes in liver enzymes. In experimental studies, it has been given in an oral capsule, but bioavailability is only 30% to 40% (Fumoleau *et al.*, 1993). As with the other vincas, doses should be reduced in patients with elevated bilirubin or with >75% liver replacement by metastatic disease.

Taxanes

The first compound of this series, paclitaxel (TAXOL), was isolated from the bark of the Western yew tree in 1971 (Wani *et al.*, 1971). It and its congenic, the semisynthetic docetaxel (TAXOTERE), exhibit unique pharmacological actions as inhibitors of mitosis, differing from the vinca alkaloids and colchicine derivatives in that they bind to a different site on β-tubulin and promote rather than inhibit microtubule formation. The drugs have a central role in the therapy of ovarian, breast, lung, esophageal, bladder, and head and neck cancers (Rowinsky and Donehower, 1995). Their optimal dose, schedule, and use in drug combinations still are evolving.

Chemistry. Paclitaxel is a diterpenoid compound that contains a complex 8-member taxane ring as its nucleus (Figure 51–14). The

side chain linked to the taxane ring at C13 is essential for its antitumor activity. Modification of the side chain has led to identification of the more potent analog, docetaxel (Figure 51–14), which shares the same spectrum of clinical activity as paclitaxel, but differs in its spectrum of toxicity. Originally purified as the parent molecule from yew bark, paclitaxel now can be obtained for commercial purposes by semisynthesis from 10-desacetylbaccatin, a precursor found in yew leaves. It also has been successfully synthesized (Nicolaou *et al.*, 1994) in a complex series of reactions. Paclitaxel has very limited solubility and must be administered in a vehicle of 50% ethanol and 50% polyethoxylated castor oil (CREMOPHOR EL), a formation likely responsible for a high rate of hypersensitivity reactions. Patients receiving this formulation are protected by pretreatment with a histamine H₁ receptor antagonist such as *diphenhydramine*, an H₂ receptor antagonist such as *cimetidine* (*see* Chapter 24), and a glucocorticoid such as dexamethasone (*see* Chapter 59).

Docetaxel, somewhat more soluble, is administered in polysorbate 80 and causes a lower incidence of hypersensitivity reactions. Pretreatment with dexamethasone is required to prevent progressive, and often disabling, fluid retention. A variety of new taxanes, including some with oral bioavailability, are undergoing clinical testing.

Mechanism of Action. Interest in paclitaxel was stimulated by the finding that the drug possessed the unique ability to promote microtubule formation at cold temperatures and in the absence of GTP. It binds specifically to the β-tubulin subunit of microtubules and antagonizes the disassembly of this key cytoskeletal protein, with the result that bundles of microtubules and aberrant struc-

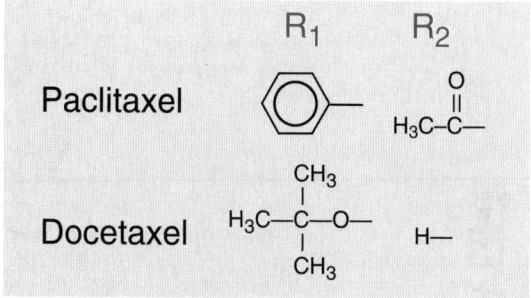

Figure 51–14. Chemical structures of paclitaxel and its more potent analog, docetaxel.

tures derived from microtubules appear in the mitotic phase of the cell cycle. Arrest in mitosis follows. Cell killing is dependent on both drug concentration and duration of cell exposure. Drugs that block cell-cycle progression prior to mitosis antagonize the toxic effects of taxanes.

Schedules for optimal use alone or in combination with other drugs, including doxorubicin and cisplatin, still are evolving. Drug interactions have been noted; the sequence of cisplatin preceding paclitaxel decreases paclitaxel clearance and produces greater toxicity than the opposite schedule (Rowinsky and Donehower, 1995). Paclitaxel decreases doxorubicin clearance and enhances cardiotoxicity, while docetaxel has no apparent effect on anthracycline pharmacokinetics (Holmes and Rowinsky, 2001).

In cultured tumor cells, resistance to taxanes is associated in some lines with increased expression of the *mdr*-1 gene and its product, the P-glycoprotein; other resistant cells have β-tubulin mutations, and these latter cells may display heightened sensitivity to vinca alkaloids (Cabral, 1983). Other cell lines display an increase in survivin, an anti-apoptotic factor (Zaffaroni *et al.*, 2002) or aurora kinase, an enzyme that promotes completion of mitosis (Anand *et al.*, 2003). The basis of clinical drug resistance is not known. Cell death occurs by apoptosis, but the effectiveness of paclitaxel against experimental tumors does not depend on an intact p53 gene product.

Absorption, Fate, and Excretion. Paclitaxel is administered as a 3-hour infusion of 135 to 175 mg/m^2 every 3 weeks, or as a weekly 1-hour infusion of 80 to 100 mg/m^2. Longer infusions (96 hours) have yielded significant response rates in breast cancer patients in preliminary trials (Wilson *et al.*, 1994), but this form of treatment has serious practical limitations. The drug undergoes extensive CYP-mediated hepatic metabolism (primarily CYP2C8 with a contribution of CYP3A4), and less than 10% of a dose is excreted in the urine intact. The primary metabolite identified thus far is 6-OH paclitaxel, which is inactive, but multiple additional hydroxylation products are found in plasma (Cresteil *et al.*, 1994).

Paclitaxel clearance is nonlinear and decreases with increasing dose or dose rate, possibly related to its dissolution in the vehicle of 50% ethanol and 50% polyethoxylated castor oil, and the nonlinearity of concentrations of the diluent (Henningsson *et al.*, 2001). In studies of 96-hour infusion of 35 mg/m^2 per day, the presence of hepatic metastases greater than 2 cm in size decreased clearance and led to high drug concentrations in plasma and greater myelosuppression. Paclitaxel disappears from the plasma compartment with a half-life of 10 to 14 hours and a clearance of 15 to 18 L/hour per square meter. The critical plasma concentration for inhibiting bone marrow elements depends on duration of exposure, but likely lies in the range of 50 to 100 nM (Huizing *et al.*, 1993).

Docetaxel pharmacokinetics are similar to those of paclitaxel. Its elimination half-life is approximately 12 hours, and its clear-

ance is 22 L/hour per square meter. Clearance is primarily through CYP3A4- and CYP3A5-mediated hydroxylation, leading to inactive metabolites (Clark and Rivory, 1999). In contrast to paclitaxel, the pharmacokinetics or docetaxel are linear up to doses of 115 mg/m^2.

Dose reductions in patients with abnormal hepatic function have been suggested and 50% to 75% doses of taxanes should be used in the presence of hepatic metastases >2 cm in size or in patients with abnormal serum bilirubin. Drugs that induce CYP2C8 or CYP3A4, such as phenytoin and phenobarbital, or those that inhibit the same cytochromes, such as antifungal imidazoles, significantly alter drug clearance and toxicity.

Paclitaxel clearance is markedly delayed by *cyclosporine A* and a number of other drugs employed experimentally as inhibitors of the P-glycoprotein. This inhibition may be due to a block of CYP-mediated metabolism or effects on biliary excretion of parent drug or metabolites (Kang *et al.*, 2001).

Therapeutic Uses. Docetaxel and paclitaxel have become central components of regimens for treating metastatic ovarian, breast, lung, and head and neck cancers (McGuire *et al.*, 1996; Seidman, 1998). Docetaxel has significant activity with *estramustine* for treatment of hormone-refractory prostate cancer. In current regimens, either drug is administered once weekly or once every 3 weeks, with comparable response rates and somewhat different patterns of toxicity. Docetaxel produces greater leukopenia and peripheral edema, while paclitaxel causes a higher incidence of hypersensitivity, muscle aching, and neuropathy (particularly when used in combination with a platinum analog). The optimal schedule of taxane administration, alone or in combination with other drugs, is still under evaluation.

Clinical Toxicities. Paclitaxel exerts its primary toxic effects on the bone marrow. Neutropenia usually occurs 8 to 11 days after a dose and reverses rapidly by days 15 to 21. Used with *filgrastim* (granulocyte-colony stimulating factor; G-CSF), doses as high as 250 mg/m^2 over 24 hours are well tolerated, and peripheral neuropathy becomes dose limiting (Kohn *et al.*, 1994). Many patients experience myalgias for several days after receiving paclitaxel. In high-dose schedules, or with prolonged use, a stocking-glove sensory neuropathy can be disabling, particularly in patients with underlying diabetic alcoholic neuropathy or concurrent cisplatin therapy. Mucositis is prominent in 72- or 96-hour infusions and in the weekly schedule.

Hypersensitivity reactions occurred in patients receiving paclitaxel infusions of short duration (1 to 6 hours), but have largely been averted by pretreatment with dexamethasone, diphenhydramine, and histamine H$_2$ receptor antagonists, as noted above. Premedication is not necessary with 96-hour infusions. Many patients experience asymptomatic bradycardia, and occasional episodes of silent ventricular tachycardia also occur and resolve spontaneously during 3- or 24-hour infusions.

Docetaxel tends to cause more severe, but short-lived, neutropenia than does paclitaxel. It causes less severe peripheral neuropathy and asthenia, and less frequent hypersensitivity. Fluid retention is a progressive problem with multiple cycles of therapy, leading to peripheral edema, pleural and peritoneal fluid, and pulmonary edema in extreme cases. Oral dexamethasone, 8 mg/day, begun 1 day prior to drug infusion and continuing for 3 days, greatly ameliorates fluid retention. In rare cases, docetaxel may cause a progressive interstitial pneumonitis, with respiratory failure supervening if the drug is not discontinued (Read *et al.*, 2002).

CAMPTOTHECIN ANALOGS

The camptothecins are potent, cytotoxic antineoplastic agents that target the nuclear enzyme topoisomerase I. The lead compound in this class, *camptothecin,* was isolated from the Chinese tree *Camptotheca acuminata* in 1966. Initial efforts to develop the compound as a sodium salt were compromised, despite evidence of promising preclinical and clinical antitumor activity, by severe and unpredictable toxicity, principally myelosuppression and hemorrhagic cystitis. Elucidation of the mechanism of action and a better understanding of its physicochemical properties during the 1980s led to the development of more soluble and less toxic analogs. Irinotecan and *topotecan,* currently the only camptothecin analogs approved for clinical use, have established activity in colorectal, ovarian, and small cell lung cancer (Garcia-Carbonero and Supko, 2002).

Chemistry. All camptothecins have a fused five-ring backbone beginning with a weakly basic quinoline moiety and terminating with a lactone ring (Figure 51–15). The hydroxyl group and S-conformation of the chiral center at C20 in the lactone ring to which it is attached are absolute requirements for biological activity. Appropriate substitutions on the A and B rings of the quinoline subunit can enhance water solubility and increase potency for inhibiting topoisomerase I. Topotecan [(S)-9-dimethylaminoethyl-10-hydroxy-camptothecin hydrochloride] is a semisynthetic molecule with a basic dimethylamino group that increases its water solubility. Irinotecan (7-ethyl-10-[4-(1-piperidino)-1-piperidino]carbonyloxycamptothecin, or CPT-11) differs from topotecan in that it is a prodrug. The carbamate bond between the camptothecin moiety and the dibasic bispiperidine side chain at position C10, which makes the molecule water soluble, is cleaved by a carboxylesterase to form the biologically active metabolite known as SN-38.

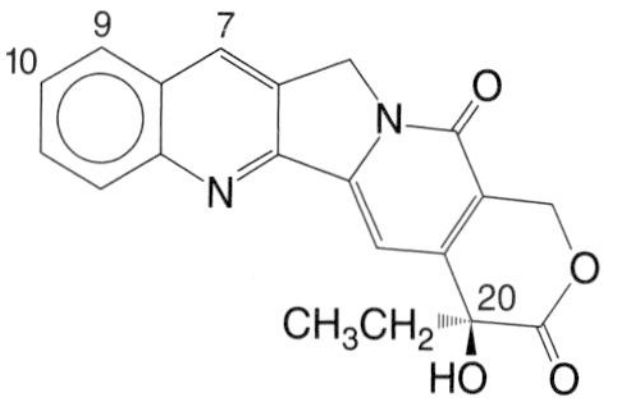

	C-10	C-9	C-7
Camptothecin	H	H	H
Topotecan	OH	(CH₃)₂NHCH₂	H
Irinotecan	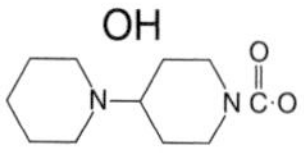	H	CH₂CH₃

Figure 51–15. Chemical structures of camptothecin and its analogs.

Although an intact lactone ring is necessary for the biological activity of the camptothecins, it is nevertheless unstable, undergoing reversible, nonenzymatic, pH-dependent hydrolysis in aqueous solution. Consequently, the camptothecins exist as an equilibrium mixture of the intact lactone and opened-ring carboxylate forms in biological fluids. Substituents on the A and B rings can modulate the equilibrium position between the closed and opened lactone ring forms of the molecule through effects on their relative affinities for binding to plasma proteins. For instance, the carboxylate form of camptothecin binds to serum albumin with a 200 times greater affinity than the intact lactone, and it is the predominant form in plasma and whole blood. In contrast, the lactone form of SN-38 binds preferentially to serum albumin, thereby shifting the equilibrium in the opposite direction.

Mechanism of Action. The DNA topoisomerases are nuclear enzymes that reduce torsional stress in supercoiled DNA, allowing selected regions of DNA to become sufficiently untangled and relaxed to permit its replication, recombination, repair, and transcription. Two classes of topoisomerase (I and II) are known to mediate DNA strand breakage and resealing, and both have become the target of cancer chemotherapies. Camptothecin analogs inhibit the function of topoisomerase I, while a number of different chemical entities (*e.g.,* anthracyclines, epipodophyllotoxins, acridines) inhibit topoisomerase II. Topoisomerase I binds covalently to double-stranded DNA through a reversible trans-esterification reaction. This reaction yields an intermediate complex in which the tyrosine of the enzyme is bound to the 3′-phosphate end of the DNA strand, creating a single-strand DNA break. This "cleavable complex" allows for relaxation of the DNA torsional strain, either by passage of the intact single-strand through the nick, or by free rotation of the DNA about the noncleaved strand. Once the DNA torsional strain has been relieved, the topoisomerase I reseals the cleavage and dissociates from the newly relaxed double helix.

The camptothecins bind to and stabilize the normally transient DNA-topoisomerase I cleavable complex (Hsiang *et al.*, 1985). Although the initial cleavage action of topoisomerase I is not affected, the religation step is inhibited, leading to the accumulation of single-stranded breaks in DNA. These lesions are reversible and not by themselves toxic to the cell. However, the collision of a DNA replication fork with this cleaved strand of DNA causes an irreversible double-strand DNA break, ultimately leading to cell death (Tsao *et al.*, 1993). Camptothecins are therefore S-phase–specific drugs, because ongoing DNA synthesis is necessary for cytotoxicity. This has important clinical implications, because S-phase–specific cytotoxic agents generally require prolonged exposures of tumor cells to drug concentrations above a minimum threshold to optimize therapeutic efficacy. In fact, preclinical studies of low-dose, protracted administration of camptothecin analogs have shown less toxicity, and equal or greater antitumor activity, than shorter more intense courses.

The precise sequence of events that lead from drug-induced DNA damage to cell death has not been fully elucidated. *In vitro* studies have shown that camptothecin-induced DNA damage abolishes the activation of the p34[cdc2]/cyclin B complex, leading to cell-cycle arrest at the G2 phase (Tsao *et al.*, 1993). It also has been observed that treatment with camptothecins can induce the transcription of *c-fos* and *c-jun* early-response genes, and this occurs in association with internucleosomal DNA fragmentation, a characteristic of programmed cell death (Kharbanda *et al.*, 1991). Interestingly, camptothecin-induced cytotoxicity also has been observed in cells not actively synthesizing DNA. Replication-independent mechanisms of cytotoxicity may involve the induction of serine proteases and endonucleases.

Mechanisms of Resistance. A variety of mechanisms of resistance to topoisomerase I–targeted agents have been characterized *in vitro,* although little is known about their significance in the clinical setting. Decreased intracellular drug accumulation has been observed in several cell lines resistant to camptothecin analogs. Topotecan, but not SN-38 or the intact lactone form of irinotecan, is a substrate for P-glycoprotein. However, the clinical relevance of P-glycoprotein–mediated efflux as a mechanism of resistance against topotecan remains unclear, as the magnitude of the effect in preclinical studies was found to be substantially lower than that observed with other MDR substrates, such as etoposide or doxorubicin. Other reports have associated topotecan or irinotecan resistance with the MRP class of transporters (Miyake *et al.*, 1999). Preclinical studies suggest drug metabolism could have a role in resistance to the prodrug irinotecan, as cell lines that lack carboxylesterase activity demonstrate resistance to irinotecan (Van Ark-Otte *et al.*, 1998), but in patients the liver and red blood cells may have sufficient carboxylesterase activity to convert irinotecan to SN-38. Camptothecin resistance also may result from decreased expression or mutation of topoisomerase I. Although a good correlation has been found in certain tumor cell lines between sensitivity to camptothecin analogs and topoisomerase I levels (Sugimoto *et al.*, 1990), clinical studies have not confirmed this association. Chromosomal deletions or hypermethylation of the topoisomerase I gene are possible mechanisms of decreased topoisomerase I expression in resistant cells. A transient downregulation of topoisomerase I has been demonstrated following prolonged exposure to camptothecins *in vitro* and *in vivo*. Moreover, an association between the degree of topoisomerase I downregulation in peripheral blood mononuclear cells and the area under the plasma concentration–time curve (AUC) or neutrophil nadir has been observed in ovarian cancer patients treated with a 21-day continuous intravenous infusion of topotecan. Mutations leading to reduced topoisomerase I enzyme catalytic activity or DNA binding affinity have been described *in vitro* in association with camptothecin resistance (Tamura *et al.*, 1991). In addition, some posttranscriptional events, such as enzyme phosphorylation (Pommier *et al.*, 1990) or poly-ADP ribosylation (Kasid *et al.*, 1989), may have a significant impact on the activity of topoisomerase I and on its susceptibility to inhibition. Finally, exposure of cells to topoisomerase I–targeted agents leads to increased expression of topoisomerase II, providing a rationale for sequential therapy with topoisomerase I and II inhibitors.

Very little is known about how the cell deals with the stabilized DNA-topoisomerase complexes. As cleavable complexes normally are present in the untreated cell, cellular repair processes may not readily recognize the drug-enzyme-DNA complex. However, an enzyme with specific tyrosyl-DNA phosphodiesterase activity may be involved in the disassembly of topoisomerase I–DNA complexes (Yang *et al.*, 1996). Since entry into S phase is required to kill tumor cells exposed to camptothecins, drugs that abolish the G_1-S checkpoint enhance lethality of camptothecins (Shao *et al.*, 1997). The fact that cell-cycle arrest in G_2 has been correlated with drug resistance to topoisomerase I–targeted drugs in colon cancer and leukemia cell lines *in vitro* suggests that enhanced DNA repair activity can lead to camptothecin resistance.

The role of p53 in mediating cell death due to camptothecins is unclear. These drugs induce p53 expression, but cells without functional p53 also can undergo apoptosis following exposure to camptothecins.

Absorption, Fate, and Excretion. *Topotecan.* Topotecan is only approved for intravenous administration. However, there has been interest in developing an oral dosage form for the drug, which has a bioavailability of 30% to 40% in cancer patients. Topotecan exhibits linear pharmacokinetics and it is rapidly eliminated from systemic circulation. The biological half-life of total topotecan, which ranges from 3.5 to 4.1 hours, is relatively short as compared with other camptothecins. Only 20% to 35% of the total drug in plasma is found to be in the active lactone form. Elimination of the lactone form appears to result mainly from rapid hydrolysis to the carboxylate species followed by renal excretion, with 30% to 40% of the administered dose excreted in the urine within 24 hours. Doses should be reduced in proportion to reductions in creatinine clearance. Although several oxidative metabolites have been identified, hepatic metabolism appears to be a relatively minor route of drug elimination. Unlike most other camptothecins considered for clinical development, plasma protein binding of topotecan is low, being only 7% to 35%, which may explain its relatively greater CNS penetration.

Irinotecan. The conversion of irinotecan to SN-38 is mediated predominantly by carboxylesterases in the liver (*see* Figure 3–5). Although SN-38 can be measured in plasma shortly after beginning an intravenous infusion of irinotecan, the AUC of SN-38 is only about 4% of the AUC of irinotecan, suggesting that only a relatively small fraction of the dose is ultimately converted to the active form of the drug. Irinotecan exhibits linear pharmacokinetics at doses evaluated in cancer patients. In comparison to topotecan, a relatively large fraction of both irinotecan and SN-38 are present in plasma as the biologically active intact lactone form. Another potential advantage of this analog is that the biological half-life of SN-38 is 11.5 hours, which is much longer than topotecan. Oral administration does not appear to be feasible because the bioavailability of irinotecan is only 8%. Plasma protein binding is at least 43% for irinotecan and 92% to 96% for SN-38. CSF penetration of SN-38 in humans has not been characterized yet, although in rhesus monkeys it is only 14%, significantly lower than that observed for topotecan.

In contrast to topotecan, hepatic metabolism represents an important route of elimination for both irinotecan and SN-38 (*see* Figures 3–7 and 3–8). Several oxidative metabolites have been identified in plasma, all of which result from CYP3A-mediated reactions directed at the bispiperidine side chain. These metabolites are not significantly converted to SN-38. The total body clearance of irinotecan was found to be two times greater in brain cancer patients who were concurrently taking antiseizure drugs that induce hepatic CYPs, further attesting to the importance of oxidative hepatic metabolism as a route of elimination for this drug (Gilbert *et al.*, 2003).

Conjugation of SN-38 with glucuronic acid, through the hydroxyl group at position C10 resulting from cleavage of the bispiperidine promoiety, is the only known metabolite of SN-38. Biliary excretion appears to be the primary elimination route of irinotecan, SN-38, and their metabolites, although urinary excretion also contributes significantly (14% to 37%). Uridine diphosphate-glucuronosyltransferase (UGT), particularly the UGT1A1 isoform, converts SN-38 to its inactive glucuronidated derivative (Iyer *et al.*, 1998). The extent of SN-38 glucuronidation has been inversely correlated with the risk of severe diarrhea after irinote-can therapy. UGT1A1 also glucuronidates bilirubin. Polymorphisms of this enzyme (*see* Figure 3–6) are associated with familial hyperbilirubinemia syndromes such as Crigler-Najjar syndrome and Gilbert syndrome. Crigler-Najjar syndrome is rare (1 in a million births), but Gilbert syndrome occurs in up to 15% of the general population, and results in a mild hyperbilirubinemia that may be clinically silent. The existence of UGT enzyme polymorphisms may have a major impact on the clinical use of irinotecan. A positive correlation has been found between baseline serum unconjugated bilirubin concentration and both severity of neutropenia and the AUC of irinotecan and SN-38 in patients treated with irinotecan. Moreover, severe irinotecan toxicity has been observed in cancer patients with Gilbert syndrome, presumably due to decreased glucuronidation of SN-38. The presence of bacterial glucuronidase in the intestinal lumen potentially can contribute to irinotecan's GI toxicity by releasing unconjugated SN-38 from the inactive glucuronide metabolite excreted in the bile.

Therapeutic Uses. **Topotecan.** Topotecan (HYCAMTIN) is indicated for previously treated patients with ovarian (Herzog, 2002) and small cell lung cancer (Huang and Treat, 2001). Its significant hematological toxicity, though, has limited its use in combination with other active agents in these diseases (*e.g.,* cisplatin). Promising antitumor activity also has been observed in hematological malignancies, particularly in CML and in myelodysplastic syndromes.

The recommended dosing regimen of topotecan is a 30-minute infusion of 1.5 mg/m² per day for 5 consecutive days every 3 weeks. Since a significant fraction of the topotecan administered is excreted in the urine, severe toxicities have been observed in patients with decreased creatinine clearance (O'Reilly *et al.*, 1996). Therefore, the dose of topotecan should be reduced to 0.75 mg/m² per day in patients with moderate renal dysfunction (creatinine clearance 20 to 40 ml/minute), and topotecan should not be administered to patients with severe renal impairment (creatinine clearance <20 ml/minute). Topotecan clearance and toxicity are not significantly altered in patients with hepatic dysfunction, and therefore no dose reduction is necessary in these patients.

Irinotecan. Approved dosage schedules of irinotecan (CAMP-TOSAR) in the United States include: 125 mg/m² as a 90-minute infusion administered weekly for 4 out of 6 weeks; 350 mg/m² given every 3 weeks; 100 mg/m² every week; or 150 mg/m² every other week. Irinotecan has significant clinical activity in patients with advanced colorectal cancer. It now is the treatment of choice in combination with fluoropyrimidines for advanced colorectal cancer in patients who have not received chemotherapy previously (Douillard *et al.*, 2000) or as a single agent following failure on a 5-FU regimen (Rothenberg, 2001). Encouraging results from different phase II studies suggest that irinotecan may have an increasing role in the treatment of other solid tumors, including small cell and non–small cell lung cancer, cervical cancer, ovarian cancer, gastric cancer, and brain tumors.

Clinical Toxicities. *Topotecan.* The dose-limiting toxicity with all schedules is neutropenia, with or without thrombocytopenia. The

incidence of severe neutropenia at the recommended phase II dose of 1.5 mg/m² daily for 5 days every 3 weeks may be as high as 81%, with a 26% incidence of febrile neutropenia. In patients with hematological malignancies, gastrointestinal side effects such as mucositis and diarrhea become dose limiting. Other less common and generally mild topotecan-related toxicities include nausea and vomiting, elevated liver transaminases, fever, fatigue, and rash.

Irinotecan. The dose-limiting toxicity with all schedules is delayed diarrhea, with or without neutropenia. In the initial studies, up to 35% of patients experienced severe diarrhea. Adoption of an intensive *loperamide* (*see* Chapter 38) regimen (4 mg of loperamide starting at the onset of any loose stool beginning more than a few hours after receiving therapy, followed by 2 mg every 2 hours) has effectively reduced this incidence by more than half. However, once severe diarrhea does occur, standard doses of antidiarrheal agents tend to be ineffective, although the diarrhea episode generally resolves within a week and, unless associated with fever and neutropenia, is rarely fatal.

The second most common irinotecan-associated toxicity is myelosuppression. Severe neutropenia occurs in 14% to 47% of the patients treated with the every-3-week schedule, and is less frequently encountered among patients treated with the weekly schedule. Febrile neutropenia is observed in 3% of patients, and may be fatal, particularly when associated with concomitant diarrhea. A cholinergic syndrome resulting from the inhibition of acetylcholinesterase activity by irinotecan may occur within the first 24 hours after irinotecan administration. Symptoms include acute diarrhea, diaphoresis, hypersalivation, abdominal cramps, visual accommodation disturbances, lacrimation, rhinorrhea, and less often, asymptomatic bradycardia. These effects are short lasting and respond within minutes to atropine. Atropine may be prophylactically administered to patients who have previously experienced a cholinergic reaction, prior to the administration of additional cycles of irinotecan. Other common and generally manageable toxicities include nausea and vomiting, fatigue, vasodilation or skin flushing, mucositis, elevation in liver transaminases, and alopecia. Finally, there have been case reports of dyspnea and interstitial pneumonitis associated with irinotecan therapy in Japanese patients with lung cancer (Fukuoka *et al.*, 1992).

ANTIBIOTICS

Dactinomycin (Actinomycin D)

The first anticancer antibiotics to be isolated from a culture broth of a species of *Streptomyces* were the series of actinomycins discovered by Waksman and colleagues in 1940. The most important of these, actinomycin D, has beneficial effects in the treatment of solid tumors in children and choriocarcinoma.

Chemistry and Structure–Activity Relationship. The actinomycins are chromopeptides. Most contain the same chromophore, the planar phenoxazone actinosin, which is responsible for their yellow-red color. The differences among naturally occurring actinomycins are confined to variations in the structure of the amino acids of the peptide side chains. By varying the amino acid content of the growth medium, it is possible to alter the types of actinomycins produced and the biological activity of the molecule (Crooke, 1983). The chemical structure of dactinomycin is as follows:

DACTINOMYCIN
(Sar = sarcosine)
(Meval = N-methylvaline)

Mechanism of Action. The capacity of actinomycins to bind with double-helical DNA is responsible for their biological activity and cytotoxicity. X-ray studies of a crystalline complex between dactinomycin and deoxyguanosine permitted formulation of a model that appears to explain the binding of the drug to DNA (Sobell, 1973). The planar phenoxazone ring intercalates between adjacent guanine–cytosine base pairs of DNA, while the polypeptide chains extend along the minor groove of the helix. The summation of these interactions provides great stability to the dactinomycin-DNA complex, and as a result of the binding of dactinomycin, the transcription of DNA by RNA polymerase is blocked. The DNA-dependent RNA polymerases are much more sensitive to the effects of dactinomycin than are the DNA polymerases. In addition, dactinomycin causes single-strand breaks in DNA, possibly through a free-radical intermediate or as a result of the action of topoisomerase II (Goldberg et al., 1977).

Cytotoxic Action. Dactinomycin inhibits rapidly proliferating cells of normal and neoplastic origin, and on a molar basis is among the most potent antitumor agents known. The drug may produce alopecia, and when extravasated subcutaneously, causes marked local inflammation. Erythema, sometimes progressing to necrosis, has been noted in areas of the skin exposed to x-ray radiation before, during, or after administration of dactinomycin.

Absorption, Fate, and Excretion. Dactinomycin is administered by intravenous injection. The drug is excreted both in bile and in the urine and disappears from plasma with a terminal half-life of 36 hours. Metabolism of the drug is minimal. Dactinomycin does not cross the blood–brain barrier.

Therapeutic Uses. The usual daily dose of dactinomycin (actinomycin D; COSMEGEN) is 10 to 15 μg/kg; this is given intravenously for 5 days; if no manifestations of toxicity are encountered, additional courses may be given at intervals of 2 to 4 weeks. In other regimens, 3 to 6 μg/kg per day, for a total of 125 μg/kg, and weekly maintenance doses of 7.5 μg/kg have been used. If infiltrated during administration, the drug is extremely corrosive to soft tissues.

The most important clinical use of dactinomycin is in the treatment of rhabdomyosarcoma and Wilms' tumor in children, where it is curative in combination with primary surgery, radiotherapy, and other drugs, particularly vincristine and cyclophosphamide (Pinkel and Howarth, 1985). Antineoplastic activity has been noted in Ewing's tumor, Kaposi's sarcoma, and soft tissue sarcomas. Dactinomycin can be effective in women with advanced cases of choriocarcinoma in combination with methotrexate. Dactinomycin also has been used as an immunosuppressant in renal transplants.

Clinical Toxicities. Toxic manifestations include anorexia, nausea, and vomiting, usually beginning a few hours after administration. Hematopoietic suppression with pancytopenia may occur in the first week after completion of therapy. Proctitis, diarrhea, glossitis, cheilitis, and ulcerations of the oral mucosa are common; dermatological manifestations include alopecia, as well as erythema, desquamation, and increased inflammation and pigmentation in areas previously or concomitantly subjected to x-ray radiation. Severe injury may occur as a result of local toxic extravasation.

Daunorubicin, Doxorubicin, Epirubicin, Idarubicin, and Mitoxantrone

These anthracycline antibiotics are among the most important antitumor agents. They are derived from the fungus *Streptococcus peucetius* var. *caesius*. *Idarubicin* and *epirubicin* are analogs of the naturally produced anthracyclines, differing only slightly in chemical structure, but having somewhat distinct patterns of clinical activity. *Daunorubicin* and idarubicin have been used primarily in the acute leukemias, whereas doxorubicin and epirubicin display broader activity against human solid tumors. These agents, which all possess potential for generating free radicals, cause an unusual and often irreversible cardiomyopathy, the occurrence of which is related to the total dose of the drug. The structurally similar agent mitoxantrone has useful activity against prostate cancer and AML, and is used in high-dose chemotherapy. Mitoxantrone, an anthracenedione, has significantly less cardiotoxicity than do the anthracyclines.

Chemistry. The anthracycline antibiotics have a tetracyclic ring structure attached to an unusual sugar, daunosamine. Cytotoxic agents of this class all have quinone and hydroquinone moieties on adjacent rings that permit the gain and loss of electrons. Although there are marked differences in the clinical use of daunorubicin and doxorubicin, their chemical structures differ only by a single hydroxyl group on C14. Idarubicin is 4-demethoxydaunorubicin, a synthetic derivative of daunorubicin, while epirubicin is an epimer at the 4'-position of the sugar. Mitoxantrone lacks a glycosidic side group. The chemical structures of doxorubicin, daunorubicin, epirubicin, and idarubicin are as follows:

	DOXORUBICIN	DAUNORUBICIN	EPIRUBICIN	IDARUBICIN
R_1 =	OCH_3	OCH_3	OCH_3	H
R_2 =	H	H	OH	H
R_3 =	OH	OH	H	OH
R_4 =	OH	H	OH	H

Mechanism of Action. A number of important biochemical effects have been described for the anthracyclines and anthracenediones, all of which could contribute to their therapeutic and toxic effects. These compounds can intercalate with DNA, directly affecting transcription and replication. A more important action is the ability of these drugs to form a tripartite complex with topoisomerase II and DNA. Topoisomerase II is an ATP-dependent enzyme that binds to DNA and produces double-strand breaks at the 3′ phosphate backbone, allowing strand passage and uncoiling of supercoiled DNA. Following strand passage, topoisomerase II religates the DNA strands. This enzymatic function is essential for DNA replication and repair. Formation of the tripartite complex with anthracyclines and with etoposide inhibits the re-ligation of the broken DNA strands, leading to apoptosis (Rubin and Hait, 2000). Defects in DNA double-strand break repair sensitize cells to damage by these drugs, while overexpression of transcription-linked DNA repair may contribute to resistance. Anthracyclines, by virtue of their quinone groups, also generate free radicals in solution and in both normal and malignant tissues (Myers, 1988; Gewirtz, 1999). Anthracyclines can form semiquinone radical intermediates, which in turn can react with oxygen to produce superoxide anion radicals. These can generate both hydrogen peroxide and hydroxyl radicals (·OH), which attack DNA (Serrano *et al.*, 1999) and oxidize DNA bases. The production of free radicals is significantly stimulated by the interaction of doxorubicin with iron (Myers, 1988). Enzymatic defenses such as superoxide dismutase and catalase are believed to have an important role in protecting cells against the toxicity of the anthracyclines, and these defenses can be augmented by exogenous antioxidants such as *alpha tocopherol* or by an iron chelator, *dexrazoxane* (ZINECARD), which protects against cardiac toxicity (Swain *et al.*, 1997).

Exposure of cells to anthracyclines leads to apoptosis; mediators of this process include the p53 DNA-damage sensor and activated caspases (proteases), although ceramide, a lipid breakdown product, and the fas receptor-ligand system also have been implicated in selected tumor cells (Friesen *et al.*, 1996; Jaffrezou *et al.*, 1996).

As discussed above, the phenomenon of multidrug resistance is observed in tumor cell populations exposed to anthracyclines. Attempts to reverse or prevent the emergence of resistance through the simultaneous use of inhibitors of the P-glycoprotein, such as calcium channel blockers, steroidal compounds, and others, have yielded inconclusive results, primarily because of the effects of these inhibitors on anthracycline pharmacokinetics and metabolism. Anthracyclines also are exported from tumor cells by members of the MRP transporter family and by the breast cancer resistance protein, a "half" transporter (Doyle *et al.*, 1998). Other biochemical changes in resistant cells include increased glutathione peroxidase activity (Sinha *et al.*, 1989), decreased activity or mutation of topoisomerase II (Jarvinen *et al.*, 1998), and enhanced ability to repair DNA strand breaks.

Absorption, Fate, and Excretion. Daunorubicin, doxorubicin, epirubicin, and idarubicin usually are administered intravenously and are cleared by a complex pattern of hepatic metabolism and biliary excretion. The plasma disappearance curve for doxorubicin is multiphasic, with elimination half-lives of 3 hours and about 30 hours. All anthracyclines are converted to an active alcohol intermediate that plays a variable role in their therapeutic activity. Idarubicin has a half-life of about 15 hours, and its active metabolite, idarubicinol, has a half-life of about 40 hours. There is rapid uptake of the drugs in the heart, kidneys, lungs, liver, and spleen. They do not cross the blood–brain barrier.

Daunorubicin and doxorubicin are eliminated by metabolic conversion to a variety of aglycones and other inactive products. Idarubicin is primarily metabolized to idarubicinol, which accumulates in plasma and likely contributes significantly to its activity. Clearance is delayed in the presence of hepatic dysfunction, and at least a 50% initial reduction in dose should be considered in patients with abnormal serum bilirubin levels (Twelves *et al.*, 1998).

Idarubicin. The recommended dosage for idarubicin (IDAMYCIN) is 12 mg/m² daily for 3 days by intravenous injection in combination with cytarabine. Slow injection with care over 10 to 15 minutes is recommended to avoid extravasation, as with other anthracyclines.

Daunorubicin. *Therapeutic Uses.* Daunorubicin (daunomycin, rubidomycin; CERUBIDINE, others) is available for intravenous use. The recommended dosage is 30 to 60 mg/m² daily for 3 days. The agent is administered with appropriate care to prevent extravasation, since severe local vesicant action may result. Total doses of greater than 1000 mg/m² are associated with a high risk of cardiotoxicity. A daunorubicin citrate liposomal product (DAUNOXOME) is indicated for the treatment of AIDS-related Kaposi's sarcoma. It is given in a dose of 40 mg/m² infused over 60 minutes and repeated every 2 weeks. Patients should be advised that the drug may impart a red color to the urine.

Daunorubicin is primarily used in the treatment of AML in combination with Ara-C and has largely been replaced by idarubicin.

Clinical Toxicities. The toxic manifestations of daunorubicin as well as idarubicin include bone marrow depression, stomatitis, alopecia, GI disturbances, and dermatological manifestations. Cardiac toxicity is a peculiar adverse effect observed with these agents. It is characterized by tachycardia, arrhythmias, dyspnea, hypotension, pericardial effusion, and congestive heart failure that is poorly responsive to digitalis (*see* below).

Doxorubicin. *Therapeutic Uses.* Doxorubicin (ADRIAMYCIN, others) is available for intravenous use. The recommended dose is 50 to 75 mg/m², administered as a single rapid intravenous infusion that is repeated after 21 days. Care should be taken to avoid extravasation, since severe local vesicant action and tissue necrosis may result. A doxorubicin liposomal product (DOXIL) is available for treatment of AIDS-related Kaposi's sarcoma and is given intravenously in a dose of 20 mg/m² over 30 minutes and repeated every 3 weeks. As for daunorubicin, patients should be advised that the drug may impart a red color to the urine.

Doxorubicin is effective in malignant lymphomas; however, in contrast to daunorubicin, it also is active in a number of solid tumors, particularly breast cancer. Used in combination with cyclophosphamide, vinca alkaloids, and other agents, it is an important ingredient for the successful treatment of lymphomas. It is a valuable component of various regimens of chemotherapy for adjuvant and metastatic carcinoma of the breast and small cell carcinoma of the lung. The drug also is particularly beneficial in a wide range of pediatric and adult sarcomas, including osteogenic, Ewing's, and soft tissue sarcomas.

Clinical Toxicities. The toxic manifestations of doxorubicin are similar to those of daunorubicin. Myelosuppression is a major dose-limiting complication, with leukopenia usually reaching a nadir during the second week of therapy and recovering by the fourth week; thrombocytopenia and anemia follow a similar pattern but usually are less pronounced. Stomatitis, GI disturbances, and alopecia are common but reversible. Erythematous streaking near the site of infusion ("ADRIAMYCIN flare") is a benign local allergic reaction and should not be confused with extravasation. Facial flushing, conjunctivitis, and lacrimation may occur rarely. The drug may produce severe local toxicity in irradiated tissues (*e.g.,* the skin, heart, lung, esophagus, and gastrointestinal mucosa). Such reactions may occur even when the two therapies are not administered concomitantly.

Cardiomyopathy is the most important long-term toxicity. Two types of cardiomyopathies may occur:

1. An acute form is characterized by abnormal electrocardiographic changes, including ST- and T-wave alterations and arrhythmias. This is brief and rarely a serious problem. An acute reversible reduction in ejection fraction is observed in some patients in the 24 hours after a single dose, and elevation of troponin T, a cardiac enzyme released with myocardial damage, is found in a minority of patients in the first few days following drug administration (Lipshultz *et al.,* 2004). An exaggerated manifestation of acute myocardial damage, the "pericarditis–myocarditis syndrome," may be characterized by severe disturbances in impulse conduction and frank congestive heart failure, often associated with pericardial effusion.

2. Chronic, cumulative dose-related toxicity (usually at or above total doses of 550 mg/m^2) is manifested by congestive heart failure that is unresponsive to digitalis. The mortality rate in patients with congestive failure approaches 50%. Total dosage of doxorubicin as low as 250 mg/m^2 can cause pathologic changes in the myocardium, as demonstrated by subendocardial biopsies. Nonspecific alterations, including a decrease in the number of myocardial fibrils, mitochondrial changes, and cellular degeneration, are visible by electron microscopy. The most promising noninvasive techniques used to detect the early development of drug-induced congestive heart failure are radionuclide cineangiography, which assesses ejection fraction, and echocardiography, which reveals abnormalities in contractility and ventricular dimensions. Sequential echocardiograms have detected structural abnormalities in 25% of children who received up to 300 mg/m^2 of doxorubicin, although fewer than 10% have clinical manifestations of cardiac disease in long-term follow-up. Although no completely practical and reliable predictive tests are available, the frequency of clinically apparent cardiomyopathy is 1% to 10% at total doses below 450 mg/m^2. The risk increases markedly (to >20% of patients) at total doses higher than 550 mg/m^2,

and this total dosage should be exceeded only under exceptional circumstances or with the concomitant use of dexrazoxane, a cardioprotective iron-chelating agent that appears not to compromise the anticancer activity of the drug (Speyer *et al.,* 1988; Swain *et al.,* 1997). Cardiac irradiation, administration of high doses of cyclophosphamide or another anthracycline, or concomitant *herceptin* (Slamon *et al.,* 2001) increases the risk of cardiotoxicity. Late-onset cardiac toxicity, with congestive heart failure years after treatment, may occur in both pediatric and adult populations (Lipshultz *et al.,* 2004). In children treated with anthracyclines, there is a three- to tenfold elevated risk of arrhythmias, congestive heart failure, and sudden death in adult life. A total dose limit of 300 mg/m^2 is advised for pediatric cases, and there is preliminary evidence that concomitant administration of dexrazoxane may reduce troponin T elevations that predict later cardiotoxicity (Lipshultz *et al.,* 2004).

Newer Analogs of Doxorubicin. Valrubicin (VALSTAR) was approved in 1998 for intravesical therapy of bacille Calmette-Guérin–refractory urinary bladder carcinoma *in situ* in patients for whom immediate cystectomy would be associated with unacceptable morbidity or mortality. Epirubicin (4′-epidoxorubicin, ELLENCE) was approved by the FDA in 1999 as a component of adjuvant therapy following resection of early lymph-node–positive breast cancer.

A related anthracenedione, mitoxantrone, has been approved for use in AML. Mitoxantrone has limited ability to produce quinone-type free radicals and causes less cardiac toxicity than does doxorubicin. It produces acute myelosuppression, cardiac toxicity, and mucositis as its major toxicities; the drug causes less nausea and vomiting and alopecia than does doxorubicin. It also is used as a component of experimental high-dose chemotherapy regimens, with uncertain efficacy.

Mitoxantrone (NOVANTRONE) is supplied for intravenous infusion. To induce remission in acute nonlymphocytic leukemia in adults, the drug is given in a daily dose of 12 mg/m^2 for 3 days as a component of a regimen that also includes cytosine arabinoside. Mitoxantrone also is used in advanced hormone-resistant prostate cancer in a dose of 12 to 14 mg/m^2 every 21 days. Mitoxantrone has been approved by the FDA for the treatment of late-stage, secondary progressive multiple sclerosis.

EPIPODOPHYLLOTOXINS

Podophyllotoxin, extracted from the mandrake plant (may-apple; *Podophyllum peltatum*), was used as a folk remedy by the American Indians and early colonists for its emetic, cathartic, and anthelmintic effects. Two of the many derivatives synthesized during the past 20 years show significant therapeutic activity in several human neoplasms, including pediatric leukemia, small cell carcinomas of the lung, testicular tumors, Hodgkin's disease, and large cell lymphomas.

These derivatives, shown below, are etoposide (VP-16-213) and *teniposide* (VM-26). Although podophyllotoxin binds to tubulin at a site distinct from that for interaction with the vinca alkaloids, etoposide and teniposide have no effect on microtubular structure or function at usual concentrations (for reviews of the epipodophyllotoxins, *see* Hande, 1998; Pommier *et al.*, 2001).

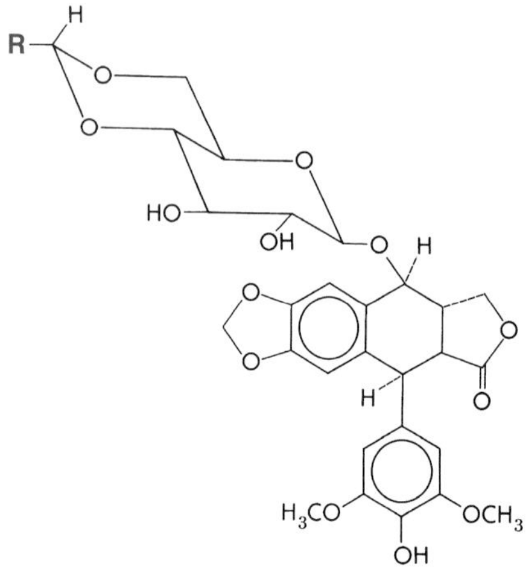

ETOPOSIDE: R = CH₃

TENIPOSIDE: R =

Mechanism of Action. Etoposide and teniposide are similar in their actions and in the spectrum of human tumors affected. Unlike podophyllotoxin, but like the anthracyclines, they form a ternary complex with topoisomerase II and DNA and prevent resealing of the break that normally follows topoisomerase binding to DNA. The enzyme remains bound to the free end of the broken DNA strand, leading to an accumulation of DNA breaks and cell death (Pommier *et al.*, 2001). Cells in the S and G_2 phases of the cell cycle are most sensitive to etoposide and teniposide. Resistant cells demonstrate amplification of the *mdr*-1 gene that encodes the P-glycoprotein drug efflux transporter, mutation or decreased expression of topoisomerase II, or mutations of the p53 tumor suppressor gene, a required component of the apoptotic pathway (Lowe *et al.*, 1993).

Etoposide

Absorption, Fate, and Excretion. Oral administration of etoposide results in variable absorption that averages about 50%. After intravenous injection, peak plasma concentrations of 30 μg/ml are achieved; there is a biphasic pattern of clearance with a terminal half-life of about 6 to 8 hours in patients with normal renal function. Approximately 40% of an administered dose is excreted intact in the urine. In patients with compromised renal function, dosage should be reduced in proportion to the reduction in creatinine clearance (Arbuck *et al.*, 1986). In patients with advanced liver disease, low serum albumin and elevated bilirubin (which displaces etoposide from albumin) tend to increase the unbound fraction of drug, increasing the toxicity of any given dose. However, guidelines for dose reduction in this circumstance have not been defined (Stewart *et al.*, 1991). Drug concentrations in the cerebrospinal fluid average 1% to 10% of those in plasma.

Therapeutic Uses. The intravenous dose of etoposide (VEPESID, TOPOSAR, ETOPOPHOS) for testicular cancer in combination therapy is 50 to 100 mg/m² for 5 days, or 100 mg/m² on alternate days for three doses. For small cell carcinoma of the lung, the dose in combination therapy is 50 to 120 mg/m² per day intravenously for 3 days, or 50 mg per day orally for 21 days. Cycles of therapy usually are repeated every 3 to 4 weeks. When given intravenously, the drug should be administered slowly during a 30- to 60-minute infusion to avoid hypotension and bronchospasm, which likely result from the additives used to dissolve etoposide, a relatively insoluble compound.

A disturbing complication of etoposide therapy has emerged in long-term follow-up of patients with childhood acute lymphoblastic leukemia, who develop an unusual form of acute nonlymphocytic leukemia with a translocation in chromosome 11 at 11q23. At this locus is found a gene(s) (the MLL or mixed-lineage leukemia gene) that regulates the proliferation of pluripotent stem cells. The leukemic cells have the cytological appearance of acute monocytic or monomyelocytic leukemia. Another distinguishing feature of etoposide-related leukemia is the short time interval between the end of treatment and onset of leukemia (1 to 3 years), as compared to the 4- to 5-year interval for secondary leukemias related to alkylating agents, and the absence of a myelodysplastic period preceding leukemia (Levine and Bloomfield, 1992; Pui *et al.*, 1995; Sandler *et al.*, 1997; Smith *et al.*, 1999). Patients receiving weekly or twice-weekly doses of etoposide, with cumulative doses above 2000 mg/m², seem to be at higher risk of leukemia.

Etoposide is used primarily for treatment of testicular tumors, in combination with bleomycin and cisplatin, and in combination with cisplatin and ifosfamide for small cell carcinoma of the lung (Nemati *et al.*, 2000). It also is active against non-Hodgkin's lymphomas, acute nonlymphocytic leukemia, and Kaposi's sarcoma associated with acquired immunodeficiency syndrome (AIDS) (Chao *et al.*, 2000; Tung *et al.*, 2000). Etoposide has a favorable toxicity profile for dose escalation in that its primary acute toxicity is myelosuppression. In combination with ifosfamide and carboplatin, it is frequently used for high-dose chemotherapy in total doses of 1500 to 2000 mg/m² (Josting *et al.*, 2000).

Clinical Toxicities. The dose-limiting toxicity of etoposide is leukopenia, with a nadir at 10 to 14 days and recovery by 3 weeks. Thrombocytopenia occurs less often and usually is not severe. Nausea, vomiting, stomatitis, and diarrhea occur in approximately 15% of patients treated intravenously and in about 55% of patients who receive the drug orally. Alopecia is common but reversible. Fever, phlebitis, dermatitis, and allergic reactions including anaphylaxis have been observed. Hepatic toxicity is particularly evident after high-dose treatment. For both etoposide and teniposide, toxicity is increased in patients with decreased serum albumin, an effect related to decreased protein binding of the drug (Stewart *et al.*, 1991).

Teniposide

Teniposide (VUMON) is administered intravenously. It has a multiphasic pattern of clearance from plasma. After distribution, half-lives of 4 hours and 10 to 40 hours are observed. Approximately 45% of the drug is excreted in the urine, but in contrast to etoposide, as much as 80% is recovered as metabolites. Anticonvulsants such as phenytoin increase the hepatic metabolism of teniposide and reduce systemic exposure (Baker *et al.*, 1992). Dosage need not be reduced for patients with impaired renal function (Pommier

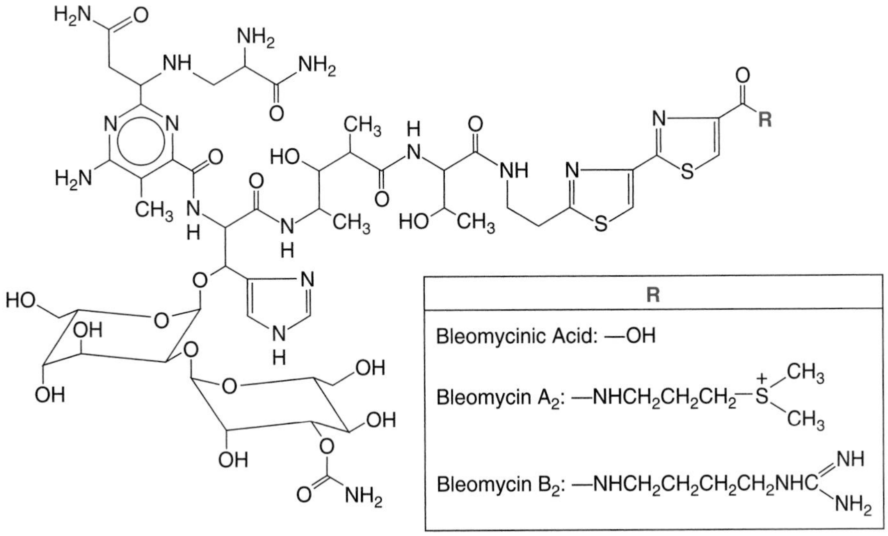

Figure 51–16. Chemical structures of bleomycin A2 and B2.

et al., 2001). Less than 1% of the drug crosses the blood–brain barrier. However, teniposide has produced responses in small cell and non–small cell lung cancer metastases in the brain (Boogerd et al., 1999).

Teniposide is available for treatment of refractory ALL in children and appears to be synergistic with cytarabine. It is administered by intravenous infusion in doses that range from 50 mg/m^2 per day for 5 days to 165 mg/m^2 per day twice weekly. The clinical spectrum of activity includes acute leukemia in children, particularly monocytic leukemia in infants, as well as glioblastoma, neuroblastoma, and brain metastases from small cell carcinomas of the lung (Odom and Gordon, 1984; Postmus et al., 1995; Boogerd et al., 1999). Myelosuppression, nausea, and vomiting are its primary toxic effects.

Bleomycins

The bleomycins are an important group of DNA-cleaving antibiotics discovered by Umezawa and colleagues as fermentation products of *Streptococcus verticillus*. The drug currently employed clinically is a mixture of the two copper-chelating peptides, bleomycins A$_2$ and B$_2$. The bleomycins differ only in their terminal amino acid (*see* below), which can be altered by the amino acids added to the fermentation medium.

Bleomycins have attracted interest both because of their significant antitumor activity against squamous carcinoma of the cervix, and against lymphomas and testicular tumors. They are minimally myelo- and immunosuppressive but cause unusual cutaneous side effects and pulmonary fibrosis. Because their toxicities do not overlap with those of other drugs, and because of their unique mechanism of action, bleomycins maintain an important role in combination chemotherapy.

Chemistry. The bleomycins are water-soluble, basic glycopeptides (Figure 51–16). The core of the bleomycin molecule is a complex metal-binding structure containing a pyrimidine chromophore linked to propionamide, a β-aminoalanine amide side chain, and the sugars L-gulose and 3-O-carbamoyl-D-mannose. Attached to this core are a tripeptide chain and a terminal bithiazole carboxylic acid; this latter segment binds to DNA. The bleomycins form equimolar complexes with metal ions, including Cu^{2+} and Fe^{2+}.

Mechanism of Action. Although bleomycin has a number of interesting biochemical properties, its cytotoxic action results from their ability to cause oxidative damage to the deoxyribose of thymidylate and other nucleotides, leading to single- and double-stranded breaks in DNA. Studies *in vitro* indicate that bleomycin causes accumulation of cells in the G$_2$ phase of the cell cycle, and many of these cells display chromosomal aberrations, including chromatid breaks, gaps, and fragments, as well as translocations (Twentyman, 1983).

Bleomycin causes scission of DNA by interacting with O$_2$ and Fe^{2+}. In the presence of O$_2$ and a reducing agent, such as dithiothreitol, the metal–drug complex becomes activated and functions mechanistically as a ferrous oxidase, transferring electrons from Fe^{2+} to molecular oxygen to produce activated species of oxygen (Burger, 1998). Metallobleomycin complexes can be activated by reaction with the flavin enzyme, NADPH-cytochrome P450 reductase. Bleomycin binds to DNA through its amino-terminal peptide, and the activated complex generates free radicals that are responsible for scission of the deoxyribose backbone of the DNA chain. Bleomycin is degraded by a specific hydrolase found in various normal tissues, including liver; however, hydrolase activity is low in skin and lung, perhaps contributing to the toxicity at those sites (Sebti et al., 1987). Some bleomycin-resistant cells contain high levels of hydrolase activity (Sebti et al., 1991). In other cell lines resistance has been attributed to decreased uptake, cleavage by the hydrolase, repair of strand breaks, or drug inactivation by thiols or thiol-rich proteins (Zuckerman et al., 1986).

Absorption, Fate, and Excretion. Bleomycin is administered parenterally, either intravenously or intramuscularly, or instilled into the bladder for local treatment of bladder cancer (Bracken *et al.*, 1977). After intravenous infusion, relatively high drug concentrations are detected in the skin and lungs of experimental animals, and these organs become major sites of toxicity. Having a high molecular mass, bleomycin crosses the blood–brain barrier poorly.

After intravenous administration of a bolus dose of 15 units/m^2, peak concentrations of 1 to 5 units/ml are achieved in plasma. The half-time for elimination is approximately 3 hours. The average steady-state concentration of bleomycin in plasma of patients receiving continuous intravenous infusions of 30 units daily for 4 to 5 days is approximately 0.15 units/ml. About two-thirds of the drug normally is excreted in the urine. Concentrations in plasma are greatly elevated if usual doses are given to patients with renal impairment, and such patients are at high risk of developing pulmonary toxicity. Doses of bleomycin should be reduced in the presence of a creatinine clearance lower than 60 ml/min (Dalgleish *et al.*, 1984).

Therapeutic Uses. The recommended dose of bleomycin (BLENOXANE, others) is 10 to 30 units/m^2 given weekly by the intravenous or intramuscular route. It also may be administered as a subcutaneous injection or as an intrapleural or intracystic instillation. Total courses exceeding 250 units should be given with great caution because of a marked increase in pulmonary toxicity above this total dose. However, pulmonary toxicity may occur at lower doses (*see* below).

Bleomycin is highly effective against germ cell tumors of the testis and ovary. In testicular cancer it is curative when used with cisplatin and vinblastine or cisplatin and etoposide. It is used as a component of the standard ABVD regimen for Hodgkin's disease, although its contribution to this curative therapy is uncertain (Duggan *et al.*, 2003). Bleomycin also is given intrapleurally (60 units) for malignant pleural effusions.

Clinical Toxicities. Because bleomycin causes little myelosuppression, it has significant advantages in combination with other cytotoxic drugs. However, it does cause significant cutaneous toxicity, including hyperpigmentation, hyperkeratosis, erythema, and even ulceration. These changes may begin with tenderness and swelling of the distal digits and progress to erythematous, ulcerating lesions over the elbows, knuckles, and other pressure areas. Skin changes often leave a residual hyperpigmentation at these points and may recur when patients are treated with other antineoplastic drugs.

The most serious adverse reaction to bleomycin is pulmonary toxicity, which begins with a dry cough, fine rales, and diffuse basilar infiltrates on x-ray and may progress to life-threatening pulmonary fibrosis. Radiologic changes may be indistinguishable from interstitial infection or tumor, but may progress to dense fibrosis, cavitation, atelectasis or lobar collapse, or even apparent consolidation. Approximately 5% to 10% of patients receiving bleomycin develop clinically apparent pulmonary toxicity, and about 1% die of this complication. Most who recover experience a significant improvement in pulmonary function, but fibrosis may be irreversible (Van Barneveld *et al.*, 1987). Pulmonary function tests are not of predictive value for detecting early onset of this complication. The CO diffusion capacity declines in patients receiving doses above 250 units. The risk is related to total dose, with a significant increase above total doses of 250 units and in patients over 70 years of age and in those with underlying pulmonary disease; single doses of 30 units/m^2 or more also are associated with an increased risk of pulmonary toxicity. Administration of high inspired oxygen concentrations during anesthesia or respiratory therapy may aggravate or precipitate pulmonary toxicity in patients previously treated with the drug. There is no known specific therapy for bleomycin lung injury except for standard symptomatic management and pulmonary care. Steroids are of uncertain benefit. The etiology of bleomycin pulmonary toxicity has been the subject of intense investigation in rodent models. These studies implicate cytokine (transforming growth factor-β [TGF-β] and tumor necrosis factor [TNF]) and chemokine (CXCLI2) secretion by macrophages in response to epithelial apoptosis in the pulmonary fibrosis (Munger *et al.*, 1999). Recruitment of bone marrow derived fibrocytes to the site of injury may contribute to the evolution of pulmonary fibrosis (Garanziotis *et al.*, 2004).

Other toxic reactions to bleomycin include hyperthermia, headache, nausea and vomiting, and a peculiar acute fulminant reaction observed in patients with lymphomas. This is characterized by profound hyperthermia, hypotension, and sustained cardiorespiratory collapse; it does not appear to be a classical anaphylactic reaction and possibly may be related to release of an endogenous pyrogen. Because this reaction has occurred in approximately 1% of patients with lymphomas and has resulted in deaths, it is recommended that patients receive a test dose of bleomycin (1 unit), followed by a 1-hour period of observation, before administration of the drug on standard dosage schedules. Unexplained exacerbations of rheumatoid arthritis also have been reported during bleomycin therapy. Raynaud's phenomenon and coronary artery occlusive events have been reported in patients with testicular tumors treated with bleomycin in combination with other chemotherapeutic agents.

Mitomycin

This antibiotic was isolated from *Streptococcus caespitosus* by Wakaki and associates in 1958. It has limited clinical utility, having been replaced by less toxic and more effective drugs in lung, colorectal, and anal cancers. However, it remains of considerable pharmacologic interest.

Mitomycin contains an azauridine group and a quinone group in its structure, as well as a mitosane ring, and each of these participates in the alkylation reactions with DNA. Its structural formula is:

MITOMYCIN

Mechanism of Action. After intracellular enzymatic or spontaneous chemical reduction of the quinone and loss of the methoxy group, mitomycin becomes a bifunctional or trifunctional alkylating agent (Verweij *et al.*, 2001). Reduction occurs preferentially in hypoxic cells in some experimental systems. The drug inhibits DNA synthesis and cross-links DNA at the N6 position of adenine and at the O^6

and N7 positions of guanine. In addition, single-strand breakage of DNA and chromosomal breaks are caused by mitomycin. Mitomycin is a potent radiosensitizer and is teratogenic and carcinogenic in rodents. Resistance has been ascribed to deficient activation, intracellular inactivation of the reduced quinone, and P-glycoprotein–mediated drug efflux (Dorr, 1988).

Absorption, Fate, and Excretion. Mitomycin is administered intravenously. It disappears rapidly from the blood after injection, with a half-life of 25 to 90 minutes. Peak concentrations in plasma are 0.4 μg/ml after doses of 20 mg/m^2 (Dorr, 1988). The drug is widely distributed throughout the body but is not detected in the CNS. Inactivation occurs by metabolism or chemical conjugation. Less than 10% of the active drug is excreted in the urine or the bile.

Therapeutic Uses. Mitomycin (mitomycin-C; MUTAMYCIN) is administered by intravenous infusion; extravasation may result in severe local injury. The usual dose (6 to 10 mg/m^2) is given as a single bolus every 6 weeks. Dosage is modified based on hematological recovery. Mitomycin also may be used by direct instillation into the bladder to treat superficial carcinomas (Boccardo et al., 1994).

Mitomycin is used with decreasing frequency in combination with 5-FU, cisplatin, or doxorubicin in carcinomas of the cervix, stomach, breast, bladder, anus, head and neck, and lung.

Clinical Toxicities. The major toxic effect is myelosuppression, characterized by marked leukopenia and thrombocytopenia; after higher doses, the nadirs may be delayed and cumulative, with recovery only after 6 to 8 weeks of pancytopenia. Nausea, vomiting, diarrhea, stomatitis, dermatitis, fever, and malaise also are observed. A hemolytic uremic syndrome represents the most dangerous toxic manifestation of mitomycin and is believed to result from drug-induced endothelial damage. Patients who have received more than 50 mg/m^2 total dose may acutely develop hemolysis, neurological abnormalities, interstitial pneumonia, and glomerular damage resulting in renal failure. The incidence of renal failure increases to 28% in patients who receive total doses of 70 mg/m^2 or higher (Valavaara and Nordman, 1985). There is no effective treatment for the disorder; blood transfusion may cause pulmonary edema. Mitomycin causes interstitial pulmonary fibrosis, and total doses above 30 mg/m^2 have infrequently led to congestive heart failure. It also may potentiate the cardiotoxicity of doxorubicin when used in conjunction with this drug.

ENZYMES

L-Asparaginase

In 1953, Kidd reported that guinea pig serum had antileukemic activity and identified L-*asparaginase* (L-asp) as the source of this activity (Kidd, 1953). Fifteen years later, the enzyme was introduced into cancer chemotherapy in an effort to exploit a distinct, qualitative difference between normal and malignant cells (Broome, 1981). It remains a standard agent for treating lymphocytic leukemia.

Mechanism of Action. While most normal tissues are able to synthesize L-asparagine in amounts sufficient for protein synthesis, some types of lymphoid malignancies derive the required amino acid from plasma. L-asp, by catalyzing the hydrolysis of circulating asparagine to aspartic acid and ammonia, deprives these malignant cells of the asparagine necessary for protein synthesis, leading to cell death. L-asp commonly is used in combination with other agents, including methotrexate, doxorubicin, vincristine, and prednisone for the treatment of ALL and for high-grade lymphomas. The sequence of drug administration in these combinations may be critical; for example, synergistic cytotoxicity results when methotrexate precedes the enzyme, but the reverse sequence leads to abrogation of methotrexate cytotoxicity. The latter outcome is a consequence of the inhibition of protein synthesis by L-asp, an effect that stops the progression of cells through the cell cycle and negates the effect of methotrexate, a drug that exerts its greatest effect during the DNA synthetic phase of the cell cycle (Capizzi and Handschumacher, 1982).

Resistance arises through induction of asparagine synthetase in tumor cells. For unknown reasons, hyperdiploid ALL cells are particularly sensitive to L-asp (Pui et al., 2004).

Absorption, Fate, Excretion, and Therapeutic Use. L-Asparaginase (ELSPAR) is given parenterally. Three different preparations of L-asp are used clinically. Their pharmacokinetics and immunogenicity differ significantly. After intravenous administration, E. coli–derived L-asp has a clearance rate from plasma of 0.035 ml/minute per kg, a volume of distribution that approximates the volume of plasma in humans, and a half-life of 14 to 24 hours (Asselin et al., 1993). It is given in doses of 6000 to 10,000 international units every third day for 3 to 4 weeks, although doses up to 25,000 international units once per week have been employed in experimental ALL protocols. Enzyme levels are maintained above 0.03 international units/ml in plasma to abolish asparagine in the bloodstream. An Erwinia preparation (see below), used in patients hypersensitive to the enzyme from E. coli, has a shorter half-life of 16 hours and thus requires administration of higher doses. Pegaspargase (PEG-L-ASPARAGINASE; ONCASPAR), is a preparation in which the enzyme is conjugated to 5000-dalton units of monomethoxy polyethylene glycol and is cleared much less rapidly. Its plasma half-life is 6 days, and it is administered in doses of 2500 international units/m^2 intramuscularly every week. Pegaspargase has much reduced immunogenicity (fewer than 20% of patients develop antibodies) (Hawkins et al., 2004).

Intermittent dosage regimens have an increased risk of inducing anaphylaxis. In hypersensitive patients, circulating antibodies lead to immediate inactivation of the enzyme and L-asp levels rapidly become immeasurable after drug administration. Not all patients with neutralizing antibodies experience hypersensitivity, although enzyme may be inactivated and therapy may be ineffective. In previously untreated ALL, pegaspargase produces more rapid clearance of lymphoblasts from bone marrow than does the E. coli preparation and circumvents the rapid antibody-mediated clearance seen with E. coli enzyme in relapsed patients (Avramis et al., 2002). Only partial depletion of CSF asparagine is achieved by the various asparaginase preparations in clinical use.

Clinical Toxicity. L-Asparaginase has minimal effects on bone marrow and gastrointestinal mucosa. Its most serious toxicities result from its antigenicity as a foreign protein and its inhibition of protein synthesis. Hypersensitivity reactions occur in 5% to 20% of patients and may be fatal. These reactions are heralded by the appearance of circulating neutralizing antibody in some, but not all, hypersensitive patients. In these patients, pegaspargase is a safe alternative, and the *Erwinia* enzyme may be used with caution.

Other toxicities result from inhibition of protein synthesis in normal tissues and include hyperglycemia due to insulin deficiency, clotting abnormalities due to deficient clotting factors, and hypoalbuminemia. The clotting problems may take the form of spontaneous thrombosis related to deficient factor S, factor C, or antithrombin III, or less frequently, hemorrhagic episodes. Thrombosis of cortical sinus vessels frequently goes unrecognized. Brain magnetic resonance imaging studies should be considered in patients treated with L-asp who present with seizures, headache, or altered mental status (Bushara and Rust, 1997). L-Asparaginase–induced thromboses occur with greater frequency in patients with underlying inherited disorders of coagulation, such as factor V Leiden, elevated serum homocysteine, protein C or S deficiency, antithrombin III deficiency, or the 620210A variant of prothrombin (Nowak-Gottl *et al.*, 1999). Intracranial hemorrhage in the first week of L-asp treatment is an infrequent but devastating complication. L-Asparaginase suppresses immune function as well.

In addition to these side effects, coma may rarely result and has been attributed to ammonia toxicity resulting from L-asparagine hydrolysis. Pancreatitis also has been observed; its cause is uncertain.

IV. MISCELLANEOUS AGENTS

HYDROXYUREA

Dresler and Stein originally synthesized hydroxyurea in 1869, but its potential biological significance was not recognized until 1928, when leukopenia and megaloblastic anemia were observed in experimental animals treated with this compound. In the 1950s, the drug was evaluated in a large number of experimental murine tumor models and was found to have broad antitumor activity against both leukemia and solid tumors. Clinical trials with hydroxyurea began in the 1960s. Since then this drug has attracted interest, as it has unique and surprisingly diverse biological effects that have led to exploration of its clinical utility as an antileukemic drug, radiation sensitizer, and an inducer of fetal hemoglobin in patients with sickle cell disease. Its use has been encouraged because the drug is orally administered and its toxicity in most patients is modest and limited to myelosuppression (Paz-Ares and Donehower, 2001). The structural formula of hydroxyurea is:

$$H_2N-\overset{\overset{\displaystyle O}{\|}}{C}-NH-OH$$

HYDROXYUREA

Cytotoxic Action. Hydroxyurea (HU) inhibits the enzyme ribonucleoside diphosphate reductase. This enzyme, which catalyzes the reductive conversion of ribonucleotides to deoxyribonucleotides, is a crucial rate-limiting step in the biosynthesis of DNA, and it represents a logical target for the design of chemotherapeutic agents. HU destroys a tyrosyl free radical that binds iron in the catalytic center of the human ribonucleotide reductase subunit hRRM2. Iron is an essential mediator of the reduction of nucleotides, providing an electron for this reaction. The drug is specific for the S phase of the cell cycle, in which concentrations of the target reductase are maximal, and causes cells to arrest at or near the G_1–S interface. Cell-cycle arrest by HU is mediated by both p53-dependent and p53-independent mechanisms (Zhou *et al.*, 2003). Since cells are highly sensitive to irradiation in the G_1–S boundary, combinations of HU and irradiation cause synergistic toxicity (Schilsky *et al.*, 1992). Through depletion of deoxynucleotides, HU also may potentiate the antiproliferative effects of DNA-damaging agents such as cisplatin, alkylating agents, or topoisomerase II inhibitors, and facilitates the incorporation of drugs such as Ara-C, gemcitabine, or fludarabine into DNA. HU also induces the expression of a number of genes (*e.g.,* TNF, interleukin-6) and accelerates the loss of extrachromosomally amplified genes present in double-minute chromosomes formed in response to methotrexate therapy. The role of nitric oxide release in its differentiating activity and in its antitumor effects is uncertain, but intriguing (Cokic *et al.*, 2003).

HU reduces vaso-occlusive events in patients with sickle cell disease. It does so *via* several potential mechanisms. Increased expression of fetal hemoglobin and synthesis of fetal hemoglobin may result from suppression of erythroid precursor proliferation with compensatory stimulation of a distinct set of fetal Hb-producing cells. An alternative mechanism (Steinberg, 2003) has been offered because of the ability of HU to generate nitric oxide both *in vitro* and *in vivo*, causing nitrosylation of small-molecular-weight GTPases that stimulate γ-globin production in erythroid precursors. Through the induction of HbF, it promotes solubility of hemoglobin within red cells. It also reduces adhesion of red cells to vascular endothelium, and by suppressing the production of neutrophils, decreases their contribution to vascular occlusion. It specifically lowers the expression of adhesion molecules such as L-selectin in neutrophils (Halsey and Roberts, 2003).

The principal mechanism by which cells achieve resistance to HU is increased synthesis of the hRRM2 subunit of ribonucleoside diphosphate reductase, thus restoring enzyme activity. HU reduces the frequency of painful events, acute chest syndrome, and secondary strokes in patients.

Absorption, Fate, and Excretion. The oral bioavailability of hydroxyurea is excellent (80% to 100%), and comparable plasma concentrations are seen after oral or intravenous dosing (Rodriguez *et al.*, 1998). Peak plasma concentrations are reached 1 to 1.5 hours after oral doses of 15 to 80 mg/kg. Hydroxyurea disappears from plasma with a half-life from 3.5 to 4.5 hours. The drug readily crosses the blood–brain barrier, and it appears in significant quantities in human breast milk. From 40% to 80% of the drug is recovered in the urine within 12 hours after either intravenous or oral administration. Although precise guidelines are not available, it seems prudent to modify doses for patients with abnormal renal function until individual tolerance can be assessed. Data from several experimental animal systems suggest that metabolism of hydroxyurea does occur, but the extent and significance of metabolism of the drug in humans have not been established.

Therapeutic Uses. In cancer treatment, two dosage schedules for hydroxyurea (HYDREA, DROXIA, others), alone or in combination with other drugs, are most commonly used in a variety of clinical situations: (1) intermittent therapy with 80 mg/kg administered orally as a single dose every third day; or (2) continuous therapy with 20 to 30 mg/kg administered as a single daily dose. In patients with essential thrombocythemia and in sickle cell disease, HU is given in daily dose of 15 to 30 mg/kg, depending on tolerance and myelosuppression (Halsey and Roberts, 2003). Dosage should be adjusted according to the number of leukocytes in the peripheral blood. Treatment is typically continued for a period of 6 weeks in malignant diseases to determine its effectiveness; if satisfactory results are obtained, therapy can be continued indefinitely, although leukocyte counts at weekly intervals are advisable.

The principal use of HU has been as a myelosuppressive agent in various myeloproliferative syndromes, particularly CML, polycythemia vera, and essential thrombocytosis. In essential thrombocythemia, it is the drug of choice for patients with a platelet count over 1.5 million cells per mm^3, or with a history of arterial or venous thrombosis. In this disease it dramatically lowers the risk of thrombosis by lowering the platelet count, but also through its effect on neutrophil and red cell counts, and by reducing expression of L-selectin and increasing nitric oxide production of neutrophils (Finazzi et al., 2003).

In CML, HU has been largely replaced by imatinib (Silver et al., 1999). Thus, HU cannot be considered to be standard therapy, although it has produced anecdotal, temporary remissions in patients with advanced cancers (e.g., head and neck or genitourinary carcinomas, melanoma). HU has been incorporated into several schedules with concurrent irradiation, as it is able to synchronize cells into a radiation-sensitive phase of the cell cycle. This combination has shown promise in several diseases, including cervical carcinoma, primary brain tumors, head and neck cancer, and non–small cell lung cancer, although it has not been proven to be superior to regimens including cisplatin and irradiation.

HU (DROXIA) has been approved by the FDA for the treatment of adult patients with sickle cell disease. Hydroxyurea also appears to be effective in children with sickle cell disease and in patients with sickle cell–α-thalassemia and sickle cell–hemoglobin C disease (Zimmerman et al., 2004).

Clinical Toxicity. Hematopoietic depression—involving leukopenia, megaloblastic anemia, and occasionally thrombocytopenia—is the major toxic effect; recovery of the bone marrow usually is prompt if the drug is discontinued for a few days. Other adverse reactions include a desquamative interstitial pneumonitis, gastrointestinal disturbances, and mild dermatological reactions; more rarely, stomatitis, alopecia, and neurological manifestations have been encountered. Increased skin and fingernail pigmentation may occur, as well as painful leg ulcers. Hydroxyurea has uncertain effect on the risk of secondary leukemia in patients with myeloproliferative disorders and should be used with caution in nonmalignant diseases. Hydroxyurea is a potent teratogen in all animal species tested and should not be used in women with childbearing potential.

DIFFERENTIATING AGENTS

One of the hallmarks of malignant transformation is a block in differentiation. In some malignancies, the trans-

forming genetic change directly confers this block, an example being the t(15;17) translocation in APL. This translocation involves the retinoic acid receptor-α, which forms a heterodimeric retinoid binding protein critical for differentiation, and the PML gene, which encodes a transcription factor important in inhibiting proliferation and promoting myeloid differentiation. The product of the new gene, a fusion protein of portions of RAR-α and PML, binds retinoids with much decreased affinity, lacks PML inhibitory function, and blocks the function of transcription factors such as C/EBP, which promote myeloid differentiation (Jing, 2003). The fusion gene also promotes expression of genes that increase leukemic stem cell renewal, and suppresses expression of DNA repair functions, thereby enhancing mutability of APL cells (Alcalay et al., 2003). A number of chemical entities, including vitamin D and its analogs, retinoids, benzamides and other inhibitors of histone deacetylase, various cytotoxics and biological agents, and inhibitors of DNA methylation, can induce differentiation in tumor cell lines in vitro. Fittingly, the first and best example of differentiating therapy has been discovered in the treatment of APL.

Retinoids

Tretinoin. The biology and pharmacology of retinoids and related compounds are discussed in detail in Chapter 62. The most important of these for cancer treatment is *tretinoin* (all-trans retinoic acid; ATRA), which induces a high rate of complete remission in APL as a single agent, and in combination with anthracyclines, has become part of a curative regimen for this disease (Huang et al., 1988).

Under physiologic conditions, the RAR-α receptor dimerizes with the retinoid X receptor to form a complex that binds ATRA tightly, displacing a repressor of differentiation. In APL cells, physiologic concentrations of retinoid are inadequate to displace the repressor. Pharmacologic concentrations, however, are effective in displacing the repressor, activating the differentiation program, and promoting degradation of the PML-RAR-α fusion gene. Resistance to ATRA arises by further mutation of the fusion gene, abolishing ATRA binding or by loss of expression of the fusion gene (Roussel and Lanotte, 2001). Sensitivity can be restored by transfection of a functional RAR-α gene.

Clinical Pharmacology. The usual dosing regimen of orally administered ATRA is 45 mg/m^2 per day until remission is achieved. ATRA as a single agent reverses the hemorrhagic diathesis associated with APL and induces a high rate of temporary remission. However, clinical trials have clearly established the benefit of giving ATRA in combination with an anthracycline for remission induction, achieving 70% or greater relapse-free long-term survival (Tallman et al., 1997, Sanz et al., 1999).

ATRA concentrations reach 400 ng/ml in plasma, and are cleared by a CYP-mediated elimination with a half-life of less than 1 hour. Treatment with inducers of CYP leads to more rapid drug disappearance, and in some patients, resistance to ATRA (Gallagher, 2002). Remission rate and time to remission induction improve with the inclusion of other chemotherapy. Corticosteroids and chemotherapy decrease the occurrence of "retinoic acid syndrome," which is characterized by fever, dyspnea, weight gain, pulmonary infiltrates, and pleural or pericardial effusions. When used as a single agent for remission induction, especially in patients with >5000 leukemic cells per mm^3 in the peripheral blood, ATRA induces an outpouring of cytokines and mature appearing neutrophils of leukemic origin. These cells express high concentrations of integrins and other adhesion molecules on their surface, and clog small vessels in the pulmonary circulation, leading to significant morbidity in 15% to 20% of patients. The syndrome includes respiratory distress, pleural and pericardial effusions, mental status changes, and death.

Toxicity. Retinoids as a class, including ATRA, cause dry skin, cheilitis, reversible hepatic enzyme abnormalities, bone tenderness, and hyperlipidemia, and as mentioned above, the retinoic acid syndrome.

Arsenic Trioxide (ATO)

Although recognized as a heavy metal toxin for centuries, *arsenic trioxide* (ATO) attracted interest as a medicinal agent nearly a century ago for syphilis and parasitic disease, and eventually CML. Through the efforts of Shen and colleagues in Shanghai (Shen *et al.*, 1997), it was shown to be a highly effective treatment for relapsed APL, producing complete responses in more than 85% of such patients. The chemistry and toxicity of arsenic is considered in detail in Chapter 65.

The mechanism of pharmacological action of ATO remains uncertain (Miller *et al.*, 2002). It causes differentiation of APL cells in culture and in clinical use, and also promotes apoptosis. ATO is highly reactive with sulfhydryls of glutathione and with cysteine-rich proteins. It generates free radicals and inhibits angiogenesis, both of which may be relevant to its antileukemic effects (Miller *et al.*, 2002). Cells exposed to ATO upregulate p53, Jun kinase, and caspases associated with the intrinsic pathway of apoptosis (Davison *et al.*, 2004). It promotes the phosphorylation, sumoylation, and the degradation of the fusion protein, as well as promoting degradation of NF-κB, a transcription factor that stimulates angiogenesis and dampens apoptotic responses in cells with DNA damage (Hayakawa and Privalsky, 2004).

Clinical Pharmacology. ATO is administered as a 2-hour intravenous infusion in doses of 0.15 mg/kg per day for up to 60 days, until remission is documented. Further consolidation therapy resumes after a 3-week break. The primary mechanism of elimination is through enzymatic methylation (Miller *et al.*, 2002). Methylated metabolites have uncertain biological effects. Peak concentrations of ATO in plasma reach 5 to 7 μM with rapid conversion to metabolites. Little drug appears in the urine. No dose reductions are indicated for hepatic or renal dysfunction.

Toxicity. Pharmacological doses of ATO are well tolerated. Patients may experience reversible side effects including hyperglycemia, hepatic enzyme elevations, fatigue, dysesthesias, and light-headedness. Ten percent or fewer of patients will experience a leukocyte maturation syndrome similar to that seen with ATRA, including pulmonary distress, effusions, and mental status changes. Oxygen, corticosteroids, and temporary discontinuation of ATO leads to full reversal of this syndrome (Soignet *et al.*, 1998). Another important and potentially dangerous side effect is lengthening of the QT interval on the electrocardiogram in 40% of patients. The basis for this conduction defect appears to be an enhancement of Ca^{2+} flux and an inhibition of K$^+$ channels in myocardial tissue by As$_2$O$_3$. This change leads to atrial or ventricular arrhythmias in a small minority of patients, but daily monitoring of the ECG and repletion of serum K$^+$ in patients with hypokalemia are standard measures in ATO therapy.

PROTEIN TYROSINE KINASE INHIBITORS

Protein kinases are ubiquitous and critical components of signal transduction pathways that transmit information concerning extracellular or cytoplasmic conditions to the nucleus, thereby influencing gene transcription and/or DNA synthesis. The human genome contains approximately 550 protein kinases and an additional 130 protein phosphatases that regulate the activity of the various protein kinases. The protein kinases can be classified into three different categories: tyrosine kinases, with specific activity for tyrosine residues only, serine/threonine kinases, with activity for serine and threonine residues only, and kinases with activity for all three residues. Tyrosine kinases can be further subdivided into proteins that have an extracellular ligand binding domain (receptor tyrosine kinases) and enzymes that are confined to the cytoplasm and/or nuclear cellular compartment (nonreceptor tyrosine kinases) (Hubbard and Till, 2000). Abnormal activation of specific protein tyrosine kinases has been demonstrated in many human neoplasms (Blume-Jensen and Hunter, 2001), making them attractive molecular targets for cancer therapy. There currently are three small-molecular-weight protein tyrosine kinase inhibitors that are FDA approved and many others are in clinical trials.

Imatinib

Chemistry. Imatinib mesylate (STI 571, GLEEVEC, GLIVEC) was identified through the combined use of high throughput screening and medicinal chemistry and is 4-[(4-methyl-1-piperazinyl)methyl]-N-[4-methyl-3-[[4-(3-pyridinyl)-2-pyrimidinyl] amino]-phenyl]benzamidemethanesulfonate. The lead compound of this series, a 2-phenylaminopyrimidine, had low potency and poor specificity, inhibiting both serine/threonine and tyrosine kinases (Buchdunger *et al.*, 2001). The addition of a 3′-pyridyl group at the 3′-position of the pyrimidine enhanced the cellular activity of the derivatives. A number of chemical modifications resulted in improved activity against the platelet-derived growth factor receptor (PDGFR) tyrosine kinase and loss of serine/threonine kinase inhibition. These compounds also were found to possess inhibitory activity toward the cytoplasmic ABL tyrosine kinase and receptor tyrosine kinase, KIT. Introduction of N-methylpiperazine as a polar side chain greatly improved water solubility and oral bioavailability, yielding imatinib, whose chemical structure is:

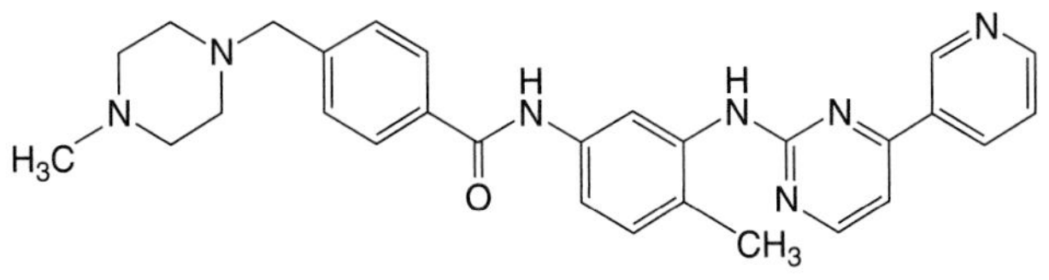

IMATINIB

Mechanism of Action. Imatinib has inhibitory activity against ABL and its activated derivatives v-ABL, BCR-ABL, and EVT6-ABL (Buchdunger *et al.*, 1996; Druker *et al.*, 1996). IC_{50} values are in the range of 0.025 μM using *in vitro* kinase assays with immunoprecipitated or purified proteins. Activity against the PDGFR and KIT are in a similar range. In contrast, the IC_{50} values for a large number of other tyrosine and serine/threonine kinases generally are at least 100 times higher, demonstrating that imatinib exhibits a high level of selectivity (Buchdunger *et al.*, 2001).

Cellular studies showed that imatinib specifically inhibited the proliferation of myeloid cell lines that express the BCR-ABL fusion protein associated with CML (Druker *et al.*, 1996). The IC_{50} for BCR-ABL phosphorylation in intact cells is between 0.25 and 0.5 μM (Buchdunger *et al.*, 2001). Complete inhibition of proliferation with cell death through apoptotic mechanisms occurs between 0.5- and 1-μM concentrations of imatinib. Similar concentrations of imatinib inhibit the proliferation of cells dependent on KIT or PDGFR for proliferation. This includes cells expressing mutant KIT isoforms associated with gastrointestinal stromal tumors (GISTs) (Heinrich *et al.*, 2000), the ETV6-PDGFR fusion associated with a subset of chronic myelomonocytic leukemia (CMML) (Carroll *et al.*, 1997), and the FIP1L1-PDGFRA fusion associated with hypereosinophilic syndrome (HES) (Cools *et al.*, 2003).

Mechanisms of Resistance. Resistance to imatinib can be primary, that is, failure to achieve a specific desired response, or secondary (acquired), that is, loss of a desired response. The acquired resistance predominantly results from mutations in the kinase domain (Shah *et al.*, 2002), although some patients have amplification of BCR-ABL (Hochhaus *et al.*, 2002). Interestingly, in CML patients in whom the malignancy is driven by the BCR-ABL tyrosine kinase, mutations have only been observed in the ABL kinase, whereas in GIST and HES, only KIT and PDGFR mutations have been observed, respectively (Cools *et al.*, 2003; Wakai *et al.*, 2004). These data demonstrate the critical tumor dependence on the specific mutated kinase. ABL mutations are scattered throughout the kinase domain and variably render the kinase less sensitive to imatinib (Corbin *et al.*, 2003). Mutations affect sites that are direct contact points between the kinase and imatinib or affect residues that are required for the kinase to adopt a conformation to which imatinib can bind (Deininger and Druker,

2004; Shah *et al.*, 2002). Alternate kinase inhibitors that can inhibit the imatinib-resistant mutations are currently in clinical development (Deininger and Druker, 2004).

In contrast to acquired resistance, the mechanisms mediating primary resistance are unknown. Hypotheses include alternate pathways that allow tumors to escape the antiapoptotic effects of an agent targeting a single pathway, quiescence of a population of cells in the tumors that are not susceptible to the antiproliferative effects of this class of agents, or inadequate drug levels due to poor tumor penetration of the drug, drug efflux, protein binding, or unappreciated mutations that affect drug sensitivity.

Pharmacokinetics. Imatinib is well absorbed after oral administration with maximum plasma concentrations (C_{max}) achieved within 2 to 4 hours (Peng *et al.*, 2004). Mean absolute bioavailability for the capsule formulation is 98%. Following oral administration in healthy volunteers, the elimination half-lives of imatinib and its major active metabolite, the N-desmethyl derivative, are approximately 18 and 40 hours, respectively. Mean imatinib AUC increases proportionally with increasing dose in the range 25 to 1000 mg (Peng *et al.*, 2004). There is no significant change in the pharmacokinetics of imatinib on repeated dosing or with administration of food. Doses >300 mg per day achieve trough levels of 1 μM, which corresponds to *in vitro* levels required to kill BCR-ABL–expressing cells. Pharmacodynamic inhibition of the BCR-ABL tyrosine kinase can be demonstrated in white blood cells from patients with CML with a plateau in inhibition between doses of 250 and 750 mg (Druker *et al.*, 2001). Nonrandomized studies suggest that improved responses may be observed with doses of 600 or 800 mg per day as opposed to 400 mg per day (Kantarjian *et al.*, 2004; Talpaz *et al.*, 2002), consistent with dose-dependent inhibition of the kinase.

CYP3A4 is the major enzyme responsible for metabolism of imatinib. Other cytochrome P450 enzymes, such as CYP1A2, CYP2D6, CYP2C9, and CYP2C19, play a minor role in its metabolism. Plasma levels of drugs that are substrates for these cytochromes may increase if coadministered with imatinib due to competition for biotransformation pathways, and those that are enzyme inhibitors or inducers may increase or decrease the plasma levels of imatinib, respectively. A single dose of *ketoconazole* increases mean C_{max} and AUC of imatinib by 26% and 40%, respectively, confirming that imatinib is a CYP3A4 substrate (Dutreix *et al.*, 2004). Imatinib increased the C_{max} and AUC of *simvastatin* by 2 and 3.5 times, respectively, indicating inhibition of CYP3A4 (O'Brien *et al.*, 2003). Coadministration with *rifampin*, an inducer of CYP3A4, reduces plasma imatinib AUC by approximately 70% (Bolton *et al.*, 2004). Elimination of imatinib occurs predominantly in the feces, mostly as metabolites.

Therapeutic Uses. Imatinib has efficacy in diseases in which the ABL, KIT, or PDGFR have dominant roles in driving the proliferation of the tumor. This dominant role is defined by the presence of a mutation that results in constitutive activation of the kinase, either by fusion with another protein or point mutations. Thus, imatinib shows remarkable therapeutic benefits in patients with CML (BCR-ABL), GIST (KIT mutation positive), CMML (EVT6-PDGFR), HES (FIP1L1-PDGFR), and dermatofibrosarcoma protuberans (constitutive production of the ligand for PDGFR) (Druker, 2004). The situation in GIST is particularly instructive, as patients with an exon 11 mutation of KIT have a significantly higher partial response rate (72%) than those with no detectable KIT mutations (9%) (Heinrich *et al.*, 2003). Thus, KIT mutational status predicts response. The currently recommended dose of imatinib is 400 to 600 mg per day.

Clinical Toxicity. The most frequently reported drug-related adverse events are nausea, vomiting, edema, and muscle cramps (Deininger *et al.*, 2003). Most events are of mild-to-moderate grade, and only 2% to 5% of patients permanently discontinue therapy, most commonly because of skin rashes and elevations of transaminases (each in <1% of patients). Edema can manifest at any site, most commonly in the ankles and periorbital tissues. Severe fluid retention (pleural effusion, pericardial effusion, pulmonary edema, and ascites) is reported in 1% to 2% of patients taking imatinib. The probability of edema increases with higher imatinib doses and in persons >65 years old. Neutropenia and thrombocytopenia are consistent findings in all studies in leukemia patients, with a higher frequency at doses ≥750 mg. The occurrence of cytopenias also is dependent on the stage of CML, with a frequency of grade 3 or 4 neutropenia and thrombocytopenia between two- and threefold higher in blast crisis and accelerated phase compared to chronic phase. In solid tumor patients, grade 4 neutropenia has been reported in <5% of patients. Thrombocytopenia is much less common.

Gefitinib

The epidermal growth factor receptor (EGFR) belongs to a family of four receptor tyrosine kinases. The EGFR type 1 (ErbB1 or HER1) is overexpressed in many common malignancies, and may be activated by autocrine loops in many others. A truncated version of the EGFR (EGFRvIII) that has lost a portion of the extracellular ligand-binding domain and is constitutively activated, is found in a subset of patients with glioblastoma. Based on these data, the EGFR is viewed as a particularly attractive molecular target for anticancer drugs (Grunwald and Hidalgo, 2003).

Chemistry. Gefitinib (ZD1839, IRESSA, [4-(3-chloro-4-fluoroanilino)-7-methoxy-6-(3-morphiolenopropoxy)quinazoline] is a low-molecular-weight quinazoline derivative discovered through the screening of a compound library with the EFGR tyrosine kinase, which identified 4-anilinoquinazolines as lead compounds (Barker *et al.*, 2001). Structure–activity relationships reveal that the quinazoline moiety was absolutely required for activity with electron-donating substituents at the 6- and 7-positions leading to increased potency. Other chemical modifications improved potency and pharmacokinetics of these compounds. A wide variety of compounds were generated from this foundation and gefitinib was selected as the lead candidate for clinical development based on its superior *in vivo* antitumor activity and pharmacokinetic properties (Barker *et al.*, 2001). The chemical structure of gefitinib is displayed below.

GEFITINIB

Mechanism of Action. Gefitinib is a specific inhibitor of the EGFR tyrosine kinase that competitively inhibits ATP binding. Gefitinib inhibits the EGFR with an IC_{50} of 2.7 nM. It is 100 times less potent against highly related tyrosine kinases such as HER2 (ErbB2/neu) and does not inhibit a variety of serine/threonine kinases (Wakeling *et al.*, 2002). Preclinical studies showed that gefitinib inhibits the growth of a variety of cell lines that are dependent on EGFR activity for growth (Baselga and Averbuch, 2000; Grunwald and Hidalgo, 2003). Treatment with gefitinib was associated with cell-cycle arrest at the G_0/G_1 boundary. *In vivo* studies showed significant antitumor activity in a variety of human xenograft tumor models with EGFR overexpression. In these preclinical studies, although gefitinib treatment resulted in rapid tumor regression, the tumors regrew when the drug was discontinued, suggesting that long-term administration would be required to maintain activity. Interestingly, in xenograft models, expression levels of EGFR did not correlate with responses, suggesting that factors other than EGFR expression may be more predictive of response. Preclinical studies showed that combinations of gefitinib with chemotherapy or radiation therapy improves therapeutic outcome (Grunwald and Hidalgo, 2003).

Mechanisms of Resistance. The predominant problem with the clinical use of gefitinib has been relatively low response rates (Dancey and Freidlin, 2003). Consistent with the preclinical studies, levels of EGFR expression do not correlate with responses. As with KIT mutational status in GIST, patients whose non–small cell lung tumors have point mutations in the EGFR respond dramatically to gefitinib (Lynch *et al.*, 2004; Paez *et al.*, 2004). Thus, primary resistance could be due to the fact that tumors are not uniquely dependent on EGFR activity for survival. Although target inhibition by gefitinib has been demonstrated in normal skin (Albanell *et al.*, 2002), it is possible that poor tumor penetration of the drug could lead to incomplete inhibition of the EGFR. Alternatively, drug efflux, unappreciated mutations that affect drug sensitivity, or a variety of other factors that could affect target inhibition may have a role in mediating lack of responsiveness.

Pharmacokinetics. Following oral administration of gefitinib, peak plasma concentrations are achieved within 3 to 7 hours (Baselga *et al.*, 2002; Ranson *et al.*, 2002). Mean absolute bioavailability of the oral formulation is 59%. Exposure to gefitinib is not significantly altered by food; however, coadministration of drugs that cause sustained elevations in gastric pH to ≥5 reduce mean gefitinib AUC by 47%. Administration of gefitinib once daily results in two- to eightfold accumulation with steady-state exposures achieved after 7 to 10 doses. At steady state, circulating plasma concentrations typically are maintained within a two- to threefold range over the 24-hour dosing interval. The mean terminal half-life is 41 hours (Thomas and Grandis, 2004).

In vitro studies showed that the metabolism of gefitinib is predominantly *via* CYP3A4 (Cohen *et al.*, 2004). The major metabolite identified in human plasma is O-desmethyl gefitinib. It is 14 times less potent than gefitinib at inhibiting EGFR-stimulated cell growth and is unlikely to contribute significantly to the clinical activity of gefitinib. Substances that are inducers of CYP3A4 activity may increase metabolism and decrease gefitinib plasma concentrations. Therefore, CYP3A4 inducers (*e.g.*, phenytoin, *carbamazepine*, rifampin, barbiturates, or *St. John's wort*) may reduce efficacy. Coadministration with *rifampin* (a known potent CYP3A4 inducer) in healthy volunteers reduced mean gefitinib AUC by 83%. Coadministration with *itraconazole* (a CYP3A4 inhibitor) resulted in an 80% increase in the mean AUC of gefitinib in healthy volunteers (Cohen *et al.*, 2004). This increase may be clinically relevant since adverse experiences are related to dose and exposure. Elimination of gefitinib is primarily by metabolism and excretion in feces.

Therapeutic Uses. Gefitinib is approved for the treatment of patients with non–small cell lung cancer who have failed standard chemotherapy. Single-agent responses in these heavily pretreated patients are in the 12% to 18% range (Fukuoka *et al.*, 2003; Kris *et al.*, 2003). However, there is a subset of patients who responded dramatically to gefitinib and these are predominantly non-smoking women with bronchoalveolar tumors (Miller *et al.*, 2004). It has been shown that this subset of patients has EGFR mutations that render the EGFR hypersensitive to ligand and to gefitinib (Lynch *et al.*, 2004; Paez *et al.*, 2004). Tumors from patients responding to other EGFR inhibitors in clinical development, such as *erlotinib* (TARCEVA), display EGFR mutations. The recommended dose of gefitinib is one 250-mg tablet daily, taken with or without food.

Clinical Toxicity. The most commonly reported adverse drug reactions are diarrhea, rash, acne, pruritus, dry skin, nausea, vomiting, and anorexia (Baselga *et al.*, 2002; Ranson *et al.*, 2002). A higher rate of most of these adverse events is observed in patients treated with 500 mg per day of gefitinib as compared to treatment with 250 mg per day. Most adverse events are of mild-to-moderate grade. Less than 2% of patients have permanently discontinued therapy. Adverse drug reactions usually occur within the first month of therapy and generally are reversible. Asymptomatic increases in liver transaminases have been observed and periodic liver function testing should be performed. Interstitial lung disease, which may be acute in onset, has been observed uncommonly in patients receiving gefitinib, and some cases have been fatal. The overall frequency of interstitial lung disease is approximately 0.3% outside of Japan (39,000 patients exposed) and approximately 2% in Japan (27,000 patients exposed) (Cohen *et al.*, 2004).

Erlotinib

Pharmacology and Cytotoxic Effects. Erlotinib (TARCEVA) is a human HER1/EGFR tyrosine kinase inhibitor with the following chemical formula: N-(3-ethynylphenyl)-6,7-bis(2-methoxyethoxy)-4-quinazolinamine. It is indicated for treatment of patients with locally advanced or metastatic non–small cell lung cancer.

FDA approval was based on a 731-patient double-blind, multinational, randomized trial comparing oral erlotinib 150 mg daily to placebo. An analysis of EGFR protein expression status on treatment survival effect was performed; however, EGFR status was known for only one-third of patients. In the EGFR-positive subgroup, erlotinib prolonged survival compared to placebo by a median of 6.9 months. No apparent survival benefit for erlotinib was observed in the EGFR-negative subgroup. However, the confidence intervals for the two subgroups did not allow an erlotinib survival

effect in the EGFR-negative subgroup to be excluded. The chemical structure of erlotinib is shown below.

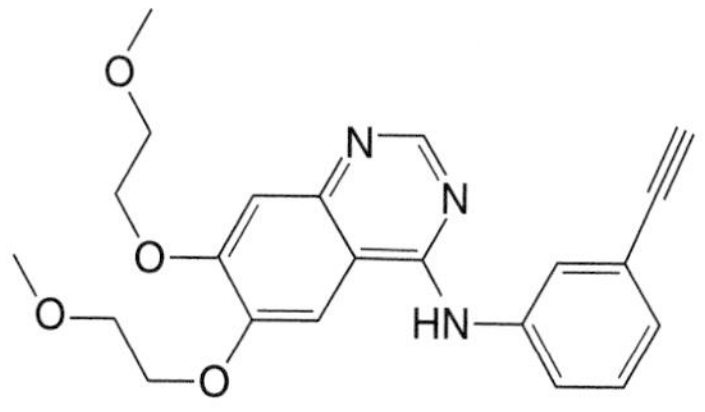

ERLOTINIB

Absorption, Fate, and Excretion. Erlotinib is about 60% absorbed after oral administration and its bioavailability is substantially increased to almost 100% by food. Peak plasma levels occur 4 hours after an oral dose. Following absorption, erlotinib is approximately 93% protein-bound to albumin and α_1-acid glycoprotein. Its half-life is ~36 hours. Erlotinib is metabolized primarily by CYP3A4 and to a lesser extent by CYP1A2 and CYP1A1.

Clinical Toxicities. The most common adverse reactions in patients receiving erlotinib were diarrhea and rash. Serious interstitial lung disease also has been reported. Other adverse effects include elevated liver enzymes and bleeding, especially in patients receiving warfarin. Coadministration of CYP3A4 inhibitors is expected to increase toxicity to erlotinib.

THALIDOMIDE

Thalidomide originally was developed in the 1950s for the treatment of pregnancy-associated morning sickness, but withdrawn from the market due to the tragic consequences of teratogenicity and dysmyelia (stunted limb growth) (Franks *et al.*, 2004). However, it has since been reintroduced to clinical practice, initially because of its clinical efficacy as an oral agent for the management of erythema nodosum leprosum, which the FDA approved in 1998 (*see* Chapter 47). Meanwhile, the realization of thalidomide's antiangiogenic and immunomodulatory effects, including the inhibition of TNF-α signaling, triggered an expansion of thalidomide uses in other disease settings, most notably multiple myeloma (MM) (Franks *et al.*, 2004). Indeed, significant clinical experience has been acquired on the activity of thalidomide in both newly diagnosed and heavily pretreated relapsed/refractory MM patients. In addition, thalidomide has shown clinical activity in patients with myelodysplastic syndromes and ongoing clinical studies are addressing the potential role of thalidomide in the therapeutic management of other neoplasias. Although the precise mechanism(s) of antitumor activity of thalidomide remain(s) to be fully elucidated, substantial insight has been generated by extensive preclinical studies in MM. New analogs derived from thalidomide now are in clinical trials for MM and myelodysplasia.

Chemistry and Pharmacology of Thalidomide and Its Derivatives. Thalidomide (Figure 51–17) exists at physiologic pH as a nonpolar racemic mixture of cell permeable and rapidly interconverting S(–) and R(+) isomers, the former being associated with the teratogenic, and the latter with the sedative properties of thalidomide. Thalidomide absorption from the GI tract is slow and highly variable (4 hours mean time to reach peak concentration [t_{max}], with a range of 1 to 7 hours) (Figg *et al.*, 1999). Thalidomide is widely distributed throughout most tissues and organs, without significant binding to plasma proteins, and with a large apparent volume of distribution (V_d). Importantly, thalidomide is detected in the semen of patients after a period of 4 weeks of therapy, with levels that correlate with serum levels. Thalidomide metabolism *via* the hepatic CYP system is limited, and no induction of its own metabolism is noted with prolonged use. However, thalidomide undergoes rapid and spontaneous nonenzymatic hydrolytic cleavage at physiologic pH, generating >50 metabolites, most of which are unstable *in vitro* or *in vivo*. Importantly, there are substantial species-specific differences in the patterns and profiles of thalidomide metabolites in mice compared with humans, which likely explains why teratogenicity of thalidomide was not detected in preclinical murine models (Lenz, 1962).

Elimination of thalidomide is mainly by spontaneous hydrolysis, which occurs in all body fluids, with an apparent mean clearance of 10 L/hour for the (R)-enantiomer and 21 L/hour for the (S)-enantiomer in adult subjects. This leads to higher blood concentrations of the (R)-enantiomer compared to those of the (S)-enantiomer. Thalidomide and its metabolites appear to be rapidly excreted in the urine, while the nonabsorbed portion of the drug is excreted unchanged in feces, but clearance is primarily nonrenal. Studies of both single and multiple dosing of thalidomide in elderly prostate cancer patients showed significantly longer half-life at higher doses (1200 mg daily) *versus* lower doses (200 mg daily) (Figg *et al.*, 1999). Conversely, no effect of increased age on elimination half-life was identified in the age range of 55 to 80 years. The impact of renal or hepatic dysfunction on thalidomide clearance remains to be fully elucidated.

Thalidomide's interactions with other drugs have not been systematically addressed, except for lack of significant interaction with oral contraceptives (Franks *et al.*, 2004) and thalidomide's effect in enhancing the sedative effects of barbiturates and alcohol and the catatonic effects of *chlorpromazine* and *reserpine*. Conversely, CNS stimulants (such as *methamphetamine* and *methylphenidate*) counteract the depressant effects of thalidomide.

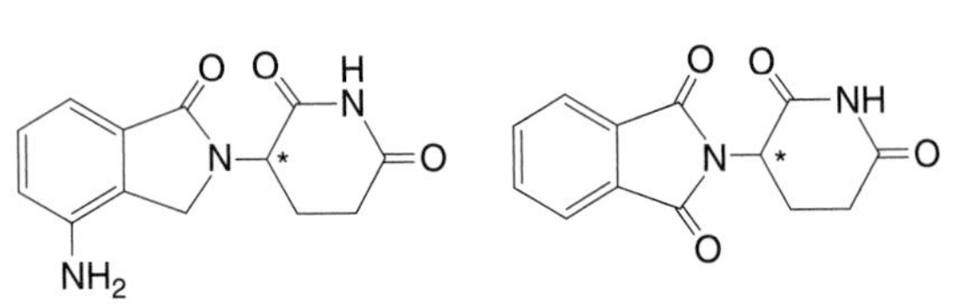

Figure 51–17. Structures of thalidomide and lenalidomide. The asterisk denotes the chiral center.

Pharmacology of Thalidomide Derivatives. *Lenalidomide* (Figure 51–17) constitutes a lead compound in the new class of immunomodulatory thalidomide derivatives (IMIDs) and exhibits a constellation of pharmacological properties, including stimulation of T cells and NK cells, inhibition of angiogenesis and tumor cell proliferation, and modulation of hematopoietic stem cell differentiation (Corral and Kaplan, 1999; Hideshima *et al.*, 2000; Davies *et al.*, 2001). This orally administered agent has been tested in MM, myelodysplastic syndrome, and an expanding array of other clinical settings, because of preclinical data suggesting more potent activity than its parent compound, as well as less toxicity and a lack of teratogenic effects as compared to thalidomide (Franks *et al.*, 2004). Lenalidomide is rapidly absorbed following oral administration, with peak plasma levels occurring between 0.6 and 1.5 hours postdose. The C_{max} and AUC values increased proportionately with increasing dose, both over a single-dose range of 5 to 400 mg and after multiple dosing with 100 mg daily. The half-life increases with dose, from approximately 3 hours at the 5-mg dose, to approximately 9 hours at the 400-mg dose (the higher dose is believed to provide a better estimate of the half-life due to the prolonged elimination phase). Approximately 70% of the orally administered dose of lenalidomide is excreted by the kidney. Ongoing studies are characterizing the adverse-effect profile of lenalidomide use and are addressing the potential for drug interactions with other agents. More extensive clinical experience is required to determine whether lenalidomide is completely devoid of some of thalidomide's side effects.

Mechanism(s) of Action of Thalidomide and Its Immunomodulatory Derivatives. The precise mechanisms responsible for thalidomide's clinical activity remain to be completely elucidated. Its enantiomeric interconversion and spontaneous cleavage to multiple short-lived and poorly characterized metabolites, as well as its species-specific *in vivo* metabolic activation, confound the interpretation of preclinical *in vitro* and *in vivo* mechanistic studies. At least four distinct, but potentially complementary, mechanisms (Figure 51–18) have been proposed to explain the antitumor activity of thalidomide and its derivatives: (1) direct antiproliferative/proapoptotic antitumor effects (Hideshima *et al.*, 2000), probably mediated by one or more metabolites of thalidomide, that include inhibition of the transcriptional activity of NF-κB and its antiapoptotic target genes, including the caspase inhibitors FLIP, cIAP-2 (cellular inhibitor of apoptosis-2), or the antiapoptotic Bcl-2 family member A1/Bfl-1 (Mitsiades *et al.*, 2002a); (2) indirect targeting of tumor cells by abrogation of the protection conferred to tumor cells by their cell adhesion molecule– or cytokine (*e.g.*, IL-6)–mediated interactions with bone marrow stromal cells (Hideshima *et al.*, 2000); (3) inhibition of cytokine production, release, and signaling, leading to antiangiogenic effects (D'Amato *et al.*, 1994); and (4) immunomodulatory effects, including enhanced natural killer (NK) cell–mediated cytotoxicity against tumor cells (Davies *et al.*, 2001), contributing to potentiated antitumor immune response. It is conceivable that because NF-κB protects MM cells from the proapoptotic effects of steroids or cytotoxic chemotherapeutics (Mitsiades *et al.*, 2002b), the inhibitory effect of thalidomide and its derivatives on NF-κB activity could account for the ability of its combination with dexamethasone or cytotoxic chemotherapeutics to achieve synergistic antitumor responses (Weber *et al.*, 2003).

Adverse Effects. Generally, thalidomide is well tolerated at doses below 200 mg daily. The most common adverse effects reported in

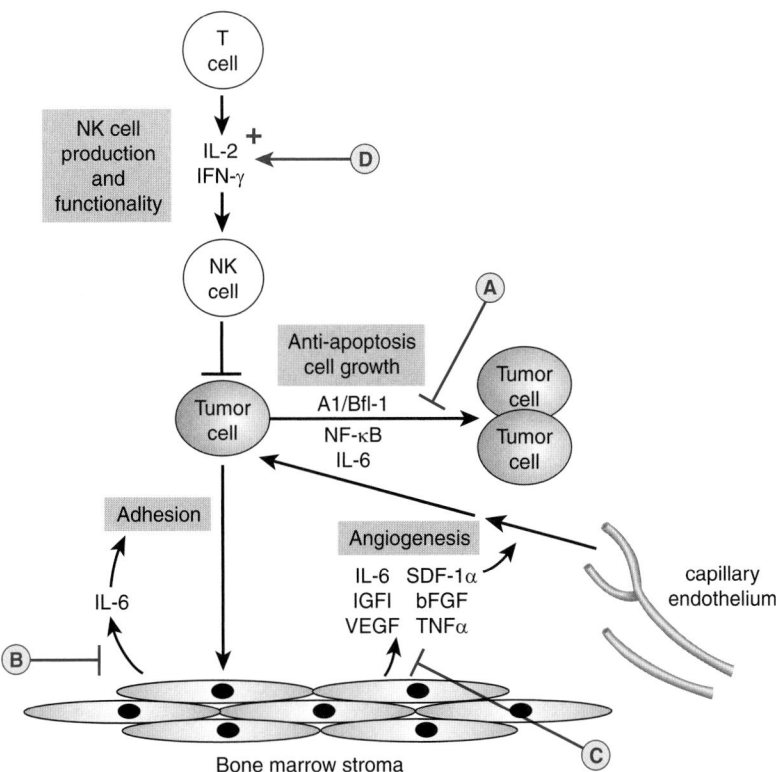

Figure 51–18. *Schematic overview of proposed mechanisms of antimyeloma activity of thalidomide and its derivatives.* Some biological hallmarks of the malignant phenotype are indicated in light gray boxes. The proposed sites of action for thalidomide (*dark blue letters within circles*) are hypothesized to be operative for thalidomide derivatives also. *A.* Direct anti-MM effect on tumor cells including G1 growth arrest and/or apoptosis, even against MM cells resistant to conventional therapy. This is due to the disruption of the anti-apoptotic effect of Bcl-2 family members, blocking NF-κB signaling, and inhibition of the production of IL-6. *B.* Inhibition of MM cell adhesion to bone marrow stromal cells due partially to the reduction in IL-6 release. *C.* Decreased angiogenesis due to the inhibition of cytokine and growth factor production and release. *D.* Enhanced T-cell production of cytokines, such as IL-2 and IFN-γ, that increase the number and cytotoxic functionality of natural killer (NK) cells.

cancer patients are sedation and constipation (Franks *et al.*, 2004), while the most serious one is treatment-emergent peripheral sensory neuropathy, which occurs in 10% to 30% of patients with MM or other malignancies in a dose- and time-dependent manner (Richardson *et al.*, 2004). Thalidomide-related neuropathy is an asymmetric, painful, peripheral paresthesia with sensory loss, commonly presenting with numbness of toes and feet, muscle cramps, weakness, signs of pyramidal tract involvement, and carpal tunnel syndrome. The incidence of peripheral neuropathy increases with higher cumulative doses of thalidomide, especially in elderly patients. Although clinical improvement typically occurs upon prompt drug discontinuation, long-standing residual sensory loss can occur. Particular caution should be applied in cancer patients with preexisting neuropathy (*e.g.*, related to diabetes) or prior exposure to drugs that can cause peripheral neuropathy (*e.g.*, vinca alkaloids or *bortezomib*), especially since there has been little progress in defining effective strategies to alleviate neuropathic symptoms. An increasing incidence of thromboembolic events in thalidomide-treated patients has been reported, but mostly in the context of thalidomide combinations with other drugs, including steroids and particularly anthracycline-based chemotherapy (Zangari *et al.*, 2001), and with very low incidence with single-agent thalidomide treatment.

ESTRAMUSTINE

Pharmacology and Cytotoxic Effects. Estramustine (EMCYT) is a combination of *estradiol* coupled to *normustine* (nornitrogen mustard) by a carbamate link. Respectively, estramustine has weaker estrogenic and antineoplastic activity than estradiol and other alkylating agents. While the intent of the combination was to enhance the uptake of the alkylating agent into estradiol-sensitive prostate cancer cells, estramustine does not appear to function *in vivo* as an alkylating agent. Rather, estramustine binds to β-tubulin and microtubule-associated proteins, causing microtubule disassembly and antimitotic actions.

Resistance to estramustine has been described (Laing *et al.*, 1998). Estramustine is used for the treatment of metastatic or progressive prostate cancer (Kitamura, 2001) at a usual initial dose of 10 to 16 mg/kg daily in three or four divided doses.

Absorption, Fate, and Excretion. Following oral administration, at least 75% of a dose of estramustine is absorbed from the gastrointestinal tract and rapidly dephosphorylated. Estramustine is found in the body mainly as its oxidized 17-keto analog isomer, estromustine; both forms accumulate in the prostate. Some hydrolysis of the carbamate linkage occurs in the liver, releasing estradiol, estrone, and the normustine group. Estramustine and estromustine have plasma half-lives of 10 to 20 hours, respectively, and are excreted with their metabolites, mainly in the feces (Bergenheim and Henriksson, 1998).

Clinical Toxicities. In addition to myelosuppression, estramustine also possesses estrogenic side effects (gynecomastia, impotence, and elevated risk of thrombosis, and fluid retention) and is associated with hypercalcemia, acute attacks of porphyria, impaired glucose tolerance, and hypersensitivity reactions including angioedema.

Bortezomib

Chemistry. Bortezomib (VELCADE) is [(1R)-3-methyl-1-[[(2S)-1-oxo-3-phenyl-2-[(pyrazinylcarbonyl)amino]propyl]amino]butyl]boronic acid, and its structure is:

BORTEZOMIB

Mechanism of Action. Bortezomib binds to the 20S core of the 26S proteasome and is a reversible inhibitor of its chymotrypsin-like activity (Orlowski *et al.*, 2002). Inhibition of the proteasome disrupts multiple signaling cascades within the cell, often leading to cell death. Most important consequences of proteasome inhibition are believed to result from downregulation of NF-κB, a key transcription factor that promotes cell survival. Generally, NF-κB is bound to IκB in the cytosol, thus preventing transfer to the nucleus and binding to DNA. In response to "environmental" stress such as hypoxia, chemotherapy, and DNA damage, IκB becomes ubiquitinated, resulting in its degradation *via* the proteasome and subsequent release of NF-κB to the nucleus. NF-κB is thought to be responsible for the activation of cell adhesion proteins E-selectin, ICAM-1, VCAM-1, and VEGF. NF-κB also activates cyclin-D1, cIAPs, IL-6, and BCL-2, promoting cell proliferation and survival (Aghajanian *et al.*, 2002). Bortezomib blocks degradation of IκB so that NF-κB is silenced. In a similar manner, bortezomib disrupts the ubiquitin-proteasome regulation of p21, p27, and p53, which are key regulatory proteins in the cell cycle and initiators of apoptosis. The antineoplastic activity of bortezomib in tumors is likely due to a greater dependence on certain cell proliferating and promoting pathways in cancer relative to normal tissues.

General Toxicity and Cytotoxic Action. Animal and human toxicity studies have shown that escalating doses of bortezomib have resulted in dose-limiting toxicities in the following organ systems: gastrointestinal, hematopoietic, lymphatic, and renal.

Absorption, Fate, and Excretion. After intravenous administration of 1 to 1.3 mg/m^2 of bortezomib in animals and patients without renal or hepatic impairment, there is a rapid distribution phase (<10 minutes), followed by a longer elimination phase of 5 to 15 hours (Papandreou *et al.*, 2001). The median peak plasma concentration was 509 ng/ml after a 1.3-mg/m^2 bolus injection. Plasma protein binding averaged 83%. The mean terminal elimination in phase I and II studies was 5.45 hours, with an average clearance of 65.9 L/hour following a 2-compartment model. Peak pharmacodynamic activity (proteasome inhibition) occurred at 1 hour with a mean of 61% inhibition and a half-life of approximately 24 hours (Aghajanian *et al.*, 2002; Orlowski *et al.*, 2002). Inhibition of the 20S subunit was 10% to 30% at 96 hours. Proteasome inhibition is very sensitive to bortezomib concentrations, inhibition being 0% to 60% over a range of concentrations of 0.5 to 2 ng/ml.

In vivo studies and work with human liver microsomes has shown that bortezomib is primarily metabolized to an inactive metabolite by the CYP system and not by glucuronidation or sulfation. Deboronation accounts for greater than 90% of total metabolism, with CYP3A4 being more active than CYP2D6. Studies in patients with hepatic or renal impairment are being conducted and should help guide dose reduction in such patients, and pathways of elimination in humans. No formal drug interaction studies have been performed, but bortezomib is known to be a poor inhibitor of human liver microsome cytochrome P450 enzymes.

Preparations. Bortezomib is available for intravenous injection only. Each vial contains 3.5 mg of bortezomib as a sterile lyophilized powder and 35 mg of mannitol. Prior to use, the contents of each vial must be reconstituted with 3.5 ml of normal (0.9%) saline. The reconstituted product should be clear and colorless, and should be administered to patients within 8 hours.

Dosage and Routes of Administration. The recommended starting dose of bortezomib is 1.3 mg/m^2 given as an intravenous bolus, and this should be given on days 1, 4, 8, and 11 of every 21-day cycle (10-day rest period per cycle). At least 72 hours should elapse between doses. For grade 3 nonhematologic toxicities and grade 4 hematologic toxicities, drug administration should be held until resolution and subsequent doses should be reduced 25%. In clinical trials some patients have received 2 mg/m^2 without severe toxicity, and extravasation of bortezomib has occurred without tissue damage.

Therapeutic Uses and Clinical Toxicity. Bortezomib was approved by the FDA in 2003 for use in patients with MM who have received two prior therapies and are progressing on their current therapy (Kane *et al.*, 2003). In a phase II trial in such patients the complete response rate was 4%, the partial response rate was 24%, and the minor response rate was 7% (Richardson *et al.*, 2003). The drug currently is being studied in combination with other drugs in MM as well as other hematologic neoplasms and solid tumors.

Toxicities from the use of bortezomib have been well characterized (Orlowski *et al.*, 2002; Richardson *et al.*, 2003). At the standard dose and schedule, grade 4 toxicities were rare (<4%) and grade 3 toxicities encountered in >5% of patients were as follows: thrombocytopenia (28%), fatigue (12%), peripheral neuropathy (12%), neutropenia (11%), anemia (8%), vomiting (8%), diarrhea (7%), limb pain (7%), dehydration (7%), nausea (6%), and weakness (5%). Peripheral neuropathy was encountered more frequently in patients with a prior history of neuropathy or preexisting numbness, pain, or burning. Dose reductions of bortezomib are recommended for these patients. Usually, the neuropathy improves or resolves completely after several months off treatment. Hypotension associated with the injection of bortezomib has been rarely encountered, and caution should be taken with patients who are volume-depleted, have a history of syncope, or who are on antihypertensive medications. Cardiac toxicity in the form of hypotension and failure has been encountered in animal studies at twice the recommended dose. Very little cardiac toxicity has been encountered in human studies.

Zoledronic Acid

Zoledronic acid (ZOMETA) is a bisphosphonate (*see* Chapter 61) indicated both for the treatment of patients with bony metastases and for patients with multiple myeloma. A direct antitumor effect on myeloma cells has been suggested (Aparicio *et al.*, 1998) and preclinical data suggest the possibility that inhibition of bone matrix–degrading proteinases may inhibit tumor cell invasion in breast and prostate cancers (Bossier *et al.*, 2000).

Mitotane

The principal application of *mitotane* (*o,p′*-DDD), a compound chemically similar to the insecticides DDT and DDD, is in the treatment of neoplasms derived from the adrenal cortex. In studies of the toxicology of related insecticides in dogs, it was noted that the adrenal cortex was severely damaged, an effect caused by the presence of the *o,p′* isomer of DDD, whose structural formula is as follows:

MITOTANE

Cytotoxic Action. The mechanism of action of mitotane has not been elucidated, but its relatively selective attack on adrenocortical cells, normal or neoplastic, is well established. Thus, administration of the drug causes a rapid reduction in the levels of adrenocorticosteroids and their metabolites in blood and urine, a response that is useful both in guiding dosage and in following the course of hyperadrenocorticism (Cushing's syndrome) resulting from an adrenal

tumor or adrenal hyperplasia. Damage to the liver, kidneys, or bone marrow has not been encountered.

Absorption, Fate, and Excretion. Approximately 40% of mitotane is absorbed after oral administration. After daily doses of 5 to 15 g, concentrations of 10 to 90 μg/ml of unchanged drug and 30 to 50 μg/ml of a metabolite are present in the blood. After discontinuation of therapy, plasma concentrations of mitotane are still measurable for 6 to 9 weeks. Although the drug is found in all tissues, fat is the primary site of storage. A water-soluble metabolite of mitotane is found in the urine; approximately 25% of an oral or parenteral dose is recovered in this form. About 60% of an oral dose is excreted unchanged in the stool.

Therapeutic Uses. Mitotane (LYSODREN) is administered in initial daily oral doses of 2 to 6 g, usually given in three or four divided portions, but the maximal tolerated dose may vary from 2 to 16 g per day. Treatment should be continued for at least 3 months; if beneficial effects are observed, therapy should be maintained indefinitely. *Spironolactone* should not be administered concomitantly, since it interferes with the adrenal suppression produced by mitotane (Wortsman and Soler, 1977).

Treatment with mitotane is indicated for the palliation of inoperable adrenocortical carcinoma, producing symptomatic benefit in 30% to 50% of such patients.

Clinical Toxicity. Although the administration of mitotane produces anorexia and nausea in approximately 80% of patients, somnolence and lethargy in about 34%, and dermatitis in 15% to 20%, these effects do not contraindicate the use of the drug at lower doses. Since this drug damages the adrenal cortex, administration of adrenocorticosteroids is indicated, particularly in patients with evidence of adrenal insufficiency, shock, or severe trauma (Hogan *et al.*, 1978).

BIOLOGICAL RESPONSE MODIFIERS

In contrast to small molecules, biological response modifiers include biological agents or approaches that beneficially affect the patient's biological response to a neoplasm. Included are agents that act indirectly to mediate their antitumor effects (*e.g.,* by enhancing the immunologic response to neoplastic cells) or directly on the tumor cells (*e.g.,* differentiating agents). Recombinant DNA technology has greatly facilitated the identification and production of a number of human proteins with potent effects on the function and growth of both normal and neoplastic cells. Proteins that currently are in clinical trials include the interferons (*see* Chapters 49 and 52), interleukins (*see* Chapter 52), hematopoietic growth factors (*see* Chapter 53) such as *erythropoietin,* filgrastim (granulocyte colony-stimulating factor [G-CSF]), and *sargramostim* (granulocyte-macrophage colony-stimulating factor [GM-CSF]), *tumor necrosis factor* (TNF), and monoclonal antibodies such as trastuzumab, *cetuximab,* and rituximab.

Among the agents now approved for clinical use because of their activity in specific neoplastic diseases are *interferon-alfa* for use in hairy cell leukemia, condylomata acuminata, CML, and Kaposi's sarcoma associated with AIDS; *interleukin-2* (IL-2) for kidney cancer; trastuzumab for breast cancer; and rituximab for B-cell lymphomas.

Interleukin-2 (IL-2, ALDESLEUKIN, PROLEUKIN)

The isolation of a cytokine initially named T-cell growth factor, subsequently renamed IL-2, allowed the first attempts to treat cancer by producing lymphocytes specifically cytolytic for the malignant cell (Morgan *et al.,* 1976). IL-2 is not directly cytotoxic; rather, it induces and expands a T-cell response cytolytic for tumor cells. Clinical trials have studied the antitumor activity of IL-2 both as a single agent and with adoptive cellular therapy using IL-2–stimulated autologous lymphocytes obtained by leukopheresis, termed *lymphokine-activated killer* (LAK) *cells.* Randomized trials have not shown that the addition of LAK cells to the treatment regimen improves overall response rates (Rosenberg *et al.,* 1989). Later studies in adoptive cellular therapy have used expanded populations of lymphocytes obtained from tumor biopsies and expanded *in vitro,* so-called tumor-infiltrating lymphocytes (Rosenberg *et al.,* 1994).

Because the half-life of IL-2 in humans is short (13 minutes for α and 85 minutes for β) (Konrad *et al.,* 1990), most clinical schedules have explored either continuous infusion or multiple intermittent dosing. Others have explored the use of liposome-encapsulated IL-2 or conjugation of IL-2 with polyethylene glycol to extend the half-life of IL-2 and to enhance its delivery to immune cells in tumors. These alternative forms of IL-2 therapy are experimental at this time (Bukowski *et al.,* 2001). The most significant antitumor activity has been demonstrated with the most intense dosing schedules: continuous intravenous infusion for 5 days every other week for 2 cycles, or intravenous bolus dosing every 8 hours daily for 5 days every other week.

The toxicities of IL-2 are likely related to the activation and expansion of cytotoxic lymphocytes in organs and within vessels, resulting in inflammation and vascular leak, and to the secondary release by activated cells of other cytokines, such as tumor necrosis factor and interferon. When given at maximally tolerated doses of 600,000 units/kg every 8 hours for up to 5 days, IL-2 causes hypotension, arrhythmias, peripheral edema, prerenal azotemia, elevated liver transaminases, anemia, thrombocytopenia, nausea, vomiting, diarrhea, confusion, and fever (Rosenberg *et al.,* 1989).

Reproducible antitumor activity has been reported in advanced MM and renal cell cancer, where response rates (partial and complete) are seen in 20% to 30% of patients. Complete responses,

seen in approximately 5% to 10% of patients, appear to be durable, with some patients now free of disease beyond 5 years of treatment.

IL-2 currently is being studied in the treatment of AML, where it is capable of inducing remission in relapsed patients (Meloni *et al.,* 1994). In some studies where IL-2 is given following bone marrow transplantation, it appears that IL-2 can lengthen the remission duration as compared to historical controls (Fefer *et al.,* 1993). Randomized trials are in progress to test this hypothesis prospectively.

Monoclonal Antibodies

Since the discovery of methods for fusing mouse myeloma cells with B lymphocytes, it has been possible to produce a single species of antibody that recognizes a specific antigen. Cancer cells express a variety of antigens that are attractive targets for monoclonal antibody–based therapy (Table 51–3). The development of monoclonal antibodies against specific targets has been largely accomplished by the empiric method of immunizing mice against human tumor cells and screening the hybridomas for antibodies of interest. This technology has led to the production of therapeutic monoclonal antibodies for the treatment of cancer. Because murine antibodies have a short half-life and induce a human anti-mouse antibody immune response, they usually are chimerized or humanized when used as therapeutic reagents. Presently, several monoclonal antibodies have received FDA approval for lymphoid and solid tumor malignancies, and include rituximab and *alemtuzumab* for lymphoid malignancies, and trastuzumab for breast cancer (Keating *et al.,* 2002; Vogel *et al.,* 2002; Cobleigh *et al.,* 1999). The nomenclature adopted for naming therapeutic monoclonal antibodies is to terminate the name in *-ximab* for chimeric antibodies and *-umab* for humanized antibodies. A variety of mechanism(s) of cell killing have been described for monoclonal antibodies, including antibody-dependent cellular cytotoxicity (ADCC), complement-dependent cytotoxicity (CDC) and direct induction of apoptosis, but the clinically relevant mechanisms remain uncertain (Shan *et al.,* 1998).

Monoclonal antibodies also may be engineered to combine the antibody with a toxin (immunotoxins), such as *gemtuzumab ozogamicin* (MYLOTARG) or *denileukin diftitox* (ONTAK), or combined with a radioactive isotope, as in the case of *90Y-ibritumomab tiuxetan* (ZEVALIN) (Table 51–3). More recently, antibodies have been engineered to contain a second specificity, known as bispecific antibodies (Onda *et al.,* 2004; Silverman *et al.,* 2004). For example, an antibody with specificity to B-cell lymphomas and to CD3, which binds to and acti-

Table 51-3

Monoclonal Antibodies Approved for Hematopoietic and Solid Tumors

ANTIGEN AND TUMOR CELL TARGETS	ANTIGEN FUNCTION	NAKED ANTIBODIES	RADIOISOTOPE-BASED ANTIBODIES	TOXIN-BASED ANTIBODIES
Antigen: CD20 Tumor type: B-cell lymphoma and CLL	Proliferation/differentiation	Rituximab (chimeric)	^{131}I-tositumomab; ^{90}Y-ibritumomab tiuxetan	None
Antigen: CD52 Tumor type: B-cell CLL and T-cell lymphoma	Unknown	Alemtuzumab (humanized)	None	None
Antigen: CD25 α subunit Tumor type: T-cell mycosis fungoides	Activation antigen	Daclizumab (humanized)	None	Denileukin diftitox (diphtheria toxin)
Antigen: CD33 Tumor type: acute myeloid leukemia	Unknown	Gemtuzumab (humanized)	None	Gemtuzumab ozogamicin
Antigen: HER2/neu (ErbB-2) Tumor type: breast cancer	Tyrosine kinase	Trastuzumab (humanized)	None	None
Antigen: EGFR (ErbB-1) Tumor type: colorectal; NSCLC; pancreatic, breast	Tyrosine kinase	Cetuximab (chimeric)	None	None
Antigen: VEGF Tumor type: colorectal cancer	Angiogenesis	Bevacizumab (humanized)	None	None

Abbreviations: CLL, chronic lymphocytic leukemia; EGFR, epidermal growth factor receptor; NSCLC, non-small cell lung cancer; VEGF, vascular-endothelial growth factor.

vates normal T cells, may enhance T-cell mediated lysis of the lymphoma cell. Monoclonal antibodies raised against the immunoglobulin idiotype on a B-cell lymphoma represent another therapeutic strategy (Miller *et al.*, 1982).

Naked Monoclonal Antibodies

Rituximab. Rituximab (RITUXAN) is a chimeric monoclonal antibody that targets the CD20 B-cell antigen (Tables 51–3 and 51–4) (Maloney *et al.*, 1997a; Maloney *et al.*, 1994; Maloney *et al.*, 1997b). CD20 is found on cells from the pre–B-cell stage through terminal differentiation to plasma cells and is expressed on 90% of B-cell neoplasms (Stashenko *et al.*, 1980; Bhan, 1981). The biological functions of CD20 are uncertain, although incubation of B cells with anti-CD20 antibody has variable effects on cell-cycle progression, depending on the monoclonal antibody type (Tedder *et al.*, 1986; Smeland *et al.*, 1985). Monoclonal antibody binding to CD20 generates transmembrane signals that produce autophosphorylation and activation of serine/tyrosine protein kinases, and induction of c-myc oncogene expression and major histocompatibility complex class II molecules (Deans *et al.*, 1993). Studies have shown that CD20 also is associated with transmembrane Ca^{2+} conductance, through its possible function as a Ca^{2+} channel (Deans *et al.*, 1993). These studies demonstrate the importance of CD20 in B-cell regulation, but do not in themselves indicate how ligation of the receptor produces cell death independent of ADCC or complement-mediated pathways.

Rituximab is the first monoclonal antibody to receive FDA approval and initially was approved for relapsed indolent lymphomas. However, it has shown activity in a wide variety of clinical settings (Coiffier *et al.*, 1998; Foran *et al.*, 2000). In the initial phase II study of rituximab in 37 patients with relapsed low-grade lymphoma, 46% responded with a median time to progression of 10 months (Maloney *et al.*, 1997a). Notably, rituximab also was shown to be effective in 40% of patients who had previously responded to rituximab, but has a longer median time to progression of 18 months (Davis *et al.*, 2000). Recent studies also have demonstrated significant activity of rituximab in mantle cell lymphoma, relapsed aggressive B-cell lymphomas, and CLL (Coiffier *et al.*, 1998; O'Brien *et al.*, 2001). The use of maintenance rituximab has gained increased acceptance, based on demonstration of delayed time to progression, but effects on survival have not been demonstrated (Hainsworth, 2004). Increasingly evident are the synergistic effects of rituximab and chemotherapy, suggesting it sensitizes lymphoma cells to the apoptotic effects of chemotherapy by directly acting on tumor cells (Maloney *et al.*, 2002). Based on *in vitro* studies showing synergistic effects of chemotherapy and rituximab, rituximab is being clinically combined with agents such as fludarabine and combinations

such as CHOP (Savage *et al.*, 2003). Of great importance is the recent finding that the addition of rituximab to CHOP chemotherapy significantly improves the event-free survival of diffuse large B-cell lymphoma (Coiffier *et al.*, 2002; Wilson *et al.*, 2003).

Rituximab demonstrates dose-dependent pharmacokinetics. At a dose of 375 mg/m^2, the mean serum half-life was 76.3 hours (range, 32 to 153 hours) after one dose and 205.8 hours (range, 84 to 407 hours) after the last dose (Maloney *et al.*, 1997a; Maloney *et al.*, 1997b). The wide range of half-lives likely reflects differences in patient tumor burden and normal B-cell populations. Rituximab toxicities are mostly related to infusion reactions, although there are increasing reports of late-onset neutropenia and rare reports of severe skin toxicity (Table 51–4) (Maloney *et al.*, 1994; Lemieux, 2004).

Alemtuzumab. Alemtuzumab (CAMPATH) is a humanized monoclonal antibody targeting the CD52 antigen present on normal neutrophils and lymphocytes as well as most B- and T-cell lymphomas (Tables 51–3 and 51–4) (Kumar *et al.*, 2003). CD52 is expressed at reasonable levels and does not modulate with antibody binding, making it a good target for unconjugated monoclonal antibodies. Mechanistically, alemtuzumab can induce tumor cell death through antibody-dependent cellular cytotoxicity (ADCC) and complement-dependent cytotoxicity (CDC) (Table 51–4) (Villamor *et al.*, 2003). Clinical activity has been demonstrated in low-grade lymphomas and CLL, including in patients with purine analog–refractory disease (Keating *et al.*, 2002; Rai *et al.*, 2002). In refractory CLL, response rates from 33% to 59% have been described, with higher rates in untreated CLL patients (Osterborg *et al.*, 1997).

Alemtuzumab demonstrates dose-dependent pharmacokinetic behavior. In clinical studies, alemtuzumab had a mean half-life of 12 days and steady-state levels were reached at approximately week 6 of treatment, although there was significant interpatient variability. The most concerning side effects are from acute infusion reactions and the depletion of hematopoietic cells and T cells (Table 51–4). Patients also may develop severe pancytopenia and death. Opportunistic infections are a serious side effect, particularly in patients who have received purine analogs, and have resulted in patient deaths (Tang *et al.*, 1996). The broad expression of CD52 in T cells has led to the testing of alemtuzumab in T-cell lymphomas. Recent studies have shown a high response rate in mycosis fungoides, and combination chemotherapy trials are being conducted in aggressive T-cell lymphomas (Kennedy *et al.*, 2003).

Trastuzumab. Trastuzumab (HERCEPTIN) is a humanized monoclonal antibody against the HER2/neu (ErbB-2) member of the epidermal growth factor family of cellular receptors (Noonberg and Benz, 2000). The internal domain of the HER2/neu glycoprotein encodes a tyrosine kinase that activates downstream signals and enhances metastatic potential and inhibits apoptosis.

Table 51–4
Dose and Toxicity of Monoclonal Antibody–Based Drugs

DRUG	MECHANISM	DOSE AND SCHEDULE	MAJOR TOXICITY
Rituximab[12, 25]	ADCC; CDC; apoptosis	375 mg/m² IV infusion weekly for 4 weeks	Infusion-related toxicity with fever, rash, and dyspnea; B-cell depletion; late-onset neutropenia
Alemtuzumab[88]	ADCC; CDC; apoptosis	Escalation 3, 10, 30 mg/m² IV 3 times per week followed by 30 mg/m² 3 times per week for 4 to 12 weeks	Infusion-related toxicity, T-cell depletion with increased infection; hematopoietic suppression; pancytopenia
Trastuzumab[3, 43]	ADCC; apoptosis; inhibition of HER2 signaling with G_1 arrest	Loading dose of 4 mg/kg infusion followed by 2 mg/kg weekly	Cardiomyopathy; infusion-related toxicity
Cetuximab[58]	Inhibition of EGFR signaling; apoptosis; ADCC	Loading dose of 400 mg/kg infusion followed by 250 mg/kg weekly	Infusion-related toxicity; skin rash in 75%
Bevacizumab[68]	Inhibition of angiogenesis/neo-vascularization	5 mg/kg IV every 14 days until disease progression	Hypertension; pulmonary hemorrhage; gastrointestinal perforation; proteinuria; congestive heart failure
Denileukin diftitox[73]	Targeted diphtheria toxin with inhibition of protein synthesis	9–18 μg/kg per day IV for the first 5 days every 3 weeks	Fever; arthralgia; asthenia; hypotension
Gemtuzumab ozogamicin[82]	Double DNA strand breaks and apoptosis	2 doses of 9 mg/m² IV separated by 14 days	Infusion-related toxicity; hematopoietic suppression; mucosal hepatic (VOD); and skin toxicity
90Y-ibritumomab tiuxetan[89]	Targeted radiotherapy	0.4 mCi/kg IV	Hematologic toxicity; myelodyplasia
131I-tositumomab[86]	Targeted radiotherapy	Patient-specific dosimetry	Hematologic toxicity; myelodyplasia

Abbreviations: ADCC, antibody-dependent cellular cytotoxicity; CDC, complement-dependent cytotoxicity; EGFR, epidermal growth factor receptor; VOD, veno-occlusive disease.

HER2/neu is overexpressed in up to 30% of breast cancers and is associated with clinical resistance to cytotoxic and hormone therapy (Slamon *et al.*, 1989). A number of mechanisms of action have been proposed, which may lead to both cytostatic and cytotoxic effects (Nahta and Esteva, 2003). Downregulation of HER2/neu expression may inhibit cell proliferation, potentially through induction of p27 and reduction of cyclin D1, and is associated with antiangiogenetic effects (Izumi *et al.*, 2002). Trastuzumab also can initiate FCγ-receptor–mediated antibody-dependent cellular cytotoxicity and directly induce apoptosis.

Trastuzumab is the first monoclonal antibody to be approved for the treatment of a solid tumor. Currently, trastuzumab is approved for HER2/neu overexpressing metastatic breast cancer in combination with paclitaxel as initial treatment or as monotherapy following chemotherapy relapse (Vogel *et al.*, 2002; Cobleigh *et al.*, 1999). Trastuzumab also is synergistic with other cytotoxic agents, but expectedly, this is only observed in HER2/neu–overexpressing cancers (Slamon *et al.*, 2001; Seidman *et al.*, 2001; Baselga *et al.*, 1998; Baselga, 2000). Phase III studies are randomizing patients between chemotherapy with or without trastuzumab to assess the optimum regimen (Hinoda *et al.*, 2004). HER2/neu expression also is found in other solid tumors and responses have been reported in colorectal and non–small cell lung cancer (Vogel *et al.*, 2002; Langer *et al.*, 2004). Clinical trials of trastuzumab in other tumors that express HER2/neu at relatively high frequency, such as pancreas and stomach, are likely.

Trastuzumab has dose-dependent pharmacokinetics with a mean half-life of 5.8 days at the 2-mg/kg maintenance dose. Steady-state levels were achieved between the 16th and the 32nd weeks with mean trough and peak concentrations of approximately 79 and 123 μg/ml, respectively (Cobleigh *et al.*, 1999; Baselga, 2000). The infusional effects of trastuzumab are typical of other monoclonal antibodies and include fever, chills, nausea, dyspnea, and rashes. Allergic reactions also may be observed. Cardiac dysfunction is an unexpected and potentially serious side effect that was observed in the pivotal trial of trastuzumab and chemotherapy (Seidman *et al.*, 2002). Left ventricular dysfunction was seen most commonly in those patients who received doxorubicin and cyclophosphamide. In a murine model, mice with a ventricular-restricted deletion of the HER2/neu gene developed cardiomyopathy, indicating that HER2/neu signaling is important for cardiac muscle (Crone *et al.*, 2002).

Cetuximab. Cetuximab (ERBITUX) is a chimeric monoclonal antibody that recognizes the epidermal growth factor receptor (EGFR; also ERBB1 or HER1) (Mendelsohn and Baselga, 2000; Grunwald and Hidalgo, 2003). Activation of EGF receptor signaling through its intercellular tyrosine kinase domain produces multiple cellular events associated with proliferation, survival, and angiogenesis (Kim *et al.*, 2001). EGFR expression is found in 60% to 75% of colorectal cancers, where it has been linked to tumor progression and a poor prognosis (Mayer *et al.*, 1993). Multiple epithelial cancers, such as breast, lung, kidney, prostate, brain, pancreas, bladder, and head and neck malignancies, also express EGFR and are potential therapeutic targets of cetuximab (Mendelsohn and Baselga, 2000; Kim *et al.*, 2001). Although the mechanism of tumor cell kill for cetuximab is uncertain, it is likely to involve inhibition of EGF binding and signaling, which may lead to inhibition of pro-angiogenic factors and apoptosis (Petit *et al.*, 1997). The role of more classical immune mechanisms, such as ADCC, is unclear.

Cetuximab was approved by the FDA in 2004 for the treatment of EGFR-positive metastatic colorectal cancer as a single agent in patients who could not tolerate irinotecan-based therapy, or in combination with irinotecan for refractory patients (Saltz *et al.*, 2004; Cunningham *et al.*, 2004). In part, this approval was based on a randomized study of cetuximab alone *versus* cetuximab and irinotecan in patients with refractory colorectal cancer. The combined therapy group had a significantly higher response rate (22.9%) compared to the monotherapy group (10.8%), and a longer median time to progression (4.1 *vs.* 1.5 months). However, the median survival times of 8.6 months and 6.9 months, respectively, were not significantly different (Cunningham *et al.*, 2004). Studies in head and neck cancer in combination with radiation therapy suggest that cetuximab improves local control.

Cetuximab displays nonlinear characteristics (Thomas and Grandis, 2004). Following the recommended dose regimen, steady-state levels were achieved by the third weekly infusion, with mean peak and trough concentrations ranging from 168 to 235 and 41 to 85 μg/mL, respectively. The mean half-life was 114 hours (range, 75 to 188 hours). Toxic side effects observed with cetuximab are typical of other monoclonal antibodies and include infusion reactions. The incidence of skin rash is significantly greater than that observed with other monoclonal antibodies; it may occur in 75% of patients, and may be severe in 16% (Saltz *et al.*, 2004). Interestingly, there is a correlation between development of a rash and its intensity with duration of benefit from cetuximab.

Bevacizumab. Bevacizumab (AVASTIN) is a humanized monoclonal antibody against vascular-endothelial growth factor (VEGF) and inhibits its interaction with the VEGFR1 and VEGFR2 receptors (Rosen, 2002). Functionally, VEGF is an angiogenic growth factor that regulates vascular proliferation and permeability and inhibits apoptosis of new blood vessels (Ferrara *et al.*, 1992; Aotake *et al.*, 1999). VEGF expression is increased in a variety of tumor types, including breast, ovarian, non–small cell lung, and colorectal cancer, and its expression correlates with neovascularization within tumor masses (Vermeulen *et al.*, 1999). Furthermore, in colorectal cancer, microvessel density is associated with progression of adenomas to carcinomas and with metastatic potential and a poor prognosis (Vermeulen, 1999; Choi *et al.*, 1998).

Bevacizumab is approved by the FDA for treatment of metastatic colorectal cancer in combination with 5-FU (Kabbinavar *et al.*, 2003; Hurwitz *et al.*, 2004). A phase III study of irinotecan/5-FU/leucovorin with or without bevacizumab for the initial treatment of advanced colorectal cancer showed a significant, albeit modest, benefit in median survival (20.3 *vs.* 15.6 months) and progression-free survival (10.6 *vs.* 6.2 months) for patients receiving bevacizumab (Hurwitz *et al.*, 2004). There also is evidence of biological activity of bevacizumab in clear-cell renal cancer as a single agent and in non–small cell lung cancer and breast cancer in combination with chemotherapy (Yang *et al.*, 2003; Cobleigh *et al.*, 2003).

The pharmacokinetics of bevacizumab vary by sex, body weight, and tumor burden. Clearance is higher in patients with greater tumor burden, but the relationship with clinical outcome has not been explored. Bevacizumab has an estimated half-life of 20 days (range, 11 to 50 days) and a predicted time to reach steady state of 100 days at the therapeutic dose (Zondor and Medina, 2004). Infusion-related toxicities are relatively uncommon. However, this agent has a number of unique and potentially serious toxicities including severe hypertension, proteinuria, and congestive heart failure (Hurwitz *et al.*, 2004). It also has been reported to cause hemorrhage and gastrointestinal perforation.

Monoclonal Antibody-Cytotoxic Conjugates

Gemtuzumab Ozogamicin. Gemtuzumab ozogamicin (MYLOTARG) comprises a humanized monoclonal antibody against CD33 that is covalently linked to a semisynthetic derivative of *calicheamicin*, a potent enediyne antitumor antibiotic (Bernstein, 2000). The CD33 antigen is found on most hematopoietic cells and on more than 80% of AML and in most myelodysplasias (Wellhausen and Peiper, 2002). However, it has little expression on other cell types, making it attractive for targeted therapy. The function of CD33 is unknown, although monoclonal antibody cross-linking inhibits normal and myeloid leukemia cell proliferation (Bernstein, 2000). Following binding to CD33, gemtuzumab ozogamicin undergoes endocytosis with cleavage of calicheamicin within the lysosome, which then enters the nucleus (van Der Velden *et al.*, 2001) and causes double-strand DNA breaks and cell death (Zein *et al.*, 1988).

Gemtuzumab ozogamicin is approved by the FDA for the treatment of CD33-positive AML in first relapse, which occurs in patients at least 60 years old and who are not candidates for conventional cytotoxic therapy. The approval was based on its single-agent activity in refractory AML, where 20% of patients had reductions in blast counts (Sievers *et al.*, 2001). However, there are no controlled studies demonstrating clinical benefit compared with other treatments. There are multiple studies exploring new roles for gemtuzumab ozogamicin, such as in combination with chemotherapy or stem cell transplant and as maintenance treatment. These studies are being conducted in a variety of clinical settings including refractory and previously untreated AML (Amadori *et al.*, 2004; Damle, 2004).

Pharmacokinetics of gemtuzumab ozogamicin at the standard 9 mg/m^2 dose showed a half-life of total and unconjugated calicheamicin of 41 and 143 hours, respectively (Dowell *et al.*, 2001). Following a second dose, the half-life increased to 64 hours and the area under the curve was twice that of the initial dose. Serious toxicities may occur with gemtuzumab ozogamicin. Like other monoclonal antibodies, infusion-related toxicities occur with the first infusion but are ameliorated by glucocorticoids. The primary toxicities are bone marrow suppression and hepatic toxicity. Hepatic toxicity can be serious and may lead to fatal veno-occlusive disease. In the phase II study, grade 3 or 4 hyperbilirubinemia was observed in 23% of patients and may represent subclinical veno-occlusive disease in some cases (Sievers *et al.*, 2001).

Radioimmuno-Conjugates

Radioimmuno-conjugates provide monoclonal antibody targeted delivery of radioactive particles to tumor cells (Tables 51–3 and 51–4) (Kaminski *et al.*, 2001). [131]Iodine (^{131}I) is a commonly used radioisotope, as it is readily available, relatively inexpensive, and easily conjugated to a monoclonal antibody. The gamma particles emitted by ^{131}I can be used for both imaging and therapy, but have the drawbacks of releasing free ^{131}I and ^{131}I-tyrosine into the blood, presenting a potential health hazard to caregivers. The β-emitter, [90]Yttrium (^{90}Y), has emerged as an attractive alternative to ^{131}I, based on its higher energy and longer path length, which may be more effective in tumors with larger diameters. It also has a short half-life and remains conjugated, even after endocytosis, providing a safer profile for outpatient use. However, disadvantages include its inability to image, limited availability, and its expense.

Clinically, radioimmuno-conjugates have been developed with murine monoclonal antibodies against CD20 conjugated with [131]I (131*I-tositumomab* or BEXXAR) and ^{90}Y-ibritumomab tiuxetan (ZEVALIN). Both drugs have shown response rates in relapsed lymphoma of 65% to 80% (Kaminski *et al.*, 2001). These agents have been well tolerated with most toxicity attributable to bone marrow suppression. However, there have been worrisome reports of secondary leukemias (Table 51–4).

Pretargeting has been used to increase the therapeutic index of radioimmuno-conjugates by taking advantage of the high binding affinity of avidin and biotin. Patients initially are treated with avidin-labeled monoclonal antibody, followed 1 to 2 days later, after maximal binding of the monoclonal antibody to the target, by administration of yttrium-conjugated biotin. This technique may improve the specificity of radioisotope delivery to tumor cells and increase the therapeutic index.

Immunotoxin

Denileukin Diftitox. Denileukin diftitox (ONTAK) is an immunotoxin made from the genetic recombination of IL-2 and the catalytically active fragment of diphtheria toxin (Foss, 2001). The human IL-2 receptor (IL-2R) consists of three discrete subunits, CD25 (α chain, Tac, p55), CD122 (β chain, p70), and CD132 (γ chain, p64), assembled as a trimolecular complex to generate the high-affinity IL-2R. CD25, the low-affinity IL-2R, is incapable of internalizing IL-2, whereas CD122, the β chain of the IL-2R, internalizes IL-2 and has an intermediate affinity. In a complex with CD25, CD122 produces the high-affinity IL-2R with an affinity 100-fold greater than that of the intermediate-affinity receptor. The high affinity IL-2R is not expressed on resting T cells, but is upregulated by antigen activation and is constitutively expressed on malignant lymphocytes of both T-cell and B-cell origin. The limited tissue expression of the high-affinity IL-2R makes this an attractive target for cancer treatments, as cells that do not express the IL-2R or express only the intermediate- or low-affinity types are significantly less sensitive to this agent.

Denileukin diftitox is FDA approved for the treatment of recurrent/refractory cutaneous T-cell lymphomas. Response rates of 30% to 37% have been achieved in such patients with denileukin diftitox, with a median response duration of 6.9 months in one study (Olsen *et al.*, 2001). A larger proportion of patients showed clinical benefit but did not meet the objective criteria for response. Denileukin diftitox is being evaluated in patients with CD25-negative tumors and modulators of CD25 expression are being combined in an attempt to increase response rates. This latter approach may allow higher levels of intracellular toxin to be delivered. *Bexarotene* increases the level of CD25 expression on malignant T cells and provides a rationale for combining these agents (Gorgun and Foss, 2002).

The systemic exposure to denileukin diftitox is variable but proportional to dose (LeMaistre *et al.*, 1998). It has a distribution half-life of 2 to 5 minutes with a terminal half-life of approximately 70 minutes. Immunologic reactivity to denileukin diftitox can be detected in virtually all patients after treatment but does not preclude clinical benefit with continued treatment. Denileukin diftitox clearance in later cycles of treatment is accelerated by two- to threefold as a result of development of antibodies, but serum levels are greater than that required to produce cell death in IL-2R–expressing cell lines (1 to 10 ng/ml for more than 90 minutes). Patients with a history of hypersensitivity reactions to diphtheria toxin or IL-2 should not be treated. Significant toxicities associated with denileukin diftitox are typically acute hypersensitivity reactions, a vascular leak syndrome, and constitutional toxicities; glucocorticoid premedication significantly decreases toxicity (Table 51–4) (Foss, 2001).

Colony-Stimulating Factors

As noted above, many agents used for cancer chemotherapy suppress the production of multiple types of hematopoietic cells, and bone marrow suppression often has limited the delivery of chemotherapy on schedule

and at prescribed doses. The availability of recombinant growth factors for erythrocytes (*i.e.,* erythropoietin), granulocytes (*i.e.,* granulocyte colony-stimulating factor), and granulocytes and macrophages (*i.e.,* granulocyte-macrophage colony-stimulating factor) have enormously advanced the ability to use combination therapy or high-dose therapy with diminished complications such as febrile neutropenia. Whether this will result in improved survival rates for specific cancers remains to be determined by clinical trials. The individual growth factors and specifics of therapy are described in detail in Chapter 53.

V. HORMONES AND RELATED AGENTS

GLUCOCORTICOIDS

The pharmacology, major therapeutic uses, and toxic effects of the glucocorticoids are discussed in Chapter 59. Only the applications of the hormones in the treatment of neoplastic disease are considered here. Because of their lympholytic effects and their ability to suppress mitosis in lymphocytes, the greatest value of these steroids as cytotoxic agents is in the treatment of acute leukemia in children and malignant lymphoma in children and adults.

In acute lymphoblastic or undifferentiated leukemia of childhood, glucocorticoids may produce prompt clinical improvement and objective hematological remissions in up to 30% of children. Although these responses frequently are characterized by complete disappearance of all detectable leukemic cells from the peripheral blood and bone marrow, the duration of remission is brief. Remissions occur more rapidly with glucocorticoids than with antimetabolites, and there is no evidence of cross-resistance to unrelated agents. For these reasons, therapy is initiated with prednisone and vincristine, often followed by an anthracycline or methotrexate, and L-asparaginase. Glucocorticoids are a valuable component of curative regimens for Hodgkin's disease and non-Hodgkin's lymphoma, as well as for treatment of multiple myeloma and CLL. Glucocorticoids are extremely helpful in controlling autoimmune hemolytic anemia and thrombocytopenia associated with CLL.

The glucocorticoids, particularly dexamethasone, are used in conjunction with radiotherapy to reduce edema related to tumors in critical areas such as the superior mediastinum, brain, and spinal cord. Doses of 4 to 6 mg every 6 hours have dramatic effects in restoring neurological function in patients with cerebral metastases, but these effects are temporary. Acute changes in dexamethasone dosage can lead to a rapid recrudescence of symptoms. Dexamethasone should not be discontinued abruptly in patients receiving radiotherapy or chemotherapy for brain metastases. Gradual tapering of the dosage may be undertaken if a clinical response to definitive antitumor therapy has been achieved. The antitumor effects of glucocorticoids are mediated by their binding to the glucocorticoid receptor, which activates a program of gene expression that leads to apoptosis.

Several glucocorticoids are available and at equivalent dosages exert similar effects (*see* Chapter 59). Prednisone, for example, usually is administered orally in doses as high as 60 to 100 mg, or even higher, for the first few days and gradually reduced to levels of 20 to 40 mg/day. A continuous attempt should be made to establish the lowest possible dosage required to control the manifestations of the disease. These agents, when used chronically, exert a wide range of side effects, including glucose intolerance, immunosuppression, osteoporosis, and psychosis (*see* Chapter 59).

PROGESTINS

Progestational agents (*see* Chapter 57) have been used as second-line hormonal therapy for metastatic hormone-dependent breast cancer and in the management of endometrial carcinoma previously treated by surgery and radiotherapy. In addition, progestins stimulate appetite and restore a sense of well-being in cachectic patients with advanced stages of cancer and AIDS. While progesterone itself is poorly absorbed when given orally and must be used with an oil carrier when given intramuscularly, there are synthetic progesterone preparations.

Hydroxyprogesterone usually is administered intramuscularly in doses of 1000 mg one or more times weekly; *medroxyprogesterone* (DEPO-PROVERA) can be administered intramuscularly in doses of 400 to 1000 mg weekly. An alternative and more commonly used oral agent is *megestrol acetate* (MEGACE, others; 40 to 320 mg daily, in divided doses). Beneficial effects have been observed in approximately one-third of patients with endometrial cancer. The response of breast cancer to megestrol is predicted by both the presence of hormonal receptors and the evidence of response to a prior hormonal treatment. The effect of progestin therapy in breast cancer appears to be dose-dependent, with patients demonstrating second responses following escalation of megestrol to 1600 mg/day. Clinical use of progestins in breast cancer has been largely superceded by the advent of the aromatase inhibitors (*see* below). Responses to progestational agents have also been reported in metastatic carcinomas of the prostate and kidney.

ESTROGENS AND ANDROGENS

Discussions of the pharmacology of the estrogens and androgens appear in Chapters 57 and 58, respectively.

They are of value in certain neoplastic diseases, notably those of the prostate and the mammary gland, because these organs are dependent upon hormones for their growth, function, and morphological integrity. Carcinomas arising from these organs often retain some of the hormonal responsiveness of their normal counterparts for varying periods of time. By changing the hormonal environment of such tumors, it is possible to alter the course of the neoplastic process.

Androgen-Control Therapy of Prostatic Carcinoma

The development of anti-androgenic therapy for prostatic carcinoma is largely the contribution of Huggins and associates. Although the hormonal treatment of metastatic prostate carcinoma is palliative, life expectancy is increased and thousands of patients have enjoyed its benefit.

Localized prostate cancer is curable with surgery or radiation therapy. However, when distant metastases already are present, hormonal therapy becomes the primary treatment. Standard approaches to reduce the concentrations of endogenous androgens or inhibit their effects include bilateral orchiectomy, antiandrogens, or most commonly, the administration of gonadotropin-releasing hormone (GnRH) agonists or antagonists with or without antiandrogens (*see* below).

Subjective and objective improvements rapidly follow the institution of androgen-control therapy of prostatic carcinoma in the majority of patients with metastatic disease, and these benefits last an average of 1 year. From the patient's point of view, the most gratifying may be relief of bone pain. This is associated with an increase in appetite, weight gain, and a feeling of well-being. Objectively, there are regressions of the primary tumor and soft tissue metastases, but neoplastic cells do not disappear completely. The concentration of prostate-specific antigen (PSA) in plasma is a useful marker of response. Eventually prostatic tumors become insensitive to androgen deprivation through loss or mutation of the androgen receptor, which in some patients recognizes androgen antagonists such as *flutamide* as agonists (*see* below and Chapter 58). In such cases, withdrawal of the antagonist may lead to a response.

Estrogens and Androgens in the Treatment of Mammary Carcinoma

Despite remissions of disease being noted with pharmacologic doses of estrogen therapy in breast cancer patients, unwanted side effects prompted the development of alternate strategies. Paradoxically, antagonizing the effects of estrogen also is frequently effective as exemplified by remission of disease achieved with oophorectomy. Thus, because of a relative paucity of side effects and equivalence of efficacy, the use of anti-estrogens such as *tamoxifen* replaced treatment with estrogens or androgens as hormonal therapy of breast cancer. The detection of the estrogen receptors (ER) and progesterone receptors (PR) by monoclonal antibodies has led to improved selection of patients for hormone therapies. A significant minority of patients with ER- or PR-positive tumors have a response to hormonal therapy, and furthermore have a better overall prognosis independent of the type of therapy. In contrast, ER- and PR-negative carcinomas do not respond to hormonal therapy.

Clinically detectable responses to hormone therapy can be slow and usually take 8 to 12 weeks to detect. If the disease responds or remains stable on a given treatment, the medication typically is continued indefinitely until the disease progresses or unwanted toxicities develop. The duration of an induced remission averages 6 to 12 months but sometimes can last for many years.

Anti-Estrogen Therapy

Anti-estrogen approaches for the therapy of hormone-receptor positive breast cancer include the use of selective estrogen-receptor modulators (SERMs), selective estrogen-receptor downregulators (SERDs), and aromatase inhibitors (AIs).

Selective Estrogen-Receptor Modulators. Tamoxifen citrate is the lead compound of the SERM class. These agents bind to the estrogen receptor and exert either estrogenic or anti-estrogenic effects depending on the specific organ. Tamoxifen is the most widely studied anti-estrogenic treatment in breast cancer. The recent decline in breast cancer mortality in Western countries is believed to be in part due to the widespread utilization of tamoxifen (Hermon and Beral, 1996). However, in addition to its estrogen antagonist effects on breast cancer, tamoxifen also exerts estrogenic agonist effects in nonbreast tissues, which influences the overall therapeutic index of the drug. Therefore several novel anti-estrogen compounds have been developed that offer the potential for enhanced efficacy and reduced toxicity compared with tamoxifen. These novel antiestrogens can be divided into tamoxifen analogues (*e.g., toremifene, droloxifene*, and *idoxifene*), "fixed ring" compounds (*e.g., raloxifene, lasofoxifene, arzoxifene, miproxifene, levormeloxifene*, and EM652), and the selective estrogen-receptor downregulators (SERDs) (*e.g., fulvestrant*, SR 16234, and ZK 191703, the latter also termed "pure antiestrogens") (Howell *et al.*, 2004a).

Tamoxifen. Tamoxifen is the most broadly used antiestrogen therapy. It was first synthesized in 1966 and initially developed as an oral contraceptive but was found to induce ovulation. For over three decades, tamoxifen has been studied and developed for use in various stages of breast cancer. Its broad use is related to its anticancer activity and good tolerability profile to allow for chronic daily dosing. Tamoxifen is prescribed for the prevention of breast cancer in high-risk patients, for the adjuvant therapy of early-stage breast cancer, and for the therapy of advanced breast cancer.

Mechanism of Action. Tamoxifen is a competitive inhibitor of estradiol binding to the ER. There are two subtypes of estrogen receptors: ER α and ER β, which have different tissue distributions and can either homodimerize or heterodimerize. Binding of estradiol and SERMs to the estrogen-binding sites of the ERs initiates a series of events that includes change in altered conformation of the ER, dissociation of heat-shock proteins, and ER dimerization. Dimerization facilitates the binding of the ER to specific DNA estrogen-response elements (EREs) in the vicinity of estrogen-regulated genes. As detailed in Chapter 57, many coregulator proteins interact with the receptor to act as corepressors or coactivators, while at least 50 transcriptional activating factors modulate the effects of estrogen on target genes. Differences in tissue distribution of ER subtypes, the function of coregulator proteins, and the various transcriptional activating factors may explain the variable response to tamoxifen in hormone-receptor positive breast cancer. Other organs that are affected by the administration of tamoxifen include the uterine endometrium (endometrial hypertrophy, vaginal bleeding, and endometrial cancer), the coagulation system (thromboembolism), bone metabolism (modulation of bone mineral density), and liver function (alterations of blood lipid profile) (Ellis and Swain, 2001).

Absorption, Fate, and Excretion. Tamoxifen is readily absorbed following oral administration, with peak concentrations measurable after 3 to 7 hours and steady-state levels being reached at 4 to 6 weeks (Jordan, 1982). The drug is metabolized predominantly to *N*-desmethyltamoxifen and to 4-hydroxytamoxifen, a more potent metabolite. Both of these metabolites can be further converted to 4-hydroxy-*N*-desmethyltamoxifen, which retains high affinity for the ER. The parent drug has a terminal half-life of 7 days, while the half-lives of *N*-desmethyltamoxifen and 4-hydroxytamoxifen are significantly longer at about 14 days (Ellis and Swain, 2001). After enterohepatic circulation, glucuronides and other metabolites are excreted in the stool; excretion in the urine is minimal.

Therapeutic Uses. The usual oral dose of tamoxifen (NOLVADEX) in the United States is 10 mg twice a day. Doses as high as 200 mg per day have been used in the therapy of breast cancer, but high doses are associated with retinal degeneration.

Tamoxifen is used for the endocrine treatment of women with ER-positive metastatic breast cancer or following primary tumor excision as adjuvant therapy, where it is used either alone or in sequence with adjuvant chemotherapy.

Tamoxifen also is used in premenopausal women with ER-positive tumors. Disease response rates are similar to those seen in postmenopausal patients. Alternative or additional antiestrogen strategies in premenopausal women include oophorectomy or gonadotropin-releasing hormone analogs (*see* Chapter 55). The combined use of tamoxifen and a gonadotropin-releasing hormone analog (to reduce high estrogen levels resulting from tamoxifen effects on the gonadal-pituitary axis) has been shown to yield better response rates and improved overall survival than has either drug alone (Klijn *et al.*, 2000).

The NOLVADEX Adjuvant Trial Organization (NATO) study indicated an overall disease-free survival advantage for patients receiving tamoxifen. Five years of adjuvant therapy with tamoxifen yielded superior results compared to 1 or 2 years of therapy (Swedish Breast Cancer Cooperative Group, 1996; Early Breast Cancer Trialists' Collaborative Group, 1998). Therefore, although the optimal duration of tamoxifen has not been fully determined, randomized trials have demonstrated superiority of 5 years over shorter durations. One clinical trial evaluating the administration of tamoxifen for more than 5 years failed to show benefit of continued therapy, and a trend toward worse outcomes in women who received a longer duration (Fisher *et al.*, 2001).

Tamoxifen also has shown effectiveness in initial trials for preventing breast cancer in women at increased risk (Strasser-Weippl and Goss, 2004). These studies were prompted by preclinical experiments showing prevention of tumors in animal models and also by the observation of reduced contralateral new primary breast tumors in women receiving adjuvant tamoxifen for early-stage breast cancer (Early Breast Cancer Trialists' Collaborative Group, 1998; Fisher *et al.*, 2001). Tamoxifen only reduces ER-positive tumors without affecting ER-negative tumors, which contribute disproportionately to breast cancer mortality. Additional clinical studies are ongoing (Riggs and Hartmann, 2003).

Clinical Toxicity. The common adverse reactions to tamoxifen include vasomotor symptoms (hot flushes), atrophy of the lining of the vagina, hair loss, nausea, and vomiting. These may occur in as many as 25% of patients and are rarely sufficiently severe to require discontinuation of therapy. Menstrual irregularities, vaginal bleeding and discharge, pruritus vulvae, and dermatitis occur frequently, depending on the menopausal state of the patient. Although side effects are common in women taking tamoxifen, overall quality of life appears not to be impaired (Day *et al.*, 1999).

Tamoxifen also increases the incidence of endometrial cancer by two- to threefold, particularly in older postmenopausal women who receive 20 mg per day for 2 years or longer. In general, tamoxifen-associated endometrial cancers are reported as low-grade and early-stage tumors (O'Regan and Jordan, 2001). Standard practice guidelines from the National Comprehensive Cancer Network recommend monitoring and reporting of abnormal vaginal bleeding with prompt evaluation for endometrial cancer in women with an intact uterus (National Comprehensive Cancer Network Clinical Practice Guidelines in Oncology, 2004).

Tamoxifen increases the risk of thromboembolic events, but this is age dependent and also frequently related to operative procedures. Hence, it is recommended to discontinue tamoxifen prior to elective surgery. Because tamoxifen is associated with thromboembolism, consideration of screening evaluation of factor V Leiden and activated protein C levels has been suggested for women considering tamoxifen, though this has not become a standard of clinical practice (Cushman *et al.*, 2003). Like estrogen, tamoxifen is a hepatic carcinogen in animals, although increases in primary hepatocellular carcinoma have not been reported in

patients on the drug. Tamoxifen causes retinal deposits, decreased visual acuity, and cataracts in occasional patients, although the frequency of these changes is uncertain.

In addition to its ability to prevent recurrence or the development of primary breast cancer, tamoxifen has other end-organ benefits related to its partial estrogenic action. For example, it may slow the development of osteoporosis in postmenopausal women (Fornander *et al.*, 1990). In addition, like certain estrogens, tamoxifen lowers total serum cholesterol, LDL cholesterol, and lipoproteins, and raises apolipoprotein A-I levels, potentially decreasing the risk of myocardial infarction (Love *et al.*, 1994).

Toremifene. Toremifene (FARESTON) is a triphenylethylene derivative of tamoxifen and has a similar pharmacological profile. Toremifene is indicated for the treatment of breast cancer in women with tumors that are ER-positive or of unknown receptor status.

In preclinical models, toremifene has activity against breast cancer cells *in vitro* and *in vivo* similar to that of tamoxifen. Unlike tamoxifen, however, toremifene is not hepatocarcinogenic in experimental animals. Two adjuvant studies were initiated to compare efficacy of these two agents, and in particular long-term tolerability and safety, in early-stage breast cancer. In the largest of these studies, 1480 postmenopausal patients with lymph node–positive disease were randomized to receive adjuvant tamoxifen (20 mg daily) or toremifene (40 mg daily) for 5 years. Although longer follow-up is needed, there were no significant differences in efficacy or tolerability after a median follow-up of 4.4 years, and the number of subsequent second cancers was similar (Howell *et al.*, 2004a). Other head-to-head comparisons of toremifene and tamoxifen in prospective, randomized clinical trials have shown that toremifene has generally similar efficacy and adverse events to tamoxifen (Riggs and Hartmann, 2003). However, *in vitro* in a low-estrogen environment, toremifene has approximately 40 times lower estrogen agonist effect than tamoxifen. This may make toremifene more effective in combination with an aromatase inhibitor than tamoxifen (Di Salle *et al.*, 1990) and this is the subject of ongoing clinical trials.

Selective Estrogen-Receptor Downregulators

SERDs, also termed "pure anti-estrogens," include compounds such as fulvestrant, RU 58668, SR 16234, ZD 164384, and ZK 191703. SERDs, unlike SERMs, are devoid of any estrogen agonist activity. The lead compound of this class currently approved for the treatment of advanced breast cancer is fulvestrant.

Fulvestrant. Fulvestrant (FASLODEX) is the first FDA approved agent in the new class of estrogen-receptor downregulators, which were hypothesized to have an improved safety profile, faster onset, and longer duration of action than the SERMs due to their pure ER antagonist activity (Robertson, 2002). Fulvestrant was approved in

2002 for postmenopausal women with hormone receptor-positive metastatic breast cancer that has progressed despite antiestrogen therapy.

Mechanism of Action. Fulvestrant is a steroidal antiestrogen that binds to the ER with an affinity more than 100 times that of tamoxifen, inhibits its dimerization, and increases its degradation. This appears to occur because fulvestrant's long, bulky side-chain at the 7α position sterically hinders receptor dimerization, leading to increased ER turnover and disruption of nuclear localization. Unlike tamoxifen, which stabilizes or even increases ER expression, fulvestrant reduces the number of ER molecules in cells, both *in vitro* and *in vivo* (Howell *et al.*, 2004b).

Preclinical studies suggest that as a consequence of this ER "downregulation," ER-mediated transcription is abolished, completely suppressing the expression of estrogen-dependent genes (Howell *et al.*, 2004b). This difference in the activity of fulvestrant likely explains why fulvestrant demonstrates efficacy against tamoxifen-resistant breast cancer. However, the hypothesis that fulvestrant provides more effective antiestrogen activity than tamoxifen was not confirmed by a clinical trial comparing fulvestrant (250 mg intramuscularly monthly) with tamoxifen (20 mg orally daily) as first-line therapy in metastatic breast cancer (Howell *et al.*, 2004a).

Absorption, Fate, and Excretion. Maximum plasma concentrations are reached about 7 days after intramuscular administration of fulvestrant and are maintained over a period of 1 month. The plasma half-life is approximately 40 days. Steady-state concentrations are reached after 3 to 6 monthly injections. There is extensive and rapid distribution, predominantly to the extravascular compartment.

Various pathways, similar to those of steroid metabolism including oxidation, aromatic hydroxylation, and conjugation, extensively metabolize fulvestrant. CYP3A4 appears to be the only CYP isoenzyme involved in the oxidation of fulvestrant. Several preclinical and clinical studies have confirmed that fulvestrant is not subject to CYP3A4 interactions that might affect the safety or efficacy of the drug. The putative metabolites possess no estrogenic activity and only the 17-keto compound demonstrates a level of antiestrogenic activity about 4.5 times less than that of fulvestrant. The major route of excretion is *via* the feces, with less than 1% being excreted in the urine (Robertson and Harrison, 2004).

Therapeutic Uses. Fulvestrant typically is administered as a 250-mg intramuscular injection at monthly intervals. It is used in postmenopausal women as antiestrogen therapy of hormone receptor-positive metastatic breast cancer after progression on first-line antiestrogen therapy such as tamoxifen (Strasser-Weippl and Goss, 2004). Fulvestrant is at least as effective in this setting as the third-generation aromatase inhibitor *anastrozole*.

Fulvestrant 250 mg (administered as a once-monthly 5-ml intramuscular injection) also has been compared with tamoxifen 20 mg (orally once daily) in a trial of postmenopausal women with ER-positive and/or progesterone receptor (PR)-positive or ER/PR-unknown metastatic breast cancer who had not previously received endocrine or chemotherapy. There was no difference between fulvestrant and tamoxifen in time to disease progression in either the entire study population or the subset of patients with ER- and/or PR-positive disease. Observed differences in other efficacy endpoints favored tamoxifen, and fulvestrant equivalence was not

demonstrated (Vergote and Robertson, 2004). The long time to steady-state plasma levels for fulvestrant has brought into question the results of existing studies, and trials are in progress to test the relative efficacy of giving an initial loading dose followed by regular monthly injections.

Clinical Toxicity. Fulvestrant generally is well tolerated with the most common adverse events being nausea, asthenia, pain, vasodilation (hot flushes), and headache. Injection site reactions, seen in about 7% of patients, are reduced by giving the injection slowly. In the study comparing anastrozole and fulvestrant, quality-of-life outcome measures were maintained over time with no significant difference between the drugs (Vergote and Robertson, 2004).

AROMATASE INHIBITORS

Aromatase is the product of the *CYP19* gene. CYP19 is highly expressed in human placenta and in granulosa cells of ovarian follicles, where its expression depends on cyclical gonadotropin stimulation. Aromatase also is present, at lower levels, in several nonglandular tissues, including subcutaneous fat, liver, muscle, brain, normal breast, and breast-cancer tissue (Smith and Dowsett, 2003). The aromatase enzyme is responsible for the conversion of androstenedione and testosterone to the estrogens, estrone (E1) and estradiol (E2), respectively. In postmenopausal women, this conversion occurs primarily in peripheral tissues while estrogen production in premenopausal women is primarily from the ovary.

Aromatase inhibitors (AIs) are a newer class of drugs that inhibit the function of the aromatase enzyme. In postmenopausal women, AIs can suppress most of the peripheral aromatase activity, leading to profound estrogen deprivation. This strategy of estrogen deprivation of ER-positive breast cancer cells is in contrast to the ER-binding antagonistic activity that SERMs and SERDs exert.

Based on when they were developed, AIs are classified as first-, second-, or third-generation. In addition, they are further classified as type 1 (steroidal aromatase inactivator) or type 2 (nonsteroidal aromatase inhibitor) inhibitors according to their mechanism of action. Type 1 inhibitors are steroidal analogs of androstenedione. Androstenedione analogs bind to the same site on the aromatase molecule, but unlike androstenedione, they bind irreversibly because of their conversion to reactive intermediates by aromatase. Thus, they commonly are known as aromatase inactivators. Type 2 inhibitors are nonsteroidal and bind reversibly to the heme group of the enzyme by way of a basic nitrogen atom (Smith and Dowsett, 2003) (Figure 51–19).

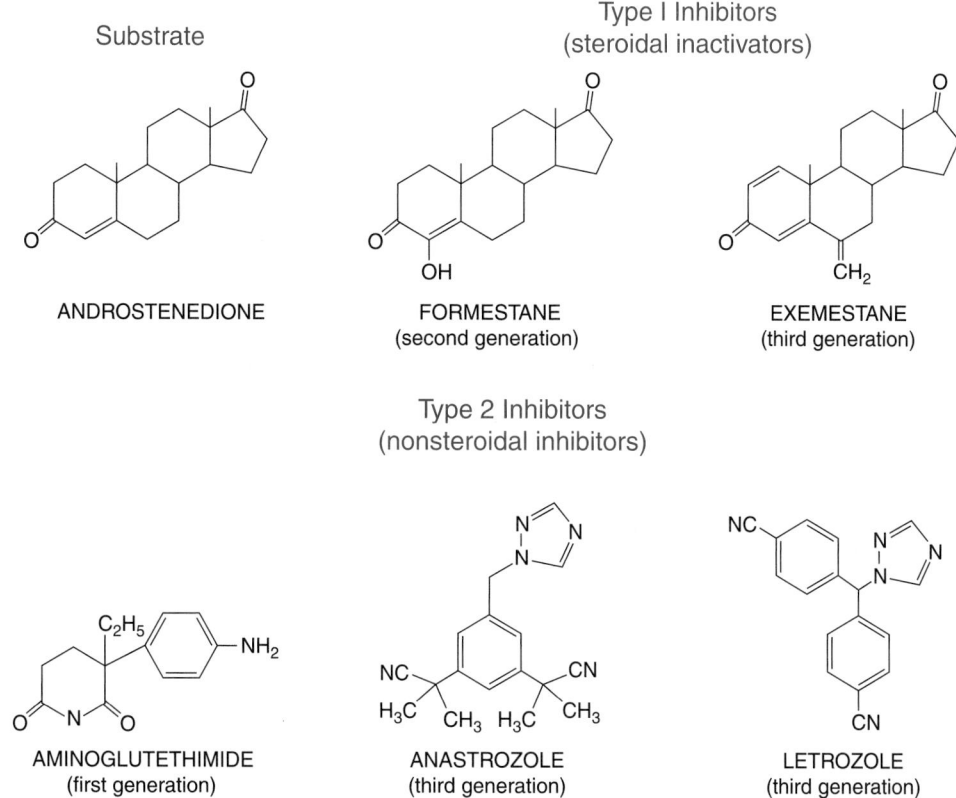

Figure 51–19. *Structure of the main aromatase inhibitors and the natural substrate androstenedione.*

First- and Second-Generation Aromatase Inhibitors

Aminoglutethimide (CYTADREN; AG), a first-generation type 2 AI, originally was developed as an anticonvulsant but was subsequently found to inhibit the synthesis of adrenocortical steroids (*see* Chapter 59). AG is a nonspecific weak AI, administered as a 250-mg dose four times daily with *hydrocortisone* supplementation because of unwanted adrenal suppression. Because of significant toxicities related to its anticonvulsant structure and its relatively weak inhibition of aromatase, its use has declined considerably with the advent of newer AIs.

Second-generation AIs include *formestane* (4-hydroxyandrostenedione; LENTARON), a type 1 steroidal inactivator; *fadrozole*, a type 2 imidazole; and *rogletimide* (pyridoglutethimide), a type 2 inhibitor structurally similar to aminoglutethimide. Formestane was the first steroidal aromatase inactivator widely used for the treatment of breast cancer patients (Goss, 1986). Because of better aromatase inhibition *in vivo* following parenteral administration, it is administered as an intramuscular depot injection. However, formestane has also been shown to be active when given orally. It suppresses plasma sex hormone–binding globulin (SHBG), which is interpreted as an androgenic side effect. The response rates in phase II and III trials were about 25% to 40%. Due to the introduction of novel compounds, especially *exemestane*, formestane is not widely used today (Geisler, 2003).

Third-Generation Aromatase Inhibitors

The third-generation inhibitors, developed in the 1990s, include the type 1 steroidal agent exemestane and the type 2 nonsteroidal imidazoles anastrozole and *letrozole*. Currently, third-generation AIs are most commonly used for the treatment of early-stage and advanced breast cancer.

Anastrozole. **Mechanism of Action.** Anastrozole is a potent and selective triazole AI. Anastrozole, like letrozole, binds competitively and specifically to the heme of the CYP19. Anastrozole 1 or 10 mg administered once daily for 28 days reduces total body aromatization by

96.7% and 98.1%, respectively. In addition, anastrozole reduces local aromatization in large, ER-positive breast tumors.

Anastrozole has no clinically significant effect on adrenal glucocorticoid or mineralocorticoid synthesis in postmenopausal women. Anastrozole also has no effect on the adrenocorticotropic hormone–stimulated release of cortisol or aldosterone, or on plasma concentrations of luteinizing hormone or follicle-stimulating hormone. Anastrozole, unlike AG, has no effect on thyroid-stimulating hormone (Wellington and Faulds, 2002).

Absorption, Fate, and Excretion. Anastrozole is absorbed rapidly after oral administration with maximal plasma concentration occurring after 2 hours. Repeated dosing increases plasma concentrations of anastrozole and steady-state is attained after 7 days. Although the rate of absorption is delayed after a high-fat breakfast, steady-state concentrations are not generally affected upon multiple dosing. Anastrozole is metabolized by *N*-dealkylation, hydroxylation, and glucuronidation. The main metabolite of anastrozole is a triazole. In addition, several other metabolites with no pharmacological activity are formed. Less than 10% of the drug is excreted as the unmetabolized parent compound. The principal excretory pathway is *via* the liver. The pharmacokinetics of anastrozole, which can be affected by drug interactions *via* the CYP system, is unaffected by coadministration of tamoxifen or cimetidine (Köberle and Thürlimann, 2001).

Therapeutic Uses. Anastrozole (ARIMIDEX), 1 mg oral daily dose, has shown efficacy in the treatment of postmenopausal women with early-stage or advanced, hormone-receptor positive breast cancer. In early-stage breast cancer, anastrozole was significantly more effective than tamoxifen in terms of time to tumor recurrence and odds of a primary contralateral tumor (Baum *et al.*, 2002).

In the setting of advanced breast cancer, the results of two large, randomized trials in postmenopausal women with disease progression while taking tamoxifen showed a statistically significant survival advantage for anastrozole 1 mg/day over megestrol acetate 40 mg four times daily. In another phase III clinical trial involving >1000 postmenopausal women with advanced breast cancer, anastrozole showed a statistically significant advantage over tamoxifen in median time to disease progression in >600 patients who were known to have ER- or PR-positive disease.

Clinical Toxicity. Anastrozole has been associated with a significantly lower incidence of vaginal bleeding, vaginal discharge, hot flushes, endometrial cancer, ischemic cerebrovascular events, venous thromboembolic events, and deep vein thrombosis, including pulmonary embolism. Tamoxifen is associated with a lower incidence of musculoskeletal disorders and fracture. In the advanced disease setting, anastrozole is as well tolerated as megestrol, while weight gain is significantly increased by megestrol compared to anastrozole. In addition, anastrozole is as well tolerated as tamoxifen, with a low rate of withdrawal due to drug-related adverse events (2%). In addition, anastrozole is associated with fewer thromboembolic events and episodes of vaginal bleeding than tamoxifen (Wellington and Faulds, 2002; Nabholtz and Reese, 2002).

Letrozole. *Mechanism of Action.* In postmenopausal women with primary breast cancer, letrozole inhibits whole body aromatization and reduces local aromatiza-

tion within the tumors. The drug has no significant effect on the synthesis of adrenal steroids or thyroid hormone and does not alter levels of a range of other hormones. Letrozole also reduces cellular markers of proliferation to a significantly greater extent than tamoxifen in human estrogen-dependent tumors that overexpress human epidermal growth factor receptors (HER)1 and/or HER2/neu.

Letrozole increases the levels of bone resorption markers in healthy postmenopausal women and in those with a history of breast disease but without current active disease. Letrozole has not demonstrated a consistent effect on serum lipid levels in healthy women or postmenopausal women with breast cancer (Simpson *et al.*, 2004).

Absorption, Fate, and Excretion. Letrozole is rapidly absorbed after oral administration and maximum plasma levels are reached about 1 hour after ingestion. Letrozole has a bioavailability of 99.9%. Steady-state plasma concentrations of letrozole are reached after 2 to 6 weeks of treatment. Following metabolism by CYP2A6 and CYP3A4, letrozole is eliminated as an inactive carbinol metabolite mainly *via* the kidneys. Due to the low total body clearance (2.21 L/h), the elimination half-life is about 40 to 42 hours (Geisler, 2003).

Therapeutic Uses. Letrozole (FEMARA), 2.5 mg administered orally once daily, has shown efficacy in the treatment of postmenopausal women with early-stage or advanced, hormone-receptor positive breast cancer.

In early-stage disease, extending adjuvant endocrine therapy with letrozole (beyond the standard 5-year period of tamoxifen) improved disease-free survival compared with placebo (Goss *et al.*, 2003) and improved overall survival in the subset of patients with positive axillary nodes (Goss *et al.*, 2004).

In advanced breast cancer, letrozole is superior to tamoxifen as first-line treatment; time to disease progression is significantly longer and objective response rate is significantly greater with letrozole, but median overall survival is similar between groups. As secondline therapy of advanced breast cancer that has progressed on antiestrogen therapy, letrozole shows efficacy equivalent to that of anastrozole and similar to or better than that of megestrol (Simpson *et al.*, 2004).

Clinical Toxicity. Similarly to tamoxifen, letrozole generally is well tolerated; the most common treatment-related adverse events are hot flushes, nausea, and hair thinning. In patients with tumors that progressed on antiestrogen therapy, letrozole was tolerated at least as well as, or better than, megestrol. In the trial of extended adjuvant therapy, adverse events reported more frequently with letrozole than placebo were hot flushes, arthralgia, myalgia, and arthritis, but cessation of letrozole was no more frequent than placebo in this double-blind trial. A greater number of new diagnoses of osteoporosis occurred among women receiving letrozole, but the long-term effects on bone mineral density or lipid metabolism have yet to be determined.

Exemestane. *Mechanism of Action.* Exemestane (AROMASIN) is a more potent, orally administered analog of the natural substrate androstenedione that lowers estrogen

levels more effectively than does formestane. In contrast to the reversible competitive inhibitors, anastrozole and letrozole, exemestane irreversibly inactivates the enzyme, and therefore is referred to as a "suicide substrate." Doses of 25 mg per day inhibit aromatase activity by 98% and lower plasma estrone and estradiol levels by about 90%. It has less androgenic activity than formestane, but otherwise has a similar toxicity profile.

Absorption, Fate, and Excretion. Exemestane is rapidly absorbed from the gastrointestinal tract, reaching maximum plasma levels after 2 hours. Its absorption is increased by 40% after a high-fat meal. Exemestane is extensively protein-bound in plasma and has a terminal half-life of approximately 24 hours. It is extensively metabolized in the liver to inactive metabolites. A key metabolite, 17-hydroxyexemestane, which is formed by reduction of the 17-oxo group *via* 17-β-hydroxysteroid dehydrogenase, has weak androgenic activity, which also could contribute to antitumor activity (Lønning *et al.*, 2000). Excretion is distributed almost equally between the urine and feces. Since significant quantities of active metabolites are excreted in the urine, exemestane doses should be adjusted in patients with renal dysfunction.

Therapeutic Uses. Exemestane has been tested in a randomized clinical trial in postmenopausal women with estrogen-receptor positive breast cancer. Women who had completed 2 to 3 years of adjuvant tamoxifen were randomized to complete a total of 5 years of adjuvant treatment with tamoxifen or exemestane (Coombes *et al.*, 2004). The unadjusted hazard ratio in the exemestane group *vs.* the tamoxifen group was 0.68, representing a 32% reduction in risk and corresponding to an absolute benefit in terms of disease-free survival of 4.7% at 3 years after randomization. Overall survival was not significantly different in the two groups.

In advanced breast cancer, exemestane has been evaluated in a phase III trial against megestrol in women with disease progressing on prior antiestrogen therapy. Patients receiving exemestane had a similar response rate but improved time to disease progression, time to treatment failure, and longer duration of survival compared with those taking megestrol acetate. Responses to treatment also have been shown in women with disease progressing on prior nonsteroidal aromatase inhibitors.

Clinical Toxicity. Exemestane generally is well tolerated. Discontinuations due to toxicity are not common (2.8%). Hot flushes, nausea, fatigue, increased sweating, peripheral edema, and increased appetite have been reported. In the trial comparing exemestane to tamoxifen in early-stage breast cancer, exemestane was associated with more frequent arthralgia and diarrhea, but gynecologic symptoms, vaginal bleeding, and muscle cramps were more frequent with tamoxifen. Visual disturbances and clinical fractures were more common with exemestane (Coombes *et al.*, 2004).

ANTI-ANDROGEN THERAPY IN PROSTATE CANCER

Carcinoma of the prostate is uniquely dependent upon hormonal stimulation with androgens. Huggins and col-

leagues pioneered the use of anti-androgenic therapy in treating prostate cancer more than half a century ago. Early studies noted that either surgical castration (bilateral orchiectomy) or the administration of injectable hormonal therapies that induced medical castration were effective forms of treatment. Androgen deprivation therapy (ADT) through either surgical or medical castration has been the mainstay of treatment for advanced prostate cancer since that time.

Among men with metastatic prostate cancer, >90% have an initial favorable response to primary hormonal therapy with ADT. This is manifest as disease regression or stabilization and relief of cancer-related symptoms. The average time to progression is 18 to 36 months, making ADT one of the longest-lasting beneficial treatments in any advanced solid tumor. A large trial found a survival benefit to ADT (Byar and Corle, 1988; Seidenfeld *et al.*, 2000). In numerous trials of ADT, its positive effects were diluted to some extent by increased cardiovascular toxicity in men receiving high doses of estrogen as the primary form of ADT (Seidenfeld *et al.*, 2000; Hedlund and Henriksson, 2000).

Disease progression after ADT signifies an androgen-independent state, with subsequent median survival of only 12 months. However, many men will respond to secondary hormonal therapy even after failure of ADT. Secondary hormonal treatments include androgen receptor (AR) blockers, adrenal androgen synthesis inhibitors, and estrogenic agents. Responses are more variable than to primary hormonal therapy, but a substantial portion of men benefit from these well-tolerated forms of treatment. When patients become refractory to any form of hormonal therapy, their management usually involves chemotherapeutic agents.

Common side effects of all forms of antiandrogen hormonal therapy include vasomotor flushing, loss of libido, gynecomastia, increased weight, loss of bone mineral density (BMD), and loss of muscle mass. There is variability to these side effects. For example, AR blockers compared with GnRH agonists cause more gynecomastia, but less bone loss, vasomotor flushing, and loss of BMD (Spetz *et al.*, 2001; Smith *et al.*, 2004). Importantly, the increased cardiovascular toxicity observed with high doses of estrogen is not observed with other forms of ADT.

Gonadotropin-Releasing Hormone Agonists and Antagonists

The most common form of ADT involves chemical suppression of the pituitary with gonadotropin-releasing hormone (GnRH) agonists. GnRH agonists cause an initial surge in levels of luteinizing hormone (LH) and follicle-stimulating hormone (FSH), followed by inhibition of gonadotropin release (*see* Chapter 55). This results in reduction of testicular production of testosterone to castrate levels. GnRH agonists in common use include *leuprolide* (LUPRON, others), *goserelin* (ZOLADEX), *triptorelin* (TRELSTAR), and *buserelin* (SUPREFACT; not available in the United States). Randomized trials have shown that GnRH analogs are as effective as *diethylstilbestrol* and bilateral orchiectomy in the treatment of men with prostate cancer (Seidenfeld *et al.*, 2000). One important side effect, a transient flare of disease, may result from the initial surge of gonadotropins, and can be avoided by temporary (2 to 4 weeks) administration of AR blockers or by the use of GnRH antagonists (*see below*).

Complete androgen blockade (CAB) refers to combination therapy with androgen-receptor blockers and GnRH agonists. However, the advantages of long-term CAB over GnRH agonists alone are questionable. Large meta-analyses of numerous trials show a small advantage to CAB that is clinically insignificant (Prostate Cancer Trialists' Collaborative Group, 2000; Samson *et al.*, 2002).

Treatment with GnRH antagonists rapidly reduces serum testosterone levels, without the transient initial increase observed after GnRH agonists (Tomera *et al.*, 2001). One such compound is *abarelix* (PLENAXIS), which effectively reduces serum testosterone to castrate levels within a week in most men (Trachtenberg *et al.*, 2002). Other than avoidance of the initial flare, GnRH antagonist therapy offers no advantage compared with GnRH agonists, and GnRH antagonists currently are available only in the 1-month depot formulation.

Androgen Receptor Blockers

Compounds that competitively inhibit the natural ligands of the androgen receptor (AR) are called AR blockers, often referred to simply as anti-androgens. As discussed above, when given with GnRH agonists, the combination therapy is called CAB, since androgens from the adrenals are blocked, in addition to gonad-derived androgens. Currently, AR blockers as monotherapy are not indicated as routine, first-line treatment for patients with advanced prostate cancer, although some evidence points to reduced adverse effects of AR blockers relative to GnRH agonists on bone density and body composition (Smith *et al.*, 2004).

From a structural standpoint, AR blockers are classified as steroidal, including *cyproterone* (ANDROCUR) and megestrol, or nonsteroidal, including flutamide (EULEXIN, others), *nilutamide* (NILANDRON), and *bicalutamide* (CASODEX) (Reid *et al.*, 1999). The nonsteroidal AR blockers (Figure 51–20) are more commonly used in clinical practice. They inhibit ligand binding and consequent AR translocation from the cytoplasm to the nucleus. Unlike

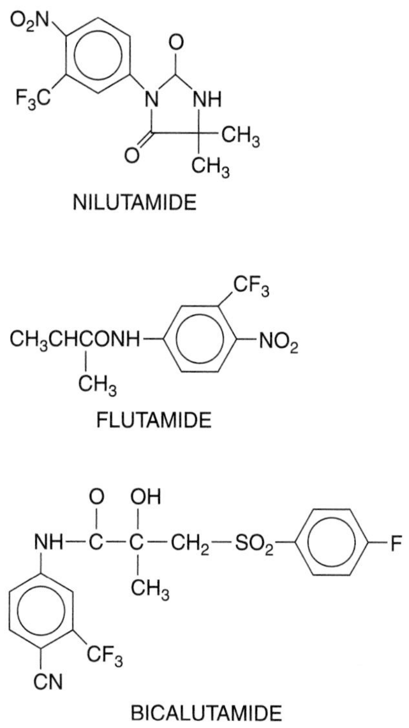

Figure 51–20. *Nonsteroidal androgen-receptor blockers.*

the steroidal agents, nonsteroidal AR blockers interrupt the negative feedback of testosterone to the pituitary-hypothalamic axis, resulting in increased serum testosterone levels, thus attenuating the loss of libido and potency (Knuth *et al.*, 1984).

All of the nonsteroidal AR blockers may cause vasomotor flushing, gynecomastia, mastodynia, and variable degrees of decreased libido and potency. Bicalutamide has a serum half-life of 5 to 6 days, and is administered at a dose of 50 mg/day when given in combination with GnRH agonist therapy. Bicalutamide is well tolerated at higher doses as well, with rare additional side effects. Both enantiomers of bicalutamide undergo glucuronidation to inactive metabolites, and the parent compounds and metabolites are eliminated in bile and urine. The elimination half-life of bicalutamide is increased in severe hepatic insufficiency and is unchanged in renal insufficiency. Flutamide is administered at 250 mg three times a day, and may cause diarrhea, nausea, and reversible liver abnormalities. It has one major metabolite, hydroxyflutamide, that is biologically active, and at least five other minor metabolites. The parent compound and metabolites are mainly excreted in the urine. Nilutamide causes less diarrhea than flutamide, but causes diminished adaptation to darkness and other visual disturbances in 25% to 40%, alcohol intolerance in 5% to 20%, and idiopathic allergic pneumonitis in 1% to 2% of patients. It is extensively metabolized, with five known metabolites. At least one of these is biologically active, and all are excreted in the urine. The elimination half-life of nilutamide is 38 to 40 hours, which allows once-daily dosing at 150 mg/day.

CLINICAL SUMMARY

The therapy of cancer has improved dramatically during the past half century. This improvement can be traced to a number of factors: a better understanding of cancer's causes and natural history, better technologies for early detection and diagnosis, improved control of primary tumors through better surgery and radiation therapy, and more effective drugs. It is instructive to remember that at the end of World War II, there were no drugs to treat this group of diseases (Chabner and Roberts, 2005). The evolution of drug therapy for cancer has progressed rapidly, from alkylating agents and antimetabolites to natural products, and most recently, molecularly targeted drugs such as imatinib and gefitinib. As our understanding of the biology of cancer improves, new targets for therapy are being identified daily, and small molecules and monoclonal antibodies are being developed to test the validity of these targets in human cancer.

Although imatinib has been a spectacular success in controlling the chronic phase of CML, it clearly does not eradicate the disease. CML cells develop resistance through point mutations in the target protein or through amplification of the expression of the target gene, the BCR-ABL kinase gene. Importantly, these resistance mutations exist prior to drug exposure and reflect the inherent mutability of cancer cells, as previously reflected in the experience with cytotoxic agents. Thus, it seems likely that single agents, whether cytotoxic or molecularly targeted, will not cure cancer. Future endeavors will include determining how to use the growing list of potential agents in combination, the only strategy that can address the inherent ability of cancer to escape single agents.

There are two challenges standing in the way of more effective cancer treatment. The first is the search for better drugs based on our rapidly evolving knowledge of cancer biology. The second challenge, one that has never been adequately addressed in the age of cytotoxic chemotherapy, is to identify the determinants of response (Roberts and Chabner, 2004) and to select drugs for individual patients. Traditionally, cytotoxic therapies were administered based on regimens devised for broad histologic categories of cancer, such as lung, breast, or colon cancer. Single-agent response rates rarely exceeded 30% for these tumors. Increasingly, however, with the advent of technologies for measurement of targets in tumor samples, it has become possible to select patients

with higher rates of response to hormonal agents, monoclonal antibodies, and now targeted therapies such as gefitinib. Thus, in the future, therapies will be selected based both on histology and on the molecular features of the tumor. Furthermore, through characterization of genetic polymorphisms, it also will be possible to predict individual susceptibility to toxicity. Thus, drug selection will be guided by molecular testing of both patient and tumor. The result will be more effective, less wasteful, and less toxic therapy for cancer.

BIBLIOGRAPHY

Abbruzzese, J.L., Grunewald, R., Weeks, E.A., *et al.* A phase I clinical, plasma, and cellular pharmacology study of gemcitabine. *J. Clin. Oncol.,* **1991,** *9:*491–498.

Aghajanian, C., Soignet, S., Dizon, D.S., *et al.* A phase I trial of the novel proteasome inhibitor PS341 in advanced solid tumor malignancies. *Clin. Cancer Res.,* **2002,** *8:*2505–2511.

Albanell, J., Rojo, F., Averbuch, S., *et al.* Pharmacodynamic studies of the epidermal growth factor receptor inhibitor ZD1839 in skin from cancer patients: histopathologic and molecular consequences of receptor inhibition. *J. Clin. Oncol.,* **2002,** *20:*110–124.

Alberts, D.S., Chang, S.Y., Chen, H.S., *et al.* Kinetics of intravenous melphalan. *Clin. Pharmacol. Ther.,* **1979,** *26:*73–80.

Alcalay, M., Meani, N., Gelmetti, V., *et al.* Acute myeloid leukemia fusion proteins deregulate genes involved in stem cell maintenance and DNA repair. *J. Clin. Invest.,* **2003,** *112:*1751–1761.

Allegra, C.J., Chabner, B.A., Tuazon, C.U., *et al.* Trimetrexate for the treatment of *Pneumocystis carinii* pneumonia in patients with acquired immunodeficiency syndrome. *N. Engl. J. Med.,* **1987a,** *317:*978–985.

Allegra, C.J., Hoang, K., Yeh, G.C., Drake, J.C., and Baram, J. Evidence for direct inhibition of de novo purine synthesis in human MCF-7 breast cells as a principal mode of metabolic inhibition by methotrexate. *J. Biol. Chem.,* **1987b,** *262:*13520–13526.

Amadori, S., Suciu, S., Willemze, R., *et al.* Sequential administration of gemtuzumab ozogamicin and conventional chemotherapy as first line therapy in elderly patients with acute myeloid leukemia: a phase II study (AML-15) of the EORTC and GIMEMA leukemia groups. *Haematologica,* **2004,** *89:*950–956.

Anand, S., Penrhyn-Lowe, S., and Venkitaraman, A.R. AURORA-A amplification overrides the mitotic spindle assembly checkpoint, inducing resistance to Taxol. *Cancer Cell,* **2003,** *3:*51–62.

Aotake, T., Lu, C.D., Chiba, Y., Muraoka, R., and Tanigawa, N. Changes of angiogenesis and tumor cell apoptosis during colorectal carcinogenesis. *Clin. Cancer Res.,* **1999,** *5:*135–142.

Aparicio A., Gardner, A., Tu, Y., *et al. In vitro* cytoreductive effects on multiple myeloma cells induced by bisphosphonates. *Leukemia,* **1998,** *12:*220–229.

Arbuck, S.G., Douglass, H.O., Crom, W.R., *et al.* Etoposide pharmacokinetics in patients with normal and abnormal organ function. *J. Clin. Oncol.,* **1986,** *4:*1690–1695.

Assaraf, Y.G., Rothem, L., Hooijberg, J.H., *et al.* Loss of multidrug resistance protein 1 expression and folate efflux activity results in a highly concentrative folate transport in human leukemia cells. *J. Biol. Chem.,* **2003,** *278:*6680–6686.

Asselin, B.L., Whitin, J.C., Coppola, D.J., *et al.* Comparative pharmacokinetic studies of three asparaginase preparations. *J. Clin. Oncol.,* **1993,** *11:*1780–1786.

Avramis, V.I., Sencer, S., Periclou, A.P., *et al.* A randomized comparison of native *Escherichia coli* asparaginase and polyethylene glycol conjugated asparaginase for treatment of children with newly diagnosed standard-risk acute lymphoblastic leukemia: a Children's Cancer Group study. *Blood,* **2002,** *99:*1986–1994.

Baker, D.K., Relling, M.V., Pui, C.H., *et al.* Increased teniposide clearance with concomitant anticonvulsant therapy. *J. Clin. Oncol.,* **1992,** *10:*311–315.

Baker, S.D., Wirth, M., Statkevich, P., *et al.* Absorption, metabolism and excretion of ^{14}C-temozolomide following oral administration to patients with advanced cancer. *Clin. Cancer Res.,* **1999,** *5:*309–317.

Barbour, K.W., Berger, S.H., and Berger, F.G. Single amino acid substitution defines a naturally occurring genetic variant of human thymidylate synthase. *Mol. Pharmacol.,* **1990,** *37:*515–518.

Barker, A.J., Gibson, K.H., Grundy, W., *et al.* Studies leading to the identification of ZD1839 (IRESSA): an orally active, selective epidermal growth factor receptor tyrosine kinase inhibitor targeted to the treatment of cancer. *Bioorg. Med. Chem. Lett.,* **2001,** *11:*1911–1914.

Baselga, J. Clinical trials of single-agent trastuzumab (Herceptin). *Semin. Oncol.,* **2000,** *27:*20–26.

Baselga, J., and Averbuch, S.D. ZD1839 ('Iressa') as an anticancer agent. *Drugs,* **2000,** *60*(Suppl. 1):33–40.

Baselga, J., Norton, L., Albanell, J., Kim, Y.M., and Mendelsohn, J. Recombinant humanized anti-HER2 antibody (Herceptin) enhances the antitumor activity of paclitaxel and doxorubicin against HER2/neu overexpressing human breast cancer xenografts. *Cancer Res.,* **1998,** *58:*2825–2831. Erratum in: *Cancer Res.,* **1999,** *59:*2020.

Baselga, J., Rischin, D., Ranson, M., *et al.* Phase I safety, pharmacokinetic, and pharmacodynamic trial of ZD1839, a selective oral epidermal growth factor receptor tyrosine kinase inhibitor, in patients with five selected solid tumor types. *J. Clin. Oncol.,* **2002,** *20:*4292–4302.

Bergenheim A.T., and Henriksson, R. Pharmacokinetics and pharmacodynamics of estramustine phosphate. *Clin. Pharmacokinet.,* **1998,** *34:*163–172.

Baum, M., Budzar, A.U., Cuzick, J., *et al.* Anastrozole alone or in combination with tamoxifen versus tamoxifen alone for adjuvant treatment of postmenopausal women with early breast cancer: first results of the ATAC randomised trial. *Lancet,* **2002,** *359:*2131–2139.

Bernstein, I.D. Monoclonal antibodies to the myeloid stem cells: therapeutic implications of CMA-676, a humanized anti-CD33 antibody calicheamicin conjugate. *Leukemia,* **2000,** *14:*474–475.

Bhan, A.K., Nadler, L.M., Stashenko, P., McCluskey, R.T., and Schlossman, S.F. Stages of B cell differentiation in human lymphoid tissue. *J. Exp. Med.,* **1981,** *154:*737–749.

Bianchi Scarra, G.L., Romani, M., Coviello, D.A., *et al.* Terminal erythroid differentiation in the K-562 cell line by 1-β-D-arabinofuranosylcytosine: accompaniment by c-myc messenger RNA decrease. *Cancer Res.,* **1986,** *46:*6327–6332.

Blakley, R.L., and Sorrentino, B.P. In vitro mutations in dihydrofolate reductase that confer resistance to methotrexate: potential for clinical application. *Hum. Mutat.,* **1998,** *11:*259–263.

Blume-Jensen, P., and Hunter, T. Oncogenic kinase signaling. *Nature,* **2001,** *411:*355–365.

Boccardo, F., Cannata, D., Rubagotti, A., *et al.* Prophylaxis of superficial bladder cancer with mitomycin or interferon alfa-2b: results of a multicentric Italian study. *J. Clin. Oncol.,* **1994,** *12:*7–13.

Bo, J., Schroder, H., Kristinsson, J., *et al.* Possible carcinogenic effect of 6-mercaptopurine on bone marrow stem cells: relation to thiopurine metabolism. *Cancer,* **1999,** *86:*1080–1086.

Bossier, S., Ferreras, M., Peyruchaud, O., *et al.* Bisphosphonates inhibit breast and prostate carcinoma cell invasion, an early event in the formation of bone metastases. *Cancer Res.,* **2000,** *60:*2949–2954.

Bollag, W. The tumor-inhibitory effects of the methylhydrazine derivative Ro 4-6467/1 (NSC-77213). *Cancer Chemother. Rep.,* **1963,** *33:*1–4.

Bolton, A.E., Peng, B., Hubert, M., *et al.* Effect of rifampicin on the pharmacokinetics of imatinib mesylate (Gleevec, STI571) in healthy subjects. *Cancer Chemother. Pharmacol.,* **2004,** *53:*102–106.

Boogerd, W., van der Sande, J.J., and van Zandwijk, N. Teniposide sometimes effective in brain metastases from non-small-cell lung cancer. *J. Neurooncol.,* **1999,** *41:*285–289.

Bracken, R.B., Johnson, D.E., Rodriquez, L., Samuels, M.L., and Ayala, A. Treatment of multiple superficial tumors of bladder with intravesical bleomycin. *Urology,* **1977,** *9:*161–163.

Breast Cancer Trials Committee, Scottish Cancer Trials Office (MRC). Adjuvant tamoxifen in the management of operable breast cancer: the Scottish Trial. Report from the Breast Cancer Trials Committee, Scottish Cancer Trials Office (MRC), Edinburgh. *Lancet,* **1987,** *2:*171–175.

Bruckner, H.W., and Schleifer, S.J. Orthostatic hypotension as a complication of hexamethylmelamine antidepressant interaction. *Cancer Treat. Rep.,* **1983,** *67:*516.

Buchdunger, E., Matter, A., and Druker, B.J. Bcr-Abl inhibition as a modality of CML therapeutics. *Biochem. Biophys. Acta,* **2001,** *1551:*M11–M18.

Buchdunger, E., Zimmermann, J., Mett, H., *et al.* Inhibition of the Abl protein-tyrosine kinase in vitro and in vivo by a 2-phenylaminopyrimidine derivative. *Cancer Res.,* **1996,** *56:*100–104.

Burger, R.M. Cleavage of nucleic acids by bleomycin. *Chem. Rev.,* **1998,** *98:*1153–1169.

Bushara, K.O., and Rust, R.S. Reversible MRI lesions due to pegaspargase treatment of non-Hodgkin's lymphoma. *Pediatr. Neurol.,* **1997,** *17:*185–187.

Byar, D.P., and Corle, D.K. Hormone therapy for prostate cancer: results of the Veterans Administration Cooperative Urologic Research Group studies. *NCI Monogr.,* **1988,** *7:*165–170.

Cabral, F.R. Isolation of Chinese hamster ovary cell mutants requiring the continuous presence of Taxol for cell division. *J. Cell Biol.,* **1983,** *97:*22–29.

Calvert, A.H., and Egorin M.J. Carboplatin dosing formulae: gender bias and the use of creatinine-based methodologies. *Eur. J. Cancer,* **2002,** *38:*11–16.

Calvert, A.H., Newell, D.R., Gumbrell, L.A., *et al.* Carboplatin dosage: prospective evaluation of a simple formula based on renal function. *J. Clin. Oncol.,* **1989,** *7:*1748–1756.

Cardoen, S., Van Den Neste, E., Small, C., *et al.* Resistance to 2-Chloro-2′-deoxyadenosine of the human B-cell leukemia cell line EHEB. *Clin. Cancer Res.,* **2001,** *7:*3559–3566.

Carroll, M., Ohno-Jones, S., Tamura, S., *et al.* CGP 57148, a tyrosine kinase inhibitor, inhibits the growth of cells expressing BCR-ABL, TEL-ABL and TEL-PDGFR fusion proteins. *Blood,* **1997,** *90:*4947–4952.

Chao, Y., Teng, H.C., Hung, H.C., *et al.* Successful initial treatment with weekly etoposide, epirubicin, cisplatin, 5-fluorouracil and leucovorin chemotherapy in advanced gastric cancer patients with disseminated intravascular coagulation. *Jpn. J. Clin. Oncol.,* **2000,** *30:*122–125.

Chen, V.J., Bewley, J.R., Andis, S.L., *et al.* Preclinical cellular pharmacology of LY231514 (MTA): a comparison with methotrexate, LY309887 and raltitrexed for their effects on intracellular folate and nucleoside triphosphate pools in CCRF-CEM cells. *Br. J. Cancer,* **1998,** *78*(Suppl. 3):27–34.

Chen, T.L., Passos-Coelho, J.L., Noe, D.A., *et al.* Nonlinear pharmacokinetics of cyclophosphamide in patients with metastatic breast cancer receiving high-dose chemotherapy followed by autologous bone marrow transplantation. *Cancer Res.,* **1995,** *55:*810–816. Erratum in: *Cancer Res.,* **1995,** *55:*1600.

Cheson, B.D., Vena, D.A., Barrett, J., and Freidlin, B. Second malignancies as a consequence of nucleoside analog therapy for chronic lymphoid leukemias. *J. Clin. Oncol.,* **1999,** *17:*2454–2460.

Choi, H.J., Hyun, M.S., Jung, G.J., Kim, S.S., and Hong, S.H. Tumor angiogenesis as a prognostic predictor in colorectal carcinoma with special reference to mode of metastasis and recurrence. *Oncology,* **1998,** *55:*575–581.

Chu, E., Koeller, D.M., Casey, J.L., *et al.* Autoregulation of human thymidylate synthase messenger RNA translation by thymidylate synthase. *Proc. Natl. Acad. Sci. U.S.A.,* **1991,** *88:*8977–8981.

Citron, M.L., Berry, D.A., Cirrincione, C., *et al.* Randomized trial of dose-dense versus conventionally scheduled and sequential versus concurrent combination chemotherapy as postoperative adjuvant treatment of node-positive primary breast cancer: first report of Intergroup Trial C9741/Cancer and Leukemia Group B Trial 9741. *J. Clin. Oncol.,* **2003,** *21:*1431–1439.

Clark, S.J., and Rivory, L.P. Clinical pharmacokinetics of docetaxel. *Clin. Pharmacokinet.,* **1999,** *36:*99–114.

Cobleigh, M.A., Langmuir, V.K., Sledge, G.W., *et al.* A phase I/II dose-escalation trial of bevacizumab in previously treated metastatic breast cancer. *Semin. Oncol.,* **2003,** *30:*117–124.

Cobleigh, M.A., Vogel, C.L., Tripathy, D., *et al.* Multinational study of the efficacy and safety of humanized anti-HER2 monoclonal antibody in women who have HER2 overexpressing metastatic breast cancer that has progressed after chemotherapy for metastatic disease. *J. Clin. Oncol.,* **1999,** *17:*2639–2648.

Cohen, M.H., Williams, G.A., Sridhara, R., *et al.* United States Food and Drug Administration drug approval summary: gefitinib (ZD1839, Iressa) tablets. *Clin. Cancer Res.,* **2004,** *10:*1212–1218.

Coiffier, B., Haioun, C., Ketterer, N., *et al.* Rituximab (anti-CD20 monoclonal antibody) for the treatment of patients with relapsing or refractory aggressive lymphoma: a multicenter phase II study. *Blood,* **1998,** *92:*1927–1932.

Coiffier, B., Lepage, E., Briere, J., *et al.* CHOP chemotherapy plus rituximab compared with CHOP alone in elderly patients with diffuse large-B-cell lymphoma. *N. Engl. J. Med.,* **2002,** *346:*235–242.

Cokic, V.P., Smith, R.D., Beleslin-Cokic, B., *et al.* Hydroxyurea induces fetal hemoglobin by the nitric oxide-dependent activation of soluble guanylyl cyclase. *J. Clin. Invest.,* **2003,** *111:*231–239.

Cole, B.F., Glantz, M.J., Jaeckle, K.A., *et al.* Quality-of-life-adjusted survival comparison of sustained-release cytosine arabinoside versus intrathecal methotrexate for treatment of solid tumor neoplastic meningitis. *Cancer,* **2003,** *97:*3053–3060.

Cools, J., DeAngelo, D.J., Gotlib, J., *et al.* A tyrosine kinase created by fusion of the PDGFRA and FIP1L1 genes as a therapeutic target of imatinib in idiopathic hypereosinophilic syndrome. *N. Engl. J. Med.,* **2003,** *348:*1201–1214.

Coombes, R.C., Hall, E., Gibson, L.J., *et al.* A randomized trial of exemestane after two to three years of tamoxifen therapy in postmenopausal women with primary breast cancer. *N. Engl. J. Med.,* **2004,** *350:*1081–1092. Erratum in: *N. Engl. J. Med.,* **2004,** *351:*2461.

Corbin, A.S., La Rosée, P., Stoffregen, E., Druker, B.J., and Deininger, M.W. Several Bcr-Abl kinase domain mutants associated with imatinib mesylate resistance remain sensitive to imatinib. *Blood,* **2003,** *101:*4611–4614.

Cornwell, G.G. III, Pajak, T.F., McIntyre, O.R., *et al.* Influence of renal failure on myelosuppressive effects of melphalan: Cancer and Leukemia Group B Experience. *Cancer Treat. Rep.,* **1982,** *66:*475–481.

Corral, L.G., and Kaplan, G. Immunomodulation by thalidomide and thalidomide analogues. *Ann. Rheum. Dis.,* **1999,** *58*(Suppl. 1):1107–1113.

Cortes, J., Kantarjian, H., Talpaz, M., *et al.* Treatment of chronic myelogenous leukemia with nucleoside analogs deoxycoformycin and fludarabine. *Leukemia,* **1997,** *11:*788–791.

Cresteil, T., Monsarrat, B., Alvinerie, P., *et al.* Taxol metabolism by human liver microsomes: identification of cytochrome P450 isozymes involved in its biotransformation. *Cancer Res.,* **1994,** *54:*386–392.

Crone, S.A., Zhao, Y.Y., Fan, L., *et al.* ErbB2 is essential in the prevention of dilated cardiomyopathy. *Nat. Med.,* **2002,** *8:*459–465.

Cunningham, D., Humblet, Y., Siena, S., *et al.* Cetuximab monotherapy and cetuximab plus irinotecan in irinotecan-refractory metastatic colorectal cancer. *N. Engl. J. Med.,* **2004,** *351:*337–345.

Curt, G.A., Jolivet, J., Carney, D.N., *et al.* Determinants of the sensitivity of human small-cell lung cancer cell lines to methotrexate. *J. Clin. Invest.,* **1985,** *76:*1323–1329.

Cushman, M., Costantino, J.P., Bovill, E.G., *et al.* Effect of tamoxifen on venous thrombosis risk factors in women without cancer: the Breast Cancer Prevention Trial. *Br. J. Haematol.,* **2003,** *120:*109–116.

Dalgleish, A.G., Woods, R.L., and Levi, J.A. Bleomycin pulmonary toxicity: its relationship to renal dysfunction. *Med. Pediatr. Oncol.,* **1984,** *12:*313–317.

D'Amato, R.J., Loughnan, M.S., Flynn, E., and Folkman, J. Thalidomide is an inhibitor of angiogenesis. *Proc. Natl. Acad. Sci. U.S.A.,* **1994,** *91:*4082–4085.

Damia, G., and D'Incalci, M. Clinical pharmacokinetics of altretamine. *Clin. Pharmacokinet.,* **1995,** *28:*439–448.

Damle, N.K. Tumor-targeted chemotherapy with immunoconjugates of calicheamicin. *Expert Opin. Biol. Ther.,* **2004,** *4:*1445–1452.

Dancey, J.E., and Freidlin, B. Targeting epidermal growth factor receptor—are we missing the mark? *Lancet,* **2003,** *362:*62–64.

Danenberg, P.V., Shea, L.C., and Danenberg, K. Effect of 5-fluorouracil substitution on the self-splicing activity of *Tetrahymena* ribosomal RNA. *Cancer Res.,* **1990,** *50:*1757–1763.

Davis, T.A., Grillo-Lopez, A.J., White, C.A., *et al.* Rituximab anti-CD20 monoclonal antibody therapy in non-Hodgkin's lymphoma: safety and efficacy of re-treatment. *J. Clin. Oncol.,* **2000,** *18:*3135–3143.

Davies, F.E., Raje, N., Hideshima, T., *et al.* Thalidomide and immunomodulatory derivatives augment natural killer cell cytotoxicity in multiple myeloma. *Blood,* **2001,** *98:*210–216.

Davison, K., Mann, K.K., Waxman, S., *et al.* JNK activation is a mediator of arsenic trioxide–induced apoptosis in acute promyelocytic leukemia cells. *Blood,* **2004,** *103:*3496–3502.

Day, R., Ganz, P.A., Costatino, J.P., *et al.* Health-related quality of life and tamoxifen in breast cancer prevention: a report from the National Surgical Adjuvant Breast and Bowel Project P-1 Study. *J. Clin. Oncol.,* **1999,** *17:*2659–2669.

DeAngelis, L.M., Tong, W.P., Lin, S., Fleisher, M., and Berting, J.R. Carboxypeptidase G2 rescue after high-dose methotrexate. *J. Clin. Oncol.,* **1996,** *14:*2145–2149.

Deans, J.P., Schieven, G.L., Shu, G.L., *et al.* Association of tyrosine and serine kinases with the B cell surface antigen CD20. Induction via CD20 of tyrosine phosphorylation and activation of phospholipase C-gamma 1 and PLC phospholipase C-gamma 2. *J. Immunol.,* **1993,** *151:*4494–4504.

Dearden, C.E., Matutes, E., Hilditch, B.L., Swansbury, G.J., and Catovsky, D. Long-term follow-up of patients with hairy cell leukemia after treatment with pentostatin or cladribine. *Br. J. Haematol.,* **1999,** *106:*515–519.

DeFronzo, R.A., Braine, H., Colvin, M., and Davis, P.J. Water intoxication in man after cyclophosphamide therapy. Time course and relation to drug activation. *Ann. Intern. Med.,* **1973,** *78:*861–869.

Deguchi, Y., Yokoyama, Y., Sakamoto, T., *et al.* Brain distribution of 6-mercaptopurine is regulated by the efflux transport system in the blood–brain barrier. *Life Sci.,* **2000,** *66:*649–662.

Deininger, M.W., and Druker, B.J. Circumventing imatinib resistance. *Cancer Cell,* **2004,** *6:*108–110.

Deininger, M.W., O'Brien, S.G., Ford, J.M., and Druker, B.J. Practical management of patients with chronic myeloid leukemia receiving imatinib. *J. Clin. Oncol.,* **2003,** *21:*1637–1647.

van Der Velden, V.H., te Marvelde, J.G., Hoogeveen, P.G., *et al.* Targeting of the CD33-calicheamicin immunoconjugate Mylotarg (CMA-676) in acute myeloid leukemia: in vivo and in vitro saturation and internalization by leukemic and normal myeloid cells. *Blood,* **2001,** *97:*3197–3204.

Di Salle, E., Zaccheo, T., and Ornati, G. Antiestrogenic and antitumor properties of the new triphenylethylene derivative toremifene in the rat. *J. Steroid Biochem.,* **1990,** *36:*203–206.

Dolan, M.E., Moschel, R.C., and Pegg, A.E. Depletion of mammalian O^6-alkylguanine-DNA alkyltransferase activity by O^6-benzylguanine provides a means to evaluate the role of this protein in protection against carcinogenic and therapeutic alkylating agents. *Proc. Natl. Acad. Sci. U.S.A.,* **1990,** *87:*5368–5372.

Douillard, J.Y., Cunningham, D., Roth, A.D., *et al.* Irinotecan combined with fluorouracil compared with fluorouracil alone as first-line treatment for metastatic colorectal cancer: a multicentre randomised trial. *Lancet,* **2000,** *355:*1041–1047.

Dowell, J.A., Korth-Bradley, J., Liu, H., King, S.P., and Berger, M.S. Pharmacokinetics of gemtuzumab ozogamicin, an antibody-targeted chemotherapy agent for the treatment of patients with acute myeloid leukemia in first relapse. *J. Clin. Pharmacol.,* **2001,** *41:*1206–1214.

Doyle, L.A., Yang, W., Abruzzo, L.V., *et al.* A multidrug resistance transporter from human MCF-7 breast cancer cells. *Proc. Natl. Acad. Sci. U.S.A.,* **1998,** *95:*15665–15670.

Druker, B.J. Imatinib as a paradigm of targeted therapies. *Adv. Cancer Res.,* **2004,** *91:*1–30.

Druker, B.J., Talpaz, M., Resta, D.J., *et al.* Efficacy and safety of a specific inhibitor of the BCR-ABL tyrosine kinase in chronic myeloid leukemia. *N. Engl. J. Med.,* **2001,** *344:*1031–1037.

Druker, B.J., Tamura, S., Buchdunger, E., *et al.* Effects of a selective inhibitor of the ABL tyrosine kinase on the growth of BCR-ABL positive cells. *Nat. Med.,* **1996,** *2:*561–566.

Duggan, D.B., Petroni, G.R., Johnson, J.L., *et al.* Randomized comparison of ABVD and MOPP/ABV hybrid for the treatment of advanced Hodgkin's disease. *J. Clin. Oncol.,* **2003,** *21:*607–614.

Dutreix, C., Peng, B., Mehring, G., *et al.* Pharmacokinetic interaction between ketoconazole and imatinib mesylate (Gleevec) in healthy subjects. *Cancer Chemother. Pharmacol.,* **2004,** *54:*290–294.

Early Breast Cancer Trialists' Collaborative Group. Effects of adjuvant tamoxifen and of cytotoxic therapy on mortality in early breast can-

cer. An overview of 61 randomized trials among 28,896 women. *N. Engl. J. Med.,* **1988,** *319:*1681–1692.

Early Breast Cancer Trialists' Collaborative Group. Tamoxifen for early breast cancer: an overview of the randomised trials. *Lancet,* **1998,** *351:*1451–1467.

Elwood, P.C. Molecular cloning and characterization of the human folate-binding protein cDNA from placenta and malignant tissue culture (KB) cells. *J. Biol. Chem.,* **1989,** *264:*14893–14901.

Emmanouilides, C., Rosen, P., Rasti, S., Territo, M., and Kunkel, L. Treatment of indolent lymphoma with fludarabine/mitoxantrone combination: a phase II trial. *Hematol. Oncol.,* **1998,** *16:*107–116.

Endicott, J.A., and Ling, V. The biochemistry of P-glycoprotein–mediated multidrug resistance. *Annu. Rev. Biochem.,* **1989,** *58:*137–171.

Erikson, J.M., Tweedie, D.J., Ducore, J.M., and Prough, R.A. Cytotoxicity and DNA damage caused by the azoxy metabolites of procarbazine in L1210 tumor cells. *Cancer Res.,* **1989,** *49:*127–133.

Esteller, M., and Herman, J.G. Generating mutations but providing chemosensitivity: the role of O^6-methylguanine DNA methyltransferase in human cancer. *Oncogene,* **2004,** *23:*1–8.

Farber, S., Diamond, L.K., Mercer, R.D., Sylvester, R.F., and Wolff, V.A. Temporary remissions in acute leukemia in children produced by folic antagonist 4-amethopteroylglutamic acid (aminopterin). *N. Engl. J. Med.,* **1948,** *238:*787–793.

Fefer, A., Benyunes, M.C., Massumoto, C., *et al.* Interleukin-2 therapy after autologous bone marrow transplantation for hematologic malignancies. *Semin. Oncol.,* **1993,** *20:*41–45.

Ferrajoli, A., O'Brien, S.M., Cortes, J.E., *et al.* Phase II study of alemtuzumab in chronic lymphoproliferative disorders. *Cancer,* **2003,** *98:*773–778.

Ferrara, N., Houck, K., Jakeman, L., and Leung, D.W. Molecular and biological properties of the vascular endothelial growth factor family of proteins. *Endocr. Rev.,* **1992,** *13:*18–32.

Figg, W.D., Raje, S., Bauer, K.S., *et al.* Pharmacokinetics of thalidomide in an elderly prostate cancer population. *J. Pharm. Sci.,* **1999,** *88:*121–125.

Fink, D., Nebel, S., Aebi, S., *et al.* The role of DNA mismatch repair in platinum drug resistance. *Cancer Res.,* **1996,** *56:*4881–4886.

Fischel, J.L., Formento, P., Ciccolini, J., *et al.* Impact of the oxaliplatin-5 fluorouracil-folinic acid combination on respective intracellular determinants of drug activity. *Br. J. Cancer,* **2002,** *86:*1162–1168.

Fisher, B., Dignam, J., Bryant, J., and Wolmark, N. Five versus more than five years of tamoxifen for lymph node–negative breast cancer: Updated findings from the National Surgical Adjuvant Breast and Bowel Project B-14 randomized trial. *J. Natl. Cancer Inst.,* **2001,** *93:*684–690.

Foran, J.M., Rohatiner, A.Z., Cunningham, D., *et al.* European phase II study of rituximab (chimeric anti-CD20 monoclonal antibody) for patients with newly diagnosed mantle-cell lymphoma and previously treated mantle-cell lymphoma, immunocytoma, and small B-cell lymphocytic lymphoma. *J. Clin. Oncol.,* **2000,** *18:*317–324.

Fornander, T., Rutqvist, L.E., Sjoberg, H.E., *et al.* Long-term adjuvant tamoxifen in early breast cancer: effect on bone mineral density in postmenopausal women. *J. Clin. Oncol.,* **1990,** *8:*1019–1024.

Foss, F.M., Bacha, P., Osann, K.E., *et al.* Biological correlates of acute hypersensitivity events with DAB(389)IL-2 (denileukin diftitox, ONTAK) in cutaneous T-cell lymphoma: decreased frequency and severity with steroid premedication. *Clin. Lymphoma,* **2001,** *1:*298–302.

Friesen, C., Herr, I., Krammer, P.H., and Debatin, K.M. Involvement of the CD95 (APO-1/FAS) receptor/ligand system in drug-induced apoptosis in leukemia cells. *Nat. Med.,* **1996,** *2:*574–577.

Fukuoka, M., Niitani, H., Suzuki, A., *et al.* A phase II study of CPT-11, a new derivative of camptothecin, for previously untreated non-small-cell lung cancer. *J. Clin. Oncol.,* **1992,** *10:*16–20.

Fukuoka, M., Yano, S., Giaccone, G., *et al.* Multi-institutional randomized phase II trial of gefitinib for previously treated patients with advanced non-small-cell lung cancer. *J. Clin. Oncol.,* **2003,** *21:*2237–2246.

Fumoleau, P., Delgado, F.M., Delozier, T., *et al.* Phase II trial of weekly intravenous vinorelbine in first-line advanced breast cancer chemotherapy. *J. Clin. Oncol.,* **1993,** *11:*1245–1252.

Gallagher, R.E. Retinoic acid resistance in acute promyelocytic leukemia. *Leukemia,* **2002,** *16:*1940–1958.

Garanziotis, S., Steele, M.P., and Schwartz, D.A. Pulmonary fibrosis: thinking outside of the lung. *J. Clin. Invest.,* **2004,** *114:*319–321.

Garcia, S.T., McQuillan, A., and Panasci, L. Correlation between the cytotoxicity of melphalan and DNA crosslinks as detected by the ethidium bromide fluorescence assay in the F_1 variant of B_{16} melanoma cells. *Biochem. Pharmacol.,* **1988,** *37:*3189–3192.

Garcia-Carbonero, R., and Supko, J.G. Current perspectives on the clinical experience, pharmacology, and continued development of the camptothecins. *Clin. Cancer Res.,* **2002,** *8:*641–661.

Gewirtz, D.A. A critical evaluation of the mechanisms of action proposed for the antitumor effects of the anthracycline antibiotics adriamycin and daunorubicin. *Biochem. Pharmacol.,* **1999,** *57:*727–741.

Gilbert, M.R., Supko, J.G., Batchelor, T., *et al.* Phase I clinical and pharmacokinetic study of irinotecan in adults with recurrent malignant glioma. *Clin. Cancer Res.,* **2003,** *9:*2940–2949.

Gilman, A., and Philips, F.S. The biological actions and therapeutic applications of the β-chlorethylamines and sulfides. *Science,* **1946,** *103:*409–415.

Giverhaug, T., Loennechen, T., and Aarbakke, J. The interaction of 6-mercaptopurine (6-MP) and methotrexate (MTX). *Gen. Pharmacol.,* **1999,** *33:*341–346.

Glantz, M.J., LaFollette, S., Jaeckle, K.A., *et al.* Randomized trial of a slow-release versus a standard formulation of cytarabine for the intrathecal treatment of lymphomatous meningitis. *J. Clin. Oncol.,* **1999,** *17:*3110–3116.

Go, R.S., and Adjei, A.A. Review of the comparative pharmacology and clinical activity of cisplatin and carboplatin. *J. Clin. Oncol.,* **1999,** *17:*409–422.

Goker, E., Waltham, M., Kheradpour, A., *et al.* Amplification of the dihydrofolate reductase gene is a mechanism of acquired resistance to methotrexate in patients with acute lymphoblastic leukemia and is correlated with p53 gene mutations. *Blood,* **1995,** *86:*677–684.

Goldberg, I.H., Beerman, T.A., and Poon, R. Antibiotics: nucleic acids as targets in chemotherapy. In, *Cancer: A Comprehensive Treatise. Vol. 5: Chemotherapy.* (Becker, F.F., ed.) Plenum Press, New York, **1977,** pp. 427–456.

Gong, J.G., Costanzo, A., Yang, H.Q., *et al.* The tyrosine kinase c-Abl regulates p73 in apoptotic response to cisplatin-induced DNA damage. *Nature,* **1999,** *399:*806–809.

Gorgun, G., and Foss, F. Immunomodulatory effects of RXR rexinoids: modulation of high-affinity IL-2R expression enhances susceptibility to denileukin diftitox. *Blood,* **2002,** *100:*1399–1403.

Goss, P.E., Ingle, J.N., Martino, S., *et al.* A randomized trial of letrozole in postmenopausal women after five years of tamoxifen therapy for early-stage breast cancer. *N. Engl. J. Med.,* **2003,** *349:*1793–1802.

Goss P.E., Ingle, J.N., Martino, S., *et al.* Updated analysis of the NCIC CTG MA.17 randomized placebo (P) controlled trial of letrozole (L) after five years of tamoxifen in postmenopausal women with early stage breast cancer. *J. Clin. Oncol.,* **2004,** *22*(Suppl. 14):847.

Goss, P.E., Powles, T.J., Dowsett, M., *et al.* Treatment of advanced postmenopausal breast cancer with an aromatase inhibitor, 4-hydroxyandrostenedione: phase II report. *Cancer Res.,* **1986,** *46:*4823–4826.

Grossman, S.A., Levin, V., Sawaya, R., *et al.* National Comprehensive Cancer Network Adult Brain Tumor Practice Guidelines. *Oncology (Huntingt.),* **1997,** *11:*237–277.

Grunewald, R., Abbruzzese, J.L., Tarassoff, P., and Plunkett, W. Saturation of 2′,2′-difluorodeoxycytidine 5′-triphosphate accumulation by mononuclear cells during a phase I trial of gemcitabine. *Cancer Chemother. Pharmacol.,* **1991,** *27:*258–262.

Grunewald, R., Kantarjian, H., Du, M., *et al.* Gemcitabine in leukemia: a phase I clinical, plasma, and cellular pharmacology study. *J. Clin. Oncol.,* **1992,** *10:*406–413.

Grunwald, V., and Hidalgo, M. Developing inhibitors of the epidermal growth factor receptor for cancer treatment. *J. Natl. Cancer Inst.,* **2003,** *95:*851–867.

Hainsworth, J.D. Prolonging remission with rituximab maintenance therapy. *Semin. Oncol.,* **2004,** *31:*17–21.

Halsey, C., and Roberts, I.A. The role of hydroxyurea in sickle cell disease. *Br. J. Haematol.,* **2003,** *120:*177–186. Erratum in: *Br. J. Haematol.,* **2003,** *121:*200.

Hande, K.R. Etoposide: four decades of development of a topoisomerase II inhibitor. *Eur. J. Cancer,* **1998,** *34:*1514–1521.

Hausknecht, R.U. Methotrexate and misoprostol to terminate early pregnancy. *N. Engl. J. Med.,* **1995,** *333:*537–540.

Hayakawa, F., and Privalsky, M.L. Phosphoration of PML by mitogen-activated protein kinases plays a key role in arsenic trioxide–mediated apoptosis. *Cancer Cell,* **2004,** *5:*389–401.

He, X., Batchelor, T.A., Grossman, S., Supko, J.G., and New Approaches to Brain Tumor Therapy (NABTT) CNS Consortium. Determination of procarbazine in human plasma by high performance liquid chromatography with electrospray ionization mass spectrometry. *J. Chromatogr. B Analyt. Technol. Biomed. Life Sci.,* **2004,** *799:*281–291.

Hedlund, P.O., and Henriksson, P. Parenteral estrogen versus total androgen ablation in the treatment of advanced prostate carcinoma: effects on overall survival and cardiovascular mortality. The Scandinavian Prostatic Cancer Group (SPCG)-5 Trial Study. *Urology,* **2000,** *55:*328–333.

Heinemann, V., Hertel, L.W., Grindey, G.B., and Plunkett, W. Comparison of the cellular pharmacokinetics and toxicity of 2′,2′-difluorodeoxycytidine and 1-β-D-arabinofuranosylcytosine. *Cancer Res.,* **1988,** *48:*4024–4031.

Heinrich, M.C., Corless, C.L., Demetri, G.D., *et al.* Kinase mutations and imatinib response in patients with metastatic gastrointestinal stromal tumor. *J. Clin. Oncol.,* **2003,** *21:*4342–4349.

Heinrich, M.C., Wait, C.L., Yee, K.W.H., and Griffith, D.J. STI571 inhibits the kinase activity of wild type and juxtamembrane c-kit mutants but not the exon 17 D816V mutation associated with mastocytosis. *Blood,* **2000,** *96:*173b.

Heizer, W.D., and Peterson, J.L. Acute myeloblastic leukemia following prolonged treatment of Crohn's disease with 6-mercaptopurine. *Dig. Dis. Sci.,* **1998,** *43:*1791–1793.

Henningsson, A., Karlsson, M.O., Vigano, L., *et al.* Mechanism-based pharmacokinetic model for paclitaxel. *J. Clin. Oncol.,* **2001,** *19:*4065–4073.

Hermon, C., and Beral, V. Breast cancer mortality rates are leveling off or beginning to decline in many western countries: analysis of time trends, age-cohort and age-period models of breast cancer mortality in 20 countries. *Br. J. Cancer,* **1996,** *73:*955–960.

Hertel, L.W., Boder, G.B., Kroin, J.S., *et al.* Evaluation of the antitumor activity of gemcitabine (2′,2′-difluoro-2′-deoxycytidine). *Cancer Res.,* **1990,** *50:*4417–4422.

Herzog, T.J. Update on the role of topotecan in the treatment of recurrent ovarian cancer. *Oncologist,* **2002,** *7*(Suppl. 5):3–10.

Hideshima, T., Chauhan, D., Shima, Y., *et al.* Thalidomide and its analogs overcome drug resistance of human multiple myeloma cells to conventional therapy. *Blood,* **2000,** *96:*2943–2950.

Hinoda, Y., Sasaki, S., Ishida, T., and Imai, K. Monoclonal antibodies as effective therapeutic agents for solid tumors. *Cancer Sci.,* **2004,** *95:*621–625.

Hochhaus, A., Kreil, S., Corbin, A.S., *et al.* Molecular and chromosomal mechanisms of resistance to imatinib (STI571) therapy. *Leukemia,* **2002,** *16:*2190–2196.

Hoffmeister, R.T. Methotrexate therapy in rheumatoid arthritis: 15 years experience. *Am. J. Med.,* **1983,** *75:*69–73.

Hogan, T.F., Citrin, D.L., Johnson, B.M., *et al.* o,p′-DDD (mitotane) therapy of adrenal cortical carcinoma: observations on drug dosage, toxicity, and steroid replacement. *Cancer,* **1978,** *42:*2177–2181.

Holmes, F.A., and Rowinsky, E.K. Pharmacokinetic profiles of doxorubicin in combination with taxanes. *Semin. Oncol.,* **2001,** *28:*8–14.

Howell, A., Robertson, J.F., Abram, P., *et al.* Comparison of fulvestrant versus tamoxifen for the treatment of advanced breast cancer in postmenopausal women previously untreated with endocrine therapy: a multinational, double-blind, randomized trial. *J. Clin. Oncol.,* **2004a,** *22:*1605–1613.

Howell, S.J., Johnston, S.R., and Howell, A. The use of selective estrogen receptor modulators and selective estrogen receptor down-regulators in breast cancer. *Best Pract. Res. Clin. Endocrinol. Metab.,* **2004b,** *18:*47–66.

Hsiang, Y.H., Hertzberg, R., Hecht, S., and Liu, L.F. Camptothecin induces protein-linked DNA breaks via mammalian DNA topoisomerase I. *J. Biol. Chem.,* **1985,** *260:*14873–14878.

Huang, C.H., and Treat, J. New advances in lung cancer chemotherapy: topotecan and the role of topoisomerase I inhibitors. *Oncology,* **2001,** *61*(Suppl. 1):14–24.

Huang, M.E., Ye, Y.C., Chen, S.R., *et al.* Use of all-trans retinoic acid as a differentiation therapy for acute promyelocytic leukemia. *Blood,* **1988,** *72:*567–572.

Hubbard, S.R., and Till, J.H. Protein tyrosine kinase structure and function. *Annu. Rev. Biochem.,* **2000,** *69:*373–398.

Huizing, M.T., Keung, A.C., Rosing, H., *et al.* Pharmacokinetics of paclitaxel and metabolites in a randomized comparative study in platinum-pretreated ovarian cancer patients. *J. Clin. Oncol.,* **1993,** *11:*2127–2135.

Humphreys, B.D., Sharman, J.P., Henderson, J.M., *et al.* Gemcitabine-associated thrombotic microangiopathy. *Cancer,* **2004,** *100:*2664–2670.

Hurwitz, H., Fehrenbacher, L., Novotny, W., *et al.* Bevacizumab plus irinotecan, fluorouracil, and leucovorin for metastatic colorectal cancer. *N. Engl. J. Med.,* **2004,** *350:*2335–2342.

Ibrado, A.M., Huang, Y., Fang, G., Liu, L., and Bhalla, K. Overexpression of Bcl-2 or Bcl-xL inhibits Ara-C-induced CPP32/Yama protease activity and apoptosis of human acute myelogenous leukemia HL-60 cells. *Cancer Res.,* **1996,** *56:*4743–4748.

Innocenti, F., Danesi, R., Di Paolo, A., *et al.* Clinical and experimental pharmacokinetic interaction between 6-mercaptopurine and methotrexate. *Cancer Chemother. Pharmacol.,* **1996,** *37:*409–414.

Ishikawa, T., Sekiguchi, F., Fukase, Y., Sawada, N., and Ishitsuka, H. Positive correlation between the efficacy of capecitabine and doxiflu-ridine and the ratio of thymidine phosphorylase to dihydropyrimidine dehydrogenase activities in tumors in human cancer xenografts. *Cancer Res.,* **1998,** *58:*685–690.

Iwasaki, H., Huang, P., Keating, M.J., and Plunkett, W. Differential incorporation of ara-C, gemcitabine, and fludarabine into replicating and repairing DNA in proliferating human leukemia cells. *Blood,* **1997,** *90:*270–278.

Iyer, L., King, C.D., Whitington, P.F., *et al.* Genetic predisposition to the metabolism of irinotecan (CPT-11). Role of uridine diphosphate glucuronosyltransferase isoform 1A1 in the glucuronidation of its active metabolite (SN-38) in human liver microsomes. *J. Clin. Invest.,* **1998,** *101:*847–854.

Izumi, Y., Xu, L., di Tomaso, E., Fukumura, D., and Jain, R.K. Tumor biology: herceptin acts as an anti-angiogenic cocktail. *Nature,* **2002,** *416:*279–280.

Jaffrezou, J.P., Levade, T., Bettaieb, A., *et al.* Daunorubicin-induced apoptosis: triggering of ceramide generation through sphingomyelin hydrolysis. *EMBO J.,* **1996,** *15:*2417–2424.

Jao, J.Y., Jusko, W.J., and Cohen, J.L. Phenobarbital effects on cyclophosphamide pharmacokinetics in man. *Cancer Res.,* **1972,** *32:*2761–2764.

Jarvinen, T.A., Holli, K., Kuukasjarvi, T., and Isola, J.J. Predictive value of topoisomerase II α and other prognostic factors for epirubicin chemotherapy in advanced breast cancer. *Br. J. Cancer,* **1998,** *77:*2267–2273.

Jing, Y. The PML-RARα Fusion protein and targeted therapy for acute promyelocytic leukemia. *Leuk. Lymphoma,* **2003,** *45:*639–648.

Jordan, V.C. Metabolites of tamoxifen in animals and man: identification, pharmacology, and significance. *Breast Cancer Res. Treat.,* **1982,** *2:*123–138.

Josting, A., Reiser, M., Wickramanayake, P.D., *et al.* Dexamethasone, carmustine, etoposide, cytarabine, and melphalan (dexa-BEAM) followed by high-dose chemotherapy and stem cell rescue—a highly effective regimen for patients with refractory or relapsed indolent lymphoma. *Leuk. Lymphoma,* **2000,** *37:*115–123.

Kabbinavar, F., Hurwitz, H.I., Fehrenbacher, L., *et al.* Phase II, randomized trial comparing bevacizumab plus fluorouracil (FU)/leucovorin (LV) with FU/LV alone in patients with metastatic colorectal cancer. *J. Clin. Oncol.,* **2003,** *21:*60–65.

Kaminski, M.S., Zelenetz, A.D., Press, O.W., *et al.* Pivotal study of iodine I 131 tositumomab for chemotherapy-refractory low-grade or transformed low-grade B-cell non-Hodgkin's lymphomas. *J. Clin. Oncol.,* **2001,** *19:*3918–3928.

Kamiya, K., Huang, P., and Plunkett, W. Inhibition of the 3′→5′ exonuclease human DNA polymerase by fludarabine-terminated DNA. *J. Biol. Chem.,* **1996,** *271:*19428–19435.

Kane, R.C., Bross, P.F., Farrell, A.T., and Pazdur, R. Velcade: U.S. FDA approval for the treatment of multiple myeloma progressing on prior therapy. *Oncologist,* **2003,** *8:*508–513.

Kang, M.H., Figg, W.D., Ando, Y., *et al.* The p-glycoprotein antagonist PSC833 increases the plasma concentrations of 6α-hydroxypaclitaxel, a major metabolite of paclitaxel. *Clin. Cancer Res.,* **2001,** *7:*1610–1617.

Kantarjian, H., Talpaz, M., O'Brien, S., *et al.* High-dose imatinib mesylate therapy in newly diagnosed Philadelphia chromosome–positive chronic phase chronic myeloid leukemia. *Blood,* **2004,** *103:*2873–2878.

Kasid, U.N., Halligan, B., Liu, L.F., Dritschilo, A., and Smulson, M. Poly(ADP-ribose)-mediated post-translational modification of chromatin-associated human topoisomerase I. Inhibitory effects on catalytic activity. *J. Biol. Chem.,* **1989,** *264:*18687–18692.

Kastan, M.B. Molecular determinants of sensitivity to antitumor agents. *Biochem. Biophys. Acta,* **1999,** *1424:*R37–R42.

Keating, M.J., Flinn, I., Jain, V., et al. Therapeutic role of alemtuzumab (Campath-1H) in patients who have failed fludarabine: results of a large international study. *Blood,* **2002,** *99:*3554–3561.

Kemeny, N., Huang, Y., Cohen, A.M., et al. Hepatic arterial infusion of chemotherapy after resection of hepatic metastases from colorectal cancer. *N. Engl. J. Med.,* **1999,** *341:*2039–2048.

Kennedy, G.A., Seymour, J.F., Wolf, M., et al. Treatment of patients with advanced mycosis fungoides and Sezary syndrome with alemtuzumab. *Eur. J. Haematol.,* **2003,** *71:*250–256.

Kharbanda, S., Rubin, E., Gunji, H., et al. Camptothecin and its derivatives induce expression of the c-jun proto-oncogene in human myeloid leukemia cells. *Cancer Res.,* **1991,** *51:*6636–6642.

Kidd, J.G. Regression of transplanted lymphomas induced in vivo by means of normal guinea pig serum. 1. Course of transplanted cancers of various kinds in mice and rats given guinea pig serum, horse serum, or rabbit serum. *J. Exp. Med.,* **1953,** *98:*565–582.

Kim, E.S., Khuri, F.R., and Herbst, R.S. Epidermal growth factor receptor biology (IMC-C225). *Curr. Opin. Oncol.,* **2001,** *13:*506–513.

Kitamura, T. Necessity of re-evaluation of estramustine phosphate sodium (EMP) as a treatment option for first-line monotherapy in advanced prostate cancer. *Int. J. Urol.,* **2001,** *8:*33–36.

Klijn, J.G., Beex, L.V., Mauriac, L., et al. Combined treatment with buserelin and tamoxifen in premenopausal metastatic breast cancer: a randomized study. *J. Natl. Cancer Inst.,* **2000,** *92:*903–911.

Knuth, U.A., Hano, R., and Nieschlag, E. Effect of flutamide or cyproterone acetate on pituitary and testicular hormones in normal men. *J. Clin. Endocrinol. Metab.,* **1984,** *59:*963–969.

Köberle, D., and Thürlimann, B. Anastrozole: pharmacological and clinical profile in postmenopausal women with breast cancer. *Expert Rev. Anticancer Ther.,* **2001,** *1:*169–176.

Kohn, E.C., Sarosy, G., Bicher, A., et al. Dose-intense taxol: high response rate in patients with platinum-resistant recurrent ovarian cancer. *J. Natl. Cancer Inst.,* **1994,** *86:*18–24.

Konrad, M.W., Hemstreet, G., Hersh, E.M., et al. Pharmacokinetics of recombinant interleukin 2 in humans. *Cancer Res.,* **1990,** *50:*2009–2017.

Korelitz, B.I., Fuller, S.R., Warman, J.I., and Goldberg, M.D. Shingles during the course of treatment with 6-mercaptopurine for inflammatory bowel disease. *Am. J. Gastroenterol.,* **1999,** *94:*424–426.

Kris, M.G., Natale, R.B., Herbst, R.S., et al. Efficacy of gefitinib, an inhibitor of the epidermal growth factor receptor tyrosine kinase, in symptomatic patients with non-small cell lung cancer: a randomized trial. *JAMA,* **2003,** *290:*2149–2158.

Krishna, R., Webb, M.S., St. Onge, G., et al. Liposomal and nonliposomal drug pharmacokinetics after administration of liposome-encapsulated vincristine and their contribution to drug tissue distribution properties. *J. Pharmacol. Exp. Ther.,* **2001,** *298:*1206–1212.

Kumar, S., Kimlinger, T.K., Lust, J.A., Donovan, K., and Witzig, T.E. Expression of CD52 on plasma cells in plasma cell proliferative disorders. *Blood,* **2003,** *102:*1075–1077.

Kuss, B.J., Deeley, R.G., Cole, S.P., et al. Deletion of gene for multidrug resistance in acute myeloid leukemia with inversion in chromosome 16: prognostic implications. *Lancet,* **1994,** *343:*1531–1534.

Laing, N.M., Belinsky, M.G., Kruh, G.D., et al. Amplification of the ATP-binding cassette 2 transporter gene is functionally linked with enhanced efflux of estramustine in ovarian carcinoma cells. *Cancer Res.,* **1988,** *58:*1332–1337.

Langer, C.J., Stephenson, P., Thor, A., Vangel, M., and Johnson, D.H. Trastuzumab in the treatment of advanced non-small-cell lung cancer:

is there a role? Focus on Eastern Cooperative Oncology Group study 2598. *J. Clin. Oncol.,* **2004,** *22:*1180–1187.

Lee, C.R., and Faulds, D. Altretamine: a review of its pharmacodynamic and pharmacokinetic properties, and therapeutic potential in cancer chemotherapy. *Drugs,* **1995,** *49:*932–953.

LeMaistre, C.F., Saleh, M.N., Kuzel, T.M., et al. Phase I trial of a ligand fusion-protein (DAB389IL-2) in lymphomas expressing the receptor for interleukin-2. *Blood,* **1998,** *91:*399–405.

Lemieux, B., Tartas, S., Traulle, C., et al. Rituximab-related late-onset neutropenia after autologous stem cell transplantation for aggressive non-Hodgkin's lymphoma. *Bone Marrow Transplant.,* **2004,** *33:*921–923.

Lenz, W. Thalidomide and congenital abnormalities. *Lancet,* **1962,** *1:*45.

Lerner, H.J. Acute myelogenous leukemia in patients receiving chlorambucil as long-term adjuvant chemotherapy for stage II breast cancer. *Cancer Treat. Rep.,* **1978,** *62:*1135–1138.

Levin, V.A., Hoffman, W., and Weinkam, R.J. Pharmacokinetics of BCNU in man: a preliminary study of 20 patients. *Cancer Treat. Rep.,* **1978,** *62:*1305–1312.

Li, W.W., Lin, J.T., Schweitzer, B.I., et al. Intrinsic resistance to methotrexate in human soft tissue sarcoma cell lines. *Cancer Res.,* **1992,** *52:*3908–3913.

Liliemark, J., and Juliusson, G. On the pharmacokinetics of 2-chloro-2′-deoxyadenosine in humans. *Cancer Res.,* **1991,** *51:*5570–5572.

Lipshultz, S.E., Rifai, N., Dalton, V.M., et al. The effect of dexrazoxane on myocardial injury in doxorubicin-treated children with acute lymphoblastic leukemia. *N. Engl. J Med.,* **2004,** *351:*145–153.

Lønning, P.E., Bajetta, E., Murray, R., et al. Activity of exemestane in metastatic breast cancer after failure of nonsteroidal aromatase inhibitors: a phase II trial. *J. Clin. Oncol.,* **2000,** *18:*2234–2244.

Loo, T.L., Housholder, G.E., Gerulath, A.H., Saunders, P.H., and Farquhar, D. Mechanism of action and pharmacology studies with DTIC (NSC-45388). *Cancer Treat. Rep.,* **1976,** *60:*149–152.

Love, R.R., Wiebe, D.A., Feyzi, J.M., Newcomb, P.A., and Chappell, R.J. Effects of tamoxifen on cardiovascular risk factors in postmenopausal women after 5 years of treatment. *J. Natl. Cancer Inst.,* **1994,** *86:*1534–1539.

Lowe, S.W., Ruley, H.E., Jacks, T., and Housman, D.E. p53-Dependent apoptosis modulates the cytotoxicity of anticancer agents. *Cell,* **1993,** *74:*957–967.

Ludlum, D.B. DNA alkylation by the haloethylnitrosoureas: nature of modifications produced and their enzymatic repair or removal. *Mutat. Res.,* **1990,** *233:*117–126.

Lynch, T.J., Bell, D.W., Sordella, R., et al. Activating mutations in the epidermal growth factor receptor underlying responsiveness of non-small-cell lung cancer to gefitinib. *N. Engl. J. Med.,* **2004,** *350:*2129–2139.

Ma, X.J., Wang, Z., Ryan, P.D., et al. A two-gene expression ratio predicts clinical outcome in breast cancer patients treated with tamoxifen. *Cancer Cell,* **2004,** *5:*607–616.

Mackey, J.R., Mani, R.S., Selner, M., et al. Functional nucleoside transporters are required for gemcitabine influx and manifestation of toxicity in cancer cell lines. *Cancer Res.,* **1998,** *58:*4349–4357.

Maloney, D.G., Grillo-Lopez, A.J., White, C.A., et al. IDEC-C2B8 (Rituximab) anti-CD20 monoclonal antibody therapy in patients with relapsed low-grade non-Hodgkin's lymphoma. *Blood,* **1997a,** *90:*2188–2195.

Maloney, D.G., Grillo-Lopez, A.J., Bodkin, D.J., et al. IDEC-C2B8: results of a phase I multiple-dose trial in patients with relapsed non-Hodgkin's lymphoma. *J. Clin. Oncol.,* **1997b,** *15:*3266–2674.

Maloney, D.G., Liles, T.M., Czerwinski, D.K., et al. Phase I clinical trial using escalating single-dose infusion of chimeric anti-CD20 monoclonal antibody (IDEC-C2B8) in patients with recurrent B-cell lymphoma. *Blood,* **1994,** *84:*2457–2466.

Maloney, D.G., Smith, B., and Rose, A. Rituximab: mechanism of action and resistance. *Semin. Oncol.,* **2002,** *29:*2–9.

Mansson, E., Flordal, E., Liliemark, J., *et al.* Down-regulation of deoxy-cytidine kinase in human leukemic cell lines resistant to cladribine and clofarabine and increased ribonucleotide reductase activity contributes to fludarabine resistance. *Biochem. Pharmacol.,* **2003,** *65:*237–247.

Marquet, P., Lachatre, G., Debord, J., *et al.* Pharmacokinetics of vinorelbine in man. *Eur. J. Clin. Pharmacol.,* **1992,** *42:*545–547.

Matherly, L.H., Taub, J.W., Wong, S.C., *et al.* Increased frequency of expression of elevated dihydrofolate reductase in T-cell versus B-precursor acute lymphoblastic leukemia in children. *Blood,* **1997,** *90:*578–589.

Matijasevic, Z., Boosalis, M., Mackay, W., *et al.* Protection against chloroethylnitrosourea cytotoxicity by eukaryotic 3-methyladenine DNA glycosylase. *Proc. Natl. Acad. Sci. U.S.A.,* **1993,** *90:*11855–11859.

Matthews, D.A., Bolin, J.T., Burridge, J.M., *et al.* Refined crystal structures of *Escherichia coli* and chicken liver dihydrofolate reductase containing bound trimethoprim. *J. Biol. Chem.,* **1985,** *260:*381–391.

Mayer, R.J., Davis, R.B., Schiffer, C.A., *et al.* Intensive postremission chemotherapy in adults with acute myeloid leukemia. Cancer and Leukemia Group B. *N. Engl. J. Med.,* **1994,** *331:*896–903.

Mayer, A., Takimoto, M., Fritz, E., *et al.* The prognostic significance of proliferating cell nuclear antigen, epidermal growth factor receptor, and mdr gene expression in colorectal cancer. *Cancer,* **1993,** *71:*2454–2460.

McGuire, W.P., Hoskins, W.J., Brady, M.F., *et al.* Cyclophosphamide and cisplatin compared with paclitaxel and cisplatin in patients with stage III and stage IV ovarian cancer. *N. Engl. J. Med.,* **1996,** *334:*1–6.

Meijer, C., Mulder, N.H., Hospers, G.A., Uges, D.R., and de Vries, E.G. The role of glutathione in resistance to cisplatin in a human small cell lung cancer cell line. *Br. J. Cancer,* **1990,** *62:*72–77.

Mello, J.A., Acharya, S., Fischel, R., *et al.* The mismatch repair protein hMSH2 binds selectively to DNA adducts of the anticancer drug cisplatin. *Chem. Biol.,* **1996,** *3:*579–589.

Meloni, G., Foa, R., Vignetti, M., *et al.* Interleukin-2 may induce prolonged remissions in advanced acute myelogenous leukemia. *Blood,* **1994,** *84:*2158–2163.

Mendelsohn, J., and Baselga, J. The EGF receptor family as targets for cancer therapy. *Oncogene,* **2000,** *19:*6550–6565.

Middleton, M.R., and Margison, G.P. Improvement of chemotherapy efficacy by inactivation of a DNA-repair pathway. *Lancet Oncol.,* **2003,** *4:*37–44.

Milano, G., Etienne, M.C., Pierrefite, V., *et al.* Dihydropyrimidine dehydrogenase deficiency and fluorouracil-related toxicity. *Br. J. Cancer,* **1999,** *79:*627–630.

Miller, V.A., Kris, M.G., Shah, N., *et al.* Bronchioloalveolar pathologic subtype and smoking history predict sensitivity to gefitinib in advanced non-small-cell lung cancer. *J. Clin. Oncol.,* **2004,** *22:*1103–1109.

Miller, R.A., Maloney, D.G., Warnke, R., and Levy, R. Treatment of B-cell lymphoma with monoclonal anti-idiotype antibody. *N. Engl. J. Med.,* **1982,** *306:*517–522.

Miller, W.H. Jr., Schipper, H.M., Lee, J.S., *et al.* Mechanisms of action of arsenic trioxide. *Cancer Res.,* **2002,** *62:*3893–3903.

Mitsiades, N., Mitsiades, C.S., Poulaki, V., *et al.* Apoptotic signaling induced by immunomodulatory thalidomide analogs in human multi-ple myeloma cells: therapeutic implications. *Blood,* **2002a,** *99:*4525–4530.

Mitsiades, N., Mitsiades, C.S., Poulaki, V., *et al.* Biologic sequelae of nuclear factor-κB blockade in multiple myeloma: therapeutic applications. *Blood,* **2002b,** *99:*4079–4086.

Miyake, K., Mickley, L., Litman, T., *et al.* Molecular cloning of cDNAs which are highly overexpressed in mitoxantrone-resistant cells: demonstration of homology to ABC transport genes. *Cancer Res.,* **1999,** *59:*8–13.

Morgan, D.A., Ruscetti, F.W., and Gallo, R. Selective in vitro growth of T lymphocytes from normal human bone marrows. *Science,* **1976,** *193:*1007–1008.

Munger, J.S., Huang, X., Kawakatsu, H., *et al.* The integrin α v β 6 binds and activates latent TGFβ_1: a mechanism for regulating pulmonary inflammation and fibrosis. *Cell,* **1999,** *96:*319–328.

Nabholtz, J.M., and Reese, D. Anastrozole in the management of breast cancer. *Expert Opin. Pharmacother.,* **2002,** *3:*1329–1339.

Nahta, R., and Esteva, F.J. HER-2-targeted therapy: lessons learned and future directions. *Clin. Cancer Res.,* **2003,** *9:*5078–5084.

National Comprehensive Cancer Network Clinical Practice Guidelines in Oncology. Breast cancer risk reduction, v.1.2004. Available at: http://www.nccn.org/professionals/physician_gls/PDF/breast_risk.pdf. Accessed January 9, 2005.

Nemati, F., Livartowski, A., De Cremoux, P., *et al.* Distinctive potentiating effects of cisplatin and/or ifosfamide combined with etoposide in human small cell lung carcinoma xenografts. *Clin. Cancer Res.,* **2000,** *6:*2075–2086.

Ng, S.F., and Waxman, D.J. N,N′,N″-triethylenethiophosphoramide (thio-TEPA) oxygenation by constitutive hepatic P450 enzymes and modulation of drug metabolism and clearance in vivo by P450-inducing agents. *Cancer Res.,* **1991,** *51:*2340–2345.

Nicolao, P., and Giometto, B. Neurological toxicity of ifosfamide. *Oncology,* **2003,** *65:*11–16.

Nicolaou, K.C., Yang, Z., Liu, J.J., *et al.* Total synthesis of Taxol. *Nature,* **1994,** *367:*630–634.

Niitsu, N., Yamaguchi, Y., Umeda, M., and Honma, Y. Human monocytoid leukemia cells are highly sensitive to apoptosis induced by 2′-deoxycoformycin and 2′-deoxyadenosine: association with dATP-dependent activation of caspase-3. *Blood,* **1998,** *92:*3368–3375.

Nilsson, C., Aschan, J., Ringden, O., *et al.* The effect of metronidazole on busulfan pharmacokinetics in patients undergoing hemapoietic stem cell transplantation. *Bone Marrow Transplant.,* **2003,** *31:*429–435.

Noonberg, S.B., and Benz, C.C. Tyrosine kinase inhibitors targeted to the epidermal growth factor receptor subfamily: role as anticancer agents. *Drugs,* **2000,** *59:*753–767.

Nowak-Gottl, U., Wermes, C., Junker, R., *et al.* Prospective evaluation of the thrombotic risk in children with acute lymphoblastic leukemia carrying the MTHFR TT 677 genotype, the prothrombin G20210A variant, and further prothrombotic risk factors. *Blood,* **1999,** *93:*1595–1599.

O'Brien, S.M., Kantarjian, H., Thomas, D.A., *et al.* Rituximab dose-escalation trial in chronic lymphocytic leukemia. *J. Clin. Oncol.,* **2001,** *19:*2165–2170.

O'Brien, S.G., Meinhardt, P., Bond, E., *et al.* Effects of imatinib mesylate (STI571, Glivec) on the pharmacokinetics of simvastatin, a cytochrome p450 3A4 substrate, in patients with chronic myeloid leukemia. *Br. J. Cancer,* **2003,** *89:*1855–1859.

O'Regan, R.M., and Jordan, V.C. Tamoxifen to raloxifene and beyond. *Semin. Oncol.,* **2001,** *28:*260–273.

O'Reilly, S., Rowinsky, E.K., Slichenmyer, W., *et al.* Phase I and pharmacologic study of topotecan in patients with impaired renal function. *J. Clin. Oncol.,* **1996,** *14:*3062–3073.

Odom, L.F., and Gordon, E.M. Acute monoblastic leukemia in infancy and early childhood: successful treatment with an epipodophyllotoxin. *Blood,* **1984,** *64:*875–882.

Oliverio, V.T., Denham, C., DeVita, V.T., and Kelly, M.G. Some pharmacologic properties of a new antitumor agent, *N*-isopropyl-α-(2-methylhydrazino)-*p*-toluamide, hydrochloride (NSC-77213). *Cancer Chemother. Rep.,* **1964,** *42:*1–7.

Olsen, E., Duvic, M., Frankel, A., *et al.* Pivotal phase III trial of two dose levels of denileukin diftitox for the treatment of cutaneous T-cell lymphoma. *J. Clin. Oncol.,* **2001,** *19:*376–388.

Onda, M., Wang, Q.C., Guo, H.F., Cheung, N.K., and Pastan, I. In vitro and in vivo cytotoxic activities of recombinant immunotoxin 8H9(Fv)-PE38 against breast cancer, osteosarcoma, and neuroblastoma. *Cancer Res.,* **2004,** *64:*1419–1424.

Orlowski, R.Z., Stinchcombe, T.E., Mitchell B.S., *et al.* Phase I trial of the proteasome inhibitor PS-341 in patients with refractory hematologic malignancies. *J. Clin. Oncol.,* **2002,** *20:*4420–4427.

Osterborg, A., Dyer, M.J., Bunjes, D., *et al.* Phase II multicenter study of human CD52 antibody in previously treated chronic lymphocytic leukemia. European Study Group of CAMPATH-1H Treatment in Chronic Lymphocytic Leukemia. *J. Clin. Oncol.,* **1997,** *15:*1567–1574.

Paez, J.G., Janne, P.A., Lee, J.C., *et al.* EGFR mutations in lung cancer: correlation with clinical response to gefitinib therapy. *Science,* **2004,** *304:*1497–1500.

Papandreou, C., Daliani, D., Millikan, R.E., *et al.* Phase I study of intravenous (I.V.) proteasome inhibitor PS-341 in patients with advanced malignancies. *Am. Soc. Clin. Oncol. Ann. Meeting,* **2001,** abstract 340.

Park, J.W., Kerbel, R.S., Kelloff, G.J., *et al.* Rationale for biomarkers and surrogate endpoints in mechanism-driven oncology drug development. *Clin. Cancer Res.,* **2004,** *10:*3885–3896.

Parker, R.J., Eastman, A., Bostick-Bruton, F., and Reed, E. Acquired cisplatin resistance in human ovarian cancer cells is associated with enhanced repair of cisplatin-DNA lesions and reduced drug accumulation. *J. Clin. Invest.,* **1991,** *87:*772–777.

Peng, B., Hayes, M., Resta, D., *et al.* Pharmacokinetics and pharmacodynamics of imatinib in a phase 1 trial with chronic myeloid leukemia patients. *J. Clin. Oncol.,* **2004,** *22:*935–942.

Petit, A.M., Rak, J., Hung, M.C., *et al.* Neutralizing antibodies against epidermal growth factor and ErbB-2/neu receptor tyrosine kinases down-regulate vascular endothelial growth factor production by tumor cells in vitro and in vivo: angiogenic implications for signal transduction therapy of solid tumors. *Am. J. Pathol.,* **1997,** *151:*1523–1530.

Pommier, Y., Kerrigan, D., Hartman, K.D., and Glazer, R.I. Phosphorylation of mammalian DNA topoisomerase I and activation by protein kinase C. *J. Biol. Chem.,* **1990,** *265:*9418–9422.

Postmus, P.E., Smit, E.F., Haaxma-Reiche, H., *et al.* Teniposide for brain metastases of small-cell lung cancer: a phase II study. European Organization for Research and Treatment of Cancer Lung Cancer Cooperative Group. *J. Clin. Oncol.,* **1995,** *13:*660–665.

Preisler, H.D., Rustum, Y., and Priore, R.L. Relationship between leukemic cell retention of cytosine arabinoside triphosphate and the duration of remission in patients with acute non-lymphocytic leukemia. *Eur. J. Cancer Clin. Oncol.,* **1985,** *21:*23–30.

Prostate Cancer Trialists' Collaborative Group. Maximum androgen blockade in advanced prostate cancer: an overview of randomised trials. *Lancet,* **2000,** *355:*1491–1498.

Pui, C.H., Relling, M.V., Rivera, G.K., *et al.* Epipodophyllotoxin-related acute myeloid leukemia: a study of 35 cases. *Leukemia,* **1995,** *9:*1990–1996.

Pullarkat, S.T., Stoehlmacher, J., Ghaderi, V., *et al.* Thymidylate synthase gene polymorphism determines response and toxicity of 5-FU chemotherapy. *Pharmacogenomics J.,* **2001,** *1:*65–70.

Rai, K.R., Freter, C.E., Mercier, R.J., *et al.* Alemtuzumab in previously treated chronic lymphocytic leukemia patients who also had received fludarabine. *J. Clin. Oncol.,* **2002,** *20:*3891–3897.

Rajapakse, R.O., Korelitz, B.I., Zlatanic, J., *et al.* Outcome of pregnancies when fathers are treated with 6-mercaptopurine for inflammatory bowel disease. *Am. J. Gastroenterol.,* **2000,** *95:*684–688.

Ramaswamy, S., Ross, K.N., Lander, E.S., and Golub, T.R. A molecular signature of metastasis in primary solid tumors. *Nat. Genet.,* **2003,** *33:*49–54.

Ranson, M., Hammond, L.A., Ferry, D., *et al.* ZD1839, a selective oral epidermal growth factor receptor-tyrosine kinase inhibitor, is well tolerated and active in patients with solid, malignant tumors: results of a phase I trial. *J. Clin. Oncol.,* **2002,** *20:*2240–2250.

Read, W.L., Mortimer, J.E., and Picus, J. Severe interstitial pneumonitis associated with docetaxel administration. *Cancer,* **2002,** *94:*847–853.

Reed, E. Platinum-DNA adduct, nucleotide excision repair and platinum based anti-cancer chemotherapy. *Cancer Treat. Rev.,* **1998,** *24:*331–344.

Reed, E., Yuspa, S.H., Zwelling, L.A., *et al.* Quantitation of cis-diamminedichloroplatinum II (cisplatin)-DNA-intrastrand adducts in testicular and ovarian cancer patients receiving cisplatin chemotherapy. *J. Clin. Invest.,* **1986,** *77:*545–550.

Reid, P., Kantoff, P., and Oh, W. Antiandrogens in prostate cancer. *Invest. New Drugs,* **1999,** *17:*271–284.

Relling, M.V., Hancock, M.L., Boyett, J.M., *et al.* Prognostic importance of 6-mercaptopurine dose intensity in acute lymphoblastic leukemia. *Blood,* **1999,** *93:*2817–2823.

Richardson, P.G., Barlogie, B., Berenson, J., *et al.* A phase 2 study of bortezomib in relapsed, refractory myeloma. *N. Engl. J. Med.,* **2003,** *348:*2609–2617.

Richardson, P., Schlossman, R., Jagannath, S., *et al.* Thalidomide for patients with relapsed multiple myeloma after high-dose chemotherapy and stem cell transplantation: results of an open-label multicenter phase 2 study of efficacy, toxicity, and biological activity. *Mayo Clin. Proc.,* **2004,** *79:*875–882.

Riggs, B.L., and Hartmann, L.C. Selective estrogen-receptor modulators—mechanisms of action and application to clinical practice. *N. Engl. J. Med.,* **2003,** *348:*618–629.

Robertson, J.F. Estrogen receptor downregulators: new antihormonal therapy for advanced breast cancer. *Clin. Ther.,* **2002,** *24:*A17–A30.

Robertson, J.F., and Harrison, M. Fulvestrant: pharmacokinetics and pharmacology. *Br. J. Cancer,* **2004,** *90:*S7–S10.

Robieux, I., Sorio, R., Borsatti, E., *et al.* Pharmacokinetics of vinorelbine in patients with liver metastases. *Clin. Pharmacol. Ther.,* **1996,** *59:*32–40.

Rodriguez, G.I., Kuhn, J.G., Weiss, G.R., *et al.* A bioavailability and pharmacokinetic study of oral and intravenous hydroxyurea. *Blood,* **1998,** *91:*1533–1541.

Rosell, R., Taron, M., Barnadas, A., *et al.* Nucleotide excision repair pathways involved in cisplatin resistance in non-small-cell lung cancer. *Cancer Control,* **2003,** *10:*297–305.

Rosen, L.S. Clinical experience with angiogenesis signaling inhibitors: focus on vascular endothelial growth factor (VEGF) blockers. *Cancer Control,* **2002,** *9:*36–44.

Rosenberg, S.A., Lotze, M.T., Yang, J.C., *et al.* Experience with the use of high-dose interleukin-2 in the treatment of 652 cancer patients. *Ann. Surg.,* **1989,** *210:*474–484.

Rosenberg, S.A., Yannelli, J.R., Yang, J.C., *et al.* Treatment of patients with metastatic melanoma with autologous tumor-infiltrating lymphocytes and interleukin 2. *J. Natl. Cancer Inst.,* **1994,** *86:*1159–1166.

Rothenberg, M.L. Irinotecan (CPT-11): recent developments and future directions—colorectal cancer and beyond. *Oncologist,* **2001,** *6:*66–80.

Roussel, M.J., and Lanotte, M. Maturation sensitive and resistant t(15,17) NB4 cell lines as tools for APL physiopathology, nomenclature of cells and repertory of their known genetic alterations and phenotypes. *Oncogene,* **2001,** *20:*7287–7291.

Saltz, L.B., Meropol, N.J., Loehrer, P.J. Sr., *et al.* Phase II trial of cetuximab in patients with refractory colorectal cancer that expresses the epidermal growth factor receptor. *J. Clin. Oncol.,* **2004,** *22:*1201–1208.

Samson, D.J., Seidenfeld, J., Schmitt, B., *et al.* Systematic review and meta-analysis of monotherapy compared with combined androgen blockade for patients with advanced prostate carcinoma. *Cancer,* **2002,** *95:*361–376.

Sandler, E.S., Friedman, D.J., Mustafa, M.M., *et al.* Treatment of children with epipodophyllotoxin-induced secondary acute myeloid leukemia. *Cancer,* **1997,** *79:*1049–1054.

Santi, D.V., McHenry, C.S., and Sommer, H. Mechanism of interaction of thymidylate synthetase with 5-fluorodeoxyuridylate. *Biochemistry,* **1974,** *13:*471–481.

Sanz, M.A., Martín, G., Rayón, C., *et al.* A modified AIDA protocol with anthracycline-based consolidation results in high antileukemic efficacy and reduced toxicity in newly diagnosed PML/RARα-positive acute promyelocytic leukemia. *Blood,* **1999,** *94:*3015–3021.

Savage, D.G., Cohen, N.S., Hesdorffer, C.S., *et al.* Combined fludarabine and rituximab for low grade lymphoma and chronic lymphocytic leukemia. *Leuk. Lymphoma,* **2003,** *44:*477–481.

Saven, A., and Burian, C. Cladribine activity in adult langerhans-cell histiocytosis. *Blood,* **1999,** *93:*4125–4130.

Sawyer, M., and Ratain, M.J. Body surface area as a determinant of pharmacokinetics and drug dosing. *Invest. New Drugs,* **2001,** *19:*171–177.

Scagliotti, G.V., Shin, D.M., Kindler, H.L., *et al.* Phase II study of pemetrexed with and without folic acid and vitamin B_{12} as front-line therapy in malignant pleural mesothelioma. *J. Clin. Oncology,* **2003,** *21:*1556–1561.

Schimke, R.T., Kaufman, R.J., Alt, F.W., and Kellems, R.F. Gene amplification and drug resistance in cultured murine cells. *Science,* **1978,** *202:*1051–1055.

Sebti, S.M., DeLeon, J.C., and Lazo, J.S. Purification, characterization, and amino acid composition of rabbit pulmonary bleomycin hydrolase. *Biochemistry,* **1987,** *26:*4213–4219.

Sebti, S.M., Jani, J.P., Mistry, J.S., Gorelik, E., and Lazo, J.S. Metabolic inactivation: a mechanism of human tumor resistance to bleomycin. *Cancer Res.,* **1991,** *51:*227–232.

Seidenfeld, J., Samson, D.J., Hasselblad, V., *et al.* Single-therapy androgen suppression in men with advanced prostate cancer: a systematic review and meta-analysis. *Ann. Intern. Med.,* **2000,** *132:*566–577.

Seidman, A.D., Fornier, M.N., Esteva, F.J., *et al.* Weekly trastuzumab and paclitaxel therapy for metastatic breast cancer with analysis of efficacy by HER2 immunophenotype and gene amplification. *J. Clin. Oncol.,* **2001,** *19:*2587–2595.

Seidman, A., Hudis, C., Pierri, M.K., *et al.* Cardiac dysfunction in the trastuzumab clinical trials experience. *J. Clin. Oncol.,* **2002,** *20:*1215–1221.

Serrano, J., Palmeira, C.M., Kuehl, D.W., and Wallace, K.B. Cardioselective and cumulative oxidation of mitochondrial DNA following subchronic doxorubicin administration. *Biochem. Biophys. Acta,* **1999,** *1411:*201–205.

Shan, D., Ledbetter, J.A., and Press, O.W. Apoptosis of malignant human B cells by ligation of CD20 with monoclonal antibodies. *Blood,* **1998,** *91:*1644–1652.

Shah, N.P., Nicoll, J.M., Nagar, B., *et al.* Multiple BCR-ABL kinase domain mutations confer polyclonal resistance to the tyrosine kinase inhibitor imatinib (STI571) in chronic phase and blast crisis chronic myeloid leukemia. *Cancer Cell,* **2002,** *2:*117–125.

Shao, R.G., Cao, C.X., Shimizu, T., O'Connor, P.M., Kohn, K.W., and Pommier, Y. Abrogation of an S-phase checkpoint and potentiation of camptothecin cytotoxicity by 7-hydroxystaurosporine (UCN-01) in human cancer cell lines, possibly influenced by p53 function. *Cancer Res.,* **1997,** *57:*4029–4035.

Shen, Z.X., Chen, G.Q., Ni, J.H., *et al.* Use of arsenic trioxide in the treatment of acute promyelocytic leukemia (APL). *Blood,* **1997,** *89:*3345–3353.

Shiba, D.A., and Weinkam, R.J. Quantitative analysis of procarbazine, procarbazine metabolites and chemical degradation products with application to pharmacokinetic studies. *J. Chromatogr.,* **1982,** *229:*397–407.

Shiba, D.A., and Weinkam, R.J. The in vivo cytotoxic activity of procarbazine and procarbazine metabolites against L1210 ascites leukemia cells in CDF1 mice and the effects of pretreatment with procarbazine, phenobarbital, diphenylhydantoin, and methylprednisolone upon in vivo procarbazine activity. *Cancer Chemother. Pharmacol.,* **1983,** *11:*124–129.

Sievers, E.L., Larson, R.A., Stadtmauer, E.A., *et al.* Efficacy and safety of gemtuzumab ozogamicin in patients with CD33-positive acute myeloid leukemia in first relapse. *J. Clin. Oncol.,* **2001,** *19:*3244–3254.

Silver, R.T., Woolf, S.H., Hehlmann, R., *et al.* An evidence-based analysis of the effect of busulfan, hydroxyurea, interferon, and allogeneic bone marrow transplantation in treating the chronic phase of chronic myeloid leukemia: developed for the American Society of Hematology. *Blood,* **1999,** *94:*1517–1536.

Silverman, D.H., Delpassand, E.S., Torabi, F., *et al.* Radiolabeled antibody therapy in non-Hodgkins lymphoma: radiation protection, isotope comparisons and quality of life issues. *Cancer Treat. Rev.,* **2004,** *30:*165–172.

Simpson, D., Curran, M.P., and Perry, C.M. Letrozole: a review of its use in postmenopausal women with breast cancer. *Drugs,* **2004,** *64:*1213–1230.

Sinha, B.K., Mimnaugh, E.G., Rajagopalan, S., and Myers, C.E. Adriamycin activation and oxygen free radical formation in human breast tumor cells: protective role of glutathione peroxidase in adriamycin resistance. *Cancer Res.,* **1989,** *49:*3844–3848.

Skinner, R. Chronic ifosfamide nephrotoxicity in children. *Med. Pediatr. Oncol.,* **2003,** *41:*190–197.

Slamon, D.J., Godolphin, W., Jones, L.A., *et al.* Studies of the HER-2/neu proto-oncogene in human breast and ovarian cancer. *Science,* **1989,** *244:*707–712.

Slamon, D.J., Leyland-Jones, B., Shak, S., *et al.* Use of chemotherapy plus a monoclonal antibody against HER2 for metastatic breast cancer that overexpresses HER2. *N. Engl. J. Med.,* **2001,** *344:*783–792.

Smeland, E., Godal, T., Ruud, E., et al. The specific induction of myc protooncogene expression in normal human B cells is not a sufficient event for acquisition of competence to proliferate. *Proc. Natl. Acad. Sci. U.S.A.,* **1985**, *82:*6255–6259.

Smith, I.E., and Dowsett, M. Aromatase inhibitors in breast cancer. *N. Engl. J. Med.,* **2003**, *348:*2431–2442.

Smith, M.R., Goode, M., Zietman, A.L., et al. Bicalutamide monotherapy versus leuprolide monotherapy for prostate cancer: effects on bone mineral density and body composition. *J. Clin. Oncol.,* **2004**, *22:*2546–2553.

Smith, M.A., Rubinstein, L., Anderson, J.R., et al. Secondary leukemia or myelodysplastic syndrome after treatment with epipodophyllotoxins. *J. Clin. Oncol.,* **1999**, *17:*569–577.

Soignet, S.L., Maslak, P., Wang, Z.G., et al. Complete remission after treatment of acute promyelocytic leukemia with arsenic trioxide. *N. Engl. J. Med.,* **1998**, *339:*1341–1348.

Sonneveld, P., Schultz, F.W., Nooter, K., and Hahlen, K. Pharmacokinetics of methotrexate and 7-hydroxy-methotrexate in plasma and bone marrow of children receiving low-dose oral methotrexate. *Cancer Chemother. Pharmacol.,* **1986**, *18:*111–116.

Souliotis, V.L., Dimopoulos, M.A., and Sfikakis, P.P. Gene-specific formation and repair of DNA monoadducts and interstrand cross-links after therapeutic exposure to nitrogen mustards. *Clin. Cancer Res.,* **2003**, *9:*4465–4474.

Souliotis, V.L., Kaila, S., Boussiotis, V.A., Pangalis, G.A., and Kyrtopoulos, S.A. Accumulation of O^6-methylguanine in human blood leukocyte DNA during exposure to procarbazine and its relationships with dose and repair. *Cancer Res.,* **1990**, *50:*2759–2764.

Spetz, A.C., Hammar, M., Lindberg, B., Spangberg, A., and Varenhorst, E. Prospective evaluation of hot flashes during treatment with parenteral estrogen or complete androgen ablation for metastatic carcinoma of the prostate. *J. Urol.,* **2001**, *166:*517–520.

Speyer, J.L., Green, M.D., Kramer, E., et al. Protective effect of the bispiperazinedione ICRF-187 against doxorubicin-induced cardiac toxicity in women with advanced breast cancer. *N. Engl. J. Med.,* **1988**, *319:*745–752.

Srimatkandada, S., Schweitzer, B.I., Moroson, B.A., Dube, S., and Bertino, J.R. Amplification of a polymorphic dihydrofolate reductase gene expressing an enzyme with decreased binding to methotrexate in a human colon carcinoma cell line, HCT-8R4, resistant to this drug. *J. Biol. Chem.,* **1989**, *264:*3524–3528.

Stashenko, P., Nadler, L.M., Hardy, R., and Schlossman, S.F. Characterization of a human B lymphocyte-specific antigen. *J. Immunol.,* **1980**, *125:*1678–1685.

Steinberg, M.H. Therapies to increase fetal hemoglobin in sickle cell disease. *Curr. Hem. Reports,* **2003**, *2:*95–101.

Steis, R.G., Urba, W.J., Kopp, W.C., et al. Kinetics of recovery of CD4+ T cells in peripheral blood of deoxycoformycin-treated patients. *J. Natl. Cancer Inst.,* **1991**, *83:*1678–1679.

Stewart, C.F., Arbuck, S.G., Fleming, R.A., and Evans, W.E. Relation of systemic exposure to unbound etoposide and hematologic toxicity. *Clin. Pharmacol. Ther.,* **1991**, *50:*385–393.

Stoica, G.S., Greenberg, H.E., and Rossoff, L.J. Corticosteroid responsive fludarabine pulmonary toxicity. *Am. J. Clin. Oncol.,* **2002**, *25:*340–341.

Stoller, R.G., Hande, K.R., Jacobs, S.A., Rosenberg, S.A., and Chabner, B.A. Use of plasma pharmacokinetics to predict and prevent methotrexate toxicity. *N. Engl. J. Med.,* **1977**, *297:*630–634.

Sugimoto, Y., Tsukahara, S., Oh-hara, T., Isoe, T., and Tsuruo, T. Decreased expression of DNA topoisomerase I in camptothecin-resistant tumor cell lines as determined by monoclonal antibody. *Cancer Res.,* **1990**, *50:*6925–6930.

Swaffar, D.S., Horstman, M.G., Jaw, J.-Y., et al. Methylazoxyprocarbazine, the active metabolite responsible for the anticancer activity of procarbazine against L1210 leukemia. *Cancer Res.,* **1989**, *49:*2442–2447.

Swain, S.M., Whaley, F.S., Gerber, M.C., et al. Cardioprotection with dexrazoxane for doxorubicin-containing therapy in advanced breast cancer. *J. Clin. Oncol.,* **1997**, *15:*1318–1332.

Swedish Breast Cancer Cooperative Group. Randomized trial of two versus five years of adjuvant tamoxifen for postmenopausal early stage breast cancer. *J. Natl. Cancer Inst.,* **1996**, *88:*1543–1549.

Takimoto, C.H., Remick, S.C., Sharma, S., et al. Dose-escalating and pharmacological study of oxaliplatin in adult cancer patients with impaired renal function: a National Cancer Institute organ dysfunction working group study. *J. Clin. Oncol.,* **2003**, *21:*2664–2672.

Tallman, M.S., Andersen, J.W., Schiffer, C.A., et al. All-trans-retinoic acid in acute promyelocytic leukemia. *N. Engl. J. Med.,* **1997**, *337:*1021–1028.

Talpaz, M., Silver, R.T., Druker, B.J., et al. Imatinib induces durable hematologic and cytogenetic responses in patients with accelerated phase chronic myeloid leukemia: results of a phase 2 study. *Blood,* **2002**, *99:*1928–1937.

Tamura, H., Kohchi, C., Yamada, R., et al. Molecular cloning of a cDNA of a camptothecin-resistant human DNA topoisomerase I and identification of mutation sites. *Nucleic Acids Res.,* **1991**, *19:*69–75.

Tang, S.C., Hewitt, K., Reis, M.D., and Berinstein, N.L. Immunosuppressive toxicity of CAMPATH1H monoclonal antibody in the treatment of patients with recurrent low grade lymphoma. *Leuk. Lymphoma,* **1996**, *24:*93–101.

Taniguchi, T., Tischkowitz, M., Ameziane, N., et al. Disruption of the Fanconi anemia–BRCA pathway in cisplatin-sensitive ovarian tumors. *Nat. Med.,* **2003**, *9:*568–574.

Taussig, D.C., Davies, A.J., Cavenagh, J.D., et al. Durable remissions of myelodysplastic syndrome and acute myeloid leukemia after reduced-intensity allografting. *J. Clin. Oncol.,* **2003**, *21:*3060–3065.

Taylor, E.C., Kuhnt, D., Shih, C., et al. A dideazatetrahydrofolate analog lacking a chiral center at C-6, N-[4-[2-(2-amino-3,4-dihydro-4-oxo-7H–pyrrolo[2,3-d]pyrimidin-5-yl)ethyl]benzoyl]-L-glutamic acid, is an inhibitor of thymidylate synthase. *J. Med. Chem.,* **1992**, *35:*4450–4454.

Tedder, T.F., Forsgren, A., Boyd, A.W., Nadler, L.M., and Schlossman, S.F. Antibodies reactive with the B1 molecule inhibit cell cycle progression but not activation of human B lymphocytes. *Eur. J. Immunol.,* **1986**, *16:*881–887.

Tempero, M., Plunkett, W., Van Haperen, V.R., et al. Randomized phase II comparison of dose-intense gemcitabine: 30-minute infusion and fixed dose rate infusion in patients with pancreatic adenocarcinoma. *J. Clin. Oncol.,* **2003**, *21:*3402–3408.

Thomas, S.M., and Grandis, J.R. Pharmacokinetic and pharmacodynamic properties of EGFR inhibitors under clinical investigation. *Cancer Treat. Rev.,* **2004**, *30:*255–268.

Thyss, A., Milano, G., Kubar, J., Namer, M., and Schneider, M. Clinical and pharmacokinetic evidence of a life-threatening interaction between methotrexate and ketoprofen. *Lancet,* **1986**, *1:*256–258.

Tomera, K., Gleason, D., Gittelman, M., et al. The gonadotropin-releasing hormone antagonist abarelix depot versus luteinizing hormone releasing hormone agonists leuprolide or goserelin: initial results of endocrinological and biochemical efficacies in patients with prostate cancer. *J. Urol.,* **2001**, *165:*1585–1589.

Tondini, C., Balzarotti, M., Rampinelli, I., *et al*. Fludarabine and cladribine in relapsed/refractory low-grade non-Hodgkin's lymphoma: a phase II randomized study. *Ann. Oncol.*, **2000**, *11*:231–233.

Trachtenberg, J., Gittleman, M., Steidle, C., *et al*. A phase 3, multicenter, open label, randomized study of abarelix versus leuprolide plus daily antiandrogen in men with prostate cancer. *J. Urol.*, **2002**, *167*:1670–1674.

Tran, H.T., Madden, T., Petropoulos, D., *et al*. Individualizing high-dose oral busulfan: prospective dose adjustment in a pediatric population undergoing allogeneic stem cell transplantation for advanced hematologic malignancies. *Bone Marrow Transplant.*, **2000**, *26*:463–470.

Travis, L.B., Holowaty, E.J., Bergfeldt, K., *et al*. Risk of leukemia after platinum-based chemotherapy for ovarian cancer. *N. Engl. J. Med.*, **1999**, *340*:351–357.

Trippett, T., Schlemmer, S., Elisseyeff, Y., *et al*. Defective transport as a mechanism of acquired resistance to methotrexate in patients with acute lymphoblastic leukemia. *Blood*, **1992**, *80*:1158–1162.

Tsao, Y.P., Russo, A., Nyamuswa, G., Silber, R., and Liu, L.F. Interaction between replication forks and topoisomerase I-DNA cleavable complexes: studies in a cell-free SV40 DNA replication system. *Cancer Res.*, **1993**, *53*:5908–5914.

Tucker, M.A., Coleman, C.N., Cox, R.S., Varghese, A., and Rosenberg, S.A. Risk of second cancers after treatment for Hodgkin's disease. *N. Engl. J. Med.*, **1988**, *318*:76–81.

Tung, N., Berkowitz, R., Matulonis, U., *et al*. Phase I trial of carboplatin, paclitaxel, etoposide, and cyclophosphamide with granulocyte colony stimulating factor as first-line therapy for patients with advanced epithelial ovarian cancer. *Gynecol. Oncol.*, **2000**, *77*:271–277.

Twelves, C.J., Dobbs, N.A., Gillies, H.C., *et al*. Doxorubicin pharmacokinetics: the effect of abnormal liver biochemistry tests. *Cancer Chemother. Pharmacol.*, **1998**, *42*:229–234.

Twelves, C., Glynne-Jones, R., Cassidy, J., *et al*. Effect of hepatic dysfunction due to liver metastases on the pharmacokinetics of capecitabine and its metabolites. *Clin. Cancer Res.*, **1999**, *5*:1696–1702.

Twentyman, P.R. Bleomycin: mode of action with particular reference to the cell cycle. *Pharmacol. Ther.*, **1983**, *23*:417–441.

Vaisman, A., Varchenko, M., Umar, A., *et al*. The role of hMLH1, hMSH3, and hMSH6 defects in cisplatin and oxaliplatin resistance: correlation with replicative bypass of platinum-DNA adducts. *Cancer Res.*, **1998**, *58*:3579–3585.

Valavaara, R., and Nordman, E. Renal complications of mitomycin C therapy with special reference to the total dose. *Cancer*, **1985**, *55*:47–50.

Van Ark-Otte, J., Kedde, M.A., van der Vijgh, W.J., *et al*. Determinants of CPT-11 and SN-38 activities in human lung cancer cells. *Br. J. Cancer*, **1998**, *77*:2171–2176.

Van Barneveld, P.W., Sleijfer, D.T., van der Mark, T.W., *et al*. Natural course of bleomycin-induced pneumonitis. A follow-up study. *Am. Rev. Respir. Dis.*, **1987**, *135*:48–51.

Van Kuilenburg, A.B., Meinsma, R., Zoetekouw, L., and Van Gennip, A.H. High prevalence of the IVS14 + 1G>A mutation in the dihydropyrimidine dehydrogenase gene of patients with severe 5-fluorouracil-associated toxicity. *Pharmacogenetics*, **2002**, *12*:555–558.

Van Moorsel, C.J., Pinedo, H.M., Veerman, G., *et al*. Mechanisms of synergism between cisplatin and gemcitabine in ovarian and non-small-cell lung cancer cell lines. *Br. J. Cancer*, **1999**, *80*:981–990.

Van Triest, B., Pinedo, H.M., Blaauwgeers, J.L., *et al*. Prognostic role of thymidylate synthase, thymidine phosphorylase/platelet-derived endo-

thelial cell growth factor, and proliferation markers in colorectal cancer. *Clin. Cancer Res.*, **2000**, *6*:1063–1072.

Vassal, G., Challine, D., Koscielny, S., *et al*. Chronopharmacology of high-dose busulfan in children. *Cancer Res.*, **1993**, *53*:1534–1537.

Vergote, I., and Robertson, J.F. Fulvestrant is an effective and well-tolerated endocrine therapy for postmenopausal women with advanced breast cancer: results from clinical trials. *Br. J. Cancer*, **2004**, *90*:S11–S14.

Vermeulen, P.B., Van den Eynden, G.G., Huget, P., *et al*. Prospective study of intratumoral microvessel density, p53 expression and survival in colorectal cancer. *Br. J. Cancer*, **1999**, *79*:316–322.

Villamor, N., Montserrat, E., and Colomer, D. Mechanism of action and resistance to monoclonal antibody therapy. *Semin. Oncol.*, **2003**, *30*:424–343.

Vogel, C.L., Cobleigh, M.A., Tripathy, D., *et al*. Efficacy and safety of trastuzumab as a single agent in first-line treatment of HER2-overexpressing metastatic breast cancer. *J. Clin. Oncol.*, **2002**, *20*:719–726.

Vogelzang, N.J., Rusthoven, J.J., Symanowski, J., *et al*. Phase III study of pemetrexed in combination with cisplatin versus cisplatin alone in patients with malignant pleural mesothelioma. *J. Clin. Oncol.*, **2003**, *21*:2636–2644.

Wakai, T., Kanda, T., Hirota, S., *et al*. Late resistance to imatinib therapy in a metastatic gastrointestinal stromal tumor is associated with a second KIT mutation. *Br. J. Cancer*, **2004**, *90*:2059–2061.

Wakeling, A.E., Guy, S.P., Woodburn, J.R., *et al*. ZD1839 (Iressa): an orally active inhibitor of epidermal growth factor signaling with potential for cancer therapy. *Cancer Res.*, **2002**, *62*:5749–5754.

Wall, S.M., Johansen, M.J., Molony, D.A., *et al*. Effective clearance of methotrexate using high-flux hemodialysis membranes. *Am. J. Kidney Dis.*, **1996**, *28*:846–854.

Wang, Z.M., Chen, Z.P., Xu, Z.Y., *et al*. In vitro evidence for homologous recombinational repair in resistance to melphalan. *J. Natl. Cancer Inst.*, **2001**, *93*:1473–1478.

Wang, Y., Zhao, R., Chattopadhyay, S., *et al*. A novel folate transport activity in human mesothelioma cell lines with high affinity and specificity for the new-generation antifolate, pemetrexed. *Cancer Res.*, **2002**, *62*:6434–6437.

Wani, M.C., Taylor, H.L., Wall, M.E., Coggon, P., and McPhail, A.T. Plant antitumor agents. VI. The isolation and structure of taxol, a novel antileukemic and antitumor agent from *Taxus brevifolia*. *J. Am. Chem. Soc.*, **1971**, *93*:2325–2327.

Washtein, W.L. Thymidylate synthetase levels as a factor in 5-fluorodeoxyuridine and methotrexate cytotoxicity in gastrointestinal tumor cells. *Mol. Pharmacol.*, **1982**, *21*:723–728.

Weber, D., Rankin, K., Gavino, M., Delasalle, K., and Alexanian, R. Thalidomide alone or with dexamethasone for previously untreated multiple myeloma. *J. Clin. Oncol.*, **2003**, *21*:16–19.

Wellhausen, S.R., and Peiper, S.C. CD33: biochemical and biological characterization and evaluation of clinical relevance. *J. Biol. Regul. Homeost. Agents*, **2002**, *16*:139–143.

Wellington, K., and Faulds, D.M. Anastrozole: in early breast cancer. *Drugs*, **2002**, *62*:2483–2490.

Westerhof, G.R., Rijnboutt, S., Schornagel, J.H., *et al*. Functional activity of the reduced folate carrier in KB, MA104, and IGROV-I cells expressing folate-binding protein. *Cancer Res.*, **1995**, *55*:3795–3802.

Widemann, B.C., Balis, F.M., Kempf-Bielack, B., *et al*. High-dose methotrexate-induced nephrotoxicity in patients with osteosarcoma. *Cancer*, **2004**, *100*:2222–2230.

Widemann, B.C., Balis, F.M., Murphy, R.F., *et al*. Carboxypeptidase-G2, thymidine, and leucovorin rescue in cancer patients with methotrexate-induced renal dysfunction. *J. Clin. Oncol.,* **1997,** *15*:2125–2134.

Wijnholds, J., Mol., C.A., van Deemter, L., *et al.* Multidrug-resistance protein 5 is a multispecific organic anion transporter able to transport nucleotide analogs. *Proc. Natl. Acad. Sci. U.S.A.,* **2000,** *97*:7476–7481.

Williams, M.E., Walker, A.N., Bracikowski, J.P., *et al.* Ascending myeloencephalopathy due to intrathecal vincristine sulfate. A fatal chemotherapeutic error. *Cancer,* **1983,** *51*:2041–2147.

Wilson, W.H., Berg, S.L., Bryant, G., *et al.* Paclitaxel in doxorubicin-refractory or mitoxantrone-refractory breast cancer: a phase I/II trial of 96-hour infusion. *J. Clin. Oncol.,* **1994,** *12*:1621–1629.

Wilson, W.H., Pittaluga, S., Gutierrez, M., *et al.* Dose-adjusted EPOCH-rituximab in untreated diffuse large B-cell lymphoma: benefit of rituximab appears restricted to tumors harboring anti-apoptotic mechanisms. *Am. Soc. Hematol. Ann. Meeting,* **2003,** abstract 356.

Witherspoon, R.P., Deeg, H.J., Storer, B., *et al.* Hematopoietic stem-cell transplantation for treatment-related leukemia or myelodysplasia. *J. Clin. Oncol.,* **2001,** *19*:2134–2141.

Wortsman, J., and Soler, N.G. Mitotane. Spironolactone antagonism in Cushing's syndrome. *JAMA,* **1977,** *238*:2527.

Xie, H.J., Yasar, U., Lundgren, S., *et al.* Role of polymorphic human CYP2B6 in cyclophosphamide bioactivation. *Pharmacogenomics,* **2003,** *3*:53–61.

Yang, S.W., Burgin, A.B. Jr., Huizenga, B.N., *et al.* A eukaryotic enzyme that can disjoin dead-end covalent complexes between DNA and type I topoisomerases. *Proc. Natl. Acad. Sci. U.S.A.,* **1996,** *93*:11534–11539.

Yang, J.C., Haworth, L., Sherry, R.M., *et al.* A randomized trial of bevacizumab, an anti–vascular endothelial growth factor antibody, for metastatic renal cancer. *N. Engl. J. Med.,* **2003,** *349*:427–434.

Zaffaroni, N., Pennati, M., Colella, G., *et al.* Expression of the anti-apoptotic gene survivin correlates with taxol resistance in human ovarian cancer. *Cell Mol. Life Sci.,* **2002,** *59*:1406–1412.

Zangari, M., Anaissie, E., Barlogie, B., *et al.* Increased risk of deep-vein thrombosis in patients with multiple myeloma receiving thalidomide and chemotherapy. *Blood,* **2001,** *98*:1614–1615.

Zein, N., Sinha, A.M., McGahren, W.J., and Ellestad, G.A. Calicheamicin gamma 1I: an antitumor antibiotic that cleaves double-stranded DNA site specifically. *Science,* **1988,** *240*:1198–1201.

Zhou, B., Liu, X., Mo, M., *et al.* The human ribonucleotide reductase subunit hRRM2 complements p53R2 in response to UV-induced DNA repair in cells with mutant p53. *Cancer Res.,* **2003,** *63*:6583–6594.

Zimmerman, S.H., Schultz, W.H., Davis, J.S., *et al.* Sustained long-term hematologic efficacy of hydroxyurea at maximum tolerated dose in children with sickle cell disease. *Blood,* **2004,** *103*:2039–2045.

Zinzani, P.L., Magagnoli, M., Bendandi, M., *et al.* Efficacy of fludarabine and mitoxantrone (FN) combination regimen in untreated indolent non-Hodgkin's lymphomas. *Ann. Oncol.,* **2000,** *11*:363–365.

Zondor, S.D., and Medina, P.J. Bevacizumab: an angiogenesis inhibitor with efficacy in colorectal and other malignancies. *Ann. Pharmacother.,* **2004,** *38*:1258–1264.

Zuckerman, J.E., Raffin, T.A., Brown, J.M., *et al.* In vitro selection and characterization of a bleomycin-resistant subline of B16 melanoma. *Cancer Res.,* **1986,** *46*:1748–1753.

MONOGRAPHS AND REVIEWS

Alberts, D.S., Chang, S.Y., Chen, H.S., Larcom, B.J., and Jones, S.E. Pharmacokinetics and metabolism of chlorambucil in man: a preliminary report. *Cancer Treat. Rev.,* **1979,** *6*(Suppl.):9–17.

Andre, T., Louvet, C., and De Gramont, A. Colon cancer: what is new in 2004? *Bull. Cancer,* **2004,** *91*:75–80.

Berlin, N.I., Rall, D., Mead, J.A., *et al.* Folic acid antagonist. Effects on the cell and the patient. Combined clinical staff conference at the National Institutes of Health. *Ann. Intern. Med.,* **1963,** *59*:931–956.

Beutler, E. Cladribine (2-chlorodeoxyadenosine). *Lancet,* **1992,** *340*:952–956.

Bleyer, W.A. The clinical pharmacology of methotrexate: new applications of an old drug. *Cancer,* **1978,** *41*:36–51.

Borst, P., and Oude Elfrink, K. Mammalian ABC transporters in health and disease. *Ann. Rev. Biochem.,* **2002,** *71*:537–592.

Broome, J.D. L-Asparaginase: discovery and development as a tumor-inhibitory agent. *Cancer Treat. Rep.,* **1981,** *65*(Suppl. 4):111–114.

Budman, D.R. Vinorelbine (Navelbine): a third-generation vinca alkaloid. *Cancer Invest.,* **1997,** *15*:475–490.

Bukowski, R.M., McLain, D., and Finke, J. Clinical pharmacokinetics of interleukin-1, interleukin-2, interleukin-3, tumor necrosis factor, and macrophage colony-stimulating factor. In, *Cancer Chemotherapy and Biotherapy: Principles and Practice,* 3rd ed. (Chabner, B.A., and Longo, D.L., eds.) Lippincott Williams & Wilkins, Philadelphia, **2001,** pp. 779–828.

Calvert, A.H., Boddy, A., Bailey, N.P., *et al.* Carboplatin in combination with paclitaxel in advanced ovarian cancer: dose determination and pharmacokinetic and pharmacodynamic interactions. *Semin. Oncol.,* **1995,** *22*:91–98. Erratum in: *Semin. Oncol.,* **1996,** *23*:781.

Canman, C.E., Lawrence, T.S., Shewach, D.S., Tang, H.Y., and Maybaum, J. Resistance to fluorodeoxyuridine-induced DNA damage and cytotoxicity correlates with an elevation of deoxyuridine triphosphatase activity and failure to accumulate deoxyuridine triphosphate. *Cancer Res.,* **1993,** *53*:5219–5224.

Capizzi, R.L., and Handschumacher, R.E. Asparaginase. In, *Cancer Medicine,* 2nd ed. (Holland, J.F., and Frei, E., eds.) Lea & Febiger, Philadelphia, **1982,** pp. 920–932.

Chabner, B.A., and Roberts, T.G. Timeline: Chemotherapy and the war on cancer. *Nat. Rev. Cancer,* **2005,** *5*:65–72.

Crooke, S.T. Antitumor antibiotics II: actinomycin D, bleomycin, mitomycin C and other antibiotics. In *The Cancer Pharmacology Annual.* (Chabner, B.A., and Pinedo, H.M., eds.) Excerpta Medica, Amsterdam, **1983,** pp. 69–79.

De Gramont, A., Louvet, C., Andre, T., Tournigand, C., and Krulik, M. A review of GERCOD trials of bimonthly leucovorin plus 5-fluorouracil 48-h continuous infusion in advanced colorectal cancer: evolution of a regimen. Groupe d'Etude et de Recherche sur les Cancers de l'Ovaire et Digestifs (GERCOD). *Eur. J. Cancer,* **1998,** *34*:619–626.

DeVita, V.T. Jr. The consequences of the chemotherapy of Hodgkin's disease: The 10th David A. Karnofsky Memorial Lecture. *Cancer,* **1981,** *47*:1–13.

Dighiero, G. Adverse and beneficial immunological effects of purine nucleoside analogs. *Hematol. Cell Ther.,* **1996,** *38*(Suppl. 2):S75–S81.

Dillman, R.O. A new chemotherapeutic agent: deoxycoformycin (pentostatin). *Semin. Hematol.,* **1994,** *31*:16–27.

Dorr, R.T. New findings in the pharmacokinetic, metabolic, and drug-resistance aspects of mitomycin C. *Semin. Oncol.,* **1988,** *15*:32–41.

Ellis, M., and Swain, S.M. Steroid hormone therapies for cancer. In, *Cancer Chemotherapy and Biotherapy: Principles and Practice,* 3rd ed. (Chabner, B.A., and Longo, D.L., eds.) Lippincott Williams & Wilkins, Philadelphia, **2001,** pp. 85–138.

Finazzi, G., Ruggeri, M., Rodeghiero, F., and Barbui, T. Efficacy and safety of long-term use of hydroxyurea in young patients with essential thrombocythemia and a high risk of thrombosis. *Blood,* **2003,** *101:*3749–3750.

Fisher, D.E. Apoptosis in cancer therapy: crossing the threshold. *Cell,* **1994,** *78:*539–542.

Fox, E., Curt, G.A., and Balis, F.M. Clinical trial design for target-based therapy. *Oncologist,* **2002,** *7:*401–409.

Franks, M.E., Macpherson, G.R., and Figg, W.D. Thalidomide. *Lancet,* **2004,** *363:*1802–1811.

Friedman, H.S., Auerbuch, S.D., and Kurtzberg, J. Nonclassic alkylating agents. In, *Cancer Chemotherapy and Biotherapy: Principles and Practice,* 3rd ed. (Chabner, B.A., and Longo, D.L., eds.) Lippincott Williams & Wilkins, Philadelphia, **2001,** pp. 415–446.

Furlanut, M., and Franceschi, L. Pharmacology of ifosfamide. *Oncology,* **2003,** *65:*2–6.

Garcia-Carbonero, R., Ryan, D.P., Chabner, B.A. Cytidine analogs. In, *Cancer Chemotherapy and Biotherapy: Principles and Practice,* 3rd ed. (Chabner, B.A., and Longo, D.L., eds.) Lippincott Williams & Wilkins, Philadelphia, **2001,** pp. 265–294.

Goldberg, R.M., Sargent, D.J., Morton, R.F., *et al.* A randomized controlled trial of fluorouracil plus leucovorin, irinotecan, and oxaliplatin combinations in patients with previously untreated metastatic colorectal cancer. *J. Clin. Oncol.,* **2004,** *22:*23–30.

Grem, J.L. 5-Fluoropyrimidines. In, *Cancer Chemotherapy and Biotherapy: Principles and Practice,* 3rd ed. (Chabner, B.A., and Longo, D.L., eds.) Lippincott Williams & Wilkins, Philadelphia, **2001,** 185–264.

Grever, M.R., Doan, C.A., and Kraut, E.H. Pentostatin in the treatment of hairy-cell leukemia. *Best Pract. Res. Clin. Haematol.,* **2003,** *16:*91–99.

Grochow, L.B. Busulfan disposition: the role of therapeutic monitoring in bone marrow transplantation induction regimens. *Semin. Oncol.,* **1993,** *20:*18–25.

Grogan, L., Sotos, G.A., and Allegra, C.J. Leucovorin modulation of fluorouracil. *Oncology (Huntingt.),* **1993,** *7:*63–72.

Hawkins, D.S., Park, J.R., Thomson, B.G., *et al.* Asparaginase pharmacokinetics following intensive polyethylene glycol conjugated L-asparaginase (PEG-ASNase) therapy for children with relapsed acute lymphoblastic leukemia. *Clin. Cancer Res.,* **2004,** *10:*5335–5341.

Huang, P., and Plunkett, W. Induction of apoptosis by gemcitabine. *Semin. Oncol.,* **1995,** *22:*19–25.

Ibrahim, A., Hirschfeld, S., Cohen, M.H., *et al.* FDA drug approval summaries: oxaliplatin. *Oncologist,* **2004,** *9:*8–12.

Kruh, G.D. Lustrous insights into cisplatin accumulation: copper transporters. *Clin. Cancer Res.,* **2003,** *9:*5807–5809.

Kufe D.W., Munroe, D., Herrick, D., *et al.* Effects of 1-β-D-arabinofuranosylcytosine incorporation on eukaryotic DNA template function. *Mol. Pharmacol.,* **1984,** *26:*128–134.

Lane, D.P., and Fischer, P.M. Turning the key on p53. *Nature,* **2004,** *427:*789–790.

Lawrence, T.S., Eisbruch, A., McGinn, C.J., *et al.* Radiosensitization by gemcitabine. *Oncology,* **1999,** *13:*55–60.

Levine, E.G., and Bloomfield, C.D. Leukemias and myelodysplastic syndromes secondary to drug, radiation, and environmental exposure. *Semin. Oncol.,* **1992,** *19:*47–84.

Malspeis, L., Grever, M.R., Staubus, A.E., and Young, D. Pharmacokinetics of 2-F-ara-A (9-β-D-arabinofuranosyl-2-fluoroadenine) in cancer patients during the phase I clinical investigation of fludarabine phosphate. *Semin. Oncol.,* **1990,** *17:*18–32.

Manegold, C. Pemetrexed: its promise in treating non-small-cell lung cancer. *Oncology (Huntingt.),* **2004,** *18:*43–48.

Myers, C.E. Role of iron in anthracycline action. In, *Organ-Directed Toxicities of Anticancer Drugs.* (Hacker, M.P., Lazo, J.S., and Tritton, T.R., eds.) Nijhoff, Boston, **1988,** pp. 17–30.

Paz-Ares, L., and Donehower, R. Hydroxyurea. In, *Cancer Chemotherapy and Biotherapy: Principles and Practice,* 3rd ed. (Chabner, B.A., and Longo, D.L., eds.) Lippincott Williams & Wilkins, Philadelphia, **2001,** 315–328.

Pinkel, D., and Howarth, C.B. Pediatric neoplasms. In, *Medical Oncology: Basic Principles and Clinical Management of Cancer.* (Calabresi, P., Schein, P.S., and Rosenberg, S.A., eds.) Macmillan, New York, **1985,** pp. 1226–1258.

Plunkett, W., and Gandhi, V. Cellular metabolism of nucleoside analogs in CLL: implications for drug development. In, *Chronic Lymphocytic Leukemia: Scientific Advances and Clinical Developments.* (Cheson, B., ed.) Marcel Dekker, New York, **1993,** p. 197.

Pommier, Y., Fesen, M.R., and Goldwasser, F. Topoisomerase II inhibitors: the epipodophyllotoxins, m-AMSA, and the ellipticine derivatives. In, *Cancer Chemotherapy and Biotherapy: Principles and Practice,* 3rd ed. (Chabner, B.A., and Longo, D.L., eds.) Lippincott Williams & Wilkins, Philadelphia, **2001,** pp. 538–578.

Pratt, W.B., Ruddon, R.W., Ensminger, W.D., and Maybaum, J. *The Anticancer Drugs,* 2nd ed. Oxford University Press, New York, **1994.**

Pui, C.H., Relling, M.V., and Downing, J.R. Mechanisms of disease: acute lymphoblastic leukemia. *N. Engl. J. Med.,* **2004,** *350:*1535–1548.

Reid, P., Kantoff, P., and Oh, W. Antiandrogens in prostate cancer. *Invest. New Drugs,* **1999,** *17:*271–284.

Richardson, P. Hemostatic complications of hematopoietic stem cell transplantation: from hemorrhage to microangiopathies and VOD. *Pathophysiol. Haemost. Thromb.,* **2003,** *33*(Suppl. 1):50–53.

Roberts, T., and Chabner, B.A. Beyond fast track for drug approvals. *N. Engl. J. Med.,* **2004,** *351:*501–505.

Rowinsky, E.K., and Donehower, R.C. Paclitaxel. *N. Engl. J. Med.,* **1995,** *332:*1004–1014.

Rubin, E.H., and Hait, W.N. Anthracyclines and DNA intercalators/epipodophyllotoxins/camptothecins/DNA topoisomerases. In, *Cancer Medicine 5.* (Bast, R.C., *et al.* eds.) B.C. Decker, New York, **2000,** pp. 670–679.

Schilsky, R.L., Ratain, M.J., Vokes, E.E., *et al.* Laboratory and clinical studies of biochemical modulation by hydroxyurea. *Semin. Oncol.,* **1992,** *19:*84–89.

Schultz, R.M., Chen, V.J., Bewley, J.R., *et al.* Biological activity of the multitargeted antifolate, MTA (LY231514), in human cell lines with different resistance mechanisms to antifolate drugs. *Semin. Oncol.,* **1999,** *26:*68–73.

Seidman, A.D. One-hour paclitaxel via weekly infusion: dose-density with enhanced therapeutic index. *Oncology (Huntingt.),* **1998,** *12:*19–22.

Smets, L.A. Programmed cell death (apoptosis) and response to anticancer drugs. *Anticancer Drugs,* **1994,** *5:*3–9.

Sobell, H.M. The stereochemistry of actinomycin binding to DNA and its implications in molecular biology. *Prog. Nucleic Acid Res. Mol. Biol.,* **1973,** *13:*153–190.

Stark, G.R., and Wahl, G.M. Gene amplification. *Annu. Rev. Biochem.,* **1984,** *53:*447–491.

Strasser-Weippl, K. and Goss, P.E. Counteracting estrogen as breast cancer prevention. In, *Cancer Chemoprevention.* (Kelloff, G.J., Hawk, E.T., and Sigman, C.C., eds.) Humana Press, Totowa, N.J., **2005,** pp. 249–264.

Tew, K., Colvin, M., and Chabner, B.A. Alkylating agents. In, *Cancer Chemotherapy and Biotherapy: Principles and Practice*, 3rd ed. (Chabner, B.A., and Longo, D.L., eds.) Lippincott Williams & Wilkins, Philadelphia, **2001,** pp. 373–414.

Van Echo, D.A., Egorin, M.J., and Aisner, J. The pharmacology of carboplatin. *Semin. Oncol.,* **1989,** *16:*1–6.

Venkitaraman, A.R. Tracing the network connecting BRCA and Fanconi anaemia proteins. *Nature Rev. Cancer,* **2004,** *4:*266–276.

Verweij, J., Sparreboom, A., and Nooter, K. Antitumor antibiotics. In, *Cancer Chemotherapy and Biotherapy: Principles and Practice,* 3rd ed. (Chabner, B.A., and Longo, D.L., eds.) Lippincott Williams & Wilkins, Philadelphia, **2001,** pp. 482–499.

Watters, J.W., and McLeod, H.L. Recent advances in the pharmacogenetics of cancer chemotherapy. *Curr. Opinion in Mol. Therapeutics,* **2002,** *4:*565–571.

Williams, S.D., and Einhorn, L.H. Neoplasms of the testis. In, *Medical Oncology: Basic Principles and Clinical Management of Cancer.* (Calabresi, P., Schein, P.S., and Rosenberg, S.A., eds.) Macmillan, New York, **1985,** pp. 1077–1088.

Zhou, X.J., and Rahmani, R. Preclinical and clinical pharmacology of vinca alkaloids. *Drugs,* **1992,** *44*(Suppl. 4):1–16.

IMMUNOSUPPRESSANTS, TOLEROGENS, AND IMMUNOSTIMULANTS

Alan M. Krensky, Flavio Vincenti, and William M. Bennett

THE IMMUNE RESPONSE

The immune system evolved to discriminate self from nonself. Multicellular organisms were faced with the problem of destroying infectious invaders (microbes) or dysregulated self (tumors) while leaving normal cells intact. These organisms responded by developing a robust array of receptor-mediated sensing and effector mechanisms broadly described as innate and adaptive. Innate, or natural, immunity is primitive, does not require priming, and is of relatively low affinity, but is broadly reactive. Adaptive, or learned, immunity is antigen-specific, depends upon antigen exposure or priming, and can be of very high affinity. The two arms of immunity work closely together, with the innate immune system being most active early in an immune response and adaptive immunity becoming progressively dominant over time. The major effectors of innate immunity are complement, granulocytes, monocytes/macrophages, natural killer cells, mast cells, and basophils. The major effectors of adaptive immunity are B and T lymphocytes. B lymphocytes make antibodies; T lymphocytes function as helper, cytolytic, and regulatory (suppressor) cells. These cells are important in the normal immune response to infection and tumors, but also mediate transplant rejection and autoimmunity (Janeway *et al.*, 2001; Paul, 1999). Immunoglobulins (antibodies) on the B lymphocyte surface are receptors for a large variety of specific structural conformations. In contrast, T lymphocytes recognize antigens as peptide fragments in the context of self major histocompatibility complex (MHC) antigens (called human leukocyte antigens [HLA] in human beings) on the surface of antigen-presenting cells, such as dendritic cells, macrophages, and other cell types expressing MHC class I (HLA-A, -B, and -C) and class II antigens (HLA-DR, -DP, and -DQ) in human beings. Once activated by specific antigen recognition *via* their respective clonally restricted cell-surface receptors, both B and T lymphocytes are triggered to differentiate and divide, leading to release of soluble mediators (cytokines, lymphokines) that perform as effectors and regulators of the immune response.

The impact of the immune system in human disease is enormous. Developing vaccines against emerging infectious agents such as human immunodeficiency virus (HIV) and Ebola virus is among the most critical challenges facing the research community. Immune system–mediated diseases are significant medical problems.

Immunological diseases are growing at epidemic proportions that require aggressive and innovative approaches to develop new treatments. These diseases include a broad spectrum of autoimmune diseases such as rheumatoid arthritis, type I diabetes mellitus, systemic lupus erythematosus, and multiple sclerosis; solid tumors and hematologic malignancies; infectious diseases; asthma; and various allergic conditions. Furthermore, one of the great therapeutic opportunities for the treatment of many disorders is organ transplantation. However, immune system–mediated graft rejection remains the single greatest barrier to widespread use of this technology. An improved understanding of the immune system has led to the development of new therapies to treat immune system–mediated diseases.

This chapter briefly reviews drugs used to modulate the immune response in three ways: immunosuppression, tolerance, and immunostimulation. Four major classes of immunosuppressive drugs are discussed: glucocorticoids (*see* Chapter 59), calcineurin inhibitors, antiproliferative and antimetabolic agents (*see* Chapter 51), and antibodies. The "holy grail" of immunomodulation is the induction and maintenance of immune tolerance, the active state of antigen-specific nonresponsiveness. Approaches expected to overcome the risks of infections and tumors with immunosuppression are reviewed. These include costimulatory blockade, donor-cell chimerism, soluble human leukocyte antigens (HLA), and antigen-based therapies. A general discussion of the limited number of immunostimulant agents is presented, followed by an overview of active and passive immunization, and concluding with a brief case study of immunotherapy for multiple sclerosis.

IMMUNOSUPPRESSION

Immunosuppressive drugs are used to dampen the immune response in organ transplantation and autoimmune disease. In transplantation, the major classes of immunosuppressive drugs used today are: (1) *glucocorticoids,* (2) *calcineurin inhibitors,* (3) *antiproliferative/antimetabolic agents,* and (4) *biologics (antibodies).* These drugs have met with a high degree of clinical success in treating conditions such as acute immune rejection of organ transplants and severe autoimmune diseases. However, such therapies require lifelong use and nonspecifically suppress the entire immune system, exposing patients to considerably higher risks of infection and cancer. The calcineurin inhibitors and glucocorticoids, in particular, are nephrotoxic and diabetogenic,

respectively, thus restricting their usefulness in a variety of clinical settings.

Monoclonal and polyclonal antibody preparations directed at reactive T cells are important adjunct therapies and provide a unique opportunity to target specifically immune-reactive cells. Finally, newer small molecules and antibodies have expanded the arsenal of immunosuppressives. In particular, mTOR (*mammalian target of rapamycin*) inhibitors (*sirolimus, everolimus*) and anti-CD25 [interleukin (IL)-2 receptor] antibodies (*basiliximab, daclizumab*) target growth factor pathways, substantially limiting clonal expansion and thus potentially promoting tolerance. Immunosuppressive drugs used more commonly today are described below. Many more selective therapeutic agents under development are expected to revolutionize immunotherapy in the next decade.

General Approach to Organ Transplantation Therapy

Organ transplant therapy is organized around five general principles. The first principle is careful patient preparation and selection of the best available ABO blood type–compatible HLA match for organ donation. Second, a multitiered approach to immunosuppressive drug therapy, similar to that in cancer chemotherapy, is employed. Several agents are used simultaneously, each of which is directed at a different molecular target within the allograft response (Table 52–1; Hong and Kahan, 2000a). Synergistic effects permit use of the various agents at relatively low doses, thereby limiting specific toxicities while maximizing the immunosuppressive effect. The third principle is that greater immunosuppression is required to gain early engraftment and/or to treat established rejection than to maintain long-term immunosuppression. Therefore, intensive induction and lower-dose maintenance drug protocols are employed. Fourth, careful investigation of each episode of transplant dysfunction is required, including evaluation for rejection, drug toxicity, and infection, keeping in mind that these various problems can and often do coexist. Organ-specific problems (*e.g.,* obstruction in the case of kidney transplants) must also be considered. The fifth principle, which is common to all drugs, is that a drug should be reduced or withdrawn if its toxicity exceeds its benefit.

Biologic Induction Therapy. Induction therapy with polyclonal and monoclonal antibodies (mAbs) has been an important component of immunosuppression dating back to the 1960s, when Starzl and colleagues demonstrated the beneficial effect of antilymphocyte globulin (ALG) in the prophylaxis of rejection in renal transplant recipients. Over the past 40 years, several polyclonal antilymphocyte preparations have been used in renal transplantation; however, only 2 preparations are currently FDA approved: *lymphocyte immune globulin* (ATGAM) and *antithymocyte globulin* (THYMOGLOBULIN) (Howard *et al.,* 1997; Monaco, 1999). Another important milestone in biologic therapy was the development of mAbs and the introduction of the murine anti-CD3 mAb (*muromonab-CD3* or OKT3) (Ortho Multicenter Transplant Study Group, 1985).

In many transplant centers, induction therapy with biologic agents is used to delay the use of the nephrotoxic calcineurin inhibitors or to intensify the initial immunosuppressive therapy in patients at high risk of rejection (*i.e.,* repeat transplants, broadly presensi-

Table 52–1
Sites of Action of Selected Immunosuppressive Agents on T-Cell Activation

DRUG	SITE OF ACTION
Glucocorticoids	Glucocorticoid response elements in DNA (regulate gene transcription)
Muromonab-CD3	T-cell receptor complex (blocks antigen recognition)
Cyclosporine	Calcineurin (inhibits phosphatase activity)
Tacrolimus	Calcineurin (inhibits phosphatase activity)
Azathioprine	Deoxyribonucleic acid (false nucleotide incorporation)
Mycophenolate Mofetil	Inosine monophosphate dehydrogenase (inhibits activity)
Daclizumab, Basiliximab	IL-2 receptor (block IL-2–mediated T-cell activation)
Sirolimus	Protein kinase involved in cell-cycle progression (mTOR) (inhibits activity)

tized patients, African-American patients, or pediatric patients). Most of the limitations of murine-based mAbs generally were overcome by the introduction of chimeric or humanized mAbs that lack antigenicity and have prolonged serum half-lives. The anti–interleukin-2 receptor (IL-2R) mAbs (frequently referred to as anti-CD25) were the first biologics proven to be effective as induction agents in randomized double-blind prospective trials (Vincenti *et al.*, 1998; Nashan *et al.*, 1997; Nashan *et al.*, 1999; Kahan *et al.*, 1999b).

Biologic agents for induction therapy in the prophylaxis of rejection currently are used in approximately 70% of *de novo* transplant patients and have been propelled by several factors, including the introduction of the safe anti–IL-2R antibodies and the emergence of antithymocyte globulin as a safer and more effective alternative to lymphocyte immune globulin or muromonab-CD3 mAb. Biologics for induction can be divided into 2 groups: the depleting agents and the immune modulators. The depleting agents consist of lymphocyte immune globulin, antithymocyte globulin, and muromonab-CD3 mAb (the latter also produces immune modulation); their efficacy derives from their ability to deplete the recipient's CD3-positive cells at the time of transplantation and antigen presentation. The second group of biologic agents, the anti–IL-2R mAbs, do not deplete T lymphocytes, but rather block IL-2–mediated T-cell activation by binding to the α chain of IL-2R.

For patients with high levels of anti-HLA antibodies, humoral rejection mediated by B cells can be modified by plasmapheresis, usually given every other day for 4 to 5 treatments followed by intravenous immunoglobulin to suppress antibody production (Akalin *et al.*, 2003; Zachary *et al.*, 2003).

Maintenance Immunotherapy. The basic immunosuppressive protocols in most transplant centers use multiple drugs simultaneously.

Therapy typically involves a calcineurin inhibitor, glucocorticoids, and mycophenolate mofetil (a purine metabolism inhibitor; *see* below), each directed at a discrete site in T-cell activation (Suthanthiran *et al.*, 1996; Perico and Remuzzi, 1997). Glucocorticoids, azathioprine, cyclosporine, tacrolimus, mycophenolate mofetil, sirolimus, and various monoclonal and polyclonal antibodies are all approved for use in transplantation. Glucocorticoid-free regimens have achieved special prominence in recent successes in using pancreatic islet transplants to treat patients with type I diabetes mellitus. Protocols employing steroid withdrawal or steroid avoidance are being evaluated in many transplant centers. Short-term results are good, but the effects on long-term graft function are unknown (Hricik *et al.*, 2003). Recent data suggest that calcineurin inhibitors may shorten graft half-life by their nephrotoxic effects (Ojo *et al.*, 2003; Colvin, 2003). Protocols under evaluation include calcineurin dose reduction or switching from calcineurin to sirolimus-based immunosuppressive therapy at 3 to 4 months (Oberbauer *et al.*, 2003).

Therapy for Established Rejection. Although low doses of prednisone, calcineurin inhibitors, purine metabolism inhibitors, or sirolimus are effective in preventing acute cellular rejection, they are less effective in blocking activated T lymphocytes, and thus are not very effective against established, acute rejection or for the total prevention of chronic rejection (Monaco *et al.*, 1999). Therefore, treatment of established rejection requires the use of agents directed against activated T cells. These include glucocorticoids in high doses (pulse therapy), polyclonal antilymphocyte antibodies, or muromonab-CD3 mAb.

Adrenocortical Steroids

The introduction of glucocorticoids as immunosuppressive drugs in the 1960s played a key role in making organ transplantation possible. Their chemistry, pharmacokinetics, and drug interactions are described in Chapter 59. Prednisone, prednisolone, and other glucocorticoids are used alone and in combination with other immunosuppressive agents for treatment of transplant rejection and autoimmune disorders.

Mechanism of Action. The immunosuppressive effects of glucocorticoids have long been known, but the specific mechanism(s) of their immunosuppressive action remains somewhat elusive. Glucocorticoids lyse (in some species) and induce the redistribution of lymphocytes, causing a rapid, transient decrease in peripheral blood lymphocyte counts. To effect longer-term responses, steroids bind to receptors inside cells; either these receptors, glucocorticoid-induced proteins, or interacting proteins regulate the transcription of numerous other genes (*see* Chapter 59). Additionally, glucocorticoid-receptor complexes increase IκB expression, thereby curtailing activation of NF-κB, which increases apoptosis of activated cells (Auphan *et al.*, 1995). Of central importance, key proinflammatory cytokines such as IL-1 and IL-6 are downregulated. T cells are inhibited from making IL-2 and proliferating. The activation of cytotoxic T lymphocytes is inhibited. Neutrophils and monocytes display poor chemotaxis and decreased lysosomal enzyme release. Therefore, glucocorticoids have broad antiinflammatory effects on multiple components of cellular immunity. In contrast, they have relatively little effect on humoral immunity.

Therapeutic Uses. There are numerous indications for glucocorticoids (Zoorob and Cender, 1998). They commonly are combined with other immunosuppressive agents to prevent and treat transplant rejection. High dose pulses of intravenous *methylprednisolone sodium succinate* (SOLU-MEDROL, A-METHAPRED) are used to reverse acute transplant rejection and acute exacerbations of selected autoimmune disorders (Shinn *et al.*, 1999; Laan *et al.*, 1999). Glucocorticoids also are efficacious for treatment of graft-*versus*-host disease in bone-marrow transplantation. Glucocorticoids are used routinely to treat autoimmune disorders such as rheumatoid and other arthritides, systemic lupus erythematosus, systemic dermatomyositis, psoriasis and other skin conditions, asthma and other allergic disorders, inflammatory bowel disease, inflammatory ophthalmic diseases, autoimmune hematologic disorders, and acute exacerbations of multiple sclerosis (*see* below). In addition, glucocorticoids limit allergic reactions that occur with other immunosuppressive agents and are used in transplant recipients to block first-dose cytokine storm caused by treatment with muromonad-CD3 and to a lesser extent thymoglobulin (*see* below).

Toxicity. Unfortunately, the extensive use of steroids often results in disabling and life-threatening adverse effects. These effects include growth retardation in children, avascular necrosis of bone, osteopenia, increased risk of infection, poor wound healing, cataracts, hyperglycemia, and hypertension (*see* Chapter 59). The advent of combined glucocorticoid/cyclosporine regimens has allowed reduced doses of steroids, but steroid-induced morbidity remains a major problem in many transplant patients.

Calcineurin Inhibitors

Perhaps the most effective immunosuppressive drugs in routine use are the calcineurin inhibitors, *cyclosporine* and *tacrolimus,* which target intracellular signaling pathways induced as a consequence of T-cell–receptor activation (Schreiber and Crabtree, 1992). Although they are structurally unrelated (Figure 52–1) and bind to distinct, albeit related molecular targets, they inhibit normal T-cell signal transduction essentially by the same mechanism (Figure 52–2). Cyclosporine and tacrolimus do not act *per se* as immunosuppressive agents. Instead, these drugs bind to an immunophilin (cyclophilin for cyclosporine or FKBP-12 for tacrolimus), resulting in subsequent interaction with calcineurin to block its phosphatase activity. Calcineurin-catalyzed dephosphorylation is required for movement of a component of the nuclear factor of activated T lymphocytes (NFAT) into the nucleus (Figure 52–2).

NFAT, in turn, is required to induce a number of cytokine genes, including that for interleukin-2 (IL-2), a prototypic T-cell growth and differentiation factor.

Cyclosporine. *Chemistry.* Cyclosporine (cyclosporin A), a cyclic polypeptide consisting of 11 amino acids, is produced by the fungus species *Beauveria nivea*. Of note, all amide nitrogens are either hydrogen bonded or methylated, the single D-amino acid is at position 8, the methyl amide between residues 9 and 10 is in the *cis* configuration, and all other methyl amide moieties are in the *trans* form (Figure 52–1). Because cyclosporine is lipophilic and highly hydrophobic, it is formulated for clinical administration using castor oil or other strategies to ensure solubilization.

Mechanism of Action. Cyclosporine suppresses some humoral immunity, but is more effective against T-cell–dependent immune mechanisms such as those underlying transplant rejection and some forms of autoimmunity (Kahan, 1989). It preferentially inhibits antigen-triggered signal transduction in T lymphocytes, blunting expression of many lymphokines including IL-2, and the expression of antiapoptotic proteins. Cyclosporine forms a complex with cyclophilin, a cytoplasmic receptor protein present in target cells. This complex binds to calcineurin, inhibiting Ca^{2+}-stimulated dephosphorylation of the cytosolic component of NFAT (Schreiber and Crabtree, 1992). When cytoplasmic NFAT is dephosphorylated, it translocates to the nucleus and complexes with nuclear components required for complete T-cell activation, including transactivation of IL-2 and other lymphokine genes. Calcineurin phosphatase activity is inhibited after physical interaction with the cyclosporine/cyclophilin complex. This prevents NFAT dephosphorylation such that NFAT does not enter the nucleus, gene transcription is not activated, and the T lymphocyte fails to respond to specific antigenic stimulation. Cyclosporine also increases expression of transforming growth factor-β (TGF-β), a potent inhibitor of IL-2–stimulated T-cell proliferation and generation of cytotoxic T lymphocytes (CTL) (Khanna *et al.*, 1994).

Disposition and Pharmacokinetics. Cyclosporine can be administered intravenously or orally. The intravenous preparation (SANDIMMUNE Injection) is provided as a solution in an ethanol-polyoxyethylated castor oil vehicle that must be further diluted in 0.9% sodium chloride solution or 5% dextrose solution before injection. The oral dosage forms include soft gelatin capsules and oral solutions. Cyclosporine supplied in the original soft gelatin capsule (SANDIMMUNE) is absorbed slowly with 20% to 50% bioavailability. A modified microemulsion formulation (NEORAL) is available (Noble and Markham, 1995). It has more uniform and slightly increased bioavailability compared to SANDIMMUNE and is provided as 25-mg and 100-mg soft gelatin capsules and a 100-mg/ml oral solution. Since SANDIMMUNE and NEORAL are not bioequivalent, they cannot be used interchangeably without supervision by a physician and monitoring of drug concentrations in plasma. Comparison of blood concentrations in published literature and in clinical practice must be performed with a detailed knowledge of the assay system employed.

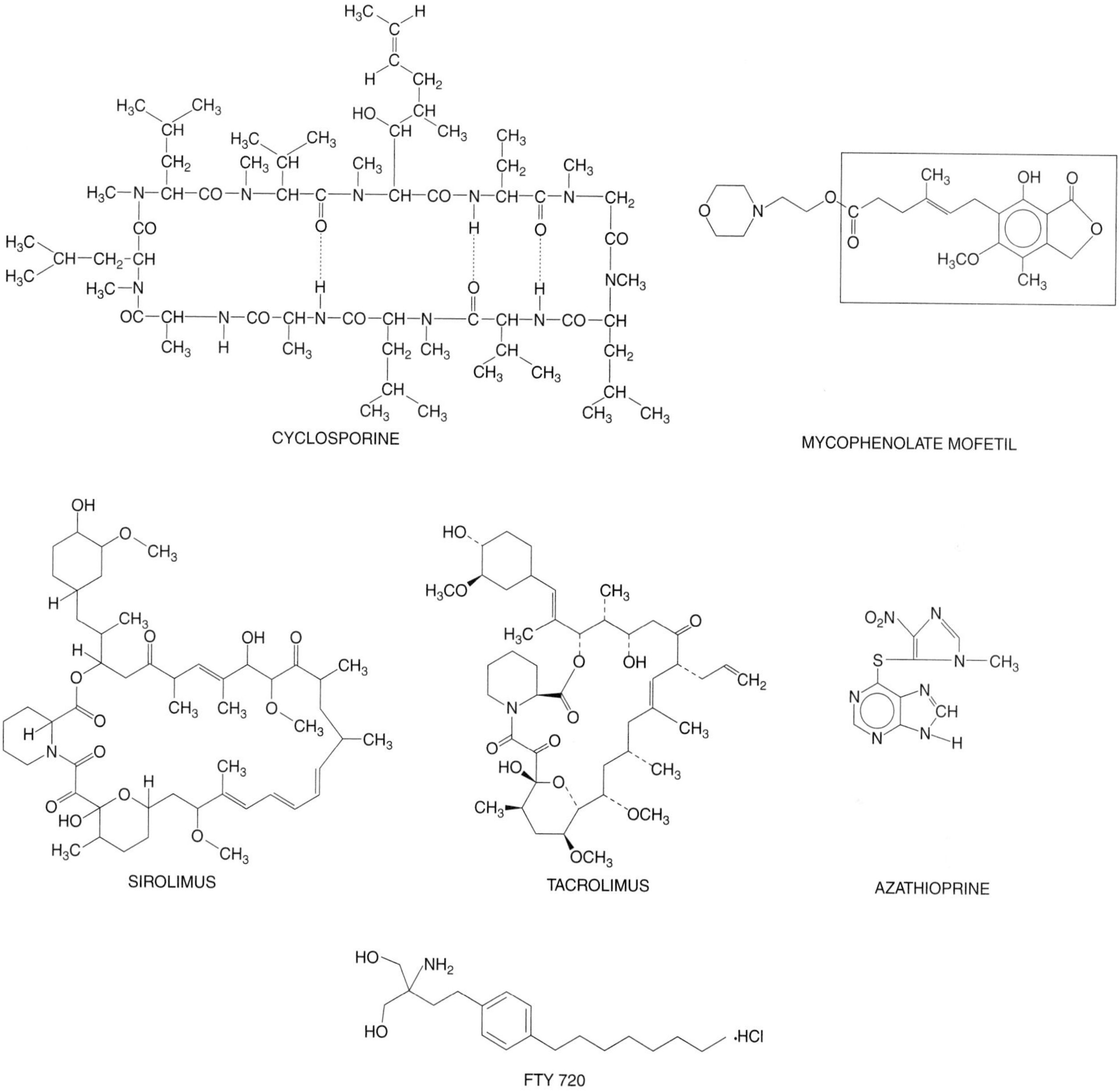

Figure 52–1. *Chemical structures of immunosuppressive drugs: azathioprine, mycophenolate mofetil, cyclosporine, tacrolimus, and sirolimus.*

Generic preparations of both NEORAL and SANDIMMUNE are available that are bioequivalent by FDA criteria. The generic preparations for NEORAL have been shown to be bioequivalent in normal volunteers, and, in some studies, also in transplant recipients. A consensus conference held under the auspices of the American Society of Transplantation recommended that generic preparations of cyclosporine could be used *de novo* in transplantation to substitute for NEORAL (Alloway *et al.*, 2003). However, when switching between generic and NEORAL formulations, increased surveillance is recommended to ensure that drug levels remain in the therapeutic range. This need for increased monitoring is based on anecdotal experience rather than validated differences. In fact the generic preparations were comparable to NEORAL for immunosuppressive purposes in most studies. *Since* SANDIMMUNE *and* NEORAL *differ in terms of their pharmacokinetics and are definitely not bioequivalent, their generic versions cannot*

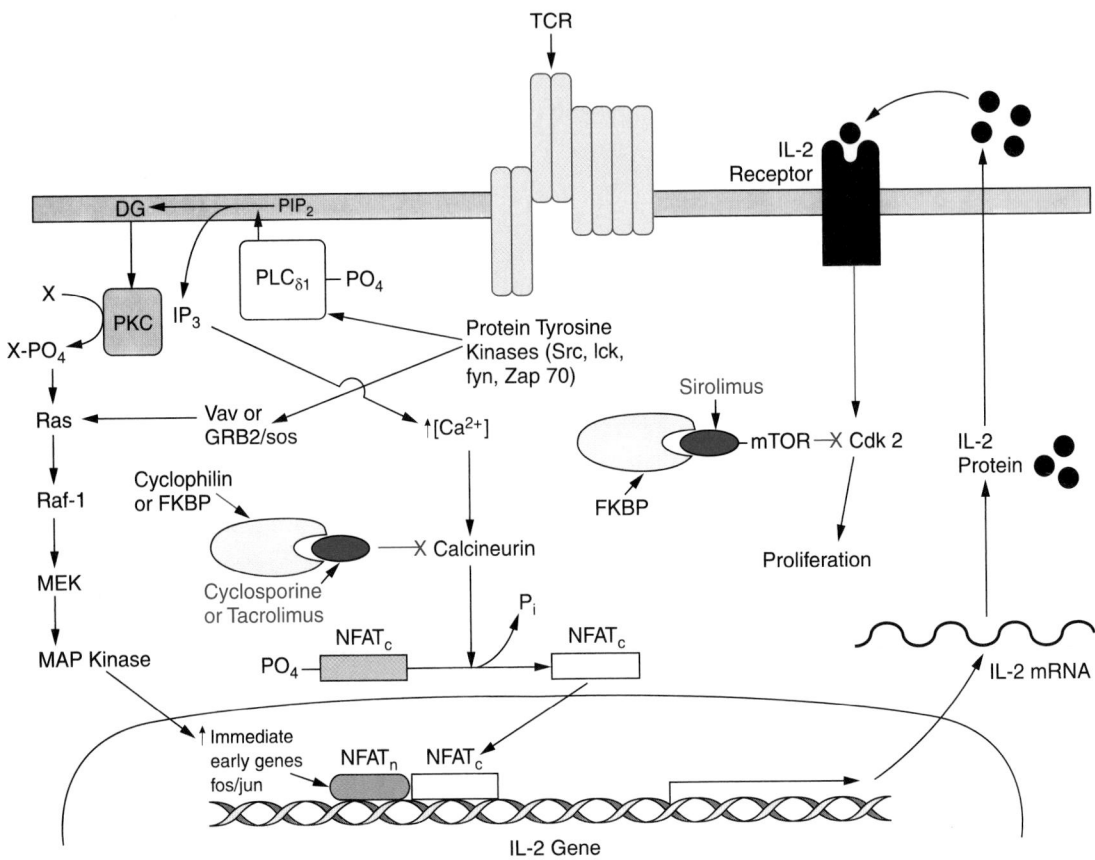

Figure 52–2. Mechanisms of action of cyclosporine, tacrolimus, and sirolimus on T cells. Both cyclosporine and tacrolimus bind to immunophilins (cyclophilin and FK506-binding protein [FKBP], respectively), forming a complex that binds the phosphatase calcineurin and inhibits the calcineurin-catalyzed dephosphorylation essential to permit movement of the nuclear factor of activated T cells (NFAT) into the nucleus. NFAT is required for transcription of interleukin-2 (IL-2) and other growth and differentiation–associated cytokines (lymphokines). Sirolimus (rapamycin) works at a later stage in T-cell activation, downstream of the IL-2 receptor. Sirolimus also binds FKBP, but the FKBP-sirolimus complex binds to and inhibits the mammalian target of rapamycin (mTOR), a kinase involved in cell-cycle progression (proliferation). TCR, T-cell receptor. (From Pattison *et al.*, 1997, with permission.)

be used interchangeably. This has been a source of confusion to pharmacists and patients. Transplant units need to educate patients that SANDIMMUNE and its generics are not the same as NEORAL and its generics, such that one preparation cannot be substituted for another without risk of inadequate immunosuppression or increased toxicity.

Both radioimmunoassays and high-performance liquid chromatography assays for cyclosporine and tacrolimus are available. Because these methods differ, the prescribing physician should ensure that the methods are consistent when monitoring an individual patient. Blood is most conveniently sampled before the next dose, namely a C_0 or trough level. While this is convenient, it has been shown repeatedly that C_0 concentrations do not reflect the area under the curve (AUC) for cyclosporine exposure in individual patients. As a practical solution to this problem and

to better measure the overall exposure of a patient to the drug, it has been proposed that levels be taken 2 hours after a dose administration, so-called C_2 levels (Cole *et al.*, 2003). Some studies have shown a better correlation of C_2 with the AUC, but no single time point can simulate the exposure as measured by more frequent drug sampling. In complex patients with delayed absorption, such as diabetics, the C_2 level may underestimate the peak cyclosporine level obtained, and in others who are rapid absorbers the C_2 level may have peaked before the blood sample is drawn. In practice if a patient has clinical signs or symptoms of toxicity, or there is unexplained rejection or renal dysfunction, a pharmacokinetic profile can be used to estimate that person's exposure to the drug. Many clinicians, particularly those caring for transplant patients some time after the transplant, monitor cyclosporine blood levels only when a clinical event (*e.g.*, renal dysfunction or rejection) occurs. In that setting, either a C_0 or C_2 level helps to ascertain whether inadequate immunosuppression or drug toxicity is present. As described above, cyclosporine absorption is incomplete following oral administration and varies with the individual patient and the formulation used. The elimination of cyclosporine from the blood is generally biphasic, with a terminal half-life of 5 to 18 hours (Faulds *et al.*, 1993; Noble and Markham, 1995). After intravenous infusion, clearance is approximately 5 to 7 ml/min per kg in adult recipients of renal transplants, but results differ by age and patient populations. For example, clearance is slower in cardiac transplant patients and more rapid in children. Thus, the intersubject variability is so large that individual monitoring is required (Faulds *et al.*, 1993; Noble and Markham, 1995).

After oral administration of cyclosporine (as NEORAL), the time to peak blood concentrations is 1.5 to 2 hours (Faulds *et al.*, 1993; Noble and Markham, 1995). Administration with food delays and decreases absorption. High- and low-fat meals consumed within 30 minutes of administration decrease the AUC by approximately 13% and the maximum concentration by 33%. This makes it imperative to individualize dosage regimens for outpatients.

Cyclosporine is distributed extensively outside the vascular compartment. After intravenous dosing, the steady-state volume of distribution is reportedly as high as 3 to 5 L/kg in solid-organ transplant recipients.

Only 0.1% of cyclosporine is excreted unchanged in urine (Faulds *et al.*, 1993). Cyclosporine is extensively metabolized in the liver by CYP3A and to a lesser degree by the gastrointestinal tract and kidneys (Fahr, 1993). At least 25 metabolites have been identified in human bile, feces, blood, and urine (Christians and Sewing, 1993). Although the cyclic peptide structure of cyclosporine is relatively resistant to metabolism, the side chains are extensively metabolized. All of the metabolites have reduced biological activity and toxicity compared to the parent drug. Cyclosporine and its metabolites are excreted principally through the bile into the feces, with only about 6% being excreted in the urine. Cyclosporine also is excreted in human milk. In the presence of hepatic dysfunction, dosage adjustments are required. No adjustments generally are necessary for dialysis or renal failure patients.

Therapeutic Uses. Clinical indications for cyclosporine are kidney, liver, heart, and other organ transplantation; rheumatoid arthritis; and psoriasis (Faulds *et al.*, 1993). Its use in dermatology is discussed in Chapter 62. Cyclosporine generally is recognized as the agent that ushered in the modern era of organ transplantation, increasing the rates of early engraftment, extending kidney graft survival, and making cardiac and liver transplantation possi-

ble. Cyclosporine usually is combined with other agents, especially glucocorticoids and either azathioprine or mycophenolate mofetil, and most recently, sirolimus. The dose of cyclosporine varies, depending on the organ transplanted and the other drugs used in the specific treatment protocol(s). The initial dose generally is not given before the transplant because of the concern about nephrotoxicity. Especially for renal transplant patients, therapeutic algorithms have been developed to delay cyclosporine introduction until a threshold renal function has been attained. The amount of the initial dose and reduction to maintenance dosing is sufficiently variable that no specific recommendation is provided here. Dosage is guided by signs of rejection (too low a dose), renal or other toxicity (too high a dose), and close monitoring of blood levels. Great care must be taken to differentiate renal toxicity from rejection in kidney transplant patients. Ultrasound-guided allograft biopsy is the best way to assess the reason for renal dysfunction. Because adverse reactions have been ascribed more frequently to the intravenous formulation, this route of administration is discontinued as soon as the patient is able to take the drug orally.

In rheumatoid arthritis, cyclosporine is used in severe cases that have not responded to *methotrexate*. Cyclosporine can be combined with methotrexate, but the levels of both drugs must be monitored closely (Baraldo *et al.*, 1999). In psoriasis, cyclosporine is indicated for treatment of adult immunocompetent patients with severe and disabling disease for whom other systemic therapies have failed (Linden and Weinstein, 1999). Because of its mechanism of action, there is a theoretical basis for the use of cyclosporine in a variety of other T-cell–mediated diseases (Faulds *et al.*, 1993). Cyclosporine reportedly is effective in Behçet's acute ocular syndrome, endogenous uveitis, atopic dermatitis, inflammatory bowel disease, and nephrotic syndrome, even when standard therapies have failed.

Toxicity. The principal adverse reactions to cyclosporine therapy are renal dysfunction, tremor, hirsutism, hypertension, hyperlipidemia, and gum hyperplasia (Burke *et al.*, 1994). Hyperuricemia may lead to worsening of gout, increased P-glycoprotein activity, and hypercholesterolemia. Nephrotoxicity occurs in the majority of patients treated and is the major indication for cessation or modification of therapy. Hypertension occurs in approximately 50% of renal transplant and almost all cardiac transplant patients. Combined use of calcineurin inhibitors and glucocorticoids is particularly diabetogenic, although this apparently is more problematic in patients treated with tacrolimus (*see* below). Especially at risk are obese patients, African-American or Hispanic recipients, or those with family history of type II diabetes or obesity. Cyclosporine, as opposed to tacrolimus, is more likely to produce elevations in LDL cholesterol (Artz *et al.*, 2003; Kramer *et al.*, 2003; Tanabe, 2003).

Drug Interactions. Cyclosporine interacts with a wide variety of commonly used drugs, and close attention must be paid to drug interactions. Any drug that affects microsomal enzymes, especially the CYP3A system, may impact cyclosporine blood concentrations (Faulds *et al.*, 1993). Substances that inhibit this enzyme can decrease cyclosporine metabolism and increase blood concentrations. These include Ca^{2+} channel blockers (*e.g., verapamil, nicardipine*), antifungal agents (*e.g., fluconazole, ketoconazole*), antibiotics (*e.g., erythromycin*), glucocorticoids (*e.g., methylprednisolone*), HIV-protease inhibitors (*e.g., indinavir*), and other drugs (*e.g., allopurinol, metoclopramide*). Grapefruit and grapefruit juice block CYP3A and the multidrug efflux pump and should be avoided by patients taking cyclosporine; these effects can increase cyclosporine blood concentrations. In contrast, drugs that induce CYP3A activity can increase cyclosporine metabolism and decrease blood concentrations. Such drugs include antibiotics (*e.g., nafcillin, rifampin*), anticonvulsants (*e.g., phenobarbital, phenytoin*), and other drugs (*e.g., octreotide, ticlopidine*). In general, close monitoring of cyclosporine blood levels and the levels of other drugs is required when such combinations are used.

Interactions between cyclosporine and sirolimus (*see* below) have led to the recommendation that administration of the two drugs be separated by time. Sirolimus aggravates cyclosporine-induced renal dysfunction, while cyclosporine increases sirolimus-induced hyperlipidemia and myelosuppression. Other drug interactions of concern include additive nephrotoxicity when cyclosporine is coadministered with nonsteroidal antiinflammatory drugs and other drugs that cause renal dysfunction; elevation of methotrexate levels when the two drugs are coadministered; and reduced clearance of other drugs, including *prednisolone, digoxin,* and statins.

Tacrolimus. Tacrolimus (PROGRAF, FK506) is a macrolide antibiotic produced by *Streptomyces tsukubaensis* (Goto *et al.*, 1987). Its formula is shown in Figure 52–1.

Mechanism of Action. Like cyclosporine, tacrolimus inhibits T-cell activation by inhibiting calcineurin (Schreiber and Crabtree, 1992). Tacrolimus binds to an intracellular protein, FK506-binding protein–12 (FKBP-12), an immunophilin structurally related to cyclophilin. A complex of tacrolimus-FKBP-12, Ca^{2+}, calmodulin, and calcineurin then forms, and calcineurin phosphatase activity is inhibited. As described for cyclosporine and depicted in Figure 52–2, the inhibition of phosphatase activity prevents dephosphorylation

and nuclear translocation of NFAT and inhibits T-cell activation. Thus, although the intracellular receptors differ, cyclosporine and tacrolimus target the same pathway for immunosuppression (Plosker and Foster, 2000).

Disposition and Pharmacokinetics. Tacrolimus is available for oral administration as capsules (0.5, 1, and 5 mg) and as a sterile solution for injection (5 mg/ml). Immunosuppressive activity resides primarily in the parent drug. Because of intersubject variability in pharmacokinetics, individualized dosing is required for optimal therapy (Fung and Starzl, 1995). Whole blood, rather than plasma, is the most appropriate sampling compartment to describe tacrolimus pharmacokinetics. For tacrolimus, the C_0 level seems to correlate better with clinical events than it does for cyclosporine. Target concentrations in many centers are 200 to 400 ng/ml in the early preoperative period and 100 to 200 ng/ml 3 months after transplantation. Unlike cyclosporine, more frequent tacrolimus dosing has not been formally evaluated. Gastrointestinal absorption is incomplete and variable. Food decreases the rate and extent of absorption. Plasma protein binding of tacrolimus is 75% to 99%, involving primarily albumin and α_1-acid glycoprotein. Its half-life is about 12 hours. Tacrolimus is extensively metabolized in the liver by CYP3A, with a half-life of ~12 hours; at least some of the metabolites are active. The bulk of excretion of the parent drug and metabolites is in the feces. Less than 1% of administered tacrolimus is excreted unchanged in the urine.

Therapeutic Uses. Tacrolimus is indicated for the prophylaxis of solid-organ allograft rejection in a manner similar to cyclosporine and as rescue therapy in patients with rejection episodes despite "therapeutic" levels of cyclosporine (Mayer *et al.*, 1997; The U.S. Multicenter FK506 Liver Study Group, 1994). The recommended starting dose for tacrolimus injection is 0.03 to 0.05 mg/kg per day as a continuous infusion. Recommended initial oral doses are 0.15 to 0.2 mg/kg per day for adult kidney transplant patients, 0.1 to 0.15 mg/kg per day for adult liver transplant patients, and 0.15 to 0.2 mg/kg per day for pediatric liver transplant patients in two divided doses 12 hours apart. These dosages are intended to achieve typical blood trough levels in the 5- to 15-ng/ml range. Pediatric patients generally require higher doses than do adults (Shapiro, 1998).

Toxicity. Nephrotoxicity, neurotoxicity (tremor, headache, motor disturbances, seizures), GI complaints, hypertension, hyperkalemia, hyperglycemia, and diabetes are all associated with tacrolimus use (Plosker and Foster, 2000). As with cyclosporine, nephrotoxicity is limiting (Mihatsch *et al.*, 1998; Henry, 1999). Tacrolimus has a negative effect on pancreatic islet beta cells, and glucose intolerance and diabetes mellitus are well-recognized complications of tacrolimus-based immunosuppression. As with other immunosuppressive agents, there is an increased risk of secondary tumors and opportunistic infections. Notably, tacrolimus does not adversely affect uric acid or LDL cholesterol.

Drug Interactions. Because of its potential for nephrotoxicity, tacrolimus blood levels and renal function should be monitored closely, especially when tacrolimus is used with other potentially nephrotoxic drugs. Coadministration with cyclosporine results in additive or synergistic nephrotoxicity; therefore a delay of at least 24 hours is required when switching a patient from cyclosporine to tacrolimus. Since tacrolimus is metabolized mainly by CYP3A, the potential interactions described above for cyclosporine also apply for tacrolimus (Venkataramanan *et al.*, 1995; Yoshimura *et al.*, 1999).

Antiproliferative and Antimetabolic Drugs

Sirolimus. Sirolimus (*rapamycin*; RAPAMUNE) is a macrocyclic lactone produced by *Streptomyces hygroscopicus* (Vezina *et al.*, 1975). Its structure is shown in Figure 52–1.

Mechanism of Action. Sirolimus inhibits T-lymphocyte activation and proliferation downstream of the IL-2 and other T-cell growth factor receptors (Figure 52–2) (Kuo *et al.*, 1992). Like cyclosporine and tacrolimus, therapeutic action of sirolimus requires formation of a complex with an immunophilin, in this case FKBP-12. However, the sirolimus–FKBP-12 complex does not affect calcineurin activity. It binds to and inhibits a protein kinase, designated *mammalian target of rapamycin* (mTOR), which is a key enzyme in cell-cycle progression (Brown *et al.*, 1994). Inhibition of mTOR blocks cell-cycle progression at the $G_1 \rightarrow S$ phase transition. In animal models, sirolimus not only inhibits transplant rejection, graft-*versus*-host disease, and a variety of autoimmune diseases, but its effect also lasts several months after discontinuing therapy, suggesting a tolerizing effect (*see* Tolerance, below; Groth *et al.*, 1999). A newer indication for sirolimus is the avoidance of calcineurin inhibitors, even when patients are stable, to protect kidney function (Stegall *et al.*, 2003).

Disposition and Pharmacokinetics. After oral administration, sirolimus is absorbed rapidly and reaches a peak blood concentration within about 1 hour after a single dose in healthy subjects and within about 2 hours after multiple oral doses in renal transplant patients (Napoli and Kahan, 1996; Zimmerman and Kahan, 1997). Systemic availability is approximately 15%, and blood concentrations are proportional to doses between 3 and 12 mg/m^2. A high-fat meal decreases peak blood concentration by 34%; sirolimus therefore should be taken consistently either with or without food, and blood levels should be monitored closely. About 40% of sirolimus in plasma is protein bound, especially to albumin. The drug partitions into formed elements of blood, with a blood-to-plasma ratio of 38 in renal transplant patients. Sirolimus is extensively metabolized by CYP3A4 and is transported by P-glycoprotein. Seven major metabolites have been identified in whole blood (Salm *et al.*, 1999). Metabolites also are detectable in feces and urine, with the bulk of total excretion being in feces. Although some of its metabolites are active, sirolimus itself is the major active component in whole blood and contributes more than 90% of the immunosuppressive effect. The blood half-life after multiple doses in stable renal transplant patients is 62 hours (Napoli and Kahan, 1996; Zimmerman and Kahan, 1997). A loading dose of three times the maintenance dose will provide nearly steady-state concentrations within 1 day in most patients.

Therapeutic Uses. Sirolimus is indicated for prophylaxis of organ transplant rejection in combination with a calcineurin inhibitor and glucocorticoids (Kahan *et al.*,

1999a). In patients experiencing or at high risk for calcineurin inhibitor–associated nephrotoxicity, sirolimus has been used with glucocorticoids and mycophenolate mofetil to avoid permanent renal damage. The initial dosage in patients 13 years or older who weigh less than 40 kg should be adjusted based on body surface area (1 mg/m^2 per day) with a loading dose of 3 mg/m^2. Data regarding doses for pediatric and geriatric patients are lacking at this time (Kahan, 1999). It is recommended that the maintenance dose be reduced by approximately one-third in patients with hepatic impairment (Watson *et al.*, 1999). Sirolimus also has been incorporated into stents to inhibit local cell proliferation and blood vessel occlusion.

Toxicity. The use of sirolimus in renal transplant patients is associated with a dose-dependent increase in serum cholesterol and triglycerides that may require treatment (Murgia *et al.*, 1996). While immunotherapy with sirolimus *per se* is not nephrotoxic, patients treated with cyclosporine plus sirolimus have impaired renal function compared to patients treated with cyclosporine and either *azathioprine* or placebo. Sirolimus also may prolong delayed graft function in deceased donor kidney transplants, presumably because of its antiproliferative action (Smith *et al.*, 2003; McTaggart *et al.*, 2003). Renal function therefore must be monitored closely in such patients. Lymphocele, a known surgical complication associated with renal transplantation, is increased in a dose-dependent fashion by sirolimus, requiring close postoperative follow-up. Other adverse effects include anemia, leukopenia, thrombocytopenia (Hong and Kahan, 2000b), hypokalemia or hyperkalemia, fever, and gastrointestinal effects. Delayed wound healing may occur with sirolimus use. As with other immunosuppressive agents, there is an increased risk of neoplasms, especially lymphomas, and infections. Prophylaxis for *Pneumocystis carinii* pneumonia and cytomegalovirus is recommended (Groth *et al.*, 1999).

Drug Interactions. Since sirolimus is a substrate for CYP3A4 and is transported by P-glycoprotein, close attention to interactions with other drugs that are metabolized or transported by these proteins is required (Yoshimura *et al.*, 1999). As noted above, cyclosporine and sirolimus interact, and their administration should be separated by time. Dose adjustment may be required when sirolimus is coadministered with *diltiazem* or rifampin. The combination of sirolimus plus tacrolimus probably is more nephrotoxic than cyclosporine plus sirolimus. Dose adjustment apparently is not required when sirolimus is coadministered with *acyclovir*, digoxin, *glyburide*, *nifedipine*, *norgestrel/ethinyl estradiol*, prednisolone, or *trimethoprim-sulfamethoxazole*. This list is incomplete, and blood levels and potential drug interactions must be monitored closely.

Everolimus. Everolimus (40-*0*-[2-hydroxy] ethyl-rapamycin) is closely related chemically and clinically to sirolimus but has distinct pharmacokinetics. The main difference is a shorter half-life and thus a shorter time to achieve steady-state concentrations of the drug. Dosage on a milligram per kilogram basis is similar to sirolimus. Aside from the shorter half-life, no studies have compared everolimus with sirolimus in standard immunosuppressive regimens (Eisen *et al.*, 2003). As with sirolimus, the combination of a calcineurin inhibitor and an mTOR inhibitor produces worse renal function at 1 year than does calcineurin inhibitor therapy alone, suggesting a drug interaction between the mTOR inhibitors and the calcineurin inhibitors to enhance toxicity and to reduce rejection. The toxicity of everolimus and the drug interactions reported to date seem to be the same as with sirolimus.

Azathioprine. Azathioprine (IMURAN) is a purine antimetabolite. It is an imidazolyl derivative of 6-mercaptopurine (Figure 52–1).

Mechanism of Action. Following exposure to nucleophiles such as glutathione, azathioprine is cleaved to 6-mercaptopurine, which in turn is converted to additional metabolites that inhibit *de novo* purine synthesis (*see* Chapter 51). 6-Thio-IMP, a fraudulent nucleotide, is converted to 6-thio-GMP and finally to 6-thio-GTP, which is incorporated into DNA. Cell proliferation is thereby inhibited, impairing a variety of lymphocyte functions. Azathioprine appears to be a more potent immunosuppressive agent than 6-mercaptopurine, which may reflect differences in drug uptake or pharmacokinetic differences in the resulting metabolites.

Disposition and Pharmacokinetics. Azathioprine is well absorbed orally and reaches maximum blood levels within 1 to 2 hours after administration. The half-life of azathioprine is about 10 minutes, while that of its metabolite 6-mercaptopurine is about an hour. Other metabolites have half-lives of up to 5 hours. Blood levels have limited predictive value because of extensive metabolism, significant activity of many different metabolites, and high tissue levels attained. Azathioprine and *mercaptopurine* are moderately bound to plasma proteins and are partially dialyzable. Both are rapidly removed from the blood by oxidation or methylation in the liver and/or erythrocytes. Renal clearance has little impact on biological effectiveness or toxicity, but the dose should be reduced in patients with renal failure.

Therapeutic Uses. Azathioprine was first introduced as an immunosuppressive agent in 1961, helping to make allogeneic kidney transplantation possible. It is indicated as an adjunct for prevention of organ transplant rejection and in severe rheumatoid arthritis (Hong and Kahan,

2000a; Gaffney and Scott, 1998). Although the dose of azathioprine required to prevent organ rejection and minimize toxicity varies, 3 to 5 mg/kg per day is the usual starting dose. Lower initial doses (1 mg/kg per day) are used in treating rheumatoid arthritis. Complete blood count and liver function tests should be monitored.

Toxicity. The major side effect of azathioprine is bone marrow suppression, including leukopenia (common), thrombocytopenia (less common), and/or anemia (uncommon). Other important adverse effects include increased susceptibility to infections (especially varicella and herpes simplex viruses), hepatotoxicity, alopecia, GI toxicity, pancreatitis, and increased risk of neoplasia.

Drug Interactions. Xanthine oxidase, an enzyme of major importance in the catabolism of azathioprine metabolites, is blocked by allopurinol. If azathioprine and allopurinol are used concurrently, the azathioprine dose must be decreased to 25% to 33% of the usual dose; it is best not to use these two drugs together. Adverse effects resulting from coadministration of azathioprine with other myelosuppressive agents or angiotensin-converting enzyme inhibitors include leukopenia, thrombocytopenia, and anemia as a result of myelosuppression.

Mycophenolate Mofetil. Mycophenolate mofetil (CELL-CEPT) is the 2-morpholinoethyl ester of mycophenolic acid (MPA) (Allison and Eugui, 1993). Its structure is shown in Figure 52–1.

Mechanism of Action. Mycophenolate mofetil is a prodrug that is rapidly hydrolyzed to the active drug, mycophenolic acid (MPA), a selective, noncompetitive, and reversible inhibitor of inosine monophosphate dehydrogenase (IMPDH) (Natsumeda and Carr, 1993), an important enzyme in the *de novo* pathway of guanine nucleotide synthesis. B and T lymphocytes are highly dependent on this pathway for cell proliferation, while other cell types can use salvage pathways; MPA therefore selectively inhibits lymphocyte proliferation and functions, including antibody formation, cellular adhesion, and migration.

Disposition and Pharmacokinetics. Mycophenolate mofetil undergoes rapid and complete metabolism to MPA after oral or intravenous administration. MPA, in turn, is metabolized to the inactive phenolic glucuronide MPAG. The parent drug is cleared from the blood within a few minutes. The half-life of MPA is about 16 hours. Negligible (<1%) amounts of MPA are excreted in the urine (Bardsley-Elliot *et al.*, 1999). Most (87%) is excreted in the urine as MPAG. Plasma concentrations of MPA and MPAG are increased in patients with renal insufficiency. In early renal transplant patients (<40 days posttransplant), plasma concentrations of MPA after a single dose of mycophenolate mofetil are about half of those found in healthy volunteers or stable renal transplant patients. Studies in children are limited, and safety and effectiveness have not been established (Butani *et al.*, 1999).

Therapeutic Uses. Mycophenolate mofetil is indicated for prophylaxis of transplant rejection, and it typically is used in combination with glucocorticoids and a calcineurin inhibitor, but not with azathioprine (Kimball *et al.*, 1995; Ahsan *et al.*, 1999; Kreis *et al.*, 2000). Combined treatment with sirolimus is possible, although potential drug interactions necessitate careful monitoring of drug levels. For renal transplants, 1 g is administered orally or intravenously (over 2 hours) twice daily (2 g per day). A higher dose, 1.5 g twice daily (3 g per day), is recommended for African-American renal transplant patients and all cardiac transplant patients. Use of mycophenolate mofetil in other clinical settings is under investigation.

Toxicity. The principal toxicities of mycophenolate mofetil are gastrointestinal and hematologic (Fulton and Markham, 1996; Bardsley-Elliot *et al.*, 1999). These include leukopenia, diarrhea, and vomiting. There also is an increased incidence of some infections, especially sepsis associated with cytomegalovirus. Tacrolimus in combination with mycophenolate mofetil has been associated with devastating viral infections including polyoma nephritis (Zavos *et al.*, 2004; Elli *et al.*, 2002).

Drug Interactions. Potential drug interactions between mycophenolate mofetil and several other drugs commonly used by transplant patients have been studied (Bardsley-Elliot *et al.*, 1999). There appear to be no untoward effects produced by combination therapy with cyclosporine, trimethoprim-sulfamethoxazole, or oral contraceptives. Unlike cyclosporine, tacrolimus delays elimination of mycophenolate mofetil by impairing the conversion of MPA to MPAG. This may enhance GI toxicity. Mycophenolate mofetil has not been tested with azathioprine. Coadministration with antacids containing aluminum or magnesium hydroxide leads to decreased absorption of mycophenolate mofetil; thus, these drugs should not be administered simultaneously. Mycophenolate mofetil should not be administered with *cholestyramine* or other drugs that affect enterohepatic circulation. Such agents decrease plasma MPA concentrations, probably by binding free MPA in the intestines. Acyclovir and *ganciclovir* may compete with MPAG for tubular secretion, possibly resulting in increased concentrations of both MPAG and the antiviral agents in the blood, an effect that may be compounded in patients with renal insufficiency.

Other Antiproliferative and Cytotoxic Agents. Many of the cytotoxic and antimetabolic agents used in cancer chemotherapy (*see* Chapter 51) are immunosuppressive due to their action on lymphocytes and other cells of the immune system. Other cytotoxic drugs that have been used as immunosuppressive agents include methotrexate, *cyclophosphamide* (CYTOXAN), *thalidomide,* and *chlorambucil* (LEUKERAN). Methotrexate is used for treatment of graft-*versus*-host disease, rheumatoid arthritis, and psoriasis, as well as in anticancer therapy (*see* Chapter 51) (Grosflam and Weinblatt, 1991). Cyclophosphamide and chlorambucil are used in treating childhood nephrotic syndrome (Neuhaus *et al.*, 1994) and a variety of malignancies (*see* Chapter 51). Cyclophosphamide also is used widely for treatment of severe systemic lupus erythematosus (Valeri *et al.*, 1994) and other vasculitides such as Wegener's granulomatosis. *Leflunomide* (ARAVA) is a pyrimidine-synthesis inhibitor indicated for the treatment of adults with rheumatoid arthritis (Prakash and Jarvis, 1999). This drug has found utility in the treatment of polyomavirus nephropathy seen in immunosuppressed renal transplant recipients and is increasingly being used for that purpose. There are no studies showing efficacy, however, compared with control patients treated with withdrawal or reduction of immunosuppression alone in BK virus nephropathy. The drug inhibits dihydroorotate dehydrogenase in the *de novo* pathway of pyrimidine synthesis. It is hepatotoxic and can cause fetal injury when administered to pregnant women.

FTY720

FTY720 (*see* Figure 52-1), an S1P receptor prodrug, is the first agent in a new class of small molecules, sphingosine 1-phosphate receptor (S1P-R) agonists, which reduce recirculation of lymphocytes from the lymphatic system to the blood and peripheral tissues, including inflammatory lesions and organ grafts.

Therapeutic Uses. FTY720 may have an important role in combination immunosuppression therapy in the prevention of acute rejection. FTY720 is not effective as monotherapy; it has demonstrated efficacy in clinical trials with cyclosporine and *prednisone* or in combination with the mTOR inhibitor everolimus and steroids. In Phase II trials with cyclosporine, FTY720 at daily doses of 2.5 and 5 mg showed comparable efficacy in the prevention of acute rejection in *de novo* renal transplant patients when compared to immunosuppression with cyclosporine, mycophenolate mofetil, and prednisone. FTY720 now is in Phase III trials.

Mechanism of Action. Unlike other immunosuppressive agents, FTY720 acts *via* "lymphocyte homing." It specifically and reversibly sequesters host lymphocytes into the lymph nodes and Peyer's patches, and thus away from the circulation. This protects the graft from T-cell–mediated attack. FTY720 sequesters lymphocytes but does not impair either T or B cell functions. FTY720 is phosphorylated by sphingosine kinase-2 and the FTY720-phosphate product is a potent agonist of S1P receptors. Altered lymphocyte traffic induced by FTY720 clearly results from its effect on S1P receptors.

Toxicity. Lymphopenia, the most common side effect of FTY720, is predicted from its pharmacologic effect and is fully reversible upon drug discontinuation. Of greater concern is the negative chronotropic effect of FTY720 on the heart, which has been observed with the first dose of FTY720 in up to 30% of patients. In most patients, the heart rate returns to baseline within 48 hours after the administration of the first dose of FTY720, with the remainder returning to baseline thereafter. The negative chronotropic effect of FTY720 likely is related to the presence of S1P-R on human atrial myocytes, thus affecting S1P signaling pathways. This effect can be functionally antagonized by β_1-receptor agonists or by the muscarinic receptor antagonist *atropine*. Importantly, cardiac rhythm was not affected in patients treated chronically with FTY720; however, the safety of the first-dose response of FTY720 on the heart rate in patients with underlying coronary artery disease remains to be determined.

Antibodies

Both polyclonal and monoclonal antibodies against lymphocyte cell-surface antigens are widely used for preven-

tion and treatment of organ transplant rejection. Polyclonal antisera are generated by repeated injections of human thymocytes (antithymocyte globulin, ATG) or lymphocytes (antilymphocyte globulin, ALG) into animals such as horses, rabbits, sheep, or goats, and then purifying the serum immunoglobulin fraction. Although highly effective immunosuppressive agents, these preparations vary in efficacy and toxicity from batch to batch. The advent of hybridoma technology to produce monoclonal antibodies was a major advance in immunology (Kohler and Milstein, 1975). It is now possible to make essentially unlimited amounts of a single antibody of a defined specificity (Figure 52–3). These monoclonal reagents have overcome the problems of variability in efficacy and toxicity seen with the polyclonal products, but they are more limited in their target specificity. The first-generation murine monoclonal antibodies have been replaced by newer chimeric or humanized monoclonal antibodies that lack antigenicity, have prolonged half-lives, and can be mutagenized to alter their affinity to Fc receptors. Thus, both polyclonal and monoclonal products have a place in immunosuppressive therapy.

Antithymocyte Globulin. Antithymocyte globulin is a purified gamma globulin from the serum of rabbits immu-

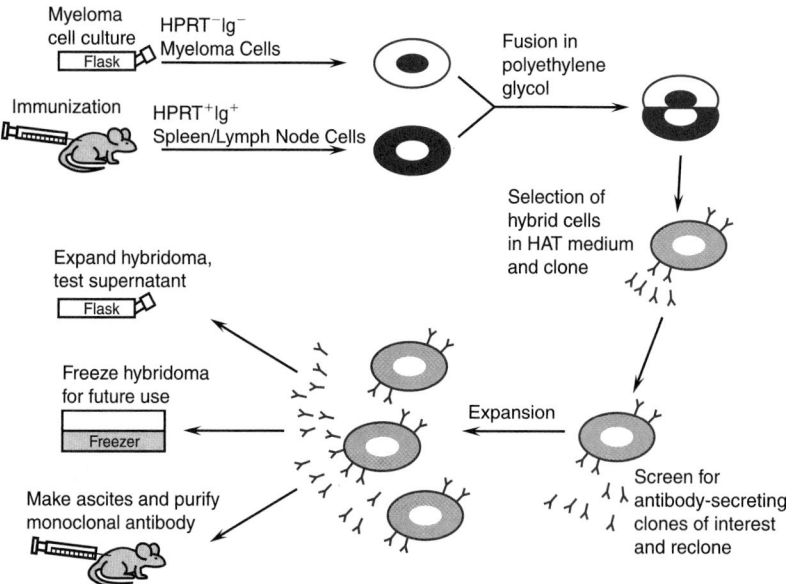

Figure 52–3. *Generation of monoclonal antibodies.* Mice are immunized with the selected antigen, and spleen or lymph node is harvested and B cells separated. These B cells are fused to a suitable B-cell myeloma that has been selected for its inability to grow in medium supplemented with hypoxanthine, aminopterin, and thymidine (HAT). Only myelomas that fuse with B cells can survive in HAT-supplemented medium. The hybridomas expand in culture. Those of interest based upon a specific screening technique are then selected and cloned by limiting dilution. Monoclonal antibodies can be used directly as supernatants or ascites fluid experimentally but are purified for clinical use. HPRT, hypoxanthine-guanine phosphoribosyl transferase. (From Krensky, 1999, with permission.)

nized with human thymocytes (Regan *et al.*, 1999). It is provided as a sterile, freeze-dried product for intravenous administration after reconstitution with sterile water.

Mechanism of Action. Antithymocyte globulin contains cytotoxic antibodies that bind to CD2, CD3, CD4, CD8, CD11a, CD18, CD25, CD44, CD45, and HLA class I and II molecules on the surface of human T lymphocytes (Bourdage and Hamlin, 1995). The antibodies deplete circulating lymphocytes by direct cytotoxicity (both complement and cell-mediated) and block lymphocyte function by binding to cell surface molecules involved in the regulation of cell function.

Therapeutic Uses. Antithymocyte globulin is used for induction immunosuppression, although the only approved indication is in the treatment of acute renal transplant rejection in combination with other immunosuppressive agents (Mariat *et al.*, 1998). Antilymphocyte-depleting agents (THYMOGLOBULIN, ATGAM, and OKT3) have been neither rigorously tested in clinical trials nor registered for use as induction immunosuppression. However, a meta-analysis (Szczech *et al.*, 1997) showed that antilymphocyte induction improves graft survival. A course of antithymocyte-globulin treatment often is given to renal transplant patients with delayed graft function to avoid early treatment with the nephrotoxic calcineurin inhibitors and thereby aid in recovery from ischemic reperfusion injury. The recommended dose for acute rejection of renal grafts is 1.5 mg/kg per day (over 4 to 6 hours) for 7 to 14 days. Mean T-cell counts fall by day 2 of therapy. Antithymocyte globulin also is used for acute rejection of other types of organ transplants and for prophylaxis of rejection (Wall, 1999).

Toxicity. Polyclonal antibodies are xenogeneic proteins that can elicit major side effects, including fever and chills with the potential for hypotension. Premedication with corticosteroids, *acetaminophen*, and/or an antihistamine and administration of the antiserum by slow infusion (over 4 to 6 hours) into a large-diameter vessel minimize such reactions. Serum sickness and glomerulonephritis can occur; anaphylaxis is a rare event. Hematologic complications include leukopenia and thrombocytopenia. As with other immunosuppressive agents, there is an increased risk of infection and malignancy, especially when multiple immunosuppressive agents are combined. No drug interactions have been described; anti-ATG antibodies develop, although they do not limit repeated use.

Monoclonal Antibodies. **Anti-CD3 Monoclonal Antibodies.** Antibodies directed at the ε chain of CD3, a trimeric molecule adjacent to the T-cell receptor on the surface of human T lymphocytes, have been used with

considerable efficacy since the early 1980s in human transplantation. The original mouse IgG_{2a} antihuman CD3 monoclonal antibody, muromonab-CD3 (OKT3, ORTHOCLONE OKT3), still is used to reverse glucocorticoid-resistant rejection episodes (Cosimi, *et al.*, 1981).

Mechanism of Action. Muromonab-CD3 binds to the ε chain of CD3, a monomorphic component of the T-cell receptor complex involved in antigen recognition, cell signaling, and proliferation (Hooks *et al.*, 1991). Antibody treatment induces rapid internalization of the T-cell receptor, thereby preventing subsequent antigen recognition. Administration of the antibody is followed rapidly by depletion and extravasation of a majority of T cells from the bloodstream and peripheral lymphoid organs such as lymph nodes and spleen. This absence of detectable T cells from the usual lymphoid regions is secondary both to cell death following complement activation and activation-induced cell death and to margination of T cells onto vascular endothelial walls and redistribution of T cells to nonlymphoid organs such as the lungs. Muromonab-CD3 also reduces function of the remaining T cells, as defined by lack of IL-2 production and great reduction in the production of multiple cytokines, perhaps with the exception of IL-4 and IL-10.

Therapeutic Uses. Muromonab-CD3 is indicated for treatment of acute organ transplant rejection (Ortho Multicenter Transplant Study Group, 1985; Woodle *et al.*, 1999; Rostaing *et al.*, 1999). Muromonab-CD3 is provided as a sterile solution containing 5 mg per ampule. The recommended dose is 5 mg/day (in adults; less for children) in a single intravenous bolus (less than 1 minute) for 10 to 14 days. Antibody levels increase over the first 3 days and then plateau. Circulating T cells disappear from the blood within minutes of administration and return within approximately 1 week after termination of therapy. Repeated use of muromonab-CD3 results in the immunization of the patient against the mouse determinants of the antibody, which can neutralize and prevent its immunosuppressive efficacy (Jaffers *et al.*, 1983). Thus, repeated treatment with the muromonab-CD3 or other mouse monoclonal antibodies generally is contraindicated. The use of muromonab-CD3 for induction and rejection therapy has diminished substantially in the past 5 years because of its toxicity and the availability of antithymocyte globulin.

Toxicity. The major side effect of anti-CD3 therapy is the "cytokine release syndrome" (Wilde and Goa, 1996; Ortho Multicenter Transplant Study Group, 1985). The syndrome typically begins 30 minutes after infusion of the antibody (but can occur later) and may persist for hours. Antibody binding to the T-cell receptor complex combined with Fc receptor (FcR)–mediated crosslinking is the basis for the initial activating properties of this agent. The syndrome is associated with and attributed to increased serum levels of cytokines (including tumor necrosis factor [TNF]-α, IL-2, IL-6, and interferon-γ), which are released by activated T cells and/or monocytes. In several studies, the production of TNF-α has been shown to be the major cause of the toxicity (Herbelin *et al.*, 1995). The symptoms usually are worst with the first dose; frequency and severity decrease with subsequent doses. Common clinical manifestations include high fever, chills/rigor, headache, tremor, nausea/vomiting, diarrhea, abdominal pain, malaise, myalgias, arthralgias, and generalized weakness. Less common complaints include skin reactions and cardiorespiratory and CNS disorders, including aseptic meningitis. Potentially fatal severe pulmonary edema, acute respiratory distress syndrome, cardiovascular collapse, cardiac arrest, and arrhythmias have been described.

Administration of glucocorticoids before the injection of muromonab-CD3 prevents the release of cytokines and reduces first-dose reactions considerably and is now a standard procedure. Volume status of patients also must be monitored carefully before therapy; steroids and other premedications should be given, and a fully competent resuscitation facility must be immediately available for patients receiving their first several doses of this therapy.

Other toxicities associated with anti-CD3 therapy include anaphylaxis and the usual infections and neoplasms associated with immunosuppressive therapy. "Rebound" rejection has been observed when muromonab-CD3 treatment is stopped (Wilde and Goa, 1996). Anti-CD3 therapies may be limited by anti-idiotypic or anti-murine antibodies in the recipient.

New-Generation Anti-CD3 Antibodies. Recently, genetically altered anti-CD3 monoclonal antibodies have been developed that are "humanized" to minimize the occurrence of antiantibody responses and mutated to prevent binding to FcRs (Friend *et al.*, 1999). The rationale for developing this new generation of anti-CD3 monoclonal antibodies is that they could induce selective immunomodulation in the absence of toxicity associated with conventional anti-CD3 monoclonal antibody therapy. In initial clinical trials, a humanized anti-CD3 monoclonal antibody that does not bind to FcRs reversed acute renal allograft rejection without causing the first-dose cytokine-release syndrome (Woodle *et al.*, 1999). Clinical efficacy of these agents in autoimmune diseases is being evaluated (Herold *et al.*, 2002).

Anti-IL-2 Receptor (Anti-CD25) Antibodies. Daclizumab (ZENAPAX), a humanized murine complementarity-determining region (CDR)/human IgG$_1$ chimeric monoclonal antibody, and basiliximab (SIMULECT), a murine-human chimeric monoclonal antibody, have been produced by recombinant DNA technology (Wiseman and Faulds, 1999). The composite daclizumab antibody consists of human (90%) constant domains of IgG$_1$ and variable framework regions of the Eu myeloma antibody and murine (10%) CDR of the anti-Tac antibody.

Mechanism of Action. Daclizumab has a somewhat lower affinity than does basiliximab, but a longer half-life (20 days). The exact mechanism of action of the anti-CD25 mAbs is not completely understood, but likely results from the binding of the anti-CD25 mAbs to the IL-2 receptor on the surface of activated, but not resting, T cells (Vincenti *et al.*, 1998; Amlot *et al.*, 1995). Significant depletion of T cells does not appear to play a major role in the mechanism of action of these mAbs. However, other mechanisms of action may mediate the effect of these antibodies. In a study of daclizumab-treated patients, there was a moderate decrease in circulating lymphocytes staining with 7G7, a fluorescein-conjugated antibody that binds a different α-chain epitope than that recognized and bound by daclizumab (Vincenti *et al.*, 1998). Similar results were obtained in studies with basiliximab (Amlot *et al.*, 1995). These findings indicate that therapy with the anti IL-2R mAbs results in a relative decrease of the expression of the α chain, either from depletion of coated lymphocytes or modulation of the α chain secondary to decreased expression or increased shedding. There is also recent evidence that the β chain may be down-regulated by the anti-CD25 antibody.

Therapeutic Uses. Anti–IL-2-receptor monoclonal antibodies are used for prophylaxis of acute organ rejection in adult patients. There are two anti–IL-2R preparations for use in clinical transplantation: daclizumab and basiliximab (Vincenti *et al.*, 1998; Nashan *et al.*, 1999). In Phase III trials, daclizumab was administered in five doses (1 mg/kg given intravenously over 15 minutes in 50 ml to 100 ml of normal saline) starting immediately preoperatively, and subsequently at biweekly intervals. The half-life of daclizumab was 20 days, resulting in saturation of the IL-2Rα on circulating lymphocytes for up to 120 days after transplantation. In these trials, daclizumab was used with maintenance immunosuppression regimens (cyclosporine, azathioprine, and steroids; cyclosporine and steroids). Subsequently, daclizumab was successfully used with a maintenance triple-therapy regimen—either with cyclosporine or tacrolimus, steroids, and mycophenolate mofetil (MMF) substituting for azathioprine (Ciancio *et al.*, 2003; Pescovitz *et al.*, 2003). In Phase III trials, basiliximab was administered in a fixed dose of 20 mg preoperatively and on days 0 and 4 after transplantation (Nashan *et al.*, 1997; Kahan *et al.*, 1999a). This regimen of basiliximab resulted in a concentration of ≥ 0.2 μg/mL, sufficient to saturate IL-2R on circulating lymphocytes for 25 to 35 days after transplantation. The half-life of basiliximab was 7 days. In the Phase III trials, basiliximab was used with a maintenance regimen consisting of cyclosporine and prednisone. In one randomized trial, basiliximab was safe and effective when used in a maintenance regimen consisting of cyclosporine, MMF, and prednisone (Lawen *et al.*, 2000).

There presently is no marker or test to monitor the effectiveness of anti–IL-2R therapy. Saturation of α chain on circulating lymphocytes during anti–IL-2R mAb therapy does not predict rejection. The duration of IL-2R blockade by basiliximab was similar in patients with or without acute rejection episodes (34 ± 14 days vs. 37 ± 14 days, mean + SD) (Kovarik et al., 1999). In another daclizumab trial, patients with acute rejection were found to have circulating and intragraft lymphocytes with saturated IL-2R (Vincenti et al., 2001). A possible explanation is that those patients who reject despite anti–IL-2R blockade do so through a mechanism that bypasses the IL-2 pathway due to cytokine-cytokine receptor redundancy (i.e., IL-7, IL-15).

Toxicity. No cytokine-release syndrome has been observed with these antibodies, but anaphylactic reactions can occur. Although lymphoproliferative disorders and opportunistic infections may occur, as with the depleting antilymphocyte agents, the incidence ascribed to anti-CD25 treatment appears remarkably low. No significant drug interactions with anti–IL-2-receptor antibodies have been described (Hong and Kahan, 1999).

Campath-1H. *Campath-1H* (ALEMTUZUMAB) is a humanized mAb that has been approved for use in chronic lymphocytic leukemia. The antibody targets CD52, a glycoprotein expressed on lymphocytes, monocytes, macrophages, and natural killer cells; thus, the drug causes extensive lympholysis by inducing apoptosis of targeted cells. It has achieved some use in renal transplantation because it produces prolonged T- and B-cell depletion and allows drug minimization. Large controlled studies of efficacy or safety are not available. Although short-term results are promising, further clinical experience is needed before Campath-1H is accepted into the clinical armamentarium for transplantation.

Anti-TNF Reagents. *Infliximab. Infliximab* (REMICADE) is a chimeric anti–TNF-α monoclonal antibody containing a human constant region and a murine variable region. It binds with high affinity to TNF-α and prevents the cytokine from binding to its receptors.

Patients with rheumatoid arthritis have elevated levels of TNF-α in their joints, while patients with Crohn's disease have elevated levels of TNF-α in their stools. In one trial, infliximab plus methotrexate improved the signs and symptoms of rheumatoid arthritis more than methotrexate alone. Patients with active Crohn's disease who had not responded to other immunosuppressive therapies also improved when treated with infliximab, including those with Crohn's-related fistulae. Infliximab is approved in the United States for treating the symptoms of rheumatoid arthritis, and is used in combination with methotrexate in patients who do not respond to methotrexate alone. Infliximab also is approved for treatment of symptoms of moderate to severe Crohn's disease in patients who have failed to respond to conventional therapy, and in treatment to reduce the number of draining fistulae in Crohn's disease patients (see Chapter 38). About 1 of 6 patients receiving infliximab experiences an infusion reaction characterized by fever, urticaria, hypotension, and dyspnea within 1 to 2 hours after antibody administration. Serious infections also have occurred in infliximab-treated patients, most frequently in the upper respiratory and urinary tracts. The development of antinuclear antibodies, and rarely a lupuslike syndrome, have been reported after treatment with infliximab.

Although not a monoclonal antibody, *etanercept* (ENBREL) is mechanistically related to infliximab because it also targets TNF-α. Etanercept contains the ligand-binding portion of a human TNF-α receptor fused to the Fc portion of human IgG$_1$, and binds to TNF-α and prevents it from interacting with its receptors. It is approved in the United States for treatment of the symptoms of rheumatoid arthritis in patients who have not responded to other treatments. Etanercept can be used in combination with methotrexate in patients who have not responded adequately to methotrexate alone. As with infliximab, serious infections have occurred after treatment with etanercept. Injection-site reactions (erythema, itching, pain, or swelling) have occurred in more than one-third of etanercept-treated patients.

Adalimimab (HUMIRA) is another anti-TNF product for intravenous use. This recombinant human IgG$_1$ monoclonal antibody was created by phage display technology and is approved for use in rheumatoid arthritis.

LFA-1 Inhibition. *Efalizumab* is a humanized IgG$_1$ mAb targeting the CD11a chain of LFA-1 (lymphocyte function associated antigen). Efalizumab binds to LFA-1 and prevents the LFA-1–ICAM (intercellular adhesion molecule) interaction to block T-cell adhesion, trafficking, and activation (Arnaout, 1990). Pretransplant therapy with anti-CD11a prolonged survival of murine skin and heart allografts and monkey heart allografts (Nakakura et al., 1996). In a randomized, multicenter trial, a murine anti–ICAM-1 mAb (ENLIMOMAB) failed to reduce the rate of acute rejection or to improve delayed graft function of cadaveric renal transplants (Salmela et al., 1999). This may have been due to either the murine nature of the mAb or the redundancy of the ICAMs. Efalizumab also is approved for use in patients with psoriasis. In a Phase I/II open-label, dose-ranging, multidose, multicenter trial, efalizumab (dose 0.5 mg/kg or 2 mg/kg) was administered subcutaneously for 12 weeks after renal transplantation (Vincenti et al., 2001). Both doses of efalizumab decreased the incidence of acute rejection. Pharmacokinetic and pharmacodynamic studies showed that efalizumab produced saturation and 80% modulation of CD11a within 24 hours of therapy. In a subset of 10 patients who received the higher dose efalizumab (2 mg/kg) with full-dose cyclosporine, MMF, and steroids, 3 patients developed posttransplant lymphoproliferative diseases. While efalizumab appears to be an effective immunosuppressive agent, it may be best used in a lower dose and with an immunosuppressive regimen that spares calcineurin inhibitors.

TOLERANCE

Immunosuppression has concomitant risks of opportunistic infections and secondary tumors. Therefore, the ultimate goal of research on organ transplantation and autoimmune diseases is to induce and maintain immunologic tolerance, the active state of antigen-specific nonresponsiveness (Krensky and Clayberger, 1994; Hackett and Dickler, 1999). Tolerance, if attainable, would represent a true cure for conditions discussed above without the side effects of the various immunosuppressive therapies. The calcineurin inhibitors prevent tolerance induction in some, but not all, preclinical models (Wood, 1991; Van Parijs and Abbas, 1998). In these same model systems, sirolimus does not prevent tolerance and may even promote tolerance induction (Li *et al.*, 1998). Several other promising approaches are being evaluated in clinical trials. Because they remain experimental, they are discussed only briefly here.

Costimulatory Blockade

Induction of specific immune responses by T lymphocytes requires two signals: an antigen-specific signal *via* the T-cell receptor and a costimulatory signal provided by the interaction of molecules such as CD28 on the T lymphocyte and CD80 and CD86 on the antigen-presenting cell (Figure 52–4; Khoury *et al.*, 1999). In preclinical studies, inhibition of the costimulatory signal can induce tolerance (Larsen *et al.*, 1996; Kirk *et al.*, 1997). Experimental approaches to inhibit costimulation include a recombinant fusion protein molecule, CTLA4Ig, and anti-CD80 and/or anti-CD86 mAbs. The antibodies h1F1 and h3D1 are humanized anti-CD80 and anti-CD-86 mAbs, respectively. *In vitro,* h1F1 and h3D1 were shown to block CD28-dependent T-cell proliferation and decrease mixed lymphocyte reactions. These mAbs must be used in tandem since either CD80 or CD86 is sufficient to stimulate T cells *via* CD28. In nonhuman primates, anti CD80 and CD86 mAbs were proven effective in renal transplantation, either as monotherapy or in combination with steroids or cyclosporine (Kirk *et al.*, 2001; Ossevoort *et al.*, 1999), but did not induce durable tolerance. A Phase I study of h1F1 and h3D1 in renal transplant recipients was performed in patients receiving maintenance therapy consisting of cyclosporine, mycophenolate

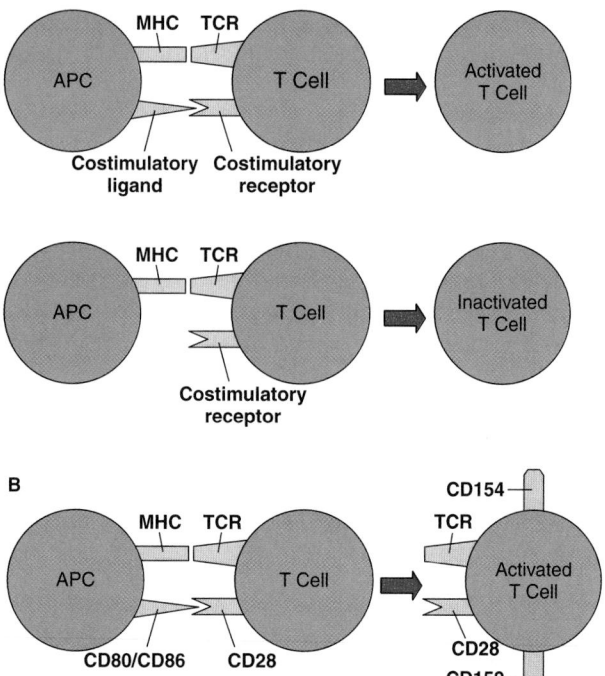

Figure 52–4. Costimulation. A. Two signals are required for T-cell activation. Signal 1 is *via* the T-cell receptor (TCR) and signal 2 is *via* a costimulatory receptor-ligand pair. Both signals are required for T-cell activation. Signal 1 in the absence of signal 2 results in an inactivated T cell. *B.* One important costimulatory pathway involves CD28 on the T cell and B7-1 (CD80) and B7-2 (CD86) on the antigen-presenting cell (APC). After a T cell is activated, it expresses additional costimulatory molecules. CD152 is CD40 ligand, which interacts with CD40 as a costimulatory pair. CD154 (CTLA4) interacts with CD80 and CD86 to dampen or down-regulate an immune response. Antibodies against CD80, CD86, and CD152 are being evaluated as potential therapeutic agents. CTLA4-Ig, a chimeric protein consisting of part of an immunoglobulin molecule and part of CD154, also has been tested as a therapeutic agent. (From Clayberger and Krensky, 2001, with permission.)

mofetil, and steroids (Vincenti, 2002). While the results of this study are as yet unpublished, the preliminary results appear to show that these mAbs are safe and possibly effective.

CTLA4Ig contains the binding region of CTLA4, which is a CD28 homolog, and the constant region of the human IgG$_1$. CTLA4Ig competitively inhibits CD28. Numerous animal studies have confirmed the efficacy of CTLA4Ig in inhibiting alloimmune responses, resulting in successful organ transplantation. More recently, CTLA4Ig was shown to be effective in the treatment of rheumatoid arthritis. However, CTLA4Ig was less effective when utilized in nonhuman primate models of renal transplantation. LEA29Y (*see* Figure 52–5) is a second-generation CTLA4Ig with two amino acid substitutions. LEA29Y has higher affinity for CD80 (twofold) and CD86 (fourfold), yielding a tenfold increase in potency *in vitro* as compared to CTLA4Ig. Preclinical

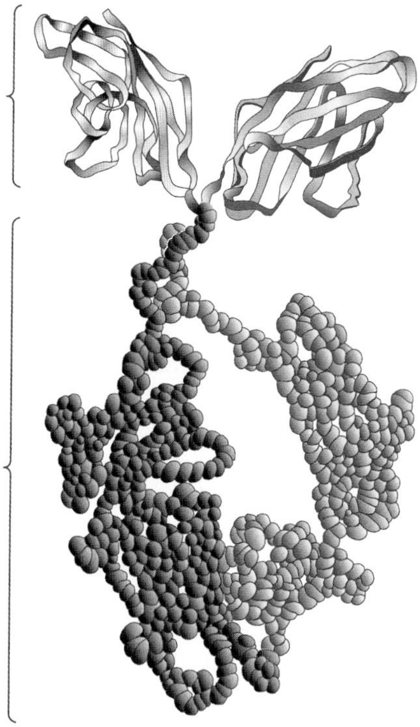

Figure 52–5. *Structure of LEA29Y, a CLTA4Ig congener.* For details, *see* text and Figure 52–4.

extracellular portion of CTLA4 (CD152)

mutations at positions 29 and 105 confer increased potency

fragment of FC domain of IgG1

renal transplant studies in nonhuman primates showed that LEA29Y did not induce tolerance but did prolong graft survival. LEA29Y (administered intravenously every 4 or 8 weeks) is undergoing clinical trials in calcineurin inhibitor–free immunosuppression regimens.

A second costimulatory pathway involves the interaction of CD40 on activated T cells with CD40 ligand (CD154) on B cells, endothelium, and/or antigen-presenting cells (Figure 52–4). Among the purported activities of anti-CD154 antibody treatment is its blockade of B7 expression induced by immune activation. Two humanized anti-CD154 monoclonal antibodies have been used in clinical trials in renal transplantation and autoimmune diseases. The development of these antibodies, however, is on hold because of associated thromboembolic events. An alternative approach to block the CD154-CD40 pathway is to target CD40 with monoclonal antibodies.

Donor Cell Chimerism

Another promising approach is induction of chimerism (coexistence of cells from two genetic lineages in a single individual) by any of a variety of protocols that first dampen or eliminate immune function in the recipient with ionizing radiation, drugs such as cyclophosphamide, and/or antibody treatment, and then provide a new source of immune function by adoptive transfer (transfusion) of bone marrow or hematopoietic stem cells (Starzl *et al.*, 1997; Fuchimoto *et al.*, 1999; Spitzer *et al.*, 1999; Hale *et al.*, 2000). Upon reconstitution of immune function, the recipient no longer recognizes new antigens provided during a critical period as "nonself." Such tolerance is long-lived and is less likely to be complicated by the use of calcineurin inhibitors. Although the most promising approaches in this arena have

been therapies that promote the development of mixed or macrochimerism, in which substantial numbers of donor cells are present in the circulation, some microchimerization approaches also have shown promise in the development of long-term unresponsiveness.

Soluble HLA

In the precyclosporine era, blood transfusions were shown to be associated with improved outcomes in renal transplant patients (Opelz and Terasaki, 1978). These findings gave rise to donor-specific transfusion protocols that improved outcomes (Opelz *et al.*, 1997). After the introduction of cyclosporine, however, these effects of blood transfusions disappeared, presumably due to the efficacy of this drug in blocking T-cell activation. Nevertheless, the existence of tolerance-promoting effects of transfusions is irrefutable. It is possible that this effect is due to HLA molecules on the surface of cells or in soluble forms. Recently, soluble HLA and peptides corresponding to linear sequences of HLA molecules have been shown to induce immunologic tolerance in animal models *via* a variety of mechanisms (Murphy and Krensky, 1999).

Antigens

Specific antigens provided in a variety of forms (generally as peptides) induce immunologic tolerance in preclinical models of diabetes mellitus, arthritis, and multiple sclerosis. Clinical trials of such approaches are under way. The past decade has witnessed a revolution in our understanding of the basis for immune tolerance. It is now well established that antigen/MHC complex binding to the T-cell-receptor/CD3 complex coupled with soluble and membrane-bound costimulatory signals initiates a cascade of signaling events that lead to productive immunity. In addition, the immune response is regulated by a number of negative signaling events that control cell survival and expansion. For the first time, *in vitro* and preclinical *in vivo* studies have demonstrated that one can selectively inhibit immune responses to specific antigens without the associated toxicity of established immunosuppressive therapies (Van Parijs and Abbas, 1998). With these new insights comes the enormous promise of specific immune therapies to treat the vast array of immune disorders from autoimmunity to transplant rejection. These new therapies will take advantage of a combination of drugs that target the primary T-cell receptor–mediated signal, either by blocking cell-surface receptor interactions or inhibiting early signal transduction events. The drugs will be combined with therapies that effectively block costimulation to prevent cell expansion and differentiation of those cells that have engaged antigen while maintaining a noninflammatory milieu.

IMMUNOSTIMULATION

General Principles

In contrast to immunosuppressive agents that inhibit the immune response in transplant rejection and autoimmunity, a few immunostimulatory drugs have been developed with applicability to infection, immunodeficiency, and cancer. Problems with such drugs include systemic (generalized) effects at one extreme or limited efficacy at the other.

Immunostimulants

Levamisole. *Levamisole* (ERGAMISOL) was synthesized originally as an anthelmintic but appears to "restore" depressed immune function of B lymphocytes, T lymphocytes, monocytes, and macrophages. Its only clinical indication is as adjuvant therapy with 5-fluorouracil after surgical resection in patients with Dukes' stage C colon cancer (Moertel *et al.*, 1990; Figueredo *et al.*, 1997), where it occasionally has been associated with fatal agranulocytosis.

Thalidomide. Thalidomide (THALOMID) is best known for the severe, life-threatening birth defects it caused when administered to pregnant women (Smithells and Newman, 1992; Lary *et al.*, 1999). For this reason, it is available only under a restricted distribution program and can be prescribed only by specially licensed physicians who understand the risk of teratogenicity if thalidomide is used during pregnancy. *Thalidomide should never be taken by women who are pregnant or who could become pregnant while taking the drug.* Nevertheless, it is indicated for the treatment of patients with erythema nodosum leprosum (Sampaio *et al.*, 1993; *see* Chapter 47) and also is used in conditions such as multiple myeloma. Its mechanism of action is unclear (Tseng *et al.*, 1996). Reported immunologic effects vary substantially under different conditions. For example, thalidomide has been reported to decrease circulating TNF-α in patients with erythema nodosum leprosum, but to increase it in patients who are HIV-seropositive (Jacobson *et al.*, 1997). Alternatively, it has been suggested that the drug affects angiogenesis (Miller and Stromland, 1999). The anti–TNF-α effect has led to its evaluation as a treatment for severe, refractory rheumatoid arthritis (Keesal *et al.*, 1999).

Bacillus Calmette-Guérin (BCG). Live *bacillus Calmette-Guérin* (BCG; TICE BCG, THERACYS) is an attenuated, live culture of the bacillus of Calmette and Guérin strain of *Mycobacterium bovis,* that induces a granulomatous reaction at the site of administration. By unclear mechanisms, this preparation is active against tumors and is indicated for treatment and prophylaxis of carcinoma *in situ* of the urinary bladder and for prophylaxis of primary and recurrent stage Ta and/or T1 papillary tumors after transurethral resection (Morales *et al.*, 1981; Paterson and Patel, 1998; Patard *et al.*, 1998). Adverse effects include hypersensitivity, shock, chills, fever, malaise, and immune complex disease.

Recombinant Cytokines. **Interferons.** Although interferons (alpha, beta, and gamma) initially were identified by their antiviral activity, these agents also have important immunomodulatory activities (Johnson *et al.*, 1994; Tilg and Kaser, 1999; Ransohoff, 1998). The interferons bind to specific cell-surface receptors that initiate a series of intracellular events: induction of certain enzymes, inhibition of cell proliferation, and enhancement of immune activities, including increased phagocytosis by macrophages and augmentation of specific cytotoxicity by T lymphocytes (Tompkins, 1999). Recombinant *interferon alfa-2b* (IFN-alpha 2, INTRON A) is obtained from *Escherichia coli* by recombinant expression. It is a member of a family of naturally occurring small proteins with molecular weights of 15,000 to 27,600 daltons, produced and secreted by cells in response to viral infections and other

inducers. Interferon alfa-2b is indicated in the treatment of a variety of tumors, including hairy cell leukemia, malignant melanoma, follicular lymphoma, and AIDS-related Kaposi's sarcoma (Punt, 1998; Bukowski, 1999; Sinkovics and Horvath, 2000). It also is indicated for infectious diseases, chronic hepatitis B, and condylomata acuminata. In addition, it is supplied in combination with *ribavirin* (REBETRON) for treatment of chronic hepatitis C in patients with compensated liver function not treated previously with interferon alfa-2b or who have relapsed after interferon alfa-2b therapy (Lo Iacono *et al.*, 2000). Flu-like symptoms, including fever, chills, and headache, are the most common adverse effects after interferon alfa-2b administration. Adverse experiences involving the cardiovascular system (hypotension, arrhythmias, and rarely cardiomyopathy and myocardial infarction) and CNS (depression, confusion) are less-frequent side effects.

Interferon gamma-1b (ACTIMMUNE) is a recombinant polypeptide that activates phagocytes and induces their generation of oxygen metabolites that are toxic to a number of microorganisms. It is indicated to reduce the frequency and severity of serious infections associated with chronic granulomatous disease. Adverse reactions include fever, headache, rash, fatigue, GI distress, anorexia, weight loss, myalgia, and depression.

Interferon beta-1a (AVONEX, REBIF), a 166–amino acid recombinant glycoprotein, and *interferon beta-1b* (BETASERON), a 165–amino acid recombinant protein, have antiviral and immunomodulatory properties. They are FDA approved for the treatment of relapsing and relapsing-remitting multiple sclerosis to reduce the frequency of clinical exacerbations (*see* below). The mechanism of their action in multiple sclerosis is unclear. Flu-like symptoms (fever, chills, myalgia) and injection-site reactions have been common adverse effects.

Further discussion of the use of these and other interferons in the treatment of viral diseases can be found in Chapter 49.

Interleukin-2. Human recombinant interleukin-2 (*aldesleukin*, PROLEUKIN; des-alanyl-1, serine-125 human IL-2) is produced by recombinant DNA technology in *E. coli* (Taniguchi and Minami, 1993). This recombinant form differs from native IL-2 in that it is not glycosylated, has no amino terminal alanine, and has a serine substituted for the cysteine at amino acid 125 (Doyle *et al.*, 1985). The potency of the preparation is represented in International Units in a lymphocyte proliferation assay such that 1.1 mg of recombinant IL-2 protein equals 18 million International Units. Aldesleukin has the following *in vitro* biologic activities of native IL-2: enhancement of lymphocyte proliferation and growth of IL-2–dependent cell lines; enhancement of lymphocyte-mediated cytotoxicity and killer cell activity; and induction of interferon-γ activity (Winkelhake *et al.*, 1990; Whittington and Faulds, 1993). *In vivo* administration of aldesleukin in animals produces multiple immunologic effects in a dose-dependent manner. Cellular immunity is profoundly activated with lymphocytosis, eosinophilia, thrombocytopenia, and release of multiple cytokines (*e.g.*, TNF, IL-1, interferon-γ). Aldesleukin is indicated for the treatment of adults with metastatic renal cell carcinoma and melanoma. Administration of aldesleukin has been associated with serious cardiovascular toxicity resulting from capillary leak syndrome, which involves loss of vascular tone and leak of plasma proteins and fluid into the extravascular space. Hypotension, reduced organ perfusion, and death may occur. An increased risk of disseminated infection due to impaired neutrophil function also has been associated with aldesleukin treatment.

Immunization

Immunization may be active or passive. Active immunization involves stimulation with an antigen to develop immunologic defenses against a future exposure. Passive immunization involves administration of preformed antibodies to an individual who is already exposed or is about to be exposed to an antigen.

Vaccines. Active immunization, vaccination, involves administration of an antigen as a whole, killed organism, attenuated (live) organism, or a specific protein or peptide constituent of an organism. Booster doses often are required, especially when killed (inactivated) organisms are used as the immunogen. In the United States, vaccination has sharply curtailed or practically eliminated a variety of major infections, including diphtheria, measles, mumps, pertussis, rubella, tetanus, *Haemophilus influenzae* type b, and pneumococcus (Dorner and Barrett, 1999; The National Vaccine Advisory Committee, 1999).

Although most vaccines have targeted infectious diseases, a new generation of vaccines may provide complete or limited protection from specific cancers or autoimmune diseases (Lee *et al.*, 1998; Del Vecchio and Parmiani, 1999; Simone *et al.*, 1999). Because T cells optimally are activated by peptides and costimulatory ligands that both are present on antigen-presenting cells (APCs), one approach for vaccination has consisted of immunizing patients with APCs expressing a tumor antigen. The first generation of anticancer vaccines used whole cancer cells or tumor-cell lysates as a source of antigen in combination with various adjuvants, relying on host APCs to process and present tumor-specific antigens (Sinkovics and Horvath, 2000).

These anticancer vaccines resulted in occasional clinical responses and are being tested in prospective clinical trials. Second generation anticancer vaccines utilized specific APCs incubated *ex vivo* with antigen or transduced to express antigen and subsequently reinfused into patients. In laboratory animals, immunization with dendritic cells previously pulsed with MHC class I–restricted peptides derived from tumor-specific antigens led to pronounced antitumor cytotoxic T-lymphocyte responses and protective tumor immunity (Tarte and Klein, 1999). Finally, multiple studies have demonstrated the efficacy of DNA vaccines in small- and large-animal models of infectious diseases and cancer (Lewis and Babiuk, 1999; Liljeqvist and Stahl, 1999). The advantage of DNA vaccination over peptide immunization is that it permits generation of entire proteins, enabling determinant selection to occur in the host without having to restrict immunization to patients bearing specific HLA alleles. However, a safety concern about this technique is the potential for integration of the plasmid DNA into the host genome, possibly disrupting important genes and thereby leading to phenotypic mutations or carcinogenicity. A final approach to generate or enhance immune responses against specific antigens consists of infecting cells with recombinant viruses that encode the protein antigen of interest. Different types of viral vectors that can infect mammalian cells, such as vaccinia, avipox, lentivirus, adenovirus or adenovirus-associated virus, have been used.

Immune Globulin. Passive immunization is indicated when an individual is deficient in antibodies because of a congenital or acquired immunodeficiency, when an individual with a high degree of risk is exposed to an agent and there is inadequate time for active immunization (*e.g.*, measles, rabies, hepatitis B), or when a disease is already present but can be ameliorated by passive antibodies (*e.g.*, botulism, diphtheria, tetanus). Passive immunization may be provided by several different products (Table 52–2). Nonspecific immunoglobulins or highly specific immunoglobulins may be provided based upon the indication. The protection provided usually lasts from 1 to 3 months. Immune globulin is derived from pooled plasma of adults by an alcohol-fractionation procedure. It contains largely IgG (95%) and is indicated for antibody-deficiency disorders, exposure to infections such as hepatitis A and measles, and specific immunologic diseases such as immune thrombocytopenic purpura and Guillain-Barré syndrome (Ballow, 1997; Jordan *et al.*, 1998a; Jordan *et al.*, 1998b). In contrast, specific immune globulins ("hyperimmune") differ from other immune globulin preparations in that donors are selected for high titers of the desired antibodies. Specific immune globulin preparations are available

Table 52–2
Selected Immune Globulin Preparations

Immune globulin intravenous	BAYGAM
	GAMMAGARD S/D
	GAMMAR-P.I.V
	IVEEGAM
	SANDOGLOBULIN I.V.
	others
Cytomegalovirus immune globulin	CYTOGAM
Respiratory syncytial virus immune globulin	RESPIGAM
Hepatitis B immune globulin	BAYHEP B
	HYPERHEP
	H-BIG
Rabies immune globulin	BAYRAB
	IMOGAM RABIS-HT
	HYPER-AB
Rho(D) immune globulin	BAY-RHO-D
	WINRHO SDF
	MICRHOGAM
	RHOGAM
	others
Tetanus immune globulin	BAYTET
	HYPERTET

for hepatitis B, rabies, tetanus, varicella-zoster, cytomegalovirus, and respiratory syncytial virus. Rho(D) immune globulin is a specific hyperimmune globulin for prophylaxis against hemolytic disease of the newborn due to Rh incompatibility between mother and fetus. All such plasma-derived products carry the theoretical risk of transmission of infectious disease.

Rho(D) Immune Globulin. The commercial forms of Rho(D) immune globulin (Table 52–2) consist of IgG containing a high titer of antibodies against the Rh(D) antigen on the surface of red blood cells. All donors are carefully screened to reduce the risk of transmitting infectious diseases. Fractionation of the plasma is performed by precipitation with cold alcohol followed by passage through a viral clearance system (Bowman, 1998; Contreras, 1998; Lee, 1998).

Mechanism of Action. Rho(D) immune globulin binds Rho antigens, thereby preventing sensitization (Peterec, 1995). Rh-negative women may be sensitized to the "foreign" Rh antigen on red blood cells *via* the fetus at the time of birth, miscarriage, ectopic pregnancy, or any transplacental hemorrhage. If the women go on to have a primary immune response, they will make antibodies to Rh antigen that can cross the placenta and damage subsequent fetuses by lysing

red blood cells. This syndrome, called hemolytic disease of the newborn, is life-threatening. The form due to Rh incompatibility is largely preventable by Rho(D) immune globulin.

Therapeutic Use. Rho(D) immune globulin is indicated whenever fetal red blood cells are known or suspected to have entered the circulation of an Rh-negative mother unless the fetus is known also to be Rh-negative. The drug is given intramuscularly. The half-life of circulating immunoglobulin is approximately 21 to 29 days.

Toxicity. Injection site discomfort and low-grade fever have been reported. Systemic reactions are extremely rare, but myalgia, lethargy, and anaphylactic shock have been reported. As with all plasma-derived products, there is a theoretical risk of transmission of infectious diseases.

Intravenous Immunoglobulin (IVIG). In recent years, indications for the use of intravenous immunoglobulin (IVIG) have expanded beyond replacement therapy for agammaglobulinemia and other immunodeficiencies to include a variety of bacterial and viral infections, and an array of autoimmune and inflammatory diseases as diverse as thrombocytopenic purpura, Kawasaki's disease, and autoimmune skin, neuromuscular, and neurologic diseases (Dalakas, 2004). Although the mechanism of action of IVIG in immune modulation remains largely unknown, proposed mechanisms include modulation of expression and function of Fc receptors on leukocytes and endothelial cells, interference with complement activation and cytokine production, provision of anti-idiotypic antibodies (Jerne network theory), and effects on the activation and effector function of T and B lymphocytes (Larroche *et al.*, 2002; Rutter and Luger, 2002). Although IVIG is effective in many autoimmune diseases, its spectrum of efficacy and appropriate dosing (especially duration of therapy) are unknown. Additional controlled studies of IVIG are needed to identify proper dosing, cost-benefit, and quality-of-life parameters.

A CASE STUDY: IMMUNOTHERAPY FOR MULTIPLE SCLEROSIS

Clinical Features and Pathology. Multiple sclerosis (MS) is a demyelinating inflammatory disease of the CNS white matter that displays a triad of pathogenic symptoms: mononuclear cell infiltration, demyelination, and scarring (gliosis). The peripheral nervous system is uninvolved. The disease, which may be episodic or progressive, occurs in early to middle adulthood with prevalence increasing from late adolescence to 35 years and then declining. MS is roughly twice as common in females as in males and occurs mainly in higher latitudes of the temperate climates. Epidemiologic studies suggest a role for environmental factors in the pathogenesis of MS; despite many suggestions, associations with infectious agents have proven inconclusive, even though several viruses can cause similar demyelinating diseases in laboratory animals and humans. A stronger linkage is the genetic one: people of Northern European origin have a higher susceptibility to MS, and studies in twins and siblings suggest a genetic component of susceptibility to MS. The genetic linkage in the pathogenesis of MS is complex. Several studies indicate that one determinant of MS may be the class II (or HLA-DR) domain of the major histocompatibility complex (MHC) on chromosome 6 that encodes the histocompatibility antigens. Other loci under study include polymorphisms for GSH transferase and CD45. There is also substantial evidence of an autoimmune component to MS: in MS patients, there are activated T cells that are reactive to different myelin antigens including myelin basic protein (MBP); in addition, there is evidence for the presence of autoantibodies to myelin oligodendrocyte glycoprotein (MOG) and to MBP that can be eluted from the CNS plaque tissue, though it appears unlikely that high-affinity autoantibodies are present in the circulation. These antibodies may act with pathogenic T cells to produce some of the cellular pathology of MS. The neurophysiological result is altered conduction (both positive and negative) in myelinated fibers within the CNS (cerebral white matter, brain stem, cerebellar tracts, optic nerves, spinal cord); some alterations appear to result from exposure of voltage-dependent K^+ channels that are normally covered by myelin.

Attacks are classified by type and severity and likely correspond to specific degrees of CNS damage and pathologic processes. Thus, physicians refer to acute MS (an acute attack), relapsing-remitting MS (the form in 85% of younger patients), secondary progressive MS (progressive neurologic deterioration following a long period of relapsing-remitting disease), and primary progressive MS (about 15% of patients, wherein deterioration with relatively little inflammation is apparent at onset). Keegan and Noseworthy (2002) have recently reviewed current concepts of the etiology, natural history, and current therapy of MS.

Pharmacotherapy for MS. Specific therapies are aimed at resolving acute attacks, reducing recurrences and exacerbations, and slowing the progression of disability (Table 52–3). Nonspecific therapies focus on maintaining function and quality of life. For acute attacks, pulse glucocorticoids are often employed (typically, 1 g/day of methylprednisolone administered intravenously for 3 to 5 days). There is no evidence that tapered doses of oral prednisone are useful or even desirable.

For relapsing-remitting attacks, immunomodulatory therapies are approved: beta-1 interferons (interferon beta-1a, interferon beta-1b, and *glatiramer acetate* [COPAXONE]). The interferons suppress the proliferation of T lymphocytes, inhibit their movement into the CNS from the periphery, and shift the cytokine profile from pro- to anti-inflammatory types.

Random polymers that contain amino acids commonly used as MHC anchors and T-cell receptor contact residues have been proposed as possible "universal APLs (altered peptide ligands)." Glatiramer acetate (GA) is a random sequence polypeptide consisting of four amino acids (alanine [A], lysine [K], glutamate [E], and tyrosine [Y] at a molar ratio of A:K:E:Y of 4.5:3.6:1.5:1) with an average length of 40 to 100 amino acids. Directly labeled GA binds efficiently to different murine H2 I-A molecules, as well as to their human counterparts, the MHC class II DR molecules, but does not bind MHC class II DQ or MHC class I molecules *in vitro*. In Phase III clinical trials, GA, administered subcutaneously to patients with relapsing-remitting MS, decreased the rate of exacerbations by about 30% (Steinman, 2004; Hafler, 2004). *In vivo* administration of GA induces highly cross-reactive CD4$^+$ T cells that are immune-deviated to secrete Th2 cytokines and prevents the appearance of new lesions detectable by MRI. This represents one of the first successful uses of an agent that ameliorates autoimmune disease by altering signals through the T-cell receptor complex (Steinman, 2004; Hafler, 2004).

For relapsing-remitting attacks and for secondary progressive MS, the alkylating agent cyclophosphamide (reviewed in Weiner, 2004) and the anthracenedionene-derivative *mitoxantrone* (NOVATRONE) are currently used in patients refractory to other immunomodulators. These agents, used primarily for cancer chemotherapy, have significant toxicities (*see* Chapter 51 for structures and pharmacology). While cyclophosphamide in patients with MS may not be limited by an accumulated dose exposure, mitoxantrone can be tolerated only up to an accumulated dose of 100 to 140 mg/m^2 (Crossley, 1984). The utility of interferon therapy in patients with secondary progressive MS is unclear. In primary progressive MS, with no discrete attacks and less observed inflammation, suppression of inflammation seems to be less helpful. A minority of patients at this stage will respond to high doses of glucocorticoids. Table 52–3 summarizes current immunomodulatory therapies for MS.

Each of the agents mentioned above has side effects and contraindications that may be limiting: infections (for glucocorticoids); hypersensitivity and pregnancy (for immunomodulators); and prior anthracycline/anthracenedione use, mediastinal irradiation, or cardiac disease (mitoxantrone). With all of these agents, it is clear that the

Table 52–3
Pharmacotherapy of Multiple Sclerosis

THERAPEUTIC AGENT	BRAND NAME (DOSE, regimen)	INDICATIONS	RESULTS	MECHANISM OF ACTION
IFNβ-1a	AVONEX (30 μg, IM, weekly) REBIFF (22 or 44 μg, SC, 3 times weekly)	Treatment of RRMS	Reduction of relapses by one-third Reduction of new MRI T2 lesions and the volume of enlarging T2 lesions Reduction in the number and volume of Gd-enhancing lesions Slowing of brain atrophy	Acts on blood–brain barrier by interfering with T-cell adhesion to the endothelium by binding VLA-4 on T cells or by inhibiting the T cell expression of MMP Reduction in T cell activation by interfering with HLA class II and costimulatory molecules B7/CD28 and CD40:CD40L Immune deviation of Th2 over Th1 cytokine profile
IFNβ-1b	BETASERON (0.3 mg, SC, every other day)	Treatment of RRMS	Same as IFNβ-1a, above	Same as IFNβ-1a, above
Glatiramer acetate	COPAXONE (20 μg, SC, daily)	Treatment of RRMS	Reduction of relapses by one-third Reduction in the number and volume of Gd-enhancing lesions	Induces T-helper type 2 cells that enter the CNS; mediates bystander suppression at sites of inflammation
Mitoxantrone	NOVANTRONE (12 mg/m^2, as short [5–15 min] IV infusion every 3 months)	Worsening forms of RRMS SPMS	Reduction in relapses by 67% Slowed progression on EDSS, ambulation index, and MRI disease activity	Intercalates DNA (*see* Chapter 51) Suppresses cellular and humoral immune response

IFN, interferon; IM, intramuscularly; RRMS, relapsing-remitting MS; SC, subcutaneously; SPMS, secondary progressive MS; IV, intravenously. Gd, gadolinium, used in Gd-enhanced MRI to assess number and size of inflammatory brain lesions; EDSS, Expanded Disability Status Scale, a neurologic assessment scale for MS pathology (*see* Ravnborg *et al.*, 2005); MMP, matrix metalloprotease.

earlier they are used, the more effective they are in preventing disease relapses. What is not clear is whether any of these agents will prevent or diminish the later onset of secondary progressive disease, which causes the more severe form of disability. Given the fluctuating nature of this disease, only long-term studies lasting decades will answer this question.

A number of other new immunomodulatory therapies are completing Phase III trials. One is a monoclonal antibody, *natalizumab* (ANTEGREN), directed against the adhesion molecule α_4 integrin; natalizumab binds to α_4 integrin and antagonizes interactions with integrin heterodimers containing α_4 integrin, such as $\alpha_4\beta_1$ integrin that is expressed on the surface of activated lymphocytes

and monocytes. Preclinical data suggest that an interaction of $\alpha_4\beta_1$ integrin with VCAM-1 (vascular cellular-adhesion molecule 1) is critical for T-cell trafficking from the periphery into the CNS (Steinman, 2004); thus, blocking this interaction would hypothetically inhibit disease exacerbations. In fact, Phase II clinical trials have demonstrated a significant decrease in the number of new lesions as determined by magnetic resonance imaging and clinical attacks in MS patients receiving natalizumab (Miller *et al.*, 2003). Monoclonal antibodies directed against the IL-2 receptor are also entering Phase III clinical trials. The pharmacotherapy of MS has been reviewed by Weiner (2004); the utility of immunotherapy for autoimmune diseases has been reviewed by Steinman (2004).

CLINICAL SUMMARY

Most transplant centers employ some combination of immunosuppressive drugs with antilymphocyte induction therapy with either a monoclonal or polyclonal antibody agent. Maintenance immunosuppression consists of a calcineurin inhibitor (cyclosporine or tacrolimus), glucocorticoids, and an antimetabolite (azathioprine or mycophenolate mofetil). Mycophenolate mofetil has largely replaced azathioprine as part of the standard immunosuppressive regimen after transplantation. At present, a number of centers are conducting trials with new drug combinations including either cyclosporine or tacrolimus in combination with glucocorticoids and mycophenolate mofetil, with or without antibody-induction therapy or FTY70 with cyclosporine. Sirolimus is being used to limit exposure to the nephrotoxic calcineurin inhibitors, while steroid avoidance or minimization strategies increasingly are used. Newer immunosuppressive agents are providing more effective control of rejection and permitting transplantation to become an accepted procedure with a number of different organs, including kidney, liver, pancreas, and heart. The apparent effectiveness of new drug combinations has resulted in a resurgence of interest in glucocorticoid withdrawal.

BIBLIOGRAPHY

Ahsan, N., Hricik, D., Matas, A., *et al*. Prednisone withdrawal in kidney transplant recipients on cyclosporine and mycophenolate mofetil—a prospective randomized study. Steroid Withdrawal Study Group. *Transplantation*, **1999**, *68:*1865–1874.

Akalin, E., Ames, S., Sehgal, V., *et al*. Intravenous immunoglobulin and thymoglobulin facilitate kidney transplantation in complement-dependent cytotoxicity B-cell and blow cytometry T- or B-cell crossmatch-positive patients. *Transplantation*, **2003**, *76:*1444–1447.

Alloway, R.R., Isaacs, R., Lake, K., *et al*. Report of the American Society of Transplantation Conference on Immunosuppressive Drugs and the use of generic immunosuppressants. *Am. J. Transplant.*, **2003**, *3:*1211–1215.

Amlot, P.L., Rawlings, E., Fernando, O.N., *et al*. Prolonged action of chimeric interleukin-2 receptor (CD25) monoclonal antibody used in cadaveric renal transplantation. *Transplantation*, **1995**, *60:*748–756.

Arnaout, M.A. Structure and function of the leukocyte adhesion molecules CD11/CD18. *Blood*, **1990**, *75:*1037–1050.

Artz, M.A., Boots, J.M.M., Ligtenberg, G., *et al*. Improved cardiovascular risk profile and renal function in renal transplant patients after randomized conversion from cyclosporine to tacrolimus. *J. Am. Soc. Nephrol.*, **2003**, *14:*1880–1888.

Auphan, N., DiDonato, J.A., Rosette, C., *et al*. Immunosuppression by glucocorticoids: inhibition of NF-κB activity through induction of I κB synthesis. *Science*, **1995**, *270:*286–290.

Ballow, M. Mechanisms of action of intravenous immune serum globulin in autoimmune and inflammatory diseases. *J. Allergy Clin. Immunol.*, **1997**, *100:*151–157.

Baraldo, M., Ferraccioli, G., Pea, F., *et al*. Cyclosporine A pharmacokinetics in rheumatoid arthritis patients after 6 months of methotrexate therapy. *Pharmacol. Res.*, **1999**, *40:*483–486.

Bourdage, J.S., and Hamlin, D.M. Comparative polyclonal antithymocyte globulin and antilymphocyte/antilymphoblast globulin anti-CD antigen analysis by flow cytometry. *Transplantation*, **1995**, *59:*1194–1200.

Bowman, J.M. RhD hemolytic disease of the newborn. *N. Engl. J. Med.*, **1998**, *339:*1775–1777.

Brown, E.J., Albers, M.W., Shin, T.B., *et al*. A mammalian protein targeted by G1-arresting rapamycin-receptor complex. *Nature*, **1994**, *369:*756–758.

Burke, J.F. Jr., Pirsch, J.D., Ramos, E.L., *et al*. Long-term efficacy and safety of cyclosporine in renal-transplant recipients. *N. Engl. J. Med.*, **1994**, *331:*358–363.

Butani, L., Palmer, J., Baluarte, H.J., and Polinsky, M.S. Adverse effects of mycophenolate mofetil in pediatric renal transplant recipients with presumed chronic rejection. *Transplantation*, **1999**, *68:*83–86.

Christians, U., and Sewing, K.F. Cyclosporin metabolism in transplant patients. *Pharmacol. Ther.*, **1993**, *57:*291–345.

Ciancio, G., Burke, G.W., Suzart, K., *et al*. Efficacy and safety of daclizumab induction for primary kidney transplant recipients in combination with tacrolimus, mycophenolate mofetil, and steroids as maintenance immunosuppression. *Transplant Proc.*, **2003**, *35:* 873–874.

Cole, E., Maham, N., Cardella, C., *et al*. Clinical benefits of Neoral C2 monitoring in the long-term management of renal transplant recipients. *Transplantation*, **2003**, *75:*2086–2090.

Colvin, R.B. Chronic allograft nephropathy. *N. Engl. J. Med.*, **2003**, *349:*2288–2290.

Contreras, M. The prevention of Rh haemolytic disease of the fetus and newborn—general background. *Br. J. Obstet. Gynaecol.*, **1998**, *105*(Suppl. 18):7–10.

Cosimi, A.B., Burton, R.C., Colvin, R.B., *et al*. Treatment of acute renal allograft rejection with OKT3 monoclonal antibody. *Transplantation*, **1981**, *32:*535–539.

Crossley, R.J. Clinical safety and tolerance of mitoxantrone. *Semin. Oncol.*, **1984**, *11:*54–58.

Dalakas, M.C. Intravenous immunoglobulin in autoimmune neuromuscular diseases. *JAMA*, **2004**, *291:*2367–2375.

Doyle M.V., Lee, M.T., and Fong, S. Comparison of the biological activities of human recombinant interleukin-2 (125) and native interleukin-2. *J. Biol. Response Mod.*, **1985**, *4:*96–109.

Eisen, H.J., Tuzcu, E.M., Dorent, R., *et al*., for the RAD B253 Study Group. Everolimus for the prevention of allograft rejection and vasculopathy in cardiac-transplant recipients. *N. Engl. J. Med.*, **2003**, *349:*847–858.

Elli, A., Banfi, G., Fogazzi, G.B., *et al*. BK polyomavirus interstitial nephritis in a renal transplant patient with no previous acute rejection episodes. *J. Nephrol.*, **2002**, *15:*313–316.

Fahr, A. Cyclosporin clinical pharmacokinetics. *Clin. Pharmacokinet.*, **1993**, *24:*472–495.

Figueredo, A., Germond, C., Maroun, J., *et al*. Adjuvant therapy for stage II colon cancer after complete resection. Provincial Gastrointestinal Disease Site Group. *Cancer Prev. Control*, **1997**, *1:*379–392.

Friend, P.J., Hale, G., Chatenoud, L., *et al*. Phase I study of an engineered aglycosylated humanized CD3 antibody in renal transplant rejection. *Transplantation*, **1999**, *68:*1632–1637.

Fuchimoto, Y., Yamada, K., Shimizu, A., *et al.* Relationship between chimerism and tolerance in a kidney transplantation model. *J. Immunol.,* **1999,** *162:*5704–5711.

Gaffney, K., and Scott, D.G. Azathioprine and cyclophosphamide in the treatment of rheumatoid arthritis. *Br. J. Rheumatol.,* **1998,** *37:*824–836.

Goto, T., Kino, T., Hatanaka, H., *et al.* Discovery of FK-506, a novel immunosuppressant isolated from *Streptomyces tsukubaensis. Transplant Proc.,* **1987,** *19:*4–8.

Groth, C.G., Backman, L., Morales, J.M., *et al.* Sirolimus (rapamycin)-based therapy in human renal transplantation: similar efficacy and different toxicity compared with cyclosporine. Sirolimus European Renal Transplant Study Group. *Transplantation,* **1999,** *67:*1036–1042.

Hafler, D.A. Multiple sclerosis. *J. Clin. Invest.,* **2004,** *113:*788–794.

Hale, D.A., Gottschalk, R., Umemura, A., *et al.* Establishment of stable multilineage hematopoietic chimerism and donor-specific tolerance without irradiation. *Transplantation,* **2000,** *69:*1242–1251.

Henry, M.L. Cyclosporine and tacrolimus (FK506): a comparison of efficacy and safety profiles. *Clin. Transplant.,* **1999,** *13:*209–220.

Herbelin, A., Chatenoud, L., Roux-Lombard, P., *et al. In vivo* soluble tumor necrosis factor receptor release in OKT3-treated patients. Differential regulation of TNF-sR55 and TNF-sR75. *Transplantation,* **1995,** *59:*1470–1475.

Herold, K.C., Hagopian, W., Auger, J.A., *et al.* Anti-CD3 Monoclonal antibody in new-onset type 1 diabetes mellitus. *N. Engl. J. Med.,* **2002,** *346:*1692–1698.

Hong, J.C., and Kahan, B.D. Sirolimus-induced thrombocytopenia and leukopenia in renal transplant recipients: risk factors, incidence, progression, and management. *Transplantation,* **2000b,** *69:*2085–2090.

Hong, J.C., and Kahan, B.D. Use of anti-CD25 monoclonal antibody in combination with rapamycin to eliminate cyclosporine treatment during the induction phase of immunosuppression. *Transplantation,* **1999,** *68:*701–704.

Howard, R.J., Condie, R.M., Sutherland, D.E., *et al.* The use of antilymphoblast globulin in the treatment of renal allograft rejection: a double-blind, randomized study. *Transplantation,* **1997,** *24:*419–423.

Hricik, D.E., Knauss, T.C., Bodziak, K.A., *et al.* Withdrawal of steroid therapy in African American kidney transplant recipients receiving sirolimus and tacrolimus. *Transplantation,* **2003,** *76:*938–942.

Jacobson, J.M., Greenspan, J.S., Spritzler, J., *et al.* Thalidomide for the treatment of oral aphthous ulcers in patients with human immunodeficiency virus infection. National Institute of Allergy and Infectious Diseases AIDS Clinical Trials Group. *N. Engl. J. Med.,* **1997,** *336:*1487–1493.

Jaffers, G.J., Colvin, R.B., Cosimi, A.B., *et al.* The human immune response to murine OKT3 monoclonal antibody. *Transplant. Proc.,* **1983,** *15:*646–648.

Jordan, S.C., Quartel, A.W., Czer, L.S., *et al.* Posttransplant therapy using high-dose human immunoglobulin (intravenous gammaglobulin) to control acute humoral rejection in renal and cardiac allograft recipients and potential mechanism of action. *Transplantation,* **1998a,** *66:*800–805.

Jordan, S.C., Tyan, D., Czer, L., and Toyoda, M. Immunomodulatory actions of intravenous immunoglobulin (IVIG): potential applications in solid organ transplant recipients. *Pediatr. Transplant.,* **1998b,** *2:*92–105.

Kahan, B.D., Julian, B.A., Pescovitz, M.D., *et al.* Sirolimus reduces the incidence of acute rejection episodes despite lower cyclosporine doses in Caucasian recipients of mismatched primary renal allografts: a phase II trial. Rapamune Study Group. *Transplantation,* **1999a,** *68:*1526–1532.

Kahan, B.D., Rajagopalan, P.R., and Hall, M. Reduction of the occurrence of acute cellular rejection among renal allograft recipients treated with basiliximab, a chimeric anti-interleukin-2-receptor monoclonal antibody. United States Simulect Renal Study Group. *Transplantation,* **1999b,** *67:*276–284.

Kahan, B.D. The potential role of rapamycin in pediatric transplantation as observed from adult studies. *Pediatr. Transplant.,* **1999,** *3:*175–180.

Keegan, B.M., and Noseworthy, J.H. Multiple sclerosis. *Annu. Rev. Med.,* **2002,** *53:*285–302.

Keesal, N., Wasserman, M.J., Bookman, A., *et al.* Thalidomide in the treatment of refractory rheumatoid arthritis. *J. Rheumatol.,* **1999,** *26:*2344–2347.

Khanna, A., Li, B., Stenzel, K.H., and Suthanthiran, M. Regulation of new DNA synthesis in mammalian cells by cyclosporine. Demonstration of a transforming growth factor beta-dependent mechanism of inhibition of cell growth. *Transplantation,* **1994,** *57:*577–582.

Kimball, J.A., Pescovitz, M.D., Book, B.K., and Norman, D.J. Reduced human IgG anti-ATGAM antibody formation in renal transplant recipients receiving mycophenolate mofetil. *Transplantation,* **1995,** *60:*1379–1383.

Kirk, A.D., Harlan, D.M., Armstrong, N.N., *et al.* CTLA4-Ig and anti-CD40 ligand prevent renal allograft rejection in primates. *Proc. Natl. Acad. Sci. U.S.A.,* **1997,** *94:*8789–8794.

Kirk, A.D., Tadaki, D.K., Celniker, A., *et al.* Induction therapy with monoclonal antibodies specific for CD80 and CD86 delays the onset of acute renal allograft rejection in non-human primates. *Transplantation,* **2001,** *72:*377–384.

Kohler, G., and Milstein, C. Continuous cultures of fused cells secreting antibody of predefined specificity. *Nature,* **1975,** *256:*495–497.

Kovarik, J.M., Kahan, B.D., Rajagopalan, P.R., *et al.* Population pharmacokinetics and exposure-response relationships for basiliximab in kidney transplantation. The U.S. Simulect Renal Transplant Study Group. *Transplantation,* **1999,** *68:*1288–1294.

Kramer, B.K., Zulke, C., Kammerl, M.C., *et al.,* and the European Tacrolimus vs. Cyclosporine Microemulsion Renal Transplantation Study Group. Cardiovascular risk factors and estimated risk for CAD in a randomized trial comparing calcineurin inhibitors in renal transplantation. *Am. J. Transplant.,* **2003,** *3:*982–987.

Kreis, H., Cisterne, J.M., Land, W., *et al.* Sirolimus in association with mycophenolate mofetil induction for the prevention of acute graft rejection in renal allograft recipients. *Transplantation,* **2000,** *69:*1252–1260.

Kuo, C.J., Chung, J., Fiorentino, D.F., *et al.* Rapamycin selectively inhibits interleukin-2 activation of p70 S6 kinase. *Nature,* **1992,** *358:*70–73.

Larroche, C., Chanseaud, Y., de la Pena-Lefebvre, G., *et al.* Mechanisms of intravenous immunoglobulin action in the treatment of autoimmune disorders. *BioDrugs,* **2002,** *16:*47–55.

Larsen, C.P., Alexander, D.Z., Hollenbaugh, D., *et al.* CD40-gp39 interactions play a critical role during allograft rejection. Suppression of allograft rejection by blockade of the CD40-gp39 pathway. *Transplantation,* **1996,** *61:*4–9.

Lary, J.M., Daniel, K.L., Erickson, J.D., *et al.* The return of thalidomide: can birth defects be prevented? *Drug Saf.,* **1999,** *21:*161–169.

Lawen, J., Davies, E., Morad, F., *et al.* Basiliximab (Simulect) is safe and effective in combination with triple therapy of Neoral, steroids and CellCept in renal transplant patients. *Transplantation,* **2000,** *69:*S260.

Lee, D. Preventing RhD haemolytic disease of the newborn. Revised guidelines advocate two doses of anti-D immunoglobulin for antenatal prophylaxis. *BMJ,* **1998,** *316:*1611.

Li, Y., Zheng, X.X., Li, X.C., *et al*. Combined costimulation blockade plus rapamycin but not cyclosporine produces permanent engraftment. *Transplantation,* **1998,** *66:*1387–1388.

Lo Iacono, O., Castro, A., Diago, M., *et al*. Interferon alfa-2b plus ribavirin for chronic hepatitis C patients who have not responded to interferon monotherapy. *Aliment. Pharmacol. Ther.,* **2000,** *14:*463–469.

Mariat, C., Alamartine, E., Diab, N., *et al*. Randomized prospective study comparing low-dose OKT3 to low-dose ATG for the treatment of acute steroid-resistant rejection episodes in kidney transplant recipients. *Transplant. Int.,* **1998,** *11:*231–236.

Mayer, A.D., Dmitrewski, J., Squifflet, J.P., *et al*. Multicenter randomized trial comparing tacrolimus (FK506) and cyclosporine in the prevention of renal allograft rejection: a report of the European Tacrolimus Multicenter Renal Study Group. *Transplantation,* **1997,** *64:*436–443.

McTaggart, R.A., Gottlieb, D., Brooks, J.H., *et al*. Sirolimus prolongs recovery from delayed graft function after cadaveric renal transplantation. *Am. J. Transplant,* **2003,** *3:*416–423.

Mihatsch, M.J., Kyo, M., Morozumi, K., *et al*. The side-effects of cyclosporine-A and tacrolimus. *Clin. Nephrol.,* **1998,** *49:*356–363.

Miller, D.H., Khan, O.A., Sheremata, W.A., *et al*. International Natalizumab Multiple Sclerosis Trial Group. A controlled trial of natalizumab for relapsing multiple sclerosis. *N. Engl. J. Med.,* **2003,** *348:*68–72.

Moertel, C.G., Fleming, T.R., Macdonald, J.S., *et al*. Levamisole and fluorouracil for adjuvant therapy of resected colon carcinoma. *N. Engl. J. Med.,* **1990,** *322:*352–358.

Monaco, A.P. A new look at polyclonal antilymphocyte antibodies in clinical transplantation. *Graft,* **1999,** *2:*S2–S5.

Morales, A., Ottenhof, P., and Emerson, L. Treatment of residual, noninfiltrating bladder cancer with bacillus Calmette-Guérin. *J. Urol.* **1981,** *125:*649–651.

Murgia, M.G., Jordan, S., and Kahan, B.D. The side effect profile of sirolimus: a phase I study in quiescent cyclosporine-prednisone-treated renal transplant patients. *Kidney Int.,* **1996,** *49:*209–216.

Nakakura, E.K., Shorthouse, R.A., Zheng, B., *et al*. Long-term survival of solid organ allografts by brief anti-lymphocyte function-associated antigen-1 monoclonal antibody monotherapy. *Transplantation,* **1996,** *62:*547–552.

Napoli, K.L., and Kahan, B.D. Routine clinical monitoring of sirolimus (rapamycin) whole-blood concentrations by HPLC with ultraviolet detection. *Clin. Chem.,* **1996,** *42:*1943–1948.

Nashan, B., Light, S., Hardie, I.R., *et al*. Reduction of acute renal allograft rejection by daclizumab. Daclizumab Double Therapy Study Group. *Transplantation,* **1999,** *67:*110–115.

Nashan, B., Moore, R., Amlot, P., *et al*. Randomized trial of basiliximab versus placebo for control of acute cellular rejection in renal allograft recipients. CHIB 201 International Study Group. *Lancet,* **1997,** *350:*1193–1198.

Oberbauer, R., Kreis, H., Johnson, R.W.G., *et al*., for the Rapamune Maintenance Regimen Study Group. Long-term improvement in renal function with sirolimus after early cyclosporine withdrawal in renal transplant recipients: 2-year results of the Rapamune Maintenance Regimen Study. *Transplantation,* **2003,** *76:*364–370.

Ojo, A.O., Held, P.J., Port, F.K., *et al*. Chronic renal failure after transplantation of a nonrenal organ. *N. Engl. J. Med.*, **2003,** *349:*931–940.

Opelz, G., and Terasaki, P.I. Improvement of kidney-graft survival with increased numbers of blood transfusions. *N. Engl. J. Med.,* **1978,** *299:*799–803.

Opelz, G., Vanrenterghem, Y., Kirste, G., *et al*. Prospective evaluation of pretransplant blood transfusions in cadaver kidney recipients. *Transplantation,* **1997,** *63:*964–967.

Ortho Multicenter Transplant Study Group. A randomized clinical trial of OKT3 monoclonal antibody for acute rejection of cadaveric renal transplants. *N. Engl. J. Med.,* **1985,** *313:*337–342.

Ossevoort, M.A., Ringers, J., Kuhn, E.-M., *et al*. Prevention of renal allograft rejection in primates by blocking the B7/CD28 pathway. *Transplantation,* **1999,** *68:*1010–1018.

Pescovitz, M.D., Bumgardner, G.L., Gaston, R.S., *et al*. Addition of daclizumab to mycophenolate mofetil, cyclosporine, and steroids in renal transplantation: pharmacokinetics, safety, and efficacy. *Clinical Transplantation,* **2003,** *17:*511-517.

Ravnborg, M., *et al*. Responsiveness of the Multiple Sclerosis Impairment Scale in comparison with the Expanded Disability Status Scale. *Mult. Scler.,* **2005,** *11:*81–84.

Regan, J.F., Campbell, K., Van Smith, L., *et al*. Sensitization following Thymoglobulin and Atgam rejection therapy as determined with a rapid enzyme-linked immunosorbent assay. US Thymoglobulin Multi-Center Study Group. *Transplant. Immunol.,* **1999,** *7:*115–121.

Rostaing, L., Chabannier, M.H., Modesto, A., *et al*. Predicting factors of long-term results of OKT3 therapy for steroid resistant acute rejection following cadaveric renal transplantation. *Am. J. Nephrol.,* **1999,** *19:*634–640.

Rutter, A., and Luger, T.A. Intravenous immunoglobulin: an emerging treatment for immune-mediated skin diseases. *Curr. Opin. Investig. Drugs.,* **2002,** *3:*713–719.

Salmela, K., Wramner, L., Ekberg, H., *et al*. A randomized multicenter trial of the anti-ICAM-1 monoclonal antibody (enlimomab) for the prevention of acute rejection and delayed onset of graft function in cadaveric renal transplantation: a report of the European Anti-ICAM-1 Renal Transplant Study Group. *Transplantation,* **1999,** *67:*729–736.

Salm, P., Taylor, P.J., and Pillans, P.I. Analytical performance of microparticle enzyme immunoassay and HPLC-tandem mass spectrometry in the determination of sirolimus in whole blood. *Clin. Chem.,* **1999,** *45:*2278–2280.

Sampaio, E.P., Kaplan, G., Miranda, A., *et al*. The influence of thalidomide on the clinical and immunologic manifestation of erythema nodosum leprosum. *J. Infect. Dis.,* **1993,** *168:*408–414.

Shinn, C., Malhotra, D., Chan, L., *et al*. Time course of response to pulse methylprednisolone therapy in renal transplant recipients with acute allograft rejection. *Am. J. Kidney Dis.,* **1999,** *34:*304–307.

Simone, E.A., Wegmann, D.R., and Eisenbarth, G.S. Immunologic "vaccination" for the prevention of autoimmune diabetes (type 1A). *Diabetes Care,* **1999,** *22*(Suppl. 2):B7–B15.

Smith, K.D., Wrenshall, L.E., Nicosia, R.F., *et al*. Delayed graft function and case nephropathy associated with tacrolimus plus rapamycin use. *J. Am. Soc. Nephrol.,* **2003,** *14:*1037–1045.

Spitzer, T.R., Delmonico, F., Tolkoff-Rubin, N., *et al*. Combined histocompatibility leukocyte antigen-matched donor bone marrow and renal transplantation for multiple myeloma with end stage renal disease: the induction of allograft tolerance through mixed lymphohematopoietic chimerism. *Transplantation,* **1999,** *68:*480–484.

Stegall, M.D., Larson, T.S., Prieto, M., *et al*. Kidney transplantation without calcineurin inhibitors using sirolimus. *Transplant Proc.,* **2003,** *35:*125S–127S.

Steinman, L. Immune therapy for autoimmune diseases. *Science,* **2004,** *305:*212–216.

Szczech, L.A., Berlin, J.A., Aradhye, S., *et al*. Effect of anti-lymphocyte induction therapy on renal allograft survival: a meta-analysis. *J. Am. Soc. Nephrol.*, **1997,** *8:*1771–1777.

Tanabe, K. Calcineurin inhibitors in renal transplantation. What is the best option? *Drugs,* **2003,** *63:*1535–1548.

The National Vaccine Advisory Committee. Strategies to sustain success in childhood immunizations. *JAMA*, **1999**, *282:*363–370.

The U.S. Multicenter FK506 Liver Study Group. A comparison of tacrolimus (FK 506) and cyclosporine for immunosuppression in liver transplantation. *N. Engl. J. Med.*, **1994**, *331:*1110–1115.

Valeri, A., Radhakrishnan, J., Estes, D., *et al.* Intravenous pulse cyclophosphamide treatment of severe lupus nephritis: a prospective five-year study. *Clin. Nephrol.*, **1994**, *42:*71–78.

Venkataramanan, R., Swaminathan, A., Prasad, T., *et al.* Clinical pharmacokinetics of tacrolimus. *Clin. Pharmacokinet.*, **1995**, *29:*404–430.

Vezina, C., Kudelski, A., and Sehgal, S.N. Rapamycin (AY-22,989), a new antifungal antibiotic. I. Taxonomy of the producing streptomycete and isolation of the active principle. *J. Antibiot. (Tokyo)*, **1975**, *28:*721–726.

Vincenti, F., Kirkman, R., Light, S., *et al.* Interleukin-2-receptor blockade with daclizumab to prevent acute rejection in renal transplantation. Daclizumab Triple Therapy Study Group. *N. Engl. J. Med.*, **1998**, *338:*161–165.

Vincenti, F., Mendez, R., Rajagopalan, P.R., *et al.* A phase I/II trial of anti-CD11a monoclonal antibody in renal transplantation. *Am. J. Transplant*, **2001**, *1*(Suppl. 1):276.

Vincenti, F. What's in the pipeline. New immunosuppressive drugs in transplantation. *Am. J. Transplant.*, **2002**, *2:*898–903.

Wall, W.J. Use of antilymphocyte induction therapy in liver transplantation. *Liver Transplant. Surg.*, **1999**, *5:*S64–S70.

Watson, C.J., Friend, P.J., Jamieson, N.V., *et al.* Sirolimus: a potent new immunosuppressant for liver transplantation. *Transplantation*, **1999**, *67:*505–509.

Weiner, H.L. Immunosuppressive treatment in multiple sclerosis. *J. Neurological Sci.*, **2004**, *223:*1–11.

Woodle, E.S., Xu, D., Zivin, R.A., *et al.* Phase I trial of a humanized, Fc receptor nonbinding OKT3 antibody, huOKT3gamma1(Ala-Ala) in the treatment of acute renal allograft rejection. *Transplantation*, **1999**, *68:*608–616.

Yoshimura, R., Yoshimura, N., Ohyama, A., *et al.* The effect of immunosuppressive agents (FK-506, rapamycin) on renal P450 systems in rat models. *J. Pharm. Pharmacol.*, **1999**, *51:*941–948.

Zachary, A.A., Montgomery, R.A., Ratner, L.E., *et al.* Specific and durable elimination of antibody to donor HLA antigens in renal-transplant patients. *Transplantation*, **2003**, *76:*1519–1525.

Zavos, G., Gazouli, M., Psimenou, E., *et al.* Polyomavirus BK infection in Greek renal transplant recipients. *Transplant Proc.*, **2004**, *36:*1413–1414.

Zimmerman, J.J., and Kahan, B.D. Pharmacokinetics of sirolimus in stable renal transplant patients after multiple oral dose administration. *J. Clin. Pharmacol.*, **1997**, *37:*405–415.

MONOGRAPHS AND REVIEWS

Allison, A.C., and Eugui, E.M. Immunosuppressive and other effects of mycophenolic acid and an ester prodrug, mycophenolate mofetil. *Immunol. Rev.*, **1993**, *136:*5–28.

Bardsley-Elliot, A., Noble, S., and Foster, R.H. Mycophenolate mofetil: a review of its use in the management of solid organ transplantation. *BioDrugs*, **1999**, *12:*363–410.

Bukowski, R.M. Immunotherapy in renal cell carcinoma. *Oncology (Huntingt.)*, **1999**, *13:*801–810.

Clayberger, C., and Krensky, A.M. Mechanisms of allograft rejection. In, *Immunologic Renal Diseases.* (Neilson, E.G., and Couser, W.G., eds.) Lippincott-Raven, Philadelphia, **2001**.

Del Vecchio, M., and Parmiani, G. Cancer vaccination. *Forum (Genova)*, **1999**, *9:*239–256.

Dorner, F., and Barrett, P.N. Vaccine technology: looking to the future. *Ann. Med.*, **1999**, *31:*51–60.

Faulds, D., Goa, K.L., and Benfield, P. Cyclosporin. A review of its pharmacodynamic and pharmacotherapeutic properties, and therapeutic use in immunoregulatory disorders. *Drugs*, **1993**, *45:*953–1040.

Fulton, B., and Markham, A. Mycophenolate mofetil. A review of its pharmacodynamic and pharmacokinetic properties and clinical efficacy in renal transplantation. *Drugs*, **1996**, *51:*278–298.

Fung, J.J., and Starzl, T.E. FK506 in solid organ transplantation. *Ther. Drug Monit.*, **1995**, *17:*592–595.

Grosflam, J., and Weinblatt, M.E. Methotrexate: mechanism of action, pharmacokinetics, clinical indications, and toxicity. *Curr. Opin. Rheumatol.*, **1991**, *3:*363–368.

Hackett, C.J., and Dickler, H.B. Immunologic tolerance for immune system-mediated diseases. *J. Allergy Clin. Immunol.*, **1999**, *103:*362–370.

Hong, J.C., and Kahan, B.D. Immunosuppressive agents in organ transplantation: past, present, and future. *Semin. Nephrol.*, **2000a**, *20:*108–125.

Hooks, M.A., Wade, C.S., and Millikan, W.J. Jr. Muromonab CD-3: a review of its pharmacology, pharmacokinetics, and clinical use in transplantation. *Pharmacotherapy*, **1991**, *11:*26–37.

Janeway, C.A., Travers, P., Walport, M., and Shlomchik M., eds. *Immunobiology: The Immune System in Health and Disease*, 5th ed. Garland, New York, **2001.**

Johnson, H.M., Bazer, F.W., Szente, B.E., and Jarpe, M.A. How interferons fight disease. *Sci. Am.*, **1994**, *270:*68–75.

Kahan, B.D. Cyclosporine. *N. Engl. J. Med.*, **1989**, *32:*1725–1738.

Khoury, S., Sayegh, M.H., and Turka, L.A. Blocking costimulatory signals to induce transplantation tolerance and prevent autoimmune disease. *Int. Rev. Immunol.*, **1999**, *18:*185–199.

Krensky, A.M., and Clayberger, C. Prospects for induction of tolerance in renal transplantation. *Pediatr. Nephrol.*, **1994**, *8:*772–779.

Krensky, A.M. Transplantation immunobiology. In, *Pediatric Nephrology*, 4th ed. (Barratt, T.M., Auner, E.D., and Harmon, W., eds.) Williams & Wilkins, Baltimore, **2001**, pp. 1289–1307.

Laan, R.F., Jansen, T.L., and van Riel, P.L. Glucocorticosteroids in the management of rheumatoid arthritis. *Rheumatology (Oxford)*, **1999**, *38:*6–12.

Lee, D.J., Corr, M., and Carson, D.A. Control of immune responses by gene immunization. *Ann. Med.*, **1998b**, *30:*460–468.

Lewis, P.J., and Babiuk, L.A. DNA vaccines: a review. *Adv. Virus Res.*, **1999**, *54:*129–188.

Liljeqvist, S., and Stahl, S. Production of recombinant subunit vaccines: protein immunogens, live delivery systems and nucleic acid vaccines. *J. Biotechnol.*, **1999**, *73:*1–33.

Linden, K.G., and Weinstein, G.D. Psoriasis: current perspectives with an emphasis on treatment. *Am. J. Med.*, **1999**, *107:*595–605.

Miller, M.T., and Stromland, K. Teratogen update: thalidomide: a review, with a focus on ocular findings and new potential uses. *Teratology*, **1999**, *60:*306–321.

Monaco, A.P., Burke, J.F. Jr., Ferguson, R.M., *et al.* Current thinking on chronic renal allograft rejection: issues, concerns, and recommendations from a 1997 roundtable discussion. *Am. J. Kidney Dis.*, **1999**, *33:*150–160.

Murphy, B., and Krensky, A.M. HLA-derived peptides as novel immunomodulatory therapeutics. *J. Am. Soc. Nephrol.*, **1999**, *10:*1346–1355.

Natsumeda, Y., and Carr, S.F. Human type I and II IMP dehydrogenases as drug targets. *Ann. N.Y. Acad. Sci.,* **1993,** *696:*88–93.

Neuhaus, T.J., Fay, J., Dillon, M.J., *et al.* Alternative treatment to corticosteroids in steroid sensitive idiopathic nephrotic syndrome. *Arch. Dis. Child,* **1994,** *71:*522–526.

Noble, S., and Markham, A. Cyclosporin. A review of the pharmacokinetic properties, clinical efficacy and tolerability of a microemulsion-based formulation (Neoral). *Drugs,* **1995,** *50:*924–941.

Patard, J.J., Saint, F., Velotti, F., *et al.* Immune response following intravesical bacillus Calmette-Guérin instillations in superficial bladder cancer: a review. *Urol. Res.,* **1998,** *26:*155–159.

Paterson, D.L., and Patel, A. Bacillus Calmette-Guérin (BCG) immunotherapy for bladder cancer: review of complications and their treatment. *Aust. N.Z. J. Surg.,* **1998,** *68:*340–344.

Pattison, J.M., Sibley, R.K., and Krensky, A.M. Mechanisms of allograft rejection. *In, Immunologic Renal Diseases.* (Neilson, E.G., and Couser, W.G., eds.) Lippincott-Raven, Philadelphia, **1997,** pp. 331–354.

Paul, W.E., ed. *Fundamental Immunology,* 4th ed. Lippincott-Raven, Philadelphia, **1999.**

Perico, N., and Remuzzi, G. Prevention of transplant rejection: current treatment guidelines and future developments. *Drugs,* **1997,** *54:*533–570.

Peterec, S.M. Management of neonatal Rh disease. *Clin. Perinatol.,* **1995,** *22:*561–592.

Plosker, G.L., and Foster, R.H. Tacrolimus: a further update of its pharmacology and therapeutic use in the management of organ transplantation. *Drugs,* **2000,** *59:*323–389.

Prakash, A., and Jarvis, B. Leflunomide: a review of its use in active rheumatoid arthritis. *Drugs,* **1999,** *58:*1137–1164.

Punt, C.J. The use of interferon-alpha in the treatment of cutaneous melanoma: a review. *Melanoma Res.,* **1998,** *8:*95–104.

Ransohoff, R.M. Cellular responses to interferons and other cytokines: the JAK-STAT paradigm. *N. Engl. J. Med.,* **1998,** *338:*616–618.

Schreiber, S.L., and Crabtree, G.R. The mechanism of action of cyclosporin A and FK506. *Immunol. Today,* **1992,** *13:*136–142.

Shapiro, R. Tacrolimus in pediatric renal transplantation: a review. *Pediatr. Transplant.,* **1998,** *2:*270–276.

Sinkovics, J.G., and Horvath, J.C. Vaccination against human cancers (review). *Int. J. Oncol.,* **2000,** *16:*81–96.

Smithells, R.W., and Newman, C.G. Recognition of thalidomide defects. *J. Med. Genet.,* **1992,** *29:*716–723.

Starzl, T.E., Demetris, A.J., Murase, N., *et al.* Chimerism after organ transplantation. *Curr. Opin. Nephrol. Hypertens.,* **1997,** *6:*292–298.

Suthanthiran, M., Morris, R.E., and Strom, T.B. Immunosuppressants: cellular and molecular mechanisms of action. *Am. J. Kidney Dis.,* **1996,** *28:*159–172.

Taniguchi, T., and Minami, Y. The IL-2/IL-2 receptor system: a current overview. *Cell,* **1993,** *73:*5–8.

Tarte, K., and Klein, B. Dendritic cell-based vaccine: a promising approach for cancer immunotherapy. *Leukemia,* **1999,** *13:*653–663.

Tilg, H., and Kaser, A. Interferons and their role in inflammation. *Curr. Pharm. Des.,* **1999,** *5:*771–785.

Tompkins, W.A. Immunomodulation and therapeutic effects of the oral use of interferon-alpha: mechanism of action. *J. Interferon Cytokine Res.,* **1999,** *19:*817–828.

Tseng, S., Pak, G., Washenik, K., *et al.* Rediscovering thalidomide: a review of its mechanism of action, side effects, and potential uses. *J. Am. Acad. Dermatol.,* **1996,** *35:*969–979.

Van Parijs, L., and Abbas, A.K. Homeostasis and self-tolerance in the immune system: turning lymphocytes off. *Science,* **1998,** *280:*243–248.

Whittington, R., and Faulds, D. Interleukin-2. A review of its pharmacological properties and therapeutic use in patients with cancer. *Drugs,* **1993,** *46:*446–514.

Wilde, M.I., and Goa, K.L. Muromonab CD3: a reappraisal of its pharmacology and use as prophylaxis of solid organ transplant rejection. *Drugs,* **1996,** *51:*865–894.

Winkelhake, J.L., and Gauny, S.S. Human recombinant interleukin-2 as an experimental therapeutic. *Pharmacol. Rev.,* **1990,** *42:*1–28.

Wiseman, L.R., and Faulds, D. Daclizumab: a review of its use in the prevention of acute rejection in renal transplant recipients. *Drugs,* **1999,** *58:*1029–1042.

Wood, K.J. Transplantation tolerance. *Curr. Opin. Immunol.,* **1991,** *3:*710–714.

Zoorob, R.J., and Cender, D. A different look at corticosteroids. *Am. Fam. Physician,* **1998,** *58:*443–450.

CHAPTER

53

HEMATOPOIETIC AGENTS
Growth Factors, Minerals, and Vitamins

Kenneth Kaushansky and Thomas J. Kipps

The finite life span of most mature blood cells requires their continuous replacement, a process termed hematopoiesis. New cell production must respond to basal needs and states of increased demand. Red blood cell production can increase more than twentyfold in response to anemia or hypoxemia, white blood cell production increases dramatically in response to a systemic infection, and platelet production can increase ten- to twentyfold when platelet consumption results in thrombocytopenia.

The regulation of blood cell production is complex. Hematopoietic stem cells are rare marrow cells that manifest self-renewal and lineage commitment, resulting in cells destined to differentiate into the nine distinct blood-cell lineages. For the most part, this process occurs in the marrow cavities of the skull, vertebral bodies, pelvis, and proximal long bones; it involves interactions among hematopoietic stem and progenitor cells and the cells and complex macromolecules of the marrow stroma, and is influenced by a number of soluble and membrane-bound hematopoietic growth factors. A number of these hormones and cytokines have been identified and cloned, permitting their production in quantities sufficient for therapeutic use. Clinical applications range from the treatment of primary hematological diseases to use as adjuncts in the treatment of severe infections and in the management of patients who are undergoing cancer chemotherapy or marrow transplantation.

Hematopoiesis also requires an adequate supply of minerals (*e.g.,* iron, cobalt, and copper) and vitamins (*e.g.,* folic acid, vitamin B_{12}, pyridoxine, ascorbic acid, and riboflavin), and deficiencies generally result in characteristic anemias, or, less frequently, a general failure of hematopoiesis (Hoffbrand and Herbert, 1999). Therapeutic correction of a specific deficiency state depends on the accurate diagnosis of the anemic state and knowledge about the correct dose, the use of these agents in various combinations, and the expected response. This chapter deals with the growth factors, vitamins, minerals, and drugs that affect the blood and blood-forming organs.

I. HEMATOPOIETIC GROWTH FACTORS

History. Modern concepts of hematopoietic cell growth and differentiation arose in the 1950s, when cells from the spleen and marrow were shown to play an important role in the restoration of hematopoietic tissue in irradiated animals. In 1961, Till and McCulloch demonstrated that individual hematopoietic cells could form macroscopic hematopoietic colonies in the spleens of irradiated mice.

Their work established the concept that there exist discrete hematopoietic stem cells, which can be experimentally identified, albeit in retrospect (*i.e.*, the presence of a multilineage clonal splenic colony appearing 11 days after transplantation implied that a single cell lodged and expanded into several cell lineages). This concept now has been expanded to include normal human marrow cells. Moreover, such cells now can be prospectively identified.

The basis for identifying soluble growth factors was provided by Sachs and independently by Metcalf, who developed clonal, *in vitro* assays for hematopoietic progenitor cells. Initially, such hematopoietic colonies developed only in the presence of conditioned culture medium from leukocytes or tumor cell lines. Individual growth factors then were isolated based on their activities in such assays. Many of these same assays were instrumental in purifying a hierarchy of progenitor cells committed to individual and combinations of mature blood cells (Kondo *et al.*, 1997; Akashi *et al.*, 2000; Sawada *et al.*, 1990; Nakorn *et al.*, 2003).

The existence of a circulating growth factor that controls red blood cell development was first suggested by the experiments of Paul Carnot in 1906. He observed an increase in the red cell count in rabbits injected with serum obtained from anemic animals and postulated the existence of a factor that he called *hemapoietine*. However, it was not until the 1950s that Reissmann, Erslev, and Jacobsen and coworkers defined the origin and actions of the hormone, now called *erythropoietin*. Subsequently, extensive studies of erythropoietin were carried out in patients with anemia and polycythemia, leading to the purification of erythropoietin from urine and the subsequent cloning of the erythropoietin gene. The high-level expression of erythropoietin in and purification from cell lines has allowed for its use in humans with anemia.

Similarly, the existence of specific leukocyte growth factors was suggested by the capacity of different conditioned culture media to induce the *in vitro* growth of colonies containing different combinations of granulocytes and monocytes. Using a multistep purification process beginning with conditioned culture medium from fibroblasts, macrophage colony–stimulating factor (M-CSF) was purified and the corresponding gene identified (Wong *et al.*, 1987). An activity that stimulated the production of both granulocytes and monocytes was purified from murine lung–conditioned medium, leading to cloning of its cDNA (Gough *et al.*, 1984), as was an activity that stimulated the exclusive production of neutrophils, permitting the cloning of granulocyte colony–stimulating factor (G-CSF) (Welte *et al.*, 1985). Most recently, a megakaryocyte colony–stimulating factor termed *thrombopoietin* was purified and cloned (Kaushansky, 1998).

The growth factors that support lymphocyte growth were not identified using *in vitro* colony-forming assays, but rather using assays that measured the capacity of the cytokine to promote lymphocyte proliferation *in vitro*. This permitted the identification of the growth-promoting properties of interleukin-7, interleukin-4, or interleukin-15 for all lymphocytes, B cells, or NK cells, respectively (Goodwin *et al.*, 1989; Yokota *et al.*, 1986; Grabstein *et al.*, 1994). Again, recombinant expression of these cDNAs permitted production of sufficient quantities of biologically active growth factors for clinical investigations, allowing for the demonstration of the potential clinical utility of such factors.

Growth Factor Physiology. Steady-state hematopoiesis encompasses the production of more than 400 billion blood cells each day. This production is tightly regulated and can be increased severalfold with increased demand. The hematopoietic organ also is unique in adult physiology

in that several mature cell types are derived from a much smaller number of multipotent progenitors, which develop from a more limited number of pluripotent hematopoietic stem cells. Such cells are capable of maintaining their own number and differentiating under the influence of cellular and humoral factors to produce the large and diverse number of mature blood cells.

Stem cell differentiation can be described as a series of steps that produce so-called burst-forming units (BFU) and colony-forming units (CFU) for each of the major cell lines (Quesenberry and Levitt, 1979). These early progenitors (BFU and CFU) are capable of further proliferation and differentiation, increasing their number by some thirtyfold. Subsequently, colonies of morphologically distinct cells form under the control of an overlapping set of additional growth factors (G-CSF, M-CSF, erythropoietin, and thrombopoietin). Proliferation and maturation of the CFU for each cell line can amplify the resulting mature cell product by another thirtyfold or more, generating more than 1000 mature cells from each committed stem cell.

Hematopoietic and lymphopoietic growth factors are glycoproteins produced by a number of marrow cells and peripheral tissues. They are active at very low concentrations and typically affect more than one committed cell lineage. Most interact synergistically with other factors and also stimulate production of additional growth factors, a process called *networking*. Growth factors generally exert actions at several points in the processes of cell proliferation and differentiation and in mature cell function (Metcalf, 1985). However, the network of growth factors that contributes to any given cell lineage depends absolutely on a nonredundant, lineage-specific factor, such that absence of factors that stimulate developmentally early progenitors is compensated for by redundant cytokines, but loss of the lineage-specific factor leads to a specific cytopenia. Some of the overlapping and nonredundant effects of the more important hematopoietic growth factors are illustrated in Figure 53–1 and listed in Table 53–1.

ERYTHROPOIETINS

While erythropoietin is not the sole growth factor responsible for erythropoiesis, it is the most important regulator of the proliferation of committed progenitors (CFU-E) and their immediate progeny. In its absence, severe anemia is invariably present. Erythropoiesis is controlled by a highly responsive feedback system in which a sensor in the kidney detects changes in oxygen delivery to modu-

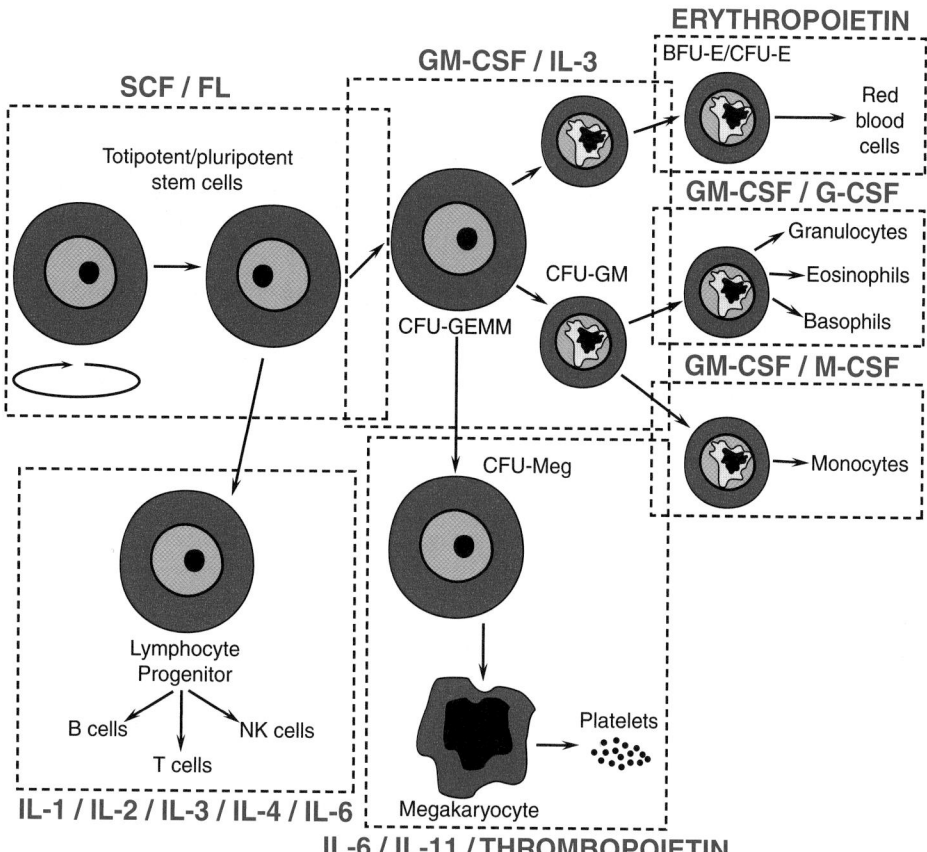

Figure 53–1. *Sites of action of hematopoietic growth factors in the differentiation and maturation of marrow cell lines.* A self-sustaining pool of marrow stem cells differentiates under the influence of specific hematopoietic growth factors to form a variety of hematopoietic and lymphopoietic cells. Stem cell factor (SCF), ligand (FL), interleukin-3 (IL-3), and granulocyte-macrophage colony-stimulating factor (GM-CSF), together with cell–cell interactions in the marrow, stimulate stem cells to form a series of burst-forming units (BFU) and colony-forming units (CFU): CFU-GEMM (granulocyte, erythrocyte, monocyte and megakaryocyte), CFU-GM (granulocyte and macrophage), CFU-Meg (megakaryocyte), BFU-E (erythrocyte), and CFU-E (erythrocyte). After considerable proliferation, further differentiation is stimulated by synergistic interactions with growth factors for each of the major cell lines—granulocyte colony–stimulating factor (G-CSF), monocyte/macrophage-stimulating factor (M-CSF), thrombopoietin, and erythropoietin. Each of these factors also influences the proliferation, maturation, and in some cases the function of the derivative cell line (*see* Table 53–1).

late the erythropoietin secretion. The sensor mechanism is now understood at the molecular level (Maxwell *et al.*, 2001). Hypoxia-inducible factor (HIF-1) is a heterodimeric (HIF-1α and HIF-1β) transcription factor that enhances expression of multiple hypoxia-inducible genes, such as vascular endothelial growth factor and erythropoietin. HIF-1α is labile due to its prolyl hydroxylation and subsequent polyubiquitination and degradation, aided by the von Hippel-Lindau (VHL) protein. During states of hypoxia, the prolyl hydroxylase is inactive, allowing the accumulation of HIF-1α and activating erythropoietin expression, which in turn stimulates a rapid expansion of erythroid progenitors. Specific alteration of VHL leads to an oxygen-sensing defect, characterized by constitutively

elevated levels of HIF-1α and erythropoietin, with a resultant polycythemia (Gordeuk *et al.*, 2004).

Erythropoietin is encoded by a gene on human chromosome 7 that is expressed primarily in peritubular interstitial cells of the kidney. Erythropoietin contains 193 amino acids, of which the first 27 are cleaved during secretion. The final hormone is heavily glycosylated and has a molecular mass of approximately 30,000 daltons. After secretion, erythropoietin binds to a receptor on the surface of committed erythroid progenitors in the marrow and is internalized. With anemia or hypoxemia, synthesis rapidly increases by one hundredfold or more, serum erythropoietin levels rise, and marrow progenitor cell survival, proliferation, and maturation are dramati-

Table 53–1
Hematopoietic Growth Factors

ERYTHROPOIETIN (EPO)
- Stimulates proliferation and maturation of committed erythroid progenitors to increase red cell production

STEM CELL FACTOR (SCF, c-kit ligand, Steel factor) and FLT-3 LIGAND (FL)
- Act synergistically with a wide range of other colony-stimulating factors and interleukins to stimulate pluripotent and committed stem cells
- FL also stimulates both dendritic and natural killer cells (anti-tumor response)
- SCF also stimulates mast cells and melanocytes

INTERLEUKINS
IL-1, IL-3, IL-5, IL-6, IL-9, and IL-11
- Act synergistically with each other and SCF, GM-CSF, G-CSF, and EPO to stimulate BFU-E, CFU-GEMM, CFU-GM, CFU-E, and CFU-Meg growth
- Numerous immunologic roles, including stimulation of B cell and T cell growth
- IL-6 stimulates human myeloma cells to proliferate
- IL-6 and IL-11 stimulate BFU-Meg to increase platelet production

IL-5
- Controls eosinophil survival and differentiation

IL-1, IL-2, IL-4, IL-7, and IL-12
- Stimulate growth and function of T cells, B cells, NK cells, and monocytes
- Co-stimulate B, T, and LAK cells

IL-8 and IL-10
- Numerous immunological activities involving B and T cell functions
- IL-8 acts as a chemotactic factor for basophils and neutrophils

GRANULOCYTE-MACROPHAGE COLONY–STIMULATING FACTOR (GM-CSF)
- Acts synergistically with SCF, IL-1, IL-3, and IL-6 to stimulate CFU-GM, and CFU-Meg to increase neutrophil and monocyte production
- With EPO may promote BFU-E formation
- Enhances migration, phagocytosis, superoxide production, and antibody-dependent cell-mediated toxicity of neutrophils, monocytes, and eosinophils
- Prevents alveolar proteinosis

GRANULOCYTE COLONY–STIMULATING FACTOR (G-CSF)
- Stimulates CFU-G to increase neutrophil production
- Enhances phagocytic and cytotoxic activities of neutrophils

MONOCYTE/MACROPHAGE COLONY–STIMULATING FACTOR (M-CSF, CSF-1)
- Stimulates CFU-M to increase monocyte precursors
- Activates and enhances function of monocyte/macrophages

MACROPHAGE COLONY–STIMULATING FACTOR (M-CSF)
- Stimulates CFU-M to increase monocyte/macrophage precursors
- Acts in concert with tissues and other growth factors to determine the proliferation, differentiation, and survival of a range of cells of the mononuclear phagocyte system

THROMBOPOIETIN (TPO, *Mpl* ligand)
- Stimulates the self-renewal and expansion of hematopoietic stem cells
- Stimulates stem cell differentiation into megakaryocyte progenitors
- Selectively stimulates megakaryocytopoiesis to increase platelet production
- Acts synergistically with other growth factors, especially IL-6 and IL-11

ABBREVIATIONS: BFU, burst-forming unit; CFU, colony-forming unit; E, erythrocyte; G, granulocyte; M, macrophage; Meg, megakaryocyte; NK cells, natural killer cells; LAK cells, lymphokine-activated killer cells.

cally stimulated. This finely tuned feedback loop can be disrupted by kidney disease, marrow damage, or a deficiency in iron or an essential vitamin. With an infection or an inflammatory state, erythropoietin secretion, iron delivery, and progenitor proliferation all are suppressed by inflammatory cytokines, but this accounts for only part of the resultant anemia; interference with iron metabolism also is an effect of inflammatory mediator effects on the hepatic protein hepcidin (Nemeth *et al.*, 2004).

Recombinant human erythropoietin (*epoetin alfa*), produced using engineered Chinese hamster ovary cells, is nearly identical to the endogenous hormone except for two subtle differences. First, the carbohydrate modification pattern of epoetin alfa differs slightly from the native protein, but this difference apparently does not alter kinetics, potency, or immunoreactivity of the drug. However, modern assays can detect these differences (Skibeli *et al.*, 2001), which is of significance for detecting athletes who use the recombinant product for "blood doping." The second difference probably is related to the manufacturing process, as one commercially available form of the drug was recently associated with the development of anti-recombinant erythropoietin antibodies that cross-react with the patient's own erythropoietin, potentially causing pure red cell aplasia (Macdougall, 2004). Most of these cases were caused by one preparation of the drug shortly after albumin was removed from the formulation (Casadevall, 2003).

Available preparations of epoetin alfa include EPOGEN, PROCRIT, and EXPREX, supplied in single-use vials of from 2000 to 40,000 units/ml for intravenous or subcutaneous administration. When injected intravenously, epoetin alfa is cleared from plasma with a half-life of 4 to 8 hours. However, the effect on marrow progenitors is sufficiently sustained that it need only be given three times a week to achieve an adequate response. Combination of the weekly dose into a single injection also can achieve virtually identical results. No significant allergic reactions have been associated with the intravenous or subcutaneous administration of epoetin alfa, and—except as noted above—antibodies have not been detected even after prolonged administration.

More recently, novel erythropoiesis-stimulating protein (NESP) or darbapoetin alfa (ARANESP) has been approved for clinical use in patients with indications similar to those for epoetin alfa. It is a genetically modified form of erythropoietin in which four amino acids have been mutated such that additional carbohydrate side chains are added during its synthesis, prolonging the circulatory survival of the drug to 24 to 26 hours (Jelkmann, 2002).

Therapeutic Uses, Monitoring, and Adverse Effects. Recombinant erythropoietin therapy, in conjunction with adequate iron intake, can be highly effective in a number of anemias, especially those associated with a poor erythropoietic response. There is a clear dose-response relationship between the epoetin alfa dose and the rise in hematocrit in anephric patients, with eradication of their anemia at higher doses (Eschbach *et al.*, 1987). Epoetin alfa also is effective in the treatment of anemias associated with surgery, AIDS, cancer chemotherapy, prematurity, and certain chronic inflammatory conditions. Darbapoetin alfa also has been approved for use in patients with anemia associated with chronic kidney disease and is under review for several other indications.

During erythropoietin therapy, absolute or functional iron deficiency may develop. Functional iron deficiency (*i.e.,* normal ferritin levels but low transferrin saturation) presumably results from the inability to mobilize iron stores rapidly enough to support the increased erythropoiesis. Virtually all patients eventually will require supplemental iron to increase or maintain transferrin saturation to levels that will adequately support stimulated erythropoiesis. Supplemental iron therapy is recommended for all patients whose serum ferritin is below 100 μg/L or whose serum transferrin saturation is less than 20% (*see* below).

During initial therapy and after any dosage adjustment, the hematocrit is determined once a week (HIV-infected and cancer patients) or twice a week (renal failure patients) until it has stabilized in the target range and the maintenance dose has been established; the hematocrit then is monitored at regular intervals. If the hematocrit increases by more than 4 points in any 2-week period, the dose should be decreased. Due to the time required for erythropoiesis and the erythrocyte half-life, hematocrit changes lag behind dosage adjustments by 2 to 6 weeks. The dose of darbepoetin should be decreased if the hemoglobin increase exceeds 1 g/dl in any two-week period because of the association of excessive rate of rise of hemoglobin with adverse cardiovascular events.

During hemodialysis, patients receiving epoetin alfa or darbepoetin may require increased anticoagulation. Serious thromboembolic events have been reported, including migratory thrombophlebitis, microvascular thrombosis, pulmonary embolism, and thrombosis of the retinal artery and temporal and renal veins. The risk of thrombotic events, including vascular access thromboses, was higher in adults with ischemic heart disease or congestive heart failure receiving epoetin alfa therapy with the goal of reaching a normal hematocrit (42%) than in those with a lower target hematocrit of 30%. The higher risk of cardiovascular events from erythropoietic therapies may be associated with higher hemoglobin or higher rates of rise of hemoglobin. The hemoglobin level should be managed to avoid exceeding a target level of 12 g/dl. Although epoetin alfa is not associated with direct pressor effects, blood pressure may rise, especially during the early phases of therapy when the hematocrit is increasing. Erythropoietins should be withheld in patients with pre-existing uncontrolled hypertension. Patients may require initiation of, or increases in, antihypertensive therapy. Hypertensive encephalopathy and seizures have occurred in chronic renal failure patients treated with epoetin alfa. The incidence of seizures appears to be higher during the first 90 days of therapy with epoetin alfa in patients on dialysis (occurring in about 2.5% of patients) when compared with subsequent 90-day periods. Headache, tachycardia, edema, shortness of breath, nausea, vomiting, diarrhea, injection site stinging, and flu-like symptoms (*e.g.,* arthralgias and myalgias) also have been reported in conjunction with epoetin alfa therapy. Pure red cell aplasia in association with neutralizing antibodies to native erythropoietin has been observed in patients treated with recombinant erythropoietins (*see* above); underlying infectious, inflammatory, or malignant processes; occult blood loss; underlying hematologic diseases (*e.g.,* thalassemia, refractory anemia, or other myelodysplastic disorders); folic acid or vitamin B$_{12}$ deficiency; hemolysis; aluminum intoxication; bone marrow fibrosis; and osteitis fibrosa cystica.

Anemia of Chronic Renal Failure. Patients with anemia secondary to chronic kidney disease are ideal candidates for epoetin alfa therapy. The response in predialysis, peritoneal dialysis, and hemodialysis patients is dependent on severity of the renal failure, the erythropoietin dose and route of administration, and iron availability (Eschbach *et al.*, 1989; Kaufman *et al.*, 1998; Besarab *et al.*, 1999). The subcutaneous route of administration is preferred over the intravenous route because absorption is slower and the amount of drug required is reduced by 20% to 40%.

The dose of epoetin alfa should be adjusted to obtain a gradual rise in the hematocrit over a 2- to 4-month period to a final hematocrit of 33% to 36%. Treatment to hematocrit levels greater than 36% is not recommended, as patients treated to a hematocrit above 40% showed a higher incidence of myocardial infarction and death (Besarab *et al.*, 1998). The drug should not be used to replace emergency transfusion in patients who need immediate correction of a life-threatening anemia.

Patients are started on doses of 80 to 120 units/kg of epoetin alfa, given subcutaneously, three times a week. It can be given on a once-a-week schedule, but somewhat more drug is required for an equivalent effect. If the response is poor, the dose should be progressively increased. The final maintenance dose of epoetin alfa can vary from as little as 10 units/kg to more than 300 units/kg, with an average dose of 75 units/kg, three times a week. Children younger than 5 years generally require a higher dose. Resistance to therapy is common in patients who develop an inflammatory illness or become iron deficient, so close monitoring of general health and iron status is essential. Less common causes of resistance include occult blood loss, folic acid deficiency, carnitine deficiency, inadequate dialysis, aluminum toxicity, and osteitis fibrosa cystica secondary to hyperparathyroidism.

The most common side effect of epoetin alfa therapy is aggravation of hypertension, which occurs in 20% to 30% of patients and most often is associated with a rapid rise in hematocrit. Blood pressure usually can be controlled either by increasing antihypertensive therapy or ultrafiltration in dialysis patients or by reducing the epoetin alfa dose to slow the hematocrit response.

Darbapoetin alfa also is approved for use in patients who are anemic secondary to chronic kidney disease. The recommended starting dose is 0.45 μg/kg administered intravenously or subcutaneously once weekly, with dose adjustments depending on the response. Like epoetin alfa, side effects tend to occur when patients experience a rapid rise in hemoglobin concentration; a rise of less than 1 g/dl every 2 weeks generally has been considered safe.

Anemia in AIDS Patients. Epoetin alfa therapy has been approved for the treatment of HIV-infected patients, especially those on *zidovudine* therapy (Fischl *et al.*, 1990). Excellent responses to doses of 100 to 300 units/kg, given subcutaneously three times a week, generally are seen in patients with zidovudine-induced anemia. In the face of advanced disease, marrow damage, and elevated serum erythropoietin levels (greater than 500 IU/L), therapy is less effective.

Cancer-Related Anemias. Epoetin alfa therapy, 150 units/kg three times a week or 450 to 600 units/kg once a week, can reduce the transfusion requirement in cancer patients undergoing chemotherapy. Evidence-based guidelines for the therapeutic use of recombinant erythropoietin in patients with cancer have been published (Rizzo *et al.*, 2002). Briefly, the guidelines recommend the use of epoetin alfa in patients with chemotherapy-associated anemia when hemoglobin levels fall below 10 g/dl, basing the decision to treat less severe anemia (hemoglobin between 10 and 12 g/dl) on clinical circumstances. For anemia associated with hematologic malignancies, the guidelines support the use of recombinant erythropoietin in patients with low-grade myelodysplastic syndrome, although the evidence that the drug is effective in anemic patients with multiple myeloma, non-Hodgkin's lymphoma, or chronic lymphocytic leukemia not receiving chemotherapy is less robust. A baseline serum erythropoietin level may help to predict the response; most patients with blood levels of more than 500 IU/L are unlikely to respond to any dose of the drug. Most patients treated with epoetin alfa experienced an improvement in their anemia, sense of well being, and quality of life (Demetri *et al.*, 1998; Littlewood *et al.*, 2001). This improved sense of well being, particularly in cancer patients, may not be solely due to the rise in the hematocrit. Erythropoietin receptors have been demonstrated in cells of the CNS, and erythropoietin has been found to act as a cytoprotectant in several models of CNS ischemia (Juul, 2002; Prass *et al.*, 2003; Martinez-Estrada *et al.*, 2003). Thus, high levels of the hormone may directly affect cancer patients' sense of well-being.

Darbopoetin alfa also has been tested in cancer patients undergoing chemotherapy (Bloomfield *et al.*, 2003; Hesketh *et al.*, 2004), and preliminary studies appear promising. However, recent case reports have suggested a direct effect of both epoetin alfa and darbopoetin alfa in stimulation of tumor cells. For example, patients with cancer of the head and neck randomized to receive recombinant erythropoietin had a statistically significant increase in likelihood of tumor progression during the duration of the study (Henke *et al.*, 2003). This finding is being evaluated by the FDA and warrants serious attention.

Surgery and Autologous Blood Donation. Epoetin alfa has been used perioperatively to treat anemia and reduce the need for transfusion. Patients undergoing elective orthopedic and cardiac procedures have been treated with 150 to 300 units/kg of epoetin alfa once daily for the 10 days preceding surgery, on the day of surgery, and for 4 days after surgery. As an alternative, 600 units/kg can be given on days –21, –14, and –7 before surgery, with an additional dose on the day of surgery. This can correct a moderately severe preoperative anemia (*i.e.,* hematocrit 30% to 36%) and reduce the need for transfusion. Epoetin alfa also has been used to improve autologous blood donation (Goodnough *et al.*, 1989). However, the potential benefit generally is small, and the expense is considerable. Patients treated for 3 to 4 weeks with epoetin alfa (300 to 600 units/kg twice a week) are able to donate only one or two more units than untreated patients, and most of the time this goes unused. Still, the ability to stimulate erythropoiesis for blood storage can be invaluable in the patient with multiple alloantibodies to red blood cells.

Other Uses. Epoetin alfa has received orphan drug status from the FDA for the treatment of the anemia of prematurity, HIV infection, and myelodysplasia. In the latter case, even very high doses of more than 1000 units/kg two to three times a week have had limited success. The utility of very high-dose therapy in other hematological disorders, such as sickle cell anemia, still is under study. Highly competitive athletes have used epoetin alfa to increase their hemoglobin levels ("blood doping") and improve performance. Unfortunately, this misuse of the drug has been implicated in the deaths of several athletes and is strongly discouraged.

MYELOID GROWTH FACTORS

The myeloid growth factors are glycoproteins that stimulate the proliferation and differentiation of one or more myeloid cell lines. They also enhance the function of mature granulocytes and monocytes. Recombinant forms of several growth factors have been produced, including GM-CSF (Wong *et al.*, 1985), G-CSF (Welte *et al.*, 1985), IL-3 (Yang *et al.*, 1986), M-CSF or CSF-1 (Kawasaki *et al.*, 1985), and SCF (Huang *et al.*, 1990) (Table 53–1).

The myeloid growth factors are produced naturally by a number of different cells, including fibroblasts, endothelial cells, macrophages, and T cells (Figure 53–2). They are active at extremely low concentrations and act *via* membrane receptors of the cytokine receptor superfamily to activate the JAK/STAT signal transduction pathway. GM-CSF is capable of stimulating the proliferation, differentiation, and function of a number of the myeloid cell lineages (Figure 53–1). It acts synergistically with other growth factors, including erythropoietin, at the level of the BFU. GM-CSF stimulates the CFU-GEMM, CFU-GM, CFU-M, CFU-E, and CFU-Meg to increase cell production. It also enhances the migration, phagocytosis, superoxide production, and antibody-dependent cell-mediated toxicity of neutrophils, monocytes, and eosinophils (Weisbart *et al.*, 1987).

The activity of G-CSF is restricted to neutrophils and their progenitors, stimulating their proliferation, differentiation, and function. It acts primarily on the CFU-G, although it also can play a synergistic role with IL-3 and GM-CSF in stimulating other cell lines. G-CSF enhances phagocytic and cytotoxic activities of neutrophils. Unlike GM-CSF, G-CSF has little effect on monocytes, macrophages, and eosinophils and reduces inflammation by inhibiting IL-1, tumor necrosis factor, and interferon gamma. G-CSF also mobilizes primitive hematopoietic cells, including hematopoietic stem cells, from the marrow into the peripheral blood (Sheridan *et al.*, 1992). This observation has virtually transformed the practice of stem cell transplantation, such that more than 90% of all such procedures today use G-CSF–mobilized peripheral blood stem cells as the donor product.

Granulocyte-Macrophage Colony-Stimulating Factor (GM-CSF). Recombinant human GM-CSF (*sargramostim*) is a 127–amino acid glycoprotein produced in yeast. Except for the substitution of a leucine in position 23 and variable levels of glycosylation, it is identical to endogenous human GM-CSF. While sargramostim, like natural GM-CSF, has a wide range of effects on cells in culture, its primary therapeutic effect is to stimulate myelopoiesis. The initial clinical application of sargramostim was in patients undergoing autologous bone marrow transplantation. By shortening the duration of neutropenia, transplant morbidity was significantly reduced without a change in long-term survival or risk of inducing an early relapse of the malignant process (Brandt *et al.*, 1988; Rabinowe *et al.*, 1993).

The role of GM-CSF therapy in allogeneic transplantation is less clear. Its effect on neutrophil recovery is less pronounced in patients receiving prophylactic treatment for graft-versus-host disease (GVHD), and studies have failed to show a significant effect on transplant mortality, long-term survival, the appearance of GVHD, or disease relapse. However, it may improve survival in transplant patients who exhibit early graft failure (Nemunaitis *et al.*, 1990). It also has been used to mobilize CD34-positive progenitor cells for peripheral blood stem cell collection for transplantation after myeloablative chemotherapy (Haas *et al.*, 1990). Sargramostim has been used to shorten the period of neutropenia and reduce morbidity in patients receiving intensive cancer chemotherapy (Gerhartz *et al.*, 1993). It also stimulates myelopoiesis in some patients with cyclic neutropenia, myelodysplasia, aplastic anemia, or AIDS-associated neutropenia (Groopman *et al.*, 1987).

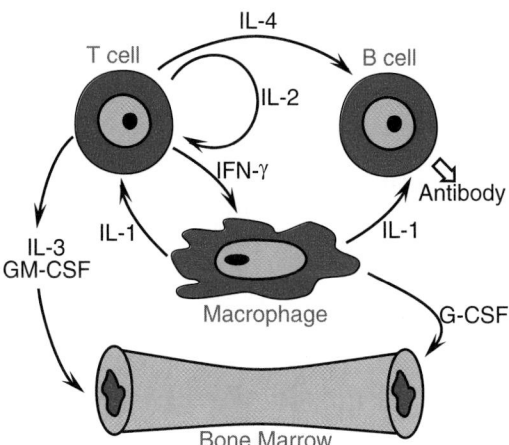

Figure 53–2. *Cytokine–cell interactions.* Macrophages, T cells, B cells, and marrow stem cells interact *via* several cytokines (IL-1, IL-2, IL-3, IL-4, IFN [interferon]-γ, GM-CSF, and G-CSF) in response to a bacterial or a foreign antigen challenge. *See* Table 53–1 for the functional activities of these various cytokines.

Sargramostim (LEUKINE) is administered by subcutaneous injection or slow intravenous infusion at doses of 125 to 500 $\mu g/$m^2 per day. Plasma levels of GM-CSF rise rapidly after subcutaneous injection and then decline with a half-life of 2 to 3 hours. When given intravenously, infusions should be maintained over 3 to 6 hours. With the initiation of therapy, there is a transient decrease in the absolute leukocyte count secondary to margination and sequestration in the lungs. This is followed by a dose-dependent, biphasic increase in leukocyte counts over the next 7 to 10 days. Once the drug is discontinued, the leukocyte count returns to baseline within 2 to 10 days. When GM-CSF is given in lower doses, the response is primarily neutrophilic, while monocytosis and eosinophilia are observed at larger doses. After hematopoietic stem cell transplantation or intensive chemotherapy, sargramostim is given daily during the period of maximum neutropenia until a sustained rise in the granulocyte count is observed. Frequent blood counts are essential to avoid an excessive rise in the granulocyte count. The dose may be increased if the patient fails to respond after 7 to 14 days of therapy. However, higher doses are associated with more pronounced side effects, including bone pain, malaise, flu-like symptoms, fever, diarrhea, dyspnea, and rash. An acute reaction to the first dose, characterized by flushing, hypotension, nausea, vomiting, and dyspnea, with a fall in arterial oxygen saturation due to granulocyte sequestration in the pulmonary circulation occurs in sensitive patients. With prolonged administration, a few patients may develop a capillary leak syndrome, with peripheral edema and pleural and pericardial effusions. Other serious side effects have included transient supraventricular arrhythmia, dyspnea, and elevation of serum creatinine, bilirubin, and hepatic enzymes.

Granulocyte Colony-Stimulating Factor (G-CSF).

Recombinant human G-CSF *filgrastim* (NEUPOGEN) is a 175–amino acid glycoprotein produced in *E. coli.* Unlike natural G-CSF, it is not glycosylated and carries an extra N-terminal methionine. The principal action of filgrastim is the stimulation of CFU-G to increase neutrophil production (Figure 53–1). It also enhances the phagocytic and cytotoxic functions of neutrophils.

Filgrastim is effective in the treatment of severe neutropenia after autologous hematopoietic stem cell transplantation and high-dose cancer chemotherapy (Lieschke and Burgess, 1992). Like GM-CSF, filgrastim shortens the period of severe neutropenia and reduces morbidity secondary to bacterial and fungal infections. When used as a part of an intensive chemotherapy regimen, it can decrease the frequency of hospitalization for febrile neutropenia and interruptions in the chemotherapy protocol; a positive impact on patient survival has not been demonstrated. G-CSF also is effective in the treatment of severe congenital neutropenias. In patients with cyclic neutropenia, G-CSF therapy will increase the level of neutrophils and shorten the length of the cycle sufficiently to prevent recurrent bacterial infections (Hammond *et al.*, 1989). Filgrastim therapy can improve neutrophil counts in some patients with myelodysplasia or marrow damage (moderately severe aplastic anemia or tumor infiltration of the marrow). The neutropenia of AIDS patients receiving zidovudine also can be partially or completely reversed. Filgrastim is routinely used in patients undergoing peripheral blood stem cell (PBSC) collection for stem cell transplantation. It promotes the release of CD34$^+$ progenitor cells from the marrow, reducing the number of collections necessary for transplant. Moreover, filgrastim-mobilized PBSCs appear more capable of rapid engraftment. PBSC-transplanted patients require fewer days of platelet and red blood cell transfusions and a shorter duration of hospitalization than do patients receiving autologous bone marrow transplants.

Filgrastim is administered by subcutaneous injection or intravenous infusion over at least 30 minutes at doses of 1 to 20 $\mu g/kg$ per day. The usual starting dose in a patient receiving myelosuppressive chemotherapy is 5 $\mu g/kg$ per day. The distribution and clearance rate from plasma (half-life of 3.5 hours) are similar for both routes of administration. As with GM-CSF therapy, filgrastim given daily after hematopoietic stem cell transplantation or intensive cancer chemotherapy will increase granulocyte production and shorten the period of severe neutropenia. Frequent blood counts should be obtained to determine the effectiveness of the treatment and guide dosage adjustment. In patients who received intensive myelosuppressive cancer chemotherapy, daily administration of G-CSF for 14 to 21 days or longer may be necessary to correct the neutropenia. With less intensive chemotherapy, fewer than 7 days of treatment may suffice. In AIDS patients on zidovudine or patients with cyclic neutropenia, chronic G-CSF therapy often is required.

One indication for G-CSF presently under investigation is its use to increase the number of peripheral blood neutrophils in leukocyte donors. For many years it had been hoped that, like platelet transfusions for the bleeding associated with severe thrombocytopenia, neutrophil transfusion could diminish the infectious complications of neutropenia. However, given the short circulatory half-life of neutrophils (~6 hours) and the need for large numbers of cells, the practical collection of sufficient cell numbers has eluded hematologists. With few complications of therapy in more than 15 years of clinical experience, G-CSF now has been used to increase peripheral neutrophil counts in prospective donors and neutrophil transfusions (Hubel *et al.*, 2002). While initial results were modest, the therapy is likely to be optimized and greater efficacy is anticipated.

Adverse reactions to filgrastim include mild to moderate bone pain in patients receiving high doses over a protracted period, local skin reactions following subcutaneous injection, and rare cutaneous necrotizing vasculitis. Patients with a history of hypersensitivity to proteins produced by *E. coli* should not receive the drug. Marked granulocytosis, with counts greater than 100,000/μl, can occur in patients receiving filgrastim over a prolonged period of time. However, this is not associated with any reported clinical morbidity or mortality and rapidly resolves once therapy is discontinued. Mild to moderate splenomegaly has been observed in patients on long-term therapy.

Pegylated recombinant human G-CSF *pegfilgrastim* (NEULASTA) is generated through conjugation of a 20,000-dalton polyethylene glycol moiety to the N-terminal methionyl residue of the 175–amino acid G-CSF glyco-protein produced in *E. coli*. The clearance of peg-filgrastim by glomerular filtration is minimized, thus making neutrophil-mediated clearance the primary route of elimination. Consequently the circulating half-life of pegfilgrastim is longer than that of filgrastim, allowing for more sustained duration of action and less frequent dosing (Waladkhani, 2004). Clinical studies suggest that neutrophil-mediated clearance of pegfilgrastim may be self-regulating and therefore specific to each patient's hematopoietic recovery (Crawford, 2002). As such, the recommended dose for pegfilgrastim is fixed at 6 mg administered subcutaneously.

The therapeutic roles of other growth factors still need to be defined, although IL-3 and IL-6 have been removed from testing due to poor efficacy and/or significant toxicity. M-CSF may play a role in stimulating monocyte and mac-rophage production, although with significant side effects, including splenomegaly and thrombocytopenia. Stem cell factor (SCF) has been shown to augment peripheral blood mobilization of primitive hematopoietic progenitor cells (Molineux *et al.*, 1991; Moskowitz *et al.*, 1997).

THROMBOPOIETIC GROWTH FACTORS

Interleukin-11. Interleukin-11 was cloned based on its activity to promote proliferation of an IL-6–dependent myeloma cell line (Du *et al.*, 1994). The 23,000-dalton cytokine contains 178 amino acids and stimulates hemato-poiesis, intestinal epithelial cell growth, and osteoclasto-genesis and inhibits adipogenesis. IL-11 enhances mega-karyocyte maturation *in vitro* (Teramura *et al.*, 1992; Debili *et al.*, 1993), and its *in vivo* administration to ani-mals modestly increases peripheral blood platelet counts (Neben *et al.*, 1993; Farese *et al.*, 1994). Clinical trials in patients who previously demonstrated significant chemo-therapy-induced thrombocytopenia demonstrated that admin-istration of the recombinant cytokine was associated with less severe thrombocytopenia and reduced use of platelet transfusion (Tepler *et al.*, 1996; Isaacs *et al.*, 1997) lead-ing to its approval for clinical use by the FDA.

Recombinant human interleukin-11 *oprelvekin* (NEU-MEGA) is a bacterially derived, 19,000-dalton polypeptide of 177 amino acids that differs from the native protein only because it lacks the amino terminal proline residue

and is not glycosylated. The recombinant protein has a 7-hour half-life after subcutaneous injection. In normal sub-jects, daily administration of oprelvekin leads to a throm-bopoietic response in 5 to 9 days.

The drug is available in single-use vials containing 5 mg and is administered to patients at 25 to 50 μg/kg per day subcutaneously. Oprelvekin is approved for use in patients undergoing chemotherapy for nonmyeloid malig-nancies that displayed severe thrombocytopenia (platelet count $<20,000/\mu l$) on a prior cycle of the same chemother-apy, and is administered until the platelet count returns to more than $100,000/\mu l$. The major complications of thera-py are fluid retention and other associated cardiac symp-toms, such as tachycardia, palpitation, edema, and short-ness of breath; this is a significant concern in elderly patients and often requires concomitant therapy with diuretics. Fluid retention reverses upon drug discontinua-tion, but volume status should be carefully monitored in elderly patients, those with a history of heart failure, or those with preexisting fluid collections in the pleura, peri-cardium, or peritoneal cavity. Also reported are blurred vision, injection-site rash or erythema, and paresthesias.

Thrombopoietin. The cloning and expression of recom-binant thrombopoietin, a cytokine that predominantly stimulates megakaryopoiesis, is potentially another mile-stone in the development of hematopoietic growth factors as therapeutic agents (Lok *et al.*, 1994; de Sauvage *et al.*, 1994; Kaushansky *et al.*, 1994) (Table 53–1). Throm-bopoietin is a 45,000- to 75,000-dalton glycoprotein con-taining 332 amino acids that is produced by the liver, marrow stromal cells, and many other organs. In both humans and mice, genetic elimination of thrombopoietin or its receptor reduces the platelet counts to 10% of nor-mal values. Moreover, blood levels of the hormone are inversely related to the blood platelet count, together indi-cating that the hormone is the primary regulator of plate-let production.

Administration of recombinant thrombopoietin leads to a log-linear increase in the platelet count in mice, rats, dogs, and nonhuman primates (Harker, 1999) that begins on the third day of administration. In a number of human preclinical trials in several models of chemotherapy- and radiation-induced myelosuppression, thrombopoietin accel-erated the recovery of platelet counts and other hematologic parameters (Kaushansky, 1998). Of note, however, the agent failed to substantially affect hematopoietic recovery when administered after myeloablative therapy and stem cell transplantation, unless given to the stem cell donor (Fibbe *et al.*, 1995).

Two forms of recombinant thrombopoietin have been developed for clinical use. One is a truncated version of the native polypeptide, termed recombinant *human mega-karyocyte growth and development factor* (rHuMGDF), which is produced in bacteria and then covalently modified with polyethylene glycol to increase the circulatory half-life. The second is the full-length polypeptide termed *recombinant human thrombopoietin* (rHuTPO), which is produced in mammalian cells. *In vitro*, both drugs are equally potent in stimulating megakaryocyte growth.

In clinical trials, both drugs are safe in the patient populations selected for study (Basser *et al.*, 1996; Fanucchi *et al.*, 1997; Vadhan-Raj *et al.*, 1997). However, efficacy results using these agents have been mixed. In a small number of patients with gynecological cancers who were receiving *carboplatin* (Vadhan-Raj *et al.*, 2000), recombinant human thrombopoietin therapy reduced the duration of severe thrombocytopenia and the need for platelet transfusions. In a similar study of patients treated with carboplatin plus *cyclophosphamide,* patients receiving a cycle of chemotherapy supplemented with G-CSF plus thrombopoietin had higher platelet counts at nadir and a shorter median duration of severe thrombocytopenia than they did after cycles of therapy supplemented only with G-CSF (Basser *et al.*, 2000). When used to augment peripheral blood counts in preparation for platelet donation, a single dose of thrombopoietin in the platelet donors tripled their platelet counts, allowed for a threefold increase in the number of platelets that could be collected in a single apheresis, and led to a fourfold increase in the mean platelet count increase noted in transfusion recipients (Kuter *et al.*, 2001). However, this particular regimen was associated with several instances of anti–recombinant thrombopoietin antibodies that cross-reacted with the native hormone, resulting in subsequent thrombocytopenia (Li *et al.*, 2001).

In several studies, although the drug was safe, rHuMGDF was not effective. In two studies of patients treated for 7 days with standard, aggressive therapy for acute leukemia, the addition of recombinant thrombopoietin failed to accelerate platelet recovery (Archimbaud *et al.*, 1999; Schiffer *et al.*, 2000). A similar lack of efficacy was seen when the drug was used following autologous peripheral blood stem cell transplantation (Bolwell *et al.*, 2000). Failure to improve hematopoiesis in some of these trials may have resulted from the dosing regimen employed; the optimal dose and schedule of administration in various clinical settings need to be established. After a single bolus injection, platelet counts showed a detectable increase by day 4, peaked by 12 to

14 days, and then returned to normal over the next 4 weeks. The peak platelet response follows a log-linear dose response. Platelet activation and aggregation are not affected, and patients are not at increased risk of thromboembolic disease, unless the platelet count is allowed to rise to very high levels. These kinetics need to be taken into account when planning therapy in cancer chemotherapy patients.

Due to concerns over the immunogenicity of these agents, and to other considerations, efforts now are under way to develop small molecular mimics of recombinant thrombopoietin, discovered either through screening of phage display peptide libraries (Broudy *et al.*, 2004) or of small organic molecules (Kimura *et al.*, 1998). Several of these agents are in clinical trials.

II. Drugs Effective in Iron Deficiency and Other Hypochromic Anemias

IRON AND IRON SALTS

Iron deficiency is the most common nutritional cause of anemia in humans. It can result from inadequate iron intake, malabsorption, blood loss, or an increased requirement, as with pregnancy. When severe, it results in a characteristic microcytic, hypochromic anemia. The impact of iron deficiency is not limited to the erythron (Dallman, 1982). Iron also is an essential component of myoglobin; heme enzymes such as the cytochromes, catalase, and peroxidase; and the metalloflavoprotein enzymes, including xanthine oxidase and the mitochondrial enzyme α-glycerophosphate oxidase. Iron deficiency can affect metabolism in muscle independently of the effect of anemia on oxygen delivery. This may reflect a reduction in the activity of iron-dependent mitochondrial enzymes. Iron deficiency also has been associated with behavioral and learning problems in children, abnormalities in catecholamine metabolism, and possibly, impaired heat production. Awareness of the ubiquitous role of iron has stimulated considerable interest in the early and accurate detection of iron deficiency and in its prevention.

History. The modern understanding of iron metabolism began in 1937 with the work of McCance and Widdowson on iron absorption and excretion and Heilmeyer and Plotner's measurement of iron in plasma (Beutler, 2002). In 1947, Laurell described a plasma iron transport protein that he called *transferrin*. Hahn and coworkers first used radioactive isotopes to quantitate iron absorption and define the role of the intestinal mucosa to regulate this function. In the next decade, Huff and associates initiated isotopic studies of internal iron metabolism. The subsequent development of practical clinical measurements of serum iron, transferrin saturation, plasma ferritin, and red cell protoporphyrin permitted the definition and detection of the body's iron store status and iron-deficient erythropoiesis.

Iron and the Environment. Iron exists in the environment largely as ferric oxide or hydroxide or as polymers. In this state, its biological availability is limited unless solubilized by acid or chelating agents. For example, bacteria and some plants produce high-affinity chelating agents that extract iron from the surrounding environment. Most mammals have little difficulty in acquiring iron; this is explained by an ample iron intake and perhaps also by a greater efficiency in absorbing iron. Humans, however, appear to be an exception. Although total dietary intake of elemental iron in human beings usually exceeds requirements, the bioavailability of the iron in the diet is limited.

Metabolism of Iron. The body store of iron is divided between essential iron-containing compounds and excess iron, which is held in storage. Quantitatively, hemoglobin dominates the essential fraction (Table 53–2). This protein, with a molecular weight of 64,500, contains four atoms of iron per molecule, amounting to 1.1 mg of iron per milliliter of red blood cells (20 mmol). Other forms of essential iron include myoglobin and a variety of heme and nonheme iron-dependent enzymes. Ferritin is a protein-iron storage complex that exists as individual molecules or as aggregates. Apoferritin has a molecular weight of about 450,000 and is composed of 24 polypeptide subunits that form an outer shell, within which resides a storage cavity for polynuclear hydrous ferric oxide phosphate. More than 30% of the weight of ferritin may be iron (4000 atoms of iron per ferritin molecule). Ferritin aggregates, referred to as *hemosiderin* and visible by light microscopy, constitute about one-third of normal stores, a fraction that increases as stores enlarge. The two predominant sites of iron storage are the reticuloendothelial system and the hepatocytes, although some storage also occurs in muscle.

Internal exchange of iron is accomplished by the plasma protein transferrin. This 76-kd β_1-glycoprotein has two binding sites for ferric iron. Iron is delivered from transferrin to intracellular sites by means of specific transferrin receptors in the plasma membrane. The iron–transferrin complex binds to the receptor, and the ternary complex is taken up by receptor-mediated endocytosis. Iron subsequently dissociates in the acidic, intracellular vesicular compartment (the endosomes), and the receptor returns the apotransferrin to the cell surface, where it is

Table 53–2
The Body Content of Iron

	MG/KG OF BODY WEIGHT	
	Male	*Female*
Essential iron		
Hemoglobin	31	28
Myoglobin and enzymes	6	5
Storage iron	13	4
Total	50	37

released into the extracellular environment (Klausner *et al.*, 1983).

Cells regulate their expression of transferrin receptors and intracellular ferritin in response to the iron supply. When iron is plentiful, the synthesis of transferrin receptors is reduced and ferritin production is increased (Rouault, 2002). Conversely, with iron deficiency, cells express a greater number of transferrin receptors and reduce ferritin concentrations to maximize uptake and prevent diversion of iron to storage forms. Apoferritin synthesis is regulated posttranscriptionally by two cytoplasmic binding proteins (IRP-1 and IRP-2) and an iron-regulating element on mRNA (IRE). When iron is in short supply, IRP binds to mRNA IRE and inhibits apoferritin translation. Conversely, when iron is abundant, binding is blocked and apoferritin synthesis increases (Klausner *et al.*, 1993).

The flow of iron through the plasma amounts to a total of 30 to 40 mg per day in the adult (about 0.46 mg/kg of body weight) (Finch and Huebers, 1982). The major internal circulation of iron involves the erythron and reticuloendothelial cells (Figure 53–3). About 80% of the iron in plasma goes to the erythroid marrow to be packaged into new erythrocytes; these normally circulate for about 120 days before being catabolized by the reticuloendothelial system. At that time, a portion of the iron is immediately returned to the plasma bound to transferrin, while another portion is incorporated into the ferritin stores of reticuloendothelial cells and returned to the circulation more gradually. Isotopic studies indicate some degree of iron wastage in this process, wherein defective cells or unused portions of their iron are transferred to the reticuloendothelial cell during maturation, bypassing the circulating blood. With abnormalities in erythrocyte maturation, the predominant portion of iron assimilated by the erythroid marrow may be rap-

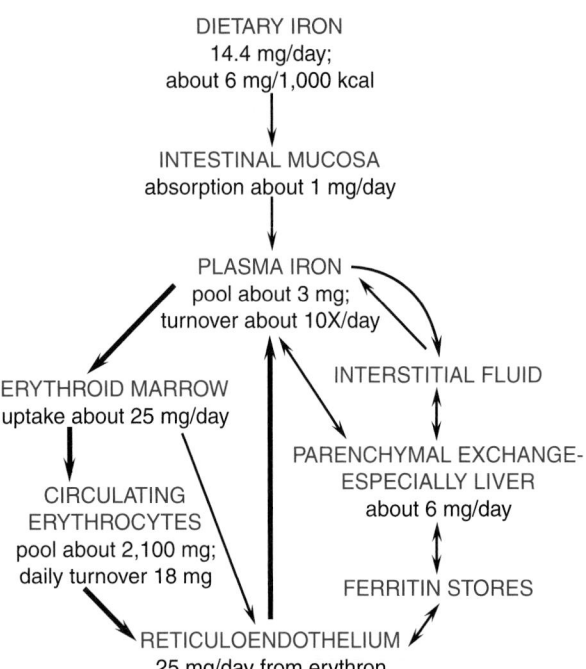

Figure 53–3. *Pathways of iron metabolism in human beings (excretion omitted).*

Table 53–3
Iron Requirements for Pregnancy

	AVERAGE, *mg*	RANGE, *mg*
External iron loss	170	150–200
Expansion of red cell mass	450	200–600
Fetal iron	270	200–370
Iron in placenta and cord	90	30–170
Blood loss at delivery	150	90–310
Total requirement[*]	980	580–1340
Cost of pregnancy[†]	680	440–1050

[*]Blood loss at delivery not included. [†]Iron lost by the mother; expansion of red cell mass not included.
SOURCE: Council on Foods and Nutrition. Iron deficiency in the United States. *JAMA* 1968, 203:407–412. Used with permission.

idly localized in the reticuloendothelial cells as defective red cell precursors are broken down; this is termed *ineffective erythropoiesis.* The rate of iron turnover in plasma may be reduced by one-half or more with red cell aplasia, with all the iron directed to the hepatocytes for storage.

The most remarkable feature of iron metabolism is the degree to which body stores are conserved. Only 10% of the total is lost per year by normal men, *i.e.,* about 1 mg per day. Two-thirds of this iron is excreted from the gastrointestinal tract as extravasated red cells, iron in bile, and iron in exfoliated mucosal cells. The other third is accounted for by small amounts of iron in desquamated skin and in the urine. Physiological losses of iron in men vary over a narrow range, from 0.5 mg in the iron-deficient individual to 1.5 to 2 mg per day when excessive iron is consumed. Additional losses of iron occur in women due to menstruation. While the average loss in menstruating women is about 0.5 mg per day, 10% of menstruating women lose more than 2 mg per day. Pregnancy and lactation impose an even greater requirement for iron (Table 53–3). Other causes of iron loss include blood donation, the use of antiinflammatory drugs that cause bleeding from the gastric mucosa, and gastrointestinal disease with associated bleeding. Two much rarer causes are the hemosiderinuria that follows

intravascular hemolysis, and pulmonary siderosis, where iron deposited in the lungs becomes unavailable to the rest of the body.

The limited physiological losses of iron point to the primary importance of absorption in determining of the body's iron content. Unfortunately, this process is understood only in general terms (Roy and Enns, 2000; Morgan and Oates, 2002). After acidification and partial digestion of food in the stomach, iron is presented to the intestinal mucosa as either inorganic iron or heme iron. These fractions are taken up by the absorptive cells of the duodenum and upper small intestine, and the iron is transported either directly into the plasma or stored as mucosal ferritin. Absorption appears to be regulated by two transporters: DCT1, which controls uptake from the intestinal lumen, and a second transporter that governs movement of mucosal cell iron across the basolateral membrane to bind to plasma protein. Mucosal cell iron transport and the delivery of iron to transferrin from reticuloendothelial stores both are determined by the HFE gene, a major histocompatibility complex class 1 molecule localized to chromosome 6 (Peters *et al.,* 1993; Beutler, 2003). Regulation is finely tuned to prevent iron overload in times of iron excess while allowing for increased absorption and mobilization of iron stores with iron deficiency (Roy and Andrews, 2001; Sheth and Brittenham, 2000). A predominant negative regulator of iron absorption in the small intestine is hepcidin, a 25-amino acid peptide made by hepatocytes (Ganz, 2003). The synthesis of hepcidin is greatly stimulated by inflammation or by iron overload. A deficient hepcidin response to iron

Table 53–4

Daily Iron Intake and Absorption

SUBJECT	IRON REQUIREMENT, *mg/kg*	AVAILABLE IRON IN POOR DIET–GOOD DIET, *mg/kg*	SAFETY FACTOR, *AVAILABLE IRON/REQUIREMENT*
Infant	67	33–66	0.5–1
Child	22	48–96	2–4
Adolescent (male)	21	30–60	1.5–3
Adolescent (female)	20	30–60	1.5–3
Adult (male)	13	26–52	2–4
Adult (female)	21	18–36	1–2
Mid-to-late pregnancy	80	18–36	0.22–0.45

loading can contribute to iron overload and one type of hemochromatosis. In anemia of chronic disease, hepcidin production can be increased up to one hundredfold, potentially accounting for characteristic features of this condition, namely poor gastrointestinal uptake and enhanced sequestration of iron in the reticuloendothelial system.

Normal iron absorption is about 1 mg per day in adult men and 1.4 mg per day in adult women; 3 to 4 mg of dietary iron is the most that normally can be absorbed. Increased iron absorption is seen whenever iron stores are depleted or when erythropoiesis is increased or ineffective. Patients with hereditary hemochromatosis due to HFE mutations demonstrate increased iron absorption and loss of the normal regulation of iron delivery to transferrin by reticuloendothelial cells (Beutler, 2003; Ajioka and Kushner, 2003). The resulting increased saturation of transferrin permits abnormal iron deposition in nonhematopoietic tissues.

Iron Requirements and the Availability of Dietary Iron. Iron requirements are determined by obligatory physiological losses and the needs imposed by growth. Thus, adult men require only 13 μg/kg per day (about 1 mg), whereas menstruating women require about 21 μg/kg per day (about 1.4 mg). In the last two trimesters of pregnancy, requirements increase to about 80 μg/kg per day (5 to 6 mg), and infants have similar requirements due to their rapid growth. These requirements (Table 53–4) must be considered in the context of the amount of dietary iron available for absorption.

In developed countries, the normal adult diet contains about 6 mg of iron per 1000 calories, providing an average daily intake for adult men of between 12 and 20 mg and for adult women of between 8 and 15 mg. Foods high in iron (>5 mg/100 g) include organ meats such as liver and heart, brewer's yeast, wheat germ, egg yolks, oysters, and certain dried beans and fruits; foods low in iron (<1 mg/100 g) include milk and milk products and most non-green vegetables. The content of iron in food is affected further by the manner of its preparation, since iron may be added from cooking in iron pots.

Although the iron content of the diet obviously is important, of greater nutritional significance is the bioavailability of iron in food. Heme iron, which constitutes only 6% of dietary iron, is far more available and is absorbed independent of the diet composition; it therefore represents 30% of iron absorbed (Conrad and Umbreit, 2002).

The nonheme fraction nonetheless represents by far the largest amount of dietary iron ingested by the economically underprivileged. In a vegetarian diet, nonheme iron is absorbed very poorly because of the inhibitory action of a variety of dietary components, particularly phosphates. Ascorbic acid and meat facilitate the absorption of nonheme iron. Ascorbate forms complexes with and/or reduces ferric to ferrous iron. Meat facilitates the absorption of iron by stimulating production of gastric acid; other effects also may be involved. Either of these substances can increase availability severalfold. Thus, assessment of available dietary iron should include both the amount of iron ingested and an estimate of its availability (Figure 53–4) (Monsen *et al.*, 1978).

A comparison of iron requirements with available dietary iron is seen in Table 53–4. Obviously, pregnancy and infancy represent periods of negative balance. Menstruating women also are at risk, whereas iron balance in adult men and nonmenstruating women is reasonably secure. The difference between dietary supply and require-

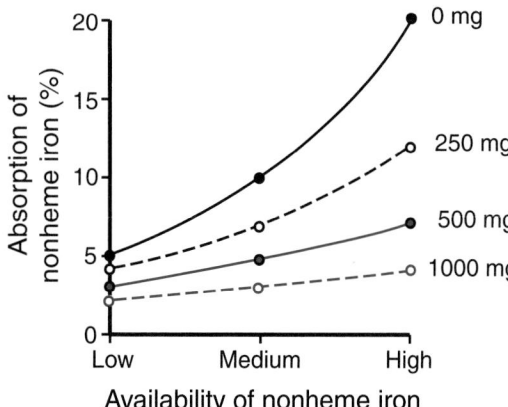

Figure 53–4. ***Effect of iron status on the absorption of*** ***nonheme iron in food.*** The percentages of iron absorbed from diets of low, medium, and high bioavailability in individuals with iron stores of 0, 250, 500, and 1000 mg are portrayed. (After Monsen *et al.*, 1978; used with permission.)

ments is reflected in the size of iron stores, which are low or absent when iron balance is precarious and high when iron balance is favorable (Table 53–2). Thus, in infants after the third month of life and in pregnant women after the first trimester, stores of iron are negligible. Menstruating women have approximately one-third the stored iron found in adult men, indicative of the extent to which the additional average daily loss of about 0.5 mg of iron affects iron balance.

Iron Deficiency. Iron deficiency is the most common nutritional disorder (World Health Organization, 2003; Hoffbrand and Herbert, 1999). The prevalence of iron-deficiency anemia in the United States is on the order of 1% to 4% (Anonymous, 2002) and depends on the economic status of the population. In developing countries, up to 20% to 40% of infants and pregnant women may be affected. Better iron balance has resulted from the practice of fortifying flour, the use of iron-fortified formulas for infants, and the prescription of medicinal iron supplements during pregnancy.

Iron-deficiency anemia results from dietary intake of iron that is inadequate to meet normal requirements (nutritional iron deficiency), blood loss, or interference with iron absorption. Most nutritional iron deficiency in the United States is mild. More severe iron deficiency is usually the result of blood loss, either from the gastrointestinal tract, or in women, from the uterus. Impaired absorption of iron from food results most often from partial gastrectomy or malabsorption in the small intestine. Finally, treatment of patients with

erythropoietin can result in a functional iron deficiency (Beutler, 2003).

Iron deficiency in infants and young children can lead to behavioral disturbances and can impair development, which may not be fully reversible. Iron deficiency in children also can lead to an increased risk of lead toxicity secondary to pica and an increased absorption of heavy metals. Premature and low-birth-weight infants are at greatest risk for developing iron deficiency, especially if they are not breast-fed and/or do not receive iron-fortified formula. After age 2 to 3, the requirement for iron declines until adolescence, when rapid growth combined with irregular dietary habits again increase the risk of iron deficiency. Adolescent girls are at greatest risk; the dietary iron intake of most girls ages 11 to 18 is insufficient to meet their requirements.

The recognition of iron deficiency rests on an appreciation of the sequence of events that lead to depletion of iron stores (Hillman and Finch, 1997; Beutler, 2003). A negative balance first results in a reduction of iron stores, and eventually a parallel decrease in red-cell iron and iron-related enzymes (Figure 53–5). In adults, depletion of iron stores may be recognized by a plasma ferritin of less than 12 $\mu g/L$ and the absence of reticuloendothelial hemosiderin in the marrow aspirate. Iron-deficient erythropoiesis is identified by a decreased saturation of transferrin to less than 16% and/or by an increase above normal in red-cell protoporphyrin. Iron-deficiency anemia is associated with a recognizable decrease in the concentration of hemoglobin in blood. However, the physiological variation in hemoglobin levels is so great that only about half the individuals with iron-deficient erythropoiesis are identified from their anemia. Moreover, "normal" hemoglobin and iron values in infancy and childhood are lower because of the more restricted supply of iron in young children (Dallman *et al.*, 1980).

In mild iron deficiency, identifying the underlying cause is more important than any symptoms related to the deficiency state. Because of the frequency of iron deficiency in infants and in menstruating or pregnant women, the need for exhaustive evaluation of such individuals usually is determined by the severity of the anemia. However, iron deficiency in men or postmenopausal women necessitates a search for a site of bleeding.

Although the presence of microcytic anemia is the most common indicator of iron deficiency, laboratory tests—such as quantitation of transferrin saturation, red cell protoporphyrin, and plasma ferritin—are required to distinguish iron deficiency from other causes of microcytosis. Such measurements are particularly useful when circulating red cells are not yet microcytic because of the recent nature of blood loss, but iron supply nonetheless limits erythropoiesis. More difficult is the differentiation of true iron deficiency from iron-deficient erythropoiesis due to inflammation. In the latter condition, iron stores actually are increased, but the release of iron from reticuloendothelial cells is blocked; the concentration of iron in plasma is decreased, and the supply of iron to the erythroid marrow becomes inadequate. The increased stores of iron in this condition may be demonstrated directly by examination of an aspirate of marrow or may be inferred from determination of an elevated plasma concentration of ferritin.

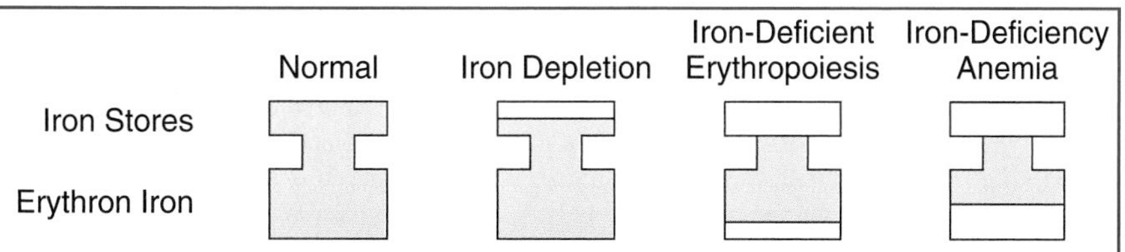

	Normal	Iron Depletion	Iron-Deficient Erythropoiesis	Iron-Deficiency Anemia
Iron Stores				
Erythron Iron				
RE marrow Fe	2–3+	0–1+	0	0
Transferrin µg/100 ml (µM)	330 ± 30 (59 ± 5)	360 (64)	390 (70)	410 (73)
Plasma ferritin, µg/l	100 ± 60	20	10	<10
Iron absorption, %	5–10	10–15	10–20	10–20
Plasma iron µg/100 ml (µM)	115 ± 50 (21 ± 9)	115 (21)	<60 (<11)	<40 (<7)
Transferrin saturation, %	35 ± 15	30	<15	<10
Sideroblasts, %	40–60	40–60	<10	<10
RBC protoporphyrin µg/100 ml RBC (µmol per liter RBC)	30 (0.53)	30 (0.53)	100 (1.8)	200 (3.5)
Erythrocytes	Normal	Normal	Normal	Microcytic/ hypochromic

Figure 53–5. Sequential changes (from left to right) in the development of iron deficiency in the adult. Rectangles enclose abnormal test results. RE marrow Fe, reticuloendothelial hemosiderin; RBC, red blood cells. (Adapted from Hillman and Finch, 1997. Used with permission.)

Treatment of Iron Deficiency

General Therapeutic Principles. The response of iron-deficiency anemia to iron therapy is influenced by several factors, including the severity of anemia, the ability of the patient to tolerate and absorb medicinal iron, and the presence of other complicating illnesses. Therapeutic effectiveness is best measured by the resulting increase in the rate of production of red cells. The magnitude of the marrow response to iron therapy is proportional to the severity of the anemia (level of erythropoietin stimulation) and the amount of iron delivered to marrow precursors.

The patient's ability to tolerate and absorb medicinal iron is a key factor in determining the rate of response to therapy. The small intestine regulates absorption, and with increasing doses of oral iron, limits the entry of iron into the bloodstream. This provides a natural ceiling on how much iron can be supplied by oral therapy. In the patient with a moderately severe iron-deficiency anemia, tolerable doses of oral iron will deliver, at most, 40 to 60 mg of iron per day to the erythroid marrow. This is an amount sufficient for production rates of two to three times normal.

Complicating illness also can interfere with the response of an iron-deficiency anemia to iron therapy.

By decreasing the number of red cell precursors, intrinsic disease of the marrow can blunt the response. Inflammatory illnesses suppress the rate of red cell production, both by reducing iron absorption and reticuloendothelial release and by direct inhibition of erythropoietin and erythroid precursors. Continued blood loss can mask the response as measured by recovery of the hemoglobin or hematocrit.

Clinically, the effectiveness of iron therapy is best evaluated by tracking the reticulocyte response and the rise in the hemoglobin or the hematocrit. An increase in the reticulocyte count is not observed for at least 4 to 7 days after beginning therapy. A measurable increase in the hemoglobin level takes even longer. A decision as to the effectiveness of treatment should not be made for 3 to 4 weeks after the start of treatment. An increase of 20 g per liter or more in the concentration of hemoglobin by that time should be considered a positive response, assuming that no other change in the patient's clinical status can account for the improvement and that the patient has not been transfused.

If the response to oral iron is inadequate, the diagnosis must be reconsidered. A full laboratory evaluation should be conducted, and poor compliance by the patient or the presence of a concurrent inflammatory disease must be explored. A source of continued bleeding obviously should be sought. If no other explanation can be found, an evaluation of the patient's ability to absorb oral iron should be considered. There is no justification for merely continuing oral iron therapy beyond 3 to 4 weeks if a favorable response has not occurred.

Once a response to oral iron is demonstrated, therapy should be continued until the hemoglobin returns to normal. Treatment may be extended if it is desirable to replenish iron stores. This may require a considerable period of time, since the rate of absorption of iron by the intestine will decrease markedly as iron stores are reconstituted. The prophylactic use of oral iron should be reserved for patients at high risk, including pregnant women, women with excessive menstrual blood loss, and infants. Iron supplements also may be of value for rapidly growing infants who are consuming substandard diets and for adults with a recognized cause of chronic blood loss. Except for infants, in whom the use of supplemented formulas is routine, the use of over-the-counter mixtures of vitamins and minerals to prevent iron deficiency should be discouraged.

Therapy with Oral Iron. Orally administered *ferrous sulfate* is the treatment of choice for iron deficiency. Ferrous salts are absorbed about three times as well as ferric salts, and the discrepancy becomes even greater at high dosages. Variations in the particular ferrous salt have relatively little effect on bioavailability, and the sulfate, fumarate, succinate, gluconate, and other ferrous salts are absorbed to approximately the same extent.

Ferrous sulfate (FEOSOL, others) is the hydrated salt, $FeSO_4 \cdot 7H_2O$, which contains 20% iron. *Dried ferrous sulfate* (32% elemental iron) is also available. *Ferrous fumarate* (FEOSTAT, others) contains 33% iron and is moderately soluble in water, stable, and almost tasteless. *Ferrous gluconate* (FERGON, others) also has been successfully used in the therapy of iron-deficiency anemia. The gluconate contains 12% iron. *Polysaccharide–iron complex* (NIFEREX, others), a compound of ferrihydrite and carbohydrate, is another preparation with comparable absorption. The effective dose of all of these preparations is based on iron content.

Other iron compounds have utility in fortification of foods. Reduced iron (metallic iron, elemental iron) is as effective as ferrous sulfate, provided that the material employed has a small particle size. Large-particle *ferrum reductum* and iron phosphate salts have a much lower bioavailability, and their use for the fortification of foods is undoubtedly responsible for some of the confusion concerning effectiveness. *Ferric edetate* has been shown to have good bioavailability and to have advantages for maintenance of the normal appearance and taste of food.

The amount of iron, rather than the mass of the total salt in iron tablets, is important. It also is essential that the coating of the tablet dissolve rapidly in the stomach. Surprisingly, since iron usually is absorbed in the upper small intestine, certain delayed-release preparations have been reported to be effective and have been said to be even more effective than ferrous sulfate when taken with meals. However, reports of absorption from such preparations vary. Because a number of forms of delayed-release preparations are on the market, and information on their bioavailability is limited, the effectiveness of most such preparations must be considered questionable.

A variety of substances designed to enhance the absorption of iron has been marketed, including surface-acting agents, carbohydrates, inorganic salts, amino acids, and vitamins. When present in an amount of 200 mg or more, ascorbic acid increases the absorption of medicinal iron by at least 30%. However, the increased uptake is associated with a significant increase in the incidence of side effects; therefore, the addition of ascorbic acid seems to have little advantage over increasing the amount of iron administered. It is inadvisable to use preparations that contain other compounds with therapeutic actions of their own, such as vitamin B_{12}, folate, or cobalt, because the patient's response to the combination cannot easily be interpreted.

The average dose for the treatment of iron-deficiency anemia is about 200 mg of iron per day (2 to 3 mg/kg), given in three equal doses of 65 mg. Children weighing 15 to 30 kg can take half the average adult dose, while small children and infants can tolerate relatively large doses of iron—for example, 5 mg/kg. The dose used is a compromise between the desired therapeutic action and the toxic effects. Prophylaxis and mild nutritional iron deficiency may be managed with modest doses. When the object is the prevention of iron deficiency in pregnant women, for example, doses of 15 to 30 mg of iron per day are adequate to meet the 3- to 6-mg daily requirement of the last two trimesters. When the purpose is to treat iron-deficiency anemia, but the circumstances do not demand haste, a total dose of about 100 mg (35 mg three times daily) may be used.

The responses expected for different dosage regimens of oral iron are given in Table 53–5. These effects are modified by the severity of the iron-deficiency anemia and by the time of ingestion of iron relative to meals. Bioavailability of iron ingested with food is probably one-half or one-third of that seen in the fasting subject (Grebe *et al.*, 1975). Antacids also reduce iron absorption if given concurrently. It is always preferable to administer iron in the fasting state, even if the dose must be reduced because of gastrointestinal side effects. For patients who require maximal therapy to encourage a rapid response or to counteract continued bleeding, as much as 120 mg of iron may be administered four times a day. Sustained high rates of red cell production require an uninterrupted supply of iron, and oral doses should be spaced equally to maintain a continuous high concentration of iron in plasma.

The duration of treatment is governed by the rate of recovery of hemoglobin and the desire to create iron stores. The former depends on the severity of the anemia. With a daily rate of repair of 2 g of hemoglobin per liter of whole blood, the red cell mass usually is reconstituted within 1 to 2 months. Thus, an individual with a hemoglobin of 50 g per liter may achieve a normal complement of 150 g per liter in about 50 days, whereas an individual

Table 53–5
Average Response to Oral Iron

TOTAL DOSE, mg of iron per day	ESTIMATED ABSORPTION		INCREASE IN HEMOGLOBIN, g/liter of blood per day
	%	mg	
35	40	14	0.7
105	24	25	1.4
195	18	35	1.9
390	12	45	2.2

with a hemoglobin of 100 g per liter may take only half that time. The creation of stores of iron requires many months of oral iron administration. The rate of absorption decreases rapidly after recovery from anemia, and after 3 to 4 months of treatment, stores may increase at a rate of not much more than 100 mg per month. Much of the strategy of continued therapy depends on the estimated future iron balance. Patients with an inadequate diet may require continued therapy with low doses of iron. If the bleeding has stopped, no further therapy is required after the hemoglobin has returned to normal. With continued bleeding, long-term, high-dose therapy clearly is indicated.

Untoward Effects of Oral Preparations of Iron.
Intolerance to oral preparations of iron primarily is a function of the amount of soluble iron in the upper GI tract and of psychological factors. Side effects include heartburn, nausea, upper gastric discomfort, and diarrhea or constipation. A good policy is to initiate therapy at a small dosage, to demonstrate freedom from symptoms at that level, and then gradually to increase the dosage to that desired. With a dose of 200 mg of iron per day divided into three equal portions, symptoms occur in approximately 25% of treated individuals *versus* 13% among those receiving placebo; this increases to approximately 40% when the dosage of iron is doubled. Nausea and upper abdominal pain are increasingly common at high dosage. Constipation and diarrhea, perhaps related to iron-induced changes in the intestinal bacterial flora, are not more prevalent at higher dosage, nor is heartburn. If a liquid is given, one can place the iron solution on the back of the tongue with a dropper to prevent transient staining of teeth.

The normal individual apparently is able to control absorption of iron despite high intake, and it is only individuals with underlying disorders that augment the absorption of iron who run the hazard of developing iron overload (hemochromatosis). However, hemochromatosis is a relatively common genetic disorder, present in 0.5% of the population.

Iron Poisoning. Large amounts of ferrous salts are toxic, but fatalities are rare in adults. Most deaths occur in children, particularly between the ages of 12 and 24 months. As little as 1 to 2 g of iron may cause death, but 2 to 10 g usually is ingested in fatal cases. The frequency of iron poisoning relates to its availability in the household, particularly the supply that remains after a pregnancy. The colored sugar coating of many of the commercially available tablets gives them the appearance of candy. *All iron preparations should be kept in childproof bottles.*

Signs and symptoms of severe poisoning may occur within 30 minutes after ingestion or may be delayed for several hours. They include abdominal pain, diarrhea, or vomiting of brown or bloody stomach contents containing pills. Of particular concern are pallor or cyanosis, lassitude, drowsiness, hyperventilation due to acidosis, and cardiovascular collapse. If death does not occur within 6

hours, there may be a transient period of apparent recovery, followed by death in 12 to 24 hours. The corrosive injury to the stomach may result in pyloric stenosis or gastric scarring. Hemorrhagic gastroenteritis and hepatic damage are prominent findings at autopsy. In the evaluation of a child thought to have ingested iron, a color test for iron in the gastric contents and an emergency determination of the concentration of iron in plasma can be performed. If the latter is less than 63 μmol (3.5 mg per liter), the child is not in immediate danger. However, vomiting should be induced when there is iron in the stomach, and an x-ray should be taken to evaluate the number of pills remaining in the small bowel (iron tablets are radiopaque). Iron in the upper GI tract can be precipitated by lavage with sodium bicarbonate or phosphate solution, although the clinical benefit is questionable. When the plasma concentration of iron is greater than the total iron-binding capacity (63 μmol; 3.5 mg per liter), *deferoxamine* should be administered; dosage and routes of administration are detailed in Chapter 65. Shock, dehydration, and acid-base abnormalities should be treated in the conventional manner. Most important is the speed of diagnosis and therapy. With early effective treatment, the mortality from iron poisoning can be reduced from as high as 45% to about 1%.

Therapy with Parenteral Iron.
When oral iron therapy fails, parenteral iron administration may be an effective alternative (Silverstein and Rodgers, 2004). The rate of response to parenteral therapy is similar to that which follows usual oral doses. Common indications are iron malabsorption (*e.g.,* sprue, short bowel syndrome), severe oral iron intolerance, as a routine supplement to total parenteral nutrition, and in patients who are receiving erythropoietin (Eschbach *et al.*, 1987). Parenteral iron also has been given to iron-deficient patients and pregnant women to create iron stores, something that would take months to achieve by the oral route. *Parenteral iron therapy should be used only when clearly indicated, since acute hypersensitivity, including anaphylactic and anaphylactoid reactions, can occur in 0.2% to 3% of patients.* The belief that the response to parenteral iron, especially *iron dextran,* is faster than oral iron is open to debate. In otherwise healthy individuals, the rate of hemoglobin response is determined by the balance between the severity of the anemia (the level of erythropoietin stimulus) and the delivery of iron to the marrow from iron absorption and iron stores. When a large intravenous dose of iron dextran is given to a severely anemic patient, the hematologic response can exceed that seen with oral iron for 1 to 3 weeks. Subsequently, however, the response is no better than that seen with oral iron.

Three preparations of iron are FDA-approved for parenteral therapy, sodium ferric gluconate complex in sucrose (FERR-LECIT), iron sucrose (SACCHARATE), and iron dextran (INFED, DEXFERRUM). Unlike iron dextran, which requires processing by macrophages that may require several weeks, approximately 80% of sodium ferric gluconate is delivered to transferrin with 24 hours. Sodium ferric gluconate also has a much lower risk of inducing serious anaphylactic reactions than iron dextran (Michael et al., 2002). No deaths were reported with 25 million infusions of sodium ferric gluconate, whereas there were 31 infusion-related deaths reported from approximately half the number of patients treated with iron dextran (Faich and Strobos, 1999). Thus, sodium ferric gluconate is the preferred agent for parenteral iron therapy. Currently, iron dextran is reserved for noncompliant patients or for those who are seriously inconvenienced by the multiple infusions that may be required for treatment with sodium ferric gluconate (Beutler, 2003). *Sodium ferric gluconate complex in sucrose* (FERRLECIT) was approved by the FDA for the treatment of iron deficiency in patients undergoing chronic hemodialysis who are receiving supplemental erythropoietin therapy (Eichbaum et al., 2003).

Iron sucrose (SACCHARATE) also is approved for use in the United States, providing yet another form of parenteral iron for treatment of patients with iron deficiency intractable to therapy with oral iron. Like sodium ferric gluconate, iron sucrose appears to be better tolerated than iron dextran (Fishbane and Kowalski, 2000; Michaud, et al., 2002). However, the experience with iron sucrose is much more limited than that with either iron dextran or sodium ferric gluconate.

Iron dextran injection (INFED, DEXFERRUM) is a colloidal solution of ferric oxyhydroxide complexed with polymerized dextran (molecular weight approximately 180,000) that contains 50 mg/ml of elemental iron. It can be administered by either intravenous (preferred) or intramuscular injection. When given by deep intramuscular injection, it is gradually mobilized *via* the lymphatics and transported to reticuloendothelial cells; the iron then is released from the dextran complex. Intravenous administration gives a more reliable response. Given intravenously in a dose of less than 500 mg, the iron dextran complex is cleared exponentially with a plasma half-life of 6 hours. When 1 g or more is administered intravenously as total dose therapy, reticuloendothelial cell clearance is constant at 10 to 20 mg/hour. This slow rate of clearance results in a brownish discoloration of the plasma for several days and an elevation of the serum iron for 1 to 2 weeks.

Once the iron is released from the dextran within the reticuloendothelial cells, it is either incorporated into stores or transported *via* transferrin to the erythroid marrow. While a portion of the processed iron is rapidly made available to the marrow, a significant fraction is only gradually converted to usable iron stores. All of the iron eventually is released, although many months are required before the process is complete. During this time, the iron dextran stores in reticuloendothelial cells can confuse the clinician who attempts to evaluate the iron status of the patient.

Intramuscular injection of iron dextran should only be initiated after a test dose of 0.5 ml (25 mg of iron). If no adverse reactions are observed, the injections can proceed. The daily dose ordinarily should not exceed 0.5 ml (25 mg of iron) for infants weighing less than 4.5 kg (10 lb), 1 ml (50 mg of iron) for children weighing less than 9 kg (20 lb), and 2 ml (100 mg of iron) for other patients. Iron dextran should be injected only into the muscle mass of the upper outer quadrant of the buttock using a z-track technique (displacement of the skin laterally before injection). However, local reactions and the concern about malignant change at the site of injection

(Weinbren et al., 1978) make intramuscular administration inappropriate except when the intravenous route is inaccessible.

A test injection of 0.5 ml of undiluted iron dextran or an equivalent amount (25 mg of iron) diluted in saline also should precede intravenous administration of a therapeutic dose of iron dextran. The patient should be observed for signs of immediate anaphylaxis, and for an hour after injection for any signs of vascular instability or hypersensitivity, including respiratory distress, hypotension, tachycardia, or back or chest pain. When widely spaced, total-dose infusion therapy is given, a test dose injection should be given before each infusion because hypersensitivity can appear at any time. Furthermore, the patient should be monitored closely throughout the infusion for signs of cardiovascular instability. Delayed hypersensitivity reactions also are observed, especially in patients with rheumatoid arthritis or a history of allergies. Fever, malaise, lymphadenopathy, arthralgias, and urticaria can develop days or weeks following injection and last for prolonged periods of time. Therefore, iron dextran should be used with extreme caution in patients with rheumatoid arthritis or other connective tissue diseases, and during the acute phase of an inflammatory illness. Once hypersensitivity is documented, iron dextran therapy must be abandoned.

Before initiating iron dextran therapy, the total dose of iron required to repair the patient's iron-deficient state should be calculated. Relevant factors are the hemoglobin deficit, the need to reconstitute iron stores, and continued excess losses of iron, as seen with hemodialysis and chronic GI bleeding. Iron dextran solution (50 mg/ml of elemental iron) can be administered undiluted in daily doses of 2 ml until the total dose is reached or given as a single total-dose infusion. In the latter case, the iron dextran should be diluted in 250 to 1000 ml of 0.9% saline and infused over an hour or more.

When hemodialysis patients are started on erythropoietin, oral iron therapy alone generally is insufficient to guarantee an optimal hemoglobin response. It therefore is recommended that sufficient parenteral iron be given to maintain a plasma ferritin level between 100 and 800 $\mu g/L$ and a transferrin saturation of between 20% and 50% (Goodnough et al., 2000). One approach is to administer an initial intravenous dose of 200 to 500 mg, followed by weekly or every-other-week injections of 25 to 100 mg of iron dextran to replace ongoing blood loss (Besarab et al., 1999). With repeated doses of iron dextran—especially multiple, total-dose infusions such as those sometimes used in the treatment of chronic GI blood loss—accumulations of slowly metabolized iron dextran stores in reticuloendothelial cells can be impressive. The plasma ferritin level also can rise to levels associated with iron overload. While disease-related hemochromatosis has been associated with an increased risk of infections and cardiovascular disease, this has not been shown to be true in hemodialysis patients treated with iron dextran (Owen, 1999). It seems prudent, however, to withhold the drug whenever the plasma ferritin rises above 800 $\mu g/L$.

Reactions to intravenous iron include headache, malaise, fever, generalized lymphadenopathy, arthralgias, urticaria, and in some patients with rheumatoid arthritis, exacerbation of the disease. Phlebitis may occur with prolonged infusions of a concentrated solution or when an intramuscular preparation containing 0.5% phenol is used in error. Of greatest concern is the rare anaphylactic reaction, which may be fatal despite treatment (Faich and Strobos, 1999).

COPPER

Copper deficiency is extremely rare because the amount present in food is more than adequate to provide the needed body complement of slightly more than 100 mg. There is no evidence that copper ever needs to be added to a normal diet, either prophylactically or therapeutically. Even in clinical states associated with hypocupremia (sprue, celiac disease, and nephrotic syndrome), effects of copper deficiency usually are not demonstrable. Anemia due to copper deficiency has been described in individuals who have undergone intestinal bypass surgery (Zidar *et al.*, 1977), in those who are receiving parenteral nutrition (Dunlap *et al.*, 1974), in malnourished infants (Graham and Cordano, 1976), and in patients ingesting excessive amounts of zinc (Hoffman *et al.*, 1988). While an inherited disorder affecting the transport of copper in human beings (Menkes' disease; steely hair syndrome) is associated with reduced activity of several copper-dependent enzymes, this disease is not associated with hematological abnormalities.

Copper deficiency in experimental animals interferes with the absorption of iron and its release from reticuloendothelial cells (Lee *et al.*, 1976). The associated microcytic anemia is related to a decrease in the availability of iron to the normoblasts, and perhaps even more importantly, to decreased mitochondrial production of heme. It may be that the specific defect in the latter case is a decrease in the activity of cytochrome oxidase. Other pathological effects involving the skeletal, cardiovascular, and nervous systems have been observed in copper-deficient experimental animals. In human beings, the outstanding findings have been leukopenia, particularly granulocytopenia, and anemia. Concentrations of iron in plasma are variable, and the anemia is not always microcytic. When a low plasma copper concentration is determined in the presence of leukopenia and anemia, a therapeutic trial with copper is appropriate. Daily doses up to 0.1 mg/kg of *cupric sulfate* have been given by mouth, or 1 to 2 mg per day may be added to the solution of nutrients for parenteral administration.

PYRIDOXINE

Harris and associates first described pyridoxine-responsive anemia in 1956. Subsequent reports suggested that the vitamin might improve hematopoiesis in up to 50% of patients with either hereditary or acquired sidero-

blastic anemia. These patients characteristically have impaired hemoglobin synthesis and accumulate iron in the perinuclear mitochondria of erythroid precursor cells, so-called ringed sideroblasts. Hereditary sideroblastic anemia is an X-linked recessive trait with variable penetrance and expression that results from mutations in the erythrocyte form of δ-aminolevulinate synthase. Affected men typically show a dual population of normal red cells and microcytic, hypochromic cells in the circulation. In contrast, idiopathic acquired sideroblastic anemia and the sideroblastic anemias associated with a number of drugs, inflammatory states, neoplastic disorders, and preleukemic syndromes show a variable morphological picture. Moreover, erythrokinetic studies demonstrate a spectrum of abnormalities, from a hypoproliferative defect with little tendency to accumulate iron to marked ineffective erythropoiesis with iron overload of the tissues (Solomon and Hillman, 1979a).

Oral therapy with pyridoxine is of proven benefit in correcting the sideroblastic anemias associated with the antituberculosis drugs *isoniazid* and *pyrazinamide,* which act as vitamin B_6 antagonists. A daily dose of 50 mg of pyridoxine completely corrects the defect without interfering with treatment, and routine supplementation of pyridoxine often is recommended (*see* Chapter 47). In contrast, if pyridoxine is given to counteract the sideroblastic abnormality associated with administration of levodopa, the effectiveness of levodopa in controlling Parkinson's disease is decreased. Pyridoxine therapy does not correct the sideroblastic abnormalities produced by chloramphenicol or lead.

Patients with idiopathic acquired sideroblastic anemia generally fail to respond to oral pyridoxine, and those individuals who appear to have a pyridoxine-responsive anemia require prolonged therapy with large doses of the vitamin, 50 to 500 mg per day. Unfortunately, the early enthusiasm for treatment with pyridoxine was not reinforced by results of later studies (Chillar *et al.*, 1976; Solomon and Hillman, 1979a). Moreover, even when a patient with sideroblastic anemia responds, the improvement is only partial because both the ringed sideroblasts and the red cell defect persist, and the hematocrit rarely returns to normal. Nonetheless, in view of the low toxicity of oral pyridoxine, a therapeutic trial with pyridoxine is appropriate.

As shown in studies of normal subjects, oral pyridoxine in a dosage of 100 mg three times daily produces a maximal increase in red cell pyridoxine kinase and the major pyridoxal phosphate–dependent enzyme glutamic-aspartic aminotransferase (Solomon and Hillman, 1978). For an adequate therapeutic trial, the drug is administered for at least 3 months while the response is monitored by measuring the reticulocyte index and the hemoglobin concentration. The occasional patient who is refractory to oral pyridoxine may respond to parenteral administration of pyridoxal phosphate. However, oral pyridoxine in doses of 200 to 300 mg per day produces intracellular concentrations of pyridoxal phosphate equal to or greater than those generated by therapy with the phosphorylated vitamin (Solomon and Hillman, 1979b).

RIBOFLAVIN

Pure red cell aplasia that responded to the administration of riboflavin was reported in patients with protein depletion and complicating infections. Lane and associates induced riboflavin deficiency in human beings and demonstrated that a hypoproliferative anemia resulted within a month. The spontaneous appearance in human beings of red cell aplasia due to riboflavin deficiency undoubtedly is rare, if it occurs at all. It has been described in combination with infection and protein deficiency, both of which are capable of producing a hypoproliferative anemia. However, it seems reasonable to include riboflavin in the nutritional management of patients with gross, generalized malnutrition.

III. Vitamin B₁₂, Folic Acid, and the Treatment of Megaloblastic Anemias

Vitamin B₁₂ and *folic acid* are dietary essentials. A deficiency of either vitamin impairs DNA synthesis in any cell in which chromosomal replication and division are taking place. Since tissues with the greatest rate of cell turnover show the most dramatic changes, the hematopoietic system is especially sensitive to deficiencies of these vitamins. An early sign of deficiency is megaloblastic anemia. Abnormal macrocytic red blood cells are produced, and the patient becomes severely anemic. Recognized in the 19th century, this pattern of abnormal hematopoiesis, termed *pernicious anemia*, spurred investigations that ultimately led to the discovery of vitamin B₁₂ and folic acid. Even today, the characteristic abnormality in red blood cell morphology is important for diagnosis and as a therapeutic guide following administration of the vitamins.

History. The discovery of vitamin B₁₂ and folic acid is a dramatic story that started more than 180 years ago and includes two Nobel prize–winning discoveries. The first descriptions of what must have been megaloblastic anemias came from the work of Combe and Addison, who published a series of case reports beginning in 1824. It still is common practice to describe megaloblastic anemia as Addisonian pernicious anemia. Although Combe suggested that the disorder might have some relationship to digestion, it was Austin Flint who in 1860 first described the severe gastric atrophy and called attention to its possible relationship to the anemia.

After the observation by Whipple in 1925 that liver is a source of a potent hematopoietic substance for iron-deficient dogs, Minot

and Murphy carried out Nobel Prize–winning experiments that demonstrated the effectiveness of the feeding of liver to reverse pernicious anemia. Soon thereafter, Castle defined the need for both intrinsic factor, a substance secreted by the parietal cells of the gastric mucosa, and extrinsic factor, the vitamin-like material provided by crude liver extracts. Nearly 20 years passed before Rickes and coworkers and Smith and Parker isolated and crystallized vitamin B₁₂; Dorothy Hodgkin received the Nobel Prize for determining its x-ray crystal structure.

As attempts were being made to purify extrinsic factor, Wills and her associates described a macrocytic anemia in women in India that responded to a factor present in crude liver extracts but not in the purified fractions known to be effective in pernicious anemia. This factor, first called Wills' factor and later vitamin M, is now known to be folic acid. The term folic acid was coined by Mitchell and coworkers in 1941, after its isolation from leafy vegetables.

More recent work has shown that neither vitamin B₁₂ nor folic acid as purified from foodstuffs is the active coenzyme for human beings. During extraction, active, labile forms are converted to stable congeners of vitamin B₁₂ and folic acid, *cyanocobalamin* and *pteroylglutamic acid,* respectively. These congeners must then be modified *in vivo* to be effective. While a great deal has been learned about the intracellular metabolic pathways in which these vitamins function as required cofactors, many questions remain. The most important of these is the relationship of vitamin B₁₂ deficiency to the neurological abnormalities that occur with this disorder (Chanarin *et al.*, 1985).

Relationships Between Vitamin B₁₂ and Folic Acid. The major roles of vitamin B₁₂ and folic acid in intracellular metabolism are summarized in Figure 53–6. Intracellular vitamin B₁₂ is maintained as two active coenzymes: methylcobalamin and deoxyadenosylcobalamin. Deoxyadenosylcobalamin (deoxyadenosyl B₁₂) is a cofactor for the mitochondrial mutase enzyme that catalyzes the isomerization of L-methylmalonyl CoA to succinyl CoA, an important reaction in carbohydrate and lipid metabolism. This reaction has no direct relationship to the metabolic pathways that involve folate. In contrast, methylcobalamin (CH₃B₁₂) supports the methionine synthetase reaction, which is essential for normal metabolism of folate (Weir and Scott, 1983). Methyl groups contributed by methyltetrahydrofolate (CH₃H₄PteGlu₁) are used to form methylcobalamin, which then acts as a methyl group donor for the conversion of homocysteine to methionine. This folate–cobalamin interaction is pivotal for normal synthesis of purines and pyrimidines, and therefore of DNA. The methionine synthetase reaction is largely responsible for the control of the recycling of folate cofactors; the maintenance of intracellular concentrations of folylpolyglutamates; and, through the synthesis of methionine and its product, *S*-adenosylmethionine, the maintenance of a number of methylation reactions.

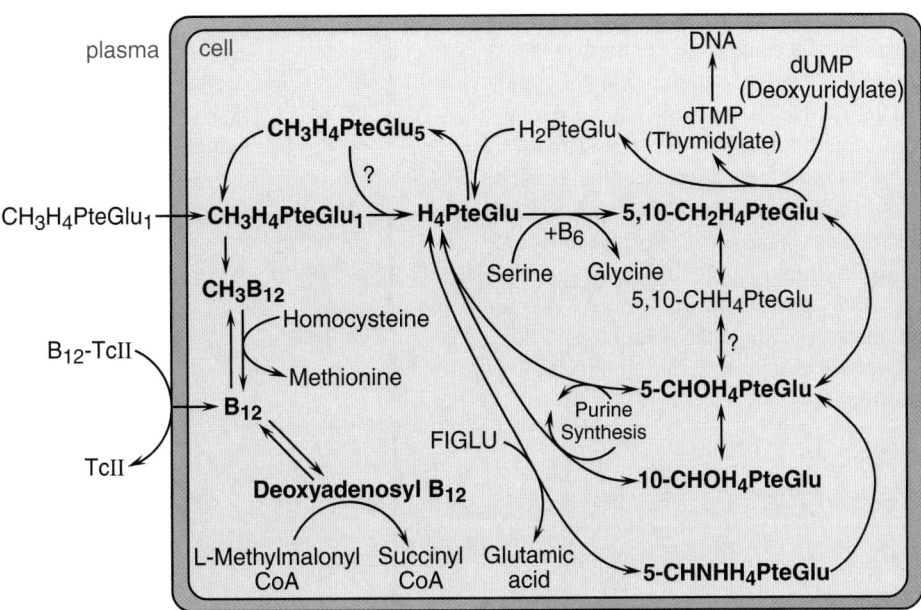

Figure 53–6. *Interrelationships and metabolic roles of vitamin B$_{12}$ and folic acid. See* text for explanation and Figure 53–9 for structures of the various folate coenzymes. FIGLU, formiminoglutamic acid, which arises from the catabolism of histidine; TcII, transcobalamin II; CH$_3$H$_4$PteGlu$_1$, methyltetrahydrofolate.

Since methyltetrahydrofolate is the principal folate congener supplied to cells, the transfer of the methyl group to cobalamin is essential for the adequate supply of tetrahydrofolate (H$_4$PteGlu$_1$), the substrate for a number of metabolic steps. Tetrahydrofolate is a precursor for the formation of intracellular folylpolyglutamates; it also acts as the acceptor of a one-carbon unit in the conversion of serine to glycine, with the resultant formation of 5,10-methylenetetrahydrofolate (5,10-CH$_2$H$_4$PteGlu). The latter derivative donates the methylene group to deoxyuridylate (dUMP) for the synthesis of thymidylate (dTMP)—an extremely important reaction in DNA synthesis. In the process, the 5,10-CH$_2$H$_4$PteGlu is converted to dihydrofolate (H$_2$PteGlu). The cycle then is completed by the reduction of the H$_2$PteGlu to H$_4$PteGlu by dihydrofolate reductase, the step that is blocked by folate antagonists such as methotrexate (*see* Chapter 51). As shown in Figure 53–6, other pathways also lead to the synthesis of 5,10-methylenetetrahydrofolate. These pathways are important in the metabolism of formiminoglutamic acid (FIGLU) and purines and pyrimidines (*see* reviews by Weir and Scott, 1983; Chanarin *et al.*, 1985).

In the presence of a deficiency of either vitamin B$_{12}$ or folate, the decreased synthesis of methionine and *S*-adenosylmethionine interferes with protein biosynthesis, a number of methylation reactions, and the synthesis of

polyamines. In addition, the cell responds to the deficiency by redirecting folate metabolic pathways to supply increasing amounts of methyltetrahydrofolate; this tends to preserve essential methylation reactions at the expense of nucleic acid synthesis. With vitamin B$_{12}$ deficiency, methylenetetrahydrofolate reductase activity increases, directing available intracellular folates into the methyltetrahydrofolate pool (not shown in Figure 53–6). The methyltetrahydrofolate then is trapped by the lack of sufficient vitamin B$_{12}$ to accept and transfer methyl groups, and subsequent steps in folate metabolism that require tetrahydrofolate are deprived of substrate. This process provides a common basis for the development of megaloblastic anemia with deficiency of either vitamin B$_{12}$ or folic acid.

The mechanisms responsible for the neurological lesions of vitamin B$_{12}$ deficiency are less well understood (Weir and Scott, 1983). Damage to the myelin sheath is the most obvious lesion in this neuropathy. This observation led to the early suggestion that the deoxyadenosyl B$_{12}$–dependent methylmalonyl CoA mutase reaction, a step in propionate metabolism, is related to the abnormality. However, other evidence suggests that the deficiency of methionine synthetase and the block of the conversion of methionine to *S*-adenosylmethionine are more likely to be responsible (Scott *et al.*, 1981).

Nitrous oxide (N_2O), used for anesthesia (*see* Chapter 13), can cause megaloblastic changes in the marrow and a neuropathy that resemble those of vitamin B_{12} deficiency (Chanarin *et al.*, 1985). Studies with N_2O have demonstrated a reduction in methionine synthetase and reduced concentrations of methionine and *S*-adenosylmethionine. The latter is necessary for methylation reactions, including those required for the synthesis of phospholipids and myelin. Significantly, the neuropathy induced with N_2O can be prevented partially by feeding methionine. A neuropathy similar to that occurring with vitamin B_{12} deficiency has been reported in dentists who are exposed to N_2O used as an anesthetic.

VITAMIN B_{12}

Chemistry. The structural formula of vitamin B_{12} is shown in Figure 53–7. The three major portions of the molecule are:

A planar group or corrin nucleus—a porphyrin-like ring structure with four reduced pyrrole rings (A to D in Figure 53–7) linked to a central cobalt atom and extensively substituted with methyl, acetamide, and propionamide residues.

A 5,6-dimethylbenzimidazolyl nucleotide, which links almost at right angles to the corrin nucleus with bonds to the cobalt atom and to the propionate side chain of the C pyrrole ring.

A variable R group—the most important of which are found in the stable compounds cyanocobalamin and *hydroxocobalamin* and the active coenzymes methylcobalamin and 5-deoxyadenosylcobalamin.

The terms *vitamin B_{12}* and *cyanocobalamin* are used interchangeably as generic terms for all of the cobamides active in humans. Preparations of vitamin B_{12} for therapeutic use contain either cyanocobalamin or hydroxocobalamin, since only these derivatives remain active after storage.

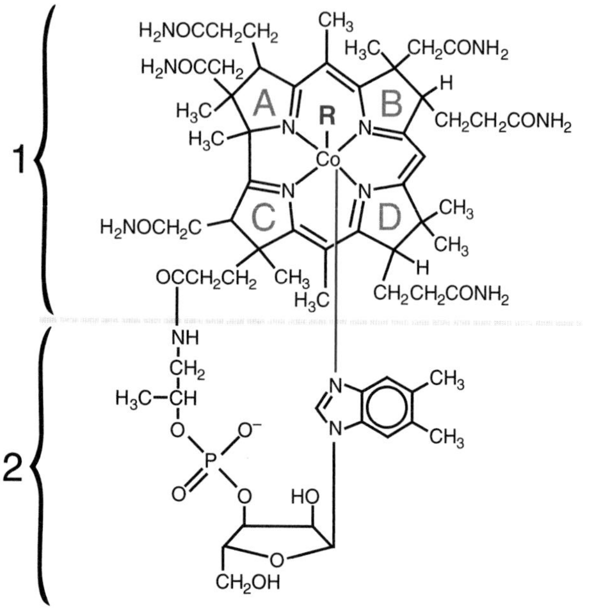

Vitamin B_{12} Congeners	
Permissive Name	**R Group**
Cyanocobalamin (Vitamin B_{12})	–CN
Hydroxocobalamin	–OH
Methylcobalamin	$-CH_3$
5'-Deoxyadenosylcobalamin	–5'-Deoxyadenosyl

Figure 53–7. ***The structures and nomenclature of vitamin B_{12} congeners.***

Metabolic Functions. The active coenzymes methylcobalamin and 5-deoxyadenosylcobalamin are essential for cell growth and replication. Methylcobalamin is required for the conversion of homocysteine to methionine and its derivative *S*-adenosylmethionine. In addition, when concentrations of vitamin B_{12} are inadequate, folate becomes “trapped” as methyltetrahydrofolate to cause a functional deficiency of other required intracellular forms of folic acid (*see* Figures 53–6 and 53–7 and discussion above). The hematological abnormalities in vitamin B_{12}–deficient patients result from this process. 5-Deoxyadenosylcobalamin is required for the isomerization of L-methylmalonyl CoA to succinyl CoA (Figure 53–6).

Sources in Nature. Humans depend on exogenous sources of vitamin B_{12}. In nature, the primary sources are certain microorganisms that grow in soil, sewage, water, or the intestinal lumen of animals that synthesize the vitamin. Vegetable products are free of vitamin B_{12} unless they are contaminated with such microorganisms, so that animals are dependent on synthesis in their own alimentary tract or the ingestion of animal products containing vitamin B_{12}. The daily nutritional requirement of 3 to 5 μg must be obtained from animal by-products in the diet. Despite this, strict vegetarians rarely develop vitamin B_{12} deficiency. Some vitamin B_{12} is available from legumes, which are contaminated with bacteria capable of synthesizing vitamin B_{12}, and vegetarians often fortify their diets with a wide range of vitamins and minerals.

Absorption, Distribution, Elimination, and Daily Requirements. In the presence of gastric acid and pancreatic proteases, dietary vitamin B_{12} is released from food and salivary binding protein and bound to gastric intrinsic factor. When the vitamin B_{12}–intrinsic factor complex reaches the ileum, it interacts with a receptor on the mucosal cell surface and is actively transported into circulation. Adequate intrinsic factor, bile, and sodium bicarbonate (to provide a suitable pH) all are required for ileal transport of vitamin B_{12}. Vitamin B_{12} deficiency in adults is rarely the result of a deficient diet *per se;* rather, it usually reflects a defect in one or another aspect of this complex sequence of absorption (Figure 53–8). Achlorhydria and decreased secretion of intrinsic factor by parietal cells secondary to gastric atrophy or gastric surgery is a common cause of vitamin B_{12} deficiency in adults. Antibodies to parietal cells or intrinsic factor complex also can play a prominent role in producing a deficiency. A number of intestinal diseases can interfere with absorption, including pancreatic disorders (loss of pancreatic protease secretion), bacterial overgrowth, intestinal parasites, sprue, and localized damage to ileal mucosal cells by disease or as a result of surgery.

Once absorbed, vitamin B_{12} binds to transcobalamin II, a plasma β-globulin, for transport to tissues. Two other transcobalamins (I and III) also are present in plasma; their concentrations are related to the rate of turnover of granulocytes. They may represent intracellular storage proteins that are released with cell death. Vitamin B_{12} bound to transcobalamin II is rapidly cleared from plasma and preferentially distributed to hepatic parenchymal cells. The liver is a storage depot for other tissues. In normal adults, as much as 90% of the body's stores of vitamin B_{12}, from 1 to 10 mg, is in the liver. Vitamin B_{12} is stored as the active coenzyme with a turnover rate of 0.5 to 8 μg per day, depending on the size of body stores. The recommended daily intake of the vitamin in adults is 2.4 μg.

Approximately 3 μg of cobalamins is secreted into bile each day, 50% to 60% of which is not destined for reabsorption. This enterohepatic cycle is important because interference with reabsorption by intestinal disease can progressively deplete hepatic stores of the vitamin. This process may help explain why patients can develop vitamin B_{12} deficiency within 3 to 4 years of major gastric surgery, even though a daily requirement of 1 to 2 μg would not be expected to deplete hepatic stores of more than 2 to 3 mg during this time.

The supply of vitamin B_{12} available for tissues is directly related to the size of the hepatic storage pool and the amount of vitamin B_{12} bound to transcobalamin II (Figure 53–8). The plasma concentration of vitamin B_{12} is the best routine measure of B_{12} deficiency, and normally ranges from 150 to 660 pmol (about 200 to 900 pg/ml). Deficiency should be suspected whenever the con-

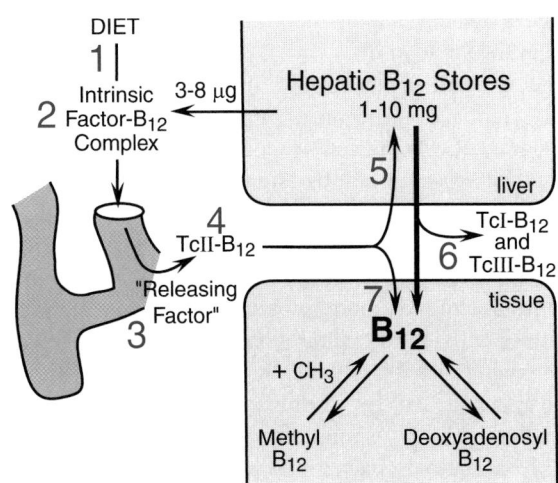

Figure 53–8. *The absorption and distribution of vitamin B_{12}.* Deficiency of vitamin B_{12} can result from a congenital or acquired defect in any one of the following: (1) inadequate dietary supply; (2) inadequate secretion of intrinsic factor (classical pernicious anemia); (3) ileal disease; (4) congenital absence of transcobalamin II (TcII); or (5) rapid depletion of hepatic stores by interference with reabsorption of vitamin B_{12} excreted in bile. The utility of measurements of the concentration of vitamin B_{12} in plasma to estimate supply available to tissues can be compromised by liver disease and (6) the appearance of abnormal amounts of transcobalamins I and III (TcI and III) in plasma. Finally, the formation of methylcobalamin requires (7) normal transport into cells and an adequate supply of folic acid as $CH_3H_4PteGlu_1$.

centration falls below 150 pmol. The correlation is excellent except when the plasma concentrations of transcobalamin I and III are increased, as occurs with hepatic disease or a myeloproliferative disorder. Inasmuch as the vitamin B_{12} bound to these transport proteins is relatively unavailable to cells, tissues can become deficient when the concentration of vitamin B_{12} in plasma is normal or even high. In subjects with congenital absence of transcobalamin II, megaloblastic anemia occurs despite relatively normal plasma concentrations of vitamin B_{12}; the anemia will respond to parenteral doses of vitamin B_{12} that exceed the renal clearance (Hakami *et al.,* 1971).

Defects in intracellular metabolism of vitamin B_{12} have been reported in children with methylmalonic aciduria and homocystinuria. Potential mechanisms include an incapacity of cells to transport vitamin B_{12} or accumulate the vitamin because of a failure to synthesize an intracellular acceptor, a defect in the formation of deoxyadenosylcobalamin, or a congenital lack of methylmalonyl CoA isomerase.

Vitamin B_{12} Deficiency. Vitamin B_{12} deficiency is recognized clinically by its impact on the hematopoietic and nervous systems. The sensitivity of the hematopoietic system relates to its high rate of cell turnover. Other tissues with high rates of cell turnover (*e.g.,* mucosa and cervical epithelium) also have high requirements for the vitamin.

As a result of an inadequate supply of vitamin B_{12}, DNA replication becomes highly abnormal. Once a hematopoietic stem cell is committed to enter a programmed series of cell divisions, the defect in chromosomal replication results in an inability of maturing cells to complete nuclear divisions while cytoplasmic maturation continues at a relatively normal rate. This results in the production of morphologically abnormal cells and death of cells during maturation, a phenomenon referred to as *ineffective hematopoiesis*. These abnormalities are readily identified by examination of the marrow and peripheral blood. Maturation of red cell precursors is highly abnormal (megaloblastic erythropoiesis). Those cells that do leave the marrow also are abnormal, and many cell fragments, poikilocytes, and macrocytes appear in the peripheral blood. The mean red cell volume increases to values greater than 110 fl. Severe deficiency affects all cell lines, and a pronounced pancytopenia results.

The diagnosis of a vitamin B_{12} deficiency usually can be made using measurements of the serum vitamin B_{12} and/or serum methylmalonic acid. The latter is somewhat more sensitive and has been used to identify metabolic deficiency in patients with normal serum vitamin B_{12} levels. As part of the clinical management of a patient with severe megaloblastic anemia, a therapeutic trial using very small doses of the vitamin can be used to confirm the diagnosis. Serial measurements of the reticulocyte count, serum iron, and hematocrit are performed to define the characteristic recovery of normal red cell production. The Schilling test can be used to quantitate the absorption of the vitamin and delineate the mechanism of the disease. By performing the Schilling test with and without added intrinsic factor, it is possible to discriminate between intrinsic factor deficiency by itself and primary ileal cell disease.

Vitamin B_{12} deficiency can irreversibly damage the nervous system. Progressive swelling of myelinated neurons, demyelination, and neuronal cell death are seen in the spinal column and cerebral cortex. This causes a wide range of neurological signs and symptoms, including paresthesias of the hands and feet, decreased vibration and position senses with resultant unsteadiness, decreased deep tendon reflexes, and in the later stages, confusion, moodiness, loss of memory, and even a loss of central vision. The patient may exhibit delusions, hallucinations, or even overt psychosis. Since the neurological damage can be dissociated from the changes in the hematopoietic system, vitamin B_{12} deficiency must be considered in elderly patients with dementia or psychiatric disorders, even if they are not anemic (Lindenbaum *et al.*, 1988).

Vitamin B_{12} Therapy. Vitamin B_{12} is available for injection or oral administration; combinations with other vitamins and minerals also can be given orally or parenterally. The choice of a preparation always depends on the cause of the deficiency. Although oral preparations may be used to supplement deficient diets, they are of limited value in the treatment of patients with deficiency of intrinsic factor or ileal disease. Even though small amounts of vitamin B_{12} may be absorbed by simple diffusion, the oral route of administration cannot be relied upon for effective therapy in the patient with a marked deficiency of vitamin B_{12} and abnormal hematopoiesis or neurological deficits. Therefore, the preparation of choice for treatment of a vitamin B_{12}–deficiency state is cyanocobalamin, and it should be administered by intramuscular or subcutaneous injection.

Cyanocobalamin injection is safe when given by the intramuscular or deep subcutaneous route, but it should never be given intravenously. There have been rare reports of transitory exanthema and anaphylaxis after injection. If a patient reports a previous sensitivity to injections of vitamin B_{12}, an intradermal skin test should be performed before the full dose is administered.

Cyanocobalamin is administered in doses of 1 to 1000 μg. Tissue uptake, storage, and utilization depend on the availability of transcobalamin II (*see* above). Doses in excess of 100 μg are cleared rapidly from plasma into the urine, and administration of larger amounts of vitamin B_{12} will not result in greater retention of the vitamin. Administration of 1000 μg is of value in the performance of the Schilling test. After isotopically labeled vitamin B_{12} is administered orally, the compound that is absorbed can be quantitatively recovered in the urine if 1000 μg of cyanocobalamin is administered intramuscularly. This unlabeled material saturates the transport system and tissue binding sites, so that more than 90% of the labeled and unlabeled vitamin is excreted during the next 24 hours.

A number of multivitamin preparations are marketed either as nutritional supplements or for the treatment of anemia. Many of these contain up to 80 μg of cyanocobalamin without or with intrinsic factor concentrate prepared from the stomachs of hogs or other domestic animals. One oral unit of intrinsic factor is defined as that amount of material that will bind and transport 15 μg of cyanocobalamin. Most multivitamin preparations supplemented with intrinsic factor contain 0.5 oral unit per tablet. While the combination of oral vitamin B_{12} and intrinsic factor would appear to be ideal for patients with an intrinsic factor deficiency, such preparations are not reliable. With prolonged therapy, some patients become refractory to oral intrinsic factor, perhaps related to production of an intraluminal antibody against the hog protein. Patients taking such preparations must be reevaluated at periodic intervals for recurrence of pernicious anemia.

Hydroxocobalamin given in doses of 100 μg intramuscularly has been reported to have a more sustained effect than cyanocobalamin, with a single dose maintaining plasma vitamin B_{12} concentrations in the normal range for up to 3 months. However, some patients show reductions of the concentration of vitamin B_{12} in plasma within 30 days, similar to that seen after cyanocobalamin. Furthermore, the administration of hydroxocobalamin has resulted in the formation of antibodies to the transcobalamin II–vitamin B_{12} complex.

Vitamin B_{12} has an undeserved reputation as a health tonic and has been used for a number of disease states. Effective use of the vitamin depends on accurate diagnosis and an understanding of the following general principles of therapy:

1. Vitamin B_{12} should be given prophylactically only when there is a reasonable probability that a deficiency exists or will exist. Dietary deficiency in the strict vegetarian, the predictable malabsorption of vitamin B_{12} in patients who have had a gastrectomy, and certain diseases of the small intestine constitute such indications. When gastrointestinal function is normal, an oral prophylactic supplement of vitamins and minerals, including vitamin B_{12}, may be indicated. Otherwise, the patient should receive monthly injections of cyanocobalamin.

2. The relative ease of treatment with vitamin B_{12} should not prevent a full investigation of the etiology of the deficiency. The initial diagnosis usually is suggested by a macrocytic anemia or an unexplained neuropsychiatric disorder. Full understanding of the etiology of vitamin B_{12} deficiency involves studies of dietary supply, gastrointestinal absorption, and transport.

3. Therapy always should be as specific as possible. While a large number of multivitamin preparations are available, the use of "shotgun" vitamin therapy in the treatment of vitamin B_{12} deficiency can be dangerous. With such therapy, there is the danger that sufficient folic acid will be given to result in a hematological recovery. This can mask continued vitamin B_{12} deficiency and permit neurological damage to develop or progress.

4. Although a classical therapeutic trial with small amounts of vitamin B_{12} can help confirm the diagnosis, acutely ill, elderly patients may not be able to tolerate the delay in the correction of a severe anemia. Such patients require supplemental blood transfusions and immediate therapy with folic acid and vitamin B_{12} to guarantee rapid recovery.

5. Long-term therapy with vitamin B_{12} must be evaluated at intervals of 6 to 12 months in patients who are otherwise well. If there is an additional illness or a condition that may increase the requirement for the vitamin (*e.g.*, pregnancy), reassessment should be performed more frequently.

Treatment of the Acutely Ill Patient. The therapeutic approach depends on the severity of the patient's illness. In uncomplicated pernicious anemia, in which the abnormality is restricted to a mild or moderate anemia without leukopenia, thrombocytopenia, or neurological signs or symptoms, the administration of vitamin B_{12} alone will suffice. Moreover, therapy may be delayed until other causes of megaloblastic anemia have been excluded and sufficient studies of gastrointestinal function have been performed to reveal the underlying cause of the disease. In this situation, a therapeutic trial with small amounts of parenteral vitamin B_{12} (1 to 10 μg per day) can confirm the presence of an uncomplicated vitamin B_{12} deficiency.

In contrast, patients with neurological changes or severe leukopenia or thrombocytopenia associated with infection or bleeding require emergency treatment. The older individual with a severe anemia (hematocrit less than 20%) is likely to have tissue hypoxia, cerebrovascular insufficiency, and congestive heart failure. Effective therapy must not wait for detailed diagnostic tests. Once the megaloblastic erythropoiesis has been confirmed and sufficient blood collected for later measurements of vitamin B_{12} and folic acid, the patient should receive intramuscular injections of 100 μg of cyanocobalamin and 1 to 5 mg of folic acid. For the next 1 to 2 weeks the patient should receive daily intramuscular injections of 100 μg of cyanocobalamin, together with a daily oral supplement of 1 to 2 mg of folic acid. Because an effective increase in red cell mass will not occur for 10 to 20 days, the patient with a markedly depressed hematocrit and tissue hypoxia also should receive a transfusion of 2 to 3 units of packed red blood cells. If congestive heart failure is present, diuretics can be administered to prevent volume overload.

Patients usually report an increased sense of well-being within the first 24 hours of the initiation of therapy. Objectively, memory and orientation can improve dramatically, although full recovery of mental function may take months, or may never occur. In addition, even before an obvious hematological response is apparent, the patient may report an increase in strength, a better appetite, and reduced soreness of the mouth and tongue.

The first objective hematological change is the disappearance of the megaloblastic morphology of the bone marrow. As the ineffective erythropoiesis is corrected, the concentration of iron in plasma falls dramatically as the metal is used in the formation of hemoglobin. This usually occurs within the first 48 hours. Full correction of precursor maturation in marrow with production of an increased number of reticulocytes begins about the second or third day and peaks 3 to 5 days later. When the anemia is moderate to severe, the maximal reticulocyte index will be between three and five times the normal value (*i.e.*, a reticulocyte count of 20% to 40%). The ability of the marrow to sustain a high rate of production determines the rate of recovery of the hematocrit. Patients with complicating iron deficiency, an infection or other inflammatory state, or renal disease may be unable to correct their anemia. Therefore it is important to monitor the reticulocyte index over the first several weeks. If it does not continue at elevated levels while the hematocrit is less than 35%, plasma concentrations of iron and folic acid should again be determined and the patient reevaluated for an illness that could inhibit the response of the marrow.

The degree and rate of improvement of neurological signs and symptoms depend on the severity and the duration of the abnormalities. Those that have been present for only a few months usually disappear relatively rapidly. When a defect has been present for many months or years, full return to normal function may never occur.

Long-Term Therapy with Vitamin B$_{12}$. Once begun, vitamin B$_{12}$ therapy must be maintained for life. This fact must be impressed upon the patient and family, and a system must be established to guarantee continued monthly injections of cyanocobalamin. Intramuscular injection of 100 μg of cyanocobalamin every 4 weeks is sufficient to maintain a normal concentration of vitamin B$_{12}$ in plasma and an adequate supply for tissues. Patients with severe neurological symptoms and signs may be treated with larger doses of vitamin B$_{12}$ in the period immediately after the diagnosis. Doses of 100 μg per day or several times per week may be given for several months with the hope of encouraging faster and more complete recovery. It is important to monitor vitamin B$_{12}$ concentrations in plasma and to obtain peripheral blood counts at intervals of 3 to 6 months to confirm the adequacy of therapy. Since refractoriness to therapy can develop at any time, evaluation must continue throughout the patient's life.

Other Therapeutic Uses of Vitamin B$_{12}$. Vitamin B$_{12}$ has been used in the therapy of a number of conditions, including trigeminal neuralgia, multiple sclerosis and other neuropathies, various psychiatric disorders, poor growth or nutrition, and as a "tonic" for patients complaining of tiredness or easy fatigue. There is no evidence for the validity of such therapy in any of these conditions. Maintenance therapy with vitamin B$_{12}$ has been used with some apparent success in the treatment of children with methylmalonic aciduria.

FOLIC ACID

Chemistry and Metabolic Functions. The structural formula of pteroylglutamic acid (PteGlu) is shown in Figure 53–9. Major portions of the molecule include a pteridine ring linked by a methylene bridge to para-aminobenzoic acid, which is joined by an amide linkage to glutamic acid. While pteroylglutamic acid is the common pharmaceutical form of folic acid, it is neither the principal folate congener in food nor the active coenzyme for intracellular metabolism. After absorption, PteGlu is rapidly reduced at the 5, 6, 7, and 8 positions to tetrahydrofolic acid (H$_4$PteGlu), which then acts as an acceptor of a number of one-carbon units. These are attached at either the 5 or the 10 position of the pteridine ring or may bridge these atoms to form a new five-membered ring. The most important forms of the coenzyme that are synthesized by these reactions are listed in Figure 53–9. Each plays a specific role in intracellular metabolism, summarized as follows (*see* "Relationships Between Vitamin B$_{12}$ and Folic Acid," above, as well as Figure 53–6):

Conversion of homocysteine to methionine. This reaction requires CH$_3$H$_4$PteGlu as a methyl donor and utilizes vitamin B$_{12}$ as a cofactor.

Conversion of serine to glycine. This reaction requires tetrahydrofolate as an acceptor of a methylene group from serine and utilizes pyridoxal phosphate as a cofactor. It results in the formation of 5,10-CH$_2$H$_4$PteGlu, an essential coenzyme for the synthesis of thymidylate.

Synthesis of thymidylate. 5,10-CH$_2$H$_4$PteGlu donates a methylene group and reducing equivalents to deoxyuridylate for the synthesis of thymidylate—a rate-limiting step in DNA synthesis.

Histidine metabolism. H$_4$PteGlu also acts as an acceptor of a formimino group in the conversion of formiminoglutamic acid to glutamic acid.

Synthesis of purines. Two steps in the synthesis of purine nucleotides require the participation of derivatives of folic acid. Glycinamide ribonucleotide is formylated by 5,10-CHH$_4$PteGlu; 5-aminoimidazole-4-carboxamide ribonucleotide is formylated by 10-CHOH$_4$PteGlu. By these reactions, carbon atoms at positions 8 and 2, respectively, are incorporated into the growing purine ring.

Utilization or generation of formate. This reversible reaction utilizes H$_4$PteGlu and 10-CHOH$_4$PteGlu.

Daily Requirements. Many food sources are rich in folates, especially fresh green vegetables, liver, yeast, and some fruits. However, lengthy cooking can destroy up to 90% of the folate content of such food. Generally, a standard United States diet provides 50 to 500 μg of absorbable folate per day, although individuals with high intakes of fresh vegetables and meats will ingest as much as 2 mg per day. In the normal adult, the recommended daily intake is 400 μg, while pregnant or lactating women and patients with high rates of cell turnover (such as patients with a hemolytic anemia) may require 500 to 600 μg or more per day. For the prevention of neural tube defects, a daily intake of at least 400 μg of folate in food or in supplements beginning a month before pregnancy and continued for at least the first trimester is recommended. Folate supplementation also is being considered in patients with elevated levels of plasma homocysteine (*see* below).

Absorption, Distribution, and Elimination. As with vitamin B$_{12}$, the diagnosis and management of deficiencies of folic acid depend on an understanding of the transport pathways and intracellular metabolism of the vitamin (Figure 53–10). Folates present in food are largely in the form of reduced polyglutamates, and absorption requires transport and the action of a pteroylglutamyl carboxypeptidase associated with mucosal cell membranes. The mucosae of the duodenum and upper part of the jejunum are rich in dihydrofolate reductase and can methylate most or all of the reduced folate that is absorbed. Since most absorption occurs in the proximal portion of the small intestine, it is not unusual for folate deficiency to occur when the jejunum is diseased. Both nontropical and tropical sprue are common causes of folate deficiency and megaloblastic anemia.

Once absorbed, folate is transported rapidly to tissues as CH$_3$H$_4$PteGlu. While certain plasma proteins do bind folate derivatives, they have a greater affinity for nonmethylated analogs. The role of such binding proteins in folate homeostasis is not well understood. An increase in binding capacity is detectable in folate deficiency and in certain disease states, such as uremia, cancer, and alcohol-

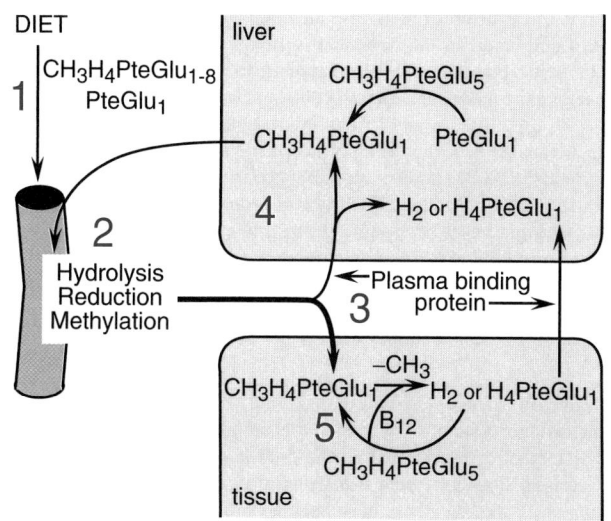

Position	Radical	Congener	
N^5	—CH_3	$CH_3H_4PteGlu$	Methyltetrahydrofolate
N^5	—CHO	$5\text{-}CHOH_4PteGlu$	Folinic acid (citrovorum factor)
N^{10}	—CHO	$10\text{-}CHOH_4PteGlu$	10-Formyltetrahydrofolate
$N^{5,10}$	—CH—	$5,10\text{-}CHH_4PteGlu$	5,10-Methenyltetrahydrofolate
$N^{5,10}$	—CH_2—	$5,10\text{-}CH_2H_4PteGlu$	5,10-Methylenetetrahydrofolate
N^5	—CHNH	$CHNHH_4PteGlu$	Formiminotetrahydrofolate
N^{10}	—CH_2OH	$CH_2OHH_4PteGlu$	Hydroxymethyltetrahydrofolate

Figure 53–9. The structures and nomenclature of pteroylglutamic acid (folic acid) and its congeners. X represents additional residues of glutamate; polyglutamates are the storage and active forms of the vitamin. The subscript that designates the number of residues of glutamate is frequently omitted because this number is variable.

Figure 53–10. Absorption and distribution of folate derivatives. Dietary sources of folate polyglutamates are hydrolyzed to the monoglutamate, reduced, and methylated to $CH_3H_4PteGlu_1$ during gastrointestinal transport. Folate deficiency commonly results from (1) inadequate dietary supply and (2) small intestinal disease. In patients with uremia, alcoholism, or hepatic disease there may be defects in (3) the concentration of folate binding proteins in plasma and (4) the flow of $CH_3H_4PteGlu_1$ into bile for reabsorption and transport to tissue (the folate enterohepatic cycle). Finally, vitamin B_{12} deficiency will (5) "trap" folate as $CH_3H_4PteGlu$, thereby reducing the availability of $H_4PteGlu_1$ for its essential roles in purine and pyrimidine synthesis.

ism, but how binding affects transport and tissue supply requires further investigation.

A constant supply of $CH_3H_4PteGlu$ is maintained by food and by an enterohepatic cycle of the vitamin. The liver actively reduces and methylates PteGlu (and H_2 or $H_4PteGlu$) and then transports the $CH_3H_4PteGlu$ into bile for reabsorption by the gut and subsequent delivery to tissues (Steinberg *et al.*, 1979). This pathway may provide 200 μg or more of folate each day for recirculation to tissues. The importance of the enterohepatic cycle is suggested by animal studies that show a rapid reduction of the plasma folate concentration after either drainage of bile or ingestion of alcohol, which apparently blocks the release of $CH_3H_4PteGlu$ from hepatic parenchymal cells (Hillman *et al.*, 1977).

Following uptake into cells, $CH_3H_4PteGlu$ acts as a methyl donor for the formation of methylcobalamin and as a source of $H_4PteGlu$ and other folate congeners, as described above. Folate is stored within cells as polyglutamates.

Folate Deficiency. Folate deficiency is a common complication of diseases of the small intestine, which interfere with the absorption of folate from food and the recirculation of folate through the enterohepatic cycle. In acute or chronic alcoholism, daily intake of folate in food may be severely restricted, and the enterohepatic cycle of the vitamin may be impaired by toxic effects of alcohol on hepatic parenchymal cells; this is the most common cause of folate-deficient megaloblastic erythropoiesis. However, it also is the most amenable to therapy, inasmuch as the reinstitution of a normal diet is sufficient to overcome the effect of alcohol. Disease states characterized by a high rate of cell turnover, such as hemolytic anemias, also may be complicated by folate deficiency. Additionally, drugs that inhibit dihydrofolate reductase (*e.g.*, methotrexate and trimethoprim) or that interfere with the absorption and storage of folate in tissues (*e.g.*, certain anticonvulsants and oral contraceptives) can lower the concentration of folate in plasma and may cause a megaloblastic anemia (Stebbins and Bertino, 1976).

Folate deficiency has been implicated in the incidence of neural tube defects, including spina bifida, encephaloceles, and anencephaly. This is true even in the absence of folate-deficient anemia or alcoholism. A less-than-adequate intake of folate also can result in elevations in plasma homocysteine (Green and Miller, 1999). Since even moderate hyperhomocysteinemia is considered an independent risk factor for coronary artery and peripheral vascular disease and for venous thrombosis, the role of folate as a methyl donor in the homocysteine-to-methionine conversion is getting increased attention. Patients who are heterozygous for one or another enzymatic defect and have high normal to moderate elevations of plasma homocysteine may improve with folic acid therapy.

Folate deficiency is recognized by its impact on the hematopoietic system. As with vitamin B_{12}, this fact reflects the increased requirement associated with high rates of cell turnover. The megaloblastic anemia that results from folate deficiency cannot be distinguished from that caused by vitamin B_{12} deficiency. This finding is to be expected because of the final common pathway of the major intracellular metabolic roles of the two vitamins. At the same time, folate deficiency is rarely if ever associated with neurological abnormalities. Thus the observation of characteristic abnormalities in vibratory and position sense and in motor and sensory pathways is incompatible with an isolated deficiency of folic acid.

After deprivation of folate, megaloblastic anemia develops much more rapidly than it does following interruption of vitamin B_{12} absorption (*e.g.*, gastric surgery). This observation reflects the fact that body stores of folate are limited. Although the rate of induction of megaloblastic erythropoiesis may vary, a folate-deficiency state may appear in 1 to 4 weeks, depending on the individual's dietary habits and stores of the vitamin.

Folate deficiency is best diagnosed from measurements of folate in plasma and in red cells. However, an empiric trial of folate in cases of suspected deficiency has been proposed as more cost effective (Robinson and Mladenovic, 2001). Indeed, the concentration of folate in plasma is extremely sensitive to changes in dietary intake of the vitamin and the influence of inhibitors of folate metabolism or transport, such as alcohol. Normal folate concentrations in plasma range from 9 to 45 nmol (4 to 20 ng/ml); below 9 nmol is considered folate deficient. The plasma folate concentration rapidly falls to values indicative of deficiency within 24 to 48 hours of steady ingestion of alcohol (Eichner and Hillman, 1971; Eichner and Hillman, 1973). The plasma folate concentration will revert quickly to normal once such ingestion is stopped, even while the marrow is still megaloblastic. Such rapid fluctuations detract from the clinical utility of the plasma folate concentration. The amount of folate in red cells or the adequacy of stores in lymphocytes (as measured by the deoxyuridine suppression test) may be used to diagnose a long-standing deficiency of folic acid. A positive result on either test shows that the deficiency must have existed for a sufficient time to allow the production of a population of cells with deficient folate stores.

Folic acid is marketed as oral tablets containing 0.4, 0.8, and 1 mg pteroylglutamic acid, as an aqueous solution for injection (5 mg/ml), and in combination with other vitamins and minerals.

Folinic acid (*leucovorin calcium, citrovorum factor*) is the 5-formyl derivative of tetrahydrofolic acid. The principal therapeutic uses of folinic acid are to circumvent the inhibition of dihydrofolate reductase as a part of high-dose methotrexate therapy and to potentiate fluorouracil in the treatment of colorectal cancer (*see* Chapter 51). It also has been used as an antidote to counteract the toxicity of folate antagonists such as pyrimethamine or trimethoprim. While it can be used to treat any folate-deficient state, folinic acid provides no advantage over folic acid, is more expensive, and therefore is not recommended. A single exception is the megaloblastic anemia associated with congenital dihydrofolate reductase deficiency. Leucovorin should never be used for the treatment of pernicious anemia or other megaloblastic anemias secondary to a deficiency of vitamin B_{12}. Just as is seen with folic acid, its use can result in an apparent response of the hematopoietic system, but neurological damage may occur or progress if already present.

Untoward Effects. There have been rare reports of reactions to parenteral injections of folic acid and leucovorin. If a patient describes a history of a reaction before the drug is given, caution should be exercised. Oral folic acid usually is not toxic. Even with doses as high as 15 mg/day, there have been no substantiated reports of side effects. Folic acid in large amounts may counteract the antiepileptic effect of *phenobarbital, phenytoin,* and *primidone,* and increase the frequency of seizures in susceptible children (Reynolds, 1968). While some studies have not supported these contentions, the FDA recommends that oral tablets of folic acid be limited to strengths of 1 mg or less.

General Principles of Therapy. The therapeutic use of folic acid is limited to the prevention and treatment of deficiencies of the vitamin. As with vitamin B_{12} therapy, effective use of the vitamin depends on accurate diagnosis and an understanding of the mechanisms that are operative in a specific disease state. The following general principles of therapy should be respected:

1. Prophylactic administration of folic acid should be undertaken for clear indications. Dietary supplementation is necessary when there is a requirement that may not be met by a "normal" diet. The daily ingestion of a multivitamin preparation containing 400 to 500 μg of folic acid has become standard practice before and during pregnancy to reduce the incidence of neural tube defects and for as long as a woman is breastfeeding. In women with a history of a pregnancy complicated by a neural tube defect, an even larger dose of 4 mg a day has been recommended (MRC Vitamin Study Research Group, 1991). Patients on total parenteral nutrition should receive folic acid supplements as part of their fluid regimen because liver folate stores are limited. Adult patients with a disease state characterized by high cell turnover (*e.g.,* hemolytic anemia) generally require larger doses, 1 mg of folic acid given once or twice a day. The 1-mg dose also has been used in the treatment of patients with elevated levels of homocysteine.

2. As with vitamin B_{12} deficiency, any patient with folate deficiency and a megaloblastic anemia should be evaluated carefully to determine the underlying cause of the deficiency state. This should include evaluation of the effects of medications, the amount of alcohol intake, the patient's history of travel, and the function of the gastrointestinal tract.

3. Therapy always should be as specific as possible. Multivitamin preparations should be avoided unless there is good reason to suspect deficiency of several vitamins.

4. *The potential danger of mistreating a patient who has vitamin B_{12} deficiency with folic acid must be kept in mind.* The administration of large doses of folic acid can result in an apparent improvement of the megaloblastic anemia, inasmuch as PteGlu is converted by dihydrofolate reductase to H_4PteGlu; this circumvents the methylfolate "trap." However, folate therapy does not prevent or alleviate the neurological defects of vitamin B_{12} deficiency, and these may progress and become irreversible.

Treatment of the Acutely Ill Patient. As described in detail in the section on vitamin B_{12}, treatment of the patient who is acutely ill with megaloblastic anemia should begin with intramuscular injections of vitamin B_{12} and folic acid. Inasmuch as the patient requires therapy before the exact cause of the disease has been defined, it is important to avoid the potential problem of a combined deficiency of vitamin B_{12} and folic acid. When the patient is deficient in both, therapy with only one vitamin will not provide an optimal response. Longstanding nontropical sprue is one example of a disease in which combined deficiency of B_{12} and folate is common. When

indicated, vitamin B_{12} (100 μg) and folic acid (1 to 5 mg) should be administered intramuscularly, and the patient should then be maintained on daily oral supplements of 1 to 2 mg of folic acid for the next 1 to 2 weeks.

Oral administration of folate generally is satisfactory for patients who are not acutely ill, regardless of the cause of the deficiency state. Even the patient with tropical or nontropical sprue and a demonstrable defect in absorption of folic acid will respond adequately to such therapy. Abnormalities in the activity of pteroyl-γ-glutamyl carboxypeptidase and the function of mucosal cells will not prevent passive diffusion of sufficient amounts of PteGlu across the mucosal barrier if the dosage is adequate, and continued ingestion of alcohol or other drugs also will not prevent an adequate therapeutic response. The effects of most inhibitors of folate transport or dihydrofolate reductase are overcome easily by administration of pharmacological doses of the vitamin. Folinic acid is the appropriate form of the vitamin for use in chemotherapeutic protocols, including "rescue" from methotrexate (*see* Chapter 51). Perhaps the only situation in which oral administration of folate will be ineffective is when vitamin C is severely deficient. Patients with scurvy may suffer from a megaloblastic anemia despite increased intake of folate and normal or high concentrations of the vitamin in plasma and cells.

The therapeutic response may be monitored by study of the hematopoietic system in a fashion identical to that described for vitamin B_{12}. Within 48 hours of the initiation of appropriate therapy, megaloblastic erythropoiesis disappears, and as efficient erythropoiesis begins, the concentration of iron in plasma falls to normal or below-normal values. The reticulocyte count begins to rise on the second or third day and reaches a peak by the fifth to seventh days; the reticulocyte index reflects the proliferative state of the marrow. Finally, the hematocrit begins to rise during the second week.

It is possible to use the pattern of recovery as the basis for a therapeutic trial. For this purpose, the patient should receive a daily parenteral injection of 50 to 100 μg of folic acid. Administration of doses in excess of 100 μg per day entails the risk of inducing a hematopoietic response in patients who are deficient in vitamin B_{12}, while oral administration of the vitamin may be unreliable because of intestinal malabsorption. A number of other complications also may interfere with the therapeutic trial. The patient with sprue and deficiencies of other vitamins or iron may fail to respond because of these inadequacies. In cases of alcoholism, the presence of hepatic disease, inflammation, or iron deficiency can blunt the proliferative response of the marrow and prevent the correction of the anemia. For these reasons, the therapeutic trial for the evaluation of the patient with a potential deficiency of folic acid has not gained great popularity.

CLINICAL SUMMARY

Several hematopoietic growth factors are available for clinical use. Recombinant erythropoietin routinely is used for patients with the anemia of renal insufficiency, inflammation, and associated with cancer or the therapy of cancer. Longer-acting growth factors that permit less frequent dosing schedules are coming into increased use. One of the first of these is novel erythropoiesis-stimulating protein (NESP), produced by the insertion of two extra N-linked sialic acid side chains into the erythropoietin molecule. Myeloid growth factors (*e.g.*, GM-CSF and G-CSF) are used to hasten the recovery of granulocytes after myelosuppressive therapy, to help mobilize hematopoietic stem cells into the peripheral blood to allow their harvest for transplantation, and to augment the number of mature leukocytes in the peripheral blood so that they can be used in patients with overwhelming infection. Finally, the development of IL-11 for use in thrombocytopenia and the investigational use of thrombopoietin or mimics of the molecule may provide many of the same therapeutic advances.

BIBLIOGRAPHY

Ajioka, R.S., and Kushner, J.P. Clinical consequences of iron overload in hemochromatosis homozygotes. *Blood,* 2003, *101:*3351–3353.

Akashi, K., Traver D., Miyamoto T., and Weissman, I.L. A clonogenic common myeloid progenitor that gives rise to all myeloid lineages. *Nature,* 2000, *404:*193–197.

Archimbaud, E., Ottmann, O., Liu Yin, J.A., *et al.* A randomised, double-blind, placebo-controlled study with pegylated recombinant human megakaryocyte growth and development factor (PEG-rHuMGDF) as an adjunct to chemotherapy for adults with de novo acute myeloid leukemia. *Blood,* 1999, *94:*3694–3701.

Basser, R.L., Rasko, J.E.J., Clarke, K., *et al.* Thrombopoietic effects of pegylated recombinant human megakaryocyte growth and development factor (PEG-rHuMGDF) in patients with advanced cancer. *Lancet,* 1996, *348:*1279–1281.

Basser, R.L., Underhill, C., Davis, I., *et al.* Enhancement of platelet recovery after myelosuppressive chemotherapy by recombinant human megakaryocyte growth and development factor in patients with advanced cancer. *J. Clin. Oncol.,* 2000, *18:*2852–2861.

Besarab, A., Bolton, W.K., Browne, J.K., *et al.* The effects of normal as compared with low hematocrit values in patients with cardiac disease who are receiving hemodialysis and epoetin. *N. Engl. J. Med.,* 1998, *339:*584–590.

Besarab, A., Kaiser, J.W., and Frinak, S. A study of parenteral iron regimens in hemodialysis patients. *Am. J. Kidney Dis.,* 1999, *34:*21–28.

Beutler, E. History of iron in medicine. *Blood Cells Mol. Dis.,* 2002, *29:*297–308.

Beutler, E. The HFE Cys282Tyr mutation as a necessary but not sufficient cause of clinical hereditary hemochromatosis. *Blood,* 2003, *101:*3347–3450.

Bloomfield, M., Jaresko, G., Zarek, J., and Dozier, N. Guidelines for using darbepoetin alfa in patients with chemotherapy-induced anemia. *Pharmacotherapy,* 2003, *23:*110S–118S.

Bolwell, B., Vredenburgh, J., Overmoyer, B., *et al.* Phase 1 study of pegylated recombinant human megakaryocyte growth and development factor (PEG-rHuMGDF) in breast cancer patients after autologous peripheral blood progenitor cell transplantation (PBPC). *Bone Marrow Transpl.,* 2000, *26:*141–145.

Brandt, S.J., Peters, W.P., Atwater, S.K., *et al.* Effect of recombinant human granulocyte-macrophage colony-stimulating factor on hematopoietic reconstitution after high-dose chemotherapy and autologous bone marrow transplantation. *N. Engl. J. Med.,* 1988, *318:*869–876.

Broudy, V.C., and Lin, N.L. AMG531 stimulates megakaryopoiesis *in vitro* by binding to Mpl. *Cytokine,* 2004, *25:*52–60.

Casadevall, N. Pure red cell aplasia and anti-erythropoietin antibodies in patients treated with epoetin. *Nephrol. Dial. Transplant.,* 2003, *18*(suppl. 8):viii, 37–41.

Chillar, R.K., Johnson, C.S., and Beutler, E. Erythrocyte pyridoxine kinase levels in patients with sideroblastic anemia. *N. Engl. J. Med.,* 1976, *295:*881–883.

Conrad, M.E., and Umbreit, J.N. Pathways of iron absorption. *Blood Cells Mol. Dis.,* 2002, *29:*336–355.

Crawford, J. Neutrophil growth factors. *Curr. Hematol. Rep.,* 2002, *1:*95–102.

Dallman, P.R., Siimes, M.A., and Stekel, A. Iron deficiency in infancy and childhood. *Am. J. Clin. Nutr.,* 1980, *33:*86–118.

Debili, N., Massé, J.M., Katz, A., *et al.* Effects of the recombinant hematopoietic growth factors interleukin-3, interleukin-6, stem cell factor, and leukemia inhibitory factor on the megakaryocytic differentiation of CD34+ cells. *Blood,* 1993, *82:*84–95.

Demetri, G.D., Kris, M., Wade, J., *et al.* Quality-of-life benefit in chemotherapy patients treated with epoetin alfa is independent of disease response or tumor type: results from a prospective community oncology study. Procrit Study Group. *J. Clin. Oncol.,* 1998, *16:*3412–3425.

Dunlap, W.M., James, G.W. III, and Hume, D.M. Anemia and neutropenia caused by copper deficiency. *Ann. Intern. Med.,* 1974, *80:*470–476.

Du, X.X., and Williams, D.A. Interleukin 11: A multifunctional growth factor derived from the hematopoietic microenvironment. *Blood,* 1994, *83:*2023–2030.

Eichbaum, Q., Foran, S., and Dzik, S. Is iron gluconate really safer than iron dextran? *Blood,* 2003, *101:*3756–3757.

Eichner, E.R., and Hillman, R.S. Effect of alcohol on serum folate level. *J. Clin. Invest.,* 1973, *52:*584–591.

Eichner, E.R., and Hillman, R.S. The evolution of anemia in alcoholic patients. *Am. J. Med.,* 1971, *50:*218–232.

Eschbach, J.W., Egrie, J.C., Downing, M.R., *et al.* Correction of the anemia of end-stage renal disease with recombinant human erythropoietin. Results of a combined phase I and II clinical trial. *N. Engl. J. Med.,* 1987, *316:*73–78.

Eschbach, J.W., Kelly, M.R., Haley, N.R., *et al.* Treatment of the anemia of progressive renal failure with recombinant human erythropoietin. *N. Engl. J. Med.,* 1989, *321:*158–163.

Faich, G., and Strobos, J. Sodium ferric gluconate complex in sucrose: safer intravenous iron therapy than iron dextran. *Am. J. Kidney Dis.,* 1999, *33:*464–470.

Fanucchi, M., Glaspy, J., Crawford, J., *et al.* Effects of polyethylene glycol-conjugated recombinant human megakaryocyte growth and development factor on platelet counts after chemotherapy for lung cancer. *N. Engl. J. Med.,* 1997, *336:*404–409.

Farese, A.M., Myers, L.A., and MacVittie, T.J. Therapeutic efficacy of recombinant human leukemia inhibitory factor in a primate model of radiation-induced marrow aplasia. *Blood,* 1994, *84:*3675–3678.

Fibbe, W.E., Heemskerk, D.P.M., Laterveer, L., *et al.* Accelerated reconstitution of platelets and erythrocytes following syngeneic transplantation of bone marrow cells derived from thrombopoietin pretreated donor mice. *Blood,* 1995, *86:*3308–3313.

Fischl, M., Galpin, J.E., Levine, J.D., *et al.* Recombinant human erythropoietin therapy for AIDS patients treated with AZT: a double-blind, placebo-controlled clinical study. *N. Engl. J. Med.,* 1990, *322:*1488–1493.

Fishbane, S., and Kowalski, E.A. The comparative safety of intravenous iron dextran, iron saccharate, and sodium ferric gluconate. *Sem. Dialysis,* 2000, *13:*381–384.

Ganz, T. Hepcidin, a key regulator of iron metabolism and mediator of anemia of inflammation. *Blood*, **2003**, *102:*783–788.

Gerhartz, H.H., Engellhard, M., Meusers, P., *et al.* Randomized, double-blind, placebo-controlled, phase III study of recombinant human granulocyte-macrophage colony-stimulating factor as adjunct to induction treatment of high-grade malignant non-Hodgkin's lymphomas. *Blood*, **1993**, *82:*2329–2339.

Goodnough, L.T., Rudnick, S., Price, T.H., *et al.* Increased preoperative collection of autologous blood with recombinant human erythropoietin therapy. *N. Engl. J. Med.,* **1989**, *321:*1163–1168.

Goodnough, L.T., Skikne, B., and Brugnara, C. Erythropoietin, iron, and erythropoiesis. *Blood*, **2000**, *96:*823–833.

Goodwin, R.G., Lupton, S., Schmierer, A., *et al.* Human interleukin 7: molecular cloning and growth factor activity on human and murine B-lineage cells. *Proc. Natl. Acad. Sci. U.S.A.,* **1989**, *86:*302–306.

Gordeuk, V.R., Sergueeva, A.I., Miasnikova, G.Y., *et al.* Congenital disorder of oxygen sensing: association of the homozygous Chuvash polycythemia VHL mutation with thrombosis and vascular abnormalities but not tumors. *Blood*, **2004**, *103:*3924–3932.

Gough, N.M., Gough, J., Metcalf, D., *et al.* Molecular cloning of cDNA encoding a murine hematopoietic growth regulator, granulocyte-macrophage colony stimulating factor. *Nature*, **1984**, *309:*763–767.

Grabstein, K.H., Eisenman, J., Shanebeck, K., *et al.* Cloning of a T cell growth factor that interacts with the β chain of the interleukin-2 receptor. *Science*, **1994**, *264:*965–968.

Grebe, G., Martinez-Torres, C., and Layrisse, M. Effect of meals and ascorbic acid on the absorption of a therapeutic dose of iron as ferrous and ferric salts. *Curr. Ther. Res. Clin. Exp.,* **1975**, *17:*382–397.

Groopman, J.E., Mitsuyasu, R.T., DeLeo, M.J., *et al.* Effect of recombinant human granulocyte macrophage colony stimulating factor on myelopoiesis in the acquired immunodeficiency syndrome. *N. Engl. J. Med.,* **1987**, *317:*593–598.

Haas, R., Ho, A.D., Bredthauer, U., *et al.* Successful autologous transplantation of blood stem cells mobilized with recombinant human granulocyte-macrophage colony-stimulating factor. *Exp. Hematol.,* **1990**, *18:*94–98.

Hakami, N., Neiman, P.E., Canellos, G.P., and Lazerson, J. Neonatal megaloblastic anemia due to inherited transcobalamin II deficiency in two siblings. *N. Engl. J. Med.,* **1971**, *285:*1163–1170.

Hammond, W.P. IV, Price, T.H., Souza, L.M., and Dale, D.C. Treatment of cyclic neutropenia with granulocyte colony-stimulating factor. *N. Engl. J. Med.,* **1989**, *320:*1306–1311.

Henke, M., Laszig, R., Rube, C., *et al.* Erythropoietin to treat head and neck cancer patients with anemia undergoing radiotherapy: randomised, double-blind, placebo-controlled trial. *Lancet*, **2003**, *18:*1255–1260.

Hesketh, P.J., Arena, F., Patel, D., *et al.* A randomized controlled trial of darbepoetin alfa administered as a fixed or weight-based dose using a front-loading schedule in patients with anemia who have nonmyeloid malignancies. *Cancer*, **2004**, *100:*859–868.

Hillman, R.S., McGuffin, R., and Campbell, C. Alcohol interference with the folate enterohepatic cycle. *Trans. Assoc. Am. Physicians,* **1977**, *90:*145–156.

Hoffbrand, A.V., and Herbert, V. Nutritional anemias. *Semin. Hematol.,* **1999**, *36:*23–23.

Hoffman, H.N. II, Phyliky, R.L., and Fleming, C.R. Zinc-induced copper deficiency. *Gastroenterology*, **1988**, *94:*508–512.

Huang, E., Nocka, K., Beier, D.R., *et al.* The hematopoietic growth factor K1 is encoded at the S1 locus and is the ligand of the c-kit receptor, the gene product of the W locus. *Cell*, **1990**, *63:*225–233.

Hubel, K., Carter, R.A., Liles, W.C., *et al.* Granulocyte transfusion therapy for infections in candidates and recipients of HPC transplanta-tion: a comparative analysis of feasibility and outcome for community donors versus related donors. *Transfusion*, **2002**, *42:*1414–1421.

Isaacs, C., Robert, N.J., Bailey, F.A., *et al.* Randomized placebo-controlled study of recombinant human interleukin-11 to prevent chemotherapy-induced thrombocytopenia in patients with breast cancer receiving dose-intensive cyclophosphamide and doxorubicin. *J. Clin. Oncol.,* **1997**, *15:*3368–3377.

Jelkmann, W. The enigma of the metabolic fate of circulating erythropoietin (Epo) in view of the pharmacokinetics of the recombinant drugs rhEpo and NESP. *Eur. J. Haematol.,* **2002**, *69:*265–274.

Juul, S. Erythropoietin in the central nervous system, and its use to prevent hypoxic-ischemic brain damage. *Acta. Paediatr. Suppl.,* **2002**, *91:*36–42.

Kaufman, J.S., Reda, D.J., Fye, C.L., *et al.* Subcutaneous compared with intravenous epoetin in patients receiving hemodialysis. Department of Veterans Affairs Cooperative Study Group on Erythropoietin in Hemodialysis Patients. *N. Engl. J. Med.,* **1998**, *339:*578–583.

Kaushansky, K., Lok, S., Holly, R.D., *et al.* Promotion of megakaryocyte progenitor expansion and differentiation by the c-Mp1 ligand thrombopoietin. *Nature*, **1994**, *369:*568–571.

Kaushansky, K. Thrombopoietin. Drug Therapy Series. *N. Engl. J. Med.,* **1998**, *339:*746–754.

Kawasaki, E.S., Ladner, M.B., Wang, A.M., *et al.* Molecular cloning of a complementary DNA encoding human macrophage-specific colony-stimulating factor (CSF-I). *Science*, **1985**, *230:*291–296.

Kimura, T., Kaburaki, H., Tsujino, T., *et al.* A non-peptide compound which can mimic the effect of thrombopoietin via c-Mpl. *FEBS Lett.,* **1998**, *428:*250–254.

Klausner, R.D., Rouault, T.A., and Harford, J.B. Regulating the fate of mRNA: the control of cellular iron metabolism. *Cell*, **1993**, *72:*19–28.

Kondo, M., Weissman, I.L., and Akashi, K. Identification of clonogenic common lymphoid progenitors in mouse bone marrow. *Cell*, **1997**, *91:*661–672.

Kuter, D.J., Goodnough, L.T., Romo, J., *et al.* Thrombopoietin therapy increases platelet yields in healthy platelet donors. *Blood*, **2001**, *98:*1339–1345.

Lindenbaum, J., Healton, E.B., Savage, D.G., *et al.* Neuropsychiatric disorders caused by cobalamin deficiency in the absence of anemia or macrocytosis. *N. Engl. J. Med.,* **1988**, *318:*1720–1728.

Littlewood, T.J., Bajetta, E., Nortier, J.W., *et al.*, and Epoetin/Alfa Study Group. Effects of epoetin alfa on hematologic parameters and quality of life in cancer patients receiving nonplatinum chemotherapy: results of a randomized, double-blind, placebo-controlled trial. *J. Clin. Oncol.,* **2001**, *19:*2865–2874.

Lok, S., Kaushansky, K., Holly, R.D., *et al.* Cloning and expression of murine thrombopoietin cDNA and stimulation of platelet production *in vivo. Nature*, **1994**, *369:*565–568.

Macdougall, I.C. Pure red cell aplasia with anti-erythropoietin antibodies occurs more commonly with one formulation of epoetin alfa than another. *Curr. Med. Res. Opin.,* **2004**, *20:*83–86.

Martinez-Estrada, O.M., Rodriguez-Millan, E., Gonzalez-De Vicente, E., *et al.* Erythropoietin protects the *in vitro* blood-brain barrier against VEGF-induced permeability. *Eur. J. Neurosci.,* **2003**, *18:*2538–2544.

Maxwell, P.H., Pugh, C.W., and Ratcliffe, P.J. The pVHL-hIF-1 system. A key mediator of oxygen homeostasis. *Adv. Exp. Med. Biol.,* **2001**, *502:*365–376.

Michael, B., Coyne, D.W., Fishbane, S., *et al.* Sodium ferric gluconate complex in hemodialysis patients: Adverse reactions compared to placebo and iron dextran. *Kid. Int.,* **2002**, *61:*1830–1839.

Michaud, L., Guimber, D., Mention, K., *et al.* Tolerance and efficacy of intravenous iron saccharate for iron deficiency anemia in children and adolescents receiving long-term parenteral nutrition. *Clin. Nut.*, **2002**, *21:*403–407.

Monsen, E.R., Hallberg, L., Layrisse, M., *et al.* Estimation of available dietary iron. *Am. J. Clin. Nutr.*, **1978**, *31:*134–141.

Morgan, E.H., and Oates, P.S. Mechanisms and regulation of intestinal iron absorption. *Blood Cells Mol. Dis.*, **2002**, *29:*384–399.

Moskowitz, C.H., Stiff, P., Gordon, M.S., *et al.* Recombinant methionyl human stem cell factor and filgrastim for peripheral blood progenitor cell mobilization and transplantation in non-Hodgkin's lymphoma patients—results of a phase I/II trial. *Blood*, **1997**, *89:*3136–3147.

Nakorn, T.N., Miyamoto, T., and Weissman, I.L. Characterization of mouse clonogenic megakaryocyte progenitors. *Proc. Natl. Acad. Sci. U.S.A.*, **2003**, *100:*205–210.

Neben, T.Y., Loebelenz, J., Hayes, L., *et al.* Recombinant human interleukin-11 stimulates megakaryocytopoiesis and increases peripheral platelets in normal and splenectomized mice. *Blood*, **1993**, *81:*901–908.

Nemeth, E., Rivera, S., Gabayan, V., *et al.* IL-6 mediates hypoferremia of inflammation by inducing the synthesis of the iron regulatory hormone hepcidin. *J. Clin. Invest.*, **2004**, *113:*1271–1276.

Nemunaitis, J., Singer, J.W., Buckner, C.D., *et al.* Use of recombinant human granulocyte-macrophage colony-stimulating factor in graft failure after bone marrow transplantation. *Blood*, **1990**, *76:*245–253.

Owen, W.F. Jr. Optimizing the use of parenteral iron in end-stage renal disease patients: focus on issues of infection and cardiovascular disease. Introduction. *Am. J. Kidney Dis.*, **1999**, *34:*S1–S2.

Peters, L.L., Andrews, N.C., Eicher, E.M., *et al.* Mouse microcytic anemia caused by a defect in the gene encoding the globin enhancer-binding protein NF-E2. *Nature*, **1993**, *362:*768–770.

Prass, K., Scharff, A., Ruscher K, *et al.* Hypoxia-induced stroke tolerance in the mouse is mediated by erythropoietin. *Stroke*, **2003**, *34:*1981–1986.

Rabinowe, S.N., Neuberg, D., Bierman, P.J., *et al.* Long-term follow-up of a phase III study of recombinant human granulocyte-macrophage colony-stimulating factor after autologous bone marrow transplantation for lymphoid malignancies. *Blood*, **1993**, *81:*1903–1908.

Reynolds, E.H. Mental effects of anticonvulsants and folic acid metabolism. *Brain*, **1968**, *91:*197–214.

Rizzo, J.D., Lichtin, A.E., Woolf, S.H., *et al.,* American Society of Clinical Oncology, American Society of Hematology. Use of epoetin in patients with cancer: evidence-based clinical practice guidelines of the American Society of Clinical Oncology and the American Society of Hematology. *Blood*, **2002**, *100:*2303–2320.

Robinson, A.R., and Mladenovic, J. Lack of clinical utility of folate levels in the evaluation of macrocytosis or anemia. *Am. J. Med.*, **2001**, *110:*88–90.

Rouault, T.A. Post-transcriptional regulation of human iron metabolism by iron regulatory proteins. *Blood Cells Mol. Dis.*, **2002**, *29:*309–314.

Roy, C.N., and Andrews, N.C. Recent advances in disorders of iron metabolism: mutations, mechanisms, and modifiers. *Hum. Mol. Genet.*, **2001**, *10:*2181–2186.

Roy, C.N., and Enns, C.A. Iron homeostasis: new tales from the crypt. *Blood*, **2000**, *96:*4020–4027.

de Sauvage, F.J., Hass, P.E., Spencer, S.D., *et al.* Stimulation of megakaryocytopoiesis and thrombopoiesis by the c-Mpl ligand. *Nature*, **1994**, *369:*533–538.

Sawada, K., Krantz, S.B., Dai, C.H., *et al.* Purification of human blood burst-forming units-erythroid and demonstration of the evolution of erythropoietin receptors. *J. Cell. Physiol.*, **1990**, *142:*219–230.

Schiffer, C.A., Miller, K., Larson, R.A., *et al.* A double-blind, placebo-controlled trial of pegylated recombinant human megakaryocyte

growth and development factor as an adjunct to induction and consolidation therapy for patients with acute myeloid leukemia. *Blood*, **2000**, *95:*2530–2535.

Scott, J.M., Dinn, J.J., Wilson, P., and Weir, D.G. Pathogenesis of subacute combined degeneration: a result of methyl group deficiency. *Lancet*, **1981**, *2:*334–337.

Sheridan, W.P., Begley, C.G., Juttner, C.A., *et al.* Effect of peripheral-blood progenitor cells mobilised by filgrastim (G-CSF) on platelet recovery after high-dose chemotherapy. *Lancet*, **1992**, *339:*640–644.

Sheth, S., and Brittenham, G.M. Genetic disorders affecting proteins of iron metabolism: clinical implications. *Annu. Rev. Med.*, **2000**, *51:*443–464.

Silverstein, S.B., and Rodgers, G.M. Parenteral iron therapy options. *Am. J. Hematol.*, **2004**, *76:*74–78.

Solomon, L.R., and Hillman, R.S. Vitamin B_6 metabolism in anaemic and alcoholic man. *Br. J. Haematol.*, **1979b**, *41:*343–356.

Solomon, L.R., and Hillman, R.S. Vitamin B_6 metabolism in human red blood cells. I. Variation in normal subjects. *Enzyme*, **1978**, *23:*262–273.

Solomon, L.R., and Hillman, R.S. Vitamin B_6 metabolism in idiopathic sideroblastic anaemia and related disorders. *Br. J. Haematol.*, **1979a**, *42:*239–253.

Steinberg, S.E., Campbell, C.L., and Hillman, R.S. Kinetics of the normal folate enterohepatic cycle. *J. Clin. Invest.*, **1979**, *64:*83–88.

Teramura, M., Kobayashi, S., Hoshino, S., *et al.* Interleukin 11 enhances human megakaryocytopoiesis *in vitro*. *Blood*, **1992**, *79:*327–331.

Vadhan-Raj, S., Vershragen, C.F., Bueso-Ramos, C., *et al.* Recombinant human thrombopoietin attenuates carboplatin-induced severe thrombocytopenia and the need for platelet transfusions in patients with gynecologic cancer. *Ann. Intern. Med.*, **2000**, *132:*364–368.

Waladkhani, A.R. Pegfilgrastim: A recent advance in the prophylaxis of chemotherapy-induced neutropenia. *Eur. J. Cancer Care*, **2004**, *13:*371–379.

Weinbren, K., Salm, R., and Greenberg, G. Intramuscular injections of iron compounds and oncogenesis in man. *Br. Med. J.*, **1978**, *1:*683–685.

Weisbart, R.H., Kwan, L., Golde, D.W., and Gasson, J.C. Human GM-CSF primes neutrophils for enhanced oxidative metabolism in response to the major physiological chemoattractants. *Blood*, **1987**, *69:*18–21.

Wong, G.G., Witek, J.S., Temple, P.A., *et al.* Human GM-CSF: molecular cloning of the complementary DNA and purification of the natural recombinant proteins. *Science*, **1985**, *228:*810–815.

Yang, Y.C., Ciarletta, A.B., Temple, P.A., *et al.* Human IL-3 (multi-CSF): identification by expression cloning of a novel hematopoietic growth factor related to murine IL-3. *Cell*, **1986**, *47:*3–10.

Zidar, B.L., Shadduck, R.K., Zeigler, Z., and Winkelstein, A. Observations on the anemia and neutropenia of human copper deficiency. *Am. J. Hematol.*, **1977**, *3:*177–185.

MONOGRAPHS AND REVIEWS

Anonymous. Iron Deficiency—United States 1999–2000. *MMWR Morb. Mortal. Wkly. Rep.*, **2002**, *51:*897–899.

Chanarin, I., Deacon, R., Lumb, M., *et al.* Cobalaminfolate interrelationships: a critical review. *Blood*, **1985**, *66:*479–489.

Dallman, P.R. Manifestations of iron deficiency. *Semin. Hematol.*, **1982**, *19:*19–30.

Finch, C.A., and Huebers, H. Perspectives in iron metabolism. *N. Engl. J. Med.*, **1982**, *306:*1520–1528.

Graham, G.G., and Cordano, A. Copper deficiency in human subjects. In, *Trace Elements in Human Health and Disease,* Vol. 1, *Zinc and Copper.* (Prasad, A.S., and Oberleas, D., eds.) Academic Press, New York, **1976,** pp. 363–372.

Green, R., and Miller, J.W. Folate deficiency beyond megaloblastic anemia: hyperhomocysteinemia and other manifestations of dysfunctional folate status. *Semin. Hematol.,* **1999,** *36:*47–64.

Harker, L.A. Physiology and clinical applications of platelet growth factors. *Curr. Opin. Hematol.,* **1999,** *6:*127–134.

Hillman, R.S., and Finch, C.A. *Red Cell Manual,* 7th ed. F.A. Davis Co., Philadelphia, **1997.**

Klausner, R.D., Ashwell, G., van Renswoude, J., *et al.* Binding of apotransferrin to k562 cells: explanation of the transferrin cycle. *Proc. Natl. Acad. Sci. U.S.A.,* **1983,** *80:*2263–2266.

Lee, G.R., Williams, D.M., and Cartwright, G.E. Role of copper in iron metabolism and heme biosynthesis. In, *Trace Elements in Human Health and Disease,* Vol. 1, *Zinc and Copper.* (Prasad, A.S., and Oberleas, D., eds.) Academic Press, New York, **1976,** pp. 373–390.

Lieschke, G.J., and Burgess, A.W. Granulocyte colony-stimulating factor and granulocyte-macrophage colony-stimulating factor (1). *N. Engl. J. Med.,* **1992,** *327:*28–35.

Li, J., Yang, C., Xia, Y., *et al.* Thrombocytopenia caused by the development of antibodies to thrombopoietin. *Blood,* **2001,** *98:*3241–3248.

Metcalf, D. The granulocyte-macrophage colony-stimulating factors. *Science,* **1985,** *229:*16–22.

Micronutrient deficiencies: Battling iron deficiency anemia. World Health Organization. Available at: http://www.who.int/nut/ida/htm. Accessed September 3, 2003.

Molineux, G., Migdalska, A., Szmitkowski, M., *et al.* The effects on hematopoiesis of recombinant stem cell factor (ligand for c-kit) administered *in vivo* to mice either alone or in combination with granulocyte colony-stimulating factor. *Blood,* **1991,** *78:*961–966.

MRC Vitamin Study Research Group. Prevention of neural tube defects: results of the Medical Research Council Vitamin Study. *Lancet,* **1991,** *338:*131–137.

Quesenberry, P., and Levitt, L. Hematopoietic stem cells. *N. Engl. J. Med.,* **1979,** *301:*755–761; 819–823; 868–872.

Skibeli, V., Nissen-Lie, G., and Torjesen, P. Sugar profiling proves that human serum erythropoietin differs from recombinant human erythropoietin. *Blood,* **2001,** *98:*3626–3634.

Stebbins, R., and Bertino, J.R. Megaloblastic anemia produced by drugs. *Clin. Haematol.,* **1976,** *5:*619–630.

Tepler, I., Elias, L., Smith, J.W. II, *et al.* A randomized placebo-controlled trial of recombinant human interleukin-11 in cancer patients with severe thrombocytopenia due to chemotherapy. *Blood,* **1996,** *87:*3607–3614.

Vadhan-Raj, S., Murray, L.J., Bueso-Ramos, C., *et al.* Stimulation of megakaryocyte and platelet production by a single dose of recombinant human thrombopoietin in cancer patients. *Ann. Intern. Med.,* **1997,** *126:*673–681.

Weir, D.G., and Scott, J.M. Interrelationships of folates and cobalamins. In, *Contemporary Issues in Clinical Nutrition,* Vol. 5, *Nutrition in Hematology.* (Lindenbaum, J., ed.) Churchill Livingstone, New York, **1983,** pp. 121–142.

Welte, K., Platzer, E., Lu, L., *et al.* Purification and biochemical characterization of human pluripotent hematopoietic colony-stimulating factor. *Proc. Natl. Acad. Sci. U.S.A.,* **1985,** *82:*1526–1530.

Wong, G.G., Temple, P.A., Leary, A.C., *et al.* Human CSF-1: Molecular cloning and expression of 4-kb cDNA encoding the urinary protein. *Science,* **1987,** *235:*1504–1508.

Wong, G.G., Witek, J.S., Temple, P.A., *et al.* Human GM-CSF: Molecular cloning of the complementary DNA and purification of the natural and recombinant proteins. *Science,* **1985,** *228:*810–815.

Yang, Y.C., Ciarletta, A.B., Temple, P.A., *et al.* Human IL-3 (multi-CSF): Identification by expression cloning of a novel hematopoietic growth factor related to murine IL-3. *Cell,* **1986,** *47:*3–10.

Yokota, T., Otsuka, T., Mosmann, T., *et al.* Isolation and characterization of a human interleukin cDNA clone, homologous to mouse B-cell stimulatory factor 1, that expresses B-cell- and T-cell-stimulating activities. *Proc. Natl. Acad. Sci. U.S.A.,* **1986,** *83:*5894–5898.

BLOOD COAGULATION AND ANTICOAGULANT, THROMBOLYTIC, AND ANTIPLATELET DRUGS

Philip W. Majerus and Douglas M. Tollefsen

The physiological systems that control blood fluidity are both complex and elegant. Blood must remain fluid within the vasculature and yet clot quickly when exposed to nonendothelial surfaces at sites of vascular injury. When intravascular thrombi do occur, a system of fibrinolysis is activated to restore fluidity. In the normal situation, a delicate balance prevents both thrombosis and hemorrhage and allows physiological fibrinolysis without excess pathological fibrinogenolysis. The drugs described in this chapter have very different mechanisms of action, but all alter the balance between procoagulant and anticoagulant reactions. With these drugs, efficacy and toxicity are necessarily intertwined. For example, the desired therapeutic effect of anticoagulation can be offset by the toxic effect of bleeding due to overdosing of anticoagulant. Similarly, overstimulation of fibrinolysis can lead to systemic destruction of fibrinogen and coagulation factors. This chapter reviews the predominant agents for controlling blood fluidity, including (1) the parenteral anticoagulant heparin and its derivatives, which stimulate a natural inhibitor of coagulant proteases; (2) the coumarin anticoagulants, which block multiple steps in the coagulation cascade; (3) fibrinolytic agents, which lyse pathological thrombi; and (4) antiplatelet agents, especially aspirin.

OVERVIEW OF HEMOSTASIS: PLATELET FUNCTION, BLOOD COAGULATION, AND FIBRINOLYSIS

Hemostasis is the cessation of blood loss from a damaged vessel. Platelets first adhere to macromolecules in the subendothelial regions of the injured blood vessel; they then aggregate to form the primary hemostatic plug. Platelets stimulate local activation of plasma coagulation factors, leading to generation of a fibrin clot that reinforces the platelet aggregate. Later, as wound healing occurs, the platelet aggregate and fibrin clot are degraded. The process of platelet aggregation and blood coagulation are summarized in Figures 54–1 and 54–2. The pathway of clot removal, fibrinolysis, is shown in Figure 54–3, along with sites of action of fibrinolytic agents.

Coagulation involves a series of zymogen activation reactions, as shown in Figure 54–2 (Mann *et al.*, 2003). At each stage, a precursor protein, or *zymogen,* is converted to an active protease by cleavage of one or more peptide bonds in the precursor molecule. The components at each stage include a protease from the preceding stage, a zymogen, a nonenzymatic protein cofactor, Ca^{2+}, and an organizing surface that is provided by a phospholipid emulsion *in vitro* or by platelets *in vivo*. The final protease generated is thrombin (factor IIa).

Conversion of Fibrinogen to Fibrin. Fibrinogen is a 330,000-dalton protein that consists of three pairs of polypeptide chains (designated Aα, Bβ, and γ covalently linked by disulfide bonds. Thrombin converts fibrinogen to fibrin monomers by cleaving fibrinopeptides A (16 amino acid residues) and B (14 amino acid residues) from the amino-terminal ends of the Aα and Bβ chains, respectively. Removal of the fibrinopeptides allows the fibrin monomers to form a gel, which is the end point of *in vitro* assays of coagulation (*see* below). Initially, the fibrin monomers are bound to each other noncovalently. Subsequently, factor XIIIa catalyzes an interchain transglutamination reaction that cross-links adjacent fibrin monomers to enhance the strength of the clot.

Structure of Coagulation Protease Zymogens. The protease zymogens involved in coagulation include factors II (prothrombin), VII, IX, X, XI, XII, and prekallikrein. About 200 amino acid residues at the car-

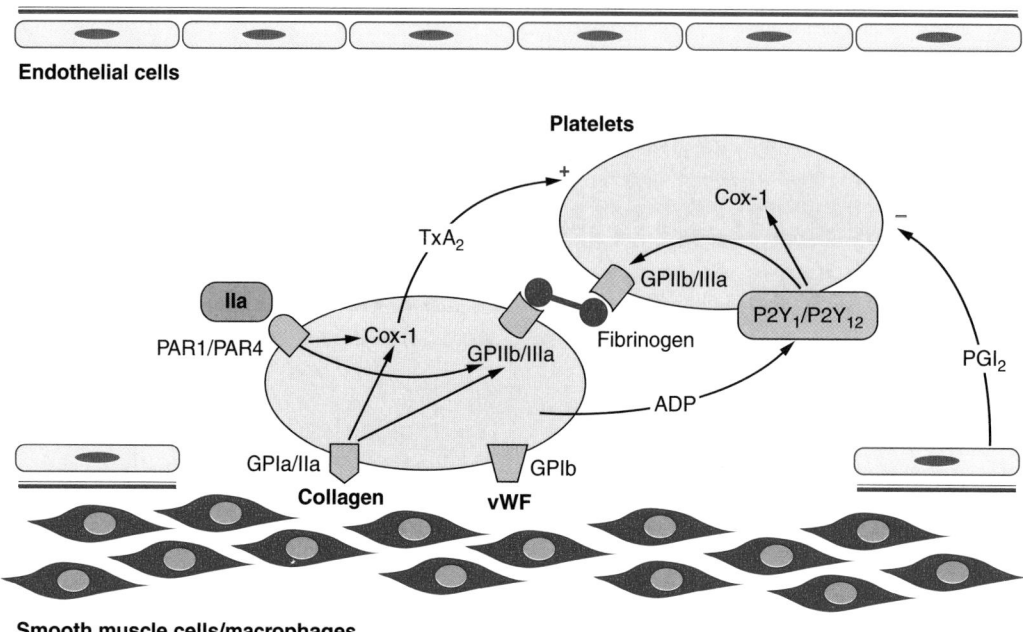

Figure 54–1. ***Platelet adhesion and aggregation.*** GPIa/IIa and GPIb are platelet membrane proteins that bind to collagen and von Willebrand factor (vWF), causing platelets to adhere to the subendothelium of a damaged blood vessel. PAR1 and PAR4 are protease-activated receptors that respond to thrombin (IIa); $P2Y_1$ and $P2Y_{12}$ are receptors for ADP (adenosine diphosphate); when stimulated by agonists, these receptors activate the fibrinogen-binding protein GPIIb/IIIa and cyclooxygenase-1 (COX-1) to promote platelet aggregation and secretion. Thromboxane A_2 (TXA_2) is the major product of COX-1 involved in platelet activation. Prostaglandin I_2 (PGI_2), synthesized by endothelial cells, inhibits platelet activation.

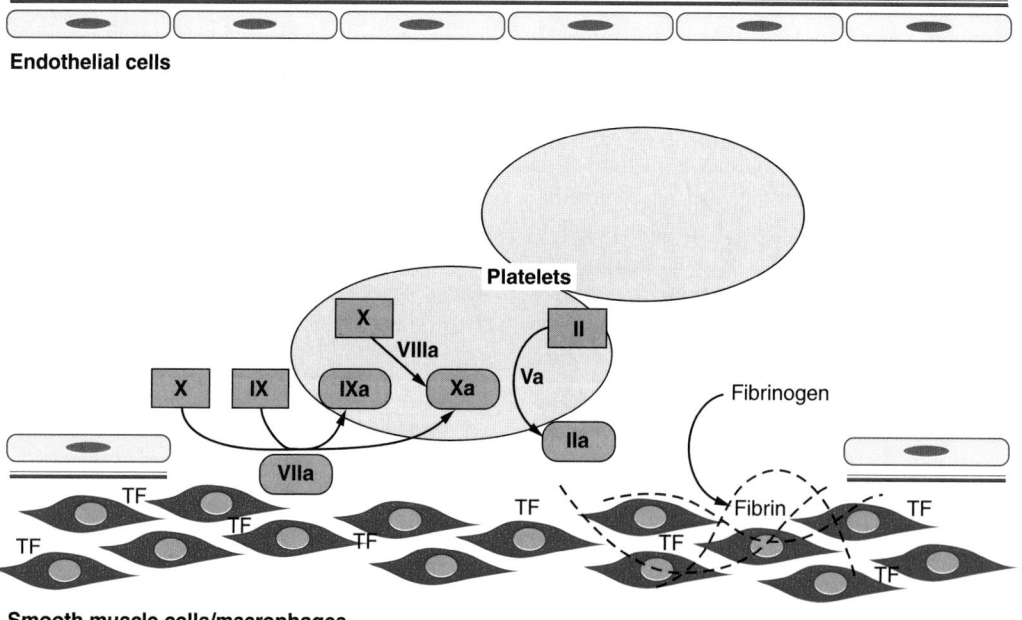

Figure 54–2. ***Major reactions of blood coagulation.*** Shown are interactions among proteins of the "extrinsic" (tissue factor and factor VII), "intrinsic" (factors IX and VIII), and "common" (factors X, V, and II) coagulation pathways that are important *in vivo.* Boxes enclose the coagulation factor zymogens (indicated by Roman numerals) and the rounded boxes represent the active proteases. TF, tissue factor; activated coagulation factors are followed by the letter "a." II, prothrombin; IIa, thrombin.

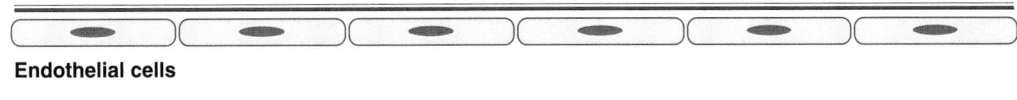

Endothelial cells

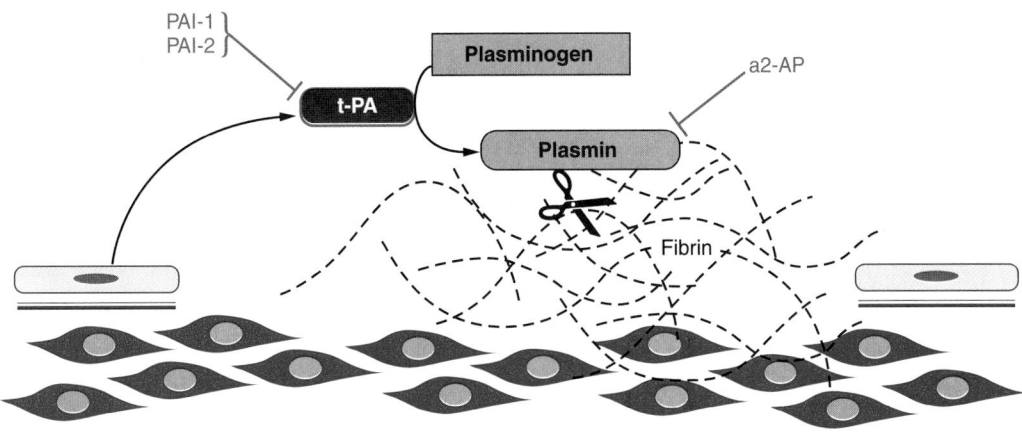

Smooth muscle cells/macrophages

Figure 54–3. Fibrinolysis. Endothelial cells secrete tissue plasminogen activator (t-PA) at sites of injury. t-PA binds to fibrin and cleaves plasminogen to plasmin, resulting in fibrin digestion. Plasminogen activator inhibitors-1 and -2 (PAI-1, PAI-2) inactivate t-PA; α_2-antiplasmin (α_2-AP) inactivates plasmin.

boxyl-terminal end of each zymogen are homologous to trypsin and contain the active site of the protease. In addition, 9 to 12 glutamate residues near the amino-terminal ends of factors II, VII, IX, and X are converted to γ-carboxyglutamate (Gla) residues during biosynthesis in the liver. The Gla residues bind Ca^{2+} and are necessary for the coagulant activities of these proteins.

Nonenzymatic Protein Cofactors. Factors V and VIII are homologous 350,000-dalton proteins. Factor VIII circulates in plasma bound to von Willebrand factor, while factor V is present both freely in plasma and as a component of platelets. Thrombin cleaves V and VIII to yield activated factors (Va and VIIIa) that have at least 50 times the coagulant activity of the precursor forms. Factors Va and VIIIa have no intrinsic enzymatic activity but serve as cofactors that increase the proteolytic efficiency of Xa and IXa, respectively. Tissue factor (TF) is a nonenzymatic lipoprotein cofactor that greatly increases the proteolytic efficiency of VIIa. It is present on the surface of cells that do not normally contact plasma (*e.g.,* macrophages and smooth muscle cells) and initiates coagulation outside a broken blood vessel. Monocytes and endothelial cells also may express tissue factor when exposed to a variety of stimuli, such as endotoxin, tumor necrosis factor, and interleukin-1. Thus these cells may be involved in thrombus formation under pathological circumstances. High-molecular-weight kininogen is a plasma protein that serves as the cofactor for XIIa when clotting is initiated *in vitro* in the activated partial thromboplastin time (aPTT) test.

Activation of Prothrombin. Factor Xa cleaves two peptide bonds in prothrombin to form thrombin. Activation of prothrombin by Xa is accelerated by Va, phospholipids, and Ca^{2+}. When these components are all present, prothrombin is activated nearly 20,000 times faster than the rate achieved by Xa and Ca^{2+} alone. The maximal rate of activation occurs only when prothrombin and Xa both contain Gla residues, and therefore have the ability to bind to phospholipids. Purified platelets can substitute for phospholipids and Va to facilitate activation of prothrombin *in vitro*, provided that the platelets are stimulated to release endogenous platelet factor Va or that factor Va is added exogenously to unstimulated platelets. The surface of platelets that are aggregated at the site of hemostasis concentrates the factors required for prothrombin activation.

Initiation of Coagulation. Coagulation is initiated *in vivo* by the extrinsic pathway. Small amounts of factor VIIa in the plasma bind to subendothelial tissue factor following vascular injury. Tissue factor accelerates activation of factor X by VIIa, phospholipids, and Ca^{2+} about 30,000-fold. VIIa also can activate IX in the presence of tissue factor, providing a convergence between the extrinsic and intrinsic pathways.

Clotting by the intrinsic pathway is initiated *in vitro* when XII, prekallikrein, and high-molecular-weight kininogen interact with kaolin, glass, or another surface to generate small amounts of XIIa. Activation of XI to XIa and IX to IXa follows. IXa then activates X in a reaction that is accelerated by VIIIa, phospholipids, and Ca^{2+}. Activation of factor X by IXa appears to occur by a mechanism similar to that for activation of prothrombin and may also be accelerated by platelets *in vivo*. Activation of factor XII is not required for hemostasis, since patients with deficiency of XII, prekallikrein, or high-molecular-weight kininogen do not bleed abnormally, even though their aPTT values are prolonged. Factor XI deficiency is associated with a variable and usually mild bleeding disorder. The mechanism for activation of factor XI *in vivo* is not known, although thrombin activates factor XI *in vitro*.

Fibrinolysis and Thrombolysis

The fibrinolytic system dissolves intravascular clots as a result of the action of plasmin, an enzyme that digests fibrin. Plasminogen, an inactive precursor, is converted to plasmin by cleavage of a single peptide bond. Plasmin is a relatively nonspecific protease; it digests fibrin clots and other plasma proteins, including several coagulation factors. Therapy with thrombolytic drugs tends to dissolve both pathological thrombi and fibrin deposits at sites of vascular injury. Therefore, the drugs are toxic, producing hemorrhage as a major side effect.

The fibrinolytic system is regulated such that unwanted fibrin thrombi are removed, while fibrin in wounds persists to maintain hemostasis (Lijnen and Collen, 2001). *Tissue plasminogen activator (t-PA)* is released from endothelial cells in response to various signals, including stasis produced by vascular occlusion. It is rapidly cleared from blood or inhibited by circulating inhibitors, plasminogen activator inhibitor-1 and plasminogen activator inhibitor-2, and thus exerts little effect on circulating plasminogen. t-PA binds to fibrin and converts plasminogen, which also binds to fibrin, to plasmin. Plasminogen and plasmin bind to fibrin at binding sites located near their amino termini that are rich in lysine residues (*see* below). These sites also are required for binding of plasmin to the inhibitor α_2-antiplasmin. Therefore, fibrin-bound plasmin is protected from inhibition. Any plasmin that escapes this local milieu is rapidly inhibited. Some α_2-antiplasmin is bound covalently to fibrin and thereby protects fibrin from premature lysis. When plasminogen activators are administered for thrombolytic therapy, massive fibrinolysis is initiated, and the inhibitory controls are overwhelmed. The pathway of fibrinolysis and sites of pharmacologic perturbation are summarized by Figure 54–3.

Coagulation In Vitro. Blood clots in 4 to 8 minutes when placed in a glass tube. Clotting is prevented if a chelating agent such as ethylenediaminetetraacetic acid (EDTA) or citrate is added to bind Ca^{2+}. Recalcified plasma clots in 2 to 4 minutes. The clotting time after recalcification is shortened to 26 to 33 seconds by the addition of negatively charged phospholipids and a particulate substance such as kaolin (aluminum silicate); this is termed

the *activated partial thromboplastin time* (aPTT). Alternatively, recalcified plasma will clot in 12 to 14 seconds after addition of "thromboplastin" (a mixture of tissue factor and phospholipids); this is termed the *prothrombin time* (PT).

Two pathways of coagulation are recognized. An individual with a prolonged aPTT and a normal PT is considered to have a defect in the *intrinsic coagulation pathway,* because all of the components of the aPTT test (except kaolin) are intrinsic to the plasma. A patient with a prolonged PT and a normal aPTT has a defect in the *extrinsic coagulation pathway,* since thromboplastin is extrinsic to the plasma. Prolongation of both the aPTT and the PT suggests a defect in a common pathway.

Natural Anticoagulant Mechanisms. Platelet activation and coagulation normally do not occur within an intact blood vessel (Edelberg *et al.,* 2001). Thrombosis is prevented by several regulatory mechanisms that require a normal vascular endothelium. Prostacyclin (prostaglandin I_2; PGI_2), a metabolite of arachidonic acid, is synthesized by endothelial cells and inhibits platelet aggregation and secretion (*see* Chapter 25). Antithrombin is a plasma protein that inhibits coagulation factors of the intrinsic and common pathways (*see* below). Heparan sulfate proteoglycans synthesized by endothelial cells stimulate the activity of antithrombin. Protein C is a plasma zymogen that is homologous to II, VII, IX, and X; its activity depends on the binding of Ca^{2+} to Gla residues within its amino-terminal domain. Activated protein C, in combination with its nonenzymatic Gla-containing cofactor (protein S), degrades cofactors Va and VIIIa and thereby greatly diminishes the rates of activation of prothrombin and factor X (Esmon, 2003). Protein C is activated by thrombin only in the presence of thrombomodulin, an integral membrane protein of endothelial cells. Like antithrombin, protein C appears to exert an anticoagulant effect in the vicinity of intact endothelial cells. Tissue factor pathway inhibitor (TFPI) is found in the lipoprotein fraction of plasma. When bound to factor Xa, TFPI inhibits factor Xa and the factor VIIa–tissue factor complex. By this mechanism, factor Xa may regulate its own production.

PARENTERAL ANTICOAGULANTS

Heparin

Biochemistry. Heparin is a glycosaminoglycan found in the secretory granules of mast cells. It is synthesized from

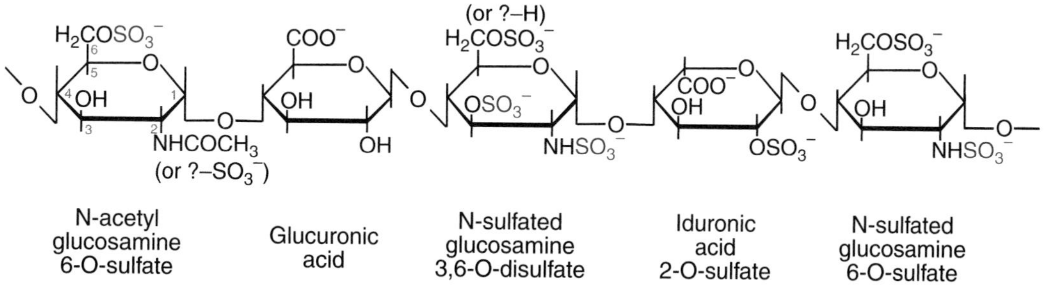

Figure 54–4. *The antithrombin-binding structure of heparin.* Sulfate groups required for binding to antithrombin are indicated in blue.

UDP-sugar precursors as a polymer of alternating D-glucuronic acid and *N*-acetyl-D-glucosamine residues (Figure 54–4) (Sugahara and Kitagawa, 2002). About 10 to 15 glycosaminoglycan chains, each containing 200 to 300 monosaccharide units, are attached to a core protein and yield a proteoglycan with a molecular mass of 750,000 to 1,000,000 daltons. The glycosaminoglycan then undergoes a series of modifications, which include the following: *N*-deacetylation and *N*-sulfation of glucosamine residues, epimerization of D-glucuronic acid to L-iduronic acid, *O*-sulfation of iduronic and glucuronic acid residues at the C2 position, and *O*-sulfation of glucosamine residues at the C3 and C6 positions. Each of these modifications is incomplete, yielding a variety of oligosaccharide structures. After the heparin proteoglycan has been transported to the mast cell granule, an endo-β-D-glucuronidase degrades the glycosaminoglycan chains to fragments of 5000 to 30,000 daltons (mean, about 12,000 daltons or 40 monosaccharide units) over a period of hours.

Heparan Sulfate. Heparan sulfate is synthesized from the same repeating disaccharide precursor (D-glucuronic acid linked to *N*-acetyl-D-glucosamine) as is heparin. However, heparan sulfate undergoes less modification of the polymer than does heparin and therefore contains higher proportions of glucuronic acid and *N*-acetylglucosamine and fewer sulfate groups. Heparan sulfate on the surface of vascular endothelial cells or in the subendothelial extracellular matrix interacts with circulating antithrombin (*see* below) to provide a natural antithrombotic mechanism. Patients with malignancies may experience bleeding related to circulating heparan sulfate or related glycosaminoglycans that probably originate from lysis of the tumor cells.

Source. Heparin is commonly extracted from porcine intestinal mucosa or bovine lung, and preparations may contain small amounts of other glycosaminoglycans. Despite the heterogeneity in composition among different commercial preparations of heparin, their biological activities are similar (about 150 USP units/mg). The USP unit is the quantity of heparin that prevents 1 ml of citrated sheep plasma from clotting for 1 hour after the addition of 0.2 ml of 1% $CaCl_2$.

Low-molecular-weight heparins (1000 to 10,000 daltons; mean, 4500 daltons, or 15 monosaccharide units) are isolated from standard heparin by gel filtration chromatography, precipitation with

ethanol, or partial depolymerization with nitrous acid and other chemical or enzymatic reagents. Low-molecular-weight heparins differ from standard heparin and from each other in their pharmacokinetic properties and mechanism of action (*see* below). The biological activity of low-molecular-weight heparin is generally measured with a factor Xa inhibition assay, which is mediated by antithrombin (*see* below).

Mechanism of Action. Heparin catalyzes the inhibition of several coagulation proteases by antithrombin, a glycosylated, single-chain polypeptide composed of 432 amino acid residues (Olson and Chuang, 2002). Antithrombin is synthesized in the liver and circulates in plasma at an approximate concentration of 2.6 μM. It inhibits activated coagulation factors of the intrinsic and common pathways, including thrombin, Xa, and IXa; however, it has relatively little activity against factor VIIa. Antithrombin is a "suicide substrate" for these proteases; inhibition occurs when the protease attacks a specific Arg-Ser peptide bond in the reactive site of antithrombin and becomes trapped as a stable 1:1 complex.

Heparin increases the rate of the thrombin-antithrombin reaction at least a thousandfold by serving as a catalytic template to which both the inhibitor and the protease bind. Binding of heparin also induces a conformational change in antithrombin that makes the reactive site more accessible to the protease. Once thrombin has become bound to antithrombin, the heparin molecule is released from the complex. The binding site for antithrombin on heparin is a specific pentasaccharide sequence that contains a 3-*O*-sulfated glucosamine residue (Figure 54–4). This structure occurs in about 30% of heparin molecules and less abundantly in heparan sulfate. Other glycosaminoglycans (*e.g.*, dermatan sulfate, chondroitin-4-sulfate, and chondroitin-6-sulfate) lack the antithrombin-binding structure and do not stimulate antithrombin. Heparin molecules containing fewer than 18 monosaccharide units (<5400 daltons) also do not catalyze inhibition of thrombin by antithrombin. Molecules of 18 monosaccharides or greater are required to bind thrombin and antithrombin simultaneously. In contrast, the pentasaccharide shown in Figure 54–4 catalyzes inhibition of factor Xa by antithrombin. In this case, catalysis may occur solely by induction of a conformational change in antithrombin that facilitates reaction with the protease. Low-molecular-weight heparin preparations produce an anticoagulant effect mainly through inhibition of Xa by antithrombin, because the majority of molecules are of insufficient length to catalyze inhibition of thrombin.

When the concentration of heparin in plasma is 0.1 to 1 units/ml, thrombin, factor IXa, and factor Xa are inhibited rapidly (half-lives less than 0.1 second) by antithrombin. This effect prolongs both the aPTT and the thrombin time (*i.e.*, the time required for plasma to clot when exogenous thrombin is added); the PT is affected to a lesser degree. Factor Xa bound to platelets in the prothrombinase complex and thrombin bound to fibrin are both protected from inhibition by antithrombin in the presence of heparin. Thus, heparin may promote inhibition of factor Xa and thrombin only after they have diffused away from these binding sites. Platelet factor 4, released from the α-granules during platelet aggregation, blocks binding of antithrombin to heparin or heparan sulfate and may promote local clot formation at the site of hemostasis.

Miscellaneous Pharmacological Effects. High doses of heparin can interfere with platelet aggregation and thereby prolong bleeding time. It is unclear to what extent the antiplatelet effect of heparin contributes to the hemorrhagic complications of treatment with the drug. Heparin "clears" lipemic plasma *in vivo* by causing the release of lipoprotein lipase into the circulation. Lipoprotein lipase hydrolyzes triglycerides to glycerol and free fatty acids. The clearing of lipemic plasma may occur at concentrations of heparin below those necessary to produce an anticoagulant effect. Rebound hyperlipemia may occur after heparin administration is stopped.

Clinical Use. Heparin is used to initiate treatment of venous thrombosis and pulmonary embolism because of its rapid onset of action (Hirsh *et al.*, 2001). An oral anticoagulant usually is started concurrently, and heparin is continued for at least 4 to 5 days to allow the oral anticoagulant to achieve its full therapeutic effect (*see* Clinical Use and Monitoring Anticoagulant Therapy). Patients who experience recurrent thromboembolism despite adequate oral anticoagulation (*e.g.*, patients with Trousseau's syndrome) may benefit from long-term heparin administration. Heparin is used in the initial management of patients with unstable angina or acute myocardial infarction, during and after coronary angioplasty or stent placement, and during surgery requiring cardiopulmonary bypass. Heparin also is used to treat selected patients with disseminated intravascular coagulation. Low-dose heparin regimens are effective in preventing venous thromboembolism in certain high-risk patients. Specific recommendations for heparin use have been reviewed (Hirsh *et al.*, 2001).

Low-molecular-weight heparin preparations were first approved for prevention of venous thromboembolism.

They are also effective in the treatment of venous thrombosis, pulmonary embolism, and unstable angina (Hirsh *et al.*, 2001). The principal advantage of low-molecular-weight heparin over standard heparin is a more predictable pharmacokinetic profile, which allows weight-adjusted subcutaneous administration without laboratory monitoring. Thus, therapy of many patients with acute venous thromboembolism can be provided in the outpatient setting. Other advantages of low-molecular-weight heparin include a lower incidence of heparin-induced thrombocytopenia and possibly lower risks of bleeding and osteopenia.

In contrast to warfarin, heparin does not cross the placenta and has not been associated with fetal malformations; therefore it is the drug of choice for anticoagulation during pregnancy. Heparin does not appear to increase the incidence of fetal mortality or prematurity. If possible, the drug should be discontinued 24 hours before delivery to minimize the risk of postpartum bleeding. The safety and efficacy of low-molecular-weight heparin use during pregnancy have not been adequately evaluated.

Absorption and Pharmacokinetics. Heparin is not absorbed through the gastrointestinal mucosa and therefore is given by continuous intravenous infusion or subcutaneous injection. Heparin has an immediate onset of action when given intravenously. In contrast, there is considerable variation in the bioavailability of heparin given subcutaneously, and the onset of action is delayed 1 to 2 hours; low-molecular-weight heparins are absorbed more uniformly.

The half-life of heparin in plasma depends on the dose administered. When doses of 100, 400, or 800 units/kg of heparin are injected intravenously, the half-lives of the anticoagulant activities are approximately 1, 2.5, and 5 hours, respectively (*see* Appendix II for pharmacokinetic data). Heparin appears to be cleared and degraded primarily by the reticuloendothelial system; a small amount of undegraded heparin also appears in the urine. The half-life of heparin may be shortened in patients with pulmonary embolism and prolonged in patients with hepatic cirrhosis or end-stage renal disease. Low-molecular-weight heparins have longer biological half-lives than do standard preparations of the drug.

Administration and Monitoring. Full-dose heparin therapy usually is administered by continuous intravenous infusion. Treatment of venous thromboembolism is initiated with a bolus injection of 5000 units, followed by 1200 to 1600 units per hour delivered by an infusion pump. Therapy routinely is monitored by the aPTT. The therapeutic range for standard heparin is considered to be that which is equivalent to a plasma heparin level of 0.3 to 0.7 units/ml as determined with an anti–factor Xa assay (Hirsh *et al.*, 2001). The aPTT value that corresponds to this range varies depending on the reagent and instrument used to perform the assay. A clotting time of 1.8 to 2.5 times the normal mean aPTT value generally is assumed to be therapeutic; however, values in this range obtained with some aPTT assays may overestimate the amount of circulating heparin, and therefore be subtherapeutic. The risk of recurrence of thromboembolism is greater in patients who do not achieve a therapeutic level of anticoagulation within the first 24 hours. Initially, the aPTT should be measured and the infusion rate adjusted every 6 hours; dose adjustments may be aided by use of a nomogram (Hirsh *et al.*, 2001). Once a steady dosage schedule has been established, daily monitoring is sufficient.

Very high doses of heparin are required to prevent coagulation during cardiopulmonary bypass. The aPTT is infinitely prolonged over the dosage range used. Another coagulation test, such as the activated clotting time, is employed to monitor therapy in this situation.

Subcutaneous administration of heparin can be used for the long-term management of patients in whom warfarin is contraindicated (*e.g.*, during pregnancy). A total daily dose of about 35,000 units administered as divided doses every 8 to 12 hours usually is sufficient to achieve an aPTT of 1.5 times the control value (measured midway between doses). Monitoring generally is unnecessary once a steady dosage schedule is established.

Low-dose heparin therapy is used prophylactically to prevent deep venous thrombosis and thromboembolism in susceptible patients. (Until recently a suggested regimen for such treatment was 5000 units of heparin given every 8 to 12 hours.) The body of evidence now suggests that this regimen is clinically less effective than giving heparin every 8 hours in hospitalized medical and surgical patients at high risk for venous thromboembolism (Cade, 1982; Gardlund, 1996; Belch *et al.*, 1981). Laboratory monitoring is unnecessary, since this regimen does not prolong the aPTT.

Low-Molecular-Weight Heparin Preparations. *Enoxaparin* (LOVENOX), *dalteparin* (FRAGMIN), *tinzaparin* (INNOHEP, others), *ardeparin* (NORMIFLO), *nadroparin* (FRAXIPARINE, others), and *reviparin* (CLIVARINE) differ considerably in composition, and it cannot be assumed that two preparations that have similar anti–factor Xa activity will produce equivalent antithrombotic effects. The more predictable pharmacokinetic properties of low-molecular-weight heparins, however, permit administration in a fixed or weight-adjusted dosage regimen once or twice daily by subcutaneous injection. Since they have a minimal effect on tests of clotting *in vitro,* monitoring is not done routinely. Patients with end-stage renal failure may require monitoring with an anti–factor Xa assay because this condition may prolong the half-life of low-molecular-weight heparin. Specific dosage recommendations for various low-molecular-weight heparins may be obtained from the manufacturer's literature. Nadroparin and reviparin are not currently available in the United States.

Synthetic Heparin Derivatives. *Fondaparinux* (ARIXTRA) is a synthetic pentasaccharide based on the structure of the antithrombin binding region of heparin. It mediates inhibition of factor Xa by antithrombin but does not cause thrombin inhibition due to its short polymer length. Fondaparinux is administered by subcutaneous injection, reaches peak plasma levels in 2 hours, and is excreted in the urine with a half-life of 17 to 21 hours. It should not be used in patients with renal failure. Because it does not interact significantly with blood cells or plasma proteins other than antithrombin, fondaparinux can be given once a day at a fixed dose without coagulation monitoring. Fondaparinux appears to be much less likely than heparin or low-molecular-weight heparin to trigger the syndrome of heparin-induced thrombocytopenia (*see* below). Fondaparinux is approved for thromboprophylaxis of patients undergoing hip or knee surgery (Buller *et al.*, 2003) and for the therapy of pulmonary embolism and deep venous thrombosis. *Idraparinux* (undergoing phase III clinical testing as of 2004) is a more highly sulfated derivative of fondaparinux that has a half-life of 5 to 6 days; the lack of a suitable antidote may limit its clinical application.

Heparin Resistance. The dose of heparin required to produce a therapeutic aPTT varies due to differences in the concentrations of heparin-binding proteins in plasma, such as histidine-rich glycoprotein, vitronectin, and platelet factor 4; these proteins competitively inhibit binding of heparin to antithrombin. Occasionally a patient's aPTT will not be prolonged unless very high doses of heparin (>50,000 units per day) are administered. Such patients may have "therapeutic" concentrations of heparin in plasma at the usual dose when values are measured by other tests (*e.g.*, anti–factor Xa activity or protamine sulfate titration). These patients may have very short aPTT values prior to treatment because of the presence of an increased concentration of factor VIII and may not be truly resistant to heparin. Other patients may require large doses of heparin because of accelerated clearance of the drug, as may occur with massive pulmonary embolism. Patients with inherited antithrombin deficiency ordinarily have 40% to 60% of the normal plasma concentration of this inhibitor and respond normally to intravenous heparin. However, acquired antithrombin deficiency (concentration less than 25% of normal) may occur in patients with hepatic cirrhosis, nephrotic syndrome, or disseminated intravascular coagulation; large doses of heparin may not prolong the aPTT in these individuals.

Toxicities. **Bleeding.** Bleeding is the primary untoward effect of heparin. Major bleeding occurs in 1% to 5% of patients treated with intravenous heparin for venous thromboembolism (Hirsh *et al.,* 2001). The incidence of bleeding is somewhat less in patients treated with low-molecular-weight heparin for this indication. Although the number of bleeding episodes appears to increase with the total daily dose of heparin and with the degree of prolongation of the aPTT, these correlations are weak, and patients can bleed with aPTT values that are within the therapeutic range. Often an underlying cause for bleeding is present, such as recent surgery, trauma, peptic ulcer disease, or platelet dysfunction.

The anticoagulant effect of heparin disappears within hours of discontinuation of the drug. Mild bleeding due to heparin usually can be controlled without the administration of an antagonist. If life-threatening hemorrhage occurs, the effect of heparin can be reversed quickly by the slow intravenous infusion of *protamine sulfate,* a mixture of basic polypeptides isolated from salmon sperm. Protamine binds tightly to heparin and thereby neutralizes its anticoagulant effect. Protamine also interacts with platelets, fibrinogen, and other plasma proteins and may cause an anticoagulant effect of its own. Therefore, one should give the minimal amount of protamine required to neutralize the heparin present in the plasma. This amount is approximately 1 mg of protamine for every 100 units of heparin remaining in the patient; it is given intravenously at a slow rate (up to 50 mg over 10 minutes).

Protamine is used routinely to reverse the anticoagulant effect of heparin following cardiac surgery and other vascular procedures. Anaphylactic reactions occur in about 1% of patients with diabetes mellitus who have received protamine-containing insulin (*NPH insulin* or *protamine zinc insulin*) but are not limited to this group. A less common reaction consisting of pulmonary vasoconstriction, right ventricular dysfunction, systemic hypotension, and transient neutropenia also may occur after protamine administration.

Heparin-Induced Thrombocytopenia. Heparin-induced thrombocytopenia (platelet count <150,000/ml or a 50% decrease from the pretreatment value) occurs in about 0.5% of medical patients 5 to 10 days after initiation of therapy with standard heparin (Warkentin, 2003). The incidence of thrombocytopenia is lower with low-molecular-weight heparin. Thrombotic complications that can be life-threatening or lead to amputation occur in about one-half of the affected heparin-treated patients and may precede the onset of thrombocytopenia. The incidence of heparin-induced thrombocytopenia and thrombosis is higher in surgical patients. Venous thromboembolism occurs most commonly, but arterial thromboses causing limb ischemia, myocardial infarction, and stroke also occur. Bilateral adrenal hemorrhage, skin lesions at the site of subcutaneous heparin injection, and a variety of systemic reactions may accompany heparin-induced thrombocytopenia. The development of IgG antibodies against complexes of heparin with platelet factor 4 (or, rarely, other chemokines) appears to cause all of these reactions. These complexes activate platelets by binding to FcγIIa receptors, which results in platelet aggregation, release of more platelet factor 4, and thrombin generation. The antibodies also may trigger vascular injury by binding to platelet factor 4 attached to heparan sulfate on the endothelium.

Heparin should be discontinued immediately if unexplained thrombocytopenia or any of the clinical manifestations mentioned above occur 5 or more days after beginning heparin therapy, regardless of the dose or route of administration. The onset of heparin-induced thrombocytopenia may occur earlier in patients who have received heparin within the previous 3 to 4 months and have residual circulating antibodies. The diagnosis of heparin-induced thrombocytopenia can be confirmed by a heparin-dependent platelet activation assay or an assay for antibodies that react with heparin/platelet factor 4 complexes. Since thrombotic complications may occur after cessation of therapy, an alternative anticoagulant such as *lepirudin, argatroban,* or *danaparoid* (*see* below) should be administered to patients with heparin-induced thrombocytopenia. Low-molecular-weight heparins should be avoided, because these drugs often cross-react with standard heparin in heparin-dependent antibody assays. Warfarin may precipitate venous limb gangrene or multicentric skin necrosis in patients with heparin-induced thrombocytopenia and should not be used until the thrombocytopenia has resolved and the patient is adequately anticoagulated with another agent.

Other Toxicities. Abnormalities of hepatic function tests occur frequently in patients who are receiving heparin intravenously or subcutaneously. Mild elevations of the activities of hepatic transaminases in plasma occur without an increase in bilirubin levels or alkaline phosphatase activity. Osteoporosis resulting in spontaneous vertebral fractures can occur, albeit infrequently, in patients who have received full therapeutic doses of heparin (greater than 20,000 units per day) for extended periods of time (*e.g.,* 3 to 6 months). Heparin can inhibit the synthesis of aldosterone by the adrenal glands and occasionally causes hyperkalemia, even when low doses are given. Allergic reactions to heparin (other than thrombocytopenia) are rare.

Other Parenteral Anticoagulants

Lepirudin. Lepirudin (REFLUDAN) is a recombinant derivative (Leu^1-Thr^2-63-desulfohirudin) of hirudin, a direct thrombin inhibitor present in the salivary glands of the medicinal leech. It is a 65-amino-acid polypeptide that binds tightly to both the catalytic site and the extended substrate recognition site (exosite I) of thrombin. Lepirudin is approved in the United States for treatment of patients with heparin-induced thrombocytopenia. It is administered intravenously at a dose adjusted to maintain the aPTT at 1.5 to 2.5 times the median of the laboratory's normal range for aPTT. The drug is excreted by the kidneys and has a half-life of about 1.3 hours. Lepirudin should be used cautiously in patients with renal failure, since it can accumulate and cause bleeding in these patients. Patients may develop antihirudin antibodies that occasionally cause a paradoxical increase in the aPTT; therefore, daily monitoring of the aPTT is recommended. There is no antidote for lepirudin.

Bivalirudin. Bivalirudin (ANGIOMAX) is a synthetic, 20-amino-acid polypeptide that directly inhibits thrombin by a mechanism similar to that of lepirudin. Bivalirudin contains the sequence Phe^1-Pro^2-Arg^3-Pro^4, which occupies the catalytic site of thrombin, followed by a polyglycine linker and a hirudin-like sequence that binds to exosite I. Thrombin slowly cleaves the Arg^3-Pro^4 peptide bond and thus regains activity. Bivalirudin is administered intravenously and is used as an alternative to heparin in patients undergoing coronary angioplasty. The half-life of bivalirudin in patients with normal renal function is 25 minutes; dosage reductions are recommended for patients with moderate or severe renal impairment.

Argatroban. Argatroban, a synthetic compound based on the structure of L-arginine, binds reversibly to the catalytic site of thrombin. It is administered intravenously and has an immediate onset of action. Its half-life is 40 to 50 minutes. Argatroban is metabolized by cytochrome P450 enzymes in the liver and is excreted in the bile; therefore dosage reduction is required for patients with hepatic insufficiency. The dosage is adjusted to maintain an aPTT of 1.5 to 3 times the baseline value. Argatroban can be used as an alternative to lepirudin for prophylaxis or treatment of patients with or at risk of developing heparin-induced thrombocytopenia.

Danaparoid. Danaparoid (ORGARAN) is a mixture of nonheparin glycosaminoglycans isolated from porcine intestinal mucosa (84% heparan sulfate, 12% dermatan sulfate, 4% chondroitin sulfate) with a mean mass of 5500 daltons. Danaparoid is approved in the United States for prophylaxis of deep venous thrombosis. It also is an effective anticoagulant for patients with heparin-induced thrombocytopenia and has a low rate of cross-reactivity with heparin in platelet-activation assays. Danaparoid mainly promotes inhibition of factor Xa by antithrombin, but it does not prolong the PT or aPTT at the recommended dosage. Danaparoid is administered subcutaneously at a fixed dose for prophylactic use and intravenously at a higher, weight-adjusted dose for full anticoagulation. Its half-life is about 24 hours. Patients with renal failure may require monitoring with an anti–factor Xa assay because of a prolonged half-life of the drug. No antidote is available. Danaparoid is no longer available in the United States.

Drotrecogin Alfa. Drotrecogin alfa (XIGRIS) is a recombinant form of human activated protein C that inhibits coagulation by proteolytic inactivation of factors Va and VIIIa. It also has antiinflammatory effects (Esmon, 2003). A 96-hour continuous infusion of drotrecogin alfa decreases mortality in adult patients who are at high risk for death from severe sepsis if given within 48 hours of the onset of organ dysfunction (*e.g.*, shock, hypoxemia, oliguria). The major adverse effect is bleeding.

ORAL ANTICOAGULANTS

Warfarin

History. Following the report of a hemorrhagic disorder in cattle that resulted from the ingestion of spoiled sweet clover silage, Campbell and Link, in 1939, identified the hemorrhagic agent as bishydroxycoumarin (dicoumarol). In 1948, a more potent synthetic congener was introduced as an extremely effective rodenticide; the compound was named *warfarin* as an acronym derived from the name of the patent holder, Wisconsin Alumni Research Foundation. Warfarin's potential as a therapeutic anticoagulant was recognized but not widely accepted, partly due to fear of unacceptable toxicity. However, in 1951, an Army inductee uneventfully survived an attempted suicide with massive doses of a preparation of warfarin intended for rodent control. Since then, these anticoagulants have become a mainstay for prevention of thromboembolic disease.

Chemistry. Numerous anticoagulants have been synthesized as derivatives of 4-hydroxycoumarin and of the related compound, indan-1,3-dione (Figure 54–5). Only the coumarin derivatives are widely used; the 4-hydroxycoumarin residue, with a nonpolar carbon substituent at the 3 position, is the minimal structural requirement for activity. This carbon is asymmetrical in warfarin (and in *phenprocoumon* and *acenocoumarol*). The enantiomers differ in anticoagulant potency, metabolism, elimination, and interactions with other drugs. Commercial preparations of these anticoagulants

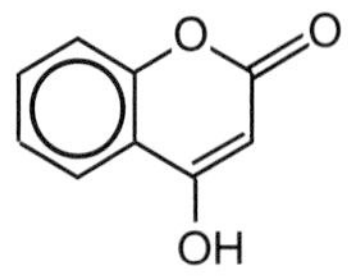

4-Hydroxycoumarin

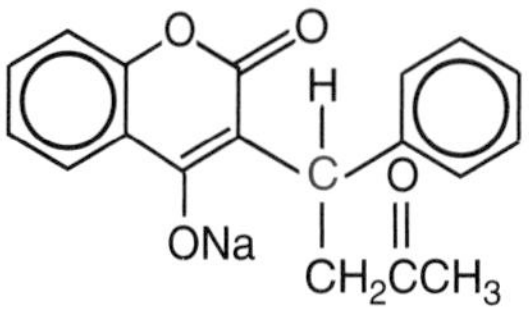

Warfarin Sodium

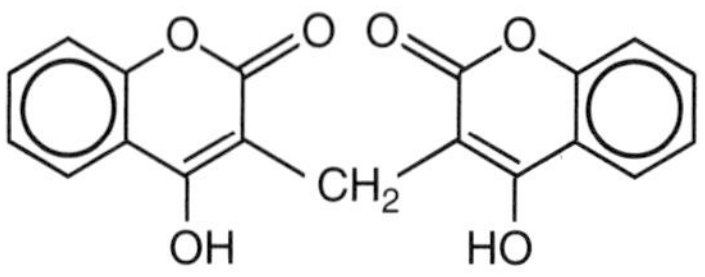

Dicumarol

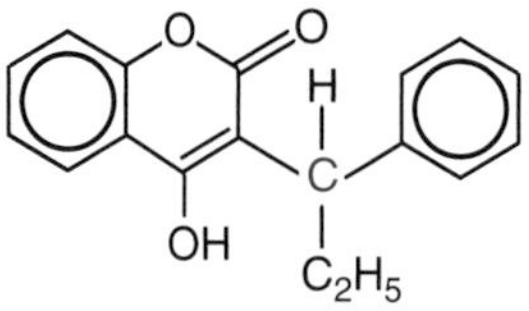

Phenprocoumon

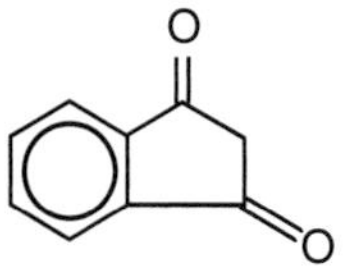

Indan-1,3-dione

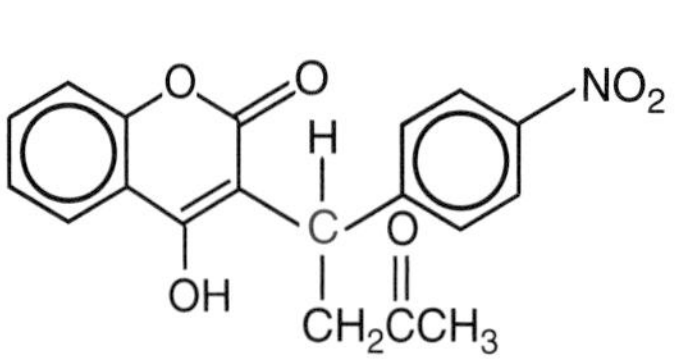

Acenocoumarol

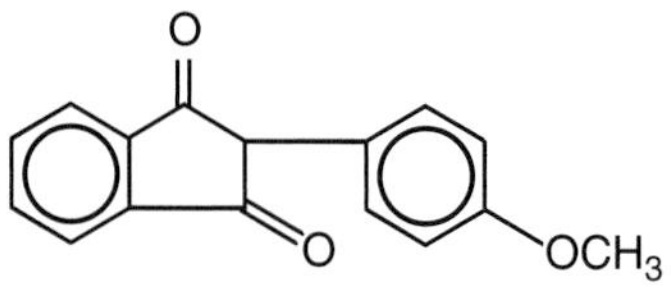

Anisindione

Figure 54–5. ***Structural formulas of the oral anticoagulants.*** 4-Hydroxycoumarin and indan-1,3-dione are the parent molecules from which the oral anticoagulants are derived. The asymmetrical carbon atoms in the coumarins are shown in blue.

are racemic mixtures. No advantage of administering a single enantiomer has been established.

Mechanism of Action. The oral anticoagulants are antagonists of vitamin K (*see* section on vitamin K, below). Coagulation factors II, VII, IX, and X and the anticoagulant proteins C and S are synthesized mainly in the liver and are biologically inactive unless 9 to 13 of the amino-terminal glutamate residues are carboxylated to form the Ca^{2+}-binding γ-carboxyglutamate (Gla) residues. This reaction of the descarboxy precursor protein requires carbon dioxide, molecular oxygen, and reduced vitamin K, and is catalyzed by γ-glutamyl carboxylase in the rough endoplasmic reticulum (Figure 54–6). Carboxylation is directly coupled to the oxidation of vitamin K to its corresponding epoxide.

Reduced vitamin K must be regenerated from the epoxide for sustained carboxylation and synthesis of biologically competent proteins. The enzyme that catalyzes this, vitamin K epoxide reductase, is inhibited by therapeutic doses of warfarin. Vitamin K (but not vitamin K epoxide) also can be converted to the corresponding hydroquinone by a second reductase, DT-diaphorase. This enzyme requires high concentrations of vitamin K and is less sensitive to coumarin drugs, which may explain why administration of sufficient vitamin K can counteract even large doses of oral anticoagulants.

Therapeutic doses of warfarin decrease by 30% to 50% the total amount of each vitamin K–dependent coagulation factor made by the liver; in addition, the secreted molecules are undercarboxylated, resulting in diminished biological activity (10% to 40% of normal). Congenital deficiencies of the procoagulant proteins to these levels cause mild bleeding disorders. Oral anticoagulants have no effect on the activity of fully carboxylated molecules in the circulation. Thus, the time required for the activity of each factor in plasma to reach a new steady state after therapy is initiated or adjusted depends on its individual

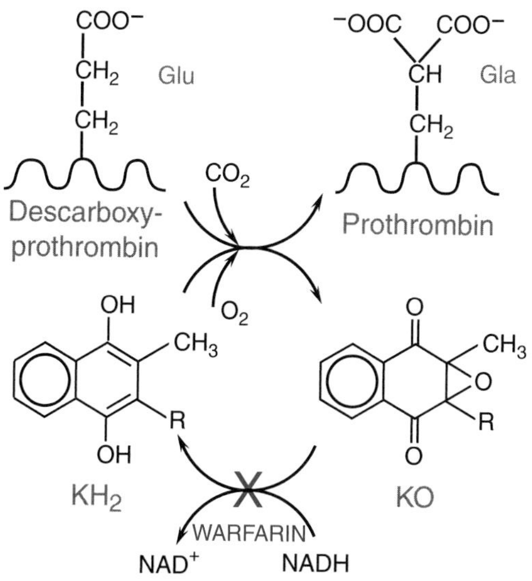

Figure 54–6. *The Vitamin K cycle: γ-glutamyl carboxylation of vitamin K–dependent proteins.* The enzyme γ-glutamyl carboxylase couples the oxidation of the reduced hydroquinone form (KH_2) of vitamin K_1 or K_2, to γ-carboxylation of Glu residues on vitamin K–dependent proteins, generating the epoxide of vitamin K (KO) and γ-carboxyglutamate (Gla) residues in vitamin K–dependent precursor proteins in the endoplasmic reticulum. A 2,3-epoxide reductase regenerates vitamin KH_2 and is the warfarin-sensitive step. The R on the vitamin K molecule represents a 20-carbon phytyl side chain in vitamin K_1 and a 5- to 65-carbon prenyl side chain in vitamin K_2.

rate of clearance. The approximate half-lives (in hours) are as follows: factor VII, 6; factor IX, 24; factor X, 36; factor II, 50; protein C, 8; and protein S, 30. Because of the long half-lives of some of the coagulation factors, in particular factor II, the full antithrombotic effect of warfarin is not achieved for several days, even though the PT may be prolonged soon after administration due to the more rapid reduction of factors with a shorter half-life, in particular factor VII. There is no obvious selectivity of the effect of warfarin on any particular vitamin K–dependent coagulation factor, although the antithrombotic benefit and the hemorrhagic risk of therapy may be correlated with the functional level of prothrombin, and to a lesser extent, factor X (Zivelin *et al.*, 1993).

Dosage. The usual adult dose of warfarin (COUMADIN) is 5 mg per day for 2 to 4 days, followed by 2 to 10 mg per day as indicated by measurements of the international normalized ratio (INR), a value derived from the patient's PT (*see* functional definition of INR in section on laboratory monitoring, below). A lower initial dose should be given to

patients with an increased risk of bleeding, including the elderly. Warfarin usually is administered orally; age correlates with increased sensitivity to oral anticoagulants. Warfarin also can be given intravenously without modification of the dose. Intramuscular injection is not recommended because of the risk of hematoma formation.

Absorption. The bioavailability of warfarin is nearly complete when the drug is administered orally, intravenously, or rectally. Bleeding has occurred from repeated skin contact with solutions of warfarin used as a rodenticide. However, different commercial preparations of warfarin tablets vary in their rate of dissolution, and this causes some variation in the rate and extent of absorption. Food in the gastrointestinal tract also can decrease the rate of absorption. Warfarin usually is detectable in plasma within 1 hour of its oral administration, and concentrations peak in 2 to 8 hours.

Distribution. Warfarin is almost completely (99%) bound to plasma proteins, principally albumin, and the drug distributes rapidly into a volume equivalent to the albumin space (0.14 L/kg). Concentrations in fetal plasma approach the maternal values, but active warfarin is not found in milk (unlike other coumarins and indandiones).

Biotransformation and Elimination. Warfarin is a racemic mixture of R (weak) and S (potent) anticoagulant enantiomers. S-warfarin is transformed into inactive metabolites by CYP2C9 and R-warfarin is transformed by CYP1A2, CYP2C19 (minor pathway), and CYP3A4 (minor pathway). The inactive metabolites of warfarin are excreted in urine and stool. The average rate of clearance from plasma is 0.045 ml/min^{-1}·kg^{-1}. The half-life ranges from 25 to 60 hours, with a mean of about 40 hours; the duration of action of warfarin is 2 to 5 days.

Drug and Other Interactions. The list of drugs and other factors that may affect the action of oral anticoagulants is prodigious and expanding (Hirsh *et al.*, 2003). Any substance or condition is potentially dangerous if it alters (1) the uptake or metabolism of the oral anticoagulant or vitamin K; (2) the synthesis, function, or clearance of any factor or cell involved in hemostasis or fibrinolysis; or (3) the integrity of any epithelial surface. Patients must be educated to report the addition or deletion of any medication, including nonprescription drugs and food supplements. Some of the more commonly described factors that cause a decreased effect of oral anticoagulants include: reduced absorption of drug caused by binding to *cholestyramine* in the gastrointestinal tract; increased volume of distribution and a short half-life secondary to hypoproteinemia, as in nephrotic syndrome; increased metabolic clearance of drug secondary to induction of hepatic enzymes, especially CYP2C9, by barbiturates, *carbamazepine*, or *rifampin*; ingestion of large amounts of vitamin K–rich foods or supplements; and increased levels of coagulation factors during pregnancy. Hence, the PT can be shortened in any of these cases.

Frequently cited interactions that enhance the risk of hemorrhage in patients taking oral anticoagulants include decreased metabolism due to CYP2C9 inhibition by *amiodarone*, azole antifungals, *cimetidine, clopidogrel, cotrimoxazole, disulfiram, fluoxetine, isoniazid, metronidazole, sulfinpyrazone, tolcapone,* or *zafirlukast*, and displacement from protein binding sites caused by loop diuretics or *valproate*. Relative deficiency of vitamin K may result from inadequate diet (*e.g.,* postoperative patients on parenteral fluids), especially when coupled with the elimination of intestinal flora by antimicrobial agents. Gut bacteria synthesize vitamin K and thus are an important source of this vitamin. Consequently, antibiotics can cause excessive PT prolongation in patients adequately controlled on warfarin. In addition to an effect on reducing intestinal flora, cephalosporins containing heterocyclic side chains also inhibit steps in the vitamin K cycle. Low concentrations of coagulation factors may result from impaired hepatic function, congestive heart failure, or hypermetabolic states, such as hyperthyroidism; generally, these conditions increase the prolongation of the PT. Serious interactions that do not alter the PT include inhibition of platelet function by agents such as *aspirin* and gastritis or frank ulceration induced by antiinflammatory drugs. Agents may have more than one effect; for example, *clofibrate* increases the rate of turnover of coagulation factors and inhibits platelet function. Elderly patients are more sensitive to oral anticoagulants.

Resistance to Warfarin. Some patients require more than 20 mg per day of warfarin to achieve a therapeutic INR. These patients often have excessive vitamin K intake from the diet or parenteral supplementation. Noncompliance and laboratory error are other causes of apparent warfarin resistance. A few patients with hereditary warfarin resistance have been reported, in whom very high plasma concentrations of warfarin are associated with minimal depression of vitamin K–dependent coagulation factor biosynthesis; mutations in the vitamin K epoxide reductase gene have been identified in some of these patients (Rost *et al.*, 2004).

Sensitivity to Warfarin. Approximately 10% of patients require less than 1.5 mg per day of warfarin to achieve an INR of 2 to 3. These patients are more likely to possess one or two variant alleles of CYP2C9, which is the major enzyme responsible for converting the S-enantiomer warfarin to its inactive metabolites (Daly and King, 2003). In comparison with the wild-type CYP2C9*1 allele, the variant alleles CYP2C9*2 and CYP2C9*3 have been shown to inactivate S-warfarin much less efficiently *in vitro*. The variant alleles are present in 10% to 20% of Caucasians, but in <5% of African-Americans or Asians.

Toxicities. **Bleeding.** Bleeding is the major toxicity of oral anticoagulant drugs (Hirsh *et al.*, 2003). The risk of bleeding increases with the intensity and duration of anticoagulant therapy, the use of other medications that interfere with hemostasis, and the presence of a potential anatomical source of bleeding. Especially serious episodes involve sites where irreversible damage may result from compression of vital structures (*e.g.,* intracranial, pericardial, nerve sheath, or spinal cord) or from massive internal blood loss that may not be diagnosed rapidly (*e.g.,* gastrointestinal, intraperitoneal, or retroperitoneal). Although the reported incidence of major bleeding episodes varies considerably, it is generally less than 5% per year in patients treated with a target INR of 2 to 3. The risk of intracranial hemorrhage increases dramatically with an INR greater than 4, especially in older patients. In a large outpatient anticoagulation clinic, the most common factors

associated with a transient elevation of the INR (>6) were use of a new medication known to potentiate warfarin (*e.g., acetaminophen*), advanced malignancy, recent diarrheal illness, decreased oral intake, and taking more warfarin than prescribed (Hylek *et al.*, 1998). Patients must be informed of the signs and symptoms of bleeding, and laboratory monitoring should be done at frequent intervals during intercurrent illnesses or any changes of medication or diet.

If the INR is above the therapeutic range but <5 and the patient is not bleeding or in need of a surgical procedure, warfarin can be discontinued temporarily and restarted at a lower dose once the INR is within the therapeutic range (Hirsh *et al.*, 2003). If the INR is ≥5, vitamin K$_1$ (*phytonadione,* MEPHYTON, AQUAMEPHYTON) can be given orally at a dose of 1 to 2.5 mg (for an INR between 5 and 9) or 3 to 5 mg (for an INR >9). These doses of oral vitamin K$_1$ generally cause the INR to fall substantially within 24 to 48 hours without rendering the patient resistant to further warfarin therapy. Higher doses may be required if more rapid correction of the INR is necessary. The effect of vitamin K$_1$ is delayed for at least several hours, because reversal of anticoagulation requires synthesis of fully carboxylated coagulation factors. If immediate hemostatic competence is necessary because of serious bleeding or profound warfarin overdosage (INR >20), adequate concentrations of vitamin K–dependent coagulation factors can be restored by transfusion of fresh frozen plasma (10 to 20 ml per kg), supplemented with 10 mg of vitamin K$_1$, given by slow intravenous infusion. Transfusion of plasma may need to be repeated, since the transfused factors (particularly factor VII) are cleared from the circulation more rapidly than the residual oral anticoagulant. Vitamin K$_1$ administered intravenously carries the risk of anaphylactoid reactions, and therefore should be used cautiously. Patients who receive high doses of vitamin K$_1$ may become unresponsive to warfarin for several days, but heparin can be used if continued anticoagulation is required.

Birth Defects. Administration of warfarin during pregnancy causes birth defects and abortion. A syndrome characterized by nasal hypoplasia and stippled epiphyseal calcifications that resemble chondrodysplasia punctata may result from maternal ingestion of warfarin during the first trimester. Central nervous system abnormalities have been reported following exposure during the second and third trimesters. Fetal or neonatal hemorrhage and intrauterine death may occur, even when maternal PT values are in the therapeutic range. Oral anticoagulants should not be used during pregnancy, but as indicated in the previous section, heparin can be used safely in this circumstance.

Skin Necrosis. Warfarin-induced skin necrosis is a rare complication characterized by the appearance of skin lesions 3 to 10 days after treatment is initiated. The lesions typically are on the extremities, but adipose tissue, the penis, and the female breast also may be involved. Lesions are characterized by widespread thrombosis of the microvasculature and can spread rapidly, sometimes becoming necrotic and requiring disfiguring débridement or occasionally amputation. Cases have been reported in subjects heterozygous for protein C or protein S deficiency. Since protein C has a shorter half-life than do the other vitamin K–dependent coagulation factors (except factor VII), its functional activity falls more rapidly in response to the initial dose of vitamin K antagonist. It has been proposed that the dermal necrosis is a manifestation of a temporal imbalance between the anticoagulant protein C and one or more of the procoagulant factors and is exaggerated in patients who are partially deficient in protein C or protein S. However, not all patients with heterozygous deficiency of protein C or protein S develop skin necrosis when treated with warfarin, and patients with normal activities of these proteins also can be affected. Morphologically similar lesions can occur in patients with vitamin K deficiency.

Other Toxicities. A reversible, sometimes painful, blue-tinged discoloration of the plantar surfaces and sides of the toes that blanches with pressure and fades with elevation of the legs (purple toe syndrome) may develop 3 to 8 weeks after initiation of therapy with warfarin; cholesterol emboli released from atheromatous plaques have been implicated as the cause. Other infrequent reactions include alopecia, urticaria, dermatitis, fever, nausea, diarrhea, abdominal cramps, and anorexia.

Warfarin appears to precipitate the syndromes of venous limb gangrene and multicentric skin necrosis that sometimes are associated with heparin-induced thrombocytopenia (Warkentin, 2003). Other anticoagulant agents, such as lepirudin or argatroban, should be used until the heparin-induced thrombocytopenia has resolved (*see* Heparin Toxicities, above).

Clinical Use

Oral anticoagulants are used to prevent the progression or recurrence of acute deep vein thrombosis or pulmonary embolism following an initial course of heparin. They also are effective in preventing venous thromboembolism in patients undergoing orthopedic or gynecological surgery and in preventing systemic embolization in patients with acute myocardial infarction, prosthetic heart valves, or chronic atrial fibrillation. Specific recommendations for oral anticoagulant use for these and other indications have been reviewed (The Sixth American College of Chest Physicians Guidelines for Antithrombotic Therapy for Prevention and Treatment of Thrombosis, 2001).

Prior to initiation of therapy, laboratory tests are used in conjunction with the patient's history and physical examination to uncover hemostatic defects that might make the use of oral anticoagulant drugs more dangerous (congenital coagulation factor deficiency, thrombocytopenia, hepatic or renal insufficiency, vascular abnormalities, *etc.*). Thereafter, the INR calculated from the patient's PT is used to monitor efficacy and compliance. Therapeutic ranges for various clinical indications have been established empirically and reflect dosages that reduce the

morbidity from thromboembolic disease while minimally increasing the risk of serious hemorrhage. For most indications the target INR is 2 to 3. A higher target INR (*e.g.,* 2.5 to 3.5) generally is recommended for patients with mechanical prosthetic heart valves (Hirsh *et al.*, 2003).

For treatment of acute venous thromboembolism, heparin usually is continued for at least 4 to 5 days after oral anticoagulation is begun and until the INR is in the therapeutic range on 2 consecutive days. This overlap allows for adequate depletion of the vitamin K–dependent coagulation factors with long half-lives, especially factor II. Daily INR measurements are indicated at the onset of therapy to guard against excessive anticoagulation in the unusually sensitive patient. The testing interval can be lengthened gradually to weekly and then to monthly for patients on long-term therapy in whom test results have been stable.

Monitoring Anticoagulant Therapy: The INR (International Normalized Ratio). To monitor therapy, a fasting blood sample is usually obtained 8 to 14 hours after the last dose of an oral anticoagulant, and the patient's PT is determined along with that of a sample of normal pooled plasma. Formerly, the results were reported as a simple ratio of the two PT values. However, this ratio can vary widely depending on the thromboplastin reagent and the instrument used to initiate and detect clot formation. The PT is prolonged when the functional levels of fibrinogen, factor V, or the vitamin K–dependent factors II, VII, or X are decreased. Reduced levels of factor IX or proteins C or S have no effect on the PT. PT measurements are converted to INR measurements by the following equation:

$$INR = \left(\frac{PT_{pt}}{PT_{ref}}\right)^{ISI} \tag{54-1}$$

where INR = International Normalized Ratio
ISI = International Sensitivity Index

The ISI value, generally supplied by the manufacturer, indicates the relative sensitivity of the PT determined with a given thromboplastin to decreases in the vitamin K–dependent coagulation factors in comparison with a World Health Organization human thromboplastin standard. Reagents with lower ISI values are more sensitive to the effects of oral anticoagulants (*i.e.,* the PT is prolonged to a greater extent in comparison with that obtained with a less sensitive reagent having a higher ISI). Ideally, the ISI value of each batch of thromboplastin should be confirmed in each clinical laboratory using a set of reference plasmas to control for local variables of sample handling and instrumentation.

The major practical consequence of standardization to the INR has been an appreciation that the commercial thromboplastins from rabbit tissue, used especially in North America, are relatively insensitive. This property led to administration of larger doses of oral anticoagulants than were considered optimal in many of the original clinical trials in which more sensitive human brain thromboplastins generally were used. Thus, the target INR of 2 to 3 corresponds to a PT ratio of 1.2 to 1.5 if rabbit thromboplastin is used or 2 to 3 if human thromboplastin is used.

The INR does not provide a reliable indication of the degree of anticoagulation in patients with the lupus anticoagulant, in whom the PT and other phospholipid-dependent coagulation tests are prolonged at baseline. In these patients, a chromogenic anti–factor Xa assay or the prothrombin-proconvertin–time assay may be used to monitor therapy (Moll and Ortel, 1997).

Other Oral Anticoagulants

Phenprocoumon and Acenocoumarol. These agents are not generally available in the United States but are prescribed in Europe and elsewhere. Phenprocoumon (MARCUMAR) has a longer plasma half-life (5 days) than warfarin, as well as a somewhat slower onset of action and a longer duration of action (7 to 14 days). It is administered in daily maintenance doses of 0.75 to 6 mg. By contrast, acenocoumarol (SINTHROME) has a shorter half-life (10 to 24 hours), a more rapid effect on the PT, and a shorter duration of action (2 days). The maintenance dose is 1 to 8 mg daily.

Indandione Derivatives. Anisindione (MIRADON) is available for clinical use in some countries. It is similar to warfarin in its kinetics of action; however, it offers no clear advantages and may have a higher frequency of untoward effects. *Phenindione* (DINDEVAN) still is available in some countries. Serious hypersensitivity reactions, occasionally fatal, can occur within a few weeks of starting therapy with this drug, and its use can no longer be recommended.

Rodenticides. Bromadiolone, brodifacoum, diphenadione, chlorophacinone, and *pindone* are long-acting agents (prolongation of the PT may persist for weeks). They are of interest because they sometimes are agents of accidental or intentional poisoning. In this setting, reversal of the coagulopathy can require very large doses of vitamin K (*i.e.*, >100 mg/day) for weeks or months.

Ximelagatran. Ximelagatran is a novel drug that is readily absorbed after oral administration and is rapidly metabolized to *melagatran*, a direct thrombin inhibitor. Therefore, its onset of action is much faster than that of warfarin. Ximelagatran is administered twice daily at a fixed dose and does not appear to require coagulation monitoring. Melagatran is excreted primarily by the kidney; therefore, dosage reduction may be necessary for patients with renal failure. Ximelagatran has been used successfully in clinical trials for prevention of venous thromboembolism (Francis *et al.*, 2003; Schulman *et al.*, 2003). Ximelagatran causes elevation of hepatic transaminases in about 6% of patients, but this side effect usually is asymptomatic and often is transient. The drug has not yet been approved for use in the United States.

FIBRINOLYTIC DRUGS

The fibrinolytic pathway is summarized by Figure 54–3. The action of fibrinolytic agents is best understood in conjunction with an understanding of the characteristics of the physiologic components.

Plasminogen. Plasminogen is a single-chain glycoprotein that contains 791 amino acid residues; it is converted to an active protease by cleavage at arginine 560. High-affinity binding sites mediate the binding of plasminogen (or plasmin) to carboxyl-terminal lysine residues in partially degraded fibrin; this enhances fibrinolysis. A plasma carboxypeptidase termed *thrombin-activatable fibrinolysis inhibitor* (TAFI) can remove these lysine residues and thereby attenuate fibrinolysis. The lysine binding sites are in the amino-terminal "kringle" domain of plasminogen between amino acids 80 and 165, and they also promote formation of complexes of plasmin with α_2-antiplasmin, the major physiological plasmin inhibitor. Plasminogen concentrations in human plasma average 2 μM. A degraded form of plasminogen termed *lys-plasminogen* binds to fibrin much more rapidly than does intact plasminogen.

α_2-Antiplasmin. α_2-*Antiplasmin* is a glycoprotein of 452 amino acid residues. It forms a stable complex with plasmin, thereby inactivating it. Plasma concentrations of α_2-antiplasmin (1 μM) are sufficient to inhibit about 50% of potential plasmin. When massive activation of plasminogen occurs, the inhibitor is depleted, and free plasmin causes a "systemic lytic state," in which hemostasis is impaired. In this state, fibrinogen is destroyed and fibrinogen degradation products impair formation of fibrin and therefore increase bleeding from wounds. α_2-Antiplasmin inactivates plasmin nearly instantaneously, as long as the lysine binding sites on plasmin are unoccupied by fibrin or other antagonists, such as *aminocaproic acid* (*see* below).

Streptokinase. Streptokinase (STREPTASE) is a 47,000-dalton protein produced by β-hemolytic streptococci. It has no intrinsic enzymatic activity, but it forms a stable, noncovalent 1:1 complex with plasminogen. This produces a conformational change that exposes the active site on plasminogen that cleaves arginine 560 on free plasminogen to form free plasmin. Streptokinase is rarely used clinically for fibrinolysis since the advent of newer agents.

Tissue Plasminogen Activator (t-PA). t-PA is a serine protease that contains 527 amino acid residues. It is a poor plasminogen activator in the absence of fibrin (Lijnen and Collen, 2001). t-PA binds to fibrin *via* lysine binding sites at its amino terminus and activates bound plasminogen several hundredfold more rapidly than it activates plasminogen in the circulation. The lysine binding sites on t-PA are in a "finger" domain that is homologous to similar sites on fibronectin. Under physiological conditions (t-PA concentrations of 5 to 10 ng/ml), the specificity of t-PA for fibrin limits systemic formation of plasmin and induction of a systemic lytic state. During therapeutic infusions of t-PA, however, concentrations rise to 300 to 3000 ng/ml. Clearance of t-PA primarily occurs by hepatic metabolism, and its half-life is 5 to 10 minutes. t-PA is effective in lysing thrombi during treatment of acute myocardial infarction. t-PA (*alteplase*, ACTIVASE) is produced by recombinant DNA technology. The currently recommended ("accelerated") regimen for coronary thrombolysis is a 15-mg intravenous bolus, followed by 0.75 mg/kg of body weight over 30 minutes (not to exceed 50 mg) and 0.5 mg/kg (up to 35 mg accumulated dose) over the following hour. Recombinant mutant variants of t-PA now are available (*reteplase*, RETAVASE and *tenecteplase*, TNKASE). They differ from native t-PA by having increased plasma half-lives that allow convenient bolus dosing (2 doses of 15 milliunits given 30 minutes apart). They also are relatively resistant to inhibition by plasma activator inhibitor-1. Despite these apparent advantages, these agents are similar to t-PA in efficacy and toxicity (GUSTO III Investigators, 1997).

Hemorrhagic Toxicity of Thrombolytic Therapy. The major toxicity of all thrombolytic agents is hemorrhage, which results from two factors: (1) the lysis of fibrin in "physiological thrombi" at sites of vascular injury; and (2) a systemic lytic state that results from systemic formation of plasmin, which produces fibrinogenolysis and destruction of other coagulation factors (especially factors V and VIII). The actual toxicity of streptokinase and t-PA is difficult to assess. In early clinical trials, many bleeding episodes resulted from the extensive invasive monitoring of therapy that was required by the protocol. Many studies to evaluate thrombolysis involved concurrent systemic heparinization, which also contributes to bleeding complications. Analysis of more recent clinical trials suggests that heparin confers no benefit in patients receiving fibrinolytic therapy plus aspirin (Collins *et al.*, 1997; Zijlstra *et al.*, 1999).

The contraindications to fibrinolytic therapy are listed in Table 54–1. Patients with these conditions should not receive such treatment, and invasive procedures (*e.g.,* cardiac catheterization and arterial blood gases) should be avoided. If heparin is used concurrently with either streptokinase or t-PA, serious hemorrhage will occur in 2% to 4% of patients. Intracranial hemorrhage is by far the most serious problem. Hemorrhagic stroke occurs with all regimens and is more common when heparin is used. In several large

Table 54–1
Contraindications to Thrombolytic Therapy

1. Surgery within 10 days, including organ biopsy, puncture of noncompressible vessels, serious trauma, cardiopulmonary resuscitation
2. Serious gastrointestinal bleeding within 3 months
3. History of hypertension (diastolic pressure >110 mm Hg)
4. Active bleeding or hemorrhagic disorder
5. Previous cerebrovascular accident or active intracranial process
6. Aortic dissection
7. Acute pericarditis

studies, t-PA was associated with an excess of hemorrhagic strokes of about 0.3% of treated patients. Based on the data of three large trials involving almost 100,000 patients, the efficacies of t-PA and streptokinase in treating myocardial infarction are essentially identical. Both agents reduce death and reinfarction by about 30% in regimens containing aspirin (Zijlstra *et al.*, 1999). Recent studies suggest that angioplasty with or without stent placement, when feasible, is superior to thrombolytic therapy, although direct comparisons using otherwise identical regimens have not been performed (Armstrong *et al.*, 2003; Andersen *et al.*, 2003).

Inhibition of Fibrinolysis

Aminocaproic Acid. Aminocaproic acid (AMICAR) is a lysine analog that competes for lysine binding sites on plasminogen and plasmin, thus blocking the interaction of plasmin with fibrin. Aminocaproic acid is thereby a potent inhibitor of fibrinolysis and can reverse states that are associated with excessive fibrinolysis. The main problem with its use is that thrombi that form during treatment with the drug are not lysed. For example, in patients with hematuria, ureteral obstruction by clots may lead to renal failure after treatment with aminocaproic acid. Aminocaproic acid has been used to reduce bleeding after prostatic surgery or after tooth extractions in hemophiliacs. Use of aminocaproic acid to treat a variety of other bleeding disorders has been unsuccessful, either because of limited benefit or because of thrombosis (*e.g.,* after subarachnoid hemorrhage). Aminocaproic acid is absorbed rapidly after oral administration, and 50% is excreted unchanged in the urine within 12 hours. For intravenous use, a loading dose of 4 to 5 g is given over 1 hour, followed by an infusion of 1 g per hour until bleeding is controlled. No more than 30 g should be given in a 24-hour period. Rarely, the drug causes myopathy and muscle necrosis.

ANTIPLATELET DRUGS

Platelets provide the initial hemostatic plug at sites of vascular injury. They also participate in pathological thromboses that lead to myocardial infarction, stroke, and peripheral vascular thromboses. Potent inhibitors of platelet function have been developed in recent years. These drugs act by discrete mechanisms, and thus in combination their effects are additive or even synergistic. Their availability has led to a revolution in cardiovascular medicine, whereby angioplasty and vascular stenting of lesions now is feasible with low rates of restenosis and thrombosis when effective platelet inhibition is employed.

Aspirin. Processes including thrombosis, inflammation, wound healing, and allergy are modulated by oxygenated metabolites of arachidonate and related polyunsaturated fatty acids that are collectively termed *eicosanoids*. Interference with the synthesis of eicosanoids is the basis for the effects of many therapeutic agents, including analgesics, antiinflammatory drugs, and antithrombotic agents (*see* Chapters 25 and 26).

In platelets, the major cyclooxygenase product is thromboxane A_2, a labile inducer of platelet aggregation and a potent vasoconstrictor. Aspirin blocks production of thromboxane A_2 by acetylating a serine residue near the active site of platelet cyclooxygenase (COX-1), the enzyme that produces the cyclic endoperoxide precursor of thromboxane A_2. Since platelets do not synthesize new proteins, the action of aspirin on platelet cyclooxygenase is permanent, lasting for the life of the platelet (7 to 10 days). Thus, repeated doses of aspirin produce a cumulative effect on platelet function. Complete inactivation of platelet COX-1 is achieved when 160 mg of aspirin is taken daily. Therefore, aspirin is maximally effective as an antithrombotic agent at doses much lower than those required for other actions of the drug. Numerous trials indicate that aspirin, when used as an antithrombotic drug, is maximally effective at doses of 50 to 320 mg per day (Antithrombotic Trialists' Collaboration, 2002; Patrono *et al.*, 2004). Higher doses do not improve efficacy; moreover, they potentially are less efficacious because of inhibition of prostacyclin production, which can be largely spared by using lower doses of aspirin. Higher doses also increase toxicity, especially bleeding.

Other NSAIDs that are reversible inhibitors of COX-1 have not been shown to have antithrombotic efficacy and in fact may even interfere with low-dose aspirin regimens.

Dipyridamole. *Dipyridamole* (PERSANTINE) is a vasodilator that, in combination with warfarin, inhibits embolization from prosthetic heart valves. Dipyridamole has little or no benefit as an antithrombotic drug. In trials in which a regimen of dipyridamole plus aspirin was compared with aspirin alone, dipyridamole provided no additional beneficial effect (Antithrombotic Trialists' Collaboration, 2002). A single study suggests that dipyridamole plus aspirin reduces strokes in patients with prior strokes or transient ischemic attack (Diener *et al.*, 1996). A formulation containing 200 mg of dipyridamole, in an extended-release form, and 25 mg of aspirin (AGGRENOX) is available. Dipyridamole interferes with platelet function by increasing the cellular concentration of adenosine $3',5'$-monophosphate (cyclic AMP). This effect is mediated by inhibition of cyclic nucleotide phosphodiesterase and/or by blockade of uptake of adenosine, which acts at adenosine A_2 receptors to stimulate platelet adenylyl cyclase. The only current recommended use of dipyridamole is in combination with warfarin for postoperative primary prophylaxis of thromboemboli in patients with prosthetic heart valves.

Ticlopidine. Purinergic receptors respond to extracellular nucleotides as agonists. Platelets contain two purinergic receptors, $P2Y_1$ and $P2Y_{12}$; both are GPCRs for ADP. The ADP-activated platelet $P2Y_1$ receptor couples to the G_q-PLC-IP_3-Ca^{2+} pathway and induces a shape change and aggregation. The $P2Y_{12}$ receptor couples to G_i and, when activated by ADP, inhibits adenylyl cyclase, resulting in lower levels of cyclic AMP and thereby less cyclic AMP–dependent inhibition of platelet activation. Based on pharmacological studies, it appears that both receptors must be stimulated to result in platelet activation (Jin and Kunapuli, 1998), and inhibition of either receptor is sufficient to block platelet activation. *Ticlopidine* (TICLID) is a thienopyridine (Figure 54–7) that inhibits the $P2Y_{12}$ receptor. Ticlopidine is a prodrug that requires conversion to the active thiol metabolite by a hepatic cytochrome P450 enzyme (Savi *et al.*, 2000). It is rapidly absorbed and highly bioavailable. It permanently inhibits the $P2Y_{12}$ receptor by forming a disulfide bridge between the thiol on the drug and a free cysteine residue in the extracellular region of the receptor and thus has a prolonged effect. Like aspirin it has a short half-life with a long duration of action, which has been termed "hit-and-run pharmacology" (Hollopeter *et al.*, 2001). Maximal inhibition of platelet aggregation is not seen until 8 to 11 days after starting therapy. Thus, "loading doses" of 500 mg sometimes are given to achieve a more rapid onset of action. The usual dose is 250 mg twice per day. Inhibition of platelet aggregation persists for a few days after the drug is stopped.

Adverse Effects. The most common side effects are nausea, vomiting, and diarrhea. The most serious is severe neutropenia (absolute neutrophil count [ANC] <1500/μL), which occurred in 2.4% of stroke patients given the drug during premarketing clinical trials. Fatal agranulocytosis with thrombopenia has occurred within the first 3 months of therapy; therefore, frequent blood counts should be obtained during the first few months of therapy, with immediate dis-

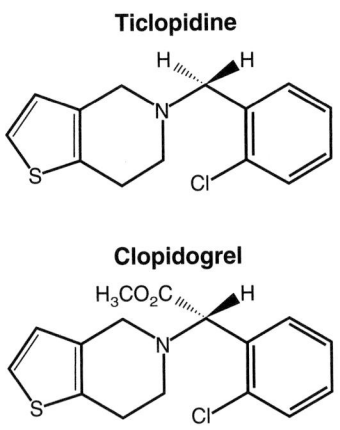

Ticlopidine

Clopidogrel

Figure 54–7. *Structure of ticlopidine and clopidogrel.*

continuation of therapy should cell counts decline. Platelet counts also should be monitored, as thrombocytopenia has been reported. Rare cases of thrombotic thrombocytopenic purpura–hemolytic uremic syndrome (TTP-HUS) have been associated with ticlopidine with a reported incidence of 1 in 1600 to 4800 patients when the drug is used after cardiac stenting; the mortality associated with these cases is reported to be as high as 18% to 57% (Bennett *et al.*, 1998; Bennett *et al.*, 1999). Remission of TTP has been reported when the drug is stopped (Quinn and Fitzgerald, 1999).

Therapeutic Uses. Ticlopidine has been shown to prevent cerebrovascular events in secondary prevention of stroke and is at least as good as aspirin in this regard (Patrono *et al.*, 1998). It also reduces cardiac events in patients with unstable angina; however, its only FDA-approved indication is to reduce the risk of thrombotic stroke in patients who have experienced stroke precursors, and in patients who have had a completed thrombotic stroke. Since ticlopidine has a mechanism of action distinct from that of aspirin, combining the drugs might be expected to provide additive or even synergistic effects. This appears to be the case, and the combination has been used in patients undergoing angioplasty and stenting for coronary artery disease, with a very low frequency of stent thrombosis occurring over a short, 30-day follow-up (<1%) (Leon *et al.*, 1998). As ticlopidine is associated with life-threatening blood dyscrasias and a relatively high rate of TTP, it is generally reserved for patients who are intolerant or allergic to aspirin or who have failed aspirin therapy.

Clopidogrel.

The thienopyridine clopidogrel (PLAVIX) is closely related to ticlopidine (Figure 54–7) and appears to have a slightly more favorable toxicity profile with less frequent thrombocytopenia and leukopenia, although thrombotic thrombocytopenic purpura has been reported (Bennett *et al.*, 2000). Clopidogrel is a prodrug with a slow onset of action. The usual dose is 75 mg per day with or without an initial loading dose of 300 mg. The drug is equivalent to aspirin in the secondary prevention of stroke, and in combination with aspirin it appears to be as effective as ticlopidine and aspirin. It is used with aspirin after angioplasty and should be continued for at least 1 year (Steinhubl *et al.*, 2002). In one study, the combination of clopidogrel and aspirin clearly was superior to aspirin alone; this finding suggests that the actions of the two drugs are synergistic, as might be expected from their distinct mechanisms of action (Yusuf *et al.*, 2001). The FDA-approved indications for clopidogrel are to reduce the rate of stroke, MI, and death in patients with recent myocardial infarction or stroke, established peripheral arterial disease, or acute coronary syndrome.

Glycoprotein IIb/IIIa Inhibitors.

Glycoprotein IIb/IIIa is a platelet-surface integrin which, by the integrin nomenclature, is designated $\alpha_{IIb}\beta_3$. This dimeric glycoprotein is a receptor for fibrinogen and von Willebrand factor, which anchor platelets to foreign surfaces and to each other, thereby mediating aggregation. The integrin heterodimer/receptor is activated by platelet agonists such as thrombin, collagen,

or thromboxane A_2 to develop binding sites for its ligands, which do not bind to resting platelets. Inhibition of binding to this receptor blocks platelet aggregation induced by any agonist. Thus, inhibitors of this receptor are potent antiplatelet agents that act by a mechanism distinct from that of aspirin or the thienopyridine platelet inhibitors. Three agents are approved for use at present, with others under development.

Abciximab.

Abciximab (REOPRO) is the Fab fragment of a humanized monoclonal antibody directed against the $\alpha_{IIb}\beta_3$ receptor. It also binds to the vitronectin receptor on platelets, vascular endothelial cells, and smooth muscle cells. The antibody is used in conjunction with percutaneous angioplasty for coronary thromboses, and when used in conjunction with aspirin and heparin, has been shown to be quite effective in preventing restenosis, recurrent myocardial infarction, and death. The reduction in total events is about 50% in various large trials (Scarborough *et al.*, 1999). The unbound antibody is cleared from the circulation with a half-life of about 30 minutes, but antibody remains bound to the $\alpha_{IIb}\beta_3$ receptor and inhibits platelet aggregation as measured *in vitro* for 18 to 24 hours after infusion is stopped. It is given as a 0.25-mg/kg bolus followed by 0.125 μg/kg per minute for 12 hours or longer.

Adverse Effects. The major side effect of abciximab is bleeding, and the contraindications to its use are similar to those for fibrinolytic agents listed in Table 54–1. The frequency of major hemorrhage in clinical trials varies from 1% to 10%, depending on the intensity of anticoagulation with heparin. Thrombocytopenia of less than 50,000 μ/L is seen in about 2% of patients and may be due to development of neo-epitopes induced by bound antibody. Since the duration of action is long, if major bleeding or emergent surgery occurs, platelet transfusions can reverse the aggregation defect, because free antibody concentrations fall rapidly after cessation of infusion. Readministration of antibody has been performed in a small number of patients without evidence of decreased efficacy or allergic reactions. The expense of the antibody limits its use.

Eptifibatide.

Eptifibatide (INTEGRILIN) is a cyclic peptide inhibitor of the fibrinogen binding site on $\alpha_{IIb}\beta_3$. It blocks platelet aggregation *in vitro* after intravenous infusion into patients. Eptifibatide is given as a bolus of 180 μg/kg followed by 2 μg/kg per minute for up to 96 hours. It is used to treat acute coronary syndrome and for angioplastic coronary interventions. In the latter case, myocardial infarction and death have been reduced by about 20%. Although the drug has not been compared directly to abciximab, it appears that its benefit is somewhat less than that obtained with the antibody, perhaps because eptifibatide is specific for $\alpha_{IIb}\beta_3$ and does not react with the vitronectin receptor. The duration of action of the drug is relatively short and platelet aggregation is restored within 6 to 12 hours after cessation of infusion. Eptifibatide generally is administered in conjunction with aspirin and heparin.

Adverse Effects. The major side effect is bleeding, as is the case with abciximab. The frequency of major bleeding in trials was about 10%, compared with about 9% in a placebo group, which included heparin. Thrombocytopenia has been seen in 0.5% to 1% of patients.

Tirofiban. Tirofiban (AGGRASTAT) is a nonpeptide, small-molecule inhibitor of $\alpha_{IIb}\beta_3$ that appears to have a similar mechanism of action as eptifibatide. Tirofiban has a short duration of action and has efficacy in non-Q-wave myocardial infarction and unstable angina. Reductions in death and myocardial infarction have been about 20% compared to placebo, results similar to those with eptifibatide. Side effects also are similar to those of eptifibatide. The agent is specific to $\alpha_{IIb}\beta_3$ and does not react with the vitronectin receptor. Meta-analysis of trials using $\alpha_{IIb}\beta_3$ inhibitors suggests that their value in antiplatelet therapy after acute myocardial infarction is limited (Boersma *et al.*, 2002). Tirofiban is administered intravenously at an initial rate of 0.4 *μ*g/kg per minute for 30 minutes, and then continued at 0.1 mg/kg per minute for 12 to 24 hours after angioplasty or atherectomy. It is used in conjunction with heparin.

THE ROLE OF VITAMIN K

Vitamin K is essential in both mammals and in photosynthetic organisms. In certain photosynthetic bacteria, vitamin K is a cofactor in the photosynthetic electron-transport system; in green plants, vitamin K_1 is a component of photosystem I, the membrane-bound macromolecular light-sensitive complex. Green plants are a nutritional source of vitamin K for humans, in whom vitamin K is an essential cofactor in the γ-carboxylation of multiple glutamate (Glu) residues of several clotting factors and anticoagulant proteins. The vitamin K–dependent formation of γ-carboxy-glutamate (Gla) residues permits the appropriate interactions of clotting factors, Ca^{2+}, and membrane phospholipids and modulator proteins (Figures 54–1, 54–2, and 54–3). Oral anticoagulant drugs (coumadin derivatives, Figure 54–5) block Gla formation and thereby inhibit clotting; excess vitamin K_1 can reverse the effects of these oral anticoagulants.

History. In 1929, Dam observed that chickens fed inadequate diets developed a deficiency disease characterized by spontaneous bleeding and reduced prothrombin in the blood. Subsequently, Dam and coworkers (1935, 1936) found that the condition could be alleviated rapidly by feeding an unidentified fat-soluble substance, named *vitamin K (Koagulation* vitamin) by Dam. Independently, Almquist

and Stokstad (1935) performed similar work. Quick and coworkers (1935) observed a coagulation defect in jaundiced individuals that was due to a decrease in the plasma concentration of prothrombin. In the same year, Hawkins and Whipple reported that animals with biliary fistulas were likely to develop excessive bleeding. Subsequently, Hawkins and Brinkhous (1936) showed that this, too, was due to a deficiency in prothrombin and that the condition could be relieved by the feeding of bile salts. The culmination of these studies came with the demonstration by Butt and coworkers (1938) and Warner and associates (1938) that combination therapy with vitamin K and bile salts was effective in the treatment of the hemorrhagic diathesis of jaundice. Thus, the relationship between vitamin K, adequate hepatic function, and the physiological mechanisms operating in the normal clotting of blood was established.

Chemistry and Occurrence. Vitamin K activity is associated with at least two distinct natural substances, designated as vitamin K_1 and vitamin K_2. Vitamin K_1, or *phylloquinone (phytonadione)*, is 2-methyl-3-phytyl-1,4-naphthoquinone; it is found in plants and is the only natural vitamin K available for therapeutic use. Vitamin K_2 is actually a series of compounds (the *menaquinones*) in which the phytyl side chain of phylloquinone has been replaced by a side chain built up of 2 to 13 prenyl units. Considerable synthesis of menaquinones occurs in gram-positive bacteria; indeed, intestinal flora synthesize the large amounts of vitamin K contained in human and animal feces (Bentley and Meganathan, 1982). In animals, menaquinone-4 can be synthesized from the vitamin precursor *menadione* (2-methyl-1,4-naphthoquinone), or vitamin K_3. Depending on the bioassay system used, menadione is at least as active on a molar basis as phylloquinone. The structures of phylloquinone and the menaquinone series are:

PHYLLOQUINONE (vitamin K_1, phytonadione)

MENAQUINONE (vitamin K_2) series

Physiological Functions and Pharmacological Actions. In normal animals and humans, phylloquinone and menaquinones are virtually devoid of pharmacodynamic activity. However, in subjects deficient in vitamin K, the vitamin performs its normal physiological function: to promote the biosynthesis of the γ-carboxy-glutamate (Gla) forms of factors II (prothrombin), VII, IX, and X, anticoagulant proteins C and S, protein Z (a cofactor to the inhibitor of Xa), the bone Gla protein osteocalcin, matrix Gla protein, growth arrest–specific protein 6 (Gas6), and four transmembrane monospans of unknown function (Brown *et al.*, 2000; Broze, 2001; Kulman *et al.*, 2001).

Figure 54–6 summarizes the coupling of the vitamin K cycle with glutamate carboxylation. Vitamin K, as KH_2, the reduced vitamin K hydroquinone, is an essential cofactor for γ-glutamyl carboxylase (Rishavy *et al.*, 2004). Using KH_2, O_2, CO_2, and the glutamate-containing substrate, the enzyme forms a γ-carboxy-glutamatyl protein (Gla protein) and concomitantly, the 2,3-epoxide of vitamin K. A coumarin-sensitive 2,3-epoxide reductase regenerates KH_2. The γ-glutamyl carboxylase and epoxide reductase are integral membrane proteins of the endoplasmic reticulum and seem to function as a multicomponent system that may include the chaperone protein, calumenin, which reportedly inhibits γ-carboxylation (Wajih *et al.*, 2004). Two natural mutations in γ-glutamyl carboxylase lead to bleeding disorders (Mutucumarana *et al.*, 2003). With respect to proteins affecting blood coagulation, these reactions occur in the liver, but γ-carboxylation of glutamate also occurs in lung, bone, and other cell types. Vitamin K epoxide reductase recently has been cloned (Rost *et al.*, 2004; Li *et al.*, 2004).

The γ-carboxylation reaction is aided by the grouping of glutamate residues in a *Gla domain* (about 45 residues in clotting factors) near the amino terminus of the nascent substrate protein; the reaction is guided by an adjacent propeptide (18 to 28 amino acids) that interacts with the carboxylase. In the case of the vitamin K–dependent clotting proteins, the Gla domain is about 45 residues long, and 9 to 13 glutamates are γ-carboxylated in the primary sequence of the Gla domain, C-terminal to the propeptide. The Glu→Gla conversion enables the factors to interact well with Ca^{2+} and thence with phospholipids of platelet membranes, positioning the factors in the proper conformations for interacting with their substrates and modulators. In the absence of vitamin K (or in the presence of a coumarin derivative), newly synthesized vitamin K–dependent clotting factors lack Gla residues and are inactive because the molecular conformations needed for their interactions are not achieved.

Human Requirements. The human requirement for vitamin K has not been defined precisely. In patients made vitamin K–deficient by a starvation diet and antibiotic therapy for 3 to 4 weeks, the minimum daily requirement is estimated to be 0.03 μg/kg of body weight (Frick, 1967) and possibly as high as 1 μg/kg, which is approximately the recommended intake for adults (70 μg/day).

Symptoms of Deficiency. The chief clinical manifestation of vitamin K deficiency is an increased tendency to bleed (*see* discussion of hypoprothrombinemia in section on oral anticoagulants, above). Ecchymoses, epistaxis, hematuria, gastrointestinal bleeding, and postoperative hemorrhage are common; intracranial hemorrhage may occur. Hemoptysis is uncommon. The discovery of a vitamin K–dependent protein in bone suggests that the fetal bone abnormalities associated with the administration of oral anticoagulants during the first trimester of pregnancy ("fetal warfarin syndrome") may be related to a deficiency of the vitamin.

Considerable evidence indicates a role for vitamin K in adult skeletal maintenance and osteoporosis. Low concentrations of the vitamin are associated with deficits in bone mineral density and fractures; vitamin K supplementation increases the carboxylation state of osteocalcin and also improves bone mineral density, but the relationship of these two effects is unclear (Feskanich *et al.*, 1999). Bone mineral density in adults is not changed by therapeutic use of oral anticoagulants (Rosen *et al.*, 1993), but new bone formation may be affected.

Toxicity. Phylloquinone and the menaquinones are nontoxic to animals, even when given at 500 times the RDA. However, menadione

and its derivatives (synthetic forms of vitamin K) have been implicated in producing hemolytic anemia and kernicterus in neonates, especially in premature infants (Diploma and Ritchie, 1997). For this reason menadione should not be used as a therapeutic form of vitamin K.

Absorption, Fate, and Excretion. The mechanism of intestinal absorption of compounds with vitamin K activity varies with their solubility. In the presence of bile salts, phylloquinone and the menaquinones are adequately absorbed from the intestine, almost entirely by way of the lymph. Phylloquinone is absorbed by an energy-dependent, saturable process in proximal portions of the small intestine; menaquinones are absorbed by diffusion in the distal portions of the small intestine and in the colon. Following absorption, phylloquinone is incorporated into chylomicrons in close association with triglycerides and lipoproteins. In a large survey, plasma phylloquinone and triglyceride concentration were well correlated (Sadowski *et al.*, 1989). The extremely low phylloquinone levels in newborns may be partly related to very low plasma lipoprotein concentrations at birth and may lead to an underestimation of vitamin K tissue stores. After absorption, phylloquinone and menaquinones are concentrated in the liver, but the concentration of phylloquinone declines rapidly. Menaquinones, produced in the lower bowel, are less biologically active than phylloquinone due to their long side chain. Very little vitamin K accumulates in other tissues.

Phylloquinone is metabolized rapidly to more polar metabolites, which are excreted in the bile and urine. The major urinary metabolites result from shortening of the side chain to five or seven carbon atoms, yielding carboxylic acids that are conjugated with glucuronate prior to excretion.

Apparently, there is only modest storage of vitamin K in the body. Under circumstances in which lack of bile interferes with absorption of vitamin K, hypoprothrombinemia develops slowly over a period of several weeks.

Therapeutic Uses. Vitamin K is used therapeutically to correct the bleeding tendency or hemorrhage associated with its deficiency. Vitamin K deficiency can result from inadequate intake, absorption, or utilization of the vitamin, or as a consequence of the action of a vitamin K antagonist.

Phylloquinone (AQUAMEPHYTON, KONAKION, MEPHYTON) is available as tablets and in a dispersion with buffered polysorbate and propylene glycol (KONAKION) or polyoxyethylated fatty acid derivatives and dextrose (AQUAMEPHYTON). KONAKION is administered only intramuscularly. AQUAMEPHYTON may be given by any parenteral route; however, subcutaneous or intramuscular injection is preferred because severe reactions resembling anaphylaxis have followed its intravenous administration.

Inadequate Intake. After infancy, hypoprothrombinemia due to dietary deficiency of vitamin K is extremely rare: The vitamin is present in many foods and also is synthesized by intestinal bacteria. Occasionally, the use of a broad-spectrum antibiotic may itself produce a hypoprothrombinemia that responds readily to small doses of vitamin K and reestablishment of normal bowel flora. Hypoprothrombinemia can occur in patients receiving prolonged intravenous alimentation. It is recommended to give 1 mg of phylloquinone per week (the equivalent of about 150 μg per day) to patients on total parenteral nutrition.

Hypoprothrombinemia of the Newborn. Healthy newborn infants show decreased plasma concentrations of vitamin K–dependent clotting factors for a few days after birth, the time required to obtain an adequate dietary intake of the vitamin and to establish a normal intestinal flora. In premature infants and in infants with hemorrhagic disease of the newborn, the concentrations of clotting factors are particularly depressed. The degree to which these changes reflect true vitamin K deficiency is controversial. Measurements of non-γ-carboxylated prothrombin suggests that vitamin K deficiency occurs in about 3% of live births (Shapiro *et al.*, 1986).

Hemorrhagic disease of the newborn has been associated with breast-feeding; human milk has low concentrations of vitamin K (Haroon *et al.*, 1982). In addition, the intestinal flora of breast-fed infants may lack microorganisms that synthesize the vitamin (Keenan *et al.*, 1971). Commercial infant formulas are supplemented with vitamin K.

In the neonate with hemorrhagic disease of the newborn, the administration of vitamin K raises the concentration of these clotting factors to the level normal for the newborn infant and controls the bleeding tendency within about 6 hours. The routine administration of 1 mg phylloquinone intramuscularly at birth is required by law in the United States. This dose may have to be increased or repeated if the mother has received anticoagulant or anticonvulsant drug therapy or if the infant develops bleeding tendencies. Alternatively, some clinicians treat mothers who are receiving anticonvulsants with oral vitamin K prior to delivery (20 mg per day for 2 weeks) (Vert and Deblay, 1982).

Inadequate Absorption. Vitamin K is poorly absorbed in the absence of bile. Thus, hypoprothrombinemia may be associated with either intrahepatic or extrahepatic biliary obstruction or a severe defect in the intestinal absorption of fat from other causes.

Biliary Obstruction or Fistula. Bleeding that accompanies obstructive jaundice or biliary fistula responds promptly to the administration of vitamin K. Oral phylloquinone administered with bile salts is both safe and effective and should be used in the care of the jaundiced patient, both preoperatively and postoperatively. In the absence of significant hepatocellular disease, the prothrombin activity of the blood rapidly returns to normal. If oral administration is not feasible, a parenteral preparation should be used. The usual dose is 10 mg of vitamin K per day.

The treatment of a patient during hemorrhage requires transfusion of fresh blood or reconstituted fresh plasma. Vitamin K also should be given. If biliary obstruction has caused hepatic injury, the response to vitamin K may be poor.

Malabsorption Syndromes. Among the disorders that result in inadequate absorption of vitamin K from the intestinal tract are: cystic fibrosis, sprue, Crohn's disease and enterocolitis, ulcerative colitis, dysentery, and extensive resection of bowel. Since drugs that greatly reduce the bacterial population of the bowel are used frequently in many of these disorders, the availability of the vitamin may be further reduced. Moreover, dietary restrictions also may limit the availability of the vitamin. For immediate correction of the deficiency, parenteral therapy should be used.

Inadequate Utilization. Hepatocellular disease may be accompanied or followed by hypoprothrombinemia. Hepatocellular damage also may be secondary to long-lasting biliary obstruction. In these conditions, the damaged parenchymal cells may not be able to produce the vitamin K–dependent clotting factors, even if excess vitamin is available. However, if an inadequate secretion of bile salts is contributing to the syndrome, some benefit may be obtained from the parenteral administration of 10 mg of phylloquinone daily. Paradoxically, the administration of large doses of vitamin K or its analogs in an attempt to correct the hypoprothrombinemia associated with severe hepatitis or cirrhosis actually may result in a further depression of the concentration of prothrombin. The mechanism for this action is unknown.

Drug-Induced Hypoprothrombinemia. Anticoagulant drugs such as warfarin and its congeners act as competitive antagonists of vitamin K and interfere with the hepatic biosynthesis of Gla-containing clotting factors. The treatment of bleeding caused by oral anticoagulants is discussed above. Vitamin K may be of help in combating the bleeding and hypoprothrombinemia that follow the bite of the tropical American pit viper or other species whose venom destroys or inactivates prothrombin.

CLINICAL SUMMARY

A variety of anticoagulant, thrombolytic, and antiplatelet agents are available and are among the most widely used drugs. Heparin and its low-molecular-weight derivatives are commonly used to treat venous thromboembolism, unstable angina, and acute myocardial infarction; these agents are also used to prevent thrombosis during and after coronary angioplasty, during surgery requiring cardiopulmonary bypass, and in certain other high-risk patients. The major toxicities of heparin are bleeding and the syndrome of heparin-induced thrombocytopenia, which often precipitates venous or arterial thrombosis. Direct thrombin inhibitors, such as lepirudin or argatroban, are indicated for patients with heparin-induced thrombocytopenia. Warfarin and other vitamin K antagonists are used to prevent the progression or recurrence of acute venous thromboembolism following an initial course of heparin. They also decrease the incidence of systemic embolization in patients with prosthetic heart valves or after acute myocardial infarction. Warfarin causes major bleeding in a significant number of patients and produces fetal abnormalities when given during pregnancy. Fibrinolytic agents, such as t-PA or streptokinase, reduce the mortality of acute myocardial infarction and are used in situations in which angioplasty is not readily available. Antiplatelet agents, including aspirin, ticlopidine, clopidogrel, and glycoprotein IIb/IIIa inhibitors, are often used to prevent restenosis and thrombosis following coronary angioplasty and in the secondary prophylaxis of myocardial infarction and stroke. Bleeding is the major toxicity of the antiplatelet agents, but thrombocytopenia and neutropenia can also occur. New agents, such as the oral direct thrombin inhibitor ximelagatran, may prove to be more effective, less toxic, and easier to use than currently available drugs.

BIBLIOGRAPHY

Almquist, H.J., and Stokstad, C.L.R. Hemorrhagic chick disease of dietary origin. *J. Biol. Chem.*, **1935,** *111:*105–113.

Andersen, H.R., Nielsen, T.T., Rasmussen, K., *et al.* DANAMI-2 Investigators. A comparison of coronary angioplasty with fibrinolytic therapy in acute myocardial infarction. *N. Engl. J. Med.*, **2003**, *349:*733–742.

Antithrombotic Trialists' Collaboration. Collaborative meta-analysis of randomised trials of antiplatelet therapy for prevention of death, myocardial infarction, and stroke in high risk patients. *BMJ*, **2002**, *324:*71–86. Erratum in: *BMJ*, **2002**, *324:*141.

Belch, J.J., Lowe, G.D., Ward, A.G., *et al.* Prevention of deep vein thrombosis in medical patients by low-dose heparin. *Scott. Med. J.*, **1981**, *26:*115–117.

Bennett, C.L., Connors, J.M., Carwile, J.M., *et al.* Thrombotic thrombocytopenic purpura associated with clopidogrel. *N. Engl. J. Med.*, **2000**, *342:*1773–1777.

Bennett, C.L., Davidson, C.J., Raisch, D.W., *et al.* Thrombotic thrombocytopenic purpura associated with ticlopidine in the setting of coronary artery stents and stroke prevention. *Arch. Intern. Med.*, **1999**, *159:*2524–2528.

Bennett, C.L., Weinberg, P.D., Rozenberg-Ben-Dror, K., *et al.* Thrombotic thrombocytopenic purpura associated with ticlopidine. A review of 60 cases. *Ann. Intern. Med.*, **1998**, *128:*541–544.

Bentley, R., and Meganathan, R. Biosynthesis of vitamin K (menaquinone) in bacteria. *Microbiol. Rev.*, **1982**, *46:*241–280.

Boersma, E., Harrington, R.A., Moliterno, D.J., *et al.* Platelet glycoprotein IIb/IIIa inhibitors in acute coronary syndromes: a meta-analysis of all major randomised clinical trials. *Lancet*, **2002**, *359:*189–198. Erratum in: *Lancet*, **2002**, *359:*2120.

Brown, M.A., Stenberg, L.M., Persson, U., and Stenflo, J. Identification and purification of vitamin K-dependent proteins and peptides with monoclonal antibodies specific for γ-carboxyglutamyl (Gla) residues. *J. Biol. Chem.*, **2000**, *275:*19795–19802.

Broze, G., Jr. Protein Z-dependent regulation of coagulation. *Thromb. Haemost.*, **2001**, *86:*1–13.

Buller, H.R., Davidson, B.L., Decousus, H., *et al.* Matisse Investigators. Subcutaneous fondaparinux versus intravenous unfractionated heparin in the initial treatment of pulmonary embolism. *N. Engl. J. Med.*, **2003**, *349:*1695–1702. Erratum in: *N. Engl. J. Med.*, **2004**, *350:*423.

Butt, H.R., Snell, A.M., and Osterberg, A.E. The use of vitamin K and bile in treatment of hemorrhagic diathesis in cases of jaundice. *Proc. Staff Meet. Mayo Clin.*, **1938**, *13:*74–80.

Cade, J.F. High risk of the critically ill for venous thromboembolism. *Crit. Care Med.*, **1982**, *10:*448–450.

Dam, H., and Schønheyder, F. The antihaemorrhagic vitamin of the chick. *Nature*, **1935**, *135:*652–653.

Dam, H., Schønheyder, F., and Tage-Hansen, E. Studies on the mode of action of vitamin K. *Biochem. J.*, **1936**, *30:*1075–1079.

Diener, H.C., Cunha, L., Forbes, C., *et al.*, European Stroke Prevention Study. 2. Dipyridamole and acetylsalicylic acid in the secondary prevention of stroke. *J. Neurol. Sci.*, **1996**, *143:*1–13.

Diploma, J.R., and Ritchie, D.M. Vitamin toxicity. *Annu. Rev. Pharmacol. Toxicol.*, **1997**, *17:*133–148.

Feskanich, D., Weber, P., Willett, W.C., *et al.* Vitamin K intake and hip fractures in women: a prospective study. *Am. J. Clin. Nutr.*, **1999**, *69:*74–79.

Francis, C.W., Berkowitz, S.D., Comp, P.C., *et al.* EXULT A Study Group. Comparison of ximelagatran with warfarin for the prevention of venous thromboembolism after total knee replacement. *N. Engl. J. Med.*, **2003**, *349:*1703–1712.

Frick, P.G., Riedler, G., and Brögli, H. Dose response and minimal daily requirement for vitamin K in man. *J. Appl. Physiol.*, **1967**, *23:*387–389.

Gardlund, B. Randomised, controlled trial of low-dose heparin for prevention of fatal pulmonary embolism in patients with infectious diseases. *Lancet*, **1996**, *347:*1357–1361.

GUSTO III (The Global Use of Strategies to Open Occluded Coronary Arteries) Investigators. A comparison of reteplase with alteplase for acute myocardial infarction. *N. Engl. J. Med.*, **1997**, *337:*1118–1123.

Haroon, Y., Shearer, M.J., Rahim, S., *et al.* The content of phylloquinone (vitamin K_1) in human milk, cows' milk, and infant formula foods determined by high-performance liquid chromatography. *J. Nutr.*, **1982**, *112:*1105–1117.

Hawkins, W.B., and Brinkhous, K.M. Prothrombin deficiency as the cause of bleeding in bile fistula dogs. *J. Exp. Med.*, **1936**, *63:*795–801.

Hollopeter, G., Jantzen, H.M., Vincent, D., *et al.* Identification of the platelet ADP receptor targeted by antithrombotic drugs. *Nature*, **2001**, *409:*202–207.

Hylek, E.M., Heiman, H., Skates, S.J., *et al.* Acetaminophen and other risk factors for excessive warfarin anticoagulation. *JAMA*, **1998**, *279:*657–662.

Jin, J., and Kunapuli, S.P. Coactivation of two different G protein-coupled receptors is essential for ADP-induced platelet aggregation. *Proc. Natl. Acad. Sci. U. S. A.*, **1998**, *95:*8070–8074.

Keenan, W.J., Jewett, T., and Glueck, H.I. Role of feeding and vitamin K in hypoprothrombinemia of the newborn. *Am. J. Dis. Child.*, **1971**, *121:*271–277.

Kulman, J.D., Harris, J.E., Xie, L., and Davie, E.W. Identification of two novel transmembrane γ-carboxyglutamic acid proteins expressed broadly in fetal and adult tissues. *Proc. Natl. Acad. Sci. U. S. A.*, **2001**, *98:*1370–1375.

Leon, M.B., Baim, D.S., Popma, J.J., *et al.* A clinical trial comparing three antithrombotic-drug regimens after coronary-artery stenting. Stent Anticoagulation Restenosis Study Investigators. *N. Engl. J. Med.*, **1998**, *339:*1665–1671.

Li, T., Chang, C.Y., Jin, D.Y., *et al.* Identification of the gene for vitamin K epoxide reductase. *Nature*, **2004**, *427:*541–544.

Moll, S., and Ortel, T.L. Monitoring warfarin therapy in patients with lupus anticoagulants. *Ann. Intern. Med.*, **1997**, *127:*177–185.

Mutucumarana, V.P., Acher, F., Straight, D.L., *et al.* A conserved region of human vitamin K-dependent carboxylase between residues 398 and 404 is important for its interaction with the glutamate substrate. *J. Biol. Chem.*, **2003**, *278:*46488–46493.

Quick, A.J., Stanley-Brown, M., and Bancroft, F.W. A study of the coagulation defect in hemophilia and in jaundice. *Am. J. Med. Sci.*, **1935**, *190:*501–511.

Rishavy, M.A., Pudota, B.N., Hallgren, K.W., *et al.* A new model for vitamin K-dependent carboxylation: The catalytic base that deprotonates vitamin K hydroquinone is not Cys but an activated amine. *Proc. Natl. Acad. Sci. U. S. A.*, **2004**, *101:*13732–13737.

Rosen, H.N., Maitland, L.A., Suttie, J.W., *et al.* Vitamin K and maintenance of skeletal integrity in adults. *Am. J. Med.*, **1993**, *94:*62–68.

Rost, S., Fregin, A., Ivaskevicius, V., *et al.* Mutations in VKORC1 cause warfarin resistance and multiple coagulation factor deficiency type 2. *Nature*, **2004**, *427:*537–541.

Sadowski, J.A., Hood, S.J., Dallal, G.E., and Garry, P.J. Phylloquinone in plasma from elderly and young adults: factors influencing its concentration. *Am. J. Clin. Nutr.*, **1989**, *50:*100–108.

Savi, P., Pereillo, J.M., Uzabiaga, M.F., *et al.* Identification and biological activity of the active metabolite of clopidogrel. *Thromb. Haemost.*, **2000**, *84:*891–896.

Schulman, S., Wahlander, K., Lundstrom, T., *et al.* THRIVE III Investigators. Secondary prevention of venous thromboembolism with the oral direct thrombin inhibitor ximelagatran. *N. Engl. J. Med.*, **2003**, *349:*1713–1721.

Shapiro, A.D., Jacobson, L.J., Armon, M.E., *et al.* Vitamin K deficiency in the newborn infant: prevalence and perinatal risk factors. *J. Pediatr.,* **1986,** *109:*675–680.

The Sixth American College of Chest Physicians Guidelines for Antithrombotic Therapy for Prevention and Treatment of Thrombosis (2000). Hirsh, J., Warkentin, T.E., Shaughnessy, S.G., *et al.* Heparin and low-molecular-weight heparin: mechanisms of action, pharmacokinetics, dosing, monitoring, efficacy, and safety. *Chest,* **2001,** *119*(1 suppl.):64S–94S.

Steinhubl, S.R., Berger, P.B., Mann, J.T. 3rd, *et al.* CREDO Investigators. Early and sustained dual oral antiplatelet therapy following percutaneous coronary intervention: a randomized controlled trial. *JAMA,* **2002,** *288:*2411–2420.

Wajih, N., Sane, D.C., Hutson S.M., and Wallin, R. The inhibitory effect of calumenin on the vitamin K-dependent γ-carboxylation system. Characterization of the system in normal and warfarin-resistant rats. *J. Biol. Chem.,* **2004,** *279:*25276–25283.

Warner, E.D., Brinkhous, K.M., and Smith, H.P. Bleeding tendency of obstructive jaundice: prothrombin deficiency and dietary factors. *Proc. Soc. Exp. Biol. Med.,* **1938,** *37:*628–630.

Yusuf, S., Zhao, F., Mehta, S.R., *et al.* Clopidogrel in Unstable Angina to Prevent Recurrent Events Trial Investigators. Effects of clopidogrel in addition to aspirin in patients with acute coronary syndromes without ST-segment elevation. *N. Engl. J. Med.,* **2001,** *345:*494–502.

Zijlstra, F., Hoorntje, J.C.A., de Boer, M.J., *et al.* Long-term benefit of primary angioplasty as compared with thrombolytic therapy for acute myocardial infarction. *N. Engl. J. Med.,* **1999,** *341:*1413–1419.

Zivelin, A., Rao, L.V., and Rapaport, S.I. Mechanism of the anticoagulant effect of warfarin as evaluated in rabbits by selective depression of individual procoagulant vitamin K-dependent clotting factors. *J. Clin. Invest.,* **1993,** *92:*2131–2140.

MONOGRAPHS AND REVIEWS

Armstrong, P.W., Collen, D., Antman, E. Fibrinolysis for acute myocardial infarction: the future is here and now. *Circulation,* **2003,** *107:*2533–2537.

Collins, R., Peto, R., Baigent, C., and Sleight, P. Aspirin, heparin, and fibrinolytic therapy in suspected acute myocardial infarction. *N. Engl. J. Med.,* **1997,** *336:*847–860.

Daly, A.K., and King, B.P. Pharmacogenetics of oral anticoagulants. *Pharmacogenetics,* **2003,** *13:*247–252.

Edelberg, J.M., Christie, P.D., and Rosenberg, R.D. Regulation of vascular bed-specific prothrombotic potential. *Circ. Res.,* **2001,** *89:*117–124.

Esmon, C.T. The protein C pathway. *Chest,* **2003,** *124*(Suppl.):26S–32S.

Hirsh, J., Anand, S.S., Halperin, J.L., and Fuster, V. Guide to anticoagulant therapy. Heparin: a statement for healthcare professionals from the American Heart Association. *Circulation,* **2001,** *103:*2994–3018.

Hirsh, J., Fuster, V., Ansell, J., and Halperin, J.L. American Heart Association/American College of Cardiology Foundation guide to warfarin therapy. *Circulation,* **2003,** *107:*1692–1711.

Lijnen, H.R., and Collen, D. Fibrinolysis and the control of hemostasis. In, *The Molecular Basis of Blood Diseases,* 3rd ed. (Stamatoyannopoulos, G., Majerus, P.W., Perlmutter, R.M., and Varmus, H., eds) W.B. Saunders Co., Philadelphia, **2001,** pp. 740–763.

Mann, K.G., Butenas, S., and Brummel, K. The dynamics of thrombin formation. *Arterioscler. Thromb. Vasc. Biol.,* **2003,** *23:*17–25.

Olson, S.T., and Chuang, Y.J. Heparin activates antithrombin anticoagulant function by generating new interaction sites (exosites) for blood clotting proteinases. *Trends Cardiovasc. Med.,* **2002,** *12:*331–338.

Patrono, C., Bachmann, F., Baigent, C., *et al.* European Society of Cardiology. Expert consensus document on the use of antiplatelet agents. The task force on the use of antiplatelet agents in patients with atherosclerotic cardiovascular disease of the European Society of Cardiology. *Eur. Heart J.,* **2004,** *25:*166–181.

Patrono, C., Coller, B., Dalen, J.E., *et al.* Platelet-active drugs: the relationships among dose, effectiveness, and side effects. *Chest,* **1998,** *114:*470S–488S.

Quinn, M.J., and Fitzgerald, D.J. Ticlopidine and clopidogrel. *Circulation,* **1999,** *100:*1667–1672.

Scarborough, R.M., Kleiman, N.S., and Phillips, D.R. Platelet glycoprotein IIb/IIIa antagonists. What are the relevant issues concerning their pharmacology and clinical use? *Circulation,* **1999,** *100:*437–444.

Sugahara, K., and Kitagawa, H. Heparin and heparan sulfate biosynthesis. *IUBMB Life,* **2002,** *54:*163–175.

Vert, P., and Deblay, M.F. Hemorrhagic disorders in infants of epileptic mothers. In, *Epilepsy, Pregnancy, and the Child.* (Janz, D., Bossi, L., Daum, M., *et al.,* eds.) Raven Press, New York, **1982,** pp. 387–388.

Warkentin, T.E. Heparin-induced thrombocytopenia: pathogenesis and management. *Br. J. Haematol.,* **2003,** *121:*535–555.

CHAPTER

55

PITUITARY HORMONES AND THEIR HYPOTHALAMIC RELEASING HORMONES

Keith L. Parker and Bernard P. Schimmer

The peptide hormones of the anterior pituitary are essential for the regulation of growth and development, reproduction, responses to stress, and intermediary metabolism. Their synthesis and secretion are controlled by hypothalamic hormones and by hormones from the peripheral endocrine organs. A large number of disease states, as well as a diverse group of drugs, also affect their secretion. The complex interactions among the hypothalamus, pituitary, and peripheral endocrine glands provide elegant examples of integrated feedback regulation. Clinically, an improved understanding of the mechanisms that underlie these interactions provides the rationale for diagnosing and treating endocrine disorders and for predicting certain side effects of drugs that affect the endocrine system. Moreover, the elucidation of the structures of the anterior pituitary hormones and hypothalamic-releasing hormones makes it possible to produce synthetic peptide agonists and antagonists that have important diagnostic and therapeutic applications.

The anterior pituitary hormones can be classified into three different groups based on their structural features (Table 55–1). *Growth hormone* (GH) and *prolactin* (PRL) belong to the somatotropic family of hormones, which in humans also includes placental lactogen. The glycoprotein hormones—*thyroid-stimulating hormone* (TSH, also called thyrotropin), *luteinizing hormone* (LH), and *follicle-stimulating hormone* (FSH)—share a common α-sub-

unit but have different β-subunits that determine their distinct biological activities. In humans, the glycoprotein hormone family also includes *human chorionic gonadotropin* (hCG). *Corticotropin* (adrenocorticotropic hormone; ACTH) and α-*melanocyte-stimulating hormone* (α-MSH) are part of a family of peptides derived from *pro-opiomelanocortin* (POMC) by proteolytic processing (*see* Chapter 59).

The synthesis and release of anterior pituitary hormones are influenced by the central nervous system. Their secretion is positively regulated by a group of peptides referred to as *hypothalamic releasing hormones*, which are released from hypothalamic neurons in the region of the median eminence and reach the anterior pituitary through the hypothalamic-adenohypophyseal portal system (Figure 55–1). The hypothalamic releasing hormones include *growth hormone–releasing hormone* (GHRH), *gonadotropin-releasing hormone* (GnRH), *thyrotropin-releasing hormone* (TRH), and *corticotropin-releasing hormone* (CRH). *Somatostatin* (SST), another hypothalamic peptide, negatively regulates pituitary secretion of growth hormone and thyrotropin. The catecholamine *dopamine* inhibits the secretion of prolactin by lactotropes.

The posterior pituitary gland, also known as the neurohypophysis, contains the endings of nerve axons arising from distinct populations of neurons in the supraoptic and

Table 55–1

Properties of the Protein Hormones of the Human Adenohypophysis and Placenta

HORMONE	MOLECULAR MASS, DALTONS	PEPTIDE CHAINS	AMINO ACID RESIDUES	CHROMOSOMAL LOCATION	COMMENTS
Somatotropic hormones					
Growth hormone (GH)	22,000	1	191	17q22-24	
Prolactin (PRL)	23,000	1	199	6p22.2-21.3	
Placental lactogen (PL)	22,125	1	190	17q22-24	
Glycoprotein hormones					
Luteinizing hormone (LH)	29,400	2	α-92	6q12.q21	
			β-121	19q13.3	Heterodimeric glycoproteins with a common α-subunit and unique β-subunits that determine biological specificity
Follicle-stimulating hormone (FSH)	32,600	2	α-92	6q12.q21	
			β-111	11p13	
Human chorionic gonadotropin (hCG)	38,600	2	α-92	6q12.q21	
			β-145	19q13.3	
Thyroid-stimulating hormone (TSH)	28,000	2	α-92	6q12.q21	
			β-118	1p13	
*POMC-derived hormones**					
Corticotropin (ACTH)	4500	1	39	2p22.3	These peptides are derived by proteolytic processing of the common precursor, pro-opiomelanocortin (POMC)
α-Melanocyte-stimulating hormone (α-MSH)	1650	1	13		

*See Chapter 59 for further discussion of POMC-derived peptides, including ACTH and α-MSH.

paraventricular nuclei that synthesize either *arginine vasopressin* or *oxytocin* (Figure 55–1). Arginine vasopressin plays an important role in water homeostasis (*see* Chapter 29); oxytocin plays important roles in labor and parturition and in milk let-down, as discussed below.

GROWTH HORMONE

The gene encoding human growth hormone (GH) resides on the long arm of chromosome 17 (17q22), which also contains three different variants of placental lactogen and a GH variant expressed in the syncytiotrophoblast (chorionic somatotropin). Secreted GH is a heterogeneous mixture of peptides; the principal 22,000-dalton form is a single polypeptide chain of 191 amino acids that has two disulfide bonds and is not glycosylated. Alternative splicing deletes residues 32 to 46 of the larger form to produce a smaller form (~20,000 daltons) with equal bioactivity that makes up 5% to 10% of circulating GH. Additional GH species, differing in size or charge, are found in

serum, but their physiological significance is unclear. In the circulation, approximately 45% of the 22,000-dalton and 25% of the 20,000-dalton GH are bound by a 55,000-dalton binding protein that contains the extracellular domain of the GH receptor and apparently arises from proteolytic cleavage. A second protein unrelated to the GH receptor also binds approximately 5% to 10% of circulating GH with lower affinity. Bound GH is cleared more slowly and has a biological half-life approximately 10 times that of unbound GH, suggesting that the binding protein may provide a GH reservoir that dampens acute fluctuations in GH levels associated with its pulsatile secretion. Alternatively, the binding protein may decrease GH bioactivity by preventing it from binding to its receptor in target tissues. Obesity and estrogen treatment increase circulating levels of GH binding proteins, and thus may affect the clinical response to exogenous GH.

Regulation of Growth Hormone Secretion

Growth hormone, the most abundant anterior pituitary hormone, is synthesized and secreted by somatotropes.

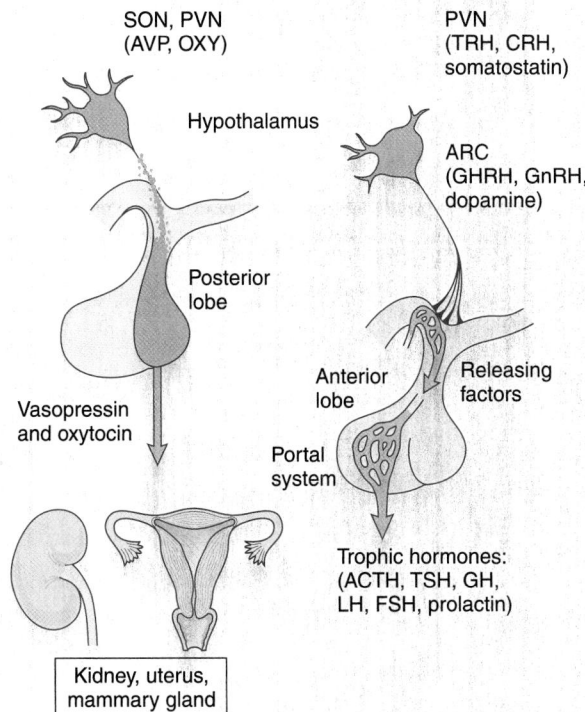

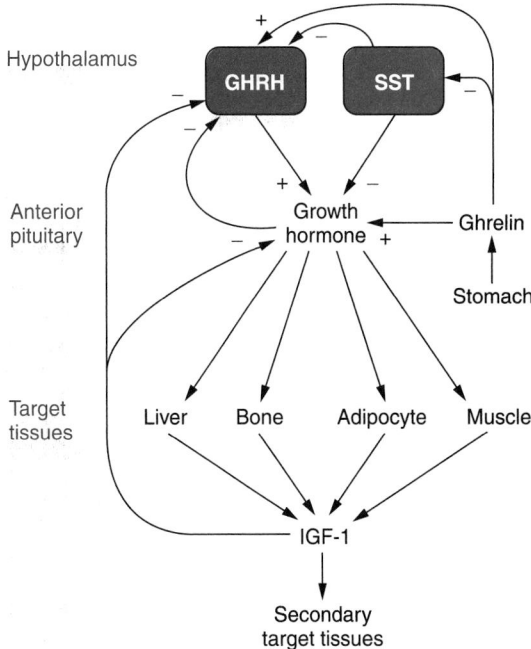

Figure 55–1. Organization of the anterior and posterior pituitary gland. Hypothalamic neurons in the supraoptic (SON) and paraventricular (PVN) nuclei synthesize arginine vasopressin (AVP) or oxytocin (OXY). Most of their axons project directly to the posterior pituitary, from which AVP and OXY are secreted into the systemic circulation to regulate their target tissues. Neurons that regulate the anterior lobe cluster in the mediobasal hypothalamus, including the PVN and the arcuate (ARC) nuclei. They secrete hypothalamic releasing hormones, which reach the anterior pituitary *via* the hypothalamic-adenohypophyseal portal system and stimulate distinct populations of pituitary cells. These cells, in turn, secrete the trophic hormones, which regulate endocrine organs and other tissues.

Figure 55–2. Secretion and actions of growth hormone. Two hypothalamic factors, growth hormone-releasing hormone (GHRH) and somatostatin (SST), act on the somatotropes in the anterior pituitary to regulate growth hormone secretion. SST also inhibits GHRH release. Growth hormone exerts direct effects on target tissues and indirect effects mediated by stimulating the release of insulin-like growth factor-1 (IGF-1). The gastric peptide ghrelin enhances growth hormone release, directly by actions at the anterior pituitary and indirectly by multiple actions on the hypothalamus. IGF-1 feeds back at the anterior pituitary to inhibit growth hormone secretion and also to inhibit further GHRH release by the hypothalamus.

The somatotropes account for about 40% of hormone-secreting cells of the anterior pituitary and cluster at the lateral wings of the gland. Daily GH secretion varies throughout life; secretion is high in children, reaches maximal levels at puberty, and then decreases in an age-related manner in adulthood. GH is secreted in discrete but irregular pulses. Between these pulses, circulating GH falls to levels that are undetectable with most current assays. The amplitude of secretory pulses is maximal at night, and the most consistent period of GH secretion is shortly after the onset of deep sleep.

The regulation of GH secretion, as illustrated in Figure 55–2, incorporates many of the features of the classic negative feedback systems seen in other endocrine axes.

GHRH, produced by hypothalamic neurons found predominantly in the arcuate nucleus, stimulates GH secretion by binding to a specific G protein–coupled receptor on somatotropes that resembles most closely the receptors for secretin, vasoactive intestinal polypeptide, pituitary adenylyl cyclase–activating peptide, glucagon, glucagon-like peptide 1, calcitonin, and parathyroid hormone. Upon binding GHRH, the GHRH receptor couples to G_s to elevate intracellular cyclic AMP and Ca^{2+} concentrations and thereby stimulates GH synthesis and secretion. Loss-of-function mutations of the GHRH receptor cause a rare form of dwarfism in human beings, thereby demonstrating the essential role of the GHRH receptor in normal GH secretion.

Typical of other endocrine systems, GH and its predominant peripheral effector, insulin-like growth factor-1 (IGF-1), act in negative feedback loops to suppress GH secretion. The negative effect of IGF-1 is predominantly through direct effects on the anterior pituitary gland. In contrast, the negative feedback action of GH is mediated in part by SST, which is synthesized by more widely distributed neurons, as well as by neuroendocrine cells in the gastrointestinal tract and pancreas.

Somatostatin is synthesized as a 92-amino-acid precursor and processed by proteolytic cleavage to generate two predominant forms: SST-14 and SST-28. The somatostatins exert their effects by binding to and activating a family of five related G protein–coupled receptors that signal through G_i to inhibit cyclic AMP accumulation and to activate K^+ channels and phosphotyrosine phosphatases. Each of the SST receptor subtypes (abbreviated SSTR or sstr) binds SST with nanomolar affinity; whereas receptor types 1 to 4 (SSTR1–4) bind the two SSTs with approximately equal affinity, type 5 (SSTR5) has a ten- to fifteenfold greater selectivity for somatostatin-28. SSTR2 and SSTR5 are the most important for regulation of GH secretion. SST exerts direct effects on somatotropes in the pituitary and indirect effects mediated *via* GHRH neurons in the arcuate nucleus. As discussed below, SST analogs play a key role in the therapy of syndromes of GH excess such as acromegaly.

Appreciation of a third regulator of GH secretion has emerged from the development of peptide and nonpeptide compounds, called GH secretagogues, that stimulate GH secretion. These secretagogues act primarily through a distinct G protein–coupled receptor, called the GH secretagogue receptor. Although GH secretagogues directly stimulate GH release by isolated somatotropes, their major action on GH secretion apparently is through actions on the GHRH neurons in the arcuate nucleus. The endogenous ligand for the GH secretagogue receptor is ghrelin, a 28-amino-acid peptide with an octanoylated serine at residue 3. Ghrelin is synthesized predominantly in endocrine cells in the fundus of the stomach, but also is produced at lower levels at a number of other sites. Both fasting and hypoglycemia stimulate circulating ghrelin levels. In human beings and experimental animals, ghrelin stimulates appetite and increases food intake, apparently by central actions on NPY and agouti-related peptide neurons in the hypothalamus. Thus ghrelin and its receptor play complex roles to integrate the gastrointestinal tract, the hypothalamus, and the anterior pituitary (Yoshihara *et al.*, 2002).

Several neurotransmitters, drugs, metabolites, and other stimuli modulate the release of GHRH and/or SST and thereby affect GH secretion. Dopamine, 5-hydroxytryptamine, and α_2 adrenergic receptor agonists stimulate GH release, as do hypoglycemia, exercise, stress, emotional excitement, and ingestion of protein-rich meals. In contrast, β adrenergic receptor agonists, free fatty acids, insulin-like growth factor-1 (IGF-1, *see* below), and GH itself inhibit release, as does the administration of glucose to normal subjects in an oral glucose tolerance test.

These observations form the basis for provocative tests to assess the ability of the pituitary to secrete GH. Provocative stimuli include arginine, glucagon, insulin-induced hypoglycemia, clonidine, and the dopamine precursor levodopa; these agents all increase circulating GH levels in normal subjects within 45 to 90 minutes. At present, insulin-induced hypoglycemia is preferred by some authorities, whereas the FDA recommends two independent tests of GH deficiency to establish the diagnosis. When excess GH secretion is suspected (*see* below), the failure of an oral glucose load to suppress GH is diagnostically useful. Finally, as described below, GH secretion in response to GHRH can be used to distinguish pituitary disease from hypothalamic disease.

Molecular and Cellular Bases of Growth Hormone Action

All of the effects of GH result from its interactions with the GH receptor, as evidenced by the severe phenotype of rare patients with homozygous mutations of the GH receptor gene (the Laron syndrome of GH-resistant dwarfism). The GH receptor is a widely distributed cell-surface receptor that belongs to the Class I cytokine receptor superfamily and thus shares structural similarity with the receptors for prolactin, erythropoietin, granulocyte-macrophage colony-stimulating factor, and several of the interleukins. Like other members of the cytokine receptor family, the GH receptor contains an extracellular domain that binds GH, a single membrane-spanning region, and an intracellular domain that mediates signal transduction. Receptor activation results from the binding of a single GH molecule to two identical receptor molecules, forming a ligand-occupied receptor dimer that presumably brings the intracellular domains of the receptor into close proximity to activate cytosolic components critical for cell signaling.

The mature human GH receptor contains 620 amino acids, ~250 of which are extracellular, 24 of which are transmembrane, and ~350 of which are cytoplasmic. The GH receptor exists as a dimer and forms a ternary complex with one molecule of GH. The formation of the GH-GH receptor ternary complex is initiated by high-affinity interaction of GH with one monomer of the GH receptor dimer (mediated by GH site 1), followed by a second interaction of GH with the GH receptor (mediated by GH site 2); these interactions induce a conformational change that activates downstream signaling. Guided by structure-function analyses, GH analogs have been engineered with a disrupted site 2; these analogs bind the receptor and induce its internalization but cannot induce a conformational change or stimulate downstream events in the signal transduction pathway. One such analog, *pegvisomant,* behaves as a GH antagonist and is used for the treatment of acromegaly (Kopchick *et al.*, 2002; *see* below).

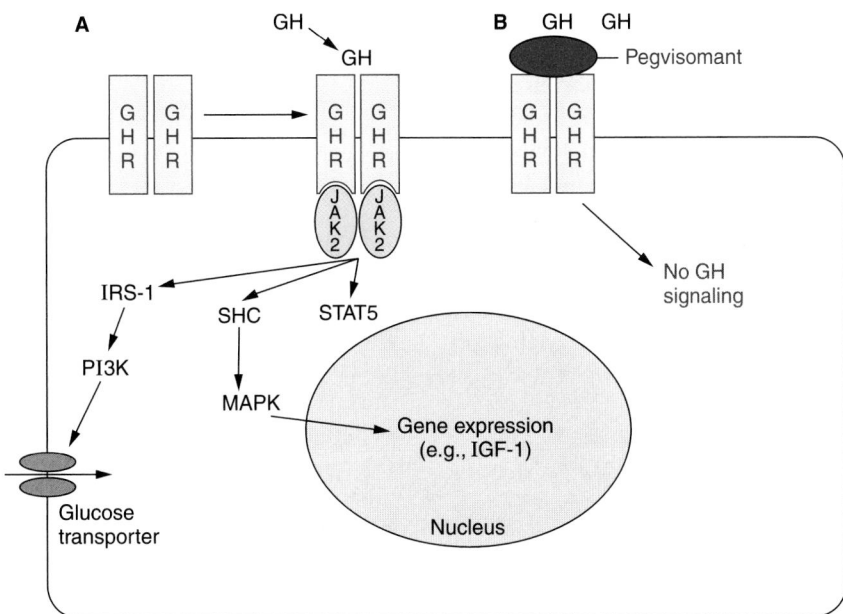

Figure 55–3. *Mechanisms of growth hormone and prolactin action and of GH receptor antagonism.* **A.** The binding of GH to two molecules of the growth hormone receptor (GHR) induces autophosphorylation of JAK2. JAK2 then phosphorylates cytoplasmic proteins that activate downstream signaling pathways, including signal transducer and activator of transcription (Stat)5 and mediators upstream of mitogen-activated protein kinase (MAPK), which ultimately modulate gene expression. The structurally related prolactin receptor also is a ligand-activated homodimer that recruits the JAK-Stat signaling pathway (*see* text for further details). The GHR also activates the insulin receptor substrate-1 (IRS-1), which may mediate the increased expression of glucose transporters on the plasma membrane. The diagram does not reflect the localization of the intracellular molecules, which presumably exist in multicomponent signaling complexes. **B.** Pegvisomant, a recombinant pegylated variant of human GH, contains mutations that increase the affinity for the GHR but do not activate downstream signaling by the GHR. It thus interferes with GH signaling in target tissues. JAK2, Janus kinase 2; IRS-1, insulin receptor substrate-1; PI3K, phosphatidyl inositol-3 kinase; STAT, signal transducer and activator of transcription; MAPK, mitogen-activated protein kinase; SHC, Src homology containing.

The ligand-occupied receptor dimer does not have inherent tyrosine kinase activity, but rather provides docking sites for two molecules of Jak2, a cytoplasmic tyrosine kinase of the Janus kinase family. The juxtaposition of two Jak2 molecules leads to *trans*-phosphorylation and autoactivation of Jak2, with consequent tyrosine phosphorylation of cytoplasmic proteins that mediate downstream signaling events (Herrington and Carter-Su, 2001). These include Stat proteins (*signal transducers and activators of transcription*), Shc (an adapter protein that regulates the Ras/MAP kinase signaling pathway), and IRS-1 and IRS-2 (insulin-receptor substrate proteins that activate the PI3 kinase regulatory pathway) (Figure 55–3).

Physiological Effects of Growth Hormone

The most striking physiological effect of GH—and the basis for its name—is the stimulation of the longitudinal growth of bones. GH also increases bone mineral density after longitudinal growth ceases and epiphyses have closed. These effects of GH involve the differentiation of prechondrocytes to chondrocytes and stimulation of osteoclast and osteoblast proliferation. Other effects of GH include the stimulation of myoblast differentiation (in experimental animals) and increased muscle mass (in human subjects with growth hormone deficiency), increased glomerular filtration rate, and stimulation of preadipocyte differentiation into adipocytes. GH has potent anti-insulin actions in both the liver and peripheral sites (*e.g.,* adipocytes and muscle) that decrease glucose utilization and increase lipolysis. Finally, GH has been implicated in the development and function of the immune system.

GH acts directly on adipocytes to increase lipolysis and on hepatocytes to stimulate gluconeogenesis, but its anabolic and growth-promoting effects are mediated indirectly through the induction of insulin-like growth factor-1 (IGF-1). Although most circulating IGF-1 is made in the liver, IGF-1 produced locally in many tissues is critical for growth, as revealed by normal growth in mice that have a hepatocyte-specific inactivation of IGF-1. Circulating IGF-1 is associated with a family of binding proteins that serve as transport proteins, which also may mediate certain aspects of IGF-1 signaling (Firth and Baxter, 2002). The essential role of IGF-1 in GH signaling is evidenced by a patient with loss-of-function mutations in both alleles of the *IGF1* gene whose severe intrauterine and postnatal growth retardation was unresponsive to GH but responsive to recombinant human IGF-1 (Comacho-Hubner *et al.*, 1999) and by the association of mutations in the IGF-1 receptor with intrauterine growth retardation (Abuzzahab *et al.*, 2003).

After its synthesis and release, IGF-1 interacts with receptors on the cell surface that mediate its biological activities. The type 1 IGF receptor is closely related to the insulin receptor, consisting of a het-ero-tetramer with intrinsic tyrosine kinase activity. This receptor is present in essentially all tissues and binds IGF-1 and the related growth factor, IGF-2, with high affinity; insulin also can activate the type 1 IGF receptor, but with an affinity approximately two orders of magnitude less than that of the IGFs. The signal transduction pathway for the insulin receptor is described in detail in Chapter 60.

Clinical Disorders of Growth Hormone

Although the manifestations vary depending on the age of onset, GH deficiency and excess are associated with defined diseases that form an important part of endocrine practice.

Diagnosis of Growth Hormone Deficiency. Clinically, children with GH deficiency present with short stature, delayed bone age, and a low age-adjusted growth velocity. Most commonly, these children have an isolated deficiency of GH without other documented pathology (*e.g.*, idiopathic, isolated GH deficiency) and are presumed to have a hypothalamic defect. *Because GH secretion is episodic, random sampling of serum GH is insufficient to diagnose GH deficiency.* Tests that provide an estimate of integrated GH levels over time (*e.g.*, IGF-1 and IGF-binding protein 3 levels) are more useful, although provocative tests usually are required. After excluding other causes of poor growth, the diagnosis of GH deficiency should be entertained in patients with height more than 2 to 2.5 standard deviations below normal, delayed bone age, a decreased growth velocity, and a predicted adult height substantially below the mean parental height (Vance and Mauras, 1999). In this setting, a serum GH level of less than 10 ng/ml following provocative testing (*e.g.*, insulin-induced hypoglycemia, arginine, levodopa, or glucagon) indicates GH deficiency; a stimulated value of less than 5 ng/ml reflects severe deficiency.

In adults, overt GH deficiency almost always results from pituitary disease due either to a functioning or nonfunctioning pituitary adenoma or secondary to surgery or radiotherapy for a pituitary or suprasellar mass. Almost all patients with multiple deficits in other pituitary hormones also will have deficient GH secretion, and some experts incorporate the number of other pituitary deficiencies into a diagnostic algorithm for diagnosing GH deficiency (Molitch, 2002b). Others will accept a serum IGF-1 level below the age- and sex-adjusted normal value as indicative of GH deficiency in a patient with known pituitary disease. Finally, some experts require an inadequate GH response to provocative testing, with either insulin-induced hypoglycemia or a combination of arginine and GHRH, as the preferred stimulus for GH secretion. The risk of false-positive provocative tests (*i.e.*, a subnormal GH response) is increased in obese subjects.

Indications for Growth Hormone Treatment. GH deficiency in children is a well-accepted cause of short stature, and replacement therapy has been used for more than 30 years to treat children with severe GH deficiency. With the advent of essentially unlimited supplies of recombinant GH, therapy has been extended to children with other conditions associated with short stature despite adequate GH production, including Turner's syndrome, Prader-Willi syndrome (in the absence of morbid obesity or obstructive sleep apnea), chronic renal insufficiency, children born small for gestational age, and children with idiopathic short stature (*i.e.*, more than 2.25 standard deviations below mean height for age and sex but normal laboratory indices of growth hormone levels).

In adults, GH deficiency is associated with a defined endocrinopathy that includes increased mortality from cardiovascular causes, probably secondary to deleterious changes in fat distribution, increases in circulating lipids, and increased inflammation; decreased muscle mass and exercise capacity; decreased bone density; and impaired psychosocial function (Cummings and Merriam, 2003). With the ready availability of recombinant human GH, attention also has shifted to the proper role of GH therapy in GH-deficient adults. While this is an area of ongoing debate, the consensus is that at least the most severely affected GH-deficient adults may benefit from GH replacement therapy. The FDA also has approved GH therapy for AIDS-associated wasting and for malabsorption associated with the short bowel syndrome. The latter indication is based on GH action to stimulate adaptation of gastrointestinal epithelial cells; in this setting, GH is administered once daily for 4 weeks.

Based on controlled clinical trials showing increased mortality, GH should not be used in patients with acute critical illness due to complications after open heart or abdominal surgery, multiple accidental trauma, or acute respiratory failure. GH also should not be used in patients who have any evidence of neoplasia, and antitumor therapy should be completed before initiation of GH therapy.

Treatment of Growth Hormone Deficiency. Humans do not respond to GH from nonprimate species. GH for therapeutic use formerly was purified from human cadaver pituitaries and thus was available in very limited quantities and carried the risk of Creutzfeldt-Jakob disease. The production of human GH by recombinant DNA technology not only increased availability of the hormone, but also eliminated the risk of disease transmission associated with the pituitary-derived hormone.

GH is used for replacement therapy in GH-deficient children, whether the deficiency is congenital or acquired (Vance and Mauras, 1999). By convention, *somatropin* refers to the many GH preparations whose sequences match that of native GH (SEROSTIM, GENOTROPIN, HUMA-TROPE, NUTROPIN, NORDITROPIN, SAIZEN), while *somatrem* refers to a derivative of GH with an additional methionine at the amino terminus (PROTROPIN). Although the microbial systems used to express the recombinant hormone subtly affect the structures of these preparations, they all have similar biological actions and potencies. To mimic the normal pattern of secretion, they typically are administered to GH-deficient children in a dose of 40 μg/kg per day subcutaneously in the evening; although the circulating half-life of GH is only 20 minutes, its biological half-life is in the range of 9 to 17 hours, and once-daily administration is sufficient. Higher daily doses (*e.g.,* 50 μg/kg) are employed for patients with Turner's syndrome, who have partial GH resistance. In children with overt GH deficiency, measurements of serum IGF-1 levels are used to monitor initial response and compliance; long-term response is monitored by close evaluation of height, sometimes in conjunction with measurements of serum IGF-1 levels. Although the most pronounced increase in growth velocity occurs within the first 2 years of therapy, GH is continued until the epiphyses are fused, and also may be extended into the transition period from childhood to adulthood (Quigley, 2003).

Newer GH formulations are supplied in prefilled syringes, which may be more convenient for the patient, or in non-needle injection systems. The FDA also has approved an encapsulated form of somatropin (NUTROPIN DEPOT) that is injected intramuscularly either monthly (1.5 mg/kg body weight) or every 2 weeks (0.75 mg/kg body weight). The depot formulation was associated with local reactions at the site of injection, and the manufacturer has announced a decision to discontinue commercialization of this product. The relative advantages of any specific formulations over others in clinical use have not been definitively established.

In addition to GH, *sermorelin acetate* (GEREF), a synthetic form of human GHRH, is FDA approved for treatment of GH deficiency (Anonymous, 1999). Sermorelin is a peptide of 29 amino acids that corresponds in sequence to the first 29 amino acids of human GHRH (a 44-amino-acid peptide) and has full biological activi-ty. Sermorelin generally is well tolerated and is less expensive than somatropin, but at recommended doses (30 μg/kg per day given subcutaneously) it has been less effective than GH in clinical trials. Moreover, this agent will not work in patients whose GH deficiency results from defects in the anterior pituitary. Therefore, a GH response (>2 ng/ml) to a test dose of sermorelin should be documented before initiating therapy, and patients must be monitored frequently to ascertain continued growth on therapy. Sermorelin also has been employed diagnostically to distinguish between pituitary and hypothalamic disease, although its clinical utility for this purpose is not fully established.

In view of the increased appreciation of the effects of GH on bone density and the manifestations of GH deficiency in adults, some experts continue therapy into adulthood for children with GH deficiency. However, many patients who clearly were GH deficient in childhood, especially those with idiopathic, isolated GH deficiency, respond normally to provocative tests as adults. Thus it is essential to confirm GH deficiency after optimal growth has been achieved so as to identify patients who will benefit from continuing GH treatment.

Growth impairment also may be associated with elevated GH levels and GH resistance, most frequently secondary to mutations in the GH receptor (Laron dwarfism). These patients can be treated effectively with recombinant human IGF-1 (IGEF), which is administered subcutaneously either once or twice daily in doses ranging from 40 to 120 μg/kg (Comacho-Hubner *et al.*, 1999). Although this therapy clearly is beneficial in promoting growth, the optimal regimen remains to be established, and novel approaches to modulate the IGF-1 pathway are under investigation (Torrado and Carrascosa, 2003).

For adults, the FDA recommends a starting dose of 3 to 4 μg/kg, given once daily by subcutaneous injection, with a maximum dose of 25 μg/kg in patients ≤35 years old and 12.5 μg/kg in older patients. Other experts recommend a starting dose of 150 to 300 μg/day regardless of body weight. Clinical response is monitored by serum IGF-1 levels, which should be restored to the mid-normal range adjusted for age and sex. Either an elevated serum IGF-1 or persistent side effects are grounds for decreasing the dose; conversely, the dose can be increased if serum IGF-1 has not reached the normal range after 2 months of GH therapy. Because estrogen increases the levels of GH binding proteins, women taking oral—but not transdermal—estrogen often require larger GH doses to achieve the target IGF-1 level. In clinical trials in the setting of AIDS-related wasting, considerably higher doses (*e.g.,* 100 μg/kg) have been used.

Based on the known age-related decline in GH levels, the use of GH therapy to ameliorate or even reverse the consequences of aging has been widely promoted. Many of the studies supporting this use were not placebo-controlled and involved small numbers of subjects. Moreover, at least one well-designed trial showed no improvement in strength or aerobic performance with GH therapy in elderly subjects. In violation of regulations and standard medical practice, some athletes also use injectable GH preparations as anabolic agents to enhance performance. In addition to the parenteral GH preparations, oral preparations containing "stacked" amino acids that reportedly stimulate GH release have been marketed as nutritional supplements. Despite the absence of validation in controlled trials, these formulations are part of multibillion dollar anti-aging and performance-enhancing programs.

Side Effects of GH Therapy. In children, GH therapy is associated with remarkably few side effects. Rarely, generally within the first 8 weeks of therapy, patients develop intracranial hypertension, with papilledema, visual changes, headache, nausea, and/or vomiting. Because of this, funduscopic examination is recommended at the initiation of therapy and at periodic intervals thereafter. Leukemia has been reported in some children receiving GH therapy; a causal relationship has not been established, and conditions associated with GH deficiency (*e.g.,* Down's syndrome, cranial irradiation for CNS tumors) probably explain the apparent increased incidence of leukemia. Despite this, the consensus is that GH should not be administered in the first year after treatment of pediatric tumors, including leukemia, or during the first 2 years after therapy for medulloblastomas or ependymomas. An increased incidence of type 2 diabetes mellitus has been reported. Finally, too-rapid growth may be associated with slipped epiphyses or scoliosis.

In adults, side effects associated with the initiation of GH therapy include peripheral edema, carpal tunnel syndrome, arthralgia, and myalgia. These symptoms, which occur most frequently in patients who are older or more obese, generally respond to a decrease in dose. Although there are potential concerns about impaired glucose tolerance secondary to anti-insulin actions of GH, this generally has not been a major problem with clinical use at the recommended doses. In fact, changes in visceral fat composition associated with GH replacement may improve insulin sensitivity in some patients.

Syndromes of GH Excess

GH excess causes distinct clinical syndromes depending on the age of the patient. If the epiphyses are unfused, GH excess causes increased longitudinal growth, resulting in gigantism. In adults, GH excess causes acromegaly. The symptoms and signs of acromegaly (*e.g.,* arthropathy, carpal tunnel syndrome, generalized visceromegaly, macroglossia, hypertension, glucose intolerance, headache, lethargy, excess perspiration, and sleep apnea) progress slowly, and

diagnosis often is delayed. Life expectancy is shortened in these patients; mortality is increased at least twofold relative to age-matched controls due to increased death from cardiovascular disease, upper airway obstruction, and gastrointestinal malignancies.

Diagnosis of GH Excess. While the diagnosis of acromegaly should be suspected in patients with the appropriate symptoms and signs, confirmation requires the demonstration of increased circulating GH or IGF-1. The gold standard diagnostic test for acromegaly is the oral glucose tolerance test. While normal subjects suppress their GH level to <1 ng/ml in response to a 75-g glucose challenge (the absolute value may vary depending on the sensitivity of the assay), patients with acromegaly either fail to suppress or show a paradoxical increase in GH level.

Treatment options in acromegaly include transsphenoidal surgery, radiation, and drugs that inhibit GH secretion or action. Pituitary surgery traditionally has been viewed as the treatment of choice. In patients with microadenomas (*i.e.,* tumors <1 cm in diameter), skilled neurosurgeons can achieve cure rates of 60% to 90%; however, the long-term success rate for patients with macroadenomas (*i.e.,* tumors ≥1 cm in diameter) typically is less than 50%. In addition, there is increasing appreciation that acromegalic patients previously considered cured by pituitary surgery actually have persistent GH excess, with its attendant complications, and that pituitary irradiation may be associated with significant long-term complications. Thus, more attention has been given to the pharmacological management of acromegaly, either as a primary treatment modality or for the treatment of persistent GH excess after transsphenoidal surgery.

Somatostatin Analogs. The development of analogs of SST (Figure 55–4) revolutionized the medical treatment of acromegaly. Based on structure-function studies of SST and its derivatives, the amino acid residues in positions 7 to 10 [FWKT] are the major determinants of biological activity. Residues W^8 and K^9 appear to be essential, whereas conservative substitutions at F^7 and T^{10} are permissible. Active SST analogs retain this core segment constrained in a cyclic structure—formed either by a disulfide bond or amide linkage that stabilizes the optimal conformation (Weckbecker *et al.*, 2003). The endogenous peptides, SST-14 and SST-28, do not show specificity for SSTR subtypes except for SSTR5, for which SST-28 shows some preference. Some of the somatostatin analogs exhibit greater selectivity. For example, the octapeptides *octreotide, lanreotide,* and *vapreotide* and the hexapeptide *seglitide* all bind to the SSTR subtypes with the following order of selectivity: SSTR2 > SSTR5 > SSTR3 >> SSTR1 and SSTR4. The octapeptide analog BIM23268 exhibits modest selectivity for SSTR5, and the undecapeptide CH275 appears to bind preferentially to SSTR1 and SSTR4. More recently, small nonpeptide agonists that exhibit high selectivity for SSTR subtypes have been isolated from combinatorial chemical libraries; these compounds may lead to a new class of highly selective, orally active somatostatin mimetics (Weckbecker *et al.*, 2003).

Somatostatin-28 (Prosomatostatin):

Ser-Ala-Asn-Ser-Asn-Pro-Ala-Met-Ala-Pro-Arg-Glu-Arg-Lys-Ala-Gly-Cys-Lys-Asn-Phe-Phe-Trp-Lys-Thr-Phe-Thr-Ser-Cys

Somatostatin-14:   Ala-Gly-Cys-Lys-Asn-Phe-Phe-Trp-Lys-Thr-Phe-Thr-Ser-Cys

Octreotide: D-Phe-Cys-Phe-D-Trp-Lys-Thr-Cys-Thr-ol

Lanreotide: D-Nal-Cys-Tyr-D-Trp-Lys-Val-Cys-Thr-NH₂

Seglitide: N-Methyl-Ala-Tyr-D-Trp-Lys-Val-Phe

Vapreotide: D-Phe-Cys-Tyr-D-Trp-Lys-Val-Cys-Trp-NH₂

Figure 55–4. *Structures of the somatostatins and clinically available analogs.* The amino acid sequences of SST-28 and SST-14 are shown. Residues that play key roles in receptor binding, as discussed in the text, are shown in blue. Also shown are the structures of the synthetic somatostatin analogs, octreotide, lanreotide, seglitide, and vapreotide. *Abbreviation:* D-Nal, 3-(2-naphthyl)-D-alanyl.

Currently, the most widely used somatostatin analog is octreotide (SANDOSTATIN), an 8-amino-acid synthetic derivative of somatostatin that has a longer half-life and binds preferentially to SSTR-2 and SSTR-5 receptors. Typically, octreotide (100 μg) is administered subcutaneously three times daily; bioactivity is virtually 100%, peak effects are seen within 30 minutes, serum half-life is approximately 90 minutes, and duration of action is approximately 12 hours. The goal of treatment is to decrease GH levels to less than 2 ng/ml after an oral glucose tolerance test and to bring IGF-1 levels to within the normal range for age and gender. Depending on the biochemical response, higher or lower octreotide doses may be used in individual patients.

In addition to its effect on GH secretion, octreotide can decrease tumor size—although tumor growth generally resumes after octreotide treatment is stopped. Octreotide also has significant inhibitory effects on thyrotropin secretion, and it is the treatment of choice for patients who have thyrotrope adenomas that oversecrete TSH and who are not good candidates for surgery. The use of octreotide in gastrointestinal disorders is discussed in Chapter 37.

Gastrointestinal side effects—including diarrhea, nausea, and abdominal pain—occur in up to 50% of patients receiving octreotide. In most patients, these symptoms diminish over time and do not require cessation of therapy. Approximately 25% of patients receiving octreotide develop gallstones, presumably due to decreased gallblad-

der contraction and gastrointestinal transit time. In the absence of symptoms, gallstones are not a contraindication to continued use of octreotide. Compared to somatostatin, octreotide reduces insulin secretion to a lesser extent and only infrequently affects glycemic control.

The need to inject octreotide three times daily poses a significant obstacle to patient compliance. A long-acting, slow-release form (SANDOSTATIN LAR) is a more convenient alternative that can be administered intramuscularly once every 4 weeks; the recommended dose is 20 or 30 mg (McKeage *et al.*, 2003). The long-acting preparation is at least as effective as the regular formulation and is used in patients who have responded favorably to a trial of the shorter-acting formulation of octreotide. Like the shorter-acting formulation, the longer-acting formulation of octreotide generally is well tolerated and has a similar incidence of side effects (predominantly gastrointestinal and/or discomfort at the injection site) that do not require cessation of therapy.

Lanreotide (SOMATULINE LA) is another long-acting octapeptide analog of somatostatin that causes prolonged suppression of GH secretion when administered in a 30-mg dose intramuscularly. Although its efficacy appears comparable to that of the long-acting formulation of octreotide, its duration of action is shorter; thus it must be administered either at 10- or 14-day intervals. A 60-mg formulation of lanreotide (SOMATULINE AUTOGEL) has recently been introduced that reduces the required dosing frequency to once every 4 weeks; current results are comparable to those with the slow-release octreotide formulation, as are the incidence and severity of side effects. Lanreotide has not been approved by the FDA for use in the United States.

Somatostatin blocks not only GH secretion, but also the secretion of other hormones, growth factors, and cytokines. Thus, octreotide and the delayed-release somatostatin analogs have been used to treat symptoms associated with metastatic carcinoid tumors (*e.g.,* flushing and diarrhea) and adenomas secreting vasoactive intestinal peptide (*e.g.,* watery diarrhea). Octreotide also is used for treatment of acute variceal bleeding, for perioperative prophylaxis in pancreatic surgery, and for TSH-secreting adenomas in patients who are not candidates for surgery. Novel uses under evaluation currently include the treatment of eye diseases associated with excessive proliferation and inflammation (*e.g.,* Graves' orbitopathy and diabetic retinopathy), diabetic nephropathy, and various systemic diseases associated with inflammation (*e.g.,* rheumatoid arthritis, inflammatory bowel disease, and psoriasis). Finally, modified forms of octreotide labeled with indium or technetium have been used for diagnostic imaging of neuroendocrine tumors such as pituitary adenomas and carcinoids; modified forms labeled with β emitters such as ^{90}Y have been used in selective destruction of SSTR-2–positive tumors.

Dopamine-Receptor Agonists. The dopamine-receptor agonists are described in more detail below in the section dealing with treatment of prolactin excess. Although dopamine-receptor agonists normally stimulate GH secretion, they paradoxically decrease GH secretion in some patients with acromegaly. The best responses have been seen in patients whose tumors secrete both GH and prolactin. The long-acting dopamine-receptor agonist *cabergoline* (DOSTINEX) may lower GH and IGF-1 levels into the target range and thus may be of value in patients who are unwilling to undergo treatment with drugs administered by injection. Doses used in treating acromegaly typically are considerably higher than those employed in prolactinomas.

Growth Hormone Antagonists. Pegvisomant (SOMAVERT) is a GH antagonist that is FDA approved for the treatment of acromegaly. Pegvisomant binds to the GH receptor but does not activate Jak-Stat signaling or stimulate IGF-1 secretion (Figure 55–3). Pegvisomant is administered subcutaneously as a 40-mg loading dose under physician supervision, followed by self-administration of 10 mg/day. Based on serum IGF-1 levels, the dose is titrated at 4- to 6-week intervals to a maximum of 40 mg/day. Liver function should be monitored in all patients, and pegvisomant should not be used in patients with elevated levels of liver transaminases. Because there are concerns that loss of negative feedback by GH and IGF-1 may increase the growth of GH-secreting adenomas, careful follow-up by pituitary MRI is mandatory. Pegvisomant differs structurally from native GH and induces the formation of specific antibodies in ~15% of patients despite the covalent coupling to lysine residues of 4 to 5 molecules of a polyethylene glycol polymer per modified GH molecule. Nevertheless, the development of tachyphylaxis due to these antibodies has not been reported.

In clinical trials, pegvisomant at higher doses significantly decreased serum IGF-1 to normal age- and sex-adjusted levels in >90% of patients, and significantly improved clinical parameters such as ring size, soft-tissue swelling, excessive perspiration, and fatigue. Thus, while its ultimate role in the management of acro-

megaly remains to be determined, pegvisomant is an exciting new pharmacologic agent, particularly for those acromegalic patients who do not respond to somatostatin analogs.

PROLACTIN

As a member of the somatotropin family, prolactin is related structurally to GH and placental lactogen (Table 55–1). Human prolactin is a 23,000-dalton protein of 199 amino acids with three intramolecular disulfide bonds. It is synthesized by lactotropes in the anterior pituitary gland, and a portion of secreted prolactin is glycosylated at a single asparagine residue. In circulation, dimeric and polymeric forms of prolactin also are found, as are degradation products of 16,000 and 18,000 daltons; the biological significance of these different forms is not known.

Secretion

Prolactin synthesis and secretion in the fetal pituitary start in the fifth week of gestation. Serum prolactin levels decline shortly after birth. Whereas serum prolactin levels remain low throughout life in normal males, they are elevated somewhat in normal cycling females. Prolactin levels rise markedly during pregnancy, reach a maximum at term, and decline thereafter unless the mother breast-feeds the child. Suckling or breast manipulation in nursing mothers stimulates circulating prolactin levels, which can rise ten- to one hundredfold within 30 minutes of stimulation. This response is transmitted from the breast to the hypothalamus *via* the spinal cord and the median forebrain bundle, and is distinct from milk let-down, which is mediated by oxytocin release by the posterior pituitary gland. The precise mechanism for suckling-induced prolactin secretion is not known but involves both decreased secretion of dopamine by tuberoinfundibular neurons and possibly increased release of factors that stimulate prolactin secretion (*see* below). The suckling response becomes less pronounced after several months of breast-feeding, and prolactin concentrations eventually decline to prepregnancy levels.

Prolactin detected in maternal and fetal blood originates from maternal and fetal pituitaries, respectively. Prolactin also is synthesized by decidual cells near the end of the luteal phase of the menstrual cycle and early in pregnancy; the latter source is responsible for the very high levels of prolactin in amniotic fluid during the first trimester.

Many of the physiological factors that influence prolactin secretion are similar to those that affect GH secre-

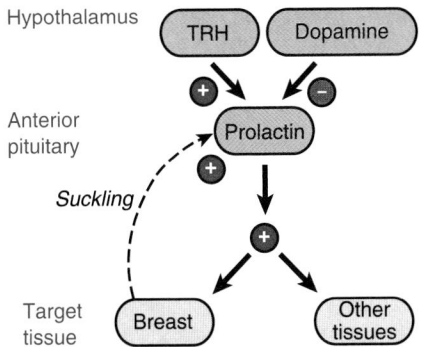

Hypothalamus

Anterior pituitary

Suckling

Target tissue

Figure 55–5. *Prolactin secretion and actions.* Prolactin is the only anterior pituitary hormone for which a unique stimulatory releasing factor has not been identified. Thyrotropin-releasing hormone (TRH), however, can stimulate prolactin release and dopamine can inhibit it. Prolactin affects lactation and reproductive functions but it also has varied effects on many other tissues. Prolactin is not under feedback control by peripheral hormones, but its secretion is induced by suckling (*see* text for further details).

tion. Thus, sleep, stress, hypoglycemia, exercise, and estrogen increase the secretion of both hormones.

Like other anterior pituitary hormones, prolactin is secreted in a pulsatile manner. Prolactin is unique among the anterior pituitary hormones in that hypothalamic regulation of its secretion is predominantly inhibitory. The major regulator of prolactin secretion is dopamine, which is released by tuberoinfundibular neurons and interacts with the D_2 receptor on lactotropes to inhibit prolactin secretion (Figure 55–5). A number of putative prolactin-releasing factors have been described, including thyrotropin-releasing hormone (TRH), vasoactive intestinal peptide, prolactin-releasing peptide, and *p*ituitary *a*denylyl cyclase–*a*ctivating *p*eptide (PACAP), but their physiological roles are unclear. Under certain pathophysiological conditions, such as severe primary hypothyroidism, persistently elevated levels of TRH can induce hyperprolactinemia and galactorrhea.

Molecular and Cellular Bases of Prolactin Action

The effects of prolactin result from interactions with specific receptors that are widely distributed among a variety of cell types within many tissues (Goffin *et al.*, 2002). The prolactin receptor is encoded by a single gene on chromosome 5. Alternative splicing of this gene gives rise to multiple forms of the receptor, including a short form of 310 amino acids, a long form of 610 amino acids, and an intermediate form of 412 amino acids. In addition, sol-

uble forms that correspond to the extracellular domain of the receptor are found in the circulation. The membrane-bound prolactin receptor is related structurally to receptors for GH and several cytokines and uses similar signaling mechanisms. Like the GH receptor, the prolactin receptor lacks intrinsic tyrosine kinase activity; prolactin induces a conformational change leading to recruitment and activation of Jak kinases (Figure 55–3). The activated Jak2 kinase, in turn, induces phosphorylation, dimerization, and nuclear translocation of the transcription factor Stat5. Unlike human GH and placental lactogen, which bind to the prolactin receptor and are lactogenic, prolactin binds specifically to the prolactin receptor and has no somatotropic (GH-like) activity.

Physiological Effects of Prolactin

A number of hormones—including estrogens, progesterone, placental lactogen, and GH—stimulate development of the breast and prepare it for lactation. Prolactin, acting *via* prolactin receptors, plays an important role in inducing growth and differentiation of the ductal and lobuloalveolar epithelium and is essential for lactation. Target genes by which prolactin induces mammary development include those encoding milk proteins (*e.g.*, caseins), genes important for intracellular structure (*e.g.*, keratins), genes important for cell-cell communication (*e.g.*, amphiregulin and Wnt4), and components of the extracellular matrix (*e.g.*, laminin and collagen).

Prolactin receptors are present in many other sites, including the hypothalamus, liver, testes, ovaries, prostate, and immune system, prompting the hypothesis that prolactin plays multiple roles outside the breast. The physiological effects of prolactin at these sites, however, remain poorly characterized. For example, a considerable body of evidence suggests that prolactin can stimulate immune function *via* effects on multiple cell types; however, knockout mice lacking either prolactin or its receptor exhibit neither immunodeficiency nor autoimmune disease. Some have therefore proposed that prolactin modulates immune function during stress rather than under normal circumstances.

Agents Used to Treat Syndromes of Prolactin Excess

Prolactin has no therapeutic uses. Hyperprolactinemia is a relatively common endocrine abnormality that can result from hypothalamic or pituitary diseases that interfere with the delivery of inhibitory dopaminergic signals, from renal failure, from primary hypothyroidism associated with increased TRH levels, or from treatment with dopamine-receptor antagonists. Most often, hyperprolactinemia is caused by prolactin-secreting pituitary adenomas—either microadenomas or macroadenomas. Manifestations of prolactin excess in women include galactorrhea, amenorrhea, and infertility. In men, hyperprolactinemia causes loss of libido, impotence, and infertility.

The therapeutic options for patients with prolactinomas include transsphenoidal surgery, radiation, and treatment with dopamine-receptor agonists that suppress prolactin production *via* activation of D_2 dopamine receptors. Inasmuch as initial surgical cure rates are only 50% to 70% with microadenomas and 30% with macroadenomas, most patients with prolactinomas ultimately require drug therapy. Thus, dopamine-receptor agonists have become the initial treatment of choice for many patients (Molitch, 2002a). These agents generally decrease both prolactin secretion and the size of the adenoma, thereby improving the endocrine abnormalities, as well as the neurological symptoms caused directly by the adenoma (including visual field deficits).

Bromocriptine. *Bromocriptine* (PARLODEL) is the dopamine-receptor agonist against which newer agents are compared. Bromocriptine is a semisynthetic ergot alkaloid that interacts with D_2 dopamine receptors to inhibit spontaneous and TRH-induced release of prolactin; to a lesser extent, it also activates D_1 dopamine receptors. Bromocriptine normalizes serum prolactin levels in 70% to 80% of patients with prolactinomas and decreases tumor size in more than 50% of patients, including those with macroadenomas. It is worth noting that bromocriptine does not cure the underlying adenoma, and hyperprolactinemia and tumor growth typically recur upon cessation of therapy.

Frequent side effects of bromocriptine include nausea and vomiting, headache, and postural hypotension—particularly on initial use. Less-frequent side effects include nasal congestion, digital vasospasm, and CNS effects such as psychosis, hallucinations, nightmares, or insomnia. These side effects can be diminished by starting at a low dose (1.25 mg) administered at bedtime with a snack. After 1 week, a morning dose of 1.25 mg can be added. If clinical symptoms persist or serum prolactin levels remain elevated, the dose can be increased gradually, every 3 to 7 days, to 5 mg twice per day or 2.5 mg three times a day as tolerated. Patients often develop tolerance to the side effects of bromocriptine. Those who do not respond to bromocriptine or who develop intractable side effects may respond to a different dopamine agonist. Although a high fraction of the oral dose of bromocriptine is absorbed, only 7% of the dose reaches the systemic circulation because of a high extraction rate and extensive first-pass metabolism in the liver. Furthermore, bromocriptine has a relatively short elimination half-life (between 2 and 8 hours). To avoid the need for frequent dosing, a slow-release oral form is available outside the United States. Bromocriptine may be administered intravaginally (2.5 mg once daily), reportedly with fewer gastrointestinal side effects. At higher concentrations, bromocriptine is used in the management of acromegaly, as noted above, and at still higher concentrations is used in the management of Parkinson's disease. A parenteral long-acting form

of bromocriptine incorporated into biodegradable microspheres (PARLODEL-LAR) has been developed, but is not available in the United States. In clinical trials, this product has produced results that are comparable to those with oral bromocriptine.

Pergolide. *Pergolide* (PERMAX), an ergot derivative approved by the FDA for treatment of Parkinson's disease, also is used "off label" to treat hyperprolactinemia. If the cost of therapy is the key consideration, pergolide is the least expensive dopamine-receptor agonist currently available. It induces many of the same side effects as does bromocriptine, but it can be given once a day, starting at 0.025 mg at bedtime and increased gradually to a maximum daily dose of 0.5 mg.

Cabergoline. Cabergoline (DOSTINEX) is an ergot derivative with a longer half-life (approximately 65 hours), higher affinity, and greater selectivity for the D_2 receptor (approximately four times more potent) than bromocriptine. It has been approved by the FDA for the treatment of hyperprolactinemia and likely will play an increasing role in the treatment of this syndrome. Compared to bromocriptine, cabergoline has a much lower tendency to induce nausea, although it still may cause hypotension and dizziness. In some clinical trials, cabergoline has been more effective than bromocriptine in decreasing serum prolactin in patients with hyperprolactinemia, although this may reflect improved adherence to therapy due to decreased side effects. Therapy is initiated at a dose of 0.25 mg twice a week or 0.5 mg once a week. If the serum prolactin remains elevated, the dose can be increased to a maximum of 1.5 to 2 mg two or three times a week as tolerated; however, the dose should not be increased more often than once every 4 weeks.

Quinagolide. *Quinagolide* (NORPROLAC) is a nonergot D_2 dopamine agonist with a half-life of 22 hours. Quinagolide is administered once daily at doses of 0.1 to 0.5 mg/day. It is not approved by the FDA but has been used extensively in Europe.

Patients with prolactinomas who wish to become pregnant comprise a special subset of hyperprolactinemic patients. In this setting, drug safety during pregnancy is an important consideration. Bromocriptine, cabergoline, and quinagolide all relieve the inhibitory effect of prolactin on ovulation and permit most patients with prolactinomas to become pregnant without apparent detrimental effects on pregnancy or fetal development. However, experience with cabergoline and quinagolide is less extensive than that with bromocriptine. Therefore, bromocriptine is recommended as the first-line treatment in this setting; this opinion may change as experience with cabergoline or quinagolide increases.

GONADOTROPIN-RELEASING HORMONE AND GONADOTROPIC HORMONES

Luteinizing hormone (LH) and follicle-stimulating hormone (FSH) were named initially based on their actions on the ovary; appreciation of their roles in male reproductive function came later. These pituitary hormones, together with the related placental hormone human chorionic gonadotropin (hCG), are collectively referred to as the gonadotropic hormones because of their actions on the gonads (Table 55–1).

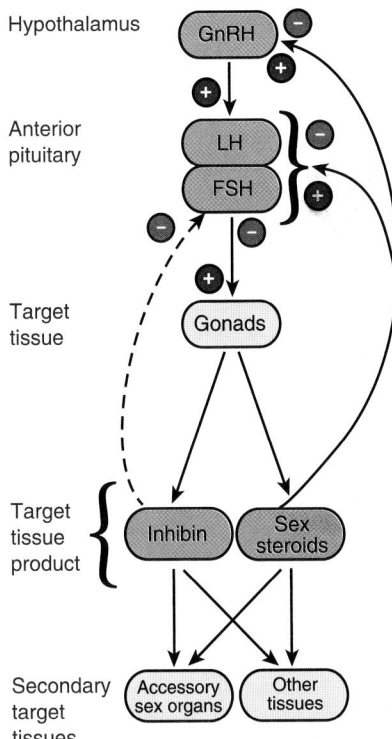

Figure 55–6. *The hypothalamic-pituitary-gonadal axis.* A single hypothalamic releasing factor, gonadotropin-releasing hormone (GnRH), controls the synthesis and release of both gonadotropins (LH and FSH) in males and females. Gonadal steroid hormones (androgens, estrogens, and progesterone) cause feedback inhibition at the level of the pituitary and the hypothalamus. The preovulatory surge of estrogen also can exert a stimulatory effect at the level of the pituitary and the hypothalamus. Inhibins, polypeptide hormones produced by the gonads, specifically inhibit FSH secretion by the pituitary.

The regulation of gonadotropin secretion is described in detail in Chapters 57 and 58. LH and FSH are synthesized and secreted by gonadotropes, which make up approximately 20% of the hormone-secreting cells in the anterior pituitary. hCG, which is produced only in primates and horses, is synthesized by syncytiotrophoblast cells of the placenta. Pituitary gonadotropin production is stimulated by GnRH and is further regulated by feedback effects of the gonadal hormones (Figure 55–6; *see also* Figure 57–2).

Regulation of Release of GnRH. GnRH is a decapeptide with blocked amino and carboxyl termini (Table 55–2) that is derived by proteolytic cleavage of a 92-amino-acid precursor peptide. GnRH release is intermittent and is governed by a neural pulse generator in the mediobasal hypothalamus, primarily in the arcuate nucleus, that controls the frequency and amplitude of GnRH release. The GnRH

pulse generator is active late in fetal life and for approximately one year after birth, but decreases considerably thereafter, presumably secondarily to CNS inhibition. Shortly before puberty, CNS inhibition decreases and the amplitude and frequency of GnRH pulses increase, particularly during sleep. As puberty progresses, the GnRH pulses increase further in amplitude and frequency until the normal adult pattern is established. The intermittent release of GnRH is crucial for the proper synthesis and release of the gonadotropins; the continuous administration of GnRH leads to desensitization and down-regulation of GnRH receptors on pituitary gonadotropes. This down-regulation forms the basis for the clinical use of long-acting GnRH analogs to suppress gonadotropin secretion (*see* below).

Molecular and Cellular Bases of GnRH Action. GnRH signals through a specific G protein–coupled receptor on gonadotropes that activates $G_{q/11}$ and stimulates the PLC-IP_3-Ca^{2+} pathway (*see* Chapter 1) resulting in increased synthesis and secretion of LH and FSH. Although cyclic AMP is not the major mediator of GnRH action, binding of GnRH to its receptor also increases adenylyl cyclase activity. GnRH receptors also are present in the ovary and testis, where their physiological significance remains to be determined.

Other Regulators of Gonadotropin Production. Gonadal steroids regulate gonadotropin production at the level of the pituitary and the hypothalamus, but effects on the hypothalamus predominate. The feedback effects of gonadal steroids are sex-, dosage-, and time-dependent. In women, low levels of estradiol and progesterone inhibit gonadotropin production, largely through opioid action on the neural pulse generator that controls GnRH secretion. Higher and more sustained levels of estradiol have positive feedback effects that ultimately result in the gonadotropin surge that precedes ovulation. In men, testosterone inhibits gonadotropin production, in part through direct actions and in part *via* its conversion to estradiol.

Gonadotropin production also is regulated by the *inhibins,* which are members of the bone morphogenetic protein family of secreted signaling proteins. Inhibins are made by granulosa cells in the ovary and Sertoli cells in the testis in response to the gonadotropins and local growth factors. They act directly in the pituitary to inhibit FSH secretion without affecting that of LH.

Molecular and Cellular Bases of Gonadotropin Action

The gonadotropins (LH, FSH, and hCG), together with TSH, constitute the glycoprotein family of pituitary hor-

Table 55–2
Structures of GnRH and Decapeptide GnRH Analogs

AMINO ACID RESIDUE	1	2	3	4	5	6	7	8	9	10	DOSAGE FORM
Agonists											
GnRH (FACTREL, LUTREPULSE)	PyroGlu	His	Trp	Ser	Tyr	Gly	Leu	Arg	Pro	Gly-NH$_2$	IV, SC
Leuprolide (LUPRON, ELIGARD, VIADUR)	—	—	—	—	—	D-Leu	—	—	Pro-NHEt		IM, SC, depot
Buserelin (SUPREFACT)	—	—	—	—	—	D-Ser(tBu)	—	—	Pro-NHEt		SC, IN
Nafarelin (SYNAREL)	—	—	—	—	—	D-Nal	—	—		Gly-NH$_2$	IN
Deslorelin	—	—	—	—	—	D-Trp	—	—	Pro-NHEt		SC, IM, depot
Histrelin (SUPPRELIN)	—	—	—	—	—	D-His(ImBzl)	—	—	Pro-NHEt		SC
Triptorelin (TRELSTAR DEPOT, LA)	—	—	—	—	—	D-Trp	—	—		Gly-NH$_2$	IM
Goserelin (ZOLADEX)	—	—	—	—	—	D-Ser(tBu)	—	—		AzGly-NH$_2$	SC implant
Antagonists											
Cetrorelix (CETROTIDE)	Ac-D-Nal	D-Cpa	D-Pal			D-Cit				D-Ala-NH$_2$	SC
Ganirelix (ANTAGON)	Ac-D-Nal	D-Cpa	D-Pal			D-hArg(Et)$_2$		D-hArg(Et)$_2$		D-Ala-NH$_2$	SC
Abarelix (PLENAXIS)	Ac-D-Nal	D-Cpa	D-Pal		Tyr(N-Me)	D-Asn		Lys(iPr)		D-Ala-NH$_2$	SC depot

ABBREVIATIONS: Ac, acetyl; EtNH$_2$, *N*-ethylamide; tBu, t butyl; D-Nal, 3-(2-naphthyl)-D-alanyl; ImBzl, imidobenzyl; Cpa, chlorophenylalanyl; Pal, 3-pyridylalanyl; AzGly, azaglycyl; hArg(Et)$_2$, ethyl homoarginine; IV, intravenous; SC, subcutaneous; IN, intranasal; IM, intramuscular.

mones. Each hormone is a glycosylated heterodimer containing a common α-subunit and a distinct β-subunit that confers specificity of action. Among the β-subunits of this family, that of hCG is most different because it contains a carboxy-terminal extension of 30 amino acids and extra carbohydrate residues. The carbohydrate residues on the gonadotropins play a role in signal transduction at the gonadotropin receptors and also influence the rates of clearance of the gonadotropins from the circulation and thus their serum half-lives; the longer half-life of hCG has some clinical relevance for its use in assisted reproduction technologies (*see* below).

The actions of LH and hCG are mediated by the LH receptor, while those of FSH are mediated by the FSH receptor. Both of these G protein–coupled receptors have large, glycosylated extracellular domains that contribute to their affinity and specificity for their ligands. The FSH and LH receptors couple to G_s to activate the adenylyl cyclase–cyclic AMP pathway. At higher ligand concentrations, the agonist-occupied gonadotropin receptors also activate protein kinase C and Ca^{2+} signaling pathways *via* G_q-mediated effects on PLCβ. Since most, if not all, of the actions of the gonadotropins can be mimicked by cyclic AMP analogs, the precise physiological role of Ca^{2+} and protein kinase C in gonadotropin action remains to be determined.

Physiological Effects of Gonadotropins

In men, LH acts on testicular Leydig cells to stimulate the *de novo* synthesis of androgens, primarily testosterone, from cholesterol. Testosterone is required for gametogenesis within the seminiferous tubules and for maintenance of libido and secondary sexual characteristics (*see* Chapter 58). FSH acts on the Sertoli cells to stimulate the production of proteins and nutrients required for sperm maturation, thereby indirectly supporting germ cell maturation.

In women, the actions of FSH and LH are more complicated. FSH stimulates the growth of developing ovarian follicles and induces the expression of LH receptors on theca and granulosa cells. FSH also regulates the activity of aromatase in granulosa cells, thereby stimulating the production of 17β-estradiol. LH acts on the theca cells to stimulate the *de novo* synthesis of androstenedione, the major precursor of ovarian 17β-estradiol in premenopausal women (*see* Figure 57–1). LH also is required for the rupture of the dominant follicle during ovulation and for the synthesis of progesterone by the corpus luteum.

Mutations in genes encoding the gonadotropin subunits or their cognate receptors impair sexual development and reproduction

(Achermann and Jameson, 1999). Women with mutations in either FSHβ or its receptor present clinically with primary amenorrhea, infertility, and the absence of breast development. Histologically, the ovarian follicles fail to mature and corpora lutea are missing. In men, mutations of FSHβ or the FSH receptor are associated with decreased testes size and oligospermia, although several subjects have been fertile.

An inactivating mutation of LHβ has been reported in a 46-year-old XY subject with Leydig cell hypoplasia, lack of spontaneous puberty, and infertility. The external genitalia were masculinized, suggesting that androgen production *in utero* was driven by hCG. In contrast, apparently complete loss-of-function mutations of the LH receptor cause phenotypes ranging from male hypogonadism to male-to-female sex reversal of the external genitalia and failure to initiate puberty. Presumably, the loss of the LH receptor leads to a combined loss of responsiveness to both hCG and LH signaling *in utero*, which prevents virilization of the external genitalia. Women with homozygous inactivating mutations of the LH receptor present with primary amenorrhea or oligomenorrhea and infertility and have cystic ovaries on histological examination.

Mutations that constitutively activate the LH receptor cause an autosomal dominant syndrome of precocious puberty in males, a condition called testotoxicosis. The excessive production of testosterone before true puberty commences induces virilization in an LH-independent manner. A subset of these LH receptor mutations that also activate the phosphoinositide pathway has been associated with familial testicular tumors.

CLINICAL USES OF GNRH

As illustrated in Table 55–2, a number of clinically useful GnRH analogs have been synthesized. These include synthetic GnRH (gonadorelin) and GnRH analogs that contain substitutions at position 6 that protect against proteolysis and substitutions at the C-terminus that improve receptor-binding affinity. The analogs exhibit enhanced potency and a prolonged duration of action compared to GnRH, which has a half-life of approximately 2 to 4 minutes.

Pure GnRH antagonists have been developed that do not cause the initial increase in gonadotropin secretion seen when long-acting GnRH agonists are used to downregulate gonadotropin secretion. The antagonists used currently elicit fewer of the manifestations of local and systemic release of histamine that hampered the development of earlier compounds for clinical use.

Diagnostic Use of GnRH. Synthetic GnRH (*gonadorelin hydrochloride;* FACTREL) is marketed for diagnostic purposes to differentiate between pituitary and hypothalamic defects in patients with hypogonadotropic hypogonadism. After a blood sample is obtained for the baseline LH value, a single 100-μg dose of GnRH is administered subcutaneously or intravenously and serum LH levels are measured over the next 2 hours (at 15, 30, 45, 60, and 120 minutes after injection). A normal LH response to >10 mIU/ml indicates the presence of functional pituitary gonadotropes and prior exposure to GnRH.

Inasmuch as the long-term absence of GnRH can result in a decreased responsiveness of otherwise normal gonadotropes, the absence of a response does not always indicate intrinsic pituitary disease. Thus, some experts advocate use of multiple doses of GnRH in an effort to restore responsiveness of the gonadotropes. GnRH-stimulation testing also is used to determine whether a subject with precocious puberty has central (*i.e.,* GnRH-dependent) or peripheral (*i.e.,* GnRH-independent) precocious puberty. A GnRH-induced rise in plasma LH to greater than 10 mIU/ml in boys or 7 mIU/ml in girls is indicative of true precocious puberty rather than a GnRH-independent process. Due to intermittent problems with gonadorelin availability, some experts have employed GnRH agonists off-label as the stimulating agent for diagnostic assessment.

Therapeutic Uses of GnRH

Management of Infertility. Until recently, synthetic GnRH (*gonadorelin acetate,* LUTREPULSE) was used to treat patients with reproductive disorders secondary to disordered secretion of GnRH or GnRH deficiency. In women, it was administered either intravenously or subcutaneously by a pump in pulses that promoted a physiological cycle, with a starting dose of 2.5 μg per pulse every 120 minutes. If necessary, the dose was increased to 10 to 20 μg per pulse until ovulation was induced. Advantages over gonadotropin therapy (*see* below) included a lower risk of multiple pregnancies and a decreased need to monitor plasma estrogen levels or follicle size by ovarian ultrasonography. Side effects generally were minimal; the most common was local irritation due to the infusion device. In women, normal cycling levels of ovarian steroids could be achieved, leading to ovulation and menstruation. Because of its complexity, this regimen was previously available only in specialized centers of reproductive endocrinology. Production was discontinued by the United States manufacturer in 2003 and GnRH is no longer available.

Two GnRH antagonists, *ganirelix* (ANTAGON) and *cetrorelix* (CETROTIDE) (Table 55–2), have been used to suppress the LH surge and thus prevent premature follicular luteinization in ovarian-stimulation protocols that are part of assisted reproduction techniques. The GnRH antagonist is given either in the follicular phase (termed the "short protocol") or in the midluteal phase (termed the "long protocol")—in conjunction with gonadotropins—to induce follicular maturation (*see* below). Ovulation is then induced with hCG or LH. Because they lack the initial stimulation of gonadotropin secretion seen with GnRH agonists, the GnRH antagonists provide a more rapid effect and are likely to become the preferred drugs in this setting.

Suppression of Gonadotropin Secretion. As noted above, long-acting GnRH analogs eventually desensitize GnRH signaling pathways, markedly inhibiting gonado-

tropin secretion and decreasing the production of gonadal steroids. This pharmacological castration is useful in disorders that respond to reductions in gonadal steroids. A clear indication for this therapy is in children with gonadotropin-dependent precocious puberty, whose premature sexual maturation can be arrested with minimal side effects by chronic administration of a GnRH agonist.

Long-acting GnRH agonists are used for palliative therapy of hormonally responsive tumors (*e.g.,* prostate or breast cancer), generally in conjunction with agents that block steroid biosynthesis or action to avoid transient increases in hormone levels (*see* Chapter 51). Because it does not transiently increase sex steroid production, an extended-release form of the GnRH antagonist *abarelix* (PLENAXIS) also is marketed for use in prostate cancer patients in whom serious adverse consequences might accompany any stimulus to tumor growth (*e.g.,* in patients with spinal cord metastases where increased tumor growth could lead to paralysis). The GnRH agonists also are used to suppress steroid-responsive conditions such as endometriosis, uterine leiomyomas, and acute intermittent porphyria. Depot preparations of *goserelin* (ZOLADEX), *leuprolide* (LUPRON DEPOT, ELEGARD) or *triptorelin* (TRELSTAR LA), which can be administered subcutaneously or intramuscularly monthly or every 3 months, can be used in these settings and may be particularly useful for pharmacological castration in disorders such as paraphilia, for which strict patient compliance is problematic.

The long-acting agonists generally are well tolerated, and side effects are those that would be predicted to occur when gonadal steroidogenesis is inhibited (*e.g.,* hot flashes, vaginal dryness and atrophy, decreased bone density). Because of these effects, therapy in non–life-threatening diseases such as endometriosis or uterine leiomyomas generally is limited to 6 months unless add-back therapy with estrogens and/or progestins is incorporated into the regimen. In addition to these predicted effects, abarelix has been associated with a significant incidence of hypersensitivity reactions, and its therapeutic role remains to be defined. For safety reasons, abarelix distribution is limited to physicians who are enrolled in the manufacturer's prescribing program.

Clinical Uses of Gonadotropins

The gonadotropins are used increasingly in the arena of reproductive endocrinology. As a result, a number of formulations are available for clinical use.

Diagnostic Uses of Gonadotropins

Diagnosis of Pregnancy. Significant amounts of hCG are present in the maternal bloodstream and urine during pregnancy and can be detected immunologically with anti-sera specific for its unique β-subunit. This provides the basis for commercial pregnancy kits that qualitatively assay for the presence or absence of hCG in the urine. These kits offer a rapid, noninvasive means of detecting pregnancy within a few days after a woman's first missed menstrual period and are widely available without a prescription.

Quantitative measurements of plasma hCG concentration are made by immunoassay. These assays typically are used to assess whether or not pregnancy is proceeding normally or to help detect the presence of an ectopic pregnancy, hydatidiform mole, or choriocarcinoma. They also are employed to follow the therapeutic response of malignancies, such as germ cell tumors, that secrete hCG.

Timing of Ovulation. Ovulation occurs approximately 36 hours after the onset of the LH surge (10 to 12 hours after the peak of LH). Therefore, urinary concentrations of LH can be used to predict the time of ovulation. Kits are available over the counter that use LH-specific antibodies to provide a semiquantitative assessment of LH levels in urine. Urine LH levels are measured every 12 to 24 hours, beginning on day 10 to 12 of the menstrual cycle (assuming a 28-day cycle), to detect the rise in LH and thus estimate the time of ovulation. Such estimates facilitate the timing of sexual intercourse to achieve pregnancy.

Differential Diagnosis of Diseases of Male and Female Reproduction. Measurements of plasma LH and FSH levels, as determined by quantitative β-subunit–specific immunoassays, are useful in the diagnosis of several reproductive disorders. Low or undetectable levels of LH and FSH are indicative of hypogonadotropic hypogonadism and suggest hypothalamic or pituitary disease, whereas high levels of gonadotropins suggest primary gonadal diseases. Therefore, in cases of amenorrhea in women or delayed puberty in men and women, measurements of plasma gonadotropins can be used to distinguish between gonadal failure and hypothalamic-pituitary failure.

The FSH level on day 3 of the menstrual cycle is useful in assessing relative fertility. An FSH level of ≥ 10 mIU/ml is associated with reduced fertility, even if a woman is menstruating normally, and predicts a lower likelihood of success in assisted reproduction techniques such as *in vitro* fertilization.

The administration of hCG also is used to stimulate testosterone production and thus to assess Leydig cell function in men suspected of having Leydig cell failure (for example, in delayed puberty). Serum testosterone levels are assayed after multiple injections of hCG. A diminished testosterone response to hCG indicates Leydig

cell failure; a normal testosterone response suggests a hypothalamic-pituitary disorder.

Therapeutic Uses of Gonadotropins

Gonadotropins are purified from human urine or prepared using recombinant DNA technology. Several preparations of urinary gonadotropins have been developed. *Chorionic gonadotropin* (PREGNYL, NOVAREL, PROFASI, others), which mimics the action of LH, is obtained from the urine of pregnant women. Urine from postmenopausal women is the source of *menotropins* (PERGONAL, REPRONEX), which contain roughly equal amounts of FSH and LH, as well as a number of other urinary proteins. Because of their relatively low purity, menotropins are administered intramuscularly to decrease the incidence of hypersensitivity reactions. *Urofollitropin* (uFSH; BRAVELLE) is a highly purified FSH prepared by immunoconcentration with monoclonal antibodies and pure enough to be administered subcutaneously.

Recombinant preparations of gonadotropins are assuming an increasing role in clinical practice. Recombinant FSH (rFSH) is prepared by expressing cDNAs encoding the α and β subunits of FSH in a mammalian cell line, yielding products whose glycosylation pattern mimics that of FSH produced by gonadotropes. The two rFSH preparations that are available (*follitropin α* [GONAL-F] and *follitropin β* [PUREGON, FOLLISTIM]) differ slightly in their carbohydrate structures; both exhibit less inter-batch variability than do preparations purified from urine and can be administered subcutaneously, since they are considerably purer. The recombinant preparations are more expensive than the naturally derived hormones, and their relative advantages (*i.e.*, efficacy, lower frequency of side effects such as ovarian hyperstimulation) have not been definitively established despite much debate in the published literature.

Recombinant forms of hCG (choriogonadotropin alfa; OVIDREL) and LH (LUVERIS, LHADI) also have been developed and are being investigated for the treatment of infertility. Providing that their cost-benefit ratios are favorable, it is likely that these recombinant gonadotropin preparations will have an increasing role in the future, possibly replacing the urinary preparations entirely. In addition, recombinant technology is likely to lead to improved forms of gonadotropins with increased half-lives or higher clinical efficacy.

Female Infertility. Infertility affects approximately 10% of couples of reproductive age. Gonadotropins are used in the treatment of infertility, either for the induction of ovulation or in conjunction with assisted reproduction technologies (Huirne *et al.*, 2004). The administration of gonadotropins in these settings should be limited to physicians experienced in the treatment of infertility or endocrine disorders. Although most clearly indicated for ovulation induction in anovulatory women with hypogonadotropic hypogonadism secondary to hypothalamic or pituitary dysfunction, gonadotropins also are used to induce ovulation in women with the polycystic ovary syndrome who do not respond to clomiphene citrate (*see* Chapter 57). Gonadotropins also are used in women who are infertile despite normal ovulation, although therapy with clomiphene citrate typically is attempted first.

The goal of ovulation induction in anovulatory women is to induce the formation and ovulation of a single dominant follicle. A typical therapeutic regimen is to administer 75 IU of FSH daily in a "low-dose, step-up protocol." This dose is given daily until cycle day 6 or 7, after which transvaginal ultrasound is used to assess the number and size of developing follicles. Scans typically are performed every 2 to 3 days and focus on identifying intermediate follicles. Although the criteria used at different centers vary, the finding of a follicle larger than 18 mm in diameter indicates that follicular development has progressed adequately. If three or more follicles >16 mm are present, gonadotropin therapy generally is stopped and pregnancy prevented by barrier contraception to decrease the likelihood of multiple pregnancies or the ovarian hyperstimulation syndrome (OHSS; *see* below). Measurements of serum estradiol levels also may be helpful. The target estradiol range is from 500 to 1500 pg/ml, with lower levels indicating inadequate gonadotropin stimulation and higher values portending an increased risk of OHSS. If laboratory assessment indicates impaired ovarian response, the dose of FSH can be increased in increments of 37.5 IU daily to a maximum range of 225 to 450 IU/day.

To complete follicular maturation and induce ovulation, hCG (5000 to 10,000 IU) is given one day after the last dose of FSH. Despite the precautions outlined above, gonadotropin-induced ovulation results in multiple births in up to 10% to 20% of cases, due to the nonphysiological development of more than one preovulatory follicle and the release of more than one ovum.

Gonadotropin induction also is used for ovarian stimulation in conjunction with *in vitro* fertilization (IVF) and intracytoplasmic sperm injection (ICSI). In this setting, larger doses of FSH (typically 225 IU/day) are administered to induce the maturation of multiple follicles, thus permitting the retrieval of multiple oocytes for IVF and intrauterine transfer. In the most common "long protocol," FSH is administered in conjunction with a GnRH analog to prevent premature ovulation. Thereafter, hCG is given to induce final oocyte development (with typical doses of 5000 to 10,000 IU of urine-derived product or 250 μg of recombinant hCG), and then the mature eggs are retrieved from the preovulatory follicles at 32 to 36 hours after hCG administration. The ova are retrieved transvaginally under ultrasound guidance, fertilized *in vitro* with sperm (IVF) or by sperm injection (ICSI), and then transferred to the uterus (IVF) or less frequently to the fallopian tubes (gamete intrafallopian transfer). With these approaches, the increased risk of multiple births is related to the number of embryos that are transferred to the woman,

and there is a trend towards decreasing the number of embryos transferred to diminish this risk.

Aside from the risk of multiple births and its attendant complications, the major side effect of gonadotropin treatment is OHSS, which is believed to result from increased ovarian secretion of substances that increase vascular permeability and is characterized by rapid accumulation of fluid in the peritoneal cavity, thorax, and even the pericardium. Signs and symptoms include abdominal pain and/or distention, nausea and vomiting, diarrhea, marked ovarian enlargement, dyspnea, and oliguria. OHSS can lead to hypovolemia, electrolyte abnormalities, abnormal fluid accumulation (*e.g.*, ascites, pleural effusions, and hemoperitoneum), acute respiratory distress syndrome, thromboembolic events, and hepatic dysfunction. If there is clinical suspicion that OHSS is developing, or if routine laboratory investigation reveals the presence of more than 2 follicles greater than 17 mm or an estrogen level of >1500 pg/ml, then hCG should be withheld. Clinical data suggest that ovulation induction with either a GnRH agonist or recombinant LH, whose half-life is considerably shorter than that of hCG, may diminish the incidence of OHSS.

Apart from OHSS, there is debate about the potential deleterious effects of gonadotropins. Some studies have suggested that gonadotropins are associated with an increased risk of ovarian cancer, but this conclusion is controversial. Similarly, although there is emerging evidence that IVF itself may be associated with abnormal imprinting that increases the risk of developmental syndromes such as Angelman and Beckwith-Wiedemann syndromes (Gosden *et al.*, 2003), there is no evidence that the gonadotropins themselves increase the rate of congenital abnormalities in babies born from stimulated oocytes.

Male Infertility. In men with impaired fertility secondary to gonadotropin deficiency, gonadotropins can establish or restore fertility. Due to expense and to the occasional development of resistance to gonadotropins with prolonged use, standard treatment is to induce sexual development with androgens, reserving gonadotropins until fertility is desired.

Treatment typically is initiated with hCG (1500 to 2000 IU intramuscularly or subcutaneously) three times per week until clinical parameters and the plasma testosterone level indicate full induction of steroidogenesis. Thereafter, the dose of hCG is reduced to 2000 IU twice a week or 1000 IU three times a week, and menotropins (FSH + LH) or recombinant FSH is injected three times a week (typical doses for menotropins range from 75 to 150 IU or 37.5 IU for rFSH) to fully induce spermatogenesis. The most common side effect of gonadotropin therapy is gynecomastia, which occurs in up to one-third of patients and presumably reflects increased production of estrogens due to the induction of aromatase. Maturation of the prepubertal testes typically requires treatment for more than 6 months, and optimal spermatogenesis in some patients may require treatment for up to 2 years. Once spermatogenesis has been initiated by this combined therapy or in patients who develop hypogonadotropic hypogonadism after sexual maturation, ongoing treatment with hCG alone usually is sufficient to support sperm production. As discussed in the section entitled "Female Infertility," regimens employing recombinant LH, FSH, and hCG very likely will play increasing clinical roles.

Cryptorchidism. Cryptorchidism, the failure of one or both testes to descend into the scrotum, affects up to 3% of full-term male infants and becomes less prevalent with advancing postnatal age. Cryptorchid testes have defective spermatogenesis and are at increased risk for developing germ cell tumors. Hence, the current approach is to reposition the testes as early as possible, typically at 1 year of age but definitely before 2 years of age. The local actions of androgens stimulate descent of the testes; thus, hCG can be used to induce testicular descent if the cryptorchidism is not secondary to anatomical blockage. Therapy usually consists of injections of hCG (3000 IU/m² body surface area) intramuscularly every other day for 6 doses. If this does not induce testicular descent, orchiopexy should be performed.

OXYTOCIN

The structures of the neurohypophyseal hormones oxytocin and arginine vasopressin (also called antidiuretic hormone, or ADH) and the physiology and pharmacology of vasopressin are presented in Chapter 29. The following discussion emphasizes the physiology of oxytocin and its use in pregnancy.

Biosynthesis of Oxytocin

Oxytocin is a cyclic nonapeptide that differs from vasopressin by only two amino acids. It is synthesized as a larger precursor molecule in cell bodies of the paraventricular nucleus, and to a lesser extent, the supraoptic nucleus in the hypothalamus. The precursor is rapidly converted by proteolysis to the active hormone and its neurophysin, packaged into secretory granules as an oxytocin-neurophysin complex, and secreted from nerve endings that terminate primarily in the posterior pituitary gland (neurohypophysis). In addition, oxytocinergic neurons that regulate the autonomic nervous system project to regions of the hypothalamus, brainstem, and spinal cord. Other sites of oxytocin synthesis include the luteal cells of the ovary, the endometrium, and the placenta.

Stimuli for oxytocin secretion include sensory stimuli arising from dilation of the cervix and vagina and from suckling at the breast. Increases in circulating oxytocin in women in labor are difficult to detect, partly because of the pulsatile nature of oxytocin secretion and partly because of the activity of circulating oxytocinase. Nevertheless, increased oxytocin in maternal circulation is detected in the second stage of labor, likely triggered by sustained distension of the uterine cervix and vagina. Estradiol stimulates oxytocin secretion, whereas the ovarian polypeptide relaxin inhibits release. The inhibitory effect of relaxin appears to be the net result of a direct stimulatory effect on oxytocin-producing cells and an inhibitory action mediated indirectly by endogenous opioids. Other factors that primarily affect vasopressin secretion also have some impact on oxytocin release (*e.g.,* ethanol inhibits release, while pain, dehydration, hemorrhage, and hypovolemia stimulate release). Although peripheral actions of oxytocin appear to play no significant role in the response to dehydration, hemorrhage, or hypovolemia, oxytocin may participate in the central regulation of blood pressure. As described below, pharmacological doses of oxytocin can inhibit free water clearance by the kidney through activity similar to that of arginine vasopressin at vasopressin V_2 receptors, occasionally causing water intoxication if administered with large volumes of hypotonic fluid.

Physiological Roles of Oxytocin

Uterus. The human uterus has a very low level of motor activity during the first two trimesters of pregnancy. During the third trimester, spontaneous motor activity increases progressively until the sharp rise that constitutes the initiation of labor. Oxytocin stimulates the frequency and force of uterine contractions. Uterine responsiveness to oxytocin roughly parallels this increase in spontaneous activity and is highly dependent on estrogen, which increases the expression of the oxytocin receptors. Progesterone antagonizes the stimulant effect of oxytocin *in vitro,* and a decline in progesterone receptor signaling in late pregnancy may contribute to the normal initiation of human parturition. Because of difficulties associated with the measurement of oxytocin levels (*see* above) and because loss of pituitary oxytocin apparently does not compromise labor and delivery, the physiological role of oxytocin in pregnancy has been highly debated. Exogenous oxytocin can initiate or enhance rhythmic contractions at any time, but a considerably higher dose is required in early pregnancy. An eightfold increase in uterine sensitivity to oxytocin occurs in the last half of pregnancy, mostly in the last 9 weeks, accompanied by a thirtyfold increase in oxytocin receptor number between early pregnancy and early labor. The finding that the oxytocin antagonist *atosiban* (TRACTOCILE) is effective in suppressing preterm labor (*see* below) further supports the physiological importance of oxytocin in this setting.

Breast. Oxytocin plays an important physiological role in milk ejection. Stimulation of the breast through suckling or mechanical manipulation induces oxytocin secretion, causing contraction of the myoepithelium that surrounds alveolar channels in the mammary gland. This action forces milk from the alveolar channels into large collecting sinuses, where it is available to the suckling infant.

Mechanism of Action

Oxytocin acts *via* specific G protein–coupled receptors closely related to the V_{1a} and V_2 vasopressin receptors. In the human myometrium, these receptors couple to G_q and G_{11}, activating the $PLC\beta$-IP_3-Ca^{2+} pathway and enhancing activation of voltage-sensitive Ca^{2+} channels. Oxytocin also increases local prostaglandin production, which further stimulates uterine contractions.

Clinical Use of Oxytocin

Induction of Labor. Uterine-stimulating agents are used most frequently to induce or augment labor in selected pregnant women. Indications for induction of labor include situations in which the risk of continued pregnancy to the mother or fetus is considered to be greater than the risks of delivery or of pharmacological induction. Such circumstances include premature rupture of the membranes, isoimmunization, fetal growth restriction, and uteroplacental insufficiency (as in diabetes, preeclampsia, or eclampsia). Before labor is induced, it is essential to verify that the fetal lungs are sufficiently mature (*i.e.,* the lecithin-sphingomyelin ratio in amniotic fluid is >2) and to exclude potential contraindications (*e.g.,* abnormal fetal position, evidence of fetal distress, placental abnormalities, or previous uterine surgery that predisposes the uterus to rupture during labor).

Oxytocin (PITOCIN, SYNTOCINON) is the drug of choice for labor induction. It is administered by intravenous infusion of a diluted solution (typically 10 mIU/mL), preferably by means of an infusion pump. Although there is continuing debate concerning the optimal dose to induce labor, some physicians use a protocol involving an initial dose of 1 mIU/minute, with dose increases of no greater than 1 mIU/minute every 30 to 40 minutes. Other authorities advocate a more aggressive approach, with starting doses of 6 mIU/minute and increases of up to 2 mIU/minute at 20-minute intervals. Some published trials have suggested that the higher-dose regimens result in a lower rate of cesarean sections. If doses of 40 mIU/minute fail to initiate satisfactory uterine contractions, higher rates of infusion are unlikely to be successful. As labor progresses, the dose of oxytocin required to maintain good uterine contractions may decrease.

During labor induction, a physician must be immediately available, and the mother and fetus should be monitored continuously to determine fetal and maternal heart rates, maternal blood pressure, and the strength of uterine contractions. If uterine hyperstimulation occurs, as evidenced by too-frequent contractions or the development of uterine tetany, the oxytocin should be discontinued immediately. The half-life of intravenous oxytocin is short (~3 minutes); thus the hyperstimulatory effects of oxytocin should resolve within several minutes after the infusion is stopped. Because of its structural similarity to vasopressin, oxytocin at higher doses has antidiuretic effects and infusions of ≥20 mIU/minute decrease free water clearance by the kidney. Particularly if hypotonic fluids (*e.g.,* dextrose in water) are infused too liberally, water intoxication may result in convulsions, coma, and even death. Vasodilating actions of oxytocin also have been noted, particularly at high doses, which may provoke hypotension and reflex tachycardia. Deep anesthesia may exaggerate the hypotensive effect of oxytocin by preventing the reflex tachycardia.

Augmentation of Labor. Because the resulting uterine hyperstimulation often is too forceful and sustained to be compatible with the safety of the mother and fetus, oxytocin generally should not be used to augment labor that is progressing normally. To augment hypotonic contractions in dysfunctional labor, it rarely is necessary to exceed an infusion rate of 10 mIU/minute, and doses of >20 mIU/minute rarely are effective when lower concentrations fail. Potential complications of overstimulation include trauma of the mother or fetus due to forced passage through an incompletely dilated cervix, uterine rupture, and compromised fetal oxygenation due to decreased uterine perfusion. In the setting of dysfunctional labor, as seen most frequently in nulliparous women, oxytocin can be used to advantage by experienced obstetricians to facilitate labor progression. Oxytocin usually is effective when there is a prolonged latent phase of cervical dilation and when, in the absence of cephalopelvic disproportion, there is an arrest of dilation or descent. Epidural anesthesia can impair the reflex stimulation of endogenous oxytocin during the second stage of labor; in this setting, the cautious administration of oxytocin may facilitate labor progression.

Third Stage of Labor and Puerperium. Postpartum hemorrhage is a significant problem in developed nations and is of even greater importance in underdeveloped countries. After delivery of the fetus or after therapeutic abortion, a firm, contracted uterus greatly reduces the incidence and extent of hemorrhage. Oxytocin (10 IU/minute intramuscularly) often is given immediately after delivery to help maintain uterine contractions and tone. Alternatively, 20 IU of oxytocin is diluted in 1 L of intravenous solution and infused at a rate of 10 ml/minute until the uterus is contracted. Then the infusion rate is reduced to 1 to 2 ml/minute until the mother is ready for transfer to the postpartum unit. If this is ineffective, ergot alkaloids such as *ergonovine maleate* (ERGOTRATE) or its methyl analog *methylergonovine maleate* (METHERGINE) or the prostaglandin analog *misoprostol* may be used in normotensive patients. The ergot alkaloids are discussed in more detail in Chapter 11; prostaglandins are discussed in Chapter 25.

Oxytocin Challenge Test. In patients whose pregnancy holds increased risk for maternal or fetal complications (*e.g.,* maternal diabetes mellitus or hypertension), an oxytocin challenge test can be used to assess fetal well-being. Oxytocin is infused intravenously, initially at a rate of 0.5 mIU/minute; this rate is increased slowly until 3 uterine contractions occur in 10 minutes. Concurrent monitoring of the fetal heart rate indicates whether or not the uterine contractions are associated with changes in fetal heart rate known to be associated with fetal distress. The outcome of the oxytocin challenge test is helpful in determining the presence of adequate placental reserve for continuation of high-risk pregnancies.

Oxytocin-Receptor Antagonists

Peptide analogs that competitively inhibit the interaction of oxytocin with its membrane receptor have been developed, and one such antagonist, atosiban, has been introduced in a number of countries for the treatment of preterm labor. In clinical trials, atosiban decreased the frequency of uterine contractions and increased the number of women who remained undelivered, with at least comparable efficacy to β adrenergic agonists but with a lower incidence of side effects (Tsatsaris *et al.*, 2004). To date, however, studies have not demonstrated a significant improvement in infant outcome. Establishing the relative roles of atosiban and other oxytocin receptor antagonists under development *versus* agents such as calcium channel blockers in premature labor remains an area of active investigation.

CLINICAL SUMMARY

We continue to make advances in the pharmacotherapy of certain endocrine and reproductive disorders. In children, the indications for growth hormone therapy have been expanded beyond patients with classic, unequivocal growth hormone deficiency, and the drug increasingly is used in conditions such as Turner's syndrome, chronic renal failure, cystic fibrosis, and other conditions associated with short stature, including idiopathic short stature. Although it remains controversial, growth hormone also is used increasingly to treat adults with growth hormone deficiency, with proposed benefits that include increased muscle mass, decreased adiposity, increased bone mineral density, and improved subjective well-being. Adverse effects occur more commonly in adults, and the dose should be adjusted so that the serum IGF-1 level is in the mid-normal range.

Pharmacotherapy also plays an important role in the treatment of functional tumors that produce growth hormone (acromegaly) or prolactin (prolactinomas). For acromegaly, sustained-release preparations of somatostatin analogs normalize growth hormone and IGF-1 levels in approximately 65% of patients. Pegvisomant, a growth hormone receptor antagonist, is even more effective, normalizing these parameters in up to 90% of patients. For prolactinomas, dopamine receptor antagonists remain the mainstay of treatment; cabergoline is preferred by many patients because of its lower incidence of side effects relative to other agents.

Another important use of the pituitary hormones is in reproductive medicine. Both GnRH receptor agonists and GnRH receptor antagonists can be used to down-regulate gonadotropin levels and block endogenous production of sex steroids. Indications include interruption of precocious puberty, therapy of cancers whose growth is stimulated by sex steroids (*e.g.,* breast, prostate), and suppression of endogenous gonadotropins in assisted reproduction technologies. Gonadotropins are frequently used in assisted reproduction technologies to stimulate follicular maturation and to induce ovulation. Although debate continues about relative efficacy and cost-benefit factors of these alternative therapies, recombinant gonadotropins largely are replacing gonadotropins purified from human urine in clinical use.

Oxytocin is used to induce labor or to augment its progression. After delivery, oxytocin also can be used to increase uterine tone and diminish postpartum hemorrhage. In contrast, the oxytocin receptor antagonist, atosiban, can be used to suppress uterine contractions in the setting of premature labor; its precise role relative to other drugs is still under evaluation.

BIBLIOGRAPHY

Abuzzahab, M.J., Schneider, A., Goddard, A., *et al.* Intrauterine Growth Retardation (IUGR) Study Group. IGF-1 receptor mutations resulting in intrauterine and postnatal growth retardation. *N. Engl. J. Med.,* **2003,** *349:*2211–2222.

Achermann, J.C., and Jameson, J.L. Fertility and infertility: genetic contributions from the hypothalamic-pituitary-gonadal axis. *Mol. Endocrinol.,* **1999,** *13:*812–818.

Anonymous. Growth-hormone-releasing factor for growth hormone deficiency. *Med. Lett. Drugs Ther.,* **1999,** *41:*2–3.

Comacho-Hubner, C., Woods, K.A., Miraki-Moud, F., *et al.* Effects of recombinant human insulin-like growth factor I (IGF-1) therapy on the growth hormone-IGF system of a patient with a partial IGF-1 gene deletion. *J. Clin. Endocrinol. Metab.,* **1999,** *84:*1611–1616.

Cummings, D.E., and Merriam, G. Growth hormone therapy in adults. *Annu. Rev. Med.,* **2003,** *54:*513–533.

Firth, S.M., and Baxter, R.C. Cellular actions of the insulin-like growth factor binding proteins. *Endocr. Rev.,* **2002,** *23:*824–854.

Goffin, V., Binart, N., Touraine, P., and Kelly, P.A. Prolactin: the new biology of an old hormone. *Annu. Rev. Physiol.*, **2002**, *64:*47–67.

Gosden, R., Trasler, J., Lucifero, D., and Faddy, M. Rare congenital disorders, imprinted genes, and assisted reproductive technology. *Lancet,* **2003**, *361:*1975–1977.

Herrington, J., and Carter-Su, C. Signaling pathway activated by the growth hormone receptor. *Trends Endocrinol. Metab.*, **2001**, *12:*252–257.

Huirne, J.A.F., Lambalk, C.B., Van Loenen, A.C., *et al.* Contemporary pharmacological manipulation in assisted reproduction. *Drugs,* **2004**, *64:*297–322.

Kopchick, J.J., Parkinson, C., Stevens, E.C., and Trainer, P.J. Growth hormone receptor antagonists: discovery, development, and use in patients with acromegaly. *Endocr. Rev.*, **2002**, *23:*623–646.

McKeage, K., Cheer, S., and Wagstaff, A.J. Octreotide long-acting release (LAR): a review of its use in the management of acromegaly. *Drugs,* **2003**, *63:*2473–2499.

Molitch, M.E. Medical management of prolactin-secreting pituitary adenomas. *Pituitary,* **2002a**, *5:*55–65.

Molitch, M.E. Diagnosis of growth hormone deficiency in adults—how good do the criteria need to be? *J. Clin. Endocrinol. Metab.*, **2002b**, *87:*473–476.

Quigley, C.A. The patient with growth hormone deficiency: issues in the transition from childhood to adulthood. *Curr. Opin. Endocrinol. Diab.*, **2003**, *10:*277–289.

Torrado, J., and Carrascosa, C. Pharmacological characteristics of parenteral IGF-1 administration. *Curr. Pharm. Biotechnol.*, **2003**, *4:*123–140.

Tsatsaris, V., Carbonne, B., and Cabrol, D. Atosiban for preterm labour. *Drugs,* **2004**, *64:*375–382.

Vance, M.L., and Mauras, N. Growth hormone therapy in adults and children. *N. Engl. J. Med.,* **1999**, *341:*1206–1216.

Weckbecker, G., Lewis, I., Albert, R., *et al.* Opportunities in somatostatin research: biological, chemical, and therapeutic aspects. *Nat. Rev. Drug Discov.*, **2003**, *2:*999–1017.

Yoshihara, F., Kojima, M., Hosoda, H., *et al.* Ghrelin: a novel peptide for growth hormone release and feeding regulation. *Curr. Opin. Clin. Nutr. Metab. Care,* **2002**, *5:*391–395.

THYROID AND ANTITHYROID DRUGS

Alan P. Farwell and Lewis E. Braverman

Thyroid hormones, the only known iodine-containing compounds with biological activity, have two important functions. In developing animals and human beings, they are crucial determinants of normal development, especially in the central nervous system (CNS). In the adult, thyroid hormones act to maintain metabolic homeostasis, affecting the function of virtually all organ systems. To meet these requirements, the thyroid gland contains large stores of preformed hormone. Metabolism of the thyroid hormones occurs primarily in the liver, although local metabolism also occurs in target tissues such as the brain. Serum concentrations of thyroid hormones are precisely regulated by the pituitary hormone, thyrotropin, in a classic negative-feedback system. The predominant actions of thyroid hormone are mediated *via* binding to nuclear thyroid hormone receptors (TRs) and modulating transcription of specific genes. In this regard, thyroid hormones share a common mechanism of action with steroid hormones, vitamin D, and retinoids, whose receptors make up a superfamily of nuclear receptors (*see* Chapter 1). As with steroid hormones, it has become clear that thyroid hormones also have diverse nongenomic actions (Yen and Chin, 2005).

Disorders of the thyroid are common. They consist of two general presentations: changes in the size or shape of the gland or changes in secretion of hormones from the gland. Thyroid nodules and goiter in the euthyroid patient are the most common endocrinopathies and can be caused by benign and malignant tumors. Overt hyper- and hypothyroidism often exhibit dramatic clinical manifestations; however, more subtle presentations require the use of biochemical tests of thyroid function. Screening of the newborn population for congenital hypothyroidism, followed by the institution of appropriate thyroid hormone replacement therapy, has dramatically decreased the incidence of mental retardation and cretinism in the United States. Congenital hypothyroidism due to iodine deficiency remains the major preventable cause of mental retardation worldwide, although much progress has been made to eradicate iodine deficiency.

Effective treatment of most thyroid disorders is readily available. Treatment of the hypothyroid patient is straightforward and consists of hormone replacement. There are more options for treatment of the hyperthyroid patient, including the use of antithyroid drugs to decrease hormone synthesis and secretion and destruction of the gland by the administration of radioactive iodine or by surgical removal. Treatment of thyroid disorders in general is extremely satisfying, as most patients can be either cured or have their diseases controlled (Braverman and Utiger, 2005).

THYROID

The thyroid gland is the source of two fundamentally different types of hormones. The iodothyronine hormones include *thyroxine* (T_4) and *3,5,3′-triiodothyronine* (T_3); they are essential for normal growth and development and play an important role in energy metabolism. The other known secretory product of the thyroid, calcitonin, is produced by the parafollicular (C–) cells and is discussed in Chapter 61.

History. The thyroid gland was described by Galen and was named "glandulae thyroidaeae" by Wharton in 1656. For two centuries thereafter, various clinicians offered opinions about the gland's function (Harington, 1935): that the viscous fluid within the follicles lubricated the trachea and that the gland was larger in women, to serve a cosmetic function in giving grace to the contour of the neck (Wharton); that the liberal blood supply of the gland provided a vascular shunt for the brain; that the larger size of the gland in women was "necessary to guard the female system from the influence of the more numerous causes of irritation and vexation of mind to which they are exposed than the male sex" (Rush), a view opposed by Hofrichter, who pointed out, "If it were indeed true that the thyroid contains more blood at some times than at others, this effect would be visible to the naked eye; in this case women would certainly have long ceased to go about with bare necks, for husbands would have learned to recognize the swelling of this gland as a danger signal of threatening trouble from their better halves." Reading this, one cannot but wonder at how future scientists will look upon some of the biomedical opinions of our own age.

The thyroid was first recognized as an organ of importance when enlargement was observed to be associated with changes in the eyes and the heart in the condition we now call *hyperthyroidism.* This condition, the manifestations of which can be as striking as any in medicine, escaped description until Parry saw his first case in 1786. Parry's account, published in 1825, was followed in 1835 and 1840 by those of Graves and Basedow, whose names became applied to the disorder. In 1874, Gull associated atrophy of the gland with the symptoms now known to be characteristic of *hypothyroidism,* also known in adults as *Gull's disease.* The term *myxedema* was applied to the clinical syndrome in 1878 by Ord in the belief that the characteristic thickening of the subcutaneous tissues was due to excessive formation of mucus.

Extirpation experiments to elucidate the function of the thyroid were at first misinterpreted because of the simultaneous removal of the parathyroids. However, Gley's research on the parathyroid glands in the late 19th century allowed the functional differentiation of these two endocrine glands. Only after calcitonin was discovered in 1961 was it realized that the thyroid also plays a role in the regulation of Ca^{2+}. In 1891, Murray first treated a case of hypothyroidism by injecting an extract of the thyroid gland; in 1892, Howitz, Mackenzie, and Fox independently discovered that thyroid tissue was fully effective when given by mouth.

Magnus-Levy discovered the effect of the thyroid on metabolic rate in 1895; he found that Gull's disease was characterized by a low rate of metabolism and that the administration of thyroid to hypothyroid or normal individuals increased oxygen consumption.

Chemistry of Thyroid Hormones. The principal hormones of the thyroid gland are the iodine-containing amino acid derivatives of thyronine—(T_4 and T_3; Figure 56–1). Thyroxine was isolated and crystallized from a hydrolysate of thyroid by Kendall in 1915; he found that the crystalline product exerted the same physiological effects as the extract from which it was obtained. Eleven years later, Harington elucidated the structural formula of thyroxine, and in 1927 Harington and Barger synthesized the hormone.

Following the isolation and the chemical identification of thyroxine, it was generally believed that all the hormonal activity of thyroid tissue could be accounted for by its content of thyroxine. However, careful studies revealed that crude thyroid preparations possessed greater calorigenic activity than could be accounted for by their thyroxine content. The enigma was resolved with the detection, isolation, and synthesis of triiodothyronine by Gross and Pitt-Rivers (1952). Triiodothyronine is qualitatively similar to thyroxine in its biological action but is much more potent on a molar basis.

Structure–Activity Relationships. The stereochemical nature of the thyroid hormones plays an important role in defining hormone activity. Myriad structural analogs of thyroxine have been synthesized to define the structure–activity relationship, to detect antagonists of thyroid hormones, and to find compounds exhibiting a desirable activity while not showing unwanted effects. The only significant success has

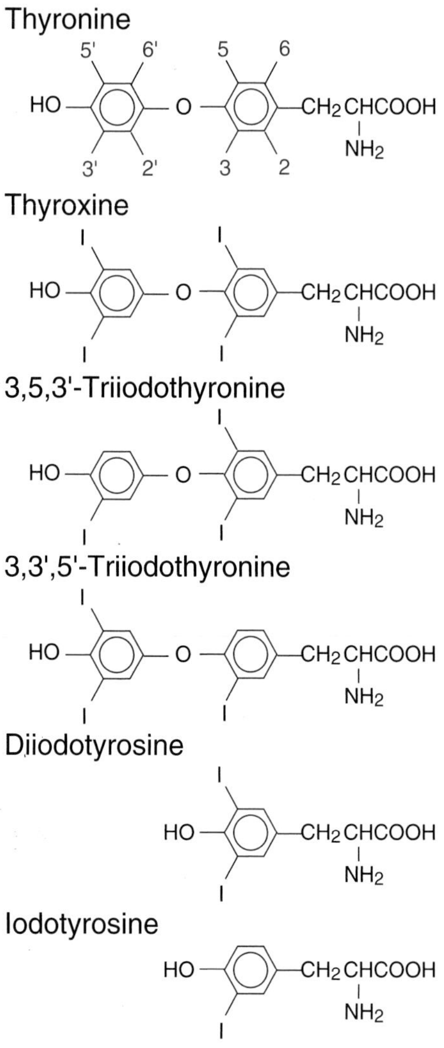

Figure 56–1. *Thyronine, thyroid hormones, and precursors.*

been the partial separation of the cholesterol-lowering action of thyroxine analogs from their calorigenic or cardiac effects. For example, introduction of specific arylmethyl groups at the 3′ position of triiodothyronine results in analogs that are liver-selective, cardiac-sparing thyromimetics (Leeson *et al.*, 1989). The D isomer of thyroxine was once used to lower the concentration of cholesterol in plasma, but cardiac side effects resulted in discontinuation of the clinical uses of this hormone. 3,5,3′-triiodothyroacetic acid (triac) has less thyromimetic activity in the heart than in other thyroid hormone–responsive tissues (Liang *et al.*, 1997). GC-1, a new thyromimetic, offers preferential binding to the β isoform of the thyroid hormone receptor (TRβ), which should result in specific metabolic effects in different target tissues (Yoshihara *et al.*, 2003).

The structural requirements for a significant degree of thyroid hormone activity have been defined (Cody, 2005; Baxter *et al.*, 2004). The 3′-monosubstituted compounds are more active than the 3′,5′-disubstituted molecules. Thus, triiodothyronine is five times more potent than thyroxine, while 3′-isopropyl-3,5-diiodothyronine has seven times the activity.

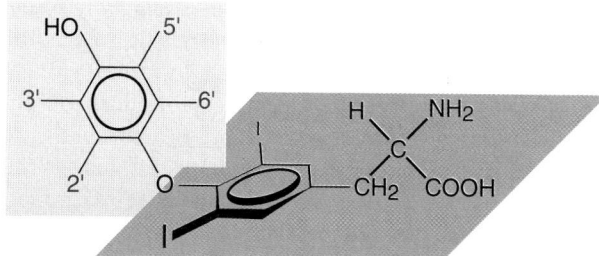

Figure 56–2. *Structural formula of 3,5-diiodothyronine, drawn to show the conformation in which the planes of the aromatic rings are perpendicular to each other.* (Adapted from Jorgensen, 1964. *See also* Cody, 2005.)

Although the chemical nature of the 3, 5, 3′, and 5′ substituents is important, their effects on the conformation of the molecule are even more so. In thyronine, the two rings are angulated at about 120° at the ether oxygen and are free to rotate on their axes. As depicted schematically in Figure 56–2, the 3,5 iodines restrict rotation of the two rings, which tend to take up positions perpendicular to one another. While not potent, even halogen-free derivatives possess some activity if they have the proper conformation. In general, the affinity of iodothyronines for the TRs parallels their biological potency (Yen and Chin, 2005), but additional factors can affect therapeutic potency, including affinity for plasma proteins, rate of metabolism, and rate of entry into cell nuclei. There are, for instance, T_4 transporters resembling the monocarboxylate transporter MCT8.

Recent structure–activity correlations indicate that certain plant flavonoids that are long-standing folk remedies can exhibit antithyroid properties, including inhibition of the enzyme that catalyzes 5′ (outer, or tyrosyl ring) deiodination of T_4 (type I iodothyronine 5′-deiodinase) (Cody, 2005). These compounds are also potent competitors of thyroxine binding to transthyretin. Computer graphic modeling suggests that the best structural homology between thyroid hormones and flavonoids involves their respective phenolic rings.

Biosynthesis of Thyroid Hormones. The synthesis of the thyroid hormones is unique, complex, and seemingly grossly inefficient. The thyroid hormones are synthesized and stored as amino acid residues of thyroglobulin, a protein constituting the vast majority of the thyroid follicular colloid. The thyroid gland is unique in storing great quantities of potential hormone in this way, and extracellular thyroglobulin can represent a large portion of the thyroid mass. Thyroglobulin is a complex glycoprotein made up of two apparently identical subunits, each of 330,000 daltons. Interestingly, molecular cloning has revealed that thyroglobulin belongs to a superfamily of serine hydrolases, including acetylcholinesterase (*see* Chapter 7).

The major steps in the synthesis, storage, release, and interconversion of thyroid hormones are the following: (1) uptake of iodide ion (I^-) by the gland; (2) oxidation of iodide and the iodination of tyrosyl groups of thyroglobulin; (3) coupling of iodotyrosine residues by ether linkage

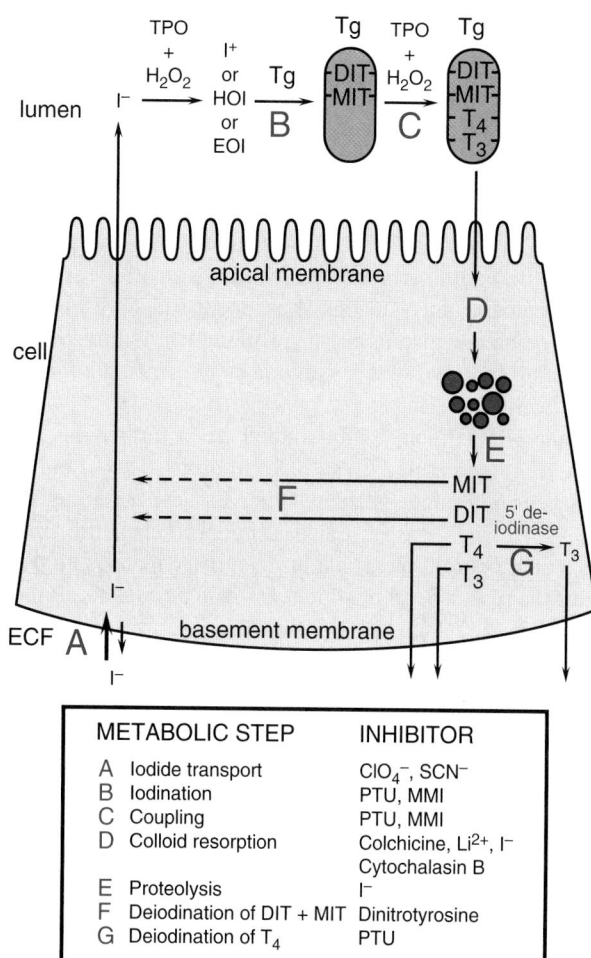

Figure 56–3. *Major pathways of thyroid hormone biosynthesis and release.* *Abbreviations:* Tg, thyroglobulin; DIT, diiodotyrosine; MIT, monoiodotyrosine; TPO, thyroid peroxidase; HOI, hypoiodous acid; EOI, enzyme-linked species; PTU, propylthiouracil; MMI, methimazole; ECF, extracellular fluid. (Adapted from Taurog, 2000, with permission.)

to generate the iodothyronines; (4) resorption of the thyroglobulin colloid from the lumen into the cell; (5) proteolysis of thyroglobulin and the release of thyroxine and triiodothyronine into the blood; (6) recycling of the iodine within the thyroid cell via de-iodination of mono- and diiodotyrosines and reuse of the I^-; and (7) conversion of thyroxine (T_4) to triiodothyronine (T_3) in peripheral tissues as well as in the thyroid. These processes are summarized in Figure 56–3 and described in the correspondingly labeled sections below.

1. Uptake of Iodide. Iodine ingested in the diet reaches the circulation in the form of iodide. Under normal circumstances, its concentration in the blood is very low (0.2 to 0.4 μg/dl; about 15 to 30 nM), but the thyroid efficiently and actively transports the ion *via* a specific, membrane-bound protein, termed the sodium-iodide symporter (NIS) (Dohan *et al.*, 2003). As a result, the ratio of thyroid to plasma iodide concentration is usually between 20 and 50 and can far exceed 100 when the gland is stimulated. The iodide transport mechanism is inhibited by a number of ions such as thiocyanate and perchlorate (Figure 56–3). Thyrotropin (thyroid-stimulating hormone [TSH]; *see* below) stimulates the NIS, which is controlled by an autoregulatory mechanism. Thus, decreased stores of thyroid iodine enhance iodide uptake, and the administration of iodide can reverse this situation by decreasing NIS protein expression (Eng *et al.*, 1999).

The NIS is more easily studied when further metabolism of I^- is inhibited by antithyroid drugs. Thus, the NIS has been identified in many other tissues, including the salivary glands, gastric mucosa, midportion of the small intestine, choroid plexus, skin, mammary gland, and perhaps the placenta, all of which maintain a concentration of iodide greater than that of the blood (Carrasco, 2005). Iodide accumulation by the placenta and mammary gland may provide adequate supplies for the fetus and infant; no obvious purpose is served by the accumulation of iodide at the other sites.

2. Oxidation and Iodination. Consistent with the conditions generally necessary for halogenation of aromatic rings, the iodination of tyrosine residues requires the iodinating species to be in a higher state of oxidation than is the anion. The exact nature of the iodinating species was uncertain for many years. However, Magnusson and coworkers (1984) have provided convincing evidence that it is hypoiodate, either as hypoiodous acid or as an enzyme-linked species.

The oxidation of iodide to its active form is accomplished by thyroid peroxidase, a heme-containing enzyme that utilizes hydrogen peroxide (H_2O_2) as the oxidant (Arvan, 2005). The peroxidase is membrane-bound and appears to be concentrated at or near the apical surface of the thyroid cell. The reaction results in the formation of monoiodotyrosyl and diiodotyrosyl residues in thyroglobulin just prior to its extracellular storage in the lumen of the thyroid follicle. The formation of the H_2O_2 that serves as a substrate for the peroxidase probably occurs near its site of utilization and is stimulated by a rise in cytosolic Ca^{2+} (Takasu *et al.*, 1987). The TSH receptor is notably promiscuous in its coupling, stimulating members of four G protein families including G_q, which couples to the PLC-IP_3-Ca^{2+} pathway (Laugwitz *et al.*, 1996); thus, a Ca^{2+}-dependent effect on H_2O_2 production may be a means by which TSH stimulates the organification of iodide in thyroid cells.

3. Formation of Thyroxine and Triiodothyronine from Iodotyrosines. The remaining synthetic step is the coupling of two diiodotyrosyl residues to form thyroxine or of monoiodotyrosyl and diiodotyrosyl residues to form triiodothyronine. These oxidative reactions apparently are catalyzed by the same peroxidase discussed above. The mechanism involves the enzymatic transfer of groups, perhaps as iodotyrosyl free radicals or positively charged ions, within thyroglobulin. Although many other proteins can serve as substrates for the peroxidase, none is as efficient as thyroglobulin in yielding thyroxine. The conformation of the protein is thus presumed to facilitate this coupling reaction. Thyroxine formation primarily occurs near the amino terminus of the protein, while most of the triiodotyrosine is synthesized near the carboxy terminus (Dunn and Dunn, 2000). The relative rates of synthetic activity at the various sites depend on the concentration of TSH and the availability of iodide. This may account, at least in part, for the long-known relationship between the proportion of thyroxine and triiodothyronine formed in the thyroid and the availability of iodide or the relative quantities of the two iodotyrosines. For example, when there is a deficiency of iodine in rat thyroid, the ratio of thyroxine to triiodothyronine decreases from 4:1 to 1:3 (Greer *et al.*, 1968). Because triiodothyronine is the transcriptionally active iodothyronine and contains only three-fourths as much iodine, a decrease in the quantity of available iodine need have little impact on the effective amount of thyroid hormone elaborated by the gland. Although a decrease in the availability of iodide and the associated increase in the proportion of monoiodotyrosine favor the formation of triiodothyronine over thyroxine, a deficiency in diiodotyrosine ultimately can impair the formation of both compounds. In addition to the coupling reaction, intrathyroidal and secreted T_3 is generated by the 5′-deiodination of thyroxine.

4. Resorption; 5. Proteolysis of Colloid; 6. Secretion of Thyroid Hormones. Since T_4 and T_3 are synthesized and stored within thyroglobulin, proteolysis is an important part of the secretory process. This process is initiated by endocytosis of colloid from the follicular lumen at the apical surface of the cell, with the participation of a thyroglobulin receptor, megalin. This "ingested" thyroglobulin appears as intracellular colloid droplets, which apparently fuse with lysosomes containing the requisite proteolytic enzymes. It is generally believed that thyroglobulin must be completely broken down into its constituent amino acids for the hormones to be released. As the molecular mass of thyroglobulin is 660,000 daltons, and the protein is made up of about 300 carbohydrate residues and 5500 amino acid residues, only two to five of which are thyrox-

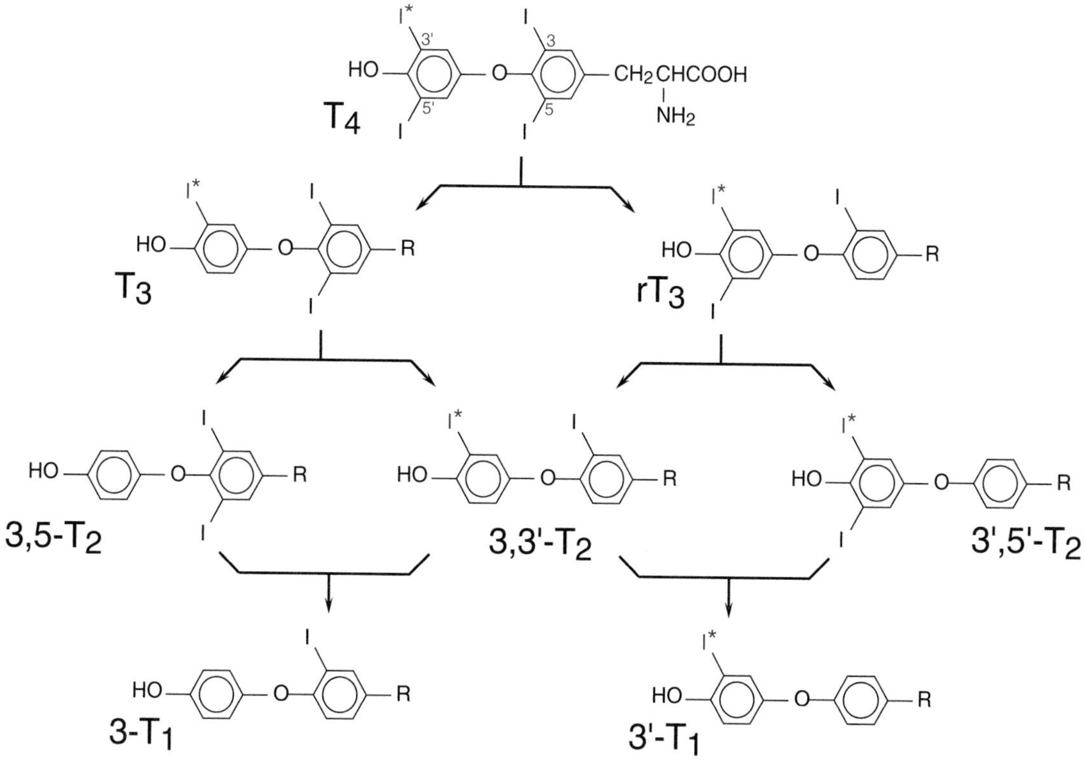

***Figure 56–4.** Pathways of iodothyronine deiodination.*

ine, this is an extravagant process. TSH appears to enhance the degradation of thyroglobulin by increasing the activity of several thiol endopeptidases of the lysosomes. The endopeptidases selectively cleave thyroglobulin, yielding hormone-containing intermediates that subsequently are processed by exopeptidases (Dunn and Dunn, 2000). The liberated hormones then exit the cell, presumably at its basal membrane. When thyroglobulin is hydrolyzed, monoiodotyrosine and diiodotyrosine also are liberated but usually do not leave the thyroid. Instead, they are selectively metabolized; the iodine, liberated in the form of iodide, is reincorporated into protein. Normally, all this iodide is reused; however, when proteolysis is activated intensely by TSH, some of the iodide reaches the circulation, at times accompanied by trace amounts of the iodotyrosines.

7. Conversion of Thyroxine to Triiodothyronine in Peripheral Tissues. The normal daily production of thyroxine is estimated to range between 70 and 90 μg, while that of triiodothyronine is between 15 and 30 μg. Although triiodothyronine is secreted by the thyroid, metabolism of thyroxine by sequential monodeiodination in the peripheral tissues accounts for about 80% of circulating triiodothyronine (Figure 56–4). Removal of the 5′-, or outer ring, iodine leads to the formation of

triiodothyronine and is the "activating" metabolic pathway. The major nonthyroidal site of conversion of T_4 to T_3 is the liver. Thus, when thyroxine is given to hypothyroid patients in doses that produce normal plasma concentrations of thyroxine, the plasma concentration of T_3 also normalizes (Braverman *et al.*, 1970). Most peripheral target tissues utilize T_3 that is derived from the circulating hormone. Notable exceptions are the brain and pituitary, where local generation of T_3 is the major source of intracellular hormone. Removal of the iodine on position 5 of the inner ring produces the metabolically inactive 3,3′,5′-triiodothyronine (reverse T_3, rT_3; Figure 56–1). Under normal conditions, about 41% of T_4 is converted to T_3, about 38% is converted to reverse T_3, and about 21% is metabolized *via* other pathways, such as conjugation in the liver and excretion in the bile. Normal circulating concentrations of T_4 in plasma range from 4.5 to 11 μg/dl, while those of T_3 are about one hundredfold less (60 to 180 ng/dl).

The enzymes that convert thyroxine to triiodothyronine are iodothyronine 5′-deiodinases, which exist as two distinct isozymes that are differentially expressed and regulated in peripheral tissues (Figure 56–5). Type I 5′-deiodinase (D1) is found in the liver, kidney, and thyroid and generates circulating T_3 that is utilized by most peripheral target tissues. Although 5′-deiodination is the major

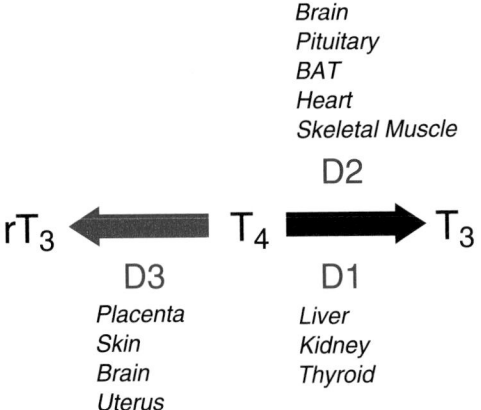

Brain
Pituitary
BAT
Heart
Skeletal Muscle

D2

rT₃ ⬅ T₄ ➡ T₃

D3   D1

Placenta   Liver
Skin   Kidney
Brain   Thyroid
Uterus

Figure 56–5. *Deiodinase isozymes. Abbreviations:* D1, type I iodothyronine 5′-deiodinase; D2, type II iodothyronine 5′-deiodinase; D3, type III iodothyronine 5-deiodinase; BAT, brown adipose tissue.

Table 56–1

Conditions and Factors That Inhibit Type I 5′-Deiodinase Activity

Acute and chronic illness
Caloric deprivation (especially carbohydrate)
Malnutrition
Glucocorticoids
β Adrenergic receptor antagonists (*e.g.*, propranolol in high doses)
Oral cholecystographic agents (*e.g.*, iopanoic acid, sodium ipodate)
Amiodarone
Propylthiouracil
Fatty acids
Fetal/neonatal period
Selenium deficiency

function of this isozyme, D1 also catalyzes 5-deiodination. D1 is inhibited by a variety of factors (Table 56–1), including the antithyroid drug *propylthiouracil* (*see* below). The decreased plasma triiodothyronine concentrations observed in nonthyroidal illnesses result from inhibition of D1 (Farwell and Dubord-Tomasetti, 1999) and decreased entrance of thyroxine into cells. D1 is up-regulated in hyperthyroidism and down-regulated in hypothyroidism. The cloning of D1 identified the enzyme as a selenoprotein that contains a selenocystine at the active site. Type II 5′-deiodinase (D2), also a selenoprotein, is distributed in the brain, pituitary, skeletal and cardiac muscle, and in the rat, in brown fat. It primarily supplies intracellular triiodothyronine to these tissues (Visser *et al.*, 1982). D2 has a much lower K_m for thyroxine than does D1 (nM *vs.* μM K_m values), and its activity is unaffected by propylthiouracil. D2 is dynamically regulated by its substrate, thyroxine, such that elevated levels of the enzyme are found in hypothyroidism and suppressed levels are found in hyperthyroidism. Thus, D2 appears to autoregulate the intracellular supply of triiodothyronine in the brain and pituitary. A D2-like selenoprotein DNA has been cloned from frog skin and from mammalian sources; however, some controversy still exists on the exact biochemical nature of D2. Inner ring- or 5-deiodination, a main inactivating pathway for T_3, is catalyzed by type III deiodinase (D3), which is found in placenta, skin, uterus, and brain. The three deiodinases comprise a family of selenoproteins encoded by different genes (Bianco and Larsen, 2005).

Transport of Thyroid Hormones in the Blood. Iodine in the circulation is normally present in several forms, with 95% as organic iodine and approximately 5% as iodide. Most organic iodine is thyroxine (90% to 95%), while triiodothyronine represents a relatively minor fraction (about 5%). The thyroid hormones are transported in the blood in strong but noncovalent association with certain plasma proteins (Benvenga, 2005).

Thyroxine-binding globulin (TBG) is the major carrier of thyroid hormones. It is an acidic glycoprotein with a molecular mass of approximately 63,000 daltons that binds one molecule of T_4 per molecule of protein with a very high affinity (the equilibration association constant, K_a, is approximately 10^{10} M^{-1}). T_3 is bound less avidly. Thyroxine, but not triiodothyronine, also is bound by transthyretin (thyroxine-binding prealbumin), a retinol-binding protein. This protein is present in higher concentration than is TBG and primarily binds thyroxine with an equilibrium association constant near 10^7 M^{-1}. Transthyretin has four apparently identical subunits but only a single high-affinity binding site. Albumin also can bind thyroxine when the more avid carriers are saturated but it is difficult to estimate its quantitative or physiological importance except in *familial dysalbuminemic hyperthyroxinemia*. This syndrome is an autosomal dominant disorder characterized by the increased affinity of albumin for thyroxine due to a point mutation in the albumin gene. Thyroxine binds also to the apolipoproteins of the high density lipoproteins, HDL₂ and HDL₃, the significance of which is unclear (Benvenga *et al.*, 1992).

Binding of thyroid hormones to plasma proteins protects the hormones from metabolism and excretion, resulting in their long half-lives in the circulation. The free (unbound) hormone is a small percentage (about 0.03% of thyroxine and about 0.3% of triiodothyronine) of the total hormone in plasma. The differential binding affinities for serum proteins also are reflected in the ten- to one hundredfold differences in circulating hormone concentrations and half-lives of T_4 and T_3.

Essential to understanding the regulation of thyroid function is the "free hormone" concept: only the unbound hormone has metabolic activity. Thus, because of the high degree of binding of thyroid hormones to plasma proteins,

Table 56–2

Factors That Alter Binding of Thyroxine to Thyroxine-Binding Globulin

INCREASE BINDING	DECREASE BINDING
Drugs	
Estrogens	Glucocorticoids
Methadone	Androgens
Clofibrate	L-Asparaginase
5-Fluorouracil	Salicylates
Heroin	Mefenamic Acid
Tamoxifen	Antiseizure medications
Selective estrogen	(phenytoin,
receptor modulators	carbamazepine)
	Furosemide
Systemic Factors	
Liver disease	Inheritance
Porphyria	Acute and chronic illness
HIV infection	
Inheritance	

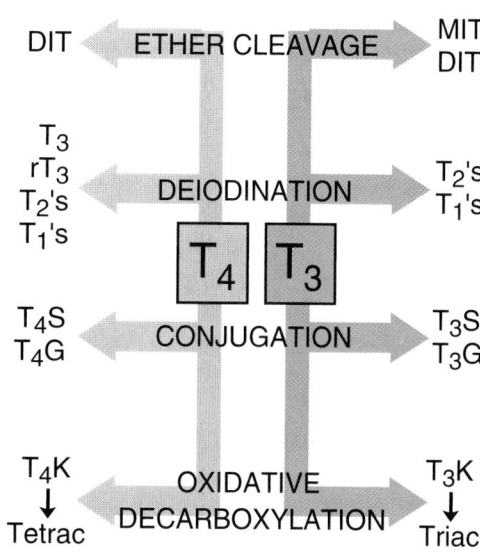

Figure 56–6. *Pathways of metabolism of thyroxine (T_4) and triiodothyronine (T_3).* Abbreviations: DIT, diiodotyrosine; MIT, monoiodotyrosine; T_4S, T_4 sulfate; T_4G, T_4 glucuronide; T_3S, T_3 sulfate; T_3G, T_3 glucuronide; T_4K, T_4 pyruvic acid; T_3K, T_3 pyruvic acid; Tetrac, tetraiodothyroacetic acid; Triac, triiodothyroacetic acid.

changes in either the concentrations of these proteins or the binding affinity of the hormones for the proteins has major effects on the total serum hormone levels. Certain drugs and a variety of pathological and physiological conditions, such as the changes in circulating concentrations of estrogens during pregnancy or during the administration of oral estrogens, can alter both the binding of thyroid hormones to plasma proteins and the amounts of these proteins (Table 56–2). However, since the pituitary responds to and regulates circulating free hormone levels, minimal changes in free hormone concentrations are seen. Therefore laboratory tests that measure only total hormone levels can be misleading. Appropriate tests of thyroid function are discussed later in this chapter.

Degradation and Excretion (Figure 56–6). Thyroxine is eliminated slowly from the body, with a half-life of 6 to 8 days. In hyperthyroidism, the half-life is shortened to 3 or 4 days, whereas in hypothyroidism it may be 9 to 10 days. These changes presumably reflect altered rates of metabolism of the hormone. In conditions associated with increased binding to TBG, such as pregnancy, clearance is retarded. The increase in TBG is due to the estrogen-induced increase in the sialic acid content of the synthesized TBG, resulting in decreased TBG clearance. The opposite effect is observed

when there is reduced protein binding of thyroid hormones or when binding to protein is inhibited by certain drugs (Table 56–2). T_3, which is less avidly bound to protein, has a half-life of approximately 1 day.

The liver is the major site of non-deiodinative degradation of thyroid hormones; T_4 and T_3 are conjugated with glucuronic and sulfuric acids through the phenolic hydroxyl group and excreted in the bile. Some thyroid hormone is liberated by hydrolysis of the conjugates in the intestine and reabsorbed. A portion of the conjugated material reaches the colon unchanged, where it is hydrolyzed and eliminated in feces as the free compounds.

As discussed above, the major route of metabolism of T_4 is deiodination to either T_3 or reverse T_3. Triiodothyronine and reverse T_3 are deiodinated to three different diiodothyronines, which are further deiodinated to two monoiodothyronines (Figure 56–4), inactive metabolites that are normal constituents of human plasma. Additional metabolites (monoiodotyrosine and diiodotyrosine) in which the diphenyl ether linkage is cleaved have been detected both *in vitro* and *in vivo*.

Regulation of Thyroid Function. Cellular changes occur in the anterior pituitary in association with endemic goiter or following thyroidectomy. The classical observations of Cushing in 1912 and of Simmonds two years later established that ablation or disease of the pituitary causes thyroid hypoplasia (Simmonds, 1914). It eventually was determined that thyrotropes of the anterior pituitary secrete *thyrotropin,* or TSH. TSH is a glycoprotein hormone with α and β subunits analogous to those of the gonadotropins. Its structure is discussed with those of other glycoprotein hormones in Chapter 55. Although there was evidence that thyroid hormone or its lack causes cellular changes in the pituitary, the control of secretion of TSH by the negative-feedback action of thyroid hormone was not appreciated fully until its central role in the pathogenesis of goiter was elucidated in the early 1940s. TSH is secreted in a pulsatile manner and circadian pattern, its levels in the circulation being highest during sleep at night. TSH secretion is precisely controlled by the hypothalamic peptide *thyrotropin-releasing hormone* (TRH) and by the concentration of free thyroid hormones in the circulation. Extra thyroid hormone inhibits transcription of both the TRH gene (Wilber and Xu, 1998) and the genes encoding the α and β subunit of thyrotropin, which suppresses the secretion of TSH and causes the thyroid to become inactive and regress. Any decrease in the normal rate of thyroid hormone secretion by the thyroid evokes an enhanced secretion of TSH in an attempt to stimulate the thyroid to secrete more hormone. Additional mechanisms of the effect of thyroid hormone on TSH secretion appear to be a reduction in TRH secretion by the hypothalamus and a reduction in the number of TRH receptors on pituitary cells. Figure 56–7 summarizes the regulation of thyroid hormone secretion.

Thyrotropin-Releasing Hormone (TRH). TRH stimulates the release of preformed TSH from secretory granules and also stimulates the subsequent synthesis of both α and β subunits of TSH. Somatostatin, dopamine, and pharmacological doses of glucocorticoids inhibit TRH-stimulated TSH secretion.

TRH is a tripeptide with both terminal amino and carboxyl groups blocked (L-pyroglutamyl-L-histidyl-L-proline amide). The mature hormone is derived from a precursor protein that contains six copies of the tripeptide flanked by dibasic residues. TRH is synthesized by the hypothalamus and released into the hypophyseal-portal circulation, where it interacts with TRH receptors on thyrotropes. The binding of TRH to its receptor, a GPCR, stimulates the G_q-PLC-IP$_3$-Ca^{2+} pathway and activates protein kinase C, ultimately stimulating the synthesis and release of TSH by the thyrotropes.

TRH also has been localized in the CNS in the cerebral cortex, circumventricular structures, neurohypophysis, pineal gland, and spinal cord. These findings, as well as its localization in nerve endings, suggest that TRH may

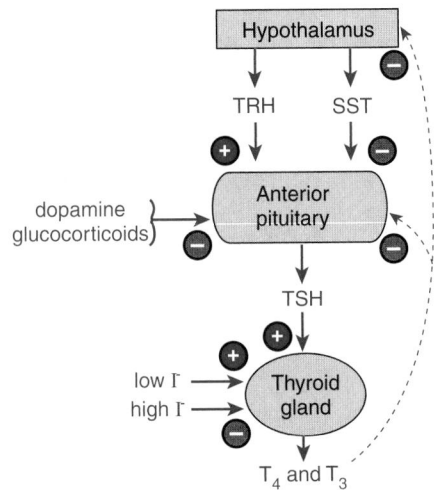

Figure 56–7. *Regulation of thyroid hormone secretion.* Myriad neural inputs influence hypothalamic secretion of thyrotropin-releasing hormone (TRH). TRH stimulates release of thyrotropin (TSH, thyroid-stimulating hormone) from the anterior pituitary; TSH stimulates the synthesis and release of the thyroid hormones T$_3$ and T$_4$. T$_3$ and T$_4$ feed back to inhibit the synthesis and release of TRH and TSH. Somatostatin (SST) can inhibit TRH action, as can dopamine and high concentrations of glucocorticoids. Low levels of I$^-$ are required for thyroxine synthesis, but high levels inhibit thyroxin synthesis and release.

act as a neurotransmitter or neuromodulator outside of the hypothalamus. Administration of TRH to animals produces CNS-mediated effects on behavior, thermoregulation, autonomic tone, and cardiovascular function, including increases in blood pressure and heart rate. TRH also has been identified in pancreatic islets, heart, testis, and parts of the gastrointestinal tract. Its physiological role in these sites is not known. TRH has been administered both intravenously and intrathecally as a therapeutic agent in refractory depression (Marangell *et al.,* 1997). TRH is no longer available in the United States.

Actions of TSH on the Thyroid. When TSH is given to experimental animals, the first measurable effect on thyroid hormone metabolism is increased secretion, which is detectable within minutes. All phases of hormone synthesis and release are eventually stimulated: iodide uptake and organification, hormone synthesis, endocytosis, and proteolysis of colloid. There is increased vascularity of the gland and hypertrophy and hyperplasia of thyroid cells.

These effects follow the binding of TSH to its receptor on the plasma membrane of thyroid cells. The TSH receptor is a GPCR that is structurally similar to the receptors for luteinizing hormone and follicle-stimulating hormone (*see* Chapter 55) (Vassart *et al.,* 2004). These receptors share significant amino acid homology and have large extracellular domains that are involved in hormone binding.

Binding of TSH to its receptor stimulates the G_s-adenylyl cyclase–cyclic AMP pathway. Higher concentrations of TSH activate the G_q-PLC pathway. Both the adenylyl cyclase and the phospholipase C signaling pathways appear to mediate effects of TSH on thyroid function in human beings (Vassart, 2005).

Multiple mutations of the TSH receptor result in clinical thyroid dysfunction (Tonacchera *et al.*, 1996b). Germline mutations can present as congenital, nonautoimmune hypothyroidism (Kopp *et al.*, 1995) or as autosomal dominant toxic thyroid hyperplasia (Tonacchera *et al.*, 1996a). Germline mutations of the TSH receptor can cause gestational hyperthyroidism due to a hypersensitivity of the receptor to HCG (Rodien *et al.*, 1998). Somatic mutations that result in constitutive activation of the receptor are associated with hyperfunctioning thyroid adenomas (Paschke *et al.*, 1994). Finally, resistance to TSH has been described, both in families with mutant TSH receptors (Sunthornthepvarakul *et al.*, 1995) and in those with no apparent mutations in either the TSH receptor or in TSH itself (Xie *et al.*, 1997).

Relation of Iodine to Thyroid Function. Normal thyroid function obviously requires an adequate intake of iodine; without it, normal amounts of hormone cannot be made, TSH is secreted in excess, and the thyroid becomes hyperplastic and hypertrophies. The enlarged and stimulated thyroid becomes remarkably efficient at extracting the residual traces of iodide from the blood, developing an iodine gradient that may be ten times normal; in mild-to-moderate iodine deficiency, the thyroid usually succeeds in producing sufficient hormone and preferentially secreting T_3. In more severe iodine deficiency, adult hypothyroidism and cretinism may occur.

In some areas of the world, simple or nontoxic goiter is prevalent because of insufficient dietary iodine (Dunn and Delange, 2005). Regions of iodine deficiency exist in Central and South America, Africa, Europe, Southeast Asia, and China. The daily requirement for iodine in adults is 1 to 2 μg/kg body weight. In the United States, recommended daily allowances for iodine range from 40 to 120 μg for children, 150 μg for adults, 220 μg for pregnancy, and 270 μg for lactation (Food and Nutrition Board, 2001). Vegetables, meat, and poultry contain minimal amounts of iodine, whereas dairy products and fish are relatively high in iodine content (Table 56–3) (Braverman, 2003). Potable water usually contains negligible amounts of iodine.

Table 56–3
Iodine Content in Some Foodstuffs in the United States (1982–1989)

FOOD	IODINE/SERVING, μg
Ready-to-eat cereals	87
Dairy-based desserts	70
Fish	57
Milk	56
Dairy products	49
Eggs	27
Bread	27
Beans, peas, tubers	17
Meat	16
Poultry	15

SOURCE: Adapted from Braverman *et al.*, 1994.

Iodine has been used empirically for the treatment of iodine-deficiency goiter for 150 years; however, its modern use evolved from extensive studies using iodine to prevent goiter in schoolchildren in Akron, Ohio, where endemic iodine-deficiency goiter was prevalent. The success of these experiments led to the adoption of iodine prophylaxis and therapy in many regions throughout the world where iodine-deficiency goiter was endemic.

The most practical method for providing small supplements of iodine for large segments of the population is the addition of iodide or iodate to table salt; iodate is now preferred. In some countries, the use of iodized salt is required by law; in others, including the United States, the use is optional. In the United States, iodized salt provides 100 μg of iodine per gram. However, while the United States population remains iodine-sufficient, iodine intake has steadily decreased over the last 20 years, a trend that needs to be monitored (Hollowell *et al.*, 1998). Other vehicles for supplying iodine to large populations who are iodine-deficient include oral or intramuscular injection of iodized oil (Elnagar *et al.*, 1995), iodized drinking water supplies, iodized irrigation systems, and iodized animal feed.

Actions of Thyroid Hormones. Although the precise biochemical mechanisms by which thyroid hormones exert their developmental and tissue-specific effects are the subject of ongoing investigation, most actions of thyroid hormones seem to be mediated by nuclear receptors (for review, *see* Yen, 2001; Yen and Chin, 2005). Triiodothyronine binds to high-affinity nuclear receptors, which then bind to specific DNA sequences (thyroid hormone response elements, TREs) in the promoter/regulato-

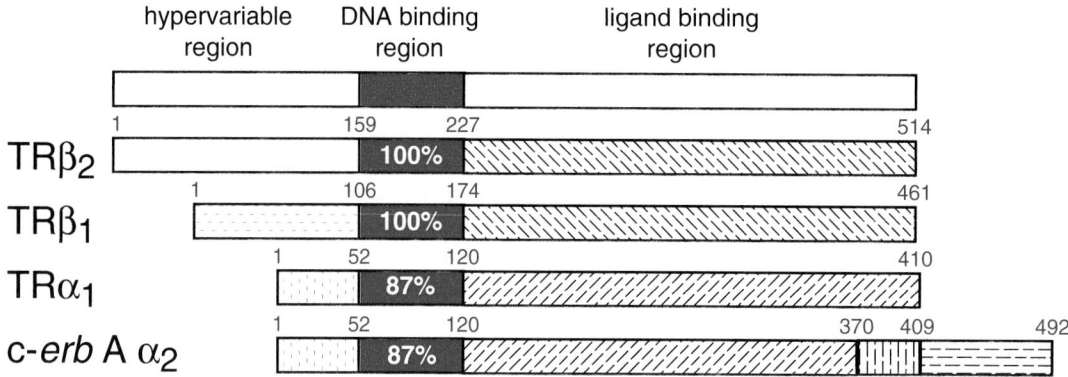

Figure 56–8. ***Thyroid hormone receptor isoforms.*** The percentage of amino acid identity in the DNA binding region is indicated. Identical patterns in the hypervariable and ligand binding regions indicate 100% homology. Three thyroid hormone receptor (TR) isoforms bind thyroid hormone (TRβ_1, TRβ_2, and TRα_1); c-*erb* A α_2 does not.

ry regions of target genes. In this fashion, triiodothyronine modulates gene transcription, and ultimately, protein synthesis. In general, the unliganded T$_3$ receptor is bound to thyroid response elements in the basal state. Typically, this represses gene transcription, although there are some examples of constitutive gene activation. Binding by T$_3$ may activate gene transcription by releasing the repression; the T$_3$-receptor complex also may have direct activation or repressive actions. T$_4$ also binds to these receptors, but with a much lower affinity than T$_3$. Despite its capacity to bind to nuclear receptors, thyroxine has not been shown to alter gene transcription. Thus, it is likely that T$_4$ serves principally as a "prohormone," with essentially all transcriptional actions of thyroid hormone caused by T$_3$.

Nuclear thyroid hormone receptors are the cellular homologs of an avian retroviral oncoprotein, denoted c-*erb* A. There is considerable homology between the thyroid hormone receptors and the steroid hormone receptors, which make up a gene superfamily that includes the retinoic acid and vitamin D receptors (*see* Chapters 1 and 61). The thyroid hormone receptors (TRs) are derived from two genes, c-*erb* A α (TRα) and c-*erb* A β (TRβ), with multiple isoforms identified (Figure 56–8) (Lazar, 1993). TRα_1 and TRβ_1 are found in virtually all tissues that respond to thyroid hormone; the other isoforms exhibit a more restricted distribution. For example, TRβ_2 is expressed solely in the anterior pituitary. c-*erb* A α_2, an isoform that binds to the TRE but does not bind T$_3$, is the most abundant isoform in the brain (Strait *et al.*, 1990). Another level of complexity in the regulation of thyroid hormone action at the transcriptional level was added with the identification of co-activators (Takeshita *et al.*, 1996) and co-repressors (Chen and Evans, 1995; Hörlein *et al.*, 1995) that are associated with the T$_3$-receptor complex and mediate hormone action (Lee and Yen, 1999). Resistance to thyroid hormone has been described in patients with mutations in the TRβ gene (Brucker-Davis *et al.*, 1995; Adams *et al.*, 1994) and in patients with defective co-activators (Weiss *et al.*, 1996).

Further insight into the mechanisms of thyroid hormone action emerged from transgenic mice lacking one or more of the thyroid hormone receptor isoforms. These knockout mice have abnormali-

ties in the auditory system, the thyroid-pituitary axis, the heart, the skeletal system, and the small intestine (Forrest *et al.*, 1996; Forrest *et al.*, 1990; Fraichard *et al.*, 1997; Wikström *et al.*, 1998). Despite the well-documented roles of thyroid hormone during brain development (Oppenheimer and Schwartz, 1997), knockout mice devoid of all known thyroid hormone receptors had few, if any, obvious abnormalities in brain development (Göthe *et al.*, 1999; Gauthier *et al.*, 2001). Since the overall deficits observed in the absence of TRs are markedly less than what one would expect if the T$_3$-binding thyroid hormone receptors were the sole mediator(s) of thyroid hormone action, the unliganded TRs may participate in this developmental program and the action of T$_3$ on target genes during brain development may be to relieve gene repression, rather than to activate gene expression (Hashimoto *et al.*, 2001; Flamant and Samarut, 2003). As noted above, the most abundant thyroid hormone receptor isoform in the brain throughout development is c-*erb* A α_2 (Strait *et al.*, 1990), which is obligatorily unliganded since it cannot bind T$_3$; this form continues to be expressed in most knockout mice due to the strategy used for thyroid hormone receptor gene deletion.

In addition to nuclear receptor–mediated actions, there are several well-characterized, nongenomic actions of thyroid hormones, including those occurring at the level of the plasma membrane and on the cellular cyto-architecture (Bassett *et al.*, 2003). In addition, there are thyroid hormone binding sites on mitochondria (Sterling, 1989). In several of these processes, thyroxine is the hormone that produces the response. Previously, the overall contribution of nongenomic actions to the general mechanism of thyroid hormone action was considered to be minor. However, at least in some species, this concept may need to be reassessed in light of the paucity of abnormalities in knockout mice, especially during brain development.

Growth and Development. Thyroid hormones seem to exert most of their effects through control of DNA transcription, and ultimately protein synthesis, profoundly influencing normal growth and development. Perhaps the most dramatic example is the tadpole, which is almost magically transformed into a frog by triiodothyronine. Not only does the animal grow limbs, lungs, and other terrestrial accoutrements, but T$_3$ also stimulates the synthesis of a host of enzymes, and in a gambit that plastic surgeons must envy, so influences the tail that it is digested away and used to build new tissue elsewhere.

Thyroid hormone plays a critical role in brain development (Bernal *et al.*, 2003; Koibuchi *et al.*, 2003). The appearance of functional, chromatin-bound thyroid hormone receptors coincides with neurogenesis in the brain (Strait *et al.*, 1990). The absence of thyroid hormone during the period of active neurogenesis (up to 6 months postpartum) leads to irreversible mental retardation (cretinism) and is accompanied by multiple morphological alterations in the brain. These severe morphological alterations result from disturbed neuronal migration, deranged axonal projections, and decreased synaptogenesis. Thyroid hormone supplementation during the first 2 weeks of life prevents the development of these disturbed morphological changes.

Myelin basic protein, a major component of myelin, is regulated by thyroid hormone during development (Farsetti *et al.*, 1991), and decreased expression of myelin basic protein in the hypothyroid brain impairs myelinization. The appearance of laminin, an extracellular matrix protein that provides key guidance signals to migrating neurons, is delayed and the content is diminished in the developing cerebellum of the hypothyroid rat (Farwell and Dubord-Tomasetti, 1999). Altered expression of laminin likely alters neuronal migration and leads to the morphological abnormalities observed in the cretinous brain. Several other brain-specific genes reportedly are developmentally regulated by thyroid hormone (Bernal *et al.*, 2003). A common characteristic of many of these proteins is that their expression appears to be merely delayed in the hypothyroid animal; normal levels are eventually achieved in the adult.

The actions of thyroid hormones on protein synthesis and enzymatic activity are certainly not limited to the brain, and a large number of tissues are affected by the administration of thyroid hormone or by its deficiency. The extensive defects in growth and development in cretins vividly illustrate the pervasive effects of thyroid hormones in normal individuals.

Cretinism is usually classified as endemic or sporadic. *Endemic cretinism* occurs in regions of endemic goiter and usually is caused by extreme iodine deficiency. Goiter may or may not be present. *Sporadic cretinism* is a consequence of failure of the thyroid to develop normally or the result of a defect in the synthesis of thyroid hormone. Goiter is present if a synthetic defect is at fault.

While detectable at birth, cretinism often is not recognized until 3 to 5 months of age. When untreated, the condition eventually leads to such gross changes as to be unmistakable: The child is dwarfed, with short extremities, mentally retarded, inactive, uncomplaining, and listless. The face is puffy and expressionless, and the enlarged tongue may protrude through the thickened lips of the half-opened mouth. The skin may have a yellowish hue and feel doughy, and dry, and cool to the touch. The heart rate is slow, the body temperature may be low, closure of the fontanels is delayed, and the teeth erupt late. Appetite is poor, feeding is slow and interrupted by choking, constipation is frequent, and there may be an umbilical hernia.

For treatment to be fully effective, the diagnosis must be made long before these changes are obvious. In regions of endemic cretinism due to iodine deficiency, iodine replacement is best instituted prior to pregnancy. However, iodine replacement given to pregnant women up to the end of the second trimester has been shown to enhance the neurological and psychological development of the children (Cao *et al.*, 1994). Screening of newborn infants for deficient thyroid function is carried out in the United States and in most industrialized countries. Concentrations of TSH and thyroxine are measured in blood from the umbilical cord or from a heel stick. The incidence of congenital dysfunction of the thyroid is about 1 per 4000 births.

Calorigenic Effects. A characteristic response of homeothermic animals to thyroid hormone is increased O_2 consumption. Most peripheral tissues contribute to this response; heart, skeletal muscle, liver, and kidney are stimulated markedly by thyroid hormone. Indeed, 30% to 40% of the thyroid hormone–dependent increase in O_2 consumption can be attributed to stimulation of cardiac contractility. Several organs, including brain, gonads, and spleen, are unresponsive to the calorigenic effects of thyroid hormone. The mechanism of the calorigenic effect of thyroid hormone has been elusive (Silva, 2003). It once was erroneously believed that thyroid hormone uncoupled mitochondrial oxidative phosphorylation. Thyroid hormone–dependent lipogenesis may constitute a quantitatively important energy sink, and studies in rats have demonstrated that about 4% of the increased caloric expenditure induced by thyroid hormone is accounted for by lipogenesis. The observation that T_3 stimulates lipolysis provides a link between lipogenesis and thermogenesis. Further, thyroid hormone induces expression of several lipogenic enzymes, including malic enzyme and fatty acid synthase. Although the entire picture is not clear, there appears to be an integrated program by which thyroid hormone regulates the set-point of energy expenditure and maintains the metabolic machinery necessary to sustain it. Indeed, even small changes in L-thyroxine replacement doses may significantly alter the set-point for resting energy expenditure in the hypothyroid patient (al-Adsani *et al.*, 1997).

Cardiovascular Effects. Thyroid hormone influences cardiac function by direct and indirect actions; changes in the cardiovascular system are prominent clinical consequences in thyroid dysfunctional states. In hyperthyroidism, there is tachycardia, increased stroke volume, increased cardiac index, cardiac hypertrophy, decreased peripheral vascular resistance, and increased pulse pressure. In hypothyroidism, there is bradycardia, decreased cardiac index, pericardial effusion, increased peripheral vascular resistance, decreased pulse pressure, and elevation of mean arterial pressure (Klein, 2005a; Klein, 2005b).

Thyroid hormones directly regulate myocardial gene expression. T_3 regulates genes encoding the isoforms of the sarcomeric myosin heavy chains by increasing the expression of the α gene and decreasing the expression of the β gene. A TRE has been located in the 5-flanking region of the α myosin heavy chain gene. T_3 also upregulates the gene encoding the sarcoplasmic reticulum Ca^{2+}–ATPase, which plays a critical role in myocardial contraction (Rohrer and Dillman, 1988). Regulation of these two genes results in altered contractility observed in hyper- and hypothyroidism. Indeed, stress echocardiography in hyperthyroid patients revealed abnormalities in cardiac contractility that reverted to normal when euthyroidism was restored (Kahaly et al., 1999). Similarly, left ventricular diastolic dysfunction in hypothyroidism was reversed with L-thyroxine replacement therapy (Biondi et al., 1999).

Observations in transgenic mice have provided insight into the action of thyroid hormone on heart rate. Previously, alterations in the sensitivity of the cardiac myocyte to catecholamines (enhanced in hyperthyroidism and depressed in hypothyroidism) were considered an indirect effect of thyroid hormone, possibly due to changes in expression of myocardial β adrenergic receptors. This is the basis for the use of β adrenergic receptor antagonists in relieving some of the cardiac manifestations in hyperthyroidism. However, basal heart rate is decreased in mice lacking the $TR\alpha_1$ gene (Johansson et al., 1998) and increased in mice lacking $TR\beta$ (Johansson et al., 1999), suggesting a more direct role for thyroid hormone in cardiac pacemaking. Finally, T_3 leads to peripheral hemodynamic effects that alter the chronotropic and inotropic state of the myocardium. Interestingly, T_3 appears to have a direct, nongenomic vasodilating effect on vascular smooth muscle (Park et al., 1997; Ojamaa et al., 1996).

Metabolic Effects. Thyroid hormones stimulate metabolism of cholesterol to bile acids, and hypercholesterolemia is a characteristic feature of hypothyroid states. Thyroid hormones increase the specific binding of low-density lipoprotein (LDL) by liver cells (Salter et al., 1988), and the concentration of hepatic receptors for LDL is decreased in hypothyroidism. The number of LDL receptors on the surface of hepatocytes is a strong determinant of the plasma cholesterol concentration (*see* Chapter 35).

Thyroid hormones enhance the lipolytic responses of fat cells to other hormones (*e.g.,* catecholamines) and elevated plasma free fatty acid concentrations are seen in hyperthyroidism. In contrast to other lipolytic hormones, thyroid hormones do not directly increase the accumulation of cyclic AMP. They may, however, regulate the capacity of other hormones to enhance cyclic AMP accumulation by decreasing the activity of a microsomal phosphodiesterase that hydrolyzes cyclic AMP. There also is evidence that thyroid hormones act to maintain normal coupling of the β adrenergic receptor to the catalytic subunit of adenylyl cyclase in fat cells. Fat cells from hypothyroid rats have increased concentrations of G proteins that inhibit adenylyl cyclase. This could account for both the decreased response to lipolytic hormones and the increased sensitivity to inhibitory regulators (*e.g.,* adenosine) that are found in hypothyroidism (Ros et al., 1988).

Thyrotoxicosis is an insulin-resistant state (Gottlieb and Braverman, 1994). Postreceptor defects in the liver and peripheral tissues, manifested by depleted glycogen stores and enhanced glucogenesis, lead to insulin insensitivity. In addition, there is increased absorption of glucose from the gut. Compensatory increases in insulin secretion result in order to maintain euglycemia. This may precipitate clinical diabetes in previously undiagnosed patients and increase insulin requirements of diabetic patients already on insulin. Conversely, hypothyroidism results in decreased absorption of glu-

cose from the gut, decreased insulin secretion, and a reduced rate of peripheral glucose uptake; however, glucose utilization by the brain is unaffected. Insulin requirements are decreased in the hypothyroid patient with diabetes.

Thyroid Hyperfunction. Thyrotoxicosis is a condition caused by elevated concentrations of circulating free thyroid hormones. Various disorders of different etiologies can result in this syndrome. The term *hyperthyroidism* is restricted to those conditions in which thyroid hormone production and release are increased due to gland hyperfunction. Iodine uptake by the thyroid gland is increased, as determined by the measurement of the percent uptake of ^{123}I or ^{131}I in a 24-hour radioactive iodine uptake (RAIU) test. In contrast, thyroid inflammation or destruction resulting in excess "leak" of thyroid hormones or excess exogenous thyroid hormone intake results in a low 24-hour RAIU. The term *subclinical hyperthyroidism* is defined as few if any symptoms with a low serum TSH and normal concentrations of T_4 and T_3.

Graves' disease, or toxic diffuse goiter, is the most common cause of high RAIU thyrotoxicosis. It accounts for 60% to 90% of cases, depending upon age and geographic region. Graves' disease is an autoimmune disorder characterized by hyperthyroidism, diffuse goiter, and IgG antibodies that bind to and activate the TSH receptor. This is a relatively common disorder, with an incidence of 0.02% to 0.4% in the United States. Endemic areas of iodine deficiency have a lower incidence of autoimmune thyroid disease. As with most types of thyroid dysfunction, women are affected more than men, with a ratio ranging from 5:1 to 7:1. Graves' disease is more common between the ages of 20 and 50, but may occur at any age. Major histocompatibility alleles (HLA) B_8 and DR_3 are associated with Graves' disease in Caucasians. Graves' disease is commonly associated with other autoimmune diseases. The characteristic exophthalmos associated with Graves' disease is an infiltrative ophthalmopathy and is considered an autoimmune-mediated inflammation of the periorbital connective tissue and extraocular muscles. This disorder is clinically evident with various degrees of severity in about 50% of patients with Graves' disease, but it is present on radiological studies, such as ultrasound or CT scan, in almost all patients. The pathogenesis of Graves' ophthalmopathy, including the role of the TSH receptor present in retro-orbital tissues, and the management of this disorder, are reviewed by Rapoport and McLachlan (2000).

Toxic uninodular/multinodular goiter accounts for 10% to 40% of cases of hyperthyroidism and is more common in older patients. Infiltrative ophthalmopathy is absent.

A low RAIU is seen in the destructive thyroiditides and in thyrotoxicosis resulting from exogenous thyroid hormone ingestion. Low RAIU thyrotoxicosis caused by subacute (painful) and silent (painless or lymphocytic) thyroiditis represents about 5% to 20% of all cases. Silent thyroiditis occurs in 7% to 10% of postpartum women in the United States (Lazarus, 2005). Other causes of thyrotoxicosis are much less common.

Most of the signs and symptoms of thyrotoxicosis stem from the excessive production of heat and from increased motor activity and increased activity of the sympathetic nervous system. The skin is flushed, warm, and moist; the muscles are weak and tremulous; the heart rate is rapid, the heartbeat is forceful, and the arterial pulses are prominent and bounding. Increased expenditure of energy gives rise to increased appetite, and if intake is insufficient, to loss of weight. There also may be insomnia, difficulty in remaining still, anxiety and apprehension, intolerance to heat, and increased frequency of bowel movements. Angina, arrhythmias, and heart failure may be present in older patients. Some individuals may show extensive muscular wasting as a result of thyroid myopathy. Patients with long-standing undiagnosed or undertreated thyrotoxicosis may develop osteoporosis due to increased bone turnover (Sheppard, 2005a; Sheppard, 2005b).

The most severe form of hyperthyroidism is thyroid storm, which is discussed below, under therapeutic uses of antithyroid drugs.

Thyroid Hypofunction. Hypothyroidism, known as myxedema when severe, is the most common disorder of thyroid function. Worldwide, hypothyroidism results most often from iodine deficiency. In nonendemic areas where iodine is sufficient, chronic autoimmune thyroiditis (Hashimoto's thyroiditis) accounts for the majority of cases. This disorder is characterized by high levels of circulating antibodies directed against thyroid peroxidase, and less commonly, thyroglobulin. In addition, blocking antibodies directed at the TSH receptor may be present, exacerbating the hypothyroidism (Botero and Brown, 1998). Finally, thyroid destruction may result from apoptotic cell death due to the interaction of Fas with the Fas ligand in the thyrocytes (Giordano *et al.*, 1997). Failure of the thyroid to produce sufficient thyroid hormone is the most common cause of hypothyroidism and is referred to as *primary hypothyroidism*. *Central hypothyroidism* occurs much less often and results from diminished stimulation of the thyroid by TSH because of pituitary failure (*secondary hypothyroidism*) or hypothalamic failure (*tertiary hypothyroidism*). Hypothyroidism present at birth (*congenital hypothyroidism*) is the most common preventable cause of mental retardation in the world. Diagnosis and early intervention with thyroid hormone replacement prevent the development of cretinism, as discussed above.

Nongoitrous hypothyroidism is associated with degeneration and atrophy of the thyroid gland. The same condition follows surgical removal of the thyroid or its destruction by radioactive iodine. Since it also may occur years after antithyroid drug therapy for Graves' disease, some have speculated that hypothyroidism can be the end stage of this disorder ("burnt-out" Graves' disease). *Goitrous hypothyroidism* occurs in Hashimoto's thyroiditis or when there is a severe defect in synthesis of thyroid hormone. When the disease is mild, it may be subtle in its presentation. By the time it has become severe, however, all of the signs are overt. The appearance of the patient is pathognomonic. The face is quite expressionless, puffy, and pallid. The skin is cold and dry, the scalp is scaly, and the hair is coarse, brittle, and sparse. The fingernails are thickened and brittle, the subcutaneous tissue appears to be thickened, and there may

be true edema. The voice is husky and low-pitched, speech is slow, hearing is often faulty, mentation is impaired, and depression may be present. The appetite is poor, gastrointestinal activity is diminished, and constipation is common. Atony of the bladder is rare and suggests that the function of other smooth muscles may be impaired. The voluntary muscles are weak and the relaxation phase of the deep-tendon reflexes is delayed. The heart can be dilated, and there is frequently a pericardial effusion, although this is rarely clinically significant. There also may be pleural effusions and ascites. Anemia, most commonly normochromic and normocytic, is often present, although menstrual irregularity with menorrhagia may result in iron deficiency anemia. Hyperlipidemia often is present in hypothyroid patients. Patients are lethargic and tend to sleep a lot and often complain of cold intolerance.

Thyroid Function Tests. The development of radioimmunoassays, and more recently, chemiluminescent and enzyme-linked immunoassays for T_4, T_3, and TSH have greatly improved the laboratory diagnosis of thyroid disorders (Demers and Spencer, 2003). However, measurement of the total hormone concentration in plasma may not give an accurate picture of the activity of the thyroid gland. The total hormone concentration changes with alterations in either the amount of TBG in plasma or the binding affinity of TBG for hormones. Although equilibrium dialysis of undiluted serum and radioimmunoassay for free thyroxine in the dialysate represent the gold standard for determining free thyroxine concentrations, this assay is typically not available in routine clinical laboratories. The free thyroxine index is an estimation of the free thyroxine concentration and is calculated by multiplying the total thyroxine concentration by the thyroid hormone binding ratio, which estimates the degree of saturation of TBG. Additional assays commonly in use for estimating the free T_4 and free T_3 concentrations employ labeled analogs of these iodothyronines in chemiluminescence and enzyme-linked immunoassays. These assays correlate well with free T_4 concentrations measured by the more cumbersome equilibrium dialysis method and are easily adaptable to routine clinical laboratory use. However, the analog assays may be affected by a wide variety of nonthyroidal disease states, including acute illness, and by certain drugs to a greater degree than are the free T_4 index and free T_4 determined by equilibrium dialysis.

Serum measurements of TSH have been available since 1965. In individuals whose pituitary function and TSH secretion are normal, serum measurement of TSH is the thyroid function test of choice (Danese *et al.*, 1996; Helfand and Redfern, 1998), because pituitary secretion of TSH is sensitively regulated in response to circulating concentrations of thyroid hormones.

The first "sensitive" TSH assay was developed in 1985, utilizing a dual-antibody approach. Application of this method resulted in the expansion of the assay detection limit below the normal range. Thus, any assay of this type is referred to as a *sensitive TSH assay* (Demers and Spencer, 2003). A major use of the sensitive TSH assay is to differentiate between normal and thyrotoxic patients, who should exhibit suppressed TSH values. Indeed, the sensitive TSH assay has replaced evaluation of the response of TSH to injection of synthetic TRH (TRH stimulation test) in the thyrotoxic patient. While the serum TSH assay is extremely useful in determining the euthyroid state and titrating the replacement dose of thyroid hormone in patients with primary hypothyroidism, abnormal serum TSH concentrations may not always indicate thyroid dysfunction. In such patients, assessment of the circulating thyroid hormone levels will further determine whether or not thyroid dysfunction is truly present. Synthetic preparations of TRH (*protirelin*, THYREL) are no longer available in the United States for the evaluation of pituitary or hypothalamic failure as a cause of secondary hypothyroidism.

Recombinant human TSH (*thyrotropin alfa*, THYROGEN) is now available as an injectable preparation to test the ability of thyroid tissue, both normal and malignant, to take up radioactive iodine and release thyroglobulin (Haugen *et al.*, 1999). This preparation replaces *bovine TSH* (THYTROPAR), which was associated with a high incidence of side effects, including anaphylaxis.

Therapeutic Uses of Thyroid Hormone. The major indications for the therapeutic use of thyroid hormone are for hormone replacement therapy in patients with hypothyroidism or cretinism and for TSH suppression therapy in patients with thyroid cancer (Mazzaferri and Kloos, 2001), and occasionally those with nontoxic goiter. While the consensus has been that thyroid hormone therapy is not indicated for treatment of the "low T_4 syndrome" ("sick euthyroid syndrome") that results from nonthyroidal illness (Brent and Hershman, 1986; Farwell, 2003), this concept has been challenged with the suggestion that severely ill patients may benefit by treatment with T_3 (DeGroot, 1999). However, there is no published evidence supporting this recommendation, which remains a minority opinion. For example, T_3 treatment does not decrease mortality in the sick euthyroid syndrome that occurs in patients undergoing coronary artery bypass surgery (Klemperer *et al.*, 1995).

The synthetic preparations of the sodium salts of the natural isomers of the thyroid hormones are available and widely used for thyroid hormone therapy. *Levothyroxine sodium* (L-T_4, SYNTHROID, LEVOXYL, LEVOTHROID, UNITHROID, others) is available in tablets and as a lyophilized powder for injection. L-thyroxine has a narrow therapeutic index, and the FDA has recently altered its recommendations for approval of the various L-thyroxine preparations to assure biological equivalence. *Liothyronine sodium* (L-T_3) is the salt of triiodothyronine and is available in tablets (CYTOMEL) and in an injectable form (TRIOSTAT). A mixture of thyroxine and triiodothyronine is marketed as *liotrix* (THYROLAR). Desiccated thyroid preparations, derived from whole animal thyroids, contain both T_3 and T_4 and have highly variable biologic activity, making these preparations much less desirable.

Thyroid Hormone Replacement Therapy. Thyroxine (levothyroxine sodium) is the hormone of choice for thyroid hormone replacement therapy because of its consistent potency and prolonged duration of action. The absorption of thyroxine occurs in the small intestine and is variable and incomplete, with 50% to 80% of the dose absorbed. Absorption is slightly increased when the hormone is taken on an empty stomach. In addition, certain drugs may interfere with absorption of levothyroxine in the gut, including *sucralfate*, *cholestyramine resin*, *iron and calcium supplements*, *aluminum hydroxide*, and certain soy products. Enhanced biliary excretion of levothyroxine occurs during the administration of drugs that induce hepatic CYPs, such as *phenytoin*, *carbamazepine*, and *rifampin*. This enhanced excretion may necessitate an increase in the dose of orally administered levothyroxine. Triiodothyronine (liothyronine sodium)

may be used occasionally when a quicker onset of action is desired, *e.g.*, in the rare presentation of myxedema coma or for preparing a patient for ^{131}I therapy for treatment of thyroid cancer. It is less desirable for chronic replacement therapy because of the requirement for more frequent dosing, higher cost, and transient elevations of serum T_3 concentrations above the normal range. Combination therapy with levothyroxine and liothyronine has been suggested for use in hypothyroid patients that remain symptomatic on levothyroxine alone and have serum TSH concentrations in the normal range (Bunevicius *et al.*, 1999). However, three recent studies have not confirmed these findings (Sawka *et al.*, 2003; Walsh *et al.*, 2003; Clyde *et al.*, 2003). Furthermore, this combination may lead to transient elevations of circulating T_3 concentrations in contrast to the steady levels of T_3 during levothyroxine administration due to conversion of T_4 to T_3 in peripheral tissues.

The average daily adult replacement dose of levothyroxine sodium in a 68-kg person is 112 μg as a single dose, while that of liothyronine sodium is 50 to 75 μg in divided doses. Institution of therapy in healthy younger individuals can begin at full replacement doses. Because of the prolonged half-life of thyroxine (7 days), new steady-state concentrations of the hormone will not be achieved until 5 half-lives have elapsed, or at least 5 weeks after a change in dose. Thus, re-evaluation with determination of serum TSH concentration should not be performed at intervals less than 6 to 8 weeks. The goal of thyroxine replacement therapy is to achieve a TSH value in the normal range, since overreplacement of thyroxine, suppressing TSH values to the subnormal range, may induce osteoporosis and cause cardiac dysfunction (Surks *et al.*, 2004). In noncompliant young patients, the cumulative weekly doses of levothyroxine may be given as a single weekly dose, which is safe, effective, and well tolerated (Grebe *et al.*, 1997). In individuals over the age of 60, institution of therapy at a lower daily dose of levothyroxine sodium (25 to 50 μg per day) is indicated to avoid exacerbation of underlying and undiagnosed cardiac disease. Death due to arrhythmias has been reported during the initiation of thyroid hormone replacement therapy in hypothyroid patients. The dose can be increased at a rate of 25 μg per day every few months until the TSH is normalized. For individuals with pre-existing cardiac disease, an initial dose of 12.5 μg per day, with increases of 12.5 to 25 μg per day every 6 to 8 weeks, is indicated. Daily doses of thyroxine may be interrupted periodically because of intercurrent medical or surgical illnesses that prohibit taking medications by mouth. Because of the 7-day half-life of T_4, a lapse of several days of hormone replacement is unlikely to have any significant metabolic consequences. However, if more prolonged interruption in oral therapy is necessary, levothyroxine may be given parenterally at a dose 25% to 50% less than the patient's daily oral requirements.

Subclinical hypothyroidism is a clinical state with few if any symptoms, characterized by elevated serum TSH concentrations (for review, *see* Surks *et al.*, 2004). Population screening has shown that subclinical hypothyroidism is very common, with a prevalence of up to 15% in some populations and up to 25% in the elderly. The decision to use levothyroxine therapy in these patients to normalize the serum TSH must be made on an individual basis, as treatment may not be appropriate for all patients. Patients with subclinical hypothyroidism who may benefit from levothyroxine therapy include those with goiter, autoimmune thyroid disease, hypercholesterolemia, cognitive dysfunction, or pregnancy (*see* below), and those patients who have symptoms of hypothyroidism.

The dose of levothyroxine in the hypothyroid patient who becomes pregnant often needs to be increased, perhaps due to the increased serum concentrations of TBG induced by estrogen and a small transplacental passage of levothyroxine from mother to fetus (Glinoer, 2005). In addition, pregnancy may "unmask" hypothyroidism in patients with pre-existing autoimmune thyroid disease or in those who reside in a region of iodine deficiency (Glinoer *et al.*, 1994). Overt hypothyroidism during pregnancy is associated with fetal distress (Wasserstrum and Anaia, 1995) and impaired psychoneural development in the progeny (Man *et al.*, 1991). In addition, studies have suggested that subclinical hypothyroidism during pregnancy is associated with mildly impaired psychomotor development in the children (Haddow *et al.*, 1999; Pop *et al.*, 1999). These findings strongly suggest that any degree of hypothyroidism, as judged by an elevated serum TSH, should be treated during pregnancy. Thus, serum TSH values should be determined in the first trimester in all patients with pre-existing hypothyroidism, as well as in those at high risk for developing hypothyroidism. Therapy with levothyroxine should be administered to keep the serum TSH in the normal range. Any adjustment of the levothyroxine dose should be re-evaluated in 4 to 6 weeks to determine if further adjustments are necessary.

Comparative Responses to Thyroid Preparations. There is no significant difference in the qualitative response of the patient with myxedema to triiodothyronine, thyroxine, or desiccated thyroid. However, there are obvious quantitative differences. Following the subcutaneous administration of a large experimental dose of T_3, a metabolic response can be detected within 4 to 6 hours, at which time the skin becomes detectably warmer and the pulse rate and temperature increase. With this dose, a 40% decrease in metabolic rate can be restored to normal in 24 hours. The maximal response occurs in 2 days or less, and the effects subside with a half-life of about 8 days. The same single dose of T_4 exerts much less effect. However, if thyroxine is given in approximately 4 times the dose of triiodothyronine, a comparable elevation in metabolic rate can be achieved. The peak effect of a single dose is evident in about 9 days, and this declines to half the maximum in 11 to 15 days. In both cases the effects outlast the presence of detectable amounts of hormone; these disappear from the blood with mean half-lives of approximately 1 day for T_3 and 7 days for T_4.

Myxedema Coma. Myxedema coma is a rare syndrome that represents the extreme expression of severe, long-standing hypothyroidism (Emerson, 2003; Farwell, 2004). It is a medical emergency, and even with early diagnosis and treatment, the mortality rate can be as high as 60%. Myxedema coma occurs most often in elderly patients during the winter months. Common precipitating factors include pulmonary infections, cerebrovascular accidents, and congestive heart failure. The clinical course of lethargy proceeding to stupor and then coma is often hastened by drugs, especially sedatives, narcotics, antidepressants, and tranquilizers. Indeed, many cases of myxedema coma have occurred in hypothyroid patients who have been hospitalized for other medical problems.

Cardinal features of myxedema coma are: (1) hypothermia, which may be profound; (2) respiratory depression; and (3) unconsciousness. Other clinical features include bradycardia, macroglossia, delayed reflexes, and dry, rough skin. Dilutional hyponatremia is common and may be severe. Elevated plasma creatine kinase (CK) and lactate dehydrogenase (LDH) concentrations, acidosis, and anemia are common findings. Lumbar puncture reveals increased opening pressure and high protein content. Hypothyroidism is confirmed by measuring serum free thyroxine index and TSH values. Ultimately, myxedema coma is a clinical diagnosis.

The mainstay of therapy is supportive care, with ventilatory support, rewarming with blankets, correction of hyponatremia, and

treatment of the precipitating incident. Because of a 5% to 10% incidence of coexisting decreased adrenal reserve in patients with myxedema coma, intravenous steroids are indicated before initiating thyroxine therapy (*see* Chapter 59). Parenteral administration of thyroid hormone is necessary due to uncertain absorption through the gut. With intravenous preparations of both levothyroxine and liothyronine now available, a reasonable approach is an initial intravenous loading dose of 200 to 300 µg of levothyroxine with a second dose of 100 µg given 24 hours later. Alternatively, a bolus of 500 µg levothyroxine given orally (by mouth or *via* nasogastric tube) may be administered to patients <50 years old without cardiac complications (Yamamoto *et al.*, 1999). Some clinicians recommend adding liothyronine (at a dose of 10 µg intravenously every 8 hours) with the initial dose of levothyroxine, until the patient is stable and conscious. The dose of thyroid hormone should be adjusted on the basis of hemodynamic stability, the presence of coexisting cardiac disease, and the degree of electrolyte imbalance. Studies suggest that overaggressive treatment with either levothyroxine (>500 µg per day) or liothyronine (>75 µg) may be associated with an increased mortality rate (Yamamoto *et al.*, 1999).

Treatment of Cretinism. Success in the treatment of cretinism depends upon the age at which therapy is started. Because of this, newborn screening for congenital hypothyroidism is routine in the United States, Canada, and many other countries around the world. In cases that do not come to the attention of physicians until retardation of development is clinically obvious, the detrimental effects of thyroid hormone deficiency on mental development will be irreversible. If, on the other hand, therapy is instituted within the first few weeks of life, normal physical and mental development is almost always achieved (Rovet, 2003; Rovet and Daneman, 2003). Prognosis also depends on the severity of the hypothyroidism at birth and may be worse for babies with thyroid agenesis. The most critical need for thyroid hormone is during the period of myelination of the central nervous system that occurs about the time of birth. To rapidly normalize the serum thyroxine concentration in the congenitally hypothyroid infant, an initial daily dose of levothyroxine of 10 to 15 µg/kg is recommended (Brown, 2005). This dose will increase the total serum thyroxine concentration to the upper half of the normal range in most infants within 1 to 2 weeks. Individual levothyroxine doses are adjusted at 4- to 6-week intervals during the first 6 months, at 2-month intervals during the 6- to 18-month period, and at 3- to 6-month intervals thereafter to maintain serum thyroxine concentrations in the 10- to 16-µg/dl range and serum TSH values in the normal range. The free thyroxine levels should be kept in the upper normal or elevated range. Assessments that are important guides for appropriate hormone replacement include physical growth, motor development, bone maturation, and developmental progress. Management of premature infants with hypothyroxinemia due to the sick euthyroid syndrome (~50% of those born at less than 30 weeks of gestation) remains a therapeutic dilemma. Despite impaired psychomotor development in these patients (Reuss *et al.*, 1996; Den Ouden *et al.*, 1996), levothyroxine therapy has not been shown to be beneficial and may be deleterious if overreplacement is administered (Den Ouden *et al.*, 1996).

Nodular Thyroid Disease. Nodular thyroid disease is the most common endocrinopathy. The prevalence of clinically apparent nodules is 4% to 7% in the United States, with the frequency increasing throughout adult life. When ultrasound and autopsy data are included, the prevalence of thyroid nodules approaches 50% by age 60. As with other forms of thyroid disease, nodules are more frequent in women. Nodules have been estimated to develop at a rate of 0.1% per year. In individuals exposed to ionizing radiation, the rate of nodule development is 20 times higher. While the presence of a nodule raises the question of a malignancy, only 8% to 10% of patients with thyroid nodules have thyroid cancer. About 22,000 new cases of thyroid cancer are diagnosed annually, with about 1000 deaths from the disease per year. However, many more people have clinically silent thyroid cancer, as up to 35% of thyroids removed at autopsy or at surgery harbor a small (<1 cm) occult papillary cancer.

The evaluation of the patient with nodular thyroid disease includes a careful physical examination, biochemical analysis of thyroid function, and assessment of the malignant potential of the nodule. If the serum TSH is normal, the most efficacious diagnostic procedure is a fine-needle aspiration biopsy. Other diagnostic measures that may be useful in the evaluation of the nodule include radioisotope scanning and ultrasound.

TSH suppressive therapy with levothyroxine is an option for the patient diagnosed with a benign solitary nodule and a normal serum TSH. The rationale behind levothyroxine therapy is that the benign nodule will either stop growing or decrease in size after TSH stimulation of the thyroid gland has been suppressed. The success rate of such therapy varies widely (Papini *et al.*, 1998; Zelmanovitz *et al.*, 1998; Gharib and Mazzaferri, 1998). Identification of those patients who are most likely to benefit from thyroid hormone therapy can be achieved through measurement of the serum TSH concentration and radioisotope scanning. Suppression therapy will be of no value if thyroid nodule autonomy exists, as evidenced by a subnormal TSH value and all, or almost all, isotope uptake in the nodule. Functioning nodules are the most likely to respond to suppression therapy. However, once TSH concentrations are suppressed, a repeat radioisotope scan (suppression scan) should be obtained. If significant uptake persists on a suppression scan, the nodule is nonsuppressible and levothyroxine therapy should be discontinued. Suppression therapy needs to be considered carefully in older patients or in those with coronary artery disease; in general, such therapy should be avoided in these patients. Hypofunctioning nodules are much less likely to respond to suppression therapy. However, a 6- to 12-month trial of levothyroxine suppression is reasonable (Hermus and Huysmans, 1998). If levothyroxine is administered, therapy should be continued for as long as the nodule is decreasing in size. Once the size of a nodule remains stable for a 6- to 12-month period, therapy may be discontinued and the nodule observed for recurrent growth. Any nodule that grows while on suppression therapy should be re-biopsied and/or surgically excised.

Thyroid Cancer. Surgery is the primary treatment for all forms of thyroid cancer, followed by levothyroxine suppression therapy (Mazzaferri and Kloos, 2001). In most patients, RAI ablation follows surgery (*see* below).

Table 56–4
Antithyroid Compounds

PROCESS AFFECTED	EXAMPLES OF INHIBITORS
Active transport of iodide	Complex anions: perchlorate, fluoborate, pertechnetate, thiocyanate
Iodination of thyroglobulin	Thionamides: propylthiouracil, methimazole, carbimazole
	Thiocyanate
	Aniline derivatives; sulfonamides
	Iodide
Coupling reaction	Thionamides
	Sulfonamides
	?All other inhibitors of iodination
Hormone release	Lithium salts
	Iodide
Iodotyrosine deiodination	Nitrotyrosines
Peripheral iodothyronine deiodination	Thiouracil derivatives
	Oral cholecystographic agents
	Amiodarone
Hormone excretion/ inactivation	Inducers of hepatic drug-metabolizing enzymes: phenobarbital, rifampin, carbamazepine, phenytoin
Hormone action	Thyroxine analogs
	Amiodarone
	?Phenytoin
	Binding in gut: cholestyramine

SOURCE: Adapted from Meier, 2005.

ANTITHYROID DRUGS AND OTHER THYROID INHIBITORS

A large number of compounds are capable of interfering, directly or indirectly, with the synthesis, release, or action of thyroid hormones (Table 56–4). Several are of great clinical value for the temporary or extended control of hyperthyroid states. The major inhibitors may be classified into four categories: (1) antithyroid drugs, which interfere directly with the synthesis of thyroid hormones; (2) ionic inhibitors, which block the iodide transport mechanism; (3) high concentrations of iodine itself, which decrease release of thyroid hormones from the gland and also may decrease hormone synthesis; and (4) radioactive iodine, which damages the gland with ionizing radiation. Adjuvant therapy with drugs that have no specific effects on thyroid gland hormonogenesis is useful in controlling the peripheral manifestations of thyrotoxicosis. These drugs include inhibitors of the peripheral deiodination of thyroxine to the active hormone, triiodothyronine; β adrenergic receptor antagonists; and Ca^{2+} channel blockers. The antithyroid drugs have been reviewed by Cooper (2003). Adrenergic receptor antagonists are discussed more fully in Chapter 10 and Ca^{2+} channel blockers in Chapters 31 and 34.

Antithyroid Drugs

The antithyroid drugs that have clinical utility are the thioureylenes, which belong to the family of thionamides. Propylthiouracil may be considered as the prototype.

History. Studies on the mechanism of the development of goiter began with the observation that rabbits fed a diet composed largely of cabbage often developed goiters. This result was probably due to the presence of precursors of the thiocyanate ion in cabbage leaves (*see* below). Later, two pure compounds were shown to produce goiter: sulfaguanidine and phenylthiourea.

Investigation of the effects of thiourea derivatives revealed that rats became hypothyroid despite hyperplastic changes in their thyroid glands that were characteristic of intense thyrotropic stimulation. After treatment was begun, no new hormone was made, and the goitrogen had no visible effect upon the thyroid gland following hypophysectomy or the administration of thyroid hormone. This suggested to Astwood that the goiter was a compensatory change resulting from the induced state of hypothyroidism and that the primary action of the compounds was to inhibit the formation of thyroid hormone. The therapeutic possibilities of such agents in hyperthyroidism were evident, and the substances so used became known as *antithyroid drugs*.

Structure–Activity Relationship. The two goitrogens found in the early 1940s proved to be prototypes of two different classes of antithyroid drugs. These two, with one later addition, made up three general categories into which the majority of the agents can be assigned: (1) *thioureylenes* include all the compounds currently used clinically (Figure 56–9); (2) *aniline derivatives,* of which the sulfonamides make up the largest number, embrace a few substances that have been found to inhibit thyroid hormone synthesis; and (3) *polyhydric phenols,* such as resorcinol, which have caused goiter in human beings when applied to the abraded skin. A few other compounds, mentioned briefly below, do not fit into any of these categories.

Thiourea and its simpler aliphatic derivatives and heterocyclic compounds containing a thioureylene group make up the majority of the known antithyroid agents that are effective in human beings. Although most of them incorporate the entire thioureylene group, in some a nitrogen atom is replaced by oxygen or sulfur so that only the thioamide group is common to all. Among the heterocyclic compounds, active representatives are the sulfur derivatives of *imidazole, oxazole, hydantoin, thiazole, thiadiazole, uracil,* and *barbituric acid.*

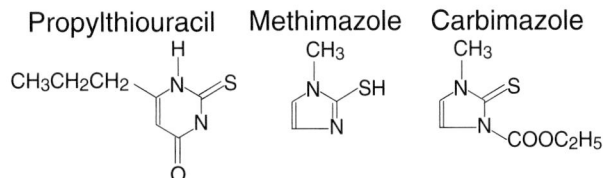

Figure 56–9. *Antithyroid drugs of the thiamide type.*

L-5-Vinyl-2-thiooxazolidone (goitrin) is responsible for the goiter that results from consuming turnips or the seeds or green parts of cruciferous plants. These plants are eaten by cows, and the compound is found in cow's milk in areas of endemic goiter in Finland; it is about as active as propylthiouracil in humans.

As the result of industrial exposure, toxicological studies, or clinical trials for various purposes, several other compounds have been noted to possess antithyroid activity (DeRosa *et al.*, 1998). *Thiopental* and oral hypoglycemic drugs of the sulfonylurea class have weak antithyroid action in experimental animals. This is not significant at usual doses in humans. However, antithyroid effects in human beings have been observed from *dimercaprol, aminoglutethimide,* and *lithium salts.* Polychlorinated biphenyls bear a striking structural resemblance to the thyroid hormones and may function as either agonists or antagonists of thyroid hormone action (DeRosa *et al.*, 1998; Zoeller *et al.*, 2000; Gauger *et al.*, 2004). *Amiodarone,* the iodine-rich drug used in the management of cardiac arrhythmias, has complex effects on thyroid function (Harjai and Licata, 1997). In areas of iodine sufficiency, amiodarone-induced hypothyroidism due to the excess iodine is not uncommon, whereas in iodine-deficient regions, amiodarone-induced thyrotoxicosis predominates, whether because of the excess iodine or the thyroiditis induced by the drug. Amiodarone and its major metabolite, desethylamiodarone, are potent inhibitors of iodothyronine deiodination, resulting in decreased conversion of thyroxine to triiodothyronine. In addition, desethylamiodarone decreases binding of triiodothyronine to its nuclear receptors. Recommendations have been made as to screening methods to identify chemicals that may alter thyroid hormone action or homeostasis (DeVito *et al.*, 1999).

Mechanism of Action. The mechanism of action of the thioureylene drugs has been thoroughly discussed by Taurog (2000). Antithyroid drugs inhibit the formation of thyroid hormones by interfering with the incorporation of iodine into tyrosyl residues of thyroglobulin; they also inhibit the coupling of these iodotyrosyl residues to form iodothyronines. This implies that they interfere with the oxidation of iodide ion and iodotyrosyl groups. Taurog (2000) proposed that the drugs inhibit the peroxidase enzyme, thereby preventing oxidation of iodide or iodotyrosyl groups to the required active state. The antithyroid drugs bind to and inactivate the peroxidase only when the heme of the enzyme is in the oxidized state. Over a period of time, the inhibition of hormone synthesis results in the depletion of stores of iodinated thyroglobulin as the protein is hydrolyzed and the hormones are released into the circulation. Only when the preformed hormone is depleted and the concentrations of circulating thyroid hormones begin to decline do clinical effects become noticeable.

There is some evidence that the coupling reaction may be more sensitive to an antithyroid drug, such as propylthiouracil, than is the iodination reaction (Taurog, 2000). This may explain why patients with hyperthyroidism respond well to doses of the drug that only partially suppress organification.

When Graves' disease is treated with antithyroid drugs, the concentration of thyroid-stimulating immunoglobulins in the circulation often decreases, prompting some to propose that these agents act as immunosuppressants. Perchlorate, which acts by an entirely different mechanism, also decreases thyroid-stimulating immunoglobulins, suggesting that improvement in hyperthyroidism may itself favorably affect the abnormal humoral immune state.

In addition to blocking hormone synthesis, propylthiouracil partially inhibits the peripheral deiodination of T_4 to T_3. *Methimazole* does not have this effect; although the quantitative significance of this inhibition has not been established, it provides a rationale for the choice of propylthiouracil over other antithyroid drugs in the treatment of severe hyperthyroid states or of thyroid storm, where a decreased rate of $T_4 \rightarrow T_3$ conversion would be beneficial.

Absorption, Metabolism, and Excretion. The antithyroid compounds currently used in the United States are propylthiouracil (6-*n*-propylthiouracil) and methimazole (1-methyl-2-mercaptoimidazole; TAPAZOLE). In Great Britain and Europe, *carbimazole* (NEO-MERCAZOLE), a carbethoxy derivative of methimazole, is available, and its antithyroid action is due to its conversion to methimazole after absorption. Some pharmacological properties of propylthiouracil and methimazole are shown in Table 56–5. Measurements of the course of organification of radioactive iodine by the thyroid show that absorption of effective amounts of propylthiouracil follows within 20 to 30 minutes of an oral dose and that the duration of action of the compounds used clinically is brief. The effect of a dose of 100 mg of propylthiouracil begins to wane in 2 to 3 hours, and even a 500-mg dose is completely inhibitory for only 6 to 8 hours. As little as 0.5 mg of methimazole similarly decreases the organification of radioactive iodine in the thyroid gland, but a single dose of 10 to 25 mg is needed to extend the inhibition to 24 hours.

The half-life of propylthiouracil in plasma is about 75 minutes, whereas that of methimazole is 4 to 6 hours. The drugs are concentrated in the thyroid, and methimazole, derived from the metabolism of carbimazole, accumulates after carbimazole is administered. Drugs and metabolites appear largely in the urine.

Table 56–5
Selected Pharmacokinetic Features of Antithyroid Drugs

	PROPYLTHIOURACIL	METHIMAZOLE
Plasma protein binding	~75%	Nil
Plasma half-life	75 minutes	~4–6 hours
Volume of distribution	~20 liters	~40 liters
Concentrated in thyroid	Yes	Yes
Metabolism of drug during illness		
Severe liver disease	Normal	Decreased
Severe kidney disease	Normal	Normal
Dosing frequency	1 to 4 times daily	Once or twice daily
Transplacental passage	Low	Low
Levels in breast milk	Low	Low

Propylthiouracil and methimazole cross the placenta equally (Mortimer *et al.*, 1997) and also can be found in milk. The use of these drugs during pregnancy is discussed below.

Untoward Reactions. The incidence of side effects from propylthiouracil and methimazole as currently used is relatively low. The overall incidence as compiled from published cases by early investigators was 3% for propylthiouracil and 7% for methimazole, with 0.44% and 0.12% of cases, respectively, developing the most serious reaction, agranulocytosis. The development of agranulocytosis with methimazole is probably dose-related, but no such relationship exists with propylthiouracil. Further observations have found little, if any, difference in side effects between these two agents and suggest that an incidence of agranulocytosis of approximately 1 in 500 is a maximal figure. Agranulocytosis usually occurs during the first few weeks or months of therapy but may occur later. Because agranulocytosis can develop rapidly, periodic white cell counts usually are of little help. Patients should immediately report the development of sore throat or fever, which usually heralds the onset of this reaction. Agranulocytosis is reversible upon discontinuation of the offending drug, and the administration of recombinant human granulocyte colony-stimulating factor may hasten recovery (Magner and Snyder, 1994). Mild granulocytopenia, if noted, may be due to thyrotoxicosis or may be the first sign of this dangerous drug reaction. Caution and frequent leukocyte counts are then required.

The most common reaction is a mild, occasionally purpuric, urticarial papular rash. It often subsides spontaneously without interrupting treatment, but it sometimes calls for the administration of an antihistamine, corticosteroids, or changing to another drug (cross-sensitivity to propylthiouracil and methimazole is uncommon). Other less frequent complications are pain and stiffness in the joints, paresthesias, headache, nausea, skin pigmentation, and loss of hair. Drug fever, hepatitis, and nephritis are rare, although abnormal liver function tests are not infrequent with higher doses of propylthiouracil. While vasculitis was previously thought to be a rare complication, antineutrophilic cytoplasmic antibodies (ANCAs) have been reported to occur in about 50% of patients receiving propylthiouracil and rarely with methimazole (Sera *et al.*, 2000; Sato *et al.*, 2000).

Therapeutic Uses. The antithyroid drugs are used in the treatment of hyperthyroidism in the following three ways: (1) as definitive treatment, to control the disorder in anticipation of a spontaneous remission in Graves' disease; (2) in conjunction with radioactive iodine, to hasten recovery while awaiting the effects of radiation; and (3) to control the disorder in preparation for surgical treatment.

The usual starting dose for propylthiouracil is 100 mg every 8 hours or 150 mg every 12 hours. When doses larger than 300 mg daily are needed, further subdivision of the time of administration to every 4 to 6 hours is occasionally helpful. Methimazole is effective when given as a single daily dose because of its relatively long plasma and intrathyroidal half-life, as well as its long duration of action. Failures of response to daily treatment with 300 to 400 mg of propylthiouracil or 30 to 40 mg of methimazole are most commonly due to noncompliance. Delayed responses also are noted in patients with very large goiters or those in whom iodine in any form has been given beforehand. Once euthyroidism is achieved, usually within 12 weeks, the dose of antithyroid drug can be reduced, but not stopped, lest an enhanced recurrence of Graves' disease occur (*see* Remissions, below).

Response to Treatment. The thyrotoxic state usually improves within 3 to 6 weeks after the initiation of antithyroid drugs. The clinical response is related to the dose of antithyroid drug, the size of the goiter, and pretreatment serum T_3 concentrations. The rate of response is determined by the quantity of stored hormone, the rate of turnover of hormone in the thyroid, the half-life of the hormone in the periphery, and the completeness of the block in synthesis imposed by the dosage given. When large doses are continued, and sometimes with the usual dose, hypothyroidism may develop as a result of overtreatment. The earliest signs of hypothyroidism call for a reduction in dose; if they have advanced to the point of discomfort, thyroid hormone in full replacement doses can be given to hasten recovery; then the lower maintenance dose of antithyroid drug

discussed above is instituted for continued therapy. Despite initial suggestions to the contrary, there is no benefit of combination levothyroxine and methimazole therapy on either remission rates (Rittmaster *et al.*, 1998) or on changes in serum concentrations of thyroid-stimulating immunoglobulins (Rittmaster *et al.*, 1996).

After treatment is initiated, patients should be examined and thyroid function tests (serum free thyroxine index and total triiodothyronine concentrations) measured every 2 to 4 months. Once euthyroidism is established, follow-up every 4 to 6 months is reasonable.

Control of the hyperthyroidism usually is associated with a decrease in goiter size, but if the thyroid enlarges, hypothyroidism probably has been induced. When this occurs, the dose of the antithyroid drug should be significantly decreased and/or levothyroxine can be added once hypothyroidism is confirmed by laboratory testing.

Remissions. The antithyroid drugs have been used in many patients to control the hyperthyroidism of Graves' disease until a remission occurs. Early investigators reported that 50% of patients so treated for 1 year remained well without further therapy for long periods, perhaps indefinitely. More recent reports have indicated that a much smaller percentage of patients sustain remissions after such treatment (Maugendre *et al.*, 1999; Benker *et al.*, 1998). Increased dietary iodine has been implicated in the latter, less favorable rates.

Unfortunately, there is no way of predicting before treatment is begun which patients will eventually achieve a lasting remission and who will relapse. It is clear that a favorable outcome is unlikely when the disorder is of long standing, the thyroid is quite large, or various forms of treatment have failed. To complicate the issue further, remission and eventual hypothyroidism may represent the natural history of Graves' disease.

During treatment, a positive sign that a remission may have taken place is reduced size of the goiter. The persistence of goiter often indicates failure, unless the patient becomes hypothyroid. Another favorable indication is continued freedom from all signs of hyperthyroidism when the maintenance dose is small. Finally, a decrease in thyroid-stimulating immunoglobulins, suppression of ^{123}I thyroid uptake when thyroxine or triiodothyronine is given, and a normal serum TSH response to TRH may be helpful in predicting a remission in some patients, although these tests are not routinely performed.

The Therapeutic Choice. Because antithyroid drug therapy, radioactive iodine, and subtotal thyroidectomy all are effective treatments for Graves' disease, there is no worldwide consensus among endocrinologists as to the best approach to therapy. Prolonged drug therapy of Graves' disease in anticipation of a remission is most successful in patients with small goiters or mild hyperthyroidism. Those with large goiters or severe disease usually require definitive therapy with either surgery or radioactive iodine (^{131}I). Radioactive iodine remains the treatment of choice of many endocrinologists in the United States. Many investigators consider coexisting ophthalmopathy to be a relative contraindication for radioactive iodine therapy, since worsening of ophthalmopathy has been reported after radioactive iodine (Bartalena *et al.*, 1998a), although this remains controversial. Others suggest that development of hypothyroidism, regardless of the treatment, is the strongest risk factor for progression of ophthalmopathy (Manso *et al.*, 1998). Smoking may also be a risk factor for worsening ophthalmopathy (Bartelena *et al.*, 1998b). In older patients, depleting the thyroid gland of preformed hormone by treatment with antithyroid drugs is advisable prior to therapy with radioactive iodine, thus preventing a severe exacerbation of the hyperthyroid state during the subsequent development of radiation thyroiditis. Subtotal thyroidectomy is advocated for Graves' disease in young patients with large goiters, children who are allergic to antithyroid drugs, pregnant women (usually in the second trimester) who are allergic to antithyroid drugs, and patients who prefer surgery over antithyroid drugs or radioactive iodine. Radioactive iodine or surgery is indicated for definitive therapy in toxic nodular goiter, since remissions following antithyroid drug therapy do not occur.

Thyrotoxicosis in Pregnancy. Thyrotoxicosis occurs in about 0.2% of pregnancies and is caused most frequently by Graves' disease. Antithyroid drugs are the treatment of choice; radioactive iodine is clearly contraindicated. Historically, propylthiouracil has been preferred over methimazole because transplacental passage was thought to be lower; however, as noted above, both propylthiouracil and methimazole cross the placenta equally (Mortimer, 1997). Current data suggest that either may be used safely in the pregnant patient (Momotani *et al.*, 1997; Mortimer *et al.*, 1997). Recent reports from Scandinavia, where carbimazole is used more frequently than propylthiouracil, have suggested that carbimazole administration is rarely associated with congenital gut abnormalities (Barwell *et al.*, 2002; Diav-Citrin and Ornoy, 2002). The antithyroid drug dosage should be minimized in order to keep the serum free thyroxine index in the upper half of the normal range or slightly elevated. As pregnancy progresses, Graves' disease often improves, and it is not uncommon for patients either to be on very low doses or off antithyroid drugs completely by the end of pregnancy. Therefore the antithyroid drug dose should be reduced, and maternal thyroid function should be frequently monitored in order to decrease chances of fetal hypothyroidism. Relapse or worsening of Graves' disease is common after delivery, and patients should be monitored closely. Propylthiouracil is the drug of choice in nursing women, since very small amounts of the drug appear in breast milk and do not appear to affect thyroid function in the suckling baby. However, doses of methimazole up to 20 mg daily in nursing mothers have been shown to have no effect on thyroid function in the baby (Azizi *et al.*, 2003).

Adjuvant Therapy. Several drugs that have no intrinsic antithyroid activity are useful in the symptomatic treatment of thyrotoxicosis. *β Adrenergic receptor antagonists* (*see* Chapter 10) are effective in antagonizing the sympathetic/adrenergic effects of thyrotoxicosis, thereby reducing the tachycardia, tremor, and stare, and relieving palpitations, anxiety, and tension. Either *propranolol*, 20 to 40 mg four times daily, or *atenolol*, 50 to 100 mg daily, is usually given initially. Propranolol or *esmolol* can be given intravenously if needed. Propranolol, in addition to its β adrenergic receptor antagonist action, has weak inhibitory effects on peripheral $T_4 \rightarrow T_3$ conversion. *Calcium channel blockers* (*diltiazem*, 60 to 120 mg four times daily) can be used to control tachycardia and decrease the incidence of supraventricular tachyarrhythmias (*see* Chapter 34). These drugs should be discontinued once the patient is euthyroid.

Other drugs that are useful in the rapid treatment of the severely thyrotoxic patient are agents that inhibit the peripheral conversion of thyroxine to triiodothyronine. *Dexamethasone* (0.5 to 1 mg two to four times daily) and the iodinated radiological contrast agents *iopanoic acid* (TELEPAQUE, 500 to 1000 mg once daily) and *sodium ipodate* (ORAGRAFIN, 500 to 1000 mg once daily) are effective in preoperative preparation. Neither iopanoic acid nor sodium ipodate is available in the United States. Cholestyramine has been used in severely toxic patients to bind thyroid hormones in the gut and thus block the enterohepatic circulation of the iodothyronines (Mercado *et al.*, 1996).

Preoperative Preparation. To reduce operative morbidity and mortality, patients must be rendered euthyroid prior to subtotal thyroidectomy as definitive treatment for hyperthyroidism. It is possible to bring virtually 100% of patients to a euthyroid state; the operative mortality in these patients in the hands of an experienced thyroid surgeon is extremely low. Prior treatment with antithyroid drugs usually is successful in rendering the patient euthyroid for surgery. Iodide is added to the regimen for 7 to 10 days prior to surgery to decrease the vascularity of the gland, making it less friable and decreasing the difficulties for the surgeon. In the patient who is either allergic to antithyroid drugs or is noncompliant, a euthyroid state usually can be achieved by treatment with iopanoic acid, dexamethasone, and propranolol for 5 to 7 days prior to surgery. All of these drugs should be discontinued after surgery.

Thyroid Storm. Thyroid storm is an uncommon but life-threatening complication of thyrotoxicosis in which a severe form of the disease is usually precipitated by an intercurrent medical problem (Safran *et al.*, 2003; Farwell, 2004). It occurs in untreated or partially treated thyrotoxic patients. Precipitating factors associated with thyrotoxic crisis include infections, stress, trauma, thyroidal or nonthyroidal surgery, diabetic ketoacidosis, labor, heart disease, and rarely, radioactive iodine treatment.

Clinical features are similar to those of thyrotoxicosis, but more exaggerated. Cardinal features include fever (temperature usually over 38.5°C) and tachycardia out of proportion to the fever. Nausea, vomiting, diarrhea, agitation, and confusion are frequent presentations. Coma and death may ensue in up to 20% of patients. Thyroid function abnormalities are similar to those found in uncomplicated hyperthyroidism. Therefore thyroid storm is primarily a clinical diagnosis.

Treatment includes supportive measures such as intravenous fluids, antipyretics, cooling blankets, and sedation. Antithyroid drugs are given in large doses. Propylthiouracil is preferred over methimazole because it also impairs peripheral conversion of $T_4 \rightarrow T_3$. The recommended initial dose of propylthiouracil is 200 to 400 mg every 4 hours. Propylthiouracil and methimazole can be administered by nasogastric tube or rectally if necessary. Neither of these preparations is available for parenteral administration in the United States.

Oral iodides are used after the first dose of an antithyroid drug has been administered (*see* below). The agents mentioned above as adjuvant therapies of thyrotoxicosis may be usefully applied. Dexamethasone (0.5 to 1 mg intravenously every 6 hours) is recommended both as an inhibitor of conversion of thyroxine to triiodothyronine and as supportive therapy of possible relative adrenal insufficiency. Finally, *treatment of the underlying precipitating illness is essential.*

Ionic Inhibitors

The term *ionic inhibitors* designates substances that interfere with the concentration of iodide by the thyroid gland. The effective agents are anions that resemble iodide: They are all monovalent, hydrated anions of a size similar to that of iodide. The most studied example, *thiocyanate,* differs from the others qualitatively; it is not concentrated by the thyroid gland, but in large amounts may inhibit the organification of iodine. Thiocyanate is produced following the enzymatic hydrolysis of certain plant glycosides. Thus, certain foods (*e.g.,* cabbage) and cigarette smoking result in an increased concentration of thiocyanate in the blood and urine, as does the administration of *sodium nitroprusside.* Indeed, cigarette smoking has been reported to worsen both subclinical hypothyroidism (Müller *et al.*, 1995) and Graves' ophthalmopathy (Bartalena *et al.*,

1998b). Dietary precursors of thiocyanate may be a contributing factor in endemic goiter in certain parts of the world, especially in Central Africa, where the intake of iodine is very low.

Among other anions, *perchlorate* (ClO_4^-) is ten times as active as thiocyanate (Wolff, 1998). Perchlorate blocks the entrance of iodide into the thyroid by competitively inhibiting the NIS (Carrasco, 2005). Although perchlorate can be used to control hyperthyroidism, it has caused fatal aplastic anemia when given in excessive amounts (2 to 3 g daily). Over the past few years, however, perchlorate in doses of 750 mg daily has been used in the treatment of Graves' disease and amiodarone-iodine–induced thyrotoxicosis. Perchlorate can be used to "discharge" inorganic iodide from the thyroid gland in a diagnostic test of iodide organification. Other ions, selected on the basis of their size, also have been found to be active; *fluoborate* (BF_4^-) is as effective as perchlorate.

Over the past few years, concern has been raised in several western states over the potential antithyroid effects of trace amounts of perchlorate contaminating the drinking water. Ammonium perchlorate is an essential oxidizer in the production of rocket fuel, and water supplies have been contaminated with perchlorate derived from these sites. However, the minute amounts detected in drinking water are far below the levels (*e.g.*, 500 μg daily for 2 weeks) that had no effect on thyroid ^{123}I uptake and thyroid function tests in normal volunteers (Greer *et al.*, 2002). Perchlorate levels in drinking water are almost always below 10 μg/L or 20 μg perchlorate daily, assuming a maximum intake of 2 L. Epidemiological studies around Redlands, California, where perchlorate has been detected in the water supply, have not found any increase in thyroid cancer (Morgan and Cassady, 2002) or elevations in neonatal serum TSH values (Kelsh *et al.*, 2003). However, one study from Arizona has reported an increase in neonatal serum TSH values in neonates in Yuma City (perchlorate found in the water supply) compared to Flagstaff (perchlorate not found) (Brechner *et al.*, 2000). The latter report has been refuted when socioeconomic factors, altitude, time of neonatal sampling, and length of stay in the hospital are accounted for by comparing neonatal serum TSH values in Yuma City with a nearby city in Yuma County where perchlorate is not detected in the water supply (Lamm, 2003). The Environmental Protection Agency and a National Academy of Sciences Committee are currently determining an allowable concentration of perchlorate in drinking water that unequivocally does not affect thyroid function.

Lithium has a multitude of effects on thyroid function; its principal effect is decreased secretion of thyroxine and triiodothyronine (Takami, 1994), which can cause overt hypothyroidism in some patients taking lithium for the treatment of mania (*see* Chapter 18).

Iodide

Iodide is the oldest remedy for disorders of the thyroid gland. Before the antithyroid drugs were used, it was the only substance available for control of the signs and symptoms of hyperthyroidism. Its use in this way is indeed paradoxical, and the explanation for this paradox is still incomplete.

Mechanism of Action. High concentrations of iodide appear to influence almost all important aspects of iodine metabolism by the thyroid gland (Roti and Vagenakis, 2005). The capacity of iodide to limit its own transport

has been mentioned above. Acute inhibition of the synthesis of iodotyrosines and iodothyronines by iodide also is well known (the *Wolff-Chaikoff effect*). This transient, 2-day inhibition is observed only above critical concentrations of intracellular rather than extracellular concentrations of iodide. With time, "escape" from this inhibition is associated with an adaptive decrease in iodide transport and a lowered intracellular iodide concentration, most likely due to a decrease in NIS mRNA and protein (Eng *et al.*, 1999). The mechanism of the acute Wolff-Chaikoff effect remains elusive and has been postulated to be due to the generation of organic iodo-compounds within the thyroid (Pisarev and Gärtner, 2000).

An important clinical effect of high $[I^-]_{plasma}$ is inhibition of the release of thyroid hormone. This action is rapid and efficacious in severe thyrotoxicosis. The effect is exerted directly on the thyroid gland and can be demonstrated in the euthyroid subject as well as in the hyperthyroid patient. Studies in a cultured thyroid cell line suggest that some of the inhibitory effects of iodide on thyrocyte proliferation may be mediated by actions of iodide on crucial regulatory points in the cell cycle (Smerdely *et al.*, 1993).

In euthyroid individuals, the administration of doses of iodide from 1.5 to 150 mg daily results in small decreases in plasma thyroxine and triiodothyronine concentrations and small compensatory increases in serum TSH values, with all values remaining in the normal range. However, euthyroid patients with a history of a wide variety of underlying thyroid disorders may develop iodine-induced hypothyroidism when exposed to large amounts of iodine present in many commonly prescribed drugs (Table 56–6), and these patients do not escape from the acute Wolff-Chaikoff effect (Roti *et al.*, 1997). Among the disorders that predispose patients to iodine-induced hypothyroidism are treated Graves' disease, Hashimoto's thyroiditis, postpartum lymphocytic thyroiditis, subacute painful thyroiditis, and lobectomy for benign nodules. The most commonly prescribed iodine-containing drugs are certain expectorants, topical antiseptics, and radiological contrast agents.

Response to Iodide in Hyperthyroidism. The response to iodides in patients with hyperthyroidism is often striking and rapid. The effect usually is discernible within 24 hours, and the basal metabolic rate may fall at a rate comparable to that following thyroidectomy. This provides evidence that the release of hormone into the circulation is rapidly blocked. Furthermore, thyroid hormone synthesis also is mildly decreased. In the thyroid gland vascularity is reduced, the gland becomes much firmer, the cells become smaller, colloid reaccumulates in the follicles, and the quantity of bound iodine increases, as though an excessive stimulus to the gland has been removed or antagonized. The maximal effect is attained after 10 to 15 days of continuous therapy, when the signs and symptoms of hyperthyroidism may have greatly improved.

Table 56–6
Commonly Used Iodine-Containing Drugs

DRUGS	IODINE CONTENT
Oral or local	
Amiodarone	75 mg/tablet
Calcium iodide (*e.g.*, CALCID-RINE SYRUP)	26 mg/ml
Iodoquinol (diiodohydroxyquin)	134–416 mg/tablet
Echothiophate iodide ophthalmic solution	5–41 μg/drop
Hydriodic acid syrup	13–15 mg/ml
Iodochlorhydroxyquin	104 mg/tablet
Iodine-containing vitamins	0.15 mg/tablet
Idoxuridine ophthalmic solution	18 μg/drop
Kelp/seaweed	0.15 mg/tablet
Lugol's solution	6.3 mg/drop
PONARIS nasal emollient	5 mg/0.8 ml
Saturated solution of potassium iodide (SSKI)	38 mg/drop
Topical antiseptics	
Iodoquinol (diiodohydroxyquin) cream	6 mg/g
Iodine tincture	40 mg/ml
Iodochlorhydroxyquin cream	12 mg/g
Iodoform gauze	4.8 mg/100 mg gauze
Povidone–iodine	10 mg/ml
Radiology contrast agents	
Diatrizoate meglumine sodium	370 mg/ml
Propyliodone	340 mg/ml
Iopanoic acid	333 mg/tablet
Ipodate	308 mg/capsule
Iothalamate	480 mg/ml
Metrizamide	483 mg/ml before dilution
Iohexol	463 mg/ml

SOURCE: Adapted from Roti *et al.*, 1997.

Unfortunately, iodide therapy usually does not completely control the manifestations of hyperthyroidism, and after a variable period of time, the beneficial effect disappears. With continued treatment, the hyperthyroidism may return in its initial intensity or may become even more severe than it was at first.

Therapeutic Uses. The uses of iodide in the treatment of hyperthyroidism are in the preoperative period in preparation for thyroidecto-

my, and in conjunction with antithyroid drugs and propranolol, in the treatment of thyrotoxic crisis. Prior to surgery, iodide is sometimes employed alone, but more frequently it is used after the hyperthyroidism has been controlled by an antithyroid drug. It is then given for 7 to 10 days immediately preceding the operation. Optimal control of hyperthyroidism is achieved if antithyroid drugs are first given alone. If iodine also is given from the beginning, variable responses are observed; sometimes the effect of iodide predominates, storage of hormone is promoted, and prolonged antithyroid treatment is required before the hyperthyroidism is controlled. These clinical observations may be explained by the capacity of iodide to prevent the inactivation of thyroid peroxidase by antithyroid drugs (Taurog, 2000).

Another use of iodide is to protect the thyroid from radioactive iodine fallout following a nuclear accident. Because the uptake of radioactive iodine is inversely proportional to the serum concentration of stable iodine, the administration of 30 to 100 mg of iodide daily will markedly decrease the thyroid uptake of radioisotopes of iodine. Following the Chernobyl nuclear reactor accident in 1986, approximately 10 million children and adults in Poland were given stable iodide to block the thyroid exposure to radioactive iodine from the atmosphere and from dairy products from cows that ate contaminated grass (Nauman and Wolff, 1993). This prevented the occurrence of radiation-induced thyroid cancer, as observed in children residing near Chernobyl.

The dosage or form in which iodide is administered bears little relationship to the response achieved in hyperthyroidism, provided that not less than the minimal effective amount is given; this dosage is 6 mg of iodide per day in most, but not all, patients. *Strong iodine solution* (Lugol's solution) is widely used and consists of 5% iodine and 10% potassium iodide, which yields a dose of 6.3 mg of iodine per drop. The iodine is reduced to iodide in the intestine before absorption. *Saturated solution of potassium iodide* (SSKI) also is available, containing 38 mg per drop. Typical doses include 3 to 5 drops of Lugol's solution or 1 to 3 drops of SSKI three times a day. These doses have been determined empirically and are far in excess of that needed.

Untoward Reactions. Occasional individuals show marked sensitivity to iodide or to organic preparations that contain iodine when they are administered intravenously. The onset of an acute reaction may occur immediately or several hours after administration. Angioedema is the outstanding symptom, and laryngeal edema may lead to suffocation. Multiple cutaneous hemorrhages may be present. Also, manifestations of the serum-sickness type of hypersensitivity—such as fever, arthralgia, lymph node enlargement, and eosinophilia—may appear. Thrombotic thrombocytopenic purpura and fatal periarteritis nodosa attributed to hypersensitivity to iodide also have been described.

The severity of symptoms of chronic intoxication with iodide (*iodism*) is related to the dose. The symptoms start with an unpleasant brassy taste and burning in the mouth and throat as well as soreness of the teeth and gums. Increased salivation is noted. Coryza, sneezing, and irritation of the eyes with swelling of the eyelids are commonly observed. Mild iodism simulates a "head cold." The patient often complains of a severe headache that originates in the frontal sinuses. Irritation of the mucous glands of the respiratory tract causes a productive cough. Excess transudation into the bronchial tree may lead to pulmonary edema. In addition, the parotid and submaxillary glands may become enlarged and tender, and the syndrome may be mistaken for mumps parotitis. There also may be inflammation of the pharynx, larynx, and tonsils. Skin lesions are common and vary in type and intensity. They usually are mildly acneform and distributed in the seborrheic areas. Rarely, severe and sometimes fatal eruptions (ioderma) may occur after the prolonged use of iodides. The lesions are bizarre; they resemble those caused by bromism, a rare problem, and as a rule involute quickly when iodide is withdrawn. Symptoms of gastric irritation are common, and diarrhea, which is sometimes bloody, may occur. Fever is occasionally observed, and anorexia and depression may be present.

Fortunately, the symptoms of iodism disappear spontaneously within a few days after stopping the administration of iodide. The renal excretion of I⁻ can be increased by procedures that promote Cl⁻ excretion (*e.g.,* osmotic diuresis, chloruretic diuretics, and salt loading). These procedures may be useful when the symptoms of iodism are severe.

Radioactive Iodine

Chemical and Physical Properties. Although iodine has several radioactive isotopes, greatest use has been made of ^{131}I. It has a half-life of 8 days; therefore, more than 99% of its radiation is expended within 56 days. Its radioactive emissions include both γ rays and β particles. The short-lived radionuclide of iodine, ^{123}I, is primarily a γ-emitter with a half-life of only 13 hours. This permits a relatively brief exposure to radiation during thyroid scans.

Effects on the Thyroid Gland. The chemical behavior of the radioactive isotopes of iodine is identical to that of the stable isotope, ^{127}I. ^{131}I is rapidly and efficiently trapped by the thyroid, incorporated into the iodoamino acids, and deposited in the colloid of the follicles, from which it is slowly liberated. Thus, the destructive β particles originate within the follicle and act almost exclusively upon the parenchymal cells of the thyroid, with little or no damage to surrounding tissue. The γ radiation passes through the tissue and can be quantified by external detection. The effects of the radiation depend on the dosage. When small tracer doses of ^{131}I are administered, thyroid function is not disturbed. However, when large amounts of radioactive iodine gain access to the gland, the characteristic cytotoxic actions of ionizing radiation are observed. Pyknosis and necrosis of the follicular cells are followed by disappearance of colloid and fibrosis of the gland. With properly selected doses of ^{131}I, it is possible to destroy the thyroid gland completely without detectable injury to adjacent tissues. After smaller doses, some of the follicles, usually in the periphery of the gland, retain their function.

Therapeutic Uses. Radioactive iodine finds its widest use in the treatment of hyperthyroidism and in the diagnosis of disorders of thyroid function. *Sodium iodide* ^{131}I (IODOTOPE THERAPEUTIC) is available as a solution or in capsules containing essentially carrier-free ^{131}I suitable for oral administration. Sodium iodide ^{123}I is available for scanning procedures. Discussion here is limited to the uses of ^{131}I.

Hyperthyroidism. Radioactive iodine is highly useful in the treatment of hyperthyroidism; in many circumstances it is regarded as the therapeutic procedure of choice for this condition (Leslie *et al.,* 2003). The use of stable iodide as treatment for hyperthyroidism, however, may preclude treatment and certain imaging studies with radioactive iodine for weeks after the iodide has been discontinued.

Dosage and Technique. ^{131}I, 7000 to 10,000 rads per gram of thyroid tissue, is administered orally. The effective dose for a given patient depends primarily upon the size of the thyroid, the iodine uptake of the gland, and the rate of release of radioactive iodine from the gland subsequent to the nuclide's deposition in the colloid. Comparison studies have shown little advantage of a standard individualized dose, based on gland weight and radioactive iodine uptake, over a fixed dose (Jarløv *et al.,* 1995; de Bruin *et al.,* 1994; Leslie *et al.,* 2003). For these reasons, the optimal dose of ^{131}I, expressed in terms of microcuries taken up per gram of thyroid tissue, varies in different laboratories from 80 to 150 μCi. The usual total dose is 4 to 15 mCi. The incidence of hypothyroidism in the early years after doses on the lower side is reduced; however, many patients with late hypothyroidism may go undetected. Therefore, the ultimate incidence of hypothyroidism is probably no less than with the larger doses. In addition, relapse of the hyperthyroid state, or initial failure to alleviate the hyperthyroid state, is increased in patients receiving lower doses of ^{131}I. Thus, many endocrinologists recommend initial treatment with thyroid ablative doses of ^{131}I, with subsequent treatment for hypothyroidism. There also is evidence that pretreatment with propylthiouracil reduces the therapeutic efficacy of ^{131}I, necessitating a higher dose for a desired effect (Imseis *et al.,* 1998; Tuttle *et al.,* 1995). Methimazole appears not to share this effect of propylthiouracil (Imseis *et al.,* 1998).

Course of Disease. The course of hyperthyroidism in a patient who has received an optimal dose of ^{131}I is characterized by progressive recovery. Beginning a few weeks after treatment, the symptoms of hyperthyroidism gradually abate over a period of 2 to 3 months. If therapy has been inadequate, the necessity for further treatment is apparent within 6 to 12 months. It is not uncommon, however, for the serum TSH to remain low for several months after ^{131}I therapy, especially if the patient was not rendered euthyroid prior to receiving the radioactive iodine (Uy *et al.,* 1995). Occasionally, this delayed recovery of the hypothalamic-pituitary-thyroid axis results in a picture of central hypothyroidism, with low circulating thyroid hormones. Thus, assessing radioactive iodine failure based on TSH concentrations alone may be misleading and should always be accompanied by determination of free T_4 and serum T_3 concentrations. Furthermore, transient hypothyroidism, lasting up to 6 months, may occur in up to 50% of patients receiving a dose of ^{131}I calculated to result in euthyroidism (Aizawa *et al.,* 1997). This is less of a problem if the patient receives a higher, ablative dose of ^{131}I, since hypothyroidism occurs far more frequently and persists.

Depending to some extent upon the dosage schedule adopted, one-half to two-thirds of patients are cured by a single dose, one-third to one-fifth require two doses, and the remainder require three or more doses before the disorder is controlled. Patients treated with larger doses of ^{131}I almost always develop hypothyroidism within a few months.

β Adrenergic antagonists, antithyroid drugs, or both, or stable iodide, can be used to hasten the control of hyperthyroidism while awaiting the full effects of the radioactive iodine. However, the antithyroid drugs should be withheld for a few days before and after the therapeutic dose of [131]I.

Advantages. The advantages of radioactive iodine in the treatment of Graves' disease are many. No death as a direct result of the use of the isotope has been reported. There have been reports of increased mortality from cardiovascular and cerebrovascular disease in the first year after radioactive iodine therapy (Franklyn *et al.*, 1998); however, there is no evidence that the increased mortality was related to the radioactive iodine itself, and long-term follow-up of radioactive iodine therapy for Graves' disease has demonstrated no increase in overall cancer mortality in patients treated with [131]I (Ron *et al.*, 1998). In the nonpregnant patient, no tissue other than the thyroid is exposed to sufficient ionizing radiation to be detectably altered. Nevertheless, continuing concern about potential effects of radiation on germ cells prompts some endocrinologists to advocate antithyroid drugs or surgery in younger patients who are acceptable operative risks. Hypoparathyroidism is a small risk of surgery. With radioactive iodine treatment, the patient is spared the risks and discomfort of surgery. The cost is low, hospitalization is not required in the United States, and patients can indulge in their customary activities during the entire procedure.

Disadvantages. The chief disadvantage of the use of radioactive iodine is the high incidence of delayed hypothyroidism that is induced. Even when elaborate procedures are used to estimate iodine uptake and gland size, a certain percentage of patients will be overtreated. A distressing feature of this complication is its rising prevalence with the passage of time; the longer the interval after treatment, the higher the incidence. Several analyses of groups of patients treated 10 or more years previously suggest that the eventual rate may exceed 80%. However, it now appears that the incidence of hypothyroidism also increases progressively after subtotal thyroidectomy or after antithyroid drug therapy, and such failure of glandular function is probably part of the natural progression of Graves' disease, no matter what the therapy.

Although it is often said that hypothyroidism is not a serious complication because it can be treated so easily with thyroid hormone, its onset may be insidious and overlooked for some time. Also, once diagnosed, it is difficult to ensure that patients who need the hormone actually take it. Since the health risks of untreated subclinical hypothyroidism are becoming increasingly evident (Surks *et al.*, 2004), hypothyroidism, either subclinical or overt, requires long-term follow-up to ensure that optimal replacement therapy is provided.

Another disadvantage of radioactive iodine therapy is the long period of time that is sometimes required before the hyperthyroidism is controlled. When a single dose is effective, the response is most satisfactory; however, when multiple doses are needed, it may be many months or a year or more before the patient is well. This disadvantage can be largely overcome if the initial dose is sufficiently large. Other disadvantages include possible worsening of ophthalmopathy after treatment, although this is controversial (DeGroot *et al.*, 1995). Although extremely rare, thyroid storm has occurred after therapy with ^{131}I, usually in patients who did not receive pretreatment with antithyroid drugs. Finally, salivary gland dysfunction may be seen, especially after the higher doses used for the treatment of thyroid cancer (*see* below) (Caglar *et al.*, 2002).

Indications. The clearest indication for this form of treatment is hyperthyroidism in older patients and in those with heart disease. Radioactive iodine also is the best form of treatment when Graves' disease has persisted or recurred after subtotal thyroidectomy and when prolonged treatment with antithyroid drugs has not led to

remission. Finally, radioactive iodine is indicated in patients with toxic nodular goiter, since the disease does not go into spontaneous remission. The risk of inducing hypothyroidism is less in nodular goiter than in Graves' disease, perhaps because of the normal progression of the latter and the preservation of nonautonomous thyroid tissue in the former. Usually, larger doses of radioactive iodine are required in the treatment of toxic nodular goiter than in the treatment of Graves' disease. Radioactive iodine has been used to decrease the size of large, nontoxic, multinodular goiters that are causing compressive symptoms in patients who are otherwise poor operative risks. While surgery remains the treatment of choice for the young patient with compressive multinodular goiters, radioactive iodine therapy may benefit elderly patients, especially those with cardiopulmonary disease.

Contraindications. The main contraindication for the use of ^{131}I therapy is pregnancy. After the first trimester, the fetal thyroid will concentrate the isotope and thus suffer damage; even during the first trimester, radioactive iodine is best avoided because there may be adverse effects of radiation on fetal tissues. The risk of causing neoplastic changes in the thyroid gland has been an ongoing concern since radioactive iodine was first introduced, and only small numbers of children have been treated in this way. Indeed, many clinics have declined to treat younger patients for fear of causing cancer and have reserved radioactive iodine for patients over some arbitrary age, such as 25 or 30 years. Since experience with ^{131}I is now vast, these age limits are lower than they were in the past. The most recent report by the Cooperative Thyrotoxicosis Therapy Follow-up Study Group shows no increase in total cancer mortality following ^{131}I treatment for Graves' disease (Ron *et al.*, 1998). Furthermore, there was no increase in the occurrence of leukemia following large-dose ^{131}I therapy for thyroid cancer, although there was an increase in colorectal cancers in this population (de Vathaire *et al.*, 1997). These data strongly suggest that laxatives be given to all patients receiving ^{131}I therapy for treatment of thyroid cancer to decrease the risk of future digestive tract malignancies. Transient abnormalities in testicular function have been reported following ^{131}I therapy for treatment of thyroid cancer, but no long-term effects on fertility in either men or women have been demonstrated (Pacini *et al.*, 1994b; Dottorini *et al.*, 1995).

Thyroid Carcinoma. While most well-differentiated thyroid carcinomas accumulate very little iodine, stimulation of iodine uptake with TSH often is used effectively to treat metastases. Follicular carcinomas, which account for 10% to 15% of thyroid malignancies, are especially amenable to this treatment. Currently, endogenous TSH stimulation is evoked by withdrawal of thyroid hormone replacement therapy in patients previously treated with near-total thyroidectomy with or without radioactive ablation of residual thyroid tissue. Total body ^{131}I scanning and measurement of serum thyroglobulin when the patient is hypothyroid (TSH >35 milliunits/L) should be performed to identify metastatic disease or residual thyroid bed tissue. Depending upon the residual uptake or the presence of metastatic disease, an ablative dose of ^{131}I ranging from 30 to 150 mCi is administered, and a repeat total body scan is obtained 1 week later. The precise amount of ^{131}I needed to treat residual tissue and metastases is controversial. *Recombinant human TSH* (THYROGEN) is now available to test the ability of thyroid tissue, both normal and malignant, to take up radioactive iodine and to secrete thyroglobulin (Haugen *et al.*, 1999). The major advantage to the use of this medication is that patients do not have to stop their suppressive levothyroxine therapy and become clinically hypothyroid for the presence of persistent or metastatic disease to be assessed. While recombinant human TSH is not yet approved for treatment prior to therapeutic administration of ^{131}I, trials are ongoing to assess this therapeutic indication (Robbins *et al.*, 2002; Robbins and Robbins, 2003).

TSH-suppressive therapy with levothyroxine is indicated in all patients after treatment for thyroid cancer. The goal of therapy usually is to keep serum TSH levels in the subnormal range (Burmeister *et al.*, 1992). Follow-up evaluation every 6 months is reasonable, along with determination of serum thyroglobulin concentrations. A rise in serum thyroglobulin concentration is often the first indication of recurrent disease. Prognosis in patients with thyroid cancer depends upon the pathology and size of the tumor and is generally worse in the elderly. Overall, the vast majority of patients with thyroid cancer will not die of their disease. Papillary cancer is not aggressive; the 10-year survival rate exceeds 40%. Follicular cancer is more aggressive and can metastasize *via* the bloodstream. Still, prognosis is fair and long-term survival is common. Even in patients with metastatic, differentiated thyroid cancer, ^{131}I therapy is very effective and may be even curative (Pacini *et al.*, 1994a). Anaplastic cancer is the exception, as it is highly malignant with survival usually less than 1 year. Medullary thyroid carcinomas do not accumulate I$^-$ and cannot usually be treated with [131]I.

Diagnostic Uses. Measurement of the thyroidal accumulation of a tracer dose is helpful in the differential diagnosis of thyrotoxicosis and nodular goiter. The response of the thyroid to TSH-suppressive doses of thyroid hormone can be evaluated in this way. Following the administration of a tracer dose, the pattern of localization in the thyroid gland can be depicted by a special scanning apparatus, and this technique is sometimes useful in defining thyroid nodules as functional ("hot") or nonfunctional ("cold") and in finding ectopic thyroid tissue and occasionally metastatic thyroid tumors.

CLINICAL SUMMARY

Replacement therapy for hypothyroidism typically uses oral L-thyroxine given once daily, with the goal of restoring the serum TSH concentrations to the mid-normal or low-normal range. This usually is possible and most patients are treated successfully. Based on the prolonged half-life of thyroxine, at least 6 to 8 weeks are required before a new steady-state level is reached following initiation of therapy or adjustment of dose. Special cases of hypothyroidism include patients following surgical resection of differentiated thyroid carcinoma and pregnancy. In the former setting, the goal is to suppress the TSH level to below normal, thereby removing the potential effect of TSH to stimulate proliferation of the cancer cells. In pregnant patients, the standard replacement dose generally must be increased due to higher levels of TBG and small amounts of thyroxine crossing the placenta to reach the fetus. Realizing the effects of even relatively mild hypothyroidism on neurological development of the fetus, it is especially important to carefully monitor thyroid function tests during pregnancy.

Options available for treating hyperthyroid patients include antithyroid drugs (*e.g.*, propylthiouracil and methimazole), radioactive iodine ablation, and surgery. The preferred therapy differs among endocrinologists and regions. Special circumstances such as the presence of coexisting ophthalmopathy in patients with Graves' disease also may influence the choice of therapy; radioactive iodine may aggravate the ophthalmopathy. Although younger patients with hyperthyroidism often can be treated effectively with radioactive iodine, medical therapy with antithyroid drugs to reduce the levels of thyroid hormone may be preferred. In younger patients with very large goiters, thyroidectomy is a viable alternative. In older patients or those with cardiac disease, radioactive iodine usually is recommended after the patient has been rendered euthyroid with antithyroid medication. Recombinant human TSH is available for stimulation of radioactive iodine uptake and release of thyroglobulin in patients with thyroid cancer after thyroidectomy. It essentially has replaced induced hypothyroidism after thyroid hormone withdrawal for most patients who are having a total body scan and serum thyroglobulin measurement to determine the presence of residual tissue.

BIBLIOGRAPHY

Adams, M., Matthews, C., Collingwood, T.N., *et al.* Genetic analysis of 29 kindreds with generalized and pituitary resistance to thyroid hormone. Identification of thirteen novel mutations in the thyroid hormone receptor beta gene. *J. Clin. Invest.,* **1994,** *94:*506–515.

al-Adsani, H., Hoffer, L.J., and Silva, J.E. Resting energy expenditure is sensitive to small dose changes in patients on chronic thyroid hormone replacement. *J. Clin. Endocrinol. Metab.,* **1997,** *82:*1118–1125.

Aizawa, Y., Yoshida, K., Kaise, N., *et al.* The development of transient hypothyroidism after iodine-131 treatment in hyperthyroid patients with Graves' disease: prevalence, mechanism and prognosis. *Clin. Endocrinol. (Oxf.),* **1997,** *46:*1–5.

Astwood, E.B. Chemotherapy of hyperthyroidism. *Harvey Lect.,* **1945,** *40:*195–235.

Azizi, F., Bahrainian, M., Khamseh, M.E., and Khoshniat, M. Intellectual development and thyroid function in children who were breast-fed by thyrotoxic mothers taking methimazole. *J. Pediatr. Endocrinol. Metab.,* **2003,** *16:*1239–1243.

Bartalena, L., Marcocci, C., Bogazzi, F., *et al.* Relation between therapy for hyperthyroidism and the course of Graves' ophthalmopathy. *N. Engl. J. Med.,* **1998a,** *338:*73–78.

Bartalena, L., Marcocci, C., Tanda, M.L., *et al.* Cigarette smoking and treatment outcomes in Graves' ophthalmopathy. *Ann. Intern. Med.,* **1998b,** *129:*632–635.

Barwell, J., Fox, G.F., Round, J., and Berg, J. Choanal atresia: the result of maternal thyrotoxicosis or fetal carbimazole? *Am. J. Med. Genet.,* **2002,** *111:*55–56.

Baxter, J.D., Webb, P., Grover, G., and Scanlan, T.S. Selective activation of thyroid hormone signaling pathways by GC-1: a new approach to controlling cholesterol and body weight. *Trends Endocrinol. Metab.*, **2004,** *15:*154–157.

Benker, G., Reinwein, D., Kahaly, G., *et al.* Is there a methimazole dose effect on remission rate in Graves' disease? Results from a long-term prospective study. The European Multicentre Trial Group of the Treatment of Hyperthyroidism with Antithyroid Drugs. *Clin. Endocrinol. (Oxf.),* **1998,** *49:*451–457.

Benvenga, S., Cahnmann, H.J., Rader, D., *et al.* Thyroxine binding to the apolipoproteins of high-density lipoproteins HDL_2 and HDL_3. *Endocrinology,* **1992,** *131:*2805–2811.

Biondi, B., Fazio, S., Palmieri, E.A., *et al.* Left ventricular diastolic dysfunction in patients with subclinical hypothyroidism. *J. Clin. Endocrinol. Metab.,* **1999,** *84:*2064–2067.

Botero, D., and Brown, R.S. Bioassay of thyrotropin receptor antibodies with Chinese hamster ovary cells transfected with recombinant human thyrotropin receptor: clinical utility in children and adolescents with Graves' disease. *J. Pediatr.,* **1998,** *132:*612–618.

Braverman, L.E., Ingbar, S.H., and Sterling, K. Conversion of thyroxine (T_4) to triiodothyronine (T_3) in athyreotic human subjects. *J. Clin. Invest.,* **1970,** *49:*855–864.

Brechner, R.J., Parkhurst, G.D., Humble, W.O., *et al.* Ammonium perchlorate contamination of Colorado River drinking water is associated with abnormal thyroid function in newborns in Arizona. *J. Occup. Environ. Med.,* **2000,** *42:*777–782.

Brent, G.A., and Hershman, J.M. Thyroxine therapy in patients with severe nonthyroidal illnesses and low serum thyroxine concentration. *J. Clin. Endocrinol. Metab.,* **1986,** *63:*1–8.

Brucker-Davis, F., Skarulis, M.C., Grace, M.B., *et al.* Genetic and clinical features of 42 kindreds with resistance to thyroid hormone. The National Institutes of Health Prospective Study. *Ann. Intern. Med.,* **1995,** *123:*572–583.

de Bruin, T.W., Croon, C.D., de Klerk, J.M., and van Isselt, J.W. Standardized radioiodine therapy in Graves' disease: the persistent effect of thyroid weight and radioiodine uptake on outcome. *J. Intern. Med.,* **1994,** *236:*507–513.

Bunevicius, R., Kazanavicius, G., Zalinkevicius, R., and Prange, A.J. Jr. Effects of thyroxine as compared with thyroxine plus triiodothyronine in patients with hypothyroidism. *N. Engl. J. Med.,* **1999,** *340:*424–429.

Burmeister, L.A., Goumaz, M.O., Mariash, C.N., and Oppenheimer, J.H. Levothyroxine dose requirements for thyrotropin suppression in the treatment of differentiated thyroid cancer. *J. Clin. Endocrinol. Metab.,* **1992,** *75:*344–350.

Caglar, M., Tuncel, M., and Alpar, R. Scintigraphic evaluation of salivary gland dysfunction in patients with thyroid cancer after radioiodine treatment. *Clin. Nucl. Med.,* **2002,** *27:*767–771.

Cao, X.Y., Jiang, X.M., Dou, Z.H., *et al.* Timing of vulnerability of the brain to iodine deficiency in endemic cretinism. *N. Engl. J. Med.,* **1994,** *331:*1739–1744.

Chen, J.D, and Evans, R.M. A transcriptional co-repressor that interacts with nuclear hormone receptors. *Nature,* **1995,** *377:*454–457.

Clyde, P.W., Harari, A.E., Getka, E.J., and Shakir, K.M. Combined levothyroxine plus liothyronine compared with levothyroxine alone in primary hypothyroidism: a randomized controlled trial. *JAMA,* **2003,** *290:*2952–2958.

Danese, M.D., Powe, N.R., Sawin, C.T., and Ladenson, P.W. Screening for mild thyroid failure at the periodic health examination: a decision and cost-effectiveness analysis. *JAMA,* **1996,** *276:*285–292.

DeGroot, L.J. Dangerous dogmas in medicine: the nonthyroidal illness syndrome. *J. Clin. Endocrinol. Metab.,* **1999,** *84:*151–164.

DeGroot, L.J., Gorman, C.A., Pinchera, A., *et al.* Therapeutic controversies. Retro-orbital radiation and radioactive iodide ablation of the thyroid may be good for Graves' ophthalmopathy. *J. Clin. Endocrinol. Metab.,* **1995,** *80:*339–340.

Den Ouden, A.L., Kok, J.H., Verkerk, P.H., Brand, R., and Verloove-Vanhorick, S.P. The relation between neonatal thyroxine levels and neurodevelopmental outcome at age 5 and 9 years in a national cohort of very preterm and/or very low birth weight infants. *Pediatr. Res.,* **1996,** *39:*142–145.

DeRosa, C., Richter, P., Pohl, H., and Jones, D.E. Environmental exposures that affect the endocrine system: public health implications. *J. Toxicol. Environ. Health. B. Crit. Rev.,* **1998,** *1:*3–26.

Dottorini, M.E., Lomuscio, G., Mazzucchelli, L., *et al.* Assessment of female fertility and carcinogenesis after iodine-131 therapy for differentiated thyroid carcinoma. *J. Nucl. Med.,* **1995,** *36:*21–27.

Elnagar, B., Eltom, M., Karlsson, F.A., *et al.* The effects of different doses of oral iodized oil on goiter size, urinary iodine, and thyroid-related hormones. *J. Clin. Endocrinol. Metab.,* **1995,** *80:*891–897.

Eng, P.H., Cardona, G.R., Fang, S.L., *et al.* Escape from the acute Wolff-Chaikoff effect is associated with a decrease in thyroid sodium/iodide symporter messenger ribonucleic acid and protein. *Endocrinology,* **1999,** *140:*3404–3410.

Farsetti, A., Mitsuhashi, T., Desvergne, B., *et al.* Molecular basis of thyroid hormone regulation of myelin basic protein gene expression in rodent brain. *J. Biol. Chem.,* **1991,** *266:*23226–23232.

Farwell, A.P., and Dubord-Tomasetti, S.A. Thyroid hormone regulates the expression of laminin in the developing rat cerebellum. *Endocrinology,* **1999,** *140:*4221–4227.

Forrest, D., Erway, L.C., Ng, L., *et al.* Thyroid hormone receptor β is essential for development of auditory function. *Nat. Genet.,* **1996,** *13:*354–357.

Forrest, D., Sjoberg, M., and Vennström, B. Contrasting developmental and tissue-specific expression of α and β thyroid hormone receptor genes. *EMBO J.,* **1990,** *9:*1519–1528.

Fraichard, A., Chassande, O., Plateroti, M., *et al.* The T3R α gene encoding a thyroid hormone receptor is essential for post-natal development and thyroid hormone production. *EMBO J.,* **1997,** *16:*4412–4420.

Franklyn, J.A., Maisonneuve, P., Sheppard, M.C., *et al.* Mortality after the treatment of hyperthyroidism with radioactive iodine. *N. Engl. J. Med.,* **1998,** *338:*712–718.

Giordano, C., Stassi, G., De Maria, R., *et al.* Potential involvement of Fas and its ligand in the pathogenesis of Hashimoto's thyroiditis. *Science,* **1997,** *275:*960–963.

Gauger, K.J., Kato, Y., Haraguchi, K., *et al.* Polychlorinated biphenyls (PCBs) exert thyroid hormone-like effects in the fetal rat brain but do not bind to thyroid hormone receptors. *Environ. Health Perspect.,* **2004,** *112:*516–523.

Gauthier, K., Plateroti, M., Harvey, C.B., *et al.* Genetic analysis reveals different functions for the products of the thyroid hormone receptor α locus. *Mol. Cell. Biol.,* **2001,** *21:*4748–4760.

Glinoer, D., Riahi, M., Grun, J.P., and Kinthaert, J. Risk of subclinical hypothyroidism in pregnant women with asymptomatic autoimmune thyroid disorders. *J. Clin. Endocrinol. Metab.,* **1994,** *79:*197–204.

Göthe, S., Wang, Z., Ng, L., *et al.* Mice devoid of all known thyroid hormone receptors are viable but exhibit disorders of the pituitary-thyroid axis, growth, and bone maturation. *Genes Dev.,* **1999,** *13:*1329–1341.

Grebe, S.K., Cooke, R.R., Ford, H.C., *et al.* Treatment of hypothyroidism with once weekly thyroxine. *J. Clin. Endocrinol. Metab.,* **1997,** *82:*870–875.

Greer, M.A., Goodman, G., Pleus, R.C. and Greer, S.E. Health effects assessment for environmental perchlorate contamination: The dose response for inhibition of thyroidal radioiodine uptake in humans. *Environ. Health Perspect.* **2002,** *110:*927–937.

Greer, M.A., Grimm, Y., and Studer, H. Qualitative changes in the secretion of thyroid hormones induced by iodine deficiency. *Endocrinology,* **1968,** *83:*1193–1198.

Gross, J., and Pitt-Rivers, R. The identification of 3:5:3´-L-triiodothyronine in human plasma. *Lancet,* **1952,** *1:*439–441.

Haddow, J.E., Palomaki, G.E., Allan, W.C., *et al.* Maternal thyroid deficiency during pregnancy and subsequent neuropsychological development of the child. *N. Engl. J. Med.,* **1999,** *341:*549–555.

Harington, C.R. Biochemical basis of thyroid function. *Lancet,* **1935,** *1:*1199–1204, 1261–1266.

Hashimoto, K., Curty, F.H., Borges, P.P., *et al.* An unliganded thyroid hormone receptor causes severe neurological dysfunction. *Proc. Natl. Acad. Sci. U. S. A.,* **2001,** *98:*3998–4003.

Haugen, B.R., Pacini, F., Reiners, C., *et al.* A comparison of recombinant human thyrotropin and thyroid hormone withdrawal for the detection of thyroid remnant or cancer. *J. Clin. Endocrinol. Metab.,* **1999,** *84:*3877–3885.

Hollowell, J.G., Staehling, N.W., Hannon, W.H., *et al.* Iodine nutrition in the United States. Trends and public health implications: iodine excretion data from National Health and Nutrition Examination Surveys I and III (1971–1974 and 1988–1994). *J. Clin. Endocrinol. Metab.,* **1998,** *83:*3401–3408.

Hörlein, A.J., Näär, A.M., Heinzel, T., *et al.* Ligand-independent repression by the thyroid hormone receptor mediated by a nuclear receptor co-repressor. *Nature,* **1995,** *377:*397–404.

Imseis, R.E., Vanmiddlesworth, L., Massie, J.D., *et al.* Pretreatment with propylthiouracil but not methimazole reduces the therapeutic efficacy of iodine-131 in hyperthyroidism. *J. Clin. Endocrinol. Metab.,* **1998,** *83:*685–687.

Jarløv, A.E., Hegedus, L., Kristensen, L.O., *et al.* Is calculation of the dose in radioiodine therapy of hyperthyroidism worth while? *Clin. Endocrinol. (Oxf.),* **1995,** *43:*325–329.

Johansson, C., Göthe, S., Forrest, D., *et al.* Cardiovascular phenotype and temperature control in mice lacking thyroid hormone receptor-β or both α1 and β. *Am. J. Physiol.,* **1999,** *276:*H2006–H2012.

Johansson, C., Vennström, B., and Thorén, P. Evidence that decreased heart rate in thyroid hormone receptor-α1–deficient mice is an intrinsic defect. *Am. J. Physiol.,* **1998,** *275:*R640–R646.

Jorgensen, E.C. Stereochemistry of thyroxine and analogues. *Mayo Clin. Proc.,* **1964,** *39:*560–568.

Kahaly, G.J., Wagner, S., Nieswandt, J., *et al.* Stress echocardiography in hyperthyroidism. *J. Clin. Endocrinol. Metab.,* **1999,** *84:*2308–2313.

Kelsh, M.A., Buffler, P.A., Daaboul, J.J., *et al.* Primary congenital hypothyroidism, newborn thyroid function, and environmental perchlorate exposure among residents of a Southern California community. *J. Occup. Environ. Med.,* **2003,** *45:*1116–1127.

Klemperer, J.D., Klein, I., Gomez, M., *et al.* Thyroid hormone treatment after coronary-artery bypass surgery. *N. Engl. J. Med.,* **1995,** *333:*1522–1527.

Kopp, P., van Sande, J., Parma, J., *et al.* Brief report: congenital hyperthyroidism caused by a mutation in the thyrotropin-receptor gene. *N. Engl. J. Med.,* **1995,** *332:*150–154.

Lamm, S.H. Perchlorate exposure does not explain differences in neonatal thyroid function between Yuma and Flagstaff [Letter]. *J. Occup. Environ. Med.,* **2003,** *45:*1131–1132.

Laugwitz, K-L., Allgeier, A., Offermanns, S., *et al.* The human thyrotropin receptor: A heptahelical receptor capable of stimulating members of all four G protein families. *Proc. Natl. Acad. Sci. U. S. A.,* **1996,** *93:*116–120.

Leeson, P.D., Emmett, J.C., Shah, V.P., *et al.* Selective thyromimetics. Cardiac-sparing thyroid hormone analogues containing 3´-arylmethyl substituents. *J. Med. Chem.,* **1989,** *32:*320–336.

Leslie, W.D., Ward, L., Salamon, E.A., Ludwig, S., Rowe, R.C., and Cowden, E.A. A randomized comparison of radioiodine doses in Graves' hyperthyroidism. *J. Clin. Endocrinol. Metab.,* **2003,** *88:*978–983.

Liang, H., Juge-Aubry, C.E., O'Connell, M., and Burger, A.G. Organ-specific effects of 3,5,3´-triiodothyroacetic acid in rats. *Eur. J. Endocrinol.,* **1997,** *137:*537–544.

Magner, J.A., and Snyder, D.K. Methimazole-induced agranulocytosis treated with recombinant human granulocyte colony-stimulating factor (G-CSF). *Thyroid,* **1994,** *4:*295–296.

Magnusson, R.P., Taurog, A., and Dorris, M.L. Mechanisms of thyroid peroxidase- and lactoperoxidase-catalyzed reactions involving iodide. *J. Biol. Chem.,* **1984,** *259:*13783–13790.

Man, E.B., Brown, J.F., and Serunian, S.A. Maternal hypothyroxinemia: psychoneurological deficits of progeny. *Ann. Clin. Lab. Sci.,* **1991,** *21:*227–239.

Manso, P.G., Furlanetto, R.P., Wolosker, A.M., *et al.* Prospective and controlled study of ophthalmopathy after radioiodine therapy for Graves' hyperthyroidism. *Thyroid,* **1998,** *8:*49–52.

Marangell, L.B., George, M.S., Callahan, A.M., *et al.* Effects of intrathecal thyrotropin-releasing hormone (protirelin) in refractory depressed patients. *Arch. Gen. Psychiatry,* **1997,** *54:*214–222.

Maugendre, D., Gatel, A., Campion, L., *et al.* Antithyroid drugs and Graves' disease—prospective randomized assessment of long-term treatment. *Clin. Endocrinol. (Oxf.),* **1999,** *50:*127–132.

Mercado, M., Mendoza-Zubieta, V., Bautista-Osorio, R., and Espinoza-de los Monteros, A.L. Treatment of hyperthyroidism with a combination of methimazole and cholestyramine. *J. Clin. Endocrinol. Metab.,* **1996,** *81:*3191–3193.

Momotani, N., Noh, J.Y., Ishikawa, N., and Ito, K. Effects of propylthiouracil and methimazole on fetal thyroid status in mothers with Graves' hyperthyroidism. *J. Clin. Endocrinol. Metab.,* **1997,** *82:*3633–3636.

Morgan, J.W., and Cassady, R.E. Community cancer assessment in response to long-time exposure to perchlorate and trichloroethylene in drinking water. *J. Occup. Environ. Med.,* **2002,** *44:*616–621.

Mortimer, R.H., Cannell, G.R., Addison, R.S., *et al.* Methimazole and propylthiouracil equally cross the perfused human term placental lobule. *J. Clin. Endocrinol. Metab.,* **1997,** *82:*3099–3102.

Müller, B., Zulewski, H., Huber, P., *et al.* Impaired action of thyroid hormone associated with smoking in women with hypothyroidism. *N. Engl. J. Med.,* **1995,** *333:*964–969.

Nauman, J., and Wolff, J. Iodide prophylaxis in Poland after the Chernobyl reactor accident: benefits and risks. *Am. J. Med.,* **1993,** *94:*524–532.

Ojamaa, K., Klemperer, J.D., and Klein, I. Acute effects of thyroid hormone on vascular smooth muscle. *Thyroid,* **1996,** *6:*505–512.

Pacini, F., Cetani, F., Miccoli, P., *et al.* Outcome of 309 patients with metastatic differentiated thyroid carcinoma treated with radioiodine. *World J. Surg.,* **1994a,** *18:*600–604.

Pacini, F., Gasperi, M., Fugazzola, L., *et al.* Testicular function in patients with differentiated thyroid carcinoma treated with radioiodine. *J. Nucl. Med.,* **1994b,** *35:*1418–1422.

Papini, E., Petrucci, L., Guglielmi, R., *et al.* Long-term changes in nodular goiter: a 5-year prospective randomized trial of levothyroxine suppressive therapy for benign cold thyroid nodules. *J. Clin. Endocrinol. Metab.,* **1998,** *83:*780–783.

Park, K.W., Dai, H.B., Ojamaa, K., *et al.* The direct vasomotor effect of thyroid hormones on rat skeletal muscle resistance arteries. *Anesth. Analg.,* **1997,** *85:*734–738.

Paschke, R., Tonacchera, M., Van Sande, J., *et al.* Identification and functional characterization of two new somatic mutations causing constitutive activation of the thyrotropin receptor in hyperfunctioning autonomous adenomas of the thyroid. *J. Clin. Endocrinol. Metab.,* **1994,** *79:*1785–1789.

Pop, V.J., Kuijpens, J.L., van Baar, A.L., *et al.* Low maternal free thyroxine concentrations during early pregnancy are associated with impaired psychomotor development in infancy. *Clin. Endocrinol. (Oxf.),* **1999,** *50:*149–155.

Reuss, M.L., Paneth, N., Pinto-Martin, J.A., *et al.* The relation of transient hypothyroxinemia in preterm infants to neurologic development at two years of age. *N. Engl. J. Med.,* **1996,** *334:*821–827.

Rittmaster, R.S., Abbott, E.C., Douglas, R., *et al.* Effect of methimazole, with or without L-thyroxine, on remission rates in Graves' disease. *J. Clin. Endocrinol. Metab.,* **1998,** *83:*814–818.

Rittmaster, R.S., Zwicker, H., Abbott, E.C., *et al.* Effect of methimazole with or without exogenous L-thyroxine on serum concentrations of thyrotropin (TSH) receptor antibodies in patients with Graves' disease. *J. Clin. Endocrinol. Metab.,* **1996,** *81:*3283–3288.

Robbins, R.J., Larson, S.M., Sinha, N., *et al.* A retrospective review of the effectiveness of recombinant human TSH as a preparation for radioiodine thyroid remnant ablation. *J. Nucl. Med.,* **2002,** *43:*1482–1488.

Rohrer, D., and Dillmann, W.H. Thyroid hormone markedly increases the mRNA coding for sarcoplasmic reticulum Ca^{2+}–ATPase in the rat heart. *J. Biol. Chem.,* **1988,** *263:*6941–6944.

Ron, E., Doody, M.M., Becker, D.V., *et al.* Cancer mortality following treatment for adult hyperthyroidism. Cooperative Thyrotoxicosis Therapy Follow-up Study Group. *JAMA,* **1998,** *280:*347–355.

Ros, M., Northup, J.K., and Malbon, C.C. Steady-state levels of G proteins and β-adrenergic receptors in rat fat cells. Permissive effects of thyroid hormones. *J. Biol. Chem.,* **1988,** *263:*4362–4368.

Roti, E., Cozani, R., and Braverman, L.E. Adverse effects of iodine on the thyroid. *Endocrinologist,* **1997,** *7:*245–254.

Rovet, J. Long-term follow-up of children born with sporadic congenital hypothyroidism. *Ann. Endocrinol. (Paris),* **2003,** *64:*58–61.

Salter, A.M., Fisher, S.C., and Brindley, D.N. Interactions of triiodothyronine, insulin, and dexamethasone on the binding of human LDL to rat hepatocytes in monolayer culture. *Atherosclerosis,* **1988,** *71:*77–80.

Sato, H., Hattori, M., Fujieda, M., *et al.* High prevalence of antineutrophil cytoplasmic antibody positivity in childhood onset Graves' disease treated with propylthiouracil. *J. Clin. Endocrinol. Metab.,* **2000,** *85:*4270–4273.

Sawka, A.M., Gerstein, H.C., Marriott, M.J., MacQueen, G.M., and Joffe, R.T. Does a combination regimen of thyroxine (T4) and 3,5,3′-triiodothyronine improve depressive symptoms better than T4 alone in patients with hypothyroidism? Results of a double-blind, randomized, controlled trial. *J. Clin. Endocrinol. Metab.,* **2003,** *88:*4551–4555.

Sera, N., Ashizawa, K., Ando, T., *et al.* Treatment with propylthiouracil is associated with appearance of antineutrophil cytoplasmic antibodies in some patients with Graves' disease. *Thyroid,* **2000,** *10:*595–599.

Simmonds, M. Ueber Hypophysisschwund mit todlichem Ausang. *Dtsch. Med. Wochenschr.,* **1914,** *40:*322–323.

Smerdely, P., Pitsiavas, V., and Boyages, S.C. Evidence that the inhibitory effects of iodide on thyroid cell proliferation are due to arrest of the cell cycle at G0G1 and G2M phases. *Endocrinology,* **1993,** *133:*2881–2888.

Sterling, K. Direct triiodothyronine (T_3) action by a primary mitochondrial pathway. *Endocr. Res.,* **1989,** *15:*683–715.

Strait, K.A., Schwartz, H.L., Perez-Castillo, A., and Oppenheimer, J.H. Relationship of c-*erb*-A mRNA content to tissue triiodothyronine nuclear binding capacity and function in developing and adult rats. *J. Biol. Chem.,* **1990,** *265:*10514–10521.

Sunthornthepvarakul, T., Gottschalk, M.E., Hayashi, Y., and Refetoff, S. Brief report: resistance to thyrotropin caused by mutations in the thyrotropin-receptor gene. *N. Engl. J. Med.,* **1995,** *332:*155–160.

Takami, H. Lithium in the preoperative preparation of Graves' disease. *Int. Surg.,* **1994,** *79:*89–90.

Takasu, N., Yamada, T., and Shimizu, Y. Generation of H_2O_2 is regulated by cytoplasmic free calcium in cultured porcine thyroid cells. *Biochem. Biophys. Res. Commun.,* **1987,** *148:*1527–1532.

Takeshita, A., Yen, P.M., Misiti, S., *et al.* Molecular cloning and properties of a full-length putative thyroid hormone receptor coactivator. *Endocrinology,* **1996,** *137:*3594–3597.

Tonacchera, M., Van Sande, J., Cetani, F., *et al.* Functional characteristics of three new germline mutations of the thyrotropin receptor gene causing autosomal dominant toxic thyroid hyperplasia. *J. Clin. Endocrinol. Metab.,* **1996a,** *81:*547–554.

Tuttle, R.M., Patience, T., and Budd, S. Treatment with propylthiouracil before radioactive iodine therapy is associated with a higher treatment failure rate than therapy with radioactive iodine alone in Graves' disease. *Thyroid,* **1995,** *5:*243–247.

Uy, H.L., Reasner, C.A., and Samuels, M.H. Pattern of recovery of the hypothalamic-pituitary-thyroid axis following radioactive iodine therapy in patients with Graves' disease. *Am. J. Med.,* **1995,** *99:*173–179.

de Vathaire, F., Schlumberger, M., Delisle, M.J., *et al.* Leukaemias and cancers following iodine-131 administration for thyroid cancer. *Br. J. Cancer,* **1997,** *75:*734–739.

Visser, T.J., Leonard, J.L., Kaplan, M.M., and Larsen, P.R. Kinetic evidence suggesting two mechanisms for iodothyronine 5′-deiodination in rat cerebral cortex. *Proc. Natl. Acad. Sci. United States A.,* **1982,** *79:*5080–5084.

Walsh, J.P., Shiels, L., Lim, E.M., *et al.* Combined thyroxine/liothyronine treatment does not improve well-being, quality of life, or cognitive function compared to thyroxine alone: a randomized controlled trial in patients with primary hypothyroidism. *J. Clin. Endocrinol. Metab.,* **2003,** *88:*4543–4550.

van Wassenaer, A.G., Kok, J.H., de Vijlder, J.J., *et al.* Effects of thyroxine supplementation on neurologic development in infants born at less than 30 weeks' gestation. *N. Engl. J. Med.,* **1997,** *336:*21–26.

Wasserstrum, N., and Anania, C.A. Perinatal consequences of maternal hypothyroidism in early pregnancy and inadequate replacement. *Clin. Endocrinol. (Oxf.),* **1995,** *42:*353–358.

Weiss, R.E., Hayashi, Y., Nagaya, T., *et al.* Dominant inheritance of resistance to thyroid hormone not linked to defects in the thyroid hormone receptor α or β genes may be due to a defective cofactor. *J. Clin. Endocrinol. Metab.,* **1996,** *81:*4196–4203.

Wikström, L., Johansson, C., Saltó, C., *et al.* Abnormal heart rate and body temperature in mice lacking thyroid hormone receptor alpha 1. *EMBO J.,* **1998,** *17:*455–461.

Wilber, J.F., and Xu, A.H. The thyrotropin-releasing hormone gene 1998: cloning, characterization, and transcriptional regulation in the central nervous system, heart, and testis. *Thyroid,* **1998,** *8:*897–901.

Xie, J., Pannain, S., Pohlenz, J., *et al.* Resistance to thyrotropin (TSH) in three families is not associated with mutations in the TSH receptor or TSH. *J. Clin. Endocrinol. Metab.,* **1997,** *82:*3933–3940.

Yamamoto, T., Fukuyama, J., and Fujiyoshi, A. Factors associated with mortality of myxedema coma: report of eight cases and literature survey. *Thyroid,* **1999,** *9:*1167–1174.

Yoshihara, H.A., Apriletti, J.W., Baxter, J.D., and Scanlan, T.S. Structural determinants of selective thyromimetics. *J. Med. Chem.,* **2003,** *46:*3152–3161.

Zelmanovitz, F., Genro, S., and Gross, J.L. Suppressive therapy with levothyroxine for solitary thyroid nodules: a double-blind controlled clinical study and cumulative meta-analyses. *J. Clin. Endocrinol. Metab.,* **1998,** *83:*3881–3885.

Zoeller, R.T., Dowling, A.L., and Vas, A.A. Developmental exposure to polychlorinated biphenyls exerts thyroid hormone-like effects on the expression of RC3/neurogranin and myelin basic protein messenger ribonucleic acids in the developing rat brain. *Endocrinology,* **2000,** *141:*181–189.

MONOGRAPHS AND REVIEWS

Arvan, P. Thyroglobulin: Chemistry, biosynthesis and secretion. In, *Werner and Ingbar's The Thyroid,* 9th ed. (Braverman, L.E., and Utiger, R.D., eds.) Lippincott Williams & Wilkins, New York, **2005.**

Bassett, J.H., Harvey, C.B., and Williams, G.R. Mechanisms of thyroid hormone receptor-specific nuclear and extra nuclear actions. *Mol. Cell. Endocrinol.,* **2003,** *213:*1–11.

Benvenga, S. Thyroid hormone transport proteins and the physiology of hormone binding. In, *Werner and Ingbar's The Thyroid,* 9th ed. (Braverman, L.E., and Utiger, R.D., eds.) Lippincott Williams & Wilkins, New York, **2005.**

Bernal, J., Guadano-Ferraz, A., and Morte, B. Perspectives in the study of thyroid hormone action on brain development and function. *Thyroid,* **2003,** *13:*1005–1012.

Bianco, A.C., and Larsen, P.R. Intracellular pathways of iodothyronine metabolism. In, *Werner and Ingbar's The Thyroid,* 9th ed. (Braverman, L.E., and Utiger, R.D., eds.) Lippincott Williams & Wilkins, New York, **2005.**

Braverman, L.E., Eber, O., and Langsteger, W. *Heart and Thyroid.* Blackwell-MZV, Vienna, **1994.**

Braverman, L.E., and Utiger, R.D., eds. *Werner and Ingbar's The Thyroid,* 8th ed. Lippincott Williams & Wilkins, New York, **2000,** pp. 578–589.

Brown, R. Thyroid physiology in the perinatal period and during childhood. In, *Werner and Ingbar's The Thyroid,* 9th ed. (Braverman, L.E., and Utiger, R.D., eds.) Lippincott Williams & Wilkins, Philadelphia, **2005.**

Carrasco, N. Thyroid iodine transport. In, *Werner and Ingbar's The Thyroid,* 9th ed. (Braverman, L.E., and Utiger, R.D., eds.) Lippincott Williams & Wilkins, New York, **2005.**

Cody, V. Thyroid hormone structure and function. In, *Werner and Ingbar's The Thyroid,* 9th ed. (Braverman, L.E., and Utiger, R.D., eds.) Lippincott Williams & Wilkins, New York, **2005.**

Cooper, D.S. Antithyroid drugs in the management of patients with Graves' disease: an evidence-based approach to therapeutic controversies. *J. Clin. Endocrinol. Metab.,* **2003,** *88:*3474–3481.

Demers, L.M., and Spencer, C.A. Laboratory medicine practice guidelines: laboratory support for the diagnosis and monitoring of thyroid disease. *Clin. Endocrinol. (Oxf.),* **2003,** *58:*138–140.

DeVito, M., Biegel, L., Brouwer, A., *et al.* Screening methods for thyroid hormone disruptors. *Environ. Health. Perspect.,* **1999,** *107:*407–415.

Diav-Citrin, O., and Ornoy, A. Teratogen update: antithyroid drugs-methimazole, carbimazole, and propylthiouracil. *Teratology,* **2002,** *65:*38–44.

Dohan, O., De la Vieja, A., Paroder, V., *et al.* The sodium/iodide symporter (NIS): characterization, regulation, and medical significance. *Endocr. Rev.,* **2003,** *24:*48–77.

Dunn, J.T., and Delange, F.M. Iodine deficiency. In, *Werner and Ingbar's The Thyroid,* 9th ed. (Braverman, L.E., and Utiger, R.D., eds.) Lippincott Williams & Wilkins, New York, **2005.**

Dunn, J.T., and Dunn, A.D. Thyroglobulin: chemistry, biosynthesis, and proteolysis. In, *Werner and Ingbar's The Thyroid,* 8th ed. (Braverman, L.E., and Utiger, R.D., eds.) Lippincott Williams & Wilkins, New York, **2000,** pp. 91–104.

Emerson, C.H. Myxedema coma. In, *Intensive Care Medicine.* (Irwin, R.S., Cerra, F.B., and Rippe, J.M., eds.) Lippincott-Raven, Boston, **2003,** pp. 1171–1173.

Farwell, A.P. Sick euthyroid syndrome in the intensive care unit. In, *Intensive Care Medicine,* 5th ed. (Irwin, R.S., and Rippe, J.M., eds.) Lippincott Williams & Wilkins, Philadelphia, **2003,** pp. 1205–1216.

Farwell, A.P. Thyroid gland disorders. In, *Textbook of Critical Care.* (Fink, M., Abraham, E., Vincent, J.L., eds.) Elsevier Science, Philadelphia, **2004.**

Flamant, F., and Samarut, J. Thyroid hormone receptors: lessons from knockout and knock-in mutant mice. *Trends Endocrinol. Metab.,* **2003,** *14:*85–90.

Food and Nutrition Board. *Dietary Reference Intakes.* National Academy Press, Washington, DC, **2001.**

Gharib, H., and Mazzaferri, E.L. Thyroxine suppressive therapy in patients with nodular thyroid disease. *Ann. Intern. Med.,* **1998,** *128:*386–394.

Glinoer, D. Thyroid disease during pregnancy. In, *Werner and Ingbar's The Thyroid,* 9th ed. (Braverman, L.E., and Utiger, R.D., eds.) Lippincott Williams & Wilkins, Philadelphia, **2005.**

Gottlieb, P.A., and Braverman, L.E. The effect of thyroid disease on diabetes. *Clin. Diabetes,* **1994,** *12:*15–18.

Harjai, K.J., and Licata, A.A. Effects of amiodarone on thyroid function. *Ann. Intern. Med.,* **1997,** *126:*63–73.

Helfand, M., and Redfern, C.C. Clinical guideline, part 2. Screening for thyroid disease: an update. American College of Physicians. *Ann. Intern. Med.,* **1998,** *129:*144–158.

Hermus, A.R., and Huysmans, D.A. Treatment of benign nodular thyroid disease. *N. Engl. J. Med.,* **1998,** *338:*1438–1447.

Klein, I. The cardiovascular system in hypothyroidism. In, *Werner and Ingbar's The Thyroid,* 9th ed. (Braverman, L.E., and Utiger, R.D., eds.) Lippincott Williams & Wilkins, New York, **2005a.**

Klein, I. The cardiovascular system in thyrotoxicosis. In, *Werner and Ingbar's The Thyroid,* 9th ed. (Braverman, L.E., and Utiger, R.D., eds.) Lippincott Williams & Wilkins, New York, **2005b.**

Koibuchi, N., Jingu, H., Iwasaki, T., and Chin, W.W. Current perspectives on the role of thyroid hormone in growth and development of cerebellum. *Cerebellum,* **2003,** *2:*279–289.

Lazar, M.A. Thyroid hormone receptors: multiple forms, multiple possibilities. *Endocr. Rev.,* **1993,** *14:*184–193.

Lee, H., and Yen, P.M. Recent advances in understanding thyroid hormone receptor coregulators. *J. Biomed. Sci.,* **1999,** *6:*71–78.

Lazarus, J.H. Sporadic and postpartum thyroiditis. In, *Werner and Ingbar's The Thyroid,* 9th ed. (Braverman, L.E., and Utiger, R.D., eds.) Lippincott Williams & Wilkins, Philadelphia, **2005.**

Mazzaferri, E.L., and Kloos, R.T. Clinical review 128: Current approaches to primary therapy for papillary and follicular thyroid cancer. *J. Clin. Endocrinol. Metab.,* **2001,** *86:*1447–1463.

Meier, C.A. Effects of drugs and other substances on thyroid hormone synthesis and metabolism. In, *Werner and Ingbar's The Thyroid,* 9th ed. (Braverman, L.E., and Utiger, R.D., eds.) Lippincott Williams & Wilkins, New York, **2005.**

Oppenheimer, J.H., and Schwartz, H.L. Molecular basis of thyroid hormone-dependent brain development. *Endocr. Rev.,* **1997,** *18:*462–475.

Pisarev, M.A., and Gärtner, R. Autoregulatory actions of iodine. In, *Werner and Ingbar's The Thyroid,* 8th ed. (Braverman, L.E., and Utiger, R.D., eds.) Lippincott Williams & Wilkins, New York, **2000,** pp. 85–90.

Rapoport, B., and McLachlan, S. *Endocrine Updates: Graves' Disease.* Kluwer Academic Publishers, The Netherlands, **2000.**

Robbins, R.J., and Robbins, A.K. Clinical review 156: Recombinant human thyrotropin and thyroid cancer management. *J. Clin. Endocrinol. Metab.,* **2003,** *88:*1933–1938.

Rodien, P., Bremont, C., Sanson, M.L., *et al.* Familial gestational hyperthyroidism caused by a mutant thyrotropin receptor hypersensitive to human chorionic gonadotropin. *N. Engl. J. Med.,* **1998,** *339:*1823–1826.

Roti, E., and Vagenakis, A.G. Effect of excess iodide. In, *Werner and Ingbar's The Thyroid,* 9th ed. (Braverman, L.E., and Utiger, R.D., eds.) Lippincott Williams & Wilkins, Philadelphia, **2005.**

Rovet, J., and Daneman, D. Congenital hypothyroidism: a review of current diagnostic and treatment practices in relation to neuropsychologic outcome. *Paediatr. Drugs,* **2003,** *5:*141–149.

Safran, M., Abend, A.L., *et al.* Thyroid storm. In, *Intensive Care Medicine,* 4th ed. (Irwin, R.S., Cerra, F.B., and Rippe, J.M.) Lippincott-Raven, Philadelphia, **2003,** pp. 1167–1170.

Sheppard, M. The skeletal system in hypothyroidism. In, *Werner and Ingbar's The Thyroid,* 9th ed. (Braverman, L.E., and Utiger, R.D., eds.) Lippincott Williams & Wilkins, New York, **2005a.**

Sheppard, M. The skeletal system in thyrotoxicosis. In, *Werner and Ingbar's The Thyroid,* 9th ed. (Braverman, L.E., and Utiger, R.D., eds.) Lippincott Williams & Wilkins, New York, **2005b.**

Silva, J.E. The thermogenic effect of thyroid hormone and its clinical implications. *Ann. Intern. Med.,* **2003,** *139:*205–213.

Spencer, C.A. Clinical utility and cost-effectiveness of sensitive thyrotropin assays in ambulatory and hospitalized patients. *Mayo Clin. Proc.,* **1988,** *63:*1214–1222.

Surks, M.I., Ortiz, E., Daniels, G.H., *et al.* Subclinical thyroid disease: scientific review and guidelines for diagnosis and management. *JAMA,* **2004,** *291:*228–238.

Taurog, A. Hormone synthesis: thyroid iodine metabolism. In, *Werner and Ingbar's The Thyroid,* 8th ed. (Braverman, L.E., and Utiger, R.D., eds.) Lippincott Williams & Wilkins, New York, **2000,** pp. 61–84.

Tonacchera, M., Van Sande, J., Parma, J., *et al.* TSH receptor and disease. *Clin. Endocrinol. (Oxf.),* **1996b,** *44:*621–633.

Vassart, G., Pardo, L., and Costagliola, S. A molecular dissection of the glycoprotein hormone receptors. *Trends Biochem. Sci.,* **2004,** *29:*119–126.

Vassart, G. The thyrotropin receptor. In, *Werner and Ingbar's The Thyroid,* 9th ed. (Braverman, L.E., and Utiger, R.D., eds.) Lippincott Williams & Wilkins, New York, **2005.**

Wolff, J. Perchlorate and the thyroid gland. *Pharmacol. Rev.,* **1998,** *50:*89–105.

Yen, P.M., and Chin, W.W. Genomic and nongenomic actions of thyroid hormone. In, *Werner and Ingbar's The Thyroid,* 9th ed. (Braverman, L.E., and Utiger, R.D., eds.) Lippincott Williams & Wilkins, New York, **2005.**

Yen, P.M. Physiological and molecular basis of thyroid hormone action. *Physiol. Rev.,* **2001,** *81:*1097–1142.

ESTROGENS AND PROGESTINS

David S. Loose and George M. Stancel

Estrogens and *progestins* are endogenous hormones that produce numerous physiological actions. In women, these include developmental effects, neuroendocrine actions involved in the control of ovulation, the cyclical preparation of the reproductive tract for fertilization and implantation, and major actions on mineral, carbohydrate, protein, and lipid metabolism. Estrogens also have important actions in males, including effects on bone, spermatogenesis, and behavior.

The biosynthesis, biotransformation, and disposition of estrogens and progestins are well established. Two well-characterized nuclear receptors are present for each hormone. This knowledge provides a firm conceptual basis for understanding the actions of both steroids.

The therapeutic use of estrogens and progestins largely reflects extensions of their physiological activities. The most common uses of these agents are menopausal hormone therapy and contraception in women, but the specific compounds and dosages used in these two settings differ substantially.

Estrogen- and progesterone-receptor antagonists also are available. The main uses of anti-estrogens are treatment of hormone-responsive breast cancer and infertility. Selective estrogen receptor modulators (SERMs) that display tissue-selective agonist or antagonist activities are increasing in number. The main use of anti-progestins has been for medical abortion, but other uses are theoretically possible.

A number of naturally occurring and synthetic environmental chemicals mimic, antagonize, or otherwise affect the actions of estrogens in experimental test systems. The precise effect of these agents on humans is unknown, but this is an area of active investigation. Cancer chemotherapeutic strategies based on blockade of estrogen- and/or progesterone-receptor functions are considered in further detail in Chapter 51. Complementary therapeutic strategies based on suppression of gonadotropin secretion by long-acting gonadotropin-releasing hormone agonists are discussed in Chapter 55.

History. The hormonal nature of the ovarian control of the female reproductive system was firmly established in 1900 by Knauer when he found that ovarian transplants prevented the symptoms of gonadectomy, and by Halban, who showed that normal sexual development and function occurred when glands were transplanted. In 1923, Allen and Doisy devised a bioassay for ovarian extracts based upon the vaginal smear of the rat. Frank and associates in 1925 detected an active sex principle in the blood of sows in estrus, and Loewe and Lange discovered in 1926 that a female sex hormone varied in the urine of women throughout the menstrual cycle. The excretion of estrogen in the urine during pregnancy also was reported by Zondek in 1928 and enabled Butenandt and Doisy in 1929 to crystallize an active substance.

Early investigations indicated that the ovary secretes two substances. Beard had postulated in 1897 that the corpus luteum serves a necessary function during pregnancy, and Fraenkel showed in 1903 that destruction of the corpora lutea in pregnant rabbits caused abortion. Several groups then isolated progesterone from mammalian corpora lutea in the 1930s.

In the early 1960s, pioneering studies by Jensen and colleagues suggested the presence of intracellular receptors for estrogens in target tissues. This was the first demonstration of receptors of the steroid/thyroid superfamily and provided techniques to identify receptors for the other steroid hormones. A second estrogen receptor was identified in 1996 and termed *estrogen receptor β* (ER β) to distinguish it from the receptor identified by Jensen and others, termed *estrogen receptor α* (ER α). Two protein isoforms, A and B, of the progesterone receptor arise from a single gene by transcription initiation from different promoters. (*Note:* For the primary literature references about the history of this subject, consult the ninth and tenth editions of this volume.)

ESTROGENS

Chemistry. Many steroidal and nonsteroidal compounds, some of which are shown in Table 57–1 and Figure 57–1, possess estrogenic activity. The most potent naturally occurring estrogen in humans, for

Table 57–1
Structural Formulas of Selected Estrogens

STEROIDAL ESTROGENS				NONSTEROIDAL COMPOUNDS WITH ESTROGENIC ACTIVITY

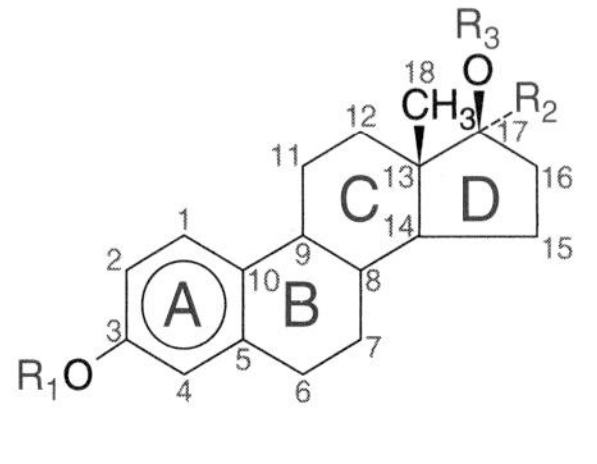

Derivative	R_1	R_2	R_3
Estradiol	—H	—H	—H
Estradiol valerate	—H	—H	$-\overset{\overset{\text{O}}{\|}}{\text{C}}(CH_2)_3CH_3$
Ethinyl estradiol	—H	—C≡CH	—H
Mestranol	—CH$_3$	—C≡CH	—H
Estrone sulfate	—SO$_3$H	–*	=O*
Equilin[†]	—H	–*	=O*

Diethylstilbestrol

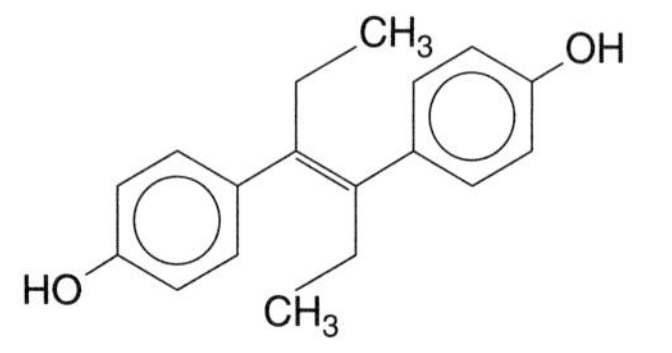

Bisphenol A

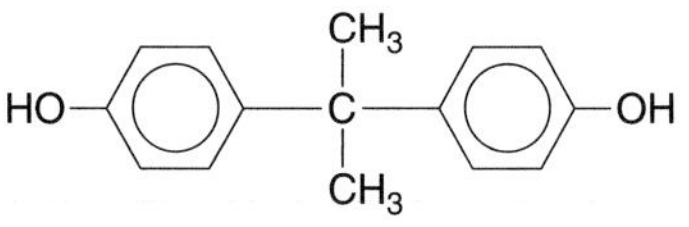

Genistein

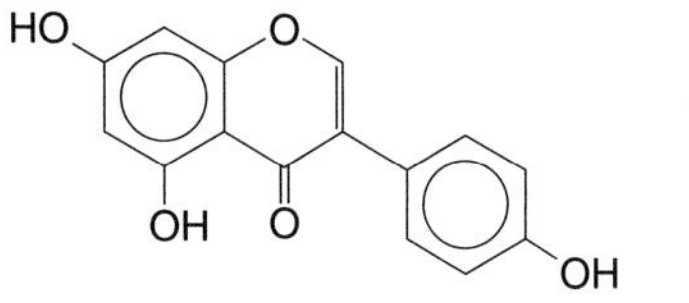

*Designates C17 ketone. [†]Also contains 7, 8 double bond.

both ER α- and β-mediated actions, is 17β-estradiol, followed by *estrone* and *estriol*. Each contains a phenolic A ring with a hydroxyl group at carbon 3, and a β-OH or ketone in position 17 of ring D.

The phenolic A ring is the principal structural feature responsible for selective, high-affinity binding to both receptors. Most alkyl substitutions on the A ring impair binding, but substitutions on ring C or D may be tolerated. Ethinyl substitutions at the C17 position greatly increase oral potency by inhibiting first-pass hepatic metabolism. Models for the ligand-binding sites of both estrogen receptors have been determined from structure–activity relationships (Harrington *et al.*, 2003) and structural analysis (Pike *et al.*, 2000).

Diethylstilbestrol (DES), which is structurally similar to *estradiol* when viewed in the *trans* conformation, binds with high affinity to both estrogen receptors and is as potent as estradiol in most assays, but has a much longer half-life. DES no longer has widespread use, but it was important historically as an inexpensive, orally active estrogen.

Selective ligands for ER α and ER β are available for experimental studies but are not yet used therapeutically (Harrington *et al.*, 2003).

Nonsteroidal compounds with estrogenic or anti-estrogenic activity—including flavones, isoflavones (*e.g.,* genistein), and coumestan derivatives—occur in plants and fungi. Synthetic agents—including

pesticides (*e.g., p,p´*-DDT), plasticizers (*e.g.,* bisphenol A), and a variety of other industrial chemicals (*e.g.,* polychlorinated biphenyls)—also have hormonal or antihormonal activity. While their affinity is relatively weak, their large number, bioaccumulation, and persistence in the environment have raised concerns about their potential toxicity in humans and wildlife (Mäkelä *et al.*, 1999). Over-the-counter and prescription preparations containing naturally occurring, estrogenlike compounds from plants (*i.e.,* phytoestrogens) now are available (Fitzpatrick, 2003).

Biosynthesis. Steroidal estrogens arise from androstenedione or testosterone (Figure 57–1) by aromatization of the A ring. The reaction is catalyzed by a cytochrome P450 monooxygenase enzyme complex (aromatase or CYP19) that uses NADPH and molecular oxygen as co-substrates. A ubiquitous flavoprotein, NADPH–cytochrome P450 reductase, also is essential. Both proteins are localized in the endoplasmic reticulum of ovarian granulosa cells, testicular Sertoli and Leydig cells, adipose stroma, placental syncytiotrophoblasts, preimplantation blastocysts, bone, various brain regions, and many other tissues (Simpson *et al.*, 2002).

The ovaries are the principal source of circulating estrogen in premenopausal women, with estradiol being the main secretory product. Gonadotropins, acting via receptors that couple to the G_s-

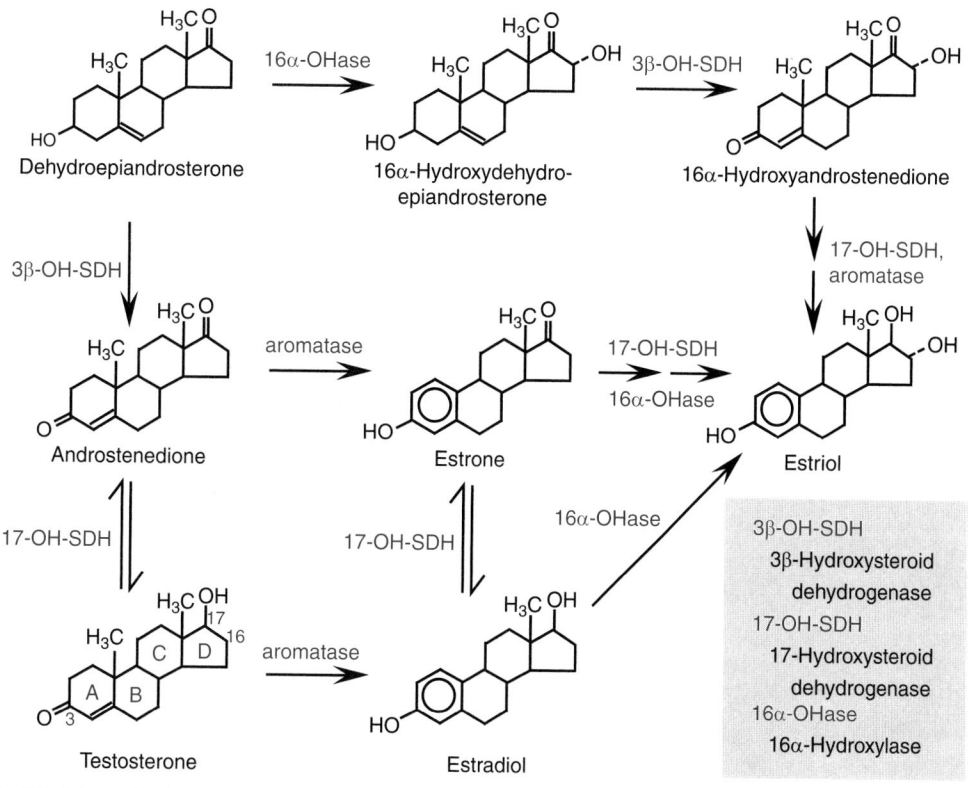

Figure 57–1. *The biosynthetic pathway for the estrogens.*

adenylyl cyclase–cyclic AMP pathway, increase the activities of aromatase and the cholesterol side-chain cleavage enzyme and facilitate the transport of cholesterol (the precursor of all steroids) into the mitochondria of cells that synthesize steroids. The ovary contains a form of 17β-hydroxysteroid dehydrogenase (type I) that favors the production of testosterone and estradiol from androstenedione and estrone, respectively. However, in the liver, another form of this enzyme (type II) favors oxidation of circulating estradiol to estrone (Peltoketo *et al.*, 1999), and both of these steroids are then converted to estriol (Figure 57–1). All three of these estrogens are excreted in the urine along with their glucuronide and sulfate conjugates.

In postmenopausal women, the principal source of circulating estrogen is adipose tissue stroma, where estrone is synthesized from dehydroepiandrosterone secreted by the adrenals. In men, estrogens are produced by the testes, but extragonadal production by aromatization of circulating C19 steroids (*e.g.*, androstenedione and dehydroepiandrosterone) accounts for most circulating estrogens. Thus, the level of estrogens is regulated in part by the availability of androgenic precursors (Simpson, 2003).

Estrogenic effects most often have been attributed to circulating hormones, but locally produced estrogens also may have important actions (Simpson *et al.*, 2002). For example, estrogens may be produced from androgens by the actions of aromatase or from estrogen conjugates by hydrolysis. Such local production of estrogens could play a causal role in the development of certain diseases such as breast cancer, since mammary tumors contain both aromatase and hydrolytic enzymes. Estrogens also may be produced from androgens *via* aromatase in the central nervous system (CNS) and other

tissues and exert local effects near their production site (*e.g.*, in bone they affect bone mineral density).

The placenta uses fetal dehydroepiandrosterone and its 16α-hydroxyl derivative to produce large amounts of estrone and estriol. Human urine during pregnancy is thus an abundant source of natural estrogens, and pregnant mare's urine is the source of *conjugated equine estrogens*, which have been widely used therapeutically for many years.

Physiological and Pharmacological Actions

Developmental Actions. Estrogens are largely responsible for pubertal changes in girls and secondary sexual characteristics. They cause growth and development of the vagina, uterus, and fallopian tubes, and contribute to breast enlargement. They also contribute to molding the body contours, shaping the skeleton, and causing the pubertal growth spurt of the long bones and epiphyseal closure. Growth of axillary and pubic hair, pigmentation of the genital region, and the regional pigmentation of the nipples and areolae that occur after the first trimester of pregnancy are also estrogenic actions. Androgens may also play a secondary role in female sexual development (*see* Chapter 58).

Estrogens appear to play important developmental roles in males. In boys, estrogen deficiency diminishes the puber-

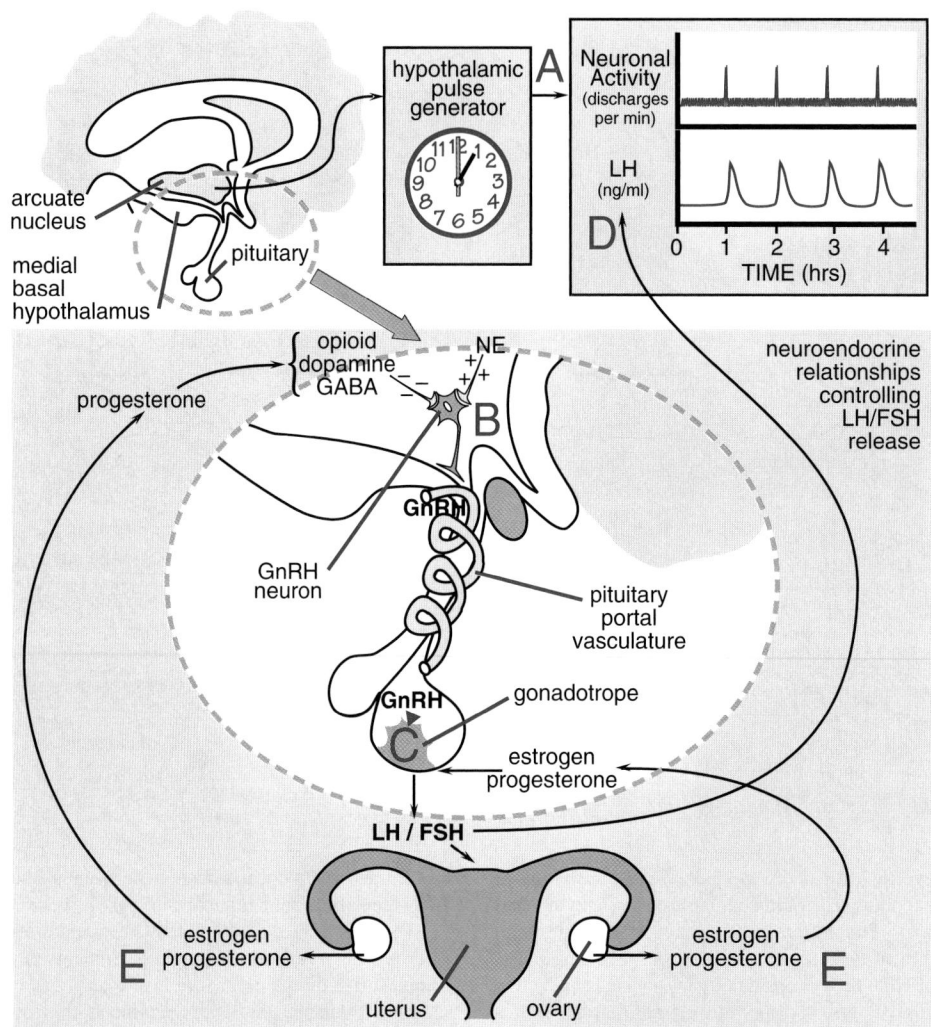

Figure 57–2. ***Neuroendocrine control of gonadotropin secretion in females.*** The hypothalamic pulse generator located in the arcuate nucleus of the hypothalamus functions as a neuronal "clock" that fires at regular hourly intervals (***A***). This results in the periodic release of gonadotropin-releasing hormone (GnRH) from GnRH-containing neurons into the hypothalamic-pituitary portal vasculature (***B***). GnRH neurons (***B***) receive inhibitory input from opioid, dopamine, and GABA neurons and stimulatory input from noradrenergic neurons (NE, norepinephrine). The pulses of GnRH trigger the intermittent release of luteinizing hormone (LH) and follicle-stimulating hormone (FSH) from pituitary gonadotropes (***C***), resulting in the pulsatile plasma profile (***D***). FSH and LH regulate ovarian production of estrogen and progesterone, which exert feedback controls (***E***). (*See* text and Figure 57–3 for additional details.)

tal growth spurt and delays skeletal maturation and epiphyseal closure so that linear growth continues into adulthood. Estrogen deficiency in men leads to elevated gonadotropins, macroorchidism, and increased testosterone levels and also may affect carbohydrate and lipid metabolism and fertility in some individuals (Grumbach and Auchus, 1999).

Neuroendocrine Control of the Menstrual Cycle. A neuroendocrine cascade involving the hypothalamus, pituitary, and ovaries controls the menstrual cycle (Figure 57–2). A neuronal oscillator or "clock" in the hypothalamus fires

at intervals that coincide with bursts of gonadotropin-releasing hormone (GnRH) release into the hypothalamic-pituitary portal vasculature (*see* Chapter 55). GnRH interacts with its cognate receptor on pituitary gonadotropes to cause release of luteinizing hormone (LH) and follicle-stimulating hormone (FSH). The frequency of the GnRH pulses, which varies in the different phases of the menstrual cycle (*see* below), controls the relative synthesis of the unique β subunits of FSH and LH.

The gonadotropins (LH and FSH) regulate the growth and maturation of the graafian follicle in the ovary and the ovarian production of estrogen and progesterone, which exert feedback regulation on the pituitary and hypothalamus.

Because the release of GnRH is intermittent, LH and FSH secretion is pulsatile. The pulse *frequency* is determined by the neural "clock" (Figure 57–2), termed the *hypothalamic GnRH pulse generator* (Knobil, 1981), but the amount of gonadotropin released in each pulse (*i.e.,* the pulse *amplitude*) is largely controlled by the actions of estrogens and progesterone on the pituitary. The intermittent, *pulsatile* nature of hormone release is essential for the maintenance of normal ovulatory menstrual cycles, since constant infusion of GnRH results in a cessation of gonadotropin release and ovarian steroid production (*see* Chapter 55). The pulse generator resides in the arcuate nucleus of the hypothalamus, which also contains the highest concentration of GnRH neurons; considerable evidence suggests that these GnRH neurons collectively form the pulse generator.

The precise mechanism that regulates the timing of GnRH release (*i.e.,* pulse frequency) is unclear, but these cells appear to have an intrinsic ability to release GnRH episodically. The overall pattern of GnRH release likely is regulated by the interplay of intrinsic mechanism(s) and extrinsic synaptic inputs from opioid, catecholamine, and GABAergic neurons (Figure 57–2). Ovarian steroids, primarily progesterone, regulate the frequency of GnRH release, but the cellular and molecular mechanisms of this regulation are not well established. Some GnRH cells appear to contain immunoreactive steroid receptors. Some nerve cells that synapse with GnRH neurons contain steroid receptors, and neighboring glial cells also may contain estrogen and progesterone receptors. Steroids may thus directly and indirectly modulate GnRH neuronal function.

At puberty the pulse generator is activated and establishes cyclic profiles of pituitary and ovarian hormones. While the mechanism of activation is not entirely established, it may involve increases in circulating IGF-1 and leptin levels, the latter acting to inhibit neuropeptide Y (NPY) in the arcuate nucleus to relieve an inhibitory effect on GnRH neurons.

Figure 57–3 provides a schematic diagram of the profiles of gonadotropin and gonadal steroid levels in the menstrual cycle. The "average" plasma levels of LH throughout the cycle are shown in panel *A* of Figure 57–3; inserts illustrate the pulsatile patterns of LH during the proliferative and secretory phases in more detail. The average LH levels are similar throughout the early (follicular) and late (luteal) phases of the cycle, but the frequency and amplitude of the LH pulses are quite different in the two phases. This characteristic pattern of hormone secretions results from complex positive and negative feedback mechanisms (Hotchkiss and Knobil, 1994).

In the early follicular phase of the cycle: (1) the pulse generator produces bursts of neuronal activity with a frequency of about one per hour that correspond with pulses of GnRH secretion; (2) these

cause a corresponding pulsatile release of LH and FSH from pituitary gonadotropes; and (3) FSH in particular causes the graafian follicle to mature and secrete estrogen. The effects of estrogens on the pituitary are inhibitory at this time and cause the amount of LH and FSH released from the pituitary to decline (*i.e.,* the amplitude of the LH pulse decreases), so gonadotropin levels gradually fall, as seen in Figure 57–3. Inhibin, produced by the ovary, also exerts a negative feedback to selectively decrease serum FSH at this time (*see* Chapter 55). Activin and follistatin, two other peptides released from the ovary, may also regulate FSH production and secretion to a lesser extent, although their levels do not vary appreciably during the menstrual cycle.

At mid-cycle, serum estradiol rises above a threshold level of 150 to 200 pg/ml for approximately 36 hours. This sustained elevation of estrogen no longer inhibits gonadotropin release but exerts a brief positive feedback effect on the pituitary to trigger the preovulatory surge of LH and FSH. This effect primarily involves a change in pituitary responsiveness to GnRH. In some species, estrogens may also exert a positive effect on hypothalamic neurons that contributes to a mid-cycle "surge" of GnRH release; this is not yet established in humans. Progesterone may contribute to the mid-cycle LH surge.

The mid-cycle surge in gonadotropins stimulates follicular rupture and ovulation within 1 to 2 days. The ruptured follicle then develops into the corpus luteum, which produces large amounts of progesterone and lesser amounts of estrogen under the influence of LH during the second half of the cycle. In the absence of pregnancy, the corpus luteum ceases to function, steroid levels drop, and menstruation occurs. When steroid levels drop, the pulse generator reverts to a firing pattern characteristic of the follicular phase, the entire system then resets, and a new ovarian cycle occurs.

Regulation of the frequency and amplitude of gonadotropin secretions by steroids may be summarized as follows: Estrogens act primarily on the pituitary to control the amplitude of gonadotropin pulses, and may also contribute to the amplitude of GnRH pulses secreted by the hypothalamus.

In the follicular phase of the cycle, estrogens inhibit gonadotropin release, but then have a brief mid-cycle stimulatory action that increases the amount released and causes the LH surge. Progesterone, acting on the hypothalamus, exerts the predominant control of the frequency of LH release. It decreases the firing rate of the hypothalamic pulse generator, an action thought to be mediated largely *via* inhibitory opioid neurons (containing progesterone receptors) that synapse with GnRH neurons. Progesterone also exerts a direct effect on the pituitary to oppose the inhibitory actions of estrogens and thus enhance the amount of LH released (*i.e.,* to increase the amplitude of the LH pulses). These steroid feedback effects, coupled with the intrinsic activity of the hypothalamic GnRH pulse generator, lead to relatively frequent LH pulses of small amplitude in the follicular phase of the cycle, and less frequent pulses of larger amplitude in the luteal phase. Studies in knockout mice indicate that ER α (Hewitt and Korach, 2003) and the progesterone receptor PR-A (Conneely *et al.,* 2002) mediate the major actions of estrogens and progestins, respectively, on the hypothalamic-pituitary axis.

In males, testosterone regulates the hypothalamic-pituitary-gonadal axis at both the hypothalamic and pituitary levels, and its negative feedback effect is mediated to a substantial degree by estrogen formed *via* aromatization. Thus, exogenous estrogen administration decreases LH and testosterone levels in men, and anti-estrogens such as *clomiphene* cause an elevation of serum LH, which can be used to evaluate the male reproductive axis.

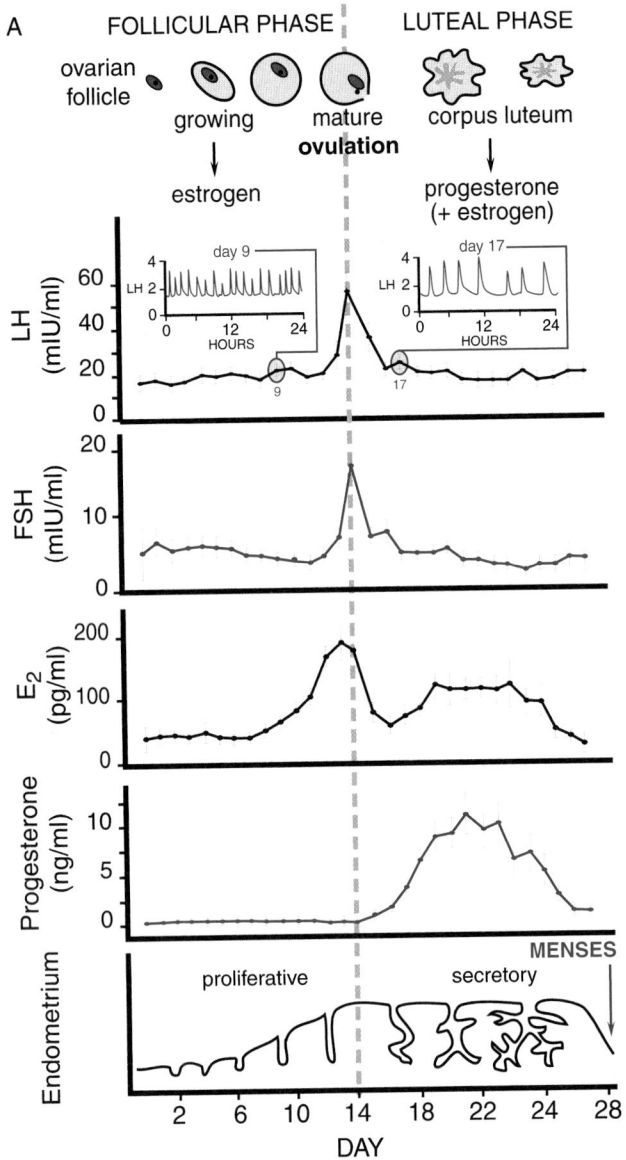

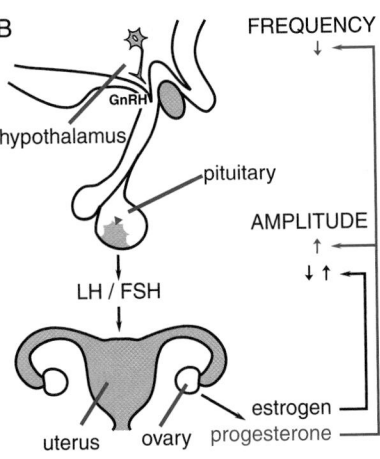

Figure 57–3. Hormonal relationships of the human menstrual cycle. A. Average daily values of LH, FSH, estradiol (E₂), and progesterone in plasma samples from women exhibiting normal 28-day menstrual cycles. Changes in the ovarian follicle (*top*) and endometrium (*bottom*) also are illustrated schematically.

Frequent plasma sampling reveals pulsatile patterns of gonadotropin release. Characteristic profiles are illustrated schematically for the follicular phase (day 9, inset on left) and luteal phase (day 17, inset on right). Both the frequency (number of pulses per hour) and amplitude (extent of change of hormone release) of pulses vary throughout the cycle. (Redrawn with permission from Thorneycroft *et al.*, 1971).
B. Major regulatory effects of ovarian steroids on hypothalamic-pituitary function. Estrogen decreases the amount of follicle-stimulating hormone (FSH) and luteinizing hormone (LH) released (*i.e.*, gonadotropin pulse amplitude) during most of the cycle and triggers a surge of LH release only at mid-cycle. Progesterone decreases the frequency of GnRH release from the hypothalamus and thus decreases the frequency of plasma gonadotropin pulses. Progesterone also increases the amount of LH released (*i.e.*, the pulse amplitude) during the luteal phase of the cycle.

When the ovaries are removed or cease to function, there is overproduction of FSH and LH, which are excreted in the urine. Measurement of urinary or plasma LH is valuable to assess pituitary function and the effectiveness of therapeutic doses of estrogen. Although FSH levels will also decline upon estrogen administration, they do not return to normal, secondary to production of inhibin by the ovary (*see* Chapter 55). Consequently, the measurement of FSH levels as a means to monitor the effectiveness of hormone therapy is not clinically useful. Additional features of the regulation of gonadotropin secretion and actions are discussed in Chapters 55 and 58.

Effects of Cyclical Gonadal Steroids on the Reproductive Tract. The cyclical changes in estrogen and progesterone production by the ovaries regulate corresponding events in the fallopian tubes, uterus, cervix, and vagina. Physiologically, these changes prepare the uterus for implantation, and the proper timing of events in these tissues is essential for pregnancy. If pregnancy does not occur, the endometrium is shed as the menstrual discharge.

The uterus is composed of an endometrium and a myometrium. The endometrium contains an epithelium lining the uterine cavity and an underlying stroma; the myometrium is the smooth muscle component responsible for uterine contractions. These cell layers, the fallopian tubes, cervix, and vagina display a characteristic set of responses to both estrogens and progestins. The changes typically associated with menstruation occur largely in the endometrium (Figure 57–3).

The luminal surface of the endometrium is a layer of simple columnar epithelial secretory and ciliated cells that is continuous with the openings of numerous glands that extend through the underlying stroma to the myometrial border. Fertilization normally occurs in the fallopian tubes, so ovulation, transport of the fertilized ovum through the fallopian tube, and preparation of the endometrial surface must be temporally coordinated for successful implantation.

The endometrial stroma is a highly cellular connective-tissue layer containing a variety of blood vessels that undergo cyclic changes associated with menstruation. The predominant cells are fibroblasts, but macrophages, lymphocytes, and other resident and migratory cell types also are present.

Menstruation marks the start of the menstrual cycle. During the follicular (or proliferative) phase of the cycle, estrogen begins the rebuilding of the endometrium by stimulating proliferation and differentiation. Numerous mitoses become visible, the thickness of the layer increases, and characteristic changes occur in the glands and blood vessels. In rodent models, ER α mediates the uterotrophic effects of estrogens (Hewitt and Korach, 2003). The overall endometrial response involves estrogen- and progesterone-mediated expression of peptide growth factors and receptors, cell cycle genes, and other regulatory signals. An important response to estrogen in the endometrium and other tissues is induction of the progesterone receptor (PR), which enables cells to respond to this hormone during the second half of the cycle.

In the luteal (or secretory) phase of the cycle, elevated progesterone limits the proliferative effect of estrogens on the endometrium by stimulating differentiation. Major effects include stimulation of epithelial secretions important for implantation of the blastocyst and the characteristic growth of the endometrial blood vessels seen at this time. These effects are mediated by PR-A in animal models (Conneely et al., 2002). Progesterone is thus important in preparation for implantation and for the changes that take place in the uterus at the implantation site (i.e., the decidual response). There is a narrow "window of implantation," spanning days 19 to 24 of the endometrial cycle, when the epithelial cells of the endometrium are receptive to blastocyst implantation. Since endometrial status is regulated by estrogens and progestins, the efficacy of some contraceptives may be due in part to production of an endometrial surface that is not receptive to implantation. If pregnancy does not occur, the corpus luteum regresses due to lack of continued LH secretion, estrogen and progesterone levels fall, and the endometrium is shed (Figure 57–3).

If implantation occurs, human chorionic gonadotropin (hCG) (see Chapter 55), produced initially by the trophoblast and later by the placenta, interacts with the LH receptor of the corpus luteum to maintain steroid hormone synthesis during the early stages of pregnancy. In later stages the placenta itself becomes the major site of estrogen and progesterone synthesis.

Estrogens and progesterone have important effects on the fallopian tube, myometrium, and cervix. In the fallopian tube, estrogens stimulate proliferation and differentiation, whereas progesterone inhibits these processes. Also, estrogens increase and progesterone decreases tubal muscular contractility, which affects transit time of the ovum to the uterus. Estrogens increase the amount of cervical mucus and its water content to facilitate sperm penetration of the cervix, whereas progesterone generally has opposite effects. Estrogens favor rhythmic contractions of the uterine myometrium, while progesterone diminishes contractions. These effects are physiologically important and may also play a role in the action of some contraceptives.

Metabolic Effects. Estrogens affect many tissues and have many metabolic actions in human beings and animals. It is not clear in all cases if effects result directly from hormone actions on the tissue in question or secondarily from actions at other sites. Many nonreproductive tissues, including bone, vascular endothelium, liver, CNS, immune system, gastrointestinal tract, and heart, express low levels of both estrogen receptors, and the ratio of ER α to ER β varies in a cell-specific manner. Many metabolic effects of estrogens result directly from receptor-mediated events in affected organs. The effects of estrogens on selected aspects of mineral, lipid, carbohydrate, and protein metabolism are particularly important for understanding their pharmacological actions.

It long has been recognized that estrogens have positive effects on bone mass (reviewed by Riggs et al., 2002). Bone is continuously remodeled at sites called "bone-remodeling units" by the resorptive action of osteoclasts and the bone-forming action of osteoblasts (see Chapter 61). Maintenance of total bone mass requires equal rates of formation and resorption as occurs in early adulthood (18 to 40 years); thereafter resorption predominates. Osteoclasts and osteoblasts express both ER α and ER β, with the former apparently playing a greater role. Bone also expresses both androgen and progesterone receptors. Based on animal models, the actions of ER α predominate in bone. Estrogens directly regulate osteoblasts and increase the synthesis of type I collagen, osteocalcin, osteopontin, osteonectin, alkaline phosphatase, and other markers of differentiated osteoblasts. Estrogens also increase osteocyte survival by inhibiting apoptosis. However, the major effect of estrogens is to decrease the number and activity of osteoclasts. Much of the action of estrogens on osteoclasts appears to be mediated by altering cytokine (both paracrine and autocrine) signals from osteoblasts. Estrogens decrease osteoblast and stromal cell production of the osteoclast-stimulating cytokines interleukin (IL)-1, IL-6, and tumor necrosis factor (TNF)-α and increase the production of insulin-like growth factor (IGF)-1, bone morphogenic protein (BMP)-6, and transforming growth factor (TGF)-β, which are anti-resorptive (reviewed by Spelsberg et al., 1999). Estrogens also increase osteoblast production of the cytokine osteoprotegrin (OPG), a soluble non–membrane-bound member of the TNF superfamily (see Chapter 61). OPG acts as a "decoy" receptor that antagonizes the binding of OPG-ligand (OPG-L) to its receptor (termed RANK, or receptor activator of NF-κB) and prevents the differentiation of osteoclast precursors to mature osteoclasts. Estrogens increase osteoclast apoptosis, either directly or by increasing OPG. Estrogens have anti-apoptotic effects on both osteoblasts and osteocytes in animal models, and this action may be mediated by nongenomic mechanisms (Kousteni *et al.*, 2002). Estrogens affect bone growth and epiphyseal closure in both sexes. The importance of estrogen in the male skeleton is illustrated by a man with a completely defective ER who had osteoporosis, unfused epiphyses, increased bone turnover, and delayed bone age (Smith *et al.*, 1994), and by the observation that male idiopathic osteoporosis is associated with reduced ER α expression in both osteocytes and osteoblasts (Braidman *et al.*, 2000).

Estrogens have many effects on lipid metabolism; of major interest are their effects on serum lipoprotein and triglyceride levels (Walsh *et al.*, 1994). In general, estrogens slightly elevate serum triglycerides and slightly reduce total serum cholesterol levels. More important, they increase HDL levels and decrease the levels of LDL and Lp(a) (*see* Chapter 35). This beneficial alteration of the ratio of HDL to LDL is an attractive effect of estrogen therapy in postmenopausal women; however, the conclusion from two large clinical trials—the Heart and Estrogen/progestin Replacement Study, or HERS (Hulley *et al.*, 1998), and the Women's Health Initiative or WHI (Rossouw *et al.*, 2002; Anderson *et al.*, 2004)—is that estrogen-progestin or estrogen-only regimens *do not provide any protection from cardiovascular disease*. The presence of estrogen receptors in the liver suggests that the beneficial effects of estrogen on lipoprotein metabolism are due partly to direct hepatic actions, but other sites of action cannot be excluded. Estrogens also alter bile composition by increasing cholesterol secretion and decreasing bile acid secretion. This leads to increased saturation of bile with cholesterol and appears to be the basis for increased gallstone formation in some women receiving estrogens. The decline in bile acid biosynthesis may contribute to the decreased incidence of colon cancer in women receiving combined estrogen-progestin treatment.

Estrogen alone slightly decreases fasting levels of glucose and insulin but does not have major effects on carbohydrate metabolism. Some older studies of combined oral contraceptives (which contained higher levels of both estrogens and progestins than contraceptives do today) suggested that estrogens might impair glucose tolerance, but it is uncertain whether these effects were due to the progestin or the estrogen component of those oral contraceptives.

Estrogens affect many serum proteins, particularly those involved in hormone binding and clotting cascades. In general, estrogens increase plasma levels of cortisol-binding globulin, thyroxine-binding globulin, and sex hormone–binding globulin (SHBG), which binds both androgens and estrogens.

Estrogens alter a number of metabolic pathways that affect the cardiovascular system (Mendelsohn and Karas, 1999). Systemic effects include changes in lipoprotein metabolism and in hepatic production of plasma proteins. Estrogens cause a small increase in coagulation factors II, VII, IX, X, and XII, and decrease the anticoagulation factors protein C, protein S, and antithrombin III (*see* Chapter 54). Fibrinolytic pathways also are affected, and several studies of women treated with estrogen alone or estrogen with a progestin have demonstrated decreased levels of plasminogen-activator inhibitor protein-1 (PAI-1) with a concomitant increase in fibrinolysis (Koh *et al.*, 1997). Thus, estrogens increase both coagulation and fibrinolytic pathways, and imbalance in these two opposing activities may cause adverse effects. At relatively high concentrations, estrogens have antioxidant activity and may inhibit the oxidation of LDL by affecting superoxide dismutase. Long-term administration of estrogen is associated with decreased plasma renin, angiotensin-converting enzyme, and endothelin-1; expression of the AT_1 receptor for angiotensin II is also decreased. Estrogen actions on the vascular wall include increased production of NO, which occurs within minutes *via* a mechanism involving activation of Akt (also known as protein kinase B) (Simoncini *et al.*, 2000), and induction of inducible NO synthase and increased production of prostacyclin. All of these changes promote vasodilation. Estrogens also promote endothelial cell growth while inhibiting the proliferation of vascular smooth muscle cells.

Estrogen Receptors

Estrogens exert their effects by interaction with receptors that are members of the superfamily of nuclear receptors. The two estrogen receptor genes are located on separate chromosomes: ESR1 encodes ER α, and ESR2 encodes ER β. Both ERs are estrogen-dependent nuclear transcription factors that have different tissue distributions and transcriptional regulatory effects on a wide number of target genes (reviewed by Hanstein *et al.*, 2004). Ligands that discriminate between ER α and ER β have been developed (Harrington *et al.*, 2003) but are not yet in clinical use. Both ER α and ER β exist as multiple mRNA isoforms due to differential promoter use and alternative splicing (reviewed by Kos *et al.*, 2001; Lewandowski *et al.*, 2002). The two human ERs are 44% identical in overall amino-acid sequence and share the domain structure common to members of this family. The estrogen receptor is divided into six functional domains: the NH_2-terminal A/B domain contains the activation function-1 (AF-1) segment, which can activate transcription independently of ligand; the highly conserved C domain comprises the DNA-binding domain, which contains 4 cysteines arranged in 2 zinc fingers; the D domain, frequently called the "hinge region," contains the nuclear localization signal; and the E/F domain has multiple functions, including ligand binding, dimerization, and ligand-dependent transactivation, mediated by the AF-2 domain. There are significant differences between the two receptor isoforms in the ligand-binding domains and in both transactivation domains. Human ER β does not appear to contain a functional AF-1 domain. The receptors appear to have different biological functions and respond differently to various estrogenic compounds (Kuiper *et al.*, 1997). However, their high homology in the DNA-binding domains suggests that both receptors recognize similar DNA sequences and hence regulate many of the same target genes.

ER α, the first discovered, is expressed most abundantly in the female reproductive tract—especially the uterus, vagina, and ovaries—as well as in the mammary gland, the hypothalamus, endothelial cells, and vascular smooth muscle. ER β is expressed most highly in the prostate and ovaries, with lower expression in lung, brain, bone, and vasculature. Many cells express both ER α and ER β, which can form either homo- or heterodimers. When co-expressed, in many cases ER β inhibits ER α–mediated transcriptional activation (Hall and McDonnell, 1999). Polymorphic variants of ER have been identified, but attempts to correlate specific polymorphisms with the frequency of breast cancer (Han *et al.*, 2003), bone mass (Vandevyver *et al.*, 1999; Kurabayashi *et al.*, 2004), endometrial cancer (Weiderpass *et al.*, 2000), or cardiovascular disease (Herrington and Howard, 2003) have led to contradictory results.

Mechanism of Action

Both estrogen receptors (ERs) are ligand-activated transcription factors that increase or decrease the transcription of target genes (Figure 57–4). After entering the cell by passive diffusion through the plasma membrane, the hormone binds to an ER in the nucleus. In the nucleus, the ER is present as an inactive monomer bound to heat-shock proteins, and upon binding estrogen, a change in ER conformation dissociates the heat-shock proteins and causes receptor dimerization, which increases the affinity and the rate of receptor binding to DNA (Cheskis *et al.*, 1997). Homodimers of ER α or ER β and ER α/ER β heterodimers can be produced depending on the receptor complement in a given cell. The concept of ligand-mediated changes in ER conformation is central to understanding the mechanism of action of estrogen agonists and antagonists. The ER dimer binds to estrogen response elements (EREs), typically located in the promoter region of target genes with the consensus sequence GGTCANNNT-GACC, but several similar sequences can act as estrogen

response elements in a promoter-specific context. The type of ERE with which ERs interact also regulates the three-dimensional structure of the activated receptor (Hall *et al.*, 2002).

The ER/DNA complex recruits a cascade of co-activator and other proteins to the promoter region of target genes (Figure 57–4B). There are three families of proteins that interact with ERs. The first of these has the ability to modify nucleosome structure either in an ATP-dependent manner, like SWI/Snf, or by histone methyl-transferase (HMT) activity, as in proteins such as PRMT1. The second family comprises the p160/SRC proteins and includes SRC-1 (steroid-receptor co-activator-1), SRC-2, and SRC-3. The third family includes p300/CBP (cyclic AMP response-element binding protein), co-activators that are targets of several signal transduction cascades and may integrate function among diverse pathways and the basal transcriptional apparatus. Agonist-bound ERs appear initially to recruit SWI/Snf and HMT members that modify nucleosome structure and facilitate the subsequent recruitment of p160 members and p300 proteins (Metivier *et al.*, 2003). The co-activators and p300 proteins have histone acetylase (HAT) activity. Acetylation of histones further alters chromatin structure in the promoter region of target genes and allows the proteins that make up the general transcription apparatus to assemble and initiate transcription.

Interaction of ERs with antagonists also promotes dimerization and DNA binding. However, an antagonist produces a conformation of ER that is different from the agonist-occupied receptor (Wijayaratne *et al.*, 1999; Smith and O'Malley, 2004). The antagonist-induced conformation facilitates binding of co-repressors such as NcoR/SMRT (nuclear hormone receptor co-repressor/silencing mediator of retinoid and thyroid receptors) (Figure 57–4C). The co-repressor/ER complex then further recruits other proteins with histone deacetylase activity such as HDAC1. Deacetylation of histones alters chromatin conformation and reduces the ability of the general transcription apparatus to form initiation complexes.

Besides co-activators and co-repressors, both ER α and ER β can interact physically with other transcription factors such as Sp1 (Saville *et al.*, 2000) or AP-1 (Paech *et al.*, 1997), and these protein-protein interactions provide an alternate mechanism of action. In these circumstances, ER-ligand complexes interact with Sp1 or AP-1 that is already bound to its specific regulatory element, such that the ER complex does not interact directly with an ERE. This may explain how estrogens are able to regulate genes that lack a consensus ERE. Responses to agonists and antagonists mediated by these protein-protein interactions also are ER isoform- and promoter-specific. For example, 17β-estradiol induces transcription of a target gene controlled by an AP-1 site in the presence of an ER α/AP-1 complex, but inhibits transcription in the presence of an ER β/AP-1

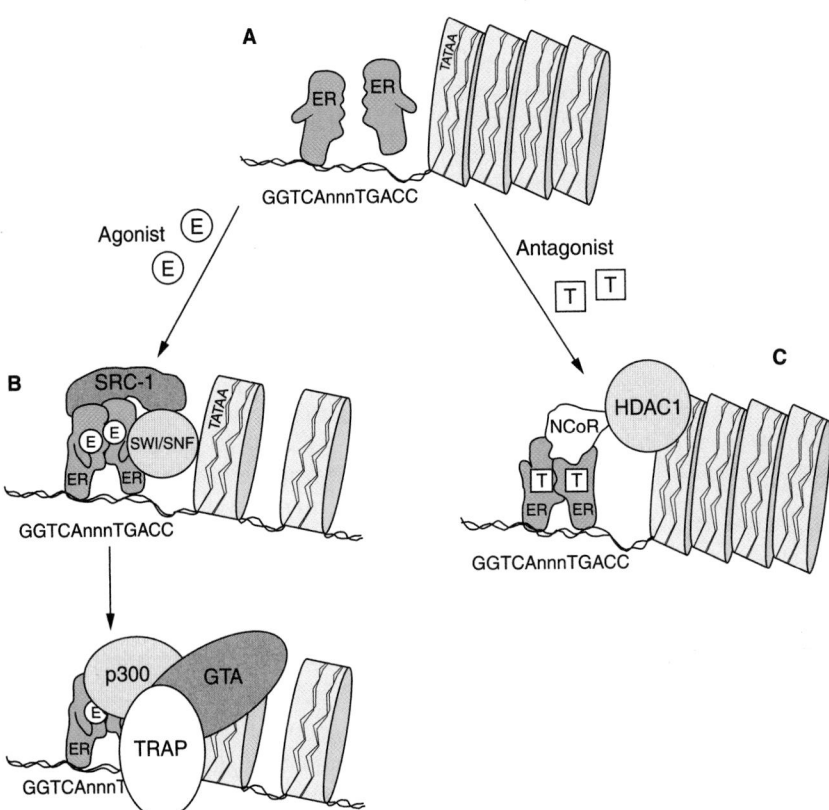

Figure 57–4. ***Molecular mechanism of action of nuclear estrogen receptor.*** ***A.*** Unliganded estrogen receptor (ER) exists as a monomer within the nucleus. ***B.*** Agonists such as 17β-estradiol (ⓔ) bind to the ER and cause a ligand-directed change in conformation that facilitates dimerization and interaction with specific estrogen response element (ERE) sequences in DNA. The ER-DNA complex recruits co-activators such as SWI/SNF that modify chromatin structure, and co-activators such as steroid-receptor co-activator-1 (SRC-1) that has histone acetyltransferase (HAT) activity that further alters chromatin structure. This remodeling facilitates the exchange of the recruited proteins such that other co-activators (*e.g.*, p300 and the TRAP complex) associate on the target gene promoter and proteins that comprise the general transcription apparatus (GTA) are recruited, with subsequent synthesis of mRNA. ***C.*** Antagonists such as tamoxifen (Ⓣ) also bind to the ER but produce a different receptor conformation. The antagonist-induced conformation also facilitates dimerization and interaction with DNA, but a different set of proteins called co-repressors, such as nuclear-hormone receptor co-repressor (NcoR), are recruited to the complex. NcoR further recruits proteins such as histone deacetylase I (HDAC1) that act on histone proteins to stabilize nucleosome structure and prevent interaction with the GTA.

complex. Conversely, anti-estrogens are potent activators of ER β/AP-1 but not of ER α/AP-1 complexes.

Other signaling systems may activate nuclear ER by ligand-independent mechanisms. Phosphorylation of ER α at serine 118 by MAP kinase activates the receptor (Kato *et al.*, 1995). Similarly, PI-3-kinase–activated Akt directly phosphorylates ER α, causing ligand-independent activation of estrogen-target genes (Simoncini *et al.*, 2000). This provides a means of cross-talk between membrane-bound receptor pathways (*i.e.*, EGF/IGF-1) that activate MAPK and the nuclear ER. In a reciprocal fashion ER may interact directly with members of the Src-Shc/Erk signaling pathway. Activation of Erk by the novel ER and androgen receptor (AR) agonist estren is thought to be responsible for the anti-apoptotic action of this drug in bone (reviewed in Manolagas *et al.*, 2002).

Several studies have suggested that some estrogen receptors are located on the plasma membrane of cells. It appears that this form of the ER is encoded by the same gene that encodes ER α, but it is

transported to the plasma membrane, mainly in caveolae (reviewed by Zhu and Smart, 2003). These membrane-localized ERs mediate the rapid activation of some proteins such as MAPK, which is phosphorylated in several cell types within 5 to 10 minutes of 17β-estradiol addition (Endoh *et al.*, 1997), or the rapid increase in cyclic AMP caused by the hormone (Aronica and Katzenellenbogen, 1993). The finding that MAPK is activated by estradiol provides an additional level of cross-talk with growth factors, such as IGF-1 and EGF, that activate this kinase pathway.

Absorption, Fate, and Elimination

Various estrogens are available for oral, parenteral, transdermal, or topical administration (Table 57–1). Given the lipophilic nature of estrogens, absorption generally is good with the appropriate preparation. Aqueous or oil-based esters of estradiol and estrone are available for intramuscular injection, ranging in frequency from every several days to once per month. Transdermal patches that are changed once or twice weekly deliver estradiol continuously through the skin. Preparations are available for topical use in the vagina or creams applied to the skin. For many uses, preparations are available as an estrogen alone or in combination with a progestin.

Oral administration is common and may utilize estradiol, conjugated estrogens, esters of estrone and other estrogens, and *ethinyl estradiol*. A special micronized preparation of estradiol (ESTRACE, others) that yields a large surface for rapid absorption is required for oral administration, although high doses must be used because absolute bioavailability remains low due to first-pass metabolism (Fotherby, 1996). Ethinyl estradiol is used orally, as the ethinyl substitution in the C17 position inhibits first-pass hepatic metabolism. Other common oral preparations contain conjugated equine estrogens (PREMARIN), which are primarily the sulfate esters of estrone, equilin, and other naturally occurring compounds; *esterified esters*; or mixtures of conjugated estrogens prepared from plant-derived sources (CENESTIN). These are hydrolyzed by enzymes present in the lower gut that remove the charged sulfate groups and allow absorption of estrogen across the intestinal epithelium. In another oral preparation, *estropipate* (ORTHO-EST, OGEN), estrone is solubilized as the sulfate and stabilized with piperazine. Due largely to differences in metabolism, the potencies of various oral preparations differ widely; ethinyl estradiol, for example, is much more potent than conjugated estrogens.

A number of foodstuffs and plant-derived products, largely from soy, are available as nonprescription items and often are touted as providing benefits similar to those from compounds with established estrogenic activity. These products may contain flavonoids such as genistein (Table 57–1), which display estrogenic activity in laboratory tests, albeit generally much less than that of estradiol. In theory, these preparations could produce appreciable estrogenic effects, but their efficacy at relevant doses has not been established in human trials (Mäkelä *et al.*, 1999; Fitzpatrick, 2003).

Administration of estradiol *via* transdermal patches (ESTRADERM, VIVELLE, ALORA, CLIMARA, others) provides slow, sustained release of the hormone, systemic distribution, and more constant blood levels than oral dosing. Estradiol is also available as a topical cream (ESTRASORB) that is applied to the upper thigh and calf, or as a gel (ESTROGEL) that is applied once daily to the arm. The transdermal route does not lead to the high level of the drug that enters the liver *via* the portal circulation after oral administration, and is thus expected to minimize hepatic effects of estrogens (*e.g.*, on hepatic protein synthesis, lipoprotein profiles, and triglyceride levels).

Other preparations are available for intramuscular injection. When dissolved in oil and injected, esters of estradiol are well absorbed. The aryl and alkyl esters of estradiol become less polar as the size of the substituents increases; correspondingly, the rate of absorption of oily preparations is progressively slowed, and the duration of action can be prolonged. A single therapeutic dose of compounds such as *estradiol valerate* (DELESTROGEN) or *estradiol cypionate* (DEPO-ESTRADIOL) may be absorbed over several weeks following a single intramuscular injection. Suspensions containing estrone or a combination of esters (primarily estrone and equilin sulfates) also may be given *via* intramuscular injection.

Preparations of estradiol and conjugated estrogen creams are available for topical administration to the vagina. These are effective locally, but systemic effects also are possible due to significant absorption. A 3-month vaginal ring (ESTRING, FEMRING) may be used for slow release of estradiol, and tablets are also available for vaginal use (VAGIFEM).

Estradiol, ethinyl estradiol, and other estrogens are extensively bound to plasma proteins. Estradiol and other naturally occurring estrogens are bound mainly to sex hormone–binding globulin (SHBG) and to a lesser degree to serum albumin. In contrast, ethinyl estradiol is bound extensively to serum albumin but not SHBG. Due to their size and lipophilic nature, unbound estrogens distribute rapidly and extensively.

Variations in estradiol metabolism occur and depend upon the stage of the menstrual cycle, menopausal status, and several genetic polymorphisms (Herrington and Klein, 2001). In general, the hormone undergoes rapid hepatic biotransformation, with a plasma half-life measured in minutes. Estradiol is converted primarily by 17β-hydroxysteroid dehydrogenase to estrone, which undergoes conversion by 16α-hydroxylation and 17-keto reduction to estriol, the major urinary metabolite. A variety of sulfate and glucuronide conjugates also are excreted in the urine. Lesser amounts of estrone or estradiol are oxidized to the 2-hydroxycatechols by CYP3A4 in the liver and by CYP1A in extrahepatic tissues or to 4-hydroxycatechols by CYP1B1 in extrahepatic sites, with the 2-hydroxycatechol being formed to a greater extent. The 2- and 4-hydroxycatechols are largely inactivated by catechol-*O*-methyl transferases (COMTs). However, smaller amounts may be converted by CYP- or peroxidase-catalyzed reactions to yield semiquinones or quinones that are capable of forming DNA adducts or of generating (*via* redox cycling) reactive oxygen species that could oxidize DNA bases (Yue *et al.*, 2003).

Estrogens also undergo enterohepatic recirculation *via* (1) sulfate and glucuronide conjugation in the liver, (2) biliary secretion of the conjugates into the intestine, and (3) hydrolysis in the gut (largely by bacterial enzymes) followed by reabsorption.

Many other drugs and environmental agents (*e.g.*, cigarette smoke) act as inducers or inhibitors of the various enzymes that metabolize estrogens, and thus have the potential to alter their clearance. Consideration of the impact of these factors on efficacy and untoward effects is increasingly important with the decreased doses of estrogens currently employed for both menopausal hormone therapy and contraception.

Ethinyl estradiol is cleared much more slowly than is estradiol due to decreased hepatic metabolism, and the elimination-phase half-life in various studies ranges from 13 to 27 hours. Unlike estradiol, the primary route of biotransformation of ethinyl estradiol is *via* 2-hydroxylation and subsequent formation of the corresponding 2- and 3-methyl ethers. *Mestranol*, another semisynthetic estrogen and a component of some combination oral contraceptives, is the 3-methyl ether of ethinyl estradiol. In the body it undergoes rapid hepatic demethylation to ethinyl estradiol, which is its active form (Fotherby, 1996).

Untoward Responses

Estrogens are highly efficacious, but they do carry a number of risks as well. Many concerns arose initially from studies of early oral contraceptives, which contained high doses of estrogens, but the amount of estrogens (and progestins) in oral contraceptives has been markedly decreased, which has significantly diminished the risks associated with their use. Nevertheless, major concerns about the use of estrogens remain today, especially regarding cancer, thromboembolic disease, increased risk of cardiovascular disease, altered cognition, changes in carbohydrate and lipid metabolism, hypertension, gallbladder disease, nausea, migraine, changes in mood, and several lesser side effects.

Concern about Carcinogenic Actions. The possibility of developing cancer is probably the major concern for the use of estrogens and oral contraceptives. Early studies established that estrogens can induce tumors of the breast, uterus, testis, bone, kidney, and several other tissues in various animal species. These early studies disseminated a fear of cancer resulting from estrogen use.

In later reports (Greenwald *et al.*, 1971; Herbst *et al.*, 1971), an increased incidence of vaginal and cervical adenocarcinoma was noted in female offspring of mothers who had taken diethylstilbestrol (DES) during the first trimester of pregnancy. The incidence of clear-cell vaginal and cervical adenocarcinoma in women who were exposed to DES *in utero* was 0.01% to 0.1% (Food and Drug Administration, 1985); these findings established for the first time that developmental exposure to estrogens was associated with an increase in a human cancer. Estrogen use during pregnancy also can increase the incidence of nonmalignant genital abnormalities in both male and female offspring. Thus, pregnant patients should not be given estrogens because of the possibility of such reproductive tract toxicities.

Other studies established that the use of unopposed estrogen for hormone treatment in postmenopausal women increases the risk of endometrial carcinoma by five- to fifteenfold (Shapiro *et al.*, 1985). This increased risk can be prevented if a progestin is co-administered with the estrogen (Pike *et al.*, 1997), and this is now standard practice.

The association between estrogen and/or estrogen-progestin use and breast cancer continues to be of great concern and debate. The results of two very large, randomized, clinical trials of estrogen-progestin and estrogen-only (*i.e.*, the two arms of The Women's Health Initiative or WHI) use in postmenopausal women have clearly established a small but significant increase in the risk of breast cancer, apparently due to the medroxyprogesterone (Rossouw *et al.*, 2002; Anderson *et al.*, 2004). In the WHI study, an estrogen-progestin combination increased the total risk of breast cancer by 24%; the absolute increase in attributable cases of disease was 6 per 1000 women and required 3 or more years of treatment. In women without a uterus who received estrogen alone, the relative risk of breast cancer was actually decreased by 23%, and the decrease only narrowly missed reaching statistical significance.

The Million Women Study (MWS) in the United Kingdom was a cohort study rather than a clinical trial (Beral *et al.*, 2003). It surveyed over one million women, about half receiving some type of hormone treatment and half had never used them. Those receiving an estrogen-progestin combination had an increased relative risk of invasive breast cancer of 2, and those receiving estrogen alone had an increased relative risk of 1.3, but the increase in actual attributable cases of the disease was again small.

Both the WHI and MWS data are thus consistent with earlier studies indicating that the progestin component (*e.g.*, medroxyprogesterone) in hormone-replacement therapy plays a major role in this increased risk of breast cancer (Schairer *et al.*, 2000; Ross *et al.*,

2000). Importantly, although long-term data have not accumulated for the WHI trials, the available data suggest that the excess risk of breast cancer associated with menopausal hormone use appears to abate 5 years after discontinuing therapy.

Historically, the carcinogenic actions of estrogens were thought to be related to their trophic effects. An increase in cell proliferation would be expected to cause an increase in spontaneous errors associated with DNA replication, and estrogens would then enhance the growth of clones with mutations introduced by this or other mechanisms (*e.g.*, chemical carcinogens). More recently, another mechanism has been proposed. If catechol estrogens, especially the 4-hydroxycatechols, are converted to semiquinones or quinones prior to "inactivation" by COMT, these products, or reactive oxygen species generated during subsequent biotransformations, may cause direct chemical damage to DNA bases (Yue *et al.*, 2003). In this regard, CYP1B1, which has specific estrogen-4-hydroxylase activity, is present in tissues such as uterus, breast, ovary, and prostate, which often give rise to hormone-responsive cancers (Yue *et al.*, 2003).

Metabolic and Cardiovascular Effects. Although they may slightly elevate plasma triglycerides, estrogens themselves generally have favorable overall effects on plasma lipoprotein profiles. However, as noted in a later section dealing with hormone-replacement regimens, progestins may reduce the favorable actions of estrogens. In contrast, estrogens do increase cholesterol levels in bile and cause a relative two- to threefold increase in gallbladder disease. Currently prescribed doses of estrogens do not increase the risk of hypertension.

A number of observational studies, clinical trials using intermediate markers of cardiovascular disease, and numerous animal studies suggested that estrogen therapy in postmenopausal women would reduce the risk of cardiovascular disease by 35% to 50% (Manson and Martin, 2001). However, two recent randomized clinical trials have not found such protection. The Heart and Estrogen/progestin Replacement Study, or HERS (Hulley *et al.*, 1998), followed women with established coronary heart disease (CHD) and found that estrogen plus a progestin increased the relative risk of nonfatal myocardial infarction or CHD death within 1 year of treatment, and found no overall change in 5 years. The HERS II follow-up (Grady *et al.*, 2002) found no overall change in the incidence of CHD after 6.8 years of the treatment. A similar conclusion was reached in the WHI trials for women *without* existing CHD treated with an estrogen plus progestin (Rossouw *et al.*, 2002). These studies establish unequivocally that the estrogen-progestin combination used does not protect against CHD. However, only conjugated equine estrogens (CEE) or CEE plus medroxyprogesterone acetate (MPA) were examined in these studies, and only a single dose was used in a relatively old patient population (*e.g.*, average age approximately 60 years). It thus remains unclear whether these conclusions can be globally extended to other preparations, doses, and patient populations (*e.g.*, women closer to age 50 who typically initiate hormone therapy for relief of vasomotor symptoms).

It is clear, however, that oral estrogens increase the risk of thromboembolic disease in healthy women and in women with pre-existing cardiovascular disease (Grady *et al.*, 2000). The increase in absolute risk is small but significant. In the WHI, for example, an estrogen-progestin combination led to an increase in 8 attributable cases of stroke per 10,000 women and a similar increase in pulmonary embolism (Rossouw *et al.*, 2002).

Effects on Cognition. Several retrospective studies had suggested that estrogens had beneficial effects on cognition and delayed the onset of Alzheimer's disease (Green and Simpkins, 2000). However, the Women's Health Initiative Memory Study (WHIMS) of a group of women aged 65 or older (Shumaker *et al.*, 2003) found that estrogen-progestin therapy was associated with a doubling in the number of women diagnosed with probable dementia, and no benefit of hormone treatment on global cognitive function was observed (Rapp *et al.*, 2003). Women in the estrogen-only arm also showed a comparable decrease in cognitive function (Espeland *et al.*, 2004), implicating estrogens in these cognitive changes.

Other Potential Untoward Effects. Nausea and vomiting are an initial reaction to estrogen therapy in some women, but these effects may disappear with time and may be minimized by taking estrogens with food or just prior to sleeping. Fullness and tenderness of the breasts and edema may occur but sometimes can be diminished by lowering the dose. A more serious concern is that estrogens may cause severe migraine in some women. Estrogens also may reactivate or exacerbate endometriosis.

Therapeutic Uses

The two major uses of estrogens are as components of combination oral contraceptives (*see* below) and for menopausal hormone therapy (MHT). The pharmacological considerations for their use and the specific drugs and doses used differ in these settings. Historically, conjugated estrogens have been the most common agents for postmenopausal use (0.625 mg/day most often used). In contrast, most combination oral contraceptives in current use employ 20 to 35 μg/day of ethinyl estradiol. These preparations differ widely in their oral potencies; *e.g.*, a dose of 0.625 mg of conjugated estrogens generally is considered equivalent to 5 to 10 μg of ethinyl estradiol. Thus, the "effective" dose of estrogen used for MHT is less than that in oral contraceptives when one considers potency. Furthermore, in the last two decades the doses of estrogens employed in both settings have decreased substantially. The untoward effects of the 20- to 35-μg doses now commonly used thus have a lower incidence and severity than those reported in older studies (*e.g.*, with oral contraceptives that contained 50 to 150 μg of ethinyl estradiol or mestranol).

Menopausal Hormone Therapy. The established benefits of estrogen therapy in postmenopausal women include amelioration of vasomotor symptoms and the prevention of bone fractures and urogenital atrophy.

Vasomotor Symptoms. The decline in ovarian function at menopause is associated with vasomotor symptoms in most women. The characteristic hot flashes may alternate with chilly sensations, inappropriate sweating, and (less commonly) paresthesias. Treatment with estrogen is specific and is the most efficacious pharmacotherapy for these symptoms (Belchetz, 1994). If estrogen is contraindicated or otherwise undesirable, other options may be considered.

Medroxyprogesterone acetate (discussed in the later section on progestins) may provide some relief of vasomotor symptoms for certain patients, and the α_2 adrenergic agonist *clonidine* diminishes vasomotor symptoms in some women, presumably by blocking the CNS outflow that regulates blood flow to cutaneous vessels. In many women, hot flashes diminish within several years; when prescribed for this purpose the dose and duration of estrogen use should thus be the minimum necessary to provide relief.

Osteoporosis. Osteoporosis is a disorder of the skeleton associated with the loss of bone mass (*see* Chapter 61). The result is thinning and weakening of the bones and an increased incidence of fractures, particularly compression fractures of the vertebrae and minimal-trauma fractures of the hip and wrist. The frequency and severity of these fractures and their associated complications (*e.g.*, death and permanent disability) are a major public health problem, especially as the population continues to age. Osteoporosis is an indication for estrogen therapy, which clearly is efficacious in decreasing the incidence of fractures. However, because of the risks associated with estrogen use, first-line use of other drugs should be carefully considered (*see* Chapter 61). Nevertheless, it is important to note that the majority of fractures in the postmenopausal period occur in women without a prior history of osteoporosis, and estrogens are the most efficacious agents available for prevention of fractures at all sites in such women (Rossouw *et al.*, 2002; Anderson *et al.*, 2004).

The primary mechanism by which estrogens act is to decrease bone resorption; consequently, estrogens are more effective at preventing rather than restoring bone loss (Prince *et al.*, 1991; Belchetz, 1994). Estrogens are most effective if treatment is initiated before significant bone loss occurs, and their maximal beneficial effects require continuous use; bone loss resumes when treatment is discontinued. An appropriate diet with adequate intake of Ca^{2+} and vitamin D and weight-bearing exercise enhance the effects of estrogen treatment. Public health efforts to improve diet and exercise patterns in girls and young women also are rational approaches to increase bone mass.

Vaginal Dryness and Urogenital Atrophy. Loss of tissue lining the vagina or bladder leads to a variety of symptoms in many postmenopausal women (Robinson and Cardozo, 2003). These include dryness and itching of the vagina, dyspareunia, swelling of tissues in the genital region, pain during urination, a need to urinate urgently or often, and sudden or unexpected urinary incontinence. When estrogens are being used solely for relief of vulvar and vaginal atrophy, local administration as a vaginal cream, ring device, or tablets may be considered.

Cardiovascular Disease. The incidence of cardiovascular disease is low in premenopausal women, rising rapidly after menopause, and epidemiological studies consistently showed an association between estrogen use and reduced cardiovascular disease in postmenopausal women. Furthermore, estrogens produce a favorable lipoprotein profile, promote vasodilation, inhibit the response to vascular injury, and reduce atherosclerosis. Studies such as these led to the widespread use of estrogen for prevention of cardiovascular disease in postmenopausal women (Mendelsohn and Karas, 1999). As discussed above, several randomized, prospective studies (Rossouw *et al.*, 2002; Grady *et al.*, 2002) unexpectedly indicated that the incidence of heart disease and stroke in older postmenopausal women treated with conjugated estrogens and a progestin was initially increased, although the trend reversed with time. While it is not clear if similar results would occur with different drugs/doses or in different patient populations (Turgeon *et al.*, 2004), estrogens (alone or in combination with a progestin) should *not* be used for the treatment or prevention of cardiovascular disease.

Other Therapeutic Effects. Many other changes occur in postmenopausal women, including a general thinning of the skin; changes in the urethra, vulva, and external genitalia; and a variety of changes including headache, fatigue, and difficulty concentrating, many of which may be due to the chronic lack of sleep created by hot flashes and other vasomotor symptoms. Estrogen replacement may help alleviate or lessen some of these *via* direct actions (*e.g.,* improvement of vasomotor symptoms) or secondary effects resulting in an improved feeling of well-being (Belchetz, 1994).

The Women's Health Initiative also demonstrated that a conjugated estrogen in combination with a progestin reduces the risk of colon cancer by roughly one-half in postmenopausal women (Rossouw *et al.*, 2002).

Menopausal Hormone Regimens. In the 1960s and 1970s there was an increase in *estrogen-replacement therapy,* or ERT (*i.e.,* estrogens alone), in postmenopausal women, primarily to reduce vasomotor symptoms, vaginitis, and osteoporosis. About 1980, epidemiological studies indicated that this treatment increased the incidence of endometrial carcinoma. This led to the use of *hormone-replacement therapy,* or HRT, that includes a progestin to limit estrogen-related endometrial hyperplasia. While the actions of progesterone on the endometrium are complex, its effects on estrogen-induced hyperplasia may involve a decrease in estrogen receptor content, increased local conversion of estradiol to the less potent estrone *via* the induction of 17β-hydroxysteroid dehydrogenase in the tissue, and/or the conversion of the endometrium from a proliferative to a secretory state. "Hormone-replacement" therapy (now generally referred to as "menopausal hormone" therapy) with both an estrogen and progestin now is recommended for postmenopausal women with a uterus (Belchetz, 1994). For women who have undergone a hysterectomy, endometrial carcinoma is not a concern, and estrogen alone avoids the possible deleterious effects of progestins previously discussed.

Conjugated estrogens and medroxyprogesterone acetate (MPA) historically have been used most commonly in menopausal hormone regimens, although estradiol, estrone, and estriol have been used as estrogens, and *norethindrone, norgestimate, levonorgestrel, norethisterone,* and *progesterone* also have been widely used (especially in Europe). Various "continuous" or "cyclic" regimens have been used; the latter regimens include drug-free days. An example of a cyclic regimen is as follows: (1) administration of an estrogen for 25 days; (2) the addition of MPA for the last 12 to 14 days of estrogen treatment; and (3) 5 to 6 days with no hormone treatment, during which withdrawal bleeding normally occurs due to breakdown and shedding of the endometrium. Continuous administration of combined estrogen plus progestin does not lead to regular, recurrent endometrial shedding, but may cause intermittent spotting or bleeding, especially in the first year of use. Other regimens include a progestin intermittently (*e.g.,* every third month), but the long-term endometrial safety of these regimens remains to be firmly established. PREMPRO (conjugated estrogens plus MPA given as a fixed dose daily) and PREMPHASE (conjugated estrogens given for 28 days plus MPA given for 14 out of

28 days) are widely used combination formulations. Other combination products available in the United States are FEMHRT (ethinyl estradiol plus *norethindrone acetate*), ACTIVELLA (estradiol plus norethindrone), and PREFEST (estradiol and norgestimate). Doses and regimens are usually adjusted empirically based on control of symptoms, patient acceptance of bleeding patterns, and/or other untoward effects.

Another pharmacological consideration is the route of estrogen administration. Oral administration exposes the liver to higher concentrations of estrogens than transdermal administration. Either route effectively relieves vasomotor symptoms and protects against bone loss. Oral but not transdermal estrogen may increase SHBG, other binding globulins, and angiotensinogen; the oral route might be expected to cause greater increases in the cholesterol content of the bile. Transdermal estrogen appears to cause smaller beneficial changes in LDL and HDL profiles (approximately 50% of those seen with the oral route) (Walsh *et al.*, 1994), but may be preferred in women with hypertriglyceridemia.

Tibolone (LIVIAL) is widely used in Europe for treatment of vasomotor symptoms and prevention of osteoporosis but is not currently approved in the United States. The parent compound itself is devoid of activity, but it is metabolized in a tissue-selective manner to three metabolites that have predominantly estrogenic, progestogenic, and androgenic activities. The drug appears to increase bone mineral density and decrease vasomotor symptoms without stimulating the endometrium, but its effects on fractures, breast cancer, and long-term outcomes remain to be established (Modelska and Cummings, 2002).

Regardless of the specific agent or regimen, menopausal hormone therapy with estrogens should use the lowest dose and shortest duration necessary to achieve an appropriate therapeutic goal.

Estrogen Treatment in the Failure of Ovarian Development. In several conditions (*e.g.,* Turner's syndrome), the ovaries do not develop and puberty does not occur. Therapy with estrogen at the appropriate time replicates the events of puberty, and androgens (*see* Chapter 58) and/or growth hormone (*see* Chapter 55) may be used concomitantly to promote normal growth. While estrogens and androgens promote bone growth, they also accelerate epiphyseal fusion, and their premature use can thus result in a shorter ultimate height.

SELECTIVE ESTROGEN RECEPTOR MODULATORS (SERMS) AND ANTI-ESTROGENS

In the past, estrogen pharmacology was based on a simple model of an agonist binding to a single ER that subsequently affected transcription by the same molecular mechanism in all target tissues, and of antagonists that acted by simple competition with agonists for binding. This simple concept is no longer valid. By altering the conformation of the two different ERs and thereby changing interactions with co-activators and co-repressors in a cell- and promoter-specific context, ligands may have a broad spectrum of activities from purely anti-estrogenic in all tissues, to partially estrogenic in some tissues with anti-estrogenic or no activities in others, to purely estrogenic activities in all tissues. The elucidation of these concepts has been a major breakthrough in estrogen pharmacology and should permit the rational design of drugs with very selective patterns of estrogenic activity (Smith and O'Malley, 2004).

SERMs: Tamoxifen, Raloxifene, and Toremifene. Selective estrogen receptor modulators, or SERMs, are compounds with tissue-selective actions. The pharmacological goal of these drugs is to produce beneficial estrogenic actions in certain tissues (*e.g.,* bone, brain, and liver) during postmenopausal hormone therapy, but antagonist activity in tissues such as breast and endometrium, where estrogenic actions (*e.g.,* carcinogenesis) might be deleterious. Currently approved drugs in the United States in this class are *tamoxifen citrate* (NOLVADEX, OTHERS), *raloxifene hydrochloride* (EVISTA), and *toremifene* (FARESTON), which is chemically related and has similar actions to tamoxifen. Tamoxifen and toremifene are used for treatment of breast cancer, and raloxifene is used primarily for prevention and treatment of osteoporosis.

Anti-estrogens: Clomiphene and Fulvestrant. These compounds are distinguished from the SERMs in that they are pure antagonists in all tissues studied. Clomiphene (CLOMID, SEROPHENE, others) is approved for the treatment of infertility in anovulatory women, and *fulvestrant* (FASLODEX, ICI 182,780) is used for the treatment of breast cancer in women with disease progression after tamoxifen.

Chemistry. The structures of the *trans*-isomer of tamoxifen, and of raloxifene, *trans*-clomiphene (enclomiphene), and fulvestrant are as follows:

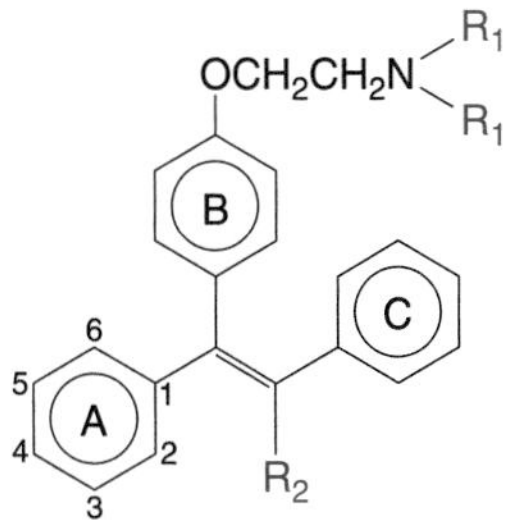

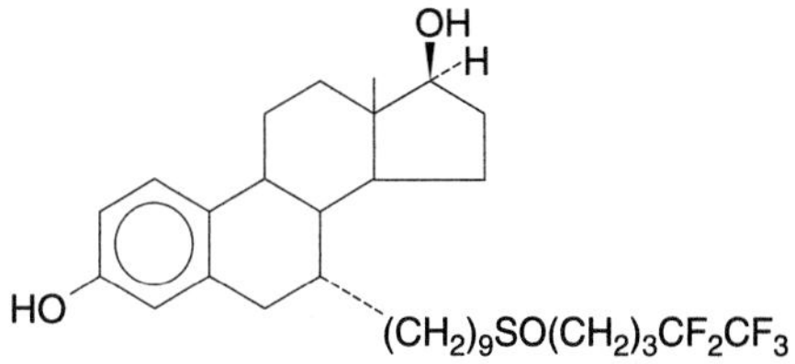

FULVESTRANT (ICI 182, 780)

Tamoxifen is a triphenylethylene with the same stilbene nucleus as diethylstilbestrol; compounds of this class display a variety of estrogenic and anti-estrogenic activities. In general, the *trans* conformations have anti-estrogenic activity, whereas the *cis* conformations display estrogenic activity. However, the pharmacological activity of the *trans* compound depends on the species, target tissue, and gene. Hepatic metabolism produces primarily *N*-desmethyltamoxifen, which has affinity for ER comparable to that of tamoxifen, and lesser amounts of the highly active 4-hydroxy metabolite, which has a 25 to 50 times higher affinity for both ER α and ER β than does tamoxifen (Kuiper *et al.,* 1997). Tamoxifen is marketed as the pure *trans*-isomer. Toremifene is a triphenylethylene with a chlorine substitution at the R2 position.

Raloxifene is a polyhydroxylated nonsteroidal compound with a benzothiophene core. Raloxifene binds with high affinity for both ER α and ER β (Kuiper *et al.,* 1997).

Clomiphene citrate is a triphenylethylene; its two isomers, zuclomiphene (*cis*-clomiphene) and enclomiphene (*trans*-clomiphene), are a weak estrogen agonist and a potent antagonist, respectively. Clomiphene binds to both ER α and ER β, but the individual isomers have not been examined (Kuiper *et al.,* 1997).

Fulvestrant is a 7α-alkylamide derivative of estradiol that interacts with both ER α and ER β (Van Den Bemd *et al.,* 1999).

Pharmacological Effects

Tamoxifen exhibits anti-estrogenic, estrogenic, or mixed activity depending on the species and target gene measured. In clinical tests or laboratory studies with human cells, the drug's activity depends on the tissue and endpoint measured. For example, tamoxifen inhibits the proliferation of cultured human breast cancer cells and reduces tumor size and number in women (reviewed in Jaiyesimi *et al.,* 1995), and yet it stimulates proliferation of endometrial cells and causes endometrial thickening (Lahti *et al.,* 1993). The drug has an antiresorptive effect on bone, and in humans it decreases total cholesterol, LDL, and lipoprotein (a), but does not increase HDL and triglycerides (Love *et al.,* 1994). Tamoxifen treatment causes a two- to threefold increase in the relative risk of deep vein thrombosis and pulmonary embolism and a roughly twofold increase in endometrial carcinoma (Smith, 2003). Tamoxifen produces hot flashes and other adverse effects, including cataracts and nausea. Due to its agonist activity in bone, it does not increase the incidence of fractures when used in this setting.

ENCLOMIPHENE   TAMOXIFEN

	ENCLOMIPHENE	TAMOXIFEN
R_1:	—CH$_2$CH$_3$	—CH$_3$
R_2:	—Cl	—CH$_2$CH$_3$

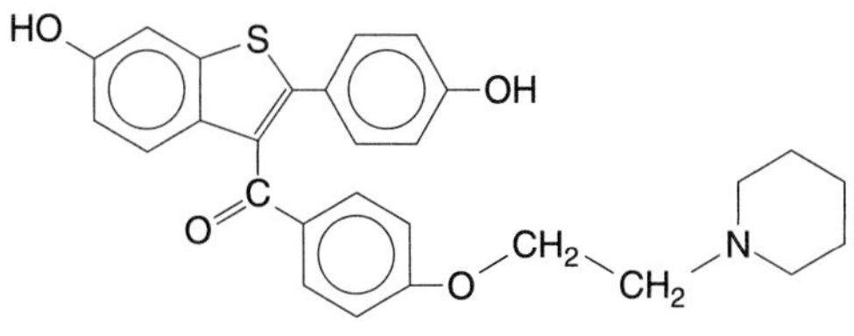

RALOXIFENE

Raloxifene is an estrogen agonist in bone, where it exerts an antiresorptive effect. It reduces the number of vertebral fractures by up to 50% in a dose-dependent manner (Delmas *et al.*, 1997; Ettinger *et al.*, 1999). The drug also acts as an estrogen agonist in reducing total cholesterol and LDL, but it does not increase HDL or normalize plasminogen-activator inhibitor 1 in postmenopausal women (Walsh *et al.*, 1998). Raloxifene does not cause proliferation or thickening of the endometrium. Preclinical studies indicate that raloxifene has an antiproliferative effect on ER-positive breast tumors and on proliferation of ER-positive breast cancer cell lines (Hol *et al.*, 1997) and significantly reduces the risk of ER-positive but not ER-negative breast cancer (Cummings *et al.*, 1999). Raloxifene does not alleviate the vasomotor symptoms associated with menopause. Adverse effects include hot flashes and leg cramps and a threefold increase in deep vein thrombosis and pulmonary embolism (Cummings *et al.*, 1999).

Initial animal studies with clomiphene showed slight estrogenic activity and moderate anti-estrogenic activity, but the most striking effect was the inhibition of pituitary gonadotropes. In contrast, the most prominent effect in women was enlargement of the ovaries, and the drug induced ovulation in many patients with amenorrhea, polycystic ovarian syndrome, and dysfunctional bleeding with anovulatory cycles. This is the basis for clomiphene's major pharmacological use: to induce ovulation in women with a functional hypothalamic-hypophyseal-ovarian system and adequate endogenous estrogen production. In some cases, clomiphene is used in conjunction with human gonadotropins (*see* Chapter 55) to induce ovulation.

Fulvestrant and its less potent forerunner ICI 164,384 have been purely anti-estrogenic in studies to date. *In vitro*, fulvestrant was more potent than 4-hydroxytamoxifen (DeFriend *et al.*, 1994) in inhibiting proliferation of breast cancer cells, and in clinical trials it is efficacious in treating tamoxifen-resistant breast cancers (Robertson *et al.*, 2003).

All of these agents bind to the ligand-binding pocket of both ER α and ER β and competitively block estradiol binding. However, the conformation of the ligand-bound ERs is different with different ligands (Smith and O'Malley, 2004), and this has two important mechanistic consequences. The distinct ER-ligand conformations recruit different co-activators and co-repressors onto the promoter of a target gene by differential protein-protein interactions at the receptor surface. The tissue-specific actions of SERMs thus can be explained in part by the distinct conformation of the ER when occupied by different ligands, in combination with different co-activator and co-repressor levels in different cell types that together affect the nature of ER complexes formed in a tissue-selective fashion.

The conformation of ERs, especially in the AF-2 domain, determines whether a co-activator or a co-repressor will be recruited to the ER-DNA complex (Smith and O'Malley, 2004). While 17β-estradiol induces a conformation that recruits co-activators to the receptor, tamoxifen induces a conformation that permits the recruitment of the co-repressor to both ER α and ER β. The agonist activity of tamoxifen seen in tissues such as the endometrium is mediated by the ligand-independent AF-1 transactivation domain of ER α; since ER β does not contain a functional AF-1 domain, tamoxifen does not activate ER β (McInerney *et al.*, 1998).

Raloxifene acts as a partial agonist in bone but does not stimulate endometrial proliferation in postmenopausal women. Presumably this is due to some combination of differential expression of transcription factors in the two tissues and the effects of this SERM on ER conformation. Raloxifene induces a configuration in ER α that is distinct from that of tamoxifen-ER β (Tamrazi *et al.*, 2003), suggesting that a different set of co-activators/co-repressors may interact with ER-raloxifene compared to ER-tamoxifen.

Clomiphene increases gonadotropin secretion and stimulates ovulation. It increases the amplitude of LH and FSH pulses without changing pulse frequency (Kettel *et al.*, 1993). This suggests that the drug is acting largely at the pituitary level to block inhibitory actions of estrogen on gonadotropin release from the gland, and/or is somehow causing the hypothalamus to release larger amounts of GnRH per pulse.

Fulvestrant binds to ER α and ER β with a high affinity comparable to estradiol, but represses transactivation. It also increases dramatically the intracellular proteolytic degradation of ER α, while apparently protecting ER β from degradation (Van Den Bemd *et al.*, 1999). This effect on ER α protein levels may explain its efficacy in tamoxifen-resistant breast cancer.

Absorption, Fate, and Excretion

Tamoxifen is given orally, and peak plasma levels are reached within 4 to 7 hours after treatment. This drug displays two elimination phases with half-lives of 7 to 14 hours and 4 to 11 days. Due to the prolonged half-life, 3 to 4 weeks of treatment are required to reach steady-state plasma levels. The parent drug is converted largely to metabolites within 4 to 6 hours after oral administration. Tamoxifen is metabolized in humans by multiple hepatic CYPs, some of which it also induces (Sridar *et al.*, 2002). In human beings and other species, 4-hydroxytamoxifen is produced *via* hepatic metabolism, and this compound is considerably more potent than the parent drug as an anti-estrogen. The major route of elimination from the body involves *N*-demethylation and deamination. The drug undergoes enterohepatic circulation, and excretion is primarily in the feces as conjugates of the deaminated metabolite.

Raloxifene is absorbed rapidly after oral administration and has an absolute bioavailability of about 2%. The drug has a half-life of about 28 hours and is eliminated primarily in the feces after hepatic glucuronidation; it does not appear to undergo significant biotransformation by CYPs.

Clomiphene is well absorbed following oral administration, and the drug and its metabolites are eliminated primarily in the feces and to a lesser extent in the urine. The long plasma half-life (5 to 7 days) is due largely to plasma-protein binding, enterohepatic circulation, and accumulation in fatty tissues. Other active metabolites with long half-lives also may be produced.

Fulvestrant is administered monthly by intramuscular depot injections. Plasma concentrations reach maximal levels in 7 days and are maintained for a month. Numerous metabolites are formed *in vivo*, possibly by pathways similar to endogenous estrogen metabolism, but the drug is eliminated primarily (90%) *via* the feces in humans.

Therapeutic Uses

Breast Cancer. Tamoxifen is highly efficacious in the treatment of breast cancer. It is used alone for palliation of advanced breast cancer in women with ER-positive tumors, and it is now indicated as the hormonal treatment of choice for both early and advanced breast cancer in women of all ages (Jaiyesimi *et al.*, 1995). Response rates are approximately 50% in women with ER-positive tumors and 70% for ER- and PR-positive tumors. Tamoxifen increases disease-free survival and overall survival; treatment for 5 years reduces cancer recurrence by 50% and death by 27% and is more efficacious than shorter 1- to 2-year treatment periods. Tamoxifen reduces the risk of developing contralateral breast cancer and is approved for primary prevention of breast cancer in women at high risk, in whom it causes a 50% decrease in the development of new tumors. Prophylactic treatment should be limited to 5 years, as effectiveness decreases thereafter. The most frequent side effect is hot flashes. Tamoxifen has estrogenic activity in the uterus, increases the risk of endometrial cancer by two- to threefold, and also causes a comparable increase in the risk of thromboembolic disease that leads to serious risks for women receiving anticoagulant therapy (Smith, 2003).

Toremifene has therapeutic actions similar to tamoxifen, and fulvestrant may be efficacious in women who become resistant to tamoxifen. Untoward effects of fulvestrant include hot flashes, GI symptoms, headache, back pain, and pharyngitis.

Osteoporosis. Raloxifene reduces the rate of bone loss and may increase bone mass at certain sites. In a large clinical trial, raloxifene increased spinal bone mineral density by more than 2% and reduced the rate of vertebral fractures by 30% to 50%, but did not significantly reduce nonvertebral fractures (Ettinger *et al.*, 1999; Delmas *et al.*, 2002). Raloxifene does not appear to increase the risk of developing endometrial cancer. The drug has beneficial actions on lipoprotein metabolism, reducing both total cholesterol and LDL; however, HDL is not increased. Adverse effects include hot flashes, deep vein thrombosis, and leg cramps.

Infertility. Clomiphene is used primarily for treatment of female infertility due to anovulation. By increasing gonadotropin levels, primarily FSH, it enhances follicular recruitment. It is relatively inexpensive, orally active, and

requires less extensive monitoring than do other treatment protocols. However, the drug may exhibit untoward effects, including ovarian hyperstimulation, increased incidence of multiple births, ovarian cysts, hot flashes, and blurred vision. In addition, clomiphene-induced cycles have a relatively high incidence of luteal phase dysfunction due to inadequate progesterone production, and prolonged use (*e.g.*, 12 or more cycles) may increase the risk of ovarian cancer. The drug should not be administered to pregnant women due to reports of teratogenicity in animals, but there is no evidence of this when the drug has been used to induce ovulation. Clomiphene also may be used to evaluate the male reproductive system, since testosterone feedback on the hypothalamus and pituitary is mediated to a large degree by estrogens formed from aromatization of the androgen.

Experimental SERM-Estrogen Combinations. There is considerable interest in menopausal hormone therapy using combinations of a pure estrogen agonist (*e.g.*, estradiol) with a SERM that has predominantly antagonist activity in the breast and endometrium, but does not distribute to the CNS. The strategy is to obtain the beneficial actions of the agonist (*e.g.*, prevention of hot flashes and bone loss), while the SERM blocks unwanted agonist action at peripheral sites (*e.g.*, proliferative effects in breast and endometrium), but does not enter the brain to cause hot flashes. Animal studies have been encouraging (Labrie *et al.*, 2003), but clinical efficacy and safety of this approach remain to be established.

Estrogen-Synthesis Inhibitors

Several agents can be used to block estrogen biosynthesis. Continual administration of GnRH agonists prevents ovarian synthesis of estrogens but not their peripheral synthesis from adrenal androgens (*see* Chapter 55). *Aminoglutethimide* inhibits aromatase activity, but its use is limited by lack of selectivity (*see* Chapters 51 and 59).

The recognition that locally produced, as well as circulating, estrogens may play a significant role in breast cancer has greatly stimulated interest in the use of aromatase inhibitors to selectively block production of estrogens (*see* Chapter 51). Both steroidal (*e.g., formestane* and *exemestane* [AROMASIN]) and nonsteroidal agents (*e.g., anastrozole* [ARIMIDEX], *letrozole* [FEMARA], and *vorozole*) are available. Steroidal, or type I, agents are substrate analogs that act as suicide inhibitors to irreversibly inactivate aromatase, while the nonsteroidal, or type II, agents interact reversibly with the heme groups of CYPs (Haynes *et al.*, 2003). Exemestane, letrozole, and anastrozole are currently approved in the United States for the treatment of breast cancer. The structures of exemestane and anastrozole are as follows:

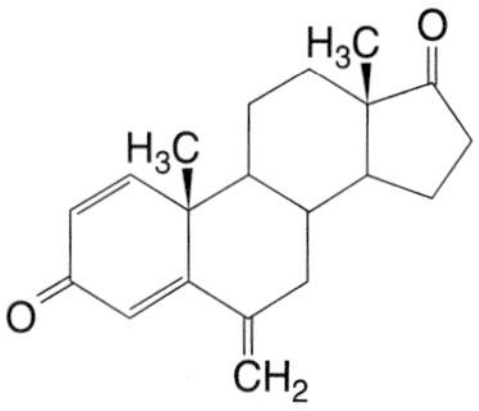

EXEMESTANE

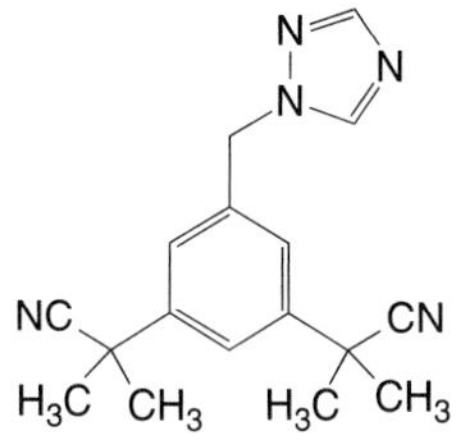

ANASTROZOLE

As discussed in Chapter 51, these agents may be used as first-line treatment of breast cancer or as second-line drugs after tamoxifen. They are highly efficacious and actually superior to tamoxifen in some adjuvant settings (Coombes *et al.*, 2004), but unlike tamoxifen, they do not increase the risk of uterine cancer or venous thromboembolism. Because they dramatically reduce circulating as well as local levels of estrogens, they produce hot flashes. Their potential long-term effects on bone and plasma lipids remain to be established.

There is also great interest in the potential use of aromatase inhibitors for the chemoprevention of breast cancer. These agents decrease estrogen levels and thus block hormonal effects as tumor promoters (*i.e.*, by stimulating cell proliferation), but would also prevent actions of locally produced estrogens to initiate tumors (*i.e.*, *via* formation of DNA-adducts). This would provide a theoretical advantage over tamoxifen, which would only be expected to decrease actions of estrogens as tumor promoters.

PROGESTINS

Compounds with biological activities similar to those of progesterone have been variously referred to in the literature as progestins, progestational agents, progestagens, progestogens, gestagens, or gestogens. The progestins (Figure 57–5) include the naturally occurring hormone progesterone, 17α-acetoxyprogesterone derivatives in the

pregnane series, 19-nortestosterone derivatives (estranes), and *norgestrel* and related compounds in the gonane series. Medroxyprogesterone acetate (MPA) and *megestrol acetate* are C21 steroids with selective activity very similar to that of progesterone itself. MPA and oral micronized progesterone are widely used with estrogens for menopausal hormone therapy and other situations in which a selective progestational effect is desired, and a depot form of MPA is used as a long-acting injectable contraceptive. The 19-nortestosterone derivatives were developed for use as progestins in oral contraceptives, and while their predominant activity is progestational, they exhibit androgenic and other activities. The gonanes are a more recently developed series of "19-nor" compounds, containing an ethyl rather than a methyl substituent in the 13-position, and they have diminished androgenic activity. These two classes of 19-nortestosterone derivatives are the progestational components of all oral and some long-acting injectable contraceptives.

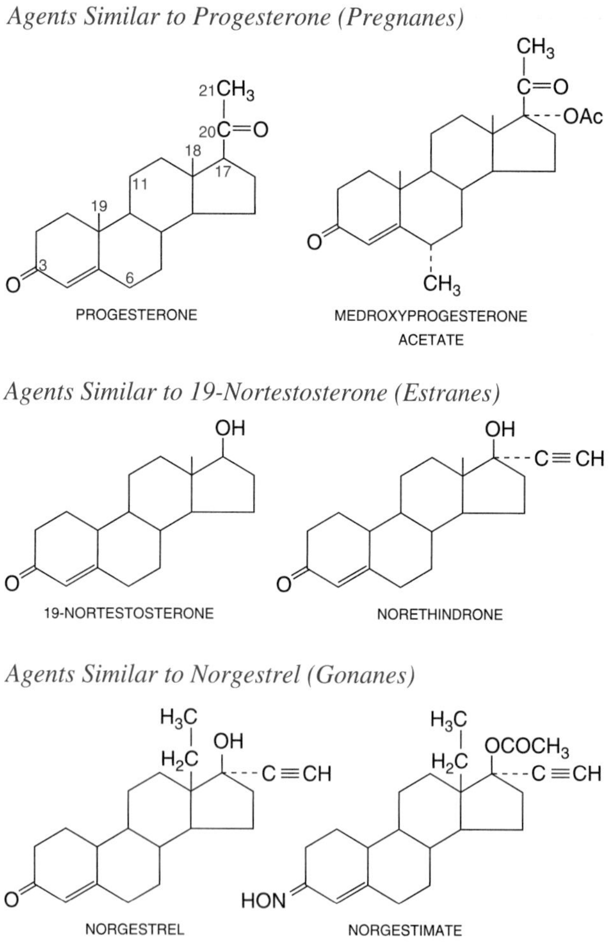

Agents Similar to Progesterone (Pregnanes)

PROGESTERONE   MEDROXYPROGESTERONE ACETATE

Agents Similar to 19-Nortestosterone (Estranes)

19-NORTESTOSTERONE   NORETHINDRONE

Agents Similar to Norgestrel (Gonanes)

NORGESTREL   NORGESTIMATE

Figure 57–5. *Structural features of various progestins.*

History. Corner and Allen originally isolated a hormone in 1933 from the corpora lutea of sows and named it "progestin." The next year, several European groups independently isolated the crystalline compound and called it "luteo-sterone," unaware of the previous name. This difference in nomenclature was resolved in 1935 at a garden party in London given by Sir Henry Dale, who helped persuade all parties that the name "progesterone" was a suitable compromise.

Two major advances overcame the early difficulties and astronomical expense of obtaining progesterone from animal sources. The first was the synthesis of progesterone by Russel Marker from the plant product diosgenin in the 1940s, which provided relatively inexpensive and highly pure product. The second was the synthesis of 19-nor compounds, the first orally active progestins, in the early 1950s by Carl Djerassi, who synthesized norethindrone at Syntex, and Frank Colton, who synthesized the isomer *norethynodrel* at Searle. These advances led to the development of effective oral contraceptives.

Chemistry. Unlike the ER, which requires a phenolic A ring for high-affinity binding, the progesterone receptor (PR) favors a Δ^4-3-one A-ring structure in an inverted 1β, 2α-conformation (Duax *et al.*, 1988). Other steroid hormone receptors also bind this nonphenolic A-ring structure, although the optimal conformation differs from that for the PR. Thus, some synthetic progestins (especially the 19-nor compounds) display limited binding to glucocorticoid, androgen, and mineralocorticoid receptors, a property that probably accounts for some of their nonprogestational activities. The spectrum of activities of these compounds is highly dependent upon specific substituent groups, especially the nature of the C17 substituent in the D ring, the presence of a C19 methyl group, and the presence of an ethyl group at position C13.

One major class of agents is similar to progesterone and its metabolite 17α-hydroxyprogesterone (Figure 57–5). Compounds such as hydroxyprogesterone caproate have progestational activity but must be used parenterally due to first-pass hepatic metabolism. However, further substitutions at the 6-position of the B ring yield orally active compounds such as medroxyprogesterone acetate and megestrol acetate with selective progestational activity.

The second major class of agents is 19-nor testosterone derivatives. These testosterone derivatives, lacking the C19 methyl group, display primarily progestational rather than androgenic activity. An ethinyl substituent at C17 decreases hepatic metabolism and yields orally active 19-nortestosterone analogs such as norethindrone, norethindrone acetate, norethynodrel, and *ethynodiol diacetate*. The activity of the latter three compounds is due primarily to their rapid *in vivo* conversion to norethindrone. These compounds are less selective than the 17α-hydroxyprogesterone derivatives mentioned above and have varying degrees of androgenic activity, and to a lesser extent, estrogenic and anti-estrogenic activities.

Replacement of the 13-methyl group of norethindrone with a 13-ethyl substituent yields the gonane *norgestrel,* which is a more potent progestin than the parent compound but has less androgenic activity. Norgestrel is a racemic mixture of an inactive dextrorotatory isomer and the active levorotatory isomer, levonorgestrel. Preparations containing half as much levonorgestrel as norgestrel thus have equivalent pharmacological activity. Other gonanes—including norgestimate, *desogestrel,* and *gestodene* (not available in the United States)—are reported to have very little if any androgenic activity at therapeutic doses (Rebar and Zeserson, 1991).

Newer steroidal progestins include the gonane *dienogest*; 19-nor-progestin derivatives (*e.g., nomegestrol, nestorone,* and *trimegestone*), which have increased selectivity for the progesterone receptor and less androgenic activity than estranes; and the spironolactone derivative *drospirenone*, which is used in a combination oral contraceptive. Like spironolactone, drospirenone is also a mineralocorticoid receptor antagonist. In addition, efforts are currently underway to develop novel, nonsteroidal progestins, as these may have less affinity for other steroid receptors.

Synthesis and Secretion. Progesterone is secreted by the ovary, mainly from the corpus luteum, during the second half of the menstrual cycle (Figure 57–3). The stimulatory effect of LH on progesterone synthesis and secretion is mediated by a receptor that couples to the G_s–adenylyl cyclase–cyclic AMP pathway (*see* Chapter 55).

After fertilization, the trophoblast secretes hCG into the maternal circulation to sustain the corpus luteum. During the second or third month of pregnancy, the developing placenta begins to secrete estrogen and progesterone in collaboration with the fetal adrenal glands, and thereafter the corpus luteum is not essential to continued gestation. Estrogen and progesterone continue to be secreted in large amounts by the placenta up to the time of delivery.

Physiological and Pharmacological Actions

Neuroendocrine Actions. As discussed previously, progesterone produced in the luteal phase of the cycle has several physiological effects including decreasing the frequency of GnRH pulses, which is the major mechanism of action of progestin-containing contraceptives.

Reproductive Tract. Progesterone decreases estrogen-driven endometrial proliferation and leads to the development of a secretory endometrium (Figure 57–3), and the abrupt decline in progesterone at the end of the cycle is the main determinant of the onset of menstruation. If the duration of the luteal phase is artificially lengthened, either by sustaining luteal function or by treatment with progesterone, decidual changes in the endometrial stroma similar to those seen in early pregnancy can be induced. Under normal circumstances, estrogen antecedes and accompanies progesterone in its action upon the endometrium and is essential to the development of the normal menstrual pattern.

Progesterone also influences the endocervical glands, and the abundant watery secretion of the estrogen-stimulated structures is changed to a scant, viscid material. As noted previously, these and other effects of progestins decrease penetration of the cervix by sperm.

The estrogen-induced maturation of the human vaginal epithelium is modified toward the condition of pregnancy by the action of progesterone, a change that can be detected in cytological alterations in the vaginal smear. If the quantity of estrogen concurrently acting is known to be adequate, or if it is assured by giving estrogen, the cytological response to a progestin can be used to evaluate its progestational potency.

Progesterone is very important for the maintenance of pregnancy. Progesterone suppresses menstruation and uterine contractility, but other effects also may be important. These effects to maintain pregnancy led to the historical use of progestins to prevent threatened abortion. However, such treatment is of questionable benefit, probably because spontaneous abortion infrequently results from diminished progesterone. Based on a recent report that premature labor in high-risk mothers was diminished by weekly intramuscular administration of *17-hydroxy-progesterone* (DELALUTIN), this indication is being re-evaluated (Meis *et al.*, 2003).

Mammary Gland. Development of the mammary gland requires both estrogen and progesterone. During pregnancy and to a minor degree during the luteal phase of the cycle, progesterone, acting with estrogen, brings about a proliferation of the acini of the mammary gland. Toward the end of pregnancy, the acini fill with secretions and the vasculature of the gland notably increases; however, only after the levels of estrogen and progesterone decrease at parturition does lactation begin.

During the normal menstrual cycle, mitotic activity in the breast epithelium is very low in the follicular phase and then peaks in the luteal phase. This pattern is due to progesterone, which triggers a *single* round of mitotic activity in the mammary epithelium. This effect is transient, however, and continued exposure to the hormone is rapidly followed by arrest of growth of the epithelial cells. As described above, progesterone may be responsible for the increased risk of breast cancer associated with estrogen-progestin use in postmenopausal women (Anderson *et al.*, 2004; Rossouw *et al.*, 2002).

CNS Effects. During a normal menstrual cycle, an increase in basal body temperature of about 0.6°C (1°F) may be noted at mid-cycle; this correlates with ovulation. This increase is due to progesterone, but the exact mechanism of this effect is unknown. Progesterone also increases the ventilatory response of the respiratory centers to carbon dioxide and leads to reduced arterial and alveolar P_{CO_2} in the luteal phase of the menstrual cycle and during pregnancy. Progesterone also may have depressant and hypnotic actions in the CNS, possibly accounting for reports of drowsiness after hormone administration. This potential untoward effect may be abrogated by giving progesterone preparations at bedtime, which may even help some patients sleep.

Metabolic Effects. Progestins have numerous metabolic actions. Progesterone itself increases basal insulin levels and the rise in insulin after carbohydrate ingestion, but it does not normally alter glucose tolerance. However, long-term administration of more potent progestins, such as norgestrel, may decrease glucose tolerance. Progesterone stimulates lipoprotein lipase activity and seems to enhance fat deposition. Progesterone and analogs such as MPA have been reported to increase LDL and cause either no effects or modest reductions in serum HDL levels. The 19-norprogestins may have more pronounced effects on plasma lipids because of their androgenic activity. In this regard, a large prospective study has shown that MPA decreases the favorable HDL increase caused by conjugated estrogens during postmenopausal hormone replacement, but does not significantly affect the beneficial effect of estrogens to lower LDL. In contrast, micronized progesterone does not significantly affect beneficial estrogen effects on either HDL or LDL profiles (Writing Group for the PEPI Trial, 1995). Progesterone also may diminish the effects of aldosterone in the renal tubule and cause a decrease in sodium reabsorption that may increase mineralocorticoid secretion from the adrenal cortex.

Mechanism of Action

There is a single gene that encodes two isoforms of the progesterone receptor (PR): PR-A and PR-B. The first 164 N-terminal amino acids of PR-B are missing from PR-A; this occurs by use of two distinct estrogen-dependent promoters in the PR gene (Giangrande and McDonnell, 1999). The ratios of the individual isoforms vary in reproductive tissues as a consequence of tissue type, developmental status, and hormone levels. Both PR-A and PR-B have AF-1 and AF-2 transactivation domains, but the longer PR-B also contains an additional AF-3 that contributes to its cell- and promoter-specific activity. Since the ligand-binding domains of the two PR isoforms are identical, there is no difference in ligand binding. In the absence of ligand, PR is present in the nucleus in an inactive monomeric state bound to heat-shock proteins (HSP-90, HSP-70, and p59). Upon binding progesterone, the heat-shock proteins dissociate, and the receptors are phosphorylated and subsequently form dimers (homo- and heterodimers) that bind with high selectivity to PREs (progesterone response elements) located on target genes (Giangrande and McDonnell, 1999). Transcriptional activation by PR occurs primarily *via* recruitment of co-activators such as SRC-1, NcoA-1, or NcoA-2 (Collingwood *et al.*, 1999). The receptor–co-activator complex then favors further interactions with additional proteins such as CBP and p300, which have histone acetylase activity. Histone acetylation causes a remodeling of chromatin that increases the accessibility of general transcriptional proteins, including RNA polymerase II, to the target promoter. Progesterone antagonists also facilitate receptor dimerization and DNA binding, but, as with ER, the conformation of antagonist-bound PR is different from that of agonist-bound PR. This different conformation favors PR interaction with co-repressors such as NcoR/SMRT, which recruit histone deacetylases. Histone deacetylation increases DNA interaction with nucleosomes and renders a target promoter inaccessible to the general transcription apparatus.

The biological activities of PR-A and PR-B are distinct and depend on the target gene in question. In most cells, PR-B mediates the stimulatory activities of progesterone; PR-A strongly inhibits this action of PR-B (Vegeto *et al.*, 1993) and is also a transcriptional inhibitor of other steroid receptors (McDonnell and Goldman, 1994). Current data suggest that co-activators and co-repressors interact differentially with PR-A and PR-B, *e.g.*, the co-repressor SMRT binds much more tightly to PR-A than to PR-B (Giangrande *et al.*, 2000), and this may account, at least in part, for the differential activities of the two isoforms. Female PR-A knockout mice are infertile, with impaired ovulation and defective decidualization and implantation. Several uterine genes appear to be regulated exclusively by PR-A, including calcitonin and amphiregulin (Mulac-Jericevic *et al.*, 2000), and the antiproliferative effect of progesterone on the estrogen-stimulated endometrium is lost in PR-A knockout mice. In contrast, knockout studies suggest that PR-B is largely responsible for mediating hormone effects in the mammary gland (Mulac-Jericevic *et al.*, 2003).

Certain effects of progesterone, such as increased Ca^{2+} mobilization in sperm, can be seen in as little as 3 minutes (Blackmore, 1999), and these effects are caused by nongenomic mechanisms involving membrane-bound progesterone receptors that are not derived from the gene encoding PR-A/PR-B (Losel *et al.*, 2004). The pharmacological importance of these membrane-bound receptors has not been determined.

Absorption, Fate, and Excretion

Progesterone undergoes rapid first-pass metabolism, but high-dose (*e.g.*, 100 to 200 mg) preparations of micronized progesterone (PROMETRIUM) are available for oral use. Although the absolute bioavailability of these preparations is low (Fotherby, 1996), efficacious plasma levels nevertheless may be obtained. Progesterone also is available in oil solution for injection, as a vaginal gel (CRINONE, PROCHIEVE), and as a slow-release intrauterine device (PROGESTA-SERT) for contraception.

Esters such as *hydroxyprogesterone caproate* (HYALUTIN) and MPA (DEPO-PROVERA) are available for intramuscular administration, and MPA (PROVERA, others) and megestrol acetate (MEGACE) may be used orally due to decreased hepatic metabolism. The 19-nor steroids have good oral activity because the ethinyl substituent at C17 significantly slows hepatic metabolism. Implants and depot preparations of synthetic progestins are available in many countries for release over very long periods of time (*see* later section on contraceptives).

In the plasma, progesterone is bound by albumin and corticosteroid-binding globulin, but is not appreciably bound to SHBG. 19-Nor compounds, such as norethindrone, norgestrel, and desogestrel, bind to SHBG and albumin, and esters such as MPA bind primarily to albumin. Total binding of all these synthetic compounds to plasma proteins is extensive, 90% or more, but the proteins involved are compound-specific.

The elimination half-life of progesterone is approximately 5 minutes, and the hormone is metabolized primarily in the liver to hydroxylated metabolites and their sulfate and glucuronide conjugates, which are eliminated in the urine. A major metabolite specific for progesterone is pregnane-3α, 20α-diol; its measurement in urine and plasma is used as an index of endogenous progesterone secretion. The synthetic progestins have much longer half-lives, *e.g.*, approximately 7 hours for norethindrone, 16 hours for norgestrel, 12 hours for gestodene, and 24 hours for MPA. The metabolism of synthetic progestins is thought to be primarily hepatic, and elimination is generally *via* the urine as conjugates and various polar metabolites, although their metabolism is not as clearly defined as that of progesterone.

Therapeutic Uses

The two most frequent uses of progestins are for contraception, either alone or with an estrogen (*see* below), and in combination with estrogen for hormone therapy of postmenopausal women (*see* above).

Progestins also are used for secondary amenorrhea, abnormal uterine bleeding in patients without underlying organic pathology (*e.g.*, fibroids or cancer), luteal-phase support to treat infertility, and premature labor. Among the oral progestins used besides MPA in these settings is norethindrone acetate (AYGESTIN). In general, these uses of oral progestins are extensions of the physiological actions of progesterone on the neuroendocrine control of ovarian function and on the endometrium.

Progesterone can be used diagnostically to test for estrogen secretion and for responsiveness of the endometrium. After administration of progesterone to amenorrheic women for 5 to 7 days, withdrawal bleeding will occur if the endometrium has been stimulated by endogenous estrogens. Combinations of estrogens and progestins also can be used to test endometrial responsiveness in patients with amenorrhea.

As described above, progestins are highly efficacious in decreasing the occurrence of endometrial hyperplasia and carcinoma caused by unopposed estrogens; when used in this setting, there appears to be less irregular uterine bleeding with sequential rather than continuous administration. When used to decrease estrogen-induced endometrial hyperplasia, local intrauterine application *via* a hormone-releasing IUD would be a rational approach to prevent untoward effects (*e.g.*, unfavorable lipid profiles and incidence of breast cancer) of systemically administered progestins. Progestins are also used as a palliative measure for metastatic endometrial carcinoma, but adjuvant therapy after surgery does not significantly reduce cancer-related deaths; megestrol acetate is used as a second-line treatment for breast cancer. Megestrol acetate is also used off-label for AIDS-related wasting.

ANTI-PROGESTINS AND PROGESTERONE-RECEPTOR MODULATORS

The first report of an anti-progestin, RU 38486 (often referred to as RU-486) or *mifepristone,* appeared in 1981;

this drug is available for the termination of pregnancy (Christin-Maitre *et al.*, 2000). Anti-progestins also have several other potential applications, including uses as contraceptives, to induce labor, and to treat uterine leiomyomas, endometriosis, meningiomas, and breast cancer (Spitz and Chwalisz, 2000).

Mifepristone

Chemistry. Mifepristone is a derivative of the 19-norprogestin norethindrone containing a dimethyl-aminophenol substituent at the 11β-position. It effectively competes with both progesterone and glucocorticoids for binding to their respective receptors. Mifepristone was initially thought to be a pure anti-progestin; this is its predominant activity in most situations, but it also has some agonist activity. Thus it is now considered a progesterone-receptor modulator (PRM) due to its context-dependent activity.

Other PRMs and pure progesterone antagonists now have been synthesized, and most contain an 11β-aromatic group. Another widely studied anti-progestin is *onapristone* (or ZK 98299), which is similar in structure to mifepristone but contains a methyl substituent in the 13α rather than 13β orientation. More selective progesterone-receptor modulators, such as *asoprisnil*, are being studied experimentally (DeManno *et al.*, 2003). Mifepristone and onapristone have the following structures:

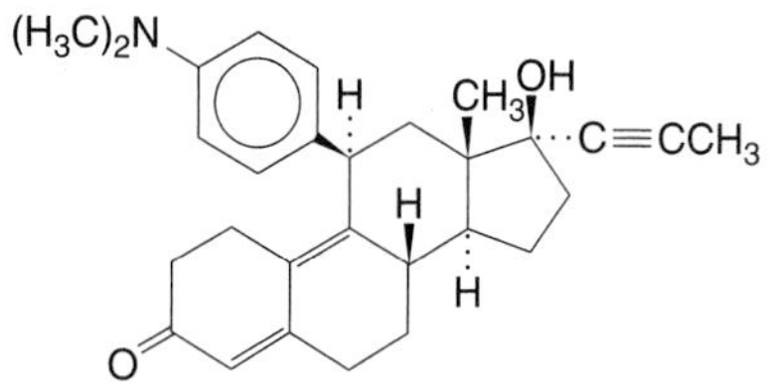

MIFEPRISTONE

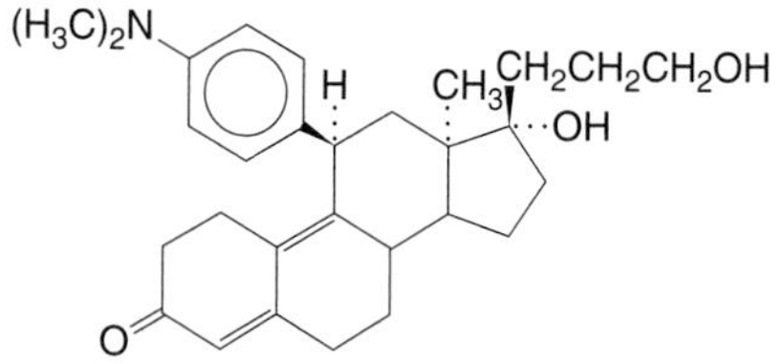

ONAPRISTONE

Pharmacological Actions. In the presence of progestins, mifepristone acts as a competitive receptor antagonist for both progesterone receptors. While mifepristone acts primarily as an antagonist *in vivo,* it exhibits some agonist activity in certain *in vivo* and *in vitro* contexts. In contrast, onapristone appears to be a pure progesterone antagonist both *in vivo* and *in vitro.* PR complexes of both compounds antagonize the actions of progesterone-PR complexes and also appear to preferentially recruit co-repressors (Leonhardt and Edwards, 2002).

When administered in the early stages of pregnancy, mifepristone causes decidual breakdown by blockade of uter-

ine progesterone receptors. This leads to detachment of the blastocyst, which decreases hCG production. This in turn causes a decrease in progesterone secretion from the corpus luteum, which further accentuates decidual breakdown. Decreased endogenous progesterone coupled with blockade of progesterone receptors in the uterus increases uterine prostaglandin levels and sensitizes the myometrium to their contractile actions. Mifepristone also causes cervical softening, which facilitates expulsion of the detached blastocyst.

Mifepristone can delay or prevent ovulation depending upon the timing and manner of administration. These effects are due largely to actions on the hypothalamus and pituitary rather than the ovary, although the mechanisms are unclear.

If administered for one or several days in the mid- to late luteal phase, mifepristone impairs the development of a secretory endometrium and produces menses. Progesterone-receptor blockade at this time is the pharmacological equivalent of progesterone withdrawal, and bleeding normally ensues within several days and lasts for 1 to 2 weeks after anti-progestin treatment.

Mifepristone also binds to glucocorticoid and androgen receptors and exerts anti-glucocorticoid and anti-androgenic actions. A predominant effect in humans is blockade of the feedback inhibition by cortisol of ACTH secretion from the pituitary, thus increasing both corticotropin and adrenal steroid levels in the plasma (*see* Chapter 59 for further discussion of effects on the hypothalamic-pituitary-adrenal axis). Onapristone also binds to both glucocorticoid and androgen receptors, but has less anti-glucocorticoid activity than does mifepristone.

Absorption, Fate, and Excretion. Mifepristone is orally active with good bioavailability. Peak plasma levels occur within several hours, and the drug is slowly cleared with a plasma half-life of 20 to 40 hours. In plasma, it is bound by α_1-acid glycoprotein, which contributes to its long half-life. Metabolites are primarily the mono- and di-demethylated products (which are thought to have pharmacological activity) formed *via* CYP3A4-catalyzed reactions, and to a lesser extent, hydroxylated compounds. The drug undergoes hepatic metabolism and enterohepatic circulation, and metabolic products are found predominantly in the feces (Jang and Benet, 1997).

Therapeutic Uses and Prospects. Mifepristone (MIFEPREX), in combination with *misoprostol* or other prostaglandins (*see* below), is available for the termination of early pregnancy. When mifepristone is used to produce a medical abortion, a prostaglandin is given 48 hours after the anti-progestin to further increase myometrial contractions and ensure expulsion of the detached blastocyst. Intramuscular *sulprostone,* intravaginal *gemeprost,* and oral misoprostol have been used. The success rate with such regimens is >90% among women with pregnancies of 49 days' duration or less. The most severe untoward effect is vaginal bleeding, which most often lasts from 8 to 17 days, but is only rarely (0.1% of patients) severe enough to require blood transfusions. High percentages of women also have experienced abdominal pain and uterine cramps, nausea, vomiting, and diarrhea due to the prostaglandin. Women receiving chronic glucocorticoid therapy should not be given mifepristone because of its anti-glucocorticoid activity, and the drug should be used very cautiously in women who are anemic or receiving anticoagulants. Women over 35 years old with cardiovascular risk factors should not be given sulprostone because of possible heart failure (Christin-Maitre *et al.*, 2000).

Other investigational or potential uses for mifepristone that are under development include the induction of labor after fetal death; the induction of labor at the end of the third trimester; treatment of endometriosis, leiomyomas, breast cancer, and meningiomas; and as a postcoital or luteal-phase contraceptive (Spitz and Chwalisz, 2000). A major concern about long-term use is the possibility of unopposed estrogenic effects, but this concern could be allayed by further development of selective progesterone-receptor modulators.

HORMONAL CONTRACEPTIVES

Oral contraceptives are among the most widely used agents in the United States and throughout the world and have had a revolutionary impact on global society. For the first time in history, they provided a convenient, affordable, and completely reliable means of contraception for family planning and the avoidance of unplanned pregnancies.

It is important to consider several key points as a prelude to the pharmacology of specific hormonal contraceptives: (1) A variety of agents with substantially different components, doses, and side effects are available and provide real therapeutic options; (2) In addition to contraceptive actions, these agents have substantial health benefits; (3) Because of differences in doses and specific compounds used, it is not appropriate to extrapolate directly untoward effects of hormonal contraceptives to menopausal hormone therapy, or *vice versa*. Oral contraceptives are now extremely effective and have a low incidence of untoward effects for most women.

History. Around the beginning of the twentieth century, a number of European scientists including Beard, Prenant, and Loeb developed the concept that secretions of the corpus luteum suppressed ovulation during pregnancy. The Austrian physiologist Haberlandt then produced temporary sterility in rodents in 1927 by feeding ovarian and placental extracts—a clear example of an oral contraceptive! In 1937 it was shown by Makepeace and colleagues that pure progesterone blocked ovulation in rabbits, and Astwood and Fevold found a similar effect in rats in 1939.

In the 1950s, Pincus, Garcia, and Rock found that progesterone and 19-nor progestins prevented ovulation in women. Ironically, this finding grew out of their attempts to treat infertility with progestins or estrogen-progestin combinations. The initial findings were that either treatment effectively blocked ovulation in the majority of women. However, concern about cancer and other possible side effects of the estrogen they used (*i.e.,* diethylstilbestrol) led to the use of a progestin alone in their studies.

One of the compounds used was norethynodrel, and early batches of this compound were contaminated with a small amount of mestranol. When mestranol was removed, it was noted that treatment with pure norethynodrel led to increased breakthrough bleeding and less consistent inhibition of ovulation. Mestranol was thus re-incorporated into the preparation, and this combination was employed in the first large-scale clinical trial of combination oral contraceptives.

Clinical studies in the 1950s in Puerto Rico and Haiti established the virtually complete contraceptive success of the norethynodrel-mestranol combination. In late 1959, ENOVID (norethynodrel plus mestranol; no longer marketed in the United States) was the first "Pill" approved by the FDA for use as a contraceptive agent in the United States; this was followed in 1962 by approval for ORTHO-NOVUM (norethindrone plus mestranol). By 1966 numerous preparations utilizing either mestranol or ethinyl estradiol with a 19-nor progestin were available. In the 1960s, the progestin-only minipill and long-acting injectable preparations were developed and introduced.

Millions of women began using oral contraceptives, and frequent reports of untoward effects began appearing in the 1970s (Kols *et al.*, 1982). The recognition that these side effects were dose-dependent and the realization that estrogens and progestins synergistically inhibited ovulation led to the reduction of doses and the development of so-called low-dose or second-generation contraceptives. The increasing use of biphasic and triphasic preparations throughout the 1980s further reduced steroid dosages; it may be that currently used doses are the lowest that will provide reliable contraception. In the 1990s, the "third-generation" oral contraceptives, containing progestins with reduced androgenic activity (*e.g.,* norgestimate [CYCLEN, ORTHO TRI-CYCLEN LO] and desogestrel [DESOGEN]), became available in the United States after being used in Europe. Products containing gestodene as a progestin with reduced androgenic activity also are available in Europe. Another major development in the 1980s was the widespread realization that oral contraceptives have a number of substantial health benefits. More recently, a variety of contraceptive formulations have become available and now include pills, injections providing 1 or 3 months of contraceptive coverage, skin patches, subcutaneous implants, vaginal rings, and intrauterine devices that release hormones.

Types of Hormonal Contraceptives

Combination Oral Contraceptives. The most frequently used agents in the United States are combination oral contraceptives containing both an estrogen and a progestin. Their theoretical efficacy generally is considered to be 99.9%. Ethinyl estradiol and mestranol are the two estrogens used (with ethinyl estradiol being much more frequently used); several progestins currently are used, with levonorgestrel probably being the most common worldwide. The progestins are 19-nor compounds in the estrane or gonane series, and each has varying degrees of androgenic, estrogenic, and anti-estrogenic activities that may be responsible for some of their side effects. Compounds such as desogestrel and norgestimate are the most recently developed and have less androgenic activity than other 19-nor compounds.

Combination oral contraceptives are available in many formulations. Monophasic, biphasic, or triphasic pills are generally provided in 21-day packs. For the monophasic agents, fixed amounts of the estrogen and progestin are present in each pill, which is taken daily for 21 days, followed by a 7-day "pill-free" period. (Virtually all preparations come as 28-day packs, with the pills for the last 7 days containing only inert ingredients.) The biphasic and triphasic preparations provide two or three different pills containing varying amounts of active ingredients, to be taken at different times during the 21-day cycle. This reduces the total amount of steroids administered and more closely approximates the estrogen-to-progestin ratios that occur during the menstrual cycle. With these preparations, predictable menstrual bleeding generally occurs during the 7-day "off" period each month. In 2003, the FDA approved a norgestrel–ethinyl estradiol combination (SEASONALE) that is taken continuously for 84 days followed by 7 days of placebo tablets; this reduces menstrual bleeding to once every 13 weeks. Additional options include a once-monthly medroxyprogesterone–estradiol cypionate injectable (LUNELLE), an ethinyl estradiol–*norelgestromin* (the active metabolite of norgestimate) patch (ORTHO EVRA) applied weekly, and an ethinyl estradiol–*etonogestrel* (the active metabolite of desogestrel) flexible vaginal ring (NUVARING) used for 3 weeks (followed by a removal for 1 week that leads to menstrual bleeding).

The estrogen content of current preparations ranges from 20 to 50 μg; the majority contain 30 to 35 μg. Preparations containing 35 μg or less of an estrogen are generally referred to as "low-dose" or "modern" pills. The dose of progestin is more variable because of differences in potency of the compounds used. For example, monophasic pills currently available in the United States contain 0.4 to 1 mg of norethindrone, 0.1 to 0.15 mg of levonorgestrel, 0.3 to 0.5 mg of norgestrel, 1 mg of ethynodiol diacetate, 0.25 mg of norgestimate, and 0.15 mg of desogestrel, with slightly different dose ranges in biphasic and triphasic preparations. In contrast, most first-generation preparations (circa 1966) contained 50 to 100 μg of an estrogen and 2 to 10 mg of a progestin. These large differences in doses complicate extrapolation of data from early epidemiological studies on the side effects of "high-dose" oral contraceptives to the "low-dose" preparations now used.

Progestin-Only Contraceptives. Several agents are available for progestin-only contraception. They are only slightly less efficacious than combination oral contraceptives, with reports of theoretical efficacy of 99%. Specific preparations include the "minipill"; low doses of progestins (*e.g.*, 350 μg of norethindrone [NOR-QD, MICRONOR] or 75 μg of norgestrel [OVRETTE]) taken daily without interruption; subdermal implants of 216 mg of norgestrel (NOR-PLANT II, JADELLE) for slow release and resultant long-term contraceptive action (*e.g.*, up to 5 years); and crystalline suspensions of medroxyprogesterone acetate (DEPO-PROVERA) for intramuscular injection of 150 mg of drug, which provides effective contraception for 3 months.

An intrauterine device (PROGESTASERT) that releases low amounts of progesterone locally is available for insertion on a yearly basis. Its effectiveness is considered to be 97% to 98%, and contraceptive action probably is due to local effects on the endometrium. Another intrauterine device (MIRENA) releases levonorgestrel for up to 5 years. It inhibits ovulation in some women but is thought to act primarily by producing local effects.

Postcoital or Emergency Contraceptives. High doses of diethylstilbestrol and other estrogens once were used

for postcoital contraception (the "morning-after pill") but never received FDA approval for this indication. The FDA has now approved two preparations for postcoital contraception. PLAN-B is two doses of the "minipill" (0.75 mg levonorgestrel per pill) separated by 12 hours. PREVEN is two 2-pill doses of a high-dose oral contraceptive (0.25 mg of levonorgestrel and 0.05 mg of ethinyl estradiol per pill) separated by 12 hours. This is sometimes referred to as the "Yuzpe" method after the Canadian physician who pioneered its use. The FDA also has declared other products with the same or very similar composition safe and effective for use as emergency contraceptive pills.

The first dose of such preparations should be taken anytime within 72 hours after intercourse, and this should be followed 12 hours later by a second dose. This treatment reduces the risk of pregnancy following unprotected intercourse by approximately 60% for the Yuzpe method and 80% for levonorgestrel alone. With either preparation, effectiveness appears to increase the sooner after intercourse the pills are taken (Task Force on Postovulatory Methods of Fertility Regulation, 1998).

Mechanism of Action

Combination Oral Contraceptives. Combination oral contraceptives act by preventing ovulation (Lobo and Stanczyk, 1994). Direct measurements of plasma hormone levels indicate that LH and FSH levels are suppressed, a mid-cycle surge of LH is absent, endogenous steroid levels are diminished, and ovulation does not occur. While either component alone can be shown to exert these effects in certain situations, the combination synergistically decreases plasma gonadotropin levels and suppresses ovulation more consistently than either alone.

Given the multiple actions of estrogens and progestins on the hypothalamic-pituitary-ovarian axis during the menstrual cycle and the extraordinary efficacy of these agents, several effects probably contribute to the blockade of ovulation.

Hypothalamic actions of steroids play a major role in the mechanism of oral contraceptive action. Progesterone clearly diminishes the frequency of GnRH pulses. Since the proper frequency of LH pulses is essential for ovulation, this effect of progesterone likely plays a major role in the contraceptive action of these agents. In monkeys and women with normal menstrual cycles, estrogens do not affect the frequency of the pulse generator. However, in the prolonged absence of a menstrual cycle (e.g., in ovariectomized monkeys and postmenopausal women; Hotchkiss and Knobil, 1994), estrogens markedly diminish pulse-generator frequency, and progesterone enhances this effect. In theory, this hypothalamic effect of estrogens could come into play when oral contraceptives are used for extended time periods.

Multiple pituitary effects of both estrogen and progestin components are thus likely to contribute to oral contraceptive action. Oral contraceptives seem likely to decrease pituitary responsiveness to GnRH. Estrogens also suppress FSH release from the pituitary during the follicular phase of the menstrual cycle, and this effect seems likely to contribute to the lack of follicular development in oral contraceptive users. Pharmacologically, the progestin component may also inhibit the estrogen-induced LH surge at mid-cycle. Other effects may contribute to a minor extent to the extraordinary efficacy of oral contraceptives. Transit of sperm, the egg, and fertilized ovum are important to establish pregnancy, and steroids are likely to affect transport in the fallopian tube. In the cervix, progestin effects also are likely to produce a thick, viscous mucus to reduce sperm penetration and in the endometrium to produce a state that is not receptive to implantation. However, it is difficult to assess quantitatively the contributions of these effects because the drugs block ovulation so effectively.

Progestin-Only Contraceptives. Progestin-only pills and levonorgestrel implants are highly efficacious but block ovulation in only 60% to 80% of cycles. Their effectiveness is thus thought to be due largely to a thickening of cervical mucus, which decreases sperm penetration, and to endometrial alterations that impair implantation; such local effects account for the efficacy of intrauterine devices that release progestins. Depot injections of MPA are thought to exert similar effects, but they also yield plasma levels of drug high enough to prevent ovulation in virtually all patients, presumably by decreasing the frequency of GnRH pulses.

Emergency Contraceptive Pills. Multiple mechanisms are likely to contribute to the efficacy of these agents, but their precise contributions are unknown (Glasier, 1997). Some studies have shown that ovulation is inhibited or delayed, but additional mechanisms thought to play a role include alterations in endometrial receptivity for implantation; interference with functions of the corpus luteum that maintain pregnancy; production of a cervical mucus that decreases sperm penetration; alterations in tubular transport of sperm, egg, or embryo; or effects on fertilization. However, emergency contraceptives do not interrupt pregnancy after implantation.

Untoward Effects

Combination Oral Contraceptives. Shortly after the introduction of oral contraceptives, reports of adverse side effects associated with their use began to appear. Many of the side effects were found to be dose dependent, and this led to the development of current low-dose preparations. Untoward effects of early hormonal contraceptives fell into several major categories: adverse cardiovascular effects, including hypertension, myocardial infarction, hemorrhagic or ischemic stroke, and venous thrombosis and embolism; breast, hepatocellular, and cervical cancers; and a number of endocrine and metabolic effects. The current consensus is that low-dose preparations pose minimal health risks in women who have no predisposing

risk factors, and these drugs also provide many beneficial health effects (Burkman *et al.*, 2004).

Cardiovascular Effects. The question of cardiovascular side effects has been re-examined for the newer low-dose oral contraceptives (Sherif, 1999; Burkman *et al.*, 2004). For nonsmokers without other risk factors such as hypertension or diabetes, there is no significant increase in the risk of myocardial infarction or stroke. There is a 28% increase in relative risk for venous thromboembolism, but the estimated absolute increase is very small because the incidence of these events in women without other predisposing factors is low (*e.g.,* roughly half that associated with the risk of venous thromboembolism in pregnancy). Nevertheless, the risk is significantly increased in women who smoke or have other factors that predispose to thrombosis or thromboembolism (Castelli, 1999). Early high-dose combination oral contraceptives caused hypertension in 4% to 5% of normotensive women and increased blood pressure in 10% to 15% of those with pre-existing hypertension. This incidence is much lower with newer, low-dose preparations, and most reported changes in blood pressure are not significant. The cardiovascular risk associated with oral contraceptive use does not appear to persist after use is discontinued. As noted previously, estrogens increase serum HDL and decrease LDL levels, and progestins tend to have the opposite effect. Recent studies of several low-dose preparations have not found significant change in total serum cholesterol or lipoprotein profiles, although slight increases in triglycerides have been reported.

Cancer. Given the growth-promoting effects of estrogens, there has been a long-standing concern that oral contraceptives might increase the incidence of endometrial, cervical, ovarian, breast, and other cancers. These concerns were further heightened in the late 1960s by reports of endometrial changes caused by sequential oral contraceptives, which have since been removed from the market in the United States. However, it is now clear that there is *not* a widespread association between oral contraceptive use and cancer (Westhoff, 1999; Burkman *et al.*, 2004).

Recent epidemiological evidence suggests that combined oral contraceptive use may increase the risk of cervical cancer by about twofold, but only in long-term users (>5 years) with persistent human papilloma virus infection (Moodley, 2004).

There have been reports of increases in the incidence of hepatic adenoma and hepatocellular carcinoma in oral contraceptive users. Current estimates indicate that there is about a doubling in the risk of liver cancer after 4 to 8 years of use. However, these are rare cancers and the absolute increases are small.

The major present concern about the carcinogenic effects of oral contraceptives is focused on breast cancer. Numerous studies have dealt with this issue, and the following general picture has emerged. The risk of breast cancer in women of childbearing age is very low, and current oral contraceptive users in this group have only a very small increase in relative risk of 1.1 to 1.2, depending on other variables. This small increase is not substantially affected by duration of use, dose or type of component, age at first use, or parity. Importantly, 10 years after discontinuation of oral contraceptive use, there is no difference in breast cancer incidence between past users and never users. In addition, breast cancers diagnosed in women who have ever used oral contraceptives are more likely to be localized to the breast and thus easier to treat, *i.e.,* are less likely to have spread to other sites (Westhoff, 1999). Thus, overall there is no significant difference in the cumulative risk of breast cancer between those who have ever used oral contraceptives and those who have never used them.

Combination oral contraceptives do *not* increase the incidence of endometrial cancer, but actually cause a 50% *decrease* in the incidence of this disease, which lasts 15 years after the pills are stopped. This is thought to be due to the inclusion of a progestin, which opposes estrogen-induced proliferation, throughout the entire 21-day cycle of administration. These agents also decrease the incidence of ovarian cancer, and decreased ovarian stimulation by gonadotropins provides a logical basis for this effect. There are accumulating data that oral contraceptive use decreases the risk of colorectal cancer (Fernandez *et al.*, 2001).

Metabolic and Endocrine Effects. The effects of sex steroids on glucose metabolism and insulin sensitivity are complex (Godsland, 1996) and may differ among agents in the same class (*e.g.,* the 19-nor progestins). Early studies with high-dose oral contraceptives generally reported impaired glucose tolerance as demonstrated by increases in fasting glucose and insulin levels and responses to glucose challenge. These effects have decreased as steroid dosages have been lowered, and current low-dose combination contraceptives may even improve insulin sensitivity. Similarly, the high-dose progestins in early oral contraceptives did raise LDL and reduce HDL levels, but modern low-dose preparations do not produce unfavorable lipid profiles (Sherif, 1999). There also have been periodic reports that oral contraceptives increase the incidence of gallbladder disease, but any such effect appears to be weak and limited to current or very long-term users (Burkman, 2004).

The estrogenic component of oral contraceptives may increase hepatic synthesis of a number of serum proteins, including those that bind thyroid hormones, glucocorticoids, and sex steroids. While physiological feedback mechanisms generally adjust hormone synthesis to maintain normal "free" hormone levels, these changes can affect the interpretation of endocrine function tests that measure *total* plasma hormone levels, and may necessitate dose adjustment in patients receiving thyroid-hormone replacement.

The ethinyl estradiol present in oral contraceptives appears to cause a dose-dependent increase in several serum factors known to increase coagulation. However, in healthy women who do not smoke, there also is an increase in fibrinolytic activity, which exerts a counter effect so that overall there is a minimal effect on hemostatic balance. In women who smoke, however, this compensatory effect is diminished, which may shift the hemostatic profile toward a hypercoagulable condition (Fruzzetti, 1999).

Miscellaneous Effects. Nausea, edema, and mild headache occur in some individuals, and more severe migraine headaches may be precipitated by oral contraceptive use in a smaller fraction of women. Some patients may experience breakthrough bleeding during the 21-day cycle when the active pills are being taken. Withdrawal bleeding may fail to occur in a small fraction of women during the 7-day "off" period, thus causing confusion about a possible pregnancy. Acne and hirsutism are thought to be mediated by the androgenic activity of the 19-nor progestins.

Progestin-Only Contraceptives. Episodes of irregular, unpredictable spotting and breakthrough bleeding are the most frequently encountered untoward effect and the major reason women discontinue use of all three types of progestin-only contraceptives. With time, the incidence of these bleeding episodes decreases, especially with the long-acting preparations, and amenorrhea becomes common after a year or more of use.

There is no evidence that the progestin-only minipill preparations increase thromboembolic events, which are thought to be related to the estrogenic component of combination preparations; blood pressure does not appear to be elevated, and nausea and breast tenderness do not occur. Acne may be a problem, however, because of the androgenic activity of norethindrone-containing preparations. These preparations may be attractive for nursing mothers because they do not decrease lactation as do products containing estrogens.

Aside from bleeding irregularities, headache is the most commonly reported untoward effect of depot MPA (medroxyprogesterone acetate). Mood changes and weight gain also have been reported, but controlled clinical studies of these effects are not available. It is of more concern that many studies have found decreases in HDL levels and increases in LDL levels and that there have been several reports of decreased bone density. These effects may be due to reduced endogenous estrogens because depot MPA is particularly effective in lowering gonadotropin levels. Numerous human studies have not found any increases in breast, endometrial, cervical, or ovarian cancer in women receiving MPA (Westhoff, 2003). Because of the time required to completely eliminate the drug, the contraceptive effect of this agent may remain for 6 to 12 months after the last injection.

Implants of norethindrone may be associated with infection, local irritation, pain at the insertion site, and rarely, expulsion of the inserts. Headache, weight gain, and mood changes have been reported, and acne is seen in some patients. A number of metabolic studies have been performed in NORPLANT (no longer marketed in the United States) users, and in most cases only minimal changes have been observed in lipid, carbohydrate, and protein metabolism. In women desiring pregnancy, ovulation occurs fairly soon after implant removal, reaching 50% in 3 months and almost 90% within 1 year.

Emergency Contraceptive Pills. Nausea and vomiting are the main untoward effects, with an incidence of roughly 50% and 20%, respectively, for combined estrogen-levonorgestrel combinations and 23% and 6% for levonorgestrel alone (Task Force on Postovulatory Methods of Fertility Regulation, 1998). No changes in clotting factors have been reported for the combined regimen, but based on concerns with combination oral contraceptives, levonorgestrel alone might be considered for women who smoke or have a history of blood clots. *Emergency contraceptive pills are contraindicated in cases of confirmed pregnancy.*

Contraindications

While the use of modern oral contraceptives is considered generally safe in most healthy women, *these agents can contribute to the incidence and severity of certain diseases if other risk factors are present.* The following conditions are thus considered absolute contraindications for combination oral contraceptive use: the presence or history of thromboembolic disease, cerebrovascular disease, myocardial infarction, coronary artery disease, or congenital hyperlipidemia; known or suspected carcinoma of the breast, carcinoma of the female reproductive tract, or other hormone-dependent/responsive neoplasias; abnormal undiagnosed vaginal bleeding; known or suspected pregnancy; and past or present liver tumors or impaired liver function. *The risk of serious cardiovascular side effects is particularly marked in women over 35 years of age who smoke heavily (e.g., over 15 cigarettes per day); even low-dose oral contraceptives are contraindicated in such patients.*

Several other conditions are relative contraindications and should be considered on an individual basis. These include migraine headaches, hypertension, diabetes mellitus, obstructive jaundice of pregnancy or prior oral contraceptive use, and gallbladder disease. If elective surgery is planned, many physicians recommend discontinuation of oral contraceptives for several weeks to a month to minimize the possibility of thromboembolism after surgery. These agents should be used with care in women with prior gestational diabetes or uterine fibroids, and low-dose pills should generally be used in such cases.

Progestin-only contraceptives are contraindicated in the presence of undiagnosed vaginal bleeding, benign or malignant liver disease, and known or suspected breast cancer. Depot medroxyprogesterone acetate and levonorgestrel inserts are contraindicated in women with a history or predisposition to thrombophlebitis or thromboembolic disorders.

Choice of Contraceptive Preparations

Many preparations that differ substantially in dose and specific components are available, providing the option to select the preparation best suited to each individual. Treatment should generally begin with preparations containing the minimum dose of steroids that provides effective contraceptive coverage. This is typically a pill with 30 to 35 μg of estrogen, but preparations with 20 μg may be adequate for lighter women or those over 40 with perimenopausal symptoms, while a preparation containing 50 μg of estrogen may be required for heavier women. Breakthrough bleeding may occur if the estrogen-to-progestin ratio is too low to produce a stable endometrium, and this may be prevented by switching to a pill with a higher ratio.

In women for whom estrogens are contraindicated or undesirable, progestin-only contraceptives may be an option. The progestin-only minipill may have enhanced effectiveness in several such types of women (e.g., nursing mothers and women over 40, in whom fertility may be decreased).

Another consideration is the concomitant administration of medications that may increase metabolism of estrogens (e.g., *rifampicin*, barbiturates, and *phenytoin*) or reduce their enterohepatic recycling (e.g., tetracyclines and *ampicillin* decrease intestinal bacteria that produce enzymes required for hydrolysis and reuptake of conjugated metabolites). In these situations, a low-dose pill may *not* be 99.9% effective due to increased steroid metabolism.

The choice of a preparation also may be influenced by the specific 19-nor progestin component, since this component may have varying degrees of androgenic and other activities. The androgenic activity of this component may contribute to untoward effects such as weight gain, acne due to increased sebaceous gland secretions, and unfavorable lipoprotein profiles. These side effects are greatly reduced in newer, low-dose contraceptives, but any patients exhibiting such side effects may benefit by switching to pills that contain a progestin with less androgenic activity. Of the progestins commonly found in oral contraceptives, norgestrel is generally considered to have the most androgenic activity; norethindrone and ethynodiol diacetate to have more moderate androgenic activity; and desogestrel, norgestimate, and drospirenone to have the least androgenic activity.

The FDA has approved a triphasic, low-dose combination oral contraceptive (ORTHO TRI-CYCLEN) containing ethinyl estradiol and norgestimate for the treatment of moderate acne vulgaris. Similar preparations (DEMULEN 1/35, DESOGEN, others) also are effective. The mechanism appears to be a decrease in free plasma testosterone due to an increase in plasma SHBG, since total testosterone levels are unchanged (Redmond *et al.*, 1997).

In summary, for a given individual, both the efficacy and side effects of hormonal contraceptives may vary considerably among preparations. A number of choices are available to counter the development of side effects and improve patient tolerance, both in terms of specific components and routes of administration, without decreasing contraceptive efficacy.

Noncontraceptive Health Benefits

It is generally accepted that combination oral contraceptives have substantial health benefits unrelated to their contraceptive use. Oral contraceptives significantly reduce the incidence of ovarian and endometrial cancer within 6 months of use, and the incidence is decreased 50% after 2 years of use. Depot MPA injections also reduce very substantially the incidence of uterine cancer. Furthermore, this protective effect persists for up to 15 years after oral contraceptive use is discontinued. These agents also decrease the incidence of ovarian cysts and benign fibrocystic breast disease.

Oral contraceptives have major benefits related to menstruation in many women. These include more regular menstruation, reduced menstrual blood loss and less iron-deficiency anemia, and decreased frequency of dysmenorrhea. There also is a decreased incidence of pelvic inflammatory disease and ectopic pregnancies, and endometriosis may be ameliorated. Some women also may obtain these benefits with progestin-only contraceptives. There are suggestions that MPA may improve hematological parameters in women with sickle-cell disease (Cullins, 1996).

There is now a consensus that combination oral contraceptives prevent thousands of deaths, episodes of various diseases, and cases of hospitalization each year in the United States alone. From a purely statistical perspective, fertility regulation by oral contraceptives is substantially safer than pregnancy or childbirth for most women, even without considering the additional health benefits of these agents.

CLINICAL SUMMARY

Estrogens are most commonly used to treat vasomotor disturbances ("hot flashes") in postmenopausal women. Other important benefits are amelioration of the effects of urogenital atrophy, a decreased incidence of colon cancer, and prevention of bone loss. Estrogens have proven efficacy for prevention of bone fractures at all sites in normal women, although when used solely for this purpose they should not be considered first-line because of possible untoward side effects including breast cancer, stroke, and coronary heart disease (CHD). Estrogens should *not* be prescribed for treatment or prevention of CHD or other cardiovascular diseases, or to prevent neurodegenerative disease. A variety of preparations, including oral, transdermal, and vaginal, are available. *Regardless of the specific drug(s) selected, treatment should use the minimum dose and duration for the desired therapeutic endpoint.*

In postmenopausal women with an intact uterus, a progestin is included to prevent endometrial cancer. Medroxyprogesterone acetate is frequently used in the United States and micronized progesterone is available; norethindrone and norgestrel/levonorgestrel are also commonly used. As progestins may contribute to untoward effects, especially breast cancer and CHD, women without a uterus are administered estrogen alone. Postmenopausal hormone therapy and contraception are the most frequent uses of progestins.

Tamoxifen, a selective estrogen receptor modulator or SERM, is widely used for the adjuvant treatment of breast cancer and for prophylaxis of the disease in high-risk women, but treatment should be limited to 5 years. The drug is most effective in the treatment of estrogen-receptor positive disease, and untoward effects include hot flashes as well as an increase in blood clots and uterine cancer. Another SERM, raloxifene, is used to prevent osteoporosis and decreases the incidence of vertebral fractures in postmenopausal women. Raloxifene does not increase the risk of uterine cancer, but does increase the incidence of thromboembolic events and hot flashes.

The pure estrogen antagonist fulvestrant is also used to treat breast cancer, especially in patients who become refractory to tamoxifen. Another estrogen antagonist, clomiphene, is used to treat infertility in anovulatory women. Both compounds may cause hot flashes.

Aromatase inhibitors, including letrozole, anastrozole, and exemestane, are also highly effective for the adjuvant treatment of breast cancer, and their prophylactic use is being explored. Untoward effects include hot flashes; potential long-term effects of these agents on osteoporosis and bone fractures remain to be established.

Mifepristone is used therapeutically as an anti-progestin for medical abortion, and is administered with a prostaglandin for this purpose.

Estrogens and progestins are widely used as "combination" contraceptives and are 99% effective in preventing ovulation. These combinations are most often used orally, although transdermal preparations, once-monthly injections, and vaginal rings are available. Ethinyl estradiol (or mestranol) and 19-nor steroids such as norgestrel/

levonorgestrel, norethindrone, or another synthetic progestin are commonly used. The greatest concern with these agents is the risk of stroke or other thromboembolic events; consequently, they should not be used in older women (over 35) who smoke or have other risk factors (*e.g.*, hypertension) for cardiovascular disease.

Several progestin-only contraceptives are available, including low-dose pills, long-lasting (*e.g.*, 3-month) depot injections, and subdermal implants (not available in the United States). These agents are also highly efficacious and exert a number of actions, including decreased frequency of ovulation, and effects on cervical mucus, ovum transport, and implantation. They may be used in nursing mothers and in some women with contraindications for combined estrogen-progestin combinations. The most common untoward effect is unpredictable vaginal bleeding.

A levonorgestrel-only pill and high-dose estrogen-progestin oral contraceptives are available and effective for postcoital or emergency contraception within 72 hours of unprotected intercourse. These preparations are ineffective in cases of established pregnancy and should not be used to terminate pregnancy.

BIBLIOGRAPHY

Anderson, G.L., Limacher, M., Assaf, A.R., *et al.* for The Women's Health Initiative Steering Committee. Effects of conjugated equine estrogen in postmenopausal women with hysterectomy: The Women's Health Initiative randomized controlled trial. *JAMA,* **2004,** *291:*1701–1712.

Aronica, S.M., and Katzenellenbogen, B.S. Stimulation of estrogen receptor-mediated transcription and alteration in the phosphorylation state of the rat uterine estrogen receptor by estrogen, cyclic adenosine monophosphate, and insulin-like growth factor-I. *Mol. Endocrinol.,* **1993,** *7:*743–52.

Beral, V., for the Million Women Study Collaborators. Breast cancer and hormone-replacement therapy in the Million Women Study. *Lancet,* **2003,** *362:*419–427.

Blackmore, P.F. Extragenomic actions of progesterone in human sperm and progesterone metabolites in human platelets. *Steroids,* **1999,** *64:*149–156.

Braidman, I., Baris, C., Wood, L., *et al.* Preliminary evidence for impaired estrogen receptor-α protein expression in osteoblasts and osteocytes from men with idiopathic osteoporosis. *Bone,* **2000,** *26:*423–427.

Cheskis, B.J., Karathanasis, S., and Lyttle, C.R. Estrogen receptor ligands modulate its interaction with DNA. *J. Biol. Chem.,* **1997,** *272:*11384–11391.

Coombes, R.C., Hall, E., Gibson, L.J., *et al.*, for the Intergroup Exemestane Study. A randomized trial of exemestane after two to three years of tamoxifen therapy in postmenopausal women with primary breast cancer. *N. Engl. J. Med.,* **2004,** *350:*1081–1092.

Cummings, S.R., Eckert, S., Krueger, K.A., *et al.* The effect of raloxifene on risk of breast cancer in postmenopausal women: results from the MORE randomized trial. Multiple Outcomes of Raloxifene Evaluation. *JAMA*, **1999**, *281:*2189–2197.

DeFriend, D.J., Anderson, E., Bell, J., *et al*. Effects of 4-hydroxytamoxifen and a novel pure antioestrogen (ICI 182780) on the clonogenic growth of human breast cancer cells in vitro. *Br. J. Cancer*, **1994**, *70:*204–211.

Delmas, P.D., Bjarnason, N.H., Mitlak, B.H., *et al*. Effects of raloxifene on bone mineral density, serum cholesterol concentrations, and uterine endometrium in postmenopausal women. *N. Engl. J. Med.,* **1997**, *337:*1641–1647.

Delmas, P.D., Ensrud, K.E., Adachi, J.D., *et al*. Multiple Outcomes of Raloxifene Evaluation (MORE) Investigators. Efficacy of raloxifene on vertebral fracture risk reduction in postmenopausal women with osteoporosis: four-year results from a randomized clinical trial. *J. Clin. Endocrinol. Metab.*, **2002**, *87:*3609–3617.

DeManno, D., Elger, W., Garg, R., *et al*. Asoprisnil (J867): a selective progesterone receptor modulator for gynecological therapy. *Steroids*, **2003**, *68:*1019–1032.

Endoh, H., Sasaki, H., Maruyama, K., *et al*. Rapid activation of MAP kinase by estrogen in the bone cell line. *Biochem. Biophys. Res. Commun.,* **1997**, *235:*99–102.

Espeland, M.A., Rapp, S.R., Shumaker, S.A., *et al.,* for the Women's Health Initiative Memory Study. Conjugated equine estrogens and global cognitive function in postmenopausal women: Women's Health Initiative Memory Study. *JAMA*, **2004**, *291:*2959–2968.

Ettinger, B., Black, D.M., Mitlak, B.H., *et al*. Reduction of vertebral fracture risk in postmenopausal women with osteoporosis treated with raloxifene: results from a 3-year randomized clinical trial. Multiple Outcomes of Raloxifene Evaluation (MORE) Investigators. *JAMA*, **1999**, *282:*637–645.

Food and Drug Administration. Recommendations of DES Task Force. *FDA Drug Bull.*, **1985**, *15:*40–42.

Giangrande, P.H., Kimbrel, E.A., Edwards, D.P., and McDonnell, D.P. The opposing transcriptional activities of the two isoforms of the human progesterone receptor are due to differential cofactor binding. *Mol. Cell Biol.,* **2000**, *20:*3102–3115.

Grady, D., Herrington, D., Bittner, V., *et al.,* for the HERS Research Group. Cardiovascular disease outcomes during 6.8 years of hormone therapy: Heart and Estrogen/progestin Replacement Study follow-up (HERS II). *JAMA*, **2002**, *288:*49–57.

Grady, D., Wenger, N.K., Herrington, D., *et al*. Postmenopausal hormone therapy increases risk for venous thromboembolic disease. Heart and Estrogen/progestin Replacement Study. *Ann. Intern. Med.*, **2000**, *132:*689–696.

Greenwald, P., Barlow, J.J., Nasca, P.C., and Burnett, W.S. Vaginal cancer after maternal treatment with synthetic estrogens. *N. Engl. J. Med.,* **1971**, *285:*390–392.

Hall, J.M., and McDonnell, D.P. The estrogen receptor *β*-isoform (ER *β*) of the human estrogen receptor modulates ER *β* transcriptional activity and is a key regulator of the cellular response to estrogens and antiestrogens. *Endocrinology*, **1999**, *140:*5566–5578.

Hall, J.M., McDonnell, D.P., and Korach, K.S. Allosteric regulation of estrogen receptor structure, function, and co-activator recruitment by different estrogen response elements. *Mol. Endocrinol.*, **2002**, *16:*469–486.

Han, W., Kang, D., Lee, K.M., *et al*. Full sequencing analysis of estrogen receptor-*α* gene polymorphism and its association with breast cancer risk. *Anticancer Res.*, **2003**, *23:*4703–4707.

Harrington, W.R., Sheng, S., Barnett, D.H., *et al*. Activities of estrogen receptor *α*- and *β*-selective ligands at diverse estrogen responsive gene sites mediating transactivation or transrepression. *Mol. Cell Endocrinol.*, **2003**, *206:*13–22.

Herbst, A.L., Ulfelder, H., and Poskanzer, D.C. Adenocarcinoma of the vagina. Association of maternal stilbestrol therapy with tumor appearance in young women. *N. Engl. J. Med.,* **1971**, *284:*878–881.

Herrington, D.M., and Howard, T.D. ER-*α* variants and the cardiovascular effects of hormone replacement therapy. *Pharmacogenomics,* **2003**, *4:*269–277.

Hewitt, S.C., and Korach K.S. Oestrogen receptor knockout mice: roles for oestrogen receptors *α* and *β* in reproductive tissues. *Reproduction,* **2003**, *125:*143–149.

Hulley, S., Grady, D., Bush, T., *et al*. Randomized trial of estrogen plus progestin for secondary prevention of coronary heart disease in postmenopausal women. Heart and Estrogen/progestin Replacement Study (HERS) Research Group. *JAMA*, **1998**, *280:*605–613.

Kato, S., Endoh, H., Masuhiro, Y., *et al*. Activation of the estrogen receptor through phosphorylation by mitogen-activated protein kinase. *Science,* **1995**, *270:*1491–1494.

Kettel, L.M., Roseff, S.J., Berga, S.L., *et al*. Hypothalamic-pituitary-ovarian response to clomiphene citrate in women with polycystic ovary syndrome. *Fertil. Steril.,* **1993**, *59:*532–538.

Knobil, E. Patterns of hypophysiotropic signals and gonadotropin secretion in the rhesus monkey. *Biol. Reprod.,* **1981**, *24:*44–49.

Koh, K.K., Mincemoyer, R., Bui, M.N., *et al*. Effects of hormone-replacement therapy on fibrinolysis in postmenopausal women. *N. Engl. J. Med.,* **1997**, *336:*683–690.

Kousteni, S., Chen, J.R., Bellido, T., *et al*. Reversal of bone loss in mice by nongenotropic signaling of sex steroids. *Science,* **2002**, *298:*843–846.

Kuiper, G.G., Carlsson, B., Grandien, K., *et al*. Comparison of the ligand binding specificity and transcript tissue distribution of estrogen receptors ER *α* and *β. Endocrinology*, **1997**, *138:*863–870.

Kurabayashi, T., Matsushita, H., Tomita, M., *et al*. Association of vitamin D and estrogen receptor gene polymorphism with the effects of long term hormone replacement therapy on bone mineral density. *J. Bone Miner. Metab.*, **2004**, *22:*241–247.

Labrie, F., El-Alfy, M., Berger, L., *et al*. The combination of a novel selective estrogen receptor modulator with an estrogen protects the mammary gland and uterus in a rodent model: the future of postmenopausal women's health? *Endocrinology*, **2003**, *144:*4700–4706.

Lahti, E., Blanco, G., Kauppila, A., *et al*. Endometrial changes in postmenopausal breast cancer patients receiving tamoxifen. *Obstet. Gynecol.,* **1993**, *81:*660–664.

Losel, R., Dorn-Beineke, A., Falkenstein, E., *et al*. Porcine spermatozoa contain more than one membrane progesterone receptor. *Int. J. Biochem. Cell Biol.*, **2004**, *36:*1532–1541.

Love, R.R., Wiebe, D.A., Feyzi, J.M., *et al*. Effects of tamoxifen on cardiovascular risk factors in postmenopausal women after 5 years of treatment. *J. Natl. Cancer Inst.*, **1994**, *86:*1534–1539.

McDonnell, D.P., and Goldman, M.E. RU486 exerts antiestrogenic activities through a novel progesterone receptor A form-mediated mechanism. *J. Biol. Chem.*, **1994**, *269:*11945–11949.

McInerney, E.M., Weis, K.E., Sun, J., *et al*. Transcription activation by the human estrogen receptor subtype *β* (ER *β*) studied with ER *β* and ER *α* receptor chimeras. *Endocrinology*, **1998**, *139:*4513–4522.

Meis, P.J., Klebanoff, M., Thom, E., *et al*. Prevention of recurrent preterm delivery by 17 *α*-hydroxyprogesterone caproate. *N. Engl. J. Med.*, **2003**, *348:*2379–2385.

Metivier, R., Penot, G., Hubner, M.R., *et al*. Estrogen receptor-*α* directs ordered, cyclical, and combinatorial recruitment of cofactors on a natural target promoter. *Cell,* **2003**, *115:*751–763.

Modelska, K., and Cummings, S. Tibolone for postmenopausal women: systematic review of randomized trials. *J. Clin. Endocrinol. Metab.*, **2002**, *87:*16–23.

Moodley, J. Combined oral contraceptives and cervical cancer. *Curr. Opin. Obstet. Gynecol.*, **2004**, *16:*27–29.

Mulac-Jericevic, B., Lydon, J.P., DeMayo, F.J., and Conneely, O.M. Defective mammary gland morphogenesis in mice lacking the progesterone receptor B isoform. *Proc. Natl. Acad. Sci. U. S. A.*, **2003**, *100:*9744–9749.

Mulac-Jericevic, B., Mullinax, R.A., DeMayo, F.J., *et al.* Subgroup of reproductive functions of progesterone mediated by progesterone receptor-B isoform. *Science*, **2000**, *289:*1751–1754.

Paech, K., Webb, P., Kuiper, G.G., *et al.* Differential ligand activation of estrogen receptors ERα and ERβ at AP1 sites. *Science,* **1997**, *277:*1508–1510.

Pike, M.C., Peters, R.K., Cozen, W., *et al.* Estrogen-progestin replacement therapy and endometrial cancer. *J. Natl. Cancer Inst.,* **1997**, *89:*1110–1116.

Prince, R.L., Smith, M., Dick, I.M., *et al.* Prevention of postmenopausal osteoporosis. A comparative study of exercise, calcium supplementation, and hormone-replacement therapy. *N. Engl. J. Med.,* **1991**, *325:*1189–1195.

Rapp, S.R., Espeland, M.A., Shumaker, S.A., *et al.*, for the WHIMS Investigators. Effect of estrogen plus progestin on global cognitive function in postmenopausal women: the Women's Health Initiative Memory Study: a randomized controlled trial. *JAMA*, **2003**, *289:*2663–2672.

Redmond, G.P., Olson, W.H., Lippman, J.S., *et al.* Norgestimate and ethinyl estradiol in the treatment of acne vulgaris: a randomized, placebo-controlled trial. *Obstet. Gynecol.,* **1997**, *89:*615–622.

Robertson, J.F., Osborne, C.K., Howell, A., *et al.* Fulvestrant versus anastrozole for the treatment of advanced breast carcinoma in postmenopausal women: a prospective combined analysis of two multicenter trials. *Cancer*, **2003**, *98:*229–238.

Rossouw, J.E., Anderson, G.L., Prentice, R.L., *et al.,* for the Writing Group for the Women's Health Initiative Investigators. Risks and benefits of estrogen plus progestin in healthy postmenopausal women: principal results from the Women's Health Initiative randomized controlled trial. *JAMA*, **2002**, *288:*321–333.

Ross, R.K., Paganini-Hill, A., Wan, P.C., and Pike, M.C. Effect of hormone replacement therapy on breast cancer risk: estrogen versus estrogen plus progestin. *J. Natl. Cancer Inst.,* **2000**, *92:*328–332.

Saville, B., Wormke, M., Wang, F., *et al.* Ligand-, cell-, and estrogen receptor subtype (α/β)-dependent activation at GC-rich (Sp1) promoter elements. *J. Biol. Chem.,* **2000**, *275:*5379–5387.

Schairer, C., Lubin, J., Troisi, R., *et al.* Menopausal estrogen and estrogen-progestin replacement therapy and breast cancer risk. *JAMA,* **2000**, *283:*485–491.

Shapiro, S., Kelly, J.P., Rosenberg, L., *et al.* Risk of localized and widespread endometrial cancer in relation to recent and discontinued use of conjugated estrogens. *N. Engl. J. Med.,* **1985**, *313:*969–972.

Shumaker, S.A., Legault, C., Rapp, S.R., *et al.*, for the WHIMS Investigators. Estrogen plus progestin and the incidence of dementia and mild cognitive impairment in postmenopausal women: the Women's Health Initiative Memory Study: a randomized controlled trial. *JAMA*, **2003**, *289:*2651–2662.

Simoncini, T., Hafezi-Moghadam, A., Brazil, D.P., *et al.* Interaction of oestrogen receptor with the regulatory subunit of phosphatidylinositol-3-OH kinase. *Nature*, **2000**, *407:*538–541.

Smith, E.P., Boyd, J., Frank, G.R., *et al.* Estrogen resistance caused by a mutation in the estrogen-receptor gene in a man. *N. Engl. J. Med.,* **1994**, *331:*1056–1061.

Sridar, C., Kent, U.M., Notley, L.M., *et al.* Effect of tamoxifen on the enzymatic activity of human cytochrome CYP2B6. *J. Pharmacol. Exp. Ther.*, **2002**, *301:*945–952.

Tamrazi, A., Carlson, K.E., and Katzenellenbogen, J.A. Molecular sensors of estrogen receptor conformations and dynamics. *Mol. Endocrinol.*, **2003**, *17:*2593–2602.

Task Force on Postovulatory Methods of Fertility Regulation. Randomised controlled trial of levonorgestrel versus the Yuzpe regimen of combined oral contraceptives for emergency contraception. *Lancet,* **1998**, *352:*428–433.

Thorneycroft, I.H., Mishell, D.R. Jr., Stone, S.C., *et al.* The relation of serum 17-hydroxyprogesterone and estradiol-17β levels during the human menstrual cycle. *Am. J. Obstet. Gynecol.*, **1971**, *111:*947–951.

Van Den Bemd, G.J., Kuiper, G.G., Pols, H.A., and Van Leeuwen, J.P. Distinct effects on the conformation of estrogen receptor α and β by both the antiestrogens ICI 164,384 and ICI 182,780 leading to opposite effects on receptor stability. *Biochem. Biophys. Res. Commun.,* **1999**, *261:*1–5.

Vandevyver, C., Vanhoof, J., Declerck, K., *et al.* Lack of association between estrogen receptor genotypes and bone mineral density, fracture history, or muscle strength in elderly women. *J. Bone Miner. Res.,* **1999**, *14:*1576–1582.

Vegeto, E., Shahbaz, M.M., Wen, D.X., *et al.* Human progesterone receptor A form is a cell- and promoter-specific repressor of human progesterone receptor B function. *Mol. Endocrinol.,* **1993**, *7:*1244–1255.

Walsh, B.W., Kuller, L.H., Wild, R.A., *et al.* Effects of raloxifene on serum lipids and coagulation factors in healthy postmenopausal women. *JAMA*, **1998**, *279:*1445–1451.

Walsh, B.W., Li, H., and Sacks, F.M. Effects of postmenopausal hormone replacement with oral and transdermal estrogen on high density lipoprotein metabolism. *J. Lipid Res.,* **1994**, *35:*2083–2093.

Weiderpass, E., Persson, I., Melhus, H., *et al.* Estrogen receptor α gene polymorphisms and endometrial cancer risk. *Carcinogenesis,* **2000**, *21:*623–627.

Wijayaratne, A.L., Nagel, S.C., Paige, L.A., *et al.* Comparative analyses of mechanistic differences among antiestrogens. *Endocrinology,* **1999**, *140:*5828–5840.

Writing Group for the PEPI Trial. Effects of estrogen or estrogen/progestin regimens on heart disease risk factors in postmenopausal women. The Postmenopausal Estrogen/Progestin Interventions (PEPI) Trial. *JAMA*, **1995**, *273:*199–208.

Yue, W., Santen, R.J., Wang, J.P., *et al.* Genotoxic metabolites of estradiol in breast: potential mechanism of estradiol induced carcinogenesis. *J. Steroid Biochem. Mol. Biol.*, **2003**, *86:*477–486.

MONOGRAPHS AND REVIEWS

Belchetz, P.E. Hormonal treatment of postmenopausal women. *N. Engl. J. Med.,* **1994**, *330:*1062–1071.

Burkman, R., Schlesselman, J.J., and Zieman, M. Safety concerns and health benefits associated with oral contraception. *Am. J. Obstet. Gynecol.,* **2004**, *190*(suppl 4):S5–S22.

Castelli, W.P. Cardiovascular disease: pathogenesis, epidemiology, and risk among users of oral contraceptives who smoke. *Am. J. Obstet. Gynecol.,* **1999**, *180:*349S–356S.

Christin-Maitre, S., Bouchard, P., and Spitz, I.M. Medical termination of pregnancy. *N. Engl. J. Med.,* **2000**, *342:*946–956.

Collingwood, T.N., Urnov, F.D., and Wolffe, A.P. Nuclear receptors: co-activators, co-repressors and chromatin remodeling in the control of transcription. *J. Mol. Endocrinol.,* **1999**, *23:*255–275.

Conneely, O.M., Mulac-Jericevic, B., DeMayo, F., *et al.* Reproductive functions of progesterone receptors. *Recent Prog. Horm. Res.,* **2002**, *57:*339–355.

Cullins, V.E. Noncontraceptive benefits and therapeutic uses of depot medroxyprogesterone acetate. *J. Reprod. Med.,* **1996**, *41*(suppl 5):428–433.

Duax, W.L., Griffin, J.F., Weeks, C.M., and Wawrzak, Z. The mechanism of action of steroid antagonists: insights from crystallographic studies. *J. Steroid Biochem.,* **1988**, *31*:481–492.

Fernandez, E., La Vecchia, C., Balducci, A., *et al.* Oral contraceptives and colorectal cancer risk: a meta-analysis. *Br. J. Cancer,* **2001**, *84*:722–727.

Fitzpatrick, L.A. Soy isoflavones: hope or hype? *Maturitas,* **2003**, *44*(suppl 1):S21–S29.

Fotherby, K. Bioavailability of orally administered sex steroids used in oral contraception and hormone replacement therapy. *Contraception,* **1996**, *54*:59–69.

Fruzzetti, F. Hemostatic effects of smoking and oral contraceptive use. *Am. J. Obstet. Gynecol.,* **1999**, *180*:S369–S374.

Giangrande, P.H., and McDonnell, D.P. The A and B isoforms of the human progesterone receptor: two functionally different transcription factors encoded by a single gene. *Recent Prog. Horm. Res.,* **1999**, *54*:291–313.

Glasier, A. Emergency postcoital contraception. *N. Engl. J. Med.,* **1997**, *337*:1058–1064

Godsland, I.F. The influence of female sex steroids on glucose metabolism and insulin action. *J. Intern. Med. Suppl.,* **1996**, *738*:1–60.

Green, P.S., and Simpkins, J.W. Neuroprotective effects of estrogens: potential mechanisms of action. *Int. J. Dev. Neurosci.,* **2000**, *18*:347–358.

Grumbach, M.M., and Auchus, R.J. Estrogen: consequences and implications of human mutations in synthesis and action. *J. Clin. Endocrinol. Metab.,* **1999**, *84*:4677–4694.

Hanstein, B., Djahansouzi, S., Dall, P., *et al.* Insights into the molecular biology of the estrogen receptor define novel therapeutic targets for breast cancer. *Eur. J. Endocrinol.,* **2004**, *150*:243–255.

Haynes, B.P., Dowsett, M., Miller, W.R., *et al.* The pharmacology of letrozole. *J. Steroid Biochem. Mol. Biol.,* **2003**, *87*:35–45.

Herrington, D.M., and Klein, K.P. Pharmacogenetics of estrogen replacement therapy. *J. Appl. Physiol.,* **2001**, *91*:2776–2784.

Hol, T., Cox, M.B., Bryant, H.U., and Draper, M.W. Selective estrogen receptor modulators and postmenopausal women's health. *J. Womens Health,* **1997**, *6*:523–531.

Hotchkiss, J., and Knobil, E. The menstrual cycle and its neuroendocrine control. In, *The Physiology of Reproduction,* 2nd ed. (Knobil, E., and Neill, J.D., eds.) Raven Press, New York, **1994**, pp. 711–749.

Jaiyesimi, I.A., Buzdar, A.U., Decker, D.A., and Hortobagyi, G.N. Use of tamoxifen for breast cancer: twenty-eight years later. *J. Clin. Oncol.,* **1995**, *13*:513–529.

Jang, G.R., and Benet, L.Z. Antiprogestin pharmacodynamics, pharmacokinetics, and metabolism: implications for their long-term use. *J. Pharmacokinet. Biopharm.,* **1997**, *25*:647–672.

Jordan, V.C., and Murphy, C.S. Endocrine pharmacology of antiestrogens as antitumor agents. *Endocr. Rev.,* **1990**, *11*:578–610.

Kos, M., Reid, G., Denger, S., and Gannon, F. Minireview: genomic organization of the human ERα gene promoter region. *Mol Endocrinol.,* **2001**, *15*:2057–2063.

Leonhardt, S.A., and Edwards, D.P. Mechanism of action of progesterone antagonists. *Exp. Biol. Med.,* **2002**, *227*:969–980.

Lewandowski, S., Kalita, K., and Kaczmarek, L. Estrogen receptor β. Potential functional significance of a variety of mRNA isoforms. *FEBS Lett.,* **2002**, *524*:1–5.

Lobo, R.A., and Stanczyk, F.Z. New knowledge in the physiology of hormonal contraceptives. *Am. J. Obstet. Gynecol.,* **1994**, *170*:1499–1507.

Mäkelä, S., Hyder, S.M., and Stancel, G.M. Environmental estrogens. In, *Handbook of Experimental Pharmacology,* Vol. 135, part II: *Estrogens and Antiestrogens.* (Oettel, M., and Schillinger, E., eds.) Springer-Verlag, Berlin, **1999**, pp. 613–663.

Manolagas, S.C., Kousteni, S., and Jilka, R.L. Sex steroids and bone. *Recent Prog. Horm. Res.,* **2002**, *57*:385–409.

Manson, J.E., and Martin, K.A. Clinical practice. Postmenopausal hormone-replacement therapy. *N. Engl. J. Med.,* **2001**, *345*:34–40.

Mendelsohn, M.E., and Karas, R.H. The protective effects of estrogen on the cardiovascular system. *N. Engl. J. Med.,* **1999**, *340*:1801–1811.

Peltoketo, H., Vihko, P., and Vihko, R. Regulation of estrogen action: role of 17 β-hydroxysteroid dehydrogenases. *Vitam. Horm.,* **1999**, *55*:353–398.

Pike, A.C., Brzozowski, A.M., and Hubbard, R.E. A structural biologist's view of the oestrogen receptor. *J. Steroid Biochem. Mol. Biol.,* **2000**, *74*:261–268.

Riggs, B.L., Khosla, S., and Melton, L.J. III. Sex steroids and the construction and conservation of the adult skeleton. *Endocr. Rev.,* **2002**, *23*:279–302.

Robinson, D., and Cardozo, L.D. The role of estrogens in female lower urinary tract dysfunction. *Urology,* **2003**, *62*(suppl 4A):45–51.

Sherif, K. Benefits and risks of oral contraceptives. *Am. J. Obstet. Gynecol.,* **1999**, *180*:S343–S348.

Simpson, E.R., Clyne, C., Rubin, G., *et al.* Aromatase—A brief overview. *Annu. Rev. Physiol.,* **2002**, *64*:93–127.

Simpson, E.R. Sources of estrogen and their importance. *J. Steroid Biochem. Mol. Biol.,* **2003**, *86*:225–230.

Smith, C.L., and O'Malley, B.W. Coregulator function: a key to understanding tissue specificity of selective receptor modulators. *Endocr. Rev.,* **2004**, *25*:45–71.

Smith, R.E. A review of selective estrogen receptor modulators and national surgical adjuvant breast and bowel project clinical trials. *Semin. Oncol.,* **2003**, *30*(5 suppl 16):4–13.

Spelsberg, T.C., Subramaniam, M., Riggs, B.L., and Khosla, S. The actions and interactions of sex steroids and growth factors/cytokines on the skeleton. *Mol. Endocrinol.,* **1999**, *13*:819–828.

Spitz, I.M., and Chwalisz, K. Progesterone receptor modulators and progesterone antagonists in women's health. *Steroids,* **2000**, *65*:807–815.

Turgeon, J.L., McDonnell, D.P., Martin, K.A., and Wise, P.M. Hormone therapy: physiological complexity belies therapeutic simplicity. *Science,* **2004**, *304*:1269–1273.

Westhoff, C.L. Breast cancer risk: perception versus reality. *Contraception,* **1999**, *59*(suppl):25S–28S.

Westhoff, C. Depot-medroxyprogesterone acetate injection (Depo-Provera): a highly effective contraceptive option with proven long-term safety. *Contraception,* **2003**, *68*:75–87.

Zhu, W., and Smart, E.J. Caveolae, estrogen and nitric oxide. *Trends Endocrinol. Metab.,* **2003**, *14*:114–117.

ANDROGENS

Peter J. Snyder

TESTOSTERONE AND OTHER ANDROGENS

Synthesis of Testosterone. In men, testosterone is the principal secreted androgen. The Leydig cells synthesize the majority of testosterone by the pathways shown in Figure 58–1. In women, testosterone also is probably the principal androgen and is synthesized both in the corpus luteum and the adrenal cortex by similar pathways. The testosterone precursors androstenedione and dehydroepiandrosterone are weak androgens that can be converted peripherally to testosterone.

Secretion and Transport of Testosterone. The magnitude of testosterone secretion is greater in men than in women at almost all stages of life, a difference that explains almost all other differences between men and women. In the first trimester *in utero,* the fetal testes begin to secrete testosterone, which is the principal factor in male sexual differentiation, probably stimulated by human chorionic gonadotropin (hCG) from the placenta. By the beginning of the second trimester, the value is close to that of midpuberty, about 250 ng/dl (Figure 58–2) (Dawood and Saxena, 1977; Forest, 1975). Testosterone production then falls by the end of the second trimester, but by birth the value is again about 250 ng/dl (Dawood and Saxena, 1977; Forest, 1975), possibly due to stimulation of the fetal Leydig cells by luteinizing hormone (LH) from the fetal pituitary gland. The testosterone value falls again in the first few days after birth, but it rises and peaks again at about 250 ng/dl at 2 to 3 months after birth and falls to <50 ng/dl by 6 months, where it remains until puberty (Forest, 1975). During puberty, from about age 12 to 17 years, the serum testosterone concentration in males increases to a much greater degree than in females, so that by early adulthood the serum testosterone concentration is 500 to 700 ng/dl in men, compared to 30 to 50 ng/dl in women.

The magnitude of the testosterone concentration in the male is responsible for the pubertal changes that further differentiate men from women. As men age, their serum testosterone concentrations gradually decrease, which may contribute to other effects of aging in men.

LH, secreted by the pituitary gonadotropes (*see* Chapter 55), is the principal stimulus of testosterone secretion in men, perhaps potentiated by follicle-stimulating hormone (FSH), also secreted by gonadotropes. The secretion of LH by gonadotropes is positively regulated by hypothalamic gonadotropin-releasing hormone (GnRH), while testosterone directly inhibits LH secretion in a negative feedback loop (*see* Chapter 55). LH is secreted in pulses, which occur approximately every 2 hours and are greater in magnitude in the morning. The pulsatility appears to result from pulsatile secretion of GnRH from the hypothalamus. Pulsatile administration of GnRH to men who are hypogonadal due to hypothalamic disease results in normal LH pulses and testosterone secretion, but continuous administration does not (Crowley *et al.,* 1985). Testosterone secretion is likewise pulsatile and diurnal, with the highest plasma concentrations occurring at about 8 A.M. and the lowest at about 8 P.M. The morning peaks diminish as men age (Bremner *et al.,* 1983).

In women, LH stimulates the corpus luteum (formed from the follicle after release of the ovum) to secrete testosterone. Under normal circumstances, however, estradiol and progesterone, not testosterone, are the principal inhibitors of LH secretion in women. Sex hormone–binding globulin (SHBG) binds about 40% of circulating testosterone with high affinity. Because of this high affinity, testosterone bound to SHBG is unavailable for biological effects. Albumin binds almost 60% of circulating testosterone with low affinity, leaving approximately 2% unbound or free. In some testosterone assays, the latter two components are considered as "bioavailable" testosterone.

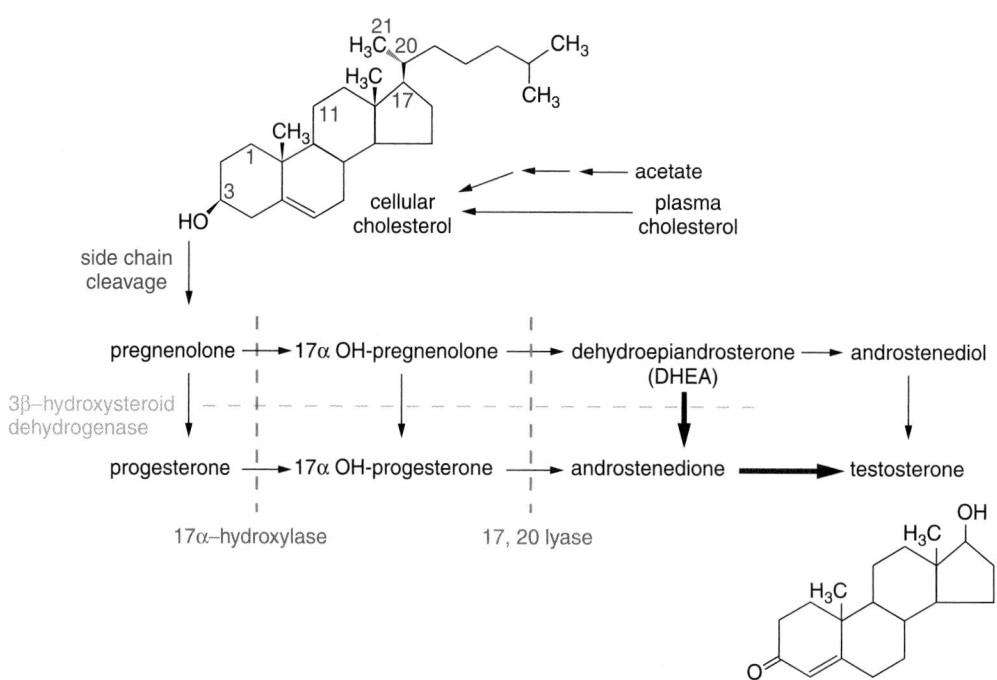

Figure 58–1. *Pathway of synthesis of testosterone in the Leydig cells of the testes.* In Leydig cells, the 11 and 21 hydroxylases (present in adrenal cortex) are absent but CYP17 (17 α-hydroxylase) is present. Thus, androgens and estrogens are synthesized; corticosterone and cortisol are not formed (*see* Figure 59–3). Bold arrows indicate favored pathways.

Metabolism of Testosterone to Active and Inactive Compounds.

Testosterone has many different effects in tissues. One of the mechanisms by which the varied effects are mediated is the metabolism of testosterone to two other active steroids, dihydrotestosterone and estradiol (Figure 58–3). Some effects of testosterone appear to be mediated by testosterone itself, some by dihydrotestosterone, and others by estradiol.

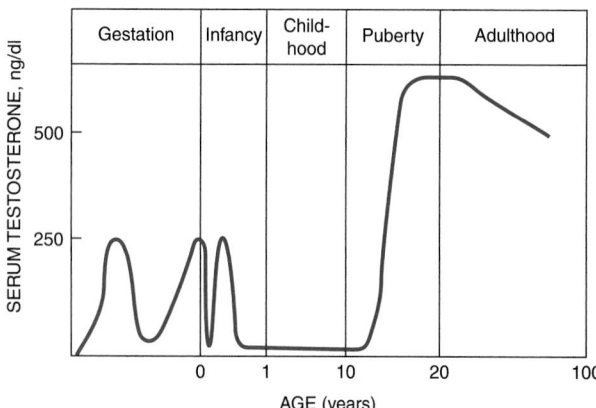

Figure 58–2. *Schematic representation of the serum testosterone concentration from early gestation to old age.*

The enzyme 5α-reductase catalyzes the conversion of testosterone to dihydrotestosterone. Although both testosterone and dihydrotestosterone act *via* the androgen receptor, dihydrotestosterone binds with higher affinity (Wilbert *et al.*, 1983) and activates gene expression more efficiently (Deslypere *et al.*, 1992). As a result, testosterone, acting *via* dihydrotestosterone, is able to have effects in tissues that express 5α-reductase that it could not have if it were present only as testosterone. Two forms of 5α-reductase have been identified: type I, which is found predominantly in non-genital skin, liver, and bone, and type II, which is found predominantly in urogenital tissue in men and genital skin in men and women. The effects of dihydrotestosterone in these tissues are described below.

The enzyme complex aromatase (CYP19), which is present in many tissues, especially the liver and adipose tissue, catalyzes the conversion of testosterone to estradiol. This conversion results in approximately 85% of circulating estradiol in men; the remainder is secreted directly by the testes, probably the Leydig cells (MacDonald *et al.*, 1979). The effects of testosterone thought to be mediated *via* estradiol are described below.

Testosterone is metabolized in the liver to androsterone and etiocholanolone (Figure 58–3), which are biologically inactive. Dihydrotestosterone is metabolized to androsterone, androstanedione, and androstanediol.

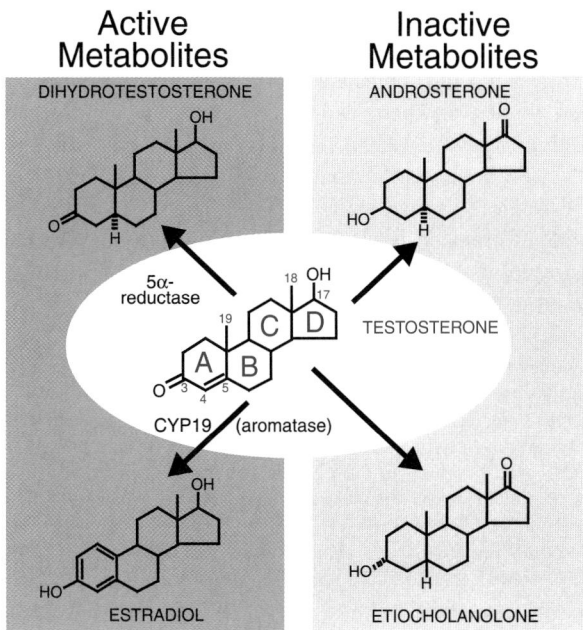

Active Metabolites

DIHYDROTESTOSTERONE

ESTRADIOL

Inactive Metabolites

ANDROSTERONE

ETIOCHOLANOLONE

5α-reductase

CYP19 (aromatase)

TESTOSTERONE

Figure 58–3. Metabolism of testosterone to its major active and inactive metabolites.

Physiological and Pharmacological Effects of Androgens

The biological effects of testosterone can be considered by the receptor it activates and by the tissues in which effects occur at various stages of life. Testosterone can act as an androgen either directly, by binding to the androgen receptor, or indirectly by conversion to dihydrotestosterone, which binds to the androgen receptor even more avidly than testosterone. Testosterone also can act as an estrogen by conversion to estradiol, which binds to the estrogen receptor (Figure 58–4).

Effects That Occur via the Androgen Receptor. Testosterone and dihydrotestosterone act as androgens *via* a single androgen receptor (Figure 58–5). The androgen receptor—officially designated NR3A—is a member of the nuclear receptor superfamily (steroid hormone receptors, thyroid hormone receptors, and orphan receptors). The androgen receptor is comprised of an amino-terminal domain, a DNA-binding domain, and a ligand-binding domain. Testosterone and dihydrotestosterone bind to the ligand-binding domain, causing a conformational change in the receptor that allows the ligand-receptor complex to translocate to the nucleus and bind *via* the DNA-binding domain to androgen response elements on certain responsive genes. The ligand-receptor complex acts as a transcription factor complex and stimulates expression of those genes (Brinkman and Trapman, 2000).

The mechanisms by which androgens have different actions in diverse tissues have become clearer in recent years. One mechanism is the higher affinity with which dihydrotestosterone binds to and activates the androgen

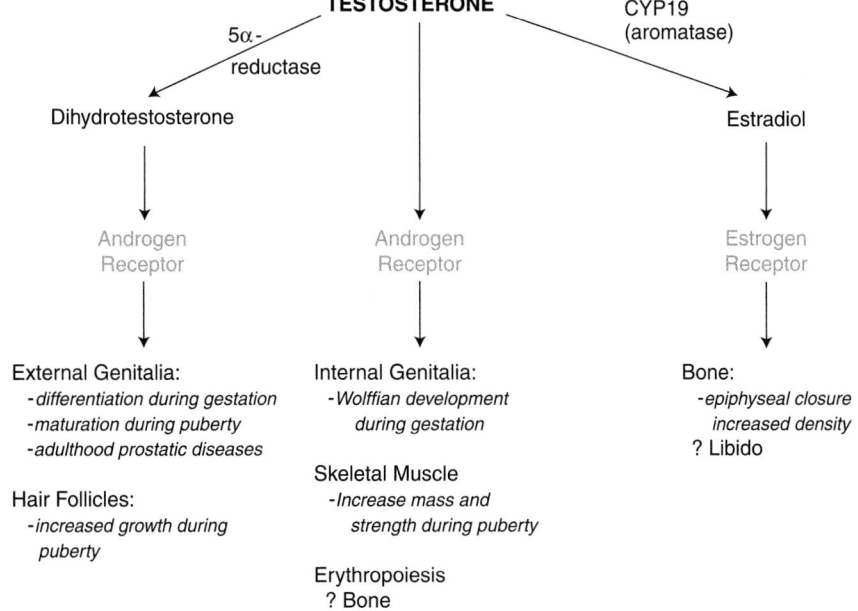

*Figure 58–4. Direct effects of testosterone and effects mediated indirectly **via** dihydrotestosterone or estradiol.*

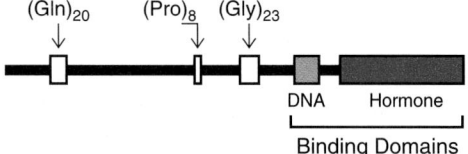

Figure 58–5. *Structure of the androgen receptor.*

receptor compared to testosterone (Deslypere *et al.*, 1992; Wilbert *et al.*, 1983). Another mechanism involves transcription co-factors, both co-activators and co-repressors, which are tissue-specific. At this time, the roles of co-factors are better described for other nuclear receptors than for the androgen receptor (Smith and O'Malley, 2004).

The importance of the androgen receptor is illustrated by the consequences of its mutations. Predictably, mutations that either alter the primary sequence of the protein or cause a single amino-acid substitution in the hormone- or DNA-binding domains result in resistance to the action of testosterone, beginning *in utero* (McPhaul and Griffin, 1999). Male sexual differentiation therefore is incomplete, as is pubertal development.

Another kind of mutation occurs in patients who have spinal and bulbar muscular atrophy, known as Kennedy's disease. These patients have an expansion of the CAG repeat, which codes for glutamine, at the amino terminus of the molecule (Walcott and Merry, 2002). The result is very mild androgen resistance, manifest principally by gynecomastia (Dejager *et al.*, 2002), but progressively severe motor neuron atrophy. The mechanism by which the neuron atrophy occurs is unknown, but similar trinucleotide repeats are associated with a number of other neurological disorders (Masino and Pastore, 2002).

Other kinds of androgen receptor mutations may explain why prostate cancer that is treated by androgen deprivation eventually becomes androgen-independent. Prostate cancer is initially at least partially androgen-sensitive, which is the basis for the initial treatment of metastatic prostate cancer by androgen deprivation. Metastatic prostate cancer often regresses initially in response to this treatment, but then becomes unresponsive to continued deprivation. The androgen receptor not only continues to be expressed in androgen-independent prostate cancer, but its signaling remains active, as indicated by expression of the androgen receptor–dependent prostate-specific antigen. It has been postulated that these observations can be explained by mutations in the androgen receptor gene or changes in androgen receptor co-regulatory proteins (Heinlein and Chang, 2004; Taplin and Balk, 2004).

Effects That Occur via the Estrogen Receptor.

The effects of testosterone on at least one tissue are mediated by its conversion to estradiol, catalyzed by the CYP19 enzyme complex (Figures 58–3 and 58–4). In the rare cases in which a male does not express CYP19 (Carani *et al.*, 1997; Morishma *et al.*, 1995) or the estrogen receptor (Smith *et al.*, 1994), the epiphyses do not fuse and long-bone growth continues indefinitely. In addition, the patients are osteoporotic. Administration of estradiol cor-

rects the bone abnormalities in patients with CYP19 deficiency (Bilizekian *et al.*, 1998), but not in those with an estrogen-receptor defect. Because men have larger bones than women, and bone cells express the androgen receptor (Colvard *et al.*, 1989), testosterone also may have an effect on bone *via* the androgen receptor. Administration of estradiol to a man with CYP19 deficiency increased his libido (Carani *et al.*, 1997), suggesting that the effect of testosterone on male libido may be mediated by conversion to estradiol.

Effects of Androgens at Different Stages of Life. *In Utero.* When the fetal testes, stimulated by human chorionic gonadotropin, begin to secrete testosterone at about the eighth week of gestation, the high local concentration of testosterone around the testes stimulates the nearby wolffian ducts to differentiate into the male internal genitalia: the epididymis, vas deferens, and seminal vesicles. Farther away, in the anlage of the external genitalia, testosterone is converted to dihydrotestosterone, which causes the development of the male external genitalia—the penis, scrotum—and the prostate. The increase in testosterone at the end of gestation may result in further phallic growth.

Infancy. The consequences of the increase in testosterone secretion by the testes during the first few months of life are not yet known.

Puberty. Puberty in the male begins at a mean age of 12 years with an increase in the secretion of FSH and LH from the gonadotropes, stimulated by increased secretion of GnRH from the hypothalamus. The increased secretion of FSH and LH stimulates the testes, so, not surprisingly, the first sign of puberty is an increase in testicular size. The increase in testosterone production by Leydig cells, along with the effect of FSH on the Sertoli cells, stimulates the development of the seminiferous tubules, which eventually produce mature sperm. Increased secretion of testosterone into the systemic circulation affects many tissues simultaneously, and the changes in most of them occur gradually during the course of several years. The phallus enlarges in length and width, the scrotum becomes rugated, and the prostate begins secreting the fluid it contributes to the semen. The skin becomes coarser and oilier due to increased sebum production, which contributes to the development of acne. Sexual hair begins to grow, initially pubic and axillary hair, then hair on the lower legs, and finally other body hair and facial hair. Full development of the latter two may not occur until 10 years after the start of puberty and marks the completion of puberty. Muscle mass and strength increase, especially of the shoulder girdle, and subcutaneous fat decreases. Epiphyseal bone growth accelerates, resulting in the pubertal growth spurt, but epiphyseal maturation leads eventually to a slowing and then cessation of growth. Bones also become thicker. The increase in the mass of muscle and bone results in a pronounced increase in body weight. Erythropoiesis increases, resulting in higher hematocrit and hemoglobin concentrations in men than boys or women. The larynx thickens, resulting in a lower voice. Libido develops.

Other changes may result from the increase in testosterone during puberty. Men tend to have a better sense of spatial relations than do women and to exhibit behavior that differs in some ways from that of women, including being more aggressive.

Adulthood. The serum testosterone concentration and the characteristics of the adult male are largely maintained during early adulthood and midlife. One change during this time is the gradual development of male pattern baldness, beginning with recession of hair at the temples and the vertex.

Two changes that can occur in the prostate gland during adulthood are of much greater medical significance. One is the gradual development of benign prostatic hyperplasia, which occurs to a variable degree in almost all men, sometimes obstructing urine outflow by compressing the urethra as it passes through the prostate. This development is mediated by the conversion of testosterone to dihydrotestosterone by 5α-reductase II within prostatic cells (Wilson, 1980).

The other change that can occur in the prostate during adulthood is the development of cancer. Although no direct evidence suggests that testosterone causes the disease, prostate cancer is dependent on testosterone, at least to some degree and at some time in its course. This dependency is the basis of treating metastatic prostate cancer by lowering the serum testosterone concentration (Iversen *et al.*, 1990) or by blocking its action.

Senescence. As men age, the serum testosterone concentration gradually declines (Figure 58–2), and the sex hormone–binding globulin concentration gradually increases, so that by age 80, the total testosterone concentration is approximately 80% and the free testosterone is approximately 40% of that present at age 20 (Harman *et al.*, 2001). This fall in serum testosterone could contribute to several other changes that occur with increasing age in men, including decreases in energy, libido, muscle mass (Forbes, 1976) and strength (Murray *et al.*, 1980), and bone mineral density (Riggs *et al.*, 1982). A causal role is suggested by the occurrence of similar changes seen in men who develop hypogonadism due to disease at a younger age, as discussed below.

Consequences of Androgen Deficiency

The consequences of androgen deficiency depend on the stage of life during which the deficiency first occurs and on the degree of the deficiency.

During Fetal Development. Testosterone deficiency in a male fetus during the first trimester *in utero* causes incomplete sexual differentiation. Testosterone deficiency in the first trimester results only from testicular disease, such as deficiency of CYP17 (17α-hydroxylase); deficiency of LH secretion because of pituitary or hypothalamic disease does not result in testosterone deficiency during the first trimester, presumably because Leydig cell secretion of testosterone at that time is regulated by placental hCG. Complete deficiency of testosterone secretion results in entirely female external genitalia; less severe testosterone deficiency results in incomplete virilization of the external genitalia proportionate to the degree of deficiency. Testosterone deficiency at this stage of development also leads to failure of the wolffian ducts to differentiate into the male internal genitalia, such as the vas deferens and seminal vesicles, but the müllerian ducts do not differentiate into the female internal genitalia as long as testes are present and secrete müllerian inhibitory substance. Similar changes occur if testosterone is secreted normally, but its action is

diminished because of an abnormality of the androgen receptor or of 5α-reductase. Abnormalities of the androgen receptor can have quite varied effects. The most severe form results in complete absence of androgen action and a female phenotype; moderately severe forms result in partial virilization of the external genitalia; and the mildest forms permit normal virilization *in utero* and result only in impaired spermatogenesis in adulthood (McPhaul and Griffin, 1999). Abnormal 5α-reductase results in incomplete virilization of the external genitalia *in utero* but normal development of the male internal genitalia, which requires only testosterone (Wilson *et al.*, 1993).

Testosterone deficiency during the third trimester, caused either by a testicular disease or a deficiency of fetal LH secretion, has two known consequences. First, the phallus fails to grow normally. The result, called microphallus, is a common occurrence in boys later discovered to be unable to secrete LH due to abnormalities of GnRH synthesis. Second, the testes fail to descend into the scrotum; this condition, called cryptorchidism, occurs commonly in boys whose LH secretion is subnormal (*see* Chapter 55).

Before Completion of Puberty. When a boy can secrete testosterone normally *in utero* but loses the ability to do so before the anticipated age of puberty, the result is failure to complete puberty. All of the pubertal changes described above, including those of the external genitalia, sexual hair, muscle mass, voice, and behavior, are impaired to a degree proportionate to the abnormality of testosterone secretion. In addition, if growth hormone secretion is normal when testosterone secretion is subnormal during the years of expected puberty, the long bones continue to lengthen because the epiphyses do not close. The result is longer arms and legs relative to the trunk; these proportions are referred to as eunuchoid. Another consequence of subnormal testosterone secretion during the age of expected puberty is enlargement of glandular breast tissue (gynecomastia).

After Completion of Puberty. When testosterone secretion becomes impaired after puberty is completed, regression of the pubertal effects of testosterone depends on both the degree and the duration of testosterone deficiency. When the degree of testosterone deficiency is substantial, libido and energy decrease within a week or two, but other testosterone-dependent characteristics decline more slowly. A clinically detectable decrease in muscle mass in an individual does not occur for several years. A pronounced decrease in hematocrit and hemoglobin will occur within several months. A decrease in bone mineral density probably can be detected by dual-energy x-ray absorptiometry within 2 years, but an increase in fracture incidence would not be likely to occur for many years. A loss of sexual hair takes many years.

In Women. Loss of androgen secretion in women results in a decrease in sexual hair, but not for many years. Androgens may have other important effects in women, and the loss of androgens (especially with the severe loss of ovarian and adrenal androgens that occurs in panhypopituitarism) would result in the loss of these effects. Testosterone preparations that can yield serum testosterone concentrations in the physiological range in women currently are being developed. The availability of such preparations will allow clinical trials to determine if testosterone replacement in androgen-deficient women improves their libido, energy, muscle mass and strength, and bone mineral density.

Therapeutic Androgen Preparations

The need for a creative approach to pharmacotherapy with androgens arises from the fact that ingestion of testosterone is not an effective means of replacing testosterone deficiency. Even though ingested testosterone is readily absorbed into the hepatic circulation, rapid hepatic metabolism ensures that hypogonadal men generally cannot ingest testosterone in sufficient amounts and with sufficient frequency to maintain a normal serum concentration. Therefore most pharmaceutical preparations of androgens are designed to bypass hepatic metabolism of testosterone.

Testosterone Esters. Esterifying a fatty acid to the 17α hydroxyl group of testosterone creates a compound that is even more lipophilic than testosterone itself. When an ester, such as *testosterone enanthate (heptanoate)* (Figure 58–6) or *cypionate (cyclopentylpropionate)* is dissolved in oil and administered intramuscularly every 2 weeks to hypogonadal men, the ester hydrolyzes *in vivo* and results in serum testosterone concentrations that range from higher-than-normal in the first few days after the injection to low-normal just before the next injection (Snyder and Lawrence, 1980) (Figure 58–7). Attempts to decrease the frequency of injections by increasing the amount of each injection result in wider fluctuations and poorer therapeutic outcomes. The undecanoate ester of testosterone (Figure 58–6), when dissolved in oil and ingested orally, is absorbed into the lymphatic circulation, thus bypassing initial hepatic metabolism. *Testosterone undecanoate* in oil also can be injected and produces stable serum testosterone concentrations for a month (Zhang *et al.*, 1998). The undecanoate ester of testosterone is not currently marketed in the United States.

Alkylated Androgens. Adding an alkyl group to the 17α position of testosterone (Figure 58–6) retards hepatic metabolism of the compound. Consequently, 17α-alkylated androgens are androgenic when administered orally;

however, they are less androgenic than testosterone itself, and they cause hepatotoxicity (Cabasso, 1994; Petera *et al.*, 1962), whereas native testosterone does not.

Transdermal Delivery Systems. Recent attempts to avoid the first-pass inactivation of testosterone by the liver have employed novel delivery systems; chemicals called excipients are used to facilitate the absorption of native testosterone across the skin in a controlled fashion. These transdermal preparations provide more stable serum testosterone concentrations than do injections of testosterone esters. The first such preparations were patches, one of which (ANDRODERM) is still available (Dobs *et al.*, 1999). Newer preparations include gels (ANDROGEL, TESTIM) (Marbury *et al.*, 2003; Swerdloff *et al.*, 2000) and a buccal tablet (STRIANT). These preparations produce mean serum testosterone concentrations within the normal range in hypogonadal men (Figure 58–7).

Attempts to Design Selective Androgens

Alkylated Androgens. Decades ago, investigators attempted to synthesize analogs of testosterone that possessed greater anabolic effects than androgenic effects compared to native testosterone. Several compounds appeared to have such differential effects, based on a greater effect on the levator ani muscle compared to the ventral prostate of the rat. These compounds were called anabolic steroids, and most are 17α-alkylated androgens. None of these compounds, however, has been convincingly demonstrated to have such a differential effect in human beings. Nonetheless, they have enjoyed popularity among athletes who seek to enhance their performance, as described below. Another alkylated androgen, 7α-methyl-19-nortestosterone, is poorly converted to dihydrotestosterone (Kumar *et al.*, 1992).

Selective Androgen Receptor Modulators. Stimulated by the development of selective estrogen receptor modulators, which have estrogenic effects in some tissues but not others (*see* Chapter 57), investigators are attempting to develop selective androgen receptor modulators. Indeed, it would be desirable to produce effects of testosterone in some tissues, such as muscle and bone, while avoiding the undesirable effects in other tissues, such as the prostate. Nonsteroidal molecules have been developed that bind to the androgen receptor, and when administered to castrated rats, stimulate the growth of the levator ani more than the prostate (Hanada *et al.*, 2003; Yin *et al.*, 2003). One molecule also improved several properties of bone (Hanada *et al.*, 2003). No human studies have yet been reported.

Therapeutic Uses of Androgens

Male Hypogonadism. The best-established indication for administration of androgens is for the treatment of

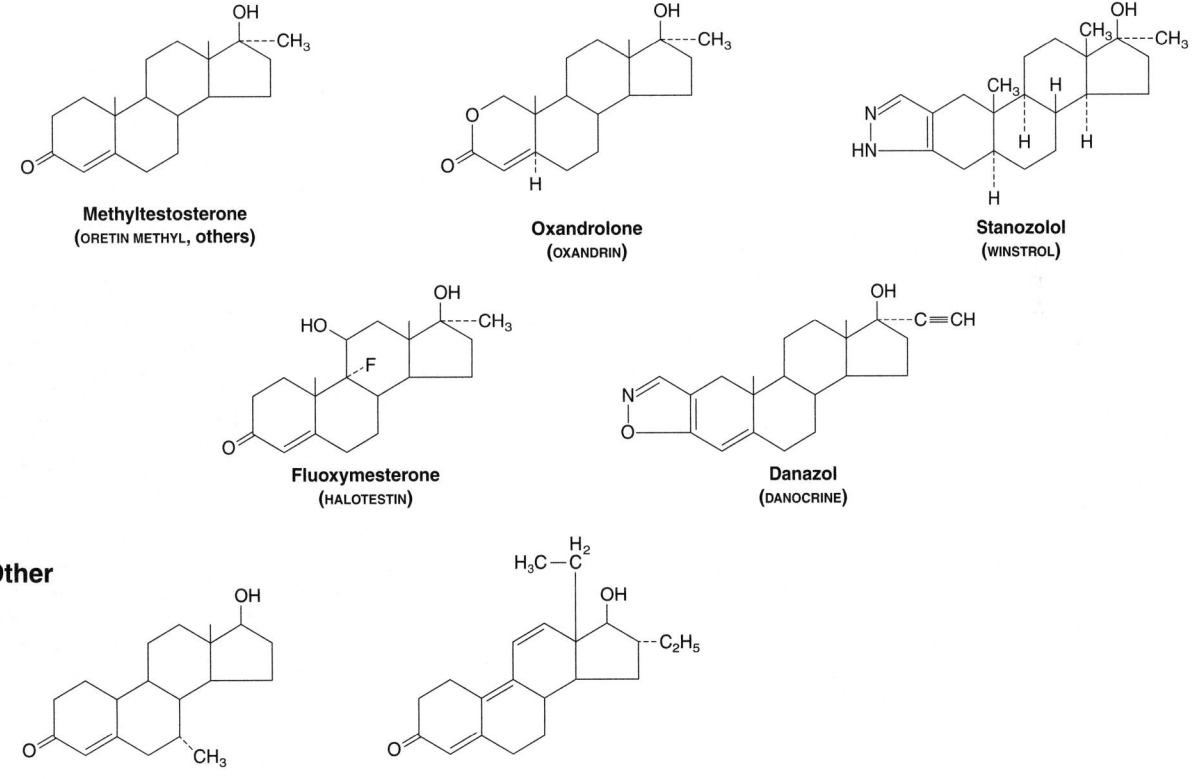

Figure 58–6. *Structures of some androgens available for therapeutic use.*

male hypogonadism (testosterone deficiency in men). Any of the transdermal testosterone preparations or testosterone esters described above can be used to treat testosterone deficiency. Monitoring treatment for beneficial and deleterious effects differs somewhat in adolescents and the elderly from that in other men.

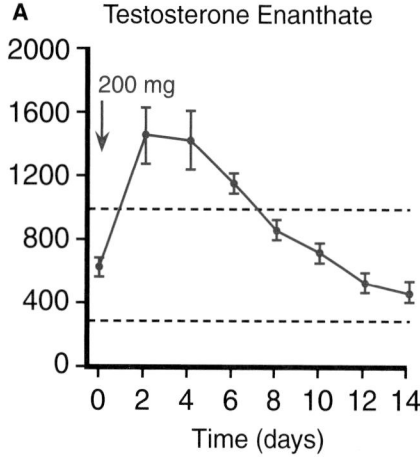

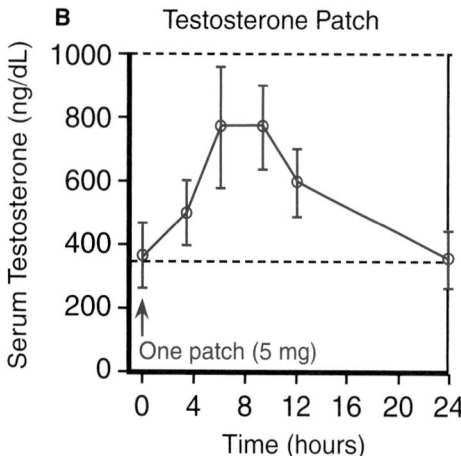

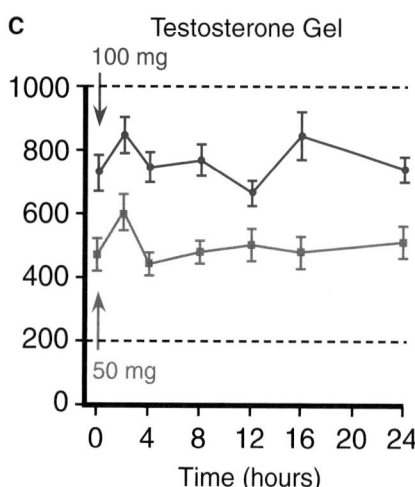

Figure 58–7. Pharmacokinetic profiles of three testosterone preparations during their chronic administration to hypogonadal men. Doses of each were given at time 0. Dashed lines indicate range of normal levels. (*A.* Adapted from Snyder and Lawrence, 1980; *B.* Dobs *et al.*, 1999; and *C.* Swerdloff *et al.*, 2000.)

Monitoring for Efficacy. The goal of testosterone therapy for a hypogonadal man is to mimic as closely as possible the normal serum concentration; therefore, serum testosterone concentration must be monitored during treatment. When the serum testosterone concentration is measured depends on the testosterone preparation used. With transdermal patches (*e.g.*, ANDRODERM), the serum testosterone concentration fluctuates during the 24-hour wearing period, with a peak value 6 to 9 hours after application and a nadir (about 50% of the peak) just before the next patch is applied (Dobs *et al.*, 1999). With testosterone gels, the mean serum testosterone concentration is relatively constant from one application to the next (Marbury *et al.*, 2003; Swerdloff *et al.*, 2000). Occasional random fluctuations can occur, however, so measurements should be repeated for any dose. When the enanthate or cypionate esters of testosterone are administered once every 2 weeks, the serum testosterone concentration measured midway between doses should be normal; if not, the dosage schedule should be adjusted accordingly. If testosterone deficiency results from testicular disease, as indicated by an elevated serum LH concentration, adequacy of testosterone treatment also can be judged indirectly by the normalization of LH within 2 months of treatment initiation (Findlay *et al.*, 1989; Snyder and Lawrence, 1980).

Normalization of the serum testosterone concentration induces normal virilization in prepubertal boys and restores virilization in men who became hypogonadal as adults. Within a few months, and often sooner, libido, energy, and hematocrit return to normal. Within 6 months, muscle mass increases and fat mass decreases. Bone density, however, continues to increase for 2 years (Snyder *et al.*, 2000).

Monitoring for Deleterious Effects. When testosterone itself is administered, as in one of the transdermal preparations or as an ester that is hydrolyzed to testosterone, it has no "side effects" (*i.e.*, no effects that endogenously secreted testosterone does not have), as long as the dose is not excessive. Modified testosterone compounds, such as the 17α-alkylated androgens, do have undesirable effects even when dosages are targeted at physiologic replacement. Some of these undesirable effects occur shortly after testosterone administration is initiated, whereas others usually do not occur until administration has been continued for many years. Raising the serum testosterone concentration from prepubertal or midpubertal levels to that of an adult male at any age can result in undesirable effects similar to those that occur during puberty, including acne, gynecomastia, and more aggressive sexual behavior. Physiological amounts of testosterone do not appear to affect serum lipids or apolipoproteins. Replacement of physiological levels of testosterone may occasionally have undesirable effects in the presence of concomitant illnesses. For example, stimulation of erythropoiesis would increase the hematocrit from subnormal to normal in a healthy man, but would raise the hematocrit above normal in a man with a predisposition to erythrocytosis, such as in chronic pulmonary disease. Similarly, the mild degree of sodium and water retention seen with testosterone replacement would have no clinical effect in a healthy man, but would exacerbate pre-existing congestive heart failure. If the testosterone dose is excessive, erythrocytosis, and uncommonly, salt and water retention and peripheral edema occur, even in men who have no predisposition to these conditions. When a man's serum testosterone concentration has been in the normal adult male range for many years, whether from endogenous secretion or exogenous administration, and he is older than 40, he is subject to certain testosterone-dependent diseases, including benign prostatic hyperplasia and prostate cancer.

The principal side effects of the 17α-alkylated androgens are hepatic, including cholestasis, and uncommonly, peliosis hepatis, blood-filled hepatic cysts. Hepatocellular cancer has been reported rarely. Case reports of cancer regression after androgen cessation suggest a possible causal role, but an etiologic link is unproven. The

17α-alkylated androgens, especially in large amounts, may lower serum HDL cholesterol.

Monitoring at the Anticipated Time of Puberty. Administration of testosterone to testosterone-deficient boys at the anticipated time of puberty should be guided by the considerations above, but also by the fact that testosterone accelerates epiphyseal maturation, leading initially to a growth spurt but then to epiphyseal closure and permanent cessation of linear growth. Consequently, the height and growth-hormone status of the boy must be considered. Boys who are short because of growth-hormone deficiency should be treated with growth hormone before their hypogonadism is treated with testosterone.

Male Senescence. Preliminary evidence suggests that increasing the serum testosterone concentration of men whose serum levels are subnormal for no reason other than their age will increase their bone mineral density and lean mass and decrease their fat mass (Amory *et al.*, 2004; Kenny *et al.*, 2001; Snyder *et al.*, 1999a; Snyder *et al.*, 1999b). However, it is entirely uncertain at this time if such treatment will worsen benign prostatic hyperplasia or increase the incidence of clinically detectable prostate cancer.

Female Hypogonadism. It remains to be determined if increasing the serum testosterone concentrations of women whose serum testosterone concentrations are below normal will improve their libido, energy, muscle mass and strength, or bone mineral density.

Enhancement of Athletic Performance. Some athletes take drugs, including androgens, to attempt to improve their performance. Because androgens taken for this purpose usually are taken surreptitiously, information about their possible effects is not as reliable as that for androgens taken for treatment of male hypogonadism.

Kinds of Androgens Used. Virtually all androgens produced for human or veterinary purposes have been taken by athletes. When use by athletes began more than two decades ago, the favored compounds were 17α-alkylated androgens and other compounds that were thought to have greater anabolic effects than androgen effects relative to testosterone (so-called "anabolic steroids"). Because these compounds can be detected readily by organizations that govern athletic competitions, preparations that increase the serum concentration of testosterone itself, such as the testosterone esters or human chorionic gonadotropin, have increased in popularity. Testosterone precursors, such as androstenedione and dehydroepiandrosterone (DHEA), also have increased in popularity recently because they are considered nutritional supplements and thus are not regulated by national governments or athletic organizations.

A new development in use of androgens by athletes is represented by tetrahydrogestrinone (THG), a potent androgen (Death *et al.*, 2004) that appears to have been designed and synthesized in order to avoid detection by anti-doping laboratories on the basis of its novel structure (Figure 58–6) and rapid metabolism.

Efficacy. There have been few controlled studies of the effects of pharmacological doses of androgens on muscle strength. In one controlled study, 43 normal young men were randomized to one of four groups: strength training with either 600 mg of testosterone enanthate once a week (more than six times the replacement dose) or placebo; or no exercise with either testosterone or placebo. The men who received testosterone experienced an increase in muscle strength compared to those who received placebo, and the men who exercised simultaneously experienced even greater increases (Bhasin *et al.*, 1996). In another study, normal young men were treated with a GnRH analog to reduce endogenous testosterone secretion severely and in a random, blinded fashion, weekly doses of testosterone enanthate from 25 mg to 600 mg. There was a dose-dependent effect of testosterone on muscle strength (Bhasin *et al.*, 2001).

In a double-blind study of androstenedione, men who took 100 mg three times a day for 8 weeks did not experience an increase in muscle strength compared to men who took placebo. Failure of this treatment to increase muscle strength is not surprising, because it also did not increase the mean serum testosterone concentration (King *et al.*, 1999).

Side Effects. All androgens suppress gonadotropin secretion when taken in high doses and thereby suppress endogenous testicular function. This decreases endogenous testosterone and sperm production, resulting in diminished fertility. If administration continues for many years, testicular size may diminish. Testosterone and sperm production usually return to normal within a few months of discontinuation but may take longer. High doses of androgens also cause erythrocytosis (Drinka *et al.*, 1995).

When administered in high doses, androgens that can be converted to estrogens, such as testosterone, cause gynecomastia. Androgens whose A rings have been modified so that they cannot be aromatized, such as dihydrotestosterone, do not cause gynecomastia, even in high doses.

The 17α-alkylated androgens are the only androgens that cause hepatotoxicity. When administered at high doses, these androgens are more likely than others to affect serum lipid concentrations, specifically to decrease high-density lipoprotein (HDL) cholesterol and increase low-density lipoprotein (LDL) cholesterol. Other side effects have been suggested by many anecdotes but have not been confirmed, including psychological disorders and sudden death due to cardiac disease, possibly related to changes in lipids or to coagulation activation.

Certain side effects occur specifically in women and children. Both experience virilization, including facial and body hirsutism, temporal hair recession in a male pattern, and acne. Boys experience phallic enlargement, and women experience clitoral enlargement. Boys and girls whose epiphyses have not yet closed experience premature closure and stunting of linear growth.

Male Contraception. As discussed above, androgens inhibit LH secretion by the pituitary and thereby decrease endogenous testosterone production. Based on these observations, scientists have tried for more than a decade to use androgens—either alone or in combination with other drugs—as a male contraceptive. Because the concentration of testosterone within the testes, approximately one hundred times that in the peripheral circulation, is necessary for spermatogenesis, suppression of endogenous testosterone production greatly diminishes spermatogenesis. Initial use of testosterone alone, however, required supraphysiologic doses, and addition of GnRH agonists required daily injections. A more promising approach is the combination of a progestin with a physiological dose of testosterone to suppress LH secretion and spermatogenesis, but provide a normal serum testosterone concentration (Bebb *et al.*, 1996). A recent trial employed injections of testosterone undecanoate with a depot progestin every 2 months (Gu *et al.*, 2004). Another androgen being tested as part of a male contraceptive regimen is 7α-methyl-19-nortestosterone, a synthetic androgen that cannot be metabolized to dihydrotestosterone (Cummings *et al.*, 1998).

Catabolic and Wasting States. Testosterone, because of its anabolic effects, has been used in attempts to ameliorate catabolic and muscle-wasting states, but this has not been generally effective. One exception is in the treatment of muscle wasting associated with acquired immunodeficiency syndrome (AIDS), which often is accompanied by hypogonadism. Treatment of men with AIDS-related muscle wasting and subnormal serum testosterone concentrations increases their muscle mass and strength (Bhasin *et al.*, 2000).

Angioedema. Chronic androgen treatment of patients with angioedema effectively prevents attacks. The disease is caused by hereditary impairment of C1-esterase inhibitor or acquired development of antibodies against it (Cicardi *et al.*, 1998). The 17α-alkylated androgens, such as *stanozolol* and *danazol*, stimulate the hepatic synthesis of the esterase inhibitor. In women, virilization is a potential side effect. In children, virilization and premature epiphyseal closure prevent chronic use of androgens for prophylaxis, although they are used occasionally to treat acute episodes.

Blood Dyscrasias. Androgens once were employed to attempt to stimulate erythropoiesis in patients with anemias of various etiologies, but the availability of erythropoietin has supplanted that use. Androgens such as danazol still are used occasionally as adjunctive treatment for hemolytic anemia and idiopathic thrombocytopenic purpura that are refractory to first-line agents.

ANTI-ANDROGENS

Because some effects of androgens are undesirable, at least under certain circumstances, agents have been developed specifically to inhibit androgen synthesis or effects. Other drugs, originally developed for different purposes, have been accidentally found to be anti-androgens and now are used intentionally for this indication.

Inhibitors of Testosterone Secretion. Both agonists and antagonists of the GnRH receptor are used to reduce testosterone secretion. Analogs of GnRH effectively inhibit testosterone secretion by inhibiting LH secretion. GnRH "superactive" analogs, given repeatedly, down-regulate the GnRH receptor and are available for treatment of prostate cancer. An extended-release form of the GnRH antagonist *abarelix* (PLENAXIS) is approved for treating prostate cancer (Trachtenberg *et al.*, 2002). Because abarelix does not transiently increase sex steroid production, this preparation may be especially useful in prostate cancer patients in whom any stimulus to tumor growth might have serious adverse consequences, such as patients

with spinal cord metastases in whom increased tumor growth could cause paralysis (*see* Chapter 55).

Some antifungal drugs of the imidazole family, such as ketoconazole (*see* Chapter 48), inhibit CYPs and thereby block the synthesis of steroid hormones, including testosterone and cortisol. Because they may induce adrenal insufficiency and are associated with hepatotoxicity, these drugs generally are not used to inhibit androgen synthesis, but sometimes are employed in cases of glucocorticoid excess (*see* Chapter 59).

Inhibitors of Androgen Action

These drugs inhibit the binding of androgens to the androgen receptor or inhibit 5α-reductase.

Androgen Receptor Antagonists. **Flutamide, Bicalutamide, and Nilutamide.** These relatively potent androgen receptor antagonists have limited efficacy when used alone because the increased LH secretion stimulates higher serum testosterone concentrations. They are used primarily in conjunction with a GnRH analog in the treatment of metastatic prostate cancer. In this situation, they block the action of adrenal androgens, which are not inhibited by GnRH analogs. Survival rates in groups of patients with metastatic prostate cancer treated with a combination of a GnRH agonist and *flutamide* (EULEXIN), *bicalutamide* (CASODEX), or *nilutamide* (NILANDRON) are similar to one another (Schellhammer *et al.*, 1995) and to survival rates in those treated by castration (Iversen *et al.*, 1990). Bicalutamide is replacing flutamide for this purpose because it appears to have less hepatotoxicity and is taken once a day instead of three times a day. Nilutamide appears to have worse side effects than flutamide and bicalutamide (Dole and Holdsworth, 1997). Flutamide also has been used to treat hirsutism in women, and it appears to be as effective as any other treatment for this purpose (Venturoli *et al.*, 1999). However, the association with hepatotoxicity warrants cautions against its use for this cosmetic purpose.

Flutamide

Bicalutamide

Nilutamide

Spironolactone. *Spironolactone* (ALDACTONE) (*see* Chapter 28) is an inhibitor of aldosterone that also is a weak antagonist at the androgen receptor and a weak inhibitor of testosterone synthesis, apparently inhibiting CYP17. When used to treat fluid retention or hypertension in men, gynecomastia is a common side effect (Caminos-Torres *et al.*, 1977). In part because of this adverse effect, the selective mineralocorticoid receptor antagonist *epleronone* (INSPIRA) recently was launched in the United States. Spironolactone is approved by the FDA for treating hirsutism in women, for which it is moderately effective (Cumming *et al.*, 1982); however, it may cause irregular menses.

Cyproterone Acetate. *Cyproterone acetate* is a progestin and a weak anti-androgen by virtue of binding to the androgen receptor. It is moderately effective in reducing hirsutism alone or in combination with an oral contraceptive (Venturoli *et al.*, 1999), but it is not approved for use in the United States.

5α-Reductase Inhibitors. *Finasteride* (PROSCAR) is an antagonist of 5α-reductase, especially type II; *dutasteride* (AVODART) is an antagonist of types I and II; both drugs block the conversion of testosterone to dihydrotestosterone, especially in the male external genitalia. These agents were developed to treat benign prostatic hyperplasia, and they are approved in the United States and many other countries for this purpose. When they are administered to men with moderately severe symptoms due to obstruction of urinary tract outflow, serum and prostatic concentrations of dihydrotestosterone decrease, prostatic volume decreases, and urine flow rate increases (McConnell *et al.*, 1998; Roehrborn *et al.*, 2004; Clark *et al.*, 2004). Impotence is a well-documented, albeit infrequent, side effect of this use, although the mechanism is not understood. Finasteride also is approved for use in the treatment of male pattern baldness under the trade name PROPECIA, even though that effect is presumably mediated *via* type I 5α-reductase. Finasteride appears to be as effective as flutamide and the combination of estrogen and cyproterone in the treatment of hirsutism (Venturoli *et al.*, 1999).

Finasteride

BIBLIOGRAPHY

Amory, J.K., Watts, N.B., Easley K.A., *et al.* Exogenous testosterone or testosterone with finasteride increases bone mineral density in older men with low serum testosterone. *J. Clin. Endocrinol. Metab.*, **2004**, *89*:503–510.

Bebb, R.A., Anawalt, B., Christensen, R.B., *et al.* Combined administration of levonorgestrel and testosterone induces a more rapid and effective suppression of spermatogenesis than testosterone alone: a promising male contraceptive approach. *J. Clin. Endocrinol. Metab.*, **1996**, *81*:757–762.

Bhasin, S., Storer, T.W., Berman, N., *et al.* The effects of supraphysiologic doses of testosterone on muscle size and strength in normal men. *N. Engl. J. Med.*, **1996**, *335*:1–7.

Bhasin, S., Storer, T.W., Javanbakht, M., *et al.* Testosterone replacement and resistance exercise in HIV-infected men with weight loss and low testosterone levels. *JAMA*, **2000**, *283*:763–770.

Bhasin, S., Woodhouse, L., Casaburi, R., *et al.* Testosterone dose-response relationships in healthy young men. *Am. J. Physiol. Endocrinol. Metab.*, **2001**, *281*:E1172–E1181.

Bilizekian, J., Morishima, A., Bell, J., and Grumbach, M.M. Estrogen markedly increases bone mass in an estrogen-deficient young man with aromatase deficiency. *N. Engl. J. Med.*, **1998**, *339*:599–603.

Bremner, W.J., Vitiello, V., and Prinz, P.N. Loss of circadian rhythmicity in blood testosterone levels with aging in normal men. *J. Clin. Endocrinol. Metab.* **1983**, *56*:1278–1280.

Brinkman, A.O., and Trapman, J. Genetic analysis of androgen receptors in development and disease. *Adv. Pharmacol.*, **2000**, *47*:317–341.

Cabasso, A. Peliosis hepatis in a young adult bodybuilder. *Med. Sci. Sports Exerc.*, **1994**, *26*:2–4.

Caminos-Torres, R., Ma, L., and Snyder, P.J. Gynecomastia and semen abnormalities induced by spironolactone in normal men. *J. Clin. Endocrinol. Metab.*, **1977**, *45*:255–260.

Carani, C., Qin, K., Simoni, M., *et al.* Effect of testosterone and estradiol in a man with aromatase deficiency. *N. Engl. J. Med.*, **1997**, *337*:91–95.

Cicardi, M., Bergamaschini, L., Cugno, M., *et al.* Pathogenetic and clinical aspects of C1 esterase inhibitor deficiency. *Immunobiology*, **1998**, *199*:366–376.

Clark, R.V., Hermann, D.J., Cunningham, G.R., *et al.* Marked suppression of dihydrotestosterone in men with benign prostatic hypertrophy by dutasteride, a dual 5α-reductase inhibitor. *J. Clin. Endocrinol. Metab.*, **2004**, *89*:2179–2184.

Colvard, D.S., Eriksen, E.F., Keeting, P.E., *et al.* Identification of androgen receptors in normal human osteoblast-like cells. *Proc. Natl. Acad. Sci. U.S.A.*, **1989**, *86*:854–857.

Crowley, W.F., Filicori, M., Spratt, D.I., and Santoro, N.F. The physiology of gonadotropin-releasing hormone secretion in men and women. *Recent Prog. Horm. Res.*, **1985**, *41*:473–531.

Cumming, D.C., Yang, J.C., Rebar, R.W., and Yen, S.C. Treatment of hirsutism with spironolactone. *JAMA*, **1982**, *247*:1295–1298.

Cummings, D.E., Kumar, N., Bardin, C.W., *et al.* Prostate-sparing effects in primates of the potent androgen 7α-methyl-19-nortestosterone: a potential alternative to testosterone for androgen replacement and male contraception. *J. Clin. Endocrinol. Metab.*, **1998**, *84*:4212–4219.

Dawood, M.Y., and Saxena, B.B. Testosterone and dihydrotestosterone in maternal and cord blood and in amniotic fluid. *Am. J. Obstet. Gynecol.*, **1977**, *129*:37–42.

Death, A.K., McGrath, K.C., Kazlauskas, R., and Handelsman, D.J. Tetrahydrogestrinone is a potent androgen and progestin. *J. Clin. Endocrinol. Metab.,* **2004,** *89:*2498–2500.

Dejager, S., Bry-Gauillard, H., Bruckert, E., *et al.* A comprehensive endocrine description of Kennedy's disease revealing androgen insensitivity linked to CAG repeat length. *J. Clin. Endocrinol. Metab.,* **2002,** *87:*3893–3901.

Deslypere, J.P., Young, M., Wilson, J.D., and McPhaul, M.J. Testosterone and 5α-dihydrotestosterone interact differently with the androgen receptor to enhance transcription of the MMTV-CAT reporter gene. *Mol. Cell. Endocrinol.,* **1992,** *88:*15–22.

Dobs, A.S., Meikle, A.W., Arver, S., *et al.* Pharmacokinetics, efficacy, and safety of a permeation-enhanced testosterone transdermal system in comparison with bi-weekly injections of testosterone enanthate for the treatment of hypogonadal men. *J. Clin. Endocrinol. Metab.,* **1999,** *84:*3469–3478.

Dole, E.J., and Holdsworth, M.T. Nilutamide: an antiandrogen for the treatment of prostate cancer. *Ann. Pharmacother.,* **1997,** *31:*65–75.

Drinka, P.J., Jochen, A.L., Cuisiner, M., *et al.* Polycythemia as a complication of testosterone replacement therapy in nursing home men with low testosterone levels. *J. Am. Geriatr. Soc.,* **1995,** *43:*899–901.

Findlay, J.C., Place, V.A., and Snyder, P.J. Treatment of primary hypogonadism in men by the transdermal administration of testosterone. *J. Clin. Endocrinol. Metab.,* **1989,** *68:*369–373.

Forbes, G.B. The adult decline in lean body mass. *Hum. Biol.,* **1976,** *48:*161–173.

Forest, M.G. Differentiation and development of the male. *Clin. Endocrinol. Metab.,* **1975,** *4:*569–596.

Gu, Y.Q., Tong, J.S., Ma, D.Z., *et al.* Male hormonal contraception: effects of injections of testosterone undecanoate and depot medroxyprogesterone acetate at eight-week intervals in Chinese men. *J. Clin. Endocrinol. Metab.,* **2004,** *89:*2254–2262.

Hanada, K., Furuya, K., Yamamoto, N., *et al.* Bone anabolic effects of S-40503, a novel nonsteroidal selective androgen receptor modulator (SARM), in rat models of osteoporosis. *Biol. Pharm. Bull.,* **2003,** *26:*1563–1569.

Harman, S.M., Metter, E.J., Tobin, J.D., *et al.* Longitudinal effects of aging on serum total and free testosterone levels in healthy men. Baltimore Longitudinal Study of Aging. *J. Clin. Endocrinol. Metab.,* **2001,** *86:*724–731.

Heinlein, C.A., and Chang, C. Androgen receptor in prostate cancer. *Endocr. Rev.,* **2004,** *25:*276–308.

Iversen, P., Christenson, M.G., Friis, E., *et al.* A phase III of zoladex and flutamide versus orchiectomy in the treatment of patients with advanced carcinoma of the prostate. *Cancer,* **1990,** *66:*1058–1066.

Kenny, A.M., Prestwood, K.M., Gruman, C.A., *et al.* Effects of transdermal testosterone on bone and muscle in older men with low bioavailable testosterone levels. *J. Gerontol. A. Biol. Sci. Med. Sci.,* **2001,** *56:*M266–M272.

King, D.S., Sharp, R.L., Vukovich, M.D., *et al.* Effect of oral androstenedione on serum testosterone and adaptation to resistance training in young men: a randomized controlled trial. *JAMA,* **1999,** *281:*2020–2028.

Kumar, N., Didolkar, A.K., Monder, C., *et al.* The biological activity of 7α-methyl-19-nortestosterone is not amplified in male reproductive tract as is that of testosterone. *Endocrinology,* **1992,** *130:*3677–3683.

McConnell, J.D., Bruskewitz, R., Walsh, P., *et al.* The effect of finasteride on the risk of acute urinary retention and the need for surgical treatment among men with benign prostatic hyperplasia. Finasteride

Long-Term Efficacy and Safety Study Group. *N. Engl. J. Med.,* **1998,** *338:*557–563.

MacDonald, P.C., Madden, J.D., Brenner, P.F., *et al.* Origin of estrogen in normal men and in women with testicular feminization. *J. Clin. Endocrinol. Metab.,* **1979,** *49:*905–917.

McPhaul, M.J., and Griffin, J.E. Male pseudohermaphroditism caused by mutations of the human androgen receptor. *J. Clin. Endocrinol. Metab.,* **1999,** *84:*3435–3441.

Marbury, T., Hamill, E., Bachand, R., *et al.* Evaluation of the pharmacokinetic profiles of the new testosterone topical gel formulation, Testim, compared to AndroGel. *Biopharm. Drug Dispos.,* **2003,** *24:*115–120.

Masino, L., and Pastore, A. Glutamine repeats: structural hypotheses and neurodegeneration. *Biochem. Soc. Trans.,* **2002,** *30:*548–551.

Morishma, A., Grumbach, M.M., Simpson, E.R., *et al.* Aromatase deficiency in male and female siblings caused by a novel mutation and the physiological role of estrogens. *J. Clin. Endocrinol. Metab.,* **1995,** *80:*3689–3698.

Murray, M.P., Gardner, G.M., Mollinger, L.A., and Sepic, S.B. Strength of isometric and isokinetic contractions: knee muscles and of men aged 20–86. *Phys. Ther.,* **1980,** *60:*412–419.

Petera, V., Bobeck, K., and Lahn, V. Serum transaminase (GOT < GPT) and lactic dehydrogenase activity during treatment with methyltestosterone. *Clin. Chem. Acta.,* **1962,** *7:*604–606.

Riggs, B.L., Wahner, H.W., Seeman, E., *et al.* Changes in bone mineral density of the proximal femur and spine with aging. *J. Clin. Invest.,* **1982,** *70:*716–723.

Roehrborn, C.G., Marks, L.S., Fenter, T., *et al.* Efficacy and safety of dutasteride in the four-year treatment of men with benign prostatic hyperplasia. *Urology,* **2004,** *63:*709–715.

Schellhammer, P., Sharifi, R., Block N., *et al.* A controlled trial of bicalutamide versus flutamide, each in combination with luteinizing hormone releasing hormone analogue therapy, in patients with advanced prostate cancer. *Urology,* **1995,** *45:*745–752.

Smith, C.L., and O'Malley, B.W. Coregulator function: a key to understanding tissue specificity of selective receptor modulators. *Endocr. Rev.,* **2004,** *25:*45–71.

Smith, E.P., Boyd, J., Frank, G.R., *et al.* Estrogen resistance caused by a mutation in the estrogen-receptor gene in a man. *N. Engl. J. Med.,* **1994,** *331:*1056–1061.

Snyder, P.J., and Lawrence, D.A. Treatment of male hypogonadism with testosterone enanthate. *J. Clin. Endocrinol. Metab.,* **1980,** *51:*1335–1339.

Snyder, P.J., Peachey, H., Berlin, J.A., *et al.* Effects of testosterone replacement in hypogonadal men. *J. Clin. Endocrinol. Metab.,* **2000,** *85:*2670–2677.

Snyder, P.J., Peachey, H., Hannoush, P., *et al.* Effect of testosterone treatment on body composition and muscle strength in men over 65 years of age. *J. Clin. Endocrinol. Metab.,* **1999b,** *84:*2647–2653.

Snyder, P.J., Peachey, H., Hannoush, P., *et al.* Effect of testosterone treatment on bone mineral density in men over 65 years of age. *J. Clin. Endocrinol. Metab.,* **1999a,** *84:*1966–1972.

Swerdloff, R.S., Wang, C., Cunningham, G., *et al.* Long-term pharmacokinetics of transdermal testosterone gel in hypogonadal men. *J. Clin. Endocrinol. Metab.,* **2000,** *85:*4500–4510.

Taplin, M.E., and Balk, S.P. Androgen receptor: a key molecule in the progression of prostate cancer to hormone independence. *J. Cell. Biochem.,* **2004,** *91:*483–490.

Trachtenberg, J., Gittleman, M., Steidle, C., *et al.* A phase 3, multicenter, open label, randomized study of abarelix versus leuprolide plus daily antiandrogen in men with prostate cancer. *J. Urol.,* **2002,** *167:*1670–1674.

Venturoli, S., Marescalchi, O., Colombo, F.M., *et al.* A prospective randomized trial comparing low-dose flutamide, finasteride, ketoconazole, and cyproterone acetate-estrogen regimens in the treatment of hirsutism. *J. Clin. Endocrinol. Metab.,* **1999,** *84:*1304–1310.

Walcott, J.L., and Merry, D.E. Trinucleotide repeat disease. The androgen receptor in spinal and bulbar muscular atrophy. *Vitam. Horm.,* **2002,** *65:*127–147.

Wilbert, D.M., Griffin, J.E., and Wilson, J.D. Characterization of the cytosol androgen receptor of the human prostate. *J. Clin. Endocrinol. Metab.,* **1983,** *56:*113–120.

Wilson, J.D., Griffin, J.E., and Russell, D.W. Steroid 5 α-reductase 2 deficiency. *Endocr. Rev.,* **1993,** *14:*577–593.

Wilson, J.D. The pathogenesis of benign prostatic hyperplasia. *Am. J. Med.,* **1980,** *68:*745–756.

Yin, D., Gao, W., Kearbey, J.D., Xu, H., *et al.* Pharmacodynamics of selective androgen receptor modulators. *J. Pharmacol. Exp. Ther.,* **2003,** *304:*1334–1340.

Zhang, G.Y., Gu, Y.Q., Wang, X.H., *et al.* A pharmacokinetic study of injectable testosterone undecanoate in hypogonadal men. *J. Androl.,* **1998,** *19:*761–768.

ADRENOCORTICOTROPIC HORMONE; ADRENOCORTICAL STEROIDS AND THEIR SYNTHETIC ANALOGS; INHIBITORS OF THE SYNTHESIS AND ACTIONS OF ADRENOCORTICAL HORMONES

Bernard P. Schimmer and Keith L. Parker

Adrenocorticotropic hormone (ACTH, also called corticotropin) and the steroid hormone products of the adrenal cortex are considered together because the major physiological and pharmacological effects of ACTH result from its action to increase the circulating levels of adrenocortical steroids. Synthetic derivatives of ACTH are used principally in the diagnostic assessment of adrenocortical function. Because all known therapeutic effects of ACTH can be achieved with corticosteroids, synthetic steroid hormones generally are used therapeutically instead of ACTH.

Corticosteroids and their biologically active synthetic derivatives differ in their metabolic (glucocorticoid) and electrolyte-regulating (mineralocorticoid) activities. These agents are employed at physiological doses for replacement therapy when endogenous production is impaired. In addition, glucocorticoids potently suppress inflammation, and their use in a variety of inflammatory and autoimmune diseases makes them among the most frequently prescribed classes of drugs. Because they exert effects on almost every organ system, the clinical use of and withdrawal from corticosteroids are complicated by a number of serious side effects, some of which are life-threatening. Therefore, the decision to institute therapy with corticosteroids always requires careful consideration of the relative risks and benefits in each patient.

Agents that inhibit steps in the steroidogenic pathway and thus alter the biosynthesis of adrenocortical steroids are discussed, as are synthetic steroids that inhibit glucocorticoid action. Agents that inhibit the action of aldosterone are presented in Chapter 28; agents used to inhibit growth of steroid-dependent tumors are discussed in Chapter 51.

History. Addison described fatal outcomes in patients with adrenal destruction in a presentation to the South London Medical Society in 1849. These studies were soon extended when Brown-Séquard demonstrated that bilateral adrenalectomy was fatal in laboratory animals. It later was shown that the adrenal cortex, rather than the medulla, was essential for survival in these experiments. Further studies demonstrated that the adrenal cortex regulated both carbohydrate metabolism and fluid and electrolyte balance. Studies of the factors that regulated carbohydrate metabolism (termed *glucocorticoids*) culminated with the synthesis of *cortisone,* the first pharmacologically effective glucocorticoid to become readily available. Subsequently, Tate and colleagues isolated and characterized a distinct corticosteroid, *aldosterone,* which potently affected fluid and electrolyte balance and therefore was termed a *mineralocorticoid.* The isolation of distinct corticosteroids that regulated carbohydrate metabolism or fluid and electrolyte balance led to the concept that the adrenal cortex comprises two largely independent units: an outer zone that produces mineralocorticoids and an inner region that synthesizes glucocorticoids and androgen precursors.

Studies of adrenocortical steroids also played a key part in delineating the role of the anterior pituitary in endocrine function. As early as 1912, Cushing described patients with hypercorticism, and later recognized that pituitary basophilism caused the adrenal overactivity, thus establishing the link between the anterior pituitary and adrenal function. These studies led to the purification of ACTH and the determination of its chemical structure. ACTH was further shown to be essential for maintaining the structural integrity and steroidogenic capacity of the inner cortical zones. Harris established the role of the hypothalamus in pituitary control and postulated that a soluble factor produced by the hypothalamus activated ACTH release. These investigations culminated with the determination of the structure of corticotropin-releasing hormone (CRH), a hypothalamic peptide that regulates secretion of ACTH from the pituitary.

Shortly after synthetic cortisone became available, Hench and colleagues demonstrated its dramatic effect in the treatment of rheumatoid arthritis. These studies set the stage for the clinical use of corticosteroids in a wide variety of diseases, as discussed below.

ADRENOCORTICOTROPIC HORMONE (ACTH; CORTICOTROPIN)

As summarized in Figure 59–1, ACTH is synthesized as part of a larger precursor protein, pro-opiomelanocortin (POMC), and is liberated from the precursor through proteolytic cleavage at dibasic residues by the enzyme prohormone convertase 1 (*see* Chapter 21). Impaired processing of POMC due to a mutation in prohormone convertase 1 has been implicated in the pathogenesis of a human disorder that presents with adrenal insufficiency, childhood obesity, hypogonadotropic hypogonadism, and diabetes. A number of other biologically important peptides, including endorphins, lipotropins, and the melanocyte-stimulating hormones (MSH), also are produced from the same POMC precursor.

Human ACTH is a peptide of 39 amino acids (Figure 59–1). Whereas removal of a single amino acid at the amino terminus considerably impairs biological activity, a number of amino acids can be removed from the carboxyl-terminal end without a marked effect. The structure–activity relationships of ACTH have been studied extensively, and it is believed that a stretch of four basic amino acids at positions 15 to 18 is an important determinant of high-affinity binding to the ACTH receptor, whereas amino acids 6 to 10 are important for receptor activation.

The actions of ACTH and the other melanocortins liberated from POMC are mediated by their specific interactions with five melanocortin receptor (MCR) subtypes comprising a distinct subfamily of G protein–coupled receptors. The well-known effects of MSH on pigmentation result from interactions with the MC1R on melanocytes. MC1Rs also are found on cells of the immune system and are thought to mediate the antiinflammatory effects of α-MSH in experimental models of inflammation. ACTH, which is identical to α-MSH in its first 13 amino acids (Ser-Tyr-Ser-Met-Glu-His-Phe-Arg-Trp-Gly-Lys-Pro-Val), exerts its effects on the adrenal cortex through the MC2R. ACTH has a much higher affinity for the MC2R than for the MC1R; however, under pathological conditions in which ACTH levels are

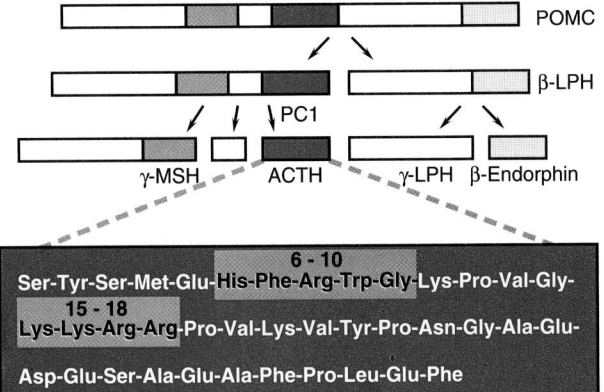

Figure 59–1. *Processing of pro-opiomelanocortin to adrenocorticotropic hormone and the sequence of adrenocorticotropic hormone.* The pathway by which pro-opiomelanocortin (POMC) is converted to adrenocorticotropic hormone (ACTH) and other peptides in the anterior pituitary is depicted. The amino acid sequence of human ACTH is shown. The light blue boxes behind the ACTH structure indicate regions identified as important for steroidogenic activity (residues 6–10) and binding to the ACTH receptor (15–18). α-Melanocyte-stimulating hormone also derives from the POMC precursor and contains the first 13 residues of ACTH. LPH, lipotropin; MSH, melanocyte-stimulating hormone; PC1, prohormone convertase 1. For additional information on peptide hormones derived from POMC, *see* Table 55–1.

persistently elevated, such as primary adrenal insufficiency, ACTH can signal through the MC1R and cause hyperpigmentation. Recent studies have defined a key role for α-MSH acting *via* the MC3R and MC4R receptors in the hypothalamic regulation of appetite and body weight (Wardlaw, 2001), and they therefore are the subject of considerable investigation as possible targets for drugs that affect appetite. The role of MC5R is less well defined, but studies in rodents suggest that MSH stimulates LH secretion and triggers aggressive, pheromone-related behavior *via* the MC5R.

Actions on the Adrenal Cortex. Acting *via* MC2R, ACTH stimulates the adrenal cortex to secrete glucocorticoids, mineralocorticoids, and the androgen precursor dehydroepiandrosterone (DHEA) that can be converted peripherally into more potent androgens. The adrenal cortex histologically and functionally can be separated into three zones that produce different steroid products under different regulatory influences. The outer zona glomerulosa secretes the mineralocorticoid aldosterone, the middle zona fasciculata secretes the glucocorticoid cortisol, and the inner zona reticularis secretes DHEA and its sulfated derivative (Figure 59–2).

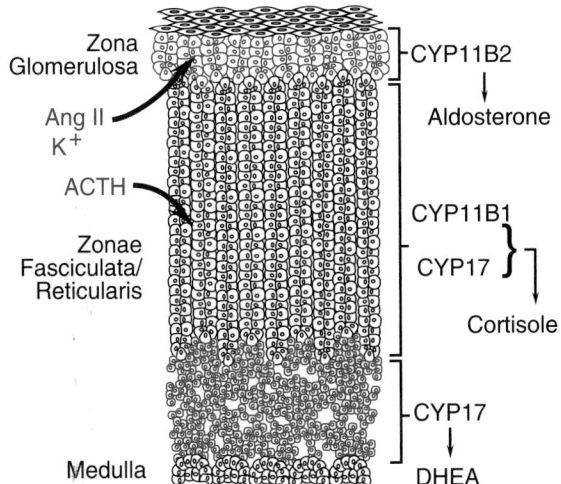

Figure 59–2. *The adrenal cortex contains three anatomically and functionally distinct compartments.* The major functional compartments of the adrenal cortex are shown, along with the steroidogenic enzymes that determine the unique profiles of corticosteroid products. Also shown are the predominant physiologic regulators of steroid production: angiotensin II (Ang II) and K+ for the zona glomerulosa and ACTH for the zona fasciculata. The physiological regulator(s) of dehydroepiandrosterone (DHEA) production by the zona reticularis are not known, although ACTH acutely increases DHEA biosynthesis.

Cells of the outer zone have receptors for angiotensin II and express aldosterone synthase (CYP11B2), an enzyme that catalyzes the terminal reactions in mineralocorticoid biosynthesis. Although ACTH acutely stimulates mineralocorticoid production by the zona glomerulosa, this zone is regulated predominantly by angiotensin II and extracellular K+ (*see* Chapter 30) and does not undergo atrophy in the absence of ongoing stimulation by the pituitary gland. In the setting of persistently elevated ACTH, mineralocorticoid levels initially increase and then return to normal (a phenomenon termed *ACTH escape*).

In contrast, cells of the zona fasciculata have fewer receptors for angiotensin II and express two enzymes, steroid 17α-hydroxylase (CYP17) and 11β-hydroxylase (CYP11B1), which catalyze the production of glucocorticoids. In the zona reticularis, CYP17 carries out a second C 17-20 lyase reaction that converts C 21 corticosteroids to C 19 androgen precursors.

In the absence of the anterior pituitary, the inner zones of the cortex atrophy, and the production of glucocorticoids and adrenal androgens is markedly impaired.

Persistently elevated levels of ACTH, due either to repeated administration of large doses of ACTH or to excessive endogenous production, induce hyperplasia and hypertrophy of the inner zones of the adrenal cortex, with overproduction of cortisol and adrenal androgens. Adrenal hyperplasia is most marked in congenital disorders of steroidogenesis, in which ACTH levels are continuously elevated as a secondary response to impaired cortisol biosynthesis. There is some debate regarding the relative roles of ACTH versus other POMC-derived peptides in stimulating adrenal growth, but the essential role of the anterior pituitary in maintaining the integrity of the zona fasciculata is indisputable.

Mechanism of Action. ACTH stimulates the synthesis and release of adrenocortical hormones. As specific mechanisms for steroid hormone secretion have not been defined and since steroids do not accumulate appreciably in the gland, it is believed that the actions of ACTH to increase steroid hormone production are mediated predominantly at the level of *de novo* biosynthesis.

ACTH, binding to MC2R, activates the G protein Gα_s to stimulate adenylyl cyclase, increase intracellular cyclic AMP content, and activate PKA. Cyclic AMP is an obligatory second messenger for most, if not all, effects of ACTH on steroidogenesis. Mutations in the ACTH receptor are one of the causes of the rare syndrome of familial resistance to ACTH (Clark and Weber, 1998).

Temporally, the response of adrenocortical cells to ACTH has two phases. The acute phase, which occurs within seconds to minutes, largely reflects increased supply of cholesterol substrate to the steroidogenic enzymes. The chronic phase, which occurs over hours to days, results largely from increased transcription of the steroidogenic enzymes. A summary of the pathways of adrenal steroid biosynthesis and the structures of the major steroid intermediates and products of the human adrenal cortex are shown in Figure 59–3. The rate-limiting step in steroid hormone production is the conversion of cholesterol to pregnenolone, a reaction catalyzed by CYP11A1, the cholesterol side-chain cleavage enzyme. Most of the enzymes required for steroid hormone biosynthesis, including CYP11A1, are members of the cytochrome P450 superfamily of mixed-function oxidases that play important roles in the metabolism of xenobiotics such as drugs and environmental pollutants, as well as in the biosynthesis of such endogenous compounds as steroid hormones, vitamin D, bile acids, fatty acids, prostaglandins, and biogenic amines (*see* Chapter 3). The rate-limiting components in this reaction regulate the mobilization of substrate cholesterol and its delivery to CYP11A1 in the inner mitochondrial matrix.

To ensure an adequate supply of substrate for steroidogenesis, the adrenal cortex uses multiple sources of cholesterol, including: (1) circulating cholesterol and cholesterol esters taken up *via* the low-density lipoprotein and high-density lipoprotein receptor pathways; (2) liberation of cholesterol from endogenous cholesterol ester stores *via* activation of cholesterol esterase; and (3) increased *de novo* biosynthesis.

The mechanisms by which ACTH stimulates the translocation of cholesterol to the inner mitochondrial matrix are not fully defined. A 30,000-dalton phosphoprotein—designated the steroidogenic

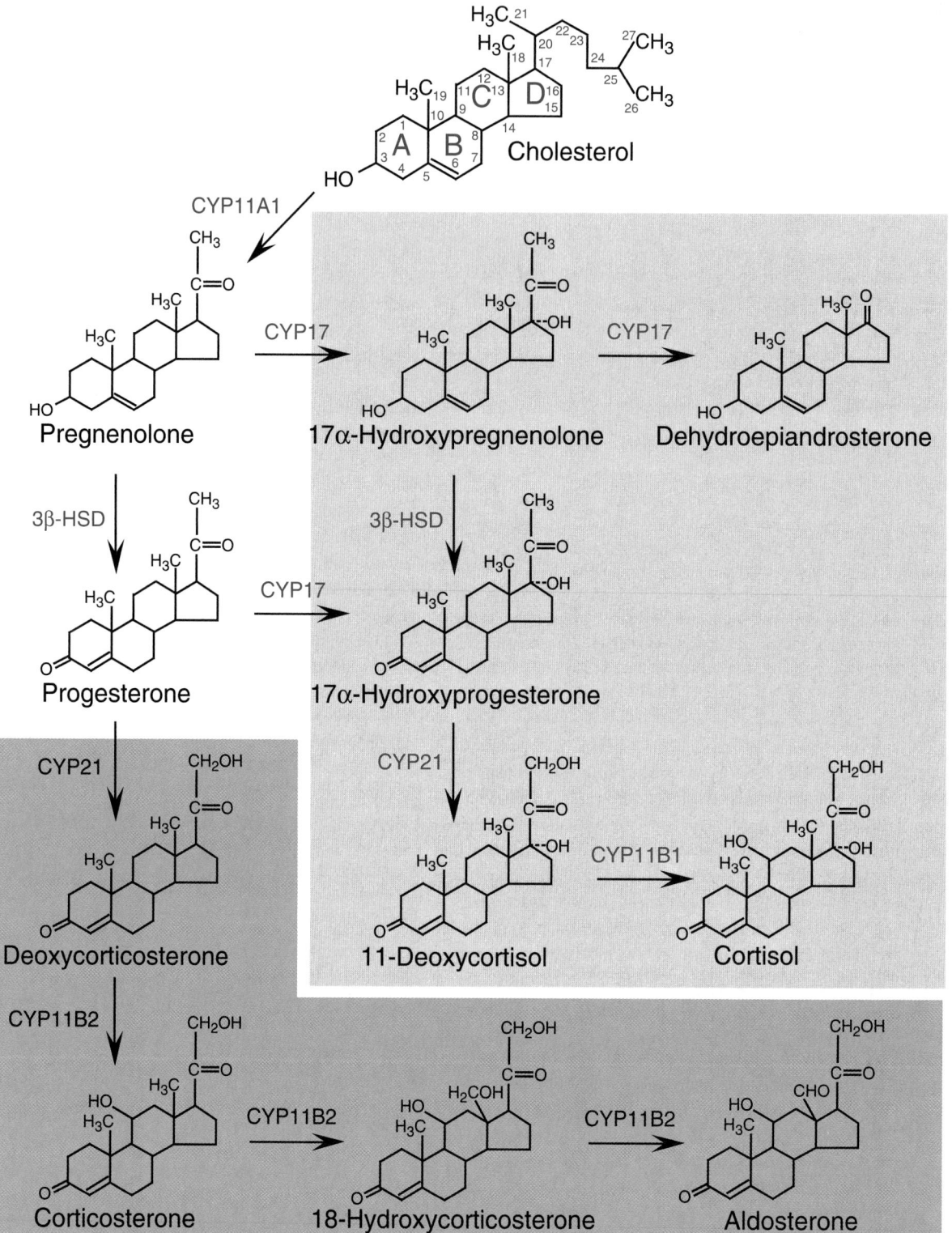

Figure 59–3. Pathways of corticosteroid biosynthesis. The steroidogenic pathways used in the biosynthesis of the corticosteroids are shown, along with the structures of the intermediates and products. The pathways that are unique to the zona glomerulosa are shown in blue, whereas those that occur in the inner zona fasciculata and zona reticularis are shown in gray. The zona reticularis does not express 3β-HSD, and thus preferentially synthesizes DHEA. CYP11A1, cholesterol side-chain cleavage enzyme; 3β-HSD, 3β-hydroxysteroid dehydrogenase; CYP17, steroid 17α-hydroxylase; CYP21, steroid 21-hydroxylase; CYP11B2, aldosterone synthase; CYP11B1, steroid 11β-hydroxylase.

acute regulatory protein—clearly plays essential roles in cholesterol delivery. Mutations in the gene encoding this phosphoprotein are found in patients with congenital lipoid adrenal hyperplasia, a rare congenital disorder in which adrenal cells become engorged with cholesterol deposits secondary to an inability to synthesize any steroid hormones. An important component of the trophic effect of ACTH is the enhanced transcription of genes that encode the individual steroidogenic enzymes, with associated increases in the steroidogenic capacity of the gland. A variety of transcriptional regulators mediate the induction of steroid hydroxylases by ACTH, and concerted mechanisms that coordinate the expression of the different genes have not been defined.

Extra-adrenal Effects of ACTH. In large doses, ACTH causes a number of metabolic changes in adrenalectomized animals, including ketosis, lipolysis, hypoglycemia (immediately after treatment), and resistance to insulin (later after treatment). Because of the large doses of ACTH required, the physiological significance of these extra-adrenal effects is questionable. ACTH also improves learning in experimental animals; this latter effect appears to be non-endocrine and mediated *via* distinct receptors in the central nervous system.

Regulation of ACTH Secretion. **Hypothalamic-Pituitary-Adrenal Axis.** The rate of glucocorticoid secretion is determined by fluctuations in the release of ACTH by the pituitary corticotropes. These corticotropes, in turn, are regulated by corticotropin-releasing hormone (CRH), a peptide hormone released by CRH neurons of the endocrine hypothalamus. These three organs collectively are referred to as the hypothalamic-pituitary-adrenal (HPA) axis, an integrated system that maintains appropriate levels of glucocorticoids (*see* Figure 59–4 for a schematic overview). There are three characteristic modes of regulation of the HPA axis: diurnal rhythm in basal steroidogenesis, negative feedback regulation by adrenal corticosteroids, and marked increases in steroidogenesis in response to stress. The diurnal rhythm is entrained by higher neuronal centers in response to sleep-wake cycles, such that levels of ACTH peak in the early morning hours, causing the circulating glucocorticoid levels to peak at approximately 8 A.M. As discussed below, negative feedback regulation occurs at multiple levels of the HPA axis and is the major mechanism that maintains circulating glucocorticoid levels in the appropriate range. Stress can override the normal negative feedback control mechanisms, leading to marked increases in plasma concentrations of glucocorticoids.

Central Nervous System. The central nervous system integrates a number of positive and negative influences on ACTH secretion that are conveyed by several neurotransmitters (Figure 59–4). These signals converge on the CRH neurons, which are clustered largely in the

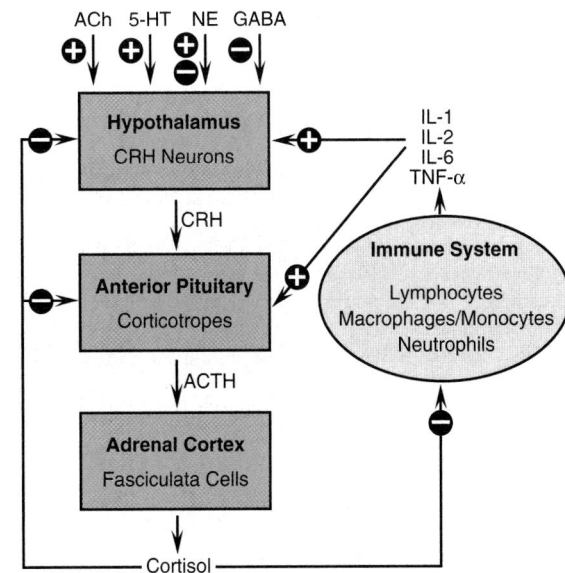

Figure 59–4. *Overview of the hypothalamic-pituitary-adrenal (HPA) axis and the immune inflammatory network.* Also shown are inputs from higher neuronal centers that regulate CRH secretion. + indicates a positive regulator, – indicates a negative regulator, +/– indicates a mixed effect. IL-1, interleukin-1; IL-2, interleukin-2; IL-6, interleukin-6; TNF-α, tumor necrosis factor-α; CRH, corticotropin-releasing hormone; ACh, acetylcholine; 5-HT, 5-hydroxytryptamine (serotonin); NE, norepinephrine; GABA, γ-aminobutyric acid.

parvocellular region of the paraventricular hypothalamic nucleus and make axonal connections to the median eminence of the hypothalamus (*see* Chapter 12). Following release into the hypophyseal plexus, CRH is transported *via* this portal system to the anterior pituitary, where it binds to specific membrane receptors on corticotropes. Upon CRH binding, the CRH receptor activates the G_s-adenylyl cyclase–cyclic AMP pathway within corticotropes, ultimately stimulating both ACTH biosynthesis and secretion. CRH and CRH-related peptides called urocortins also are produced at other sites, including the amygdala and hindbrain, gut, skin, adrenal gland, adipose tissue, placenta, and other sites in the periphery (Bale and Vale, 2004). The classical CRH receptor, now designated CRF_1 receptor, belongs to the class II family of G protein–coupled receptors that includes receptors for calcitonin, parathyroid hormone, growth hormone–releasing hormone, secretin, glucagon, and glucagon-like peptide. A second CRH receptor, designated CRF_2 receptor, shares 70% homology at the amino-acid level. These two receptors differentially bind CRH and the urocortins, providing a highly complex neural network that modulates the adaptive response to stress. The complex relationships between stress and mood have stimulated considerable interest in the possible use of CRH antagonists in disorders such as anxiety and depression.

Arginine Vasopressin. Arginine vasopressin (AVP) also acts as a secretagogue for corticotropes, significantly potentiating the effects of CRH. Animal studies suggest that the potentiation of CRH action by AVP probably contributes to the full magnitude of the stress response *in vivo*. Like CRH, AVP is produced in the parvocellular neurons of the paraventricular nucleus and secreted into the pituitary plexus from the median eminence. After binding to V_{1b} receptors, AVP activates the G_q-PLC-IP$_3$-Ca^{2+} pathway to enhance the release of ACTH. In contrast to CRH, AVP apparently does not increase ACTH synthesis.

Negative Feedback of Glucocorticoids. Glucocorticoids inhibit ACTH secretion *via* direct and indirect actions on CRH neurons to decrease CRH mRNA levels and CRH release and *via* direct effects on corticotropes. The inhibition of CRH release may be mediated by specific corticosteroid receptors in the hippocampus. At lower cortisol levels, the mineralocorticoid receptor (MR), which has a higher affinity for glucocorticoids and is the predominant form found in the hippocampus, is the major receptor species occupied. As glucocorticoid concentrations rise and exceed the capacity of the MR, the glucocorticoid receptor (GR) also becomes occupied. Both classes of receptor apparently control the basal activity of the HPA axis, whereas feedback inhibition by glucocorticoids predominantly involves the GR.

In the pituitary, glucocorticoids act through the GR to inhibit the release of ACTH from corticotropes and the expression of POMC. These effects are both rapid (occurring within seconds to minutes and possibly mediated by glucocorticoid receptor–independent mechanisms) and delayed (requiring hours and involving changes in gene transcription mediated through the GR).

The Stress Response. Stress overcomes negative feedback regulation of the HPA axis, leading to a marked rise in corticosteroid production. Examples of stress signals include injury, hemorrhage, severe infection, major surgery, hypoglycemia, cold, pain, and fear. Although the precise mechanisms that underlie this stress response and the essential actions played by corticosteroids are not fully defined, it is clear that their increased secretion is vital to maintain homeostasis in these stressful settings. As discussed below, complex interactions between the HPA axis and the immune system may be a fundamental physiological component of this stress response (Sapolsky *et al.*, 2000).

Assays for ACTH.

Initially, ACTH levels were assessed by bioassays that measured induced steroid production or the depletion of adrenal ascorbic acid. Radioimmunoassays that subsequently were developed to quantitate ACTH levels in individual patients were not always reproducible and did not clearly differentiate between low and normal levels of ACTH. Immunochemiluminescent assays that use two separate antibodies directed at distinct epitopes on the ACTH molecule now are widely available. These assays increase considerably the ability to differentiate patients with primary hypoadrenalism due to intrinsic adrenal disease, who have high ACTH levels due to the loss of normal glucocorticoid feedback inhibition, from those with secondary forms of hypoadrenalism, due to low ACTH levels resulting from hypothalamic or pituitary disorders. The immunochemiluminescent ACTH assays also are useful in differentiating between ACTH-dependent and ACTH-independent forms of hypercorticism: High ACTH levels are seen when the hypercorticism results from pituitary adenomas (*e.g.*, Cushing's disease) or nonpituitary tumors that secrete ACTH (*e.g.*, the syndrome of ectopic ACTH), whereas low ACTH levels are seen in patients with exces-

sive glucocorticoid production due to primary adrenal disorders. Despite their considerable utility, one problem with the immunoassays for ACTH is that their specificity for intact ACTH can lead to falsely low values in patients with ectopic ACTH secretion; these tumors can secrete aberrantly processed forms of ACTH that have biological activity but do not react in the antibody assays.

Therapeutic Uses and Diagnostic Applications of ACTH.

There are anecdotal reports that selected conditions respond better to ACTH than to corticosteroids (*e.g.*, multiple sclerosis), and some clinicians continue to advocate therapy with ACTH. Despite this, ACTH currently has only limited utility as a therapeutic agent. Therapy with ACTH is less predictable and less convenient than therapy with corticosteroids. In addition, ACTH stimulates mineralocorticoid and adrenal androgen secretion and may therefore cause acute retention of salt and water, as well as virilization. While ACTH and the corticosteroids are not pharmacologically equivalent, all proven therapeutic effects of ACTH can be achieved with appropriate doses of corticosteroids with a lower risk of side effects.

Testing the Integrity of the HPA Axis. The major clinical use of ACTH is in testing the integrity of the HPA axis. Other tests used to assess the HPA axis include the insulin tolerance test (*see* Chapter 55) and the metyrapone test (discussed later in this chapter). *Cosyntropin* (CORTROSYN, SYNACTHEN) is a synthetic peptide that corresponds to residues 1 to 24 of human ACTH. At the considerably supraphysiological dose of 250 μg, cosyntropin maximally stimulates adrenocortical steroidogenesis. In the standard cosyntropin stimulation test, 250 μg of cosyntropin is administered either intramuscularly or intravenously, with cortisol measured just before administration (baseline) and 30 to 60 minutes after cosyntropin administration. An increase in the circulating cortisol to a level greater than 18 to 20 μg/dl indicates a normal response. Others also have included an increase of 7 μg/dl over the baseline value as a positive response, although this is less widely accepted. In patients with pituitary or hypothalamic disease of recent onset or shortly after surgery for pituitary tumors, the standard cosyntropin stimulation test may be misleading, as the duration of ACTH deficiency may have been insufficient to cause significant adrenal atrophy with frank loss of steroidogenic capacity. For these patients, some experts advocate a "low-dose" cosyntropin stimulation test, in which 1 μg of cosyntropin is administered intravenously, and cortisol is measured just before and 30 minutes after cosyntropin administration; the cutoff for a normal response is the same as that for the standard test. Because cosyntropin is not generally available in a 1-μg dose, the standard ampule of cosyntropin (250 μg) is diluted to permit accurate delivery of the 1-μg challenge dose. Care must be taken to avoid adsorption of the cosyntropin to plastic tubing and to measure the plasma cortisol precisely at 30 minutes after the cosyntropin injection. Although some studies indicate that the low-dose test is more sensitive than the standard 250-μg test, others report that this test also may fail to detect secondary adrenal insufficiency.

As noted above, primary adrenocortical insufficiency and secondary adrenocortical insufficiency are reliably distinguished using available sensitive assays for ACTH. Thus, longer-course ACTH stimulation tests rarely are used to differentiate between these disorders.

CRH Stimulation Test. Ovine CRH (*corticorelin* [ACTHREL]) and human CRH are available for diagnostic testing of the HPA axis, with the former used in the United States and the latter preferred in Europe. In patients with documented ACTH-dependent hypercortisism, CRH testing may help differentiate between a pituitary source (*i.e.,* Cushing's disease) and an ectopic source of ACTH. After two baseline blood samples are obtained 15 minutes apart, CRH (1 μg/kg body weight) is administered intravenously over a 30- to 60-second interval, and peripheral blood samples are obtained at 15, 30, and 60 minutes for ACTH measurement. It is important that the blood samples be handled as recommended for the ACTH assay. At the recommended dose, CRH generally is well tolerated, although flushing may occur, particularly if the dose is administered as a bolus. Patients with Cushing's disease respond to CRH with either a normal or an exaggerated increase in ACTH, whereas ACTH levels do not increase in patients with ectopic sources of ACTH. It should be noted that this test is not perfect: ACTH levels are induced by CRH in occasional patients with ectopic ACTH, whereas approximately 5% to 10% of patients with Cushing's disease fail to respond.

To improve the diagnostic accuracy of the CRH stimulation test, many authorities advocate sampling of blood from the inferior petrosal sinuses and the peripheral circulation after peripheral administration of CRH as above. In this test, an inferior petrosal/peripheral ratio of >2.5 supports a pituitary source of ACTH. When performed by a skilled neuroradiologist, this procedure increases diagnostic accuracy with a tolerable risk of complications from the catheterization procedure (Arnaldi *et al.*, 2003).

Absorption and Fate. ACTH is readily absorbed from parenteral sites. The hormone rapidly disappears from the circulation after intravenous administration; in humans, the half-life in plasma is about 15 minutes, primarily due to rapid enzymatic hydrolysis.

Toxicity of ACTH. Aside from rare hypersensitivity reactions, the toxicity of ACTH is primarily attributable to the increased secretion of corticosteroids. Cosyntropin generally is less antigenic than native ACTH; thus cosyntropin is the preferred agent for clinical use.

ADRENOCORTICAL STEROIDS

The adrenal cortex synthesizes two classes of steroids: the *corticosteroids* (glucocorticoids and mineralocorticoids), which have 21 carbon atoms, and the *androgens,* which have 19 (Figure 59–3). The actions of corticosteroids historically were described as glucocorticoid (carbohydrate metabolism–regulating) and mineralocorticoid (electrolyte balance–regulating), reflecting their preferential activities. In humans, *cortisol* (*hydrocortisone*) is the main glucocorticoid and aldosterone is the main mineralocorticoid. The mechanisms by which glucocorticoid biosynthesis is regulated by ACTH are discussed above, and the regulation of aldosterone production is described in Chapter 30. Table 59–1 shows typical rates of secretion of cortisol and aldosterone, as well as their normal circulat-

Table 59–1
Normal Daily Production Rates and Circulating Levels of the Predominant Corticosteroids

	CORTISOL	ALDOSTERONE
Rate of secretion under optimal conditions	10 mg/day	0.125 mg/day
Concentration in peripheral plasma:		
8 A.M.	16 μg/100 ml	0.01 μg/100 ml
4 P.M.	4 μg/100 ml	0.01 μg/100 ml

ing concentrations. Earlier studies had suggested that cortisol was produced at a daily rate of 20 mg, but more recent studies indicate that the actual rate is closer to 10 mg/day.

Although the adrenal cortex is an important source of androgen precursors in women, patients with adrenal insufficiency can be restored to normal life expectancy by replacement therapy with glucocorticoids and mineralocorticoids. Nevertheless, some recent studies have shown that addition of DHEA to the standard replacement regimen in women with adrenal insufficiency improved subjective well-being and sexuality (Allolio and Arlt, 2002). While adrenal androgens are not essential for survival, the levels of dehydroepiandrosterone (DHEA) and its sulfated derivative DHEA-S peak in the third decade of life and decline progressively thereafter. Moreover, patients with a number of chronic diseases have very low DHEA levels, leading some to propose that DHEA treatment might at least partly alleviate the adverse consequences of aging. These findings have prompted considerable discussion about uses of DHEA, which despite the absence of definitive data is widely used as a nutritional supplement for its alleged health benefits.

Physiological Functions and Pharmacological Effects

Physiological Actions. The effects of corticosteroids are numerous and widespread, and include alterations in carbohydrate, protein, and lipid metabolism; maintenance of fluid and electrolyte balance; and preservation of normal function of the cardiovascular system, the immune system, the kidney, skeletal muscle, the endocrine system, and the nervous system. In addition, corticosteroids endow the organism with the capacity to resist such

Table 59–2
Relative Potencies and Equivalent Doses of Representative Corticosteroids

COMPOUND	ANTIINFLAMMATORY POTENCY	Na$^+$-RETAINING POTENCY	DURATION OF ACTION*	EQUIVALENT DOSE,† MG
Cortisol	1	1	S	20
Cortisone	0.8	0.8	S	25
Fludrocortisone	10	125	I	‡
Prednisone	4	0.8	I	5
Prednisolone	4	0.8	I	5
6α-Methylprednisolone	5	0.5	I	4
Triamcinolone	5	0	I	4
Betamethasone	25	0	L	0.75
Dexamethasone	25	0	L	0.75

*S, short (*i.e.*, 8–12 hour biological half-life); I, intermediate (*i.e.*, 12–36 hour biological half-life); L, long (*i.e.*, 36–72 hour biological half-life).
†These dose relationships apply only to oral or intravenous administration, as glucocorticoid potencies may differ greatly following intramuscular or intraarticular administration. ‡This agent is not used for glucocorticoid effects.

stressful circumstances as noxious stimuli and environmental changes. In the absence of the adrenal cortex, survival is made possible only by maintaining an optimal environment, including adequate and regular feedings, ingestion of relatively large amounts of sodium chloride, and maintenance of an appropriate environmental temperature; stresses such as infection and trauma in this setting can be life-threatening.

Until recently, corticosteroid effects were viewed as physiological (reflecting actions of corticosteroids at doses corresponding to normal daily production levels) or pharmacological (representing effects seen only at doses exceeding the normal daily production of corticosteroids). More recent concepts suggest that the antiinflammatory and immunosuppressive actions of corticosteroids—one of the major "pharmacological" uses of this class of drugs—also provide a protective mechanism in the physiological setting. Many of the immune mediators associated with the inflammatory response decrease vascular tone and could lead to cardiovascular collapse if unopposed by the adrenal corticosteroids. This hypothesis is supported by the fact that the daily production rate of cortisol can rise at least tenfold in the setting of severe stress. In addition, as discussed below, the pharmacological actions of corticosteroids in different tissues and their physiological effects are mediated by the same receptor. Thus, the various glucocorticoid derivatives used as pharmacological agents generally have side effects on physiological processes that parallel their therapeutic effectiveness.

The actions of corticosteroids are interrelated to those of other hormones. For example, in the absence of lipolytic

hormones, cortisol has virtually no effect on the rate of lipolysis by adipocytes. Likewise, in the absence of glucocorticoids, epinephrine and norepinephrine have only minor effects on lipolysis. Administration of a small dose of glucocorticoid, however, markedly potentiates the lipolytic action of these catecholamines. Those effects of corticosteroids that involve concerted actions with other hormonal regulators are termed *permissive* and most likely reflect steroid-induced changes in protein synthesis that, in turn, modify tissue responsiveness to other hormones.

Corticosteroids are grouped according to their relative potencies in Na$^+$ retention, effects on carbohydrate metabolism (*i.e.*, hepatic deposition of glycogen and gluconeogenesis), and antiinflammatory effects. In general, potencies of steroids as judged by their ability to sustain life in adrenalectomized animals closely parallel those determined for Na$^+$ retention, while potencies based on effects on glucose metabolism closely parallel those for antiinflammatory effects. The effects on Na$^+$ retention and the carbohydrate/antiinflammatory actions are not closely related and reflect selective actions at distinct receptors, as noted above.

Based on these differential potencies, the corticosteroids traditionally are divided into mineralocorticoids and glucocorticoids. Estimates of potencies of representative steroids in these actions are listed in Table 59–2. Some steroids that are classified predominantly as glucocorticoids (*e.g.*, cortisol) also possess modest but significant mineralocorticoid activity and thus may affect fluid and electrolyte handling in the clinical setting. At doses used for replacement therapy in patients with primary adrenal insufficiency (*see* below), the mineralocorticoid effects of these "glucocorticoids" are insufficient to replace that of aldosterone, and concurrent therapy with a more potent mineralocorticoid generally is needed. In contrast, aldosterone is exceedingly potent with respect to Na⁺ retention, but has only modest potency for effects on carbohydrate metabolism. At normal rates of secretion by the adrenal cortex or in doses that maximally affect electrolyte balance, aldosterone has no significant glucocorticoid activity and thus acts as a pure mineralocorticoid.

General Mechanisms for Corticosteroid Effects. Corticosteroids interact with specific receptor proteins in target tissues to regulate the expression of corticosteroid-responsive genes, thereby changing the levels and array of proteins synthesized by the various target tissues (Figure 59–5). As a consequence of the time required to modulate gene expression and protein synthesis, most effects of corticosteroids are not immediate but become apparent after several hours. This fact is of clinical significance, because a delay generally is seen before beneficial effects of corticosteroid therapy become manifest. Although corticosteroids predominantly act to increase expression of target genes, there are well-documented examples in which glucocorticoids decrease transcription of target genes (De Bosscher *et al.*, 2003), as discussed below. In addition to these genomic effects, some immediate actions of corticosteroids may be mediated by membrane-bound receptors (Norman *et al.*, 2004).

The receptors for corticosteroids are members of the nuclear receptor family of transcription factors that transduce the effects of a diverse array of small, hydrophobic ligands, including the steroid hormones, thyroid hormone, vitamin D, and retinoids. These receptors share two highly conserved domains: a region of approximately 70 amino acids forming two zinc-binding domains, called *zinc fingers,* that are essential for the interaction of the receptor with specific DNA sequences, and a region at the carboxyl terminus that interacts with ligand (the ligand-binding domain).

Although complete loss of glucocorticoid receptor (GR) function apparently is lethal, mutations leading to partial loss of GR function have been identified in rare patients with generalized glucocorticoid resistance (Bray and Cotton, 2003). These patients harbor mutations in the GR that impair glucocorticoid binding and decrease transcriptional activation. As a consequence of these mutations, cortisol levels that normally mediate feedback inhibition fail to suppress the HPA axis completely. In this setting of partial loss of GR function, the HPA axis resets to a higher level to provide compensatory increases in ACTH and cortisol secretion. Because the GR defect is partial, adequate compensation for the end-organ insensitivity can result from the elevated cortisol level, but the excess ACTH secretion also stimulates the production of mineralocorticoids and adrenal androgens. Because the mineralocorticoid receptor (MR) and the androgen receptor are intact, these subjects present with manifestations of mineralocorticoid excess (hypertension and hypokalemic alkalosis) and/or of increased androgen levels (acne, hirsutism, male

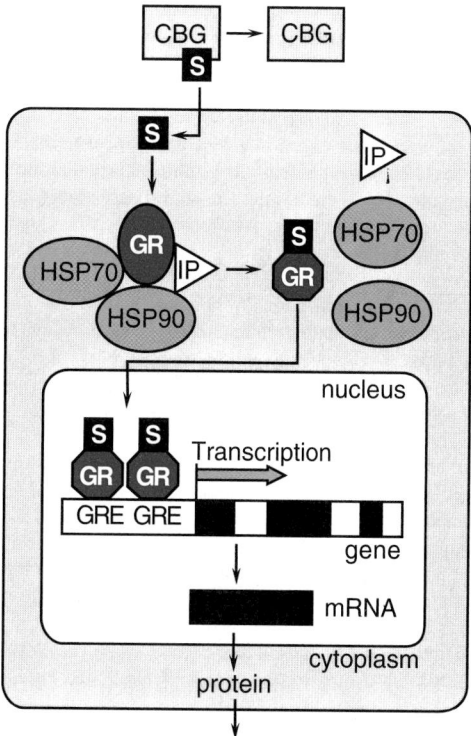

Figure 59–5. *Intracellular mechanism of action of the glucocorticoid receptor.* The figure shows the molecular pathway by which cortisol (labeled S) enters cells and interacts with the glucocorticoid receptor (GR) to change GR conformation (indicated by the change in shape of the GR), induce GR nuclear translocation, and activate transcription of target genes. The example shown is one in which glucocorticoids activate expression of target genes; the expression of certain genes, including pro-opiomelanocortin (POMC) expression by corticotropes, is inhibited by glucocorticoid treatment. CBG, corticosteroid-binding globulin; GR, glucocorticoid receptor; S, steroid hormone; HSP90, the 90-kd heat-shock protein; HSP70, the 70-kd heat-shock protein; IP, the 56-kd immunophilin; GRE, glucocorticoid-response elements in the DNA that are bound by GR, thus providing specificity to induction of gene transcription by glucocorticoids. Within the gene are introns (*unshaded*) and exons (*shaded*); transcription and mRNA processing leads to splicing and removal of introns and assembly of exons into mRNA.

pattern baldness, menstrual irregularities, anovulation, and infertility). In children, the excess adrenal androgens can cause precocious sexual development.

Glucocorticoid Receptor. The GR resides predominantly in the cytoplasm in an inactive form until it binds glucocorticoids (Figure 59–5). Steroid binding results in receptor activation and translocation to the nucleus. The inactive GR is complexed with other proteins, including heat-shock protein (HSP) 90, a member of the heat-shock family of stress-induced proteins; HSP70; and a 56,000-dalton immunophilin, one of the group of intracellular proteins that bind the immunosuppressive agents *cyclosporine* and *tacrolimus* (*see* Chapter 52 for a discussion of these agents). HSP90, through interactions with the steroid-binding domain, may facilitate folding of the GR into an appropriate conformation that permits ligand binding.

Regulation of Gene Expression by Glucocorticoids. After ligand binding, the GR dissociates from its associated proteins and translocates to the nucleus. There, it interacts with specific DNA sequences within the regulatory regions of affected genes. The short DNA sequences that are recognized by the activated GR are called *glucocorticoid responsive elements* (GREs) and provide specificity to the induction of gene transcription by glucocorticoids. The consensus GRE sequence is an imperfect palindrome (GGTACAnnnTGTTCT, where n is any nucleotide) to which the GR binds as a receptor dimer. The mechanisms by which GR activates transcription are complex and not completely understood, but they involve the interaction of the GR with transcriptional coactivators and with proteins that make up the basal transcription apparatus. Genes that are negatively regulated by glucocorticoids also have been identified. One well-characterized example is the pro-opiomelanocortin gene, whose negative regulation in corticotropes by glucocorticoids is an important part of the negative feedback regulation of the HPA axis. In this case, the GR appears to inhibit transcription by a direct interaction with a GRE in the *POMC* promoter. Other genes negatively regulated by glucocorticoids include genes for cyclooxygenase-2 (COX-2), inducible nitric oxide synthase (NOS2), and inflammatory cytokines.

Although glucocorticoids and the GR are essential for survival, interactions of the GR with specific GREs apparently are not. These conclusions are supported by the findings that genetically engineered mice completely lacking GR function die immediately after birth, whereas mice harboring a mutated GR incapable of binding to DNA are viable. These observations imply that the critical function of GR involves protein–protein interactions with other transcription factors. Indeed, protein–protein interactions have been observed between the GR and the transcription factors NF-κB and AP-1, which regulate the expression of a number of components of the immune system (De Bosscher *et al.*, 2003). Such interactions repress the expression of genes encoding a number of cytokines—regulatory molecules that play key roles in the immune and inflammatory networks—and enzymes, such as collagenase and stromelysin, that are proposed to play key roles in the joint destruction seen in inflammatory arthritis. Thus, these negative effects on gene expression appear to contribute significantly to the antiinflammatory and immunosuppressive effects of the glucocorticoids.

The recognition that the metabolic effects of glucocorticoids generally are mediated by transcriptional activation, while the antiinflammatory effects largely are mediated by transrepression, suggests that selective GR ligands may maintain the antiinflammatory actions while lessening the metabolic side effects (Coghlan *et al.*, 2003). Recent reports describe steroidal and nonsteroidal compounds that exhibit antiinflammatory actions but have little effect on blood glucose, suggesting that such selective glucocorticoid agonists may emerge from ongoing research.

Regulation of Gene Expression by Mineralocorticoids. Like the GR, MR also is a ligand-activated transcription factor and binds to a very similar, if not identical, hormone-responsive element. Although its actions have been studied in less detail than the GR, the basic principles of action appear to be similar; in particular, the MR also associates with HSP90 and activates the transcription of discrete sets of genes within target tissues. Studies have not yet identified differences

in the DNA recognition motifs for the GR and the MR that would explain their differential capacities to activate discrete sets of target genes. The GR and MR differ in their ability to inhibit AP-1–mediated gene activation, suggesting that differential interactions with other transcription factors may underlie their distinct effects on cell function. In addition, unlike the GR, the MR has a restricted expression: It is expressed principally in the kidney (distal cortical tubule and cortical collecting duct), colon, salivary glands, sweat glands, and hippocampus.

Aldosterone exerts its effects on Na^+ and K^+ homeostasis primarily *via* its actions on the principal cells of the distal renal tubules and collecting ducts, while the effects on H^+ secretion largely are exerted in the intercalated cells. After binding to the MR, aldosterone initiates a sequence of events that includes the rapid induction of serum- and glucocorticoid-regulated kinase, which in turn phosphorylates and activates amiloride-sensitive epithelial Na^+ channels in the apical membrane. Thereafter, increased Na^+ influx stimulates the Na^+,K^+-ATPase in the basolateral membrane. In addition to these rapid actions, aldosterone also increases the synthesis of the individual components of these membrane proteins.

Further insights into the roles of the MR and its target genes in fluid and electrolyte balance have emerged from analyses of patients with rare genetic disorders of mineralocorticoid action, such as *pseudohypoaldosteronism* and *pseudoaldosteronism.* Despite elevated levels of mineralocorticoids, patients with pseudohypoaldosteronism present with clinical manifestations suggestive of deficient mineralocorticoid action (*i.e.,* volume depletion, hypotension, hyperkalemia, and metabolic acidosis). Molecular analyses have defined discrete subpopulations of patients with this disorder. One form is an autosomal recessive disease resulting from loss-of-function mutations in genes encoding subunits of the amiloride-sensitive epithelial sodium channel. A second, autosomal dominant form of pseudohypoaldosteronism is caused by mutations in the MR that impair its activity. Pseudoaldosteronism, also termed Liddle's syndrome, is an autosomal dominant disease that results from mutations in subunits of the amiloride-sensitive Na^+ channel that interfere with its down-regulation. The constitutive activity of this channel leads to hypertension, hypokalemia, and metabolic alkalosis, despite low levels of plasma renin and aldosterone.

Receptor-Independent Mechanism for Corticosteroid Specificity. The availability of cloned genes encoding the GR and MR led to the surprising finding that aldosterone (a classic mineralocorticoid) and cortisol (generally viewed as predominantly glucocorticoid) binds the MR with equal affinity. This raised the question of how the apparent specificity of the MR for aldosterone was maintained in the face of much higher circulating levels of glucocorticoids. We now know that the type 2 isozyme of 11β-hydroxysteroid dehydrogenase (11βHSD2) plays a key role in corticosteroid specificity, particularly in the kidney, colon, and salivary glands (Sandeep and Walker, 2001). This enzyme metabolizes glucocorticoids such as cortisol to receptor-inactive 11-keto derivatives such as cortisone (Figure 59–6). Because its predominant form in physiological settings is the hemiacetal derivative (Figure 59–7), which is resistant to 11βHSD action, aldosterone escapes this inactivation and maintains mineralocorticoid activity. In the absence of 11βHSD2, as occurs in an inherited disease called the *syndrome of apparent mineralocorticoid excess,* the MR is swamped by cortisol, leading to severe hypokalemia and mineralocorticoid-related hypertension. A state of mineralocorticoid excess also can be induced by inhibiting 11βHSD with *glycyrrhizic acid,* a component of licorice implicated in licorice-induced hypertension.

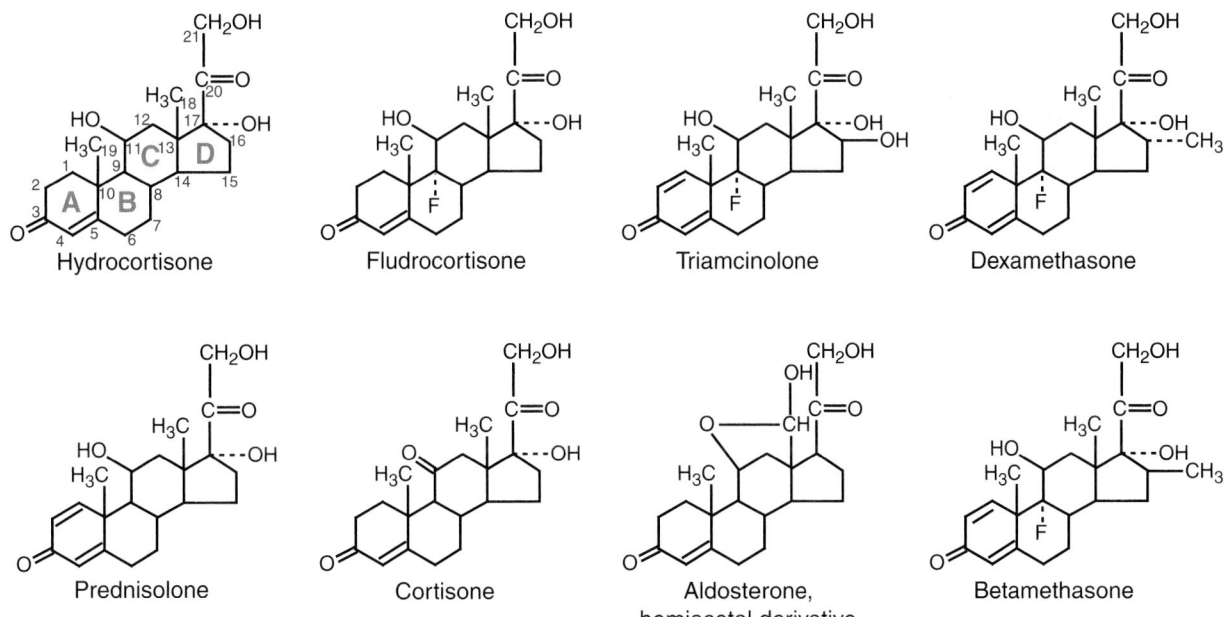

Cortisol — Active (binds to MR and GR)

Cortisone — Inactive (binds to neither MR nor GR)

Figure 59–6. *Receptor-independent mechanism by which 11β-hydroxysteroid dehydrogenase confers specificity of corticosteroid action.* By converting cortisol, which binds to both the mineralocorticoid receptor (MR) and the glucocorticoid receptor (GR), to cortisone, which binds to neither MR nor GR, the type 2 isozyme of 11β-hydroxysteroid dehydrogenase (11β-HSD2) protects the MR from the high circulating concentrations of cortisol. This inactivation allows specific responses to aldosterone in sites such as the distal nephron. The reverse reaction is catalyzed by the type 1 isozyme of 11β-HSD, which converts inactive cortisone to active cortisol in such tissues as liver and fat.

Carbohydrate and Protein Metabolism. Corticosteroids profoundly affect carbohydrate and protein metabolism. Teleologically, these effects of glucocorticoids on intermediary metabolism can be viewed as protecting glucose-dependent tissues (*e.g.,* the brain and heart) from starvation. They stimulate the liver to form glucose from amino acids and glycerol and to store glucose as liver glycogen. In the periphery, glucocorticoids diminish glucose utilization, increase protein breakdown and the synthesis of glutamine, and activate lipolysis, thereby providing amino acids and glycerol for gluconeogenesis. The net result is to increase blood glucose levels. Because of their effects on glucose metabolism, glucocorticoids can worsen glycemic control in patients with overt diabetes and can precipitate the onset of hyperglycemia in patients who are otherwise predisposed.

The mechanisms by which glucocorticoids inhibit glucose utilization in peripheral tissues are not fully understood. Glucocorticoids decrease glucose uptake in adipose tissue, skin, fibroblasts, thymocytes, and polymorphonuclear leukocytes; these effects are postulated to result from translocation of the glucose transporters from the plasma membrane to an intracellular location. These peripheral effects are associated with a number of catabolic actions, including atrophy of lymphoid tissue, decreased muscle mass, negative nitrogen balance, and thinning of the skin.

Similarly, the mechanisms by which the glucocorticoids promote gluconeogenesis are not fully defined. Amino acids mobilized from a number of tissues in response to glucocorticoids reach the liver and provide substrate for the production of glucose and glycogen. In the liver, glucocorticoids induce the transcription of a number of

Figure 59–7. *Structure and nomenclature of corticosteroid products and selected synthetic derivatives.* The structure of hydrocortisone is represented in two dimensions. It should be noted that the steroid ring system is not completely planar and that the orientation of the groups attached to the steroid rings is an important determinant of the biological activity. The methyl groups at C18 and C19 and the hydroxyl group at C11 project upward (*forward* in the two-dimensional representation and shown by a solid line connecting the atoms) and are designated β. The hydroxyl at C17 projects below the plane (*behind* in the two-dimensional representation, and represented by the dashed line connecting the atoms) and is designated α.

enzymes involved in gluconeogenesis and amino acid metabolism, including phosphoenolpyruvate carboxykinase (PEPCK), glucose-6-phosphatase, and the bi-functional enzyme fructose-2,6-bisphosphatase. Analyses of the molecular basis for regulation of PEPCK gene expression have identified complex regulatory influences involving an interplay among glucocorticoids, insulin, glucagon, and catecholamines. The effects of these hormones and amines on PEPCK gene expression mirror the complex regulation of gluconeogenesis in the intact organism.

Lipid Metabolism. Two effects of corticosteroids on lipid metabolism are firmly established. The first is the dramatic redistribution of body fat that occurs in settings of endogenous or pharmacologically induced hypercorticism, such as Cushing's syndrome. The other is the permissive facilitation of the lipolytic effect of other agents, such as growth hormone and β adrenergic receptor agonists, resulting in an increase in free fatty acids after glucocorticoid administration. With respect to fat distribution, there is increased fat in the back of the neck ("buffalo hump"), face ("moon facies"), and supraclavicular area, coupled with a loss of fat in the extremities.

One hypothesis for this redistribution is that peripheral and truncal adipocytes differ in their relative sensitivities to insulin and to glucocorticoid-facilitated lipolytic effects, that truncal adipocytes respond predominantly to elevated levels of insulin resulting from glucocorticoid-induced hyperglycemia, whereas peripheral adipocytes are less sensitive to insulin and respond mostly to the glucocorticoid-facilitated effects of other lipolytic hormones. This differential sensitivity may reflect differences in the expression of the type 1 isozyme of 11βHSD that converts inactive cortisone into active cortisol in target tissues (Figure 59–6). Consistent with this idea, overexpression of 11βHSD1 in adipocytes causes obesity in a transgenic mouse model. The potential role of this enzyme in adipocyte function has prompted speculation that 11βHSD1 inhibitors may have a role in the treatment of obesity.

Electrolyte and Water Balance. Aldosterone is by far the most potent endogenous corticosteroid with respect to fluid and electrolyte balance. Thus, electrolyte balance is relatively normal in patients with adrenal insufficiency due to pituitary disease, despite the loss of glucocorticoid production by the inner cortical zones. Mineralocorticoids act on the distal tubules and collecting ducts of the kidney to enhance reabsorption of Na^+ from the tubular fluid; they also increase the urinary excretion of K^+ and H^+. Conceptually, it is useful to think of aldosterone as stimulating a renal exchange between Na^+ and K^+ or H^+, although this does not involve a simple 1:1 exchange of cations in the renal tubule.

These actions on electrolyte transport, in the kidney and in other tissues (*e.g.,* colon, salivary glands, and sweat glands), appear to account for the physiological and pharmacological activities that are characteristic of mineralo-

corticoids. Thus, the primary features of hyperaldosteronism are positive Na^+ balance with consequent expansion of extracellular fluid volume, normal or slight increases in plasma Na^+ concentration, hypokalemia, and alkalosis. Mineralocorticoid deficiency, in contrast, leads to Na^+ wasting and contraction of the extracellular fluid volume, hyponatremia, hyperkalemia, and acidosis. Chronically, hyperaldosteronism can cause hypertension, whereas aldosterone deficiency can lead to hypotension and vascular collapse. Because of the effects of mineralocorticoids on electrolyte handling by sweat glands, patients who are adrenal insufficient are especially predisposed to Na^+ loss and volume depletion through excessive sweating in hot environments.

Glucocorticoids also exert effects on fluid and electrolyte balance, largely due to permissive effects on tubular function and actions that maintain glomerular filtration rate. Glucocorticoids play a permissive role in the renal excretion of free water; the ability to excrete a water challenge was used at one time to diagnose adrenal insufficiency. In part, the inability of patients with glucocorticoid deficiency to excrete free water results from the increased secretion of AVP, which stimulates water reabsorption in the kidney.

In addition to their effects on monovalent cations and water, glucocorticoids also exert multiple effects on Ca^{2+} metabolism. Steroids interfere with Ca^{2+} uptake in the gut and increase Ca^{2+} excretion by the kidney. These effects collectively lead to decreased total body Ca^{2+} stores.

Cardiovascular System. The most striking effects of corticosteroids on the cardiovascular system result from mineralocorticoid-induced changes in renal Na^+ excretion, as is evident in primary aldosteronism. The resultant hypertension can lead to a diverse group of adverse effects on the cardiovascular system, including increased atherosclerosis, cerebral hemorrhage, stroke, and hypertensive cardiomyopathy. Consistent with the known actions of mineralocorticoids in the kidney, restriction of dietary Na^+ can lower the blood pressure considerably in mineralocorticoid excess.

Studies also have shown direct effects of aldosterone on the heart and vascular lining; aldosterone induces hypertension and interstitial cardiac fibrosis in animal models. The increased cardiac fibrosis is proposed to result from direct mineralocorticoid actions in the heart rather than from the effect of hypertension, because treatment with spironolactone, a MR antagonist, blocked the fibrosis without altering blood pressure. Similar effects of mineralocorticoids on cardiac fibrosis in human beings may explain, at least in part, the beneficial effects of spironolactone in patients with congestive heart failure (*see* Chapter 33).

The second major action of corticosteroids on the cardiovascular system is to enhance vascular reactivity to other vasoactive substances. Hypoadrenalism is associated with reduced response to vasoconstrictors such as norepinephrine and angiotensin II, perhaps due to decreased expression of adrenergic receptors in the vascular wall. Conversely, hypertension is seen in patients with excessive glucocorticoid secretion, occurring in most patients with Cushing's syndrome and in a subset of patients treated with synthetic glucocorticoids (even those lacking any significant mineralocorticoid action).

The underlying mechanisms in glucocorticoid-induced hypertension also are unknown; in hypertension related to the endogenous secretion of cortisol, as seen in patients with Cushing's syndrome, it is not known if the effects are mediated by the GR or MR. Unlike hypertension caused by high aldosterone levels, the hypertension secondary to excess glucocorticoids is generally resistant to Na+ restriction.

Skeletal Muscle. Permissive concentrations of corticosteroids are required for the normal function of skeletal muscle, and diminished work capacity is a prominent sign of adrenocortical insufficiency. In patients with Addison's disease, weakness and fatigue are frequent symptoms that may reflect an inadequacy of the circulatory system. Excessive amounts of either glucocorticoids or mineralocorticoids also impair muscle function. In primary aldosteronism, muscle weakness results primarily from hypokalemia rather than from direct effects of mineralocorticoids on skeletal muscle. In contrast, glucocorticoid excess over prolonged periods, either secondary to glucocorticoid therapy or endogenous hypercorticism, causes skeletal muscle wasting. This effect, termed *steroid myopathy,* accounts in part for weakness and fatigue in patients with glucocorticoid excess and is discussed in more detail below.

Central Nervous System. Corticosteroids exert a number of indirect effects on the CNS, through maintenance of blood pressure, plasma glucose concentrations, and electrolyte concentrations. Increasingly, direct effects of corticosteroids on the CNS have been recognized, including effects on mood, behavior, and brain excitability.

Patients with adrenal insufficiency exhibit a diverse array of psychiatric manifestations, including apathy, depression, and irritability; some patients are frankly psychotic. Appropriate replacement therapy corrects these abnormalities. Conversely, glucocorticoid administration can induce multiple CNS reactions. Most patients respond with mood elevation, which may impart a sense of well-being despite the persistence of underlying disease. Some patients exhibit more pronounced behavioral changes, such as euphoria, insomnia, restlessness, and increased motor activity. A smaller but significant percentage of patients treated with glucocorticoids becomes anxious, depressed, or overtly psychotic. A high incidence of neuroses and psychoses is seen in patients with Cushing's syndrome. These abnormalities usually disappear after cessation of glucocorticoid therapy or treatment of the Cushing's syndrome.

The mechanisms by which corticosteroids affect neuronal activity are unknown, but it has been proposed that steroids produced locally in the brain (termed *neurosteroids*) may regulate neuronal excitability. Studies in rodent models indicated that glucocorticoids deleteriously affect survival and function of hippocampal neurons, and that these changes are associated with diminished memory. In one study, basal cortisol levels in human beings correlated directly with hippocampal atrophy and memory deficits. To the extent that these results are confirmed, they have important prognostic implications for age-related memory decline, and they suggest therapeutic approaches directed at diminishing the negative effects of glucocorticoids on hippocampal neurons with aging.

Formed Elements of Blood. Glucocorticoids exert minor effects on hemoglobin and erythrocyte content of blood, as evidenced by the frequent occurrence of polycythemia in Cushing's syndrome and of normochromic, normocytic anemia in adrenal insufficiency. More profound effects are seen in the setting of autoimmune hemolytic anemia, in which the immunosuppressive effects of glucocorticoids can diminish the self-destruction of erythrocytes.

Corticosteroids also affect circulating white blood cells. Addison's disease is associated with an increased mass of lymphoid tissue and lymphocytosis. In contrast, Cushing's syndrome is characterized by lymphocytopenia and decreased mass of lymphoid tissue. The administration of glucocorticoids leads to a decreased number of circulating lymphocytes, eosinophils, monocytes, and basophils. A single dose of hydrocortisone leads to a decline of these circulating cells within 4 to 6 hours; this effect persists for 24 hours and results from the redistribution of cells away from the periphery rather than from increased destruction. In contrast, glucocorticoids increase circulating polymorphonuclear leukocytes as a result of increased release from the marrow, diminished rate of removal from the circulation, and increased demargination from vascular walls. Finally, certain lymphoid malignancies are destroyed by glucocorticoid treatment, an effect that may relate to the ability of glucocorticoids to activate programmed cell death.

Antiinflammatory and Immunosuppressive Actions. In addition to their effects on lymphocyte number, corticosteroids profoundly alter the immune responses of lymphocytes. These effects are an important facet of the antiinflammatory and immunosuppressive actions of the glucocorticoids. Glucocorticoids can prevent or suppress

Table 59–3
Effects of Glucocorticoids on Components of Inflammatory/Immune Responses

CELL TYPE	FACTOR	COMMENTS
Macrophages and monocytes	Arachidonic acid and its metabolites (prostaglandins and leukotrienes)	Mediated by glucocorticoid inhibition of cyclooxygenase–2 and phospholipase A_2.
	Cytokines, including: interleukin (IL)-1, IL-6, and tumor necrosis factor-α (TNF-α)	Production and release are blocked. The cytokines exert multiple effects on inflammation (*e.g.*, activation of T cells, stimulation of fibroblast proliferation).
	Acute phase reactants	These include the third component of complement.
Endothelial cells	Endothelial leukocyte adhesion molecule-1 (ELAM-1) and intracellular adhesion molecule-1 (ICAM-1)	ELAM-1 and ICAM-1 are intracellular adhesion molecules that are critical for leukocyte localization.
	Acute phase reactants	Same as above, for macrophages and monocytes.
	Cytokines (*e.g.*, IL-1)	Same as above, for macrophages and monocytes.
	Arachidonic acid derivatives	Same as above, for macrophages and monocytes.
Basophils	Histamine, leukotriene C4	IgE-dependent release inhibited by glucocorticoids.
Fibroblasts	Arachidonic acid metabolites	Same as above for macrophages and monocytes. Glucocorticoids also suppress growth factor–induced DNA synthesis and fibroblast proliferation.
Lymphocytes	Cytokines (IL-1, IL-2, IL-3, IL-6, TNF-α, GM-CSF, interferon-γ)	Same as above for macrophages and monocytes.

inflammation in response to multiple inciting events, including radiant, mechanical, chemical, infectious, and immunological stimuli. Although the use of glucocorticoids as antiinflammatory agents does not address the underlying cause of the disease, the suppression of inflammation is of enormous clinical utility and has made these drugs among the most frequently prescribed agents. Similarly, glucocorticoids are of immense value in treating diseases that result from undesirable immune reactions. These diseases range from conditions that predominantly result from humoral immunity, such as urticaria (*see* Chapter 62), to those that are mediated by cellular immune mechanisms, such as transplantation rejection (*see* Chapter 52). The immunosuppressive and antiinflammatory actions of glucocorticoids are inextricably linked, perhaps because they both involve inhibition of leukocyte functions.

Multiple mechanisms are involved in the suppression of inflammation by glucocorticoids. It is now clear that glucocorticoids inhibit the production by multiple cells of factors that are critical in generating the inflammatory response. As a result, there is decreased release of vasoactive and chemoattractive factors, diminished secretion of lipolytic and proteolytic enzymes, decreased extravasation of leukocytes to areas of injury, and ultimately, decreased fibrosis. Glucocorticoids can also reduce expression of proinflammatory cytokines, such as COX-2 and NOS2. Some of the cell types and mediators that are inhibited by

glucocorticoids are summarized in Table 59–3. The net effect of these actions on various cell types is to diminish markedly the inflammatory response.

The influence of stressful conditions on immune defense mechanisms is well documented, as is the contribution of the HPA axis to the stress response (Sapolsky *et al.*, 2000). This has led to a growing appreciation of the importance of glucocorticoids as physiological modulators of the immune system, where glucocorticoids appear to protect the organism against life-threatening consequences of a full-blown inflammatory response (Chrousos, 1995).

Stresses such as injury, infection, and disease result in the increased production of cytokines, a network of signaling molecules that integrate actions of macrophages/monocytes, T lymphocytes, and B lymphocytes in mounting immune responses. Among these cytokines, interleukin (IL)-1, IL-6, and tumor necrosis factor-α (TNF-α) stimulate the HPA axis, with IL-1 having the broadest range of actions. IL-1 stimulates the release of CRH by hypothalamic neurons, interacts directly with the pituitary to increase the release of ACTH, and may directly stimulate the adrenal gland to produce glucocorticoids. As detailed above, the increased production of glucocorticoids, in turn, profoundly inhibits the immune system at multiple sites. Factors that are inhibited include components of the cytokine network, including interferon-γ (IFN-γ), granulocyte-macrophage colony-stimulating factor (GM-CSF), interleukins (IL-1, IL-2, IL-3, IL-6, IL-8, and IL-12), and TNF-α. Thus, the HPA axis and the immune system are capable of bidirectional interactions in response to stress, and these interactions appear to be important for homeostasis (Chrousos, 1995).

Absorption, Transport, Metabolism, and Excretion

Absorption. Hydrocortisone and numerous congeners, including the synthetic analogs, are orally effective. Certain water-soluble esters of hydrocortisone and its synthetic congeners are administered intravenously to achieve high concentrations of drug rapidly in body fluids. More prolonged effects are obtained by intramuscular injection of suspensions of hydrocortisone, its esters, and congeners. Minor changes in chemical structure may markedly alter the rate of absorption, time of onset of effect, and duration of action.

Glucocorticoids also are absorbed systemically from sites of local administration, such as synovial spaces, the conjunctival sac, skin, and respiratory tract. When administration is prolonged, when the site of application is covered with an occlusive dressing, or when large areas of skin are involved, the absorption may be sufficient to cause systemic effects, including suppression of the HPA axis.

Transport, Metabolism, and Excretion. After absorption, 90% or more of cortisol in plasma is reversibly bound to protein under normal circumstances. Only the fraction of corticosteroid that is unbound can enter cells to mediate corticosteroid effects. Two plasma proteins account for almost all of the steroid-binding capacity: corticosteroid-binding globulin (CBG; also called transcortin), and albumin. CBG is an α-globulin secreted by the liver that has high affinity (estimated association constant of approximately 7.6×10^7 M^{-1}) for steroids but relatively low total binding capacity, whereas albumin, also produced by the liver, has low affinity (estimated association constant of 1×10^3 M^{-1}) but relatively large binding capacity. At normal or low concentrations of corticosteroids, most of the hormone is protein-bound. At higher steroid concentrations, the capacity of protein binding is exceeded, and a greater fraction of the steroid exists in the free state. Corticosteroids compete with each other for binding sites on CBG. CBG has relatively high affinity for cortisol and most of its synthetic congeners and low affinity for aldosterone and glucuronide-conjugated steroid metabolites; thus, greater percentages of these latter steroids are found in the free form.

A special state of physiological hypercorticism occurs during pregnancy. The elevated circulating estrogen levels induce CBG production, and CBG and total plasma cortisol increase severalfold. The physiological significance of these changes remains to be established.

All of the biologically active adrenocortical steroids and their synthetic congeners have a double bond in the 4,5 position and a ketone group at C 3 (Figure 59–7). As a general rule, the metabolism of steroid hormones involves sequential additions of oxygen or hydrogen atoms, followed by conjugation to form water-soluble derivatives. Reduction of the 4,5 double bond occurs at both hepatic and extrahepatic sites, yielding inactive compounds. Subsequent reduction of the 3-ketone substituent to the 3-hydroxyl derivative, forming tetrahydrocortisol, occurs only in the liver. Most of these A ring–reduced steroids are conjugated through the 3-hydroxyl group with sulfate or glucuronide by enzymatic reactions that take place in the liver, and to a lesser extent in the kidney. The resultant sulfate esters and glucuronides are water-soluble and are the predominant forms excreted in urine. Neither biliary nor fecal excretion is of quantitative importance in humans.

Synthetic steroids with an 11-keto substituent, such as cortisone and *prednisone*, must be enzymatically reduced to the corresponding 11β-hydroxy derivative before they are biologically active. The type 1 isozyme of 11β-hydroxysteroid dehydrogenase catalyzes this reduction, predominantly in the liver, but also in specialized sites such as adipocytes, bone, eye, and skin. In settings in which this enzymatic activity is impaired, it is prudent to use steroids that do not require enzymatic activation (*e.g.*, hydrocortisone and *prednisolone* rather than cortisone or prednisone). Such settings include severe hepatic failure and patients with the rare condition of cortisone reductase deficiency, who are unable to activate the 11-keto steroids because of a partial loss of 11βHSD1 activity and a relative deficiency in the enzyme hexose-6-phosphate dehydrogenase, which supplies reducing equivalents to the 11β-hydroxysteroid dehydrogenase.

Structure–Activity Relationships

Chemical modifications to the cortisol molecule have generated derivatives with greater separations of glucocorticoid and mineralocorticoid activity; for a number of synthetic glucocorticoids, the effects on electrolytes are minimal even at the highest doses used (Table 59–2). In addition, these modifications have led to derivatives with greater potencies and with longer durations of action. A vast array of steroid preparations is available for oral, parenteral, and topical use. Some of these agents are summarized in Table 59–4. None of these currently available derivatives effectively separates antiinflammatory effects from effects on carbohydrate, protein, and fat metabolism, or from suppressive effects on the HPA axis, as discussed above.

The structures of hydrocortisone (cortisol) and some of its major derivatives are shown in Figure 59–7. Changes in chemical structure may alter the specificity and/or potency due to changes in affinity and intrinsic activity at corticosteroid receptors, and alterations in absorption, protein binding, rate of metabolic transformation, rate of excretion, or membrane permeability. The effects of various substitutions on glucocorticoid and mineralocorticoid activity and on duration of action are summarized in Table 59–2. The 4,5 double bond and the 3-keto group on ring A are essential for glucocorticoid and mineralocorticoid activity; an 11β-hydroxyl group on ring C is required for glucocorticoid activity but not mineralocorticoid activity; a hydroxyl group at C 21 on ring D is present on all natural corti-

Table 59–4
Available Preparations of Adrenocortical Steroids and Their Synthetic Analogs

NONPROPRIETARY NAME (TRADE NAME)	TYPES OF PREPARATIONS	NONPROPRIETARY NAME (TRADE NAME)	TYPES OF PREPARATIONS
Alclometasone dipropionate (ACLOVATE)	Topical	Cortisol (hydrocortisone) valerate (WESTCORT)	Topical
Amcinonide (CYCLOCORT)	Topical	Cortisone acetate (CORTONE ACETATE)	Oral, injectable
Beclomethasone dipropionate (BECLOVENT, VANCERIL, others)	Inhalation	Desonide (DESOWEN, TRIDESILON)	Topical
Betamethasone (CELESTONE)	Oral	Desoximetasone (TOPICORT)	Topical
Betamethasone dipropionate (DIPROSONE, others)	Topical	Dexamethasone (DECADRON, others)	Oral, topical
Betamethasonesodium phosphate (CELESTONE PHOSPHATE, others)	Injectable	Dexamethasone acetate (DECADRON-LA, others)	Injectable
Betamethasonesodium phosphate and acetate (CELESTONE SOLUSPAN)	Injectable	Dexamethasonesodium phosphate (DECADRON PHOSPHATE, HEXADROL PHOSPHATE, others)	Topical, ophthalmic, otic, injectable
Betamethasone valerate (BETA-VAL, VALISONE, others)	Topical	Diflorasone diacetate (FLORONE, MAXIFLOR)	Topical
Budesonide (PULMICORT, RHINOCORT)	Inhalation	Fludrocortisone acetate* (FLORINEF)	Oral
Clobetasol propionate (TEMOVATE)	Topical	Flunisolide (AEROBID, NASALIDE)	Inhalation
Clocortolone pivalate (CLODERM)	Topical	Fluocinolone acetonide (FLUONID, SYNALAR, others)	Topical
Cortisol (hydrocortisone) (CORTEF, HYDROCORTONE, others)	Topical, enema, otic solutions, oral, injectable	Fluocinonide (LIDEX)	Topical
		Fluorometholone (FLUOR-OP, FML, LIQUIFILM)	Ophthalmic
Cortisol (hydrocortisone) acetate (HYDROCORTONE ACETATE others)	Topical, suppositories, rectal foam, injectable	Fluorometholone acetate (FLAREX)	Ophthalmic
Cortisol (hydrocortisone) butyrate (LOCOID)	Topical	Flurandrenolide (CORDRAN)	Topical
		Halcinonide (HALOG)	Topical
Cortisol (hydrocortisone) cypionate (CORTEF)	Oral	Medrysone (HMS LIQUIFILM)	Ophthalmic
		Methylprednisolone (MEDROL)	Oral
Cortisol (hydrocortisone) sodium phosphate (HYDROCORTONE PHOSPHATE)	Injectable	Methylprednisolone acetate (DEPO-MEDROL, MEDROL ACETATE, others)	Topical, injectable
Cortisol (hydrocortisone) sodium succinate (A-HYDROCORT, SOLU-CORTEF)	Injectable	Methylprednisolone sodium succinate (A-METHAPRED, SOLU-MEDROL)	Injectable
Mometasone furoate (ELOCON)	Topical	Prednisone (DELTASONE, others)	Oral
Prednisolone (DELTA-CORTEF)	Oral	Triamcinolone (ARISTOCORT, KENACORT)	Oral
Prednisolone acetate (ECONOPRED, others)	Ophthalmic, injectable	Triamcinolone acetonide (KENALOG, others)	Topical, inhalation, injectable
Prednisolone sodium phosphate (PEDIAPRED, others)	Oral, ophthalmic, injectable	Triamcinolone diacetate (ARISTOCORT, KENACORT DIACETATE, others)	Oral, injectable
Prednisolone tebutate (HYDELTRA-T.B.A., others)	Injectable	Triamcinolone hexacetonide (ARISTOSPAN)	Injectable

*Fludrocortisone acetate is intended for use as a mineralocorticoid. *Note: Topical* preparations include agents for application to skin or mucous membranes in creams, solutions, ointments, gels, pastes (for oral lesions), and aerosols; *ophthalmic* preparations include solutions, suspensions, and ointments; inhalation preparations include agents for nasal or oral inhalation.

costeroids and on most of the active synthetic analogs and seems to be an absolute requirement for mineralocorticoid activity, but not for glucocorticoid activity. The 17α-hydroxyl group on ring D is a substituent on cortisol and on all of the currently used synthetic glucocorticoids. While steroids without the 17α-hydroxyl group (*e.g.*, *corticosterone*) have appreciable glucocorticoid activity, the 17α-hydroxyl group gives optimal potency.

Introduction of an additional double bond in the 1,2 position of ring A, as in prednisolone or prednisone, selectively increases glucocorticoid activity (approximately fourfold compared to hydrocortisone), resulting in an enhanced glucocorticoid/mineralocorticoid potency ratio. This modification also results in compounds that are metabolized more slowly than hydrocortisone.

Fluorination at the 9α position on ring B enhances both glucocorticoid and mineralocorticoid activity, possibly related to an electron-withdrawing effect on the nearby 11β-hydroxyl group. *Fludrocortisone* (9α-fluorocortisol) has enhanced activity at the GR (10 times relative to cortisol) but even greater activity at the MR (125 times relative to cortisol). It is used in mineralocorticoid replacement therapy (*see* below) and has no appreciable glucocorticoid effect at usual daily doses of 0.05 mg to 0.2 mg. When combined with the 1,2 double bond in ring A and other substitutions at C 16 on ring D (Figure 59–7), the 9α-fluoro derivatives formed (*e.g.*, *triamcinolone*, *dexamethasone*, and *betamethasone*) have marked glucocorticoid activity. The substitutions at C 16 virtually eliminate mineralocorticoid activity.

Other Substitutions. 6α Substitution on ring B has somewhat unpredictable effects. 6α-Methylcortisol has increased glucocorticoid and mineralocorticoid activity, whereas 6α-methylprednisolone has somewhat greater glucocorticoid activity and somewhat less mineralocorticoid activity than prednisolone. A number of modifications convert the glucocorticoids to more lipophilic molecules with enhanced topical/systemic potency ratios. Examples include the introduction of an acetonide between hydroxyl groups at C 16 and C 17, esterification of the hydroxyl group with valerate at C 17, esterification of hydroxyl groups with propionate at C 17 and C 21, and substitution of the hydroxyl group at C 21 with chlorine. Other approaches to achieve local glucocorticoid activity while minimizing systemic effects involve the formation of analogs that are rapidly inactivated after absorption; examples include C 21 carboxylate or carbothioate glucocorticoid esters, which are rapidly metabolized to inactive 21-carboxylic acids.

Toxicity of Adrenocortical Steroids

Two categories of toxic effects result from the therapeutic use of corticosteroids: those resulting from withdrawal of steroid therapy and those resulting from continued use at supraphysiological doses. The side effects from both categories are potentially life-threatening and mandate a careful assessment of the risks and benefits in each patient.

Withdrawal of Therapy. The most frequent problem in steroid withdrawal is flare-up of the underlying disease for which steroids were prescribed. There are several other complications associated with steroid withdrawal. The most severe complication of steroid cessation, acute adrenal insufficiency, results from overly rapid withdrawal of

corticosteroids after prolonged therapy has suppressed the HPA axis. The therapeutic approach to acute adrenal insufficiency is detailed below. There is significant variation among patients with respect to the degree and duration of adrenal suppression after glucocorticoid therapy, making it difficult to establish the relative risk in any given patient. Many patients recover from glucocorticoid-induced HPA suppression within several weeks to months; however, in some individuals the time to recovery can be one year or longer.

In an effort to diminish the risk of iatrogenic acute adrenal insufficiency, protocols for discontinuing corticosteroid therapy in patients receiving long-term treatment with corticosteroids have been proposed, generally without rigorous documentation of their efficacy. Patients who have received supraphysiological doses of glucocorticoids for a period of 2 to 4 weeks within the preceding year should be considered to have some degree of HPA impairment in settings of acute stress and should be treated accordingly.

In addition to this most severe form of withdrawal, a characteristic glucocorticoid withdrawal syndrome consists of fever, myalgias, arthralgias, and malaise, which may be difficult to differentiate from some of the underlying diseases for which steroid therapy was instituted. Finally, *pseudotumor cerebri*, a clinical syndrome that includes increased intracranial pressure with papilledema, is a rare condition that sometimes is associated with reduction or withdrawal of corticosteroid therapy.

Continued Use of Supraphysiological Glucocorticoid Doses. Besides the consequences that result from the suppression of the HPA axis, there are a number of other complications that result from prolonged therapy with corticosteroids. These include fluid and electrolyte abnormalities, hypertension, hyperglycemia, increased susceptibility to infection, osteoporosis, myopathy, behavioral disturbances, cataracts, growth arrest, and the characteristic habitus of steroid overdose, including fat redistribution, striae, and ecchymoses.

Fluid and Electrolyte Handling. Alterations in fluid and electrolyte handling can cause hypokalemic alkalosis, edema, and hypertension, particularly in patients with primary hyperaldosteronism secondary to an adrenal adenoma or in patients treated with potent mineralocorticoids. Similarly, hypertension is a relatively common manifestation in patients with endogenous glucocorticoid excess and can even be seen in patients treated with glucocorticoids lacking appreciable mineralocorticoid activity.

Metabolic Changes. The effects of glucocorticoids on intermediary metabolism have been described above. Hyperglycemia with glycosuria usually can be managed with diet and/or insulin, and its occurrence should not be a major factor in the decision to continue corticosteroid therapy or to initiate therapy in diabetic patients.

Immune Responses. Because of their multiple effects to inhibit the immune system and the inflammatory response, glucocorticoid use is associated with an increased susceptibility to infection and a risk for reactivation of latent tuberculosis. In the presence of known infections of some consequence, glucocorticoids should be administered only if absolutely necessary and concomitantly with appropriate and effective antimicrobial or antifungal therapy.

Possible Risk of Peptic Ulcers. There is considerable debate about the association between peptic ulcers and glucocorticoid therapy. The possible onset of hemorrhage and perforation in these ulcers and their insidious onset make peptic ulcers serious therapeutic problems (*see* Chapter 36); estimating the degree of risk from corticosteroids has received much study. Most patients who develop gastrointestinal bleeding while receiving corticosteroids also received nonsteroidal antiinflammatory agents, which are known to promote ulceration, such that the pathogenic role of corticosteroids remains open to debate. Nonetheless, it is prudent to be especially vigilant for peptic ulcer formation in patients receiving therapy with corticosteroids, especially when administered concomitantly with nonsteroidal antiinflammatory drugs.

Myopathy. Myopathy, characterized by weakness of proximal limb muscles, can occur in patients taking large doses of corticosteroids and also is part of the clinical picture in patients with endogenous Cushing's syndrome. It can be of sufficient severity to impair ambulation and is an indication for withdrawal of therapy. Attention also has focused on steroid myopathy of the respiratory muscles in patients with asthma or chronic obstructive pulmonary disease (*see* Chapter 27); this complication can diminish respiratory function. Recovery from the steroid myopathies may be slow and incomplete.

Behavioral Changes. Behavioral disturbances are common after administration of corticosteroids and in patients who have Cushing's syndrome secondary to endogenous hypercorticism; these disturbances may take many forms, including nervousness, insomnia, changes in mood or psyche, and overt psychosis. Suicidal tendencies are not uncommon. A history of previous psychiatric illness does not preclude the use of steroids in patients for whom they are otherwise indicated. Conversely, the absence of a history of previous psychiatric illness does not guarantee that a given patient will not develop psychiatric disorders while on steroids.

Cataracts. Cataracts are a well-established complication of glucocorticoid therapy and are related to dosage and duration of therapy. Children appear to be particularly at risk. Cessation of therapy may not lead to complete resolution of opacities, and the cataracts may progress despite reduction or cessation of therapy. Patients on long-term glucocorticoid therapy at doses of prednisone of 10 to 15 mg/day or greater should receive periodic slit-lamp examinations to detect glucocorticoid-induced posterior subcapsular cataracts.

Osteoporosis. Osteoporosis, a frequent serious complication of glucocorticoid therapy, occurs in patients of all ages and is related to dosage and duration of therapy (Saag, 2003). A reasonable estimate is that 30% to 50% of all patients who receive chronic glucocorticoid therapy ultimately will develop osteoporotic fractures. Glucocorticoids preferentially affect trabecular bone and the cortical rim of the vertebral bodies; the ribs and vertebrae are the most frequent sites of fracture. Glucocorticoids decrease bone density by multiple mechanisms, including inhibition of gonadal steroid hormones, diminished gastrointestinal absorption of Ca^{2+}, and inhibition of bone formation due to suppressive effects on osteoblasts and stimulation of resorption due to effects on osteoclasts mediated by changes in the production of osteoprotegerin and RANK ligand. In addition, glucocorticoid inhibition of intestinal Ca^{2+} uptake may lead to secondary increases in parathyroid hormone, thereby increasing bone resorption.

The considerable morbidity of glucocorticoid-related osteoporosis has led to efforts to identify patients at risk for fractures and to prevent or reverse bone loss in patients requiring chronic glucocorticoid

therapy. The initiation of glucocorticoid therapy is considered an indication for bone densitometry, preferably with techniques such as dual-energy x-ray absorptiometry of the lumbar spine and hip that most sensitively detect abnormalities in trabecular bone. Because bone loss associated with glucocorticoids predominantly occurs within the first 6 months of therapy, densitometric evaluation and prophylactic measures should be initiated with therapy or shortly thereafter. Most authorities advocate maintaining a Ca^{2+} intake of 1500 mg/day by diet plus Ca^{2+} supplementation and vitamin D intake of 400 IU/day, assuming that these measures do not increase urinary calcium excretion above the normal range. Although gonadal hormone replacement therapy has been widely used in specific groups of patients receiving chronic glucocorticoid therapy, this is the subject of considerable debate based on recently published results from randomized, placebo-controlled trials (*see* Chapter 57). Recombinant parathyroid hormone recently has received considerable attention as a potential therapy of glucocorticoid-induced osteoporosis.

The most important advance to date in the prevention of glucocorticoid-related osteoporosis is the successful use of bisphosphonates, which have been shown to decrease the decline in bone density and the incidence of fractures in patients receiving glucocorticoid therapy. Additional discussion of these issues is found in Chapters 57 and 61.

Osteonecrosis. Osteonecrosis (also known as avascular or aseptic necrosis) is a relatively common complication of glucocorticoid therapy. The femoral head is affected most frequently, but this process also may affect the humeral head and distal femur. Joint pain and stiffness usually are the earliest symptoms, and this diagnosis should be considered in patients receiving glucocorticoids who abruptly develop hip, shoulder, or knee pain. Although the risk increases with the duration and dose of glucocorticoid therapy, osteonecrosis also can occur when high doses of glucocorticoids are given for short periods of time. Osteonecrosis generally progresses, and most affected patients ultimately require joint replacement.

Regulation of Growth and Development. Growth retardation in children can result from administration of relatively small doses of glucocorticoids. Although the precise mechanism is unknown, there are reports that collagen synthesis and linear growth in these children can be restored by treatment with growth hormone; further studies are needed to define the role of concurrent treatment with growth hormone in this setting. Further studies also are needed to explore the possible effects of exposure to corticosteroids *in utero*. Studies in experimental animals have shown that antenatal exposure to glucocorticoids is clearly linked to cleft palate and altered neuronal development, ultimately resulting in complex behavioral abnormalities. Thus, although the actions of glucocorticoids to promote cellular differentiation play important physiological roles in human development in the neonatal period (*e.g.,* induction of the hepatic gluconeogenic enzymes and surfactant production in the lung), the possibility remains that antenatal steroids can lead to subtle abnormalities in fetal development.

Therapeutic Uses

With the exception of replacement therapy in deficiency states, the use of glucocorticoids largely is empirical. Based on extensive clinical experience, a number of therapeutic principles can be proposed. Given the number and severity of potential side effects, the decision to institute therapy with glucocorticoids always requires a careful consideration of the relative risks and benefits in each patient. For any disease and in any patient, the appropriate dose to achieve a given therapeutic effect must be determined by trial and error and must be re-evaluated periodically as the activity of the underlying disease changes or as complications of therapy arise. A single dose of glucocorticoid, even a large one, is virtually without harmful effects, and a short course of therapy (up to one week), in the absence of specific contraindications, is unlikely to be harmful. As the duration of glucocorticoid therapy is increased beyond one week, there are time- and dose-related increases in the incidence of disabling and potentially lethal effects. Except in patients receiving replacement therapy, glucocorticoids are neither specific nor curative; rather, they are palliative by virtue of their antiinflammatory and immunosuppressive actions. Finally, abrupt cessation of glucocorticoids after prolonged therapy is associated with the risk of adrenal insufficiency, which may be fatal.

These principles have several implications for clinical practice. When glucocorticoids are to be given over long periods, the dose must be determined by trial and error and must be the smallest one that will achieve the desired effect. When the therapeutic goal is relief of painful or distressing symptoms not associated with an immediately life-threatening disease, complete relief is not sought, and the steroid dose is reduced gradually until worsening symptoms indicate that the minimal acceptable dose has been found. Where possible, the substitution of other medications, such as nonsteroidal antiinflammatory drugs, may facilitate the tapering process once the initial benefit of glucocorticoid therapy has been achieved. When therapy is directed at a life-threatening disease (e.g., pemphigus or lupus cerebritis), the initial dose should be a large one aimed at achieving rapid control of the crisis. If some benefit is not observed quickly, then the dose should be doubled or tripled. After initial control in a potentially lethal disease, dose reduction should be carried out under conditions that permit frequent, accurate observations of the patient. It is always essential to weigh carefully the relative dangers of therapy and of the disease being treated.

The lack of demonstrated deleterious effects of a single dose of glucocorticoids within the conventional therapeutic range justifies their administration to critically ill patients who may have adrenal insufficiency. If the underlying condition does result from deficiency of glucocorticoids, then a single intravenous injection of a soluble glucocorticoid may prevent immediate death and allow time for a definitive diagnosis to be made. If the underlying disease is not adrenal insufficiency, the single dose will not harm the patient.

In the absence of specific contraindications, short courses of high-dose, systemic glucocorticoids also may be given for diseases that are not life-threatening, but the general rule is that long courses of therapy at high doses should be reserved for life-threatening disease. In selected settings, as when a patient is threatened with permanent disability, this rule is justifiably violated.

In an attempt to dissociate therapeutic effects from undesirable side effects, various regimens of steroid administration have been utilized. To diminish HPA axis suppression, the intermediate-acting steroid preparations (e.g., prednisone or prednisolone) should be given in the morning as a single dose. Alternate-day therapy with the same glucocorticoids also has been employed, as certain patients obtain adequate therapeutic responses on this regimen. Alternatively, pulse therapy with higher glucocorticoid doses (e.g., doses as high as 1 to 1.5 g/day of methylprednisolone for 3 days) frequently is used to initiate therapy in patients with fulminant, immunologically related disorders such as acute transplantation rejection, necrotizing glomerulonephritis, and lupus nephritis. The benefit of such pulse therapy in long-term maintenance regimens remains to be defined.

Replacement Therapy.

Adrenal insufficiency can result from structural or functional lesions of the adrenal cortex (primary adrenal insufficiency or Addison's disease) or from structural or functional lesions of the anterior pituitary or hypothalamus (secondary adrenal insufficiency). In developed countries, primary adrenal insufficiency most frequently is secondary to autoimmune adrenal disease, whereas tuberculous adrenalitis is the most frequent etiology in underdeveloped countries. Other causes include adrenalectomy, bilateral adrenal hemorrhage, neoplastic infiltration of the adrenal glands, acquired immunodeficiency syndrome, inherited disorders of the steroidogenic enzymes, and X-linked adrenoleukodystrophy (Carey, 1997). Secondary adrenal insufficiency resulting from pituitary or hypothalamic dysfunction generally presents in a more insidious manner than does the primary disorder, probably because mineralocorticoid biosynthesis is preserved.

Acute Adrenal Insufficiency. This life-threatening disease is characterized by gastrointestinal symptoms (nausea, vomiting, and abdominal pain), dehydration, hyponatremia, hyperkalemia, weakness, lethargy, and hypotension. It usually is associated with disorders of the adrenal rather than the pituitary or hypothalamus, and sometimes follows abrupt withdrawal of glucocorticoids used at high doses or for prolonged periods.

The immediate management of patients with acute adrenal insufficiency includes intravenous therapy with isotonic sodium chloride solution supplemented with 5% glucose and corticosteroids and appropriate therapy for precipitating causes such as infection, trauma, or hemorrhage. Because cardiovascular function often is reduced in the setting of adrenocortical insufficiency, the patient should be monitored for evidence of volume overload such as rising central venous pressure or pulmonary edema. After an initial intravenous bolus of 100 mg, hydrocortisone (cortisol) should be given by continuous infusion at a rate of 50 to 100 mg every 8 hours. At this dose, which approximates the maximum daily rate of cortisol secretion in response to stress, hydrocortisone alone has sufficient mineralocorticoid activity to meet all requirements. As the patient stabilizes, the hydrocortisone dose may be decreased to 25 mg every 6 to 8 hours. Thereafter, patients are treated in the same fashion as those with chronic adrenal insufficiency (*see* below).

For the treatment of suspected but unconfirmed acute adrenal insufficiency, 4 mg of *dexamethasone sodium phosphate* can be substituted for hydrocortisone, since dexamethasone does not cross-react in the cortisol assay and will not interfere with the measurement of cortisol (either basally or in response to the cosyntropin stimulation test). A failure to respond to cosyntropin in this setting is diagnostic of adrenal insufficiency. Often, a sample for the measurement of plasma ACTH also is obtained, as it will provide information about the underlying etiology if the diagnosis of adrenocortical insufficiency is established.

Chronic Adrenal Insufficiency. Patients with chronic adrenal insufficiency present with many of the same manifestations seen in adrenal crisis, but with lesser severity. These patients require daily treatment with corticosteroids (Coursin and Wood, 2002). Traditional replacement regimens have used hydrocortisone in doses of 20 to 30 mg/day. *Cortisone acetate*, which is inactive until converted to cortisol by 11βHSD, also has been used in doses ranging from 25 to 37.5 mg/day. In an effort to mimic the normal diurnal rhythm of cortisol secretion, these glucocorticoids generally have been given in divided doses, with two-thirds of the dose given in the morning and one-third given in the afternoon. Based on revised estimates of daily cortisol production and clinical studies showing that subtle degrees of glucocorticoid excess can decrease bone density in patients on conventional replacement regimens, many authorities advocate a lower daily hydrocortisone dose of 15 to 20 mg/day divided into either two doses (*e.g.,* 10 to 15 mg on awakening and 5 mg in late afternoon) or three doses (*e.g.,* 10 mg on awakening, 5 mg at lunch, and 5 mg in late afternoon). Others prefer to use intermediate- (*e.g.,* prednisone) or long-acting (*e.g.,* dexamethasone) glucocorticoids, since no regimen employing shorter-acting steroids can reproduce the peak serum glucocorticoid levels that normally occur before awakening in the morning. The superiority of any one of these regimens has not been rigorously demonstrated. Although some patients with primary adrenal insufficiency can be maintained on hydrocortisone and liberal salt intake, most of these patients also require mineralocorticoid replacement; *fludrocortisone acetate* generally is used in doses of 0.05 to 0.2 mg/day. For patients with

secondary adrenal insufficiency, the administration of a glucocorticoid alone is generally adequate, as the zona glomerulosa, which makes mineralocorticoids, is intact. When initiating treatment in patients with panhypopituitarism, it is important to administer glucocorticoids before initiating treatment with thyroid hormone, because the administration of thyroid hormone may precipitate acute adrenal insufficiency by increasing the metabolism of cortisol.

The adequacy of corticosteroid replacement therapy is judged by clinical criteria and biochemical measurements. The subjective well-being of the patient is an important clinical parameter in primary and secondary disease. In primary adrenal insufficiency, the disappearance of hyperpigmentation and the resolution of electrolyte abnormalities are valuable indicators of adequate replacement. Overtreatment may cause manifestations of Cushing's syndrome in adults and decreased linear growth in children. Plasma ACTH levels may be used to monitor therapy in patients with primary adrenal insufficiency; the early-morning ACTH level should not be suppressed, but should be less than 100 pg/ml (20 pmol/L). Although advocated by some endocrinologists, assessments of daily profiles of cortisol based on multiple blood samples or measurements of urinary free cortisol have been used more frequently as research tools than as a routine part of clinical practice.

Standard doses of glucocorticoids often must be adjusted upward in patients who also are taking drugs that increase their metabolic clearance (*e.g.,* phenytoin, barbiturates, or rifampin). Dosage adjustments also are needed to compensate for the stress of intercurrent illness, and proper patient education is essential for the execution of these adjustments. All patients with adrenal insufficiency should wear a medical alert bracelet or tag that lists their diagnosis and carries information about their steroid regimen. During minor illness, the glucocorticoid dose should be doubled. Patients should be instructed to contact their physician if nausea and vomiting preclude the retention of oral medications. The patient and family members should also be trained to administer parenteral dexamethasone (4 mg subcutaneously or intramuscularly) in the event that severe nausea or vomiting precludes the oral administration of medications; they then should seek medical attention immediately. Based largely on empirical data, glucocorticoid doses also are adjusted when patients with adrenal insufficiency undergo either elective or emergency surgery (Axelrod, 2003). In this setting, the doses are designed to approximate or exceed the maximal cortisol secretory rate of 200 mg/day; a standard regimen is hydrocortisone, 100 mg parenterally every 8 hours. Following surgery, the dose is halved each day until it is reduced to routine maintenance levels. Although some data suggest that increases in dose to this degree are not essential for survival even in major surgery, this approach remains the standard clinical practice.

Congenital Adrenal Hyperplasia. This term denotes a group of genetic disorders in which the activity of one of the several enzymes required for the biosynthesis of glucocorticoids is deficient. The impaired production of cortisol and the consequent lack of negative feedback inhibition lead to increased release of ACTH. As a result, other hormonally active steroids that are proximal to the enzymatic block in the steroidogenic pathway are produced in excess. Congenital adrenal hyperplasia (CAH) includes a spectrum of disorders whose precise clinical presentation, laboratory findings, and treatment depend on which of the steroidogenic enzymes is deficient.

In approximately 90% of patients, CAH results from mutations in CYP21, the enzyme that carries out the 21-hydroxylation reaction (Figure 59–3). Clinically, patients are divided into those with classic CAH, who have severe defects in enzymatic activity and first present during childhood, and those with nonclassic CAH, who present after puberty with signs and symptoms of mild androgen excess such as hirsutism, amenorrhea, infertility, and acne. Female patients with classic CAH, if not treated *in utero* with glucocorticoids, frequently are born with virilized external genitalia (female pseudohermaphroditism), which results from elevated production of adrenal androgen precursors at critical stages of sexual differentiation *in utero.* Males appear normal at birth and later may have precocious development of secondary sexual characteristics (isosexual precocious puberty). In both sexes, linear growth is accelerated in childhood, but the adult height is reduced by premature closure of the epiphyses.

In a subset of patients with classical CAH, the enzymatic deficiency is sufficiently severe to compromise aldosterone production. Such patients are unable to conserve Na^+ normally and thus are called "salt wasters." These patients can present with cardiovascular collapse secondary to volume depletion. In an effort to prevent such life-threatening events, especially in males who appear normal at birth, many centers routinely screen all newborn babies for elevated levels of 17-hydroxyprogesterone, the immediate steroid precursor to the enzymatic block.

All patients with classical CAH require replacement therapy with hydrocortisone or a suitable congener, and those with salt wasting also require mineralocorticoid replacement. The goals of therapy are to restore levels of physiological steroid hormones to the normal range and to suppress ACTH and thereby abrogate the effects of overproduction of adrenal androgens. The typical oral dose of hydrocortisone is approximately 0.6 mg/kg daily in two or three divided doses. The mineralocorticoid used is fludrocortisone acetate (0.05 to 0.2 mg/day). Many experts also administer table salt to infants (one-fifth of a teaspoon dis-

solved in formula daily) until the child is eating solid food. Therapy is guided by gain in weight and height, by plasma levels of 17-hydroxyprogesterone, and by blood pressure. Elevated plasma renin activity suggests that the patient is receiving an inadequate dose of mineralocorticoid. Sudden spurts in linear growth often indicate inadequate pituitary suppression and excessive androgen secretion, whereas growth failure suggests overtreatment with glucocorticoid.

The ability to detect classical CAH (21-hydroxylase deficiency) prenatally has made possible the treatment of affected females with glucocorticoids *in utero,* potentially eliminating the need for genital surgery to correct the virilization of the external genitalia. To effectively suppress fetal adrenal androgen production and consequent virilization, glucocorticoid therapy (*e.g.,* dexamethasone, 20 µg/kg taken daily orally by mothers at risk) must be initiated before 10 weeks' gestation, before a definitive diagnosis of CAH can be made. The genotype and sex of the fetus then are determined and steroid therapy is stopped if the sex is male or there is at least one wild-type allele for 21-hydroxylase. If genotyping reveals an affected female, steroid therapy is continued until delivery. Potential maternal side effects include hypertension, weight gain, edema, and mood changes. Although exposure to glucocorticoids *in utero* may have developmental consequences, adverse effects of this regimen have not yet been described.

Therapeutic Uses in Nonendocrine Diseases. Outlined below are important uses of glucocorticoids in diseases that do not directly involve the HPA axis. The disorders discussed are not inclusive; rather, they illustrate the principles governing glucocorticoid use in selected diseases for which glucocorticoids are more frequently employed. The dosage of glucocorticoids varies considerably depending on the nature and severity of the underlying disorder. For convenience, approximate doses of a representative glucocorticoid (generally prednisone) are provided. This choice is not an endorsement of one particular glucocorticoid preparation over other congeners but is made for illustrative purposes only.

Rheumatic Disorders. Glucocorticoids are used widely in the treatment of a variety of rheumatic disorders and are a mainstay in the treatment of the more serious inflammatory rheumatic diseases, such as systemic lupus erythematosus, and a variety of vasculitic disorders, such as polyarteritis nodosa, Wegener's granulomatosis, Churg-Strauss syndrome, and giant cell arteritis. For these more serious disorders, the starting dose of glucocorticoids should be sufficient to suppress the disease rapidly and minimize resultant tissue damage. Initially, prednisone (1 mg/kg per day in divided doses) often is used, generally followed by consolidation to a single daily dose, with subsequent tapering to a minimal effective dose as determined by clinical variables.

While they are an important component of treatment of rheumatic diseases, glucocorticoids are often used in conjunction with other immunosuppressive agents such as *cyclophosphamide* and *methotrexate,* which offer better long-term control than steroids alone. The exception is giant cell arteritis, for which glucocorticoids remain superior to other agents. Caution should be exercised in the use of glucocorticoids in some forms of vasculitis (*e.g.,* polyarteritis nodosa), for which underlying infections with hepatitis viruses may play a pathogenetic role. Although glucocorticoids are indicated in these cases, there is at least a theoretical concern that glucocorticoids may complicate the course of the viral infection by suppressing the immune system. To facilitate drug tapering and/or conversion to alternate-day treatment regimens, the intermediate-acting glucocorticoids such as prednisone and methylprednisolone are generally preferred over longer-acting steroids such as dexamethasone.

In rheumatoid arthritis, because of the serious and debilitating side effects associated with chronic use, glucocorticoids are used as temporizing agents for progressive disease that fails to respond to first-line treatments such as physiotherapy and nonsteroidal antiinflammatory agents. In this case, glucocorticoids provide relief until other, slower-acting anti-rheumatic drugs, such as methotrexate or newer agents targeted at tumor necrosis factor take effect. A typical starting dose is 5 to 10 mg of prednisone per day. In the setting of an acute exacerbation, higher doses of glucocorticoids may be employed (typically 20 to 40 mg/day of prednisone or equivalent), with rapid taper thereafter. Complete relief of symptoms is not sought, and the symptomatic effect of small reductions in dose (decreases of perhaps 1 mg/day of prednisone every 2 to 3 weeks) should be tested frequently, while concurrent therapy with other measures is continued, to maintain the lowest possible prednisone dose. Alternatively, patients with major symptomatology confined to one or a few joints may be treated with intra-articular steroid injections. Depending on joint size, typical doses are 5 to 20 mg of *triamcinolone acetonide* or its equivalent.

In noninflammatory degenerative joint diseases (*e.g.,* osteoarthritis) or in a variety of regional pain syndromes (*e.g.,* tendinitis or bursitis), glucocorticoids may be administered by local injection for the treatment of episodic disease flare-up. It is important to minimize the frequency of local steroid administration whenever possible. In the case of repeated intra-articular injection of steroids, there is a significant incidence of painless joint destruction, resembling Charcot's arthropathy. It is recommended that intra-articular injections be performed with intervals of at least 3 months to minimize complications.

Renal Diseases. Patients with nephrotic syndrome secondary to minimal change disease generally respond well to steroid therapy, and glucocorticoids clearly are the first-line treatment in both adults and children. Initial daily doses of prednisone are 1 to 2 mg/kg for 6 weeks, followed by a gradual tapering of the dose over 6 to 8 weeks, although some nephrologists advocate alternate-day therapy. Objective evidence of response, such as diminished proteinuria, is seen within 2 to 3 weeks in 85% of patients, and more than 95% of patients will have remission within 3 months. Cessation of steroid therapy frequently is complicated by disease relapse, as manifested by recurrent proteinuria. Patients who relapse repeatedly are termed *steroid-resistant* and often are treated with other immunosuppressive drugs such as *azathioprine* or cyclophosphamide. Patients with renal disease secondary to systemic lupus erythematosus also are generally given a therapeutic trial of glucocorticoids.

Studies with other forms of renal disease, such as membranous and membranoproliferative glomerulonephritis and focal sclerosis,

have provided conflicting data on the role of glucocorticoids. In clinical practice, patients with these disorders often are given a therapeutic trial of glucocorticoids with careful monitoring of laboratory indices of response. In the case of membranous glomerulonephritis, many nephrologists recommend a trial of alternate-day glucocorticoids for 8 to 10 weeks (*e.g.,* prednisone, 120 mg every other day), followed by a 1- to 2-month period of tapering.

Allergic Disease. The onset of action of glucocorticoids in allergic diseases is delayed, and patients with severe allergic reactions such as anaphylaxis require immediate therapy with epinephrine: for adults, 0.3 to 0.5 ml of a 1:1000 solution intramuscularly or subcutaneously (repeated as often as every 15 minutes for up to three additional doses if necessary). The manifestations of allergic diseases of limited duration—such as hay fever, serum sickness, urticaria, contact dermatitis, drug reactions, bee stings, and angioneurotic edema—can be suppressed by adequate doses of glucocorticoids given as supplements to the primary therapy. In severe disease, intravenous glucocorticoids (methylprednisolone 125 mg intravenously every 6 hours, or equivalent) are appropriate. In less severe disease, antihistamines are the drugs of first choice. In allergic rhinitis, intranasal steroids are now viewed as the drug of choice by many experts.

Bronchial Asthma and Other Pulmonary Conditions. Corticosteroids frequently are used in bronchial asthma (*see* Chapter 27). They sometimes are employed in chronic obstructive pulmonary disease (COPD), particularly when there is some evidence of reversible obstructive disease. Data supporting the efficacy of corticosteroids are much more convincing for bronchial asthma than for COPD. The increased use of corticosteroids in asthma reflects an increased appreciation of the role of inflammation in the immunopathogenesis of this disorder. In severe asthma attacks requiring hospitalization, aggressive treatment with parenteral glucocorticoids is considered essential, even though their onset of action is delayed for 6 to 12 hours. Intravenous administration of 60 to 120 mg of methylprednisolone (or equivalent) every 6 hours is used initially, followed by daily oral doses of prednisone (30 to 60 mg) as the acute attack resolves. The dose then is tapered gradually, with withdrawal planned for 10 days to 2 weeks after initiation of steroid therapy. In general, patients subsequently can be managed on their prior medical regimen.

Less severe, acute exacerbations of asthma (as well as acute flares of COPD) often are treated with brief courses of oral glucocorticoids. In adult patients, 30 to 60 mg of prednisone is administered daily for 5 days; an additional week of therapy at lower doses also may be required. Upon resolution of the acute exacerbation, the glucocorticoids generally can be rapidly tapered without significant deleterious effects. Any suppression of adrenal function usually dissipates within 1 to 2 weeks. In the treatment of severe chronic bronchial asthma (or, less frequently, COPD) that is not controlled by other measures, the long-term administration of glucocorticoids may be necessary. As with other long-term uses of these agents, the lowest effective dose is used, and care must be exercised when withdrawal is attempted. Given the risks of long-term treatment with glucocorticoids, it is especially important to document objective evidence of a response (*e.g.,* an improvement in pulmonary function tests). In addition, these risks dictate that long-term glucocorticoid therapy be reserved for those patients who have failed to respond to adequate regimens of other medications (*see* Chapter 27).

In many patients, inhaled steroids (*e.g., beclomethasone dipropionate* [VANCERIL]*,* triamcinolone acetonide [AZMACORT]*, fluticasone* [FLOVENT]*, flunisolide* [AEROBID]*,* or *budesonide* [PULMICORT]) can either reduce the need for oral corticosteroids or replace them entirely. Many physicians prefer inhaled glucocorticoids over previously recommended oral *theophylline* in the treatment of children with moderately severe asthma, in part because of the behavioral toxicity associated with chronic theophylline administration (*see* Chapter 27). When used as recommended, inhaled glucocorticoids are effective in reducing bronchial hyperreactivity with less suppression of adrenal function than with oral glucocorticoids. Dysphonia or oropharyngeal candidiasis may develop, but the incidence of such side effects can be reduced substantially by maneuvers that reduce drug deposition in the oral cavity, such as spacers and mouth rinsing. The status of glucocorticoids in asthma therapy is discussed in detail in Chapter 27.

Antenatal glucocorticoids are used frequently in the setting of premature labor, decreasing the incidence of respiratory distress syndrome, intraventricular hemorrhage, and death in babies delivered prematurely. Betamethasone (12 mg intramuscularly every 24 hours for two doses) or dexamethasone (6 mg intramuscularly every 12 hours for four doses) are administered to women with premature labor between 27 and 34 weeks' gestation. Due to evidence of decreased birth weight and adrenal suppression in babies whose mothers were given repeated courses of glucocorticoids, only a single course of glucocorticoids should be administered.

Infectious Diseases. Although the use of immunosuppressive glucocorticoids in infectious diseases may seem paradoxical, there are a limited number of settings in which they are indicated in the therapy of specific infectious pathogens. One dramatic example of such beneficial effects is seen in AIDS patients with *Pneumocystis carinii* pneumonia and moderate to severe hypoxia; addition of glucocorticoids to the antibiotic regimen increases oxygenation and lowers the incidence of respiratory failure and mortality. Similarly, glucocorticoids clearly decrease the incidence of long-term neurological impairment associated with *Haemophilus influenzae* type b meningitis in infants and children 2 months of age or older.

A long-standing controversy in medicine is the use of glucocorticoids in septic shock (Annane and Cavaillon, 2003). Although studies initially suggested a benefit from the routine administration of glucocorticoids to subjects with septic shock associated with gram-negative bacteremia, subsequent studies showed that glucocorticoid therapy in supraphysiologic doses was actually associated with increased mortality. Several recent trials have shown benefit in subjects treated early in their course with intermediate doses of glucocorticoids (*e.g.,* 100 mg hydrocortisone every 8 hours). Of note, in one multicenter, randomized, placebo-controlled trial, beneficial effects were seen only in subjects who failed to increase their serum cortisol level by >9 μg/dl during the rapid cosyntropin stimulation test. To the extent that these results are confirmed, they suggest that glucocorticoid therapy may be beneficial in septic shock, presumably by damping the effects of cytokines that are induced by the disease.

Ocular Diseases. Ocular pharmacology, including some consideration of the use of glucocorticoids, is discussed in Chapter 63. Glucocorticoids frequently are used to suppress inflammation in the eye and can preserve sight when used properly. They are administered topically for diseases of the outer eye and anterior segment and attain therapeutic concentrations in the aqueous humor after instillation into the conjunctival cul-de-sac. For diseases of the posterior segment, systemic administration is required. Generally, ocular use of glucocorticoids should be supervised by an ophthalmologist.

A typical prescription is 0.1% dexamethasone sodium phosphate solution (ophthalmic), 2 drops in the conjunctival sac every 4 hours

while awake, and 0.05% dexamethasone sodium phosphate ointment (ophthalmic) at bedtime. For inflammation of the posterior segment, typical doses are 30 mg of prednisone or equivalent per day, administered orally in divided doses.

Topical glucocorticoid therapy frequently increases intraocular pressure in normal eyes and exacerbates intraocular hypertension in patients with antecedent glaucoma. The glaucoma is not always reversible on cessation of glucocorticoid therapy. Intraocular pressure should be monitored when glucocorticoids are applied to the eye for more than 2 weeks.

Topical administration of glucocorticoids to patients with bacterial, viral, or fungal conjunctivitis can mask evidence of progression of the infection until sight is irreversibly lost. Glucocorticoids are contraindicated in herpes simplex keratitis, because progression of the disease may lead to irreversible clouding of the cornea. Topical steroids should not be used in treating mechanical lacerations and abrasions of the eye because they delay healing and promote the development and spread of infection.

Skin Diseases. Glucocorticoids are remarkably efficacious in the treatment of a wide variety of inflammatory dermatoses. As a result, a large number of different preparations and concentrations of topical glucocorticoids of varying potencies are available. A typical regimen for an eczematous eruption is 1% hydrocortisone ointment applied locally twice daily. Effectiveness is enhanced by application of the topical steroid under an occlusive film, such as plastic wrap; unfortunately, the risk of systemic absorption also is increased by occlusive dressings, and this can be a significant problem when the more potent glucocorticoids are applied to inflamed skin. Glucocorticoids are administered systemically for severe episodes of acute dermatologic disorders and for exacerbations of chronic disorders. The dose in these settings is usually 40 mg/day of prednisone. Systemic steroid administration can be lifesaving in pemphigus, which may require daily doses of up to 120 mg of prednisone. Further discussion of the treatment of skin diseases is given in Chapter 62.

Gastrointestinal Diseases. Glucocorticoid therapy is indicated in selected patients with inflammatory bowel disease (chronic ulcerative colitis and Crohn's disease; *see* Chapter 38). Patients who fail to respond to more conservative management (*i.e.,* rest, diet, and *sulfasalazine*) may benefit from glucocorticoids; steroids are most useful for acute exacerbations. In mild ulcerative colitis, hydrocortisone (100 mg) can be administered as a retention enema with beneficial effects. In more severe acute exacerbations, oral prednisone (10 to 30 mg/day) frequently is employed. For severely ill patients—with fever, anorexia, anemia, and impaired nutritional status—larger doses should be used (40 to 60 mg prednisone per day). Major complications of ulcerative colitis or Crohn's disease may occur despite glucocorticoid therapy, and glucocorticoids may mask signs and symptoms of complications such as intestinal perforation and peritonitis.

Budesonide, a highly potent synthetic glucocorticoid that is inactivated by first-pass hepatic metabolism, reportedly has diminished systemic side effects commonly associated with glucocorticoids. Oral administration of budesonide in delayed-release capsules (ENTOCORT, 9 mg/day) facilitates drug delivery to the ileum and ascending colon; the drug also has been used as a retention enema in the treatment of ulcerative colitis.

Hepatic Diseases. The use of corticosteroids in hepatic disease has been highly controversial. Glucocorticoids clearly are of benefit in autoimmune hepatitis, where as many as 80% of patients show histological remission when treated with prednisone (40 to 60 mg daily initially, with tapering to a maintenance dose of 7.5 to

10 mg daily after serum transaminase levels fall). The role of corticosteroids in alcoholic liver disease is not fully defined; the most recent studies, including meta-analysis of previously published reports, suggest a beneficial role of prednisolone (40 mg/day for 4 weeks) in patients with severe disease indicators (*e.g.,* hepatic encephalopathy) without active gastrointestinal bleeding. Further studies are needed to confirm or refute the role of steroids in this setting. In the setting of severe hepatic disease, prednisolone should be used instead of prednisone, which requires hepatic conversion to be active.

Malignancies. Glucocorticoids are used in the chemotherapy of acute lymphocytic leukemia and lymphomas because of their anti-lymphocytic effects. Most commonly, glucocorticoids are one component of combination chemotherapy administered under scheduled protocols. Further discussion of the chemotherapy of malignant disease is given in Chapter 51. Glucocorticoids once were frequently employed in the setting of hypercalcemia of malignancy, but more effective agents, such as the bisphosphonates, now are the preferred therapy.

Cerebral Edema. Corticosteroids are of value in the reduction or prevention of cerebral edema associated with parasites and neoplasms, especially those that are metastatic. Although corticosteroids are frequently used for the treatment of cerebral edema caused by trauma or cerebrovascular accidents, controlled clinical trials do not support their use in these settings.

Miscellaneous Diseases and Conditions. Sarcoidosis. Sarcoidosis is treated with corticosteroids (approximately 1 mg/kg per day of prednisone, or equivalent dose of alternative steroids) to induce remission. Maintenance doses, which often are required for long periods of time, may be as low as 10 mg/day of prednisone. These patients, like all patients who require chronic glucocorticoid therapy at doses exceeding the normal daily production rate, are at increased risk for secondary tuberculosis; therefore, patients with a positive tuberculin reaction or other evidence of tuberculosis should receive prophylactic antituberculosis therapy.

Thrombocytopenia. In thrombocytopenia, prednisone (0.5 mg/kg) is used to decrease the bleeding tendency. In more severe cases, and for initiation of treatment of idiopathic thrombocytopenia, daily doses of prednisone (1 to 1.5 mg/kg) are employed. Patients with refractory idiopathic thrombocytopenia may respond to pulsed, high-dose glucocorticoid therapy.

Autoimmune Destruction of Erythrocytes. Patients with autoimmune destruction of erythrocytes (*i.e.,* hemolytic anemia with a positive Coombs test) are treated with prednisone (1 mg/kg per day). In the setting of severe hemolysis, higher doses may be used, with tapering as the anemia improves. Small maintenance doses may be required for several months in patients who respond.

Organ Transplantation. In organ transplantation, high doses of prednisone (50 to 100 mg) are given at the time of transplant surgery, in conjunction with other immunosuppressive agents, and most patients are kept on a maintenance regimen that includes lower doses of glucocorticoids (*see* Chapter 52). Of note, success rates for islet transplantation in type 1 diabetes mellitus have increased considerably following the use of immunosuppressive regimens that do not include glucocorticoids.

Spinal Cord Injury. Multicenter trials have shown significant decreases in neurological defects in patients with acute spinal cord injury treated within 8 hours of injury with large doses of methylprednisolone (30 mg/kg initially followed by an infusion of 5.4 mg/kg per hour for 23 hours). The ability of corticosteroids at these high doses to decrease neurological injury may reflect inhibition of free radical–mediated cellular injury, as occurs following ischemia and reperfusion.

Diagnostic Applications of Adrenocortical Steroids

In addition to their therapeutic uses, glucocorticoids also are used for diagnostic purposes. To determine if patients with clinical manifestations suggestive of hypercortisolism have biochemical evidence of increased cortisol biosynthesis, an overnight dexamethasone test has been devised. Patients are given 1 mg of dexamethasone orally at 11 P.M., and cortisol is measured at 8 A.M. the following morning. Suppression of plasma cortisol to less than 1.8 μg/dl suggests strongly that the patient does not have Cushing's syndrome (Arnaldi *et al.,* 2003).

The formal dexamethasone suppression test is used in the differential diagnosis of biochemically documented Cushing's syndrome. Following determination of baseline cortisol levels for 48 hours, dexamethasone (0.5 mg every 6 hours) is administered orally for 48 hours. This dose markedly suppresses cortisol levels in normal subjects, including those who have nonspecific elevations of cortisol due to obesity or stress, but does not suppress levels in patients with Cushing's syndrome. In the high-dose phase of the test, dexamethasone is administered orally at 2 mg every 6 hours for 48 hours. Patients with pituitary-dependent Cushing's syndrome (*i.e.,* Cushing's disease) generally respond with decreased cortisol levels. In contrast, patients with ectopic production of ACTH or with adrenocortical tumors generally do not exhibit decreased cortisol levels. Despite these generalities, dexamethasone may suppress cortisol levels in some patients with ectopic ACTH production, particularly with tumors such as bronchial carcinoids, and many experts prefer to use inferior petrosal sinus sampling after CRH administration to make this distinction.

INHIBITORS OF THE BIOSYNTHESIS AND ACTION OF ADRENOCORTICAL STEROIDS

Five pharmacologic agents are useful inhibitors of adrenocortical secretion. *Mitotane* (o,p'-DDD), an adrenocorticolytic agent, is discussed in Chapter 51. The other inhibitors of steroid hormone biosynthesis—*metyrapone, aminoglutethimide, ketoconazole,* and *trilostane*—are discussed here. Metyrapone, aminoglutethimide, and ketoconazole inhibit cytochrome P450 enzymes involved in adrenocorticosteroid biosynthesis. Differential selectivity of these agents for the different steroid hydroxylases provides some degree of specificity to their actions. Trilostane is a competitive inhibitor of the conversion of pregnenolone to progesterone, a reaction catalyzed by 3β-hydroxysteroid dehydrogenase. In addition, agents that act as glucocorticoid receptor antagonists (anti-glucocorticoids) are discussed here (mineralocorticoid antagonists are discussed in Chapter 28). All of these agents pose the common risk of precipitating acute adrenal insufficiency; thus, they must be used in appropriate doses, and the status of the patient's HPA axis must be carefully monitored.

Aminoglutethimide. Aminoglutethimide (α-ethyl-*p*-aminophenyl-glutarimide; CYTADREN) primarily inhibits CYP11A1, which catalyzes the initial and rate-limiting step in the biosynthesis of all physiological steroids. As a result, the production of all classes of steroid hormones is impaired. Aminoglutethimide also inhibits CYP11B1 and the enzyme aromatase, which converts androgens to estrogens. Aminoglutethimide has been used to decrease hypersecretion of cortisol in patients with Cushing's syndrome secondary to autonomous adrenal tumors and hypersecretion associated with ectopic production of ACTH. Because of its actions to inhibit aromatase, aminoglutethimide also has been evaluated as a therapeutic agent for the treatment of hormonally responsive tumors such as prostate and breast cancer, although more effective agents such as *tamoxifen* and the aromatase inhibitors are preferred. Dose-dependent gastrointestinal and neurological side effects are relatively common, as is a transient, maculopapular rash. The usual dose is 250 mg every 6 hours, with gradual increases of 250 mg per day at 1- to 2-week intervals until the desired biochemical effect is achieved, side effects prohibit further increases, or a daily dose of 2 g is reached. Because aminoglutethimide can cause frank adrenal insufficiency, glucocorticoid replacement therapy is necessary, and mineralocorticoid supplements also may be indicated. Aminoglutethimide accelerates the metabolism of dexamethasone, and this steroid therefore should not be used for glucocorticoid replacement in this setting.

Ketoconazole. Ketoconazole (NIZORAL) is an antifungal agent, and this remains its most important clinical role (*see* Chapter 48). In doses higher than those employed in antifungal therapy, it is an effective inhibitor of adrenal and gonadal steroidogenesis, primarily because of its inhibition of the activity of CYP17 (17α-hydroxylase). At even higher doses, ketoconazole also inhibits CYP11A1, effectively blocking steroidogenesis in all primary steroidogenic tissues. Ketoconazole is the most effective inhibitor of steroid hormone biosynthesis in patients with Cushing's disease. In most cases, a dosage regimen of 600 to 800 mg/day (in two divided doses) is required, and some patients may require up to 1200 mg/day given in two to three doses. Side effects include hepatic dysfunction, which ranges from asymptomatic elevations of transaminase levels to severe hepatic injury. The potential of ketoconazole to interact with CYP isoforms can lead to drug interactions of serious consequence (*see* Chapter 3). Further studies are needed to define the precise role of ketoconazole in the medical management of patients with excessive steroid

hormonal production, and the FDA has not approved this indication for ketoconazole use.

Metyrapone. Metyrapone (METOPIRONE) is a relatively selective inhibitor of CYP11B1 (11β-hydroxylase), which converts 11-deoxycortisol to cortisol in the terminal reaction of the glucocorticoid biosynthetic pathway. Because of this inhibition, the biosynthesis of cortisol is markedly impaired, and the levels of steroid precursors (*e.g.,* 11-deoxycortisol) are markedly increased. Although the biosynthesis of aldosterone also is impaired, the elevated levels of 11-deoxycortisol sustain mineralocorticoid-dependent functions. In a diagnostic test of the entire HPA axis, metyrapone (30 mg/kg, maximum dose of 3 g) is administered orally with a snack at midnight, and plasma cortisol and 11-deoxycortisol are measured at 8 A.M. the next morning. A plasma cortisol of less than 8 μg/dl validates adequate inhibition of CYP11B1; in this setting, an 11-deoxycortisol level of less than 7 μg/dl is highly suggestive of impaired hypothalamic-pituitary-adrenal function. An abnormal response does not identify the site of the defect—hypothalamic CRH release, ACTH production, or adrenal biosynthetic capacity could be impaired. Some authorities avoid overnight metyrapone testing in outpatients thought to have a reasonable probability of impaired HPA function, as there is some risk of precipitating acute adrenal insufficiency. Others believe that the ability to assess the entire HPA axis with a relatively easy test justifies the use of metyrapone testing in outpatients.

Metyrapone also is used to diagnose patients with Cushing's syndrome who respond equivocally to the formal dexamethasone suppression test. Those with pituitary-dependent Cushing's syndrome exhibit a normal response, whereas those patients with ectopic secretion of ACTH exhibit no changes in ACTH or 11-deoxycortisol levels.

Therapeutically, metyrapone has been used to treat the hypercorticism resulting from either adrenal neoplasms or tumors producing ACTH ectopically. Maximal suppression of steroidogenesis requires doses of 4 g/day. More frequently, metyrapone is used as adjunctive therapy in patients who have received pituitary irradiation or in combination with other agents that inhibit steroidogenesis. In this setting, a dose of 500 to 750 mg three or four times daily is employed. The use of metyrapone in the treatment of Cushing's syndrome secondary to pituitary hypersecretion of ACTH is more controversial. Chronic administration of metyrapone can cause hirsutism, which results from increased synthesis of adrenal androgens upstream from the enzymatic block, and hypertension, which results from elevated levels of 11-deoxycortisol. Other side effects include nausea, headache, sedation, and rash.

Metyrapone is not available from pharmacy sources in the United States, but can be obtained directly from Novartis for compassionate use.

ANTI-GLUCOCORTICOIDS

The progesterone receptor antagonist *mifepristone* [RU-486; (11β-4-dimethylaminophenyl)-17β-hydroxy-7α-(propyl-1-ynyl)estra-4,9-dien-3-one] has received considerable attention because of its use as an antiprogestagen that can terminate early pregnancy (*see* Chapter 57). At higher doses, mifepristone also inhibits the GR, blocking feedback regulation of the HPA axis and secondarily increasing endogenous ACTH and cortisol levels. Because of its ability to inhibit glucocorticoid action, mifepristone also has been studied as a potential therapeutic agent in patients with hypercorticism, although it currently can be recommended only for patients with inoperable causes of cortisol excess that have not responded to other agents.

CLINICAL SUMMARY

Glucocorticoids are administered in multiple formulations (*e.g.,* oral, parenteral, and topical) for disorders that share an inflammatory or immunological basis. Except in patients receiving replacement therapy for adrenal insufficiency, glucocorticoids are neither specific nor curative, but rather are palliative because of their antiinflammatory and immunosuppressive actions. Given the number and severity of potential side effects, the decision to institute therapy with glucocorticoids always requires a careful consideration of the relative risks and benefits in each patient. After therapy is initiated, the minimal dose needed to achieve a given therapeutic effect must be determined by trial and error and must be re-evaluated periodically as the activity of the underlying disease changes or as complications of therapy arise. A single dose of glucocorticoid, even a large one, is virtually without harmful effects, and a short course of therapy (up to 1 week) is unlikely to cause harm in the absence of specific contraindications. As the duration of glucocorticoid therapy increases beyond 1 week, adverse effects increase in a time- and dose-related manner. Finally, abrupt cessation of glucocorticoids after prolonged therapy is associated with the risk of adrenal insufficiency due to suppression of the HPA axis, which may be fatal.

BIBLIOGRAPHY

Allolio, B., and Arlt, W. DHEA treatment: myth or reality? *Trends Endocrinol. Metab.,* **2002,** *341:*288–294.

Annane, D., and Cavaillon, J.C. Corticosteroids in sepsis: from bench to bedside? *Shock,* **2003,** *20:*197–207.

Arnaldi, G., Angeli, A., Atkinson, A.B., *et al.* Diagnosis and complications of Cushing's syndrome: a consensus statement. *J. Clin. Endocrinol. Metab.,* **2003,** *88:*5593–5602.

Axelrod, L. Perioperative management of patients treated with glucocorticoids. *Endocrinol. Metab. Clin. North Am.,* **2003,** *32:*367–383.

Bale, T.L., and Vale W. CRF and CRF receptors: role in stress responsivity and other behaviors. *Annu. Rev. Pharmacol. Toxicol.,* **2004,** *44:*525–557.

Bray, P.J., and Cotton, R.G. Variations of the human glucocorticoid receptor gene (NR3C1): pathological and in vitro mutations and polymorphisms. *Hum. Mutat.,* **2003,** *21:*557–568.

Carey, R.M. The changing clinical spectrum of adrenal insufficiency. *Ann. Intern. Med.,* **1997,** *127:*1103–1105.

Chrousos, G.P. The hypothalamic–pituitary–adrenal axis and immune-mediated inflammation. *N. Engl. J. Med.,* **1995,** *332:*1351–1362.

Clark, A.J.L., and Weber, A. Adrenocorticotropin insensitivity syndromes. *Endocr. Rev.,* **1998,** *19:*828–844.

Coghlan, M.J., Elmore, S.W., Kym, P.R., and Kort, M.E. The pursuit of differentiated ligands for the glucocorticoid receptor. *Curr. Top. Med. Chem.,* **2003,** *3:*1617–1635.

Coursin, D.B., and Wood K.E. Corticosteroid supplementation for adrenal insufficiency. *JAMA,* **2002,** *287:*236–240.

De Bosscher, K., Vanden Berghe, W., and Haegeman, G. The interplay between the glucocorticoid receptor and nuclear factor-κB or activator protein-1: molecular mechanisms for gene repression. *Endocr. Rev.,* **2003,** *24:*488–522.

Norman, A.W., Mizwicki, M.T., and Norman, D.P. Steroid-hormone rapid actions, membrane receptors, and a conformational ensemble model. *Nat. Rev. Drug Discov.,* **2004,** *3:*27–41.

Saag, K.G. Glucocorticoid-induced osteoporosis. *Endocrinol. Metab. Clin. North Am.,* **2003,** *32:*135–157.

Sandeep, T.C., and Walker, B.R. Pathophysiology of modulation of local glucocorticoid levels by 11β-hydroxysteroid dehydrogenases. *Trends Endocrinol. Metab.,* **2001,** *12:*446–453.

Sapolsky, R.M., Romero, L.M., and Munck, A.U. How do glucocorticoids influence stress responses? Integrating permissive, suppressive, stimulatory, and preparative actions. *Endocr. Rev.,* **2000,** *21:*55–89.

Wardlaw, S.L. Obesity as a neuroendocrine disease: lessons to be learned from proopiomelanocortin and melanocortin receptor mutations in mice and men. *J. Clin. Endocrinol. Metab.,* **2001,** *86:*1442–1446.

INSULIN, ORAL HYPOGLYCEMIC AGENTS, AND THE PHARMACOLOGY OF THE ENDOCRINE PANCREAS

Stephen N. Davis

INSULIN

In recent years, developed nations have witnessed an explosive increase in the prevalence of diabetes mellitus (DM) predominantly related to lifestyle changes and the resulting surge in obesity. The metabolic consequences of prolonged hyperglycemia and dyslipidemia, including accelerated atherosclerosis, chronic kidney disease, and blindness, pose an enormous burden on patients with diabetes mellitus and on the public health system. Improvements in our understanding of the pathogenesis of diabetes and its complications and in the therapy and prevention of diabetes are critical to meeting this health care challenge.

History. Few events in the history of medicine are more dramatic than the discovery of insulin. Although the discovery is appropriately attributed to Banting and Best, others provided important observations and techniques that made it possible. In 1869, a German medical student, Paul Langerhans, noted that the pancreas contains two distinct groups of cells—the acinar cells, which secrete digestive enzymes, and cells that are clustered in islands, or islets, which he suggested served a second function. Direct evidence for this function came in 1889, when Minkowski and von Mering showed that pancreatectomized dogs exhibit a syndrome similar to diabetes mellitus in humans.

There were numerous attempts to extract the pancreatic substance responsible for regulating blood glucose. In the early 1900s, Gurg Zuelzer, an internist in Berlin, attempted to treat a dying diabetic patient with extracts of pancreas. Although the patient improved temporarily, he sank back into a coma and died when the supply of extract was exhausted. E.L. Scott, a student at the University of Chicago, made another early attempt to isolate an active principle in 1911. Using alcoholic extracts of the pancreas (not so different from those eventually used by Banting and Best), Scott treated several diabetic dogs with encouraging results; however, he lacked clear measures of control of blood glucose concentrations, and his professor considered the experiments inconclusive at best. Between 1916 and 1920, the Romanian physiologist Nicolas Paulesco found that injections of pancreatic extracts reduced urinary sugar and ketones in diabetic dogs. Although he published the results of his experiments, their significance was fully appreciated only years later.

Unaware of much of this work, Frederick Banting, a young Canadian surgeon, convinced J.J.R. Macleod, a professor of physiology in Toronto, to allow him access to a laboratory to search for the antidiabetic principle of the pancreas. Banting assumed that the islets secreted insulin but that the hormone was destroyed by proteolytic digestion prior to or during extraction. Together with Charles Best, a fourth-year medical student, he attempted to overcome the problem by ligating the pancreatic ducts. The acinar tissue degenerated, leaving the islets undisturbed; the remaining tissue then was extracted with ethanol and acid. Banting and Best thus obtained a pancreatic extract that decreased the concentration of blood glucose in diabetic dogs.

The first patient to receive the active extracts prepared by Banting and Best was Leonard Thompson, aged 14. He presented at the Toronto General Hospital with a blood glucose level of 500 mg/dl (28 mM). Despite rigid control of his diet (450 kcal/day), he continued to excrete large quantities of glucose, and without insulin, the most likely outcome would be death after a few months. The administration of Banting and Best's extracts reduced the plasma concentration and urinary excretion of glucose. Daily injections were given. Glucose excretion was reduced from over 100 to as little as 7.5 g/day, and the patient demonstrated marked clinical improvement. Thus replacement therapy with the newly discovered hormone, insulin, had interrupted what was clearly an otherwise fatal metabolic disorder. Banting and Best faced many trials and tribulations during the subsequent year. It was difficult to obtain active extracts reproducibly. This led to a greater involvement of Macleod; Banting also sought help from J.B. Collip, a chemist with expertise in extraction and purification of epinephrine. Stable extracts eventually were

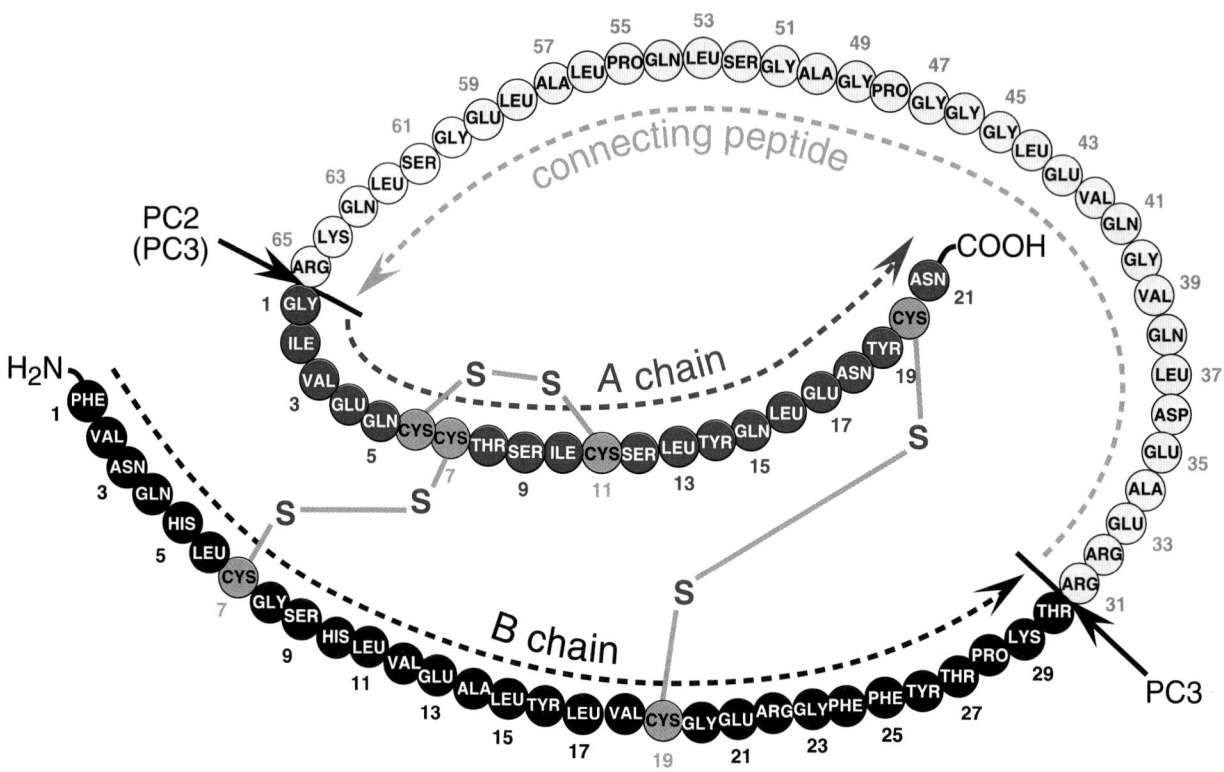

Figure 60–1. *Human proinsulin and its conversion to insulin.* The amino acid sequence of human proinsulin is shown. By proteolytic cleavage, four basic amino acids (residues 31, 32, 64, and 65) and the connecting peptide are removed, converting proinsulin to insulin. The sites of action of the endopeptidases PC2 and PC3 are shown.

obtained, and patients in many parts of North America soon were being treated with insulin from porcine and bovine sources. Now, as a result of recombinant DNA technology, human insulin is used for therapy.

The Nobel Prize in medicine and physiology was awarded to Banting and Macleod with remarkable rapidity in 1923, and a furor over credit followed immediately. Banting announced that he would share his prize with Best; Macleod did the same with Collip.

Chemistry. Insulin was purified and crystallized by Abel within a few years of its discovery. Sanger established the amino acid sequence of insulin in 1960, the protein was synthesized in 1963, and Hodgkin and coworkers elucidated insulin's three-dimensional structure in 1972. Insulin was the hormone for which Yalow and Berson first developed the radioimmunoassay (Kahn and Roth, 2004).

The β (or B) cells of pancreatic islets synthesize insulin from a single-chain precursor of 110 amino acids termed *preproinsulin.* After translocation through the membrane of the rough endoplasmic reticulum, the 24-amino-acid N-terminal signal peptide of preproinsulin is cleaved rapidly to form proinsulin (Figure 60–1). Thereafter, proinsulin folds, and the disulfide bonds form. During conversion of human proinsulin to insulin, four basic amino acids and the remaining connector or C peptide are removed by proteolysis. This gives rise to the A and B peptide chains of the insulin molecule, which contains one intrasubunit and two intersubunit disulfide bonds. The A chain usually is composed of 21 amino acid residues, and the B

chain has 30; the molecular mass is thus about 5734 daltons. Although the amino acid sequence of insulin has been highly conserved in evolution, there are significant variations that account for differences in both biological potency and immunogenicity (De Meyts, 1994). There is a single insulin gene and a single protein product in most species. However, rats and mice have two genes that encode insulin and synthesize two molecules that differ at two amino acid residues in the B chain.

The crystal structure reveals that the two chains of insulin form a highly ordered structure with α-helical regions in each of the chains. The isolated chains of insulin are inactive. In solution, insulin can exist as a monomer, dimer, or hexamer. Two molecules of Zn^{2+} are coordinated in the hexamer, and this form of insulin presumably is stored in the granules of the pancreatic β cell. It is believed that Zn^{2+} has a functional role in the hexamer formation and that this process facilitates the conversion of proinsulin to insulin and storage of the hormone. Traditional insulin is hexameric in most of the highly concentrated preparations used for therapy. When the hormone is absorbed and the concentration falls to physiological levels (nanomolar), the hormone dissociates into monomers, and the monomer is most likely the biologically active form of insulin. Monomeric insulin is now available for therapy.

Substantial information about the structure–activity relationship of insulin has been obtained by study of insulins purified from a wide variety of species and by modification of the molecule. A dozen invariant residues in the A and B chains form a surface that interacts with the insulin receptor (Figure 60–2). These residues—

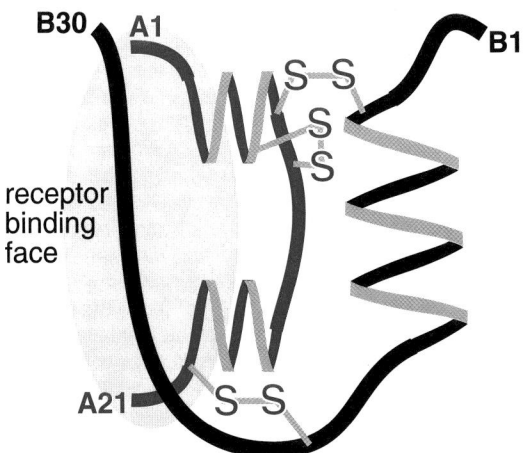

B30 A1 B1

S—S
S
S

receptor
binding
face

A21 S—S

Figure 60–2. *Model of the three-dimensional structure of insulin.* The shaded area indicates the receptor-binding face of the insulin molecule.

Gly^{A1}, Glu^{A4}, Gln^{A5}, Tyr^{A19}, Asn^{A21}, Val^{B12}, Tyr^{B16}, Gly^{B23}, Phe^{B24}, Phe^{B25}, and Tyr^{B26}—overlap with domains that also are involved in insulin dimerization (De Meyts, 1994). The Leu^{A13} and Leu^{B17} residues may form part of a second binding surface. Insulin binds to surfaces located at the N- and C-terminal regions of the α subunit of the receptor, including a cysteine-rich region in the receptor α chain. In most cases, the affinity of insulin for the insulin receptor correlates closely with its potency for eliciting effects on glucose metabolism. Human, bovine, and porcine insulins are equipotent; South American guinea pig insulin is much less potent, whereas certain avian insulins are significantly more so.

Insulin is a member of a family of related peptides termed *insulinlike growth factors* (IGFs). The two IGFs (IGF-1 and IGF-2) have molecular masses of about 7500 daltons and structures that are homologous to that of proinsulin. However, the short equivalents of the C peptide in proinsulin are not removed from the IGFs. In contrast with insulin, the IGFs are produced in many tissues, and they may serve a more important function in the regulation of growth than in the regulation of metabolism. These peptides, particularly IGF-1, are the presumed mediators of the action of growth hormone, and they originally were called *somatomedins*. The uterine hormone *relaxin* also may be a distant relative of this family of polypeptides, although the relaxin receptor clearly is distinct from those for insulin and IGF-1.

The receptors for insulin and IGF-1 are also closely related (Nakae *et al.*, 2001). Thus, insulin can bind to the receptor for IGF-1 with low affinity and *vice versa*. The growth-promoting actions of insulin appear to be mediated in part through the IGF-1 receptor, and there may be discordance between the metabolic potency of an insulin analog and its ability to promote growth. For example, proinsulin has only 2% of the metabolic potency of insulin *in vitro*, but it is half as potent as insulin in stimulating mitogenesis.

Synthesis, Secretion, Distribution, and Degradation of Insulin

Insulin Production. The molecular and cellular events involved in the synthesis, storage, and secretion of insulin

by the β cell and ultimate degradation of the hormone by its target tissues have been studied in great detail and have served as a model for study of other cell types in the pancreatic islet. The islet of Langerhans is composed of four types of cells, each of which synthesizes and secretes a distinct polypeptide hormone: insulin in the β (B) cell, *glucagon* in the α (A) cell, *somatostatin* in the δ (D) cell, and pancreatic polypeptide in the PP or F cell. The β cells make up 60% to 80% of the islet and form its central core. The α, δ, and F cells form a discontinuous mantle, one to three cells thick, around this core.

The cells in the islet are connected by tight junctions that allow small molecules to pass and facilitate coordinated control of groups of cells. Arterioles enter the islets and branch into a glomerularlike capillary mass in the β-cell core. Capillaries then pass to the rim of the islet and coalesce into collecting venules. Blood flows in the islet from the β cells to α and δ cells. Thus, the β cell is the primary glucose sensor for the islet, and the other cell types presumably are exposed to particularly high concentrations of insulin.

As noted earlier, insulin is synthesized as a single-chain precursor in which the A and B chains are connected by the C peptide. The initial translation product, preproinsulin, contains a sequence of 24 primarily hydrophobic amino acid residues attached to the N terminus of the B chain. This signal sequence is required for the association and penetration of nascent preproinsulin into the lumen of the rough endoplasmic reticulum. This sequence is cleaved rapidly, and proinsulin is then transported in small vesicles to the Golgi complex. Here, proinsulin is packaged into secretory granules along with the enzyme(s) responsible for its conversion to insulin.

The conversion of proinsulin to insulin begins in the Golgi complex, continues in the secretory granules, and is nearly complete at the time of secretion. Thus, equimolar amounts of C peptide and insulin are released into the circulation. The C peptide has no known biological function but serves as a useful index of insulin secretion in distinguishing between patients with factitious insulin injection and insulin-producing tumors. Small quantities of proinsulin and des-31,32 proinsulin also are released from β cells. This presumably reflects either exocytosis of granules in which the conversion of proinsulin to insulin is not complete or secretion by another pathway. Since the half-life of proinsulin in the circulation is much longer than that of insulin, up to 20% of immunoreactive insulin in plasma is, in reality, proinsulin and intermediates.

Two distinct Ca^{2+}-dependent endopeptidases, which are found in the islet cell granules and in other neuroendocrine cells, are responsible for the conversion of proinsulin to insulin. These endoproteases, PC2 and PC3, have catalytic domains related to that of subtilisin and cleave at Lys–Arg or Arg–Arg sequences (Steiner *et al.*, 1996). PC2 selectively cleaves at the C peptide–A chain junction (Figure 60–1). PC3 preferentially cleaves at the C peptide–B chain junction but has some action at the A chain junction as well. Although there are at least two other members of the family of endoproteases (PC1 and furin), PC2 and PC3 appear to be the enzymes responsible for processing proinsulin to insulin.

Regulation of Insulin Secretion. Insulin secretion is a tightly regulated process designed to provide stable concentrations of glucose in blood during both fasting and feeding. This regulation is achieved by the coordinated interplay of various nutrients, gastrointestinal hormones, pancreatic hormones, and autonomic neurotransmitters. Glucose, amino acids, fatty acids, and ketone bodies promote the secretion of insulin. The islets of Langerhans are richly innervated by both adrenergic and cholinergic nerves. Stimulation of α_2 adrenergic receptors inhibits insulin secretion, whereas β_2 adrenergic receptor agonists and vagal nerve stimulation enhance release. In general, any condition that activates the sympathetic branch of the autonomic nervous system (such as hypoxia, hypoglycemia, exercise, hypothermia, surgery, or severe burns) suppresses the secretion of insulin by stimulation of α_2 adrenergic receptors. Predictably, α_2 adrenergic receptor antagonists increase basal concentrations of insulin in plasma, and β_2 adrenergic receptor antagonists decrease them.

Glucose is the principal stimulus to insulin secretion in human beings and is an essential permissive factor for the actions of many other secretagogues (Matschinsky, 1996). The sugar is more effective in provoking insulin secretion when taken orally than when administered intravenously because the ingestion of glucose (or food) induces the release of gastrointestinal hormones and stimulates vagal activity. Several gastrointestinal hormones promote the secretion of insulin. The most potent of these are gastrointestinal inhibitory peptide (GIP) and glucagonlike peptide 1 (GLP-1). Insulin release also is stimulated by gastrin, secretin, cholecystokinin, vasoactive intestinal peptide, gastrin-releasing peptide, and enteroglucagon.

When evoked by glucose, insulin secretion is biphasic: The first phase reaches a peak after 1 to 2 minutes and is short-lived; the second phase has a delayed onset but a longer duration.

Recent research has provided an outline of how glucose stimulates insulin secretion. Basically, the resting β cell is hyperpolarized, and its depolarization leads to the secretion of insulin. A rising plasma glucose concentration initiates a series of events that leads to depolarization. Glucose enters the β cell by facilitated transport, which is mediated by GLUT2, a specific subtype of glucose transporter, whereupon the sugar is phosphorylated to glucose-6-phosphate (G-6-P) by glucokinase. The increase in oxidizable substrate (glucose and G-6-P) enhances adenosine triphosphate (ATP) production, thereby increasing the ATP–adenosine diphosphate (ADP) ratio and inhibiting an ATP-sensitive K$^+$ channel. This decrease in K$^+$ conductance causes E_m to rise, opening a voltage-sensitive Ca^{2+} channel.

Intracellular Ca^{2+} acts as the insulin secretagogue, as it does for the secretion of many vesicular products. The influx of Ca^{2+} also activates several phospholipases, leading to the production of eicosanoids and IP$_3$ and the mobilization of intracellular Ca^{2+} stores.

The ATP-sensitive K$^+$ channel in insulin-secreting cells is an octamer composed of four Kir 6.2 and four SUR1 subunits. Both types of subunits contain nucleotide-binding domains; Kir 6.2 appears to mediate the inhibitory response to ATP; SUR1 binds ADP, the channel activator *diazoxide,* and the channel inhibitors (and promoters of insulin secretion) sulfonylureas and meglitinide. Mutations in the channel proteins can lead to altered insulin secretion (*see* Proks *et al.,* 2004).

Elevation of free Ca^{2+} concentrations also occurs in response to stimulation of phospholipase C by acetylcholine and cholecystokinin and by hormones that increase intracellular concentrations of cyclic AMP. In the β cell, G protein–coupled receptors (GPCRs) for glucagon, GIP, and GLP-1 couple to G$_s$ to stimulate adenylyl cyclase; somatostatin and α_2 adrenergic receptor agonists couple to G$_i$ to reduce cellular cyclic adenosine monophosphate (AMP) production.

The hexokinase involved in this process is a specific isoform, glucokinase, whose expression is limited primarily to cells and tissues involved in the regulation of glucose metabolism, such as the liver and pancreatic cells. Its relatively high K_m (10 to 20 mM) gives it an important regulatory role at physiological concentrations of glucose. The capacity of sugars to undergo phosphorylation and subsequent glycolysis correlates closely with their ability to stimulate insulin release. The role of glucokinase as a glucose sensor was inferred from the association of mutations of the glucokinase gene with a form of maturity-onset diabetes of the young (MODY2; *see* below), a rare genetic form of diabetes. These mutations, which compromise the ability of glucokinase to phosphorylate glucose, raise the threshold for glucose-stimulated insulin release.

Most of the nutrients and hormones that stimulate insulin secretion also enhance its biosynthesis. Although there is a close correlation between the two processes, some factors affect one pathway but not the other. For example, lowering extracellular concentrations of Ca^{2+} inhibits secretion of insulin without affecting biosynthesis.

There usually is a reciprocal relationship between the rates of secretion of insulin and glucagon from the pancreatic islet. This reciprocity reflects both the influence of insulin on the α cell and the level of glucose and other substrates (*see* below). In addition, somatostatin, a third islet cell hormone, can modulate the secretion of both hormones (*see* below). Glucagon stimulates the release of somatostatin, which may suppress the secretion of insulin but is not a major physiological influence. Since the blood supply in the islet flows from the β-cell core to the α and δ cells, insulin can inhibit glucagon release in a paracrine manner, but somatostatin must pass through the circulation to reach the α and β cells. Thus, while insulin affects the secretion of glucagon and pancreatic polypeptide, the paracrine of islet somatostatin is not clear.

Distribution and Degradation of Insulin. Insulin circulates in blood as the free monomer, and its volume of distribution approximates the volume of extracellular fluid. Under fasting conditions, the pancreas secretes about 40 μg (1 unit) of insulin per hour into the portal vein to achieve a concentration of insulin in portal blood of 2 to 4 ng/ml (50 to 100 μunits/ml) and in the peripheral circulation of 0.5 ng/ml (12 μunits/ml) or about 0.1 nM. After ingestion of a meal, there is a rapid rise in the concentration of insulin in portal blood, followed by a parallel but smaller rise in the peripheral circulation. A goal of insulin therapy is to mimic this pattern, but this is difficult to achieve with subcutaneous injections.

The half-life of insulin in plasma is about 5 to 6 minutes in normal subjects and patients with uncomplicated diabetes. This value may be increased in diabetics who develop anti-insulin antibodies. The half-life of proinsulin is longer than that of insulin (about 17 minutes), and this protein usually accounts for about 10% of the immunoreactive "insulin" in plasma. In patients with insulinoma, the percentage of proinsulin in the circulation usually is increased and may be as much as 80% of immunoreactivity. Since proinsulin is only about 2% as potent as insulin, the biologically effective concentration of insulin is somewhat lower than estimated by immunoassay. C peptide is secreted in equimolar amounts with insulin; however, its molar concentration in plasma is higher because of its lower hepatic clearance and considerably longer half-life (about 30 minutes). C peptide serves as a marker for acute insulin secretion.

Degradation of insulin occurs primarily in liver, kidney, and muscle (Duckworth, 1988). About 50% of the insulin that reaches the liver *via* the portal vein is destroyed and never reaches the general circulation. Insulin is filtered by the renal glomeruli and is reabsorbed by the tubules, which also degrade it. Severe impairment of renal function appears to affect the rate of disappearance of circulating insulin to a greater extent than does hepatic disease. Hepatic degradation of insulin operates near its maximal capacity and cannot compensate for diminished renal breakdown of the hormone. Peripheral tissues such as fat also inactivate insulin, but this is of less significance quantitatively.

Proteolytic degradation of insulin in the liver occurs primarily after internalization of the hormone and its receptor and, to a lesser extent, at the cell surface. The primary pathway for internalization is receptor-mediated endocytosis. The complex of insulin and its receptor is internalized into small vesicles termed *endosomes,* where degradation is initiated (Duckworth, 1988). Some insulin also is delivered to lysosomes for degradation.

The extent to which internalized insulin is degraded by the cell varies considerably with the cell type. In hepatocytes, over 50% of the internalized insulin is degraded, whereas most internalized insulin is released intact from endothelial cells. In the latter case, this finding appears to be related to the role of these cells in transcytosis of insulin molecules from the intravascular to the extracellular space. Transcytosis has an important role in the delivery of insulin to its target cells in tissues where endothelial cells form tight junctions, including skeletal muscle and adipose tissue.

Several enzymes have been implicated in insulin degradation. The primary insulin-degrading enzyme is a thiol metalloproteinase. It is localized primarily in hepatocytes, but immunologically related molecules also have been found in muscle, kidney, and brain (Duckworth, 1988). Most insulin-degrading enzyme activity appears to be cytosolic, raising the question of how the internalized vesicular insulin becomes associated with the degrading enzyme, although this activity also has been found in endosomes. A second insulin-degrading enzyme also has been described (Authier *et al.,* 1994), but the relative roles of these enzymes have not been established. Insulin-degrading enzyme also may have a role in the degradation of other hormones, including glucagon.

Cellular Actions of Insulin. Insulin elicits a remarkable array of biological responses. The important target tissues for regulation of glucose homeostasis by insulin are liver, muscle, and fat, but insulin exerts potent regulatory effects on other cell types as well. Insulin is the primary hormone responsible for controlling the uptake, use, and storage of cellular nutrients. Insulin's anabolic actions include the stimulation of intracellular use and storage of glucose, amino acids, and fatty acids, whereas it inhibits catabolic processes such as the breakdown of glycogen, fat, and protein. It accomplishes these general purposes by stimulating the

transport of substrates and ions into cells, promoting the translocation of proteins between cellular compartments, activating and inactivating specific enzymes, and changing the amounts of proteins by altering the rates of gene transcription and specific mRNA translation (Figure 60–3).

Some effects of insulin occur within seconds or minutes, including the activation of glucose and ion transport systems, the covalent modification (*i.e.,* phosphorylation or dephosphorylation) of enzymes, and some effects on gene transcription (*i.e.,* inhibition of the phosphoenolpyruvate carboxykinase gene) (O'Brien and Granner, 1996). Other effects, such as those on protein synthesis and gene transcription, may take a few hours. Effects of insulin on cell proliferation and differentiation may take days. It is not clear whether these kinetic differences result from the use of different mechanistic pathways or from the intrinsic kinetics of the various processes.

Regulation of Glucose Transport. Stimulation of glucose transport into muscle and adipose tissue is a crucial component of the physiological response to insulin. Glucose enters cells by facilitated diffusion through one of a family of glucose transporters. Five of these (GLUT1 through GLUT5) are thought to be involved in Na^+-independent facilitated diffusion of glucose into cells (Shepherd and Kahn, 1999). The glucose transporters are integral membrane glycoproteins with molecular masses of about 50,000 daltons, and each has 12 membrane-spanning α-helical domains. Insulin stimulates glucose transport at least in part by promoting translocation of intracellular vesicles that contain the GLUT4 and GLUT1 glucose transporters to the plasma membrane (Figure 60–3). This effect is reversible; the transporters return to the intracellular pool on removal of insulin. Faulty regulation of this process may contribute to the pathophysiology of type 2 DM (Shepherd and Kahn, 1999).

Regulation of Glucose Metabolism. The facilitated diffusion of glucose into cells along a downhill gradient is ensured by glucose phosphorylation. This enzymatic reaction, the conversion of glucose to glucose-6-phosphate (G-6-P), is accomplished by one of a family of hexokinases. Like the glucose transporters described earlier, the four hexokinases (I through IV) are distributed differently in tissues, and two are regulated by insulin. Hexokinase IV, a 50,000-dalton enzyme more commonly known as *glucokinase,* is found in association with GLUT2 in liver and pancreatic β cells. There is one glucokinase gene, but different first exons and promoters are employed in the two tissues (Printz *et al.,* 1993). The liver glucokinase gene is regulated by insulin. Hexokinase II, a 100,000-dalton enzyme, is found in associa-

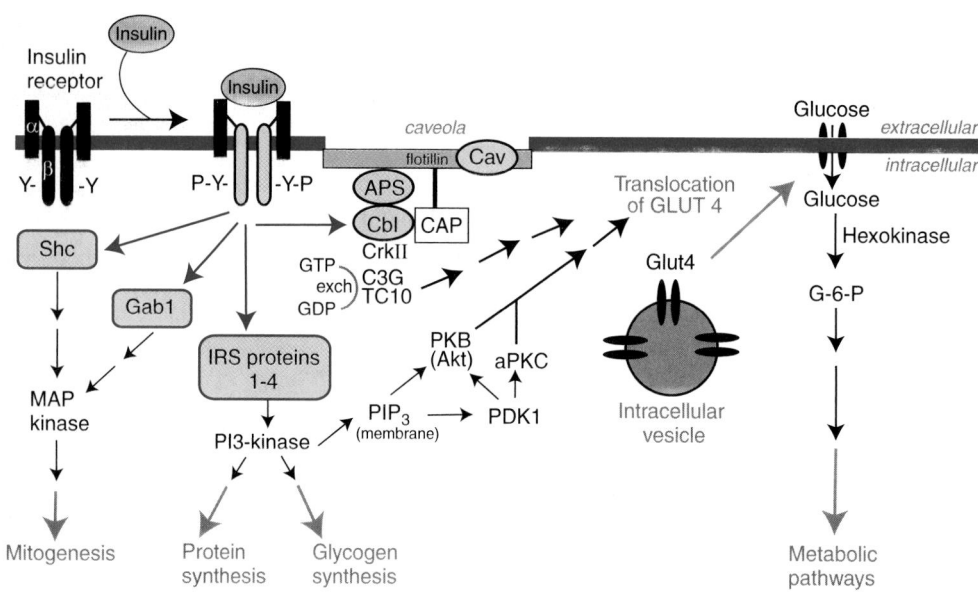

Figure 60–3. *Pathways of insulin signaling.* The binding of insulin to its plasma membrane receptor activates a cascade of downstream signaling events. Insulin binding activates the intrinsic tyrosine kinase activity of the receptor dimer, resulting in the tyrosine phosphorylation (Y-P) of the receptor's β subunits and a small number of specific substrates (light blue shapes): the Insulin Receptor Substrate (IRS) proteins, Gab-1 and SHC; within the membrane, a caveolar pool of insulin receptor phosphorylates caveolin (Cav), APS, and Cbl. These tyrosine-phosphorylated proteins interact with signaling cascades via SH2 and SH3 domains to mediate the effects of insulin, with specific effects of insulin resulting from each pathway. In target tissues such as skeletal muscle and adipocytes, a key event is the translocation of the Glut4 glucose transporter from intracellular vesicles to the plasma membrane; this translocation is stimulated by both the caveolar and non-caveolar pathways. In the non-caveolar pathway, the activation of PI3K is crucial, and PKB/Akt (anchored at the membrane by PIP3) and/or an atypical form of PKC is involved. In the caveolar pathway, the caveolar protein flotillin localizes the signaling complex to the caveola; the signaling pathway involves series of SH2 domain interactions that add the adaptor protein CrkII, the guanine nucleotide exchange protein C3G, and small GTP-binding protein, TC10. The pathways are inactivated by specific phosphoprotein phosphatases (eg, PTB1B) and possibly by actions of ser/thr protein kinases. In addition to the actions shown, insulin also stimulates the plasma membrane Na^+,K^+-ATPase by a mechanism that is still being elucidated; the result is an increase in pump activity and a net accumulation of K^+ in the cell. Abbreviations: APS, adaptor protein with PH and SH2 domains; CAP, Cbl associated protein; CrkII, chicken tumor virus regulator of kinase II; Glut4, glucose transporter 4; Gab-1, Grb-2 associated binder; MAP kinase, mitogen-activated protein kinase; PDK, phosphoinositide-dependent kinase; PI3 kinase, phosphatidylinositol-3-kinase; PIP3, phosphatidylinositol trisphosphate; PKB, protein kinase B (also called Akt); aPKC, atypical isoform of protein kinase C; Y, tyrosine residue; Y-P, phosphorylated tyrosine residue.

tion with GLUT4 in skeletal and cardiac muscle and in adipose tissue. Like GLUT4, hexokinase II is regulated transcriptionally by insulin.

G-6-P is a branch-point substrate that can enter several pathways. Thus, following isomerization to G-1-P, G-6-P can be stored as glycogen (insulin enhances the activity of glycogen synthase); G-6-P can enter the glycolytic pathway (leading to ATP production); and G-6-P can also enter the pentose phosphate pathway (providing NADPH for reductive syntheses, for the xenobiotic metabolizing activities of CYPs, and for maintenance of reduced glutathione). Effects of insulin on cellular metabolic enzymes are myriad and generally are mediated via the activities of protein kinases and phosphoprotein phosphatases that are enhanced following insulin treatment. Figure 60–3 shows the initial signaling events following the binding of insulin to its membrane receptor.

Regulation of Gene Transcription. A major action of insulin is the regulation of transcription of specific genes. More than a hundred genes are known to be regulated by insulin (O'Brien and Granner, 1996), although the mechanisms of regulation are still being worked out. As an example, insulin inhibits the transcription of phosphoenolpyruvate carboxykinase, contributing to insulin's inhibition of gluconeogenesis; this effect of insulin may explain why the liver overproduces glucose in the insulin-resistant state that is characteristic of type 2 DM.

The Insulin Receptor. Insulin initiates its actions by binding to a cell-surface receptor. Such receptors are present in virtually all mammalian cells, including not only the classic targets for insulin action (*i.e.,* liver, muscle, and fat) but also such nonclassic targets as circulating blood cells, neurons, and gonadal cells. The number of receptors varies from as few as 40 per cell on erythrocytes to 300,000 per cell on adipocytes and hepatocytes.

The insulin receptor is a large transmembrane glycoprotein composed of two 135,000-dalton α subunits (719 or 731 amino acids, depending on whether a 12-amino-acid insertion has occurred through alternate RNA splicing) and two 95,000-dalton β subunits (620 amino acids); the subunits are linked by disulfide bonds to form a β-α-α-β heterotetramer (Figure 60–3) (Virkamäki *et al.*, 1999). Both subunits are derived from a single-chain precursor molecule that contains the entire sequence of the α and β subunits separated by a processing site consisting of four basic amino acid residues. The α subunits are entirely extracellular and contain the insulin-binding domain (*see* above), whereas the β subunits are transmembrane proteins that possess tyrosine protein kinase activity. After insulin is bound, receptors aggregate and are internalized rapidly. Since bivalent (but not monovalent) anti-insulin receptor antibodies cross-link adjacent receptors and mimic the rapid actions of insulin, it has been suggested that receptor dimerization is essential for signal transduction. After internalization, the receptor may be degraded or recycled back to the cell surface.

Tyrosine Phosphorylation and the Insulin Action Cascade. Receptors for insulin and IGF-1 belong to the family of receptor tyrosine kinases, in common with many growth factor receptors.

The activated receptors undergo autophosphorylation, which seems to activate their tyrosine kinase activity toward other substrates, principally the four insulin receptor substrates IRS-1 through 4 and Shc (White, 2002). The tyrosine phosphorylated IRS proteins direct the recruitment of signaling cascades *via* the interaction of SH2 domains with phosphotyrosines, recruiting such proteins as SHP2, Grb2, and SOS and resulting in the activation of MAP kinases and PI$_3$-kinase, which transduce many of insulin's cellular effects.

Insulin signaling is complicated by the fact that the IGF-1 receptor resembles the insulin receptor and uses similar signaling pathways; furthermore, the two receptors bind each other's ligand, albeit with lower affinity. In addition, IGF-1 and insulin-receptor heterodimers can combine to form hybrid heterotetramers.

The tyrosine kinase activity of the insulin receptor is required for signal transduction. Mutation of the insulin receptor with modification of the ATP-binding site or replacement of the tyrosine residues at major sites of autophosphorylation decreases both insulin-stimulated kinase activity and the cellular response to insulin. An insulin receptor incapable of autophosphorylation is biologically inert. A polymorphism in the human IRS-1, G972R, is associated with insulin resistance and increased risk of type 2 DM; this polymorphic IRS-1 appears to act as an inhibitor of the insulin-receptor tyrosine kinase (McGettrick *et al.*, 2005). In intact cells, the insulin receptor also is phosphorylated on serine and threonine residues, presumably by protein kinase C (PKC) and protein kinase A (PKA). Such phosphorylation inhibits the tyrosine kinase activity of the insulin receptor.

Diabetes Mellitus and the Physiological Effects of Insulin

Diabetes mellitus (DM) consists of a group of syndromes characterized by hyperglycemia; altered metabo-

lism of lipids, carbohydrates, and proteins; and an increased risk of complications from vascular disease. Most patients can be classified clinically as having either type 1 or type 2 DM (Expert Committee on the Diagnosis and Treatment of Diabetes Mellitus, 2003). DM or carbohydrate intolerance also is associated with certain other conditions or syndromes (Table 60–1). Criteria for the diagnosis of DM have been proposed by several medical organizations. The American Diabetes Association (ADA) criteria include symptoms of DM (*e.g.*, polyuria, polydipsia, and unexplained weight loss) and a random plasma glucose concentration of greater than 200 mg/dl (11.1 mM), a fasting plasma glucose concentration of greater than 126 ml/dl (7 mM), or a plasma glucose concentration of greater than 200 mg/dl (11 mM) 2 hours after the ingestion of an oral glucose load (Expert Committee on the Diagnosis and Treatment of Diabetes Mellitus, 2003).

The incidence of each type of diabetes varies widely throughout the world. In the United States, about 5% to 10% of all diabetic patients have type 1 DM, with an incidence of 18 per 100,000 inhabitants per year. A similar incidence is found in the United Kingdom. The incidence of type 1 DM in Europe varies with latitude. The highest rates occur in northern Europe (Finland, 43 per 100,000) and the lowest in the south (France and Italy, 8 per 100,000). The one exception to this rule is the small island of Sardinia, close to Italy, which has an incidence of 30 per 100,000. However, even the relatively low incidence rates of type 1 DM in southern Europe are far higher than the rates in Japan (1 per 100,000 inhabitants).

The vast majority of diabetic patients have type 2 DM. In the United States, about 90% of all diabetic patients have type 2 DM. Incidence rates of type 2 DM increase with age, with a mean rate of about 440 per 100,000 per year by the sixth decade in males in the United States. Ethnicity within a country also can influence the incidence of type 2 DM; the mean rate in African-American males is 540 per 100,000, and that in Pima Indians is about 5000 per 100,000. Unlike those for type 1 DM, the incidence rates for type 2 DM are lower in northern Europe (100 to 250 per 100,000) than in the south (800 per 100,000). Although prevalence data exist for type 2 DM, these numbers almost certainly are underestimates because 33% of all cases are undiagnosed.

There are more than 125 million persons with diabetes in the world today, and by 2010, this number is expected to approach 220 million (Amos *et al.*, 1997). Both type 1 and type 2 DM are increasing in frequency. The reason for the increase of type 1 DM is not known. The genetic basis for type 2 DM cannot change in such a short time; thus other contributing factors, including increasing age, obesity, sedentary lifestyle, and low birth weight, must account for this dramatic increase. In addition, type 2 DM is being diagnosed with remarkable frequency in preadolescents and adolescents. Up to 45% of newly diagnosed children and adolescents have type 2 DM.

In certain tropical countries, the most common cause of diabetes is chronic pancreatitis associated with nutritional or toxic factors (a form of secondary diabetes). Very rarely, diabetes results from point mutations in the insulin gene (Chan *et al.*, 1987). Amino acid substi-

Table 60–1
Different Forms of Diabetes Mellitus

General—genetic and other factors not precisely defined

Type 1 diabetes mellitus (formerly called insulin-dependent diabetes mellitus)

Autoimmune type 1 diabetes mellitus (type 1A)

Non-autoimmune or idiopathic type 1 diabetes mellitus (type 1B)

Type 2 diabetes mellitus (formerly called non-insulin-dependent diabetes mellitus)

Specific—defined gene mutations

Maturity-onset diabetes of youth (MODY)

MODY 1 hepatic nuclear factor 4α (*HNF4A*) gene mutations

MODY 2 glucokinase (*GCK*) gene mutations

MODY 3 hepatic nuclear factor 1α (*TCF1*) gene mutations

MODY 4 insulin promoter factor 1 (*IPF1*) gene mutations

MODY 5 hepatic nuclear factor 1β (*HNF1β*) gene mutations

MODY 6 neurogenic differentiation 1 (*NEUROD1*) gene mutation

MODY X unidentified gene mutation(s)

Maternally inherited diabetes and deafness (MIDD)

Mitochondrial leucine tRNA gene mutations

Insulin gene mutations

Insulin receptor gene mutations

Diabetes secondary to pancreatic disease

Chronic pancreatitis

Surgery

Tropical diabetes (chronic pancreatitis associated with nutritional and/or toxic factors)

Diabetes secondary to other endocrinopathies

Cushing's disease

Glucocorticoid administration

Acromegaly

Diabetes secondary to immune suppression

Diabetes associated with genetic syndromes; *e.g.*, Prader-Willi syndrome

Diabetes associated with drug therapy (*see* Table 60–5)

tutions from such mutations may result in insulins with lower potency or may alter the processing of proinsulin to insulin (*see* above). Other single-gene mutations cause the several types of MODY (Hattersley, 1998) and maternally inherited diabetes and deafness (van den Ouwenland *et al.*, 1992) (Table 60–1).

There are genetic and environmental components that affect the risk of developing either type 1 or type 2 DM. A positive family history of type 2 DM is predictive for the disease. Studies of identical twins show 70% to 80% concordance for developing type 2 DM. Furthermore, there is a high prevalence of type 2 DM in offspring of parents with the disease (up to 70%) as well as in siblings of affected individuals. Persons more than 20% over their ideal body weight also have a greater risk of developing type 2 DM. In fact, 80% to 90% of type 2 DM subjects in the United States are obese. Certain ethnic groups have a higher incidence of type 2 DM (*e.g.*, American Indians, African-Americans, Hispanics, and Polynesian Islanders). In addition, previously identified impaired glucose tolerance, gestational diabetes, hypertension, or significant hyperlipidemia is associated with an increased risk of type 2 DM. These data suggest a strong genetic basis for type 2 DM, but the genetic mechanism(s) involved are not known. A pancreatic β-cell defect and a reduction in tissue sensitivity to insulin both are required before overt type 2 DM is apparent. However, type 2 DM is an extremely heterogeneous disease, and it is likely that a number of different genes are involved. In addition, environmental factors may play a role. Type 2 DM thus is a multifactorial disease. Any combination of genetic and environmental factors that exceeds a threshold can result in type 2 DM. The genetic basis for type 2 DM in a small subset of patients has been established. MODY2 is a rare disorder that is inherited as an autosomal dominant trait and is caused by mutations of the glucokinase gene. Because of decreased glucokinase activity, these patients have an increased glycemic threshold for insulin release that results in persistent mild hyperglycemia. This and other rare genetic forms of MODY are quite distinct from the usual type 2 DM (Table 60–1).

With type 1 DM, the concordance rate for identical twins is only 25% to 50%; this suggests that environmental as well as genetic influences have an important role in the disease. However, the known genetic factors in type 1 DM relate to the genes that control the immune response. There is considerable evidence that type 1 DM involves an autoimmune attack on the pancreatic β cell. Antibodies to islet cell antigens are detected in up to 80% of patients with type 1 DM shortly after diagnosis or even prior to the onset of clinical disease. The antibodies are directed at both cytoplasmic and membrane-bound antigens and include islet cell antibodies and antibodies directed against insulin (IAAs), glutamic acid decarboxylase-65 and -67 (GAD-65 and -67), heat-shock protein 65 (HSP-65), and tyrosine phosphatase–like protein (IA-2 or IA-2B).

Although these autoantibodies are correlated with the clinical expression of type 1 DM, it is controversial whether they can predict the development of clinical diabetes. Most prospective studies designed to determine if type 1 DM can be predicted on the basis of antibodies have been performed in healthy first-degree relatives of diabetic patients. These studies have determined that the presence of IAAs confers only a small risk for the development of type 1 DM. On the other hand, the presence of high-titer islet-cell antibodies (ICAs) and GAD antibodies or ICAs combined with IAAs confers a very high risk for the development of type 1 DM in first-degree relatives (Verge *et al.*, 1996).

Since most of the studies aimed at predicting the development of type 1 DM have been carried out in first-degree relatives of diabetic patients, it is not known whether the occurrence of ICAs in individuals from the general population confers a similar risk for development of clinical diabetes. Most available data indicate that the presence of ICAs in individuals from the general population is associated with a lower risk of developing type 1 DM. However, as in first-degree relatives of type 1 DM patients, it may be that the presence of more than one form of autoantibody in individuals from the general population is a more powerful predictor of the development of clinical diabetes. Individuals with type 1 DM also tend to have antibodies directed toward other endocrine tissues, including the adrenal, parathyroid, and thyroid glands, and have an increased incidence of other autoimmune diseases.

Type 1 DM is associated with specific human leukocyte antigen (HLA) alleles, especially at the B and DR loci (Florez *et al.*, 2003). Approximately 90% of patients with type 1 DM are positive for HLA-DR3 or -DR4, as compared with only 40% of the general population. Compound heterozygotes appear to be at particular risk. In contrast, the haplotype HLA-DR2 appears to be negatively associated with the occurrence of the disease. A polymorphism of the HLA-DQβ chain at position 57 correlates even more closely with susceptibility to diabetes (Todd *et al.*, 1987). Type 1 DM is associated with alleles coding for alanine, valine, or serine at position 57 in the HLA-DQβ chain, whereas aspartic acid in this position is negatively correlated with the disease in Caucasians. These findings implicate both humoral and cell-mediated immune mechanisms in the etiology of type 1 DM.

The trigger for the immune response remains unknown. The identification of triggering agents is difficult because autoimmune destruction of pancreatic β cells may occur over a period of many months or several years before the onset of overt disease. In about 10% of new cases of type 1 DM, there is no evidence of autoimmune insulitis (Imagawa *et al.*, 2000). The ADA and the World Health Organization (WHO) therefore subdivide this disease into autoimmune (1A) and idiopathic (1B) subtypes. Whatever the causes, the final result in type 1 DM is an extensive and selective loss of pancreatic β cells and a state of absolute insulin deficiency.

The situation in type 2 DM is not so clear-cut. Most studies indicate that there is reduced β-cell mass in type 2 DM patients. Obesity, duration of diabetes, and prevailing hyperglycemia potentially can confound interpretation of data, but studies that have controlled for these variables have reported an approximately 50% reduction in β-cell volume in type 2 DM patients compared with nondiabetic control subjects. Owing to the heterogeneous nature of type 2 DM, mean 24-hour plasma concentrations of insulin in patients have been reported to vary from low to even normal relative to values in control subjects. Of note, standard insulin radioimmunoassays detect proinsulin and processing intermediates. Studies in which specific insulin and proinsulin assays have been used (Temple *et al.*, 1989) have revealed that "true" insulin values in "hyperinsulinemic" type 2 DM patients are either no greater or distinctly less than values in control subjects. Therefore, increased amounts of proinsulin have confounded the appreciation of subnormal insulin levels in type 2 DM patients. Furthermore, even apparently "normal" values of plasma insulin in a hyperglycemic type 2 DM patient are considerably reduced relative to the insulin levels that would be observed in a similarly hyperglycemic nondiabetic individual.

In healthy persons, the contribution of proinsulin to basal immunoreactive insulin levels is low. Proinsulin intermediates make up about 10% of the total immunoreactive insulin in the portal vein. However, owing to its long half-life (about 44 minutes) and tenfold slower metabolic clearance, proinsulin and intermediates make up about 20% of circulating immunoreactive insulin. This amount is physiologically trivial because proinsulin has only

about 5% of the metabolic effect of insulin (Davis *et al.*, 1991). Nevertheless, plasma proinsulinlike molecules are increased in type 2 DM to about 20% or more of total immunoreactive insulin. Furthermore, proinsulin levels increase in response to any β-cell stimulation.

Type 2 DM also is associated with several distinct defects in insulin secretion. At diagnosis, virtually all persons with type 2 DM have a profound defect in first-phase insulin secretion in response to an intravenous glucose challenge. The responses to other secretagogues (*e.g.*, isoproterenol or arginine) are preserved, although there is less potentiation by glucose. Some of these β-cell abnormalities in type 2 DM may be secondary to desensitization by chronic hyperglycemia. The relationship between fasting glycemia and insulinemia in type 2 DM subjects is complex. Patients who have fasting blood glucose levels of 6 to 10 mM (108 to 180 mg/dl) have fasting and stimulated insulin values equal to those of euglycemic control subjects. More severely hyperglycemic subjects are frankly hypoinsulinemic.

Virtually all forms of DM are caused by a decrease in the circulating concentration of insulin (insulin deficiency) and a decrease in the response of peripheral tissues to insulin (insulin resistance). These abnormalities lead to alterations in the metabolism of carbohydrates, lipids, ketones, and amino acids; the central feature of the syndrome is hyperglycemia (Figure 60–4).

Insulin lowers the concentration of glucose in blood by inhibiting hepatic glucose production and by stimu-

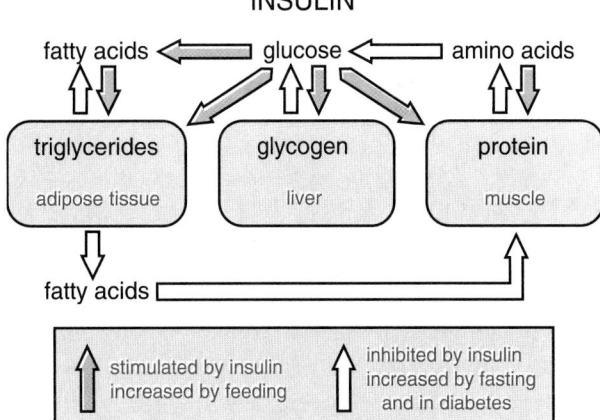

Figure 60–4. Overview of insulin action. Insulin stimulates glucose storage in the liver as glycogen and in adipose tissue as triglycerides and amino acid storage in muscle as protein; it also promotes utilization of glucose in muscle for energy. These pathways, which also are enhanced by feeding, are indicated by the solid blue arrows. Insulin inhibits the breakdown of triglycerides, glycogen, and protein and the conversion of amino acids to glucose (gluconeogenesis), as indicated by the white arrows. These pathways are increased during fasting and in diabetic states. The conversion of amino acids to glucose and of glucose to fatty acids occurs primarily in the liver.

Table 60–2
Hypoglycemic Actions of Insulin

LIVER	MUSCLE	ADIPOSE TISSUE
Inhibits hepatic glucose production (decreases gluconeogenesis and glycogenolysis)	Stimulates glucose uptake	Stimulates glucose uptake (amount is small compared to muscle)
Stimulates hepatic glucose uptake	Inhibits flow of gluconeogenic precursors to the liver (*e.g.*, alanine, lactate, and pyruvate)	Inhibits flow of gluconeogenic precursor to liver (glycerol) and reduces energy substrate for hepatic gluconeogenesis (nonesterfied fatty acids)

lating the uptake and metabolism of glucose by muscle and adipose tissue (Table 60–2). These two important effects occur at different concentrations of insulin. Production of glucose is inhibited half maximally by an insulin concentration of about 20 μunits/ml, whereas glucose utilization is stimulated half maximally at about 50 μunits/ml.

In both types of diabetes, glucagon (the levels of which are elevated in untreated patients) opposes the hepatic effects of insulin by stimulating glycogenolysis and gluconeogenesis, but it has relatively little effect on peripheral utilization of glucose. Thus, in the diabetic patient with insulin deficiency or insulin resistance and hyperglucagonemia, there is an increase in hepatic glucose production, a decrease in peripheral glucose uptake, and a decrease in the conversion of glucose to glycogen in the liver (DeFronzo *et al.*, 1992).

Alterations in secretion of insulin and glucagon also profoundly affect lipid, ketone, and protein metabolism. At concentrations below those required to stimulate glucose uptake, insulin inhibits the hormone-sensitive lipase in adipose tissue and thus inhibits the hydrolysis of triglyceride stores. This counteracts the lipolytic action of catecholamines, cortisol, and growth hormone and reduces the concentrations of glycerol (a substrate for gluconeogenesis) and free fatty acids (a substrate for production of ketone bodies and a necessary fuel for gluconeogenesis). These actions of insulin are deficient in the diabetic patient, leading to increased gluconeogenesis and ketogenesis.

The liver produces ketone bodies by oxidation of free fatty acids to acetyl CoA, which then is converted to acetoacetate and β-hydroxybutyrate. The initial step in fatty acid oxidation is transport of the fatty acid into the mitochondria. This involves the interconversion of the coenzyme A (CoA) and carnitine esters of fatty acids by the enzyme acylcarnitine transferase. The activity of this enzyme is inhibited by intramitochondrial malonyl CoA, one of the products of fatty acid synthesis. Under normal conditions, insulin inhibits lipolysis, stimulates fatty acid synthesis (thereby increasing the concentration of malonyl CoA), and decreases the hepatic concentration of carnitine; these factors all decrease the production of ketone bodies. Conversely, glucagon stimulates ketone body production by increasing fatty acid oxidation and decreasing concentrations of malonyl CoA. In the diabetic patient, particularly the patient with type 1 DM, the consequences of insulin deficiency and glucagon excess provide a hormonal milieu that favors ketogenesis and, in the absence of appropriate treatment, may lead to ketonemia and acidosis.

Insulin also enhances the transcription of lipoprotein lipase in the capillary endothelium. This enzyme hydrolyzes triglycerides present in very low density lipoproteins (VLDL) and chylomicrons, resulting in release of intermediate-density lipoprotein (IDL) particles (*see* Chapter 35). The IDL particles are converted by the liver to the more cholesterol-rich low-density lipoproteins (LDL). Thus, in the untreated or undertreated diabetic patient, hypertriglyceridemia and hypercholesterolemia often occur. In addition, deficiency of insulin may be associated with increased production of VLDL.

The important role of insulin in protein metabolism usually is evident clinically only in diabetic patients with persistently poor control of their disease. Insulin stimulates amino acid uptake and protein synthesis and inhibits protein degradation in muscle and other tissues; it thus causes a decrease in the circulating concentrations of most amino acids. Glutamine and alanine are the major amino acid precursors for gluconeogenesis. Insulin lowers alanine concentrations during hyperinsulinemic euglycemic conditions. The rate of appearance of alanine is maintained in part by the enhanced rate of transamination of pyruvate to alanine. However, alanine utilization greatly exceeds production (owing to increased hepatic uptake and fractional extraction of the amino acid), and this results in a fall of peripheral alanine levels. In poorly controlled diabetics, there is increased conversion of alanine to glucose, contributing to the enhanced rate of gluconeogenesis. The increased conversion of amino acids to glucose also results in increased production and excretion of urea and ammonia. In addition, there are increased circulating concentrations of branched-chain amino acids as a result of increased proteolysis, decreased protein synthesis, and increased release of branched-chain amino acids from the liver.

A nearly pathognomonic feature of diabetes mellitus is thickening of the capillary basement membrane and other vascular changes that occur during the course of the disease. The cumulative effect is progressive narrowing of the vessel lumina, causing inadequate perfusion of critical regions of certain organs. The matrix is expanded in many vessel walls, in the basement membrane of the retina, and in the mesangial cells of the renal glomerulus (McMillan, 1997). Cellular proliferation in many large vessels further contributes to luminal narrowing. These pathological changes contribute to some of the major complications of diabetes, including premature atherosclerosis, intercapillary glomerulosclerosis, retinopathy, neuropathy, and ulceration and gangrene of the extremities.

It is hypothesized that the factor responsible for the development of most complications of diabetes is the prolonged exposure of tissues to elevated concentrations of glucose. Prolonged hyperglycemia results in the formation of advanced glycation end products (Beisswenger *et al.*, 1995). These macromolecules are thought to induce many of the vascular abnormalities that result in the complications of diabetes (Brownlee, 1995). The results from the Diabetes Control and Complications Trial (DCCT) definitively answered this question: Most diabetic complications arise from prolonged exposure of tissue to elevated glucose concentrations.

The DCCT (DCCT Research Group, 1993) was a multicenter, randomized clinical trial designed to compare intensive and conventional diabetes therapies with regard to their effects on the development and progression of the early vascular and neurologic complications of type 1 DM. The intensive therapy regimen was designed to achieve blood glucose values as close to the normal range as possible with three or more daily insulin injections or with an external insulin pump. Conventional therapy consisted of one or two insulin

injections daily. Two groups of patients were studied to answer separate but related questions. The first question was whether or not intensive therapy could prevent the development of diabetic complications such as retinopathy, nephropathy, and neuropathy (primary prevention). The second was whether or not intensive therapy could slow the progression of existing complications of diabetes (secondary intervention).

In the primary prevention group, intensive therapy reduced the mean risk for the development of retinopathy by 76% compared with conventional therapy. In the secondary intervention group, intensive therapy slowed the progression of retinopathy by 54%. Intensive therapy reduced the risk of nephropathy by 34% in the primary prevention group and by 43% in the secondary intervention group. Similarly, neuropathy was reduced by about 60% in both the primary prevention and secondary intervention groups. Intensive therapy reduced the development of hypercholesterolemia by 34% overall. Because of the relative youth of the patients, it was predicted that the detection of treatment-related differences in rates of macrovascular events would be unlikely. However, intensive therapy reduced the risk of macrovascular disease by 41% in the combined groups. These results established unequivocally that improving day-to-day glycemic control in type 1 DM patients can reduce and slow the development of diabetic complications dramatically. A follow-up study showed that the reduction in the risk of progressive retinopathy and nephropathy persists for at least 4 years, even if tight glycemic control was not maintained (DCCT Research Group, 2000).

A serious complication of intensive therapy was an increased incidence of severe hypoglycemia. Patients receiving intensive therapy had a threefold greater incidence of severe hypoglycemia (blood glucose concentration below 50 mg/dl or 2.8 mM and needing external resuscitative assistance) and hypoglycemic coma than did conventionally treated subjects. Therefore, the present guidelines for treatment given by the ADA include a contraindication for implementing tight metabolic control in infants younger than 2 years old and an extreme caution in children between 2 and 7 years of age because hypoglycemia may impair brain development. Older patients with significant arteriosclerosis also may be vulnerable to permanent injury from hypoglycemia.

The DCCT was performed in relatively young type 1 DM patients. The question was asked whether intensive therapy would provide similar benefits to typical middle-aged or elderly patients with type 2 DM. The results of the DCCT indeed also apply to patients with type 2 DM (U.K. Prospective Diabetes Study Group, 1998a, 1998b). The eye, kidney, and nerve abnormalities appear similar in type 1 and type 2 DM, and it is likely that the same or similar underlying mechanisms of disease apply. However, because of a higher prevalence of macrovascular disease, older patients with type 2 DM may be more vulnerable to serious consequences of hypoglycemia. Thus, as is the case for everyone with diabetes, treatment of type 2 DM patients must be tailored to the individual. Nevertheless, the results of the DCCT and U.K. Prospective Diabetes Study (UKPDS) suggest that many otherwise healthy patients with type 2 DM should attempt to achieve tight metabolic control.

The toxic effects of hyperglycemia may be the result of accumulation of non-enzymatically glycosylated products and osmotically active sugar alcohols such as sorbitol in tissues; the effects of glucose on cellular metabolism also may be responsible (Brownlee, 1995). The covalent reaction of glucose with hemoglobin provides a convenient method to determine an integrated index of the glycemic state. Hemoglobin undergoes glycosylation on its aminoterminal valine residue to form the glucosyl valine adduct of hemoglobin, termed *hemoglobin* A_{1c} (Brownlee, 1995). The half-life of the modified hemoglobin is equal to that of the erythrocyte (about 120 days). Since the amount of glycosylated protein formed is proportional to the glucose concentration and the time of exposure of the protein to glucose, the concentration of hemoglobin A_{1c} in the circulation reflects the severity of the glycemic state over an extended period (4 to 12 weeks) prior to sampling. Thus a rise in hemoglobin A_{1c} from 5% to 10% suggests a prolonged doubling of the mean blood glucose concentration. Although this assay is used widely, measurement of the glycosylation of proteins with somewhat shorter survival times (*e.g.,* albumin) also has proven useful in the management of pregnant diabetic patients.

Glycosylated products accumulate in tissues and eventually may form cross-linked proteins termed *advanced glycosylation end products* (Beisswenger *et al.,* 1995). Such nonenzymatic glycosylation may be directly responsible for expansion of the vascular matrix and the vascular complications of diabetes. This process also may explain the modified cellular proliferative activity in vascular lesions of diabetic patients because macrophages appear to have receptors for advanced glycosylation end products. Binding of such proteins to macrophages in these lesions may stimulate the production of cytokines such as tumor necrosis factor α and interleukin 1 (IL-1), which, in turn, induce degradative and proliferative cascades in mesenchymal and endothelial cells, respectively.

Other explanations for the toxic manifestations of hyperglycemia may exist. Intracellular glucose is reduced to its corresponding sugar alcohol, sorbitol, by the enzyme aldose reductase, and the rate of production of sorbitol is determined by the ambient glucose concentration. This is particularly true in tissues such as the lens, retina, arterial wall, and Schwann cells of peripheral nerves. In diabetic human beings and rodents, these tissues have increased intracellular concentrations of sorbitol, which may contribute to an increased osmotic effect and tissue damage. Inhibitors of aldose reductase currently are being evaluated for treatment of diabetic neuropathy and retinopathy. The results of studies with these agents thus far have been somewhat conflicting and inconclusive (reviewed by Frank, 1994).

In neural tissue and perhaps in other tissues, glucose competes with myoinositol for transport into cells. Reduc-

tion of cellular concentrations of myoinositol may contribute to altered nerve function and neuropathy. Hyperglycemia also may enhance the *de novo* synthesis of diacylglycerol, which could facilitate persistent activation of protein kinase C.

Insulin Therapy

Insulin is the mainstay for treatment of virtually all type 1 DM and many type 2 DM patients. When necessary, insulin may be administered intravenously or intramuscularly; however, long-term treatment relies predominantly on subcutaneous injection of the hormone. Subcutaneous administration of insulin differs from physiological secretion of insulin in at least two major ways: The kinetics do not reproduce the normal rapid rise and decline of insulin secretion in response to ingestion of nutrients, and the insulin diffuses into the peripheral circulation instead of being released into the portal circulation; the direct effect of secreted insulin on hepatic metabolic processes thus is eliminated. Nonetheless, when such treatment is performed carefully, considerable success is achieved.

Preparations of insulin can be classified according to their duration of action into short, intermediate, and long acting and by their species of origin—human or porcine. Human insulin (HUMULIN, NOVOLIN) is now widely available as a result of its recombinant production. Porcine insulin differs from human insulin by one amino acid (alanine instead of threonine at the carboxy terminal of the B chain, *i.e.,* in position B30. Prior to the mid-1970s, commercially available insulin preparations contained proinsulin or glucagonlike substances, pancreatic polypeptide, somatostatin, and vasoactive intestinal peptides. These contaminants were avoided with the advent of monocomponent porcine insulins. During the late 1970s, intense work was carried out on the development of biosynthetic human insulin. During the last decade, human insulin rapidly has become the standard form of therapy, and beef insulin products have been discontinued in the United States.

The physicochemical properties of human and porcine insulins differ owing to their different amino acid sequences. Human insulin, produced using recombinant DNA technology, is more soluble than porcine insulin in aqueous solution owing to the presence of threonine (instead of alanine), with its extra hydroxyl group. The vast majority of preparations now are supplied at neutral pH, which improves stability and permits storage for several days at a time at room temperature.

Table 60–3
Properties of Currently Available Insulin Preparations

TYPE	APPEARANCE	ADDED PROTEIN	ZINC CONTENT, mg/100 units	BUFFER*	Action, Hours†		
					ONSET	PEAK	DURATION
Rapid							
Regular soluble (crystalline)	Clear	None	0.01–0.04	None	0.5–0.7	1.5–4	5–8
Lispro	Clear	None	0.02	Phosphate	0.25	0.5–1.5	2–5
Aspart	Clear	None	0.0196	Phosphate	0.25	0.6–0.8	3–5
Glulisine	Clear	None	None	None	—	0.5–1.5	1–2.5
Intermediate							
NPH (isophane)	Cloudy	Protamine	0.016–0.04	Phosphate	1–2	6–12	18–24
Lente	Cloudy	None	0.2–0.25	Acetate	1–2	6–12	18–24
Slow							
Ultralente	Cloudy	None	0.2–0.25	Acetate	4–6	16–18	20–36
Protamine zinc	Cloudy	Protamine	0.2–0.25	Phosphate	4–6	14–20	24–36
Glargine	Clear	None	0.03	None	2–5	5–24	18–24

*Most insulin preparations are supplied at pH 7.2–7.4. Glargine is supplied at a pH of 4.0. †These are approximate figures. There is considerable variation from patient to patient and from time to time in a given patient.

Unitage. For therapeutic purposes, doses and concentrations of insulin are expressed in units. This tradition dates to the time when preparations of the hormone were impure, and it was necessary to standardize them by bioassay. One unit of insulin is equal to the amount required to reduce the concentration of blood glucose in a fasting rabbit to 45 mg/dl (2.5 mM). The current international standard is a mixture of bovine and porcine insulins and contains 24 units/mg. Homogeneous preparations of human insulin contain between 25 and 30 units/mg. Almost all commercial preparations of insulin are supplied in solution or suspension at a concentration of 100 units/ml, which is about 3.6 mg insulin per milliliter (0.6 mM). Insulin also is available in a more concentrated solution (500 units/ml) for patients who are resistant to the hormone.

Classification of Insulins. *Short-* and *rapid-acting insulins* are solutions of *regular, crystalline zinc insulin (insulin injection)* dissolved usually in a buffer at neutral pH. These preparations have the most rapid onset of action but the shortest duration (Table 60–3). Short-acting insulin (*i.e.*, regular or soluble) usually should be injected 30 to 45 minutes before meals. Regular insulin also may be given intravenously or intramuscularly. After intravenous injection, there is a rapid fall in the blood glucose concentration, which usually reaches a nadir in 20 to 30 minutes. In the absence of a sustained infusion of insulin, the hormone is cleared rapidly, and counter-regulatory hormones (*e.g.,* glucagon, epinephrine, norepinephrine, cortisol, and growth hormone) restore plasma glucose to baseline in 2 to 3 hours. In the absence of a normal counter-regulatory response (*e.g.,* in diabetic patients with autonomic neuropathy), plasma glucose will remain suppressed

for many hours following an insulin bolus of 0.15 units/kg because the cellular actions of insulin are prolonged far beyond its clearance from plasma. Intravenous infusions of insulin are useful in patients with ketoacidosis or when requirements for insulin may change rapidly, such as during the perioperative period, during labor and delivery, and in intensive care situations (*see* below).

When metabolic conditions are stable, regular insulin usually is given subcutaneously in combination with an intermediate- or long-acting preparation. Short-acting insulin is the only form of the hormone that can be used in subcutaneous infusion pumps. Special buffered formulations of regular insulin have been made for the latter purpose that are less likely to crystallize in the tubing during the slow infusion associated with this type of therapy.

The native insulin monomers are associated as hexamers in currently available insulin preparations. These hexamers slow the absorption and reduce postprandial peaks of subcutaneously injected insulin. These pharmacokinetics stimulated the development of short-acting insulin analogs that retain a monomeric or dimeric configuration. A number of compounds have been investigated, and two, insulin *lispro* (HUMALOG) and insulin *aspart* (NOVOLOG), are available for clinical use (Hirsch, 2005). These analogs are absorbed three times more rapidly from subcutaneous sites than is human insulin. Consequently, there is a more rapid increase in plasma insulin concentrations and an earlier hypoglycemic response. Injection of the analogs 15 minutes before a meal affords glycemic control similar to that from an injection of human insulin given 30 minutes before the meal. The first commercially available short-acting analog was human insulin lispro. This analog is identical to human insulin except at positions B28 and B29, where the sequence of the two residues has been reversed to match the sequence in IGF-1, which does not self-associate. Like regular insulin, lispro exists as a hexamer in commercially available formulations. Unlike regular insulin, lispro dissociates into monomers almost instantaneously following injection. This property results in the characteristic rapid absorption and shorter duration of action compared with regular insulin. Two therapeutic advantages have emerged with lispro as compared with regular insulin. First, the prevalence of hypoglycemia is reduced by 20% to 30% with lispro; second, glucose control, as assessed by hemoglobin A_{1c}, is modestly but significantly improved (0.3% to 0.5%) with lispro as compared with regular insulin.

Insulin aspart is formed by the replacement of proline at B28 with aspartic acid. This reduces self-association to that observed with lispro. Like lispro, insulin aspart dissociates rapidly into monomers following injection. Comparison of a single subcutaneous dose of aspart and lispro in a group of type 1 DM patients revealed similar plasma insulin profiles. In clinical trials, insulin aspart and insulin lispro have had similar effects on glucose control and hypoglycemia frequency, with lower rates of nocturnal hypoglycemia as compared with regular insulin (reviewed by Hirsh, 2005).

A third rapid-acting insulin analog called insulin *glulysine* has been approved for clinical use in the United States. In this compound, glutamic acid replaces lysine at B29, and lysine replaces asparagine at B23. Similar to the other two available rapid-acting analogs, this causes a reduction in self-association and rapid dissociation into active monomers. The time–action profile of insulin glulysine is similar to that of insulin aspart and lispro. Similar to insulin aspart, glulysine has been approved by the Food and Drug Administration (FDA) for continuous subcutaneous insulin infusion (CSII) pump use. Owing to their rapid onset, the fast-acting insulin analogs all may be injected immediately before or after a meal, which may confer considerable clinical advantages. Many individuals with diabetes consume smaller amounts of food than originally planned. This, in the presence of a previously injected dose of insulin that was based on a larger meal, could result in postprandial hypoglycemia. Thus, in patients who have gastroparesis or loss of appetite, injection of a rapid-acting analog postprandially, based on the amount of food actually consumed, may provide smoother glycemic control.

Clinical trials of inhaled insulin are underway in a number of countries. Early results demonstrate that inhaled insulin and short-acting subcutaneously-injected insulin provide similar postprandial glycemic control in patients with type 1 and type 2 DM. Patient satisfaction is uniformly high with inhaled insulin, and the prevalence of hypoglycemia is no higher (and may even be reduced) compared with regular (soluble) insulin. Smoking increases and asthma decreases absorption of inhaled insulin. Long-term safety data are awaited before registration approval of the compound will be given.

Intermediate-acting insulins are formulated to dissolve more gradually when administered subcutaneously; thus their durations of action are longer. The two preparations used most frequently are *neutral protamine Hagedorn (NPH) insulin (isophane insulin suspension)* and *lente insulin (insulin zinc suspension)*. NPH insulin is a suspension of insulin in a complex with zinc and protamine in a phosphate buffer. Lente insulin is a mixture of crystallized (ultralente) and amorphous (semilente) insulins in an acetate buffer, which minimizes the solubility of insulin. The pharmacokinetic properties of human intermediate-acting insulins are slightly different from those of porcine preparations. Human insulins have a

more rapid onset and shorter duration of action than do porcine insulins. This difference may be related to the more hydrophobic nature of human insulin, or human and porcine insulins may interact differently with protamine and zinc crystals. This difference may create a problem with optimal timing for evening therapy; human insulin preparations taken before dinner may not have a duration of action sufficient to prevent hyperglycemia by morning. It should be noted that there is no evidence that lente or NPH insulin has different pharmacodynamic effects when used in combination with regular (soluble) insulin in a twice-a-day dosage regimen. Intermediate-acting insulins usually are given either once a day before breakfast or twice a day. In patients with type 2 DM, intermediate-acting insulin given at bedtime may help normalize fasting blood glucose. When lente insulin is mixed with regular insulin, some of the regular insulin may form a complex with the protamine or Zn^{2+} after several hours, and this may slow the absorption of the fast-acting insulin. NPH insulin does not retard the action of regular insulin when the two are mixed vigorously by the patient or when they are available commercially as a mixture (Davis *et al.*, 1991) (*see* below).

Ultralente insulin (extended insulin zinc suspension) and protamine zinc insulin suspension are long-acting insulins; they have a slower onset and a prolonged peak of action. These insulins have been advocated to provide a low basal concentration of insulin throughout the day. The long half-life of ultralente insulin makes it difficult to determine the optimal dosage because several days of treatment are required before a steady-state concentration of circulating insulin is achieved. Doses given once or twice daily are adjusted according to the fasting blood glucose concentration. Protamine zinc insulin is used rarely today because of its very unpredictable and prolonged course of action, and it is no longer available in the United States. Preparations of insulin that are available for clinical use in the United States are shown in Table 60–4.

In the vast majority of patients, insulin-replacement therapy includes intermediate- or long-acting insulin. A search for the ideal intermediate-acting insulin identified *human proinsulin* (HPI) as a promising candidate. Animal studies using *porcine proinsulin* indicated that the compound was a soluble intermediate-acting insulin agonist that had a greater suppressive effect on hepatic glucose production than on stimulation of peripheral glucose disposal. This profile of action appeared favorable for clinical use in diabetic subjects because unrestrained hepatic glucose production is a hallmark of the disease, and a liver-specific insulin would tend to reduce peripheral hyperinsulinemia and the attendant risk of hypoglycemia. Early studies with HPI in human beings confirmed its relatively specific action on hepatocytes and demonstrated that its duration of action was similar to that of NPH insulin. Preliminary results from clinical trials, however, indicated that HPI conferred no additional benefit over currently available human insulins, and all clinical studies soon were suspended because of a high incidence of myocardial infarction in HPI-treated subjects.

The pharmacokinetic limitations of ultralente insulin have prompted efforts to develop an insulin analog that does not have a significant peak in its action. Considerable research has been directed to the development of such a product. Insulin *glargine* (LANTUS) is the first long-acting analog of human insulin to be approved for clinical use in the United States and Europe. Insulin glargine is produced following two alterations of human insulin (Hirsch, 2005). Two arginine residues are added to the C terminus of the B chain, and an asparagine molecule in position A21 on the A chain is

Table 60–4
Insulin Preparations Available in the United States

TYPE	HUMAN	PORCINE
Rapid		
Insulin injection (regular)	R, C	P, S
Lispro	R	—
Aspart	R	—
Glulisine	R	—
Intermediate		
Isophane insulin suspen- sion (NPH)	R	P
Insulin zinc suspension (lente)	R	P
Slow		
Extended insulin zinc sus- pension (ultralente)	R	—
Insulin glargine	R	—
Mixtures		
70% NPH/30% Regular	R	—
50% NPH/50% Regular	R	—
75% Lispro Protamine/ 25% Lispro	R	—
70% Aspart Protamine/ 30% Aspart	R	—

ABBREVIATIONS: S, standard insulins; P, purified insulins; C, concentrated insulin; R, recombinant or semisynthetic human insulins.

replaced with glycine. Glargine is a clear solution with a pH of 4.0. This pH stabilizes the insulin hexamer and results in a prolonged and predictable absorption from subcutaneous tissues. Owing to insulin glargine's acidic pH, it cannot be mixed with currently available short-acting insulin preparations (*i.e.,* regular insulin, aspart, or lispro) that are formulated at a neutral pH. In clinical studies, insulin glargine results in less hypoglycemia, has a sustained "peakless" absorption profile, and provides a better once-daily 24-hour insulin coverage than ultralente or NPH insulin. Glargine may be administered at any time during the day with equivalent efficacy and no difference in the frequency of hypoglycemic episodes. Glargine does not accumulate after several injections. A recent study has demonstrated that duration of action remains at approximately 24 hours and intersubject variability actually improves after seven as compared to one injection.

Insulin glargine can be combined with various oral antihyperglycemic agents (*see* below) to effectively lower plasma glucose levels. Combination of glargine with *sulfonylureas* and/or *metformin* can reduce both fasting (basal) and postprandial glucose levels. It should be noted that the use of a long-acting basal insulin alone will not control postprandial glucose elevations in insulin-deficient type 1 or type 2 DM. Glargine has been shown in clinical studies to normalize fasting (postabsorptive) glucose levels following once-daily administration in patients with type 2 DM.

Rarely, splitting the dose of glargine may be needed in very lean, insulin-sensitive type 1 DM patients in order to achieve good fasting (basal) glucose levels. Unlike traditional insulin preparations that are absorbed more rapidly from the abdomen than from the arm or leg, the site of administration does not influence the time–action profile of glargine. Similarly, exercise does not influence glargine's unique absorption kinetics, even when the insulin is injected into a working limb. Glargine binds with a slightly greater affinity to IGF-1 receptors as compared with human insulin. However, this slightly increased binding is still approximately two log scales lower than that of IGF-1. The deterioration of retinopathy in a few patients with type 2 DM in early clinical studies with glargine led to a concern that it might be involved in the development of retinopathy. However, none of the patients had optic disc swelling, which is pathognomonic of IGF-1 effects, suggesting that the finding was probably due to the well-recognized "glucose reentry phenomenon" that occurs with improvement of glycemic control rather than the insulin *per se.*

Other approaches to prolong the action of soluble insulin analogs are under investigation. One approach is the addition of a saturated fatty acid to the ε amino group of LysB29, yielding a myristoylated insulin called *insulin detemir* (Hirsch, 2005).

When insulin detemir is injected subcutaneously, it binds to albumin *via* its fatty acid chain. Clinical studies in patients with type 1 DM have demonstrated that when insulin detemir is administered twice a day, it has a smoother time–action profile and a reduced prevalence of hypoglycemia as compared with NPH insulin. Additional clinical studies are currently in progress with the aim of submitting insulin detemir for registration in the United States.

The wide variability in the kinetics of insulin action between and even within individuals must be emphasized. The time to peak hypoglycemic effect and insulin levels can vary by 50%. This variability is caused, at least in part, by large variations in the rate of subcutaneous absorption and often has been said to be more noticeable with the intermediate- and long-acting insulins. However, the administration of regular insulin can result in similar variability. When this variability is coupled with normal variations in diet and exercise, it is sometimes surprising how many patients do achieve good control of blood glucose concentrations.

Indications and Goals for Therapy. Subcutaneous administration of insulin is the primary treatment for all patients with type 1 DM, for patients with type 2 DM that is not controlled adequately by diet and/or oral hypoglycemic agents, and for patients with postpancreatectomy diabetes or gestational diabetes (American Diabetes Association, 1999). In addition, insulin is critical for the management of diabetic ketoacidosis, and it has an important role in the treatment of hyperglycemic, nonketotic coma and in the perioperative management of both type 1 and type 2 DM. In all cases, the goal is to normalize not only blood glucose but also all aspects of metabolism; the latter is difficult to achieve. Optimal treatment requires a coordinated approach to diet, exercise, and the administration of insulin. A brief overview of the principles of therapy is given below. (For a more detailed description, *see* LeRoith *et al.,* 2000.)

Near-normoglycemia can be attained in patients with multiple daily doses of insulin or with infusion pump therapy. The goal is to achieve a fasting blood glucose concentration of between 90 and 120 mg/dl (5 to 6.7 mM) and a 2-hour postprandial value below 150 mg/dl (8.3 mM). Goal hemoglobin A_{1C} values should be below 7% and are advocated by some authorities to be below 6.5%. In less disciplined patients, or in those with defective responses of counter-regulatory hormones, it may be necessary to accept higher fasting [*e.g.,* 140 mg/dl (7.8 mM)] and 2-hour postprandial [*e.g.,* 200 to 250 mg/dl (11.1 to 13.9 mM)] blood glucose concentrations.

Daily Requirements. Insulin production by a normal, thin, healthy person is between 18 and 40 units/day or about 0.2 to 0.5 units/kg of body weight per day. About half this amount is secreted in the basal state and about half in response to meals. Thus, basal secretion is about 0.5 to 1 units/h; after an oral glucose load, insulin secretion may increase to 6 units/h. In nondiabetic, obese, and insulin-resistant individuals, insulin secretion may be increased fourfold or more. Insulin is secreted into the portal circulation, and about 50% is destroyed by the liver before reaching the systemic circulation.

In a mixed population of type 1 DM patients, the average dose of insulin is usually 0.6 to 0.7 units/kg body weight per day, with a range of 0.2 to 1 units/kg per day. Obese patients generally require more (about 2 units/kg per day) because of resistance of peripheral tissues to insulin. Patients who require less insulin than 0.5 units/ kg per day may have some endogenous production of insulin or may be more sensitive to the hormone because of good physical conditioning. As in nondiabetics, the daily requirement for insulin can be divided into basal and postprandial needs. The basal dose suppresses lipolysis, proteolysis, and hepatic glucose production; it is usually 40% to 60% of the total daily dose. The dose necessary for disposition of nutrients after meals usually is given before meals. Insulin often has been administered as a single daily dose of intermediate-acting insulin, alone or in combination with regular insulin. This is rarely sufficient to achieve true euglycemia; since hyperglycemia is the major determinant of long-term complications of diabetes, more complex regimens that include combinations of intermediate- or long-acting insulins with regular insulin are used to reach this goal.

A number of commonly used dosage regimens that include mixtures of insulin given in two or three daily injections are depicted in Figure 60–5 (LeRoith *et al.,* 2000). The most frequently used is the so-called split-mixed regimen involving the prebreakfast and presupper injection of a mixture of regular and intermediate-acting insulins (Figure 60–5A). When the presupper NPH or lente insulin is not sufficient to control hyperglycemia throughout the night, the evening dose may be divided into a presupper dose of regular insulin followed by NPH or lente insulin at bedtime (Figure 60–5B). Both normal and diabetic individuals have an increased requirement for insulin in the early morning; this is termed the *dawn phenomenon* and makes the kinetics and timing of the evening dose of insulin extremely important.

An alternative regimen that is gaining widespread use involves multiple daily injections consisting of basal administration of long-acting insulin (*e.g.,* insulin glargine) either before breakfast or at bedtime and preprandial injections of a short-acting insulin (Figure

60–5C). This method is called *basal/bolus* and is very similar to the pattern of insulin administration achieved with a subcutaneous infusion pump (Figure 60–5E). Following the successful demonstration that intensive glycemic control can reduce the risk of micro- and macrovascular complications in patients with type 2 DM, there has been increased interest in using insulin earlier in the treatment of these patients. Data from the UKPDS indicate that 50% of relative β-cell insulin secretory capacity is lost for every 6 years of type 2 DM. This progressive insulin deficiency as type 2 DM progresses makes it increasingly difficult to achieve tight glycemic control (hemoglobin $A_{1C} < 7.0\%$) with oral antihyperglycemic agents. One way to improve control in this setting is to introduce basal-acting insulin in combination with oral hypoglycemic agents. The exact combination of therapies should be guided by the β-cell secretory reserve in each patient. Thus, in an individual with some exogenous insulin secretory capacity (*i.e.,* a measurable circulating C peptide level), combining an oral insulin secretagogue (*see* below) with basal insulin may provide smooth and efficient glycemic control. The addition of a second oral agent, such as an insulin sensitizer (*see* below), either alone or in combination with an oral insulin secretagogue, also may provide good therapeutic results. This combination allows the oral agents to provide postprandial glycemic control while the basal insulin provides the foundation for normalizing fasting or "basal" glucose levels.

In all patients, careful monitoring of therapeutic end points directs the insulin dose used. This approach is facilitated by the use of home glucose monitors and measurements of hemoglobin A_{1c}. Special care must be taken when the patient has other underlying diseases, deficiencies in other endocrine systems (*e.g.,* adrenocortical or pituitary failure), or substantial resistance to insulin.

Factors That Affect Insulin Absorption. The degree of control of plasma glucose may be modified by changes in insulin absorption, factors that alter insulin action, diet, exercise, and other factors. Factors that determine the rate of absorption of insulin after subcutaneous administration include the site of injection, the type of insulin, subcutaneous blood flow, smoking, regional muscular activity at the site of the injection, the volume and concentration of the injected insulin, and depth of injection (insulin has a more rapid onset of action if delivered intramuscularly rather than subcutaneously).

When insulin is injected subcutaneously, there can be an initial "lag phase" followed by a slow but steadily increasing rate of absorption. The initial lag phase almost disappears when a reduced concentration or volume of insulin is injected.

Insulin usually is injected into the subcutaneous tissues of the abdomen, buttock, anterior thigh, or dorsal arm. Absorption is usually most rapid from the abdominal wall, followed by the arm, buttock, and thigh. Rotation of insulin injection sites traditionally has been advocated to avoid lipohypertrophy or lipoatrophy, although these conditions are less likely to occur with highly purified preparations of insulin. If a patient is willing to inject into the abdomen, injections can be rotated

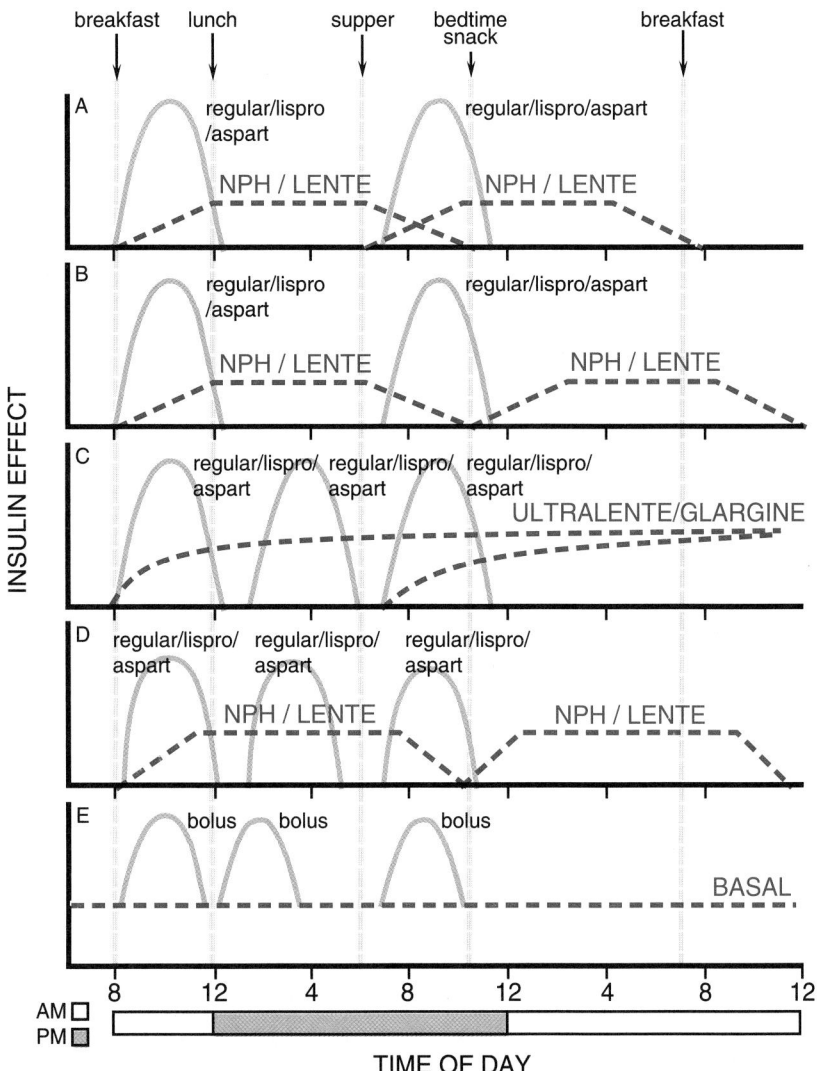

Figure 60–5. ***Common multidose insulin regimens.*** ***A.*** Typical split-mixed regimen consisting of twice-daily injections of a mixture of regular (regular/lispro/aspart) and intermediate-acting (NPH or lente) insulin. ***B.*** A variation in which the evening dose of intermediate-acting insulin is delayed until bedtime to increase the amount of insulin available the next morning. ***C.*** A regimen that incorporates ultralente or glargine insulin. ***D.*** A variation that includes premeal short-acting insulin with intermediate-acting insulin at breakfast and bedtime. ***E.*** Patterns of insulin administration with a regimen of continuous subcutaneous insulin infusion.

throughout the entire area, thereby eliminating the injection site as a cause of variability in the rate of absorption. The abdomen currently is the preferred site of injection in the morning because insulin is absorbed about 20% to 30% faster from that site than from the arm. If the patient refuses to inject into the abdominal area, it is preferable to select a consistent injection site for each component of insulin treatment (*e.g.,* prebreakfast dose into the thigh, evening dose into the arm).

Several other factors may affect the absorption of insulin. In a small group of patients, subcutaneous degradation of insulin has been observed, and this has necessitated the injection of large amounts of insulin for adequate metabolic control. Increased subcutaneous blood flow (brought about by massage, hot baths, or exercise) increases the rate of absorption. In the upright posture, subcutaneous blood flow diminishes considerably in the legs and to a lesser extent in the abdominal wall. An altered volume or concentration of injected insulin affects the rate of absorption and the duration of action. When regular insulin is mixed with lente insulin, some of the regular insulin becomes modified, causing a partial loss of the rapidly acting component. This problem is even more severe if regular insulin is mixed with ultralente insulin. Injections of mixtures of insulin preparations thus should be made without delay. There is less delay in absorption of regular insulin when it is mixed with NPH insulin. Stable, mixed combinations of NPH and regular insulin in proportions of 50:50, 60:40, 70:30, and 80:20, respectively, are available commercially; in the United States, only the 70:30 and 50:50 combinations are available. Combinations of lispro protamine-Lispro (75/25, HUMALOG MIX) and aspart protamine-aspart (70/30, NOVOLOG MIX) are also available in the United States (Table 60–4). "Pen devices" containing prefilled regular, lispro, NPH, glargine, or premixed regular-NPH, lispro protamine-lispro, or apsart protamine-aspart combinations have proven to be popular with many diabetic patients.

Jet injector systems that enable patients to receive subcutaneous insulin "injections" without a needle are available. These devices are rather expensive and cumbersome but are preferred by some patients. Dispersal of insulin throughout an area of subcutaneous tissue theoretically should increase the rate of absorption of both regular and intermediate-acting insulins; however, this result has not always been observed.

Subcutaneous insulin administration results in anti-insulin IgG antibody formation. Older, impure preparations of animal insulins were far more antigenic than the more recent purified porcine and recombinant human preparations. It is disputed whether chronic therapy with human insulin reduces antibody production compared with monocomponent porcine insulin. Regardless, it is clear that human insulin is immunogenic. In the vast majority of patients receiving insulin treatment, circulating anti-insulin antibodies do not alter the pharmacokinetics of the injected hormone.

In rare patients who have a high titers of anti-insulin antibodies, the kinetics of action of regular insulin may resemble those of an intermediate-acting insulin, which itself may become longer acting. Such effects could lead to increased postprandial hyperglycemia (owing to decreased action of regular insulin) but nighttime hypoglycemia (owing to the prolonged action of intermediate insulin).

IgG antibodies can cross the placenta, raising the possibility that anti-insulin antibodies could cause fetal hyperglycemia by neutralizing fetal insulin. On the other hand, fetal or neonatal hypoglycemia could result from the undesirable and unpredictable release of insulin from insulin–antibody complexes. Switching from bovine/porcine to monocomponent insulin preparations has been shown to reduce anti-insulin antibodies, leading to the recommendation that only human insulin be used during pregnancy.

Continuous Subcutaneous Insulin Infusion. A number of pumps are available for continuous subcutaneous

insulin infusion (CSII) therapy. CSII, or "pump," therapy is not suitable for all patients because it demands considerable attention, especially during the initial phases of treatment. However, for patients interested in intensive insulin therapy, a pump may be an attractive alternative to several daily injections. Most modern pumps provide a constant basal infusion of insulin and have the option of different infusion rates during the day and night to help avoid the dawn phenomenon and bolus injections that are programmed according to the size and nature of a meal.

Pump therapy presents some unique problems. Since all the insulin used is short acting and there is a minimal amount of insulin in the subcutaneous pool at any given time, insulin deficiency and ketoacidosis may develop rapidly if therapy is interrupted accidentally. Although modern pumps have warning devices that detect changes in line pressure, mechanical problems such as pump failure, dislodgement of the needle, aggregation of insulin in the infusion line, or accidental kinking of the infusion catheter may occur. There also is a possibility of subcutaneous abscesses and cellulitis. Selection of the most appropriate patients is extremely important for success with pump therapy. Offsetting these potential problems, pump therapy is capable of producing a more physiological profile of insulin replacement during exercise (where insulin production is decreased) and therefore less hypoglycemia than do traditional subcutaneous insulin injections.

Adverse Reactions. *Hypoglycemia.* The most common adverse reaction to insulin is hypoglycemia. This may result from an inappropriately large dose, from a mismatch between the time of peak delivery of insulin and food intake, or from superimposition of additional factors that increase sensitivity to insulin (*e.g.,* adrenal or pituitary insufficiency) or that increase insulin-independent glucose uptake (*e.g.,* exercise). The more vigorous the attempt to achieve euglycemia, the more frequent are the episodes of hypoglycemia. In the DCCT, the incidence of severe hypoglycemic reactions was three times higher in the intensive insulin therapy group than in the conventional therapy group (DCCT Research Group, 1993). Milder but significant hypoglycemic episodes were much more common than were severe reactions, and their frequency also increased with intensive therapy. Hypoglycemia is the major risk that always must be weighed against benefits of intensive therapy.

There is a hierarchy of physiological responses to hypoglycemia. The first response is a reduction of endogenous insulin secretion, which occurs at a plasma glucose level of about 70 mg/dl (3.9 mM); thereafter, the counter-regulatory hormones—epinephrine, glucagon, growth hormone, cortisol, and norepinephrine—are released. Symptoms of hypoglycemia are first discerned at a plasma glucose level of 60 to 80 mg/dl (3.3 to 4.4 mM). Sweating, hunger, paresthesias, palpitations, tremor, and anxiety, principally of autonomic origin, usually are seen first. Difficulty in concentrating, confusion, weakness, drowsiness, a feeling of warmth, dizziness, blurred vision, and loss of consciousness (*i.e.,* the *neuroglycopenic symptoms*) usually occur at lower plasma glucose levels than do autonomic symptoms. In a normal individual, plasma glucose levels are tightly regulated, and it is only under rare conditions that hypoglycemia occurs.

Glucagon and epinephrine are the predominant counter-regulatory hormones in acute hypoglycemia in newly diagnosed type 1 DM patients and normal subjects. In patients with type 1 DM of longer duration, the glucagon secretory response to hypoglycemia becomes deficient, but effective glucose counter-regulation still occurs because epinephrine plays a compensatory role. Patients with type 1 DM thus become dependent on epinephrine for counter-regulation, and if this mechanism becomes deficient, the incidence of severe hypoglycemia increases. This occurs in patients with diabetes of long duration who have autonomic neuropathy. The absence of both glucagon and epinephrine can lead to prolonged hypoglycemia, particularly during the night, when some individuals can have extremely low plasma glucose levels for several hours. Severe hypoglycemia can lead to convulsions and coma.

In addition to autonomic neuropathy, several related syndromes of defective counter-regulation contribute to the increased incidence of severe hypoglycemia in intensively treated type 1 DM patients. These include hypoglycemic unawareness, altered thresholds for release of counter-regulatory hormones, and deficient secretion of counter-regulatory hormones (reviewed by Cryer 1993).

With the ready availability of home glucose monitoring, hypoglycemia can be documented in most patients who experience suggestive symptoms. Hypoglycemia that occurs during sleep may be difficult to detect but should be suspected from a history of morning headaches, night sweats, or symptoms of hypothermia. Nocturnal hypoglycemia has been proposed as a cause of morning hyperglycemia in type 1 DM patients. This syndrome, known as the *Somogyi phenomenon,* was reputedly due to an elevation of counter-regulatory hormones in response to nocturnal hypoglycemia, but several groups of investigators have been unable to reproduce it. Moreover, neuroendocrine counter-regulatory responses are severely diminished with disease duration and intensive control. Therefore, it is unlikely that in patients

with reduced neuroendocrine responses to hypoglycemia, nocturnal counter-regulatory responses to hypoglycemia could be responsible for morning hyperglycemia. The practice of reducing nighttime insulin doses in type 1 DM subjects with morning hyperglycemia thus cannot now be recommended. Rather, the current recommended therapeutic approach to treating morning hyperglycemia is to administer more long- or intermediate-acting insulin the night before, perhaps at bedtime, or to increase the basal rate of a CSII pump between the hours of 3 and 7 A.M.

All diabetic patients who receive insulin should be aware of the symptoms of hypoglycemia, carry some form of easily ingested glucose, and carry an identification card or bracelet containing pertinent medical information. When possible, patients who suspect that they are experiencing hypoglycemia should document the glucose concentration with a measurement. Mild-to-moderate hypoglycemia may be treated simply by ingestion of glucose. When hypoglycemia is severe, it should be treated with intravenous glucose or an injection of glucagon (*see* below).

Insulin Allergy and Resistance. Although there has been a dramatic decrease in the incidence of resistance and allergic reactions to insulin with the use of recombinant human insulin or highly purified preparations of the hormone, these reactions still occur as a result of reactions to the small amounts of aggregated or denatured insulin in all preparations, to minor contaminants, or because of sensitivity to one of the components added to insulin in its formulation (protamine, Zn^{2+}, phenol, *etc.*). The most frequent allergic manifestations are IgE-mediated local cutaneous reactions, although on rare occasions patients may develop life-threatening systemic responses or insulin resistance owing to IgG antibodies. Attempts should be made to identify the underlying cause of the hypersensitivity response by measuring insulin-specific IgG and IgE antibodies. Skin testing also is useful; however, many patients exhibit positive reactions to intradermal insulin without experiencing any adverse effects from subcutaneous insulin. If patients have allergic reactions to porcine insulin, human insulin should be used. If allergy persists, desensitization may be attempted; it is successful in about 50% of cases. Antihistamines may provide relief in patients with cutaneous reactions, whereas glucocorticoids have been used in patients with resistance to insulin or more severe systemic reactions.

Lipoatrophy and Lipohypertrophy. Atrophy of subcutaneous fat at the site of insulin injection (lipoatrophy) is probably a variant of an immune response to insulin, whereas lipohypertrophy (enlargement of subcutaneous fat depots) has been ascribed to the lipogenic action of high local concentrations of insulin (LeRoith *et al.,* 2000). Both problems may be related to some contaminant in insulin and are rare with more purified preparations. However, hypertrophy occurs frequently with human insulins if patients inject themselves repeatedly in the same site. When these problems occur, they may cause irregular absorption of insulin, as well as a cosmetic problem. The recommended treatment is to avoid the hypertrophic areas by using other injection sites and to inject insulin into the periphery of the atrophic sites in an attempt to restore the subcutaneous adipose tissue.

Insulin Edema. Some degree of edema, abdominal bloating, and blurred vision develops in many diabetic patients with severe hyperglycemia or ketoacidosis that is brought under control with insulin. This is associated with a weight gain of 0.5 to 2.5 kg. The edema usually disappears spontaneously within several days to a week unless there is underlying cardiac or renal disease. Edema is attributed primarily to retention of Na^+, although increased capillary permeability associated with inadequate metabolic control also may contribute.

Insulin Treatment of Ketoacidosis and Other Special Situations.

Acutely ill diabetic patients may have metabolic disturbances that are sufficiently severe or labile to justify intravenous administration of insulin. Such treatment is most appropriate in patients with ketoacidosis. Although there has been some controversy over appropriate dosage, infusion of a relatively low dose of insulin (0.1 units/kg per hour) will produce plasma concentrations of insulin of about 100 μunits/ml—a level sufficient to inhibit lipolysis and gluconeogenesis completely and to produce near-maximal stimulation of glucose uptake in normal individuals. In most patients with diabetic ketoacidosis, blood glucose concentrations will fall by about 10% per hour; the acidosis is corrected more slowly. As treatment proceeds, it often is necessary to administer glucose along with the insulin to prevent hypoglycemia but to allow clearance of all ketones. Some physicians prefer to initiate therapy with a loading dose of insulin, but this tactic appears unnecessary because steady-state concentrations of the hormone are achieved within 30 minutes with a constant infusion. Patients with nonketotic hyperglycemic coma typically are more sensitive to insulin than are those with ketoacidosis. Appropriate replacement of fluid and electrolytes is an integral part of the therapy in both situations because there is always a major deficit. Regardless of the exact insulin regimen, the key to effective therapy is careful and frequent monitoring of the patient's clinical status, glucose, and electrolytes. A frequent error in the management of such patients is the failure to administer insulin subcutaneously at least 30 minutes before intravenous therapy is discontinued. This is necessary because of the very short half-life of insulin.

Intravenous administration of insulin also is well suited to the treatment of diabetic patients during the perioperative period and during childbirth (Jacober and Sower, 1999). There is debate, however, about the optimal route of insulin administration during surgery. Although some clinicians advocate subcutaneous insulin administration, most recommend intravenous insulin infusion. The two most widely used protocols for intravenous insulin administration are the variable-rate regimen and the glucose–insulin–potassium (GIK) infusion method (*see* LeRoith *et al.,* 2000). Both protocols provide stable plasma glucose, fluid, and electrolyte levels during the operative and postoperative period. Despite this, many physicians give patients half their normal daily dose of insulin as intermediate-acting insulin subcutaneously on the morning of an operation and then administer 5% dextrose infusions during surgery to maintain glucose concentrations. This approach provides less minute-to-minute control than is possible with intravenous regimens and also may increase the likelihood of hypogly-

cemia. Newer subcutaneously administered basal and rapid-acting analogs may provide smoother glycemic control without the drawback of hypoglycemia. Recent multicenter trials have demonstrated dramatic improvement in patient outcome, including significant reductions in mortality, when intensive insulin regimens (predominantly intravenous) have been used to reduce glycemia after myocardial infarction or surgery (Malmberg *et al.,* 1995; Davies and Lawrence, 2002; van den Berghe *et al.,* 2001; van den Berghe 2004).

Drug Interactions and Glucose Metabolism. A large number of drugs can cause hypoglycemia or hyperglycemia or may alter the response of diabetic patients to their existing therapeutic regimens. Some drugs with hypoglycemic or hyperglycemic effects and their presumed sites of action are listed in Table 60–5.

Aside from insulin and oral hypoglycemic drugs, the most common drug-induced hypoglycemic states are those caused by *ethanol, β adrenergic receptor antagonists,* and *salicylates.* The primary action of ethanol is to inhibit gluconeogenesis. This is not an idiosyncratic reaction but is observed in all individuals. In diabetic patients, β adrenergic receptor antagonists pose a risk of hypoglycemia because of their capacity to inhibit the effects of catecholamines on gluconeogenesis and glycogenolysis. These agents also may mask the sympathetically mediated symptoms associated with the fall in blood glucose (*e.g.,* tremor and palpitations). Salicylates, on the other hand, exert their hypoglycemic effect by enhancing pancreatic β-cell sensitivity to glucose and potentiating insulin secretion. These agents also have a weak insulinlike action in the periphery. *Pentamidine,* an antiprotozoal agent used for the treatment of infections caused by *Pneumocystis carinii,* apparently can cause both hypoglycemia and hyperglycemia. The hypoglycemic effect results from destruction of β cells and release of insulin; continued use may cause secondary hypoinsulinemia and hyperglycemia. A number of drugs have no direct hypoglycemic action but may potentiate the actions of sulfonylureas (*see* below).

An equally large number of drugs may cause hyperglycemia in normal individuals or impair metabolic control in diabetic patients. Many of these agents have direct effects on peripheral tissues that counter the actions of insulin; examples include epinephrine, glucocorticoids, atypical antipsychotic drugs such as *clozapine* and *olanzapine,* and drugs used in highly active antiretroviral therapy (HAART) of HIV-1 infection (especially the protease inhibitors). Other drugs cause hyperglycemia by inhibiting insulin secretion directly (*e.g.,* phenytoin, clonidine, and Ca^{2+}-channel blockers) or indirectly *via* depletion of K^+ (diuretics). It is important to be aware of such interactions and to modify treatment regimens for diabetic patients accordingly.

New Forms of Insulin Therapy. There are a number of experimental approaches to insulin delivery, including the use of new insulins, new routes of administration, intraperitoneal delivery devices, implantable pellets, the closed-loop artificial pancreas, islet cell and pancreatic transplantation, and gene therapy.

New Routes of Delivery. Attempts have been made to administer insulin orally, nasally, rectally, by inhalation, and by subcutaneous implantation of pellets. The most promising of these alternatives is by inhalation, which can be achieved by addition of various adjuvants such as *mannitol, glycine,* and *sodium citrate* to insulin to increase its absorption through the pulmonary mucosa (Skyler *et al.,* 2001; Cefalu *et al.,* 2001). Absorption is rapid and approaches the

Table 60–5
Some Drugs That Cause Hypoglycemia or Hyperglycemia

DRUG	POSSIBLE SITE OF ACTION			
	Pancreas	Liver	Periphery	Other
Drugs with Hypoglycemic Effects				
β Adrenergic receptor antagonists		+	+	+
Salicylates	+			
Indomethacin*				
Naproxen*				
Ethanol		+		+
Clofibrate			+	
Angiotensin-converting enzyme inhibitors			+	
Li^+		+	+	
Theophylline	+			
Ca^{2+}	+			
Bromocriptine			+	
Mebendazole	+			
Sulfonamides				+
Sulbactam–ampicillin*				
Tetracycline*				
Pyridoxine		+		
Pentamidine†	+			
Drugs with Hyperglycemic Effects				
Epinephrine	+	+	+	
Glucocorticoids		+	+	
Diuretics	+		+	
Atypical antipsychotics‡			+	+
HIV-1 protease inhibitors§				
Diazoxide	+			
$β_2$ Adrenergic receptor agonists	+	+	+	
Ca^{2+}-channel blockers	+			
Phenytoin	+			
Clonidine	+			+
H_2-receptor blockers	+			
Pentamidine†				+
Morphine	+			
Heparin				+
Nalidixic acid				?
Sulfinpyrazone*				
Marijuana				+
Nicotine*				

*Although these drugs are reported to have an effect on control of diabetes, there are no conclusive data about their effects on carbohydrate metabolism. †Short-term effect is insulin release and hypoglycemia. ‡Atypical antipsychotics: clozapine, olanzapine, risperidone. §HIV-1 protease inhibitors: ritonavir, lopinavir, aprenavir, nelfinavir, indinavir, saquinavir. SOURCE: Adapted from Koffler *et al.*, 1989, with permission.

rate achieved with subcutaneous administration of regular insulin. Further work is under way with the aim of reducing the size and increasing the convenience of the inhaled delivery systems. Implantable pellets have been designed to release insulin slowly over days or weeks. Although oral delivery of insulin would be preferred by patients and would provide higher relative concentrations of insulin in the portal circulation, attempts to increase intestinal absorption of the hormone have met with only limited success. Efforts have focused on protection of insulin by encapsulation or incorporation into liposomes. Intraperitoneal infusion of insulin into the portal circulation has been used experimentally in human subjects for periods of several months.

Transplantation and Gene Therapy. Transplantation and gene therapy are provocative approaches to insulin replacement. Segmental pancreatic transplantation has been employed successfully in hundreds of patients (Sutherland *et al.*, 2004). However, the surgery is technically complex and usually is considered only in patients with advanced disease and complications. The best-documented benefits have been in patients who also require a kidney transplant for diabetic nephropathy. Islet cell transplants theoretically are less complicated. Successful protocols for islet cell transplants were based on advances in islet preparation and a novel glucocorticoid-free immunosuppressive regimen (Robertson, 2004). The precise role of islet cell transplantation is debated, and the supply of available islet preparations remains very limited. In rodents, gene therapy using transcription factors that regulate β-cell function has been used to transdifferentiate hepatocytes into a functional endocrine pancreas, eliminating the need for insulin therapy for months in experimental models of diabetes mellitus (Meivar-Levy and Ferber, 2004).

ORAL HYPOGLYCEMIC AGENTS

History. In contrast to the systematic studies that led to the isolation of insulin, the *sulfonylureas* were discovered accidentally. In 1942, Janbon and colleagues noted that some sulfonamides caused hypoglycemia in experimental animals. Soon thereafter, *1-butyl-3-sulfonylurea (carbutamide)* became the first clinically useful sulfonylurea for the treatment of diabetes. Although later withdrawn because of adverse effects on the bone marrow, this compound led to the development of the entire class of sulfonylureas. Clinical trials of *tolbutamide,* the first widely used member of this group, were instituted in patients with type 2 DM in the early 1950s. Since that time, approximately 20 different agents of this class have been in use worldwide.

In 1997, *repaglinide,* the first member of a new class of oral insulin secretagogues called *meglitinides* (benzoic acid derivatives), was approved for clinical use; this agent has gained acceptance as a fast-acting premeal therapy to limit postprandial hyperglycemia.

The goat's rue plant (*Galega officinalis*), used to treat diabetes in Europe in medieval times, was found in the early twentieth century to contain *guanidine.* Guanidine has hypoglycemic properties but was too toxic for clinical use. During the 1920s, *biguanides* were investigated for use in diabetes, but they were overshadowed by the discovery of insulin. Later, the antimalarial agent *chloroguanide* was found to have weak hypoglycemic action. Shortly after the introduction of the sulfonylureas, the first

biguanides became available for clinical use. However, *phenformin*, the primary drug in this group, was withdrawn from the market in the United States and Europe because of an increased frequency of lactic acidosis associated with its use. Another biguanide, metformin, has been used extensively in Europe without significant adverse effects and was approved for use in the United States in 1995.

Thiazolidinediones were introduced in 1997 as the second major class of "insulin sensitizers." These agents bind to peroxisome proliferator–activated receptors (principally PPARγ), resulting in increased glucose uptake in muscle and reduced endogenous glucose production. The first of these agents, *troglitazone,* was withdrawn from use in the United States in 2000 because of an association with hepatic toxicity. Two other agents of this class, *rosiglitazone* and *pioglitazone,* have not been associated with widespread liver toxicity and are used worldwide.

Sulfonylureas

Chemistry. The sulfonylureas are divided into two groups or generations of agents. Their structural relationships are shown in Table 60–6. All members of this class of drugs are substituted arylsulfonylureas. They differ by substitutions at the *para* position on the benzene ring and at one nitrogen residue of the urea moiety. The first group of sulfonylureas includes tolbutamide, *acetohexamide, tolazamide,* and *chlorpropamide.* A second, more potent generation of hypoglycemic sulfonylureas has emerged, including *glyburide (glibenclamide), glipizide, gliclazide,* and *glimepiride.*

Mechanism of Action. Sulfonylureas cause hypoglycemia by stimulating insulin release from pancreatic β cells. Their effects in the treatment of diabetes, however, are more complex. The acute administration of sulfonylureas to type 2 DM patients increases insulin release from the pancreas. Sulfonylureas also may further increase insulin levels by reducing hepatic clearance of the hormone. In the initial months of sulfonylurea treatment, fasting plasma insulin levels and insulin responses to oral glucose challenges are increased. With chronic administration, circulating insulin levels decline to those that existed before treatment, but despite this reduction in insulin levels, reduced plasma glucose levels are maintained. The explanation for this is not clear, but it may relate to reduced plasma glucose allowing circulating insulin to have more pronounced effects on its target tissues and to the fact that chronic hyperglycemia *per se* impairs insulin secretion (glucose toxicity).

The absence of acute stimulatory effects of sulfonylureas on insulin secretion during chronic treatment is attributed to down-regulation of cell surface receptors for sulfonylureas on the pancreatic β cell. If chronic sulfonylurea therapy is discontinued, pancreatic β-cell response to acute administration of the drug is restored. Sulfonylureas also stimulate release of somatostatin, and they may suppress the secretion of glucagon slightly.

Table 60–6
Structural Formulas of the Sulfonylureas

GENERAL FORMULA:

First-Generation Agents	R_1	R_2
Tolbutamide (ORINASE, others)	H_3C-	$-C_4H_9$
Chlorpropamide (DIABINESE, others)	$Cl-$	$-C_3H_7$
Tolazamide (TOLINASE, others)	H_3C-	(azepane ring)
Acetohexamide (DYMELOR, others)	H_3CCO-	(cyclohexyl ring)

Second-Generation Agents	R_1	R_2
Glyburide (Glibenclamide, MICRONASE, DIABETA, others)	$-CONH(CH_2)_2-$ (chloro-, methoxy-substituted phenyl)	(cyclohexyl ring)
Glipizide (GLUCOTROL, others)	H_3C- pyrazine $-CONH(CH_2)_2-$	(cyclohexyl ring)
Gliclazide (DIAMICRON, others; unavailable in the U.S.)	H_3C-	(bicyclic N ring)
Glimepiride (AMARYL)	pyrroline ring $-CONH-CH_2-CH_2-$	(methylcyclohexyl ring)

Sulfonylureas bind to the SUR1 subunits and block the ATP-sensitive K^+ channel (Aguilar-Bryan *et al.*, 1995; Philipson and Steiner, 1995). The drugs thus resemble physiological secretagogues (*e.g.*, glucose, leucine), which also lower the conductance of this channel. Reduced K^+ conductance causes membrane depolarization and influx of Ca^{2+} through voltage-sensitive Ca^{2+} channels.

There has been controversy about whether or not sulfonylureas have clinically significant extrapancreatic effects. In general, attempts to ascribe the long-term blood glucose-lowering effects of sulfonylureas to specific changes in insulin action on target tissues are confounded by the effects of a lower prevailing blood glucose level. Although extrapancreatic effects of sulfonylureas can be demonstrated, they are of minor clinical significance in the treatment of type 2 DM patients.

Absorption, Fate, and Excretion. The sulfonylureas have similar spectra of activities; thus their pharmacokinetic properties are their most distinctive characteristics (*see* Appendix II). Although the rates of absorption of the different sulfonylureas vary, all are effectively absorbed from the gastrointestinal tract. However, food and hyperglycemia can reduce the absorption of sulfonylureas. Hyperglycemia *per se* inhibits gastric and intestinal motility and thus can retard the absorption of many drugs. In view of the time required to reach an optimal concentration in plasma, sulfonylureas with short half-lives may be more effective when given 30 minutes before eating. Sulfonylureas in plasma are largely (90% to 99%) bound to protein, especially albumin; plasma protein binding is least for chlorpropamide and greatest for glyburide. The volumes of distribution of most of the sulfonylureas are about 0.2 L/kg.

The first-generation sulfonylureas vary considerably in their half-lives and extents of metabolism. The half-life of acetohexamide is short, but the drug is reduced to an active compound whose half-life is similar to those of tolbutamide and tolazamide (4 to 7 hours). It may be necessary to take these drugs in divided daily doses. Chlorpropamide has a long half-life (24 to 48 hours). The second-generation agents are approximately 100 times more potent than are those in the first group. Although their half-lives are short (3 to 5 hours), their hypoglycemic effects are evident for 12 to 24 hours, and they often can be administered once daily. The reason for the discrepancies between their half-lives and duration of action is not clear.

All the sulfonylureas are metabolized by the liver, and the metabolites are excreted in the urine. Metabolism of chlorpropamide is incomplete, and about 20% of the drug is excreted unchanged. Thus sulfonylureas should be administered with caution to patients with either renal or hepatic insufficiency.

Adverse Reactions. Adverse effects of the sulfonylureas are infrequent, occurring in about 4% of patients taking first-generation drugs and perhaps slightly less often in patients receiving second-generation agents. Not unexpectedly, sulfonylureas may cause hypoglycemic reactions, including coma. This is a particular problem in elderly patients with impaired hepatic or renal function who are taking longer-acting sulfonylureas. Sulfonylureas can be ranked in order of decreasing risk of causing hypoglycemia. It used to be thought that longer-acting sulfonylureas resulted in a greater prevalence of hypoglycemia. That is certainly the case when comparing the older preparations such as chlorpropamide (long acting) against tolbutamide (short acting). However, more recent second-generation sulfonylureas have very differing incidences of causing hypoglycemia despite similar half-lives. Thus glyburide (glibenclamide) has been reported to result in hypoglycemia in up to 20% to 30% of users, whereas another long-acting sulfonylurea, glimepiride, results in hypoglycemia in only 2% to 4% of users. A modified long-acting version of glipizide also results in a lower hypoglycemia frequency relative to gliburide.

Recent studies have provided an insight into the physiological basis for the differing rates of hypoglycemia occurring with these long-acting sulfonylureas. As described earlier for insulin, the ability of the body to inhibit endogenous insulin secretion is central to the homeostatic defense against hypoglycemia. This glucose-dependent inhibition of insulin secretion during hypoglycemia occurs with glimepiride but not with glyburide. Additionally, the major anti-insulin counter-regulatory hormone glucagon appears to be reduced by glyburide during hypoglycemia but is preserved during glimepiride therapy.

Severe hypoglycemia in the elderly can present as an acute neurological emergency that may mimic a cerebrovascular accident. Thus, it is important to check the plasma glucose level of any elderly patient presenting with acute neurological symptoms. Because of the long half-life of some sulfonylureas, it may be necessary to treat elderly hypoglycemic patients for 24 to 48 hours with an intravenous glucose infusion.

Many other drugs may potentiate the effects of the sulfonylureas, particularly the first-generation agents, by inhibiting their metabolism or excretion. Some drugs also displace the sulfonylureas from binding proteins, thereby transiently increasing the free concentration. These include other sulfonamides, *clofibrate,* and salicylates. Other drugs, especially ethanol, may enhance the action of sulfonylureas by causing hypoglycemia.

Other side effects of sulfonylureas include nausea and vomiting, cholestatic jaundice, agranulocytosis, aplastic and hemolytic anemias, generalized hypersensitivity reactions, and dermatological reactions. About 10% to 15% of patients who receive these drugs, particularly chlorpropamide, develop an alcohol-induced flush similar to that caused by *disulfiram* (*see* Chapter 23). Sulfonylureas, especially chlorpropamide, also may induce hyponatremia by potentiating the effects of antidiuretic hormone on the renal collecting duct (*see* Chapter 29). This undesirable side effect occurs in up to 5% of all patients; it is less frequent with glyburide, glipizide, and glimepiride. This effect on water retention has been used to therapeutic advantage in patients with mild forms of central diabetes insipidus.

A long-running debate centered on whether treatment with sulfonylureas is associated with increased cardiovascular mortality; this possibility was suggested by a large multicenter trial [the University Group Diabetes Program (UGDP)]. The UGDP was designed to compare the effect of diet, oral agents (tolbutamide or phenformin), and fixed-dose insulin therapy on the development of vascular complications in type 2 DM. During an 8-year period of observation, patients who received tolbutamide had a twofold higher rate of cardiovascular death than patients treated with placebo or insulin (Meinert *et al.*, 1970). A 10-year debate followed on the validity of this conclusion because the observation was unexpected, the study had not been designed to test this question, and all the excess mortality occurred in only three centers. The recent UKPDS (U.K. Prospective Diabetes Study Group, 1998a) clearly demonstrated no excess cardiovascular mortality over a 14-year period in patients receiving first- or second-generation sulfonylureas. It is worth noting that some of the newer sulfonylurea agents may confer even greater cardiovascular benefits compared with earlier second-generation compounds. Glimepiride, the most recent sulfonylurea, exerts beneficial effects with regard to ischemic preconditioning as compared with glyburide. The physiological response to an ischemic event in the coronary vasculature is a reflex vasodilation to a subsequent ischemic episode. This reflex appears to be preserved with glimepiride but reduced with glyburide.

Therapeutic Uses. Sulfonylureas are used to control hyperglycemia in type 2 DM patients who cannot achieve appropriate control with changes in diet alone. In all patients, continued dietary restrictions are essential to maximize the efficacy of the sulfonylureas. Contraindications to the use of these drugs include type 1 DM, pregnancy, lactation, and for the older preparations, significant hepatic or renal insufficiency.

Between 50% and 80% of properly selected patients will respond initially to an oral hypoglycemic agent. All the drugs appear to be equally efficacious. Concentrations of glucose often are lowered sufficiently to relieve symptoms of hyperglycemia but may not reach normal levels. To the extent that complications of diabetes are related to hyperglycemia, the goal of treatment should be normalization of both fasting and postprandial glucose concentrations. About 5% to 10% of patients per year who respond initially to a sulfonylurea become secondary failures, as defined by unacceptable levels of hyperglycemia. This may occur as a result

of a change in drug metabolism, progression of β-cell failure, change in dietary compliance, or misdiagnosis of a patient with slow-onset type 1 DM. Additional oral agent(s) can produce a satisfactory response, but most of these patients eventually will require insulin.

The usual initial daily dose of tolbutamide is 500 mg, and 3000 mg is the maximally effective total dose. Tolazamide and chlorpropamide usually are initiated in a daily dose of 100 to 250 mg, with maximal doses of 1000 (tolazamide) or 750 mg (chlorpropamide). Tolbutamide and tolazamide often are taken twice daily 30 minutes before breakfast and dinner. The initial daily dose of glyburide is 2.5 to 5 mg, and daily doses of more than 20 mg are not recommended. Therapy with glipizide usually is initiated with 5 mg given once daily. The maximal recommended daily dose is 40 mg; daily doses of more than 15 mg should be divided. The starting dose of gliclazide is 40 to 80 mg/day, and the maximal daily dose is 320 mg. Glimepiride therapy can begin with doses as low as 0.5 mg once per day. The maximal effective daily dose of the agent is 8 mg. Treatment with the sulfonylureas must be guided by the patient's response, which must be monitored frequently.

Combinations of insulin and sulfonylureas have been used in some patients with type 1 and type 2 DM. Studies in type 1 DM patients have provided no evidence that glucose control is improved by combination therapy. The results in type 2 DM patients have shown significant improvements in metabolic control. A prerequisite for a beneficial effect of combination therapy is residual β-cell activity; a short duration of diabetes also may predict a good response.

Repaglinide

Repaglinide (PRANDIN) is an oral insulin secretagogue of the meglitinide class. This agent is a derivative of benzoic acid, and its structure (shown below) is unrelated to that of the sulfonylureas.

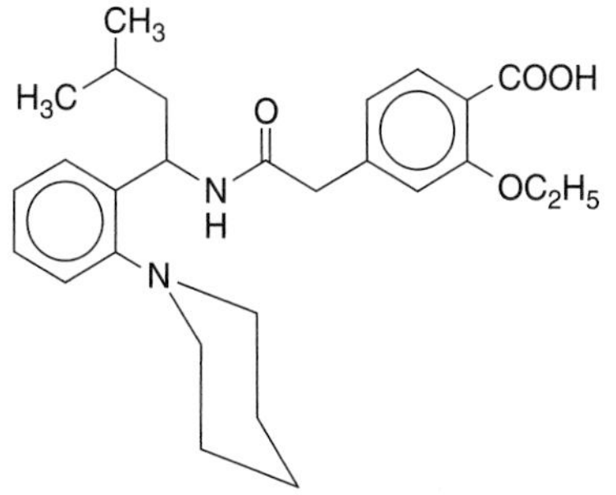

REPAGLINIDE

Like sulfonylureas, repaglinide stimulates insulin release by closing ATP-dependent potassium channels in pancreatic β cells. The drug is absorbed rapidly from the gastrointestinal tract, and peak blood levels are obtained within 1 hour. The half-life of the drug is about 1 hour. These features of the drug allow for multiple preprandial use as compared with the classical once- or twice-daily dosing of sulfonylureas. Repaglinide is metabolized primarily by the liver to inactive derivatives. Repaglinide should be used cautiously in patients with hepatic insufficiency. Because a small proportion (about 10%) of repaglinide is metabolized by the kidney, increased dosing of the drug in patients with renal insufficiency also should be performed cautiously. As with sulfonylureas, the major side effect of repaglinide is hypoglycemia.

Nateglinide

Nateglinide (STARLIX) is an orally effective insulin secretagogue derived from D-phenylalanine. Like sulfonylureas and repaglinide, nateglinide stimulates insulin secretion by blocking ATP-sensitive potassium channels in pancreatic β cells. Nateglinide promotes a more rapid but less sustained secretion of insulin than do other available oral antidiabetic agents (Kalbag *et al.*, 2001). The drug's major therapeutic effect is reducing postprandial glycemic elevations in type 2 DM patients. Nateglinide is approved by the FDA for use in type 2 DM and is most effective if administered in a dose of 120 mg 1 to 10 minutes before a meal. Nateglinide is metabolized primarily by the liver and thus should be used cautiously in patients with hepatic insufficiency. About 16% of an administered dose is excreted by the kidney as unchanged drug. Dosage adjustment is unnecessary in renal failure. Nateglinide therapy may produce fewer episodes of hypoglycemia than most other currently available oral insulin secretagogues including repaglinide (Horton *et al.*, 2001).

Biguanides

Metformin (GLUCOPHAGE, others) and phenformin were introduced in 1957, and *buformin* was introduced in 1958. The latter was of limited use, but metformin and phenformin were used widely. Phenformin was withdrawn in many countries during the 1970s because of an association with lactic acidosis. Metformin has been associated only rarely with that complication and has been used widely in Europe and Canada; it became available in the United States in 1995. Metformin given alone or in combination with a sulfonylurea improves glycemic control and lipid concentrations in patients who respond poorly to diet or to a sulfonylurea alone (DeFronzo *et al.*, 1995).

Mechanism of Action. Metformin is antihyperglycemic, not hypoglycemic (*see* Bailey, 1992). It does not cause insulin release from the pancreas and generally does not cause hypoglycemia,

even in large doses. Metformin has no significant effects on the secretion of glucagon, cortisol, growth hormone, or somatostatin. Metformin reduces glucose levels primarily by decreasing hepatic glucose production and by increasing insulin action in muscle and fat. At a molecular level, these actions are mediated at least in part by activation of the cellular kinase AMP-activated protein kinase (AMP kinase) (*see* below and Zhou *et al.*, 2001). The mechanism by which metformin reduces hepatic glucose production is controversial, but most data indicate an effect on reducing gluconeogenesis (Stumvoll *et al.*, 1995). Metformin also may decrease plasma glucose by reducing the absorption of glucose from the intestine, but this action has not been shown to have clinical relevance.

Absorption, Excretion, and Dosing. Metformin is absorbed mainly from the small intestine. The drug is stable, does not bind to plasma proteins, and is excreted unchanged in the urine. It has a half-life of about 2 hours. The maximum recommended daily dose of metformin in the United States is 2.5 g given in three doses with meals.

Precautions and Adverse Effects. Patients with renal impairment should not receive metformin. Other contraindications include hepatic disease, a past history of lactic acidosis (of any cause), cardiac failure requiring pharmacological therapy, or chronic hypoxic lung disease. The drug also should be discontinued temporarily prior to the administration of intravenous *contrast media* and prior to any surgical procedure. The drug should not be readministered any sooner than 48 hours after such procedures and should be withheld until renal function is determined to be normal. These conditions all predispose to increased lactate production and hence to the potentially fatal complication of lactic acidosis. The reported incidence of lactic acidosis during metformin treatment is less than 0.1 cases per 1000 patient-years, and the mortality risk is even lower.

Acute side effects of metformin, which occur in up to 20% of patients, include diarrhea, abdominal discomfort, nausea, metallic taste, and anorexia. These usually can be minimized by increasing the dosage of the drug slowly and taking it with meals. Intestinal absorption of *vitamin B_{12}* and *folate* often is decreased during chronic metformin therapy, and calcium supplements reverse the effect of metformin on vitamin B_{12} absorption.

Consideration should be given to stopping treatment with metformin if the plasma lactate level exceeds 3 mM or in the setting of decreased renal or hepatic function. It also is prudent to stop metformin if a patient is undergoing a prolonged fast or is treated with a very low calorie diet. Myocardial infarction or septicemia mandates immediate drug discontinuation. Metformin usually is administered in divided doses two or three times daily. The maximum effective dose is 2.5 g/day. Metformin lowers hemoglobin A_{1c} values by about 2%, an effect comparable with that of the sulfonylureas. Metformin does not promote weight gain and can reduce plasma triglycerides by 15% to 20%. There is a strong consensus that reduction in hemoglobin A_{1c} by any therapy (insulin or oral agents) diminishes microvascular complications. Metformin, however, is the only therapeutic agent that has been demonstrated to reduce macrovascular events in type 2 DM (U.K. Prospective Diabetes Study Group, 1998b). Metformin can be administered in combination with sulfonylureas, thiazolizinediones, and/or insulin. Fixed-dose combinations containing metformin and glyburide (GLUCOVANCE, others), glipizide (METAGLIP), and rosiglitazone (AVANDAMET) are available.

Thiazolidinediones

Three thiazolidinediones have been used in clinical practice (troglitazone, rosiglitazone, and pioglitazone); however, troglitazone was withdrawn from use because it was associated with severe hepatic toxicity. Rosiglitazone and pioglitazone can lower hemoglobin A_{1c} levels by 1% to 1.5% in patients with type 2 DM. These drugs can be combined with insulin or other classes of oral glucose-lowering agents. The thiazolidinediones tend to increase high-density lipoprotein (HDL) cholesterol but have variable effects on triglycerides and low-density lipoprotein (LDL) cholesterol. The structures of rosiglitazone and pioglitazone are:

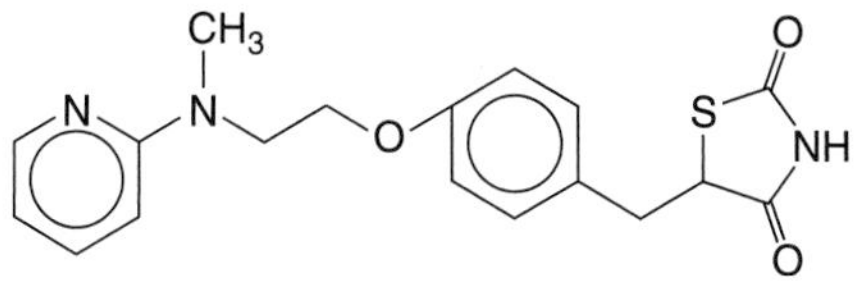

ROSIGLITAZONE

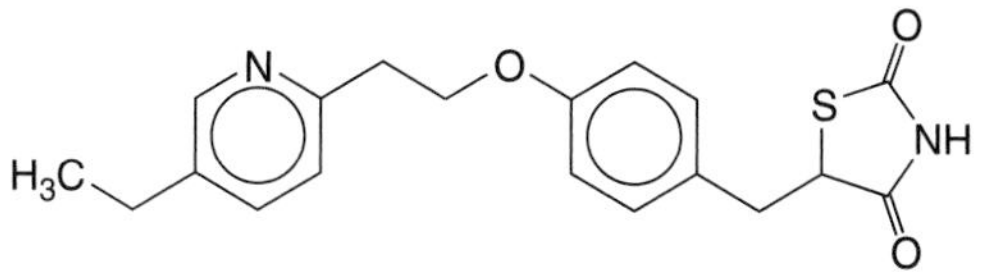

PIOGLITAZONE

Mechanism of Action. Thiazolidinediones are selective agonists for nuclear peroxisome proliferator–activated receptor-γ (PPARγ). These drugs bind to PPARγ, which activates insulin-responsive genes that regulate carbohydrate and lipid metabolism. Thiazolidinediones require insulin to be present for their action. Thiazolidinediones exert their principal effects by increasing insulin sensitivity in peripheral tissue but also may lower glucose production by the liver. Thiazolidinediones increase glucose transport into muscle and adipose tissue by enhancing the synthesis and translocation of specific forms of the glucose transporters. The thiazolidinediones also can activate genes that regulate fatty acid metabolism in peripheral tissue. Although muscle is a major insulin-sensitive tissue, PPARγ is virtually absent in skeletal muscle. This has provoked questions as to how thiazo-

lidinediones can reduce peripheral insulin resistance. One suggestion is that activation of PPARγ in adipose tissue reduces the flux of fatty acids into muscle, thereby lowering insulin resistance. Other suggestions include the activation of adipocyte hormones and/or adipokines, the most promising of which is adiponectin. Adiponectin is associated with increased insulin sensitivity and reportedly increases insulin sensitivity by elevating AMP kinase, which stimulates glucose transport into muscle and increases fatty acid oxidation (Havel, 2003). Because the actions of both metformin and the thiazolidinediones apparently converge on AMP kinase, it has emerged as an attractive target for drug development (Ruderman and Prentki, 2004).

Absorption, Excretion, and Dosing. Rosiglitazone (AVANDIA) and pioglitazone (ACTOS) are taken once a day. Both agents are absorbed within about 2 hours, but the maximum clinical effect is not observed for 6 to 12 weeks. The thiazolidinediones are metabolized by the liver and may be administered to patients with renal insufficiency but should not be used if there is active hepatic disease or significant elevations of serum liver transaminases.

Rosiglitazone is metabolized by hepatic cytochrome P450 (CYP) 2C8, whereas pioglitazone is metabolized by CYP3A4 and CYP2C8. As discussed in Chapter 3, other drugs that induce or inhibit these enzymes can cause drug interactions. Clinically significant interactions between the available thiazolidinediones and other drug classes have not yet been described, but further studies are in progress.

Precautions and Adverse Effects. Liver function should be monitored in patients receiving thiazolidinediones, even though pioglitazone and rosiglitazone rarely have been associated with hepatotoxicity (12 cases up to July 2004). This lower hepatotoxicity has been attributed to the lack of the tocopherol side chain that was included in the troglitazone molecule. Additionally, the rare cases of hepatotoxicity occurring with second-generation thiazolidinediones appear to be less severe than those occurring with troglitazone. Hepatotoxicity can occur several months after initiation of the drugs. Any patient who has suffered any hepatotoxicity (even abnormal liver function tests) while on a thiazolidinediones should not receive any drugs in this class. Thiazolidinediones also have been reported to cause anemia, weight gain, edema, and plasma volume expansion. Edema is more likely to occur when these agents are combined with insulin; these drugs should not be used in patients with New

York Heart Association class 3 or 4 heart failure. Fluid retention and even overt heart failure usually occur within 6 months of thiazolidinedione therapy. In most cases, the subjects had no past history of heart failure, but all had underlying abnormal cardiac function. Obese hypertensive individuals and those with cardiac diastolic dysfunction are at greatest risk for fluid retention with thiazolidinediones. Thiazolidinediones also can induce peripheral edema independent of heart failure; proposed mechanisms include an increase in weight, an expansion of plasma volume following a reduction in renal sodium excretion, or a direct effect to increase vascular permeability. Exacerbations of fluid retention and/or heart failure should be treated, and the thiazolidinedione should be discontinued.

The availability of thiazolidinediones as powerful PPARγ ligands has sparked a number of novel avenues of clinical research. Studies have investigated whether thiazolidinediones can improve insulin sensitivity in HIV-associated lipodystrophy (*see* Chapter 50). Studies also are underway to explore the effects of thiazolidinediones on nonalcoholic hepatic steatosis. Finally, small single-site studies have investigated whether rosiglitazone can slow the progression of atheromatous lesions in carotid and coronary arteries in both nondiabetic and type 2 DM patients. Results to date have been mixed, and further multicenter studies are ongoing.

α-Glucosidase Inhibitors

α-Glucosidase inhibitors reduce intestinal absorption of starch, dextrin, and disaccharides by inhibiting the action of α-glucosidase in the intestinal brush border. Inhibition of this enzyme slows the absorption of carbohydrates; the postprandial rise in plasma glucose is blunted in both normal and diabetic subjects.

α-Glucosidase inhibitors do not stimulate insulin release and therefore do not result in hypoglycemia. These agents may be considered as monotherapy in elderly patients or in patients with predominantly postprandial hyperglycemia. α-Glucosidase inhibitors typically are used in combination with other oral antidiabetic agents and/or insulin. The drugs should be administered at the start of a meal. They are poorly absorbed.

Acarbose (PRECOSE), an oligosaccharide of microbial origin, and *miglitol* (GLYSET), a desoxynojirimycin derivative, also competitively inhibit glucoamylase and sucrase but have weak effects on pancreatic α-amylase. They reduce postprandial plasma glucose levels in type 1 and type 2 DM subjects. α-Glucosidase inhibitors can significantly improve hemoglobin A_{1c} levels in severely hyper-

glycemic type 2 DM patients. However, in patients with mild-to-moderate hyperglycemia, the glucose-lowering potential of α-glucosidase inhibitors (assessed by hemoglobin A_{1c} levels) is about 30% to 50% of that of other oral antidiabetic agents.

α-Glucosidase inhibitors cause dose-related malabsorption, flatulence, diarrhea, and abdominal bloating. Titrating the dose of drug slowly (25 mg at the start of a meal for 4 to 8 weeks, followed by increases at 4- to 8-week intervals to a maximum of 75 mg before each meal) reduces gastrointestinal side effects. Smaller doses are given with snacks. Acarbose is most effective when given with a starchy, high-fiber diet with restricted amounts of glucose and sucrose. If hypoglycemia occurs when α-glucosidase inhibitors are used with insulin or an insulin secretagogue, glucose rather than sucrose, starch, or maltose should be administered.

Reduction in the Incidence of Type 2 DM

Type 2 DM is a rapidly expanding worldwide health problem. In addition, the number of individuals who have impaired glucose tolerance (often termed *prediabetes*) may be equal to or even higher than the number of people with diabetes. In the United States, nearly 20 million individuals are diagnosed with diabetes, but perhaps twice that number have *impaired glucose tolerance* (IGT), which is defined as a fasting plasma glucose concentration of between 100 and 126 mg/dl (5.6 to 7 mM) or 2-hour values in the oral glucose tolerance test of between 140 and 199 mg/dl (7.8 to 11 mM) (Expert Committee on the Diagnosis and Classification of Diabetes, 2003). The rate of progression of IGT to overt diabetes ranges from 9% to 15% worldwide. A major factor in this increased incidence of diabetes is obesity. In the United States, approximately 60% of the population is overweight or obese. Particularly troubling is the rapid increase of obesity in children. Owing to the deleterious effects of obesity and decreased physical activity on insulin sensitivity, the incidence of type 2 DM in U.S. children has increased by tenfold over the last generation. Several large multicenter studies have investigated the effects of lifestyle and/or differing pharmacologic agents on reducing the incidence of type 2 DM. In the Diabetes Prevention Program study (Diabetes Prevention Program Research Group, 2002), a lifestyle intervention consisting of 150 minutes of exercise per week and a 7% weight loss over 2.8 years reduced the incidence of type 2 DM by 58% compared with placebo. Metformin (1700 mg/day) reduced the progression by 31%. Interestingly, when metformin was stopped, its protective effect in preventing diabetes dissipated rapidly. In the Tripod study, troglitazone (400 mg/day) for 30 months reduced the progression of type 2 DM by 55% in insulin-resistant high-risk Hispanic women (Buchanan *et al.*, 2002). This protective effect of troglitazone was maintained for at least 8 months after the drug was stopped. In the Stop-NIDDM study, acarbose (100 mg/three times a day) was given over a period of 3 years and produced a 25% reduction in the progression to type 2 DM (Chiasson *et al.*, 2002). *Orlistat,* a gastrointestinal lipase inhibitor used for weight loss, was administered over a 4-year period and resulted in a 37% reduction in the progression of type 2 DM in a group of insulin-resistant obese patients (Torgerson *et al.*, 2004). Finally, although the mechanisms are poorly understood, there are reports that angiotensin-converting enzyme inhibitors are associated with a decreased incidence of diabetes mellitus in high-risk patients (Scheen, 2004).

Based on the evidence that a variety of pharmacological agents can delay—and perhaps prevent—the onset of type 2 DM, multiple studies are underway investigating the effects of a range of pharmacologic agents in the prevention of type 2 DM.

Glucagon-like Peptide 1

Over four decades ago, McIntyre and colleagues reported that oral as compared with intravenous delivery of glucose produced a greater release of insulin. Subsequent work identified two hormones—*glucose-dependent insulinotropic polypeptide* (GIP) and *glucagon-like peptide* (GLP-1)—that are released from the upper and lower bowel that augment glucose-dependent insulin secretion. These hormones are termed *incretins.* The two incretins differentially stimulate insulin secretion. GIP has little effect on augmenting insulin secretion in type 2 DM, whereas GLP-1 significantly augments glucose-dependent insulin secretion. Consequently, GLP-1 has become an attractive target for therapeutic development in type 2 DM. GLP-1 also reduces glucagon secretion, slows gastric emptying, and decreases appetite. Thus, the compound may have unique properties to reduce postprandial glucose excursions (*i.e.,* increase in insulin, reduction of glucagon, slowing of gastric emptying) and also to induce weight loss. Offsetting these advantages, circulating GLP-1 is rapidly (1 to 2 minutes) inactivated by the dipeptidyl peptidase IV enzyme (DPP-IV). Thus, GLP-1 must be infused continuously to have therapeutic benefits. Consequently, considerable work has been performed to produce GLP-1 receptor agonists that maintain the physiologic effects of the native incretin but are resistant to the actions of DPP-IV. To date, two synthet-

ic GLP-1 analogs have entered clinical trials. Exendin-4 is derived from the salivary gland of the Gila monster and has 53% homology with human GLP-1. Exendin-4 is resistant to DPP-IV and has full agonist activity at GLP-1 receptors. Several clinical studies have demonstrated that *exendin-4 (exenatide,* BYETTA) is effective in lowering hemoglobin A_{1c} (approximately 1% to 1.3%) and also promotes weight loss in type 2 DM. The compound is administered as twice-daily injections, although studies are planned to test a weekly or perhaps even a longer-acting formulation. Based on results of clinical trials, the FDA recently approved exenatide for twice-daily injection in combination therapy with other agents in subjects with type 2 DM. Reported exendin-4 side effects include a self-limiting nausea in 15% to 30% of patients; hypoglycemia can occur when GLP-1 agonists are used in conjunction with oral insulin secretagogues. A second long-acting analog of GLP-1, known as *NN2211,* is also in clinical trials. NN2211 contains a fatty acid moiety (hexadeconyl residue) covalently linked to GLP-1. NN2211 is resistant to the action of DPP-IV but also must be injected. Early clinical studies show that NN2211 is effective in lowering hemoglobin A_{1c} but may not induce as much weight loss as exendin-4. Nausea and hypoglycemia also occur with NN2211 when used with oral hypoglycemic agents.

An alternative approach to GLP-1 therapy is to inactivate the DPP-IV protease, thereby increasing endogenous circulating GLP-1 levels. A number of orally effective DPP-IV inhibitors have entered clinical trials. One study in type 2 DM reported similar reductions in hemoglobin A_{1c} as compared with the GLP-1 receptor analogs. These agents are well tolerated and appear to result in less nausea than the GLP-1 analogs. However, since DPP-IV can metabolize a wide range of peptides, there is a theoretical concern about the long-term safety of these compounds. Furthermore, the potency of the DPP-IV inhibitors may be limited by the amount of endogenous production of GLP-1. In contrast, pharmacological amounts of the injectable GLP-1 analogs can be administered with possibly increased therapeutic effect. Ongoing studies are currently being performed to further delineate the therapeutic effects of these agents, which offer promise for a novel pharmacotherapy in type 2 DM.

GLUCAGON

History. Distinct populations of cells were identified in the islets of Langerhans before the discovery of insulin. Glucagon was dis-

$$NH_2$$
$$|$$
H–HIS–SER–GLU–GLY–THR–PHE–THR–SER–ASP–TYR–

$$NH_2$$
$$|$$
SER–LYS–TYR–LEU–ASP–SER–ARG–ARG–ALA–GLU–

$$NH_2 \qquad\qquad NH_2$$
$$| \qquad\qquad\quad |$$
ASP–PHE–VAL–GLU–TRP–LEU–MET–ASP–THR–OH

Figure 60–6. *The amino acid sequence of glucagon.*

covered by Murlin and Kimball in 1923, less than 2 years after the discovery of insulin. In contrast to the excitement caused by the discovery of insulin, few were interested in glucagon, and it was not recognized as an important hormone for more than 40 years. Glucagon has significant physiological roles in the regulation of glucose and ketone body metabolism but is only of minor therapeutic interest for the short-term management of hypoglycemia. It also is used in radiology for its inhibitory effects on intestinal smooth muscle.

Chemistry. Glucagon is a single-chain polypeptide of 29 amino acids (Figure 60–6). It has significant homology with several other polypeptide hormones, including secretin, vasoactive intestinal peptide, and gastrointestinal inhibitory polypeptide. The primary sequence of glucagon is identical in human beings, cattle, pigs, and rats.

Glucagon is synthesized from preproglucagon, a 180-amino-acid precursor with five separately processed domains. An amino-terminal signal peptide is followed by glicentin-related pancreatic peptide, glucagon, GLP-1, and glucagon-like peptide-2. Processing of the protein is sequential and occurs in a tissue-specific fashion; this results in different secretory peptides in pancreatic α cells and intestinal α-like cells (termed *L cells*). *Glicentin,* a major processing intermediate, consists of glicentin-related pancreatic polypeptide at the amino terminus and glucagon at the carboxyl terminus, with an Arg–Arg pair between. *Enteroglucagon* (or *oxyntomodulin*) consists of glucagon and a carboxyl-terminal hexapeptide linked by an Arg–Arg pair.

The highly controlled nature of the processing suggests that these peptides may have distinct biological functions. In the pancreatic α cell, the granule consists of a central core of glucagon surrounded by a halo of glicentin. Intestinal L cells contain only glicentin and presumably lack the enzyme required to process this precursor to glucagon. Enteroglucagon binds to hepatic glucagon receptors and stimulates adenylyl cyclase with 10% to 20% of the potency of glucagon. GLP-1 is an extremely potent potentiator of insulin secretion (*see* above), although it apparently lacks significant hepatic actions. Glicentin, enteroglucagon, and the glucagon-like peptides are found predominantly in the intestine, and their secretion continues after total pancreatectomy.

Regulation of Secretion. Glucagon secretion is regulated by dietary glucose, insulin, amino acids, and fatty acids. As in insulin secretion, glucose is a more effective inhibitor of glucagon secretion when taken orally than when administered intravenously, suggesting a possible role for gastrointestinal hormones in the response. The effect of glucose is lost in untreated or undertreated type 1 DM patients and in isolated pancreatic α cells, indicating that at least part of the effect is sec-

ondary to stimulation of insulin secretion. Somatostatin also inhibits glucagon secretion, as do free fatty acids and ketones.

Most amino acids stimulate the release of both glucagon and insulin. This coordinated response to amino acids may prevent insulin-induced hypoglycemia in individuals who ingest a meal of pure protein. Like glucose, amino acids are more potent when taken orally and thus may exert some of their effects *via* gastrointestinal hormones. Secretion of glucagon also is regulated by the autonomic innervation of the pancreatic islet. Stimulation of sympathetic nerves or administration of sympathomimetic amines increases glucagon secretion. *Acetylcholine* has a similar effect.

Glucagon in Diabetes Mellitus. Plasma concentrations of glucagon are elevated in poorly controlled diabetic patients. Because it enhances gluconeogenesis and glycogenolysis, glucagon exacerbates the hyperglycemia of diabetes. However, this abnormality of glucagon secretion appears to be secondary to the diabetic state and is corrected with improved control of the disease. The importance of the hyperglucagonemia in diabetes has been evaluated by administration of *somatostatin*. Although somatostatin does not restore glucose metabolism to normal, it significantly slows the rate of development of hyperglycemia and ketonemia in insulin-deficient subjects with type 1 DM. In normal individuals, glucagon secretion increases in response to hypoglycemia, but this important defense mechanism against insulin-induced hypoglycemia is lost in type 1 DM.

Degradation. Glucagon is degraded extensively in liver, kidney, plasma, and other sites of action. Its half-life in plasma is approximately 3 to 6 minutes. Proteolytic removal of the amino-terminal histidine residue leads to loss of biological activity.

Cellular and Physiological Actions. Glucagon interacts with a glycoprotein GPCR on the plasma membrane of target cells that signals through G_s (Mayo *et al.*, 2003) (*see* Chapter 1). The primary effects of glucagon on the liver are mediated by cyclic AMP. In general, modifications of the amino-terminal region of glucagon (*e.g.*, [Phe^1]glucagon and des-His$_1$-[Glu^9]glucagon amide) result in molecules that behave as partial agonists that retain some affinity for the glucagon receptor but have a markedly reduced capacity to stimulate adenylyl cyclase.

Glucagon activates phosphorylase, the rate-limiting enzyme in glycogenolysis, *via* cyclic AMP–stimulated phosphorylation, whereas concurrent phosphorylation of glycogen synthase inactivates the enzyme; glycogenolysis is enhanced, and glycogen synthesis is inhibited. Cyclic AMP also stimulates transcription of the gene for phosphoenolpyruvate carboxykinase, a rate-limiting enzyme in gluconeogenesis. These effects normally are opposed by insulin, and insulin is dominant when maximal concentrations of both hormones are present.

Cyclic AMP also stimulates phosphorylation of the bifunctional enzyme 6-phosphofructo-2-kinase/fructose-2,6-bisphosphatase. This enzyme determines the cellular concentration of fructose-2,6-bisphosphate, which acts as a potent regulator of gluconeogenesis and glycogenolysis. When the concentration of glucagon is high relative to that of insulin, this enzyme is phosphorylated and acts as a phosphatase, reducing the concentration of fructose-2,6-bisphosphate in the liver. When the concentration of insulin is high relative to that of glucagon, the dephosphorylated enzyme acts as a kinase, raising fructose-2,6-bisphosphate concentrations. Fructose-2,6-bisphosphate interacts allosterically with phosphofructokinase-1, the rate-limiting enzyme in glycolysis, increasing its activity. Thus, when glucagon concentrations are high, glycolysis is inhibited, and gluconeogenesis is stimulated. This also leads to a decrease in the concentration of malonyl CoA, stimulation of fatty acid oxidation, and production of ketone bodies. Conversely, when insulin concentrations are high, glycolysis is stimulated, and gluconeogenesis and ketogenesis are inhibited (*see* Foster, 1984).

Glucagon exerts effects on tissues other than liver, especially at higher concentrations. In adipose tissue, it stimulates adenylyl cyclase and increases lipolysis. In the heart, glucagon increases the force of contraction. Glucagon has relaxant effects on the gastrointestinal tract; this has been observed with analogs that apparently do not stimulate adenylyl cyclase. Some tissues (including liver) possess a second type of glucagon receptor that is linked to generation of IP_3, diacylglycerol, and Ca^{2+}. The role of this receptor in metabolic regulation remains uncertain.

Therapeutic Use. Glucagon is used to treat severe hypoglycemia, particularly in diabetic patients when intravenous glucose is not available; it also is used by radiologists for its inhibitory effects on the gastrointestinal tract.

All glucagon used clinically is extracted from bovine and porcine pancreas; its sequence is identical to that of the human hormone. For hypoglycemic reactions, 1 mg is administered intravenously, intramuscularly, or subcutaneously. The first two routes are preferred in an emergency. Clinical improvement is sought within 10 minutes to minimize the risk of neurological damage from hypoglycemia. The hyperglycemic action of glucagon is transient and may be inadequate if hepatic stores of glycogen are depleted. After the initial response to glucagon, patients should be given glucose or urged to eat to prevent recurrent hypoglycemia. Nausea and vomiting are the most frequent adverse effects.

Glucagon also is used to relax the intestinal tract to facilitate radiographic examination of the upper and lower gastrointestinal tract with barium and retrograde ileography and in magnetic resonance imaging of the gastrointestinal tract. Glucagon has been used to treat the spasm associated with acute diverticulitis and disorders of the biliary tract and sphincter of Oddi, as an adjunct in basket retrieval of biliary calculi, and for impaction of the esophagus and intussusception. Finally, it has been used diagnostically to distinguish obstructive from hepatocellular jaundice.

Glucagon releases catecholamines from pheochromocytomas and has been used experimentally as a diagnostic test for this disorder. Based on this effect, glucagon therapy is contraindicated in known pheochromocytoma. The hormone also has been used as a cardiac inotropic agent for the treatment of shock, particularly when prior administration of a β adrenergic receptor antagonist has rendered β adrenergic receptor agonists ineffective.

SOMATOSTATIN

Somatostatin was first isolated in 1973, following a search for hypothalamic factors that might regulate secretion of growth hormone from the pituitary gland (*see* Chapter 5). A potential physiological role for somatostatin in the islet was suggested by the observation that somatostatin inhibits secretion of insulin and glucagon. The peptide subsequently was identified in the δ cells of the pancreatic islet, in similar cells of the gastrointestinal tract, and in the central nervous system.

Somatostatin, the name originally given to a cyclic peptide containing 14 amino acids, is now known to be one of a group of related peptides. These include the original somatostatin (S-14), an extended 28-amino-acid peptide molecule (S-28), and a fragment containing the initial 12 amino acids of somatostatin-28 [S-28(1–12)]. S-14 is the predominant form in the brain, whereas S-28 is the main form in the gut. Acting *via* a family of GPCRs (*see* Chapter 55), somatostatin inhibits the release of thyroid-stimulating hormone and growth hormone from the pituitary gland; of gastrin, motilin, VIP, glicentin, and gastrointestinal polypeptide from the gut; and of insulin, glucagon, and pancreatic polypeptide from the pancreas.

Somatostatin secreted from the pancreas can regulate pituitary function, thereby acting as a true endocrine hormone. In the gut, however, somatostatin acts as a paracrine agent that influences the functions of adjacent cells. It also can act as an autocrine agent by inhibiting its own release in the pancreas. As the last cell to receive blood flow in the islets, the δ cell is downstream of the β and α cells. Thus, somatostatin may regulate the secretion of insulin and glucagon only *via* the systemic circulation.

Somatostatin is released in response to many of the nutrients and hormones that stimulate insulin secretion, including glucose, arginine, leucine, glucagon, VIP, and cholecystokinin. The physiological role of somatostatin has not been defined precisely. When administered in pharmacological doses, somatostatin inhibits virtually all endocrine and exocrine secretions of the pancreas, gut, and gallbladder. Somatostatin also can inhibit secretion of the salivary glands and, under some conditions, can block parathyroid, calcitonin, prolactin, and adrenocorticotropic hormone (ACTH) secretion. The α cell is about 50 times more sensitive to somatostatin than is the β cell, but inhibition of glucagon secretion is more transient. Somatostatin also inhibits nutrient absorption from the intestine, decreases intestinal motility, and reduces splanchnic blood flow.

Therapeutic uses of somatostatin are confined mainly to blocking hormone release in endocrine-secreting tumors, including insulinomas, glucagonomas, VIPomas, carcinoid tumors, and growth hormone–secreting adenomas (causing acromegaly). Because of its short half-life (3 to 6 minutes), substantial effort has been directed toward the production of longer-acting analogs. One such agent, *octreotide* (SANDOSTATIN), is available in the United States for treatment of carcinoid tumors, glucagonomas, VIPomas, and acromegaly. Another agent, *lanreotide,* is available in Europe. A depot form of octreotide administered intramuscularly every 4 weeks (SANDOSTATIN LAR) may be particularly suitable for chronic administration (*see* Chapter 55). Octreotide or lanreotide successfully controls excess secretion of growth hormone in most patients, and both have been reported to reduce the size of pituitary tumors in about one-third of cases. Octreotide also has been used to reduce the disabling form of diarrhea that occasionally occurs in diabetic autonomic neuropathy. Since octreotide also can decrease blood flow to the gastrointestinal tract, it has been used to treat bleeding esophageal varices, peptic ulcers, and postprandial orthostatic hypotension.

Gallbladder abnormalities (stones and biliary sludge) occur frequently with chronic use of the somatostatin analogs, as do gastrointestinal symptoms. Hypoglycemia, hyperglycemia, hypothyroidism, and goiter have been reported in patients being treated with octreotide for acromegaly.

DIAZOXIDE

Diazoxide is an antihypertensive, antidiuretic benzothiadiazine derivative with potent hyperglycemic actions when given orally (*see*

Chapter 32). Hyperglycemia results primarily from inhibition of insulin secretion. Diazoxide interacts with the ATP-sensitive K^+ channel on the β-cell membrane and either prevents its closing or prolongs the open time; this effect is opposite to that of the sulfonylureas. The drug does not inhibit insulin synthesis, and thus there is an accumulation of insulin within the β cell. Diazoxide also has a modest capacity to inhibit peripheral glucose utilization by muscle and to stimulate hepatic gluconeogenesis.

Diazoxide (PROGLYCEM) has been used to treat patients with various forms of hypoglycemia. The usual oral dose is 3 to 8 mg/kg per day in adults and 8 to 15 mg/kg per day in infants and neonates. The drug can cause nausea and vomiting and thus usually is given in divided doses with meals. Diazoxide circulates largely bound to plasma proteins and has a half-life of about 48 hours. Thus, the patient should be maintained at any dosage for several days before evaluating the therapeutic result.

Diazoxide has a number of adverse effects, including retention of Na^+ and fluid, hyperuricemia, hypertrichosis (especially in children), thrombocytopenia, and leucopenia, which sometimes limit its use. Despite these side effects, the drug may be quite useful in patients with inoperable insulinomas and in children with hyperinsulinism owing to nesidioblastosis.

BIBLIOGRAPHY

Aguilar-Bryan, L., Nichols, C., Wechsler, S., *et al.* Cloning of the beta cell high-affinity sulfonylurea receptor: A regulator of insulin secretion. *Science,* **1995,** *268*:423–426.

American Diabetes Association. Consensus statement on pharmacologic treatment. *Diabetes Care,* **1999,** *22*:S1–114.

Authier, F., Rachubinski, R.A., Posner, B.I., and Bergeron, J.J. Endosomal proteolysis of insulin by an acidic thiol metalloprotease unrelated to insulin degrading enzyme. *J. Biol. Chem.,* **1994,** *269*:3010–3016.

Beisswenger, P.J., Makita, Z., Curphey, T.J., *et al.* Formation of immunochemical advanced glycosylation end products precedes and correlates with early manifestations of renal and retinal disease in diabetes. *Diabetes,* **1995,** *44*:824–829.

Buchanan, T.A., Xiang, A.H., Peters, R.K., *et al.* Preservation of pancreatic β-cell function and prevention of type 2 diabetes by pharmacological treatment of insulin resistance in high-risk Hispanic women. *Diabetes,* **2002,** *51*:2796–2803.

Cefalu, W.T., Skyler, J.S., Kourides, I.A., *et al.* Inhaled human insulin treatment in patients with type 2 diabetes mellitus. *Ann. Intern. Med.,* **2001,** *134*:203–207.

Chan, S.J., Seino, S., Gruppuso, P.A., Schwartz, R., and Steiner, D.F. A mutation in the B chain coding region is associated with impaired proinsulin conversion in a family with hyperproinsulinemia. *Proc. Natl. Acad. Sci. U.S.A.,* **1987,** *84*:2194–2197.

Chiasson, J.L., Josse, R.G., Gomis, R., *et al.* STOP-NIDDM Trail Research Group. Acarbose for prevention of type 2 diabetes mellitus: The STOP-NIDDM randomised trial. *Lancet,* **2002,** *359*:2072–2077.

Davis, S.N., Butler, P.C., Brown, M., *et al.* The effects of human proinsulin on glucose turnover and intermediary metabolism. *Metabolism,* **1991,** *40*:953–961.

Davis, S.N., Thompson, C.J., Brown, M.D., Home, P.D., and the DCCT Research Group. The effect of intensive treatment of diabetes on the development and progression of long-term complications in insulin-dependent diabetes mellitus. The Diabetes Control and Complications Trial Research Group. *New Engl. J. Med.,* **1993,** *329*: 977–986.

DCCT Research Group. Retinopathy and nephropathy in patients with type 1 diabetes four years after a trial of intensive therapy. The Diabetes Control and Complications Trial/Epidemiology of Diabetes Interventions and Complications Research Group. *New Engl. J. Med.,* **2000,** *342*:381–389.

Diabetes Prevention Program Research Group. Reduction in the incidence of type 2 diabetes with lifestyle intervention or metformin. *New Engl. J. Med.,* **2002,** *346*:393–403.

DeFronzo, R.A., and Goodman, A.M. Efficacy of metformin in patients with non-insulin-dependent diabetes mellitus. The Multicenter Metformin Study Group. *New Engl. J. Med.,* **1995,** *333*:541–549.

De Meyts, P. The structural basis of insulin and insulin-like growth factor-I receptor binding and negative co-operativity, and its relevance to mitogenic versus metabolic signalling. *Diabetologia,* **1994,** *37*:S135–148.

Expert Committee on the Diagnosis and Classification of Diabetes Mellitus. *Diabetes Care,* **2003,** *26*:3160–3167.

Hirsch, I.B. Insulin analogs. *New Engl. J. Med.,* **2005,** *352*:174–183.

Horton, E.S., Clinkingbeard, C., Gatlin, M., *et al.* Nateglinide alone and in combination with metformin improves glycemic control by reducing mealtime glucose levels in type 2 diabetes. *Diabetes Care,* **2000,** *23*:1660–1665.

Imagawa, A., Hanafusa, T., Miyagawa, J., and Matsuzawa, Y. A novel subtype of type 1 diabetes mellitus characterized by a rapid onset and an absence of diabetes-related antibodies. Osaka IDDM Study Group. *New Engl. J. Med.,* **2000,** *342*:301–307.

Kahn, C.R., and Roth, J. Berson, Yalow, and the JCI: The agony and the ecstasy. *J. Clin. Invest.,* **2004,** 114:1051–1054.

Kalbag, J.B., Walter, Y.H., Nedelman, J.R., and McLeod, J.F. Mealtime glucose regulation with nateglinide in healthy volunteers: comparison with repaglinide and placebo. *Diabetes Care,* **2001,** *24*:73–77.

Malmberg, K., Ryden, L, Efendic, S., *et al.* Randomized trial of insulin-glucose infusion followed by subcutaneous insulin treatment in diabetic patients with acute myocardial infarction (DIGAMI study): Effects on mortality at one year. *J. Am. Coll. Cardiol.,* **1995,** *26*:57–65.

McGettrick, A.J., Feener, E.P., and Kahn, C.R. Human IRS-1 polymorphism, G972R, causes IRS-1 to associate with the insulin receptor and inhibit receptor autophosphorylation. *J. Biol. Chem.,* **2005,** *8*:6441–6446

Meinert, C.L., Knatterud, G.L., Prout, T.E., and Klimt, C.R. A study of the effects of hypoglycemic agents on vascular complications in patients with adult-onset diabetes: II. Mortality results. *Diabetes,* **1970,** *19*:789–830.

Philipson, L.H., and Steiner, D.F. Pas de deux or more: the sulfonylurea receptor and K^+ channels. *Science,* **1995,** *268*:372–373.

Printz, R.L., Koch, S., Potter, L.R., *et al.* Hexokinase II mRNA and gene structure, regulation by insulin, and evolution. *J. Biol. Chem.,* **1993,** *268*:5209–5219.

Proks, P., Antcliff, J.F., Lippiat, J., *et al.* Molecular basis of Kir6.2 mutations associated with neonatal diabetes or neonatal diabetes plus neurological features. *Proc. Natl. Acad. Sci. U.S.A.,* **2004,** *101*:17539–17544.

Skyler, J.S., Cefalu, W.T., Kourides, I.A., *et al.* Efficacy of inhaled human insulin in type 1 diabetes mellitus: A randomised proof-of-concept study. *Lancet,* **2001,** *357*:331–335.

Srikanta, S., Ganda, O.P., Jackson, R.A., *et al.* Type I diabetes mellitus in monozygotic twins: Chronic progressive beta cell dysfunction. *Ann. Intern. Med.,* **1983,** 99:320–326.

Stumvoll, M., Nurjhan, N., Perriello, G., Dailey, G., and Gerich, J.E. Metabolic effects of metformin in non-insulin-dependent diabetes mellitus. *New Engl. J. Med.,* **1995,** *333*:550–554.

Temple, R.C., Carrington, C.A., Luzio, S.D., *et al.* Insulin deficiency in non-insulin-dependent diabetes. *Lancet,* **1989,** *1*:293–295.

Todd, J.A., Bell, J.F., and McDevitt, H.O. HLA-DQβ gene contributes to susceptibility and resistance to insulin-dependent diabetes mellitus. *Nature,* **1987,** *329*:599–604.

Torgerson, J.S., Hauptman, J., Boldrin, M.N., and Sjostrom, L. XENical in the prevention of Diabetes in Obese Subjects (XENDOS) study: A randomized study of orlistat as an adjunct to lifestyle changes for the prevention of type 2 diabetes in obese patients. *Diabetes Care,* **2004,** *27*:155–161.

U.K. Prospective Diabetes Study Group. Intensive blood-glucose control with sulphonylureas or insulin compared with conventional treatment and risk of complications in patients with type 2 diabetes (UKPDS 33). *Lancet,* **1998a,** *352*:837–853.

U.K. Prospective Diabetes Study Group. Effect of intensive blood-glucose control with metformin on complications in overweight patients with type 2 diabetes (UKPDS 34). *Lancet,* **1998b,** *352*:854–865.

van Den Berghe, G. How does blood glucose control with insulin save lives in intensive care? *J. Clin. Invest.,* **2004,** *114*:1187–1195.

Van Den Berghe, G., Wouters, P., Weekers, F., *et al.* Intensive insulin therapy in the critically ill patients. *New Engl. J. Med.,* **2001,** *345*:1359–1367.

van den Ouwenland, J.M., Lemkes, H.H., Ruitenbeek, W., *et al.* Mutation in mitochondrial tRNA (Leu) (UUR) gene in a large pedigree with maternally transmitted type II diabetes mellitus and deafness. *Nature Genet.,* **1992,** *1*:368–371.

Verge, C.F., Gianani, R., Kawasaki, E., *et al.* Prediction of type I diabetes in first-degree relatives using a combination of insulin, GAD, and ICA512bdc/IA-2 autoantibodies. *Diabetes,* **1996,** *45*:926–933.

Zhou, G., Myers, R., Li, Y., *et al.* Role of AMP-activated protein kinase in mechanism of metformin action. *J. Clin. Invest.,* **2001,** *108*:1167–1174.

MONOGRAPHS AND REVIEWS

Amos, A.F., McCarty, D.J., and Zimmet, P. The rising global burden of diabetes and its complications: Estimates and projections to the year 2010. *Diabet. Med.,* **1997,** *14*:S1–85.

Bailey, C.J. Biguanides and NIDDM. *Diabetes Care,* **1992,** *15*:755–772.

Brownlee, M. The pathological implications of protein glycation. *Clin. Invest. Med.,* **1995,** *18*:275–281.

Cryer, P.E. Hypoglycemia begets hypoglycemia in IDDM. *Diabetes,* **1993,** *42*:1691–1693.

Davies, M.J., and Lawrence, I.G. DIGAMI (diabetes mellitus, insulin glucose infusion in acute myocardial infarction): Theory and practice. *Diabetes Obes. Metab.,* **2002,** *4*:289–295.

Duckworth, W.C. Insulin degradation: Mechanisms, products, and significance. *Endocr. Rev.,* **1988,** *9*:319–345.

Florez, J.C., Hirschhorn, J., and Altshuler, D. The inherited basis of diabetes mellitus: Implications for the genetic analysis of complex traits. *Ann. Rev. Genomics Hum. Genet.,* **2003,** *4*:257–291.

Foster, D.W. Banting lecture 1984. From glycogen to ketones—and back. *Diabetes,* **1984,** *33*:1188–1199.

Frank, R.N. The aldose reductase controversy. *Diabetes,* **1994,** *43*:169–172.

Granner, D.K. Hormones of the pancreas and gastrointestinal tract. In, *Harper's Biochemistry,* 25th ed. (Murray, R.K., Granner, D.K., Mayes, P.A., and Rodwell, V.W., eds.) Appleton & Lange, Stamford, CT, **2000,** pp. 610–626.

Hattersley, A.T. Maturity-onset diabetes of the young: Clinical heterogeneity explained by genetic heterogeneity. *Diabet. Med.,* **1998,** *15*:15–24.

Havel, P.J. Update on adipocyte hormones: Regulation of energy balance and carbohydrate/lipid metabolism. *Diabetes,* **2004,** *53*:S143–151.

Jacober, S.J., and Sowers, J.R. An update on the perioperative management of diabetes. *Arch. Intern. Med.,* **1999;** *159*:2405–2411.

Leahy, J.L. Natural history of β-cell dysfunction in NIDDM. *Diabetes Care,* **1990,** *13*:992–1010.

LeRoith, D., Taylor, S.I., and Olefsky, J.M. (eds.). *Diabetes Mellitus: A Fundamental and Clinical Text,* 2d ed. Lippincott Williams & Wilkins, Philadelphia, **2000.**

Matchinsky, F.M. Banting Lecture 1995. A lesson in metabolic regulation inspired by the glucokinase glucose sensor paradigm. *Diabetes,* **1996,** *45*:223–241.

Mayo, K.E., Miller, L.J., Bataille, D., *et al.* International Union of Pharmacology: The glucagon receptor family. *Pharmacol. Rev.,* **2003,** *55*:167–194.

McMillan, D.E. Development of vascular complications in diabetes. *Vasc. Med.,* **1997,** *2*:132–142.

Meivar-Levy, I., and Ferber, S. New organs from our own tissues: Liver-to-pancreas transdifferentiation. *Trends Endocrinol. Metab.,* **2003,** *14*:460–466.

Nakae, J., Kido, Y., and Accili, D. Distinct and overlapping functions of insulin and IGF-I receptors. *Endocr. Rev.,* **2001,** *22*:818–835.

O'Brien, R.M., and Granner, D.K. The regulation of gene expression by insulin. *Physiol. Rev.,* **1996,** *76*:1109–1161.

Printz, R.L., Magnuson, M.A., and Granner, D.K. Mammalian glucokinase. *Annu. Rev. Nutr.,* **1993,** *13*:463–496.

Robertson R.P. Islet transplantation as a treatment for diabetes: A work in progress. *New Engl. J. Med.,* **2004,** *350*:694–705.

Ruderman, N., and Prentki, M. AMP kinase and malonyl-CoA: Targets for therapy of the metabolic syndrome. *Nature Rev. Drug Discov.,* **2004,** *3*:340–351.

Scheen, A.J. Prevention of type 2 diabetes mellitus through inhibition of the renin–angiotensin system. *Drugs,* **2004,** *64*:2537–2565.

Shepherd, P.R., and Kahn, B.B. Glucose transporters and insulin action: Implications for insulin resistance and diabetes mellitus. *New Engl. J. Med.,* **1999,** *341*:248–256.

Steiner, D.F., Rouille, Y., Gong, Q., *et al.* The role of prohormone convertases in insulin biosynthesis: Evidence for inherited defects in their action in man and experimental animals. *Diabetes Metab.,* **1996,** *22*:94–104.

Sutherland, D.E., Gruessner, A., and Herin, B.J. Beta-cell replacement therapy (pancreas and islet transplantation) for the treatment of diabetes mellitus: An integrated approach. *Endocrinol. Metab. Clin. North Am.* **2004,** *33*:135–148.

Virkamäki, A., Ueki, K., and Kahn, C.R. Protein–protein interaction in insulin signaling and the molecular mechanisms of insulin resistance. *J. Clin. Invest.,* **1999,** *103*:931–943.

White, M.F. IRS proteins and the common path to diabetes. *Am. J. Physiol. Endocrinol. Metab.,* **2002,** *283*:E413–422.

AGENTS AFFECTING MINERAL ION HOMEOSTASIS AND BONE TURNOVER

Peter A. Friedman

PHYSIOLOGY OF MINERAL HOMEOSTASIS AND BONE METABOLISM

Calcium

Ca^{2+}, the ionized form of elemental calcium, is essential for the Ca^{2+} component of current flow across excitable membranes, fusion and release of storage vesicles, and muscle contraction. Intracellular Ca^{2+} also acts in the submicromolar range as a critical second messenger (*see* Chapter 1). In extracellular fluid, millimolar concentrations of calcium promote blood coagulation (Figure 61–3) (*see* below) and support the formation and continuous remodeling of the skeleton.

Ca^{2+} has an adaptable coordination sphere that facilitates binding to the irregular geometry of proteins. The capacity of an ion to cross-link two proteins requires a high coordination number, which dictates the number of electron pairs that can be formed and generally is six to eight for Ca^{2+}. Unlike disulfide or sugar–peptide cross-links, Ca^{2+} linking is readily reversible. Cross-linking of structural proteins in bone matrix is enhanced by the relatively high extracellular concentration of calcium.

In the face of millimolar extracellular Ca^{2+}, intracellular free Ca^{2+} is maintained at a low level, approximately 100 nM in cells in their basal state, by active extrusion by Ca^{2+}–ATPases and by Na^+/Ca^{2+} exchange. As a consequence, changes in cytosolic Ca^{2+} (whether released from intracellular stores or entering *via* membrane Ca^{2+} channels) can modulate effector targets, often by interacting with the Ca^{2+}-binding protein calmodulin. The rapid association–dissociation kinetics of Ca^{2+} and the relatively high affinity and selectivity of

Ca^{2+}-binding domains permit effective regulation of Ca^{2+} over the 100 nM to 1 μM range.

Healthy adult men and women possess about 1300 and 1000 g of calcium, respectively, of which more than 99% is in bone and teeth. Ca^{2+} is the major extracellular divalent cation. Although the absolute amount of calcium in extracellular fluids is small, this fraction is stringently regulated within narrow limits. In adult humans, the normal serum calcium concentration ranges from 8.5 to 10.4 mg/dl (4.25 to 5.2 mEq/L, 2.1 to 2.6 mM) and includes three distinct chemical forms of Ca^{2+}: ionized (50%), protein-bound (40%), and complexed (10%). Thus, whereas total plasma calcium concentration is approximately 2.54 mM, the concentration of ionized Ca^{2+} in human plasma is approximately 1.2 mM.

The various pools of calcium are illustrated schematically in Figure 61–1. Only diffusible calcium, *i.e.*, ionized plus complexed, can cross cell membranes. Of the serum calcium bound to plasma proteins, albumin accounts for some 90%. Smaller percentages are bound, albeit with greater affinity, to β-globulin, α_2-globulin, α_1-globulin, and γ-globulin. The remaining 10% of the serum calcium is complexed in ion pairs with small polyvalent anions, primarily phosphate and citrate. The degree of complex formation depends on the ambient pH and the concentrations of ionized calcium and complexing anions. As the physiologically relevant component, it is ionized Ca^{2+} that exerts biological effects and, when perturbed, produces the characteristic signs and symptoms of hypo- or hypercalcemia.

The total plasma calcium concentration can be interpreted only by correcting for the concentration of plasma proteins. A change in plasma albumin concentration of 1.0 g/dl from the normal value of 4.0 g/dl can be expected to alter total calcium concentration by approximately 0.8 mg/dl.

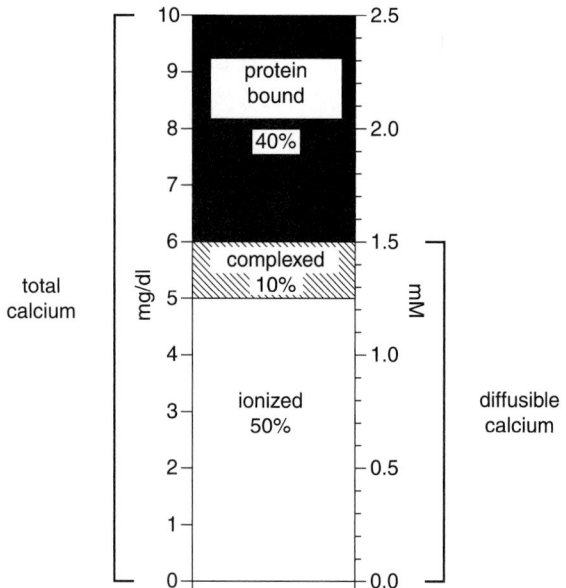

Figure 61–1. *Pools of calcium in serum.* Concentrations are expressed as mg/dl on the left-hand axis and as mM on the right. The total serum calcium concentration is 10 mg/dl or 2.5 mM, divided into three pools: protein-bound (40%), complexed with small anions (10%), and ionized calcium (50%). The complexed and ionized pools represent the diffusable forms of calcium.

The extracellular Ca^{2+} concentration is tightly controlled by hormones that affect its entry at the intestine and its exit at the kidney; when needed, these same hormones regulate withdrawal from the large skeletal reservoir.

Calcium Stores. The skeleton contains 99% of total body calcium in a crystalline form resembling the mineral hydroxyapatite $[Ca_{10}(PO_4)_6(OH)_2]$; other ions, including Na^+, K^+, Mg^{2+}, and F^-, also are present in the crystal lattice. The steady-state content of calcium in bone reflects the net effect of bone resorption and bone formation, coupled with aspects of bone remodeling (*see* below). In addition, a labile pool of bone Ca^{2+} exchanges readily with interstitial fluid. This exchange is modulated by hormones, vitamins, drugs, and other factors that directly alter bone turnover or that influence the Ca^{2+} level in interstitial fluid.

Calcium Absorption and Excretion. In the United States, about 75% of dietary calcium is obtained from milk and dairy products. The adequate intake value for calcium is 1300 mg/day in adolescents and 1000 mg/day in adults. After age 50, the adequate intake is 1200 mg/day. This contrasts with median intakes of calcium for boys and girls aged 9 years and older of 865 and 625 mg, respec-

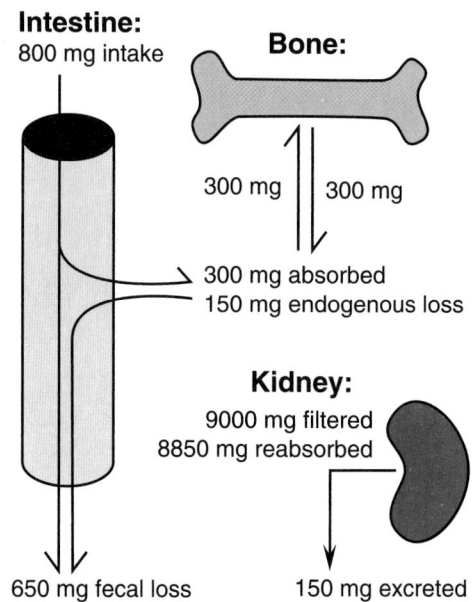

Figure 61–2. *Schematic representation of the whole body daily turnover of calcium. (Adapted with permission from Yanagawa and Lee, 1992.)*

tively, and a median daily calcium intake of 517 mg for women after age 50.

Figure 61–2 illustrates the components of whole-body daily calcium turnover. Ca^{2+} enters the body only through the intestine. *Active vitamin D–dependent transport* (*see* below) occurs in the proximal duodenum, whereas *facilitated diffusion* throughout the small intestine accounts for the majority of total Ca^{2+} uptake. This uptake is counterbalanced by an obligatory daily intestinal calcium loss of about 150 mg/day that reflects the mineral contained in mucosal and biliary secretions and in sloughed intestinal cells.

The efficiency of intestinal Ca^{2+} absorption is inversely related to calcium intake. Thus, a diet low in calcium leads to a compensatory increase in fractional absorption owing partly to activation of vitamin D. In older persons, this response is considerably less robust. Disease states associated with steatorrhea, diarrhea, or chronic malabsorption promote fecal loss of calcium, whereas drugs such as *glucocorticoids* and *phenytoin* depress intestinal Ca^{2+} transport.

Urinary Ca^{2+} excretion is the net difference between the quantity filtered at the glomerulus and the amount reabsorbed. About 9 g of Ca^{2+} is filtered each day. Tubular reabsorption is very efficient, with more than 98% of filtered Ca^{2+} returned to the circulation. The efficiency of reabsorption is highly regulated by parathyroid hormone (PTH) but also is influenced by filtered Na^+, the presence of nonreabsorbed anions, and diuretic agents (*see* Chapter 28). Sodium intake, and therefore sodium excretion, is directly related to urinary calcium excretion. Diuretics that act on the ascending limb of the loop of Henle (*e.g.,* *furosemide*) increase calcium excretion. By contrast, *thiazide diuretics* uncouple the relationship between Na^+ and Ca^{2+} excretion, increasing sodium excretion but diminishing calcium excretion (Friedman and Bushinsky, 1999). Dietary protein is directly related to urine Ca^{2+} excretion, presumably owing to the effect of sulfur-containing amino acids on renal tubular function.

Phosphate

In addition to its roles as a dynamic constituent of intermediary and energy metabolism and as a key regulator of enzyme activity when transferred by protein kinases from ATP to phosphorylatable serine, threonine, and tyrosine residues, phosphate is an essential component of all body tissues, being present in plasma, extracellular fluid, cell membrane phospholipids, intracellular fluid, collagen, and bone tissue. More than 80% of total body phosphorus is found in bone, and about 15% is in soft tissue.

Biologically, phosphorus (P) exists in both organic and inorganic forms. Organic forms include phospholipids and various organic esters. In extracellular fluid, the bulk of phosphorus exists as inorganic phosphate in the form of NaH_2PO_4 and Na_2HPO_4; the ratio of disodium to monosodium phosphate at pH 7.40 is 4:1, so plasma phosphate has an intermediate valence of 1.8. Owing to its relatively low concentration in extracellular fluid, phosphate contributes little to buffering capacity. The aggregate level of inorganic phosphate (P_i) modifies tissue concentrations of Ca^{2+} and plays a major role in renal H^+ excretion. Within bone, phosphate is complexed with calcium as hydroxyapatites having the general formula $Ca_{10}(PO_4)_6(OH)_2$ and as calcium phosphate.

Absorption, Distribution, and Excretion. Phosphate is absorbed from and to a limited extent secreted into the gastrointestinal tract. Phosphate is a ubiquitous component of ordinary foods; thus, an inadequate diet rarely causes phosphate depletion. Transport of phosphate from the intestinal lumen is an active, energy-dependent process that is regulated by several factors, including vitamin D, which stimulates absorption. In adults, about two-thirds of ingested phosphate is absorbed and is excreted almost entirely into the urine. In growing children, phosphate balance is positive, and plasma concentrations of phosphate are higher than in adults.

Phosphate excretion in the urine represents the difference between the amount filtered and that reabsorbed. More than 90% of plasma phosphate is freely filtered at the glomerulus, and 80% is actively reabsorbed, predominantly in the initial segment of the proximal convoluted tubule but also in the proximal straight tubule (pars recta). Renal phosphate absorption is regulated by a variety of hormones and other factors; the most important are PTH and dietary phosphate, with extracellular volume and acid–base status playing lesser roles. Dietary phosphate deficiency up-regulates renal phosphate transporters and decreases excretion, whereas a high-phosphate diet increases phosphate excretion; these changes are independent of any effect on plasma P_i, Ca^{2+}, or PTH. PTH increases urinary phosphate excretion by blocking phosphate absorption. Expansion of plasma volume increases urinary phosphate excretion. Effects of vitamin D and its metabolites on proximal tubular phosphate are modest at best.

Role of Phosphate in Urine Acidification. Despite the fact that the concentration and buffering capacity of phosphate in extracellular fluid are low, phosphate is concentrated progressively in the renal tubule and becomes the most abundant buffer system in the distal tubule and terminal nephron. The exchange of H^+ and Na^+ in the tubular urine converts disodium hydrogen phosphate (Na_2HPO_4) to sodium dihydrogen phosphate (NaH_2PO_4), permitting the excretion of large amounts of acid without lowering the urine pH to a degree that would block H^+ transport.

Actions of Phosphate Ion. If large amounts of phosphate are introduced into the gastrointestinal tract by oral administration or enema, a cathartic action will result. Thus phosphate salts are employed as mild laxatives (*see* Chapter 37). If excessive phosphate salts are introduced either intravenously or orally, they may reduce the concentration of Ca^{2+} in the circulation and induce precipitation of calcium phosphate in soft tissues.

PHYSIOLOGY OF CALCIUM AND PHOSPHATE REGULATION

A number of hormones interact to regulate the calcium and phosphate ions. The most important are parathyroid hormone (PTH) and 1,25-dihydroxyvitamin D (*calcitriol*), which regulate mineral homeostasis by effects on the kidney, intestine, and bone (Figure 61–3).

Parathyroid Hormone (PTH)

PTH is a polypeptide hormone that helps to regulate plasma Ca^{2+} by affecting bone resorption/formation, renal Ca^{2+} excretion/reabsorption, and calcitriol synthesis (thus gastrointestinal Ca^{2+} absorption).

History. Sir Richard Owen, the curator of the British Museum of Natural History, discovered the parathyroid glands in 1852 while dissecting a rhinoceros that had died in the London Zoo. Credit for discovery of the human parathyroid glands usually is given to Sandstrom, a Swedish medical student who published an anatomical report in 1890. In 1891, von Recklinghausen reported a new bone disease, which he termed "osteitis fibrosa cystica," which Askanazy subsequently described in a patient with a parathyroid tumor in

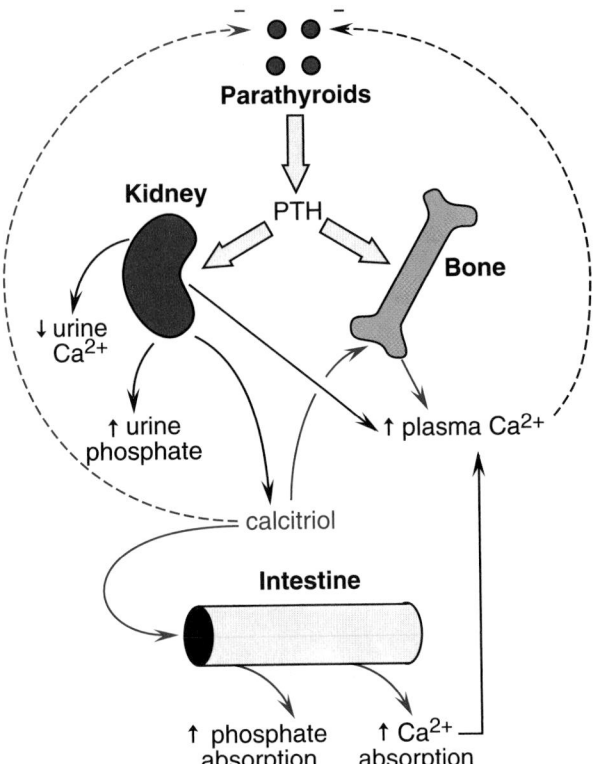

Figure 61–3. *Calcium homeostasis and its regulation by parathyroid hormone (PTH) and 1,25-dihydroxyvitamin D.* PTH has stimulatory effects on bone and kidney, including the stimulation of 1α-hydroxylase activity in kidney mitochondria leading to the increased production of 1,25-dihydroxyvitamin D (calcitriol) from 25-hydroxycholecalciferol, the monohydroxylated vitamin D metabolite (*see* Figure 61–6). Calcitriol is the biologically active metabolite of vitamin D. Solid lines indicate a positive effect; dashed lines refer to negative feedback.

1904. The glands were rediscovered a decade later by Gley, who determined the effects of their extirpation with the thyroid. Vassale and Generali then successfully removed only the parathyroids and noted that tetany, convulsions, and death quickly followed unless calcium was given postoperatively.

MacCallum and Voegtlin first noted the effect of parathyroidectomy on plasma Ca^{2+}. The relation of low plasma Ca^{2+} concentration to symptoms was quickly appreciated, and a comprehensive picture of parathyroid function began to form. Active glandular extracts alleviated hypocalcemic tetany in parathyroidectomized animals and raised the level of plasma Ca^{2+} in normal animals. For the first time, the relation of clinical abnormalities to parathyroid hyperfunction was appreciated.

While American and British investigators used physiological approaches to explore the function of the parathyroid glands, German and Austrian pathologists related the skeletal changes of osteitis fibrosa cystica to the presence of parathyroid tumors; these two diverse types of investigations finally arrived at the same con-

clusions. Much of the history of the parathyroid has been recounted by Carney (1996).

Chemistry. Human, bovine, and porcine PTH molecules are all single polypeptide chains of 84 amino acids with molecular masses of approximately 9500 daltons. Biological activity is associated with the N-terminal portion of the peptide; residues 1 to 27 are required for optimal binding to the PTH receptor and hormone activity. Derivatives lacking the first or second residue bind to PTH receptors but do not activate the cyclic AMP or IP_3–Ca^{2+} signaling pathways. The PTH fragment lacking the first six amino acids inhibits PTH action.

Synthesis, Secretion, and Immunoassay. PTH is synthesized as a 115-amino-acid translation product called *preproparathyroid hormone*. This single-chain peptide is converted to proparathyroid hormone by cleavage of 25 amino-terminal residues as the peptide is transferred to the intracisternal space of the endoplasmic reticulum. Proparathyroid hormone then moves to the Golgi complex, where it is converted to PTH by cleavage of six amino acids. PTH(1–84) resides within secretory granules until it is discharged into the circulation. Neither preproparathyroid hormone nor proparathyroid hormone appears in plasma. The synthesis and processing of PTH have been reviewed (Jüppner *et al.*, 2001).

A major proteolytic product of PTH is PTH(7–84). PTH(7–84) and other amino-truncated PTH fragments accumulate significantly during renal failure in part because they are cleared from the circulation predominantly by the kidneys, whereas intact PTH is also removed by extrarenal mechanisms. Rather than competitively displacing PTH(1–84), PTH(7–84) may inhibit the PTH receptor by causing it to internalize from the plasma membrane in a cell-specific manner (Sneddon *et al.*, 2003).

During periods of hypocalcemia, more PTH is secreted and less is hydrolyzed. In this setting, PTH(7–84) release is augmented. In prolonged hypocalcemia, PTH synthesis also increases, and the gland hypertrophies.

PTH(1–84) has a half-life in plasma of 2 to 5 minutes; removal by the liver and kidney accounts for about 90% of its clearance. As noted earlier, metabolism of PTH generates smaller fragments [*e.g.*, PTH(7–84)] that also circulate in blood and are measured by standard immunoradiometric assays (IRMAs) using two monoclonal antibodies, one directed toward but not at the amino terminus and the other directed toward the carboxyl-terminal portion of the hormone. Large amino-terminal PTH fragments such as PTH(7–84) also react with antibodies prepared against the intact hormone and are measured by standard IRMAs. Therefore, second-generation PTH assays have been developed that differentiate between PTH(1–84), or whole PTH, and "intact" PTH [PTH(1–84) and PTH(7–84)]. The ability to measure whole PTH separately from large amino-terminally truncated PTH fragments has increased the accuracy of laboratory testing of parathyroid and bone status in patients with renal failure (Monier-Faugere *et al.*, 2001).

Physiological Functions. The primary function of PTH is to maintain a constant concentration of Ca^{2+} in the extracellular fluid. The principal processes regulated are renal Ca^{2+} absorption and mobilization of bone Ca^{2+} (Figure 61–3). PTH also affects a variety of nonclassical target tissues that include cartilage, vascular smooth muscle, placenta, liver, pancreatic islets, brain, dermal fibroblasts, and lymphocytes (Tian *et al.*, 1993; Urena *et al.*, 1993). The actions of PTH on its target tissues are mediated by at least two receptors. The PTH-1 receptor (PTH1R or PTH/PTHrP receptor) also binds PTH-related protein (PTHrP), and the PTH-2 receptor, found in vascular tissues, brain, pancreas, and placenta, binds only PTH. Both of these are G protein–coupled receptors that can couple with G_s and G_q in cell-type specific manners; thus, cells may show one, the other, or both types of responses. There is also evidence that PTH can activate phospholipase D through a $G_{12/13}$–RhoA pathway (Singh *et al.*, 2005). A third receptor, designated the CPTH receptor, interacts with forms of PTH that are truncated in the amino-terminal region but that contain most of the carboxy terminus.

Regulation of Secretion. Plasma Ca^{2+} is the major factor regulating PTH secretion. As the concentration of Ca^{2+} diminishes, PTH secretion increases. Sustained hypocalcemia induces parathyroid hypertrophy and hyperplasia. Conversely, if the concentration of Ca^{2+} is high, PTH secretion decreases. Studies of parathyroid cells in culture show that amino acid transport, nucleic acid and protein synthesis, cytoplasmic growth, and PTH secretion are all stimulated by low concentrations of Ca^{2+} and suppressed by high concentrations. Thus, Ca^{2+} itself appears to regulate parathyroid gland growth as well as hormone synthesis and secretion.

Changes in plasma Ca^{2+} regulate PTH secretion by the plasma membrane–associated calcium-sensing receptor (CaSR) on parathyroid cells (Brown and MacLeod, 2001). The CaSR is a GPCR that couples with G_q–PLC and G_i. Occupancy of the CaSR by Ca^{2+} inhibits PTH secretion, whereas reduced CaSR occupancy promotes hormone secretion. Thus, the extracellular concentration of Ca^{2+} is controlled by a classical negative-feedback system, the afferent limb of which is sensitive to the ambient activity of Ca^{2+} and the efferent limb of which releases PTH. Acting *via* the CaSR, hypercalcemia reduces intracellular cyclic AMP content and protein kinase C (PKC) activity, whereas hypocalcemia leads to activation of PKC. However, the precise links between these changes and alterations in PTH secretion remain to be defined. Other agents that increase parathyroid cell cyclic AMP levels, such as β adrenergic receptor agonists and *dopamine,* also increase PTH secretion, but the magnitude of response is far less than that seen with hypocalcemia. The active vitamin D metabolite, 1,25-dihydroxyvitamin D (calcitriol), directly suppresses PTH gene expression. There appears to be no relation between physiological concentrations of extracellular phosphate and PTH secretion, except insofar as changes in phosphate concentration alter circulating Ca^{2+}. Severe hypermagnesemia or hypomagnesemia can inhibit PTH secretion.

Effects on Bone. PTH increases bone resorption and thereby increases Ca^{2+} delivery to the extracellular fluid.

This process involves the release of organic and mineral matrix components (*see* below). The apparent skeletal target cell for PTH is the osteoblast, although evidence for the presence of PTH receptors on mammalian osteoblasts is limited (Manen *et al.*, 1998). PTH also recruits osteoclast precursor cells to form new bone remodeling units (*see* below). Sustained increases in circulating PTH cause characteristic histological changes in bone that include an increase in the prevalence of osteoclastic resorption sites and in the proportion of bone surface that is covered with unmineralized matrix (Martin and Ng, 1994).

Direct effects of PTH on osteoblasts *in vitro* generally are inhibitory and include reduced formation of type I collagen, alkaline phosphatase, and osteocalcin. However, the response to PTH *in vivo* reflects not only hormone action on individual cells but also the increased total number of active osteoblasts owing to initiation of new remodeling units. Thus plasma levels of osteocalcin and alkaline phosphatase activity actually may be increased. No simple model can fully explain the molecular basis of PTH effects on bone. PTH stimulates cyclic AMP production in osteoblasts, but there also is evidence that intracellular Ca^{2+} mediates some PTH actions.

Effects on Kidney. In the kidney, PTH enhances the efficiency of Ca^{2+} reabsorption, inhibits tubular reabsorption of phosphate, and stimulates conversion of vitamin D to its biologically active form, calcitriol (Figure 61–3; *see* below). As a result, filtered Ca^{2+} is avidly retained, and its concentration increases in plasma, whereas phosphate is excreted, and its plasma concentration falls. Newly synthesized calcitriol interacts with specific high-affinity receptors in the intestine to increase the efficiency of intestinal Ca^{2+} absorption, thereby also increasing the plasma Ca^{2+} concentration.

Calcium. PTH increases tubular reabsorption of Ca^{2+} with concomitant decreases in urinary Ca^{2+} excretion. The effect occurs at distal nephron sites (Friedman, 1999). This action, along with mobilization of calcium from bone and increased absorption from the gut, increases the concentration of Ca^{2+} in plasma. Eventually, the increased glomerular filtration of Ca^{2+} overwhelms the stimulatory effect of PTH on tubular reabsorption, and hypercalciuria ensues. Conversely, reduction of serum PTH depresses tubular reabsorption of Ca^{2+} and thereby increases urinary Ca^{2+} excretion. When the plasma Ca^{2+} concentration falls below 7 mg/dl (1.75 mM), Ca^{2+} excretion decreases as the filtered load of Ca^{2+} reaches the point where the cation is almost completely reabsorbed despite reduced tubular capacity.

Phosphate. PTH increases renal excretion of inorganic phosphate by decreasing its reabsorption. This action is mediated by retrieval of the luminal membrane Na–P_i cotransport protein rather than an effect on its activity. Patients with primary hyperparathyroidism therefore typically have low tubular phosphate reabsorption.

Cyclic AMP apparently mediates the renal effects of PTH on proximal tubular phosphate reabsorption. PTH-sensitive adenylyl cyclase is located in the renal cortex, and cyclic AMP synthesized in response to the hormone affects tubular transport mechanisms. A portion of the cyclic AMP synthesized at this site, so-called nephrogenous cyclic AMP, escapes into the urine; measurement of urinary cyclic AMP is used as a surrogate for parathyroid activity and renal responsiveness.

Other Ions. PTH reduces renal excretion of Mg^{2+}. This effect reflects the net result of increased renal Mg^{2+} reabsorption and increased mobilization of the ion from bone (Quamme, 1997). PTH increases excretion of water, amino acids, citrate, K^+, bicarbonate, Na^+, Cl^-, and SO_4^{2-}, whereas it decreases the excretion of H^+.

Calcitriol Synthesis. The final step in the activation of vitamin D to calcitriol occurs in kidney proximal tubule cells. Three primary regulators govern the activity of the 25-hydroxyvitamin D_3-1α-hydroxylase that catalyzes this step: P_i, PTH, and Ca^{2+}(*see* below for further discussion). Reduced circulating or tissue phosphate content rapidly increases calcitriol production, whereas hyperphosphatemia or hypercalcemia suppresses it. PTH powerfully stimulates calcitriol synthesis. Thus, when hypocalcemia causes a rise in PTH concentration, both the PTH-dependent lowering of circulating P_i and a more direct effect of the hormone on the 1α-hydroxylase lead to increased circulating concentrations of calcitriol.

Integrated Regulation of Extracellular Ca^{2+} Concentration by PTH.

Even modest reductions of serum Ca^{2+} stimulate PTH secretion. For minute-to-minute regulation of Ca^{2+}, adjustments in renal Ca^{2+} handling more than suffice to maintain plasma calcium homeostasis. With more prolonged hypocalcemia, the renal 1α-hydroxylase is induced, enhancing the synthesis and release of calcitriol that directly stimulates intestinal calcium absorption (Figure 61–3). In addition, delivery of calcium from bone into the extracellular fluid is stimulated. In the face of prolonged and severe hypocalcemia, new bone remodeling units are activated to restore circulating Ca^{2+} concentrations, albeit at the expense of skeletal integrity.

When plasma Ca^{2+} activity rises, PTH secretion is suppressed, and tubular Ca^{2+} reabsorption decreases. The reduction in circulating PTH promotes renal phosphate conservation, and both the decreased PTH and the increased phosphate reduce calcitriol production and thereby decrease intestinal Ca^{2+} absorption. Finally, bone remodeling is suppressed. These integrated physiological events ensure a coherent response to positive or negative excursions of plasma Ca^{2+} concentration. In human beings, the importance of other hormones, such as calcitonin, to this scheme remains unsettled, but it is likely that these modulate the Ca^{2+}–parathyroid–vitamin D axis rather than serving as primary regulators.

Vitamin D

Vitamin D traditionally was viewed as a permissive factor in calcium metabolism because it was thought to permit efficient absorption of dietary calcium and to allow full expression of the actions of PTH. We now know that vitamin D exerts a more active role in calcium homeostasis. Vitamin D is actually a hormone rather than a vitamin; it is synthesized in mammals and, under ideal conditions, probably is not required in the diet. Receptors for the activated form of vitamin D are expressed in many cells that are not involved in calcium homeostasis, including hematopoietic cells, lymphocytes, epidermal cells, pancreatic islets, muscle, and neurons.

History. Vitamin D is the name applied to two related fat-soluble substances, *cholecalciferol* and *ergocalciferol* (Figure 61–4), that share the capacity to prevent or cure rickets. Prior to the discovery of vitamin D, a high percentage of urban children living in temperate zones developed rickets. Some researchers believed that the disease was due to lack of fresh air and sunshine; others claimed a dietary factor was responsible. Mellanby and Huldschinsky showed both notions to be correct; addition of cod liver oil to the diet or exposure to sunlight prevented or cured the disease. In 1924, it was found that ultraviolet irradiation of animal rations was as efficacious at curing rickets as was irradiation of the animal itself. These observations led to the elucidation of the structures of chole- and ergocalciferol and eventually to the discovery that these compounds require further processing in the body to become active. The discovery of metabolic activation is attributable primarily to studies conducted in the laboratories of DeLuca (DeLuca and Schnoes, 1976) and Kodicek (Mason *et al.*, 1974).

Chemistry and Occurrence. Ultraviolet irradiation of several animal and plant sterols results in their conversion to compounds possessing vitamin D activity. The principal provitamin found in animal tissues is 7-dehydrocholesterol, which is synthesized in the skin. Exposure of the skin to sunlight converts 7-dehydrocholesterol to cholecalciferol (vitamin D_3) (Figure 61–4). Ergosterol, which is present only in plants, is the provitamin for vitamin D_2 (ergocalciferol). Ergosterol and vitamin D_2 differ from 7-dehydrocholesterol and vitamin D_3, respectively, by the presence of a double bond between C22 and C23 and a methyl group at C24. Vitamin D_2 is the active constituent of a number of commercial vitamin preparations, and is in irradiated bread and irradiated milk. In humans there is no practical difference between the antirachitic potencies of vitamin D_2 and vitamin D_3. Therefore, "vitamin D" will be used here as a collective term for vitamins D_2 and D_3.

Human Requirements and Units.

Although sunlight provides adequate vitamin D supplies in the equatorial belt, in temperate climates insufficient cutaneous solar radiation in winter may necessitate dietary vitamin D supplementation. It was assumed that vitamin D deficiency had been eliminated as a significant problem in the United States. However, recent evidence points to low circulating levels of vitamin D with a reemergence of vitamin D–

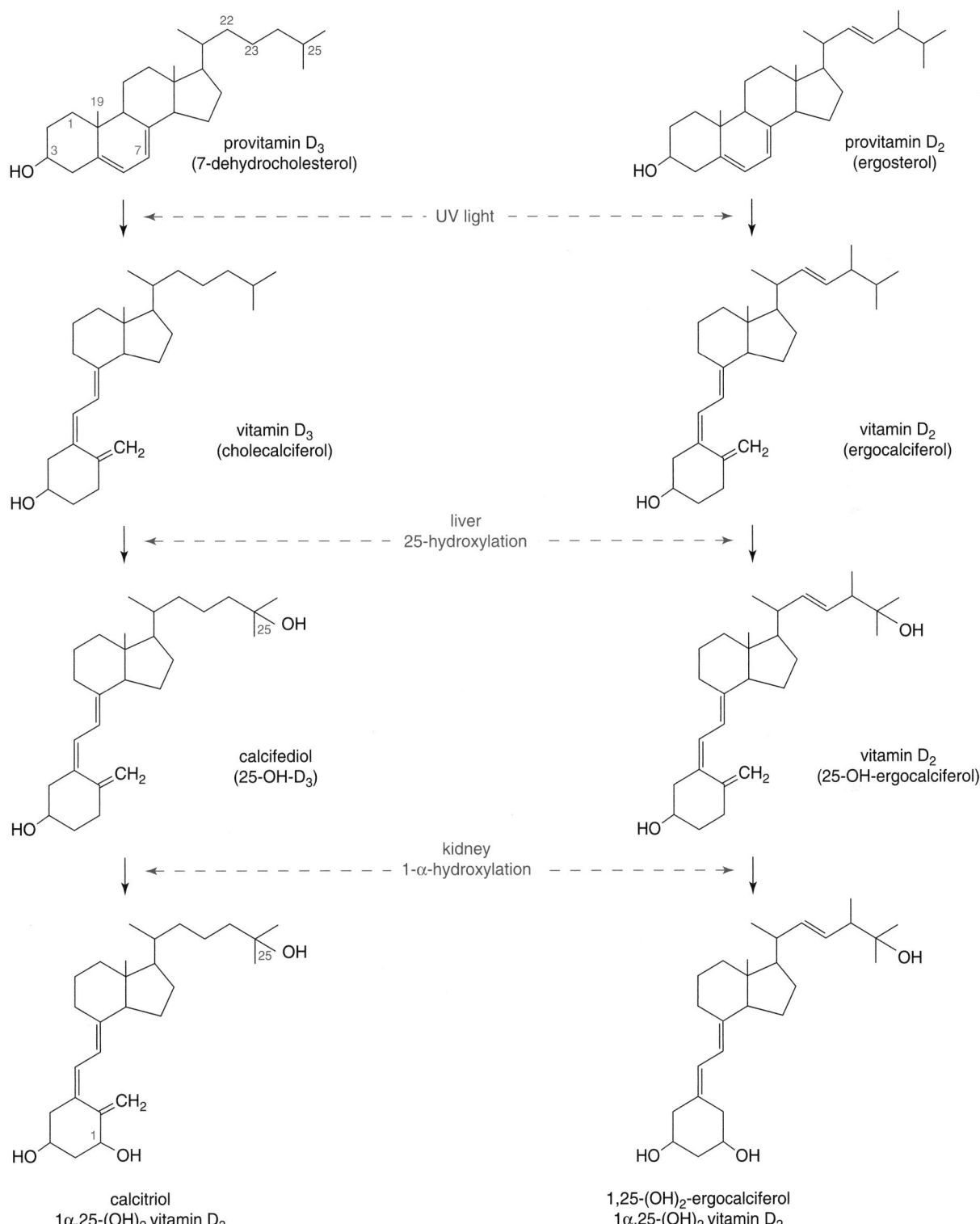

Figure 61–4. ***Photobiology and metabolic pathways of vitamin D production and metabolism.*** Numbering for select positions discussed in the text is shown.

dependent rickets. Potential factors contributing to the rise in vitamin D deficiency include diminished intake of vitamin D–fortified foods owing to concerns about fat intake; reduced intake of calcium-rich foods, including milk, in adolescents and young women of reproductive age; increased use of sunscreens and decreased exposure to sunlight to reduce the risk of skin cancer and prevent premature aging owing to exposure to ultraviolet radiation; and an increased prevalence and duration of exclusive breast-feeding (the combination of human milk, a poor source of vitamin D, and the high prevalence of low circulating vitamin D levels in U.S. women, particularly African-American mothers) (Nesby-O'Dell *et al.*, 2002; Stokstad, 2003; Holick *et al.*, 2005).

There is no consensus regarding optimal vitamin D intake, and determination of vitamin D requirements is remarkably unsupported by clinical measurements. The recommended dietary allowance of vitamin D for infants and children is 400 IU, or 10 μg. The basis for this dose was that it approximates that in a teaspoon (5 ml) of cod liver oil, which had long been considered safe and effective in preventing rickets (Vieth, 1999). On the basis that adults require less vitamin D than infants, the adult dose was set arbitrarily at 200 IU.

There are no recommended dietary allowances for vitamin D. However, the Food and Nutrition Board of the Institute of Medicine has developed Dietary Reference Intakes (DRI) for vitamins (Institute of Medicine, 2003). In both premature and normal infants, intake of 200 units per day of vitamin D from any source is considered adequate for optimal growth. During adolescence and beyond, this amount probably is also sufficient. There is some evidence that vitamin D requirements increase during pregnancy and lactation (Hollis and Wagner, 2004), where vitamin D doses of less than 1000 IU/day may be inadequate to maintain normal circulating 25-hydroxyvitamin D concentrations. Doses of 10,000 IU/day or less of vitamin D for up to 5 months do not elevate circulating 25-hydroxyvitamin D to concentrations greater than 90 ng/ml.

Absorption, Fate, and Excretion. Both vitamins D_2 and D_3 are absorbed from the small intestine, although vitamin D_3 may be absorbed more efficiently. Most of the vitamin appears first within chylomicrons in lymph. Bile is essential for adequate absorption of vitamin D; deoxycholic acid is the major constituent of bile in this regard (*see* Chapter 37). The primary route of vitamin D excretion is the bile; only a small percentage is found in the urine. Patients who have intestinal bypass surgery or otherwise have severe shortening or inflammation of the small intestine may fail to absorb vitamin D sufficiently to maintain normal levels; hepatic or biliary dysfunction also may seriously impair vitamin D absorption.

Absorbed vitamin D circulates in the blood in association with vitamin D–binding protein, a specific α-globu-

lin. The vitamin disappears from plasma with a half-life of 19 to 25 hours but is stored in fat depots for prolonged periods.

Metabolic Activation. Whether derived from diet or endogenously synthesized, vitamin D requires modification to become biologically active. The primary active metabolite of the vitamin is calcitriol [1α,25-dihydroxyvitamin D, 1,25(OH)$_2$D], the product of two successive hydroxylations of vitamin D (Figure 61–4).

25-Hydroxylation of Vitamin D. The initial step in vitamin D activation occurs in the liver, where cholecalciferol and ergocalciferol are hydroxylated in the 25-position to generate 25-OH-cholecalciferol (25-OHD, or calcifediol) and 25-OH-ergocalciferol, respectively. 25-OHD is the major circulating form of vitamin D$_3$; it has a biological half-life of 19 days, and normal steady-state concentrations are 15 to 50 ng/ml. Reduced extracellular Ca^{2+} levels stimulate 1α-hydroxylation of 25-OHD, increasing the formation of biologically active 1,25(OH)$_2$D$_3$. In contrast, when Ca^{2+} concentrations are elevated, 25-OHD is inactivated by 24-hydroxylation. Similar reactions occur with 25-OH-ergocalciferol. Normal steady-state concentrations of 25-OHD in human beings are 15 to 50 ng/ml, although concentrations below 25 ng/ml may be associated with increased circulating PTH and greater bone turnover.

1α-Hydroxylation of 25-OHD. After production in the liver, 25-OHD enters the circulation and is carried by vitamin D–binding globulin. Final activation to calcitriol occurs primarily in the kidney but also takes place in other sites, including keratinocytes and macrophages (Hewison *et al.*, 2004). The enzyme system responsible for 1α-hydroxylation of 25-OHD (CYP1α, 25-hydroxyvitamin D$_3$-1α-hydroxylase, 1α-hydroxylase) is associated with mitochondria in proximal tubules.

Vitamin D 1α-hydroxylase is subject to tight regulatory controls that result in changes in calcitriol formation appropriate for optimal calcium homeostasis. Dietary deficiency of vitamin D, calcium, or phosphate enhances enzyme activity. 1α-Hydroxylase is potently stimulated by PTH and probably also by prolactin and estrogen. Conversely, high calcium, phosphate, and vitamin D intakes suppress 1α-hydroxylase activity. Regulation (Figure 61–5) is both acute and chronic, the latter owing to changes in protein synthesis. PTH increases calcitriol production rapidly *via* a cyclic AMP–dependent pathway. Hypocalcemia can activate the hydroxylase directly in addition to affecting it indirectly by eliciting PTH secretion (Bland *et al.*, 1999). Hypophosphatemia greatly increases 1α-hydroxylase activity (Haussler and McCain, 1977; Yoshida *et al.*, 2001). Calcitriol controls 1α-hydroxylase activity by a negative-feedback mechanism that involves a direct action on the kidney, as well as inhibition of PTH secretion. The plasma half-life of calcitriol is estimated to be between 3 and 5 days in humans.

24-Hydroxylase. Calcitriol and 25-OHD are hydroxylated to 1,24,25(OH)$_2$D and 24,25(OH)$_2$D, respectively, by another renal enzyme, 24-hydroxylase, whose expression is induced by calcitriol and suppressed by factors that stimulate the 25-OHD-1α-hydroxylase. Both 24-hydroxylated compounds are less active than calcitriol and presumably represent metabolites destined for excretion.

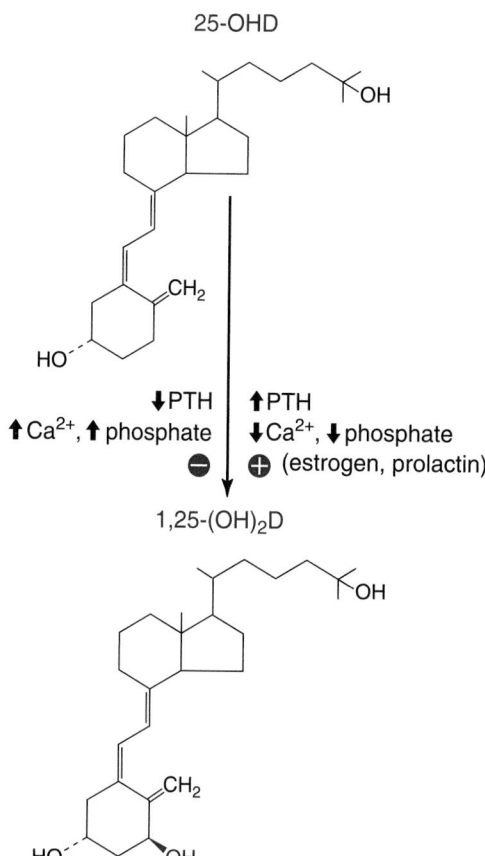

25-OHD

↓PTH | ↑PTH
↑Ca²⁺, ↑ phosphate | ↓Ca²⁺, ↓phosphate
⊖ | ⊕ (estrogen, prolactin)

1,25-(OH)₂D

Figure 61–5. ***Regulation of 1α-hydroxylase activity.*** Changes in the plasma levels of PTH, Ca²⁺, and phospate modulate the hydroxylation of 25-OH vitamin D to the active form, 1,25,dihydroxyvitamin D. 25-OHD, 25-hydroxycholecalciferol; 1,25-(OH)₂-D, calcitriol; PTH, parathyroid hormone.

Physiological Functions and Mechanism of Action.

Calcitriol augments absorption and retention of Ca²⁺ and phosphate. Although regulation of Ca²⁺ homeostasis is considered to be its primary function, accumulating evidence underscores the importance of calcitriol in a number of other processes (*see* below).

Calcitriol acts to maintain normal concentrations of Ca²⁺ and phosphate in plasma by facilitating their absorption in the small intestine, by interacting with PTH to enhance their mobilization from bone, and by decreasing their renal excretion. It also exerts direct physiological and pharmacological effects on bone mineralization (Suda *et al.*, 2003).

The mechanism of action of calcitriol is mediated by the interaction of calcitriol with the vitamin D receptor (VDR). Calcitriol binds to cytosolic VDRs within target cells, and the receptor–hormone complex translocates to

the nucleus and interacts with DNA to modify gene transcription. The VDR belongs to the steroid and thyroid hormone receptor supergene family (Christakos *et al.*, 2003). Calcitriol also exerts nongenomic effects (Farach-Carson and Nemere, 2003) that may require the presence of a functional VDR (Zanello and Norman, 2004).

Intestinal Absorption of Calcium. Calcium is absorbed predominantly in the duodenum, with progressively smaller amounts in the jejunum and ileum. Studies of Ca²⁺ uptake by isolated cells reflect these differences and suggest that elevated amounts of transport are likely due to greater transport by each duodenal cell. The colon also contributes to calcium absorption because ileostomy reduces absorption.

In the absence of calcitriol, calcium absorption is inefficient and proceeds in a thermodynamically passive manner through the lateral intercellular spaces (paracellular pathway). Calcitriol increases the transcellular movement of Ca²⁺ from the mucosal to the serosal surface of the duodenum. Transcellular Ca²⁺ movement involves three processes: Ca²⁺ entry across the mucosal surface, diffusion through the cell, and energy-dependent extrusion across the serosal cell membrane. Calcium is also secreted from serosal to mucosal compartments. Thus net calcium absorption is the difference between the two oppositely oriented vectorial processes. The complex mechanisms and the proteins mediating calcium absorption are still incompletely understood (Bronner, 2003). Evidence implicates TRPV6 Ca²⁺ channels in mediating mucosal calcium entry in the intestine (Nijenhuis *et al.*, 2003). In humans, TRPV6 is expressed in the duodenum and proximal jejunum (Barley *et al.*, 2001). A calcium-poor diet up-regulates intestinal TRPV6 expression in mice (Van Cromphaut *et al.*, 2001). This effect is greatly reduced in VDR knockout mice, suggesting that TRPV6 mediates calcium entry and is vitamin D–dependent. Calcitriol also up-regulates the calcium-binding protein calbindin-D₉ₖ.

Ca²⁺ absorption is potently augmented by calcitriol. It is likely that calcitriol enhances all three steps involved in intestinal Ca²⁺ absorption: entry across mucosal brush border membranes, diffusion through the enterocytes, and active extrusion across serosal plasma membranes (Bronner, 2003). Calcitriol up-regulates the synthesis of calbindin-D₉ₖ and calbindin-D₂₈ₖ and the serosal plasma membrane Ca–ATPase. Calbindin-D₉ₖ enhances the extrusion of Ca²⁺ by the Ca–ATPase, whereas the precise function of calbindin-D₂₈ₖ is unsettled.

Mobilization of Bone Mineral. Although vitamin D–deficient animals show obvious deficits in bone mineral, there is little evidence that calcitriol directly promotes mineralization. Thus, although VDR knockout mice exhibit severely impaired bone formation and mineralization, these deficiencies can be entirely corrected by a high-calcium diet. These results support the view that the primary role of calcitriol is to stimulate intestinal absorption of calcium, which, in turn, indirectly promotes bone mineralization. Indeed, children with rickets caused by mutations of the VDR have been treated successfully with intravenous infusions of Ca²⁺ and phosphate (*see* below). In contrast, physiological doses of vitamin D promote mobilization of Ca²⁺ from bone, and large doses cause excessive bone turnover. Although calcitriol-induced bone resorption may be reduced in parathyroidectomized animals, the response is restored when hyperphosphatemia is corrected. Thus, PTH and calcitriol act independently to enhance bone resorption.

Calcitriol increases bone turnover by multiple mechanisms (*see* Suda *et al.*, 2003). Mature osteoclasts apparently lack the VDR. Acting by a non-VDR mechanism, calcitriol promotes the recruitment of osteoclast precursor cells to resorption sites, as well as the development of differentiated functions that characterize mature osteoclasts.

Osteoblasts, the cells responsible for bone formation, express the VDR, and calcitriol induces their production of several proteins, including osteocalcin, a vitamin K–dependent protein that contains γ-carboxyglutamic acid residues, and interleukin-1 (IL-1), a lymphokine that promotes bone resorption (Spear *et al.*, 1988). Thus, the current view is that calcitriol is a bone-mobilizing hormone but not a bone-forming hormone. Osteoporosis is a disease in which osteoclast responsiveness to calcitriol or other bone-resorbing agents is profoundly impaired, leading to deficient bone resorption.

Renal Retention of Calcium and Phosphate. The effects of calcitriol on the renal handling of Ca^{2+} and phosphate are of uncertain importance. Calcitriol increases retention of Ca^{2+} independently of phosphate. The effect on Ca^{2+} is thought to proceed in distal tubules, whereas enhanced phosphate absorption occurs in proximal tubules.

Other Effects of Calcitriol. It now is evident that the effects of calcitriol extend beyond calcium homeostasis. Receptors for calcitriol are distributed widely throughout the body (*see* Pike, 1997). Calcitriol affects maturation and differentiation of mononuclear cells and influences cytokine production and immune function (Hayes *et al.*, 2003). One focus of research is the potential use of calcitriol to inhibit proliferation and to induce differentiation of malignant cells (*see* van den Bemd *et al.*, 2000). The possibility of dissociating the hypercalcemic effect of calcitriol from its actions on cell differentiation has encouraged the search for analogs that might be useful in cancer therapy. Calcitriol inhibits epidermal proliferation and promotes epidermal differentiation and therefore is a potential treatment for psoriasis vulgaris (Kragballe and Iversen, 1993) (*see* Chapter 62). Calcitriol also affects the function of skeletal muscle and brain (Carswell, 1997).

Calcitonin

Calcitonin is a hypocalcemic hormone whose actions generally oppose those of PTH.

History and Source. Copp observed in 1962 that perfusion of canine parathyroid and thyroid glands with hypercalcemic blood caused a transient hypocalcemia that occurred significantly earlier than that caused by total parathyroidectomy. He concluded that the parathyroid glands secreted a calcium-lowering hormone (calcitonin) in response to hypercalcemia and in this way normalized plasma Ca^{2+} concentrations. The physiological relevance of calcitonin has been challenged vigorously: Calcitonin normally circulates at remarkably low levels; surgical removal of the thyroids has no appreciable effect on calcium metabolism; and conditions associated with profound elevations of serum calcitonin concentration are not accompanied by hypocalcemia (Hirsch and Baruch, 2003). The primary interest in calcitonin arises from its pharmacologic use in treating Paget's disease and hypercalcemia and in its diagnostic use as a tumor marker for medullary carcinoma of the thyroid (*see* below).

The thyroid parafollicular C cells are the site of production and secretion of calcitonin. Human C cells, which are derived from neural crest ectoderm, are distributed widely in the thyroid, parathyroid, and thymus. In nonmammalian vertebrates, calcitonin is found in ultimobranchial bodies, which are separate organs from the thyroid gland.

The calcitonin gene is localized on human chromosome 11p and contains six exons (Figure 61–6). The primary transcript is alternatively spliced in a tissue-specific manner. In *thyroid C cells*, the calcitonin/calcitonin gene-related peptide (CGRP) pre-mRNA is processed primarily with common exons 2 and 3 to include exon 4. This leads to production of the 32-amino-acid peptide calcitonin, along with a flanking 21-amino-acid peptide called *katacalcin*, whose physiological significance is unknown. In *neuronal cells,* on the other hand, most of the calcitonin/CGRP pre-mRNA, is processed to exclude exon 4, resulting in inclusion of exons 5 and 6 with common exons 2 and 3, which ultimately gives rise to CGRP. This results in the production of the 37-amino-acid CGRP. Calcitonin is the most potent peptide inhibitor of osteoclast-mediated bone resorption and helps to protect the skeleton during periods of "calcium stress," such as growth, pregnancy, and lactation. CGRP and the closely related peptide adrenomedullin, are potent endogenous vasodilators.

Chemistry and Immunoreactivity. Calcitonin is a single-chain peptide of 32 amino acids with a disulfide bridge linking the cysteine residues in positions 1 and 7 (Figure 61–7). In all species, 8 of the 32 residues are invariant, including the disulfide bridge and a carboxyl-terminal proline amide; both structural features are essential for biological activity. The residues in the middle portion of the molecule (positions 10 to 27) are more variable and apparently influence potency and/or duration of action. Calcitonins derived from salmon and eel differ from the human hormone by 13 and 16 amino acid residues, respectively, and are more potent than mammalian calcitonin. Salmon calcitonin is used therapeutically in part because it is cleared more slowly from the circulation (*see* below).

Regulation of Secretion. The biosynthesis and secretion of calcitonin are regulated by the plasma Ca^{2+} concentration. Calcitonin secretion increases when plasma Ca^{2+} is high and decreases when plasma Ca^{2+} is low. Multiple forms of calcitonin are found in plasma, including high-molecular-weight aggregates or cross-linked products. Assays for the intact monomeric peptide are now available. The circulating concentrations of calcitonin are low, normally less than 15 and 10 pg/ml for males and females, respectively. The circulating half-life of calcitonin is about 10 minutes. Abnormally elevated levels of calcitonin are characteristic of thyroid C-cell hyperplasia and medullary thyroid carcinoma.

Calcitonin secretion is stimulated by a number of agents, including catecholamines, glucagon, gastrin, and cholecystokinin, but there is little evidence for a physiological role for secretion in response to these stimuli.

Mechanism of Action. Calcitonin actions are mediated by the calcitonin receptor (CTR), which is a member of

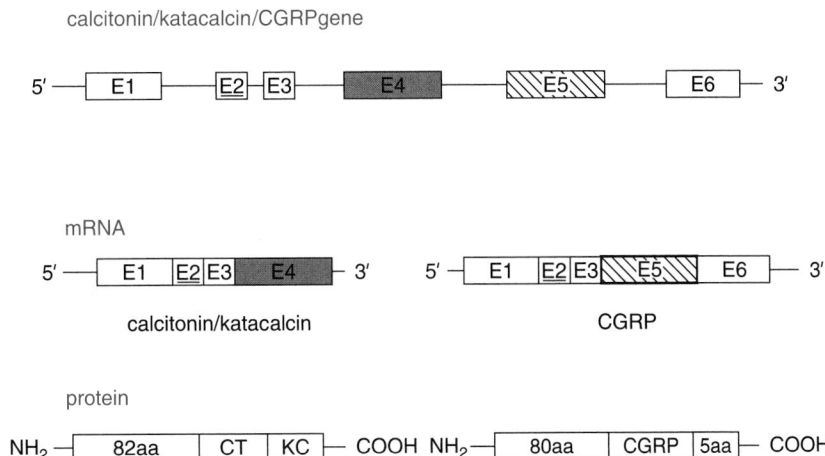

Figure 61–6. *Alternative splicing of calcitonin/calcitonin gene–related peptide (CGRP).*

the PTH/secretin subfamily of GPCRs (Lin *et al.*, 1991). Six human CTR subtypes occur through alternative splicing of coding and noncoding exons (Galson and Goldring, 2002). These isoforms exhibit distinct ligand-binding specificity and/or signal-transduction pathways and are distributed in a tissue-specific pattern. Of the most abundant isoforms, hCTRI1⁻ preferentially couples with the Gₛ–adenylyl cyclase pathway (Gorn *et al.*, 1995). The hCTRI1⁺ isoform does not couple with phospholipase C (Naro *et al.*, 1998) and therefore does not activate protein kinase C or trigger an increase in Ca²⁺. Calcitonin receptors can dimerize with modulatory proteins to create receptors with high affinity for amylin (Hay *et al.*, 2005).

The hypocalcemic and hypophosphatemic effects of calcitonin are caused predominantly by direct inhibition of osteoclastic bone resorption. Although calcitonin inhibits the effects of PTH on osteolysis, it inhibits neither PTH activation of bone cell adenylyl cyclase nor PTH-induced uptake of Ca²⁺ into bone. Calcitonin interacts directly with receptors on osteoclasts to produce a rapid

and profound decrease in ruffled border surface area, thereby diminishing resorptive activity.

Depressed bone resorption reduces urinary excretion of Ca²⁺, Mg²⁺, and hydroxyproline. Plasma phosphate concentrations are lowered owing also to increased urinary phosphate excretion. Direct renal effects of calcitonin vary with species. Acute administration of pharmacological doses of calcitonin increases urinary calcium excretion, whereas calcitonin inhibits renal calcium excretion at physiological concentrations. In humans, calcitonin increases fractional urinary calcium excretion in a dose-dependent manner in subjects given a modest calcium load (Carney, 1997).

BONE PHYSIOLOGY

The skeleton is the primary structural support for the body and also provides a protected environment for hematopoiesis. It contains both a large mineralized matrix and a highly active cellular compartment.

	1	2	3	4	5	6	7	8	9	10	11	12	13	14	15	16	17	18	19	20	21	22	23	24	25	26	27	28	29	30	31	32
human	cys	gly	asn	leu	ser	thr	cys	met	leu	gly	thr	tyr	thr	gln	asp	phe	asn	lys	phe	his	thr	phe	pro	gln	thr	ala	ile	gly	val	gly	ala	pro
mouse																										lys			ser		glu	
porcine								val			ser	ala	tyr	trp	arg	asn	leu	asn	asn	phe	his	arg	phe	ser	gly	met	gly	phe		pro	glu	thr
salmon		ser						val			gly	lys	leu	ser	gln	glu	leu	his	lys	leu	gln	thr	tyr	pro	arg	thr	asn	thr		ser	gly	thr
eel								val			lys	leu	ser	gln	glu	leu	his	lys	leu	gln	thr	tyr	pro	arg	thr	asp	val		ala	gly	thr	

(Disulfide bond between residues 1 and 7; S—S bridge)

Figure 61–7. *Comparison of calcitonins from several species.* Calcitonin is a 32-amino-acid polypeptide with a disulfide bond between residues 1 and 7 and a proline-amide at the C-terminus. The figure highlights the differences in amino acid seqence between human calcitonin and calcitonins of other species; lack of an entry indicates identity with human calcitonin. Salmon calcitonin is ~20 times more potent in humans than is human calcitonin.

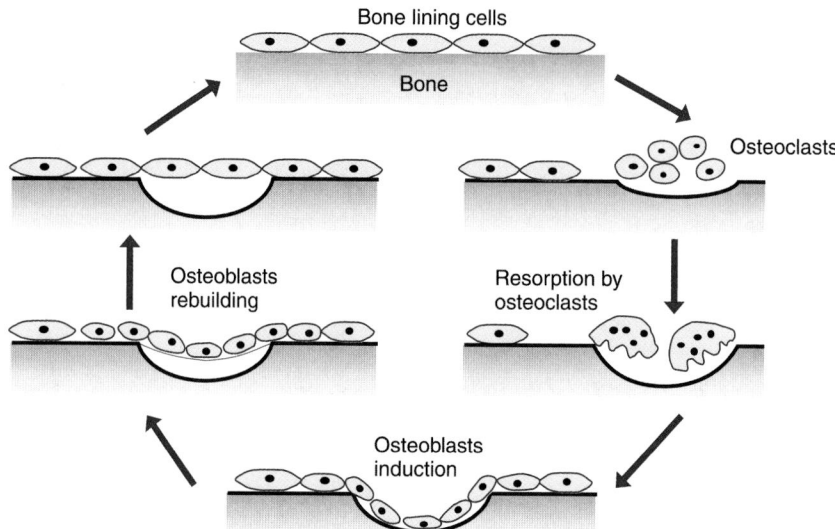

Figure 61–8. *The bone remodeling cycle.* Osteoclast precursors fuse and are activated to resorb a lacuna in a previously quiescent surface. These cells are replaced by osteoblasts that deposit new bone to restore the integrity of the tissue. (*Adapted from Skerry and Gowen, 1995.*)

Skeletal Organization. Because their bone turnover rates differ, it is useful to consider the *appendicular*, or *peripheral*, skeleton as separate from the *axial*, or *central*, skeleton. Appendicular bones make up 80% of bone mass and are composed predominantly of compact cortical bone. Axial bones, such as the spine and pelvis, contain substantial amounts of trabecular bone within a thin cortex. Trabecular bone consists of highly connected bony plates that resemble a honeycomb. The intertrabecular interstices contain bone marrow and fat. *Alterations in bone turnover are observed first and foremost in axial bone* both because bone surfaces, where bone remodeling occurs, are more densely distributed in trabecular bone and because marrow precursor cells that ultimately participate in bone turnover lie in close proximity to trabecular surfaces.

Bone Mass. Bone mineral density (BMD) and fracture risk in later years reflect the maximal bone mineral content at skeletal maturity (peak bone mass) and the subsequent rate of bone loss. Major increases in bone mass, accounting for about 60% of final adult levels, occur during adolescence, mainly during years of highest growth velocity. Bone acquisition is largely complete by age 17 in girls and by age 20 in boys. Inheritance accounts for much of the variance in bone acquisition; other factors include circulating estrogen and androgens, physical activity, and dietary calcium.

Bone mass peaks during the third decade, remains stable until age 50, and then declines progressively. Similar trajectories occur for men and women of all ethnic groups. The fundamental accuracy of this model has been amply confirmed for cortical bone, although trabecular bone loss at some sites probably begins prior to age 50. In women, loss of estrogen at menopause accelerates the rate of bone loss. *Primary regulators of adult bone mass include physical activity, reproductive endocrine status, and calcium intake. Optimal maintenance of BMD requires sufficiency in all three areas, and deficiency in one area is not compensated by excessive attention to another.*

Bone Remodeling. Growth and development of endochondral bone are driven by a process called *modeling*. Once new bone is laid down,

it is subject to a continuous process of breakdown and renewal called *remodeling,* by which bone mass is adjusted throughout adult life (Ballock and O'Keefe, 2003). Remodeling is carried out by myriad independent "bone remodeling units" throughout the skeleton (Figure 61–8). Remodeling proceeds on bone surfaces, about 90% of which are normally inactive, covered by a thin layer of lining cells. In response to physical or biochemical signals, recruitment of marrow precursor cells to the bone surface results in their fusion into the characteristic multinucleated osteoclasts that resorb, or excavate, a cavity into the bone.

Osteoclast production is regulated by osteoblast-derived cytokines such as IL-1 and IL-6. Studies have begun to clarify the mechanisms through which osteoclast production is regulated (*see* Suda *et al.*, 1999). The receptor for activating NFκB (RANK) is an osteoclast protein whose expression is required for osteoclastic bone resorption. Its natural ligand, RANK ligand (RANKL; previously called *osteoclast differentiation factor*), is a membrane-spanning osteoblast protein. On binding to RANK, RANKL induces osteoclast formation (Khosla, 2001) (Figure 61–9). RANKL initiates the activation of mature osteoclasts, as well as the differentiation of osteoclast precursors. Osteoblasts produce osteoprotegerin (OPG), which acts as a decoy ligand for RANKL. Under conditions favoring increased bone resorption, such as estrogen deprivation, OPG is suppressed, RANKL binds to RANK, and osteoclast production increases. When estrogen sufficiency is reestablished, OPG increases and competes effectively with RANKL for binding to RANK. In certain model systems, OPG is superior to bisphosphonates in suppressing bone resorption and hypercalcemia (Morony, *et al.*, 2005).

Completion of the resorption phase is followed by ingress of preosteoblasts derived from marrow stroma into the base of the resorption cavity. These cells develop the characteristic osteoblastic phenotype and begin to replace the resorbed bone by elaborating new bone matrix constituents, such as collagen and osteocalcin. Once the newly formed osteoid reaches a thickness of about 20 μm, mineralization begins. A complete remodeling cycle normally requires about 6 months.

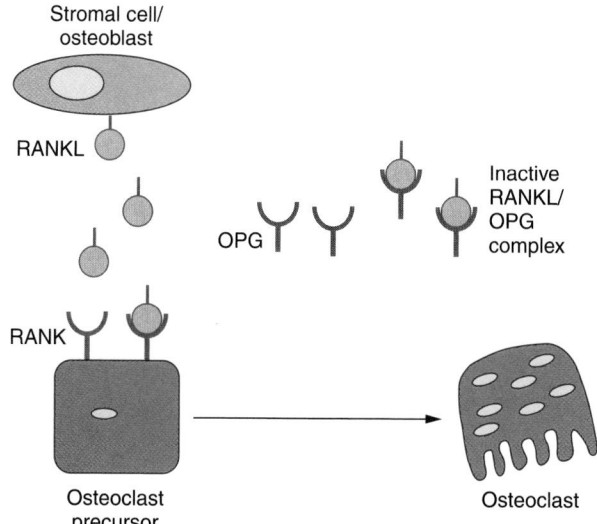

Figure 61–9. *RANK ligand and osteoclast formation.*
RANKL, acting on RANK, promotes osteoclast formation and subsequent resorption of bone matrix. OPG binds to RANKL, inhibiting its binding to RANK and thereby inhibiting osteoclast differentiation.

If the replacement of resorbed bone matched the amount that was removed, remodeling would not change net bone mass. However, small bone deficits persist on completion of each cycle, reflecting inefficient remodeling dynamics. Consequently, lifelong accumulation of remodeling deficits underlies the well-documented phenomenon of age-related bone loss, a process that begins shortly after growth stops. *Alterations in remodeling activity represent the final pathway through which diverse stimuli, such as dietary insufficiency, hormones, and drugs, affect bone balance.* Changes in hormonal milieu often lead to an increase in the activation, or birth rate, of remodeling units. Examples include hyperthyroidism, hyperparathyroidism, and hypervitaminosis D. Other factors may impair osteoblast function, such as high doses of *corticosteroids* or *ethanol*. Finally, estrogen deficiency augments osteoclastic resorptive capacity by a proapoptotic action (Manolagas *et al.*, 2002).

At any given time, a transient deficit in bone, the remodeling space, represents sites of bone resorption that have not yet filled in. Stimuli that alter the rate of emergence of new remodeling units will either increase or decrease the remodeling space until a new steady-state is established at an increased or decreased bone mass.

DISORDERS OF MINERAL HOMEOSTASIS AND BONE

Abnormal Calcium Metabolism

Hypercalcemia. Moderate elevations of the concentration of Ca^{2+} in the extracellular fluid may have no clinically detectable effects. The degree of hypercalcemia and the rate of onset of the elevation in the serum calcium concentration

largely dictate the extent of symptoms. Chronic elevation of serum Ca^{2+} to 12 to 14 mg/dl (3 to 3.5 mmol/L) generally causes few manifestations, whereas an acute rise to the same levels may cause marked neuromuscular manifestations owing to an increased threshold for excitation of nerve and muscle. Symptoms include fatigue, muscle weakness, anorexia, depression, diffuse abdominal pain, and constipation.

Hypercalcemia can result from a number of conditions. Ingestion of large quantities of calcium by itself generally does not cause hypercalcemia; exceptions are hyperthyroid subjects, who absorb Ca^{2+} with increased efficiency (Benker *et al.*, 1988), and subjects with the uncommon *milk-alkali syndrome*, a condition caused by concurrent ingestion of large quantities of milk and absorbable alkali, resulting in impaired renal Ca^{2+} excretion and attendant hypercalcemia.

In an outpatient setting, the most common cause of hypercalcemia is primary hyperparathyroidism, which results from hypersecretion of PTH by one or more parathyroid glands. Secondary hyperparathyroidism, in contrast, arises as a compensation for reductions of circulating Ca^{2+} and is not associated with hypercalcemia.

Symptoms and signs of primary hyperparathyroidism include fatigue, exhaustion, weakness, polydipsia, polyuria, joint pain, bone pain, constipation, depression, anorexia, nausea, heartburn, nephrolithiasis, and hematuria. This condition frequently is accompanied by significant hypophosphatemia owing to the effects of PTH in diminishing renal tubular phosphate reabsorption. Some patients have renal calculi and peptic ulceration, and a few display classical parathyroid skeletal disease. However, most patients show few, if any, symptoms, and those that are present are often vague and nonspecific. Contemporary IRMAs that distinguish between full-length PTH(1–84) and "intact" PTH [PTH(1–84) + PTH(7–84)] obviate many of the difficulties with previous assays and, in conjunction with an elevated serum calcium, possess a diagnostic accuracy of greater than 90% (Gao *et al.*, 2001; Jüppner and Potts, 2002; Silverberg *et al.*, 2003).

Familial benign hypercalcemia (or *familial hypocalciuric hypercalcemia*) is a genetic disorder generally accompanied by extremely low urinary calcium excretion. Familial benign hypercalcemia results from heterozygous mutations in the Ca^{2+}-sensing receptor (Pollak *et al.*, 1996). Hypercalcemia usually is mild, and circulating PTH often is normal to slightly elevated. The importance of making this diagnosis lies in the fact that patients mistakenly diagnosed as having primary hyperparathyroidism may undergo surgical exploration without discovery of an adenoma and without therapeutic benefit. Patients do not experience long-term clinical consequences, except for homozygous infants, who may have severe, even lethal, hypercalcemia. Diagnosis is established by demonstrating hypercalcemia in first-degree family members and a decreased fractional excretion of calcium.

Newly diagnosed hypercalcemia in hospitalized patients is caused most often by a systemic malignancy, either with or without bony metastasis. PTH-related protein (PTHrP) is a primitive, highly conserved protein that may be abnormally expressed in malignant tissue, particularly by squamous cell and other epithelial cancers. The substantial sequence homology of the amino-terminal portion of PTHrP with that of native PTH permits it to interact with the PTH-1 receptor in target tissues, thereby causing the hypercalcemia and hypophosphatemia seen in humoral hypercalcemia of malignancy (Grill *et al.*, 1998). Other tumors release cytokines or prostaglandins that stimulate bone resorption. In some patients with lymphomas, hypercalcemia results from overproduction of 1,25-dihydroxyvitamin D by the tumor cells owing to expression of 1α-hydroxylase. A similar mechanism underlies the hypercalcemia that is seen occasionally in sarcoidosis and other granulomatous disorders.

Hypercalcemia associated with malignancy generally is more severe than in primary hyperparathyroidism (frequently with calcium levels that exceed 13 mg/dl) and may be associated with lethargy, weakness, nausea, vomiting, polydipsia, and polyuria. Assays for PTHrP may aid diagnosis.

Vitamin D excess may cause hypercalcemia if sufficient 25-hydroxyvitamin D is present to stimulate intestinal Ca^{2+} hyperabsorption, leading to hypercalcemia and suppressing PTH and 1,25-dihydroxyvitamin D levels. Measurement of 25-hydroxyvitamin D is diagnostic. Occasional patients with *hyperthyroidism* show mild hypercalcemia, presumably owing to increased bone turnover. *Immobilization* may lead to hypercalcemia in growing children and young adults but rarely causes hypercalcemia in older individuals unless bone turnover is already increased, as in Paget's disease or hyperthyroidism. Hypercalcemia sometimes is noted in adrenocortical deficiency, as in Addison's disease, or following removal of a hyperfunctional adrenocortical tumor. Hypercalcemia occurs following renal transplantation owing to persistent hyperfunctioning parathyroid tissue that resulted from the previous renal failure.

The differential diagnosis of hypercalcemia may pose difficulties, but advances in serum assays for PTH, PTHrP, and 25-hydroxy- and 1,25-dihydroxyvitamin D permit accurate diagnosis in the great majority of cases.

Hypocalcemia. Mild hypocalcemia [*i.e.*, reduction in ionized serum Ca^{2+} concentrations from normal to concentrations above 3.2 mg/dl (0.8 mM), approximately equal to a total serum Ca^{2+} concentration of 8 to 8.5 mg/dl (2 to 2.1 mM)] is usually asymptomatic. Again, the rapidity of change affects the clinical picture because patients exhibit greater signs and symptoms if the hypocalcemia develops acutely. The signs and symptoms of hypocalcemia include tetany and related phenomena such as paresthesias, increased neuromuscular excitability, laryngospasm, muscle cramps, and tonic-clonic convulsions. In chronic hypoparathyroidism, ectodermal changes—consisting of loss of hair, grooved and brittle fingernails, defects of dental enamel, and cataracts—are encountered; calcification in the basal ganglia may be seen on routine skull radiographs. Psychiatric symptoms such as emotional lability, anxiety, depression, and delusions often are present.

Combined deprivation of Ca^{2+} and vitamin D, as observed with malabsorption states or dietary deficiency, readily promotes hypocalcemia. When caused by malabsorption, hypocalcemia is accompanied by low concentrations of phosphate, total plasma proteins, and magnesium. Mg^{2+} deficiency may accentuate the hypocalcemia by diminishing the secretion and action of PTH. In infants with malabsorption or inadequate calcium intake, Ca^{2+} concentrations usually are depressed, with attendant hypophosphatemia resulting in rickets.

Hypoparathyroidism is most often a consequence of thyroid or neck surgery but also may be due to genetic or autoimmune disorders. In hypoparathyroidism, hypocalcemia is accompanied by hyperphosphatemia, reflecting decreased PTH action on renal phosphate transport.

Pseudohypoparathyroidism is a diverse family of hypocalcemic and/or hyperphosphatemic disorders. Pseudohypoparathyroidism results from resistance to PTH rather than PTH deficiency; this resistance is not due to mutations of the PTH receptor but rather to mutations in $G_s\alpha$ (*GNAS1*), which normally mediates hormone-induced adenylyl cyclase activation (Yu *et al.*, 1999). The variable phenotypes arising from *GNAS1* defects apparently are due to differential genomic imprinting of the maternal and paternal alleles (Levine *et al.*, 2003). Multiple hormonal abnormalities have been associated with the *GNAS1* mutation, but none is as severe as the deficient response to PTH.

Hypocalcemia is not unusual in the first several days following removal of a parathyroid adenoma. If hyperphosphatemia is also present, the condition is one of functional hypothyroidism owing to temporary failure of the remaining parathyroid glands to compensate for the missing adenomatous tissue. In patients with parathyroid bone disease, postoperative hypocalcemia associated with hypophosphatemia may reflect rapid uptake of calcium into bone, the "hungry bone" syndrome. In this setting, persistent, severe hypocalcemia may require administration of vitamin D and supplemental calcium for several months.

Neonatal tetany resulting from hypocalcemia sometimes occurs in infants of mothers with *hyper*parathyroidism; indeed, the tetany may call attention to the mother's disorder. This problem disappears when the infant's own parathyroid glands develop sufficiently to respond appropriately.

Hypocalcemia is associated with advanced renal insufficiency accompanied by hyperphosphatemia. Many patients with this condition do not develop tetany unless the accompanying acidosis is treated, which decreases the ionized calcium. High concentrations of phosphate in plasma inhibit the conversion of 25-hydroxycholecalciferol to 1,25-dihydroxycholecalciferol. Hypocalcemia also can occur following massive transfusions with citrated blood, which chelates calcium.

Disturbed Phosphate Metabolism

Dietary inadequacy very rarely causes phosphate depletion. Sustained use of antacids, however, can severely limit phosphate absorption and result in clinical phosphate depletion, manifest as malaise, muscle weakness, and osteomalacia (*see* Chapter 36). *Osteomalacia*, as described further below, is characterized by undermineralized bone matrix and may occur when sustained phosphate depletion is caused by inhibiting its absorption in the gastrointestinal tract (as with aluminum-containing antacids) or by excess renal excretion owing to PTH action.

Hyperphosphatemia is an important component of the bone disease seen in chronic renal failure. In this condition, phosphate retention is primary and reflects the degree of renal compromise. The increased phosphate level reduces the serum Ca^{2+} concentration, which, in turn, activates the parathyroid gland calcium-sensing receptor, stimulates

PTH secretion, and exacerbates the hyperphosphatemia. The continuing hyperphosphatemia may be modified by vigorous administration of aluminum hydroxide gel or calcium carbonate supplements. As discussed below, the Food and Drug Administration (FDA) recently approved therapeutic use of the calcium-sensing receptor agonist *cinacalcet* to suppress PTH secretion.

Disorders of Vitamin D

Hypervitaminosis D. The acute or long-term administration of excessive amounts of vitamin D or enhanced responsiveness to normal amounts of the vitamin leads to derangements in calcium metabolism. The responses to vitamin D reflect endogenous vitamin D production, tissue reactivity, and vitamin D intake. Some infants may be hyperreactive to small doses of vitamin D. In adults, hypervitaminosis D results from overtreatment of *hypo*parathyroidism or secondary *hyper*parathyroidism of renal osteodystrophy and from faddist use of excessive doses. Toxicity in children also may occur following accidental ingestion of adult doses.

The amount of vitamin D necessary to cause hypervitaminosis varies widely. As a rough approximation, continued daily ingestion of 50,000 units or more by a person with normal parathyroid function and sensitivity to vitamin D may result in poisoning. Hypervitaminosis D is particularly dangerous in patients who are receiving digoxin because the toxic effects of the cardiac glycosides are enhanced by hypercalcemia (*see* Chapters 33 and 34).

The initial signs and symptoms of vitamin D toxicity are those associated with hypercalcemia (*see* above). Since hypercalcemia in vitamin D intoxication generally is due to very high circulating levels of 25-OHD, the plasma concentrations of PTH and calcitriol typically (but not uniformly) are suppressed. In children, a single episode of moderately severe hypercalcemia may arrest growth completely for 6 months or more, and the deficit in height may never be fully corrected. Vitamin D toxicity in the fetus is associated with excess maternal vitamin D intake or extreme sensitivity and may result in congenital supravalvular aortic stenosis. In infants, this anomaly frequently is associated with other stigmata of hypercalcemia.

Vitamin D Deficiency. Vitamin D deficiency results in inadequate absorption of Ca^{2+} and phosphate. The consequent decrease of plasma Ca^{2+} concentration stimulates PTH secretion, which acts to restore plasma Ca^{2+} at the expense of bone. Plasma concentrations of phosphate remain subnormal because of the phosphaturic effect of increased circulating PTH. In children, the result is a failure to mineralize newly formed bone and cartilage matrix, causing the defect in growth known as *rickets*. As a consequence of inadequate calcification, bones of individuals with rickets are soft, and the stress of weight bearing gives rise to bowing of the long bones.

In adults, vitamin D deficiency results in osteomalacia, a disease characterized by generalized accumulation of undermineralized bone matrix. Severe osteomalacia may be associated with extreme bone pain and tenderness. Muscle weakness, particularly of large proximal muscles, is typical and may reflect both hypophosphatemia and inadequate vitamin D action on muscle. Gross deformity of bone occurs only in advanced stages of the disease. Circulating 25-OHD concentrations below 8 ng/ml are highly predictive of osteomalacia.

Metabolic Rickets and Osteomalacia. These disorders are characterized by abnormalities in calcitriol synthesis or response.

Hypophosphatemic vitamin D–resistant rickets, in its most common form, is an X-linked disorder (XLH) of calcium and phosphate metabolism. Calcitriol levels are inappropriately normal for the observed degree of hypophosphatemia. Patients experience clinical improvement when treated with large doses of vitamin D, usually in combination with inorganic phosphate. Even with vitamin D treatment, calcitriol concentrations may remain lower than expected. The genetic basis for XLH has been defined (HYP Consortium, 1995). The affected protein, a phosphate-regulating gene with homologies to endopeptidases on the X chromosome (PHEX), is a neutral endoprotease. The substrate for this enzyme likely is involved in renal phosphate transport. Syndromes closely related to XLH, in which phosphate levels are altered without significant net changes in serum concentrations of calcium, PTH, or $1,25(OH)_2D_3$, include *hereditary hypophosphatemic rickets with hypercalciuria* (HHRH) and *autosomal dominant hypophosphatemic rickets.* The latter disorder maps to chromosome 12p13.3 (Econs *et al.*, 1997) and is associated with mutations in the gene encoding fibroblast growth factor 23 (White *et al.*, 2001).

Vitamin D–dependent rickets (also called *vitamin D–dependent rickets type I*) is an autosomal recessive disease caused by an inborn error of vitamin D metabolism involving defective conversion of 25-OHD to calcitriol owing to mutations in CYP1α (1α-hydroxylase). The condition responds to physiological doses of calcitriol.

Hereditary 1,25-dihydroxyvitamin D resistance (also called *vitamin D–dependent rickets type II*) is an autosomal recessive disorder that is characterized by hypocalcemia, osteomalacia, rickets, and total alopecia. Mutations of the vitamin D receptor cause vitamin D–dependent rickets type II (Malloy *et al.*, 1999). Absolute hormone resistance results from premature stop mutations or missense mutations in the zinc finger DNA-binding domain. Several missense mutations in the ligand-binding domain also have been described that result in partial or complete hormone resistance. These mutations alter ligand binding or heterodimerization with the retinoid X receptor (RXR).

Serum abnormalities include low serum concentrations of calcium and phosphate and elevated serum alkaline phosphatase activity. The hypocalcemia leads to secondary hyperparathyroidism with elevated PTH levels and hypophosphatemia. The 25(OH)-vitamin D values are normal, whereas $1,25(OH)_2$-vitamin D levels are elevated in type II vitamin D–dependent rickets. This clinical feature distinguishes hereditary vitamin D–dependent rickets type II from CYP1α deficiency (vitamin D–dependent rickets type I), where serum $1,25(OH)2$-vitamin D values are depressed. Children affected by vitamin D–

dependent rickets type II are refractory even to massive doses of vitamin D and calcitriol, and they may require prolonged treatment with parenteral Ca^{2+}. Some remission of symptoms has been observed during adolescence, but the basis of remission is unknown.

Renal osteodystrophy (renal rickets) is associated with chronic renal failure and is characterized by decreased conversion of 25-OHD to calcitriol. Phosphate retention decreases plasma Ca^{2+} concentrations, leading to secondary hyperparathyroidism. In addition, calcitriol deficiency impairs intestinal Ca^{2+} absorption and mobilization from bone. Hypocalcemia commonly results (although in some patients, prolonged and severe hyperparathyroidism eventually may lead to hypercalcemia). Aluminum deposition in bone also may play a role in the genesis of the skeletal disease.

SPECIFIC DISORDERS OF BONE

Osteoporosis

Osteoporosis is a condition of low bone mass and microarchitectural disruption that results in fractures with minimal trauma. Osteoporosis is a major and growing public health problem in developed nations. Between 30% and 50% of women and between 15% and 30% of men suffer a fracture related to osteoporosis. Characteristic sites of fracture include vertebral bodies, the distal radius, and the proximal femur, but osteoporotic individuals have generalized skeletal fragility, and fractures at sites such as ribs and long bones also are common. Fracture risk increases exponentially with age and is associated with reduced survival after any type of fracture (Center *et al.*, 1999).

Osteoporosis can be categorized as *primary* or *secondary*. In 1948, Albright and Reifenstein concluded that primary osteoporosis included two separate entities: one related to menopausal estrogen loss and the other to aging. This concept was extended by the proposal that primary osteoporosis represents two fundamentally different conditions: *type I osteoporosis,* characterized by loss of trabecular bone owing to estrogen lack at menopause, and *type II osteoporosis,* characterized by loss of cortical and trabecular bone in men and women owing to long-term remodeling inefficiency, dietary inadequacy, and activation of the parathyroid axis with age. It is not clear, however, that these two entities are truly distinct. Although many osteoporotic women undoubtedly have experienced excessive menopausal bone loss, it may be more appropriate to consider osteoporosis as the result of multiple physical, hormonal, and nutritional factors acting alone or in concert.

Secondary osteoporosis is due to systemic illness or medications such as glucocorticoids or phenytoin. The most successful approach to secondary osteoporosis is prompt resolution of the underlying cause or drug discontinuation. Whether primary or secondary, osteoporosis is associated with characteristic disordered bone remodeling, so the same therapies can be used.

Paget's Disease. Paget's disease is characterized by single or multiple foci of disordered bone remodeling. The etiology of the disease is uncertain but is thought to be the result of infection with the measles virus of the paramyxovirus family (Kurihara *et al.*, 2000). It affects up to 2% to 3% of the population over age 60. The primary pathologic abnormality is increased bone resorption followed by exuberant new bone formation. However, the newly formed bone is disorganized and of poor quality, resulting in characteristic bowing, stress fractures, and arthritis of joints adjoining the involved bone. Pagetic lesions contain many abnormal multinucleated osteoclasts associated with a disordered mosaic pattern of bone formation. Pagetic bone is thickened and has abnormal microarchitecture. The altered bone structure can produce secondary problems, such as deafness, spinal cord compression, high-output cardiac failure, and pain. Malignant degeneration to osteogenic sarcoma is a rare but lethal complication of Paget's disease.

Renal Osteodystrophy. Bone disease is a frequent consequence of chronic renal failure and dialysis. Pathologically, lesions are typical of hyperparathyroidism (osteitis fibrosa), deficiency of vitamin D (osteomalacia), or a mixture of both. The underlying pathophysiology reflects increased phosphate and decreased calcium, leading to secondary events that strive to preserve circulating levels of mineral ions at the expense of bone.

PHARMACOLOGICAL TREATMENT OF DISORDERS OF MINERAL ION HOMEOSTASIS AND BONE METABOLISM

Hypercalcemia. Hypercalcemia can be life-threatening. Such patients frequently are severely dehydrated because hypercalcemia compromises renal concentrating mechanisms. Thus, fluid resuscitation with large volumes of isotonic saline must be early and aggressive (6 to 8 L/day). Agents that augment Ca^{2+} excretion, such as loop diuretics (*see* Chapter 28), may help to counteract the effect of plasma volume expansion by saline but are contraindicated until volume is repleted because they otherwise will aggravate volume depletion and hypercalcemia.

Corticosteroids administered at high doses (*e.g.,* 40 to 80 mg/day of *prednisone*) may be useful when hypercalcemia results from sarcoidosis, lymphoma, or hypervitaminosis D (*see* Chapter 59). The response to steroid therapy is slow; from 1 to 2 weeks may be required before plasma Ca^{2+} concentration falls.

Calcitonin (CALCIMAR, MIACALCIN) may be useful in managing hypercalcemia. Reduction in Ca^{2+} can be rapid, although "escape" from the hormone commonly occurs within several days. The recommended starting dose is 4 units/kg of body weight administered subcutaneously every 12 hours; if there is no response within 1 or 2 days, the dose may be increased to a maximum of 8 units/kg every 12 hours. If the response after 2 more days still is unsatisfactory, the dose may be increased to a maximum of 8 units/kg every 6 hours.

Plicamycin (*mithramycin*, MITHRACIN) is a cytotoxic antibiotic that also decreases plasma Ca^{2+} concentrations by inhibiting bone resorption. Reduction in plasma Ca^{2+} concentrations occurs within 24 to 48 hours when a relatively low dose of this agent is given (15 to 25 $\mu g/kg$ of body weight) to minimize the high systemic toxicity of the drug.

Intravenous *bisphosphonates* (*pamidronate, zoledronate*) have proven very effective in the management of hypercalcemia (*see* below for further discussion of bisphosphonates). These agents potently inhibit osteoclastic bone resorption. Oral bisphosphonates are less effective for treating hypercalcemia. Therefore, pamidronate (AREDIA) is given as an intravenous infusion of 60 to 90 mg over 4 to 24 hours. With pamidronate, resolution of hypercalcemia occurs over several days, and the effect usually persists for several weeks.

Oral *sodium phosphate* lowers plasma Ca^{2+} concentrations and may offer short-term calcemic control of some patients with primary hyperparathyroidism who are awaiting surgery. However, the risk of precipitating calcium phosphate salts in soft tissues throughout the body is of concern. In light of satisfactory responses to other agents, administration of intravenous sodium phosphate is not recommended as a treatment for hypercalcemia.

Once the hypercalcemic crisis has resolved or in patients with milder calcium elevations, therapy turns to more durable resolution of the hypercalcemic state. Parathyroidectomy remains the only definitive treatment for primary hyperparathyroidism. Specific indications for surgery have been proposed (Bilezikian *et al.*, 2002). In the hands of a skilled parathyroid surgeon, resection of a single adenoma (about 80% of cases) or of the hyperplastic glands (about 15% of cases) cures hyperparathyroidism. Complications include transient postoperative hypocalcemia, which may reflect temporary disruption of blood supply to the remaining parathyroid tissue or skeletal avidity for calcium, and permanent hypoparathyroidism. As described below, a calcium mimetic that stimulates the calcium-sensing receptor is a promising new therapy for hyperparathyroidism that may be used increasingly in the future.

Therapy of hypercalcemia of malignancy ideally is directed at the underlying cancer. When this is not possible, parenteral bisphosphonates often will maintain calcium levels within an acceptable range.

Hypocalcemia and Other Therapeutic Uses of Calcium. Hypoparathyroidism is treated primarily with vitamin D (*see* below). Dietary supplementation with Ca^{2+} also may be necessary.

Calcium is used in the treatment of calcium deficiency states and as a dietary supplement. Ca^{2+} salts are specific in the immediate treatment of hypocalcemic tetany regardless of etiology. In severe tetany, symptoms are best brought under control by intravenous medication. *Calcium chloride* ($CaCl_2 \cdot 2H_2O$) contains 27% Ca^{2+}; it is valuable in the treatment of hypocalcemic tetany and laryngospasm. The salt is given intravenously and *must never be injected into tissues*. Injections of calcium chloride are accompa-

nied by peripheral vasodilation and a cutaneous burning sensation. The salt usually is given intravenously in a concentration of 10% (equivalent to 1.36 mEq Ca^{2+}/ml). The rate of injection should be slow (not over 1 ml/min) to prevent cardiac arrhythmias from a high concentration of Ca^{2+}. The injection may induce a moderate fall in blood pressure owing to vasodilation. Since calcium chloride is an acidifying salt, it is usually undesirable in the treatment of the hypocalcemia caused by renal insufficiency. *Calcium gluceptate* injection (a 22% solution; 18 mg or 0.9 mEq of Ca^{2+}/ml) is administered intravenously at a dose of 5 to 20 ml for the treatment of severe hypocalcemic tetany; the injection produces a transient tingling sensation when given too rapidly. When the intravenous route is not possible, injections may be given intramuscularly in the gluteal region at a dose of up to 5 ml. A mild local reaction may result. *Calcium gluconate* injection (a 10% solution; 9.3 mg of Ca^{2+}/ml) given intravenously is the treatment of choice for severe hypocalcemic tetany. Patients with moderate-to-severe hypocalcemia may be treated by intravenous infusion of calcium gluconate at a dose of 10 to 15 mg of Ca^{2+}/kg of body weight over 4 to 6 hours. Since the usual 10-ml vial of a 10% solution contains only 93 mg Ca^{2+}, many vials are needed. The intramuscular route should not be employed because abscess formation at the injection site may result.

For control of milder hypocalcemic symptoms, oral medication suffices, frequently in combination with vitamin D or one of its active metabolites. Calcium salts are acidifying, and different forms can be interchanged to avoid gastric irritation. Available Ca^{2+} salts include calcium carbonate, lactate, gluconate, phosphate, citrate, and hydroxyapatite. Calcium carbonate is prescribed most frequently, whereas calcium citrate may be absorbed more efficiently than other salts. However, absorption efficiency for most commonly prescribed calcium products is reasonable, and for many patients, cost and palatability outweigh modest differences in efficacy. Average doses for hypocalcemic patients are calcium gluconate, 15 g/day in divided doses; calcium lactate, 7.7 g plus 8 g lactose with each meal; and calcium carbonate or calcium phosphate, 1 to 2 g with meals.

Calcium carbonate and calcium acetate are used to restrict phosphate absorption in patients with chronic renal failure and oxalate absorption in patients with inflammatory bowel disease. Acute administration of calcium may be life-saving in patients with extreme hyperkalemia (serum K^+ > 7 mEq/L). Calcium gluconate (10 to 30 ml of a 10% solution) can reverse some of the cardiotoxic effects of hyperkalemia, providing time while other efforts are taken to lower the plasma K^+ concentration.

Additional FDA-approved uses of calcium include intravenous treatment for black widow spider envenomation and management of magnesium toxicity. Use of supplemental calcium in the prevention and treatment of osteoporosis is discussed below.

THERAPEUTIC USES OF VITAMIN D

Specific Forms of Vitamin D. Calcitriol (1,25-dihydroxycholecalciferol; CALCIJEX, ROCALTROL) is available for oral administration or injection. Several derivatives of vitamin D (Figure 61–10) are of considerable experimental and therapeutic interest.

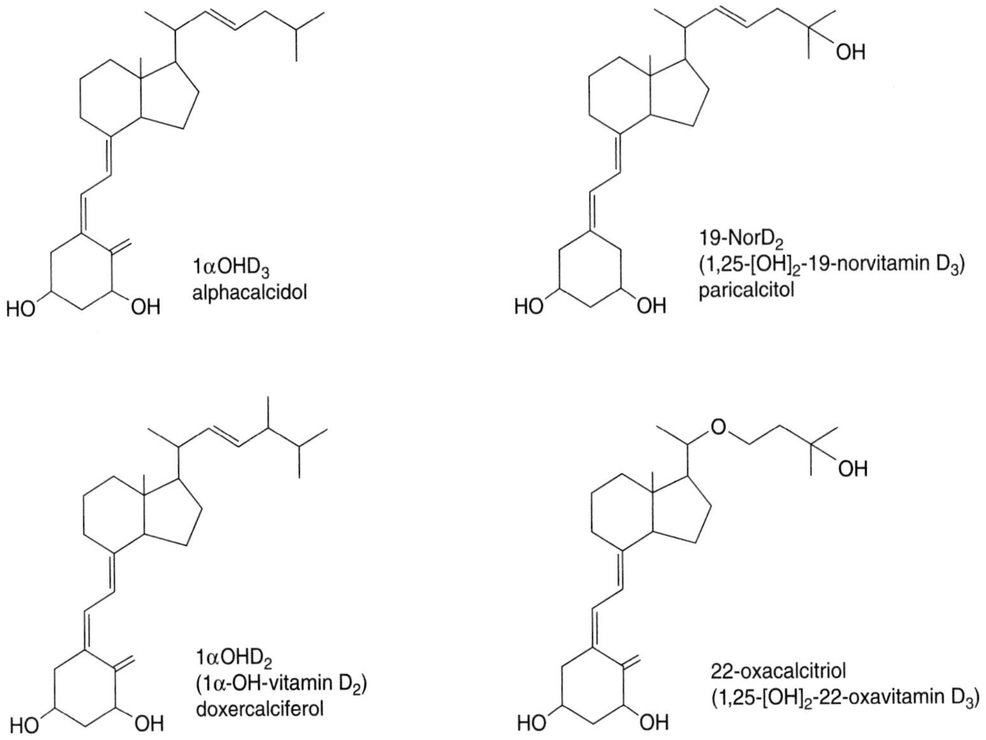

Figure 61–10. *Vitamin D analogs.*

Doxercalciferol (1α-hydroxyvitamin D₂, HECTOROL) is a pro-drug that first must be activated by hepatic 25-hydroxylation to generate the biologically active compound, $1\alpha,25\text{-(OH)}_2D_2$ (Figure 61–10). The FDA has approved oral and intravenous preparations of 1α-hydroxyvitamin D₂ for use in treating secondary hyperparathyroidism, starting at 10 mg three times per week.

Dihydrotachysterol (DHT, ROXANE) is a reduced form of vitamin D₂. DHT is converted in the liver to its active form, 25-hydroxydihydrotachysterol. DHT is less than 1% as active as calcitriol in antirachitic assays but is much more effective in mobilizing bone mineral at high doses; it therefore can be used to maintain plasma Ca^{2+} in hypoparathyroidism. DHT is well absorbed from the gastrointestinal tract and maximally increases serum calcium concentration after 2 weeks of daily administration. The hypercalcemic effects typically persist for 2 weeks but can last for up to 1 month. DHT is available for oral administration in doses ranging from 0.2 to 1 mg/day (average 0.6 mg/day).

1α-Hydroxycholecalciferol (1-OHD₃, *alphacalcidol*; ONE-ALPHA) was introduced as a substitute for $1,25\text{(OH)}_2D_3$; alphacalcidol is a synthetic vitamin D₃ derivative that is already hydroxylated in the 1α position and is rapidly hydroxylated by 25-hydroxylase to form $1,25\text{-(OH)}_2D_3$. It is equal to calcitriol in assays for stimulation of intestinal absorption of Ca^{2+} and bone mineralization and does not require renal activation. It therefore has been used to treat renal osteodystrophy and is available in the United States for experimental purposes.

Ergocalciferol (*calciferol*, DRISDOL) is pure vitamin D₂. It is available for oral, intramuscular, or intravenous administration. Ergocalciferol is indicated for the prevention of vitamin D deficiency and the treatment of familial hypophosphatemia, hypopar-athyroidism, and vitamin D–resistant rickets type II, typically in doses of 50,000 to 200,000 units/day in conjunction with calcium supplements.

Analogs of Calcitriol. Several vitamin D analogs (Figure 61–10) suppress PTH secretion by the parathyroid glands but have less or negligible hypercalcemic activity. They therefore offer a safer and more effective means of controlling secondary hyperparathyroidism.

Calcipotriol (*calcipotriene*) is a synthetic derivative of calcitriol with a modified side chain that contains a 22–23 double bond, a 24(S)-hydroxy functional group, and carbons 25 to 27 incorporated into a cyclopropane ring. Calcipotriol has comparable affinity with calcitriol for the vitamin D receptor, but it is less than 1% as active as calcitriol in regulating calcium metabolism. This reduced calcemic activity largely reflects the pharmacokinetics of calcipotriol (Kissmeyer and Binderup, 1991). Calcipotriol has been studied extensively as a treatment for psoriasis (*see* Chapter 62), although its mode of action is not known; a topical preparation (DOVONEX) is available for that purpose. In clinical trials, topical calcipotriol has been found to be slightly more effective than glucocorticoids with a good safety profile.

Paricalcitol (1,25-dihydroxy-19-norvitamin D₂, ZEMPLAR) is a synthetic calcitriol derivative that lacks the exocyclic C19 and has a vitamin D₂ rather than a vitamin D₃ side chain (Figure 61–10). It reduces serum PTH levels without producing hypercalcemia or altering serum phosphorus (Martin *et al.*, 1998). In an animal model, paricalcitol prevented or reversed PTH-induced high-turnover bone disease (Slatopolsky *et al.*, 2003). Paricalcitol administered intravenously is FDA approved for treating secondary hyperparathyroidism in patients with chronic renal failure.

22-Oxacalcitriol (1,25-dihydroxy-22-oxavitamin D$_3$, OCT, *maxicalcitol*, OXAROL) differs from calcitriol only in the substitution of C-22 with an oxygen atom. Oxacalcitriol has a low affinity for vitamin D–binding protein; as a result, more of the drug circulates in the free (unbound) form, allowing it to be metabolized more rapidly than calcitriol with a consequent shorter half-life. Oxacalcitriol is a potent suppressor of PTH gene expression and shows very limited activity on intestine and bone. It is a useful compound in patients with overproduction of PTH in chronic renal failure or even with primary hyperparathyroidism (Cunningham, 2004).

Indications for Therapy with Vitamin D

The major therapeutic uses of vitamin D may be divided into four categories: (1) prophylaxis and cure of nutritional rickets; (2) treatment of metabolic rickets and osteomalacia, particularly in the setting of chronic renal failure; (3) treatment of hypoparathyroidism; and (4) prevention and treatment of osteoporosis (discussed in the section on osteoporosis).

Nutritional Rickets. Nutritional rickets results from inadequate exposure to sunlight or deficiency of dietary vitamin D. The condition, once extremely rare in the United States and other countries where food fortification with the vitamin is practiced, is now increasing. Infants and children receiving adequate amounts of vitamin D–fortified food do not require additional vitamin D; however, breast-fed infants or those fed unfortified formula should receive 400 units of vitamin D daily as a supplement. The usual practice is to administer vitamin A in combination with vitamin D. A number of balanced vitamin A and D preparations are available for this purpose. *Since the fetus acquires more than 85% of its calcium stores during the third trimester, premature infants are especially susceptible to rickets and may require supplemental vitamin D.*

Treatment of fully developed rickets requires a larger dose of vitamin D than that used prophylactically. One thousand units daily will normalize plasma Ca^{2+} and phosphate concentrations in approximately 10 days, with radiographic evidence of healing within about 3 weeks. However, a larger dose of 3000 to 4000 units daily often is prescribed for more rapid healing, particularly when respiration is compromised by severe thoracic rickets.

Vitamin D may be given prophylactically in conditions that impair its absorption (*e.g.*, diarrhea, steatorrhea, and biliary obstruction). Parenteral administration also may be used in such cases.

Treatment of Osteomalacia and Renal Osteodystrophy. Osteomalacia, distinguished by undermineralization of bone matrix, occurs commonly during sustained phosphate depletion. Patients with chronic renal disease are at risk for developing osteomalacia but also may develop a complex bone disease called *renal osteodystrophy*. In this setting, bone metabolism is stimulated by an increase in PTH and by a delay in bone mineralization that is due to decreased renal synthesis of calcitriol. In renal osteodystrophy, low bone mineral density may be accompanied by high-turnover bone lesions typically seen in patients with uncontrolled hyperparathyroidism or by low bone remodeling activity seen in patients with adynamic bone disease. The therapeutic approach to the patient with renal osteodystrophy depends on its specific type. In high-turnover (hyperparathyroid) or mixed high-turnover disease with deficient mineralization, dietary phosphate restriction, generally in combination with a phosphate binder, is recommended because phosphate restriction is limited by the need to provide adequate protein intake to maintain nitrogen balance. Although highly effective, *aluminum* is no longer used as a phosphate binder because it promotes adynamic bone disease, anemia, myopathy, and occasionally dementia. Calcium-containing phosphate binders along with calcitriol administration may contribute to oversuppression of PTH secretion and likewise result in adynamic bone disease and an increased incidence of vascular calcification. Highly effective non-calcium-containing phosphate binders have been developed. *Sevelamer hydrochloride* (RENAGEL), a nonabsorbable phosphate-binding polymer, effectively lowers serum phosphate concentration in hemodialysis patients, with a corresponding reduction in the calcium × phosphate product. Sevelamer hydrochloride consists of cross-linked poly[allylamine hydrochloride] that is resistant to digestive degradation. Partially protonated amines spaced one carbon from the polymer backbone chelate phosphate ions by ionic and hydrogen bonding. Side effects of sevelamer include vomiting, nausea, diarrhea, and dyspepsia. Sevelamer does not affect the bioavailability of *digoxin, warfarin, enalapril*, or *metoprolol*.

Renal osteodystrophy associated with low bone turnover (adynamic bone disease) is increasingly common and may be due to oversuppression of PTH with aggressive use of either calcitriol or other vitamin D analogs. While PTH levels generally are low (<100 pg/ml), a high PTH level does not exclude the presence of adynamic bone disease, especially with PTH assays that do not distinguish between biologically active and inactive PTH fragments (Monier-Faugere *et al.*, 2001). Current guidelines suggest that treatment with an active vitamin D preparation is indicated if serum 25-OHD levels are less than 30 ng/ml and serum calcium is less than 9.5 mg/dl (2.37 mM). However, if 25-OHD and serum calcium levels are elevated, vitamin D supplementation should be discontinued. If the serum calcium level is less than 9.5 mg/dl, treatment with a vitamin D analog is warranted irrespective of the 25-OHD level (Eknoyan *et al.*, 2003).

Hypoparathyroidism. Vitamin D and its analogs are a mainstay of the therapy of hypoparathyroidism. Dihydrotachysterol (DHT) has a faster onset, shorter duration of action, and a greater effect on bone mobilization than does vitamin D and traditionally has been a preferred agent. Calcitriol also is effective in the management of hypoparathyroidism and certain forms of pseudohypoparathyroidism in which endogenous levels of calcitriol are abnormally low. However, most hypoparathyroid patients respond to any form of vitamin D. Calcitriol may be preferred for temporary treatment of hypocalcemia while awaiting effects of a slower-acting form of vitamin D.

Miscellaneous Uses of Vitamin D. Vitamin D is used to treat hypophosphatemia associated with Fanconi syndrome. Large doses of vitamin D (over 10,000 units/day) are not useful in patients with osteoporosis and even can be dangerous. However, administration of 400 to 800 units/day of vitamin D to frail, elderly men and women has been shown to suppress bone remodeling, protect bone mass, and reduce fracture incidence (*see* later section on osteoporosis). Clinical trials suggest that calcitriol may become an important agent for the treatment of psoriasis (Kowalzick, 2001). As such nontraditional uses of vitamin D are discovered, it will become important to develop noncalcemic analogs of calcitriol that achieve effects on cellular differentiation without the risk of hypercalcemia.

Adverse Effects of Vitamin D Therapy

The primary toxicity associated with calcitriol reflects its potent effect to increase intestinal calcium and phosphate absorption, along with the potential to mobilize osseous calcium and phosphate. Hypercalcemia, with or without hyperphosphatemia, commonly complicates calcitriol therapy and may limit its use at doses that effectively suppress PTH secretion. As described earlier, noncalcemic vitamin D analogs provide alternative interventions, although they do not obviate the need to monitor serum calcium and phosphorus concentrations.

Hypervitaminosis D is treated by immediate withdrawal of the vitamin, a low-calcium diet, administration of glucocorticoids, and vigorous fluid support. As noted earlier under hypercalcemia, forced saline diuresis with loop diuretics is also useful. With this regimen, the plasma Ca^{2+} concentration falls to normal, and Ca^{2+} in soft tissue tends to be mobilized. Conspicuous improvement in renal function occurs unless renal damage has been severe.

CALCITONIN

Diagnostic Uses of Calcitonin

Calcitonin is a sensitive and specific marker for the presence of medullary thyroid carcinoma (MTC), a neuroendocrine malignancy originating in thyroid parafollicular C cells. MTC can be hereditary (25%) or sporadic (75%) and is present in all patients with the multiple endocrine neoplasia type 2 (MEN2) syndromes. Because one form of MEN2 is inherited as a dominant trait, relatives of patients should be examined repeatedly by calcitonin measurements from early childhood. Because calcitonin levels may be low in early tumor stages or in premalignant C-cell hyperplasia, pentagastrin-induced calcitonin provides greater sensitivity and increased MTC detection (Karanikas *et al.*, 2004). The identification of discrete mutations in the *RET* protooncogene in subjects with MEN2 offers hope that genetic screening will supplant reliance on testing serum calcitonin, which can give spurious results.

Therapeutic Uses. Calcitonin lowers plasma Ca^{2+} and phosphate concentrations in patients with hypercalcemia; this effect results from decreased bone resorption and is greater in patients in whom bone turnover rates are high. Although calcitonin is effective for up to 6 hours in the initial treatment of hypercalcemia, patients become refractory after a few days. This is likely due to receptor down-regulation (Takahashi *et al.*, 1995). Use of calcitonin does not substitute for aggressive fluid resuscitation, and the bisphosphonates are the preferred agents (*see* above on hypercalcemia).

Calcitonin is effective in disorders of increased skeletal remodeling, such as Paget's disease, and in some patients with osteoporosis. In Paget's disease, chronic use of calcitonin produces long-term reductions of serum alkaline phosphatase activity and symptoms. Development of antibodies to calcitonin occurs with prolonged therapy, but this is not necessarily associated with clinical resistance. Side effects of calcitonin include nausea, hand swelling, urticaria, and rarely, intestinal cramping. Side effects appear to occur with equal frequency with human and salmon calcitonin. *Salmon calcitonin* is approved for clinical use. The latter product also is available as a nasal spray, introduced for once-daily treatment of postmenopausal osteoporosis (*see* below). For Paget's disease, calcitonin generally is administered by subcutaneous injection because intranasal delivery is relatively ineffective owing to limited bioavailability. After initial therapy at 100 units/day, the dose typically is reduced to 50 units three times a week.

BISPHOSPHONATES

Bisphosphonates are analogs of pyrophosphate (Figure 61–11) that contain two phosphonate groups attached to a geminal (central) carbon that replaces the oxygen in pyrophosphate. Because they form a three-dimensional structure capable of chelating divalent cations such as Ca^{2+}, the bisphosphonates have a strong affinity for bone, targeting especially bone surfaces undergoing remodeling. Accordingly, they are used extensively in conditions characterized by osteoclast-mediated bone resorption, including osteoporosis, steroid-induced osteoporosis, Paget's disease, tumor-associated osteolysis, breast and prostate cancer, and hypercalcemia. Recent evidence suggests that second- and third-generation bisphosphonates also may be effective anticancer drugs (*see* below). For a review of the basic and clinical pharmacology of bisphosphonates, *see* Licata (2005).

The clinical utility of bisphosphonates resides in their direct inhibition of bone resorption. First-generation bisphosphonates contain minimally modified side chains

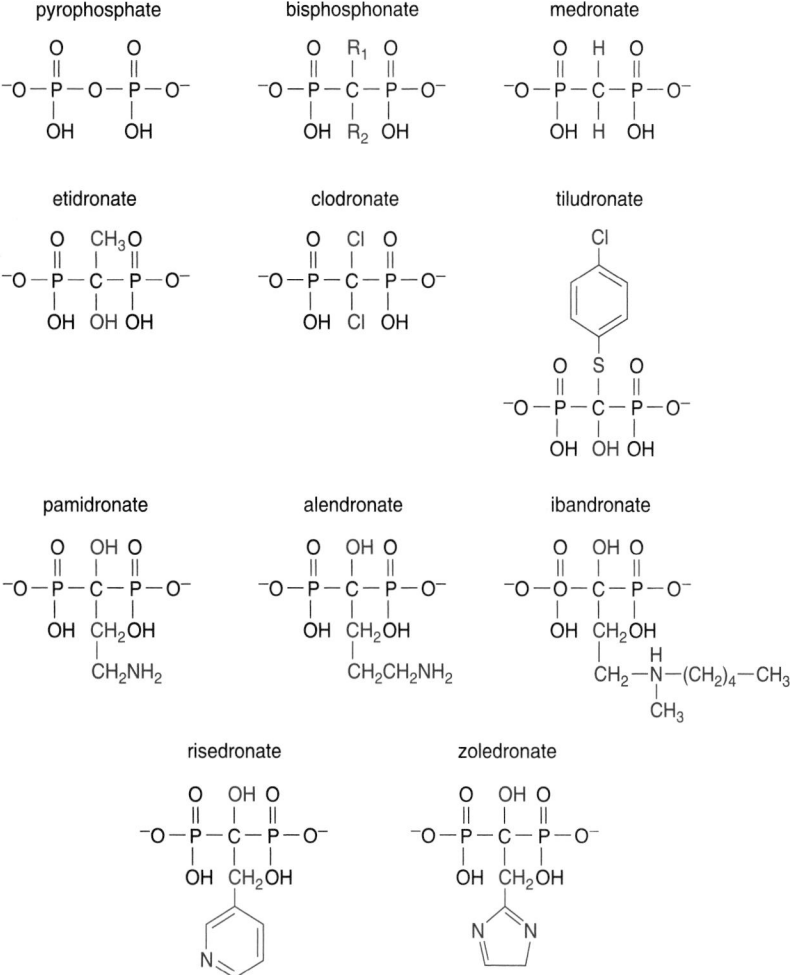

Figure 61–11. *Structures of pyrophosphate and bisphosphonates.* The substituents (R_1 and R_2) on the central carbon of the bisphosphonate parent structure are shown in blue.

(R1, R2) (*medronate, clodronate,* and *etidronate*) or contain a chlorophenyl group (*tiludronate*) (Figure 61–11). They are the least potent and in some instances cause bone demineralization. Second-generation aminobisphosphonates (*e.g., alendronate* and *pamidronate*) contain a nitrogen group in the side chain. They are 10 to 100 times more potent than first-generation compounds. Third-generation bisphosphonates (*e.g., risedronate* and *zoledronate*) contain a nitrogen atom within a heterocyclic ring and are up to 10,000 times more potent than first-generation agents.

Bisphosphonates concentrate at sites of active remodeling. Because they are highly negatively charged, bisphosphonates are membrane impermeable but are incorporated into the bone matrix by fluid-phase endocytosis (Stenbeck and Horton, 2000). Bisphosphonates remain in the matrix until the bone is remodeled and then are released in the acid environment of the resorption lacunae beneath the osteoclast as the overlying mineral matrix is dissolved. The importance of this process for the antiresorptive effect of bisphosphonates is evidenced by the fact that calcitonin blocks the antiresorptive action.

Although bisphosphonates prevent hydroxyapatite dissolution, their antiresorptive action is due to direct inhibitory effects on osteoclasts rather than strictly physiochemical effects. The antiresorptive activity apparently involves two primary mechanisms: osteoclast apoptosis and inhibition of components of the cholesterol biosynthetic pathway.

The current model is that apoptosis accounts for the antiresorptive effect of first-generation bisphosphonates, whereas the inhibitory action of aminobisphosphonates proceeds through the latter mechanism. Consistent with this view, the antiresorptive effect of aminobisphosphonates such as alendronate and risedronate, but not of clodronate or etidronate, persists when apoptosis is suppressed (Halasy-Nagy *et al.*, 2001). First-generation bisphosphonates are metabolized into a nonhydrolyzable ATP analog (AppCCl$_2$p) that accumulates within osteoclasts and induces apoptosis (Rogers, 2003). In contrast, the aminobisphosphonates such as alendronate and *ibandronate* directly inhibit multiple steps in the pathway from mevalonate to cholesterol and isoprenoid lipids, such as geranylgeranyl diphosphate, that are required for the prenylation of proteins that are important for osteoclast function. The potency of aminobisphosphonates for inhibiting farnesyl synthase correlates directly with their antiresorptive activity (Dunford *et al.*, 2001).

Available Bisphosphonates

Several bisphosphonates are available in the United States (Figure 61–11). Etidronate sodium (DIDRONEL) is used for treatment of Paget's disease and may be used parenterally to treat hypercalcemia. Since etidronate is the only bisphosphonate that inhibits mineralization, it has been supplanted largely by pamidronate and zoledronate for treating hypercalcemia. Pamidronate (AREDIA) is approved for management of hypercalcemia but also is effective in other skeletal disorders. Pamidronate is available in the United States only for parenteral administration. For treatment of hypercalcemia, pamidronate may be given as an intravenous infusion of 60 to 90 mg over 4 to 24 hours.

Several newer bisphosphonates have been approved for treatment of Paget's disease. These include tiludronate (SKELID), alendronate (FOSAMAX), and risedronate (ACTONEL). Although the drug is approved only for treating hypercalcemia of malignancy, a single injection of zoledronate (ZOMETA) decreased bone turnover markers for 90 days in patients with Paget's disease (Buckler *et al.*, 1999). Tiludronate and the potent bisphosphonate ibandronate currently are under development for treatment of women with osteoporosis, with encouraging preliminary results.

Absorption, Fate, and Excretion. All oral bisphosphonates are very poorly absorbed from the intestine and have remarkably limited bioavailability [<1% (alendronate, risedronate) to 6% (etidronate tiludronate)]. Thus these drugs should be administered with a full glass of water following an overnight fast and at least 30 minutes before breakfast. Oral bisphosphonates have not been used widely in children or adolescents because of uncertainty of long-term effects of bisphosphonates on the growing skeleton.

Bisphosphonates are excreted primarily by the kidneys. Adjusted doses for patients with diminished renal function have not been determined; bisphosphonates currently are not recommended for patients with a creatinine clearance of less than 30 ml/min.

Adverse Effects. As noted earlier, the first-generation bisphosphonate etidronate was associated with osteomalacia. This adverse effect, coupled with its relatively low efficacy, has limited its current use. Although alendronate and risedronate were well tolerated in clinical trials, some patients experience symptoms of esophagitis. Symptoms often abate when patients fastidiously take the medication with water and remain upright. Esophageal complications are infrequent when the drug is taken as described. If symptoms persist despite these precautions, use of a proton pump inhibitor at bedtime may be helpful (*see* Chapter 36). Both drugs may be better tolerated on a once-weekly regimen with no reduction of efficacy. Patients with active upper gastrointestinal disease should not be given oral bisphosphonates.

Mild fever and aches may attend the first parenteral infusion of pamidronate, likely owing to cytokine release. These symptoms are short-lived and generally do not recur with subsequent administration.

Zoledronate has been associated with renal toxicity, deterioration of renal function, and potential renal failure. Thus, the infusion should be given over at least 15 minutes, and the dose should be 4 mg. Patients who receive zoledronate should have standard laboratory and clinical parameters of renal function assessed prior to treatment and periodically after treatment to monitor for deterioration in renal function.

Therapeutic Uses

Hypercalcemia. The use of pamidronate in the management of malignancy-associated hypercalcemia was described earlier. Zoledronate appears to be more effective than pamidronate and at least as safe and can be infused over 15 minutes rather than 2 to 4 hours. It therefore has received FDA approval for this indication.

Postmenopausal Osteoporosis. Much interest is focused on the role of bisphosphonates in the treatment of osteoporosis (*see* "Osteoporosis," below). Clinical trials show that treatment is associated with increased bone mineral density and protection against fracture.

Cancer. Bisphosphonates also may act as anticancer drugs by inhibiting the activation of cancer-associated proteins, such as Ras, through suppression of geranylgeranylation and farnesylation. Second- and third-generation bisphosphonates inhibit the proliferation of some cancer cells by preventing post-translational prenylation of Ras-related proteins. Zoledronate has been used successfully as an adjunct in treating Philadelphia chromosome–positive chronic myelogenous leukemia.

PARATHYROID HORMONE (PTH)

Continuous administration of PTH or high circulating PTH levels achieved in primary hyperparathyroidism causes bone demineralization and osteopenia. However, *intermittent* PTH administration promotes bone growth. Selye first described the anabolic action of PTH some 80 years ago, but this observation was largely ignored and generally forgotten. Beginning in the 1970s, studies focused on the anabolic action of PTH, culminating with FDA approval of synthetic human 34-amino-acid amino-terminal PTH fragment [hPTH(1–34), *teriparatide*] for use in treating severe osteoporosis (Hodsman *et al.*, 2005). Full-length PTH(1–84) is likely to be approved in the near future; its benefits over PTH(1–34) are unclear.

Absorption, Fate, and Excretion. Pharmacokinetics and systemic actions of teriparatide on mineral metabolism are the same as for PTH. Teriparatide is administered by once-daily subcutaneous injection of 20 μg into the thigh or abdomen. With this regimen, serum PTH concentrations peak at 30 minutes after the injection and decline to undetectable concentrations within 3 hours, whereas the serum calcium concentration peaks at 4 to 6 hours after administration. Based on aggregate data from different dosing regimens, teriparatide bioavailability averages 95%. Teriparatide clearance averages 62 L/hour in women and 94 L/hour in men, which exceeds normal liver plasma flow, consistent with both hepatic and extrahepatic PTH removal. The serum half-life of teriparatide is approximately 1 hour when administered subcutaneously *versus* 5 minutes when administered intravenously. The longer half-life following subcutaneous administration reflects the time required for absorption from the injection site. The elimination of PTH(1–34) and full-length PTH proceeds by nonspecific enzymatic mechanisms in the liver, followed by renal excretion.

Clinical Effects. In postmenopausal women with osteoporosis, teriparatide increases BMD and reduces the risk of vertebral and nonvertebral fractures. Several laboratories have examined the effects of intermittent PTH on BMD in patients with osteoporosis. In these studies, teriparatide increased axial bone mineral, although initial reports of effects on cortical bone were disappointing. Coadministration of hPTH(1–34) with estrogen or synthetic androgen led to impressive gains in vertebral bone mass or trabecular bone. However, in some early studies there was only maintenance or even loss of cortical bone. Vitamin D insufficiency in patients at baseline or pharmacokinetic differences involving bioavailability or circulating half-life may have contributed to observed differences on cortical bone. The most comprehensive studies to date established the value of daily hPTH(1–34) administration on total BMD, with significant elevations of BMD in lumbar spine and femoral neck and with significant reductions of vertebral and nonvertebral fracture risk in osteoporotic women (Neer *et al.*, 2001) and men (Finkelstein *et al.*, 2003).

Candidates for teriparatide treatment include women who have a history of osteoporotic fracture, who have multiple risk factors for fracture, or who failed or are intolerant of previous osteoporosis therapy.

Adverse Effects. In rats, teriparatide increased the incidence of bone tumors, including osteosarcoma (Vahle *et al.*, 2004). The clinical relevance of this finding is unclear, especially since patients with primary hyperparathyroidism have considerably higher elevations of serum PTH without a greater incidence of osteosarcoma. Nonetheless, teriparatide should not be used in patients who are at increased baseline risk for osteosarcoma (including those with Paget's disease of bone, unexplained elevations of alkaline phosphatase, open epiphyses, or prior radiation therapy involving the skeleton). Full-length PTH(1–84), which is in clinical trials, has not been associated with osteosarcomas. Other adverse effects have included exacerbation of nephrolithiasis and elevation of serum uric acid levels.

CALCIUM SENSOR MIMETICS: CINACALCET

Calcimimetics are drugs that mimic the stimulatory effect of calcium to inhibit PTH secretion by the parathyroid glands. By enhancing the sensitivity of the CaSR to extracellular Ca^{2+}, calcimimetics lower the concentration of Ca^{2+} at which PTH secretion is suppressed. The type II calcimimetics are phenylalkylamine derivatives that allosterically modulate the CaSR. *Cinacalcet* (SENSIPAR) (Figure 61–12) is FDA approved for the treatment of secondary hyperparathyroidism owing to chronic renal disease and for patients with hypercalcemia associated with parathyroid carcinoma. Cinacalcet lowers serum PTH levels in patients with normal or reduced renal function (Block *et al.*, 2004; Barman Balfour and Scott, 2005). In clinical trials, cinacalcet at 20- to 100-mg doses lowered PTH levels in a concentration-dependent manner by 15% to 50% and serum calcium $\times$ phosphate product by 7% compared with placebo (Franceschini *et al.*, 2003). Cinacalcet also effectively reduced PTH in patients with primary hyperparathyroidism and provided sustained normalization of serum calcium without altering bone mineral density (Shoback *et al.*, 2003). Long-term control

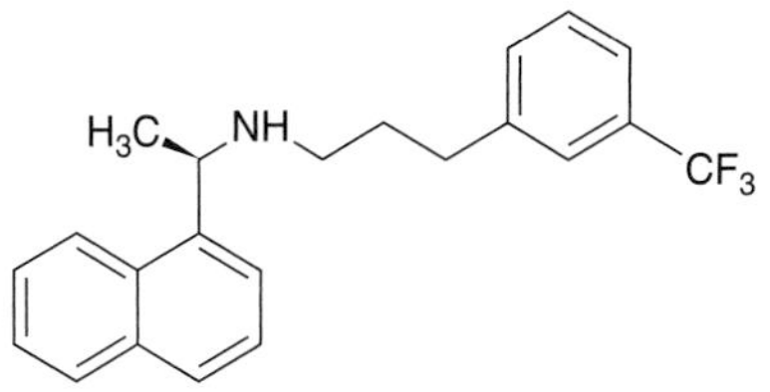

Figure 61–12. Structure of cinacalcet. Cinacalcet exists as optical isomers. The *R*-enantiomer, which is more active, is shown.

of PTH levels was achieved during a 2-year study of cinacalcet, suggesting that resistance does not develop. There currently is insufficient information to know whether reducing serum PTH levels with cinacalcet improves outcomes such as risk of cardiovascular events, bone disease, or mortality.

Absorption, Fate, and Excretion. Cinacalcet (αR)-(–)-α-methyl-N-[3-[3-[trifluoromethylphenyl]propyl]-1-napthalenemethanamine hydrochloride) exhibits first-order absorption, with maximal serum concentrations achieved 2 to 6 hours after oral administration. Maximal effects, as defined by the nadir of serum PTH, occur 2 to 4 hours after administration. After absorption, plasma concentrations of cinacalcet decrease with a half-life of 30 to 40 hours. Cinacalcet is eliminated primarily by renal excretion, with some 85% recovered in the urine after oral administration; the drug is also metabolized by multiple hepatic cytochromes, including CYP3A4, CYP2D6, and CYP1A2.

Cinacalcet is available in 30-, 60-, and 90-mg tablets. Optimal doses have not been defined. The recommended starting dose for treatment of secondary hyperparathyroidism in patients with chronic kidney disease on dialysis is 30 mg once daily, with a maximum of 180 mg/day. For treatment of parathyroid carcinoma, a starting dose of 30 mg twice daily is recommended, with a maximum of 90 mg four times daily. The starting dose is titrated upward every 2 to 4 weeks to maintain the PTH level between 150 and 300 pg/ml (secondary hyperparathyroidism) or to normalize serum calcium (parathyroid carcinoma).

Adverse Reactions. The principal adverse event with cinacalcet is hypocalcemia. Thus, the drug should not be used if the initial serum calcium concentration is less than 8.4 mg/dl; serum calcium and phosphorus concentrations should be measured within 1 week, and PTH should be measured within 4 weeks after initiating therapy or after changing dosage.

Hypocalcemia can be diminished by initiating therapy with a low dose and gradually titrating it as necessary or adjusting the dose when vitamin D and/or phosphate binders are administered concomitantly. Patients on hemodialysis with low-calcium dialysate need to be monitored closely for hypocalcemia. Seizure threshold is lowered by significant reductions in serum Ca^{2+}, so patients with a history of seizure disorders should be monitored especially closely. Finally, adynamic bone disease may develop if the PTH level is less than 100 pg/ml, and the drug should be discontinued or the dose decreased if the PTH level falls below 150 pg/ml.

Drug Interactions. Potential drug interactions can be anticipated with drugs that interfere with calcium homeostasis or that hinder cinacalcet absorption. Based on these considerations, potentially interfering drugs may include vitamin D analogs, phosphate binders, bisphosphonates, calcitonin, glucocorticoids, *gallium,* and *cisplatin.* The other category of drug interactions is for compounds metabolized by CYPs. Caution is recommended when cinacalcet is coadministered with inhibitors of CYP3A4 (*e.g.,* ketoconazole, erythromycin, or itraconazole), CYP2D6 (many β adrenergic receptor blockers, *flecainide, vinblastine,* and most *tricyclic antidepressants*), and many other drugs.

INTEGRATED APPROACH TO OSTEOPOROSIS PREVENTION AND TREATMENT

Osteoporosis is a major and growing public health problem in developed nations, causing fractures in 30% to 50% of women and 15% to 30% of men. Important reductions in fracture risk can be achieved with appropriate lifelong attention to prevention. Regular physical activity of reasonable intensity is endorsed at all ages. For children and adolescents, adequate dietary calcium is important if peak bone mass is to reach the level appropriate for genetic endowment. Attention to nutritional status (*i.e.,* increased dietary calcium or calcium and/or vitamin D supplements) also may be required in the seventh decade and beyond. Although the administration of estrogen to women at menopause is a powerful intervention to preserve bone and protect against fracture, the detrimental effects of hormone-replacement therapy (HRT) have mandated a major reexamination on treatment options (*see* below and Chapter 57).

Pharmacological agents used to manage osteoporosis act by decreasing the rate of bone resorption and thereby slowing the rate of bone loss (antiresorptive therapy) or by promoting bone formation (anabolic therapy). Since bone remodeling is a coupled process, antiresorptive drugs ultimately decrease the rate of bone formation and therefore do not promote substantial gains in BMD. They nonetheless reduce fracture risk, particularly in the spine but also in the hip (for alendronate and risedronate). Increases in BMD during the first years of antiresorptive therapy represent a constriction of the remodeling space to a new steady-state level, after which BMD reaches a plateau (Figure 61–13). One consequence of this phenomenon is that therapeutic trials in osteoporosis must be of sufficient duration (*i.e.,* at least 2 years) to determine whether an increase in BMD represents anything more than a simple reduction in remodeling space.

Pharmacologic treatment of osteoporosis is aimed at restoring bone strength and preventing fractures. The long-standing centerpiece of this approach has been antiresorptive drugs such as the bisphosphonates, *estrogen,* or the selective estrogen receptor modulator (SERM) *raloxifene* and, to some extent, calcitonin. These drugs inhibit osteoclast-mediated bone loss, thereby reducing bone turnover.

Until recently, antiresorptives were the only drugs approved in the United States for treating osteoporosis. The increase in bone density that they produce is variable

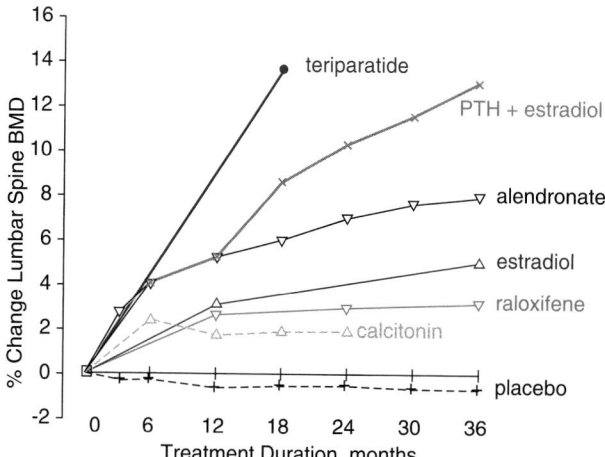

Figure 61–13. *Relative efficacy of different therapeutic interventions on bone mineral density of the lumbar spine.* Teriparatide (40 μg) (Neer *et al.*, 2001), PTH (25 μg) + estradiol (Lindsay *et al.*, 1997), alendronate (10 mg) (Liberman *et al.*, 1995), estradriol (0.625 mg/day) (Writing Group for the PEPI Trial, 1996), raloxifene (120 mg) (Ettinger *et al.*, 1999), calcitonin (200 IU) (Reginster *et al.*, 1995). Typical results with placebo treatment underscore the inexorable bone loss without intervention. Some of the indicated treatment interventions involved combination therapy, and absolute comparisons should not be made.

and depends on the site and the particular drug; generally, the increase is less than 10% after 3 years (Figure 61–12). This situation changed in 2002 when the FDA approved the biologically active PTH fragment PTH(1–34) (*teriparatide*, FORTEO) for use in treating postmenopausal women with osteoporosis and to increase bone mass in men with primary or hypogonadal osteoporosis. For a review and proposed guidelines for teriparatide/PTH use, see Hodsman *et al.* (2005). Therapeutic approaches likely will evolve considerably as newer treatment paradigms are developed and combinations of antiresorptive agents and PTH are introduced, and as the molecular physiology of osteoblast and osteoclast function is elucidated (Grey and Reid, 2005).

Antiresorptive Agents. Bisphosphonates. Bisphosphonates have emerged as the most effective drugs currently approved for prevention and treatment of osteoporosis. Second- and third-generation oral bisphosphonates alendronate and risedronate have sufficient potency to suppress bone resorption at doses that do not inhibit mineralization.

Alendronate is approved for prevention (5 mg daily, 35 mg once weekly) and treatment (10 mg daily, 70 mg once weekly) of

osteoporosis and for the treatment of glucocorticoid-associated osteoporosis. In fact, 3-, 7-, and 10-year studies of daily treatment with alendronate established its efficacy to increase bone mineral density, decrease bone turnover, and reduce the risk of vertebral fracture among women with osteoporosis (Bone *et al.*, 2004; Liberman *et al.*, 1995; Tonino *et al.*, 2000; Tucci *et al.*, 1996). The results of 10-year daily treatment with 10 mg of alendronate (with 500 mg of supplemental calcium) reported a 14% increase of lumbar spine BMD, with smaller increments at the trochanter, total hip, and femoral neck (Bone *et al.*, 2004). On reduction and discontinuation of treatment, BMD at the lumbar spine was maintained. Although significant decreases of BMD occurred at the total hip, femoral neck, and forearm, BMD at the lumbar spine, trochanter, total hip, and total body remained significantly above baseline values at year 10.

Alendronate conserves BMD in recently menopausal women (Hosking *et al.*, 1998), as well as in men, and also improves BMD in patients receiving glucocorticoids (Saag *et al.*, 1998).

For patients in whom oral bisphosphonates cause severe esophageal distress despite countermeasures, intravenous pamidronate (AREDIA) offers skeletal protection without causing adverse GI effects. For treatment of osteoporosis, pamidronate is given as a 3-hour infusion, 30 mg every 3 months. Oral pamidronate (150 or 300 mg daily) has been evaluated for treatment of postmenopausal osteoporosis. Both doses are effective; however, gastrointestinal side effects are frequent with the 300-mg dose. Oral risedronate has been approved for treatment of postmenopausal osteoporosis (5 mg daily or 35 mg once weekly) and glucocorticoid-induced osteoporosis. Risedronate improves BMD and reduces vertebral fracture incidence in postmenopausal women. Combined analysis of four placebo-controlled, randomized trials with risedronate in women with low bone density but no previous vertebral fracture displayed increases of lumbosacral and femoral neck BMD with a significant reduced risk of first vertebral compression fracture (Heaney *et al.*, 2002).

Thiazide Diuretics. Although not strictly antiresorptive, *thiazides* reduce urinary Ca^{2+} excretion and constrain bone loss in patients with hypercalciuria. Whether they will prove to be useful in patients who are not hypercalciuric is not clear, but data suggest that they reduce hip fracture risk. No sustained effect is observed (Schoofs *et al.*, 2003). *Hydrochlorothiazide*, 25 mg once or twice daily, may reduce urinary Ca^{2+} excretion substantially. Effective doses of thiazides for reducing urinary Ca^{2+} excretion generally are lower than those necessary for blood pressure control. For a more detailed discussion of thiazide diuretics, *see* Chapter 28.

Calcium. The physiological roles of Ca^{2+} and its use in the treatment of hypocalcemic disorders were discussed earlier. The rationale for using supplemental calcium to protect bone varies with time of life.

For preteens and adolescents, adequate substrate calcium is required for bone accretion. Controlled trials indicate that supplemental calcium promotes adolescent bone acquisition (Johnston *et al.*, 1992), but its impact on peak bone mass is not known. Higher calcium intake during the third decade of life is positively related to the final phase of bone acquisition (Recker *et al.*, 1992). There is controversy about the role of calcium during the early years after menopause, when the primary basis for bone loss is estrogen withdrawal. Although little effect of calcium on trabecular bone has been reported, reduction in cortical bone loss with calcium supplementation has been observed, even in populations with high dietary calcium intake. In elderly subjects, supplemental calcium suppresses bone turnover, improves BMD, and decreases the incidence of fracture (Dawson-Hughes *et al.*, 1997).

Patients who are unable or unwilling to increase calcium by dietary means alone may choose from many palatable, low-cost calcium preparations. As noted previously, numerous oral calcium preparations are available, the most frequently prescribed being carbonate. Traditional dosing of calcium is about 1000 mg/day, nearly the amount present in a quart of milk. Added to the 500 to 600 mg of dietary calcium that typifies the diet of elderly men and women, this provides a total daily intake of about 1500 mg. More may be necessary to overcome endogenous intestinal calcium losses, but daily intakes of 2000 mg or more frequently are reported to be constipating. Calcium supplements are taken most often with meals to improve absorption.

Vitamin D and Its Analogs. Modest supplementation with vitamin D (400 to 800 IU/day) may improve intestinal Ca^{2+} absorption, suppress bone remodeling, and improve BMD in individuals with marginal or deficient vitamin D status. Although supplemental vitamin D appeared to reduce fracture incidence in several trials, a prospective study found that neither dietary calcium nor vitamin D intake was of major importance for the primary prevention of osteoporotic fractures in women (Michaelsson *et al.*, 2003). Nonetheless, because women commonly consume less than the recommended intake of vitamin D, use of supplemental vitamin D or increased consumption of such vitamin D–rich foods as dark fish may be prudent.

The use of calcitriol to treat osteoporosis is distinct from ensuring vitamin D nutritional adequacy. Here, the rationale is to suppress parathyroid function directly and reduce bone turnover. Calcitriol and the polar vitamin D metabolite 1α-hydroxycholecalciferol are used frequently in Japan and other countries, but experience in the United States has been mixed. Higher doses of calcitriol appear to be more likely to improve BMD, but at the risk of hypercalciuria and hypercalcemia; therefore, close scrutiny of patients and dose modification are required. Restriction of dietary calcium may reduce toxicity during calcitriol therapy (Gallagher and Goldgar, 1990). A low incidence of hypercalciuric and hypercalcemic complications of therapy in Japan may reflect relatively poor calcium intakes in that country.

Estrogen. There is an unambiguous relationship between estrogen deficiency and osteoporosis. Postmenopausal status or estrogen deficiency at any age significantly increases a patient's risk for osteoporosis and

fractures. Likewise, overwhelming evidence supports the positive impact of estrogen replacement on the conservation of bone and protection against osteoporotic fracture after menopause (Rosen and Kessenich, 1997) (*see* Chapter 57). The outcome of the Women's Health Initiative (WHI) studies, however, has strikingly altered the view of the therapeutic use of HRT for long-term prevention or treatment of osteoporosis. Significantly increased risks of heart disease and breast cancer were found (Anderson *et al.*, 2004; Cauley *et al.*, 2003). The consensus among experts now is to reserve HRT only for the short-term relief of vasomotor symptoms associated with menopause. HRT should be limited to osteoporosis prevention in women with significant ongoing vasomotor symptoms who are not at an increased risk for cardiovascular disease. An annual individualized risk-benefit reassessment should be performed on these patients.

Selective Estradiol Receptor Modulators (SERMs). Considerable work has been undertaken to develop estrogenic compounds with tissue-selective activities. One of these, raloxifene (EVISTA), acts as an estrogen agonist on bone and liver, is inactive on the uterus, and acts as an antiestrogen on the breast (*see* Chapter 57). In postmenopausal women, raloxifene stabilizes and modestly increases BMD and has been shown to reduce the risk of vertebral compression fracture (Ettinger *et al.*, 1999). Raloxifene is approved for both the prevention and treatment of osteoporosis. With the decreased use of estrogen for treating osteoporosis, the SERM raloxifene would seem to be an ideal alternative to HRT because raloxifene reduces the risk of vertebral fractures (albeit without a positive effect on nonvertebral fractures), breast cancer, and coronary events (coronary death, nonfatal myocardial infarction, and hospitalized acute coronary syndromes other than myocardial infarction) (Clemett and Spencer, 2000). The major drawback of raloxifene is that it can worsen vasomotor symptoms.

Calcitonin. Calcitonin inhibits osteoclastic bone resorption and modestly increases bone mass in patients with osteoporosis (Civitelli *et al.*, 1988); the largest increases occurred in patients with high intrinsic rates of bone turnover. One study showed that calcitonin nasal spray (200 units/day) reduced the incidence of vertebral compression fractures by about 40% in osteoporotic women (Chesnut *et al.*, 2000).

Combination Therapies

Because teriparatide stimulates bone formation, whereas bisphosphonates reduce bone resorption, it was predicted that therapy combining the two would enhance the effect on BMD more than treatment with either one alone. However, addition of alendronate to PTH treatment provided no additional benefit for BMD and reduced the anabolic effect of PTH in both women and men (Black *et al.*, 2003; Body *et al.*, 2002; Finkelstein *et al.*, 2003). Sequential treatment with PTH(1–84) followed by alendronate increased vertebral BMD to a greater degree than alendronate or estrogen alone (Rittmaster *et al.*, 2000). Recent work underscores the beneficial action of alendronate in consolidating the gains in lumbar spine BMD achieved by antecedent teriparatide treatment in men.

Paget's Disease. Although most patients with Paget's disease require no treatment, factors such as severe pain, neural compression, progressive deformity, hypercalcemia, high-output congestive heart failure, and repeated fracture risk are considered indications for treatment. Bisphosphonates and calcitonin decrease the elevated biochemical markers of bone turnover, such as plasma alkaline phosphatase activity and urinary excretion of hydroxyproline. An initial course of bisphosphonate typically is given once daily or once weekly for 6 months. With treatment, most patients experience a decrease in bone pain over several weeks. Such treatment may induce long-lasting remission. If symptoms recur, additional courses of therapy can be effective. When etidronate is given at higher doses (10 to 20 mg/kg per day) or continuously for longer than 6 months, there is a substantial risk for osteomalacia. At lower doses (5 to 7.5 mg/kg per day), focal osteomalacia has been observed occasionally. Defective mineralization has not been observed with other bisphosphonates or with calcitonin.

Choice of optimal therapy for Paget's disease varies among patients. Bisphosphonates are the standard therapy. Intravenous pamidronate induces long-term remission following a single infusion. Zoledronate seems to exhibit greater response rates and a longer median duration of complete response (Major *et al.*, 2001). Compared with calcitonin, bisphosphonates have the advantage of oral administration, lower cost, lack of antigenicity, and generally fewer side effects. Resistance to calcitonin develops in most patients. However, calcitonin is highly reliable and may have a distinct skeletal analgesic property. Mithramycin (plicamycin) has been used in difficult cases of Paget's disease that do not respond to bisphosphonates or calcitonin. Therapeutic utility of this agent is limited by a high potential for hemorrhagic and other toxicities, and it is not generally recommended.

FLUORIDE

Fluoride is discussed because of its toxic properties and its effect on dentition and bone.

Absorption, Distribution, and Excretion. Human beings obtain fluoride predominantly from the ingestion of plants and water, with most absorption taking place in the intestine. The degree of fluoride absorption correlates with its water solubility. Relatively soluble compounds, such as sodium fluoride, are absorbed almost completely, whereas relatively insoluble compounds, such as cryolite

(Na_3AlF_6) and the fluoride found in bone meal (*fluoroapatite*) are absorbed poorly. A second route of absorption is through the lungs, and inhalation of fluoride present in dusts and gases constitutes the major route of industrial exposure.

Fluoride is distributed widely in organs and tissues but is concentrated in bone and teeth, and the skeletal burden is related to intake and age. Bone deposition reflects skeletal turnover; growing bone shows greater deposition than mature bone.

The kidneys are the major site of fluoride excretion. Small amounts of fluoride also appear in sweat, milk, and intestinal secretions; in a very hot environment, sweat can account for nearly 50% of total fluoride excretion.

Pharmacological Actions and Uses. Because it is concentrated in the bone, the radionuclide ^{18}F has been used in skeletal imaging. Sodium fluoride enhances osteoblast activity and increases bone volume. These effects may be bimodal, with low doses stimulating and higher doses suppressing osteoblasts; if true, this may account for the poorly mineralized and mechanically defective bone seen in some studies. In doses of 30 to 60 mg/day, fluoride increases trabecular bone mineral density in many, but not all, patients. In one controlled trial, fluoride increased lumbar spine density (cancellous bone) but decreased cortical bone mineral density; these changes were associated with a significant increase in peripheral fractures and stress fractures (Riggs *et al.*, 1990). In one study, sustained-release fluoride, which provided lower blood fluoride levels, increased bone mineral density and decreased fractures (Pak *et al.*, 1994). Intermittent courses of slow-release fluoride also have been evaluated. When the total fluoride dose was kept constant (Balena *et al.*, 1998), there was no difference in outcome between continuous and intermittent fluoride treatment; notably, both regimens increased cancellous and trabecular thickness to the same extent. *Unfortunately, increased bone mass is not synonymous with increased bone strength* (Riggs *et al.*, 1990). Thus, the apparent effects of fluoride in osteoporosis are slight compared with those achieved with PTH or other agents.

Other pharmacological actions of fluoride can be classified as toxic, as described below. Fluoride inhibits several enzyme systems and diminishes tissue respiration and anaerobic glycolysis.

Acute Poisoning. Acute fluoride poisoning usually results from accidental ingestion of fluoride-containing insecticides or rodenticides. Initial symptoms (salivation, nausea, abdominal pain, vomiting, and diarrhea) are secondary to the local action of fluoride on the intestinal mucosa. Systemic symptoms are varied and severe: increased irritability of the central nervous system consistent with the Ca^{2+}-binding effect of fluoride and the resulting hypocalcemia; hypotension, presumably owing to central vasomotor depression as well as direct cardiotoxicity; and stimulation and then depression of respiration. Death can result from respiratory paralysis or cardiac failure. The lethal dose of sodium fluoride for human beings is about 5 g, although there is considerable variation. Treatment includes the intravenous administration of glucose in saline and gastric lavage with lime water (0.15% calcium hydroxide solution) or other Ca^{2+} salts to precipitate the fluoride. Calcium gluconate is given intravenously for tetany; urine volume is kept high with vigorous fluid resuscitation.

Chronic Poisoning. In human beings, the major manifestations of chronic ingestion of excessive fluoride are osteosclerosis and mottled enamel. Osteosclerosis is characterized by increased bone density secondary both to elevated osteoblastic activity and to the replacement of hydroxyapatite by the denser fluoroapatite. The degree of skeletal involvement varies from changes that are barely detectable radiologically to marked cortical thickening of long bones, numerous exostoses scattered throughout the skeleton, and calcification of ligaments, tendons, and muscle attachments. In its severest form, it is a disabling and crippling disease.

Mottled enamel, or dental fluorosis, was first described more than 60 years ago. In very mild mottling, small, opaque, paper-white areas are scattered irregularly over the tooth surface. In severe cases, discrete or confluent, deep brown- to black-stained pits give the tooth a corroded appearance. Mottled enamel results from a partial failure of the enamel-forming ameloblasts to elaborate and lay down enamel. Since mottled enamel is a developmental injury, fluoride ingestion following the eruption of teeth has no effect. Mottling is one of the first visible signs of excess fluoride intake during childhood. Continuous use of water containing about 1 ppm of fluoride may result in very mild mottling in 10% of children; at 4 to 6 ppm the incidence approaches 100%, with a marked increase in severity.

Severe dental fluorosis formerly occurred in regions where local water supplies had a very high fluoride content (*e.g.*, Pompeii, Italy, and Pike's Peak, Colorado). Current regulations in the United States require lowering the fluoride content of the water supply or providing an alternative source of acceptable drinking water for affected communities. Sustained consumption of water with a fluoride content of 4 mg/L (4 ppm) is associated with deficits in cortical bone mass and increased rates of bone loss over time (Sowers *et al.*, 1991).

Fluoride and Dental Caries. After a new water supply was established, children in Bauxite, Arkansas, had a much higher incidence of caries than those who had been exposed to the former fluoride-containing water. Subsequent studies established definitely that supplementation of water fluoride content to 1.0 ppm is a safe and practical intervention that substantially reduces the incidence of caries in permanent teeth.

There are partial benefits for children who begin drinking fluoridated water at any age; however, optimal benefits are obtained at ages before permanent teeth erupt. Topical application of fluoride solutions by dental personnel appears to be particularly effective on newly erupted teeth and can reduce the incidence of caries by 30% to 40%. Dietary fluoride supplements should be considered for children younger than age 12 years whose drinking water contains less than 0.7 ppm fluoride. Conflicting results have been reported from studies of fluoride-containing toothpastes.

Adequate incorporation of fluoride into teeth hardens the outer layers of enamel and increases resistance to demineralization. Fluoride deposition apparently involves exchange with hydroxyl or citrate anions in the enamel apatite crystal surface. The mechanism by which fluoride prevents caries is not completely understood. There is no convincing evidence that fluoride from any source reduces the development of caries after the permanent teeth are completely formed (usually about age 14).

The fluoride salts usually employed in dentifrices are *sodium fluoride* and *stannous fluoride.* Sodium fluoride also is available in a variety of preparations for oral and topical use, including tablets, drops, rinses, and gels.

Since its inception, regulation of the fluoride concentration of community water supplies periodically has encountered vocal opposition, including allegations of putative adverse health consequences of fluoridated water. Careful examination of these issues indicates that cancer and all-cause mortalities do not differ significantly between communities with fluoridated and nonfluoridated water (Richmond, 1985).

CLINICAL SUMMARY

Increasing evidence supports the concept that regular physical activity, adequate calcium intake, and lifestyle changes have a positive impact on bone remodeling, constrain bone loss, and reduce fracture risk. Antiresorptive agents such as bisphosphonates, estrogen, selective estrogen response modulators (SERMs), and calcium, will slow bone resorption. Recombinant human PTH has been approved for the treatment of osteoporosis and provides significant intervention for restoring normal bone mass.

Cinacalcet, a drug that acts directly on the parathyroid calcium-sensing receptor, also has been approved, providing a novel approach to decreasing PTH secretion in secondary hyperparathyroidism and parathyroid carcinoma. Improved assays for measuring biologically active and inactive forms of PTH likely will facilitate the diagnosis and treatment of diseases associated with PTH resistance.

Estrogen-replacement therapy, once a mainstay treatment for osteoporosis in women, has been curtailed by the findings of the Women's Health Initiative: Despite estrogen's beneficial effects on bone and fracture risk, alone or in combination with *progestin,* estrogen promotes an array of serious adverse cardiovascular consequences. The FDA now recommends that estrogen be reserved for women at significant risk of osteoporosis who cannot take other medications.

BIBLIOGRAPHY

Anderson, G.L., Limacher, M., Assaf, A.R., *et al.* Effects of conjugated equine estrogen in postmenopausal women with hysterectomy: the Women's Health Initiative randomized controlled trial. *JAMA,* **2004,** *291*:1701–1712.

Balena, R., Kleerekoper, M., Foldes, J.A., *et al.* Effects of different regimens of sodium fluoride treatment for osteoporosis on the structure, remodeling and mineralization of bone. *Osteoporos. Int.*, **1998**, *8*:428–435.

Ballock, R.T., and O'Keefe, R.J. The biology of the growth plate. *J. Bone Joint Surg.*, **2003**, *85A*:715–726.

Barley, N.F., Howard, A., O'Callaghan, D., Legon, S., and Walters, J.R. Epithelial calcium transporter expression in human duodenum. *Am. J. Physiol. Gastrointest. Liver Physiol.*, **2001**, *280*:G285–G290.

Barman Balfour, J., and Scott, L. Cinacalcet hydrochloride. *Drugs*, **2005**, *65*:271–281.

Benker, G., Breuer, N., Windeck, R., and Reinwein, D. Calcium metabolism in thyroid disease. *J. Endocrinol. Invest.*, **1988**, *11*:61–69.

Bilezikian, J.P., Potts, J.T., Jr., Fuleihan, Gel-H., *et al.* Summary statement from a workshop on asymptomatic primary hyperparathyroidism: A perspective for the 21st century. *J. Bone Miner. Res.*, **2002**, *17*(suppl. 2):N2–N11.

Black, D.M., Greenspan, S.L., Ensrud, K.E., *et al.* The effects of parathyroid hormone and alendronate alone or in combination in postmenopausal osteoporosis. *New Engl. J. Med.*, **2003**, *349*:1207–1215.

Bland, R., Walker, E.A., Hughes, S.V., Stewart, P.M., and Hewison, M. Constitutive expression of 25-hydroxyvitamin D_3-1α-hydroxylase in a transformed human proximal tubule cell line: Evidence for direct regulation of vitamin D metabolism by calcium. *Endocrinology*, **1999**, *140*:2027–2034.

Block, G.A., Martin, K.J., de Francisco, A.L., *et al.* Cinacalcet for secondary hyperparathyroidism in patients receiving hemodialysis. *New Engl. J. Med.*, **2004**, *350*:1516–1525.

Body, J.J., Gaich, G.A., Scheele, W.H., *et al.* A randomized, double-blind trial to compare the efficacy of teriparatide [recombinant human parathyroid hormone (1–34)] with alendronate in postmenopausal women with osteoporosis. *J. Clin. Endocrinol. Metab.*, **2002**, *87*:4528–4535.

Bone, H.G., Hosking, D., Devogelaer, J.P., *et al.* Ten years' experience with alendronate for osteoporosis in postmenopausal women. *New Engl. J. Med.*, **2004**, *350*:1189–1199.

Bronner, F. Mechanisms of intestinal calcium absorption. *J. Cell. Biochem.*, **2003**, *88*:387–393.

Brown, E.M., and MacLeod, R.J. Extracellular calcium sensing and extracellular calcium signaling. *Physiol. Rev.*, **2001**, *81*:239–297.

Buckler, H., Fraser, W., Hosking, D., *et al.* Single infusion of zoledronate in Paget's disease of bone: A placebo-controlled, dose-ranging study. *Bone*, **1999**, *24*:81S–85S.

Carney, J.A. The glandulae parathyroideae of Ivar Sandstrom: Contributions from two continents. *Am. J. Surg. Pathol.*, **1996**, *20*:1123–1144.

Carney, S.L. Calcitonin and human renal calcium and electrolyte transport. *Miner. Electrolyte Metab.*, **1997**, *23*:43–47.

Carswell, S. Vitamin D in the nervous system: Action and therapeutic potential. In, *Vitamin D* (Feldman, D., Glorieux, F.H., and Pike, J.W., eds.) Academic Press, San Diego, **1997**, pp. 1197–1212.

Cauley, J.A., Robbins, J., Chen, Z., *et al.* Effects of estrogen plus progestin on risk of fracture and bone mineral density: the Women's Health Initiative randomized trial. *JAMA*, **2003**, *290*:1729-1738.

Center, J.R., Nguyen, T.V., Schneider, D., Sambrook, P.N., and Eisman, J.A. Mortality after all major types of osteoporotic fracture in men and women: An observational study. *Lancet*, **1999**, *353*:878–882.

Chesnut, C.H., 3d, Silverman, S., Andriano, K., *et al.* A randomized trial of nasal spray salmon calcitonin in postmenopausal women with established osteoporosis: The prevent recurrence of osteoporotic fractures study. PROOF Study Group. *Am. J. Med.*, **2000**, *109*:267–276.

Christakos, S., Dhawan, P., Liu, Y., Peng, X., and Porta, A. New insights into the mechanisms of vitamin D action. *J. Cell. Biochem.*, **2003**, *88*:695–705.

Civitelli, R., Gonnelli, S., Zacchei, F., *et al.* Bone turnover in postmenopausal osteoporosis: Effect of calcitonin treatment. *J. Clin. Invest.*, **1988**, *82*:1268–1274.

Clemett, D., and Spencer, C.M. Raloxifene: A review of its use in postmenopausal osteoporosis. *Drugs*, **2000**, *60*:379–411.

Cunningham, J. New vitamin D analogues for osteodystrophy in chronic kidney disease. *Pediatr. Nephrol.*, **2004**, *19*:705–708.

Dawson-Hughes, B., Harris, S.S., Krall, E.A., and Dallal, G.E. Effect of calcium and vitamin D supplementation on bone density in men and women 65 years of age or older. *New Engl. J. Med.*, **1997**, *337*:670–676.

DeLuca, H.F., and Schnoes, H.K. Metabolism and mechanism of action of vitamin D. *Annu. Rev. Biochem.*, **1976**, *45*:631–666.

Dunford, J.E., Thompson, K., Coxon, F.P., *et al.* Structure-activity relationships for inhibition of farnesyl diphosphate synthase in vitro and inhibition of bone resorption in vivo by nitrogen-containing bisphosphonates. *J. Pharmacol. Exp. Ther.*, **2001**, *296*:235–242.

Econs, M.J., McEnery, P.T., Lennon, F., and Speer, M.C. Autosomal dominant hypophosphatemic rickets is linked to chromosome 12p13. *J. Clin. Invest.*, **1997**, *100*:2653–2657.

Eknoyan, G., Levin, A., and Levin, N.W. Bone metabolism and disease in chronic kidney disease. *Am. J. Kidney Dis.*, **2003**, *42*(4 suppl. 3):1–201.

Ettinger, B., Black, D.M., Mitlak, B.H., *et al.* Reduction of vertebral fracture risk in postmenopausal women with osteoporosis treated with raloxifene: Results from a 3-year randomized clinical trial. Multiple Outcomes of Raloxifene Evaluation (MORE) Investigators. *JAMA*, **1999**, *282*:637–645.

Farach-Carson, M.C., and Nemere, I. Membrane receptors for vitamin D steroid hormones: Potential new drug targets. *Curr. Drug Targets*, **2003**, *4*:67–76.

Finkelstein, J.S., Hayes, A., Hunzelman, J.L., *et al.* The effects of parathyroid hormone, alendronate, or both in men with osteoporosis. *New Engl. J. Med.*, **2003**, *349*:1216–1226.

Franceschini, N., Joy, M.S., and Kshirsagar, A. Cinacalcet HCl: A calcimimetic agent for the management of primary and secondary hyperparathyroidism. *Expert Opin. Investig. Drugs*, **2003**, *12*:1413–1421.

Friedman, P.A. Calcium transport in the kidney. *Curr. Opin. Nephrol. Hypertens.*, **1999**, *8*:589–595.

Friedman, P.A., and Bushinsky, D.A. Diuretic effects on calcium metabolism. *Semin. Nephrol.*, **1999**, *19*:551–556.

Gallagher, J.C., and Goldgar, D. Treatment of postmenopausal osteoporosis with high doses of synthetic calcitriol: A randomized, controlled study. *Ann. Intern. Med.*, **1990**, *113*:649–655.

Galson, D.L., and Goldring, S.R. The structure and molecular biology of the calcitonin receptor. In, *Endocrinology.* (Bilezikian, J.P., Raisz, L.G., and Rodan, G., eds.) Academic Press, New York, 2002, pp. 603–617.

Gao, P., Scheibel, S., D'Amour, P., *et al.* Development of a novel immunoradiometric assay exclusively for biologically active whole parathyroid hormone 1–84: implications for improvement of accurate assessment of parathyroid function. *J. Bone Miner. Res.*, **2001**, *16*:605–614.

Gorn, A.H., Rudolph, S.M., Flannery, M.R., *et al.* Expression of two human skeletal calcitonin receptor isoforms cloned from a giant cell tumor of bone: The first intracellular domain modulates ligand binding and signal transduction. *J. Clin. Invest.*, **1995**, *95*:2680–2691.

Grey, A., and Reid, I. Emerging and potential therapies for osteoporosis. *Expert Opin. Investig. Drugs*, **2005**, *14*:265–278.

Grill, V., Rankin, W., and Martin, T.J. Parathyroid hormone–related protein (PTHrP) and hypercalcaemia. *Eur. J. Cancer*, **1998**, *34*:222–229.

Halasy-Nagy, J.M., Rodan, G.A., and Reszka, A.A. Inhibition of bone resorption by alendronate and risedronate does not require osteoclast apoptosis. *Bone*, **2001**, *29*:553–559.

Haussler, M.R., and McCain, T.A. Basic and clinical concepts related to vitamin D metabolism and action. *New Engl. J. Med.*, **1977**, *297*:1041–1050.

Hay, D., Christopoulos, G., Christopoulos, A., Poyner, D., and Sexton, P. Pharmacologic discrimination of calcitonin receptor: Receptor activity modifying complexes. *Mol. Pharmacol.*, **2005**, *67*:1655–1665.

Hayes, C.E., Nashold, F.E., Spach, K.M., and Pedersen, L.B. The immunological functions of the vitamin D endocrine system. *Cell. Mol. Biol.*, **2003**, *49*:277–300.

Heaney, R.P., Zizic, T.M., Fogelman, I., *et al.* Risedronate reduces the risk of first vertebral fracture in osteoporotic women. *Osteoporos. Int.*, **2002**, *13*:501–505.

Hewison, M., Zehnder, D., Chakraverty, R., and Adams, J.S. Vitamin D and barrier function: A novel role for extra-renal 1α-hydroxylase. *Mol. Cell. Endocrinol.*, **2004**, *215*:31–38.

Hirsch, P.F., and Baruch, H. Is calcitonin an important physiological substance? *Endocrine*, **2003**, *21*:201–208.

Hodsman, A., Bauer, D., Dempster, D., *et al.* Parathyroid hormone and teriparatide for the treatment of osteoporosis: A review of the evidence and suggested guidelines for its use. *Endocr. Rev.*, **2005**, *26*: Epub ahead of print.

Hollis, B.W., and Wagner, C.L. Assessment of dietary vitamin D requirements during pregnancy and lactation. *Am. J. Clin. Nutr.*, **2004**, *79*:717–726.

Holick, M., Siris, E., Binkley, N., *et al.* Prevalence of vitamin D inadequacy among postmenopausal North American women receiving osteoporosis therapy. *J. Clin. Endocrinol. Metab.*, **2005**, *90*: Epub ahead of print.

Hosking, D., Chilvers, C.E., Christiansen, C., *et al.* Prevention of bone loss with alendronate in postmenopausal women under 60 years of age. Early Postmenopausal Intervention Cohort Study Group. *New Engl. J. Med.*, **1998**, *338*:485–492.

HYP Consortium. A gene (*PEX*) with homologies to endopeptidases is mutated in patients with X-linked hypophosphatemic rickets. *Nature Genet.*, **1995**, *11*:130–136.

Johnston, C.C., Jr., Miller, J.Z., Slemenda, C.W., *et al.* Calcium supplementation and increases in bone mineral density in children. *New Engl. J. Med.*, **1992**, *327*:82–87.

Institute of Medicine (U.S.). Subcommittee on Interpretation and Uses of Dietary Reference Intakes. Standing Committee on the Scientific Evaluation of Dietary Reference Intakes. *Dietary Reference Intakes: Applications in Dietary Planning.* National Academy Press, Washington, **2003**, p. 237.

Jüppner, H., and Potts, J.T., Jr. Immunoassays for the detection of parathyroid hormone. *J. Bone Miner. Res.*, **2002**, *17*(suppl. 2):N81–N86.

Jüppner, H.W., Gardella, T.J., Brown, E.M., Kronenberg, H.M., and Potts, J.T., Jr. Parathyroid hormone and parathyroid hormone–related peptide in the regulation of calcium homeostasis and bone development. In, *Endocrinology.* (DeGroot, L.J., and Jameson, J.L., eds.) Saunders, Philadelphia, **2001**, pp. 969–998.

Karanikas, G., Moameni, A., Poetzi, C., *et al.* Frequency and relevance of elevated calcitonin levels in patients with neoplastic and nonneoplastic thyroid disease and in healthy subjects. *J. Clin. Endocrinol. Metab.*, **2004**, *89*:515–519.

Khosla, S. Minireview: The OPG/RANKL/RANK system. *Endocrinology*, **2001**, *142*:5050–5055.

Kissmeyer, A.M., and Binderup, L. Calcipotriol (MC 903): Pharmacokinetics in rats and biological activities of metabolites. A comparative study with 1,25(OH)$_2$D$_3$. *Biochem. Pharmacol.*, **1991**, *41*:1601–1606.

Kowalzick, L. Clinical experience with topical calcitriol (1,25-dihydroxyvitamin D$_3$) in psoriasis. *Br. J. Dermatol.*, **2001**, *144*(suppl. 58).

Kragballe, K., and Iversen, L. Calcipotriol: A new topical antipsoriatic. *Dermatol. Clin.*, **1993**, *11*:137–141.

Kurihara, N., Reddy, S.V., Menaa, C., Anderson, D., and Roodman, G.D. Osteoclasts expressing the measles virus nucleocapsid gene display a Pagetic phenotype. *J. Clin. Invest.*, **2000**, *105*:607–614.

Levine, M.A., Germain-Lee, E., and Jan de Beur, S. Genetic basis for resistance to parathyroid hormone. *Horm. Res.*, **2003**, *60*(suppl. 3):87–95.

Liberman, U.A., Weiss, S.R., Broll, J., *et al.* Effect of oral alendronate on bone mineral density and the incidence of fractures in postmenopausal osteoporosis. The Alendronate Phase III Osteoporosis Treatment Study Group. *New Engl. J. Med.*, **1995**, *333*:1437–1443.

Licata, A. Discovery, clinical development and therapeutic uses of bisphosphonates. *Ann. Pharmacotherap.*, **2005**, *39*:668–677.

Lin, H.Y., Harris, T.L., Flannery, M.S., *et al.* Expression cloning of an adenylate cyclase–coupled calcitonin receptor. *Science*, **1991**, *254*:1022–1024.

Lindsay, R., Nieves, J., Formica, C., *et al.* Randomised, controlled study of effect of parathyroid hormone on vertebral bone mass and fracture incidence among postmenopausal women on oestrogen with osteoporosis. *Lancet*, **1997**, *350*:550–555.

Major, P., Lortholary, A., Hon, J., *et al.* Zoledronic acid is superior to pamidronate in the treatment of hypercalcemia of malignancy: A pooled analysis of two randomized, controlled clinical trials. *J. Clin. Oncol.*, **2001**, *19*:558–567.

Malloy, P.J., Pike, J.W., and Feldman, D. The vitamin D receptor and the syndrome of hereditary 1,25-dihydroxyvitamin D–resistant rickets. *Endocr. Rev.*, **1999**, *20*:156–188.

Manen, D., Palmer, G., Bonjour, J.P., and Rizzoli, R. Sequence and activity of parathyroid hormone/parathyroid hormone–related protein receptor promoter region in human osteoblast-like cells. *Gene*, **1998**, *218*:49–56.

Manolagas, S.C., Kousteni, S., and Jilka, R.L. Sex steroids and bone. *Recent Prog. Horm. Res.*, **2002**, *57*:385–409.

Martin, K.J., Gonzalez, E.A., Gellens, M., *et al.* 19-Nor-1-α-25-dihydroxyvitamin D$_2$ (paricalcitol) safely and effectively reduces the levels of intact parathyroid hormone in patients on hemodialysis. *J. Am. Soc. Nephrol.*, **1998**, *9*:1427–1432.

Martin, T.J., and Ng, K.W. Mechanisms by which cells of the osteoblast lineage control osteoclast formation and activity. *J. Cell. Biochem.*, **1994**, *56*:357–366.

Mason, J.B., Hay, R.W., Leresche, J., Peel, S., and Darley, S. The story of vitamin D: From vitamin to hormone. *Lancet*, **1974**, *1*:325–329.

Michaelsson, K., Melhus, H., Bellocco, R., and Wolk, A. Dietary calcium and vitamin D intake in relation to osteoporotic fracture risk. *Bone*, **2003**, *32*:694–703.

Monier-Faugere, M.C., Geng, Z., Mawad, H., *et al.* Improved assessment of bone turnover by the PTH(1–84)/large C-PTH fragments ratio in ESRD patients. *Kidney Int.*, **2001**, *60*:1460–1468.

Morony, S., Warmington, K., Adamu, S., *et al.* The RANKL inhibitor osteoprotegerin (OPG) causes greater suppression of bone resorption and hypercalcemia compared to bisphosphonates in two models of humoral hypercalcemia of malignancy. *Endocrinology*, **2005**, *146*: Epub ahead of print.

Naro, F., Perez, M., Migliaccio, S., *et al.* Phospholipase D– and protein kinase C isoenzyme–dependent signal transduction pathways activated by the calcitonin receptor. *Endocrinology*, **1998**, *139*:3241–3248.

Neer, R.M., Arnaud, C.D., Zanchetta, J.R., *et al.* Effect of parathyroid hormone (1–34) on fractures and bone mineral density in postmenopausal women with osteoporosis. *New Engl. J. Med.,* **2001**, *344*:1434–1441.

Nesby-O'Dell, S., Scanlon, K.S., Cogswell, M.E., *et al.* Hypovitaminosis D prevalence and determinants among African American and white women of reproductive age: Third National Health and Nutrition Examination Survey, 1988–1994. *Am. J. Clin. Nutr.,* **2002**, *76*:187–192.

Nijenhuis, T., Hoenderop, J.G., Nilius, B., and Bindels, R.J. (Patho)physiological implications of the novel epithelial Ca^{2+} channels TRPV5 and TRPV6. *Pflugers Arch.,* **2003**, *446*:401–409.

Pak, C.Y., Sakhaee, K., Piziak, V., *et al.* Slow-release sodium fluoride in the management of postmenopausal osteoporosis: A randomized, controlled trial. *Ann. Intern. Med.,* **1994**, *120*:625–632.

Pike, J.W. The vitamin D receptor and its gene. In, *Vitamin D.* (Feldman, D., Glorieux, F.H., and Pike, J.W., eds.) Academic Press, San Diego, **1997**, pp. 105–125.

Pollak, M.R., Seidman, C.E., and Brown, E.M. Three inherited disorders of calcium sensing. *Medicine,* **1996**, *75*:115–123.

Quamme, G.A. Renal magnesium handling: New insights in understanding old problems. *Kidney Int.,* **1997**, *52*:1180–1195.

Recker, R.R., Davies, K.M., Hinders, S.M., *et al.* Bone gain in young adult women. *JAMA,* **1992**, *268*:2403–2408.

Reginster, J.Y., Deroisy, R., Lecart, M.P., *et al.* A double-blind, placebo-controlled, dose-finding trial of intermittent nasal salmon calcitonin for prevention of postmenopausal lumbar spine bone loss. *Am. J. Med.,* **1995**, *98*:452–458.

Richmond, V.L. Thirty years of fluoridation: A review. *Am. J. Clin. Nutr.,* **1985**, *41*:129–138.

Riggs, B.L., Hodgson, S.F., O'Fallon, W.M., *et al.* Effect of fluoride treatment on the fracture rate in postmenopausal women with osteoporosis. *New Engl. J. Med.,* **1990**, *322*:802–809.

Rittmaster, R.S., Bolognese, M., Ettinger, M.P., *et al.* Enhancement of bone mass in osteoporotic women with parathyroid hormone followed by alendronate. *J. Clin. Endocrinol. Metab.,* **2000**, *85*:2129–2134.

Rogers, M.J. New insights into the molecular mechanisms of action of bisphosphonates. *Curr. Pharm. Des.,* **2003**, *9*:2643–2658.

Rosen, C.J., and Kessenich, C.R. The pathophysiology and treatment of postmenopausal osteoporosis: An evidence-based approach to estrogen replacement therapy. *Endocrinol. Metab. Clin. North Am.,* **1997**, *26*:295–311.

Saag, K.G., Emkey, R., Schnitzer, T.J., *et al.* Alendronate for the prevention and treatment of glucocorticoid-induced osteoporosis. Glucocorticoid-Induced Osteoporosis Intervention Study Group. *New Engl. J. Med.,* **1998**, *339*:292–299.

Schoofs, M.W., van der Klift, M., Hofman, A., *et al.* Thiazide diuretics and the risk for hip fracture. *Ann. Intern. Med.,* **2003**, *139*:476–482.

Shoback, D.M., Bilezikian, J.P., Turner, S.A., *et al.* The calcimimetic cinacalcet normalizes serum calcium in subjects with primary hyperparathyroidism. *J. Clin. Endocrinol. Metab.,* **2003**, *88*:5644–5649.

Silverberg, S.J., Gao, P., Brown, I., *et al.* Clinical utility of an immunoradiometric assay for parathyroid hormone (1–84) in primary hyperparathyroidism. *J. Clin. Endocrinol. Metab.,* **2003**, *88*:4725–4730.

Singh, A., Gilchrist, A., Voyono-Yasenetskaya, T., Radeff-Huang, J., and Stern, P. $G_{\alpha12}$ and $G_{\alpha13}$ subunits of heterotrimeric G proteins mediate

parathyroid hormone activation of phospholipase D in UMR-106 osteoblastic cells. *Endocrinology*, **2005**, *146*: Epub ahead of print.

Skerry, T.M., and Gowen, M. Bone cells and bone in remodelling in rheumatoid arthritis. In, *Mechanisms and Models in Rheumatoid Arthritis.* (Henderson, B., Edwards, J.C.W., and Pettipher, E.R., eds.) Academic Press, London, **1995**, pp. 205–220.

Slatopolsky, E., Cozzolino, M., Lu, Y., *et al.* Efficacy of 19-nor-1,25-$(OH)_2D_2$ in the prevention and treatment of hyperparathyroid bone disease in experimental uremia. *Kidney Int.,* **2003**, *63*:2020–2027.

Sneddon, W.B., Syme, C.A., Bisello, A., *et al.* Activation-independent parathyroid hormone receptor internalization is regulated by NHERF1 (EBP50). *J. Biol. Chem.,* **2003**, *278*:43787–43796.

Sowers, M.F., Clark, M.K., Jannausch, M.L., and Wallace, R.B. A prospective study of bone mineral content and fracture in communities with differential fluoride exposure. *Am. J. Epidemiol.,* **1991**, *133*:649–660.

Spear, G.T., Paulnock, D.M., Helgeson, D.O., and Borden, E.C. Requirement of differentiative signals of both interferon-gamma and 1,25-dihydroxyvitamin D_3 for induction and secretion of interleukin-1 by HL-60 cells. *Cancer Res.,* **1988**, *48*:1740–1744.

Stenbeck, G., and Horton, M.A. A new specialized cell-matrix interaction in actively resorbing osteoclasts. *J. Cell Sci.,* **2000**, *113*:1577–1587.

Stokstad, E. Nutrition. The vitamin D deficit. *Science,* **2003**, *302*:1886–1888.

Suda, T., Takahashi, N., Udagawa, N., *et al.* Modulation of osteoclast differentiation and function by the new members of the tumor necrosis factor receptor and ligand families. *Endocr. Rev.,* **1999**, *20*:345–357.

Suda, T., Ueno, Y., Fujii, K., and Shinki, T. Vitamin D and bone. *J. Cell. Biochem.,* **2003**, *88*:259–266.

Takahashi, S., Goldring, S., Katz, M., *et al.* Down-regulation of calcitonin receptor mRNA expression by calcitonin during human osteoclast-like cell differentiation. *J. Clin. Invest.,* **1995**, *95*:167–171.

Tian, J., Smogorzewski, M., Kedes, L., and Massry, S.G. Parathyroid hormone–parathyroid hormone–related protein receptor messenger RNA is present in many tissues besides the kidney. *Am. J. Nephrol.,* **1993**, *13*:210–213.

Tonino, R.P., Meunier, P.J., Emkey, R., *et al.* Skeletal benefits of alendronate: 7-year treatment of postmenopausal osteoporotic women. Phase III Osteoporosis Treatment Study Group. *J. Clin. Endocrinol. Metab.,* **2000**, *85*:3109–3115.

Tucci, J.R., Tonino, R.P., Emkey, R.D., *et al.* Effect of three years of oral alendronate treatment in postmenopausal women with osteoporosis. *Am. J. Med.,* **1996**, *101*:488–501.

Urena, P., Kong, X.F., Abou-Samra, A.B., *et al.* Parathyroid hormone (PTH)/PTH–related peptide receptor messenger ribonucleic acids are widely distributed in rat tissues. *Endocrinology,* **1993**, *133*:617–623.

Vahle, J.L., Long, G.G., Sandusky, G., *et al.* Bone neoplasms in F344 rats given teriparatide [rhPTH(1–34)] are dependent on duration of treatment and dose. *Toxicol. Pathol.,* **2004**, *32*:426–438.

Van Cromphaut, S.J., Dewerchin, M., Hoenderop, J.G., *et al.* Duodenal calcium absorption in vitamin D receptor knockout mice: Functional and molecular aspects. *Proc. Natl. Acad. Sci. U.S.A.,* **2001**, *98*:13324–13329.

van den Bemd, G.J., Pols, H.A., and van Leeuwen, J.P. Anti-tumor effects of 1,25-dihydroxyvitamin D_3 and vitamin D analogs. *Curr. Pharm. Des.,* **2000**, *6*:717–732.

Vieth, R. Vitamin D supplementation, 25-hydroxyvitamin D concentrations, and safety. *Am. J. Clin. Nutr.,* **1999**, *69*:842–856.

White, K.E., Jonsson, K.B., Carn, G., *et al.* The autosomal dominant hypophosphatemic rickets (*ADHR*) gene is a secreted polypeptide overexpressed by tumors that cause phosphate wasting. *J. Clin. Endocrinol. Metab.,* **2001,** *86*:497–500.

Writing Group for the PEPI Trial. Effects of hormone replacement therapy on endometrial histology in postmenopausal women. The Postmenopausal Estrogen/Progestin Interventions (PEPI) Trial. *JAMA,* **1996,** *275*:370–375.

Yanagawa, N., and Lee, D.B.N. Renal handling of calcium and phosphorus. *In, Disorders of Bone and Mineral Metabolism.* (Coe, F.L., and Favus, M.J., eds.) Raven Press Ltd., New York, **1992,** pp. 3–40.

Yoshida, T., Yoshida, N., Monkawa, T., Hayashi, M., and Saruta, T. Dietary phosphorus deprivation induces 25-hydroxyvitamin D_3 1α-hydroxylase gene expression. *Endocrinology,* **2001,** *142*:1720–1726.

Yu, D., Yu, S., Schuster, V., *et al.* Identification of two novel deletion mutations within the $G_s\alpha$ gene (*GNAS1*) in Albright hereditary osteodystrophy. *J. Clin. Endocrinol. Metab.,* **1999,** *84*:3254–3259.

Zanello, L.P., and Norman, A.W. Rapid modulation of osteoblast ion channel responses by $1\alpha,25(OH)_2$-vitamin D_3 requires the presence of a functional vitamin D nuclear receptor. *Proc. Natl. Acad. Sci. U.S.A.,* **2004,** *101*:1589–1594.

CHAPTER

62

DERMATOLOGICAL PHARMACOLOGY

Lindy P. Fox, Hans F. Merk, and David R. Bickers

The skin has many essential functions, including protection, thermoregulation, immune responsiveness, biochemical synthesis, sensory detection, and social and sexual communication. Therapy to correct dysfunction in any of these activities may employ chemical agents that can be delivered systemically, intralesionally, or topically and physical agents to which the skin can be exposed, including ultraviolet and ionizing radiation.

A unique aspect of dermatological pharmacology is the direct accessibility of the skin as a target organ for diagnosis and treatment (Figure 62–1). Topical agents are employed alone or in conjunction with phototherapy and/or systemic medications in the management of most dermatological conditions. Therapeutic agents can reach epidermal keratinocytes and immunocompetent cells in the epidermis and the underlying dermis that are involved in the pathogenesis of numerous cutaneous diseases. Topical agents can be applied directly to the skin but must penetrate into the tissue to achieve efficacy. Appropriate use of topical agents requires an appreciation of the factors that influence percutaneous absorption.

Antibacterial, antiviral, and antifungal agents are employed widely both topically and systemically. Oral antimalarial, cytotoxic, and immunosuppressive agents and antihistamines frequently are used for treatment of dermatological diseases. *Calcipotriene*, a vitamin D analog, is used topically for psoriasis. Ultraviolet radiation

therapy is a frequent mode of treatment that can be administered independently or in combination with photosensitizers. The pathogenetic role of ultraviolet radiation in cutaneous cancers has led to the development of sunscreens to reduce or prevent premalignant and malignant skin lesions. An improved understanding of the pathogenesis of immunologic disorders has led to a number of novel biological agents that hold considerable promise to match the efficacy of *glucocorticoids* and other immunosuppressive agents in dermatologic diseases, possibly with fewer serious adverse effects.

THE STRUCTURE AND FUNCTION OF SKIN

The skin acts as a two-way barrier to prevent absorption or loss of water and electrolytes. The barrier resides in the outermost layer of the epidermis, the stratum corneum, as evidenced by approximately equal rates of penetration of chemicals through isolated stratum corneum or whole skin. Having lost their nuclei and cytoplasmic organelles, the corneocytes of the stratum corneum are nonviable. The cells are flattened, and the fibrous keratins are aligned into disulfide cross-linked macrofibers in association with filaggrin, the major protein component of the keratohyalin granule. Each cell develops a cornified enve-

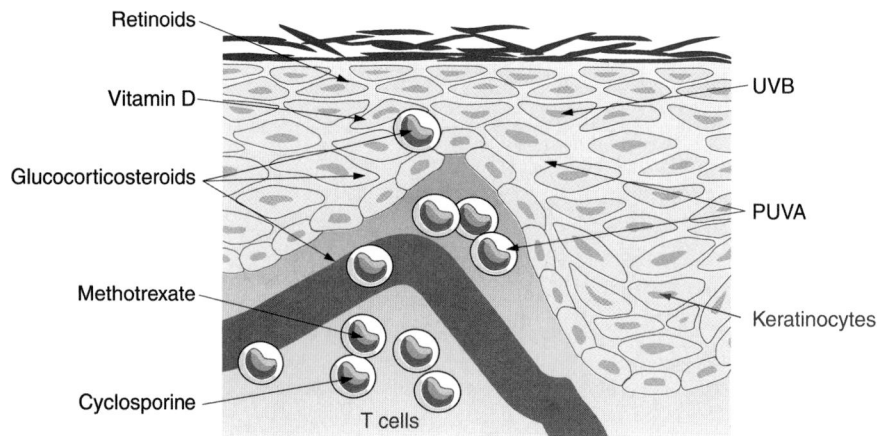

Figure 62–1. *Skin as a pharmacological target.* The skin is a multicellular organ containing numerous indigenous cells and structures as well as circulating cells that are potential targets for pharmacological intervention (*black arrows*). UVB, ultraviolet radiation (290–320 nm); PUVA, psoralen activated by UVA radiation (320–400 nm).

lope resulting from cross-linking of involucrin and keratohyalin, forming an insoluble exoskeleton that acts as a rigid scaffold for the internal keratin filaments. The intercellular spaces are filled with hydrophobic lamellar lipids derived from membrane-coating granules. The combination of hydrophilic cornified cells in hydrophobic intercellular material provides a barrier to both hydrophilic and hydrophobic substances (Ebling, 1993). In dermatological diseases, the thickened epidermis may further diminish the penetration of pharmacological agents into the dermis.

DRUG DELIVERY IN DERMATOLOGICAL DISEASES

Topical Preparations

Molecules can penetrate the skin by three routes: through intact stratum corneum, through sweat ducts, or through the sebaceous follicle. The surface of the stratum corneum presents more than 99% of the total skin surface available for percutaneous drug absorption. Passage through this outermost layer is the rate-limiting step for percutaneous absorption. The major steps involved in percutaneous absorption include the establishment of a concentration gradient, which provides the driving force for drug movement across the skin; release of drug from the vehicle (partition coefficient); and drug diffusion across the layers of the skin (diffusion coefficient). Preferable characteristics of topical drugs include low molecular mass (600 Da), adequate solubility in oil and water, and a high partition coefficient (Barry, 2004). Except for very small particles, water-soluble

ions and polar molecules do not penetrate intact stratum corneum. The relationship of these factors to one another is summarized in the following equation:

$$J = C_{veh} \cdot K_m \cdot D/x$$

where J is the rate of absorption, C_{veh} is the concentration of drug in vehicle, K_m is the partition coefficient, D is the diffusion coefficient, and x is the thickness of stratum corneum (Piacquadio and Kligman, 1998).

Metabolism

The viable epidermis contains a variety of enzyme systems capable of metabolizing drugs that reach this compartment, including CYPs, epoxide hydrolase, transferases such as *N*-acetyl-transferases, and diverse enzymes including glucuronyl transferases and sulfatases (Baron *et al.*, 2001; Du *et al.*, 2004). A specific CYP isoform, CYP26A1, metabolizes retinoic acid and may control its level in the skin (White *et al.*, 1997; Baron *et al.*, 2001). In addition, transporter proteins that influence influx (OATP) or efflux (MRD and LRD) of certain xenobiotics are present in human keratinocytes (Baron *et al.*, 2001). While substrate turnover is considerably less than that for hepatic CYPs, these enzymes influence concentrations of xenobiotics in the skin.

General Guidelines for Topical Therapy

Dosage. An amount of topical medication sufficient to cover affected body surfaces in repeated applications must be dispensed to the patient. A general rule is that approximately 30 g is required to cover the body surface.

Regional Anatomic Variation. Permeability generally is inversely proportional to the thickness of the stratum corneum. Drug penetration is higher on the face, in intertriginous areas, and especially in the perineum. Consequently, the skin in these regions may be more susceptible to irritant and allergic contact reactions. Skin sites that are naturally occluded by apposing surfaces, such as the axillae, groin, and inframammary areas, also may be vulnerable to drug-related toxicity such as atrophy from potent topical glucocorticoids.

Altered Barrier Function. In many dermatological diseases, such as psoriasis, the stratum corneum is abnormal, and barrier function is compromised. In these settings, percutaneous absorption may be increased to the point that standard drug doses can result in systemic toxicity (*e.g.,* hypothalamic–pituitary–adrenal axis suppression can result from systemic absorption of potent topical glucocorticoids).

Hydration. Drug absorption is increased with *hydration,* defined as an increase in the water content of the stratum corneum that is produced by inhibiting transepidermal loss of water. Methods of hydration include occlusion with an impermeable film, application of lipophilic occlusive vehicles such as ointments, and soaking dry skin before occlusion.

Vehicle. Many factors influence the rate and extent to which topical medications are absorbed. Most topical medications are incorporated into bases or vehicles that are applied directly to the skin. The chosen vehicle can influence drug absorption and provide therapeutic efficacy; for example, an ointment is more occlusive and has superior emollient properties than a cream or a lotion base.

Newer vehicles include liposomes and microgel formulations. Liposomes are concentric spherical shells of phospholipids in an aqueous medium that may enhance percutaneous absorption. Variations in size, charge, and lipid content can influence liposome function substantially. Liposomes penetrate compromised epidermal barriers more efficiently (Korting *et al.,* 1991). Microgels are polymers that may enhance solubilization of certain drugs, thereby enhancing penetration and diminishing irritancy.

Transfersomes are a drug-delivery technology based on highly deformable, ultraflexible lipid vesicles that penetrate the skin when applied nonocclusively (Barry, 2004). Finally, pressure waves generated by intense laser radiation can permeabilize the stratum corneum and may provide a novel system for transdermal drug delivery.

Age. Children have a greater ratio of surface area to mass than adults, so a given amount of topical drug results in a greater systemic dose. Based on transepidermal water loss and percutaneous absorption studies, term infants seem to possess a stratum corneum with barrier properties comparable with adults.

Application Frequency. Topical agents often are applied twice daily. For certain drugs, once-daily application of a larger dose may be equally effective as more frequent applications of smaller doses. The stratum corneum may act as a drug reservoir that allows gradual penetration into the viable skin layers over a prolonged period. Intermittent pulse therapy—treatment for several days or weeks alternating with treatment-free periods—may prevent development of tachyphylaxis associated with drugs such as topical glucocorticoids.

Intralesional Administration. Intralesional drug administration is used mainly for inflammatory lesions but also can be used for treatment of warts and selected neoplasms. Medications injected intralesionally have the advantages of direct contact with the underlying pathologic process, no first-pass metabolism, and the formation of a slowly absorbed depot of drug. In considering the use of intralesional medications, it is important to be cognizant of the possibility of systemic absorption of the medication.

Systemic Administration. Systemic administration of medication in dermatology usually involves oral ingestion but also can involve intramuscular (*e.g., methotrexate* and glucocorticoids), intravenous (*e.g., immunoglobulin* and *alefacept*), or subcutaneous administration (e.g., *efalizumab* and *etanercept*).

GLUCOCORTICOIDS

Glucocorticoids are prescribed frequently for their immunosuppressive and antiinflammatory properties. They are administered locally, through topical and intralesional routes, and systemically, through intramuscular, intravenous, and oral routes. Mechanisms of glucocorticoid action are numerous, as discussed in Chapter 59. These include apoptosis of lymphocytes, inhibitory effects on the arachidonic acid cascade, depression of production of many cytokines, and myriad effects on inflammatory cells.

Shortly after the synthesis of *hydrocortisone* in 1951, topical glucocorticoids were recognized as effective agents for the treatment of skin disease. With the development of appropriate vehicles, these agents rapidly became the mainstay of therapy for many inflammatory skin diseases.

Topical glucocorticoids have been grouped into seven classes in order of decreasing potency (Table 62–1); many of the more potent drugs have a fluorinated hydrocortisone backbone. Potency traditionally is measured using a vasoconstrictor assay in which an agent is applied to skin under occlusion, and the area of skin blanching is assessed. Vasoconstriction-induced blanching can be readily quantified by this methodology, which has been verified using laser–Doppler perfusion imaging (Sommer *et*

Table 62–1
Potency of Selected Topical Glucocorticoids

CLASS OF DRUG*	GENERIC NAME, FORMULATION	TRADE NAME
1	Betamethasone dipropionate cream, ointment 0.05% (in optimized vehicle)	DIPROLENE
	Clobetasol propionate cream, ointment 0.05%	TEMOVATE
	Diflorasone diacetate ointment 0.05%	PSORCON
	Halobetasol propionate ointment 0.05%	ULTRAVATE
2	Amcinonide ointment 0.1%	CYCLOCORT
	Betamethasone dipropionate ointment 0.05%	DIPROSONE, others
	Desoximetasone cream, ointment 0.25%, gel 0.05%	TOPICORT
	Diflorasone diacetate ointment 0.05%	FLORONE, MAXIFLOR
	Fluocinonide cream, ointment, gel 0.05%	LIDEX, LIDEX-E, FLUONEX
	Halcinonide cream, ointment 0.1%	HALOG, HALOG-E
3	Betamethasone dipropionate cream 0.05%	DIPROSONE, others
	Betamethasone valerate ointment 0.1%	BETATREX, others
	Diflorasone diacetate cream 0.05%	FLORONE, MAXIFLOR
	Triamcinolone acetonide ointment 0.1%, cream 0.5%	ARISTOCORT A, others
4	Amcinonide cream 0.1%	CYCLOCORT
	Desoximetasone cream 0.05%	TOPICORT LP
	Fluocinolone acetonide cream 0.2%	SYNALAR-HP
	Fluocinolone acetonide ointment 0.025%	SYNALAR
	Flurandrenolide ointment 0.05%, tape 4 μg/cm^2	CORDRAN
	Hydrocortisone valerate ointment 0.2%	WESTCORT
	Triamcinolone acetonide ointment 0.1%	KENALOG, ARISTOCORT
	Mometasone furoate cream, ointment 0.1%	ELOCON
5	Betamethasone dipropionate lotion 0.05%	DIPROSONE, others
	Betamethasone valerate cream, lotion 0.1%	BETATREX, others
	Fluocinolone acetonide cream 0.025%	SYNALAR
	Flurandrenolide cream 0.05%	CORDRAN SP
	Hydrocortisone butyrate cream 0.1%	LOCOID
	Hydrocortisone valerate cream 0.2%	WESTCORT
	Triamcinolone acetonide cream, lotion 0.1%	KENALOG
	Triamcinolone acetonide cream 0.025%	ARISTOCORT
6	Aclometasone dipropionate cream, ointment 0.05%	ACLOVATE
	Desonide cream 0.05%	TRIDESILON, DESOWEN
	Fluocinolone acetonide cream, solution 0.01%	SYNALAR
7	Dexamethasonesodium phosphate cream 0.1%	DECADRON
	Hydrocortisone cream, ointment, lotion 0.5%, 1.0%, 2.5%	HYTONE, NUTRICORT, PENECORT

*Class 1 is most potent; class 7 is least potent. Adapted from Arndt, K.A. *Manual of Dermatologic Therapeutics*, 4th ed. Little, Brown, and Company, Boston, 1989, p. 234, with permission.

al., 1998). Other assays of glucocorticoid potency involve suppression of erythema and edema after experimentally induced inflammation and the psoriasis bioassay, in which the effect of steroid on psoriatic lesions is quantified.

Therapeutic Uses. Many inflammatory skin diseases respond to topical or intralesional administration of glucocorticoids. Absorption varies among body areas; the steroid is selected on the basis of its potency, the site of involvement, and the severity of the skin disease. Often, a more potent steroid is used initially, followed by a less potent agent. Most practitioners become familiar with one glucocorticoid in each class so as to select the appropriate strength of drug. Twice-daily application is sufficient, and more frequent application does not improve response (Yohn and Weston, 1990). In general, only nonfluorinated glucocorticoids should be used on the face or in occluded areas such as the axillae or groin.

Intralesional preparations of glucocorticoids include insoluble preparations of *triamcinolone acetonide* (KENALOG-10 and others) and *triamcinolone hexacetonide* (KENALOG-40 AND ARISTOSPAN), which solubilize gradually and therefore have a prolonged duration of action.

Toxicity and Monitoring. Chronic use of class I topical glucocorticoids can cause skin atrophy, striae, telangiectasias, purpura, and acneiform eruptions. Because perioral dermatitis and rosacea can develop after the use of fluorinated compounds on the face, they should not be used in this site.

Systemic Glucocorticoids

Therapeutic Uses. Systemic glucocorticoid therapy is used for severe dermatological illnesses. In general, it is best to reserve this method for allergic contact dermatitis to plants (*e.g.*, poison ivy) and for life-threatening vesiculobullous dermatoses such as pemphigus vulgaris and bullous pemphigoid. Chronic administration of oral glucocorticoids is problematic, given the side effects associated with their long-term use (*see* Chapter 59).

Daily morning dosing with *prednisone* generally is preferred, although divided doses are used occasionally to enhance efficacy. Fewer side effects are seen with alternate-day dosing, and if required for chronic therapy, prednisone is tapered to every other day as soon as it is practical. Pulse therapy using large intravenous doses of *methylprednisolone sodium succinate* (SOLU-MEDROL) is an option for severe resistant pyoderma gangrenosum, pemphigus vulgaris, systemic lupus erythematosus with multisystem disease, and dermatomyositis (Werth, 1993). The dose usually is 0.5 g to 1 g given over 2 to 3 hours. More rapid infusion has been associated with increased rates of hypotension, electrolyte shifts, and cardiac arrhythmias.

Toxicity and Monitoring. Oral glucocorticoids have numerous systemic effects, as discussed in Chapter 59. Most side effects are dose-dependent. Long-term use is associated with a number of complications, including psy-

chiatric problems, cataracts, myopathy, osteoporosis, avascular bone necrosis, glucose intolerance or overt diabetes mellitus, and hypertension. In addition, psoriatic patients treated with parenteral or topical glucocorticoids may have a pustular flare, particularly if the steroid is tapered rapidly.

RETINOIDS

Retinoids include natural compounds and synthetic derivatives of retinol that exhibit vitamin A activity. Retinoids have many important functions throughout the body, including roles in vision, regulation of cell proliferation and differentiation and bone growth, immune defense, and tumor suppression (Chandraratna, 1998). Because vitamin A affects normal epithelial differentiation, it was investigated as a treatment for cutaneous disorders but was abandoned initially because of unfavorable side effects. Molecular modifications yielded compounds with vastly improved margins of safety. First-generation retinoids include *retinol, tretinoin* (all-*trans*-retinoic acid), *isotretinoin* (13-*cis*-retinoic acid), and *alitretinoin* (9-*cis*-retinoic acid). Second-generation retinoids, also known as *aromatic retinoids,* were created by alteration of the cyclic end group and include *acitretin*. Third-generation retinoids contain further modifications and are called *arotinoids*. Members of this generation include *tazarotene* and *bexarotene. Adapalene,* a derivative of naphthoic acid with retinoid-like properties, does not fit precisely into any of the three generations.

Retinoic acid (RA) exerts its effects on gene expression by activating two families of receptors—*retinoic acid receptors* (RARs) and the *retinoid X receptors* (RXRs)—that are members of the thyroid/steroid hormone receptor superfamily (Winterfield *et al.*, 2003). Retinoids (ligands) bind transcription factors (nuclear receptors), and the ligand–receptor complex then binds to the promoter regions of target genes to regulate their expression (Saurat, 1999). The gene products formed contribute to the desirable pharmacological effects of these drugs and their unwanted side effects (Shroot, 1998). Additional complexity arises because each receptor has three isoforms (α, β, and γ) that form homo- and heterodimers. Retinoid-responsive tissues express one or more RAR and RXR subtypes in various combinations that determine activity locally (Petkovich, 2001). Human skin contains mainly RARα and RARβ.

First- and second-generation retinoids can bind to several retinoid receptors because of the flexibility imparted by their alternating single and double bonds. This relative lack of receptor specificity may lead to greater side effects. The structures of third-generation retinoids are much less flexible than those of earlier-generation retinoids and therefore interact with fewer retinoid receptors (Chandraratna, 1998).

Acute retinoid toxicity is similar to vitamin A intoxication. Side effects of retinoids include dry skin, nosebleeds from dry mucous membranes, conjunctivitis, and hair loss. Less frequently, musculoskeletal pain, pseudotumor cerebri, and mood alterations occur. Oral retinoids are potent teratogens and cause severe fetal malformations. Because of this, *systemic retinoids should be used with great caution in females of childbearing potential.*

Retinoids are used in the treatment of diverse diseases and are effective in the treatment of inflammatory skin disorders, skin malignancies, hyperproliferative disorders, photoaging, and many other disorders. Topical retinoids can normalize disordered keratinization in sebaceous follicles and reduce inflammation, and they may enhance the penetration of other topical medications. Specific retinoids and their uses in the treatment of dermatologic disorders are discussed below.

Tretinoin

Tretinoin (RETIN-A, others) has been used in the treatment of acne vulgaris for almost four decades. A primary use for tretinoin is to reduce the hyperkeratinization that leads to microcomedone formation, the initial lesion in acne. Follicular corneocytes become less cohesive as a result of shedding of desmosomes, decreasing tonofilaments and increasing keratinocyte autolysis and intracellular deposition of glycogen (Wolff *et al.*, 1975).

In addition to treating acne, tretinoin improves photodamaged human skin (Kligman *et al.*, 1986). Epidermal effects include increased epidermal and granular layer thickness, decreased melanocytic activity, and increased secretion of a glycosaminoglycan-like substance into the intercellular space. In the dermis, blood vessel vasodilation and angiogenesis and increased papillary dermal collagen synthesis have been documented. Clinically, this translates to modest attenuation of fine and coarse wrinkling, smoother texture, increased pinkness, and diminished hyperpigmentation (Green *et al.*, 1993). In clinical trials, wrinkling, mottled hyperpigmentation, and roughness improved in most patients treated with retinoids, a response rate roughly twice that of control subjects who used sunscreens and emollients (Stern, 2004). Ultraviolet radiation also activates growth factor and cytokine receptors on epidermal keratinocytes and dermal cells. These receptors stimulate mitogen-activated protein kinases (MAP kinases), which, in turn, induce c-Jun

expression. This transcription factor heterodimerizes with c-Fos to form activated AP-1 complexes that induce the transcription of metalloproteinases that degrade dermal collagens and other proteins (Fisher and Voorhees, 1998).

Tretinoin is approved for the treatment of acne vulgaris and as an adjunctive agent for treating photoaging. Topical preparations contain from 0.01% to 0.1% tretinoin in cream, gel, and solution formulations. Initiation of therapy with lower-strength preparations and progression to higher strengths may be useful because individual sensitivity is unpredictable. Tretinoin formulations with a cream base are indicated for dry skin, whereas gel-based formulations are indicated for oily skin. The medication is applied once daily before bedtime to minimize photodegradation. Maximum clinical response in acne may require several months, and maintenance therapy is necessary. A formulation of tretinoin with active drug incorporated into microsponges (RETIN-A MICRO) has been developed (Gollnick and Krautheim, 2003). The microsponges not only decrease irritation by slowing the release of the medication but also may enhance efficacy by targeting delivery to the sebaceous follicle (Webster, 1998).

A 0.5% emollient cream formulation of tretinoin (RENOVA) is one formulation approved for treatment of photoaged skin. Nightly application produces maximum response within 1 year, and application one to three times weekly is said to maintain improvement (Green *et al.*, 1993). Treatment must be combined with a rigorous program of photoprotection, including sunscreens, sun avoidance, and photoprotective clothing.

Adapalene

Adapalene (DIFFERIN), a derivative of naphthoic acid, is a synthetic retinoid-like compound that is available in solution, cream, and gel formulations for topical use. In addition to displaying typical retinoid effects, it also has antiinflammatory properties. Adapalene has similar efficacy to tretinoin, but unlike tretinoin, it is stable in sunlight (Weiss and Shavin, 1998) and tends to be less irritating. The structure for adapalene is shown below.

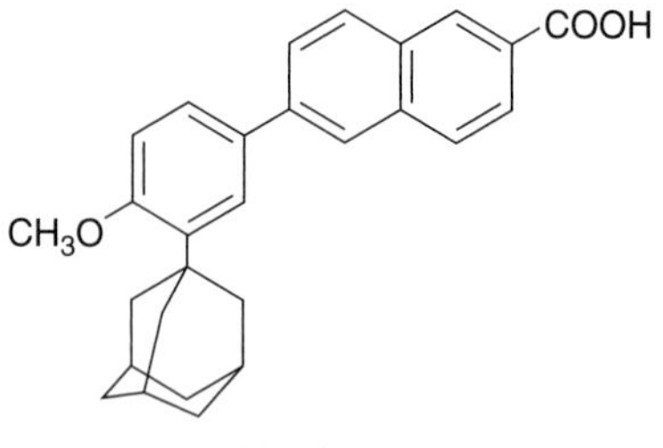

ADAPALENE

Tazarotene

Tazarotene (TAZORAC) is a third-generation retinoid approved for the treatment of psoriasis and acne vulgaris (Duvic and Marks, 1998). This retinoid binds to all three RARs. In mice, tazarotene blocks ornithine decarboxylase activity, which is associated with cell proliferation and hyperplasia. In cell culture, it suppresses markers of epidermal inflammation and inhibits cornification of the keratinocyte.

Tazarotene gel, applied once daily to dry skin, may be used as monotherapy or in combination with other medications, such as topical corticosteroids, for the treatment of localized plaque psoriasis. This is the first topical retinoid approved by the Food and Drug Administration (FDA) for the treatment of psoriasis. Side effects of burning, itching, and skin irritation are relatively common, and patients should avoid sun exposure.

Alitretinoin

Alitretinoin (PANRETIN) is a retinoid that binds all types of retinoid receptors and is approved only for treatment of the skin manifestations of Kaposi's sarcoma. Approximately 50% of patients in an open-label trial responded positively to topical application of this drug (Walmsley *et al.*, 1999).

Toxicity and Monitoring. Adverse effects of all topical retinoids include erythema, desquamation, burning, and stinging. These effects often decrease spontaneously with time and are lessened by concomitant use of emollients. Photosensitivity can occur as a result of epidermal thinning, with a resulting greater potential for phototoxic reactions such as sunburn. Although there is little systemic absorption of tretinoin and no alteration in plasma vitamin A levels with its use as a topical agent, most physicians do not prescribe tretinoin during pregnancy, and the FDA lists it as category X for pregnant women.

Isotretinoin

Oral isotretinoin (ACCUTANE) is approved for the treatment of severe nodulocystic acne vulgaris. The drug has remarkable efficacy in severe acne and may induce prolonged remissions after a single course of therapy. It normalizes keratinization in the sebaceous follicle, reduces sebocyte number with decreased sebum synthesis, and reduces *Propionibacterium acnes,* the organism that produces inflammation in acne (Layton and Cunliffe, 1992; Harper and Thiboutot, 2003).

Therapeutic Uses. Isotretinoin is administered orally. The recommended dose is 0.5 to 2 mg/kg per day for 15 to 20 weeks. Lower doses are effective but are associated with shorter remissions. The cumulative dose also is important, so smaller doses for longer periods can be used to achieve a total dose in the range of 120 mg/kg (Smith, 1999). Approximately 40% of patients will relapse, usually within 3 years of therapy, and may require retreatment (Layton *et al.*, 1993). Preteens and patients with acne conglobata or androgen excess are at increased risk of relapse. However, mild relapses may respond to conventional management with topical and systemic antiacne agents.

Isotretinoin is prescribed for severe, recalcitrant nodular acne, moderate acne unresponsive to oral antibiotics, and acne that produces scarring. It also is used commonly for other related disorders, such as gram-negative folliculitis, acne rosacea, and hidradenitis suppurativa (Leyden, 1988).

Toxicity and Monitoring. A consensus statement regarding the safe and optimal use of isotretinoin has been published (Goldsmith *et al.*, 2004). Dose-dependent adverse effects on the skin and mucous membranes are observed most commonly, including cheilitis, mucous membrane dryness, epistaxis, dry eyes, blepharoconjunctivitis, erythematous eruptions, and xerosis. Alteration of epidermal surfaces may facilitate *Staphylococcus aureus* colonization and, rarely, subsequent infection. Hair loss, exuberant granulation tissue formation, photosensitivity, and dark adaptation dysfunction are rarer occurrences.

Systemic side effects generally are less significant with short-term therapy. Transitory elevations in serum transaminases occur rarely. Hyperlipidemia is frequent, with 25% of patients developing increased triglyceride levels and, less frequently, increased cholesterol and low-density lipoproteins and decreased high-density lipoproteins (Bershad *et al.*, 1985). Myalgia and arthralgia are common complaints. Headaches occur and rarely are a symptom of pseudotumor cerebri. Use of isotretinoin concomitantly with *tetracycline* antibiotics may increase the risk of pseudotumor cerebri. Controversy exists regarding the potential linking of isotretinoin to depression, suicidal thoughts, and suicide. Epidemiological studies to date have not shown an association between isotretinoin and depression or suicide, perhaps because acne itself may be a risk factor for depression. Some physicians have proposed a causal relationship with mood changes and depression in a limited number of patients. These uncontrolled clinical observations have not been examined in a rigorous, prospective manner. In addition, there is a paucity of data on the effect of retinoids on adult brain function (Goldsmith *et al.*, 2004). Long-term therapy may produce skeletal side effects, including diffuse idiopathic skeletal hyperostoses, extraskeletal ossification (particularly at tendinous insertions), and premature epiphyseal closure in children (DiGiovanna, 2001).

Teratogenicity is a major problem; it occurs if the drug is given within the first 3 weeks of gestation and is not dose-related. Teratogenic effects include CNS, cardiac, thymus, and craniofacial abnormalities. Spontaneous abortion occurs in one-third of patients (Lammer *et al.,* 1985). *Pregnancy is an absolute contraindication to the use of isotretinoin.* Females of childbearing potential should initiate therapy at the beginning of a normal menstrual period after giving informed consent and obtaining two negative pregnancy tests. Two forms of birth control (one of which must be surgical or hormonal) must be practiced during therapy and for 1 month both before beginning therapy and after completion of therapy; pregnancy tests should be repeated monthly. Patients should not donate blood for transfusion during treatment and for 1 month after treatment.

Other laboratory evaluations should include a complete blood count, liver function tests, and fasting lipid determination before initiating therapy. Testing should be repeated after 1 month of therapy and thereafter only as abnormalities indicate.

Acitretin

Acitretin (SORIATANE) is the major metabolite of *etretinate,* an aromatic retinoid that formerly was approved for psoriasis but withdrawn from the market because of its undesirable pharmacokinetics. Acitretin has an elimination half-life of 2 to 3 days.

Acitretin is readily esterified *in vivo* to produce etretinate, especially in the presence of *ethanol* (Katz *et al.,* 1999). The optimal dosing range for acitretin in adults is 25 to 50 mg/day, providing efficacy with an acceptable level of side effects. Improvement of plaque psoriasis requires up to 3 to 6 months for optimal results. As monotherapy, acitretin has an overall rate of complete remission of less than 50% (Ling, 1999); response rates are higher when the drug is combined with other modalities (Lebwohl, 1999; Lebwohl *et al.,* 2004). At doses of 10 to 25 mg/day, both pustular and erythrodermic psoriasis usually respond more rapidly than common plaque psoriasis. Excellent control of these conditions usually can be achieved with acitretin (Goldfork and Ellis, 1998). Common side effects include dry skin and mucous membranes, xerophthalmia, and hair thinning. Less frequently, arthralgias and decreased night vision have been noted. Serious side effects (*e.g.,* hepatotoxicity or pseudotumor cerebri) are rare (Katz *et al.,* 1999). *Acitretin is a potent teratogen and should not be used by females who intend to become pregnant during therapy or at any time for at least 3 years following discontinuation of therapy.*

The same precautions regarding blood donation described earlier for isoretinoin should be followed. Laboratory monitoring should include a baseline pregnancy test in all female patients and a complete blood count, lipid profile, and hepatic profile in all patients. Serial follow-up of laboratory tests should be conducted every 1 to 2 weeks until stable and thereafter as clinically indicated.

Bexarotene

Bexarotene (TARGRETIN) is a retinoid that selectively binds RXRs. Bexarotene has been used in patients with cutaneous T-cell lymphoma with a suggested dose of 300 mg/m^2 per day. Because it is metabolized by CYP3A4, inhibitors of CYP3A4 (*e.g., imidazole antifungals* and *macrolide antibiotics*) will increase and inducers of the CYP3A4 system will decrease plasma levels of bexarotene. Side effects include lipid abnormalities, hypothyroidism secondary to a reversible RXR-mediated suppression of *TSH* gene expression (Sherman, 2003), pancreatitis, leukopenia, and gastrointestinal symptoms. Blood lipids and thyroid function should be measured before initiating therapy and periodically thereafter.

Cancer Chemoprevention with Retinoids. The association of vitamin A deficiency with squamous metaplasia, increased cell proliferation, hyperkeratosis, and carcinoma suggested that retinoids might be valuable in the treatment and prevention of cutaneous premalignant and malignant disorders. Clinical trials indicate that retinoids have significant activity in the reversal of oral, skin, and cervical premalignancies and in the prevention of head and neck, lung, and skin primary tumors. As with the treatment of other dermatological diseases, individual retinoids show selectivity in tumor prevention and treatment.

Systemic and topical retinoids have been used successfully to treat premalignant skin conditions and may have a role in chemoprevention of skin malignancies. High-dose isotretinoin (2 mg/kg per day) has suppressed skin cancers in patients with increased risk of skin malignancy from congenital disorders such as xeroderma pigmentosa and nevoid basal cell carcinoma syndrome. To achieve an anticancer effect, toxic doses of retinoids generally are required. Acitretin at a dose of 25 mg/day or more appears to reduce the risk of skin cancer by about 25% among patients with psoriasis who are at high risk for squamous cell carcinoma because of prior use of 8-methoxypsoralen and ultraviolet radiation or other carcinogenic modalities for psoriasis (Nijsten and Stern, 2003). Tretinoin cream applied once or twice daily decreased the size and number of actinic keratoses by 50% in one multicenter study.

High doses of isotretinoin produce partial regression of multiple basal cell carcinomas (Peck *et al.*, 1988) but are more effective in suppressing the formation of new tumors, as demonstrated in patients with xeroderma pigmentosum (Kraemer *et al.*, 1988). Isotretinoin also prevents second primary tumors in patients who have had a previous squamous cell carcinoma of the head and neck (Hong *et al.*, 1990). Isotretinoin also is effective for oral leukoplakia (Hong *et al.*, 1986). Topical tazarotene has shown efficacy in some basal cell carcinomas (Peris *et al.*, 1999). Cutaneous T-cell lymphoma has been shown to respond to several types of topical and systemic retinoids, including bexarotene (Zhang and Duvic, 2003). The benefits of long-term retinoid use in malignant lymphomas such as cutaneous T-cell lymphoma must be balanced by appreciation of retinoid toxicity and the chronicity of the disease.

β-Carotene. *β-Carotene* (SOLATENE, others) is a precursor of vitamin A that is present in green and yellow vegetables. The drug is used in dermatology to reduce skin photosensitivity in patients with erythropoietic protoporphyria. The mechanism of action is controversial but may involve an antioxidant effect that decreases the production of free radicals or singlet oxygen (Harber and Bickers, 1989). While this concept has led to the use of β-carotene as a chemopreventative agent, current evidence indicates that this compound has no discernible cancer chemoprevention effects in human skin cancer (Darlington *et al.*, 2003).

PHOTOCHEMOTHERAPY

Electromagnetic radiation is defined by its wavelength and frequency; for convenience, it can be classified into different regions based on its photon energy. For therapeutic purposes, dermatologists are most concerned with the ultraviolet (UV) B (290 to 320 nm), A-I (320 to 340 nm), and A-II (340 to 400 nm) and visible (400 to 800 nm) portions of the solar spectrum. UVC (100 to 290 nm) is absorbed by stratospheric ozone, does not reach earth's surface, and is no longer used therapeutically. UVB is the most erythrogenic and melanogenic type of radiation. It is the major action spectrum for sunburn, tanning, skin cancer, and photoaging. The longer wavelengths of UVA are a thousand times less erythrogenic than UVB; however, they penetrate more deeply into the skin and contribute substantially to photoaging and photosensitivity diseases. They also enhance UVB-induced erythema and increase the risk of skin carcinogenesis. Visible radiation may augment the severity of some photosensitive eruptions. Electromagnetic radiation has proven to be highly efficacious in the treatment of numerous dermatologic diseases (Scheinfeld and Deleo, 2003; Lebwohl *et al.*, 2004). Phototherapy and photochemotherapy are treatment methods in which ultraviolet or visible radiation is used to induce a therapeutic response either alone or in the presence of a photosensitizing drug. Phototherapy using broad-band (290 to 320 nm) or narrow-band (311 to 313 nm) UVB or high-dose UVA-I is efficacious in selected dermatological diseases. To be effective, the incident radiation must be absorbed by a target or chromophore in the skin—which in phototherapy is endogenous and in photochemotherapy must be admin-

istered exogenously. Patients treated with these modalities should be monitored for concomitant use of other potential photosensitizing medications before initiation of therapy. Such drugs include *phenothiazines, thiazides, sulfonamides, nonsteroidal antiinflammatory agents, sulfonylureas,* tetracyclines, and *benzodiazepines.*

PUVA: Psoralens and UVA

Photochemotherapy with *psoralen*-containing plant extracts was employed for the treatment of vitiligo in Egypt and India as early as 1500 B.C. Orally administered *8-methoxypsoralen* followed by UVA (PUVA) is FDA approved for the treatment of vitiligo, psoriasis, and cutaneous T-cell lymphoma.

Chemistry. Psoralens belong to the furocoumarin class of compounds, which are derived from the fusion of a furan with a coumarin. They occur naturally in many plants, including limes, lemons, figs, and parsnips. Two psoralens, 8-methoxypsoralen (*methoxsalen*) and 4, 5, 8-trimethylpsoralen (*trioxsalen*, TRISORALEN) are available in the United States. Methoxsalen is used primarily because of its superior gastrointestinal absorption. Structures of the two psoralens are:

METHOXSALEN   TRIOXSALEN

Pharmacokinetics. The psoralens are absorbed rapidly after oral administration. Photosensitivity typically is maximal 1 to 2 hours after ingestion of methoxsalen. There is significant but saturable first-pass elimination in the liver, which may account for variations in plasma levels among individuals after a standard dose. Methoxsalen has a serum half-life of approximately 1 hour, but the skin remains sensitive to light for 8 to 12 hours. Despite widespread drug distribution throughout the body, it is photoactivated only in the skin where the UVA penetrates.

Mechanism of Action. The mechanism by which PUVA induces photosensitivity is not known. The action spectrum for oral PUVA is between 320 and 400 nm. Two distinct photoreactions take place. Type I reactions involve the oxygen-independent formation of mono- and bifunctional adducts in DNA. Type II reactions are oxygen-dependent and involve sensitized transfer of energy to molecular oxygen. The therapeutic effects of PUVA in psoriasis may result from a decrease in DNA-dependent proliferation after adduct formation. Perhaps more important, PUVA can alter cytokine profiles and cause immunocyte apoptosis, thereby interrupting immunopathologic processes (Godar, 1999).

PUVA promotes melanogenesis in normal skin. Increased pigmentation results from augmented transfer of melanosomes from melanocytes to keratinocytes; however, there is no change in the size of melanosomes or in their distribution pattern.

Therapeutic Uses. Methoxsalen is supplied in soft gelatin capsules (OXSORALEN-ULTRA) and hard gelatin capsules (8-MOP). The dose is 0.4 mg/kg for the soft capsule and 0.6 mg/kg for the hard capsule taken 1.5 to 2 hours before UVA exposure. A lotion containing 1% methoxsalen (OXSORALEN) also is available for topical application. It can be diluted for use in bath water to minimize systemic absorption. The risk of phototoxicity is increased with topical PUVA therapy. In U.S. and European multicenter cooperative studies of PUVA for the treatment of psoriasis, initial clearance rates approaching 90% were achieved (Melski *et al.*, 1977; Henseler *et al.*, 1981). Relapse occurs within 6 months of cessation of treatment in many patients, which has prompted efforts to design maintenance protocols.

PUVA also is used to repigment the leukoderma of vitiligo. Success rates are highest in young individuals with recent onset of disease involving nonacral areas. Localized vitiligo can be treated with topical PUVA and more extensive disease with systemic administration. PUVA also is employed in the treatment of cutaneous T-cell lymphoma, atopic dermatitis, alopecia areata, lichen planus, urticaria pigmentosa, and as a preventive modality in some forms of photosensitivity.

Toxicity and Monitoring. The major acute side effects of PUVA include nausea, blistering, and painful erythema. PUVA-induced redness and blistering generally peak within 48 to 72 hours.

Chronic PUVA therapy accelerates photoaging and the development of actinic keratoses, nonmelanoma skin cancer, and melanoma. Squamous cell carcinomas occur at 10 times the expected frequency. In patients receiving 250 or more treatments, there is an increased risk of melanoma. Careful monitoring of patients for cutaneous carcinoma therefore is essential.

Photopheresis. Extracorporeal photopheresis (ECP) is a form of pheresis therapy that has proven effective in the treatment of cutaneous T-cell lymphoma (Edelson *et al.*, 1987). After oral administration of methoxsalen, leukocytes are separated from whole blood using an extracorporeal pheresis device and then exposed to UVA radiation. The irradiated cells then are returned to the patient. Multiple mechanisms probably contribute to the effectiveness of this procedure. ECP simultaneously and efficiently induces apoptosis of disease-causing T cells and con-

version of monocytes to functional dendritic cells. By processing and presenting the unique antigenic determinants of pathogenic T-cell clones, the dendritic cells can either initiate a clinically relevant anti–cutaneous T-cell lymphoma cytotoxic response or suppress the activity of autoreactive T-cell clones (Bisaccia *et al.*, 2000; Knobler and Girardi, 2001).

Initially, patients receive therapy monthly on two consecutive days. Treatment intervals are increased as the patient improves. Patients with Sézary syndrome or those with the plaque stage of cutaneous T-cell lymphoma who have atypical peripheral blood cells are most responsive to the therapy. For patients with disease parameters suggesting a low probability of response to photopheresis alone, adjuvant therapy with interferon-α or superficial electron-beam irradiation is employed. Prolonged clinical remissions can occur in patients with Sézary syndrome. Favorable results also have been obtained in pemphigus vulgaris, scleroderma (Sapadin and Fleischmajer, 2002), and graft-versus-host disease (Coyle *et al.*, 2004). Clinical trials are being conducted in patients undergoing allogeneic organ transplantation.

Photodynamic Therapy (PDT). This modality combines the use of photosensitizing drugs and visible light for the treatment of various dermatological disorders, particularly nonmelanoma skin cancer and precancerous actinic keratoses (Kalka *et al.*, 2000; Lopez *et al.*, 2004; Taub 2004). The concept is predicated on the insight that tumor tissue selectively absorbs greater amounts of porphyrins than surrounding nontumor tissue. The agents most widely employed in PDT are *porphyrins,* their precursors, or derivatives thereof. The photosensitized chemical reaction is oxygen-dependent. Light delivered to the skin is absorbed by porphyrin molecules. These molecules transfer their energy to oxygen, forming reactive oxygen species that result in injury or destruction of lipid-rich membranes and subsequent tissue damage.

Early studies with PDT employed complex mixtures of poorly defined porphyrins known as *hematoporphyrin derivative* (PHOTO-FRIN I) or a partially purified mixture known as *porfimer sodium* (PHOTOFRIN II) that was administered parenterally with subsequent irradiation using polychromatic light sources. The major problem with this approach was the prolonged period (4 to 6 weeks) of photosensitivity caused by skin retention of the porphyrin formulations. This led to a search for compounds that could be administered topically and that were eliminated more readily from the skin. The porphyrin precursor δ-aminolevulinic acid (ALA) is converted to various porphyrins, particularly *protoporphyrin* (PROTO), in tissues including the skin (*see* below). Protoporphyrin subsequently is eliminated rapidly from the body, thereby minimizing the period of skin photosensitivity to a few hours. Topically applied ALA HCl (20% w/v) and, more recently, the methyl ester of ALA have been used successfully for the PDT of various types of nonmelanoma skin cancers and premalignant lesions (Lopez *et al.*, 2004; Taub, 2004).

8 × ALA ⟶ Protoporphyrin IX

Incoherent (nonlaser) and laser light sources have been used for PDT. The wavelengths chosen must include those within the action spectrum of protoporphyrin and ideally those that permit maximum skin penetration. Light sources in use emit energy predominantly in the blue portion (maximum porphyrin absorption) or the red portion (better tissue penetration) of the visible spectrum. Nonhypertrophic actinic keratoses (Piacquadio *et al.*, 2004) and superficial basal cell carcinomas and Bowen's disease seem to respond best to PDT. Topical ALA products for PDT approved by the FDA include LEVULAN KERASTICK, BLU-U blue light, and METVIX.

ANTIHISTAMINES

Histamine is a potent vasodilator, bronchial smooth muscle constrictor, and stimulant of nociceptive itch nerves (Repka-Ramirez and Baraniuk, 2002). In addition to histamine, multiple chemical itch mediators can act as pruritogens on C-fibers, including *neuropeptides, prostaglandins, serotonin, acetylcholine,* and *bradykinin* (Stander *et al.*, 2003). Furthermore, new receptor systems such as vanilloid, opioid, and cannabinoid receptors on cutaneous sensory nerve fibers that may modulate itch offer novel targets for antipruritic therapy.

Histamine is in mast cells, basophils, and platelets. Human skin mast cells express H_1, H_2, and H_4 receptors but not H_3 receptors (Lippert *et al.*, 2004). H_1 and H_2 receptors are involved in wheal formation and erythema, whereas only H_1 receptor agonists cause pruritus. Complete blockade of H_1 receptors does not totally relieve itching, and combinations of H_1 and H_2 blockers may be superior to H_1 blockers alone.

Oral *antihistamines,* particularly H_1-receptor antagonists, have some anticholinergic activity and are sedating (*see* Chapter 24), making them useful for the control of pruritus. First-generation sedating H_1-receptor antagonists include *hydroxyzine hydrochloride* (ATARAX), which is given in a dose of 0.5 mg/kg every 6 hours; *diphenhydra-*

mine (BENADRYL; others); *promethazine* (PHENERGAN); and *cyproheptadine* (PERIACTIN). *Doxepin* (ADAPIN, SINEQUAN)*,* which has tricyclic antidepressant and sedative antihistamine effects (*see* Chapter 17), is a good alternative for severe pruritus. A topical formulation of doxepin also is available as a 5% cream (ZONALON), which can be used in conjunction with low- to moderate-potency topical glucocorticoids. The systemic effect from topical doxepin is comparable with that of low-dose oral therapy.

Second-generation H_1-receptor antagonists lack anticholinergic side effects and are described as nonsedating largely because they do not cross the blood–brain barrier. They include *cetirizine* (ZYRTEC), *loratadine* (CLARITIN), *desloratidine* (CLARINEX), and *fexofenadine hydrochloride* (ALLEGRA). While second-generation nonsedating H_1-receptor blockers are as effective as the first-generation H_1 blockers (Monroe, 1993), they are metabolized by CYP3A4 and, to a lesser extent, by CYP2D6 and should not be coadministered with medications that inhibit these enzymes (*e.g.,* imidazole antifungals and macrolide antibiotics).

H_2-receptor blockers include *cimetidine* (TAGAMET), *ranitidine* (ZANTAC)*, famotidine (*PEPCID), and *nizatidine* (AXID). Besides their use in combination with H_1-receptor blockers for pruritus, the H_2-receptor blockers have immunomodulating effects, and this property has been exploited in children to treat warts (Orlow and Paller, 1993).

ANTIMICROBIAL AGENTS

Antibiotics

These drugs are used commonly to treat superficial cutaneous infections (pyoderma) and noninfectious diseases. Topical agents are very effective for the treatment of superficial bacterial infections and acne vulgaris. Systemic antibiotics also are prescribed commonly for acne and for deeper bacterial infections. The pharmacology of individual antibacterial agents is discussed in Section VIII, Chemotherapy of Microbial Diseases. Only the topical and systemic antibacterial agents principally used in dermatology are discussed here.

Acne vulgaris is the most common dermatologic disorder treated with either topical or systemic antibiotics. The anaerobe *Propionibacterium acnes* is a component of normal skin flora that proliferates in the obstructed, lipid-rich lumen of the pilosebaceous unit, where O_2 tension is low. *P. acnes* generates free fatty acids that are irritants and may lead to microcomedo formation and result in the inflammatory lesions of acne. Suppression of cutaneous

P. acnes with antibiotic therapy is correlated with clinical improvement (Tan, 2003).

Resistant strains of *P. acnes* are emerging that may respond to judicious use of retinoids in combination with antibiotics (Leyden, 2001). Commonly used topical antimicrobials in acne include *erythromycin, clindamycin* (CLEOCIN-T), and *benzoyl peroxide* and antibiotic–benzoyl peroxide combinations (BENZAMYCIN, BENZACLIN, others). Other antimicrobials used in treating acne include *sulfacetamide* (KLARON), *sulfacetamide/sulfur combinations* (SULFACET-R), *metronidazole* (METROCREAM, METROGEL, NORITATE), and *azelaic acid* (AZELEX). *Systemic therapy* is prescribed for patients with more extensive disease and acne that is resistant to topical therapy. Effective agents include tetracycline (SUMYCIN, others), *minocycline* (MINOCIN, others), erythromycin (ERYC, others), clindamycin (CLEOCIN), and *trimethoprim–sulfamethoxazole* (BACTRIM, others). Antibiotics usually are administered twice daily, and doses are tapered after control is achieved. Tetracycline is the most commonly employed antibiotic because it is inexpensive, safe, and effective. The initial daily dose is usually 1 g in divided doses. Although tetracycline is an antimicrobial agent, its efficacy in acne may be more dependent on its antiinflammatory activity.

Minocycline has better gastrointestinal absorption than tetracycline and may be less photosensitizing than either tetracycline or doxycycline. Side effects of minocycline include dizziness and hyperpigmentation of the skin and mucosa, serum-sickness-like reactions, and drug-induced lupus erythematosus. With all the tetracyclines, vaginal candidiasis is a common complication that is readily treated with local administration of antifungal drugs.

In healthy individuals taking oral antibiotics for acne, laboratory monitoring is not necessary. Orally administered antibiotics also may be indicated in other noninfectious conditions, including acne rosacea, perioral dermatitis, hidradenitis suppurativa, autoimmune blistering diseases, sarcoidosis, and pyoderma gangrenosum (Carter, 2003).

Cutaneous Infections. Gram-positive organisms, including *Staphylococcus aureus* and *Streptococcus pyogenes*, are the most common cause of pyoderma. Skin infections with gram-negative bacilli are rare, although they can occur in diabetics and patients who are immunosuppressed; appropriate parenteral antibiotic therapy is required for their treatment.

Topical therapy frequently is adequate for impetigo, the most superficial bacterial infection of the skin caused by *S. aureus* and *S. pyogenes*. *Pseudomonic acid* (MUPIROCIN, BACTROBAN*),* produced by *Pseudomonas fluorescens,* is effective for such localized infections. It inhibits protein synthesis by binding to bacterial isoleucyl-tRNA synthetase. Mupirocin is highly active against staphylococci and all streptococci except those of group D. It is less active against

gram-negative organisms, but it has *in vitro* activity against *Haemophilus influenzae, Neisseria gonorrhoeae, Pasteurella multocida, Moraxella catarrhalis,* and *Bordetella pertussis.* Mupirocin is inactive against normal skin flora (Leyden, 1992). Its antibacterial activity is enhanced by the acid pH of the skin surface. Mupirocin is available as a 2% ointment or cream (BACTODERM, BACTROBAN, BACTROBAN NASAL, EISMYCIN) and is applied three times daily.

Topical therapy often is employed for prophylaxis of superficial infections caused by wounds and injuries. *Neomycin* is active against staphylococci and most gram-negative bacilli. It may cause allergic contact dermatitis, especially on disrupted skin. *Bacitracin* inhibits staphylococci, streptococci, and gram-positive bacilli. *Polymyxin B* is active against aerobic gram-negative bacilli. Bacitracin and polymyxin B are combined in a number of over-the-counter preparations.

Deeper bacterial infections of the skin include folliculitis, erysipelas, cellulitis, and necrotizing fasciitis. Since streptococcal and staphylococcal species also are the most common causes of deep cutaneous infections, *penicillins* (especially β-lactamase-resistant β-lactams) and *cephalosporins* are the systemic antibiotics used most frequently in their treatment (Carter, 2003) (*see* Chapter 44). A growing concern is the increased incidence of skin and soft tissue infections with hospital- and community-acquired methicillin-resistant *S. aureus* (MRSA) and drug-resistant pneumococci. Infection with community-acquired MRSA often is susceptible to trimethoprim–sulfamethoxazole (Cohen and Grossman, 2004).

Novel antibacterial agents such as *linezolid, quinupristin–dalfopristin,* and *daptomycin* (*see* Chapter 46) have been approved for the treatment of complicated skin and skin-structure infections (Schweiger and Weinberg, 2004).

Antifungal Agents

Fungal infections are among the most common causes of skin disease in the United States, and numerous effective topical and oral antifungal agents have been developed. *Griseofulvin,* topical and oral *imidazoles, triazoles,* and *allylamines* are the most effective agents available. The pharmacology, uses, and toxicities of antifungal drugs are discussed in Chapter 48. This section will address the management of common cutaneous fungal diseases. Recommendations for cutaneous antifungal therapy are summarized in Table 62–2.

The azoles *miconazole* (MICATIN, others) and *econazole* (SPECTRAZOLE, others) and the allylamines *naftifine* (NAFTIN) and *terbinafine* (LAMISIL, others) are effective topical agents for the treatment of localized tinea corporis and uncomplicated tinea pedis. Topical therapy with the azoles is preferred for localized cutaneous candidiasis and tinea versicolor.

Systemic therapy is necessary for the treatment of tinea capitis. Oral griseofulvin (FULVICIN V/F, P/G, others) has been the traditional medication for treatment of tinea capitis. Oral terbinafine is a safe and effective alternative to griseofulvin in treating tinea capitis in children (Moosavi *et al.,* 2001).

Table 62–2
Recommended Cutaneous Antifungal Therapy

CONDITION	TOPICAL THERAPY	ORAL THERAPY
Tinea corporis, localized	Azoles, allylamines	—
Tinea corporis, widespread	—	Griseofulvin, terbinafine, itraconazole, fluconazole
Tinea pedis	Azoles, allylamines	Griseofulvin, terbinafine, itraconazole, fluconazole
Onychomycosis	—	Griseofulvin, terbinafine, itraconazole, fluconazole
Candidiasis, localized	Azoles	—
Candidiasis, widespread and mucocutaneous	—	Ketaconazole, itraconazole, fluconazole
Tinea versicolor, localized	Azoles, allylamines	
Tinea versicolor, widespread	—	Ketaconazole, itraconazole, fluconazole

Tinea Pedis. Topical therapy with the azoles and allylamines is effective for tinea pedis. Macerated toe web disease may require the addition of antibacterial therapy. *Econazole nitrate*, which has a limited antibacterial spectrum, can be useful in this situation. Systemic therapy with griseofulvin, terbinafine, or *itraconazole* (SPORANOX, others) is used for more extensive tinea pedis. It should be recognized that long-term topical therapy may be necessary in some patients after courses of systemic antifungal therapy.

Onychomycosis. Fungal infection of the nails is caused most frequently by dermatophytes and *Candida*. Mixed infections are common. The nail must be cultured or clipped for histological examination before initiating therapy because up to a third of dystrophic nails that appear clinically to be onychomycosis are actually due to psoriasis or other conditions.

Systemic therapy is necessary for effective management of onychomycosis. Treatment of onychomycosis of toenails with griseofulvin for 12 to 18 months produces a cure rate of 50% and a relapse rate of 50% after 1 year. Terbinafine and itraconazole offer significant potential advantages. They quickly produce high drug levels in the nail, which persist after therapy is discontinued. Additional advantages include a broader spectrum of coverage with itraconazole and few drug interactions with terbinafine. Treatment of toenail onychomycosis requires 3 months with terbinafine (250 mg/day) or itraconazole (pulsed dosing 1 week per month for 3 months). Cure rates of 75% or greater have been achieved with both drugs (Gupta *et al.*, 1994a, 1994b; Darkes *et al.*, 2003).

Ciclopirox topical (PENLAC) solution is a nail lacquer that is FDA approved for the treatment of onychomycosis but demonstrates low complete cure rates (5.5% to 8.5%).

Antiviral Agents

Viral infections of the skin are very common and include verrucae [human papillomavirus (HPV)], herpes simplex (HSV), condyloma acuminatum (HPV), molluscum contagiosum (poxvirus), and chicken pox [varicella-zoster virus (VZV)]. *Acyclovir* (ZOVIRAX), *famciclovir* (FAMVIR), and *valacyclovir* (VALTREX) frequently are used systemically to treat herpes simplex and varicella infections (*see* Chapter 49). *Cidofovir* (VISTIDE) may be useful in treating acyclovir-resistant HSV or VZV and other cutaneous viral infections (Anonymous, 2002a). Topically, acyclovir, *docosanol* (ABREVA), and *penciclovir* (DENAVIR) are available for treating mucocutaneous HSV. *Podophyllin* (25% solution) and *podofilox* (CONDYLOX; 0.5% solution) are used to treat condylomata. The immune response modifier *imiquimod* (ALDARA) is discussed below. Interferons α-2b (INTRON-A), α-n1 (not commercially available in the United States), and α-n3 (ALFERON N) may be useful for treating refractory or recurrent warts (Carter *et al.*, 2004).

Agents Used to Treat Infestations

Infestations with ectoparasites such as body lice and scabies are common throughout the world. These conditions have a significant impact on public health in the form of disabling pruritus, secondary infection, and in the case of the body louse, transmission of life-threatening illnesses such as typhus. Topical and oral medications are available to treat these infestations.

Perhaps the best known anti-ectoparasitic medication is 1% *γ-benzene hexachloride* lotion, also known as *lindane*. Its chemical structure is:

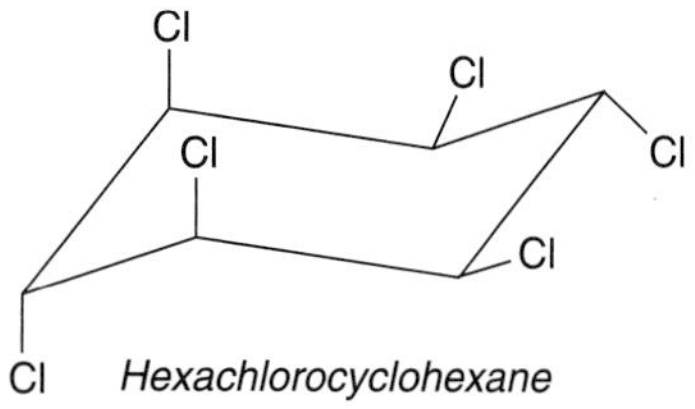

Hexachlorocyclohexane

Lindane has been used as a commercial insecticide as well as a topical medication. It is highly effective in the treatment of ectoparasites. Neurotoxicity, although a concern with the use of lindane, is a rare side effect when the medication is used correctly. However, the FDA has defined lindane as a second-line drug in treating pediculosis and scabies and has highlighted the potential for neurotoxicity in children and adults weighing less than 110 pounds (FDA, 2003). The lotion is applied in a thin layer from the neck down, left in place for 8 to 12 hours or overnight, and removed by thorough washing at the end of the 8- to 12-hour period. The treatment may be repeated in 1 week. To avoid problems with neurotoxicity, the lotion should be applied only in a thin coat to dry skin, should not be applied immediately after bathing, and should be kept away from the eyes, mouth, and open cuts or sores. A 1% lindane shampoo also is available for head and body lice.

A second topical agent that is very useful in the treatment of ectoparasites is *permethrin*. Its structure is:

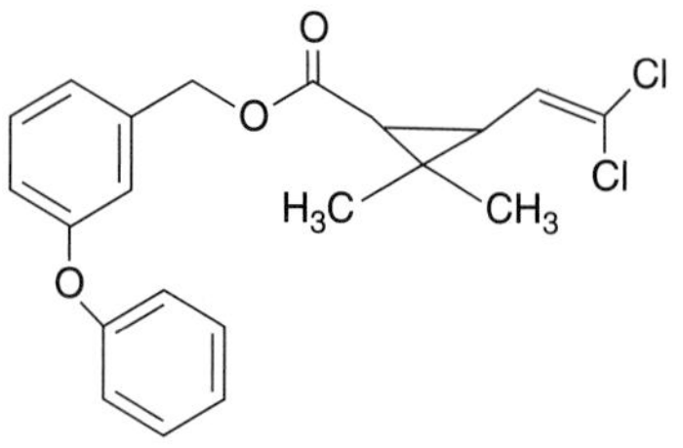

PERMETHRIN

Permethrin is a synthetic derivative of the insecticide pyrethrum, which was obtained originally from *Chrysanthemum cinerariaefolium*. Neurotoxicity associated with this compound is extremely rare. A 5% cream (ACTICIN, ELIMITE, others) is available for the treatment of scabies. This is used as an 8- to 12-hour or overnight application. A 1% permethrin cream rinse (NIX) also is available for the treatment of lice.

Ivermectin (STROMECTOL), an anthelmintic drug (*see* Chapter 41) used traditionally to treat onchocerciasis, also is effective in the off-label treatment of scabies. Its structure is:

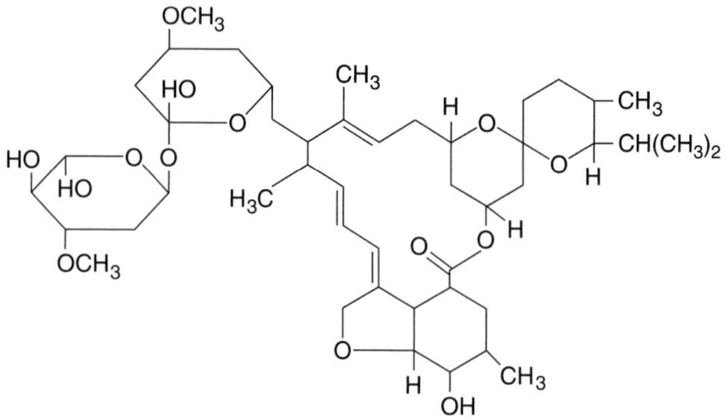

IVERMECTIN

Because ivermectin does not cross the blood–brain barrier, there is no major CNS toxicity. Ivermectin, available as a 6-mg tablet, is given at a dose of 250 to 400 μg/kg, which is repeated in a week. Cure rates of 70% after one dose and 95% after two doses given 2 weeks apart have been achieved (Usha *et al.*, 2000). For treatment of scabies outbreaks in large groups, this drug has obvious advantages as compared with topical therapy.

Other, less effective topical treatments for scabies include 10% *crotamiton* cream and lotion (EURAX) and 5% precipitated *sulfur* in petrolatum. Crotamiton and sulfur typically are considered for use in patients in whom lindane or permethrin may be contraindicated.

ANTIMALARIAL AGENTS

The major antimalarials used commonly in dermatology include *chloroquine* (ARALEN), *hydroxychloroquine* (PLAQUENIL), and to a lesser extent, *quinacrine* (no longer available in the United States); all three drugs are useful because of their antiinflammatory effects, especially in connective tissue disorders and photosensitivity diseases (*see* Chapter 39).

The mechanism of action of antimalarials is controversial, but there are immunological and antiinflammatory effects. Likely mechanisms of action include inhibition of phospholipase A_2, inhibition of platelet aggregation, a range of lysosomal effects (*e.g.*, an increase in pH, membrane stabilization, and inhibition of release and activity of lysosomal enzymes), inhibition of phagocytosis, an increase in intracellular pH in cytoplasmic vacuoles leading to decreased stimulation of autoimmune CD4+ T cells, decreased cytokine release from lymphocytes and stimulated monocytes, inhibition of immune complex formation, and antioxidant activity (Van Beek and Piette, 2001; Callen and Camisa, 2001). In patients with porphyria cutanea tarda, chloroquine and hydroxychloroquine bind to porphyrins and/or iron to facilitate their hepatic clearance. The ability to bind to melanin and other pigments may contribute to the retinal toxicity seen occasionally when antimalarial agents are used.

Therapeutic Uses. FDA-approved dermatological uses of hydroxychloroquine include treatment of discoid and systemic lupus erythematosus. Unapproved but first-line uses include treatment of dermatomyositis, porphyria cutanea tarda, polymorphous light eruption, sarcoidosis, eosinophilic fasciitis, lymphocytic infiltrate of Jessner, lymphocytoma cutis, solar urticaria, granuloma annulare, and some forms of panniculitis.

The usual doses of antimalarials are hydroxychloroquine, 200 mg twice a day; chloroquine, 250 to 500 mg/day; and quinacrine, 100 to 200 mg/day. Usually, hydroxychloroquine is started first, and if no improvement is noted in 3 months, quinacrine is added. Alternatively, chloroquine is used as a single agent. Dosing should be adjusted for low-weight individuals so that chloroquine dosing is 2.5 mg/kg per day and hydroxychloroquine is 6.5 mg/kg per day. Antimalarial agents are the treatment of choice for widespread forms of cutaneous lupus that do not respond to topical glucocorticoids and sunscreens. Clinical improvement may be delayed for several months.

Porphyria cutanea tarda, characterized by fluid-filled vesicles and bullae on sun-exposed areas, can be either genetic or associated with alcohol abuse or hepatitis C. Although the associated iron overload is treated with phlebotomy, the dermatologic manifestations sometimes are treated with antimalarial agents. These patients require reduced doses because of the potential for hepatotoxicity, as manifested by elevated transaminase levels, and the rapid excretion of large amounts of uroporphyrins in the urine that can occur with usual doses. Low-dose twice-weekly administration is effective and avoids these side effects.

Toxicity and Monitoring. The toxic effects of antimalarial agents are described in Chapter 39. The incidence of retinopathy from chloroquine and hydroxychloroquine is low, as long as the doses are within the above-mentioned guidelines and the medication is used for less than 10 years in patients with normal renal function (Callen and Camisa, 2001).

Quinacrine does not cause retinopathy. Current recommendations for ophthalmological supervision may be overly cautious, and eye examinations every 6 months or even yearly after a baseline examination probably are sufficient, provided dosing guidelines are followed. Although caution is required, there is evidence that antimalarial agents probably are safe in pregnancy and in children (Parke, 1993; Callen and Camisa, 2001).

Rare hematological side effects include agranulocytosis, aplastic anemia, and hemolysis in patients with glucose-6-phosphatase deficiency. Liver function tests and complete blood counts should be performed monthly at the start of therapy and at least every 4 to 6 months throughout treatment.

CYTOTOXIC AND IMMUNOSUPPRESSANT DRUGS

Cytotoxic and immunosuppressive drugs are used in dermatology for immunologically mediated diseases such as psoriasis, the autoimmune blistering diseases, and leukocytoclastic vasculitis. These agents are discussed in detail in Chapters 51 and 52.

Antimetabolites

Methotrexate. The antimetabolite methotrexate is a folic acid analog that competitively inhibits dihydrofolate reductase. Methotrexate has been used for moderate-to-severe psoriasis since 1951. It suppresses immunocompetent cells in the skin, and it also decreases the expression of cutaneous lymphocyte-associated antigen (CLA)–positive T cells and endothelial cell E-selectin, which may account for its efficacy in psoriasis (Sigmundsdottir *et al.*, 2004). It is useful in treating a number of other dermatological conditions, including pityriasis lichenoides et varioliformis, lymphomatoid papulosis, sarcoidosis, pemphigus vulgaris, pityriasis rubra pilaris, lupus erythematosus, dermatomyositis, and cutaneous T-cell lymphoma.

Despite its widespread acceptance for decades as a first-line systemic monotherapy for the treatment of psoriasis, methotrexate (RHEUMATREX, others) was subjected only recently to a randomized, controlled clinical trial comparing its efficacy with that of orally administered *cyclosporine* for the treatment of moderate to severe chronic plaque psoriasis (Heydendael *et al.*, 2003). Both medications were equally effective in achieving partial or complete clearing of psoriasis. Methotrexate is used often in combination with phototherapy and photochemotherapy or other systemic agents, and it also may be useful in combination with the biologics (Saporito and Menter, 2004) (*see* Biological Agents, below).

A usual starting dose for methotrexate therapy is 5 to 7.5 mg/week (maximum of 15 mg/week). This dose may be increased gradually to 20 to 30 mg/week if needed. Widely used regimens include three oral doses given at 12-hour intervals once weekly or weekly intramuscular injections. Doses must be decreased for patients with impaired renal clearance. *Methotrexate should never be coadministered with trimethoprim–sulfamethoxazole, probenecid, salicylates, or other drugs that can compete with it for protein binding and thereby raise plasma concentrations to levels that may result in bone marrow suppression.* Fatalities have occurred because of concurrent treatment with methotrexate and nonsteroidal antiinflammatory agents. Methotrexate exerts significant antiproliferative effects on the bone marrow; therefore, complete blood counts should be monitored serially. Physicians administering methotrexate should be familiar with the use of *folinic acid (leucovorin)* to rescue patients with hematologic crises caused by methotrexate-induced bone marrow suppression. Careful monitoring of liver function tests is necessary but may not be adequate to identify early hepatic fibrosis in patients receiving chronic methotrexate therapy. Some believe that methotrexate-induced hepatic fibrosis occurs more commonly in patients with psoriasis than in those with rheumatoid arthritis. Consequently, liver biopsy is recommended when the cumulative dose reaches 1 to 1.5 g. A baseline liver biopsy also is recommended for patients with increased potential risk for hepatic fibrosis, such as a history of alcohol abuse or infection with hepatitis B or C. Patients with significantly abnormal liver function tests, symptomatic liver disease, or evidence of hepatic fibrosis should not use this drug. Pregnancy and lactation are absolute contraindications to methotrexate use (Roenigk *et al.*, 1998).

Azathioprine (IMURAN) is discussed in detail in Chapters 38 and 52. In dermatologic practice, the drug is used as a steroid-sparing agent for autoimmune and inflammatory dermatoses, including pemphigus vulgaris, bullous pemphigoid, dermatomyositis, atopic dermatitis, chronic actinic dermatitis, lupus erythematosus, psoriasis, pyoderma gangrenosum, and Behçet's disease (Silvis, 2001). The usual starting dose is 1 to 2 mg/kg per day. Since it often takes 6 to 8 weeks to achieve therapeutic effect, azathioprine often is started early in the course of disease management. Careful laboratory monitoring is important (Silvis, 2001). The enzyme thiopurine *S*-methyltransferase is critical for the metabolism of azathioprine to nontoxic metabolites. Homozygous deficiency of this enzyme may raise plasma levels of the drug and cause myelosuppression, and some experts advocate measuring this enzyme before initiating azathioprine therapy (*see* Chapter 38).

Fluorouracil (5-FU) interferes with DNA synthesis by blocking the methylation of deoxyuridylic acid to thymidylic acid (Dinehart, 2000). Topical formulations (CARAC, EFUDEX, FLUOROPLEX) are used in multiple actinic keratoses, actinic cheilitis, Bowen's disease, and superficial basal cell carcinomas not amenable to other treatments.

Fluorouracil is applied twice daily for 2 to 4 weeks. The treated areas may become severely inflamed during treatment, but the inflammation subsides after the drug is stopped. Intralesional injection of 5-FU has been used for keratoacanthomas, warts, and porokeratoses.

Alkylating Agents. *Cyclophosphamide* (CYTOXAN, NEOSAR) is an effective cytotoxic and immunosuppressive agent.

Both oral and intravenous preparations of cyclophosphamide are used in dermatology (Fox and Pandya, 2000). Cyclophosphamide is FDA approved for treatment of advanced cutaneous T-cell lymphoma. Other uses include treatment of pemphigus vulgaris, bullous pemphigoid, cicatricial pemphigoid, paraneoplastic pemphigus, pyoderma gangrenosum, toxic epidermal necrolysis, Wegener's granulomatosis, polyarteritis nodosa, Churg-Strauss angiitis, Behçet's disease, scleromyxedema, and cytophagic histiocytic panniculitis (Ho and Zloty, 1993; Silvis, 2001). The usual oral dose is 2 to 3 mg/kg per day in divided doses, and there is often a 4- to 6-week delay in onset of action. Alternatively, intravenous pulse administration of cyclophosphamide may offer advantages, including lower cumulative dose and a decreased risk of bladder cancer (Fox and Pandya, 2000; Silvis, 2001).

Cyclophosphamide has many adverse effects, including the risk of secondary malignancy and myelosuppression, and thus is used only in the most severe, recalcitrant dermatological diseases. The secondary malignancies have included bladder, myeloproliferative, and lymphoproliferative malignancies and have been seen with the use of cyclophosphamide alone or in combination with other antineoplastic drugs.

Mechlorethamine hydrochloride (MUSTARGEN) and *carmustine* (*bischloronitrosourea,* BCNU, BICNU) are used topically to treat cutaneous T-cell lymphoma. Both can be applied as a solution or in ointment form. It is important to monitor complete blood counts and liver function tests because systemic absorption can cause bone marrow suppression and hepatitis. Other side effects include allergic contact dermatitis, irritant dermatitis, secondary cutaneous malignancies, and pigmentary changes. Carmustine also can cause erythema and posttreatment telangiectasias (Zackheim *et al.*, 1990).

Calcineurin Inhibitors. Cyclosporine (SANDIMMUNE, NEORAL, SANGCYA) is a potent immunosuppressant isolated from the fungus *Tolypocladium inflatum*. It inhibits calcineurin, a phosphatase that normally dephosphorylates the cytoplasmic subunit of nuclear factor of activated T cells (NFAT), thus permitting NFAT to translocate to the nucleus and augment transcription of numerous cytokines.

In T-lymphocytes, calcineurin inhibition blocks interleukin 2 (IL-2) gene transcription and release and ultimately results in inhibition of T-cell activation (Cather *et al.*, 2001). The presence of calcineurin in Langerhans' cells, mast cells, and keratinocytes may further explain the therapeutic efficacy of cyclosporine and the other calcineurin inhibitors (*e.g., tacrolimus* and *pimecrolimus; see* below) (Reynolds and Al-Daraji, 2002). Cyclosporine has FDA approval for the treatment of psoriasis. Other cutaneous disorders that typically respond well to cyclosporine are atopic dermatitis (Czech *et al.*, 2000), alopecia areata, epidermolysis bullosa acquisita, pemphigus vulgaris, bullous pemphigoid, lichen planus, and pyoderma gangrenosum. The usual initial oral dose is 3 to 5 mg/kg per day given in divided doses.

Hypertension and renal dysfunction are the major adverse effects associated with the use of cyclosporine. These risks can be minimized by monitoring serum creatinine (which should not rise more than 30% above baseline), calculating creatinine clearance or glomerular filtration rate in patients on long-term therapy or with a rising creatinine, maintaining a daily dose of less than 5 mg/kg, and regular monitoring of blood pressure (Cather *et al.*, 2001). Alternation with other therapeutic modalities may diminish cyclosporine toxicity (Shupack *et al.*, 1997). *Laboratory monitoring during therapy is essential.* Cyclosporine is not mutagenic. However, as with other immunosuppressive agents, patients with psoriasis treated with cyclosporine are at increased risk of cutaneous, solid organ, and lymphoproliferative malignancies (Flores and Kerdel, 2000). The risk of cutaneous malignancies is compounded if patients have received phototherapy with PUVA.

Tacrolimus (FK506, PROGRAF), a metabolite of *Streptomyces tsukubaensis*, was discovered in 1984. The structure of tacrolimus is:

TACROLIMUS

It is a potent macrolide immunosuppressant traditionally used to prevent kidney, liver, and heart allograft rejection. Like cyclosporine, tacrolimus works mainly by inhibiting early activation of T-lymphocytes, thereby inhibiting the release of IL-2, suppressing humoral and cell-mediated immune responses, and suppressing mediator release from mast cells and basophils (Anonymous, 2001; Assmann and Ruzicka, 2002). In contrast to cyclosporine, this effect is mediated by binding to the intracellular protein FK506-binding protein 12, generating a complex that inhibits the phosphatase activity of calcineurin.

Tacrolimus is available in oral and topical forms for the treatment of skin disease. Systemic tacrolimus has shown some efficacy in the treatment of inflammatory skin diseases such as psoriasis, pyoderma gangrenosum, and Behçet's disease (Dé Tran *et al.*, 2001; Assmann and Ruzicka, 2002). When administered systemically, the most common side effects are hypertension, nephrotoxicity, neurotoxicity, gastrointestinal symptoms, hyperglycemia, and hyperlipidemia. Topical formulations of tacrolimus penetrate into the epidermis.

In commercially available topical formulations (0.03% and 0.1%), tacrolimus ointment (PROTOPTIC) is effective in and approved for the treatment of atopic dermatitis in adults (0.03% and 0.1%) and children (0.03%). Other uses in dermatology include intertriginous psoriasis, vitiligo, mucosal lichen planus, graft-versus-host disease, allergic contact dermatitis, and rosacea (Ngheim *et al.*, 2002). It is applied to the affected area twice a day and generally is well tolerated.

A major benefit of topical tacrolimus compared with topical glucocorticoids is that tacrolimus does not cause skin atrophy and therefore can be used safely in locations such as the face and intertriginous areas. Common side effects at the site of application are transient erythema, burning, and pruritus, which tend to improve with continued treatment. Other reported adverse effects include skin tingling, flu-like symptoms, headache, alcohol intolerance, folliculitis, acne, and hyperesthesia (Ngheim *et al.*, 2002). Skin infections have been reported, although whether an increased risk truly exists relative to age-matched controls is uncertain (Anonymous, 2001). Systemic absorption generally is very low and decreases with resolution of the dermatitis. However, topical tacrolimus should be used with extreme caution in patients with Netherton's syndrome because these patients have been shown to develop elevated blood levels of the drug after topical application (Assmann and Ruzicka, 2002). Mice treated with 0.1% topical tacrolimus had a higher incidence of lymphoma and, after exposure to UV radiation, showed decreased time to skin tumor formation. It therefore is recommended that patients using tacrolimus use sunscreen and avoid excessive UV exposure. The risk of lymphoma development in humans is uncertain (Anonymous, 2001).

Pimecrolimus 1% cream (ELIDEL), a macrolide derived from ascomycin, is FDA approved for the treatment of atopic dermatitis in patients older than 2 years of age. The structure of pimecrolimus is:

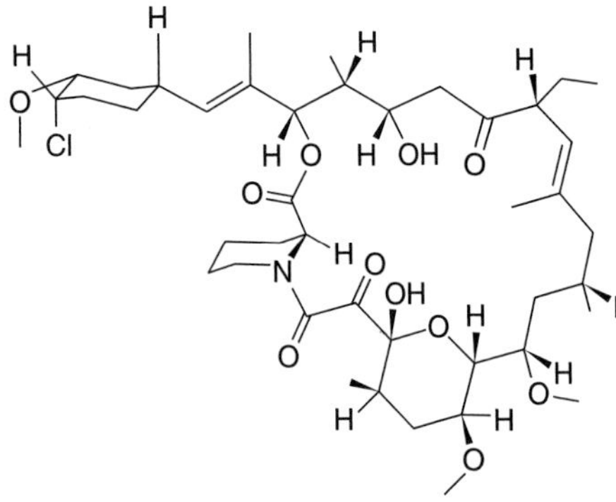

PIMECROLIMUS

Its mechanism of action and side-effect profile are similar to those of tacrolimus. Burning, while occurring in some patients, appears to be less common with pimecrolimus than with tacrolimus (Ngheim *et al.*, 2002). In addition, pimecrolimus has less systemic absorption. Similar precautions with regard to UV exposure should be taken during treatment with pimecrolimus (Anonymous, 2002b).

MISCELLANEOUS IMMUNOSUPPRESSANT AND ANTIINFLAMMATORY AGENTS

Mycophenolate mofetil (CELLCEPT) is an immunosuppressant approved for prophylaxis of organ rejection in patients with renal, cardiac, and hepatic transplants (*see* Chapter 52). Mycophenolic acid, the active derivative of mycophenolate mofetil, inhibits the enzyme inosine monophosphatase dehydrogenase (IMPDH), thereby depleting guanosine nucleotides essential for DNA and RNA synthesis (Frieling and Luger, 2002). Moreover, mycophenolic acid is a fivefold more potent inhibitor of the type II isoform of IMPDH found in activated B- and T-lymphocytes and thus functions as a specific inhibitor of T- and B-lymphocyte activation and proliferation. The drug also may enhance apoptosis.

Mycophenolate mofetil is used increasingly to treat inflammatory and autoimmune diseases in dermatology (Carter *et al.*, 2004) in doses ranging from 1 to 2 g/day

orally. Mycophenolate mofetil is particularly useful as a corticosteroid-sparing agent in the treatment of autoimmune blistering disorders, including pemphigus vulgaris, bullous pemphigoid, cicatricial pemphigoid, and pemphigus foliaceus. It also has been used effectively in the treatment of inflammatory diseases such as psoriasis, atopic dermatitis, and pyoderma gangrenosum.

Imiquimod (ALDARA) is a synthetic imidazoquinoline amine believed to exert immunomodulatory effects by acting as a ligand at toll-like receptors in the innate immune system and inducing the cytokines interferon-α (IFN-α), tumor necrosis factor-α (TNF-α), and IL-1, IL-6, IL-8, IL-10, and IL-12. The structure of imiquimod is:

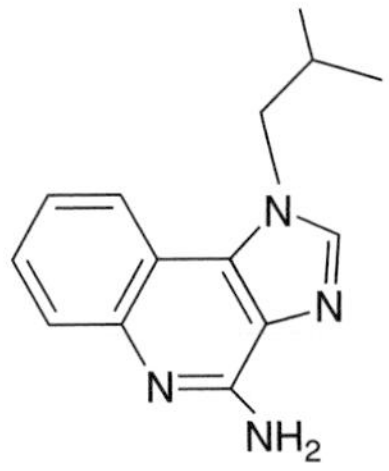

IMIQUIMOD

Approved for the treatment of genital warts since 1997, imiquimod is applied to genital or perianal lesions three times a week usually for a 16-week period that may be repeated as necessary. Imiquimod also has been approved recently for the treatment of actinic keratoses. In this capacity, imiquimod is applied three times a week for 16 weeks to the face, scalp, and arms (Anonymous, 2004). Phase II trials evaluating imiquimod for the treatment of nodular and superficial basal cell carcinomas (BCC) suggest that imiquimod may prove useful when applied daily over a 6- to 12-week period (Salasche and Shumack, 2003), and the drug is approved for this indication by the FDA. Off-label applications include the treatment of non-genital warts, molluscum contagiosum, extramammary Paget's disease, and Bowen's disease. Irritant reactions occur in virtually all patients, and some develop edema, vesicles, erosions, or ulcers. It appears that the degree of inflammation parallels therapeutic efficacy. No systemic effects have been reported.

Systemic *vinblastine* (VELBAN, others) is approved for use in Kaposi's sarcoma and advanced cutaneous T-cell lymphoma. Intralesional vinblastine also is used to treat Kaposi's sarcoma (Hengge *et al.*, 2002). Intralesional *bleomycin* (BLENOXANE, others) is used for recalcitrant warts and has cytotoxic and proinflammatory effects (Templeton *et al.*, 1994). Intralesional injection of bleomycin into the digits has been associated with a vasospastic response that mimics Raynaud's phenomenon, local skin necrosis, and flagellate hyperpigmentation (Abess *et al.*, 2003). Intralesional bleomycin has been used for palliative treatment of squamous cell carcinoma. Systemic bleomycin has been used for Kaposi's sarcoma (*see* Chapter 51 for a more complete discussion of these agents). Liposomal anthracyclines [specifically *doxorubicin* (DOXIL, CAE-LYX)] may provide first-line monotherapy for advanced Kaposi's sarcoma (Hengge *et al.*, 2002).

Dapsone (4,4′-diaminodiphenylsulfone) has been in clinical use for almost 50 years. Its structure is:

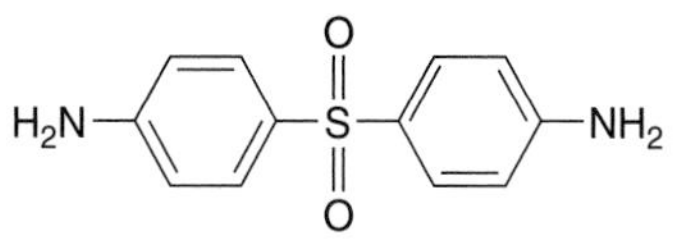

DAPSONE

Dapsone is used in dermatology for its antiinflammatory properties, particularly in sterile (noninfectious) pustular diseases of the skin. Dapsone prevents the respiratory burst from myeloperoxidase, suppresses neutrophil migration by blocking integrin-mediated adherence, inhibits adherence of antibodies to neutrophils, and decreases the release of eicosanoids and blocks their inflammatory effects; all these actions are likely to be important in autoimmune skin diseases (Booth *et al.*, 1992; Thuong-Nguyen *et al.*, 1993; Zhu and Stiller, 2001).

Dapsone is approved for use in dermatitis herpetiformis and leprosy. It is particularly useful in the treatment of linear immunoglobulin A (IgA) dermatosis, bullous systemic lupus erythematosus, erythema elevatum diutinum, and subcorneal pustular dermatosis. In addition, reports indicate efficacy in patients with acne fulminans, pustular psoriasis, lichen planus, Hailey–Hailey disease, pemphigus vulgaris, bullous pemphigoid, cicatricial pemphigoid, leukocytoclastic vasculitis, Sweet's syndrome, granuloma faciale, relapsing polychondritis, Behçet's disease, urticarial vasculitis, pyoderma gangrenosum, and granuloma annulare (Paniker and Levine, 2001).

An initial dose of 50 mg/day is prescribed, followed by increases of 25 mg/day at weekly intervals, always with appropriate laboratory testing. Potential side effects of dapsone include methemoglobinemia and hemolysis. The glucose-6-phosphate dehydrogenase (G6PD) level should be checked in all patients before initiating dapsone therapy because dapsone hydroxylamine, the toxic metabolite of dapsone formed by hydroxylation, depletes glutathione within G6PD-deficient cells. The nitroso derivative then causes peroxidation reactions, leading to rapid hemolysis. A maximum dose of 150 to 300 mg/day should be given

in divided doses to minimize the risks of methemoglobinemia. The H_2 blocker cimetidine, at a dose of 400 mg three times daily, alters the degree of methemoglobinemia by competing with dapsone for CYPs. Toxicities include agranulocytosis, peripheral neuropathy, and psychosis.

Thalidomide (THALOMID) is an antiinflammatory, immunomodulating, antiangiogenic agent experiencing resurgence in the treatment of dermatologic diseases (*see* Chapter 52). Its structure is:

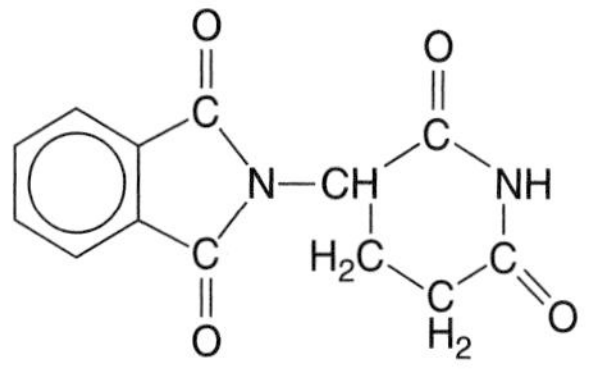

THALIDOMIDE

The mechanisms that underlie the pharmacologic properties of thalidomide are not clear, although modulation of inflammatory cytokines such as TNF-α, IFN-α, IL-10, IL-12, cyclooxygenase 2, and possibly nuclear factor κB (NF-κB) may be involved (Franks *et al.*, 2004). It also can modulate T cells by altering their patterns of cytokine release and can increase keratinocyte migration and proliferation (Wines *et al.*, 2002).

Thalidomide is FDA approved for the treatment of erythema nodosum leprosum. There are reports suggesting its efficacy in actinic prurigo, aphthous stomatitis, Behçet's disease, Kaposi's sarcoma, and the cutaneous manifestations of lupus erythematosus, as well as prurigo nodularis and uremic prurigo. Thalidomide has been associated with increased mortality when used to treat toxic epidermal necrolysis. The drug always will be infamous for its association with limb abnormalities (phocomelia), as well as other congenital anomalies. It also may cause an irreversible neuropathy. *Because of its teratogenic effects, thalidomide use is restricted to specially licensed physicians who fully understand the risks. Thalidomide should never be taken by women who are pregnant or who could become pregnant while taking the drug.*

BIOLOGICAL AGENTS

Biological agents (*see* Chapters 38 and 52) are highly specialized systemic therapies that target specific mediators of the immunologic/inflammatory reactions that are, at least in part, responsible for the clinical manifestations of a disease. The rapidly advancing knowledge of cutaneous immunolo-

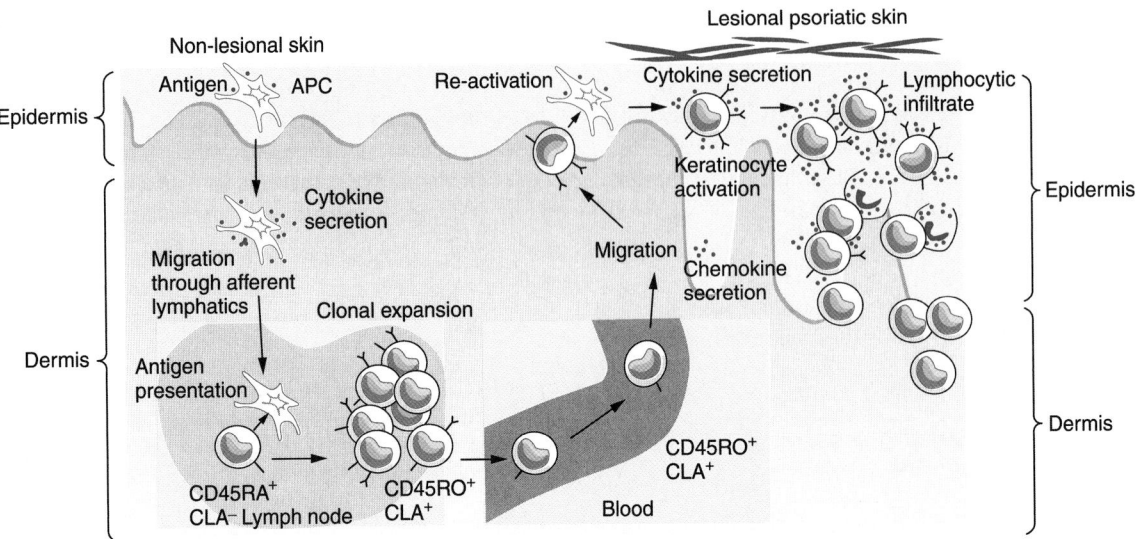

Figure 62–2. ***Immunopathogenesis of psoriasis.*** Psoriasis is a prototypical inflammatory skin disorder in which specific T-cell populations are stimulated by as yet undefined antigen(s) presented by antigen-presenting cells. The T cells release proinflammatory cytokines such as TNF-α and IFN-γ that induce keratinocyte and endothelial cell proliferation.

gy has brought with it equally impressive innovations in the therapy of malignant disorders such as cutaneous T-cell lymphoma and immunologic diseases such as psoriasis and psoriatic arthritis. Investigational studies are evaluating a variety of biological agents for the treatment of malignancy and autoimmune diseases. This section will focus on agents that have been well studied or applied widely to the treatment of dermatological disease.

Once thought to be primarily a disorder of keratinocyte hyperproliferation, psoriasis now is known to be an autoimmune process mediated by T-lymphocytes that can react with epidermal keratinocytes (Figure 62–2). The mechanism of biological therapies in psoriasis can be illustrated by a conceptual model that outlines four strategies in the treatment of psoriasis: (1) reduction of pathogenic T cells; (2) inhibition of T-cell activation; (3) immune deviation (from a T_H1 to a T_H2 immune response); and (4) blockade of the activity of inflammatory cytokines (Weinberg, 2003).

Although there are limited long-term data regarding the efficacy and safety of biological agents solely for the treatment of psoriasis, similar, if not identical, therapies have been used extensively in the treatment of rheumatoid arthritis and Crohn's disease. The major advantage of biological agents in the treatment of psoriasis appears to be that they specifically target the activity of T-lymphocytes and cytokines that mediate inflammation with fewer side effects than traditional systemic immunosuppressive/cytotoxic agents.

When evaluating the efficacy of biological agents, it is important to understand the standard measurement of efficacy in psoriasis treatment, the Psoriasis Area Severity Index (PASI). The PASI

quantitates the extent and severity of skin involvement in different body regions as a score from 0 (no lesions) to 72 (severe disease). To gain FDA approval for the treatment of psoriasis, a biological agent must decrease the PASI by 75%. While such quantitation is an essential element in controlled clinical trials, many patients in practice may gain clinically significant benefit from biological treatment without achieving this degree of PASI improvement.

Alefacept (AMEVIVE) was the first immunobiological agent approved for the treatment of moderate-to-severe psoriasis in patients who are candidates for systemic therapy. Alefacept consists of a recombinant fully human fusion protein composed of the binding site of the leukocyte function–associated antigen 3 (LFA-3) protein and a human IgG1 Fc domain. The LFA-3 portion of the alefacept molecule binds to CD2 on the surface of T cells, thus blocking a necessary costimulation step in T-cell activation (Figure 62–3). Importantly, since CD2 is expressed preferentially on memory-effector T cells, naive T cells largely are unaffected by alefacept. A second important action of alefacept is its ability to induce apoptosis of memory-effector T cells through simultaneous binding of its IgG1 portion to immunoglobulin receptors on cytotoxic cells and its LFA-3 portion to CD2 on T cells, thus inducing granzyme-mediated apoptosis of memory-effector T cells.

Alefacept is administered by in-office intramuscular injection at a dose of 15 mg/week for 12 weeks. An additional 12-week course can be initiated if required, and a continuous 24-week regimen is under investigation. In an international randomized, double-blind, placebo-controlled phase III trial of intramuscular alefacept (15 mg once weekly for 12 weeks, 10 mg once weekly for 12 weeks, or placebo), 21% of patients receiving the 15-mg dose showed a 75%

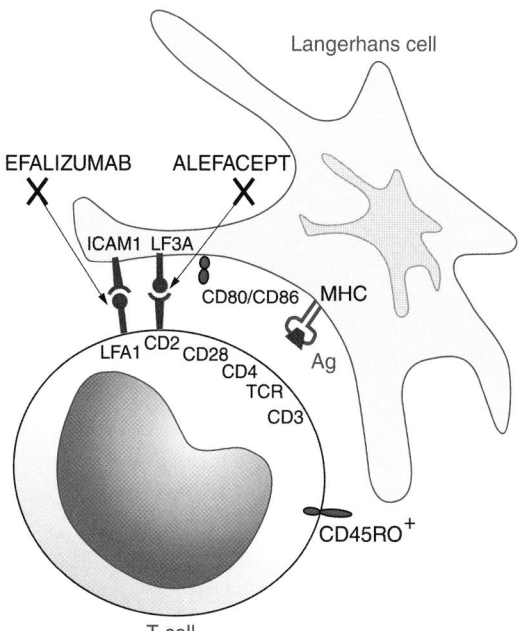

Figure 62–3. *Mechanisms of action of selected biological agents in psoriasis.* Newer biological agents can interfere with one or more steps in the pathogenesis of psoriasis, resulting in clinical improvement. *See* text for details.

reduction in PASI, and 42% of patients showed a 50% decrease in PASI at week 14. Of those patients who achieved a 75% PASI reduction at week 14, 71% maintained a minimum PASI improvement of 50% throughout the 12-week follow-up period (Lebwohl *et al.*, 2004), suggesting that alefacept may induce longer remissions than do other biological agents. Adverse effects include a reduction in CD4+ lymphocyte counts, requiring a baseline T-lymphocyte count before initiating alefacept and weekly monitoring of T cells during therapy.

Efalizumab (RAPTIVA) is a humanized monoclonal antibody against the CD11a molecule of LFA-1. By binding to CD11a on T cells, efalizumab prevents binding of LFA-1 to intercellular adhesion molecule 1 (ICAM-1) on the surface of antigen-presenting cells, vascular endothelial cells, and cells in the dermis and epidermis (*see* Figure 62–3), thereby interfering with T-cell activation and migration and cytotoxic T-cell function (Weinberg, 2003). Efalizumab is FDA approved for the treatment of moderate-to-severe psoriasis in patients who are candidates for systemic therapy.

The drug is administered by subcutaneous injection once a week at a dose of 1 mg/kg, usually for 12 or 24 weeks. In a phase III, multicenter, randomized, placebo-controlled, double-blind trial, at a dose of 1 mg/kg per week, 52% and 22% of patients achieved reductions in their PASI scores of 50 and 75, respectively. At a dose of 2 mg/kg, 57% and 28% of patients achieved PASI reductions of 50 and 75, respectively. In patients who achieved PASI reductions

of 75 or greater at week 12 and were treated through week 24 with 2 mg/kg every other week, 78% and 95% of patients achieved PASI reductions of 50 and 75, respectively (Lebwohl *et al.*, 2004). After discontinuation of therapy, patients may experience rebound of disease. It is recommended that periodic evaluation of platelet levels be performed during therapy. Side effects generally are mild, and there is no evidence to date of increased risk of malignancy, infection, or end-organ toxicity (Weinberg, 2003).

Etanercept (ENBREL) is FDA approved for the treatment of psoriasis, psoriatic arthritis, rheumatoid arthritis, juvenile rheumatoid arthritis, and ankylosing spondylitis. Etanercept is a soluble, recombinant, fully human TNF receptor fusion protein consisting of two molecules of the ligand-binding portion of the TNF receptor fused to the Fc portion of IgG1. As a dimeric molecule, it can bind two molecules of TNF. Etanercept binds soluble and membrane-bound TNF, thereby inhibiting the action of TNF (Krueger and Callis, 2004).

Etanercept is administered by subcutaneous injection at doses of either 25 or 50 mg twice a week. In a phase III, placebo-controlled, double-blind, parallel-group study, 34% and 44% of patients receiving the 25-mg dose reached PASI reductions of 75% at 12 and 24 weeks, respectively, and 58% and 70% of patients achieved PASI reductions of 50% at 12 and 24 weeks, respectively. At the 50-mg dose, 49% and 59% reached PASI reduction of 75% at 12 and 24 weeks, respectively, and 74% and 77% reached PASI reductions of 50% at 12 and 24 weeks, respectively. Except for injection-site reactions, the drug is well tolerated. Monthly complete blood counts with a differential should be monitored for the first 3 months of treatment. Potential side effects include aplastic anemia, increased risk of infection, and exacerbation of congestive heart failure and demyelinating disorders. The risk of malignancy is unknown but may be increased with the use of etanercept.

Infliximab (REMICADE) is a mouse–human chimeric monoclonal antibody that binds to soluble and membrane-bound TNF-α and inhibits binding with its receptors (Krueger and Callis, 2004). Infliximab is a complement-fixing antibody that induces complement-dependent and cell-mediated lysis when bound to cell-surface-bound TNF-α. It also induces proinflammatory cytokines, such as IL-1 and IL-6, and enhances leukocyte migration. Infliximab is FDA approved for the treatment of Crohn's disease and rheumatoid arthritis, but it is also in phase III trials for the treatment of psoriasis.

Infliximab is administered by intravenous infusion over 2 hours at doses of 3 or 5 mg/kg, usually at weeks 0, 2, and 6. In a phase II trial, 82% and 72% of patients given the 3 mg/kg dose for 10 weeks achieved PASI reductions of 50% and 75%, respectively, whereas 97% and 75% of those receiving the 5 mg/kg dose achieved PASI reductions of 50% and 75%, respectively (Weinberg, 2003). Complications of therapy include infusion reactions, reactivation of latent tuberculosis infection, exacerbation of congestive heart failure, and multiple sclerosis–like syndromes. Purified protein derivative (PPD) testing is required before initiating therapy. Neutralizing antibodies to

infliximab may develop, and concomitant administration of methotrexate or glucocorticoids may suppress antibody formation.

Denileukin diftitox or DAB$_{389}$–IL-2, (ONTAK) is a fusion
protein composed of diphtheria toxin fragments A and B
and the receptor-binding portion of IL-2. DAB$_{389}$–IL-2 is
indicated for advanced cutaneous T-cell lymphoma in
patients with more than 20% of T cells expressing the surface marker CD25. The IL-2 portion of the fusion protein
binds the CD25 marker on the T cell and promotes destruction of the T cell by the cytocidal action of diphtheria toxin.

In a phase III trial consisting of 9 or 18 μg/kg per day of
DAB$_{389}$–IL-2 given as an intravenous infusion for 5 consecutive
days every 3 weeks for up to 6 months or eight courses, the overall
response rate was 36% with 18 μg/kg per day and 23% with 9 μg/kg
per day. Adverse effects included pain, fevers, chills, nausea, vomiting, and diarrhea. Immediate hypersensitivity manifested by
hypotension, back pain, dyspnea, and chest pain occurred in 60% of
patients within 24 hours of drug administration; other serious side
effects of DAB$_{389}$–IL-2 are the capillary leak syndrome (*i.e.*, edema,
hypoalbuminemia, and/or hypotension), occurring in 20% to 30% of
patients, and elevated blood levels of hepatic transaminases (Olsen
et al., 2001; Apisarnthanarax *et al.*, 2002).

INTRAVENOUS IMMUNOGLOBULIN IN DERMATOLOGY

Intravenous immunoglobulin (IVIG) is prepared from frac-
tionated pooled human sera derived from thousands of donors
with various antigenic exposures (*see* Chapter 52). Commercial preparations of IVIG are composed mainly of IgG with
minimal amounts of IgA. There is a risk of anaphylaxis if
IgA-deficient patients receive IVIG that is not IgA-poor.
Although the mechanism of action of IVIG is not understood
fully, proposed mechanisms include anti-idiotype interactions,
Fc receptor modulation, cytokine inhibition, neutralization of
causative microbes or toxins, superantigen neutralization, and
acceleration of IgG catabolism (Colsky, 2000). While mostly
anecdotal, reports of successful use of IVIG in the treatment
of autoimmune and inflammatory dermatoses are accumulating. IVIG has been used to treat dermatomyositis, chronic recalcitrant urticaria/angioedema, atopic dermatitis, systemic lupus erythematosus, and autoimmune blistering disorders.

A multicenter retrospective analysis of 48 cases of
toxic epidermal necrolysis (TEN) treated with IVIG at a
dose of 1 g/kg per day for 3 days demonstrated remarkably rapid cessation of cutaneous and mucosal blistering
and improved survival (Prins *et al.*, 2003). A subsequent
retrospective chart review that compared the outcome of
24 TEN patients treated with IVIG with 21 patients who
did not receive IVIG found no improvement in mortality

but rather a possible detrimental trend in treated patients
(Brown *et al.*, 2004). Clearly, a multicenter, prospective,
double-blind, randomized trial is needed to determine the
usefulness of IVIG in the treatment of TEN.

SUNSCREENS

Photoprotection from the acute and chronic effects of sun
exposure is readily available with sunscreens. The major
active ingredients of available sunscreens include chemical
agents that absorb incident solar radiation in the UVB and/or
UVA ranges and physical agents that contain particulate
materials that can block or reflect incident energy and reduce
its transmission to the skin. Many of the sunscreens available
are mixtures of organic chemical absorbers and particulate
physical substances. Ideal sunscreens provide a broad spectrum of protection and are formulations that are photostable
and remain intact for sustained periods on the skin. They also
should be nonirritating, invisible, and nonstaining to clothing. No single sunscreen ingredient possesses all these desirable properties, but many are quite effective nonetheless.

UVA Sunscreen Agents

Currently available UVA filters in the United States include (1) *avoben-
zone,* also known as *Parsol 1789;* (2) *oxybenzone* (2-hydroxy-4-meth-
oxy-benzophenone); (3) *titanium dioxide;* and (4) *zinc oxide.* Additional
UVA sunscreens, including *ecamsule* (MEXORYL SX and XL), *bisethylhex-
yloxyphenol methoxyphenyl triazine* (TINOSORB S), and *methylene bisben-
zotriazolyl tetramethylbutylphenol* (TINSORB M), are available in Europe
and elsewhere but not in the United States.

UVB Sunscreen Agents

There are numerous UVB filters, including (1) PABA esters (*e.g.,
padimate O*); (2) cinnamates (*octinoxate*); (3) *octocrylene* (2-ethyl-
hexyl-2-cyano-3,3 diphenylacrylate); and (4) salicylates (*octisalate*).

The major measurement of sunscreen photoprotection is the *sun
protection factor* (SPF), which defines a ratio of the minimal dose of
incident sunlight that will produce erythema or redness (sunburn) on
skin with the sunscreen in place (protected) and the dose that evokes
the same reaction on skin without the sunscreen (unprotected). The
SPF provides valuable information regarding UVB protection but is
useless in documenting UVA efficacy because no standard systems
have been developed to measure UVA protection. Such protocols are
needed because more than 85% of solar ultraviolet radiation reaching
earth's surface is UVA, which penetrates more deeply into human
skin than does UVB and appears to play an important role in photoaging and photocarcinogenesis. Despite their universal availability, a
major problem with sunscreens is the fact that people do not use them
on a regular basis. In a population study evaluating the use of sunscreens in northern England, it was reported that only 35% of females
and 8% of males regularly used sunscreens (Ling *et al.*, 2003). Furthermore, 22% of those surveyed used no sunscreen at all, and 34%
recalled at least one sunburn reaction in the previous 2 years.

There is evidence that the regular use of sunscreens can reduce the risk of actinic keratoses (Thompson *et al.*, 1993) and squamous cell carcinomas (SCCs) of the skin. One study noted a 46% decrease in the incidence of SCCs in people who used sunscreen regularly for 4.5 years (Green *et al.*, 1999).

Except for total sun avoidance, sunscreens are the best single method of protection from UV-induced damage to the skin. There is a need for more definitive answers to questions related to the efficacy of sunscreens in reducing skin cancer risk. Prospects for more effective photoprotection are excellent as better sunscreen components are developed and as more careful evaluations are performed (Rigel, 2002).

THE TREATMENT OF PRURITUS

The term *pruritus* is derived from the Latin *prurire,* which means "to itch." Pruritus is a symptom unique to skin that occurs in a multitude of dermatologic disorders, including dry skin or xerosis, atopic eczema, urticaria, and infestations. Itching also may be a sign of internal disorders, including malignant neoplasms, chronic renal failure, and hepatobiliary disease. The treatment of pruritus varies greatly depending on the underlying disorder.

General measures employing copious application of emollients usually are sufficient for xerosis. Inflammatory disorders such as atopic dermatitis, contact dermatitis, and lichen simplex chronicus may respond better to potent topical glucocorticoids and oral doses of sedating antihistamines. Antihistamines are useful in histamine-induced pruritus and in other pruritic disorders in which the sedating effects of these drugs facilitate sleep and reduce scratching at night, when most pruritic disorders are more symptomatic.

Cholestasis-associated pruritus may respond to *cholestyramine* (QUESTRAN, others; *see* Chapter 35), *ursodeoxycholic acid* (ACTIGALL, others; *see* Chapter 37), *ondansetron* (ZOFRAN; *see* Chapter 37), or *rifampin* (*see* Chapter 47). Recently, *nalmefene* (REVEX) (20 mg twice per day; *see* Chapter 21) has been shown to be effective in cholestatic pruritus (Bergasa *et al.*, 1999).

The pruritus of uremia is treated most effectively with UVB radiation. Prurigo, a ubiquitous disorder associated with itchy nodules of the skin, is notoriously difficult to treat. In addition to topical and intralesional steroids, prurigo may respond to the opioid antagonist *naltrexone* (*see* Chapter 21) at a dose of 50 mg/day (Metze *et al.*, 1999) or to the proton pump inhibitor *omeprazole* (*see* Chapter 36).

MISCELLANEOUS DRUGS

Azelaic acid (AZELEX, FINACEA) is a naturally occurring dicarboxylic acid used for the treatment of acne and pigmentary disorders such as melasma and postinflammatory hyperpigmentation. Its structure is:

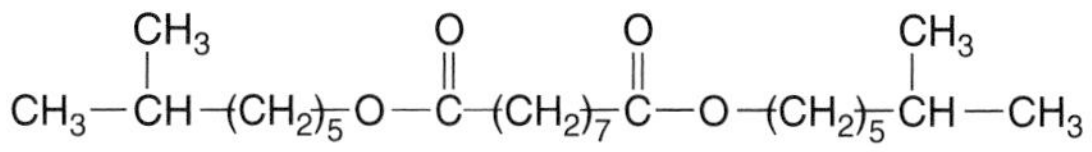

AZELAIC ACID

In the United States, azelaic acid is available as a 20% cream. Azelaic acid has been used for the treatment of pigmentary disorders because of its inhibition of tyrosinase, the rate-limiting enzyme in the synthesis of melanin (Hsu and Quan, 2001). Azelaic acid also possesses comedolytic and antimicrobial activity and may have additional antiinflammatory properties. Applied topically twice a day, azelaic acid is effective for the treatment of acne. In patients with papulopustular rosacea, 15% azelaic acid gel was superior to metronidazole gel (0.75%) in the treatment of inflammatory lesions and erythema; neither medication improved the telangiectatic blood vessels that frequently accompany rosacea (Elewski *et al.*, 2003).

Calcipotriene (DOVONEX) is a vitamin D analog that is used in the treatment of psoriasis. Its structure is:

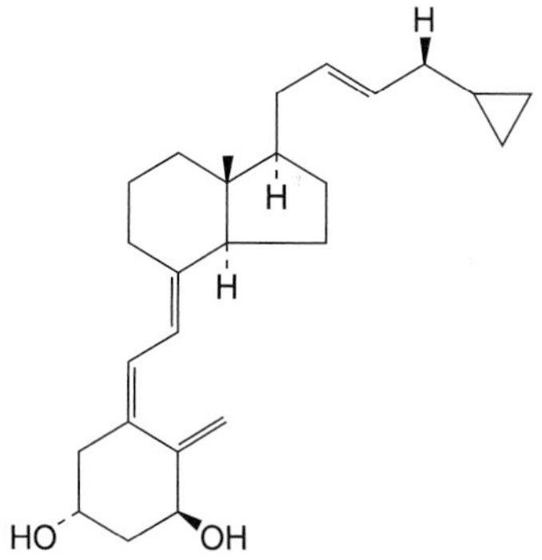

CALCIPOTRIENE

It was developed after the fortuitous observation of improved psoriasis in a patient with osteoporosis receiving an oral derivative of 1,25-dihydroxyvitamin D_3 [1,25-$(OH)_2D_3$], the active form of vitamin D (Morimoto and Kumahara, 1985) (*see* Chapter 61). 1,25-$(OH)_2D_3$ plays a major role in calcium homeostasis by activating the vitamin D receptor, which belongs to the steroid/thyroid hormone receptor superfamily. The receptor–vitamin D complex binds to DNA and modulates the transcription of genes related to cell proliferation and differentiation.

Calcipotriene is applied twice daily to plaque psoriasis on the body. Improvement is detectable within 1 to 2 weeks, and maximum clinical response occurs within 6 to 8 weeks. Most patients show some improvement, but complete resolution occurs in no more than 15%. Maintenance therapy usually is necessary, and tachyphylaxis does not occur (Kragballe, 1992). Reports of hypercalcemia with calcipotriene are rare (Hardman *et al.*, 1993).

DRUGS FOR HYPERKERATOTIC DISORDERS

Keratolytic agents—including *lactic acid, glycolic acid, salicylic acid, urea,* and *sulfur*—are employed to treat various forms of hyperkeratosis ranging from calluses and verrucae to severe xerosis. Lactic and glycolic acid are α-hydroxy acids that are thought to disrupt ionic bonds and thus diminish corneocyte cohesion (Van Scott and Yu, 1984).

Salicylic acid is a β-hydroxy acid that is thought to function through solubilization of intercellular cement, again reducing corneocyte adhesion. It appears to eliminate the stratum corneum layer by layer from the outermost level downward. This contrasts with the α-hydroxy acids, which preferentially diminish cellular cohesion between the corneocytes at the lowest levels of the stratum corneum.

Urea is an antimicrobial agent that denatures and dissolves proteins and increases skin absorption and retention of water (Hessel *et al.*, 2001). Sulfur is antiseptic, antiparasitic, antiseborrheic, and keratolytic, accounting for its myriad uses in dermatology.

Keratolytics are available in a multitude of formulations for treating skin diseases. Prolonged use of salicylic acid preparations over large areas, especially in children and patients with renal and hepatic impairment, can result in salicylism. Irritation is a common side effect with higher concentrations. Lactic acid (LAC-HYDRIN, others) is an emollient that contains 12% lactic acid that is an effective moisturizer indicated for the treatment of xerosis and ichthyosis vulgaris.

Glycolic acid is marketed in multiple cosmetic preparations (4% to 10%) and is used for the treatment of xerosis, ichthyosis, and photoaging.

Destructive Agents

Podophyllin (podophyllum resin) is a mixture of chemicals from the plant *Podophyllum peltatum* (mandrake or May apple). The major constituent of the resin is podophyllotoxin (podofilox). It binds to microtubules and causes mitotic arrest in metaphase. Podophyllum resin (10% to 40%) is applied by a physician and left in place for 2 to 6 hours weekly for the treatment of anogenital warts. Irritation and ulcerative local reactions are the major side effects. It should not be used in the mouth or during pregnancy. Podofilox (CONDYLOX, others) is available as a 0.5% solution for application twice daily for 3 consecutive days. Weekly cycles may be repeated.

DRUGS FOR ANDROGENETIC ALOPECIA

Androgenetic alopecia, commonly known as male and female pattern baldness, is the most common cause of hair loss in adults older than age 40. Up to 50% of men and women are affected. Androgenetic alopecia is a genetically inherited trait with variable expression. In susceptible hair follicles, dihydrotestosterone binds to the androgen receptor, and the hormone–receptor complex activates the genes responsible for the gradual transformation of large terminal follicles into miniaturized vellus follicles. Treatment of androgenetic areata is aimed at reducing hair loss and maintaining existing hair. The capacity to stimulate substantial regrowth of human hair remains a formidable pharmacological challenge.

Minoxidil (ROGAINE) was first developed as an antihypertensive agent (*see* Chapter 32) and was noted to be associated with hypertrichosis in some patients. A topical formulation of minoxidil then was developed to exploit this side effect. The structure of minoxidil is:

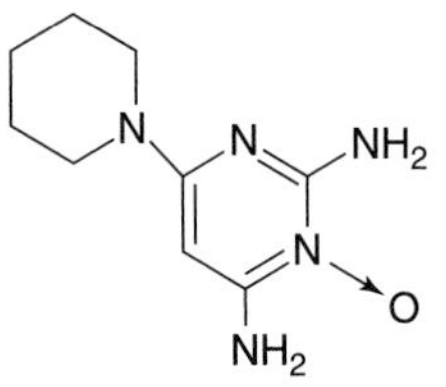

MINOXIDIL

Topical minoxidil is available as a 2% solution (ROGAINE) and a 5% solution (ROGAINE EXTRA STRENGTH FOR MEN). Minoxidil enhances follicular size, resulting in thicker hair shafts, and stimulates and prolongs the anagen phase of the hair cycle, resulting in longer and increased numbers of hairs (Fiedler, 1999). Treatment must be continued, or any drug-induced hair growth will be lost. Allergic and irritant contact dermatitis can occur, and care should be taken in applying the drug because hair growth may emerge in undesirable locations. This is reversible on stopping the drug. Patients should be instructed to wash their hands after applying minoxidil.

Finasteride (PROPECIA) inhibits the type II isozyme of 5α-reductase, the enzyme that converts testosterone to dihydrotestosterone (*see* Chapter 58). The structure of finasteride is:

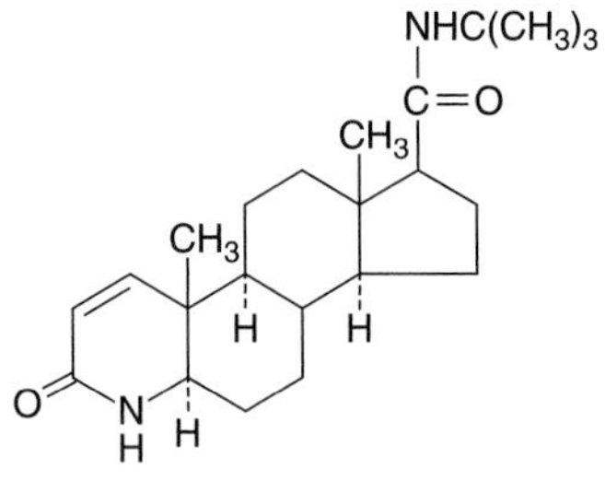

FINASTERIDE

The type II 5α-reductase is found in hair follicles. Balding areas of the scalp are associated with increased dihydrotesterone levels and smaller hair follicles than nonbalding areas. Orally administered finasteride (1 mg/day) has been shown to variably increase hair growth in men over a 2-year period, increasing hair counts in the vertex and the frontal scalp (Leyden *et al.*, 1999). Finasteride is approved for use only in men. Pregnant women should not be exposed to the drug because of the potential for inducing genital abnormalities in male fetuses. Adverse effects of finasteride include decreased libido, erectile dysfunction, ejaculation disorder, and decreased ejaculate volume. Each of these occurs in less than 2% of patients (Kaufman *et al.*, 1998). Like minoxidil, treatment with finasteride must be continued, or any new hair growth will be lost.

TREATMENT OF HYPERPIGMENTATION

Hyperpigmentation is treated with products containing *hydroquinone* that produce reversible depigmentation of the skin by inhibiting the enzymatic oxidation of tyrosine to 3,4-dihydroxyphenyalanine and also inhibiting other melanocyte metabolic processes. It is indicated for the gradual bleaching of hyperpigmented skin in conditions such as melasma, freckles, and solar lentigines. Concomitant application of SPF 15 to 30 sunscreens and meticulous photoprotection are essential to minimize sun-induced exacerbation of hyperpigmentation. Numerous preparations are available (SOLAQUIN FORTE, others). The structure of hydroquinone is:

HYDROQUINONE

MISCELLANEOUS AGENTS

Capsaicin is a naturally occurring substance derived from hot chili peppers of the genus *Capsicum*. Its structure is:

CAPSAICIN

Capsaicin interacts with the vanilloid receptor (VR1) on sensory afferents. VR1 is a gated cation channel of the TRP family, modulated by a variety of noxious stimuli (Caterina and Julius, 2001). Chronic exposure to capsaicin stimulates and desensitizes this channel. Capsaicin also causes local depletion of substance P, an endogenous neuropeptide involved in sensory perception and pain transmission. Capsaicin is available as a 0.025% cream (ZOSTRIX, others) and a 0.075% cream (ZOSTRIX HP, others) to be applied three to four times daily. Capsaicin is FDA approved for the treatment of postherpetic neuralgia and painful diabetic neuropathy, although its efficacy in relieving pain is debatable.

Masoprocol, a dicatechol compound with an aliphatic spacer, is derived from the plant *Larrea divaricata;* it is a potent 5-lipoxygenase inhibitor with anti-tumor activity. It is effective for the topical therapy of actinic keratoses (Olsen *et al.*, 1991). Masoprocol is available as a cream (ACTINEX) and is applied twice daily for approximately 1 month. Common side effects include redness, scaling, and pruritus.

BIBLIOGRAPHY

Anonymous. Topical tacrolimus for the treatment of atopic dermatitis. *Med. Lett.*, **2001,** *43*:33–34.

Anonymous. Drugs for non-HIV viral infections. *Med. Lett.*, **2002a,** *44*:9–16.

Anonymous. Topical pimecrolimus (ELIDEL) for the treatment of atopic dermatitis. *Med. Lett.*, **2002b,** *44*:48–50.

Anonymous. Imiquimod (ALDARA) for actinic keratoses. *Med. Lett.* **2004,** *46*:42–44.

Apisarnthanarax, N., Talpur, R., and Duvic, M. Treatment of cutaneous T cell lymphoma: Current status and future directions. *Am. J. Clin. Dermatol.*, **2002,** *3*:193–215.

Barry, B.W. Breaching the skin's barrier to drugs. *Nature Biotech.*, **2004,** *22*:165–167

Bergasa, N.V., Alling, D.W., Talbot, T.L., *et al.* Oral nalmefene therapy reduces scratching activity due to the pruritus of cholestasis: A controlled study. *J. Am. Acad. Dermatol.*, **1999,** *41*:431–434.

Bershad, S., Rubinstein, A., Paterniti, J.R., *et al.* Changes in plasma lipids and lipoproteins during isotretinoin therapy for acne. *New Engl. J. Med.*, **1985,** *313*:981–985.

Bisaccia, E., Gonzalez, J., Palangio, M., *et al.* Extracorporeal photochemotherapy alone or with adjuvant therapy in the treatment of cutaneous T-cell lymphoma: A 9-year retrospective study at a single institution. *J. Am. Acad. Dermatol.*, **2000,** *43*:263–271.

Booth, S.A., Moody, C.E., Dahl, M.V., *et al.* Dapsone suppresses integrin-mediated neutrophil adherence function. *J. Invest. Dermatol.*, **1992,** *98*:135–140.

Brown, K.M., Silver, G.M., Halerz, M., *et al.* Toxic epidermal necrolysis: Does immunoglobulin make a difference? *J. Burn Care Rehabil.*, **2004,** *25*:81–88.

Callen, J.P., and Camisa, C. Antimalarial agents. In, *Comprehensive Dermatologic Drug Therapy*. (Wolverton, S.E., ed.) Saunders, Philadelphia, **2001,** pp. 251–268.

Carter, E.L., Chren, M.M., and Bickers, D.R. Drugs used in dermatological disorders. In, *Modern Pharmacology with Clinical Applications*, 6th ed. (Craig, C.R., and Stitzel, R.E., eds.) Lippincott Williams & Wilkins, Baltimore, **2004,** pp. 484–498.

Chandraratna, R.A. Rational design of receptor-selective retinoids. *J. Am. Acad. Dermatol.,* **1998,** *39*:S124–128.

Cohen, P.R., and Grossman, M.E. Management of cutaneous lesions associated with an emerging epidemic: Community-acquired methicillin-resistant *Staphylococcus aureus* skin infections. *J. Am. Acad. Dermatol.,* **2004,** *51*:132–135.

Coyle, T.S., Nam, T.K, Camouse, M.M., *et al.* Steroid-sparing effect of extracorporeal photopheresis in the treatment of graft-vs-host disease. *Arch. Dermatol.,* **2004,** *140*:763–764.

Czech, W., Brautigam, M., Weidinger, G., and Schopf, E. A body-weight-independent dosing regimen of cyclosporine microemulsion is effective in severe atopic dermatitis and improves quality of life. *J. Am. Acad. Dermatol.,* **2000,** *42*:653–659.

Darkes, M.J., Scott, L.J., and Goa, K.L. Terbinafine: A review of its use in onychomycosis in adults. *Am. J. Clin. Dermatol.,* **2003,** *4*:39–65.

Darlington S., Williams G., Neale R., *et al.* A randomized, controlled trial to assess sunscreen application and β-carotene supplementation in the prevention of solar keratoses. *Arch. Dermatol.,* **2003,** *139*:451–455.

Dé Tran, Q.H., Guay, E., Charier, S., and Tousignant, J. Tacrolimus in dermatology. *J. Cutan. Med. Surg.,* **2001,** *5*:329–335.

DiGiovanna, J. Isotretinoin effects on bone. *J. Am. Acad. Dermatol.,* **2001,** *45*:S176–182.

Dinehart, S.M. The treatment of actinic keratoses. *J. Am. Acad. Dermatol.,* **2000,** *42*:25–28.

Duvic, M., and Marks, R. Tazarotene: Optimizing the therapeutic benefits of a new topical receptor-selective retinoid. Proceedings of a symposium held during the 19th World Congress of Dermatology, Sydney, Australia, 1997. *J. Am. Acad. Dermatol.,* **1998,** *39*:S123–152.

Edelson, R., Berger, C., Gasparro F., *et al.* Treatment of cutaneous T-cell lymphoma by extracorporeal photochemotherapy: Preliminary results. *New Engl. J. Med.,* **1987,** *316*:297–303.

Elewski, B.E., Fleischer, A.B., Jr., and Pariser, D.M. A comparison of 15% azelaic acid gel and 0.75% metronidazole gel in the topical treatment of papulopustular rosacea: Results of a randomized trial. *Arch. Dermatol.,* **2003,** *139*:1444–1450.

Food and Drug Administration (FDA). *FDA Public Health Advisory: Safety of Topical Lindane Products for the Treatment of Scabies and Lice.* Center for Drug Evaluation and Research, U.S. Food and Drug Administration, Rockville, MD, **2003.**

Fiedler, V.C. Understanding the causes of androgenetic alopecia. *Skin Aging,* March **1999,** pp. 72–80.

Fisher, G.J., and Voorhees, J.J. Molecular mechanisms of photoaging and its prevention by retinoic acid: Ultraviolet radiation induces MAP kinase signal transduction cascades that induce Ap-1 regulated matrix metalloproteinases that degrade human skin *in vivo. J. Invest. Dermatol. Symp. Proc.,* **1998,** *3*:61–68.

Frieling, U., and Luger, T.A. Mycophenolate mofetil and leflunomide: Promising compounds for the treatment of skin diseases. *Clin. Exp. Dermatol.,* **2002,** *27*:562–570.

Godar, D.E. Light and death: photons and apoptosis. *J. Invest. Dermatol. Symp. Proc.,* **1999,** *4*:17–23.

Goldsmith, L.A., Bolognia, J.L., Callen, J.P., *et al.* American Academy of Dermatology Consensus Conference on the safe and optimal use of isotretinoin: Summary and recommendations. *J. Am. Acad. Dermatol.,* **2004,** *50*:900–906.

Gollnick, H.P., and Krautheim, A. Topical treatment in acne: Current status and future aspects. *Dermatology,* **2003,** *206*:29–36.

Green, A., Williams, G., and Neal, R. Daily sunscreen application and β-carotene supplementation in prevention of basal cell and squamous

cell carcinomas of the skin: A randomized, controlled trial. *Lancet,* **1999,** *354*:723–729.

Hardman, K.A., Heath, D.A., and Nelson, H.M. Hypercalcaemia associated with calcipotriol (DOVONEX) treatment. *Br. Med. J.,* **1993,** *306*:896.

Hengge, U.R., Ruzicka, T., Tyring, S.K., *et al.* Update on Kaposi's sarcoma and other HHV8-associated diseases: 1. Epidemiology, environmental predispositions, clinical manifestations, and therapy. *Lancet Infect. Dis.,* **2002,** *2*:281–292.

Henseler, T., Wolff, K., Honigsmann, H., and Christophers, E. Oral 8-methoxypsoralen photochemotherapy of psoriasis. The European PUVA study: A cooperative study among 18 European centers. *Lancet,* **1981,** *1*:853–857.

Hessel, A.B., Cruz-Ramon, J.C., and Lin, A.N. Agents used for the treatment of hyperkeratosis. In, *Comprehensive Dermatologic Drug Therapy.* (Wolverton, S.E., ed.) Saunders, Philadelphia, **2001,** pp. 671–684.

Heydendael, V.M.R., Spuls, P.I., Opmeer, B.C., *et al.* Methotrexate versus cyclosporine in moderate-to-severe chronic plaque psoriasis. *New Engl. J. Med.,* **2003,** *349*:658–665.

Hong, W.K., Endicott, J., Itri, L.M., *et al.* 13-*cis*-Retinoic acid in the treatment of oral leukoplakia. *New Engl. J. Med.,* **1986,** *315*:1501–1505.

Hong, W.K., Lippman, S.M., Itri, L.M., *et al.* Prevention of second primary tumors with isotretinoin in squamous cell carcinoma of the head and neck. *New Engl. J. Med.,* **1990,** *323*:795–801.

Hsu, S., and Quan, L.T. Topical antibacterial agents. In, *Comprehensive Dermatologic Drug Therapy.* (Wolverton, S.E., ed.) Saunders, Philadelphia, **2001,** pp. 472–496.

Kalka, K., Merk, H., and Mukhtar, J. Photodynamic therapy in dermatology. *J. Am. Acad. Dermatol.,* **2000,** *42*:389–413.

Kaufman, K.D., Olsen, E.A., Whiting, D., *et al.* Finasteride in the treatment of men with androgenetic alopecia. Finasteride Male Pattern Hair Loss Study Group. *J. Am. Acad. Dermatol.,* **1998,** *39*:578–589.

Kligman, A.M., Grove, G.L., Hirose, R., and Leyden, J.J. Topical tretinoin for photoaged skin. *J. Am. Acad. Dermatol.,* **1986,** *15*:836–859.

Knobler, R., and Girardi, M. Extracorporeal photochemoimmunotherapy in cutaneous T-cell lymphomas. *Ann. N.Y. Acad. Sci.,* **2001,** *941*:123–38.

Korting, H.C., Blecher, P., Schafer-Korting, M., and Wendel, A. Topical liposome drugs to come: what the patent literature tells us: A review. *J. Am. Acad. Dermatol.,* **1991,** *25*:1068–1071.

Kraemer, K.H., DiGiovanna, J.J., Moshell, A.N., *et al.* Prevention of skin cancer in xeroderma pigmentosum with the use of oral isotretinoin. *New Engl. J. Med.,* **1988,** *318*:1633–1637.

Kragballe, K. Treatment of psoriasis with calcipotriol and other vitamin D analogues. *J. Am. Acad. Dermatol.,* **1992,** *27*:1001–1008.

Lammer, E.J., Chen, D.T., Hoar, R.M., *et al.* Retinoic acid embryopathy. *New Engl. J. Med.,* **1985,** *313*:837–841.

Lebwohl, M. Acitretin in combination with UVB or PUVA. *J. Am. Acad. Dermatol.,* **1999,** *41*:S22–24.

Lebwohl, M., Menter, A., Koo, J., and Feldman, S.R. Combination therapy to treat moderate to severe psoriasis. *J. Am. Acad. Dermatol.* **2004,** *50*:416–430.

Leyden, J.J. Current issues in antimicrobial therapy for the treatment of acne. *J. Eur. Acad. Dermatol. Venereol.,* **2001,** *15*(suppl. 3):51–55.

Leyden, J., Dunlap, F., Miller, B., *et al.* Finasteride in the treatment of men with frontal male pattern hair loss. *J. Am. Acad. Dermatol.,* **1999,** *40*:930–937.

Ling, M.R. Acitretin: Optimal dosing strategies. *J. Am. Acad. Dermatol.,* **1999,** *41*:S13–17.

Ling, T.C., Faulkner, C., and Rhodes, L.E. A questionnaire survey of attitudes to and usage of sunscreens in northwest England. *Photodermatol. Photoimmunol. Photomed.,* **2003,** *19*:98–101.

Lippert, U., Artuc, M., Grutzkau, A., *et al.* Human skin mast cells express H_2 and H_4, but not H_3 receptors. *J. Invest. Dermatol.,* **2004,** *123*:116–123.

Melski, J.W., Tanenbaum, L., Parrish, J.A., *et al.* Oral methoxsalen photochemotherapy for the treatment of psoriasis: A cooperative clinical trial. *J. Invest. Dermatol.,* **1977,** *68*:328–335.

Metze, D., Reimann, S., Biessert, S., and Luger, T. Efficacy and safety of naltrexone, an oral opiate receptor antagonist, in the treatment of pruritus in internal and dermatological diseases. *J. Am. Acad. Dermatol.,* **1999,** *41*:533–539.

Morimoto, S., and Kumahara, Y. A patient with psoriasis cured by 1-α-hydroxyvitamin D_3. *Med. J. Osaka Univ.,* **1985,** *35*:51–54.

Ngheim, P., Pearson, G., and Langley, R.G. Tacrolimus and pimecrolimus: From clever prokaryotes to inhibiting calcineurin and treating atopic dermatitis. *J. Am. Acad. Dermatol.,* **2002,** *46*:228–241.

Nijsten, T.E., and Stern, R.S. Oral retinoid use reduces cutaneous squamous cell carcinoma risk in patients with psoriasis treated with psoralen–UVA: A nested cohort study. *J. Am. Acad. Dermatol.,* **2003,** *49*:644–650.

Olsen, A.E., Abernethy, M.L., Kulp-Shorten, C., *et al.* A double-blind, vehicle-controlled study evaluating masoprocol cream in the treatment of actinic keratoses on the head and neck. *J. Am. Acad. Dermatol.,* **1991,** *24*:738–743.

Olsen, E., Duvic, M., Frankel, A., *et al.* Pivotal phase III trial of two dose levels of denileukin diftitox for the treatment of cutaneous T-cell lymphoma. *J. Clin. Oncol.,* **2001,** *19*:376–388.

Orlow, S.J., and Paller, A. Cimetidine therapy for multiple viral warts in children. *J. Am. Acad. Dermatol.,* **1993,** *28*:794–796.

Peck, G.L., DiGiovanna, J.J., Sarnoff, D.S., *et al.* Treatment and prevention of basal cell carcinoma with oral isotretinoin. *J. Am. Acad. Dermatol.,* **1988,** *19*:176–185.

Petkovich, M. Retinoic acid metabolism. *J. Am. Acad. Dermatol.,* **2001,** *45*:136–142.

Piacquadio, D., and Kligman, A. The critical role of the vehicle to therapeutic efficacy and patient compliance. *J. Am. Acad. Dermatol.,* **1998,** *39*:S67–73.

Piacquadio, D.J., Chen, D.M., Farber, H.F., *et al.* Photodynamic therapy with aminolevulinic acid topical solution and visible blue light in the treatment of multiple actinic keratoses of the face and scalp: investigator-blinded, phase 3, multicenter trials. *Arch Dermatol.,* **2004,** *140*:41–46.

Prins, C., Kerdel, F.A., Padilla, S., *et al.* Treatment of toxic epidermal necrolysis with high-dose intravenous immunoglobulins: Multicenter retrospective analysis of 48 consecutive cases. *Arch. Dermatol.,* **2003,** *139*:26–32.

Repka-Ramirez, M.S., and Baraniuk, J.N. Histamine in health and disease. *Clin. Allergy Immunol.,* **2002,** *17*:1–25.

Rigel, D.S. The effect of sunscreen on melanoma risk. *Dermatol. Clin.,* **2002,** *20*:601–606.

Roenigk, H.H., Auerbach, R., Maibach, H., *et al.* Methotrexate in psoriasis: Consensus conference. *J. Am. Acad. Dermatol.,* **1998,** *38*:478–485.

Sapadin, A.N., and Fleischmajer, R. Treatment of scleroderma. *Arch. Dermatol.,* **2002,** *138*:99–105.

Saporito, F.C., and Menter, M.A. Methotrexate and psoriasis in the era of new biologic agents. *J. Am. Acad. Dermatol.,* **2004,** *50*:301–309.

Saurat, J.H. Retinoids and psoriasis: Novel issues in retinoid pharmacology and implications for psoriasis treatment. *J. Am. Acad. Dermatol.,* **1999,** *41*:S2–S6.

Sherman, S.I. Etiology, diagnosis, and treatment recommendations for central hypothyroidism associated with bexarotene therapy for cutaneous T-cell lymphoma. *Clin. Lymphoma,* **2003,** *3*:249–252.

Shroot, B. Pharmacodynamics and pharmacokinetics of topical adapalene. *J. Am. Acad. Dermatol.,* **1998,** *39*:S17–24.

Shupack, J., Abel, E., Bayer, E., *et al.* Cyclosporine as maintenance therapy in patients with severe psoriasis. *J. Am. Acad. Dermatol.,* **1997,** *36*:423–432.

Sigmundsdottir, H., Johnston A., Gudjonsson, J.E., *et al.* Methotrexate markedly reduces the expression of vascular E-selectin, cutaneous lymphocyte-associated antigen and the numbers of mononuclear leucocytes in psoriatic skin. *Exp. Dermatol.,* **2004,** *13*:426–434.

Sommer, A., Veraart, J., Neumann, M., and Kessels, A. Evaluation of the vasoconstrictive effects of topical steroids by laser–Doppler perfusion imaging. *Acta Derm. Venereol.,* **1998,** *78*:15–18.

Tan, H.H. Antibacterial therapy for acne: A guide to selection and use of systemic agents. *Am. J. Clin. Dermatol.,* **2003,** *4*:307–314.

Templeton, S.F., Solomon, A.R., and Swerlick, R.A. Intradermal bleomycin injections into normal human skin: A histologic and immunopathologic study. *Arch. Dermatol.,* **1994,** *130*:577–583.

Thompson, S.C., Jolley, D., and Marks, R. Reduction of solar keratoses by regular sunscreen use. *New Engl. J. Med.,* **1993,** *329*:1147–1151.

Thuong-Nguyen, V., Kadunce, D.P., Hendrix, J.D., *et al.* Inhibition of neutrophil adherence to antibody by dapsone: A possible therapeutic mechanism of dapsone in the treatment of IgA dermatoses. *J. Invest. Dermatol.,* **1993,** *100*:349–355.

Usha, V., Gopalakrishnan, T.V., and Nair, T.V. A comparative study of oral ivermectin and topical permethrin cream in the treatment of scabies. *J. Am. Acad. Dermatol.,* **2000,** *42*:236–240.

Van Scott, E.J., and Yu, R.J. Hyperkeratinization, corneocyte cohesion and α-hydroxy acids. *J. Am. Acad. Dermatol.,* **1984,** *11*:867–879.

Walmsley, S., Northfelt, D.W., Melosky, B., *et al.* Treatment of AIDS-related cutaneous Kaposiís sarcoma with topical alitretinoin (9-*cis*-retinoic acid) gel. Panretin Gel North American Study Group. *J. Acquir. Immune Defic. Syndr.,* **1999,** *22*:235–246.

Webster, G.F. Topical tretinoin in acne therapy. *J. Am. Acad. Dermatol.,* **1998,** *39*:S38–44.

Weiss, J.S., and Shavin, J.S. Adapalene for the treatment of acne vulgaris. *J. Am. Acad. Dermatol.,* **1998,** *39*:S50–54.

White, J.A., Beckett-Jones, B., Guo, Y.D., *et al.* cDNA cloning of human retinoic acid–metabolizing enzyme (hP450RAI) identifies a novel family of cytochromes P450. *J. Biol. Chem.,* **1997,** *272*:18538–18541.

Wolff, H.H., Plewig, G., and Braun-Falco, O. Ultrastructure of human sebaceous follicles and comedones following treatment with vitamin A acid. *Acta. Dermatol. Venereol.,* **1975,** *55*:S99–110

Zackheim, H.S., Epstein, E.H., Jr., and Crain, W.R. Topical carmustine (BCNU) for cutaneous T-cell lymphoma: A 15-year experience in 143 patients. *J. Am. Acad. Dermatol.,* **1990,** *22*:802–810.

MONOGRAPHS AND REVIEWS

Abess, A., Keel, D.M., and Graham, B.S. Flagellate hyperpigmentation following intralesional bleomycin treatment of verruca plantaris. *Arch. Dermatol.,* **2003,** *139*:337–339.

Assmann, T., and Ruzicka, T. New immunosuppressive drugs in dermatology (mycophenolate mofetil, tacrolimus): unapproved uses, dosages, or indications. *Dermatol. Clin.,* **2002,** *20*:505–514.

Baron, J.M., Holler, D., Schiffer, R., *et al.* Expression of multiple cytochrome P450 enzymes and multidrug resistance–associated transport proteins in human skin keratinocytes. *J. Invest. Dermatol.,* **2001,** *116*:541–548.

Carter, E.L. Antibiotics in cutaneous medicine: An update. *Semin. Cutan. Med. Surg.,* **2003,** *22*:196–211.

Caterina, M., and Julius, D. The vanilloid receptor: A molecular gateway to the pain pathway. *Annu. Rev. Neurosci.,* **2001,** *24*:487–517.

Cather, J.C., Abramovits, W., and Menter, A. Cyclosporine and tacrolimus in dermatology. *Dermatol. Clin.,* **2001,** *19*:119–137.

Colsky, A.S. Intravenous immunoglobulin in autoimmune and inflammatory dermatoses: A review of the proposed mechanisms of action and therapeutic applications. *Dermatol. Clin.,* **2000,** *18*:447–457.

Du, L., Hoffman, S.M.G., and Keeney, D.S. Epidermal CYP2 family cytochrome P450. *Toxicol. Appl. Pharmacol.,* **2004,** *195*:278–287.

Ebling, F.J.G. Functions of the skin. In, *Rook, Wilkinson, Ebling Textbook of Dermatology,* 5th ed. (Champion, R.H., Burton, J.L., Ebling, F.J.G., eds.) Blackwell Scientific Publications, Oxford, England, **1993,** pp. 125–155.

Flores, F., and Kerdel, F.A. Other novel immunosuppressants. *Dermatol. Clin.,* **2000,** *18*:475–483.

Fox, L.P., and Pandya, A G. Pulse intravenous cyclophosphamide therapy for dermatologic disorders. *Dermatol. Clin.,* **2000,** *18*:459–473.

Franks, M.E., Macpherson, G.R., and Figg, W.D. Thalidomide. *Lancet,* **2004,** *363*:1802–1811.

Goldfork, M.T., and Ellis, C. Clinical uses of etretinate and acitretin. In, *Psoriasis,* 3d ed. (Roenigk, H.H., Jr., and Maibach, H.I., eds.) Marcel Dekker, New York, **1998,** pp. 663–670.

Green, L.J., McCormick, A., and Weinstein, G.D. Photoaging and the skin: The effects of tretinoin. *Dermatol. Clin.,* **1993,** *11*:97–105.

Gupta, A.K., Sauder, D.N., and Shear, N.H. Antifungal agents: An overview, part I. *J. Am. Acad. Dermatol.,* **1994a,** *30*:677–698.

Gupta, A.K., Sauder, D.N., and Shear, N.H. Antifungal agents: An overview, part II. *J. Am. Acad. Dermatol.,* **1994b,** *30*:911–933.

Harber, L.C., and Bickers, D.R. *Photosensitivity Diseases: Principles of Diagnosis and Treatment,* 2d ed. B.C. Decker, Philadelphia, **1989.**

Harper, J.C., and Thiboutot, D.M. Pathogenesis of acne: Recent research advances. *Adv Dermatol.,* **2003,** *19*:1–10.

Ho, V.C., and Zloty, D.M. Immunosuppressive agents in dermatology. *Dermatol. Clin.,* **1993,** *11*:73–85.

Katz, H.I., Waalen, J., and Leach, E.E. Acitretin in psoriasis: An overview of adverse effects. *J. Am. Acad. Dermatol.,* **1999,** *41*:S7–12.

Krueger, G. and Callis, K. Potential of tumor necrosis factor inhibitors in psoriasis and psoriatic arthritis. *Arch. Dermatol.,* **2004,** *140*:218–225.

Layton, A.M., and Cunliffe, W.J. Guidelines for optimal use of isotretinoin in acne. *J. Am. Acad. Dermatol.,* **1992,** *27*: S2–7.

Layton, A.M., Knaggs, H., Taylor, J., and Cunliffe, W.J. Isotretinoin for acne vulgaris 10 years later: A safe and successful treatment. *Br. J. Dermatol.,* **1993,** *129*:292–296.

Leyden, J.J. Retinoids and acne. *J. Am. Acad. Dermatol.,* **1988,** *19*:164–168.

Leyden, J.J. Review of mupirocin ointment in the treatment of impetigo. *Clin. Pediatr.,* **1992,** *31*:549–553.

Lopez, R.F., Lange, N., Guy. R, and Bentley, M.V. Photodynamic therapy of skin cancer: Controlled drug delivery of 5-ALA and its esters. *Adv. Drug Deliv. Rev.,* **2004,** *56*:77–94.

Monroe, E.W. Nonsedating H_1 antihistamines in chronic urticaria. *Ann. Allergy,* **1993,** *71*:585–591.

Moosavi, M., Bagheri, B., and Scher, R. Systemic antifungal therapy. *Dermatol. Clin.,* **2001,** *19*:35–52.

Paniker, U., and Levine, N. Dapsone and sulfapyridine. *Dermatol. Clin.,* **2001,** *19*:79–86.

Parke, A.L. Antimalarial drugs, pregnancy and lactation. *Lupus,* **1993,** *2*:S21–23.

Peris, K., Fargnoli, M.C., and Chimenti, S. Preliminary observations on the use of topical tazarotene to treat basal cell carcinoma. *New Engl. J. Med.,* **1999,** *341*:1767–1768.

Reynolds, N.J., and Al-Daraji, W.I. Calcineurin inhibitors and sirolimus: Mechanisms of action and applications in dermatology. *Clin. Exp. Dermatol.,* **2002,** *27*:555–561.

Salasche, S., and Shumack, S. A review of imiquimod 5% cream for the treatment of various dermatological conditions. *Clin. Exp. Dermatol.,* **2003,** *28*(suppl.):1–3.

Scheinfeld, N., and Deleo, V. A review of studies that have utilized different combinations of psoralen and ultraviolet B phototherapy and ultraviolet A phototherapy. *Dermatol. Online J.,* **2003,** *9*:7.

Schweiger, E.S., and Weinberg, J.M. Novel antibacterial agents for skin and skin structure infections. *J. Am. Acad. Dermatol.,* **2004,** *50*:331–340.

Silvis, N.G. Antimetabolites and cytotoxic drugs. *Dermatol. Clin.,* **2001,** *19*:105–118.

Smith, K. Expert advice on using Accutane. *Skin Aging,* October **1999,** pp. 62–70.

Stander, S., Steinhoff, M., Schmelz, M., *et al.* Neurophysiology of pruritus: Cutaneous elicitation of itch. *Arch. Dermatol.,* **2003,** *139*:1463–1470.

Stern, R.S. Treatment of photoaging. *New Eng. J. Med.,* **2004,** *350*:1526–1534.

Taub, A.F. Photodynamic therapy in dermatology: history and horizons. *J. Drugs Dermatol.,* **2004,** *3*(suppl. 1):S8–25.

Van Beek, M.J. and Piette, W.W. Antimalarials. *Dermatol. Clin.,* **2001,** *19*:147–160.

Weinberg, J.M. An overview of infliximab, etanercept, efalizumab, and alefacept as biologic therapy for psoriasis. *Clin. Ther.,* **2003,** *25*:2487–24505

Werth, V.P. Management and treatment with systemic glucocorticoids. *Adv. Dermatol.,* **1993,** *8*:81–103.

Wines, N.Y., Cooper, A.J., and Wines, M.P. Thalidomide in dermatology. *Austral. J. Dermatol.,* **2002,** *45*:229–240.

Winterfield, L., Cather, J., Cather, J. and Menter, A. Changing paradigms in dermatology: Nuclear hormone receptors. *Clin. Dermatol.,* **2003,** *21*:447–454.

Yohn, J.J., and Weston, W.L. Topical glucocorticoids. *Curr. Probl. Dermatol.,* **1990,** *11*:37–63.

Zhang, C., and Duvic, M.P. Retinoids: Therapeutic applications and mechanisms of action in cutaneous T-cell lymphoma. *Dermatol. Ther.,* **2003,** *16*:322–330.

Zhu, Y.I., and Stiller, M.J. Dapsone and sulfones in dermatology: Overview and update. *J. Am. Acad. Dermatol.,* **2001,** *45*:420–434.

OCULAR PHARMACOLOGY

Jeffrey D. Henderer and Christopher J. Rapuano

OVERVIEW OF OCULAR ANATOMY, PHYSIOLOGY, AND BIOCHEMISTRY

The eye is a specialized sensory organ that is relatively secluded from systemic access by the blood–retinal, blood–aqueous, and blood–vitreous barriers; as a consequence, the eye exhibits some unusual pharmacodynamic and pharmacokinetic properties. Because of its anatomical isolation, the eye offers a unique, organ-specific pharmacological laboratory to study the autonomic nervous system and effects of inflammation and infectious diseases. No other organ in the body is so readily accessible or as visible for observation; however, the eye also presents some unique opportunities as well as challenges for drug delivery (Robinson, 1993).

Extraocular Structures

The eye is protected by the eyelids and by the orbit, a bony cavity of the skull that has multiple fissures and foramina that conduct nerves, muscles, and vessels (Figure 63–1). In the orbit, connective (*i.e.,* Tenon's capsule) and adipose tissues and six extraocular muscles support and align the eyes for vision. The retrobulbar region lies immediately behind the eye (or *globe*). Understanding ocular and orbital anatomy is important for safe periocular drug delivery, including subconjunctival, sub-Tenon's, and retrobulbar injections.

The eyelids serve several functions. Foremost, their dense sensory innervation and eyelashes protect the eye from mechanical and chemical injuries. Blinking, a coordinated movement of the orbicularis oculi, levator palpebrae, and Müller's muscles, serves to distribute tears over the cornea and conjunctiva. In humans, the average blink rate is 15 to 20 times per minute. The external surface of the eyelids is covered by a thin layer of skin; the internal surface is lined with the palpebral portion of the conjunctiva, which is a vascularized mucous membrane continuous with the bulbar conjunctiva. At the reflection of the palpebral and bulbar conjunctivae is a space called the fornix, located superiorly and inferiorly behind the upper and lower lids, respectively. Topical medications usually are placed in the inferior fornix, also known as the inferior cul-de-sac.

The lacrimal system consists of secretory glandular and excretory ductal elements (Figure 63–2). The secretory system is composed of the main lacrimal gland, which is located in the temporal outer portion of the orbit, and accessory glands, also known as the glands of Krause and Wolfring (Figure 63–1), located in the conjunctiva. The lacrimal gland is innervated by the autonomic nervous system (Table 63–1 and Chapter 6). The parasympathetic innervation is clinically relevant since a patient may complain of dry eye symptoms while taking medications with anticholinergic side effects, such as tricyclic antidepressants (*see* Chapter 17), antihistamines (*see* Chapter 25),

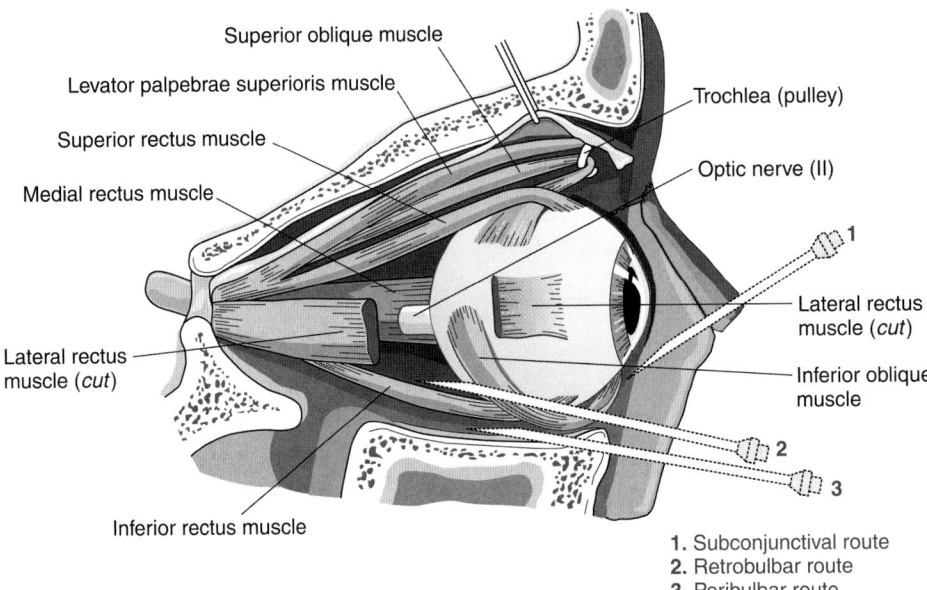

1. Subconjunctival route
2. Retrobulbar route
3. Peribulbar route

Figure 63–1. Anatomy of the globe in relationship to the orbit and eyelids. Various routes of administration of anesthesia are demonstrated by the blue needle pathways.

and drugs used in the management of Parkinson's disease (*see* Chapter 20). Located just posterior to the eyelashes are meibomian glands (Figure 63–1), which secrete oils that retard evaporation of the tear film. Abnormalities in gland function, as in acne rosacea and meibomitis, can greatly affect tear film stability.

Conceptually, tears constitute a trilaminar lubrication barrier covering the conjunctiva and cornea. The anterior layer is composed primarily of lipids secreted by the meibomian glands. The middle aqueous layer, produced by the main lacrimal gland and accessory lacrimal glands

(*i.e.,* Krause and Wolfring glands), constitutes about 98% of the tear film. Adherent to the corneal epithelium, the posterior layer is a mixture of mucins produced by goblet cells in the conjunctiva. Tears also contain nutrients, enzymes, and immunoglobulins to support and protect the cornea.

The tear drainage system starts through small puncta located on the medial aspects of both the upper and lower eyelids (Figure 63–2). With blinking, tears enter the puncta and continue to drain through the canaliculi, lacrimal sac, nasolacrimal duct, and then into the nose. The nose is

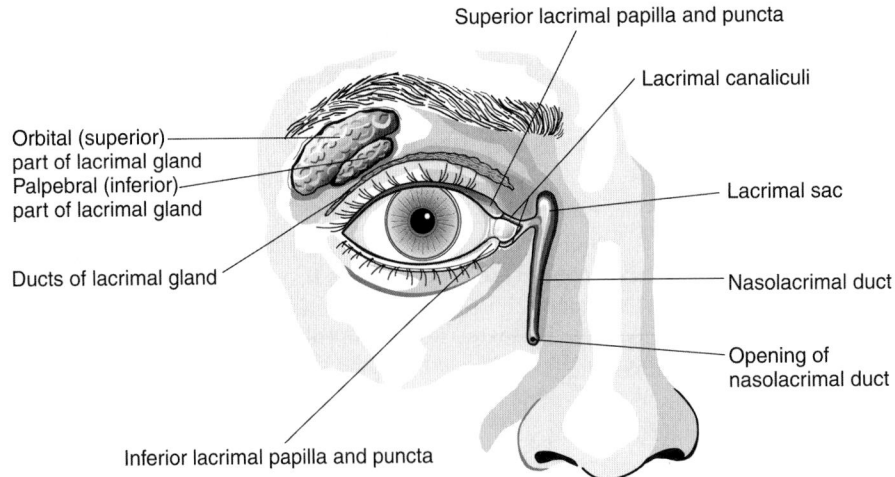

Figure 63–2. Anatomy of the lacrimal system.

Table 63–1

Autonomic Pharmacology of the Eye and Related Structures

TISSUE	Adrenergic Receptors			Cholinergic Receptors	
	SUBTYPE	RESPONSE		SUBTYPE	RESPONSE
Corneal epithelium	β_2	Unknown		M[†]	Unknown
Corneal endothelium	β_2	Unknown		Undefined	Unknown
Iris radial muscle	α_1	Mydriasis			
Iris sphincter muscle				M_3	Miosis
Trabecular meshwork	β_2	Unknown			
Ciliary epithelium[‡]	α_2/β_2	Aqueous production			
Ciliary muscle	β_2	Relaxation[§]		M_3	Accommodation
Lacrimal gland	α_1	Secretion		M_2, M_3	Secretion
Retinal pigment epithelium	α_1/β_2	H_2O transport/unknown			

[†]Although acetylcholine and choline acetyltransferase are abundant in corneal epithelium of most species, the function of this neurotransmitter in this tissue is unknown. [‡]The ciliary epithelium is also the target of carbonic anhydrase inhibitors. Carbonic anhydrase isoenzyme II is localized to both the pigmented and nonpigmented ciliary epithelium. [§]Although β_2 adrenergic receptors mediate ciliary body smooth muscle relaxation, there is no clinically significant effect on accommodation.

lined by a highly vascular mucosal epithelium; consequently, topically applied medications that pass through this nasolacrimal system have direct access to the systemic circulation.

Ocular Structures

The eye is divided into anterior and posterior segments (Figure 63–3A). Anterior segment structures include the cornea, limbus, anterior and posterior chambers, trabecular meshwork, Schlemm's canal, iris, lens, zonule, and ciliary body. The posterior segment comprises the vitreous, retina, choroid, sclera, and optic nerve.

Anterior Segment. The cornea is a transparent and avascular tissue organized into five layers: epithelium, Bowman's membrane, stroma, Descemet's membrane, and endothelium (Figure 63–3B).

Representing an important barrier to foreign matter, including drugs, the hydrophobic epithelial layer comprises five to six cell layers. The basal epithelial cells lie on a basement membrane that is adjacent to Bowman's membrane, a layer of collagen fibers. Constituting approximately 90% of the corneal thickness, the stroma, a hydrophilic layer, is uniquely organized with collagen lamellae synthesized by keratocytes. Beneath the stroma lies Descemet's membrane, the basement membrane of the corneal endothelium. Lying most posteriorly, the endothelium is a monolayer of cells adhering to each other by tight junctions. These cells maintain corneal integrity by active transport processes and serve as a hydrophobic barrier. Hence, drug absorption across the cornea requires penetration of the trilaminar hydrophobic-hydrophilic-hydrophobic domains of the various anatomical layers.

At the periphery of the cornea and adjacent to the sclera lies a transitional zone (1 to 2 mm wide) called the limbus. Limbal structures include the conjunctival epithelium, which contains the stem cells, Tenon's capsule, episclera, corneoscleral stroma, Schlemm's canal, and trabecular meshwork (Figure 63–3B). Limbal blood vessels, as well as the tears, provide important nutrients and immunological defense mechanisms for the cornea. The anterior chamber holds approximately 250 μl of aqueous humor. The peripheral anterior chamber angle is formed by the cornea and the iris root. The trabecular meshwork and canal of Schlemm are located just above the apex of this angle. The posterior chamber, which holds approximately 50 μl of aqueous humor, is defined by the boundaries of the ciliary body processes, posterior surface of the iris, and lens surface.

Aqueous Humor Dynamics and Regulation of Intraocular Pressure. Aqueous humor is secreted by the ciliary processes and flows from the posterior chamber, through the pupil, into the anterior chamber, and leaves the eye primarily by the trabecular meshwork and canal of Schlemm. From the canal of Schlemm, aqueous humor drains into an episcleral venous plexus and into the systemic circulation. This conventional pathway accounts for 80% to 95% of aqueous humor outflow and is the main target for cholinergic drugs used in glaucoma therapy. Another outflow pathway is the uveoscleral route (*i.e.,* fluid flows through the ciliary muscles and into the suprachoroidal space), which is the target of selective prostanoids (*see* Chapter 25 and later in this chapter).

The peripheral anterior chamber angle is an important anatomical structure for differentiating two forms of glaucoma: open-angle glaucoma, which is by far the most common form of glaucoma in the United States, and angle-closure glaucoma. Current medical therapy of *open-angle glaucoma* is aimed at decreasing aqueous humor production and/or increasing aqueous outflow. The preferred management for *angle-closure glaucoma* is surgical iridectomy, either by laser or by incision, but short-term medical management

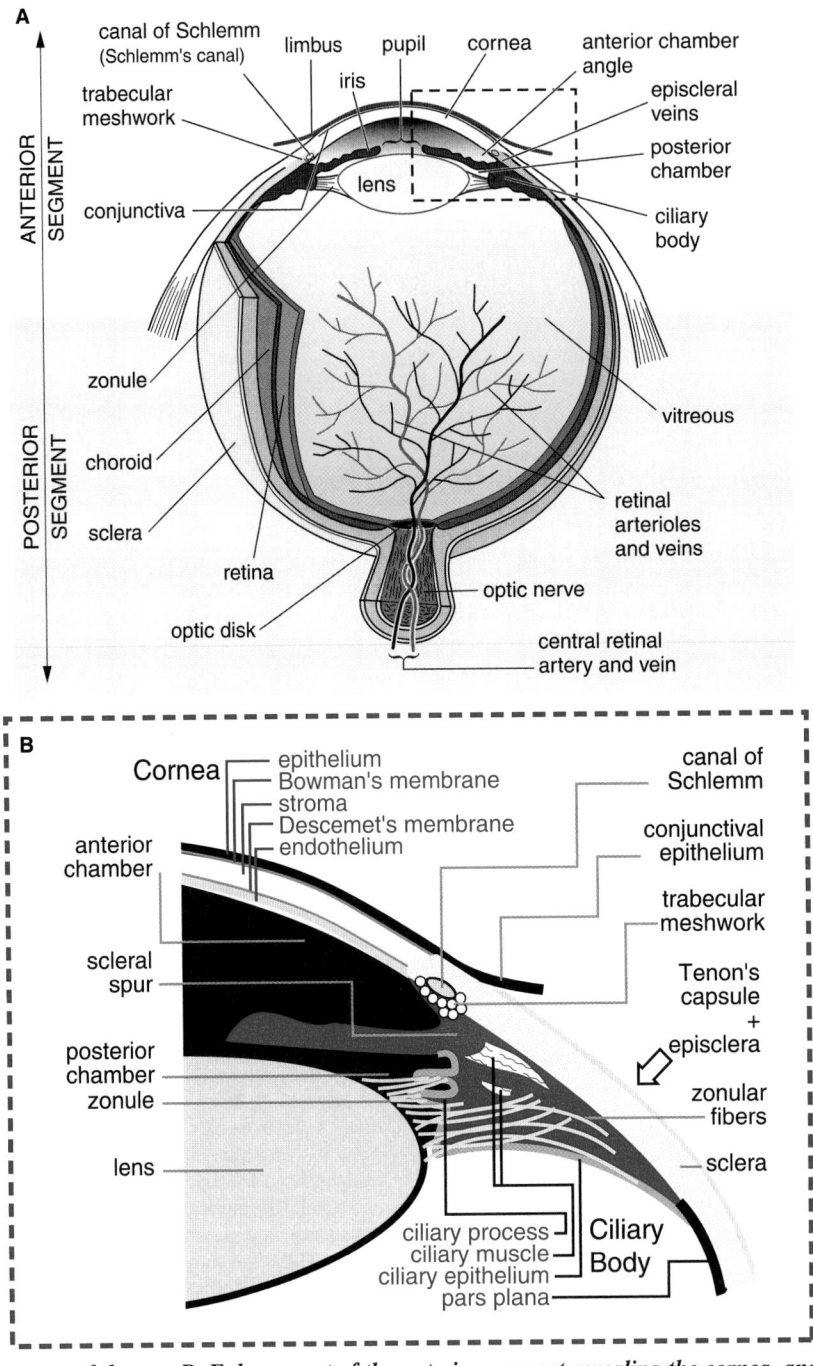

Figure 63–3. *A. Anatomy of the eye. B. Enlargement of the anterior segment revealing the cornea, angle structures, lens, and ciliary body.* (*B.* Adapted with permission from Riordan-Eva, P., Tabbara, K.F. Anatomy and embryology of the eye. In, *General Ophthalmology*, 13th ed. (Vaughan, D., Asbury, T., Riordan-Eva, P., eds.) Appleton & Lange, Stamford, CT, **1992.**)

may be necessary to reduce the acute intraocular pressure elevation and to clear the cornea prior to surgery. Long-term intraocular pressure reduction may be necessary, especially if the peripheral iris has permanently covered the trabecular meshwork. Acute angle-closure glaucoma may be induced rarely in anatomically predisposed eyes

by anticholinergic, sympathomimetic, and antihistaminic agents. Interestingly, however, individuals with susceptible angles are not aware of a risk of angle-closure glaucoma. Unfortunately, drug warning labels do not always specify the type of glaucoma for which this rare risk exists. Thus, unwarranted concern is raised among patients who have open-angle glaucoma who need not be concerned about taking these drugs. In any event, in anatomically susceptible eyes, anticholinergic, sympathomimetic, and antihistaminic drugs can lead to partial dilation of the pupil and a change in the vectors of force between the iris and the lens. The aqueous humor then is prevented from passing through the pupil from the posterior chamber to the anterior chamber. The result is known as an acute attack of pupillary-block angle-closure glaucoma. The change in the lens-iris relationship leads to an increase in pressure in the posterior chamber, causing the iris base to be pushed against the angle wall, thereby closing the filtration angle and markedly elevating the intraocular pressure.

Iris and Pupil. The iris is the most anterior portion of the uveal tract, which also includes the ciliary body and choroid. The anterior surface of the iris is the stroma, a loosely organized structure containing melanocytes, blood vessels, smooth muscle, and parasympathetic and sympathetic nerves. Differences in iris color reflect individual variation in the number of melanocytes located in the stroma. Individual variation may be an important consideration for ocular drug distribution due to drug-melanin binding (*see* "Distribution," below). The posterior surface of the iris is a densely pigmented bilayer of epithelial cells. Anterior to the pigmented epithelium, the dilator smooth muscle is oriented radially and is innervated by the sympathetic nervous system (Figure 63–4) which causes mydriasis (dilation). At the pupillary margin, the sphincter smooth muscle is organized in a circular band with parasympathetic innervation, which when stimulated causes miosis (constriction). The use of pharmacological agents to dilate normal pupils (*i.e.*, for clinical purposes such as examining the ocular fundus) and to evaluate the pharmacological response of the pupil (*e.g.*, unequal pupils, or anisocoria, seen in Horner's syndrome or Adie's pupil) is summarized in Table 63–2. Figure 63–5 provides a flowchart for the diagnostic evaluation of anisocoria.

Ciliary Body. The ciliary body serves two very specialized roles in the eye: secretion of aqueous humor by the epithelial bilayer and accommodation by the ciliary muscle. The anterior portion of the ciliary body, called the pars plicata, is composed of 70 to 80 ciliary processes with intricate folds. The posterior portion is the pars plana. The ciliary muscle is organized into outer longitudinal, middle radial, and inner circular layers. Coordinated contraction of this smooth muscle apparatus by the parasympathetic nervous system causes the zonule suspending the lens to relax, allowing the lens to become more convex and to shift slightly forward. This process, known as *accommodation*, permits focusing on near objects and may be pharmacologically blocked by muscarinic cholinergic antagonists, through the process called *cycloplegia*. Contraction of the ciliary muscle also puts traction on the scleral spur, and

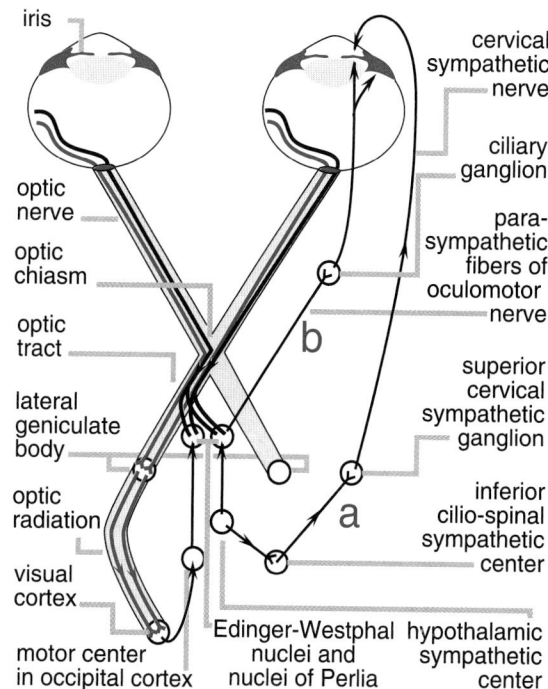

Figure 63–4. *Autonomic innervation of the eye by the sympathetic (a) and parasympathetic (b) nervous systems.* (Adapted with permission from Wybar, K.C., Karr Muir, M. *Baillière's Concise Medical Textbooks, Ophthalmology,* 3rd ed. Baillière Tindall, New York, 1984.)

hence widens the spaces within the trabecular meshwork. This latter effect accounts for at least some of the intraocular pressure–lowering effect of both directly acting and indirectly acting parasympathomimetic drugs.

Lens. The lens, a transparent biconvex structure, is suspended by *zonules,* specialized fibers emanating from the ciliary body. The lens is approximately 10 mm in diameter and is enclosed in a capsule. The bulk of the lens is composed of fibers derived from proliferating lens epithelial cells located under the anterior portion of the lens capsule. These lens fibers are continuously produced throughout life. Aging, in addition to certain medications, such as corticosteroids, and certain diseases, such as diabetes mellitus, cause the lens to become opacified, which is termed a *cataract*.

Posterior Segment. Because of the anatomical and vascular barriers to both local and systemic access, drug delivery to the eye's posterior pole is particularly challenging.

Sclera. The outermost coat of the eye, the sclera, covers the posterior portion of the globe. The external surface of the scleral shell is covered by an episcleral vascular coat, by Tenon's capsule, and by the conjunctiva. The ten-

Table 63–2
Effects of Pharmacological Agents on the Pupil

CLINICAL SETTING	DRUG*	PUPILLARY RESPONSE
Normal	Sympathomimetic drugs	Dilation (mydriasis)
Normal	Parasympathomimetic drugs	Constriction (miosis)
Horner's syndrome	Cocaine 4–10%	No dilation
Preganglionic Horner's	Hydroxyamphetamine 1%	Dilation
Postganglionic Horner's	Hydroxyamphetamine 1%	No dilation
Adie's pupil	Pilocarpine 0.05–0.1%†	Constriction
Normal	Opioids (oral or intravenous)	Pinpoint pupils

*Topically applied ophthalmic drugs unless otherwise noted. †This percentage of pilocarpine is not commercially available and usually is prepared by the physician administering the test or by a pharmacist. This test also requires that no prior manipulation of the cornea (*i.e.*, tonometry for measuring intraocular pressure or testing corneal sensation) be done so that the normal integrity of the corneal barrier is intact. Normal pupils will not respond to this weak dilution of pilocarpine; however, an Adie's pupil manifests a denervation supersensitivity and is, therefore, pharmacodynamically responsive to this dilute cholinergic agonist.

dons of the six extraocular muscles insert into the superficial scleral collagen fibers. Numerous blood vessels pierce the sclera through emissaria to supply as well as drain the choroid, ciliary body, optic nerve, and iris.

Inside the scleral shell, the vascular choroid nourishes the outer retina by a capillary system in the choriocapillaris. Between the outer retina and the choriocapillaris lie Bruch's membrane and the retinal pigment epithelium, whose tight junctions provide an outer barrier between the retina and the choroid. The retinal pigment epithelium serves many functions, including vitamin A metabolism, phagocytosis of the rod outer segments, and multiple transport processes.

Retina. The retina is a thin, transparent, highly organized structure of neurons, glial cells, and blood vessels. Of all structures within the eye, the neurosensory retina has been the most widely studied. The unique organization and biochemistry of the photoreceptors have provided a superb system for investigating signal transduction mechanisms. The wealth of information about rhodopsin has made it an excellent model for the G protein–coupled signal transduc-

tion. Such detailed understanding holds promise for targeted therapy for some of the hereditary retinal diseases.

Vitreous. Approximately 80% of the eye's volume is the vitreous, which is a clear medium containing collagen type II, hyaluronic acid, proteoglycans, a variety of macromolecules including glucose, ascorbic acid, amino acids, and a number of inorganic salts. Glutamate in the vitreous has been suspected to have a possible relationship to glaucoma. The ganglion cells appear to die in glaucoma *via* a process of apoptosis (Quigley *et al.*, 1995; Wax *et al.*, 1998) and glutamate has been shown to induce apoptosis *via* NMDA-receptor excitotoxicity (Sucher *et al.*, 1997). Elevated glutamate levels have been noted in experimental animal models (Dreyer *et al.*, 1996; Yoles and Schwartz, 1998) and in humans with glaucoma (Dreyer *et al.*, 1996), although this has been questioned (Levkovitch-Verbin *et al.*, 2002). *Memantine*, an uncompetitive NMDA-receptor antagonist (Vorwerk *et al.*, 1996; Chen and Lipton, 1997), is currently being investigated clinically as a possible treatment for glaucoma.

Optic Nerve. The optic nerve is a myelinated nerve conducting the retinal output to the central nervous system. It is composed of (1) an intraocular portion, which is visible as the 1.5-mm optic disk in the retina; (2) an intraorbital portion; (3) an intracanalicular portion; and (4) an intracranial portion. The nerve is ensheathed in meninges continuous with the brain. At present, pharmacological treatment of some optic neuropathies is based on management of the underlying disease. For example, optic neuritis may be treated best with intravenous glucocorticoids (Beck *et al.*, 1992; Beck *et al.*, 1993); glaucomatous optic neuropathy is medically managed by decreasing intraocular pressure.

PHARMACOKINETICS AND TOXICOLOGY OF OCULAR THERAPEUTIC AGENTS

Drug Delivery Strategies

Properties of varying ocular routes of administration are outlined in Table 63–3. A number of delivery systems have been developed for treating ocular diseases. Most ophthalmic drugs are delivered in solutions, but for compounds with limited solubility, a suspension form facilitates delivery.

Several formulations prolong the time a drug remains on the surface of the eye. These include gels, ointments, solid inserts, soft contact lenses, and collagen shields. *Prolonging the time in the cul-de-sac facilitates drug*

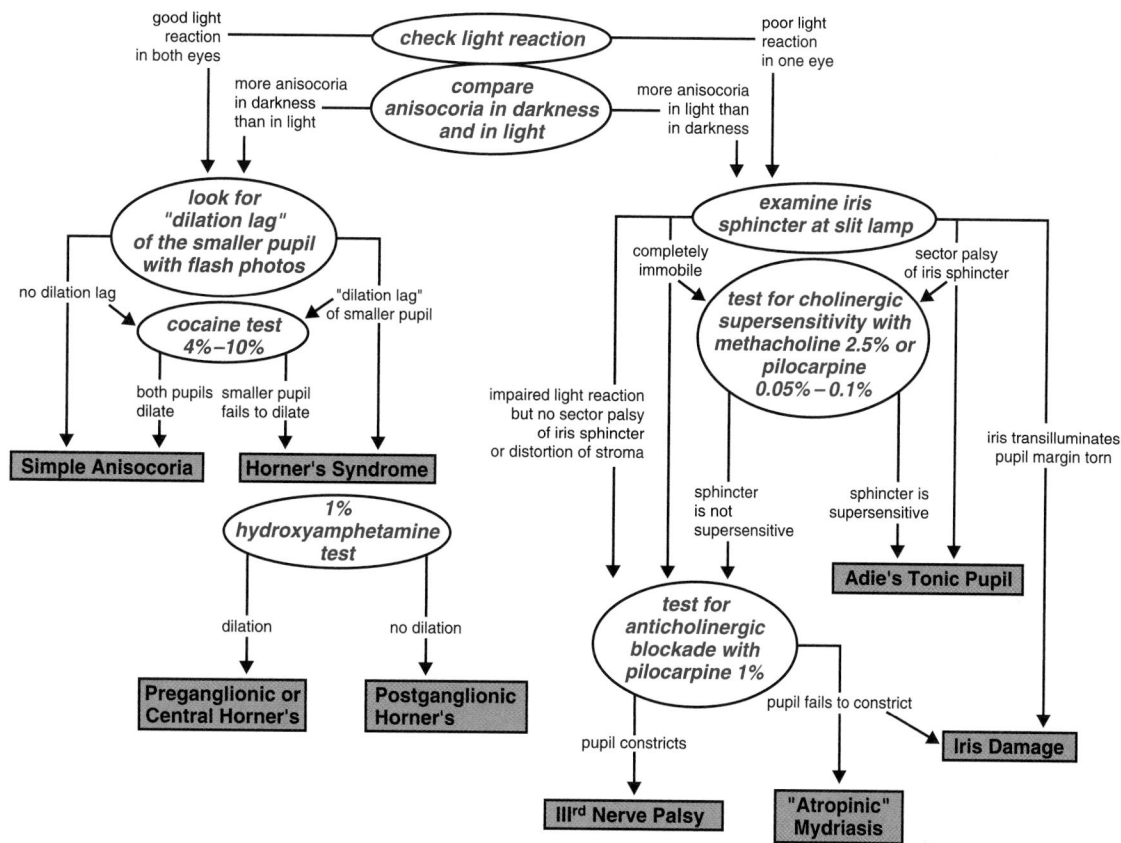

Figure 63–5. *Anisocoria evaluation flowsheet.* (Adapted with permission from Thompson and Pilley, 1976.)

absorption. Ophthalmic gels (*e.g., pilocarpine* 4% gel) release drugs by diffusion following erosion of soluble polymers. The polymers used include cellulosic ethers, polyvinyl alcohol, carbopol, polyacrylamide, polymethylvinyl ether–maleic anhydride, poloxamer 407, and puronic acid. Ointments usually contain mineral oil and a petrolatum base and are helpful in delivering antibiotics, cycloplegic drugs, or miotic agents. Solid inserts, such as the *ganciclovir* intravitreal implant, provide a *zero-order* rate of delivery by steady-state diffusion, whereby drug is released at a more constant rate over a finite period of time rather than as a bolus. This surgical implant has been used to deliver anti-cytomegalovirus medication in proximity to the retinal infection (Marx *et al.*, 1996). The intent is to deliver a sustained dose of medication over several months with reduced spikes in drug delivery (Kunou *et al.*, 2000) independent of patient compliance.

Pharmacokinetics

Classical pharmacokinetic theory based on studies of systemically administered drugs (*see* Chapter 1) does not

fully apply to all ophthalmic drugs (Kaur and Kanwar, 2002). Although similar principles of absorption, distribution, metabolism, and excretion determine the fate of drug disposition in the eye, alternative routes of drug administration, in addition to oral and intravenous routes, introduce other variables in compartmental analysis (Table 63–3 and Figure 63–6). Most ophthalmic medications are formulated to be applied topically. Drugs also may be injected by subconjunctival, sub-Tenon's, and retrobulbar routes (Figure 63–1 and Table 63–3). For example, anesthetic agents are administered commonly by injection for surgical procedures and antibiotics and glucocorticoids also may be injected to enhance their delivery to local tissues. The antimetabolite *5-fluorouracil* and the DNA alkylating agent *mitomycin C* may be administered subconjunctivally to retard the fibroblast proliferation related to scarring after glaucoma surgery. Mitomycin C also can be applied to the cornea to prevent scarring after corneal surgery. Intraocular (*i.e.,* intravitreal) injections of antibiotics are considered in instances of endophthalmitis, a severe intraocular infection. The sensitivities of the organisms to the antibiotic and the retinal

Table 63–3
Some Characteristics of Ocular Routes of Drug Administration*

ROUTE	ABSORPTION PATTERN	SPECIAL UTILITY	LIMITATIONS AND PRECAUTIONS
Topical	Prompt, depending on formulation	Convenient, economical, relatively safe	Compliance, corneal and conjunctival toxicity, nasal mucosal toxicity, systemic side effects from nasolacrimal absorption
Subconjunctival, sub-Tenon's, and retrobulbar injections	Prompt or sustained, depending on formulation	Anterior segment infections, posterior uveitis, cystoid macular edema	Local toxicity, tissue injury, globe perforation, optic nerve trauma, central retinal artery and/or vein occlusion, direct retinal drug toxicity with inadvertent globe perforation, ocular muscle trauma, prolonged drug effect
Intraocular (intracameral) injections	Prompt	Anterior segment surgery, infections	Corneal toxicity, intraocular toxicity, relatively short duration of action
Intravitreal injection or device	Absorption circumvented, immediate local effect, potential sustained effect	Endophthalmitis, retinitis	Retinal toxicity

*See text for more complete discussion of individual routes.

toxicity threshold may be nearly the same for some antibiotics; hence, the antibiotic dose injected intravitreally must be carefully titrated. Intraocular inserts are used to treat intraocular viral infections. The ganciclovir implant is indicated to treat cytomegalovirus retinitis in patients with AIDS.

Unlike clinical pharmacokinetic studies on systemic drugs, where data are collected relatively easily from blood samples, there is significant risk in obtaining tissue and fluid samples from the human eye. Consequently, animal models, frequently rabbits, are studied to provide pharmacokinetic data on ophthalmic drugs.

Absorption. After topical instillation of a drug, the rate and extent of absorption are determined by the time the drug remains in the cul-de-sac and precorneal tear film, elimination by nasolacrimal drainage, drug binding to tear proteins, drug metabolism by tear and tissue proteins, and diffusion across the cornea and conjunctiva (Lee, 1993). A drug's residence time may be prolonged by changing its formulation. Residence time also may be extended by blocking the egress of tears from the eye by closing the tear drainage ducts with plugs or cautery. Nasolacrimal drainage contributes to systemic absorption of topically administered ophthalmic medications. Absorption from the nasal mucosa avoids so-called first-pass metabolism by the liver (*see* Chapter 1), and consequently significant systemic side effects may be caused by topical medications, especially when used chronically. Possible absorption pathways of an ophthalmic drug following topical application to the eye are shown schematically in Figure 63–6.

Transcorneal and transconjunctival/scleral absorption are the desired routes for localized ocular drug effects. The time period

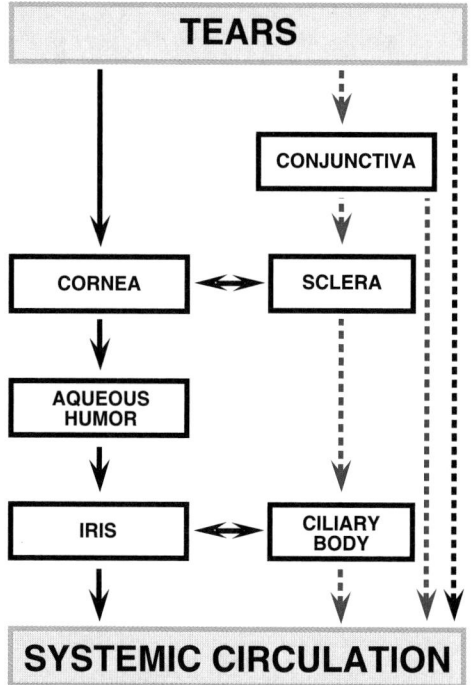

Figure 63–6. *Possible absorption pathways of an ophthalmic drug following topical application to the eye.* Solid black arrows represent the corneal route; dashed blue arrows represent the conjunctival/scleral route; the black dashed line represents the nasolacrimal absorption pathway. (Adapted with permission from Chien *et al.*, 1990.)

between drug instillation and its appearance in the aqueous humor is defined as the *lag time*. The drug concentration gradient between the tear film and the cornea and conjunctival epithelium provides the driving force for passive diffusion across these tissues. Other factors that affect a drug's diffusion capacity are the size of the molecule, chemical structure, and steric configuration. Transcorneal drug penetration is conceptualized as a differential solubility process; the cornea may be thought of as a trilamellar "fat-water-fat" structure corresponding to the epithelial, stromal, and endothelial layers. The epithelium and endothelium represent barriers for hydrophilic substances; the stroma is a barrier for hydrophobic compounds. Hence, a drug with both hydrophilic and lipophilic properties is best suited for transcorneal absorption.

Drug penetration into the eye is approximately linearly related to its concentration in the tear film. Certain disease states, such as corneal ulcers and other corneal epithelial defects, may alter drug penetration. Medication absorption usually is increased when an anatomic barrier is compromised or removed. Experimentally, drugs may be screened for their potential clinical utility by assessing their corneal permeability coefficients. These pharmacokinetic data combined with the drug's octanol/water partition coefficient (for lipophilic drugs) or distribution coefficient (for ionizable drugs) yield a parabolic relationship that is a useful parameter for predicting ocular absorption. Of course, such *in vitro* studies do not account for other factors that affect corneal absorption, such as epithelial integrity, blink rate, dilution by tear flow, nasolacrimal drainage, drug binding to proteins and tissue, and transconjunctival absorption; hence, these studies have limitations in predicting ocular drug absorption *in vivo*.

Distribution. Topically administered drugs may undergo systemic distribution primarily by nasal mucosal absorption and possibly by local ocular distribution by transcorneal/transconjunctival absorption. Following transcorneal absorption, the aqueous humor accumulates the drug, which then is distributed to intraocular structures as well as potentially to the systemic circulation *via* the trabecular meshwork pathway (Figure 63–3B). Melanin binding of certain drugs is an important factor in some ocular compartments. For example, the mydriatic effect of α adrenergic receptor agonists is slower in onset in human volunteers with darkly pigmented irides compared to those with lightly pigmented irides. In rabbits, radiolabeled *atropine* binds significantly to melanin granules in irides of nonalbino animals. This finding correlates with the fact that atropine's mydriatic effect lasts longer in nonalbino rabbits than in albino rabbits, and suggests that drug–melanin binding is a potential reservoir for sustained drug release. Another clinically important consideration for drug–melanin binding involves the retinal pigment epithelium. In the retinal pigment epithelium, accumulation of *chloroquine* (*see* Chapter 39) causes a toxic retinal lesion known as a "bull's-eye" maculopathy, which is associated with a decrease in visual acuity.

Metabolism. Enzymatic biotransformation of ocular drugs may be significant since a variety of enzymes, including esterases, oxidoreductases, lysosomal enzymes, peptidases, glucuronide and sulfate transferases, glutathione-conjugating enzymes, catechol-*O*-methyl-transferase, monoamine oxidase, and 11β-hydroxysteroid dehydrogenase are found in the eye. The esterases have been of particular interest because of the development of prodrugs for enhanced corneal permeability; for example, *dipivefrin hydrochloride* is a prodrug for *epinephrine*, and *latanoprost* is a prodrug for *prostaglandin* $F_{2\alpha}$; both drugs are used for glaucoma management. Topically

applied ocular drugs are eliminated by the liver and kidney after systemic absorption, but enzymatic transformation of systemically administered drugs also is important in ophthalmology.

Toxicology. All ophthalmic medications are potentially absorbed into the systemic circulation (Figure 63–6), so undesirable systemic side effects may occur. Most ophthalmic drugs are delivered locally to the eye, and the potential local toxic effects are due to hypersensitivity reactions or to direct toxic effects on the cornea, conjunctiva, periocular skin, and nasal mucosa. Eyedrops and contact lens solutions commonly contain preservatives such as benzalkonium chloride, chlorobutanol, chelating agents, and thimerosal for their antimicrobial effectiveness. In particular, benzalkonium chloride may cause a punctate keratopathy or toxic ulcerative keratopathy (Grant and Schuman, 1993). Thimerosal currently is used rarely due to a high incidence of hypersensitivity reactions.

THERAPEUTIC AND DIAGNOSTIC APPLICATIONS OF DRUGS IN OPHTHALMOLOGY

Chemotherapy of Microbial Diseases in the Eye

Antibacterial Agents. **General Considerations.** A number of antibiotics have been formulated for topical ocular use (Table 63–4). The pharmacology, structures, and kinetics of individual drugs have been presented in detail in Section VIII. Appropriate selection of antibiotic and route of administration is dependent on the patient's symptoms, the clinical examination, and the culture/sensitivity results. Specially formulated antibiotics also may be extemporaneously prepared by qualified pharmacists for serious eye infections such as corneal infiltrates or ulcers and endophthalmitis.

Therapeutic Uses. Infectious diseases of the skin, eyelids, conjunctivae, and lacrimal excretory system are encountered regularly in clinical practice. Periocular skin infections are divided into preseptal and postseptal or orbital cellulitis. Depending on the clinical setting (*i.e.,* preceding trauma, sinusitis, age of patient, relative immunocompromised state), oral or parenteral antibiotics are administered. The microbiological spectrum for orbital cellulitis is changing; for example, there has been a sharp decline in *Haemophilus influenzae* after the introduction in 1985 of the *H. influenzae* vaccine (Ambati *et al.,* 2000).

Dacryoadenitis, an infection of the lacrimal gland, is most common in children and young adults. It may be bacterial (typically *Staphylococcus aureus, Streptococcus* species) or viral (most commonly seen in mumps, infectious mononucleosis, influenza, and herpes zoster). When bacterial infection is suspected, systemic antibiotics usually are indicated.

Table 63–4
*Topical Antibacterial Agents Commercially Available for Ophthalmic Use**

GENERIC NAME (TRADE NAME)	FORMULATION†	TOXICITY†	INDICATIONS FOR USE
Bacitracin zinc (AK-TRACIN)	500 units/g ointment	H	Conjunctivitis, blepharitis
Chloramphenicol (AK-CHLOR, CHLORO-MYCETIN, CHLOROPTIC)	0.5% solution 1% ointment	H, BD	Conjunctivitis, keratitis
Ciprofloxacin hydrochloride (CILOXAN)	0.3% solution 0.3% ointment	H, D-RCD	Conjunctivitis, keratitis
Erythromycin (ILOTYCIN)	0.5% ointment	H	Blepharitis, conjunctivitis
Gatifloxacin (ZYMAR)	0.3% solution	H	Conjunctivitis
Gentamicin sulfate (GARAMYCIN, GENOPTIC, GENT-AK, GENTACIDIN)	0.3% solution 0.3% ointment	H	Conjunctivitis, blepharitis, keratitis
Levofloxacin (QUIXIN)	0.5% solution	H	Conjunctivitis
Levofloxacin (IQUIX)	1.5% solution	H	Conjunctivitis, keratitis
Moxifloxacin (VIGAMOX)	0.5% solution	H	Conjunctivitis
Ofloxacin (OCUFLOX)	0.3% solution	H	Conjunctivitis, keratitis
Sulfacetamide sodium (BLEPH-10, CETA-MIDE, SULF-10, ISOPTO CETAMIDE, SULAMYD SODIUM, others)	10, 15, 30% solution 10% ointment	H, BD	Conjunctivitis, keratitis
Polymyxin B combinations‡	Various solutions Various ointments		Conjunctivitis, blepharitis, keratitis
Tobramycin sulfate (TOBREX, AKTOB)	0.3% solution 0.3% ointment	H	Conjunctivitis, blepharitis, keratitis

*For specific information on dosing, formulation, and trade names, refer to the *Physician's Desk Reference for Ophthalmology*, which is published annually. †*Abbreviations*: H, hypersensitivity; BD, blood dyscrasia; D-RCD, drug-related corneal deposits. ‡Polymyxin B is formulated for delivery in combination with bacitracin, neomycin, gramicidin, oxytetracycline, or trimethoprim. *See* Chapters 43 through 46 for further discussion of these antibacterial agents.

Dacryocystitis is an infection of the lacrimal sac. In infants and children, the disease usually is unilateral and secondary to an obstruction of the nasolacrimal duct. In adults, dacryocystitis and canalicular infections may be caused by *Staphylococcus aureus, Streptococcus* species, *Diptheroids, Candida* species, and *Actinomyces israelii.* Any discharge from the lacrimal sac should be sent for smears and cultures. Systemic antibiotics typically are indicated.

Infectious processes of the lids include *hordeolum* and *blepharitis.* A hordeolum, or stye, is an infection of the meibomian, Zeis, or Moll glands at the lid margins. The typical offending bacterium is *S. aureus,* and the usual treatment consists of warm compresses and topical antibiotic ointment. Blepharitis is a common bilateral inflammatory process of the eyelids characterized by irritation and burning, and it also is usually associated with a *Staphylococcus* species. Local hygiene is the mainstay of therapy; topical antibiotics frequently are used, usually in ointment form, particularly when the disease is accompanied

by conjunctivitis and keratitis. Systemic *tetracycline, doxycycline, minocycline,* and *erythromycin* often are effective in reducing severe eyelid inflammation, but must be used for weeks to months.

Conjunctivitis is an inflammatory process of the conjunctiva that varies in severity from mild hyperemia to severe purulent discharge. The more common causes of conjunctivitis include viruses, allergies, environmental irritants, contact lenses, and chemicals. The less common causes include other infectious pathogens, immune-mediated reactions, associated systemic diseases, and tumors of the conjunctiva or eyelid. The more commonly reported infectious agents are adenovirus and herpes simplex virus, followed by other viral (*e.g.,* enterovirus, coxsackievirus, measles virus, varicella zoster virus, and vaccinia-variola virus) and bacterial sources (*e.g., Neisseria* species, *Streptococcus pneumoniae, Haemophilus* species, *S. aureus, Moraxella lacunata,* and chlamydial species). *Rickettsia,* fungi, and parasites, in both cyst and trophozoite form, are rare causes of conjunctivitis. Effective management is based on selection of an appropriate antibiotic for suspected bacterial pathogens. Unless an unusual causative organism is suspected, bacterial conjunctivitis is treated empirically with a broad-spectrum topical antibiotic without obtaining a culture.

Keratitis, or corneal inflammation, can occur at any level of the cornea (*e.g.,* epithelium, subepithelium, stroma, and endothelium). It can be due to noninfectious or infectious causes. Numerous microbial agents have been identified as causes of infectious keratitis, including bacteria, viruses, fungi, spirochetes, and cysts and trophozoites. Severe infections, with tissue loss (corneal ulcers), generally are treated more aggressively than infections without tissue loss (corneal infiltrates). The mild, small, more peripheral infections usually are not cultured and the eyes are treated with broad-spectrum topical antibiotics. In more severe, central, or larger infections, corneal scrapings for smears, cultures, and sensitivities are performed and the patient is immediately started on intensive hourly, around-the-clock topical antibiotic therapy. The goal of treatment is to eradicate the infection and reduce the amount of corneal scarring and the chance of corneal perforation and severe decreased vision or blindness. The initial medication selection and dosage are adjusted according to the clinical response and culture and sensitivity results.

Endophthalmitis is a potentially severe and devastating inflammatory, and usually infectious, process involving the intraocular tissues. When the inflammatory process encompasses the entire globe, it is called *panophthalmitis*. Endophthalmitis is usually caused by bacteria or fungi, or rarely by spirochetes. The typical case occurs during the early postoperative course (*e.g.,* after cataract, glaucoma, cornea, or retinal surgery), following trauma, or by endogenous seeding in the immunocompromised host or intravenous drug user. Acute postoperative endophthalmitis requires a prompt vitreous tap for smears and cultures and empirical injection of intravitreal antibiotics. Immediate vitrectomy (*i.e.,* specialized surgical removal of the vitreous) is beneficial for patients who have light perception–only vision (Endophthalmitis Vitrectomy Study Group, 1995). Vitrectomy for other causes of endophthalmitis (*e.g.,* glaucoma bleb–related, posttraumatic, or endogenous) may be beneficial. In cases of endogenous seeding, parenteral antibiotics have a role in eliminating the infectious source, but the efficacy of systemic antibiotics with trauma is not well established.

Antiviral Agents. General Considerations. The various antiviral drugs currently used in ophthalmology are summarized in Table 63–5 (*see* Chapter 49 for additional details about these agents).

Table 63–5
Antiviral Agents for Ophthalmic Use*

GENERIC NAME (TRADE NAME)	ROUTE OF ADMINISTRATION	OCULAR TOXICITY†	INDICATION FOR USE
Trifluridine (VIROPTIC)	Topical (1% solution)	PK, H	Herpes simplex keratitis Herpes simplex conjunctivitis
Vidarabine (VIRA-A)	Topical (3% ointment)	PK, H	Herpes simplex keratitis Herpes simplex conjunctivitis
Acyclovir (ZOVIRAX)	Oral, intravenous (200-mg capsules, 400- and 800-mg tablets)		Herpes zoster ophthalmicus Herpes simplex iridocyclitis
Valacyclovir (VALTREX)	Oral (500-mg, 1000-mg tablets)		Herpes simplex keratitis Herpes zoster ophthalmicus
Famciclovir (FAMVIR)	Oral (125-mg, 250-mg, 500-mg tablets)		Herpes simplex keratitis Herpes zoster ophthalmicus
Foscarnet (FOSCAVIR)	Intravenous Intravitreal		Cytomegalovirus retinitis
Ganciclovir (CYTOVENE) (VITRASERT)	Intravenous, oral Intravitreal implant		Cytomegalovirus retinitis
Formivirsen (VITRAVENE)	Intravitreal injection		Cytomegalovirus retinitis
Cidofovir (VISTIDE)	Intravenous		Cytomegalovirus retinitis

*For additional details, *see* Chapter 49. †*Abbreviations*: PK, punctate keratopathy; H, hypersensitivity.

Therapeutic Uses. The primary indications for the use of antiviral drugs in ophthalmology are viral keratitis, herpes zoster ophthalmicus (Liesegang, 1999; Chern and Margolis, 1998), and retinitis. There currently are no antiviral agents for the treatment of viral conjunctivitis caused by adenoviruses, which usually has a self-limited course and typically is treated by symptomatic relief of irritation.

Viral keratitis, an infection of the cornea that may involve either the epithelium or stroma, is most commonly caused by herpes simplex type I and varicella zoster viruses. Less common viral etiologies include herpes simplex type II, Epstein-Barr virus, and cytomegalovirus. Topical antiviral agents are indicated for the treatment of epithelial disease due to herpes simplex infection. *When treating viral keratitis topically, there is a very narrow margin between the therapeutic topical antiviral activity and the toxic effect on the cornea;* hence, patients must be followed very closely. The role of oral *acyclovir* and glucocorticoids in herpetic corneal and external eye disease has been examined in the Herpetic Eye Disease Study (Herpetic Eye Disease Study Group, 1997a; Herpetic Eye Disease Study Group, 1998). Topical glucocorticoids are contraindicated in herpetic epithelial keratitis due to active viral replication. In contrast, for herpetic disciform keratitis, which predominantly is presumed to involve a cell-mediated immune reaction, topical glucocorticoids accelerate recovery (Wilhelmus *et al.*, 1994). For recurrent herpetic stromal keratitis, there is clear benefit from treatment with oral acyclovir in reducing the risk of recurrence (Herpetic Eye Disease Study Group, 1998).

Herpes zoster ophthalmicus is a latent reactivation of a varicella zoster infection in the first division of the trigeminal cranial nerve. Systemic acyclovir, *valacyclovir,* and *famciclovir* are effective in reducing the severity and complications of herpes zoster ophthalmicus (Colin *et al.*, 2000). Currently, there are no ophthalmic preparations of acyclovir approved by the FDA, although an ophthalmic ointment is available for investigational use.

Viral retinitis may be caused by herpes simplex virus, cytomegalovirus (CMV), adenovirus, and varicella zoster virus. With the highly active antiretroviral therapy (HAART; *see* Chapter 50), CMV retinitis does not appear to progress when specific anti-CMV therapy is discontinued, but some patients develop an immune recovery uveitis (Jacobson *et al.*, 2000; Whitcup, 2000). Treatment usually involves long-term parenteral administration of antiviral drugs. Intravitreal administration of ganciclovir has been found to be an effective alternative to the systemic route (Sanborn *et al.*, 1992). Acute retinal necrosis and progressive outer retinal necrosis, most often caused by varicella zoster virus, can be treated by various combinations of oral, intravenous,

intravitreal injection, and intravitreal implantation of antiviral medications (Roig-Melo *et al.*, 2001).

Antifungal Agents. ***General Considerations.*** The only currently available topical ophthalmic antifungal preparation is a polyene, *natamycin* (NATACYN), which has the following structure:

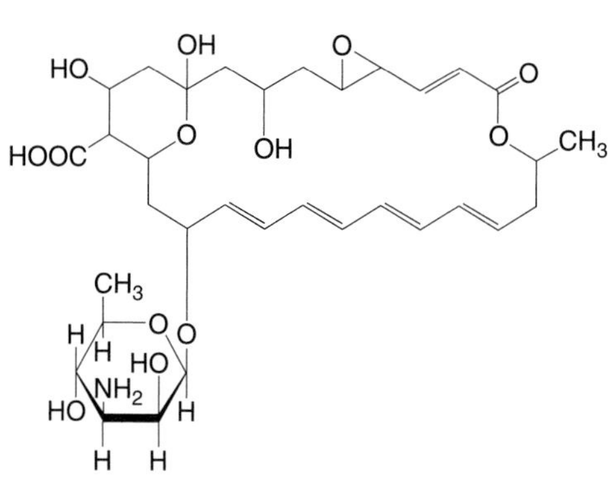

NATAMYCIN

Other antifungal agents may be extemporaneously compounded for topical, subconjunctival, or intravitreal routes of administration (Table 63–6). The pharmacology and structures of available antifungal agents are given in Chapter 48.

Therapeutic Uses. As with systemic fungal infections, the incidence of ophthalmic fungal infections has risen with the growing number of immunocompromised hosts. Ophthalmic indications for antifungal medications include fungal keratitis, scleritis, endophthalmitis, mucormycosis, and canaliculitis. Risk factors for fungal keratitis include trauma, chronic ocular surface disease, and immunosuppression (including topical steroid use). When fungal infection is suspected, samples of the affected tissues are obtained for smears, cultures, and sensitivities, and this information is used for drug selection.

Antiprotozoal Agents. ***General Considerations.*** Parasitic infections involving the eye usually manifest themselves as a form of *uveitis,* an inflammatory process of either the anterior or posterior segments, and less commonly as conjunctivitis, keratitis, and retinitis.

Therapeutic Uses. In the United States, the most commonly encountered protozoal infections include *Acanthamoeba* and *Toxoplasma gondii.* In contact-lens wearers who develop keratitis, physicians should be highly suspicious of the presence of *Acanthamoeba* (McCulley *et al.*, 2000). Additional risk factors for *Acanthamoeba* keratitis include poor contact lens hygiene, wearing contact lenses in a pool or hot tub, and ocular trauma. Treatment usually consists of a combination topical antibiotic, such as *poly-*

Table 63–6
*Antifungal Agents for Ophthalmic Use**

DRUG CLASS/AGENT	METHOD OF ADMINISTRATION	INDICATIONS FOR USE
Polyenes		
Amphotericin B	0.1–0.5% (typically 0.15%) topical solution	Yeast and fungal keratitis and endophthalmitis
	0.8–1 mg subconjunctival	Yeast and fungal endophthalmitis
	5-μg intravitreal injection	Yeast and fungal endophthalmitis
	intravenous	Yeast and fungal endophthalmitis
Natamycin	5% topical suspension	Yeast and fungal blepharitis, conjunctivitis, keratitis
Imidazoles		
Fluconazole	oral, intravenous	Yeast keratitis and endophthalmitis
Itraconazole	oral	Yeast and fungal keratitis and endophthalmitis
Ketoconazole	oral	Yeast keratitis and endophthalmitis
Miconazole	1% topical solution	Yeast and fungal keratitis
	5–10 mg subconjunctival	Yeast and fungal endophthalmitis
	10 μg intravitreal injection	Yeast and fungal endophthalmitis

*Only natamycin (NATACYN) is commercially available for ophthalmic use. The other antifungal drugs must be formulated for the given method of administration. For further dosing information, refer to the *Physicians' Desk Reference for Ophthalmology*. For additional discussion of these antifungal agents, *see* Chapter 48.

myxin B sulfate, bacitracin zinc, and *neomycin sulfate* (*e.g.,* NEOSPORIN), and sometimes an imidazole (*e.g., clotrimazole, miconazole,* or *ketoconazole*). In the United Kingdom, the aromatic diamidines (*i.e., propamidine isethionate* in both topical aqueous and ointment forms, BROLENE) have been used successfully to treat this relatively resistant infectious keratitis (Hargrave *et al.,* 1999). The cationic antiseptic agent *polyhexamethylene biguanide* (PHMB) also is typically used in drop form for acanthamoeba keratitis, although this is not an FDA-approved antiprotozoal agent. Topical *chlorhexidine* can be used as an alternative to PHMB. Oral itraconazole or ketoconazole often are used in addition to the topical medications. Resolution of *Acanthamoeba* keratitis may require many months of treatment.

Toxoplasmosis may present as a posterior (*e.g.,* focal retinochoroiditis, papillitis, vitritis, or retinitis) or occasionally as an anterior uveitis. Treatment is indicated when inflammatory lesions encroach upon the macula and threaten central visual acuity. Several regimens have been recommended with concurrent use of systemic steroids: (1) *pyrimethamine, sulfadiazine,* and *folinic acid (leucovorin);* (2) pyrimethamine, sulfadiazine, *clindamycin,* and folinic acid; (3) sulfadiazine and clindamycin; (4) clindamycin; and (5) *trimethoprim-sulfamethoxazole* with or without clindamycin.

Other protozoal infections (*e.g.,* giardiasis, leishmaniasis, and malaria) and helminths are less common eye pathogens in the United States. Systemic pharmacological management as well as vitrectomy may be indicated for selected parasitic infections.

In the eye, infections can occur in a variety of locations, such as the cornea, sclera, vitreous and retina, and can be due to bacteria, viruses, fungi, and parasites. Treatment is based on severity of infection, location, and the class of infectious agent. Within each group of microbial cause, different organisms are treated with different medications. Gram-positive bacteria respond to certain antibiotics and gram-negative bacteria to others. Some organisms are quite susceptible to many antimicrobial agents, while others are not. Still others may have been susceptible in the past but have become resistant. The task of staying ahead of the rapidly developing resistances is becoming increasingly difficult. In ophthalmology, fortunately, newer-generation topical fluoroquinolones recently were brought to market, which have at least temporarily helped stem the tide of resistant infections. Additional topical fluoroquinolones are in development.

While the selection of topical antiviral agents is rather limited, two new systemic antiviral agents have become available in the past decade. Similarly, there is only one commercially available topical antifungal medication, but there are numerous systemic agents, several of them new in the past few years. Potentially, some of these systemic medications could be modified for topical use or even formulated as intraocular implants, greatly expanding our options in the treatment of many ophthalmic infectious diseases.

Use of Autonomic Agents in the Eye

General Considerations. General autonomic pharmacology has been discussed extensively in Chapters 6 through 10. The autonomic agents used in ophthalmology as well as the responses (*i.e.,* mydriasis and cycloplegia) to muscarinic cholinergic antagonists are summarized in Table 63–7.

Therapeutic Uses. Autonomic drugs are used extensively for diagnostic and surgical purposes and for the treatment of glaucoma, uveitis, and strabismus.

Table 63–7
Autonomic Drugs for Ophthalmic Use[*]

DRUG CLASS (TRADE NAME)	FORMULATION	INDICATIONS FOR USE	OCULAR SIDE EFFECTS
Cholinergic agonists			
Acetylcholine (MIOCHOL-E)	1% solution	Intraocular use for miosis in surgery	Corneal edema
Carbachol (MIOSTAT, ISOPTO CARBACHOL, others)	0.01 to 3% solution	Intraocular use for miosis in surgery, glaucoma	Corneal edema, miosis, induced myopia, decreased vision, brow ache, retinal detachment
Pilocarpine (AKARPINE, ISOPTO CARPINE, PILOCAR, PILAGAN, PILOPINE-HS, PILOPTIC, PILOSTAT, others)	0.25–10% solution, 4% gel	Glaucoma	Same as for carbachol
Anticholinesterase agents			
Physostigmine (ESERINE)	0.25% ointment	Glaucoma, accommodative esotropia, louse and mite infestation of lashes	Retinal detachment, miosis, cataract, pupillary block glaucoma iris cysts, brow ache, punctal stenosis of the nasolacrimal system
Echothiophate (PHOSPHOLINE IODIDE)	0.125% solution	Glaucoma, accommodative esotropia	Same as for physostigmine
Muscarinic antagonists			
Atropine (ATROPISOL, ATROPINE-CARE, ISOPTO ATROPINE)	0.5–2% solution, 1% ointment	Cycloplegic retinoscopy, dilated funduscopic exam, cycloplegia[†]	Photosensitivity, blurred vision
Scopolamine (ISOPTO HYOSCINE)	0.25% solution	Same as for atropine	Same as for atropine
Homatropine (ISOPTO HOMATROPINE)	2 & 5% solution	Same as for atropine	Same as for atropine
Cyclopentolate (AK-PENTOLATE, CYCLOGYL, PENTOLAIR)	0.5, 1, & 2% solution	Same as for atropine	Same as for atropine
Tropicamide (MYDRIACYL, TROPICACYL, OPTICYL)	0.5 & 1% solution	Same as for atropine	Same as for atropine
Sympathomimetic agents			
Dipivefrin (PROPINE, AKPRO)	0.1% solution	Glaucoma	Photosensitivity, conjunctival hyperemia, hypersensitivity

(Continued)

Table 63–7

*Autonomic Drugs for Ophthalmic Use** (Continued)*

DRUG CLASS (TRADE NAME)	FORMULATION	INDICATIONS FOR USE	OCULAR SIDE EFFECTS
Epinephrine (EPINAL, EPIFRIN, GLAUCON)	0.1, 0.5, 1, & 2% solution	Glaucoma	Same as for dipivefrin
Phenylephrine (AK-DILATE, MYDFRIN, NEO-SYNEPHRINE, others)	0.12, 2.5, & 10% solution	Mydriasis	Same as for dipivefrin
Apraclonidine (IOPIDINE)	0.5 & 1% solution	Glaucoma, pre- & postlaser prophylaxis of intraocular pressure spike	Same as for dipivefrin
Brimonidine (ALPHAGAN)	0.15 and 0.2% solution	Glaucoma	Same as for dipivefrin
Cocaine	1–4% solution	Topical anesthesia, evaluate anisocoria (*see* Figure 63–5)	
Hydroxyamphetamine (PAREDRINE)	1% solution	Evaluate anisocoria (*see* Figure 63–5)	
Naphazoline (AK-CON, ALBALON, CLEAR EYES, NAPHCON, VASOCLEAR, VASOCON REGULAR, others)	0.012 to 0.1% solution	Decongestant	Same as for dipivefrin
Tetrahydrozoline (COLLYRIUM FRESH, MURINE PLUS, VISINE MOISTURIZING, others)	0.05% solution	Decongestant	Same as for dipivefrin
α & β Adrenergic antagonists			
Dapiprazole (α) (REV-EYES)	0.5% solution	Reverse mydriasis	Conjunctival hyperemia
Betaxolol (β_1-selective) (BETOPTIC, BETOPTIC-S)	0.25 & 0.5% suspension	Glaucoma	
Carteolol (β) (OCUPRESS)	1% solution	Glaucoma	
Levobunolol (β) (BETAGAN, AKBETA)	0.25 & 0.5% solution	Glaucoma	
Metipranolol (β) (OPTIPRANOLOL)	0.3% solution	Glaucoma	
Timolol (β) (TIMOPTIC, TIMOPTIC XE, BETIMOL)	0.25 & 0.5% solution & gel	Glaucoma	

*Refer to *Physicians' Desk Reference for Ophthalmology* for specific indications and dosing information. †Mydriasis and cycloplegia, or paralysis of accommodation, of the human eye occurs after one drop of atropine 1%, scopolamine 0.5%, homatropine 1%, cyclopentolate 0.5% or 1%, and tropicamide 0.5% or 1%. Recovery of mydriasis is defined by return to baseline pupil size to within 1 mm. Recovery of cycloplegia is defined by return to within two diopters of baseline accommodative power. The maximal mydriatic effect of homatropine is achieved with a 5% solution, but cycloplegia may be incomplete. Maximal cycloplegia with tropicamide may be achieved with a 1% solution. Times to development of maximal mydriasis and to recovery, respectively, are: for *atropine*, 30 to 40 minutes and 7 to 10 days; for *scopolamine*, 20 to 130 minutes and 3 to 7 days; for *homatropine*, 40 to 60 minutes and 1 to 3 days; for *cyclopentolate*, 30 to 60 minutes and 1 day; for *tropicamide*, 20 to 40 minutes and 6 hours. Times to development of maximal cycloplegia and to recovery, respectively, are: for *atropine*, 60 to 180 minutes and 6 to 12 days; for *scopolamine*, 30 to 60 minutes and 3 to 7 days; for *homatropine*, 30 to 60 minutes and 1 to 3 days; for *cyclopentolate*, 25 to 75 minutes and 6 hours to 1 day; for *tropicamide*, 30 minutes and 6 hours.

Glaucoma. In the United States, glaucoma is the second leading cause of blindness in African-Americans, the third leading cause in Caucasians, and the leading cause in Hispanic-Americans (Congdon *et al.*, 2004). African-Americans have three times the age-adjusted prevalence of glaucoma compared to Caucasians (Friedman *et al.*, 2004). Characterized by progressive optic nerve cupping and visual field loss, glaucoma is responsible for the bilateral blindness of 90,000 Americans (half of whom are African-American or Hispanic) (Congdon *et al.*, 2004), and about 2.2 million have the disease (1.86% of the population over age 40). This number is expected to increase by 50% by the year 2020 (Friedman *et al.*, 2004). Risk factors associated with glaucomatous nerve damage include increased intraocular pressure (IOP), positive family history of glaucoma, African-American heritage, and possibly myopia and hypertension. The production and regulation of aqueous humor have been discussed in an earlier section of this chapter. Previously an intraocular pressure of greater than 21 was considered abnormal. This, however, is incorrect, as intraocular pressure is not an accurate indicator of disease. Nonetheless, elevated intraocular pressure is a risk factor for glaucoma. Several randomized, controlled trials have determined that reducing intraocular pressure can delay glaucomatous nerve or field damage (Fluorouracil Filtering Surgery Study Group, 1996; AGIS Investigators, 2000; Heijl *et al.*, 2002). Although markedly elevated intraocular pressures (*e.g.*, greater than 30 mm Hg) usually will lead to optic nerve damage, the optic nerves in certain patients apparently can tolerate intraocular pressures in the mid-to-high twenties. These patients are referred to as *ocular hypertensives.* A recent prospective multicenter trial found that prophylactic medical reduction of intraocular pressure reduced the risk of progression to glaucoma from about 10% to about 5% (Kass *et al.*, 2002). Other patients have progressive glaucomatous optic nerve damage despite having intraocular pressures in the normal range, and this form of the disease sometimes is called *normal-* or *low-tension* glaucoma. A reduction of intraocular pressure by 30% reduces disease progression from about 35% to about 10%, even for normal-tension glaucoma patients (Collaborative Normal-Tension Glaucoma Study Group, 1998a; Collaborative Normal-Tension Glaucoma Study Group, 1998b). Despite overwhelming evidence that intraocular pressure reduction is a helpful treatment, at present the pathophysiological processes involved in glaucomatous optic nerve damage and the relationship to aqueous humor dynamics are not understood.

Current pharmacotherapies are targeted to decrease the production of aqueous humor at the ciliary body and to increase outflow through the trabecular meshwork and uveoscleral pathways. There is no consensus on the best intraocular pressure–lowering technique for glaucoma therapy. Currently, a National Eye Institute–sponsored clinical trial, the Collaborative Initial Glaucoma Treatment Study (CIGTS), aims to determine whether it is best, in terms of preservation of visual function and quality of life, to treat patients newly diagnosed with open-angle glaucoma with filtering surgery or with medication. Initial results show no difference in disease progression rates between the two treatment groups at 5 years (Lichter *et al.*, 2001), but the study is ongoing.

The CIGTS study aside, a stepped medical approach depends on the patient's health, age, and ocular status. Some general principles prevail in patient management: (1) asthma and chronic obstructive pulmonary disease with a bronchospastic component are relative contraindications to the use of topical β adrenergic receptor antagonists because of the risk of significant side effects from systemic absorption *via* the nasolacrimal system; (2) some cardiac dysrhythmias (*i.e.*, bradycardia and heart block) also are relative contraindications to β adrenergic antagonists for similar reasons; (3) history of nephrolithiasis, or kidney stones, sometimes is a contraindication for carbonic anhydrase inhibitors; (4) young patients usually are intolerant of miotic therapy secondary to visual blurring from induced myopia; (5) direct miotic agents are preferred over cholinesterase inhibitors in "phakic" patients (*i.e.*, those patients who have their own crystalline lens), since the latter drugs can promote cataract formation; and (6) in patients who have an increased risk of retinal detachment, miotics should be used with caution, since they have been implicated in promoting retinal tears in susceptible individuals; such tears are thought to be due to altered forces at the vitreous base produced by ciliary body contraction induced by the drug.

The goal is to prevent progressive glaucomatous optic-nerve damage with minimum risk and side effects from either topical or systemic therapy. With these general principles in mind, a stepped medical approach may begin with a topical prostaglandin analog. Due to their once-daily dosing, low incidence of systemic side effects, and potent intraocular pressure lowering effect, prostaglandin analogs have largely replaced β adrenergic receptor antagonists as first-line medical therapy for glaucoma. The prostaglandin analogs consist of latanoprost (XALATAN), *travoprost* (TRAVATAN), *bimatoprost* (LUMIGAN), and *unoprostone* (RESCULA). The chemical structure of latanoprost is shown below.

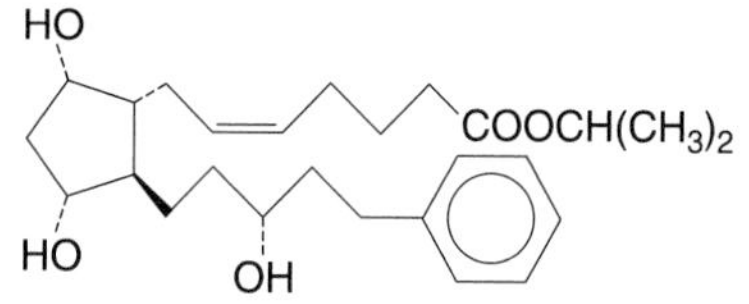

LATANOPROST

Prostaglandin $PGF_{2\alpha}$ was found to reduce IOP but has intolerable local side effects. Modifications to the chemical structure of $PGF_{2\alpha}$ have produced a number of analogs with a more acceptable side-effect profile. In primates and humans, $PGF_{2\alpha}$ analogs appear to lower intraocular pressure by facilitating aqueous outflow through the accessory uveoscleral outflow pathway. The mechanism by which this occurs is unclear. $PGF_{2\alpha}$ and its analogs (prodrugs that are hydrolyzed to $PGF_{2\alpha}$) bind to FP receptors that link to G_{q11} and thence to the $PLC–IP_3–Ca^{2+}$ pathway. This pathway is active in isolated human ciliary muscle cells. Other cells in the eye also may express FP receptors. Theories of IOP lowering by $PGF_{2\alpha}$ range from altered ciliary muscle tension to effects on trabecular mesh-work cells to release of matrix metalloproteases and digestion of extracellular matrix materials that may impede outflow tracts. There also is less myocilin protein noted in monkey smooth muscle after $PGF_{2\alpha}$ treatment (Lindsey *et al.*, 2001).

The β-receptor antagonists now are the next most common topical medical treatment. There are two classes of topical β blockers. The nonselective ones bind to both β_1 and β_2 receptors and include *timolol maleate* and *hemihydrate, levobunolol, metipranolol,* and *carteolol.* There is one β_1-selective antagonist, *betaxolol,* available for ophthalmic use, but it is less efficacious than the nonselective β blockers since the β receptors of the eye are largely of the β_2 subtype. However, because the β_1 receptors are found preferentially in the heart while the β_2 receptors are found in the lung, betaxolol is less likely to cause breathing difficulty. In the eye, the targeted tissues are the ciliary body epithelium and blood vessels, where β_2 receptors account for 75% to 90% of the total population. How β blockade leads to decreased aqueous production and reduced IOP is uncertain. Production of aqueous humor seems to be activated by a β-receptor–mediated cyclic AMP–PKA pathway; β blockade blunts adrenergic activation of this pathway by preventing catecholamine stimulation of the β receptor, thereby decreasing intracellular cAMP. Another hypothesis is that β blockers decrease ocular blood flow, which decreases the ultrafiltration responsible for aqueous production (Juzych and Zimmerman, 1997).

When there are medical contraindications to the use of prostaglandin analogs or β-receptor antagonists, other agents, such as an α_2 adrenergic receptor agonist or topical carbonic anhydrase inhibitor may be used as first-line therapy. The α_2 adrenergic agonists improve the pharmacologic profile of the nonselective sympathomimetic agent epinephrine and its derivative, dipivefrin (PROPINE). Epinephrine stimulates both α and β adrenergic receptors. The drug appears to decrease IOP by enhancing both conventional (*via* a β_2-receptor mechanism) and uveoscleral outflow (perhaps *via* prostaglandin production) from the eye. Although effective, epinephrine is poorly tolerated, principally due to localized irritation and hyperemia. Dipivefrin is an epinephrine prodrug that is converted into epinephrine by esterases in the cornea. It is much better tolerated, but still is prone to cause epinephrine-like side effects (Fang and Kass, 1997). The α_2 adrenergic agonist *clonidine* is effective at reducing IOP, but also readily crosses the blood–brain barrier and causes systemic hypotension; as a result it no longer is used for glaucoma. In contrast, *apraclonidine* (IOPIDINE) is a relatively selective α_2 adrenergic agonist that is highly ionized at physiologic pH and therefore does not cross the blood–brain barrier. *Brimonidine* (ALPHAGAN, others) is also a selective α_2 adrenergic agonist, but is lipophilic, enabling easy corneal penetration. Both apraclonidine and brimonidine reduce aqueous production and may enhance some uveoscleral outflow. Both appear to bind to pre- and postsynaptic α_2 receptors. By binding to the presynaptic receptors, the drugs reduce the amount of neurotransmitter release from sympathetic nerve stimulation and thereby lower IOP. By binding to postsynaptic α_2 receptors, these drugs stimulate the G_i pathway, reducing cellular cyclic AMP production, thereby reducing aqueous humor production (Juzych *et al.*, 1997).

The development of a topical carbonic anhydrase inhibitor took many years but was an important event because of the poor side-effect profile of oral carbonic anhydrase inhibitors (CAIs). *Dorzolamide* (TRUSOPT) and *brinzolamide* (AZOPT) both work by inhibiting carbonic anhydrase (isoenzyme II), which is found in the ciliary body epithelium. This reduces the formation of bicarbonate ions, which reduces fluid transport and thus IOP (Sharir, 1997).

Any of these four drug classes can be used as additive second- or third-line therapy. In fact, the β-receptor antagonist timolol has been combined with the carbonic anhydrase inhibitor dorzolamide (*see* structure below) in a single medication (COSOPT).

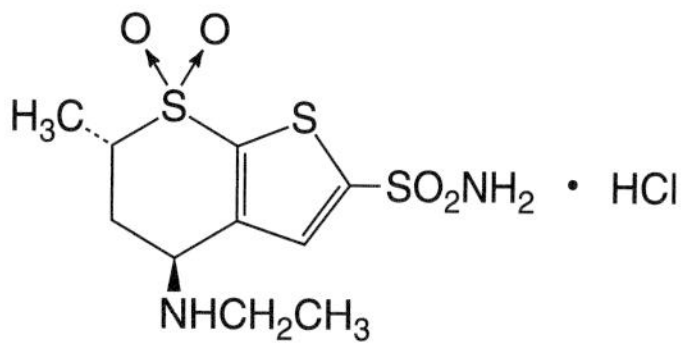

DORZOLAMIDE

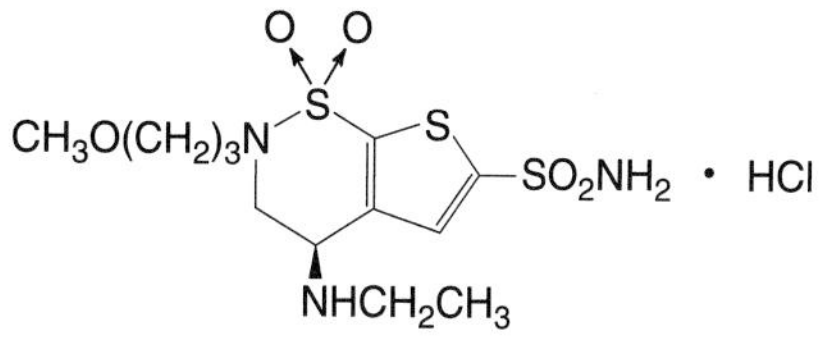

BRINZOLAMIDE

Such combinations reduce the number of drops needed and may improve compliance. Other combination products involving prostaglandin analogs and β blockers are in development.

Topical miotic agents are historically important glaucoma medications but are less commonly used today. Miotics lower IOP by causing muscarinic-induced contraction of the ciliary muscle, which facilitates aqueous outflow. They do not affect aqueous production. Multiple miotic agents have been developed. Pilocarpine and *carbachol* are cholinomimetics that stimulate muscarinic receptors. *Echothiophate* (PHOSPHOLINE IODIDE) is an organophosphate inhibitor of acetylcholinesterase; it is relatively stable in aqueous solution, and by virtue of its quaternary ammonium structure, is positively charged and poorly absorbed. The usefulness of these medicines is lessened by their numerous side effects and the need to use them three to four times a day (Kaufman and Gabelt, 1997).

If combined topical therapy fails to achieve the target intraocular pressure or fails to halt glaucomatous optic nerve damage, then systemic therapy with carbonic anhydrase inhibitors is a final medication option before resorting to laser or incisional surgical treatment. The best-tolerated oral preparation is *acetazolamide* in sustained-release capsules (*see* Chapter 28), followed by *methazolamide.* The least well-tolerated are acetazolamide tablets.

Toxicity of Agents in Treatment of Glaucoma. Ciliary body spasm is a muscarinic cholinergic effect that can lead to induced myopia and a changing refraction due to iris and ciliary body contraction as the drug effect waxes and wanes between doses. Headaches can occur from the iris and ciliary body contraction. Epinephrine-related compounds, effective in intraocular pressure reduction, can cause a vasoconstriction-vasodilation rebound phenomenon leading to a red eye. Ocular and skin allergies from topical epinephrine, related prodrug formulations, apraclonidine, and brimonidine are common. Brimonidine is less likely to cause ocular allergy and is therefore more commonly used. These agents can cause CNS depression and apnea in neonates and are contraindicated in children under the age of 2.

Systemic absorption of epinephrine-related drugs and β adrenergic antagonists can induce all the side effects found with direct systemic administration. The use of carbonic anhydrase inhibitors systematically may give some patients significant problems with malaise, fatigue, depression, paresthesias, and nephrolithiasis; the topical CAIs may minimize these relatively common side effects. These medical strategies for managing glaucoma do help to slow the progression of this disease, yet there are potential risks from treatment-related side effects, and treatment effects on quality of life must be recognized.

Uveitis. Inflammation of the uvea, or uveitis, has both infectious and noninfectious causes, and medical treatment of the underlying cause (if known) is essential in addition to the use of topical therapy. *Cyclopentolate,* or sometimes even longer-acting antimuscarinic agents such as atropine, *scopolamine,* and *homatropine* frequently are used to prevent posterior synechia formation between the lens and iris margin and to relieve ciliary muscle spasm that is responsible for much of the pain associated with anterior uveitis. If posterior synechiae already have formed, an α adrenergic agonist may be used to break the synechiae by enhancing pupillary dilation. A solution containing scopolamine 0.3% in combination with 10% *phenylephrine* is available for this purpose. Topical steroids usually are adequate to decrease inflammation, but sometimes they must be supplemented by systemic steroids.

Strabismus. Strabismus, or ocular misalignment, has numerous causes and may occur at any age. Besides causing *diplopia* (double vision), in children, strabismus may lead to *amblyopia* (reduced vision). Nonsurgical efforts to treat amblyopia include occlusion therapy, orthoptics, optical devices, and pharmacological agents. An eye with *hyperopia,* or farsightedness, must accommodate to focus distant images. In some hyperopic children, the synkinetic accommodative-convergence response leads to excessive convergence and a manifest *esotropia* (turned-in eye). The brain rejects diplopia and suppresses the image from the deviated eye. If proper vision is not restored by about the age of 7, the brain never learns to process visual information from that eye. The result is that the eye appears structurally normal but does not develop normal visual acuity and is therefore amblyopic. Unfortunately this is a fairly common cause of visual disability. In this setting, atropine (1%) instilled in the preferred seeing eye produces cycloplegia and the inability of this eye to accommodate, thus forcing the child to use the amblyopic eye (Pediatric Eye Disease Investigator Group, 2002; Pediatric Eye Disease Investigator Group, 2003). Echothiophate iodide also has been used in the setting of accommodative strabismus. Accommodation drives the near reflex, the triad of miosis, accommodation, and convergence. An irreversible cholinesterase inhibitor such as echothiophate causes miosis and an accommodative change in the shape of the lens; hence, the accommodative drive to initiate the near reflex is reduced, and less convergence will occur.

Surgery and Diagnostic Purposes. For certain surgical procedures and for clinical funduscopic examination, it is desirable to maximize the view of the retina and lens. Muscarinic cholinergic antagonists and α_2 adrenergic agonists frequently are used singly or in combination for this purpose (Table 63–7).

Intraoperatively, there are circumstances when miosis is preferred, and two cholinergic agonists are available for intraocular use, *acetylcholine* and carbachol. Patients with myasthenia gravis may first present to an ophthalmologist with complaints of double vision (diplopia) or lid droop (ptosis); the *edrophonium test* is helpful in diagnosing these patients (*see* Chapter 8).

Use of Immunomodulatory Drugs for Ophthalmic Therapy

Glucocorticoids. Glucocorticoids have an important role in managing ocular inflammatory diseases; their chemistry and pharmacology are described in Chapter 59.

Therapeutic Uses. Currently the glucocorticoids formulated for topical administration to the eye are *dexamethasone* (DECADRON, others), *prednisolone* (PRED FORTE, others), *fluorometholone* (FML, others), *loteprednol* (ALREX, LOTEMAX), *medrysone* (HMS), and *rimexolone* (VEXOL). Because of their antiinflammatory effects, topical corticosteroids are used in managing significant ocular allergy, anterior uveitis, external eye inflammatory diseases associated with some infections and ocular cicatricial pemphigoid, and postoperative inflammation following refractive, corneal, and intraocular surgery. After glaucoma filtering surgery, topical steroids can delay the wound-healing process by decreasing fibroblast infiltration, thereby reducing potential scarring of the surgical site (Araujo *et al.*, 1995). Steroids are commonly given systemically and by sub-Tenon's capsule injection to manage posterior uveitis. Intravitreal injection of steroids now is being used to treat a variety of retinal conditions including age-related macular degeneration, diabetic retinopathy, and cystoid macular edema. Parenteral steroids followed by tapering oral doses are the preferred treatment for optic neuritis (Kaufman *et al.*, 2000; Trobe *et al.*, 1999).

Toxicity of Steroids. Steroid drops, pills, and creams are associated with ocular problems, as are intravitreal and intravenous steroids. Ocular complications include the development of posterior subcapsular cataracts, secondary infections (*see* Chapter 59), and secondary open-angle glaucoma (Becker and Mills, 1963). There is a significant increase in risk for developing secondary glaucoma when there is a positive family history of glaucoma. In the absence of a family history of open-angle glaucoma, only about 5% of normal individuals respond to topical or long-term systemic steroids with a marked increase in intraocular pressure. With a positive family history, however, moderate to marked steroid-induced intraocular pressure elevations may occur in up to 90% of patients. The pathophysiology of steroid-induced glaucoma is not fully understood, but there is evidence that the *GLCIA* gene may be involved (Stone *et al.*, 1997). Typically, steroid-induced elevation of intraocular pressure is reversible once administration of the steroid ceases. However, intraocular or sub-Tenon's steroid-related pressure elevation may persist for months and may require treatment with glaucoma medication or even filtering surgery. Newer topical steroids, so called "soft steroids" (*e.g.*, loteprednol), have been developed that reduce, but do not eliminate, the risk of elevated intraocular pressure.

Nonsteroidal Antiinflammatory Agents. **General Considerations.** Nonsteroidal drug therapy for inflammation is discussed in Chapter 26. Nonsteroidal antiinflammatory drugs (NSAIDs) now are being applied to the treatment of ocular disease.

Therapeutic Uses. Currently, there are three topical NSAIDs approved for ocular use: *diclofenac* (VOLTAREN), *flurbiprofen* (OCUFEN), and *ketorolac* (ACULAR). Diclofenac and flurbiprofen are discussed in Chapter 26; the chemical structure of ketorolac, a pyrrolo-pyrolle derivative, is shown below:

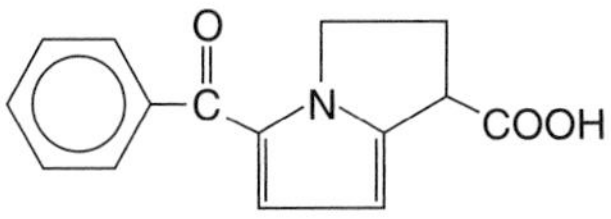

KETOROLAC

Flurbiprofen is used to counter unwanted intraoperative miosis during cataract surgery. Ketorolac is given for seasonal allergic conjunctivitis. Diclofenac is used for postoperative inflammation. Both ketorolac (Weisz *et al.*, 1999) and diclofenac have been found to be effective in treating cystoid macular edema occurring after cataract surgery. In patients treated with prostaglandin analogs such as latanoprost or bimatoprost, ketorolac and diclofenac may help decrease postoperative inflammation. They also are useful in decreasing pain after corneal refractive surgery. Topical NSAIDs occasionally have been associated with sterile corneal melts and perforations, especially in older patients with ocular surface disease, such as dry eye syndrome.

Antihistamines and Mast-Cell Stabilizers. *Pheniramine* (*see* Chapter 24) and *antazoline,* both H_1-receptor antagonists, are formulated in combination with *naphazoline,* a vasoconstrictor, for relief of allergic conjunctivitis. The chemical structure of antazoline is:

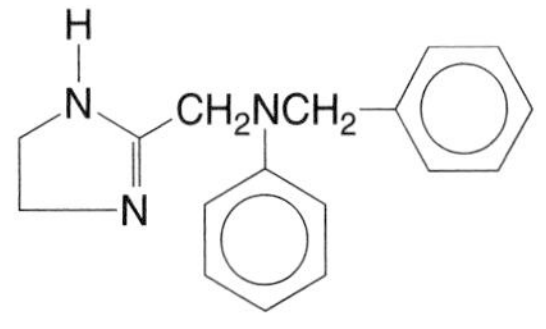

ANTAZOLINE

Topical antihistamines include *emedastine difumarate* (EMADINE) and *levocabastine hydrochloride* (LIVOSTIN).

Cromolyn sodium (CROLOM), which prevents the release of histamine and other autacoids from mast cells (*see* Chapter 27), has found limited use in treating conjunctivitis that is thought to be allergen-mediated, such as vernal conjunctivitis. *Lodoxamide tromethamine* (ALOMIDE) and *pemirolast* (ALAMAST), mast-cell stabilizers, also are available for ophthalmic use. *Nedocromil* (ALOCRIL) also is primarily a mast-cell stabilizer with some antihistamine properties. *Olopatadine hydrochloride* (PATANOL), *ketotifen fumarate* (ZADITOR), and *azelastine* (OPTIVAR) are H_1 antagonists with mast cell–stabilizing properties. *Epinastine* (ELESTAT) antagonizes H_1 and H_2 receptors and exhibits mast cell–stabilizing activity.

Immunosuppressive and Antimitotic Agents. **General Considerations.** The principal application of immunosuppressive and antimitotic agents to ophthalmology relates to the use of 5-fluorouracil and mitomycin C in corneal and glaucoma surgeries. Interferon alpha-2b also has occasionally been used. Certain systemic diseases with serious vision-threatening ocular manifestations— such as Behçet's disease, Wegener's granulomatosis, rheumatoid arthritis, and Reiter's syndrome—require systemic immunosuppression (*see* Chapter 52).

Therapeutic Uses. In glaucoma surgery, both fluorouracil and mitomycin (MUTAMYCIN), which also are antineoplastic agents (*see* Chapter 51), improve the success of filtration surgery by limiting the postoperative wound-healing process. Mitomycin is used intraoperatively as a single subconjunctival application at the trabeculectomy site. Meticulous care is used to avoid intraocular penetration, since mitomycin is extremely toxic to intraocular structures. Fluorouracil may be used intraoperatively at the trabeculectomy site and/or subconjunctivally during the postoperative course (Fluorouracil Filtering Surgery Study Group, 1989). Although both agents work by limiting the healing process, sometimes this can result in thin, ischemic, avascular tissue that is prone to breakdown. The resultant leaks can cause hypotony (low intraocular pressure) and increase the risk of infection.

In cornea surgery, mitomycin has been used topically after excision of pterygium, a fibrovascular membrane that can grow onto the cornea. Mitomycin can be used to reduce the risk of scarring after certain procedures to remove corneal opacities and also prophylactically to prevent corneal scarring after excimer laser surface ablation (photorefractive and phototherapeutic keratectomy). Mitomycin also is used to treat certain conjunctival and corneal tumors. Interferon alpha-2b has been used in the treatment of conjunctival papilloma and certain conjunctival tumors. Although the use of mitomycin for both corneal surgery and glaucoma filtration surgeries augments the success of these surgical procedures, caution is advocated in light of the potentially serious delayed ocular complications (Rubinfeld *et al.*, 1992; Hardten and Samuelson, 1999).

Immunomodulatory Agent. Topical *cyclosporine* (RESTASIS) is approved for the treatment of chronic dry eye associated with inflammation. Cyclosporine is an immunomodulatory agent that inhibits activation of T cells. Use of cyclosporine is associated with decreased inflammatory markers in the lacrimal gland, increased tear production, and improved vision and comfort (Sall *et al.*, 2000).

Drugs and Biological Agents Used in Ophthalmic Surgery

Adjuncts in Anterior Segment Surgery. Viscoelastic substances assist in ocular surgery by maintaining spaces, moving tissue, and protecting surfaces. These substances are prepared from hyaluronate, chondroitin sulfate, or hydroxypropylmethylcellulose and share the following important physical characteristics: viscosity, shear flow, elasticity, cohesiveness, and coatability. Various viscoelastic agents emphasize certain features that are broadly characterized as dispersive or cohesive. They are used almost exclusively in anterior segment surgery. Complications associated with viscoelastic substances are related to transient elevation of intraocular pressure after the surgical procedure.

Ophthalmic Glue. Cyanoacrylate tissue adhesive (ISODENT, DERMABOND, HISTOACRYL), while not FDA approved for the eye, is widely used in the management of corneal ulcerations and perforations. It is applied in liquid form and polymerized into a solid plug.

Fibrinogen glue (TISSEEL) is increasingly being used on the ocular surface to secure tissue such as conjunctiva, amniotic membrane, and lamellar corneal grafts. It is FDA approved for use in cardiac and gastrointestinal surgery, but not for the eye.

Corneal Band Keratopathy. Edetate disodium (disodium EDTA; ENDRATE) is a chelating agent that can be used to remove a band keratopathy (*i.e.*, a calcium deposit at the level of Bowman's membrane on the cornea). After the overlying corneal epithelium is removed, it is applied topically to chelate the calcium deposits from the cornea.

Anterior Segment Gases. Sulfur hexafluoride (SF_6) and perfluoropropane gases have long been used as vitreous substitutes during retinal surgery. In the anterior segment they are used in nonexpansile concentrations to treat Descemet's detachments, typically after cataract surgery. These detachments can cause mild to severe corneal edema. The gas is injected into the anterior chamber to push Descemet's membrane up against the stroma, where ideally it reattaches and clears the corneal edema.

Vitreous Substitutes. The primary use of vitreous substitutes is reattachment of the retina following vitrectomy and membrane-peeling procedures for complicated proliferative vitreoretinopathy and traction retinal detachments. Several compounds are available, including gases, perfluorocarbon liquids, and silicone oil (Table 63–8). With the exception of air, the gases expand because of interaction with systemic oxygen, carbon dioxide, and nitrogen, and this property makes them desirable to temporarily tamponade areas of the retina. However, use of these expansile gases carries the risk of complications from elevated intraocular pressure, subretinal gas, corneal edema, and cataract formation. The gases are absorbed over a time period of days (for air) to 2 months (for perfluoropropane).

The liquid perfluorocarbons, with specific gravities between 1.76 and 1.94, are denser than vitreous and are helpful in flattening the retina when vitreous is present. If a lens becomes dislocated into the vitreous, a perfluorocarbon liquid injection posteriorly will float the lens anteriorly, leading to easier surgical retrieval. This liquid can be an important tool for flattening and unrolling severely detached and contorted retinas such those found in giant retinal tears and proliferative vitreoretinopathy. This liquid is potentially toxic if it remains in chronic contact with the retina.

Silicone oil has had extensive use both in Europe and in the United States for long-term tamponade of the retina. Complications from silicone oil use include glaucoma,

Table 63–8
*Vitreous Substitutes**

VITREOUS SUBSTITUTE	CHEMICAL STRUCTURE	CHARACTERISTICS (DURATION OR VISCOSITY)
Nonexpansile gases		
Air		Duration of 5–7 days
Argon		
Carbon dioxide		
Helium		
Krypton		
Nitrogen		
Oxygen		
Xenon		Duration of 1 day
Expansile gases		
Sulfur hexafluoride (SF_6)		Duration of 10–14 days
Octafluorocyclobutane (C_4F_8)		
Perfluoromethane (CF_4)		Duration of 10–14 days
Perfluoroethane (C_2F_6)		Duration of 30–35 days
Perfluoropropane (C_3F_8)		Duration of 55–65 days
Perfluoro-*n*-butane (C_4F_{10})		
Perfluoropentane (C_5F_{12})		
Silicone oils		
Nonfluorinated silicone oils	$(CH_3)_3SiO[(CH_3)_2SiO]_nSi(CH_3)_3$	Viscosity range from 1000–30,000 cs
Fluorosilicone	$(CH_3)_3SiO[(C_3H_4F_3)(CH_3)SiO]_nSi(CH_3)_3$	Viscosity range from 1000–10,000 cs
"High-tech" silicone oils	$(CH_3)_3SiO[(C_6H_5)(CH_3)SiO]_nSi(CH_3)_3$	May terminate as trimethylsiloxy (shown) or polyphenylmethyl-siloxane, viscosity not reported

*See Parel and Villain, 1994, and Chang, 1994, for further details. cs, centistoke (unit of viscosity).

cataract formation, corneal edema, corneal band keratopathy, and retinal toxicity.

Surgical Hemostasis and Thrombolytic Agents.
Hemostasis has an important role in most surgical procedures and usually is achieved by temperature-mediated coagulation. In some intraocular surgeries, thrombin has a valuable role in hemostasis. Intravitreal administration of thrombin can assist in controlling intraocular hemorrhage during vitrectomy. When used intraocularly, a potentially significant inflammatory response may occur, but this reaction can be minimized by thorough irrigation after hemostasis is achieved. This coagulation factor also may be applied topically *via* soaked sponges to exposed conjunctiva and sclera, where hemostasis may be a challenge due to the rich vascular supply.

Topical *aminocaproic acid* (CAPROGEL) has been advocated to prevent rebleeding after traumatic *hyphema* (blood in the anterior chamber), but recent clinical trials report mixed success (Karkhaneh *et al.*, 2003; Pieramici *et al.*, 2003).

Depending on the intraocular location of a clot, there may be significant problems relating to intraocular pressure, retinal degeneration, and persistent poor vision. *Tissue plasminogen activator* (t-PA) (*see* Chapter 54) has been used during intraocular surgeries to assist evacuation of a hyphema, subretinal clot, or nonclearing vitreous hemorrhage. t-PA also has been administered subconjunctivally and intracamerally (*i.e.,* controlled intraocular administration into the anterior segment) to lyse blood clots obstructing a glaucoma filtration site. The main complication related to the use of t-PA is bleeding.

Botulinum Toxin Type A in the Treatment of Strabismus, Blepharospasm, and Related Disorders.
Botulinum toxin type A (BOTOX) has been used to treat strabismus, blepharospasm, Meige's syndrome, spasmodic torticollis hemifacial spasm, facial wrinkles, and certain migraine headaches (Tsui, 1996; Price *et al.*, 1997) (*see also* Chapter 9). By preventing acetylcholine release at the neuromuscular junction, botulinum toxin A usually causes a temporary paralysis of the locally injected muscles. The variability in duration of paralysis may be related to the rate of developing antibodies to the toxin, upregulation of nicotinic cholinergic postsynaptic receptors, and aberrant regeneration of motor nerve fibers at the neuromuscular junction. Complications related to this toxin include double vision (diplopia) and lid droop (ptosis).

Blind and Painful Eye.
Retrobulbar injection of either absolute or 95% ethanol may provide relief from chronic pain associated with a blind and painful eye. Retrobulbar chlorpromazine also has been used. This treatment is preceded by administration of local anesthesia. Local infiltration of the ciliary nerves provides symptomatic relief from pain, but other nerve fibers may be damaged, causing paralysis of the extraocular muscles, including those in the eyelids, or neuroparalytic keratitis. The sensory fibers of the ciliary nerves may regenerate, and repeated injections sometimes are needed to control pain.

Systemic Agents with Ocular Side Effects.
Just as certain systemic diseases have ocular manifestations, certain systemic drugs have ocular side effects. These can range from mild and inconsequential to severe and vision threatening.

Retina. Numerous drugs have toxic side effects on the retina. The antiarthritis and antimalarial medicines *hydroxychloroquine* (PLAQUENIL) and chloroquine can cause a central retinal toxicity by an unknown mechanism. With normal dosages, toxicity does not appear until about 6 years after the drug is started. Stopping the drug will not reverse the damage, but will prevent further toxicity. *Sildenafil* (VIAGRA) inhibits PDE5 in the corpus cavernosum for the purpose of helping to achieve and maintain penile erection. The drug also mildly inhibits PDE6, which controls the levels of cyclic GMP in the retina. Visually, this can result in seeing a blueish haze or experiencing light sensitivity. Although no retinal damage has been reported, no long-term studies have been reported (Marmor and Kessler, 1999). Two new phosphodiesterase inhibitors, *vardenafil* and *tadalafil,* also are associated with similar visual disturbances.

Optic Nerve. Multiple medications can cause a toxic optic neuropathy characterized by gradually progressive bilateral central scotomas and vision loss. There can be accompanying optic nerve pallor. These medicines include *ethambutol, chloramphenicol,* and *rifampin.* Systemic or ocular steroids can cause elevated IOP and glaucoma. If the steroids cannot be stopped, glaucoma medications, and even filtering surgery, often are required.

Anterior Segment. Steroids also have been implicated in cataract formation. If vision is reduced, cataract surgery may be necessary. *Rifabutin,* if used in conjunction with *clarithromycin* or *fluconazole* for treatment of *Mycobacterium avium complex* (MAC) opportunistic infections in HIV-positive persons, is associated with an iridocyclitis and even hypopyon. This will resolve with steroids or by stopping the medication.

Ocular Surface. *Isotretinoin* (ACCUTANE) has a drying effect on mucous membranes and is associated with dry eye.

Corneal Side Effects of Systemic Medications. The cornea, conjunctiva, and even eyelids can be affected by systemic medications. One of the most common drug deposits found in the cornea is from the cardiac medication *amiodarone.* It deposits in the inferior and central cornea in a whorl-like pattern termed *cornea verticillata.* It appears as fine tan or brown pigment in the epithelium. Fortunately, the deposits seldom affect vision and, therefore, this is rarely a cause to discontinue the medication. The deposits disappear slowly if the medication is stopped. Other medications can cause a similar pattern, including *indomethacin, atovaquone,* chloroquine, and hydroxychloroquine.

The phenothiazines, including *chlorpromazine* and *thioridazine,* can cause brown pigmentary deposits in the cornea, conjunctiva, and eyelids. The deposits generally are found in Descemet's membrane and the posterior cornea. They typically do not affect vision. The ocular deposits generally persist after discontinuation of the medication and can even worsen, perhaps because the medication deposits in the skin are slowly released and accumulate in the eye.

Gold treatments for arthritis (now rarely used) can lead to gold deposition in the cornea and conjunctiva, which are termed *chrysiasis* and are gold to violet in color. With lower cumulative doses (1 to 2 g) the deposits are found primarily in the epithelium and anterior stroma. These deposits usually disappear with discontinuation of the medication. With higher doses, the gold is deposited in Descemet's membrane and posterior stroma and can involve the entire stroma. These changes can be permanent. The deposits generally do not affect vision and are not a reason to stop gold therapy.

Tetracyclines can cause a yellow discoloration of the light-exposed conjunctiva. Systemic minocycline can induce a blue-gray scleral pigmentation that is most prominent in the interpalpebral zone (Morrow and Abbott, 1998).

Agents Used to Assist in Ocular Diagnosis

A number of agents are used in an ocular examination (*e.g.,* mydriatic agents and topical anesthetics, and dyes to evaluate corneal surface integrity), to facilitate intraocular surgery (*e.g.,* mydriatic and miotic agents, topical and local anesthetics), and to help in making a diagnosis in cases of anisocoria (Figure 63–5) and retinal abnormalities (*e.g.,* intravenous contrast agents). The autonomic agents have been discussed earlier. The diagnostic and therapeutic uses of topical and intravenous dyes and of topical anesthetics are discussed below.

Anterior Segment and External Diagnostic Uses. Epiphora (excessive tearing) and surface problems of the cornea and conjunctiva are commonly encountered external ocular disorders. The dyes *fluorescein, rose bengal,* and *lissamine green* are used in evaluating these problems. Available both as a 2% alkaline solution and as an impregnated paper strip, fluorescein reveals epithelial defects of the cornea and conjunctiva and aqueous humor leakage that may occur after trauma or ocular surgery. In the setting of epiphora, fluorescein is used to help determine the patency of the nasolacrimal system. In addition, this dye is used as part of the procedure of *applanation tonometry* (intraocular pressure measurement) and to assist in determining the proper fit of rigid and semirigid contact lenses. Fluorescein in combination with *proparacaine* or *benoxinate* is available for procedures in which a disclosing agent is needed in conjunction with a topical anesthetic. *Fluorexon* (FLUORESOFT), a high-molecular-weight fluorescent solution, is used when fluorescein is contraindicated (as when soft contact lenses are in place).

Rose bengal and lissamine green, which also are available as a 1% solution and as saturated paper strips, stain devitalized tissue on the cornea and conjunctiva.

Posterior Segment Diagnostic and Therapeutic Uses. The integrity of the blood–retinal and retinal pigment epithelial barriers may be examined directly by retinal angiography using intravenous administration of either *fluorescein sodium* or *indocyanine green* (structures shown below). These agents commonly cause nausea and may precipitate serious allergic reactions in susceptible individuals.

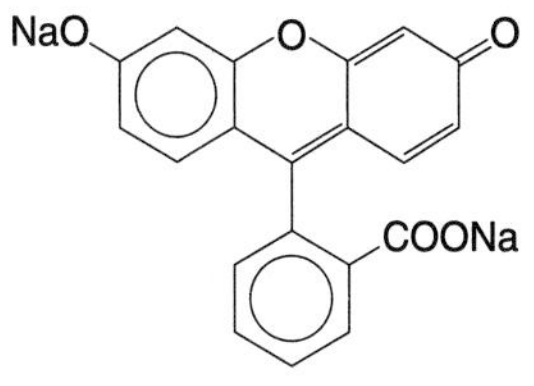

FLUORESCEIN SODIUM

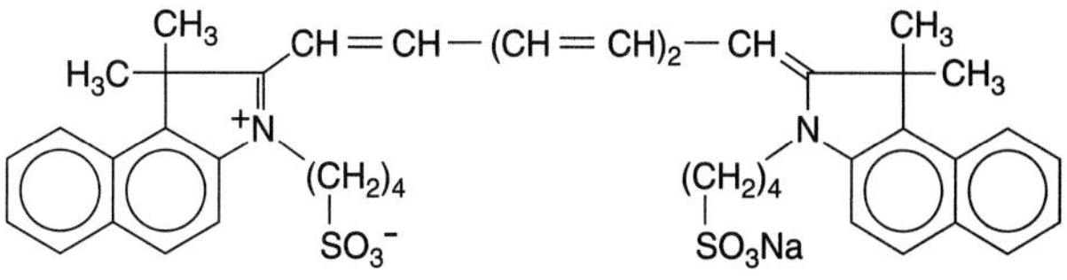

INDOCYANINE GREEN

Verteporfin (VISUDYNE) is approved for photodynamic therapy of the exudative form of age-related macular degeneration with predominantly classic choroidal neovascular membranes (Fine *et al.*, 2000). Verteporfin also is used in the treatment of predominantly classic choroidal neovascularization caused by conditions such as pathological myopia and presumed ocular histoplasmosis syndrome. The chemical structure of verteporfin, which is a mixture of two regioisomers (I and II), is shown below:

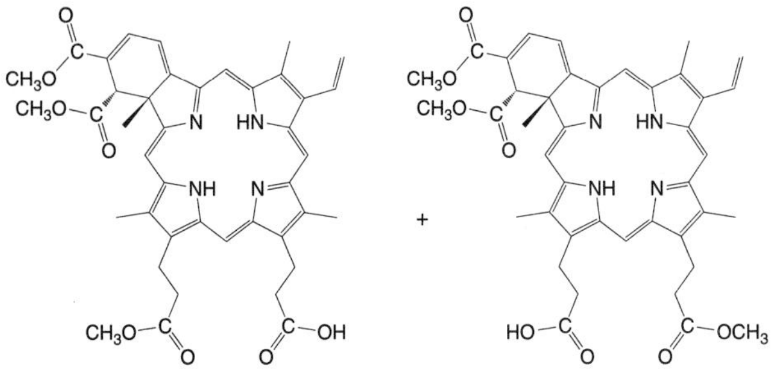

VERTEPORFIN REGIOISOMERS

Verteporfin is administered intravenously, and once it reaches the choroidal circulation, the drug is light-activated by a nonthermal laser source. Depending on the size of the neovascular membrane and concerns of occult membranes and recurrence, multiple photodynamic treatments may be necessary. Activation of the drug in the presence of oxygen generates free radicals, which cause vessel damage and subsequent platelet activation, thrombosis, and occlusion of choroidal neovascularization. The half-life of the drug is 5 to 6 hours. It is eliminated predominantly in the feces. The potential side effects include headache, injection site reactions, and visual disturbances. The drug causes temporary photosensitization, and patients must avoid exposure of skin or eyes to direct sunlight or bright indoor lights for 5 days after receiving it.

Use of Anesthetics in Ophthalmic Procedures

Topical anesthetic agents used clinically in ophthalmology include *cocaine,* proparacaine, and *tetracaine* drops and *lidocaine* gel (*see* Chapter 14). Proparacaine and tetracaine are used topically to perform tonometry, to remove foreign bodies on the conjunctiva and cornea, to perform superficial corneal surgery, and to manipulate the nasolacrimal canalicular system. They also are used topically to anesthetize the ocular surface for refractive surgery using either the excimer laser or placement of intrastromal corneal rings. Cocaine may be used intranasally in combination with topical anesthesia for cannulating the nasolacrimal system.

Lidocaine and *bupivacaine* are used for infiltration and retrobulbar block anesthesia for surgery. Potential complications and risks relate to allergic reactions, globe perforation, hemorrhage, and vascular and subdural injections. Both preservative-free lidocaine (1%), which is introduced into the anterior chamber, and lidocaine jelly (2%), which is placed on the ocular surface during preoperative patient preparation, are used for cataract surgery performed under topical anesthesia. This form of anesthesia eliminates the risks of the anesthetic injection and allows for more rapid visual recovery after surgery. General anesthetics and sedation are important adjuncts for patient care for surgery and examination of the eye, especially in children and uncooperative adults. Most inhalational agents and central nervous system depressants are associated with a reduction in intraocular pressure. An exception is *ketamine,* which has been associated with an elevation in intraocular pressure. In the setting of a patient with a ruptured globe, the anesthesia should be selected carefully to avoid agents that depolarize the extraocular muscles, which may result in expulsion of intraocular contents.

Other Agents for Ophthalmic Therapy

Vitamins and Trace Elements. *General Considerations.* Table 63–9 summarizes the current understanding of vitamins related to eye function and disease, especially the biochemistry of vitamin A.

Although vitamin A must be supplied from the environment, most actions of vitamin A, like those of vitamin D, are exerted through hormone-like receptors. Vitamin A has diverse actions in cellular regulation and differentiation that go far beyond its classically defined function in vision. Analogs of vitamin A, because of their prominent effects on epithelial differentiation, have found important therapeutic applications in the treatment of a variety of dermatological conditions and are being evaluated in cancer chemoprevention.

History. The relationship of night blindness to nutritional deficiency was definitively recognized in the 1800s. Ophthalmia brasiliana (keratomalacia), a disease of the eyes that afflicted primarily poorly nourished slaves, was first described in 1865. Later it was observed that the nurslings of mothers who fasted were prone to develop spontaneous sloughing of the cornea. Other reports of nutritional keratomalacia soon followed from all parts of the world.

Experimental rather than clinical observations, however, led to the discovery of vitamin A. In 1913, McCollum and Davis, and Osborne and Mendel independently reported that animals fed artificial diets with lard as the sole source of fat developed a nutritional deficiency that could be corrected by the addition to the diet of a factor contained in butter, egg yolk, and cod liver oil. An outstanding symptom of this experimental nutritional deficiency was xerophthalmia (dryness and thickening of the conjunctiva). Clinical and experimental vitamin A deficiencies were recognized to be related during World War I, when it became apparent that xerophthalmia in human beings was a result of a decrease in the amount of butterfat in the diet.

Chemistry and Terminology. Retinoid refers to the chemical entity retinol and other closely related naturally occurring derivatives. Retinoids, which exert most of their effects by binding to specific nuclear receptors and modulating gene expression, also include structurally related synthetic analogs that need not have retinol-like (vitamin A) activity (Evans and Kaye, 1999).

Table 63–9
Ophthalmic Effects of Selected Vitamin Deficiencies and Zinc Deficiency

DEFICIENCY	EFFECTS IN ANTERIOR SEGMENT	EFFECTS IN POSTERIOR SEGMENT
Vitamin		
A (retinol)	Conjunctiva (Bitot's spots, xerosis) Cornea (keratomalacia; punctate keratopathy)	Retina (nyctalopia; impaired rhodopsin synthesis); retinal pigment epithelium (hypopigmentation)
B_1 (thiamine)		Optic nerve (temporal atrophy with corresponding visual field defects)
B_6 (pyridoxine)	Cornea (neovascularization)	Retina (gyrate atrophy)
B_{12} (cyanocobalamin)		Optic nerve (temporal atrophy with corresponding visual field defects)
C (ascorbic acid)	Lens (?cataract formation)	
E (tocopherol)		Retina and retinal pigment epithelium (?macular degeneration)
Folic acid		Vein occlusion
K	Conjunctiva (hemorrhage) Anterior chamber (hyphema)	Retina (hemorrhage)
Zinc		Retina and retinal pigment epithelium (?macular degeneration)

See Chambers, 1994.

The purified plant pigment carotene (provitamin A) is a remarkably potent source of vitamin A. β-Carotene, the most active carotenoid found in plants, has the structural formula shown in Figure 63–7A. The structural formulas for the vitamin A family of retinoids are shown in Figure 63–7B.

Retinol, a primary alcohol, is present in esterified form in the tissues of animals and saltwater fish, mainly in the liver.

A number of *cis-trans* isomers exist because of the unsaturated carbons in the retinol side chain. Fish liver oils contain mixtures of the stereoisomers; synthetic retinol is the all-*trans* isomer. Interconversion between isomers readily takes place in the body. In the visual cycle, the reaction between retinal (vitamin A aldehyde) and opsin to form rhodopsin occurs only with the 11-*cis* isomer. Ethers and esters derived from the alcohol also show activity *in vivo*. The ring structure of retinol (β-ionone), or the more unsaturated ring in 3-dehydroretinol (dehydro-β-ionone), is essential for activity; hydrogenation destroys biological activity. Of all known derivatives, all-*trans*-retinol and its aldehyde, retinal, exhibit the greatest biological potency *in vivo;* 3-dehydroretinol has about 40% of the potency of all-*trans*-retinol.

Retinoic acid, in which the alcohol moiety has been oxidized, shares some but not all of the actions of retinol. Retinoic acid is ineffective in restoring visual or reproductive function in certain species where retinol is effective. However, retinoic acid is very potent in promoting growth and controlling differentiation and maintenance of epithelial tissue in vitamin A–deficient animals. Indeed, all-*trans*-retinoic acid (*tretinoin*) appears to be the active form of vitamin A in all tissues except the retina, and is ten- to one hundredfold more potent than retinol in various systems *in vitro*. Isomerization of this compound in the body yields 13-*cis*-retinoic acid (*isotretinoin*), which is nearly as potent as tretinoin in many of its actions on epithelial tissues, but may be only one-fifth as potent in producing the toxic symptoms of hypervitaminosis A.

Many retinoic acid analogs have been synthesized, including the prodrug *etretinate,* which is the ethyl ester of the active compound *acitretin*. These compounds are representative of the "second-generation" retinoids, in which the β-ionone ring is aromatized; they are more active than tretinoin in some systems but are less active in others. The highly potent "third-generation" retinoids feature two aromatic rings that serve to restrict the flexibility of the polyenoic side chain. This class of aromatic retinoids has been called *arotinoids,* and includes the carboxylic acid Ro 13-7410, and the ethyl sulfone Ro 15-1570.

Physiological Functions and Pharmacological Actions. Vitamin A plays an essential role in the function of the retina, is necessary for growth and differentiation of epithelial tissue, and is required for growth of bone, reproduction, and embryonic development. Together with certain carotenoids, vitamin A enhances immune function, reduces the consequences of some infectious diseases, and may protect against the development of certain malignancies. As a result, there is considerable interest in the pharmacological use of retinoids for cancer prophylaxis and for treating various premalignant conditions. Because of the effects of vitamin A on epithelial tissues, retinoids and their analogs are used to treat a number of skin diseases, including some of the consequences of aging and prolonged exposure to the sun (*see* Chapter 62).

The functions of vitamin A are mediated by different forms of the molecule. In vision, the functional vitamin is retinal. Retinoic acid appears to be the active form in functions associated with growth, differentiation, and transformation.

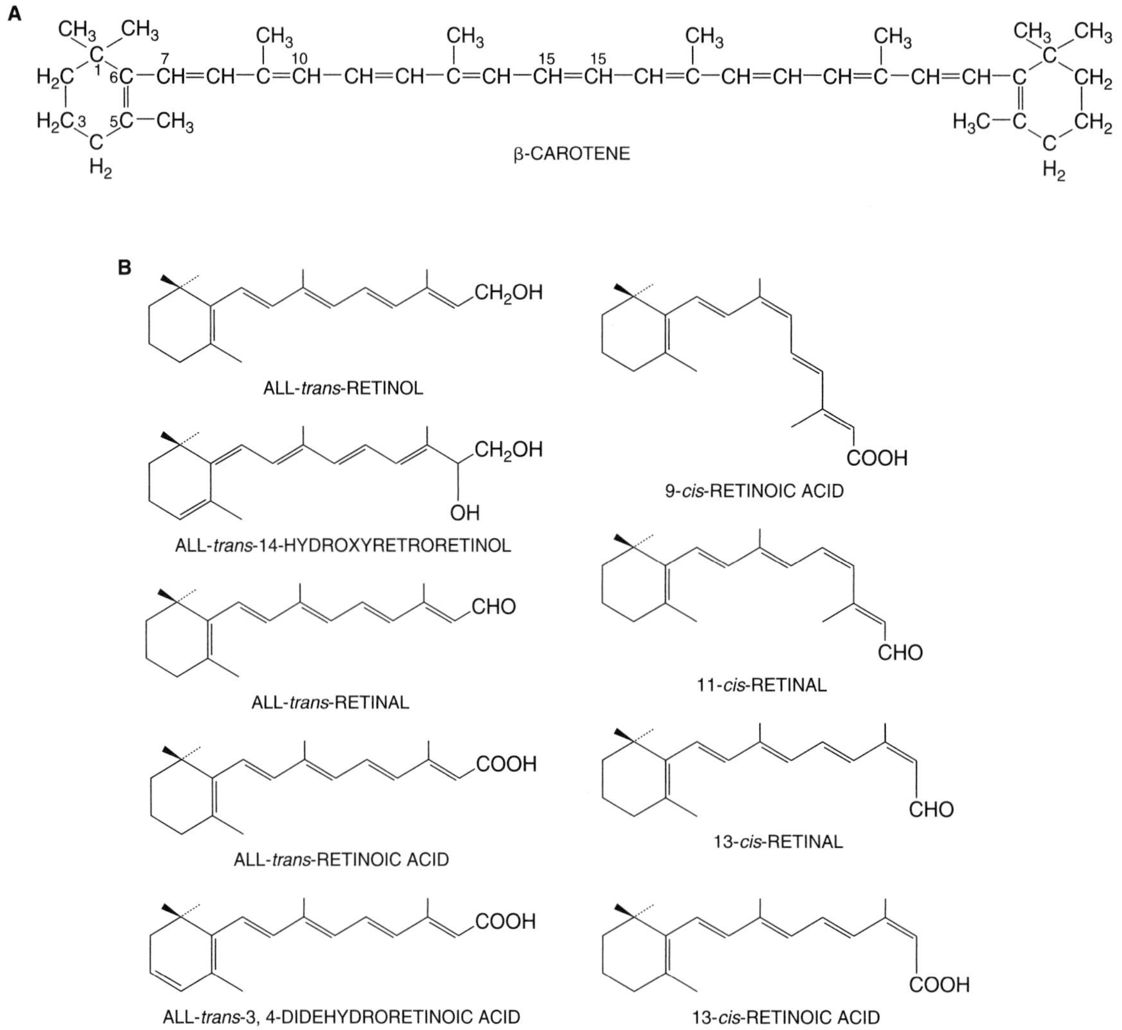

A

β-CAROTENE

B

ALL-*trans*-RETINOL

ALL-*trans*-14-HYDROXYRETRORETINOL

ALL-*trans*-RETINAL

ALL-*trans*-RETINOIC ACID

ALL-*trans*-3, 4-DIDEHYDRORETINOIC ACID

9-*cis*-RETINOIC ACID

11-*cis*-RETINAL

13-*cis*-RETINAL

13-*cis*-RETINOIC ACID

Figure 63–7. *A. Structural formula for β-Carotene. B. Structural formulas for the vitamin A family of retinoids.*

Retinal and the Visual Cycle. Vitamin A deficiency interferes with vision in dim light, a condition known as *night blindness* (nyctalopia).

Photoreception is accomplished by two types of specialized retinal cells, termed *rods* and *cones*. Rods are especially sensitive to light of low intensity; cones act as receptors of high-intensity light and are responsible for color vision. The initial step is the absorption of light by a chromophore attached to the receptor protein. The chromophore of both rods and cones is 11-*cis*-retinal. The holoreceptor in rods is termed *rhodopsin*—a combination of the protein opsin and 11-*cis*-retinal attached as a prosthetic group. The three different types of cone cells (red, green, and blue) contain individual, related photoreceptor proteins and respond optimally to light of different wavelengths.

In the synthesis of rhodopsin, 11-*cis*-retinol is converted to 11-*cis*-retinal in a reversible reaction that requires pyridine nucleotides. 11-*cis*-Retinal then combines with the ε-amino group of a specific lysine residue in opsin to form rhodopsin. Most rhodopsin is located in the membranes of the discs situated in the outer segments of the rods. The polypeptide chain of the protein spans the membrane seven times, a characteristic shared by all receptors whose functions are transduced *via* G proteins.

The visual cycle, depicted in Figure 63–8, is initiated by the absorption of a photon of light, followed by the photodecomposition, or bleaching, of rhodopsin through a cascade of unstable conformational states, leading ultimately to the isomerization of 11-*cis*-retinal to the all-*trans* form and dissociation of the opsin moiety. Activated rhodopsin interacts rapidly with another protein of the retinal rod outer segment, a G protein termed *transducin* or G_t. Transducin stimulates a cyclic GMP–specific phosphodiesterase (Figure 63–9). The resultant decline in cyclic GMP concentration causes a decreased conductance of cyclic GMP–gated Na^+ channels in the plasma membrane and an increased transmembrane potential (Figure 63–10). After processing within the retinal circuitry, this primary receptor potential ultimately leads to the generation of action potentials that travel to the brain *via* the optic nerve (Stryer, 1991). All-*trans*-retinal can isomerize to 11-*cis*-retinal, which then may

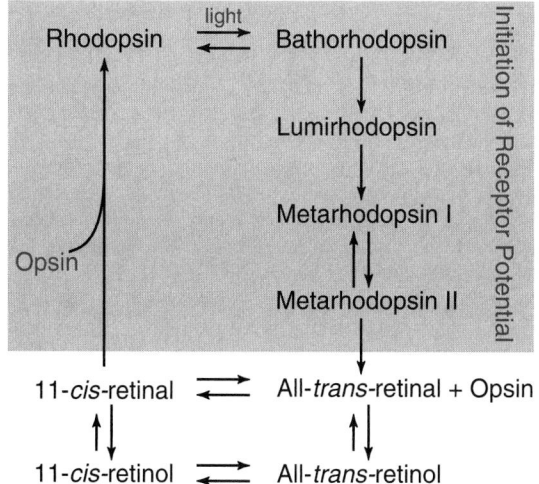

Figure 63–8. *The visual cycle.*

recombine with opsin to form rhodopsin. Alternatively, all-*trans*-retinal can cycle through all-*trans*-retinol and 11-*cis*-retinol to 11-*cis*-retinal, which combines with opsin to regenerate rhodopsin (Figure 63–8).

Humans deficient in vitamin A lose their ability for dark adaptation. Rod vision is affected more than cone vision. Upon depletion of retinol from liver and blood, usually at plasma concentrations of retinol of less than 0.2 mg/liter (0.70 μM), the concentrations of retinol and rhodopsin in the retina fall. Unless the deficiency is overcome, opsin, lacking the stabilizing effect of retinal, decays and anatomical deterioration of the rods' outer segments takes place. In rats maintained on a vitamin A–deficient diet, irreversible ultrastructural changes leading to blindness then supervene, a process that takes approximately 10 months.

Following short-term deprivation of vitamin A, dark adaptation can be restored to normal by the addition of retinol to the diet. However, vision does not return to normal for several weeks after adequate amounts of retinol have been supplied. The reason for this delay is unknown.

Vitamin A and Epithelial Structures. The functional and structural integrity of epithelial cells throughout the body is dependent upon an adequate supply of vitamin A. The vitamin plays a major role in the induction and control of epithelial differentiation in mucus-secreting or keratinizing tissues. In the presence of retinol or retinoic acid, basal epithelial cells are stimulated to produce mucus. Excessive concentrations of the retinoids lead to the production of a thick layer of mucin, the inhibition of keratinization, and the display of goblet cells.

In the absence of vitamin A, goblet mucous cells disappear and are replaced by basal cells that have been stimulated to proliferate. These undermine and replace the original epithelium with a stratified, keratinizing epithelium. The suppression of normal secretions leads to irritation and infection. Reversal of these changes is achieved by the administration of retinol, retinoic acid, or other retinoids. When this process happens in the cornea, severe hyperkeratinization (xerophthalmia) may lead to permanent blindness. Worldwide, xerophthalmia remains one of the most common causes of blindness.

Mechanism of Action. In isolated fibroblasts or epithelial tissue, retinoids enhance the synthesis of some proteins (*e.g.,* fibronectin) and reduce the synthesis of others (*e.g.,* collagenase, certain species of keratin), and molecular evidence suggests that these actions can be entirely accounted for by changes in nuclear transcription (Mangelsdorf *et al.*, 1994). Retinoic acid appears to

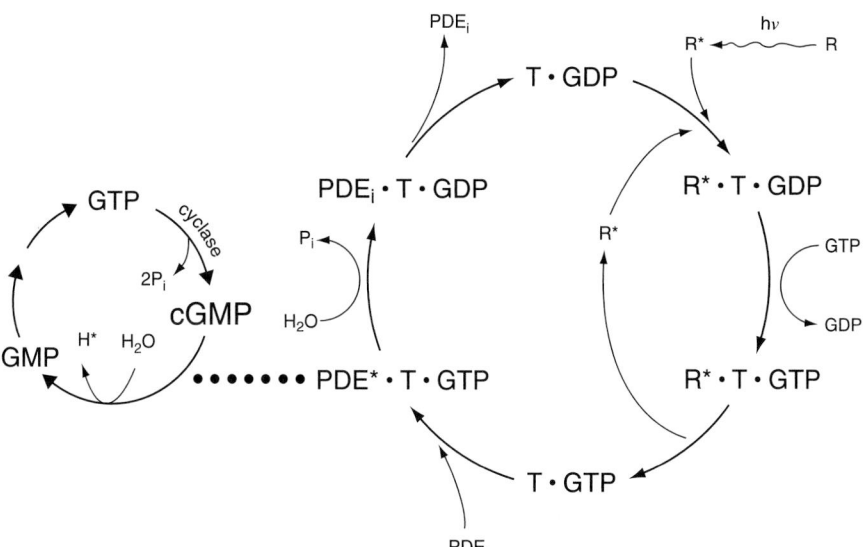

Figure 63–9. *The cGMP cascade of phototransduction.* The cycle on the right shows the steps by which the absorption of light by rhodopsin leads to the activation of a phosphodiesterase (PDE) hydrolyzing cGMP. T represents the GTP-binding protein transduction. (Reproduced with permission from Falk, G. Retinal physiology. In, (Heckenlively, J.R., and Arden, G.B., eds.) *Principles and Practice of Clinical Electrophysiology of Vision.* Mosby Year Book, New York, 1991.)

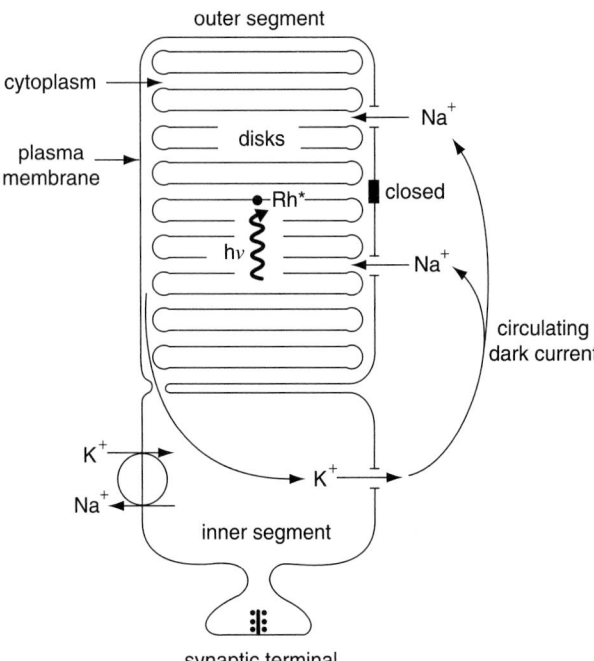

Figure 63–10. Ion movements across the surface membrane of a rod. In the dark there is a circulating current as cations, mainly Na ions, cross the outer segment membrane while K ions exit from the inner segment. Rhodopsin is embedded in stacks of disc membranes that are separated from each other and from the surface membrane. Light, absorbed by rhodopsin, leads to a change in the concentration of a diffusible substance and the closure of ion channels in the outer segment surface membrane, and this reduces the circulating current. (Reproduced with permission from Lamb, T.D. Transduction in vertebrate photoreceptors: the roles of cyclic GMP and calcium. *Trends Neurosci.*, **1986,** *9:*224–228.)

be considerably more potent than retinol in mediating these effects.

Retinoic acid influences gene expression by combining with nuclear receptors. Multiple retinoid receptors have been described. These are grouped into two families. One family, the retinoic acid receptors (RARs), designated α, β, and γ, are derived from genes localized to human chromosomes 17, 3, and 12, respectively. The second family, the retinoid X receptors (RXRs), also is composed of α, β, and γ receptor isoforms (Chambon, 1995). The retinoid receptors show extensive sequence homology to each other in both their DNA and hormone-binding domains and belong to a receptor superfamily that includes receptors for steroid and thyroid hormones and calcitriol (Mangelsdorf *et al.,* 1994). Cellular responses to thyroid hormones, calcitriol, and retinoic acid are enhanced by the presence of RXR. Gene activation involves binding of the hormone-receptor complex to promoter elements in target genes, followed by dimerization with an RXR-ligand complex. The endogenous RXR ligand is 9-*cis*-retinoic acid (Heyman *et al.,* 1992; Levin *et al.,* 1992). No comparable receptor for retinol has been identi-

fied; retinol may need to be oxidized to retinoic acid to produce its effects within target cells.

Retinoids can influence the expression of receptors for certain hormones and growth factors, and thus can influence the growth, differentiation, and function of target cells by both direct and indirect actions (Love and Gudas, 1994).

Therapeutic Uses. Nutritional vitamin A deficiency causes *xerophthalmia,* a progressive disease characterized by *nyctalopia* (night blindness), *xerosis* (dryness), and *keratomalacia* (corneal thinning) which may lead to perforation; xerophthalmia may be reversed with vitamin A therapy (WHO/UNICEF/IVAGG Task Force, 1988). However, rapid, irreversible blindness ensues once the cornea perforates. Vitamin A also is involved in epithelial differentiation and may have some role in corneal epithelial wound healing. Currently, there is no evidence to support using topical vitamin A for keratoconjunctivitis sicca in the absence of a nutritional deficiency. The current recommendation for retinitis pigmentosa is to administer 15,000 IU of vitamin A palmitate daily under the supervision of an ophthalmologist and to avoid high-dose vitamin E.

The recent Age-Related Eye Disease Study (AREDS) found a reduction in the risk of progression of some types of age-related macular degeneration for those randomized to receive high-doses of vitamins C (500 mg), E (400 IU), β-carotene (15 mg), cupric oxide (2 mg), and zinc (80 mg) (Age-Related Eye Disease Study Research Group, 2001b). Interestingly, zinc has been found to be neuroprotective in a rat model of glaucoma. The mechanism appears to be mediated by heat shock proteins and may represent a novel treatment strategy for glaucoma (Park *et al.,* 2001).

Wetting Agents and Tear Substitutes. *General Considerations.* The current management of dry eyes usually includes instilling artificial tears and ophthalmic lubricants. In general, tear substitutes are hypotonic or isotonic solutions composed of electrolytes, surfactants, preservatives, and some viscosity-increasing agent that prolongs the residence time in the cul-de-sac and precorneal tear film. Common viscosity agents include cellulose polymers (*e.g., carboxymethylcellulose, hydroxyethyl cellulose, hydroxypropyl cellulose, hydroxypropyl methylcellulose,* and *methylcellulose*), *polyvinyl alcohol, polyethylene glycol, polysorbate, mineral oil, glycerin,* and *dextran.* The tear substitutes are available as preservative-containing or preservative-free preparations. The viscosity of the tear substitute depends on its exact formulation and can range from watery to gel-like. Some tear formulations also are combined with a vasoconstrictor, such as naphazoline, phenylephrine, or *tetrahydrozoline.* In other countries, *hyaluronic acid* sometimes is used as a viscous agent; *hyaluronate* has not been approved for use in the United States.

The lubricating ointments are composed of a mixture of white petrolatum, mineral oil, liquid or alcohol lanolin, and sometimes a preservative. These highly viscous formulations cause considerable blurring of vision, and consequently they are used primarily at bedtime, in critically ill patients, or in very severe dry eye conditions.

Such aqueous and ointment formulations are only fair substitutes for the precorneal tear film, which is truly a poorly understood lipid, aqueous, and mucin trilaminar barrier (*see* above).

Therapeutic Uses. Many local eye conditions and systemic diseases may affect the precorneal tear film. Local eye disease, such as blepharitis, ocular rosacea, ocular pemphigoid, chemical burns, or corneal dystrophies, may alter the ocular surface and change the tear composition. Appropriate treatment of the symptomatic dry eye includes treating the accompanying disease and possibly the addition of tear substitutes. There also are a number of systemic conditions that may manifest themselves with symptomatic dry eyes, including Sjögren's syndrome, rheumatoid arthritis, vitamin A deficiency, Stevens-Johnson syndrome, and trachoma. Treating the systemic disease may not eliminate the symptomatic dry eye complaints; chronic therapy with tear substitutes or surgical occlusion of the lacrimal drainage system may be indicated.

Osmotic Agents and Drugs Affecting Carbonic Anhydrase. *General Considerations.* The main osmotic drugs for ocular use include *glycerin, mannitol* (*see* Chapter 28), and *hypertonic saline.* With the availability of these agents, the use of urea for management of acutely elevated intraocular pressure is nearly obsolete.

Therapeutic Uses. Ophthalmologists occasionally use glycerin and mannitol for short-term management of acute rises in intraocular pressure. Sporadically, these agents are used intraoperatively to dehydrate the vitreous prior to anterior segment surgical procedures. Many patients with acute glaucoma do not tolerate oral medications because of nausea; therefore, intravenous administration of mannitol and/or acetazolamide may be preferred over oral administration of glycerin. These agents should be used with caution in patients with congestive heart failure or renal failure.

Corneal edema is a clinical sign of corneal endothelial dysfunction, and topical osmotic agents may effectively dehydrate the cornea. Identifying the cause of corneal edema will guide therapy, and topical osmotic agents, such as hypertonic saline, may temporize the need for surgical intervention in the form of a corneal transplant. Sodium chloride is available in either aqueous or ointment formulations. Topical glycerin also is available; however, because it causes pain upon contact with the cornea and conjunctiva, its use is limited to urgent evaluation of filtration-angle structures. In general, when corneal edema occurs secondary to acute glaucoma, the use of an oral osmotic agent to help reduce intraocular pressure is preferred to topical glycerin, which simply clears the cornea temporarily. Reducing the intraocular pressure will help clear the cornea more permanently to allow both a view of the filtration angle by gonioscopy and a clear view of the iris as required to perform laser iridotomy.

BIBLIOGRAPHY

Age-Related Eye Disease Study Research Group. A randomized, placebo-controlled, clinical trial of high-dose supplementation with vitamins C and E, β carotene, and zinc for age-related macular degeneration and vision loss: AREDS report no. 8. *Arch Ophthalmol.,* **2001b,** *119:*1417–1436.

AGIS Investigators. The Advanced Glaucoma Intervention Study (AGIS): 7. The relationship between control of intraocular pressure and visual field deterioration. *Am J Ophthalmol.,* **2000,** *130:*429–440.

Ambati, B.K., Ambati, J., Azar, N., Stratton, L., and Schmidt, E.V. Periorbital and orbital cellulitis before and after the advent of *Haemophilus influenzae* type B vaccination. *Ophthalmology,* **2000,** *107:*1450–1453.

Araujo, S., Spaeth, G., Roth, S., and Starita, R. A 10-year follow-up on a prospective, randomized trial of postoperative corticosteroids after trabeculectomy. *Ophthalmology,* **1995,** *102:*1753–1759.

Becker, B., and Mills, D.W. Corticosteroids and intraocular pressure. *Arch. Ophthalmol.,* **1963,** *70:*500–507.

Beck, R.W., Cleary, P.A., Anderson, M.M., Jr., *et al.* A randomized, controlled trial of corticosteroids in the treatment of acute optic neuritis. The Optic Neuritis Study Group. *N. Engl. J. Med.,* **1992,** *326:*581–588.

Beck, R.W., Cleary, P.A., Trobe, J.D., *et al.* The effect of corticosteroids for acute optic neuritis on the subsequent development of multiple sclerosis. The Optic Neuritis Study Group. *N. Engl. J. Med.,* **1993,** *329:*1764–1769.

Chambon, P. The molecular and genetic dissection of the retinoid signaling pathway. *Recent Prog. Horm. Res.,* **1995,** *50:*317–332.

Chen, H.S., and Lipton, S.A. Mechanism of memantine block of NMDA-activated channels in rat retinal ganglion cells: uncompetitive antagonism. *J. Physiol. (Lond).,* **1997,** *499:*27–46.

Chien, D.S., Homsy, J.J., Gluchowski, C., and Tang-Liu, D.D. Corneal and conjunctival/scleral penetration of *p*-aminoclonidine, AGN 190342, and clonidine in rabbit eyes. *Curr. Eye Res.,* **1990,** *9:*1051–1059.

Colin, J., Prisant, O., Cochener, B., *et al.* Comparison of the efficacy and safety of valacyclovir and acyclovir for the treatment of herpes zoster ophthalmicus. *Ophthalmology,* **2000,** *107:*1507–1511.

Collaborative Normal-Tension Glaucoma Study Group. Comparison of glaucomatous progression between untreated patients with normal-tension glaucoma and patients with therapeutically reduced intraocular pressures. *Am. J. Ophthalmol.,* **1998a,** *126:*487–497.

Collaborative Normal-Tension Glaucoma Study Group. The effectiveness of intraocular pressure reduction in the treatment of normal-tension glaucoma. *Am. J. Ophthalmol.,* **1998b,** *126:*498–505.

Congdon, N., O'Colmain, B., Klaver, C.C., *et al.* Causes and prevalence of visual impairment among adults in the United States. *Arch Ophthalmol.,* **2004,** *122:*477–485.

Dreyer, E.B., Zurakowski, D., Schumer, R.A., *et al.* Elevated glutamate levels in the vitreous body of humans and monkeys with glaucoma. *Arch. Ophthalmol.,* **1996,** *114:*299–305.

Endophthalmitis Vitrectomy Study Group. Results of the Endophthalmitis Vitrectomy Study. A randomized trial of immediate vitrectomy and of intravenous antibiotics for the treatment of postoperative bacterial endophthalmitis. *Arch. Ophthalmol.,* **1995,** *113:*1479–1496.

Fluorouracil Filtering Surgery Study Group. Five-year follow-up of the fluorouracil filtering surgery study. *Am. J.Ophthalmol.,* **1996,** *121:*349–366.

Fluorouracil Filtering Surgery Study Group. Fluorouracil Filtering Surgery Study: one-year follow-up. *Am. J. Ophthalmol.,* **1989,** *108:*625–635.

Friedman, D.S., Wolfs, R.C., O'Colmain, B.J., *et al.* Prevalence of open-angle glaucoma among adults in the United States. *Arch. Ophthalmol.,* **2004,** *122:*532–538.

Hargrave, S.L., McCulley, J.P., and Husseini, Z. Results of a trial of combined propamidine isethionate and neomycin therapy for *Acanthamoeba* keratitis. Brolene Study Group. *Ophthalmology,* **1999,** *106:*952–957.

Heijl, A., Leske, M.C., Bengtsson, B., Hyman, L., and Hussein, M. Reduction of intraocular pressure and glaucoma progression: results from the Early Manifest Glaucoma Trial. *Arch. Ophthalmol.,* **2002,** *120:*1268–1279.

Herpetic Eye Disease Study Group. Acyclovir for the prevention of recurrent herpes simplex virus eye disease. *N. Engl. J. Med.,* **1998,** *339:*300–306.

Herpetic Eye Disease Study Group. A controlled trial of oral acyclovir for the prevention of stromal keratitis or iritis in patients with herpes simplex virus epithelial keratitis. The Epithelial Keratitis Trial. *Arch.*

Ophthalmol., **1997a,** *115:*703–712. [Published erratum appears in *Arch. Ophthalmol.,* **1997,** *115:*1196.]

Heyman, R.A., Mangelsdorf, D.J., Dyck, J.A., *et al.* 9-*cis* retinoic acid is a high affinity ligand for the retinoid X receptor. *Cell,* **1992,** *68:*397–406.

Karkhaneh, R., Naeeni, M., Chams, H., *et al.* Topical aminocaproic acid to prevent rebleeding in cases of traumatic hyphema. *Eur. J. Ophthalmol.,* **2003,** *13:*57–61.

Kass, M.A., Heuer, D.K., Higginbotham, E.J., *et al.* The Ocular Hypertension Treatment Study: a randomized trial determines that topical ocular hypotensive medication delays or prevents the onset of primary open-angle glaucoma. *Arch. Ophthalmol.,* **2002,** *120:*701–713; discussion 829–730.

Kaufman, D.I., Trobe, J.D., Eggenberger, E.R., and Whitaker, J.N. Practice parameter: the role of corticosteroids in the management of acute monosymptomatic optic neuritis. Report of the Quality Standards Subcommittee of the American Academy of Neurology. *Neurology,* **2000,** *54:*2039–2044.

Kunou, N., Ogura, Y., Yasukawa, T., *et al.* Long-term sustained release of ganciclovir from biodegradable scleral implant for the treatment of cytomegalovirus retinitis. *J. Control Release.,* **2000,** *68:*263–271.

Levin, A.A., Sturzenbecker, L.J., Kazmer, S., *et al.* 9-*Cis* retinoic acid stereoisomer binds and activates the nuclear receptor RXRα. *Nature,* **1992,** *355:*359–361.

Levkovitch-Verbin, H., Martin, K.R., Quigley, H.A., *et al.* Measurement of amino acid levels in the vitreous humor of rats after chronic intraocular pressure elevation or optic nerve transection. *J. Glaucoma,* **2002,** *11:*396–405.

Lichter, P.R., Musch, D.C., Gillespie, B.W., *et al.* Interim clinical outcomes in the Collaborative Initial Glaucoma Treatment Study comparing initial treatment randomized to medications or surgery. *Ophthalmology,* **2001,** *108:*1943–1953.

Lindsey, J.D., Gaton, D.D., Sagara, T., *et al.* Reduced TIGR/myocilin protein in the monkey ciliary muscle after topical prostaglandin F(2α) treatment. *Invest. Ophthalmol. Vis. Sci.,* **2001,** *42:*1781–1786.

Marx, J.L., Kapusta, M.A., Patel, S.S., *et al.* Use of the ganciclovir implant in the treatment of recurrent cytomegalovirus retinitis. *Arch. Ophthalmol.,* **1996,** *114:*815–820.

Morrow, G.L., and Abbott, R.L. Minocycline-induced scleral, dental, and dermal pigmentation. *Am. J. Ophthalmol.,* **1998,** *125:*396–397.

Park, K.H., Cozier, F., Ong, O.C., and Caprioli, J. Induction of heat shock protein 72 protects retinal ganglion cells in a rat glaucoma model. *Invest. Ophthalmol. Vis. Sci.,* **2001,** *42:*1522–1530.

Pediatric Eye Disease Investigator Group. A comparison of atropine and patching treatments for moderate amblyopia by patient age, cause of amblyopia, depth of amblyopia, and other factors. *Ophthalmology,* **2003,** *110:*1632–1638.

Pediatric Eye Disease Investigator Group. A randomized trial of atropine vs. patching for treatment of moderate amblyopia in children. *Arch. Ophthalmol.,* **2002,** *120:*268–278.

Pieramici, D.J., Goldberg, M.F., Melia, M., *et al.* A phase III, multicenter, randomized, placebo-controlled clinical trial of topical aminocaproic acid (Caprogel) in the management of traumatic hyphema. *Ophthalmology,* **2003,** *110:*2106–2112.

Price, J., Farish, S., Taylor, H., and O'Day, J. Blepharospasm and hemifacial spasm. Randomized trial to determine the most appropriate location for botulinum toxin injections. *Ophthalmology,* **1997,** *104:*865–868.

Quigley, H.A., Nickells, R.W., Kerrigan, L.A., *et al.* Retinal ganglion cell death in experimental glaucoma and after axotomy occurs by apoptosis. *Invest. Ophthalmol. Vis. Sci.,* **1995,** *36:*774–786.

Roig-Melo, E.A., Macky, T.A., Heredia-Elizondo, M.L., and Alfaro, D.V. 3rd. Progressive outer retinal necrosis syndrome: successful treatment with a new combination of antiviral drugs. *Eur. J. Ophthalmol.,* **2001,** *11:*200–202.

Rubinfeld, R.S., Pfister, R.R., Stein, R.M., *et al.* Serious complications of topical mitomycin-C after pterygium surgery. *Ophthalmology,* **1992,** *99:*1647–1654.

Sall, K., Stevenson, O.D., Mundorf, T.K., and Reis, B.L. Two multicenter, randomized studies of the efficacy and safety of cyclosporine ophthalmic emulsion in moderate to severe dry eye disease. CsA Phase 3 Study Group. *Ophthalmology,* **2000,** *107:*631–639.

Sanborn, G.E., Anand, R., Torti, R.E., *et al.* Sustained-release ganciclovir therapy for treatment of cytomegalovirus retinitis. Use of an intravitreal device. *Arch. Ophthalmol.,* **1992,** *110:*188–195.

Stone, E.M., Fingert, J.H., Alward, W.L.M., *et al.* Identification of a gene that causes primary open angle glaucoma. *Science,* **1997,** *275:*668–670.

Trobe, J.D., Sieving, P.C., Guire, K.E., and Fendrick, A.M. The impact of the optic neuritis treatment trial on the practices of ophthalmologists and neurologists. *Ophthalmology,* **1999,** *106:*2047–2053.

Vorwerk, C.K., Lipton, S.A., Zurakowski, D., *et al.* Chronic low-dose glutamate is toxic to retinal ganglion cells: toxicity blocked by memantine. *Invest. Ophthalmol. Vis. Sci.,* **1996,** *37:*1618–1624.

Wax, M.B., Tezel, G., and Edward, D. Clinical and ocular histopathological findings in a patient with normal-pressure glaucoma. *Arch. Ophthalmol.,* **1998,** *116:*993–1001.

Weisz, J.M., Bressler, N.M., Bressler, S.B., and Schachat, A.P. Ketorolac treatment of pseudophakic cystoid macular edema identified more than 24 months after cataract extraction. *Ophthalmology,* **1999,** *106:*1656–1659.

Wilhelmus, K.R., Gee, L., Hauck, W.W., *et al.* Herpetic Eye Disease Study. A controlled trial of topical corticosteroids for herpes simplex stromal keratitis. *Ophthalmology,* **1994,** *101:*1883–1895.

Yoles, E., and Schwartz, M. Elevation of intraocular glutamate levels in rats with partial lesion of the optic nerve. *Arch. Ophthalmol.,* **1998,** *116:*906–910.

MONOGRAPHS AND REVIEWS

Chambers, R.B. Vitamins. In, *Havener's Ocular Pharmacology,* 6th ed. (Mauger, T.F., and Craig, E.L., eds.) Mosby, St. Louis, **1994,** pp. 510–519.

Chang, S. Intraocular gases. In, *Retina,* Vol. 3: *Surgical Retina.* (Ryan, S.R., ed. in chief, Glaser B.M., section ed.) Mosby, St. Louis, **1994,** pp. 2115–2129.

Chern, K.C., and Margolis, T.P. Varicella zoster virus ocular disease. *Int. Ophthalmol. Clin.,* **1998,** *38:*149–160.

Evans, T.R., and Kaye, S.B. Retinoids: present role and future potential. *Br. J. Cancer,* **1999,** *80:*1–8.

Fang, E.N., and Kass, M.A. Epinephrine and dipivefrin. In, *Textbook of Ocular Pharmacology,* (Zimmerman, T.J., *et al.,* eds.) Lippincott-Raven, Philadelphia, **1997,** pp. 239–246.

Fine, S.L., Berger, J.W., Maguire, M.G., and Ho, A.C. Age-related macular degeneration. *N. Engl. J. Med.,* **2000,** *342:*483–492.

Grant, W.M., and Schuman, J.S. *Toxicology of the Eye,* 4th ed. Charles C. Thomas, Springfield, IL, **1993.**

Hardten, D.R., and Samuelson, T.W. Ocular toxicity of mitomycin-C. *Int. Ophthalmol. Clin.,* **1999,** *39:*79–90.

Jacobson, M.A., Stanley, H., Holtzer, C., *et al.* Natural history and outcome of new AIDS-related cytomegalovirus retinitis diagnosed in the era of highly active antiretroviral therapy. *Clin. Infect. Dis.,* **2000,** *30:*231–233.

Juzych, M.S., and Zimmerman, T.J. *β*-Blockers. In, *Textbook of Ocular Pharmacology.* (Zimmerman, T.J., *et al.,* eds.) Lippincott-Raven, Philadelphia, **1997,** pp. 261–275.

Juzych, M.S., Robin, A.L., and Novak, G.D. *α*-2 Agonists in glaucoma therapy. In, *Textbook of Ocular Pharmacology.* (Zimmerman, T.J., ed.) Lippincott-Raven, Philadelphia, **1997,** pp. 247–254.

Kaufman, P.L., and Gabelt, B.A.T. Direct, indirect, and dual-action parasympathetic drugs. In, *Textbook of Ocular Pharmacology.* (Zimmerman, T.J., ed.) Lippincott-Raven, Philadelphia, **1997,** pp. 221–238.

Kaur, I.P., and Kanwar, M. Ocular preparations: the formulation approach. *Drug Dev. Ind. Pharm.,* **2002,** *28:*473–493.

Lee, V.H.L. Precorneal, corneal, and postcorneal factors. In, *Ophthalmic Drug Delivery Systems.* (Mitra, A.K., ed.) Marcel Dekker, New York, **1993,** pp. 59–82.

Liesegang, T.J. Varicella-zoster virus eye disease. *Cornea,* **1999,** *18:*511–531.

Love, J.M., and Gudas, L.J. Vitamin A, differentiation and cancer. *Curr. Opin. Cell. Biol.,* **1994,** *6:*825–831.

Mangelsdorf, D.J., Umesomo, K., and Evans, R.M. The retinoid receptors. In, *The Retinoids: Biology, Chemistry, and Medicine,* 2nd ed. (Sporn, M.B., Roberts, A.B., and Goodman, D.S., eds.) Raven Press, New York, **1994,** pp. 319–349.

Marmor, M.F., and Kessler, R. Sildenafil (Viagra) and ophthalmology. *Surv. Ophthalmol.,* **1999,** *44:*153–162.

McCulley, J.P., Alizadeh, H., and Niederkorn, J.Y. The diagnosis and management of *Acanthamoeba* keratitis. *CLAO J.,* **2000,** *26:*47–51.

Parel, J. -M., and Villain, F. Silicone oils: physicochemical properties. In, *Retina,* Vol. 3: *Surgical Retina.* (Ryan, S.R., ed. in chief, Glaser, B.M., section ed.) Mosby, St. Louis, **1994,** pp. 2131–2149.

Physicians' Desk Reference for Ophthalmology, 28th ed. Medical Economics, Oradell, NJ, **2000.**

Robinson, J.C. Ocular anatomy and physiology relevant to ocular drug delivery. In, *Ophthalmic Drug Delivery Systems.* (Mitra, A.K., ed.) Marcel Dekker, New York, **1993,** pp. 29–58.

Sharir, M. Topical carbonic anhydrase inhibitors. In, *Textbook of Ocular Pharmacology,* (Zimmerman, T.J., ed.) Lippincott-Raven, Philadelphia, **1997,** pp. 287–290.

Stryer, L. Visual excitation and recovery. *J. Biol. Chem.,* **1991,** *266:*10711–10714.

Sucher, N.J., Lipton, S.A., and Dreyer, E.B. Molecular basis of glutamate toxicity in retinal ganglion cells. *Vision Res.,* **1997,** *37:*3483–3493.

Thompson, S., and Pilley, S.F. Unequal pupils. A flow chart for sorting out the anisocorias. *Surv. Ophthalmol.,* **1976,** *21:*45–48.

Tsui, J.K. Botulinum toxin as a therapeutic agent. *Pharmacol. Ther.,* **1996,** *72:*13–24.

Whitcup, S.M. Cytomegalovirus retinitis in the era of highly active antiretroviral therapy. *JAMA,* **2000,** *283:*653–657.

WHO/UNICEF/IVAGG Task Force. *Vitamin A Supplements: A Guide to Their Use in the Treatment and Prevention of Vitamin A Deficiency and Xerophthalmia.* World Health Organization, Geneva, **1988.**

SECTION XV
Toxicology

PRINCIPLES OF TOXICOLOGY AND TREATMENT OF POISONING

Curtis D. Klaassen

Toxicology is the science of the adverse effects of chemicals, including drugs, on living organisms. The discipline often is divided into several major areas. The *descriptive toxicologist* performs toxicity tests (*see* below) to obtain information that can be used to evaluate the risk that exposure to a chemical poses to humans and to the environment. The *mechanistic toxicologist* attempts to determine how chemicals exert deleterious effects on living organisms. Such studies are essential for the development of tests for the prediction of risks, for facilitating the search for safer chemicals, and for rational treatment of the manifestations of toxicity. The *regulatory toxicologist* judges whether a drug or other chemical has a low enough risk to justify making it available for its intended purpose. Two specialized areas of toxicology are particularly important for medicine. *Forensic toxicology,* which combines analytical chemistry and fundamental toxicology, is concerned with the medicolegal aspects of chemicals. Forensic toxicologists assist in postmortem investigations to establish the cause or circumstances of death. *Clinical toxicology* focuses on diseases that are caused by or are uniquely associated with toxic substances. Clinical toxicologists treat patients who are poisoned by drugs and other chemicals and develop new techniques for the diagnosis and treatment of such intoxications.

The clinician must evaluate the possibility that a patient's signs and symptoms may be caused by toxic chemicals present in the environment or administered as therapeutic agents. Many of the adverse effects of drugs mimic symptoms of disease. Appreciation of the principles of toxicology is necessary for the recognition and management of such clinical problems.

DOSE–RESPONSE RELATIONSHIP

Evaluation of the dose–response or the dose–effect relationship is crucially important to toxicologists. There is a graded dose–response relationship in an *individual* and a quantal dose–response relationship in the *population* (*see* Chapters 1 and 5). Graded doses of a drug given to an individual usually result in a greater magnitude of response as the dose is increased. In a quantal dose–response relationship, the percentage of the population affected increases as the dose is raised; the relationship is quantal in that the effect is specified to be either present or absent in a given individual (*see* Figure 5–4). This quantal dose–response phenomenon is extremely important in toxicology and is used to determine the *median lethal dose* (LD_{50}) of drugs and other chemicals.

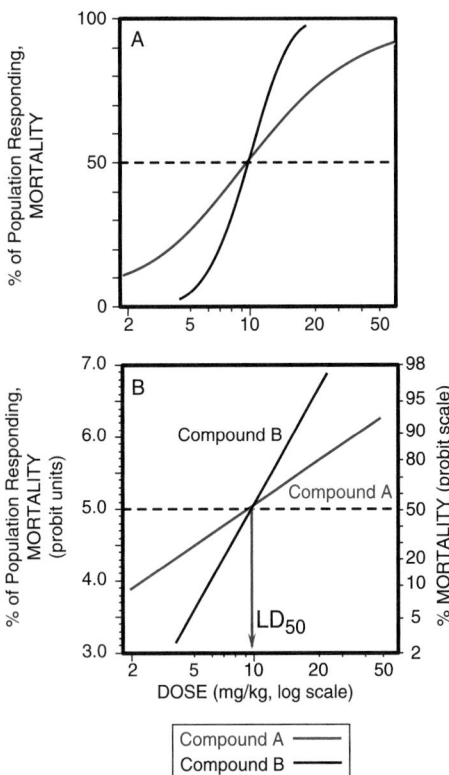

Figure 64–1. *Dose–response relationships.* **A.** The toxic response to a chemical is evaluated at several doses in the toxic or lethal range. The midpoint of the curve representing percent of population responding (response here is DEATH) *versus* dose (log scale) represents the LD_{50}, or the concentration of drug that is lethal in 50% of the population. **B.** A linear transformation of the data in *A* is provided by plotting the log of the dose administered *versus* the percent of the population killed in probit units.

The LD_{50} of a compound is determined experimentally, usually by administration of the chemical to mice or rats (orally or intraperitoneally) at several doses (usually four or five) in the lethal range (Figure 64–1A). To linearize such data, the response (death) can be converted to units of *deviation from the mean,* or *probits (probability units).* The probit designates the deviation from the median; a probit of 5 corresponds to a 50% response, and because each probit equals one standard deviation, a probit of 4 equals 16% and a probit of 6 equals 84%. A plot of the percentage of the population responding, in probit units, against log dose yields a straight line (Figure 64–1B). The LD_{50} is determined by drawing a vertical line from the point on the line where the probit unit equals 5 (50% mortality). The slope of the dose–effect curve also is important. The LD_{50} for both compounds depicted in Figure 64–1 is the same (10 mg/kg). However, the slopes of the dose–response curves are quite different. At a dose equal to one-half the LD_{50} (5 mg/kg), less than 5% of the animals exposed to compound B would die, but 30% of the animals given compound A would die.

The quantal, or "all-or-none," response is not limited to lethality. As described in Chapters 1 and 5, similar dose–effect curves can be constructed for any effect produced by chemicals.

RISK AND ITS ASSESSMENT

There are marked differences in the LD_{50} values of various chemicals. Some result in death at doses of a fraction of a microgram (LD_{50} for botulinum toxin equals 10 pg/kg); others may be relatively harmless in doses of several grams or more. While categories of toxicity that are of some practicality have been devised based on the amount required to produce death, often it is not easy to distinguish between toxic and nontoxic chemicals. Paracelsus (1493–1541) noted: "All substances are poisons; there is none which is not a poison. The right dose differentiates a poison and a remedy." It is simply not possible to categorize all chemicals as either safe or toxic. The real concern is the *risk* associated with use of the chemical. In the assessment of risk, one must consider concentration or dose as well as the harmful effects of the chemical accrued directly or indirectly through adverse effects on the environment when used in the quantity and in the manner proposed. Depending on the use and disposition of a chemical, a very toxic compound ultimately may be less harmful than a relatively nontoxic one.

At present, there is much concern about the risk from exposure to chemicals that have produced cancer in laboratory animals. For most of these chemicals, it is not known if they also produce cancer in humans. Regulatory agencies take one of three approaches to potential chemical carcinogens. For food additives, the U.S. Food and Drug Administration (FDA) is very cautious because large numbers of people are likely to be exposed to the chemicals, and they are not likely to have beneficial effects to individuals. For drugs, the FDA weighs the relative risks and benefits of the drugs for patients. Thus it is unlikely that the FDA will approve the use of a drug that produces tumors in laboratory animals for a mild ailment, but it may approve its use for a serious disease. In fact, most cancer chemotherapeutic drugs also are chemical carcinogens.

In the regulation of environmental carcinogens, government agencies, such as the U.S. Environmental Protection Agency (EPA), attempt to limit lifetime exposure such that the incidence of cancer due to the chemical would be no more than one in a million people. To determine the daily allowable exposure for humans, mathematical models are used to extrapolate doses of chemicals that produce a particular incidence of tumors in laboratory animals (often in the range of 10% to 20%) to those that should produce cancer in no more than one person in a million. The models used are conservative and are thought to provide adequate protection from undue risks from exposure to potential carcinogens. As discussed in Chapter 3, variations in drug metabolism often result in substantial differences between the biological responses of humans and rodents.

Acute versus Chronic Exposure. Effects of acute exposure to a chemical often differ from those that follow chronic exposure. Acute exposure occurs when a dose is delivered as a single event. Chronic exposure is likely to be to small quantities of a substance over a long period of time, which often results in slow accumulation of the compound in the body. Evaluation of *cumulative* toxic effects is receiving increased attention because of chronic exposure to low concentrations of various natural and synthetic chemical substances in the environment.

Chemical Forms of Drugs That Produce Toxicity. The "parent" drug administered to the patient often is the chemical form producing the desired therapeutic effect; the parent drug also may produce the toxic effects of drug. However, both therapeutic and toxic effects also can be due to metabolites of the drug produced by enzymes, light, or reactive oxygen species. In considering the toxicity of drugs and chemicals, it is important to understand their metabolism, activation, or decomposition.

Toxic Metabolites. The metabolites of many chemicals are responsible for their toxicities. Most organophosphate insecticides are biotransformed by cytochrome P450 enzymes (CYPs) to produce the active toxin. For example, parathion is biotransformed to paraoxon (Figure 64–2). Paraoxon is a stable metabolite that binds to and inactivates cholinesterase. Some drug metabolites are not chemically stable and are referred to as *reactive intermediates*. An example of a toxic reactive intermediate is the metabolite of *acetaminophen* (Figure 64–3), which is very reactive and binds to nucleophiles such as glutathione; when cellular glutathione is depleted, the metabolite binds to cellular macromolecules, the mechanism by which acetaminophen kills liver cells (*see* Chapter 26). Both parathion and acetaminophen are more toxic under conditions in which CYPs are increased, such as following *ethanol* or *phenobarbital* exposure, because CYPs produce the toxic metabolites (*see* Chapter 3).

  Phototoxic and Photoallergic Reactions. Many chemicals are activated to toxic metabolites by hepatic enzymatic biotransformation. However, some chemicals can be activated in the skin by ultraviolet and/or visible radiation. In photoallergy, radiation absorbed by a drug, such as a *sulfonamide*, results in its conversion to a product that is a more potent allergen than the parent compound. Phototoxic reactions to drugs, in contrast to photoallergic ones, do not have an immunological component. Drugs that are either absorbed locally into the skin or have reached the skin through the systemic circulation may be the object of photochemical reactions within the skin; this can lead directly either to chemically induced photosensitivity reactions or to enhancement of the usual effects of sunlight. *Tetracyclines,* sulfonamides, *chlorpro-*

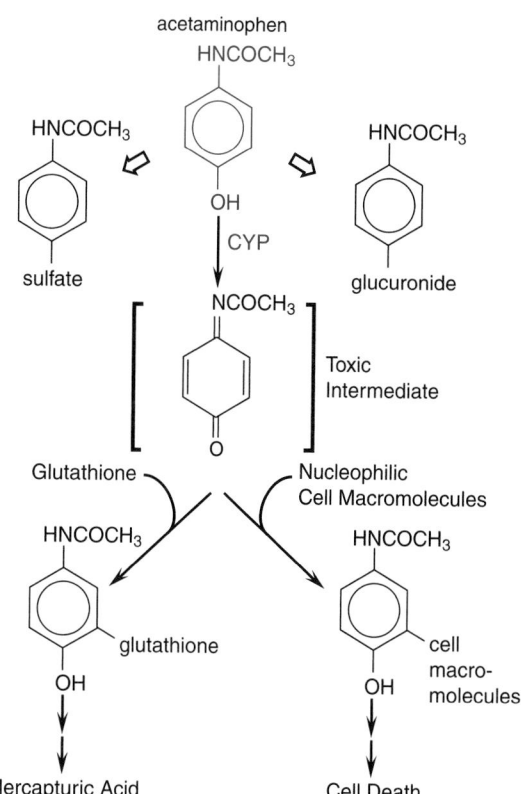

Figure 64–3. *Pathways of acetaminophen metabolism.*

mazine, and *nalidixic acid* are examples of phototoxic chemicals; generally, they are innocuous to skin if not exposed to light.

  Reactive Oxygen Species. Paraquat is an herbicide that produces severe lung injury. Its toxicity is not due to paraquat or its metabolites but rather to reactive oxygen species formed during one-electron reduction of paraquat paired with an electron donation to oxygen (Figure 64–4).

SPECTRUM OF UNDESIRED EFFECTS

The spectrum of undesired effects of chemicals may be broad and ill defined (Figure 64–5). In therapeutics, a

Figure 64–2. *Biotransformation of parathion.*

Figure 64–4. *Biotransformation of paraquat.*

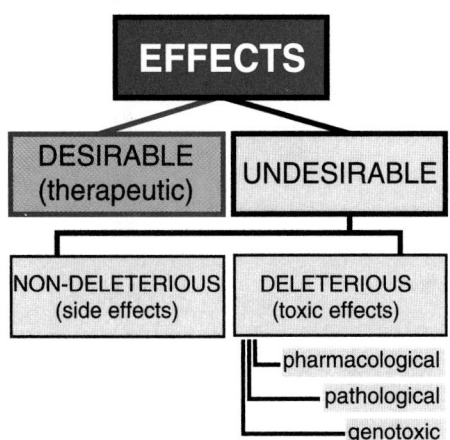

Figure 64–5. *Classification of the effects of chemicals.*

drug typically produces numerous effects, but usually only one is sought as the primary goal of treatment; most of the other effects are referred to as *undesirable effects* of that drug for that therapeutic indication. *Side effects* of drugs usually are nondeleterious; they include effects such as dry mouth occurring with tricyclic antidepressant therapy. Some side effects may be *adverse* or *toxic*. Mechanistic categorization of *toxic* effects is a necessary prelude to their avoidance or, if they occur, to effect their rational and successful management.

Types of Toxic Reactions. Toxic effects of drugs may be classified as pharmacological, pathological, or genotoxic (alterations of DNA), and their incidence and seriousness are related, at least over some range, to the concentration of the toxic chemical in the body. An example of a pharmacological toxicity is excessive depression of the central nervous system (CNS) by barbiturates; of a pathological effect, hepatic injury produced by acetaminophen; of a genotoxic effect, a neoplasm produced by a *nitrogen mustard*. If the concentration of chemical in the tissues does not exceed a critical level, the effects usually will be reversible. The pharmacological effects usually disappear when the concentration of drug or chemical in the tissues is decreased by biotransformation or excretion from the body. Pathological and genotoxic effects may be repaired. If these effects are severe, death may ensue within a short time; if more subtle damage to DNA is not repaired, cancer may appear in a few months or years in laboratory animals or in a decade or more in humans.

Local versus Systemic Toxicity. Local toxicity occurs at the site of first contact between the biological system and the toxicant. Local effects can be caused by ingestion of caustic substances or

inhalation of irritant materials. Systemic toxicity requires absorption and distribution of the toxicant; most substances, with the exception of highly reactive chemical species, produce systemic toxic effects. The two categories are not mutually exclusive. Tetraethyl lead, for example, injures skin at the site of contact and deleteriously affects the CNS after it is absorbed into the circulation (*see* Chapter 65).

Most systemic toxicants predominantly affect one or a few organs. The target organ of toxicity is not necessarily the site of accumulation of the chemical. For example, lead is concentrated in bone, but its primary toxic action is on soft tissues; DDT (chlorophenothane) is concentrated in adipose tissue but produces no known toxic effects there.

The CNS is involved in systemic toxicity most frequently because many compounds with prominent effects elsewhere also affect the brain. Next in order of frequency of involvement in systemic toxicity are the circulatory system; the blood and hematopoietic system; visceral organs such as liver, kidney, and lung; and the skin. Muscle and bone are least often affected. With substances that have a predominantly local effect, the frequency of tissue reaction depends largely on the portal of entry (skin, gastrointestinal tract, or respiratory tract).

Reversible and Irreversible Toxic Effects. The effects of drugs on humans, whenever possible, must be reversible; otherwise, the drugs would be prohibitively toxic. If a chemical produces injury to a tissue, the capacity of the tissue to regenerate or recover largely will determine the reversibility of the effect. Injuries to a tissue such as liver, which has a high capacity to regenerate, usually are reversible; injury to the CNS is largely irreversible because the highly differentiated neurons of the brain have a more limited capacity to divide and regenerate.

Delayed Toxicity. Most toxic effects of drugs occur at a predictable (usually short) time after administration. However, such is not always the case. For example, aplastic anemia caused by *chloramphenicol* may appear weeks after the drug has been discontinued. Carcinogenic effects of chemicals usually have a long latency period: 20 to 30 years may pass before tumors are observed. Because such delayed effects cannot be assessed during any reasonable period of initial evaluation of a chemical, there is an urgent need for reliably predictive short-term tests for such toxicity, as well as for systematic surveillance of the long-term effects of marketed drugs and other chemicals (*see* Chapter 5).

Chemical Carcinogens. Chemical carcinogens are classified into two major groups, *genotoxic* and *nongenotoxic*. Genotoxic carcinogens interact with DNA, whereas nongenotoxic carcinogens do not. Chemical carcinogenesis is a multistep process. Most genotoxic carcinogens are themselves unreactive (*procarcinogens* or *proximate carcinogens*) but are converted to *primary* or *ultimate carcinogens* in the body. The drug-metabolizing enzymes often convert the proximate carcinogens to reactive electron-deficient intermediates (electrophiles). These reactive intermediates can interact with electron-rich (nucleophilic) centers in DNA to produce a mutation. Such interaction of the ultimate carcinogen with DNA in a cell is thought to be the initial step in chemical carcinogenesis. The DNA may revert to normal if DNA repair mechanisms operate successfully; if not, the transformed cell may grow into a tumor that becomes apparent clinically.

Nongenotoxic carcinogens, also referred to as *promoters,* do not produce tumors alone but do potentiate the effects of genotoxic carcinogens. Promotion involves facilitation of the growth and development of so-called dormant or latent tumor cells. The time from initiation to the development of a tumor probably depends on the presence of such promoters; for many human tumors, the latent period is 15 to 45 years.

To determine whether a chemical is potentially carcinogenic to humans, two main types of laboratory tests are conducted. One type of study is performed to determine whether the chemical is mutagenic because many carcinogens are also mutagens. These studies often use assays such as the Ames test (*see* below), which can be completed within a few days and can detect genotoxic carcinogens but not promoters. The second type of study to detect chemical carcinogens consists of feeding laboratory animals (mice and rats) the chemical at high dosages for their entire life span, after which autopsies and histopathological examinations are performed on each animal. The incidence of tumors in control animals and animals fed the chemical are compared to determine whether the chemical produces an increased incidence of tumors. This latter study can detect both promoters and genotoxic carcinogens.

Allergic Reactions. *Chemical allergy* is an adverse reaction that results from previous sensitization to a particular chemical or to one that is structurally similar. Such reactions are mediated by the immune system. The terms *hypersensitivity* and *drug allergy* often are used to describe the allergic state.

For a low-molecular-weight chemical to cause an allergic reaction, it or its metabolic product usually acts as a hapten, combining with an endogenous protein to form an antigenic complex. Such antigens induce the synthesis of antibodies, usually after a latent period of at least 1 or 2 weeks. Subsequent exposure of the organism to the chemical results in an antigen–antibody interaction that provokes the typical manifestations of allergy. Dose–response relationships usually are not apparent for the provocation of allergic reactions.

Allergic responses have been divided into four general categories based on the mechanism of immunological involvement (Coombs and Gell, 1975). Type I, or anaphylactic, reactions, are mediated by IgE antibodies. The Fc portion of IgE can bind to receptors on mast cells and basophils (*see* Chapter 27). If the Fab portion of the antibody molecule then binds antigen, various mediators (*e.g.,* histamine, leukotrienes, and prostaglandins) are released and cause vasodilation, edema, and an inflammatory response. The main targets of this type of reaction are the gastrointestinal tract (food allergies), the skin (urticaria and atopic dermatitis), the respiratory system (rhinitis and asthma), and the vasculature (anaphylactic shock). These responses tend to occur quickly after challenge with an antigen to which the individual has been sensitized and are termed *immediate hypersensitivity reactions.*

Type II, or cytolytic, reactions are mediated by both IgG and IgM antibodies and usually are attributed to their ability to activate the complement system. The major target tissues for cytolytic reactions are the cells in the circulatory system. Examples of type II allergic responses include *penicillin*-induced hemolytic anemia, *methyldopa*-induced autoimmune hemolytic anemia, *quinidine*-induced thrombocytopenic purpura, and sulfonamide-induced granulocytopenia. Fortunately, these autoimmune reactions to drugs usually subside within several months after removal of the offending agent.

Type III, or Arthus, reactions are mediated predominantly by IgG; the mechanism involves the generation of antigen–antibody complexes that subsequently fix complement. The complexes are deposited in the vascular endothelium, where a destructive inflammatory response called *serum sickness* occurs. This phenomenon contrasts with the type II reaction, in which the inflammatory response is induced by antibodies directed against tissue antigens. The clinical symptoms of serum sickness include urticarial skin eruptions, arthralgia or arthritis, lymphadenopathy, and fever. These reactions usually last for 6 to 12 days and then subside after the offending agent is eliminated. Several drugs (*e.g.,* sulfonamides, penicillins, certain *anticonvulsants,* and *iodides*) can induce serum sickness. Stevens-Johnson syndrome, such as that caused by sulfonamides, is a more severe form of immune vasculitis. Manifestations of this reaction include erythema multiforme, arthritis, nephritis, CNS abnormalities, and myocarditis.

Type IV, or delayed-hypersensitivity, reactions are mediated by sensitized T-lymphocytes and macrophages. When sensitized cells come in contact with antigen, an inflammatory reaction is generated by the production of lymphokines and the subsequent influx of neutrophils and macrophages. An example of type IV or delayed hypersensitivity is the contact dermatitis caused by poison ivy.

Idiosyncratic Reactions. *Idiosyncrasy* is an abnormal reactivity to a chemical that is peculiar to a given individual. The idiosyncratic response may take the form of extreme sensitivity to low doses or extreme insensitivity to high doses of chemicals. We now know that certain idiosyncratic reactions can result from genetic polymorphisms that cause individual differences in drug pharmacokinetics; for example, an increased incidence of peripheral neuropathy is seen in patients with inherited deficiencies in acetylation when *isoniazid* is used to treat tuberculosis. The polymorphisms also can be due to pharmacodynamic factors such as drug-receptor interactions (Evans and Relling, 1999). For example, many black males (about 10%) develop a serious hemolytic anemia when they receive *primaquine* as an antimalarial therapy. Such individuals have a deficiency of erythrocyte glucose-6-phosphate dehydrogenase (*see* Chapter 39). Genetically determined resistance to the anticoagulant action of *warfarin* is due to an alteration in the vitamin K epoxide reductase (*see* Chapter 54). The use of genetic information to explain interindividual differences in drug responses or to individualize dosages of drugs for patients with known genetic polymorphisms is referred to as *pharmacogenomics* (*see* Chapters 3 and 4).

Interactions between Chemicals. The existence of numerous toxicants requires consideration of their potential interactions (Figure 64–6). Concurrent exposures may alter the pharmacokinetics of drugs by changing rates of absorption, the degree of protein binding, or the rates of biotransformation or excretion of one or both interacting compounds. The pharmacodynamics of chemicals can be altered by competition at the receptor; for example, *atropine* is used

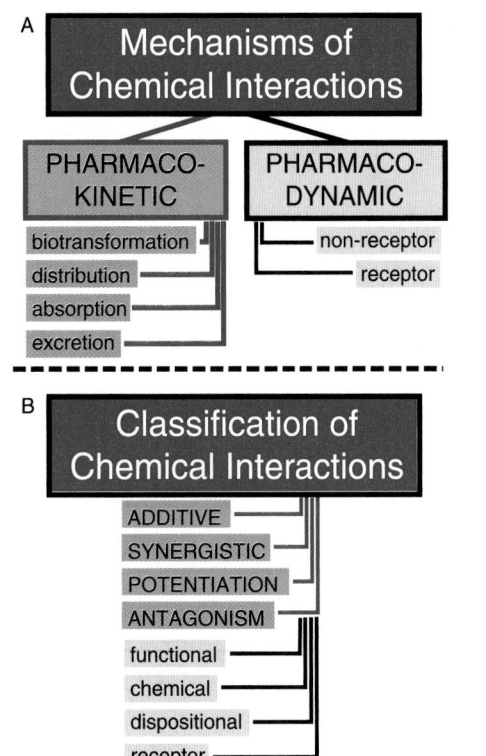

Figure 64–6. *Mechanisms and classifications of chemical interactions.*

to treat organophosphate insecticide toxicity because it blocks muscarinic cholinergic receptors and prevents their stimulation by the excess acetylcholine accruing from inhibition of acetylcholinesterase by the insecticide. Nonreceptor pharmacodynamic drug interactions also can occur when two drugs have different mechanisms of action: *Aspirin* and *heparin* given together can cause unexpected bleeding. The response to combined toxicants thus may be equal to, greater than, or less than the sum of the effects of the individual agents.

Numerous terms describe pharmacological and toxicological interactions (Figure 64–6B). An *additive* effect describes the combined effect of two chemicals that equals the sum of the effect of each agent given alone; the additive effect is the most common. A *synergistic* effect is one in which the combined effect of two chemicals exceeds the sum of the effects of each agent given alone. For example, both carbon tetrachloride and ethanol are hepatotoxins, but together they produce much more injury to the liver than expected from the sum of their individual effects. *Potentiation* is the increased effect of a toxic agent acting simultaneously with a nontoxic one. *Isopropanol* alone, for example, is not hepatotoxic; however, it greatly increases the hepatotoxicity of carbon tetrachloride. *Antagonism* is the interference of one chemical with the action of another. An antagonistic agent is often desirable as an antidote. *Functional* or *physiological antagonism* occurs when two chemicals produce opposite effects on the same physiological function. For example, this principle is applied to the use of intravenous infusion of dopamine to maintain perfusion of vital organs during certain severe intoxications characterized by marked hypotension. *Chemical antagonism* or *inactivation* is a reaction between two chemicals to neutralize their effects. For example, *dimercaprol* chelates various metals to decrease their toxicity (*see*

Chapter 65). *Dispositional antagonism* is the alteration of the disposition of a substance (its absorption, biotransformation, distribution, or excretion) so that less of the agent reaches the target organ or its persistence there is reduced (*see* below). *Antagonism* at the *receptor* for the chemical entails the blockade of the effect of an agonist with an appropriate antagonist that competes for the same site. For example, the antagonist *naloxone* is used to treat respiratory depression produced by opioids (*see* Chapter 21).

DESCRIPTIVE TOXICITY TESTS IN ANIMALS

Two main principles underlie all descriptive toxicity tests performed in animals. First, effects of chemicals produced in laboratory animals, when properly qualified, apply to human toxicity. When calculated on the basis of dose per unit of body surface, toxic effects in human beings usually are encountered in the same range of concentrations as those in experimental animals. On the basis of body weight, human beings generally are more vulnerable than experimental animals. Such information is used to select dosages for clinical trials of candidate therapeutic agents and to attempt to set limits on permissible exposure to environmental toxicants.

Second, exposure of experimental animals to toxic agents in high doses is a necessary and valid method to discover possible hazards to human beings who are exposed to much lower doses. This principle is based on the quantal dose–response concept. As a matter of practicality, the number of animals used in experiments on toxic materials usually will be small compared with the size of human populations potentially at risk. For example, 0.01% incidence of a serious toxic effect (such as cancer) represents 25,000 people in a population of 250 million. Such an incidence is unacceptably high. Yet, detecting an incidence of 0.01% experimentally probably would require a minimum of 30,000 animals. To estimate risk at low dosage, large doses must be given to relatively small groups. The validity of the necessary extrapolation is clearly a crucial question.

Chemicals are first tested for toxicity by estimation of the LD_{50} in two animal species by two routes of administration; one of these is the expected route of exposure of human beings to the chemical being tested. The number of animals that die in a 14-day period after a single dose is recorded. The animals also are examined for signs of intoxication, lethargy, behavioral modification, and morbidity.

The chemical is next tested for toxicity by repeat exposure, usually for 90 days. This study is performed most often in two species by the route of intended use or exposure with at least three doses. A number of parameters are monitored during this period, and at the end of the study, organs and tissues are examined by a pathologist.

Long-term or chronic studies are carried out in animals at the same time that clinical trials are undertaken. For drugs, the length of exposure depends somewhat on the intended clinical use. If the drug normally would be used for short periods under medical supervision, as would an antimicrobial agent, a chronic exposure of animals for 6 months might suffice. If the drug would be used in human beings for longer periods, a study of chronic use for 2 years may be required.

Studies of chronic exposure often are used to determine the carcinogenic potential of chemicals. These studies usually are performed in rats and mice for the average lifetime of the species. Other tests are designed to evaluate teratogenicity (congenital malformations), perinatal and postnatal toxicity, and effects on fertility. Teratogenicity studies usually are performed by administering drugs to pregnant rats and rabbits during the period of organogenesis.

In addition to chronic studies for evaluation of carcinogenic potential or teratogenicity, drugs often are tested for *mutagenic* potential. The most popular such test currently available, the reverse mutation test developed by Ames and colleagues (Ames *et al.*, 1975), uses a strain of *S. typhimurium* that has a mutant gene for the enzyme phosphoribosyl adenosine triphosphate (ATP) synthetase. This enzyme is required for histidine synthesis, and the bacterial strain is unable to grow in a histidine-deficient medium unless a reverse mutation is induced. Because many chemicals are not mutagenic or carcinogenic unless activated by enzymes on the endoplasmic reticulum, rat hepatic microsomes usually are added to the medium containing the mutant bacteria and the drug. The Ames test is rapid and sensitive. Its usefulness for the prediction of genotoxic carcinogens is widely accepted, but it does not detect nongenotoxic carcinogens (promoters).

INCIDENCE OF ACUTE POISONING

The true incidence of poisoning in the United States is not known, but in 2003, nearly 2.4 million cases were voluntarily reported to the American Association of Poison Control Centers. The number of actual poisonings almost certainly exceeds by far the number reported.

Deaths in the United States owing to poisoning number more than 1100 per year. The incidence of poisoning in children younger than 5 years of age has decreased dramatically over the past four decades. For example, there were no reported childhood deaths owing to aspirin in 2003, compared with about 140 deaths per year in the early 1960s. This favorable trend probably is due to safety packaging of drugs, drain cleaners, turpentine, and other household chemicals; improved medical training and care; and increased public awareness of potential poisons.

The substances involved most frequently in human poison exposures are shown in Table 64–1. Analgesic drugs lead the list, followed by two nondrug entries, cleaning agents and cosmetics. However, the top five categories of substances that produce deaths are drugs (Table 64–2). The categories most commonly associated with fatalities are analgesics (*e.g.,* acetaminophen and salicylates), sedative-hypnotics/antipsychotics, antidepressants, stimulants and street drugs (including *opiates* and *cocaine*), and cardiovascular drugs (including *digoxin* and Ca^{2+} channel blockers). The most

Table 64–1
Substances Most Frequently Involved in Human Poison Exposures in the United States

SUBSTANCE	NUMBER	%*
Analgesics	256,843	10.8
Cleaning substances	225,578	9.5
Cosmetics and personal care products	219,877	9.2
Foreign bodies	110,000	5.0
Sedatives/hypnotics/ antipsychotics	111,001	4.7
Topicals	105,815	4.4
Cough and cold preparations	100,612	4.2
Antidepressants	99,800	4.2
Bites/envenomations	98,585	4.1
Pesticides	96,112	4.0
Plants	84,578	3.6
Food products, food poisoning	75,813	3.2
Alcohols	69,215	2.9
Antihistamines	69,107	2.9
Antimicrobials	63,372	2.7
Cardiovascular drugs	61,056	2.6
Hydrocarbons	59,132	2.5
Chemicals	54,623	2.3

NOTE: Despite a high frequency of involvement, these substances are not necessarily the most toxic, but rather may only be the most readily accessible. *Percentages are based on total number of known ingested substances in the United States rather than the total number of human exposure cases. SOURCE: From Watson *et al.,* 2004. Courtesy of the *American Journal of Emergency Medicine.*

common categories of nonpharmaceutical poisons were alcohols (particularly methanol) and fumes (principally carbon monoxide). Most of the people who die from poisoning are adults, and the deaths often result from intentional rather than accidental exposure. Children younger than 6 years of age account for 52% of the poisoning incidents reported but only 3% of the deaths. Children between 1 and 2 years of age have the highest incidence of accidental poisoning. Fortunately, most of the substances available to these young children are not highly toxic. Iron and pesticides are the leading cause of pediatric accidental poisoning fatalities.

The incidence of serious and fatal adverse drug reactions in U.S. hospitals is extremely high (Lazarou *et al.,* 1998; Institute of Medicine, 1999). It is estimated that about 2 million hospitalized patients have serious adverse drug reactions each year, and about 100,000 have fatal adverse drug reactions. If this estimate is correct, then more people die annually from medication errors than from highway

Table 64–2
Categories with Largest Numbers of Deaths*

CATEGORY	NUMBER	% OF ALL EXPOSURES
Analgesics	659	0.257
Sedative/hypnotics/ antipsychotics	364	0.328
Antidepressants	318	0.316
Stimulants and street drugs	242	0.528
Cardiovascular drugs	181	0.295
Alcohols	139	0.200
Chemicals	50	0.091
Anticonvulsants	65	0.181
Gases and fumes	44	0.106
Antihistamines	71	0.103
Muscle relaxants	52	0.260
Hormones and hor- mone antagonists	33	0.062
Cleaning substances	33	0.013
Automotive products	30	0.213
Cough and cold prep- arations	22	0.022
Pesticides	18	0.019

**This list is for deaths in the United States. SOURCE: From Watson *et al.,* 2004. Courtesy of the *American Journal of Emergency Medicine.*

accidents, breast cancer, or the acquired immune deficiency syndrome (AIDS).

MAJOR SOURCES OF INFORMATION ON POISONING

Pharmacology textbooks are a good source of information on the treatment of poisoning by drugs, but they usually say little about other chemicals. Additional information on drugs and other chemicals can be found in books on poisoning (Ellenhorn, 1997; Goldfrank *et al.,* 2002; Haddad *et al.,* 1998; Klaassen, 2001). A popular computerized system for information on toxic substances is POISIN-DEX (Micromedex, Inc., Denver, CO).

The Web site of the American Association of Poison Control Centers (*http://www.aapcc.org/*) lists 78 members, including 11 regional centers. Valuable information can be obtained from these centers by telephone (800-222-1222). The National Library of Medicine maintains a very informative Web site on toxicology and environmental health (*http://sis.nlm.nih.gov/Tox/ToxMain.html*), including a link to ToxNet (*http://toxnet.nlm.nih.gov/*), a cluster of databases on toxicology, hazardous chemicals, and related areas.

PREVENTION AND TREATMENT OF POISONING

Many acute poisonings from drugs could be prevented if physicians provided common-sense instructions about the storage of drugs and other chemicals and if patients or parents of patients accepted this advice. These instructions are so widely publicized that they need not be repeated here.

For clinical purposes, all toxic agents can be divided into two classes: those for which a specific treatment or antidote exists and those for which there is no specific treatment. For the vast majority of drugs and other chemicals, there is no specific treatment; symptomatic medical care that supports vital functions is the only strategy.

As in other medical emergencies, supportive therapy is the mainstay of the treatment of drug poisoning. The adage, "Treat the patient, not the poison," remains the most basic and important principle of clinical toxicology. Maintenance of respiration and circulation takes precedence. Serial measurement and charting of vital signs and important reflexes help to judge the progress of intoxication, response to therapy, and need for additional treatment. This monitoring usually requires hospitalization. The classification in Table 64–3 often is used to indicate the severity of CNS intoxication. Treatment with large doses of stimulants and sedatives often causes more harm than the poison. Chemical antidotes should be used judiciously; heroic measures seldom are necessary.

Treatment of acute poisoning must be prompt. The first goal is to maintain the vital functions if their impairment is imminent. The second goal is to keep the concentration of poison in the crucial tissues as low as possible by preventing absorption and enhancing elimination. The third goal is to combat the pharmacological and toxicological effects at the effector sites.

Prevention of Further Absorption of Poison

Emesis. Historically, emesis was one of the major tools of gastric decontamination in the management of acute poi-

Table 64–3
Signs and Symptoms of CNS Intoxication

DEGREE OF SEVERITY	CHARACTERISTICS
Depressants	
0	Asleep, but can be aroused and can answer questions
I	Semicomatose, withdraws from painful stimuli, reflexes intact
II	Comatose, does not withdraw from painful stimuli, no respiratory or circulatory depression, most reflexes intact
III	Comatose, most or all reflexes absent, but without depression of respiration or of circulation
IV	Comatose, reflexes absent, respiratory depression with cyanosis or circulatory failure and shock, or both
Stimulants	
I	Restlessness, irritability, insomnia, tremor, hyperreflexia, sweating, mydriasis, flushing
II	Confusion, hyperactivity, hypertension, tachypnea, tachycardia, extrasystoles, sweating, mydriasis, flushing, mild hyperpyrexia
III	Delirium, mania, self-injury, marked hypertension, tachycardia, arrhythmias, hyperpyrexia
IV	As in III, plus convulsions, coma, and circulatory collapse

soning. However, its routine use in the emergency room is declining. According to the annual report of the Toxic Exposure Surveillance System (TESS) (Watson *et al.*, 2004), emesis accounted for only 0.7% of the therapy provided in human exposure cases in 2003 compared with 7.5% in 1993 (Litovitz *et al.*, 1994) and 13.8% in 1983 (Veltri *et al.*, 1984). Although emesis still may be indicated for immediate intervention after poisoning by oral ingestion of chemicals, it is contraindicated in certain situations: (1) If the patient has ingested a corrosive poison, such as a strong acid or alkali (*e.g.,* drain cleaners), emesis increases the likelihood of gastric perforation and further necrosis of the esophagus; (2) if the patient is comatose or in a state of stupor or delirium, emesis may cause aspiration of the gastric contents; (3) if the patient has ingested a CNS stimulant,

further stimulation associated with vomiting may precipitate convulsions; and (4) if the patient has ingested a petroleum distillate (*e.g.,* kerosene, gasoline, or petroleum-based liquid furniture polish), regurgitated hydrocarbons can be aspirated readily and cause chemical pneumonitis (Ervin, 1983). In contrast, emesis should be considered if the ingested solution contains potentially dangerous compounds, such as pesticides.

There are marked differences in the capabilities of various petroleum distillates to produce hydrocarbon pneumonia, which is an acute hemorrhagic necrotizing process. In general, the ability of various hydrocarbons to produce pneumonitis is inversely proportional to their viscosity: If the viscosity is high, as with oils and greases, the risk is limited; if the viscosity is low, as with mineral seal oil found in liquid furniture polishes, the risk of aspiration is high.

Vomiting can be induced mechanically by stroking the posterior pharynx. However, this technique is not as effective as the administration of *ipecac* or *apomorphine*.

Ipecac. The most common household emetic is syrup of ipecac (not ipecac fluid extract, which is 14 times more potent and may cause fatalities). Syrup of ipecac is available in 0.5- and 1-fluid ounce containers (approximately 15 and 30 ml), which may be purchased without prescription. The drug can be given orally, but it takes 15 to 30 minutes to produce emesis; this compares favorably with the time usually required for adequate gastric lavage. The oral dose is 15 ml in children from 6 months to 12 years of age and 30 ml in older children and adults. Because emesis may not occur when the stomach is empty, administration of ipecac should be followed by a drink of water.

In 2004, the American Academy of Clinical Toxicology and the European Association of Poisons Control Centers and Clinical Toxicologists issued position papers on the use of ipecac syrup in poisonings (Anonymous, 2004). *After careful review of the medical literature, these groups concluded that syrup of ipecac should not be administered routinely in the management of poisoned patients.* In studies with various marker substances, the beneficial effects of ipecac-induced emesis were highly variable and diminished rapidly with time. Another concern was that initial use of ipecac in fact may be counterproductive by reducing the efficacy of other, later, and presumably more effective treatments such as use of activated charcoal, oral antidotes, and whole-bowel irrigation. Ipecac may be indicated when it can be administered to conscious, alert patients within 60 minutes of poisoning.

Ipecac acts as an emetic because of its local irritant effect on the enteric tract and its effect on the chemoreceptor trigger zone (CTZ) in the area postrema of the medulla. Syrup of ipecac may be effective even when antiemetic drugs (such as *phenothiazines*) have been ingested. Ipecac can produce toxic effects on the heart because of its content of emetine, but this usually is not a problem with the dose used for emesis. If emesis does not occur, ipecac should be removed by gastric lavage. Chronic abuse of ipecac for weight reduction can result in cardiomyopathy, ventricular fibrillation, and death.

Apomorphine. Apomorphine stimulates the CTZ and causes emesis. The drug is unstable in solution and must be prepared just prior to use and thus is not often readily available. Apomorphine is not effective orally and must be given parenterally, usually by the subcutaneous route, 6 mg for adults and 0.06 mg/kg for children (Goldfrank *et al.*, 2002). However, this can be an advantage over ipecac in that it can be administered to an uncooperative patient and produces vomiting in 3 to 5 minutes. Because apomorphine is a respiratory depressant, it should not be used if the patient has been poisoned by a CNS depressant or if the patient's respiration is slow and labored. At present, apomorphine is used rarely as an emetic.

Gastric Lavage. Gastric lavage is accomplished by inserting a tube into the stomach and washing the stomach with water, normal saline, or one-half normal saline to remove the unabsorbed poison. The procedure should be performed as soon as possible, but only if vital functions are adequate or supportive procedures have been implemented. The contraindications to this procedure generally are the same as for emesis, and there is the additional potential complication of mechanical injury to the throat, esophagus, and stomach. A position statement on the use of gastric lavage by American and European clinical toxicologists (Anonymous, 1997) concluded that *gastric lavage should not be used routinely in the management of the poisoned patient but should be reserved for patients who have ingested a potentially life-threatening amount of poison and when the procedure can be undertaken within 60 minutes of ingestion.*

The only equipment needed for gastric lavage is a tube and a large syringe. The tube should be as large as possible so that the wash solution, food, and poison (whether in the form of a capsule, pill, or liquid) will flow freely, and lavage can be accomplished quickly. A 36-French tube or larger should be used in adults and a 24-French tube or larger in children. Orogastric lavage is preferred over nasogastric lavage because a larger tube can be employed. To prevent aspiration, an endotracheal tube with an inflatable cuff should be positioned before lavage is initiated if the patient is comatose, having seizures, or has lost the gag reflex. During gastric lavage, the patient should be placed on his or her left side because of the anatomical asymmetry of the stomach, with the head hanging face down over the edge of the examining table. If possible, the foot of the table should be elevated. This technique minimizes chances of aspiration.

The contents of the stomach should be aspirated with an irrigating syringe and saved for chemical analysis. The stomach then may be washed with saline solution. Saline solution is safer than water in young children because of the risk of water intoxication, manifested by tonic-clonic seizures and coma. Only small volumes (120 to 300 ml) of lavage solution should be instilled into the stomach at one time so that the poison is not pushed into the intestine. Lavage is

repeated until the returns are clear, which usually requires 10 to 12 washings and a total of 1.5 to 4 L of lavage fluid. When the lavage is complete, the stomach may be left empty, or an antidote may be instilled through the tube. If no specific antidote for the poison is known, an aqueous suspension of activated charcoal and a cathartic often is given.

Chemical Adsorption. Activated charcoal avidly adsorbs drugs and chemicals on the surfaces of the charcoal particles, thereby preventing absorption and toxicity. Many, but not all, chemicals are adsorbed by charcoal. For example, alcohols, hydrocarbons, metals, and corrosives are not well adsorbed by activated charcoal, and charcoal therefore is of little value in treating these poisonings. The effectiveness of charcoal also depends on the time since the ingestion and on the dose of charcoal; one should attempt to achieve a charcoal–drug ratio of at least 10:1. Activated charcoal also can interrupt the enterohepatic circulation of drugs and enhance the net rate of diffusion of the chemical from the body into the gastrointestinal tract. For example, serial doses of activated charcoal have been shown to enhance the elimination of *theophylline* and phenobarbital.

During the last two decades, there has been an increase in the use of activated charcoal and a corresponding decrease in the use of ipecac-induced emesis and gastric lavage in the treatment of poisoning. Studies in patients with drug overdoses and in normal subjects fail to show a benefit of treatment with ipecac or lavage plus activated charcoal as compared with charcoal alone. Based on these findings, American and European clinical toxicologists issued a position paper in 1999 on the use of multidose activated charcoal in treatment of acute poisoning (Anonymous, 1999). They concluded that while experimental and clinical trials demonstrate that elimination of some drugs can be enhanced by treatment with activated charcoal in volunteer studies, rarely has it been demonstrated to reduce morbidity or mortality in a controlled study. The position paper recommends consideration of activated charcoal treatment only if a patient has ingested a life-threatening amount of *carbamazepine, dapsone,* phenobarbital, *quinine,* or theophylline. Even then, there are certain contraindications, such as an unprotected airway, the presence of intestinal obstruction, or if the gastrointestinal tract is not intact or there is decreased peristalsis. There is a need for ongoing study of the efficacy of this treatment for other drugs and to establish optimal dosage regimens.

Activated charcoal usually is prepared as a mixture of at least 50 g (about 10 heaping tablespoons) in a glass of water. The mixture is then administered either orally or *via* a gastric tube. Because most poisons do not appear to desorb from the charcoal if charcoal is present in excess, the adsorbed poison need not be removed from the gastrointestinal tract. Activated charcoal should not be used simultaneously with ipecac because charcoal can adsorb the emetic agent in ipecac and thus reduce the drug's emetic effect. Charcoal also may adsorb and decrease the effectiveness of specific antidotes.

Activated charcoal must be distinguished from the so-called universal antidote, which consists of two parts burned toast (not activated charcoal), one part tannic acid (strong tea), and one part magnesium oxide. In practice, the universal antidote is ineffective.

As mentioned earlier, the presence of an adsorbent in the intestine may interrupt enterohepatic circulation of a toxicant, thus enhancing its excretion. Activated charcoal is useful in interrupting the enterohepatic circulation of drugs such as tricyclic antidepressants and *glutethimide*. A nonabsorbable *polythiol resin* has been used to treat poisoning by methylmercury owing to its capacity to bind mercury excreted into the bile (*see* Chapter 65). *Cholestyramine* hastens the elimination of cardiac glycosides by a similar mechanism.

Chemical Inactivation. Antidotes can change the chemical nature of a poison by rendering it less toxic or preventing its absorption. Formaldehyde poisoning can be treated with ammonia to form hexamethylenetetramine; sodium formaldehyde sulfoxylate can convert mercuric ion to the less soluble metallic mercury; and sodium bicarbonate converts ferrous iron to ferrous carbonate, which is poorly absorbed. Chemical inactivation techniques seldom are used today, however, because valuable time may be lost, whereas emetics, activated charcoal, and gastric lavage are rapid and effective.

In the past, neutralization was the usual treatment of poisoning with acids or bases. Vinegar, orange juice, or lemon juice has been used often for the patient who has ingested alkali, and various antacids often have been advocated for treatment of acid burns. The use of neutralizing agents is controversial because they may produce excessive heat. Carbon dioxide gas produced from bicarbonates used to treat oral poisoning with acids can cause gastric distension and even perforation. The treatment of choice for ingestion of either acids or alkalis is dilution with water or milk. Similarly, burns produced by acid or alkali on the skin should be treated with copious amounts of water.

Purgation. The rationale for using an osmotic cathartic is to minimize absorption by hastening the passage of the toxicant through the gastrointestinal tract. Few, if any, controlled clinical data are available on the effectiveness of cathartics in the treatment of poisoning. Cathartics generally are considered harmless unless the poison has injured the gastrointestinal tract. Cathartics are indicated after the ingestion of enteric-coated tablets, when the time after ingestion is greater than 1 hour, and for poisoning by volatile hydrocarbons. *Sorbitol* is the most effective, but *sodium sulfate* and *magnesium sulfate* also are used; all act promptly and usually have minimal toxicity. However, magnesium sulfate should be used cautiously in patients with renal failure or in those likely to develop renal dysfunction, and Na$^+$-containing cathartics should be avoided in patients with congestive heart failure.

Whole-bowel irrigation (WBI) is a technique that not only promotes defecation but also eliminates the entire contents of the intestines. This technique uses a high-molecular-weight *polyethylene glycol* and *isosmolar electrolyte* solution (PEG-E S) that does not alter serum electrolytes. It is available commercially as GOLYTELY and COLYTE. A position statement on WBI, issued by the American Academy of Clinical Toxicology and the European Association of Poisons Centres and Clinical Toxicologists, indicates that *WBI should not be used routinely in the management of the poisoned patient*. Even though volunteer studies have shown substantial decreases in the bioavailability of certain ingested drugs, evidence from controlled clinical trials is lacking. WBI may be considered in cases of acute poisoning by sustained-release or enteric-coated drugs and possibly toxic ingestions of iron, lead, zinc, or packets of illicit drugs.

Inhalation and Dermal Exposure to Poisons. When a poison has been inhaled, the first priority is to remove the patient from the source of exposure. Similarly, if the skin has had contact with a poison, it should be washed thoroughly with water. Contaminated clothing should be removed. Initial treatment of all types of chemical injuries to the eye must be rapid; thorough irrigation of the eye with water for 15 minutes should be performed immediately.

Enhanced Elimination of the Poison

Biotransformation. Once a chemical has been absorbed, procedures sometimes can be employed to enhance its rate of elimination. Many drugs are metabolized by hepatic CYPs, and components of this system can be induced by a number of compounds (*see* Chapter 3). However, induction of these oxidative enzymes is too slow (days) to be valuable in the treatment of acute poisoning by most chemical agents.

Many chemicals are toxic because they are biotransformed into more toxic chemicals. Thus inhibition of biotransformation should decrease the toxicity of such drugs. For example, ethanol is used to inhibit the conversion of methanol to its highly toxic metabolite, formic acid, by alcohol dehydrogenase (*see* Chapter 22). Acetaminophen is converted by the CYP system to an electrophilic metabolite that is detoxified by glutathione, a cellular nucleophile (Figure 64–3). Acetaminophen does not cause hepatotoxicity until glutathione is depleted, whereupon the reactive metabolite binds to essential macromolecular constituents of the hepatocyte, resulting in cell death. The liver can be protected by maintenance of the concentration of glutathione, and this can be accomplished by the administration of *N*-acetylcysteine (*see* Chapter 26).

Some drugs are detoxified by conjugation with glucuronic acid or sulfate before elimination from the body, and the availability of the endogenous cosubstrates for conjugation may limit the rate of elimination; such is the case in the detoxication of acetaminophen. Methods to replete these compounds will provide an additional mechanism to treat poisoning. Similarly, detoxication of cyanide by conversion to thiocyanate can be accelerated by the administration of *thiosulfate*.

Biliary Excretion. The liver excretes many drugs and other foreign chemicals into bile, but little is known about efficient ways to enhance biliary excretion of xenobiotics for the treatment of acute poisoning. Inducers of microsomal enzyme activity enhance biliary excretion of some xenobiotics, but the effect is slow in onset.

Urinary Excretion. Drugs and poisons are excreted into the urine by glomerular filtration and active tubular secretion (*see*

Chapter 28); they can be reabsorbed into the blood if they are in a lipid-soluble form that will penetrate the tubule or if there is an active mechanism for their transport.

There are no methods known to accelerate the active transport of poisons into urine, and enhancement of glomerular filtration is not a practical means to facilitate elimination of toxicants. However, passive reabsorption from the tubular lumen can be altered. Diuretics inhibit reabsorption by decreasing the concentration gradient of the drug from the lumen to the tubular cell and by increasing flow through the tubule. *Furosemide* is used most often, but osmotic diuretics also are employed (*see* Chapter 28). Forced diuresis should be used with caution, especially in patients with renal, cardiac, or pulmonary complications.

Nonionized compounds are reabsorbed far more rapidly than ionized polar molecules; therefore, a shift from the nonionized to the ionized species of the toxicant by alteration of the pH of the tubular fluid may hasten elimination (*see* Chapter 1). Acidic compounds such as phenobarbital and salicylates are cleared much more rapidly in alkaline than in acidic urine. In 2004, American and European clinical toxicologists issued a position paper on the use of urine alkalinization in treatment of acute poisoning (Proudfoot *et al.*, 2004). Urine alkalinization increases the urine elimination of *chlorpropamide, 2,4-dichlorophenoxyacetic acid, diflunisal, fluoride, mecoprop, methotrexate,* phenobarbital, and salicylate. However, urine alkalinization is recommended as first-line treatment only for patients with moderately severe salicylate poisoning who do not meet the criteria for hemodialysis. Urine alkalinization and high urine flow (approximately 600 ml/h) should also be considered in patients with severe 2,4-dichlorophenoxyacetic acid and mecoprop poisoning. Even though it has been shown to be effective in enhancing elimination of phenobarbital (Figure 64–7), urine alkalinization is not recommended as first-line treatment in cases of phenobarbital poisoning because multiple-dose activated charcoal has been shown to be superior. Urine alkalinization is contraindicated in the case of compromised renal function or failure. Hypokalemia is the most common complication but can be corrected by giving potassium supplements.

Intravenous sodium bicarbonate is used to alkalinize the urine. Renal excretion of basic drugs such as *amphetamine* theoretically can be enhanced by acidification of the urine. Acidification can be accomplished by the administration of ammonium chloride or ascorbic acid. Urinary excretion of an acidic compound is particularly sensitive to changes in urinary pH if its pK_a is within the range of 3.0 to 7.5; for bases, the corresponding range is 7.5 to 10.5.

Dialysis. Hemodialysis or hemoperfusion usually has limited use in the treatment of intoxication with chemicals. However, under cer-

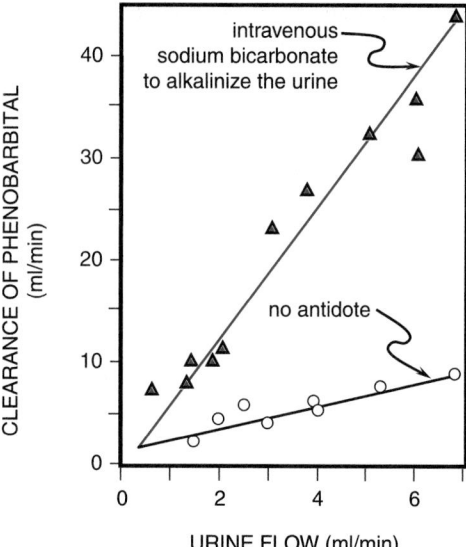

Figure 64–7. *Renal clearance of phenobarbital in the dog as related to urinary pH and the rate of urine flow.* The values designated by circles are from experiments in which diuresis was induced by administration of water orally or Na$_2$SO$_4$ intravenously and the urinary pH was below 7.0. The values designated by triangles are from experiments in which NaHCO$_3$ was administered intravenously and in which the urinary pH was 7.8 to 8.0. (After Waddell and Butler, 1957. Courtesy of *Journal of Clinical Investigation.*)

tain circumstances, such procedures can be lifesaving. The utility of dialysis depends on the amount of poison in the blood relative to the total-body burden. Thus, if a poison has a large volume of distribution, as is the case for the tricyclic antidepressants, the plasma will contain too little of the compound for effective removal by dialysis. Extensive binding of the compound to plasma proteins impairs dialysis greatly. The elimination of a toxicant by dialysis also depends on dissociation of the compound from binding sites in tissues; for some chemicals, this rate may be slow and limiting.

Although peritoneal dialysis requires a minimum of personnel and can be started as soon as the patient is admitted to the hospital, it is too inefficient to be of value for the treatment of acute intoxications. Hemodialysis (extracorporeal dialysis) is much more effective than peritoneal dialysis and may be essential in a few life-threatening intoxications, such as with methanol, ethylene glycol, and salicylates.

Passage of blood through a column of charcoal or adsorbent resin (hemoperfusion) is a technique for the extracorporeal removal of a poison (Winchester, 1983). Because of the high adsorptive capacity and affinity of the material in the column, some chemicals that are bound to plasma proteins can be removed. The principal side effect of hemoperfusion is depletion of platelets.

Antagonism or Chemical Inactivation of an Absorbed Poison. The functional and pharmacological antagonism of the effects of absorbed toxicants was discussed earlier. If a patient is poisoned with a compound that acts as an agonist at a receptor for which a specific blocking agent is available, administration of the receptor antagonist may be highly effective. Functional antagonism also can be valuable for support of the patient's vital functions. For example, anticonvulsant drugs are used to treat chemically induced convulsions. However, drugs that stimulate antagonistic physiological mechanisms are not always of clinical value and may even decrease survival because it often is difficult to titrate the effect of one drug against another when the two act on opposing systems. An example of such a complication is the use of CNS stimulants to attempt to reverse respiratory depression. Convulsions are a typical complication of such therapy, and mechanical support of respiration is preferred. In addition, the duration of action of the poison and the antidote may differ, sometimes leading to poisoning with the antidote.

Specific chemical antagonists of a toxicant, such as opioid antagonists (*see* Chapter 21) and *atropine* as an antagonist of pesticide-induced acetylcholine excess (*see* Chapter 7), are valuable but unfortunately rare. A recently approved antagonist is *fomepizole*, an inhibitor of alcohol dehydrogenase, approved for treatment for poisoning by ethylene glycol and methanol (Barceloux *et al.*, 1999; Mycyk and Leikin, 2003). Chelating agents with high selectivity for certain metal ions are used more commonly (*see* Chapter 65). Antibodies offer the potential for the production of specific antidotes for a host of common poisons and for drugs that frequently are abused or misused. A notable example of such success is the use of purified digoxin-specific Fab fragments of antibodies in the treatment of potentially fatal cases of poisoning with digoxin (*see* Chapter 33). The development of human monoclonal antibodies directed against specific toxins has significant potential therapeutic value.

BIBLIOGRAPHY

Ames, B.N., McCann, J., and Yamasaki, E. Methods for detecting carcinogens and mutagens with the *Salmonella*/mammalian microsome mutagenicity test. *Mutat. Res.,* **1975,** *31*:347–364.

Anonymous. Position statement: Gastric lavage. American Academy of Clinical Toxicology; European Association of Poison Centres and Clinical Toxicologists. *J. Toxicol. Clin. Toxicol.,* **1997,** *35*:711–719.

Anonymous. Position statement and practice guidelines on the use of multi-dose activated charcoal in the treatment of acute poisoning. American Academy of Clinical Toxicology; European Association of Poisons Centres and Clinical Toxicologists. *J. Toxicol. Clin. Toxicol.,* **1999,** *37*:731–751.

Anonymous. Position paper: Ipecac syrup. *J. Toxicol. Clin. Toxicol.,* **2004,** *42*:133–143.

Barceloux, D.G., Krenzelok, E.P., Olson, K., and Watson W. American Academy of Clinical Toxicology practice guidelines on the treatment of ethylene glycol poisoning. Ad Hoc Committee. *J. Toxicol. Clin. Toxicol.,* **1999,** *37*:537–560.

Evans, W.E., and Relling, M.V. Pharmacogenomics: Translating functional genomics into rational therapeutics. *Science,* **1999,** *286*:487–491.

Lazarou, J., Pomeranz, B.H., and Corey, P.N. Incidence of adverse drug reactions in hospitalized patients: A meta-analysis of prospective studies. *JAMA,* **1998,** *279*:1200–1205.

Litovitz, T.L., Clark, L.R., and Soloway, R.A. 1993 annual report of the American Association of Poison Control Centers Toxic Exposure Surveillance System. *Am. J. Emerg. Med.,* **1994,** *12*:546–584.

Mycyk, M.B., and Leikin, J.B. Antidote review: Fomepizole for methanol poisoning. *Am. J. Ther.,* **2003,** *10*:68–70.

Proudfoot, A.T., Krenzelok, E.P., and Vale, J.A. Position paper on urine alkalinization. *J.Toxicol. Clin. Toxicol.,* **2004,** *42*:1–26.

Veltri, J.C., and Litovitz, T.L. 1983 Annual Report of the American Association of Poison Control Centers National Data Collection System. *Am. J. Emerg. Med.,* **1984,** *2*:420–443.

Waddell, W.J., and Butler, T.C. The distribution and excretion of phenobarbital. *J. Clin. Invest.,* **1957,** *36*:1217–1226.

Watson, W.A., Litovitz, T.L., Klein-Schwartz, W., *et al.* 2003 Annual Report of the American Association of Poison Control Centers Toxic Exposure Surveillance System. *Am. J. Emerg. Med.,* **2004,** *22*:335–404.

MONOGRAPHS AND REVIEWS

Coombs, R.R.A., and Gell, P.G.H. Classification of allergic reactions responsible for clinical hypersensitivity and disease. In, *Clinical Aspects of Immunology.* (Gell, P.G.H., Coombs, R.R.A., and Lachmann, P.J., eds.) Blackwell Scientific Publications, Oxford, England, **1975,** pp. 761–781.

Ellenhorn, M.J. *Ellenhorn's Medical Toxicology,* 2d ed. Williams & Wilkins, Baltimore, **1997.**

Ervin, M.E. Petroleum distillates and turpentine. In, *Clinical Management of Poisoning and Drug Overdose.* (Haddad, L.M., and Winchester, J.F., eds.) Saunders, Philadelphia, **1983,** pp. 771–779.

Goldfrank, L.R., Flomenbaum, N.E., Lewin, N.A., *et al. Goldfrank's Toxicologic Emergencies,* 7th ed. McGraw-Hill, New York, **2002.**

Haddad, L.M., Shannon, M.W., and Winchester, J.F., eds. *Clinical Management of Poisoning and Drug Overdose,* 3d ed. Saunders, Philadelphia, **1998.**

Institute of Medicine. *To Err Is Human: Building a Safer Health System.* National Academy Press, Washington, DC, **1999.**

Klaassen, C.D., ed. *Casarett and Doull's Toxicology: The Basic Science of Poisons,* 6th ed. McGraw-Hill, New York, **2001.**

Winchester, J.F. Active methods for detoxification: Oral sorbents, forced diuresis, hemoperfusion, and hemodialysis. In, *Clinical Management of Poisoning and Drug Overdose.* (Haddad, L.M., and Winchester, J.F., eds.) Saunders, Philadelphia, **1983,** pp. 154–169.

HEAVY METALS AND HEAVY-METAL ANTAGONISTS

Curtis D. Klaassen

People continue to be exposed to heavy metals in the environment. Metals contaminate water and food in some areas. Metals also leach from eating utensils and cookware. The emergence of the industrial age and large-scale mining brought occupational diseases caused by various toxic metals. Metallic constituents of pesticides and even therapeutic agents (*e.g.,* antimicrobials) have been additional sources of hazardous exposure. The burning of fossil fuels containing heavy metals, the addition of tetraethyl lead to gasoline, and the increase in industrial applications of metals have made environmental pollution the major source of heavy-metal poisoning. The first part of this chapter covers the toxic properties of lead, mercury, arsenic, and cadmium, as well as radioactive heavy metals, and treatment of the consequences of toxic exposure to these metals. The second part of the chapter covers the chemical properties and therapeutic uses of several heavy-metal antagonists.

Heavy metals exert their toxic effects by combining with one or more reactive groups (ligands) essential for normal physiological functions. Heavy-metal antagonists (chelating agents) are designed specifically to compete with these groups for the metals and thereby prevent or reverse toxic effects and enhance the excretion of metals. Heavy metals, particularly those in the transition series, may react in the body with ligands containing oxygen ($-OH$, $-COO-$, $-OPO_3H^-$, $>C=O$), sulfur ($-SH, -S-S-$), and nitrogen ($-NH_2$ and $>NH$). The resulting metal complex (or coordination compound) is formed by a coordinate bond in which both electrons are contributed by the ligand.

THE IDEAL CHELATOR

The heavy-metal antagonists discussed in this chapter share the capacity to form complexes with heavy metals and thereby prevent or reverse the binding of metallic cations to body ligands. These drugs are referred to as *chelating agents*. A *chelate* is a complex formed between a metal and a compound that contains two or more potential ligands. The product of such a reaction is a heterocyclic ring. Five- and six-membered chelate rings are the most stable, and a polydentate (multiligand) chelator typically is designed to form such a highly stable complex, far more stable than when a metal is combined with only one ligand atom.

The stability of chelates varies with the metal and the ligand atoms. For example, lead and mercury have greater affinities for sulfur and nitrogen than for oxygen ligands; calcium, however, has a greater affinity for oxygen than for sulfur and nitrogen. These differences in affinity serve as the basis of selectivity of action of a chelating agent in the body.

The effectiveness of a chelating agent for the treatment of poisoning by a heavy metal depends on several factors, including the relative affinity of the chelator for the heavy metal as compared with essential body metals, the distribution of the chelator in the body as compared with the distribution of the metal, and the capacity of the chelator to mobilize the metal from the body once chelated.

An ideal chelating agent would have the following properties: high solubility in water, resistance to biotransformation, ability to reach sites of metal storage, capacity to form nontoxic complexes with toxic metals, ability to retain chelating activity at the pH of body fluids, and ready excretion of the chelate. A low affinity for Ca^{2+} also is desirable because Ca^{2+} in plasma is readily available for chelation, and a drug might produce hypocalcemia despite high affinity for heavy metals. The most important property of a therapeutic chelating agent is greater affinity for the metal than that of the endogenous ligands. The large number of ligands in the body is a formidable barrier to the effectiveness of a chelating agent. Observations *in vitro* on chelator–metal interactions provide only a rough guide to the treatment of heavy-metal poisoning. Empirical observations *in vivo* are necessary to determine the clinical utility of a chelating agent.

Lead

Through natural occurrence and its industrial use, lead is ubiquitous in the environment. The decreased addition of tetraethyl lead to gasoline over the past two decades has resulted in decreased concentrations of lead in blood in humans. The primary sources of environmental exposure to lead are leaded paint and drinking water; most of the overt toxicity from lead results from environmental and industrial exposures.

Acidic foods and beverages—including tomato juice, fruit juice, carbonated beverages, cider, and pickles—can dissolve the lead when packaged or stored in improperly glazed containers. Foods and beverages thus contaminated have caused fatal human lead poisoning. Lead poisoning in children is a common result of their ingestion of paint chips from old buildings. Paints applied to dwellings before World War II, when lead carbonate (white) and lead oxide (red) were common constituents of interior and exterior house paints, are primarily responsible. In such paint, lead may constitute 5% to 40% of dried solids. Young children are poisoned most often by nibbling sweet-tasting paint chips and dust from lead-painted windowsills and door frames. The American Standards Association specified in 1955 that paints for toys, furniture, and the interior of dwellings should not contain more than 1% lead in the final dried solids of fresh paint, and in 1978, the Consumer Product Safety Commission (CPSC) banned paint containing more than 0.06% lead for use in and around households. Renovation or demolition of older homes, using a physical process that would cause an airborne dispersion of lead dust or fumes, may cause substantial contamination and lead poisoning. Lead poisoning from the use of discarded automobile-battery casings made of wood and vulcanite and used as fuel during times of economic distress, such as during World Wars I and II, has been reported. Sporadic cases of lead poisoning have been traced to miscellaneous sources such as lead toys, retained bullets, drinking water that is conveyed through lead pipes, artists' paint pigments, ashes and fumes of painted wood, jewelers' wastes, home battery manufacture, and lead type. Finally, lead also is a common contaminant of illicitly distilled whiskey ("moonshine") because automobile radiators frequently are used as condensers and other components of the still are connected by lead solder.

Occupational exposure to lead has decreased markedly because of appropriate regulations and programs of medical surveillance. Workers in lead smelters have the highest potential for exposure because fumes are generated, and dust containing lead oxide is deposited in their environment. Workers in storage-battery factories face similar risks.

Dietary intake of lead also has decreased since the 1940s, when the estimate of intake was about 500 μg/day in the U.S. population, to less than 20 μg/day in 2000. This decrease has been due largely to (1) a decrease in the use of lead-soldered cans for food and beverages; (2) a decrease in the use of lead pipes and lead-soldered joints in water distribution systems; (3) the introduction of lead-free gasoline; and (4) public awareness of the hazards of indoor leaded paint (NRC, 1993). A decline in blood levels from 13 μg/dl in the 1980s to less than 5 μg/dl has been observed in the general U.S. population (Pirkle *et al.*, 1998). However, many children living in central portions of large cities still have blood lead concentrations over 10 μg/dl.

Absorption, Distribution, and Excretion. The major routes of absorption of lead are from the gastrointestinal (GI) tract and the respiratory system. GI absorption of lead varies with age; adults absorb approximately 10% of ingested lead, whereas children absorb up to 40%. Little is known about lead transport across the GI mucosa; lead and Ca^{2+} may compete for a common transport mechanism because there is a reciprocal relationship between the dietary content of Ca^{2+} and lead absorption. Iron deficiency also enhances intestinal absorption of lead apparently because in the absence of iron, the divalent metal transporter (DMT) can readily transport lead in place of iron. Absorption of inhaled lead varies with the form (vapor *versus* particle) as well as with concentration. Approximately 90% of inhaled lead particles from ambient air are absorbed (Goyer and Clarkson, 2001).

After absorption, about 99% of lead in the bloodstream binds to hemoglobin in erythrocytes. Only 1% to 3% of the circulating blood lead is in the serum available to the tissues. Inorganic lead initially distributes in the soft tissues, particularly the tubular epithelium of the kidney and in the liver. In time, lead is redistributed and deposited in bone, teeth, and hair. About 95% of the body burden of lead eventually is found in bone. Only small quantities of inorganic lead accumulate in the brain, mostly in gray matter and the basal ganglia.

The deposition of Pb^{2+} in bone closely resembles that of Ca^{2+}, but Pb^{2+} is deposited as tertiary lead phosphate, which does not contribute to toxicity. After a recent exposure, the concentration of lead often is higher in the flat bones than in the long bones, although, as a general rule, the long bones contain more lead. In the early period of deposition, the concentration of lead is highest in the epiphyseal portion of the long bones. This is especially true in growing bones, where deposits may be detected by radiography as rings of increased density in the ossification centers of the epiphyseal cartilage and as a series of transverse lines in the diaphyses, so-called lead lines. Such findings are of diagnostic significance in children.

Factors that affect the distribution of calcium similarly affect that of lead. Thus a high intake of phosphate favors skeletal storage of lead and a lower concentration in soft tissues. Conversely, a low phosphate intake mobilizes lead in bone and elevates its content in soft tissues. High intake of calcium in the absence of elevated intake of phosphate has a similar effect owing to competition with lead for available phosphate. Vitamin D tends to promote lead deposition in bone if sufficient phosphate is available; otherwise, Ca^{2+} deposition preempts that of Pb^{2+}. Parathyroid hormone mobilizes lead from the skeleton and augments the concentration of lead in blood and the rate of its excretion in urine.

In experimental animals, lead is excreted in bile, and much more lead is excreted in feces than in urine, whereas urinary excretion is a more important route of excretion in humans (Kehoe, 1987). The concentration of lead in urine is directly proportional to that in plasma, but because most lead in blood is in the erythrocytes, only a small quantity of lead is filtered. Lead also is excreted in milk and sweat and is deposited in hair and nails. Placental transfer of lead also occurs.

The half-life of lead in blood is 1 to 2 months, and a steady state thus is achieved in about 6 months. After establishment of a steady state early in human life, the daily intake of lead normally approximates the output, and concentrations of lead in soft tissues are relatively constant. However, the concentration of lead in bone apparently increases, and its half-life in bone is estimated to be 20 to 30 years. Because the capacity for lead excretion is limited, even a slight increase in daily intake may produce a positive lead balance. The average daily intake of lead is approximately 0.2 mg; positive lead balance begins at a daily intake of about 0.6 mg, an amount that ordinarily will not produce overt toxicity within a lifetime. However, the time to accumulate toxic amounts shortens disproportionately as the amount ingested increases. For example, a daily intake of 2.5 mg lead requires nearly 4 years for the accumulation of a toxic burden, whereas a daily intake of 3.5 mg requires but a few months because deposition in bone is too slow to protect the soft tissues during rapid accumulation.

Acute Lead Poisoning. Acute lead poisoning is relatively infrequent and follows ingestion of acid-soluble lead compounds or inhalation of lead vapors. Local actions in the mouth produce marked astringency, thirst, and a metallic taste. Nausea, abdominal pain, and vomiting ensue. The vomitus may be milky from the presence of lead chloride. Although the abdominal pain is severe, it is unlike that of chronic poisoning. Stools may be black from lead sulfide, and there may be diarrhea or constipation. If large amounts of lead are absorbed rapidly, a shock syndrome may develop as the result of massive GI loss of fluid. Acute central nervous system (CNS) symptoms include paresthesias, pain, and muscle weakness. An acute hemolytic crisis sometimes causes severe anemia and hemoglobinuria. The kidneys are damaged, and oliguria and urinary changes are evident. Death may occur in 1 or 2 days. If the patient survives the acute episode, characteristic signs and symptoms of chronic lead poisoning are likely to appear.

Chronic Lead Poisoning. The medical term for lead poisoning is *plumbism,* after the Latin word for lead, *plumbum.* The chemical symbol for lead, Pb, also is derived from this Latin root, as is the modern word *plumber,* which reflects the significant prior use of metallic lead in pipes, fixtures, and gutters. Signs and symptoms of plumbism can be divided into six categories: GI, neuromuscular, CNS, hematological, renal, and other. They may occur separately or in combination. The neuromuscular and CNS syndromes usually result from intense exposure, whereas the GI syndrome more commonly reflects a very slowly and insidiously developing intoxication. The CNS syndrome is more common among children, whereas the GI syndrome is more prevalent in adults.

Gastrointestinal Effects. Lead affects the smooth muscle of the gut, producing intestinal symptoms that are an important early sign of exposure to the metal. The abdominal syndrome often begins with vague symptoms, such as anorexia, muscle discomfort, malaise, and headache. Constipation usually is an early sign, especially in adults, but diarrhea occurs occasionally. A persistent metallic taste appears early in the course of the syndrome. As intoxication advances, anorexia and constipation become more marked. Intestinal spasm, which causes severe abdominal pain (*lead colic*), is the most distressing feature of the advanced abdominal syndrome. The attacks are paroxysmal and generally excruciating. The abdominal muscles become rigid, and tenderness is especially manifested in the region of the umbilicus. In cases where colic is not severe, removal of the patient from the environment of exposure may be sufficient for relief of symptoms. *Calcium gluconate* administered intravenously is recommended for relief of pain and usually is more effective than *morphine.*

Neuromuscular Effects. The neuromuscular syndrome (*lead palsy*) occurs with repeated lead exposure, as characterized by the house painter and other workers with excessive occupational exposure to lead more than a half century ago; it now is rare in the United States. Muscle weakness and easy fatigue occur long before actual paralysis and may be the only symptoms. Weakness or palsy may not become evident until after extended muscle activity. The muscle groups involved usually are the most active ones (extensors of the forearm, wrist, and fingers and extraocular muscles). Wrist drop and, to a lesser extent, foot drop with the appropriate history of exposure are almost pathognomonic for lead poisoning. There usually is no sensory involvement. Degenerative changes in the motoneurons and their axons have been described.

CNS Effects. The CNS syndrome, or *lead encephalopathy,* is the most serious manifestation of lead poisoning and is much more common in children than in adults. The early signs of the syndrome include clumsiness, vertigo, ataxia, falling, headache, insomnia, restlessness, and irritability. As the encephalopathy develops, the patient may first become excited and confused; delirium with repetitive tonic-clonic convulsions or lethargy and coma follow. Vomiting, a common sign, usually is projectile. Visual disturbances also are present. Although the signs and symptoms are characteristic of increased intracranial pressure, craniotomy to relieve intracranial pressure is not beneficial. However, treatment for cerebral edema may become necessary. There may be a proliferative meningitis, intense edema, punctate hemorrhages, gliosis, and areas of focal necrosis. Demyelination has been observed in nonhuman primates. The mortality rate among patients who develop cerebral involvement is about 25%. When chelation therapy is begun after the symptoms of acute encephalopathy appear, approximately 40% of survivors have neurological sequelae such as mental retardation, electroencephalographic abnormalities or frank seizures, cerebral palsy, optic atrophy, or dystonia musculorum deformans (Chisolm and Barltrop, 1979).

Exposure to lead occasionally produces clear-cut progressive mental deterioration in children. The history of these children indicates normal development during the first 12 to 18 months of life or longer, followed by a steady loss of motor skills and speech. They may have severe hyperkinetic and aggressive behavior disorders and a poorly controllable convulsive disorder. The lack of sensory perception severely impairs learning. Concentrations of lead in whole blood exceed 60 μg/dl (2.9 μM), and X-rays may show multiple heavy bands of increased density in the growing long bones. It once was thought that such exposure to lead was restricted largely to children in inner-city slums. However, all children are exposed chronically to low levels of lead in their diets, in the air they breathe, and in the dirt and dust in their play areas. This is reflected in elevated concentrations of lead in the blood of many children and may be a cause of subtle CNS toxicity, including learning disabilities, lowered IQ, and behavioral abnormalities. An increased incidence of hyperkinetic behavior and a statistically significant, although modest, decrease in IQ have been shown in children with higher blood lead concentrations (Needleman *et al.*, 1990; Baghurst *et al.*, 1992; Banks *et al.*, 1997; Bellinger *et al.*, 1992). Increased blood lead levels in infancy and early childhood later may be manifested as decreased attention span, reading disabilities, and failure to graduate from high school. Most studies report a 2- to 4-point IQ deficit for each microgram per deciliter increase in blood lead within the range of 5 to 35 μg/dl. As a result, the Centers for Disease Control and Prevention (CDC) considers a blood lead concentration of 10 μg/dl or greater to indicate excessive absorption of lead in children and to constitute grounds for environmental assessment, cleanup, and/or intervention. Chelation therapy should be considered when blood lead concentrations exceed 25 μg/dl. The CDC recommends universal screening of children beginning at 6 months of age.

Hematological Effects. When the blood lead concentration is near 80 μg/dl or greater, basophilic stippling occurs in erythrocytes; this is not pathognomonic of lead poisoning.

A more common hematological manifestation of chronic lead intoxication is a hypochromic microcytic anemia, which is observed more frequently in children and is morphologically similar to that resulting from iron deficiency. The anemia is thought to result from two factors: a decreased life span of the erythrocytes and an inhibition of heme synthesis.

Very low concentrations of lead influence the synthesis of heme. The enzymes necessary for heme synthesis are distributed widely in mammalian tissues, and each cell probably synthesizes its own heme for incorporation into such proteins as hemoglobin, myoglobin, cytochromes, and catalases. Lead inhibits heme formation at several points, as shown in Figure 65–1. Inhibition of δ-aminolevulinate (δ-ALA) dehydratase and ferrochelatase, which are sulfhydryl-dependent enzymes, is well documented. Ferrochelatase is the enzyme responsible for incorporating the ferrous ion into protoporphyrin to form heme. When ferrochelatase is inhibited by lead, excess protoporphyrin takes the place of heme in the hemoglobin molecule. Zinc is incorporated into the protoporphyrin molecule, resulting in the formation of zinc-protoporphyrin, which is intensely fluorescent and may be used to diagnose lead toxicity. Lead poisoning in both humans and experimental animals is characterized by accumulation of protoporphyrin IX and nonheme iron in red blood cells, by accumulation of δ-ALA in plasma, and by increased urinary excretion of δ-ALA. There also is increased urinary excretion of coproporphyrin III (the oxidation product of coproporphyrinogen III), but it is not clear whether this is due to inhibition of enzymatic activity or to other factors. Increased excretion of porphobilinogen and uroporphyrin has been reported only in severe cases. The pattern of excretion of pyrroles in lead poisoning differs from that characteristic of symptomatic episodes of acute intermittent porphyria and other hepatocellular disorders (Table 65–1). The increase in δ-ALA synthase activity is due to reduction of the cellular concentra-

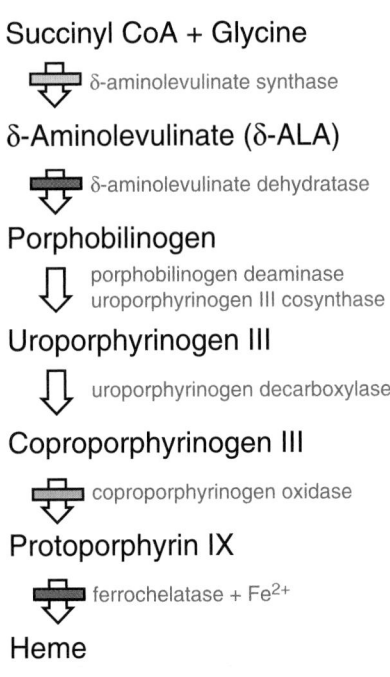

Figure 65–1. Lead interferes with the biosynthesis of heme at several enzymatic steps. Steps that definitely are inhibited by lead are indicated by blue blocks. Steps at which lead is thought to act but where evidence for this is inconclusive are indicated by gray blocks.

Table 65–1
Patterns of Increased Excretion of Pyrroles in Urine of Acutely Symptomatic Patients

	PYRROLES*			
DISEASE	δ-ALA	PBG	URO	COPRO
Lead poisoning	+++	0	±	+++
Acute intermittent porphyria	++++	++++	+ to ++++	+ to +++
Acute hepatitis	0	0	0	+ to +++
Acute alcoholism	0	0	±	+ to +++

*0, normal; + to ++++, degree of increase; δ-ALA, δ-aminolevulinic acid; PBG, porphobilinogen; URO, uroporphyrin; COPRO, coproporphyrin. SOURCE: Modified from Chisolm, 1967.

tion of heme, which regulates the synthesis of δ-ALA synthase by feedback inhibition.

Measurement of heme precursors provides a sensitive index of recent absorption of inorganic lead salts. δ-ALA dehydratase activity in hemolysates and δ-ALA in urine are sensitive indicators of exposure to lead but are not as sensitive as quantification of blood lead concentrations.

Renal Effects. Although less dramatic than those in the CNS and GI tract, renal effects do occur. Renal toxicity occurs in two forms: a reversible tubular disorder (usually seen after acute exposure of children to lead) and an irreversible interstitial nephropathy (observed more commonly in long-term industrial lead exposure) (Goyer and Clarkson, 2001). Clinically, a Fanconi-like syndrome is seen with proteinuria, hematuria, and casts in the urine (Craswell, 1987; Bernard and Becker, 1988). Hyperuricemia with gout occurs more frequently in the presence of chronic lead nephropathy than in any other type of chronic renal disease. Histologically, lead nephropathy is revealed by characteristic nuclear inclusion bodies composed of a lead–protein complex; they appear early and resolve after chelation therapy. Such inclusion bodies have been reported in the urine sediment of workers exposed to lead in an industrial setting (Schumann *et al.*, 1980).

Other Effects. Other signs and symptoms of lead poisoning are an ashen color of the face and pallor of the lips; retinal stippling; appearance of "premature aging," with stooped posture, poor muscle tone, and emaciation; and a black, grayish, or blue-black "lead line" along the gingival margin. The lead line, a result of periodontal deposition of lead sulfide, may be removed by good dental hygiene. Similar pigmentation may result from the absorption of mercury, bismuth, silver, thallium, or iron. There is a relationship between the concentration of lead in blood and blood pressure, and it has been suggested that this may be due to subtle changes in calcium metabolism or renal function (Staessen, 1995). Lead also interferes with vitamin D metabolism

(Rosen *et al.*, 1980; Mahaffey *et al.*, 1982). A decreased sperm count in lead-exposed males has been described (Lerda, 1992). The human carcinogenicity of lead is not well established but has been suggested (Cooper and Gaffey, 1975), and case reports of renal adenocarcinoma in lead workers have been published.

Diagnosis of Lead Poisoning. In the absence of a positive history of abnormal exposure to lead, the diagnosis of lead poisoning is missed easily because the signs and symptoms of lead poisoning are shared by other diseases. For example, the signs of encephalopathy may resemble those of various degenerative conditions. Physical examination does not easily distinguish lead colic from other abdominal disorders. Clinical suspicion should be confirmed by determinations of the concentration of lead in blood and protoporphyrin in erythrocytes. As noted earlier, lead at low concentrations decreases heme synthesis at several enzymatic steps. This leads to buildup of the diagnostically important substrates δ-ALA, coproporphyrin (both measured in urine), and zinc protoporphyrin (measured in the red cell as erythrocyte protoporphyrin). For children, the erythrocyte protoporphyrin level is insufficiently sensitive to identify children with elevated blood lead levels below about 25 μg/dl, and the screening test of choice is blood lead measurement.

Since lead has been removed from paints and gasoline, the mean blood levels of lead in children in the United States have decreased from 17 μg/dl in the 1970s to 6 μg/dl in the 1990s (Schoen, 1993). The concentration of lead in blood is an indication of recent absorption of the metal (Figure 65–2). Children with concentrations of lead in blood above 10 μg/dl are at risk of developmental disabilities. Adults with concentrations below 30 μg/dl exhibit no known functional injury or symptoms; however, they will have a definite decrease in δ-ALA dehydratase activity, a slight increase in urinary excretion of δ-ALA, and an increase in erythrocyte protoporphyrin. Patients with a blood lead concentration of 30 to 75 μg/dl have all

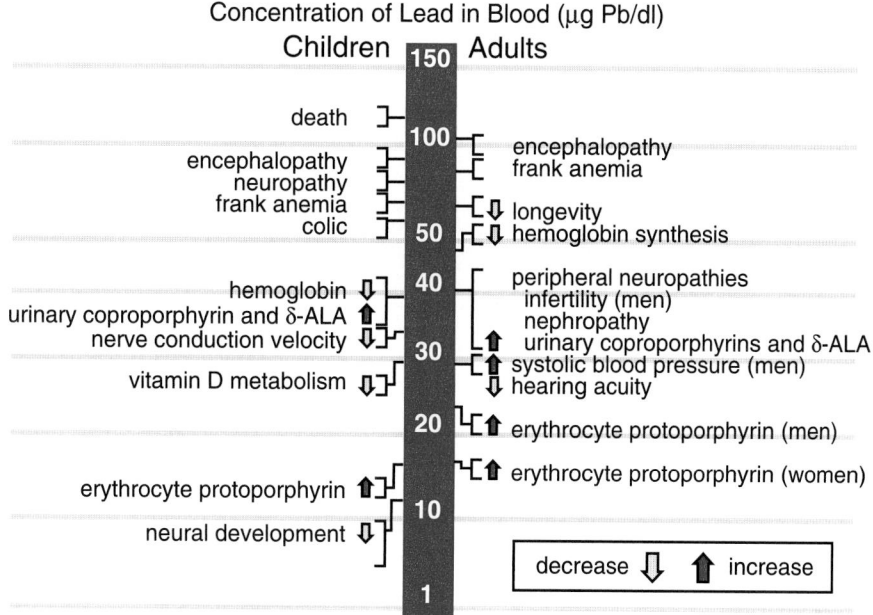

Figure 65–2. *Manifestations of lead toxicity associated with varying concentrations of lead in blood of children and adults.* δ-ALA = δ-aminolevulinate.

the preceding laboratory abnormalities and, usually, nonspecific, mild symptoms of lead poisoning. Clear symptoms of lead poisoning are associated with concentrations that exceed 75 μg/dl of whole blood, and lead encephalopathy usually is apparent when lead concentrations are greater than 100 μg/dl. In persons with moderate-to-severe anemia, interpretation of the significance of concentrations of lead in blood is improved by correcting the observed value to approximate that which would be expected if the patient's hematocrit were within the normal range.

The urinary concentration of lead in normal adults generally is less than 80 μg/L (0.4 μM). Most patients with lead poisoning show concentrations of lead in urine of 150 to 300 μg/L (0.7 to 1.4 μM). However, in persons with chronic lead nephropathy or other forms of renal insufficiency, urinary excretion of lead may be within the normal range, even though blood lead concentrations are significantly elevated.

Because the onset of lead poisoning usually is insidious, it often is desirable to estimate the body burden of lead in individuals who are exposed to an environment that is contaminated with the metal. In the past, the edetate calcium disodium (CaNa$_2$EDTA) provocation test was used to determine whether there is an increased body burden of lead in those for whom exposure occurred much earlier. The provocation test is performed by intravenous administration of a single dose of CaNa$_2$EDTA (50 mg/kg), and urine is collected for 8 hours. The test is positive for children when the lead excretion ratio (micrograms of lead excreted in the urine per milligram of CaNa$_2$EDTA administered) is greater than 0.6; it also may be useful for therapeutic chelation in children with blood levels of 25 to 45 μg/dl. This test is not used in symptomatic patients or in those whose concentration of lead in blood is greater than 45 μg/dl because these patients require the proper therapeutic regimen with chelating agents (*see* below). Neutron activation analysis or fluorometric assays, available only as research methods, may offer a unique *in vivo* approach to the diagnosis of lead burden in the future.

Organic Lead Poisoning. Tetraethyl lead and tetramethyl lead are lipid-soluble compounds that are absorbed readily from the skin, GI tract, and lungs. The toxicity of tetraethyl lead is believed to be due to its metabolic conversion to triethyl lead and inorganic lead.

The major symptoms of intoxication with tetraethyl lead are referable to the CNS: insomnia, nightmares, anorexia, nausea and vomiting, diarrhea, headache, muscular weakness, and emotional instability (Seshia *et al.*, 1978). Subjective CNS symptoms such as irritability, restlessness, and anxiety are next evident, usually accompanied by hypothermia, bradycardia, and hypotension. With continued exposure, or in the case of intense short-term exposure, CNS manifestations progress to delusions, ataxia, exaggerated muscular movements, and finally, a maniacal state.

The diagnosis of poisoning by tetraethyl lead is established by relating these signs and symptoms to a history of exposure. The urinary excretion of lead may increase markedly, but the concentration of lead in blood remains nearly normal. Anemia and basophilic stippling of erythrocytes are uncommon in organic lead poisoning. There is little effect on the metabolism of porphyrins, and erythrocyte protoporphyrin concentrations are inconsistently elevated (Garrettson, 1983). In the case of severe exposure, death may occur within a few hours or may be delayed for several weeks. If the patient survives the acute phase of organic lead poisoning, recovery usually is complete; however, instances of residual CNS damage have been reported.

Treatment of Lead Poisoning. Initial treatment of the acute phase of lead intoxication involves supportive measures. Prevention of further exposure is important. Seizures are treated with *diazepam* or *phenytoin* (*see* Chapter 19), fluid and electrolyte balances must be maintained, and cerebral edema is treated with *mannitol* and *dexamethasone* or controlled hyperventilation. The concentration of lead in blood should be determined or at least a blood sample obtained for analysis prior to initiation of chelation therapy.

Chelation therapy is indicated in symptomatic patients or in patients with a blood lead concentration in excess of 50 to 60 μg/dl (about 2.5 μM). Four chelators are employed: *edetate calcium disodium* (CaNa$_2$EDTA), *dimercaprol* [British antilewisite (BAL)], D-*penicillamine,* and *succimer* [2,3–dimercaptosuccinic acid (DMSA), CHEMET]. CaNa$_2$EDTA and dimercaprol usually are used in combination for lead encephalopathy.

CaNa*$_2$*EDTA. CaNa$_2$EDTA is initiated at a dose of 30 to 50 mg/kg per day in two divided doses either by deep intramuscular injection or slow intravenous infusion for up to 5 consecutive days. The first dose of CaNa$_2$EDTA should be delayed until 4 hours after the first dose of dimercaprol. An additional course of CaNa$_2$EDTA may be given after an interruption of 2 days. Each course of therapy with CaNa$_2$EDTA should not exceed a total dose of 500 mg/kg. Urine output must be monitored because the chelator–lead complex is believed to be nephrotoxic. Treatment with CaNa$_2$EDTA can alleviate symptoms quickly. Colic may disappear within 2 hours; paresthesia and tremor cease after 4 or 5 days; and coproporphyrinuria, stippled erythrocytes, and gingival lead lines tend to decrease in 4 to 9 days. Urinary elimination of lead usually is greatest during the initial infusion.

Dimercaprol. Dimercaprol is given intramuscularly at a dose of 4 mg/kg every 4 hours for 48 hours, then every 6 hours for 48 hours, and finally, every 6 to 12 hours for an additional 7 days. *The combination of dimercaprol and CaNa$_2$EDTA is more effective than is either chelator alone* (Chisolm, 1973).

D-Penicillamine. In contrast to CaNa$_2$EDTA and dimercaprol, penicillamine is effective orally and may be included in the regimen at a dosage of 250 mg given four times daily for 5 days. During chronic therapy with penicillamine, the dose should not exceed 40 mg/kg per day.

Succimer. Succimer is the first orally active lead chelator available for children, with a safety and efficacy profile that surpasses that of D-penicillamine. Succimer usually is given every 8 hours (10 mg/kg) for 5 days and then every 12 hours for an additional 2 weeks.

General Principles. In any chelation regimen, the blood lead concentration should be reassessed 2 weeks after the regimen has been completed; an additional course of therapy may be indicated if blood lead concentrations rebound.

Treatment of organic lead poisoning is symptomatic. Chelation therapy will promote excretion of the inorganic lead produced from the metabolism of organic lead, but the increase is not dramatic.

Mercury

Mercury was an important constituent of drugs for centuries as an ingredient in many diuretics, antibacterials, antiseptics, skin ointments, and laxatives. More specific, effective, and safer modes of therapy now have replaced the mercurials, and drug-induced mercury poisoning has become rare. However, mercury has a number of impor-

Table 65-2
Occupational and Environmental Exposure to Mercury

INDUSTRIAL USES OF MERCURY	% OF TOTAL MERCURY EXPOSURE
Chloralkali, *e.g.*, bleach	25
Electrical equipment	20
Paints	15
Thermometers	10
Dental	3
Laboratory	2

tant industrial uses (Table 65–2), and poisoning from occupational exposure and environmental pollution continues to be an area of concern. There have been epidemics of mercury poisoning among wildlife and human populations in many countries. With very few exceptions and for numerous reasons, such outbreaks were misdiagnosed for months or even years. Reasons for these tragic delays included the insidious onset of the affliction, vagueness of early clinical signs, and the medical profession's unfamiliarity with the disease (Gerstner and Huff, 1977).

Chemical Forms and Sources of Mercury. With regard to the toxicity of mercury, three major chemical forms of the metal must be distinguished: mercury vapor (elemental mercury), salts of mercury, and organic mercurials. Table 65–3 indicates the estimated daily retention of various forms of mercury from various sources.

Elemental mercury is the most volatile of the metal's inorganic forms. Human exposure to mercury vapor is mainly occupational. Extraction of gold with mercury and then heating the amalgam to drive off the mercury is a technique that has been used extensively by gold miners and still is used today in some developing countries.

Chronic exposure to mercury in ambient air after inadvertent mercury spills in poorly ventilated rooms, often scientific laboratories, can produce toxic effects. Mercury vapor also can be released from silver–amalgam dental restorations. In fact, this is the main source of mercury exposure to the general population, but the amount of mercury released does not appear to be of significance for human health (Eley and Cox, 1993) except for allergic contact eczema seen in a few individuals.

Salts of mercury exist in two states of oxidation—as monovalent mercurous salts or as divalent mercuric salts. Mercurous chloride (Hg_2Cl_2), or *calomel*, the best-known mercurous compound, was used in some skin creams as an antiseptic and was employed as a diuretic and cathartic. Mercuric salts are the more irritating and acutely toxic form of the metal. Mercuric nitrate was a common industrial hazard in the felt-hat industry more than 400 years ago. Occupational exposure produced neurological and behavioral changes depicted by the Mad Hatter in Lewis Carroll's *Alice's Adventures in Wonderland*. Mercuric chloride (Hg_2Cl_2), once a widely used antiseptic, also was used commonly for suicidal purposes. Mercuric salts still are employed widely in industry, and industrial discharge into rivers has introduced mercury into the environment in many parts of the world. The main industrial uses of inorganic mercury today are in chloralkali production and in electronics. Other uses of the metal include the manufacturing of plastics, fungicides, and germicides and the formulation of amalgams in dentistry.

The organomercurials in use today contain mercury with one covalent bond to a carbon atom. Members of this heterogeneous group of compounds have varying abilities to produce toxic effects. The alkylmercury salts are by far the most dangerous of these compounds; methylmercury is the most common. Alkylmercury salts have been used widely as fungicides and have produced toxic effects in humans. Major incidents of human poisoning from the inadvertent consumption of mercury-treated seed grain have occurred in Iraq, Pakistan, Ghana, and Guatemala. The most catastrophic outbreak occurred in Iraq in 1972. During the fall of 1971, Iraq imported large quantities of seed (wheat and barley) treated with methylmercury and distributed the grain for spring planting. Despite official warnings, the grain was ground into flour and made into bread. As a result, 6530 victims were hospitalized, and 500 died (Bakir *et al.*, 1973, 1980).

Table 65-3
Estimated Average Daily Retention of Total Mercury and Mercury Compounds in the General Population Not Occupationally Exposed to Mercury

EXPOSURE	ESTIMATED MEAN DAILY RETENTION OF MERCURY COMPOUNDS, μg MERCURY/DAY		
	Mercury Vapor	Inorganic Mercury Salts	Methylmercury
Air	0.024	0.001	0.0064
Food			
Fish	0.0	0.04	2.3
Nonfish	0.0	0.25	0.0
Drinking water	0.0	0.0035	0.0
Dental amalgams	3–17	0.0	0.0
Total	3–17	0.3	2.31

Minamata disease also was due to methylmercury. In the Japanese town of Minamata, the major industry was a chemical plant that emptied its effluent directly into Minamata Bay. The chemical plant used inorganic mercury as a catalyst, and some of it was methylated before it entered the bay. In addition, microorganisms can convert inorganic mercury to methylmercury; the compound then is taken up rapidly by plankton algae and is concentrated in fish *via* the food chain. Residents of Minamata who consumed fish as a large portion of their diet were the first to be poisoned. Eventually, 121 persons were poisoned, and 46 died (McAlpine and Araki, 1958; Smith and Smith, 1975; Tamashiro *et al.*, 1985). In the United States, human poisonings have resulted from ingestion of meat from pigs fed grain treated with an organomercurial fungicide. Because of concerns about methylmercury accumulation in fish, the Food and Drug Administration (FDA) recommends that pregnant or nursing women, women of childbearing age, and young children avoid eating large fish (*e.g.*, shark, swordfish, king mackerel, and tilefish) and limit their intake of albacore tuna to 6 ounces per week.

In other instances, exposure to mercury was intentional. For example, thimerosal (CH_3CH_2—Hg—S—C_6H_4—COOH) has been used as an antibacterial additive to biologics and vaccines since the 1930s. However, concerns about the possibility of health risks from thimerosal in vaccines have been debated, especially the possibility that the ethylmercury thiosalicylate preservative in hepatitis B immunoglobulin (HBIG) could release ethylmercury and cause severe mercury intoxication (Lowell *et al.*, 1996; Ball *et al.*, 2001). These concerns were based on the assumption that ethylmercury, for which there is limited toxicologic information, is toxicologically similar to its close chemical relative, methyl mercury (CH_3—Hg^+), about which much is known (Clarkson, 2002).

A study by the FDA determined that that there is a significant safety margin incorporated into all the acceptable mercury exposure limits. Furthermore, there are no data or evidence of any harm caused by the level of exposure that some children may have encountered in following the existing immunization schedule. Nevertheless, the availability of vaccines with alternate preservatives led to a statement calling for removal of all vaccines containing thimerosal (Joint Statement of the American Academy of Pediatrics and the United States Public Health Service, 1999; Ball *et al.*, 2001). This practice remains in place today, even though subsequent studies have failed to demonstrate any health risk associated with vaccines containing thiomerosal (Verstraeten *et al.*, 2003; Heron *et al.*, 2004).

Chemistry and Mechanism of Action. Mercury readily forms covalent bonds with sulfur, and it is this property that accounts for most of the biological properties of the metal. When the sulfur is in the form of sulfhydryl groups, divalent mercury replaces the hydrogen atom to form mercaptides, X—Hg—SR and Hg(SR)$_2$, where X is an electronegative radical and R is protein. Organic mercurials form mercaptides of the type R—Hg—SR'. Even in low concentrations, mercurials are capable of inactivating sulfhydryl groups of enzymes and thus interfering with cellular metabolism and function. The affinity of mercury for thiols provides the basis for treatment of mercury poisoning with such agents as dimercaprol and penicillamine. Mercury also combines with phosphoryl, carboxyl, amide, and amine groups.

Absorption, Biotransformation, Distribution, and Excretion. *Elemental Mercury.* Elemental mercury is not particularly toxic when ingested because of very low absorption from the GI tract; this is due to the formation of droplets and because the metal in this form

cannot react with biologically important molecules. However, inhaled mercury vapor is completely absorbed by the lung and then is oxidized to the divalent mercuric cation by catalase in the erythrocytes (Magos *et al.*, 1978). Within a few hours, the deposition of inhaled mercury vapor resembles that after ingestion of mercuric salts, with one important difference: Because mercury vapor crosses membranes much more readily than does divalent mercury, a significant amount of the vapor enters the brain before it is oxidized. CNS toxicity is thus more prominent after exposure to mercury vapor than to divalent forms of the metal.

Inorganic Salts of Mercury. The soluble inorganic mercuric salts (Hg^{2+}) gain access to the circulation when taken orally. GI absorption is approximately 10% to 15% of that ingested, and a considerable portion of the Hg^{2+} may remain bound to the alimentary mucosa and the intestinal contents. Insoluble inorganic mercurous compounds, such as calomel (Hg_2Cl_2), may undergo some oxidation to soluble compounds that are more readily absorbed. Inorganic mercury has a markedly nonuniform distribution after absorption. The highest concentration of Hg^{2+} is found in the kidneys, where the metal is retained longer than in other tissues. Concentrations of inorganic mercury are similar in whole blood and plasma. Inorganic mercurials do not readily pass across the blood–brain barrier or the placenta. The metal is excreted in the urine and feces with a half-life of about 60 days (Friberg and Vostal, 1972); studies in laboratory animals indicate that fecal excretion is quantitatively more important (Klaassen, 1975).

Organic Mercurials. Organic mercurials are absorbed more completely from the GI tract than are the inorganic salts because they are more lipid soluble and less corrosive to the intestinal mucosa. Their uptake and distribution are depicted in Figure 65–3A. More than 90% of methylmercury is absorbed from the human GI tract. The organic mercurials cross the blood–brain barrier and the placenta and thus produce more neurological and teratogenic effects than do the inorganic salts. Methylmercury combines with cysteine to form a structure similar to methionine, and the complex is transported by the large neutral amino acid carrier present in capillary endothelial cells (Clarkson, 1987) (Figure 65–3B). Organic mercurials are distributed more uniformly to the various tissues than are the inorganic salts (Klaassen, 1975). A significant portion of the body burden of organic mercurials is in the red blood cells. The ratio of the concentration of organomercurial in erythrocytes to that in plasma varies with the compound; for methylmercury, it approximates 20:1 (Kershaw *et al.*, 1980). Mercury concentrates in hair because of its high sulfhydryl content. The carbon–mercury bond of some organic mercurials is cleaved after absorption; with methylmercury, the cleavage is quite slow, and the inorganic mercury formed is not thought to play a major role in methylmercury toxicity. Aryl mercurials, such as mercurophen, usually contain a labile mercury–carbon bond; their toxicity is similar to that of inorganic mercury. Methylmercury in humans is excreted mainly in the feces in the form of a glutathione conjugate; less than 10% of a dose appears in urine (Bakir *et al.*, 1980). The half-life of methylmercury in the blood of humans is between 40 and 105 days (Bakir *et al.*, 1973).

Toxicity. *Elemental Mercury.* Short-term exposure to the vapor of elemental mercury may produce symptoms within several hours, including weakness, chills, metallic taste, nausea, vomiting, diarrhea, dyspnea, cough, and a feeling of tightness in the chest. Pulmonary toxicity may progress to an interstitial pneumonitis with severe compromise of respiratory function. Recovery, although usually complete, may be complicated by residual interstitial fibrosis.

A Intestinal uptake and distribution of organic mercurials

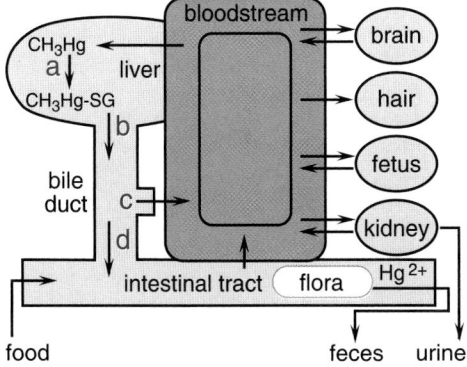

B Uptake of methylmercury complex by capillaries

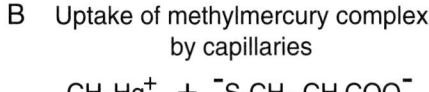

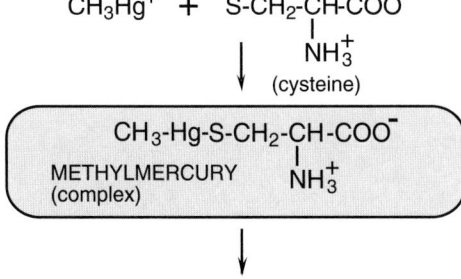

Figure 65–3. *Uptake and relative distribution of organic mercurials.* **A.** The intestinal uptake and subsequent distribution of organic mercurials, such as methylmercury, throughout the body. *a.* Conjugation with glutathione (GSH), shown as CH_3—Hg—SG. *b.* Secretion of conjugate into bile. *c.* Reabsorption in gallbladder. *d.* Remaining Hg enters intestinal tract. **B.** Uptake of the methylmercury complex by capillaries. The ability of organic mercurials to cross the blood–brain barrier and the placenta contributes to their greater neurological and teratogenic effects when compared with inorganic mercury salts. Note the structural similarity of the methylmercury complex to methionine, $CH_3SCH_2CH_2$—$CH(NH_3^+)COO^-$.

Chronic exposure to mercury vapor produces a more insidious form of toxicity that is dominated by neurological effects (Friberg and Vostal, 1972). The syndrome, termed the *asthenic vegetative syndrome,* consists of neurasthenic symptoms in addition to three or more of the following findings: goiter, increased uptake of radioiodine by the thyroid, tachycardia, labile pulse, gingivitis, dermographia, and increased mercury in the urine (Goyer and Clarkson, 2001). With continued exposure to mercury vapor, tremor becomes noticeable, and psychological changes consist of depression, irritability, excessive shyness, insomnia, reduced self-confidence, emotional instability, forgetfulness, confusion, impatience, and vasomotor disturbances (such as excessive perspiration and

uncontrolled blushing, which together are referred to as *erethism*). Common features of intoxication from mercury vapor are severe salivation and gingivitis. The triad of increased excitability, tremors, and gingivitis has been recognized historically as the major manifestation of exposure to mercury vapor when mercury nitrate was used in the fur, felt, and hat industries. Renal dysfunction also has been reported to result from long-term industrial exposure to mercury vapor. The concentrations of mercury vapor in the air and mercury in urine that are associated with the various effects are shown in Figure 65–4.

Inorganic Salts of Mercury. Inorganic ionic mercury (*e.g.,* mercuric chloride) can produce severe acute toxicity. Precipitation of mucous membrane proteins by mercuric salts results in an ashengray appearance of the mucosa of the mouth, pharynx, and intestine and also causes intense pain, which may be accompanied by vomiting. The vomiting is perceived to be protective because it removes unabsorbed mercury from the stomach; assuming that the patient is awake and alert, vomiting should not be inhibited. The local corrosive effect of ionic inorganic mercury on the GI mucosa results in severe hematochezia with evidence of mucosal sloughing in the stool. Hypovolemic shock and death can occur in the absence of proper treatment, which can overcome the local effects of inorganic mercury.

Systemic toxicity may begin within a few hours of exposure to mercury and last for days. A strong metallic taste is followed by stomatitis with gingival irritation, foul breath, and loosening of the teeth. The most serious and frequent systemic effect of inorganic mercury is renal toxicity. Acute tubular necrosis occurs after short-term exposure, leading to oliguria or anuria. Renal injury also follows long-term exposure to inorganic mercury, where glomerular injury predominates. This results from direct effects on the glomerular basement membrane and later indirect effects mediated by immune complexes (Goyer and Clarkson, 2001).

The symptom complex of acrodynia (pink disease) also commonly follows chronic exposure to inorganic mercury ions. Acrodynia is an erythema of the extremities, chest, and face with photophobia, diaphoresis, anorexia, tachycardia, and either constipation or diarrhea. This symptom complex is seen almost exclusively after ingestion of mercury and is believed to be the result of a hypersensitivity reaction (Matheson *et al.,* 1980).

Organic Mercurials. Most human toxicological data about organic mercury concern methylmercury and have been collected as the unfortunate result of large-scale accidental exposures. Symptoms of exposure to methylmercury are mainly neurological and consist of visual disturbance (scotoma and visual-field constriction), ataxia, paresthesias, neurasthenia, hearing loss, dysarthria, mental deterioration, muscle tremor, movement disorders, and with severe exposure, paralysis and death (Table 65–4). Effects of methylmercury on the fetus can occur even when the mother is asymptomatic; mental retardation and neuromuscular deficits have been observed.

Diagnosis of Mercury Poisoning. A history of exposure to mercury, either industrial or environmental, is obviously valuable in making the diagnosis of mercury poisoning. Otherwise, clinical suspicions can be confirmed by laboratory analysis. The upper limit of a nontoxic concentration of mercury in blood generally is considered to be 3 to 4 μg/dl (0.15 to 0.20 μM). A concentration of mercury in blood in excess of 4 μg/dl (0.20 μM) is unexpected in normal, healthy adults and suggests the need for environmental evaluation and medical examination to assess the possibility of adverse health effects. Because methylmercury is concentrated in erythrocytes and inorganic mercury is not, the

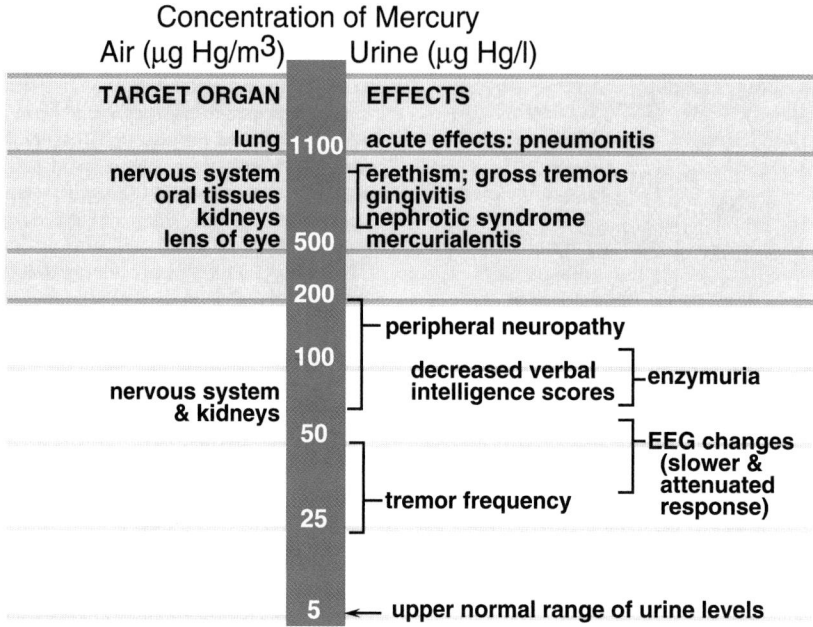

Figure 65–4. *The concentration of mercury vapor in the air and related concentrations of mercury in urine associated with a variety of toxic effects.*

distribution of total mercury between red blood cells and plasma may indicate whether the patient has been poisoned with inorganic or organic mercury. Measurement of total mercury in red blood cells gives a better estimate of the body burden of methylmercury than it does for inorganic mercury. A rough guide to the relationship between concentrations of mercury in blood and the frequency of symptoms that result from exposure to methylmercury is shown in Table 65–4. Concentrations of mercury in plasma provide a better index of the body burden of inorganic mercury, but the relationship between body burden and the concentration of inorganic mercury in plasma is not well documented. This may relate to the importance of timing of measurement of the blood sample relative to the last expo-

sure to mercury. The relationship between the concentration of inorganic mercury in blood and toxicity also depends on the form of exposure. For example, exposure to vapor results in concentrations in brain approximately 10 times higher than those that follow an equivalent dose of inorganic mercuric salts.

The concentration of mercury in the urine also has been used as a measure of the body burden of the metal. The normal upper limit for excretion of mercury in urine is 5 μg/L. There is a linear relationship between plasma concentration and urinary excretion of mercury after exposure to vapor; in contrast, the excretion of mercury in urine is a poor indicator of the amount of methylmercury in the blood because it is eliminated mainly in feces (Bakir *et al.*, 1980).

Table 65–4
Frequency of Symptoms of Methylmercury Poisoning in Relation to Concentration of Mercury in Blood

CONCENTRATION OF MERCURY IN BLOOD, μg/ml (μM)	CASES WITH SYMPTOMS (%)					
	Paresthesias	*Ataxia*	*Visual Defects*	*Dysarthria*	*Hearing Defects*	*Death*
0.1–0.5 (0.5–2.5)	5	0	0	5	0	0
0.5–1 (2.5–5)	42	11	21	5	5	0
1–2 (5–10)	60	47	53	24	5	0
2–3 (10–15)	79	60	56	25	13	0
3–4 (15–20)	82	100	58	75	36	17
4–5 (20–25)	100	100	83	85	66	28

SOURCE: Based on data in Bakir *et al.*, 1973.

Hair is rich in sulfhydryl groups, and the concentration of mercury in hair is about 300 times that in blood. Human hair grows about 20 cm a year, and a history of exposure may be obtained by analysis of different segments of hair.

Treatment of Mercury Poisoning. Measurement of the concentration of mercury in blood should be performed as soon as possible after poisoning with any form of the metal.

Elemental Mercury Vapor. Therapeutic measures include immediate termination of exposure and close monitoring of pulmonary status. Short-term respiratory support may be necessary. Chelation therapy, as described below for inorganic mercury, should be initiated immediately and continued as indicated by the clinical condition and the concentrations of mercury in blood and urine.

Inorganic Mercury. Prompt attention to fluid and electrolyte balance and hematological status is of critical importance in moderate-to-severe oral exposures. Emesis can be induced if the patient is awake and alert, although emesis should not be induced where there is corrosive injury. If ingestion of mercury is more than 30 to 60 minutes before treatment, emesis may have little efficacy. With corrosive agents, endoscopic evaluation may be warranted, and coagulation parameters are important. *Activated charcoal* is recommended by some, although it lacks proven efficacy. Administration of charcoal may make endoscopy difficult or impossible.

Chelation Therapy. Chelation therapy with dimercaprol (for high-level exposures or symptomatic patients) or penicillamine (for low-level exposures or asymptomatic patients) is used routinely to treat poisoning with either inorganic or elemental mercury. Recommended treatment includes dimercaprol 5 mg/kg intramuscularly initially, followed by 2.5 mg/kg intramuscularly every 12 to 24 hours for 10 days. Penicillamine (250 mg orally every 6 hours) may be used alone or following treatment with dimercaprol. The duration of chelation therapy will vary, and progress can be monitored by following concentrations of mercury in urine and blood. The orally effective chelator succimer appears to be an effective chelator for mercury (Campbell *et al.*, 1986; Fournier *et al.*, 1988; Bluhm *et al.*, 1992), although it has not been approved by the FDA for this purpose.

The dimercaprol–mercury chelate is excreted into both bile and urine, whereas the penicillamine–mercury chelate is excreted only into urine. Thus penicillamine should be used with extreme caution when renal function is impaired. In fact, hemodialysis may be necessary in the poisoned patient whose renal function declines. Chelators still may be used because the dimercaprol–mercury complex is removed by dialysis (Giunta *et al.*, 1983).

Organic Mercury. The short-chain organic mercurials, especially methylmercury, are the most difficult forms of mercury to mobilize from the body presumably because of their poor reactivity with chelating agents. Dimercaprol is contraindicated in methylmercury poisoning because it increases brain concentrations of methylmercury in experimental animals. Although penicillamine facilitates the removal of methylmercury from the body, it is not clinically efficacious, and large doses (2 g/day) are needed (Bakir *et al.*, 1980). During the initial 1 to 3 days of administration of penicillamine, the concentration of mercury in the blood increases before it decreases, probably reflecting the mobilization of metal from tissues to blood at a rate more rapid than that for excretion of mercury into urine and feces.

Methylmercury compounds undergo extensive enterohepatic recirculation in experimental animals. Therefore, introduction of a nonabsorbable mercury-binding substance into the intestinal tract should facilitate their removal from the body. A *polythiol resin* has been used for this purpose in humans and appears to be effective

(Bakir *et al.*, 1973). The resin has certain advantages over penicillamine. It does not cause redistribution of mercury in the body with a subsequent increase in the concentration of mercury in blood, and it has fewer adverse effects than do sulfhydryl agents that are absorbed. Clinical experience with various treatments for methylmercury poisoning in Iraq indicates that penicillamine, *N*-acetylpenicillamine, and an oral nonabsorbable thiol resin all can reduce blood concentrations of mercury; however, clinical improvement was not clearly related to reduction of the body burden of methylmercury (Bakir *et al.*, 1980).

Conventional hemodialysis is of little value in the treatment of methylmercury poisoning because methylmercury concentrates in erythrocytes, and little is contained in the plasma. However, it has been shown that L-*cysteine* can be infused into the arterial blood entering the dialyzer to convert methylmercury into a diffusible form. Both free cysteine and the methylmercury–cysteine complex form in the blood and then diffuse across the membrane into the dialysate. This method has been shown to be effective in humans (Al-Abbasi *et al.*, 1978). Studies in animals indicate that succimer may be more effective than cysteine in this regard (Kostyniak, 1982).

Arsenic

Arsenic was used more than 2400 years ago in Greece and Rome as a therapeutic agent and as a poison. The foundations of many modern concepts of chemotherapy derive from Ehrlich's early work with organic arsenicals, and such drugs once were a mainstay of chemotherapy. Although use of arsenicals as chemotherapeutics has declined, reports still emerge about their effectiveness, as shown by the use of *arsenic trioxide* in the treatment of acute promyelocytic leukemia (Chen *et al.*, 1996; Soignet *et al.*, 1998) (*see* Chapter 51). Arsenicals also remain important in the treatment of certain tropical diseases, such as African trypanosomiasis (*see* Chapter 40). In the United States, the impact of arsenic on health is predominantly from industrial and environmental exposures. (For a review, *see* NRC, 1999.)

Arsenic is found in soil, water, and air as a common environmental toxicant. Well water in sections of Argentina, Chile, and Taiwan has especially high concentrations of arsenic, which results in widespread poisoning. Large numbers of people in Bangladesh and West Bengal, India, are exposed to high concentrations of arsenic in their well water used for drinking. There also are high concentrations of arsenic in the water in many parts of the western United States. The element usually is not mined as such but is recovered as a by-product from the smelting of copper, lead, zinc, and other ores. This can release arsenic into the environment. Mineral-spring waters and the effluent from geothermal power plants leach arsenic from soils and rocks containing high concentrations of the metal. Arsenic also is present in coal at variable concentrations and is released into the environment during combustion. Application of pesticides and herbicides containing arsenic has increased its environmental dispersion. The major source of occupational exposure to arsenic-containing compounds is from the manufacture of arsenical herbicides and pesticides (Landrigan, 1981). Fruits and vegetables sprayed with arsenicals may be a source of this element, and it is concentrated in many species of fish and shellfish. Arsenicals sometimes are added to the feed of poultry and other livestock to promote growth. The average daily human intake of arsenic is about 10 μg. Almost all this is ingested with food and water.

Arsenic is used as arsine and as arsenic trioxide in the manufacture of most computer chips using silicon-based technology. Gallium arsenide is used in the production of compound (types III to V) semiconductors that are used for making light-emitting diodes (LEDs), as well as laser and solar devices. In the manufacture of both computer chips and semiconductors, metallic arsenic also may be used or produced as a by-product of the reaction chambers. Chromated copper arsenate (CCA) was used as a common treatment for outdoor lumber until 2004, although this should not pose a health risk unless treated wood is burned in fireplaces or woodstoves (Hall, 2002).

Chemical Forms of Arsenic. The arsenic atom exists in the elemental form and in trivalent and pentavalent oxidation states. The toxicity of a given arsenical is related to the rate of its clearance from the body and therefore to its degree of accumulation in tissues. In general, toxicity increases in the sequence of organic arsenicals $< As^{5+} < As^{3+} <$ arsine (AsH_3).

The organic arsenicals contain arsenic covalently linked to a carbon atom, where arsenic exists in the trivalent or pentavalent state. Arsphenamine contains trivalent arsenic; sodium arsanilate contains arsenic in the pentavalent form. The organic arsenicals usually are excreted more rapidly than are the inorganic forms.

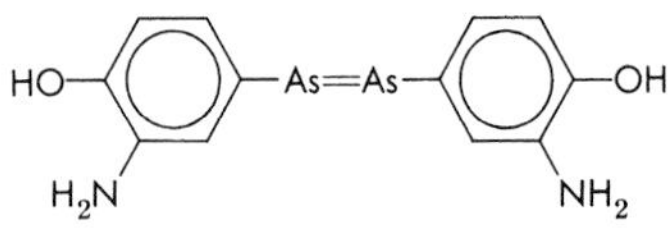

ARSPHENAMINE

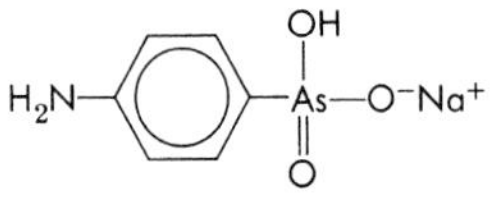

SODIUM ARSANILATE

The pentavalent oxidation state is found in arsenates (such as lead arsenate, $PbHAsO_4$), which are salts of arsenic acid, H_3AsO_4. The pentavalent arsenicals have very low affinity for thiol groups, in contrast to the trivalent compounds, and are much less toxic. The arsenites [*e.g.*, potassium arsenite ($KAsO_2$)] and salts of arsenious acid contain trivalent arsenic. Arsine (AsH_3) is a gaseous hydride of trivalent arsenic; it produces toxic effects that are distinct from those of the other arsenic compounds.

Mechanism of Action. Arsenate (pentavalent) uncouples mitochondrial oxidative phosphorylation. The mechanism is thought to be related to competitive substitution of arsenate for inorganic phosphate in the formation of adenosine triphosphate, with subsequent formation of an unstable arsenate ester that is hydrolyzed rapidly. This process is termed *arsenolysis*.

Trivalent arsenicals, including inorganic arsenite, are regarded primarily as sulfhydryl reagents. As such, trivalent arsenicals inhibit many enzymes by reacting with biological ligands containing available —SH groups. The pyruvate dehydrogenase system is especially sensitive to trivalent arsenicals because of their interaction with two sulfhydryl groups of lipoic acid to form a stable six-membered ring, as shown below:

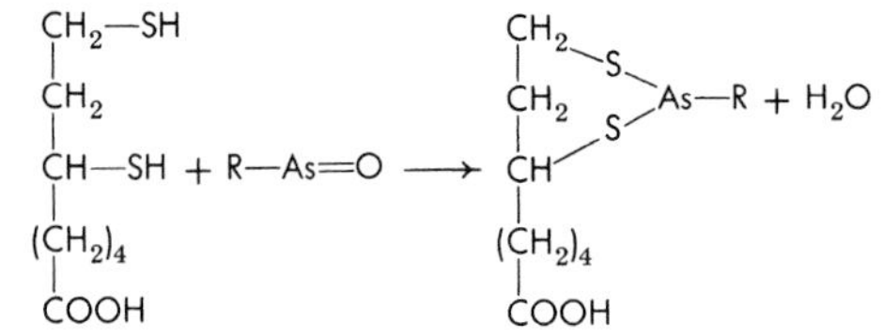

Absorption, Distribution, and Excretion. The absorption of poorly water-soluble arsenicals, such as As_2O_3, depends on the physical state of the compound. Coarsely powdered material is less toxic because it can be eliminated in feces before it dissolves. The arsenite salts are more soluble in water and are better absorbed than the oxide. Experimental evidence has shown a high degree of GI absorption (80% to 90%) of both trivalent and pentavalent forms of arsenic.

The distribution of arsenic depends on the duration of administration and the particular arsenical involved. Arsenic is stored mainly in liver, kidney, heart, and lung. Much smaller amounts are found in muscle and neural tissue. Because of the high sulfhydryl content of keratin, the highest concentrations of arsenic are found in hair and nails. Deposition in hair starts within 2 weeks of administration, and arsenic stays fixed at this site for years. Because of its chemical similarity to phosphorus, it is deposited in bone and teeth and is retained there for long periods. Arsenic readily crosses the placenta, and fetal damage has been reported. Concentrations of arsenic in human umbilical cord blood are equivalent to those in the maternal circulation.

Arsenic is readily biotransformed in both laboratory animals and humans (Figure 65–5). The pentavalent arsenic (arsenate) is coupled to the oxidation of glutathione (GSH) to GSSG to form the trivalent arsenic (arsenite). Arsenite undergoes oxidative methylation to pentavalent methylarsonic acid (MMA^V) catalyzed by arsenite methyltransferase. MMA^V is reduced by MMA^V reductase to trivalent monomethyl arsonous acid (MMA^{III}), which can undergo further oxidative methylation *via* MMA methyltransferase to dimethylarsenic acid (DMA^V).

Arsenic is eliminated by many routes (*e.g.*, feces, urine, sweat, milk, hair, skin, and lungs), although most is excreted in urine in humans. The half-life for the urinary excretion of arsenic is 3 to 5 days, much shorter than those of the other metals discussed. While it once was thought that the methylated forms of arsenic are less reactive with tissue constituents, less cytotoxic, and more readily excreted in urine than inorganic arsenic, studies have shown that methylation to monomethylarcenous (III) acid or reduction of dimethyl arsenic acid to its trivalent state actually increases the toxicity and carcinogenicity of arsenic owing to increased affinity for sulfhydryl groups (Petrick *et al.*, 2000; Thomas *et al.*, 2001). In humans, the urinary content of metabolites is 10% to 30% inorganic arsenic, 10% to 20% monomethylarsenite, and 60% to 80% dimethylarsenite (Vahter and Concha, 2001). Formation of trivalent mono- or dimethyl arsenic metabolites promotes biliary rather than renal excretion (Gregus *et al.*, 2000).

Pharmacological and Toxicological Effects of Arsenic. Arsenicals have varied effects on many organ systems, as summarized below.

Cardiovascular System. Acute and subacute doses of inorganic arsenic induce mild vasodilation. This may lead to an occult edema,

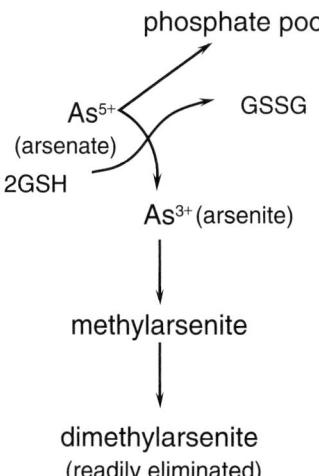

phosphate pool

As⁵⁺ (arsenate)

2GSH

GSSG

As³⁺ (arsenite)

methylarsenite

dimethylarsenite
(readily eliminated)

Figure 65–5. *The biotransformation of arsenic in human beings.*

particularly facial, which has been mistaken for a healthy weight gain and misinterpreted as a "tonic" effect of arsenic. Larger acute and subacute doses evoke capillary dilation; increased capillary permeability may occur in all capillary beds but is most pronounced in the splanchnic area. Transudation of plasma also may occur, and the decrease in intravascular volume may be significant. Serious cardiovascular effects include hypotension, congestive heart failure, and cardiac arrhythmias. Long-term exposure results in peripheral vascular disease (Engel *et al.*, 1994), more specifically gangrene of the extremities, especially of the feet, often referred to as *blackfoot disease*. Myocardial damage and hypotension may become evident after more prolonged exposure to arsenic.

Gastrointestinal Tract. Acute or subacute exposure to arsenic can produce GI disturbances that range from mild abdominal cramping and diarrhea to severe hemorrhagic gastroenteritis associated with shock. With chronic exposure to arsenic, GI effects usually are not observed. Small doses of inorganic arsenicals, especially the trivalent compounds, cause mild splanchnic hyperemia. Capillary transudation of plasma, resulting from larger doses, produces vesicles under the GI mucosa. These eventually rupture, epithelial fragments slough off, and plasma is discharged into the lumen of the intestine, where it coagulates. Tissue damage and the bulk cathartic action of the increased fluid in the lumen lead to increased peristalsis and characteristic watery diarrhea. Normal proliferation of the epithelium is suppressed, which accentuates the damage. Soon the feces become bloody. Damage to the upper GI tract usually results in hematemesis. Stomatitis also may be evident. The onset of GI symptoms may be so gradual that the possibility of arsenic poisoning may be overlooked.

Kidneys. The action of arsenic on the renal capillaries, tubules, and glomeruli may cause severe renal damage. Initially, the glomeruli are affected, and proteinuria results. Varying degrees of tubular necrosis and degeneration occur later. Oliguria with proteinuria, hematuria, and casts frequently results from arsenic exposure.

Skin. Skin is a major target organ of arsenic. Diffuse or spotted hyperpigmentation over the trunk and extremities usually is the first effect observed with chronic arsenic ingestion. Depending on the amount of exposure to arsenic, hyperpigmentation can be observed within 6 months. The hyperpigmentation of chronic arsenic expo-

sure commonly appears in a finely freckled "raindrop" pattern, progressing within a period of years to palmar-plantar hyperkeratosis. Long-term ingestion of low doses of inorganic arsenicals causes cutaneous vasodilation and a "milk and roses" complexion. Eventually, skin cancer is observed, as described below.

Nervous System. High-dose acute or subacute exposure to arsenic can cause encephalopathy; however, the most common arsenic-induced neurological lesion is a peripheral neuropathy with a stocking/glove distribution of dysesthesia. The syndrome is similar to acute inflammatory demyelinating polyradiculoneuropathy (Guillain-Barré syndrome) (Donofrio *et al.*, 1987). This is followed by muscular weakness in the extremities, and with continued exposure, deep-tendon reflexes diminish, and muscular atrophy follows. The cerebral lesions are mainly vascular in origin and occur in both the gray and white matter; characteristic multiple symmetrical foci of hemorrhagic necrosis occur.

Blood. Inorganic arsenicals affect the bone marrow and alter the cellular composition of the blood. Hematological evaluation usually reveals anemia with slight-to-moderate leukopenia; eosinophilia also may be present. Anisocytosis becomes evident with increasing exposure to arsenic. The vascularity of the bone marrow is increased. Some of the chronic hematological effects may result from impaired absorption of folic acid. Serious, irreversible blood and bone marrow disturbances from organic arsenicals are rare.

Liver. Inorganic arsenicals and a number of now-obsolete organic arsenicals are particularly toxic to the liver and produce fatty infiltration, central necrosis, and cirrhosis. The damage may be mild or so severe that death may ensue. The injury generally is to the hepatic parenchyma, but in some cases the clinical picture may closely resemble occlusion of the common bile duct, the principal lesions being pericholangitis and bile thrombi in the finer biliary radicles.

Carcinogenesis. The association of arsenic exposure and skin tumors was noted more than 100 years ago in patients treated with arsenicals. The International Agency for Research on Cancer concluded that inorganic arsenic is a skin and lung (*via* inhalation) carcinogen in humans (International Agency for Research on Cancer, 1980). Studies indicate that in Taiwan, Argentina, and Chile, where drinking water contained very high concentrations of arsenic (at least several hundred micrograms per deciliter), an increased incidence of bladder and lung cancer was due to arsenic exposure. Increased risks of other cancers, such as kidney and liver cancer, also have been reported, but the association with arsenic is not as high as for the tumors just noted.

Other. Apart from the various direct toxicities already mentioned, epidemiological studies demonstrate that inorganic arsenic exerts other adverse effects, examined in a variety of population-based epidemiological studies and clinical reports, including diseases of the cerebrovascular systems and hypertension. Chronic exposure to arsenic has been associated with increased prevalence of diabetes mellitus, goiter, hepatomegaly, and respiratory system dysfunctions (Thomas *et al.*, 2001).

Acute Arsenic Poisoning. Federal restrictions on the allowable content of arsenic in food and in the occupational environment not only have improved safety procedures and decreased the number of intoxications but also have decreased the amount of arsenic in use; only the annual production of arsenic-containing herbicides is increasing.

The incidence of accidental, homicidal, and suicidal arsenic poisoning has diminished greatly in recent decades. Previously, arsenic in the form of As₂O₃ was a common cause of poisoning because it was readily available, practically tasteless, and had the appearance of sugar.

GI discomfort usually is experienced within an hour after intake of an arsenical, although it may be delayed as much as 12 hours after oral ingestion if food is in the stomach. Burning lips, constriction of the throat, and difficulty in swallowing may be the first symptoms, followed by excruciating gastric pain, projectile vomiting, and severe diarrhea. Oliguria with proteinuria and hematuria usually is present; eventually, anuria may occur. The patient often complains of marked skeletal muscle cramps and severe thirst. As the loss of fluid proceeds, symptoms of shock appear. Hypoxic convulsions may occur terminally; coma and death ensue. In severe poisoning, death can occur within an hour, but the usual interval is 24 hours. With prompt application of corrective therapy, patients may survive the acute phase of the toxicity only to develop neuropathies and other disorders. In a series of 57 such patients, 37 had peripheral neuropathy, and 5 had encephalopathy. The motor system appears to be spared only in the mildest cases; severe crippling is common (Jenkins, 1966).

Chronic Arsenic Poisoning. The most common early signs of chronic arsenic poisoning are muscle weakness and aching, skin pigmentation (especially of the neck, eyelids, nipples, and axillae), hyperkeratosis, and edema. GI involvement is less prominent in long-term exposures. Other signs and symptoms that should arouse suspicion of arsenic poisoning include garlic odor of the breath and perspiration, excessive salivation and sweating, stomatitis, generalized itching, sore throat, coryza, lacrimation, numbness, burning or tingling of the extremities, dermatitis, vitiligo, and alopecia. Poisoning may begin insidiously with symptoms of weakness, languor, anorexia, occasional nausea and vomiting, and diarrhea or constipation. Subsequent symptoms may simulate acute coryza. Dermatitis and keratosis of the palms and soles are common features. Mee's lines are found characteristically in the fingernails (white transverse lines of deposited arsenic that usually appear 6 weeks after exposure). Because the fingernail grows at a rate of 0.1 mm/day, the approximate time of exposure can be determined. Desquamation and scaling of the skin may initiate an exfoliative process involving many epithelial structures of the body. The liver may enlarge, and obstruction of the bile ducts may result in jaundice. Eventually cirrhosis may occur from the hepatotoxic action. Renal dysfunction also may be encountered. As intoxication advances, encephalopathy may develop. Peripheral neuritis results in motor and sensory paralysis of the extremities; in contrast to lead palsy, the legs usually are more severely affected than the arms. The bone marrow is seriously damaged by arsenic, and all hematological elements may be affected with severe exposure.

Treatment of Arsenic Poisoning. After short-term exposure to arsenic, routine measures are taken to stabilize the patient and prevent further absorption of the poison. In particular, attention is directed to the intravascular volume status because the effects of arsenic on the GI tract can result in fatal hypovolemic shock. Hypotension requires fluid replacement and may necessitate pharmacological support with pressor agents such as *dopamine*.

Chelation Therapy. Chelation therapy often is begun with dimercaprol (3 to 4 mg/kg intramuscularly every 4 to 12 hours) until abdominal symptoms subside and charcoal (if given initially) is passed in the feces. Oral treatment with penicillamine then may be substituted for dimercaprol and continued for 4 days. Penicillamine is given in four divided doses to a maximum of 2 g/day. If symptoms recur after cessation of chelation therapy, a second course of penicillamine may be instituted. Succimer (2,3-dimercaptosuccinic acid), a derivative of dimercaprol, is efficacious in the treatment of arsenic

poisoning (Graziano *et al.*, 1978; Lenz *et al.*, 1981; Fournier *et al.*, 1988) but is approved by the FDA only for lead chelation in children.

After long-term exposure to arsenic, treatment with dimercaprol and penicillamine also may be used, but oral penicillamine alone usually is sufficient. The duration of therapy is determined by the clinical condition of the patient, and the decision is aided by periodic determinations of urinary arsenic concentrations. Adverse effects of the chelating agents may limit the usefulness of therapy (*see* below). Dialysis may become necessary with severe arsenic-induced nephropathy; successful removal of arsenic by dialysis has been reported (Vaziri *et al.*, 1980).

Arsine. Arsine gas, generated by electrolytic or metallic reduction of arsenic in nonferrous metal products, is a rare cause of industrial intoxication. Rapid and often fatal hemolysis is a unique characteristic of arsine poisoning and probably results from arsine combining with hemoglobin and then reacting with oxygen to cause hemolysis. A few hours after exposure, headache, anorexia, vomiting, paresthesia, abdominal pain, chills, hemoglobinuria, bilirubinemia, and anuria occur. The classic arsine triad of hemolysis, abdominal pain, and hematuria is noteworthy. Jaundice appears after 24 hours. A coppery skin pigmentation is observed frequently and is thought to be due to methemoglobin. Kidneys of persons poisoned by arsine characteristically contain hemoglobin casts, and there is cloudy swelling and necrosis of the cells of the proximal tubule. If the patient survives the severe hemolysis, death may result from renal failure. Because the hemoglobin–arsine complex cannot be dialyzed, *exchange transfusion* is recommended in severe cases; *forced alkaline diuresis* also may be employed (*see* Chapter 64). Dimercaprol has no effect on the hemolysis, and beneficial effects on renal function have not been established; it therefore is not recommended.

It should be noted that arsenic is a trace contaminant of other metals, such as lead; contact of these unrefined metals with acid may produce arsine (and/or stilbine from antimony).

Cadmium

Cadmium ranks close to lead and mercury as a metal of current toxicological concern. It occurs in nature in association with zinc and lead, and extraction and processing of these metals often lead to environmental contamination with cadmium. The element was discovered in 1817 but was seldom used until its valuable metallurgical properties were discovered approximately 50 years ago. A high resistance to corrosion, valuable electrochemical properties, and other useful chemical properties account for cadmium's wide applications in electroplating and galvanization and its use in plastics, paint pigments (cadmium yellow), and nickel–cadmium batteries. Applications for and production of cadmium will continue to increase. Because less than 5% of the metal is recycled, environmental pollution is an important consideration. Coal and other fossil fuels contain cadmium, and their combustion releases the element into the environment.

Workers in smelters and other metal-processing plants may be exposed to high concentrations of cadmium in the air; however, for most of the population, food is the major source of cadmium. Uncontaminated foodstuffs contain less than 0.05 μg cadmium per gram wet weight, and the average daily intake is about 50 μg. Cereal grains, such as rice and wheat, concentrate cadmium; thus, when they are grown in soils with naturally high concentrations of cadmium or polluted with cadmium, these grains can have high cadmium content. Drinking water normally does not contribute significantly to cadmium intake, but cigarette smoking does because the tobacco plant also concentrates cadmium. One cigarette contains 1 to 2 μg cadmium, and with even 10% pulmonary absorption (Elinder *et al.*, 1983), the smoking of one pack of cigarettes per day results in a dose of approximately 1 mg cadmium per year from smoking alone. Shellfish and animal liver and kidney can have concentrations of cadmium higher than 0.05 μg/g, even under normal circumstances. When foods such as rice and wheat are contaminated by cadmium in soil and water in which they grew, the concentration of the metal may increase considerably (1 μg/g).

Absorption, Distribution, and Excretion. Cadmium occurs only in one valency state (2$^+$) and does not form stable alkyl compounds or other organometallic compounds of known toxicological significance.

Cadmium is absorbed poorly from the GI tract, in the range of 1.5% to 5% (Engstrom and Nordberg, 1979; Rahola *et al.*, 1972). Absorption from the respiratory tract is higher; cigarette smokers may absorb 10% to 40% of inhaled cadmium (Friberg *et al.*, 1974). Cadmium absorption is higher in pregnant than nonpregnant rats apparently owing to an increased expression of divalent metal transporter 1 (DMT-1). The main function of DMT-1 is to facilitate iron absorption, so its levels increase during pregnancy owing to an increased need for iron. However, DMT-1 also is capable of transporting cadmium, which explains the observed increase in cadmium absorption (Leazer *et al.*, 2002).

After absorption, cadmium is transported in blood, bound mainly to blood cells and albumin. Cadmium initially is distributed to the liver and then redistributes slowly to the kidney as cadmium–metallothionein (Cd–MT). After distribution, approximately 50% of the total-body burden is found in the liver and kidney. Metallothionein is a low-molecular-weight protein with high affinity for metals such as cadmium and zinc. One-third of its amino acid residues are cysteines. Metallothionein is inducible by exposure to several metals, including cadmium, and elevated concentrations of this metal-binding protein protect against cadmium toxicity by preventing the interaction of cadmium with other functional macromolecules (Klaassen *et al.*, 1999).

The half-life of cadmium in the body is 10 to 30 years. Thus the metal is prone to accumulation, and with continuous environmental exposure, tissue concentrations of the metal increase throughout life. The body burden of cadmium in a 50-year-old adult in the United States is about 30 mg. Overall, fecal elimination of the metal, which is quantitatively more important than urinary excretion, becomes significant only after substantial renal toxicity has occurred (*see* Goering and Klaassen, 1984).

Acute Cadmium Poisoning. Acute poisoning usually results from inhalation of cadmium dusts and fumes (usually cadmium oxide) or from the ingestion of cadmium salts. The early toxic effects are due to local irritation. In the case of oral intake, these include nausea, vomiting, salivation, diarrhea, and abdominal cramps; the vomitus and diarrhea often are bloody. In the short term, inhaled cadmium is more toxic. Signs and symptoms, which appear within a few hours, include irritation of the respiratory tract with severe, early pneumo-

nitis, chest pains, nausea, dizziness, and diarrhea. Toxicity may progress to fatal pulmonary edema or residual emphysema with peribronchial and perivascular fibrosis (Zavon and Meadows, 1970).

Chronic Cadmium Poisoning. The toxic effects of long-term exposure to cadmium differ somewhat with the route of exposure. The kidney is affected following either pulmonary or GI exposure; marked effects are observed in the lungs only after exposure by inhalation.

Kidney. Figure 65–6 illustrates how cadmium is thought to produce renal toxicity. Although some cadmium is excreted with the bile, a cadmium–metallothionein complex can transport cadmium to the kidney, where it is released as inorganic cadmium. A sufficient concentration (200 μg/g) damages the cells of the proximal tubule, resulting in proteinuria (Dudley *et al.*, 1985). With more severe exposure, glomerular injury occurs, filtration is decreased, and aminoaciduria, glycosuria, and proteinuria occur. The nature of the glomerular injury is unknown but may involve an autoimmune component.

Excretion of β_2-microglobulin in urine is a sensitive but not specific index of cadmium-induced nephrotoxicity (Piscator and Pettersson, 1977; Lauwerys *et al.*, 1979). Although measurement of urine β_2-microglobulin is part of the Occupational Safety and Health Administration (OSHA) standard for monitoring cadmium poisoning, the concentration of β_2-microglobulin in the urine may not be the best marker for exposure. Retinol-binding protein may be a better marker, but its measurement generally is not available.

Lung. The consequence of excessive inhalation of cadmium fumes and dusts is loss of ventilatory capacity, with a corresponding increase in residual lung volume. Dyspnea is the most frequent complaint of patients with cadmium-induced lung disease. The pathogenesis of cadmium-induced emphysema and pulmonary fibrosis is not well understood (Davison *et al.*, 1988); however, cadmium specifically inhibits the synthesis of plasma α_1-antitrypsin (Chowdhury and Louria, 1976), and severe α_1-antitrypsin deficiency of genetic origin is associated with emphysema in humans.

Cardiovascular System. Perhaps the most controversial issue concerning the effects of cadmium on human beings is the suggestion that the metal plays a significant causal role in hypertension (Schroeder, 1965). An initial epidemiological study indicated that individuals dying from hypertension had significantly higher concentrations of cadmium and higher cadmium-to-zinc ratios in their kidneys than people dying of other causes. Others have found similar correlations (Thind and Fischer, 1976). However, consistent effects of cadmium on the blood pressure of experimental animals have not been observed, and hypertension is not prominent in industrial cadmium poisoning.

Bone. There may be an interaction among cadmium, nutrition, and bone disease. Body stores of calcium have been found to be decreased in subjects exposed to cadmium occupationally (Scott *et al.*, 1980). This presumed effect of cadmium may be due to interference with renal regulation of calcium and phosphate balance.

Testis. Testicular necrosis, a common characteristic of short-term exposure to cadmium in experimental animals, is uncommon with long-term low-level exposure (Kotsonis and Klaassen, 1978) and has not been observed in men.

Cancer. Cadmium produces tumors in a number of organs when administered to laboratory animals (Waalkes *et al.*, 1992). Evidence that cadmium is a human carcinogen is based mainly on epidemiological studies from workers exposed occupationally to cadmium. These investigations primarily have identified tumors of the lungs and, to a lesser extent, prostate, kidney, and stomach. The Interna-

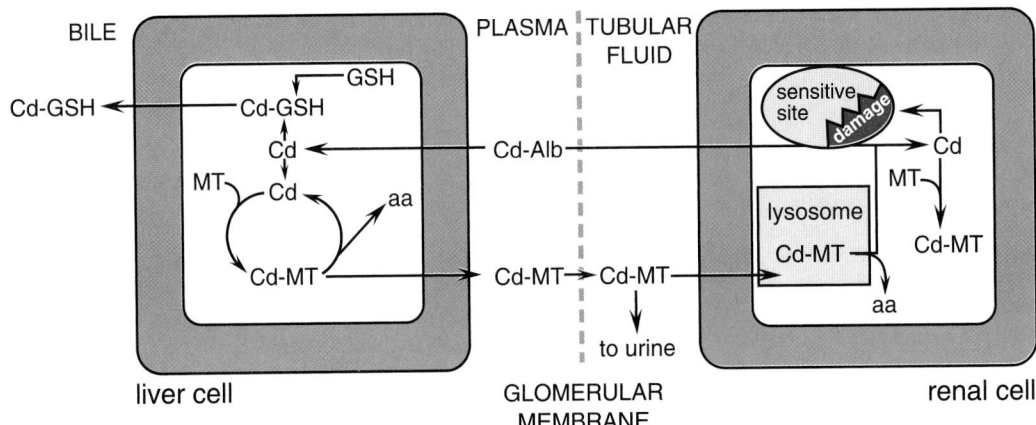

Figure 65–6. *Postulated mechanisms contributing to cadmium-induced renal toxicity.* Cadmium (Cd) taken up by the liver can combine with glutathione (GSH) and be excreted into the bile or can bind to metallothionein (MT), creating a storage form for cadmium. Some cadmium–metallothionein complex (Cd–MT) leaks into the plasma. When taken up by kidney cells, Cd–MT enters the lysosomes, the MT is degraded to its component amino acids (aa), and the cadmium is released from the lysosomes into the cytosol. At concentrations of 200 μg/g or higher, cadmium damages kidney tissue and results in proteinuria (Dudley *et al.*, 1985). Alb, albumin.

tional Agency for Cancer Research (1993) has concluded that the data are sufficient to classify cadmium as a human carcinogen.

Treatment of Cadmium Poisoning. Effective therapy for cadmium poisoning is difficult to achieve. After short-term inhalation, the patient must be removed from the source, and pulmonary ventilation should be monitored carefully. Respiratory support and steroid therapy may become necessary.

Chelation Therapy. Although there is no proven benefit, some clinicians recommend chelation therapy with $CaNa_2EDTA$. The dose of $CaNa_2EDTA$ is 75 mg/kg per day in three to six divided doses for 5 days. After a minimum of 2 days without treatment, a second 5-day course is given. The total dose of $CaNa_2EDTA$ per 5-day course should not exceed 500 mg/kg. Animal studies suggest that chelation therapy should be instituted as soon as possible after cadmium exposure because a rapid decrease in effectiveness of chelation therapy occurs in parallel with distribution to sites inaccessible to the chelators (Cantilena and Klaassen, 1982a). The use of dimercaprol and substituted dithiocarbamates appears promising for individuals chronically exposed to cadmium (Jones *et al.*, 1991).

Iron

Although iron is not an environmental poison, accidental intoxication with ferrous salts used to treat iron deficiency is a frequently encountered source of poisoning in young children. Iron is discussed further in Chapter 53.

Radioactive Heavy Metals

The widespread production and use of radioactive heavy metals for nuclear generation of electricity, nuclear weapons, laboratory research, manufacturing, and medical diagnosis have generated unique problems in dealing with accidental poisoning by such metals. Because the toxicity of radioactive metals is almost entirely a consequence of ionizing radiation, the therapeutic objective follow-

ing exposure is not only chelation of the metals but also their removal from the body as rapidly and completely as possible.

Treatment of the acute radiation syndrome is largely symptomatic. Attempts have been made to investigate the effectiveness of organic reducing agents, such as *mercaptamine (cysteamine)*, administered to prevent the formation of free radicals. Success has been limited.

Major products of a nuclear accident or the use of nuclear weapons include ^{239}Pu, ^{137}Cs, ^{144}Ce, and ^{90}Sr. Isotopes of strontium and radium are extremely difficult to remove from the body with chelating agents. Several factors are involved in the relative resistance of radioactive metals to chelation therapy; these include the affinity of these particular metals for individual chelators and the observation that radiation from Sr and Ra in bone destroys nearby capillaries, thereby decreasing blood flow and isolating the radioisotopes. Many chelating agents have been used experimentally, including $CaNa_3DTPA$ (*pentetic acid; see* below), which has been shown to be effective against ^{239}Pu (Jones *et al.*, 1986). One gram of $CaNa_3DTPA$, administered by slow intravenous drip on alternate days three times per week has enhanced excretion fifty to one hundredfold in animals and in human subjects exposed in accidents. As is seen commonly with heavy-metal poisoning, effectiveness of treatment diminishes very rapidly with an increasing delay between exposure and the initiation of therapy.

HEAVY-METAL ANTAGONISTS

Edetate Calcium Disodium

Ethylenediaminetetraacetic acid (EDTA), its sodium salt (*edetate disodium*, Na_2EDTA), and a number of closely related compounds chelate many divalent and trivalent metals. The cation used to make a water-soluble salt of EDTA has an important role in the toxicity of the chelator. Na_2EDTA causes hypocalcemic tetany. However, *edetate calcium disodium* ($CaNa_2EDTA$) can be used for treatment of poisoning by metals that have higher affinity for the chelating agent than does Ca^{2+}.

Chemistry and Mechanism of Action. The structure of $CaNa_2EDTA$ is as follows:

EDETATE CALCIUM DISODIUM

The pharmacological effects of $CaNa_2EDTA$ result from formation of chelates with divalent and trivalent metals in the body. Accessible metal ions (both exogenous and endogenous) with a higher affinity for $CaNa_2EDTA$ than Ca^{2+} will be chelated, mobilized, and usually excreted. Because EDTA is charged at physiological pH, it does not significantly penetrate cells; its volume of distribution approximates extracellular fluid space. Experimental studies in mice have shown that administration of $CaNa_2EDTA$ mobilizes several endogenous metallic cations, including those of zinc, manganese, and iron (Cantilena and Klaassen, 1982b). The main therapeutic use of $CaNa_2EDTA$ is in the treatment of metal intoxications, especially lead intoxication.

$CaNa_2EDTA$ is available as edetate calcium disodium (CAL-CIUM DISODIUM VERSENATE). Intramuscular administration of $CaNa_2EDTA$ results in good absorption, but pain occurs at the injection site; consequently, the chelator injection often is mixed with a local anesthetic or administered intravenously. For intravenous use, $CaNa_2EDTA$ is diluted in either 5% dextrose or 0.9% saline and is administered slowly by intravenous drip. A dilute solution is necessary to avoid thrombophlebitis. To minimize nephrotoxicity, adequate urine production should be established prior to and during treatment with $CaNa_2EDTA$. However, in patients with lead encephalopathy and increased intracranial pressure, excess fluids must be avoided. In such cases, conservative replacement of fluid is advised, and intramuscular administration of $CaNa_2EDTA$ is recommended.

Lead Poisoning. The successful use of $CaNa_2EDTA$ in the treatment of lead poisoning is due, in part, to the capacity of lead to displace calcium from the chelate. Enhanced mobilization and excretion of lead indicate that the metal is accessible to EDTA. Bone provides the primary source of lead that is chelated by $CaNa_2EDTA$. After such chelation, lead is redistributed from soft tissues to the skeleton.

Mercury poisoning, by contrast, does not respond to the drug despite the fact that mercury displaces calcium from $CaNa_2EDTA$ *in vitro*. Mercury is unavailable to the chelate perhaps because it is too tightly bound by sulfhydryl groups or sequestered in body compartments that are not penetrated by $CaNa_2EDTA$.

Suggestions appeared in the lay press in the 1980s that chelation therapy with $CaNa_2EDTA$ could minimize development of atherosclerotic plaques, which can accumulate calcium deposits; such use of $CaNa_2EDTA$ is without therapeutic rationale and not efficacious (Guldager *et al.*, 1992; Elihu *et al.*, 1998; Villarruz *et al.*, 2002).

Absorption, Distribution, and Excretion. Less than 5% of $CaNa_2EDTA$ is absorbed from the GI tract. After intravenous administration, $CaNa_2EDTA$ disappears from the circulation with a half-life of 20 to 60 minutes. In blood, all the drug is found in plasma. About 50% is excreted in urine in 1 hour and more than 95% in 24 hours. For this reason, adequate renal function is necessary for successful therapy. Renal clearance of the compound in dogs equals that of inulin, and glomerular filtration accounts entirely for urinary excretion. Altering either the pH or the rate of flow of urine has no effect on the rate of excretion. There is very little metabolic degradation of EDTA. The drug is distributed mainly in the extracellular fluids, but very little gains access to the spinal fluid (5% of the plasma concentration).

Toxicity. Rapid intravenous administration of Na_2EDTA causes hypocalcemic tetany. However, a slow infusion (<15 mg/minute) administered to a normal individual elicits no symptoms of hypocalcemia because of the ready availability of extracirculatory stores of Ca^{2+}. In contrast, $CaNa_2EDTA$ can be administered intravenously in relatively large quantities with no untoward effects because the change in the concentration of Ca^{2+} in the plasma and total body is negligible.

Renal Toxicity. The principal toxic effect of $CaNa_2EDTA$ is on the kidney. Repeated large doses of the drug cause hydropic vacuolization of the proximal tubule, loss of the brush border, and eventually, degeneration of proximal tubular cells (Catsch and Harmuth-Hoene, 1979). Changes in distal tubules and glomeruli are less conspicuous. The early renal effects usually are reversible, and urinary abnormalities disappear rapidly on cessation of treatment.

Renal toxicity may be related to the large amounts of chelated metals that transit the renal tubule in a relatively short period during drug therapy. Some dissociation of chelates may occur because of competition for the metal by physiological ligands or because of pH changes in the cell or the lumen of the tubule. However, a more likely mechanism of toxicity may be interaction between the chelator and endogenous metals in proximal tubular cells.

Other Side Effects. Other less serious side effects have been reported with use of $CaNa_2EDTA$, including malaise, fatigue, and excessive thirst, followed by the sudden appearance of chills and fever. This, in turn, may be followed by severe myalgia, frontal headache, anorexia, occasional nausea and vomiting, and rarely, increased urinary frequency and urgency. Other possible undesirable effects include sneezing, nasal congestion, and lacrimation; glycosuria; anemia; dermatitis with lesions strikingly similar to those of vitamin B_6 deficiency; transitory lowering of systolic and diastolic blood pressures; prolonged prothrombin time; and T-wave inversion on the electrocardiogram.

Pentetic Acid (DTPA)

Diethylenetriaminepentaacetic acid (DTPA), like EDTA, is a polycarboxylic acid chelator, but it has somewhat greater affinity for most heavy metals. Many investigations in animals have shown that the spectrum of clinical effectiveness of DTPA is similar to that of EDTA. Because of its relatively greater affinity for metals, DTPA has been tried in cases of heavy-metal poisoning that do not respond to EDTA, particularly poisoning by radioactive metals. Unfortunately, success has been limited probably because DTPA also has limited access to intracellular sites of metal storage. Because DTPA rapidly binds Ca^{2+}, $CaNa_3DTPA$ is employed. The use of DTPA is investigational.

Dimercaprol

Dimercaprol was developed during World War II as an antidote to lewisite, a vesicant arsenical war gas, hence its alternative name, *British antilewisite* (BAL). Arsenicals would form a very stable and relatively nontoxic chelate ring with the dimercaprol (2,3-dimercaptopropanol). Pharmacological investigations revealed that this compound would protect against the toxic effects of other heavy metals as well.

Chemistry. Dimercaprol has the following structure:

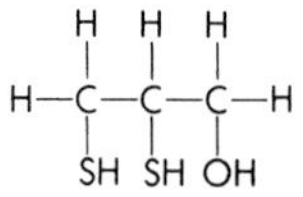

DIMERCAPROL

It is an oily fluid with a pungent, disagreeable odor typical of mercaptans. Because of its instability in aqueous solutions, peanut oil is the solvent employed in pharmaceutical preparations. Dimercaprol and related thiols are readily oxidized.

Mechanism of Action. The pharmacological actions of dimercaprol result from formation of chelation complexes between its sulfhydryl groups and metals. The molecular properties of the dimercaprol–metal chelate have considerable practical significance. With metals such as mercury, gold, and arsenic, the strategy is to attain a stable complex to promote elimination of the metal. Dissociation of the complex and oxidation of dimercaprol can occur *in vivo*. Furthermore, the sulfur–metal bond may be labile in the acidic tubular urine, which may increase delivery of metal to renal tissue and increase toxicity. The dosage regimen therefore is designed to maintain a concentration of dimercaprol in plasma adequate to favor the continuous formation of the more stable 2:1 (BAL–metal) complex and its rapid excretion. However, because of pronounced and dose-related side effects, excessive plasma concentrations must be avoided. The concentration in plasma therefore must be maintained by repeated fractional dosage until the offending metal can be excreted.

Dimercaprol is much more effective when given as soon as possible after exposure to the metal because it is more effective in preventing inhibition of sulfhydryl enzymes than in reactivating them. Dimercaprol antagonizes the biological actions of metals that form mercaptides with essential cellular sulfhydryl groups, principally arsenic, gold, and mercury. It also is used in combination with $CaNa_2EDTA$ to treat lead poisoning, especially when evidence of lead encephalopathy exists. Intoxication by selenites, which also oxidize sulfhydryl enzymes, is not influenced by dimercaprol.

Absorption, Distribution, and Excretion. Dimercaprol cannot be administered orally; it is given by deep intramuscular injection as a 100 mg/ml solution in peanut oil, and thus it should not be used in patients who are allergic to peanuts or peanut products. Peak concentrations in blood are attained in 30 to 60 minutes. The half-life is short, and metabolic degradation and excretion are essentially complete within 4 hours.

Toxicity. In humans, the administration of dimercaprol produces a number of side effects that usually are more alarming than serious. Reactions to dimercaprol occur in approximately 50% of subjects receiving 5 mg/kg intramuscularly. The effects of repeated administration of this dose are not cumulative if an interval of at least 4 hours elapses between injections. One of the most consistent responses to dimercaprol is a rise in systolic and diastolic arterial pressures, accompanied by tachycardia. The rise in pressure may be as great as 50 mmHg in response to the second of two doses (5 mg/kg) given 2 hours apart. The pressure rises immediately but returns to normal within 2 hours.

Other signs and symptoms of dimercaprol toxicity, many of which tend to parallel the change in blood pressure in time and intensity, are the following, listed in approximate order of frequency: nausea and vomiting; headache; a burning sensation in the lips, mouth, and throat and a feeling of constriction, sometimes pain, in the throat, chest, or hands; conjunctivitis, blepharospasm, lacrimation, rhinorrhea, and salivation; tingling of the hands; a burning sensation in the penis; sweating of the forehead, hands, and other areas; abdominal pain; and the occasional appearance of painful sterile abscesses at the injection site. Symptoms often are accompanied by a feeling of anxiety and unrest. Because the dimercaprol–metal complex breaks down easily in an acidic medium, production of an alkaline urine protects the kidney during therapy. Children react as do adults, although approximately 30% also may experience a fever that disappears on withdrawal of the drug. A transient reduction in the percentage of polymorphonuclear leukocytes may be observed. Dimercaprol also may cause hemolytic anemia in patients deficient in glucose-6-phosphate dehydrogenase. Dimercaprol is contraindicated in patients with hepatic insufficiency, except when this is a result of arsenic poisoning.

Succimer

Succimer (2,3-dimercaptosuccinic acid, CHEMET) is an orally effective chelator that is chemically similar to dimercaprol but contains two carboxylic acids that modify both the distribution and chelating spectrum of the drug. Succimer has the following structure:

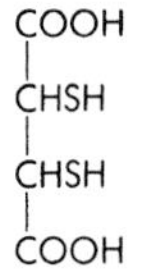

$$
\begin{array}{c}
\text{COOH} \\
|\\
\text{CHSH} \\
|\\
\text{CHSH} \\
|\\
\text{COOH}
\end{array}
$$

SUCCIMER

After its absorption in humans, succimer is biotransformed to a mixed disulfide with cysteine (Aposhian and Aposhian, 1990), the structure of which is as follows:

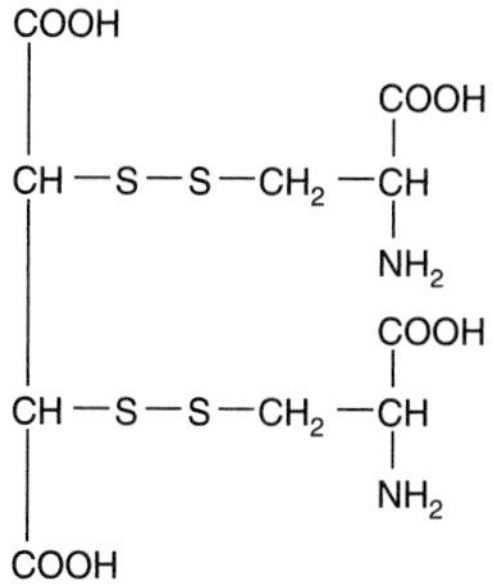

Succimer produces a lead diuresis with a subsequent lowering of blood lead levels and attenuation of the untoward biochemical effects of lead, manifested by normalization of δ-ALA dehydrase activity (Graziano *et al.*, 1992). The succimer–lead chelate also is eliminated in bile; the fraction eliminated undergoes enterohepatic circulation.

A desirable feature of succimer is that it does not significantly mobilize essential metals such as zinc, copper, or iron. Animal studies suggest that succimer is effective as a chelator of arsenic, cadmium, mercury, and other metals (Aposhian and Aposhian, 1990).

Toxicity with succimer is less than that with dimercaprol perhaps because its relatively lower lipid solubility minimizes its uptake into cells. Nonetheless, transient elevations in hepatic transaminases are observed following treatment with succimer. The most commonly reported adverse effects of succimer treatment are nausea, vomiting, diarrhea, and loss of appetite. Rashes also have been reported that may necessitate discontinuation of therapy.

Succimer has been approved in the United States for treatment of children with blood lead levels in excess of 45 μg/dl.

Penicillamine

Penicillamine was first isolated in 1953 from the urine of patients with liver disease who were receiving penicillin. Discovery of its chelating properties led to its use in patients with Wilson's disease and heavy-metal intoxications.

Chemistry. Penicillamine is D-β,β-dimethylcysteine. Its structure is as follows:

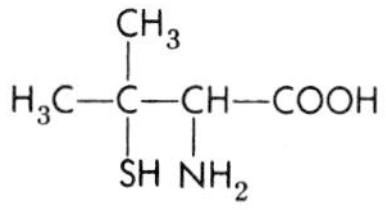

PENICILLAMINE

The D-isomer is used clinically, although the L-isomer also forms chelation complexes. Penicillamine is an effective chelator of copper, mercury, zinc, and lead and promotes the excretion of these metals in the urine.

Absorption, Distribution, and Excretion. Penicillamine is well absorbed (40% to 70%) from the GI tract and therefore has a decided advantage over many other chelating agents. Food, antacids, and iron reduce its absorption. Peak concentrations in blood are obtained between 1 and 3 hours after administration (Netter *et al.*, 1987). Unlike cysteine, its nonmethylated parent compound, penicillamine is somewhat resistant to attack by cysteine desulfhydrase or L-amino acid oxidase. As a result, penicillamine is relatively stable *in vivo*. Hepatic biotransformation is responsible for most of the degradation of penicillamine, and very little is excreted unchanged. Metabolites are found in both urine and feces (Perrett, 1981).

Therapeutic Uses. Penicillamine (CUPRIMINE, DEPEN) is available for oral administration. For chelation therapy, the usual adult dose is 1 to 1.5 g/day in four divided doses (*see* sections under individual metals). The drug should be given on an empty stomach to avoid interference by metals in food. In addition to its use as a chelating agent for the treatment of copper, mercury, and lead poisoning, penicillamine is used in Wilson's disease (hepatolenticular degeneration owing to an excess of copper), cystinuria, and rheumatoid arthritis (rarely). For the treatment of Wilson's disease, 1 to 2 g/day usually is administered in four doses. The urinary excretion of copper should be monitored to determine whether the dosage of penicillamine is adequate.

N-Acetylpenicillamine is more effective than penicillamine in protecting against the toxic effects of mercury presumably because it is even more resistant to metabolism.

The rationale for the use of penicillamine in cystinuria is that penicillamine reacts with the poorly soluble cysteine in a thiol–disulfide exchange reaction and forms a relatively water-soluble cysteine–penicillamine mixed disulfide. In cystinuria, the urinary excretion of cystine is used to adjust dosage, although 2 g/day in four divided doses usually is employed.

The mechanism of action of penicillamine in rheumatoid arthritis remains uncertain, although suppression of the disease may result from marked reduction in concentrations of IgM rheumatoid factor. A single daily dose of 125 to 250 mg usually is used to initiate therapy, with dosage increases at intervals of 1 to 3 months as necessary to a typical range of 500 to 750 mg/day. Because of toxicity, the drug is used rarely today in this setting.

Other experimental uses of penicillamine include the treatment of primary biliary cirrhosis and scleroderma. The mechanism of action of penicillamine in these diseases also may involve effects on immunoglobulins and immune complexes (Epstein *et al.*, 1979).

Toxicity. With long-term use, penicillamine induces several cutaneous lesions, including urticaria, macular or papular reactions, pemphigoid lesions, lupus erythematosus, dermatomyositis, adverse effects on collagen, and other less serious reactions, such as dryness and scaling. Cross-reactivity with penicillin may be responsible for some episodes of urticarial or maculopapular reactions with generalized edema, pruritus, and fever that occur in as many as one-third of patients taking penicillamine. For a detailed review of the adverse dermatological effects of penicillamine, *see* Levy and coworkers (1983).

The hematological system also may be affected severely; reactions include leukopenia, aplastic anemia, and agranulocytosis. These may occur at any time during therapy, and they may be fatal. Patients obviously must be monitored carefully.

Renal toxicity induced by penicillamine usually is manifested as reversible proteinuria and hematuria, but it may progress to the nephrotic syndrome with membranous glomerulopathy. More rarely, fatalities have been reported from Goodpasture's syndrome (Hill, 1979).

Toxicity to the pulmonary system is uncommon, but severe dyspnea has been reported from penicillamine-induced bronchoalveolitis. Myasthenia gravis also has been induced by long-term therapy with penicillamine (Gordon and Burnside, 1977). Less serious side effects include nausea, vomiting, diarrhea, dyspepsia, anorexia, and a transient loss of taste for sweet and salt, which is relieved by supplementation of the diet with copper. Contraindications to penicillamine therapy include pregnancy, a previous history of penicillamine-induced agranulocytosis or aplastic anemia, or the presence of renal insufficiency.

Trientine

Penicillamine is the drug of choice for treatment for Wilson's disease. However, the drug produces undesirable effects, as discussed earlier, and some patients become intolerant. For these individuals, *trientine* (triethylenetetramine dehydrochloride, CUPRID) is an acceptable alternative. Trientine is an effective cupriuretic agent in patients with Wilson's disease, although it may be less potent than penicillamine. The drug is effective orally. Maximal daily doses of 2 g for adults or 1.5 g for children are taken in two to four divided portions on an empty stomach. Trientine may cause iron deficiency; this can be overcome with short courses of iron therapy, but iron and trientine should not be ingested within 2 hours of each other.

Deferoxamine

Deferoxamine is isolated as the iron chelate from *Streptomyces pilosus* and is treated chemically to obtain the metal-free ligand. Deferoxamine has the desirable properties of a remarkably high affinity for ferric iron ($Ka = 10^{31}$) coupled with a very low affinity for calcium ($K_a = 10^2$). Studies *in vitro* have shown that it removes iron from hemosiderin and ferritin and, to a lesser extent, from transferrin. Iron in hemoglobin or cytochromes is not removed by deferoxamine. The structure of deferoxamine is

DEFEROXAMINE

Deferoxamine (*deferoxamine mesylate,* DESFERAL MESYLATE) is poorly absorbed after oral administration, and parenteral administration is required in most cases. For severe iron toxicity (serum iron levels greater than 500 μg/dl), the intravenous route is preferred. The drug is administered at 10 to 15 mg/kg per hour by constant infusion. Faster rates of infusion (45 mg/kg per hour) have been used in a few cases; rapid boluses usually are associated with hypotension. Deferoxamine may be given intramuscularly in moderately toxic cases (serum iron 350 to 500 μg/dl) at a dose of 50 mg/kg with a maximum dose of 1 g. Hypotension also can occur with the intramuscular route.

For chronic iron intoxication (*e.g.,* thalassemia), an intramuscular dose of 0.5 to 1.0 g/day is recommended, although continuous subcutaneous administration (1 to 2 g/day) is almost as effective as intravenous administration (Propper *et al.*, 1977). When blood is being transfused to patients with thalassemia, 2.0 g deferoxamine (per unit of blood) should be given by slow intravenous infusion (rate not to exceed 15 mg/kg per hour) during the transfusion but not by the same intravenous line. Deferoxamine is not recommended in primary hemochromatosis; phlebotomy is the treatment of choice. Deferoxamine also has been used for the chelation of aluminum in dialysis patients (Swartz, 1985).

Deferoxamine is metabolized principally by plasma enzymes, but the pathways have not yet been defined. The drug also is excreted readily in the urine.

Deferoxamine causes a number of allergic reactions, including pruritus, wheals, rash, and anaphylaxis. Other adverse effects include dysuria, abdominal discomfort, diarrhea, fever, leg cramps, and tachycardia. Occasional cases of cataract formation have been reported. Deferoxamine may cause neurotoxicity during long-term, high-dose therapy for transfusion-dependent thalassemia major; both visual and auditory changes have been described (Olivieri *et al.*, 1986). A "pulmonary syndrome" has been associated with high-dose (10 to 25 mg/kg per hour) deferoxamine therapy (Freedman *et al.*, 1990; Castriota-Scanderbeg *et al.*, 1990); tachypnea, hypoxemia, fever, and eosinophilia are prominent symptoms. Contraindications to the use of deferoxamine include renal insufficiency and anuria; during pregnancy, the drug should be used only if clearly indicated.

An orally effective iron chelator now under clinical investigation, *deferiprone* (1,2-dimethyl-3-hydroxypyridin-4-one), may be of value in patients with thalassemia major who are unable or unwilling to receive deferoxamine (Olivieri *et al.*, 1995). Combination therapy with deferoxamine also is under investigation.

BIBLIOGRAPHY

Al-Abbasi, A.H., Kostyniak, P.J., and Clarkson, T.W. An extracorporeal complexing hemodialysis system for the treatment of methylmercury poisoning: III. Clinical applications. *J. Pharmacol. Exp. Ther.*, **1978**, *207*:249–254.

Baghurst, P.A., McMichael, A.J., Wigg, N.R., *et al.* Environmental exposure to lead and children's intelligence at the age of seven years. The Port Pirie Cohort Study. *New Engl. J. Med.*, **1992**, *327*:1279–1284.

Bakir, F., Damluji, S.F., Amin-Zaki, L., *et al.* Methylmercury poisoning in Iraq. *Science*, **1973**, *181*:230–241.

Bakir, F., Rustam, H., Tikriti, S., *et al.* Clinical and epidemiological aspects of methylmercury poisoning. *Postgrad. Med. J.*, **1980**, *56*:1–10.

Ball L.K., Ball R., and Pratt R.D., An assessment of thimerosal use in childhood vaccines. *Pediatrics*, **2001**, *107*:1147–1154.

Banks, E.C., Ferretti, L.E., and Shucard, D.W. Effects of low level lead exposure on cognitive function in children: A review of behavioral, neuropsychological and biological evidence. *Neurotoxicology*, **1997**, *18*:237–281.

Bellinger, D.C., Stiles, K.M., and Needleman, H.L. Low-level lead exposure, intelligence and academic achievement: A long-term follow-up study. *Pediatrics*, **1992**, *90*:855–861.

Bluhm, R.E., Bobbitt, R.G., Welch, L.W., *et al.* Elemental mercury vapour toxicity, treatment, and prognosis after acute, intensive exposure in chloralkali plant workers: I. History, neuropsychological findings and chelator effects. *Hum. Exp. Toxicol.*, **1992**, *11*:201–210.

Campbell, J.R., Clarkson, T.W., and Omar, M.D. The therapeutic use of 2,3-dimercaptopropane-1-sulfonate in two cases of inorganic mercury poisoning. *JAMA*, **1986**, *256*:3127–3130.

Cantilena, L.R., Jr., and Klaassen, C.D. Decreased effectiveness of chelation therapy with time after acute cadmium poisoning. *Toxicol. Appl. Pharmacol.*, **1982a**, *63*:173–180.

Cantilena, L.R., Jr., and Klaassen, C.D. The effect of chelating agents on the excretion of endogenous metals. *Toxicol. Appl. Pharmacol.*, **1982b**, *63*:344–350.

Castriota-Scanderbeg, A., Izzi, G.C., Butturini, A., and Benaglia, G. Pulmonary syndrome and intravenous high-dose desferrioxamine. *Lancet*, **1990**, *336*:1511.

Chen, G.Q., Zhu, J., Shi, X.G., *et al.* In vitro studies on cellular and molecular mechanisms of arsenic trioxide (As_2O_3) in the treatment of acute promyelocytic leukemia: As_2O_3 induces NB_4 cell apoptosis with downregulation of Bcl-2 expression and modulation of PML-RARα/PML proteins. *Blood*, **1996**, *88*:1052–1061.

Chisolm, J.J., Jr. Management of increased lead absorption and lead poisoning in children. *New Engl. J. Med.*, **1973**, *289*:1016–1018.

Chisolm, J.J., Jr., and Barltrop, D. Recognition and management of children with increased lead absorption. *Arch. Dis. Child.*, **1979**, *54*:249–262.

Chowdhury, P., and Louria, D.B. Influence of cadmium and other trace metals on human α_1-antitrypsin: An *in vitro* study. *Science*, **1976**, *191*:480–481.

Clarkson, T.W. Metal toxicity in the central nervous system. *Environ. Health Perspect.*, **1987**, *75*:59–64.

Clarkson T.W. The three modern faces of mercury. *Environ. Health Perspect.*, **2002**, *110*:11–23.

Cooper, W.C., and Gaffey, W.R. Mortality of lead workers. *J. Occup. Med.*, **1975**, *17*:100–107.

Davison, A.G., Fayers, P.M., Taylor, A.J., *et al.* Cadmium fume inhalation and emphysema. *Lancet*, **1988**, *1*:663–667.

Donofrio, P.D., Wilbourn, A.J., Albers, J.W., *et al.* Acute arsenic intoxication presenting as Guillain-Barré-like syndrome. *Muscle Nerve*, **1987**, *10*:114–120.

Dudley, R.E., Gammal, L.M., and Klaassen, C.D. Cadmium-induced hepatic and renal injury in chronically exposed rats: Likely role of hepatic cadmium-metallothionein in nephrotoxicity. *Toxicol. Appl. Pharmacol.*, **1985**, *77*:414–426.

Eley, B.M., and Cox, S.W. The release, absorption and possible health effects of mercury from dental amalgam: A review of recent findings. *Br. Dent. J.*, **1993**, *175*:355–362.

Elinder, C.G., Kjellstrom, T., Lind, B., *et al.* Cadmium exposure from smoking cigarettes: variations with time and country where purchased. *Environ. Res.*, **1983**, *32*:220–227.

Engstrom, B., and Nordberg, G.F. Dose dependence of gastrointestinal absorption and biological half-time of cadmium in mice. *Toxicology*, **1979**, *13*:215–222.

Epstein, O., De Villiers, D., Jain, S., *et al.* Reduction of immune complexes and immunoglobulins induced by D-penicillamine in primary biliary cirrhosis. *New Engl. J. Med.*, **1979**, *300*:274–278.

Fournier, L., Thomas, G., Garnier, R., *et al.* 2,3-Dimercaptosuccinic acid treatment of heavy metal poisoning in humans. *Med. Toxicol. Adverse Drug Exp.*, **1988**, *3*:499–504.

Freedman, M.H., Grisaru, D., Olivieri, N., *et al.* Pulmonary syndrome in patients with thalassemia major receiving intravenous deferoxamine infusions. *Am. J. Dis. Child.*, **1990**, *144*:565–569.

Gerstner, H.B., and Huff, J.E. Clinical toxicology of mercury. *J. Toxicol. Environ. Health*, **1977**, *2*:491–526.

Giunta, F., Di Landro, D., Chiaranda, M., *et al.* Severe acute poisoning from the ingestion of a permanent wave solution of mercuric chloride. *Hum. Toxicol.*, **1983**, *2*:243–246.

Goering, P.L., and Klaassen, C.D. Tolerance to cadmium-induced hepatotoxicity following cadmium pretreatment. *Toxicol. Appl. Pharmacol.*, **1984**, *74*:308–313.

Gordon, R.A., and Burnside, J.W. D-Penicillamine-induced myasthenia gravis in rheumatoid arthritis. *Ann. Intern. Med.*, **1977**, *87*:578–579.

Graziano, J.H., Cuccia, D., and Friedham, E. The pharmacology of 2,3-dimercaptosuccinic acid and its potential use in arsenic poisoning. *J. Pharmacol. Exp. Ther.*, **1978**, *207*:1051–1055.

Graziano, J.H., Lolacono, N.J., Moulton, T., *et al.* Controlled study of meso-2,3-dimercaptosuccinic acid for the management of childhood lead intoxication. *J. Pediatr.*, **1992**, *120*:133–139.

Gregus Z., Gyurasics A., and Csanaky I. Biliary and urinary excretion of inorganic arsenic: Monomethylarsonous acid as a major biliary metabolite in rats. *Toxicol. Sci.*, **2000**, *56*:18–25.

Guldager, B., Jelnes, R., Jørgensen, S.J., *et al.* EDTA treatment of intermittent claudication: A double-blind, placebo-controlled study. *J. Intern. Med.*, **1992**, *231*:261–267.

Hall A.H. Chronic arsenic poisoning. *Toxicol. Lett.*, **2002**, *128*:69–72.

Heron J., Golding J., and the ALSPAC Study Team. Thimerosal exposure in infants and developmental disorders: A prospective cohort study in the United Kingdom does not support a causal association. *Pediatrics,* **2004,** *114*:577–583.

Hill, H.F. Penicillamine in rheumatoid arthritis: Adverse effects. *Scand. J. Rheumatol. Suppl.,* **1979,** *28*:94–99.

Hutchinson, J. Arsenic cancer. *Br. Med. J.,* **1887,** *2*:1280–1281.

Jenkins, R.B. Inorganic arsenic and the nervous system. *Brain,* **1966,** *89*:479–498.

Joint Statement of the American Academy of Pediatrics (AAP) and the United States Public Health Service (USPHS). *Pediatrics,* **1999,** *104*:568–569.

Jones, C.W., Mays, C.W., Taylor, G.N., *et al.* Reducing the cancer risk of ^{239}Pu by chelation therapy. *Radiat. Res.,* **1986,** *107*:296–306.

Jones, M.M., Cherian, M.G., Singh, P.K., *et al.* A comparative study of the influence of vicinal dithiols and a dithiocarbamate on the biliary excretion of cadmium in rat. *Toxicol. Appl. Pharmacol.,* **1991,** *110*:241–250.

Kehoe, R.A. Studies of lead administration and elimination in adult volunteers under natural and experimentally induced conditions over extended periods of time. *Food Chem. Toxicol.,* **1987,** *25*:425–453.

Kershaw, T.G., Clarkson, T.W., and Dhahir, P.H. The relationship between blood levels and dose of methylmercury in man. *Arch. Environ. Health,* **1980,** *35*:28–36.

Klaassen, C.D. Biliary excretion of mercury compounds. *Toxicol. Appl. Pharmacol.,* **1975,** *33*:356–365.

Kostyniak, P.J. Mobilization and removal of methylmercury in the dog during extracorporeal complexing hemodialysis with 2,3-dimercaptosuccinic acid (DMSA). *J. Pharmacol. Exp. Ther.,* **1982,** *221*:63–68.

Kotsonis, F.N., and Klaassen, C.D. The relationship of metallothionein to the toxicity of cadmium after prolonged oral administration to rats. *Toxicol. Appl. Pharmacol.,* **1978,** *46*:39–54.

Landrigan, P.J. Arsenic: State of the art. *Am. J. Ind. Med.,* **1981,** *2*:5–14.

Lauwerys, R.R., Roels, H.A., Buchet, J.P., *et al.* Investigations on the lung and kidney function in workers exposed to cadmium. *Environ. Health Perspect.,* **1979,** *28*:137–146.

Leazer, T.M., Liu, Y., and Klaassen, C.D. Cadmium absorption and its relationship to divalent metal transporter-1 in the pregnant rat. *Toxicol Appl Pharmacol,* **2002,** *185*:18–24.

Lenz, K., Hruby, K., Druml, W., *et al.* 2,3-Dimercaptosuccinic acid in human arsenic poisoning. *Arch. Toxicol.,* **1981,** *47*:241–243.

Lerda, D. Study of sperm characteristics in persons occupationally exposed to lead. *Am. J. Ind. Med.,* **1992,** *22*:567–571.

Lowell, J.A., Burgess, S., Shenoy, S., *et al.* Mercury poisoning associated with hepatitis-B immunoglobulin. *Lancet,* **1996,** 347:480.

McAlpine, D., and Araki, S. Minimata disease: An unusual neurological disorder caused by contaminated fish. *Lancet,* **1958,** *2*:629–631.

Magos, L., Halbach, S., and Clarkson, T.W. Role of catalase in the oxidation of mercury vapor. *Biochem. Pharmacol.,* **1978,** *27*:1373–1377.

Mahaffey, K.R., Rosen, J.F., Chesney, R.W., *et al.* Association between age, blood lead concentration, and serum 1,25-dihydroxycholecalciferol levels in children. *Am. J. Clin. Nutr.,* **1982,** *35*:1327–1331.

Matheson, D.S., Clarkson, T.W., and Gelfand, E.W. Mercury toxicity (acrodynia) induced by long-term injection of gammaglobulin. *J. Pediatr.,* **1980,** *97*:153–155.

Needleman, H.L., Schell, A., Bellinger, D., *et al.* The long-term effects of exposure to low doses of lead in childhood: An 11-year follow-up report. *New Engl. J. Med.,* **1990,** *322*:83–88.

Netter, P., Bannwarth, B., Pere, P., and Nicolas, A. Clinical pharmacokinetics of D-penicillamine. *Clin. Pharmacokinet.,* **1987,** *13*:317–333.

NRC (National Research Council). *Arsenic in Drinking Water.* National Academy Press, Washington, DC, **1999.**

NRC (National Research Council). *Measuring Lead in Infants, Children, and Other Sensitive Populations.* National Academy Press, Washington, DC, **1993.**

Olivieri, N.F., Brittenham, G.M., Matsui, D., *et al.* Iron-chelation therapy with oral deferiprone in patients with thalassemia major. *New Engl. J. Med.,* **1995,** *332*:918–922.

Olivieri, N.F., Buncic, J.R., Chew, E., *et al.* Visual and auditory neurotoxicity in patients receiving subcutaneous deferoxamine infusions. *New Engl. J. Med.,* **1986,** *314*:869–873.

Perrett, D. The metabolism and pharmacology of D-penicillamine in man. *J. Rheumatol. Suppl.,* **1981,** *7*:41–50.

Petrick, J.S., Ayala-Fierro, F., Cullen, W.R., *et al.* Monomethylarsonous acid [MMA(III)] is more toxic than arsenite in Chang human hepatocytes. *Toxicol. Appl. Pharmacol.,* **2000,** *163*:203–207.

Pirkle, J.L., Kaufmann, R.B., Brody, D.J., *et al.* Exposure of the U.S. population to lead, 1991–1994. *Environ. Health Perspect.,* **1998,** *106*:745–750.

Propper, R.D., Cooper, B., Rufo, R.R., *et al.* Continuous subcutaneous administration of deferoxamine in patients with iron overload. *New Engl. J. Med.,* **1977,** *297*:418–423.

Rahola, T., Aaran, R.K., and Mietinen, J.K. Half-time studies of mercury and cadmium by whole body counting. International Atomic Energy Agency symposium on the assessment of radioactive organ and body burdens. In, *Assessment of Radioactive Contamination in Man.* International Atomic Energy Agency, Vienna, **1972.**

Rosen, J.F., Chesney, R.W., Hamstra, A., *et al.* Reduction in 1,25-dihydroxyvitamin D in children with increased lead absorption. *New Engl. J. Med.,* **1980,** *302*:1128–1131.

Schoen, E.J. Childhood lead poisonings: Definitions and priorities. *Pediatrics,* **1993,** *91*:504–505.

Schroeder, H.A. Cadmium as a factor in hypertension. *J. Chronic Dis.,* **1965,** *18*:647–656.

Schumann, G.B., Lerner, S.I., Weiss, M.A., *et al.* Inclusion-bearing cells in industrial workers exposed to lead. *Am. J. Clin. Pathol.,* **1980,** *74*:192–196.

Scott, R., Haywood, J.K., Boddy, K., *et al.* Whole body calcium deficit in cadmium-exposed workers with hypercalciuria. *Urology,* **1980,** *15*:356–359.

Seshia, S.S., Rjani, K.R., Boeckx, R.L., and Chow, P.N. The neurological manifestations of chronic inhalation of leaded gasoline. *Dev. Med. Child Neurol.,* **1978,** *20*:323–334.

Soignet S.L., Maslak P., Wang Z.G., *et al.* Complete remission after treatment of acute promyelocytic leukemia with arsenic trioxide. *New Engl. J. Med.,* **1998,** *339*:1341–1348.

Staessen, J. Low-level lead exposure, renal function and blood pressure. *Verh. K. Acad. Geneeskd. Belg.,* **1995,** *57*:527–574.

Swartz, R.D. Deferoxamine and aluminum removal. *Am. J. Kidney Dis.,* **1985,** *6*:358–364.

Tamashiro, H., Arakaki, M., Akagi, H., *et al.* Mortality and survival for Minamata disease. *Int. J. Epidemiol.,* **1985,** *14*:582–588.

Thind, G.S., and Fischer, G.M. Plasma cadmium and zinc in human hypertension. *Clin. Sci. Mol. Med.,* **1976,** *51*:483–486.

Thomas, D.J., Styblo, M., and Lin, S. The cellular metabolism and systemic toxicity of arsenic. *Toxicol. Appl. Pharmacol.,* **2001,** *176*:127–144.

Vahter, M., and Concha, G. Role of metabolism in arsenic toxicity. *Pharmacol. Toxicol.,* **2001,** *89*:1–5.

Vaziri, N.D., Upham, T., and Barton, C.H. Hemodialysis clearance of arsenic. *Clin. Toxicol.,* **1980,** *17*:451–456.

Verstraeten, T., Davis, R.L., DeStefano, F., *et al.* Safety of thimerosal-containing vaccines: A two-phased study of computerized health maintenance organization databases. *Pediatrics,* **2003,** *112*:1039–1048.

Villarruz, M.V., Dans, A., and Tan, F. Chelation therapy for atherosclerotic cardiovascular disease. *Cochrane Database Syst. Rev.,* **2002,** 4:CD002785.

Waalkes, M.P., Coogan, T.P., and Barter, R.A. Toxicological principles of metal carcinogenesis with special emphasis on cadmium. *Crit. Rev. Toxicol.,* **1992,** *22*:175–201.

Zavon, M.R., and Meadows, C.D. Vascular sequelae to cadmium fume exposure. *Am. Ind. Hyg. Assoc. J.,* **1970,** *31*:180–182.

MONOGRAPHS AND REVIEWS

Aposhian, H.V., and Aposhian, M.M. meso-2,3-Dimercaptosuccinic acid: Chemical, pharmacological and toxicological properties of an orally effective metal chelating agent. *Annu. Rev. Pharmacol. Toxicol.,* **1990,** *30*:279–306.

Bernard, B.P., and Becker, C.E. Environmental lead exposure and the kidney. *J. Toxicol. Clin. Toxicol.,* **1988,** *26*:1–34.

Catsch, A., and Harmuth-Hoene, A.-E. Pharmacology and therapeutic applications of agents used in heavy metal poisoning. In, *The Chelation of Heavy Metals.* (Levine, W.G., ed.) Pergamon Press, Oxford, England, **1979,** pp. 116–124.

Craswell, P.W. Chronic lead nephropathy. *Annu. Rev. Med.,* **1987,** *38*:169–173.

Elihu, N., Anandasbapathy, S., and Frishman, W.H. Chelation therapy in cardiovascular disease: Ethylenediaminetetraacetic acid, deferoxamine, and dexrazoxane. *J. Clin. Pharmacol.,* **1998,** *38*:101–105.

Engel, R.R., Hopenhayn-Rich, C., Receveur, O., and Smith, A.H. Vascular effects of chronic arsenic exposure: A review. *Epidemiol. Rev.,* **1994,** *16*:184–209.

Friberg, L., Piscator, M., Nordberg, G.F., and Kjellstrom, T. *Cadmium in the Environment,* 2d ed. CRC Press, Cleveland, **1974.**

Friberg, L., and Vostal, J. *Mercury in the Environment: An Epidemiological and Toxicological Appraisal.* CRC Press, Cleveland, **1972.**

Garrettson, L.K. Lead. In, *Clinical Management of Poisoning and Drug Overdose.* (Haddad, L.M., and Winchester, J.F., eds.) Saunders, Philadelphia, **1983,** pp. 649–655.

Goyer, R.A., and Clarkson, T.W. Toxic effects of metals. In, *Casarett and Doull's Toxicology: The Basic Science of Poisons,* 6th ed. (Klaassen, C.D., ed.) McGraw-Hill, New York, **2001.**

International Agency for Research on Cancer (IARC). Some metals and metallic compounds. In, *IARC Monographs on the Evaluation of Carcinogenic Risks to Humans,* Vol. 23. International Agency for Research on Cancer, Lyon, France, **1980.**

International Agency for Research on Cancer (IARC). Beryllium, cadmium, mercury, and exposures in the glass manufacturing industry: Working Group views and expert opinions, Lyon, 9–16 February 1993. In, *IARC Monographs on the Evaluation of Carcinogenic Risks to Humans,* Vol. 58. International Agency for Research on Cancer, Lyon, France, **1993.**

Klaassen, C.D., Liu, J., and Choudhuri, S. Metallothionein: An intracellular protein to protect against cadmium toxicity. *Annu. Rev. Pharmacol. Toxicol.,* **1999,** *39*:267–294.

Levy, R.S., Fisher, M., and Alter, J.N. Penicillamine: Review and cutaneous manifestations. *J. Am. Acad. Dermatol.,* **1983,** *8*:548–558.

Piscator, M., and Pettersson, B. Chronic cadmium poisoning: Diagnosis and prevention. In, *Clinical Chemistry and Chemical Toxicology of Metals.* (Brown, S.S., ed.) Elsevier/North Holland Biomedical Press, Amsterdam, **1977,** pp. 143–155.

Smith, W.E., and Smith, A.M. *Minamata.* Holt, Rinehart & Winston, New York, **1975.**

Winship, K.A. Toxicity of inorganic arsenic salts. *Adverse Drug React. Acute Poisoning Rev.,* **1984,** *3*:129–160.

PRINCIPLES OF PRESCRIPTION ORDER WRITING AND PATIENT COMPLIANCE

Iain L. O. Buxton

When the physician's treatment plan for the patient involves the prescribing of one or more medications, Robert Burns' law too often prevails: "The best-laid schemes o' mice an' men gang aft a-gley." From the wrong drug prescribed to the wrong dosage or administration schedule advised, dispensed, or administered, the impact of medication misadventures are a tremendously costly problem. This appendix provides a primer on the proper approach to the medication prescription and order process and a resource for practitioners in effectively providing pharmaceutical care for their patients.

THE MECHANICS OF PRESCRIPTION ORDER WRITING

History. Knowledge of ancient prescriptions can be found in both Chinese (Chen and Qian, 1989) and Egyptian writings (Karenberg and Leitz, 2001). The use of the symbol Rx to denote the modern prescription is rooted in ancient alchemical practice of obscure origin. Rx may be derived from the Egyptian "Eye of Horus" symbol (👁) denoting health, or may be a symbolic appeal by physicians to the god Jupiter for a prescription's success. More commonly, Rx is said to be an abbreviation for the Latin word *recipere*, meaning "take" or "take thus" as a direction to a pharmacist, preceding the physician's "recipe" for preparing a medication. What is clear is the origin of the abbreviation "*Sig*" for the Latin "*Signatura*," used on the prescription to mark the directions for administration of the medication.

Early medicines were made up of multiple ingredients requiring complex preparation, and Latin was adopted as the standard language of the prescription to ensure understanding and consistency. Latin is no longer the international language of medicine, but a number of commonly used abbreviations derive from old Latin usage.

Current Practice. Today, the prescription consists of the superscription, the inscription, the subscription, the signa, and the name and signature of the prescriber, all contained on a single form (Figure AI–1).

The *superscription* includes the date the prescription order is written; the name, address, weight, and age of the patient; and the Rx. The body of the prescription, or *inscription*, contains the name and amount or strength of the drug to be dispensed, or the name and strength of each ingredient to be compounded. The *subscription* is the instruction to the pharmacist, usually consisting of a short sentence such as: "make a solution," "mix and place into 30 capsules," or "dispense 30 tablets." The *signa* or "*Sig*" is the instruction for the patient as to how to take the prescription, interpreted and transposed onto the prescription label by the pharmacist. In the United States these should always be written in English. Many physicians continue to use Latin abbreviations; for example, "1 cap tid pc," will be interpreted by the pharmacist as "take one capsule three times daily after meals." However, the use of Latin abbreviations for these directions only mystifies the prescription. This can be a hindrance to proper patient-physician communication and is an otherwise unnecessary source of potential dispensing errors. Since the pharmacist always writes the label in English (or as appropriate in the language of the patient), the use of such abbreviations or symbols is unnecessary and discouraged.

The instruction "take as directed" is not satisfactory and should be avoided by the physician. Such directions assume an understanding on the part of the patient that may not be realized and inappropriately exclude the pharmacist from the pharmaceutical care process. Such directions can only be seen as inadequate by the pharmacist, who must determine the intent of the physi-

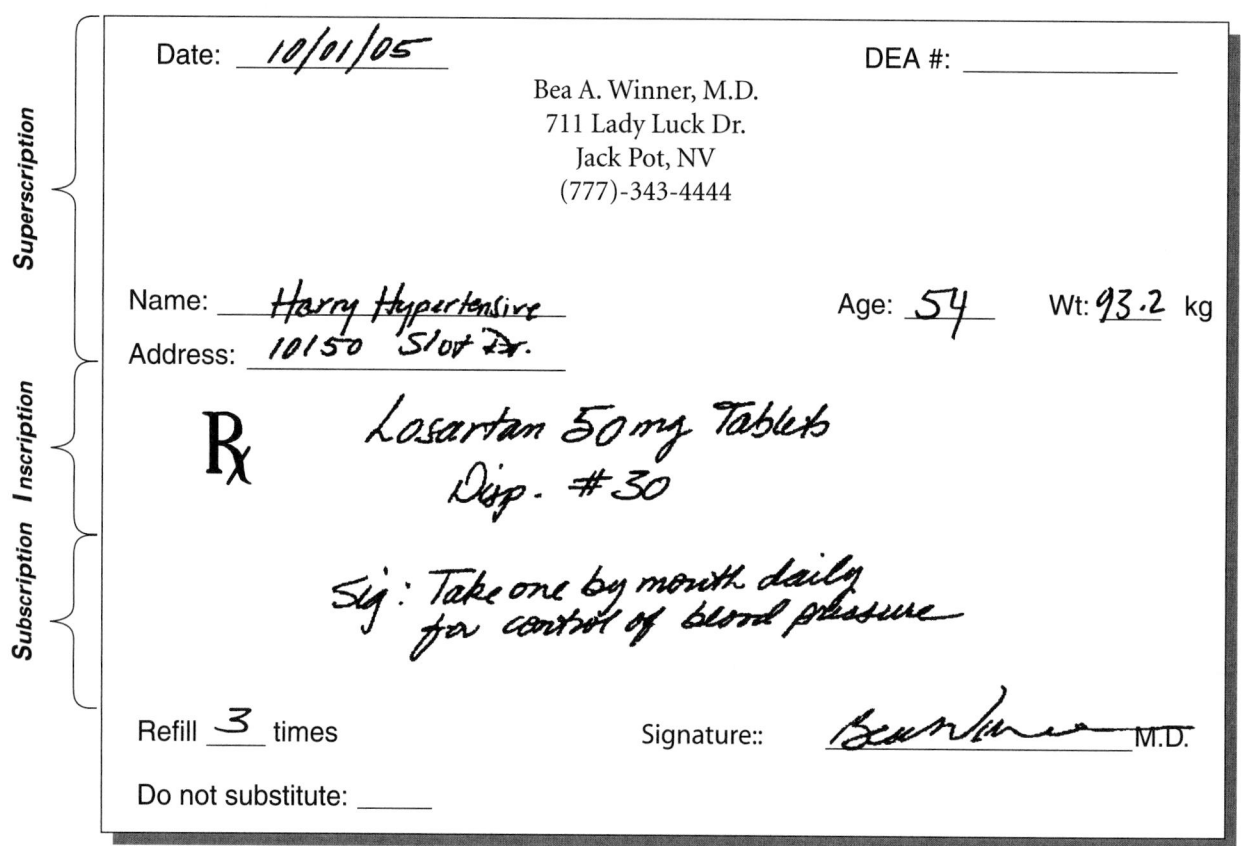

Figure AI–1. The prescription. The prescription must be carefully prepared to identify the patient and the medication to be dispensed, as well as the manner in which the drug is to be administered. Accuracy and legibility are essential. Use of abbreviations, particularly Latin, is discouraged, as it leads to dispensing errors. Inclusion of the purpose of the medication in the *subscription* (*e.g.*, "*for control of blood pressure*") can prevent errors in dispensing. For example, the use of losartan for the treatment of hypertension may require 100 mg/day (1.4 mg/kg per day), whereas treatment of congestive heart failure with this angiotensin II–receptor antagonist should not generally exceed 50 mg/day. Including the purpose of the prescription can also assist patients in organizing and understanding their medications. Including the patient's weight on the prescription can be useful in avoiding dosing errors, particularly when drugs are administered to children.

cian before dispensing the medication, and who shares the responsibility for safe and proper use of the medication by the patient. The best directions to the patient will include a reminder of the intended purpose of the medication by including such phrases as "for relief of pain," or "to relieve itching." The correct route of administration is reinforced by the choice of the first word of the directions. For an oral dosage form, the directions would begin with "take" or "give"; for externally applied products, the word "apply"; for suppositories, "insert"; and for eye, ear, or nose drops, "place" is preferable to "instill."

Prescriptive Authority. In many states in the United States, health care practitioners other than M.D. and D.O. physicians can write prescriptions. Licensed physician's

assistants (P.A.), nurse practitioners, and pharmacists can prescribe medications under various circumstances.

Avoiding Confusion. Units of measure can lead to confusion and medication errors. Older systems of measure such as minims for volume (15 minims = 1 ml) and grains for weight (1 grain = 60 mg) are obscure and should not be used. Doses always should be listed by metric weight of active ingredient; doses for liquid medications should include the volume. Writing "μg" for micrograms can very easily be misinterpreted as milligrams (mg). Thus, if abbreviated, micrograms should be written "mcg" and milligrams as "mg"; a zero should be used before a decimal (0.X mg, rather than .X mg) but not after (use X mg rather than X.0 mg). The metric system should be used in place of common household measurements such as "dropperful" and "teaspoon" in the directions for the patient, and both the doctor and the pharmacist should be sure that the patient understands the measurement prescribed. For medical purposes, a "teaspoon" or "teaspoonful" dose is considered to be equivalent to 5 ml and a "tablespoon" to 15 ml, but the actual volumes held by ordinary household teaspoons and tablespoons are far too variable to be used reliably for measurement of medications. Prescribing oral medications in "drops" likewise can cause problems when accuracy of dose is important unless the patient understands that only the calibrated dropper provided by the manufacturer or pharmacist should be used to dispense the medication. Thus, one possible dosage for a pediatric iron product would be more accurately written "15 mg (0.6 ml) three times daily" instead of "one dropperful three times daily," because a true dropperful could result in iron overdose.

Abbreviations are known to lead to dispensing errors (Teichman and Caffee, 2002). A prescription intending every-other-day dosing (qod) may be miswritten as "od" by the physician for "other-day dosing"; the pharmacist will interpret "od" as the abbreviation of the Latin for "right eye." Once-daily dosing at bedtime (qhs) may be misinterpreted as "qhr" for every hour. The use of slash marks (/) to separate names and doses can result in the incorrect drug or dose being dispensed; the slash mark may be interpreted as a letter or number. When medications are measured in units, or international units, the abbreviation "U" or "IU" must NOT be used, as it leads to errors such as misinterpretation of "U" as zero or four, or "IU" as 10 or 14. The word "unit" should be written as such. Drug products available in the Unites States that are dosed in units (*e.g.*, *corticotropin*) or international unit measures are "harmonized" by those responsible for drug standardization to avoid errors in dosing (*see* Drug Standards and Classification, below). Examples of confusion in the interpretation of a physician order abound (Kohn, 2001) and are considered further below. *The critical message is that practitioners in the United States must write out the Rx fully in English if errors are to be avoided.*

Proper Patient Information. The patient's name and address are needed on the order to assure that the correct medication goes to the correct patient and also for identification and recordkeeping purposes. For medications whose dosage involves a calculation, a patient's pertinent factors such as weight, age, or body surface area also should be listed on the prescription.

Prescribers often commit errors in dosage calculations (Lesar *et al.*, 1997) that can be prevented (Kuperman *et al.*, 2001). When prescribing a drug whose dosage involves a calculation based on body weight or surface area, it is good practice to include both the calculated dose and the dosage formula used, such as "240 mg every 8 hours (40 mg/kg per day)" to allow another health care professional to double-check the prescribed dosage. Pharmacists always should recalculate dosage equations when filling these prescriptions. Medication orders in hospitals and some clinic settings, such as those for antibiotics or antiseizure medications that are sometimes difficult to adequately dose (*e.g.*, *phenytoin*), can specify the patient diagnosis and desired drug and request dosing by the clinical pharmacist.

All prescriptions should be written in ink; this practice is compulsory for schedule II prescriptions under the Controlled Substances Act of 1970, as erasures on a prescription easily can lead to dispensing errors or diversion of controlled substances.

Prescription pad blanks normally are imprinted with a heading that gives the name of the physician and the address and phone number of the practice site (Figure AI–1). When using institutional blanks that do not bear the physician's information, the physician always should print his or her name and phone number on the face of the prescription to clearly identify the prescriber and facilitate communication with other health care professionals if questions arise. United States law requires that prescriptions for controlled substances include the name, address, and Drug Enforcement Agency (DEA) registration number of the physician.

The date of the prescription is an important part of the patient's medical record, and it can assist the pharmacist in recognizing potential problems. For example, when an opioid is prescribed for pain due to an injury, and the prescription is presented to a pharmacist 2 weeks after issuance, the drug may no longer be indicated. Compliance behavior also can be estimated using the dates when a prescription is filled and refilled. The United States Controlled Substances Act requires that all orders for controlled substances (Table AI–1) be dated as of, and signed on, the day issued, and prohibits filling or refilling orders for substances in schedules III and IV more than 6 months after their date of issuance. When writing the original prescription, the physician should designate the number of refills he or she wishes the patient to have. For maintenance medications without abuse potential, it is reasonable to write for a 1-month supply and to mark the prescription form for refills to be dispensed over a period sufficient to supply the patient until the next scheduled visit to the physician. A statement such as "refill prn" (refill as needed) is not appropriate, as it could allow the patient to misuse the medicine or neglect medical appointments. If no refills are

Table AI–1
Controlled Substance Schedules

Schedule I (examples: heroin, methylene dioxymethamphetamine, lysergic acid diethylamide, mescaline, and all salts and isomers thereof):
1. High potential for abuse.
2. No accepted medical use in the United States or lacks accepted safety for use in treatment in the United States. May be used for research purposes by properly registered individuals.

Schedule II (examples: morphine, oxycodone, fentanyl, meperidine, dextroamphetamine, cocaine, amobarbital):
1. High potential for abuse.
2. Has a currently accepted medical use in the United States.
3. Abuse of substance may lead to severe psychological or physical dependence.

Schedule III (examples: anabolic steroids, nalorphine, ketamine, certain schedule II substances in suppositories, mixtures, or limited amounts per dosage unit):
1. Abuse potential less than substances in schedule I or schedule II.
2. Has a currently accepted medical use in the United States.
3. Abuse of substance may lead to moderate or low physical dependence or high psychological dependence.

Schedule IV (examples: alprazolam, phenobarbital, meprobamate, modafinil):
1. Abuse potential less than substances in schedule III.
2. Has a currently accepted medical use in the United States.
3. Abuse of substance may lead to limited physical or psychological dependence relative to substances in schedule III.

Schedule V (examples: buprenorphine, products containing a low dose of an opioid plus a nonnarcotic ingredient such as codeine and guaifenesin cough syrup or diphenoxylate and atropine tablets):
1. Low potential for abuse relative to schedule IV.
2. Has a currently accepted medical use in the United States.
3. Some schedule V products may be sold in limited amounts without a prescription at the discretion of the pharmacist; however, if a physician wishes a patient to receive one of these products, it is preferable to provide a prescription.

desired, "zero" (not 0) should be written in the refill space to prevent alteration of the doctor's intent. Refills for controlled substances are discussed below.

Concern about the rising cost of health care has favored the dispensing of so-called "generic" drugs. A drug is called by its generic name (in the United States this is the U.S. Adopted Name or USAN) or the manufacturer's proprietary name, called the trademark, trade name, or brand name. In most states in the United States, pharmacists have the authority to dispense generic drugs rather than brand name medications. The physician can request that the pharmacist not substitute a generic for a branded medication by indicating this on the prescription ("do not substitute"), although this is generally unnecessary since the FDA requires that generic medications meet the same bioequivalence standards as their brand-named counterparts. In some jurisdictions, prescriptions may not be filled with a generic substitution unless specifically permitted as stated on the prescription. Occasions when substituting generic medications is discouraged are limited to products with specialized release systems and narrow therapeutic indices, or when substantial patient confusion and potential noncompliance may be associated with substitution.

Choice of Drug Product. Inappropriate choice of drugs by physicians has been noted as a problem in prescribing. As learned recently with the cyclooxygenase 2 inhibitors, it cannot be assumed that a drug's therapeutic promise or popularity is proof of its overall clinical superiority or safety (Topol, 2004). Physicians must rely on unbiased sources when seeking drug information that will influence their prescribing habits.

The amount to be dispensed should be clearly stated and should be only that needed by the patient. Excessive amounts should never be dispensed, as this is not only expensive to the patient, but may lead to accumulation of medicines, which can lead to harm to the patient or members of the patient's family. It is far better to have several refills of a prescription than to have more than necessary prescribed at one time.

The Prescription as a Commodity. Prescribers must be aware that patients may visit their doctor to "get" a prescription. Indeed, in an era when the time spent between physician and patient is ever shorter due to limits and pressures of physician reimbursements, patients often feel that a trip to the doctor that does not result in a new prescription is somehow a failed visit or a lost opportunity. Similarly, physicians may feel that they have fulfilled their role if the patient leaves with a prescription. Physicians must be careful to educate their patients about the importance of viewing medicines as only to be used when really needed and that remaining on a particular medicine when their condition is stable is far preferable to seeking the newest medications available.

Prescription Drug Advertising. The Federal Food, Drug, and Cosmetic Act as amended (Federal Food and Drug Administration Modernization Act of 1997) permits the use of print and television advertising of prescription drugs. The same statute and regulations apply regardless of the audience targeted by a prescription drug advertisement. The law requires that all drug advertisements contain (among other things) information in a brief summary relating to side effects, contraindications, and effectiveness. The current advertising regulations specify that this information disclosure needs to include all the risk information in a product's approved labeling or must direct consumers to health care professionals to obtain this information. (Typically, print advertisements will include a reprinting of the risk-related sections of the product's approved labeling [package insert], while television advertising will not.) In addition, advertisements cannot be false or misleading or omit material facts. They also must present a fair balance between effectiveness and risk information. It may be that the dramatizations employed by television commercials are a disservice to the physician's ability to educate and care for the patient if such advertisements only create brand loyalty. Alternatively, patients who learn about drugs on television may interact more effectively with their health care providers by asking questions about the medicines they take.

The benefits of these types of direct-to-consumer (DTC) advertising, including internet advertising, are controversial (Findlay, 2001). Prescription drug advertising has alerted consumers to the existence of new drugs and the conditions they treat, but it has also increased consumer demand for drugs. This demand has increased the number of prescriptions being dispensed (raising sales revenues) and has contributed to the higher pharmaceutical costs borne by health insurers, government, and consumers. In the face of a growing demand for particular brand name drugs driven by advertising, physicians and pharmacists must be able to counsel patients effectively and provide evidence-based drug information to their patients.

ERRORS IN DRUG ORDERS

The Institute of Medicine (IOM) estimates that the number of medical errors in the United States annually that result in death is between 44,000 and 98,000 (Kohn *et al.*,

1999). While there is some controversy about the IOM's estimates (Sox and Woloshin, 2000), it is clear that the large number of medical errors includes medication errors resulting in adverse events, including death (Mangino, 2004). Databases of anonymously reported errors are maintained jointly by the Institute for Safe Medication Practices (ISMP), the United States Pharmacopeia Medication Errors Reporting Program (USP MERP), and the FDA's MedWatch program. Adverse drug events occur in approximately 3% of hospitalizations, and this number is larger for special populations such as those in pediatric and neonatal intensive care units (Mangino, 2004).

By examining aspects of prescription writing that can cause errors and by modifying prescribing habits accordingly, the physician can improve the chance that the patient will receive the correct prescription, whether in a hospital or an outpatient setting. By being alert to common problems that can occur with medication orders, and communicating with the patient's physician, pharmacists and other healthcare professionals can assist in reducing medication errors. Areas of particular concern in the preparation of medication orders in both the institutional and outpatient settings can be summarized as follows:

- All orders should be written using metric measurements of weight and volume.
- Arabic (decimal) numerals are preferable to Roman numerals, and in some instances it is preferable for numbers to be spelled out.
- Use leading zeros (0.125 mg, not .125 mg); never use trailing zeros (5 mg, not 5.0 mg).
- Avoid abbreviating drug names since this leads to numerous errors due to sound-alike names. For instance, NEUMEGA, an interleukin-11 product abbreviated IL-11, can be dispensed as PROLEUKIN, an interleukin-2 derivative, if Roman rather than Arabic numerals are used.
- Avoid abbreviating directions for drug administration; write directions out clearly in English.
- Some drug names sound alike when spoken and may look alike when spelled out. The United States Pharmacopeial Convention Medication Error Reporting Program maintains a current list of drug names that can be confused (http://www.usp.org). The list of alliterative drug names currently contains over 750 pairs of potentially confusing names that could lead to prescribing or dispensing errors harmful to patients. The alliterative drug names can be particularly problematic when giving verbal orders to pharmacists or other healthcare providers.
- The single most important measure to prevent dispensing errors based on sound-alike or look-alike drug names is for the physician to provide the patient's diag-

nosis on the prescription order. For instance, an order for administration of *magnesium sulfate* must not be abbreviated "MS," as this may result in administration of morphine sulfate. Including the therapeutic purpose and/or the patient's diagnosis can prevent this error.

- Poor handwriting is a well-known and preventable cause of dispensing errors. Both physician and pharmacist share in the responsibility to prevent adverse drug events by writing prescriptions clearly and questioning intent whenever an order is ambiguous or potentially ambiguous.

CONTROLLED SUBSTANCES

The Drug Enforcement Agency (DEA), an agency in the Department of Justice, is responsible for the enforcement of the Federal Controlled Substances Act (CSA). The DEA regulates each step of the handling of controlled substances from manufacture to dispensing. The act provides a system that is intended to prevent diversion of controlled substances from legitimate uses. State agencies may impose additional regulations such as requiring that prescriptions for controlled substances be printed on triplicate or state-issued prescription pads or restricting the use of a particular class of drugs for specific indications. The most stringent law always takes precedence, whether it is federal, state, or local. Substances that come under the jurisdiction of the CSA are divided into five schedules (Table AI–1), but practitioners should note that individual states may have additional schedules. Criminal offenses and penalties for misuse generally depend on the schedule of a substance as well as the amount of drug in question.

Physicians must be authorized to prescribe controlled substances by the jurisdiction in which they are licensed and they must be registered with the DEA or exempted from registration as defined under the CSA. The number on the certificate of registration must be indicated on all prescription orders for controlled substances.

Prescription Orders for Controlled Substances. To be valid, a prescription for a controlled substance must be issued for a *legitimate medical purpose* by an *individual practitioner* acting in the *usual course of his or her professional practice.* An order that does not meet these criteria, such as a prescription issued as a means to obtain controlled substances for the doctor's office use or to maintain addicted individuals is not considered a legitimate prescription within the meaning of the law, and thus does not protect either the physician who issued it or the

pharmacist who dispensed it. Most states prohibit physicians from prescribing controlled substances for themselves; it is prudent to comply with this guideline even if it is not mandated by law.

Execution of the Order. Prescriptions for controlled substances should be dated and signed on the day of their issuance and must bear the full name and address of the patient and the printed name, address, and DEA number of the practitioner and should be signed the way one would sign a legal document. Preprinted orders are not allowed in most states, and presigned blanks are prohibited by federal law. When oral orders are not permitted (schedule II), the prescription must be written with ink or typewritten. The order may be prepared by a member of the physician's staff, but the prescriber is responsible for the signature and any errors that the order may contain.

Oral Order. Prescriptions for schedule III, IV, and V medications may be telephoned to a pharmacy by a physician or by trusted staff in the same manner as a prescription for a noncontrolled substance, although it is in the physician's best interest to keep his or her DEA number as private as reasonably possible (*see* Preventing Diversion, below). Schedule II prescriptions may be telephoned to a pharmacy only in *emergency* situations. To be an emergency: (1) immediate administration is necessary; (2) no appropriate alternative treatment is available; and (3) it is not reasonably possible for the physician to provide a written prescription prior to the dispensing.

For an emergency prescription, the quantity must be limited to the amount adequate to treat the patient during the emergency period, and the physician must have a written prescription delivered to the pharmacy for that emergency within 72 hours. If mailed, the prescription must be postmarked within 72 hours. The pharmacist must notify the DEA if this prescription is not received.

Refills. No prescription order for a schedule II drug may be refilled under any circumstance. For schedule III and IV drugs, refills may be issued either orally or in writing, not to exceed five refills or 6 months after the issue date, whichever comes first. Beyond this time, a new prescription must be ordered. For schedule V drugs, no restrictions are placed on the number of refills allowed, but if no refills are noted at the time of issuance, a new prescription must be made for additional drug to be dispensed.

Preventing Diversion. Prescription blanks often are stolen and used to sustain abuse of controlled substances and to divert legitimate drug products to the illicit market. To prevent this type of diversion, prescription pads should be protected in the same manner as one would protect a personal checkbook. A prescription blank should never be presigned for a staff member to fill in at a later time. Also, a minimum number of pads should be stocked, and they should be kept in a locked, secure location except when in use. If a pad or prescription is missing, it should be reported immediately to local authorities and pharmacies; some areas have systems in place to allow the rapid dissemination of such information. Ideally, the physician's full DEA number should not be preprinted on the prescription pad, because most prescriptions will not be for controlled substances and will not require the registration number, and anyone in possession of a valid DEA number may find it easier to commit prescription fraud. Some physicians may intentionally omit part or all of their DEA number on a prescription and instead write "pharmacist call to verify" or "call for registration number." This practice works only when the pharmacist may independently verify the authenticity of the prescription, and patients must be advised to fill the prescription during the prescriber's office hours. Pharmacists can ascertain the likely authenticity of a physician's DEA number using an algorithm.

Another method employed by the drug-seeker is to alter the face of a valid prescription to increase the number of units or refills. By spelling out the number of units and refills authorized instead of giving numerals, the prescriber essentially removes this option for diversion. Controlled substances should not be prescribed excessively or for prolonged periods, as the continuance of a patient's addiction is not a legitimate medical purpose.

DRUG STANDARDS AND CLASSIFICATION

The United States Pharmacopeial Convention, Inc. is a nongovernmental organization that promotes the public health and benefits practitioners and patients by disseminating authoritative standards and information on medicines and other health care technologies. This organization is home to the United States Pharmacopeia (USP), which together with the FDA, the pharmaceutical industry, and health professions, establishes authoritative drug standards. These standards are enforceable by the FDA and the governments of other countries, and are recognized worldwide. Drug monographs are published in the USP/National Formulary (USP-NF), the official drug

standards compendia that organize drugs into categories based on pharmacological actions and therapeutic uses. The USP also provides chemical reference standards to carry out the tests specified in the USP-NF. For example, a drug to be manufactured and labeled in units must comply with the USP standard for units of that compound. Such standards are essential for agents possessing biological activity such as insulin.

The USP is also home to the USAN (The USP Dictionary of *U.S. Adopted Names* and International Drug Names). This compendium is recognized throughout the healthcare industry as the authoritative dictionary of drugs. Entries include one or more of the following: U.S. Adopted Names, official drug names for the NF (National Formulary), previously used official names, international and nonproprietary names, British Approved Names, Japanese Approved Names, trade names, and other synonyms. In addition to names, the records in this file contain other substance information such as Chemical Abstract Society (CAS), Registry Number (RN), molecular formula, molecular weight, pharmacological and/or therapeutic category, drug sponsor, reference information, and structure diagram, if available. The USP maintains an electronic Web site that can be accessed for useful drug naming, classification, and standards information (http://www.usp.org).

In the United States, drug products are also coded under the National Drug Code. The NDC System was originally established as an essential part of out-of-hospital drug reimbursement under Medicare. In the United States, the NDC serves as a universal product identifier for drugs used in humans. The current edition of the National Drug Code Directory is limited to prescription drugs and a few selected over-the-counter products. Each drug product listed under the Federal Food, Drug, and Cosmetic Act is assigned a unique 10-digit, 3-segment number. This number, known as the National Drug Code (NDC) number, identifies the labeler/vendor, product, and package size. The labeler code is assigned by the FDA. The second segment, the product code, identifies a specific strength, dosage form, and formulation for a particular drug company. The third segment, the package code, identifies package sizes. Both the product and package codes are assigned by the manufacturer.

In addition to classification of drugs by therapeutic category, drugs are also grouped by control schedule. Drug schedules in the United States are listed in Table AI–1 from schedule I to schedule V, and are discussed above as controlled substances. Drugs are also grouped by their potential for misuse under British and United Nations legal classifications as class A, B, or C. The classes are linked to maximum legal penalties in a descending order of severity, from A to C.

COMPLIANCE

Compliance may be defined as the extent to which the patient follows a regimen prescribed by a healthcare professional. The assumption that the doctor tells the patient what to do and then the patient meticulously follows orders is unrealistic. It must be recognized that the patient is the final and most important determinant of how successful a therapeutic regimen will be and should be engaged as an active participant who has a vested interest in its success. Whatever term is used—*compliance, adherence, therapeutic alliance,* or *concordance*—physicians must promote a collaborative interaction between doctor and patient in which each brings an expertise that helps to determine the course of therapy. The doctor is the medical expert; the patient is the expert on himself and his beliefs, values, and lifestyle. The patient's quality-of-life beliefs may differ from the clinician's therapeutic goals, and the patient will have the last word every time when there is an unresolved conflict.

Even the most carefully prepared prescription for the ideal therapy will be useless if the patient's level of compliance is not adequate. Noncompliance may be manifest in drug therapy as intentional or accidental errors in dosage or schedule, overuse, underuse, early termination of therapy, or not having a prescription filled (Hagstrom *et al.*, 2004). Therapeutic failures can result from patient noncompliance (Hobbs, 2004). Noncompliance always should be considered in evaluating potential causes of inconsistent or nonexistent response to therapy.

The reported incidence of patient noncompliance varies widely but is usually in the range of 30% to 60% (Zyczynski and Coyne, 2000); the rate for long-term regimens is approximately 50% and tends to increase over time (Sackett and Snow, 1979). Although they complain about the illogical nature of their patients' noncompliance, healthcare professionals seem to have as much difficulty as the rest of the population in following health-related orders (Michalsen *et al.*, 1997).

Direct costs associated with noncompliance have been estimated at $8.5 to $50 billion. Hundreds of variables have been identified that may influence compliance behavior in a specific patient or condition. A few of the most frequently cited are discussed here along with some suggestions for improving compliance, although none provides 100% compliance (Table AI–2).

Table AI–2
Suggestions for Improving Patient Compliance

Provide respectful communication; ask patient how they take medicine.

Develop satisfactory, collaborative relationship between doctor and patient; encourage pharmacist involvement.

Provide and encourage use of medication counseling.

Give precise, clear instructions, with most important information given first.

Support oral instructions with easy-to-read written information.

Simplify whenever possible.

Use mechanical compliance aids as needed (sectioned pill boxes or trays, compliance packaging, color-coding).

Use optimal dosage form and schedule for the individual patient.

Assess patient's literacy and comprehension and modify educational counseling as needed. Don't rely on patient knowledge about his or her disease, alone, to improve compliance.

Find solutions when physical or sensory disabilities are present (use nonsafety caps on bottles, use large type on labels and written material, place tape marks on syringes).

Enlist support and assistance from family or caregivers.

Use behavioral techniques such as goal setting, self-monitoring, cognitive restructuring, skills training, contracts, and positive reinforcement.

SOURCE: Table based upon suggestions by DiMatteo, 1995; Feldman and DeTullio, 1994; Kehoe and Katz, 1998; Martin and Mead, 1982; Meichenbaum and Turk, 1987; and Salzman, 1995.

The Patient–Provider Relationship. Patient satisfaction with the physician has a significant impact on compliance behavior and is one of few factors that the physician can directly influence. Patients are more likely to follow instructions and recommendations when their expectations for the patient–provider relationship and for their treatment are met. These expectations include not only clinical but also interpersonal competence, so cultivating good interpersonal and communication skills is essential.

When deciding upon a course of therapy, it can be useful to discuss a patient's habits and daily routine as well as the therapeutic options with the patient. This information can help suggest cues for remembrance, such as storing a once-daily medicine atop the books on the bedside table for a patient who reads nightly, or in the cabinet with the coffee cups if it is to be taken in the morning (noting that the bathroom can be the worst place to store a medication in terms of its physical and chemical preservation). The information also can help tailor the regimen to the patient's lifestyle. A lack of information about a patient's lifestyle can lead to situations such as prescribing a medication to be taken with meals three times daily for a patient who only eats twice a day or who works a night shift and sleeps during the day. Rarely is there only one treatment option for a given problem, and it may be better to prescribe an adequate regimen that the patient will follow instead of an ideal regimen that the patient will not. Involving patients in the control of any appropriate aspects of their therapy may improve compliance, not only by aiding memory and making the dosage form or schedule more agreeable or convenient, but also by giving patients a feeling of empowerment and emphasizing their responsibility for the treatment outcome.

It is not unreasonable for the physician to ask the patient whether he or she intends to adhere to the prescribed therapy and to negotiate to get a commitment to do so. Attempts should be made to resolve collaboratively any conflicts that may hinder compliance.

Patients and Their Beliefs. Behavioral models suggest that patients are more likely to be compliant when they *perceive* that they are susceptible to the disease, that the disease may have serious negative impact, that the therapy will be effective, that the benefits outweigh the costs, and they believe in their own efficacy to execute the therapy. From the standpoint of compliance, the *actual* severity of and susceptibility to an illness is not necessarily an issue; rather, the patient's perception of severity affects compliance (Buckalew and Buckalew, 1995). Education of the patient about his or her condition alone will not improve compliance (Sackett *et al.*, 1975).

Patients' beliefs can lead them to deliberately alter their therapy, whether for convenience, personal experiments, a desire to remove themselves from the sick role, a means to exercise a feeling of control over their situation, or other reasons. This reinforces the need for excellent communication and a good patient–provider relationship to facilitate the provision of additional or corrective education when the beliefs would suggest poor compliance as an outcome.

It is difficult to predict whether a particular patient will be compliant, as there is no consistent relationship with isolated demographic variables such as age, sex, education level, intelligence, personality traits, and income. Certain of these variables have been implicated in specific situations, but they cannot be applied to the population as a whole. Social isolation generally has been found to be associated with poor compliance, although family members or other people close to the patient can undermine compliance as easily as support it. As noted above, the actual severity of the patient's disease is not predictive of compliance behavior, but characteristics of the disease can make adherence less likely, as with certain neurodegenerative or psychiatric illnesses.

Pharmacists have a legal and professional responsibility to offer medication counseling in many situations—even though practice environments are not always conducive to its provision—and can educate and support patients by discussing prescribed medications and their use. Because they often see the patient more frequently than does the physician, pharmacists who take the time to inquire about a patient's therapy can help identify compliance and other problems and notify the physician as appropriate.

Elderly patients often face a number of barriers to compliance related to their age. Such barriers include increased forgetfulness and confusion; altered drug disposition and higher sensitivity to some drug effects; decreased social and financial support; decreased dexterity, mobility, or sensory abilities; and an increased number of concurrent medicines used (both prescription and over-the-counter), whose attendant toxicities and interactions may cause decreased mental alertness or intolerable side effects. There are drugs known to be inappropriate to prescribe to elderly patients (Curtis *et al.*, 2004; Fick *et al.*, 2003) and some that may adversely impact compliance. Despite these obstacles, evidence does not show that elderly patients in general are significantly more noncompliant than any other age group. Still, the United States population is aging, and elderly patients consume a disproportionate amount of medicines and health care resources, so there is great opportunity and motivation to improve their drug-taking habits. Physicians must be careful in choosing medications for the elderly (Fick *et al.*, 2003); pharmacists must pay particular attention to thorough and compassionate counseling for elderly patients and should assist patients in finding practical solutions when problems, such as polypharmacy, are noted.

The Therapy. Increased complexity and duration of therapy are perhaps the best-documented barriers to compliance. The patient for whom multiple drugs are prescribed for a given disease or who has multiple illnesses that require drug therapy will be at higher risk for noncompliance, as will the patient whose disease is chronic.

The frequency of dosing of individual medications also can affect compliance behavior. Simplification, whenever possible and appropriate, is desirable.

The effects of the medication can make adherence less likely, as in the case of patients whose medicines cause confusion or other altered mental states. Unpleasant side effects from the medicine may influence compliance in some patients but are not necessarily predictive, especially if patient beliefs or other positive factors would tend to reinforce adherence to the regimen. A side effect that is intolerable to one patient may be of minor concern to another.

For most patients the cost of the medicine does not appear to be a major determinant of compliance (Buckalew and Buckalew, 1995), and even receiving free medicine does not guarantee clinically adequate adherence (Chisholm *et al.*, 2000). However, the cost of medicine can be a heavy burden for patients with limited economic resources, and health care providers should be sensitive to this fact. While physicians often state that drug cost is an important factor in prescribing, their actual knowledge about prices is generally low (Reichert *et al.*, 2000), even for products that they commonly prescribe (Hoffman *et al.*, 1995). The availability of this information on hand-held medical PDAs (personal digital assistants) and from dispensing pharmacists now makes it convenient for physicians to include cost as a factor and to permit appropriate generic substitution when choosing therapy for their patients. A number of other useful sources of drug information are detailed in Chapter 5.

BIBLIOGRAPHY

Buckalew, L.W., and Buckalew, N.M. Survey of the nature and prevalence of patients' noncompliance and implications for intervention. *Psychol. Rep.,* **1995,** *76:*315–321.

Chen, X.Q., and Qian, S.C. Great achievements in ancient Chinese pharmacy. *J. Tradit. Chin. Med.,* **1989,** *9:*230–232.

Chisholm, M.A., Vollenweider, L.J., Mulloy, L.L., *et al.* Renal transplant patient compliance with free immunosuppressive medications. *Transplantation,* **2000,** *70:*1240–1244.

Curtis, L.H., Ostbye, T., Sendersky, V., *et al.* Inappropriate prescribing for elderly Americans in a large outpatient population. *Arch. Intern. Med.,* **2004,** *164:*1621–1625.

DiMatteo, M.R. Patient adherence to pharmacotherapy: the importance of effective communication. *Formulary,* **1995,** *30:*596–598, 601–602, 605.

Feldman, J.A., and DeTullio, P.L. Medication compliance: an issue to consider in the drug selection process. *Hosp. Formul.,* **1994,** *29:*204–211.

Fick, D.M., Cooper, J.W., Wade, W.E., *et al.* Updating the Beers criteria for potentially inappropriate medication use in older adults: results of a US consensus panel of experts. *Arch. Intern. Med.,* **2003,** *163:*2716–2724.

Findlay, S.D. Direct-to-consumer promotion of prescription drugs. Economic implications for patients, payers and providers. *Pharmacoeconomics,* **2001,** *19:*109–119.

Hagstrom, B., Mattsson, B., Rost, I.M., and Gunnarsson, R.K. What happened to the prescriptions? A single, short, standardized telephone call may increase compliance. *Fam. Pract.,* **2004,** *21:*46–50.

Hobbs, R.E. Guidelines for the diagnosis and management of heart failure. *Am. J. Ther.,* **2004,** *11:*467–472.

Hoffman, J., Barefield, F.A., and Ramamurthy, S. A survey of physician knowledge of drug costs. *J. Pain Symptom. Manage.,* **1995,** *10:*432–435.

Karenberg, A., and Leitz, C. Headache in magical and medical papyri of ancient Egypt. *Cephalalgia,* **2001,** *21:*911–916.

Kehoe, W.A., and Katz, R.C. Health behaviors and pharmacotherapy. *Ann. Pharmacother.,* **1998,** *32:*1076–1086.

Kohn, L.T. The Institute of Medicine report on medical error: overview and implications for pharmacy. *Am. J. Health Syst. Pharm.,* **2001,** *58:*63–66.

Kohn, L.T., Findlay, S.D., and Donaldson, M.S. To Err Is Human: Building a Safer Health System (2000). Washington, DC, National Academy Press, Institute of Medicine (U.S.) Committee on Quality of Health Care in America, **1999.**

Kuperman, G.J., Teich, J.M., Gandhi, T.K., and Bates, D.W. Patient safety and computerized medication ordering at Brigham and Women's Hospital. *Jt. Comm. J. Qual. Improv.,* **2001,** *27:*509–521.

Lesar, T.S., Briceland, L., and Stein, D.S. Factors related to errors in medication prescribing. *JAMA,* **1997,** *277:*312–317.

Mangino, P.D. Role of the pharmacist in reducing medication errors. *J. Surg. Oncol.,* **2004,** *88:*189–194.

Martin, D.C., and Mead, K. Reducing medication errors in a geriatric population. *J. Am. Geriatr. Soc.,* **1982,** *4:*258–260.

Meichenbaum, D., and Turk, D.C. *Facilitating Treatment Adherence.* Plenum Press, New York, **1987.**

Michalsen, A., Delclos, G.L., and Felknor, S.A. Compliance with universal precautions among physicians. *J. Occup. Environ. Med.,* **1997,** *39:*130–137.

Reichert, S., Simon, T., and Halm, E.A. Physicians' attitudes about prescribing and knowledge of the costs of common medications. *Arch. Intern. Med.,* **2000,** *160:*2799–2803.

Sackett, D.L., Haynes, R.B., Gibson, E.S., *et al.* Randomised clinical trial of strategies for improving medication compliance in primary hypertension. *Lancet,* **1975,** *1:*1205–1207.

Sackett, D.L., and Snow, J.C. The magnitude of compliance and noncompliance. In, *Compliance in Health Care.* (Haynes, R.B. ed.) Johns Hopkins University Press, Baltimore, **1979,** pp. 11–22.

Salzman, C. Medication compliance in the elderly. *J. Clin. Psychiatry,* **1995,** *56*(suppl 1):18–22.

Sox, N.C., and Woloshin, S. How many deaths are due to medical error? Getting the number right. *Effective Clinical Practice,* **2000,** *3:*277–283.

Teichman, P.G., and Caffee, A.E. Prescription writing to maximize patient safety. *Fam. Pract. Manag.,* **2002,** *9:*27–30.

Topol, E.J. Failing the public health—rofecoxib, Merck, and the FDA. *N. Engl. J. Med.,* **2004,** *351:*1707–1709.

Zyczynski, T.M., and Coyne, K.S. Hypertension and current issues in compliance and patient outcomes. *Curr. Hypertens. Rep.,* **2000,** *2:*510–514.

DESIGN AND OPTIMIZATION OF DOSAGE REGIMENS: PHARMACOKINETIC DATA

Kenneth E. Thummel, Danny D. Shen, Nina Isoherranen, Helen E. Smith

This appendix provides a summary of basic pharmacokinetic information pertaining to drugs that are in common clinical use and are delivered to the systemic circulation by parenteral or nonparenteral administration. Drugs designed exclusively for topical administration and those that are not significantly absorbed into the bloodstream (*e.g.,* ophthalmic and some dermal applications) are not included (*see* Chapters 62 and 63). Pharmacokinetic data for many older drugs not included in this appendix can be found in earlier editions of this book.

A major objective of this appendix is to present pharmacokinetic data in a format that informs the clinician of the essential characteristics of drug disposition that form the basis of drug-dosage regimen design. Table A–II–1 contains quantitative information about the absorption, distribution, and elimination of drugs and the effects of disease states on these processes as well as information about the correlation of efficacy and toxicity with drug concentrations in blood/plasma. The general principles that underlie the design of appropriate maintenance dose and dosing interval (and, where appropriate, the loading dose) for the average patient are described in Chapter 1. Their application using the data in Table A–II–1 for individualization of dosage regimens is presented here.

To use the data that are presented, one must understand clearance concepts and their application to drug-dosage regimens. One also must know average values of clearance as well as some measures of the extent and kinetics of drug absorption and distribution. The text below defines the eight basic parameters that are listed in the tabular material for each drug and key factors that influence these values both in normal subjects and in patients with renal or liver disease. It obviously would be more straightforward if there were a consensus on a standard

value for a given pharmacokinetic parameter; instead, literature estimates usually vary over a wide range, and a consensus set of pharmacokinetic values has been reached for only a limited number of drugs.

In Table A–II–1, a single set of values for each parameter and its variability in a relevant population has been selected from the literature, based on the scientific judgment of the authors. Most data are in the form of a study population mean value ± 1 standard deviation. However, some data are presented as mean and range of values (in parentheses) observed for the study population, *i.e.*, the lowest and highest value reported. There are times when data are reported as a geometric mean with 95% confidence interval. If sufficient data were available, we present a range of mean values obtained from different studies of similar design in parentheses, sometimes below the primary study data. Occasionally, only a single mean value for the study population was available in the literature and is reported as such. Finally, some drugs can be administered intravenously in an unmodified form and orally as a prodrug. When relevant information about both the prodrug and the active molecule are needed, we have included both, using an abbreviation to indicate the species that was measured, followed by another abbreviation in parentheses to indicate the species that was dosed (*e.g.,* G (V) indicates a parameter for ganciclovir after valganciclovir administration).

A number of recently approved drugs are actually the active metabolite or stereoisomer of a previously marketed drug. For example, desloratidine is the *O*-desmethyl-metabolite of loratidine, and esomperazole is the active S-enantiomer of omeprazole. Instead of presenting the pair of drugs in separate tables, only the more established or more commonly used drug is listed, and relevant information on its alternate active form is presented in the same table. This approach has permitted us to include more drugs in the Appendix, hopefully without undue confusion. The only exception is with prednisone and prednisolone, which undergo inter-conversion in the body. We have also adopted this practice for inclusion of protein-based drugs (*e.g.*, pegfilgrastim and darbepoetin) that have been modified to enhance the pharmacokinetic properties of the originally developed molecule.

Unless otherwise indicated in footnotes, data reported in the table are those determined in healthy adults. The direction of change for these values in particular disease states is noted below the average value. One or more references are provided for each of the established drugs, typically a paper or review on its clinical pharmacokinetics, which can then serve as a source for a broader range of papers for the interested reader. In some instances, we have relied on unpublished data provided by the drug sponsor in their package labeling.

TABULATED PHARMACOKINETIC PARAMETERS

Each of the eight parameters presented in Table A–II–1 has been discussed in detail in Chapter 1. The following discussion focuses on the format in which the values are presented as well as on factors (physiological or pathological) that influence the parameters.

Bioavailability. The extent of oral bioavailability is expressed as a percentage of the administered dose. This value represents the percent of administered dose that is available to the systemic circulation—the fraction of the oral dose that reaches the arterial blood in an active or prodrug form. *Fractional availability* (*F*), which appears elsewhere in this appendix, denotes the same parameter; this value varies from 0 to 1. Measures of both the *extent* and *rate* (*see* T_{max}) of availability are presented in the table. The extent of availability is needed for the design of an oral dosage regimen to achieve a specific target blood concentration. Values for multiple routes of administration are provided, when appropriate and available. In most cases, the tabulated value represents an absolute oral bioavailability that has been determined from a comparison of area under the plasma drug concentration time curve between the oral dose and an intravenous reference dose. For those drugs where intravenous administration is not feasible, an approximate estimate of oral bioavailability based on secondary information (*e.g.,* urinary excretion of unchanged drug) is presented, or the column is left blank

[denoted by a long dash (—)]. A dash will also appear when a drug is given by parenteral administration only.

A low bioavailability may result from a poorly formulated dosage form that fails to disintegrate or dissolve in the gastrointestinal fluids, degradative loss of drug in the gastrointestinal fluid, poor mucosal permeability, first-pass metabolism during transit through the intestinal epithelium, active efflux transport of drug back into the lumen, and first-pass hepatic metabolism or biliary excretion (*see* Chapter 1). In the case of drugs with extensive first-pass metabolism, hepatic disease may increase oral availability because hepatic metabolic capacity decreases and/or because vascular shunts develop around the liver.

Urinary Excretion of Unchanged Drug. The second parameter in Table A–II–1 is the amount of drug eventually excreted unchanged in the urine, expressed as a percentage of the administered dose. Values represent the percentage expected in a healthy young adult (creatinine clearance $\geq$ 100 ml/minute). When possible, the value listed is that determined after bolus intravenous administration of the drug, for which bioavailability is 100%. If the drug is given orally, this parameter may be underestimated due to incomplete absorption of the dose; such approximated values are indicated with a footnote. The parameter obtained after intravenous dosing is of greater utility because it reflects the relative contribution of renal clearance to total body clearance irrespective of bioavailability.

Renal disease is the primary factor that causes changes in this parameter. This is especially true when alternate pathways of elimination are available; thus, as renal function decreases, a greater fraction of the dose is available for elimination by other routes. Because renal function generally decreases as a function of age, the percentage of drug excreted unchanged also decreases with age when alternate pathways of elimination are available. In addition, for a number of weakly acidic and basic drugs with pK_a values within the normal range for urine pH, changes in urine pH will affect their rate or extent of urinary excretion (*see* Chapter 1).

Binding to Plasma Proteins. The tabulated value is the percentage of drug in the plasma that is bound to plasma proteins at concentrations of the drug that are achieved clinically. In almost all cases, the values are from measurements performed *in vitro* (rather than from *ex vivo* measurements of binding to proteins in plasma obtained from patients to whom the drug had been administered). When a single mean value is presented, it signifies that there is no apparent change in percent bound over the range of plasma drug concentrations resulting from the usual clinical doses. In cases in which saturation of binding to plasma proteins is approached within the therapeutic range of plasma drug concentrations, a range of bound percentages is provided for concentrations at the lower and upper limits of the range. For some drugs, there is disagreement in the literature about the extent of plasma protein binding; in those cases, the range of reported values is given.

Plasma protein binding is affected primarily by disease states, notably hepatic disease, renal failure, and inflammatory diseases, that alter the concentration of albumin, α_1-acid glycoprotein, or other proteins in plasma that bind drugs. Uremia also changes the binding affinity of albumin for some drugs. Disease-induced changes in plasma protein binding can dramatically affect the volume of distribution, clearance, and elimination half-life of a drug.

Plasma Clearance. Total systemic clearance of drug from plasma or blood [*see* Equations (1–5) and (1–6), Chapter 1] is given in Table A–II–1. Clearance varies as a function of body size and, therefore, is presented most frequently in the table in units of ml · min^{-1} · kg^{-1} of body weight. Normalization to measures of body size other than weight may at times be more appropriate, such as normalization to body surface area in infants to better reflect the growth and development of the liver and kidneys. However, weight is easy to obtain, and its use often offsets any small loss in accuracy of clearance estimate, especially in adults. Exceptions to this rule are the anticancer drugs, for which dosage normalization to body surface area is conventionally used. When unit conversion was necessary, we used individual or mean body weight or body surface area (when appropriate) from the cited study, or if this was not available, we assumed a body mass of 70 kg or a body surface area of 1.73 m^2 for healthy adults.

In some cases, separate values for renal and nonrenal clearance also are provided. For some drugs, particularly those that are excreted predominantly unchanged in the urine, equations are given that relate total or renal clearance to creatinine clearance (also expressed as ml · min^{-1} · kg^{-1}). For drugs that exhibit saturation kinetics, K_m and V_{max} are given and represent, respectively, the plasma concentration at which half of the maximal rate of elimination is reached (in units of mass/volume) and the maximal rate of elimination (in units of mass·time^{-1}·kg^{-1} of body weight). K_m must be in the same units as the concentration of drug in plasma (C_p).

Intrinsic clearance from blood is the maximal possible clearance by the organ responsible for elimination when blood flow (delivery) of drug is not limiting. When expressed in terms of unbound drug, intrinsic clearance reflects clearance from intracellular water.

Intrinsic clearance is tabulated for a few drugs. It is also mathematically related to the biochemical intrinsic clearance [$V_{max}/(K_m + C)$] determined *in vitro*. In almost all cases, clearances based on plasma concentration data are presented in Table A–II–1, because drug analysis is most often performed on plasma samples. The few exceptions where clearance from blood is presented are indicated by footnote. Clearance estimates based on blood concentration may be useful when a drug concentrates in the erythrocytes.

To be accurate, clearances must be determined after intravenous drug administration. When only nonparenteral data are available, the ratio of *CL/F* is given; values offset by the fraction availability (*F*) are indicated in a footnote. When a drug, or its active isomer for racemic compounds, is a substrate for a CYP or drug transporter, this information is provided in a footnote. This information is becoming increasingly important to understand pharmacokinetic variability due to genetic polymorphisms and to predict metabolically based drug-drug interactions. [For more extensive coverage of this topic, *see* Chapters 2, 3, and 4 and *Metabolic Drug Interactions.* (Levy, R.H., *et al.,* eds.) Lippincott Williams & Wilkins, Philadelphia, 2000.]

Volume of Distribution. The total body volume of distribution at steady state (V_{ss}) is given in Table A–II–1 and is expressed in units of l/kg or in units of l/m^2 for some anticancer drugs. Again, when unit conversion was necessary, we used individual or mean body weights or body surface area (when appropriate) from the cited study, or if such data were not available, we assumed a body mass of 70 kg or a body surface area of 1.73 m^2 for healthy adults.

When estimates of V_{ss} were not available, values for V_{area} were provided. V_{area} represents the volume at equilibrated distribution during the terminal elimination phase (*see* Equation 1-12). Unlike V_{ss}, this volume term varies when drug elimination changes, even though there is no change in the distribution space. Because we may wish to know whether a particular disease state influences either the clearance or the tissue distribution of the drug, it is preferable to define volume in terms of V_{ss}, a parameter that is theoretically independent of changes in the rate of elimination. Occasionally, the condition under which the distribution volume was obtained was not specified in the primary reference; this is denoted by the absence of a subscript.

As with clearance, V_{ss} usually is defined in the table in terms of concentration in plasma rather than blood. Further, if data were not obtained after intravenous administration of the drug, a footnote will make clear that the apparent volume estimate, V_{ss}/F, is offset by the fractional availability.

Half-Life. Half-life ($t_\frac{1}{2}$) is the time required for the plasma concentration to decline by one-half when elimination is first-order. It also governs the rate of approach to steady state and the degree of drug accumulation during multiple dosing or continuous infusion. For example, at a fixed dosing interval, the patient will be at 50% of steady state after one half-life, 75% of steady state after two half-lives, 93.75% of steady state after four half-lives, etc. Determination of half-life is straightforward when drug elimination follows a monoexponential pattern (*i.e., one-compartment model*). However, for a number of drugs, plasma concentration follows a multiexponential pattern of decline over time. The mean value listed in Table A–II–1 corresponds to an effective rate of elimination that covers the clearance of a major fraction of the absorbed dose from the body. In many cases, this half-life refers to the rate of elimination in the terminal exponential phase. For a number of drugs, however, the half-life of an earlier phase is presented, even though a prolonged half-life may be observed at very low plasma concentrations when extremely sensitive analytical techniques are used. If the latter component accounts for 10% or less of the total area under the plasma concentration-time curve (*AUC*), predictions of drug accumulation in plasma during continuous or repetitive dosing will be in error by no more than 10% if this longer half-life is ignored. The clinician should know the half-life that will best predict drug accumulation in the patient, which will be the appropriate half-life to use for estimating the rate constant in Equations (1–19) through (1–21) (*see* Chapter 1) to predict time to steady state. It is this half-life of accumulation during multiple dosing that is given in Table A–II–1.

Half-life is usually independent of body size because it is a function of the ratio of two parameters, clearance and volume of distribution, each of which is proportional to body size. It should also be noted that the half-life is preferably obtained from intravenous studies, if feasible, because the half-life of decline in plasma drug concentration after oral dosing can be influenced by prolonged absorption, such as when slow release formulations are given. If the half-life is derived from an oral dose, this will be indicated in a footnote of Table A–II–1.

Time to Peak Concentration. Because clearance concepts are used most often in the design of multiple dosage regimens, the extent rather than the rate of availability is more critical to estimate the average steady-state concentration of drug in the body. In some circumstances, the degree of fluctuation in plasma drug concentration, *i.e.,* peak and trough concentrations, which govern drug efficacy and side effects, can be greatly influenced by modulation of drug absorption rate through the use of sustained- or extended-release formulations. Controlled-release formulations often permit a reduction in dosing frequency from 3 or 4 times daily to once or twice daily. There also are drugs that are given on an acute basis, *e.g.,* for the relief of breakthrough pain or to induce sleep, for which the rate of drug absorption is a critical determinant of onset of effect. Thus, information about the expected average time to achieve maximal plasma or blood concentration and the degree of interindividual variability in that parameter have been included in Table A–II–1.

The time required to achieve a maximal concentration (T_{max}) depends on the rate of drug absorption into blood from the site of administration and the rate of elimination. From mass balance principles, T_{max} occurs when the rate of absorption equals the rate of elimination from the reference compartment. Prior to this time, absorption rate exceeds elimination rate, and the plasma concentration of drug increases. After the peak is reached, elimination rate exceeds the absorption rate and, at some point, defines the terminal elimination phase of the concentration-time profile.

The rate of drug absorption following oral administration will depend on the formulation and physicochemical properties of the drug, its permeability across the mucosal barrier, and the intestinal villous blood flow. For an oral dose, some absorption may occur very rapidly within the buccal cavity, esophagus, and stomach, or absorption may be delayed until the drug reaches the small intestine or until the local pH in the intestine permits drug release from the dosage formulation. In the most extreme case, the rate of absorption can be sufficiently controlled by the drug formulation to permit sustained or extended delivery as the dosage form traverses the entire length of the gastrointestinal tract. In some instances, the terminal elimination of drug from the body following a peak concentration reflects the slower rate of absorption and not elimination.

When more than one type of drug formulation is available commercially, we have provided absorption information for both the immediate- and sustained-release formulations. Not surprisingly, the presence of food in the gastrointestinal tract can alter both the rate and extent of drug availability. We have indicated with footnotes when the consumption of food near the time of drug ingestion may have a significant effect on the drug bioavailability.

Peak Concentration. There is no general agreement about the best way to describe the relationship between the concentration of drug in plasma and its effect. Many different kinds of data are present in the literature, and use of a single effect parameter or effective concentration is difficult. This is particularly true for antimicrobial agents because the effective concentration depends on the identity of the microorganism causing the infection. It also is important to recognize that concentration-effect relationships are most easily obtained at steady state or during the terminal log-linear phase of the concentration-time curve, when the drug concentration(s) at the site(s) of action are expected to parallel those in plasma. Thus, when attempting to correlate a blood or plasma level to effect, the temporal aspect of distribution of drug to its site of action must be taken into account.

Despite these limitations, it is possible to define the minimum effective or toxic concentrations for some of the drugs currently in clinical use. However, in reviewing the list of drugs approved within the last five years, it is rare to find a declaration of an *effective concentration range,* even in the manufacturer's package labeling. Thus, it is necessary to infer therapeutic concentrations from concentrations observed following *effective dosage* regimens. For a given dosage regimen, a time-averaged steady-state blood or plasma concentration (*i.e.,* $\overline{C}_{ss}$ as estimated by dividing the mean *AUC* by the duration of the dosing interval) and the associated interindividual variability might be one appropriate parameter to report; however, such data often are not available. Also, $\overline{C}_{ss}$ does not take into account the onset and offset of effect during fluctuation of plasma drug concentration over a dosing interval. In some instances, drug efficacy may be more closely linked with peak concentration than with the average or trough concentration, and differences in peak concentration for special populations (*e.g.,* elderly) sometimes are associated with increased incidence of drug toxicity.

For practical reasons, the most commonly reported parameter, C_{max} (peak concentration), is presented in Table A–II–1, rather than effective or toxic concentrations. This provides a more consistent body of information about drug exposure from which one can infer, if appropriate, efficacious or toxic blood levels. While the value reported is the highest that would be encountered in a given dose interval, C_{max} can be related to the trough concentration (C_{min}) through appropriate mathematical predictions (*see* Equation 1–21). Because peak levels will vary with dose, we have attempted to present concentrations observed with a customary dose regimen that is recognized to be effective in the majority of patients. When a higher or lower dose rate is used, the expected peak level can be adjusted by assuming dose proportionality, unless nonlinear kinetics are indicated. In some instances, only limited data pertaining to multiple dosing are available, so single-dose peak concentrations are presented. When specific information is available about an effective therapeutic range of concentrations or about concentrations at

which toxicity occurs, it has been incorporated in a footnote. For individual drugs, the reader also is referred to the index to highlight pages where more detailed information is provided.

It is important to recognize that significant differences in C_{max} will occur when comparing similar daily-dose regimens for an immediate-release and sustained-release product. Indeed, the sustained-release product sometimes is administered to reduce peak-trough fluctuations during the dosing interval and to minimize swings between potentially toxic or ineffective drug concentrations. Again, we report C_{max} for both immediate-release and extended-release formulations, when available. In addition to parent drug concentrations, we have included information on any active metabolite that circulates at a concentration that may contribute to the overall pharmacological effect, particularly those active metabolites that accumulate with multiple dosing. Likewise, for chiral drugs whose stereoisomers differ in their pharmacological activity and clearance characteristics, we present information on the pharmacokinetics of the individual enantiomers or the active enantiomer that contributes most to the drug's efficacy.

Although total drug or metabolite concentrations are reported, it is important to recognize that the concentration of *unbound drug* often determines the degree of pharmacological effect. Accordingly, changes in protein binding due to disease may be expected to cause changes in the total plasma concentration associated with desired or unwanted effects. However, the clinical outcome is not always affected because an increase in free fraction will also increase the apparent clearance of an orally administered drug and of a low extraction drug dosed intravenously. Under such a scenario, the mean unbound plasma concentration at steady state will not change with reduced or elevated plasma protein binding, despite a significant change in mean total drug concentration.

ALTERATIONS OF PARAMETERS IN THE INDIVIDUAL PATIENT

Dose adjustments for an individual patient should be made according to the manufacturer's recommendation in the package labeling when available. This information is generally available when disease, age, or race has a significant impact on drug disposition, particularly for drugs that have been introduced within the last 10 years. In some cases, a significant difference in drug disposition from the "average" adult can be expected but may not require dose adjustment because of a sufficiently broad therapeutic index. In other cases, dose adjustment may be necessary, but no specific information is available. Under these circumstances, an estimate of the appropriate dosing regimen can be obtained based on pharmacokinetic principles described in Chapter 1.

Unless otherwise specified, the values in Table A–II–2 represent mean values for populations of normal adults; it may be necessary to modify them for calculation of dosage regimens for individual patients. The fraction available (*F*) and clearance (CL) also must be estimated to compute a maintenance dose necessary to achieve a desired average steady-state concentration. To calculate the loading dose, knowledge of the volume of distribution is needed. The estimated half-life is used in deciding a dosing interval that provides an acceptable peak-trough fluctuation; note, this may be the apparent half-life following dosing of a slowly absorbed formulation. The values reported in the table and the adjustments apply only to adults; exceptions are footnoted. Although the values at times may be applied to children who weigh more than about 30 kg (after proper adjustment for size; *see* below), it is best to consult pediatrics textbooks or other sources for definitive advice.

For each drug, changes in the parameters caused by certain disease states are noted within the eight segments of the table. In all cases, the qualitative direction of changes is noted, such as "↓ LD," which indicates a significant decrease in the parameter in a patient with liver disease. The relevant literature and the package label should be consulted for more definitive, quantitative information for dosage adjustment recommendations.

Plasma Protein Binding. Most acidic drugs that are extensively bound to plasma proteins are bound to albumin. Basic lipophilic drugs, such as propranolol, often bind to other plasma proteins (*e.g.,* α_1-acid glycoprotein and lipoproteins). The degree of drug binding to proteins will differ in pathophysiological states that cause changes in plasma-protein concentrations. Significant pharmacokinetic effects from a change in plasma protein binding will be denoted under clearance or volume of distribution.

Clearance. For drugs that are partly or predominantly eliminated by renal excretion, plasma clearance changes in accordance with the renal function of an individual patient. This necessitates dosage adjustment that is dependent on the fraction of normal renal function remaining and the fraction of drug normally excreted unchanged in the urine. The latter quantity appears in the table; the former can be estimated as the ratio of the patient's creatinine clearance (CL_{cr}) to a normal value (100 ml/minute

per 70 kg body weight). If urinary creatinine clearance has not been measured, it may be estimated from the concentration of creatinine in serum (C_{cr}). In men:

$$CL_{cr}(\text{ml} \cdot \text{min}^{-1}) = \frac{[140 - \text{age (yr)}] \cdot [\text{weight (kg)}]}{72 \cdot [CL_{cr}(\text{mg/dl})]} \quad (\text{A–1})$$

For women, the estimate of CL_{cr} by the above equation should be multiplied by 0.85 to reflect their smaller muscle mass. The fraction of normal renal function (rfx_{pt}) is estimated from the following:

$$rfx_{pt} = \frac{CL_{cr, pt}}{100 \text{ ml} \cdot \text{min}^{-1}} \quad (\text{A–2})$$

A more accurate measure of rfx_{pt} is seldom necessary because, given the considerable degree of interindividual variation in nonrenal clearance, the adjustment of clearance is an approximation. The following equation for adjustment of clearance uses the quantities discussed:

$$rf_{pt} = 1 - [fe_{nl} \cdot (1 - rfx_{pt})] \quad (\text{A–3})$$

where fe_{nl} is the fraction of systemic drug excreted unchanged in normal individuals (*see* Table A–II–1). The renal factor (rf_{pt}) is the value that, when multiplied by normal total clearance (CL_{nl}) from the table, gives the total clearance of the drug adjusted for the impairment in renal function.

Example. The clearance of vancomycin in a patient with reduced renal function (creatinine clearance = 25 ml/min per 70 kg) may be estimated as follows:

$$rfx_{pt} = \frac{25 \text{ ml/min}}{100 \text{ ml/min}} = 0.25$$

$fe_{nl} = 0.79$ (*see* listing for vancomycin)
$rf_{pt} = 1 - [0.79 \cdot (1 - 0.25)] = 0.41$
$CL_{pt} = (1.4 \text{ ml/minute per kg}) \cdot 0.41$
  $= 0.57 \text{ ml/minute per kg}$

Importantly, such a clearance adjustment should be regarded only as an initial step in optimizing the dosage regimen; depending on the patient's response to the drug, further individualization may be necessary.

Conventionally, clearance is adjusted for the size of the patient to reflect a difference in the mass of the eliminating organ. For orally administered drugs, the applicability of such an adjustment may be limited by the available dosage strengths of commercial formulations. In some cases, scored tablets can be split or commercial tablet splitters are used to increase the range of available dosage strengths. However, this practice should be followed only with the recommendation of the drug manufacturer because splitting a tablet sometimes can compromise the bioavailability of a product.

With the exception of certain oncolytic agents, the data presented in the table are normalized to weight. Thus, interindividual variability in the weight-normalized clearance reflects a variation in the intrinsic metabolic or transport clearance and not the size of the organ. Further, these differences can be attributed to variable expression/function of metabolic enzymes or transporters. However, it is important to recognize that liver mass and total enzyme/transporter content may not increase or decrease in proportion to weight in obese or malnourished individuals. Alternative approaches such as normalization by body surface area or other measures of body mass may be more appropriate. For example, many of the drugs used to treat cancer are dosed according to body surface area (*see* Chapter 51). In the tabulation, if the literature reported dose per body surface area, we present the data in the same unit. If the cited clearance data were not normalized, but the preponderance of the literature utilized body surface area, we followed the practice of using values of body surface area from the literature source or a standard of 1.73 m² for a healthy adult.

Volume of Distribution. Volume of distribution should be adjusted for the modifying factors indicated in Table A–II–1 as well as for body size. Again, the data in the table most often are normalized to weight. Unlike clearance, volume of distribution in an individual is most often proportional to weight itself. Whether this applies to a specific drug depends on the actual sites of distribution of drug; no absolute rule applies.

Whether or not to adjust volume of distribution for changes in binding to plasma proteins cannot be decided in general; the decision depends critically on whether or not the factors that alter binding to plasma proteins also alter binding to tissue proteins. Qualitative changes in volume of distribution, when they occur, are indicated in the table.

Half-Life. Half-life may be estimated from the adjusted values of clearance (CL_{pt}) and volume of distribution (V_{pt}) for the patient:

$$t_{\frac{1}{2}} = \frac{0.693 \cdot V_{pt}}{CL_{pt}} \tag{A–4}$$

Because half-life has been the parameter most often measured and reported in the literature, qualitative changes for this parameter are almost always given in the table.

INDIVIDUALIZATION OF DOSAGE

By using the parameters for the individual patient, calculated as described above, initial dosing regimens may be chosen. The maintenance dosage rate may be calculated with Equation (1–18) using the estimated values for *CL* and *F* for the individual patient. As described above, the target concentration may have to be adjusted for changes in plasma protein binding in the patient, as described above. The loading dose may be calculated using Equation (1–22) and estimates for V_{ss} and *F*. A particular dosing interval may be chosen; the maximal and minimal steady-state concentrations can be calculated by using Equations (1–20) and [(1–19) or (1–21)], and these can be compared with the known efficacious and toxic concentrations for the drug. As with the target concentration, these values may need to be adjusted for changes in the extent of plasma protein binding. Use of Equations (1–19) and (1–20) also requires estimates of values for *F*, V_{ss}, and *K* ($K = 0.693/t_{\frac{1}{2}}$) for the individual patient.

Note that these adjustments of pharmacokinetic parameters for an individual patient are suggested for the rational choice of initial dosing regimen. As indicated in Chapter 1, steady-state measurement of drug concentrations in the patient then can be used as a guide to further adjust the dosage regimen. However, optimization of a dosage regimen for an individual patient ultimately will depend on the clinical response produced by the drug.

Table A–II–1 Pharmacokinetic Data

AVAILABILITY (ORAL) (%)	URINARY EXCRETION (%)	BOUND IN PLASMA (%)	CLEARANCE $(ml \cdot min^{-1} \cdot kg^{-1})$	VOL. DIST. (liters/kg)	HALF-LIFE (hours)	PEAK TIME (hours)	PEAK CONCENTRATIONS
ACETAMINOPHEN[a] (Chapter 26)							
88 ± 15 ↔ Child	3 ± 1 ↔ Neo, Child	<20	5.0 ± 1.4[b] ↓ Hep[c] ↔ Aged, Child ↑ Obes, HTh, Preg	0.95 ± 0.12[b] ↔ Aged, Hep[c] LTh, HTh, Child	2.0 ± 0.4 ↔ RD, Obes, Child ↑ Neo, Hep[c] ↓ HTh, Preg	0.33–1.4[d]	20 μg/ml[e]

*Reference: Forrest, J.A., Clements, J.A., and Prescott, L.F. Clinical pharmacokinetics of paracetamol. Clin. Pharmacokinet., **1982**, 7:93–107.*

[a]Values reported are for doses less than 2 g; drug exhibits concentration-dependent kinetics above this dose. [b]Assuming a 70 kg body weight; reported range, 65–72 kg. [c]Acetaminophen-induced hepatic damage or acute viral hepatitis. [d]Absorption rate, but not extent, depends on gastric emptying; hence, it is slowed after food as well as in some disease states and co-treatment with drugs that cause gastroparesis. [e]Mean concentration following a 20-mg/kg oral dose. Hepatic toxicity associated with levels >300 μg/ml at 4 hours after an overdose.

ACETYLSALICYLIC ACID[a] (Chapters 26, 54)							
68 ± 3 ↔ Aged, Cirr	1.4 ± 1.2 ↓ RD	49 ↓ RD	9.3 ± 1.1 ↔ Aged, Cirr	0.15 ± 0.03	0.25 ± 0.03 ↔ Hep	0.39 ± 0.21[b] ↔ Hep	24 ± 4 μg/ml[b]

*Reference: Roberts, M.S., Rumble, R.H., Wanwimolruk, S., Thomas, D., and Brooks, P.M. Pharmacokinetics of aspirin and salicylate in elderly subjects and in patients with alcoholic liver disease. Eur. J. Clin. Pharmacol., **1983**, 25:253–261.*

[a]Values given are for unchanged parent drug. Acetylsalicylic acid is converted to salicylic acid during and after absorption (CL and $t_{\frac{1}{2}}$ of salicylate are dose-dependent; $t_{\frac{1}{2}}$ varies between 2.4 hours after a 300 mg dose to 19 hours when there is intoxication). [b]Following a single 1.2 g oral dose given to adults.

ACYCLOVIR (Chapter 49)							
15–30[a]	75 ± 10	15 ± 4	$CL = 3.37CL_{cr} + 0.41$ ↓ Neo ↔ Child	0.69 ± 0.19 ↓ Neo ↔ RD	2.4 ± 0.7 ↑ RD, Neo ↔ Child	1.5–2[b]	3.5–5.4 μM[b]

*Reference: Laskin, O.L. Clinical pharmacokinetics of acyclovir. Clin. Pharmacokinet., **1983**, 8:187–201.*

[a]Decreases with increasing dose. [b]Range of steady-state concentrations following a 400-mg given orally every 4 hours to steady state.

ADALIMUMAB[a] (Chapter 52)

| — | — | 0.0026 ± 0.0005 | 0.082 ± 0.014 | 389 ± 71 | 131 ± 56[c] | 4.7 ± 1.6 µg/ml[c] |

[a]Data from patients with rheumatoid arthritis. No significant gender differences. [b]Parenteral use only; mean bioavailability following SC administration is 64%. [c]Following a single 40 mg SC dose.

References: Physicians' Desk Reference, 58th ed. Medical Economics Co., Montvale, NJ, **2004**, p. 470. Weisman, M.H., Moreland, L.W., *et al.* Efficacy, pharmacokinetic, and safety assessment of adalimumab, a fully human anti-tumor necrosis factor-alpha monoclonal antibody, in adults with rheumatoid arthritis receiving concomitant methotrexate: a pilot study. *Clin. Ther.*, **2003**, 25:1700–1721.

ALBENDAZOLE[a] (Chapter 41)

| — | <1 | 70 | 10.5–30.7[c] | — | 8 (6–15)[d] | 2–4[e] | 0.50–1.8 µg/ml[e] |
| ↑ Food | | | | | | | |

[a]Oral albendazole undergoes rapid and essentially complete first-pass metabolism to albendazole sulfoxide (ALBSO), which is pharmacologically active. Pharmacokinetic data for ALBSO in male and female adults are reported. [b]The absolute bioavailability of ALBSO is not known but is increased by high-fat meals. [c]CL/F following twice daily oral dosing to steady state. Chronic albendazole treatment appears to induce the metabolism of ALBSO. [d]$t_{1/2}$ reportedly shorter in children with neurocysticercosis, compared with adults; may need to be dosed more frequently (three times a day) in children, rather than twice a day as in adults. [e]Following a 7.5 mg/kg oral dose given twice daily for 8 days to adults.

References: Marques, M.P., Takayanagui, O.M., Bonato, P.S., Santos, S.R., and Lanchote, V.L. Enantioselective kinetic disposition of albendazole sulfoxide in patients with neurocysticercosis. *Chirality*, **1999**, *11*:218–223. *Physicians' Desk Reference*, 58th ed. Medical Economics Co., Montvale, NJ, **2004**, p. 1422. Sanchez, M., Suastegui, R., Gonzalez-Esquivel, D., Sotelo, J., and Jung, H. Pharmacokinetic comparison of two albendazole dosage regimens in patients with neurocysticercosis. *Clin. Neuropharmacol.* **1993**, *16*:77–82. Sotelo, J., and Jung, H. Pharmacokinetic optimisation of the treatment of neurocysticercosis. *Clin. Pharmacokinet.*, **1998**, *34*:503–515.

ALBUTEROL[a] (Chapters 10, 27)

PO, R: 30 ± 7	R/S: 7 ± 1	R: 46 ± 8	R: 10.3 ± 3.0	R: 2.00 ± 0.70	R: 2.00 ± 0.49	R: 1.5[c]	R: 3.6 (1.9–5.9) ng/ml[c]
PO, S: 71 ± 9		S: 55 ± 11	S: 6.5 ± 2.0	S: 1.77 ± 0.69	S: 2.85 ± 0.85	S: 2.0[c]	S: 11.4 (7.1–16.2) ng/ml[c]
IH, R: 25			↓ RD[b]	↓ RD[b]			
IH, S: 47							

[a]Data from healthy subjects for R and S enantiomers. No major gender differences. No kinetic differences in asthmatics. β Adrenergic activity resides primarily with R-enantiomer. PO, oral; IH, inhalation. Oral dose undergoes extensive first-pass sulfation at the intestinal mucosa. [b]CL/F reduced, moderate renal impairment. [c]Median (range) following a single 4 mg oral dose of racemic (R/S)-albuterol.

References: Boulton, D.W., and Fawcett, J.P. Enantioselective disposition of albuterol in humans. *Clin. Rev. Allergy Immunol.*, **1996**, *14*:115–138. Mohamed, M.H., Lima, J.J., Eberle, L.V., Self, T.H., and Johnson, J.A. Effects of gender and race on albuterol pharmacokinetics. *Pharmacotherapy*, **1999**, *19*:157–161.

Key: Unless otherwise indicated by a specific footnote, the data are presented for the study population as a mean value ± 1 standard deviation, a mean and range (lowest–highest in parenthesis) of values, a range of the lowest–highest values, or a single mean value. ADH = alcohol dehydrogenase; Aged = aged; AIDS = acquired immunodeficiency syndrome; Alb = hypoalbuminemia; Atr Fib = atrial fibrillation; AVH = acute viral hepatitis; Burn = burn patients; C_{max} = peak concentration; CAD = coronary artery disease; Celiac = celiac disease; CF = cystic fibrosis; CHF = congestive heart failure; Child = children; Cirr = hepatic cirrhosis; COPD = chronic obstructive pulmonary disease; CP = cor pulmonale; CPBS = cardiopulmonary bypass surgery; CRI = chronic respiratory insufficiency; Crohn = Crohn's disease; Cush = Cushing's syndrome; CYP = cytochrome P450; Fem = female; Hep = hepatitis; HIV = human immunodeficiency virus; HL = hyperlipoproteinemia; HTh = hyperthyroid; IM = intramuscular; Inflam = inflammation; IV = intravenous; LD = chronic liver disease; LTh = hypothyroid; MAO = monoamine oxidase; MI = myocardial infarction; NAT = N-acetyltransferase; Neo = neonate; NIDDM = non-insulin-dependent diabetes mellitus; NS = nephrotic syndrome; Obes = obese; Pneu = pneumonia; Preg = pregnant; Prem = premature infants; RA = rheumatoid arthritis; RD = renal disease (including uremia); SC = subcutaneous; Smk = smoking; ST = sulfotransferase; T_{max} = peak time; Tach = ventricular tachycardia; UGT = UDP-glucuronosyl transferase; Ulcer = ulcer patients. Other abbreviations are defined in the text section of this appendix.

Table A–II–1 *Pharmacokinetic Data (Continued)*

AVAILABILITY (ORAL) (%)	URINARY EXCRETION (%)	BOUND IN PLASMA (%)	CLEARANCE $(ml \cdot min^{-1} \cdot kg^{-1})$	VOL. DIST. (liters/kg)	HALF-LIFE (hours)	PEAK TIME (hours)	PEAK CONCENTRATIONS
ALENDRONATE[a] (Chapter 61)							
<0.7[b] ↓ Food	44.9 ± 9.3	78	1.11 (1.00–1.22)[c] ↔ RD[e]	0.44 (0.34–0.55)[c]	~1.0[d]	IV: 2[f]	IV: ~275 ng/ml[f] Oral: <5–8.4 ng/ml[f]

[a]Data from healthy post-menopausal female subjects. [b]Based on urinary recovery; reduced when taken <1 hour before or up to 2 hours after a meal. [c]CL and V_{ss} values represent mean and 90% CI. [d]The $t_{\frac{1}{2}}$ for release from bone is ~11.9 years. [e]Mild-to-moderate renal impairment. [f]Following a single 10 mg IV infusion over 2 hours and a 10 mg oral dose daily for >3 years.

References: Cocquyt, V., Kline, W.F., *et al.* Pharmacokinetics of intravenous alendronate. *J. Clin. Pharmacol.,* **1999**, *39*:385–393. Porras, A.G., Holland, S.D., and Gertz, B.J. Pharmacokinetics of alendronate. *Clin. Pharmacokinet.,* **1999**, *36*:315–328.

AVAILABILITY (ORAL) (%)	URINARY EXCRETION (%)	BOUND IN PLASMA (%)	CLEARANCE	VOL. DIST.	HALF-LIFE	PEAK TIME	PEAK CONCENTRATIONS
ALFENTANIL (Chapters 13, 21)							
—	<1	92 ± 2 ↓ Cirr	6.7 ± 2.4[a] ↓ Aged, Cirr ↔ CPBS	0.8 ± 0.3 ↔ Aged ↑ CPBS ↓ Cirr	1.6 ± 0.2 ↑ Aged, Cirr, CPBS	—	100–200 ng/ml[b] 310–340 ng/ml[c]

[a]Metabolically cleared by CYP3A. [b]Provides adequate anesthesia for superficial surgery. [c]Provides adequate anesthesia for abdominal surgery.

Reference: Bodenham, A., and Park, G.R. Alfentanil infusions in patients requiring intensive care. *Clin. Pharmacokinet.,* **1988**, *15*:216–226.

AVAILABILITY (ORAL) (%)	URINARY EXCRETION (%)	BOUND IN PLASMA (%)	CLEARANCE	VOL. DIST.	HALF-LIFE	PEAK TIME	PEAK CONCENTRATIONS
ALLOPURINOL[a] (Chapters 26, 51)							
53 ± 13	12	—	9.9 ± 2.4[b] RD, Aged[b]	0.87 ± 0.13	A: 1.2 ± 0.3 O: 24 ± 4.5	A: 1.7 ± 1.0[c] O: 4.1 ± 1.4[c]	A: 1.4 ± 0.5 μg/ml[c] O: 6.4 ± 0.8 μg/ml[c]

[a]Data from healthy male and female subjects. Allopurinol (A) is rapidly metabolized to the pharmacologically active oxypurinol (O). [b]Increased oxypurinol *AUC* during renal impairment and in the elderly. [c]Following a single 300 mg oral dose.

References: Physicians' Desk Reference, 54th ed. Medical Economics Co. Montvale, NJ, **2000**, p. 1976. Turnheim, K., Krivanek, P., and Oberbauer, R. Pharmacokinetics and pharmacodynamics of allopurinol in elderly and young subjects. *Br. J. Clin. Pharmacol.,* **1999**, *48*:501–509.

AVAILABILITY (ORAL) (%)	URINARY EXCRETION (%)	BOUND IN PLASMA (%)	CLEARANCE	VOL. DIST.	HALF-LIFE	PEAK TIME	PEAK CONCENTRATIONS
ALPRAZOLAM (Chapter 17)							
88 ± 16	20	71 ± 3 ↑ Cirr ↔ Obes, Aged	0.74 ± 0.14[a] ↓ Obes, Cirr, Aged[b] ↔ RD	0.72 ± 0.12 ↔ Obes, Cirr, Aged	12 ± 2 ↑ Obes, Cirr, Aged[b] ↔ RD	1.5 (0.5–3.0)[c]	21 (15–32) ng/ml[c]

[a]Metabolically cleared by CYP3A and other CYPs. [b]Data from male subjects only. [c]Mean (range) from 19 studies following a single 1 g oral dose given to adults.

Reference: Greenblatt, D.J. and Wright, C.E. Clinical pharmacokinetics of alprazolam. Therapeutic implications. *Clin. Pharmacokinet.,* **1993**, *24*:453–471.

AVAILABILITY (ORAL) (%)	URINARY EXCRETION (%)	BOUND IN PLASMA (%)	CLEARANCE	VOL. DIST.	HALF-LIFE	PEAK TIME	PEAK CONCENTRATIONS
ALTEPLASE (t-PA) (Chapter 54)							
—	Low	—	10 ± 4	0.10 ± 0.01	0.08 ± 0.04[a]	—	973 ± 133 ng/ml[b]

[a]Initial $t_{\frac{1}{2}}$ is dominant; terminal $t_{\frac{1}{2}}$ is 0.43 ± 0.17 hours. [b]Following a single 50 mg IV dose of t-PA infused over 30 min to healthy adults.

Reference: Seifried, E., Tanswell, P., Rijken, D.C., *et al.* Pharmacokinetics of antigen and activity of recombinant tissue-type plasminogen activator after infusion in healthy volunteers. *Arzneimittelforschung,* **1988,** 38:418–422.

AMIKACIN (Chapters 45, 47)

—	98	4 ± 8[a]	1.3 ± 0.6 $CL = 0.6CL_{cr} + 0.14$ ↓ Obes ↑ CF	0.27 ± 0.06 ↔ Aged, Child, CF ↓ Obes ↑ Neo	2.3 ± 0.4 ↑ RD ↔ Obes ↓ Burn, Child, CF	—	26 ± 4 µg/ml[b]

[a]At a serum concentration of 15 µg/ml. [b]Following a 1 hour IV infusion of a 6.3 ± 1.4 mg/kg given three times a day to steady state in patients without renal disease.

Reference: Bauer, L.A. and Blouin, R.A. Influence of age on amikacin pharmacokinetics in patients without renal disease. Comparison with gentamicin and tobramycin. *Eur. J. Clin. Pharmacol.,* **1983,** 24:639–642.

AMIODARONE[a] (Chapter 34)

46 ± 22	0	99.98 ± 0.01	1.9 ± 0.4[b] ↔ Aged, Fem, CHF, RD	66 ± 44	25 ± 12 days[c] ↔ Aged, Fem, RD	2–10[d]	1.5–2.4 µg/ml[d]

[a]Significant plasma concentrations of an active desethyl metabolite are observed (ratio of drug/metabolite ~1); $t_{\frac{1}{2}}$ for metabolite = 61 days. [b]Metabolized by CYP3A. [c]Longer $t_{\frac{1}{2}}$ noted in patients (53 ± 24 days); all reported $t_{\frac{1}{2}}$s may be underestimated because of insufficient length of sampling. [d]Following a 400 mg/day oral dose to steady state in adult patients.

Reference: Gill, J., Heel, R.C., and Fitton, A. Amiodarone. An overview of its pharmacological properties, and review of its therapeutic use in cardiac arrhythmias. *Drugs,* **1992,** 43:69–110.

AMITRIPTYLINE[a] (Chapter 17)

48 ± 11 ↔ Aged	<2 ↔ Aged	94.8 ± 0.8 ↔ Aged ↑ HL	11.5 ± 3.4[b] ↔ Aged, Smk	15 ± 3[b] ↑ Aged	21 ± 5 ↑ Aged	3.6 ± 1.4[c] ↑ Aged	64 ± 35 ng/ml[c]

[a]Active metabolite is nortriptyline, listed below. [b]Blood *CL* and V_{ss} reported; formation of nortriptyline is catalyzed by CYP2C19 (polymorphic), CYP3A4, and other CYPs; formation of 10-hydroxy metabolite is catalyzed by CYP2D6 (polymorphic). [c]Following a 100 mg/day dose to steady state in adults. The nortriptyline/amitriptyline concentration ratio = 1.1 ± 0.6. Optimal range of nortriptyline + amitriptyline is 60 to 220 ng/ml. Toxic effects occur at total concentrations >1 µg/ml.

Reference: Schulz, P., Dick, P., Blaschke, T.F., and Hollister, L. Discrepancies between pharmacokinetic studies of amitriptyline. *Clin. Pharmacokinet.,* **1985,** 10:257–268.

Table A-II-1 Pharmacokinetic Data (Continued)

AVAILABILITY (ORAL) (%)	URINARY EXCRETION (%)	BOUND IN PLASMA (%)	CLEARANCE ($ml \cdot min^{-1} \cdot kg^{-1}$)	VOL. DIST. (liters/kg)	HALF-LIFE (hours)	PEAK TIME (hours)	PEAK CONCENTRATIONS
AMLODIPINE[a] (Chapters 31, 32)							
74 ± 17 ↔ Aged	10	93 ± 1 ↔ Aged	5.9 ± 1.5 ↔ RD, ↓ Aged, Hep	16 ± 4 ↔ Aged	39 ± 8 ↔ RD, ↑ Aged, Hep	5.4–8.0[b]	18.1 ± 7.1 ng/ml[b] ↑ Aged

[a]Racemic mixture; in young, healthy subjects, there are no apparent differences between the kinetics of the more active R-enantiomer and S-enantiomer. [b]Following a 10 mg oral dose given once daily for 14 days to healthy male adults.

Reference: Meredith, P.A. and Elliott, H.L. Clinical pharmacokinetics of amlodipine. *Clin. Pharmacokinet.*, **1992**, *22*:22–31.

AVAILABILITY (ORAL) (%)	URINARY EXCRETION (%)	BOUND IN PLASMA (%)	CLEARANCE ($ml \cdot min^{-1} \cdot kg^{-1}$)	VOL. DIST. (liters/kg)	HALF-LIFE (hours)	PEAK TIME (hours)	PEAK CONCENTRATIONS
AMOXICILLIN (Chapter 44)							
93 ± 10[a]	86 ± 8	18	2.6 ± 0.4 ↔ Child, ↓ RD, Aged[b]	0.21 ± 0.03 ↔ RD, Aged	1.7 ± 0.3 ↔ Child, ↑ RD, Aged[b]	1–2	IV: 46 ± 12 µg/ml[c] Oral: 5 µg/ml[c]

[a]Dose-dependent; value shown is for a 375 mg dose; decreases to about 50% at 3000 mg. [b]No change if renal function is not decreased. [c]Following a single 500 mg IV bolus dose in healthy elderly adults or a single 500 mg oral dose in adults.

References: Hoffler, D. [The pharmacokinetics of amoxicillin.] *Adv. Clin. Pharmacol.*, **1974**, *7*:28–30. Sjovall, J., Alvan, G., and Huitfeldt, B. Intra- and inter-individual variation in pharmacokinetics of intravenously infused amoxicillin and ampicillin to elderly volunteers. *Br. J. Clin. Pharmacol.*, **1986**, *21*:171–181.

AVAILABILITY (ORAL) (%)	URINARY EXCRETION (%)	BOUND IN PLASMA (%)	CLEARANCE ($ml \cdot min^{-1} \cdot kg^{-1}$)	VOL. DIST. (liters/kg)	HALF-LIFE (hours)	PEAK TIME (hours)	PEAK CONCENTRATIONS
AMPHOTERICIN B[a] (Chapter 48)							
<5	2–5	>90	0.46 ± 0.20[b] ↔ RD, Prem	0.76 ± 0.52[c]	18 ± 7[d]	—	1.2 ± 0.33 µg/ml[e]

[a]Data for amphotericin B shown. Also formulated by liposomal encapsulation (ABELCET and AMBISOME); the distribution and CL properties of these products are different from the nonencapsulated form; a terminal $t_{\frac{1}{2}}$ of 173 ± 78 and 110 to 153 hours, respectively; however, an effective steady-state concentration can be achieved within 4 days. [b]Data for eight children (age 8 months to 14 years) yield a linear regression with CL decreasing with age: $CL = -0.046 \cdot$ age (years) + 0.86. Newborns show highly variable CL values. [c]Volume of central compartment. V_{ss} increases with dose from 3.4 l/kg for single 0.25 mg/kg doses to 8.9 l/kg for 1.5 mg/kg doses. [d]$t_{\frac{1}{2}}$ for multiple dosing. In single-dose studies, a prolonged dose-dependent $t_{\frac{1}{2}}$ is seen. [e]Following 0.5 mg/kg IV dose of amphotericin B given as a 1-hour infusion, once daily for 3 days. Whole blood concentrations (free and liposome encapsulated) of 1.7 ± 0.8 µg/ml and 83 ± 35 µg/ml were reported following a 5 mg · kg⁻¹ · day⁻¹ IV dose (presumed 60- to 120-min infusion) of ABELCET and AMBISOME, respectively.

References: Gallis, H.A., Drew, R.H., and Pickard, W.W. Amphotericin B: 30 years of clinical experience. *Rev. Infect. Dis.*, **1990**, *12*:308–329. *Physicians' Desk Reference*, 54th ed. Medical Economics Co., Montvale, NJ, **2000**, pp. 1090–1091, 1654.

	Oral Bioavailability (%)	Urinary Excretion (%)	Bound in Plasma (%)	Clearance	Volume of Distribution	Half-Life	Peak Time	Peak Concentration
ANASTROZOLE[a] (Chapters 51, 57)	80	<10	~40	− ↓LD[b]	—	50	≤2[c]	46 ng/ml[c]
APREPITANT[a] (Chapter 37)	60–65[b]	Negligible	>95	0.89–1.29[b]	1.0	9–13	4[c]	1.6 μg/ml[c]
ARIPIPRAZOLE[a] (Chapter 18)	87	<1	>99	0.83 ± 0.17[b]	4.9[b]	47 ± 10	3.0 ± 0.6[c]	242 ± 36 ng/ml[c]
ATAZANAVIR[a] (Chapter 50)	−[b] ↑Food	7	86	3.4 ± 1.0[c] ↓LD	1.6–2.7[c]	7.9 ± 2.9 ↑LD	2.5[d]	5.4 ± 1.4 μg/ml[d]

ANASTROZOLE

[a]Data from healthy pre- and postmenopausal female subjects. Metabolized by CYPs and UGTs. [b]CL/F reduced, stable alcoholic cirrhosis. [c]C_{max} and T_{max} following a single 3 mg oral dose. Accumulates three- to fourfold from single to multiple daily dosing.

References: Lonning, P.E., Geisler, J., and Dowsett, M. Pharmacological and clinical profile of anastrozole. *Breast Cancer Res. Treat.* **1998,** *49*(suppl 1):S53–S57; discussion S73–S77. *Physicians' Desk Reference,* 54th ed. Medical Economics Co., Montvale, NJ, **2000,** p. 537. Plourde, P.V., Dyroff, M., Dowsett, M., *et al.* ARIMIDEX: a new oral, once-a-day aromatase inhibitor. *J. Steroid Biochem. Mol. Biol.* **1995,** *53*:175–179.

APREPITANT

[a]Extensively metabolized, primarily by CYP3A4. No significant gender differences. [b]Exhibits a slightly disproportional increase in AUC with increasing oral dose. [c]Following a single 125 mg oral dose.

References: Physicians' Desk Reference, 58th ed. Medical Economics Co., Montvale, NJ, **2004,** pp. 1980–1981. Sanchez, R.I., Wang, R.W., *et al.* Cytochrome P450 3A4 is the major enzyme involved in the metabolism of the substance P receptor antagonist aprepitant. *Drug Metab. Dispos.,* **2004,** *32*:1287–1292.

ARIPIPRAZOLE

[a]Eliminated primarily by CYP2D6- and CYP3A4-dependent metabolism. The major metabolite, dehydro-aripiprazole, has affinity for D_2 receptors similar to parent drug; found at 40% of parent drug concentration in plasma; $t_{\frac{1}{2}}$ is 94 hrs. CYP2D6 poor metabolizers exhibit increased exposure (80%) to parent drug but reduced exposure (30%) to the active metabolite. No significant gender differences. [b]CL/F and V/F at steady state reported. [c]Following a 15 mg oral dose given once daily for 14 days.

References: DeLeon, A., Patel, N.C., and Crismon, M.L. Aripiprazole: a comprehensive review of its pharmacology, clinical efficacy, and tolerability. *Clin. Ther.,* **2004,** *26*:649–666. Mallikaarjun, S., Salazar, D.E., and Bramer, S.L. Pharmacokinetics, tolerability, and safety of aripiprazole following multiple oral dosing in normal healthy volunteers. *J. Clin. Pharmacol.,* **2004,** *44*:179–187. *Physicians' Desk Reference,* 58th ed. Medical Economics Co., Montvale, NJ, **2004,** pp. 1034–1035.

ATAZANAVIR

[a]Undergoes extensive hepatic metabolism, primarily by CYP3A. Pharmacokinetic data reported for healthy adults. No significant gender or age differences. [b]Absolute bioavailability is not known, but food enhances the extent of absorption. [c]CL/F and V/F reported. Metabolic elimination affected by inhibitors and inducers of CYP3A. Co-administration with low-dose ritonavir increases systemic atazanavir exposure. [d]Following a 400 mg oral dose given with a light meal once daily to steady state.

References: Orrick, J.J., and Steinhart, C.R. Atazanavir. *Ann. Pharmacother.,* **2004,** *38*:1664–1674. *Physicians' Desk Reference,* 58th ed. Medical Economics Co., Montvale, NJ, **2004,** p. 1081.

Table A–II–1 Pharmacokinetic Data (Continued)

AVAILABILITY (ORAL) (%)	URINARY EXCRETION (%)	BOUND IN PLASMA (%)	CLEARANCE ($ml \cdot min^{-1} \cdot kg^{-1}$)	VOL. DIST. (liters/kg)	HALF-LIFE (hours)	PEAK TIME (hours)	PEAK CONCENTRATIONS
ATENOLOL[a] (Chapters 30, 31, 32)							
58 ± 16	94 ± 8	<5	2.4 ± 0.3 ↓ Aged	1.3 ± 0.5[b]	6.1 ± 2.0[c] ↑ RD, Aged	3.3 ± 1.3[d]	0.28 ± 0.09 $\mu g/ml$[d]

[a]Atenolol is administered as a racemic mixture. No significant differences in the pharmacokinetics of the enantiomers. [b]V_{area} reported. [c]$t_\frac{1}{2}$ of d- and l- atenolol are similar. [d]Following a single 50 mg oral dose.

References: Boyd, R.A., Chin, S.K., Don-Pedro, O., Williams, R.L., and Giacomini, K.M. The pharmacokinetics of the enantiomers of atenolol. *Clin. Pharmacol. Ther.*, **1989,** *45:*403–410. Mason, W.D., Winer, N., Kochak, G., Cohen, I., and Bell. R. Kinetics and absolute bioavailability of atenolol. *Clin. Pharmacol. Ther.*, **1979,** *25:*408–415.

AVAILABILITY (ORAL) (%)	URINARY EXCRETION (%)	BOUND IN PLASMA (%)	CLEARANCE	VOL. DIST.	HALF-LIFE	PEAK TIME	PEAK CONCENTRATIONS
ATOMOXETINE[a] (Chapter 10)							
EM: 63[b] PM: 94[b]	1–2%	98.7 ± 0.3	EM: 6.2[b] PM: 0.60[b] EM: ↓ LD	EM: 2.3[b] PM: 1.1[b]	EM: 5.3[b] PM: 20[b]	EM/PM: 2[c]	EM: 160 ng/ml[c] PM: 915 ng/ml[c]

[a]Metabolized by CYP2D6 (polymorphic). Poor metabolizers (PM) exhibit a higher oral bioavailability, higher C_{max}, lower *CL*, and longer $t_\frac{1}{2}$ than extensive metabolizers (EM). No differences between adults and children over 6 years old. [b]*CL/F, V/F,* and $t_\frac{1}{2}$ measured at steady state. [c]Following a 20 mg oral dose given twice daily for 5 days.

References: Sauer, J.M., Ponsler, G.D., Mattiuz, E.L., Long, A.J., Witcher, J.W., Thomasson, H.R., and Desante, K.A. Disposition and metabolic fate of atomoxetine hydrochloride: the role of CYP2D6 in human disposition and metabolism. *Drug Metab. Dispos.,* **2003,** *31:*98–107. Simpson, D., and Plosker, G.L. Atomoxetine: a review of its use in adults with attention deficit hyperactivity disorder. *Drugs,* **2004,** *64:*205–222.

AVAILABILITY (ORAL) (%)	URINARY EXCRETION (%)	BOUND IN PLASMA (%)	CLEARANCE	VOL. DIST.	HALF-LIFE	PEAK TIME	PEAK CONCENTRATIONS
ATORVASTATIN[a] (Chapter 35)							
12	<2	≥98	29[b] ↓ Cirr[c], Aged ↔ RD	~5.4[b]	19.5 ± 9.6 ↑ Cirr[b], Aged	2.3 ± 0.96[d]	14.9 ± 1.8 ngEq/ml[d]

[a]Data from healthy adult male and female subjects. No clinically significant gender differences. Atorvastatin undergoes extensive CYP3A-dependent first-pass metabolism. Metabolites are active and exhibit a longer $t_\frac{1}{2}$ (20 to 30 hours) than parent drug. [b]Mean *CL/F* parameter calculated from reported *AUC* data at steady state after a once-a-day 20 mg oral dose, assuming a 70 kg body weight. [c]*AUC* following oral administration increased, mild-to-moderate hepatic impairment. [d]Following a 20 mg oral dose, once daily, for 14 days.

References: Gibson, D.M., Bron, N.J., *et al.* Effect of age and gender on pharmacokinetics of atorvastatin in humans. *J. Clin. Pharmacol.,* **1996,** *36:*242–246. Lea, A.P., and McTavish, D. Atorvastatin. A review of its pharmacology and therapeutic potential in the management of hyperlipidaemias. *Drugs,* **1997,** *53:*828–847. *Physicians' Desk Reference,* 54th ed. Medical Economics Co., Montvale, NJ, **2000,** p. 2254.

AVAILABILITY (ORAL) (%)	URINARY EXCRETION (%)	BOUND IN PLASMA (%)	CLEARANCE	VOL. DIST.	HALF-LIFE	PEAK TIME	PEAK CONCENTRATIONS
ATROPINE[a] (Chapter 7)							
50[b]	57 ± 8	14–22 ↔ Aged	8 ± 4[c] ↓ Aged	2.0 ± 1.1 ↑ Child	3.5 ± 1.5 ↑ Aged, Child	0.15 ± 0.04[d]	2.6 ± 0.5 ng/ml[d]

[a]Racemic mixture of active *l*-hyoscyamine and inactive *d*-hyoscyamine. [b]IM injection. [c]*l*-Hyoscyamine *CL* after an IM dose is threefold greater than that for *d*-hyoscyamine. [d]Mean for *l*-hyoscyamine after a single 0.02 mg/kg IM dose given to healthy adults

Reference: Kentala, E., Kaila, T., Iisalo, E., and Kanto, J. Intramuscular atropine in healthy volunteers: a pharmacokinetic and pharmacodynamic study. *Int. J. Clin. Pharmacol. Ther. Toxicol.,* **1990,** *28:* 399–404.

AZATHIOPRINE[a] (Chapters 51, 52)

60 ± 31[b]	<2	57 ± 31[c]	0.81 ± 0.65[c]	0.16 ± 0.07[c] ↔ RD	—	MP: 1–2[d]	MP: 20–90 ng/ml[d]

[a]Kinetic values are for IV azathioprine. Azathioprine is metabolized to mercaptopurine (MP), listed below. [b]Determined as the bioavailability of mercaptopurine; intact azathioprine is undetectable after oral administration because of extensive first-pass metabolism. [c]Data from kidney transplant patients. [d]Mercaptopurine concentration following a 135 ± 34 mg oral dose of azathioprine given daily to steady state in kidney transplant patients.

Reference: Lin, S.N., Jessup, K., *et al.* Quantitation of plasma azathioprine and 6-mercaptopurine levels in renal transplant patients. *Transplantation,* **1980,** 29:290–294.

AZITHROMYCIN (Chapter 46)

34 ± 19 ↓ Food (capsules) ↑ Food (suspension)	12	7–50[a]	9	31	40[b] ↔ Cirr	2–3[c]	0.4 µg/ml[c]

[a]Dose-dependent plasma binding. The bound fraction is 50% at 50 ng/ml and 12% at 500 ng/ml. [b]A longer terminal plasma $t_{\frac{1}{2}}$ of 68 ± 8 hours, reflecting release from tissue stores, overestimates the multiple-dosing $t_{\frac{1}{2}}$. [c]Following a 250 mg/day oral dose to adult patients with an infection.

Reference: Lalak, N.J., and Morris, D.L. Azithromycin clinical pharmacokinetics. *Clin. Pharmacokinet.,* **1993,** 25:370–374.

BACLOFEN[a] (Chapter 20)

>70[b]	69 ± 14	31 ± 11	2.72 ± 0.93[c] ↓ RD[d]	0.81 ± 0.12[c]	3.75 ± 0.96[c]	1.0 (0.5–4)[e]	160 ± 49 ng/ml[e]

[a]Data from healthy adult male subjects. [b]Bioavailability estimate based on urine recovery of unchanged drug after oral dose. [c]CL/F, V_{area}/F reported for intestinal infusion of drug. [d]Limited data suggest CL/F reduced with renal impairment. [e]Following a single 10 mg oral dose.

References: Kochak, G.M., Rakhit, A., *et al.* The pharmacokinetics of baclofen derived from intestinal infusion. *Clin. Pharmacol. Ther.,* **1985,** 38:251–257. Wuis, E.W., Dirks, M.J., *et al.* Plasma and urinary excretion kinetics of oral baclofen in healthy subjects. *Eur. J. Clin. Pharmacol.,* **1989,** 37:181–184.

BENAZEPRIL[a] (Chapter 30)

≥18[a]	B:<1 BT: 18[b,c]	B: 97 BT: 95[b] ↔ Aged, Hep	BT: 0.3–0.4[b,d]	BT: 0.12[b,d]	B: 0.7 BT: 10–11[b] ↔ Aged	B: 0.5–1.0[e] BT: 1–1.5[e]	B: ~300 nM[e] BT: ~500 nM[e]

[a]Benazepril (B) is a prodrug for the active metabolite, benazeprilat (BT). Minimum bioavailability of BT based on urinary recovery data. [b]Data for active metabolite; terminal $t_{\frac{1}{2}}$ ~22 hours. [c]Following an oral dose of benazepril. BT is cleared by renal and biliary excretion. [d]CL/F and V_{area}/F reported. [e]Following a single 10 mg oral dose given to healthy adults. C_{max} calculated from original data assuming a plasma density of 1 g/ml.

Reference: Balfour, J.A. and Goa, K.L. Benazepril. A review of its pharmacodynamic and pharmacokinetic properties, and therapeutic efficacy in hypertension and congestive heart failure. *Drugs,* **1991,** 42:511–539.

Table A–II–1 *Pharmacokinetic Data (Continued)*

	AVAILABILITY (ORAL) (%)	URINARY EXCRETION (%)	BOUND IN PLASMA (%)	CLEARANCE (ml · min⁻¹ · kg⁻¹)	VOL. DIST. (liters/kg)	HALF-LIFE (hours)	PEAK TIME (hours)	PEAK CONCENTRATIONS
BICALUTAMIDE[a] (Chapters 51, 58)	—	1.7 ± 0.3	96	R: 0.043 ± 0.013[b] S: 7.3 ± 4.0[b] ↔LD, RD, Aged	—	R: 139 ± 32 S: 29 ± 8.6 ↑LD[c]	R: 23.4[d] S: 20.7[d]	SD, R: 734 ng/ml[d] SD, S: 84 ng/ml[d] MD, R/S: 8.9 ± 3.5 µg/ml

[a]Data from healthy male subjects. Exhibits stereoselective metabolism—S-enantiomer, primarily glucuronidation; R-enantiomer, primarily oxidation. [b]CL/F reported for oral dose. [c]Increased $t_{\frac{1}{2}}$ of R-enantiomer, severe liver disease. [d]Following a single (SD) 50 mg oral dose (tablet) and 50 mg once-a-day oral dose (MD) to steady state.

References: Cockshott, I.D., Oliver, S.D., Young, J.J., Cooper, K.J., and Jones, D.C. The effect of food on the pharmacokinetics of the bicalutamide ("Casodex") enantiomers. *Biopharm. Drug Dispos.,* **1997,** *18*:499–507. McKillop, D., Boyle, G.W., *et al.* Metabolism and enantioselective pharmacokinetics of Casodex in man. *Xenobiotica,* **1993,** *23*:1241–1253. *Physicians' Desk Reference,* 54th ed. Medical Economics Co., Montvale, NJ, **2000,** p. 538.

	AVAILABILITY (ORAL) (%)	URINARY EXCRETION (%)	BOUND IN PLASMA (%)	CLEARANCE (ml · min⁻¹ · kg⁻¹)	VOL. DIST. (liters/kg)	HALF-LIFE (hours)	PEAK TIME (hours)	PEAK CONCENTRATIONS
BUPIVACAINE (Chapter 14)	—	2 ± 2	95 ± 1[a] ↓Neo	7.1 ± 2.8[b] ↑Child ↓Aged	0.9 ± 0.4[b] ↑Child	2.4 ± 1.2 ↔ Aged, Child	0.17–0.5[c]	0.8 µg/ml[c]

[a]Increased postoperatively with increased concentration of α_1-acid glycoprotein. [b]Blood *CL* and *V* reported; blood-to-plasma concentration ratio = 0.73 ± 0.05. [c]Following a single 100 mg epidural dose (20 ml of 0.5%) given to adult patients.

Reference: Mather, L.E., and Cousins, M.J. Local anaesthetics and their current clinical use. *Drugs,* **1979,** *18*:185–205.

	AVAILABILITY (ORAL) (%)	URINARY EXCRETION (%)	BOUND IN PLASMA (%)	CLEARANCE (ml · min⁻¹ · kg⁻¹)	VOL. DIST. (liters/kg)	HALF-LIFE (hours)	PEAK TIME (hours)	PEAK CONCENTRATIONS
BUPRENORPHINE[a] (Chapters 21, 23)	IM: 40->90 SL: 51 ± 30 BC: 28 ± 9	Negligible	96	13.3 ± 0.59 ↑Child[b]	1.44 ± 0.11 ↑Child[b]	2.33 ± 0.24 ↓Child	IM: 0.08[c] SL: 0.7 ± 0.1[c] BC: 0.8 ± 0.2[c]	IM: 3.6 ± 3.0 ng/ml[c] SL: 3.3 ± 0.8 ng/ml[c] BC: 2.0 ± 0.6 ng/ml[c]

[a]Data from male and female subjects undergoing surgery. Buprenorphine is metabolized in the liver by both oxidative (N-dealkylation) and conjugative pathways. [b]*CL,* 60 ± 19 ml · min⁻¹ · kg⁻¹; V_{ss}, 3.2 l/kg; $t_{\frac{1}{2}}$, 1.03 ± 0.22 hour; children 4 to 7 years of age. [c]Following a 0.3 mg IM, 4 mg sublingual (SL), 4 mg buccal (BC) dose.

References: Bullingham, R.E., McQuay, H.J., Moore, A., and Bennett, M.R. Buprenorphine kinetics. *Clin. Pharmacol. Ther.,* **1980,** 28:667–672. Cone, E.J., Gorodetzky, C.W., *et al.* The metabolism and excretion of buprenorphine in humans. *Drug Metab. Dispos.,* **1984,** *12:*577–581. Kuhlman, J.J., Lalani, S., *et al.* Human pharmacokinetics of intravenous, sublingual, and buccal buprenorphine. *J. Anal. Toxicol.,* **1996,** 20:369–378. Olkkola, K.T., Maunuksela, E.L., and Korpela, R. Pharmacokinetics of intravenous buprenorphine in children. *Br. J. Clin. Pharmacol.* **1989,** 28:202–204.

	AVAILABILITY (ORAL) (%)	URINARY EXCRETION (%)	BOUND IN PLASMA (%)	CLEARANCE (ml · min⁻¹ · kg⁻¹)	VOL. DIST. (liters/kg)	HALF-LIFE (hours)	PEAK TIME (hours)	PEAK CONCENTRATIONS
BUPROPION[a] (Chapters 17, 23)	—	<1	>80%	36.0 ± 2.2[b] ↓ Aged, Cirr[c] ↔ Alcohol	18.6 ± 1.2[b] ↔ Alcohol	11 ± 1[b] (7.9–18.4) ↑ Aged, Cirr[c] ↔ Alcohol	IR: 1.6 ± 0.1[d] SR: 3.1 ± 0.3[d]	IR: 141 ± 19 ng/ml[d] SR: 142 ± 28 ng/ml[d]

References: DeVane, C.L., Laizure, S.C., *et al.* Disposition of bupropion in healthy volunteers and subjects with alcoholic liver disease. *J. Clin. Psychopharmacol.*, **1990,** *10:*328–332. Hsyu, P.H., Singh, A., *et al.* Pharmacokinetics of bupropion and its metabolites in cigarette smokers versus nonsmokers. *J. Clin. Pharmacol.*, **1997,** *37:*737–743. *Physicians' Desk Reference,* 54th ed. Medical Economics Co., Montvale, NJ, **2000,** p. 1301. Posner, J., Bye, A., Dean, K., Peck, A.W., and Whiteman, P.D. The disposition of bupropion and its metabolites in healthy male volunteers after single and multiple doses. *Eur. J. Clin. Pharmacol.*, **1985,** *29:*97–103. Posner, J., Bye, A., Jeal, S., Peck, A.W., and Whiteman, P. Alcohol and bupropion pharmacokinetics in healthy male volunteers. *Eur. J. Clin. Pharmacol.*, **1984,** *26:*627–630.

^aData from healthy adult male volunteers. Bupropion appears to undergo extensive first-pass metabolism by CYP2B6 and other CYP isozymes. Some metabolites accumulate in blood and are active. ^bCL/F, V_{ss}/F, and $t_{\frac{1}{2}}$ reported for oral dose. Mean terminal $t_{\frac{1}{2}}$ from four different studies shown in parentheses. ^cCL/F reduced, alcoholic liver disease. ^dFollowing a single 100 mg immediate release (IR) or 150 mg sustained release (SR) dose.

BUSPIRONE^a (Chapters 11, 17)

3.9 ± 4.3 ↑Food^b	<0.1	28.3 ± 10.3 ↓Cirr^c, RD^d	>95	5.3 ± 2.6	2.4 ± 1.1 ↑Cirr, RD	0.71 ± 0.06^e	1.66 ± 0.21 ng/ml^e

^aData from healthy adult male subjects. No significant gender differences. Undergoes extensive CYP3A-dependent first-pass metabolism. The major metabolite (1-pyrimidinyl piperazine) is active in some behavioral tests in animals (one-fifth potency) and accumulates in blood to levels severalfold higher than buspirone. ^bBioavailability increased ~84%; appears to be secondary to reduced first-pass metabolism. ^cCL/F reduced, hepatic cirrhosis. ^dCL/F reduced, mild renal impairment; unrelated to CL_{cr}. ^eFollowing a single 20 mg oral dose.

References: Barbhaiya, R.H., Shukla, U.A., *et al.* Disposition kinetics of buspirone in patients with renal or hepatic impairment after administration of single and multiple doses. *Eur. J. Clin. Pharmacol.*, **1994,** *46:*41–47. Gammans, R.E., Mayol, R.F., and LaBudde, J.A. Metabolism and disposition of buspirone. *Am. J. Med.*, **1986,** *80:*41–51.

BUSULFAN (Chapter 51)

70 (44–94)	1	2.7–14	4.5 ± 0.9^a	0.99 ± 0.23^a	2.6 ± 0.5	2.6 ± 1.5	Low: 65 ± 27 ng/ml^b High: 949 ± 278 ng/ml^b

^aCL/F and V_{area}/F reported. ^bFollowing a single 4 mg oral dose (Low) given to patients with chronic myelocytic leukemia or a single 1 mg/kg oral dose (High) given as ablative therapy to patients undergoing bone marrow transplantation.

References: Ehrsson, H., Hassan, M., Ehrnebo, M., and Beran, M. Busulfan kinetics. *Clin. Pharmacol. Ther.*, **1983,** *34:*86–89. Schuler, U.S., Ehrsam, M., Schneider, A., Schmidt, H., Deeg, J., and Ehninger, G. Pharmacokinetics of intravenous busulfan and evaluation of the bioavailability of the oral formulation in conditioning for haematopoietic stem cell transplantation. *Bone Marrow Transplant.*, **1998,** *22:*241–244.

BUTORPHANOL^a (Chapter 21)

TN: 70 ± 20^b ↑LD	1.9 ± 1.5	80–83	40 ± 10 ↓LD^c, RD^d ↔Aged	12 ± 4 ↑LD	4.8 ± 1.6 ↑LD, RD	0.38 (0.25–1)^e	1.4 ± 0.6 ng/ml^e

^aData from healthy adult male and female subjects. Oral butorphanol undergoes extensive first-pass metabolism catalyzed by CYPs and UGT (F ~5% to 17%). ^bTransnasal spray (TN). ^cCL reduced, hepatic cirrhosis. ^dTransnasal CL/F reduced, moderate-to-severe renal impairment. ^eMean (range) following 1 mg transnasal spray.

References: Ramsey, R., Higbee, M., Maesner, J., and Wood, J. Influence of age on the pharmacokinetics of butorphanol. *Acute Care,* **1988,** *12*(suppl 1):8–16. Shyu, W.C., Morgenthien, E.A., and Barbhaiya, R.H. Pharmacokinetics of butorphanol nasal spray in patients with renal impairment. *Br. J. Clin. Pharmacol.*, **1996,** *41:*397–402. Vachharajani, N.N., Shyu, W.C., Garnett, W.R., Morgenthien, E.A., and Barbhaiya, R.H. The absolute bioavailability and pharmacokinetics of butorphanol nasal spray in patients with hepatic impairment. *Clin. Pharmacol. Ther.*, **1996,** *60:*283–294.

Table A–II–1 *Pharmacokinetic Data (Continued)*

AVAILABILITY (ORAL) (%)	URINARY EXCRETION (%)	BOUND IN PLASMA (%)	CLEARANCE $(ml \cdot min^{-1} \cdot kg^{-1})$	VOL. DIST. (liters/kg)	HALF-LIFE (hours)	PEAK TIME (hours)	PEAK CONCENTRATIONS
CALCITRIOL[a] (Chapter 61)							
Oral: ~61 IP: ~67	<10%	99.9	0.43 ± 0.04	—	16.5 ± 3.1[b] ↑Child[c]	Oral: 3–6[d] IP: 2–3[d]	IV: ~460 pg/ml[d] Oral: ~90 pg/ml[d] IP: ~105 pg/ml[d]

[a]Data from young (15 to 22 years) patients on peritoneal dialysis. Metabolized by 23-, 24-, and 26-hydroxylases and also excreted into bile as its glucuronide. [b]Calcitriol $t_{\frac{1}{2}}$ is 5 to 8 hours in healthy adult subjects. [c]Oral dose $t_{\frac{1}{2}} = 27 \pm 12$ hours, children 2 to 16 years. [d]Following a single 60 ng/kg IV, intraperitoneal (IP) dialysate, or oral dose. Baseline plasma levels were <10 pg/ml.

References: Jones, C.L., Vieth, R., *et al.* Comparisons between oral and intraperitoneal 1,25-dihydroxyvitamin D₃ therapy in children treated with peritoneal dialysis. *Clin. Nephrol.,* **1994,** *42*:44–49. *Physicians' Desk Reference,* 54th ed. Medical Economics Co. Montvale, NJ, **2000,** p. 2650. Salusky, I.B., Goodman, W.G., *et al.* Pharmacokinetics of calcitriol in continuous ambulatory and cycling peritoneal dialysis patients. *Am. J. Kidney Dis.,* **1990,** *16*:126–132. Taylor, C.A., Abdel-Rahman, E., Zimmerman, S.W., and Johnson, C.A. Clinical pharmacokinetics during continuous ambulatory peritoneal dialysis. *Clin. Pharmacokinet.,* **1996,** *31*:293–308.

AVAILABILITY (ORAL) (%)	URINARY EXCRETION (%)	BOUND IN PLASMA (%)	CLEARANCE $(ml \cdot min^{-1} \cdot kg^{-1})$	VOL. DIST. (liters/kg)	HALF-LIFE (hours)	PEAK TIME (hours)	PEAK CONCENTRATIONS
CANDESARTAN[a] (Chapters 30, 32)							
42 (34–56)	52	99.8	0.37 (0.31–0.47) ↓RD[b], ↔LD[c]	0.13 (0.09–0.17)	9.7 (4.8–13) ↑RD, ↔LD[c]	4.0 ± 1.3	119 ± 43 ng/ml[d]

[a]Data from healthy adult male subjects. Candesartan cilexetil is rapidly and completely converted to candesartan through the action of gut wall esterases. Mean (range) for candesartan reported. No significant gender or age differences. [b]*CL/F* reduced, mild renal disease. [c]Trend for longer $t_{\frac{1}{2}}$ and increased accumulation at steady state; moderate hepatic impairment. [d]Mean following a 16 mg oral dose (tablet) given daily for 7 days.

References: Hubner, R., Hogemann, A.M., Sunzel, M., and Riddell, J.G. Pharmacokinetics of candesartan after single and repeated doses of candesartan cilexetil in young and elderly healthy volunteers. *J. Hum. Hypertens.,* **1997,** *11*(suppl 2):S19–S25. Stoukides, C.A., McVoy, H.J., and Kaul, A.F. Candesartan cilexetil: an angiotensin II receptor blocker. *Ann. Pharmacother.,* **1999,** *33*:1287–1298. van Lier, J.J., van Heiningen, P.N., and Sunzel, M. Absorption, metabolism and excretion of ¹⁴C-candesartan and ¹⁴C-candesartan cilexetil in healthy volunteers. *J. Hum. Hypertens.,* **1997,** *11*(suppl 2):S27–S28.

AVAILABILITY (ORAL) (%)	URINARY EXCRETION (%)	BOUND IN PLASMA (%)	CLEARANCE $(ml \cdot min^{-1} \cdot kg^{-1})$	VOL. DIST. (liters/kg)	HALF-LIFE (hours)	PEAK TIME (hours)	PEAK CONCENTRATIONS
CAPECITABINE[a] (Chapter 51)							
— ↓Food[e]	3	<60	145(34%) 1 hour⁻¹ (m²)⁻¹ [b,c] ↓LD[d]	270 l/m² [b,c]	C: 1.3 (146%)[b] 5-FU: 0.72 (16%)[b]	C: 0.5 (0.5–1)[f] 5-FU: 0.5 (0.5–2.1)[f] ↓Food	C: 6.6 ± 6.0 μg/ml[f] 5-FU: 0.47 ± 0.47 μg/ml[f]

[a]Data from male and female patients with cancer. Capecitabine (C) is a prodrug for 5-FU (active), listed below. It is well absorbed, and bioactivation is sequential in liver and tumor. [b]Geometric mean (coefficient of variation). [c]*CL/F* and V_{area}/F reported for oral dose. [d]*CL/F* reduced with liver metastasis. [e]*AUC* for C and 5-FU decreased. [f]Following 1255 mg/m².

References: Dooley, M. and Goa, K.L. Capecitabine. *Drugs,* **1999,** *58*:69–76; discussion 77–78. Reigner, B., Verweij, J., *et al.* Effect of food on the pharmacokinetics of capecitabine and its metabolites following oral administration in cancer patients. *Clin. Cancer Res.,* **1998,** *4*:941–948.

CARBAMAZEPINE[a] (Chapter 19)

Bioavailability (Oral) (%)	Urinary Excretion (%)	Bound in Plasma (%)	Clearance (ml·min⁻¹·kg⁻¹)	Vol. Dist. (liters/kg)	Half-Life (hours)	Peak Time (hours)	Peak Concentration
>70	<1	74 ± 3 ↔ RD, Cirr, Preg	13 ± 0.5[b,c] ↑ Preg ↔ Child, Aged, Smk	1.4 ± 0.4[b] ↔ Child, Neo, Aged	15 ± 5[b,c] ↔ Child, Neo, Aged	4–8[d]	9.3 (2–18) μg/ml[d]

[a] A metabolite, carbamazepine-10,11-epoxide, is equipotent in animal studies. Its formation is catalyzed primarily by CYP3A and secondarily by CYP2C8. Values are CL/F and V_{area}/F. [b] Data from multiple-dose regimen. Carbamazepine induces its own metabolism; for a single dose, $CL/F = 0.36 \pm 0.07$ ml · min⁻¹ · kg⁻¹ and $t_{\frac{1}{2}} = 36 \pm 5$ hours. CL also increases with dose. [c] Data from oral, multiple-dose regimen; values are CL/F and V_{area}/F. [d] Mean (range) steady-state concentration following a daily 18.4-mg/kg oral dose (immediate release) given to adult patients with epilepsy. Therapeutic range for control of psychomotor seizures is 4–10 μg/ml.

References: Bertilsson, L., and Tomson, T. Clinical pharmacokinetics and pharmacological effects of carbamazepine and carbamazepine-10,11-epoxide. An update. *Clin. Pharmacokinet.,* **1986,** *11*:177–198. Troupin, A., Ojemann, L.M., *et al.* Carbamazepine—a double-blind comparison with phenytoin. *Neurology,* **1977,** *27*:511–519.

CARBIDOPA[a] (Chapter 20)

Bioavailability (Oral) (%)	Urinary Excretion (%)	Bound in Plasma (%)	Clearance (ml·min⁻¹·kg⁻¹)	Vol. Dist. (liters/kg)	Half-Life (hours)	Peak Time (hours)	Peak Concentration
—[b]	5.3 ± 2.1	—	18 ± 7[c]	—	~2	2.1 ± 1.0	S: 165 ± 77 ng/ml S-CR: 81 ± 28 ng/ml[d]

[a] Data from healthy adult subjects. Combined with levodopa for treatment of Parkinson's disease. [b] Absolute bioavailability is unknown, but it is presumably low based on a high value for CL/F. Bioavailability of SINEMET CR (S-CR) is 55% of standard SINEMET (S). [c] CL/F reported for 2 tablets of SINEMET 25/100. [d] Following a single oral dose of 2 tablets SINEMET 25/100 or 1 tablet SINEMET CR 50/200.

Reference: Yeh, K.C., August, T.F., Bush, D.F., Lasseter, K.C., Musson, D.G., Schwartz, S., Smith, M.E., and Titus, D.C. Pharmacokinetics and bioavailability of Sinemet CR: a summary of human studies. *Neurology,* **1989,** *39*:25–38.

CARBOPLATIN[a] (Chapter 51)

Bioavailability (Oral) (%)	Urinary Excretion (%)	Bound in Plasma (%)	Clearance (ml·min⁻¹·kg⁻¹)	Vol. Dist. (liters/kg)	Half-Life (hours)	Peak Time (hours)	Peak Concentration
—	77 ± 5	0	1.5 ± 0.3 ↓ RD	0.24 ± 0.03	2 ± 0.2 ↑ RD	0.5[b]	39 ± 17 μg/ml[b]

[a] Measure of ultrafilterable platinum, which is essentially unchanged carboplatin. [b] Following a single 170–500 mg/m² IV dose (30 minute infusion) given to adult patients with ovarian cancer.

Reference: Gaver, R.C., Colombo, N., *et al.* The disposition of carboplatin in ovarian cancer patients. *Cancer Chemother. Pharmacol.,* **1988,** *22*:263–270.

CARVEDILOL[a] (Chapters 31, 32, 33)

Bioavailability (Oral) (%)	Urinary Excretion (%)	Bound in Plasma (%)	Clearance (ml·min⁻¹·kg⁻¹)	Vol. Dist. (liters/kg)	Half-Life (hours)	Peak Time (hours)	Peak Concentration
25 *S*-(−): 15 *R*-(+): 31 ↑ Cirr	<2	95[b]	8.7 ± 1.7 ↓ Cirr ↔ RD, Aged	1.5 ± 0.3	2.2 ± 0.3[c] ↑, ↔ Cirr ↔ RD, Aged	1.3 ± 0.3[d]	105 ± 12 ng/ml[d]

[a] Racemic mixture: *S*-(−) enantiomer responsible for β_1 adrenergic receptor blockade. *R*-(+) and *S*-(−) enantiomers have nearly equivalent α_1-receptor blocking activity. [b] *R*-(+) enantiomer is more tightly bound than the *S*-(−) antipode. [c] Longer $t_{\frac{1}{2}}$s of about 6 hours have been measured at lower concentrations. [d] Following a 12.5 mg oral dose given twice a day for 2 weeks to healthy young adults.

References: Morgan, T. Clinical pharmacokinetics and pharmacodynamics of carvedilol. *Clin. Pharmacokinet.,* **1994,** *26*:335–346. Morgan, T., Anderson, A., Cripps, J., and Adam, W. Pharmacokinetics of carvedilol in older and younger patients. *J. Hum. Hypertens.,* **1990,** *4*:709–715.

Table A–II–1 *Pharmacokinetic Data (Continued)*

	AVAILABILITY (ORAL) (%)	URINARY EXCRETION (%)	BOUND IN PLASMA (%)	CLEARANCE $(ml \cdot min^{-1} \cdot kg^{-1})$	VOL. DIST. (liters/kg)	HALF-LIFE (hours)	PEAK TIME (hours)	PEAK CONCENTRATIONS
CASPOFUNGIN (Chapter 48)								
	—[a]	~2	96.5	0.16 (0.14–0.18) ↓LD	0.12[b]	9.6 ± 0.8[b]	—	8.7 (7.9–9.6) μg/ ml[c]

[a]Caspofungin is available for IV administration only. [b]Initial distribution volume and $t_{\frac{1}{2}}$ reported. Exhibits biphasic elimination with a larger V_{area} (0.3–2.1 l/kg) and longer (>25 hours) terminal $t_{\frac{1}{2}}$; the terminal phase accounts for a small fraction of the dose. [c]Following a 50 mg, 1 hour IV infusion given once daily for 14 days.

References: Stone, J.A., Holland, S.D., *et al.* Single- and multiple-dose pharmacokinetics of caspofungin in healthy men. *Antimicrob. Agents Chemother.,* **2002,** *46:*739–745. Stone, J.A., Xu, X., Winchell, G.A., Deutsch, P.J., Pearson, P.G., Migoya, E.M., Mistry, G.C., Xi, L., Miller, A., Sandhu, P., Singh, R., deLuna, F., Dilzer, S.C., and Lasseter, K.C. Disposition of caspofungin: role of distribution in determining pharmacokinetics in plasma. *Antimicrob. Agents Chemother.,* **2004,** *48:*815–823.

CEFAZOLIN (Chapter 44)								
	>90	80 ± 16	89 ± 2 ↓RD, Cirr, CPBS, Neo, Child	0.95 ± 0.17 ↓RD, CPBS ↑Preg ↔Neo, Obes, Child, Cirr	0.19 ± 0.06[a] ↑RD, Neo ↔Preg, Obes, Child Cirr	2.2 ± 0.02 ↑RD, Neo, CPBS ↓Preg, Cirr ↔Obes, Child	IM: 1.7 ± 0.7[b]	IV: 237 ± 285 μg/ ml[b] IM: 42 ± 9.5 μg/ ml[b]

[a]V_{area} reported. [b]Following a single 1 g IV (model-fitted C_{max}) or IM dose to healthy adults.

Reference: Scheld, W.M., Spyker, D.A., *et al.* Moxalactam and cefazolin: comparative pharmacokinetics in normal subjects. *Antimicrob. Agents Chemother.,* **1981,** *19:*613–619.

CEFDINIR (Chapter 44)								
	CAP: 16–21[a] SUSP: 25[a] ↓Iron	13–23[b]	89[c] ↓RD	11–15[d]	1.6–2.1[d]	1.4–1.5	CAP: 3 ± 0.7[e] SUSP: 2 ± 0.4[e]	CAP: 2.9 ± 1.0 μg/ ml[e] SUSP: 3.9 ± 0.6 μg/ml[e]

[a]Bioavailability following ingestion of a capsule (CAP) or suspension (SUSP) formulated spectrum cephalosporin. *Pediatr. Infect. Dis. J.,* **2000,** *19:*S141–S146. *Physicians' Desk Reference,* 58th ed. Medical Economics Co., Montvale, NJ, **2004,** p. 503. Tomino, Y., Fukui, M., Hamada, C., Inoue, S., and Osada, S. Pharmacokinetics of cefdinir and its transfer to dialysate in patients with chronic renal failure undergoing continuous ambulatory peritoneal dialysis. *Arzneimittelforschung,* **1998,** *48:*862–867.

[a]Bioavailability following ingestion of a capsule (CAP) or suspension (SUSP) formulated dose. [b]Determined after a single oral dose. [c]Lower plasma protein binding (71–74%) reported in patients undergoing dialysis. [d]CL/F and V/F reported. [e]Following ingestion of a single 600 mg capsule given to adults or a 14 mg/kg suspension dose given to children (6 months to 12 years). No accumulation after multiple dosing.

References: Guay, D.R. Pharmacodynamics and pharmacokinetics of cefdinir, an oral extended

CEFEPIME[a] (Chapter 44)

Drug								
	—	80	16–19	1.8 (1.7–2.5)[b] ↓RD[d]	0.26 (0.24–0.31)[c]	2.1 (1.3–2.4)[b] ↑RD[d]	—	65 ± 7 μg/ml[e]

[a]Data from healthy adult patients. Available only in parenteral form. [b]Median (range) of reported CL and $t_{1/2}$ values from 16 single-dose studies. [c]Median (range) of reported V_{ss} from 6 single-dose studies. [d]Mild renal impairment. [e]Following a 1 g IV dose.

References: Okamoto, M.P., Nakahiro, R.K., Chin, A., and Bedikian, A. Cefepime clinical pharmacokinetics. Clin. Pharmacokinet., 1993, 25:88–102. Rybak, M. The pharmacokinetic profile of a new generation of parenteral cephalosporin. Am. J. Med., 1996, 100:39S–44S.

CEFIXIME (Chapter 44)

Drug								
	47 ± 15	41 ± 7	67 ± 1	1.3 ± 0.2 ↓RD	0.30 ± 0.03	3.0 ± 0.4 ↑RD	3–4[a]	1.7–2.9 μg/ml[a]

[a]Range of mean data from different studies following a single 200 mg oral dose (capsule) given to healthy adults. Minimal accumulation with twice-a-day dosing.

Reference: Brogden, R.N. and Campoli-Richards, D.M. Cefixime. A review of its antibacterial activity. Pharmacokinetic properties and therapeutic potential. Drugs, 1989, 38:524–550.

CEFOTETAN (Chapter 44)

Drug								
	—	67 ± 11	85 ± 4 ↔CF	$CL = 0.23CL_{cr} + 0.14$ ↓RD	0.14 ± 0.03 ↔RD	3.6 ± 1.0 ↑RD	IM: 1.5–3[a]	IV, B: 336–491 μg/ml[a] / IV, I: 38 μg/ml[a] / IM: 91 μg/ml[a]

[a]Range of mean C_{max} from different studies following a single 2-g IV bolus (IV, B) dose or mean C_{max} and T_{max} following a single 2 g IM dose. Mean C_{ss} was 38 μg/ml following a 12-hour, 76 mg/hour constant rate IV infusion (IV, I) in healthy adults.

Reference: Martin, C., Thomachot, L., and Albanese, J. Clinical pharmacokinetics of cefotetan. Clin. Pharmacokinet., 1994, 26:248–258.

CEFTAZIDIME (Chapter 44)

Drug								
	— / IM: 91	84 ± 4 ↔CF	21 ± 6	$CL = 1.05CL_{cr} + 0.12$ ↔CF, Burn	0.23 ± 0.02 ↔RD, CF ↑Aged, Burn	1.6 ± 0.1 ↑RD, Prem, Neo, Aged ↔CF	IM: 0.7–1.3[a]	IV: 119–146 μg/ml[a] / IM: 29–39 μg/ml[a]

[a]Range of mean data from different studies following a 1 g bolus IV or IM dose given to healthy adults.

Reference: Balant, L., Dayer, P., and Auckenthaler, R. Clinical pharmacokinetics of the third generation cephalosporins. Clin. Pharmacokinet., 1985, 10:101–143

CEFUROXIME (Chapter 44)

Drug								
	32 (21–44)[a] ↑Food	96 ± 10	33 ± 6	$CL = 0.94CL_{cr} + 0.28$	0.20 ± 0.04 ↔RD, Aged	1.7 ± 0.6 ↑RD ↔Child	2–3[b]	7–10 μg/ml[b]

[a]Cefuroxime axetil, a prodrug of cefuroxime. [b]Range of data following a single 500 mg oral dose of cefuroxime axetil given to healthy adults.

References: Emmerson, A.M. Cefuroxime axetil. J. Antimicrob. Chemother., 1988, 22:101–104. Williams, P.E., and Harding, S.M. The absolute bioavailability of oral cefuroxime axetil in male and female volunteers after fasting and after food. J. Antimicrob. Chemother., 1984, 13:191–196.

Table A–II–1 Pharmacokinetic Data (Continued)

AVAILABILITY (ORAL) (%)	URINARY EXCRETION (%)	BOUND IN PLASMA (%)	CLEARANCE (ml·min⁻¹·kg⁻¹)	VOL. DIST. (liters/kg)	HALF-LIFE (hours)	PEAK TIME (hours)	PEAK CONCENTRATIONS
CELECOXIB[a] (Chapter 26)							
— ↑Food[b]	<3	~97	6.60 ± 1.85 ↓ Aged, LD[c] ↑ RD[d]	6.12 ± 2.08	11.2 ± 3.47	2.8 ± 1.0[e] ↑ Food	705 ± 268 ng/ml[e]

[a]Data from healthy subjects. Cleared primarily by CYP2C9 (polymorphic). [b]High-fat meal. Absolute bioavailability is unknown. [c]CL/F reduced, mild or moderate hepatic impairment. [d]CL/F increased, moderate renal impairment, but unrelated to CL_{cr}. [e]Following a single 200 mg oral dose.

References: Goldenberg, M.M. Celecoxib, a selective cyclooxygenase-2 inhibitor for the treatment of rheumatoid arthritis and osteoarthritis. *Clin. Ther.,* **1999,** *21*:1497–1513; discussion 1427–1428. *Physicians' Desk Reference,* 54th ed. Medical Economics Co., Montvale, NJ, **2000,** p. 2334.

AVAILABILITY (ORAL) (%)	URINARY EXCRETION (%)	BOUND IN PLASMA (%)	CLEARANCE (ml·min⁻¹·kg⁻¹)	VOL. DIST. (liters/kg)	HALF-LIFE (hours)	PEAK TIME (hours)	PEAK CONCENTRATIONS
CEPHALEXIN[a] (Chapter 44)							
90 ± 9	91 ± 18	14 ± 3	4.3 ± 1.1[a] ↓ RD	0.26 ± 0.03[a] ↔ RD	0.90 ± 0.18 ↑ RD	1.4 ± 0.8[b]	28 ± 6.4 µg/ml[b]

[a]Assuming 70 kg body weight. [b]Following a single 500 mg oral dose given to healthy male adults.

Reference: Spyker, D.A., Thomas, B.L., Sande, M.A., and Bolton, W.K. Pharmacokinetics of cefaclor and cephalexin: dosage nomograms for impaired renal function. *Antimicrob. Agents Chemother.,* **1978,** *14*:172–177.

AVAILABILITY (ORAL) (%)	URINARY EXCRETION (%)	BOUND IN PLASMA (%)	CLEARANCE (ml·min⁻¹·kg⁻¹)	VOL. DIST. (liters/kg)	HALF-LIFE (hours)	PEAK TIME (hours)	PEAK CONCENTRATIONS
CETIRIZINE[a] (Chapter 24)							
>70	70.9 ± 7.8	98.8 ± 0.8[b]	0.74 ± 0.19[c] ↓ LD,[d] RD,[e] Aged ↑ Child[f]	0.58 ± 0.16[c]	9.42 ± 2.4 ↑ LD, RD, Aged ↓ Child	0.9 ± 0.2[g]	313 ± 45 ng/ml[g]

[a]Data from healthy male and female subjects. [b]f_b also reported as ~93%. [c]CL/F, V_d/F reported for oral dose. [d]CL/F reduced, hepatocellular and cholestatic liver disease. [e]CL/F reduced, moderate-to-severe renal impairment. [f]CL/F increased, 2-5 years of age. [g]Following a single 10 mg oral dose.

References: Horsmans, Y., Desager, J.P., Hulhoven, R., and Harvengt, C. Single-dose pharmacokinetics of cetirizine in patients with chronic liver disease. *J. Clin. Pharmacol.,* **1993,** *33*:929–932. Matzke, G.R., Yeh, J., Awni, W.M., Halstenson, C.E., and Chung, M. Pharmacokinetics of cetirizine in the elderly and patients with renal insufficiency. *Ann. Allergy,* **1987,** *59*:25–30. *Physicians' Desk Reference,* 54th ed. Medical Economics Co., Montvale, NJ, **2000,** p. 2404. Spicak, V., Dab, I., *et al.* Pharmacokinetics and pharmacodynamics of cetirizine in infants and toddlers. *Clin. Pharmacol. Ther.,* **1997,** *61*:325–330.

AVAILABILITY (ORAL) (%)	URINARY EXCRETION (%)	BOUND IN PLASMA (%)	CLEARANCE (ml·min⁻¹·kg⁻¹)	VOL. DIST. (liters/kg)	HALF-LIFE (hours)	PEAK TIME (hours)	PEAK CONCENTRATIONS
CHLOROQUINE[a] (Chapters 39, 40)							
~80	52–58[b]	(S): 66.6 ± 3.3[c] (R): 42.7 ± 2.1 ↔ RD	3.7–13[b]	132–261[b]	10–24 days[b,d]	IM: 0.25[e] Oral: 3.6 ± 2[e]	IV: 837 ± 248 ng/ml[c] IM: 57–480 ng/ml Oral: 76 ± 14 ng/ml

References: Krishna, S., and White, N.J. Pharmacokinetics of quinine, chloroquine and amodiaquine. Clinical implications. *Clin. Pharmacokinet.,* **1996,** *30:*263–299. White, N.J. Clinical pharmacokinetics of antimalarial drugs. *Clin. Pharmacokinet.,* **1985,** *10:*187–215.

[a] Active metabolite, desethylchloroquine, accounts for 20 ± 3% of urinary excretion; $t_\frac{1}{2}$ = 15 ± 6 days. Racemic mixture; kinetic parameters for the two isomers are slightly different (*e.g.,* mean residence time = 16.2 days and 11.3 days for the (*R*)-isomer and (*S*)-isomer, respectively). [b] Range of mean values from different studies (IV administration). [c] Concentrates in red blood cells. Blood-to-plasma concentration ratio for racemate = 9. [d] A longer $t_\frac{1}{2}$ (41 ± 14 days) has been reported with extended blood sampling. [e] Following a single 300 mg IV (24 minute infusion) of chloroquine HCl, or IM or oral dose of chloroquine phosphate given to healthy adults. Effective concentrations against *Plasmodium vivax* and *Plasmodium falciparum* are 15 ng/ml and 30 ng/ml, respectively. Diplopia and dizziness can occur above 250 ng/ml.

CHLORPHENIRAMINE[a] (Chapter 24)

41 ± 16	0.3–26[b]	70 ± 3	1.7 ± 0.1 ↑Child	3.2 ± 0.3 ↔Child	20 ± 5 ↓Child	IR: 2–3 / SR: 5.7–8.1[c]	IR: 16–71 ng/ml[c] / SR: 17–76 ng/ml[c]

[a] Administered as a racemic mixture; reported parameters are for racemic drug. Activity comes predominantly from *S*-(+) enantiomer, which has a 60% longer $t_\frac{1}{2}$ than the *R*-(−) enantiomer. [b] Renal elimination increases with increased urine flow and lower pH. [c] Range of data from different studies following a 4 mg oral immediate release (IR) dose given every 4 to 6 hours to steady state or following an 8 mg oral sustained release (SR) dose given every 12 hours to steady state, both in healthy adults.

Reference: Rumore, M.M. Clinical pharmacokinetics of chlorpheniramine. *Drug Intell. Clin. Pharm.,* **1984,** *18:*701–707.

CHLORPROMAZINE[a] (Chapters 18, 37)

32 ± 19[b]	<1	95–98 ↔RD	8.6 ± 2.9[c] ↓Child[d] ↔Cirr	21 ± 9[c]	30 ± 7[c]	1–4[e]	25–150 ng/ml[e]

[a] Active metabolites, 7-hydroxychlorpromazine ($t_\frac{1}{2}$ = 25 ± 15 hours) and possibly chlorpromazine *N*-oxide, yield *AUC*s comparable to the parent drug (single doses). [b] After single dose. Bioavailability may decrease to about 20% with repeated dosing. [c] *CL/F*, V_{area}, and terminal $t_\frac{1}{2}$ following IM administration. [d] Following a 100 mg oral dose given twice a day for 33 days to adult patients. Neurotoxicity (tremors and convulsions) occurs at concentrations of 750–1000 ng/ml.

Reference: Dahl, S.G., and Strandjord, R.E. Pharmacokinetics of chlorpromazine after single and chronic dosage. *Clin. Pharmacol. Ther.,* **1977,** *21:*437–448.

CHLORTHALIDONE (Chapter 28)

64 ± 10	65 ± 9[a] ↓Aged	75 ± 1	0.04 ± 0.01[a] ↓Aged	0.14 ± 0.07	47 ± 22[b] ↑Aged	13.8 ± 6.3[c]	3.7 ± 0.9 μg/ml[c]

[a] Value is for 50 and 100 mg doses; renal *CL* is decreased at an oral dose of 200 mg, and there is a concomitant decrease in the percentage excreted unchanged. [b] Chlorthalidone is sequestered in erythrocytes. $t_\frac{1}{2}$ is longer if blood, rather than plasma, is analyzed. Parameters reported based on blood concentrations. [c] Following a single 50 mg oral dose (tablet) given to healthy male adults.

Reference: Williams, R.L., Blume, C.D., Lin, E.T., Holford, N.H., and Benet, L.Z. Relative bioavailability of chlorthalidone in humans: adverse influence of polyethylene glycol. *J. Pharm. Sci.,* **1982,** *71:*533–535.

Table A–II–1 Pharmacokinetic Data (Continued)

AVAILABILITY (ORAL) (%)	URINARY EXCRETION (%)	BOUND IN PLASMA (%)	CLEARANCE ($ml \cdot min^{-1} \cdot kg^{-1}$)	VOL. DIST. (liters/kg)	HALF-LIFE (hours)	PEAK TIME (hours)	PEAK CONCENTRATIONS
CIDOFOVIR[a] (Chapter 49)							
SC: 98±10 Oral: <5	70.1±21.4[b]	<6	2.1±0.6[b] ↓RD[c]	0.36±0.13[b]	2.3±0.5[b] ↑RD	—	19.6±7.2 µg/ml[d]

[a]Data from patients with HIV infection and positive for CMV. Cidofovir is activated intracellularly by phosphokinases. For parenteral use. [b]Parameters reported for a dose given in the presence of probenecid. [c]CL reduced, mild renal impairment (cleared by high flux hemodialysis). [d]Following a single 5 mg/kg IV infusion given over 1 hour, with concomitant oral probenecid and active hydration.

References: Brody, S.R., Humphreys, M.H., et al. Pharmacokinetics of cidofovir in renal insufficiency and in continuous ambulatory peritoneal dialysis or high-flux hemodialysis. Clin. Pharmacol. Ther., **1999**, 65:21–28. Cundy, K.C., Petty, B.G., et al. Clinical pharmacokinetics of cidofovir in human immunodeficiency virus-infected patients. Antimicrob. Agents Chemother., **1995**, 39:1247–1252. Physicians' Desk Reference, 54th ed. Medical Economics Co., Montvale, NJ, **2000**, p. 1136. Wachsman, M., Petty, B.G., et al. Pharmacokinetics, safety and bioavailability of HPMPC (cidofovir) in human immunodeficiency virus-infected subjects. Antiviral Res., **1996**, 29:153–161.

AVAILABILITY (ORAL) (%)	URINARY EXCRETION (%)	BOUND IN PLASMA (%)	CLEARANCE ($ml \cdot min^{-1} \cdot kg^{-1}$)	VOL. DIST. (liters/kg)	HALF-LIFE (hours)	PEAK TIME (hours)	PEAK CONCENTRATIONS
CIMETIDINE (Chapter 36)							
60±23[a]	62±20[a] ↔Cirr, CF	19 (13–25)[a]	8.3±2.0 ↓RD, Aged ↔Ulcer, Cirr ↑Burn, CF	1.0±0.2 ↔RD, Cirr, Ulcer, Burn ↑CF	2.0±0.3 ↑RD ↔Ulcer, Cirr, CF ↓Burn	0.5–1.5[b] ↑Food	2–3 µg/ml[b]

[a]Patients with peptic ulcer disease. [b]Following a single 400 mg oral dose given after an overnight fast to healthy adults. A second peak (2 to 4 hours) is often observed when cimetidine is given after fasting but not when given with food. A concentration of 0.5–0.9 µg/ml will suppress >80% of basal acid secretion and >50% of food or gastrin-stimulated secretion and will maintain gastric pH ≥4 in patients with active peptic ulcer disease.

References: Grahnen, A., von Bahr, C., Lindstrom, B., and Rosen, A. Bioavailability and pharmacokinetics of cimetidine. Eur. J. Clin. Pharmacol., **1979**, 16:335–340. Schentag, J.J., Cerra, F.B., et al. Age, disease, and cimetidine disposition in healthy subjects and chronically ill patients. Clin. Pharmacol. Ther., **1981**, 29:737–743. Somogyi, A., Rohner, H.G., and Gugler, R. Pharmacokinetics and bioavailability of cimetidine in gastric and duodenal ulcer patients. Clin. Pharmacokinet., **1980**, 5:84–94.

AVAILABILITY (ORAL) (%)	URINARY EXCRETION (%)	BOUND IN PLASMA (%)	CLEARANCE ($ml \cdot min^{-1} \cdot kg^{-1}$)	VOL. DIST. (liters/kg)	HALF-LIFE (hours)	PEAK TIME (hours)	PEAK CONCENTRATIONS
CINACALCET[a] (Chapters 51, 61)							
~20 ↑Food	—[b]	93–97	~18 ↓LD	~17.6	34±9 ↑LD	2–6	10.6±2.8 ng/ml[c]

[a]Cinacalcet is a chiral molecule; the R-enantiomer is more potent than the S-enantiomer and is thought to be responsible for the drug's pharmacological activity. Cinacalcet is metabolized primarily by CYP3A4, CYP2D6, and CYP1A2. [b]Unreported, but presumably negligible. [c]Following a single 75 mg oral dose.

References: Joy, M.S., Kshirsagar, A.V., and Franceschini, N. Calcimimetics and the treatment of primary and secondary hyperparathyroidism. Ann. Pharmacother., **2004**, 38:1871–1880. Kumar, G.N., Sproul, C., et al. Metabolism and disposition of calcimimetic agent cinacalcet HCl in humans and animal models. Drug Metab. Dispos., **2004**, 32:1491–1500. Pharmacology and Toxicology Review of NDA. Application 21-688. U.S. FDA, CDER Available at: http://www.fda.gov/cder/foi/nda/2004/21-688.pdf_Sensipar_Pharmr_P1.pdf. Accessed October 27, 2004.

CIPROFLOXACIN (Chapter 43)

60 ± 12	50 ± 5	40	7.6 ± 0.8[a] ↓ RD, Aged ↑ CF	2.2 ± 0.4[a] ↓ Aged ↔ CF	3.3 ± 0.4 ↑ RD ↔ Aged ↓ CF	0.6 ± 0.2[b]	2.5 ± 1.1 µg/ml[b]

[a]V_{area} reported. [b]Following a 500 mg oral dose given twice daily for 3 or more days to patients with chronic bronchitis or bronchiectasis.

References: Begg, E.J., Robson, R.A., *et al.* The pharmacokinetics of oral fleroxacin and ciprofloxacin in plasma and sputum during acute and chronic dosing. *Br. J. Clin. Pharmacol.,* **2000,** *49:*32–38. Sorgel, F., Jaehde, U., Naber, K., and Stephan, U. Pharmacokinetic disposition of quinolones in human body fluids and tissues. *Clin. Pharmacokinet.,* **1989,** *16*(suppl 1):5–24.

CISPLATIN (Chapter 51)

—	2.3 ± 9	—[b]	6.3 ± 1.2	0.28 ± 0.07	0.53 ± 0.10	—	2Hr: 3.4 ± 1.1 µg/ml[c] 7Hr: 1.0 ± 0.4 µg/ml[c]

[a]Early studies measured total platinum, rather than the parent compound; values reported here are for parent drug in seven patients with ovarian cancer (mean $CI_{cr} = 66 ± 27$ ml/minute). [b]Platinum will form a tight complex with plasma proteins (90%). [c]Following a single 100 mg/m² IV dose given as a ~2- or 7-hour infusion to ovarian cancer patients.

Reference: Reece, P.A., Stafford, I., Davy, M., and Freeman, S. Disposition of unchanged cisplatin in patients with ovarian cancer. *Clin. Pharmacol. Ther.,* **1987,** *42:*320–325.

CITALOPRAM (Chapter 17)

Rac: 80 ± 13	Rac: 10.5 ± 1.4 Es: 8	Rac: 80 Es: 56	Rac: 4.3 ± 1.2[b] Es: 8.8 ± 3.2[b,c] ↓ Aged, LD[d]	Rac: 12.3 ± 2.3 Es: 15.4 ± 2.4[c]	Rac: 33 ± 4[b] Es: 22 ± 6[b] ↑ Aged, LD[d], RD[e]	Rac/Es: 4–5[f]	Rac: 50 ± 9 ng/ml[f] Es: 21 ± 4 ng/ml[f]

[a]Citalopram is available either as a racemic mixture or as the pure active S-enantiomer escitalopram. Pharmacokinetic data after dosing of the racemate (Rac) and escitalopram (Es) are reported. No significant gender differences. Citalopram is metabolized by CYP2C19 (polymorphic) and CYP3A4 to desmethylcitalopram. [b]Data from CYP2C19 extensive metabolizers. CYP2C19 poor metabolizers exhibit a lower (~44%) CL/F and longer $t_{\frac{1}{2}}$ than extensive metabolizers. [c]CL/F and V/F for escitalopram reported. [d]Alcoholic, viral, or biliary cirrhosis. [e]Moderate renal impairment. [f]Following a single 40 mg (Rac) or 20 mg (Es) oral dose.

References: Gutierrez, M.M., Rosenberg, J., and Abramowitz, W. An evaluation of the potential for pharmacokinetic interaction between escitalopram and the cytochrome P450 3A4 inhibitor ritonavir. *Clin. Ther.,* **2003,** *25:*1200–1210. Joffe, P., Larsen, F.S., *et al.* Single-dose pharmacokinetics of citalopram in patients with moderate renal insufficiency or hepatic cirrhosis compared with healthy subjects. *Eur. J. Clin. Pharmacol.* **1998,** *54:*237–242. *Physicians' Desk Reference,* 58th ed. Medical Economics Co., Montvale, **2004,** pp. 1292, 1302–1303. Sidhu, J., Priskorn, M., *et al.* Steady-state pharmacokinetics of the enantiomers of citalopram and its metabolites in humans. *Chirality,* **1997,** *9:*686–692. Sindrup, S.H., Brosen, K., *et al.* Pharmacokinetics of citalopram in relation to the sparteine and the mephenytoin oxidation polymorphisms. *Ther. Drug Monit.,* **1993,** *15:*11–17.

Table A–II–1 Pharmacokinetic Data (Continued)

AVAILABILITY (ORAL) (%)	URINARY EXCRETION (%)	BOUND IN PLASMA (%)	VOL. DIST. (liters/kg)	CLEARANCE ($ml \cdot min^{-1} \cdot kg^{-1}$)	HALF-LIFE (hours)	PEAK TIME (hours)	PEAK CONCENTRATIONS
CLARITHROMYCIN[a] (Chapter 46)							
55 ± 8[b]	36 ± 7[b] ↔ Aged	42–50	2.6 ± 0.5 ↔ Aged ↑ Cirr	7.3 ± 1.9[b] ↓ Aged, RD ↔ Cirr	3.3 ± 0.5[b] ↑ Aged, RD, Cirr	C: 2.8[c] HC: 3[c]	C: 2.4 μg/ml[c] HC: 0.7 μg/ml[c]

[a]Active metabolite, 14(R)-hydroxyclarithromycin. [b]Data generated for a 250 mg oral dose. At higher doses, metabolic *CL* saturates, resulting in increases in the % urinary excretion and $t_\frac{1}{2}$ and decrease in *CL*. [c]Mean data for clarithromycin (C) and 14-hydroxyclarithromycin (HC), following a 500 mg oral dose given twice daily to steady state in healthy adults.

Reference: Fraschini, F., Scaglione, F., and Demartini, G. Clarithromycin clinical pharmacokinetics. *Clin. Pharmacokinet.*, **1993**, 25:189–204.

AVAILABILITY (ORAL) (%)	URINARY EXCRETION (%)	BOUND IN PLASMA (%)	VOL. DIST. (liters/kg)	CLEARANCE ($ml \cdot min^{-1} \cdot kg^{-1}$)	HALF-LIFE (hours)	PEAK TIME (hours)	PEAK CONCENTRATIONS
CLINDAMYCIN (Chapter 46)							
~87[a] Topical: 2	13	93.6 ± 0.2	1.1 ± 0.3[b] ↔ RD, Child	4.7 ± 1.3 ↔ Child	2.9 ± 0.7 ↔ Child, RD, Preg ↑ Prem	—	IV: 17.2 ± 3.5 μg/ml[c] Oral: 2.5 μg/ml[d]

[a]Clindamycin hydrochloride given orally. [b]V_{area} reported. [c]Following a 1200 mg IV dose (30 minute infusion) of clindamycin phosphate (prodrug) given twice daily to steady state in healthy male adults. [d]Following a single 150 mg oral dose of clindamycin hydrochloride to adults.

References: Physicians' Desk Reference, 54th ed. Medical Economics Co., Montvale, NJ, **2000**, p. 2421. Plaisance, K.I., Drusano, G.L., Forrest, A., Townsend, R.J., and Standiford, H.C. Pharmacokinetic evaluation of two dosage regimens of clindamycin phosphate. *Antimicrob. Agents Chemother.*, **1989**, 33:618–620.

AVAILABILITY (ORAL) (%)	URINARY EXCRETION (%)	BOUND IN PLASMA (%)	VOL. DIST. (liters/kg)	CLEARANCE ($ml \cdot min^{-1} \cdot kg^{-1}$)	HALF-LIFE (hours)	PEAK TIME (hours)	PEAK CONCENTRATIONS
CLONAZEPAM (Chapters 16, 17)							
98 ± 31	<1	86 ± 0.5 ↓ Neo	3.2 ± 1.1	1.55 ± 0.28[a,b]	23 ± 5	Oral: 2.5 ± 1.3[c]	IV: 3–29 ng/ml[c] Oral: 17 ± 5.4 ng/ml[c]

[a]*CL/F* reported; this value is consistent for a number of studies but is higher than the *CL* determined in a single study of IV administration. [b]Metabolized by CYP3A. [c]Range of C_{max} values following a single 2 mg IV dose (model-fitted for bolus dose) or mean following a 2 mg oral dose (tablet) given to healthy adults. Most patients, including children, whose seizures are controlled by clonazepam have steady-state concentrations in the range of 5 to 70 ng/ml. However, patients who do not respond and those with side effects achieve similar levels.

Reference: Berlin, A., and Dahlstrom, H. Pharmacokinetics of the anticonvulsant drug clonazepam evaluated from single oral and intravenous doses and by repeated oral administration. *Eur. J. Clin. Pharmacol.*, **1975**, 9:155–159.

AVAILABILITY (ORAL) (%)	URINARY EXCRETION (%)	BOUND IN PLASMA (%)	VOL. DIST. (liters/kg)	CLEARANCE ($ml \cdot min^{-1} \cdot kg^{-1}$)	HALF-LIFE (hours)	PEAK TIME (hours)	PEAK CONCENTRATIONS
CLONIDINE (Chapter 32)							
Oral: 95 TD: 60	62 ± 11	20	2.1 ± 0.4	3.1 ± 1.2 ↓ RD	12 ± 7 ↑ RD	Oral: 2[a] TD: 72[a]	Oral: 0.8 ng/ml[a] TD: 0.3–0.4 ng/ml[a]

Reference: Lowenthal, D.T., Matzek, K.M., and MacGregor, T.R. Clinical pharmacokinetics of clonidine. *Clin. Pharmacokinet.,* **1988,** *14:*287–310

[a]Mean data following a 0.1-mg oral dose given twice a day to steady state or C_{ss} following a 3.5 cm² transdermal (TD) patch administered to normotensive male adults. Concentrations of 0.2 to 2 ng/ml are associated with a reduction in blood pressure; >1 ng/ml will cause sedation and dry mouth.

CLORAZEPATE[a] (Chapters 16, 19)

N: 91 ± 6[a]	N: <1	N: 97.5 ↓ RD ↔ Obes, Aged[c]	N: 0.17 ± 0.02[b] ↑ Smk ↓ Hep, Cirr, Obes, Aged[c]	N: 1.24 ± 0.09[b] ↑ Obes, Preg ↔ Hep, Cirr, Aged	N: 93 ± 11[b] ↑ Obes, Preg, Aged[c] ↓ Hep, Cirr, Smk	N: 0.72 ± 0.01[a,d]	N: 275 ± 27 ng/ml[a,d]

[a]Clorazepate is essentially a prodrug for nordiazepam (N). Bioavailability, peak time, and peak concentration values for N were derived after oral administration of clorazepate. [b]CL, V_{ss}, and $t_{\frac{1}{2}}$ values are for IV nordiazepam. [c]Significantly different for male subjects only. [d]Data for nordiazepam following a 20 mg IM dose of clorazepate given to nonpregnant women.

References: Greenblatt, D.J., Divoll, M.K., *et al.* Desmethyldiazepam pharmacokinetics: studies following intravenous and oral desmethyldiazepam, oral clorazepate, and intravenous diazepam. *J. Clin. Pharmacol.,* **1988,** 28:853–859. Rey, E., d'Athis, P., *et al.* Pharmacokinetics of clorazepate in pregnant and non-pregnant women. *Eur. J. Clin. Pharmacol.,* **1979,** *15:*175–180.

CLOZAPINE (Chapter 18)

55 ± 12	<1	>95	6.1 ± 1.6	5.4 ± 3.5	12 ± 4	1.9 ± 0.8[a]	546 ± 307 ng/ml[a]

[a]Following titration up to a 150 mg oral dose (tablet) given twice daily for 7 days to adult chronic schizophrenics.

References: Choc, M.G., Lehr, R.G., *et al.* Multiple-dose pharmacokinetics of clozapine in patients. *Pharm. Res.,* **1987,** *4:*402–405. Jann, M.W., Ereshefsky, L., and Saklad, S.R. Clinical pharmacokinetics of the depot antipsychotics. *Clin. Pharmacokinet.,* **1985,** *10:*315–333.

CODEINE[a] (Chapter 21)

50 ± 7[b]	Negligible	7	11 ± 2[c]	2.6 ± 0.3[c]	2.9 ± 0.7	C: 1.0 ± 0.5[d] M: 1.0 ± 0.4[d]	C: 149 ± 60 ng/ml[d] M: 3.8 ± 2.4 ng/ml[d]

[a]Codeine is metabolized by CYP2D6 (polymorphic) to morphine. Analgesic effect is thought to be due largely to derived morphine. [b]Oral/IM bioavailability reported. [c]CL/F and V_{area}/F reported. [d]Data for codeine (C) and morphine (M) following a 60 mg oral codeine dose given three times daily for 7 doses to healthy male adults.

Reference: Quiding, H., Anderson, P., Bondesson, U., Boreus, L.O., and Hynning, P.A. Plasma concentrations of codeine and its metabolite, morphine, after single and repeated oral administration. *Eur. J. Clin. Pharmacol.,* **1986,** *30:*673–677.

CYCLOPHOSPHAMIDE[a] (Chapters 51, 52)

74 ± 22	6.5 ± 4.3	13	1.3 ± 0.5 ↑ Child ↓ Cirr ↔ RD	0.78 ± 0.57 ↔ Child	7.5 ± 4.0 ↓ Child ↑ Cirr	—	121 ± 21 μM[b]

[a]Cyclophosphamide is primarily activated by CYP2C9 to hydroxycyclophosphamide. The metabolite is further converted to the active alkylating species, phosphoramide mustard ($t_{\frac{1}{2}}$ = 9 hours) and nornitrogen mustard (apparent $t_{\frac{1}{2}}$ = 3.3 hours). Kinetic parameters are for cyclophosphamide. [b]Following a 600 mg/m² IV (bolus) dose given to breast cancer patients.

References: Grochow, L.B., and Colvin, M. Clinical pharmacokinetics of cyclophosphamide. *Clin. Pharmacokinet.,* **1979,** *4:*380–394. Moore, M.J., Erlichman, C., *et al.* Variability in the pharmacokinetics of cyclophosphamide, methotrexate and 5-fluorouracil in women receiving adjuvant treatment for breast cancer. *Cancer Chemother. Pharmacol.,* **1994,** *33:*472–476.

Table A-II-1 *Pharmacokinetic Data (Continued)*

	AVAILABILITY (ORAL) (%)	URINARY EXCRETION (%)	BOUND IN PLASMA (%)	CLEARANCE (ml · min⁻¹ · kg⁻¹)	VOL. DIST. (liters/kg)	HALF-LIFE (hours)	PEAK TIME (hours)	PEAK CONCENTRATIONS
CYCLOSPORINE (Chapter 52)								
	SI: 28 ± 18[a,b]	<1	93 ± 2	5.7 (0.6–24)[b,c] ↓ Hep, Cirr, Aged ↔ RD ↑ Child	4.5 (0.12–15.5)[b] ↓ Aged ↑ Child	10.7 (4.3–53)[b] ↓ Child ↔ Aged	NL: 1.5–2[d] SI: 4.0 ± 1.8[d]	NL: 1333 ±469 ng/ml[d] SI: 1101 ±570 ng/ml[d]

[a]NEORAL (NL) exhibits a more uniform and slightly greater (125% to 150%) relative oral bioavailability than the SANDIMMUNE (SI) formulation. [b]Pharmacokinetic parameters based on measurements in blood with a specific assay. Data from renal transplant patients shown. [c]Metabolized by CYP3A to three major metabolites, which are subsequently biotransformed to numerous secondary and tertiary metabolites. [d]Steady-state C_{max} following a 344 ± 122 mg/day oral dose (divided into two doses) of cyclosporine (NL, soft gelatin capsule) or a 14 mg/kg per day (range 6–22 mg/kg per day) oral dose of cyclosporine (SI) given to adult renal transplant patients in stable condition. Mean trough concentration after NL was 251 ± 116 ng/ml; therapeutic range (trough) is 150–400 ng/ml.

References: Fahr, A. Cyclosporin clinical pharmacokinetics. *Clin. Pharmacokinet.*, **1993**, *24*:472–495. *Physicians' Desk Reference*, 54th ed. Medical Economics Co., Montvale, NJ, **2000**, pp. 2034–2035. Pollak, R., Wong, R.L., and Chang, C.T. Cyclosporine bioavailability of Neoral and Sandimmune in white and black de novo renal transplant recipients. Neoral Study Group. *Ther. Drug Monit*, **1999**, *21*:661–663. Ptachcinski, R.J., Venkataramanan, R., *et al.* Cyclosporine kinetics in renal transplantation. *Clin. Pharmacol. Ther.*, **1985**, *38*:296–300.

	AVAILABILITY (ORAL) (%)	URINARY EXCRETION (%)	BOUND IN PLASMA (%)	CLEARANCE (ml · min⁻¹ · kg⁻¹)	VOL. DIST. (liters/kg)	HALF-LIFE (hours)	PEAK TIME (hours)	PEAK CONCENTRATIONS
CYTARABINE[a] (Chapter 51)								
	<20	11 ± 8	13	13 ± 4	3.0 ± 11.9[b]	2.6 ± 0.6	—	IV, B: ~5 µg/ml[c] IV, I: 0.05–0.1 µg/ml[c]

[a]Liposome formulation of cytarabine given intrathecally. Cerebrospinal fluid $t_{\frac{1}{2}}$ = 100 to 263 hours for liposome formulation (compared to 3.4 hours for intrathecal dose of free drug). [b]V_{area} reported. [c]C_{max} following a single 200 mg/m² IV bolus (IV, B) dose or steady-state plasma concentration following a 112 mg/m² per day constant-rate IV infusion (IV, I) given to patients with leukemia, malignant melanoma, or solid tumors.

References: Ho, D.H., and Frie, E.I. Clinical pharmacology of 1-β-D-arabinofuranosyl cytosine. *Clin. Pharmacol. Ther.*, **1971**, *12*:944–954. Wan, S.H., Huffman, D.H., Azarnoff, D.L., Hoogstraten, B., and Larsen, W.E. Pharmacokinetics of 1-β-D-arabinofuranosylcytosine in humans. *Cancer Res.*, **1974**, *34*:392–397.

	AVAILABILITY (ORAL) (%)	URINARY EXCRETION (%)	BOUND IN PLASMA (%)	CLEARANCE (ml · min⁻¹ · kg⁻¹)	VOL. DIST. (liters/kg)	HALF-LIFE (hours)	PEAK TIME (hours)	PEAK CONCENTRATIONS
DAPSONE (Chapters 47, 62)								
	93 ± 8[a]	5–15[b]	73 ± 1 ↔ RD, Cirr	0.60 ± 0.17[c] ↔ Cirr, Child ↑ Neo	1.0 ± 0.1 ↔ Cirr	22.4 ± 5.6 ↔ Cirr, Child	SD: 2.1 ± 0.8[d]	SD: 1.6 ± 0.4 µg/ml[d] MD: 3.3 µg/ml[d]

[a]Decreased in severe leprosy (70–80); estimates based on urinary recovery of radioactive dose. [b]Urine pH = 6–7. [c]Undergoes reversible metabolism to a monoacetyl metabolite; the reaction is catalyzed by NAT2 (polymorphic); also undergoes N-hydroxylation (CYP3A, CYP2C9). [d]Following a single 100 mg oral dose (SD) or a 100 mg oral dose given once daily to steady state (MD) in healthy adults.

| — | 47 ± 12 | 92 | 0.14 ± 0.01 ↓RD[b] | 7.8 ± 1.0 ↑RD[b] | — | 99 ± 12 µg/ml[c] |

References: Mirochnick, M., Cooper, E., *et al.* Pharmacokinetics of dapsone administered daily and weekly in human immunodeficiency virus-infected children. *Antimicrob. Agents Chemother.,* **1999,** *43*:2586–2591. Pieters, F.A., and Zuidema, J. The pharmacokinetics of dapsone after oral administration to healthy volunteers. *Br. J. Clin. Pharmacol.,* **1986,** *22*:491–494. Venkatesan, K. Clinical pharmacokinetic considerations in the treatment of patients with leprosy. *Clin. Pharmacokinet.,* **1989,** *16*:365–386. Zuidema, J., Hilbers-Modderman, E.S., and Merkus, F.W. Clinical pharmacokinetics of dapsone. *Clin. Pharmacokinet.,* **1986,** *11*:299–315.

DAPTOMYCIN (Chapter 46)

| —[a] | | | 0.096 ± 0.009 ↑RD[b] | 7.8 ± 1.0 ↑RD[b] | — | 99 ± 12 µg/ml[c] |

[a]Available for IV administration only. [b]Changes reported for patients with severe renal impairment. [c]Peak concentration at the end of a 30 minute IV infusion of a 6 mg/kg dose given once daily for 7 days. No significant accumulation with multiple dosing.

References: Dvorchik, B.H., Brazier, D., DeBruin, M.F., and Arbeit, R.D. Daptomycin pharmacokinetics and safety following administration of escalating doses once daily to healthy subjects. *Antimicrob. Agents Chemother.,* **2003,** *47*:1318–1323. Product Information: Cubicin™ (daptomycin for injection). Cubist Pharmaceuticals, Lexington, MA, **2004.**

DEXTROAMPHETAMINE[a] (Chapter 10)

| —[b] | Rac: 23–26 / Dextro: 3.4–7.7[d] acidic urine / Dextro: 0.23–1.71[d] alkaline urine | Rac: 14.5[c] | Rac: 6.11 ± 0.22 / Rac: 3.5–4.2[d] acidic urine / Rac: 14–22[d] alkaline urine / Dextro: 6.8 ± 0.5[e] uncontrolled urine pH | Dextro: 3.1 ± 1.1[f] | | Dextro: 61 ± 20 ng/ml[f] |

[a]Amphetamine is available as a racemate (Rac), dextro-isomer (Dextro), and a mixture of the two, in both immediate- and extended-release formulations. Pharmacokinetic data on both racemic and dextroamphetamine are presented. [b]Absolute bioavailability not reported; > 55% based on urine recovery of unchanged drug under acidic urine pH conditions. [c]Measured under uncontrolled urinary pH condition. Renal CL of amphetamine is dependent on urine pH. Acidification of urine results in increased urinary excretion, up to 55%. [d]CL/F and $t_{\frac{1}{2}}$ following oral dose to adults is reported. [e]$t_{\frac{1}{2}}$ in children reported. [f]Following a 20 mg immediate-release oral dose given once daily for more than a week. An extended-release formulation consisting of a mixture of dextroamphetamine and amphetamine salts (ADDERALL XR®) exhibits a delayed t_{max} of ~7 hours.

References: Busto, U., Bendayan, R., and Sellers, E.M. Clinical pharmacokinetics of non-opiate abused drugs. *Clin. Pharmacokinet.,* **1989,** *16*:1–26. Helligrel, E.T., Arora, S., Nelson, M., and Robertson, P. Steady-state pharmacokinetics and tolerability of modafinil administered alone or in combination with dextroamphetamine in healthy volunteers. *J. Clin. Pharmacol.,* **2002,** *42*:450–460. McGough, J.J., Biederman, J., *et al.* Pharmacokinetics of SLI381 (ADDERALL XR), an extended-release formulation of adderall. *J. Am. Acad. Adolesc. Psychiatry,* **2003,** *42*:684–691.

Table A–II–1 *Pharmacokinetic Data (Continued)*

AVAILABILITY (ORAL) (%)	URINARY EXCRETION (%)	BOUND IN PLASMA (%)	CLEARANCE $(ml \cdot min^{-1} \cdot kg^{-1})$	VOL. DIST. (liters/kg)	HALF-LIFE (hours)	PEAK TIME (hours)	PEAK CONCENTRATIONS
DEXTROMETHORPHAN[a] (Chapter 21)							
—	EM: 0.19 ± 0.21 PM: 11.1 ± 3.0	—	EM: 1575 ± 658^{b} PM: $\sim 3.9 \pm 1.4^{b}$	—	EM: 3.4 ± 0.5^{b} PM: 29.5 ± 8.4^{b}	2–2.5	EM: 5.2 ± 1.8 ng/ml[c] PM: 33 ± 8.2 ng/ml[c]

[a]Data from healthy subjects. Extensive CYP2D6-dependent first-pass metabolism to dextrorphan (pharmacologically active). Data for extensive (EM) and poor (PM) metabolizers shown. [b]CL/F and $t_{\frac{1}{2}}$ reported for oral dose. [c]Following a single 60 mg oral dose to presumed EM or 30 mg to PM. C_{max} for dextrorphan was 879 ± 60 ng/ml in EMs and undetected in PMs.

References: Schadel, M., Wu, D., Otton, S.V., Kalow, W., and Sellers, E.M. Pharmacokinetics of dextromethorphan and metabolites in humans: influence of the CYP2D6 phenotype and quinidine inhibition. *J. Clin. Psychopharmacol.,* **1995,** *15:*263–269. Silvasti, M., Karttunen, P., *et al.* Pharmacokinetics of dextromethorphan and dextrorphan: a single dose comparison of three preparations in human volunteers. *Int. J. Clin. Pharmacol. Ther. Toxicol.,* **1987,** *25:*493–497.

AVAILABILITY (ORAL) (%)	URINARY EXCRETION (%)	BOUND IN PLASMA (%)	CLEARANCE $(ml \cdot min^{-1} \cdot kg^{-1})$	VOL. DIST. (liters/kg)	HALF-LIFE (hours)	PEAK TIME (hours)	PEAK CONCENTRATIONS
DIAZEPAM[a] (Chapters 16, 17)							
Oral: 100 ± 14 Rectal: 90	<1	98.7 ± 0.2 ↓ RD, Cirr, NS, Preg, Neo, Alb, Burn, Aged ↔ HTh	0.38 ± 0.06^{a} ↑ Alb ↓ Cirr ↔ Aged, Smk, HTh	1.1 ± 0.3 ↑ Cirr, Aged, Alb ↔ RD, HTh	43 ± 13^{a} ↑ Aged, Cirr ↔ HTh	Oral: 1.3 ± 0.2^{b} Rectal: 1.5^{b}	IV: 400–500 ng/ml[b] Oral: 317 ± 27 ng/ml[b] Rectal: ~ 400 ng/ml[b]

[a]Active metabolites, desmethyldiazepam and oxazepam, formed by CYP2C19 (polymorphic) and CYP3A. [b]Range of data following a single 5–10 mg IV dose (15-30 second bolus) or mean data following a single 10 mg oral or 15 mg rectal dose given to healthy adults. A concentration of 300 to 400 ng/ml provides anxiolytic effect, and >600 ng/ml provides control of seizures.

References: Friedman, H., Greenblatt, D.J., *et al.* Pharmacokinetics and pharmacodynamics of oral diazepam: effect of dose, plasma concentration, and time. *Clin. Pharmacol. Ther.,* **1992,** *52:*139–150. Greenblatt, D.J., Allen, M.D., Harmatz, J.S., and Shader, R.I. Diazepam disposition determinants. *Clin. Pharmacol. Ther.,* **1980,** *27:*301–312. *Physicians' Desk Reference,* 54th ed. Medical Economics Co, Montvale, NJ, **2000,** p. 1012.

AVAILABILITY (ORAL) (%)	URINARY EXCRETION (%)	BOUND IN PLASMA (%)	CLEARANCE $(ml \cdot min^{-1} \cdot kg^{-1})$	VOL. DIST. (liters/kg)	HALF-LIFE (hours)	PEAK TIME (hours)	PEAK CONCENTRATIONS
DICLOFENAC (Chapter 26)							
54 ± 2	<1	>99.5	4.2 ± 0.9^{a} ↓ Aged ↔ RD, Cirr, RA	0.17 ± 0.11^{b} ↑ RA	1.1 ± 0.2 ↔ RA	EC: 2.5 (1.0–4.5)[c] SR: 5.3 ± 1.5^{c}	EC: 2.0 (1.4–3.0) μg/ml[c] SR: 0.42 ± 0.17 μg/ml[c]

[a]Cleared primarily by CYP2C9-catalyzed 4'-hydroxylation; urine and biliary metabolites account for 30% and 10–20% of dose, respectively. [b]V_{area} reported. [c]Following a single 50 mg enteric-coated tablet (EC) or 100 mg of sustained-release tablet (SR) given to healthy adults.

References: Tracy, T. Nonsteroidal antiinflammatory drugs. In, *Metabolic Drug Interactions.* (Levy, R.H., Thummel, K.T., Trager, W.F., Hansten, P.D., and Eichelbaum, M., eds.) Lippincott Williams & Wilkins, Philadelphia, **2000,** pp. 457–468. Willis, J.V., Kendall, M.J., Flinn, R.M., Thornhill, D.P., and Welling, P.G. The pharmacokinetics of diclofenac sodium following intravenous and oral administration. *Eur. J. Clin. Pharmacol.,* **1979,** *16:*405–410.

DICLOXACILLIN (Chapter 44)

50–85	60±7	95.8±0.2 ↓RD, Aged, Cirr ↔CF	1.6±0.3[a] ↓RD ↑CF[b]	0.086±0.017 ↑RD, CF	0.70±0.07 ↑RD ↔CF	0.5–1.6[c]	47–91 μg/ml[c]

[a]Possible saturation of renal CL at doses of 1–2 g. [b]Concomitant increase in CL of both dicloxacillin and creatinine. [c]Estimated range of data following a single 2 g oral dose given to healthy (fasted) adults.

Reference: Nauta, E.H., and Mattie, H. Dicloxacillin and cloxacillin: pharmacokinetics in healthy and hemodialysis subjects. *Clin. Pharmacol. Ther.*, **1976**, *20*:98–108.

DIDANOSINE (Chapter 51)

38±15 ↓Child, Food[a]	36±9 ↔Child	<5	16±7 ↔Child	1.0±0.2	1.4±0.3	B: 0.67 (0.33–1.33)[b] EC: 2.0 (1.0–5.0)[b]	B: 1.5±0.7 μg/ml[a] EC: 0.93±0.43 μg/ml[b] ↓Food[a]

[a]The magnitude of the food effect may depend on the product used (Videx® vs generic didanosine), the type of meal consumed (light vs high-fat) and whether or not didanosine is coadministered with tenofovir, an inhibitor of didanosine metabolism. [b]Following a single 400-mg oral dose of didanosine formulated as a buffered tablet (B) solution or enteric-coated beads (EC), taken after a fast by patients with HIV infection.

References: Knupp, C.A., Shyu, W.C., *et al.* Pharmacokinetics of didanosine in patients with acquired immunodeficiency syndrome or acquired immunodeficiency syndrome-related complex. *Clin. Pharmacol. Ther.*, **1991**, *49*:523–535. Damle, B.D., Kaul, S., Behr, D., and Knupp C. Bioequivalence of two formulations of didanosine, encapsulated enteric-coated beads and buffered tablet, in healthy volunteers and HIV-infected subjects. *J. Clin. Pharmacol.*, **2002**, *42*:791–797. Pecora Fulco, P., and Kirian, M.A. Effect of tenofovir on didanosine absorption. *Ann. Pharmacother.*, **2003**, *37*:1325–1328.

DIGOXIN (Chapters 33, 34)

70±13[a,c] ↔RD, MI, CHF, LTh, HTh, Aged	60±11 ↓RD	25±5 ↓RD	$CL = (0.88CL_{cr} + 0.33)^{b,c}$ ↓LTh ↑HTh, Neo, Child, Preg	$V = (3.12CL_{cr} + 3.84)$ ↓LTh ↑HTh ↔CHF	39±13 ↓HTh ↑RD, CHF, Aged, LTh ↔Obes	1–3[d]	NT: 1.4±0.7 ng/ml[d] T: 3.7±1.0 ng/ml[d]

[a]LANOXIN tablets; digoxin solutions, elixirs, and capsules may be absorbed more completely. [b]Equation applies to patients with some degree of heart failure. If heart failure is not present, the coefficient of CL_{cr} is 1.0. Units of CL_{cr} must be ml·min⁻¹·kg⁻¹. [c]In the occasional patient, digoxin is metabolized to an inactive metabolite, dihydrodigoxin, by gut flora. This results in a reduced oral bioavailability. [d]Following an oral dose of 0.31 ± 0.19 mg/day or 0.36 ± 0.19 mg/day in patients with congestive heart failure who exhibited no signs of digitalis toxicity (NT) or signs of toxicity (T), respectively. Concentrations >0.8 ng/ml are associated with inotropic effect. Concentrations of 1.7, 2.5, and 3.3 ng/ml are associated with a 10%, 50%, and 90% probability of digoxin-induced arrhythmias, respectively.

References: Mooradian, A.D. Digitalis. An update of clinical pharmacokinetics, therapeutic monitoring techniques and treatment recommendations. *Clin. Pharmacokinet.*, **1988**, *15*:165–179. Smith, T.W. and Haber, E. Digoxin intoxication: the relationship of clinical presentation to serum digoxin concentration. *J. Clin. Invest*, **1970**, *49*:2377–2386.

Table A–II–1 *Pharmacokinetic Data (Continued)*

	AVAILABILITY (ORAL) (%)	URINARY EXCRETION (%)	BOUND IN PLASMA (%)	CLEARANCE (ml · min⁻¹ · kg⁻¹)	VOL. DIST. (liters/kg)	HALF-LIFE (hours)	PEAK TIME (hours)	PEAK CONCENTRATIONS
DILTIAZEM[a] (Chapters 31, 32, 34)	38 ± 11	<4	78 ± 3	11.8 ± 2.2[b] ↔ Aged ↓ RD	3.3 ± 1.2 ↔ Aged ↓ RD	4.4 ± 1.3[c] ↔ RD, Aged	4.0 ± 0.4[d]	151 ± 46 ng/ml[d]
DIPHENHYDRAMINE (Chapter 24)	72 ± 26	1.9 ± 0.8 ↔ Cirr	78 ± 3 ↓ Cirr	6.2 ± 1.7[a] ↔ Cirr ↑ Child ↓ Aged	4.5 ± 2.8[a,b] ↔ Cirr	8.5 ± 3.2[a] ↑ Cirr, Aged ↓ Child	Oral: 2.3 ± 0.64[c]	IV: ~230 ng/ml[c] Oral: 66 ± 22 ng/ml[c]
DOCETAXEL[a] (Chapter 51)	—	2.1 ± 0.2	94	22.6 ± 7.7 liters·h⁻¹·(m²)⁻¹ ↓ LD[b]	72 ± 24 l/m²	13.6 ± 6.1	—	2.4 ± 0.9 µg/ml[c]
DOFETILIDE[a] (Chapter 34)	96 (83–108)	52 ± 2[b]	64	5.23 ± 0.30 ↓ RD[b]	3.44 ± 0.25	7.5 ± 0.4 ↑ RD[b]	1–2.5	2.3 ± 1.1 ng/ml[c]

DILTIAZEM

[a]Active metabolites, desacetyldiltiazem ($t_{\frac{1}{2}}$ = 9 ± 2 hours) and *N*-desmethyldiltiazem ($t_{\frac{1}{2}}$ = 7.5 ± 1 hours). Formation of desmethyl metabolite (major pathway of *CL*) catalyzed primarily by CYP3A. [b]More than a twofold decrease with multiple dosing. [c]$t_{\frac{1}{2}}$ for oral dose is 5 to 6 hours; does not change with multiple dosing. [d]Following single 120 mg oral dose to healthy adults.

Reference: Echizen, H., and Eichelbaum, M. Clinical pharmacokinetics of verapamil, nifedipine and diltiazem. *Clin. Pharmacokinet.* **1986**, *11*:425–449.

DIPHENHYDRAMINE

[a]Increased *CL*, decreased *V*, and no change in $t_{\frac{1}{2}}$ in Asians, presumably due to decreased plasma protein binding. [b]V_{area} reported. [c]Following a single 50 mg dose of diphenhydramine hydrochloride (44 mg base) given IV or orally to fasted healthy adults. Levels >25 ng/ml provide antihistaminic effect, whereas levels >60 ng/ml are associated with drowsiness and mental impairment.

Reference: Blyden, G.T., Greenblatt, D.J., Scavone, J.M., and Shader, R.I. Pharmacokinetics of diphenhydramine and a demethylated metabolite following intravenous and oral administration. *J. Clin. Pharmacol.* **1986**, *26*:529–533.

DOCETAXEL

[a]Data from male and female patients treated for cancer. Metabolized by CYP3A and excreted into bile. Parenteral administration. [b]Mild-to-moderate liver impairment. [c]Following IV infusion of 85 mg/m² over 1.6 hours.

References: Clarke, S.J., and Rivory, L.P. Clinical pharmacokinetics of docetaxel. *Clin. Pharmacokinet.* **1999**, *36*:99–114. Extra, J.M., Rousseau, F., *et al.* Phase I and pharmacokinetic study of Taxotere (RP 56976; NSC 628503) given as a short intravenous infusion. *Cancer Res.* **1993**, *53*:1037–1042. *Physicians' Desk Reference*, 54th ed. Medical Economics Co., Montvale, NJ, **2000**, p. 2578.

DONEPEZIL[a] (Chapter 20)

—[b]	10.6 ± 2.7	92.6 ± 0.9[c]	2.90 ± 0.74[d] ↓ LD[e] ↔ RD	14.0 ± 2.42[d] ↑ Aged	59.7 ± 16.1[d] ↑ Aged	3–4[f]	30.8 ± 4.2 ng/ml[f]

[a]Data from healthy male subjects. Metabolized by CYP3A4. [b]CL/F reduced with renal impairment. [c]Following a single 0.55 mg oral dose.

References: Kalus, J.S., and Mauro, V.F. Dofetilide: a class III-specific antiarrhythmic agent. Ann. Pharmacother., 2000, 34:44–56. Smith, D.A., Rasmussen, H.S., Stopher, D.A., and Walker, D.K. Pharmacokinetics and metabolism of dofetilide in mouse, rat, dog and man. Xenobiotica, 1992, 22:709–719. Tham, T.C., MacLennan, B.A., Burke, M.T., and Harron, D.W. Pharmacodynamics and pharmacokinetics of the class III antiarrhythmic agent dofetilide (UK-68,798) in humans. J. Cardiovasc. Pharmacol., 1993, 21:507–512.

DOXEPIN[a] (Chapter 17)

30 ± 10[b]	~0	82 (75–89)	14 ± 3[c]	24 ± 7[c,d]	18 ± 5	D: 0.5–1 DD: 4–12	D: 28 ± 11 ng/ml[e] DD: 39 ± 19 ng/ml[e]

[a]Data from young, healthy male and female subjects. No significant gender differences. Metabolized by CYP2D6, CYP3A4, UGT. [b]Absolute bioavailability is unknown, but the oral dose is reportedly well absorbed. [c]Af_b of 96% has also been reported. [d]CL/F, V_{ss}/F, and $t_{\frac{1}{2}}$ reported for oral dose. [e]CL/F reduced slightly (~20%), alcoholic cirrhosis. [f]Following a 5 mg oral dose given once daily to steady state.

Reference: Ohnishi, A., Mihara, M., et al. Comparison of the pharmacokinetics of E2020, a new compound for Alzheimer's disease, in healthy young and elderly subjects. J. Clin. Pharmacol., 1993, 33:1086–1091. Physicians' Desk Reference, 54th ed. Medical Economics Co., Montvale, NJ, 2000, p. 2323.

[a]Active metabolite, desmethyldoxepin, has a longer $t_{\frac{1}{2}}$ (37 ± 15 hours). [b]Calculated from results of oral administration only, assuming complete absorption, elimination by the liver, hepatic blood flow of 1.5 l/min, and equal partition between plasma and erythrocytes. [c]Calculated assuming $F = 0.30$. [d]V_{area} reported. [e]Trough concentrations of doxepin (D) and desmethyldoxepin (DD) following a 150 mg oral dose given once daily for 3 weeks to patients with depression. Peak/trough ratio <2.

Reference: Faulkner, R.D., Pitts, W.M., Lee, C.S., Lewis, W.A., and Fann, W.E. Multiple-dose doxepin kinetics in depressed patients. Clin. Pharmacol. Ther., 1983, 34:509–515.

DOXORUBICIN[a] (Chapter 51)

5	<7	76	666 ± 339 ml · min⁻¹ · (m²)⁻¹ ↑ Child ↓ Cirr, Obes	682 ± 433 l/m² ↔ Cirr	26 ± 17[b] ↔ RD ↑ Cirr	—	High Dose[c] D: ~950 ng/ml DL: 30–1008 ng/ml Low Dose[c] D: 6.0 ± 3.2 ng/ml DL: 5.0 ± 3.5 ng/ml

[a]Active metabolites; $t_{\frac{1}{2}}$ for doxorubicinol is 29 ± 16 hours. [b]Prolonged when plasma bilirubin concentration is elevated; undergoes biliary excretion. [c]Mean data for doxorubicin (D) and range of data for doxorubicinol (DL). High dose: a single 45–72 mg/m² high-dose 1 hour IV infusion given to patients with small cell lung cancer. Low dose: continuous IV infusion at a rate of 3.9 ± 0.65 mg/m² per day for 12.4 (2 to 50) weeks to patients with advanced cancer.

References: Ackland, S.P., Ratain, M.J., et al. Pharmacokinetics and pharmacodynamics of long-term continuous-infusion doxorubicin. Clin. Pharmacol. Ther., 1989, 45:340–347. Piscitelli, S.C., Rodvold, K.A., Rushing, D.A., and Tewksbury, D.A. Pharmacokinetics and pharmacodynamics of doxorubicin in patients with small cell lung cancer. Clin. Pharmacol. Ther., 1993, 53:555–561.

Table A–II-1 Pharmacokinetic Data (Continued)

AVAILABILITY (ORAL) (%)	URINARY EXCRETION (%)	BOUND IN PLASMA (%)	CLEARANCE ($ml \cdot min^{-1} \cdot kg^{-1}$)	VOL. DIST. (liters/kg)	HALF-LIFE (hours)	PEAK TIME (hours)	PEAK CONCENTRATIONS
DOXYCYCLINE (Chapter 46)							
93	41 ± 19	88 ± 5 ↓ RD[a]	0.53 ± 0.18 ↓ HL, Aged ↔ RD	0.75 ± 0.32 ↓ HL, Aged	16 ± 6 ↔ RD, HL, Aged	Oral: 1–2[b]	IV: 2.8 μg/ml[b] Oral: 1.7–2 μg/ml[b]

[a]Decreases in plasma protein binding to 71 ± 3% in patients with uremia. [b]Mean data following a single 100 mg IV dose (1-hour infusion) or range of mean data following a 100 mg oral dose given to adults.

Reference: Saivin, S., and Houin, G. Clinical pharmacokinetics of doxycycline and minocycline. *Clin. Pharmacokinet.,* **1988,** *15:*355–366.

AVAILABILITY (ORAL) (%)	URINARY EXCRETION (%)	BOUND IN PLASMA (%)	CLEARANCE ($ml \cdot min^{-1} \cdot kg^{-1}$)	VOL. DIST. (liters/kg)	HALF-LIFE (hours)	PEAK TIME (hours)	PEAK CONCENTRATIONS
EFAVIRENZ[a] (Chapter 50)							
—[b] ↑ Food	<1	99.5–99.75	3.1 ± 1.2[c] ↔ Child[d]	—	SD: 52–76[c] MD: 40–55[c]	4.1 ± 1.7[e]	4.0 ± 1.7 μg/ml[e]

[a]Data from patients with HIV infection. No significant gender differences. Metabolized primarily by CYP3A4. [b]Absolute oral bioavailability is unknown. Oral *AUC* increased 50% by high-fat meal. [c]*CL/F* and $t_{\frac{1}{2}}$ reported single (SD) and multiple (MD) for oral dose. Efavirenz is a weak inducer of CYP3A4 and its own metabolism. [d]3 to 16 years of age, no difference in weight-adjusted *CL/F* compared to adult. [e]Following a 600 mg oral dose given daily to steady state.

References: Adkins, J.C., and Noble, S. Efavirenz. *Drugs,* **1998,** *56:*1055–1064. *Physicians' Desk Reference,* 54th ed. Medical Economics Co., Montvale, NJ, **2000,** p. 981. Villani, P., Regazzi, M.B., *et al.* Pharmacokinetics of efavirenz (EFV) alone and in combination therapy with nelfinavir (NFV) in HIV-1 infected patients. *Br. J. Clin. Pharmacol.,* **1999,** *48:*712–715.

AVAILABILITY (ORAL) (%)	URINARY EXCRETION (%)	BOUND IN PLASMA (%)	CLEARANCE ($ml \cdot min^{-1} \cdot kg^{-1}$)	VOL. DIST. (liters/kg)	HALF-LIFE (hours)	PEAK TIME (hours)	PEAK CONCENTRATIONS
ENALAPRIL[a] (Chapters 30, 31, 32)							
41 ± 15 ↓ Cirr	88 ± 7[b] ↓ Cirr	50–60	4.9 ± 1.5[c] ↓ RD, Aged, CHF, Neo ↑ Child ↔ Fem	1.7 ± 0.7[c]	11[d] ↑ RD, Cirr	3.0 ± 1.6[e]	69 ± 37 ng/ml[e]

[a]Hydrolyzed by esterases to active metabolite, enalaprilic acid (enalaprilat); pharmacokinetic values and disease comparisons are for enalaprilat, following oral enalapril administration. [b]For IV enalaprilat. [c]*CL/F* and V_{ss}/F after multiple oral doses of enalapril. Values after single IV dose of enalaprilat are misleading because binding to ACE leads to a prolonged $t_{\frac{1}{2}}$, which does not represent a significant fraction of the *CL* upon multiple dosing. [d]Estimated from the approach to steady state during multiple dosing. [e]Mean values for enalaprilat following a 10 mg enalapril oral dose given daily for 8 days to healthy young adults. The EC_{50} for ACE inhibition is 5–20 ng/ml enalaprilat.

References: Lees, K.R., and Reid, J.L. Age and the pharmacokinetics and pharmacodynamics of chronic enalapril treatment. *Clin. Pharmacol. Ther.,* **1987,** *41:*597–602. MacFadyen, R.J., Meredith, P.A., and Elliott, H.L. Enalapril clinical pharmacokinetics and pharmacodynamic-pharmacodynamic relationships. An overview. *Clin. Pharmacokinet.,* **1993,** *25:*274–282.

1820

ENOXAPARIN[a] (Chapter 54)

SC: 92	—[b]	0.3 ± 0.1[c] ↓RD	0.12 ± 0.04[c] ↔RD	3.8 ± 1.3[d] ↑RD	3[e]	ACLM: 145 ± 45 ng/ml[e] BCLM: 414 ± 87 ng/ml[e]

References: Bendetowicz, A.V., Beguin, S., Caplain, H., and Hemker, H.C. Pharmacokinetics and pharmacodynamics of a low molecular weight heparin (enoxaparin) after subcutaneous injection, comparison with unfractionated heparin—a three way cross over study in human volunteers. *Thromb. Haemost.* **1994,** *71:*305–313. *Physicians' Desk Reference,* 54th ed. Medical Economics Co, Montvale, NJ, **2000,** p. 2561.

[a]Enoxaparin consists of low-molecular-weight heparin fragments of varying lengths. [b]43% is recovered in urine when administered as ^{99}Tc-labeled enoxaparin; 8% to 20% anti–Factor Xa activity. [c]F, CL/F, and V_{area}/F for SC dose measured by functional assay for anti–Factor Xa activity. [d]Measured by functional assay of anti–Factor Xa activity. Using anti–Factor Xa activity or displacement binding assay gives a $t_{\frac{1}{2}}$ of approximately 1 to 2 hours. [e]Following a single 40 mg SC dose to healthy adult subjects. High affinity antithrombin III molecules: ACLM, above critical length molecules (anti–Factor Xa and IIa activity); BCLM, below critical length molecules (anti–Factor Xa activity).

ENTACAPONE[a] (Chapter 20)

42 ± 9[b] ↑LD[c]	Negligible	98	10.3 ± 1.74 ↔RD, LD	0.40 ± 0.16	0.28 ± 0.06[d]	0.8 ± 0.2[e]	4.3 ± 2.0 μg/ml[e]

References: Holm, K.J., and Spencer, C.M. Entacapone. A review of its use in Parkinson's disease. *Drugs,* **1999,** *58:*159–177. Keranen, T., Gordin, A., *et al.* Inhibition of soluble catechol-O-methyltransferase and single-dose pharmacokinetics after oral and intravenous administration of entacapone. *Eur. J. Clin. Pharmacol.* **1994,** *46:*151–157.

[a]Data from healthy male subjects. Eliminated primarily by biliary excretion. [b]The bioavailability of entacapone appears to be dose-dependent (increases from 29% to 46% over a 50–800 mg dose range). [c]Increased bioavailability, moderate hepatic impairment with cirrhosis. [d]Value represents the $t_{\frac{1}{2}}$ for the initial distribution phase during which 90% of a dose is eliminated. The terminal $t_{\frac{1}{2}}$ is 2.9 ± 2.0 hours. [e]Following a single 400 mg oral dose. No accumulation with multiple dosing.

EPLERENONE[a] (Chapters 28, 31, 32)

—	7[b]	33–60[c]	2.4[d] ↓CHF, LD	0.6–1.3[d]	4–6	1.8 ± 0.7[e]	1.0 ± 0.3 μg/ml[e]

References: Clinical Pharmacology and Biopharmaceutics Review. Application 21-437/S-002. U.S. Food and Drug Administration Center for Drug Evaluation and Research. Available at: http://www.fda/gov/cder/foi/nda/2002/21-437/S-002_inspra.htm. Accessed November 1, 2004. Cook, C.S., Berry, L.M., *et al.* Pharmacokinetics and metabolism of [14C]eplerenone after oral administration to humans. *Drug Metab. Dispos.,* **2003,** *31:*1448–1455. Product Information: Inspra™ (eplerenone tablets). Pfizer, Chicago, IL, **2004.**

[a]Eplerenone is converted (reversibly) to an inactive ring-open hydroxy acid. Both eplerenone (E) and the hydroxy acid (EA) circulate in plasma; concentrations of E are much higher than EA. Irreversible metabolism is catalyzed predominantly by CYP3A4. Data for E in healthy male and female volunteers reported; no significant gender differences. [b]Recovered as E and EA following an oral dose. [c]Protein binding is concentration-dependent over the therapeutic range; lower at the highest concentration. [d]CL/F and V_{ss}/F reported. [e]Following a 50 mg oral dose given once daily for 7 days.

Table A–II–1 Pharmacokinetic Data (Continued)

AVAILABILITY (ORAL) (%)	URINARY EXCRETION (%)	BOUND IN PLASMA (%)	VOL. DIST. (liters/kg)	CLEARANCE (ml · min⁻¹ · kg⁻¹)	HALF-LIFE (hours)	PEAK TIME (hours)	PEAK CONCENTRATIONS
EPOETIN ALFA[a] (Chapter 53)							
—[b]	E: <3	—	E: 0.033–0.075 DE: 0.054 (0.045–0.063)	E: 0.047–0.092 DE: 0.028 (0.02–0.03)	E: 4.0–11.2 DE: 24 (19–28)	E: 18[c] DE: 54 ± 5[d]	E: 176 ± 75 U/l[c] DE: 0.94 ± 0.1 ng/ml[d]

[a]Epoetin alfa (E) data from male and female patients receiving continuous ambulatory peritoneal dialysis. Data shown are mean results from four different IV dosing studies. Darbepoetin alfa (DE) is a new analogue of E containing five rather than three N-linked carbohydrate chains. It is cleared more slowly from the body than E. DE data shown are for dialysis patients receiving IV darbepoetin once a week to steady state. [b]For parenteral administration only. Bioavailability following SC administration is 22 (11–36) and 37 (30–50)% for E and DE, respectively. [c]Following a single 120 units/kg SC dose of E. [d]Following a single SC DE dose consisting of a peptide mass equivalent to 100 units/kg of E.

References: Allon, M. Kleinman, K., *et al.* Pharmacokinetics and pharmacodynamics of darbepoetin alfa and epoetin in patients undergoing dialysis. *Clin. Pharmacol. Ther.*, **2002**, *72:*546–555. Macdougall, I.C. Roberts, D.E., Coles, G.A., and Williams, J.D. Clinical pharmacokinetics of epoetin (recombinant human erythropoietin). *Clin. Pharmacokinet.*, **1991**, *20:*99–113. Macdougall, I.C., Gray, S.J., *et al.* Pharmacokinetics of novel erythropoiesis stimulating protein compared with epoetin alfa in dialysis patients. *J. Am. Soc. Nephrol.*, **1999**, *10:*2392–2395.

AVAILABILITY (ORAL) (%)	URINARY EXCRETION (%)	BOUND IN PLASMA (%)	VOL. DIST. (liters/kg)	CLEARANCE (ml · min⁻¹ · kg⁻¹)	HALF-LIFE (hours)	PEAK TIME (hours)	PEAK CONCENTRATIONS
ERYTHROMYCIN (Chapter 46)							
35 ± 25[a] ↓ Preg[b]	12 ± 7	84 ± 3[c] ↔ RD	0.78 ± 0.44 ↑ RD	9.1 ± 4.1[d] ↔ RD	1.6 ± 0.7 ↑ Cirr ↔ RD	B: 2.1–3.9[e] S: 2–3[e]	B: 0.9–3.5 µg/ml[e] S: 0.5–1.4 µg/ml[e]

[a]Value for enteric-coated erythromycin base. [b]Decreased concentrations in pregnancy possibly due to decreased bioavailability (or increased *CL*). [c]Erythromycin base. [d]Erythromycin is a CYP3A substrate; *N*-demethylation. It is also transported by P-glycoprotein, which may contribute to biliary excretion of parent drug and metabolites. [e]Range of mean values from studies following a 250 mg oral enteric-coated free base in a capsule (B) given four times daily for 5 to 13 doses or a 250-mg film-coated tablet or capsule of erythromycin stearate (S) given four times daily for 5 to 12 doses.

Reference: Periti, P., Mazzei, T., Mini, E., and Novelli, A. Clinical pharmacokinetic properties of the macrolide antibiotics. Effects of age and various pathophysiological states (Part I). *Clin. Pharmacokinet.*, **1989**, *16:*193–214.

AVAILABILITY (ORAL) (%)	URINARY EXCRETION (%)	BOUND IN PLASMA (%)	VOL. DIST. (liters/kg)	CLEARANCE (ml · min⁻¹ · kg⁻¹)	HALF-LIFE (hours)	PEAK TIME (hours)	PEAK CONCENTRATIONS
ESOMEPRAZOLE[a] (Chapter 36)							
Es: 89 (81–98)[b] Rac: 53 ± 29[b]	Es/Rac: <1	Es/Rac: 95–97	Es: 0.25 (0.23–0.27) Rac: 0.34 ± 0.09	Es: 4.1 (3.3–5.0)[c,d] Rac: 7.5 ± 2.7[c] ↓LD[e]	Es: 0.9 (0.7–1.0)[d] Rac: 0.7 ± 0.5 ↑LD[e]	Es: 1.5 (1.3–1.7)[f] Rac, EM: ~1[g] Rac, PM: ~3–4[g]	Es: 4.5 (3.8–5.7) µM[f] Rac, EM: 0.68 ± 0.43 µM[g] Rac, PM: 3.5 ± 1.4 µM[g]

References: Andersson, T., Hassan-Alin, M., Hasselgren, G., Rohss, K., and Weidolf, L. Pharmacokinetic studies with esomeprazole, the (S)-isomer of omeprazole. *Clin. Pharmacokinet.*, **2001**, *40*:411–426. Chang, M., Tybring, G., Dahl, M.L., Gotharson, E., Sagar, M., Seensalu, R., and Bertilsson, L. Interphenotype differences in disposition and effect on gastrin levels of omeprazole—suitability of omeprazole as a probe for CYP2C19. *Br. J. Clin. Pharmacol.*, **1995**, *39*:511–518.

[a]Esomeprazole is the S-enantiomer of omeprazole. Both esomeprazole (Es) and racemic omeprazole (Rac) are available. Data for both formulations are reported. [b]Bioavailability determined after multiple dosing. Lower Es values 64% (54–75%) reported for single dose. [c]The metabolic CL of the Es is slower than that of the R-enantiomer. Both Es and Rac are metabolized by CYP2C19 (polymorphic) and CYP3A4. CL of Es and Rac is decreased and $t_{\frac{1}{2}}$ increased in CYP2C19 poor metabolizers. [d]Following a single 40 mg IV dose. CL of Es decreases and $t_{\frac{1}{2}}$ increases with multiple dosing. [e]Reduced CL and increased $t_{\frac{1}{2}}$ in patients with severe (Childs Pugh Class C) hepatic insufficiency. [f]Following a 40 mg oral dose of Es given once daily for 5 days to healthy subjects of unspecified CYP2C19 phenotype. [g]Following a 20 mg oral dose of Rac given twice daily for 4 days to healthy subjects phenotyped as CYP2C19 extensive (EM) and poor (PM) metabolizers.

ETANERCEPT[a] (Chapter 52)

SC: 58	Negligible	—	0.02	~0.11[b]	IV: 72 SC-SD: 92[c]	SC-SD: 72 (48–96)[c]	IV: 2.32 µg/ml[c] SC-SD: 1.2 µg/ml[c] SC-MD: 3 µg/ml[c]

[a]Data from healthy adult subjects. No significant gender differences in weight-normalized kinetics. Etanercept is a recombinant human fusion protein–TNF receptor and Fc portion of IgG$_1$. [b]The volume of distribution (V_{area}) was estimated from reported CL and $t_{\frac{1}{2}}$ values. [c]Following a single 10 mg IV dose and single (SC-SD) or multiple (SC-MD) subcutaneous doses, 25 mg, twice weekly for 6 months.

References: Goldenberg, M.M. Etanercept, a novel drug for the treatment of patients with severe, active rheumatoid arthritis. *Clin. Ther.*, **1999**, *21*:75–87. Moreland, L.W., Margolies, G., *et al.* Recombinant soluble tumor necrosis factor receptor (p80) fusion protein: toxicity and dose finding trial in refractory rheumatoid arthritis. *J. Rheumatol.*, **1996**, *23*:1849–1855. *Physicians' Desk Reference*, 54th ed. Medical Economics Co, Montvale, NJ, **2000**, p. 1414.

ETHAMBUTOL (Chapter 47)

77 ± 8	79 ± 3	6–30	8.6 ± 0.8	1.6 ± 0.2	3.1 ± 0.4 ↑ RD	2–4[a]	2–5 µg/ml

[a]Following a single 800 mg oral dose to healthy subjects. Concentrations >10 µg/ml can adversely affect vision. No accumulation with once-a-day dosing in patients with normal renal function.

Reference: Holdiness, M.R. Clinical pharmacokinetics of the antituberculosis drugs. *Clin. Pharmacokinet.*, **1984**, *9*:511–544.

ETOPOSIDE (Chapter 51)

52 ± 17[a]	35 ± 5	96 ± 0.4[b] ↓ Alb	0.68 ± 0.23[c] ↔ Child, Cirr ↓ RD	0.36 ± 0.15 ↔ Child, Cirr	8.1 ± 4.3 ↑ RD ↔ Child, Cirr	1.3	NT: 2.7 µg/ml[d] T: 4.7 µg/ml[d]

[a]Decreases at oral doses greater than 200 mg. [b]Decreases with hyperbilirubinemia. [c]Metabolized by CYP3A; also a substrate for P-glycoprotein. [d]Mean C_{max} for patients without (NT) and with (T) serious hematological toxicity following a 75 to 200 mg/m^2 dose given as a 72-hour continuous IV infusion.

References: Clark, P.I., and Slevin, M.L. The clinical pharmacology of etoposide and teniposide. *Clin. Pharmacokinet.*, **1987**, *12*:223–252. McLeod, H.L., and Evans, W.E. Clinical pharmacokinetics and pharmacodynamics of epipodophyllotoxins. *Cancer Surv.*, **1993**, *17*:253–268.

Table A–II–1 *Pharmacokinetic Data (Continued)*

	AVAILABILITY (ORAL) (%)	URINARY EXCRETION (%)	BOUND IN PLASMA (%)	CLEARANCE (ml·min⁻¹·kg⁻¹)	VOL. DIST. (liters/kg)	HALF-LIFE (hours)	PEAK TIME (hours)	PEAK CONCENTRATIONS

EZETIMIBE[a] (Chapter 35)

—	~2	>90[b]	6.6[c] ↓ Aged, RD, LD	1.5[c]	28–30[d]	1[e]	122 ng/ml[e]

References: Mauro, V.F., and Tuckerman, C.E. Ezetimibe for management of hypercholesterolemia. *Ann. Pharmacother.,* **2003,** *37:*839–848. Patrick, J.E., Kosoglou, T., *et al.* Disposition of the selective cholesterol absorption inhibitor ezetimibe in healthy male subjects. *Drug Metab. Dispos.,* **2002,** *30:*430–437. *Physicians' Desk Reference,* 58th ed. Medical Economics Co., Montvale, **2004,** pp. 3085–3086.

[a]Ezetimibe is extensively metabolized to a glucuronide, which is more active than ezetimibe in inhibiting cholesterol absorption. Clinical effects are related to the total plasma concentration of ezetimibe and ezetimibe-glucuronide, with ezetimibe concentrations being only 10% of the total. [b]For ezetimibe and ezetimibe-glucuronide. [c]CL/F and V_d/F for total (unconjugated and glucuronide conjugate) ezetimibe reported. [d]Ezetimibe undergoes significant enterohepatic recycling leading to multiple secondary peaks. An effective $t_{\frac{1}{2}}$ is estimated. [e]Total (unconjugated and glucuronide conjugate) ezetimibe following a 10 mg oral dose given once daily for 10 days.

FELODIPINE[a] (Chapter 32)

15 ± 8 ↔ Aged, Cirr ↑ Food	<1	99.6 ± 02 ↓ RD, Cirr ↔ Aged	12 ± 5[b] ↓ Aged, Cirr, CHF[c]	10 ± 3 ↔ Aged ↓ Cirr	14 ± 4 ↑ Aged, CHF[c] ↔ Cirr	IR: 0.9 ± 0.4[d] ER: 3.7 ± 0.9[d]	IR: 34 ± 26 nM[d] ER: 9.1 ± 7.3 nM[d]

Reference: Dunselman, P.H. and Edgar, B. Felodipine clinical pharmacokinetics. *Clin. Pharmacokinet.,* **1991,** *21:*418–430.

[a]Racemic mixture; S-(–)-enantiomer is active Ca^{+2} channel blocker; different enantiomer pharmacokinetics result in S-(–)-enantiomer concentrations about twofold higher than those of R-(+)-isomer. [b]Undergoes significant CYP3A-dependent first-pass metabolism in the intestine and liver. [c]May be age-related rather than CHF-related. [d]Following a 10 mg oral immediate- (IR) or extended-release (ER) tablet given twice daily to steady state in healthy subjects. EC_{50} for diastolic pressure decrease is 8 ± 5 nM in patients with hypertension.

FENOFIBRATE[a] (Chapter 35)

—[b] ↑ Food	0.1–10[c]	>99	0.45[d] ↓ RD	0.89[d]	20–27 ↑RD	IR: 6–8[e] Mic: 4–6[f]	IR: 8.6 ± 0.9 μg/ml[e] Mic: 10.8 ± 0.6 μg/ml[f]

References: Balfour, J.A., McTavish, D., and Heel, R.C. Fenofibrate. A review of its pharmacodynamic and pharmacokinetic properties and therapeutic use in dyslipidaemia. *Drugs,* **1990,** *40:*260–290. Miller, D.B., and Spence, J.D. Clinical pharmacokinetics of fibric acid derivatives (fibrates). *Clin. Pharmacokinet.,* **1998,** *34:*155–162.

[a]Fenofibrate is a prodrug that is hydrolyzed by esterases to fenofibric acid, the pharmacologically active compound. All values reported are for fenofibric acid. [b]Absolute bioavailability is not known. Recovery of radiolabeled dose in urine as fenofibric acid and its glucuronide is 60%. Immediate-release tablet and micronized capsule are bioequivalent. Bioavailability is increased when taken with a standard meal. [c]Recovery following oral dose. [d]CL/F and V/F reported. [e]Following a 300 mg immediate-release (IR) fenofibrate tablet given once daily to steady state. [f]Following a 200 mg micronized (Mic) capsule given once daily to steady state.

FENTANYL (Chapters 13, 21)

TM: ~50	8	84 ± 2	13 ± 2[a] ↓ Aged ↔ Prem, Child ↑ Neo	4.0 ± 0.4 ↑ CPBS, Aged, Prem ↔ Child	3.7 ± 0.4	TD: 35 ± 15[b] TM: 0.4 (0.3–6)[b]	TD: 1.4 ± 0.5 ng/ml[b] TM: 0.8 ± 0.3 ng/ml[b]

[a]Metabolically cleared primarily by CYP3A to norfentanyl and hydroxy metabolites. [b]Following a 5 mg transdermal (TD) dose administered at 50 μg/hour through a DURAGESIC system or a single 400-μg transmucosal (TM) dose. Postoperative and intraoperative analgesia occurs at plasma concentrations of 1 ng/ml and 3 ng/ml, respectively. Respiratory depression occurs above 0.7 ng/ml.

References: Olkkola, K.T., Hamunen, K., and Maunuksela, E.L. Clinical pharmacokinetics and pharmacodynamics of opioid analgesics in infants and children. *Clin. Pharmacokinet.*, **1995,** 28:385–404. *Physicians' Desk Reference*, 54th ed. Medical Economics Co., Montvale, NJ, **2000,** pp. 405 and 1445.

FEXOFENADINE[a] (Chapter 24)

—[a]	12	60–70	9.4 ± 4.2[b]	—	1.3 ± 0.6[d]	14 ± 6[b] ↑ RD[c] ↔ LD	286 ± 143 ng/ml[d]

[a]Data from healthy adult male subjects. Absolute bioavailability is unknown. Negligible metabolism with 85% of a dose recovered in feces unchanged; a substrate for hepatic and intestinal P-glycoprotein efflux transporter. [b]CL/F and $t_{\frac{1}{2}}$ reported for oral dose. [c]Mild renal impairment. [d]Following a 60 mg oral dose twice a day to steady state.

References: Markham, A., and Wagstaff, A.J. Fexofenadine. *Drugs*, **1998,** 55:269–274; discussion 275–276. Robbins, D.K., Castles, M.A., Pack, D.J., Bhargava, V.O., and Weir, S.J. Dose proportionality and comparison of single and multiple dose pharmacokinetics of fexofenadine (MDL 16455) and its enantiomers in healthy male volunteers. *Biopharm. Drug Dispos.*, **1998,** 19:455–463.

FILGRASTIM[a] (Chapter 53)

—[b]	F: —[c] PF: negligible	F/PF: —	F: 0.5–0.7[d] ↓ RD PF: 0.23 (0.07–0.26)[e]	F: 0.15 PF: 0.48[e]	F: 3.4–4.7 ↑ RD PF: 33 (30–54)	F: 8[f] PF: 72 (24–96)[f]	F: 11 (9–16) ng/ml[f] PF: 114 (58–203) ng/ml[f]

[a]Filgrastim (F) is a recombinant form of human G-CSF; it has an extra methionine residue and is non-glycosylated. A polyethyleneglycol conjugated analog, pegfilgrastim (PF), is also available for clinical use. In general, it is eliminated from the body more slowly than F by non-renal routes. Data from healthy male and female adults and patients with cancer following IV or SC administration. [b]For parenteral use only. Bioavailability of F following SC dosing is 49% ± 9%. No data available for PF. [c]F is filtered, reabsorbed, and catabolized in the kidney. It also is eliminated through binding to neutrophil receptors, endocytosis, and proteolytic degradation. In contrast, PF does not undergo renal elimination, presumably because of its larger hydrodynamic size; elimination of PF occurs primarily through neutrophil-mediated CL. [d]CL/F of F reported for single dose at or below 4 μg/kg. CL of F increases with dose (>4 μg/kg) and with time (up to 10-fold) as absolute neutrophil count increases. [e]CL/F, V_{area}/F, and $t_{\frac{1}{2}}$ of PF from SC dose reported. CL/F of PF decreases with increasing dose but increases over time with increased neutrophil counts. [f]Following a single 5 μg/kg SC dose of F or a single 100 μg/kg SC dose of PF given 24 hours after chemotherapy.

References: Borleffs, J.C., Bosschaert, M., *et al.* Effect of escalating doses of recombinant human granulocyte colony-stimulating factor (filgrastim) on circulating neutrophils in healthy subjects. *Clin. Ther.*, **1998,** 20:722–736. *Physicians' Desk Reference*, 58th ed. Medical Economics Co., Montvale, **2004,** pp. 587–591. Stute, N., Santana, V.M., *et al.* Pharmacokinetics of subcutaneous recombinant human granulocyte colony-stimulating factor in children. *Blood*, **1992,** 79:2849–2854. Sugiura, M., Yamamoto, K., Sawada, Y., and Iga. T. Pharmacokinetic/pharmacodynamic analysis of neutrophil proliferation induced by recombinant granulocyte colony-stimulating factor (rhG-CSF): comparison between intravenous and subcutaneous administration. *Biol. Pharm. Bull.*, **1997,** 20:684–689. Zamboni, W.C. Pharmacokinetics of pegfilgrastim. *Pharmacotherapy*, **2003,** 23(8 Pt 2):9S–14S.

Table A–II–1 Pharmacokinetic Data (Continued)

AVAILABILITY (ORAL) (%)	URINARY EXCRETION (%)	BOUND IN PLASMA (%)	CLEARANCE (ml·min⁻¹·kg⁻¹)	VOL. DIST. (liters/kg)	HALF-LIFE (hours)	PEAK TIME (hours)	PEAK CONCENTRATIONS
FINASTERIDE (Chapter 58)							
63 ± 21	<1	90	2.3 ± 0.8 ↔ RD, Aged	1.1 ± 0.2	7.9 ± 2.5 ↔ RD, Aged	1–2[a]	37 (27→49) ng/ml[a]
FLECAINIDE[a] (Chapter 34)							
70 ± 11	43 ± 3 ↓ MI	61 ± 10	5.6 ± 1.3[b] ↓ RD, Cirr, CHF ↑ Child	4.9 ± 0.4[c] ↑ Cirr	11 ± 3[b] ↑ RD, Cirr, CHF ↓ Child	~3 (1–6)[d]	458 ± 100 ng/ml[d]
FLUCONAZOLE (Chapter 48)							
>90	75 ± 9	11 ± 1	0.27 ± 0.07 ↔ AIDS, Neo ↓ RD, Prem	0.60 ± 0.11 ↔ RD ↑ Prem, Neo	32 ± 5 ↑ Cirr, RD, Prem ↓ Child	1.7–4.3[a]	10.6 ± 0.4 μg/ml[a]
FLUDARABINE[a] (Chapter 51)							
—	24 ± 3	—	3.7 ± 1.5 ↓ RD	2.4 ± 0.6	10–30	—	0.57 μg/ml[b]

[a]Following a single 5 mg oral dose given to healthy adults. Drug accumulates twofold with once daily dosing.

Reference: Sudduth, S.L., and Koronkowski, M.J. Finasteride: the first 5α-reductase inhibitor. *Pharmacotherapy,* **1993,** *13:*309–325; discussion 325–329.

[a]Racemic mixture: enantiomers exert similar electrophysiological effects. [b]Metabolized by CYP2D6 (polymorphic); except for a shortened elimination $t_{\frac{1}{2}}$ and nonlinear kinetics in extensive metabolizers, CYP2D6 phenotype had no significant influence on flecainide pharmacokinetics or pharmacodynamics. [c]V_{area} reported. [d]Following a 100 mg oral dose given twice daily for 5 days in healthy adults. Similar levels for CYP2D6 extensive and poor metabolizers.

Reference: Funck-Brentano, C., Becquemont, L., *et al.* Variable disposition kinetics and electrocardiographic effects of flecainide during repeated dosing in humans: contribution of genetic factors, dose-dependent clearance, and interaction with amiodarone. *Clin. Pharmacol. Ther.,* **1994,** *55:*256–269.

[a]Following a 200 mg oral dose given twice a day for 4 days to healthy adults.

References: Debruyne, D., and Ryckelynck, J.P. Clinical pharmacokinetics of fluconazole. *Clin. Pharmacokinet.,* **1993,** *24:*10–27. Varhe, A., Olkkola, K.T., and Neuvonen, P.J. Effect of fluconazole dose on the extent of fluconazole-triazolam interaction. *Br. J. Clin. Pharmacol.,* **1996,** *42:*465–470.

[a]Data from male and female adult cancer patients following IV administration. Fludarabine is rapidly dephosphorylated to 2-fluoro-arabinoside-A (F-ara-A), transported into cells, and phosphorylated to the active triphosphate metabolite. Pharmacokinetics of F-ara-A are reported. [b]Following a single 25 mg/m² IV dose of fludarabine (30 minute infusion); no accumulation after 5 daily doses.

References: Hersh, M.R., Kuhn, J.G., *et al.* Pharmacokinetic study of fludarabine phosphate (NSC 312887). *Cancer Chemother. Pharmacol.,* **1986,** *17:*277–280. *Physicians' Desk Reference,* 54th ed. Medical Economics Co., Montvale, NJ, **2000,** p. 764. Plunkett, W., Gandhi, V., *et al.* Fludarabine: pharmacokinetics, mechanisms of action, and rationales for combination therapies. *Semin. Oncol.,* **1993,** *20:*2–12.

FLUMAZENIL (Chapter 16)

16[a]	<0.2	40 (36–46)	9.9 ± 3.1 ↓LD[b]	0.63 ± 0.18	0.9 ± 0.2 ↑LD[b]	—	10–20 ng/ml[c]

[a]Because of the need for rapid onset of action and short elimination $t_{1/2}$, flumazenil is normally given intravenously. [b]In patients with moderate-to-severe liver disease. [c]Clinically effective plasma concentrations that can be maintained for 1 to 2 hours following an IV bolus of 2.5 mg.

References: Janssen, U., Walker, S., Maier, K., von Gaisberg, U., and Klotz, U. Flumazenil disposition and elimination in cirrhosis. *Clin. Pharmacol. Ther.,* **1989,** *46:*317–323. Klotz, U., and Kanto, J. Pharmacokinetics and clinical use of flumazenil (Ro 15-1788). *Clin. Pharmacokinet.,* **1988,** *14:*1–12.

5-FLUOROURACIL (Chapter 51)

28 (0–80)[a]	<10	8–12	16 ± 7	0.25 ± 0.12	11 ± 4 min[b]	—	11.2 μM[c]

[a]Higher *F* with rapid absorption and lower *F* with slower absorption, due to a saturable first-pass effect. [b]A much longer (~20 hours) terminal $t_{1/2}$ has been reported representing a slow redistribution of drug from tissues. [c]Steady-state concentration following a continuous IV infusion of 300 to 500 mg/m² per day to cancer patients.

Reference: Diasio, R.B., and Harris, B.E. Clinical pharmacology of 5-fluorouracil. *Clin. Pharmacokinet.,* **1989,** *16:*215–237.

FLUOXETINE[a] (Chapter 17)

—[a]	<2.5	94 ↔ Cirr, RD	9.6 ± 6.9[b,c] ↔ RD, Aged, Obes ↓ Cirr	35 ± 21[d] ↔ RD, Cirr	53 ± 41[e] ↑ Cirr ↔ RD, Aged, Obes	F: 6–8[f]	F: 200–531 ng/ml[f] NF: 103–465 ng/ml[f]

[a]Active metabolite, norfluoxetine; $t_{1/2}$ of norfluoxetine is 6.4 ± 2.5 days (12 ± 2 days in cirrhosis). Absolute bioavailability is unknown, but ≥80% of dose is absorbed. [b]Reduced *CL* with repetitive dosing (~2.6 ml·min⁻¹·kg⁻¹) and with increasing dose between 40 mg and 80 mg. [c]*CL/F* reported; fluoxetine is a CYP2D6 substrate and inhibitor. [d]V_{area}/F reported. [e]Longer $t_{1/2}$ with repetitive dosing and with increasing doses. [f]Range of data for fluoxetine (F) and norfluoxetine (NF) following a 60 mg oral dose given daily for 1 week. NF continues to accumulate for several weeks.

Reference: Altamura, A.C., Moro, A.R., and Percudani, M. Clinical pharmacokinetics of fluoxetine. *Clin. Pharmacokinet.,* **1994,** *26:*201–214.

FLUPHENAZINE[a] (Chapter 18)

Oral: 2.7 (1.7–4.5)[b] SC or IM: 3.4 (2.5–5.0)[b]	Negligible	—	10 ± 7	11 ± 10	IV: 12 ± 4[c] IR: 14.4 ± 7.8[c] SR: 20.3 ± 7.9[c]	IV: 2.8 ± 2.1[d] DN: 24–48[d] EN: 48–72[d]	IR: 2.3 ± 2.1 ng/ml[d] DN: 1.3 ng/ml[d] EN: 1.1 ng/ml[d]

[a]Data from healthy males and females. Fluphenazine is extensively metabolized. [b]Available in immediate-release oral and IM formulations and depot SC or IM injections as the enanthate (EN) or decanoate (DN) esters. Geometric mean (90% CI). [c]Reported $t_{1/2}$ for a single IV dose and apparent $t_{1/2}$ following oral administration of immediate- (IR) and slow-release (SR) formulations. Longer apparent $t_{1/2}$s with oral dosing reflect an absorption-limited elimination. [d]Following single 12 mg oral dose (IR) or 5 mg IM injections of DN and EN.

References: Jann, M.W., Ereshefsky, L., and Saklad, S.R. Clinical pharmacokinetics of the depot antipsychotics. *Clin. Pharmacokinet.,* **1985,** *10:*315–333. Koytchev, R., Alken, R.G., McKay, G., and Katzarov, T. Absolute bioavailability of oral immediate and slow release fluphenazine in healthy volunteers. *Eur. J. Clin. Pharmacol.,* **1996,** *51:*183–187.

Table A–II–1 *Pharmacokinetic Data (Continued)*

AVAILABILITY (ORAL) (%)	URINARY EXCRETION (%)	BOUND IN PLASMA (%)	CLEARANCE ($ml \cdot min^{-1} \cdot kg^{-1}$)	VOL. DIST. (liters/kg)	HALF-LIFE (hours)	PEAK TIME (hours)	PEAK CONCENTRATIONS
FLUTAMIDE[a] (Chapters 51, 58)							
—	<1	F: 94–96 HF: 92–94	280[b] ↔RD	—	F: 7.8[b] HF: 8.1[b]	F: 1.3 ± 0.7[c] HF: 1.9 ± 0.6[c]	F: 0.11 ± 0.21 μg/ml[c] HF: 1.6 ± 0.59 μg/ml[c]

[a]Data obtained primarily from elderly men. Flutamide (F) is metabolized rapidly to a number of metabolites, which are mainly excreted in urine. One major metabolite, 2-hydroxyflutamide (HF), is biologically active (equal potency); formation is catalyzed primarily by CYP1A2. [b]CL/F and $t_{\frac{1}{2}}$ (terminal) reported for oral dose. [c]Data for F and HF following a 250 mg oral dose given three times daily to steady state in healthy geriatric males.

References: Anjum, S., Swan, S.K., *et al.* Pharmacokinetics of flutamide in patients with renal insufficiency. *Br. J. Clin. Pharmacol.,* **1999,** *47:*43–47. *Physicians' Desk Reference,* 54th ed. Medical Economics Co, Montvale, NJ, **2000,** p. 2798. Radwanski, E., Perentesis, G., Symchowicz, S., and Zampaglione, N. Single and multiple dose pharmacokinetic evaluation of flutamide in normal geriatric volunteers. *J. Clin. Pharmacol.,* **1989,** *29:*554–558.

FOSCARNET[a] (Chapter 49)							
9 ± 2	95 ± 5	14–17	1.6 ± 0.2 ↓RD[a]	0.35	5.7 ± 0.2 ↑RD[a]	1.4 ± 0.6[b]	86 ± 36 μM[b]

[a]In patients with moderate to severe renal disease. [b]Following an 8 mg/kg oral dose given once daily for 8 days to HIV-seropositive patients.

References: Aweeka, F.T., Jacobson, M.A., *et al.* Effect of renal disease and hemodialysis on foscarnet pharmacokinetics and dosing recommendations. *J. Acquir. Immune Defic. Syndr. Hum. Retrovirol.,* **1999,** *20:*350–357. Noormohamed, F.H., Youle, M.S., *et al.* Pharmacokinetics and absolute bioavailability of oral foscarnet in human immunodeficiency virus-seropositive patients. *Antimicrob. Agents Chemother,* **1998,** *42:*293–297.

FULVESTRANT[a] (Chapters 51, 57)							
—[b]	<1	99	9.3–14.3	3.0–5.3	14–19[c]	167[d]	8.2 ± 5.2 ng/ml[d]

[a]Eliminated by conjugation (sulfate and glucuronide) and CYP3A4-mediated oxidation. Data reported for men and women; no significant gender differences. [b]For parenteral administration only. Bioavailability following IM injection has not been reported. [c]Elimination $t_{\frac{1}{2}}$ following IM administration. The apparent $t_{\frac{1}{2}}$ following IM dosing is approximately 40 days due to very prolonged absorption. [d]Following a single 250 mg IM dose given to post-menopausal women with breast cancer.

References: Physicians' Desk Reference, 58th ed. Medical Economics Co., Montvale, **2004,** pp. 669–670. Robertson, J.F., Erikstein, B., *et al.* Pharmacokinetic profile of intramuscular fulvestrant in advanced breast cancer. *Clin. Pharmacokinet.,* **2004,** *43:*529–538. Robertson, J.F., and Harrison, M. Fulvestrant: pharmacokinetics and pharmacology. *Br. J. Cancer,* **2004,** *90*(suppl):S7–S10.

FUROSEMIDE[a] (Chapter 28)							
71 ± 35 (43–73)	71 ± 10 (50–80)	98.6 ± 0.4 (96–99)	1.66 ± 0.58 (1.5–3.0)	0.13 ± 0.06 (0.09–0.17)	1.3 ± 0.8 (0.5–2.0)	1.4 ± 0.8[c]	1.7 ± 0.9 μg/ml[c]

	Oral Bioavailability (%)	Urinary Excretion (%)	Bound in Plasma (%)	Clearance (ml·min⁻¹·kg⁻¹)	Vol. Dist. (liters/kg)	Half-Life (hours)	Peak Time (hours)	Peak Concentration
	↔ CHF, Cirr, CRI	↓ CF ↔ Aged	↓ RD, NS, Cirr, Alb, Aged ↔ CHF, SmK	↓ Aged, RD,[b] CHF, Neo, Prem ↔ Cirr ↑ CF	↑ NS, Neo, Prem, Cirr ↔ RD, CHF, Aged, Smk	↑ Aged, RD,[b] CHF, Prem, Neo, Cirr ↔ NS		

[a]Data from healthy adult male subjects. No significant gender differences described. Range of mean values from multiple studies shown in parentheses. [b]CL/F reduced, mild renal impairment. Aged: CL/F reduced with declining renal function. [c]Following a single 40 mg oral dose (tablet). Ototoxicity occurs at concentrations above 25 µg/ml.

References: Andreasen, F., Hansen, U., Husted, S.E., and Jansen, J.A. The pharmacokinetics of frusemide are influenced by age. Br. J. Clin. Pharmacol., **1983**, 16:391–397. Ponto, L.L., and Schoenwald, R.D. Furosemide (frusemide). A pharmacokinetic/pharmacodynamic review (Part I). Clin. Pharmacokinet., **1990**, 18:381–408. Waller, E.S.. Hamilton, S.F., et al. Disposition and absolute bioavailability of furosemide in healthy males. J. Pharm. Sci., **1982**, 71:1105–1108.

GABAPENTIN (Chapter 19)

	Oral Bioavailability (%)	Urinary Excretion (%)	Bound in Plasma (%)	Clearance (ml·min⁻¹·kg⁻¹)	Vol. Dist. (liters/kg)	Half-Life (hours)	Peak Time (hours)	Peak Concentration
	60[a]	64–68	<3	1.6 ± 0.3 ↓ Aged, RD	0.80 ± 0.09	6.5 ± 1.0 ↑ RD	2–3[b]	4 µg/ml[b]

[a]Decreases with increasing dose. Value for 300–600 mg dose reported. [b]Following an 800 mg oral dose given three times daily to steady state in healthy adults. Efficacious at concentrations >2 µg/ml.

References: Bialer, M. Comparative pharmacokinetics of the newer antiepileptic drugs. Clin. Pharmacokinet., **1993**, 24:441–452. McLean, M.J. Gabapentin. In, The Treatment of Epilepsy: Principles and Practice, 2nd ed. (Wyllie, E., ed.) Williams & Wilkins, Baltimore, **1997**, pp. 884–898.

GALANTAMINE[a] (Chapter 20)

	Oral Bioavailability (%)	Urinary Excretion (%)	Bound in Plasma (%)	Clearance (ml·min⁻¹·kg⁻¹)	Vol. Dist. (liters/kg)	Half-Life (hours)	Peak Time (hours)	Peak Concentration
	100 (91–110)	20 (18–22)	18	5.7 (5.0–6.3)[b] ↓ RD,[c] LD[c]	2.6 (2.4–2.9)	5.7 (5.2–6.3)	2.6 ± 1.0[d]	96 ± 29 ng/ml[d]

[a]Primarily metabolized by CYP2D6, CYP3A4, and glucuronidation. [b]CYP2D6 poor metabolizers show a lower CL, but dose adjustment is not required. [c]In patients with mild-to-moderate hepatic or renal insufficiency. [d]Following a 12 mg oral dose given twice daily for 7 days

References: Bickel, U., Thomsen, T., et al. Pharmacokinetics of galanthamine in humans and corresponding cholinesterase inhibition. Clin. Pharmacol. Ther., **1991**, 50:420–428. Huang, F., Lasseter, K.C., et al. Pharmacokinetic and safety assessments of galantamine and risperidone after the two drugs are administered alone and together. J. Clin. Pharmacol., **2002**, 42:1341–1351. Scott, L.J., and Goa, K.L. Galantamine: a review of its use in Alzheimer's disease. Drugs, **2000**, 60:1095–1122.

GANCICLOVIR (Chapter 49)

	Oral Bioavailability (%)	Urinary Excretion (%)	Bound in Plasma (%)	Clearance (ml·min⁻¹·kg⁻¹)	Vol. Dist. (liters/kg)	Half-Life (hours)	Peak Time (hours)	Peak Concentration
	3–5 ↑ Food	91 ± 5	1–2	3.4 ± 0.5 ↓ RD	1.1 ± 0.2	3.7 ± 0.6 ↑ RD	Oral: 3.0 ± 0.6[a]	IV: 6.6 ± 1.8 µg/ml[a] Oral: 1.2 ± 0.4 µg/ml[a] ↑ Food

[a]Following a single 6 mg/kg IV dose (1-hour infusion) or a 1000 mg oral dose given with food three times a day to steady state.

References: Aweeka, F.T., Gambertoglio, J.G., et al. Foscarnet and ganciclovir pharmacokinetics during concomitant or alternating maintenance therapy for AIDS-related cytomegalovirus retinitis. Clin. Pharmacol. Ther., **1995**, 57:403–412. Physicians' Desk Reference, 54th ed. Medical Economics Co, Montvale, NJ, **2000**, p. 2624.

Table A–II–1 *Pharmacokinetic Data (Continued)*

	AVAILABILITY (ORAL) (%)	URINARY EXCRETION (%)	BOUND IN PLASMA (%)	CLEARANCE (ml · min⁻¹ · kg⁻¹)	VOL. DIST. (liters/kg)	HALF-LIFE (hours)	PEAK TIME (hours)	PEAK CONCENTRATIONS
GEFITINIB[a] (Chapter 51)	60	<1	90	7.3 (2.8–21)[b]	20 (12–39)	48 (10–136)	5 (3–7)[c]	341 ± 208 ng/ml[c]
GEMCITABINE[a] (Chapter 51)	—	<10	Negligible	37.8 ± 19.4[b] ↓Aged	1.4 ± 1.3[c]	0.63 ± 0.48[c] ↑Aged	—	26.9 ± 9 μM[d]
GEMFIBROZIL (Chapter 35)	98 ± 1	<1	97	1.7 ± 0.4 ↔Cirr, RD	0.14 ± 0.03	1.1 ± 0.2 ↔RD	1–2[a]	15–25 μg/ml[a]
GENTAMICIN (Chapter 45)	IM: ~100	>90	<10	CL = 0.82CL$_{cr}$ + 0.11 ↓Obes	0.31 ± 0.10 ↔RD, Aged, CF, Child ↓Obes ↑Neo	2–3[a]	IV: 1[b] IM: 0.3–0.75[b]	IV: 4.9 ± 0.5 μg/ml[b] IM: 5.0 ± 0.4 μg/ml[b]

[a]Eliminated primarily by CYP3A4-dependent metabolism. A major circulating metabolite, O-demethyl gefitinib, has pharmacological activity and may contribute to the efficacy. No apparent age or gender differences. Data from patients with cancer reported. [b]CL can be increased and decreased by CYP3A inducers and inhibitors, respectively. [c]Following a 225 mg oral dose given once daily for 14 days in patients with cancer.

References: Nakagawa, K., Tamura, T., *et al.* Phase I pharmacokinetic trial of the selective oral epidermal growth factor receptor tyrosine kinase inhibitor ('Iressa', ZD1839) in Japanese patients with solid malignant tumors. *Ann. Oncol.* **2003**, *14:922–930. Physicians' Desk Reference,* 58th ed. Medical Economics Co., Montvale, NJ, **2004,** p. 672. Swaisland, H., Laight, A., *et al.* Pharmacokinetics and tolerability of the orally active selective epidermal growth factor receptor tyrosine kinase inhibitor ZD1839 in healthy volunteers. *Clin. Pharmacokinet.* **2001,** *40:297–306.* Wolf, M., Swaisland, H., and Averbuch, S. Development of the novel biologically targeted anticancer agent gefitinib: determining the optimum dose for clinical efficacy. *Clin. Cancer Res.* **2004,** *10:4607–4613.*

[a]Data from patients with leukemia. Rapidly metabolized intracellularly to di- and triphosphate active products; IV administration. [b]Weight-normalized CL is ~25% lower in women, compared to men. [c]V$_d$ and t$_{\frac{1}{2}}$ are reported to increase with long duration of IV infusion. [d]Steady-state concentration during a 10 mg/m² per min infusion for 120–640 minutes.

References: Grunewald, R., Kantarjian, H., *et al.* Gemcitabine in leukemia: a phase I clinical, plasma, and cellular pharmacology study. *J. Clin. Oncol.* **1992,** *10:406–413. Physicians' Desk Reference,* 54th ed. Medical Economics Co., Montvale, NJ, **2000,** p. 1586.

[a]Following a 600 mg oral dose given twice daily to steady state.

Reference: Todd, P.A., and Ward, A. Gemfibrozil. A review of its pharmacodynamic and pharmacokinetic properties, and therapeutic use in dyslipidaemia. *Drugs,* **1988,** *36:314–339.*

[a]Gentamicin has a very long terminal $t_{1/2}$ of 53 ± 25 hours (slow release from tissues), which accounts for urinary excretion for up to 3 weeks after a dose. [b]Following a single 100 mg IV infusion (1 hour) or IM injection given to healthy adults.

References: Matzke, G.R., Yeh, J., Awni, W.M., Halstenson, C.E., and Chung, M. Pharmacokinetics of cetirizine in the elderly and patients with renal insufficiency. Ann. Allergy, 1987, 59:25–30. Regamey, C., Gordon, R.C., and Kirby, W.M. Comparative pharmacokinetics of tobramycin and gentamicin. Clin. Pharmacol. Ther., 1973, 14:396–403.

GLIMEPIRIDE[a] (Chapter 60)

Bioavailability	Urinary Excretion	Bound in Plasma	Clearance	Vol. Dist.	Half-Life	Peak Time	Peak Concentration
~100	<0.5	>99.5	0.62 ± 0.26 ↑RD[b]	0.18 ↑RD[b]	3.4 ± 2.0 ↔RD[b]	2–3[c]	359 ± 98 ng/ml[c]

[a]Data from healthy male subjects. No significant gender differences. Glimepiride is metabolized by CYP2C9 to an active (~one-third potency) metabolite, M1. [b]CL/F, V_d/F and $t_{1/2}$ unchanged, moderate-to-severe renal impairment; presumably mediated through an increase in plasma free fraction. M1 AUC also increased. [c]Following a single 3 mg oral dose.

References: Badian, M., Korn, A., Lehr, K.H., Malerczyk, V., and Waldhäusl, W. Determination of the absolute bioavailability of glimepiride (HOE 490), a new sulphonylurea. Int. J. Clin. Pharmacol. Ther. Toxicol., 1992, 30:481–482. Physicians' Desk Reference, 54th ed. Medical Economics Co., Montvale, NJ, 2000, pp. 1346–1349. Rosenkranz, B., Profozic, V., et al. Pharmacokinetics and safety of glimepiride at clinically effective doses in diabetic patients with renal impairment. Diabetologia, 1996, 39:1617–1624.

GLIPIZIDE (Chapter 60)

Bioavailability	Urinary Excretion	Bound in Plasma	Clearance	Vol. Dist.	Half-Life	Peak Time	Peak Concentration
95	<5	98.4	0.52 ± 0.18[a] ↔RD, Aged	0.17 ± 0.02[a] ↔Aged	3.4 ± 0.7 ↔RD, Aged	2.1 ± 0.9[b]	465 ± 139 ng/ml[b]

[a]CL/F and V_{ss}/F reported. [b]Following a single 5 mg oral dose (immediate-release tablet) given to healthy young adults. An extended-release formulation exhibits a delayed T_{max} of 6–12 hours.

Reference: Kobayashi, K.A., Bauer, L.A., Horn, J.R., Opheim, K., Wood, F., and Kradjan, W.A. Glipizide pharmacokinetics in young and elderly volunteers. Clin. Pharm., 1988, 7:224–228.

GLYBURIDE (Chapter 60)

Bioavailability	Urinary Excretion	Bound in Plasma	Clearance	Vol. Dist.	Half-Life	Peak Time	Peak Concentration
G: 90–100[a] M: 64–90[a]	Negligible	99.8 ↓Aged	1.3 ± 0.5 ↓Cirr	0.20 ± 0.11	4 ± 1[b] ↑Cirr, NIDDM	G: ~1.5[c] M: 2–4[c]	G: 106 ng/ml[c] M: 104 ng/ml[c]

[a]Data for GLYNASE PRESTAB micronized tablet (G) and MICRONASE tablet (M). [b]$t_{1/2}$ for micronized formulation reported. $t_{1/2}$ for nonmicronized formulation is 6 to 10 hours, reflecting absorption rate limitation. A long terminal $t_{1/2}$ (15 hours), reflecting redistribution from tissues, has been reported. [c]Following a 3 mg oral GLYNASE tablet taken with breakfast or a 5 mg oral MICRONASE tablet given to healthy adult subjects.

References: Jonsson, A., Rydberg, T., Ekberg, G., Hallengren, B., and Melander, A. Slow elimination of glyburide in NIDDM subjects. Diabetes Care, 1994, 17:142–145. Physicians' Desk Reference, 54th ed. Medical Economics Co., Montvale, NJ, 2000, p. 2457.

GRANISETRON (Chapter 37)

Bioavailability	Urinary Excretion	Bound in Plasma	Clearance	Vol. Dist.	Half-Life	Peak Time	Peak Concentration
~60	16 ± 14	65 ± 9 ↔RD	11 ± 9 ↓Aged, Cirr ↔RD	3.0 ± 1.5 ↔RD	5.3 ± 3.5 ↑Aged, Cirr ↔RD	—	IV: 64(18–176) ng/ml[a] Oral: 6.0 (0.6–31) ng/ml[a]

[a]Following a 40 μg/kg IV dose (5-minute infusion) given to patients with cancer or a single 1 mg oral dose given twice daily for 7 days.

References: Allen, A., Asgill, C.C., Pierce, D.M., Upward, J., and Zussman, B.D. Pharmacokinetics and tolerability of ascending intravenous doses of granisetron, a novel 5-HT$_3$ antagonist, in healthy human subjects. Eur. J. Clin. Pharmacol., 1994, 46:159–162. Physicians' Desk Reference, 54th ed. Medical Economics Co., Montvale, NJ, 2000, pp. 3016 and 3018.

Table A–II–1 *Pharmacokinetic Data (Continued)*

AVAILABILITY (ORAL) (%)	URINARY EXCRETION (%)	BOUND IN PLASMA (%)	CLEARANCE ($ml \cdot min^{-1} \cdot kg^{-1}$)	VOL. DIST. (liters/kg)	HALF-LIFE (hours)	PEAK TIME (hours)	PEAK CONCENTRATIONS
HALOPERIDOL[a] (Chapter 18)							
60 ± 18	1	92 ± 2 ↑ Cirr ↔ Aged, Child	11.8 ± 2.9[b] ↑ Child, Smk ↓ Aged	18 ± 7	18 ± 5[b] ↓ Child	IM: 0.6 ± 0.1[c] Oral: 1.7 ± 3.2[c]	IM: 22 ± 18 ng/ml[c] Oral: 9.2 ± 4.4 ng/ml[c]

[a] Undergoes reversible metabolism to a less active reduced haloperidol. [b] Represents net *CL* of parent drug; reduced haloperidol $CL = 10 ± 5$ ml · min^{-1} · kg^{-1} and $t_{\frac{1}{2}} = 67 ± 51$ hours. Slow conversion from reduced haloperidol to parent compound probably responsible for prolonged terminal $t_{\frac{1}{2}}$ (70 hours) for haloperidol observed with 7-day oral sampling. [c] Following a single 20 mg oral dose or 10 mg IM dose. Effective concentrations are 4–20 ng/ml.

Reference: Froemming, J.S., Lam, Y.W., Jann, M.W., and Davis, C.M. Pharmacokinetics of haloperidol. *Clin. Pharmacokinet.*, **1989**, *17*:396–423.

AVAILABILITY (ORAL) (%)	URINARY EXCRETION (%)	BOUND IN PLASMA (%)	CLEARANCE ($ml \cdot min^{-1} \cdot kg^{-1}$)	VOL. DIST. (liters/kg)	HALF-LIFE (hours)	PEAK TIME (hours)	PEAK CONCENTRATIONS
HEPARIN (Chapter 54)							
—	Negligible	Extensive	$1/(0.65 + 0.008D)$ ± 0.1[a] ↓ Fem	0.058 ± 0.11[b]	$(26 + 0.323D)$ ± 12 min[a] ↓ Smk	3[c]	70 ± 39 ng/ml[c]

[a] Dose (D) is in IU/kg. *CL* and $t_{\frac{1}{2}}$ are dose-dependent, perhaps due to saturable metabolism with end-product inhibition. [b] V_{area} reported. [c] Mean of above critical length molecules following a single 5000 IU dose (unfractionated) given by SC injection.

References: Bendetowicz, A.V., Beguin, S., Caplain, H., and Hemker, H.C. Pharmacokinetics and pharmacodynamics of a low molecular weight heparin (enoxaparin) after subcutaneous injection, comparison with unfractionated heparin—a three way cross over study in human volunteers. *Thromb. Haemost.*, **1994**, *71*:305–313. Estes, J.W. Clinical pharmacokinetics of heparin. *Clin. Pharmacokinet.*, **1980**, *5*:204–220.

AVAILABILITY (ORAL) (%)	URINARY EXCRETION (%)	BOUND IN PLASMA (%)	CLEARANCE ($ml \cdot min^{-1} \cdot kg^{-1}$)	VOL. DIST. (liters/kg)	HALF-LIFE (hours)	PEAK TIME (hours)	PEAK CONCENTRATIONS
HYDROCHLOROTHIAZIDE (Chapter 28)							
71 ± 15	>95	58 ± 17	4.9 ± 1.1[a] ↓ RD, CHF,[b] Aged	0.83 ± 0.31[c] ↓ Aged	2.5 ± 0.2[d] ↑ RD, CHF,[b] Aged	SD: 1.9 ± 0.5[e] MD: 2[e]	SD: 75 ± 17 ng/ml[e] MD: 91 ± 0.2 ng/ml[e]

[a] Renal *CL* reported, which should approximate total plasma *CL*; calculated assuming a 70 kg body weight. [b] Changes may reflect decreased renal function. [c] Calculated from individual values of renal *CL*, terminal $t_{\frac{1}{2}}$, and fraction of drug excreted unchanged; 70 kg body weight assumed. [d] Longer terminal $t_{\frac{1}{2}}$s of 8 ± 2.8 hours have been reported with a corresponding increase in V_{area} to 2.8 l/kg. [e] Following a single (SD) or multiple (MD) 12.5 mg oral dose of hydrochlorothiazide; MD given once daily for 5 days to healthy adults.

References: Beermann, B., and Groschinsky-Grind, M. Pharmacokinetics of hydrochlorothiazide in man. *Eur. J. Clin. Pharmacol.*, **1977**, *12*:297–303. Jordo, L., Johnsson, G., *et al.* Bioavailability and disposition of metoprolol and hydrochlorothiazide combined in one tablet and of separate doses of hydrochlorothiazide. *Br. J. Clin. Pharmacol.*, **1979**, *7*:563–567. O'Grady, P., Yee, K.F., Lins, R., and Mangold, B. Fosinopril/hydrochlorothiazide: single dose and steady-state pharmacokinetics and pharmacodynamics. *Br. J. Clin. Pharmacol.*, **1999**, *48*:375–381.

AVAILABILITY (ORAL) (%)	URINARY EXCRETION (%)	BOUND IN PLASMA (%)	CLEARANCE ($ml \cdot min^{-1} \cdot kg^{-1}$)	VOL. DIST. (liters/kg)	HALF-LIFE (hours)	PEAK TIME (hours)	PEAK CONCENTRATIONS
HYDROCODONE[a] (Chapter 21)							
—	EM: 10.2 ± 1.8 PM: 18.1 ± 4.5	—	EM: 11.1 ± 3.57[b] PM: 6.54 ± 1.25[b]	—	EM: 4.24 ± 0.99 PM: 6.16 ± 1.97[b]	EM: 0.72 ± 0.46[c] PM: 0.93 ± 0.59[c]	EM: 30 ± 9.4 ng/ml[c] PM: 27 ± 5.9 ng/ml[c]

HYDROMORPHONE[a] (Chapter 21)

Oral: 42 ± 23 SC: ~80	6	7.1	14.6 ± 7.6	2.90 ± 1.31[b]	2.4 ± 0.6	IV: —[c] Oral: 1.1 ± 0.2[c]	IV: 242 ng/ml[c] Oral: 11.8 ± 2.6 ng/ml[c]

[a]Data from healthy male and female subjects. The metabolism of hydrocodone to hydromorphone (more active) is catalyzed by CYP2D6. Subjects were phenotyped as extensive (EM) and poor (PM) metabolizers. [b]CL/F and $t_{\frac{1}{2}}$ reported for oral dose. [c]Following a 10 mg oral dose (syrup). Maximal hydromorphone concentrations are higher in EMs than PMs (5.2 vs. 1.0 ng/ml).

Reference: Otton, S.V., Schadel, M., et al. CYP2D6 phenotype determines the metabolic conversion of hydrocodone to hydromorphone. Clin. Pharmacol. Ther., **1993**, 54:463–472.

---

[a]Data from healthy male subjects. Extensively metabolized. The principal metabolite, 3-glucuronide, accumulates to much higher (27-fold) levels than parent drug and may contribute to some side effects (not antinociceptive). [b]V_{area} reported. [c]Following a single 2 mg IV (bolus, sample at 3 minutes) or 4 mg oral dose.

References: Hagen, N., Thirlwell, M.P., et al. Steady-state pharmacokinetics of hydromorphone and hydromorphone-3-glucuronide in cancer patients after immediate and controlled-release hydromorphone. J. Clin. Pharmacol. **1995**, 35:37–44. Moulin, D.E., Kreeft, J.H., Murray-Parsons, N., and Bouquillon, A.I. Comparison of continuous subcutaneous and intravenous hydromorphone infusions for management of cancer pain. Lancet, **1991**, 337:465–468. Parab, P.V., Ritschel, W.A., Coyle, D.E., Gregg, R.V., and Denson, D.D. Pharmacokinetics of hydromorphone after intravenous, peroral and rectal administration to human subjects. Biopharm. Drug Dispos. **1988**, 9:187–199.

HYDROXYUREA[a] (Chapter 51)

108 ± 18 (79–108)	35.8 ± 14.2	Negligible	72 ± 17 ml · min⁻¹ (m²)⁻¹[b] (36.2–72.3)	19.7 ± 4.6 l/m²	3.4 ± 0.7 (2.8–4.5)	IV: 0.5[c] Oral: 1.2 ± 1.2[c]	IV: 1007 ± 371 μM[c] Oral: 794 ± 241 μM[c]

[a]Data from male and female patients treated for solid tumors. A range of mean values from multiple studies is shown in parentheses. [b]Nonrenal elimination of hydroxyurea is thought to exhibit saturable kinetics through a 10–80 mg/kg dose range. [c]Following a single 2 g, 30 minute IV infusion or oral dose.

References: Gwilt, P.R., and Tracewell, W.G. Pharmacokinetics and pharmacodynamics of hydroxyurea. Clin. Pharmacokinet. **1998**, 34:347–358. Rodriguez, G.I., Kuhn, J.G., et al. A bioavailability and pharmacokinetic study of oral and intravenous hydroxyurea. Blood, **1998**, 91:1533–1541.

HYDROXYZINE[a] (Chapters 17, 24, 37)

—	—	A: 9.8 ± 3.3[b] C: 32 ± 11[b]	A: 16 ± 3[b] C: 19 ± 9[b] ↑ Aged	A: 20 ± 4[b] C: 7.1 ± 2.3[b,c] ↑ Aged, LD	A: 2.1 ± 0.4[d] C: 2.0 ± 0.9[d]	A: 72 ± 11 ng/ml[d] C: 47 ± 17 ng/ml[d]

[a]Hydroxyzine is metabolized to an active metabolite, cetirizine. Plasma concentrations of cetirizine exceed those of parent drug; its $t_{\frac{1}{2}}$ is similar to that of hydroxyzine when formed from parent drug. Hydroxyzine data for adults (A) and children (C) are reported. [b]CL/F, V_d/F, and $t_{\frac{1}{2}}$ after oral dose reported. [c]$t_{\frac{1}{2}}$ increases with increasing age (1–15 years of age). [d]Following a single 0.7 mg/kg oral dose given to healthy adults and children.

References: Paton, D.M., and Webster, D.R. Clinical pharmacokinetics of H1-receptor antagonists (the antihistamines). Clin. Pharmacokinet. **1985**, 10:477–497. Simons, F.E., Simons, K.J., Becker, A.B., and Haydey, R.P. Pharmacokinetics and antipruritic effects of hydroxyzine in children with atopic dermatitis. J. Pediatr. **1984**, 104:123–127. Simons, F.E., Simons, K.J., and Frith, E.M. The pharmacokinetics and antihistaminic of the H1 receptor antagonist hydroxyzine. J. Allergy Clin. Immunol. **1984**, 73:69–75. Simons, F.E., Watson, W.T., Chen, X.-Y., Minuk, G.Y., and Simons, K.J. The pharmacokinetics and pharmacodynamics of hydroxyzine in patients with primary biliary cirrhosis. J. Clin. Pharmacol. **1989**, 29:809–815. Simons, K.J., Watson, W.T., Chen, X.Y., and Simons, F.E. Pharmacokinetic and pharmacodynamic studies of the H1-receptor antagonist hydroxyzine in the elderly. Clin. Pharmacol. Ther. **1989**, 45: 9–14.

Table A–II–1 Pharmacokinetic Data (Continued)

	AVAILABILITY (ORAL) (%)	URINARY EXCRETION (%)	BOUND IN PLASMA (%)	CLEARANCE (ml·min⁻¹·kg⁻¹)	VOL. DIST. (liters/kg)	HALF-LIFE (hours)	PEAK TIME (hours)	PEAK CONCENTRATIONS
IBUPROFEN[a] (Chapter 26)	>80	<1	>99[b] ↔ RA, Alb	0.75 ± 0.20[b,c] ↑ CF ↔ Child, RA	0.15 ± 0.02[c] ↑ CF	2 ± 0.5[b] ↔ RA, CF, Child ↑ Cirr	1.6 ± 0.3[d]	61.1 ± 5.5 μg/ml[d]

[a]Racemic mixture. Kinetic parameters for the active S-(+)-enantiomer do not differ from those for the inactive R-(−)-enantiomer when administered separately; 63 ± 6% of the R-(−)-enantiomer undergoes inversion to the active isomer. [b]Unbound percent of S-(+)-ibuprofen (0.77 ± 0.20%) is significantly greater than that of R-(−)-ibuprofen (0.45 ± 0.06%). Binding of each enantiomer is concentration-dependent and is influenced by the presence of the optical antipode, leading to nonlinear elimination kinetics. [c]CL/F and V_{ss}/F reported. [d]Following a single 800 mg dose of racemate. A level of 10 μg/ml provides antipyresis in febrile children.

References: Lee, E.J., Williams, K., Day, R., Graham, G., and Champion, D. Stereoselective disposition of ibuprofen enantiomers in man. *Br. J. Clin. Pharmacol.,* **1985,** *19:*669–674. Lockwood, G.F., Albert, K.S., *et al.* Pharmacokinetics of ibuprofen in man. I. Free and total area/dose relationships. *Clin. Pharmacol. Ther.,* **1983,** *34:*97–103.

	AVAILABILITY (ORAL) (%)	URINARY EXCRETION (%)	BOUND IN PLASMA (%)	CLEARANCE (ml·min⁻¹·kg⁻¹)	VOL. DIST. (liters/kg)	HALF-LIFE (hours)	PEAK TIME (hours)	PEAK CONCENTRATIONS
IDARUBICIN[a] (Chapter 51)	I: 28 ± 4	<5	I: 97 IL: 94	29 ± 10 ↓ RD[b]	24.7 ± 5.9	I: 15.2 ± 3.7 IL: 41 ± 10 IL: ↑ RD[b]	I: 5.4 ± 2.4[c] IL: 7.9 ± 2.3[c]	I: 6.9 ± 0.1 ng/ml[c] IL: 22 ± 4 ng/ml[c]

[a]Data from male and female patients with cancer. Idarubicin (I) undergoes rapid metabolism to a major active (equipotent) metabolite, idarubicinol (IL). [b]Mild to moderate renal impairment. [c]Following a single 30–35 mg/m² oral dose.

References: Camaggi, C.M., Strocchi, E., *et al.* Idarubicin metabolism and pharmacokinetics after intravenous and oral administration in cancer patients: a crossover study. *Cancer Chemother. Pharmacol.,* **1992,** *30:*307–316. Robert, J. Clinical pharmacokinetics of idarubicin. *Clin. Pharmacokinet.,* **1993,** *24:*275–288. Tamassia, V., Pacciarini, M.A., *et al.* Pharmacokinetic study of intravenous and oral idarubicin in cancer patients. *Int. J. Clin. Pharmacol. Res.,* **1987,** *7:*419–426.

	AVAILABILITY (ORAL) (%)	URINARY EXCRETION (%)	BOUND IN PLASMA (%)	CLEARANCE (ml·min⁻¹·kg⁻¹)	VOL. DIST. (liters/kg)	HALF-LIFE (hours)	PEAK TIME (hours)	PEAK CONCENTRATIONS
IFOSFAMIDE[a] (Chapter 51)	92	Low: 12–18 High: 53.1 ± 9.6	Negligible	Low: 63 ml · min⁻¹ · (m²)⁻¹ b High: 6.2 ± 1.9 ml · min⁻¹ · (m²)⁻¹ ↔ Aged	Low: – High: 12.5 ± 3.6 l/ m² ↑ Aged	Low: 5.6 High: 15.2 ± 3.6 ↑ Aged	Oral: 0.5–1.0[c]	IV: 203 (168–232) μM[c] Oral: 200 (163– 245) μM[c]

[a]Data from male and female patients treated for advanced cancers. Administered IV with mesna to avoid hemorrhagic cystitis. Exhibits dose-dependent kinetics, with apparent saturation of hepatic metabolism. Metabolic activation to 4-hydroxyifosfamide catalyzed by CYP3A and CYP2C. Parameters reported for a 1.5 g/m² (Low) or 5 g/m² (High) IV dose and 1.5 g/m² oral dose. [b]CL reported to increase with daily dosing. [c]Geometric mean (range) following a single 1.5 g/m² IV infusion over 20 minutes or 1.5 g/m² oral dose.

References: Allen, L.M., and Creaven, P.J. Pharmacokinetics of ifosfamide. *Clin. Pharmacol. Ther.,* **1975,** *17:*492–498. Kurowski, V., Cerny, T., Kupfer, A., and Wagner, T. Metabolism and pharmacokinetics of oral and intravenous ifosfamide. *J. Cancer Res. Clin. Oncol.,* **1991,** *117*(suppl. 4):S148–S153. Lind, M.J., Margison, J.M., Cerny, T., Thatcher, N., and Wilkinson, P.M. The effect of age on the pharmacokinetics of ifosfamide. *Br. J. Clin. Pharmacol.,* **1990,** *30:*140–143. *Physicians' Desk Reference,* 54th ed. Medical Economics Co., Montvale, NJ, **2000,** pp. 866–867.

IMATINIB[a] (Chapter 51)

98 (87–111)	5	95	3.3 ± 1.2	6.2 ± 2.2	22 ± 4	3.3 ± 1.1[b]	2.6 ± 0.8 μg/ml[b]

[a]Imatinib is metabolized primarily by CYP3A4. [b]Following a 400 mg oral dose given once daily to steady state.

References: Peng, B., Dutreix, C., *et al.* Absolute bioavailability of imatinib (Glivec) orally versus intravenous infusion. *J. Clin. Pharmacol.*, **2004**, *44*:158–162. Peng, B., Hayes, M., *et al.* Pharmacokinetics and pharmacodynamics of imatinib in a phase I trial with chronic myeloid leukemia patients. *J. Clin. Oncol.*, **2004**, *22*:935–942. Product Information: Gleevec™ (imatinib mesylate). Novartis, Basel, Switzerland, **2004.**

IMIPENEM/CILASTATIN[a] (Chapter 44)

Imipenem —	69 ± 15 ↓Neo, Inflam ↔Child, CF	<20	2.9 ± 0/3 ↑Child ↓RD ↔CF, Inflam, Neo, Aged, Burn, Prem	0.23 ± 0.05 ↑Neo, Child, Prem ↔CF, RD, Aged	0.9 ± 0.1 ↑Neo, RD, Prem ↔CF, Child, Aged	IM: 1–2[b]	IV: 60–70 μg/ml[b] IM: 8.2–12 μg/ml[b]
Cilastatin —	70 ± 3 ↓Neo ↔CF	~35	3.0 ± 0.3 ↑Child ↓Neo, RD, Prem ↔CF, Aged	0.20 ± 0.03 ↔Neo, RD, CF, Aged ↑Prem	0.8 ± 0.1 ↑Neo, Prem ↔CF, Aged		

[a]Formulated as a 1:1 (mg/mg) mixture for parenteral administration; cilastatin inhibits the metabolism of imipenem by the kidney, increasing concentrations of imipenem in the urine; cilastatin does not change imipenem plasma concentrations appreciably. [b]Plasma C_{max} of imipenem following a single 1 g IV infusion over 30 minutes or 750 mg administered IM.

Reference: Buckley, M.M., Brogden, R.N., Barradell, L.B., and Goa, K.L. Imipenem/cilastatin. A reappraisal of its antibacterial activity, pharmacokinetic properties and therapeutic efficacy. *Drugs*, **1992**, *44*:408–444.

IMIPRAMINE[a] (Chapter 17)

42 ± 3	<2	90.1 ± 1.4 ↑HL, MI, Burn ↔RA, Aged	13 ± 1.7[b] ↓Aged ↑Smk ↔Child	18 ± 2[c] ↔Aged, Child	16 ± 1.3 ↑Aged ↔Child	2–6[d]	200 ± 137 ng/ml[d]

[a]Active metabolite, desipramine. [b]Undergoes *N*-demethylation to desipramine, catalyzed by CYP2C19 (polymorphic), CYP1A2, and others; 2-hydroxylation is catalyzed by CYP2D6 (polymorphic). [c]V_{area} reported. [d]Following a 200 mg oral dose given daily for 4 weeks. Steady-state concentration reported is the sum of imipramine and desipramine (DMI/IMI = 1.4). Efficacy reported at combined levels of 100–300 ng/ml, and toxicity at combined levels >1 μg/ml.

Reference: Sallee, F.R., and Pollock, B.G. Clinical pharmacokinetics of imipramine and desipramine. *Clin. Pharmacokinet.*, **1990**, *18*:346–364.

INDOMETHACIN (Chapter 26)

~100	90 ↔Alb, Prem, Neo	1.4 ± 0.2 ↓Prem, Neo, Aged	0.29 ± 0.04 ↔Aged	2.4 ± 0.2[a] ↔RA, RD ↑Neo, Prem, Aged	~1.3[b]	~2.4 μg/ml[b]	

[a]There is significant enterohepatic recycling (~50% after an IV dose). [b]Following a single 50 mg oral dose given after a standard breakfast. Effective at concentrations of 0.3–3 μg/ml and toxic at >5 μg/ml.

Reference: Oberbauer, R., Krivanek, P., and Turnheim, K. Pharmacokinetics of indomethacin in the elderly. *Clin. Pharmacokinet.*, **1993**, *24*:428–434.

Table A–II–1 Pharmacokinetic Data (Continued)

AVAILABILITY (ORAL) (%)	URINARY EXCRETION (%)	BOUND IN PLASMA (%)	CLEARANCE ($ml \cdot min^{-1} \cdot kg^{-1}$)	VOL. DIST. (liters/kg)	HALF-LIFE (hours)	PEAK TIME (hours)	PEAK CONCENTRATIONS
INTERFERON ALFA[a] (Chapters 49, 51, 62)							
I - SC: 90	—[b]	—	I: 2.8 ± 0.6[c] PI_{12kD}: 0.17 PI_{40kD}: 0.014 – 0.024	I: 0.40 ± 0.19[c] PI_{12kD}: 0.44 – 1.04 PI_{40kD}: 0.11 – 0.17	I: 0.67[d] PI_{12kD}: 37 (22 – 60) PI_{40kD}: 65	I: 7.3[e] PI_{12kD}: 22[f] PI_{40kD}: 80[g]	I: 1.7 (1.2 – 2.3) ng/ml[e] PI_{12kD}: 0.91 ± 0.33 ng/ml[f] PI_{40kD}: 26 ± 8.8 ng/ml[g]

References: Glue, P., Fang, J.W.S., *et al.* Pegylated interferon-2b: pharmacodynamics, safety, and preliminary efficacy data. *Clin. Pharmacol. Ther.*, **2000**, *68*:556–567. Harris, J.M., Martin, N.E., and Modi, M. Pegylation: a novel process for modifying pharmacokinetics. *Clin. Pharmacokinet.*, **2001**, *40*:539–551. *Physicians' Desk Reference*, 54th ed. Medical Economics Co., Montvale, NJ, **2000**, p. 2654. Wills, R.J. Clinical pharmacokinetics of interferons. *Clin. Pharmacokinet.*, **1990**, *19*:390–399.

[a]Values for recombinant interferon alfa-2a (I) and its 40 kDa pegylated form (PI_{40kD}) and the 12kDa pegylated form of interferon alfa-2b (PI_{12kD}) are reported. [b]I undergoes renal filtration, tubular reabsorption, and proteolytic degradation within tubular epithelial cells. Renal elimination of PI forms is much less significant than that of I, although not negligible. [c]CL values in 4 patients with leukemia were more than halved (1.1 ± 0.3 ml · min⁻¹ · kg⁻¹), while V_{ss} increased more than 20-fold (9.5 ± 3.5 l/kg) and terminal $t_{\frac{1}{2}}$ changed only minimally (7.3 ± 2.4 hours). [d]A terminal $t_{\frac{1}{2}}$ of 5.1 ± 1.6 hours accounts for 23% of the CL of I. [e]Following a single 36×10^6 units SC dose of I. [f]Following 4 weeks of multiple SC dosing of 1 μg/kg PI_{12kD}. [g]Following 48 weekly SC doses of 180 μg of PI_{40kD}.

AVAILABILITY (ORAL) (%)	URINARY EXCRETION (%)	BOUND IN PLASMA (%)	CLEARANCE ($ml \cdot min^{-1} \cdot kg^{-1}$)	VOL. DIST. (liters/kg)	HALF-LIFE (hours)	PEAK TIME (hours)	PEAK CONCENTRATIONS
INTERFERON BETA[a] (Chapters 49, 52)							
SC: 51 ± 17	—[a]	—	13 ± 5[a]	2.9 ± 1.8	4.3 ± 2.3	SC: 1–8[b]	IV: 1491 ± 659 IU/ml[b] SC: 40 ± 20 IU/ml[b]

Reference: Chiang, J., Gloff, C.A., Yoshizawa, C.N., and Williams, G.J. Pharmacokinetics of recombinant human interferon-β_{ser} in healthy volunteers and its effect on serum neopterin. *Pharm. Res.*, **1993**, *10*:567–572.

[a]Undergoes renal filtration, tubular reabsorption, and renal catabolism, but hepatic uptake and catabolism are thought to dominate systemic CL. [b]Concentration at 5 minutes following a single 90×10^6 IU IV dose or following a single 90×10^6 IU SC dose of recombinant interferon beta-1b.

AVAILABILITY (ORAL) (%)	URINARY EXCRETION (%)	BOUND IN PLASMA (%)	CLEARANCE ($ml \cdot min^{-1} \cdot kg^{-1}$)	VOL. DIST. (liters/kg)	HALF-LIFE (hours)	PEAK TIME (hours)	PEAK CONCENTRATIONS
IRBESARTAN[a] (Chapters 30, 32)							
60–80	2.2 ± 0.9	90	2.12 ± 0.54 ↓ Aged[b] ↔ RD, Cirr	0.72 ± 0.20	13 ± 6.2	1.2 (0.7–2)[c]	1.3 ± 0.4 μg/ml[c]

References: Gillis, J.C., and Markham, A. Irbesartan. A review of its pharmacodynamic and pharmacokinetic properties and therapeutic use in the management of hypertension. *Drugs*, **1997**, *54*:885–902. *Physicians' Desk Reference*, 54th ed. Medical Economics Co., Montvale, NJ, **2000**, p. 818. Vachharajani, N.N., Shyu, W.C., *et al.* Oral bioavailability and disposition characteristics of irbesartan, an angiotensin antagonist, in healthy volunteers. *J. Clin. Pharmacol.*, **1998**, *38*:702–707.

[a]Data from healthy male subjects. No significant gender differences. Metabolized by UGT and CYP2C9. [b]CL/F reduced; no dose adjustment required. [c]Following a single 50 mg oral dose (capsule).

IRINOTECAN[a] (Chapter 51)

—	I: 16.7 ± 1.0	I: 30–68 SN-38: 95	I: 14.8 ± 41 · h^{-1} · (m^2)$^{-1}$	150 ± 49 l/m^2	I: 10.8 ± 0.5 SN-38: 10.4 ± 3.1	I: 0.5[b] SN-38: ≤1[b]	I: 1.7 ± 0.8 μg/ml[b] SN-38: 26 ± 12 ng/ml[b]

[a]Data from male and female patients with malignant solid tumors. No significant gender differences. Irinotecan (I) is metabolized to an active metabolite, SN-38 (100-fold more potent but with lower blood levels). [b]Following a 125 mg/m^2 IV infusion over 30 minutes.

References: Chabot, G.G., Abigerges, D., *et al.* Population pharmacokinetics and pharmacodynamics of irinotecan (CPT-11) and active metabolite SN-38 during phase 1 trials. *Ann. Oncol.,* **1995,** 6:141–151. *Physicians' Desk Reference,* 54th ed. Medical Economics Co., Montvale, NJ, **2000,** pp. 2412–2413.

ISONIAZID[a] (Chapter 47)

—[b] ↓ Food	RA: 7 ± 2[c] SA: 29 ± 5[c]	~0	RA: 7.4 ± 2.0[d] SA: 3.7 ± 1.1[d] ↔ Aged ↓ RD[e]	0.67 ± 0.15[d] ↔ Aged, RD	RA: 1.1 ± 0.1 SA: 3.1 ± 1.1 ↑ AVH, Cirr, Neo, RD ↔ Aged, Obes, Child, HTh	RA: 1.1 ± 0.5[f] SA: 1.1 ± 0.6[f]	RA: 5.4 ± 2.0 μg/ml[f] SA: 7.1 ± 1.9 μg/ml[f]

[a]Metabolized by *N*-acetyltransferase 2 (polymorphic). Data for slow acetylators (SA) and rapid acetylators (RA) reported. [b]It is usually stated that isoniazid is completely absorbed; however, good estimates of possible loss due to first-pass metabolism are not available. Absorption is decreased by food and antacids. [c]Recovery after oral administration; assay includes unchanged drug and acid-labile hydrazones. Higher percentages have been noted after IV administration, suggesting significant first-pass metabolism. [d]CL/F and V_{ss}/F reported. [e]Decrease in CL_{NR}/F as well as CL_R. [f]Following a single 400 mg oral dose to healthy rapid and slow acetylators.

Reference: Kim, Y.G., Shin, J.G., *et al.* Decreased acetylation of isoniazid in chronic renal failure. *Clin. Pharmacol. Ther.,* **1993,** 54:612–620.

ISOSORBIDE DINITRATE[a] (Chapter 31)

Oral: 22 ± 14[b,c] SL: 45 ± 16[b] PC: 33 ± 17[b]	<1	28 ± 12	46(38–59)[d] ↓ Cirr ↔ Smk, RD, Fem, CHF	3.1 (2.2–8.6)	0.7 (0.6–2.0)[d] ↔ RD, Fem	IR[e] ISDN: 0.3 (0.2–0.5) IS-2-MN: 0.6 (0.2–1.6) IS-5-MN: 0.7 (0.3–1.9)	IR[e] ISDN: 42 (59–166) nM IS-2-MN: 207 (197–335) nM IS-5-MN: 900 (790–1080) nM

Table A–II–1 *Pharmacokinetic Data (Continued)*

AVAILABILITY (ORAL) (%)	URINARY EXCRETION (%)	BOUND IN PLASMA (%)	CLEARANCE ($ml \cdot min^{-1} \cdot kg^{-1}$)	VOL. DIST. (liters/kg)	HALF-LIFE (hours)	PEAK TIME (hours)	PEAK CONCENTRATIONS
ISOSORBIDE DINITRATE[a] *(continued)*							
						SR[e] ISDN: ~0 IS-2-MN: 2.8 (2.7–3.7) IS-5-MN: 5.1 (4.2–6.6)	SR[e] ISDN: ~0 IS-2-MN: 28 (23–33) nM IS-5-MN: 175 (154–267) nM

[a]Isosorbide dinitrate is metabolized to the 2- and 5-mononitrates. Both metabolites and the parent compound are thought to be active. Data for the dinitrate are reported except where indicated. [b]Bioavailability calculations from single dose. SL, sublingual; PC, percutaneous. [c]↔ CHF, RD, Smk; ↑ Cirr. [d]CL may be decreased and $t_\frac{1}{2}$ prolonged after chronic dosing. [e]Mean (range) for isosorbide dinitrate (ISDN) and isosorbide-5-mononitrate (IS-5-MN) following a single 20 mg oral immediate release (IR) and sustained release (SR) dose.

References: Abshagen, U., Betzien, G., Endele, R., Kaufmann, B., and Neugebauer, G. Pharmacokinetics and metabolism of isosorbide-dinitrate after intravenous and oral administration. *Eur. J. Clin. Pharmacol.,* **1985,** 27:637–644. Fung, H.L. Pharmacokinetics and pharmacodynamics of organic nitrates. *Am. J. Cardiol.,* **1987,** 60:4H–9H.

ISOSORBIDE 5-MONONITRATE[a] **(ISOSORBIDE NITRATE) (Chapter 31)**

AVAILABILITY (ORAL) (%)	URINARY EXCRETION (%)	BOUND IN PLASMA (%)	CLEARANCE ($ml \cdot min^{-1} \cdot kg^{-1}$)	VOL. DIST. (liters/kg)	HALF-LIFE (hours)	PEAK TIME (hours)	PEAK CONCENTRATIONS
93 ± 13 ↔ Cirr, RD, Aged, CAD	<5	0	1.80 ± 0.24 ↔ Cirr, RD, Aged, CAD	0.73 ± 0.09 ↔ Cirr, RD, MI, Aged, CAD	4.9 ± 0.8 ↔ Cirr, RD, MI, Aged, CAD	1–1.5[b]	314–2093 nM[b]

[a]Active metabolite of isosorbide dinitrate. [b]Following a 20 mg oral dose given by asymmetric dosing (0 and 7 hours) for 4 days. Effective concentration is ~500 nM.

Reference: Abshagen, U.W. Pharmacokinetics of isosorbide mononitrate. *Am. J. Cardiol.,* **1992,** 70:61G–66G.

ISOTRETINOIN[a] **(Chapter 62)**

AVAILABILITY (ORAL) (%)	URINARY EXCRETION (%)	BOUND IN PLASMA (%)	CLEARANCE ($ml \cdot min^{-1} \cdot kg^{-1}$)	VOL. DIST. (liters/kg)	HALF-LIFE (hours)	PEAK TIME (hours)	PEAK CONCENTRATIONS
40[b] ↑ Food	negligible	>99	5.5 (0.9–11.1)[c]	5 (1–32)[c]	17 (5–167)[d]	I: 4.5 ± 3.4[e] 4-oxo: 6.8 ± 6.5[e]	I: 208 ± 92 ng/ml[e] 4-oxo: 473 ± 171 ng/ml[e]

[a]Isotretinoin (I) is eliminated through metabolic oxidations catalyzed by multiple CYPs (2C8, 2C9, 3A4, 2B6). The 4-oxo-isotretinoin metabolite (4-oxo) is active and is found at higher concentrations than parent drug at steady state. [b]Bioavailability when taken with food is reported. [c]*CL/F* and *V/F* reported. [d]4-oxo has an apparent mean $t_\frac{1}{2}$ of 29 ± 6 hours. [e]Values for I and 4-oxo following a 30 mg oral dose given once daily to steady state.

References: Larsen, F.G., Nielsen-Kudsk, F., Jakobsen, P., Weismann, K., and Kragballe, K. Pharmacokinetics and therapeutic efficacy of retinoids in skin diseases. *Clin. Pharmacokinet.,* **1992,** 23:42–61. Nulman, I., Berkovitch, M., *et al.* Steady-state pharmacokinetics of isotretinoin and its 4-oxo metabolite: implications for fetal safety. *J. Clin. Pharmacol.,* **1998,** 38:926–930. Wiegand, U.W., and Chou, R.C. Pharmacokinetics of oral isotretinoin. *J. Am. Acad. Dermatol.,* **1998,** 39:S8–S12.

ITRACONAZOLE[a] (Chapter 48)

55 ↑Food ↓HIV[b]	<1	99.8	23 ± 10[c]	14 ± 5[d]	21 ± 6[e]	3–5[f]	649 ± 289 ng/ml[f] ↑Food

[a]Metabolized predominantly by CYP3A4 to an active metabolite, hydroxyitraconazole, and other sequential metabolites. [c]CL/F reported. CL is concentration-dependent; the value given is for CL/F in the nonsaturable range. $K_m = 330 \pm 200$ ng/ml, $V_{max} = 2.2 \pm 0.8$ pg·ml⁻¹·min⁻¹·kg⁻¹. Apparent CL/F at steady state reported to be 5.4 ml·min⁻¹·kg⁻¹. [d]V_{area}/F reported. [b]Relative to oral dosing with food. [e]$t_{\frac{1}{2}}$ for the non-saturable concentration range. $t_{\frac{1}{2}}$ at steady state reported to be 64 hours. [f]Following a 200 mg oral dose given daily for 4 days to adults.

References: Heykants, J., Michiels, M., *et al.* The pharmacokinetics of itraconazole in animals and man. An overview. In, *Recent Trends in the Discovery, Development and Evaluation of Antifungal Agents.* (Fromtling, R.A., ed.) Prous Science Publisher, Barcelona, **1987**, pp. 223–249. Jalava, K.M., Olkkola, K.T., and Neuvonen, P.J. Itraconazole greatly increases plasma concentrations and effects of felodipine. *Clin. Pharmacol. Ther.,* **1997**, *61*:410–415.

IVERMECTIN[a] (Chapter 41)

—	<1		2.06 ± 0.81[b]	9.91 ± 2.67[b]	56.5 ± 7.5[b]	4.7 ± 0.5[c]	38.2 ± 5.8 ng/ml[c]

[a]Data from male and female patients treated for onchocerciasis. Metabolized by hepatic enzymes and excreted into bile. [b]CL/F, V_{area}/F, and other parameters reported for oral dose. Terminal $t_{\frac{1}{2}}$ reported. [c]Following a single 150 μg/kg oral dose (tablet).

References: Okonkwo, P.O., Ogbuokiri, J.E., Ofoegbu, E., and Klotz, U. Protein binding and ivermectin estimations in patients with onchocerciasis. *Clin. Pharmacol. Ther.*, **1993**, *53*:426–430. *Physicians' Desk Reference*, 54th ed. Medical Economics Co., Montvale, NJ, **2000**, p. 1886.

KETOCONAZOLE (Chapter 48)

—[a]	<1	99.0 ± 0.1	8.4 ± 4.1[b]	2.4 ± 1.6[b]	3.3 ± 1.0[b,c]	1–3[d]	3.2 (1.4–4.5) μM[d]

[a]Unknown because of lack of IV formulation. Bioavailability is diminished by hypochlorhydria (e.g., use of antacids, H_2-receptor antagonists). [b]CL/F, V_{area}/F, and $t_{\frac{1}{2}}$ reported for 200 mg daily doses given for more than 1 month. With single dose, CL/F and V_{area}/F are lower, and $t_{\frac{1}{2}}$ is about 8 hours. [c]Conflicting data from normal subjects suggest increased $t_{\frac{1}{2}}$ with increasing dose and repeated dose. [d]Following a 200 mg oral dose given once daily to steady state in patients with recalcitrant superficial mycotic infection. Average concentration at steady state was 0.51 ± 0.26 μM.

Reference: Badcock, N.R., Bartholomeusz, F.D., Frewin, D.B., Sansom, L.N., and Reid, J.G. The pharmacokinetics of ketoconazole after chronic administration in adults. *Eur. J. Clin. Pharmacol.*, **1987**, *33*:531–534.

KETOROLAC[a] (Chapter 26)

100 ± 20	5–10	99.2 ± 0.1	0.50 ± 0.15 ↓Aged, RD[b] ↔Cirr	0.21 ± 0.04	5.3 ± 1.2 ↑Aged, RD[b] ↔Cirr	IM: 0.7–0.8[c] Oral: 0.3–0.9[c]	IM: 2.2–3.0 μg/ml[c] Oral: 0.8–0.9 μg/ml[c]

[a]Racemic mixture; S-(−)-enantiomer is much more active than the R-(+)-enantiomer. Following IM injection, the mean AUC ratio for S/R enantiomers was 0.44 ± 0.04, indicating a higher CL and shorter $t_{\frac{1}{2}}$ for the S-(−)-enantiomer. Values reported are for the racemate. [b]Probably due to the accumulation of glucuronide metabolite, which is hydrolyzed back to parent drug. [c]Range of mean C_{max} and T_{max} from different studies following a single 30 mg IM or 10 mg oral dose in healthy adults.

Reference: Brocks, D.R., and Jamali, F. Clinical pharmacokinetics of ketorolac tromethamine. *Clin. Pharmacokinet.*, **1992**, *23*:415–427.

Table A–II–1 Pharmacokinetic Data (Continued)

	AVAILABILITY (ORAL) (%)	URINARY EXCRETION (%)	BOUND IN PLASMA (%)	CLEARANCE ($ml \cdot min^{-1} \cdot kg^{-1}$)	VOL. DIST. (liters/kg)	HALF-LIFE (hours)	PEAK TIME (hours)	PEAK CONCENTRATIONS
LAMIVUDINE[a] (Chapter 50)	86 ± 17 ↓ Food[b]	49–85	<36	4.95 ± 0.75 ↓ RD[b] ↔ Cirr ↑ Child[c]	1.30 ± 0.36	9.11 ± 5.09 ↑ RD[b] ↓ Child[c]	0.5–1.5[d]	1.0 (0.86–1.2) µg/ml[d]
LAMOTRIGINE[a] (Chapter 19)	97.6 ± 4.8	10	56	0.38–0.61[b,c] ↓ LD,[d] RD[e]	0.87–1.2	24–35[c] ↑ LD,[d] RD[e]	2.2 ± 1.2[f]	2.5 ± 0.4 µg/ml[f]
LANSOPRAZOLE[a] (Chapter 36)	81 ± 22 ↓ Food[b]	<1	97 ↓ RD[c]	6.23 ± 1.60 ↓ Aged,[d] LD[e]	0.35 ± 0.05	0.90 ± 0.44 ↑ Aged, LD	1.3 ± 0.6[f]	248 ± 140 ng/ml[f] ↓ Food[b]

[a]Data from healthy male subjects. No significant gender differences. [b]CL/F decreased, moderate and severe renal impairment. [c]Weight-normalized CL/F increased in children <12 years of age. [d]Following a single 100 mg oral dose (tablet).

References: Heald, A.E., Hsyu, P.H., et al. Pharmacokinetics of lamivudine in human immunodeficiency virus-infected patients with renal dysfunction. Antimicrob. Agents Chemother.. 1996, 40:1514–1519. Johnson, M.A., Moore, K.H., Yuen, G.J., Bye, A., and Pakes, G.E. Clinical pharmacokinetics of lamivudine. Clin. Pharmacokinet. 1999, 36:41–66. Physicians' Desk Reference, 54th ed. Medical Economics Co., Montvale, NJ, 2000, p. 1172. Yuen, G.J., Morris, D.M.. et al. Pharmacokinetics, absolute bioavailability, and absorption characteristics of lamivudine. J. Clin. Pharmacol., 1995, 35:1174–1180.

[a]Lamotrigine is eliminated primarily by glucuronidation. The parent-metabolite pair may undergo enterohepatic recycling. Data from healthy adults and patients with epilepsy. Range of mean values from multiple studies reported. [b]CL/F increases slightly with multiple-dose therapy. [c]CL/F increased and $t_{\frac{1}{2}}$ decreased in patients receiving enzyme-inducing anticonvulsant drugs. [d]CL/F reduced, moderate-to-severe hepatic impairment. [e]CL/F reduced, severe renal disease. [f]Following a single 200 mg oral dose to healthy adults.

References: Chen, C., Casale, E.J., Duncan, B., Culverhouse, E.H., and Gilman, J. Pharmacokinetics of lamotrigine in children in the absence of other antiepileptic drugs. Pharmacotherapy, 1999, 19:437–441. Garnett, W.R. Lamotrigine: pharmacokinetics. J. Child Neurol. 1997, 12(suppl 1):S10–S15. Physicians' Desk Reference, 54th ed. Medical Economics Co., Montvale, NJ, 2000, p. 1209. Wootton, R., Soul-Lawton, J., et al. Comparison of the pharmacokinetics of lamotrigine in patients with chronic renal failure and healthy volunteers. Br. J. Clin. Pharmacol.. 1997, 43:23–27.

References: Delhotal-Landes, B., Flouvat, B., *et al.* Pharmacokinetics of lansoprazole in patients with renal or liver disease of varying severity. *Eur. J. Clin. Pharmacol.,* **1993,** *45:*367–371. Gerloff, J., Mignot, A., Barth, H., and Heintze, K. Pharmacokinetics and absolute bioavailability of lansoprazole. *Eur. J. Clin. Pharmacol.,* **1996,** *50:*293–297. *Physicians' Desk Reference,* 54th ed. Medical Economics Co., Montvale, NJ, **2000,** pp. 3105–3106.

LEFLUNOMIDE[a] (Chapters 51, 52)

| —[b] | negligible | 99.4 ↓RD | 0.012[c] ↑RD | 0.18 (0.09–0.44)[c] ↑RD | 377 (336–432)[d] ↔RD | 6–12[e] | 35 μg/ml[e] |

[a]Leflunomide is a prodrug that is converted almost completely (~95%) to an active metabolite A77-1726 (2-cyano-3-hydroxy-N-(4-trifluoromethylphenyl)-crotonamide). All pharmacokinetic data reported are for the active metabolite. [b]Absolute bioavailability is not known; parent drug/metabolite are well-absorbed. [c]Apparent CL/F and V/F in healthy volunteers reported. Both parameters are a function of the bioavailability of leflunomide and the extent of its conversion to A77-1726. [d]In patients with rheumatoid arthritis. [e]Following a 20 mg oral dose given once daily to steady state in patients with rheumatoid arthritis.

[a]Data from healthy male subjects. No significant gender differences. [b]Food effect when taken 30 minutes after a meal. [c]Increased free fraction, severe renal impairment. No dose change with once-daily dosing. [d]CL/F reduced in elderly; no dose change required with once daily administration. [e]CL/F reduced, severe hepatic impairment. [f]Following a single 15 mg oral dose.

Reference: Rozman, B. Clinical pharmacokinetics of leflunomide. *Clin. Pharmacokinet.,* **2002,** *41:*421–430.

LETROZOLE[a] (Chapters 51, 57)

| 99.9 ± 16.3 | 3.9 ± 1.4 | 60 | 0.58 ± 0.21 ↓LD[b] | 1.87 ± 0.46 | 45 ± 16 | 1.0[c] | 115 nM[c] |

[a]Data from healthy postmenopausal female subjects. Metabolized by CYP3A4 and CYP2A6. [b]CL/F reduced, severe hepatic impairment. [c]Following a single 2.5 mg oral dose (tablet).

References: Lamb, H.M., and Adkins, J.C. Letrozole. A review of its use in postmenopausal women with advanced breast cancer. *Drugs,* **1998,** *56:*1125–1140. Sioufi, A., Gauducheau, N., *et al.* Absolute bioavailability of letrozole in healthy postmenopausal women. *Biopharm. Drug Dispos.,* **1997,** *18:*779–789.

LEVETIRACETAM[a] (Chapter 19)

| ~100 | 66 | <10 | 0.96 ↓ RD,[b] Aged, LD[c] ↑ Child[d] | 0.5–0.7 | 7 ± 1 ↑ RD,[b] Aged | 0.5–1.0[e] | ~10 μg/ml[e] |

[a]Data from healthy adults and patients with epilepsy. No significant gender differences. [b]CL/F reduced, mild renal impairment (cleared by hemodialysis). [c]CL/F reduced, severe hepatic impairment. [d]CL/F increased, 6 to 12 years of age. [e]Following a single 500 mg dose given to healthy adults.

Reference: Physicians' Desk Reference, 55 ed. Medical Economics Co., Montvale, NJ, **2001,** pp. 3206–3207.

Table A–II–1 *Pharmacokinetic Data (Continued)*

AVAILABILITY (ORAL) (%)	URINARY EXCRETION (%)	BOUND IN PLASMA (%)	CLEARANCE ($ml \cdot min^{-1} \cdot kg^{-1}$)	VOL. DIST. (liters/kg)	HALF-LIFE (hours)	PEAK TIME (hours)	PEAK CONCENTRATIONS
LEVODOPA[a] (Chapter 20)							
41±16 ↑Aged	<1	—	23±4 ↓Aged	1.7±0.4 ↓Aged	1.4±0.4 ↔Aged	Y: 1.4±0.7[c]	Y: 1.7±0.8 μg/ml[c]
86±19[b] ↔Aged			9±1[b] ↓Aged	0.9±0.2[b] ↓Aged	1.5±0.3[b] ↔Aged	E: 1.4±0.7[c]	E: 1.9±0.6 μg/ml[c]

[a]Naturally occurring precursor to dopamine. [b]Values obtained with concomitant carbidopa (inhibitor of dopa decarboxylase). [c]Following a single 125 mg oral dose of levodopa given with carbidopa (100 mg 1 hour prior to and 50 mg 6 hours after levodopa) in young (Y) and elderly (E) subjects.

Reference: Robertson, D.R., Wood, N.D., *et al.* The effect of age on the pharmacokinetics of levodopa administered alone and in the presence of carbidopa. *Br. J. Clin. Pharmacol.,* **1989,** 28:61–69.

AVAILABILITY (ORAL) (%)	URINARY EXCRETION (%)	BOUND IN PLASMA (%)	CLEARANCE ($ml \cdot min^{-1} \cdot kg^{-1}$)	VOL. DIST. (liters/kg)	HALF-LIFE (hours)	PEAK TIME (hours)	PEAK CONCENTRATIONS
LEVOFLOXACIN[a] (Chapter 43)							
99±10	61–87	24–38	2.52±0.45 ↓RD[b]	1.36±0.21	7±1 ↑RD[b]	1.6±0.8[c]	4.5±0.9 μg/ml[c]

[a]Data from healthy adult male subjects. Gender and age differences related to renal function. [b]CL/F reduced, mild to severe renal impairment (not cleared by hemodialysis). [c]Following a single 500 mg oral dose. No significant accumulation with once-daily dosing.

References: Chien, S.C., Rogge, M.C., *et al.* Pharmacokinetic profile of levofloxacin following once-daily 500-milligram oral or intravenous doses. *Antimicrob. Agents Chemother.,* **1997,** 41:2256–2260. Fish, D.N., and Chow, A.T. The clinical pharmacokinetics of levofloxacin. *Clin. Pharmacokinet.,* **1997,** 32:101–119. *Physicians' Desk Reference,* 54th ed. Medical Economics Co., Montvale, NJ, **2000,** p. 2157.

AVAILABILITY (ORAL) (%)	URINARY EXCRETION (%)	BOUND IN PLASMA (%)	CLEARANCE ($ml \cdot min^{-1} \cdot kg^{-1}$)	VOL. DIST. (liters/kg)	HALF-LIFE (hours)	PEAK TIME (hours)	PEAK CONCENTRATIONS
LIDOCAINE[a] (Chapters 14, 34)							
35±11[b] ↑Cirr, Aged	2±1 ↑Neo	70±5 ↓Neo ↑MI, CPBS, Aged, RD ↔NS, Smk, Child	9.2±2.4[c] ↓CHF, Cirr, CPBS,[d] Obes, Aged[f] ↑Smk ↔RD, AVH,[e] Neo	1.1±0.4 ↓CHF, CPBS,[d] Cirr, Neo ↔RD, Aged, Obes	1.8±0.4 ↑Cirr, MI,[g] Neo, Obes ↔RD, CPBS CHF[h]	—	2–5 μg/ml[i]

[a]Active metabolite, monoethylglycylxylidide (MEGX), is 60% to 80% as potent as lidocaine; concentrations reach 36 ± 26% of those of parent drug, but it is only 15 ± 3% protein bound. [b]Preparations available only for parenteral administration because of extensive and variable first-pass metabolism. [c]Formation of MEGX is catalyzed predominantly by CYP3A. [d]Decrease (~40%) on day 3 after surgery; returns to normal by day 7. [e]During acute phase, blood CL was 13 ± 4 ml · min⁻¹ · kg⁻¹, which increased to 20 ± 4 ml · min⁻¹ · kg⁻¹ after recovery. [f]Decreased CL with increasing age noted in patients with MI. [g]$t_{1/2}$ increased when infused longer than 24 hours, probably related to increased plasma protein binding. [h]Short term, no change; long term, marked increase. [i]Therapeutic range of blood concentrations for control of ventricular arrhythmias. Levels of 6–10 and >10 μg/ml cause occasional and frequent toxicity, respectively.

Reference: Nattel, S., Gagne, G., and Pineau, M. The pharmacokinetics of lignocaine and β-adrenoceptor antagonists in patients with acute myocardial infarction. *Clin. Pharmacokinet.*, **1987**, *13*:293–316.

LINEZOLID (Chapter 46)

100	35	31	2.1 ± 0.8 ↑Child	0.57–0.71	5.2 ± 1.7 ↓Child	PO: 1.4 ± 0.5[a]	PO: 16 ± 4 μg/ml[a] IV: 15 ± 3 μg/ml[b]

[a]Following a 600 mg oral dose given twice daily to steady state. [b]Following a 30 minute IV infusion of a 600 mg dose given twice daily to steady state in patients with gram-positive infection.

References: MacGowan, A.P. Pharmacokinetic and pharmacodynamic profile of linezolid in healthy volunteers and patients with Gram-positive infections. *J. Antimicrob. Chemother.*, **2003**, *51*(suppl 2):ii17–ii25. Stalker, D.J., and Jungbluth, G.L. Clinical pharmacokinetics of linezolid, a novel oxazolidinone antibacterial. *Clin. Pharmacokinet.*, **2003**, *42*:1129–1140.

LISINOPRIL (Chapters 30, 31, 32, 33)

25 ± 20 ↓CHF	88–100	0	4.2 ± 2.2[a] ↓CHF, RD, Aged ↔Fem	2.4 ± 1.4[a] ↔Aged, RD	12[b] ↑Aged, RD	~7[c]	50 (6.4–343) ng/ml[c]

[a]CL/F and V_{area}/F reported. [b]Effective $t_{1/2}$ to predict steady-state accumulation upon multiple dosing; a terminal $t_{1/2}$ (tissue efflux) of 30 hours reported. [c]Following a 2.5–40 mg oral dose given daily to steady state in elderly patients with hypertension and varying degrees of renal function. EC_{90} for angiotensin converting enzyme inhibition is 27 ± 10 ng/ml.

Reference: Thomson, A.H., Kelly, J.G., and Whiting, B. Lisinopril population pharmacokinetics in elderly and renal disease patients with hypertension. *Br. J. Clin. Pharmacol.*, **1989**, *27*:57–65.

LITHIUM (Chapter 18)

100[a]	95 ± 15	0	0.35 ± 0.11[b] ↓RD, Aged ↑Preg ↔Obes	0.66 ± 0.16 ↓Obes	22 ± 8[c] ↑RD, Aged ↓Obes	IR: 0.5–3[d] SR: 2–6[d]	IR: 1–2 mM[d] SR: 0.7–1.2 mM[d]

[a]Values as low as 80% reported for some prolonged-release preparations. [b]Renal CL of Li⁺ parallels that of Na⁺. The ratio of CLs of Li⁺ and creatinine is about 0.2 ± 0.03. [c]The distribution $t_{1/2}$ is 5.6 ± 0.5 hours; this influences drug concentrations for at least 12 hours. [d]Following a single 0.7 mmol/kg oral dose of immediate release (IR) lithium carbonate and sustained release (SR) tablets.

Reference: Ward, M.E., Musa, M.N., and Bailey, L. Clinical pharmacokinetics of lithium. *J. Clin. Pharmacol.*, **1994**, *34*:280–285.

Table A–II–1 *Pharmacokinetic Data (Continued)*

	AVAILABILITY (ORAL) (%)	URINARY EXCRETION (%)	BOUND IN PLASMA (%)	CLEARANCE ($ml \cdot min^{-1} \cdot kg^{-1}$)	VOL. DIST. (liters/kg)	HALF-LIFE (hours)	PEAK TIME (hours)	PEAK CONCENTRATIONS
LOPINAVIR[a] (Chapter 50)	—[b] ↑food	<3	98–99	1.2[c]	0.6[c]	5.3 ± 2.5	4.4 ± 2.4[d]	9.8 ± 3.7 µg/ml[d]
LORATADINE[a] (Chapter 24)	L: —[b] DL: —[b]	L: Negligible DL: —	L: 97 DL: 82–87[c]	L: 142 ± 57[d] ↔ RD, ↓ LD DL: 14–18[d] ↓ RD, LD	L: 120 ± 80[d] ↔ RD DL: 26[d]	L: 8 ± 6 ↔ RD, ↑ LD DL: 21–24	L: 2.0 ± 0[e] DL(L): 2.6 ± 2.9[e] DL: 3.2 ± 1.8[f] HDL (DL): 4.8 ± 1.9[f]	L: 3.4 ± 3.4 ng/ml[e] DL(L): 4.1 ± 2.6 ng/ml[e] DL: 4.0 ± 2.1 ng/ml[f] HDL (DL): 2.0 ± 0.6 ng/ml[f]

[a]Currently formulated in combination with ritonavir (Kalletra®). Ritonavir inhibits the CYP3A-dependent metabolism of lopinavir, enhancing its bioavailability, increasing plasma concentrations (50- to 100-fold), and extending its $t_{\frac{1}{2}}$. Pharmacokinetic data from male and female patients with HIV are reported. [b]Absolute bioavailability is not known; the relative bioavailability increases with a high-fat meal. [c]CL/F and V_{area}/F reported; calculated from steady-state AUC data. [d]Following a 400/100 mg lopinavir/ritonavir oral dose given twice daily in combination with stavudine and lamivudine to steady state.

References: Boffito, M., Hoggard, P.G., *et al.* Lopinavir protein binding in vivo through the 12-hour dosing interval. *Ther. Drug Monit.*, **2004**, *26*:35–39. Corbett, A.H., Lim, M.L., and Kashuba, A.D. Kaletra (lopinavir/ritonavir). *Ann. Pharmacother.*, **2002**, *36*:1193–1203. Eron, J.J., Feinberg, J., *et al.* Once-daily versus twice-daily lopinavir/ritonavir in antiretroviral-naive HIV-positive patients: a 48-week randomized clinical trial. *J. Infect. Dis.*, **2004**, *189*:265–272. King, J.R., Wynn, H., Brundage, R., and Acosta, E.P. Pharmacokinetic enhancement of protease inhibitor therapy. *Clin. Pharmacokinet.*, **2004**, *43*:291–310.

[a]Loratadine (L) is converted to a major active metabolite, desloratadine (DL). Almost all patients achieve higher plasma concentrations of DL than of L. Desloratadine (Clarinex®) was recently approved for similar clinical indications as L. It too is eliminated by metabolism to an active metabolite, 3-hydroxydesloratadine (HDL), but the responsible enzyme(s) is not known. Approximately 7–20% of patients are slow metabolizers of DL; frequency varies with ethnicity. [b]Bioavailability of L and DL is not known; L is probably low due to extensive first-pass metabolism. [c]Plasma protein binding of HDL is 85–89%. [d]CL/F and V_{area}/F reported. For DL, oral CL/F calculated from AUC data following single 5–20 mg oral doses given to healthy adults. [e]Mean for L and DL following a 10 mg oral L dose (CLARITIN-D 24 HOUR) given once daily for 7 days to healthy adults. [f]Mean for DL and HDL following a 5 mg oral DL dose (CLARINEX®) given once daily for 10 days to healthy adults.

References: Affrime, M., Gupta, S., Banfield, C., and Cohen, A. A pharmacokinetic profile of desloratadine in healthy adults, including elderly. *Clin. Pharmacokinet.*, **2002**, *41*(suppl):13–19. Gupta, S., Banfield, C., *et al.* Desloratadine demonstrates dose proportionality in healthy adults after single doses. *Clin. Pharmacokinet.*, **2002**, *41*(suppl):1–6. Haria, M., Fitton, A., and Peters, D.H. Loratadine. A reappraisal of its pharmacological properties and therapeutic use in allergic disorders. *Drugs*, **1994**, *48*:617–637. Kosoglou, T., Radwanski, E., *et al.* Pharmacokinetics of loratadine and pseudoephedrine following single and multiple doses of once- versus twice-daily combination tablet formulations in healthy adult males. *Clin. Ther.*, **1997**, *19*:1002–1012. *Physicians' Desk Reference*, 58th ed. Medical Economics Co., Montvale, NJ, **2004**, p. 3044.

LORAZEPAM (Chapters 16, 17, 19)

93 ± 10	<1	1.1 ± 0.4[a] ↔ Aged, Cirr, AVH, Smk, RD ↑ Burn, CF	91 ± 2 ↓ Cirr, RD ↔ Aged, Burn	1.3 ± 0.2[b] ↑ Cirr, Burn, CF, RD ↔ Aged, AVH	14 ± 5 ↑ Cirr, Neo, RD ↔ Aged, CPBS, AVH ↓ Burn	IM: 1.2[c] Oral: 1.2–2.6[c]	IV: ~75 ng/ml[c] IM: ~30 ng/ml[c] Oral: ~28 ng/ml[c]

[a]Eliminated primarily by glucuronidation. [b]V_{area} reported. [c]Following a single 2 mg IV bolus dose, IM dose, or oral dose given to healthy adults.

Reference: Greenblatt, D.J. Clinical pharmacokinetics of oxazepam and lorazepam. *Clin. Pharmacokinet.*, **1981**, 6:89–105.

LOSARTAN[a] (Chapters 30, 32, 33)

L: 35.8 ± 15.5	L: 98.7 LA: 99.8	L: 8.1 ± 1.8 ↓ RD,[b] LD[c]	L: 12 ± 2.8	L: 0.45 ± 0.24	L: 2.5 ± 1.0 LA: 5.4 ± 2.3	L: 1.0 ± 0.5[d] LA: 4.1 ± 1.6[d]	L: 296 ± 217 ng/ml[d] LA: 249 ± 74 ng/ml[d]

[a]Data from healthy male subjects. Losartan (L) is metabolized primarily by CYP2C9 to an active 5-carboxylic acid metabolite (LA). [b]CL/F for L but not LA decreased, severe renal impairment (L/LA not removed by hemodialysis). No dose adjustment required. [c]CL/F for L reduced, mild-to-moderate hepatic impairment. LA AUC also increased. [d]Following a single 50 mg oral dose (tablet). Higher plasma levels of L but not LA in female subjects than in male subjects.

References: Lo, M.W., Goldberg, M.R., *et al.* Pharmacokinetics of losartan, an angiotensin II receptor antagonist, and its active metabolite EXP3174 in humans. *Clin. Pharmacol. Ther.*, **1995**, 58:641–649. *Physicians' Desk Reference*, 54th ed. Medical Economics Co., Montvale, NJ, **2000**, pp. 1809–1812.

LOVASTATIN[a] (Chapter 35)

≤5 ↑ Food	10	4.3–18.3[b] ↓ RD	>95	—	1–4	AI: 2.0 ± 0.9[c] TI: 3.1 ± 2.9[c]	AI: 41 ± 6 ng-Eq/ml[c] TI: 50 ± 8 ng-Eq/ml[c]

[a]Lovastatin is an inactive lactone that is metabolized to the corresponding active β-hydroxy acid. Pharmacokinetic values are based on the sum of HMG-CoA reductase inhibition activity by the β-hydroxy acid and other less potent metabolites. [b]The lactone (in equilibrium with β-hydroxy acid metabolite) is metabolized by CYP3A. [c]Following an 80 mg oral dose or dose given once daily for 17 days. Peak levels represent total active inhibitors (AI) and total inhibitors (TI) of HMG-CoA reductase.

References: Corsini, A., Bellosta, S., *et al.* New insights into the pharmacodynamic and pharmacokinetic properties of statins. *Pharmacol. Ther.*, **1999**, 84:413–428. Desager, J.P., and Horsmans, Y. Clinical pharmacokinetics of 3-hydroxy-3-methylglutaryl-coenzyme A reductase inhibitors. *Clin. Pharmacokinet.*, **1996**, 31:348–371. McKenney, J.M. Lovastatin: a new cholesterol-lowering agent. *Clin. Pharm.*, **1988**, 7:21–36.

MEFLOQUINE[a] (Chapter 39)

—[b]	98.2	0.43 ± 0.14[c] ↑ Preg ↔ Child	19 ± 6[c]	20 ± 4 days ↓ Preg ↔ Child	<1	SD: 7–19.6[d] MD: 12 ± 8[d]	SD: 800–1020 ng/ml[d] MD: 420 ± 141 ng/ml[d]

[a]Racemic mixture; no information on relative kinetics of the enantiomers. [b]Absolute bioavailability is not known; reported values of >85% represent comparison of oral tablet to solution. [c]CL/F and V_{ss}/F reported. [d]Range of mean values from different studies following a single 1000 mg oral dose (SD) and mean following a 250 mg oral dose given once weekly for 4 weeks (MD).

Reference: Karbwang, J., and White, N.J. Clinical pharmacokinetics of mefloquine. *Clin. Pharmacokinet.*, **1990**, 19:264–279.

Table A–II–1 Pharmacokinetic Data (Continued)

AVAILABILITY (ORAL) (%)	URINARY EXCRETION (%)	BOUND IN PLASMA (%)	CLEARANCE ($ml \cdot min^{-1} \cdot kg^{-1}$)	VOL. DIST. (liters/kg)	HALF-LIFE (hours)	PEAK TIME (hours)	PEAK CONCENTRATIONS
MELOXICAM[a] (Chapter 26)							
97	<1	~99.4	0.10–0.12	0.15–0.16	15–18	5–9[b]	1.9 ± 0.6 μg/ml[b]
MELPHALAN (Chapter 51)							
71 ± 23 ↑ Cirr	12 ± 7	90 ± 5[a]	5.2 ± 2.9 ↔ Child	0.45 ± 0.15 ↔ Child	1.4 ± 0.2[b] ↔ Child	Oral: 0.75 ± 0.24[c]	IV: 1.3 ± 0.95 μg/ml[c] Oral: 0.31 ± 0.15 μg/ml[c]
MEPERIDINE[a] (Chapter 21)							
52 ± 3 ↑ Cirr	~5 (1–25)[b] ↓ Aged, RD ↔ Cirr	58 ± 9[c] ↓ Aged, Prem ↔ Cirr	17 ± 5 ↓ AVH, Cirr, RD, Prem, Neo ↔ Aged, Preg, Smk	4.4 ± 0.9 ↑ Aged, Prem ↔ Cirr, Preg, RD	3.2 ± 0.8[d] ↑ AVH, Cirr, Prem, Neo, Aged, RD ↔ Preg	IM: <1[e]	IV: 0.67 μg/ml[e] IM: ~0.7 μg/ml[e]

[a]Primarily metabolized by CYP2C9, with minor contribution by CYP3A4. Data from men and women reported; no significant gender differences. [b]Following a 15 mg oral capsule given once daily for one week.

References: Euller-Ziegler, L., Velicitat, P., *et al.* Meloxicam: a review of its pharmacokinetics, efficacy and tolerability following intramuscular administration. *Inflamm. Res.*, **2001**, *50*(suppl):S5–S9. Hanft, G., Turck, D., Scheuerer, S., and Sigmund, R. Meloxicam oral suspension: a treatment alternative to solid meloxicam formulations. *Inflamm. Res.*, **2001**, *50*(suppl):S35–S37. *Physicians' Desk Reference*, 58th ed. Medical Economics Co., Montvale, NJ, **2004**, p. 1017.

[a]Decreases to 80 ± 5% after high doses (180 mg/m²). [b]Approximately equal to the $t_{\frac{1}{2}}$ of melphalan *in vitro* in human plasma at 37°C. [c]Following a single 0.5 mg/kg IV or 25 mg oral dose in cancer patients.

Reference: Loos, U., Musch, E., *et al.* The pharmacokinetics of melphalan during intermittent therapy of multiple myeloma. *Eur. J. Clin. Pharmacol.*, **1988**, 35:187–193.

[a]Meperidine undergoes P450-dependent *N*-demethylation to normeperidine. Metabolite is not an analgesic but is a potent CNS-excitatory agent and is associated with adverse side effects of meperidine. [b]Meperidine is a weak base ($pK_a = 8.6$) and is excreted to a greater extent in the urine at low urinary pH and to a lesser extent at high urinary pH. [c]Correlates with the concentration of α_1-acid glycoprotein. [d]A longer $t_{\frac{1}{2}}$ (7 hours) is also observed. [e]Following a continuous 24 mg/hr IV infusion or 100 mg IM injection every 4 hours to steady state. Postoperative analgesia occurs at 0.4–0.7 μg/ml.

Reference: Edwards, D.J., Svensson, C.K., Visco, J.P., and Lalka, D. Clinical pharmacokinetics of pethidine: 1982. *Clin. Pharmacokinet.*, **1982**, 7:421–433.

MERCAPTOPURINE[a] (Chapter 51)

12 ± 7[b]	22 ± 12	19	0.90 ± 0.37	11 ± 4[c]	0.56 ± 0.38	Oral (−): 2.4 ± 0.4[d] Oral (+): 2.8 ± 0.4[d]	IV: 6.9 μM[d] Oral (−): 0.74 ± 0.28 μM[d] Oral (+): 3.7 ± 0.6 μM[d]

[a]Inactive prodrug is metabolized intracellularly to 6-thioinosinate. Pharmacokinetic values for mercaptopurine are reported. [b]Increases to 60% when first-pass metabolism is inhibited by allopurinol (100 mg, three times daily). [c]Metabolically cleared by xanthine oxidase and thiopurine methyltransferase (polymorphic). Despite inhibition of intrinsic CL by allopurinol, hepatic metabolism is limited by blood flow, and CL is thus little changed by allopurinol. [d]Following an IV infusion of 50 mg/m² per hour to steady state in children with refractory cancers or a single oral dose of 75 mg/m² with (+) or without (−) allopurinol pretreatment.

References: Lennard, L. The clinical pharmacology of 6-mercaptopurine. *Eur. J. Clin. Pharmacol.*, **1992**, *43*:329–339. *Physicians' Desk Reference*, 54th ed. Medical Economics Co., Montvale, NJ, **2000**, p. 1255.

METAXALONE (Chapter 20)

—[a]	—[b]	—	—	14 ± 7[c]	Fasted: 9.2 ± 4.8[d] Fed: 2.4 ± 1.2[d]	Fasted: 3.0 ± 1.2[e] Fed: 4.9 ± 2.3[e]	Fasted: 1.7 μg/ml[e] Fed: 4.9 μg/ml[e]

[a]Absolute bioavailability is not known. [b]Unknown, but probably negligible, as the drug is extensively metabolized. [c]CL/F reported; data collected following a single 400 mg oral dose taken with a meal. [d]Apparent $t_{\frac{1}{2}}$ following a 400 mg oral dose. The drug may exhibit an absorption-limited terminal $t_{\frac{1}{2}}$ in the fasted state. A value of ~2.4 hours is seen after drug administration with a high-fat meal and may represent the true systemic elimination $t_{\frac{1}{2}}$. [e]Following a single 800 mg oral dose in the fasted and fed state.

Reference: *Physicians' Desk Reference*, 58th ed., Medical Economics Co., Montvale, NJ, **2004**, p. 2181.

METFORMIN[a] (Chapter 60)

52 ± 5 (40–55)	99.9 ± 0.5 (79–100)	Negligible	7.62 ± 0.30 (6.3–10.1) ↓RD,[b] Aged	1.12 ± 0.08[c] (0.9–3.94)	1.74 ± 0.20[c] (1.5–4.5) ↑RD,[b] Aged	1.9 ± 0.4[d] (1.5–3.5)[d]	1.6 ± 0.2 μg/ml[d] (1.0–3.1 μg/ml)[d]

[a]Data from healthy male and female subjects. No significant gender differences. Shown in parentheses are mean values from different studies. [b]CL/F reduced, mild to severe renal impairment. [c]Larger volume of distribution (4 l/kg) and longer $t_{\frac{1}{2}}$ (4.5 hours) also reported. [d]Following a single 0.5 g oral dose (tablet) and range for a 0.5–1.5 g oral dose.

References: Harrower, A.D. Pharmacokinetics of oral antihyperglycaemic agents in patients with renal insufficiency. *Clin. Pharmacokinet.*, **1996**, *31*:111–119. Pentikainen, P.J., Neuvonen, P.J., and Penttila, A. Pharmacokinetics of metformin after intravenous and oral administration to man. *Eur. J. Clin. Pharmacol.*, **1979**, *16*:195–202. *Physicians' Desk Reference*, 54th ed. Medical Economics Co., Montvale, NJ, **2000**, pp. 831–835. Scheen, A.J. Clinical pharmacokinetics of metformin. *Clin. Pharmacokinet.*, **1996**, *30*:359–371.

Table A–II–1 *Pharmacokinetic Data (Continued)*

AVAILABILITY (ORAL) (%)	URINARY EXCRETION (%)	BOUND IN PLASMA (%)	CLEARANCE (ml · min⁻¹ · kg⁻¹)	VOL. DIST. (liters/kg)	HALF-LIFE (hours)	PEAK TIME (hours)	PEAK CONCENTRATIONS
METHADONE[a] (Chapters 21, 23)							
92 ± 21	24 ± 10^{b}	89 ± 2.9	1.7 ± 0.9^{b} ↑ Burn, Child	3.6 ± 1.2^{c}	27 ± 12^{d} ↓ Burn, Child	$\sim 3^{e}$	IV: 450–550 ng/ml[e] Oral: 69–980 ng/ml[e]

[a]Racemic mixture; except for protein-binding measures (*d*-methadone slightly higher % bound), no kinetic parameters reported for individual enantiomers. [b]Inversely correlated with urine pH. [c]V_{area} reported. Directly correlated with urine pH. [d]Directly correlated with urine pH. [e]Following a single 10-mg IV bolus dose in patients with chronic pain or a 0.12–1.9 mg/kg oral dose, once daily for at least 2 months in subjects with opioid dependency. Levels >100 ng/ml prevent withdrawal symptoms; EC_{50} for pain relief and sedation in cancer patients is 350 ± 180 ng/ml.

References: Dyer, K.R., Foster, D.J., *et al.* Steady-state pharmacokinetics and pharmacodynamics in methadone maintenance patients: comparison of those who do and do not experience withdrawal and concentration–effect relationships. *Clin. Pharmacol. Ther.,* **1999,** *65:*685–694. Inturrisi, C.E., Colburn, W.A., Kaiko, R.E., Houde, R.W., and Foley, K.M. Pharmacokinetics and pharmacodynamics of methadone in patients with chronic pain. *Clin. Pharmacol. Ther.,* **1987,** *41:*392–401.

AVAILABILITY (ORAL) (%)	URINARY EXCRETION (%)	BOUND IN PLASMA (%)	CLEARANCE (ml · min⁻¹ · kg⁻¹)	VOL. DIST. (liters/kg)	HALF-LIFE (hours)	PEAK TIME (hours)	PEAK CONCENTRATIONS
METHOTREXATE[a] (Chapters 51, 52, 62)							
$70 \pm 27^{b,c}$	81 ± 9	46 ± 11	2.1 ± 0.8 ↓ RD ↑, ↔ Child ↔ RA	0.55 ± 0.19 ↔ Child	7.2 ± 2.1^{d} ↔ RA	SC: 0.9 ± 0.2^{e}	SC: $1.1 \pm 0.2 \; \mu M^{e}$ IV: 37–99 μM^{e}

[a]The 7-hydroxy metabolite exhibits plasma concentrations approaching that of parent drug. Metabolite may have both therapeutic and toxic effects. [b]Bioavailability may be as low as 20% when doses exceed 80 mg/m². [c]IM bioavailability is only slightly higher. [d]Exhibits triexponential elimination kinetics. A shorter $t_{\frac{1}{2}}$ (2 hours) is seen initially, and a longer (52 hours) terminal $t_{\frac{1}{2}}$ has been observed with increased assay sensitivity. [e]Following a 15 mg SC dose given once weekly to steady state in adult patients with inflammatory bowel disease. Initial steady-state concentrations in young (1.5–22 years old) leukemia patients receiving a 500 mg/m² loading dose given over 1 hour followed by an infusion of 196 mg/m² per hour for 5 hours. Bone marrow toxicity associated with concentrations >10 μM at 24 hours, >1 μM at 48 hours, or >0.1 μM at 72 hours after the dose.

References: Egan, L.J., Sandborn, W.J., *et al.* Systemic and intestinal pharmacokinetics of methotrexate in patients with inflammatory bowel disease. *Clin. Pharmacol. Ther.,* **1999,** *65:*29–39. Tracy, T.S. Worster, T., Bradley, J.D., Greene, P.K., and Brater, D.C. Methotrexate disposition following concomitant administration of ketoprofen, piroxicam and flurbiprofen in patients with rheumatoid arthritis. *Br. J. Clin. Pharmacol.* **1994,** *37:*453–456. Wall, A.M., Gajjar, A., *et al.* Individualized methotrexate dosing in children with relapsed acute lymphoblastic leukemia. *Leukemia,* **2000,** *14:*221–225.

AVAILABILITY (ORAL) (%)	URINARY EXCRETION (%)	BOUND IN PLASMA (%)	CLEARANCE (ml · min⁻¹ · kg⁻¹)	VOL. DIST. (liters/kg)	HALF-LIFE (hours)	PEAK TIME (hours)	PEAK CONCENTRATIONS
METHYLPHENIDATE[a] (Chapter 10)							
(+): 22 ± 8 (−): 5 ± 3	(+): 1.3 ± 0.5 (−): 0.6 ± 0.3	(+/−): 15–16	(+): 6.7 ± 2.0^{b} (−): 12 ± 4.7^{b}	(+): 2.7 ± 1.1 (−): 1.8 ± 0.9	(+): 6.0 ± 1.7^{c} (−): 3.6 ± 1.1	(+): $2.4 \pm 0.8^{c,d}$ (−): 2.1 ± 0.6^{d}	(+): 18 ± 4.3 ng/ml[d] (−): 3.0 ± 0.9 ng/ml[d]

[a]Methylphenidate is available as a racemate and the active (+)-dextro-enantiomer, dexmethylphenidate. Methylphenidate and dexmethylphenidate are extensively metabolized, primarily through ester hydrolysis to ritalinic acid. Data are those of enantiomers following racemate administration to healthy adult male subjects. No significant gender differences. [b]The (+)-enantiomer exhibits dose-dependent kinetics at high doses of racemate, with a ~ 50% reduction in *CL/F* between a 10–40-mg dose. [c]When dexmethylphenidate is given alone, its $t_{\frac{1}{2}}$ is 2.2 hours, and peak time is 1–1.5 hours. [d]Following a single 40 mg oral dose (immediate release). Longer peak time (3–5 hours) and lower peak concentration reported for sustained-released oral formulation.

References: Aoyama, T., Kotaki, H., *et al.* Nonlinear kinetics of threo-methylphenidate enantiomers in a patient with narcolepsy and in healthy volunteers. *Eur. J. Clin. Pharmacol.,* **1993,** *44:*79–84. Keating, G.M., and Figgitt, D.P. Dexmethylphenidate. *Drugs,* **2002,** *62:*1899–1904; discussion 1905–1908. Kimko, H.C., Cross, J.T., and Abernethy, D.R. Pharmacokinetics and clinical effectiveness of methylphenidate. *Clin. Pharmacokinet.,* **1999,** *37:*457–470. *Physicians' Desk Reference,* 58th ed. Medical Economics Co, Montvale, **2004,** pp. 2265, 2297–2298. Srinivas, N.R., Hubbard, J.W., Korchinski, E.D., and Midha, K.K. Enantioselective pharmacokinetics of dl-threo-methylphenidate in humans. *Pharm. Res,* **1993,** *10:*14–21.

METHYLPREDNISOLONE (Chapter 59)

82 ± 13[a]	4.9 ± 2.3 ↔ Cirr	78 ± 3 ↔ Fem ↓ Cirr	6.2 ± 0.9 ↔ NS, RA, CRI, Cirr ↓ Obes ↑ Fem	1.2 ± 0.2 ↔ NS, RD, RA, CRI, Fem, Cirr ↓ Obes	2.3 ± 0.5 ↔ NS, RD, RA, CRI, Cirr ↑ Obes ↓ Fem	Oral: 1.64 ± 0.64[b]	IV: 225 ± 44 ng/ml[b] Oral: 178 ± 44 ng/ml[b]

[a]May be decreased to 50% to 60% with high doses. [b]Mean at 1 hour following a 28 mg IV infusion over 20 minutes given twice daily for 6 ± 4 days during the perioperative period following kidney transplantation. Mean following a 24 mg oral dose given twice daily for 3 days in healthy adult male subjects. IC_{50} for basophil (histamine) trafficking is 14 ± 11 ng/ml; IC_{50} for helper T-cell trafficking is 20 ± 15 ng/ml.

References: Lew, K.H., Ludwig, E.A., et al. Gender-based effects on methylprednisolone pharmacokinetics and pharmacodynamics. Clin. Pharmacol. Ther., **1993**, *54*:402–414. Rohatagi, S., Barth, J., et al. Pharmacokinetics of methylprednisolone and prednisolone after single and multiple oral administration. J. Clin. Pharmacol., **1997**, *37*:916–925. Tornatore, K.M., Reed, K.A., and Venuto, R.C. Methylprednisolone and cortisol metabolism during the early post-renal transplant period. Clin. Transplant., **1995**, *9*:427–432.

METOCLOPRAMIDE (Chapter 37)

76 ± 38 ↔ Aged, Cirr	20 ± 9 ↔ RD	40 ± 4 ↔ RD	6.2 ± 1.3 ↓ RD, Cirr ↑ Neo ↔ Aged	3.4 ± 1.3 ↔ RD, Cirr, Aged ↑ Neo	5.0 ± 1.4 ↑ RD, Cirr ↔ Aged	A: ≤1[a] I: 2.5 ± 0.7[a]	A: 80 ng/ml[a] I: 18 ± 6.2 ng/ml[a]

[a]Following a single 20 mg oral dose given to healthy adults (A) or an oral (nasogastric) dose of 0.10 to 0.15 mg/kg given four times daily to steady state to premature infants (I), 1 to 7 weeks of age (26 to 36 weeks, postconceptional).

References: Kearns, G.L., van den Anker, J.N., Reed, M.D., and Blumer, J.L. Pharmacokinetics of metoclopramide in neonates. J. Clin. Pharmacol., **1998**, *38*:122–128. Lauritsen, K., Laursen, L.S., and Rask-Madsen, J. Clinical pharmacokinetics of drugs used in the treatment of gastrointestinal diseases (Part I). Clin. Pharmacokinet., **1990**, *19*:11–31. Rotmensch, H.H., Mould, G.P., et al. Comparative central nervous system effects and pharmacokinetics of neo-metoclopramide and metoclopramide in healthy volunteers. J. Clin. Pharmacol., **1997**, *37*:222–228.

METOPROLOL[a] (Chapters 31, 32, 33)

38 ± 14[b] ↑ Cirr ↓ Preg	10 ± 3[b] ↔ Preg	11 ± 1 ↔ Preg	15 ± 3[b] ↑ HTh, Preg ↔ Aged, Smk ↓ Fem	4.2 ± 0.7 ↑ Preg ↓ Fem	3.2 ± 0.2[b] ↑ Cirr, Neo ↔ Aged, HTh, Preg, Smk	EM: ~2[c] PM: ~3[c]	EM: 99 ± 53 ng/ml[c] PM: 262 ± 29 ng/ml[c]

[a]Data for racemic mixture reported. Metabolism of less active $R-$ (+)-enantiomer ($CL/F = 28$ ml · min⁻¹ · kg⁻¹; $V_{area}/F = 7.6$ l/kg; $t_{1/2} = 2.7$ hours) is slightly faster than that of more active $S-$(–)-enantiomer ($CL/F = 20$ ml · min⁻¹ · kg⁻¹; $V_{area}/F = 5.5$ l/kg; $t_{1/2} = 3$ hours). [b]Metabolically cleared by CYP2D6 (polymorphic). Compared to extensive metabolizers, individuals who are poor metabolizers will have an increased oral bioavailability, a lower CL, and a longer $t_{1/2}$ (15 ± 7 *vs.* 2.8 ± 1.2 hours) and will excrete more unchanged drug in urine (15 ± 7 *vs.* 3.2 ± 3%) due to reduced hepatic metabolism. [c]$C_{3\ hours}$ following a single 100 mg oral dose in CYP2D6 extensive (EM) and poor (PM) metabolizer patients with hypertension. Plasma concentrations of the more active S-enantiomer are ~35% higher than the R-antipode in CYP2D6 EM. No stereochemical difference was observed in PM subjects. EC_{50} for decreased heart rate during peak submaximal exercise testing was 16 ± 7 ng/ml; EC_{50} for decreased systolic blood pressure during exercise testing was 25 ± 18 ng/ml.

References: Dayer, P., Leemann, T., Marmy, A., and Rosenthaler, J. Interindividual variation of beta-adrenoceptor blocking drugs, plasma concentration and effect: influence of genetic status on behaviour of atenolol, bopindolol and metoprolol. Eur. J. Clin. Pharmacol., **1985**, *28*:149–153. Lennard, M.S., Silas, J.H., et al. Oxidation phenotype—a major determinant of metoprolol metabolism and response. N. Engl. J. Med., **1982**, *307*:1558–1560. McGourty, J.C., Silas, J.H., Lennard, M.S., Tucker, G.T., and Woods, H.F. Metoprolol metabolism and debrisoquine oxidation polymorphism—population and family studies. Br. J. Clin. Pharmacol., **1985**, *20*:555–566.

Table A–II–1 Pharmacokinetic Data (Continued)

AVAILABILITY (ORAL) (%)	URINARY EXCRETION (%)	BOUND IN PLASMA (%)	CLEARANCE ($ml \cdot min^{-1} \cdot kg^{-1}$)	VOL. DIST. (liters/kg)	HALF-LIFE (hours)	PEAK TIME (hours)	PEAK CONCENTRATIONS
METRONIDAZOLE[a] (Chapter 40)							
99 ± 8^b ↔ Crohn	10 ± 2	11 ± 3	1.3 ± 0.3 ↓ Cirr, Neo ↔ Preg, RD, Crohn, Aged	0.74 ± 0.10 ↔ RD, Crohn, Cirr	8.5 ± 2.9 ↑ Neo, Cirr ↔ Preg, RD, Crohn, Child	Oral: 2.8^c VA: 11 ± 2^c	IV: 27 (11–41) µg/ml^c Oral: 19.8 µg/ml^c VA: 1.9 ± 0.2 µg/ml^c

[a]Active hydroxylated metabolite accumulates in renal failure. [b]Bioavailability is 67% to 82% for rectal suppositories and 53 ± 16% for intravaginal gel. [c]Following a single 100 mg dose of vaginal (VA) cream, a 100 mg IV infusion over 20 minutes three times daily to steady state, or a 100 mg oral dose three times daily to steady state.

Reference: Lau, A.H., Lam, N.P., Piscitelli, S.C., Wilkes, L., and Danziger, L.H. Clinical pharmacokinetics of metronidazole and other nitroimidazole anti-infectives. *Clin. Pharmacokinet.,* **1992,** *23:*328–364.

AVAILABILITY (ORAL) (%)	URINARY EXCRETION (%)	BOUND IN PLASMA (%)	CLEARANCE	VOL. DIST. (liters/kg)	HALF-LIFE (hours)	PEAK TIME (hours)	PEAK CONCENTRATIONS
MIDAZOLAM (Chapters 13, 16)							
44 ± 17^a ↑ Cirr	<1%	98 ↓ Aged, RD ↔ Smk, Cirr	6.6 ± 1.8 ↑ RD^c ↓ Cirr, Neo ↔ Obes, Smk, Child	1.1 ± 0.6 ↑ Obes ↔ Cirr ↓ Neo	1.9 ± 0.6 ↑ Aged, Obes, Cirr ↔ Smk	Oral: $0.67 \pm$ 0.45^d	IV: 113 ± 16 ng/ml^d Oral: 78 ± 27 ng/ml^d

[a] Metabolically cleared exclusively by CYP3A. [b]Undergoes extensive first-pass metabolism by intestinal and hepatic CYP3A. Bioavailability appears to be dose-dependent; 35% to 67% at 15 mg, 28% to 36% at 7.5 mg, and 12% to 47% at 2 mg oral dose, possibly due to saturable first-pass intestinal metabolism. [c]Increased *CL* due to increased plasma free fraction; unbound *CL* is unchanged. [d]Following a single 5 mg IV bolus dose or 10 mg oral dose.

References: Garzone, P.D., and Kroboth, P.D. Pharmacokinetics of the newer benzodiazepines. *Clin. Pharmacokinet.,* **1989,** *16:*337–364. Thummel, K.E., O'Shea, D., *et al.* Oral first-pass elimination of midazolam involves both gastrointestinal and hepatic CYP3A-mediated metabolism. *Clin. Pharmacol. Ther.,* **1996,** *59:*491–502.

AVAILABILITY (ORAL) (%)	URINARY EXCRETION (%)	BOUND IN PLASMA (%)	CLEARANCE	VOL. DIST. (liters/kg)	HALF-LIFE (hours)	PEAK TIME (hours)	PEAK CONCENTRATIONS
MIRTAZAPINE[a] (Chapter 17)							
50 ± 10	—	85	9.12 ± 1.14^b ↓ LD,^{d} RD^e	4.5 ± 1.7	$16.3 \pm 4.6^{b,c}$ ↑ LD,^{d} RD^e	1.5 ± 0.7^f	41.8 ± 7.7 ng/ml^f

[a]Data from healthy adult subjects. Metabolized by CYP2D6 and CYP1A2 (8-hydroxy) and CYP3A (N-desmethyl, N-oxide). [b]Women of all ages exhibit lower *CL/F* and longer $t_{\frac{1}{2}}$ than men. [c]The $t_{\frac{1}{2}}$ of the (–)-enantiomer is approximately twice as long as the (+)-antipode; ~threefold higher blood concentrations (+ *vs.* –) are achieved. [d]*CL/F* reduced, hepatic impairment. [e]*CL/F* reduced, moderate-to-severe renal impairment. [f]Following a 15 mg oral dose given once daily to steady state.

References: Fawcett, J., and Barkin, R.L. Review of the results from clinical studies on the efficacy, safety and tolerability of mirtazapine for the treatment of patients with major depression. *J. Affect. Disord.,* **1998,** *51:*267–285. *Physicians' Desk Reference,* 54th ed. Medical Economics Co., Montvale, NJ, **2000,** p. 2109.

AVAILABILITY (ORAL) (%)	URINARY EXCRETION (%)	BOUND IN PLASMA (%)	CLEARANCE	VOL. DIST. (liters/kg)	HALF-LIFE (hours)	PEAK TIME (hours)	PEAK CONCENTRATIONS
MITOXANTRONE[a] (Chapters 51, 52)							
—^{b}	~2	97	13 ± 8 LD ↓	90 ± 42^c	β-phase: 1.1 ± 1.1^d γ-phase: 72 ± 40^d LD ↑	—	308 ± 133 ng/ml^e

[a]Data reported for patients treated for cancer. Information from older literature confounded by nonspecific assays. [b]For parenteral administration only; usually given as rapid IV infusion every 3 months. [c]Reflects distribution into a "deep" tissue compartment. V_c is 0.3 ± 0.21 l/kg. [d]$t_{\frac{1}{2}}$ for the β-phase predicts time to steady state for short-term IV infusions. $t_{\frac{1}{2}}$ for the γ-phase predicts long-term persistence in the body. [e]Following a single 30 minute IV infusion of 12-14 mg/m².

References: Ehninger, G., Schuler, U., Proksch, B., Zeller, K.P., and Blanz, J. Pharmacokinetics and metabolism of mitoxantrone. A review. Clin. Pharmacokinet., 1990, 18:365–380. Hu, O.Y., Chang, S.P., Law, C.K., Jian, J.M., and Chen, K.Y. Pharmacokinetic and pharmacodynamic studies with mitoxantrone in the treatment of patients with nasopharyngeal carcinoma. Cancer, 1992, 69:847–853.

MONTELUKAST[a] (Chapter 27)

62	<0.2	>99	0.70 ± 0.17 ↓ Cirr[b] ↔ Child[c]	0.15 ± 0.02 ↑ Cirr[b]	3.0 ± 1.0[d]		542 ± 173 ng/ml[d]

[a]Data from healthy adult subjects. No significant gender differences. Montelukast is metabolized by CYP3A4 and CYP2C9. [b]CL/F reduced by 41%, mild to moderate hepatic impairment with cirrhosis. [c]Similar plasma profile with 5 mg chewable vs. 10 mg tablet in adults. [d]Following a single 10 mg oral dose.

References: Physicians' Desk Reference, 54th ed. Medical Economics Co., Montvale, NJ, 2000, p. 1882. Zhao, J.J., Rogers, J.D., et al. Pharmacokinetics and bioavailability of montelukast sodium (MK-0476) in healthy young and elderly volunteers. Biopharm. Drug Dispos., 1997, 18:769–777.

MORPHINE[a] (Chapter 21)

Oral: 24 ± 12 IM: ~100	4 ± 5 14 ± 7[a]	35 ± 2 ↓ AVH, Cirr, Alb	24 ± 10 ↔ Aged, Cirr, Child[b] ↓ Neo, Burn, RD, Prem	3.3 ± 0.9 ↔ Cirr, Neo ↓ RD	1.9 ± 0.5 ↔ Cirr, RD, Child ↑ Neo, Prem	IM: 0.2–0.3[c] PO-IR: 0.5–1.5[c] PO-SR: 3–8[c]	IV: 200–400 ng/ml[c] IM: ~70 ng/ml[c] PO-IR: 10 ng/ml[c] PO-SR: 7.4 ng/ml[c]

[a]Active metabolite, morphine-6-glucuronide; $t_{\frac{1}{2}} = 4.0 \pm 1.5$ hours. Steady-state ratio of active metabolite to parent after oral dosing $= 4.9 \pm 3.8$. In renal failure, $t_{\frac{1}{2}}$ increases to 50 ± 37 hours, resulting in significant accumulation of active glucuronide metabolite. [b]Decreased in children undergoing cardiac surgery requiring inotropic support. [c]Following a single 10 mg IV dose (bolus with 5-minute blood sample), a 10 mg/70 kg IM, a 10 mg/70 kg immediate-release oral (PO-IR) dose, or a 50 mg sustained-release oral dose (PO-SR). Minimum analgesic concentration is 15 ng/ml.

References: Berkowitz, B.A. The relationship of pharmacokinetics to pharmacological activity: morphine, methadone and naloxone. Clin. Pharmacokinet., 1976, 1:219–230. Glare, P.A., and Walsh, T.D. Clinical pharmacokinetics of morphine. Ther. Drug Monit., 1991, 13:1–23.

MOXIFLOXACIN[a] (Chapter 43)

86 ± 1	21.9 ± 3.6	39.4 ± 2.4	2.27 ± 0.24	2.05 ± 1.15	15.4 ± 1.2	2.0 (0.5–6.0)[b]	2.5 ± 1.3 μg/ml[b]

[a]Data from healthy adult male subjects. Moxifloxacin is metabolized by ST and UGT. [b]Following a single oral 400 mg dose.

Reference: Stass, H., and Kubitza, D. Pharmacokinetics and elimination of moxifloxacin after oral and intravenous administration in man. J. Antimicrob. Chemother., 1999, 43(suppl B):83–90.

Table A–II–1 *Pharmacokinetic Data (Continued)*

AVAILABILITY (ORAL) (%)	URINARY EXCRETION (%)	BOUND IN PLASMA (%)	CLEARANCE (ml · min⁻¹ · kg⁻¹)	VOL. DIST. (liters/kg)	HALF-LIFE (hours)	PEAK TIME (hours)	PEAK CONCENTRATIONS
MYCOPHENOLATE[a] (Chapter 52)							
MM: ~0 MPA: 94	MPA: <1	MPA: 97.5 ↓RD[c]	MM: 120–163 MPA: 2.5±0.4[b] ↓RD[c] ↔LD	MPA: 3.6–4[b]	MM: <0.033 MPA: 16.6±5.8	MPA: 1.1–2.2[d]	MPA: 8–19 μg/ml[d]

References: Bullingham, R.E., Nicholls, A.J., and Kamm, B.R. Clinical pharmacokinetics of mycophenolate mofetil. *Clin. Pharmacokinet.*, **1998,** 34:429–455. Bullingham, R., Shah, J., Goldblum, R., and Schiff, M. Effects of food and antacid on the pharmacokinetics of single doses of mycophenolate mofetil in rheumatoid arthritis patients. *Br. J. Clin. Pharmacol.,* **1996,** 41:513–516. Kriesche, H.U.M., Kaplan, B., *et al.* MPA protein binding in uremic plasma: prediction of free fraction. *Clin. Pharmacol. Ther.,* **1999,** 65:184. *Physicians' Desk Reference,* 54th ed. Medical Economics Co., Montvale, NJ, **2000,** pp. 2617–2618.

[a]Data from healthy adult male and female subjects and organ transplant patients. No significant gender differences. Mycophenolate mofetil (MM) is rapidly converted to the active mycophenolic acid (MPA) after IV and oral doses. Kinetic parameters refer to MM and MPA after a dose of MM. MPA metabolized by UGT to MPAG. MPA undergoes enterohepatic recycling; MPAG is excreted into bile and presumably is hydrolyzed by gut flora and reabsorbed as MPA. [b]CL/F and V_{area}/F reported for MPA. [c]Accumulation of MPA and MPAG and increased unbound MPA; severe renal impairment. [d]Range of mean MPA C_{max} and T_{max} from different studies following a 1–1.75 g oral dose given twice daily to steady state in renal transplant patients.

AVAILABILITY (ORAL) (%)	URINARY EXCRETION (%)	BOUND IN PLASMA (%)	CLEARANCE (ml · min⁻¹ · kg⁻¹)	VOL. DIST. (liters/kg)	HALF-LIFE (hours)	PEAK TIME (hours)	PEAK CONCENTRATIONS
NALMEFENE[a] (Chapter 21)							
40	9.6±4.9	34.4±13.6	15±4.5 ↓LD, RD[c]	8.0±1.8 ↑RD[c]	8.0±2.2 ↑LD,[b] RD[c]	Oral: 2.5±0.58[d]	IV: 17±6.3 ng/ml[d] Oral: 24±11 ng/ml[d]

References: Dixon, R., Gentile, J., *et al.* Nalmefene: safety and kinetics after single and multiple oral doses of a new opioid antagonist. *J. Clin. Pharmacol.* **1987,** 27:233–239. Frye, R.F., Matzke, G.R., Schade, R., Dixon, R., and Rabinovitz, M. Effects of liver disease on the disposition of the opioid antagonist nalmefene. *Clin. Pharmacol. Ther.,* **1997,** 61:15–23.

[a]Data from healthy adult male and female subjects. Metabolized primarily by UGT. [b]Moderate-to-severe hepatic impairment. [c]End-stage renal impairment. [d]Following a single 2 mg IV dose and a single 50 mg oral dose in healthy men.

AVAILABILITY (ORAL) (%)	URINARY EXCRETION (%)	BOUND IN PLASMA (%)	CLEARANCE (ml · min⁻¹ · kg⁻¹)	VOL. DIST. (liters/kg)	HALF-LIFE (hours)	PEAK TIME (hours)	PEAK CONCENTRATIONS
NALOXONE (Chapter 21)							
~2[a]	Negligible	—	22 ↑Neo ↔RD	2.1 ↑Neo	1.1±0.6[b] ↔Neo	—	10±1 ng/ml[c]

References: Handal, K.A., Schauben, J.L., and Salamone, F.R. Naloxone. *Ann. Emerg. Med.* **1983,** 12:438–445. Ngai, S.H., Berkowitz, B.A., Yang, J.C., Hempstead, J., and Spector, S. Pharmacokinetics of naloxone in rats and in man: basis for its potency and short duration of action. *Anesthesiology,* **1976,** 44:398–401.

[a]Absorption is relatively complete (91%), but most of the dose is subject to hepatic first-pass metabolism. [b]Short distribution $t_{\frac{1}{2}}$ of 4.8 (2 to 10) minutes may limit the duration of effect. [c]Following a single 0.4 mg IV bolus dose (sample at 2 minutes) given to healthy adults.

AVAILABILITY (ORAL) (%)	URINARY EXCRETION (%)	BOUND IN PLASMA (%)	CLEARANCE (ml · min⁻¹ · kg⁻¹)	VOL. DIST. (liters/kg)	HALF-LIFE (hours)	PEAK TIME (hours)	PEAK CONCENTRATIONS
NAPROXEN[a] (Chapter 26)							
99[b]	5–6	99.7±0.1[c] ↑RD, Aged,[d] Cirr ↓RA, Alb	0.13±0.02[e] ↓RD ↔Aged,[d] Cirr,[d] Child ↑RA	0.16±0.02[e] ↑RD, RA, Child ↔Aged, Child	14±1 ↔RD, RA, Child ↑Aged[d]	T-IR: 2–4[f] T-CR: 5[f] S: 2.2±2.1[f]	T-IR: 37[f] T-CR: 94[f] S: 55±14 μg/ml[f]

NELFINAVIR[a] (Chapter 51)

20–80[b] ↑Food	1–2	98–99	12.0 ± 7.2[c] ↑Child[d]	2–7[c]	3–5[c]	3.0 ± 1.1[e]	3.2 ± 1.2 μg/ml[e] ↑Food

[a]Metabolically cleared by CYP2C9 (polymorphic) and CYP1A2. [b]Estimated bioavailability. [c]Saturable plasma protein binding yields apparent nonlinear elimination kinetics. [d]No change in total CL, but significant (50%) decrease in CL of unbound drug; it is thus suggested that dosing rate be decreased. A second study in elderly patients found decreased CL and increased $t_{\frac{1}{2}}$ with no change in percent bound. [e]CL/F and V_{area}/F reported. [f]Following a single 250 mg dose of suspension (S) given orally to pediatric patients or a 250 mg immediate-release tablet (T-IR) or a 500 mg controlled-release tablet (T-CR) given to adults.

Reference: Wells, T.G., Mortensen, M.E., *et al.* Comparison of the pharmacokinetics of naproxen tablets and suspension in children. *J. Clin. Pharmacol.,* **1994,** *34:*30–33.

[a]Data from healthy subjects and patients with HIV infection. No significant gender differences. Nelfinavir is metabolized by multiple cytochrome CYP isozymes, including CYP3A4. [b]Absolute bioavailability is unknown; reported to vary between 20% and 80% when taken without or with food. [c]CL/F, V_{ss}/F, and $t_{\frac{1}{2}}$ reported for oral dose. [d]CL/F increased, children 2 to 7 years and 7 to 13 years of age. [e]Following a 750 mg dose given three times daily for 28 days in adults.

References: Barry, M., Mulcahy, F., Merry, C., Gibbons, S., and Back, D. Pharmacokinetics and potential interactions amongst antiretroviral agents used to treat patients with HIV infection. *Clin. Pharmacokinet.,* **1999,** *36:*289–304. Pai, V.B., and Nahata, M.C. Nelfinavir mesylate: a protease inhibitor. *Ann. Pharmacother.,* **1999,** *33:*325–339. *Physicians' Desk Reference,* 54th ed. Medical Economics Co, Montvale, NJ, **2000,** p. 483.

NEOSTIGMINE (Chapter 8)

—[a]	67	—	16.7 ± 5.4 ↓RD	—	1.4 ± 0.5	1.3 ± 0.8 ↑RD	200–350 ng/ml[b]

[a]Absorption is presumed to be less than complete because oral dose must greatly exceed IV dose to achieve a similar effect. Nasal absorption is greater than oral absorption. [b]Following a single dose of 0.07 mg/kg IV (sample at 2 minutes) to surgical patients.

Reference: Cronnelly, R., Stanski, D.R., Miller, R.D., Sheiner, L.B., and Sohn, Y.J. Renal function and the pharmacokinetics of neostigmine in anesthetized man. *Anesthesiology,* **1979,** *51:*222–226.

NEVIRAPINE[a] (Chapter 50)

93 ± 9	<3%	SD: 0.23–0.77[b] MD: 0.89[b] ↑Child[c]	60	SD: 1.2 ± 0.09[b] MD: 1.2[b]	SD: 45[b] MD: 25–35[b]	2–4[d]	SD: 2 ± 0.4 μg/ml[d] MD: 4.5 ± 1.9 μg/ml[d]

[a]Data from healthy adult and HIV-infected subjects. No significant gender differences. Metabolized by CYP3A. [b]Range of CL/F and V/F reported. Nevirapine appears to autoinduce its own metabolism. CL/F increases and $t_{\frac{1}{2}}$ decreases from a single dose (SD) to multiple doses (MD). [c]Patients <8 years. [d]Following a single 200 mg oral dose (SD) and 200 mg given twice daily to steady state (MD).

References: Cheeseman, S.H., Hattox, S.E., *et al.* Pharmacokinetics of nevirapine: initial single-rising-dose study in humans. *Antimicrob. Agents Chemother.,* **1993,** *37:*178–182. Luzuriaga, K., Bryson, Y., *et al.* Pharmacokinetics, safety, and activity of nevirapine in human immunodeficiency virus type 1-infected children. *J. Infect. Dis.,* **1996,** *174:*713–721. *Physicians' Desk Reference,* 54th ed. Medical Economics Co., Montvale, NJ, **2000,** p. 2721. Zhou, X.J., Sheiner, L.B., *et al.* Population pharmacokinetics of nevirapine, zidovudine, and didanosine in human immunodeficiency virus-infected patients. The National Institute of Allergy and Infectious Diseases AIDS Clinical Trials Group Protocol 241 Investigators. *Antimicrob. Agents Chemother.,* **1999,** *43:*121–128.

Table A–II–1 Pharmacokinetic Data (Continued)

AVAILABILITY (ORAL) (%)	URINARY EXCRETION (%)	BOUND IN PLASMA (%)	CLEARANCE ($ml \cdot min^{-1} \cdot kg^{-1}$)	VOL. DIST. (liters/kg)	HALF-LIFE (hours)	PEAK TIME (hours)	PEAK CONCENTRATIONS
NIACIN[a] (Chapter 35)							
—[b] ↑ Food	12[c]	—	14.6 ± 5.0[d]	—	~ 0.15–0.25[e]	ER: 4–5[f]	ER (1g): 0.6 µg/ml[f] ER (2g): 15.5 µg/ml[f]

[a]Niacin (nicotinic acid) is metabolized to nicotinamide, which in turn is converted to the coenzyme NAD and other inactive metabolites. It also undergoes direct glycine conjugation to nicotinuric acid. [b]The absolute bioavailability is not known. Niacin is well-absorbed but undergoes first-pass metabolism. Absorption is improved when taken with a low-fat meal. [c]Recovery of unchanged drug after multiple oral dose administration. [d]CL calculated from C_{ss} (6.6 ± 2.4 µg/ml) during an IV infusion of niacin. Niacin metabolic CL appears to be saturable. [e]Estimated from the terminal log-linear portion of a disappearance curve following the end of a 0.1 mg·kg⁻¹·min⁻¹ IV infusion in two subjects. [f]Following a single 1 g or 2 g oral dose of extended-release (ER) NIASPAN®. Markedly disproportional increases in plasma concentrations with increasing dose.

References: Ding, R.W., Kolbe, K., et al. Pharmacokinetics of nicotinic acid-salicylic acid interaction. Clin. Pharmacol. Ther., 1989, 46:642–647. Physicians' Desk Reference, 58th ed. Medical Economics Co., Montvale, NJ, 2004, p. 1797. Piepho, R.W. The pharmacokinetics and pharmacodynamics of agents proven to raise high-density lipoprotein cholesterol. Am. J. Cardiol., 2000, 86(12A):35L–40L.

AVAILABILITY (ORAL) (%)	URINARY EXCRETION (%)	BOUND IN PLASMA (%)	CLEARANCE ($ml \cdot min^{-1} \cdot kg^{-1}$)	VOL. DIST. (liters/kg)	HALF-LIFE (hours)	PEAK TIME (hours)	PEAK CONCENTRATIONS
NIFEDIPINE[a] (Chapters 31, 32)							
50 ± 13 ↑ Cirr, Aged ↔ RD	~0	96 ± 1 ↓ Cirr, RD	7.0 ± 1.8 ↓ Cirr, Aged ↔ RD, Smk	0.78 ± 0.22 ↑ Cirr, RD, Aged ↔ Smk	1.8 ± 0.4[b] ↑ Cirr, RD, Aged ↔ Smk	IR: 0.5 ± 0.2[c] ER: ~6[c]	IR: 79 ± 44 ng/ml[c] ER: 35–49 ng/ml[c]

[a]Metabolically cleared by CYP3A; undergoes significant first-pass metabolism. [b]Longer apparent $t_{\frac{1}{2}}$ after oral administration because of absorption limitation, particularly for extended-release formulations. [c]Mean following a single 10 mg immediate-release (IR) capsule given to healthy male adults or a range of steady-state concentrations following a 60 mg extended-release (ER) tablet given daily to healthy male adults. Levels of 47 ± 20 ng/ml were reported to decrease diastolic pressure in hypertensive patients.

References: Glasser, S.P., Jain, A., et al. The efficacy and safety of once-daily nifedipine: the coat-core formulation compared with the gastrointestinal therapeutic system formulation in patients with mild-to-moderate diastolic hypertension. Nifedipine Study Group. Clin. Ther., 1995, 17:12–29. Renwick, A.G., Robertson, D.R., et al. The pharmacokinetics of oral nifedipine—a population study. Br. J. Clin. Pharmacol., 1988, 25:701–708. Soons, P.A., Schoemaker, H.C., Cohen, A.F., and Breimer, D.D. Intraindividual variability in nifedipine pharmacokinetics and effects in healthy subjects. J. Clin. Pharmacol., 1992, 32:324–331.

AVAILABILITY (ORAL) (%)	URINARY EXCRETION (%)	BOUND IN PLASMA (%)	CLEARANCE ($ml \cdot min^{-1} \cdot kg^{-1}$)	VOL. DIST. (liters/kg)	HALF-LIFE (hours)	PEAK TIME (hours)	PEAK CONCENTRATIONS
NITROFURANTOIN (Chapter 43)							
87 ± 13	47 ± 13 ↑ Alkaline Urine	62 ± 4	9.9 ± 0.9 ↑ Alkaline Urine	0.58 ± 0.12	1.0 ± 0.2 ↔ Alkaline Urine	2.3 ± 1.4[a]	428 ± 146 ng/ml[a]

[a]Following a single 50 mg oral dose (tablet) given to fasted healthy adults. No changes when taken with a meal.

Reference: Hoener, B., and Patterson, S.E. Nitrofurantoin disposition. Clin. Pharmacol. Ther., 1981, 29:808–816.

NITROGLYCERIN[a] (Chapters 31, 32)

Oral: <1 SL: 38 ± 26[b] Top: 72 ± 20	<1	195 ± 86[c]	—	3.3 ± 1.2[c,d]	2.3 ± 0.6 min	SL: 0.09 ± 0.03[e] Top: 3–4[e] TD: 2[e]	IV: 3.4 ± 1.7 ng/ml[e] SL: 1.9 ± 1.6 ng/ml[e]

[a]Dinitrate metabolites have weak activity compared to nitroglycerin (<10%), but because of prolonged $t_{\frac{1}{2}}$ (~40 min), they may accumulate during administration of sustained-release preparations to yield concentrations in plasma 10- to 20-fold greater than parent drug. [b]Following sublingual dose rinsed out of mouth after 8 minutes. Rinse contained 31 ± 19% of the dose. [c]Following a 40–100 minute IV infusion. $^dV_{area}$ reported. [e]Steady-state concentration following a 20–54 μg/min IV infusion over 40–100 minutes or a 0.4 mg sublingual (SL) dose. Levels of 1.2 to 11 ng/ml associated with a 25% drop in capillary wedge pressure in patients with CHF. T_{max} for topical (Top) and transdermal (TD) preparations also reported.

References: Physicians' Desk Reference, 54th ed. Medical Economics Co., Montvale, NJ, **2000**, p. 1474. Noonan, P.K., and Benet, L.Z. Incomplete and delayed bioavailability of sublingual nitroglycerin. *Am. J. Cardiol.* **1985**, *55*:184–187. Thadani, U., and Whitsett, T. Relationship of pharmacokinetic and pharmacodynamic properties of the organic nitrates. *Clin. Pharmacokinet.* **1988**, *15*:32–43.

NORTRIPTYLINE[a] (Chapter 17)

51 ± 5	2 ± 1	92 ± 2 ↑HL	7.2 ± 1.8[b] ↓ Aged, Inflam ↔ Smk, RD	18 ± 4[c]	31 ± 13[b] ↑ Aged ↔ RD	7–10	138 (40–350) nM[d]

[a]Active metabolite, 10-hydroxynortriptyline, accumulates to twice the concentration of nortriptyline in extensive metabolizers. Formation of 10-hydroxynortriptyline is catalyzed by CYP2D6 (polymorphic). [b]For poor metabolizers, *CL/F* is lower (5.3 *vs.* 19.3 ml · min⁻¹ · kg⁻¹) and $t_{\frac{1}{2}}$ longer (54 *vs.* 21 hours) than that of extensive metabolizers. $^cV_{area}$ reported. ^{d}Mean following a 125 mg oral dose given once daily to healthy adults to steady state. Antidepressant effect observed at plasma concentrations of 190 to 570 nM. Appears less effective at plasma concentrations above 570 nM.

References: Dalen, P., Dahl, M.L., Ruiz, M.L., Nordin, J., and Bertilsson, L. 10-Hydroxylation of nortriptyline in white persons with 0, 1, 2, 3, and 13 functional CYP2D6 genes. *Clin. Pharmacol. Ther.,* **1998**, *63*:444–452. Jerling, M., Merle, Y., Mentre, F., and Mallet, A. Population pharmacokinetics of nortriptyline during monotherapy and during concomitant treatment with drugs that inhibit CYP2D6—an evaluation with the nonparametric maximum likelihood method. *Br. J. Clin. Pharmacol.* **1994**, *38*:453–462. Ziegler, V.E., Clayton, P.J., Taylor, J.R., Tee, B., and Biggs, J.T. Nortriptyline plasma levels and therapeutic response. *Clin. Pharmacol. Ther.,* 1976, *20*:458–463.

OLANZAPINE[a] (Chapter 18)

~60[b]	7.3	93	6.2 ± 2.9[c] ↔ RD, Cirr	16.4 ± 5.1[c]	33.1 ± 10.3 ↑ Aged	6.1 ± 1.9[d]	12.9 ± 7.5 ng/ml[d]

[a]Data from male and female schizophrenic patients. Metabolized primarily by UGT, CYP1A2, and flavin-containing monooxygenase. [b]Bioavailability estimated from parent-metabolite recovery data. [c]Summary of *CL/F* and V_{area}/F for 491 subjects receiving an oral dose. *CL/F* segregates by sex (F/M) and smoking status (NS/S): M, S > F, S > M, NS > F, NS. [d]Following a single 9.5 ± 4 mg oral dose to healthy males; $C_{max,ss}$ ~ 20 ng/ml following a 10 mg oral dose given once daily.

References: Callaghan, J.T., Bergstrom, R.F., Ptak, L.R., and Beasley, C.M. Olanzapine. Pharmacokinetic and pharmacodynamic profile. *Clin. Pharmacokinet.,* **1999**, *37*:177–193. Kassahun, K., Mattiuz, E., *et al.* Disposition and biotransformation of the antipsychotic agent olanzapine in humans. *Drug Metab. Dispos.,* **1997**, *25*:81–93. *Physicians' Desk Reference,* 54th ed. Medical Economics Co., Montvale, NJ, **2000**, p. 1649.

Table A–II–1 Pharmacokinetic Data (Continued)

AVAILABILITY (ORAL) (%)	URINARY EXCRETION (%)	BOUND IN PLASMA (%)	CLEARANCE ($ml \cdot min^{-1} \cdot kg^{-1}$)	VOL. DIST. (liters/kg)	HALF-LIFE (hours)	PEAK TIME (hours)	PEAK CONCENTRATIONS
ONDANSETRON (Chapter 37)							
62 ± 15^a ↑ Aged, Cirr, Fem	5 ↑ Aged, Cirr, Fem	73 ± 2	5.9 ± 2.6 ↓ Aged, Cirr, Fem ↑ Child	1.9 ± 0.05 ↔ Aged, Cirr	3.5 ± 1.2 ↑ Aged, Cirr ↓ Child	Oral: 1.0 (0.8–1.5)^b	IV: 102 (64–136) ng/ml^b Oral: 39 (31–48) ng/ml^b

^{a}In 26 cancer patients (62 ± 10 years), F = 86 ± 26%. ^{b}Mean (95% CI) values following a single dose of 0.15 mg/kg IV or an oral dose of 8 mg given three times daily for 5 days to healthy adults.

Reference: Roila, F., and Del Favero, A. Ondansetron clinical pharmacokinetics. *Clin. Pharmacokinet,* **1995,** 29:95–109.

AVAILABILITY (ORAL) (%)	URINARY EXCRETION (%)	BOUND IN PLASMA (%)	CLEARANCE ($ml \cdot min^{-1} \cdot kg^{-1}$)	VOL. DIST. (liters/kg)	HALF-LIFE (hours)	PEAK TIME (hours)	PEAK CONCENTRATIONS
OXALIPLATIN^a (Chapter 51)							
—^{b}	—^{c}	90^d	49 (41–64)^e	1.5 (1.1–2.1)	0.32 (0.27–0.46)^f	—	Ox: 0.33 (0.28–0.38) μg Pt/ml^g PtDC: 0.008 (0.004–0.014) μg Pt/ml^g

^{a}Oxaliplatin is an organoplatinum complex; Pt is coordinated with diaminocyclohexane (DACH) and an oxalate ligand as a leaving group. Oxaliplatin (Ox) undergoes nonenzymatic biotransformation to reactive derivatives, notably Pt(DACH)Cl$_2$ (PtDC). Antitumor activity and toxicity are thought to relate to the concentration of oxaliplatin and PtDC in plasma ultrafiltrate (*i.e,* unbound concentration). ^{b}For IV administration only. ^{c}Approximately 54% of the platinum eliminated is recovered in urine. ^{d}Binding to plasma proteins is irreversible. ^{e}CL of total platinum is much lower; ~2–4 ml·min^{-1}·kg^{-1}. ^{f}The elimination of platinum species in plasma follows a triexponential pattern. The quoted $t_{\frac{1}{2}}$ reflects the $t_{\frac{1}{2}}$ of the first phase, which is the clinically relevant phase. The $t_{\frac{1}{2}}$ for the slower two phases are 17 and 391 hours. ^{g}Steady-state plasma ultrafiltrate concentration of Ox and PtDC after an 85 mg/m^2 IV infusion over 2 hours during cycles 1 and 2.

Reference: Physicians' Desk Reference, 58th ed. Medical Economics Co., Montvale, NJ, **2004,** pp. 3024–3025. Shord, S.S., Bernard, S.A., *et al.* Oxaliplatin biotransformation and pharmacokinetics: a pilot study to determine the possible relationship to neurotoxicity. *Anticancer Res.,* **2002,** 22:2301–2309.

AVAILABILITY (ORAL) (%)	URINARY EXCRETION (%)	BOUND IN PLASMA (%)	CLEARANCE ($ml \cdot min^{-1} \cdot kg^{-1}$)	VOL. DIST. (liters/kg)	HALF-LIFE (hours)	PEAK TIME (hours)	PEAK CONCENTRATIONS
OXCARBAZEPINE^a (Chapter 19)							
—	O: <1 HC: 27	— HC: 45	O: 67.4^b HC: ↓ RD,^{c} Aged HC: ↑ Child^d	—	O: ~2 HC: 8–15 HC: ↑ RD, Aged	HC: 2–4^e	HC: 8.5 ± 2.0 μg/ml^e

aData from healthy adult male subjects. No significant gender differences. Oxcarbazepine (O) undergoes extensive first-pass metabolism to an active metabolite, 10-hydroxycarbamazepine (HC). Reduction by cytosolic enzymes is stereoselective (80% S-enantiomer, 20% R-enantiomer), but both show similar pharmacological activity. bCL/F for O reported. HC eliminated by glucuronidation. cAUC for HC increased, moderate-to-severe renal impairment. dAUC for HC decreased, children <6 years of age. eFollowing a 300 mg oral oxcarbazepine dose given twice daily for 12 days.

References: Battino, D., Estienne, M., and Avanzini, G. Clinical pharmacokinetics of antiepileptic drugs in paediatric patients. Part II. Phenytoin, carbamazepine, sulthiame, lamotrigine, vigabatrin, oxcarbazepine and felbamate. Clin. Pharmacokinet., 1995, 29:341–369. Lloyd, P., Flesch, G., and Dieterle, W. Clinical pharmacology and pharmacokinetics of oxcarbazepine. Epilepsia, 1994, 35(suppl 3):S10–S13. Rouan, M.C., Lecaillon, J.B., et al. The effect of renal impairment on the pharmacokinetics of oxcarbazepine and its metabolites. Eur. J. Clin. Pharmacol., 1994, 47:161–167. van Heiningen, P.N., Eve, M.D., et al. The influence of age on the pharmacokinetics of the antiepileptic agent oxcarbazepine. Clin. Pharmacol. Ther., 1991, 50:410–419.

OXYBUTYNIN[a] (Chapter 7)

1.6–10.9	<1	8.1 ± 2.3^b	—	1.3 ± 0.4^b	IV: $1.9 \pm 0.35^{b,c}$	IR: 5.0 ± 4.2^d XL: 5.2 ± 3.7^d	IR: 12.4 ± 4.1 ng/ml^d XL: 4.2 ± 1.6 ng/ml^d

aData from healthy female subjects. No significant gender differences. Racemic mixture; anticholinergic activity resides predominantly with R-enantiomer; no stereoselectivity exhibited for antispasmodic activity. Oxybutynin undergoes extensive first-pass metabolism to N-desethyloxybutynin (DEO), an active, anticholinergic metabolite. Metabolized primarily by intestinal and hepatic CYP3A. Racemic oxybutynin kinetic parameters reported. bData reported for a 1 mg IV dose, assuming a 70 kg body weight. A larger volume (2.8 l/kg) and longer $t_{\frac{1}{2}}$ (5.3 hours) reported for 5 mg IV dose. cExhibits a longer apparent $t_{\frac{1}{2}}$ following oral dosing due to absorption rate-limited kinetics: immediate-release (IR) $t_{\frac{1}{2}} = 9 \pm 2$ hours; extended-release (XL) $t_{\frac{1}{2}} = 14 \pm 3$ hours. The apparent $t_{\frac{1}{2}}$ for DEO was 4.0 ± 1.4 hours and 8.3 ± 2.5 hours for IR and XL formulations, respectively. dFollowing a dose of 5 mg immediate-release (IR) given three times daily or 15 mg extended-release (XL) given once daily for 4 days. Peak DEO levels at steady state were 45 and 23 ng/ml for IR and XL, respectively.

References: Gupta, S.K., and Sathyan, G. Pharmacokinetics of an oral once-a-day controlled-release oxybutynin formulation compared with immediate-release oxybutynin. J. Clin. Pharmacol., 1999, 39:289–296. Physicians' Desk Reference, 54th ed. Medical Economics Co., Montvale, NJ, 2000, p. 507.

OXYCODONE[a] (Chapter 21)

CR: 60–87^b IR: 42 ± 7^b	—^{c}	45	12.4 (9.2–15.4)	2.0 (1.1–2.9)	2.6 (2.1–3.1)^d	CR: 3.2 ± 2.2^e IR: 1.6 ± 0.8^e	CR: 15.1 ± 4.7 ng/ml^e IR: 15.5 ± 4.5 ng/ml^e

aOxycodone is metabolized primarily by CYP3A4/5, with a minor contribution from CYP2D6. Oxymorphone is an active metabolite produced by CYP2D6-mediated O-dealkylation. The circulating concentrations of oxymorphone are too low to contribute significantly to the opioid effects of oxycodone. Data from healthy males and females reported. bValues reported for OxyContin® (oxycodone controlled release) and immediate-release tablets. Up to 19% excreted unchanged after an oral dose. dThe apparent $t_{\frac{1}{2}}$ for controlled-release oral formulation is ~5 hours; most likely reflects absorption-limited terminal elimination kinetics. eFollowing 10 mg of OxyContin® (CR) given twice daily to steady state or a 5 mg immediate-release tablet (IR) given every 6 hours to steady state.

References: Benziger, D.P., Kaiko, R.F., et al. Differential effects of food on the bioavailability of controlled-release oxycodone tablets and immediate-release oxycodone solution. J. Pharm. Sci., 1996, 85:407–410. Physicians' Desk Reference, 58th ed. Medical Economics Co., Montvale, NJ, 2004, pp. 2854–2855. Takala, A., Kaasalainen, V., Seppala, T., Kalso, E., and Olkkola, K.T. Pharmacokinetic comparison of intravenous and intranasal administration of oxycodone. Acta. Anaesthesiol. Scand., 1997, 41:309–312.

Table A–II–1 *Pharmacokinetic Data (Continued)*

AVAILABILITY (ORAL) (%)	URINARY EXCRETION (%)	BOUND IN PLASMA (%)	CLEARANCE (ml · min⁻¹ · kg⁻¹)	VOL. DIST. (liters/kg)	HALF-LIFE (hours)	PEAK TIME (hours)	PEAK CONCENTRATIONS

PACLITAXEL[a] (Chapter 51)

| Low | 5 ± 2 | $88–98$[b] | 5.5 ± 3.5
 $\leftrightarrow$ Child | 2.0 ± 1.2
 $\leftrightarrow$ Child | 3 ± 1[c] | — | $0.85 \pm 0.21 \ \mu M$[d] |

[a]Metabolized by CYP2C8 and CYP3A, and substrate for P-glycoprotein. [b]Binding of drug to dialysis filtration devices may lead to overestimation of protein binding fraction (88% suggested). [c]Average accumulation $t_{\frac{1}{2}}$; longer terminal $t_{\frac{1}{2}}$s up to 30 hours are reported. [d]Steady-state concentration during a 250 mg/m² IV infusion given over 24 hours to adult cancer patients.

Reference: Sonnichsen, D.S., and Relling, M.V. Clinical pharmacokinetics of paclitaxel. *Clin. Pharmacokinet.*, **1994,** *27:256–269.*

PANCURONIUM (Chapter 9)

| — | 67 ± 18
 $\leftrightarrow$ CPBS | 7 ± 2
 $\leftrightarrow$ Neo, Fem, Preg, RD | 1.8 ± 0.4
 $\downarrow$ Aged, RD
 $\leftrightarrow$ Cirr, CPBS | 0.26 ± 0.07
 $\leftrightarrow$ Aged, RD, CPBS
 $\uparrow$ Cirr | 2.3 ± 0.4
 $\uparrow$ Aged, RD, Cirr
 $\downarrow$ Aged, RD
 $\leftrightarrow$ CPBS | — | $0.67 \ \mu g/ml$[a] |

[a]Estimated mean C_{max} following a single bolus dose of 0.1 mg/kg IV given to surgical patients. Levels of $0.25 \pm 0.07 \ \mu g/ml$ and $0.4 \ \mu g/ml$ elicit 50% and 95% decreases in twitch tension, respectively.

Reference: Shanks, C.A. Pharmacokinetics of the nondepolarizing neuromuscular relaxants applied to calculation of bolus and infusion dosage regimens. *Anesthesiology,* **1986,** *64:72–86.*

PAROXETINE (Chapter 17)

| Dose-dependent[a] | <2 | 95 | 8.6 ± 3.2[a,b]
 $\downarrow$ Cirr, Aged | 17 ± 10[c] | 17 ± 3[d]
 $\uparrow$ Cirr, Aged | 5.2 ± 0.5[e] | EM: ~130 nM[e]
 PM: ~220 nM[e] |

[a]Metabolized by CYP2D6 (polymorphic); undergoes time- and dose-dependent autoinhibition of metabolic CL in extensive metabolizers. [b]CL/F reported for multiple dosing in extensive metabolizers. Single dose data are significantly higher. In CYP2D6 poor metabolizers, CL/F $= 5.0 \pm 2.1 \ ml \cdot min^{-1} \cdot kg^{-1}$ for multiple dosing. [c]V_{area}/F reported. [d]Data reported for multiple dose in extensive metabolizers. In poor metabolizers, $t_{\frac{1}{2}} = 41 \pm 8$ hours. [e]Estimated mean C_{max} following a 30 mg oral dose given once daily for 14 days to adults phenotyped as CYP2D6 extensive (EM) and poor (PM) metabolizers. There is a significant disproportional accumulation of drug in blood when going from single to multiple dosing due to autoinactivation of CYP2D6.

References: Physicians' Desk Reference, 54th ed. Medical Economics Co., Montvale, NJ, **2000,** p. 3028. Sindrup, S.H., Brosen, K., *et al.* The relationship between paroxetine and the sparteine oxidation polymorphism. *Clin. Pharmacol. Ther.,* **1992,** *51:278–287.*

PENICILLIN G[a] (Chapter 44)

30[b]	79	60 (48–68)	0.5 ± 0.1[c] ↑RD	0.33	5–9 ↓RD	24 ± 5[a] ↔ Cirr, AVH	100 ± 11	PO: 0.28–1.2 μg/ml[d]; IM, SA: 12 μg/ml[d]; IM, Pro: 0.94 μg/ml[d]; IM, Benz: 0.16 μg/ml[d]
								PO: 0.5–1[d]; IM, SA: 0.5[d]; IM, Pro: 1–3[d]; IM, Benz: 12–24[d]

[a]Penicillin G (Pen G) available in various very soluble (short acting, SA) and less soluble (long acting, LA) salt forms. Procaine and benzathine salts are two long-acting forms. Data are from adults and older children. [b]Oral absorption of Pen G is irregular and variable due to its instability in stomach acid and inactivation during first-pass through the liver. Value is the maximum fraction recovered unchanged in urine following oral administration. [c]Tri-exponential elimination; $t_{\frac{1}{2}}$ is ~3 hours and most likely reflects slow redistribution from tissues. [d]Following single 180 mg oral suspension of Pen G (SA), 187.5 mg IM dose of procaine Pen G (Pro), and 750 mg IM dose of benzathine Pen G (Benz).

References: Dittert, L.W., Griffen, W.O., Jr., LaPiana, J.C., Shainfeld, F.J., and Dolusio, J.T. Pharmacokinetic interpretation of penicillin levels in serum and urine after intravenous administration. *Antimicrobial. Agents Chemother.,* **1969,** *9:*42–48. Ebert, S.C. Leggett, J., Vogelman, B., and Craig, W.A. Evidence for a slow elimination phase for penicillin G. *J. Infect. Dis.,* **1988,** *158:*200–202. Kucers, A., and Bennett, N.M. *The Use of Antibiotics,* 4th ed. J.B. Lippincott Company, Philadelphia, **1987.** McDermott, W., Bunn, P.A., Benoit, M., DuBois, R., and Reynolds, M.E. The absorption, excretion, and destruction of orally administered penicillin. *J. Clin. Invest.,* **1946,** *25:*190–210.

PHENOBARBITAL (Chapters 16, 19)

100 ± 11	51 ± 3 ↓ Neo ↔ Preg, Aged	0.062 ± 0.013 ↑ Preg, Child, Neo ↔ Smk	0.54 ± 0.03 ↑ Neo	99 ± 18 ↑ Cirr, Aged ↓ Child ↔ Epilep, Neo	2–4[b]	13.1 ± 4.5 μg/ml[b]

[a]Phenobarbital is a weak acid (pK_a = 7.3); urinary excretion is increased at an alkaline pH; it also is reduced with decreased urine flow. [b]Mean steady-state concentration following a 90 mg oral dose given daily for 12 weeks to patients with epilepsy. Levels of 10–25 μg/ml provide control of tonic-clonic seizures and 15 μg/ml for control of febrile convulsions in children. Levels >40 μg/ml can cause toxicity; 65–117 μg/ml produce stage III anesthesia—comatose but reflexes present; 100–134 μg/ml produce stage IV anesthesia—no deep-tendon reflexes.

References: Bourgeois, B.F.D. Phenobarbital and primidone. In, *The Treatment of Epilepsy: Principles and Practice,* 2nd ed. (Wyllie, E., ed.) Williams & Wilkins, Philadelphia, **1997,** pp. 845–855. Browne, T.R., Evans, J.E., Szabo, G.K., Evans, B.A., and Greenblatt, D.J. Studies with stable isotopes II: Phenobarbital pharmacokinetics during monotherapy. *J. Clin. Pharmacol.,* **1985,** *25:*51–58.

Table A–II–1 *Pharmacokinetic Data (Continued)*

AVAILABILITY (ORAL) (%)	URINARY EXCRETION (%)	BOUND IN PLASMA (%)	CLEARANCE (ml · min⁻¹ · kg⁻¹)	VOL. DIST. (liters/kg)	HALF-LIFE (hours)	PEAK TIME (hours)	PEAK CONCENTRATIONS
PHENYTOIN[a] (Chapters 19, 34)							
90 ± 3	2 ± 8	89 ± 23 ↓ RD, Hep, Alb, Neo, AVH, Cirr, NS, Preg, Burn ↔ Obes, Smk, Aged	V_{max} = 5.9 ± 1.2 mg · kg⁻¹ · day⁻¹ ↓ Aged; ↑ Child K_m = 5.7 ± 2.9 mg/l[b] ↔ Aged; ↓ Child ↑c NS, RD ↓c Prem ↔c AVH, LTh, HTh, Smk	0.64 ± 0.04[d] ↑ Neo, NS, RD ↔ AVH, LTh, HTh	6–24[e] ↑c Prem ↓c RD ↔c AVH, LTh, HTh, Smk	3–12[f]	0–5 µg/ml (27%)[f] 5–10 µg/ml (30%)[f] 10–20 µg/ml (29%)[f] 20–30 µg/ml (10%)[f] >30 µg/ml (6%)[f]

[a]Metabolized predominantly by CYP2C9 (polymorphic) and also by CYP2C19 (polymorphic); exhibits saturable kinetics with therapeutic doses. [b]Significantly decreased in the Japanese population. [c]Comparison of CLs and $t_{\frac{1}{2}}$s with similar doses in normal subjects and patients; nonlinear kinetics not considered. [d]V_{area} reported. [e]Apparent $t_{\frac{1}{2}}$ is dependent on plasma concentration. [f]Population frequency of total phenytoin concentrations following a 300 mg oral dose (capsule) given daily to steady state. Total levels >10 µg/ml associated with suppression of tonic-clonic seizures. Nystagmus can occur at levels >20 µg/ml and ataxia at levels >30 µg/ml.

References: Eldon, M.A., Loewen, G.R., *et al.* Pharmacokinetics and tolerance of fosphenytoin and phenytoin administered intravenously to healthy subjects. *Can. J. Neurol. Sci.,* **1993,** *20*(suppl 4):S180. Levine, M., and Chang, T. Therapeutic drug monitoring of phenytoin. Rationale and current status. *Clin. Pharmacokinet.,* **1990,** *19*:341–358. Tozer, T.N., and Winter, M.E. Phenytoin. In, *Applied Pharmacokinetics: Principles of Therapeutic Drug Monitoring,* 3rd ed. (Evans, W.E., Schentag, J.J., and Jusko, W.J., eds.) Applied Therapeutics, Vancouver, WA, **1992,** pp. 25-1–25-44.

AVAILABILITY (ORAL) (%)	URINARY EXCRETION (%)	BOUND IN PLASMA (%)	CLEARANCE (ml · min⁻¹ · kg⁻¹)	VOL. DIST. (liters/kg)	HALF-LIFE (hours)	PEAK TIME (hours)	PEAK CONCENTRATIONS
PIOGLITAZONE[a] (Chapter 60)							
—	Negligible	>99	1.2 ± 1.7[b]	0.63 ± 0.41[b]	11 ± 6[c]	P: 3.5 (1–4)[d] M-III: 11 (2–48)[d] M-IV: 11 (4–16)[d]	P: 1.6 ± 0.2 µg/ml[d] M-III: 0.4 ± 0.2 µg/ml[d] M-IV: 1.4 ± 0.5 µg/ml[d]

[a]Data from healthy male and female subjects and patients with type 2 diabetes. Pioglitazone (P) is metabolized extensively by CYP2C8, CYP3A4, and other CYP isozymes. Two major metabolites (M-III and M-IV) accumulate in blood and contribute to the pharmacological effect. [b]CL/F and V_{area}/F reported. CL/F is lower in women than in men. [c]Steady-state $t_{\frac{1}{2}}$ of M-III and M-IV is 29 and 27 hours, respectively. [d]Following a 45 mg oral dose given once daily for 10 days.

References: Budde, K., Neumayer, H.H., *et al.* The pharmacokinetics of pioglitazone in patients with impaired renal function. *Br. J. Clin. Pharmacol.,* **2003,** *55*:368–374. *Physicians' Desk Reference,* 58th ed. Medical Economics Co., Montvale, NJ, **2004,** p. 3186.

AVAILABILITY (ORAL) (%)	URINARY EXCRETION (%)	BOUND IN PLASMA (%)	CLEARANCE (ml · min⁻¹ · kg⁻¹)	VOL. DIST. (liters/kg)	HALF-LIFE (hours)	PEAK TIME (hours)	PEAK CONCENTRATIONS
PRAMIPEXOLE[a] (Chapter 20)							
>90[b]	~90	15	8.2 ± 1.4[b] ↓ Aged, RD[c], PD[d]	7.3 ± 1.7[b]	11.6 ± 2.57 ↑ Aged, RD	1–2	M: 1.6 ± 0.23 ng/ml[e] F: 2.1 ± 0.25 ng/ml[e]

a Data from healthy adult male and female subjects. No significant gender differences. *b* Bioavailability estimated from urinary recovery of unchanged drug. CL/F and V_{area}/F reported. *c* CL/F reduced, moderate-to-severe renal impairment. *d* Parkinson's disease (PD); CL/F reduced with declining renal function. *e* Following a 0.5 mg oral dose given three times daily for 4 days to male (M) and female (F) adults.

References: Lam, Y.W. Clinical pharmacology of dopamine agonists. *Pharmacotherapy,* **2000,** *20:*175–25S. *Physicians' Desk Reference,* 54th ed. Medical Economics Co., Montvale, NJ, **2000,** p. 2468. Wright, C.E., Sisson, T.L., Ichhpurani, A.K., and Peters, G.R. Steady-state pharmacokinetic properties of pramipexole in healthy volunteers. *J. Clin. Pharmacol.,* **1997,** *37:*520–525.

PRAVASTATIN (Chapter 35)

Availability (%)	Urinary Excretion (%)	Bound in Plasma (%)	Clearance (ml/min/kg)	Vol. Dist. (liters/kg)	Half-Life (hours)	Peak Time (hours)	Peak Concentration
18 ± 8	47 ± 7	43–48	13.5 ± 2.4 ↓Cirr ↔ Aged, RD[a]	0.46 ± 0.04	0.8 ± 0.2[b] ↔ Aged, RD[a]	1–1.4[c]	28–38 ng/ml[c]

a Although renal CL decreases with reduced renal function, no significant changes in CL/F or $t_{1/2}$ are seen following oral dosing as a result of the low and highly variable bioavailability. *b* A longer $t_{1/2}$ = 1.8 ± 0.8 hour reported for oral dosing; probably rate-limited by absorption. *d* Range of mean values from different studies following a single 20 mg oral dose.

References: Corsini, A., Bellosta, S., *et al.* New insights into the pharmacodynamic and pharmacokinetic properties of statins. *Pharmacol. Ther.,* **1999,** *84:*413–428. Desager, J.P., and Horsmans, Y. Clinical pharmacokinetics of 3-hydroxy-3-methylglutaryl-coenzyme A reductase inhibitors. *Clin. Pharmacokinet.,* **1996,** *31:*348–371. Quion, J.A., and Jones, P.H. Clinical pharmacokinetics of pravastatin. *Clin. Pharmacokinet.,* **1994,** *27:*94–103.

PRAZIQUANTEL[a] (Chapter 41)

Availability (%)	Urinary Excretion (%)	Bound in Plasma (%)	Clearance (ml/min/kg)	Vol. Dist. (liters/kg)	Half-Life (hours)	Peak Time (hours)	Peak Concentration
—[b]	Negligible	80–85	5 mg/kg: 467[c]; 40–60 mg/kg: 57–222[c] ↓LD[d]	5 mg/kg: 9.55 ± 2.86	5 mg/kg: 0.8–1.5[c]; 40–60 mg/kg: 1.7–3.0[c] ↑LD	1.5–1.8[e]	0.8–6.3 µg/ml[e]

a Data from male and female patients with schistosomiasis. *b* Absolute bioavailability is not known. Praziquantel is well absorbed (80%) but undergoes significant first-pass metabolism (hydroxylation), the extent of which appears to be dose-dependent. *c* CL/F and V_{ss}/F reported. *d* CL/F reduced, moderate-to-severe hepatic impairment. *e* Range of mean values from different studies following single 40–60 mg/kg oral dose.

References: Edwards, G., and Breckenridge, A.M. Clinical pharmacokinetics of anthelmintic drugs. *Clin. Pharmacokinet.,* **1988,** *15:*67–93. el Guiniady, M.A., el Touny, M.A., Abdel-Bary, M.A., Abdel-Fatah, S.A., and Metwally, A. Clinical and pharmacokinetic study of praziquantel in Egyptian schistosomiasis patients with and without liver cell failure. *Am. J. Trop. Med. Hyg.,* **1994,** *51:*809–818. Jung, H., Vazquez, M.L., Sanchez, M., Penagos, P., and Sotelo, J. Clinical pharmacokinetics of praziquantel. *Proc. West Pharmacol. Soc.,* **1991,** *34:*335–340. Sotelo, J., and Jung, H. Pharmacokinetic optimisation of the treatment of neurocysticercosis. *Clin. Pharmacokinet.,* **1998,** *34:*503–515. Watt, G., White, N.J., *et al.* Praziquantel pharmacokinetics and side effects in *Schistosoma japonicum*–infected patients with liver disease. *J. Infect. Dis.,* **1988,** *157:*530–535.

PRAZOSIN (Chapters 10, 32)

Availability (%)	Urinary Excretion (%)	Bound in Plasma (%)	Clearance (ml/min/kg)	Vol. Dist. (liters/kg)	Half-Life (hours)	Peak Time (hours)	Peak Concentration
68 ± 17	<4	95 ± 1 ↓Cirr, Alb, RD ↔ CHF	3.0 ± 0.3 ↓CHF, Preg ↔ RD	0.60 ± 0.13[a] ↓CHF, Preg ↔ RD	2.9 ± 0.8 ↑CHF, Preg ↔ RD	2.2 ± 1.1[a]	36 ± 17 ng/ml[a]

a Following a single 5 mg oral dose given to patients with hypertension.

References: Hobbs, D.C., Twomey, T.M., and Palmer, R.F. Pharmacokinetics of prazosin in man. *J. Clin. Pharmacol.,* **1978,** *18:*402–406. Vincent, J., Meredith, P.A., Reid, J.L., Elliott, H.L., and Rubin, P.C. Clinical pharmacokinetics of prazosin—1985. *Clin. Pharmacokinet.,* **1985,** *10:*144–154.

Table A–II–1 Pharmacokinetic Data *(Continued)*

	AVAILABILITY (ORAL) (%)	URINARY EXCRETION (%)	BOUND IN PLASMA (%)	CLEARANCE (ml · min⁻¹ · kg⁻¹)	VOL. DIST. (liters/kg)	HALF-LIFE (hours)	PEAK TIME (hours)	PEAK CONCENTRATIONS
PREDNISOLONE (Chapter 59)								
	82 ± 13[a] ↔ Hep, Cush, RD, Crohn, Celiac, Smk, Aged ↓ HTh	26 ± 9[a] ↓ Aged, HTh	90–95 (<200 ng/ml)[b] ~70 (>1 µg/ml) ↓ Alb, NS, Aged, HTh, Cirr ↔ Hep	1.0 ± 0.16[c] ↔ Hep, Cush, Smk, CRI, NS,[e] HTh[e] ↓ Aged,[e] Cirr[e]	0.42 ± 0.11[d] ↔ Hep, Cush, Smk, RD, CRI, NS[e] ↓ HTh,[e] Aged,[e] Obes	2.2 ± 0.5 ↔ Hep, Cush, Smk, RD, CRI, NS[e] ↓ HTh[e] ↑ Aged[e]	1.5 ± 0.5[f]	458 ± 150 ng/ml[f]

[a]Prednisolone and prednisone are interconvertible; an additional 3% ± 2% is excreted as prednisone. [b]Extent of binding to plasma proteins is dependent on concentration over range encountered. [c]Total *CL* increases as protein binding is saturated. *CL* of unbound drug increases slightly but significantly with increasing dose. [d]*V* increases with dose due to saturable protein binding. [e]Changes are for unbound drug. [f]Following a 30 mg oral dose given twice daily for 3 days to healthy male adults. The ratio of prednisolone/prednisone is dose-dependent and can vary from 3 to 26 over a prednisolone concentration range of 50–800 ng/ml.

References: Frey, B.M., and Frey, F.J. Clinical pharmacokinetics of prednisone and prednisolone. *Clin. Pharmacokinet.,* **1990,** *19:*126–146. Rohatagi, S., Barth, J., *et al.* Pharmacokinetics of methylprednisolone and prednisolone after single and multiple oral administration. *J. Clin. Pharmacol.,* **1997,** *37:*916–925.

	AVAILABILITY (ORAL) (%)	URINARY EXCRETION (%)	BOUND IN PLASMA (%)	CLEARANCE (ml · min⁻¹ · kg⁻¹)	VOL. DIST. (liters/kg)	HALF-LIFE (hours)	PEAK TIME (hours)	PEAK CONCENTRATIONS
PREDNISONE (Chapter 59)								
	80 ± 11[a] ↔ Hep, Cush, RD, Crohn, Celiac, Smk, Aged	3 ± 2[b] ↔ HTh	75 ± 2[c]	3.6 ± 0.8[d] ↔ Hep	0.97 ± 0.11[d] ↔ Hep	3.6 ± 0.4[d] ↔ Smk, Hep	P: 2.1–3.1[e] PL: 1.2–2.6[e]	P: 62–81 ng/ml[e] PL: 198–239 ng/ml[e]

[a]Measured relative to equivalent IV dose of prednisolone. [b]An additional 15% ± 5% excreted as prednisolone. [c]In contrast to prednisolone, there is no dependence on concentration. [d]Kinetic values for prednisone are often reported in terms of values for prednisolone, its active metabolite. However, the values cited here pertain to prednisone. [e]Range of mean data for prednisone (P) and its active metabolite, prednisolone (PL) following a single 10 mg oral dose given as different proprietary formulations to healthy adults.

References: Gustavson, L.E., and Benet, L.Z. The macromolecular binding of prednisone in plasma of healthy volunteers including pregnant women and oral contraceptive users. *J. Pharmacokinet. Biopharm.,* **1985,** *13:*561–569. Pickup, M.E. Clinical pharmacokinetics of prednisone and prednisolone. *Clin. Pharmacokinet.,* **1979,** *4:*111–128. Sullivan, T.J., Hallmark, M.R., *et al.* Comparative bioavailability: eight commercial prednisone tablets. *J. Pharmacokinet. Biopharm.,* **1976,** *4:*157–172.

	AVAILABILITY (ORAL) (%)	URINARY EXCRETION (%)	BOUND IN PLASMA (%)	CLEARANCE (ml · min⁻¹ · kg⁻¹)	VOL. DIST. (liters/kg)	HALF-LIFE (hours)	PEAK TIME (hours)	PEAK CONCENTRATIONS
PROCAINAMIDE[a] (Chapter 34)								
	83 ± 16 ↓ CHF, COPD, CP, Cirr	67 ± 8 ↓ CHF, COPD, CP, Cirr	16 ± 5	$CL = 2.7CL_{cr} + 1.7$ + 3.2 (fast)[b] or + 1.1 (slow)[b] ↑ Child ↓ MI ↔ CHF, Tach, Neo	1.9 ± 0.3 ↓ Obes ↔ RD, Child, Tach, CHF	3.0 ± 0.6 ↑ RD,[c] MI ↓ Child, Neo ↔ Obes, Tach, CHF	M: 3.6[d] F: 3.8[d]	M: 2.2 µg/ml[d] F: 2.9 µg/ml[d]

[a]Active metabolite, N-acetylprocainamide (NAPA); $CL = 3.1 \pm 0.4$ ml · min⁻¹ · kg⁻¹, $V = 1.4 \pm 0.2$ l/kg, and $t_{\frac{1}{2}} = 6.0 \pm 0.2$ hours. [b]CL calculated using units of ml · min⁻¹ · kg⁻¹ for CL_{cr}. CL depends on NAT2 acetylation phenotype. Use a mean value of 2.2 if phenotype unknown. [c]$t_{\frac{1}{2}}$ for procainamide and NAPA increased in patients with renal disease. [d]Least square mean values following 1000 mg oral dose, given twice daily to steady state in male (M) and female (F) adults. Mean peak NAPA concentrations were 2.0 and 2.2 μg/ml for male and female adults, respectively; $t_{max} = 4.1$ and 4.2 hours.

References: Benet, L.Z., and Ding, R.W. Die renale Elimination von Procainamide: Pharmacokinetik bei Niereninsuffizienz. In, Die Behandlung von Herzrhythmusstorungen bei Nierenkranken. (Braun, J., Pilgrim, R., Gessler, U., and Seybold, D., eds.) Karger, Basel, 1984, pp. 96–111. Koup, J.R., Abel, R.B., Smithers, J.A., Eldon, M.A., and de Vries, T.M. Effect of age, gender, and race on steady state procainamide pharmacokinetics after administration of procainamide and NAPA increased in patients with renal disease. bid sustained-release tablets. Ther. Drug Monit., 1998, 20:73–77.

PROPOFOL [a] (Chapter 13)

—[b]		98.3–98.8[c]	27 ± 5 ↑Child[d] ↓Aged[e] ↔LD	1.7 ± 0.7[f] ↑Child[d] ↓Aged[e]	3.5 ± 1.2[f]	—	SS: 3.5 ± 0.06 μg/ml[g] E: 1.1 ± 0.4 μg/ml[g]

[a]Data from patients undergoing elective surgery and healthy volunteers. Propofol is extensively metabolized by UGTs. [b]For IV administration only. [c]Fraction bound in whole blood. Concentration-dependent; 98.8% at 0.5 μg/ml and 98.3 at 32 μg/ml. [d]CL and central volume increased in children 1 to 3 years of age. [e]CL and central volume decreased in elderly. [f]V_{area} is much larger than V_{ss}. A much longer terminal $t_{\frac{1}{2}}$ reported following prolonged IV infusion. [g]Concentration producing anesthesia after infusion to steady state (SS) and at emergence (E) from anesthesia.

References: Mazoit, J.X., and Samii, K. Binding of propofol to blood components: implications for pharmacokinetics and for pharmacodynamics. Br. J. Clin. Pharmacol., 1999, 47:35–42. Murat, I., Billard, V., et al. Pharmacokinetics of propofol after a single dose in children aged 1–3 years with minor burns. Comparison of three data analysis approaches. Anesthesiology, 1996, 84:526–532. Servin, F., Cockshott, I.D., et al. Pharmacokinetics of propofol infusions in patients with cirrhosis. Br. J. Anaesth., 1990, 65:177–183.

PROPRANOLOL [a] (Chapters 10, 31, 32, 34)

26 ± 10 ↑Cirr	<0.5	87 ± 6[b] ↑Inflam, Crohn, Preg, Obes ↔RD, Fem, Aged ↓Cirr	16 ± 5[c,d] ↑Smk, HTh ↓Hep, Cirr, Obes, Fem ↔Aged, RD	4.3 ± 0.6[c] ↑Hep, HTh, Cirr ↓Crohn ↔Aged, RD, Obes, Fem, Preg	3.9 ± 0.4[c] ↓Hep, Cirr, Obes, Fem ↔Aged, RD, Smk, Preg	P: 1.5[e] HP: 1.0[e]	P: 49 ± 8 ng/ml[e] HP: 37 ± 9 ng/ml[e]

[a]Racemic mixture. For S-(−)-enantiomer (100-fold more active) compared to R-(+)-enantiomer, CL is 19% lower and V_{area} is 15% lower, because of a higher degree of protein binding (18% less free drug), and no difference in $t_{\frac{1}{2}}$. Active metabolite, 4-hydroxypropranolol (HP). [b]Drug is bound primarily to α_1-acid glycoprotein, which is elevated with a number of inflammatory conditions. [c]Based on blood measurements; blood-to-plasma concentration ratio = 0.89 ± 0.03. [d]CYP2D6 catalyzes the formation of 4-hydroxy metabolite; CYP1A2 is responsible for most of the N-desisopropyl metabolite; UGT catalyzes major conjugation pathway of elimination. [e]Following a single 80 mg oral dose given to healthy adults. Plasma accumulation factor was 3.6-fold after 80 mg four times daily to steady state. A concentration of 20 ng/ml gave a 50% decrease in exercise-induced cardioacceleration. Antianginal effects are manifest at 15 to 90 ng/ml. A concentration up to 1000 ng/ml may be required for control of ventricular arrhythmias.

References: Colangelo, P.M., Blouin, R.A., et al. Age and propranolol stereoselective disposition in humans. Clin. Pharmacol. Ther., 1992, 51:489–494. Walle, T., Conradi, E.C., Walle, U.K., Fagan, T.C., and Gaffney, T.E. 4-Hydroxypropranolol and its glucuronide after single and long-term doses of propranolol. Clin. Pharmacol. Ther., 1980, 27:22–31.

Table A–II–1 Pharmacokinetic Data (Continued)

AVAILABILITY (ORAL) (%)	URINARY EXCRETION (%)	BOUND IN PLASMA (%)	CLEARANCE ($ml \cdot min^{-1} \cdot kg^{-1}$)	VOL. DIST. (liters/kg)	HALF-LIFE (hours)	PEAK TIME (hours)	PEAK CONCENTRATIONS
PSEUDOEPHEDRINE[a] (Chapter 10)							
~100	43–96[b]	—	7.33[b,c]	2.64–3.51[c]	4.3–8[b,c]	IR: 1.4–2[d] CR: 3.8–6.1[d]	IR: 177–360 ng/ml[d] CR: 265–314 ng/ml[d]

[a]Data from healthy adult male and female subjects. [b]At a high urine pH (>7.0), pseudoephedrine is extensively reabsorbed; $t_{1/2}$ increases and CL decreases. [c]CL/F, V/F, and $t_{1/2}$ reported for oral dose. [d]Range of mean values from different studies following a single 60 mg immediate-release tablet or syrup (IR), or 120 mg controlled-release capsule (CR) oral dose.
Reference: Kanfer, I., Dowse, R., and Vuma, V. Pharmacokinetics of oral decongestants. *Pharmacotherapy,* **1993**, *13:*116S–128S.

AVAILABILITY (ORAL) (%)	URINARY EXCRETION (%)	BOUND IN PLASMA (%)	CLEARANCE	VOL. DIST.	HALF-LIFE	PEAK TIME	PEAK CONCENTRATIONS
PYRAZINAMIDE[a] (Chapter 47)							
—[b]	4–14[c]	10	1.1 (0.2–2.3)[d] ↑ Child	0.57 (0.13–1.04)[d]	6 (2–23) ↓ Child	1–2[e]	35 (19–103) µg/ml[e]

[a]Pyrazinamide is hydrolyzed in the liver to an active metabolite, 2-pyrazinoic acid. Reported peak 2-pyrazinoic acid concentrations range from 0.1- to 1-fold that of parent drug. Pyrazinamide data reported are for male and female adults with tuberculosis. [b]Absolute bioavailability is not known, but the drug is well absorbed based on recovery of parent drug and metabolites (70%). [c]Recovery unchanged following an oral dose; the recovery of pyrazinoic acid is 37 ± 5%. [d]CL/F and V_{area}/F reported. [e]Following a 15–53 mg/kg daily oral dose to steady state.
References: Bareggi, S.R., Cerutti, R., Pirola, R., Riva, R., and Cisternino, M. Clinical pharmacokinetics and metabolism of pyrazinamide in healthy volunteers. *Arzneimittelforschung,* **1987,** *37:*849–854. Lacroix, C., Hoang, T.P., *et al.* Pharmacokinetics of pyrazinamide and its metabolites in healthy subjects. *Eur. J. Clin. Pharmacol.* **1989,** *36:*395–400. *Physicians' Desk Reference,* 58th ed. Medical Economics Co., Montvale, **2004,** p. 766. Zhu, M., Starke, J.R., *et al.* Population pharmacokinetic modeling of pyrazinamide in children and adults with tuberculosis. *Pharmacotherapy,* **2002,** *22:*686–695.

AVAILABILITY (ORAL) (%)	URINARY EXCRETION (%)	BOUND IN PLASMA (%)	CLEARANCE	VOL. DIST.	HALF-LIFE	PEAK TIME	PEAK CONCENTRATIONS
QUETIAPINE[a] (Chapter 18)							
9 ↑ Food	<1%	83	19 ↓ Aged ↔ RD ↓ LD	10 ± 4	6	1–1.8	278 ng/ml[b]

[a]No significant gender differences. Extensively metabolized through multiple pathways, including sulfoxidation, N- and O-dealkylation catalyzed by CYP3A4. Two minor active metabolites. [b]Following a 250 mg oral dose given daily for 23 days in patients with schizophrenia.
References: Goren, J.L., and Levin, G.M. Quetiapine, an atypical antipsychotic. *Pharmacotherapy,* **1998,** *18:*1183–1194. *Physicians' Desk Reference,* 54th ed. Medical Economics Co., Montvale, NJ, **2000,** p. 563.

AVAILABILITY (ORAL) (%)	URINARY EXCRETION (%)	BOUND IN PLASMA (%)	CLEARANCE	VOL. DIST.	HALF-LIFE	PEAK TIME	PEAK CONCENTRATIONS
QUINAPRIL[a] (Chapters 30, 32, 33)							
QT (Q): 52 ± 15[b] QT (QT): 96[d]	Q (Q): 3.1 ± 1.2[c]	Q/QT: 97	QT (QT): 0.98 ± 0.22[d] ↓ RD	QT (QT): 0.19 ± 0.04[d] ↓ RD	Q (Q): 0.8–0.9[c] QT (QT): 2.1–2.9[d] ↑ RD	Q (Q): 1.4 ± 0.8[e] QT (QT): 2.3 ± 0.9[e]	Q (Q): 207 ± 89 ng/ml[e] QT (Q): 923 ± 277 ng/ml[e]

References: Breslin, E., Posvar, E., Neub, M., Trenk, D., and Jahnchen, E. A pharmacodynamic and pharmacokinetic comparison of intravenous quinaprilat and oral quinapril. *J. Clin. Pharmacol.* **1996,** 36:414–421. Olson, S.C., Horvath, A.M., *et al.* The clinical pharmacokinetics of quinapril. *Angiology,* **1989,** 40:351–359. *Physicians' Desk Reference,* 58th ed. Medical Economics Co. Montvale, **2004,** p. 2516.

[a]Hydrolyzed to its active metabolite, quinaprilat. Pharmacokinetic data for quinapril (Q) and quinaprilat (QT) following oral Q and IV QT administration are presented. [b]Absolute bioavailability based on plasma QT concentrations. [c]Data for Q following a 2.5–80 mg oral Q dose. [d]Data for QT following a 2.5 mg IV QT dose. The $t_{1/2}$ of QT after dosing Q is similar. [e]Following a single 40 mg oral Q dose. No accumulation of QT with multiple dosing.

QUINIDINE[a] (Chapter 34)

Sulfate: 80 ± 15 Gluconate: 71 ± 17	18 ± 5 ↔CHF	87 ± 3 ↓Cirr, Hep, Neo, Preg ↔RD, CRI, HL, Aged	4.7 ± 1.8[b] ↓CHF, Aged ↔Cirr, Smk	2.7 ± 1.2 ↓CHF ↑Cirr ↔Aged	6.2 ± 1.8 ↑Aged, Cirr ↔CHF, RD	IR: 1–3[c] ER: 6.3 ± 3.2[c]	IV: 2.9 ± 1.0 μg/ml[c] IR: ~1.3 μg/ml[c] ER: 0.53 ± 0.22 μg/ml[c]

[a]Active metabolite, 3-hydroxyquinidine ($t_{1/2}$ = 12 ± 3 hours; percent bound in plasma = 60 ± 10). [b]Metabolically cleared primarily by CYP3A. [c]Following a 400 mg IV dose (22-minute infusion) of quinidine gluconate or a single 400 mg oral dose of immediate-release (IR) quinidine sulfate or a 300 mg dose of extended-release (ER) quinidine sulfate (QUINIDEX) to healthy adults. Specific assay methods for quinidine show >75% reduction in frequency of premature ventricular contractions at levels of 0.7–5.9 μg/ml, but active metabolite was not measured; therapeutic levels of 2–7 μg/ml reported for nonspecific assays.

References: Brosen, K., Davidsen, F., and Gram, L.F. Quinidine kinetics after a single oral dose in relation to the sparteine oxidation polymorphism in man. *Br. J. Clin. Pharmacol.* **1990,** 29:248–253. Sawyer, W.T., Pulliam, C.C., *et al.* Bioavailability of a commercial sustained-release quinidine tablet compared to oral quinidine solution. *Biopharm. Drug Dispos.,* **1982,** 3:301–310. Ueda, C.T., Williamson, B.J., and Dzindzio, B.S. Absolute quinidine bioavailability. *Clin. Pharmacol. Ther.,* **1976,** 20:260–265.

QUININE[a] (Chapter 39)

76 ± 11	N-A: 12–20 M-A: 33 ± 18	N-A: ~85–90[b] M-A: 93–95[b] ↓Neo ↔Preg	N-A: 1.9 ± 0.5 M-A: 0.9–1.4 M-C: 0.4–1.4 ↔Preg,[c] RD[c] ↑Smk ↓Aged	N-A: 1.8 ± 0.4 M-A: 1.0–1.7 M-C: 1.2–1.7 ↓Preg[c] ↔RD[c]	N-A: 11 ± 2 M-A: 11–18 M-C: 12–16 ↓Preg,[c] Smk ↔RD[c] ↑Hep, Aged	PO: 3.5–8.4[d]	Adults IV: 11 ± 2 μg/ml[d] PO: 7.3–9.4 μg/ml[d] Children IV: 8.7–9.4 μg/ml[d] PO: 7.3 ± 1.1 μg/ml[d]

[a]Data from normal adults (N-A) and range of means from different studies of adults (M-A) or children (M-C) with malaria reported. [b]Correlates with serum α_1-acid glycoprotein levels. Binding is increased in severe malaria. [c]From patients with malaria. [d]Following single 10 mg/kg dose given as a 0.5–4 hour IV infusion or orally (PO) to children or adults with malaria. A level >0.2 μg/ml for unbound drug is targeted for treatment of *falciparum* malaria. Oculotoxicity and hearing loss/tinnitus associated with unbound concentrations >2 μg/ml.

References: Edwards, G., Winstanley, P.A., and Ward, S.A. Clinical pharmacokinetics in the treatment of tropical diseases. Some applications and limitations. *Clin. Pharmacokinet.* **1994,** 27:150–165. Krishna, S., and White, N.J. Pharmacokinetics of quinine, chloroquine and amodiaquine. Clinical implications. *Clin. Pharmacokinet.* **1996,** 30:263–299.

Table A–II–1 *Pharmacokinetic Data (Continued)*

AVAILABILITY (ORAL) (%)	URINARY EXCRETION (%)	BOUND IN PLASMA (%)	CLEARANCE (ml · min⁻¹ · kg⁻¹)	VOL. DIST. (liters/kg)	HALF-LIFE (hours)	PEAK TIME (hours)	PEAK CONCENTRATIONS
RALOXIFENE[a] (Chapters 57, 61)							
2[b]	<0.2	>95	735 ± 338[c] ↔ RD, Aged ↓ Cirr	2348 ± 1220[c]	28 (11–273)	6[d]	0.5 ± 0.3 ng/ml[d]

[a]Data from postmenopausal women. Undergoes extensive first-pass metabolism (UGT-catalyzed) and enterohepatic recycling. [b]Approximately 60% absorption from the gastrointestinal tract; not significantly affected by food. [c]CL/F and V/F reported for an oral dose. [d]Following a single 1 mg/kg oral dose.

References: Hochner-Celnikier, D. Pharmacokinetics of raloxifene and its clinical application. *Eur. J. Obstet. Gynecol. Reprod. Biol.*, **1999**, *85*:23–29. *Physicians' Desk Reference*, 54th ed. Medical Economics Co., Montvale, NJ, **2000**, p. 1583.

AVAILABILITY (ORAL) (%)	URINARY EXCRETION (%)	BOUND IN PLASMA (%)	CLEARANCE (ml · min⁻¹ · kg⁻¹)	VOL. DIST. (liters/kg)	HALF-LIFE (hours)	PEAK TIME (hours)	PEAK CONCENTRATIONS
RAMIPRIL[a] (Chapters 30, 31, 32)							
R (R): 28[b] RT (R): 48[b]	R (R): <2[c] RT (R): 13 ± 6[c]	R: 73 ± 2 RT: 56 ± 2	R (R): 23[d] RT: —[e]	—	R (R): 5 ± 2 RT (R): 9–18[f] ↑ RD	R (R): 1.2 ± 0.3[g] RT (R): 3.0 ± 0.7[g]	R (R): 43.3 ± 10.2 ng/ml[g] RT (R): 24.1 ± 5.6 ng/ml[g]

[a]Hydrolyzed to its active metabolite, ramiprilat. Pharmacokinetic data for ramapril (R) and ramaprilat (RT) following oral and IV ramapril administration are presented. [b]Based on plasma AUC of R and RT after IV and oral R administration. [c]Following an oral dose of R. [d]CL/F of R calculated from reported AUC data. [e]No data available; mean renal CL of RT is ~1.1 ml·min⁻¹·kg⁻¹. [f]$t_\frac{1}{2}$ for the elimination phase reported. A longer terminal $t_\frac{1}{2}$ of ~120 hours most likely corresponds to the release of drug from ACE; contributes to the duration of effect, but does not contribute to systemic drug accumulation. [g]Following a single 10 mg oral dose.

References: Eckert, H.G., Badian, M.J., Gantz, D., Kellner, H.M., and Volz, M. Pharmacokinetics and biotransformation of 2-[N-[(S)-1-ethoxycarbonyl-3-phenylpropyl]-L-alanyl]-(1S,3S, 5S)-2-azabicyclo [3.3.0]octane-3-carboxylic acid (Hoe 498) in rat, dog and man. *Arzneimittelforschung*, **1984**, *34*:1435–1447. Meisel, S., Shamiss, A., and Rosenthal, T. Clinical pharmacokinetics of ramipril. *Clin. Pharmacokinet.*, **1994**, *26*:7–15. *Physicians' Desk Reference*, 58th ed. Medical Economics Co., Montvale, **2004**, p. 2142. Song, J.C., and White, C.M. Clinical pharmacokinetics and selective pharmacodynamics of new angiotensin converting enzyme inhibitors: an update. *Clin. Pharmacokinet.*, **2002**, *41*:207–224. Thuillez, C., Richer, C., and Giudicelli, J.F. Pharmacokinetics, converting enzyme inhibition and peripheral arterial hemodynamics of ramipril in healthy volunteers. *Am. J. Cardiol.*, **1987**, *59*:38D–44D.

AVAILABILITY (ORAL) (%)	URINARY EXCRETION (%)	BOUND IN PLASMA (%)	CLEARANCE (ml · min⁻¹ · kg⁻¹)	VOL. DIST. (liters/kg)	HALF-LIFE (hours)	PEAK TIME (hours)	PEAK CONCENTRATIONS
RANITIDINE (Chapter 36)							
52 ± 11 ↑ Cirr ↔ RD	69 ± 6 ↓ RD	15 ± 3	10.4 ± 1.1 ↓ RD, Aged ↑ Burn	1.3 ± 0.4 ↔ Cirr, RD ↑ Burn	2.1 ± 0.2 ↑ RD, Cirr, Aged ↔ Burn	2.1 ± 0.31[a]	462 ± 54 ng/ml[a]

[a]Following a single 150 mg oral dose given to healthy adults. IC_{50} for inhibition of gastric acid secretion is 100 ng/ml.

Reference: Gladziwa, U., and Klotz, U. Pharmacokinetics and pharmacodynamics of H_2-receptor antagonists in patients with renal insufficiency. *Clin. Pharmacokinet.*, **1993**, *24*:319–332.

REMIFENTANIL[a] (Chapters 13, 21)

—[b]	Negligible	92	40–60 ↔ RD, Cirr ↓ Aged[c]	0.3–0.4 ↓ Aged[c] ↔ RD, Cirr	0.13–0.33 ↔ RD, Cirr	—	~20 ng/ml[d]

[a]Data from healthy adult male subjects and patients undergoing elective surgery. Undergoes rapid inactivation by esterase-mediated hydrolysis; resulting carboxy-metabolite has low activity. [b]For IV administration only. [c]CL and V decreased slightly in the elderly. [d]Mean $C_{1\,min}$ following a 5 μg/kg IV dose (1-min infusion). Cp_{50} for skin incision is 2 ng/ml (determined in the presence of nitrous oxide).

References: Egan, T.D., Huizinga, B., et al. Remifentanil pharmacokinetics in obese versus lean patients. Anesthesiology, 1998, 89:562–573. Glass, P.S., Gan, T.J., and Howell, S. A review of the pharmacokinetics and pharmacodynamics of remifentanil. Anesth. Analg, 1999, 89:S7–S14.

REPAGLINIDE[a] (Chapter 62)

56 ± 7	0.3–2.6	97.4	9.3 ± 6.8 ↓ RD, [b] LD[c]	0.52 ± 0.17	0.8 ± 0.2 ↑ LD	0.25–0.75[d]	47 ± 24 ng/ml[d]

[a]Data from healthy adult male subjects. Undergoes extensive oxidative and conjugative metabolism; CYP3A4 has been implicated in the formation of the major (60% of dose) metabolite. [b]CL/F reduced, severe renal impairment. [c]CL/F reduced, moderate to severe chronic liver disease. [d]Following a single 4 mg oral dose (tablet).

References: Hatorp, V., Oliver, S., and Su, C.A. Bioavailability of repaglinide, a novel antidiabetic agent, administered orally in tablet or solution form or intravenously in healthy male volunteers. Int. J. Clin. Pharmacol. Ther., 1998, 36:636–641. Hatorp, V., Walther, K.H., Christensen, M.S., and Haug-Pihale, G. Single-dose pharmacokinetics of repaglinide in subjects with chronic liver disease. J. Clin. Pharmacol., 2000, 40:142–152. Marbury, T.C., Ruckle, J.L., et al. Pharmacokinetics of repaglinide in subjects with renal impairment. Clin. Pharmacol. Ther., 2000, 67:7–15. van Heiningen, P.N., Hatorp, V., et al. Absorption, metabolism and excretion of a single oral dose of ^{14}C-repaglinide during repaglinide multiple dosing. Eur. J. Clin. Pharmacol, 1999, 55:521–525.

RIBAVIRIN[a] (Chapter 49)

45 ± 5	35 ± 8	0[b]	5.0 ± 1.0[c]	9.3 ± 1.5	28 ± 7[c]	RT: 3 ± 1.8[d]	R: 11.1 ± 1.2 μM[d] RT: 15.1 ± 12.8 μM[d]

[a]Values reported for studies conducted in asymptomatic HIV-positive men. [b]At steady state, red blood cell-to-plasma concentration ratio is ~60. [c]Following multiple oral dosing, CL/F decreases more than 50%, and a long terminal $t_{\frac{1}{2}}$ of 150 ± 50 hours is observed. [d]Following a 1200 mg oral ribavirin capsule (R) given daily for 7 days to adult subjects seropositive for HIV or a 600 mg oral REBETRON (RT) dose given twice daily to steady state to adults with hepatitis C infection.

References: Morse, G.D., Fischl, M.A., et al. Single-dose pharmacokinetics of delavirdine mesylate and didanosine in patients with human immunodeficiency virus infection. Antimicrob. Agents Chemother., 1997, 41:169–174. Physicians' Desk Reference, 54th ed. Medical Economics Co., Montvale, NJ, 2000, p. 2836. Roberts, R.B., Laskin, O.L., et al. Ribavirin pharmacodynamics in high-risk patients for acquired immunodeficiency syndrome. Clin. Pharmacol. Ther., 1987, 42:365–373.

Table A–II–1 Pharmacokinetic Data (Continued)

	AVAILABILITY (ORAL) (%)	URINARY EXCRETION (%)	BOUND IN PLASMA (%)	CLEARANCE (ml · min⁻¹ · kg⁻¹)	VOL. DIST. (liters/kg)	HALF-LIFE (hours)	PEAK TIME (hours)	PEAK CONCENTRATIONS
RIFAMPIN[a] (Chapter 47)								
	—[b]	7 ± 3 ↑ Neo	60–90	3.5 ± 1.6[d] ↑ Neo ↓ RD[c] ↔ Aged	0.97 ± 0.36 ↑ Neo ↔ Aged	3.5 ± 0.8[d] ↑ Hep, Cirr, AVH, RD[c] ↔ Child, Aged	1–3[e]	6.5 ± 3.5 µg/ml[e]

[a]Active desacetyl metabolite. [b]Absolute bioavailability is not unknown, although some studies indicate complete absorption. Such reports presumably refer to rifampin plus its desacetyl metabolite because considerable first-pass metabolism is expected. [c]Not observed with 300 mg doses, but pronounced differences with 900 mg doses. [d]$t_{\frac{1}{2}}$ is shorter (1.7 ± 0.5) and CL/F is higher after repeated administration. Rifampin is a potent enzyme (CYP3A and others) inducer and appears to autoinduce its own metabolism. [e]Following a 600 mg dose given once daily for 15 to 18 days to patients with tuberculosis.

Reference: Israili, Z.H., Rogers, C.M., and El-Attar, H. Pharmacokinetics of antituberculosis drugs in patients. *J. Clin. Pharmacol.*, **1987**, *27*:78–83.

	AVAILABILITY (ORAL) (%)	URINARY EXCRETION (%)	BOUND IN PLASMA (%)	CLEARANCE (ml · min⁻¹ · kg⁻¹)	VOL. DIST. (liters/kg)	HALF-LIFE (hours)	PEAK TIME (hours)	PEAK CONCENTRATIONS
RILUZOLE[a] (Chapter 20)								
	64 (30–100) ↓ Food[b]	<1	98	5.5 ± 0.9 LD ↓	3.4 ± 0.6	14 ± 6	0.8 ± 0.5[c]	173 ± 72 ng/ml[c]

[a]Eliminated primarily by CYP1A2-dependent metabolism; metabolites are inactive. Involvement of CYP1A2 may contribute to ethnic (lower CL/F in Japanese) and gender (lower CL in women) differences and inductive effects of smoking (higher CL in smokers). [b]High-fat meal. [c]Following a 50 mg oral dose taken twice daily to steady state.

References: Bruno, R., Vivier, N., *et al.* Population pharmacokinetics of riluzole in patients with amyotrophic lateral sclerosis. *Clin. Pharmacol. Ther.*, **1997**, *62*:518–526. Le Liboux, A., Lefebvre, P., *et al.* Single- and multiple-dose pharmacokinetics of riluzole in white subjects. *J. Clin. Pharmacol.*, **1997**, *37*:820–827. *Physicians' Desk Reference*, 58th ed., Medical Economics Co., Montvale, NJ, **2004**, p. 769. Wokke, J. Riluzole. *Lancet*, **1996**, *348*:795–799.

	AVAILABILITY (ORAL) (%)	URINARY EXCRETION (%)	BOUND IN PLASMA (%)	CLEARANCE (ml · min⁻¹ · kg⁻¹)	VOL. DIST. (liters/kg)	HALF-LIFE (hours)	PEAK TIME (hours)	PEAK CONCENTRATIONS
RISEDRONATE (Chapter 61)								
	<1[a]	87 (73–102)	24	1.5 (1.2–1.9) ↓ RD	6.3 ± 1.5	200 (183–218)[b]	1.7 ± 1.2[c]	2.8 ± 0.3 ng/ml[c]

[a]Food affects the extent of bioavailability; recommended to be taken 30 minutes prior to the first meal of the day. Data from healthy men and women reported; no significant gender differences. [b]Exhibits multi-exponential elimination. The plasma $t_{\frac{1}{2}}$ for the first and second exponential phases is 0.9 and 13 hours, respectively. The longer terminal $t_{\frac{1}{2}}$ reported is thought to represent dissociation of risedronate from the surface of bone. [c]Following a 5 mg oral dose given once daily to healthy men.

References: Mitchell, D.Y., Barr, W.H., *et al.* Risedronate pharmacokinetics and intra- and inter-subject variability upon single-dose intravenous and oral administration. *Pharm. Res.*, **2001**, *18*:166–170. Ogura, Y., Gonsho, A., Cyong, J.C., and Orimo, H. Clinical trial of risedronate in Japanese volunteers: single and multiple oral dose studies. *J. Bone Miner. Metab.*, **2004**, *22*:111–119. *Physicians' Desk Reference*, 58th ed., Medical Economics Co., Montvale, NJ, **2004**, p. 2825.

RISPERIDONE[a] (Chapter 18)

Oral: 66 ± 28[b] IM: 103 ± 13	3 ± 2[b]	89[c] ↓ Cirr	5.4 ± 1.4[b] ↓ RD,[a] Aged[d]	1.1 ± 0.2	3.2 ± 0.8[a,b] ↑ RD,[a] Aged[d]	R: ~1[e]	R: 10 ng/ml[e] TA: 45 ng/ml[e]

[a]Active metabolite, 9-hydroxyrisperidone, is the predominant circulating species in extensive metabolizers and is equipotent to parent drug. 9-Hydroxyrisperidone has a $t_{\frac{1}{2}}$ of 20 ± 3 hours. In extensive metabolizers, 35% ± 7% of an IV dose is excreted as this metabolite; its elimination is primarily renal and therefore correlates with renal function. [b]Formation of 9-hydroxyrisperidone is catalyzed by CYP2D6. Parameters reported for extensive metabolizers. In poor metabolizers, F is higher; about 20% of an IV dose is excreted unchanged, 10% as the 9-hydroxy metabolite; CL is slightly less than 1 ml · min⁻¹ · kg⁻¹, and $t_{\frac{1}{2}}$ is similar to that of the active metabolite, about 20 hours. [c]77% for 9-hydroxyrisperidone. [d]Changes in elderly due to decreased renal function affecting the elimination of the active metabolite. [e]Mean steady-state trough concentration for risperidone (R) and total active (TA) drug, risperidone + 9-OH-risperidone, following a 3 mg oral dose given twice daily to patients with chronic schizophrenia. No difference in total active drug levels between CYP2D6 extensive and poor metabolizers.

References: Cohen, L.J. Risperidone. *Pharmacotherapy*, **1994**, *14*:253–265. Heykants, J., Huang, M.L., *et al.* The pharmacokinetics of risperidone in humans: a summary. *J. Clin. Psychiatry*, **1994**, *55*(suppl):13–17.

RITONAVIR[a] (Chapter 50)

—[b] ↑ Food	98–99	3.5 ± 1.8	SD: 1.2 ± 0.4[c] MD: 2.1 ± 0.8[c] ↑ Child ↓ LD[d]	0.41 ± 0.25[c]	3–5[c] ↑ LD[d]	2–4[e]	11 ± 4 μg/ml[e]

[a]Ritonavir is extensively metabolized primarily by CYP3A4. It also appears to induce its own CL with single- (SD) to multiple-dose (MD) administration. Also used in combination with saquinavir; saquinavir has no significant effect on the pharmacokinetics of ritonavir. [b]Absolute bioavailability unknown (>60% absorbed); food elicits a 15% increase in oral AUC for capsule formulation. [c]CL/F, V_{area}/F, and $t_{\frac{1}{2}}$ reported for oral dose. [d]CL/F reduced slightly and $t_{\frac{1}{2}}$ increased slightly, moderate liver impairment. [e]Following a 600 mg oral dose given twice daily to steady state.

References: Hsu, A., Granneman, G.R., and Bertz, R.J. Ritonavir. Clinical pharmacokinetics and interactions with other anti-HIV agents. *Clin. Pharmacokinet*, **1998**, *35*:275–291. *Physicians' Desk Reference*, 54th ed. Medical Economics Co., Montvale, NJ, **2000**, p. 465.

RIVASTIGMINE[a] (Chapter 20)

72 (22–119)[b] ↑ Food, Dose	40	negligible	13 ± 4[c]	1.5 ± 0.6[c]	1.4 ± 0.4[c,d]	1.2 ± 1.0[c] ↑ Food	26 ± 10 ng/ml[e] ↓ Food

[a]Rivastigmine is metabolized by cholinesterase. No apparent gender differences. [b]Following a 6-mg oral dose. Bioavailability increases with dose; following a 3-mg dose, the median bioavailability is 36%. [c]IV dose of 2 mg. [d]The pharmacodynamic $t_{\frac{1}{2}}$ is approximately 10 hours due to tight binding to acetylcholinesterase. [e]Following oral administration of 6 mg capsule. Peak concentrations increase more than proportionally at doses above 3 mg.

References: Hossain, M., Jhee, S.S., *et al.* Estimation of the absolute bioavailability of rivastigmine in patients with mild to moderate dementia of the Alzheimer's type. *Clin. Pharmacokinet.*, **2002**, *41*:225–234. Williams, B.R., Nazarians, A., and Gill, M.A. A review of rivastigmine: a reversible cholinesterase inhibitor. *Clin. Ther.*, **2003**, *25*:1634–1653.

Table A–II–1 *Pharmacokinetic Data (Continued)*

AVAILABILITY (ORAL) (%)	URINARY EXCRETION (%)	BOUND IN PLASMA (%)	CLEARANCE $(ml \cdot min^{-1} \cdot kg^{-1})$	VOL. DIST. (liters/kg)	HALF-LIFE (hours)	PEAK TIME (hours)	PEAK CONCENTRATIONS

RIZATRIPTAN[a] (Chapter 11)

| 47 | F: 28 ± 9[b] M: 29[b] | 14 | F: 12.3 ± 1.4[b] M: 18.9 ± 2.8[b] ↓ LD,[c] RD[d] | F: 1.5 ± 0.2 M: 2.2 ± 0.4 | F: 2.2 M: 2.4 | SD: 0.9 ± 0.4[e] MD: 4.8 ± 0.7[e] | SD: 20 ± 4.9 ng/ml[e] MD: 37 ± 13 ng/ml[e] |

[a]Data from healthy adult male (M) and female (F) subjects. Oxidative deamination catalyzed by MAO-A is the primary route of elimination. *N*-desmethyl rizatriptan (DMR) is a minor metabolite (~14%) that is active and accumulates in blood. [b]Evidence of minor dose-dependent metabolic CL and urinary excretion. [c]*CL/F* reduced, moderate hepatic impairment. [d]*CL/F* reduced, severe renal impairment. [e]Following a 10 mg single (SD) and multiple (MD: 10 mg every 2 hours × 3 doses × 4 days) oral dose. DMR peak concentration is 8.5 and 26.2 ng/ml with SD and MD, respectively.

References: Goldberg, M.R. Lee, Y., *et al.* Rizatriptan, a novel 5-HT$_{1B/1D}$ agonist for migraine: single- and multiple-dose tolerability and pharmacokinetics in healthy subjects. *J. Clin. Pharmacol.,* **2000**, *40*:74–83. Lee, Y., Ermlich, S.J., *et al.* Pharmacokinetics and tolerability of intravenous rizatriptan in healthy females. *Biopharm. Drug Dispos.,* **1998**, *19*:577–581. *Physicians' Desk Reference,* 54th ed. Medical Economics Co., Montvale, NJ, **2000**, p. 1912. Vyas, K.P., Halpin, R.A., *et al.* Disposition and pharmacokinetics of the antimigraine drug, rizatriptan, in humans. *Drug Metab. Dispos.,* **2000**, 28:89–95.

ROCURONIUM[a] (Chapter 9)

| —[b] | 12–22 | 25 | 3.3–5.2[c] ↑ Child[d], ↔ LD | 0.19–0.31[c] ↑ LD | 1.2–2.2[c] ↓ Child[d], ↑ LD[e] | — | 0.8–1.4 μg/ml[f] |

[a]Eliminated primarily by biliary excretion. No significant gender differences. [b]For IV administration only. [c]Mean values from different studies reported. [d]Higher CL and shorter $t_{\frac{1}{2}}$ in pediatric (3 months to <8 years) patients. [e]Duration of clinical effect prolonged by 50%. [f]EC$_{50}$ for neuromuscular blockade (adductor pollicis and vocal cords).

References: Atherton, D.P., and Hunter, J.M. Clinical pharmacokinetics of the newer neuromuscular blocking drugs. *Clin. Pharmacokinet.,* **1999**, *36*:169–189. Khuenl-Brady, K.S., and Sparr, H. Clinical pharmacokinetics of rocuronium bromide. *Clin. Pharmacokinet.,* **1996**, *31*:174–183. *Physicians' Desk Reference,* 58th ed. Medical Economics Co., Montvale, NJ, **2004**, pp. 2394–2395.

ROPINIROLE[a] (Chapter 20)

| 55 | <10 | ~40 | 11.2 ± 5.0[b] ↓ Aged[c] ↔ RD | 7.5 ± 2.4[b] | 6[b] | 1.0 (0.5–6.0)[d] ↑ Food | 7.4 (2.4–13) ng/ml[d] ↓ Food |

[a]Data from male and female patients with Parkinson's disease. Metabolized primarily by CYP1A2 to inactive *N*-deisopropyl and hydroxy metabolites. [b]*CL/F, V$_d$/F,* and $t_{\frac{1}{2}}$ reported for oral dose. [c]*CL/F* reduced but dose titrated to desired effect. [d]Following 2 mg oral dose given three times daily to steady state.

References: Bloomer, J.C., Clarke, S.E., and Chenery, R.J. In vitro identification of the P450 enzymes responsible for the metabolism of ropinirole. *Drug Metab. Dispos.,* **1997**, *25*:840–844. *Physicians' Desk Reference,* 54th ed. Medical Economics Co., Montvale, NJ, **2000**, p. 3037. Taylor, A.C., Beerahee, A., *et al.* Lack of a pharmacokinetic interaction at steady state between ropinirole and L-dopa in patients with Parkinson's disease. *Pharmacotherapy,* **1999**, *19*:150–156.

ROPIVACAINE[a] (Chapter 14)

—[b]	1	90–94	5.5–7.1[c]	0.54–0.86[c]	1.6–2.0[c,d]	E: 0.7 ± 0.2[e]	E: 1.1 ± 0.2 μg/ml[e]
						BP: 0.9 ± 0.4[e]	BP: 2.3 ± 0.8 μg/ml[e]

[a]S-(−) enantiomer (N-propyl homolog of bupivacaine); eliminated primarily by CYP1A2-dependent metabolism to 3-hydroxyropivacaine. [b]For parenteral administration only. [c]Mean values from different studies reported. [d]Apparent $t_{\frac{1}{2}}$ is longer (4 to 7 hours) after epidural and brachial plexus administration; most likely reflects a slow absorption process. [e]Following a single 150 mg epidural (E) dose or a 300 mg dose to the brachial plexus (BP).

References: McClellan, K.J., and Faulds, D. Ropivacaine: an update of its use in regional anaesthesia. Drugs, 2000, 60:1065–1093. Physicians' Desk Reference, 58th ed., Medical Economics Co. Montvale, NJ, 2004, p. 618. Thomas, J.M., and Schug, S.A. Recent advances in the pharmacokinetics of local anaesthetics. Long-acting amide enantiomers and continuous infusions. Clin. Pharmacokinet., 1999, 36:67–83.

ROSIGLITAZONE[a] (Chapter 60)

99	Negligible	99.8	0.25 ± 0.08[b]	0.68 ± 0.16[b]	3–4[b]	1.0[d]	598 ± 117 ng/ml[d]
		↓LD[c]	(0.21)	(0.49)	↑LD		
			↓LD[c] ↔RD	↓LD[c] ↔RD			

[a]Data from male and female patients with NIDDM (type 2 diabetes). No significant gender differences. Metabolized primarily by CYP2C8. [b]CL/F, V_d/F, and $t_{\frac{1}{2}}$ reported for oral dose. Shown in parentheses are mean values from a population pharmacokinetic analysis. [c]Reduced CL/F and $CL/F_{unbound}$ moderate-to-severe liver impairment. [d]Following a single 8 mg oral dose.

References: Baldwin, S.J., Clarke, S.E., and Chenery, R.J. Characterization of the cytochrome P450 enzymes involved in the in vitro metabolism of rosiglitazone. Br. J. Clin. Pharmacol., 1999, 48:424–432. Patel, B.R., Dringer, K., et al. Population pharmacokinetics of rosiglitazone (R) in phase III clinical trials. Clin. Pharmacol. Ther., 2000, 67:123. Physicians' Desk Reference, 54th ed. Medical Economics Co., Montvale, NJ, 2000, p. 2981. Thompson, K., Zussman, B., Miller, A., Jorkasky, D., and Freed, M. Pharmacokinetics of rosiglitazone are unaltered in hemodialysis patients. Clin. Pharmacol. Ther., 1999, 65:186.

ROSUVASTATIN[a] (Chapter 35)

20 (17–23)	30 ± 7	88	10.5 ± 4.7	1.7 ± 0.5	20 ± 6	3 (1–6)[c]	4.6 ± 2.1 ng/ml[c]
			↓RD[b]				

[a]Eliminated primarily by biliary excretion; also appears to be actively transported into the liver by an organic anion transport protein (OATP2/SLC21A6). Data from healthy men reported; no significant gender or age differences. [b]Reduced CL/F in patients with severe renal impairment. [c]Following a 10 mg oral dose taken once daily for 10 days.

References: Martin, P.D., Mitchell, P.D., and Schneck, D.W. Pharmacodynamic effects and pharmacokinetics of a new HMG-CoA reductase inhibitor, rosuvastatin, after morning or evening administration in healthy volunteers. Br. J. Clin. Pharmacol., 2002, 54:472–477. Martin, P.D., Warwick, M.J., Dane, A.L., Brindley, C., and Short, T. Absolute oral bioavailability of rosuvastatin in healthy white adult male volunteers. Clin. Ther., 2003, 25:2553–2563. Product Labeling: Crestor® tablets (rosuvastatin calcium), Astra-Zeneca Pharmaceuticals LP, Wilmington, DE, 2003. Schneck, D.W., Birmingham, B.K., et al. The effect of gemfibrozil on the pharmacokinetics of rosuvastatin. Clin. Pharmacol. Ther., 2004, 75:455–463.

Table A–II-1 *Pharmacokinetic Data (Continued)*

AVAILABILITY (ORAL) (%)	URINARY EXCRETION (%)	BOUND IN PLASMA (%)	CLEARANCE (ml · min⁻¹ · kg⁻¹)	VOL. DIST. (liters/kg)	HALF-LIFE (hours)	PEAK TIME (hours)	PEAK CONCENTRATIONS
SELEGILINE[a] (Chapter 20)							
Negligible[b]	Negligible	94[c]	~1500[b] / 160[d]	1.9	1.9 ± 1.0[e]	S: 0.7 ± 0.4[f] / DS: ~1 h	S: 1.1 ± 0.4 ng/ml[f] / DS: ~15 ng/ml[f]

[a]MAO-B active metabolite: *l*-(−)-desmethylselegiline. [b]Extensive first-pass metabolism; estimate of *CL/F* reported. [c]Blood-to-plasma concentration ratio = 1.3–2.2 for parent drug and ~0.55 for *N*-desmethyl metabolite. [d]*CL/F* for *N*-desmethylselegiline assuming quantitative conversion of parent to this metabolite. [e]For parent and *N*-desmethyl metabolite. $t_{\frac{1}{2}}$ for methamphetamine (major plasma species) and amphetamine are 21 and 18 hours, respectively. [f]Mean data for selegiline (S) and its active metabolite, *N*-desmethylselegiline (DS), following a single 10 mg oral dose given to adults.

Reference: Heinonen, E.H., Anttila, M.I., and Lammintausta, R.A. Pharmacokinetic aspects of *l*-deprenyl (selegiline) and its metabolites. *Clin. Pharmacol. Ther.,* **1994,** *56:*742–749.

AVAILABILITY (ORAL) (%)	URINARY EXCRETION (%)	BOUND IN PLASMA (%)	CLEARANCE (ml · min⁻¹ · kg⁻¹)	VOL. DIST. (liters/kg)	HALF-LIFE (hours)	PEAK TIME (hours)	PEAK CONCENTRATIONS
SERTRALINE[a] (Chapter 17)							
—[a]	<1	98–99	38 ± 14[b] / ↓ Aged, Cirr	—	23 / ↑ Aged, Cirr	M: 6.9 ± 1.0[c] / F: 6.7 ± 1.8[c]	M: 118 ± 22 ng/ml[c] / F: 166 ± 65 ng/ml[d] / ↔ Aged

[a]Absolute bioavailability is not known (>44% absorbed); undergoes extensive first-pass metabolism to essentially inactive metabolites; catalyzed by multiple cytochrome P450 isoforms. [b]*CL/F* reported. [c]Following a dose titration up to 200 mg given once daily for 30 days to healthy male (M) and female (F) adults.

References: van Harten, J. Clinical pharmacokinetics of selective serotonin reuptake inhibitors. *Clin. Pharmacokinet.,* **1993,** *24:*203–220. Warrington, S.J. Clinical implications of the pharmacology of sertraline. *Int. Clin. Psychopharmacol.,* **1994,** *6*(suppl 2):11–21.

AVAILABILITY (ORAL) (%)	URINARY EXCRETION (%)	BOUND IN PLASMA (%)	CLEARANCE (ml · min⁻¹ · kg⁻¹)	VOL. DIST. (liters/kg)	HALF-LIFE (hours)	PEAK TIME (hours)	PEAK CONCENTRATIONS
SILDENAFIL[a] (Chapter 33)							
38	0	96	6.0 ± 1.1 / ↓ LD,[b] RD,[c] Aged	1.2 ± 0.3	2.4 ± 1.0	1.2 ± 0.3[e]	212 ± 59 ng/ml[e] / ↑ Aged[d]

[a]Data from healthy male subjects. Sildenafil is metabolized primarily by CYP3A and secondarily by CYP2C9. Piperazine *N*-desmethyl metabolite is active (~50% parent) and accumulates in plasma (~40% parent). [b]*CL/F* reduced, mild to moderate hepatic impairment. [c]*CL/F* reduced, severe renal impairment. [d]Increased unbound concentrations. [e]Following a single 50 mg oral (solution) dose.

References: Physicians' Desk Reference, 54th ed. Medical Economics Co., Montvale, NJ, **2000,** p. 2382. Walker, D.K., Ackland, M.J., *et al.* Pharmacokinetics and metabolism of sildenafil in mouse, rat, rabbit, dog and man. *Xenobiotica,* **1999,** *29:*297–310.

AVAILABILITY (ORAL) (%)	URINARY EXCRETION (%)	BOUND IN PLASMA (%)	CLEARANCE (ml · min⁻¹ · kg⁻¹)	VOL. DIST. (liters/kg)	HALF-LIFE (hours)	PEAK TIME (hours)	PEAK CONCENTRATIONS
SIMVASTATIN[a] (Chapter 35)							
≤5	Negligible	94	7.6[b]	—	2–3	AI: 1.4 ± 1.0[c] / TI: 1.4 ± 1.0[c]	AI: 46 ± 20 ngEq/ml[c] / TI: 56 ± 25 ngEq/ml[c]

References: Corsini, A., Bellosta, S., *et al.* New insights into the pharmacodynamic and pharmacokinetic properties of statins. *Pharmacol. Ther.,* **1999,** *84:*413–428. Desager, J.P., and Horsmans, Y. Clinical pharmacokinetics of 3-hydroxy-3-methylglutaryl-coenzyme A reductase inhibitors. *Clin. Pharmacokinet.,* **1996,** *31:*348–371. Mauro, V.F. Clinical pharmacokinetics and practical applications of simvastatin. *Clin. Pharmacokinet.,* **1993,** *24:*195–202.

[a]Simvastatin is a lactone prodrug that is hydrolyzed to the active corresponding β-hydroxy acid. Values reported are for the disposition of the acid. [b]The β-hydroxy acid can be reconverted back to the lactone; irreversible oxidative metabolites are generated by CYP3A. [c]Data for active inhibitors (AI, ring-opened molecule) and total inhibitors (TI) following a 40 mg oral dose given once daily for 17 days to healthy adults.

SIROLIMUS[a] (Chapter 52)

Oral Bioavail.	Urinary Excr.	Bound in Plasma	Clearance	Vol. Dist.	Half-Life	Peak Time	Peak Concentration
~15[b] ↑Food[b]	—	40[c]	3.47 ± 1.58[d]	12 ± 4.6[d]	62.3 ± 16.2[d]	SD: 0.81 ± 0.17[e] MD: 1.4 ± 1.2[e]	SD: 67 ± 23 ng/ml[e] MD: 94–210 ng/ml[e]

[a]Data from male and female renal transplant patients. All subjects were on a stable cyclosporine regimen. Sirolimus is metabolized primarily by CYP3A and is a substrate for P-glycoprotein. Several sirolimus metabolites are pharmacologically active. [b]Cyclosporine coadministration increases sirolimus bioavailability. F increased by high-fat meal. [c]Concentrates in blood cells; blood-to-plasma concentration ratio ~38 ± 13. [d]Blood CL/F, V_{ss}/F, and $t_{1/2}$ reported for oral dose. [e]Following a single 15 mg oral dose (SD) in healthy subjects and 4–6.5 mg/m² oral dose (with cyclosporine) given twice daily to steady state (MD) in renal transplant patients.

References: Kelly, P.A., Napoli, K., and Kahan, B.D. Conversion from liquid to solid rapamycin formulations in stable renal allograft transplant recipients. *Biopharm. Drug Dispos.,* **1999,** *20:*249–253. Zimmerman, J.J., Ferron, G.M., Lim, H.K., and Parker, V. The effect of a high-fat meal on the oral bioavailability of the immunosuppressant sirolimus (rapamycin). *J. Clin. Pharmacol.,* **1999,** *39:*1155–1161. Zimmerman, J.J., and Kahan, B.D. Pharmacokinetics of sirolimus in stable renal transplant patients after multiple oral dose administration. *J. Clin. Pharmacol.,* **1997,** *37:*405–415.

SPIRONOLACTONE[a] (Chapter 28)

Oral Bioavail.	Urinary Excr.	Bound in Plasma	Clearance	Vol. Dist.	Half-Life	Peak Time	Peak Concentration
—[b] ↑Food	<1[c]	>90[d]	93[e]	10[e]	S: 1.3 ± 0.3[f] C: 11.2 ± 2.3[f] TS: 2.8 ± 0.4[f] HTS: 10.1 ± 2.3[f] ↑LD[g]	S: 1.0[f] C: 2.9 ± 0.6[f] TS: 1.8 ± 0.5[f] HTS: 3.1 ± 0.9[f]	S: 185 ± 51 ng/ml[f] C: 231 ± 49 ng/ml[f] TS: 571 ± 74 ng/ml[f] HTS: 202 ± 54 ng/ml[f]

[a]Spironolactone (S) is extensively metabolized; it has three known active metabolites: canrenone (C), 7α-thiomethylspironolactone (TS), and 6β-hydroxy-7α-thiomethylspironolactone (HTS). [b]Absolute bioavailability is not known; likely to exhibit first-pass metabolism. *AUC* of parent drug and metabolites increased when spironolactone taken with food. [c]Measured after an oral dose. [d]Binding of spironolactone and its active metabolites. [e]CLF and V_{area}/F; calculated from reported *AUC* and $t_{1/2}$ data. [f]Following a single 200 mg oral dose of spironolactone. [g]Canrenone accumulates 2.5-fold with multiple spironolactone dosing. [g]$t_{1/2}$ of parent drug and metabolites increased in patients with cirrhosis.

References: Ho, P.C., Bourne, D.W., Triggs, E.J., and Heazlewood, V. Pharmacokinetics of canrenone and metabolites after base hydrolysis following single and multiple oral administration of spironolactone. *Eur. J. Clin. Pharmacol.,* **1984,** *27:*441–446. Overdiek, H.W., Hermens, W.A., and Merkus, F.W. New insights into the pharmacokinetics of spironolactone. *Clin. Pharmacol. Ther.,* **1985,** *38:*469–474. Overdiek, H.W., and Merkus, F.W. Influence of food on the bioavailability of spironolactone. *Clin. Pharmacol. Ther.,* **1986,** *40:*531–536. *Physicians' Desk Reference,* 54th ed., Medical Economics Co, Montvale, NJ, **2000,** p. 2883. Sungaila, I., Bartle, W.R., *et al.* Spironolactone pharmacokinetics and pharmacodynamics in patients with cirrhotic ascites. *Gastroenterology,* **1992,** *102:*1680–1685.

STREPTOKINASE[a] (Chapter 54)

Oral Bioavail.	Urinary Excr.	Bound in Plasma	Clearance	Vol. Dist.	Half-Life	Peak Time	Peak Concentration
—	0	—	1.7 ± 0.7	0.08 ± 0.04[b]	0.61 ± 0.24	0.9 ± 0.21[c]	188 ± 58 IU/ml[c]

[a]Values obtained from acute myocardial infarction patients using a function bioassay. [b]V_{area} reported. [c]Following a single 1.5×10^6 IU IV dose given as a 60-minute infusion to patients with acute myocardial infarction.

Reference: Gemmill, J.D., Hogg, K.J., *et al.* A comparison of the pharmacokinetic properties of streptokinase and anistreplase in acute myocardial infarction. *Br. J. Clin. Pharmacol.,* **1991,** *31:*143–147.

Table A–II–1 Pharmacokinetic Data (Continued)

AVAILABILITY (ORAL) (%)	URINARY EXCRETION (%)	BOUND IN PLASMA (%)	CLEARANCE $(ml \cdot min^{-1} \cdot kg^{-1})$	VOL. DIST. (liters/kg)	HALF-LIFE (hours)	PEAK TIME (hours)	PEAK CONCENTRATIONS

SULFAMETHOXAZOLE (Chapter 43)

AVAILABILITY (ORAL) (%)	URINARY EXCRETION (%)	BOUND IN PLASMA (%)	CLEARANCE	VOL. DIST.	HALF-LIFE	PEAK TIME	PEAK CONCENTRATIONS
~100	14 ± 2	53 ± 5 ↓ RD, Alb ↔ Aged, CF	$0.31 \pm 0.07^{a,b}$ ↔ RD ↑ CF	0.26 ± 0.04^{a} ↑ RD ↔ Child, CF	10.1 ± 2.6^{a} ↑ RD ↔ Child ↓ CF	4^{b}	$37.1 \ \mu g/ml^{b}$

[a]Studies include concurrent administration of trimethoprim and variation in urinary pH; these factors had no marked effect on the CL of sulfamethoxazole. Metabolically cleared primarily by N_4-acetylation. [b]Following a single 1000 mg oral dose given to healthy adults.

References: Hutabarat, R.M., Unadkat, J.D., *et al.* Disposition of drugs in cystic fibrosis. I. Sulfamethoxazole and trimethoprim. *Clin. Pharmacol. Ther.,* **1991,** *49:*402–409. Welling, P.G., Craig, W.A., Amidon, G.L., and Kunin, C.M. Pharmacokinetics of trimethoprim and sulfamethoxazole in normal subjects and in patients with renal failure. *J. Infect. Dis.,* **1973,** *128*(suppl):556–566.

SUMATRIPTAN (Chapter 11)

AVAILABILITY (ORAL) (%)	URINARY EXCRETION (%)	BOUND IN PLASMA (%)	CLEARANCE	VOL. DIST.	HALF-LIFE	PEAK TIME	PEAK CONCENTRATIONS
Oral: 14 ± 5 SC: 97 ± 16	22 ± 4	14–21	22 ± 5.4	2.0 ± 0.34	1.0 ± 0.3^{a}	SC: 0.2 (0.1–0.3)[b] Oral: ~1.5[b]	SC: 72 (55–108) ng/ml[b] Oral: 54 (27–137) ng/ml[b]

[a]An apparent $t_{\frac{1}{2}}$ of ~2 hours reported for SC and oral doses. [b]Following a single 6 mg SC or 100 mg oral dose given to young healthy adults.

References: Scott, A.K. Sumatriptan clinical pharmacokinetics. *Clin. Pharmacokinet.,* **1994,** *27:*337–344. Scott, A.K., Grimes, S., *et al.* Sumatriptan and cerebral perfusion in healthy volunteers. *Br. J. Clin. Pharmacol.,* **1992,** *33:*401–404.

TACROLIMUS (Chapter 52)

AVAILABILITY (ORAL) (%)	URINARY EXCRETION (%)	BOUND IN PLASMA (%)	CLEARANCE	VOL. DIST.	HALF-LIFE	PEAK TIME	PEAK CONCENTRATIONS
$25 \pm 10^{a,b}$ ↔ RD ↓ Food	<1	75–99^{c}	0.90 ± 0.29^{a} ↔ RD, Cirr	$0.91 \pm 0.29^{a,d}$ ↔ RD ↑ Cirr	12 ± 5^{a} ↔ RD ↑ Cirr	1.4 ± 0.5^{e}	$31.2 \pm 10.1 \ ng/ml^{e}$

[a]Drug disposition parameters calculated from blood concentrations. Data from liver transplant patients reported. Metabolized by CYP3A; also a substrate for P-glycoprotein. [b]A similar bioavailability ($F = 21 \pm 19\%$) reported for kidney transplant patients; $F = 16 \pm 7\%$ for normal subjects. Low oral bioavailability likely due to incomplete intestinal availability. [c]Different values for plasma protein binding reported. Concentrates in blood cells; blood-to-plasma concentration ratio = 35 (12–67). [d]Slightly higher V_{ss} and $t_{\frac{1}{2}}$ reported for kidney transplant patients. Because of the very high and variable blood-to-plasma concentration ratio, markedly different V_{ss} values are reported for parameters based on plasma concentrations. [e]Following a single 7 mg oral dose given to healthy adults. Consensus target trough concentrations at steady state are 5–20 ng/ml.

References: Bekersky, I., Dressler, D., and Mekki, Q.A. Dose linearity after oral administration of tacrolimus 1-mg capsules at doses of 3, 7, and 10 mg. *Clin. Ther.,* **1999,** *21:*2058–2064. Jusko, W.J., Piekoszewski, W., *et al.* Pharmacokinetics of tacrolimus in liver transplant patients. *Clin. Pharmacol. Ther.,* **1995,** *57:*281–290. *Physicians' Desk Reference,* 54th ed. Medical Economics Co., Montvale, NJ, **2000,** pp. 1098–1099.

TADALAFIL[a] (Chapter 33)

—		94	0.59[b] ↓RD[c]	0.89[b] ↓RD[c]	17.5	2[d]	378 ng/ml[d]

[a] Eliminated primarily by CYP3A4-dependent metabolism. [b] CL/F and V/F reported. [c] AUC increased in patients with mild or moderate (twofold) and severe (fourfold) renal insufficiency. [d] Following a single 20-mg oral dose.

References: Curran, M., and Keating, G. Tadalafil. *Drugs,* **2003,** *63:*2203–2212; discussion 2213–2214. Product Labeling: Cialis® (tadalafil tablets), Lilly Icos, Bothell, WA, **2004.**

TAMOXIFEN[a] (Chapters 51, 57)

—	<1	>98	1.4[b,c]	50–60[b]	4–11 days[d]	5 (3–7)	120 (67–183) ng/ml[d]

[a] Has active metabolites; 4-hydroxytamoxifen and 4-hydroxy-*N*-desmethyltamoxifen are minor metabolites that exhibit affinity for the estrogen receptor that is greater than that of parent *trans*-tamoxifen. The $t_{\frac{1}{2}}$ of all metabolites are rate-limited by tamoxifen elimination. [b] CL/F and V_{area}/F reported. [c] The major pathway of elimination, *N*-demethylation, is catalyzed by CYP3A. [d] $t_{\frac{1}{2}}$ consistent with accumulation and approach to steady state. Significantly longer terminal $t_{\frac{1}{2}}$s are observed. [e] Average concentration (C_{ss}) following a 10 mg oral dose given twice daily to steady state.

Reference: Lønning, P.E., Geisler, J., and Dowsett, M. Pharmacological and clinical profile of anastrozole. *Breast Cancer Res. Treat.* **1998,** *49(suppl 1)*:S53–S57. *Physicians' Desk Reference,* 54th ed. Medical Economics Co., Montvale, NJ, **2000,** p. 557.

TAMSULOSIN[a] (Chapter 10)

100 ↓ Food	12.7 ± 3.0 ↓ Food	99 ± 1 ↑ RD	0.62 ± 0.31 ↓ RD[b], Aged	0.20 ± 0.06	6.8 ± 3.5[c] ↑ RD, Aged	5.3 ± 0.7[d] ↑ Food	16 ± 5 ng/ml[d] ↓ Food

[a] Data from healthy male subjects. Metabolized primarily by CYP3A and CYP2D6. [b] CL/F reduced, moderate renal impairment. Unbound *AUC* relatively unchanged. [c] Apparent $t_{\frac{1}{2}}$ after oral dose in patients is ~14 to 15 hours, reflecting controlled release from modified-release granules. [d] Following a single 0.4 mg modified-release oral dose in healthy subjects.

References: Matsushima, H., Kamimura, H., *et al.* Plasma protein binding of tamsulosin hydrochloride in renal disease: role of α_1-acid glycoprotein and possibility of binding interactions. *Eur. J. Clin. Pharmacol.,* **1999,** *55:*437–443. van Hoogdalem, E.J., Soeishi, Y., Matsushima, H., and Higuchi, S. Disposition of the selective $\alpha_{1,A}$-adrenoceptor antagonist tamsulosin in humans: comparison with data from interspecies scaling. *J. Pharm. Sci.,* **1997,** *86:*1156–1161. Wolzt, M., Fabrizii, V., *et al.* Pharmacokinetics of tamsulosin in subjects with normal and varying degrees of impaired renal function: an open-label single-dose and multiple-dose study. *Eur. J. Clin. Pharmacol.,* **1998,** *4:*367–373.

TEGASEROD[a] (Chapter 37)

11 ± 2 ↓ Food	Negligible[b]	98	18 ± 4	5.2 ± 3.2	11 ± 5	0.8[c]	2.7 ± 1.2 ng/ml[c]

[a] Eliminated primarily by metabolism (presystemic acid catalyzed hydrolysis in the stomach and direct glucuronidation). Data reported for healthy men and women; no significant gender or age differences. [b] Reported for oral dose. [c] Following a 6 mg oral dose taken twice daily to steady state.

Reference: Appel-Dingemanse, S. Clinical pharmacokinetics of tegaserod, a serotonin 5-HT(4) receptor partial agonist with promotile activity. *Clin. Pharmacokinet.,* **2002,** *41:*1021–1042.

Table A–II–1 Pharmacokinetic Data *(Continued)*

AVAILABILITY (ORAL) (%)	URINARY EXCRETION (%)	BOUND IN PLASMA (%)	CLEARANCE $(ml \cdot min^{-1} \cdot kg^{-1})$	VOL. DIST. (liters/kg)	HALF-LIFE (hours)	PEAK TIME (hours)	PEAK CONCENTRATIONS
TELITHROMYCIN[a] (Chapter 46)							
57 (41–112)	23 (19–27)	70	14 (12–16) ↓RD[b]	3.0 (2.1–4.5)	12 (7–23)	1.0 (0.5–3.0)[c]	2.23 μg/ml[c]

[a]Approximately 35% of the dose is metabolized by CYP3A4. [b]*CL/F* reduced in patients with severe renal impairment. [c]Following an 800 mg oral dose given once daily for 7 days.

References: Namour, F., Wessels, D.H., *et al.* Pharmacokinetics of the new ketolide telithromycin (HMR 3647) administered in ascending single and multiple doses. *Antimicrob. Agents Chemother.*, **2001**, *45*:170–175. Perret, C., Lenfant, B., *et al.* Pharmacokinetics and absolute oral bioavailability of an 800-mg oral dose of telithromycin in healthy young and elderly volunteers. *Chemotherapy*, **2002**, *48*:217–223. Zhanel, G.G., Walters, M., *et al.* The ketolides: a critical review. *Drugs*, **2002**, *62*:1771–1804.

AVAILABILITY (ORAL) (%)	URINARY EXCRETION (%)	BOUND IN PLASMA (%)	CLEARANCE $(ml \cdot min^{-1} \cdot kg^{-1})$	VOL. DIST. (liters/kg)	HALF-LIFE (hours)	PEAK TIME (hours)	PEAK CONCENTRATIONS
TENOFOVIR[a] (Chapter 50)							
25[b] ↑Food	82 ± 13	<1	2.6 ± 0.9[c] ↓RD	0.6 ± 0.1[c]	8.1 ± 1.8[c,d] ↑RD	2.3[e]	326 ng/ml[e]

[a]Tenofovir is formulated as an ester prodrug, Viread® (tenofovir disoproxil fumarate), for oral administration. [b]Bioavailability under fasted state reported; increased to 39% with high-fat meal. [c]Data reported for steady-state 3 mg/kg IV dose given once a day for 2 weeks to HIV-1 infected male and female adults. Slightly higher *CL* with single IV dose. [d]Longer apparent plasma $t_{\frac{1}{2}}$ (17 hours) reported for steady-state oral dosing; this may reflect a longer duration of blood sampling; also, phosphorylated 'active' metabolite exhibits a longer intracellular $t_{\frac{1}{2}}$ (60 hours). [e]Following a 300 mg oral dose given once a day with a meal to steady state.

References: Barditch-Crovo, P., Deeks, S.G., *et al.* Phase i/ii trial of the pharmacokinetics, safety, and antiretroviral activity of tenofovir disoproxil fumarate in human immunodeficiency virus-infected adults. *Antimicrob. Agents Chemother.*, **2001**, *45*:2733–2739. Deeks, S.G., Barditch-Crovo, P., *et al.* Safety, pharmacokinetics, and antiretroviral activity of intravenous 9-[2-(R)-(Phosphonomethoxy)propyl]adenine, a novel anti-human immunodeficiency virus (HIV) therapy, in HIV-infected adults. *Antimicrob. Agents Chemother.*, **1998**, *42*:2380–2384. Kearney, B.P., Flaherty, J.F., and Shah, J. Tenofovir disoproxil fumarate: clinical pharmacology and pharmacokinetics. *Clin. Pharmacokinet.*, **2004**, *43*:595–612.

AVAILABILITY (ORAL) (%)	URINARY EXCRETION (%)	BOUND IN PLASMA (%)	CLEARANCE $(ml \cdot min^{-1} \cdot kg^{-1})$	VOL. DIST. (liters/kg)	HALF-LIFE (hours)	PEAK TIME (hours)	PEAK CONCENTRATIONS
TERAZOSIN (Chapters 10, 32)							
82	11–14	90–94	1.1–1.2[a]	1.1	9–12	1.7[b]	16 ng/ml[b]

[a]Plasma *CL* reportedly reduced in patients with hypertension. [b]Following a 1 mg oral dose (tablet) given to healthy volunteers.

References: Sennello, L.T. Sonders, R.C., *et al.* Effect of age on the pharmacokinetics of orally and intravenously administered terazosin. *Clin. Ther.*, **1988**, *10*:600–607. Sonders, R.C. Pharmacokinetics of terazosin. *Am. J. Med.*, **1986**, *80*:20–24.

AVAILABILITY (ORAL) (%)	URINARY EXCRETION (%)	BOUND IN PLASMA (%)	CLEARANCE $(ml \cdot min^{-1} \cdot kg^{-1})$	VOL. DIST. (liters/kg)	HALF-LIFE (hours)	PEAK TIME (hours)	PEAK CONCENTRATIONS
TETRACYCLINE (Chapter 46)							
77	58 ± 8	65 ± 3	1.67 ± 0.24	1.5 ± 0.1[a]	10.6 ± 1.5	Oral: 4	IV: 16.4 ± 1.2 μg/ml[b] Oral: 2.3 ± 0.2 μg/ml[b]

[a]V_{area} reported. [b]Following a single 10 mg/kg IV dose or a single 250 mg oral dose (taken after a fast and with water).

References: Garty, M., and Hurwitz, A. Effect of cimetidine and antacids on gastrointestinal absorption of tetracycline. Clin. Pharmacol. Ther., 1980, 28:203–207. Raghuram, T.C., and Krishnaswamy, K. Pharmacokinetics of tetracycline in nutritional edema. Chemotherapy, 1982, 28:428–433.

THALIDOMIDE[a] (Chapters 26, 47, 52)

—[b]	<1	—	2.2 ± 0.4[c]	1.1 ± 0.3[c]	6.2 ± 2.6[c]	3.2 ± 1.4[d] ↑HD, Food	2.0 ± 0.6 μg/ml[d] ↑HD

[a]Data from healthy male subjects. Similar data reported for asymptomatic patients with HIV. No age or gender differences. Thalidomide undergoes spontaneous hydrolysis in blood to multiple metabolites. [b]Absolute bioavailability is not known. Altered absorption rate and extent, Hansen's disease (HD). [c]CL/F, V_{area}/F, and $t_{\frac{1}{2}}$ reported for oral dose. [d]Following a single 200 mg oral dose.

References: Noormohamed, F.H., Youle, M.S., et al. Pharmacokinetics and hemodynamic effects of single oral doses of thalidomide in asymptomatic human immunodeficiency virus–infected subjects. AIDS Res. Hum. Retrovir., 1999, 15:1047–1052. Physicians' Desk Reference, 54th ed. Medical Economics Co., Montvale, NJ, 2000, p. 912. Teo, S.K., Colburn, W.A., and Thomas, S.D. Single-dose oral pharmacokinetics of three formulations of thalidomide in healthy male volunteers. J. Clin. Pharmacol., 1999, 39:1162–1168.

THEOPHYLLINE (Chapter 28)

96 ± 8	18 ± 3	56 ± 4	0.65 ± 0.20[a,b]	0.50 ± 0.16	9.0 ± 2.1[b]	A: ~1.5[c] TD: 11.5 ± 7.5[c] T24: 11.3 ± 4.8[c]	A: 7.9 ± 0.6 μg/ml[c] TD: 15 ± 2.8 μg/ml[c] T24: 14 ± 3.7 μg/ml[c]
	↑Neo, Prem ↔CF, Aged	↓Aged, Cirr, Neo, Preg, Obes ↔CF	↓Neo, Prem, Cirr, CHF, CP, Hep, LTh, Obes, Pneu ↑Smk, CF, HTh, Child ↔Aged, Preg, RD, COPD	↓Obes ↑Prem, CF ↔Aged, Preg, Cirr, HTh, LTh, RD	↓Smk, CF, HTh ↑Prem, Neo, Cirr, CHF, Hep, CP, LTh ↔Aged, RD		

[a]Nonlinear kinetics due to saturable metabolism, especially in children at steady state. Ratio of percent increase in steady-state concentration to percent increase in dose was >1.5 in 15% of children changed to a higher dose. Metabolically cleared primarily by CYP1A2 and by CYP3A4 to a lesser extent. [b]CL increased and $t_{\frac{1}{2}}$ decreased as a result of enzyme induction by antiepileptic drugs. [c]Following a 200 mg oral dose (aminophylline) given three times daily for 5 days, a 400 mg oral dose (THEO-DUR) given twice daily for 5 days, or a 800 mg oral dose (THEO-24) given once daily for 5 days, all to healthy adults. Sustained release formulations were taken 1 hour prior to a high-fat meal. Levels of 5 to 15 μg/ml are considered therapeutic; a level >20 μg/ml is potentially toxic.

References: Dockhorn, R.J., Cefali, E.A., and Straughn, A.B. Comparative steady-state bioavailability of Theo-24 and Theo-Dur in healthy men. Ann. Allergy, 1994, 72:218–222. Taburet, A.M., and Schmit, B. Pharmacokinetic optimisation of asthma treatment. Clin. Pharmacokinet., 1994, 26:396–418. Vestal, R.E., Thummel, K.E., Mercer, G.D., and Koup, J.R. Comparison of single and multiple dose pharmacokinetics of theophylline using stable isotopes. Eur. J. Clin. Pharmacol., 1986, 30:113–120.

Table A–II–1 Pharmacokinetic Data (Continued)

AVAILABILITY (ORAL) (%)	URINARY EXCRETION (%)	BOUND IN PLASMA (%)	CLEARANCE ($ml \cdot min^{-1} \cdot kg^{-1}$)	VOL. DIST. (liters/kg)	HALF-LIFE (hours)	PEAK TIME (hours)	PEAK CONCENTRATIONS
TIAGABINE[a] (Chapter 19)							
~90	1–2	96	2.0 ± 0.4^{b} ↑ Epilep[c], Child[d] ↓ LD[e] ↔ RD	1.3 ± 0.4^{b}	$7–9^{b}$ ↑LD	SD: 0.9 ± 0.5^{f} MD: 1.5 ± 1.0^{f}	SD: 122 ± 36 ng/ml[f] MD: 69 ± 22 ng/ml[f]

[a]Data from healthy adult male and female subjects and patients with epilepsy. Metabolized primarily by UGT and CYP3A. [b]CL/F, V_{area}/F, and $t_{\frac{1}{2}}$ reported for oral dose. [c]CL/F increased in adult and pediatric patients receiving enzyme-inducing antiepileptic drugs. [d]Weight-adjusted CL/F higher in children (3 to 10 years of age) than in adults. [e]CL/F reduced, moderate hepatic impairment. [f]Following a single 8 mg oral dose (SD) or a 3 mg oral dose given three times daily for 4 days (MD). Diurnal variation (lower C_{max} in P.M. than A.M.).

References: Gustavson, L.E., Boellner, S.W., *et al.* A single-dose study to define tiagabine pharmacokinetics in pediatric patients with complex partial seizures. *Neurology*, **1997,** 48:1032–1037. Lau, A.H., Gustavson, L.E., *et al.* Pharmacokinetics and safety of tiagabine in subjects with various degrees of hepatic function. *Epilepsia,* **1997,** 38:445–451. *Physicians' Desk Reference,* 54th ed. Medical Economics Co., Montvale, NJ, **2000,** p. 451. Snel, S., Jansen, J.A., Mengel, H.B., Richens, A., and Larsen, S. The pharmacokinetics of tiagabine in healthy elderly volunteers and elderly patients with epilepsy. *J. Clin. Pharmacol.,* **1997,** 37:1015–1020.

AVAILABILITY (ORAL) (%)	URINARY EXCRETION (%)	BOUND IN PLASMA (%)	CLEARANCE ($ml \cdot min^{-1} \cdot kg^{-1}$)	VOL. DIST. (liters/kg)	HALF-LIFE (hours)	PEAK TIME (hours)	PEAK CONCENTRATIONS
TIMOLOL[a] (Chapters 10, 31, 32, 63)							
61 ± 6	8 ± 4^{b}	<10	$7.7 \pm 1.2^{c,d}$	$1.7 \pm 0.2^{c,d}$	$2.7 \pm 0.5^{c,d}$	EM: 1.2 ± 0.4 PM: 1.8 ± 0.8	EM: 61 ± 39 ng/ml[e] PM: 114 ± 21 ng/ml[e]

[a]Timolol is metabolized primarily by the polymorphic enzyme CYP2D6. [b]Recovery following an oral dose in extensive metabolizers reported. [c]From a group of subjects with unknown CYP2D6 genotype or phenotype. [d]CYP2D6 poor metabolizers (PM) exhibited a lower CL/F (3.1 ± 1.8 vs 11.5 ± 5.5 ml·min⁻¹·kg⁻¹) and a longer apparent $t_{\frac{1}{2}}$ (7.5 ± 3.0 vs 3.7 ± 1.7 hour) for a 20 mg oral dose than extensive metabolizers (EM). [e]Following a single 20 mg oral dose given to EM and PM subjects.

References: McGourty, J.C., Silas, J.H., Fleming, J.J., McBurney, A., and Ward, J.W. Pharmacokinetics and beta-blocking effects of timolol in poor and extensive metabolizers of debrisoquin. *Clin. Pharmacol. Ther.,* **1985,** 38:409–413. *Physicians' Desk Reference,* 58th ed., Medical Economics Co., Montvale, NJ, **2004,** p. 1934. Wilson, T.W., Firor, W.B., *et al.* Timolol and propranolol: bioavailability, plasma concentrations, and beta blockade. *Clin. Pharmacol. Ther.,* **1982,** 32:676–685.

AVAILABILITY (ORAL) (%)	URINARY EXCRETION (%)	BOUND IN PLASMA (%)	CLEARANCE ($ml \cdot min^{-1} \cdot kg^{-1}$)	VOL. DIST. (liters/kg)	HALF-LIFE (hours)	PEAK TIME (hours)	PEAK CONCENTRATIONS
TOLBUTAMIDE (Chapter 61)							
$80–90^{a}$	~0.1	91–96 ↓ AVH, Aged	$0.22 \pm 0.06^{b,c}$ ↑ AVH	0.12 ± 0.02^{b} ↔ AVH	5.9 ± 1.4^{b} ↓ AVH, CRI ↔ Aged, RD	3.1 ± 1.5^{d}	53 ± 12 μg/ml[d]

References: Balant, L. Clinical pharmacokinetics of sulphonylurea hypoglycaemic drugs. *Clin. Pharmacokinet.,* **1981,** *6:*215–241. Matin, S.B., Wan, S.H., and Karam, J.H. Pharmacokinetics of tolbutamide: prediction by concentration in saliva. *Clin. Pharmacol. Ther.,* **1974,** *16:*1052–1058. Peart, G.F., Boutagy, J., and Shenfield, G.M. Lack of relationship between tolbutamide metabolism and debrisoquine oxidation phenotype. *Eur. J. Clin. Pharmacol.,* **1987,** *33:*397–402. Veronese, M.E., Miners, J.O., Randles, D., Gregov, D., and Birkett, D.J. Validation of the tolbutamide metabolic ratio for population screening with use of sulfaphenazole to produce model phenotypic poor metabolizers. *Clin. Pharmacol. Ther.,* **1990,** *47:*403–411. Williams, R.L., Blaschke, T.F., Meffin, P.J., Melmon, K.L., and Rowland, M. Influence of acute viral hepatitis on disposition and plasma binding of tolbutamide. *Clin. Pharmacol. Ther.,* **1977,** *21:*301–309.

[a]Bioavailability estimate based on recovery of oral dose in urine and expected negligible first-pass metabolism. [b]CL/F, V/F, and $t_{1/2}$ reported for oral dose. [c]Metabolized primarily by CYP2C9 (polymorphic). [d]Following a single 500 mg oral dose. A level of 80–240 μg/ml associated with a >25% decrease in blood glucose concentration.

TOLTERODINE[a] (Chapter 7)

EM: 26 ± 18	EM: negligible	T: 96.3	EM: 9.6 ± 2.8	EM: 1.7 ± 0.4	EM: 2.3 ± 0.3	EM: 1.2 ± 0.5[c]	EM: 5.2 ± 5.7 ng/ml[c]
PM: 91 ± 40	PM: <2.5	5-HM: 64	PM: 2.0 ± 0.3	PM: 1.5 ± 0.4	PM: 9.2 ± 1.2	PM: 1.9 ± 1.0[c]	PM: 38 ± 15 ng/ml[c]
EM: ↑ Food			↓ LD[b]		↑ LD		

[a]Data from healthy adult male subjects. No significant gender differences. Tolterodine (T) is metabolized primarily by CYP2D6 to an active (100% potency) metabolite, 5-hydroxymethyl tolterodine (5-HM), in extensive metabolizers (EM); $t_{1/2}$ 5-HM = 2.9 ± 0.4 hours. Also metabolized by CYP3A to an *N*-desalkyl product, particularly in poor metabolizers (PM). [b]CL/F reduced and AUC 5-HM$_{unbound}$ increased, hepatic cirrhosis. [c]Following a 4 mg oral dose given twice daily for 8 days. Peak concentration of 5-HM was 5 ± 3 ng/ml for EM.

References: Brynne, N., Dalen, P., Alvan, G., Bertilsson, L., and Gabrielsson, J. Influence of CYP2D6 polymorphism on the pharmacokinetics and pharmacodynamic of tolterodine. *Clin. Pharmacol. Ther.,* **1998,** *63:*529–539. Hills, C.J., Winter, S.A., and Balfour, J.A. Tolterodine. *Drugs,* **1998,** *55:*813–820. *Physicians' Desk Reference,* 54th ed. Medical Economics Co., Montvale, NJ, **2000,** p. 2439.

TOPIRAMATE[a] (Chapter 19)

≥70[b]	13–17	70–97	0.31–0.51[c]	0.6–0.8[c]	19–23[c]	1.7 ± 0.6[f]	5.5 ± 0.6 μg/ml[f]
			↑ Child[d]		↑ RD		
			↓ RD[e]				

[a]Data from healthy adult male and female subjects and patients with partial epilepsy. [b]Estimate of bioavailability based on urine recovery of unchanged drug. [c]CL/F, V_{area}/F, and $t_{1/2}$ reported for oral dose. Patients receiving concomitant therapy with enzyme-inducing anticonvulsant drugs exhibit increased CL/F, decreased $t_{1/2}$. [d]CL/F increased, <4 years (substantially), and 4 to 17 years of age. [e]CL/F reduced, moderate-to-severe renal impairment (drug cleared by hemodialysis). [f]Following a 400 mg oral dose given twice daily to steady state in patients with epilepsy.

References: Glauser, T.A., Miles, M.V., *et al.* Topiramate pharmacokinetics in infants. *Epilepsia,* **1999,** *40:*788–791. *Physicians' Desk Reference,* 54th ed. Medical Economics Co, Montvale, NJ, **2000,** p. 2209. Rosenfeld, W.E. Topiramate: a review of preclinical, pharmacokinetic, and clinical data. *Clin. Ther.,* **1997,** *19:*1294–1308. Sachdeo, R.C., Sachdeo, S.K., *et al.* Steady-state pharmacokinetics of topiramate and carbamazepine in patients with epilepsy during monotherapy and concomitant therapy. *Epilepsia,* **1996,** *37:*774–780.

Table A–II–1 *Pharmacokinetic Data (Continued)*

AVAILABILITY (ORAL) (%)	BOUND IN PLASMA (%)	URINARY EXCRETION (%)	CLEARANCE ($ml \cdot min^{-1} \cdot kg^{-1}$)	VOL. DIST. (liters/kg)	HALF-LIFE (hours)	PEAK TIME (hours)	PEAK CONCENTRATIONS
TOPOTECAN[a] (Chapter 51)							
32 ± 12	L: 21.3 A: 6.6	40[b]	28.6 ± 4.1 liters $\cdot$ h^{-1} $\cdot$ (m^2)$^{-1}$ [b] ↑RD[c] ↔Child, Cirr	74 ± 21 liters/m^2 [b]	2.4 ± 0.4[b] ↑RD	Oral, L: 0.92 ± 0.61[d] Oral, A: $1.5–2$[d]	IV, L: 38 ± 8 ng/ml[d] IV, A: 19 ± 2 ng/ml[d] Oral, L: 5.9 ± 0.8 ng/ml[d] Oral, A: 7.5 ± 2.6 ng/ml[d]

[a]Data from adult male and female patients (mean age, 62 years) with solid tumors. Topotecan is converted under physiological pH from a lactone (L) to a ring-opened carboxylic acid (A). Topotecan is active, but the acid metabolite is in equilibrium with parent drug. [b]CL and V_{ss} calculated assuming a 1.73 m^2 body surface area. There is considerable variability in the mean parameter reported from different IV studies: urinary excretion = 23% to 93%; $CL = 19$ to 35 liters $\cdot$ h^{-1} $\cdot$ (m^2)$^{-1}$; $V_{ss} = 61$ to 563 liters/m^2; $t_{\frac{1}{2}} = 2.9$ to 8.4 hours. [c]CL of topotecan reduced, moderate renal impairment. [d]Following a single 1.5 mg/m^2 IV or oral dose.

References: Furman, W.L., Baker, S.D., *et al.* Escalating systemic exposure of continuous infusion topotecan in children with recurrent acute leukemia. *J. Clin. Oncol.* **1996,** *14:*1504–1511. Herben, V.M., ten Bokkel Huinink, W.W., and Beijnen, J.H. Clinical pharmacokinetics of topotecan. *Clin. Pharmacokinet.* **1996,** *31:*85–102. *Physicians' Desk Reference,* 54th ed. Medical Economics Co., Montvale, NJ, **2000,** p. 3007. Schellens, J.H., Creemers, G.J., *et al.* Bioavailability and pharmacokinetics of oral topotecan: a new topoisomerase I inhibitor. *Br. J. Cancer,* **1996,** *73:*1268–1271.

AVAILABILITY (ORAL) (%)	BOUND IN PLASMA (%)	URINARY EXCRETION (%)	CLEARANCE	VOL. DIST.	HALF-LIFE	PEAK TIME	PEAK CONCENTRATIONS
TOREMIFENE[a] (Chapters 51, 57)							
—	99.7	Negligible	2.6 ± 1.2 l $\cdot$ h^{-1} $\cdot$ (m^2)$^{-1b}$ ↓LD[c] ↔RD	479 ± 154 l/m^2 [b] ↑Aged	T: 148 ± 53[b] DMT: 504 ± 578[b] ↑Aged, LD	T: $1.5–3$[d] DMT: $3–6$[d]	T: $1.1–1.3$ μg/ml[d] DMT: $2.7–5.8$ μg/ml[d]

[a]Data from healthy adult male and female subjects and female patients with breast cancer. Toremifene (T) is metabolized by CYP3A to *N*-desmethyltoremifene (DMT), a metabolite that accumulates in blood and has anti-estrogenic activity. Toremifene appears to undergo enterohepatic recycling, prolonging its apparent $t_{\frac{1}{2}}$. [b]CL/F, V_{area}/F, and $t_{\frac{1}{2}}$ reported for oral dose. [c]CL/F reduced, hepatic cirrhosis or fibrosis. [d]Following a 60 mg oral dose given once daily to steady state in patients with breast cancer.

References: Anttila, M., Laakso, S., Nylanden, P., and Sotaniemi, E.A. Pharmacokinetics of the novel antiestrogenic agent toremifene in subjects with altered liver and kidney function. *Clin. Pharmacol. Ther.* **1995,** *57:*628–635. Bishop, J., Murray, R., *et al.* Phase I clinical and pharmacokinetics study of high-dose toremifene in postmenopausal patients with advanced breast cancer. *Cancer Chemother. Pharmacol.,* **1992,** *30:*174–178. Wiebe, V.J., Benz, C.C., Shemano, I., Cadman, T.B., and DeGregorio, M.W. Pharmacokinetics of toremifene and its metabolites in patients with advanced breast cancer. *Cancer Chemother. Pharmacol.,* **1990,** *25:*247–251.

AVAILABILITY (ORAL) (%)	BOUND IN PLASMA (%)	URINARY EXCRETION (%)	CLEARANCE	VOL. DIST.	HALF-LIFE	PEAK TIME	PEAK CONCENTRATIONS
TRAMADOL[a] (Chapter 21)							
$70–75$	20	$10–30$[b]	8 $(6–12)$ ↓LD, RD	2.7 $(2.3–3.9)$	5.5 $(4.5–7.5)$ ↑RD, LD	T: 2.3 ± 1.4[c] M1: 2.4 ± 1.1[c]	T: 592 ± 178 ng/ml[c] M1: 110 ± 32 ng/ml[c]

[a]Tramadol is available as a racemic mixture. At steady state, the plasma concentration of (+) (1R,2R)-tramadol is ~30% higher than that of (−) (1S,2S)-tramadol. Both isomers contribute to analgesia. Data reported are for total (+ and −) tramadol. Tramadol (T) is metabolized by CYP2D6 to an active O-desmethyl-metabolite (M1); there are other CYP-catalyzed metabolites. [b]Recovery following an oral dose reported. [c]Following a 100 mg immediate-release tablet given every 6 hours for 7 days.

References: Klotz, U. Tramadol—the impact of its pharmacokinetic and pharmacodynamic properties on the clinical management of pain. *Arzneimittelforschung,* **2003,** *53:*681–687. *Physicians' Desk Reference,* 58th ed. Medical Economics Co., Montvale, NJ, **2004,** p. 2494.

TRAZODONE[a] (Chapter 17)

81 ± 6	93	2.1 ± 0.1	<1	1.0 ± 0.1[d]	5.9 ± 0.4	2.0 ± 1.5[e]	1.5 ± 0.2 μg/ml[e]
↔ Aged, Obes		↓ Aged,[b] Obes[c]		↑ Aged, Obes	↑ Aged, Obes		

[a]Active metabolite, *m*-chlorophenylpiperazine, is a tryptaminergic agonist; formation catalyzed by CYP3A. [b]Significant for male subjects only. [c]No difference when *CL* is normalized to ideal body weight. [d]V_{area} reported. [e]Following a single 100 mg oral dose (capsule) given with a standard breakfast to healthy adults.

References: Greenblatt, D.J., Friedman, H., *et al.* Trazodone kinetics: effect of age, gender, and obesity. *Clin. Pharmacol. Ther.,* **1987,** *42:*193–200. Nilsen, O.G., and Dale, O. Single dose pharmacokinetics of trazodone in healthy subjects. *Pharmacol. Toxicol.,* **1992,** *71:*150–153.

TRIAMTERENE[a] (Chapter 28)

51 ± 18[b]	52 ± 10[b]	61 ± 2[d]	63 ± 20[f]	13.4 ± 4.9	4.2 ± 0.7[g]	T: 2.9 ± 1.6[h]
	↓ Cirr[c]	↑ HL	↓ Cirr, RD,[e] Aged[e]		↑ RD[e]	TS: 4.1 ± 2.0[b]
	↔ Aged[b]	↓ RD, Alb, Cirr[e]				

Y, T: 26.4 ± 17.7 ng/ml[h]
Y, TS: 779 ± 310 ng/ml[h]
E, T: 84 ± 91 ng/ml[h]
E, TS: 526 ± 388 ng/ml[h]

[a]Active metabolite, hydroxytriamterene sulfuric acid ester. [b]Triamterene plus active metabolite. [c]Decreased active metabolite; increased parent drug. [d]For metabolite, percent bound = 90.4 ± 1.3. [e]Active metabolite. [f]Because triamterene is predominantly present in plasma as the active metabolite, this value is deceptively high. CL_{renal} = 2.3 ± 0.6 for the metabolite. [g]Metabolite $t_{\frac{1}{2}}$ = 3.1 ± 1.2 hours. [h]Data for triamterene (T) and hydroxytriamterene sulfate ester (TS) following a single 50 mg oral dose taken after a fast by young healthy volunteers (Y) and elderly patients requiring diuretic therapy (E).

References: Gilfrich, H.J., Kremer, G., Mohrke, W., Mutschler, E., and Volger, K.D. Pharmacokinetics of triamterene after i.v. administration to man: determination of bioavailability. *Eur. J. Clin. Pharmacol.* **1983,** *25:*237–241. Muhlberg, W., Spahn, H., Platt, D., Mutschler, E., and Jung, R. Pharmacokinetics of triamterene in geriatric patients—influence of piretanide and hydrochlorothiazide. *Arch. Gerontol. Geriatr.,* **1989,** *8:*73–85.

TRIMETHOPRIM (Chapter 43)

>63	63 ± 10	37 ± 5	1.9 ± 0.3[a]	1.6 ± 0.2[a]	10 ± 2[a]	2[b]	1.2 μg/ml[b]
↔ CF	↔ CF	↔ RD, Alb, CF	↓ RD	↔ RD, CF	↑ RD		
			↑ CF, Child	↑ Neo	↓ Child, CF		
				↓ Child			

[a]Studies included concurrent administration of sulfamethoxazole and variation in urinary pH; these factors had no marked effect on the *CL*, distribution and $t_{\frac{1}{2}}$ of trimethoprim. [c]Following a single 160 mg oral dose given to healthy adults.

References: Hutabarat, R.M., Unadkat, J.D., *et al.* Disposition of drugs in cystic fibrosis. I. Sulfamethoxazole and trimethoprim. *Clin. Pharmacol. Ther.,* **1991,** *49:*402–409. Welling, P.G., Craig, W.A., Amidon, G.L., and Kunin, C.M. Pharmacokinetics of trimethoprim and sulfamethoxazole in normal subjects and in patients with renal failure. *J. Infect. Dis.,* **1973,** *128*(suppl):556–566.

Table A–II–1 *Pharmacokinetic Data (Continued)*

AVAILABILITY (ORAL) (%)	URINARY EXCRETION (%)	BOUND IN PLASMA (%)	CLEARANCE $(ml \cdot min^{-1} \cdot kg^{-1})$	VOL. DIST. (liters/kg)	HALF-LIFE (hours)	PEAK TIME (hours)	PEAK CONCENTRATIONS
VALACYCLOVIR[a] (Chapter 49)							
V: very low A: 54 (42–73)[b]	V: <1 A: 44 ± 10[c]	V: 13.5–17.9 A: 22–33	V: — A: ↓ RD[d]	—	V: — A: 2.5 ± 0.3 A: ↑ RD	V: 1.5 A: 1.9 ± 0.6[e]	V: ≤0.56 μg/ml[e] A: 4.8 ± 1.5 μg/ml[e]

[a]Data from healthy male and female adults. Valacyclovir is a L-valine prodrug of acyclovir. Extensive first-pass conversion by intestinal (gut wall and lumenal) and hepatic enzymes. Parameters refer to acyclovir (A) and valacyclovir (V) following valacyclovir administration. See Acyclovir for its systemic disposition parameters. [b]Bioavailability of acyclovir based on *AUC* of acyclovir following IV acyclovir and oral 1 g dose of valacyclovir. [c]Urinary recovery of acyclovir is dose-dependent (76% and 44% following 100 mg and 1000 mg oral doses of valacyclovir, and 87% following IV acyclovir). [d]*CL/F* reduced, end-stage renal disease (drug cleared by hemodialysis). [e]Following a single 1 g oral dose of valacyclovir.

References: Perry, C.M., and Faulds, D. Valaciclovir. A review of its antiviral activity, pharmacokinetic properties and therapeutic efficacy in herpesvirus infections. *Drugs*, **1996**, *52*:754–772. Soul-Lawton, J., Seaber, E., *et al.* Absolute bioavailability and metabolic disposition of valaciclovir, the L-valyl ester of acyclovir, following oral administration to humans. *Antimicrob. Agents Chemother.*, **1995**, *39*:2759–2764. Weller, S., Blum, M.R., *et al.* Pharmacokinetics of the acyclovir pro-drug valaciclovir after escalating single- and multiple-dose administration to normal volunteers. *Clin. Pharmacol. Ther.*, **1993**, *54*:595–605.

AVAILABILITY (ORAL) (%)	URINARY EXCRETION (%)	BOUND IN PLASMA (%)	CLEARANCE $(ml \cdot min^{-1} \cdot kg^{-1})$	VOL. DIST. (liters/kg)	HALF-LIFE (hours)	PEAK TIME (hours)	PEAK CONCENTRATIONS
VALGANCICLOVIR[a] (Chapter 49)							
G (V): 61 ± 9[b] ↑ Food	—	—	—	—	V (V): 0.5 ± 0.2 G (V): 3.7 ± 0.6 ↑RD[c]	V (V): 0.5 ± 0.3[d] G (V): 1–3[e]	V (V): 0.20 ± 0.07 μg/ml[d] G (V): 5.6 ± 1.5 μg/ml[e]

[a]Valganciclovir (V) is an ester prodrug for ganciclovir (G). It is rapidly hydrolyzed with a plasma $t_{\frac{1}{2}} = 0.5$ hour. G and V data following oral valganciclovir dosing to male and female patients with viral infections are reported. See Ganciclovir for its systemic disposition parameters. [b]Increased and more predictable bioavailability of G when V is taken with a high-fat meal. [c]The apparent $t_{\frac{1}{2}}$ of G is increased in patients with renal impairment. [d]Following a single 360-mg oral dose of V taken without food. [e]Following a 900-mg oral dose taken once daily with food to steady state.

References: Cocohoba, J.M., and McNicholl, I.R. Valganciclovir: an advance in cytomegalovirus therapeutics. *Ann. Pharmacother.*, **2002**, *36*:1075–1079. Jung, D., and Dorr, A. Single-dose pharmacokinetics of valganciclovir in HIV- and CMV-seropositive subjects. *J. Clin. Pharmacol.*, **1999**, *39*:800–804. *Physicians' Desk Reference*, 58th ed. Medical Economics Co., Montvale, **2004**, pp. 2895, 2971.

AVAILABILITY (ORAL) (%)	URINARY EXCRETION (%)	BOUND IN PLASMA (%)	CLEARANCE $(ml \cdot min^{-1} \cdot kg^{-1})$	VOL. DIST. (liters/kg)	HALF-LIFE (hours)	PEAK TIME (hours)	PEAK CONCENTRATIONS
VALPROIC ACID[a] (Chapter 19)							
100 ± 10	1.8 ± 2.4	93 ± 1[b] ↓ RD, Cirr, Preg, Aged, Neo, Burn, Alb	0.11 ± 0.02[c,d] ↑ Child ↔ Cirr, Aged	0.22 ± 0.07[c,d] ↑ Cirr, Neo ↔ Aged, Child	14 ± 3[c,d] ↑ Cirr, Neo ↓ Child ↔ Aged	1–4[e]	34 ± 8 μg/ml[e]

References: Dean, J.C. Valproate. In, *The Treatment of Epilepsy*, 2nd ed. (Wyllie, E., ed.) Williams & Wilkins, Baltimore, **1997**, pp. 824–832. Pollack, G.M., McHugh, W.B., Gengo, F.M., Ermer, J.C., and Shen, D.D. Accumulation and washout kinetics of valproic acid and its active metabolites. *J. Clin. Pharmacol,* **1986**, *26:*668–676. Zaccara, G., Messori, A., and Moroni, F. Clinical pharmacokinetics of valproic acid—1988. *Clin. Pharmacokinet.,* **1988**, *15:*367–389.

[a]Active metabolites. [b]Dose-dependent; value shown for daily doses of 250 and 500 mg. At 1 g daily, % bound = 90 ±2. [c]Data for multiple dosing (500 mg daily) reported. Single dose value: 0.14 ± 0.04 ml · min⁻¹ · kg⁻¹; $t_{\frac{1}{2}} = 9.8 \pm 2.6$ hours. Total CL the same at 100 mg daily, although CL of free drug increases with multiple dosing. [d]Increased CL and decreased $t_{\frac{1}{2}}$ from enzyme induction following concomitant administration of other antiepileptic drugs. [e]C_{ave} following a 250 mg oral dose (capsule, DEPAKENE) given twice daily for 15 days to healthy male adults. A therapeutic range of 50 to 150 μg/ml is reported. T_{max} is 3 to 8 hours for enteric-coated tablets (DEPAKOTE) and 7 to 14 hours for extended-release tablet (DEPAKOTE-ER).

VALSARTAN[a] (Chapters 30, 32, 33)

Oral Avail.	Urinary Excr.	Bound	Clearance	Vol. Dist.	Half-Life	Peak Time	Peak Conc.
23 ± 7 ↓ Food	29.0 ± 5.8	95	0.49 ± 0.09 ↓ Aged, LD[b] ↔ RD	0.23 ± 0.09	9.4 ± 3.8 ↑ Aged	2 (1.5–3)[c]	1.6 ± 0.6 µg/ml[c]

[a]Data from healthy adult male subjects. No significant gender differences. Valsartan is cleared primarily by biliary excretion. [b]CL/F reduced, mild-to-moderate hepatic impairment and biliary obstruction. [c]Following a single 80 mg oral dose (capsule).

References: Brookman, L.J., Rolan, P.E., *et al.* Pharmacokinetics of valsartan in patients with liver disease. *Clin. Pharmacol. Ther.,* **1997**, *62:*272–278. Flesch, G., Muller, P., and Lloyd, P. Absolute bioavailability and pharmacokinetics of valsartan, an angiotensin II receptor antagonist, in man. *Eur. J. Clin. Pharmacol.,* **1997**, *52:*115–120. Muller, P., Flesch, G., de Gasparo, M., Gasparini, M., and Howald, H. Pharmacokinetics and pharmacodynamic effects of the angiotensin II antagonist valsartan at steady state in healthy, normotensive subjects. *Eur. J. Clin. Pharmacol.,* **1997**, *52:*441–449. *Physicians' Desk Reference*, 54th ed. Medical Economics Co., Montvale, NJ, **2000**, p. 2015.

VANCOMYCIN (Chapter 46)

Oral Avail.	Urinary Excr.	Bound	Clearance	Vol. Dist.	Half-Life	Peak Time	Peak Conc.
—[a]	79 ± 11 ↔ RD	30 ± 11 ↔ RD	$CL = 0.79 CL_{cr} + 0.22$ ↓ RD, Aged, Neo ↔ Obes, CPBS ↑ Burn	0.39 ± 0.06 ↓ Obes ↔ RD, CPBS	5.6 ± 1.8 ↑ RD, Aged ↓ Obes	—	18.5 (15–25) µg/ml[b]

[a]Very poorly absorbed after oral administration, but used by this route to treat *Clostridium difficile* and staphylococcal enterocolitis. [b]Following a dose of 1000 mg IV (1-hour infusion) given twice daily or a 7.5 mg/kg IV (1-hour infusion) given four times daily to adult patients with staphylococcal or streptococcal infections. Levels of 37–152 μg/ml have been associated with ototoxicity.

Reference: Leader, W.G., Chandler, M.H., and Castiglia, M. Pharmacokinetic optimisation of vancomycin therapy. *Clin. Pharmacokinet.,* **1995**, *28:*327–342.

Table A–II–1 *Pharmacokinetic Data (Continued)*

	AVAILABILITY (ORAL) (%)	URINARY EXCRETION (%)	BOUND IN PLASMA (%)	VOL. DIST. (liters/kg)	CLEARANCE (ml · min⁻¹ · kg⁻¹)	HALF-LIFE (hours)	PEAK TIME (hours)	PEAK CONCENTRATIONS
VECURONIUM[a] (Chapter 9)	—[b]	20	69	0.19–0.51[c]	3.0–6.4[c] ↓ LD	0.6–2.8[c] ↑ LD	—	130 ± 20 ng/ml[d]
VENLAFAXINE[a] (Chapter 17)	10–45	V: 4.6 ± 3.0 DV: 29 ± 7[b]	V: 27 ± 2 DV: 30 ± 12[b]	7.5 ± 3.7[c] ↔ Aged, Fem, Cirr, RD	22 ± 10[c] ↔ Aged, Fem ↓ Cirr, RD	4.9 ± 2.4 10.3 ± 4.3[b] ↔ Aged, Fem ↑ Cirr, RD	V: 2.0 ± 0.4[d] DV: 2.8 ± 0.8[d]	V: 167 ± 55 ng/ml[d] DV: 397 ± 81 ng/ml[d]
VERAPAMIL[a,b] (Chapters 31, 32, 34)	Oral: 22 ± 8 SL: 35 ± 13 ↑ Cirr ↔ RD	<3	90 ± 2 ↑ Cirr ↔ RD, Atr Fib, Aged	5.0 ± 2.1 ↑ Cirr ↑, ↔ Atr Fib ↔ RD, Aged, Obes	15 ± 6[c,d] ↑ Cirr, Aged, Obes ↑, ↔ Atr Fib ↔ RD, Child	4.0 ± 1.5[c] ↑ Cirr, Aged, Obes ↑, ↔ Atr Fib ↔ RD, Child	IR: 1.1[e] XR: 5.6–7.7[e]	IR: 272 ng/ml[e] XR: 118–165 ng/ml[e]

[a]Eliminated primarily by hepatic uptake, metabolism, and biliary excretion. [b]For IV administration only. [c]Range of mean data from different studies. [d]Plasma concentration associated with a 25% recovery of maximal muscle twitch height in patients with normal renal function; higher (210 ng/ml) in patients with renal failure.

References: Agoston, S., Vandenbrom, R.H., and Wierda, J.M. Clinical pharmacokinetics of neuromuscular blocking drugs. *Clin. Pharmacokinet.*, **1992**, 22:94–115. Bencini, A.F., Scaf, A.H., *et al.* Disposition and urinary excretion of vecuronium bromide in anesthetized patients with normal renal function or renal failure. *Anesth. Analg.*, **1986**, 65:245–251. Cameron, M., Donati, F., and Varin, F. In vitro plasma protein binding of neuromuscular blocking agents in different subpopulations of patients. *Anesth. Analg.*, **1995**, 81:1019–1025.

[a]Racemic mixture; antidepressant activity resides with the *l*-(−)-enantiomer and its equipotent *O*-desmethyl metabolite (formation catalyzed by CYP2D6—polymorphic). [b]Values for *O*-desmethylvenlafaxine after venlafaxine dosing. [c]*CL/F* and *V$_{ss}$/F* reported. [d]Mean data for venlafaxine (V) and *O*-desmethylvenlafaxine (DV), following a 75 mg oral dose (immediate-release tablet) given three times daily for 3 days to healthy adults. T_{max} for an extended-release formulation is 5.5 (V) and 9 (DV) hours.

References: Klamerus, K.J., Maloney, K., *et al.* Introduction of a composite parameter to the pharmacokinetics of venlafaxine and its active *O*-desmethyl metabolite. *J. Clin. Pharmacol.,* **1992**, 32:716–724. *Physicians' Desk Reference*, 54th ed. Medical Economics Co., Montvale, NJ, **2000**, p. 3237.

[a]Racemic mixture; (−)-enantiomer is more active. Bioavailability of (+)-verapamil is 2.5-fold greater than that for (−)-verapamil because of a lower CL (10 ± 2 vs. 18 ± 3 ml · min⁻¹ · kg⁻¹). Relative concentration of the enantiomers changes as a function of route of administration. [b]Active metabolite, norverapamil, is a vasodilator but has no direct effect on heart rate or P-R interval. At steady state (oral dosing), AUC is equivalent to that of parent drug ($t_{\frac{1}{2}} = 9 \pm 3$ hours). [c]Multiple dosing causes greater than twofold decrease in CL/F and prolongation of $t_{\frac{1}{2}}$ in some studies, but no change of $t_{\frac{1}{2}}$ in others. [d]Verapamil is a substrate for CYP3A4, CYP2C9, and other CYPs. [e]Mean data following a 120 mg oral conventional tablet (IR) given twice daily or range of data following a 240 mg oral extended release (XR) dose given once daily, both for 7 to 10 days to healthy adults. EC_{50} for prolongation of P-R interval after oral dose of racemate is 120 ± 20 ng/ml; value for IV administration is 40 ± 25 ng/ml. After oral administration, racemate concentrations above 100 ng/ml cause more than 25% reduction in heart rate in atrial fibrillation, more than 10% prolongation of P-R interval, and more than 50% increase in duration of exercise in angina patients. A level of 120 ± 40 ng/ml (after IV administration) was found to terminate reentrant supraventricular tachycardias.

Reference: McTavish, D., and Sorkin, E.M. Verapamil. An updated review of its pharmacodynamic and pharmacokinetic properties, and therapeutic use in hypertension. *Drugs*, **1989**, *38*:19–76.

VINCRISTINE[a] (Chapter 51)

| — | Low | 10–20 | $4.92 \pm 3.01 \cdot \text{h}^{-1} \cdot (\text{m}^2)^{-1}$ ↓ LD[b] ↔ Child | 22.6 ± 16.7[c] ↑ LD[b] | 96.9 ± 55.7 l/m²[c] | ~250–425 nM[d] |

[a]Data from adult male and female cancer patients. Metabolized by CYP3A and excreted unchanged into bile (substrate for P-glycoprotein). [b]CL reduced, cholestatic liver disease. [c]CL and V_γ for deep compartment. Longer $t_{\frac{1}{2}}$ (~85 ± 69 hours) also reported. [d]Following a 2 mg IV bolus dose.

References: Gelmon, K.A., Tolcher, A., *et al.* Phase 1 study of liposomal vincristine. *J. Clin. Oncol.*, **1999**, *17*:697–705. Rahmani, R., and Zhou, X.J. Pharmacokinetics and metabolism of vinca alkaloids. *Cancer Surv.*, **1993**, *17*:269–281. Sethi, V.S., Jackson, D.V., *et al.* Pharmacokinetics of vincristine sulfate in adult cancer patients. *Cancer Res.*, **1981**, *41*:3551–3555. Sethi, V.S., and Kimball, J.C. Pharmacokinetics of vincristine sulfate in children. *Cancer Chemother. Pharmacol.*, **1981**, *6*:111–115. van den Berg, H.W., Desai, Z.R., *et al.* The pharmacokinetics of vincristine in man: reduced drug clearance associated with raised serum alkaline phosphatase and dose-limited elimination. *Cancer Chemother. Pharmacol.*, **1982**, *8*:215–219.

VINORELBINE (Chapter 51)

| 27 ± 12[a] | 87 (80–91) | 11 | 21 ± 7 ↓LD | 42 ± 21[b] | 76 ± 41[b] | 1.5 ± 1.0[c] | 114 ± 43 ng/ml[c] ; 1130 ± 636 ng/ml[d] |

[a]For liquid-filled gelatin capsules. [b]Elimination kinetics of vinorelbine follow a three-compartment model with extensive tissue distribution. Values for the terminal elimination phase are reported. [c]Following a single 100 mg/m² oral dose (gel capsule). [d]Following a single 30 mg/m² 15 min IV infusion.

Reference: Leveque, D., and Jehl, F. Clinical pharmacokinetics of vinorelbine. *Clin. Pharmacokinet.*, **1996**, *31*:184–197.

Table A–II–1 *Pharmacokinetic Data (Continued)*

AVAILABILITY (ORAL) (%)	URINARY EXCRETION (%)	BOUND IN PLASMA (%)	VOL. DIST. (liters/kg)	CLEARANCE (ml · min⁻¹ · kg⁻¹)	HALF-LIFE (hours)	PEAK TIME (hours)	PEAK CONCENTRATIONS
VORICONAZOLE[a] (Chapter 48)							
96 ↓ Food	<2	58	1.6[b]	3.8[b] ↓ LD[c]	6.7[b]	PO: 1.1[d] ↑ Food	PO: 2356 ng/ml[d] ↓ Food / IV: 3621 ng/ml[e]

[a]Metabolized mainly to an inactive N-oxide by CYP2C19 (major), CYP3A4, and CYP2C9. [b]Elimination is dose- and time-dependent. Pharmacokinetic parameters determined at steady state are reported. Mean CL was reduced (64%), V_{ss} reduced (32%), and $t_{\frac{1}{2}}$ increased (16%) with 12 days of twice daily 3 mg/kg IV administration. Also, CL decreased 41% when dose was increased from 200 to 300 mg twice daily. [c]CL reduced in patients with mild-to-moderate hepatic insufficiency. [d]Following a 3 mg/kg oral dose given twice daily for 12 days. [e]Following a 3 mg/kg 1 hour IV infusion given twice daily for 12 days.

References: Boucher, H.W., Groll, A.H., Chiou, C.C., and Walsh, T.J. Newer systemic antifungal agents: pharmacokinetics, safety and efficacy. *Drugs*, **2004,** *64:*1997–2020. Purkins, L., Wood, N., Greenhalgh, K., Allen, M.J., and Oliver, S.D. Voriconazole, a novel wide-spectrum triazole: oral pharmacokinetics and safety. *Br. J. Clin. Pharmacol.,* **2003,** *56*(suppl):10–16. Purkins, L., Wood, N., *et al.* The pharmacokinetics and safety of intravenous voriconazole—a novel wide-spectrum antifungal agent. *Br. J. Clin. Pharmacol.* **2003,** *56*(suppl):2–9.

AVAILABILITY (ORAL) (%)	URINARY EXCRETION (%)	BOUND IN PLASMA (%)	VOL. DIST. (liters/kg)	CLEARANCE (ml · min⁻¹ · kg⁻¹)	HALF-LIFE (hours)	PEAK TIME (hours)	PEAK CONCENTRATIONS
WARFARIN[a] (Chapter 54)							
93 ± 8	<2	99 ± 1[b] ↓ RD ↔ Preg	0.14 ± 0.06[b,d] ↔ Aged, AVH	0.045 ± 0.024[c,d,e] ↔ Aged, AVH, CF	37 ± 15[f] ↔ Aged, AVH	<4[g]	R: 0.9 ± 0.4 µg/ml[g] / S: 0.5 ± 0.2 µg/ml[g]

[a]Values are for racemic warfarin; the *S*-(−)-enantiomer is three- to fivefold more potent than the *R*-(+)-enantiomer. [b]No difference between enantiomers in plasma protein binding or V_{area}. [c]CL of the *R*-enantiomer is about 70% of that of the antipode (0.043 *vs.* 0.059 ml · min⁻¹ · kg⁻¹). [d]Conditions leading to decreased binding (*e.g.*, uremia) presumably increase CL and V. [e]The *S*-enantiomer is metabolically cleared by CYP2C9 (polymorphic). [f]$t_{\frac{1}{2}}$ of the *R*-enantiomer is longer than that of the *S*-enantiomer (43 ± 14 *vs.* 32 ± 12 hours). [g]Mean steady-state, 12-hour postdose, concentrations of warfarin enantiomers following a daily oral dose of 6.1 ± 2.3 mg of racemic warfarin given to patients with stabilized (1 to 5 months) anticoagulant therapy.

Reference: Chan, E., McLachlan, A.J., *et al.* Disposition of warfarin enantiomers and metabolites in patients during multiple dosing with rac-warfarin. *Br. J. Clin. Pharmacol.,* **1994,** *37:*563–569.

AVAILABILITY (ORAL) (%)	URINARY EXCRETION (%)	BOUND IN PLASMA (%)	VOL. DIST. (liters/kg)	CLEARANCE (ml · min⁻¹ · kg⁻¹)	HALF-LIFE (hours)	PEAK TIME (hours)	PEAK CONCENTRATIONS
ZALEPLON[a] (Chapter 16)							
31 ± 10[b]	<1	60 ± 15	1.3 ± 0.2	15.7 ± 3.3 ↔ Aged ↓ Cirr[c]	1.0 ± 0.1 ↑ Cirr	1.1 ± 0.2[e] ↑ Food[d]	26 ± 4.4 ng/ml[e] ↓ Food[d]

[a]Data from healthy adult male and female subjects. No significant gender differences. [b]Zaleplon is well absorbed but undergoes extensive first-pass metabolism, primarily by aldehyde oxidase and also CYP3A. [c]CL/F reduced, compensated and decompensated hepatic cirrhosis. [d]High-fat, high-calorie meal. [e]Following a single 10 mg oral dose.

References: Greenblatt, D.J., Harmatz, J.S., *et al.* Comparative kinetics and dynamics of zaleplon, zolpidem, and placebo. *Clin. Pharmacol. Ther.,* **1998,** *64:*553–561. *Physicians' Desk Reference,* 54th ed. Medical Economics Co., Montvale, NJ, **2000,** pp. 3319–3320. Rosen, A.S., Fournie, P., Darwish, M., Danjou, P., and Troy, S.M. Zaleplon pharmacokinetics and absolute bioavailability. *Biopharm. Drug Dispos.* **1999,** *20:*171–175.

ZIDOVUDINE (Chapter 50)

63 ± 10 ↑ Neo ↔ Preg	18 ± 5	<25	26 ± 6[a] ↓ RD,[b] Neo, Cirr[b] ↔ Child, Preg	1.4 ± 0.4 ↓ RD,[b] Cirr,[b] ↔ Child, Preg	1.1 ± 0.2 ↔ RD, Preg ↑ Neo, Cirr	0.5–1[c]	IV: 2.6 µg/ml[c] Oral: 1.6 µg/ml[c]

[a]Formation of 5-O-glucuronide is the major route of elimination (68%). [b]A change in CL/F and V_{area}/F reported. [c]Following a 5 mg/kg IV or oral dose given every 4 hours to steady state.

References: Blum, M.R., Liao, S.H., Good, S.S., and de Miranda, P. Pharmacokinetics and bioavailability of zidovudine in humans. *Am. J. Med.,* **1988,** *85:*189–194. Morse, G.D., Shelton, M.J., and O'Donnell, A.M. Comparative pharmacokinetics of antiviral nucleoside analogues. *Clin. Pharmacokinet.,* **1993,** *24:*101–123.

ZIPRASIDONE[a] (Chapter 18)

PO: 59 ↑ Food IM: 100	99.9 ± 0.08	<1[b]	11.7	2.3	2.9[c]	PO: 4 ± 1[d] IM: 0.7[e]	PO: 68 ± 20 ng/ml[d] IM: 156 ng/ml[e]

[a]Approximately one third of the dose is oxidized by CYP3A4, and the remainder undergoes reduction. [b]Recovery following oral administration. [c]A longer $t_{\frac{1}{2}}$ after oral administration is rate-limited by absorption; food decreases apparent $t_{\frac{1}{2}}$. In the elderly, the $t_{\frac{1}{2}}$ is slightly longer. [d]Following a 20 mg oral dose given twice daily for 8 days. [e]Following a single 10 mg IM dose.

References: Gunasekara, N.S., Spencer, C.M., and Keating, G.M. Ziprasidone: a review of its use in schizophrenia and schizoaffective disorder. *Drugs,* **2002,** *62:* 1217–1251. Miceli, J.J., Wilner, K.D., *et al.* Single- and multiple-dose pharmacokinetics of ziprasidone under non-fasting conditions in healthy male volunteers. *Br. J. Clin. Pharmacol.,* **2000,** *49*(suppl):5S–13S. *Physicians' Desk Reference,* 58th ed. Medical Economics Co., Montvale, **2004,** p. 2598. Wilner, K.D., Tensfeldt, T.G., *et al.* Single- and multiple-dose pharmacokinetics of ziprasidone in healthy young and elderly volunteers. *Br. J. Clin. Pharmacol.,* **2000,** *49*(suppl):15S–20S.

ZOLPIDEM (Chapter 16)

72 ± 7	92 ↓ RD, Cirr	<1	4.5 ± 0.7[a] ↔ RD ↓ Cirr, Aged ↑ Child	0.68 ± 0.06 ↑ RD	1.9 ± 0.2 ↑ Aged, Cirr ↔ RD ↓ Child	1.0–2.6[b] ↑ Food	76–139 ng/ml[b] ↓ Food

[a]Metabolically cleared predominantly by CYP3A4. [b]Following a single 10 mg oral dose given to young adults. No accumulation of drug with once daily dosing.

References: Greenblatt, D.J., Harmatz, J.S., *et al.* Comparative kinetics and dynamics of zaleplon, zolpidem, and placebo. *Clin. Pharmacol. Ther.,* **1998,** *64:*553–561. Patat, A., Trocherie, S., *et al.* EEG profile of intravenous zolpidem in healthy volunteers. *Psychopharmacology (Berl.),* **1994,** *114:*138–146. Salva, P., and Costa, J. Clinical pharmacokinetics and pharmacodynamics of zolpidem. Therapeutic implications. *Clin. Pharmacokinet.,* **1995,** *29:*142–153.

Table A–II–1 Pharmacokinetic Data (Continued)

AVAILABILITY (ORAL) (%)	URINARY EXCRETION (%)	BOUND IN PLASMA (%)	CLEARANCE $(ml \cdot min^{-1} \cdot kg^{-1})$	VOL. DIST. (liters/kg)	HALF-LIFE (hours)	PEAK TIME (hours)	PEAK CONCENTRATIONS
ZONISAMIDE[a] (Chapter 19)							
—[b]	29–48[c]	38–40[d]	0.13[e]	1.2–1.8[f]	63 ± 14	1.8 ± 0.4[g]	28 ± 4 $\mu g/ml$[g]

[a]Primary routes of metabolism involve reductive cleavage of the isoxazole ring (CYP3A4) and N-acetylation. [b]Absolute bioavailability is not known; presumably urine recovery after an oral dose. [c]Recovery following an oral dose. [d]Concentrates in erythrocytes to as much as eightfold. [e]Steady-state *CL/F* for a 400 mg once daily dose reported. [f]*V/F* for a single dose is reported; *AUC* increases disproportionately when the dose is increased from 400-800 mg. [g]Following a 400 mg oral dose given once daily to steady state in healthy adults.

References: Kochak, G.M., Page, J.G., Buchanan, R.A., Peters, R., and Padgett, C.S. Steady-state pharmacokinetics of zonisamide, an antiepileptic agent for treatment of refractory complex partial seizures. *J. Clin. Pharmacol.* **1998**, 38:166–171. Peters, D.H., and Sorkin, E.M. Zonisamide. A review of its pharmacodynamic and pharmacokinetic properties, and therapeutic potential in epilepsy. *Drugs*, **1993**, 45:760–787. *Physicians' Desk Reference*, 58th ed. Medical Economics Co., Montvale, **2004**, p. 1232.

Key: Unless otherwise indicated by a specific footnote, the data are presented for the study population as a mean value ± 1 standard deviation, a mean and range (lowest–highest in parenthesis) of values, a range of the lowest–highest values, or a single mean value. ACE = angiotensin converting enzyme; ADH = alcohol dehydrogenase; Aged = aged; AIDS = acquired immunodeficiency syndrome; Alb = hypoalbuminemia; Atr Fib = atrial fibrillation; AVH = acute viral hepatitis; Burn = burn patients; C_{max} = peak concentration; CAD = coronary artery disease; Celiac = celiac disease; CF = cystic fibrosis; CHF = congestive heart failure; Child = children; Cirr = hepatic cirrhosis; COPD = chronic obstructive pulmonary disease; CP = cor pulmonale; CPBS = cardiopulmonary bypass surgery; CRI = chronic respiratory insufficiency; Crohn = Crohn's disease; Cush = Cushing's syndrome; CYP = cytochrome P450; Fem = female; Hep = hepatitis; HIV = human immunodeficiency virus; HL = hyperlipoproteinemia; HTh = hyperthyroid; IM = intramuscular; Inflam = inflammation; IV = intravenous; LD = chronic liver disease; LTh = hypothyroid; MAO = monoamine oxidase; MI = myocardial infarction; NAT = N-acetyltransferase; Neo = neonate; NIDDM = non-insulin-dependent diabetes mellitus; NS = nephrotic syndrome; Obes = obese; Pneu = pneumonia; Preg = pregnant; Prem = premature; RA = rheumatoid arthritis; RD = renal disease (including uremia); SC = subcutaneous; Smk = smoking; ST = sulfotransferase; T_{max} = peak time; Tach = ventricular tachycardia; UGT = UDP-glucuronosyl transferase; Ulcer = ulcer patients. Other abbreviations are defined in the text section of this appendix.

INDEX

Page numbers followed by *f* or *t* denote figures or tables, respectively. Proprietary (brand) names are listed in small capital letters. More complete information is provided under nonproprietary (generic) names, which appear in parentheses after proprietary names.